VOLPE'S
Neurology of the
Newborn

Volpe's Neurology of the Newborn

Sixth Edition

EDITOR-IN-CHIEF

Joseph J. Volpe, MD
Bronson Crothers Professor of Neurology, Emeritus
Harvard Medical School
Neurologist-in-Chief, Emeritus
Boston Children's Hospital
Boston, Massachusetts

EDITORS

Terrie E. Inder, MBChB, MD
Mary Ellen Avery Professor of Pediatrics in
 the Field of Newborn Medicine
 Harvard Medical School
Chair, Department of Pediatrics/Newborn Medicine
 Brigham and Women's Hospital
 Boston, Massachusetts

Basil T. Darras, MD
Joseph J. Volpe Chair in Neurology
 Harvard Medical School
Associate Neurologist-in-Chief
Chief, Division of Clinical Neurology
 Boston Children's Hospital
 Boston, Massachusetts

Linda S. de Vries, MD, PhD
Consultant Neonatologist
 Wilhelmina Children's Hospital
Professor in Neonatal Neurology
 University Medical Center Utrecht
 Utrecht, The Netherlands

Adré J. du Plessis, MBChB, MPH
Division of Fetal and Transitional Medicine
Fetal Medicine Institute
 Children's National Medical Center
 Washington, District of Columbia

Jeffrey J. Neil, MD, PhD
Professor of Neurology
 Department of Neurology
 Boston Children's Hospital
 Boston, Massachusetts

Jeffrey M. Perlman, MBChB
Professor of Pediatrics
Department of Pediatrics
 Weill Cornell Medical College
Division Chief, Newborn Medicine
 New York Presbyterian Hospital
 New York, New York

ELSEVIER

ELSEVIER

1600 John F. Kennedy Blvd.
Ste 1800
Philadelphia, PA 19103-2899

VOLPE'S NEUROLOGY OF THE NEWBORN, SIXTH EDITION   ISBN: 978-0-323-42876-7

Notices

Knowledge and best practice in this field are constantly changing. As new research and experience broaden our understanding, changes in research methods, professional practices, or medical treatment may become necessary.

Practitioners and researchers must always rely on their own experience and knowledge in evaluating and using any information, methods, compounds, or experiments described herein. In using such information or methods they should be mindful of their own safety and the safety of others, including parties for whom they have a professional responsibility.

With respect to any drug or pharmaceutical products identified, readers are advised to check the most current information provided (i) on procedures featured or (ii) by the manufacturer of each product to be administered, to verify the recommended dose or formula, the method and duration of administration, and contraindications. It is the responsibility of practitioners, relying on their own experience and knowledge of their patients, to make diagnoses, to determine dosages and the best treatment for each individual patient, and to take all appropriate safety precautions.

To the fullest extent of the law, neither the Publisher nor the authors, contributors, or editors, assume any liability for any injury and/or damage to persons or property as a matter of products liability, negligence or otherwise, or from any use or operation of any methods, products, instructions, or ideas contained in the material herein.

Previous editions copyrighted 2008 and 2001.

Library of Congress Cataloging-in-Publication Data

Names: Volpe, Joseph J., editor. | Preceded by (work): Volpe, Joseph J.
    Neurology of the newborn.
Title: Volpe's neurology of the newborn / editors, Joseph J. Volpe [and 6 others].
Other titles: Neurology of the newborn
Description: Sixth edition. | Philadelphia, PA : Elsevier, [2018] | Preceded
    by Neurology of the newborn / Joseph J. Volpe. 5th ed. c2008. | Includes
    bibliographical references and index.
Identifiers: LCCN 2017036645 | ISBN 9780323428767 (hardcover : alk. paper)
Subjects: | MESH: Nervous System Diseases | Infant, Newborn, Diseases |
    Infant, Newborn
Classification: LCC RJ290 | NLM WS 340 | DDC 618.92/01–dc23
LC record available at https://lccn.loc.gov/2017036645

Executive Content Strategist: Kate Dimock
Senior Content Development Specialist: Janice Gaillard
Publishing Services Manager: Patricia Tannian
Senior Project Manager: Claire Kramer
Designer: Bridget Hoette

Printed in China

Last digit is the print number: 9 8 7 6 5 4 3 2 1

Working together to grow libraries in developing countries

www.elsevier.com • www.bookaid.org

To my wife,
Sara,
for her love and understanding,
without which this book would not be possible

Contributors

Nicholas S. Abend, MD

Associate Professor of Neurology
Children's Hospital of Philadelphia
Perelman School of Medicine
University of Pennsylvania
Philadelphia, Pennsylvnania

Stephen A. Back, MD, PhD

Professor of Pediatrics and Neurology
Clyde and Elda Munson Professor of Pediatric Research
Director, Neuroscience Section
Papé Family Pediatric Research Institute
Oregon Health and Science University
Portland, Oregon

Basil T. Darras, MD

Joseph J. Volpe Chair in Neurology
Harvard Medical School
Associate Neurologist-in-Chief
Chief, Division of Clinical Neurology
Boston Children's Hospital
Boston, Massachusetts

Linda S. de Vries, MD, PhD

Consultant Neonatologist
Wilhelmina Children's Hospital
Professor in Neonatal Neurology
University Medical Center Utrecht
Utrecht, The Netherlands

Adré J. du Plessis, MBChB, MPH

Division of Fetal and Transitional Medicine
Fetal Medicine Institute
Children's National Medical Center
Washington, District of Columbia

Christopher M. Elitt, MD, PhD

Assistant in Neurology
Department of Neurology
Fetal-Neonatal Neurology Program
Boston Children's Hospital
Instructor of Neurology
Harvard Medical School
Boston, Massachusetts

Partha S. Ghosh, MD

Assistant Professor
Department of Neurology
Harvard Medical School
Director, EMG Laboratory
Boston Children's Hospital
Boston, Massachsuetts

Petra S. Hüppi, MD

Professor of Pediatrics
Chief, Division of Development and Growth
Chilren's Hospital
University of Geneva
Geneva, Switzerland

Terrie E. Inder, MBChB, MD

Mary Ellen Avery Professor of Pediatrics in the Field of
    Newborn Medicine
Harvard Medical School
Chair, Department of Pediatrics/Newborn Medicine
Brigham and Women's Hospital
Boston, Massachusetts

Frances E. Jensen, MD, FACP

Professor of Neurology
Department of Neurology
Hospital of the University of Pennsylvania
Perelman School of Medicine
University of Pennsylvania
Philadelphia, Pennsylvania

Hannah C. Kinney, MD

Department of Pathology
Boston Children's Hospital
Harvard Medical School
Boston, Massachusetts

Catherine Limperopoulos, PhD

Director, The Developing Brain Research Program
Vice-Chair, Radiology Research
Diagnostic Imaging and Radiology
Children's National Health System
Washington, District of Columbia

Christopher C. McPherson, PharmD
Assistant Professor of Pediatrics and Clinical Pharmacist
Departments of Pediatrics and Pharmacy
Washington University School of Medicine and St. Louis
    Children's Hospital
St. Louis, Missouri

Jeffrey J. Neil, MD, PhD
Professor of Neurology
Department of Neurology
Boston Children's Hospital
Boston, Massachusetts

Jeffrey M. Perlman, MBChB
Professor of Pediatrics
Department of Pediatrics
Weill Cornell Medical College
Division Chief, Newborn Medicine
New York Presbyterian Hospital
New York, New York

Annapurna Poduri, MD
Department of Neurology
Harvard Medical School and Epilepsy Genetics Program
Department of Neurology
Boston Children's Hospital
Boston, Massachusetts

Shenandoah Robinson, MD, FAAP, FACS
Professor of Neurosurgery and Neurology - PAR
Division of Pediatric Neurosurgery
Johns Hopkins University School of Medicine
Baltimore, Maryland

Joseph J. Volpe, MD
Bronson Crothers Professor of Neurology, Emeritus
Harvard Medical School
Neurologist-in-Chief, Emeritus
Boston Children's Hospital
Boston, Massachusetts

Lianne J. Woodward, PhD
Professor of Pediatrics
Pediatric Newborn Medicine
Harvard Medical School
Brigham and Women's Hospital
Boston, Massachsuetts

Preface to the Sixth Edition

In the preface to the first edition of this book, published more than 35 years ago, I expressed the view that the neurology of the newborn "should be viewed as a discipline in its own right." Over the decades, through four subsequent editions, the evolution of this discipline has been extraordinary. Work relevant to neonatal neurology now is abundant in clinical journals in the fields of pediatrics, neurology, neonatology, perinatology, and obstetrics, among others, and in multiple scientific journals of the many neurobiological disciplines. The explosion of information in the field led me to conclude several years ago that single authorship is no longer feasible, especially if the quality of the book is to be at the highest level. With the prompting of Kate Dimock and others of the Elsevier team, I decided to embark on a multiauthored effort. Thus this edition has been updated and revised with remarkable efforts from 5 editors and 12 additional authors. The editors and authors are particularly meaningful to me because they are former trainees, current colleagues, or both. They are truly experts and in this edition have tolerated my compulsive editing and sometimes incessant suggestions for each chapter. In addition to their great skills as scholars, they have proven to be markedly resilient and tolerant of my often intrusive role in each chapter.

The organization of the sixth edition is identical to that of previous editions. However, in addition to extensive updating, revising, and rewriting, many original chapters have been split into multiple chapters. The first eight chapters constitute the unit on human brain development, which were previously contained in two chapters. Particular expansion of this unit reflects new insights into the neurobiology of brain development, fetal diagnosis, intrauterine interventions, and molecular genetics. A major expansion of the discussion of brain organizational events of the third trimester of gestation was undertaken to accommodate the explosion of brain information from advanced neuroimaging of normal cerebral cortical and white matter development and derangements thereof in the human premature infant. Unit II, concerning the neurological evaluation, was expanded to describe new methodologies, especially advanced MRI techniques, to study the newborn brain. A new chapter on neurodevelopmental follow-up was added to this unit. My longstanding devotion to the neurological examination and the importance thereof is reflected in its own dedicated chapter. Unit III, which focuses on neonatal seizures, serves as an effective bridge between the initial chapters and the later, diseased-focused chapters because neonatal seizure is a key manifestation of many of the neurological disorders dealt with later in the book. The discussion of neonatal seizures reflects the impact of new neurobiological insights (e.g., chloride channels, GABA excitation) and their importance for understanding the newborn's propensity to seizures, the impact on subsequent brain development, and the effects of anticonvulsant medications. Unit IV, concerned with hypoxic-ischemic and related disorders, the largest unit of the book, was

increased from four to nine chapters. The principal changes involved separation of the discussions of the preterm and term infant because the etiologies, neuropathology, pathophysiology, and clinical features exhibit many differences and unique aspects. The chapters on neuropathology, especially, reflect new insights gained by application of advanced neuropathological techniques, those on pathophysiology, the impact of many relevant neurobiological and clinical research studies, and those on clinical features, the knowledge gained from advanced neuroimaging and the remarkable advances in therapeutic interventions. Unit V, concerned with intracranial hemorrhage, includes a separate chapter on cerebellar hemorrhage and the impact thereof on cognitive and related outcomes. The chapter on intraventricular hemorrhage and posthemorrhagic hydrocephalus in the preterm infant expands on previous discussions, especially of management, that are based on recent clinical investigations. Unit VI, concerned with metabolic encephalopathies, includes insights from clinical and basic research into hypoglycemia and hyperbilirubinemia, particularly management thereof, as well as important updates on neonatal amino acid and organic acid disorders. Unit VII is a single chapter on degenerative disorders, specifically those that present clinically in the newborn period. Insights obtained from recent studies of molecular genetics, clinical features, and novel interventions are emphasized. Unit VIII, which covers neuromuscular disorders, has been expanded to four chapters, with a new chapter on arthrogryposis. These chapters reflect the enormous advances in this field in delineation of phenotypes, diagnosis, and interventions. The roles of molecular genetics in disease characterization and gene manipulation therapies in interventions are among the new areas of emphasis in neuromuscular disorders. Unit IX, which covers intracranial infections, remains as two chapters, but they have been expanded considerably. Important insights provided by modern neuroimaging and the advent of new therapies are emphasized. Unit X, which is on perinatal trauma, remains a single chapter about injuries of extracranial, cranial, intracranial, spinal cord, and peripheral nervous system structures, expanded by insights obtained from modern neuroimaging. Unit XI, which is about intracranial mass lesions, includes a chapter on brain tumors and vein of Galen malformations that provides new insights into molecular characterization of tumors, clinical features, and advances in management. Unit XII, which covers drugs and the developing nervous system, remains a single chapter, with particularly new insights into clinical features and treatment. The impact of recent surges in opioid abuse and the effects on the newborn are among the areas of special emphasis.

Concerning the specific editors and authors who contributed to the sixth edition of *Volpe's Neurology of the Newborn,* the critical first unit, as noted earlier, was expanded from two to eight chapters. The first four of these chapters were updated and revised by one of my first neonatal neurology fellows at

Washington University in St. Louis and later a faculty member in neonatal neurology with me in Boston, Dr. Adré du Plessis, who has developed especial expertise in disorders of neural tube formation, prosencephalic development, fetal ventriculomegaly, and cerebellar development and the clinical impact of defects thereof. Dr. Annapurna Poduri, a child neurology resident and later member of the faculty in the Department of Neurology that I led at Boston Children's Hospital, is an accomplished expert in cerebral cortical development, especially proliferative and migrational defects, and genetic disorders thereof. Dr. Hannah Kinney, a distinguished neuropathologist and my longtime colleague at Boston Children's Hospital, is a pioneer in the application of advanced neuropathological techniques to the study of organizational events and myelination of the brain, especially premature and early infant brain.

Particularly involved in the update/revision of Unit II was Dr. Jeffrey Neil, a former child neurology resident and fellow during my years at Washington University in St. Louis. Dr. Neil, who is now a colleague in Neurology at Boston Children's Hospital, is internationally recognized for his expertise and innovation in advanced MR methodologies, especially as applied to premature infants. The only new chapter in the book, which is on neurodevelopmental follow-up, was prepared by Dr. Petra Huppi, a neonatal neurology fellow with me in Boston at the turn of the century when she carried out pioneering research on the application of MR methodologies to the study of the premature brain and who is currently a leading figure in neurodevelopment, and by Dr. Lianne Woodward, an esteemed colleague in the Department of Pediatric Newborn Medicine at Harvard Medical School.

Especially involved in the update/revision of Unit III was a former colleague in my Department of Neurology at Boston Children's Hospital, Dr. Frances Jensen (currently Chair of Neurology at the University of Pennsylvania). Her work on the pathophysiology of neonatal seizures has been seminal. Her colleague, also formerly with us in Boston, Dr. Nicholas Abend, contributed importantly to the update. Dr. Terrie Inder (see later) my former trainee and current colleague, also contributed in a major way to this chapter.

Unit IV, the largest unit of the book, now includes nine chapters. The update/revisions were led by Dr. Inder (see later), Dr. Kinney, Dr. Neil, and Dr. Back. The first three are current colleagues in Boston, and Dr. Stephen Back, currently at Oregon Health Sciences University, was a former child neurology resident and postdoctoral fellow with us at Boston Children's Hospital. He is now recognized as a world leader in the pathophysiology of brain injury in the premature infant. Exceptional expertise also is apparent in relation to clinical features (Dr. Inder), neuroimaging (Dr. Neil), and neuropathology (Dr. Kinney).

Unit V includes major efforts by Dr. Terrie Inder (see later), Dr. Catherine Limperopoulos, and Dr. Jeff Perlman (see later). Dr. Limperopoulos was a fellow in neonatal neurology in my Department of Neurology at Boston Children's Hospital, when I had the privilege of working with her during her initial work on the developing cerebellum. She has established her own program at George Washington University and has developed greatly her widely recognized research in the study of the cerebellum.

The four-chapter Unit VI was updated by Dr. Jeffrey Perlman. Dr. Perlman was my first fellow in neonatal neurology (then at Washington University in St. Louis) and as a brilliant clinician and clinical investigator taught me a great deal about the critical nonneurological aspects of the sick newborn and the importance thereof in the genesis of neurological illness. Over the years he has been an admired colleague who now leads a major neonatology program at Cornell University in New York.

Unit VII was updated with the help of Dr. Christopher Elitt, a fellow in neonatal neurology with me at Boston Children's Hospital and now a junior faculty member here. The final product in this important area reflects his strong background in neuroscience and molecular genetics and his ability to tolerate my incessant critiquing of his generally fine work in updating this chapter.

Unit VIII was updated and revised by Dr. Basil Darras, my closest colleague at Boston Children's Hospital during my tenure as Chair of Neurology from 1990–2005. I am especially proud that he holds a Neurology Chair in my name. He remains an esteemed colleague and a trusted friend. His stature in the neuromuscular field is recognized internationally and is reflected in part by his leading role in the outstanding book *Neuromuscular Disorders of Infancy, Childhood and Adolescence*.

Unit IX on intracranial infections, constituting two chapters, was updated by Dr. Linda de Vries. She is an admired leader in our field, with whom I have had the privilege of previously coauthoring. Her great expertise in neuroimaging and all aspects of clinical research in neonatal neurology is reflected in the two chapters.

Unit XI is a single chapter that was greatly enriched by the work of my former colleague at Boston Children's Hospital, Dr. Shenandoah (Dody) Robinson. As a leading pediatric neurosurgeon, she enhanced the chapter with new insights into surgical approaches and results, as well as molecular aspects of tumor classification and clinical characteristics.

The final unit consists of a single chapter updated by Dr. Lianne Woodward and Dr. Christopher McPherson. The latter, a particular expert on the pharmacology of drugs in the developing fetus and newborn, was a colleague during his recent period on the faculty in Pediatric Newborn Medicine at the Brigham and Women's Hospital.

Particular recognition should be accorded to Dr. Terrie Inder who has authored/coauthored multiple chapters and, importantly, has interacted copiously with Elsevier concerning myriad details involved in generating a finished product. After completing her training in neonatology in New Zealand, Terrie trained with me in Boston in the late 1990s as a resident in child neurology and then as a fellow in neonatal neurology. During that period she spearheaded seminal studies of preterm brain by advanced MR techniques, which she used also in subsequent years with distinguished academic positions in New Zealand, Australia, and St. Louis and finally as Chair of Pediatric Newborn Medicine here (Brigham and Women's Hospital and Harvard Medical School).

My colleagues in this undertaking have been aided immeasurably by many people. My assistant for the past 25 years, Irene Miller, typed manuscripts, prepared tables, manipulated thousands of references, checked and double-checked table and figure numbering, and tolerated my obsessive pursuit of perfection, as she has over three previous editions of this book. Shaye Moore, leader of the Medical Writing Team of the Department of Neurology, dealt with such complex issues of digital manuscript preparation (multiplied by 38 chapters), that I cannot begin to understand or explain. No challenge was too great for her to confront and overcome. The Elsevier team, particularly Kate Dimock and Janice Gaillard, struck a remarkable balance of guidance, patience, efficiency, and implementation in bringing this project to fruition. All the editors and authors agree that we could not have had a better publishing group.

Joseph J. Volpe, MD
Boston, Massachusetts

Preface to the First Edition

The neurology of the newborn is a topic of major importance because of the preeminence of neurological disorders in neonatology today. The advent of modern perinatal medicine, accompanied by striking improvements in obstetrical and neonatal care, has changed the spectrum of neonatal disease drastically. Many previously dreaded disorders such as respiratory disease have been controlled to a major degree. At the same time, certain beneficial results of improved care, for example, markedly decreased mortality rates for premature infants, have been accompanied by neurological disorders that would not have had time to evolve in past years.

This major importance of neonatal neurological disease has stimulated efforts by workers in many disciplines to recognize, understand, treat, and ultimately prevent such disease. This book is an attempt to bring together the knowledge gained from these efforts and to present my current understanding of the neurology of the newborn. Because of the diversity of knowledge that I have attempted to bring to bear upon the problems discussed in this book, I may have oversimplified in certain areas and displayed my own ignorance in others. Nevertheless, I have written the material in the hope that it will be of value to all health professionals involved in the care and follow-up of the newborn infant with neurological disease.

The prime focus of the discussions of neonatal neurological disease throughout this book is the clinical evaluation of the infant, that is, what we can learn from observation of the setting and mode of presentation of the disease and the disturbances of neurological function apparent on careful examination. The theme that recurs most often is that careful clinical assessment, in the traditional sense, is the prerequisite and the essential foundation for understanding the neurological disorders of the newborn. The infant does not advertise his or her neurological disorder with the drama that older children and adults exhibit, but with patience and diligence we can discover a treasure of important clinical clues when we elicit a complete history and perform a careful physical examination. It is this quality of discovery with simple techniques that has made the neurology of the newborn so stimulating for me, and I hope that this book can lead the reader to similar discoveries.

With accomplishment of the essential first step of definition of the clinical problem, we can turn in a rational way to the increasingly sophisticated means of studying the infant's deranged neural structure and function. Although my emphasis is, first, on the simplest and least invasive techniques for providing us with the necessary information, we are in an era when sophisticated and informative procedures such as imaging the brain itself can be done in a safe and effective way.

The final process in our understanding the infant with a neurological disorder requires an awareness of a burgeoning corpus of information derived from studies in human and experimental pathology, physiology, biochemistry, and related fields. Of necessity, often we must extrapolate to our newborn patient data obtained from animals. Such extrapolation must always be made cautiously, and yet we cannot ignore the many lessons learned from the laboratory that have proved invaluable in our understanding of neonatal neurological disease. In this book, on the one hand, I attempt to synthesize in a comprehensible manner relevant material from a diversity of disciplines and, on the other hand, try very hard not to oversimplify what are clearly very complex issues.

I believe that the neurology of the newborn has come of age and, indeed, should be viewed as a discipline in its own right. I hope that in some way this book will contribute to establishing that status. My most fervent hope is that this discipline excites the interests and efforts of others concerned with the neonatal patient and that, through concerted actions, the greatest possible benefits accrue to the infant with neurological disease.

Joseph J. Volpe, MD

Acknowledgments

It is with pleasure and eagerness that I acknowledge with gratitude the help of so many over the years. I am grateful to Dr. Raymond Adams, who introduced me to neurology and neuropathology and provided a model of scholarship in medicine that I have since striven to achieve; to Dr. C. Miller Fisher, who taught me the inestimable value of looking carefully at the patient and never denying observations that did not fit preconceived notions; and Dr. E. P. Richardson, Jr., who taught me neuropathology and provided a framework for study on which I remain dependent.

I owe enormous gratitude to Dr. Philip Dodge, who stimulated me to study pediatric neurology and, after my training, guided me to the neurology of the newborn. To this day he has been a continual source of support and inspiration.

I gratefully acknowledge the help and contributions of many investigators with an interest in the newborn. Their work is included on many of the pages of this book, and although acknowledgment is made in those places, I take this particular opportunity to thank them again for their generosity. Many other physicians involved in the care of newborns have shared their unusual and interesting cases with me; I thank them for their stimulation and education. Many faculty, fellows, and house officers at St. Louis Children's Hospital and Boston Children's Hospital have helped me immeasurably in the study of neonatal patients. My collaborators in clinical and basic research have been wonderful partners in our pursuit of discovery and creativity in the study of the newborn brain.

For this edition I acknowledge with great pride and gratitude the work of my former trainees and current esteemed colleagues who served as editors and authors. They are distinguished and dedicated scholars in their own right, and their efforts in bringing to fruition this sixth edition were prodigious indeed.

Joseph J. Volpe, MD

Contents

Video Contents

UNIT I

HUMAN BRAIN DEVELOPMENT

Neural Tube Development

Adré J. du Plessis • Joseph J. Volpe

An understanding of the development of the nervous system is essential for an understanding of fetal and neonatal neurology. An obvious reason for this contention is the wide variety of disturbances of neural development that are flagrantly apparent in the neonatal period and increasingly diagnosed in the fetal period. In addition, all the insults that affect the fetus and newborn, and that are the subject matter of most of this book, exert their characteristic effects in part because the brain is developing in many distinctive ways and at a very rapid rate. As discussed further in Chapter 14, a strong likelihood exists that many of these common insults exert deleterious and far-reaching effects on certain aspects of neural development—effects that until now have escaped detection by available techniques.

In Chapters 1, 2, and 4 we emphasize the aspect of normal development that has been deranged, the structural characteristics of the abnormality, and the neurological consequences. It is least profitable to attempt to characterize exhaustively all the presumed *causes* of these abnormalities of the developmental program. Although a few examples of environmental agents that insult the developing human nervous system at specific time periods and produce a defect are recognized, few of these agents leave an identifying stamp. This obtains particularly because, in the first two trimesters of gestation, the developing brain is not capable of generating the glial and other reactions to injury that serve as useful clues to environmental insults that occur at later time periods. The occasional example of a virus, chemical, drug, or other environmental agent that has been shown to produce a disorder of brain development is mentioned only in passing. However, we emphasize genetic considerations whenever possible because of their importance in parental counseling. Therefore the organizational framework is the chronology of normal development of the human nervous system. A brief review of the major developmental events that occur most prominently during each time period is presented, followed by a discussion of the disorders that result when such development is deranged.

This chapter is devoted to the first major process in human brain development: the formation of the neural tube. These early events culminate in formation of the fundamental central neuroaxis. Development of the neural tube and the subsequent development of the prosencephalon (discussed in the next chapter) can be considered the neural components of *embryogenesis*. In subsequent chapters we discuss later *fetal* developmental events that lead to the intrinsic structural development of the central nervous system (CNS).

NORMAL DEVELOPMENT OF THE FUNDAMENTAL CENTRAL NEUROAXIS

Developments in recent years have required a reevaluation of conventional paradigms for developmental disorders of the central neuroaxis. A variety of traditional classification systems have been unsatisfactory, and the persistent inconsistent use of terminology has compromised the diagnostic and prognostic accuracy in clinical practice. New insights from animal models, advanced fetal imaging, and fetal intervention trials for neural tube disorders have led to the notion of primary and secondary consequences of these conditions. For example, the *unifying hypothesis* for open neural tube defects proposes that the primary failure of spinal closure leads to cerebrospinal fluid (CSF) leakage, which in turn leads to the secondary consequences of posterior fossa underdevelopment, hindbrain herniation, and the development of hydrocephalus.[1] More precise diagnostic paradigms consider the germ cell layers involved (i.e., ectodermal, neuroectodermal, or mesodermal) in the primary dysgenetic lesion, as well as the secondary effects of trauma, *toxicity*, and mechanical disruption of subsequent development. For example, it is now proposed that the primary defect in anencephaly is likely not failure of neurulation but rather failure of normal cutaneous and mesenchymal development (skin, bone and dural coverings), with a secondary degeneration of the exposed neural tissue. Similarly, lesions such as meningoceles with no neural involvement are often still classified as "closed neural tube defects," although their etiology is unrelated to neurulation.

Milestones of Major Events

The major developmental events and their peak times of occurrence are shown in Table 1.1. The time periods are those during which the *most rapid progression* of the developmental event occurs. Although some overlap exists among these time periods, it is valid and convenient to consider the overall maturational process in terms of a sequence of individual events. In a discussion of the timing of the disorders, the time periods shown in Table 1.1 are obviously of major importance. Nonetheless, it is necessary to recognize that an aberration of a developmental event need not be caused by an insult impinging *at the time of the event*. Thus a given malformation may not have its onset after the developmental event is completed, but the developmental program may be disturbed *at any time before* the event is under way. The concept of a *termination stage* refers to the time in the development of an organ after which a specific

TABLE 1.1   Major Events in Human Brain Development and Peak Times of Occurrence

MAJOR DEVELOPMENTAL EVENT	PEAK TIME OF OCCURRENCE
Primary neurulation	3–4 weeks of gestation
Prosencephalic development	2–3 months of gestation
Neuronal proliferation	3–4 months of gestation
Neuronal migration	3–5 months of gestation
Organization	5 months of gestation to years postnatally
Myelination	Birth to years postnatally

TABLE 1.2   Development of the Fundamental Craniospinal Axis—Major Phases and Peak Times of Occurrence

MAJOR DEVELOPMENTAL PHASE	PEAK TIME OF OCCURRENCE
1. Gastrulation	16–18 days p/c
2. Primary neurulation	18–26 days p/c
Neural plate formed	18 days p/c
First fusion of neural folds	22 days p/c
Anterior neuropore closes	24 days p/c
Posterior neuropore closes	26 days p/c
3. Secondary neurulation	26 days p/c—postnatal
Vacuolation-canalization	26 days—7 weeks p/c
Retrogressive differentiation	7 weeks p/c—postnatal
4. Disjunction and fusion of mesodermal-cutaneous structures	Tracks regional neural tube closure

BOX 1.1   Primary Neurulation

Peak Time Period
3–4 weeks of gestation
Major Events
Notochord, chordal mesoderm → neural plate → neural tube, neural crest cells
Neural tube → brain and spinal cord → dura, axial skeleton (cranium, vertebrae), dermal covering
Neural crest → dorsal root ganglia, sensory ganglia of cranial nerves, autonomic ganglia, and so forth

malformation cannot occur by any teratogenic mechanism.[2] Thus, in the discussion of timing of malformations, we state that the onset of a given defect could occur *no later than* a given time. Note that in this text the timing of events is based on the postconceptional (p/c) age, rather than the postmenstrual or gestational age.

Formation of the Neural Tube

Formation of the neural tube and its coverings proceeds through four phases (Table 1.2)—namely gastrulation, primary neurulation, secondary neurulation, and dorsal midline closure of the mesodermal-cutaneous ectodermal layers. *Gastrulation* is the fundamental formation of the trilaminar plate between days 16 and 18 p/c during which the endodermal, mesodermal, and ectodermal layers of the embryo become distinct. The ectodermal layer differentiates into cutaneous and neural ectoderm. The neural ectoderm develops in the longitudinal plane along the dorsal surface of the embryo as the neural plate. *Neurulation* refers to the inductive events that occur in the neural plate that result in formation of the neural tube, which ultimately gives rise to the entire CNS. Neurulation can be divided into *primary neurulation* (i.e., formation of brain and spinal cord down to the sacral level) and *secondary neurulation* (i.e., events related to the later formation of the sacrococcygeal

segments of the spinal cord). With fusion of the neural folds, there is separation of the cutaneous and neural ectoderm, with the ingrowth of the mesodermal layers between them; the timing of these events closely follows the progressive closure of the neural tube. Primary neurulation and secondary neurulation are discussed separately.

Primary Neurulation

By the end of gastrulation, the most anterior part of the axial mesoderm is the prechordal plate, a critical ventral patterning center for the developing forebrain, while the more posterior parts of the axial mesoderm are made up of the notochord. Primary neurulation is a series of events in the dorsal neural ectoderm of the embryo culminating in formation of the neural tube—rostral to the upper sacral level—and its separation from the other germ cell layers.[3,4] The critical events are summarized in Box 1.1. By 18 days p/c the neural plate has been formed by differentiation of the dorsal neural ectoderm from the original ectodermal layer. Next the lateral edges of the neural plate become elevated into neural folds, and the midline of the neural plate invaginates (Fig. 1.1). The neural folds continue to elevate in a dorsomedial direction, until the edges meet in the midline to begin closure of the neural tube. In the human embryo, the first fusion of the neural folds is at the level of the future hindbrain-cervical junction (foramen magnum), which occurs at 22 p/c days. Closure generally proceeds rostrally to form the anterior neural tube (and then the brain) and caudally to form the posterior neural tube (and then the spinal cord), although it is not a simple, zipper-like process.[5-13] The anterior neuropore of the neural tube closes at approximately 24 days, and the posterior neuropore closes at approximately 26 days, at which point primary neurulation is complete. During closure of the neural tube, cells from the dorsal-most region become separated from the neural tube to form the neural crest, which in turn gives rise to the future craniofacial bony structures, dorsal root ganglia, sensory ganglia of the cranial nerves, autonomic ganglia, Schwann cells, and cells of the pia and arachnoid (as well as melanocytes, cells of the adrenal medulla, and certain skeletal elements of the head and face).[11] Finally, the neural tube becomes physically separated from the meso-endoderm and cutaneous ectoderm, a process called disjunction (see Table 1.2). Ongoing interaction between the neural tube and surrounding mesoderm gives rise to the dura and axial skeleton (i.e., the skull and the vertebrae). Understanding this sequence of normal differentiation of the different germ cell layers is critical to an understanding of the different features of cranial and spinal dysraphism.

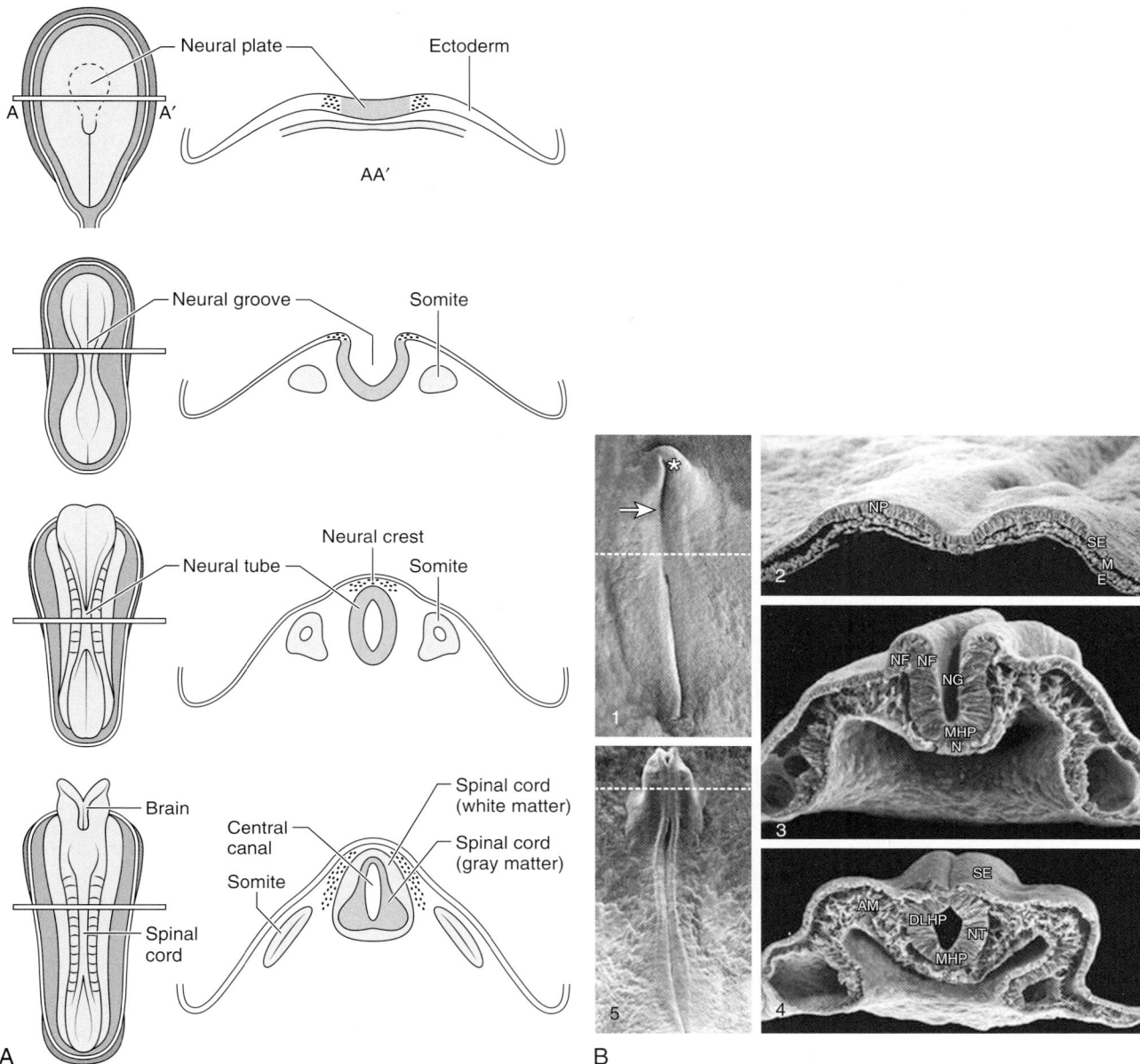

Figure 1.1 Primary neurulation. *Schematic depiction* (A) *of the developing embryo*: external view *(left)* and corresponding cross-sectional view[407] at about the middle of the future spinal cord. Note the formation of the neural plate, neural tube, and neural crest cells. (B) *Neurulation in the chick embryo.* Dorsal view showing cranial-to-caudal neural plate formation at the level of the line in *panel 1.* More cranially *(arrow)*, the neural plate is shaping, and still more cranially, the neural plate is bending *(asterisk)*, and a neural groove and paired neural folds have formed. *Panel 2:* Transverse section through the neural plate. *Panel 3:* Transverse section through neural groove at the future midbrain level. *Panel 4:* Dorsal view during closure of the neural groove. groove. *Panel 5:* Transverse section through the incipient neural tube. *DLHP,* Dorsolateral hinge point; *E,* endoderm; *M,* mesoderm; *MHP,* median hinge point; *N,* notochord; *NF,* neural fold; *NG,* neural groove; *NP,* neural plate; *NT,* neural tube; *SE,* surface ectoderm. (A, From Cowan WM. The development of the brain. *Sci Am.* 1979;241:113–133. B, From Schoenwolf GC, PhD, *Larsen's Human Embryology,* Chapter 4, 82–107. Copyright © 2015, 2009 by Churchill Livingstone, an imprint of Elsevier Inc.)

Cellular and Molecular Mechanisms of Primary Neurulation. Primary neurulation occurs under the induction of the underlying notochord and chordal mesoderm during the third and fourth weeks p/c (see Box 1.1 and Fig. 1.1).[11] The neural plate deformations required for development of the neural folds, and subsequently the neural tube, are mediated by a variety of cellular and molecular mechanisms,[5,6,9,12-33] the most important of which involve the cytoskeletal network of microtubules and microfilaments. Under the influence of vertically oriented microtubules, cells of the developing neural plate elongate, while contraction of actin microfilaments arranged circumferentially around the apical portions of the cells results in cells with a

BOX 1.2 Secondary Neurulation (Caudal Neural Tube Formation)

Peak Time Period
Canalization: 4–7 weeks of gestation
Retrogressive differentiation: 7 weeks of gestation to after birth
Major Events
Canalization: undifferentiated cells (caudal cell mass) → vacuoles → coalescence → contact central canal of rostral neural tube
Retrogressive differentiation: regression of caudal cell mass → ventriculus terminalis, filum terminale

broad base and narrow apex. These forces on the neural plate result in invagination of its midline, dorsomedial folding of its edges, and closure to form the neural tube (see Fig. 1.1). The process of neural fold bending in a dorsomedial direction also appears to involve differential proliferation and translocation of the neuroepithelial cells.[34] Surface glycoproteins, especially cell adhesion molecules important for cell-cell recognition, as well as adhesive interactions with extracellular matrix, mediate fusion of the opposing neural folds. Other critical molecular events include action of the products of certain regional patterning genes (especially bone morphogenetic proteins and sonic hedgehog), homeobox genes, surface receptors, and transcription factors.

Secondary Neurulation (Caudal Neural Tube Formation)

Secondary neurulation is the process of caudal neural tube formation, which commences at completion of primary neurulation (i.e., on closure of the posterior neuropore around the S2 spinal level, on day 26 p/c; Box 1.2).[35,36] Secondary neurulation occurs in the caudal cell mass and, by forming the remaining sacrococcygeal neural tube, completes neural tube formation. Secondary neurulation gives rise to the conus medullaris, cauda equina, as well as components of the genitourinary tract and hindgut. Starting between 28 and 32 days p/c, the caudal cell mass undergoes vacuolation, coalescence, and canalization, processes that culminate by 7 weeks p/c.[18,37,38] At this point the vacuoles connect to the central canal of the neural tube previously formed by primary neurulation.[3] Not infrequently, accessory lumens remain and may be important in the genesis of certain anomalies of neural tube formation (discussed later). Following canalization, the caudal cell mass undergoes retrogressive differentiation between 7 weeks p/c and into postnatal life (see Box 1.2). At 8 weeks p/c the spinal cord tissue extends the entire length of the spinal column. Subsequent disproportionate growth of the spinal column results in relative ascent of the conus medullaris (which contains the ventriculus terminalis), leaving the filum terminale in its wake. As a result the conus ascends to the level of L3 by 40 weeks,[39] reaching its final level of L1–L2 by 3 months postnatal.

DISORDERS OF CRANIOSPINAL DEVELOPMENT

The terminology used to describe embryonic anomalies of craniospinal development is inconsistent and often imprecise, which in turn has compromised diagnosis and counseling. To remedy this situation, we first review the definitions and

categorization to be used in this text.[40,41] The term *dysraphism* is best understood by considering its root (i.e., raphe), which is defined as a line of union between two contiguous bilaterally symmetric structures. Dysraphism is therefore a failure of this process, and in its broadest sense includes any incomplete midline closure of the developing head and spine, and may involve the mesenchymal and ectodermal structures individually or in combination. Embryologically, dysraphic states of the central neuroaxis can be divided into those that occur (1) pre-neurulation (during gastrulation) and involve the neurenteric canal; (2) during primary neurulation, forming the vast majority of open neural tube defects; (3) during secondary neurulation with disturbed development of the caudal cell mass, which is responsible for most closed neural tube defects; or (4) during midline closure of the mesoderm and cutaneous ectoderm. *Spina bifida* refers only to defects of vertebral arch formation (described later); subtyping of spina bifida is based on the presence and nature of associated neuroectodermal malformations. Isolated vertebral arch dysraphism without underlying neural defects or cystic evagination of the meninges or cord results in true *spina bifida occulta*.

Neural tube defects refer to a disturbance in neuroectodermal development, defined embryologically as defects of primary or secondary neurulation. Anatomically, neural tube defects can be further categorized by their location relative to the first fusion point of the neural tube, at the level of the future foramen magnum. Lesions of the anterior neural tube (rostral to the foramen magnum) lead to cranial dysraphism, while those of the posterior neural tube (caudal to the foramen magnum) lead to spinal dysraphism. The distinction between open or closed dysraphic lesions is important for understanding the primary lesion and its secondary complications. *Open* neural tube defects have at least some continuity between the external surface of the fetus and the underlying neural tissue and at least intermittent CSF leakage. In addition, open neural tube defects are usually associated with other CNS anomalies, including hindbrain, callosal, and cerebral cortical malformations. *Closed* neural tube defects are skin covered, with no exposed neural tissue and no CSF leak; the defect is confined to the spine, and other associated CNS anomalies are rare.[42] As a general rule, most open neural tube defects result from disturbed primary neurulation, while most closed neural tube defects result from disturbed secondary neurulation. However, there are exceptions to this rule. For example, higher (thoracic and cervical) myelomeningoceles may be skin covered (see the discussion of cervical myelocystoceles later on in this chapter), and sacral lesions are occasionally open.[43]

Disorders of primary neurulation are discussed in order of decreasing severity, starting with complete failure of neural tube formation (craniorachischisis totalis), followed by disorders of anterior neural tube formation (cranial dysraphism) and disorders of posterior neural tube formation (spinal dysraphism).

Craniocerebral Dysraphism (Box 1.3)
Craniorachischisis Totalis

Anatomical Abnormality. Craniorachischisis totalis (see Box 1.3) results from essentially total failure of neurulation at a very early stage, leaving an exposed neural plate–like structure (with no overlying axial skeleton or dermal covering) running down the entire dorsal extent of the central neuroaxis (Fig. 1.2).[44,45] Because the neural plate is formed by 18 days p/c,

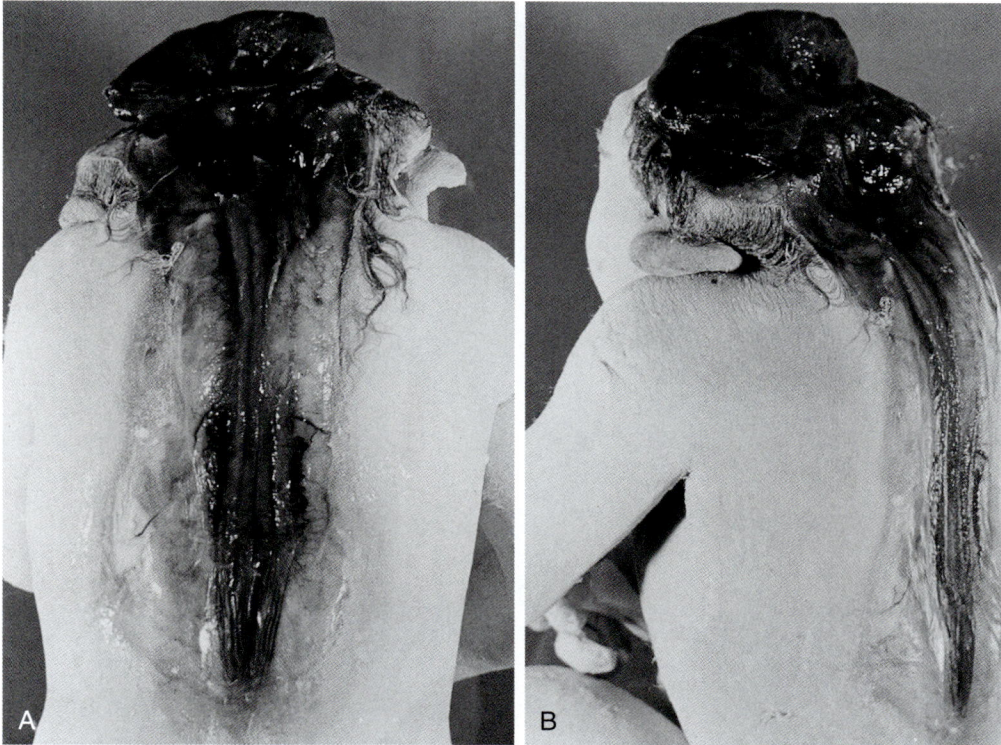

Figure 1.2 Craniorachischisis. Dorsal (A) and dorsolateral (B) views of a human fetus. (Courtesy Dr. Ronald Lemire.)

BOX 1.3   Cranial and Spinal Dysraphism

Order of Decreasing Severity
Craniorachischisis totalis
Anencephaly
Encephalocele
Myelomeningocele, Chiari type II malformation
Myeloschisis

---

and first point of closure of the neural tube occurs at 22 days p/c, the onset of craniorachischisis totalis is estimated to be no later than 20 to 22 days of gestation.[3] The precise incidence of this lesion is unknown because most cases are aborted spontaneously in early pregnancy, and only a few have survived to early fetal stages.

Anencephaly

Anatomical Abnormality. Anencephaly (see Box 1.3 and Fig. 1.3) has traditionally been classified as an anterior neural tube defect. However, based on human and animal observations,[46] some consider this lesion to be a primary defect in the formation of the cranial vault and its coverings, with secondary degeneration of the cranial neural contents. Specifically, it is proposed that anencephaly results primarily from (partial) absence of the cranial vault (acrania), with initial protrusion of the early fetal brain above the remaining skull bones (exencephaly), and subsequent degeneration of the underlying telencephalic mantle due to direct exposure to the amniotic fluid.[46] According to this viewpoint, anencephaly is not a true neural tube defect, because the primary lesion results from a skeletal (mesodermal)

defect. Instead the underlying pathogenetic mechanism of anencephaly invokes a *two-hit* hypothesis similar to that discussed for myelomeningoceles later in this chapter. This notion that anencephaly is not a true neural tube defect is not universally held.[47] The cranial defect usually involves the frontal bones above the supraciliary ridge, the parietal bones, and the squamous part of the occipital bone, and in the most severe cases, the cranial vault abnormality extends back to or through (holoacrania or holoanencephaly) the foramen magnum.[3,45] Defects stopping short of the foramen magnum are known as meroacrania or meroanencephaly. The underlying neural tissue defect in anencephaly most commonly involves the forebrain and variable amounts of upper brain stem (Fig. 1.4; see also Fig. 1.3), leaving a residual degenerated mass of hemorrhagic, fibrotic, and neuroglial tissue with little definable structure. Onset of anencephaly is estimated to be no later than 24 days of gestation.[3] Polyhydramnios is a frequent feature.[48]

Timing and Clinical Aspects. Approximately 75% of anencephalic infants are stillborn, and the remainder die in the neonatal period. The disorder is not rare, and epidemiological studies reveal striking variations in prevalence as a function of geographical location, sex, ethnic group, race, season of the year, maternal age, social class, and history of affected siblings.[45,49-53] The risk increases with decreasing social class and with a history of affected siblings in the family. Since the late 1970s, the incidence of anencephaly in the United States, like that of myelomeningocele (discussed later), declined to approximately 0.2 per 1000 live births in 1989, remaining relatively stable since then,[53,54] with the most recent estimates (2009–2011) being 0.28/1000 live births.[55] Both genetic and

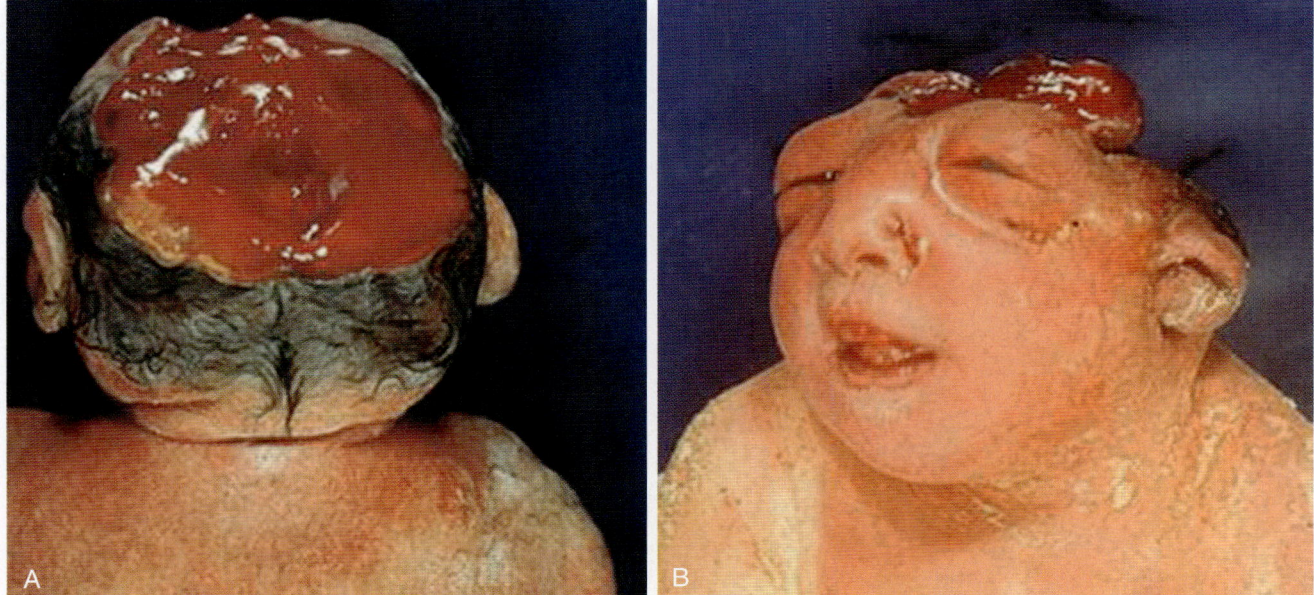

Figure 1.3 Anencephaly. Dorsal (A) and frontal (B) views. Note the absence of scalp, calvarium, and almost the entire brain, with the characteristic facies, including absent forehead giving the eyes an appearance of bulging. The lack of cranial bones causes the cranial cavity to be completely open. There is no discernible brain grossly; however, there is sometimes a small mass of neurovascular tissue (area cerebrovasculosa) in the base of the cranium. Rarely, there can be acrania without anencephaly in which the calvarium is absent, but with significant development of brain.

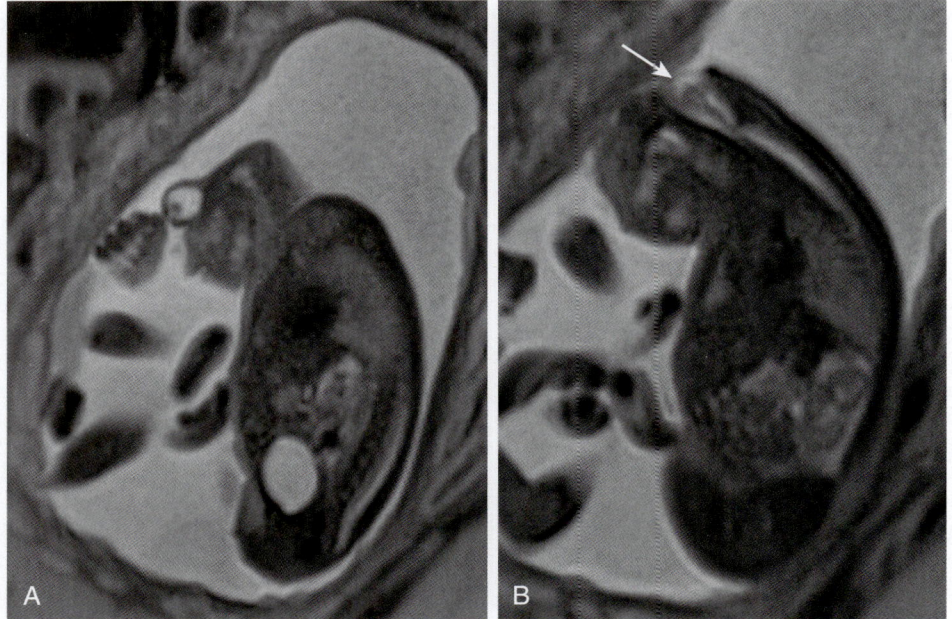

Figure 1.4 Fetal magnetic resonance imaging showing anencephaly. Note abrupt ending of brain parenchyma at the rostral end of the rudimentary brain stem *(arrow)*.

environmental influences appear to operate in the genesis of anencephaly (see later discussion of myelomeningocele). Recently, maternal use during pregnancy of the selective serotonin reuptake inhibitor paroxetine has been implicated in the development of anencephaly.[56]

Diagnosis. The skull bones begin to ossify around 11 weeks p/c, making the cranial defect readily identifiable by second trimester fetal ultrasound.[57] In fact, the proportion of anencephaly detected prenatally has been reported to be as high as 96% to 100%.[58,59] Systematic prenatal detection and elective termination

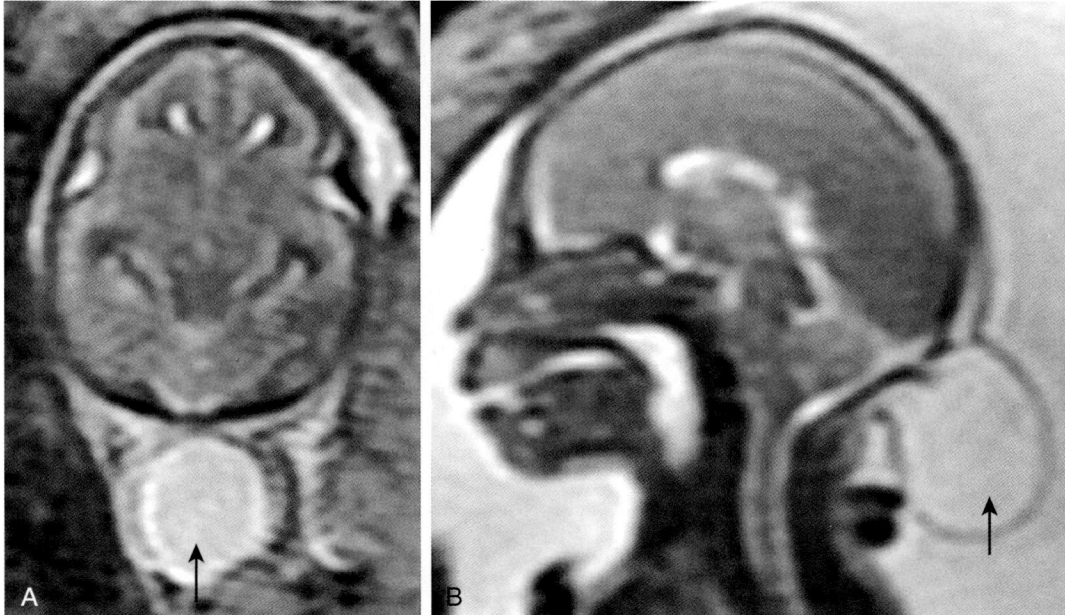

Figure 1.5 Fetal magnetic resonance imaging (MRI) showing occipital meningocele. T2-weighted fetal MRI axial (A) and sagittal (B) views showing cerebrospinal fluid-filled cystic lesion (*arrows*) apparently devoid of brain parenchymal tissue.

of pregnancy complicated by anencephaly have resulted in a sharp decline in the number of live-born cases.[60,61]

Encephaloceles

Anatomical Abnormality. Encephaloceles (see Box 1.3) were previously considered a restricted disorder of neurulation involving anterior neural tube closure, although the precise pathogenesis of these lesions remains unknown. It may be better to consider these lesions as developmental disorders of cranial mesoderm in which the cranial defect is associated with a cystic extracranial extension of meninges, neural tissue, and CSF. The notion that encephaloceles are not disorders of primary neurulation is supported by the fact that the herniated brain parenchyma is relatively normal and shows no evidence of defective neurulation.[47] Many encephaloceles are skin-covered (i.e., *closed*) lesions. When the cystic lesion includes parts of the ventricular system, the term meningoencephalocystocele is used. Lesions that involve primarily or only the overlying meninges or skull,[45] without obvious inclusion of neural elements, are called cranial meningoceles (Fig. 1.5); these are thought to be later in onset and account for up to 20% of cystic occipital lesions. Encephaloceles occur most commonly (70%–80%) in the occipital region (Fig. 1.6),[62-66] less commonly in the frontal region (Fig. 1.7), and least commonly in the temporal and parietal regions.[67] Frontal encephaloceles may protrude into the nasal cavity (frontoethmoidal encephaloceles). In the typical occipital encephalocele, the protruding brain is usually derived from the occipital lobe and may be accompanied by dysraphic disturbances involving cerebellum and superior mesencephalon. The neural tissue in an encephalocele usually connects to the underlying CNS through a narrow neck of tissue. The protruding mass is usually represented by a closed neural tube with cerebral cortex, exhibiting a normal gyral

pattern, and subcortical white matter. As many as 50% of cases are complicated by hydrocephalus.[68] Encephaloceles located in the low occipital (below the inion) or high cervical regions and combined with deformities of lower brain stem and of base of skull and upper cervical vertebrae characteristic of the Chiari type II malformation (associated with myelomeningocele [discussed later]) comprise the Chiari type III malformation.[69] This type of encephalocele contains cerebellum in virtually all cases and occipital lobes in approximately one-half of cases (Fig. 1.8).[69] Partial or complete agenesis of the corpus callosum occurs in two-thirds of cases. Venous structures may be included in the cyst, and anomalous venous drainage (aberrant sinuses and deep veins) is present in about one-half of patients and may complicate the surgical approach to these lesions.[69]

Timing and Clinical Aspects. Onset of the most severe lesions is probably no later than the approximate time of anterior neural tube closure (24 days), or shortly thereafter. Infants with encephaloceles not uncommonly exhibit associated malformations.[62,70] A frequently co-occurring CNS anomaly is subependymal nodular heterotopia.[71] The most commonly recognized syndromes associated with encephalocele are Meckel syndrome (characterized by occipital encephalocele, microcephaly, microphthalmia, cleft lip and palate, polydactyly, polycystic kidneys, ambiguous genitalia, and other deformities)[72] and Walker-Warburg syndrome (see Chapters 6 and 33). These disorders, as well as several other less common syndromes associated with encephalocele, are inherited in an autosomal recessive manner.[62,70,73] Maternal hyperthermia between 20 and 28 days of gestation has been associated with an increased incidence of occipital encephalocele,[70] as well as with other neural tube defects (discussed later).

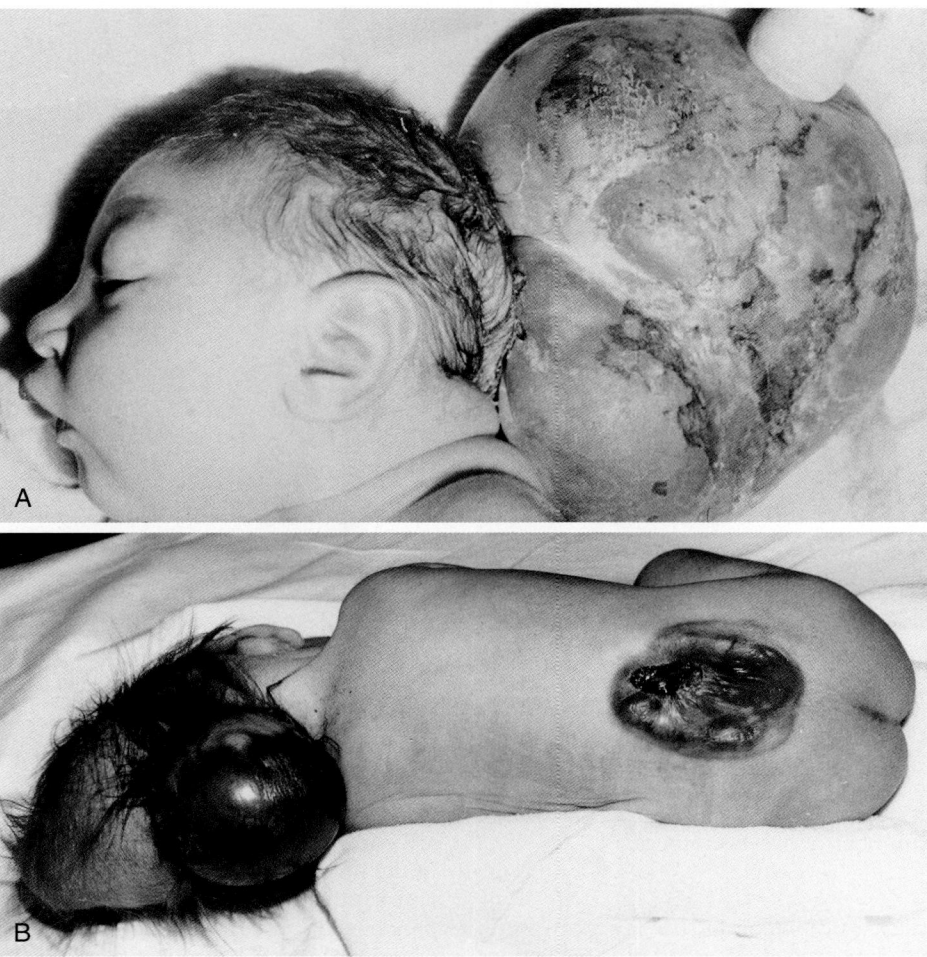

Figure 1.6 **Encephalocele.** (A) Newborn with a large occipital encephalocele. (B) Newborn with both an occipital encephalocele and a thoracolumbar myelomeningocele. (Courtesy Dr. Marvin Fishman.)

Diagnosis. Skin-covered encephaloceles have normal maternal serum and amniotic fluid AFP levels. Diagnosis by fetal ultrasonography in the second trimester has been well documented.[74-78] As with myelomeningoceles, *open* encephaloceles are often associated with decreased extraaxial CSF spaces by fetal imaging. Diagnosis before fetal viability has been followed by elective termination; later diagnosis may require delivery by cesarean section.

Management and Outcome. Neurosurgical intervention is indicated in most patients.[62,64] Exceptions include those with massive lesions and marked microcephaly. Surgery is necessary in the neonatal period for ulcerated lesions that are leaking CSF. An operation can be deferred if adequate skin covering is present. Preoperative evaluation has been facilitated by the use of computed tomography (CT) and especially magnetic resonance imaging (MRI) scans.[69,79,80] The outcome is difficult to determine precisely because of variability in selection for surgical treatment. In a combined surgical series of 40 infants,[64,65] 15 infants (38%) died, many

of whose complications can be managed more effectively now in neurosurgical facilities. Of the 25 survivors, 14 (56%) were of normal intelligence, although often with motor deficits, and 11 (44%) exhibited both impaired intellect and motor deficits. Not surprisingly, prognosis varies inversely with the extent of herniated neural tissue, with cranial meningoceles (i.e., no obvious neural tissue in the cyst) having the best prognosis. Outcome is more favorable for infants with anterior encephaloceles than those with posterior encephaloceles. Thus, in one series of 34 cases, mortality was 45% for infants with posterior defects and 0% for those with anterior defects. Normal outcome occurred in 14% of the total group with posterior defects and in 42% of those with anterior defects.[62]

Spinal Dysraphism

In the following we first consider disorders of primary neurulation, usually open neural tube defects, because these originate earlier in embryonic development and are by far the most common and clinically relevant spinal dysraphic

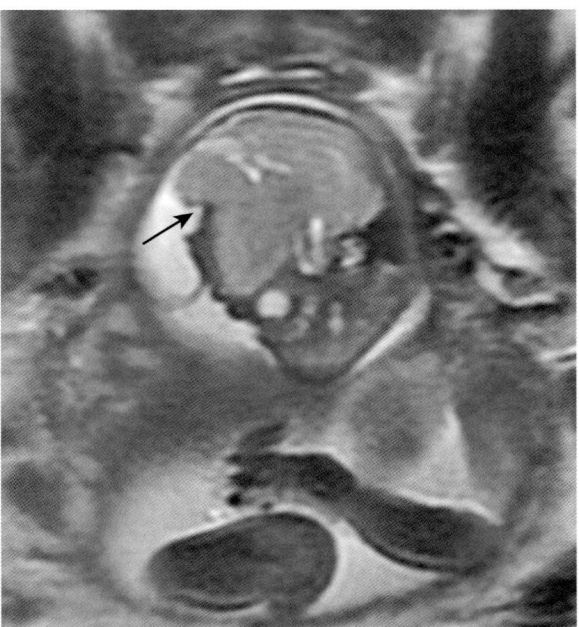

Figure 1.7 Frontoparietal encephalocele. Fetal magnetic resonance imaging (T2-weighted) angled sagittal view showing herniation of brain parenchyma through cranial defect *(arrow)*.

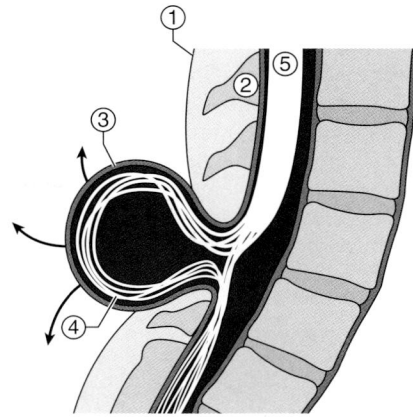

① Skin
② Bony spinal element
③ Dysplastic meningeal tissue
④ Herniating neural tissue
⑤ Spinal cord

Figure 1.9 Diagram of myelomeningocele. Note herniation of neural tissue through the bony spinous defect, dorsal displacement of the cord by ventral cerebrospinal fluid (CSF) collection, cyst covered by dysplastic meningeal tissue, leakage of CSF, and lack of skin coverage.

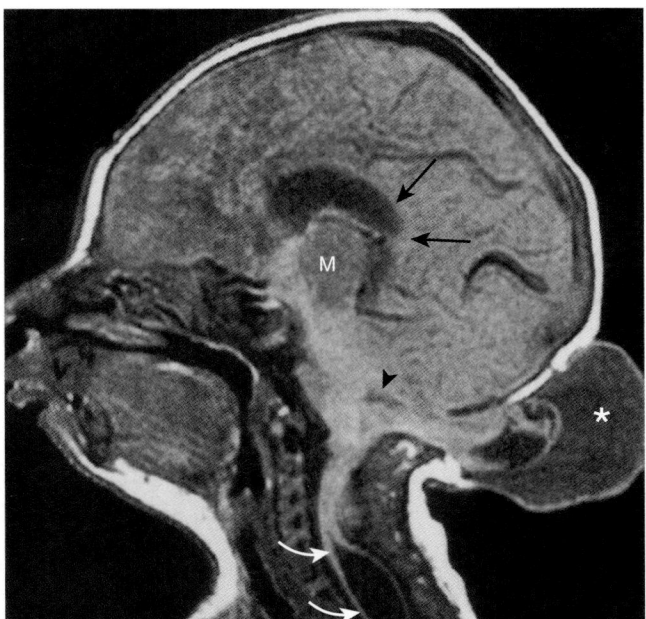

Figure 1.8 Fetal magnetic resonance imaging (MRI) showing occipital encephalocele. Midline sagittal spin echo 700/20 MRI scan demonstrates a low occipital encephalocele containing cerebellar tissue. The cystic portions *(asterisk)* within the herniated cerebellum are of uncertain origin. The posterior aspect of the corpus callosum *(straight black arrows)* is not clear and is probably dysgenetic. The third ventricle is not seen, but the massa intermedia (M) is very prominent. The tectum is deformed and is not readily identified. The fourth ventricle *(arrowhead)* is deformed and displaced posteriorly. A syrinx *(curved white arrows)* is present in the middle to lower cervical spinal cord. (From Castillo M, Quencer RM, Dominguez R. Chiari III malformation: imaging features. *AJNR Am J Neuroradiol.* 1992;13:107–113.)

conditions. Thereafter we discuss disorders of secondary neurulation, which more commonly result in closed neural tube defects.

Disorders of Primary Neurulation in the Spine

There are two major disorders of primary neurulation above the sacral level, namely, myelomeningocele and myeloschisis. The essential difference between these two lesions is that a cystic component is present in myelomeningocele (at least initially), consisting of dysplastic meningeal tissue usually leaking CSF, whereas in myeloschisis the neural placode is completely exposed, with no cystic meningeal or cutaneous covering and often continuous CSF leakage from the spinal central canal. Myelomeningoceles are usually displaced in a dorsal direction beyond the level of the surrounding skin, by a collection of CSF ventral to the cord (Fig. 1.9). Conversely, myeloschisis lesions are usually adherent to the anterior wall of the vertebral canal and are therefore either flush with, or below, the plane of the surrounding skin (discussed later). The terminology used for both these lesions has been inconsistent. Some authors use the term *myelomeningocele* for cystic lesions that contain abnormal neural tissue, even if the cystic lesion is skin covered (i.e., a closed defect).[81,82] The term *myeloschisis* has also been applied inconsistently, with some authors using the term for open lesions extending down most of the neural tube, a lesion that others refer to as rachischisis.[72] Myelomeningoceles are the most common open dysraphic lesion of the spinal cord by far, have been subject to the most investigation, and have shown some response to medical and surgical intervention (discussed later). In addition, most cases of myelomeningocele now survive. For these reasons, the following discussion focuses largely on myelomeningocele.

Myelomeningocele

Anatomical Abnormality. The essential neural defect in myelomeningocele is restricted failure of primary neurulation with varying degrees of posterior neural tube closure. Approximately 80% of lesions occur in the lumbar (thoracolumbar, lumbar, lumbosacral) area, presumably because this is the last area of the neural tube to close.[64] Myelomeningoceles are represented by a neural plate or abortive neural tube–like structure (placode) in which the ventral half of the cord is relatively less affected than the dorsal. Most of the lesions are associated with dorsal protrusion of the neural tissue, such that a sac is created on the back (Figs. 1.10 and 1.11; see also Fig. 1.9). Bony effects of the overlying tissue include failure (lack of fusion or an absence) of vertebral arch development (spina bifida), with bilateral broadening of the vertebrae and lateral displacement of pedicles, leading to a widened vertebral canal.[29] The caudal extent of the vertebral changes is usually considerably greater than the extent of the neural lesion. Soft-tissue covering consists

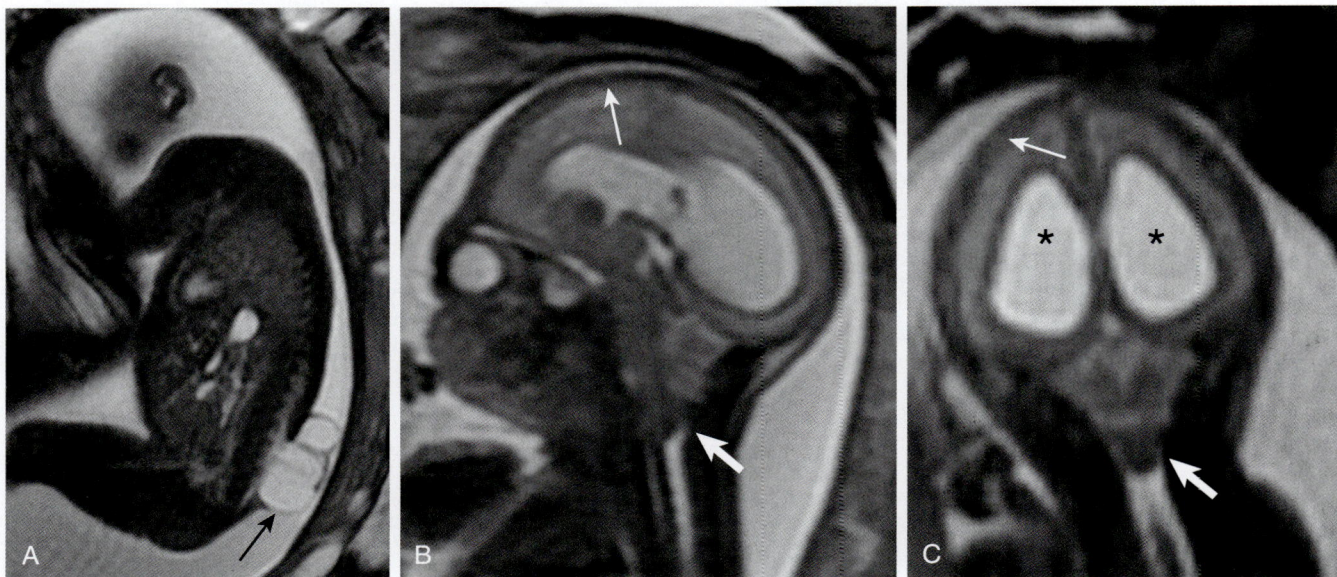

Figure 1.10 Lumbar myelomeningocele. T2-weighted fetal magnetic resonance imaging showing (A) sagittal view of the lumbar myelomeningocele *(arrow)*; (B) sagittal and (C) coronal views of the crowded posterior fossa with downward herniation of the brain stem and cerebellum (Chiari II) *(black arrow)*, paucity of extraaxial cerebrospinal fluid *(thin arrows)* around the brain, and moderate hydrocephalus (*).

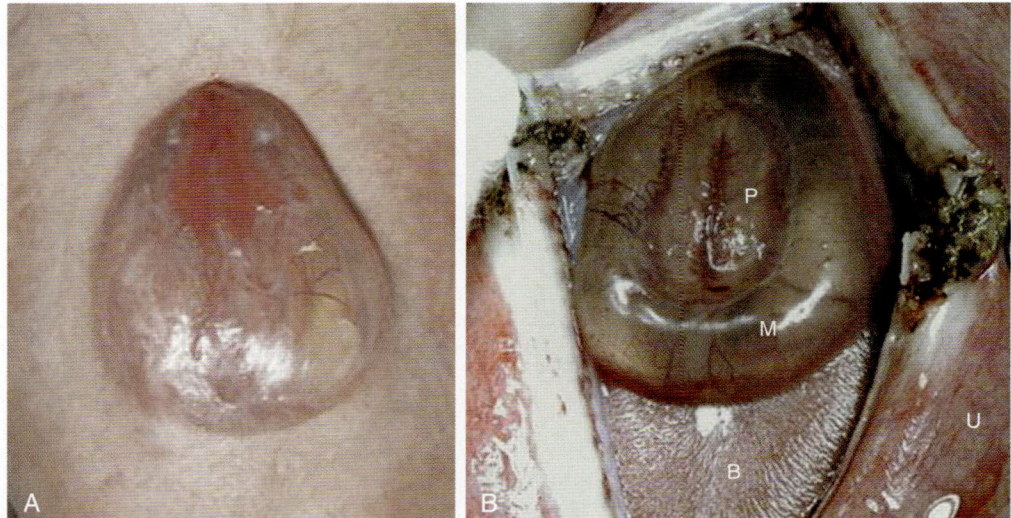

Figure 1.11 Myelomeningocele. Thoracolumbar myelomeningocele (A) in newborn. (B) Lumbar myelomeningocele exposed and viewed through hysterotomy site (B) during fetal repair. Note neural placode rising above the level of the surrounding skin. (*U*, uterus; *B*, fetal back; *M*, MMC sac; *P*, exposed neuroplacode). (A, Madan SS. Paralytic conditions in childhood. *Surgery.* 2004; 25:166–170. Copyright © 2007. B, Danzer E, Johnson MP. Fetal surgery for neural tube defects. *Semin Fetal Neonatal Med* 2014;19:2–8. Copyright © 2013 Elsevier Ltd.)

of a porous cystic sac of dysplastic meningeal tissue and a deficient skin cover.

Cervical myelomeningoceles are rare and differ in embryology, prognosis, and management from myelomeningoceles at lower spinal levels (discussed later).[43,83] These lesions are cystic and meet criteria as myelomeningoceles because they contain neuroglial tissue and CSF. However, unlike lower myelomeningoceles, the spinal cord is normal or near normal and remains within the spinal column. A stalk of neuroglial of fibrovascular tissue extends through a small midline gap between the dorsal columns of the spinal cord, passes through the bony spinous defect, and across the CSF-filled cyst to attach to the cyst wall, thereby tethering the spinal cord.[82,83] Unlike most other myelomeningoceles, these cervical lesions are almost always covered by full-thickness skin (i.e., *closed*) without CSF leakage.[81,84] Cervical myelomeningoceles are commonly associated with occult spinal lesions in other areas, such as hemivertebra, syringomyelia, and diastematomyelia (discussed later). Chiari II lesions are common in cervical myelomeningoceles, but intracranial neural lesions commonly associated with more caudal myelomeningoceles (such as fused thalami, callosal anomalies, and cortical malformations) are rare.

Timing. The onset of a typical myelomeningocele is probably no later than 26 days of gestation,[3] when the posterior neuropore closes.

Etiological Considerations. Prevention of myelomeningocele and other neural tube defects necessitates understanding of their causes. Recognized causes of such defects include (1) multifactorial inheritance, (2) single mutant genes (e.g., the autosomal recessively inherited Meckel syndrome), (3) chromosomal abnormalities (e.g., trisomies of chromosomes 2, 7, 9, 13, 14, 15, 16, 18, and 21 and duplications of chromosomes 1, 2, 3, 6, 7, 8, 9, 11, 13, 16, 20, and X), (4) certain rare syndromes of uncertain modes of transmission, (5) specific teratogens (e.g., aminopterin, thalidomide, valproic acid, carbamazepine), and (6) specific phenotypes of unknown causes (e.g., cloacal exstrophy and myelocystocele).[50,85-89] In rodent models of neural tube defects, more than 240 gene mutations have been identified.[90] Recent human studies suggest that a variety of genetic mutations may play a role, likely through complex polygenic interactions, possibly with superimposed epigenetic influences to produce the different neural tube defect phenotypes.[47,91] Of defects resulting from these causes, most cases (≈80%) are encompassed within the group in which the neural tube defect is the only major congenital abnormality and inheritance is multifactorial (i.e., dependent on a genetic predisposition that is polygenic and influenced by minor additive genetic variations at several gene loci).[92,93] Overall, genetic factors are thought to play a role in 60% to 70% of these cases. Environmental influences may play an important role on this substrate. Less than 10% of neural tube defects are part of syndromic conditions.[94]

Factors establishing the combined influence of both genetic and environmental influences are summarized in Tables 1.3 and 1.4. Factors establishing the *genetic role* include (1) a preponderance in female patients, (2) ethnic differences that persist after geographical migration, (3) increased incidence with parental consanguinity, (4) increased rate of concordance in apparently monozygotic twin pairs, and (5) increased incidence in siblings (as well as in second-degree and, to a lesser extent, third-degree relatives) and in children

TABLE 1.3	Factors Influencing Differences in Prevalence of Myelomeningocele		
FACTOR		**TIME PERIOD**	**PREVALENCE**
Country			
England/Wales		1996	0.32
Finland		1996	0.41
Norway		1996	0.57
Northern Netherlands		1996	0.63
Region of country			
Northern China		1992–1993	2.92
Southern China		1992–1993	0.26
Time period			
Eastern Ireland		1980	2.7
Eastern Ireland		1984	0.6
Ethnic/racial (California)			
Non-Hispanic white		1990–1994	0.47
Hispanic		1990–1994	0.42
African American		1990–1994	0.33
Asian		1990–1994	0.20
Prenatal diagnosis and elective termination (England/Wales)			
Live and stillbirths		1996	0.09
Live and stillbirths and terminations		1996	0.31

Data from Mitchell LE, Adzick NS, Melchionne J, Pasquariello PS, et al. Spina bifida. *Lancet.* 2004;364:1885–1895.

TABLE 1.4	Maternal Risk Factors for Myelomeningocele	
FACTOR		**RELATIVE RISK**
Previous affected pregnancy (same partner)		30
Inadequate intake of folic acid		2–8
Pregestational diabetes		2–10
Intake of valproic acid or carbamazepine		10–20
Low vitamin B_{12}		3
Obesity		1.5–3.5
Hyperthermia		2

Data from Mitchell LE, Adzick NS, Melchionne J, Pasquariello PS, et al. Spina bifida. *Lancet.* 2004;364:1885–1895.

of affected patients.[51,85-87,92,93,95-101] The possibility of important *environmental influences* is suggested particularly by large variations in incidence as a function of geographical location and time period of study (see Table 1.3). Particularly potent data to suggest environmental influences relate to long-term trends in incidence. For example, in the northeastern United States, an epidemic period could be defined between approximately 1920 and 1949, with a peak between 1929 and 1932.[102] Since the late 1980s, a prominent steady decline in incidence has occurred in both the United States and Great Britain (see earlier).[a] The *interaction of environmental and genetic influences* has been

_____
[a]References 50, 51, 53, 87, 100, and 103-107.

TABLE 1.5   Correlations Among Motor, Sensory, and Sphincter Function, Reflexes, and Segmental Innervation

MAJOR SEGMENTAL INNERVATION[a]	MOTOR FUNCTION	CUTANEOUS SENSATION	SPHINCTER FUNCTION	REFLEX
L1–L2	Hip flexion	Groin (L1) Anterior, upper thigh (L2)	—	—
L3–L4	Hip adduction Knee extension	Anterior, lower thigh and knee (L3) Medial leg (L4)	—	Knee jerk
L5–S1	Knee flexion Ankle dorsiflexion Ankle plantar flexion	Lateral leg and medial foot (L5) Sole of foot (S1)	—	Ankle jerk
S1–S4	Toe flexion	Posterior leg and thigh (S2) Middle of buttock (S3) Medial buttock (S4)	Bladder and rectal function	Anal wink

[a]Segmental innervation for motor and sensory functions overlaps considerably; correlations shown are approximate.

demonstrated in experimental studies of the curly-tail mouse, in which a neural tube defect is inherited as an autosomal recessive trait.[9,108] Among *specific environmental influences*, a particularly important role for *folate deficiency* during the period of neural tube formation is suggested by experimental and clinical studies (discussed later). Other environmental factors, such as prenatal exposure to maternal hyperthermia, maternal diabetes mellitus, valproic acid (see Chapter 38), carbamazepine (see Chapter 38), maternal obesity, and low maternal vitamin B_{12} concentrations, also are of varying importance (see Table 1.4).[51,89,93,109-125]

The increased incidence of neural tube defects in siblings of index cases has had major importance for *genetic counseling.* Recurrence risks for neural tube defects are around 3% after a single affected pregnancy, increasing to 12% after two affected pregnancies.[126] However, precise estimates of risks in subsequent siblings must take into account the population under study (see Table 1.3). A striking relationship between recurrence risk and the level of the myelomeningocele in the index case has been shown.[97] Thus the risk for recurrence in a sibling was 7.8% if the index case had a lesion at T11 or above, but only 0.7% if the lesion was below T11. A decline in the risk of neural tube defect as birth order increases also has been defined[99,127]; for example, in a study in Albany, New York, the risk for subsequent affected siblings (1.4%) was significantly less than for previously affected siblings (3.1%).[98]

Maternal diabetes is associated with a threefold increase in birth defects, but this risk increases to 5.4-fold for neural tube defects and 170-fold for caudal cell mass dysplasias (discussed later).[128] At highest risk are pregnancies complicated by hyperglycemia around the time of conception (pregestational diabetes). Pregestational obesity is also a risk factor for neural tube defects. In one large population-based study, there was a fourfold increase in neural tube defects in women with body mass index (BMI) greater than 40.[129] Other studies have shown a significantly increased risk for neural tube defects when maternal pregestational BMI exceeds 30.[130,131] The association between neural tube defects and obesity is significantly stronger for spina bifida than for anencephaly.[132] Recent reports suggest that obesity-related neural tube defects are folate unresponsive.[133]

Clinical Aspects. The precise incidence of myelomeningocele is difficult to establish, in part because of differences in the terminology used in reports. The populations included in these studies are variable, with some including anencephaly, some only open neural tube defects, or some with a broad spectrum of neural tube defects.[134,135] Although there is a wide variation between[50,51] and within countries,[53,100] it is generally agreed that the incidence of neural tube defects has been decreasing in developed countries for the past three decades, even before the advent of folic acid supplementation (discussed later).[a] Factors implicated in this decline include dietary folate supplementation, improved antenatal diagnosis and, in some areas, elective termination.[139] Nonetheless, the global burden of neural tube defects (mostly anencephaly and myelomeningocele) remains high and estimated to exceed 300,000 cases per year, with highest prevalences in low- and middle-income populations.[140] At the same time, there has been a steady increase in the survival of myelomeningocele, with one study reporting survival rates of 71%, 69%, and 66% at 1, 10, and 20 years, respectively.[141]

Neurological Features. The clinical features of myelomeningocele relate primarily to the nature of the primary spinal lesion, as well as the presence and severity of associated complications, such as hindbrain herniation, hydrocephalus, and other intracranial developmental lesions.

The disturbances of neurological function, of course, depend on the level of the spinal lesion. Particular attention should be paid to examination of motor, sensory, and sphincter function. Moreover, in the first days of life, motor function subserved by segments caudal to the level of the lesion is common but then generally disappears after the first postnatal week.[142] Table 1.5 lists some of the important correlations among motor, sensory, and sphincter function, reflexes, and segmental innervation. Assessment of the functional level of the lesion allows reasonable estimates of potential future capacities. Thus most patients with lesions below S1 ultimately are able to walk unaided, whereas those with lesions above L2 usually are wheelchair dependent for at least a major portion of their activities.[143-148] Approximately one-half of patients with intermediate lesions are ambulatory (L4, L5) or primarily ambulatory (L3) with braces or other specialized devices and crutches. Considerable variability exists between subsequent ambulatory status and apparent neurological segmental level, especially in patients

---

[a]References 50, 51, 53, 54, 61, 87, 93, 103-105, 107, 109, and 13-138.

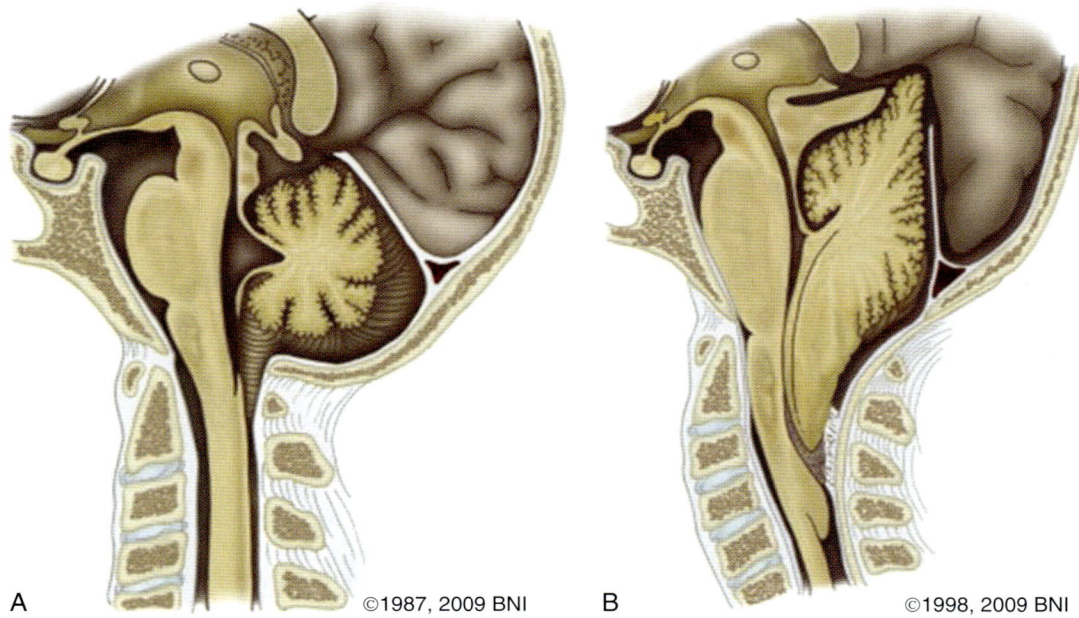

©1987, 2009 BNI   ©1998, 2009 BNI

Figure 1.12 Diagrams of (A) normal posterior fossa and (B) Chiari II malformation. (Used with permission from Barrow Neurological Institute; Upper Cervical and Craniocervical Decompression. Gantwerker BR, Spine Surgery, Chapter 37, 377–388. Copyright © 2012, 2005, 1999 by Saunders, an imprint of Elsevier Inc.)

with midlumbar lesions.[144,149,150] Good strength of iliopsoas (hip flexion) and of quadriceps (knee extension) muscles is an especially important predictor of ambulatory potential rather than wheelchair dependence.[149,150] Deterioration to a lower level of ambulatory function than that expected from segmental level occurs over years, and this tendency is worse in the absence of careful management. In addition, patients with lesions as high as thoracolumbar levels, at least as young children, can use standing braces or other specialized devices to be upright and can be taught to *swivel walk*.[151,152] Indeed, continuing improvements in ambulatory aids and their use are constantly increasing the chances for ambulation in children with higher lesions (see Results of Therapy). Segmental level also is an important determinant of the likelihood of the development of scoliosis. Most patients with lesions above L2 ultimately exhibit significant scoliosis, whereas this complication is unusual in patients with lesions below S1.

Cervical myelomeningoceles are almost always associated with a normal neurological outcome if surgical detethering is performed in infancy.[81,153] Significant primary motor, sensory, bowel, and bladder deficits are rare.[43,83] Delayed or incomplete surgical detethering may result in progressive neurological deficits over time.

Associated Anomalies and Putative Mechanisms

Chiari Type II Malformation. The Chiari II malformation (Fig. 1.12) is a virtually ubiquitous complication of thoracolumbar, lumbar, and lumbosacral myelomeningocele. The central feature of this complex anomaly is a small posterior fossa, the contents of which are crowded and distorted.[79] A Chiari II malformation involves the midbrain and hindbrain (pons, medulla, and cerebellum) and cervical spinal cord and its components and associations are listed in Box 1.4. Features of the Chiari II

malformation may be explained by the *unified theory*,[154,155] in which the ongoing spinal CSF leak results in failure of CSF *support* of the ventricles, including the fourth ventricle, which in turn leads to an underdeveloped small posterior fossa (with a low-set torcular and incomplete bony growth). The principles of the unified theory are supported by studies of fetal myelomeningocele repair showing reduced hindbrain herniation[156-158] and reduced brain stem compression.[159] The degree of hindbrain herniation does not appear to be related to the level of the spinal lesion.[154] However, some degree of hindbrain herniation is almost universally present in open myelomeningocele and remains the leading cause of death in the first 5 years of life.[160] The cerebellar hemispheres are underdeveloped,[158,161] but the cerebellar dysmorphology does not affect all cerebellar regions equally.[162] Compared with controls and corrected for reduced global volume, the anterior lobe is enlarged while the posterior lobe is reduced in size. Absence of brain stem nuclei, including the basal pontine and olivary nuclei, are also seen; these nuclei and the cerebellum have a common origin in the alar plate of the rhombencephalon.[163]

The *Chiari type II malformation* is responsible for both brain stem dysfunction (a serious complication in a minority of patients with myelomeningocele) and hydrocephalus, a serious complication in most patients with myelomeningocele (see earlier). Hydrocephalus associated with the Chiari type II malformation probably results primarily from one or both of two basic causes (see Box 1.4). The first is the hindbrain malformation that blocks either the fourth ventricular CSF outflow or the CSF flow through the posterior fossa. The second is at the aqueductal level, with aqueductal stenosis present in approximately 40% to 75%, and aqueductal atresia in an additional 10% of cases with Chiari II malformations.[127,163,164] Studies of human embryos

BOX 1.4   Complications of Myelomeningocele

Chiari II Malformation
Ubiquitous with lumbar-sacral myelomeningoceles

Temporal Features
Usually present by 2nd trimester

Etiological Features
Small posterior fossa is the fundamental mechanism; due to CSF leak from spinal lesion
Crowded and distorted contents

Anatomic Features
Small posterior fossa
Low-set torcular caudal herniation through foramen magnum (medulla, 4th ventricle, inferior vermis)
Rostral herniation through the tentorial notch (superior vermis)
Pressure/traction effects
Elongation and thinning of upper medulla and pons
Persistence of embryonic flexure
Cerebellar hemispheres may wrap around brain stem
Hydrocephalus due to disturbed flow dynamics from aqueduct, 4th ventricle, and subarachnoid space compression
Bony defects of foramen magnum, occiput and upper cervical vertebrae
Associated features of uncertain pathogenesis
Cerebellar dysplasia, hypoplasia or agenesis
Significant reduction of Purkinje cells
Absence of brain stem nuclei (basal pontine, olivary, other)

Clinical Importance
Stridor, apnea, cyanotic spells, and dysphagia may develop
Role in development of hydrocephalus

Hydrocephalus
Develops in 85%–90% of lumbar-sacral myelomeningoceles

Temporal Features
Most rapid progression occurring in first postnatal month
Dilation of ventricles before rapid head growth or before signs of increased intracranial pressure or both

Etiological Features
Chiari type II with obstruction of fourth ventricular outflow
Aqueductal stenosis
Impaired CSF flow through narrowed subarachnoid spaces and crowded posterior fossa

Importance
Requirement for shunt and its complications (especially infection) are a major cause of neurologic morbidity.

TABLE 1.6   Relation of Brain Stem Dysfunction to Mortality in Myelomeningocele

CLINICAL FEATURES	NUMBER	MORTALITY
Stridor	10	0
Stridor and apnea	4	25%
Stridor, apnea, cyanotic spells, and dysphagia	5	60%
Total	19	21%

Effective control correlated with ultimate neurological function.
Adapted from Charney EB, Rorke LB, Sutton LN, Schut L. Management of Chiari II complications in infants with myelomeningocele. *J Pediatr.* 1987;111:364–371.

flow, and reduced need for ventriculoperitoneal shunting for hydrocephalus (discussed later; see Fig. 1.10).[157,166]

Clinical features directly referable to the hindbrain anomaly of the Chiari type II malformation (i.e., not to hydrocephalus) are probably more common than is recognized. In one carefully studied series of 200 infants, one-third exhibited feeding disturbances (associated with reflux and aspiration), laryngeal stridor, or apneic episodes (or all three). In one-third of these affected infants, death was "directly or indirectly attributed to these problems." Indeed, in this and similar series, at least one-half of the deaths of infants with myelomeningocele can be attributed to the hindbrain anomaly (despite treatment of the back lesion and hydrocephalus).[160,167,168] In a cumulative series of 142 infants, the median age at onset of symptoms referable to brain stem compromise was 3.2 months.[160] The clinical syndromes of brain stem dysfunction and their relation to mortality are presented in Table 1.6.[160,170,171] The 19 affected infants represented 13% of those with myelomeningocele. The principal clinical abnormalities in this and related studies reflect lower brain stem dysfunction and include vocal cord paralysis with stridor, abnormalities of ventilation of both obstructive and central types (especially during sleep), cyanotic spells, and dysphagia.[167-170,172-179] The full constellation of stridor, apnea, cyanotic spells, and dysphagia is associated with a high mortality (see Table 1.6). Such sensitive assessments of brain stem function as brain stem auditory-evoked responses, polysomnography, pneumographic ventilatory studies, and somatosensory-evoked responses are abnormal in approximately 60% in infants with myelomeningocele and are the neurophysiological analogues of the clinical deficits.[167,180-184]

The clinical abnormalities of brain stem function have three primary causes. First, they relate in part to the brain stem malformations, which involve cranial nerve and other nuclei, and are present in most cases at autopsy (Table 1.7).[163] Second, compression and traction of the anomalous caudal brain stem by hydrocephalus and increased intracranial pressure may play a role, especially in the vagal nerve disturbance that results in the vocal cord paralysis and stridor. Third, ischemic and hemorrhagic necrosis of brain stem is often present and may result from the disturbed arterial architecture of the caudally displaced vertebrobasilar circulation.[170]

Hydrocephalus. Several clinical features are helpful in evaluating the possibility of hydrocephalus. First, on examination, *the status of the anterior fontanelle and the cranial*

and fetuses with myelomeningocele support the concept that the Chiari type II hindbrain malformation is a primary defect and not a result of hydrocephalus.[165]

Moreover, studies of a mutant mouse with defective neurulation (*Splotch*) provide insight into the mechanism by which myelomeningocele may lead to the Chiari type II malformation. Thus, in this model, it is clear that the Chiari type II malformation results from growth of the hindbrain in a posterior fossa that is too small. Hydrocephalus then results from the Chiari type II malformation, as described earlier. Additional support for this formulation is the demonstration that closure of the myelomeningocele in the second trimester of fetal life, before the most rapid growth of the cerebellum, results in upward displacement of the inferiorly herniated cerebellar vermis, expansion of the posterior fossa, improvement in CSF

TABLE 1.7	Brain Stem Malformations in Myelomeningocele	
Total With Brain Stem Malformation		76%
Defective myelination		44%
Hypoplasia of cranial nerve nuclei		20%
Hypoplasia or aplasia of olives		20%
Hypoplasia or aplasia of basal pontine nuclei		16%
Hypoplasia of tegmentum		4%

Adapted from Gilbert JN, Jones KL, Rorke LB, Chernoff GF, et al. Central nervous system anomalies associated with meningomyelocele, hydrocephalus, and the Arnold-Chiari malformation: reappraisal of theories regarding the pathogenesis of posterior neural tube closure defects. *Neurosurgery.* 1986;18:559–564.

TABLE 1.8	Cerebral Cortical Malformations in Myelomeningocele	
Total with Cerebral Cortex Dysplasia		92%
Neuronal heterotopias		44%
Polymicrogyria (with disordered lamination)		40%
Disordered lamination only		24%
Microgyria, normal lamination		12%
Profound migrational disturbances		24%

Adapted from Gilbert JN, Jones KL, Rorke LB, Chernoff GF, et al. Central nervous system anomalies associated with meningomyelocele, hydrocephalus, and the Arnold-Chiari malformation: reappraisal of theories regarding the pathogenesis of posterior neural tube closure defects. *Neurosurgery.* 1986;18:559–564.

sutures should be noted. A full anterior fontanelle and split cranial sutures are helpful signs for the diagnosis of increased intracranial pressure. CSF leakage from the myelomeningocele provides decompression in this situation, and the signs of increased intracranial pressure may be absent or delayed. *Evaluation of the head size* provides useful information. If the head circumference is more than the 90th percentile, approximately a 95% chance exists that appreciable ventricular enlargement is present.[185] If the head circumference is less than the 90th percentile, an approximately 65% chance of hydrocephalus still exists.[185] The *site of the lesion* is also helpful in predicting the presence or imminent development of hydrocephalus. With occipital, cervical, thoracic, or sacral lesions, the incidence of hydrocephalus is approximately 60%; with thoracolumbar, lumbar, or lumbosacral lesions, the incidence of hydrocephalus is approximately 85% to 90%.[84,185,186]

Signs of increased intracranial pressure are not prerequisites for the diagnosis of hydrocephalus in the newborn and indeed are observed in only approximately 15% of newborns with myelomeningocele.[164] Serial ultrasound scans are important because progressive ventricular dilation, without rapid head growth or signs of increased intracranial pressure, occurs in infants with myelomeningocele[164,187] in a manner analogous to the development of hydrocephalus after intraventricular hemorrhage (see Chapter 24). The most common time for hydrocephalus with myelomeningocele to be accompanied by overt clinical signs is 2 to 3 weeks after birth; more than 80% of infants who have hydrocephalus with myelomeningocele and who do not undergo shunting procedures exhibit such clinical signs by 6 weeks of age.[152]

Other Central Nervous System Anomalies. Other anomalies of the CNS associated with myelomeningocele and the Chiari II lesion include cerebral cortical anomalies, callosal defects, small posterior fossa, with decreased size of the cerebellum. Perhaps most important of these are abnormalities of cerebral cortical development. In earlier studies, the pathological finding of microgyria was described in 55% to 95% of cases.[188,189] Whether this finding reflected a true cortical dysgenesis was not clear, but its presence was of major potential importance because of a relationship with the intellectual deficits that occur in a minority of these patients. Moreover, the occurrence of seizures in approximately 20% to 25% of children with myelomeningocele may be accounted

for in part by such cortical dysgenesis.[190-192] This issue was clarified considerably by a careful neuropathological study of 25 cases of myelomeningocele (Table 1.8). Fully 92% of the brains showed evidence of cerebral cortical dysplasia, and 40% had overt polymicrogyria.[163] Thus impaired neuronal migration was a common feature. In addition, callosal anomalies, including hypoagenesis (reduced ventrodorsal extent) and hypoplasia (reduced thickness), are thought to occur to some degree in almost all cases of myelomeningocele.[193] In callosal hypogenesis, the rostrum, splenium, and posterior body are the most commonly missing elements.[79] Even when present, the posterior elements (i.e., isthmus and splenium) are the most commonly hypoplastic regions.[194] Thoracic myelomeningoceles are twofold more likely to have splenial agenesis than lower myelomeningoceles.[193] Up to 44% of myelomeningocele cases have callosal hypoplasia, in which the callosum is present in its entire rostrocaudal extent but is thinned.[195] More recent MRI studies using surface area and diffusion tensor analyses support the notion that the thinner corpus callosum results from fewer crossing axons.[196] Several studies have suggested that volume of the entire corpus callosum, as well as specifically the genu and splenium,[194,197] correlate with cognitive outcome.

Other anomalous features, such as cranial lacunae, hypoplasia of the falx and tentorium, low placement of the tentorium, anomalies of the septum pellucidum, anterior and inferior *pointing* of the frontal horns, thickened interthalamic connections, and widened foramen magnum, are of uncertain clinical significance. However, they are visualized readily to varying degrees with CT, MRI, and cranial ultrasonography.[72,198-200] Midbrain anomalies include tectal *beaking*, which is due to fusion of the colliculi and is evident in about 65% of cases. Anomalies in position of the cerebellum are observable in utero by ultrasonography or MRI.[201,202] Cerebellar dysplasia, including heterotopias, is definable neuropathologically in 72% of cases.[163]

Diagnosis. Maternal serum alpha-fetoprotein (AFP) levels and ultrasonography are the primary screening techniques for the prenatal diagnosis of neural tube defects. *AFP* is the major protein component of human fetal serum (Fig. 1.13) and can be detected 30 days after conception, peaking at between 10 and 13 weeks of gestation. Current recommendations are for maternal serum AFP testing between 15 and 20 weeks' gestation.[203] Increased levels of AFP in the amniotic fluid occur with open neural tube defects and anencephaly; the mechanism for the elevated levels is thought to represent transudation of the protein from the membranes covering the lesion (see Figs. 1.9 and 1.11).[204] Positive maternal serum AFP testing should be repeated, since false positive tests are not uncommon.[205] Conversely, there are conditions other than open neural tube defects that may elevate maternal serum and amniotic fluid AFP levels, including abdominal wall defects such as omphalocele or gastroschisis. Until the mid-1980s, amniocentesis for detection of elevated levels of AFP in amniotic

fluid was the most common, albeit invasive, procedure for suspicion of an open neural tube defect. Several reports in the late 1970s indicated that determination of *maternal serum AFP levels* was useful for screening for neural tube defects.[206-210] The largest study involved measurements in more than 18,000 pregnant women in the United Kingdom.[210] The optimal time for measurement was shown to be 16 to 18 weeks of pregnancy. Subsequent experience in Scotland,[206] Sweden,[211] Wales,[212] and the United States[213,214] confirmed the high sensitivity of the analysis of AFP in serum, and large-scale screening programs are now well established.[93,212,214,215] In situations where the origin of elevated maternal serum AFP remains in question, amniotic fluid levels of AFP should be tested and, if elevated, should be followed by acetylcholinesterase (AChE; primarily neuronal in origin) levels. Elevation of both AFP and AChE in the amniotic fluid confirms a neural origin for the elevated AFP.[216]

The diagnosis and anatomical details of a fetal neural tube defect are confirmed by ultrasonography and MRI.[77,78,93,212,217-221] The earliest ultrasonographic features include changes in the configuration of the posterior fossa, in addition to the lesion itself. After 12 weeks' gestation the cranial markers of myelomeningocele (i.e., banana and lemon signs [Fig. 1.14], decreased extraaxial CSF, and small cisterna magna) become detectable by ultrasound and are useful supportive findings. Fetal MRI is the diagnostic study of choice in the fetal period and best delineates the anatomical details (see Fig. 1.10).

Management. The management of myelomeningocele has undergone major changes in recent decades, both in terms of primary prevention, as well as lesion repair in the newborn, and more recently in the fetus. The following briefly reviews current concepts in management.

Primary Prevention. Management of the patient with myelomeningocele, or of any patient with a neural tube defect,

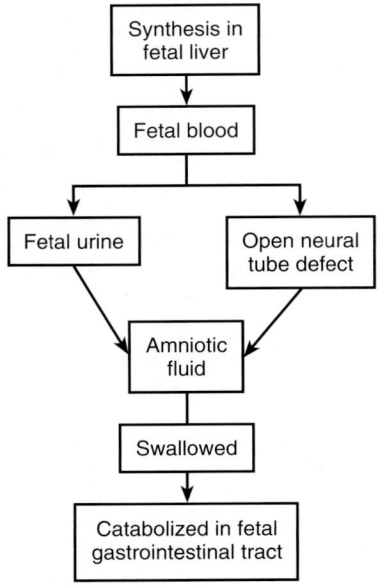

Figure 1.13 Physiology and pathophysiology of alpha-fetoprotein in utero.

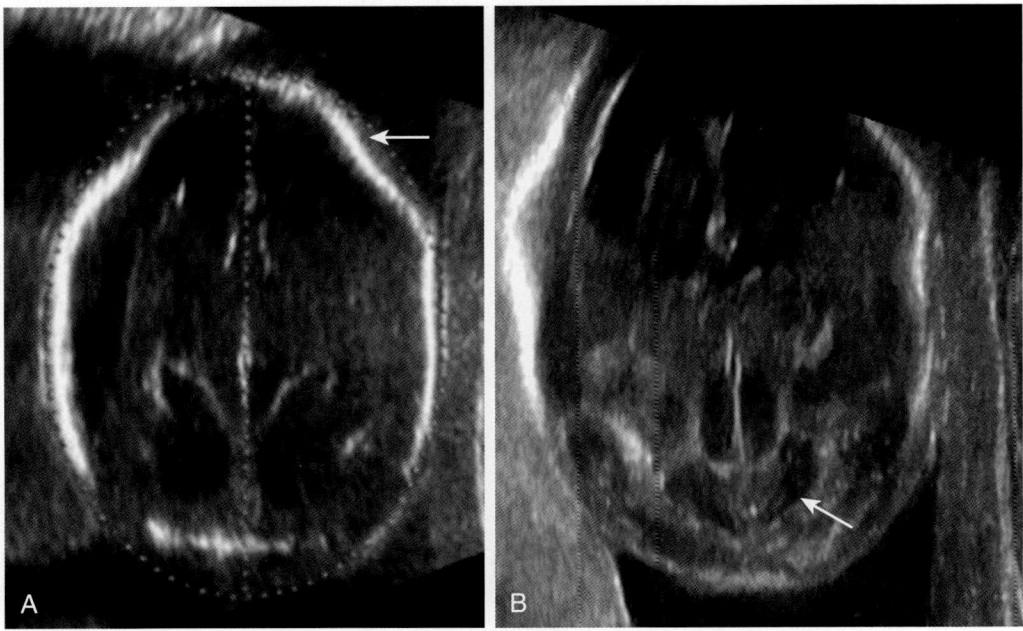

Figure 1.14 Fetal cranial ultrasound features associated with open neural tube defects. (A) The "lemon-shaped" cranium due to frontal bone scalloping *(arrow)*. (B) The "banana sign" of the compressed cerebellum *(arrow).* (From Coady AM. *Twining's Textbook of Fetal Abnormalities.* Chapter 11, 223–263 Copyright © 2015, 2007, 2000 by Churchill Livingstone, an imprint of Elsevier Limited. All rights reserved.)

BOX 1.5   The Role of Folate in Neural Tube Defects

- 1959: Failed abortions using an FA antagonist were associated with an increase in NTDs.[423]
- 1965: Embryopathy of maternal FA deficiency includes NTD.[424]
- 1980–1983: MVI supplementation reduced NTD risk.[254-257,425]
- 1989: MVI supplementation beneficial effect corroborated.[258]
- 1989: Noncontrolled study of MVI/FA supplementation in early pregnancy leads to decrease in NTD.[245]
- 1991: Medical Research Council (United Kingdom) Vitamin Study. Large RCT of FA supplementation (4 mg/day) in women with previous NTD fetus showed an 83% reduction.[246]
- 1992: RCT of FA supplementation (0.8 mg/day) from I month preconception through first 8 weeks of pregnancy reduced the risk of a first NTD-affected fetus.[228]
- 1992: Centers for Disease Control and Prevention (United States) recommended FA supplementation (0.4 mg/day) for all women of childbearing age capable of becoming pregnant in the United States.[267]
- 1997: Despite increased public awareness, supplementation campaign proved disappointing; <1/3 women compliant and >50% of pregnancies in United States are unplanned.
- 1998: Fortification campaign implemented in the United States with goal of ensuring that women of childbearing age received the daily recommended dose of 400 µg/day
- 2002–2003: Several Canadian reports describe a 32%–54% decrease in NTD since dietary FA fortification.[275,426]
- 2010: United States report ~20% decrease in NTD since dietary FA fortification.
- 2015: Late high-dose (5 mg/day) rescue FA after early pregnancy diagnosis may be protective.[286]
- Currently: More than 75 countries have mandatory FA fortification programs.

FA, Folic acid; *MVI*, multivitamins; *NTD*, neural tube defect; *RCT*, randomized clinical trial.

should begin with the following question: How could this have been prevented? Indeed, *prevention* must be considered the primary goal for the future. Major advances have been made in this direction. Prenatal diagnosis of neural tube defects and termination of pregnancy involving an affected fetus are effective methods of *secondary* prevention. However, a method of primary prevention would be more widely acceptable. Evidence now shows that folate *supplementation* around the time of conception, and therefore neural tube closure, has a major preventive effect on the occurrence of neural tube defects.[a]

The effect of *multivitamin supplementation* (Box 1.5) before and during early pregnancy on recurrence of neural tube defects was first studied definitively by Smithells and colleagues[254-257,264] in a recruited series of women with histories of births of one or more previously affected children. The multivitamin supplement contained *physiological* quantities of vitamins, such as folate, riboflavin, ascorbic acid, and vitamin A. The results of the study were striking. Of 454 women taking supplements, only 3 (0.7%) had recurrences, whereas of 519 women not taking supplements, 24 (4.7%) had recurrences. Although the study was criticized for several methodological issues,[265,266] the data were promising. A subsequent study by Smithells and coworkers[258] showed a

similarly striking effect. A noncontrolled study in the United States on women identified largely by elevated serum AFP levels, measured in a single regional laboratory, confirmed the beneficial role of folate-containing multivitamins.[245] Moreover, the beneficial effect of folate was related clearly to the time during pregnancy when neural tube closure occurs.

After the aforementioned study, the British Medical Research Council completed an extremely important multicenter study (Box 1.5).[246] Women were assigned randomly to four groups allocated to receive one of the following regimens of supplementation: folate and a multivitamin supplementation of "other vitamins," folate alone, "other vitamins" alone, or no folate or "other vitamins." The results were decisive in demonstrating the preventive effect and the specific role of folate (vs. other components of the previously used multivitamin preparations). The overall reduction in neural tube defects was 83%. The findings clearly had major implications for the primary prevention of neural tube defects. On the basis of this study, the US Centers for Disease Control and Prevention (CDC) recommended an increase in folic acid intake by 0.4 mg/day for women from the time they plan to become pregnant through the first 3 months of pregnancy.[246a] The folate was not recommended to be administered as a multivitamin preparation because of the potential danger for toxicity from excessive amounts of other vitamins in the multivitamin preparation. Because of the uncertainty of the degree of risk from the folate supplementation, the initial recommendations were directed only to women who had had a previous pregnancy complicated by a neural tube defect, as in the British study. Subsequently, two studies showed a preventive effect of periconceptional folic acid exposure on the occurrence of neural tube defects in populations of women without a prior affected child.[228,263] These observations were followed by the recommendation of the US Public Health Service and the American Academy of Pediatrics that "all women capable of becoming pregnant consume 0.4 mg of folic acid daily to prevent neural tube defects."[268]

The optimal methods of folate supplementation and dose of the supplement are not totally clarified.[269,270] Public educational campaigns, albeit useful, have not been entirely successful, especially because as many as 50% of pregnancies are unplanned, and only a few of the *nonplanners* are reached by such campaigns.[269,271] In 1998 the US Food and Drug Administration mandated fortification of all enriched grain products with folate (0.14 mg/100 g), which resulted in a 30% decrease in neural tube defects.[272] Similar programs have been instituted in many other countries and have resulted in an approximately 50% reduction in prevalence of neural tube defects.[a] However, the British Medical Research Council study used a 4 mg (rather than 0.4 mg) daily folate dose and achieved an 83% reduction in prevalence of lesions. Thus one expert in the field recommended a public health policy that includes "both the mandatory fortification of flour and a recommendation that all women planning a pregnancy take 5 mg of folic acid per day."[261]

Together these studies have led to the conclusion that folate supplementation was capable of reducing but not eradicating neural tube defects, giving rise to the notion of "folic acid–preventable spina bifida and anencephaly" (FAPSBA).

---

[a]References 9, 50, 51, 93, 103, 106, and 222-263.

[a]References 103, 106, 241, 244, 251, 259, and 273-276.

It is estimated that 50% to 72% of neural tube defects are preventable through folate supplementation.[277,278] The reduction in anencephaly and facial defects has been less striking than that of spina bifida.[279,280] In addition, in the postfortification era the initial decrease in neural tube defects has been sustained without further decline. In the United States, Hispanics continue to have the highest rate, whereas non-Hispanic blacks have the lowest rate. The decreases in prevalence of neural tube defects following fortification have been associated with increasing levels of serum and red blood cell (RBC) folate levels in the population and an almost complete eradication of folate deficiency. Recent studies have suggested that the majority of FAPSBA in the United States is prevented by fortification; however, more than 20% of women of childbearing age still do not attain the RBC folate levels known to decrease the risk of neural tube defects.[281,282] This has in turn led to recommendations for strategies that target specific RBC folate levels.[283]

The CDC has released a series of updates on global prevention of FAPSBA, as more countries instituted fortification programs. In 2006 the decrease in FAPSBA through fortification programs around the world was estimated at 6.8%,[284] in 2008 it was estimated at 9.1%, and in 2012 estimates ranged from 15.6% to 25.5%. The higher number of 25% is based on recent reports, suggesting that the threshold dose of folate necessary to prevent FAPSBA was lower than the originally proposed 0.4 mg/day. In addition, two recent case-control studies suggested that (1) full protection against FAPSBA was attained at levels lower than 0.4 mg/day, and (2) folate supplementation was no longer adding further protection against FAPSBA since the introduction of fortification.[272,285] Together, these studies suggested that most of the FAPSBA prevention in the United States was through fortification and that the vast majority of FAPSBA around the world could be prevented with fortification programs alone.

A population-based study in Denmark investigated the effects of two public health measures on the incidence of myelomeningocele, specifically recommendations for folic acid supplementation and second trimester (18–19 week gestation) fetal ultrasound screening.[139] The study concluded that recommendations for folate supplementation had no significant effect on the incidence of myelomeningocele because of lack of compliance. However, the second trimester prenatal ultrasound screening program was associated with a significant decrease in the rate of live-born babies with myelomeningocele.[139] Data from a large study in China suggest that late administration of folate might have a protective role against neural tube defects.[277] A strategy of high-dose (5 mg/day) folic acid rescue (to achieve rapid fetal levels) has been proposed for cases in which pregnancy is diagnosed before or in the provided time frame in women not taking folate supplementation.[286]

The mechanism of the beneficial effect of folate is not established. One report raised the possibility that autoantibodies against folate receptors are present in as many as 75% of women who have had a pregnancy complicated by a neural tube defect.[287] The autoantibody-mediated block of cellular folate uptake by folate receptors could be bypassed by administered folate, because the latter is reduced and methylated in vivo and is transported into cells by the reduced folate carrier. A related possibility is that the beneficial effect of folate could involve *the metabolism of homocysteine to methionine*, a reaction catalyzed by methionine synthase and necessitating a metabolite of folic acid (5-methyltetrahydrofolate).[a]

A critical enzyme in the synthesis of 5-methyltetrahydrofolate, *methylenetetrahydrofolate reductase*, is defective in 12% to 20% of cases of neural tube defects.[230,288] One biochemical result of this disturbance is an elevation of homocysteine, which has been shown to produce neural tube defects in avian embryos.[289] Another potential mechanism of a defect in homocysteine conversion to methionine is a disturbance in methylation reactions, for which methionine is crucial.[224,230] Transmethylations of DNA, proteins, and lipids have far-reaching metabolic consequences.[224,230]

Because some neural tube defects appear to be folate nonresponsive, other potential forms of nutritional supplementation have been explored. Inositol deficiency is the only known nutritional deficiency known to cause neural tube defects in mouse models.[292] In addition, inositol blood levels are significantly lower in pregnant women carrying a fetus with a neural tube defect.[293] Initial data from a randomized trial of periconceptional inositol supplementation in women with previous pregnancies complicated by neural tube defects are encouraging.[294]

Management After Fetal Diagnosis. The *two-hit* hypothesis for factors that determine the ultimate postnatal neurologic function of myelomeningocele survivors has significantly influenced fetal and delivery management of myelomeningocele. This hypothesis proposes that long-term neurologic function depends not only on the primary spinal defect but also on the accumulation of secondary, potentially treatable complications, including progressive injury to the exposed spinal neural tissue and the development of Chiari II lesions and hydrocephalus.[201,296,297] In fact, several lines of evidence have implicated these secondary insults in the majority of the ultimate deficit. Specifically, earlier studies showed preservation of exposed neural elements and absence of both hindbrain herniation and hydrocephalus in autopsies of early but not later gestation fetuses with myelomeningoceles.[298,299] Subsequent studies in midgestation fetuses showed loss of normal neural tissue at the level of the exposed tissue but not proximally.[300,301] In addition to direct trauma, noxious substances in the amniotic fluid, including meconium, have been implicated.[302] In myelomeningocele there is typically an accumulation of CSF in the subarachnoid space ventral to the cord at the level of the lesion (see Fig. 1.9); it has been suggested that the dorsal displacement of the cord exerts pressure on the dorsal cord neural elements by compression against the spinous defect.[303] Clinically, these observations are supported by the fact that fetal leg movements are often noted earlier in gestation in areas where they are lost after birth. Other studies in rodent and ovine models[304,305] suggested that secondary neural injury could be prevented or markedly attenuated and that normal hindbrain anatomy could be established after fetal closure of the spinal defect.[306,307]

On the basis of these experimental data, initial nonrandomized clinical studies of intrauterine intervention were performed in human fetuses with myelomeningocele.[156,157,166,308-311] These earlier studies reported a number of promising outcomes,

---

[a]References 9, 50, 222, 226, 230, 231, and 288-291.

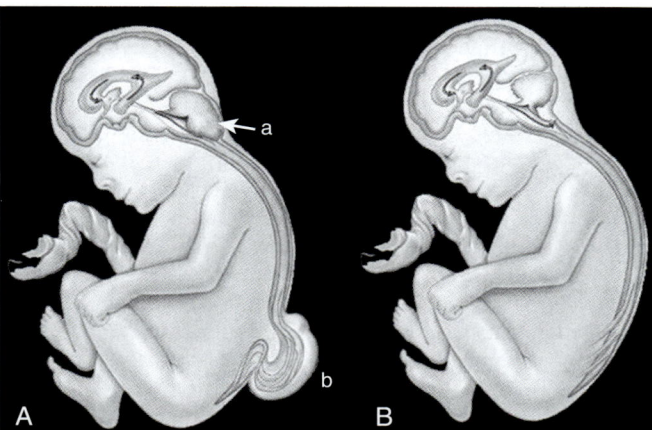

Figure 1.15 Pathogenetic formulation for the Chiari type II malformation and the effect of treatment. See text for details. In (A) Chiari malformation (a) and the open myelomeningocele (b) are shown. The negative pressure generated from drainage of cerebrospinal fluid from the open myelomeningocele (b) results in the inferior displacement of the cerebellum (a) and thereby the Chiari type II malformation. (B) After fetal closure, positive back pressure reduces the cerebellar hernia and expands the posterior fossa. (From Sutton LN, Adzick NS, Bilaniuk LT, Johnson MP, et al. Improvement in hindbrain herniation demonstrated by serial fetal magnetic resonance imaging following fetal surgery for myelomeningocele. *JAMA.* 1999;282:1826–1831.)

BOX 1.6   Outcome of Fetal Versus Neonatal Myelomeningocele Repair

Nonrandomized Studies—Prenatal Repair Associated With
- lower extremity function better than expected for anatomical level
- decreased hydrocephalus and need for VP shunt
- reversal of hindbrain herniation
- decreased brain stem dysfunction

10-Year Follow-up (n = 54)
- 79% community ambulators
- 9% household ambulators
- 14% wheelchair dependent
- 26% normal bladder function

Randomized Clinical Trial (MoM Study)—Prenatal Repair Group Had
- decreased need for VP shunt by 12 months (40% vs. 82%)
- improved motor and mental function by 30 months (25% vs. 67%)
- decreased moderate-severe Chiari II malformations (25% vs. 67%)
- increased independent orthotic-free ambulation (42%–21%)
- anatomical remodeling of posterior fossa
- increased rate of prematurity, chorionic membrane separation, and premature rupture of membranes
- increased need for postnatal cord untethering
- threatened or partial dehiscence of hysterotomy site (25%)

---

including lower extremity function better than predicted from the anatomical level of the lesion,[166] a significant decrease in hydrocephalus,[166,312,313] and the need for postnatal shunt placement.[166,311] Initial clinical reports also corroborated earlier experimental findings by showing reversal of hindbrain herniation as early as three weeks after human fetal myelomeningocele closure (possibly underlying the decreased need for shunt placement), as well as significantly fewer functional brain stem deficits (Box 1.6).[159,166] On the basis of these experimental and preliminary clinical results, a three-center randomized clinical trial of open prenatal versus conventional postnatal myelomeningocele repair was performed, in which the fetal surgery group with spinal lesions between the T1 and S1 levels underwent open surgical repair of the spinal lesion before 26 weeks' gestation. The trial was terminated early for demonstrated benefit in the experimental fetal surgery group.[314] Specifically, the fetal repair group required significantly fewer (40% vs. 82%) ventriculoperitoneal shunt procedures by 12 months of age, improved motor and mental composite scores at 30-month follow-up, and fewer (25% vs. 67%) moderate to severe Chiari II malformations (Fig. 1.15). There was an overall improvement in the functional versus anatomical spinal level, as well as an increased incidence of ambulation without orthotic devices in the fetal surgery group. Specifically, 42% versus 21% of fetal surgery cases were walking independently at follow-up (Box 1.6). However, the fetal repair group had a significantly higher rate of prematurity, chorionic membrane separation, and premature rupture of membranes, especially among those performed before 23 weeks' gestation,[315] and required more postnatal surgical untethering of the spinal cord. In addition, although no uterine ruptures occurred, 25% of women in this group had threatened or partial dehiscence

of the hysterotomy site. Subsequent reports from the same center have corroborated those from the clinical trial but have shown that fewer than 30% of cases referred for evaluation actually underwent fetal myelomeningocele repair.[316]

Measurements of the posterior fossa and its contents in three groups—(1) normal controls and cases with myelomeningocele undergoing (2) fetal repair and (3) postnatal repair—provided evidence that the fetal repair group underwent postoperative anatomical remodeling of the posterior fossa that approached that of the normal controls, whereas postnatal repair cases failed to do so.[317]

Long-term follow-up at a median age of 10 years of 54 patients who underwent fetal myelomeningocele repair *before* the MoMS (Management of Myelomeningocele Study) clinical trial showed that 79% were community ambulators, 9% were household ambulators only, 14% were wheelchair dependent, and 26% had normal bladder function (Box 1.6).[318]

Earlier attempts at endoscopic closure were abandoned for an open hysterotomy approach, used during the MoMS trial. Following reports of the maternal and pregnancy complications of open hysterotomy, such as premature labor and uterine scar dehiscence, endoscopic approach was reexplored. However, the technical approach to the fetal spinal closure was significantly more challenging and associated with a paradoxical increase in prematurity and mortality.[319,320] Most recently, a phase 1 trial (10 cases) of endoscopic fetal myelomeningocele repair, in which a biocellulose patch is used to seal the CSF leakage, obviated the need for dural repair.[321] Initial results are promising, especially in the reversal of hindbrain herniation; the need for postnatal CSF shunting for hydrocephalus was similar to that in the MoMS trial. Clearly larger studies are needed to perform side-by-side comparisons of the open versus endoscopic approaches to fetal repair of myelomeningocele.[314,321] Other experimental approaches are currently being investigated, including in utero stem cell transplantation,[323,324] but these have to date not entered into clinical care.

Management of Labor and Delivery. The optimal route for delivery of the fetus with an open neural tube defect remains controversial.[325] Proponents of the *two-hit hypothesis* argue that both labor and passage through the birth canal are likely to cause secondary traumatic neural injury. Consistent with the possibility of mechanical injury during labor, the results of a retrospective review of 160 carefully studied cases of myelomeningocele suggest that *delivery by cesarean section* before the onset of labor may result in better subsequent motor function than vaginal delivery or delivery by cesarean section after a period of labor.[325] Overall, infants delivered by cesarean section before the onset of labor had a mean level of paralysis 3.3 segments below the anatomical level of the spinal lesion, compared with 1.1 and 0.9 for infants delivered vaginally or delivered by cesarean section after the onset of labor, respectively. This variance is large enough to make the difference between the child's being ambulatory or wheelchair bound. Thus scheduled delivery by cesarean section before the onset of labor should be considered for the fetus with myelomeningocele, particularly if prenatal ultrasonography and karyotyping rule out the presence of severe hydrocephalus, chromosomal abnormality, or multiple systemic anomalies. Unfortunately there have been no prospective randomized trials comparing vaginal versus abdominal delivery to date, and in studies suggesting the benefit of cesarean delivery, comparison has been to historical controls.[325,326] As such, the mode of delivery currently remains the obstetrician's preference.

Postnatal Management. In developed countries with antenatal screening programs, most cases of myelomeningocele are diagnosed in the fetal period. Fetal imaging with ultrasound and/or MRI may allow for meaningful assessment of both acute neurological function at birth as well as long-term neurodevelopmental prognosis of the infant. Although most newborns with myelomeningocele are able to maintain vital functions, there is a higher than usual risk of cardiorespiratory failure that may require a period of extraordinary life support. In severe cases of hydrocephalus, Chiari II malformation, or associated malformations, it is reasonable to initiate discussions during pregnancy that allow the family to consider the level of intervention they would wish for their child if extraordinary life support is needed. The next step is to decide whether the newborn with myelomeningocele should receive anything more than conservative, supportive care (e.g., tender nursing care and oral feedings). Most neurosurgeons in the United States would advise early closure of the back lesion and, if needed, a CSF-diversion shunt.[160,327,328] Although the therapies are best discussed by the appropriate surgical specialists, a brief review is necessary here.

Early Postnatal Management. The prevalent notion is that *early closure of the back lesion* (within the first 24–72 hours) is optimal. The rationale for this approach has been the prevention of infection and the loss of motor function that may occur after the first days of life (see earlier). The prevention of infection is supported by several studies.[329,330] Conversely, in a large study of 110 infants with myelomeningocele, there was no significant difference in the rate of ventriculitis or lower extremity paralysis between infants undergoing early (first 48 hours) versus late

(3–7 days) closure of the back lesion.[331] On balance, it would appear most prudent to close the back as promptly as possible (within the first 24–72 hours) but not to feel compelled to proceed so rapidly as to interfere with rational decision making. In addition, value for the use of prophylactic antibiotics from the first 24 hours of life to the time of surgery is suggested by the results of two studies.[331,332] In the later and larger study, ventriculitis developed in only 1 of 73 infants (1%) receiving broad-spectrum antibiotic prophylactic therapy, compared with 5 of 27 (19%) who did not receive antibiotics.[332]

Details of the operative repair of myelomeningocele are discussed in other sources.[327,333,334] Techniques to minimize the risk of subsequent development of tethered cord are important.

Long-Term Management of Associated Lesions

Management of Hydrocephalus. The management of the commonly associated hydrocephalus depends, first, on identification of the condition in the affected child. The findings of rapid head growth, bulging anterior fontanelle, and split cranial sutures are obvious, and an ultrasound scan can define the severity and the pattern of the ventricular dilation. More difficult is identification of low-grade hydrocephalus, often with no clinical signs, with CSF pressure in the normal range and with ventricles that are moderately dilated but not necessarily increasing disproportionately in size (often called *arrested* hydrocephalus). Later observations of similar patients have demonstrated a discrepancy in performance versus verbal intelligence quotient (IQ) scores, with the latter higher than the former. This discrepancy is considered consistent with a hydrocephalic state, which benefits from placement of a shunt.[335,336] Studies suggest that earlier use of shunt placement with resulting decreased ventricular size is associated with improved performance scores, especially in the cognitive domain (see the next section).[336]

Ventriculoperitoneal shunts are the primary form of the CSF-diversion technique used currently.[168,337] Although randomized controlled studies are not available, current evidence suggests that intelligence is better preserved if ventriculoperitoneal shunts are performed more liberally.[338,339] Such an apparent benefit for the early treatment of hydrocephalus is supported by data suggesting that the degree of ventriculomegaly identified in utero or the size of the cerebral mantle in the first week of life correlates significantly with subsequent intelligence if the hydrocephalus is treated.[340,341] This conclusion must be interpreted with the awareness that the incidence of shunt complications varies depending on the clinical circumstances and that shunt complications have a major deleterious effect on intellectual outcome.[185,342,343]

The dominant deleterious shunt complication is *infection*. In a study of 167 infants with myelomeningocele, the mean IQ of infants with shunt placement for hydrocephalus complicated by infection was 73; with shunt placement for hydrocephalus and no infection, the mean IQ was 95.[344] The mean IQ in infants with myelomeningocele but no hydrocephalus was 102. The similarity of IQ in infants with and without hydrocephalus suggests that the hydrocephalus per se, if adequately treated and not complicated by infection, does not have a major deleterious effect on intellectual outcome.

Management of Brain Stem Dysfunction Associated With the Chiari Type II Malformation. Management of the clinical abnormalities of brain stem dysfunction (see Table 1.6) associated with the Chiari II malformation is difficult. Infants with stridor and obstructive apnea generally respond effectively to improved control of hydrocephalus; any additional benefit for cervical decompression is less clear.[170,172] However, infants with severe symptoms, especially cyanotic episodes related to expiratory apnea of central origin, do not respond effectively to current modes of therapy.[170,172] With progression of the condition, mortality rates in such infants exceed 50%. In a study of 17 infants who had brain stem signs in the first month of life (swallowing difficulty, 71%; stridor, 59%; apneic spells, 29%; weak cry, 18%; aspiration, 12%), and in whom functioning shunts were in place, decompressive upper cervical laminectomy resulted in complete resolution of signs in 15 (two infants died).[179] Postoperative morbidity was least when surgery was carried out within weeks rather than months after clinical presentation.

Management of Orthopedic, Bowel, and Urinary Tract Complications. Myelomeningocele is almost invariably complicated by disturbances in urinary and bowel function, as well as orthopedic complications. The management of these groups of complications is a major problem after the newborn period and is discussed in greater detail elsewhere.[345-350] Of note, orthopedic and urinary tract difficulties are very important determinants of patient and family perceptions of quality of life in adolescence[351]; careful discussion of these complications is important during prenatal counseling, since they are issues that factor significantly into parental decision making.[340,350] Dysfunction of the lower urinary tract (urethral sphincter and bladder), particularly the inability to accommodate and eliminate urine at low pressures, presents a major risk for the subsequent development of vesicoureteral reflux, ascending dysfunction of the upper urinary tract, and eventually renal dysfunction.[345,352] Mechanisms for this disturbance include dyssynergy between contracting/relaxing muscular function of the bladder and urethral sphincter, and fibrosis and irreversible hypertrophy of bladder musculature. Indeed, in a study of 36 infants, 13 of 16 who had subsequent deterioration of the urinary tract had incoordination of the detrusor-external urethral sphincter in the newborn period. This incoordination was followed by such deterioration in 72% of the newborns. Thus urodynamic evaluation in the newborn provides critical information about the urinary tract and helps determine the optimal type and frequency of follow-up management. Early evaluation and aggressive surveillance of bladder function, together with clean intermittent catheterization and antimuscarinic medications, decrease the need for future bladder surgery[353] and result in continence in up to 85% of patients.[144,345-347,350]

Ongoing monitoring of urinary function is important, since postoperative adhesions between the lower spinal cord and the repaired dural linings (often in association with dermoid inclusion cysts)[354] may result in cord tethering and stretch with progressive neurologic and urologic dysfunction. Such secondary cord tethering has been reported in up to 25% of repaired myelomeningocele cases by the age of 8 years.[355,356] In one study, more than 30% of children with normal bladder function in early infancy subsequently developed urological dysfunction requiring cord detethering.[357] Of note, fetal repair of myelomeningocele does not appear to have any beneficial effect over postnatal repair in the long-term requirement for bladder catheterization, anticholinergic, or antibiotic use.[358,359] Other techniques currently being evaluated are microsurgery to create a somatic-autonomic reflex that can be activated by

---

BOX 1.7   Outcome of Myelomeningocele as a Function of Therapeutic Approach[a]

"Conservative" Therapy: 1950s
Mortality: 85%–90% by 10 years
Survivors: 70% ambulatory; mean IQ, 89

"Aggressive" Therapy (Unselected Early Closure of Primary Lesion and Treatment of Hydrocephalus): 1960s
Mortality: 40%–50% by 16 years
Survivors: 45% ambulatory; mean IQ, 77

"Selective" Therapy (Selected Early Closure of Primary Lesion and Treatment of Hydrocephalus): Early 1970s
Mortality: 55% (most were selected for no early closure)
Survivors: 80% ambulatory; 85% IQ >75

"Aggressive-Selective" Therapy: Late 1970s to Present
Mortality: 14% by 3–7 years
Survivors: 74% ambulatory; 73% IQ >80

[a]See text for references.
IQ, Intelligence quotient.

---

cutaneous stimulation,[360] as well as Botox injections into the bladder muscle.[361]

Upper limb dysfunction is not uncommon in cases of myelomeningocele and hydrocephalus and includes spasticity and/or cerebellar signs unilaterally or bilaterally. Such dysfunction may be present in up to two-thirds of myelomeningocele cases. Upper extremity dysfunction also may result from associated cortical, brain stem, cerebellar, and callosal anomalies[362] or progressive severe Chiari II lesions.

Results of Therapy. Results of therapy are difficult to establish because of the wide-ranging spectrum of approaches that have been taken over the past 70 years, and until recently no randomized clinical trials were available.[314] Over the same time span, the overall supportive management of the newborn has advanced dramatically, making historical comparisons difficult. The approaches have been as disparate as the proposal of active neonatal euthanasia in the Netherlands (in the wake of the Groningen Protocol)[363,364] as recently as 2004 to in utero repair of the spinal lesion.[314] In the 1950s *conservative therapy* (i.e., no early surgery) was the standard of care and provided an approximate measure of the natural history of the disorder (Box 1.7).[365] Approximately 50% of patients managed conservatively were dead by 2 months of age, 80% by 1 year, and 85% to 90% by 10 years. Of the survivors, 70% were ambulatory (with or without aids), and their mean IQ was 89.

In the 1960s *aggressive therapy* became the standard, with the advent of early closure of the myelomeningocele and improved techniques of dealing with the hydrocephalus, which included unselective early operation of the primary lesion. The results of this approach were, in some ways, disappointing (Box 1.7).[144,365-367] Although mortality decreased markedly (40%–50% of patients were alive at age 16 years), the quality of life suffered notably. Of the larger number of survivors, 55% were confined to wheelchairs, and most of these children were incontinent, with a mean IQ of 77.[365] Approximately 30% of survivors exhibited epilepsy.[366]

Because the policy of unselective early operation appeared to cause a larger number of severely handicapped children who required an enormous amount of medical supervision and in-hospital therapy, and whose families required a great deal of social support, Lorber[367] advocated *selective therapy*, the use of strict criteria for treatment. The criteria were designed to exclude patients who would die despite therapy or, if they survived, would be very severely handicapped. Adverse prognostic criteria were identified as follows: (1) severe paraplegia (no lower limb function other than hip flexors, adductors, and quadriceps), (2) gross enlargement of the head, (3) kyphosis, (4) associated gross congenital anomalies, and (5) major birth injury. Shortly after the published recommendation to use such criteria, Stark and Drummond[339] reported their experience with 163 patients with myelomeningocele at a medical center (Edinburgh) that had been using criteria comparable to those recommended by Lorber for 7 years (1965–1971; see Box 1.7). Approximately 50% of the Edinburgh patients were considered to have the most favorable prognosis and were selected for early closure of the back lesion and subsequent vigorous therapy. The more severely affected 50% were given only symptomatic therapy. More than 70% of the treated patients were alive at 6 years of age, whereas more than 80% of the untreated patients were dead by 3 months of age. Of treated patients, approximately 80% were ambulatory with or without aids, and 87% were free of upper urinary tract disease. The level of intelligence was higher in the selectively treated patients than in the previously reported, unselectively treated patients.[368] Thus only 15% of patients selected for therapy exhibited an IQ of less than 75, whereas 33% of patients unselectively treated had an IQ of less than 75. The improvement in intellectual function was associated with a more liberal use of shunting procedures for hydrocephalus, a relationship noted by others.[338] In later series of children similarly selected for therapy, treated survivors exhibited a similarly better outcome than with earlier *aggressive* therapy.[369-371]

The use of selective criteria for the institution of therapy for myelomeningocele in the newborn period presented at least *two major problems*. First, some infants who could possibly have had a favorable outcome were excluded and were allowed to experience a poor outcome or to die. Second, some infants who were selected for early vigorous therapy had a poor outcome.

Perhaps in part because of the problems encountered with the use of selective criteria, as just noted, *aggressive therapy* has been favored *in the past 2–3 decades* in most centers in North America. Moreover, results of such therapy appear to be superior to those reported previously for selective therapy (see Box 1.7). For example, in one series of 200 consecutive unselected infants who were treated aggressively, mortality was only 14% after 3 to 7 years of follow-up. Of the survivors, 74% were ambulatory at least a portion of the time, and 87% were continent of urination. The apparent improvement in outcome relative to the earlier results of aggressive therapy relates to several factors, including improvements in diagnosis and monitoring of hydrocephalus (e.g., brain imaging), improvements in management of CSF shunts, more effective therapy of infections, and improvements in braces and other aids for ambulation.[160,168,372,373]

A largely *aggressive approach* that appears to *combine a degree of selection* (e.g., advising against early surgery for infants with major cerebral anomalies, hemorrhage, or infection; high cord lesions and *cord paralysis*; and advanced hydrocephalus) has yielded results similar to those just recorded for aggressive therapy.[168] Indeed, in a study of this *aggressive-selective* approach, fully 71% of infants were selected for early surgery because of the absence of the adverse initial findings noted. Of these infants,

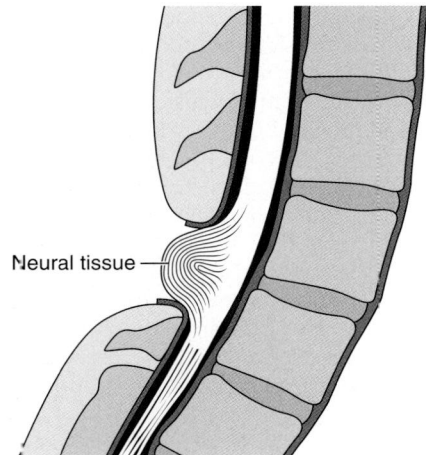

Figure 1.16 Diagram of myeloschisis. Note the ventral displacement of the underlying cord, the neural placode recessed below the cutaneous surface, and the lack of meningeal and cutaneous cover.

79% of survivors exhibited *normal* cognitive development, and 72% were ambulatory.[168]

Conclusions. No easy answers exist to the questions of when and how to treat the newborn infant who has myelomeningocele. Advances in prenatal diagnosis and the option of pregnancy termination, especially in the presence of associated severe cerebral or systemic anomalies, will continue to alter the spectrum of infants observed in neonatal units. The initial results of fetal surgery, as noted earlier, is already having a significant impact on decision making.[314,374,375] Currently, concerning the newborn with the lesion in the absence of major irreversible parenchymal injury (e.g., complicating major hypoxic-ischemic encephalopathy or serious associated cerebral anomaly), the likelihood for intellectual impairment seems low, and aggressive therapy directed toward the back lesion and the hydrocephalus seems indicated to us. Indeed, even in the infant with major parenchymal disease, closure of the back lesion and placement of a shunt for hydrocephalus for the purposes of the infant's comfort and nursing care are reasonable. Although undue delay in onset of therapy is inappropriate, time for rational discussions with the family can be taken and should not compromise outcome. However, little enthusiasm can be marshaled for delaying decisions for management. Not only does delay lead to compromise in outcome for many patients, but it also puts the parents in an uncertain and nearly intolerable position. It is not trite to conclude that management of each patient must be determined individually. Perhaps no other problem in neonatal medicine necessitates as much perception and sensitivity on the part of primary physicians. They must be able to make as precise a prognostic formulation as possible in the context of current medical knowledge and the facilities available to them and the patient's family. Of equal importance, physicians must have the sensitivity toward the family and the patient that is needed to estimate the impact of the disease on everyone concerned.

Myeloschisis. Although far less common than myelomeningocele, a brief review of myeloschisis is warranted (Fig. 1.16).

Anatomical Abnormality. This form of open neural tube defect differs from myelomeningocele in several ways, including

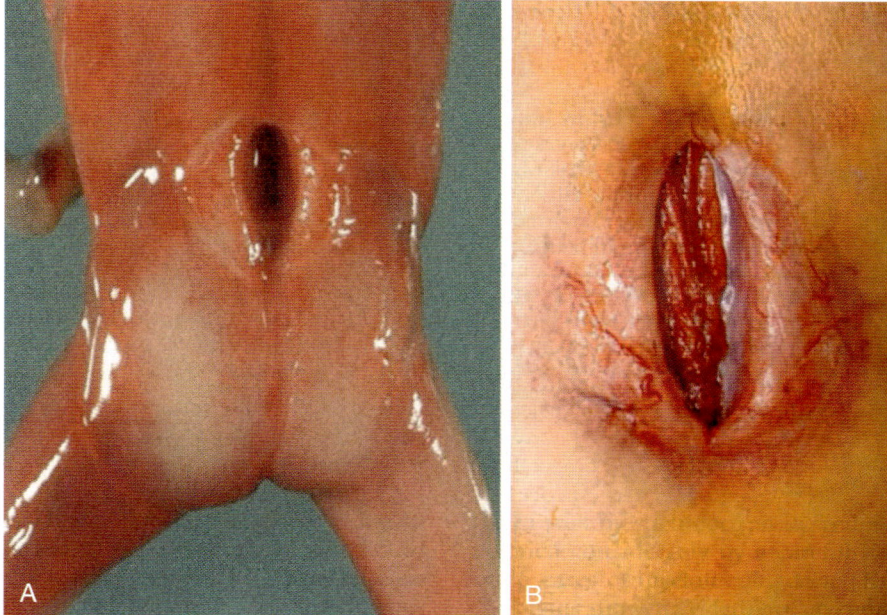

Figure 1.17 Myeloschisis. (A) Dorsal view of a 19-week fetus with myeloschisis and (B) close-up view of myeloschisis lesion. Note the absence of a cystic covering, direct exposure of the neural placode, which is recessed below the surrounding skin surface, and cerebrospinal fluid leakage from the central spinal canal. (A, Courtesy Dr. Joseph R. Siebert, Children's Hospital and Regional Medical Center, Seattle, WA; B from Moore KL. *The Developing Human.* 17, 379-416.e1; Copyright © 2016 by Elsevier, Inc. All rights reserved.)

a lack of an overlying cyst of dysplastic meningeal tissue; consequently, the spinal central canal continuously leaks CSF (Fig. 1.17). Therefore it is not surprising that myeloschisis is almost universally complicated by a Chiari malformation and hydrocephalus. The lack of redundant tissue also makes closure of myeloschisis more difficult. The neural placode is level with the overlying skin or even recessed (see Fig. 1.17) because, unlike most myelomeningoceles, myeloschisis lesions are not displaced dorsally by a ventral pocket of CSF but rather are displaced ventrally by tethering to the anterior wall of the vertebral canal.

Timing. Onset of myeloschisis is no later than 24 to 26 days p/c.[2]

Disorders of Secondary Neurulation
Occult (Closed) Spinal Dysraphism
Anatomical Abnormality. Occult dysraphic states are characterized by overt abnormalities involving vertebral overlying dermal structures or both and by neural lesions that are often subtle or even nonexistent (Fig. 1.18 and Box 1.8). The term *closed neural tube defect* is often used interchangeably with *spina bifida occulta* and considered synonymous with disorders of secondary neurulation. These disorders are distinguished from the disorders of primary neurulation not only by their usual caudal locus but also particularly by the presence of intact skin over the lesions. However, these closed or *occult* lesions may occur at spinal levels above those normally formed by secondary neurulation. A basic relation to disorders of primary neurulation is indicated by the finding that 4.1% of siblings of patients with occult dysraphic states exhibit disorders of primary neurulation, most often myelomeningocele or anencephaly.[376]

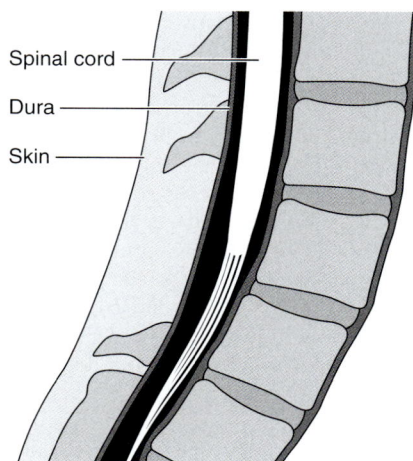

Spinal cord

Dura

Skin

Figure 1.18 Diagram of spina bifida. Spina bifida refers only to the bony midline defect.

BOX 1.8   Neonatal Clinical Features Most Suggestive of Occult Dysraphic State

Abnormal collection of hair
Subcutaneous mass
Cutaneous abnormalities (hemangioma, skin tag, cutis aplasia, pigmented macule)
Cutaneous dimples or tracts

The *principal developmental abnormality* involves the separation of overlying ectoderm from the developing neural tube, a developmental event often termed *disjunction* (see Table 1.2 and see earlier). Failure of this separation impairs the insertion of mesoderm between the ectoderm and neural tube and, as a consequence, results in disturbed development of vertebrae and related mesodermal tissue. Although disturbances in disjunction may occur at any level of the neuraxis, they are most common in the region of the caudal neural tube and are thus often classified among disorders of caudal neural tube formation.[377] The disjunctional failure results most conspicuously in ectodermal abnormalities, dermal tracts and sinuses, abnormalities of mesodermally derived tissue (e.g., vertebral defects, lipomatous masses), and caudal neural tube abnormalities. Of note, unlike disorders of primary neurulation, the incidence of closed spinal dysraphism has not decreased since the recommendation for antenatal folate supplementation.

Because caudal neural tube formation by the processes of canalization and retrogressive differentiation results in the conus medullaris and filum terminale, it is not surprising that almost invariable and unifying findings in these disorders are abnormalities of the conus and filum. The conus is usually prolonged, and the filum terminale is thickened. Moreover, these structures frequently are *tethered* or fixed at their caudal end by fibrous bands, lipoma, extension of dermal sinus, or related lesions. This fixation is thought to impair the normal mobility of the lower spinal cord, and as a consequence, movements of the trunk such as flexion and extension transmit tension through the prolonged conus to the spinal cord and cause injury.[378-380] This explanation of the neural injury complements the *traction* concept (i.e., because of its tethered caudal end, the cord sustains a traction injury caused by the differential growth of the vertebral column and the neural tissue). This latter concept of differential growth as the sole cause of the injury is contradicted by the finding that differential growth is slight between approximately the 26th week of gestation, when the cord is at the level of the third lumbar segment, and maturity, when the cord is at the level of the first or second lumbar segment.[165,381] Nevertheless, contributory importance for traction associated with tethering in the genesis of the injury is indicated by studies of the mitochondrial oxidative metabolism of the cord in vivo in affected patients by dual-wavelength reflection spectrophotometry.[382] Thus distinct disturbances observed intraoperatively improved markedly on release of the tethered cord.

With the occult dysraphic states, as noted earlier, the neural lesion is often rather subtle, and the major overt abnormality involves mesodermally derived structures (especially the vertebrae), the overlying dermal structures, or both. Thus vertebral defects occur in 85% to 90% of cases and consist most commonly of laminar defects over several segments; other skeletal abnormalities include a widened vertebral canal and sacral deformities.[3,64,79,378,380,383-385] Approximately 80% of affected infants exhibit a dermal lesion in the lumbosacral area, consisting of abnormal collections of *hair*, cutaneous *dimples* or *tracts*, superficial cutaneous *abnormalities* (e.g., hemangioma), or a subcutaneous *mass* (Box 1.8; discussed later).

Timing. The neural lesions, in approximate order of time of origin during neural development, are myelocystocele, diastematomyelia-diplomyelia (Fig. 1.19), meningocele-lipomeningocele (Fig. 1.20), lipoma (other tumors), dermal

---

BOX 1.9 Disorders of Caudal Neural Tube Formation: Occult Dysraphic States

Order of Time of Origin During Development
Myelocystocele
Meningocele-lipomeningocele
Diastematomyelia-diplomyelia
Lipoma, teratoma, other tumors
Dermal sinus with or without "dermoid" or "epidermoid" cyst
"Tethered cord" (without any of the above)

---

sinus with or without *dermoid* or *epidermoid* cyst, and *tethered cord* alone (Box 1.9). Less common (although related) lesions include anterior dysraphic disturbances, such as neurenteric cyst and anterior meningocele, and the *caudal regression syndrome*. This latter rare disorder is characterized by dysraphic changes primarily of the sacrum and coccyx, with atrophic changes of muscles and bones of the legs; the neural anomalies range from minor fusion of spinal nerves and sensory ganglia to agenesis of the distal spinal cord.[386] Approximately 15% to 20% of patients are infants of diabetic mothers, and approximately 0.3% of infants of diabetic mothers exhibit the lesion.[387-391] (Infants of diabetic mothers also exhibit a 15- to 20-fold increased risk, relative to infants of nondiabetic mothers, of anencephaly or myelomeningocele.)[388] Because the lower genitourinary tract and anorectal structures are developing simultaneously and in close proximity to the caudal neural tube, lesions of the caudal neural tube are not uncommonly associated with anorectal and genitourinary abnormalities.[79] One such clustering of malformations is the omphalocele-exstrophy-imperforate anus-spinal defect (OEIS) complex, which includes an omphalocele, cloacal extrophy, imperforate anus, and spinal defects.[392] Indeed, the presence of such lesions should be considered in infants with abnormalities of caudal neural tube formation.

Myelocystocele

Anatomical Abnormality. Myelocystocele is a localized CSF-containing cystic herniation of a distended central spinal canal that extends beyond the vertebral canal, while the spinal cord itself stays within the vertebral canal (see Box 1.9; Fig. 1.21). The lesion has two sacs, an ependymal-lined sac emanating from a ballooning hydromyelic central canal and an outer dural sac containing neural and fibrotic tissue. Myelocystoceles are most common in the cervical and lumbosacral regions. Lumbar or *terminal myelocystoceles* (see Fig. 1.21) are of caudal mass origin and may be associated with other features of the caudal regression syndrome, such as severe vertebral defects and other elements of the OEIS complex (discussed previously), making them among the most severe malformations of the newborn period.[3] Severe bladder, bowel, and lower extremity motor deficits are frequent complications of terminal myelocystoceles, and Chiari II malformations may develop later in gestation. These lesions need to be distinguished from sacrococcygeal teratomas (Fig. 1.22), OEIS complex, and myelomeningocele. Lumbosacral lesions may be part of a broader caudal regression syndrome, when they may be associated. The onset of this lesion is estimated to be 28 days of gestation.

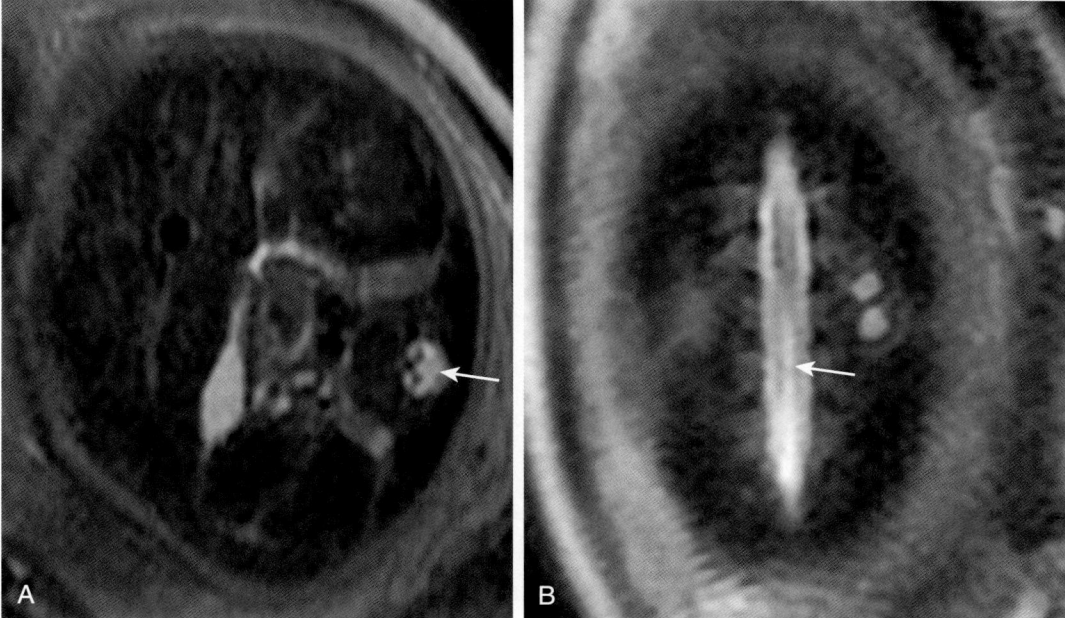

Figure 1.19 Diastematomyelia. Fetal magnetic resonance imaging (T2 weighted) showing axial (A) and coronal (B) views through the spine. Note the bifid shape of the spinal cord in both views *(arrows)*.

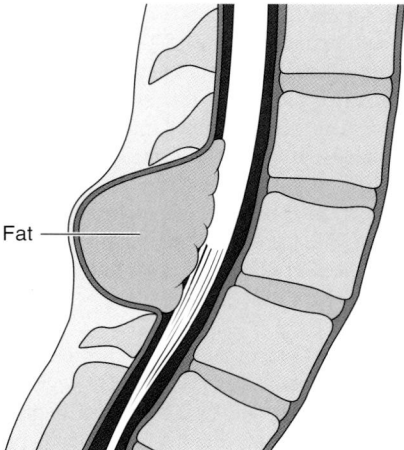

Figure 1.20 Diagram of lipomeningocele. Note skin and dural covering, with bone defect and lipomatous mass adherent to the spinal cord elements.

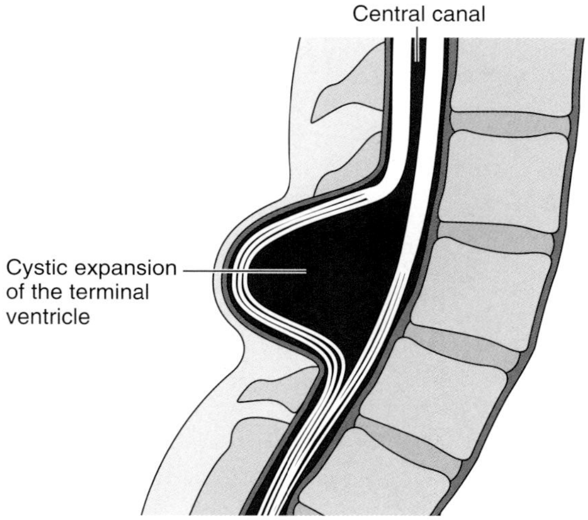

Figure 1.21 Diagram of a terminal myelocystocele. Note the expanded ventriculus terminalis and central canal protruding through the bony defect, which is covered by meningeal and cutaneous layers.

Meningoceles

Anatomical Abnormality. The fundamental abnormality in meningoceles is confined to the vertebral arches, with varying degrees of meningeal herniation (see Box 1.9; Fig. 1.23). The CSF-filled meningeal sac is covered by skin and usually contains no obvious neural elements. The underlying spinal cord is usually intact and remains within the vertebral canal. However, the cord may be malformed into a placode, and fragments of neural tissue may be present in the cyst. In addition, other occult spinal lesions may be present, and cord tethering may develop. By definition, meningoceles are skin covered and have no CSF leak. Lumbosacral meningoceles result from disturbances in secondary neurulation, while the embryology for cervical and thoracic meningoceles remains poorly understood. Posterior cervical meningoceles occur in the zone of primary neurulation but may involve more than one type of neurulation abnormality. It has been postulated that posterior cervical meningoceles are of preneurulation origin, starting during gastrulation when an abnormal endomesenchymal tract bisects the notochord and neural plate, causing a secondary disturbance in primary neurulation.[393] In this manner a midline attachment between the neural and cutaneous ectoderm persists after fusion of the neural tube.[393] The term *limited dorsal myeloschisis*[393,394] has been proposed for closed neural tube defects with a fibroneural

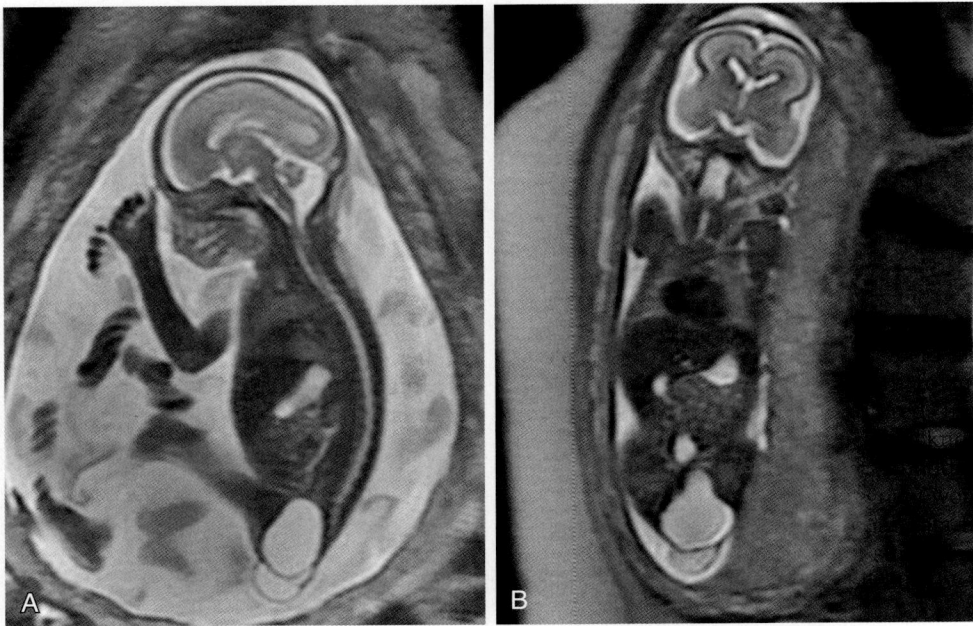

Figure 1.22 Sacrococcygeal teratoma. Fetal magnetic resonance imaging (T2 weighted) in the sagittal (A) and coronal (B) planes showing sacrococcygeal teratoma in a 24-week fetus.

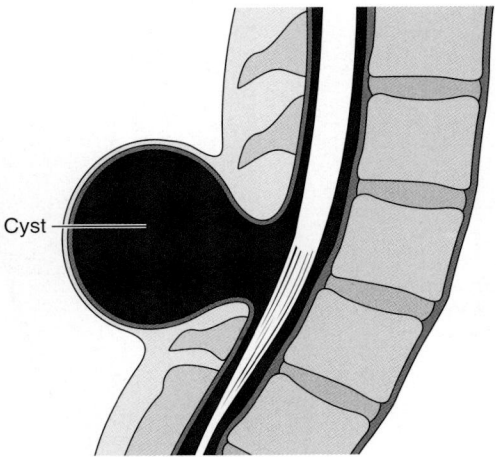

Figure 1.23 Diagram of meningocele. Note the herniation of a meningeal sac through the bony defect, without neural tissues entering into the cystic lesion. Note skin covering is intact, and hence there is no cerebrospinal fluid leak.

stalk (with or without dysplastic glial elements) that connects the spinal cord to the dome of the skin-covered meningeal sac.[395,396] In another variant, a cervical myelocystocele, the spinal cord remains in the vertebral canal, but a diverticulum of the central spinal canal extends into the meningocele. These lesions may be skin covered, partially covered, or open; when open, they are often associated with a Chiari II lesion. Unlike myelomeningoceles, which are most common in the lumbar region, meningoceles are most common in the thoracic spine. When meningoceles occur in the lumbar region, they are thought to result from abnormal secondary neurulation.[397] Lumbar meningoceles are rarely isolated and are not associated

with hydrocephalus or neurological deficits, unlike disorders of primary neurulation.[3,385]

The neurological outcome of infants with meningoceles is usually normal or near normal, especially in early childhood. Later complications of cord tethering, such as disturbances in continence and ambulation, may develop. In a minority of meningoceles with placodes and neural elements in the sac (considered myelomeningoceles by some), as well as Chiari II malformations, the outcome is significantly worse. More cases are associated with infiltration of fibro fatty tissue that is contiguous with a subcutaneous lipoma (i.e., lipomeningocele).[3,398,399]

Diastematomyelia. The spinal cord in diastematomyelia is bifid.[a] The lesion is most common in the lumbar region. In some cases, the spinal cord is separated by a bony, cartilaginous, or fibrous septum protruding from the dorsal surface of the vertebral body, whereas in other cases no septum is present. (The term *diplomyelia* is sometimes used for the latter cases.) Because many types of duplications of the developing caudal neural tube may occur during canalization, it is postulated that persistence of these tubes could result in diastematomyelia. The duplications may occur because of splitting of the notochord with impaired induction of both the neural tube and the vertebrae.

Other Lesions (See Box 1.9). *Subcutaneous lipomata* with intradural extension are more common without an accompanying meningocele. Less commonly, other *tumors* may be observed.[402-405] By far the most common of these tumors is teratoma, although neuroblastoma, ganglioneuroma, hemangioblastoma, and related neoplasms, presumably originating from germinative tissue in the primitive caudal cell

---

[a]References 3, 79, 380, 384, 385, 400, and 401.

mass, or arteriovenous malformation, may occur. Congenital *dermal sinus* consists usually of a dimple in the lumbosacral region from which a small sinus tract proceeds inwardly and rostrally. The tract may enlarge subcutaneously into a cyst that contains predominantly dermal structures (*dermoid*) or epidermal structures (*epidermoid*). Extension of the tract into the vertebral canal may cause neurological symptoms as a result of compression, tethering, or infection. These lesions result from an invagination of ectoderm that is carried by the canalized neural tube as it separates from the surface.[2,3] With *tethered cord*, the conus is prolonged, the filum abnormal, and the caudal end of the cord fixed by fibrous bands.[3,79,378,380,385]

Relative Frequency.

The relative frequency of the several occult dysraphic states differs somewhat, according to the source of the cases. Thus, in one large surgical series of 73 patients, dermal sinus with or without cyst accounted for approximately 35% of cases; lipoma accounted for approximately 30% of cases. Diastematomyelia and anterior meningocele were much less common.[383] Very frequent accompanying features, and sometimes the sole and predominant abnormalities, were the prolongation of the conus and a defective filum terminale. In a series of 144 cases of caudal lesions observed in a children's hospital, as in the surgical series, lipoma was similarly common (40% of cases), and diastematomyelia was similarly uncommon (4% of cases), but dermal sinus with or without cyst accounted for only 10% of cases.[404] Sacrococcygeal teratoma comprised 12% and myelocystocele 8% of cases in this less selected series. In another children's hospital–based series of 104 cases, data were similar, except that diastematomyelia accounted for approximately 25% of cases.[385]

Clinical Aspects.

In the newborn period, the clinical features most suggestive of an occult dysraphic state are the *dermal stigmata* (see Box 1.8). Thus abnormal collections of hair, subcutaneous mass, superficial cutaneous abnormalities, (e.g., hemangioma, skin tag, cutis aplasia, pigmented macule), or cutaneous dimples or tracts should raise suspicion of a disorder of caudal neural tube formation.[378,380,385,402,406-413] The incidence of associated spinal dysraphism with various cutaneous stigmata in one large series was as follows: "hairy patch," 4 of 10; subcutaneous mass, 6 of 6; hemangioma, 2 of 11; skin tag, 1 of 7; cutis aplasia, 1 of 1; "simple dimple" (midline, <5 mm, and <2.5 cm above the anus), 0 of 160; atypical dimples, 3 of 13; and atypical dimples and other skin lesions, 5 of 7.[410] Although neurological deficits are most unusual in the newborn, motor or sensory disturbances in the legs or feet or sphincter abnormalities occasionally may be detected.

The most common clinical presentations for occult dysraphic states later in infancy include delay in development of sphincter control, delay in walking, asymmetry of legs or abnormalities of feet (e.g., pes cavus and pes equinovarus), and pain in the back or lower extremities. Recurrent meningitis is an uncommon, although dangerous, feature. Similarly, rapid neurological deterioration, although unusual, may occur (discussed later). In the older child or adolescent, the major clinical features are gait disturbance, abnormality of sphincter function, development of a foot deformity, and scoliosis.

Management.

Management of the newborn with a skin lesion suggestive of an occult dysraphic state usually includes radiography of the spine. However, before the age of 1 year, ossification of the posterior spinal elements is insufficient to be certain that no abnormality is present. Moreover, even in older infants and children, 10% to 15% of patients with occult dysraphic states have normal spine radiographs. An important noninvasive initial evaluation is ultrasonography, a procedure made possible in the newborn in part because of the poor ossification of posterior spinal elements.[414-416] Visualization of the spinal cord, subarachnoid space, conus medullaris, and filum terminalis and real-time ultrasonographic observation of the mobility of the cord have allowed identification of a variety of occult dysraphic states.[415,416] If both radiography and ultrasonography findings of the spine are normal, no neurological signs exist, and the only clinical finding is a simple dimple or flat hemangioma, many clinicians consider further radiological study to be unnecessary in the neonatal period and clinical follow-up appropriate. Our inclination most often, however, is to perform an MRI.

If a skeletal abnormality or other abnormality is present on the radiographs or sonogram, or if the findings are equivocal, MRI is clearly indicated. MRI has added enormously to assessment (Fig. 1.24).[79,401,407,417,418] MRI is especially valuable for demonstrating the sagittal and coronal topography of the intravertebral and extravertebral components; only bony lesions are not as effectively visualized by MRI as by CT. Indeed, CT is especially useful in demonstrating anomalous bony structures and diastematomyelia spurs.[385,411]

Surgery is performed primarily to *prevent* the development of neurological deficits.[385,400,406,411] The optimal timing of surgery in the infant with few or even no neurological signs is controversial, but the combination of excellent preoperative imaging with MRI, microsurgical techniques, and intraoperative monitoring of cord function by evoked potentials has so decreased morbidity that treatment in the neonatal period before the onset of symptoms has been recommended.[380,419,420] Moreover, neurological deficits may develop in young infants suddenly, and these deficits may persist partially or totally, despite prompt surgical treatment.[378,380,421,422] The mechanism of this sudden deterioration may represent vascular insufficiency produced by tension on a tethered cord, angulation of the cord around fibrous or related structures, or a direct effect of a tumor (e.g., lipoma) or cyst. Surgical release of the tethered cord combined with removal of the tumor or cyst will prevent such deterioration and may partially reverse deficits recently acquired.

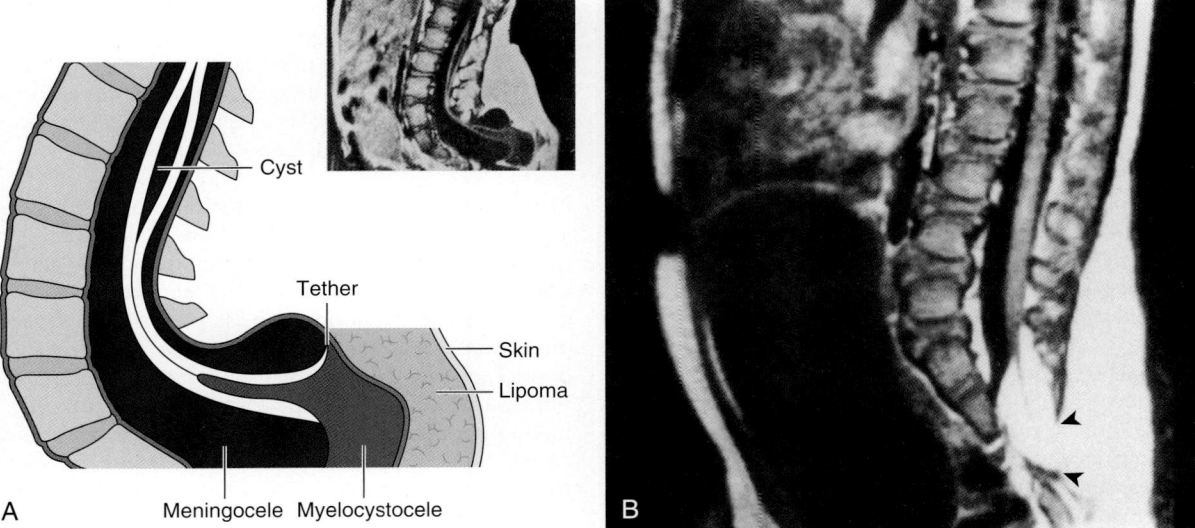

Figure 1.24 Disorders of caudal neural tube formation (A) Myelocystocele: artist's drawing of the meningocele surrounding the myelocystocele and related abnormalities. *Inset:* T1-weighted magnetic resonance imaging (MRI), sagittal view, showing a T12–L3 intramedullary cyst, terminal myelocystocele, meningocele, and lipoma dorsal and superior to the meningocele and myelocystocele. (B) Lipomyelomeningocele with tethered cord. Sagittal, partial saturation (T1-weighted) MRI, 5-mm-thick section shows spinal cord to extend to level of S1 and S2. At this level, a fatty mass envelops the distal spinal cord. The fatty mass extends through a vertebral defect *(arrowheads)* into subcutaneous soft tissues that are enlarged by the lipoma. (A, From Peacock WJ, Murovic JA. Magnetic resonance imaging in myelocystoceles: report of two cases. *J Neurosurg.* 1989;70:804–807. B, From Packer RJ, Zimmerman RA, Sutton LN, et al. Magnetic resonance imaging of spinal cord disease of childhood. *Pediatrics.* 1986;78:251–256.)

KEY REFERENCES

1. McLone DG, Knepper PA. The cause of Chiari II malformation: a unified theory. *Pediatr Neurosci.* 1989;15:1-12.
2. Warkany J. *Congenital Malformations.* Chicago: Mosby; 1971.
3. Lemire RJ, Loeser JD, Leech RW, et al. *Normal and Abnormal Development of the Human Nervous System.* Hagerstown: Harper & Row; 1975.
4. Monsoro-Burq AH, Bontoux M, Vincent C, et al. The developmental relationships of the neural tube and the notochord: short and long term effects of the notochord on the dorsal spinal cord. *Mech Dev.* 1995;53:157-170.
5. Copp AJ, Greene NDE, Murdoch JN. Dishevelled: linking convergent extension with neural tube closure. *Trends Neurosci.* 2003;28: 453-456.
6. Detrait ER, George TM, Etchevers HC, et al. Human neural tube defects: developmental biology, epidemiology, and genetics. *Neurotoxicol Teratol.* 2005;27:515-524.
8. Golden JA, Chernoff GF. Multiple sites of anterior neural tube closure in humans: evidence from anterior neural tube defects (anencephaly). *Pediatrics.* 1995;95:506-510.
10. Seller MJ. Sex, neural tube defects, and multisite closure of the human neural tube. *Am J Med Genet.* 1995;58:332-336.
11. Richtsmeier JT, Flaherty K. Hand in glove: brain and skull in development and dysmorphogenesis. *Acta Neuropathol.* 2013;125: 469-489.
14. Boyles AL, Hammock P, Speer MC. Candidate gene analysis in human neural tube defects. *Am J Med Genet Part C Semin Med Genet.* 2005;135C:9-23.
15. Chen WH, Morrisskay GM, Copp AJ. Genesis and prevention of spinal neural tube defects in the curly tail mutant mouse: involvement of retinoic acid and its nuclear receptors RAR-beta and RAR-gamma. *Development.* 1995;121:681-691.
20. Hol FA, Geurds MPA, Chatkupt S, et al. PAX genes and human neural tube defects: an amino acid substitution in PAX1 in a patient with spina bifida. *J Med Genet.* 1996;33:655-660.
25. LeDouarin NM, Halpern ME. Discussion point. Origin and specification of the neural tube floor plate: insights from the chick and zebrafish. *Curr Opin Neurobiol.* 2000;10:23-30.

26. Milunsky A. Congenital defects, folic-acid, and homoeobox genes. *Lancet.* 1996;348:419-420.
28. Nagele RG, Bush KT, Kosciuk MC, et al. Intrinsic and extrinsic factors collaborate to generate driving forces for neural tube formation in the chick: a study using morphometry and computerized three-dimensional reconstruction. *Dev Brain Res.* 1989;50:101-111.
29. Sadler TW. Mechanisms of neural tube closure and defects. *Ment Retard Dev Disabil Res Rev.* 1998;4:247-253.
30. Schorle H, Mejer P, Buchert M, et al. Transcription factor AP-2 essential for cranial closure and craniofacial development. *Nature.* 1996;381:235-238.
31. Smith JL, Schoenwolf GC. Neurulation: coming to closure. *Trends Neurosci.* 1997;20:510-517.
35. Müller F, O'Rahilly R. The development of the human brain from a closed neural tube at stage 13. *Anat Embryol.* 1988;177:203-224.
36. Nakatsu T, Uwabe C, Shiota K. Neural tube closure in humans initiates at multiple sites: evidence from human embryos and implications for the pathogenesis of neural tube defects. *Anat Embryol (Berl).* 2000;201:455-466.
39. Arthurs OJ, Thayyil S, Wade A, et al. Normal ascent of the conus medullaris: a post-mortem foetal MRI study. *J Matern Fetal Neonatal Med.* 2013;26:697-702.
40. Jeelani Y, McComb JG. Congenital hydrocephalus associated with myeloschisis. *Childs Nerv Syst.* 2011;27:1585-1588.
41. McComb JG. A practical clinical classification of spinal neural tube defects. *Childs Nerv Syst.* 2015;31:1641-1657.
42. Copp AJ, Greene ND. Neural tube defects—disorders of neurulation and related embryonic processes. *Wiley Interdiscip Rev Dev Biol.* 2013;2:213-227.
45. Lemire RJ, Siebert JR. Anencephaly: its spectrum and relationship to neural tube defects. *J Craniofac Genet Dev Biol.* 1990;10:163-174.
50. Mitchell LE. Epidemiology of neural tube defects. *Am J Med Genet Part C Semin Med Genet.* 2005;135C:88-94.
52. Nakano KK. Anencephaly: a review. *Dev Med Child Neurol.* 1973;15: 383-400.
54. Roberts HE, Moore CA, Cragan JD, et al. Impact of prenatal diagnosis on the birth prevalence of neural tube defects, Atlanta, 1990-1991. *Pediatrics.* 1995;96:880-883.

55. Williams J, Mai CT, Mulinare J, et al. Updated estimates of neural tube defects prevented by mandatory folic acid fortification - United States, 1995-2011. *MMWR Morb Mortal Wkly Rep.* 2015;64: 1-5.

57. Goldstein RB, Filly RA. Prenatal diagnosis of anencephaly: spectrum of sonographic appearances and distinction from the amniotic band syndrome. *AJR Am J Roentgenol.* 1988;151:547-550.

59. Obeidi N, Russell N, Higgins JR, et al. The natural history of anencephaly. *Prenat Diagn.* 2010;30:357-360.

66. Rowland CA, Correa A, Cragan JD, et al. Are encephaloceles neural tube defects? *Pediatrics.* 2006;118:916-923.

72. Friede RL. *Developmental Neuropathology.* 2nd ed. New York: Springer-Verlag; 1989.

75. Chervenak FA, Berkowitz RL, Tortora M, et al. The management of fetal hydrocephalus. *Am J Obstet Gynecol.* 1985;151:933-942.

76. Chervenak FA, Isaacson G, Mahoney MJ, et al. The obstetric significance of holoprosencephaly. *Obstet Gynecol.* 1984;63:115-121.

78. Nadel AS, Green JK, Holmes LB, et al. Absence of need for amniocentesis in patients with elevated levels of maternal serum alpha-fetoprotein and normal ultrasonographic examinations. *N Engl J Med.* 1990;323:557-561.

81. Kiymaz N, Yilmaz N, Gudu BO, et al. Cervical spinal dysraphism. *Pediatr Neurosurg.* 2010;46:351-356.

82. Salomao JF, Cavalheiro S, Matushita H, et al. Cystic spinal dysraphism of the cervical and upper thoracic region. *Childs Nerv Syst.* 2006;22:234-242.

83. Huang SL, Shi W, Zhang LG. Characteristics and surgery of cervical myelomeningocele. *Childs Nerv Syst.* 2010;26:87-91.

85. Hall JG, Solehdin F. Genetics of neural tube defects. *Ment Retard Dev Disabil Res Rev.* 1998;4:269-281.

86. Holmes LB, Driscoll SG, Atkins L. Etiologic heterogeneity of neural-tube defects. *N Engl J Med.* 1976;294:365-369.

87. Lemire RJ. Neural tube defects. *JAMA.* 1988;259:558-562.

88. Lynch SA. Syndromes associated with neural tube defects. *Am J Med Genet Part C Semin Med Genet.* 2005;9999:1-8.

99. Lorber J. The family history of spina bifida cystica. *Pediatrics.* 1965;35:598.

103. Gucciardi E, Pietrusiak MA, Reynolds DL, et al. Incidence of neural tube defects in Ontario 1986-1999. *Can Med Assoc J.* 2002; 167:237-240.

106. Stevenson RE, Allen WP, Pai GS, et al. Decline in prevalence of neural tube defects in a high-risk region of the United States. *Pediatrics.* 2000;106:677-683.

111. Greene MF. Diabetic embryopathy 2001: moving beyond the "diabetic milieu". *Teratology.* 2001;63:116-118.

112. Hernandez-Diaz S, Werler MM, Walker AM, et al. Neural tube defects in relation to use of folic acid antagonists during pregnancy. *Am J Epidemiol.* 2001;153:961-968.

114. Matalon S, Schechtman S, Goldzweig G, et al. The teratogenic effect of carbamazepine: a meta-analysis of 1255 exposures. *Reprod Toxicol.* 2002;16:9-17.

115. Milunsky A, Morris JS, Jick H, et al. Maternal zinc and fetal neural tube defects. *Teratology.* 1992;46:341-348.

117. Rosa FW. Spina bifida in infants of women treated with carbamazepine during pregnancy. *N Engl J Med.* 1991;324:674-677.

122. Smith MS, Upfold JB, Edwards MJ, et al. The induction of neural tube defects by maternal hyperthermia: a comparison of the guinea-pig and human. *Neuropathol Appl Neurobiol.* 1992;18: 71-80.

124. Watkins ML, Rasmussen SA, Honein MA, et al. Maternal obesity and risk for birth defects. *Pediatrics.* 2003;111:1152-1158.

128. Bell R, Glinianaia SV, Tennant PW, et al. Peri-conception hyperglycaemia and nephropathy are associated with risk of congenital anomaly in women with pre-existing diabetes: a population-based cohort study. *Diabetologia.* 2012.

129. Blomberg MI, Kallen B. Maternal obesity and morbid obesity: the risk for birth defects in the offspring. *Birth Defects Res A Clin Mol Teratol.* 2010;88:35-40.

130. Anderson JL, Waller DK, Canfield MA, et al. Maternal obesity, gestational diabetes, and central nervous system birth defects. *Epidemiology.* 2005;16:87-92.

131. Waller DK, Shaw GM, Rasmussen SA, et al. Prepregnancy obesity as a risk factor for structural birth defects. *Arch Pediatr Adolesc Med.* 2007;161:745-750.

134. Au KS, Ashley-Koch A, Northrup H. Epidemiologic and genetic aspects of spina bifida and other neural tube defects. *Dev Disabil Res Rev.* 2010;16:6-15.

137. Olney R, Mulinare J. Epidemiology of neural tube defects. *Ment Retard Dev Disabil Res Rev.* 1998;4:241-246.

139. Clemmensen D, Thygesen M, Rasmussen MM, et al. Decreased incidence of myelomeningocele at birth: effect of folic acid recommendations or prenatal diagnostics? *Childs Nerv Syst.* 2011;27: 1951-1955.

141. Tennant PW, Pearce MS, Bythell M, et al. 20-year survival of children born with congenital anomalies: a population-based study. *Lancet (London, England).* 2010;375:649-656.

143. Coniglio SJ, Anderson SM, Ferguson JEI. Functional motor outcome in children with myelomeningocele: correlation with anatomic level on prenatal ultrasound. *Dev Med Child Neurol.* 1996;38:675-680.

144. Hunt GM, Poulton A. Open spina bifida: a complete cohort reviewed 25 years after closure. *Dev Med Child Neurol.* 1995;37: 19-29.

147. Verhoef M, Barf HA, Post MW, et al. Functional independence among young adults with spina bifida, in relation to hydrocephalus and level of lesion. *Dev Med Child Neurol.* 2006;48:114-119.

149. McDonald CM, Jaffe KM, Mosca VS, et al. Ambulatory outcome of children with myelomeningocele: effect of lower-extremity muscle strength. *Dev Med Child Neurol.* 1991;33:482-490.

153. Mirzai H, Ersahin Y, Mutluer S, et al. Outcome of patients with meningomyelocele: the Ege University experience. *Childs Nerv Syst.* 1998;14:120-123.

154. McLone DG, Dias MS. The Chiari II malformation: cause and impact. *Childs Nerv Syst.* 2003;19:540-550.

157. Sutton LN, Adzick NS, Bilaniuk LT, et al. Improvement in hindbrain herniation demonstrated by serial fetal magnetic resonance imaging following fetal surgery for myelomeningocele. *JAMA.* 1999;282:1826-1831.

158. Danzer E, Johnson MP, Bebbington M, et al. Fetal head biometry assessed by fetal magnetic resonance imaging following in utero myelomeningocele repair. *Fetal Diagn Ther.* 2007;22:1-6.

159. Danzer E, Finkel RS, Rintoul NE, et al. Reversal of hindbrain herniation after maternal-fetal surgery for myelomeningocele subsequently impacts on brain stem function. *Neuropediatrics.* 2008;39:359-362.

162. Juranek J, Dennis M, Cirino PT, et al. The cerebellum in children with spina bifida and Chiari II malformation: quantitative volumetrics by region. *Cerebellum.* 2010;9:240-248.

163. Gilbert JN, Jones KL, Rorke LB, et al. Central nervous system anomalies associated with meningomyelocele, hydrocephalus, and the Arnold-Chiari malformation: reappraisal of theories regarding the pathogenesis of posterior neural tube closure defects. *Neurosurgery.* 1986;18:559-564.

166. Johnson MP, Sutton LN, Rintoul N, et al. Fetal myelomeningocele repair: short-term clinical outcomes. *Am J Obstet Gynecol.* 2003;189:482-487.

167. Kirk VG, Morielli A, Brouillette RT. Sleep-disordered breathing in patients with myelomeningocele: the missed diagnosis. *Dev Med Child Neurol.* 1999;41:40-43.

178. Swaminathan S, Paton JY, Davidson Ward SL, et al. Abnormal control of ventilation in adolescents with myelodysplasia. *J Pediatr.* 1989;115:898-903.

181. Petersen MC, Wolraich M, Sherbondy A, et al. Abnormalities in control of ventilation in newborn infants with myelomeningocele. *J Pediatr.* 1995;126:1011-1015.

183. Waters KA, Forbes P, Morielli A, et al. Sleep-disordered breathing in children with myelomeningocele. *J Pediatr.* 1998;132:672-681.

186. Rintoul NE, Sutton LN, Hubbard AM, et al. A new look at myelomeningoceles: functional level, vertebral level, shunting, and the implications for fetal intervention. *Pediarics.* 2002;109:409-413.

192. Talwar D, Baldwin M, Horbatt CI. Epilepsy in children with meningomyelocele. *Pediatr Neurol.* 1995;13:29-32.

193. Hannay HJ, Dennis M, Kramer L, et al. Partial agenesis of the corpus callosum in spina bifida meningomyelocele and potential compensatory mechanisms. *J Clin Exp Neuropsychol.* 2009;31:180-194.

194. Crawley JT, Hasan K, Hannay HJ, et al. Structure, integrity, and function of the hypoplastic corpus callosum in spina bifida myelomeningocele. *Brain Connect.* 2014;4:608-618.

195. Fletcher JM, Copeland K, Frederick JA, et al. Spinal lesion level in spina bifida: a source of neural and cognitive heterogeneity. *J Neurosurg.* 2005;102:268-279.

196. Herweh C, Akbar M, Wengenroth M, et al. DTI of commissural fibers in patients with Chiari II-malformation. *Neuroimage.* 2009;44:306-311.

202. Benacerraf BR, Stryker J, Frigoletto FD Jr. Abnormal US appearance of the cerebellum (banana sign): indirect sign of spina bifida. *Radiology.* 1989;171:151-153.

203. Shaer CM, Chescheir N, Schulkin J. Myelomeningocele: a review of the epidemiology, genetics, risk factors for conception, prenatal diagnosis, and prognosis for affected individuals. *Obstet Gynecol Surv.* 2007;62:471-479.

216. Loft AG. Immunochemical determination of amniotic fluid acetylcholinesterase in the antenatal diagnosis of open neural tube defects. *Dan Med Bull.* 1995;42:54-70.

222. Barber RC, Lammer EJ, Shaw GM, et al. The role of folate transport and metabolism in neural tube defect risk. *Mol Genet Metabol.* 1999;66:1-9.

224. Blom HJ, Shaw GM, den Heijer M, et al. Neural tube defects and folate: case far from closed. *Nat Rev Neurosci.* 2006;7:724-731.

226. Copp AJ, Fleming A, Greene NDE. Embryonic mechanisms underlying the prevention of neural tube defects by vitamins. *Ment Retard Dev Disabil Res Rev.* 1998;4:264-268.

229. Daly S, Mills JL, Molloy AM, et al. Minimum effective dose of folic acid for food fortification to prevent neural-tube defects. *Lancet.* 1997;350:1666-1669.

230. Eskes TKAB. Neural tube defects, vitamins and homocysteine. *Eur J Pediatr.* 1998;157:S139-S141.

231. Finnell RH, Greer KA, Barber RC, et al. Neural tube and craniofacial defects with special emphasis on folate pathway genes. *Crit Rev Oral Biol Med.* 1998;9:38-53.

236. Honein MA, Paulozzi LJ, Mathews TJ, et al. Impact of folic acid fortification of the US food supply on the occurrence of neural tube defects. *JAMA.* 2001;285:2981-2986.

251. Ray JG, Meier C, Vermeulen MJ, et al. Association of neural tube defects and folic acid food fortification in Canada. *Lancet.* 2002;360:2047-2048.

254. Smithells RW. Neural tube defects: prevention by vitamin supplements. *Pediatrics.* 1982;69:498-499.

255. Smithells RW, Nevin NC, Seller MJ, et al. Further experience of vitamin supplementation for prevention of neural tube defect recurrences. *Lancet.* 1983;1:1027-1031.

261. Wald NJ. Folic acid and the prevention of neural-tube defects. *N Engl J Med.* 2004;350:101-103.

270. Rader JI, Schneeman BO. Prevalence of neural tube defects, folate status, and folate fortification of enriched cereal-grain products in the United States. *Pediatrics.* 2006;117:1394-1399.

272. Mosley BS, Cleves MA, Siega-Riz AM, et al. Neural tube defects and maternal folate intake among pregnancies conceived after folic acid fortification in the United States. *Am J Epidemiol.* 2009;169:9-17.

273. Cortes F, Mellado C, Pardo RA, et al. Wheat flour fortification with folic acid: changes in neural tube defects rates in Chile. *Am J Med Genet A.* 2012;158A:1885-1890.

274. Orioli IM, Lima do Nascimento R, Lopez-Camelo JS, et al. Effects of folic acid fortification on spina bifida prevalence in Brazil. *Birth Defects Res A Clin Mol Teratol.* 2011;91:831-835.

275. De Wals P, Tairou F, Van Allen MI, et al. Reduction in neural-tube defects after folic acid fortification in Canada. *N Engl J Med.* 2007;357:135-142.

276. Klusmann A, Heinrich B, Stopler H, et al. A decreasing rate of neural tube defects following the recommendations for periconceptional folic acid supplementation. *Acta Paediatr.* 2005;94:1538-1542.

281. Crider KS, Devine O, Hao L, et al. Population red blood cell folate concentrations for prevention of neural tube defects: Bayesian model. *BMJ.* 2014;349:g4554.

282. Pfeiffer CM, Hughes JP, Lacher DA, et al. Estimation of trends in serum and RBC folate in the U.S. population from pre- to postfortification using assay-adjusted data from the NHANES 1988-2010. *J Nutr.* 2012;142:886-893.

283. Tinker SC, Cogswell ME, Devine O, et al. Folic acid intake among U.S. women aged 15-44 years, National Health and Nutrition Examination Survey, 2003-2006. *Am J Prev Med.* 2010;38:534-542.

284. Bell KN, Oakley GP Jr. Tracking the prevention of folic acid-preventable spina bifida and anencephaly. *Birth Defects Res A Clin Mol Teratol.* 2006;76:654-657.

285. Ahrens K, Yazdy MM, Mitchell AA, et al. Folic acid intake and spina bifida in the era of dietary folic acid fortification. *Epidemiology.* 2011;22:731-737.

302. Danzer E, Ernst LM, Rintoul NE, et al. In utero meconium passage in fetuses and newborns with myelomeningocele. *J Neurosurg Pediatr.* 2009;3:141-146.

303. Danzer E, Adzick NS. Fetal surgery for myelomeningocele: patient selection, perioperative management and outcomes. *Fetal Diagn Ther.* 2011;30:163-173.

307. Bouchard S, Davey MG, Rintoul NE, et al. Correction of hindbrain herniation and anatomy of the vermis after in utero repair of myelomeningocele in sheep. *J Pediatr Surg.* 2003;38:451-458, discussion 451-458.

309. Bruner JP, Tulipan N, Reed G, et al. Intrauterine repair of spina bifida: preoperative predictors of shunt-dependent hydrocephalus. *Am J Obstet Gynecol.* 2004;190:1305-1312.

313. Tulipan N, Sutton LN, Bruner JP, et al. The effect of intrauterine myelomeningocele repair on the incidence of shunt-dependent hydrocephalus. *Pediatr Neurosurg.* 2003;38:27-33.

314. Adzick NS, Thom EA, Spong CY, et al. A randomized trial of prenatal versus postnatal repair of myelomeningocele. *N Engl J Med.* 2011;364:993-1004.

316. Moldenhauer JS, Soni S, Rintoul NE, et al. Fetal myelomeningocele repair: the post-MOMS experience at the Children's Hospital of Philadelphia. *Fetal Diagn Ther.* 2015;37:235-240.

317. Grant RA, Heuer GG, Carrion GM, et al. Morphometric analysis of posterior fossa after in utero myelomeningocele repair. *J Neurosurg Pediatr.* 2011;7:362-368.

318. Danzer E, Thomas NH, Thomas A, et al. Long-term neurofunctional outcome, executive functioning, and behavioral adaptive skills following fetal myelomeningocele surgery. *Am J Obstet Gynecol.* 2016;214(269):e261-e268.

320. Verbeek RJ, Heep A, Maurits NM, et al. Fetal endoscopic myelomeningocele closure preserves segmental neurological function. *Dev Med Child Neurol.* 2012;54:15-22.

323. Li H, Gao F, Ma L, et al. Therapeutic potential of in utero mesenchymal stem cell (MSCs) transplantation in rat foetuses with spina bifida aperta. *J Cell Mol Med.* 2012;16:1606-1617.

324. Saadai P, Wang A, Nout YS, et al. Human induced pluripotent stem cell-derived neural crest stem cells integrate into the injured spinal cord in the fetal lamb model of myelomeningocele. *J Pediatr Surg.* 2013;48:158-163.

345. Kasabian NG, Bauer SB, Dyro FM, et al. The prophylactic value of clean intermittent catheterization and anticholinergic medication in newborns and infants with myelodysplasia at risk of developing urinary tract deterioration. *Am J Dis Child.* 1992;146:840-843.

351. Bier JA, Prince A, Tremont M, et al. Medical, functional, and social determinants of health-related quality of life in individuals with myelomeningocele. *Dev Med Child Neurol.* 2005;47:609-612.

352. Bauer SB, Hallett M, Khoshbin S, et al. Predictive value of urodynamic evaluation in newborns with myelodysplasia. *JAMA.* 1984;252:650-652.

353. Kessler TM, Lackner J, Kiss G, et al. Early proactive management improves upper urinary tract function and reduces the need for surgery in patients with myelomeningocele. *Neurourol Urodyn.* 2006;25:758-762.

354. Danzer E, Adzick NS, Rintoul NE, et al. Intradural inclusion cysts following in utero closure of myelomeningocele: clinical implications and follow-up findings. *J Neurosurg Pediatr.* 2008;2:406-413.

355. Bowman RM, Mohan A, Ito J, et al. Tethered cord release: a long-term study in 114 patients. *J Neurosurg Pediatr.* 2009;3:181-187.

358. Clayton DB, Tanaka ST, Trusler L, et al. Long-term urological impact of fetal myelomeningocele closure. *J Urol.* 2011;186:1581-1585.

359. Lee NG, Gomez P, Uberoi V, et al. In utero closure of myelomeningocele does not improve lower urinary tract function. *J Urol.* 2012;188:1567-1571.

363. de Jong THR. Deliberate termination of life of newborns with spina bifida, a critical reappraisal. *Childs Nerv Syst.* 2008;24:13-28.

364. Eduard Verhagen AA. Neonatal euthanasia: lessons from the Groningen Protocol. *Semin Fetal Neonatal Med*. 2014;19:296-299.

366. Hunt GM. Open spina bifida: outcome for a complete cohort treated unselectively and followed into adulthood. *Dev Med Child Neurol*. 1990;32:108-118.

367. Lorber J. Spina bifida cystica. Results of treatment of 270 consecutive cases with criteria for selection for the future. *Arch Dis Child*. 1972;47:854-873.

369. Evans RC, Tew B, Thomas MD, et al. Selective surgical management of neural tube malformations. *Arch Dis Child*. 1985;60:415-419.

374. Danzer E, Johnson MP. Fetal surgery for neural tube defects. *Semin Fetal Neonatal Med*. 2014;19:2-8.

375. Grivell RM, Andersen C, Dodd JM. Prenatal versus postnatal repair procedures for spina bifida for improving infant and maternal outcomes. *Cochrane Database Syst Rev*. 2014;(10):CD008825.

380. McLone DG, La Marca F. The tethered spinal cord: diagnosis, significance, and management. *Semin Pediatr Neurol*. 1997;4:192-208.

388. Becerra JE, Khoury MJ, Cordero JF, et al. Diabetes mellitus during pregnancy and the risks for specific birth defects: a population-based case-control study. *Pediatrics*. 1990;85:1-9.

392. Carey JC. Exstrophy of the cloaca and the OEIS complex: one and the same. *Am J Med Genet*. 2001;99:270.

393. Pang D, Zovickian J, Wong ST, et al. Limited dorsal myeloschisis: a not-so-rare form of primary neurulation defect. *Childs Nerv Syst*. 2013;29:1459-1484.

394. Steinbok P, Cochrane DD. Cervical meningoceles and myelocystoceles: a unifying hypothesis. *Pediatr Neurosurg*. 1995;23:317-322.

395. Friszer S, Dhombres F, Morel B, et al. Limited dorsal myeloschisis: a diagnostic pitfall in the prenatal ultrasound of fetal dysraphism. *Fetal Diagn Ther*. 2016.

396. Pang D, Zovickian J, Oviedo A, et al. Limited dorsal myeloschisis: a distinctive clinicopathological entity. *Neurosurgery*. 2010;67:1555-1579, discussion 1579-1580.

407. Albright AL, Gartner JC, Wiener ES. Lumbar cutaneous hemangiomas as indicators of tethered spinal cords. *Pediatrics*. 1989;83:977-980.

414. Lowe LH, Johanek AJ, Moore CW. Sonography of the neonatal spine: part 2, Spinal disorders. *AJR Am J Roentgenol*. 2007;188:739-744.

420. Naidich TP, McLone DG, Mutluer S. A new understanding of dorsal dysraphism with lipoma (lipomyeloschisis): radiologic evaluation and surgical correction. *AJR Am J Roentgenol*. 1983;140:1065-1078.

422. Pasternak JF, Volpe JJ. Lumbosacral lipoma with acute deterioration during infancy. *Pediatrics*. 1980;66:125-128.

Full references for this chapter can be found on www.expertconsult .com.

Prosencephalic Development

Adré J. du Plessis ◆ *Joseph J. Volpe*

NORMAL PROSENCEPHALIC DEVELOPMENT

Prosencephalic development, the major event following neurulation, results in structures most recognizable as the essential form of the central nervous system. Thus, these structures rostral to the other major vesicles of the brain, that is, the midbrain (mesencephalon) and hindbrain (rhombencephalon), will ultimately form the cerebral hemispheres and diencephalic (e.g., thalamus, hypothalamus) structures. Prosencephalic development peaks between the second and third months of gestation, with the earliest prominent phases in the fifth and sixth weeks of gestation (Box 2.1). The major inductive relationship of concern is between the notochord-prechordal mesoderm and the forebrain (see Box 2.1).[4] This interaction occurs ventrally at the rostral end of the embryo; thus the term *ventral induction* is sometimes used. The inductive interaction influences formation of much of the *face* as well as the *forebrain*; hence severe disorders of brain development at this time also usually result in striking facial anomalies. Development of the prosencephalon is considered best in terms of three sequential events (i.e., *prosencephalic formation, prosencephalic cleavage*, and *prosencephalic midline development*) (Box 2.1). *Prosencephalic formation* begins at the rostral end of the neural tube at the end of the first month and the beginning of the second month, shortly after the anterior neuropore closes. *Prosencephalic cleavage* occurs most actively in the fifth and sixth weeks of gestation and includes three basic cleavages of the prosencephalon: (1) horizontally, to form the paired optic vesicles, olfactory bulbs, and tracts; (2) transversely, to separate the telencephalon from the diencephalon; and (3) sagittally, to form, from the telencephalon, the paired cerebral hemispheres, lateral ventricles, and basal ganglia (Box 2.1). The third event, *prosencephalic midline development*, occurs from the latter half of the second month through the third month, when three crucial thickenings or plates of tissue become apparent (Fig. 2.1); from dorsally to ventrally, these are the commissural, chiasmatic, and hypothalamic plates. These structures are important in the formation, respectively, of the corpus callosum and the septum pellucidum, the optic nerve chiasm, and the hypothalamic structures. The most prominent of these midline developments is formation of the corpus callosum, the earliest components of which appear at approximately 9 weeks (Fig. 2.2). Initial development of the corpus callosum is dependent on support of the receding mesenchymal tissue of the meninx primitiva, which initially encases the entire forebrain. At 10 weeks'

gestation, glial cells begin to migrate from the subventricular zone toward the medial surface of the developing cerebral hemispheres. At 12 weeks, these glial fibers cross the midline through the meninx primitiva to form a transient *glial sling* across the future interhemispheric fissure. Between weeks 12 and 13, the first pioneer axons from the cingulate cortex cross through this glial sling.[5-7] The early cortical axons are attracted to the midline by specialized glial cells that express chemoattractants of the Netrin family. This interhemispheric migration is orchestrated by a complex system of cellular and molecular chemoattractant and repellent signals. After crossing, these axons do not recross because of the expression of the chemorepellent protein Slit, which activates the Roundabout (Robo) receptor.[7] By 14 weeks, all the individual components of the corpus callosum are formed. At this point there are essentially two distinct segments of the corpus callosum (anterior and posterior), which eventually fuse at the isthmus. With massive expansion of especially the frontal neocortex, the corpus callosum expands in the rostrocaudal axis with backward displacement of the splenium.

This development is followed by formation of the genu and finally, posteriorly, the splenium. The basic structure is completed by approximately 20 weeks of gestation.[3,5-9] Subsequent thickening of this structure occurs as a result of the growth of crossing fibers during organizational events (see later).

Prosencephalic development occurs by inductive interactions primarily between the notochord-prechordal mesoderm and the forebrain (Box 2.1). This inductive interaction influences formation of much of the *face* as well as the *forebrain*; hence severe disorders of brain development at this time may result in striking facial anomalies. Major insights into the molecular genetic determinants of forebrain development have been gained in recent years.[5,6,10-16] The genes involved are crucial for dorsoventral patterning in the developing forebrain. Three signaling pathways play a prominent role in forebrain development—that is, Sonic hedgehog (*Shh*), Nodal, and retinoic acid pathways.[4,17] There is significant cross-regulation between these pathways, which has important implications for forebrain development. The major events are regulated through the opposing ventralizing (*Shh*) and dorsalizing (*Notch*) influences of this interaction. In addition, forebrain development and cleavage is dependent on a delicate balance between *Shh* and fibroblast growth factor (*Fgf*) expression.

The Shh signaling pathway is the most important molecular pathway in prosencephalic development and induces developmental events through critical ventralizing molecules.[18] *Shh* is initially secreted by the notochord and prechordal mesoderm to induce ventral patterning of the developing neural tube. Before secretion, cholesterol is required to modify *Shh* at its C-terminus (an event relevant to causes of holoprosencephaly; see later). Secreted *Shh* activates the *Patch* receptor, which, in turn, leads to activation of several other genes (e.g., *GLI2*) and transcription factors that enter the nucleus to modify gene transcription.

A second major molecular pathway, the so-called *nodal pathway*, is initiated by bone morphogenetic proteins, which are key dorsalizing molecules. The transcriptional regulators induced in this pathway include *TGIF, TDGFI,* and *FASTI.* Additional genes, such as *ZIC2,* may also play a role in prosencephalic formation. The clinical relevance of these insights includes the importance of performing mutation analysis of these genes in selected patients with disorders of prosencephalic development.

DISORDERS OF PROSENCEPHALIC DEVELOPMENT

Disorders of prosencephalic development are considered best in terms of the three major events described earlier (i.e., prosencephalic formation from the rostral end of the neural tube, prosencephalic cleavage, and midline prosencephalic development) (Box 2.2). The spectrum of pathology varies from a profound derangement (e.g., aprosencephaly) to certain disturbances of midline prosencephalic development (e.g., isolated agenesis of the corpus callosum) that may be detected only incidentally by brain imaging or autopsy.

BOX 2.1   Prosencephalic Development

Peak Time Period
2–3 months
Major Events
Prechordal mesoderm → face and forebrain
Prosencephalic development
   Prosencephalic formation
   Prosencephalic cleavage
      Paired optic and olfactory structures
      Telencephalon → cerebral hemispheres
      Diencephalon → thalamus, hypothalamus
   Midline prosencephalic development
      Corpus callosum, septum pellucidum, optic nerves (chiasm),
        hypothalamus

BOX 2.2   Disorders of Prosencephalic Development

Prosencephalic Formation
Aprosencephaly/atelencephaly
Prosencephalic Cleavage
Holoprosencephaly/holotelencephaly
Midline Prosencephalic Development
Agenesis of corpus callosum
Agenesis of septum pellucidum (with or without cerebral clefts)
Septo-optic dysplasia
Septo-optic–hypothalamic dysplasia

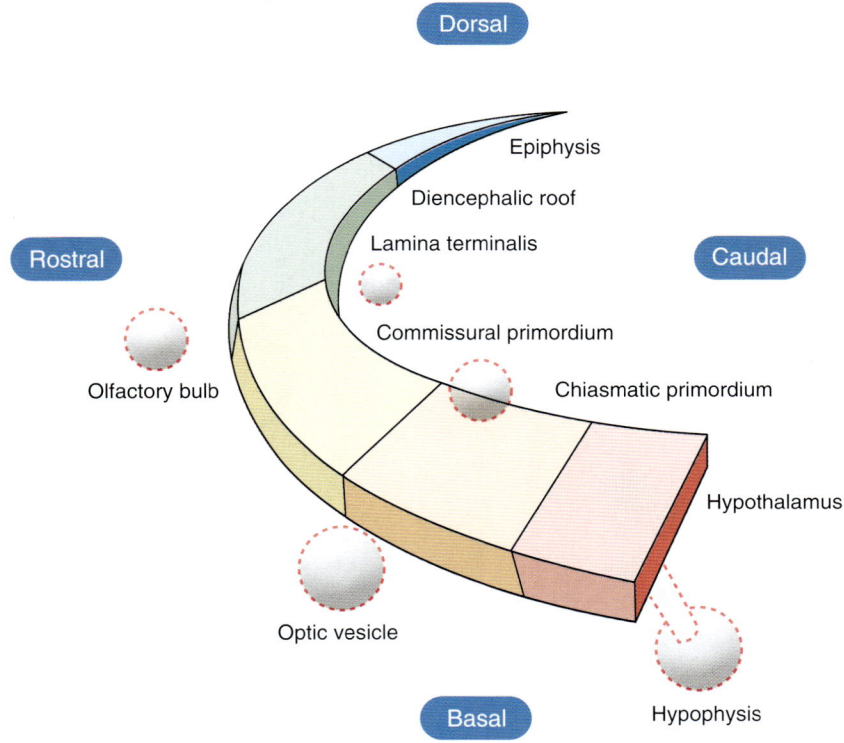

Figure 2.1 **Prosencephalic midline is represented by a series of independent but closely related segments.**
Note particularly the commissural, chiasmatic, and hypothalamic primordia or plates. (From Leech RW, Shuman RM. Holoprosencephaly and related cerebral midline anomalies: a review. *J Child Neurol.* 1986;1:3–18.)

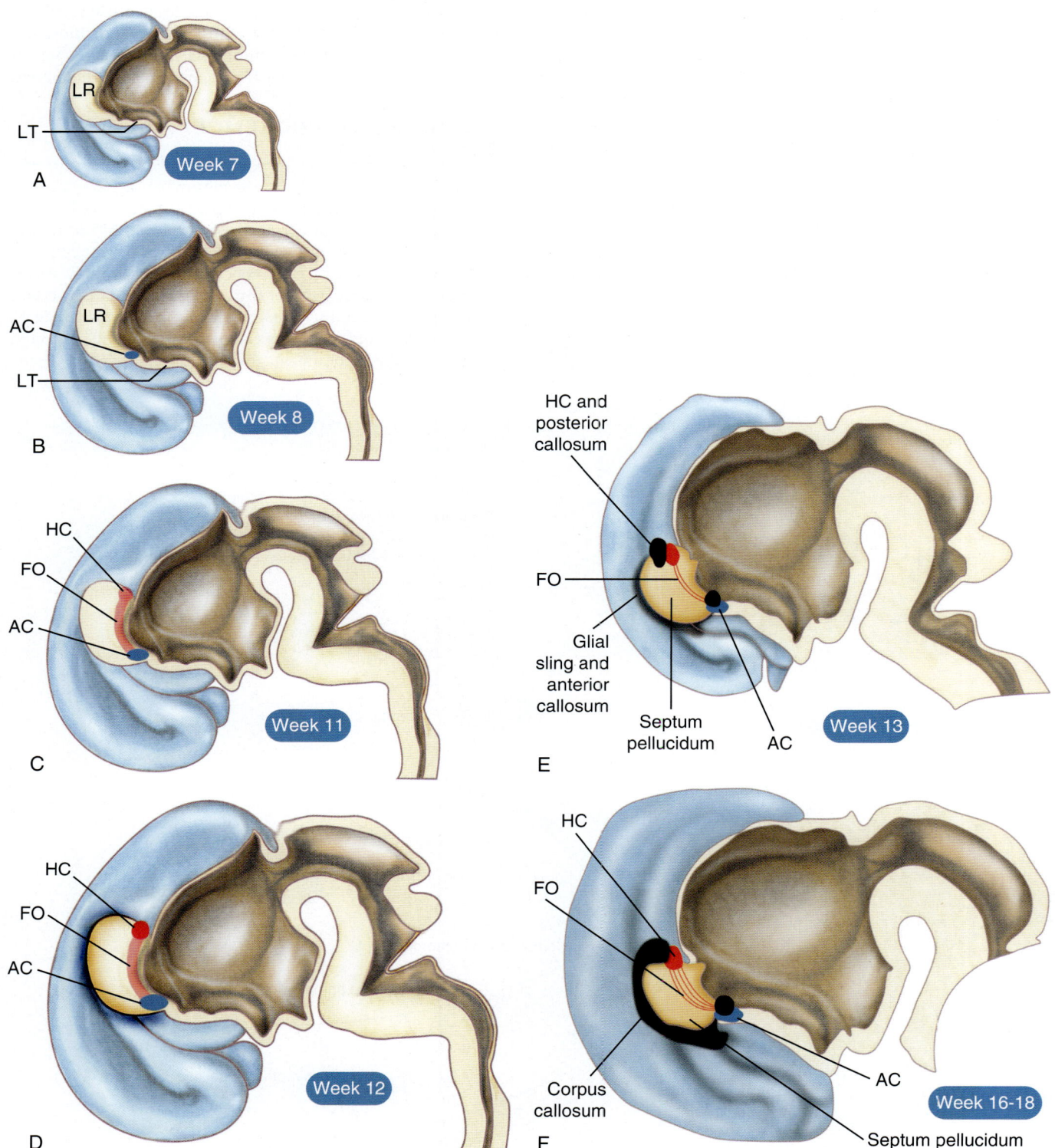

Figure 2.2 Development of the lamina reuniens and of the corpus callosum, sagittal midline. (A) During week 7, the upper portion of the lamina terminalis (LT), which connects the hemispheres across the midline, thickens and forms the lamina reuniens (LR) of His. (B) In the following week, olfactory commissural fibers cross the midline through the ventral aspect of the LR to form the anterior commissure (AC). (C) In the following weeks, fibers develop between the anterior mediobasal cortex (septal nuclei) and the future hippocampus to form the ipsilateral fornix (FO); about week 11, some forniceal fibers cross the midline in the dorsal portion of the lamina reuniens and form the hippocampal commissure (HC). (D) During week 12, the corticoseptal boundary becomes defined at the medial edge of the future neocortex and a glial sling forms along this boundary. (E) By week 13, three commissural sites have been established: anterior commissure, hippocampal commissure, and glial sling. Depending on their origin, early neocortical commissural fibers cross the midline along the anterior commissure (temporo-occipital fibers), the glial sling (frontal fibers), or the hippocampal commissure (parieto-occipitotemporal fibers). (F) The corpus callosum grows by adding further commissural fibers and forms a single continuous structure stretched between the anterior commissure and the hippocampal commissure; it circumscribes the future septum pellucidum. Later, the prominent development of the frontal lobes results in posterior growth of the anterior corpus callosum, which displaces the hippocampal commissure and the splenium backward above the velum interpositum (roof above the third ventricle), stretching the body of the fornix. (Modified from Barkovich AJ, Raybaud C. *Pediatric Neuroimaging*, 5th ed. Philadelphia: LWW; 2012:371–372.)

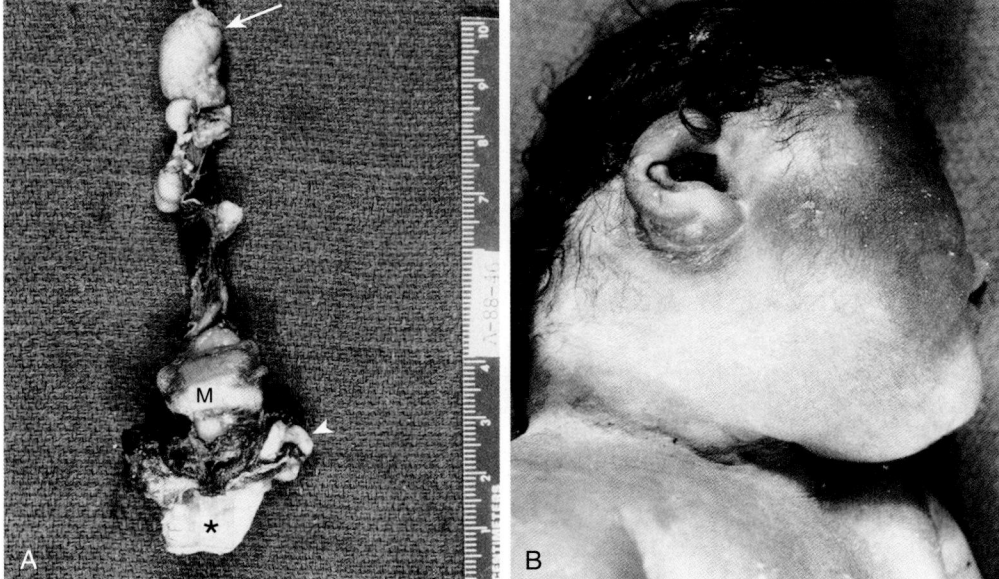

Figure 2.3 Aprosencephaly. (A) Gross photograph of the dorsal surface of the intracranial contents showing near-total absence of prosencephalon with rudimentary ball-like structures *(arrow)*, cysts (the largest cyst was ruptured during fixation), malformed midbrain (M), and relatively normal-appearing lower brain stem *(medulla, asterisk)*. The cerebellum is a vestigial remnant *(arrowhead)*. (B) Lateral view of the head in aprosencephaly. Note evidence of minimal cranial volume above the ears and supraorbital regions, as in anencephaly, but with normal hair and dermal covering. (From Kim TS, Cho S, Dickson DW. Aprosencephaly: review of the literature and report of a case with cerebellar hypoplasia, pigmented epithelial cyst and Rathke's cleft cyst. *Acta Neuropathol.* 1990;79:424–431.)

Disorders of Prosencephalic Formation

Aprosencephaly and Atelencephaly

Anatomical Abnormality. Aprosencephaly and atelencephaly are the most severe of the disorders of prosencephalic development.[19-25] In *aprosencephaly*, the entire process fails to occur, and the result is an absence of formation of both the telencephalon and diencephalon, with a prosencephalic remnant located at the rostral end of a rudimentary brain stem (Fig. 2.3A). In *atelencephaly*, the anomaly is less severe in that the diencephalon is relatively preserved. The findings of calcific vasculopathy and calcification in the remaining neural tissue have led to the suggestion that, in some cases, these disorders may result from an encephaloclastic event shortly after neurulation. These anomalies are distinguishable from anencephaly most readily by the presence of an intact although flattened skull and intact scalp (Fig. 2.3B).

Timing. The disorders presumably have their origin no later than the onset of prosencephalic development at the beginning of the second month of gestation. A slightly later time of origin may be operative in cases that appear to be related to a destructive process.

Clinical Aspects. Aprosencephaly-atelencephaly is characterized by a strikingly small cranium with little volume apparent above the supraorbital ridges (Fig. 2.3B). However, as noted earlier, distinction from anencephaly is based easily on the intact skull and dermal covering. Facial anomalies (including cyclopia or absence of eyes) that bear similarities to those associated with holoprosencephaly (see later) are associated much more commonly with aprosencephaly than with atelencephaly.

Similarly, anomalies of external genitalia and limbs are more common with aprosencephaly than with atelencephaly.

Prognosis. Aprosencephaly is a lethal condition; most examples have been fetal specimens or involved patients who died in the neonatal period. Survival for approximately a year with little neurological function except breathing has been observed with atelencephaly.

Disorders of Prosencephalic Cleavage

Holoprosencephalies

Anatomical Abnormality. The holoprosencephalic spectrum of disorders comprises the next most severe derangements of prosencephalic development and specifically involves prosencephalic cleavage (Box 2.2). In this category of disorders, the forebrain malformation may be so severe that there is marked disturbance of formation of both the telencephalon and diencephalon, in which case the term *holoprosencephaly* is most appropriate. However, in general, the term *holoprosencephaly* is used for the entire spectrum of cleavage disorders. The essential abnormality is failure of horizontal, transverse, and sagittal cleavage of the prosencephalon.

In the original neuropathological classification of the holoprosencephaly spectrum, De Myer described three entities, based principally on the severity of the cleavage abnormality in the cerebral hemispheres and deep nuclear structures.[26] The major neuropathological features of the most severe disturbance, appropriately characterized as *alobar holoprosencephaly*, include a single-sphered cerebral structure with a common ventricle, fusion of basal ganglia and thalamus, a membranous roof over the third ventricle that is often distended into a large

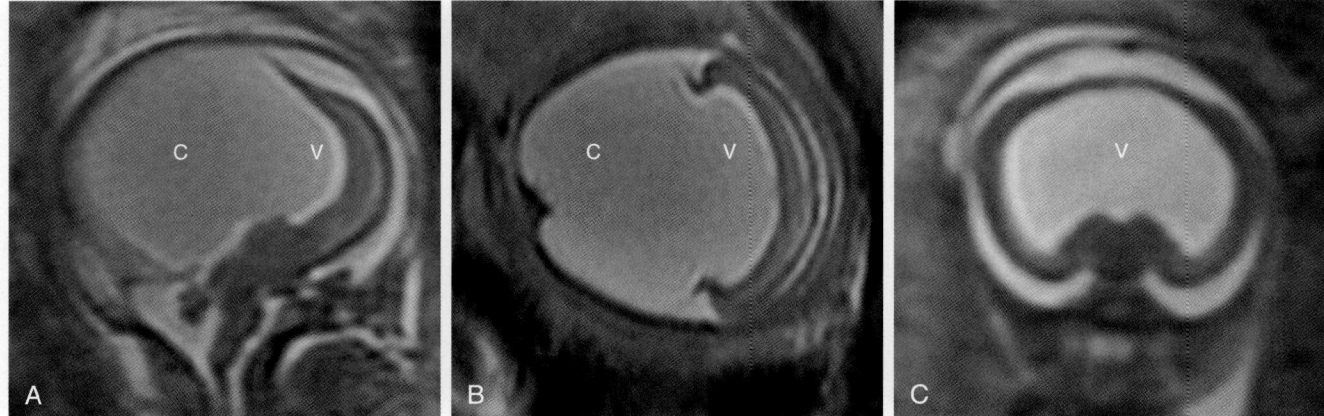

Figure 2.4 Alobar holoprosencephaly. Fetal MRI (T2-weighted) sagittal (A), axial (B), and coronal (C) views showing monoventricle (V) and dorsal cyst (C).

cyst posteriorly (Fig. 2.4), absence of the corpus callosum as well as of the olfactory bulbs and tracts, and hypoplasia of the optic nerves or the presence of only a single optic nerve (Figs. 2.5 and 2.6).[a] The cerebral cortex surrounding the single ventricle exhibits the cytoarchitecture of the hippocampus and other limbic structures, and the most striking abnormality is the essentially total failure of development of the supralimbic cortex, the hallmark of the human cerebrum (Fig. 2.5).[3] The cortical mantle often shows heterotopias and other signs of subsequently disordered neuronal migration.[32,33,40] In *semilobar holoprosencephaly*, there is failure of separation of the anterior hemispheres with presence of a posterior portion of the interhemispheric fissure and less severe fusion of deep nuclear structures (Fig. 2.7). In this form, the *anterior* portion of the corpus callosum is absent, a finding that differs from all other types of callosal hypoplasia, in which the posterior callosum is absent or deficient (see later). In *lobar holoprosencephaly*, the cerebral hemispheres are nearly fully separated, deep nuclear structures are nearly or totally separated (by brain imaging), and the posterior callosum is well developed, although the anterior callosum may be somewhat underdeveloped (Fig. 2.8). Microcephaly is present in the majority of infants with semilobar and lobar holoprosencephaly. Hydrocephalus is present in the majority of infants with alobar holoprosencephaly, usually in association with a large dorsal cyst of the third ventricle secondary to marked fusion of thalamus and impaired egress of cerebrospinal fluid (CSF) through the aqueduct (Figs. 2.4 and 2.15). Dorsal cysts are seen in 92% of alobar, 28% of semilobar, and 9% of lobar holoprosencephaly cases.[41]

Following de Myer's earlier classification, several increasingly milder variants of holoprosencephaly have been described (Table 2.1). In *syntelencephaly*, or the middle interhemispheric variant, only the posterior frontal and parietal regions fail to separate, leaving only the body of the corpus callosum deficient, with the genu, rostrum, and splenium preserved (Fig. 2.9).[26] More recently, a mild holoprosencephaly subtype has been described in which nonseparation is confined to the septal (subcallosal) and/or preoptic regions.[41] This *septopreoptic form* is associated with mild midline craniofacial anomalies (single

midline maxillary incisor, nasal piriform aperture stenosis); as a result, severe endocrine disturbances may develop (Fig. 2.10). In addition, the corpus callosum may be thickened, possibly due to heterotopic cingulate fibers.[42] The classic forms of holoprosephaly uniformly have some degree of failed hypothalamic separation.[43] On this basis, the *interhypothalamic adhesion* (IHA) lesion described recently has been proposed as an even milder *forme fruste* variant of holoprosencephaly, especially since it is often accompanied by other midline defects, including agenesis of the corpus callosum (Fig. 2.11).[44] The IHA variant is also commonly associated with hippocampal dysgenesis and white matter lesions.[44] Unlike the classic forms of holoprosencephaly, the septum pellucidum may be intact in both the septopreoptic and IHA variants.

Not surprisingly, a range of ventricular anomalies have been described in the holoprosencephaly spectrum, from the striking monoventricle of alobar holoprosencephaly to the relatively normal ventricular configuration of milder lobar holoprosencephaly and the septopreoptic and IHA variants. Several reports have described absence of lateral and third ventricles[45,46] or of the entire ventricular system[47] associated with abnormal midline fusion (fused hemispheres and thalami, rhombencephalosynapsis) and agenesis of the corpus callosum.[45-48] Some have proposed that aventriculi is a distinct variant of holoprosencephaly.[48,49]

Timing. Onset of the holoprosencephalies is no later than the fifth and sixth weeks of gestation. A particularly critical impaired event (i.e., the evagination of the cerebral hemispheres through sagittal cleavage of the prosencephalon) occurs at approximately 35 days of gestation.[2] The olfactory bulbs and tracts are not discernible until approximately 42 days of gestation; thus the frequent absence of olfactory structures is understandable.

Clinical Aspects. The frequency of holoprosencephaly is approximately 1 in 10,000 live births.[19,28,30,35] The incidence is more than 60-fold greater (i.e., 1/250) in studies of aborted human embryos, a finding indicating that most cases are eliminated prenatally.[28,50]

Facial anomalies are present in up to 80% to 90% of holoprosencephaly cases, although the severity is variable. In the most severe cases the facial anomaly is represented by a single median eye (*cyclops*) or even no eye at all and a rudimentary nasal structure, the proboscis, often located above the midline

---

[a]References 2, 12, 13, 19, 27-39.

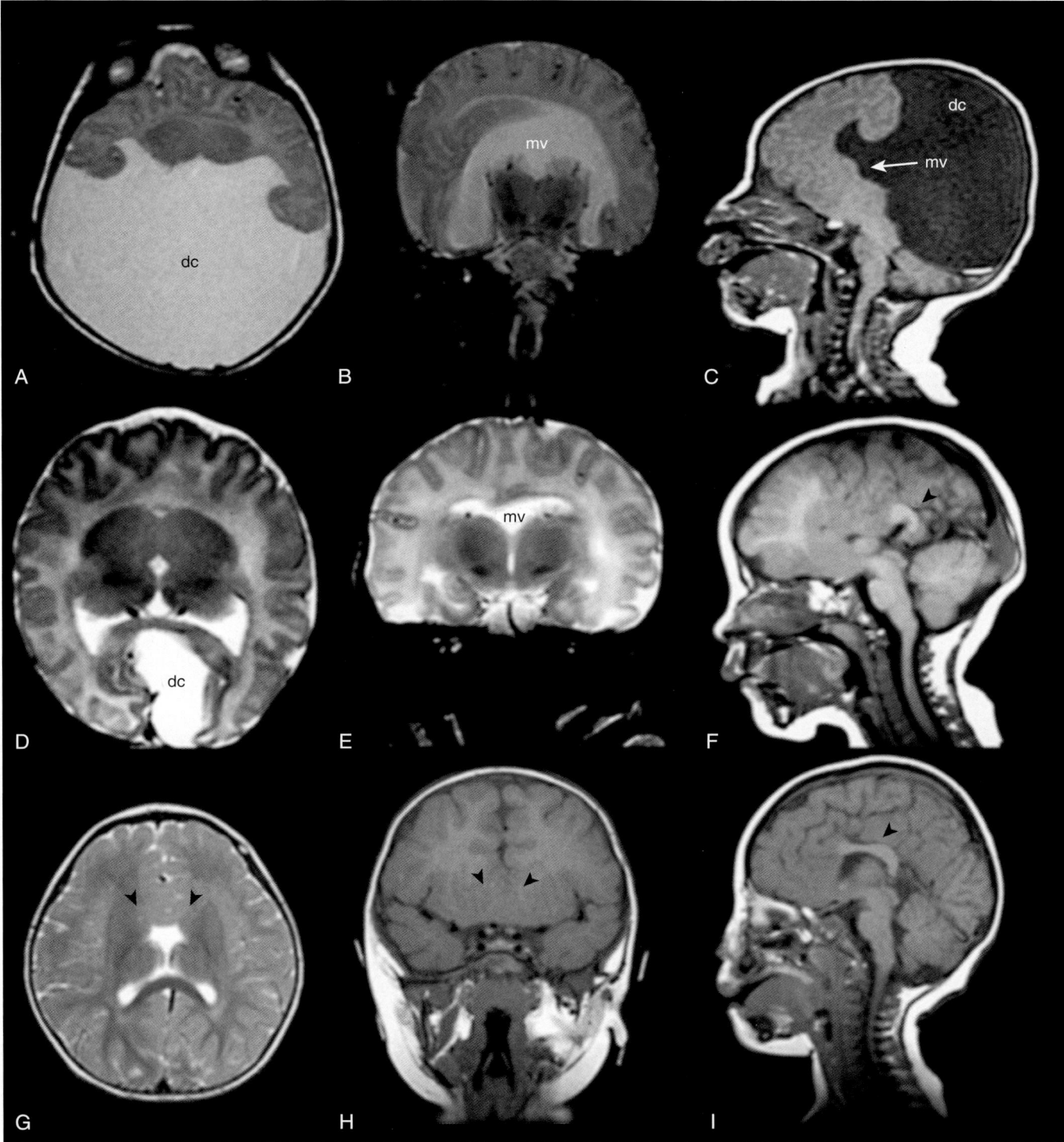

Figure 2.5 (A to C) Magnetic resonance imaging (MRI) of a newborn with alobar holoprosencephaly (HPE). Axial T2-weighted image (A) demonstrates failure of separation of the two hemispheres and thalami, and a large dorsal cyst (dc). Coronal T2-weighted image (B) shows a continuity of gray matter in the midline without an interhemispheric fissure. The ventricular system is composed of a single midline monoventricle (mv). Sagittal T1-weighted image (C) shows absence of the corpus callosum and a monoventricle that communicates with the dorsal cyst. (D to F) MRI of a 3-year-old patient with *semilobar* HPE. Axial T2-weighted image (D) shows absence of interhemispheric fissure anteriorly. The posterior hemispheres are well separated, and the posterior horns of the lateral ventricles are well formed. A dorsal cyst is present (dc). Coronal T2-weighted image (E) of the same patient shows a monoventricle (mv) and partial nonseparation of the thalamic nuclei. A sagittal T1-weighted image (F) of a different patient with semilobar HPE demonstrates absence of the genu and body of the corpus callosum, but presence of the splenium (*arrowhead*). (G to I) MRI of a 16-month-old infant with *lobar* HPE. Axial T2-weighted image (G) shows cerebral hemispheres that are fairly well separated both anteriorly and posteriorly. The fontal horns are underdeveloped (*arrowheads*). Coronal T1-weighted image (H) shows failure of complete separation of the frontal lobes with continuity of gray matter in the inferior frontal regions (*arrowheads*). A sagittal T1-weighted image (I) demonstrates that the body and splenium of the corpus callosum are present (*arrowhead*), but the genu is not developed. (From Hahn JS, Barkovich AJ, Stashinko EE, Kinsman SL, et al. Factor analysis of neuroanatomical and clinical characteristics of holoprosencephaly, *Brain Dev.* 2006;28:413–419.)

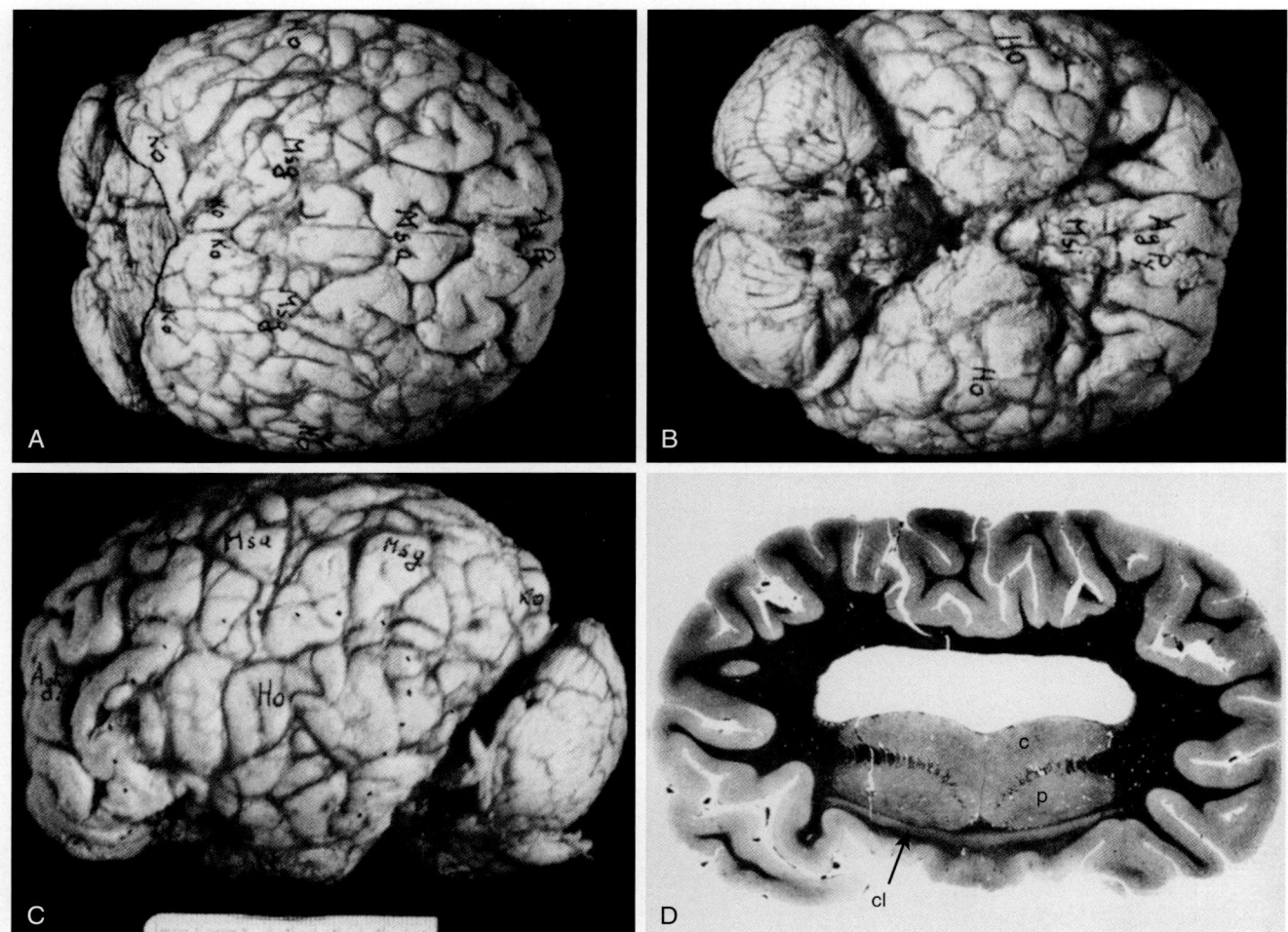

Figure 2.6 Holoprosencephaly. (A to D) Note the single-sphered forebrain. (D) Basal ganglia fused in the midline are caudate (c), putamen (p), and claustrum (cl). (Courtesy Dr. Paul Yakovlev.)

orbit.[a] There may be no nasal structure at all. Less severe facial deformities include marked ocular hypotelorism with or without a proboscis (ethmocephaly) and ocular hypotelorism with a flat, single-nostril nose (cebocephaly [i.e., facial appearance of the *Cebus* monkey]) (Figs. 2.12 and 2.13). Still less severe deformities include mild to moderate ocular hypotelorism (less commonly, ocular hypertelorism), a flat but double-nostril nose, and median cleft lip and palate, often with an absent philtrum and similar features with bilateral cleft lip and palate.[28,29,35] In the least affected cases, the facial deformity may be difficult to detect or there may be no facial deformity at all. Cases with severe facial malformations are consistently associated with severe holoprosencephaly, but the converse is not true; alobar holoprosencephaly is unassociated with a significant facial abnormality in approximately 10% of cases.[35] Abnormalities of other organ systems occur in approximately 75% of cases of holoprosencephaly and consist primarily of disturbances of cardiac, skeletal, genitourinary, and gastrointestinal development, understandable in view of the similar time periods of rapid development.[2]

Neurological features in the most severe cases are obvious from the neonatal period. Infants exhibit frequent apneic spells, stimulus-sensitive tonic spasms, various abnormalities of hypothalamic function (e.g., poikilothermia, diabetes insipidus, or inappropriate antidiuretic hormone secretion), and virtually total failure of neurological development.[19,28,29,40,51] Seizures occur in a large minority; especially in infants with cytogenetic abnormalities, the most severe forms of holoprosencephaly result in death in the first year. However, prolonged survival is common with the less severe forms of holoprosencephaly. Subsequent neurological deficits relate to the nature of the neuropathological features.[19,36,52] The degree of failure of cerebral cleavage correlates with the cognitive deficits, hypothalamic cleavage with the endocrinopathies, and basal ganglia and thalamic cleavage with dystonia and impaired motor function. Still less severely affected children may escape clinical detection until later in infancy or childhood.[a]

Etiology. Chromosomal, genetic, and environmental factors have been implicated in the pathogenesis of holoprosencephaly. Some have proposed that the majority of holoprosencephalies are

[a]References 13, 26, 28, 29, 35, 39.

[a]References 13, 19, 26, 28, 29, 31, 36, 39, 40, 50-54.

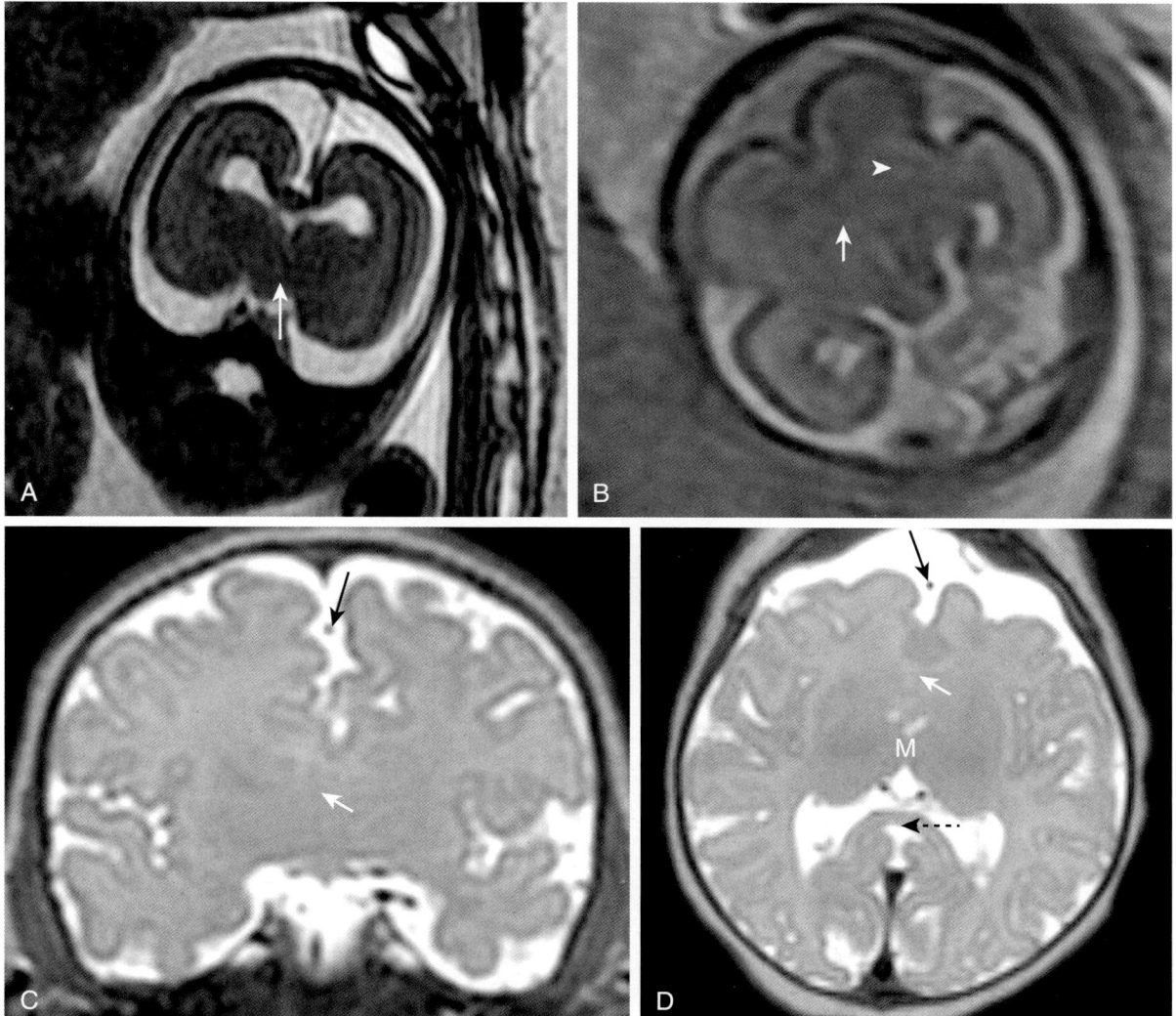

Figure 2.7 Semilobar holoprosencephaly. Fetal magnetic resonance imaging (MRI) (T2-weighted coronal views) showing fused basal frontal lobes and deep gray nuclei *(white arrow)* in a fetus of 20 weeks' gestation (A). The 25-week fetus in (B) shows midline fusion of the basal forebrain and deep nuclei *(white arrow)*, with absence of the frontal horns of lateral ventricles *(arrowhead)*. Neonatal MRI (T2-weighted) coronal (C) and axial (D) views show midline continuity of the frontal lobes *(white arrow)*, caudate nuclei, and thickened thalamic massa intermedia (M). There is absence of the genu and body (not shown) but presence of the splenium of the corpus callosum *(dashed black arrow)*. There is absence of the anterior falx cerebri and septum pellucidum as well as of the frontal horns of the lateral ventricles. Note the single (azygos) anterior cerebral artery *(solid black arrow)* in (C) and (D).

multifactorial (the "multiple-hit" hypothesis), resulting from a combination of genetic and environmental factors.[55,56]

Chromosomal causes of holoprosencephaly account for 60% of cases, of which trisomy 13 accounts for approximately half (Box 2.3).[35] The relative distribution of these causes varies considerably with the method of case ascertainment. The following discussion represents a general consensus of available data. Additional chromosomal abnormalities have involved chromosome 18 in particular.[13,28,29,35,57-59] These data may provide additional prognostic data; in one study, only 2% of cases with cytogenetic abnormalities survived to 1 year of age, compared to 30% to 54% of those without cytogenetic abnormalities.[60]

Monogenic syndromic disorders account for approximately 25% of cases (Box 2.3),[61] with Smith-Lemli-Opitz (SLO) syndrome, a disorder of cholesterol biosynthesis, being especially noteworthy, given the importance of cholesterol for the *Shh* signaling pathway (see earlier discussion). These syndromic disorders are inherited as autosomal recessive (SLO syndrome, pseudotrisomy 13, Meckel syndrome) or autosomal dominant (Pallister-Hall syndrome, velocardiofacial syndrome) traits. The Pallister-Hall syndrome results from a GLI3 mutation and is associated with hypothalamic hamartoma, bifid epiglottis, polydactyly, anal atresia, and holoprosencephaly. Panhypopituitarism with adrenal insufficiency is an important complication.

Monogenic nonsyndromic disorders account for approximately 15% to 20% of cases of holoprosencephaly (Box 2.3). The genes discussed earlier regarding prosencephalic development have been implicated.[62] Mutations in the SHH gene (located on chromosome 7q36) are the most common monogenic mutations found in holoprosencephaly (13%), with ZIC2 mutations being second most common (4% to 9%).[55,63] Holoprosencephaly due to ZIC2 mutation tends to have severe brain involvement with mild to absent facial anomalies. SIX3 mutations have been reported in 5% of holoprosencephaly cases and have a variable phenotype.[55]

Mutations in SHH are rare causes of sporadic holoprosencephaly (4%), but account for 17% of familial cases.[64] Of the monogenic nonsyndromic forms, SHH mutation is the most common (37%) and involves autosomal dominant inheritance. In these cases, considerable intrafamilial variability of the phenotype can occur, and genotype-phenotype correlations are not established. Parents may exhibit relatively inconspicuous features, such as hypotelorism, iris coloboma, hyposmia, single maxillary central incisor (Fig. 2.14), absent frenulum, microcephaly, or mild cognitive deficits. *Clearly careful examination of the parents (and other family members) is essential.* The phenotypic variability seen in cases with specific gene mutations makes single-gene haploinsufficiency an unlikely sole cause of holoprosencephaly. A *multihit* mechanism or multigenic mutations seem more likely.

Environmental teratogenic influences can be operative, although the extent of their role in pathogenesis requires

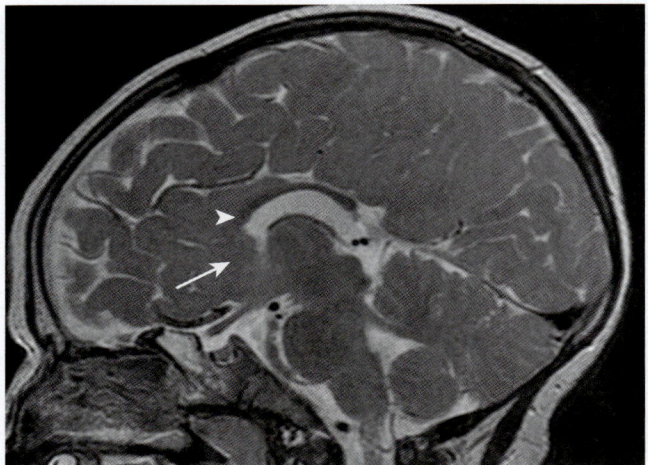

Figure 2.8 Lobar holoprosencephaly. Neonatal brain magnetic resonance imaging (T2-weighted midline sagittal) showing fusion of the basal forebrain *(arrow)* and absence of the rostrum, genu, and anterior body of the corpus callosum *(arrowhead)* but an intact splenium.

BOX 2.3   Etiological Background of Holoprosencephaly[a]

Chromosomal (~60% of All Holoprosencephalies)
Chromosome 13: (~50% of chromosomal causes) trisomy 13, ring 13, deletion 13
Chromosome 18: trisomy 18, ring 18, deletion 18
Chromosomes 2,3,7,21: deletions, trisomies
Monogenic Syndromic (~25% of All Holoprosencephalies)
Smith-Lemli-Opitz (AR)
Pseudotrisomy 13 (AR)
Monogenic Nonsyndromic (~13% of All Holoprosencephalies)
Mutations in SHH, PTCH, GLI2, SIX3, TGIF, TDGF1, FAST1, ZIC2, DLL1, DISP1, FOXH1
Teratogenic Agents
Meckel (AR)
Velocardiofacial (AD)
Pallister-Hall (AD)
Maternal diabetes
Impaired cholesterol biosynthesis
Others
Sporadic

[a]See text for references.

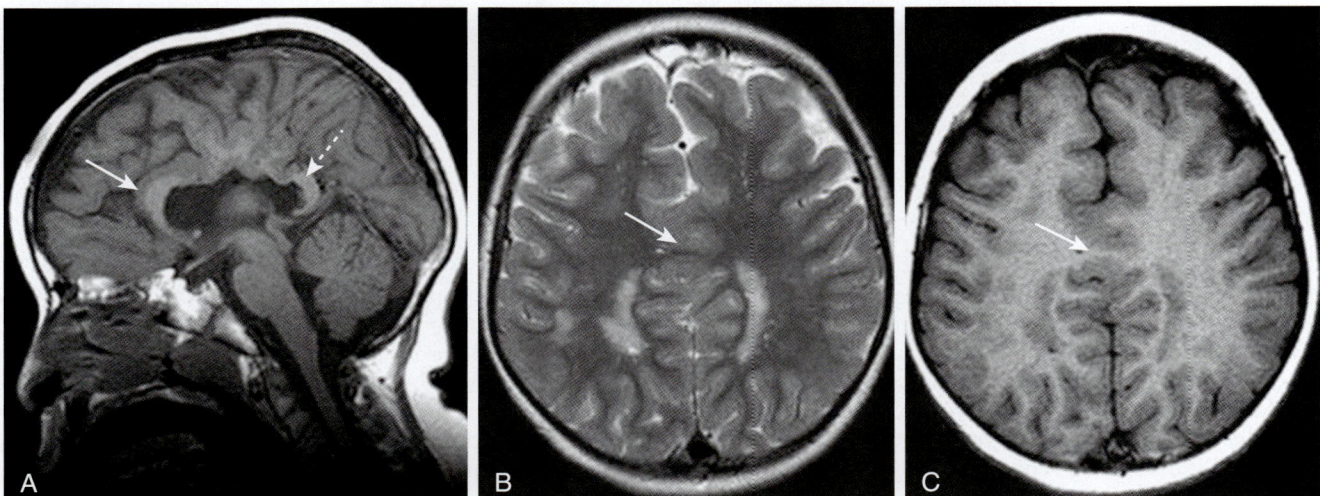

Figure 2.9 Syntelencephaly (A) T1-weighted sagittal view showing absence of the body of the corpus callosum, with genu *(solid arrow)* and splenium *(dashed arrow)* present. (B) T2-weighted and (C) T1-weighted axial images showing continuity of gray and white matter across the midline *(arrows)* connecting the hemispheres. (From Bou-Haidar PB, Lacerda S, Law M: Epilepsy. In Law M, Som PM, Naidich TP. *Problem Solving in Neuroradiology*, Philadelphia: Elsevier; 2011:507–532.)

TABLE 2.1 Magnetic Resonance Imaging Features of Holoprosencephaly Subtypes

	ALOBAR	SEMILOBAR	LOBAR	MIH
Cerebral non-separation	Diffuse (holosphere)	Frontal	Rostroventral frontal	Posterior frontal and parietal
Corpus callosum	Absent	Splenium present Rostrum, genu, and body absent	Splenium present Rostrum and genu absent Anterior body variably present	Splenium present Body absent Genu variably present
IHF and falx	Completely absent	Absent anteriorly Present posteriorly	Hypoplastic anteriorly Present posteriorly	Absent in posterior frontal and parietal region
Ventricles	Monoventricle communicating widely with dorsal cyst	Anterior horns absent Posterior horns present Small third ventricle	Anterior horns rudimentary Third ventricle formed	Anterior horns normal or hypoplastic Third ventricle formed
Dorsal cyst	Usually present	Variably present	Absent	Present in 25%
Septum pellucidum	Absent	Absent	Absent or dysplastic	Absent
Thalamus	Often fused	Partial fusion	Usually fully separated	Fused in 30%–50%
Basal ganglia	Often fused (may be single mass with thalami)	Partial fusion (especially head of caudate)	Variable degree of fusion	Separated
Hypothalamus	Fused always	Fused very often	Fused often	Separated
Sylvian fissure	Often absent	Anteromedially displaced (wide sylvian fissure) Fused frontal lobe	Anteromedially displaced (wide sylvian fissure) Small frontal lobes	Often connect across the midline over the vertex
Dysplastic/heterotopic gray matter	Diffuse broad gyri with too few sulci	Occasional broad gyri with too few sulci	Rare midline subcortical heterotopias in frontal regions	Very common
Cerebral vasculature	Vascular rete branching from internal cerebral arteries	Azygos anterior cerebral artery	Azygos anterior cerebral artery	Azygos anterior cerebral artery

	SEPTOPREOPTIC VARIANT	INTERHYPOTHALAMIC ADHESION
Cerebral nonseparation	Fusion of septal cortex	Separated
Corpus callosum	Rostrum absent/hypoplastic Genu hypoplastic Body/splenium present May be thickened	Formed in most (may be absent as an associated midline defect) (Fig. 2.11)
IHF and falx	Present anteriorly/posteriorly	Present anteriorly/posteriorly
Ventricles	Frontal horns normal or small Third ventricle formed	Normal lateral and third ventricles
Dorsal cyst	Absent	Absent
Septum pellucidum	Present/dysplastic	Present
Thalamus	Fused in some	Separated
Basal ganglia	Separated	Separated
Hypothalamus	Anterior often fused	Fused across anteroinferior third ventricle
Sylvian fissure	Present/normal	Present/normal
Dysplastic/heterotopic gray matter	Rare	Hippocampal dysgenesis common Periventricular heterotopias occasional
Cerebral vasculature	Azygos anterior cerebral artery	Normal

IHF, Interhemispheric fissure; *MIH*, middle interhemispheric variant.

Adapted from Blaas HK. Holoprosencephaly. In: Copel JA, D'Alton ME, Gratacós E et al. eds. *Obstetric Imaging*, Philadelphia: Elsevier; 2012;219-234 and Hahn JS, Barnes PD, Clegg NJ, Stashinko EE. Septopreoptic holoprosencephaly: a mild subtype associated with midline craniofacial anomalies. *AJNR Am J Neuroradiol.* 2010;31:1596–1601.

further study. Holoprosencephaly occurs in as many as 1% to 2% of infants of diabetic mothers, including gestational diabetics.[28,29,65] Holoprosencephaly has been reported in infants with prenatal exposure to antiepileptic drugs, alcohol, retinoic acid, and cytomegalovirus infection, but the extent of the role of these factors in origin remains unclear. Moreover, the occurrence of holoprosencephaly in lambs born to ewes that ingested a toxic plant alkaloid raises the possibility of environmental etiological factors. Because this alkaloid appears to alter cholesterol metabolism by inhibiting the function of 7 dehydrocholesterol reductase (DHCR7)—and, as noted earlier, cholesterol is involved in *Shh* signaling, crucial for forebrain development—a pathogenetic mechanism is suggested.[12,15] *Cholesterol-related mechanisms* of holoprosencephaly include both environmental and genetic factors. In a review of 228 cases of human HPE, almost 10% had evidence of impaired cholesterol biosynthesis.[66,67] The autosomal-recessive SLO syndrome, which results from a DHCR7 mutation, has a 5% incidence

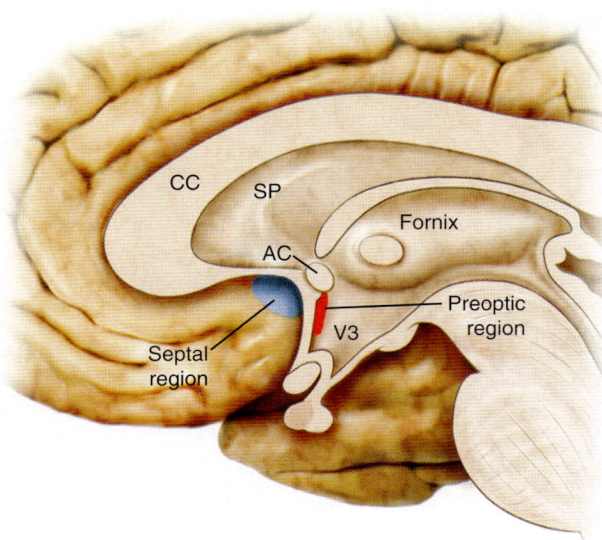

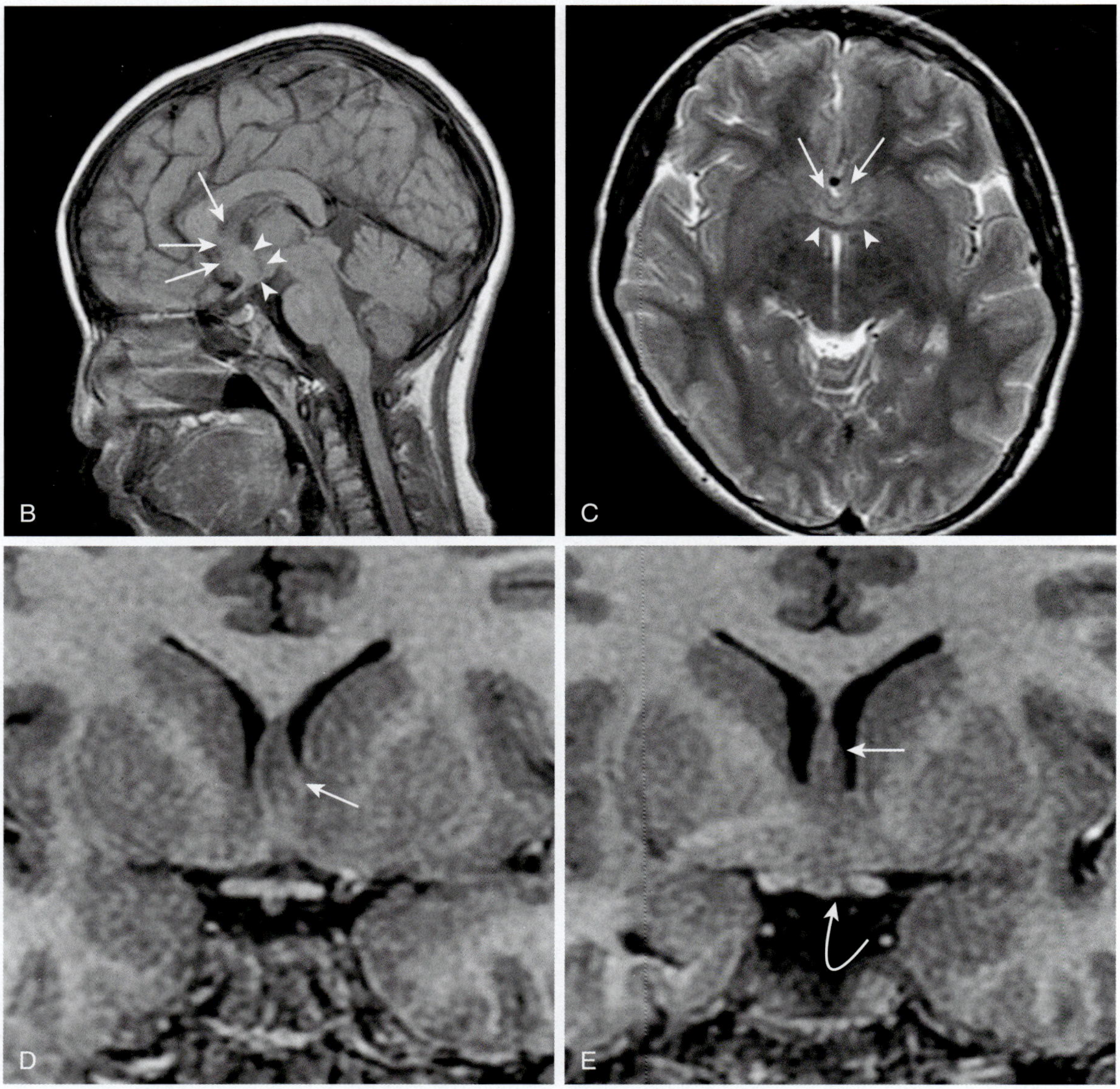

Figure 2.10 (A) Diagram of the sagittal midline brain showing septopreoptic areas (shaded). (B to E) Brain magnetic resonance imaging in a 10-year-old boy with learning disabilities, a single midline maxillary incisor, precocious puberty, and other endocrinopathies. (B) T1-weighted midline sagittal view showing a hypoplastic rostrum, a rectangular subcallosal area of septopreoptic holoprosencephaly *(arrowheads)*, and a dysplastic fornix *(arrows)*. (C) T2-weighted axial view showing well-defined anterior and posterior interhemispheric fissures, a single (azygos) anterior cerebral artery, dysplastic fornices *(arrows)*, and an abnormal area of midline fusion *(arrowheads)*. (D) Coronal spoiled gradient recalled (SPGR) image showing an area of fusion in the septal region *(arrow)*. (E) Coronal SPGR image showing dysplastic, thickened fornices *(arrow)* and an area of midline fusion in the preoptic region and basal structures *(curved arrow)*. *AC,* Anterior commissure; *CC,* corpus callosum; *SP,* septum pellucidum; *V3,* third ventricle.

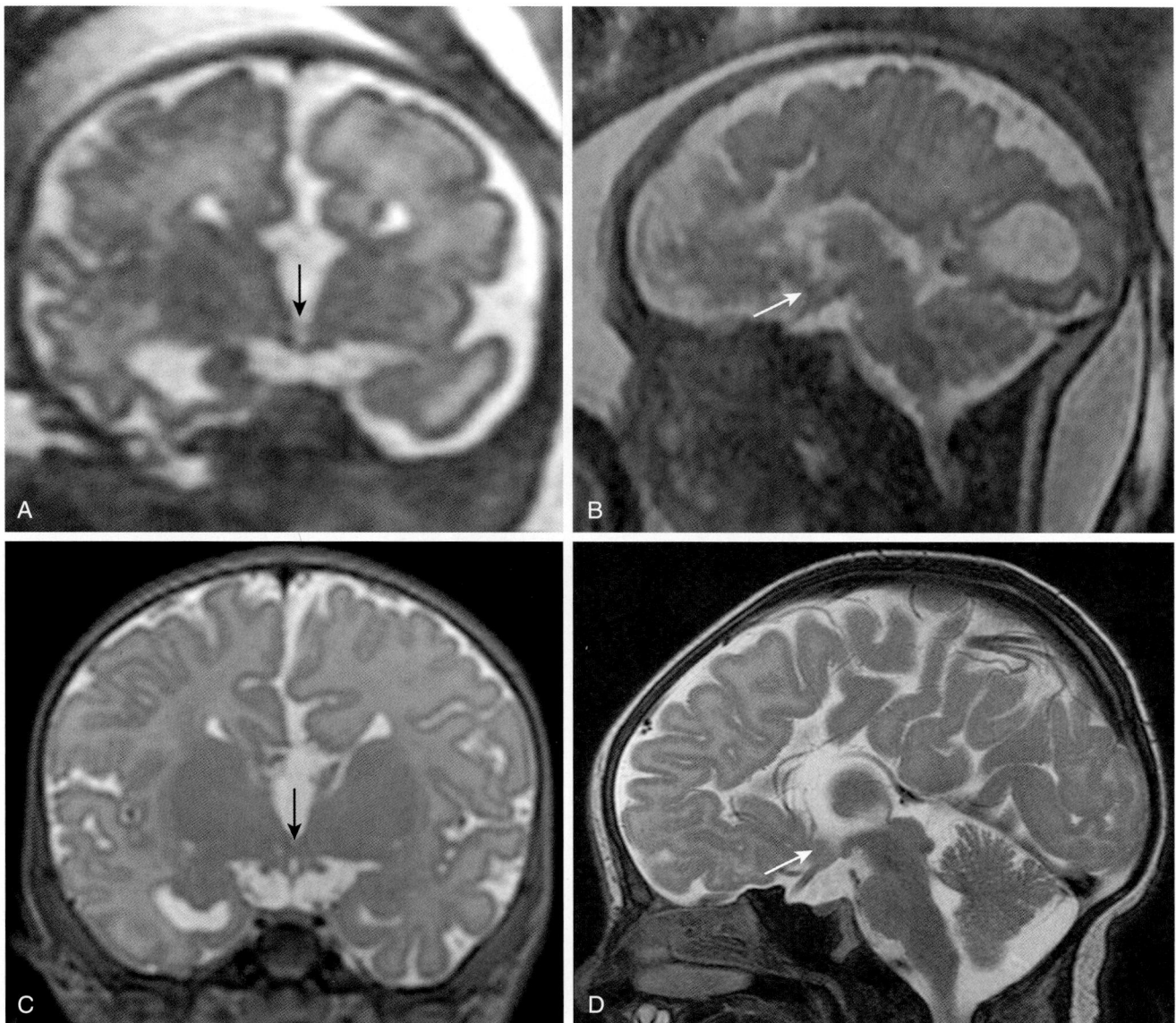

Figure 2.11 Interhypothalamic adhesion form of holoprosencephaly. T2-weighted magnetic resonance imaging studies in the fetal (A and B) and newborn periods (C and D). Interhypothalamic adhesion shown on coronal views (*black arrows* in A and C) and midline sagittal (*white arrows* in B and D). Note the additional midline defect of a complete agenesis of the corpus callosum. (Courtesy Dr. Mathew Whitehead.)

of holoprosencephaly,[68] in addition to microcephaly, mental retardation, ptosis, strabismus, anteverted nares, micrognathia, cleft palate, syndactyly, polydactyly, renal anomalies, and ambiguous genitalia. Whether agents that perturb cholesterol biosynthesis (e.g., statin drugs) play an etiological role remains to be determined.

Diagnosis

Prenatal diagnosis of alobar holoprosencephaly can be made by prenatal ultrasound (US) (especially high-frequency transvaginal transducers) during the first trimester, usually on the basis of fused thalami and a crescentic monoventricle (Fig. 2.15).[69] In a recent study, fetal diagnosis of holoprosencephaly by US was made in more than half the cases before 15 weeks of gestation.[70-72] In lobar holoprosencephaly and some cases of semilobar holoprosencephaly, fetal US may show a transverse orientation of the choroid plexus, crossing the midline (Fig. 2.16). However, the smaller the cleavage defect, the more challenging the US diagnosis becomes. Not infrequently the referral diagnosis includes such associated features as facial anomalies, absent cavum septi pellucidi, or hydrocephalus. In lobar holoprosencephaly, fetal Doppler studies may show the anterior cerebral arteries running along the surface of the fused frontal lobes. Otherwise the only fetal US finding in lobar holoprosencephaly may be absence of the cavum septi pellucidi. For this (and other) reason, fetal MRI is recommended for nonvisualization of the cavum septi pellucidi by fetal US. Detection of chromosomal abnormalities or genetic mutations by preimplantation diagnosis has been reported.[73]

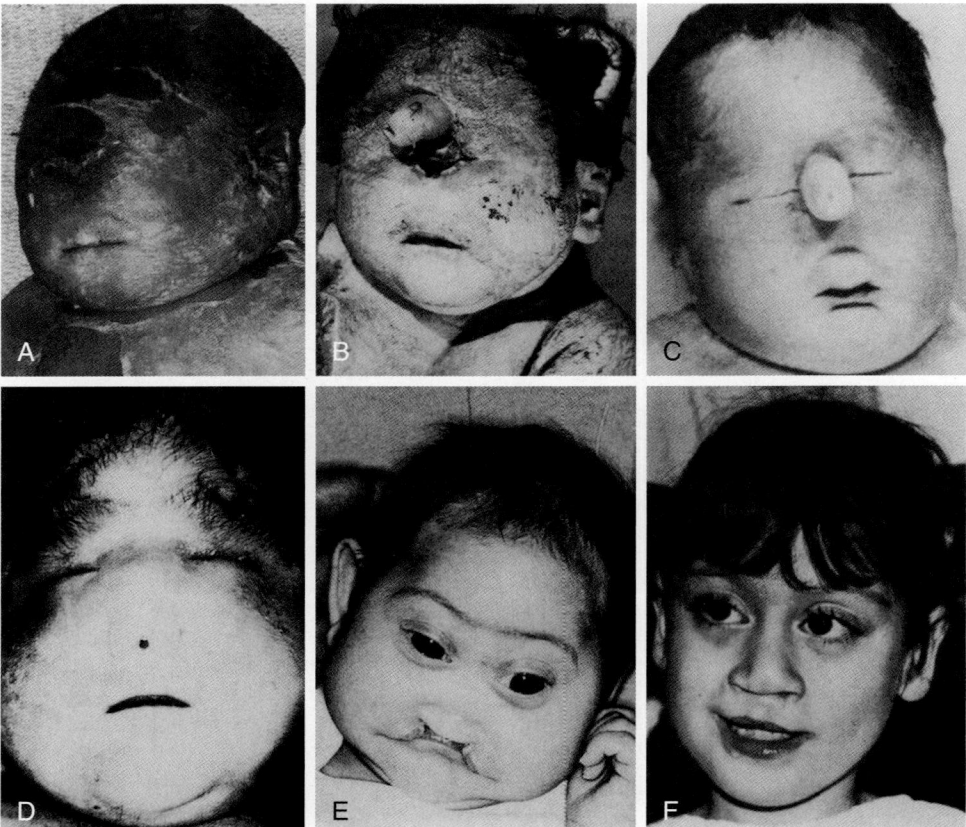

Figure 2.12 Spectrum of dysmorphic faces associated with variable degrees of holoprosencephaly. (A) Cyclopia without proboscis formation. Note the single central eye. (B) Cyclopia with proboscis. (C) Ethmocephaly. Ocular hypotelorism with the proboscis located between the eyes. (D) Cebocephaly. Ocular hypotelorism with a single-nostril nose. (E) Median cleft lip, flat nose, and ocular hypotelorism. (F) Ocular hypotelorism and surgically repaired cleft lip. (From Cohen MM Jr. Perspectives on holoprosencephaly. I. Epidemiology, genetics, and syndromology. *Teratology.* 1989;40:211–235.)

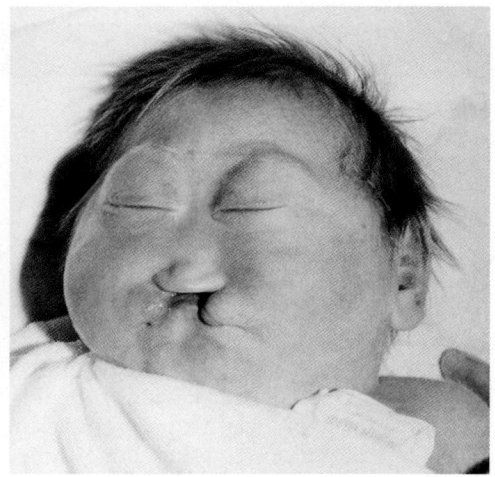

Figure 2.13 Newborn with holoprosencephaly. Note the ocular hypotelorism, flat single-nostril nose, and severe median cleft lip and palate. (Courtesy Dr. Marvin Fishman.)

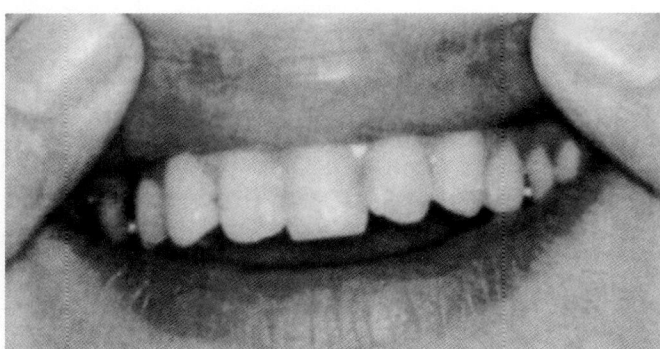

Figure 2.14 Autosomal dominant holoprosencephaly. Mother of an infant with alobar holoprosencephaly. Note the single central maxillary incisor. Computed tomography scan of the mother was normal, and she had normal intelligence. (From Hennekam RCM, Noort GV, de la Fuente FA, Norbruis OF. Agenesis of the nasal septal cartilage: another sign in autosomal dominant holoprosencephaly. *Am J Med Genet.* 1991;39:121–122.)

Genetic Diagnosis. Recent noninvasive testing for cell-free fetal DNA in maternal blood (also known as noninvasive prenatal testing, or NIPT) is able to detect fetal trisomy, including trisomy 18, with sensitivity between 91.6% and 99.3% and specificity in excess of 99%.[74,75] In cases with fetal imaging suggestive of holoprosencephaly, full gene sequence testing is available; in cases with a known mutation, specific testing for amniotic fluid or chorionic villus samples can be analyzed for mutations in the *SHH*, *SIX3*, *TGIF*, and *ZIC2* genes.[76] In cases of holoprosencephaly with multisystem anomalies, testing for monogenic syndromic disorders should be targeted toward the suspected syndromic condition(s).

Disorders of Midline Prosencephalic Development

The principal disorders of midline prosencephalic development are considered best in terms of the normal events centered around the commissural, chiasmatic, and hypothalamic plates. The abnormalities of midline prosencephalic development can be considered the least severe of the spectrum of abnormalities of prosencephalic development (Fig. 2.17). The specific disorders observed according to the plate most affected are shown in Table 2.2. The midline disorders are discussed best in terms of two broad disorders, abnormalities of the corpus callosum and of the septum pellucidum.

Agenesis of the Corpus Callosum
Anatomical Abnormality

Commissural agenesis may involve any or all three commissures. However, from a clinical perspective, agenesis of the corpus callosum is the most important by far. Strictly speaking, callosal agenesis is not a true agenesis but a form of heterotopism,[77] since axons that fail to cross the midline become rerouted to form heterotopic pathways, such as the Probst bundles (see later). However, the corpus callosum per se does not form; thus *agenesis* is a reasonable designation.

Broadly speaking, callosal agenesis can be classified as partial or complete and isolated or complex (associated with other central nervous system [CNS] anomalies, dysmorphic syndromes, chromosomal or genetic defects, or acquired infectious or vascular lesions).[1,5-7,78-83] The term *callosal hypoplasia*

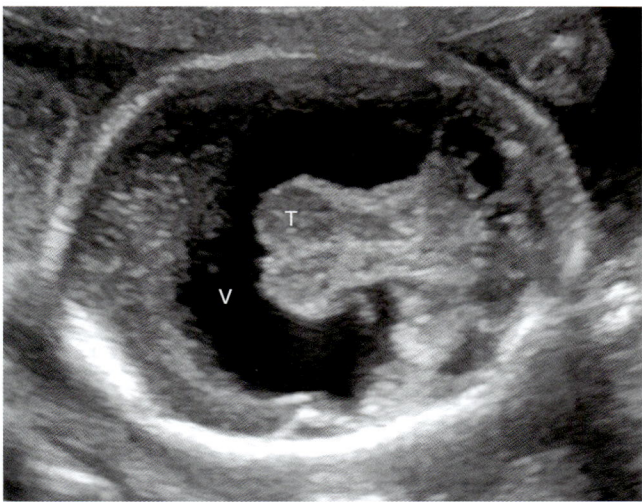

Figure 2.15 Alobar holoprosencephaly. Fetal ultrasound (axial view) showing fused thalami (T) and monoventricle (V).

TABLE 2.2 Disorders of Midline Prosencephalic Development

REGION AFFECTED	DISORDER
Commissural plate	Agenesis of corpus callosum and/or septum pellucidum
Commissural and chiasmatic plates	Septo-optic dysplasia
Commissural, chiasmatic, and hypothalamic plates	Septo-optic–hypothalamic dysplasia

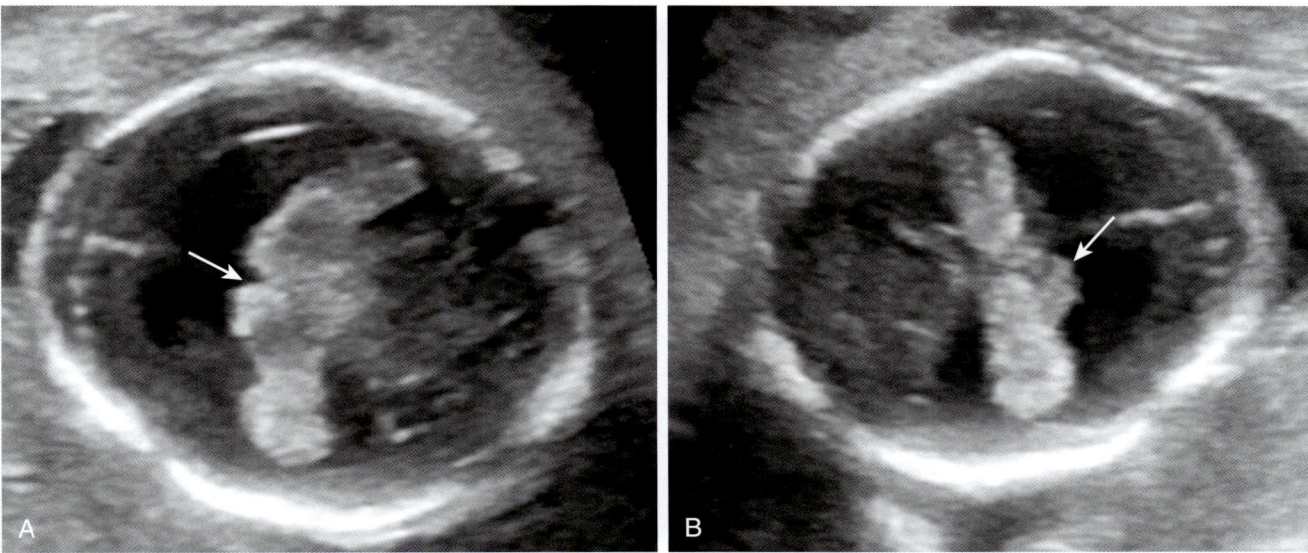

Figure 2.16 Semilobar holoprosencephaly. (A and B) Fetal ultrasound (axial) showing two examples of semilobar holoprosencephaly with transverse orientation of the choroid plexus (*arrows*) across the midline.

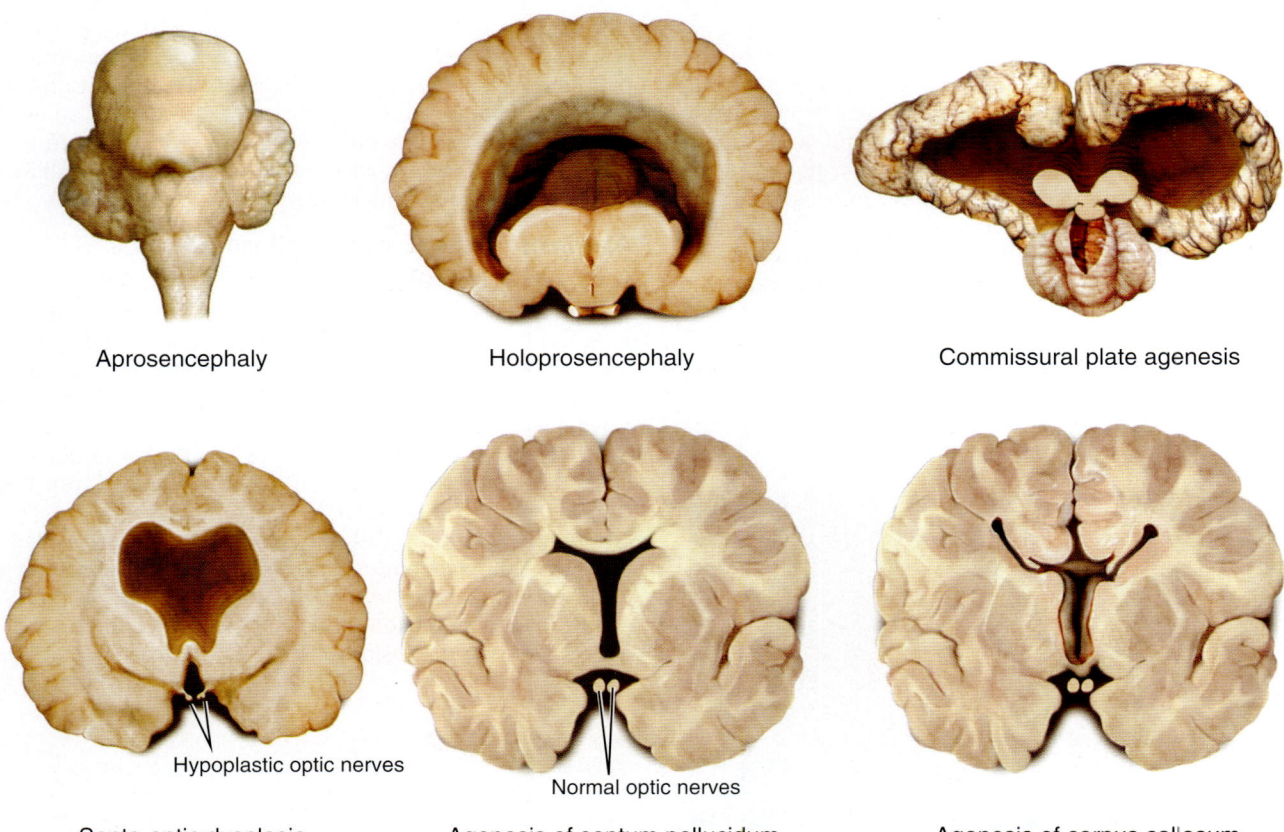

Aprosencephaly   Holoprosencephaly   Commissural plate agenesis

Hypoplastic optic nerves

Normal optic nerves

Septo-optic dysplasia   Agenesis of septum pellucidum   Agenesis of corpus callosum

Figure 2.17 Schematic depiction of the spectrum of defects of prosencephalic development. (From Leech RW, Shuman RM. Holoprosencephaly and related cerebral midline anomalies: a review. *J Child Neurol.* 1986;1:3–18.)

is sometimes used to describe a corpus callosum that is full in its rostrocaudal extent but narrow or *thin* in cross-section, presumably due to decreased numbers of crossing axons.

Complex forms of callosal agenesis are those with *associated brain findings and/or syndromic, chromosomal, or genetic conditions*. These associated conditions are important to identify since they are usually associated with a significantly worse prognosis. An extensive literature review found that coexisting anomalies occurred in 46% of cases and chromosomal abnormalities in 18%.[84] These numbers are probably inflated because many cases of isolated callosal agenesis likely escape detection. Chromosomal anomalies are rare in cases of *isolated* callosal agenesis.[84] In an autopsy review (and hence likely biased) of neuropathology from 50 abortuses with callosal anomalies, syndromic conditions were identified in 68% of cases and encephaloclastic lesions in 8%; only 10% were truly isolated.[85] Nearly 190 different syndromes have been reported in association with agenesis or hypoplasia of the corpus callosum with partial or complete callosal agenesis (Box 2.4).[77] Examples of these syndromes include autosomal recessive disorders (Walker-Warburg syndrome, Fukuyama muscular dystrophy, Joubert syndrome, Andermann syndrome, Meckel syndrome), autosomal dominant disorders (familial septo-optic dysplasia, Sotos syndrome, Rubinstein-Taybi syndrome, lissencephaly type 1 [LIS1], X-linked lissencephaly with ambiguous genitalia [XLAG], X-linked lissencephaly [XLIS], Aicardi syndrome, and

metabolic disorders (nonketotic hyperglycinemia, pyruvate dehydrogenase complex deficiency, fumarase deficiency). Callosal agenesis is also part of the **c**allosal agenesis, **r**etardation, **a**dducted thumbs, **s**huffling gait, **h**ydrocephalus syndrome (CRASH) spectrum of disorders resulting from mutations in the *L1CAM* gene,[86] including hydrocephalus due to stenosis of the aqueduct of Sylvius (HSAS) and mental retardation, aphasia, shuffling gait, and adducted thumbs (MASA) syndromes.[87]

Agenesis of the corpus callosum in *selected* series, identified by MRI, has been associated with other brain anomalies in most cases[5-7,78,81,83,88-90]; the most commonly associated anomalies are myelomeningocele with Chiari II malformation, cerebellar vermian hypoplasia, and disorders of neuronal migration (schizencephaly, lissencephaly, pachygyria, polymicrogyria, marked neuronal heterotopias). The incidence of callosal agenesis in myelomeningocele approaches 60% in some reports[91]; in this context the callosal agenesis is partial. In three large series, approximately 25% to 45% of cases were accompanied by migrational disorder.[81,83,88] The association with disorders of neuronal migration may relate to the finding that callosal development and neuronal migration occur concurrently in human brain development. The coexistence of callosal agenesis and lesions such as the Dandy-Walker syndrome is interesting since the development of both the corpus callosum and the fourth ventricular roof plate occurs through dorsalizing patterning. One important disorder characterized by agenesis

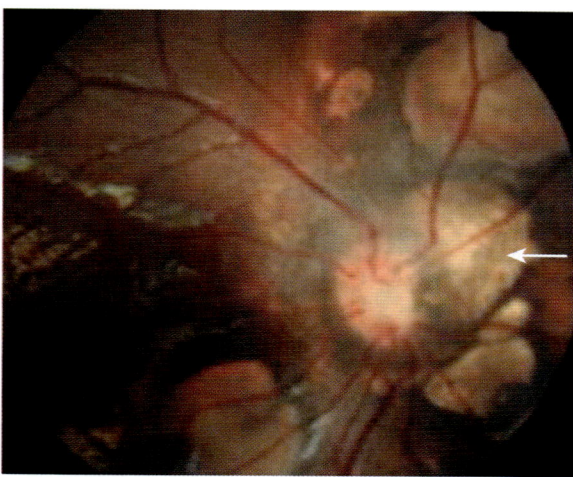

Figure 2.18 Retinal image in patient with Aicardi syndrome showing choroidal lacunae (*arrow*).

interhemispheric cysts and lipomas. Two types of midline cysts are seen with callosal agenesis (Fig. 2.19). Type 1 cysts are unilocular and represent a diverticulation of the tela choroidea from the third and both lateral ventricles[79] rather than an upward expansion of the third ventricle; they communicate with the rest of the ventricular system. These are not mesenchymal in origin and not associated with cortical dysplasia. Type 2 cysts are multilocular and do not communicate with the ventricular system. Like the lipomas, type 2 cysts result from mesenchymal dysplasia and are commonly associated with cortical malformations, including polymicrogyria and heterotopias. For these reasons, the neurodevelopmental outcome in callosal agenesis with type 2 cysts is significantly worse. The association between type 2 cysts and cortical dysplasia is interesting given the role that mesenchymal signaling is now known to have on brain development.[100] By MRI, the signal characteristics of type 2 cysts differ from those of CSF. These cysts may increase in size during pregnancy. Hydrocephalus is a common complication. Type 2 cysts are seen in Aicardi syndrome. Midline lipomas are another form of meningeal dysplasia and are usually deep within the interhemispheric fissure, where they may extend into the choroid plexuses.[101] They may calcify over time.

Timing. Complete agenesis of the corpus callosum has its origin no later than 12 weeks of gestation. Partial forms may originate as late as 20 weeks of gestation. The septum pellucidum develops with the anterior callosum and is in place by 14 weeks of gestation. It is assumed that developmental absence of the septal leaflets would occur before that time, although destructive lesions could occur later.

Clinical Aspects. *Agenesis of the corpus callosum* without other recognized abnormality of the CNS can be asymptomatic or can at least necessitate sophisticated neuropsychological tests of interhemispheric processing to detect an abnormality.[82,83,102]

Most cases reported in hospital- or clinic-based series are associated with other anomalies of the nervous system (see earlier).[7,78,80-83,88,103] Not surprisingly, the neurological features of large *hospital-based* series of infants and children with agenesis (complete or partial) of the corpus callosum are not subtle. In one study (*n* = 63), 85% had cognitive deficits, and more than 90% had neuromotor disturbances.[88] Rarely, massive dorsal

of the corpus callosum, not discussed elsewhere in this book, is the *Aicardi syndrome.*[92-99] This syndrome is believed to result from an X-linked dominant, male-lethal mutation, and the moderate degree of phenotypic variability appears to be related to nonrandom X-inactivation.[96] The phenotypic features include partial or complete callosal agenesis with multiple (type 2) dysplastic meningeal cysts (see below), cortical dysplasia (often unlayered polymicrogyria), periventricular nodular heterotopias, choroid plexus cysts, and ocular findings including choroidal lacunae or colobomata (Box 2.5 and Fig. 2.18). The neurological features (e.g., infantile spasms, other seizures, and cognitive deficits) are related principally to accompanying defects of neuronal migration. At least 80% of affected infants subsequently exhibit severe mental retardation.

Agenesis of the corpus callosum may also be associated with *midline mesenchymal (meningeal) dysplasia,* including

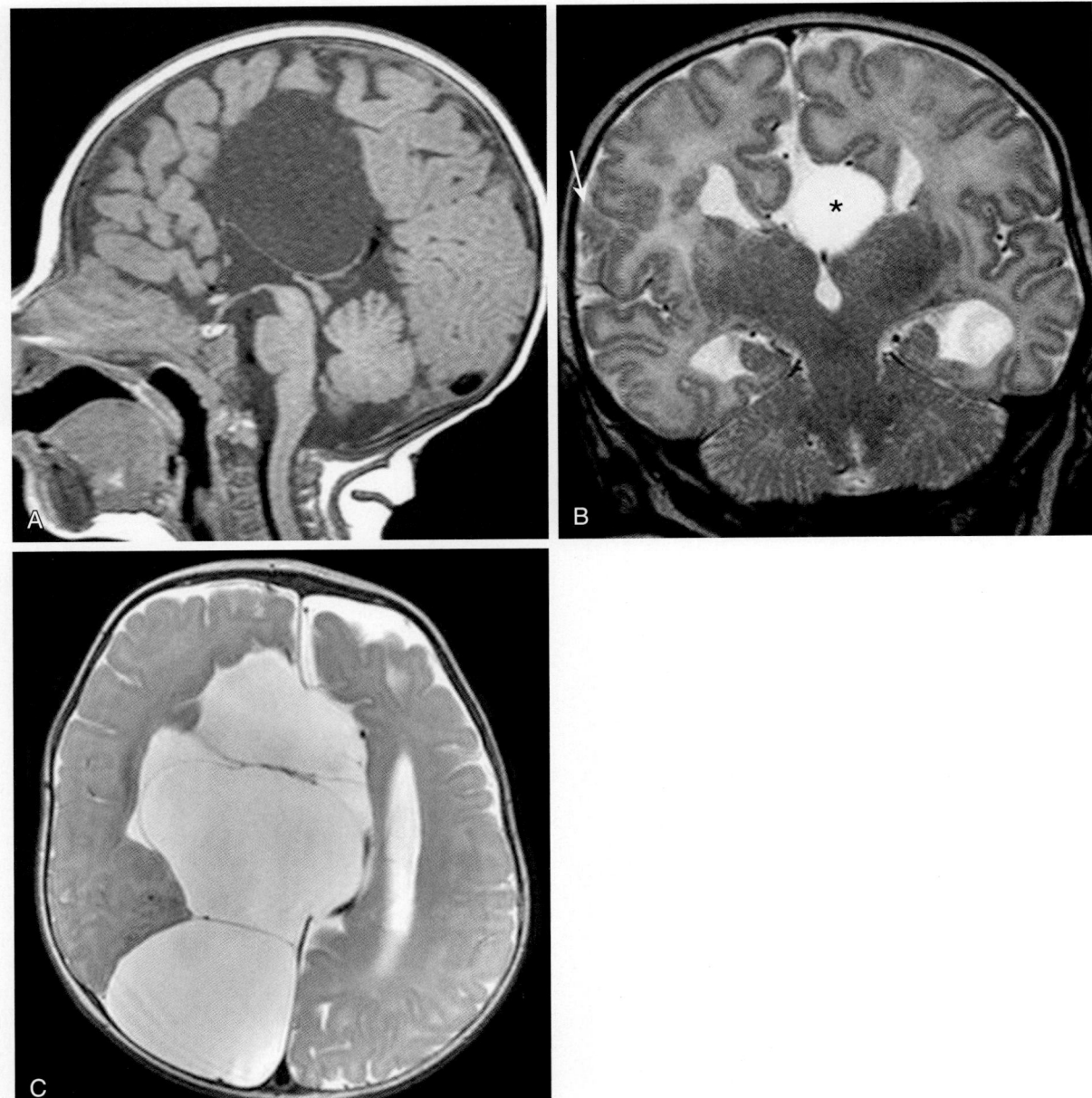

Figure 2.19 Magnetic resonance imaging of dorsal cysts in association with agenesis of the corpus callosum. T1-sagittal (A) and T2-coronal (B) images of a unilocular (type 1) cyst (asterisk in B). Note incidental area of dysplastic cortex *(arrow)*. T2-weighted axial view (C) of a multilocular type 2 dorsal cyst.

cystic expansion of the third ventricle occurs and produces hydrocephalus.[79,104] The associated anomalies determine the major features of the clinical syndrome.

Diagnosis

The diagnostic approach to agenesis of the corpus callosum should include careful evaluation of the entire commissural system as well as a detailed search for additional intra- and extracranial anomalies.

Prenatal Diagnosis. Fetal US scanning is the standard screening technique for detection of fetal anatomical anomalies. Factors such as fetal position and maternal obesity may make diagnosis

by abdominal US challenging, especially for the inexperienced scanner. In these cases, transvaginal US may improve detection. Callosal agenesis is associated with colpocephaly, which describes a teardrop shape of the lateral ventricles with the atria relatively or absolutely enlarged (see later). In one large study of 430 cases referred for ventriculomegaly and diagnosed by fetal MRI, 58 cases (13%) were associated with callosal agenesis, which was isolated in 14 of 58 (24%).[105] Good-quality and well-aligned midline sagittal and coronal views by fetal US will show the corpus callosum as two echodense lines separated by the hypodense callosum. Even when direct visualization of the corpus callosum is difficult, a number of indirect clues that emanate from the rearrangement of structures around

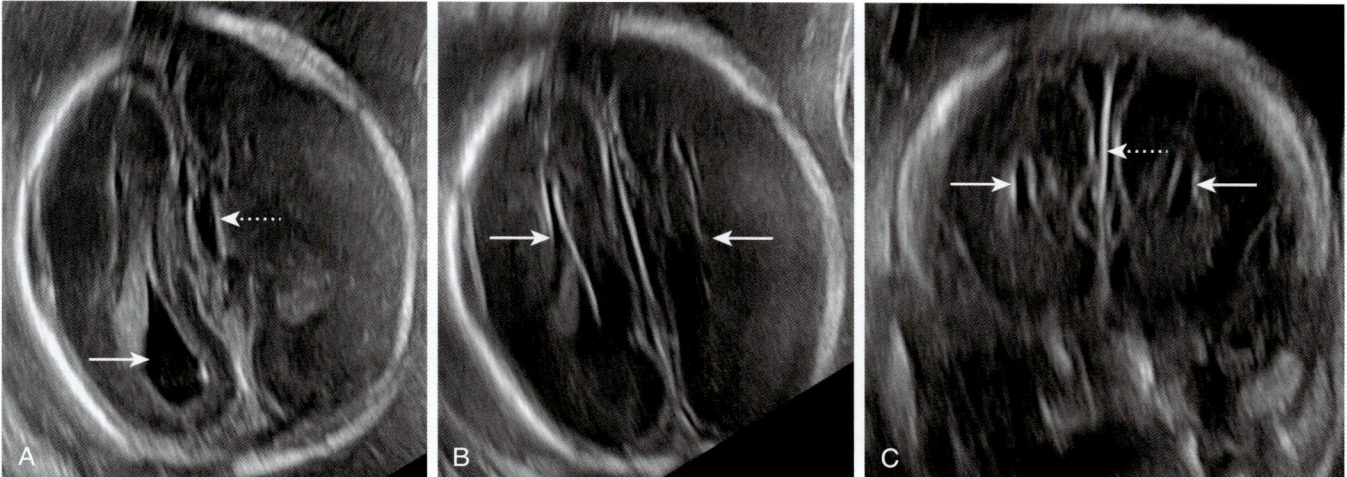

Figure 2.20 Fetal ultrasound images of agenesis of the corpus callosum. (A) Axial view showing high-riding third ventricle *(broken arrow)* and colpocephaly *(solid arrow)*. (B) Axial view showing parallel alignment of the lateral ventricles *(arrows)*. (C) Coronal view showing falx cerebri *(broken arrow)* and absence of the corpus callosum, with parallel alignment of the lateral ventricles. (Courtesy Dr. Dorothy Bulas.)

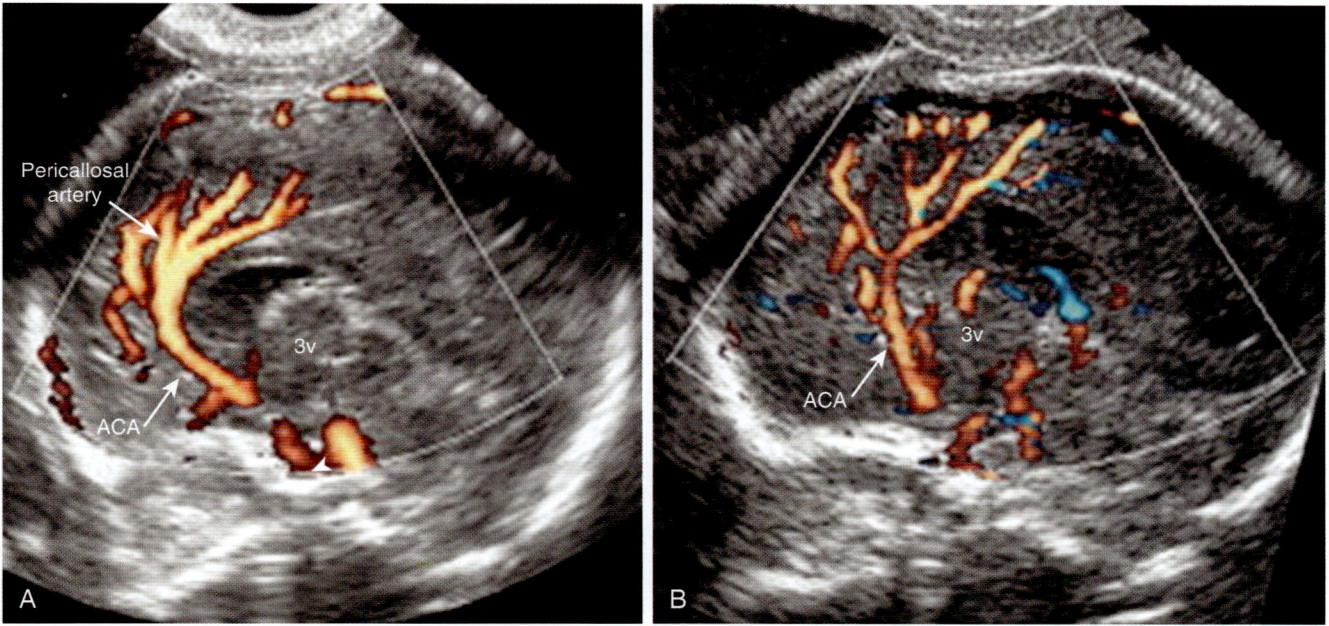

Figure 2.21 Doppler images of the anterior cerebral artery (ACA) and its branches in a normal subject (A) and an infant with agenesis of the corpus callosum (B). In callosal agenesis the ACA and its branches pass almost directly upward (B), as opposed to the curved path of the ACA around the normal genu and body of the corpus callosum (A). *3v*, Third ventricle.

the missing corpus callosum help point to the diagnosis (Fig. 2.20). The cerebral hemispheres are widely separated. The cavum septi pellucidi is absent. The lateral ventricles are widely separated, have a "steer-horn" configuration (the Probst bundles running in the medial walls of the lateral ventricles), and a parallel alignment in the axial view. In addition, the lateral ventricles have a colpocephalic shape and abnormal extension of the temporal horn into the parahippocampal gyrus. The third ventricle extends upward, unconfined by the missing callosum. These features are more helpful in

cases of complete agenesis of the corpus callosum.[106-108] In partial callosal agenesis, a more reliable sign is an abnormally wide anterior cavum septi pellucidi.[106] The pericallosal artery develops in close association with the corpus callosum. In callosal agenesis, Doppler US of the pericallosal artery shows loss of the normal semicircular arc of the artery and linear ascent of the anterior cerebral artery branches. In partial callosal agenesis, the pericallosal artery initially follows the arc of the existing corpus callosum but then courses upward and posteriorly (Fig. 2.21).

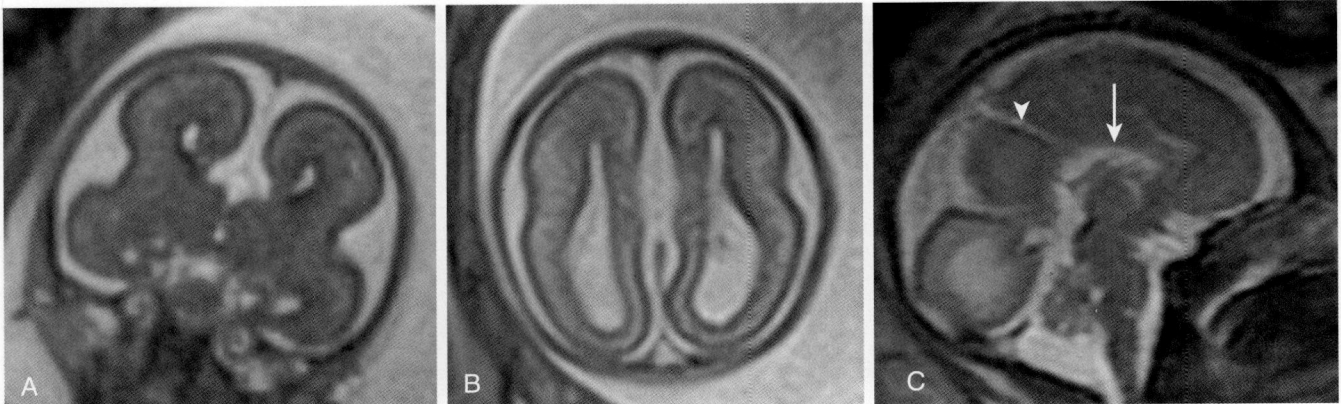

Figure 2.22 Agenesis of the corpus callosum. T2-weighted fetal magnetic resonance imaging. Coronal view (A) shows absence of the corpus callosum across the midline and a widened interhemispheric space. Axial view (B) shows parallel alignment teardrop shape (colpocephaly) of the lateral hemispheres. Midline sagittal view (C) showing absence of the corpus callosum (*white arrow*) and extension of the gyrus from the convexity surface to the third ventricle (*arrowhead*).

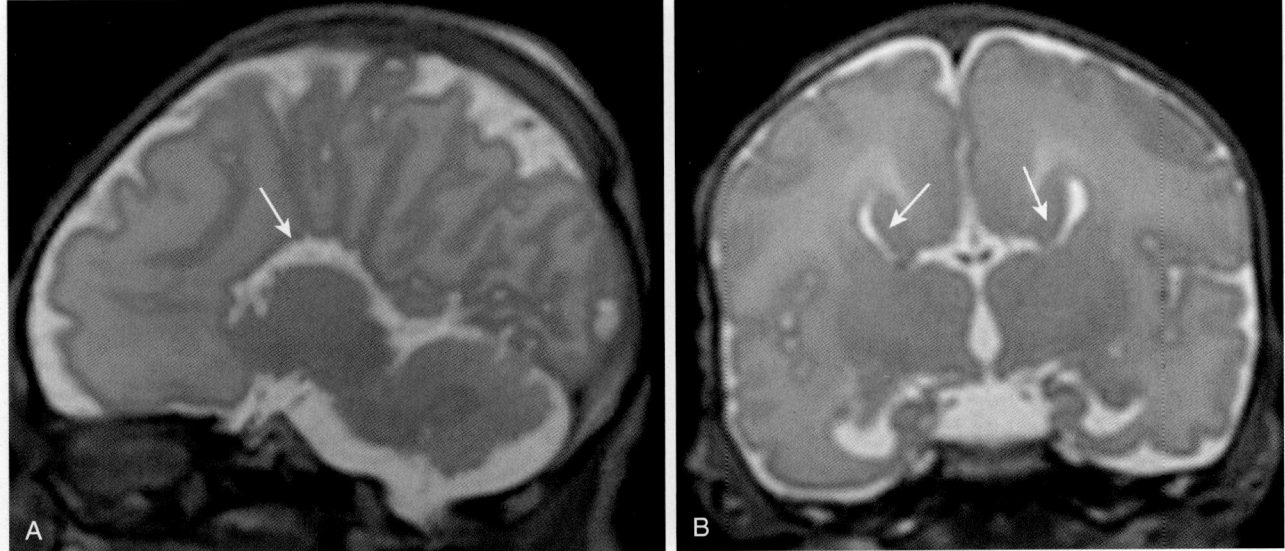

Figure 2.23 Complete agenesis of the corpus callosum (T2-weighted magnetic resonance imaging). Sagittal view (A) showing radial (sunburst) alignment of the gyral pattern, with absence of the corpus callosum and cingulate gyrus (*arrow*), allowing extension of the gyri to the edge of the third ventricle. Coronal view (B) showing the "steer horn" configuration and indentation of the medial walls of the lateral ventricles by the bundles of Probst (*arrows*).

Antenatal US has a false-positive rate of up to 20% for the diagnosis of callosal agenesis.[89,109-111] Prenatal US screening is less sensitive to associated findings and isolated callosal agenesis is misdiagnosed in 5% to 20% of cases.[111-113] When fetal US suggests callosal agenesis, an MRI is indicated (see later), to minimize the limitations of fetal US (Fig. 2.22). Prenatal MRI has been shown to increase the detection of associated abnormalities in more than 20% of cases.[114]

Postnatal Diagnosis. Callosal agenesis may be diagnosed by postnatal cranial US,[115,116] but the definitive diagnosis of the callosal and associated lesions is by brain MRI (Fig. 2.23). In addition to the features already described, postnatal MRI shows a radial gyral pattern on the medial hemispheric surface (instead of the normal horizontal orientation), producing a *sunburst* appearance, with gyri running down to the third ventricular roof unimpeded by the absent corpus callosum. On coronal views, postnatal MRI more clearly shows structures like the Probst bundles (Figs. 2.23 and 2.24). Postnatal MRI also provides greater tissue resolution, thereby allowing more detailed assessment of the entire commissural system and its constituents, namely the anterior commissure, anterior corpus callosum, hippocampal commissure–associated splenium, and the septum pellucidum. This is particularly valuable for defining what components of the structure are deficient in partial callosal agenesis.

Prognosis. The range of reported neurodevelopment outcomes for callosal agenesis is broad and inconsistent, in all likelihood owing to differences in reported populations, diagnostic tools,

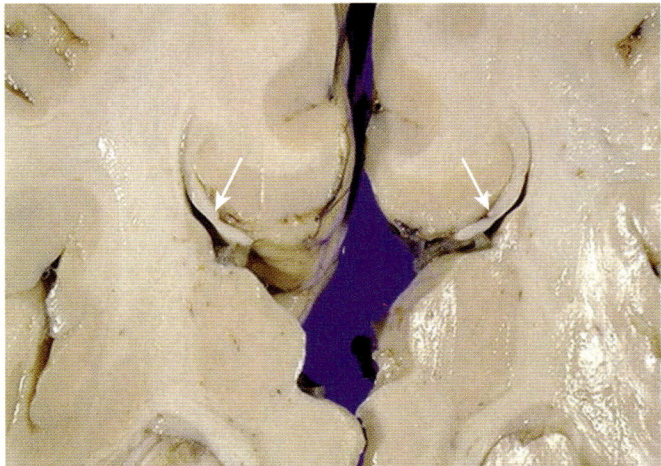

Figure 2.24 Gross coronal anatomy of the interhemispheric region. Agenesis of the corpus callosum with the heterotopic bundles of Probst on the medial surface of the lateral ventricles *(arrows)*.

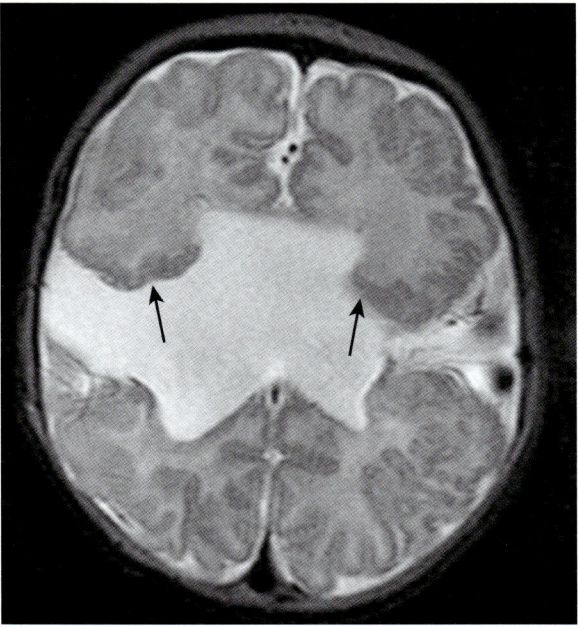

Figure 2.25 Absence of the cavum septi pellucidi and bilateral open-lipped schizencephaly. Axial T2-weighted magnetic resonance imaging in a newborn infant. Note the polymicrogyria along the edges of the bilateral clefts *(arrows)*.

and the classification systems used. A large review of 132 cases diagnosed in the fetal period showed no significant difference in neurodevelopmental outcome between isolated partial and isolated complete agenesis of the corpus callosum.[114] The outcome of isolated complete callosal agenesis, based on MRI diagnosis and standardized outcome measures, was normal in 84%, associated with mild to moderate disability in 8%, and with severe disability in 8%. In other studies up to 73% to 85% of cases of isolated callosal agenesis had favorable outcomes[84,111,117,118]; in these studies no significant differences in outcome were identified between isolated partial or complete callosal agenesis. In a large study of fetal ventriculomegaly using MRI and standardized neurodevelopmental testing, normal outcomes were seen in 67% of cases of isolated callosal agenesis compared with 7% in cases of complex callosal agenesis.[105] In a 10-year follow-up of 11 patients diagnosed prenatally with isolated callosal agenesis and evaluated by standardized neuropsychological testing,[119] 8 of 11 had normal cognitive scores (although shifted down) and 3 of 11 had borderline intelligence. Almost 50% of these cases had behavioral difficulties.

Conversely, other reports describe a high risk of neurodevelopmental disability in isolated callosal agenesis.[110,120,121]

Anomalies of the Cavum Septi Pellucidi

Developmental anomalies of the cavum septi pellucidi include absence (complete or partial) and persistent enlargement. The septum pellucidum has similar embryonic origins to the anterior corpus callosum, both being derived from the commissural plate. The space between the septal leaflets is one cavity, which is divided into the cavum septi pellucidi anterior to the foramen of Monro and the cavum vergae behind it. In most cases the septal leaflets fuse into a single septum, obliterating the cavum by 6 months postnatal. Before this time, partial or complete absence of the septal leaflets leads to the more commonly used term of *absence of the cavum septi pellucidi*. At later postnatal stages, the term *absence of the septum pellucidum* is more appropriate. Since the septum pellucidum is a critical relay structure within the limbic system, it is not surprising that anomalies in this structure are associated with neuropsychiatric disorders.

Absence of the Septum Pellucidum
Anatomical Abnormalities

Like agenesis of the corpus callosum, absence of the cavum septi pellucidi (or of the septum pellucidum postnatally) is an important clue to the presence of other, clinically more serious abnormalities of prosencephalic development or of concomitant developmental events (e.g., neuronal migration).[1,122-131] In addition, the septum pellucidum can be destroyed by concomitant hydrocephalus or by contiguous ischemic lesions (e.g., porencephaly). Thus it is understandable that in one large MRI series of absence of the septum pellucidum this anomaly was never seen as an isolated finding; it was associated with holoprosencephaly, agenesis of the corpus callosum, septo-optic dysplasia, schizencephaly (Fig. 2.25), basilar encephalocele, hydrocephalus (as a result of aqueductal stenosis or the Chiari II malformation), and porencephaly-hydranencephaly.[78] One prominent example of these disorders is the *syndrome of absence of septum pellucidum with schizencephaly* (often mistakenly termed *porencephaly*) (Fig. 2.25 and Box 2.6).[78,123,132,133] Absence of the cavum septi pellucidi is present in about two thirds of patients with schizencephaly (usually frontoparietal).

The clinical features and long-term neurodevelopmental outcome of *absence of septum pellucidum*, as with agenesis of the corpus callosum, depend principally on the associated disorders (see the earlier discussion of anatomical abnormality). In fact, some consider *isolated* absence of the cavum septi pellucidi a normal variant. In general, the associated disorders (see earlier) are detected best by MRI. One report has identified a patient with mitochondrial complex III deficiency.[130] A rare autosomal recessive form has been shown to be related to a mutation in *HESX1*, a homeobox gene crucial for the development of forebrain, eyes, and pituitary gland.[132] One series emphasized the association of craniofacial dysmorphisms, brain abnormalities (callosal agenesis, schizencephaly, heterotopias), and endocrinopathies.[128]

The syndrome of *septo-optic dysplasia* was first described by De Morsier in 1953[134] as the association between an absent cavum septi pellucidi and optic nerve hypoplasia. Subsequently disturbances of hypothalamic-pituitary function[122,128,131,133,135] became a diagnostic criterion. Consequently the diagnosis may be suspected in the fetus on the basis of absent septal leaflets (and possibly detection of optic nerve hypoplasia), but it is confirmed only postnatally on the basis of hypothalamic-pituitary dysfunction. In one selected series of infants referred to an endocrine clinic, approximately 60% exhibited diabetes insipidus, 80% had multiple pituitary hormone deficiencies, 60% had genital anomalies resulting from hypogonadotrophic hypogonadism, and, importantly, 75% had persistent *neonatal hypoglycemia*.[131] In a large selected series of children with optic nerve hypoplasia reported from a pediatric ophthalmology clinic, although only a minority had absence of the septum pellucidum, fully 72% had endocrinopathy, especially disturbances of growth hormone homeostasis.[122] Indeed, optic nerve hypoplasia and septo-optic dysplasia should be considered on a continuum of a heterogeneous group of disorders of midline development. Thus these disorders, related to defective development of the commissural and chiasmatic plates, often also involve the hypothalamic plate. Other associated defects have been described, including schizencephaly and bilateral polymicrogyria without schizencephaly. Moreover, seizure disorders and cognitive deficits, perhaps related to accompanying errors in neuronal migration, may also occur. Clearly, the clinical aspects of these several disorders of midline prosencephalic development (Table 2.2) overlap and merge with the clinical features of migrational defects discussed in Chapter 6.

Diagnosis. Absence of the cavum septi pellucidi is associated with such a broad range of forebrain anomalies that it has become a cardinal anatomical structure for identification in prenatal imaging. Its absence is considered a marker for abnormal forebrain development rather than a fundamental malformation. Nonvisualization of the cavum septi pellucidi during prenatal US screening is rarely isolated; rather, it is associated with a variety of anomalies including callosal agenesis, schizencephaly, septo-optic dysplasia, holoprosencephaly, chronic hydrocephalus, and acquired fetal brain injury. Fetal MRI detects abnormalities of the septal leaflets reliably, and detects *additional* brain anomalies not evident on fetal US in

52% cases.[136] In addition, fetal US is prone to false-positive identification of the cavum septi pellucidi when the columns of the fornix (which are embryologically distinct from the corpus callosum and cavum septi pellucidi) course together,[137] and in cases of callosal agenesis, when the "high-riding" third ventricle may be mistaken for the cavum septi pellucidi.

Enlarged Cavum Septi Pellucidi

The cavum septi pellucidi is a normal developmental structure in fetal life and early infancy. All premature infants exhibit an ultrasonographically demonstrable cavum up to 34 weeks of gestation, and 36% of term infants still have a small (mean, 0.5 cm) cavum.[125] Nevertheless, a large cavum septi pellucidi (>1 cm) in a term newborn should be viewed with suspicion. By 6 months postnatal age the septal leaflets are fused, obliterating the cavum, in about 85% of subjects.[138] A persistently enlarged cavum septi pellucidi has been associated with long-term neuropsychiatric complications.[125,126,129,139-143] In cases of bipolar disorder, a 20% rate of enlarged (>5 mm) cavum septi pellucidi has been reported, and in these cases the onset of bipolar manifestations is significantly earlier.[142] Previous suggestions of a relatively high association with subsequent cognitive deficits appear to be related largely to selection bias.[139]

REFERENCES

1. Leech RW, Shuman RM. Holoprosencephaly and related midline cerebral anomalies: a review. *J Child Neurol.* 1986;1:3-18.
2. Lemire RJ, Loeser JD, Leech RW, et al. *Normal and Abnormal Development of the Human Nervous System.* Hagerstown: Harper & Row; 1975.
3. Yakovlev PI. Pathoarchitectonic studies of cerebral malformations. I. Arrhinencephalies (holotelencephalies). *J Neuropathol Exp Neurol.* 1959;18:22.
4. Gongal PA, French CR, Waskiewicz AJ. Aberrant forebrain signaling during early development underlies the generation of holoprosencephaly and coloboma. *Biochim Biophys Acta.* 2011;1812:390-401.
5. Paul LK, Brown WS, Adolphs R, et al. Agenesis of the corpus callosum: genetic, developmental and functional aspects of connectivity. *Nat Rev Neurosci.* 2007;8:287-299.
6. Ren T, Anderson A, Shen WB, et al. Imaging, anatomical, and molecular analysis of callosal formation in the developing human fetal brain. *Anat Rec A Discov Mol Cell Evol Biol.* 2006;288:191-204.
7. Richards LJ, Plachez C, Ren T. Mechanisms regulating the development of the corpus callosum and its agenesis in mouse and human. *Clin Genet.* 2004;66:276-289.
8. Kier EL, Truwit CL. The normal and abnormal genu of the corpus callosum: an evolutionary, embryologic, anatomic, and MR analysis. *AJNR Am J Neuroradiol.* 1996;17:1631-1641.
9. Kier EL, Truwit CL. The lamina rostralis: modification of concepts concerning the anatomy, embryology, and MR appearance of the rostrum of the corpus callosum. *AJNR Am J Neuroradiol.* 1997;18:715-722.
10. Belloni E, Muenke M, Roessler E, et al. Identification of sonic hedgehog as a candidate gene responsible for holoprosencephaly. *Nature.* 1996;14:353-356.
11. El-Jaick KB, Powers SE, Bartholin L, et al. Functional analysis of mutations in TGIF associated with holoprosencephaly. *Mol Genet Metab.* 2007;90:97-111.
12. Golden JA. Holoprosencephaly: a defect in brain patterning. *J Neuropathol Exp Neurol.* 1998;57:991-999.
13. Muenke M. Holoprosencephaly as a genetic model for normal craniofacial development. *Dev Biol.* 1994;5:294-301.
14. Roessler E, Belloni E, Gaudenz K, et al. Mutations in sonic hedgehog gene cause holoprosencephaly. *Nat Genet.* 1996;14:357-360.
15. Rubenstein JL, Shimamura K, Martinez S, et al. Regionalization of the prosencephalic neural plate. *Annu Rev Neurosci.* 1998;21:445-477.

16. Sarnat HB, Flores-Sarnat L. Neuropathologic research strategies in holoprosencephaly. *J Child Neurol.* 2001;16:918-931.

17. Xavier GM, Seppala M, Barrell W, et al. Hedgehog receptor function during craniofacial development. *Dev Biol.* 2016;415:198-215.

18. Choudhry Z, Rikani AA, Choudhry AM, et al. Sonic hedgehog signalling pathway: a complex network. *Ann Neurosci.* 2014;21:28-31.

19. Hahn JS, Barkovich AJ, Stashinko EE, et al. Factor analysis of neuroanatomical and clinical characteristics of holoprosencephaly. *Brain Dev.* 2006;28:413-419.

20. Harris CP, Townsend JJ, Norman MG, et al. Atelencephalic aprosencephaly. *J Child Neurol.* 1994;9:412-416.

21. Iivanainen M, Haltia M, Lydecken K. Atelencephaly. *Dev Med Child Neurol.* 1977;19:663-668.

22. Kakita A, Hayashi S, Arakawa M, et al. Aprosencephaly: histopathological features of the rudimentary forebrain and retina. *Acta Neuropathol.* 2001;102:110-116.

23. Kim TS, Cho S, Dickson DW. Aprosencephaly: review of the literature and report of a case with cerebellar hypoplasia, pigmented epithelial cyst and Rathke's cleft cyst. *Acta Neuropathol.* 1990;79:424-431.

24. Lurie IW, Nedzved MK, Lazjuk GI, et al. Aprosencephaly-atelencephaly and the aprosencephaly (XK) syndrome. *Am J Med Genet.* 1979;3:301-309.

25. Siebert JR, Kokich VG, Warkany J, et al. Atelencephalic microcephaly: craniofacial anatomy and morphologic comparisons with holoprosencephaly and anencephaly. *Teratology.* 1987;36:279-285.

26. DeMyer W, Zeman W, Palmer CG. The face predicts the brain: diagnostic significance of median facial anomalies for holoprosencephaly (arrhinencephaly). *Pediatrics.* 1964;34:256.

27. Barkovich AJ, Raybaud C. *Pediatric Neuroimaging.* 5th ed. Philadelphia: Lippincott Williams & Wilkins; 2012.

28. Cohen MM Jr. Perspectives on holoprosencephaly: Part I. Epidemiology, genetics, and syndromology. *Teratology.* 1989;40:211-235.

29. Cohen MM Jr. Perspectives on holoprosencephaly: Part III. Spectra, distinctions, continuities, and discontinuities. *Am J Med Genet.* 1989;34:271-288.

30. Friede RL. *Developmental Neuropathology.* 2nd ed. New York: Springer-Verlag; 1989.

31. Lewis AJ, Simon EM, Barkovich AJ, et al. Middle interhemispheric variant of holoprosencephaly. A distinct cliniconeuroradiologic subtype. *Neurology.* 2002;59:1860-1865.

32. Mizuguchi M, Morimatsu Y. Histopathological study of alobar holoprosencephaly. 2. Marginal glioneural heterotopia and other gliomesenchymal abnormalities. *Acta Neuropathol.* 1989;78:183-188.

33. Mizuguchi M, Morimatsu Y. Histopathological study of alobar holoprosencephaly. 1. Abnormal laminar architecture of the telencephalic cortex. *Acta Neuropathol.* 1989;78:176-182.

34. Oba H, Barkovich AJ. Holoprosencephaly: an analysis of callosal formation and its relation to development of the interhemispheric fissure. *AJNR Am J Neuroradiol.* 1995;16:453-460.

35. Olsen CL, Hughes JP, Youngblood LG, et al. Epidemiology of holoprosencephaly and phenotypic characteristics of affected children: New York State, 1984–1989. *Am J Med Genet.* 1997;73:217-226.

36. Plawner LL, Delgado MR, Miller VS, et al. Neuroanatomy of holoprosencephaly as predictor of function. Beyond the face predicting the brain. *Neurology.* 2002;59:1058-1066.

37. Rössing R, Friede RL. Holoprosencephaly with retroprosencephalic extracerebral cyst. *Dev Med Child Neurol.* 1992;34:177-181.

38. Simon EM, Hevner R, Pinter JD, et al. Assessment of the deep gray nuclei in holoprosencephaly. *AJNR Am J Neuroradiol.* 2000;21:1955-1961.

39. Yamada S, Uwabe C, Fujii S, et al. Phenotypic variability in human embryonic holoprosencephaly in the Kyoto collection. *Birth Defects Res Part A Clin Mol Teratol.* 2004;70:495-508.

40. Takahashi S, Miyamoto A, Saino T, et al. Alobar holoprosencephaly with diabetes insipidus and neuronal migration disorder. *Pediatr Neurol.* 1995;13:175-177.

41. Hahn JS, Barnes PD, Clegg NJ, et al. Septopreoptic holoprosencephaly: a mild subtype associated with midline craniofacial anomalies. *AJNR Am J Neuroradiol.* 2010;31:1596-1601.

42. Koob M, Weingertner AS, Gasser B, et al. Thick corpus callosum: a clue to the diagnosis of fetal septopreoptic holoprosencephaly? *Pediatr Radiol.* 2012;42:886-890.

43. Simon EM, Goldstein RB, Coakley FV, et al. Fast MR imaging of fetal CNS anomalies in utero. *AJNR Am J Neuroradiol.* 2000;21:1688-1698.

44. Whitehead MT, Vezina G. Interhypothalamic adhesion: a series of 13 cases. *AJNR Am J Neuroradiol.* 2014;35:2002-2006.

45. Kumar S, Jaiswal AK, Rastogi M. Aventriculi associated with holoprosencephaly. *J Clin Neurosci.* 2006;13:378-380.

46. Sener RN. Aventriculi associated with holoprosencephaly. *Comput Med Imaging Graph.* 1998;22:345-347.

47. Garfinkle WB. Aventriculy: a new entity? *AJNR Am J Neuroradiol.* 1996;17:1649-1650.

48. Ciftcioglu E, Ozyurek H, Nural MS, et al. Absence of the lateral and third ventricles associated with holoprosencephaly. *Anat Cell Biol.* 2015;48:222-224.

49. Sener RN, Jones AO, Roebuck DJ, et al. Midline interhemispheric fusion associated with atypical callosal dysgenesis: a mild type of holoprosencephaly. *Austral Radiol.* 1996;40:357-359.

50. Matsunaga E, Shiota K. Holoprosencephaly in human embryos: epidemiologic studies of 150 cases. *Teratology.* 1977;16:261-272.

51. Hasegawa Y, Hasegawa T, Yokoyama T, et al. Holoprosencephaly associated with diabetes insipidus and syndrome of inappropriate secretion of antidiuretic hormone. *J Pediatr.* 1990;117:756-758.

52. Roesler CP, Paterson SJ, Flax J, et al. Links between abnormal brain structure and cognition in holoprosencephaly. *Pediatr Neurol.* 2006;35:387-394.

53. Biancheri R, Rossi A, Tortori-Donati P, et al. Middle interhemispheric variant of holoprosencephaly: a very mild clinical case. *Neurology.* 2004;63:2194-2196.

54. Shanks DE, Wilson WG. Lobar holoprosencephaly presenting as spastic diplegia. *Dev Med Child Neurol.* 1988;30:383-386.

55. Cohen MM Jr. Hedgehog signaling update. *Am J Med Genet A.* 2010;152A:1875-1914.

56. Roessler E, Ouspenskaia MV, Karkera JD, et al. Reduced NODAL signaling strength via mutation of several pathway members including FOXH1 is linked to human heart defects and holoprosencephaly. *Am J Hum Genet.* 2008;83:18-29.

57. Estabrooks LL, Rao KW, Donahue RP, et al. Holoprosencephaly in an infant with a minute deletion of chromosome 21(q22.3). *Am J Med Genet.* 1990;36:306-309.

58. Hamada H, Arinami T, Koresawa M, et al. A case of trisomy 21 with holoprosencephaly: the fifth case. *Jpn J Hum Genet.* 1991;36:159-163.

59. Münke M. Clinical, cytogenetic, and molecular approaches to the genetic heterogeneity of holoprosencephaly. *Am J Med Genet.* 1989;34:237-245.

60. Croen LA, Shaw GM, Lammer EJ. Risk factors for cytogenetically normal holoprosencephaly in California: a population-based case-control study. *Am J Med Genet.* 2000;90:320-325.

61. Lazaro L, Dubourg C, Pasquier L, et al. Phenotypic and molecular variability of the holoprosencephalic spectrum. *Am J Med Genet Part A.* 2004;129A:21-24.

62. Paulussen AD, Schrander-Stumpel CT, Tserpelis DC, et al. The unfolding clinical spectrum of holoprosencephaly due to mutations in SHH, ZIC2, SIX3 and TGIF genes. *Eur J Hum Genet.* 2010;18:999-1005.

63. Dubourg C, Lazaro L, Pasquier L, et al. Molecular screening of SHH, ZIC2, SIX3, and TGIF genes in patients with features of holoprosencephaly spectrum: mutation review and genotype-phenotype correlations. *Hum Mutat.* 2004;24:43-51.

64. Bertolacini CD, Richieri-Costa A, Ribeiro-Bicudo LA. Sonic hedgehog (SHH) mutation in patients within the spectrum of holoprosencephaly. *Brain Dev.* 2010;32:217-222.

65. Barr M Jr, Hanson JW, Currey K, et al. Holoprosencephaly in infants of diabetic mothers. *J Pediatr.* 1983;102:565-568.

66. Haas D, Morgenthaler J, Lacbawan F, et al. Abnormal sterol metabolism in holoprosencephaly: studies in cultured lymphoblasts. *J Med Genet.* 2007;44:298-305.

67. Haas D, Muenke M. Abnormal sterol metabolism in holoprosencephaly. *Am J Med Genet C Semin Med Genet.* 2010;154C:102-108.

68. Kelley RL, Roessler E, Hennekam RC, et al. Holoprosencephaly in RSH/Smith-Lemli-Opitz syndrome: does abnormal cholesterol

metabolism affect the function of Sonic Hedgehog? *Am J Med Genet.* 1996;66:478-484.

69. Bronshtein M, Wiener Z. Early transvaginal sonographic diagnosis of alobar holoprosencephaly. *Prenat Diagn.* 1991;11:459-462.

70. Hayashi Y, Suzumori N, Sugiura T, et al. Prenatal findings of holoprosencephaly. *Congenit Anom (Kyoto).* 2015;55:161-163.

71. Chervenak FA, Isaacson G, Hobbins JC, et al. Diagnosis and management of fetal holoprosencephaly. *Obstet Gynecol.* 1985;66: 322-326.

72. McGahan JP, Nyberg DA, Mack LA. Sonography of facial features of alobar and semilobar holoprosencephaly. *AJR Am J Roentgenol.* 1990;154:143-148.

73. Verlinsky Y, Rechitsky S, Verlinsky O, et al. Preimplantation diagnosis for sonic hedgehog mutation causing familial holoprosencephaly. *N Engl J Med.* 2003;348:1449-1454.

74. Committee Opinion No. 640: cell-Free DNA screening for fetal aneuploidy. *Obstet Gynecol.* 2015;126:e31-e37.

75. Cuckle H, Benn P, Pergament E. Cell-free DNA screening for fetal aneuploidy as a clinical service. *Clin Biochem.* 2015;48:932-941.

76. Roessler E, Velez JI, Zhou N, et al. Utilizing prospective sequence analysis of SHH, ZIC2, SIX3 and TGIF in holoprosencephaly probands to describe the parameters limiting the observed frequency of mutant genexgene interactions. *Mol Genet Metab.* 2012;105:658-664.

77. Raybaud C. The corpus callosum, the other great forebrain commissures, and the septum pellucidum: anatomy, development, and malformation. *Neuroradiology.* 2010;52:447-477.

78. Barkovich AJ, Norman D. Absence of the septum pellucidum: a useful sign in the diagnosis of congenital brain malformations. *AJNR Am J Neuroradiol.* 1988;9:1107-1114.

79. Barkovich AJ, Simon EM, Walsh CA. Callosal agenesis with cyst. A better understanding and new classification. *Neurology.* 2001;56:220-227.

80. Nissenkorn A, Michelson M, Ben-Zeev B, et al. Inborn errors of metabolism. A cause of abnormal brain development. *Neurology.* 2001;56:1265-1272.

81. Sztriha L. Spectrum of corpus callosum agenesis. *Pediatr Neurol.* 2005;32:94-101.

82. Taylor M, David AS. Agenesis of the corpus callosum: a United Kingdom series of 56 cases. *J Neurol Neurosurg Psychiatr.* 1998;64: 131-134.

83. Utsunomiya H, Ogasawara T, Hayashi T, et al. Dysgenesis of the corpus callosum and associated telencephalic anomalies: MRI. *Neuroradiology.* 1997;39:302-310.

84. Santo S, D'Antonio F, Homfray T, et al. Counseling in fetal medicine: agenesis of the corpus callosum. *Ultrasound Obstet Gynecol.* 2012;40:513-521.

85. Kidron D, Shapira D, Ben Sira L, et al. Agenesis of the corpus callosum. An autopsy study in fetuses. *Virchows Arch.* 2016;468:219-230.

86. Schmid RS, Maness PF. L1 and NCAM adhesion molecules as signaling coreceptors in neuronal migration and process outgrowth. *Curr Opin Neurobiol.* 2008;18:245-250.

87. Yamasaki M, Thompson P, Lemmon V. CRASH syndrome: mutations in L1CAM correlate with severity of the disease. *Neuropediatrics.* 1997;28:175-178.

88. Bedeschi MF, Bonaglia MC, Grasso R, et al. Agenesis of the corpus callosum: clinical and genetic study in 63 young patients. *Pediatr Neurol.* 2006;34:186-193.

89. Fratelli N, Papageorghiou AT, Prefumo F, et al. Outcome of prenatally diagnosed agenesis of the corpus callosum. *Prenat Diagn.* 2007;27:512-517.

90. Hetts SW, Sherr EH, Chao S, et al. Anomalies of the corpus callosum: an MR analysis of the phenotypic spectrum of associated malformations. *AJR Am J Roentgenol.* 2006;187:1343-1348.

91. Miller E, Widjaja E, Blaser S, et al. The old and the new: supratentorial MR findings in Chiari II malformation. *Childs Nerv Syst.* 2008;24:563-575.

92. Aicardi J. Aicardi syndrome. *Brain Dev.* 2005;27:164-171.

93. Donnenfeld AE, Packer RJ, Zackai EH, et al. Clinical, cytogenetic, and pedigree findings in 18 cases of Aicardi syndrome. *Am J Med Genet.* 1989;32:461-467.

94. Hamano S, Yagishita S, Kawakami M, et al. Aicardi syndrome: postmortem findings. *Pediatr Neurol.* 1989;5:259-261.

95. Menezes AV, MacGregor DL, Buncic JR. Aicardi syndrome: natural history and possible predictors of severity. *Pediatr Neurol.* 1994;11:313-318.

96. Neidich JA, Nussbaum RL, Packer RJ, et al. Heterogeneity of clinical severity and molecular lesions in Aicardi syndrome. *J Pediatr.* 1990;116:911-917.

97. Nielsen KB, Anvret M, Flodmark O, et al. Aicardi syndrome: early neuroradiological manifestations and results of DNA studies in one patient. *Am J Med Genet.* 1991;38:65-68.

98. Palmer L, Zetterlund B, Hard AL, et al. Aicardi syndrome: presentation at onset in Swedish children born in 1975-2002. *Neuropediatrics.* 2006;37:154-158.

99. Rosser TL, Acosta MT, Packer RJ. Aicardi syndrome: spectrum of disease and long-term prognosis in 77 females. *Pediatr Neurol.* 2002;27:343-346.

100. Haldipur P, Gillies GS, Janson OK, et al. Foxc1 dependent mesenchymal signalling drives embryonic cerebellar growth. *eLife.* 2014;3:doi:10.7554/eLife.03962.

101. Truwit CL, Barkovich AJ. Pathogenesis of intracranial lipoma: an MR study in 42 patients. *Am J Roentgenol.* 1990;155:855-864.

102. Friefeld S, MacGregor DL, Chuang S, et al. Comparative study of inter- and intrahemispheric somatosensory functions in children with partial and complete agenesis of the corpus callosum. *Dev Med Child Neurol.* 2000;42:831-838.

103. Hartmann H, Uyanik G, Gross C, et al. Agenesis of the corpus callosum, abnormal genitalia and intractable epilepsy due to a novel familial mutation in the aristaless-related homeobox gene. *Neuropediatrics.* 2004;35:157-160.

104. Young JN, Oakes WJ, Hatten HP. Dorsal third ventricular cyst: an entity distinct from holoprosencephaly. *J Neurosurg.* 1992;77:556-561.

105. Li Y, Estroff JA, Khwaja O, et al. Callosal dysgenesis in fetuses with ventriculomegaly: levels of agreement between imaging modalities and postnatal outcome. *Ultrasound Obstet Gynecol.* 2012;40:522-529.

106. Ghi T, Carletti A, Contro E, et al. Prenatal diagnosis and outcome of partial agenesis and hypoplasia of the corpus callosum. *Ultrasound Obstet Gynecol.* 2010;35:35-41.

107. Paladini D, Pastore G, Cavallaro A, et al. Agenesis of the fetal corpus callosum: sonographic signs change with advancing gestational age. *Ultrasound Obstet Gynecol.* 2013;42:687-690.

108. Shen O, Gelot AB, Moutard ML, et al. Abnormal shape of the cavum septi pellucidi: an indirect sign of partial agenesis of the corpus callosum. *Ultrasound Obstet Gynecol.* 2015;46:595-599.

109. Glenn OA, Goldstein RB, Li KC, Young SJ, Norton ME, Busse RF, Goldberg JD, Barkovich AJ. Fetal magnetic resonance imaging in the evaluation of fetuses referred for sonographically suspected abnormalities of the corpus callosum. *J Ultrasound Med.* 2005;24:791-804.

110. Pilu G, Sandri F, Perolo A, Pittalis MC, Grisolia G, Cocchi G, Foschini MP, Salivioli GP, Bovicelli L. Sonography of fetal agenesis of the corpus callosum: a survey of 35 cases. *Ultrasound Obstet Gynecol.* 1993;3:318-329.

111. Volpe P, Paladini D, Resta M, et al. Characteristics, associations and outcome of partial agenesis of the corpus callosum in the fetus. *Ultrasound Obstet Gynecol.* 2006;27:509-516.

112. Rapp B, Perrotin F, Marret H, Sembeley-Taveau C, Lansac J, Body G. Interet de l'IRM cerebrale foetale pour le diagnostic et le pronostic prenatal des agenesies du corps calleux. *J Gynecol Obstet Biol Reprod.* 2002;31:173-182.

113. Warren DJ, Connolly DJ, Griffiths PD. Assessment of sulcation of the fetal brain in cases of isolated agenesis of the corpus callosum using in utero MR imaging. *AJNR Am J Neuroradiol.* 2010;31:1085-1090.

114. Sotiriadis A, Makrydimas G. Neurodevelopment after prenatal diagnosis of isolated agenesis of the corpus callosum: an integrative review. *Am J Obstet Gynecol.* 2012;206(337):e331-e335.

115. Atlas SW, Shkolnik A, Naidich TP. Sonographic recognition of agenesis of the corpus callosum. *AJR Am J Roentgenol.* 1985;145: 167-173.

116. Fawer C-L, Calame A, Anderegg A, et al. Agenesis of the corpus callosum: real-time ultrasonographic diagnosis and autopsy findings. *Helv Paediatr Acta.* 1985;40:371-380.

117. Gupta JK, Lilford RJ. Assessment and management of fetal agenesis of the corpus callosum. *Prenat Diagn.* 1995;15:301-312.

118. Mangione R, Fries N, Godard P, et al. Neurodevelopmental outcome following prenatal diagnosis of an isolated anomaly of the corpus callosum. *Ultrasound Obstet Gynecol.* 2011;37:290-295.
119. Moutard ML, Kieffer V, Feingold J, et al. Isolated corpus callosum agenesis: a ten-year follow-up after prenatal diagnosis (how are the children without corpus callosum at 10 years of age?). *Prenat Diagn.* 2012;32:277-283.
120. Goodyear PWA, Bannister CM, Russell S, et al. Outcome in prenatally diagnosed fetal agenesis of the corpus callosum. *Fetal Diagn Ther.* 2001;16:139-145.
121. Moutard ML, Kieffer V, Feingold J, et al. Agenesis of corpus callosum: prenatal diagnosis and prognosis. *Childs Nerv Syst.* 2003;19:471-476.
122. Ahmad T, Garcia-Filion P, Borchert M, et al. Endocrinological and auxological abnormalities in young children with optic nerve hypoplasia: a prospective study. *J Pediatr.* 2006;148:78-84.
123. Aicardi J, Goutières F. The syndrome of absence of the septum pellucidum with porencephalies and other developmental defects. *Neuropediatrics.* 1981;12:319-329.
124. Barkovich AJ, Fram EK, Norman D. Septo-optic dysplasia: MR imaging. *Radiology.* 1989;171:189-192.
125. Bodensteiner JB, Schaefer GB. Wide cavum septum pellucidum: a marker of disturbed brain development. *Pediatr Neurol.* 1990;6:391-394.
126. Breeding LM, Bodensteiner JB, Cowan L, et al. The cavum septi pellucidi: a magnetic resonance imaging study of prevalence and clinical associations in a pediatric population. *J Neuroimaging.* 1991;1:115-118.
127. Miller SP, Shevell MI, Patenaude Y, et al. Septo-optic dysplasia plus: a spectrum of malformations of cortical development. *Neurology.* 2000;54:1701-1703.
128. Polizzi A, Pavone P, Iannetti P, et al. Septo-optic dysplasia complex: a heterogeneous malformation syndrome. *Pediatr Neurol.* 2006;34:66-71.
129. Schaefer GB, Bodensteiner JB, Thompson JN. Subtle anomalies of the septum pellucidum and neurodevelopmental deficits. *Dev Med Child Neurol.* 1994;36:554-559.
130. Schuelke M, Krude H, Finckh B, et al. Septo-optic dysplasia associated with a new mitochondrial *cytochrome b* mutation. *Ann Neurol.* 2002;51:388-392.
131. Traggiai C, Stanhope R. Endocrinopathies associated with midline cerebral and cranial malformations. *J Pediatr.* 2002;140:252-255.
132. Dattani MT, Martinez-Barbera JP, Thomas PQ, et al. Molecular genetics of septo-optic dysplasia. *Horm Res.* 2000;53:26-33.
133. Kuriyama M, Shigematsu Y, Konishi K, et al. Septo-optic dysplasia with infantile spasms. *Pediatr Neurol.* 1988;4:62-65.
134. De Morsier G. Etudes sur les dysraphies cranio-encephaliques. III. Agenesie du septum lucidum avec malformation du tractus optique. La dysplasie septo-optique. *Schweizer Archiv Neurol Psychiatr.* 1956;77:267-292.
135. Hellstrom A, Wiklund LM, Svensson E, et al. Midline brain lesions in children with hormone insufficiency indicate early prenatal damage. *Acta Paediatr.* 1998;87:528-536.
136. Li Y, Sansgiri R, Estroff J, et al. Outcome of fetuses with cerebral ventriculomegaly and septum pellucidum leaflet abnormalities. *AJR Am J Roentgenol.* 2011;196:W83-W92.
137. Callen PW, Callen AL, Glenn OA, et al. Columns of the fornix, not to be mistaken for the cavum septi pellucidi on prenatal sonography. *J Ultrasound Med.* 2008;27:25-31.
138. Sarwar M. The septum pellucidum: normal and abnormal. *AJNR Am J Neuroradiol.* 1989;10:989-1005.
139. Pauling KJ, Bodensteiner JB, Hogg JP, et al. Does selection bias determine the prevalence of the cavum septi pellucidi? *Pediatr Neurol.* 1998;19:195-198.
140. Brisch R, Bernstein HG, Krell D, et al. Volumetric analysis of septal region in schizophrenia and affective disorder. *Eur Arch Psychiatry Clin Neurosci.* 2007;257:140-148.
141. Jurjus GJ, Nasrallah HA, Olson SC, et al. Cavum septum pellucidum in schizophrenia, affective disorder and healthy controls: a magnetic resonance imaging study. *Psychol Med.* 1993;23:319-322.
142. Kim MJLI, Dager SR, Friedman SD, et al. The occurrence of cavum septi pellucidi enlargement is increased in bipolar disorder patients. *Bipolar Disord.* 2007;9:274-280.
143. Kwon JSSM, Hirayasu Y, et al. MRI study of cavum septi pellucidi in schizophrenia, affective disorder, and schizotypal personality disorder. *Am J Psychiatry.* 1998;155:509-515.

Congenital Hydrocephalus

Adré J. du Plessis ◆ *Shenandoah Robinson* ◆ *Joseph J. Volpe*

The terms *ventriculomegaly* and *hydrocephalus* are often used inconsistently and imprecisely in the literature. In this discussion we use *ventriculomegaly* as an overarching term to describe excessive cerebrospinal fluid (CSF) within enlarged cerebral ventricles without reference to etiopathogenesis, natural history, or outcome. Ventriculomegaly may be subcategorized in a number of ways, based on the underlying pathogenetic mechanism, clinical course, and associated features (Fig. 3.1). *Hydrocephalus* is one major category of ventriculomegaly that results from distention of the ventricles by CSF that accumulates because of an imbalance in CSF production and absorption. Ex vacuo ventriculomegaly is a second major category that is not related to the hydrocephalic state (see later and Fig. 3.1). This discussion addresses those forms of ventriculomegaly-hydrocephalus that have their mechanistic *origin in the fetal period*, even when development of hydrocephalus is delayed until after birth, for example in some cases of myelomeningocele and the Dandy-Walker malformation. Conversely, causes of neonatal ventriculomegaly-hydrocephalus with postnatal origins, such as neonatal meningitis and intracranial hemorrhage, are discussed in subsequent chapters.

FETAL VENTRICULOMEGALY

Understanding of the prevalence, natural history, and outcome of fetal ventriculomegaly has advanced significantly in recent decades. This advance is in large part due to widespread implementation in developed countries of standardized ultrasound screening protocols during pregnancy. As a consequence, fetal ventriculomegaly is now identified in up to 1% of all pregnancies, making it the leading referral diagnosis for fetal neurological consultation in larger clinical programs.[1-3]

Classification of Fetal Ventriculomegaly

Fetal ventriculomegaly has been classified by a number of different criteria (Box 3.1).[2,4-7] These criteria include *severity* (mild, moderate, or severe); *evolution* (transient, stable, or progressive); *laterality* (unilateral or bilateral); *symmetry* (symmetrical or asymmetrical); and *association with other findings* (isolated or complex).

Severity of Fetal Ventriculomegaly

This is broadly classified as mild (≤15 mm) or severe (> 15 mm), with some authors further categorizing the milder form into mild (10 to 12 mm) and moderate (13 to 15 mm) categories. Milder forms of ventriculomegaly (bilateral, unilateral, or asymmetrical) are far more common than severe forms and have a reported prevalence that varies widely from 1 to 22/1000 births.[8-10] Conversely, severe ventriculomegaly is uncommon.[1,4,11,12] Although, in one large study with an overall fetal ventriculomegaly incidence of 3.8/1000 births, the incidence of severe ventriculomegaly was 2/1000 births.[3] In some studies the percentage of fetal ventriculomegaly in the severe range (>15 mm) was as high as 53% to 55%.[3,13] Mild isolated ventriculomegaly is unilateral in 28% to 33% of cases.[14] Severe unilateral ventriculomegaly is rare and suggests either occlusion of the foramen of Monro or hemispheric tissue loss. One large recent study of 432 cases[15] included a "gray zone" group with ventricles between 7 and 10 mm, and found that only 2.8% of these cases progressed to ventriculomegaly (>10 mm).

Evolution of Fetal Ventriculomegaly (Box 3.2)

The terms stable, transient, or progressive have been used to describe the evolution of ventriculomegaly across gestation. The evolution of ventriculomegaly (i.e., the rates of progression, stabilization, and resolution) during fetal life *varies widely in different reports*.[2,3,5,14,16] The most common scenario is that of milder forms of ventriculomegaly, often unilateral or asymmetrical, that remain stable or are transient, normalizing on follow-up studies. Among cases of isolated mild-moderate ventriculomegaly (<15 mm) a small minority (11% to 16%) progress to the severe category,[5] while 43% to 75% stabilize, and 14% to 62% normalize their ventricular size.[2,5,9,10,14] In the mild-moderate group of isolated ventriculomegaly, reported spontaneous resolution rates range from 53% to 64% in the 10- to 12-mm group and from 6% to 47% in the 13- to 15-mm category.[3,5,14] Conversely, severe ventriculomegaly (>15 mm) is rare and has a low likelihood of spontaneous resolution. The unusual cases of progressive ventriculomegaly are usually severe at time of the standard mid-gestation anatomical survey.

Isolated Versus Complex Fetal Ventriculomegaly (Box 3.3)

Isolated ventriculomegaly refers to cases with *no other anomalies or risk factors* and occurs in 0.39 to 0.87 per 1000 births.[17] In most, but not all, reports[10] the rate of associated anomalies is low when the maximum ventricular diameter is less than 15 mm.[18-20] Conversely, one large review of 355 fetuses with ventriculomegaly less than 15 mm found a 55% incidence of complex ventriculomegaly, with fetal anomalies in 43% overall.[10] Within the less than 15 mm ventriculomegaly group, the associated central nervous system (CNS) anomaly rate has ranged from 6% to 41% in the 10- to 12-mm group,[10,18,21] and between 32% and 76% in the 13- to 15-mm group.[10,18,21]

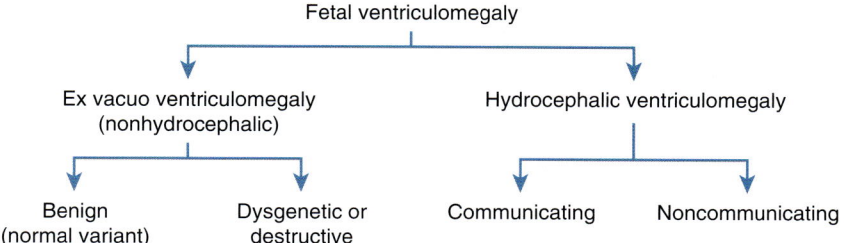

Figure 3.1 Classification of fetal ventriculomegaly.

BOX 3.1   Classification of Fetal Ventriculomegaly

Severity
- ◆ Mild (10–12 mm)
- ◆ Moderate (13–15 mm)
- ◆ Severe (>15 mm)

Evolution
- ◆ Transient
- ◆ Stable
- ◆ Progressive

Laterality
- ◆ Unilateral
- ◆ Bilateral

Associated Findings
- ◆ Isolated
- ◆ Complex

BOX 3.2   Evolution of Isolated Mild-Moderate (≤15 mm) Fetal Ventriculomegaly

Evolution	%
Normalize	**14–62**
10–12 mm	53–64
13–15 mm	6–47
Stabilize	**43–75**
Progress to Severe	**11–16**

BOX 3.3   Reported Rates of Complex Fetal Ventriculomegaly Vary Widely

Ventricle Size ≤15 mm
- ◆ 10–12 mm 6%–41% associated with CNS anomalies
- ◆ 13–15 mm 32%–72% associated with CNS anomalies
- ◆ 1%–5% associated with congenital infections

Ventricle Size >15 mm
- ◆ 32%–60% associated with CNS anomalies
- ◆ 10%–20% associated with congenital infections

CNS, Central nervous system.

BOX 3.4   Rates of Congenital Infections in Fetal Ventriculomegaly

	%
Mild Ventriculomegaly	**1–5**
10–12 mm	0.4
12–15 mm	1.5
Severe Ventriculomegaly	**10–20**

32% to 60% when ventricles are greater than 15 mm.[3,11,18,22-24] Most, but not all, studies[18,20] report a low rate of associated anomalies when ventricles are less than 15 mm. This wide variation in the presence of associated anomalies results in large part from the differences in timing and modality of fetal imaging. *Dysmorphic ventriculomegaly* is a form of complex ventriculomegaly best exemplified by agenesis of the corpus callosum with its characteristic ventricular morphology, that is, retention of the tear-drop-shaped fetal configuration posteriorly (colpocephaly) and a steer-horn configuration anteriorly (see Chapter 2).[25] In one large prospective study,[26] agenesis of the corpus callosum was diagnosed in 13% of fetal ventriculomegaly cases. Of note, before 24 weeks' gestation, the lateral ventricles may normally have a mild colpocephalic shape,[27] although the ventricular axes should not be parallel.

Congenital infections, another type of complex ventriculomegaly, are an important prognostic consideration in fetal ventriculomegaly, especially those with brain involvement. However, the positive detection rate based on maternal serology testing is highly variable, and depends on the timing, geographical and social setting, and specific testing performed in each of the studies.[18,20,28,29] The reported incidence of congenital infections in cases of severe fetal ventriculomegaly ranges from 10% to 20%,[18,28] but only from 1% to 5% in mild ventriculomegaly cases.[10,18,20,28,29] In one review,[30] evidence of congenital infection was present in 0.4% of mild ventriculomegaly (10 to 12 mm) and 1.5% of moderate ventriculomegaly (12 to 15 mm). Cerebral ventriculomegaly identified by fetal ultrasonography (US) is present almost 20% of cases of fetal cytomegalovirus encephalitis, and approximately half the cases appear isolated (Box 3.4).[2]

Diagnosis of Fetal Ventriculomegaly: Imaging Modalities

Fetal ultrasound is the standard prenatal screening modality for identifying fetal ventriculomegaly, and has become an important tool for monitoring ventricular size, configuration, and evolution over gestation.[4] Widespread clinical use over more than four decades has provided a wealth of experience and a large body of population-based normative data. By convention, fetal ventricular size is measured by ultrasound

Complex ventriculomegaly refers to cases with associated anomalies including other malformations of the fetal brain or body, chromosomal anomalies, or signs of acquired factors that may affect outcome, such as CNS infection, intracranial hemorrhage, and hypoxia-ischemia. *The incidence of associated brain malformations increases with increasing ventricular size, reaching*

TABLE 3.1 Apparent Isolated Mild Ventriculomegaly at Initial Diagnosis: Timing and Imaging Modalities for Identification of Associated Anomalies

INITIAL DIAGNOSIS TIMING AND MODALITY	REPEAT IMAGING TIMING AND MODALITY	INCREASED DETECTION OF ASSOCIATED ANOMALIES (REFS)
Second trimester US	Third trimester US	13% (16)
Second trimester US	Second trimester MRI	5%–60% (11, 38, 39)
Second trimester US	Third trimester MRI	Minimal increase (14)
Fetal MRI	Postnatal MRI	10%–28% (11, 19, 20, 22, 29, 40)

MRI, Magnetic resonance imaging; *US,* ultrasound.

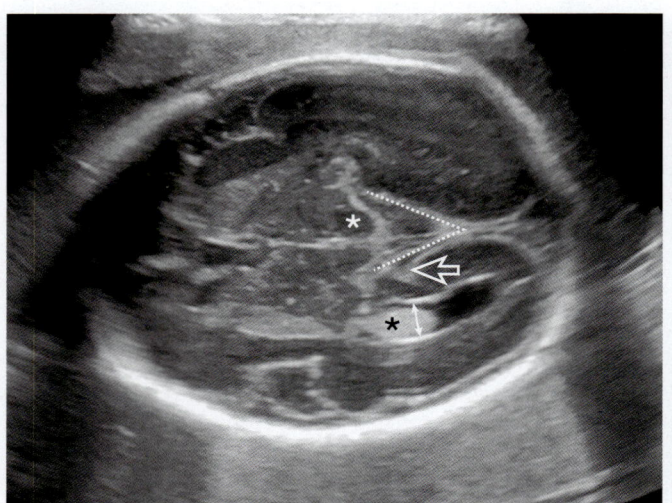

Figure 3.2 Axial view of fetal US at the level of the cerebral peduncles (*white asterisk*), the ambient cistern (*V-shaped dotted lines*), cavum septi pellucidi, and the glomus of the choroid plexus (*black asterisk*). The double-headed white arrow indicates the standard location for measurement of the lateral ventricular atrium diameter directly in line with the parieto-occipital sulcus (*open block arrow*). (Image courtesy Dr. Dorothy Bulas.)

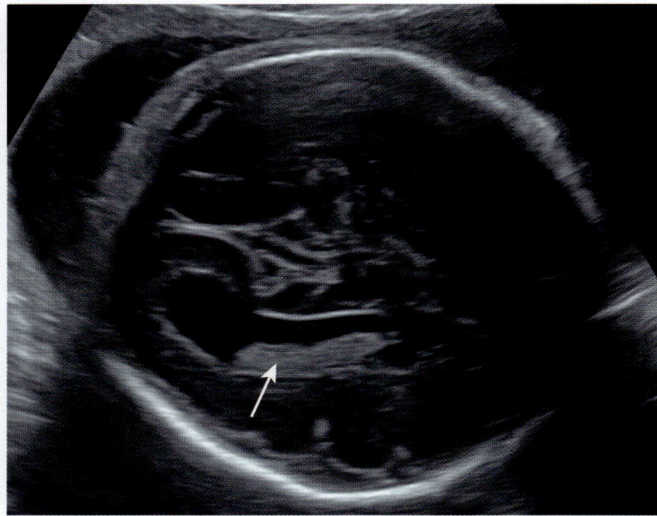

Figure 3.3 Fetal cranial US axial view showing mild ventriculomegaly with a "dangling choroid" sign. Arrow shows dependent position of the choroid plexus with increased space between the choroid and medial wall of the lateral ventricle.

as the diameter of the lateral ventricular atrium on an axial view (Fig. 3.2), at the level of the thalami or the glomus of the choroid plexus. Using this approach, the ventricular size remains relatively stable at around 6 to 7 mm during normal development between 14 weeks and term.[31] A widely used criterion for diagnosing ventriculomegaly is ventricular diameter of ≥10 mm (>4 standard deviations above the mean) at the axial level discussed earlier.[32] Fetal US can also identify other features of ventriculomegaly, such as the "dangling choroid" sign (Fig. 3.3), and may help to distinguish hydrocephalic from nonhydrocephalic ventriculomegaly. Specifically, large ventricles and a large head circumference suggest fetal hydrocephalus, while large ventricles and a small head are more suggestive of *ex vacuo* ventriculomegaly. Fetal US may also show increased echogenicity of the ventricular lining when ependymitis results from intraventricular hemorrhage or infection. Informed prognostication in cases of ventriculomegaly (see later) is based on more than ventricular size, and includes the association with other brain lesions. The limited spatial resolution of fetal US may result in false negative studies for associated brain lesions in 10% to 40% of cases.[19,33,34] Although fetal US may only detect the larger associated brain lesions, fetal MRI (see

later and Chapter 10) has superior soft tissue resolution and sensitivity to smaller lesions.

Fetal MRI has played a major role in the advancement of fetal neurology as a discipline and is discussed in more detail in Chapter 10. The primary added value of MRI over the fetal US diagnosis of ventriculomegaly is its enhanced resolution; the improved contrast allows for more precision in measurement and increases the detection of associated lesions.[35] The superior soft tissue resolution of fetal brain MRI supports prognostication (see later) in fetal ventriculomegaly by providing important etiological data and detecting associated anomalies.[18,36] In studies comparing the detection rate of associated lesions between these two imaging techniques, fetal MRI detects associated brain lesions in anywhere from 5% to 60% of cases previously diagnosed as isolated ventriculomegaly by fetal US (Table 3.1).[11,37-39] In cases where *fetal* MRI detects isolated ventriculomegaly, repeat MRI in the *postnatal* period provides an additional 10% to 28% yield for associated anomalies[a]; this increase relates not only to the increased sensitivity of ex utero MRI, but also to disturbances in late gestation brain

---

[a]References 11, 19, 20, 22, 29, and 40.

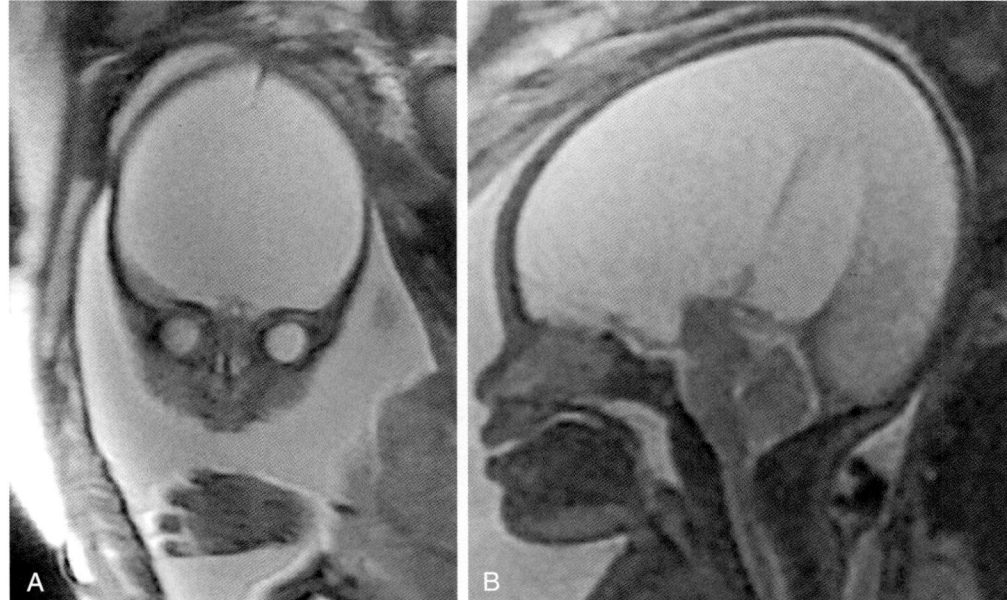

Figure 3.4 Massive hydranencephaly in fetus. Fetal magnetic resonance imaging T2-weighted. (A) Coronal view. (B) Midline sagittal view. (Reproduced from du Plessis AJ, Johnston MJ. Fetal neurology. In: Arzimanoglou A, O'Hare A, Johnston MV, Ouvrier R, eds. *Aicardi's Diseases of the Nervous System in Childhood*, 4th ed, London: Mac Keith Press [www.mackeith.co.uk]; 2017:27)

development occurring after the fetal MRI. Of note, conventional clinical fetal MRI relies heavily on subjective pattern recognition and 2-dimensional measurements, features that have left it prone to differences in interpretation.[41] The application of more advanced quantitative MRI techniques to the fetus, will likely reduce these discrepancies.[42] Several authors have reported on the use of three-dimensional volumetric MRI to measure ventricular volumes rather than the use of conventional two-dimensional measures.[43,44] Andescavage et al.[45] measured fetal ventricular volumes in healthy pregnancies between 18 and 39 weeks of gestation, and established normative data for all four ventricles and the extraaxial CSF spaces. These authors described a modest 1.4-fold increase in the volume of the lateral ventricles over this gestational period; interestingly, the growth trajectories differed, with the left ventricles larger during early gestation, but ultimately reaching a similar volume to the right ventricle.[45]

In summary, fetal US is a valuable tool for diagnosing and monitoring the evolution of ventriculomegaly. The superior tissue resolution provided by fetal MRI makes it the optimal technique to exclude other brain anomalies associated with fetal ventriculomegaly, which is of great importance for prognostication. Major events in cerebral cortical development occur in the late second and third trimesters (see Chapters 6 and 7) and are readily evaluated by fetal MRI (but not fetal US). In countries where pregnancy termination is illegal beyond mid-gestation, identifying these later cortical events by fetal MRI may not directly affect management of the pregnancy. However, this information may satisfy the parent's *need-to-know* imperative and allow them to better prepare for events after birth. In one study, the rate of identifying new lesions increased by 13% when second trimester US was repeated in the third trimester.[2] In those cases with confirmed *isolated* ventriculomegaly by second trimester MRI, repeat MRI studies in the third trimester provided minimal increased yield for associated anomalies; this

finding also confirmed that delaying the first MRI study to the third trimester provides no significant benefit.[14]

Differential Diagnosis of Fetal Ventriculomegaly

Ventriculomegaly is usually readily recognized by experienced ultrasonographers, but may on occasion be mistaken for other fluid-filled supratentorial lesions, such as hydranencephaly (Fig. 3.4), holoprosencephaly (Chapter 2), or enlarged cavum septi pellucidi or cavum velum interpositum. These issues are readily resolved by fetal MRI.

Congenital Hydrocephalus

A minority of fetal ventriculomegaly cases enter a phase of progressive ventricular enlargement (which may have arrested by the time of diagnosis) because CSF production exceeds absorption and therefore meet criteria for congenital hydrocephalus, that is, hydrocephalus overt at birth. The vast majority of cases of fetal hydrocephalus is due to decreased CSF absorption which is essentially obstructive in nature. Excessive CSF production due to a choroid plexus papilloma, for example, is a rare cause of hydrocephalus (discussed later).[46] With implementation of fetal US screening programs, congenital hydrocephalus is now increasingly identified before birth; however, some cases are only detected in the early newborn period and are assumed to have fetal origins.

Anatomical Abnormalities in Congenital Hydrocephalus

Hydrocephalus of fetal onset may result from abnormalities anywhere in the CSF pathway from formation in the choroid plexus to absorption in the arachnoidal villi. The specific pattern of enlarged CSF spaces may suggest the site of obstructed CSF flow, allowing further categorization of hydrocephalus. Enlargement of any or all of the ventricles due to obstruction of CSF flow upstream or at the fourth ventricular foramina

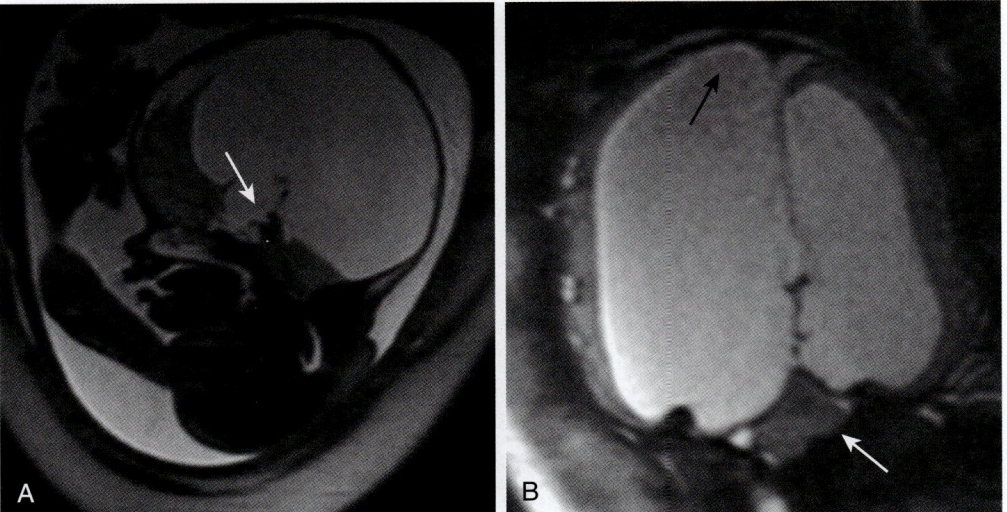

Figure 3.5 Fetus with massive hydrocephalus, aqueductal stenosis, and probable rhombencephalosynapsis.
T2-weighted magnetic resonance imaging. (A) Sagittal view showing massive hydrocephalus and V-shaped proximal opening of the aqueduct (*arrow*). (B) Coronal view showing dehiscence of the cerebral mantle (*black arrow*) and diminutive cerebellum and features of rhombencephalosynapsis (*white arrow*).

is termed *noncommunicating hydrocephalus*; in these cases the extraaxial CSF spaces appear normal or decreased in size. Impaired CSF flow distal to the fourth ventricular foramina (e.g., in the subarachnoid spaces or arachnoid granulations) results in *communicating hydrocephalus;* in which case the extraaxial CSF spaces may be enlarged. In noncommunicating hydrocephalus, the location of obstructed CSF flow is most commonly at the aqueduct of Sylvius and the fourth ventricular foramina. Aqueductal stenosis (Fig. 3.5) is inferred when the lateral and third ventricles are enlarged and the fourth ventricle is normal in size. Conversely, obstruction of fourth ventricular CSF egress through the foramina of Magendi and/or Luschka leads to tetraventricular hydrocephalus.

Etiology of Fetal Ventriculomegaly and Congenital Hydrocephalus

In the majority of *mild isolated fetal ventriculomegaly* cases, the underlying mechanism remains unknown. Some consider this a normal variant,[20,47,48] especially when the ventriculomegaly is self-resolving. Delayed fenestration of the Blake's pouch (see Chapter 4) has been suggested to underlie some of these transient forms, especially in cases with associated enlargement of the fourth ventricle.[49] Although the etiology of *congenital hydrocephalus* is heterogeneous, most cases appear to result from developmental disorders of the brain and its CSF circulatory system. The causes of fetal hydrocephalus are generally similar to those of neonatal hydrocephalus, although, not surprisingly, the severity of the hydrocephalus in fetal cases tends to be greater.[50-74] In addition, factors such as geographical location, the timing and modalities of brain imaging, and other testing underlie the considerable variance in the spectrum and prevalence of etiologies reported. The major causes of *congenital hydrocephalus*, as identified in two large series conducted in neonatal neurosurgical services, are presented in Table 3.2.[75,76] In myelomeningocele with the Chiari type II malformation (see Chapter 1; Fig. 3.6) the small and crowded posterior fossa may obstruct CSF flow at

TABLE 3.2   Major Causes of Hydrocephalus Overt at Birth in 127 Cases (n = 127)

CAUSE	%
Aqueductal stenosis	33
Myelomeningocele: Chiari type II malformation	28
"Communicating" hydrocephalus	22
Dandy-Walker malformation	7
Other	10

Data from Mealey J Jr, Gilmor RL, Bubb MP. The prognosis of hydrocephalus overt at birth, *J Neurosurg.* 1973;39:348–355; and McCullough DC, Balzer-Martin LA. Current prognosis in overt neonatal hydrocephalus. *J Neurosurg.* 1982;57:378–383.

aqueductal, foraminal, and subarachnoid levels. In these studies, *aqueductal stenosis* (see Fig. 3.5) accounted for approximately one third of cases, making it the second most common cause of fetal hydrocephalus after the Chiari II malformation.[77] The *Dandy-Walker malformation* (see Chapter 4) and *communicating hydrocephalus* account for most of the remaining cases of neonatal hydrocephalus.[75,76] In aqueductal stenosis, the lateral and third ventricular hydrocephalus tends to be severe and progressive. In severe cases, the massive ventricular distention may have destructive effects on the septal leaflets and corpus callosum. In some cases, the overlying cerebral mantle may be stretched to the point of dehiscence, most commonly in the region of the choroidal fissure. Unlike schizencephaly, the edges of the ruptured mantle are lined with white matter. Although most examples are nonfamilial, an *X-linked form of aqueductal stenosis* associated with adducted thumbs and, commonly, agenesis of the corpus callosum is important to recognize because of its consistent relationship with subsequent mental retardation (Box 3.5).[78] This disorder is related to a mutation in the L1 family of

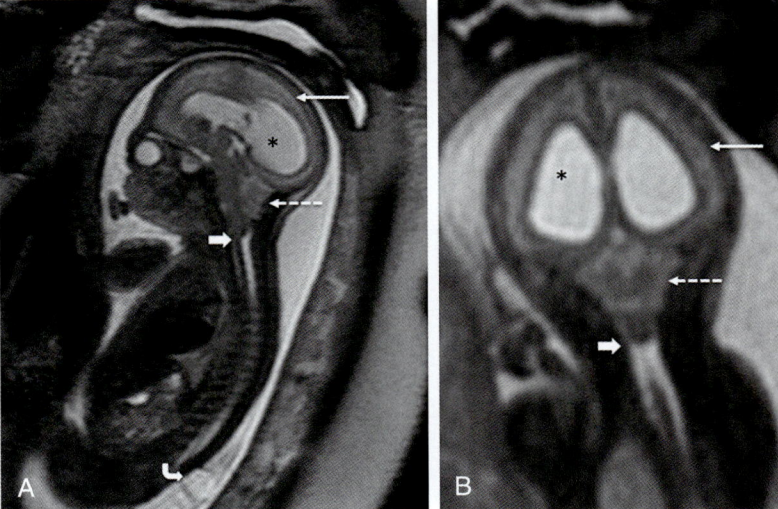

Figure 3.6 Fetal T2-weighted MRI (A) axial and (B) coronal of a 23-week-old fetus showing hydrocephalus *(asterisks)*, an open neural tube defect *(curved arrow* in A), minimal extraaxial CSF *(thin white arrows)*, crowded posterior fossa *(dashed arrows)*, and herniation of cerebellar tonsils (Chiari II) down to the midcervical level *(short white arrows)*.

BOX 3.5   Major Etiologies of Aqueductal Stenosis

Dysgenetic
- ◆ X-linked aqueductal stenosis
  - ◆ L1CAM gene mutation
  - ◆ Aqueductal stenosis
  - ◆ Hydrocephalus
  - ◆ Adducted thumbs
  - ◆ Agenesis of the corpus callosum
  - ◆ Mental retardation
  - ◆ Spastic paraplegia
- ◆ Autosomal recessive aqueductal stenosis with normal phenotype
- ◆ Autosomal recessive or X-linked aqueductal stenosis
  - ◆ VACTERL association (vertebral anomalies, anal atresia, cardiac anomalies, tracheoesophageal fistula, renal dysplasia, limb defects)
- ◆ Brain stem dysgenesis (including rhombencephalosynapsis)
- ◆ Aqueductal forking, membranes, nodules (hamartomas; Fig. 3.7).

Acquired
- ◆ Fetal intraventricular hemorrhage
- ◆ Congenital infections (toxoplasmosis, CMV)

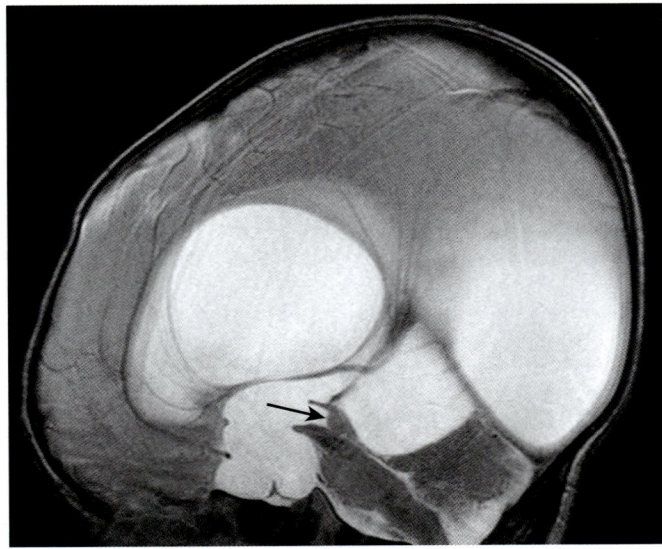

Figure 3.7 Midline sagittal T2-weighted magnetic resonance imaging in a case of severe congenital hydrocephalus due to aqueductal stenosis. The arrow indicates a nodule within the aqueduct blocking cerebrospinal fluid passage.

---

neural cell adhesion molecules (L1CAM).[78-82] These molecules play an important role in axon outgrowth, fasciculation, and neuronal migration.[15,32,82-85] The so-called CRASH syndrome results from an L1CAM mutation and is an acronym for *Corpus callosum hypoplasia, Retardation, Adducted thumbs, Spastic paraplegia,* and *Hydrocephalus.*[83] Additional genetic varieties of aqueductal stenosis included autosomal recessive inheritance, with a normal phenotype, and X-linked or autosomal recessive inheritance with the VACTERL association (vertebral anomalies, anal atresia, cardiovascular anomalies, tracheoesophageal fistula, renal dysplasia, limb defects).[86] Other etiologies may lead to aqueductal stenosis, including brain stem dysgenesis (including rhombencephalosynapsis; Chapter 4; Fig. 3.5), aqueductal forking, webs, membranes, and nodules (e.g., hamartomas; Fig. 3.7). Approximately half of rhombencephalosynapsis cases have aqueductal stenosis (see Fig. 3.5),[87] which is not surprising

given the common mesencephalic origin of the vermis and midbrain (see Chapter 4).

Chromosomal anomalies (Box 3.6), especially aneuploidy, may be associated with fetal ventriculomegaly and are important prognostic factors. In one large study of mild ventriculomegaly (<15 mm), abnormal karyotypes (most commonly trisomy 21) were detected in 11% of cases tested antenatally, and in 14% of those tested postnatally.[10] In the absence of structural anomalies, mild ventriculomegaly (≤15 mm) is associated with chromosomal anomalies in 3% to 10% cases.[10,18,26,36] Conversely, ventriculomegaly of any size associated with other fetal anomalies has an aneuploidy rate greater than 15%.[18,20,40,52] *Infectious causes* of fetal ventriculomegaly are prognostically important but relatively uncommon. Symptomatic newborns with known congenital CMV have a high incidence of mild-moderate ventriculomegaly[88]; however, ventriculomegaly is rarely the only feature of congenital CMV and is usually associated with other features such as a periventricular *halo*, calcifications, pseudocysts, intraventricular synechiae, and cortical and cerebellar malformations. Other infections may be associated with ventriculomegaly, including congenital Zika virus encephalopathy, and are discussed in Chapter 34. Toxoplasmosis is a rare cause and usually results from aqueductal stenosis.[89,90] The usual complication of fetal parvovirus B19 infection is fetal anemia, but mild ventriculomegaly has been described.[91-93] *Choroid plexus papillomas* are extremely rare in the fetus and usually present with hydrocephalus due to excessive CSF production and potentially from foraminal obstruction.[46]

Fetal intraventricular hemorrhage is increasingly detected during routine fetal imaging as a cause for fetal hydrocephalus.[94,95] *Arachnoid cysts* may interfere with CSF flow with a picture that depends on its location; posterior fossa arachnoid cysts may obstruct posterior fossa CSF egress, whereas large suprasellar cysts may compress and obstruct third ventricular CSF flow.[96] *Malformations of the vein of Galen* may result in noncommunicating hydrocephalus through aqueductal compression or communicating hydrocephalus through elevated cerebral venous pressure (see Chapter 37).[97]

Timing of Congenital Hydrocephalus

In view of the heterogeneity of causes of congenital hydrocephalus, definition of a single time of onset of the disorder is not possible. However, the most important developmental processes in this context occur at approximately 6 to 10 weeks of gestation.[2,117,118] Specifically, at this time, three events critical for the development of the CSF pathways occur: (1) development of the secretory epithelium in the choroid plexus, (2) perforation of the roof of the fourth ventricle, and (3) formation of the subarachnoid spaces. Impairments of the last two processes bear a relationship with the genesis of the hydrocephalus associated with the Dandy-Walker malformation and communicating hydrocephalus. The choroid plexuses develop between 6 and 7 weeks post-conceptual, starting in the 4th ventricle, but becoming most voluminous in the lateral ventricles. By 20 weeks the choroid plexus has an adult configuration.

The critical timing for hydrocephalus with holoprosencephaly is during this exact period. The key timing for development of aqueductal stenosis is probably later (i.e., between 15 and 17 weeks of gestation, the period of rapid elongation of the mesencephalon and evolution of the normal constriction of the aqueduct).[60] Similar timing may be appropriate for the hydrocephalus associated with the Chiari II malformation and myelomeningocele, because aqueductal stenosis is a common cause of the disturbance in CSF dynamics in this condition (see Chapter 2). Clearly, of course, the inflammatory processes that cause intrauterine onset of hydrocephalus (e.g., toxoplasmosis, intracranial hemorrhage) develop still later as a consequence of the derangement in CSF flow or absorption resulting from the associated ependymitis and arachnoiditis.

Clinical Features of Congenital Hydrocephalus

Isolated nonprogressive ventriculomegaly is clinically silent at birth. Progressive ventriculomegaly in cases of congenital hydrocephalus is now frequently known before birth through the widespread use of fetal US.[75,119-144] In cases of *fetal-onset hydrocephalus*, the ventricles dilate before 24 weeks of gestation, usually without change in biparietal diameter, and not until after 32 to 34 weeks of gestation does head growth consistently increase with progression of ventricular dilation. The most prominent additional clinical features are the occurrence of major extraneural anomalies in 40% to 50% of cases of fetal hydrocephalus, major CNS anomalies in 60% to 70%, and extraneural or CNS anomalies (or both) in 80%. These anomalies have a dominant effect on outcome (see the later prognosis section). As discussed earlier, MRI is the most sensitive imaging modality for assessment of hydrocephalus and associated CNS anomalies in the fetus, but postnatal MRI is significantly more sensitive to additional brain anomalies.

The *neonatal presentation of congenital hydrocephalus* (i.e., markedly enlarged head, full anterior fontanelle, and separated cranial sutures) is similar to, although more severe than, that described for the later postnatal development of hydrocephalus with myelomeningocele (see Chapter 1). Careful neonatal assessment should be made for signs of specific etiological types of congenital hydrocephalus, such as the flexion deformity of the thumbs (which can often be detected by fetal US) characteristic of approximately 50% of cases of X-linked aqueductal stenosis,[145-153] the occipital cranial prominence of the Dandy-Walker formation, and the chorioretinitis of intrauterine infection by toxoplasmosis or cytomegalovirus. Serial assessments of neurological status, rate of head growth, signs of increased intracranial pressure, and ventricular size (by cranial US) are of particular value in documenting the severity and rapidity of progression of the hydrocephalic process. Earlier reports noted an incidence of one or more major CNS anomalies in 84%, and non-CNS anomalies in 56%, of congenital hydrocephalus cases.[67] A careful assessment of the cerebral parenchyma by MRI is valuable for detection of the size of the cerebral mantle, associated anomalies of the cerebrum (e.g., disorder of neuronal migration), evidence of parenchymal destruction (e.g., calcification, cysts), and likely sites of disturbance of CSF dynamics (based on topographical distribution of ventricular dilation as described earlier).

MANAGEMENT OF CONGENITAL HYDROCEPHALUS

Management of infants with congenital hydrocephalus should begin, as in other infants with major neurological diseases, with the same question: Could this problem have been prevented? Unfortunately, in the large majority of cases the answer to this question remains no.

Prenatal Management of Congenital Hydrocephalus

As indicated earlier, many cases of congenital hydrocephalus in developed countries are now identified during the fetal period. In these cases of progressive fetal ventricular dilation, rational management of fetal hydrocephalus requires an understanding of the natural history.[75,154-180] In an earlier study of 47 infants with fetal ventriculomegaly more than half the cases died in utero, primarily because of elective termination provoked by the finding of serious neural or extraneural anomalies or both.[181] Among the survivors (more than half of which underwent CSF shunts) all infants with subsequent neurological deficits had additional brain anomalies. These findings suggest a limited role for intrauterine management of ventriculomegaly. This principle is illustrated by the more recent observations summarized in Table 3.3.[182]

Following earlier studies of fetal primates showing that intrauterine decompression of hydrocephalus is beneficial,[98,183-185] and in the subsequent demonstration that placement of a ventriculoamniotic shunt is possible in utero in the human fetus,[186-190] the notion of antepartum intervention for fetal hydrocephalus appeared promising. However, in a study of 41 fetuses treated with intrauterine shunting in the 1980s, the procedure-related mortality was 10%, and the outcome of survivors was not improved.[190] In a more recent series of 39 cases from Brazil the intrauterine shunting approach for fetal hydrocephalus had more promising results, with no procedure-related deaths recorded, and 67% of infants exhibiting later IQ scores higher than 70.[186] Nevertheless, it is apparent that the treated fetal cases were highly selected and were not representative of the general population of fetal hydrocephalus, because no cases of holoprosencephaly were included, infants with chromosomal defects were excluded, and approximately 50% were uncomplicated aqueductal stenosis.[186]

A reasonable and currently accepted obstetrical approach to the fetus with hydrocephalus is essentially as follows.[191-193] First, after the diagnosis of hydrocephalus is made, a thorough MRI evaluation should be directed toward measuring cortical thickness and excluding associated brain or spinal anomalies. In addition, a detailed sonographic screen for associated anomalies (e.g., open neural tube defects and renal or cardiac anomalies) is indicated. Second, amniocentesis is advisable to evaluate chromosomal abnormalities associated with hydrocephalus (e.g., trisomy 13 and trisomy 18), fetal sex (with history of X-linked aqueductal stenosis), alpha-fetoprotein levels, and cytomegalovirus or *Toxoplasma* infection (by polymerase chain reaction testing). If amniocentesis is declined, maternal blood testing is advised for cytomegalovirus and toxoplasmosis serology and cell-free fetal DNA for aneuploidy and fetal gender.

Earlier recommendations were that if the preceding evaluations did not indicate a poor prognosis, if progression of ventriculomegaly is documented, and if amniotic fluid lecithin-to-sphingomyelin ratios indicate mature fetal lungs, delivery by cesarean section might be indicated. If the fetus is too immature for delivery, close sonographic follow-up of ventricular size is important; if progression of ventricular dilation is rapid, corticosteroid therapy for induction of lung maturity and cesarean section are indicated. Delivery in a center with modern neurosurgical facilities is critical (see later), although not all infants exhibit postnatal progression and require ventriculoperitoneal shunt.[194,195] However, the decision to deliver a fetus before term has become more difficult in the context of recent evidence suggesting that even later preterm or early term delivery may be associated with adverse neurodevelopmental and behavioral outcomes.[99,100,101] Whether intrauterine shunting should be considered in selected cases, because of the possibility of injury to the cerebral mantle by progressive hydrocephalus,[196] remains unresolved. This issue is under study.[197]

Postnatal Management of Congenital Hydrocephalus

The options for postnatal treatment of symptomatic hydrocephalus are individualized to the needs of each infant, and require consideration of the comorbidities, overall prognosis, and parental preferences. Symptomatic hydrocephalus in newborns with hydrocephalus can be treated with temporary procedures such as a ventricular access device (VAD), or ventriculosubgaleal shunt (VSGS), temporary and potentially permanent interventions such as endoscopic third ventriculostomy (ETV) without or with choroid plexus coagulation (CPC), or permanent ventriculoperitoneal (VP) shunt insertion. The choice of VAD or VSGS is often influenced by institutional history, and the procedures have similar outcomes.[102] Whether a neonate with congenital hydrocephalus needs additional CSF diversion after a temporary device is unlikely to be influenced by whether a VAD or VSGS is used and is more influenced by the underlying etiology.

ETV, without or with the addition of CPC, is being used more frequently in selected neonates with favorable anatomy and other risk factors. For example, ETV can be quite effective in aqueductal stenosis and for hydrocephalus secondary to suprasellar arachnoid cysts. The role of CPC is still under evaluation. The choroid plexus cilia are important for guidance of early postnatal development, but the role the choroid plexus plays in neonates with coexisting moderate to severe CNS malformations is unknown. The rate of success of ETV+CPC varies among centers, which likely reflects regional referral patterns and selection criteria. Success, defined as shunt freedom at 1 year for all etiologies of infant hydrocephalus, has been reported in North American series as 38% in a single-center, retrospective series,[103] 57% in a single center, prospective series,[104] and 52% in a retrospective, multicenter trial.[105]

TABLE 3.3	Major Causes of Fetal Hydrocephalus ($n = 38$)	
CAUSE	**%**	**MEAN DQ/IQ**
Holoprosencephaly	45	
with myelomeningocele	27	48
without myelomeningocele	18	42
Myelomeningocele (isolated)	25	75
Dandy-Walker malformation	10	66
X-linked hydrocephalus	10	10
"Primary" hydrocephalus	10	60

DQ, Development quotient; IQ, intelligence quotient.

Data from Futagi Y, Suzuki Y, Toribe Y, Morimoto K. Neurodevelopmental outcome in children with fetal hydrocephalus. *Pediatr Neurol.* 2002;27:111–116.

Pre-pontine scarring has emerged as a factor which may be helpful in predicting ETC+CPC success in infants.[103,104] While ETV without or with CPC may provide permanent CSF diversion in only a subset of neonates, it may help temporize the insertion of a shunt until after 6 months. Shunt insertion after age 6 months is associated with better shunt survival.[106] Given that neurogenetics influences choroid plexus and ependymal cilia development, and the genetic classification of congenital hydrocephalus is rapidly expanding, we anticipate that better stratification for neonates with hydrocephalus will become available in the next several years.

Many neonates with symptomatic congenital hydrocephalus will continue to require a shunt for CSF diversion. The main complications for shunts include infections and malfunction. The risk of early shunt infection has been reduced by implementation of specific protocols and typically averages 5% to 7.5%. Late,[106] spontaneous infections without any history of shunt manipulation also occur and can be challenging to eradicate. In a recent prospective multicenter study of initial shunt insertion in children, patient-specific risk factors to shunt survival included age <6 months at insertion and cardiac comorbidity.[106] Importantly, modifications in shunt design or hardware have yet to have a significant impact on shunt survival. Any neonate who requires permanent CSF diversion with either ETV or shunt insertion typically needs long-term neurosurgical follow-up.

Prognosis of Fetal Ventriculomegaly and Congenital Hydrocephalus

Recent advances in fetal imaging and the implementation of antenatal screening programs that include fetal US have had an important impact on our understanding of fetal ventriculomegaly and hydrocephalus. Specifically, these developments have provided insight into the broader spectrum of ventriculomegaly, its natural evolution across gestation, and its association with other anomalies. Furthermore, these advances have allowed early fetal detection of more complex and severe cases, thereby enabling more informed decision-making in cases where pregnancy termination is an option. Factors to consider when formulating a prognosis during the evaluation of fetal ventriculomegaly include the ventricular size, symmetry, and progression, as well as the underlying mechanism/etiology (hydrocephalic, dysgenetic, hypoplastic/atrophic) and association with other brain or somatic anomalies (Box 3.7). Descriptions of ventriculomegaly in the literature are based primarily on features of the lateral ventricles.

Prognosis of Fetal Ventriculomegaly

The Prognostic Value of Fetal Ventricular Size. The value of ventricular size as an independent prognostic factor, especially in the most common mild cases, has been controversial. Some authors consider ventriculomegaly less than 15 mm to have no independent prognostic significance,[16] while others have suggested that long-term outcome deteriorates with increasing size of the ventricles.[29,107,108] It is important to recognize that the occurrence of increasing ventricular diameter is associated with an increasing risk of additional anomalies.[18-20] In most studies, neurodevelopmental outcome is significantly better when ventriculomegaly is less than 12 mm, is isolated, and resolves before birth.[1,2,109] In one study more than 90% of fetal ventriculomegaly cases of less than 12 mm

BOX 3.7	Factors Affecting the Prognosis of Fetal Ventriculomegaly
Ventricular Size	10–12 mm
	◆ Isolated + resolves: favorable outcome ~ 90%–100% (? normal variant)
	12–15 mm
	◆ Favorable outcome in 75%–80%
	>15 mm
	◆ Favorable outcome in ~60%
Evolution	◆ Progression from mild-moderate to >15 mm: adverse outcome in ~40%
	◆ Progressive ventriculomegaly is commonly associated with other anomalies
Associated Anomalies	◆ Associated anomalies predict adverse outcome (regardless of ventricular size)
	◆ Isolated callosal agenesis + nonhydrocephalic ventriculomegaly (colpocephaly) has favorable prognosis in ~25%
Symmetry	Mild isolated ventriculomegaly
	◆ Unilateral and bilateral have similar favorable prognosis
	Bilateral ventriculomegaly
	◆ Symmetrical: Favorable outcome in 90%
	◆ Asymmetrical: Favorable outcome in ~50%

had a normal outcome,[18] and, in another report, all cases were neurodevelopmentally normal at 10 year follow-up.[48] Consequently, some authors consider fetal ventricle size between 10 and 12 mm a normal variant.[20,47,43] At ventricular diameters between 12 and 15 mm the rate of favorable outcomes is around 75% to 80%.[18,29] When ventricular diameter exceeds 15 mm less than 60% of cases have favorable outcomes.[18,34,110] The prognosis for congenital hydrocephalus is discussed independently because it is influenced by management and its complications.

The Prognostic Value of Fetal Ventricular Symmetry. The prognostic significance of symmetry in fetal ventriculomegaly has been debated. Most cases of mild, isolated *unilateral* ventriculomegaly remain stable or transient and have a favorable neurodevelopmental outcome.[2,3,15,111,112] In mild fetal ventriculomegaly, no significant difference was noted in neurodevelopmental outcome between unilateral and bilateral cases.[2,3,16,111,112] In one cohort of mild isolated *unilateral* ventriculomegaly tested at 24 to 42 months, 15% performed at more than two standard deviations below the norm,[98] but by school age the entire cohort functioned within the normal range on the Wechsler Intelligence Scale for Children.[113] In another large study of 366 fetal cases of isolated mild ventriculomegaly[9] outcome was normal in 97% of the unilateral cases, compared to 90% of those with bilateral enlargement. Similarly, in another study of 167 fetuses with isolated mild (<15 mm) ventriculomegaly, 94% of unilateral mild (<12 mm) cases had a normal psychomotor outcome[28]; in this study, the rate of unfavorable neurological outcomes among cases of *bilateral ventriculomegaly* was 10% if the ventriculomegaly was symmetrical versus 50% when the bilateral ventriculomegaly was *asymmetrical*.[28]

The Prognostic Value of the Evolution of Fetal Ventriculomegaly.
Spontaneous resolution of ventriculomegaly occurs in almost half of cases ≤12 mm Hg, and in 25% of those between 13 and 15 mm,[2,5,16] while 16% show significant progression of ventriculomegaly.[5] Conversely, ventriculomegaly of greater than 15 mm rarely resolves spontaneously. In one study children with fetal diagnosis of mild isolated VM who had persistent ventricular enlargement at 2 years of age were at risk for mild fine motor and expressive language delay.[114] Among those mild ventriculomegaly cases that progress to greater than 15 mm, the risk of an adverse neurological outcome increases to 44%, compared to 7% among the nonprogressive cases. Perhaps not surprisingly, the risk of progressive ventriculomegaly is highest in severe cases with other brain anomalies.[3]

The Prognostic Value of Associated Anomalies. It is well recognized that the presence of *other brain or somatic anomalies or risk factors* (i.e., complex ventriculomegaly) is a significant negative prognostic indicator, regardless of ventricular size.[3,18,36] Thus in studies of isolated mild ventriculomegaly, the primary determinant of outcome is the presence or absence of associated anomalies.[19,21,52] Such associated factors could include other dysmorphic lesions, evidence of a destructive process, or genetic anomalies, and the long-term outcome is determined primarily by that of the associated factor(s). Individually, isolated forms of ventriculomegaly and isolated forms of callosal agenesis (see Chapter 2) may have a favorable prognosis. Even in combination, *nonprogressive* ventriculomegaly (colpocephaly) and callosal agenesis, in the absence of other associated factors, may be favorable. However, callosal agenesis may be complicated by *progressive* hydrocephalus, which increases the risk of an adverse outcome, as do conditions such as the X-linked CRASH syndrome (see earlier) in which hydrocephalus and callosal agenesis occur together.[83] The importance of identifying associated lesions in cases of callosal agenesis-ventriculomegaly (ACC-VM) is illustrated by one report showing normal long-term neurodevelopmental follow-up in truly isolated ACC-VM, while in cases with complex ACC-VM only 7% were normal at follow-up.[26]

In summary, most cases of mild, isolated, unilateral, nonprogressive ventriculomegaly remain stable or resolve spontaneously, have no significant associated findings, and have a favorable neurodevelopmental outcome.[2,3,16,111,112] The ability to confirm that ventriculomegaly is indeed isolated (by fetal MRI) and nonprogressive (by serial fetal US) is therefore reassuring for a favorable prognosis.

Prognosis of Congenital Hydrocephalus

The prognosis of congenital hydrocephalus is dependent on the underlying cause, the extent of secondary parenchymal brain injury, the treatment options, and the complications of intervention. Overall, the incidence of serious associated brain anomalies in fetal hydrocephalus is generally approximately 60% to 70%. For example, the prognosis of aqueductal stenosis should be guarded because the perinatal mortality is more than 20%, with an overall mortality of 40%; among survivors outcome is normal in only 10%.[66]

In earlier years, available data suggested a very unfavorable outlook for affected infants,[198] but later experience indicated a considerable improvement in prognosis with modern neurosurgery[199] and reason for a more aggressive program of intervention. This improvement relates in large part to

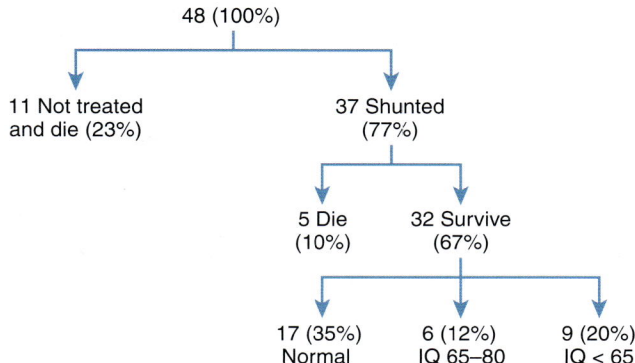

Figure 3.8 Outcome of infants with hydrocephalus identified at birth. Data are derived from a study of 48 infants. Percentage figures in parentheses are proportions of the total group of 48. *IQ*, Intelligence quotient. (From McCullough DC, Balzer-Martin LA. Current prognosis in overt neonatal hydrocephalus, *J Neurosurg.* 1982;57:378–383.)

better neonatal intensive care and neurosurgical techniques. Of 48 infants reported by McCullough and Balzer-Martin,[199] 11 were not treated, primarily because of severe neural tube defects, and died; 37 (77%) underwent shunt placement at an average age of 11 weeks (Fig. 3.8). Of the 37 infants with shunts, 86% survived. On follow-up of these survivors, 17 (46%) were normal, 6 (16%) had an IQ between 65 and 80, and 9 (24%) had an IQ less than 65. Thus, of the total group of 48 infants, only approximately one third exhibited normal intelligence. The most decisive predictors of favorable outcome were the size of the cerebral mantle before shunt placement and the origin of the hydrocephalus. Of the four major etiological categories (see Table 3.2), the mean IQ was highest for infants with communicating hydrocephalus (score of 109) and myelomeningocele (score of 108) and lowest for infants with aqueductal stenosis (score of 71) and Dandy-Walker malformation (score of 45). The poorer outlook in the last two categories may relate to associated cerebral abnormalities, especially with the Dandy-Walker malformation, consisting primarily of cerebral neuronal migrational defects and agenesis of the corpus callosum (see Chapter 4).[200-204] Later data from the same institution showed a somewhat improved outcome; 43% of infants evaluated at birth with hydrocephalus were normal on follow-up.[205] The relatively favorable results in this population of infants with hydrocephalus overt at birth (see Fig. 3.8) led to the conclusion that the infant with neonatal hydrocephalus should receive a ventriculoperitoneal shunt "except in extreme instances (severe birth defects and minimal cerebral tissue)."[206] The difficulty of using even the amount of cerebral tissue as a major criterion and the remarkable ability of neonatal hydrocephalic brain to reconstitute its cerebral mantle after ventricular decompression are illustrated by the patient whose CT scans are shown in Fig. 3.9. Indeed, rapid recovery from cortical visual impairment following correction of prolonged shunt malfunction (many months) in infants with congenital hydrocephalus attests to the potential plasticity of hydrocephalic brain.[207]

A recent retrospective series of infants with congenital hydrocephalus showed that at an average age of 5 years, 87% of children with congenital hydrocephalus could eat by mouth, 72%

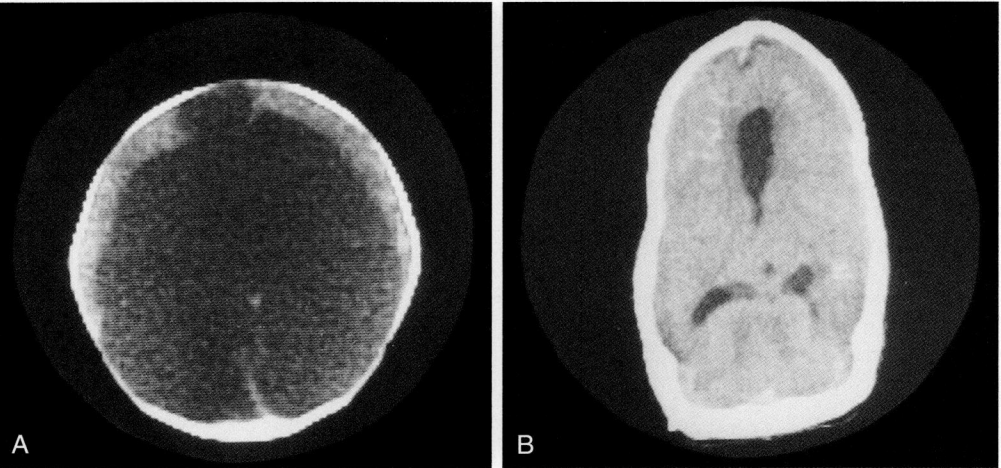

Figure 3.9 Congenital hydrocephalus: computed tomography (CT) scans. (A) On the scan performed on day 1, note the essentially total absence of recognizable cerebral mantle in the occipital region and extreme attenuation of the mantle anteriorly. (B) CT scan at 12 months (11 months after placement of ventriculoperitoneal shunt). Note the marked increase in thickness of the cerebral mantle.

were ambulatory, 18% had epilepsy, and 6% did not survive after treatment was initiated.[116] For neonates with a guarded prognosis, especially with anomalies such as severe hydranencephaly, appropriate discussions about the potential impact of CSF diversion in the context of other significant malformations should be discussed before any treatment, if possible.

REFERENCES

1. Gaglioti P, Oberto M, Todros T. The significance of fetal ventriculomegaly: etiology, short- and long-term outcomes. *Prenat Diagn.* 2009;29:381-388.
2. Melchiorre K, Bhide A, Gika AD, et al. Counseling in isolated mild fetal ventriculomegaly. *Ultrasound Obstet Gynecol.* 2009;34:212-224.
3. Weichert J, Hartge D, Krapp M, et al. Prevalence, characteristics and perinatal outcome of fetal ventriculomegaly in 29,000 pregnancies followed at a single institution. *Fetal Diagn Ther.* 2010;27:142-148.
4. Guibaud L. Fetal cerebral ventricular measurement and ventriculomegaly: time for procedure standardization. *Ultrasound Obstet Gynecol.* 2009;34:127-130.
5. Parilla BV, Endres LK, Dinsmoor MJ, et al. In utero progression of mild fetal ventriculomegaly. *Int J Gynaecol Obstet.* 2006;93:106-109.
6. Sotiriadis A, Makrydimas G. Neurodevelopment after prenatal diagnosis of isolated agenesis of the corpus callosum: an integrative review. *Am J Obstet Gynecol.* 2012;206:337.e331-337.e335.
7. Barkovich AJ, Miller SP, Bartha A, et al. MR imaging, MR spectroscopy, and diffusion tensor imaging of sequential studies in neonates with encephalopathy. *AJNR Am J Neuroradiol.* 2006;27:533-547.
8. Achiron R, Schimmel M, Achiron A, et al. Fetal mild idiopathic lateral ventriculomegaly: Is there a correlation with fetal trisomy? *Ultrasound Obstet Gynecol.* 1993;3:89-92.
9. Kelly EN, Allen VM, Seaward G, et al. Mild ventriculomegaly in the fetus, natural history, associated findings and outcome of isolated mild ventriculomegaly: a literature review. *Prenat Diagn.* 2001;21:697-700.
10. Sethna F, Tennant PW, Rankin J, et al. Prevalence, natural history, and clinical outcome of mild to moderate ventriculomegaly. *Obstet Gynecol.* 2011;117:867-876.
11. Hannon T, Tennant PW, Rankin J, et al. Epidemiology, natural history, progression, and postnatal outcome of severe fetal ventriculomegaly. *Obstet Gynecol.* 2012;120:1345-1353.

12. Glenn OA, Barkovich AJ. Magnetic resonance imaging of the fetal brain and spine: an increasingly important tool in prenatal diagnosis, part 1. *AJNR Am J Neuroradiol.* 2006;27:1604-1611.
13. Madazli R, Sal V, Erenel H, et al. Characteristics and outcome of 102 fetuses with fetal cerebral ventriculomegaly: experience of a university hospital in Turkey. *J Obstet Gynaecol.* 2011;31:142-145.
14. Griffiths PD, Morris JE, Mason G, et al. Fetuses with ventriculomegaly diagnosed in the second trimester of pregnancy by in utero MR imaging: What happens in the third trimester? *AJNR Am J Neuroradiol.* 2011;32:474-480.
15. Chiu TH, Haliza G, Lin YH, et al. A retrospective study on the course and outcome of fetal ventriculomegaly. *Taiwan J Obstet Gynecol.* 2014;53:170-177.
16. Melchiorre K, Liberati M, Celentano C, et al. Neurological outcome following isolated 10-12 mm fetal ventriculomegaly. *Arch Dis Child Fetal Neonatal Ed.* 2009;94:F311-F312.
17. Gupta JK, Bryce FC, Lilford RJ. Management of apparently isolated fetal ventriculomegaly. *Obstet Gynecol Surv.* 1994;49(10):716-721.
18. Gaglioti P, Danelon D, Bontempo S, et al. Fetal cerebral ventriculomegaly: outcome in 176 cases. *Ultrasound Obstet Gynecol.* 2005;25:372-377.
19. Goldstein RB, La Pidus AS, Filly RA, et al. Mild lateral cerebral ventricular dilatation in utero: clinical significance and prognosis. *Radiology.* 1990;176:237-242.
20. Pilu G, Falco P, Gabrielli S, et al. The clinical significance of fetal cerebral borderline ventriculomegaly: report of 31 cases and review of the literature. *Ultrasound Obstet Gynecol.* 1999;14:320-326.
21. Vergani P, Locatelli A, Strobelt N, et al. Clinical outcome of mild fetal ventriculomegaly. *Am J Obstet Gynecol.* 1998;178:218-222.
22. Breeze AC, Dey PK, Lees CC, et al. Obstetric and neonatal outcomes in apparently isolated mild fetal ventriculomegaly. *J Perinat Med.* 2005;33:236-240.
23. den Hollander NS, Vinkesteijn A, Schmitz-van Splunder P, et al. Prenatally diagnosed fetal ventriculomegaly; prognosis and outcome. *Prenat Diagn.* 1998;18:557-566.
24. Falip C, Blanc N, Maes E, et al. Postnatal clinical and imaging follow-up of infants with prenatal isolated mild ventriculomegaly: a series of 101 cases. *Pediatr Radiol.* 2007;37:981-989.
25. Pilu G. Borderline fetal cerebral ventriculomegaly—the Twilight Zone. *Ultrasound Obstet Gynecol.* 1993;3:85-87.
26. Li Y, Estroff JA, Khwaja O, et al. Callosal dysgenesis in fetuses with ventriculomegaly: levels of agreement between imaging modalities and postnatal outcome. *Ultrasound Obstet Gynecol.* 2012;40:522-529.

27. Levine D, Barnes PD. Cortical maturation in normal and abnormal fetuses as assessed with prenatal MR imaging. *Radiology.* 1999;210:751-758.
28. Ouahba J, Luton D, Vuillard E, et al. Prenatal isolated mild ventriculomegaly: outcome in 167 cases. *BJOG.* 2006;113:1072-1079.
29. Patel MD, Filly AL, Hersh DR, et al. Isolated mild fetal cerebral ventriculomegaly: clinical course and outcome. *Radiology.* 1994;192:759-764.
30. Devaseelan P, Cardwell C, Bell B, et al. Prognosis of isolated mild to moderate fetal cerebral ventriculomegaly: a systematic review. *J Perinat Med.* 2010;38:401-409.
31. Almog B, Gamzu R, Achiron R, et al. Fetal lateral ventricular width: what should be its upper limit? A prospective cohort study and reanalysis of the current and previous data. *J Ultrasound Med.* 2003;22:39-43.
32. Wyldes M, Watkinson M. Isolated mild fetal ventriculomegaly. *Arch Dis Child Fetal Neonatal Ed.* 2004;89:F9-F13.
33. Cardoza JD, Filly RA, Podrasky AE. The dangling choroid plexus: a sonographic observation of value in excluding ventriculomegaly. *AJR Am J Roentgenol.* 1988;151:767-770.
34. Filly RA. Earlier diagnosis of fetal anomalies: quo vadis? *Radiology.* 1991;181:627-628.
35. Benacerraf BR, Shipp TD, Bromley B, et al. What does magnetic resonance imaging add to the prenatal sonographic diagnosis of ventriculomegaly? *J Ultrasound Med.* 2007;26:1513-1522.
36. Nicolaides KH, Berry S, Snijders RJ, et al. Fetal lateral cerebral ventriculomegaly: associated malformations and chromosomal defects. *Fetal Diagn Ther.* 1990;5:5-14.
37. Griffiths PD, Reeves MJ, Morris JE, et al. A prospective study of fetuses with isolated ventriculomegaly investigated by antenatal sonography and in utero MR imaging. *AJNR Am J Neuroradiol.* 2010;31:106-111.
38. Morris JE, Rickard S, Paley MN, et al. The value of in-utero magnetic resonance imaging in ultrasound diagnosed foetal isolated cerebral ventriculomegaly. *Clin Radiol.* 2007;62:140-144.
39. Salomon LJ, Ouahba J, Delezoide AL, et al. Third-trimester fetal MRI in isolated 10- to 12-mm ventriculomegaly: Is it worth it? *BJOG.* 2006;113:942-947.
40. Mercier A, Eurin D, Mercier PY, et al. Isolated mild fetal cerebral ventriculomegaly: a retrospective analysis of 26 cases. *Prenat Diagn.* 2001;21:589-595.
41. Levine D, Feldman HA, Tannus JF, et al. Frequency and cause of disagreements in diagnoses for fetuses referred for ventriculomegaly. *Radiology.* 2008;247:516-527.
42. Clouchoux C, Limperopoulos C. Novel applications of quantitative MRI for the fetal brain. *Pediatr Radiol.* 2012;42:S24-S32.
43. Kazan-Tannus JF, Dialani V, Kataoka ML, et al. MR volumetry of brain and CSF in fetuses referred for ventriculomegaly. *AJR Am J Roentgenol.* 2007;189:145-151.
44. Pier DB, Levine D, Kataoka ML, et al. Magnetic resonance volumetric assessments of brains in fetuses with ventriculomegaly correlated to outcomes. *J Ultrasound Med.* 2011;30:595-603.
45. Andescavage NN, DuPlessis A, McCarter R, et al. Cerebrospinal fluid and parenchymal brain development and growth in the healthy fetus. *Dev Neurosci.* 2016;doi:10.1159/000456711.
46. Verma SK, Satyarthee GD, Sharma BS. Giant choroid plexus papilloma of the lateral ventricle in fetus. *J Pediatr Neurosci.* 2014;9:185-187.
47. Leitner Y, Stolar O, Rotstein M, et al. The neurocognitive outcome of mild isolated fetal ventriculomegaly verified by prenatal magnetic resonance imaging. *Am J Obstet Gynecol.* 2009;201:215.e211-215.e216.
48. Signorelli M, Tiberti A, Valseriati D, et al. Width of the fetal lateral ventricular atrium between 10 and 12 mm: a simple variation of the norm? *Ultrasound Obstet Gynecol.* 2004;23:14-18.
49. Robinson AJ, Goldstein R. The cisterna magna septa: vestigial remnants of Blake's pouch and a potential new marker for normal development of the rhombencephalon. *J Ultrasound Med.* 2007;26:83-95.
50. Amato M, Hüppi P, Durig P, et al. Fetal ventriculomegaly due to isolated brain malformations. *Neuropediatrics.* 1990;21:130-132.
51. Benacerraf BR. Fetal hydrocephalus: diagnosis and significance [editorial]. *Radiology.* 1988;169:858-859.
52. Bromley B, Frigoletto FD Jr, Benacerraf BR. Mild fetal lateral cerebral ventriculomegaly: clinical course and outcome. *Am J Obstet Gynecol.* 1991;164:863-867.
53. Campistol J, Poo P, Alvarez EF, et al. Parasagittal cerebral injury: magnetic resonance findings. *J Child Neurol.* 1999;14:683-685.
54. Chervenak FA, Berkowitz RL, Romero R, et al. The diagnosis of fetal hydrocephalus. *Am J Obstet Gynecol.* 1983;147:703-716.
55. Chervenak FA, Berkowitz RL, Tortora M, et al. The management of fetal hydrocephalus. *Am J Obstet Gynecol.* 1985;151:933-942.
56. Cochrane DD, Myles ST. Management of intrauterine hydrocephalus. *J Neurosurg.* 1982;57:590-596.
57. Cochrane DD, Myles ST, Nimrod C, et al. Intrauterine hydrocephalus and ventriculomegaly: associated anomalies and fetal outcome. *Can J Neurol Sci.* 1985;12:51-59.
58. Davis GH. Fetal hydrocephalus. *Clin Perinatol.* 2003;30:531-539.
59. Drugan A, Krause B, Canady A, et al. The natural history of prenatally diagnosed cerebral ventriculomegaly. *JAMA.* 1989;261:1785-1788.
60. Friedman JM, Santos-Ramos R. Natural history of X-linked aqueductal stenosis in the second and third trimesters of pregnancy. *Am J Obstet Gynecol.* 1984;150:104-106.
61. Futagi Y, Suzuki Y, Toribe Y, et al. Neurodevelopmental outcome in children with fetal hydrocephalus. *Pediatr Neurol.* 2002;27:111-116.
62. Hanigan WC, Gibson J, Kleopoulos NJ, et al. Medical imaging of fetal ventriculomegaly. *J Neurosurg.* 1986;64:575-580.
63. Hudgins RJ, Edwards MS, Goldstein R, et al. Natural history of fetal ventriculomegaly. *Pediatrics.* 1988;82:692-697.
64. Kirkinen P, Serlo W, Jouppila P, et al. Long-term outcome of fetal hydrocephaly. *J Child Neurol.* 1996;11:189-192.
65. Leidig E, Dannecker G, Pfeiffer KH, et al. Intrauterine development of posthaemorrhagic hydrocephalus. *Eur J Pediatr.* 1988;147:26-29.
66. Levitsky DB, Mack LA, Nyberg DA, et al. Fetal aqueductal stenosis diagnosed sonographically: How grave is the prognosis? *AJR Am J Roentgenol.* 1995;164:725-730.
67. Nyberg DA, Mack LA, Hirsch J, et al. Fetal hydrocephalus: sonographic detection and clinical significance of associated anomalies. *Radiology.* 1987;163:187-191.
68. Pretorius DH, Davis K, Manco-Johnson ML, et al. Clinical course of fetal hydrocephalus: 40 cases. *AJR Am J Roentgenol.* 1985;144:827-831.
69. Renier D, Flandin C, Hirsch E, et al. Brain abscesses in neonates: a study of 30 cases. *J Neurosurg.* 1988;69:877-882.
70. Renier D, Sainte-Rose C, Pierre-Kahn A, et al. Prenatal hydrocephalus: outcome and prognosis. *Childs Nerv Syst.* 1988;4:213-222.
71. Renier D, Sainte-Rose C, Pierre-Kahn A, et al. Pronostic des hydrocéphalies anténatales. *Presse Méd.* 1989;18:168-172.
72. Rosseau GL, McCullough DC, Joseph AL. Current prognosis in fetal ventriculomegaly. *J Neurosurg.* 1992;77:551-555.
73. Serlo W, Kirkinen P, Jouppila P, et al. Prognostic signs in fetal hydrocephalus. *Childs Nerv Syst.* 1986;2:93-97.
74. Stirling HF, Hendry M, Brown JK. Prenatal intracranial haemorrhage. *Dev Med Child Neurol.* 1989;31:807-811.
75. McCullough DC, Balzer-Martin LA. Current prognosis in overt neonatal hydrocephalus. *J Neurosurg.* 1982;57:378-383.
76. Mealey J Jr, Gilmor RL, Bubb MP. The prognosis of hydrocephalus overt at birth. *J Neurosurg.* 1973;39:348-355.
77. D'Addario V, Pinto V, Di Cagno L, et al. Sonographic diagnosis of fetal cerebral ventriculomegaly: an update. *J Matern Fetal Neonatal Med.* 2007;20:7-14.
78. Wong EV, Kenwrick S, Willems P, et al. Mutations in the cell adhesion molecule L1 cause mental retardation. *Trends Neurosci.* 1995;18:168-172.
79. Schrander Stumpel C, Howeler C, Jones M, et al. Spectrum of X-linked hydrocephalus (HSAS), MASA syndrome, and complicated spastic paraplegia (SPG1): clinical review with six additional families. *Am J Med Genet.* 1995;57:107-116.
80. Sztriha L, Vos YJ, Verlind E, et al. X-linked hydrocephalus: a novel missense mutation in the *L1CAM* gene. *Pediatr Neurol.* 2002;27:293-296.
81. Takahashi S, Makita Y, Okamoto N, et al. L1CAM mutation in a Japanese family with X-linked hydrocephalus: a study for genetic counseling. *Brain Dev.* 1997;19:559-562.

82. Yamasaki M, Thompson P, Lemmon V. CRASH Syndrome: mutations in L1CAM correlate with severity of the disease. *Neuropediatrics.* 1997;28:175-178.

83. Fransen E, Lemmon V, Van Camp G, et al. CRASH syndrome: clinical spectrum of corpus callosum hypoplasia, retardation, adducted thumbs, spastic paraparesis and hydrocephalus due to mutations in one single gene, L1. *Eur J Hum Genet.* 1995;3:273-284.

84. Piccione M, Matina F, Fichera M, et al. A novel L1CAM mutation in a fetus detected by prenatal diagnosis. *Eur J Pediatr.* 2010;169:415-419.

85. Schmid RS, Maness PF. L1 and NCAM adhesion molecules as signaling coreceptors in neuronal migration and process outgrowth. *Curr Opin Neurobiol.* 2008;18:245-250.

86. Haverkamp F, Wolfle J, Aretz M, et al. Congenital hydrocephalus internus and aqueduct stenosis: aetiology and implications for genetic counselling. *Eur J Pediatr.* 1999;158:474-478.

87. Ishak GE, Dempsey JC, Shaw DW, et al. Rhombencephalosynapsis: a hindbrain malformation associated with incomplete separation of midbrain and forebrain, hydrocephalus and a broad spectrum of severity. *Brain.* 2012;135(Pt 5):1370-1386.

88. De Vries LS, Gunardi H, Barth PG, et al. The spectrum of cranial ultrasound and magnetic resonance imaging abnormalities in congenital cytomegalovirus infection. *Neuropediatrics.* 2004;35:113-119.

89. Gay-Andrieu F, Marty P, Pialat J, et al. Fetal toxoplasmosis and negative amniocentesis: necessity of an ultrasound follow-up. *Prenat Diagn.* 2003;23:558-560.

90. Malinger G, Werner H, Rodriguez Leonel JC, et al. Prenatal brain imaging in congenital toxoplasmosis. *Prenat Diagn.* 2011;31:881-886.

91. Katz VL, McCoy MC, Kuller JA, et al. An association between fetal parvovirus B19 infection and fetal anomalies: a report of two cases. *Am J Perinatol.* 1996;13:43-45.

92. Hartwig NG, Vermeij-Keers C, Van Elsacker-Niele AM, et al. Embryonic malformations in a case of intrauterine parvovirus B19 infection. *Teratology.* 1989;39:295-302.

93. Weiland HT, Vermey-Keers C, Salimans MM, et al. Parvovirus B19 associated with fetal abnormality. *Lancet.* 1987;1:682-683.

94. Fusch C, Ozdoba C, Kuhn P, et al. Perinatal ultrasonography and magnetic resonance imaging findings in congenital hydrocephalus associated with fetal intraventricular hemorrhage. *Am J Obstet Gynecol.* 1997;177:512-518.

95. Ghi T, Simonazzi G, Perolo A, et al. Outcome of antenatally diagnosed intracranial hemorrhage: case series and review of the literature. *Ultrasound Obstet Gynecol.* 2003;22:121-130.

96. Bannister CM, Russell SA, Rimmer S, et al. Fetal arachnoid cysts: their site, progress, prognosis and differential diagnosis. *Eur J Pediatr Surg.* 1999;9:27-28.

97. Hirose M, Yomo H, Akiyama M, et al. In utero diagnosis of an aneurysm of the vein of Galen causing hydrocephalus and heart failure. *J Obstet Gynaecol Res.* 2003;29:343-346.

98. Sadan S, Malinger G, Schweiger A, et al. Neuropsychological outcome of children with asymmetric ventricles or unilateral mild ventriculomegaly identified in utero. *BJOG.* 2007;114:596-602.

99. Johnson S, Evans TA, Draper ES, et al. Neurodevelopmental outcomes following late and moderate prematurity: a population-based cohort study. *Arch Dis Child Fetal Neonatal Ed.* 2015;100:F301-F308.

100. Guy A, Seaton SE, Boyle EM, et al. Infants born late/moderately preterm are at increased risk for a positive autism screen at 2 years of age. *J Pediatr.* 2015;166:269-275, e263.

101. Chan E, Quigley MA. School performance at age 7 years in late preterm and early term birth: a cohort study. *Arch Dis Child Fetal Neonatal Ed.* 2014;99:F451-F457.

102. Badhiwala JH, Hong CJ, Nassiri F, et al. Treatment of posthemorrhagic ventricular dilation in preterm infants: a systematic review and meta-analysis of outcomes and complications. *J Neurosurg Pediatr.* 2015;1-11.

103. Weil AG, Westwick H, Wang S, et al. Efficacy and safety of endoscopic third ventriculostomy and choroid plexus cauterization for infantile hydrocephalus: a systematic review and meta-analysis. *Childs Nerv Syst.* 2016;32:2119-2131.

104. Stone SS, Warf BC. Combined endoscopic third ventriculostomy and choroid plexus cauterization as primary treatment for infant

hydrocephalus: a prospective North American series. *J Neurosurg Pediatr.* 2014;14:439-446.

105. Kulkarni AV, Riva-Cambrin J, Browd SR, et al. Endoscopic third ventriculostomy and choroid plexus cauterization in infants with hydrocephalus: a retrospective Hydrocephalus Clinical Research Network study. *J Neurosurg Pediatr.* 2014;14:224-229.

106. Riva-Cambrin J, Kestle JR, Holubkov R, et al. Risk factors for shunt malfunction in pediatric hydrocephalus: a multicenter prospective cohort study. *J Neurosurg Pediatr.* 2016;17:382-390.

107. Filly RA, Goldstein RB. The fetal ventricular atrium: fourth down and 10 mm to go. *Radiology.* 1994;193:315-317.

108. Bloom SL, Bloom DD, DellaNebbia C, et al. The developmental outcome of children with antenatal mild isolated ventriculomegaly. *Obstet Gynecol.* 1997;90:93-97.

109. Laskin MD, Kingdom J, Toi A, et al. Perinatal and neurodevelopmental outcome with isolated fetal ventriculomegaly: a systematic review. *J Matern Fetal Neonatal Med.* 2005;18:289-298.

110. Kennelly MM, Cooley SM, McParland PJ. Natural history of apparently isolated severe fetal ventriculomegaly: perinatal survival and neurodevelopmental outcome. *Prenat Diagn.* 2009; 29:1135-1140.

111. Pagani G, Thilaganathan B, Prefumo F. Neurodevelopmental outcome in isolated mild fetal ventriculomegaly: systematic review and meta-analysis. *Ultrasound Obstet Gynecol.* 2014;44:254-260.

112. Pasquini L, Masini G, Gaini C, et al. The utility of infection screening in isolated mild ventriculomegaly: an observational retrospective study on 141 fetuses. *Prenat Diagn.* 2014;34:1295-1300.

113. Atad-Rapoport M, Schweiger A, Lev D, et al. Neuropsychological follow-up at school age of children with asymmetric ventricles or unilateral ventriculomegaly identified in utero. *BJOG.* 2015;122:932-938.

114. Lyall AE, Woolson S, Wolfe HM, et al. Prenatal isolated mild ventriculomegaly is associated with persistent ventricle enlargement at ages 1 and 2. *Early Hum Dev.* 2012;88:691-698.

115. Deleted in review.

116. Tully HM, Ishak GE, Rue TC, et al. Two hundred thirty-six children with developmental hydrocephalus: causes and clinical consequences. *J Child Neurol.* 2016;31:309-320.

117. McComb JG. Cerebrospinal fluid physiology of the developing fetus. *AJNR Am J Neuroradiol.* 1992;13:595-599.

118. Catala M. Carbonic anhydrase activity during development of the choroid plexus in the human fetus. *Childs Nerv Syst.* 1997;13:364-368.

119. Cochrane DD, Myles ST. Management of intrauterine hydrocephalus. *J Neurosurg.* 1982;57:590-596.

120. Chervenak FA, Berkowitz RL, Romero R, et al. The diagnosis of fetal hydrocephalus. *Am J Obstet Gynecol.* 1983;147:703-716.

121. Cochrane DD, Myles ST, Nimrod C, et al. Intrauterine hydrocephalus and ventriculomegaly: associated anomalies and fetal outcome. *Can J Neurol Sci.* 1985;12:51-59.

122. Bromley B, Frigoletto FD Jr, Benacerraf BR. Mild fetal lateral cerebral ventriculomegaly: Clinical course and outcome. *Am J Obstet Gynecol.* 1991;164:863-867.

123. Amato M, Hüppi P, Durig P, et al. Fetal ventriculomegaly due to isolated brain malformations. *Neuropediatrics.* 1990;21:130-132.

124. Hudgins RJ, Edwards MS, Goldstein R, et al. Natural history of fetal ventriculomegaly. *Pediatrics.* 1988;82:692-697.

125. Pober BR, Greene MF, Holmes LB. Complexities of intraventricular abnormalities. *J Pediatr.* 1986;108:545-551.

126. Renier D, Sainte-Rose C, Pierre-Kahn A, Hirsch JF. Prognostic des hydrocéphalies anténatales. *Presse Med.* 1989;18:168-172.

127. Pretorius DH, Davis K, Manco-Johnson ML, et al. Clinical course of fetal hydrocephalus: 40 cases. *AJR Am J Roentgenol.* 1985;144:827-831.

128. Nyberg DA, Mack LA, Hirsch J, et al. Fetal hydrocephalus: Sonographic detection and clinical significance of associated anomalies. *Radiology.* 1987;163:187-191.

129. Renier D, Sainte-Rose C, Pierre-Kahn A, Hirsch JF. Prenatal hydrocephalus: outcome and prognosis. *Childs Nerv Syst.* 1988;4:213-222.

130. Drugan A, Krause B, Canady A, et al. The natural history of prenatally diagnosed cerebral ventriculomegaly. *JAMA.* 1989;261:1785-1788.

131. Stirling HF, Hendry M, Brown JK. Prenatal intracranial haemorrhage. *Dev Med Child Neurol.* 1989;31:807-811.

132. Benacerraf BR. Fetal hydrocephalus: diagnosis and significance [editorial]. *Radiology.* 1988;169:858-859.
133. Hanigan WC, Gibson J, Kleopoulos NJ, et al. Medical imaging of fetal ventriculomegaly. *J Neurosurg.* 1986;64:575-580.
134. Leidig E, Dannecker G, Pfeiffer KH, et al. Intrauterine development of posthaemorrhagic hydrocephalus. *Eur J Pediatr.* 1988;147:26-29.
135. Rosseau GL, McCullough DC, Joseph AL. Current prognosis in fetal ventriculomegaly. *J Neurosurg.* 1992;77:551-555.
136. Levitsky DB, Mack LA, Nyberg DA, et al. Fetal aqueductal stenosis diagnosed sonographically: how grave is the prognosis? *AJR Am J Roentgenol.* 1995;164:725-730.
137. Kirkinen P, Serlo W, Jouppila P, et al. Long-term outcome of fetal hydrocephaly. *J Child Neurol.* 1996;11:189-192.
138. Futagi Y, Suzuki Y, Toribe Y, Morimoto K. Neurodevelopmental outcome in children with fetal hydrocephalus. *Pediatr Neurol.* 2002;27:111-116.
139. Davis GH. Fetal hydrocephalus. *Clin Perinatol.* 2003;30:531-539.
140. Vintzileos AM, Ingardia CJ, Nochimson DJ. Congenital hydrocephalus: a review and protocol for perinatal management. *Obstet Gynecol.* 1983;62:539-549.
141. Birnholz J. Fetal neurology. In: Sanders RC, Hill M, eds. *Ultrasound Annual.* New York: Raven Press; 1984.
142. Glick PL, Harrison MR, Nakayama DK, et al. Management of ventriculomegaly in the fetus. *J Pediatr.* 1984;105:97-105.
143. Zlotogora J, Sagi M, Cohen T. Familial hydrocephalus of prenatal onset. *Am J Med Genet.* 1994;49:202-204.
144. Wyldes M, Watkinson M. Isolated mild fetal ventriculomegaly. *Arch Dis Child Fetal Neonatal Ed.* 2004;89:F9-F13.
145. Warkany J, Lemire RJ, Cohen MM Jr. *Mental Retardation and Congenital Malformations of the Central Nervous System.* Chicago: Year Book; 1981.
146. Halliday J, Chow CW, Wallace D, Danks DM. X linked hydrocephalus: a survey of a 20 year period in Victoria, Australia. *J Med Genet.* 1986;23:23-31.
147. Schrander Stumpel C, Howeler C, Jones M, et al. Spectrum of X-linked hydrocephalus (HSAS), MASA syndrome, and complicated spastic paraplegia (SPG1): clinical review with six additional families. *Am J Med Genet.* 1995;l57:107-116.
148. Yamasaki M, Thompson P, Lemmon V. CRASH Syndrome: Mutations in L1CAM correlate with severity of the disease. *Neuropediatrics.* 1997;28:175-178.
149. Takahashi S, Makita Y, Okamoto N, et al. L1CAM mutation in a Japanese family with X-linked hydrocephalus: a study for genetic counseling. *Brain Dev.* 1997;19:559-562.
150. Sztriha L, Vos YJ, Verlind E, et al. X-linked hydrocephalus: A novel missense mutation in the L1CAM gene. *Pediatr Neurol.* 2002;27:293-296.
151. Holtzman RN, Garcia L, Koenigsberger R. Hydrocephalus and congenital clasped thumbs: a case report with electromyographic evaluation. *Dev Med Child Neurol.* 1976;18:521-524.
152. Willems PJ, Vits L, Raeymaekers P, Beuten J, et al. Further localization of X-linked hydrocephalus in the chromosomal region-xq28. *Am J Hum Genet.* 1992;51:307-315.
153. Serville F, Lyonnet S, Pelet A, Reynaud M, et al. X-linked hydrocephalus-clinical heterogeneity at a single gene locus. *Eur J Pediatr.* 1992;151:515-518.
154. Cochrane DD, Myles ST. Management of intrauterine hydrocephalus. *J Neurosurg.* 1982;57:590-596.
155. Chervenak FA, Berkowitz RL, Romero R, et al. The diagnosis of fetal hydrocephalus. *Am J Obstet Gynecol.* 1983;147:703-716.
156. Cochrane DD, Myles ST, Nimrod C, et al. Intrauterine hydrocephalus and ventriculomegaly: associated anomalies and fetal outcome. *Can J Neurol Sci.* 1985;12:51-59.
157. Bromley B, Frigoletto FD Jr, Benacerraf BR. Mild fetal lateral cerebral ventriculomegaly: clinical course and outcome. *Am J Obstet Gynecol.* 1991;164:863-867.
158. Amato M, Hüppi P, Durig P, et al. Fetal ventriculomegaly due to isolated brain malformations. *Neuropediatrics.* 1990;21:130-132.
159. Hudgins RJ, Edwards MS, Goldstein R, et al. Natural history of fetal ventriculomegaly. *Pediatrics.* 1998;82:692-697.
160. Pober BR, Greene MF, Holmes LB. Complexities of intraventricular abnormalities. *J Pediatr.* 1986;108:545-551.
161. Renier D, Sainte-Rose C, Pierre-Kahn A, Hirsch JF. Prognostic des hydrocéphalies anténatales. *Presse Med.* 1989;18:168-172.
162. Pretorius DH, Davis K, Manco-Johnson ML, et al. Clinical course of fetal hydrocephalus: 40 cases. *AJR Am J Roentgenol.* 1985;144:827-831.
163. Serlo W, Kirkinen P, Jouppila P, Herva R. Prognostic signs in fetal hydrocephalus. *Childs Nerv Syst.* 1986;2:93-97.
164. Nyberg DA, Mack LA, Hirsch J, et al. Fetal hydrocephalus: sonographic detection and clinical significance of associated anomalies. *Radiology.* 1987;163:187-191.
165. Renier D, Sainte-Rose C, Pierre-Kahn A, Hirsch JF. Prenatal hydrocephalus: outcome and prognosis. *Childs Nerv Syst.* 1988;4:213-222.
166. Drugan A, Krause B, Canady A, et al. The natural history of prenatally diagnosed cerebral ventriculomegaly. *JAMA.* 1989;261:1785-1788.
167. Stirling HF, Hendry M, Brown JK. Prenatal intracranial haemorrhage. *Dev Med Child Neurol.* 1989;31:807-811.
168. Benacerraf BR. Fetal hydrocephalus: diagnosis and significance [editorial]. *Radiology.* 1988;169:858-859.
169. Leidig E, Dannecker G, Pfeiffer KH, et al. Intrauterine development of posthaemorrhagic hydrocephalus. *Eur J Pediatr.* 1988;147:26-29.
170. Rosseau GL, McCullough DC, Joseph AL. Current prognosis in fetal ventriculomegaly. *J Neurosurg.* 1992;77:551-555.
171. Levitsky DB, Mack LA, Nyberg DA, et al. Fetal aqueductal stenosis diagnosed sonographically: how grave is the prognosis? *AJR Am J Roentgenol.* 1995;164:725-730.
172. Kirkinen P, Serlo W, Jouppila P, et al. Long-term outcome of fetal hydrocephaly. *J Child Neurol.* 1996;11:189-192.
173. Futagi Y, Suzuki Y, Toribe Y, Morimoto K. Neurodevelopmental outcome in children with fetal hydrocephalus. *Pediatr Neurol.* 2002;27:111-116.
174. Davis GH. Fetal hydrocephalus. *Clin Perinatol.* 2003;30:531-539.
175. Hanigan WC, Morgan A, Shaaban A, Bradle P. Surgical treatment and long-term neurodevelopmental outcome for infants with idiopathic aqueductal stenosis. *Childs Nerv Syst.* 1991;7:386-390.
176. Vintzileos AM, Ingardia CJ, Nochimson DJ. Congenital hydrocephalus: a review and protocol for perinatal management. *Obstet Gynecol.* 1983;62:539-549.
177. Birnholz J. Fetal neurology. In: Sanders RC, Hill M, eds. *Ultrasound Annual.* New York: Raven Press; 1984.
178. Glick PL, Harrison MR, Nakayama DK, et al. Management of ventriculomegaly in the fetus. *J Pediatr.* 1984;105:97-105.
179. Wyldes M, Watkinson M. Isolated mild fetal ventriculomegaly. *Arch Dis Child Fetal Neonatal Ed.* 2004;89:F9-F13.
180. Den Hollander NS, Vinkesteijn A, Schmitz-van Splunder P, et al. Prenatally diagnosed fetal ventriculomegaly: prognosis and outcome. *Prenat Diagn.* 1998;18:557-566.
181. Hudgins RJ, Edwards MS, Goldstein R, et al. Natural history of fetal ventriculomegaly. *Pediatrics.* 1988;82:692-697.
182. Futagi Y, Suzuki Y, Toribe Y, Morimoto K. Neurodevelopmental outcome in children with fetal hydrocephalus. *Pediatr Neurol.* 2002;27:111-116.
183. Michejda M, Hodgen GD. In utero diagnosis and treatment of nonhuman primate fetal skeletal anomalies. I. Hydrocephalus. *JAMA.* 1981;246:1093-1097.
184. Michejda M, Patronas N, DiChiro G, Hodgen GD. Fetal hydrocephalus. II. Amelioration of fetal porencephaly by in utero therapy in nonhuman primates. *JAMA.* 1984;251:2548-2552.
185. Michejda M, Queenan JT, McCullough D. Present status of intrauterine treatment of hydrocephalus and its future. *Am J Obstet Gynecol.* 1986;155:873-882.
186. Cavalheiro S, Moron AF, Zymberg ST, Dastoli P. Fetal hydrocephalusprenatal treatment. *Childs Nerv Syst.* 2003;19:561-573.
187. Davis GH. Fetal hydrocephalus. *Clin Perinatol.* 2003;30:531-539.
188. Clewell WH, Johnson ML, Meier PR, et al. A surgical approach to the treatment of fetal hydrocephalus. *N Engl J Med.* 1982;306:1320-1325.
189. Bannister CM. Fetal neurosurgery: a new challenge on the horizon. *Dev Med Child Neurol.* 1984;26:827-830.
190. Manning FA, Harrison MR, Rodeck C. Catheter shunts for fetal hydronephrosis and hydrocephalus: Report of the International Fetal Surgery Registry. *N Engl J Med.* 1986;315:336-340.
191. Hudgins RJ, Edwards MS, Goldstein R, et al. Natural history of fetal ventriculomegaly. *Pediatrics.* 1988;82:692-697.
192. Davis GH. Fetal hydrocephalus. *Clin Perinatol.* 2003;30:531-539.

193. Vintzileos AM, Ingardia CJ, Nochimson DJ. Congenital hydrocephalus: a review and protocol for perinatal management. *Obstet Gynecol*. 1983;62:539-549.
194. Kirkinen P, Serlo W, Jouppila P, et al. Long-term outcome of fetal hydrocephaly. *J Child Neurol*. 1996;11:189-192.
195. Glick PL, Harrison MR, Nakayama DK, et al. Management of ventriculomegaly in the fetus. *J Pediatr*. 1984;105:97-105.
196. Oi SZ, Yamada H, Kimura M, et al. Factors affecting prognosis of intrauterine hydrocephalus diagnosed in the third trimester. *Neurol Med Chir*. 1990;30:456-461.
197. Davis GH. Fetal hydrocephalus. *Clin Perinatol*. 2003;30:531-539.
198. Mealey J Jr, Gilmor RL, Bubb MP. The prognosis of hydrocephalus overt at birth. *J Neurosurg*. 1973;39:348-355.
199. McCullough DC, Balzer-Martin LA. Current prognosis in overt neonatal hydrocephalus. *J Neurosurg*. 1982;57:378-383.
200. Warkany J, Lemire RJ, Cohen MM Jr. *Mental Retardation and Congenital Malformations of the Central Nervous System*. Chicago: Year Book; 1981.
201. Hanigan WC, Morgan A, Shaaban A, Bradle P. Surgical treatment and long-term neurodevelopmental outcome for infants with idiopathic aqueductal stenosis. *Childs Nerv Syst*. 1991;7:386-390.
202. Hart MN, Malamud N, Ellis WG. The Dandy-Walker syndrome: a clinicopathological study based on 28 cases. *Neurology*. 1972;22:771-780.
203. Tal Y, Freigang B, Dunn HG, et al. Dandy-Walker syndrome: analysis of 21 cases. *Dev Med Child Neurol*. 1980;22:189-201.
204. Hirsch JF, Pierre-Kahn A, Renier D, Sainte Rose C, et al. The Dandy-Walker malformation: A review of 40 cases. *J Neurosurg*. 1984;61:515-522.
205. Rosseau GL, McCullough DC, Joseph AL. Current prognosis in fetal ventriculomegaly. *J Neurosurg*. 1992;77:551-555.
206. McCullough DC, Balzer-Martin LA. Current prognosis in overt neonatal hydrocephalus. *J Neurosurg*. 1982;57:378-383.
207. Connolly MB, Jan JE, Cochrane DD. Rapid recovery from cortical visual impairment following correction of prolonged shunt malfunction in congenital hydrocephalus. *Arch Neurol*. 1991;48:956-957.

Chapter 4

Cerebellar Development

Adré J. du Plessis ◆ Catherine Limperopoulos ◆ Joseph J. Volpe

As is the case for development of the prosencephalic structures discussed in Chapter 2, the most critical embryonic time period for development of cerebellar form and cellular structure occurs in the second and third months of gestation. The widespread implementation of prenatal screening protocols that include fetal anatomical ultrasound surveys has made suspected posterior fossa anomalies in the fetus one of the more common indications for prenatal neurological counseling. Some of these posterior fossa anomalies are only identified, or require diagnostic confirmation or refinement, in the postnatal period. As with other developmental anomalies, a brief discussion of normal development of the major posterior fossa structures is followed by a review of the more common malformations.

NORMAL DEVELOPMENT OF THE POSTERIOR FOSSA STRUCTURES

Overview (Box 4.1)

Completion of neural tube closure toward the end of four postconceptional (p/c) weeks is followed by the development of flexures in the anterior neural tube at around 5 weeks p/c (see Chapter 1), a developmental event that plays an important role in defining the territory of the future rhombencephalic structures (Fig. 4.1). The pontine flexure causes a splaying and thinning of the dorsal hindbrain, site of the future fourth ventricular roof (see Box 4.1). Around the same time, the mesencephalic flexure appears at the border between the mesencephalon and rhombencephalon, the future midbrain-hindbrain (MHB) junction. The MHB junction defines the location of a critical *organizer* that orchestrates the patterning events required to define the territories of the cerebellar anlage and related structures. The primordia of the cerebellar hemispheres appear as bilateral thickenings in the lateral aspects of the dorsal surface of the rhombencephalon, known as the rhombic lips.[1,2] Hereafter, a series of proliferative and migratory events in the germinal matrices along the fourth ventricular surface and rhombic lips lead to development of the cerebellar hemispheres and vermis, which become apparent by 12 to 13 weeks. Although there is overlap between these processes, we review them as three broad events in temporal sequence, that is, (1) patterning of the MHB junction and cerebellar anlage; (2) development of the fourth ventricular roof; and (3) development of the cerebellar hemispheres and vermis.

Patterning events define structural domains around the midbrain-hindbrain junction (Fig. 4.2). Normal development of the cerebellum and various brain stem structures is critically dependent on a precise sequence of late first trimester events around the MHB junction. The initial critical event is the development and precise positioning of the isthmic organizer (IsO) at the MHB junction (see Fig. 4.2). This event is under the stewardship of two mutually suppressing homeobox transcription factors, *Otx2* and *Gbx2*. Specifically, the IsO develops at the interface between the expression domain of *Otx2* in the caudal midbrain and that of *Gbx2* in the rostral hindbrain. When *Otx2* expression is suppressed by *Gbx2* expression (see Fig. 4.2), the onset of cerebellar development is enabled. Conversely, suppression of *Gbx2* expression by *Otx2* permits development of the mesencephalic tectum (see Fig. 4.2). It is not surprising, therefore, that developmental anomalies in these structures may occur together (see later). Disturbed expression of either of these factors will lead to abnormal positioning of the IsO and subsequent increased or decreased growth or transformation of structures in the MHB region.[3] Once established, the IsO begins to secrete fibroblast growth factors (FGFs). Secretion of *Fgf8a* supports the development of the mesencephalic tectum,[4-6] while cerebellar development is dependent on *Fgf8b* (see Fig. 4.2). These factors set the stage for the subsequent developmental events (see later), including specific cell differentiation and migration in the mesencephalic tectum and cerebellum. Development of the medial cerebellar structures, especially the vermis, is exquisitely dependent on appropriate FGF8 expression. Consequently, lesions that include hypoplasia of the vermis likely involve early disturbances in IsO function.

Development of structures in and around the fourth ventricle roof, the second broad event in development of the cerebellum, is complex (Fig. 4.3), and developmental disturbances in this region account for many of the posterior fossa lesions seen in clinical practice. As mentioned earlier, the physical forces exerted on the neural tube during formation of the pontine flexure widen its central lumen, forming the fourth ventricle, and stretch the dorsal rhombencephalon into the thin diamond-shaped fourth ventricle roof (see Fig. 4.3). At about 10 weeks p/c, the fourth ventricle roof is transected by a transverse crease, the plica choroidea (the future fourth ventricular choroid plexus), into the anterior and posterior membranous areas (AMA and PMA, respectively). The roof of the fourth ventricle has two layers: inner ependymal and outer pial. The AMA also contains neurons while the PMA does not. During normal development, the vermis overgrows and incorporates the AMA; the PMA persists and undergoes a series of perforations.[7] Around 10 weeks p/c the outer pial layer becomes fenestrated in the midline just caudal to the plica choroidea, followed soon thereafter

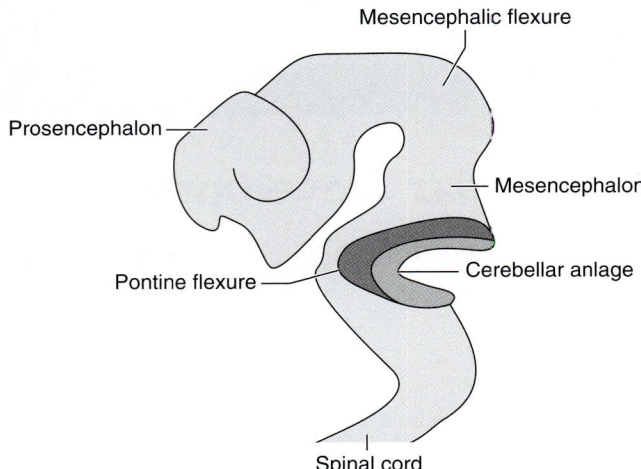

Figure 4.1   Human fetal brain stem at 7 weeks gestational age. Note the kink formed by the mesencephalic, pontine, and cervical flexures. (Image based on Stroustrup Smith et al. *J Ultrasound Med*. 2006; and image courtesy Veronika Doljenkova [Rhode Island School of Design, Providence, RI] with reference to Sarnat[1] and Sadler[2].)

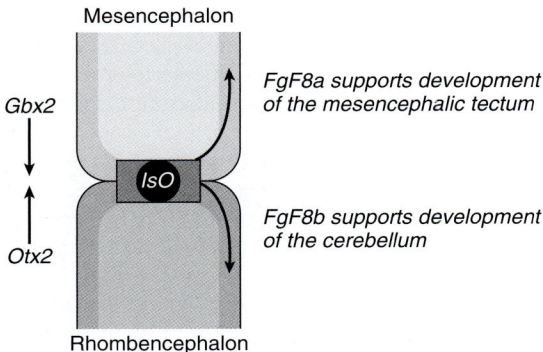

Figure 4.2   Patterning events at the developing midbrain-hindbrain junction. *IsO*, isthmic organizer; *Otx2*, homeobox protein encoded by the orthodenticle homeobox 2 (OTX2) gene; *Gbx2*, homeobox protein encoded by the gastrulation brain homeobox 2 (GBX2) gene; *FgF8a* and *b*, fibroblast 8 growth factors a and b encoded by the FgF8 gene.

BOX 4.1   Timetable of Major Developmental Events in the Posterior Fossa

Before 20 Weeks
- ◆ 4 weeks: neural tube closure
- ◆ 5 weeks: anterior neural tube flexures form
- ◆ 7–8 weeks: neuronal proliferation accelerates in dorsomedial ventricular zone—origin of all inhibitory GABAergic neurons (express *Ptf1*)
- ◆ 10 weeks: transverse crease (plica choroidea) forms in fourth ventricular roof
- ◆ 10 weeks: foramen of Magendie begins to form
- ◆ 10 weeks Blake pouch begins to perforate; by 24–26 weeks ~⅔ have resolved
- ◆ 12 weeks: neuronal proliferation accelerates in dorsolateral subventricular zone of the rhombic lips—origin of all excitatory glutamatergic neurons (express *Atoh*)
- ◆ 12–13 weeks: cerebellar hemispheres and vermis (see Box 4.2) begin to emerge
- ◆ 14–17 weeks (as late as 26 weeks): foramina of Luschka form

By 20 Weeks
- ◆ Radial migration of GABAergic interneurons from ventricular zone to form deep cerebellar nuclei and Purkinje cell layer
- ◆ Tangential migration of glutamatergic cells (1) from rostral rhombic lip to form external granular layer; (2) from caudal rhombic lip to form pontine and inferior olivary nuclei

From 20 to 30 Weeks
- ◆ Rapid expansion of external granular layer (EGL) and early foliation
- ◆ At peak thickness EGL 6–9 cells deep, divided into inner and outer layers
- ◆ 29 weeks: external granular cell precursors cover entire cerebellar surface
- ◆ EGL neurons begin inward radial migration along Bergmann glial cells to form internal granular layer (IGL)
- ◆ Purkinje cells differentiate and secrete *Shh* that stimulates proliferation of precursor cells in the EGL

From 30 to 40 Weeks
- ◆ Massive EGL proliferation and inward migration leads to fivefold volumetric growth of the cerebellum.

After 40 Weeks
- ◆ EGL gradually dissipates throughout first postnatal year and IGL cells become greatly compacted
- ◆ Purkinje cells enlarge and differentiate as major outflow to dentate nuclei
- ◆ Purkinje cell differentiation enlarges the molecular layer several fold

Modified from Table 4.1 in Volpe JJ. Cerebellum of the premature infant—rapidly developing, vulnerable, clinically important. *J Child Neurol*. 2009;24:1085–1104.

---

genes are expressed by the mesenchymal tissues, but not by the underlying rhombencephalic tissues. Nonetheless, mutations in the Forkhead box gene C1 *(Fox c1)* are associated (see later) with cerebellar hypoplasia, hypoplasia and dysplasia of the vermis, mega cisterna magna, and the Dandy-Walker syndrome.[9] Furthermore, disturbances in these signaling pathways may underlie conditions in which mesenchymal and neuroepithelial defects are associated (discussed later).

Development of the cerebellar hemispheres (see Box 4.1). Although earlier investigators proposed that up to one-third of the cerebellum derives from the rostral mesencephalon,[10] it is now known that *all cell types* composing the cerebellum are derived from the alar plate at the junction of the IsO and the *first rhombomere* (R1). With the fundamental structures of the cerebellar anlage in place, the growth and development of the cerebellar hemispheres and vermis unfold through a complex series of programmed neuronal proliferation, migration, and differentiation. The major events in cerebellar histogenesis are illustrated in Fig. 4.4.

by perforation of the underlying ependymal layer, to form the foramen of Magendie. If there is a delay in ependymal perforation, a small pouch of ependyma, the Blake pouch (a normal structure), herniates through the pial perforation,[8] and then subsequently perforates. More delayed perforation of the Blake pouch may lead to increasing encysted fluid (Blake pouch cyst) in the posterior fossa (discussed later; Figs. 4.13 to 4.15). Usually by around 14 to 17 weeks, but as late as 26 weeks, the foramina of Luschka develop in the lateral angles of the PMA (see Fig. 4.3).

Signaling support for developmental events in and around the fourth ventricular roof comes, in part, from genetic expression in the overlying mesenchyme.[9] Forkhead box (*Fox*)

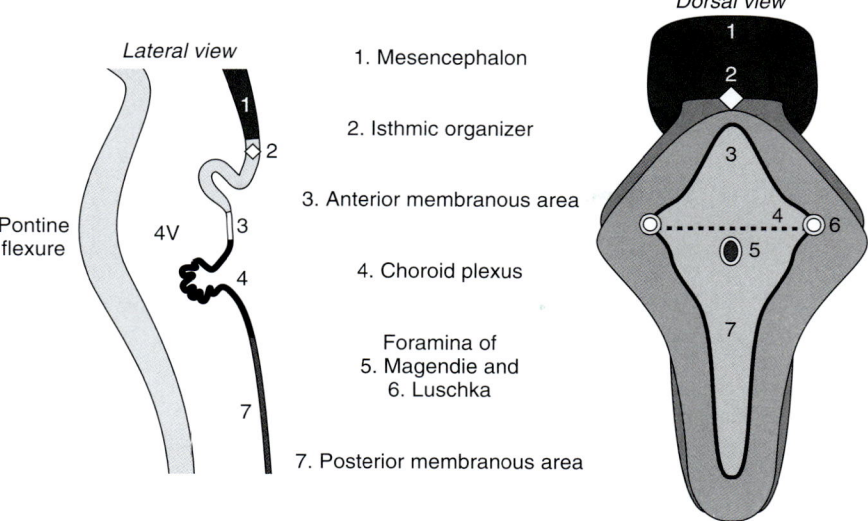

Figure 4.3 Normal landmarks of the developing fourth ventricular roof.

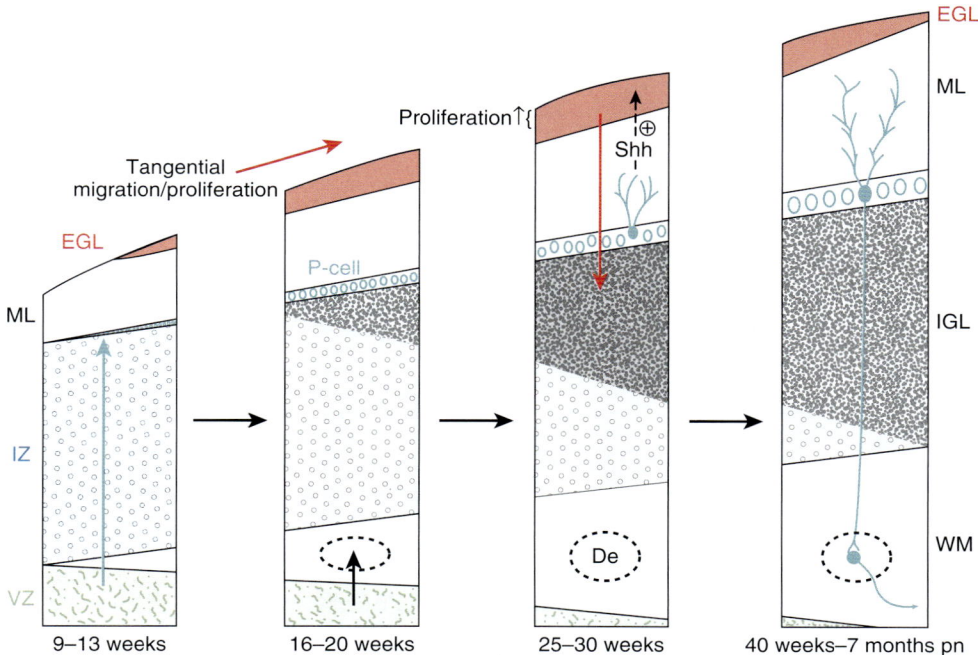

Figure 4.4 Major events in the histogenesis of the cerebellum in four major time periods from 9 weeks of gestation to 7 months postnatal (pn). The two zones of proliferation are the ventricular zone (VZ) and the external granule cell layer (EGL). Three directions of migration are indicated by arrows; that is, radial from the VZ, tangential over the surface of the cerebellum to form the EGL, and later, inward to form the internal granular layer (IGL). Proliferation in the outer half of the EGL is under positive control by Sonic hedgehog (Shh) secreted by Purkinje cells (P-cells). Note the markedly active proliferation and migration of the granule precursor cells of the EGL during the premature period. Not shown is the marked increase in size of the molecular layer (ML) during the postnatal period. *De*, dentate; *IZ*, intermediate zone; *WM*, white matter. (From Limperopoulos C, Soul JS, Gauvreau K, et al. Late gestation cerebellar growth is rapid and impeded by premature birth. *Pediatrics.* 2005;115:688-695, with permission.)

Neural progenitors originate in two proliferative zones (Fig. 4.5A).[11,12] Specifically, the *inhibitory GABAergic neurons* of the future cerebellum proliferate in the primary subependymal neuroepithelium (dorsomedial ventricular zone) around the fourth ventricle (see Fig. 4.5B). Proliferation of these inhibitory neurons and their expression of *Ptfa1* is stimulated by the diffusible mitogen, sonic hedgehog (*Shh*).[13] Neuronal proliferation in the subependymal ventricular zone accelerates around 7 to 8 weeks p/c, followed by radial migration into the body of the future cerebellar anlage[14] where these cells

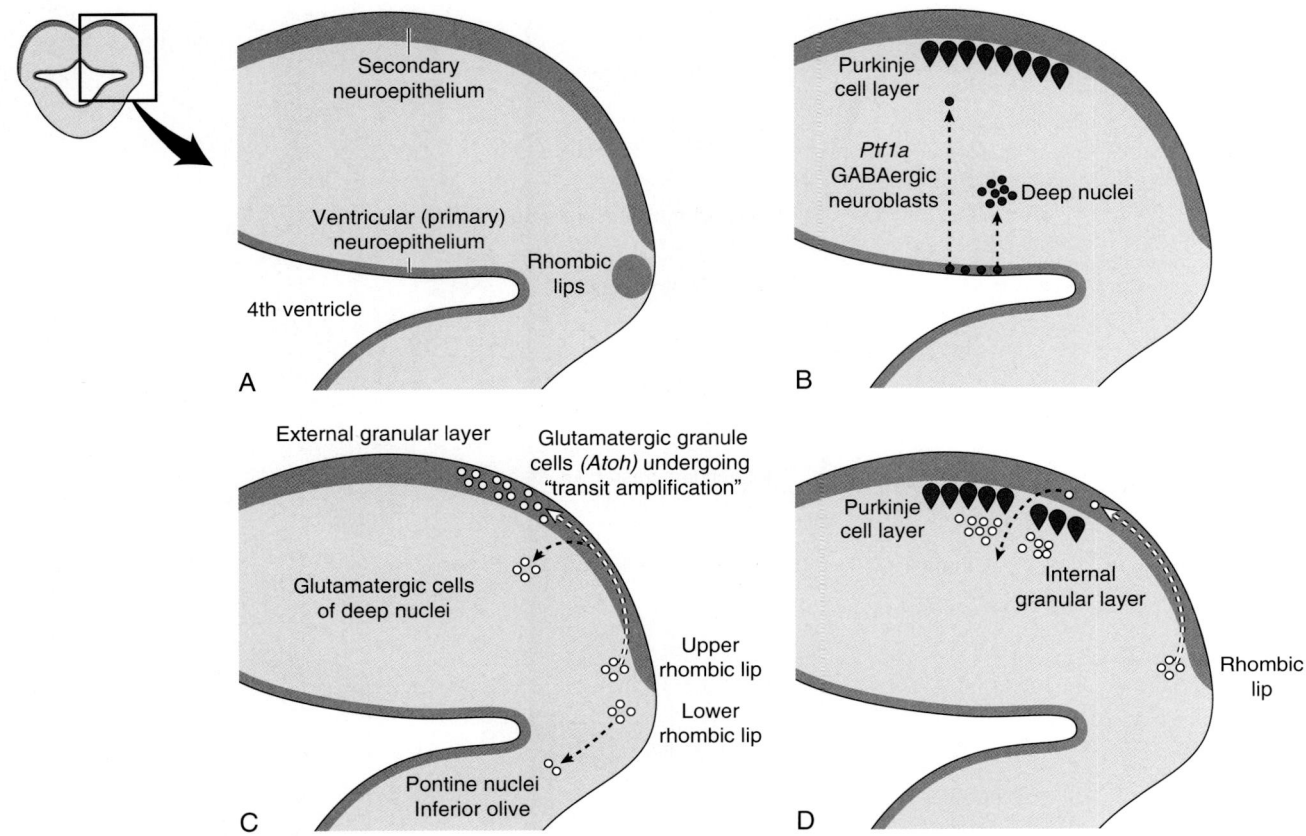

Figure 4.5 (A) Cerebellar primary and secondary neuroproliferative sites. (B) Neuronal migration of GABAergic cells from the primary ventricular neuroepithelium. (C) Neuronal proliferation and migration of glutamatergic neuronal precursors from the rhombic lips into the secondary neuroproliferative zone of the external granular layer. (D) Internal migration of the granule cells from the external granular layer through the Purkinje cell layer to form the internal granular layer.

make up the inhibitory interneurons of the deep cerebellar nuclei and the Purkinje cell layer (see Fig. 4.5B), that is, the primary efferent neurons of the cerebellum. Later, this zone generates the inhibitory GABAergic neurons that become the Golgi cells of the internal granular layer and the basket and stellate cells of the molecular layer. Proliferation of the future *excitatory glutamatergic neurons* of the cerebellum occurs in the rhombic lips (Fig. 4.5C), neuroproliferative zones along the dorsolateral margins of the fourth ventricle, comparable to the subventricular zones of the developing cerebrum (see Chapter 5).[11,12] These excitatory glutamatergic neurons express *Atoh1*. It is of interest that the origin of the glutamatergic and GABAergic neurons differs in the cerebellum and cerebrum where glutamatergic neurons originate from the ventricular zone, and the GABAergic neurons from the subventricular zone (see Chapter 5). The first cells to leave the rhombic lips are those migrating into the substance of the future cerebellum to become glutamatergic projection neurons of the cerebellar nuclei (see Fig. 4.5C).[14,15] These cells only briefly express *Atoh1* and do not have a prolonged clonal expansion phase (see the section on transit amplification later). From about 12 weeks p/c, proliferation accelerates in the dominant cell population in the rhombic lips, the granule cell precursors. The rhombic

lips are the sole source of granule cell precursors.[16] Once these cells begin expressing *Atoh1*, they leave the rhombic lips and embark on a complex tangential migration pathway over the subpial surface of the cerebellum. Given the configuration of the developing cerebellum and the fourth ventricle, the lateral subventricular zone origin of these future granule cells is in close proximity to the subpial spaces along which they migrate away from the rhombic lips.[12] By 29 weeks p/c the external granule precursors cover the entire surface of the developing cerebellum. The initial thin layer of cells undergoes waves of symmetric cell division that results in an exponential expansion of the external granular layer, a process recently termed *transit amplification*.[17] The external granular layer develops an outer zone of active proliferation and an inner zone of postmitotic cells. From the inner zone, postmitotic granule cells migrate radially into the cerebellum along the Bergmann glial cells, crossing the Purkinje cell layer to form the (internal) granular layer of the mature cerebellum (see Fig. 4.5D). During and after this inward migration, important connections are made by the granule cells. As they pass through the Purkinje cell layer they extend horizontal parallel fibers to contact the dendrites of the Purkinje cells, and soon after arrival at the internal granular layer, they link with the mossy fibers ascending from the pontine nuclei. Between 24 and 40 weeks, this external granular layer proliferation is largely responsible for the fivefold volumetric growth of the cerebellum (Fig. 4.6).[18,19] As discussed later, the close proximity of the actively proliferating outer layer of granule cells to the subarachnoid space (separated only by the thin pial layer) may expose this crucial neuroproliferative zone to potentially noxious substances circulating in the cerebrospinal fluid (CSF), including the products of prematurity-related forms of brain hemorrhage.

The dorsal rhombic lips also generate neurons that follow a different, caudal migrational path along the ventrolateral of the pons and rostral medulla to form specific brain stem nuclei, including the pontine and inferior olivary nuclei, among others. These nuclei subsequently generate important afferent input to the cerebellum, the pontine nuclei connecting to the internal granule cells through the mossy fibers, and the inferior olivary nuclei connecting to the Purkinje cells through the climbing fibers. This common origin of cellular precursors underlies the association between malformations in the cerebellum and other brain stem structures (discussed later).

Shh plays a central role in the spatial and temporal expansion of neuronal and glial cells across cerebellar development. Expressed in the choroid plexus epithelium roof plate,[13] *Shh* is released into the CSF and stimulates proliferation in the ventricular zone.[13] When *Shh* signaling is impaired, proliferation of radial glial cells, as well as their ability to generate GABAergic interneuron progenitors, fails.[13] During the phase of transit amplification, *Shh* secreted by the underlying Purkinje cells drives the rate of cell division in the overlying external granular layer.[20-22] Later, *Shh* from the Purkinje cells drives the proliferation of a secondary population of inhibitory interneurons and glial cells in the future white matter of the cerebellum. Finally, *Shh* plays an important role in the patterning of folia in the cerebellar cortex.[23]

Development of the cerebellar vermis (Box 4.2). Understanding of normal vermian development is especially important because vermian anomalies are increasingly recognized for their impact on long-term outcome. Previous understanding was that the vermis was formed by fusion of the cerebellar hemispheres. It is now known that the entire cerebellum originates from a single cerebellar anlage, rather than by fusion of the hemispheres. The vermis develops from proliferative events in a distinct region of this primordium, at the rostral midline of the first rhombomere. Initially, vermian development lags behind that of the hemispheres, but then accelerates around the late first trimester. Vermis growth is in a craniocaudal direction (Fig. 4.7); however, this is not primarily due to growth at the caudal leading edge. In fact, the caudal-most aspects of the posterior lobe of the vermis are among the earliest to develop. Rather, it is the delayed expansion of the neovermis below the primary fissure that pushes the inferior vermis caudalward; this is an important point in the terminology of vermian hypoplasia discussed later.[28] In this regard, development of the vermis resembles that of the corpus callosum (see Chapter 2). The progressive complexity of cerebellar surface growth and foliation is demonstrated in Fig. 4.8.

> ### BOX 4.2   Normal Development of the Vermis (Figs. 4.7, 4.8, and 4.9)
>
> **By 18–20 Weeks' Gestation**
> - Normal gestational age-appropriate rostrocaudal length as late as 24 weeks
> - Caudal edge covers the fourth ventricle and reaches the obex
> - Primary fissure is present between the anterior and posterior lobes of the vermis
> - Fastigium-declive line divides the vermis into anterior and posterior lobes with a 1:2 ratio.
>
> **By 27–28 Weeks' Gestation**
> - Mature pattern of vermian lobules and fissures.

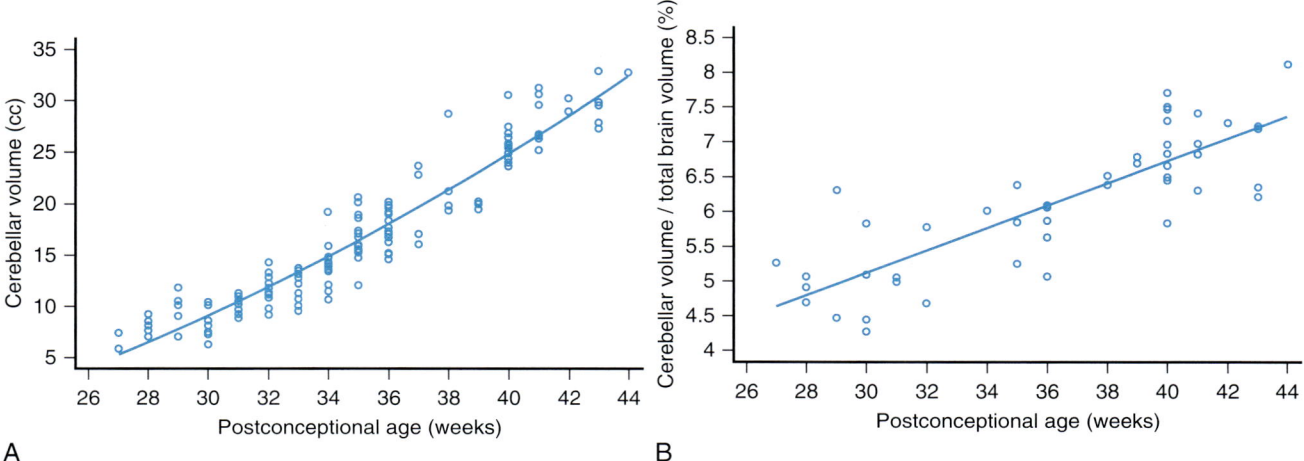

Figure 4.6 Volumetric magnetic resonance imaging studies of 169 preterm infants and 20 healthy term-born infants. Cerebellar volumetric volume (in cc) between 26 and 44 weeks (A) and cerebellar/total brain volume (%) in B. (From Limperopoulos C, Soul JS, Gauvreau K, et al. Late gestation cerebellar growth is rapid and impeded by premature birth. *Pediatrics.* 2005;115:688-695, with permission.)

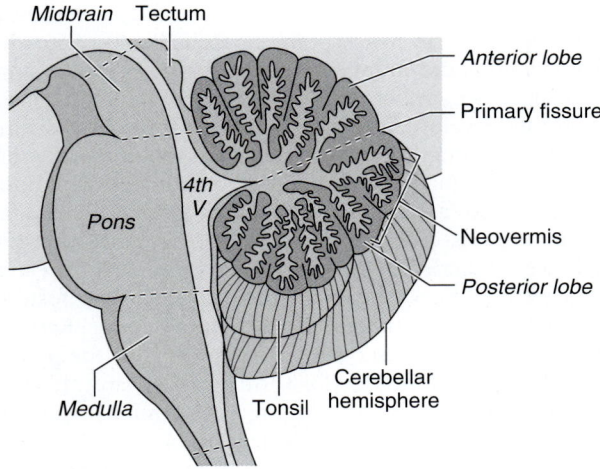

Figure 4.7 Normal mature vermis and its landmarks.

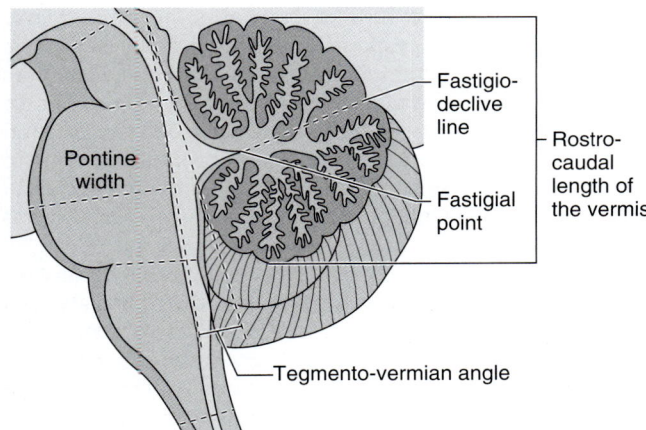

Figure 4.9 Midline sagittal landmarks of the posterior fossa.

ABNORMAL DEVELOPMENT OF THE POSTERIOR FOSSA STRUCTURES

Overview

Cerebellar malformations are diverse and extensive,[1,2,7,29] with onset in any of the major developmental events discussed earlier (Box 4.3). Because the major components of the developing cerebellum are in place by 18 to 20 weeks' gestation, most of the significant developmental lesions are now detectable during prenatal ultrasound screening, and the diagnosis confirmed by fetal or neonatal magnetic resonance imaging (MRI) testing. However, some lesions may be missed prenatally, and given their subtle or silent early postnatal clinical features, their diagnosis may be delayed. In addition, the prolonged phase of granule cell proliferation into late gestation and beyond, less severe forms of cerebellar hypoplasia may be missed by prenatal ultrasound. There is a lack of consensus about the diagnostic criteria and classification of posterior fossa malformations.

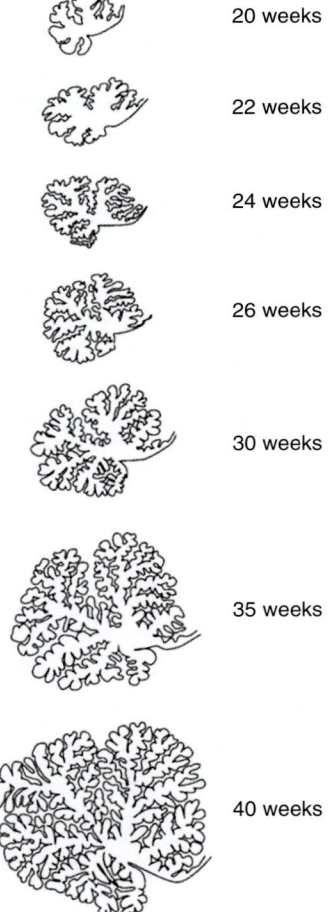

20 weeks

22 weeks

24 weeks

26 weeks

30 weeks

35 weeks

40 weeks

Figure 4.8 Growth of the cerebellar surface from 24 to 40 weeks. Drawings were made in the mid-sagittal plane. Note the extraordinary increase from 24 weeks to 40 weeks in cerebellar surface area, related primarily to increased foliation but also to increased overall cerebellar growth. (Adapted from Rakic P, Sidman RL. Histogenesis of cortical layers in human cerebellum, particularly the lamina dissecans. *J Comp Neurol.* 1970;139:473–500.)

BOX 4.3   Classification of Posterior Fossa Anomalies

Arrested Development of the Anterior Neural Tube Flexures
- *Kinked (Z-shaped) brain stem,* cerebellar hypoplasia, other brain anomalies
- Suggest arrested brain development around 7 weeks' gestation
- Some, not all, cases are in the dystroglycanopathy spectrum (e.g., Walker-Warburg syndrome)

Patterning Disorders of the Midbrain-Hindbrain Region
- Not well characterized
- Include overgrowth and undergrowth of posterior fossa structures

Developmental Disorders of the Fourth Ventricle Roof Region
- Dandy-Walker malformation
- Blake pouch cyst (persistent Blake pouch)

Disorders of Cerebellar Hemisphere and Vermis Development
- Hemispheric hypoplasia-dysplasia
- Vermis hypoplasia-dysplasia
  - Isolated vermian hypoplasia
  - Joubert syndrome–related disorders

Combined Malformations of the Midbrain-Hindbrain
- May result from patterning disorders (see above)
- Includes pontocerebellar hypoplasias
- Pontine tegmental cap dysplasia

Consistent attention to specific metrics and landmarks may lead to greater consistency in classification (Box 4.4). Some view these malformations as a continuum (Box 4.5) ranging from severe Dandy-Walker malformation (with an enlarged posterior fossa) (Figs. 4.11 and 4.12; see Box 4.5), to mild Dandy-Walker malformation (with a normal posterior fossa), Blake pouch cyst with a normal vermis (see Figs. 4.13 to 4.15; Box 4.6), isolated vermian hypoplasia (Fig. 4.16; Box 4.7), and mega cisterna magna with normal neural structures (Fig. 4.26; Box 4.12). However, this is not a uniformly accepted notion. Box 4.4 shows helpful normal landmarks for delineation of this spectrum of anomalies.

As with other regions of brain development, the earlier the onset of the disturbances in cerebellar development the more profound the subsequent deficits in development will be.

Arrested development of the anterior neural tube flexures (around 5 weeks p/c) is associated with the most fundamental malformations, leaving a *kinked brain stem* and usually major cerebellar dysgenesis (Fig. 4.10).[30] *Patterning disorders* of the hindbrain arise early, with abnormal positioning and function of the IsO (see Fig. 4.2). These lesions are currently not well characterized. Other patterning anomalies involve regional overgrowth or undergrowth of the brain stem and cerebellum (discussed later; Fig. 4.24). and are relatively rare. *Developmental disorders of the fourth ventricle roof region* include the Dandy-Walker malformation and Blake pouch cyst. The mesenchymal genes (e.g., *Foxc1*) play an important role in development of the fourth ventricular roof (see earlier) as well as in development of the meninges and skull. Therefore some authors group the developmental anomalies of the fourth ventricular roof and such lesions as mega cisterna magna (see Fig. 4.26) and arachnoid cysts (discussed later; Fig. 4.27) in the same spectrum.[3] It has been proposed that the expression of *Foxc1* dysfunction

may be related to the extent of the gene deletion, which, in turn, determines the severity of the posterior fossa anomaly.[9] These lesions are associated with *cystic* fluid collections in the posterior fossa,[9] which increases the likelihood of their detection by prenatal ultrasound surveys, making them among the more common indications for prenatal neurological counseling. *Disorders of cerebellar hemisphere and vermis development* include conditions that arise from inadequate proliferation of cells in the posterior fossa neuroepithelial zones and of

---

BOX 4.4   Important Landmarks and Metrics for Classification of Posterior Fossa Anomalies in the Fetus

Tentorium, Venous Sinuses, and Torcular Herophili
◆ Torcular Herophili is at the confluence of the major venous sinuses
◆ At the level of supraspinalis muscle insertion to occipital cranium (sagittal view)

Overall Cerebellar Size
◆ Transcerebellar diameter normal for gestational age (axial plane)[a]

Vermis Size and Development (Fig. 4.9)
◆ Rostrocaudal length of vermis normal for gestational age[a]
◆ Anterior lobe is ~50%–60% of posterior lobe (using fastigium-declive line)
◆ Fastigial point well seen
◆ Tegmento-vermian angle ≤15 degrees)
◆ Vermian foliation appropriate for gestational age

---

[a]Normative data for posterior fossa metrics are available in Barkovich AJ, Raybaud C. *Pediatric Neuroimaging.* 5th ed. Philadelphia: Lippincott, Williams, and Wilkins; 2012; Kline-Fath BM, Bulas DI, Bahado-Singh R. *Fundamental and Advanced Fetal Imaging.* Philadelphia: Wolters-Kluwer; 2015; and Timor-Tritsch IE, Monteagudo A, Pilu G, Malinger G. *Ultrasonography of the Prenatal Brain.* New York: McGraw Hill; 2012.

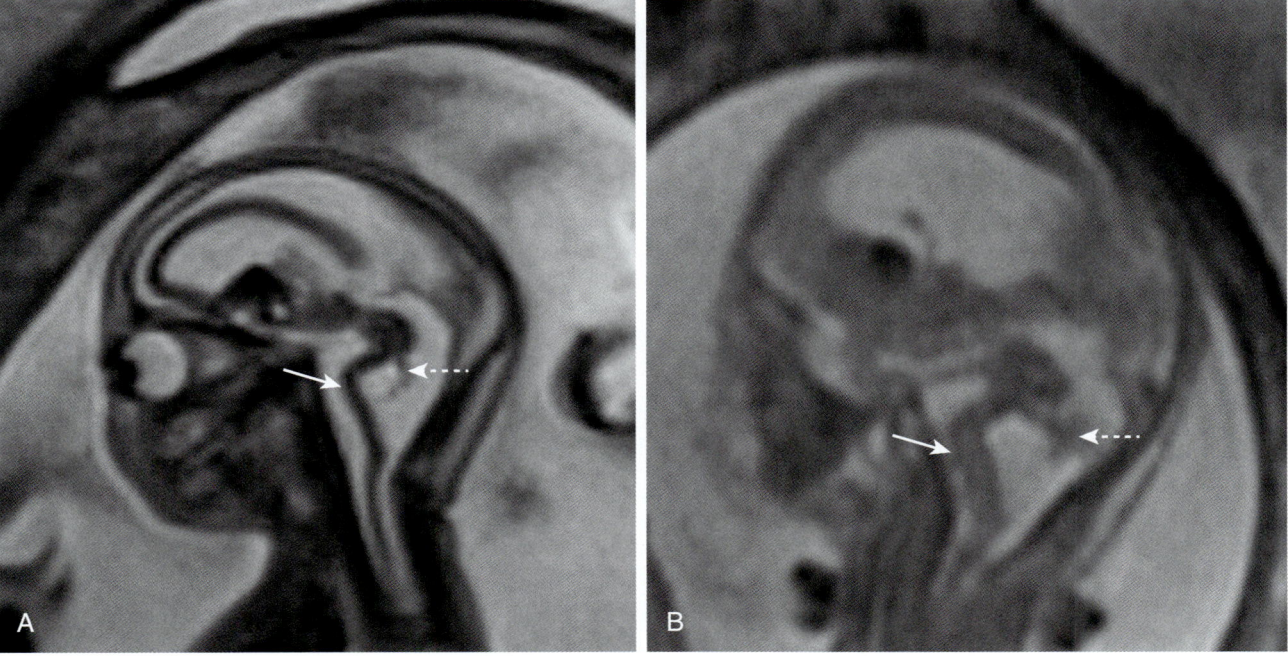

Figure 4.10 Two fetal cases with kinked brain stem with cerebellar hypoplasia. (A) and (B) Midline sagittal T2-weighted fetal magnetic resonance imaging: kinked featureless brain stem with absent ventral pons *(solid arrow),* severe cerebellar hypoplasia *(dashed arrow),* markedly hypoplastic cerebrum, and microcephaly.

their subsequent trophic support (see Fig. 4.5A–D). These disorders may result from primary disruption of proliferation in the ventricular zone, the rostral midline (vermis), and more lateral (hemispheric) rhombic lips, as well as migrational and organizational disturbances in the Purkinje cell and granule cell layers. *Foxc1* has also been shown to play an important role in the normal differentiation and migration of the rhombic lip and roof plate derivatives.[9] In addition, in Foxc1 deficient rodents there is significant expansion of the choroid plexus[9]; the resulting increase in CSF production may contribute to the cystic distention of the fourth ventricle and the development of the hydrocephalus, which often complicate Dandy-Walker malformation. Consequently, it has been suggested that defects in genes expressed solely by the cerebellar primordium result in vermian hypoplasia with or without hemispheric hypoplasia, whereas abnormal gene expression in the overlying mesenchyme results in lesions across the entire spectrum from Dandy-Walker malformation, vermian hypoplasia, and mega cisterna magna.[9]

The neurodevelopmental prognosis of rhombencephalic malformations is broad across the overall spectrum, as well as within the specific diagnostic categories.

Factors that influence outcome include the extent and topography of the lesion, associated supratentorial malformations or complications (e.g., hydrocephalus), and the presence of dysmorphic, genetic, or chromosomal syndromes. In addition, the more recent evidence for the importance of the vermis for normal cognitive-affective function has highlighted the role of vermian anomalies in the adverse outcome of rhombencephalic anomalies.[31] As discussed earlier, the AMA of the fourth ventricular roof, which normally becomes incorporated into the developing vermis, contains a neuronal population, while the PMA contains ependymal tissue but no neurons. These features may underlie the fact that children with malformations involving the AMA (Dandy-Walker malformation, vermian hypoplasia) are at higher risk for neurodevelopmental impairment than are children with PMA lesions (isolated Blake pouch cyst, mega cisterna magna) who are usually developmentally normal. In addition, the integrity of cerebellar foliation, especially of the vermis, has important prognostic value.[32]

Clinical features of rhombencephalic malformations differ in many respects from cerebellar lesions acquired later in life. Specifically, although hypotonia and motor delays are common, the classic motor signs, such as ataxia, intention tremor, nystagmus, and dysmetria, are less prominent overall. Conversely, the cognitive, affective, and behavioral consequences of early life cerebellar anomalies are now better appreciated and constitute a developmental form of the cerebellar cognitive-affective syndrome,[33] seen in older individuals with cerebellar stroke or tumor.[34] Recent studies suggest that the anatomical substrate for these *nonmotor* functions of the cerebellum is distinct closed-loop circuits, not only with the primary motor cortex, but also with many other higher cortical centers, such as the dorsolateral prefrontal cortex. The anatomical basis through which the cerebellum influences cortical activity is the ascending projections from the dentate nucleus.[28]

Specific Developmental Anomalies of the Rhombencephalon

When formulating the diagnosis of a posterior fossa anomaly, it is helpful to consider the size and configuration of specific landmarks. These are outlined in Box 4.4.

The Dandy-Walker Malformation

Anatomical Abnormality. The essential anatomical criteria for the diagnosis of Dandy-Walker malformation include (1) complete or partial agenesis of the cerebellar vermis; (2) cystic dilation of the fourth ventricle; and (3) enlargement of the posterior fossa with elevation of the tentorium, torcular Herophili, and lateral venous sinuses (see Fig. 4.11 and Box 4.5).[1-3,36,37,39,40,42-50] Although 85% of children with Dandy-Walker malformations will develop hydrocephalus by the age of 1 year (see later), this is a complication and not a diagnostic criterion. Associated central nervous system (CNS) abnormalities occur in as many as 70% of cases—the most important clinical examples being agenesis of the corpus callosum and disorders of neuronal migration (see Box 4.5). The Dandy-Walker malformation is a fundamental defect in development of the rhombencephalic roof and vermis (see Figs. 4.11 and 4.12). Abnormal rhombencephalic roof formation results from disturbances in both the AMA and PMA (see Fig. 4.12).[51] The often-massive cystic enlargement of the fourth ventricle in Dandy-Walker malformations results from a combination of failed incorporation of the AMA into the developing vermis, as well as a delay or failure in foraminal development in the PMA. Consequently, the redundant AMA billows out, possibly driven by CSF pulsations, leading to cyst formation and expansion of the posterior fossa. During development of the fourth ventricular roof, the foramen of Magendie usually opens before the foramina of Luschka. The disturbance in Dandy-Walker malformation appears to be primarily a delay or total failure of the PMA to form the foramen of Magendie (see Normal Development earlier), allowing a buildup of CSF and the development of cystic dilation of the fourth ventricle. Despite the subsequent opening of the foramina of Luschka (which are usually patent in Dandy-Walker malformation), cystic dilation of the fourth ventricle persists and CSF flow is impaired. As discussed earlier, rodent models of *Foxc1* deficiency demonstrate significant expansion of the choroid plexus,[9] which may contribute not only to the cystic distention of the fourth ventricle but also to the development of hydrocephalus. Neuropathological studies of the Dandy-Walker malformation have shown that all vermian lobules are present

---

BOX 4.5   Elements of Dandy-Walker Malformation

- Enlarged posterior fossa with elevated torcular Herophili tentorium, lateral sinuses
- Major fourth ventricle cystic distention and enlargement of tegmento-vermian angle
- Vermian hypoplasia-agenesis with absent fastigial point
- Associated anomalies
  - variable dysplasia-hypoplasia of cerebellar hemispheres
  - hydrocephalus (85%–90% by age 1 year)
  - agenesis of the corpus callosum (20%–30%)
  - inferior olivary and/or dentate anomalies (~20%)
  - cerebral neuronal heterotopias (15%)
  - occipital encephalocele (~10%–15%)
  - cerebral gyral anomalies (~10%)
  - syringomyelia (~5%–10%)
  - aqueductal stenosis (~5%–10%)
  - one or more of the above (50%–70%)
  - systemic anomalies (especially cardiac) (30%–40%)

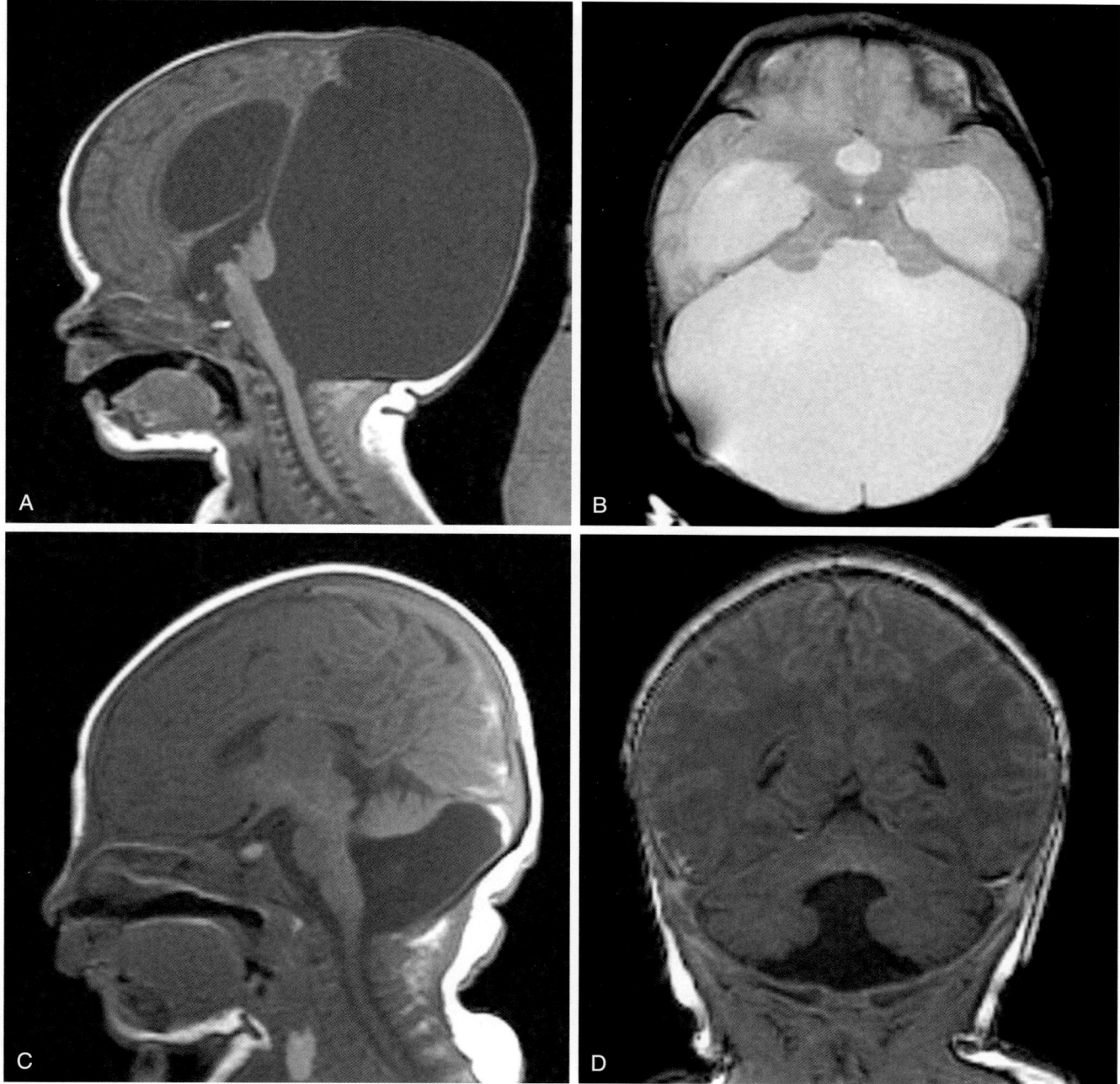

Figure 4.11 Dandy-Walker malformation. Case 1 (A and B) shows marked elevation of the tentorium and torcular Herophili, marked vermian and hemispheric hypoplasia, and hydrocephalus. Note the striking posterior bulging of the occipital cranium. Case 2 (C and D) shows mild elevation of tentorium, torcular Herophili, with milder vermian hypoplasia, relative sparing of the cerebellar hemispheres, and normal lateral ventricles.

but hypo/dysplastic, especially inferiorly, and that vermis development appears arrested at about the 12-week p/c level.[52,53] The superior-to-inferior gradient of increasing hypo/dysplasia of the vermis may result from the waning influence of the IsO with increasing distance.[54] The anomalous structures in the Dandy-Walker malformation are of rhombic lip origin, with largely normal development of the primary ventricular neuroepithelium derivatives, such as the Purkinje cells and deep cerebellar nuclei.

Timing. The timing of the development of the Dandy-Walker malformation is not entirely clear. However, the major time period of foramina development is the second and third months of gestation, that is, the peak time period of midline

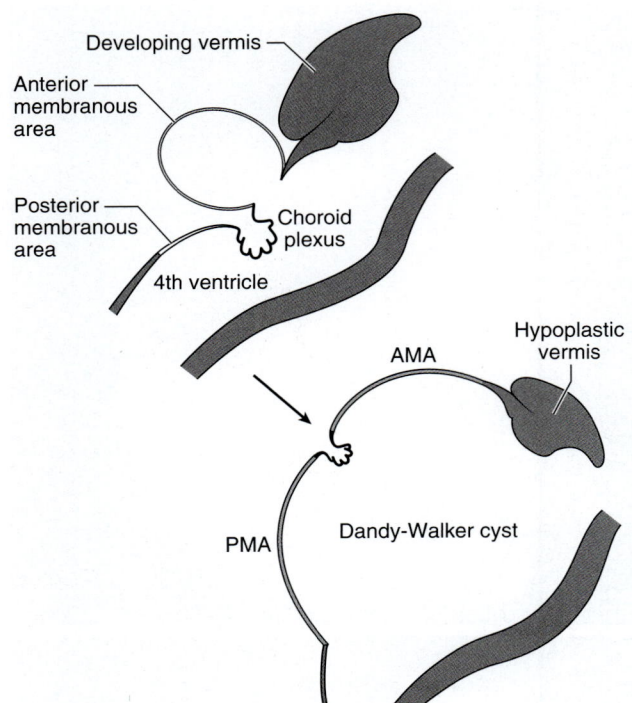

Figure 4.12 Development of the Dandy-Walker cyst. Diagram showing dorsal view of the rhombencephalon.

TABLE 4.1	Dandy-Walker Malformation: Outcome[a]	
TIME OF DIAGNOSIS	**MORTALITY (%)[b]**	**SUBNORMAL INTELLIGENCE (% OF SURVIVORS)**
Prenatal or newborn	38	75
After newborn period	10	25

[a]See text for references.
[b]Often related to systemic anomalies.

prosencephalic development (see Chapter 2).[1,55] This time period also overlaps that of neuronal migration (Chapter 6). Thus agenesis of the corpus callosum and defects of neuronal migration are not unexpected as important accompaniments to the Dandy-Walker malformation (see Box 4.5).

Clinical Aspects. The postnatal clinical spectrum of the Dandy-Walker malformation is difficult to define decisively from published writings because of inconsistent diagnostic criteria and inclusion of additional conditions. For example, in one series (*n* = 50) of fetal cases, karyotype (when available) was abnormal in 46%.[50] Moreover, the Dandy-Walker malformation is a feature of many syndromes, including Rubinstein-Taybi, Meckel-Gruber, Coffin-Siris, Ellis-van Creveld, and Smith-Lemli-Optiz, among a number of others, many of which are autosomal recessive traits. Nevertheless, certain clinical aspects are consistent.[29,36,39,50]

The *dominant clinical feature* in early infancy is the occurrence of hydrocephalus, with a striking occipital prominence to the cranium and a large cystic dilation of the fourth ventricle, enlarging the posterior fossa (see Fig. 4.11; Box 4.5). However, pronounced hydrocephalus in the neonatal period is present in only a minority of cases. Nevertheless, because of widespread prenatal and neonatal ultrasonography, more cases now are identified in utero and in the neonatal period, despite the absence of a rapidly enlarging head and overt signs of increased intracranial pressure. By 3 months, approximately 75% of cases exhibit hydrocephalus, and ultimately 90% or more have hydrocephalus. Indeed, in some cases of Dandy-Walker malformation, hydrocephalus may not develop until adulthood.

Other important clinical features include the accompanying anomalies of CNS and extraneural structures (see Box 4.5).

Systemic anomalies are present in approximately 30% to 40% of cases, and include serious cardiac and urinary tract defects.

Prognosis. Prognosis of the Dandy-Walker malformation is highly variable and related to the severity both of the malformation and the presence of associated cerebral and extracerebral anomalies, as well as the degree of hydrocephalus (Table 4.1). The degree of vermian hypo/dysplasia appears to play an important role in the long-term neurological outcome. Specifically, if anomalous brain development is confined to the posterior fossa, then the primary prognostic factor is lobulation of the vermis, with size of the cystic lesion and posterior fossa being largely irrelevant. Disturbances in vermis lobulation appear to be correlated with the intellectual impairment seen in about half of Dandy-Walker malformation cases.[32]

The severity of these features, in turn, is reflected in the usual time of diagnosis as shown in Table 4.1. For cases identified in utero or in the neonatal period, the outcome has been generally unfavorable—nearly 40% die, and 75% of survivors exhibit cognitive deficits. *However, the most fundamental determinants of outcome are the associated neural and extraneural anomalies, and if these can be excluded by imaging studies, the outcome is markedly better.*

Management. Management of the Dandy-Walker malformation is largely conservative unless significant hydrocephalus or compression effects of the posterior fossa cyst develop. Management is complicated by the presence of the cystic dilation of the fourth ventricle and by the generalized ventriculomegaly.[39,42,43] Hydrocephalus is traditionally managed by CSF diversion techniques, such as ventriculoperitoneal shunt. Direct unroofing of the fourth ventricular cyst in general is not effective.[42] Other approaches, including endoscopic third ventriculostomy with choroid plexus cauterization,[56] as well as cyst-peritoneal shunts and stents between the third ventricle and cyst, have been used.[57] Fourth ventricle shunts theoretically would be effective if the aqueduct were freely patent. Unfortunately, in Dandy-Walker malformation, the aqueduct functionally does not allow adequate flow of CSF, and thus the preferred approach is to shunt both the cyst and the lateral ventricle at the same time, connecting the two catheters by a Y-connector to the peritoneal catheter.[43] Some neurosurgeons prefer to place a ventriculoperitoneal shunt first and to later add a shunt of the posterior fossa cyst if the former shunt is not effective.[42]

The Dandy-Walker Variant

Other posterior fossa anomalies may contain elements of the Dandy-Walker malformation (see Box 4.5), such as vermian hypoplasia, fourth ventricular enlargement, or increased posterior fossa fluid spaces. The term Dandy-Walker variant has emerged to include these cases, although the existence of this as a distinct entity remains controversial. Unfortunately, the term has become the default diagnosis for a broad spectrum of posterior fossa lesions, leading to inconsistency in classification and prognostication. Consequently, use of the term Dandy-Walker variant should be discouraged. Given their significantly better prognosis, every effort should be made to distinguish conditions, such as mega cisterna magna, vermian hypoplasia, and Blake pouch cyst (see later) from the Dandy-Walker malformation. Typically, the term Dandy-Walker variant has been used when there is agenesis/hypoplasia of vermis (distinguishing it from a Blake pouch cyst), with cystic enlargement of the fourth ventricle and rotation of vermis (distinguishing it from mega cisterna magna), but with a normally sited torcular Herophili and tentorium, that is, a normal-sized posterior fossa. Previous descriptions of the Dandy-Walker variant have rarely included the development of hydrocephalus.

Blake Pouch Cyst (see Box 4.6)

Blake pouch cyst is a usually benign normal variant, which is now increasingly detected by prenatal ultrasound and MRI. As such, it frequently enters into the differential diagnosis of other posterior fossa lesions with enlarged fourth ventricles and increased fluid spaces (Box 4.11). It is likely that the vast majority of these lesions previously went undetected; therefore their natural history remains relatively undefined. There is, as yet, no consistent terminology about when the normal *pouch*

BOX 4.6   Diagnostic Criteria for a Blake Pouch Cyst

◆ Fourth ventricular enlargement
◆ Mild-moderate rotation of a normally formed vermis
◆ Widening of the tegmento-vermian angle
◆ Torcular Herophili and tentorium normally positioned
◆ Normal-sized posterior fossa
◆ *Tuft* of choroid plexus in the roof of the cyst (may need contrast)

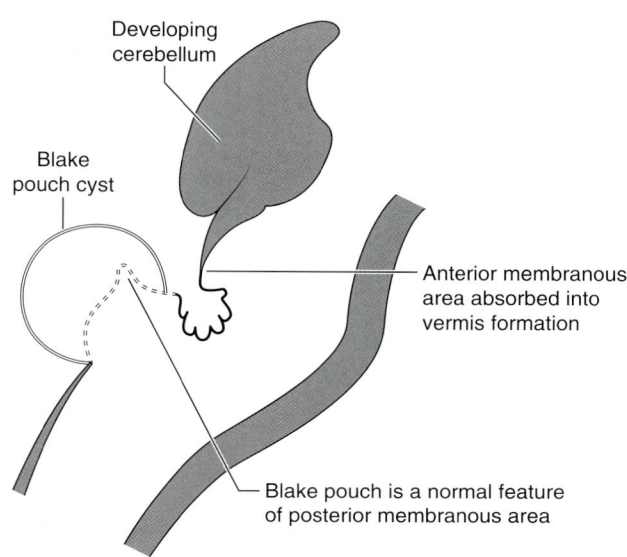

Figure 4.13 Blake pouch is a normal feature of posterior membranous area. Failure or delay of the foramen Magendie to open leads to cyst formation.

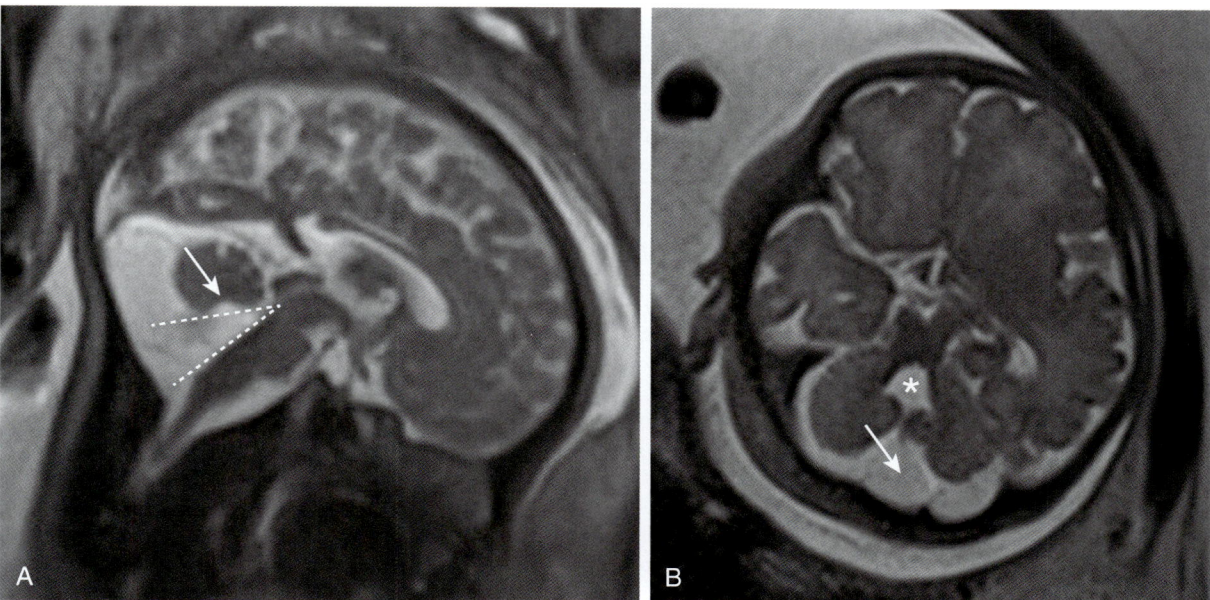

Figure 4.14 Blake pouch cyst. Fetal magnetic resonance imaging (T2-weighted) at 37 weeks' gestation. (A) Midline sagittal view showing enlarged fourth ventricle and widened tegmento-vermian angle *(dotted lines)*. Notable normal features include the size and lobulation of the vermis, torcular Herophili location, cerebellar hemispheres and brain stem, and fastigial point *(arrow)*. (B) Axial view showing enlarged fourth ventricle *(star)* with cystic lesion *(arrow)* in continuity.

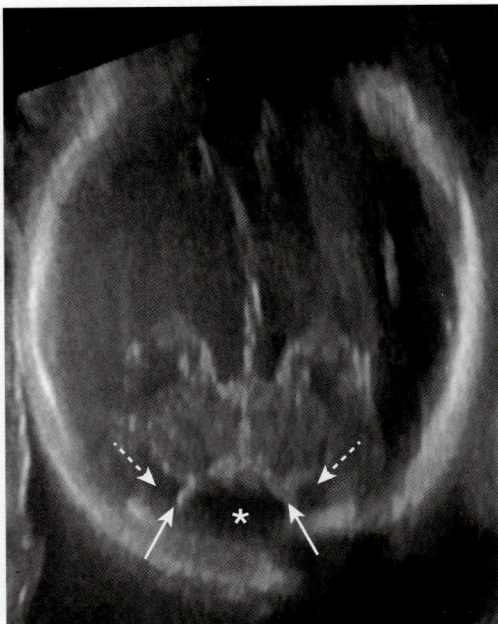

Figure 4.15 Blake pouch cyst. Fetal ultrasound axial view in a 23-week old fetus showing the septa (*solid arrows*) of the Blake pouch (*asterisk*) with the subarachnoid space on both sides (*dashed lines*). The Blake pouch cerebrospinal fluid space is usually more echolucent than the adjacent subarachnoid space, which is bridged by pial-arachnoid septations.

becomes a *cyst* and when the lesion is considered *persistent*. In this chapter, we will use the term Blake pouch cyst rather than persistent Blake pouch.

Anatomical Abnormality. The membranous roof of the fourth ventricle consists of an internal ependymal layer and an outer pial layer. Blake pouch[58] is a normal transient dorsal evagination of the fourth ventricle ependymal lining through the midline foramen of Magendie in the pial layer (see Fig. 4.13).[59] Failure or delay in perforation of the pouch leads to enlargement of the fourth ventricle, with elevation of a structurally normal vermis increasing the tegmento-vermian angle (see Figs. 4.14 and 4.15). In the subarachnoid space, the pouch forms a cyst dorsal and inferior to the vermis.[60] By fetal ultrasound (Fig. 4.15), the walls of a Blake pouch may be visible on axial views through the posterior fossa. The cyst is an extension of the fourth ventricle and is filled with clear CSF giving it a hypoechoic ultrasound appearance compared to the adjacent subarachnoid spaces (see Fig. 4.15).

Timing. Normally around 9 to 10 weeks p/c, perforation of the Blake pouch allows communication between the fourth ventricle and the subarachnoid space. More than half of Blake pouch cysts have resolved spontaneously by 24 to 26 weeks' gestation, and almost two-thirds resolve by term (presumably by delayed fenestration of the cyst), allowing the vermis to resume its normal position.[60]

Clinical Aspects. The Blake pouch cyst is usually asymptomatic with a benign long-term outcome. Diagnosis is usually incidental during fetal screening or postnatal imaging for other concerns. One of the principal clinical challenges is to distinguish the Blake pouch cyst from the Dandy-Walker malformation. Delayed, partial, or absent development of the fourth ventricular foramina plays a role in both conditions. However, these entities differ in several fundamental ways. First, the primary origin of these lesions and their cystic components are in different regions of the fourth ventricular roof. The Dandy-Walker malformation originates primarily from a developmental defect of the AMA (with contribution from delayed or failed PMA fenestration) (see Figs. 4.3 and 4.12). Specifically, the AMA fails to merge with the overlying vermis, and instead balloons out as a large cyst. Conversely, a Blake pouch cyst results from failure of ependymal perforation in the PMA (see Figs. 4.3 and 4.13). Second, although not easily seen with conventional imaging, identifying the fourth ventricle choroid plexus along the inferior surface of the vermis and the roof of the cyst is a useful diagnostic sign of a Blake pouch cyst. In the Dandy-Walker malformation, the choroid plexus is positioned in the floor of the cyst. Identifying the location of the choroid plexus may be difficult without a postnatal MRI using a contrast agent. Third, the majority of Blake pouch cysts resolve spontaneously (see earlier),[60] while spontaneous resolution of the Dandy-Walker malformation cyst does not occur. Fourth, a large majority of Dandy-Walker malformations are eventually associated with hydrocephalus. While hydrocephalus—even tetraventricular hydrocephalus—may complicate Blake pouch cysts, this is an unusual development. Unlike the Dandy-Walker malformation, Blake pouch cyst is not associated with elevation of the tentorium and torcular Herophili. Some authors consider Blake pouch cyst, Dandy-Walker variant, and mega cisterna magna part of the same spectrum, differing only in the degree and timing of cyst fenestration.[61]

Prognosis. Isolated Blake pouch cysts that are not complicated by hydrocephalus have an excellent neurodevelopmental prognosis. The outcome of more complex cases in which a Blake pouch cyst occurs in association with other cerebral or extra-cerebral conditions is determined primarily by the associated condition.

Management. Isolated Blake pouch cysts that persist rarely require active intervention. Rare cases in which significant hydrocephalus develops may warrant CSF diversion procedures.

Developmental Anomalies of the Vermis and Hemispheres
Vermian Hypoplasia (see Fig. 4.16; Box 4.7)
As discussed previously, the vermis reaches its full craniocaudal extent by 18 weeks',[24] and possibly as late as 24 weeks',[25] gestation. In one study,[62] vermian hypoplasia diagnosed before 24 weeks' gestation *resolved* by term gestation in 50% of cases, whereas those diagnosed after 24 weeks' gestation were all confirmed postnatally. The diagnosis of inferior

BOX 4.7   Diagnostic Criteria for Vermian Hypoplasia
◆ Craniocaudal and transverse extent < expected for gestational age
◆ Usually anterior:posterior lobe ratio is <1:3
◆ Fastigial point is usually present
◆ If inferior lobe is hypoplastic, tegmento-vermian angle may appear enlarged
◆ Torcular Herophili and tentorium normally positioned
◆ Normal sized posterior fossa

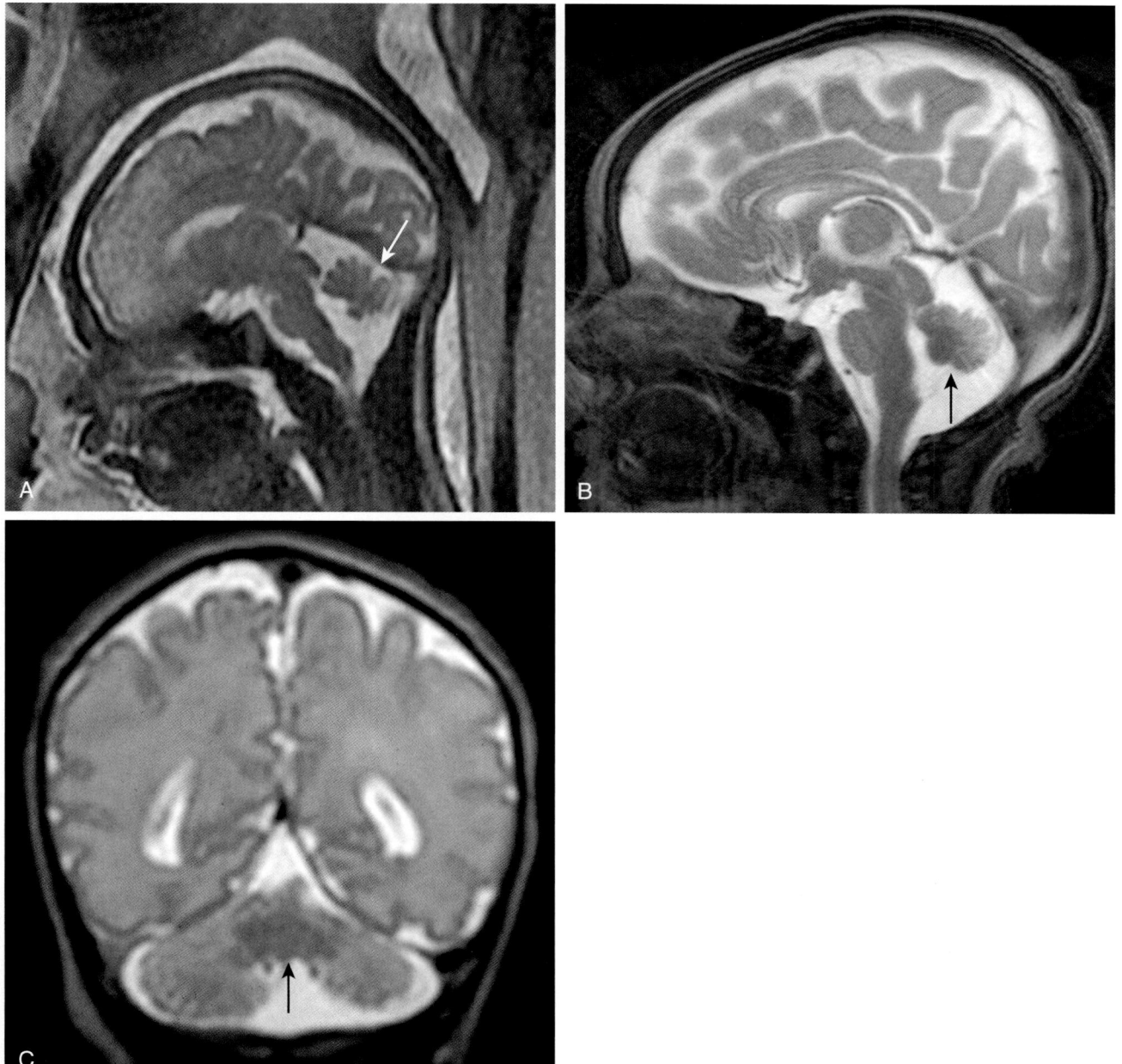

Figure 4.16 Vermian hypoplasia. MRI T2-weighted (A) Fetal MRI midline sagittal view showing primary fissure *(white arrow)*, normal anterior lobe, and hypoplastic posterior lobe. (B) Fetal MRI midline sagittal view showing vermian hypoplasia *(black arrow)*. (C) Neonatal MRI coronal view showing vermian hypoplasia/dysplasia *(black arrow)*.

vermian hypoplasia has become controversial. Because the vermis develops in a rostrocaudal direction, vermian hypoplasia usually gives the impression of failed development of the inferior leading edge. However, the inferior lobules actually develop first, and the arrested downward growth of the vermis is likely due, in most cases, to growth failure of the later-forming neovermis, located just caudal to the primary fissure (see earlier and Fig. 4.7). Even by fetal MRI it is difficult to distinguish the different vermian lobules until late gestation. Therefore unless the specific region of hypoplasia can be identified, the general term, vermian hypoplasia,

should be used. Vermian hypoplasia may be an associated finding in syndromes, such as the Joubert syndrome–related disorders.

The Joubert Syndrome–Related Disorders and the Molar Tooth Malformation

Anatomical Abnormality (Box 4.8). The *anatomical features* of the brain in these disorders commonly include the molar tooth sign, which describes the features on axial MRI at the midbrain-pontine junction (Figs. 4.17B and 4.18B). The molar tooth malformation picture results from the small, dysplastic vermis, with elongated, thick, and horizontally oriented (uncrossed) superior cerebellar peduncles (see Figs. 4.17A and 4.18A), a triangular (*bat-wing* shaped) fourth ventricle, a deep interpeduncular fossa, and variable cerebellar hemispheric findings. Additional anatomical findings include dysplasias and heterotopias of the roof nuclei, the absence of decussation of the superior cerebellar peduncles (and the pyramidal and pontine tracts), multiple brain stem nuclear abnormalities, and thinning of the pontomesencephalic junction.[1] A fundamental mechanism for this appearance relates to disturbed axonal guidance affecting midline crossing of the superior cerebellar peduncles and corticospinal tracts, although corpus callosum development is normal in the vast majority.

Clinical Aspects and Prognosis. The *clinical features* in the neonatal period most commonly include paroxysmal episodes

---

BOX 4.8   Diagnostic Criteria for Joubert Syndrome

The Molar Tooth Sign (Axial Magnetic Resonance Imaging at the Midbrain-Pontine Junction) Consists of:
◆ Small, dysplastic vermis
◆ Elongated, thick, horizontally oriented (uncrossed) superior cerebellar peduncles
◆ A triangular (*bat-wing* shaped) fourth ventricle
◆ A deep interpeduncular fossa
◆ Thinning of the pontomesencephalic junction.[1]

Associated Findings
◆ Variable cerebellar hemispheric anomalies
◆ Dysplasias and heterotopias of the roof nuclei
◆ Absent decussation of superior cerebellar peduncles, pyramidal, and pontine tracts
◆ Multiple brain stem nuclear abnormalities

---

of apnea-tachypnea, hypotonia, and an unusual craniofacial appearance (prominent forehead, high rounded eyebrows, epicanthal folds, upturned nose, and an open mouth).[2,63-65] The respiratory disturbance usually improves spontaneously over the ensuing weeks and months. Abnormal eye movements and nystagmus (*jerky* eye movements) may be apparent in the neonatal period and be replaced months later by the more characteristic oculomotor apraxia. Ataxia and cognitive deficits become apparent later. In one large series ($n = 29$) 40% attended regular school, albeit with prominent speech difficulties, and 60% had more overt cognitive disability.[65] The spectrum of cognitive developm ent is broad, ranging from apparently normal function to severe impairment.[2,63-74]

Descriptions of additional clusters of clinical features associated with the earlier phenotype led to broader designation of *Joubert syndrome and related disorders* (JSRD).[68,69] These additional clinical features include renal disease, ocular findings (retinal dystrophy, colobomas), hepatic fibrosis, oral hamartomas, occipital encephaloceles, oral-facial-digital abnormalities, hypothalamic hamartomas, and endocrine anomalies.

The JSRD spectrum has an autosomal recessive inheritance pattern. To date, more than 25 gene mutations have been implicated in JSRD.[75-77] Most of these genes are linked to primary cilia and their function, with their mutations resulting in so-called ciliopathies. It is known that the primary cilia mediate the signaling pathways that are involved in early fusion of the cerebellar anlagen.[77-79] Most animals and human postmortem studies suggest that reduced proliferation of granule cells, possibly due to impaired *Shh* signaling, is an important cause.[68,80,81] The gene mutations differ primarily in their associated systemic findings. Thus, by far the best studied mutation is *JBTS3*, which is clinically characterized by the features noted earlier as well as cerebral abnormalities,

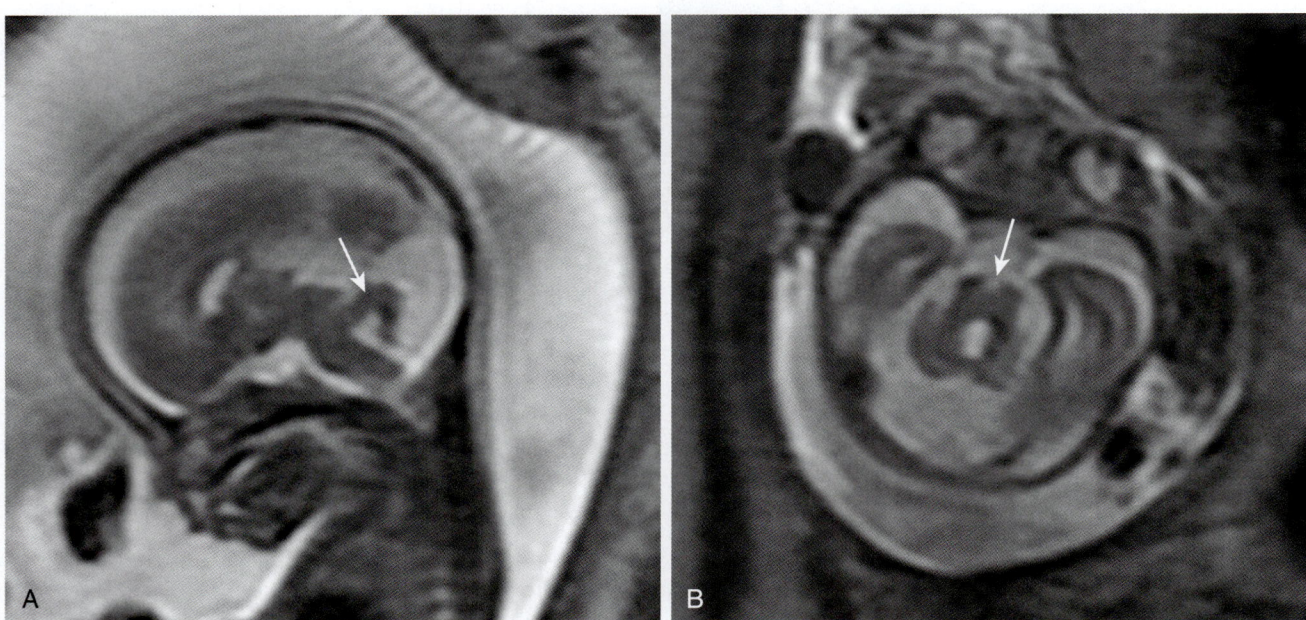

Figure 4.17 Joubert syndrome in a fetus. Fetal magnetic resonance imaging T2-weighted. (A) Sagittal view showing thick horizontally aligned superior cerebellar peduncle (*arrow*) and hypoplastic vermis. (B) Axial view and molar tooth sign with deep interpeduncular cleft (*arrow*).

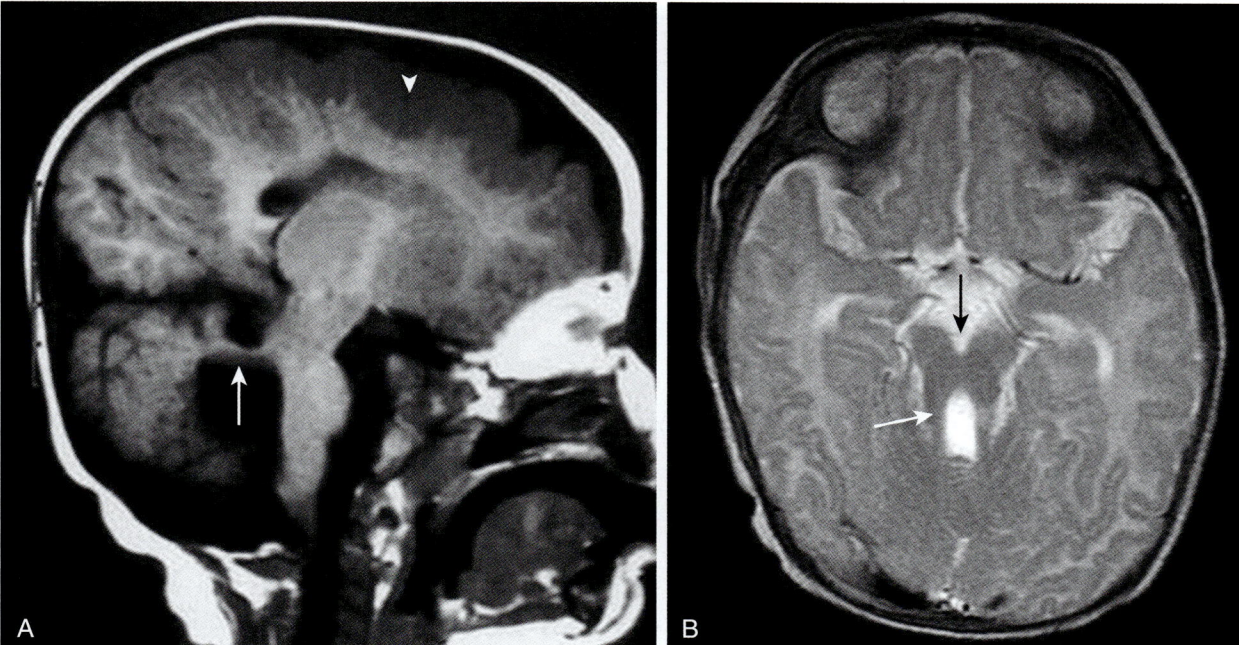

Figure 4.18 Joubert syndrome with extensive frontoparietal polymicrogyria. (A) Sagittal view magnetic resonance imaging (MRI) T1-weighted showing thickened and horizontally displaced superior cerebellar peduncle *(arrow)*, vermian hypo/dysplasia, and cerebral polymicrogyria *(arrowhead)*. (B) Axial T2-weighted MRI showing the *molar tooth sign* with a deep interpeduncular cleft *(black arrow)* with thickened superior cerebellar peduncles *(white arrow)*.

for example, polymicrogyria (see Fig. 4.18), corpus callosum abnormalities, and seizures.[68,69] The gene involved is *AHI1*, encoding the Jouberin protein, a presumed signaling molecule expressed in embryonic hindbrain and forebrain.[69,74] The developmental defect involves cerebral, brain stem, and cerebellar development, perhaps at the levels of patterning, migration, and axon pathfinding.

Rhombencephalosynapsis

Anatomical Abnormality. This rare disorder is characterized by agenesis or hypoplasia of the vermis (Box 4.9),[1,63,82-86] with *fusion* of the cerebellar hemispheres, superior cerebellar peduncles, and midline continuity of the deep cerebellar nuclei. The superior vermis is consistently absent, and the *fusion* of the hemispheres is partial (20%) or complete (80%) (Figs. 4.19 and 4.20). The anatomical features are best identified by postnatal MRI (see Fig. 4.19). The vermian agenesis and dorsal fusion of the cerebellar hemispheres are striking. Because of the fusion of the dentate nuclei, the posterior fourth ventricle has a pointed appearance, sometimes referred to as a *keyhole* (see Fig. 4.19A) or *diamond* shape on axial MRI views. Typically, the transversely oriented cerebellar folia extend across the midline uninterrupted by the vermis (see Fig. 4.19B). Ventriculomegaly is present in 80% of reported cases, often with features of aqueductal stenosis (see Fig. 4.20). A wide range of brain anomalies, often midline, are associated with rhombencephalosynapsis, including the absence of the septum pellucidum, and abnormalities of the corpus callosum, which occur in 60% to 70%. In addition, the association with holoprosencephaly, and with fused thalami and fornices, suggests a disturbance in dorsal-ventral patterning.

BOX 4.9   Diagnostic Criteria for Rhombencephalosynapsis

- Agenesis (especially superior) or hypoplasia of the vermis
- *Fusion* of the cerebellar hemispheres—partial (20%); complete (80%)
- Fusion of the dentate nuclei
- Caudal fourth ventricle has a pointed *keyhole* or *diamond* shape sometimes (axial magnetic resonance imaging views)
- Transversely oriented cerebellar folia extend uninterrupted across the midline
- Associated findings
  - aqueductal stenosis
  - ventriculomegaly (80%)
- Other midline brain anomalies
  - absence of the septum pellucidum
  - abnormalities of the corpus callosum (60%–70%)
  - holoprosencephaly, fused thalami, and fornices

Clinical Findings and Prognosis. The postnatal clinical features are usually delayed in onset. However, diagnosis is now most commonly made by fetal MRI after detection by fetal ultrasound screening of other features, such as ventriculomegaly. Most cases have some degree of neurodevelopmental impairment, but the range is very broad and often delayed in detection until later in infancy and childhood. Deficits range from mild truncal ataxia and normal cognitive abilities to severe cerebellar deficits, cerebral palsy, and intellectual disability. Progressive ventricular dilation has resulted in shunt placement in approximately 30% of cases.

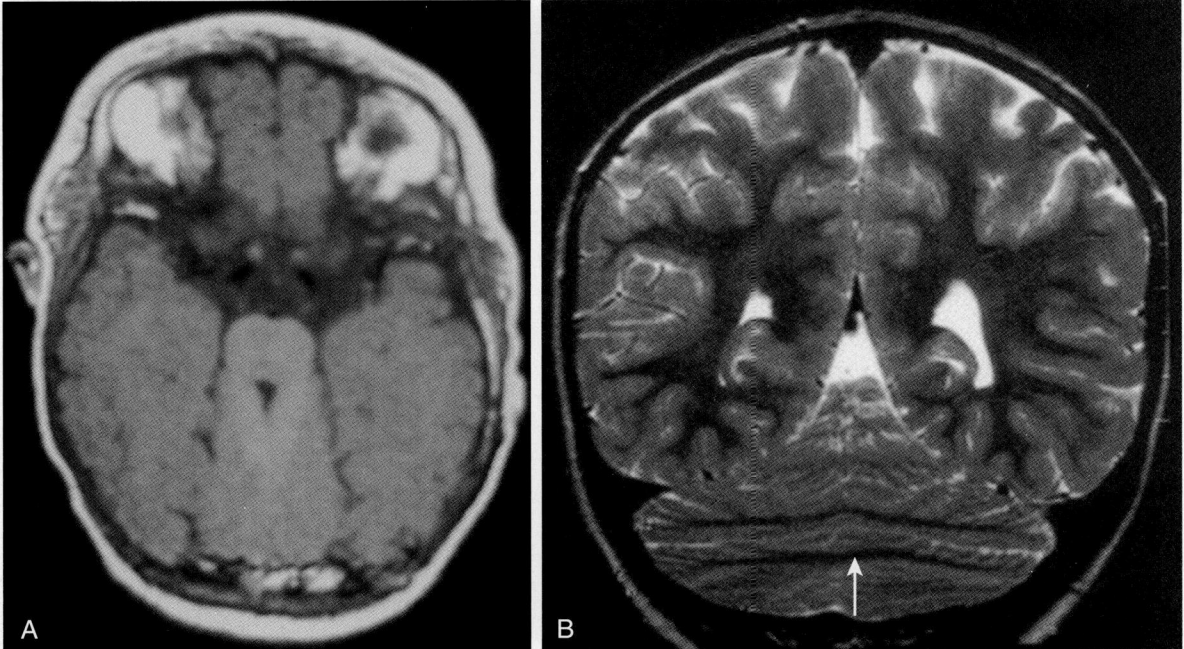

Figure 4.19 Rhombencephalosynapsis (A) Axial T1-weighted magnetic resonance imaging (MRI) study showing *fused* cerebellar hemispheres without vermis. (B) Coronal T2-weighted MRI showing absent vermis, *fused* cerebellar hemispheres with horizontal folial pattern crossing the midline *(arrow)*.

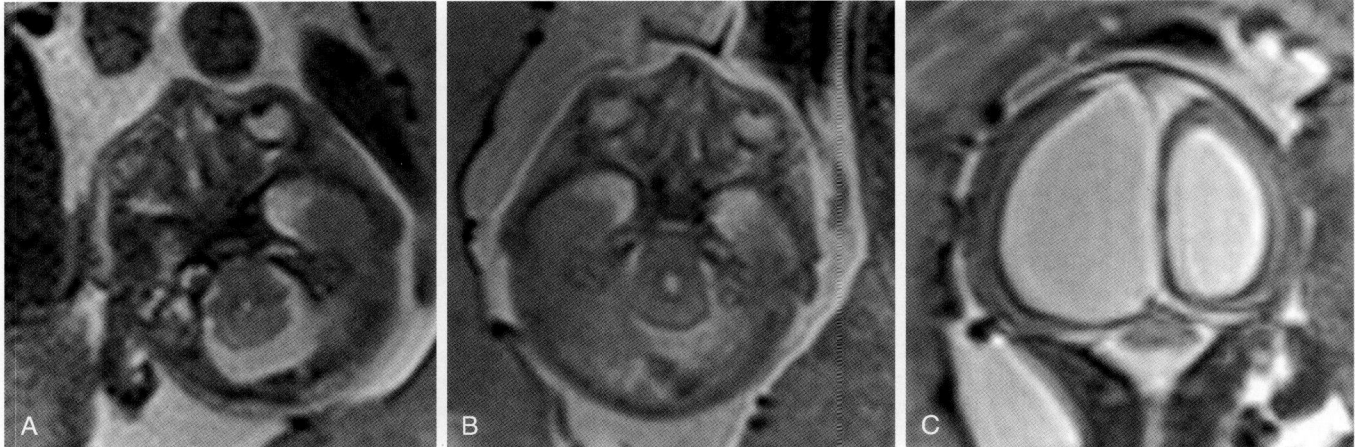

Figure 4.20 Rhombencephalosynapsis in a fetus with aqueductal stenosis and severe hydrocephalus. Fetal magnetic resonance imaging T2-weighted axial views (A and B) and coronal view (C) showing small cerebellar volume, absence of vermis and separate hemispheres, and major lateral ventricle distention.

Malformations of the Cerebellar Hemispheres

Anomalous development of the cerebellar hemispheres may result from hypoplasia, dysplasia, or disruption. It is uncommon for cerebellar hemispheric hypoplasia to be more prominent than that of the vermis, but this may be seen in the pontocerebellar hypoplasias (PCH) (see later; Fig. 4.23), or following fetal-onset insults (e.g., hemorrhage or infection) (Figs. 4.21 and 4.25). Cases of unilateral cerebellar hypoplasia are more commonly due to developmental disruptions (e.g., hemorrhage or infection) than primary dysgenesis (see Figs. 4.21 and 4.25). The two proliferative regions contribute unequal cell numbers to the

future cerebellum, the rhombic lip-derived population being far larger than that from the primary ventricular neuroepithelium. However, as discussed previously, the Purkinje cell layer (of ventricular zone origin) provides critical trophic support and stimulation (*Shh* expression)[88] for granule cell precursors (of rhombic lip origin) during their period of massive proliferation in the overlying external granular layer (see Fig. 4.5). Therefore cerebellar hypoplasia may result from impaired neuronal proliferation in either of the two major germinal zones (see Fig. 4.5A). Because granule cell proliferation continues through late gestation and into postnatal life, cerebellar hypoplasia may manifest late in development.[89] Cerebellar hypoplasia

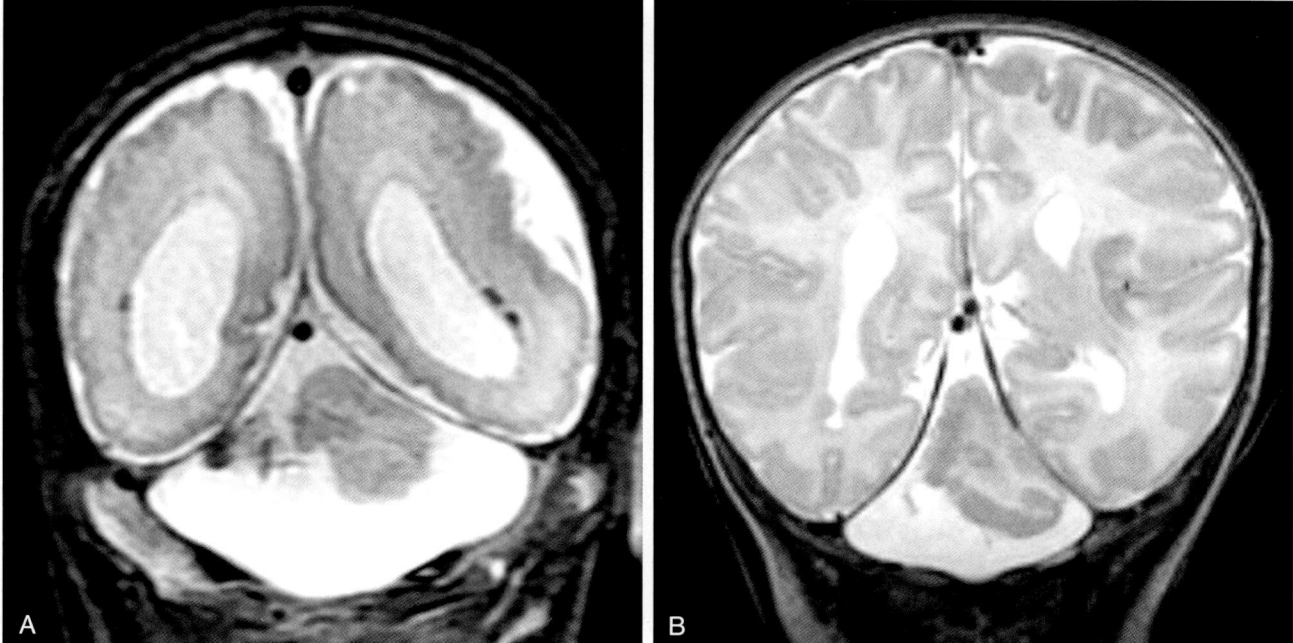

Figure 4.21 Unilateral cerebellar hypoplasia with dysplasia. (A) Coronal T2-weighted magnetic resonance imaging (MRI) showing evidence of cytomegalovirus (CMV)-encephalitis with periventricular calcifications and destructive disruptive changes in the cerebellum. (B) Coronal T2-weighted MRI showing unilateral absence of one cerebellar hemisphere and dysplastic changes in the remaining cerebellar tissue of unknown etiology.

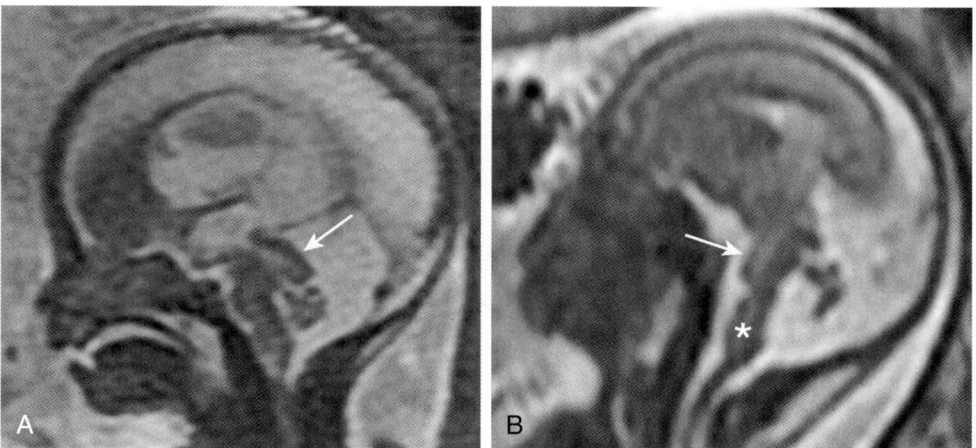

Figure 4.22 Combined midbrain-hindbrain malformations. Fetal T2-weighted magnetic resonance imaging studies. (A) Midline sagittal view with markedly abnormal and overgrown tectum *(arrow)*, with vermian hypoplasia, and severe hydrocephalus. (B) Midline sagittal view showing flat ventral pons *(arrow)*, thick medulla *(asterisk)*, and vermian hypoplasia.

resulting from *Shh* signaling defects affects the vermis and hemispheric development equally, while earlier IsO defects (see earlier) cause disproportionate vermis hypoplasia. Normal migration and organization of the Purkinje cell layer is essential for supporting later granule cell proliferation. The Bergmann glia, which originate in the ventricular zone, are responsible for guiding the migration of the Purkinje cells to their destinations. As a result, genetic mutations that disrupt normal cerebellar neuronal migration (such as *reelin* mutations) are known to cause cerebellar hypoplasia.

Combined Malformations of the Midbrain-Hindbrain

As discussed earlier, the cerebellum and certain brain stem structures share common developmental origins. Therefore it is not surprising that developmental anomalies may involve both the brain stem and the cerebellum, and lesions in the cerebellum warrant careful examination of the brain stem structures, and vice versa. As a general rule, cerebellar anomalies that have associated brain stem lesions have a significantly worse prognosis.[62] One such group of conditions is the PCH.

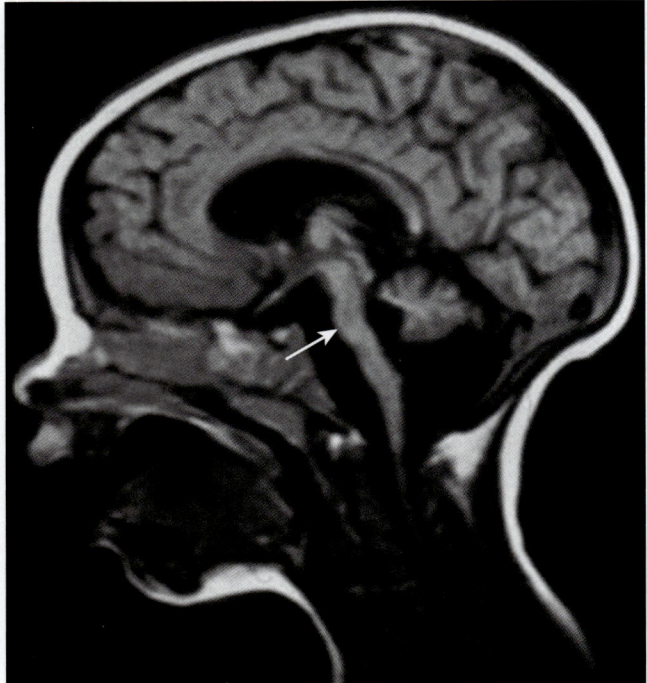

Figure 4.23 Pontocerebellar hypoplasia. T1-weighted magnetic resonance imaging midline sagittal view showing minimal ventral pons (*arrow*) with vermian hypoplasia. (From Barth PG. Pontocerebellar hypoplasias. An overview of a group of inherited neurodegenerative disorders with fetal onset. *Brain Dev.* 1993;15:411-422. With permission.)

Pontocerebellar Hypoplasias (Box 4.10; Table 4.2)

This spectrum of autosomal recessive anomalies is characterized by a small pons and varying degrees of cerebellar defect (see Fig. 4.22), and even near total absence.[90-92] Currently, 10 forms have been described, based on their clinical, imaging, and pathology findings (see Chapter 29). Some of these forms, such as types 5 and 6, are extremely rare. In PCH, the degree of vermian and hemispheric hypoplasia is similar. The two major forms are PCH1 and PCH2. All forms of PCH have some degree of supratentorial brain involvement, and microcephaly, although uncommon at birth, is a common late finding. In addition to hypoplasia of the pons (not invariable) and cerebellum (primarily Purkinje cell involvement), PCH1 also has prominent anterior horn cell degeneration, resulting in bulbar dysfunction, which manifests in the fetal period as polyhydramnios, and later contributes to the respiratory and feeding complications that lead to early death, usually before 1 year of age. About half of PCH1 cases are associated with EXOSC3 gene mutations, with TSEN54 mutations being seen in others. These infants are usually hypotonic at birth with poor feeding, and some have

---

BOX 4.10   Pontocerebellar Hypoplasias

- ◆ Spectrum of degenerative reductions in size of cerebellum and pons
- ◆ Cerebellar hemispheres more affected than vermis
- ◆ Dragonfly appearance on magnetic resonance imaging (flattened cerebellar hemispheres represent the wings, and preserved vermis represents the body)
- ◆ Associated supratentorial anomalies
  - ◆ neocortical atrophy, ventriculomegaly, and microcephaly
  - ◆ most common gene mutations are TSEN2, TSEN34, and RARS2.

TABLE 4.2   Pontocerebellar Hypoplasias

TYPE	GENE MUTATIONS	CLINICAL FEATURES
PCH1	*VRK1; EXOSC3*	Infantile onset anterior horn cell degeneration resulting in progressive muscle atrophy; resembles infantile spinal muscular atrophy.
		Cerebellar neuronal degeneration beginning at birth and resulting in decreased body tone, respiratory insufficiency, muscle atrophy, progressive microcephaly, and global developmental delay
PCH2	*TSEN54; TSEN2; TSEN34; SEPSECS; VPS53*	Profound mental retardation, progressive microcephaly, spasticity, and early-onset epilepsy
PCH3	*CLAM*	Seizures, short stature, optic atrophy, progressive microcephaly, and severe developmental delay
PCH4	*TSEN54*	Severe prenatal form of PCH2 with polyhydramnios, muscle contractures, brief involuntary muscle twitching, brief apneas, and early death
PCH5	*TSEN54*	Severe prenatal form, described in one family
PCH6	*RARS2*	Severe neonatal encephalopathy with hypotonia, intractable seizures, edema, increased lactate blood levels, and mitochondrial respiratory chain defects
PCH7	Unknown	Hypotonia, apneic episodes, seizures, and vanishing testes
PCH8	*CHMP1A*	Severe psychomotor retardation, dyskinesias, hypotonia, spasticity, and visual defects
PCH9	*AMPD2*	Severely delayed psychomotor development, progressive microcephaly, spasticity, seizures, cerebral atrophy, thin corpus callosum, and delayed myelination
PCH10	*CLP1*	Severely delayed psychomotor development, progressive microcephaly, spasticity, seizures, and brain abnormalities, including brain atrophy and delayed myelination

Modified from OMIM (https://en.wikipedia.org/wiki/Online_Mendelian_Inheritance_in_Man).

congenital muscle contractures. Intellectual disability tends to be severe, and in prolonged survivors, spasticity and epilepsy are common. PCH2 has consistent pontine hypoplasia, prominent microcephaly, and basal ganglia involvement with dyskinesias, especially chorea and dystonia. Seizures are common. The long-term prognosis for the PCH spectrum is bleak, with usually severe and progressive global delay. Death in childhood is common. Genetics evaluation in PCH2 cases indicates the involvement of transfer splicing endonuclease subunit genes, specifically TSEN54 (up to 90%), and much less commonly TSEN2, TSEN34, VPS53, and SEPSECS (see Table 4.2; Chapter 29). Unlike most other fetal rhombencephalic anomalies, the PCH spectrum of conditions has both a primary developmental defect and a subsequent progressive atrophy.

Several other disorders with a varying degree of pontocerebellar hypoplasia may be encountered in the fetal and neonatal periods (see Chapter 29). These include cerebromuscular

dystrophies (especially Walker-Warburg syndrome and muscle eye brain disease, Chapter 33), some examples of mitochondrial disorders, especially those involving the electro transport chain (see Chapters 28 and 39), loss-of-function mutations in the X-linked calcium/calmodulin-dependent serine protein kinase (CASK) (Chapter 5), and congenital disorders of glycosylation type 1a (see Chapter 29).

Pontine Tegmental Cap Dysplasia[93]

Pontine tegmental cap dysplasia is another rhombencephalic anomaly with combined brain stem and cerebellar defects. Disturbed axonal guidance has been implicated (see the section on the Joubert syndrome) in this condition, which consists of a flat ventral pons, a *cap* or beak protruding from the dorsal pons into the fourth ventricle (Fig. 4.24), and severe hypoplasia of the middle and inferior cerebellar peduncles. Pontine tegmental cap dysplasia is associated with cranial neuropathies,

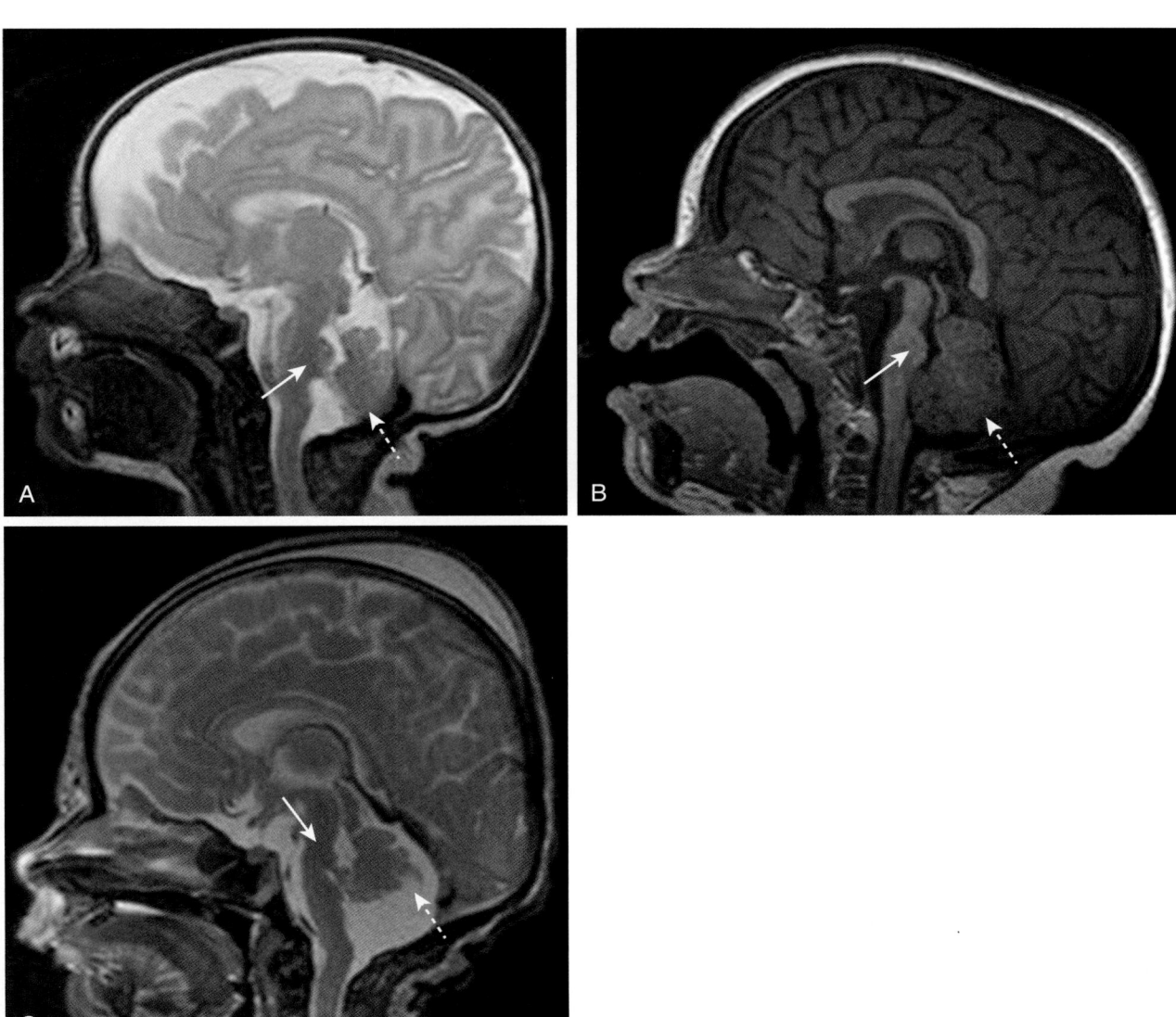

Figure 4.24 Pontine tegmental cap dysplasia. Midline sagittal magnetic resonance imaging T2-weighted (A and C) and T1-weighted (B). All views show flat ventral pons, with dorsal cap *(solid white arrows)* projecting from the dorsal tegmentum into the fourth ventricle, and dysplastic vermis *(broken white arrows)* with apparent posterior lobe overgrowth in A and B.

most commonly of the eighth nerve, with hearing loss, facial anesthesia and paralysis, and abnormal swallowing, as well as gross motor and cognitive deficits in some cases.

Other Conditions With Cerebellar and Brain Stem Abnormality

Other less commonly reported cases show evidence of combined mesencephalic-rhombencephalic anomalies often involving relative overgrowth and undergrowth of different posterior fossa structures (see Fig. 4.22). One possible mechanism for these lesions is disturbances in the early location of the IsO at the MHB junction, and abnormal patterning as a result (see earlier discussion).

Abnormalities in Posterior Fossa Cerebrospinal Fluid Spaces

The fluid spaces of the posterior fossa may be abnormally effaced or increased. Effaced CSF spaces are most commonly encountered as part of the crowded posterior fossa accompanying Chiari II lesions in cases of open neural tube defects. These are discussed in Chapter 1. Prominent posterior fossa CSF collections are a common indication for prenatal evaluation and counseling because these are relatively well detected by prenatal ultrasound. These CSF collections are best considered in three major categories (see Box 4.11): enlargement of the fourth ventricle, enlargement of the cisterna magna (mega cisterna magna), and arachnoidal cyst. An enlarged fourth ventricle is a feature especially of developmental disorders of vermian development (especially Dandy-Walker malformation and Joubert syndrome), which were discussed earlier. Only the trapped fourth ventricle will be considered here.

Trapped fourth ventricle results when both the aqueduct and the outflow of the fourth ventricle are obstructed by an inflammatory process; in the fetus this usually provoked by blood (Fig. 4.25). This striking syndrome is usually accompanied by hydrocephalus and rapidly increasing fourth ventricular size, with brain stem compression and a neurological syndrome with prominent brain stem dysfunction. Shunting of the fourth ventricle and lateral ventricles is usually indicated.

Mega cisterna magna (see Fig. 4.26; Box 4.12) is the second major category of posterior fossa CSF collections. It is separable from Dandy-Walker malformation because cystic dilation of the fourth ventricle does not exist, the cerebellar vermis is present and normal in size, and the posterior fossa is not enlarged. The cisterna magna is the space between the inferior margin of

the vermis and the posterior rim of the foramen magnum. The normal cisterna magna measures between 3 mm and 8 mm, and mega cisterna magna is diagnosed when it reaches 10 mm or more. Some propose that the mega cisterna magna is a Blake pouch cyst remnant (see Figs. 4.14 and 4.15)[61]; however, when isolated, both have an excellent prognosis.

Although developmental disturbances of the cerebellar parenchyma may result in an enlarged cisterna magna (see earlier; Box 4.12), the term mega cisterna magna is reserved for those cases in which the enlarged cisterna magna occurs in the absence of (1) volume loss of other posterior fossa elements, and (2) other cystic structures (e.g., arachnoid cysts; see later) below the vermis. An enlarged cisterna magna may be associated with other anomalies. When truly isolated, mega cisterna magna is considered by many to be an incidental normal variant. Interestingly, mega cisterna magna is commonly associated with benign infantile macrocephaly. In one study, 90% of isolated mega cisterna magna cases had normal neurological outcomes, compared to only 50% of Dandy-Walker malformation or vermian hypoplasia cases.[94] However, one large hospital-based series reported developmental and neurological abnormalities in 62% of such cases.[95]

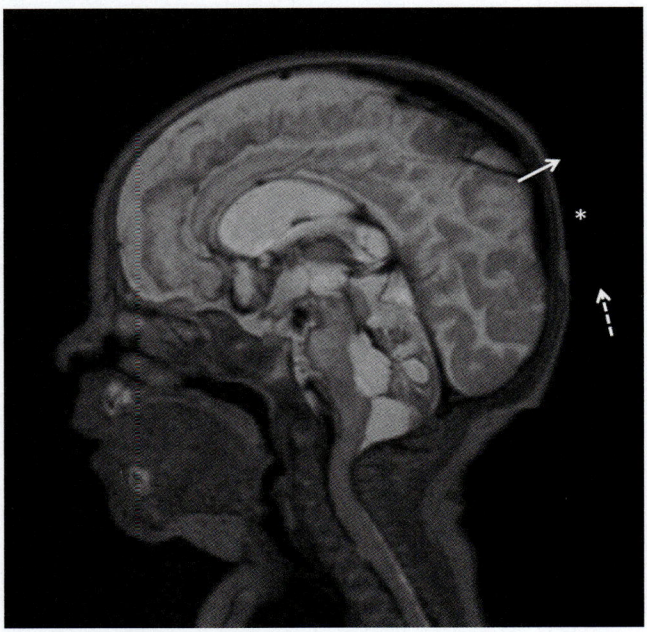

Figure 4.25 Trapped fourth ventricle Sagittal magnetic resonance imaging in 3-month-old ex-25-week premature infants with hemorrhagic brain injury, including cerebellar hemorrhage, aqueductal hemorrhagic obstruction *(arrow)*, trapped fourth ventricle *(asterisk)*, and cyst formation *(dashed arrow)* in the cisterna magna.

BOX 4.11   Categories of Enlarged Cerebrospinal Fluid Spaces

Enlarged Fourth Ventricle
- Vermian hypoplasia
- Blocked cerebrospinal fluid egress (Dandy-Walker malformation; Blake pouch cyst)
- Trapped fourth ventricle

Normal/Compressed Fourth Ventricle, Distortion/Displacement of Cerebellum-Brain Stem
- Arachnoid cyst

Normal Fourth Ventricle, Cerebellum-Brain Stem
- Mega cisterna magna

BOX 4.12   Diagnostic Criteria for Mega Cisterna Magna

- Space between inferior vermis and posterior rim of the foramen magnum is ≥10 mm (normal ~3–8 mm)
- Cerebellar hemispheres and vermis normal size (may be distorted)
- No cystic enlargement of fourth ventricle

Arachnoid cysts (see Fig. 4.27; Box 4.13) are the third major category of prominent posterior fossa CSF collections (see Box 4.11). Posterior fossa arachnoid cysts are enclosed by the pia and arachnoid layers of the meninges, and their contents have the same consistency as CSF. Such cysts do not communicate with the fourth ventricle or with the subarachnoid space in the posterior fossa. These are now more commonly detected by routine prenatal ultrasound. However, they are rarely symptomatic in the neonatal period; the usual clinical presentation is later in infancy and childhood either as a posterior fossa mass, simulating a tumor, or as a cause of hydrocephalus because of the obstruction of CSF flow in the posterior fossa or at the outflow of the fourth ventricle. Arachnoid cysts may enlarge to cause compression/distortion of the posterior fossa structures, including elevation of the vermis, and/or obstruction of CSF drainage and hydrocephalus, although they do not communicate directly with the ventricular system. Unless such complications occur, posterior arachnoid cysts may remain remarkably asymptomatic.

Impaired Cerebellar Development After Premature Birth

The cerebellum undergoes a phase of major growth and development during the second half of gestation (previously discussed),[12,17,96] which therefore represents a period of particular

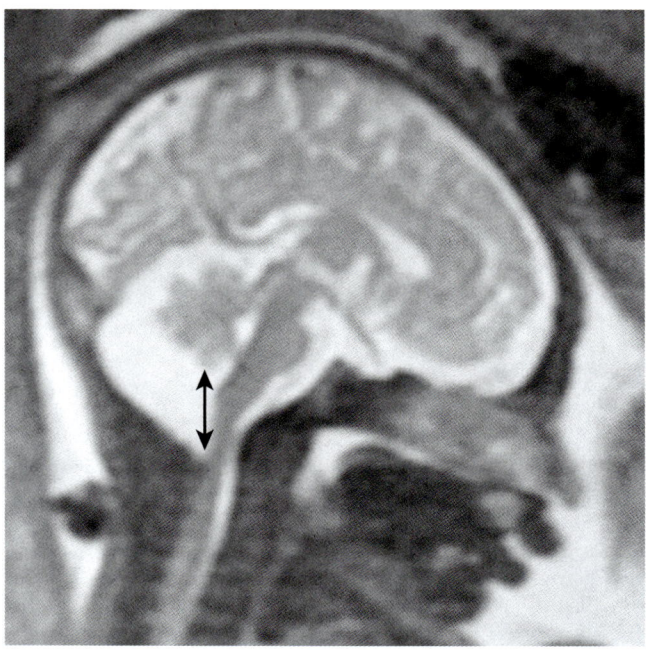

Figure 4.26 Mega cisterna magna. Fetal midline sagittal magnetic resonance imaging T2-weighted showing normal posterior parenchymal structures, including normal growth of the anterior and posterior lobes of the vermis and normal fourth ventricle and torcular Herophili with enlarged cisterna magna *(double arrow)*.

BOX 4.13   Diagnostic Criteria for Arachnoid Cysts in the Posterior Fossa

- ◆ Enclosed by the pia and arachnoid layers of the meninges
- ◆ Contents have consistency of cerebrospinal fluid (CSF)
- ◆ No communication with fourth ventricle or subarachnoid space
- ◆ Rarely symptomatic in the neonatal period
- ◆ May present later as posterior fossa mass, simulating a tumor, or
- ◆ May cause hydrocephalus by obstructing CSF flow in the posterior fossa, or
- ◆ Fourth ventricle foramina
- ◆ May cause compression/distortion of the posterior fossa structures, including elevation of the vermis

---

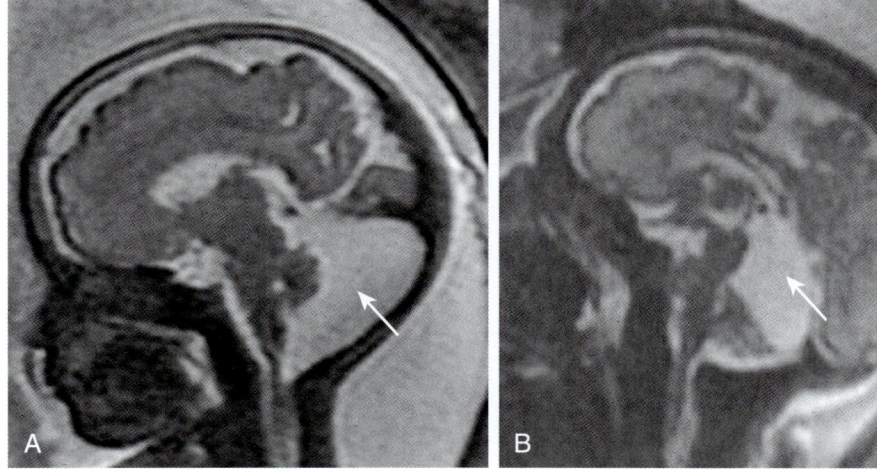

Figure 4.27 Arachnoid cysts in the posterior fossa. Fetal T2-weighted magnetic resonance imaging images from two cases of posterior fossa arachnoid cyst *(white arrows* in A and B) showing displacement and distortion of vermis and effacement of the fourth ventricle.

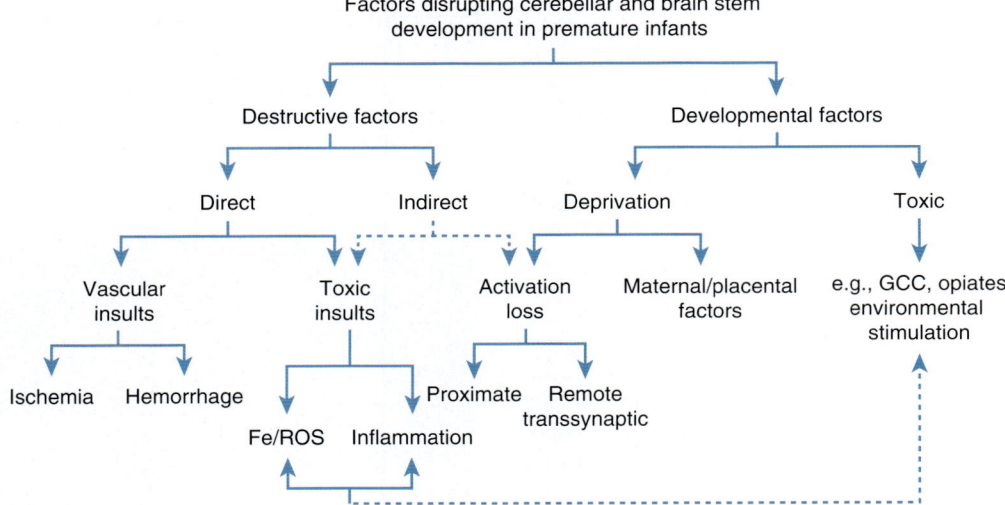

Figure 4.28 Factors disrupting cerebellar and brain stem development in premature infants. *Fe-ROS,* iron-reactive oxygen species.

vulnerability to developmental disruption. Such developmental disruption may result from factors operating in utero (e.g., placental failure) or in prematurely born infants spending part of this critical developmental period in an extrauterine environment for which they are maturationally unprepared. The effects of prematurity on cerebellar development are now increasingly recognized. A range of factors (Fig. 4.28) may conspire to cause destructive or developmental insults when the immature physiology of the premature infant is exposed to adverse conditions. *Destructive pathways* affecting cerebellar development are triggered when the immature physiology (e.g., cardiovascular) and anatomy (e.g., fragile cerebellar blood vessels) encounter environmental conditions radically different from those in the intrauterine milieu, culminating in cell death through hemorrhage or ischemia-infarction.[18,98] Destructive insults may also be mediated by exposure to toxic influences, including hemosiderin and reactive oxygen species, and infectious-inflammatory substances.[99] These pathways are discussed in greater detail in Chapter 23. It is important to note that both destructive and nondestructive influences may operate together or in sequence (see Fig. 4.28). For example, after intracranial hemorrhage, clearance of free iron from the brain and its surroundings is prolonged, resulting in potentially sustained oxidative toxicity of extravascular blood in the developing cerebellar tissue. These toxic effects may affect cerebellar maturation at several developmental steps. For example, development of the external granular layer, the major source of cerebellar growth, may be stunted by toxic blood products from direct hemorrhage into this proliferative zone or through toxic effects exerted across the pial layer by subarachnoid blood. The effects of injury-disruption in the external granular layer on overall cerebellar and brain stem development are shown in Fig. 4.29. At a subcellular level, this toxicity may limit the development of glutamate transporters in Purkinje cells and Bergmann glia. The resulting decrease in glutamate transporters may impede the clearance of extracellular glutamate, thereby promoting neuronal excitotoxicity.[100] Destructive forms of prematurity-related cerebellar injury are discussed in detail in Chapter 23.

A number of reports have described impaired volumetric growth and development of the cerebellum in premature infants,[101] which persists into adolescence,[102,103] even *in the absence of overt direct injury to the cerebellum.* Nondestructive pathways of cerebellar developmental disruption in prematurely born infants can be divided into two broad categories: toxic and deprivational (see Fig. 4.28). *Toxic* factors that may disrupt cerebellar development include iatrogenic agents (e.g., sedative-analgesics), procedural pain, and other excessive environmental stimulation (discussed later). Different *deprivational* pathways may inhibit cerebellar development, including loss of maternal-placental substances normally available in utero, and deprivation of intrinsic trophic stimulation (activation loss) from other directly injured brain regions, proximate or remote. Given the vulnerability of the immature brain to injury, common supratentorial lesions, such as cerebral white matter injury and periventricular venous infarction, may interrupt pathways that are normally crucial for the reciprocal transsynaptic activation and growth of the cerebellum.[101,105,106] The mechanisms by which premature separation from maternal and placental support might disrupt normal cerebellar development are not completely understood. However, a growing body (mainly experimental) of data have implicated a loss of endocrine factors, such as maternal thyroid hormones, and placental factors, such as allopregnanolone and other neurosteroids, in the developmental disruption of the cerebellum in premature infants.

Normal pregnancy is associated with a physiological increase in *maternal thyroid hormone* synthesis. The fetus is dependent on transplacental maternal thyroxine (T4) from which it derives tri-iodothyronine (T3). During brain development, thyroid receptors are highly expressed throughout the developing brain, including the cerebellum.[107] The thyroid hormone acts by regulating signaling pathways for gene transcription, including many of the genes involved in cerebellar development.[108] The thyroid hormone plays a wide-ranging role in neuronal migration, differentiation, and myelination,[109] and maternal hypothyroidism during pregnancy has important health effects in the offspring,[110-112] including effects on brain development.[111-113] Given the dependence of the fetus on

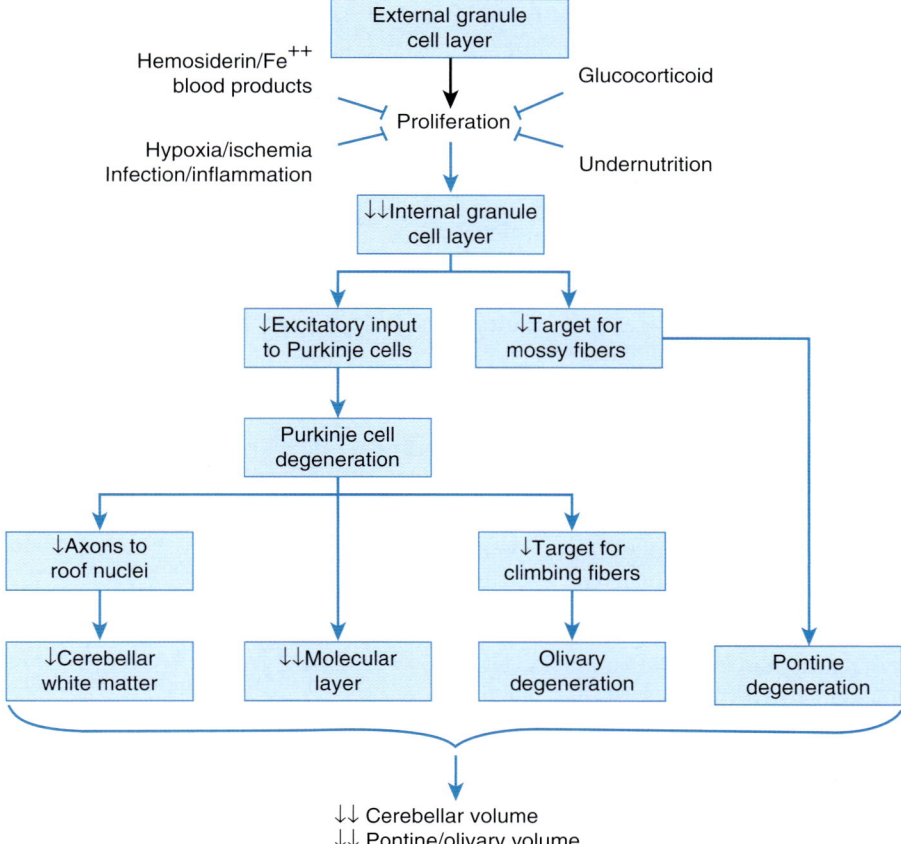

Figure 4.29 Likely mechanisms by which direct adverse effects on the external granule cell layer lead to diminished volumetric development of the cerebellum, and pontine and olivary nuclei. See text for details. (From Volpe JJ. Cerebellum of the premature infant—rapidly developing, vulnerable, clinically important. *J Child Neurol.* 2009;24:1085–1104.)

maternal thyroid hormone support during pregnancy, it is not surprising that 35% to 50% of premature infants develop neonatal hypothyroidism.[114,115] A number of earlier studies of hypothyroidism in developing rodents[116-120] showed a decrease in cerebellar weight, prolonged proliferation and delayed differentiation in the external granular layer,[116] impaired inward migration of granule cells, and disturbances in synaptogenesis and foliation.[117-120] In subsequent studies, hypothyroidism was associated with marked hypoplasia of Purkinje cell dendritic arborizations and impaired synaptogenesis with parallel fibers.[121] As discussed earlier, this decrease in Purkinje cell dendritic arborization and dendritic spine formation would be expected to have a profound impact on the development of the external granular layer and its transition to the internal granular layer.[121] More recently, hypothyroidism has been shown to result in arrested oligodendrocyte maturation and impaired myelination.[122]

The *neurosteroids*, including progesterone and its metabolite, allopregnanolone, are generated in large amounts in the maternal and placental systems throughout pregnancy. These substances cross to the fetus where they play a role in brain development, including that of the cerebellum. In rodent models, a surge in neurosteroid production coincides with the period of accelerated external granular layer development, synaptogenesis, and dendritic spine formation in Purkinje cells.[123] Allopregnanolone

exerts important effects on the $GABA_A$ receptor function and stimulates axonal and dendritic outgrowth, and myelin synthesis. In addition, allopregnanolone has important neuroprotective effects, including the inhibition of apoptosis and gliosis after insult.[124] Therefore it is to be expected that precipitous decreases in neurosteroids[123] with premature birth would not only interrupt important developmental processes (e.g., late gestation myelination),[125] but also compromise endogenous neuroprotection against encephalopathy of prematurity.[126]

Developmental toxicity to the immature cerebellum may originate from several sources, many of them iatrogenic consequences of the strategies used to support the fragile premature infant. These influences may have unintended toxic effects on cerebellar development. *Glucocorticoids* have been used prenatally for years to stimulate lung maturation in the fetus and postnatally to prevent chronic lung disease of prematurity.[127] In rodent models, *glucocorticoids* trigger a dramatic increase in apoptotic death in cerebellar neural progenitor cells. The internal granule cell layer is depleted of neurons, while the Purkinje layer is relatively spared in some,[128] but not all, reports.[129] Preceding intrauterine growth restriction from placental failure followed by premature birth may be a particularly hazardous set of risk factors for brain development in general. Postnatal glucocorticoid administration was previously widely used for the prevention of bronchopulmonary dysplasia, but has been shown to have an adverse effect on neurological outcome in premature infants.[130,131] During placental failure, the growth-restricted fetus is exposed to increased levels of cortisol,[132,133] which may play a role in brain development and neurological outcome.

The potential adverse role in cerebellar development of *procedural pain and the widespread use of sedation-analgesia* (especially opiates like morphine) to treat such discomfort has recently been raised.[134-136] These factors have been identified as independent predictors of impaired functional[135,136] and microstructural[137,138] neurodevelopment, including that of the cerebellum. Procedural pain was also shown to affect the development of specific cerebellar subregions, particularly the neocerebellar lobules VIIIA and VIIIB, in survivors of prematurity up to age 7 years.[134] It has been known for some time that opioid receptors localize at the external granule layer of the cerebellum[139,140] In other studies, the exposure of preterm infants to morphine at higher doses was associated with lower cerebellar, but not cerebral, volumes.[141,142] In rodent models, morphine is toxic to the Purkinje cell layer within a specific developmental window.[143] As discussed earlier, such injury to the Purkinje cells could impair the *Shh* stimulation of external granular layer growth and development.

Infection-inflammation is now known to be an important mediator of prematurity-related brain injury. Inflammation is a common trigger and complication of premature birth; in addition, it may cause hypothyroxinemia (discussed previously).[122] One of the proinflammatory cytokines, interleukin 1-beta, is known to cause maturational arrest in the oligodendrocyte lineage with subsequent hypomyelination. Inflammation during fetal life has been associated with altered brain development, including that of the cerebellum.[144] Postnatal infection has also been associated with impaired cerebellar growth and development in animal models[145,146] and in premature infants.[147]

In summary, a number of internal and external environmental factors are capable of causing significant disturbances in cerebellar growth and development. These influences may exert themselves in a failing intrauterine milieu, as well as during premature exposure to extrauterine life.

REFERENCE

1. Barkovich AJ. *Pediatric Neuroimaging.* 4th ed. Philadelphia: Lippincott Williams & Wilkins; 2005.
2. ten Donkelaar HJ, Lammens M, Wesseling P, et al. Development and developmental disorders of the human cerebellum. *J Neurol.* 2003;250:1025-1036.
3. Barkovich AJ, Millen KJ, Dobyns WB. A developmental and genetic classification for midbrain-hindbrain malformations. *Brain.* 2009;132:3199-3230.
4. Crossley PH, Martinez S, Martin GR. Midbrain development induced by FGF8 in the chick embryo. *Nature.* 1996;380:66-68.
5. Basson MA, Echevarria D, Ahn CP, et al. Specific regions within the embryonic midbrain and cerebellum require different levels of FGF signaling during development. *Development.* 2008;135:889-898.
6. Sgaier SK, Lao Z, Villanueva MP, et al. Genetic subdivision of the tectum and cerebellum into functionally related regions based on differential sensitivity to engrailed proteins. *Development.* 2007;134:2325-2335.
7. Patel S, Barkovich AJ. Analysis and classification of cerebellar malformations. *AJNR Am J Neuroradiol.* 2002;23:1074-1087.
8. Paladini D, Volpe P. Posterior fossa and vermian morphometry in the characterization of fetal cerebellar abnormalities: a prospective three-dimensional ultrasound study. *Ultrasound Obstet Gynecol.* 2006;27:482-489.
9. Aldinger KA, Lehmann OJ, Hudgins L, et al. FOXC1 is required for normal cerebellar development and is a major contributor to chromosome 6p25.3 Dandy-Walker malformation. *Nat Genet.* 2009;41:1037-1042.
10. Hallonet ME, Teillet MA, Le Douarin NM. A new approach to the development of the cerebellum provided by the quail-chick marker system. *Development.* 1990;108:19-31.
11. Carletti B, Rossi F. Neurogenesis in the cerebellum. *Neuroscientist.* 2008;14:91-100.
12. Volpe JJ. Cerebellum of the premature infant—rapidly developing, vulnerable, clinically important. *J Child Neurol.* 2009;24:1085-1104.
13. Huang X, Liu J, Ketova T, et al. Transventricular delivery of Sonic hedgehog is essential to cerebellar ventricular zone development. *Proc Natl Acad Sci USA.* 2010;107:8422-8427.
14. Sidman RL, Rakic P. Neuronal migration, with special reference to developing human brain: a review. *Brain Res.* 1973;62:1-35.
15. Fink AJ, Englund C, Daza RA, et al. Development of the deep cerebellar nuclei: transcription factors and cell migration from the rhombic lip. *J Neurosci.* 2006;26:3066-3076.
16. Wingate RJ, Hatten ME. The role of the rhombic lip in avian cerebellum development. *Development.* 1999;126:4395-4404.
17. Butts T, Green MJ, Wingate RJ. Development of the cerebellum: simple steps to make a 'little brain'. *Development.* 2014;141:4031-4041.
18. Limperopoulos C, Soul JS, Gauvreau K, et al. Late gestation cerebellar growth is rapid and impeded by premature birth. *Pediatrics.* 2005;115:688-695.
19. Chang CH, Chang FM, Yu CH, et al. Assessment of fetal cerebellar volume using three-dimensional ultrasound. *Ultrasound Med Biol.* 2000;26:981-988.
20. Dahmane N, Ruiz i Altaba A. Sonic hedgehog regulates the growth and patterning of the cerebellum. *Development.* 1999;126: 3089-3100.
21. Lewis PM, Gritli-Linde A, Smeyne R, et al. Sonic hedgehog signaling is required for expansion of granule neuron precursors and patterning of the mouse cerebellum. *Dev Biol.* 2004;270:393-410.
22. Wallace VA. Purkinje-cell-derived Sonic hedgehog regulates granule neuron precursor cell proliferation in the developing mouse cerebellum. *Curr Biol.* 1999;9:445-448.
23. Corrales JD, Blaess S, Mahoney EM, et al. The level of sonic hedgehog signaling regulates the complexity of cerebellar foliation. *Development.* 2006;133:1811-1821.
24. Bromley B, Nadel AS, Pauker S, et al. Closure of the cerebellar vermis: evaluation with second trimester US. *Radiology.* 1994;193(3): 761-763.
25. Bronshtein M, Zimmer EZ, Blazer S. Isolated large fourth ventricle in early pregnancy–a possible benign transient phenomenon. *Prenat Diagn.* 1998;18(10):997-1000.
26. Imamoglu EY, Gursoy T, Ovali F, et al. Nomograms of cerebellar vermis height and transverse cerebellar diameter in appropriate-for-gestational-age neonates. *Early Hum Dev.* 2013;89(12):919-923.
27. Robinson AJ, Blaser S, Toi A, et al. The fetal cerebellar vermis: assessment for abnormal development by ultrasonography and magnetic resonance imaging. *Ultrasound Q.* 2007;23(3):211-223.
28. Strick PL, Dum RP, Fiez JA. Cerebellum and nonmotor function. *Ann Rev Neurosci.* 2009;32:413-434.
29. Bordarier C, Aicardi J. Dandy-Walker syndrome and agenesis of the cerebellar vermis: diagnostic problems and genetic counselling. *Dev Med Child Neurol.* 1990;32:285-294.
30. Smith AS, Levine D, Barnes PD, et al. Magnetic resonance imaging of the kinked fetal brain stem: a sign of severe dysgenesis. *J Ultrasound Med.* 2005;24:1697-1709.
31. Bolduc ME, du Plessis AJ, Sullivan N, et al. Regional cerebellar volumes predict functional outcome in children with cerebellar malformations. *Cerebellum.* 2012;11:531-542.
32. Boddaert N, Klein O, Ferguson N, et al. Intellectual prognosis of the Dandy-Walker malformation in children: the importance of vermian lobulation. *Neuroradiology.* 2003;45:320-324.
33. Brossard-Racine M, du Plessis AJ, Limperopoulos C. Developmental cerebellar cognitive affective syndrome in ex-preterm survivors following cerebellar injury. *Cerebellum.* 2015;14:151-164.
34. Schmahmann JD, Sherman JC. Cerebellar cognitive affective syndrome. *Int Rev Neurobiol.* 1997;41:433-440.
35. Deleted in review.
36. Barkovich AJ, Kjos BO, Norman D, et al. Revised classification of posterior fossa cysts and cystlike malformations based on

the results of multiplanar MR imaging. *AJNR Am J Neuroradiol.* 1989;10:977-988.

37. Russ PD, Pretorius DH, Johnson MJ. Dandy-Walker syndrome: a review of fifteen cases evaluated by prenatal sonography. *Am J Obstet Gynecol.* 1989;161:401-406.
38. Deleted in review.
39. Maria BL, Zinreich SJ, Carson BC, et al. Dandy-Walker syndrome revisited. *Pediatr Neurosci.* 1987;13:45-51.
40. Golden JA, Rorke LB, Brucke DA. Dandy-Walker syndrome and associated anomalies. *Pediatr Neurosci.* 1987;38:38-44.
41. Deleted in review.
42. Bindal AK, Storrs BB, McLone DG. Management of the Dandy-Walker syndrome. *Pediatr Neurosurg.* 1990;16:163-169.
43. Osenbach RK, Menezes AH. Diagnosis and management of the Dandy-Walker malformation: 30 years of experience. *Pediatr Neurosurg.* 1992;18:179-189.
44. Estroff JA, Scott MR, Benacerraf BR. Dandy-Walker variant—prenatal sonographic features and clinical outcome. *Radiology.* 1992;185:755-758.
45. Strand RD, Barnes PD, Poussaint TY, et al. Cystic retrocerebellar malformations: unification of the Dandy-Walker complex and the Blake's pouch cyst. *Pediatr Radiol.* 1994;23:258-260.
46. Tortori Donati P, Fondelli MP, Rossi A, et al. Cystic malformations of the posterior cranial fossa originating from a defect of the posterior membranous area—mega cisterna magna and persisting Blake's pouch: two separate entities. *Childs Nerv Sys.* 1996;12:303-308.
47. Tan E-C, Takagi T, Karasawa K. Posterior fossa cystic lesions—magnetic resonance imaging manifestations. *Brain Dev.* 1995;17: 418-424.
48. Elterman RD, Bodensteiner JB, Barnard JJ. Sudden unexpected death in patients with Dandy-Walker malformation. *J Child Neurol.* 1995;10:382-384.
49. Ondo WG, Delong GR. Dandy-Walker syndrome presenting as opisthotonus: proposed pathophysiology. *Pediatr Neurol.* 1996;14: 165-168.
50. Ecker JL, Shipp TD, Bromley B, et al. The sonographic diagnosis of Dandy-Walker and Dandy-Walker variant: associated findings and outcomes. *Prenat Diagn.* 2000;20:328-332.
51. Deleted in review.
52. Kapur RP, Mahony BS, Finch L, et al. Normal and abnormal anatomy of the cerebellar vermis in midgestational human fetuses. *Birth Defects Res A Clin Mol Teratol.* 2009;85:700-709.
53. Russo R, Fallet-Bianco C. Isolated posterior cerebellar vermal defect: a morphological study of midsagittal cerebellar vermis in 4 fetuses—early stage of Dandy-Walker continuum or new vermal dysgenesis? *J Child Neurol.* 2007;22:492-500. discussion 501.
54. Robinson AJ. Inferior vermian hypoplasia—preconception, misconception. *Ultrasound Obstet Gynecol.* 2014;43:123-136.
55. Lemire RJ, Loeser JD, Leech RW, et al. *Normal and Abnormal Development of the Human Nervous System.* Hagerstown: Harper & Row; 1975.
56. Warf BC, Dewan M, Mugamba J. Management of Dandy-Walker complex-associated infant hydrocephalus by combined endoscopic third ventriculostomy and choroid plexus cauterization. *J Neurosurg Pediatr.* 2011;8:377-383.
57. Mohanty A. Endoscopic third ventriculostomy with cystoventricular stent placement in the management of Dandy-Walker malformation: technical case report of three patients. *Neurosurgery.* 2003;53:1223-1228. discussion 1228-1229.
58. Blake JA. The roof and lateral recesses of the fourth ventricle considered morphologically and embryologically. *J Comp Neurol.* 1900;10:79-108.
59. Strand RD, Barnes PD, Poussaint TY, et al. Cystic retrocerebellar malformations: unification of the Dandy-Walker complex and the Blake's pouch cyst. *Pediatr Radiol.* 1993;23:258-260.
60. Paladini D, Quarantelli M, Pastore G, et al. Abnormal or delayed development of the posterior membranous area of the brain: anatomy, ultrasound diagnosis, natural history and outcome of Blake's pouch cyst in the fetus. *Ultrasound Obstet Gynecol.* 2012;39:279-287.
61. Robinson AJ, Goldstein R. The cisterna magna septa: vestigial remnants of Blake's pouch and a potential new marker for normal development of the rhombencephalon. *J Ultrasound Med.* 2007;26:83-95.

62. Patek KJ, Kline-Fath BM, Hopkin RJ, et al. Posterior fossa anomalies diagnosed with fetal MRI: associated anomalies and neurodevelopmental outcomes. *Prenat Diagn.* 2012;32:75-82.
63. Boltshauser E. Cerebellum-small brain but large confusion: a review of selected cerebellar malformations and disruptions. *Am J Med Genet.* 2004;126A:376-385.
64. Maria BL, Hoang KB, Tusa RJ, et al. "Joubert Syndrome" revisited: key ocular motor signs with magnetic resonance imaging correlation. *J Child Neurol.* 1997;12:423-430.
65. Hodgkins PR, Harris CM, Shawkat FS, et al. Joubert syndrome: long-term follow-up. *Dev Med Child Neurol.* 2004;46:694-699.
66. Janecke AR, Muller T, Gassner I, et al. Joubert-like syndrome unlinked to known candidate loci. *J Pediatr.* 2004;144:264-269.
67. Morava E, Dinopoulos A, Kroes HY, et al. Mitochondrial dysfunction in a patient with Joubert syndrome. *Neuropediatrics.* 2005;36:214-217.
68. Valente EM, Marsh SE, Castori M, et al. Distinguishing the four genetic causes of Jouberts syndrome-related disorders. *Ann Neurol.* 2005;57:513-519.
69. Valente EM, Brancati F, Silhavy JL, et al. AHI1 gene mutations cause specific forms of Joubert syndrome-related disorders. *Ann Neurol.* 2006;59:527-534.
70. Joubert M, Eisenring JJ, Robb JP, et al. Familial agenesis of the cerebellar vermis. A syndrome of episodic hyperpnea, abnormal eye movements, ataxia, and retardation. *Neurology.* 1969;19:813-825.
71. Steinlin M, Schmid M, Landau K, et al. Follow-up in children with Joubert syndrome. *Neuropediatrics.* 1997;28:204-211.
72. Sztriha L, Al-Gazali LI, Aithala GR, et al. Joubert's syndrome: new cases and review of clinicopathologic correlation. *Pediatr Neurol.* 1999;20:274-281.
73. Anderson JS, Gorey MT, Pasternak JF, Trommer BL. Joubert's syndrome and prenatal hydrocephalus. *Pediatr Neurol.* 1999;20:403-405.
74. Dixon-Salazar T, Silhavy JL, Marsh SE, et al. Mutations in the AHI1 gene, encoding Jouberin, cause Joubert syndrome with cortical polymicrogyria. *Am J Human Genet.* 2004;75:979-987.
75. Romani M, Micalizzi A, Kraoua I, et al. Mutations in B9D1 and MKS1 cause mild Joubert syndrome: expanding the genetic overlap with the lethal ciliopathy Meckel syndrome. *Orphanet J Rare Dis.* 2014;9:72.
76. Romani M, Micalizzi A, Valente EM. Joubert syndrome: congenital cerebellar ataxia with the molar tooth. *Lancet Neurol.* 2013;12:894-905.
77. Bachmann-Gagescu R, Dempsey JC, Phelps IG, et al. Joubert syndrome: a model for untangling recessive disorders with extreme genetic heterogeneity. *J Med Genet.* 2015;52:514-522.
78. Lancaster MA, Gopal DJ, Kim J, et al. Defective Wnt-dependent cerebellar midline fusion in a mouse model of Joubert syndrome. *Nat Med.* 2011;17:726-731.
79. Schneider L, Clement CA, Teilmann SC, et al. PDGFR alpha signaling is regulated through the primary cilium in fibroblasts. *Curr Biol.* 2005;15:1861-1866.
80. Aguilar A, Meunier A, Strehl L, et al. Analysis of human samples reveals impaired SHH-dependent cerebellar development in Joubert syndrome/Meckel syndrome. *Proc Natl Acad Sci USA.* 2012;109:16951-16956.
81. Spassky N, Han YG, Aguilar A, et al. Primary cilia are required for cerebellar development and Shh-dependent expansion of progenitor pool. *Dev Biol.* 2008;317:246-259.
82. Toelle SP, Valcinkaya C, Kocer N, et al. Rhombencephalosynapsis: clinical findings and neuroimaging in 9 children. *Neuropediatrics.* 2002;33:209-214.
83. Odemis E, Cakir M, Aynaci FM. Rhombencephalosynapsis associated with cutaneous pretibial hemangioma in an infant. *J Child Neurol.* 2003;18:225-228.
84. Napolitano M, Righini A, Zirpoli S, et al. Prenatal magnetic resonance imaging of rhombencephalosynapsis and associated brain anomalies—report of 3 cases. *J Comput Assist Tomogr.* 2004;28: 762-765.
85. Demaerel P, Morel C, Lagae L, et al. Partial rhombencephalosynapsis. *AJNR Am J Neuroradiol.* 2004;25:29-31.
86. Chemli J, Abroug M, Tlili K, et al. Rhombencephalosynapsis diagnosed in childhood: clinical and MRI findings. *Eur J Paediatr Neurol.* 2007;11:35-38.
87. Deleted in review.

88. Hatten ME, Heintz N. Mechanisms of neural patterning and specification in the developing cerebellum. *Ann Rev Neurosci*. 1995;18:385-408.

89. Malinger G, Lev D, Lerman-Sagie T. The fetal cerebellum. Pitfalls in diagnosis and management. *Prenat Diagn*. 2009;29:372-380.

90. Barth PG. Pontocerebellar hypoplasias. An overview of a group of inherited neurodegenerative disorders with fetal onset. *Brain Dev*. 1993;15:411-422.

91. Parisi MA, Dobyns WB. Human malformations of the midbrain and hindbrain: review and proposed classification scheme. *Mol Genet Metab*. 2003;80:36-53.

92. Maricich SM, Aqeeb KA, Moayedi Y, et al. Pontocerebellar hypoplasia: review of classification and genetics, and exclusion of several genes known to be important for cerebellar development. *J Child Neurol*. 2011;26:288-294.

93. Rauscher C, Poretti A, Neuhann TM, et al. Pontine tegmental cap dysplasia: the severe end of the clinical spectrum. *Neuropediatrics*. 2009;40:43-46.

94. Gandolfi Colleoni G, Contro E, Carletti A, et al. Prenatal diagnosis and outcome of fetal posterior fossa fluid collections. *Ultrasound Obstet Gynecol*. 2012;39:625-631.

95. Bodensteiner JB, Gay CT, Marks WA, et al. Macro cisterna magna: a marker for maldevelopment of the brain? *Pediatr Neurol*. 1988;4:284-286.

96. Limperopoulos C, Soul JS, Gauvreau K, et al. Late gestation cerebellar growth is rapid and impeded by premature birth. *Pediatrics*. 2005;115:688-695.

97. Deleted in review.

98. Johnsen SD, Bodensteiner JB, Lotze TE. Frequency and nature of cerebellar injury in the extremely premature survivor with cerebral palsy. *J Child Neurol*. 2005;20:60-64.

99. Hutton LC, Yan E, Yawno T, et al. Injury of the developing cerebellum: a brief review of the effects of endotoxin and asphyxial challenges in the late gestation sheep fetus. *Cerebellum*. 2014;13: 777-786.

100. Inage YW, Itoh M, Wada K, et al. Glutamate transporters in neonatal cerebellar subarachnoid hemorrhage. *Pediatr Neurol*. 2000;23:42-48.

101. Limperopoulos C, Benson CB, Bassan H, et al. Cerebellar hemorrhage in the preterm infant: ultrasonographic findings and risk factors. *Pediatrics*. 2005;116:717-724.

102. Parker J, Mitchell AA, Kalpakidou A, et al. Cerebellar growth and behavioural and neuropsychological outcome in preterm adolescents. *Brain*. 2008;131:1344-1351.

103. Allin MP, Salaria S, Nosarti C, et al. Vermis and lateral lobes of the cerebellum in adolescents born very preterm. *Neuroreport*. 2005;16: 1821-1824.

104. Deleted in review.

105. Limperopoulos C, Chilingaryan G, Sullivan N, et al. Injury to the premature cerebellum: outcome is related to remote cortical development. *Cereb Cortex*. 2014;24:728-736.

106. Srinivasan L, Allsop J, Counsell SJ, et al. Smaller cerebellar volumes in very preterm infants at term-equivalent age are associated with the presence of supratentorial lesions. *AJNR Am J Neuroradiol*. 2006;27:573-579.

107. Koibuchi N, Jingu H, Iwasaki T, et al. Current perspectives on the role of thyroid hormone in growth and development of cerebellum. *Cerebellum*. 2003;2:279-289.

108. Anderson GW. Thyroid hormone and cerebellar development. *Cerebellum*. 2008;7:60-74.

109. Faustino LC, Ortiga-Carvalho TM. Thyroid hormone role on cerebellar development and maintenance: a perspective based on transgenic mouse models. *Front Endocrinol*. 2014;5:75.

110. Lavado-Autric R, Auso E, Garcia-Velasco JV, et al. Early maternal hypothyroxinemia alters histogenesis and cerebral cortex cytoarchitecture of the progeny. *J Clin Invest*. 2003;111:1073-1082.

111. de Escobar GM, Obregon MJ, del Rey FE. Iodine deficiency and brain development in the first half of pregnancy. *Public Health Nutr*. 2007;10:1554-1570.

112. Mannisto T, Mendola P, Reddy U, et al. Neonatal outcomes and birth weight in pregnancies complicated by maternal thyroid disease. *Am J Epidemiol*. 2013;178:731-740.

113. Koibuchi N, Chin WW. Thyroid hormone action and brain development. *Trends Endocrinol Metab*. 2000;11:123-128.

114. Berbel P, Navarro D, Auso E, et al. Role of late maternal thyroid hormones in cerebral cortex development: an experimental model for human prematurity. *Cereb Cortex*. 2010;20:1462-1475.

115. Fisher DA. Thyroid function in premature infants. The hypothyroxinemia of prematurity. *Clin Perinatol*. 1998;25:999-1014, viii.

116. Lauder JM. The effects of early hypo- and hyperthyroidism on the development of rat cerebellar cortex. III. Kinetics of cell proliferation in the external granular layer. *Brain Res*. 1977;126:31-51.

117. Nicholson JL, Altman J. The effects of early hypo- and hyperthyroidism on the development of the rat cerebellar cortex. II. Synaptogenesis in the molecular layer. *Brain Res*. 1972;44:25-36.

118. Nicholson JL, Altman J. Synaptogenesis in the rat cerebellum: effects of early hypo- and hyperthyroidism. *Science*. 1972;176: 530-532.

119. Lauder JM, Altman J, Krebs H. Some mechanisms of cerebellar foliation: effects of early hypo- and hyperthyroidism. *Brain Res*. 1974;76:33-40.

120. Lauder JM. Granule cell migration in developing rat cerebellum. Influence of neonatal hypo- and hyperthyroidism. *Dev Biol*. 1979;70:105-115.

121. Vincent J, Legrand C, Rabie A, et al. Effects of thyroid hormone on synaptogenesis in the molecular layer of the developing rat cerebellum. *J Physiol*. 1982;78:729-738.

122. Schang AL, Van Steenwinckel J, Chevenne D, et al. Failure of thyroid hormone treatment to prevent inflammation-induced white matter injury in the immature brain. *Brain Behav Immun*. 2014;37: 95-102.

123. Hirst JJ, Yawno T, Nguyen P, et al. Stress in pregnancy activates neurosteroid production in the fetal brain. *Neuroendocrinology*. 2006;84:264-274.

124. Tsutsui KM, Mellon SH. Neurosteroids in the brain neuron: biosynthesis, action and medicinal impact on neurodegenerative disease. *Cent Nerv Syst Agents Med Chem*. 2006;9:73-82.

125. Schumacher M, Akwa Y, Guennoun R, et al. Steroid synthesis and metabolism in the nervous system: trophic and protective effects. *J Neurocytol*. 2000;29:307-326.

126. Yawno T, Yan EB, Walker DW, et al. Inhibition of neurosteroid synthesis increases asphyxia-induced brain injury in the late gestation fetal sheep. *Neuroscience*. 2007;146:1726-1733.

127. Tam EW, Chau V, Ferriero DM, et al. Preterm cerebellar growth impairment after postnatal exposure to glucocorticoids. *Sci Transl Med*. 2011;3:105ra105.

128. Maloney SE, Noguchi KK, Wozniak DF, et al. Long-term effects of multiple glucocorticoid exposures in neonatal mice. *Behav Sci (Basel)*. 2011;1:4-30.

129. Pascual R, Valencia M, Larrea S, et al. Single course of antenatal betamethasone produces delayed changes in morphology and calbindin-D28k expression in a rat's cerebellar Purkinje cells. *Acta Neurobiol Exp*. 2014;74:415-423.

130. Barrington KJ. The adverse neuro-developmental effects of postnatal steroids in the preterm infant: a systematic review of RCTs. *BMC Pediatr*. 2001;1:1.

131. Murphy BP, Zientara GP, Huppi PS, et al. Line scan diffusion tensor MRI of the cervical spinal cord in preterm infants. *J Magn Reson Imaging*. 2001;13:949-953.

132. Goland RS, Jozak S, Warren WB, et al. Elevated levels of umbilical cord plasma corticotropin-releasing hormone in growth-retarded fetuses. *J Clin Endocrinol Metab*. 1993;77:1174-1179.

133. Seckl JR. Glucocorticoids, feto-placental 11 beta-hydroxysteroid dehydrogenase type 2, and the early life origins of adult disease. *Steroids*. 1997;62:89-94.

134. Ranger M, Zwicker JG, Chau CM, et al. Neonatal pain and infection relate to smaller cerebellum in very preterm children at school age. *J Pediatr*. 2015;167:292-298, e291.

135. Ranger M, Synnes AR, Vinall J, et al. Internalizing behaviours in school-age children born very preterm are predicted by neonatal pain and morphine exposure. *Eur J Pain*. 2014;18:844-852.

136. Grunau RE, Whitfield MF, Petrie-Thomas J, et al. Neonatal pain, parenting stress and interaction, in relation to cognitive and motor development at 8 and 18 months in preterm infants. *Pain*. 2009;143:138-146.

137. Brummelte S, Grunau RE, Chau V, et al. Procedural pain and brain development in premature newborns. *Ann Neurol*. 2012;71: 385-396.

138. Ranger M, Chau CM, Garg A, et al. Neonatal pain-related stress predicts cortical thickness at age 7 years in children born very preterm. *PLoS ONE*. 2013;8:e76702.

139. Kinney HC, Ottoson CK, White WF. Three-dimensional distribution of 3H-naloxone binding to opiate receptors in the human fetal and infant brainstem. *J Comp Neurol*. 1990;291:55-78.

140. Kinney HC, White WF. Opioid receptors localize to the external granular cell layer of the developing human cerebellum. *Neuroscience*. 1991;45:13-21.

141. Steinhorn R, McPherson C, Anderson PJ, et al. Neonatal morphine exposure in very preterm infants-cerebral development and outcomes. *J Pediatr*. 2015;166:1200-1207, e1204.

142. Zwicker JG, Miller SP, Grunau RE, et al. Smaller cerebellar growth and poorer neurodevelopmental outcomes in very preterm infants exposed to neonatal morphine. *J Pediatr*. 2016;172:81-87, e82.

143. Hauser KF, Gurwell JA, Turbek CS. Morphine inhibits Purkinje cell survival and dendritic differentiation in organotypic cultures of the mouse cerebellum. *Exp Neurol*. 1994;130:95-105.

144. Anblagan D, Pataky R, Evans MJ, et al. Association between preterm brain injury and exposure to chorioamnionitis during fetal life. *Sci Rep*. 2016;6:37932.

145. Biran V, Verney C, Ferriero DM. Perinatal cerebellar injury in human and animal models. *Neurol Res Int*. 2012;2012:858929.

146. Tam EW. Potential mechanisms of cerebellar hypoplasia in prematurity. *Neuroradiology*. 2013;55:41-46.

147. Lee I, Neil JJ, Huettner PC, et al. The impact of prenatal and neonatal infection on neurodevelopmental outcomes in very preterm infants. *J Perinatol*. 2014;34:741-747.

148. Barkovich AJ. *Pediatric Neuroimaging*. 5th ed. Philadelphia: Lippincott Williams & Wilkins; 2012.

149. Kline-Fath BM, Bulas D, Bahado-Singh R. *Fundamental and Advanced Fetal Imaging*. Philadelphia: Wolters-Kluwer; 2015.

150. Timor-Tritsch I, Monteagudo A, Pilu G, Malinger G. *Ultrasonography of the Prenatal Brain*. New York: McGraw Hill; 2012.

Neuronal Proliferation

Annapurna Poduri ♦ *Joseph J. Volpe*

The awesome complexity of the human brain begins its evolution after the essential external form is established by the events described in Chapters 1 and 2. The events that follow are proliferation of the brain's total complement of neurons, estimated at 86 billion,[1,2] the migration of these neurons to specific sites throughout the central nervous system (CNS), the series of organizational events that result in the intricate circuitry characteristic of the human brain, and finally the ensheathment of this circuitry with myelin, its neuron-specific membrane. These events span a period from the second month of gestation to adult life, including the perinatal period. Aberrations of brain development may be an important consequence of genetic perturbations as well as a variety of prenatal and perinatal insults at critical times during development. This chapter reviews the normal aspects of neuronal proliferation and discusses disorders encountered when normal development goes awry.

NEURONAL PROLIFERATION

Normal Development

Major proliferative events occur initially between 2 and 4 months of gestation, with the peak time period quantitatively in the third and fourth months (Box 5.1). Initially, a tangential stream of migration from the ganglionic eminence leads to the formation of the marginal zone, or preplate. All radially migrating neurons and glia are derived from the ventricular and subventricular zones, present in the subependymal location at every level of the developing nervous system.

Valuable quantitative information concerning cellular proliferation is derived from studies of the deposition of brain DNA, the chemical correlate of cell number, or from direct counting by optical and stereological methods (Fig. 5.1).[3,4] Two phases can be distinguished: the first, occurring from approximately 2 to 4 months of gestation, is associated primarily with the generation of *radial glia and neurons*, initially as neuronal-glial progenitors that over time undergo cell fate *decisions* that define them as neurons and glial cells; the second, occurring from approximately 5 months of gestation to 1 year (or more) of life, is associated primarily with *glial multiplication* (see later chapters concerning organizational events and myelination).[5] Similarly, some continued generation of neurons occurs later than 4 months of gestation, principally in the cerebral subventricular zone and the cerebellar external granule cell layer. Finally, proliferation of the *vascular tree*, arterial before venous, is particularly active during the phase

of neuronal proliferation.[6-9] Initially, a leptomeningeal plexus of vessels appears; this is followed in the third month by radially oriented, primarily unbranched vessels, which in the fourth and later months develop horizontal branching (Fig. 5.2).[7,9]

The fundamental aspects of cell proliferation in the wall of the neural tube were described first on the basis of morphological observations by Sauer in 1935.[10,11] They were then delineated further by the use of radioautography with [3H] thymidine-labeled DNA by Sidman, Rakic, Berry, and others 2 to 3 decades later and, still later, with bromodeoxyuridine-labeled DNA by Caviness, Rakic, and coworkers.[12-23] Most recently they have been demonstrated by immunocytochemistry, computer-assisted serial electron micrographic reconstruction, time-lapse multiphoton imaging, and a variety of molecular genetic techniques (Fig. 5.3).[5,24-30]

Cells at the periphery of the *ventricular zone* (VZ) were shown to replicate their DNA, migrate away from the ventricular (sometimes called *apical*) surface, and divide[31]; the two daughter cells were then noted to migrate back to the periphery of the VZ. This *to-and-fro migration*, or *interkinetic nuclear migration*, is repeated each time DNA replication and mitosis occur in the VZ. In some regions of the forebrain, a *subventricular zone* of proliferating cells can be identified (see Fig. 5.3). In the monkey cerebrum, studied in detail by Rakic and coworkers and others,[a] the VZ gives birth to most neurons, and the subventricular zone is the point of origin of some later-appearing neurons (e.g., upper layers of cerebral cortex and later subplate neurons) and most glia. When cells withdraw from the mitotic cycle and cease proliferative activity, they migrate into the intermediate zone on their way to forming the cortical plate (see later discussion). The elegant work of Caviness and coworkers defined the G_1 phase of the cell cycle as the molecular *control point* for these critical proliferative events.[23,35]

Rakic's studies of cortical development in monkeys led to the conclusion that, in the earliest phases of proliferation, progenitor cells divide *symmetrically* into two additional progenitor cells, and that *proliferative units* of neuronal progenitor cells develop in this way (see later and also Box 5.1).[19,33,34,36] This process determines the number of proliferative units in the ventricular-subventricular zones. Later, at a time comparable to the second half of the second month of gestation in the human, the number of these proliferative units becomes stable as the progenitor cells begin to divide asymmetrically (i.e., each division results in dissimilar cells, one of which is a stem cell

---

[a]References 5, 16, 19, 22, 24-26, 32-34.

BOX 5.1   Neuronal Proliferation

Peak Time Period
3–4 months
Major Events
Ventricular and subventricular zones are the sites of proliferation.
Proliferative units are produced by symmetrical divisions of progenitor
   cells.
Proliferative units later enlarge by asymmetrical divisions of progenitor
   cells before neuronal migration.

BOX 5.2   Functions of Radial Glial Cells

Progenitors for cortical neurons
Guides of neuronal migration
Progenitors for astrocytes and oligodendrocytes
Neural stem cells found in subventricular zone of adult brain

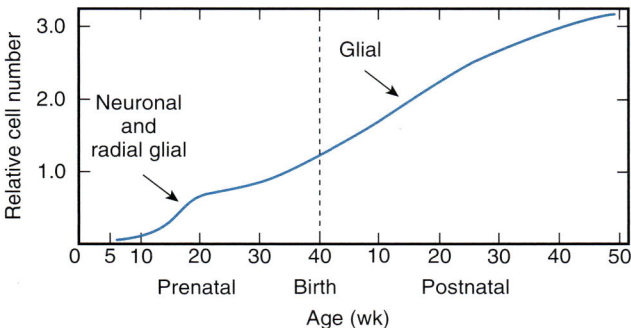

Figure 5.1 **Relative cell number in human forebrain as a function of age.** Total content of forebrain DNA is used to estimate relative cell number. Note that the curve has two phases of rapid increase in cell number. See text for details. (With permission from Dobbing J, Sands J. Quantitative growth and development of human brain. *Arch Dis Child.* 1973;48:757–767.)

and the other a postmitotic neuronal cell). These asymmetrical divisions determine the *size* of each proliferative unit (see Box 5.1). As the proliferative phase progresses, proportionately more postmitotic neuronal cells and fewer stem cells are produced.[22] Rakic concluded that the neurons of these proliferative units migrate together in a column to form the neuronal columns of the cerebral cortex (Fig. 5.4),[36] but there is also evidence, from studies in the developing ferret nervous system, that there is dispersion of cells across the would-be columnar territories arising from each neuronal-glial progenitor cell.[37,38] Other factors contribute to the complete functional organization of the cerebral cortex (see later discussion of migration), but the general principle is the generation of neuronal units in the ventricular-subventricular zones with subsequent migration of these groups. Rakic showed that the distinguishing features of the kinetics of neuronal proliferation in primates versus species with smaller neocortices are a longer cell cycle duration and, particularly, a more prolonged developmental period of neuronal proliferation.[22] Thus the total number of proliferative units of neuronal cells generated is much greater in the primate.

At *least two types of neuronal progenitors are present in the VZ:* (1) a short neural precursor that has a ventricular endfoot and a leading process of variable length and (2) the radial glial cell that spans the entire cortical plate with contacts at both the ventricular and pial surfaces (Fig. 5.5).[5,26] The former progenitor was previously considered the principal neuronal precursor cell. An exciting advance in the understanding of neuronal proliferation was the identification of the *radial glial cell as another major neuronal progenitor in the VZ.*[a] Previously,

the major roles of this cell were considered to be, initially, a glial guide for migrating neurons and, later, a source of astrocytes (see further on). However, more recent studies based on immunocytochemical and molecular techniques indicate that radial glial cells give rise to many neurons generated in the VZ, particularly radially migrating excitatory projection cortical neurons. Thus the term *radial glial cell* (which we continue to use) may ultimately be replaced by *radial glial progenitor* or *radial progenitor.* When the radial glial cell functions as a progenitor that eventually results in differentiation into a neuron, the clonally related neuron so generated then migrates along the parent radial glial fiber (see Fig. 5.5).

These elegant proliferative events involving the radial glial cell as neuronal progenitor are modulated by several key signaling pathways involving the Notch receptor, the ErbB receptor (through the ligand neuregulin), and the fibroblast growth factor receptor.[36,48,49] Other critical molecular determinants include beta-catenin, a protein that functions in the decision of progenitors to proliferate or differentiate.[50] Finally, of particular importance in the regulation of radial glial production of neurons, are calcium waves propagating through connexin channels of the radial glial cell.[45] Calcium entry is critical in the regulation of the cell cycle. Subsequent to neurogenesis, radial cells produce astrocytes and other glial cells (e.g., oligodendroglia).[5,46] In addition, it appears likely that radial glial cells also give rise to cells that persist in the subventricular zone of *adult* brain as stem cells capable of producing neurons.[46] The multiple functions of radial glial cells are summarized in Box 5.2.

The classical understanding of neuronal proliferation and migration centers on the ventricular and subventricular zones and radially migrating neurons. In addition, there are important proliferative centers in the median ganglionic eminence (MGE) that give rise to tangentially migrating cortical and striatal interneurons.[51,52] Although there was some early evidence from studies in the mouse that interneurons arising from the same MGE progenitor maintain some clustering,[53] more recent evidence suggests that many progenitors in the MGE often give rise to interneurons that disperse widely across the brain.[54] There are some important interspecies issues to consider as animal models continue to inform our understanding of human brain development, particularly regarding interneuron development and circuitry.[55] Cell lineage studies in organotypic slice cultures of human embryonic forebrain provide evidence for two GABAergic subpopulations in humans: the first, which arises from the VZ and subventricular zone (SVZ) in the dorsal telencephalon, expresses the transcription factors Dlx1/2 and Mash1 and represents about two-thirds of human neocortical GABAergic neurons; the second, which arises from the MGE of the ventral telencephalon, contains neurons that are transcriptionally distinguished from the first in that they are Dlx1/2-positive but Mash1-negative.[56]

[a]References 5, 25, 26, 29, 30, 39-48.

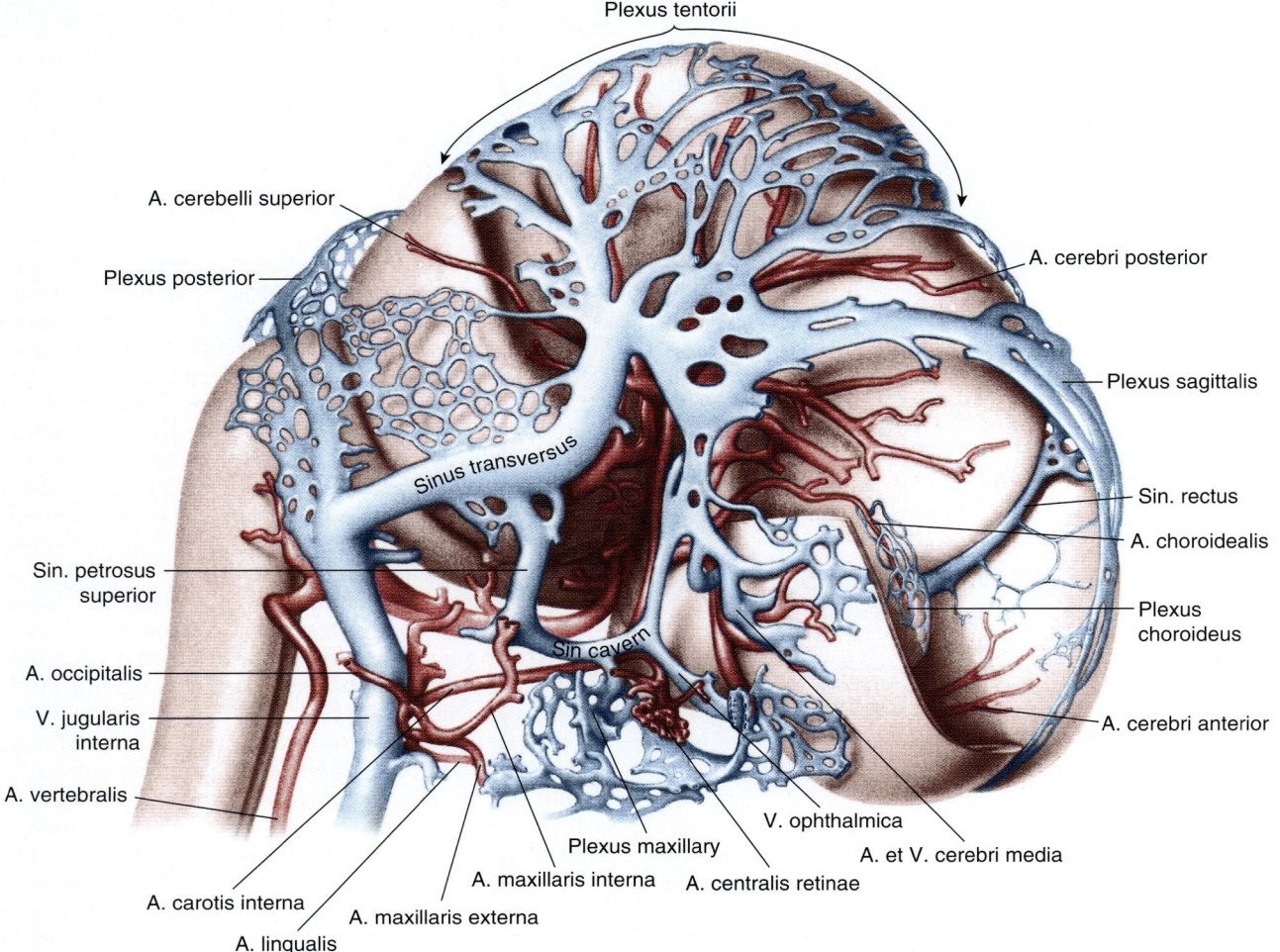

Plexus tentorii

A. cerebelli superior

Plexus posterior

Sinus transversus

Sin. petrosus superior

A. occipitalis

V. jugularis interna

A. vertebralis

A. carotis interna

A. maxillaris externa

A. lingualis

A. maxillaris interna

Plexus maxillary

Sin cavern

A. centralis retinae

V. ophthalmica

A. et V. cerebri media

A. cerebri anterior

Plexus choroideus

A. choroidealis

Sin. rectus

Plexus sagittalis

A. cerebri posterior

Figure 5.2 Reconstruction of the perineural vascular territory of the brain (intracranial vasculature) of a stage-20 human embryo (≈51 days, ≈18 to 22 mm). The dural venous sinuses, the arachnoidal arterial and venous systems, and the pial plexus that characterize the adult brain are already recognizable at this age. The wall of the cerebral cortex (cerebral vesicle) has been opened to demonstrate that, at this age, its intrinsic vascularization has not started, but that of the choroid plexus is already under way. *A,* artery; *cavern,* cavernous; *Sin,* sinus; *V,* vein. (With permission from Streeter GL. *Contributions to Embryology.* vol. 8. Carnegie Institute of Embryology; 1918.)

Disorders

Disorders of neuronal proliferation would be expected to have a major impact on CNS function. Because of difficulties in quantitating neuronal populations, however, proliferative disorders are often difficult to define by conventional neuropathological examination. Even when the disorder is so extreme that the brain is grossly undersized (as in microcephaly) or oversized (as in macrocephaly), defining the nature and severity of the proliferative derangement is also difficult by conventional techniques. (Although theoretically there is the possibility that the disorders relate to alterations in later-occurring normal apoptotic events, we consider these to be disorders of proliferation unless evidence of an apoptotic disorder is recorded.) In the following discussion, we focus on these two extremes of apparent proliferative disorders, emphasizing that conclusions about the nature of the disorders can be drawn only cautiously.

Microcephaly

Microcephaly means "small head," as opposed to *micrencephaly,* which means "small brain." We will use the former term, since head size in living patients—measured as occipitofrontal circumference—is used as an approximation of brain size. Barring severe cranial defects resulting in premature skull closure, small brain size is generally considered the reason for small head size. We distinguish *primary microcephalies,* apparently related to impaired neuronal proliferation resulting in too few neurons, from microcephalies secondary to destructive disease (Box 5.3). The latter relate to hypoxic-ischemic, infectious, metabolic, or other destructive events that usually occur *following completion* of cerebral neuronal proliferative events near the end of the fourth month of gestation (see Chapters 16, 20, 25–28, 34, and 35). The primary microcephalies that have been shown most clearly to be related to impaired neuronal proliferation include the autosomal recessively inherited disorders, often

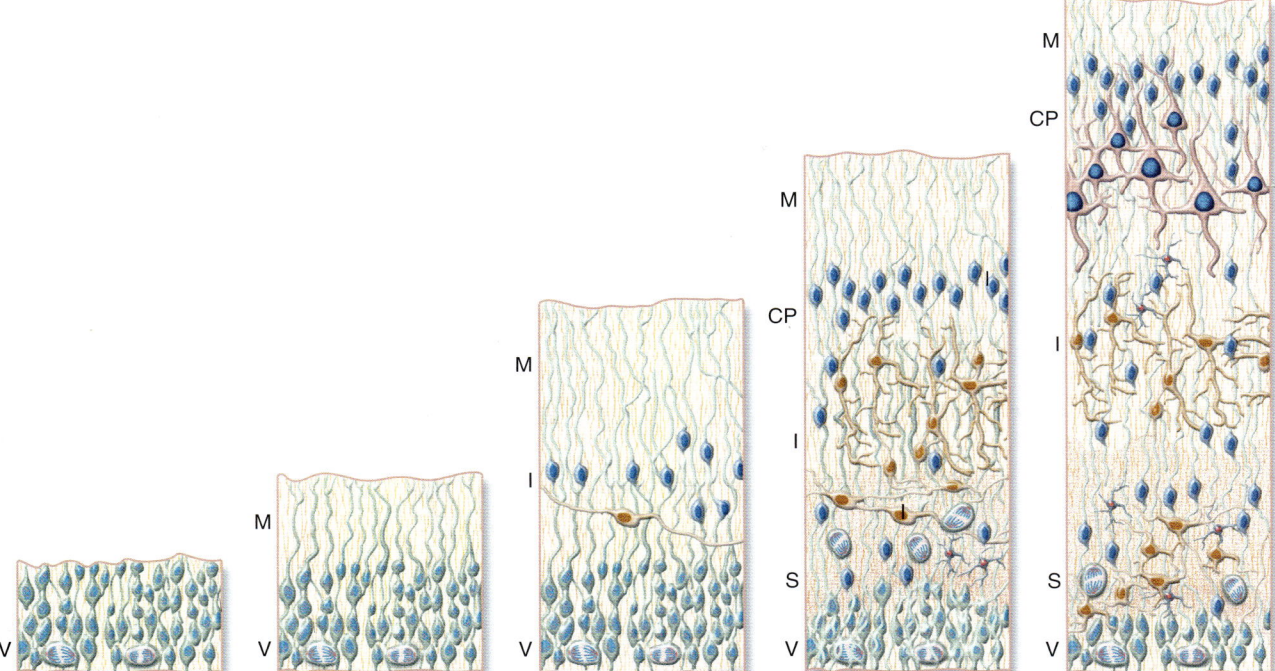

Figure 5.3 Cerebral wall during cortical plate development. Schematic drawing of the cerebral wall during development of the mammalian cortical plate (CP) to demonstrate the major zones: ventricular (V), subventricular (S), intermediate (I), and marginal (M). (With permission from Rakic P. Timing of major ontogenetic events in the visual cortex of the rhesus monkey. In Buchwald NA, Brazier MAB, eds. *Brain Mechanisms in Mental Retardation.* New York: Academic Press; 1975.)

BOX 5.3   Disorders of Neuronal Proliferation: Primary Familial Microcephaly[a]

Autosomal recessive (microcephaly vera)
Autosomal dominant
X-linked recessive
Genetics as yet undetermined
Teratogenic
Irradiation
Metabolic-toxic (e.g., fetal alcohol syndrome, related to cocaine, hyperphenylalaninemia)
Infection (rubella, cytomegalovirus, HIV, Zika virus)
Syndromic (Multiple Systemic Anomalies)
Chromosomal
Familial
Sporadic
Sporadic (Nonsyndromic)

---

[a]Excluded are cases of congenital microcephaly secondary principally to destructive disease (hypoxia-ischemia, infection) developing after the conclusion of cerebral neuronal proliferation.

---

categorized as *microcephaly vera*. Thus, in the context of this chapter, we discuss these conditions in most detail.

Microcephaly Vera. *Microcephaly vera* refers to a heterogeneous group of disorders that appear to have, as the common denominator, small brain size because of a derangement of proliferation (see Box 5.3). Thus no evidence of intrauterine destructive disease or of gross derangement of other developmental events (e.g., neurulation, prosencephalic cleavage, neuronal migration) exists, and the abnormal brain size is apparent as early as the third trimester of gestation. The brain is generally well formed, although the gyrification pattern may be simplified to a variable degree, sometimes but not always commensurate with the degree of microcephaly. We first discuss *radial microbrain*, an informative but rare and particularly severe type of microcephaly vera, and then the more common genetically determined varieties of microcephaly vera.

Anatomical Abnormality: Radial Microbrain. *Radial microbrain* is a rare disorder of particular interest because it appears to provide the first clear example of a disturbance in the number of proliferative units resulting in small brain size.[8,57] The major features of the seven cases studied carefully by Evrard et al.[8,57] are outlined in Box 5.4. The extremely small brain has no marked gyral abnormality, no evidence of a destructive process, and no disturbance of cortical lamination. The conclusion that the disturbance involves the early phase of proliferative events, by which *symmetrical* divisions of neuronal progenitors generate the *total number* of proliferative units, is based on the finding of a marked reduction in number of cortical neuronal columns but an apparent normal complement of the neurons per column (i.e., normal size of columns; Fig. 5.6).[8]

Timing and Clinical Aspects: Radial Microbrain. The presumed timing of radial microbrain is no later than the earliest phase of proliferative events in the second month of gestation. The essential abnormality involves the symmetrical divisions of progenitors to form additional progenitors and thereby the

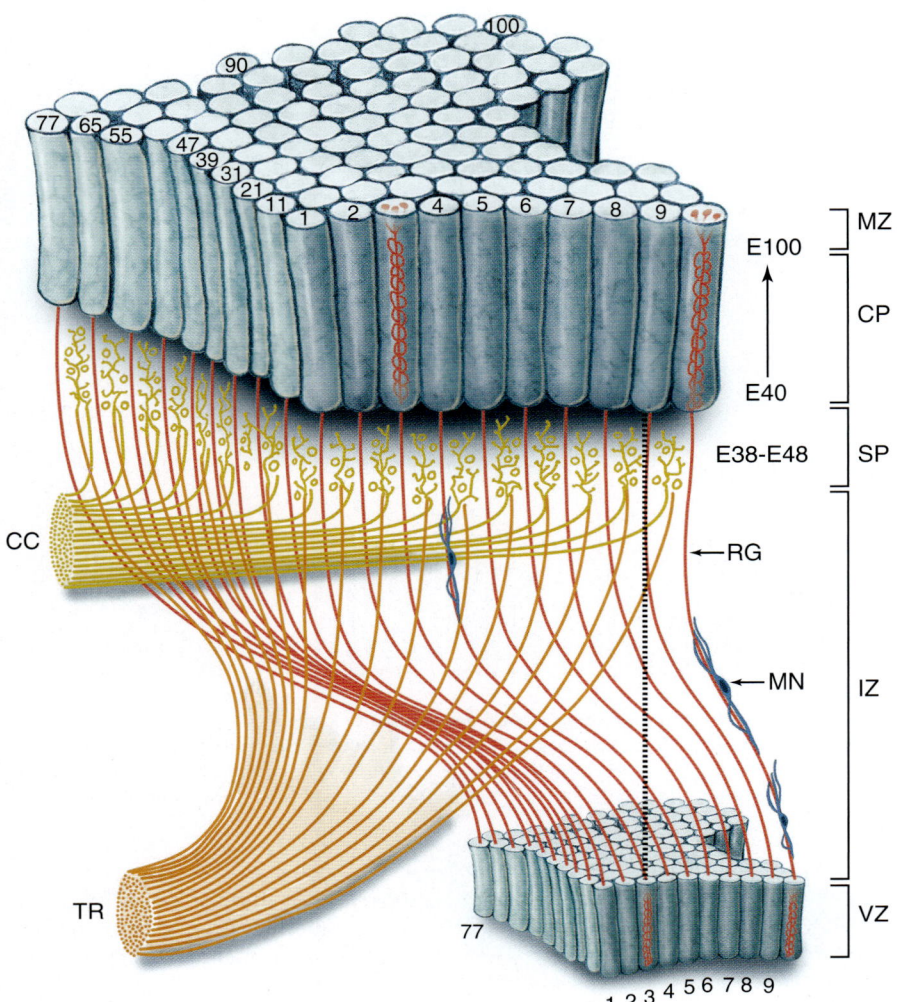

Figure 5.4 The relation between a small patch of the proliferative ventricular zone (VZ) and its corresponding area within the cortical plate (CP) in the developing cerebrum. Although the cerebral surface in primates expands and shifts during prenatal development, ontogenetic columns (outlined by cylinders) may remain attached to the corresponding proliferative units by the grid of radial glial fibers. Neurons produced between E40 and E100 by a given proliferative unit migrate in succession along the same clonally related radial glial guides (RGs) and stack up in reverse order of arrival within the same ontogenetic column. Each migrating neuron (MN) first traverses the intermediate zone (IZ) and then the subplate (SP), which contains subplate neurons and "waiting" afferents from the thalamic radiation (TR) and ipsilateral and contralateral cortico-cortical connections (CCs). After entering the cortical plate, each neuron bypasses earlier-generated neurons and settles at the interface between the CP and marginal zone (MZ). As a result, proliferative units 1 to 100 produce ontogenetic columns 1 to 100 in the same relative position to each other without a lateral mismatch (e.g., between proliferative unit 3 and ontogenetic column 9, indicated by a dashed line). Thus the specification of cytoarchitectonic areas and topographic maps depends on the spatial distribution of their ancestors in the proliferative units, whereas the laminar position and phenotype of neurons within ontogenetic columns depend on the time of their origin. Rights were not granted to include this figure in electronic media. Please refer to the printed book. (With permission from Rakic P. Specification of cerebral cortical areas. *Science.* 1988;241:170–176.)

number of proliferative units. Later proliferative events that determine the size of each column proceed normally, as evidenced not only by the normal neuronal complement of each column but also by the presence of a normal residual amount of germinal matrix at term (see Fig. 5.6).

The clinical features are not entirely clear because this anomaly is rare. The reported cases have involved full-term newborns who died in the first month of life. The distinction from anencephaly and aprosencephaly-atelencephaly is based on the presence of an intact skull and dermal covering, in contrast to anencephaly, and of a normal external appearance of cerebrum and ventricles, observable by ultrasonography, in contrast to aprosencephaly-atelencephaly. The disorder is notably familial, probably of autosomal recessive inheritance.

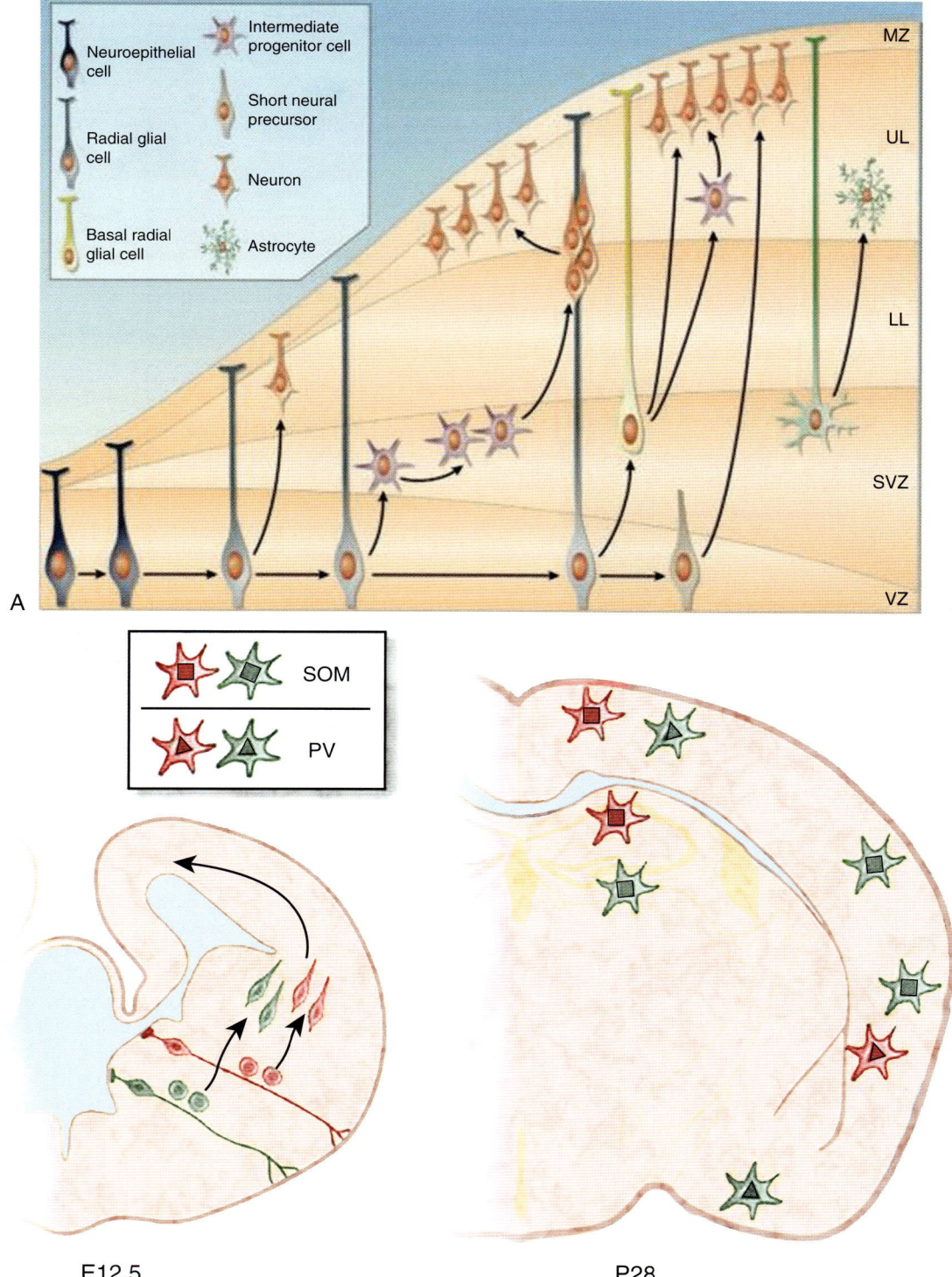

Figure 5.5 Two types of neuronal progenitors. In A, as occurs especially early in neuronal proliferation, a single neural precursor gives rise to two identical precursors, that is, a symmetrical division. In B as occurs especially later in neuronal proliferation, a radial neuronal progenitor (radial glial progenitor or radial glial cell) divides asymmetrically into dissimilar cells, that is, an identical radial progenitor and a postmitotic neuronal cell that migrates along the fiber of its clonally related radial progenitor to ultimately reach the cerebral cortex. *LL,* Lower layer; *MZ,* marginal zone; *PV,* parvalbumin; *SOM,* somatostatin; *SVZ,* subventricular zone; *UL,* upper layer; *VZ,* ventricular zone. (A, Reprinted with permission from Franco SJ, Muller U. Shaping our minds: stem and progenitor cell diversity in the mammalian neocortex. *Neuron.* 2013;77:19–34; B, reprinted with permission from Harwell CC, Fuentealba LC, Gonzalez-Cerrillo A, et al. Wide dispersion and diversity of clonally related inhibitory interneurons. *Neuron.* 2015;87:999–1007.)

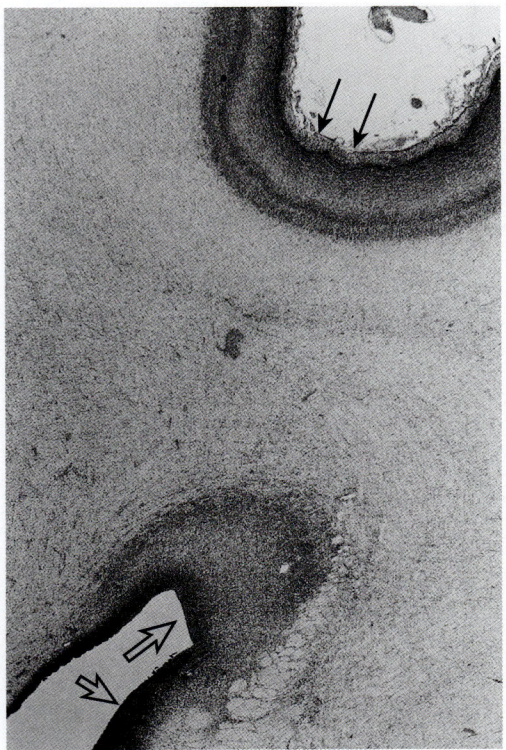

Figure 5.6 Radial microbrain. Brain of a full-term newborn with the pathological picture of radial microbrain described in the text. Note the normal cortical lamination (*long arrows*) and the normal residual germinative zone (*both open arrows*). (With permission from Evrard P, de Saint-Georges P, Kadhim HJ, et al. Pathology of prenatal encephalopathies. In French JH, Harel S, Casaer P, eds. *Child Neurology and Developmental Disabilities*, Baltimore: Paul H. Brookes; 1989.)

Anatomical Abnormality: Microcephaly Vera. As noted earlier, the designation *microcephaly vera* refers to a heterogeneous group of autosomal recessive disorders that appear to have, as the common denominator, small brain size because of a derangement of proliferation (see Box 5.3). In recent years, remarkable insights into the genetics and molecular bases of these disorders have been gained (see later).

The anatomical studies of Evrard et al.[8,57] provide insight into the fundamental disturbance in microcephaly vera, at least in a prototypical autosomal recessive variety (Box 5.5). The brain is small (clearly more than several standard deviations below the mean) but not so strikingly as in the tiny radial microbrain. Simplification of gyral pattern exists with no other external abnormality and no evidence of a destructive process. The number of cortical neuronal columns appears normal, but the neuronal complement of each column, especially the superficial cortical layers, is decreased markedly. Additional evidence of disturbance of the later proliferative events that determine size of cortical neuronal columns is the absence of residual germinal matrix in the 26-week fetal brain studied by Evrard et al. (Fig. 5.7). The deficiency in neurons of the superficial cortical layers may explain the simplification of gyral pattern (see the later discussion of gyral development in migrational disorders in Chapters 6 and 7).

Timing and Clinical Aspects: Microcephaly Vera. The presumed timing of the microcephaly vera group of disorders involves the period of later proliferative events by asymmetrical divisions of neuronal progenitors—that is, onset at approximately 6 weeks in the human—with later rapid progression until approximately 18 weeks (see earlier). The most severely undersized brains are expected to have the earliest onsets and the most marked deficiency of neurons in each cortical column.

The *clinical presentation* of infants with the prototypical autosomal recessive forms of microcephaly vera is interesting in that, with the exception of the extreme microcephaly and seizures associated with recessive mutations in the gene *PNKP*, many affected newborns do not show striking neurological deficits or seizures.[58] This presentation is in contrast with that of other varieties of microcephaly—that is, intrauterine destructive disease or other developmental derangement (e.g., migrational defect). Rare autosomal recessive forms of microcephaly with severe neuronal migrational defects (i.e., microlissencephaly) are more likely to be accompanied by neurological deficits and seizures (see the later discussion of disorders of neuronal migration in Chapter 6).

Magnetic resonance imaging (MRI) has been invaluable in the assessment of microcephaly vera, especially for evaluation of gyral development and the presence of associated migrational abnormalities.[59] Most commonly, gyral formation is variably simplified (Fig. 5.8), and the term *microcephaly with simplified gyri* is often used.[59-67] Simplification of the gyral pattern is often not obvious. Rare cases are associated with severe migrational disturbances, such as lissencephaly, periventricular heterotopia, or posterior fossa deficits, especially cerebellar hypoplasia.[62,64,65,68-70]

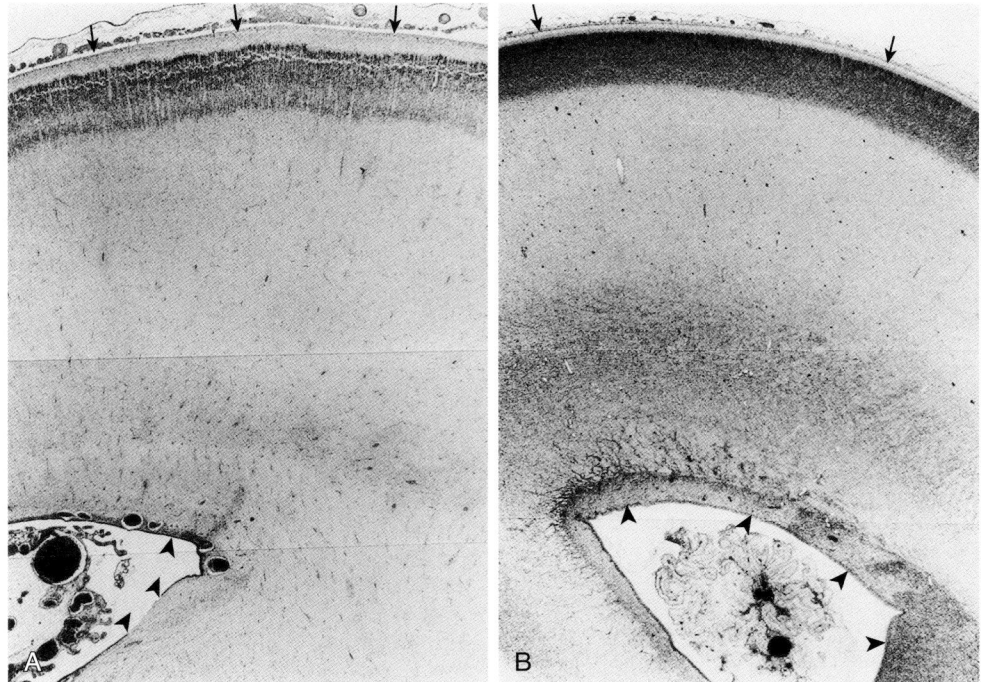

Figure 5.7 Premature exhaustion of the germinal layer in microcephaly vera. (A) Microcephaly vera, human fetal forebrain, 26 weeks of gestation. (B) Normal human fetal forebrain, 26 weeks, same cortical region for comparison. The germinal layer (*arrowheads*), cerebral cortex (*arrows*), and intervening cerebral white matter are visible. In microcephaly vera (A), the germinal layer is exhausted at this age, and the white matter is almost devoid of late migrating glial and neuronal cells. Cortical layers VI to IV are normal, whereas the two superficial layers are almost missing. (With permission from Evrard P, de Saint-Georges P, Kadhim HJ, et al. Pathology of prenatal encephalopathies. In French JH, Harel S, Casaer P, eds. *Child Neurology and Developmental Disabilities*. Baltimore, MD: Paul H. Brookes; 1989.)

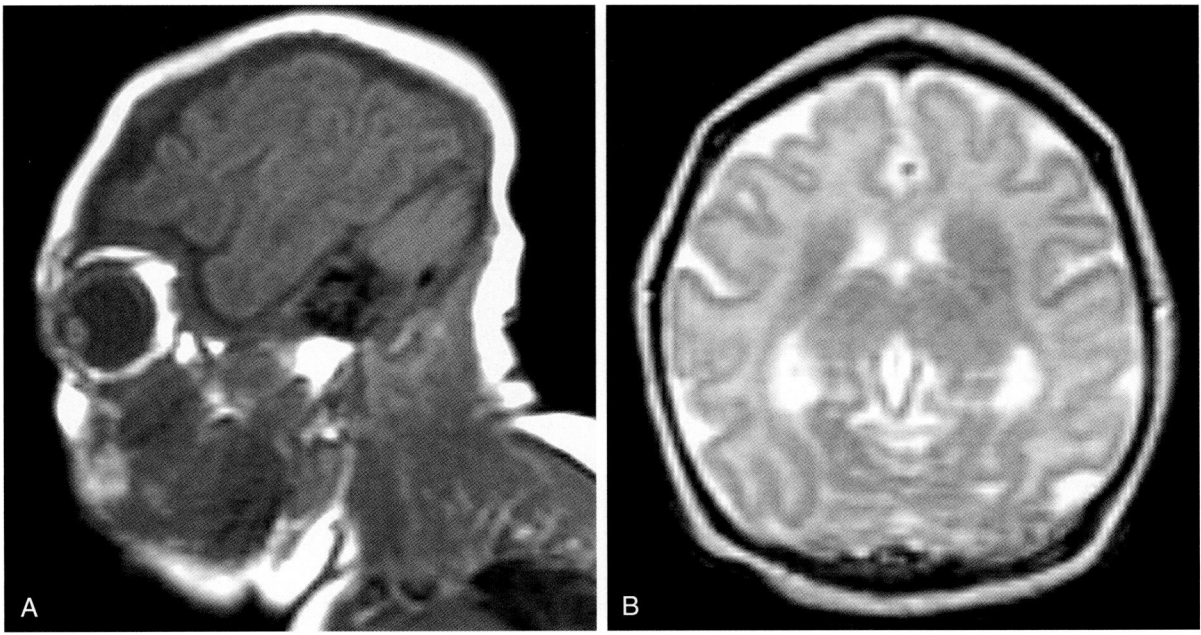

Figure 5.8 Microcephaly with simplified gyri. In A, the sagittal T1-weighted magnetic resonance image (MRI) shows marked microcephaly. In B, the axial T2-weighted MRI shows simplification of the gyral pattern. No other dysgenetic abnormalities are present, nor is there any evidence of destructive disease. (Courtesy Dr. Omar Khwaja.)

TABLE 5.1   Autosomal Recessive Primary Microcephaly (Microcephaly Vera): Molecular Genetics

LOCUS	GENE/PROTEIN	PROCESSES AFFECTED
MCPH1	MCPH1/microcephalin	Cell cycle control
MCPH2	WDR62/WD repeating-containing protein 62	Mitosis (centrosome)
MCPH3	CDK5RAP2/cyclin-dependent kinase-5 regulatory associated protein-2	Mitotic spindle formation
MCPH4	CASC5/cancer-associated candidate 5	Mitotic spindle formation
MCPH5	ASPM/abnormal spindle in microcephaly	Mitotic spindle formation
MCPH6	CENPJ/centromere-associated protein J	Mitotic spindle formation
MCPH7	STIL/SCL/Tal1 interrupting locus	Mitotic spindle formation
MCPH8	CEP135/centrosomal protein 135 kD	Mitosis (centrosome)
MCPH9	CEP152/centrosomal protein 152 kD	Mitosis (centrosome)
MCPH10	ZNF335/zinc finger protein 335	Regulation of neurogenesis

MCPH, Autosomal recessive primary microcephaly.

Etiology: Autosomal Recessive Microcephaly (Microcephaly Vera). At least 16 genetic loci have been identified for autosomal recessive primary microcephaly, or microcephaly vera. Genes have been identified for the majority of the loci, though sometimes only in one family (Table 5.1).[63,71-87] Perhaps not unexpectedly, the genes play key roles in mitosis. *Microcephalin* is crucial for cell cycle control, chromosome condensation, and DNA repair. CDK5RAP2 is a centrosomal protein involved in microtubular function necessary for formation of the mitotic spindle. ASPM also is necessary for microtubular function at the poles of the mitotic spindle, and CENPJ is similarly involved in formation of the mitotic spindle. Of all these single-gene causes of autosomal recessive microcephaly, *ASPM* appears to be the most common, and mutations have been identified in nonfamilial cases as well.

There is a group of autosomal recessive microcephalies that are associated with MRI findings suggestive of a destructive process. These include microcephaly with cerebral hemorrhage and calcification as well as congenital cataracts, associated with recessive mutations in the tight-junction protein-encoding gene *JAM3*.[88] Included in this category, which is sometimes referred to as *TORCH-like*, is also the relatively newly identified *PCDH12*-related recessive syndrome involving, progressive microcephaly with dysplasia of the hypothalamus and midbrain, the first microcephaly to be related to vascular endothelial cadherin (cell adhesion protein) dysfunction.[89]

Etiology: Other Disorders. The four major etiological categories for primary microcephaly, in addition to the autosomal recessive group just discussed, are familial, teratogenic, syndromic, and sporadic (see Box 5.3). *Familial syndromes* are most critical to detect because of implications for genetic counseling. In addition

to the autosomal recessive group (see earlier), these inherited varieties include autosomal dominant and X-linked recessive types as well as familial types with ocular abnormalities and variable genetics.[90-104] These ocular abnormalities may include chorioretinopathy, which can be confused with the chorioretinitis of intrauterine infection (see Chapter 34). One such disorder is *Cohen syndrome*, which is inherited in an autosomal recessive manner. Of the unusual cases of microcephaly with autosomal dominant inheritance, intellect is subsequently usually either spared or only mildly defective; patients generally have no facial dysmorphism, although digital anomalies and rare syndromic varieties have been reported.[101,104] X-linked recessive inheritance of microcephaly has been described, albeit less commonly than autosomal recessive inheritance.

The best-documented *teratogenic agent* producing microcephaly is irradiation, such as that due to an atomic explosion or radiation therapy for tumor or ankylosing spondylitis, particularly before 18 weeks of gestation (see Box 5.3).[105-107] The most critical gestational period in the Nagasaki-Hiroshima experience was 8 to 15 weeks.[107] Maternal alcoholism or cocaine abuse (see Chapter 38) and maternal hyperphenylalaninemia have been associated with microcephaly. Microcephaly, usually with intellectual disability, occurs in as many as 75% to 90% of (nonphenylketonuric) children of women with phenylketonuria; the risk for the fetus correlates with the severity of the maternal hyperphenylalaninemia.[108-118] With dietary treatment, the risk declines to as low as 8% when phenylalanine levels are controlled before conception and to 18% when control is achieved by 10 weeks of pregnancy.[119] When control is not achieved until 20 to 30 weeks, the incidence of microcephaly increases to 40%. Rarer intrauterine teratogens for microcephaly include anticonvulsant drugs (see Chapter 38), organic mercurials, and excessive ingestion of vitamin A or vitamin A analogues (see Chapter 38).[120] Finally, among intrauterine infections that may cause microcephaly (see Chapter 34), rubella is the best candidate for an agent that may produce microcephaly through an impairment of proliferation rather than principally through a destructive process. Cytomegalovirus infection may also act in this way, although disturbances of neuronal migration and destructive lesions contribute to the condition. Human immunodeficiency virus characteristically produces microcephaly (without major destructive lesions) after the neonatal period, although neonatal cases have been reported (see Chapter 34). Most recently, maternal infection with the Zika virus (ZIKV) has been associated with microcephaly with or without cerebral calcifications and varying degrees of intellectual disability.[121-123]

Syndromic cases, that is, those with multiple associated systemic anomalies, may be related to chromosomal disorders or monogenic (familial) defects, or they may occur sporadically (see Box 5.3). In one consecutive sample of congenital microcephaly, syndromic disorders accounted for only 6% of cases.[124] The nature of the proliferative disorder in this diverse group is generally not known, and it is not discussed further here. Clinical details are available in standard sources.[103]

Sporadic nonsyndromic cases—that is, those with no related family history, identifiable teratogen, or recognizable syndrome—are the most common varieties of microcephaly vera (see Box 5.3).[124,125] No associated systemic or other neural malformations can be identified. The nature of the proliferative disturbance is generally unknown. Any of the described autosomal dominant or X-linked conditions may also occur sporadically owing to a de novo mutation, which occurs typically during meiosis, while one of the gametes is being formed. Thus clinical genetic testing for known causes of microcephaly—for example with a gene panel—is indicated in otherwise unexplained cases.

Macrocephaly

Anatomical Abnormality. The designation *macrocephaly* signifies a large head and, by implication, a large brain. Thus the term *megalencephaly* is also often used, particularly when there is neuroimaging to support the assertion that the large head size is accompanied by, and in fact presumably caused by, large brain size. Macrocephaly is a feature of a heterogeneous group of disorders that have not been well defined from the neuropathological standpoint. Nevertheless, several entities clearly exist in which the brain is generally well formed but unusually large (Box 5.6). Genetic varieties, suggestive of a derangement in the developmental program for neuronal proliferation, have been defined (see following discussion).[126] As with microcephaly, however, the conclusion that we are dealing

---

---

with proliferative disorders can be drawn only tenuously until central neuronal populations can be quantified more accurately. This discussion *excludes* other rare disorders of macrocephaly, such as enlargement of the skull (craniometaphyseal dysplasia, hemoglobinopathy), subdural hematoma, or effusion (see Chapters 22, 35, and 36), hydrocephalus (see Chapters 3, 24, and 35), metabolic disorders (see Chapter 28), or degenerative disorders (Alexander disease, Canavan disease [see Chapter 29]).

Timing and Clinical Aspects. Although neuronal proliferation in the cerebrum is an event that occurs principally during the third and fourth months of gestation, this time period may be prolonged in disorders of excessive proliferation. Alternatively, abnormal proliferation may occur at the appropriate time during development but at an excessive rate. In addition, a later-occurring defect of normal apoptosis or programmed cell death (see later) could perhaps lead to macrocephaly. The issues of mechanism are unresolved and await development of suitable experimental models for elucidation.

The *clinical syndrome* in the several types of macrocephaly (see Box 5.6) varies from no apparent neurological deficit (e.g., autosomal dominant, isolated macrocephaly) to severe recalcitrant seizures and intellectual disability (e.g., autosomal recessive, isolated macrocephaly, or unilateral macrocephaly). In other types of the disorder, extraneural features may dominate the clinical presentation (e.g., associated growth disorders and certain neurocutaneous syndromes). Some of these individual clinical aspects are mentioned briefly in the following discussion.

Familial Isolated Macrocephaly. Perhaps the most common variety of macrocephaly occurs in the familial setting and in the absence of any other extraneural findings. For this group, we use the term *familial isolated macrocephaly*. Two genetic types can be recognized: autosomal dominant and autosomal recessive; the former is much more common.

In familial, isolated macrocephaly of the *autosomal dominant type*, the head is usually large at birth (>90th percentile in about 50%) and continues to grow postnatally at a relatively rapid rate.[127,128] Neurological deficits are rarely striking, and development and ultimate level of intelligence are in the normal range in approximately 50% to 60% of cases. Pronounced intellectual disability is present in only approximately 10%. The genetic component of this syndrome is frequently overlooked until the parents' head circumference is measured. The diagnosis of fetal macrocephaly of this type was made in the 34th week of pregnancy in a woman with benign macrocephaly.[129]

Related to autosomal dominant macrocephaly is a syndrome of macrocephaly categorized under several names: *benign enlargement of extracerebral spaces, benign subdural effusions of infancy*, and *idiopathic external hydrocephalus*.[128,130-136] The clinical features described in the previous paragraph are present, and brain imaging studies show prominent extracerebral subarachnoid spaces, particularly in the frontal regions, and a large brain (Fig. 5.9). The cisterna magna especially may be prominent. In some cases, subdural and subarachnoid fluid appears to be present; the distinction is best made by MRI.[130] Head growth in the first year is rapid, and infants not overtly macrocephalic at birth attain rates of head growth at the 97th percentile or slightly higher. Accelerating head growth ceases by approximately 1 year; over the next several years extracerebral spaces become smaller, although the brain is clearly larger than average. Because of the

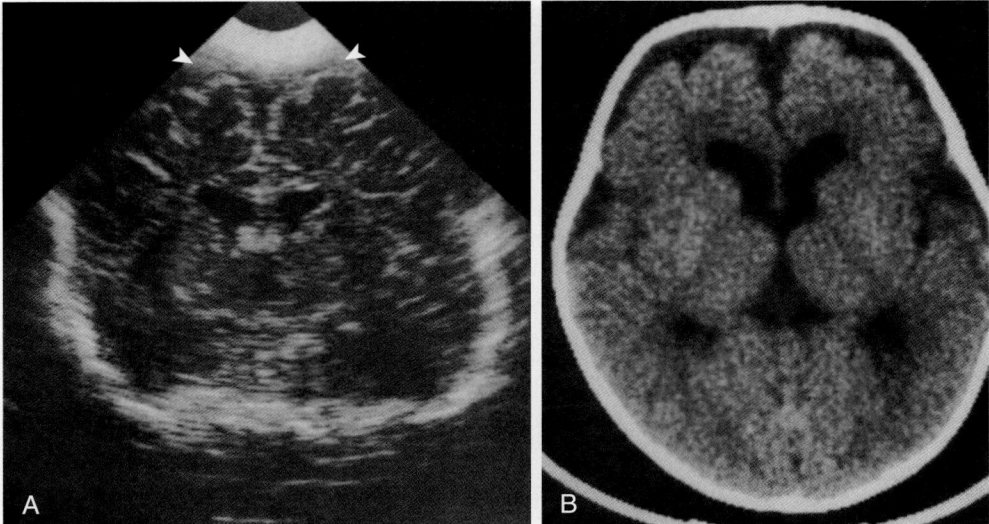

Figure 5.9 Benign macrocephaly. (A) Coronal sonogram demonstrates mild ventricular enlargement and moderate extra-axial fluid over the convexities (*arrowheads*). (B) Axial computed tomography scan shows similar findings. (With permission from Babcock DS, Han BK, Dine MS. Sonographic findings in infants with macrocrania, *AJNR Am J Neuroradiol.* 1988;9:307–313.)

large brain size, if the infant is first evaluated after the second year of life, isolated macrocephaly will be observed. Because as many as 90% of these infants have a parent with a large head, the genetic features are similar to those of autosomal dominant isolated macrocephaly. The similarity of the clinical features and genetics suggests that these may represent different forms of the same fundamental disorder. Those unusual patients with isolated macrocephaly that conforms to *autosomal recessive inheritance* are more likely to exhibit definite intellectual disability, epilepsy, and motor deficits.[120]

Sporadic Isolated Macrocephaly. Isolated macrocephaly, or megalencephaly, with no evidence of a familial disorder by history and after measurement of parental head circumference occurs only slightly less often than the autosomal dominant disorder described previously.[127,137,138] The clinical course is similar.

Associated Disturbance of Growth. Macrocephaly may be associated with generalized disorders of growth, such as achondroplasia, Beckwith syndrome, cerebral gigantism (Sotos syndrome), fragile X syndrome, Marshall-Smith syndrome, thanatophoric dysplasia, Cowden syndrome, Sotos syndrome, and Weaver syndrome (see Box 5.6).[103,126,127,139-143] Except in Beckwith syndrome, which is complicated by neonatal hypoglycemia, neurological features in the neonatal period are unusual. The precise neuropathological correlates for the macrocephaly in these disorders remain to be defined. The gene mutated or deleted in Sotos syndrome, *NSD1*, encodes a nuclear receptor binding protein that may be involved in proliferative events.[141,142]

Neurocutaneous Syndromes. Several of the neurocutaneous disorders are associated with evidence of excessive cellular proliferation within the CNS, sometimes with overt macrocephaly and evidence of excessive proliferation of mesodermal structures

(see Box 5.6). Macrocephaly occurs most consistently in this context in the multiple hemangiomatosis syndromes.[103,144-150]

In *neurofibromatosis*, an autosomal dominant disorder, the principal proliferative abnormality involves glia, particularly astrocytes. (Thus the onset of the proliferative disorder in this disease occurs primarily after the time period of neuronal proliferative events.) Approximately 40% of infants exhibit more than five café-au-lait spots larger than 5 mm at birth.[151-157] Approximately 40% to 50% of such infants have macrocephaly, usually after the neonatal period.[158,159] Consistent with the predominantly glial rather than neuronal involvement in the disorder, the megalencephaly relates primarily to increases in cerebral *white matter* volume, primarily in frontal and parietal areas.[160] Relative macrocephaly with generalized glial tumors has been documented by prenatal ultrasound.[161] Hemimegalencephaly with neonatal seizures and associated neuronal migrational defects has also been observed.[162,163] Of the glial tumors that are the hallmark of this disease, optic nerve glioma and plexiform neuroma of the eyelid have been observed in the newborn, albeit rarely.[152,157] The gene for this disorder, located on chromosome 17, *NF1*, has been shown to encode a protein involved in the negative regulation of a key signal transduction pathway, the Ras pathway, which transmits mitogenic signals to the nucleus.[155-157,164,165] Thus loss of neurofibromin, the neurofibromatosis protein, leads to increased mitogenic signaling and thereby to the proliferative abnormalities characteristic of the disorder.

In *Sturge-Weber disease*, a sporadic disorder, the principal abnormality affects leptomeningeal blood vessels. Thus the time of onset is probably coincident with that for neuronal proliferation. Data suggest that the fundamental defect in this disorder is a failure of development of superficial cortical veins, resulting in diversion of blood to the developing leptomeninges with the formation of abnormal vascular channels as a consequence.[166] Abnormalities of fibronectin in cerebral vessels may play a role in the genesis of the vascular abnormality.[167] The

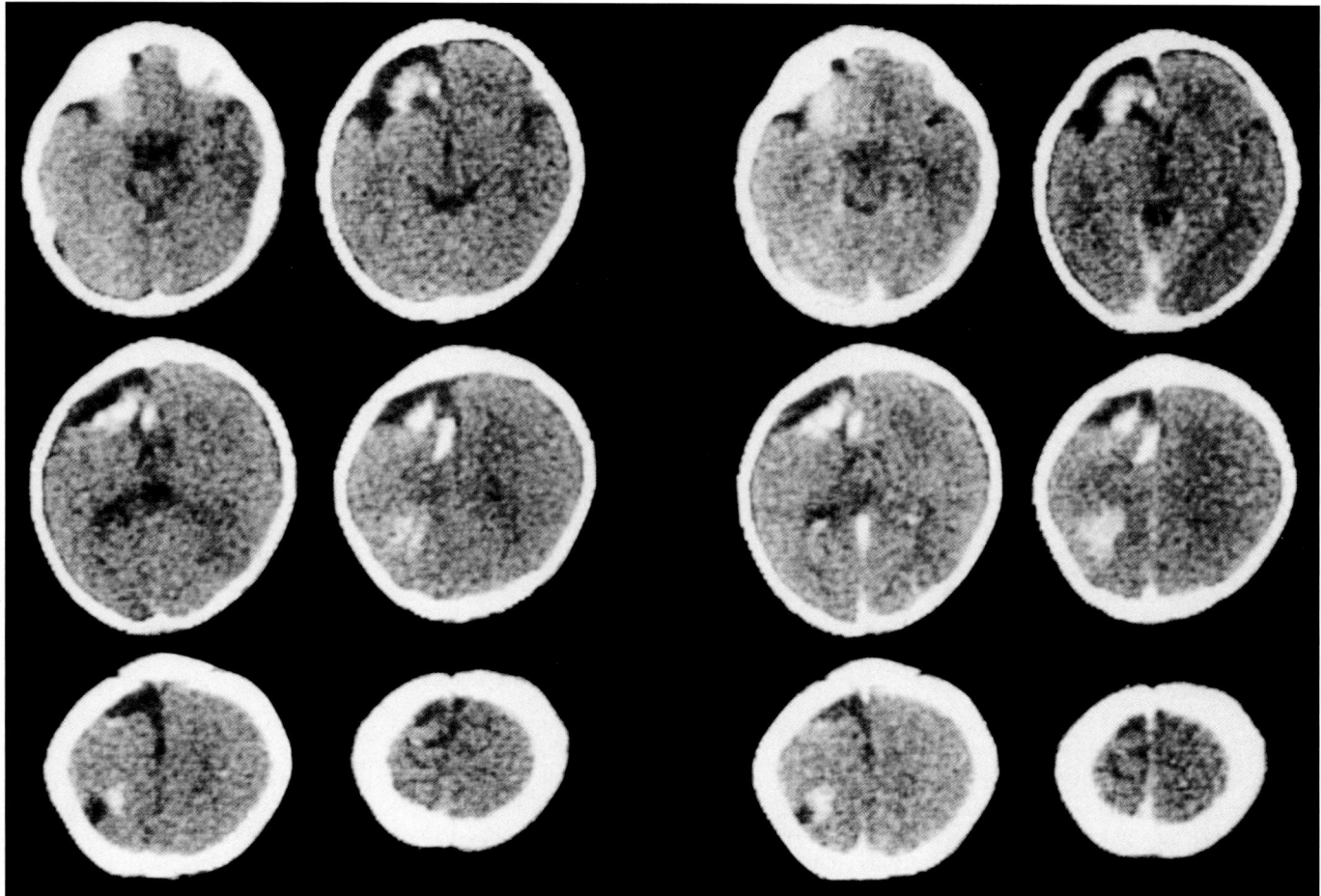

Figure 5.10 **Sturge-Weber disease, computed tomography (CT) scan.** This infant exhibited seizures on the fifth day of life. The CT scan was obtained at the age of 4 months. *Left,* Conventional CT scan. *Right,* Contrast-enhanced CT scan. Note marked atrophy and calcification in the left frontal region and, to a lesser extent, in the left parietal region. Only scant contrast enhancement is apparent. (With permission from Kitihara T, Maki U. A case of Sturge-Weber disease with epilepsy and intracranial calcification at the neonatal period. *Eur Neurol.* 1978;17:8–12.)

characteristic facial port-wine stain is described in Chapter 9; the overall incidence of clinical manifestations of Sturge-Weber disease (glaucoma or seizures) is 2% to 8% in patients with unilateral facial lesions and 24% in those with bilateral facial lesions.[166,168,169] Identification of the newborn with intracranial involvement is difficult. Seizures and cerebral calcification (identified by computed tomography [CT]) have been noted only occasionally in newborns (Fig. 5.10).[59,170-173] Cerebral calcifications most commonly appear after 6 months of age and often considerably later.[149,166,174-176] MRI is the most useful imaging study in the first year[59,149,166,169,175-178]; the principal findings are cerebral cortical and white matter changes in the region of the leptomeningeal angiomatosis, angiomatous alteration of overlying calvaria, and atypically located, congested deep cerebral veins.[149,175,177] Gadolinium-enhanced MRI is the gold standard for demonstration of the leptomeningeal vascular lesion (Fig. 5.11).[59,149,166,175-177] The choroid plexus is enlarged on the side of the leptomeningeal lesion, presumably because of the diversion of venous blood into the deep venous system as a consequence of the lack of superficial cortical venous drainage

(see earlier discussion). On studies by single photon emission tomography, decreased cortical perfusion may be observed in the region of the vascular lesion.[166,176,179,180] MRI perfusion studies also may be useful in detecting perfusion deficits.[181] Infants with Sturge-Weber syndrome who have bilateral cerebral disease have a much poorer outcome (8% with average intelligence) than those with unilateral cerebral disease (45% with average intelligence).[a] Although it has long been suspected to be a genetic syndrome, Sturge-Weber syndrome was only relatively recently associated with somatic or postzygotic mutations in the gene *GNAQ*.[184]

In *tuberous sclerosis complex (TSC)*, the principal proliferative abnormality affects both neurons and glia. The neuropathological and molecular aspects of these disorders indicate that TSC also reflects abnormal migration and differentiation (see later).[185-187] The critical neonatal cutaneous feature is a depigmented, ash leaf-shaped macule. Seizures may occur in

---

[a]References 169, 173, 179, 180, 182, 183.

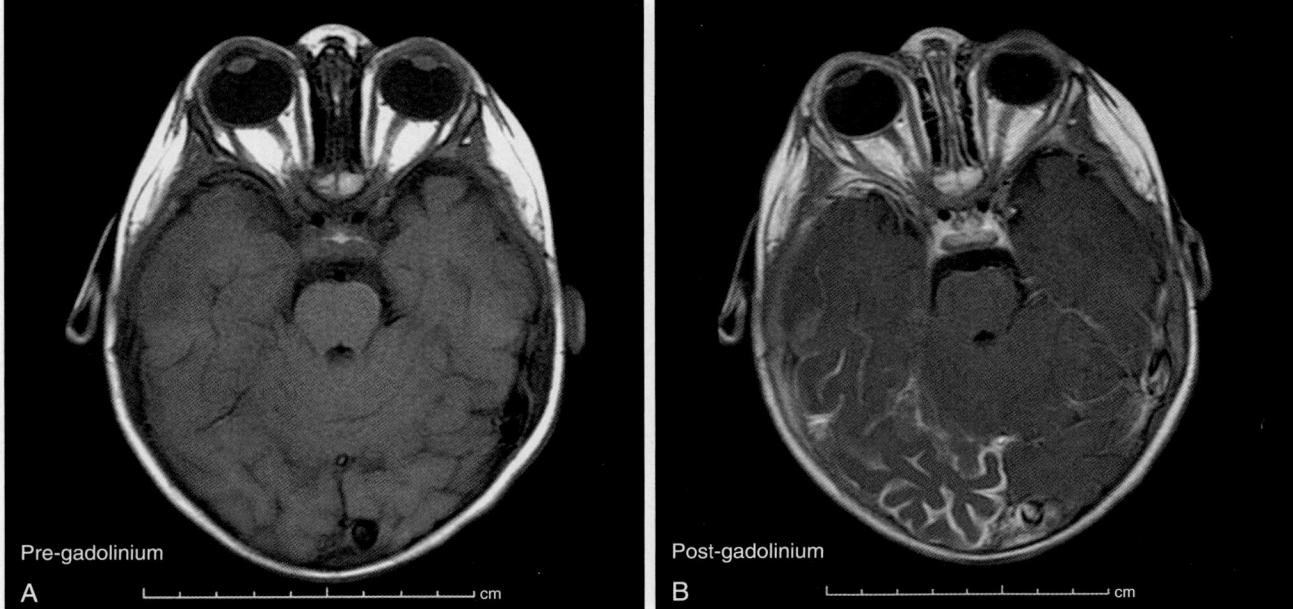

Figure 5.11 Sturge-Weber disease, gadolinium-enhanced magnetic resonance imaging (MRI) scan.
(A) Axial MRI scan before administration of gadolinium in an infant with a port-wine stain; no definite abnormality is evident. (B) The scan after gadolinium enhancement shows diffuse leptomeningeal enhancement in the right occipital and temporal regions. The findings are characteristic of Sturge-Weber disease. (Courtesy Dr. Omar Khwaja.)

the neonatal period.[185,188-191] Cardiac tumors (rhabdomyomata) are characteristic and uncommonly may lead to neurological features by causing cardiac failure, arrhythmias, or cerebral emboli (unpublished personal cases). Cardiac rhabdomyomata have been identified in affected fetuses and are usually the first clue to prenatal diagnosis.[192,193] The diagnosis of TSC is established in 80% to 95% of fetuses with cardiac rhabdomyomata.[194,195] The natural history of these tumors is favorable; virtually all regress at least partially.[195] Subependymal nodules, the most common cerebral lesion detected in utero, have been identified as early as 21 weeks.[196] Indeed, we consider the most useful *constellation of features for the diagnosis of TSC in the neonatal period* to consist of the depigmented macule, cardiac rhabdomyoma, subependymal nodule, and cortical tuber. In one large series, approximately 90% of newborns studied by MRI exhibited the last two cerebral lesions.[193]

Neuropathological features include both the characteristic subependymal and cerebral cortical-subcortical collections of abnormal neurons and glia (i.e., subependymal nodules and cortical tubers) and heterotopic collections of similar cells in the cerebral white matter, often arranged in radial bands.[197-202] The cells are often bizarre, large, and poorly differentiated, exhibiting features of both neurons and astrocytes. Subependymal giant cell astrocytoma has been reported in newborns with TSC,[193,203-205] but more typically it appears in older children. Both CT scanning and ultrasonography can be useful in diagnosis (Figs. 5.12 and 5.13).[59,188,189,206,207] However, MRI is preferred in the neonatal period and demonstrates the subependymal collections, cortical tubers, and white matter lesions especially well (Fig. 5.14).[a] Because of the unmyelinated cerebral white

matter in the newborn, the cortical tubers (hypointense on T1-weighted images, hyperintense on T2-weighted images) have signal characteristics opposite those exhibited by older children with the disorder.[59,202]

The TSC phenotype is associated with dysfunction of genes on either chromosome 9 or chromosome 16.[165,211-213] The disorder, although autosomal dominant, is associated with a high spontaneous mutation rate. Overall, approximately 80% of cases are sporadic.[186,187] The genes, *TSC1* on chromosome 9 and *TSC2* on chromosome 16, encode the respective proteins hamartin and tuberin.[186,187] Hamartin and tuberin interact to form a complex, and this complex is involved in molecular signaling critical for cell proliferation, cell growth, and cell adhesion/migration.[186,187,214] Disturbance of these processes underlies the proliferative abnormalities (subependymal nodules, astrocytomas, and cardiac, renal, and other tumors), the abnormalities of cell size (large, bizarre cells in nodules and tubers) and the radial white matter disturbances (apparent disturbances in radial migration and release of migrating cells from the radial glial progenitor). The *TSC2* mutations result in the most severe phenotypes and account for the majority of neonatal cases. Previously, diagnostic testing for mutations in the coding regions of *TSC1* and *TSC2* revealed a pathogenic mutation in 85% to 90% of individuals with TSC diagnosed clinically; the majority of the *unsolved* cases have more recently been attributed to mosaic or intronic mutations of the same two genes, providing a very tight genotype-phenotype association between the clinical syndrome and these genes.[215]

Chromosomal Disorders. The possibility that the fragile X syndrome may include a proliferative abnormality is raised by the finding of absolute or relative macrocephaly in approximately 40% of infants (see Box 5.6).[216,217] However, a disturbance

---

[a]References 59, 193, 201, 202, 204, 208-210.

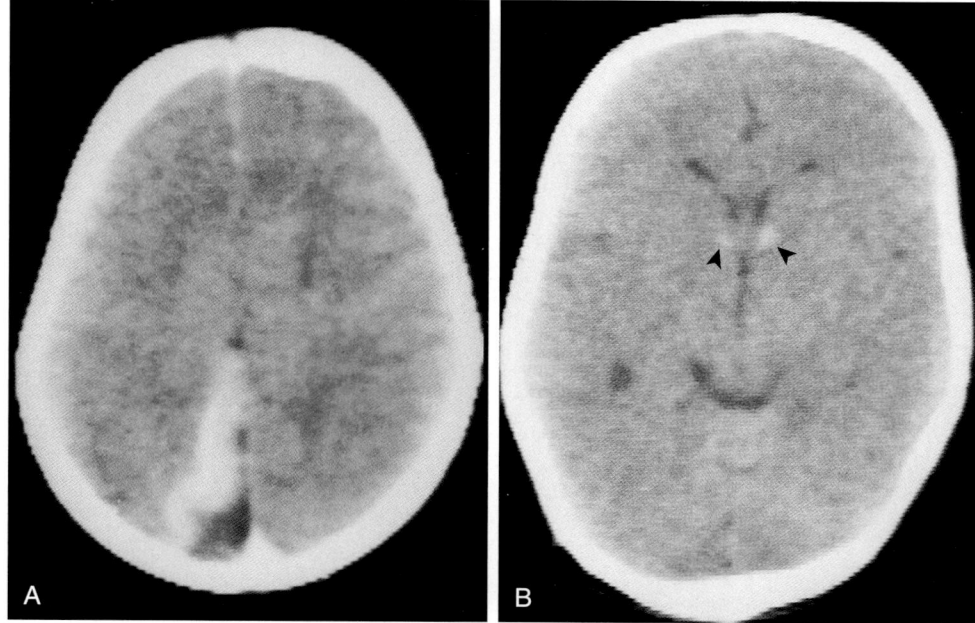

Figure 5.12 Tuberous sclerosis complex, computed tomography scan. This infant exhibited generalized seizures and depigmented macules at 4 weeks of age. Note in A, the striking cortical tuberous change in the left occipital region, and in B, the small subependymal nodules (*arrowheads*) near the heads of both caudate nuclei.

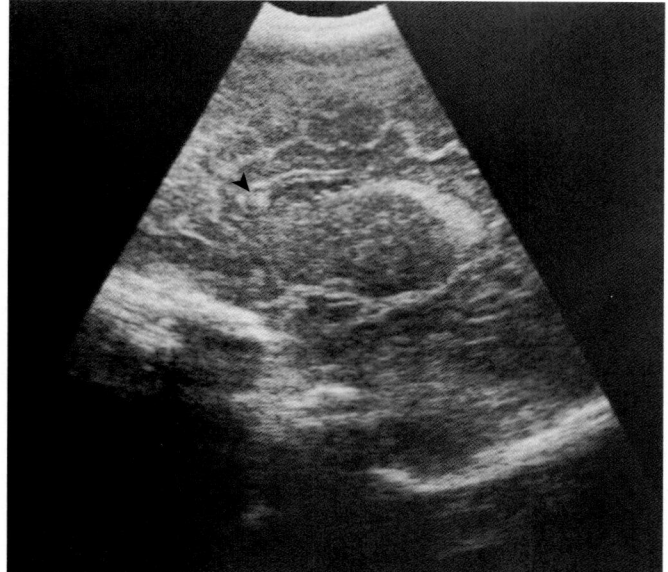

Figure 5.13 Tuberous sclerosis complex, ultrasound scan. This infant exhibited depigmented macules with myoclonic seizures at 3 weeks of age. The parasagittal ultrasound scan shows an echogenic subependymal nodule (*arrowhead*) that was also seen on a computed tomography scan.

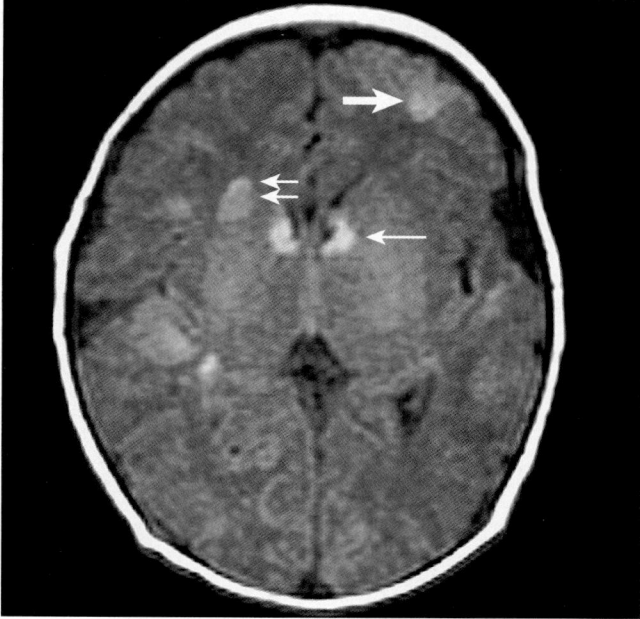

Figure 5.14 Tuberous sclerosis complex, magnetic resonance imaging (MRI). This 11-day-old infant was identified in utero with a cardiac rhabdomyoma. On this axial T1-weighted MRI, note the multiple cortical tubers (*thick arrow*), subependymal nodules (*thin arrow*), and radial cerebral white matter lesion (*double arrows*). (Courtesy Dr. Omar Khwaja.)

of cerebral organizational events appears to be the dominant neural abnormality in fragile X syndrome (see Chapter 7). Rarer chromosomal disorders with macrocephaly are Klinefelter syndrome and partial trisomy of chromosome 7.[120,218,219]

Unilateral Macrocephaly (Hemimegalencephaly).
Unilateral macrocephaly represents, at least in part, a localized disorder of cell proliferation within the CNS (see Box 5.6). The anatomical

data suggest excessive proliferation of both neurons and astrocytes but also defects in subsequent migration of neurons and cortical organization. In this disorder, enlargement of one hemisphere or a portion thereof occurs, often accompanied by abnormal cortical gyration, a disordered and unusually thick cortex, large and sometimes bizarre neurons, heterotopic neurons in subcortical white matter, and increased number and often size of astrocytes.[129,220-234]

The *clinical syndrome* in isolated and syndromic cases has consistently included severe seizures from early infancy, usually in the neonatal period, with subsequent severely disturbed neurological development.[129,231-248] The cranial asymmetry in unilateral macrocephaly may be overlooked in the newborn if the skull is not examined carefully, especially from above. CT scanning demonstrates a degree of enlargement of the hemisphere or a portion thereof that initially may be suggestive of a congenital neoplasm. MRI is preferred and is the best imaging method to demonstrate the neuronal heterotopias and abnormalities of cerebral cortical gyration (Fig. 5.15). Electroencephalography (EEG) in the infants with

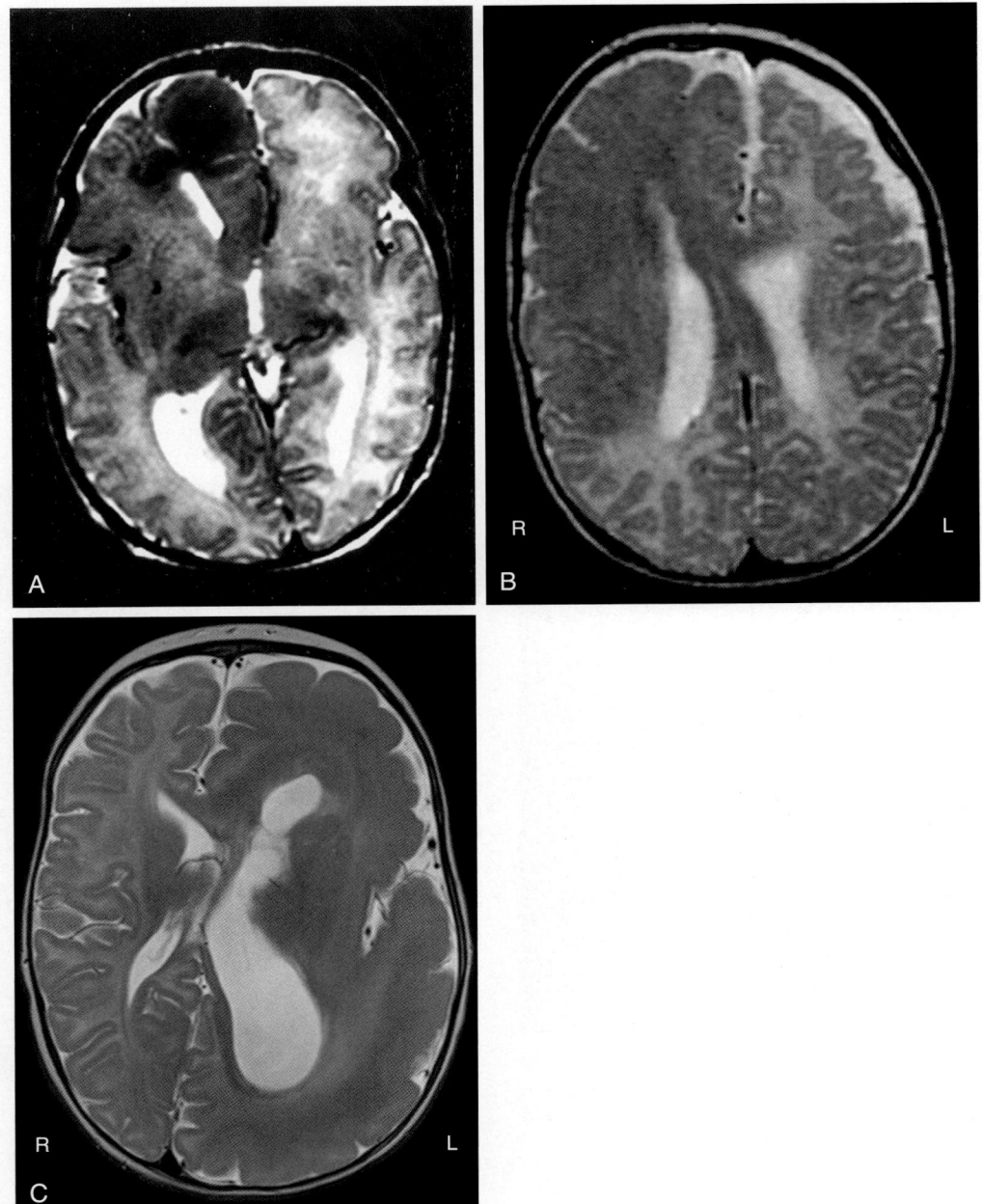

Figure 5.15 Hemimegalencephaly, magnetic resonance imaging (MRI). T2-weighted axial MRI (A) shows an enlarged right hemisphere with right frontal pachygyria. Note also the enlarged right lateral ventricle and anomalous configuration of the right frontal horn. The left hemisphere is normal. (B) Axial T2 image from a boy with hemimegalencephaly due to a postzygotic mutation in *AKT3*. The E17K mutation was reported in Poduri et al., 2012. (C) Axial T2 image from a girl with hemimegalencephaly caused by a postzygotic *PIK3CA* E545K mutation. Diagnosis was made clinically by sampling brain tissue in the course of hemispherectomy and peripheral blood leukocytes as a source of mutation-negative tissue. (A, From Flores-Sarnat L. Hemimegalencephaly. I. Genetic, clinical, and imaging aspects. *J Child Neurol.* 2002;16:373–384.)

earliest onset of seizures may demonstrate a characteristic pattern of larger-amplitude triphasic complexes. Seizures are usually recalcitrant to therapy. Hemispherectomy, as early as the first months of life, has been followed by improved outcome.[233,238-240,246,249] Prognosis after hemispherectomy depends primarily on the functional status of the contralateral hemisphere. Positron emission tomographic studies of cerebral glucose utilization showed cortical hypometabolism in the contralateral hemisphere in four of eight infants, and this abnormality correlated with a poorer outcome after hemispherectomy.[249] Related physiological studies showed that the nonmalformed hemisphere is secondarily impaired with persistent clinical and electrical seizures as early as the first months of life, and early hemispherectomy is beneficial.[250] Indeed, bilateral neuropathological changes, albeit with less severe changes in the contralateral hemisphere, have been described.[229]

Syndromic varieties of hemimegalencephaly are multiple but most commonly include epidermal nevus syndrome, Proteus syndrome, and hypomelanosis of Ito (see Box 5.6).[233] A relatively rare neurocutaneous disorder, *epidermal nevus syndrome*, is associated with hemimegalencephaly in approximately half of the cases.[233,243,251-253] The clinical neurological and neuropathological features are essentially similar to those just described for sporadic cases of hemimegalencephaly.[243,251,254-262] The characteristic cutaneous feature is illustrated in Fig. 5.16. Many infants exhibit facial hemihypertrophy as a result of lipomatous-hamartomatous lesions of the lower half of the cheek. In *Proteus syndrome*, unilateral or generalized hypertrophy of the body; thickened, hyperpigmented skin; lipomata, lymphangiomata, and hemangiomata; macrodactyly; and a curious gyriform appearance of the plantar surface of the feet may accompany the hemimegalencephaly.

Genetics of Megalencephaly, Focal Cortical Dysplasia, and Related Disorders. The association between Proteus syndrome and hemimegalencephaly has proven to have a biological basis that provides major insight to the critical role of the mTOR-AKT pathway in the regulation of cell proliferation. Thus, as somatic or postzygotic, mutations in the gene *AKT1* were identified as the cause of Proteus syndrome,[263] mutations in *AKT3*[264] and related genes in the mTOR-AKT pathway[264,265] were identified as the causes of hemimegalencephaly. These discoveries have extended to the genetics of megalencephaly as well as focal cortical dysplasia (FCD).[266,267] The dysregulation of the mTOR-AKT pathway (depicted in Fig. 5.17 and Table 5.2) in a subset of early progenitor cells can thus lead either to very focal brain lesions or very widespread overgrowth—the extent of which are mediated by the timing (germline vs. postzygotic, and if the latter, how early or late), location, and nature of the mutations.[266,268]

An early report of hemimegalencephaly genetics demonstrated that this developmental brain lesion could be related to *AKT3* mutation in mosaic form, specifically by increased copy number of *AKT3* or by point mutation resulting in a glutamate residue at amino acid position 17 being changed to lysine in the AKT3 protein (E17K).[269] The presence of mosaic mutations, present

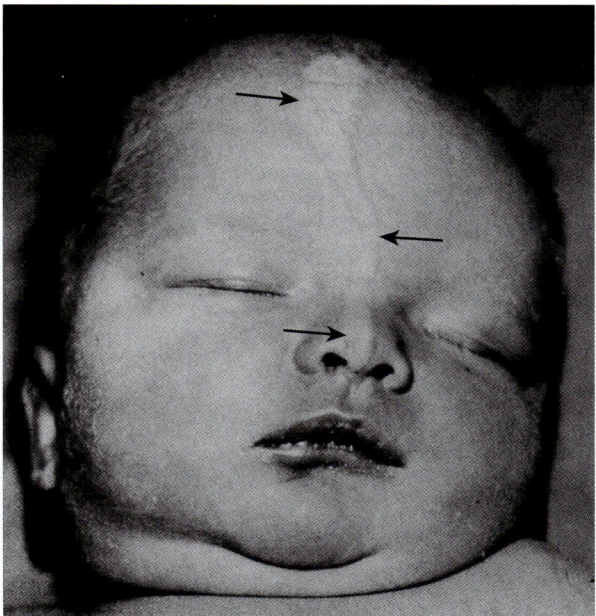

Figure 5.16 Epidermal nevus syndrome. This infant was 48 hours old. Note the midline linear nevus (*arrows*). (With permission from Chalhub EG, Volpe JJ, Gado MH. Linear nevus sebaceous syndrome associated with porencephaly and nonfunctioning major cerebral venous sinuses. *Neurology.* 1975;25:857–860.)

	BRAIN MALFORMATION/ ASSOCIATED	
GENE	**FEATURES**	**INHERITANCE**
AKT1	Hemimegalencephaly/	De novo,
AKT3	Proteus syndrome	postzygotic
CCND2	Hemimegalencephaly/FCD	De novo,
DEPDC5	Polymicrogyria/MPPH	postzygotic
MTOR	syndrome	De novo/dominant
PIK3CA	Hemimegalencephaly/FCD (also nonlesional focal epilepsy)	De novo/dominant ± postzygotic (may be inherited)
	Hemimegalencephaly/FCD	De novo,
	Hemimegalencephaly/ MCAP syndrome	postzygotic De novo,
	CLOVES and KTS	postzygotic (rare germline)
PIK3R2	MPPH syndrome	De novo/dominant
PTEN	Hemimegalencephaly/FCD Megalencephaly/autism Cowden syndrome Bannayan-Riley-Ruvalcaba syndrome	De novo/dominant (may be inherited)
TSC1/ TSC2	Hemimegalencephaly/FCD TSC	De novo/dominant ± postzygotic De novo/dominant (may be inherited)

TABLE 5.2 Brain Malformations Associated With mTOR-PI3K-AKT Pathway Mutations

CLOVES, Congenital lipomatous overgrowth syndrome; *FCD,* focal cortical dysplasia; *KTS,* Klippel-Trenaunay syndrome; *MCAP,* megalencephaly capillary malformation; *MPPH,* megalencephaly polydactyly polymicrogyria hydrocephalus; *TSC,* Tuberous sclerosis complex.

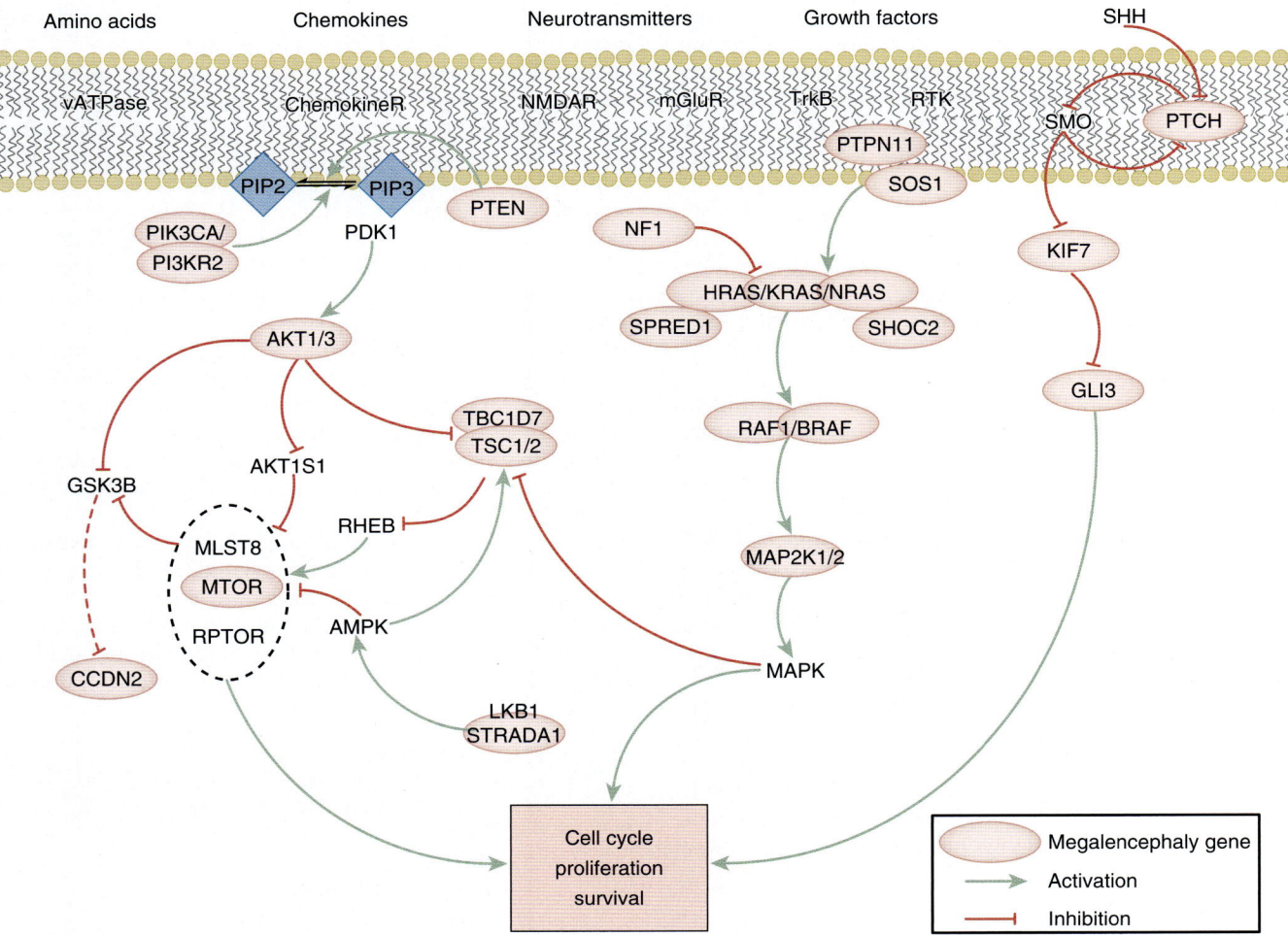

Figure 5.17 AKT-mTOR pathway. Several cases of megalencephaly, hemimegalencephaly, and focal cortical dysplasia have now been associated with genes in this pathway that are involved in growth regulation during development but also in a multitude of other processes during and after development, as shown. (Used with permission from Winden KD, Yuskaitis CJ, Poduri A. Megalencephaly and macrocephaly. *Semin Neurol.* 2015;35:277–287.)

in only a portion of the cells, indicates that a mutation arose in the postzygotic period in a progenitor cell that gives rise to a given fraction of cells in the abnormal region, depending on the timing of the mutational event.[270] Indeed, hemimegalencephaly can arise from such mutations not only at that particular locus of *AKT3* but also at other *AKT3* loci and other genes in the mTOR-AKT-PI3K pathway (see Fig. 5.17).[265,266] These initial studies have led to fascinating single-cell sequencing studies to determine the cell of origin of mutations. For example, single-cell sequencing of the case of *AKT3* E17K mutation referenced earlier was undertaken: cells were labeled for NeuN (a neuronal marker), sorted, and sequenced, revealing the *AKT3* E17K mutation in one-third of NeuN-positive cells (neurons) as well as in one-third of NeuN-negative cells (oligodendrocytes, astrocytes), indicating that a common progenitor sustained the initial mutation.[271] Another single-cell study of a case of hemimegalencephaly due to postzygotic copy number increase of the region of chromosome 1q containing *AKT3* revealed that the mutational event was a tetrasomy of this locus.[272]

FCD shares neuropathological features with tuberous sclerosis and hemimegalencephaly.[213,270,273] Because of

technical limitations that until recently limited the detection of postzygotic mutations present in a very small percentage of affected tissue, the genetics of FCD has only recently been elucidated. A recessive form of FCD was described in the Amish population, with accompanying epilepsy and intellectual disability[274] associated with mutations in the gene *CNTNAP2.* Aside from this unique recessive example, the other genetic causes of FCD are de novo and in large part postzygotic. The included genes all involve the mTOR-PI3K-AKT pathway. As with hemimegalencephaly, FCD can be associated with a mosaic increase in copy number of *AKT3*, as seen in a distal 1q duplication was reported by Conti et al.[275] More commonly, FCD has now been associated with mosaic point mutations in *AKT3*, *PIK3CA*, *MTOR*, *PTEN*, and *DEPDC5*, often with very small percentages of cells demonstrating the mutations.[267,269,276-278]

A fascinating development has been the implication of *DEPDC5*, and more recently *NPRL2* and *NPRL3*, all part of the GATOR complex upstream of mTOR, in a range of phenotypes, from FCD with epilepsy to isolated FCD to familial epilepsy in the absence of a detectable MRI lesion.[267,277,279-287] One proposed mechanism to account for the range of phenotypes is that a germline mutation is sufficient for a tendency to focal seizures but that a *second hit* in the form of a postzygotic mutation is required. This principle has been noted for TSC[288] and most recently for *DEPDC5*.[277] *Thus the study of proliferative disorders of the brain—notably megalencephaly, hemimegalencephaly, and FCD—has implicated a pathway of genes involved in growth regulation and protein synthesis, many of which are now being shown to have a role in common disorders such as non–malformation-related epilepsy.* The extent to which many focal epilepsies may be due to postzygotic mutations in this pathway of genes is one of the exciting next questions to be addressed.[270,289]

KEY REFERENCES

1. Azevedo FA, Carvalho LR, Grinberg LT, et al. Equal numbers of neuronal and nonneuronal cells make the human brain an isometrically scaled-up primate brain. *J Comp Neurol.* 2009;513: 532-541.
2. Herculano-Houzel S, Kaas JH, de Oliveira-Souza R. Corticalization of motor control in humans is a consequence of brain scaling in primate evolution. *J Comp Neurol.* 2016;524:448-455.
3. Dobbing J, Sands J. Quantitative growth and development of human brain. *Arch Dis Child.* 1973;48:757-767.
4. Samuelsen GB, Larsen KB, Bogdanovic N, et al. The changing number of cells in the human fetal forebrain and its subdivisions: a stereological analysis. *Cereb Cortex.* 2003;13:115-122.
5. Silbereis JC, Pochareddy S, Zhu Y, et al. The cellular and molecular landscapes of the developing human central nervous system. *Neuron.* 2016;89:248-268.
6. Lemire RJ, Loeser JD, Leech RW, et al. *Normal and Abnormal Development of the Human Nervous System.* Hagerstown: Harper & Row; 1975.
7. Norman MG, O'Kusky JR. The growth and development of microvasculature in human cerebral cortex. *J Neuropathol Exp Neurol.* 1986;45:222-232.
8. Evrard P, de Saint-Georges P, Kadhim HJ, et al. Pathology of prenatal encephalopathies. In: *Child Neurology and Developmental Disabilities.* Baltimore: Paul H. Brookes Publishing Co.; 1989:153-176.
9. Marin-Padilla M. Embryonic vascularization of the mammalian cerebral cortex. In: Peters A, Jones EG, eds. *Cerebral Cortex.* Vol. 7. New York: Plenum Publishing Corp.; 1988:479-509.
10. Sauer FC. The cellular structure of the neural tube. *J Comp Neurol.* 1935;63:13.
11. Sauer FC. Mitosis in the neural tube. *J Comp Neurol.* 1935;62:377.
12. Sidman RL, Miale IL, Feder N. Cell proliferation and migration in the primitive ependymal zone: an autoradiographic study of histogenesis in the nervous system. *Exp Neurol.* 1959;1:322.
13. Sidman RL, Angevine JB. Autoradiographic analysis of time of origin of nuclear versus cortical components of mouse telencephalon. *Anat Rec.* 1962;142:326.
14. Rakic P, Sidman RL. Supravital DNA synthesis in the developing human and mouse brain. *J Neuropathol Exp Neurol.* 1968;27:246-276.
15. Berry M, Rogers AW, Eayrs JF. Pattern of cell migration during cortical histogenesis. *Nature.* 1964;203:591.
16. Rakic P. Limits of neurogenesis in primates. *Science.* 1985;227:1054-1056.
17. Caviness VS, Takahashi T. Proliferative events in the cerebral ventricular zone. *Brain Dev.* 1995;17:159-163.
18. Takahashi T, Nowakowski RS, Caviness VS. Cell cycle parameters and patterns of nuclear movement in the neocortical proliferative zone of the fetal mouse. *J Neurosci.* 1993;13:820-833.
19. Rakic P. A small step for the cell, a giant leap for mankind: a hypothesis of neocortical expansion during evolution. *Trends Neurosci.* 1995;18:383-388.
20. Caviness VS, Takahashi T, Nowakowski RS. Numbers, time and neocortical neuronogenesis: a general developmental and evolutionary model. *Trends Neurosci.* 1995;18:379-383.
21. Takahashi T, Nowakowski RS, Caviness VS. The leaving or Q fraction of the murine cerebral proliferative epithelium: a general model of neocortical neuronogenesis. *J Neurosci.* 1996;16:6186-6196.
22. Kornack DR, Rakic P. Changes in cell-cycle kinetics during the development and evolution of primate neocortex. *Proc Natl Acad Sci U S A.* 1998;95:1242-1246.
23. Caviness VS, Takahashi T, Nowakowski RS. Neocortical malformation as consequence of nonadaptive regulation of neurogenetic sequence. *Ment Retard Dev Disabil Res Rev.* 2000;6: 22-33.
25. Howard B, Chen YH, Zecevic N. Cortical progenitor cells in the developing human telencephalon. *Glia.* 2006;53:57-66.
26. Gal JS, Morozov YM, Ayoub AE, et al. Molecular and morphological heterogeneity of neural precursors in the mouse neocortical proliferative zones. *J Neurosci.* 2006;26:1045-1056.
27. Miller JA, Ding SL, Sunkin SM, et al. Transcriptional landscape of the prenatal human brain. *Nature.* 2014;508:199-206.
28. Hoerder-Suabedissen A, Molnar Z. Development, evolution and pathology of neocortical subplate neurons. *Nat Rev Neurosci.* 2015;16:133-146.
29. Noctor SC, Martinez-Cerdeno V, Kriegstein AR. Contribution of intermediate progenitor cells to cortical histogenesis. *Arch Neurol.* 2007;64:639-642.
30. Mo Z, Moore AR, Filipovic R, et al. Human cortical neurons originate from radial glia and neuron-restricted progenitors. *J Neurosci.* 2007;27:4132-4145.
31. Noctor SC, Martinez-Cerdeno V, Kriegstein AR. Distinct behaviors of neural stem and progenitor cells underlie cortical neurogenesis. *J Comp Neurol.* 2008;508:28-44.
32. Rakic P. Timing of major ontogenetic events in the visual cortex of the rhesus monkey. In: Buchwald NA, Brazier M, eds. *Brain Mechanisms in Mental Retardation.* New York: Academic Press; 1975:3.
33. Rakic P. Specification of cerebral cortical areas. *Science.* 1988;241: 170-176.
34. Rakic P. Defects of neuronal migration and the pathogenesis of cortical malformations. *Prog Brain Res.* 1988;73:15-37.
35. Caviness VS, Goto T, Tarui T, et al. Cell output, cell cycle duration and neuronal specification: a model of integrated mechanisms of the neocortical proliferative process. *Cereb Cortex.* 2003;13:592-598.
36. Rakic P. Less is more: progenitor death and cortical size. *Nat Neurosci.* 2005;8:981-982.
37. Reid CB, Tavazoie SF, Walsh CA. Clonal dispersion and evidence for asymmetric cell division in ferret cortex. *Development.* 1997;124: 2441-2450.
38. Ware ML, Tavazoie SF, Reid CB, et al. Coexistence of widespread clones and large radial clones in early embryonic ferret cortex. *Cereb Cortex.* 1999;9:636-645.
39. Noctor SC, Flint AC, Weissman TA, et al. Dividing precursor cells of the embryonic cortical ventricular zone have morphological and molecular characteristics of radial glia. *J Neurosci.* 2002;22:3161-3173.
40. Kriegstein A, Parnavelas JG. Changing concepts of cortical development. *Cereb Cortex.* 2003;13:i-ii.
41. Weissman T, Noctor SC, Clinton BK, et al. Neurogenic radial glial cells in reptile, rodent and human: from mitosis to migration. *Cereb Cortex.* 2003;13:550-559.
42. Fishell G, Kriegstein AR. Neurons from radial glia: the consequences of asymmetric inheritance. *Curr Opin Neurobiol.* 2003;13:34-41.
44. Zecevic N. Specific characteristic of radial glia in the human fetal telencephalon. *Glia.* 2004;48:27-35.
46. Merkle FT, Tramontin AD, Garcia-Verdugo JM, et al. Radial glia give rise to adult neural stem cells in the subventricular zone. *Proc Natl Acad Sci U S A.* 2004;101:17528-17532.
47. Gotz M, Barde YA. Radial glial cells: defined and major intermediates between embryonic, stem cells and CNS neurons. *Neuron.* 2005;46:369-372.
48. Ever L, Gaiano N. Radial "glial" progenitors: neurogenesis and signaling. *Curr Opin Neurobiol.* 2005;15:29-33.
50. Chenn A, Walsh CA. Regulation of cerebral cortical size by control of cell cycle exit in neural precursors. *Science.* 2002;297:365-369.

51. Lavdas AA, Grigoriou M, Pachnis V, et al. The medial ganglionic eminence gives rise to a population of early neurons in the developing cerebral cortex. *J Neurosci.* 1999;19:7881-7888.

52. Villar-Cervino V, Kappeler C, Nobrega-Pereira S, et al. Molecular mechanisms controlling the migration of striatal interneurons. *J Neurosci.* 2015;35:8718-8729.

53. Brown KN, Chen S, Han Z, et al. Clonal production and organization of inhibitory interneurons in the neocortex. *Science.* 2011;334:480-486.

54. Harwell CC, Fuentealba LC, Gonzalez-Cerrillo A, et al. Wide dispersion and diversity of clonally related inhibitory interneurons. *Neuron.* 2015;87:999-1007.

55. Bystron I, Blakemore C, Rakic P. Development of the human cerebral cortex: Boulder Committee revisited. *Nat Rev Neurosci.* 2008;9:110-122.

56. Letinic K, Zoncu R, Rakic P. Origin of GABAergic neurons in the human neocortex. *Nature.* 2002;417:645-649.

57. Evrard P, Miladi N, Bonnier C, et al. Normal and abnormal development of the brain. In: Rapin I, Segalowitz SJ, eds. *Handbook of Neuropsychology, Vol. 6: Child Neuropsychology.* Amsterdam, Biomedical Division: Elsevier Science Publishers; 1992:11-44.

58. Shen J, Gilmore EC, Marshall CA, et al. Mutations in PNKP cause microcephaly, seizuresand defects in DNA repair. *Nat Genet.* 2010;42:245-249.

59. Barkovich AJ. *Pediatric Neuroimaging.* 4th ed. Philadelphia: Lippincott Williams & Wilkins; 2005.

60. Barkovich AJ, Ferriero DM, Barr RM, et al. Microlissencephaly: a heterogeneous malformation of cortical development. *Neuropediatrics.* 1998;29:113-119.

62. Dobyns WB, Barkovich AJ. Microcephaly with simplified gyral pattern (oligogyric microcephaly) and microlissencephaly: reply. *Neuropediatrics.* 2001;30:104-106.

63. Dobyns WB. Primary microcephaly: new approaches for an old disorder. *Am J Med Genet.* 2002;112:315-317.

69. Sheen VL, Ganesh VS, Topcu M, et al. Mutations in *ARFGEF2* implicate vesicle trafficking in neural progenitor proliferation and migration in the human cerebral cortex. *Nat Genet.* 2004;36:69-76.

70. Sztriha L, Johansen JG, AlGazali LI. Extreme microcephaly with agyria-pachygyria, partial agenesis of the corpus callosum, and pontocerebellar dysplasia. *J Child Neurol.* 2005;20:170-172.

73. Trimborn M, Bell SM, Felix C, et al. Mutations in microcephalin cause aberrant regulation of chromosome condensation. *Am J Hum Genet.* 2004;75:261-266.

74. Woods CG. Human microcephaly. *Curr Opin Neurobiol.* 2004;14:112-117.

75. Woods CG, Bond J, Enard W. Autosomal recessive primary microcephaly (MCPH): a review of clinical, molecular, and evolutionary findings. *Am J Hum Genet.* 2005;76:717-728.

76. Shen J, Eyaid W, Mochida GH, et al. ASPM mutations identified in patients with primary microcephaly and seizures. *J Med Genet.* 2005;42:725-729.

77. Jackson AP, Eastwood H, Bell SM, et al. Identification of microcephalin, a protein implicated in determining the size of the human brain. *Am J Hum Genet.* 2002;71:136-142.

78. Yu TW, Mochida GH, Tischfield DJ, et al. Mutations in WDR62, encoding a centrosome-associated protein, cause microcephaly with simplified gyri and abnormal cortical architecture. *Nat Genet.* 2010;42:1015-1020.

81. Bond J, Roberts E, Mochida GH, et al. ASPM is a major determinant of cerebral cortical size. *Nat Genet.* 2002;32:316-320.

82. Bond J, Roberts E, Springell K, et al. A centrosomal mechanism involving CDK5RAP2 and CENPJ controls brain size. *Nat Genet.* 2005;37:353-355.

83. Kumar A, Girimaji SC, Duvvari MR, et al. Mutations in STIL, encoding a pericentriolar and centrosomal protein, cause primary microcephaly. *Am J Hum Genet.* 2009;84:286-290.

84. Hussain MS, Baig SM, Neumann S, et al. A truncating mutation of CEP135 causes primary microcephaly and disturbed centrosomal function. *Am J Hum Genet.* 2012;90:871-878.

85. Guernsey DL, Jiang H, Hussin J, et al. Mutations in centrosomal protein CEP152 in primary microcephaly families linked to MCPH4. *Am J Hum Genet.* 2010;87:40-51.

86. Yang YJ, Baltus AE, Mathew RS, et al. Microcephaly gene links trithorax and REST/NRSF to control neural stem cell proliferation and differentiation. *Cell.* 2012;151:1097-1112.

87. Abdel-Hamid MS, Ismail MF, Darwish HA, et al. Molecular and phenotypic spectrum of ASPM-related primary microcephaly: identification of eight novel mutations. *Am J Med Genet A.* 2016;170:2133-2140.

88. Mochida GH, Ganesh VS, Felie JM, et al. A homozygous mutation in the tight-junction protein JAM3 causes hemorrhagic destruction of the brain, subependymal calcification, and congenital cataracts. *Am J Hum Genet.* 2010;87:882-889.

89. Aran A, Rosenfeld N, Jaron R, et al. Loss of function of PCDH12 underlies recessive microcephaly mimicking intrauterine infection. *Neurology.* 2016;86:2016-2024.

103. Jones KL. *Smith's Recognizable Patterns of Human Malformation.* 6th ed. Philadelphia: Elsevier Saunders; 2006.

105. Miller RW, Blot WJ. Small head size after in-utero exposure to atomic radiation. *Lancet.* 1972;2:784-787.

107. Yamazaki JN, Schull WJ. Perinatal loss and neurological abnormalities among children of the atomic bomb. Nagasaki and Hiroshima revisited, 1949 to 1989. *JAMA.* 1990;264:605-609.

108. Lenke RR, Levy HL. Maternal phenylketonuria and hyperphenylalaninemia. An international survey of the outcome of untreated and treated pregnancies. *N Engl J Med.* 1980;303:1202-1208.

111. Levy HL, Walsbren SE, Lobbregt D, et al. Maternal mild hyperphenylalaniaemia: an international survey of offspring outcome. *Lancet.* 1994;344:1589-1594.

121. Driggers RW, Ho CY, Korhonen EM, et al. Zika virus infection with prolonged maternal viremia and fetal brain abnormalities. *N Engl J Med.* 2016;374:2142-2151.

122. Mlakar J, Korva M, Tul N, et al. Zika virus associated with microcephaly. *N Engl J Med.* 2016;374:951-958.

123. Rubin EJ, Greene MF, Baden LR. Zika virus and microcephaly. *N Engl J Med.* 2016;374:984-985.

126. Mirzaa GM, Poduri A. Megalencephaly and hemimegalencephaly: breakthroughs in molecular etiology. *Am J Med Genet C Semin Med Genet.* 2014;166:156-172.

130. de Vries LS, Smet M, Ceulemans B, et al. The role of high resolution ultrasound and MRI in the investigation of infants with macrocephaly. *Neuropediatrics.* 1990;21:72-75.

139. Ott JE, Robinson A. Cerebral gigantism. *Am J Dis Child.* 1969;117:357-368.

146. Bannayan GA. Lipomatosis, angiomatosis, and macroencephalia. *Arch Pathol Lab Med.* 1971;92:1.

153. Korf BR. Diagnostic outcome in children with multiple cafe au lait spots. *Pediatrics.* 1992;90:924-927.

155. Gutmann DH, Aylsworth A, Carey JC, et al. The diagnostic evaluation and multidisciplinary management of neurofibromatosis 1 and neurofibromatosis 2. *JAMA.* 1997;278:51-57.

156. Feldkamp MM, Gutmann DH, Guha A. Neurofibromatosis type 1: piecing the puzzle together. *Can J Neurol Sci.* 1998;25:181-191.

160. Cutting LE, Cooper KL, Koth CW, et al. Megalencephaly in NF1. Predominantly white matter contribution and mitigation by ADHD. *Neurology.* 2002;59:1388-1394.

162. Cusmai R, Curatolo P, Mangano S, et al. Hemimegalencephaly and neurofibromatosis. *Neuropediatrics.* 1990;21:179-182.

164. Gutmann DH, Collins FS. Recent progress toward understanding the molecular biology of von Recklinghausen neurofibromatosis. *Ann Neurol.* 1992;31:555-561.

165. Gutmann DH. Recent insights into neurofibromatosis Type 1. Clear genetic progress. *Arch Neurol.* 1998;55:778-780.

169. Thomas-Sohl KA, Vaslow DF, Maria BL. Sturge-Weber syndrome: a review. *Pediatr Neurol.* 2004;30:303-310.

170. Nelhaus G, Haberland C, Hill BJ. Sturge-Weber disease with bilateral intracranial calcifications at birth and unusual pathologic findings. *Acta Neurol Scand.* 1967;43:314.

181. Evans AL, Widjaja E, Connolly DJ, et al. Cerebral perfusion abnormalities in children with Sturge-Weber syndrome shown by dynamic contrast bolus magnetic resonance perfusion imaging. *Pediatrics.* 2006;117:2119-2125.

184. Shirley MD, Tang H, Gallione CJ, et al. Sturge-Weber syndrome and port-wine stains caused by somatic mutation in GNAQ. *N Engl J Med.* 2013;368:1971-1979.

185. Curatolo P, Verdecchia M, Bombardieri R. Tuberous sclerosis complex: a review of neurological aspects. *Eur J Paediatr Neurol.* 2002;6:15-23.

193. Datta AN, Hahn CD, Sahin M. Clinical presentation and diagnosis of tuberous sclerosis complex in infancy. *J Child Neurol.* 2008;23:268-273.

194. Milunsky A, Shim SH, Ito M, et al. Precise prenatal diagnosis of tuberous sclerosis by sequencing the TSC2 gene. *Prenat Diagn.* 2005;25:582-585.

198. Barth PG, Stam FC, von der Harten JJ. Tuberous sclerosis and dysplasia of the corpus callosum. Case report of their combined occurrence in a newborn. *Acta Neuropathol.* 1978;42:63-64.

199. Thibault JH, Manuelidis EE. Tuberous sclerosis in a premature infant. Report of a case and review of the literature. *Neurology.* 1970;20:139-146.

202. Inoue Y, Nemoto Y, Murata R, et al. CT and MR imaging of cerebral tuberous sclerosis. *Brain Dev.* 1998;20:209-221.

205. Raju GP, Urion DK, Sahin M. Neonatal subependymal giant cell astrocytoma: new case and review of literature. *Pediatr Neurol.* 2007;36:128-131.

212. Franz DN. Diagnosis and management of tuberous sclerosis complex. *Semin Pediatr Neurol.* 1998;5:253-267.

213. Crino PB, Henske EP. New developments in the neurobiology of the tuberous sclerosis complex. *Neurology.* 1999;53:1384-1390.

214. Henske EP, Jozwiak S, Kingswood JC, et al. Tuberous sclerosis complex. *Nat Rev Dis Primers.* 2016;2:16035.

217. Chudley AE, Hagerman RJ. Fragile X syndrome. *J Pediatr.* 1987;110:821-831.

218. Budka H. Megalencephaly and chromosomal anomaly. *Acta Neuropathol.* 1978;43:263-266.

223. Townsend JJ, Nielsen SL, Malamud N. Unilateral megalencephaly: hamartoma or neoplasm? *Neurology.* 1975;25:448-453.

224. Bignami A, Palladini G, Zappella M. Unilateral megalencephaly with nerve cell hypertrophy. An anatomical and quantitative histochemical study. *Brain Res.* 1968;9:103-114.

227. Robain O, Lyon G. Familial microcephalies due to cerebral malformation. Anatomical and clinical study. *Acta Neuropathol.* 1972;20:96-109.

231. Woo CLF, Chuang SH, Becker LE, et al. Radiologic-pathologic correlation in focal cortical dysplasia and hemimegalencephaly in 18 children. *Pediatr Neurol.* 2001;25:295-303.

232. D'Agostino MD, Bastos A, Piras C, et al. Posterior quadrantic dysplasia or hemi-hemimegalencephaly: a characteristic brain malformation. *Neurology.* 2004;62:2214-2220.

233. Flores-Sarnat L. Hemimegalencephaly: part 1. Genetic, clinical, and imaging aspects. *J Child Neurol.* 2002;16:373-384.

234. Flores-Sarnat L, Sarnat HB, Davila-Gutierrez G, et al. Hemimegalencephaly: part 2. Neuropathology suggests a disorder of cellular lineage. *J Child Neurol.* 2003;18:776-785.

251. Dobyns WB, Garg BP. Vascular abnormalities in epidermal nevus syndrome. *Neurology.* 1991;41:276-278.

253. Gurecki PJ, Holden KR, Sahn EE, et al. Developmental neural abnormalities and seizures in epidermal nevus syndrome. *Dev Med Child Neurol.* 1996;38:716-723.

254. Pavone L, Curatolo P, Rizzo R, et al. Epidermal nevus syndrome: a neurologic variant with hemimegalencephaly, gyral malformation, mental retardation, seizures, and facial hemihypertrophy. *Neurology.* 1991;41:266-271.

257. Sarwar M, Schafer ME. Brain malformations in linear nevus sebaceous syndrome: an MR study. *J Comput Assist Tomogr.* 1988;12:338-340.

258. Chalhub EG, Volpe JJ, Gado MH. Linear nevus sebaceous syndrome associated with porencephaly and nonfunctioning major cerebral venous sinuses. *Neurology.* 1975;25:857-860.

262. Griffiths PD, Welch RJ, Gardner-Medwin D, et al. The radiological features of hemimegalencephaly including three cases associated with proteus syndrome. *Neuropediatrics.* 1994;25:140-144.

263. Lindhurst MJ, Sapp JC, Teer JK, et al. A mosaic activating mutation in AKT1 associated with the Proteus syndrome. *N Engl J Med.* 2011;365:611-619.

264. Lee JH, Huynh M, Silhavy JL, et al. De novo somatic mutations in components of the PI3K-AKT3-mTOR pathway cause hemimegalencephaly. *Nat Genet.* 2012;44:941-945.

265. Riviere JB, Mirzaa GM, O'Roak BJ, et al. De novo germline and postzygotic mutations in AKT3, PIK3R2 and PIK3CA cause a spectrum of related megalencephaly syndromes. *Nat Genet.* 2012;44:934-940.

266. D'Gama AM, Geng Y, Couto JA, et al. Mammalian target of rapamycin pathway mutations cause hemimegalencephaly and focal cortical dysplasia. *Ann Neurol.* 2015;77:720-725.

267. Mirzaa GM, Parry DA, Fry AE, et al. De novo CCND2 mutations leading to stabilization of cyclin D2 cause megalencephaly-polymicrogyria-polydactyly-hydrocephalus syndrome. *Nat Genet.* 2014;46:510-515.

268. Jansen LA, Mirzaa GM, Ishak GE, et al. PI3K/AKT pathway mutations cause a spectrum of brain malformations from megalencephaly to focal cortical dysplasia. *Brain.* 2015;138:1613-1628.

269. Poduri A, Evrony GD, Cai X, et al. Somatic activation of AKT3 causes hemispheric developmental brain malformations. *Neuron.* 2012;74:41-48.

270. Poduri A, Evrony GD, Cai X, et al. Somatic mutation, genomic variation, and neurological disease. *Science.* 2013;341:1237758.

271. Evrony GD, Cai X, Lee E, et al. Single-neuron sequencing analysis of L1 retrotransposition and somatic mutation in the human brain. *Cell.* 2012;151:483-496.

272. Cai X, Evrony GD, Lehmann HS, et al. Single-cell, genome-wide sequencing identifies clonal somatic copy-number variation in the human brain. *Cell Rep.* 2014;8:1280-1289.

273. Arai Y, Edwards V, Becker LE. A comparison of cell phenotypes in hemimegalencephaly and tuberous sclerosis. *Acta Neuropathol.* 1999;98:407-413.

274. Strauss KA, Puffenberger EG, Huentelman MJ, et al. Recessive symptomatic focal epilepsy and mutant contactin-associated protein-like 2. *N Engl J Med.* 2006;354:1370-1377.

275. Conti V, Pantaleo M, Barba C, et al. Focal dysplasia of the cerebral cortex and infantile spasms associated with somatic 1q21.1-q44 duplication including the AKT3 gene. *Clin Genet.* 2015;88:241-247.

276. Lim JS, Kim WI, Kang HC, et al. Brain somatic mutations in MTOR cause focal cortical dysplasia type II leading to intractable epilepsy. *Nat Med.* 2015;21:395-400.

277. Baulac S, Ishida S, Marsan E, et al. Familial focal epilepsy with focal cortical dysplasia due to DEPDC5 mutations. *Ann Neurol.* 2015;77:675-683.

278. Mirzaa GM, Campbell CD, Solovieff N, et al. Association of MTOR mutations with developmental brain disorders, including megalencephaly, focal cortical dysplasia, and pigmentary mosaicism. *JAMA Neurol.* 2016;73:836-845.

279. Korenke GC, Eggert M, Thiele H, et al. Nocturnal frontal lobe epilepsy caused by a mutation in the GATOR1 complex gene NPRL3. *Epilepsia.* 2016;57:e60-e63.

280. Weckhuysen S, Marsan E, Lambrecq V, et al. Involvement of GATOR complex genes in familial focal epilepsies and focal cortical dysplasia. *Epilepsia.* 2016;57:994-1003.

281. Ricos MG, Hodgson BL, Pippucci T, et al. Mutations in the mammalian target of rapamycin pathway regulators NPRL2 and NPRL3 cause focal epilepsy. *Ann Neurol.* 2016;79:120-131.

282. Lal D, Reinthaler EM, Schubert J, et al. DEPDC5 mutations in genetic focal epilepsies of childhood. *Ann Neurol.* 2014;75:788-792.

283. Scheffer IE, Heron SE, Regan BM, et al. Mutations in mTOR regulator DEPDC5 cause focal epilepsy with brain malformations. *Ann Neurol.* 2014;75:782-787.

284. Poduri A. DEPDC5 does it all: shared genetics for diverse epilepsy syndromes. *Ann Neurol.* 2014;75:631-633.

285. Ishida S, Picard F, Rudolf G, et al. Mutations of DEPDC5 cause autosomal dominant focal epilepsies. *Nat Genet.* 2013;45:552-555.

286. Dibbens LM, de Vries B, Donatello S, et al. Mutations in DEPDC5 cause familial focal epilepsy with variable foci. *Nat Genet.* 2013;45:546-551.

287. Sim JC, Scerri T, Fanjul-Fernandez M, et al. Familial cortical dysplasia caused by mutation in the mammalian target of rapamycin regulator NPRL3. *Ann Neurol.* 2016;79:132-137.

288. Qin W, Chan JA, Vinters HV, et al. Analysis of TSC cortical tubers by deep sequencing of TSC1, TSC2 and KRAS demonstrates that small second-hit mutations in these genes are rare events. *Brain Pathol.* 2010;20:1096-1105.

289. Lindhout D. Somatic mosaicism as a basic epileptogenic mechanism? *Brain.* 2008;131:900-901.

Full references for this chapter can be found on www.expertconsult.com

Neuronal Migration

Annapurna Poduri ◆ Joseph J. Volpe

MIGRATION

As progenitor cells proliferate and differentiate into neurons and glia (see Chapter 5), these cells migrate to form the cerebral cortex in an elaborate and still not completely understood series of genetically influenced processes. Neurodevelopmental studies as well as disorders of brain development have informed our knowledge of these processes. In fact, the period of early migration overlaps with the proliferative period, and the period of late migration overlaps with later cortical organization (see Chapter 7). The disorders referred to as *disorders of migration* are so termed if migration is thought to be the first or principal process of development affected.[1,2]

Normal Development

Neuronal migration refers to the remarkable series of events whereby millions of neurons move from their sites of origin in the ventricular and subventricular zones to the loci within the central nervous system (CNS), where they will reside for life. The *peak time period* for this occurrence is from the third to fifth months of gestation, although neuronal migration can be detected in certain areas of the cerebrum as early as the second month and after the fifth month (especially GABAergic interneurons; see later) (Table 6.1). Regulation of the timing and direction of these many simultaneous migrations must be highly ordered, but only recently has insight been gained into these control mechanisms (see later).

Radial and Tangential Migration

The major features of cell migration in the primate were defined initially, particularly by the classic studies of Sidman and Rakic,[3-9] using primarily autoradiographic, electron microscopic, and Golgi techniques. Later work used immunocytochemical and retroviral methods and the study of genetically manipulated animals to elaborate earlier observations.[7-45] *Two basic varieties* of cell migration have been delineated: *radial* and *tangential* (see Table 6.1). In the *cerebrum*, radial migration of cells from their origin in the ventricular and subventricular zones is the primary mechanism for the formation of the cortex and deep nuclear structures. *Radial migration* gives rise to the *projection neurons* of the cortex. These neurons emanate primarily from the *dorsal region of the subependymal germinative zones.*

Tangential migration of neurons generated in the dorsal and ventral telencephalon, detailed in Chapter 5, results in the *gamma-aminobutyric acid (GABA)–expressing interneurons* of the cerebral cortex.[a] These neuronal precursors migrate parallel to

the surface of the cortex and proceed in one of three streams (i.e., through the subventricular zone, the intermediate zone, or the marginal zone) before terminal radial movement to arrive in the cortical plate.

In the *cerebellum*, radial migration causes the genesis of Purkinje cells, the dentate nucleus, and other roof nuclei. Tangential migration of cells that originate in the germinal zones in the region of the rhombic lip and migrate over the surface of the cerebellum forms the well-known *external granular layer*. These cells then migrate radially inward to form the *internal granule cell layer* of the cerebellar cortex. Thus, during their journey from their point of origin in the ventricular zone, the granule cells exhibit both radial and tangential migration.

Migration to Cerebral Cortex

The basic patterns of cell migration for formation of the cerebral cortex are shown in Figs. 6.1 and 6.2. The first and earlier mechanism is movement by translocation of the cell body (i.e., somal translocation) (Table 6.2).[41,48] This mode of migration probably results in the formation of the preplate (see Fig. 6.1). This layer of neurons is later split by the arrival of the cortical plate neurons in a superficial layer nearest the pial surface, which produces the Cajal-Retzius and related neurons of the marginal zone and a deeper layer, which becomes the subplate neurons. The preplate neurons and the subsequently formed Cajal-Retzius and subplate neurons are critical for the progression of neuronal migration (see later).

The second mode of migration, leading to the formation of most of the cerebral cortex, occurs by radial migration (see Figs. 6.1 and 6.2). These cells are generated by the radial glial progenitors discussed earlier (see Chapter 5). The clonally related neuron migrates along the parental radial glial fiber, which extends to the pial surface. Initially, cells are generated in the *ventricular zone* and then migrate relatively rapidly and synchronously through the intermediate zone in waves to the developing cortical plate. At *later stages*, as shown by Rakic[3,5-9] in studies of the monkey visual cortex, the neurons are generated especially in the *subventricular zone* (see Fig. 6.1). By labeling dividing cells with [³H]thymidine at various times during development and then determining where the labeled cells appear in the cortical plate, Rakic showed that cells that migrate first take the deepest positions in the cortex, whereas those migrating later take more superficial positions. By *20 to 24 weeks* of gestation, the human cerebral cortex essentially has its *full complement* of excitatory and projection neurons, with neurons and glia having arrived from both radial and tangential migration streams and expressing various markers reflecting their neuronal identities, as schematized in Fig. 6.3.

---

[a]References 31, 32, 35, 36, 41, 42, and 45-47.

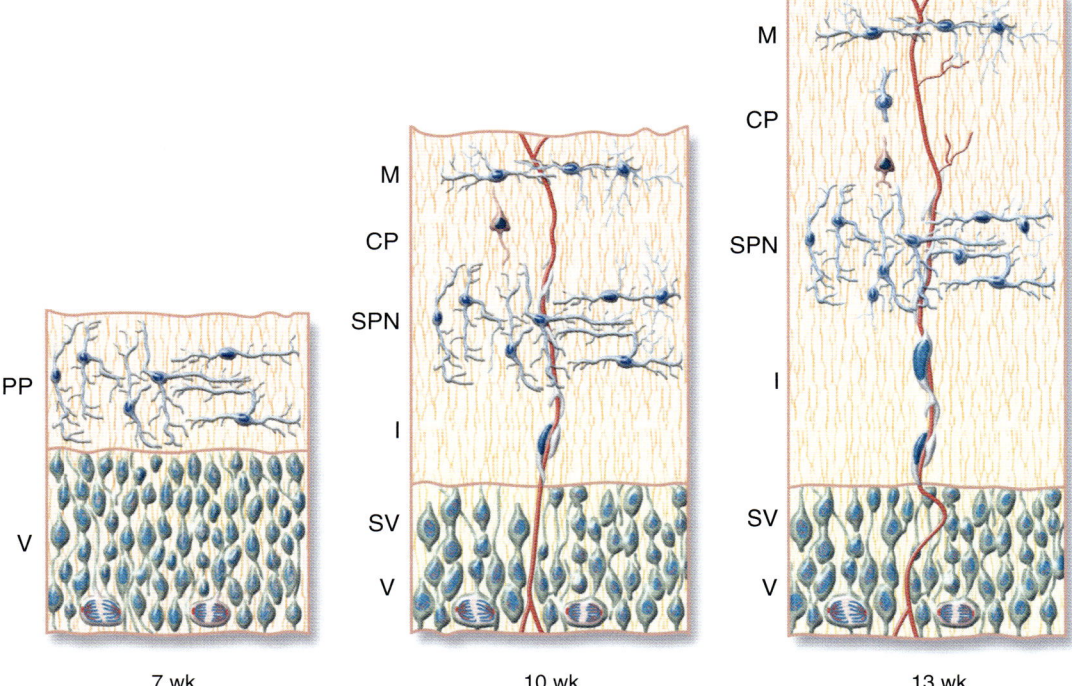

Figure 6.1 Schematic diagram of the developing human cerebral cortex at the gestational ages indicated. The pial surface is at the top and the ventricular surface at the bottom of each depiction of the cerebral wall. *CP*, Cortical plate; *I*, intermediate zone; *M*, marginal zone; *PP*, preplate zone; *SPN*, subplate neurons; *SV*, subventricular zone; *V*, ventricular zone. A radial glial fiber is shown traversing the cerebral mantle in the two right schematics and is not labeled.

TABLE 6.1   Neuronal Migration
Peak time period
3–5 months
Major events
Cerebrum
Radial migration: cerebral cortex (projection neurons), deep nuclei
Tangential migration: cerebral cortex (interneurons)
Cerebellum
Radial migration: Purkinje cells, dentate nuclei
Tangential migration: external → internal granule cells

TABLE 6.2   Migration to Cerebral Cortex
Initially, neurons migrate by translocation of the cell body (somal translocation). Later and predominantly, neurons migrate by following radial glial guides (i.e., the fibers of their clonally related radial progenitors).
Simultaneous with this radial migration, tangential migration parallel to the surface of the cortex (followed by radial migration to the cortex) results in the placement of GABA-expressing interneurons throughout the cortex.
Proliferative units of the ventricular zone migrate along the radial glial scaffolding to become the ontogenetic neuronal columns of cerebral cortex.
Migration through subplate neurons and "waiting" thalamocortical and corticocortical afferents is likely important for later neuronal development (e.g., synaptogenesis).
Early-arriving neurons take deep positions in cortex, and later-arriving neurons take superficial positions (i.e., *inside-out* pattern).
GABA, Gamma-aminobutyric acid.

A substantial proportion of GABAergic interneurons migrate in the latter months of gestation, such that by approximately term, GABAergic interneurons reach their peak density in the cortex.[49]

How do the migrating cells know how to reach where they are going? In the major process of radial migration, radial glial cells serve as the guides for the migration of young neurons from their sites of origin in the ventricular and, later, subventricular zones, across a distance that can be many times greater than the length of their leading processes, to their ultimate position in the cortical plate (see Table 6.2 and Fig. 6.4).[a] The elaboration of

the structure of the radial glial fiber system has been clarified by immunocytochemical and ultramicroscopic studies, especially by Caviness and others.[10-12,21,37,39,41] Initially, the system is uniformly radial in alignment, and in the ventricular zone the fibers appear to separate columns of germinative cells, the proliferative units described by Rakic in the primate (see Chapter 5). The radial

[a]References 6-12, 20, 21, 27, 30, 31, 33-35, 37-39, 41-43, and 50-52.

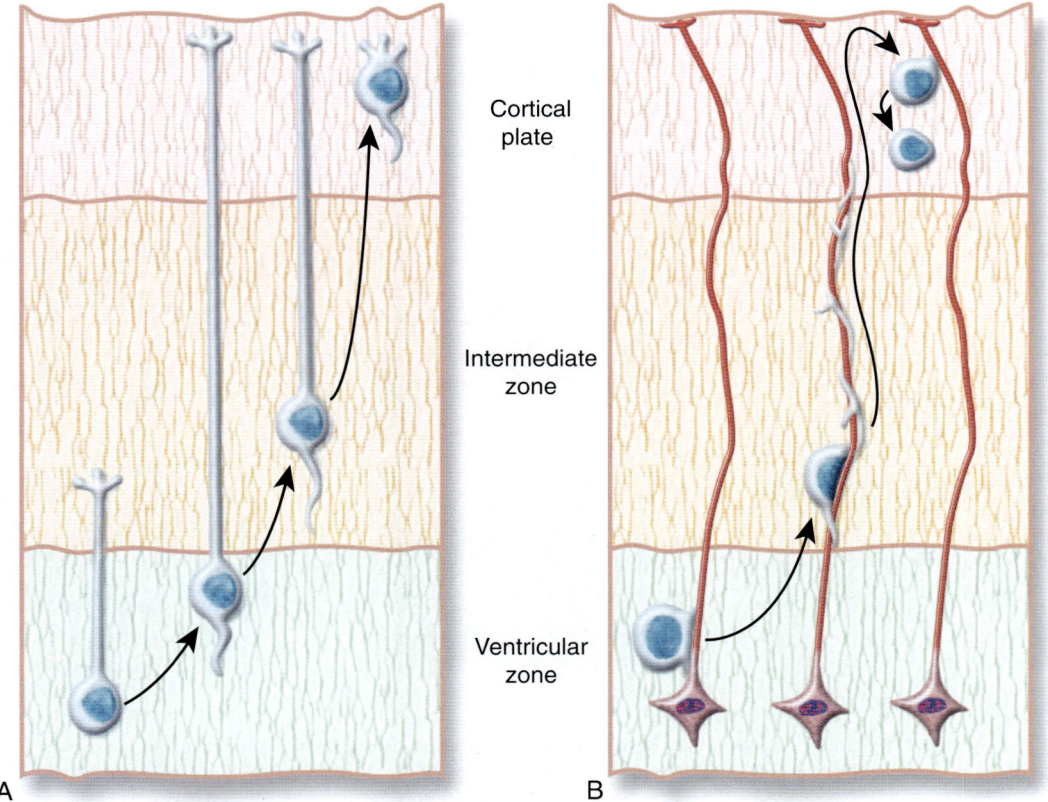

A   B

Figure 6.2 Two modes of radial neuronal migration. In (A), an early mechanism is somal translocation, in which the cell body is translocated from the point of origin in the ventricular zone to the cortical plate. In (B), a later and predominant mechanism is radial migration, in which cells are generated by radial glial progenitors and the clonally related neuron migrates along the parent radial glial fiber. Tangential migration differs from radial migration (see text).

Cortical plate

Intermediate zone

Ventricular zone

glial system in the developing cerebral wall forms fascicles of fibers rather than isolated fibers. With the rapid growth of the cerebral wall and particularly the intermediate zone, the fiber fascicles develop distinct curves with definite region-specific changes in trajectory (Fig. 6.5). Nevertheless, the dominant feature remains the migration of apparent clonally related columns of cells among the same radial glial fascicles, again likely related to the proliferative units described earlier.[18] As the migrating neurons approach the cortical plate, the radial glial fascicles begin to defasciculate, and radial fibers tend to penetrate the cortex more as single fibers.[11] This occurrence develops at the junction of the upper intermediate zone and the subplate zone, an important site for neuronal heterotopia in disorders of neuronal migration. As outlined in Chapter 5, it has long been postulated that the progeny of a single daughter cell arising from asymmetrical cell division at the ventricular zone gives rise to a column of neurons and that a columnar organization is thus established. Although this framework applies generally, there is also evidence that while some clonal populations of cells maintain regional specification, partially overlapping with other, neighboring clonal populations, other populations of neurons become widely dispersed through the cortex.[53,54]

Insights into the *key molecular determinants of neuronal migration* have been gained in recent years (Table 6.3). We present a brief discussion here of some of the best-studied molecules;

further review of molecular determinants is provided later in the discussions of the molecular aspects of individual disorders of migration. Roles for molecules on preplate neurons (and the later Cajal-Retzius and subplate neurons), radial glia, and migrating neurons have been established. From *preplate neurons and the Cajal-Retzius cells of the marginal zone*, such extracellular matrix molecules as fibronectin, chondroitin and heparan sulfate proteoglycans are clearly crucial.[13,31,55-57] The secreted glycoprotein reelin, lacking in the mutant mouse "reeler" with a neuronal migrational disorder, is an important product of the Cajal-Retzius cells.[a] Platelet-activating factor acetylhydrolase, lacking in one form of human lissencephaly (see later), suggests an important role for a molecule related to platelet-activating factor, a notion further supported by in vitro studies.[31,63-65] Neurons with GABA receptors in the preplate, Cajal-Retzius cells, and perhaps migrating neurons also now appear to be involved in migrational events.[52,66]

Important molecular determinants of migration on *radial glia* include three signaling pathways involving erb B4 receptors, Notch receptors, and brain lipid-binding protein (BLBP) (see Table 6.3).[31,33,35,67,68] The first of these are the surface ligands for neuregulin located on *migrating neurons*, which express several proteins involved in migration (see Table 6.3). An additional and well-characterized surface molecule of importance on migrating

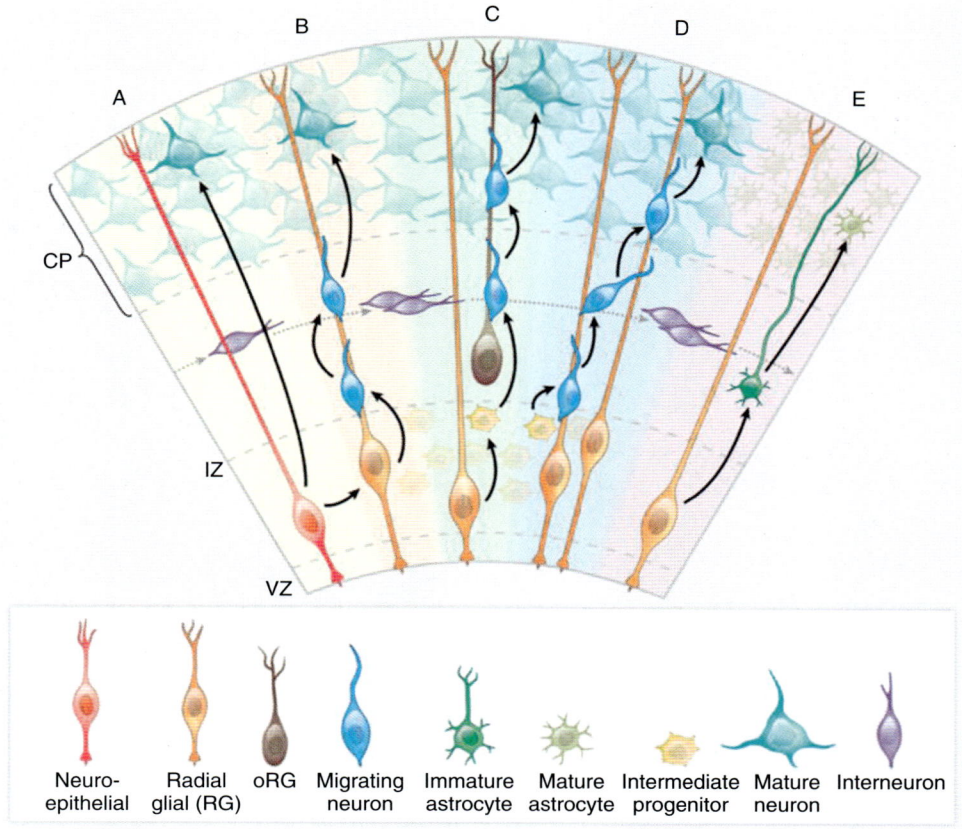

Figure 6.3 **Schematic of brain development, highlighting migration.** This figure depicts both neurons and glial cells arising from the ventricular zone (VZ) but also arriving from the medial ganglionic eminence. *CP*, Cortical plate; *IZ*, intermediate zone. (With permission from Poduri A, et al. Somatic mutation, genomic variation, and neurological disease. *Science.* 2013;341:1237758.)

neurons is the surface glycoprotein astrotactin.[69,70] Doublecortin is the product of a gene on the X chromosome and is involved in double cortex (band) heterotopia in female patients and lissencephaly in male patients, important human neuronal migration disorders (see later).[34,35,40,41,71-75] This protein, expressed in migrating neurons at their growing end, is involved in an intracellular signaling pathway important for neuronal migration. Doublecortin is a microtubule-associated protein, which plays a role in microtubule polymerization and thereby may be involved in neuronal migration by mediating the cytoskeletal changes required for such movement, including through interactions with synaptic vesicle trafficking proteins.[34,35,41,76] The gene *filamin 1* (or *FLNA*), which is responsible for the human neuronal migration disorder periventricular heterotopia, encodes a neuronal actin cross-linking protein that transduces ligand-receptor binding into actin reorganization, critical for the locomotion of many cell types.[41,77] Involvement of neuronal calcium channels, glutamate, and N-methyl-D-aspartate (NMDA) receptors is supported by the work particularly of Rakic and colleagues but also of others.[25,26,33,34,78-83] Thus selective blockage of N-type but not of L- and T-type calcium channels inhibits neuronal migration. N-type calcium channels are involved primarily in the release of neurotransmitters. That the neurotransmitter involved is glutamate, which acts on the NMDA receptor, is suggested by the demonstration that blockers of NMDA

receptors, but not of non-NMDA receptors, inhibit neuronal migration (Fig. 6.6). Axonal release of glutamate may be the source of the glutamate that acts on the migrating neuron.

Radial glial cells have *additional functions* aside from guidance of neuronal migration (see Chapter 5). Thus the initial role of these cells is as neuronal progenitors. The generation of neurons is followed by their role as radial glial guides. Still later, these cells give rise to astrocytes and oligodendroglia. Finally, the cellular progeny of the radial glial cell serves as a source of neural stem cells in the subventricular zone of the mature brain.

Disorders

Disorders of neuronal migration usually cause overt disturbances of neurological function, with clinical deficits often apparent from the first days of life. Seizures are most often the dominant early neurological sign with the more severe migrational disturbances. The advent of magnetic resonance imaging (MRI) markedly increased the ability to identify these disorders in vivo, demonstrating the relatively high prevalence of these disorders and showing their broad clinical expression (see later discussion). The major disorders are listed in Table 6.4 in order of decreasing severity. The disorders included here are considered migrational disorders conventionally, but as indicated, some have been found through molecular genetics

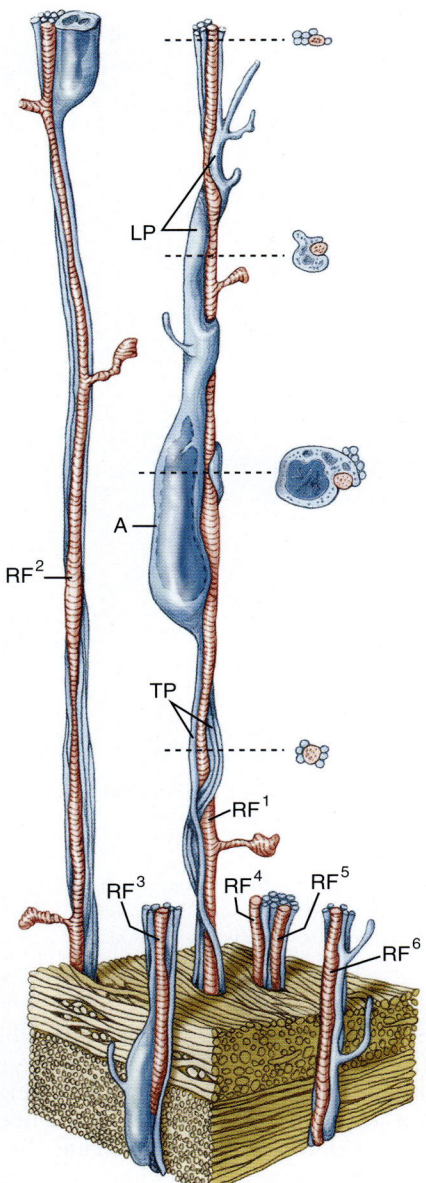

Figure 6.4 **Three-dimensional reconstruction of migrating neurons based on electron micrographs of semiserial sections.** Note the apposition of the migrating neuron (A), with its leading process (LP) and attenuated trailing process (TP), to the guiding radial glial fiber (RF). As discussed in the text, the migrating neuron and the radial glial progenitor are clonally related. (With permission from Sidman RL, Rakic P. Neuronal migration, with special reference to developing human brain: a review. *Brain Res.* 1973;62:1–35.)

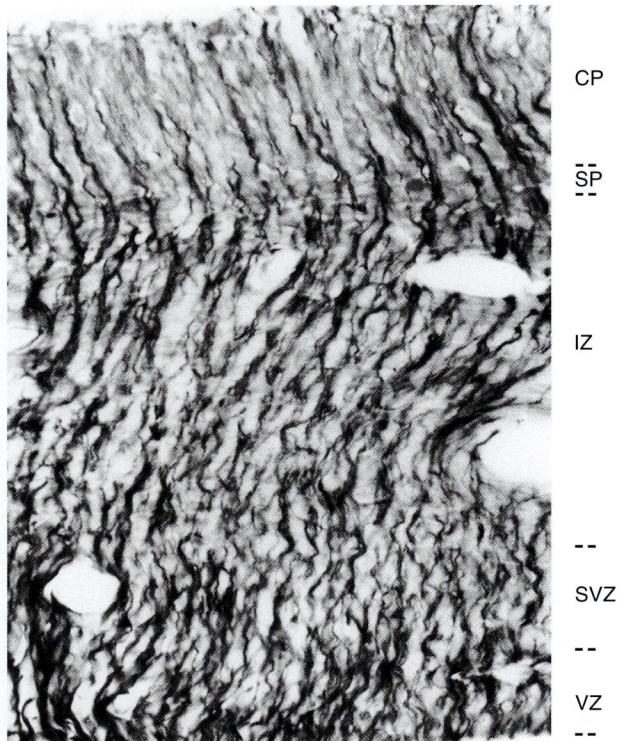

Figure 6.5 **Glial fiber alignment at E15 in the developing rat.** The glial fibers ascend almost radially through the ventricular zone (VZ) and subventricular zone (SVZ). Within the intermediate zone (IZ), the fiber fascicles become arced medially to laterally. At the level of the IZ-subplate (SP) interface, they again become inflected to a radial alignment, orthogonal to the pial surface, which is maintained across the cortical strata. This coronal 6-μm plastic section was immunostained with RC2 antibody for radial glial fibers. Bar = 20 μm; *CP,* cortical plate. (With permission from Gadisseux JF, Evrard P, Misson JP, Caviness VS. Dynamic structure of the radial glial fiber system of the developing murine cerebral wall: an immunocytochemical analysis. *Dev Brain Res.* 1989;50:55–67.)

to be due to dysfunction that begins during proliferation and continues to exact its major effects on migration as well as subsequently on cortical organization.

Gyral Abnormality in Migrational Disorders

The hallmark of the migrational disorders is an aberration of gyral development. Formation of the many secondary and tertiary gyri of the human brain occurs after neuronal migration has ceased (Fig. 6.7).[84-88] The fastest increase in number of the major gyri occurs between 26 and 28 weeks of gestation.[85]

Further elaboration of these gyri continues during the third trimester and shortly after birth.[85] The stimulus for gyral formation appears to be the remarkable increase in surface area of cerebral cortex that occurs during this period, particularly the difference in increase in surface area of the outer versus the inner cortical layers.[89] In the normal cortex, the surface area of the outer cortical layers is greater than that of the inner layers, and this discrepancy leads to compressive stresses that may lead to gyral formation. These relative increases in cortical surface area require the complement of neurons provided by migrational events. In lissencephaly, in which all cortical layers fail to receive their full complement of neurons, no gyri develop. In polymicrogyria, the surface area of outer cortical regions is much greater than that of inner cortical regions, and the result is an excess of gyri.[89] In addition, gyral development may be stimulated by the forces produced by growth of cerebral white matter axons originating in the cortex, the concept of *tension-based morphogenesis.*[90]

Corpus Callosum Defect in Migrational Disorders

In addition to gyral abnormality, a common feature of migrational disorders is hypoplasia or agenesis of the corpus callosum; occasionally, absence of the septum pellucidum

TABLE 6.3 Selected Key Molecular Determinants of Neuronal Migration

Preplate neurons (also marginal [Cajal-Retzius] zone and subplate neurons) and extracellular matrix	Fibronectin, chondroitin, and heparan sulfate Fukutin proteoglycans GABA receptors Integrins Laminin Reelin
Radial glia	erb B4 receptors Notch receptors BLBP
Migrating neurons	Neuregulin Astrotactin Doublecortin Platelet activating factor acetylhydrolase (subunit 1) Filamin 1 Cyclin-dependent kinase-5 (cdk-5) NCAM NMDA receptors Calcium channels GABA receptors

BLBP, Brain lipid binding protein; *GABA*, gamma-aminobutyric acid; *NCAM*, neural cell adhesion molecule; *NMDA*, N-methyl-D-aspartate.

TABLE 6.4 Disorders of Neuronal Migration

Order of decreasing severity
Schizencephaly
Agyria-pachygyria spectrum (e.g., lissencephaly)
Polymicrogyria
Heterotopia—periventricular, subcortical

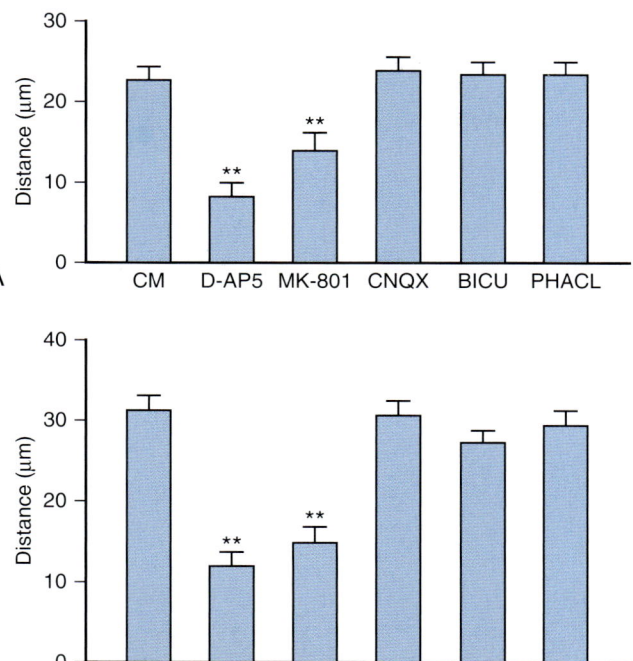

Figure 6.6 The effect of antagonists to inotropic receptors on the migration of cerebellar granule cells. All preparations were obtained from 10-day-old mice. Each column shows the mean length of the migration route for at least 100 labeled cells. The small bar is the standard error of the mean. Each antagonist to specific *N*-methyl-D-aspartate (NMDA) (D-AP5, MK-801), non-NMDA (CNQX), gamma-aminobutyric acid A (GABAA) (bicuculline [BICU]), or GABAB (phaclofen [PHACL]) receptors was added to the tissue culture medium in separate experiments 2 hours after staining, and preparations were maintained for an additional 2 hours (A) to 4 hours (B). The mean distance of cell displacement after the addition of 10 μm CNQX, 10 μm BICU, or 500 μm PHACL was not significantly different from values obtained in control slice preparations *(CM)* at each time point. However, addition of 100 μm D-AP5 or 10 μm MK-801 (NMDA antagonists) inhibited cell movement. Mean migratory distance was obtained by subtracting the mean displacement of the cell soma at 2 hours in culture from the total length of the migratory pathway. The double asterisks indicate statistical significance ($P < .01$). (With permission from Komuro H, Rakic P. Modulation of neuronal migration by NMDA receptors. *Science.* 1993;260:95–97.)

also accompanies these disorders. Development of the corpus callosum (the major interhemispheric commissure) and of the septum is associated temporally and causally with migrational events in the cerebrum (see Chapter 2). Thus the timing of these aspects of midline prosencephalic development is almost coincidental with the major neuronal migrational events for the formation of cerebral cortex. Moreover, normal elaboration of corticocortical callosal fibers requires normal progression of neuronal migration to cerebral cortex. The frequent concurrence of hypoplasia or agenesis of the callosum with the migrational disorders discussed is therefore understandable. The preponderance of cortical abnormality at times dominates to the point that the callosal defect is not initially noted; in some settings, however, the callosal defect is a key feature of the abnormality—for example, with *ARX*- and *TUBA1A*-associated lissencephaly, discussed later.

Schizencephaly

Anatomical Abnormality. *Schizencephaly* is the most severe yet restricted of the cortical malformations (see Table 6.4).[91-99] A

complete agenesis of a portion of the germinative zones and thereby the cerebral wall is believed to exist, leaving seams or clefts. The pial-ependymal seam is characteristic (Fig. 6.8). In the walls of the clefts, the cortical plate exhibits the hallmarks of migrational disturbance (e.g., a thick, microgyric cortex and large neuronal heterotopia). In bilateral lesions, schizencephaly in one hemisphere may be accompanied by polymicrogyria or focal cortical dysplasia (FCD) in the other. The lips of the clefts may become widely separated, and dilation of the lateral ventricles may occur. Hydrocephalus often complicates such open-lipped lesions, especially when they are bilateral (see later). Such bilateral open-lipped lesions may be referred to incorrectly as hydranencephaly, a later destructive lesion of the cerebral hemispheres; when they are unilateral, they may be referred to incorrectly as porencephaly, a destructive lesion of one hemisphere. Indeed, it is now clear that unilateral and bilateral schizencephalies can be familial and probably account for previous reports of "familial porencephaly."[100-108] Gray matter

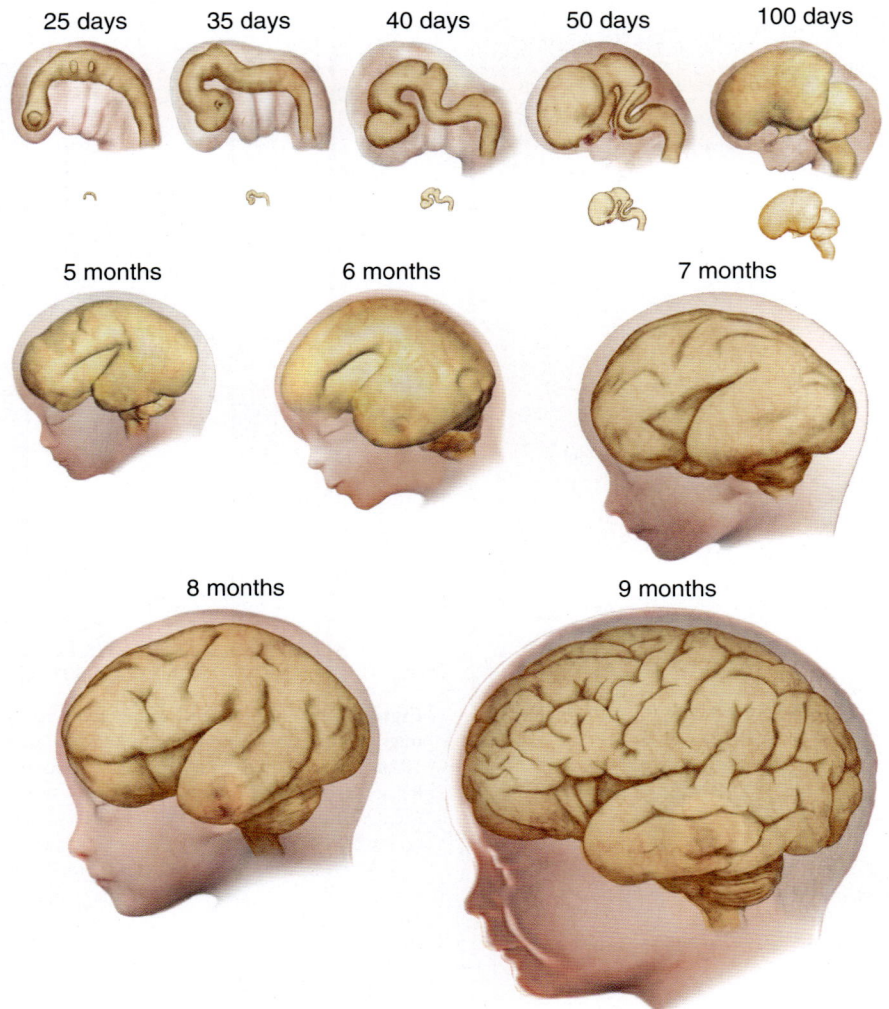

25 days   35 days   40 days   50 days   100 days

5 months   6 months   7 months

8 months   9 months

Figure 6.7 Schematic depiction of gyral development in human brain. Note the particularly prominent changes in the last 3 months of gestation. (With permission from Cowan WM. The development of the brain. *Sci Am.* 1979;241:113–133.)

(often polymicrogyric), lining the lesion and demonstrable on brain imaging, especially MRI, is the key finding indicative of schizencephaly.

The advent of MRI greatly expanded the understanding of anatomical and clinical aspects of schizencephaly (see Table 6.5). Indeed, several previous notions that were based almost exclusively on the study of autopsy cases (i.e., that schizencephaly is rare, bilateral, and associated invariably with severe neurological deficits) were shown to be incorrect. Thus, in two large series, 67 cases were collected, and schizencephaly was unilateral in 63% (see Table 6.5).[109] The clefts tended to be in the regions of the rolandic and sylvian fissures and involved predominantly frontal areas. Subsequent series confirmed these observations.[96]

Timing and Clinical Aspects. Onset of the developmental disturbance that leads to schizencephaly is considered to be no later than the beginning of migrational events in the cerebrum in the third month of gestation. The possibility that destructive lesions operate in the third or fourth month of gestation, perhaps injuring both the germinative zones and migrating neurons on radial glial fibers, is raised by multiple reports.[94,99,110-112] However, the demonstration, at least in certain rare familial cases, of a defect in the homeobox gene *EMX2* supports the notion that schizencephaly most often is a disorder of the developmental program.[34,106,113-115] This gene, specifically expressed in neuroblasts of the ventricular zone, is involved in the structural patterning of the developing forebrain, including neuronal migration. Nevertheless, a *multifactorial origin of schizencephaly* is supported by the association with fetal cytomegalovirus (CMV) infection (which can cause both dysgenetic and destructive effects) and systemic abnormalities secondary to vascular disruption.[99,116] Candidate gene sequencing for the genes *LHX2*, *HESX1*, and *SOX2*—initially thought to be associated with schizencephaly and its related condition septo-optic dysplasia—revealed that these were not common causes of the malformation.[117] To date, genetic explanations for schizencephaly remain few; one prevailing theory is that the disorder results from a disruption of vascular development during critical times of cerebral development. More recently,

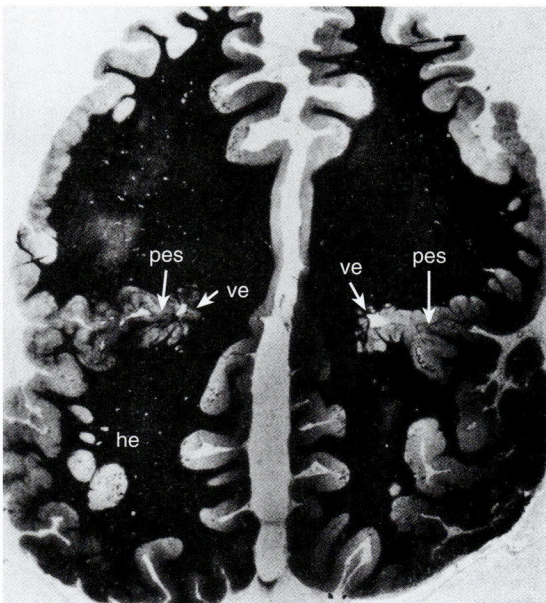

Figure 6.8 Schizencephaly. Horizontal section of the cerebrum, stained for myelin. Note the symmetrical clefts in the axis of the central fissures, pial-ependymal seams (pes), portion of lateral ventricles (ve), polymicrogyric cortex in margins of clefts, and neuronal heterotopia, especially on the left (he). (With permission from Yakovlev PI, Wadsworth RC. Schizencephalies: a study of the congenital clefts in the cerebral mantle. I. Clefts with fused lips. *J Neuropathol Exp Neurol.* 1946;5:116.)

TABLE 6.5	Schizencephaly: Anatomical (Magnetic Resonance Imaging) and Clinical Features
FEATURE	**PERCENTAGE**
Anatomical	
Unilateral	63
Bilateral	37
Closed clefts	42
Open clefts	58
Frontal	44
Frontoparietal	30
Parietal, temporal, or occipital	26
Associated septo-optic dysplasia	39
Anatomical-clinical correlates	
Cognitive disturbances (prominent)	
Bilateral	100
Unilateral	24
Motor disturbances	
Bilateral	86
Unilateral	77
Frontal	84
Not frontal	29
Open lip	94
Closed lip	22
Seizure disorder	
Bilateral	72
Unilateral	60
Hydrocephalus	
Open lip	52
Closed lip	0

Data from Barkovich AJ, Kjos BO. Schizencephaly: correlation of clinical findings with MR characteristics. *AJNR Am J Neuroradiol.* 1992;13:85–94 and Packard AM, Miller VS, Delgado MR. Schizencephaly: correlations of clinical and radiologic features. *Neurology.* 1997;48:1427–1434 and based on a cumulative series of 67 cases.

however, recessive mutations in the "microcephaly" gene *WDR62* have been shown to result not only in microcephaly but also in schizencephaly in some cases, implicating the processes underlying proliferation in the genesis of schizencephaly.[118] Another genetic cause that has emerged recently is mutation of the gene *COL4A1*, associated with schizencephaly plus a number of other features, including CNS findings (e.g., intracranial calcification, focal cortical dysgenesis, pontocerebellar hypoplasia) and extracerebral findings (e.g., hemolytic anemia).[119]

The clinical features of schizencephaly have begun to be clarified by the study of patients identified by MRI (see Table 6.5). The lesion may be suspected because of the appearance of a focal ventricular dilation on ultrasonography or CT or occasionally because of visualization of a gray matter–lined cleft on CT (Fig. 6.9A).[96,97,120,121] However, far more sensitive for identification of schizencephaly is MRI (Fig. 6.9B).[97,98,109,120,122-124] The salient feature is the lining of the cleft by cerebral cortex, often thickened by pachygyric or polymicrogyric cortex with heterotopia. The clinical spectrum is clearly broader than was previously expected. Severity relates to the extent and distribution of cerebral involvement (see Table 6.5).[96,97,109,125] In two series, prominent cognitive disturbances were present with all bilateral lesions but only 24% of unilateral lesions.[107,109] (We have seen one patient who had bilateral clefts and average intelligence.) Motor disturbances are nearly invariable with frontal and open-lipped lesions (see Table 6.5).[96,97,109] Seizures may begin as late as adult life in patients with schizencephaly.[97,107,126,127] Hydrocephalus complicates approximately 50% of open-lipped lesions (see Table 6.5), although the mechanism for the impaired cerebrospinal fluid dynamics is unclear.[107] Agenesis of the septum pellucidum occurs in 70% of cases, and accompanying septo-optic dysplasia occurs in 10% to 25% (see Chapter 1).[97] Agenesis or hypoplasia of the corpus callosum occurs in 30% of cases of schizencephaly.[97]

Lissencephaly and the Agyria-Pachygyria Spectrum

Anatomical Abnormality. In *lissencephaly* (i.e., "smooth brain"), the brain has few or no gyri.[a] Two basic anatomical types of lissencephaly can be distinguished (Tables 6.6 and 6.7). In *type I lissencephaly*, the cerebral wall is similar to that of an approximately 12-week-old fetus (Fig. 6.10A and B). The layers consist, from the pial surface, of an outermost relatively cell-poor marginal layer, a diffuse cellular layer containing primarily pyramidal and other neurons characteristic of lower layers of cortex, a zone of heterotopic neurons in columns, and an innermost band of white matter. The pathological features indicate that the diffuse cellular layer contains neurons that were destined to constitute the deep layers of cortex but were never displaced by subsequent migrations, the neurons of which constitute the heterotopic layer. In *type II lissencephaly* the appearance is quite different (see Fig. 6.10C). The cortex

---

[a]References 20, 30, 34, 35, 40, 41, 44, 46, 93, and 128-144.

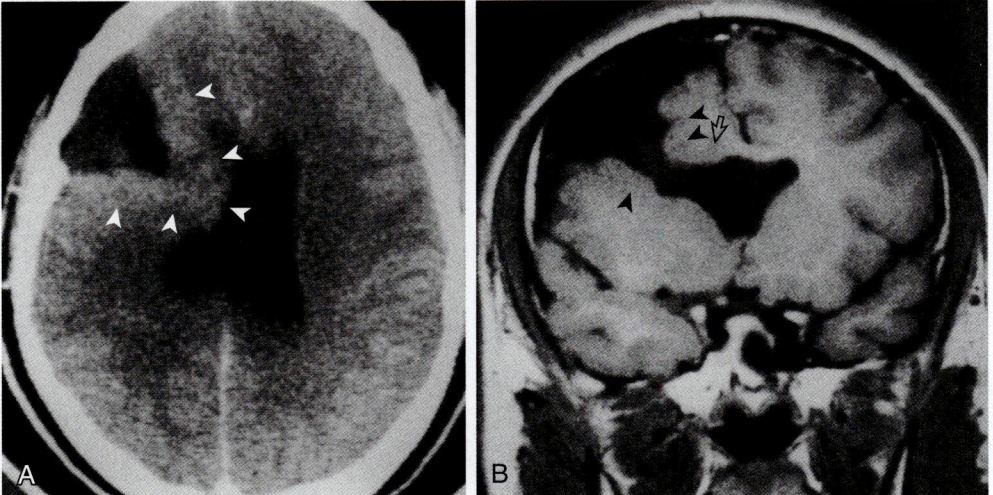

Figure 6.9 Unilateral schizencephaly with separated lips. (A) Contrast-enhanced axial computed tomography scan shows deep infolding of the cortex in the right frontal region, apparently pressing on the right lateral ventricle (*arrowheads*). (This cortical gray matter lining of the cleft is important in distinction from a destructive lesion, such as porencephaly.) (B) Coronal SE 600/20 magnetic resonance imaging scan shows the infolding to be a large cleft in apparent continuity with the lateral ventricle. (The pial-ependymal seam may not be demonstrable or may be disrupted.) Continuity of gray matter through the cleft is clearly shown (*arrowheads*), as is the focus of heterotopic gray matter along the roof of the right lateral ventricle (*open arrow*). The septum pellucidum is absent, consistent with the diagnosis of septo-optic dysplasia. (With permission from Barkovich AJ, Norman D. MR imaging of schizencephaly. *AJNR Am J Neuroradiol.* 1988;9:297–302.)

TABLE 6.6   Major Varieties of Type I Lissencephaly: Etiology/Genetics

DISORDERS	GENE LOCUS	PROTEIN	FUNCTION
Isolated lissencephaly (LIS1)	17p13.3	PAFAH1B1	Cytoskeleton (microtubules/dynein)
Miller-Dieker syndrome (LIS1)	17p13.3	PAFAH1B1	Cytoskeleton (microtubules/dynein)
		14-3-3ε	
Isolated lissencephaly (XLIS)	Xq22.3	Doublecortin	Cytoskeleton (microtubules)
XLAG	Xp22	ARX	Homeobox
LCHb	7q22	Reelin	Neuron/radial glial cell interactions

ARX, An aristaless-related homeobox transcription factor encoded by the gene *ARX*; *LCHb*, lissencephaly with cerebellar hypoplasia b; *PAFAH1B1*, platelet-activating factor acetylhydrolase; *XLAG*, X-linked lissencephaly with abnormal genitalia.

TABLE 6.7   Major Varieties of Type II ("Cobblestone") Lissencephaly: Etiology/Genetics

DISORDER	GENE LOCUS	PROTEIN	FUNCTION
Fukuyama congenital muscular dystrophy	9q31-32	Fukutin	Glycosylation
Walker-Warburg syndrome	9q34.1	POMT1	Glycosylation
Muscle-eye-brain disease	1p34	POMGnT1	Glycosylation

POMGnT1, Protein O-mannose N-acetylglucosaminyltransferase; *POMT1*, protein O-mannosyltransferase 1.

---

is represented by clusters and circular arrays of neurons, with no recognizable organization or lamination, separated by glial and vascular septa. Large heterotopic collections of neurons are prominent. Notable, however, are the protrusions over the cortical surface where neurons have migrated through the pia. These protrusions cause the cortical surface to be irregular or "pebbly" in appearance.

In *pachygyria*, the features are similar to those described for lissencephaly but are less marked.[a] The gyri are relatively few, are unusually broad, and are associated with an abnormally thick cortical plate (Fig. 6.11, parasagittal region). The microscopic features are similar to those of lissencephaly, although the

---

[a]References 20, 34, 35, 40, 41, 44, 93, 135-138, 140, 142, and 145-150.

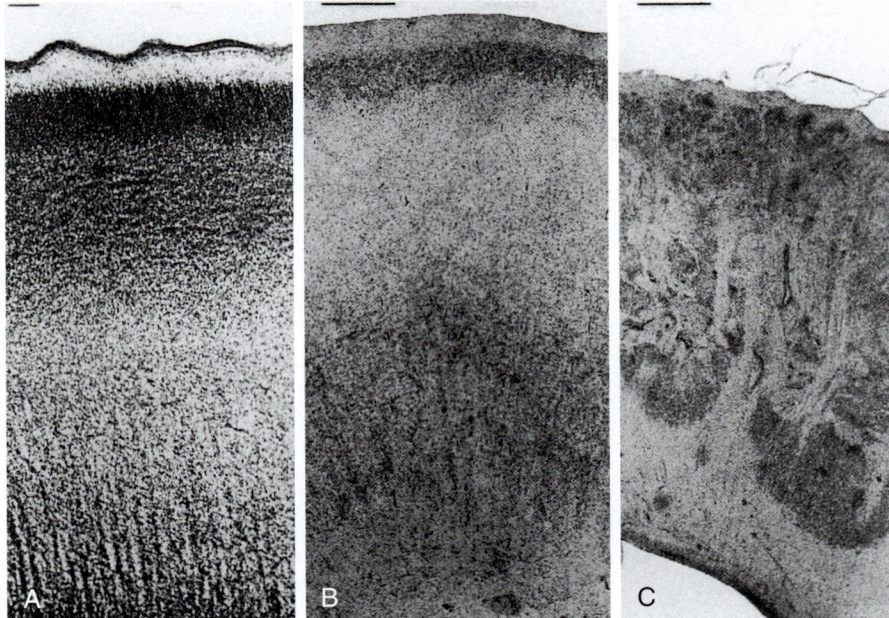

Figure 6.10 Lissencephaly types I and II. (A) Cerebral hemisphere wall of a normal 14-week human fetus. The undifferential cortical plate is bordered inferiorly by migrating neurons. In the lower part of the figure, migrating cells are seen arranged in vertical columns. The subventricular zone is seen in the lowest part (hematoxylin and eosin [H&E], bar = 0.1 mm). (B) Type I (classic) lissencephaly in a newborn. The neocortex is represented by a narrow band of (pyramidal) cells, separated by a cell-sparse zone from vertically arranged columns of neurons arrested during migration. Compare with (A) (H&E, bar = 1 mm). (C) Type II (Walker-Warburg) lissencephaly in a newborn. The neocortex is disorganized into ectopic clusters of neurons. Note the radial projection of white matter, with associated fibrovascular tissue, into the cortex between the clusters. This arrangement results in the "cobblestone" appearance on magnetic resonance imaging (H&E, bar = 1 mm). Note also the protrusion of migrating neurons through the glia limitans, leading to the uneven or *pebbly* cortical surface. (With permission from Barth PG. Disorders of neuronal migration. *Can J Neurol Sci.* 1987;14:1–16.)

abnormalities are less marked (Fig. 6.12). Pachygyria should be considered *on a continuum with lissencephaly*, because, depending on the nature of the genetic disturbance, lissencephaly syndromes may be characterized principally by pachygyria rather than by lissencephaly (see later).

Timing. The onset of lissencephaly-pachygyria is considered to be no later than the third and fourth months of gestation. This conclusion is based on the anatomical features of the lesions as well as cases in which putative teratogenic exposures could be documented.[93,137,138,151]

Clinical Aspects: Type I Lissencephaly. The clinical aspects of lissencephaly-pachygyria are considered best in terms of those disorders characterized by type I and type II disease (see Tables 6.6 and 6.7). Several genetic disorders are recognized in association with type I lissencephaly. Approximately 60% of these cases are caused by defects of the chromosome 17p13.3 gene (*LIS1*), and approximately half of the remaining cases are caused by defects of the Xq22.3 gene *XLIS* or *DCX* (see Table 6.6). (The *XLIS* cases account for nearly all the male infants in the non-*LIS1* group.) Both lissencephaly with cerebellar hypoplasia b (reelin deficiency) and X-linked lissencephaly with abnormal genitalia (XLAG), associated with mutations in the gene *ARX*,[152] are much less common. The radiographic features described with some of the newly reported "tubulinopathies" (e.g., caused by mutation in *TUBA1A*) reveal lissencephaly

TABLE 6.8	Major Neurological Features of Type I Isolated Lissencephaly

Normal head size at birth → microcephaly in the first year
Hypotonia → hypertonia later in infancy
Paucity of movement, feeding disturbance
Seizures (common evolution to infantile spasms or Lennox-Gastaut syndrome in early infancy)
Electroencephalogram severely disordered with high amplitude and rapid frequency

and pachygyria in some of these cases, often with associated abnormalities of the basal ganglia, corpus callosum, and posterior fossa.[153,154]

The *clinical features* of the major form of type I lissencephaly (*LIS1*, isolated lissencephaly related to the chromosome 17p13.3 locus) are summarized in Table 6.8.[a] Despite the major brain anomaly, microcephaly usually is *not* present at birth but characteristically develops in the first year. The craniofacial appearance is generally unremarkable except for bitemporal hollowing of the skull and a small jaw. Marked hypotonia and paucity of movement are characteristic. Spasticity does not develop until later in the first year or even after that.

---

[a]References 30, 34, 35, 40, 41, 44, 46, 138, 141, 143, and 155-169.

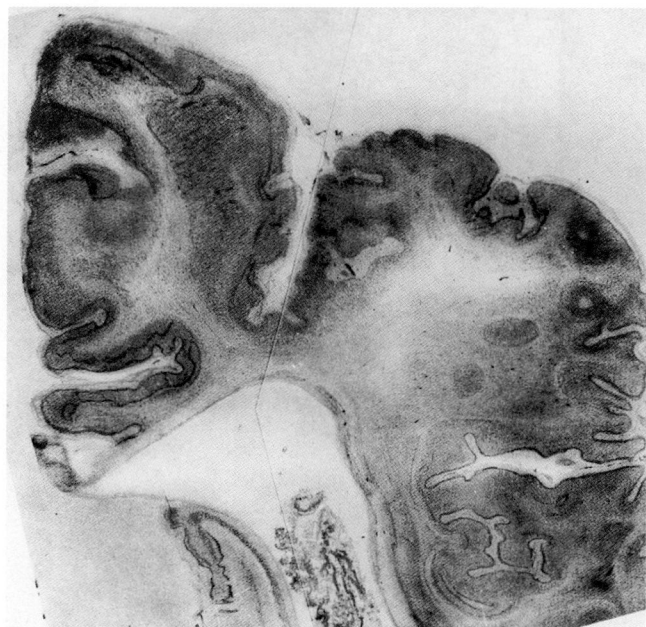

Figure 6.11 Pachygyria and polymicrogyria. Coronal section of the parietal lobe, parasagittal region, and lateral convexity from an infant with Zellweger cerebrohepatorenal syndrome (Nissl stain for cell bodies). Note the pachygyric cortex in the parasagittal region and the polymicrogyric cortex over the lateral convexity. (With permission from Volpe JJ, Adams RD. Cerebro-hepato-renal syndrome of Zellweger: an inherited disorder of neuronal migration. *Acta Neuropathol.* 1972;20:175–198.)

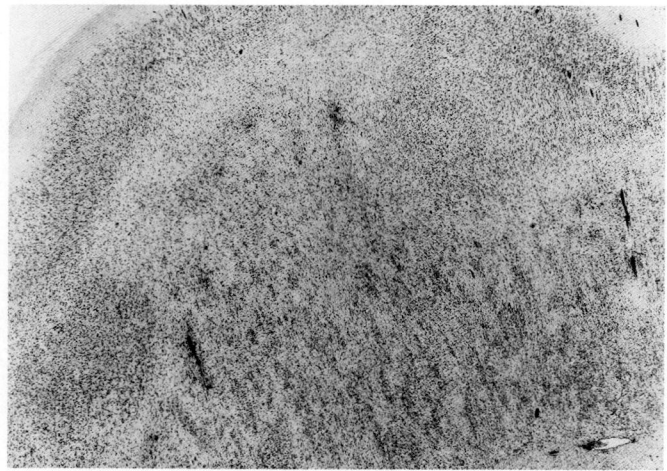

Figure 6.12 Pachygyric cortex in the specimen shown in Fig. 6.11 (Nissl stain for cell bodies). The pial surface is at the upper-left-hand corner, and the subcortical white matter is at the lower-right-hand corner. Note the broad layer of heterotopic neurons arranged in columns and nests, which is separated from the pachygyric cortex by a sparsely cellular region. The neurons of the pachygyric cortex, at higher magnification, had the characteristics of pyramidal neurons of deeper cortical layers, not displaced by subsequent migrations. (With permission from Volpe JJ, Adams RD. Cerebro-hepato-renal syndrome of Zellweger: an inherited disorder of neuronal migration. *Acta Neuropathol.* 1972;20:175–198.)

Neonatal seizures can occur, but characteristically seizures develop in the first 6 months as infantile spasms or as akinetic-myoclonic seizures with grossly disordered findings on the electroencephalogram (EEG) (Lennox-Gastaut syndrome). The EEG is always abnormal; particularly characteristic is high-amplitude, fast activity, occurring in approximately 75% of patients with type I lissencephaly. Bursts of sharp and slow-wave complexes, interspersed with periods of voltage depression, are also common features of the EEG. Infants with primarily pachygyria rather than lissencephaly have less severe clinical deficits, including occasionally only mild subsequent impairment of intellect. In general, however, neurological outcome in *LIS1* isolated lissencephaly is characterized ultimately by pronounced intellectual disability, spastic quadriparesis, and seizures.

The clinical features of the second major form of type I lissencephaly related to the chromosome 17p13.3 locus, the *Miller-Dieker syndrome*, are different from those of isolated lissencephaly because of the additional presence of craniofacial abnormalities.[a] Thus, in addition to the bitemporal hollowing and small jaw observed with isolated lissencephaly, patients have a characteristic facial appearance with a short nose with upturned nares, a long and protuberant upper lip with a thin vermilion border, and a relatively flattened midface (Fig. 6.13). Additional characteristic features of Miller-Dieker syndrome include cardiac malformations (20% to 25%), genital anomalies in male infants (70%), a sacral dimple (70%), deep palmar creases (65% to 70%), and clinodactyly (40% to 45%). Neurological features are similar to those described for isolated lissencephaly, although generally the disturbances are even more marked, consistent with the uniformly severe degree of the lissencephaly.

The *clinical aspects* of the *major X-linked form of type I lissencephaly* (i.e., those related to a defect in the *DCX* [or *XLIS*] gene), are similar to those described for isolated lissencephaly caused by *LIS1*. The clinical features, of course, occur in hemizygous male infants, whereas heterozygous female infants exhibit subcortical band heterotopia (see later).

The *clinical aspects* of the *rarer* form of X-linked lissencephaly (i.e., *XLAG*, associated with mutations in *ARX*)[152] are somewhat distinctive.[173-177] Particularly characteristic features include severe *neonatal* seizures (onset in >50% in the first hour of life and in utero in 20%), hypothermia, severe diarrhea, and ambiguous genitalia (micropenis, cryptorchidism). The epileptic syndrome is especially severe and relates to the particular involvement of GABAergic interneurons (see later). The lissencephaly, typically posterior-predominant as with *LIS1*, is accompanied also by complete agenesis of the corpus callosum. The full syndrome occurs in hemizygous male infants, although less severe phenotypes occur as a function of the severity of the genetic abnormality. Heterozygous female infants often exhibit agenesis of the corpus callosum and epilepsy.

The *clinical aspects* of *lissencephaly with cerebellar hypoplasia b*, related to a defect in *RELN*, which encodes reelin, are difficult to define decisively because of the paucity of careful clinical descriptions.[40,178-180] Perhaps most notable is the presence of microcephaly *at birth*, rather than the postnatal development of microcephaly, as in other varieties of type I lissencephaly. The term *lissencephaly with cerebellar hypoplasia b* is used to distinguish these cases from lissencephaly with cerebellar hypoplasia a.

---

[a]References 30, 40, 41, 44, 164, and 170–172.

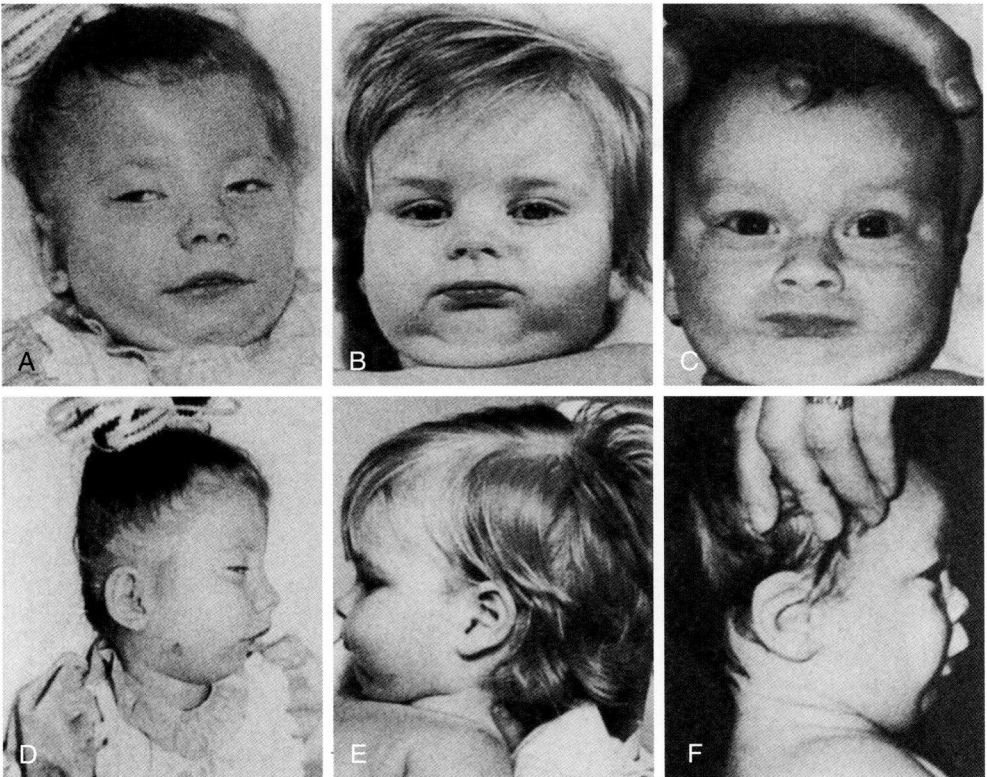

Figure 6.13 Miller-Dieker syndrome. (A to C) Frontal views of three infants. (D to F) Lateral views. See text for details. (With permission from Dobyns WB. The neurogenetics of lissencephaly. *Neurol Clin.* 1989;7:89–105.)

The latter are examples of type I lissencephaly secondary to either *LIS1* or *DCX* gene defects (see earlier), which may be accompanied by prominent hypoplasia of the cerebellar vermis and mild hypoplasia of the cerebellar hemispheres. By contrast, the reelin-related cases exhibit *severe* hypoplasia of the *entire* cerebellum, which also lacks folia.

The *radiological features* of type I lissencephaly may include a distinctive appearance on CT (Fig. 6.14). However, MRI provides superior definition of the parenchymal lesion (Figs. 6.15 and 6.16), particularly the appearance of a "cell-sparse zone" in the superficial aspect of the cortex. Indeed, insight into the likely genetic lesion can be gained by evaluating the degree of lissencephaly and pachygyria, any anteroposterior gradient, agenesis of the corpus callosum, and the degree of cerebellar hypoplasia (see Fig. 6.16).[40] Thus, among *LIS1* cases, the cortex is very thick, posterior more than anterior involvement is apparent, and Miller-Dieker cases have even more severe lissencephaly than do isolated cases. *DCX* cases have anterior more than posterior involvement. *ARX* cases have only a moderately thick cortex, posterior predominance of the abnormally thick cortex, and prominent agenesis of the corpus callosum. Reelin cases have a moderately thick, pachygyric cortex with striking cerebellar hypoplasia. A uniform accompanying feature in all genetic types is colpocephaly (i.e., dilation of the trigone, occipital horns, and temporal horns of the lateral ventricles). The ventricular dilation of colpocephaly occurs in the trigone and occipital horns because of underdevelopment of the corpus callosum and calcarine sulci and in the temporal horns because of failure of inversion of the hippocampus.[163]

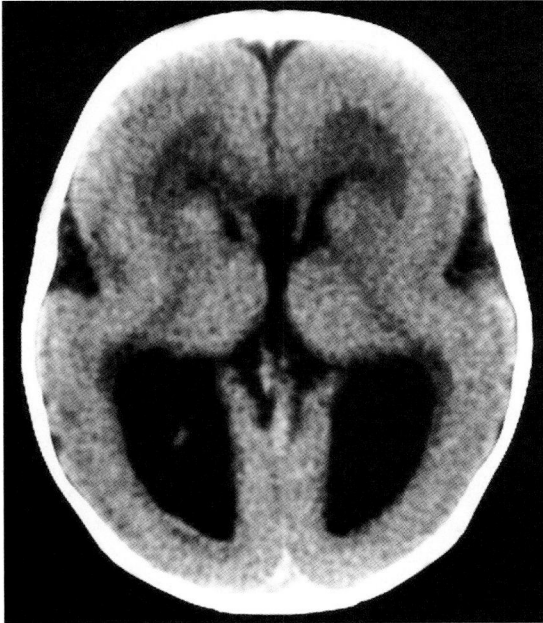

Figure 6.14 Lissencephaly type I, computed tomography scan. Note the smooth cortical surface and colpocephaly (dilation of trigone and occipital horns of lateral ventricles). (With permission from Dobyns WB. The neurogenetics of lissencephaly. *Neurol Clin.* 1989;7:89–105.)

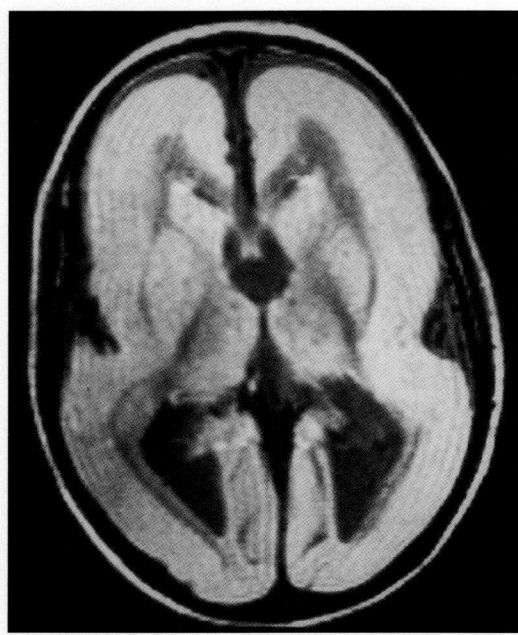

Figure 6.15 Lissencephaly type I, magnetic resonance imaging (MRI). Note the smooth cortical surface and colpocephaly, as described in the legend for Fig. 6.14. The cerebral parenchymal features are visualized better by MRI than by computed tomography.

Etiology/Genetics: Type I Lissencephaly. The major genetic varieties of type I lissencephaly appear to involve three different mechanisms of migrational failure (see Table 6.6). The *LIS1* cases, both isolated lissencephaly and Miller-Dieker syndrome, and the *DCX (XLIS)* cases have a defect in the pace of migration. The tubulinopathies likewise result from microtubule dysfunction and resultant aberrant migration.[154,181] *ARX* mutations appear to involve a defect in tangential more than radial migration. The *RELN* cases appear to be related to a defect in migrating neuron and radial glial interactions.

Isolated lissencephaly (LIS1) secondary to a deficiency in PAFAH1B1 *(LIS1)* involves a disturbance in migration because of abnormal function of the cytoskeleton.[a] This protein is the noncatalytic alpha subunit of the isoform Ib of the platelet-activating factor acetylhydrolase. This *LIS1*-encoded protein interacts with microtubules and cytoplasmic dynein motors, crucial for both somal translocation and cell motility.

Miller-Dieker syndrome, of course, shares the PAFAH defect, but because the disorder relates to a deletion, other genes are disturbed.[b] The protein 14-3-3ε appears to be the key additional defect in this more severe lissencephaly syndrome.[171] Deficiency of 14-3-3ε results in mislocalization of the *LIS1* protein; this accentuates the dynein motor disturbance and thereby neuronal migration.

Isolated lissencephaly, secondary to the X-linked DCX (XLIS) gene and deficiency of *doublecortin*, appears also to be mediated at the level of the cytoskeleton.[30,40,41,71,185-187] *Doublecortin* is a microtubule-associated protein that binds to tubulin and is necessary for microtubule polymerization. Thus, as with the

two *LIS1* disorders, a defect in the cytoskeleton and thereby in cell motility results.

XLAG involves a second mechanism of migrational disturbance.[40,41,174,176,177] The gene involved, *ARX*, is a homeobox gene that encodes a protein critical for *tangential* migration. The result of the mutation is a marked deficiency of GABAergic interneurons because, as noted earlier, tangential rather than radial migration is the principal mechanism for the movement of neurons destined to be interneurons from the ventricular zone to the cortex. The severe deficiency of GABAergic neurons likely underlies the striking clinical feature of prenatal and early neonatal seizures and intractable infantile seizures (see earlier discussion of clinical aspects).

Lissencephaly with cerebellar hypoplasia b, related to the *RELN* gene, involves a third mechanism of disturbed migration. *RELN* encodes reelin, a glycoprotein secreted by horizontally oriented Cajal-Retzius cells in the preplate and marginal zones; it is crucial for signaling to migrating neurons on radial glial cells.[40,41,44] Reelin appears to function as a stop signal and in neuronal and radial glial cell interactions. The result of reelin deficiency is a cortex that is abnormally cellular in its most superficial zone and is inverted (i.e., early migrating pyramidal cells are the uppermost layer). Preplate-like cells accumulate in the marginal zone, a finding suggesting that the preplate has not been split by the migrating cortical neurons. Related phenomena occur in cerebellum to cause the severe cerebellar hypoplasia.

The tubulinopathy family of genes frequently plays a role in lissencephaly or pachygyria, sometimes accompanied by other MRI features, as noted earlier. The genes thus far implicated include *TUBA1A*, *TUBB2B*, *TUBB3*, *TUBB5*, and *TUBA8*, typically with de novo mutations.

Other causes of type I lissencephaly, albeit rare, are worthy of note. A role for vascular insult during the third to fourth months of gestation has been suggested.[157,164,165,188] Moreover, lissencephaly/pachygyria has been documented with fetal CMV infection (see Chapter 34) and a variety of inborn errors of metabolism (e.g., pyruvate dehydrogenase deficiency, Zellweger syndrome, glutaric acidemia [type 2, nonketotic hyperglycinemia]; see Chapters 27, 28, and 29). Rare autosomal recessive forms with marked neonatal microcephaly and lissencephaly, the most severe form of microcephaly with simplified gyri discussed among proliferative disorders, have been reported (see Chapter 5).[124,142,189-191]

Recurrence risks for type 1 lissencephaly depend on the genetic type.[44] Thus, *LIS1* isolated lissencephaly, which is caused by de novo mutations, has a recurrence risk of approximately 1% to 10% (because of the theoretical risk of germline mosaicism in either parent). Miller-Dieker syndrome is related to de novo deletions in approximately 80% (recurrence risk of ≈1%); in 20%, it is related to inheritance of a deletion from a parent carrying a balanced chromosomal rearrangement. In the latter case, recurrence risk is higher and depends on the nature of the rearrangement. With *XLIS* lissencephaly, the mother may be a carrier even if the brain MRI does not show subcortical band heterotopia.[187] Even if the mother is not a carrier, the risk of harboring germline mosaicism places a recurrence risk at about 1% to 10%. With XLAG, the carrier status of the mother should be evaluated because the phenotype in girls and women can be very mild. Thus far, the few families reported with reelin deficiency lissencephaly have exhibited autosomal

---

[a]References 40, 41, 43, 46, 182, and 183.
[b]References 35, 40, 41, 164, 170, and 184.

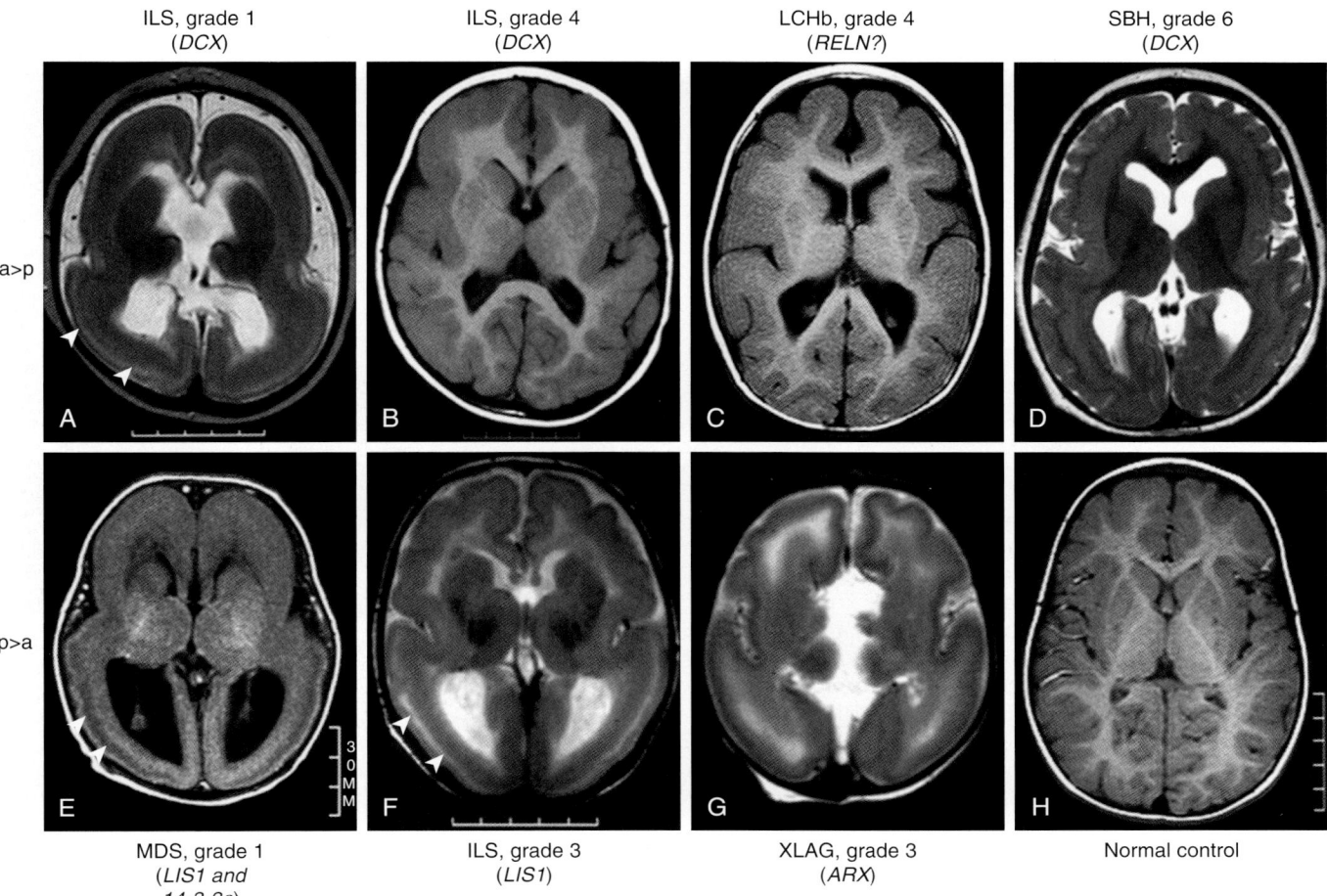

ILS, grade 1
(*DCX*)

ILS, grade 4
(*DCX*)

LCHb, grade 4
(*RELN?*)

SBH, grade 6
(*DCX*)

a>p

p>a

MDS, grade 1
(*LIS1* and
14-3-3ε)

ILS, grade 3
(*LIS1*)

XLAG, grade 3
(*ARX*)

Normal control

Figure 6.16 Lissencephaly type I, magnetic resonance imaging. In contrast to a normal control (H), all types of lissencephaly (A to G) except for subcortical band heterotopia (SBH) have absent or broad gyri and an abnormally thick cortex, resulting from a *DCX* mutation in heterozygous female infants (SBH is discussed in the text with heterotopia rather than with lissencephaly-pachygyria). The anteroposterior or rostrocaudal gradient of lissencephaly is strictly correlated with the causative gene. Specifically, mutations of *DCX* or *RELN* result in a more severe anterior than posterior (a > p) gradient (A to D), whereas mutations of *LIS1* with or without *14-3-3ε* or *ARX* lead to a more severe posterior than anterior (p > a) gradient (E to G). The absolute thickness of the cortex and the presence of a cell-sparse zone also differ based on the causative gene. In patients with mutations of *DCX* (A and B) or *LIS1* (E and F), the cortex is very thick, typically 10 to 20 mm, and prominent cell-sparse zones are seen in areas of agyria (*arrowheads* in A, E, and F). In patients with lissencephaly with cerebellar hypoplasia group b (C, which resembles patients with known *RELN* mutations, although a mutation has not been demonstrated in this patient) or *ARX* (G) mutations, the cortex is only moderately thick, typically 5 to 10 mm, and cell-sparse zones are never seen, even in areas of agyria (G). In lissencephaly with cerebellar hypoplasia group b (LCHb) with or without proven *RELN* mutations, other images depict an abnormal hippocampus and severe cerebellar hypoplasia (not shown). In male infants with X-linked lissencephaly with abnormal genitalia (XLAG) caused by *ARX* mutations, other images demonstrate poorly demarcated basal ganglia often with small cysts, immature white matter, and agenesis of the corpus callosum (not shown). In heterozygous female infants, mutations of *DCX* result in SBH (D), whereas mutations of *ARX* often result in agenesis of the corpus callosum (not shown). *ILS,* Isolated lissencephaly; *MDS,* Miller-Dieker syndrome; *XLAG,* X-linked lissencephaly with abnormal genitalia. (With permission from Kato M, Dobyns WB. Lissencephaly and the molecular basis of neuronal migration. *Hum Mol Genet.* 2003;12:R89–R96.)

recessive inheritance. The tubulinopathies are for the most part due to de novo mutations in a growing list of genes.

In cases presenting with classic patterns associated with the genes already noted, if a first attempt at genetic testing does not reveal a genetic etiology, one must consider the *possibility of a mosaic mutation* presenting with mutations that may be difficult to detect with conventional sequencing strategies but

that may be detectable as clinical testing moves to the realm of next-generation sequencing.[192]

Clinical Aspects: Type II Lissencephaly. The three disorders consistently associated with type II lissencephaly are Fukuyama congenital muscular dystrophy, Walker-Warburg syndrome, and muscle-eye-brain disease (see Table 6.7).[34,35,193-206] As noted

TABLE 6.9   Major Clinical Features of Walker-Warburg Syndrome

Macrocephaly	84%
Present at birth	58%
Develops postnatally	26%
Type II lissencephaly	100%[a]
Cerebellar malformation	100%[a]
Ventricular dilation/hydrocephalus	95%
Retinal malformation	100%[a]
Anterior chamber abnormality	76%
Congenital muscular dystrophy	100%[a]

[a]Necessary for diagnosis.
Data from Dobyns WB. The neurogenetics of lissencephaly. *Neurol Clin.* 1989;7:89–105.

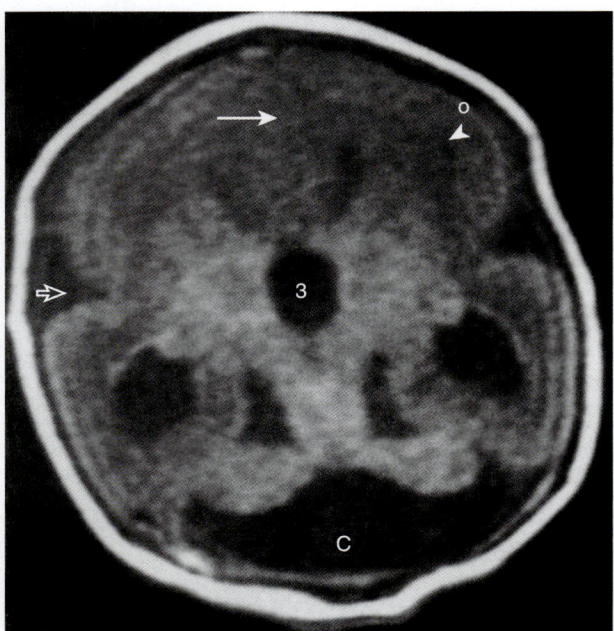

Figure 6.17 Magnetic resonance imaging, type II lissencephaly in Walker-Warburg syndrome. At the level of the third ventricle, a smooth cortical surface, open and shallow sylvian fissures *(open arrow)*, a Dandy-Walker cyst (C), and enlargement of the lateral and third (3) ventricles are demonstrated. A lack of cerebral gray-white matter interdigitation is seen (o, *arrowhead*) adjacent to a thickened cortical mantle. The *cobblestone* appearance of the cortex is faintly visible in the right frontal region and will become more apparent after the neonatal period. The anterior interhemispheric fissure is obliterated as a result of leptomeningeal thickening and proliferation *(arrow)*. The ventricular dilation and cerebellar malformation are characteristic of the syndrome (see text). (With permission from Rhodes RE. Walker-Warburg syndrome. *AJNR Am J Neuroradiol.* 1992;13:12–126.)

earlier, these disorders are characterized by lissencephaly in which protrusions of neurons are found over the surface of the brain and thereby render a *bumpy* or *pebbly* configuration to the cortical surface. In type II lissencephaly, the ectopic clusters of neurons within the cortex, separated by fibroglial vascular tissue that extends radially from the cerebral white matter, result in a typical MRI appearance, termed *cobblestone* lissencephaly (see later). The migrational defect is unique and is similar for the three disorders (see later). In addition to type II lissencephaly, these disorders also share congenital muscular dystrophy as a prominent clinical feature. Fukuyama congenital muscular dystrophy and muscle-eye-brain disease are discussed most appropriately with diseases of muscle (see Chapter 33). The clinical aspects of Walker-Warburg syndrome are described here.

The major *clinical features* of Walker-Warburg syndrome in many respects are different from those for the type I lissencephalic disorders (Table 6.9). Macrocephaly (84%), either apparent at birth (58%) or developing postnatally (26%), retinal malformations (100%), congenital muscular dystrophy (100%), cerebellar malformation (100%), and type II lissencephaly (100%) are characteristic.[193-196,204-206] Type II lissencephaly and the retinal, cerebellar, and muscular abnormalities are necessary for the diagnosis. The neurological features (e.g., severe seizure disorders and intellectual disability) are similar to those identified for type I lissencephaly. However, the severe muscle disease, accompanied by elevated serum creatine kinase, accentuates the marked hypotonia and weakness observed with lissencephaly. Death in the first year is common.

The *radiological features* are similar to those for type I lissencephaly in terms of the agyric brain and the concurrence of agenesis or hypoplasia of the corpus callosum or septum pellucidum. However, because of the different cerebrocortical microscopic pathological features (see earlier discussion), a slightly uneven cortex is apparent. Moreover, as noted earlier, irregular projections of the underlying white matter into the cortex lead to the term *cobblestone* lissencephaly (Fig. 6.17). The latter appearance is more clearly apparent after the neonatal period. The most characteristic distinguishing features of Walker-Warburg syndrome include the presence of cerebellar malformation and, invariably, vermian agenesis or hypoplasia as well as complete Dandy-Walker malformation (50%) and posterior encephalocele (25% to 35%) (Fig. 6.18; see also Fig. 6.17). The ventricular dilation (95%) can be distinguished from the colpocephaly of type I lissencephaly by involvement of the third and fourth ventricles and by the presence of the macrocephaly of hydrocephalus. Some of these distinguishing features are recalled by the eponymic designation for this syndrome: HARD ± E, *h*ydrocephalus, *a*gyria, *r*etinal *d*ysplasia, *e*ncephalocele. We suggest an alternative, CHARM ± E, to add *c*erebellar and *m*uscle.

Etiology/Genetics: Type II Lissencephaly. The autosomal recessive disorders that result in cobblestone lissencephaly occur because of a *failure of neurons to terminate their radial migration to the cerebral cortex.* Indeed, these neurons migrate through the glia limitans at the pial surface of the cortex and into the subarachnoid space.[41,201,202,206,207] The fundamental disturbance involves glycosylation of alpha-dystroglycan, a protein secreted particularly by astrocytes but also by neurons. Secreted alpha-dystroglycan interacts with beta-dystroglycan in the glial plasma membrane and with laminin of the extracellular matrix. The glia limitans consists of the apposed astrocytic end feet and the overlying extracellular matrix. Because the interactions of alpha-dystroglycan require correct glycosylation of the protein, failure of glycosylation is associated with gaps in the glia limitans, protrusion of neurons through these gaps, and failure of neurons to organize themselves within the cortical plate. The three key genes originally described, *POMT1*, *POMGnT1*, and *fukutin*, are involved in glycosylation, especially

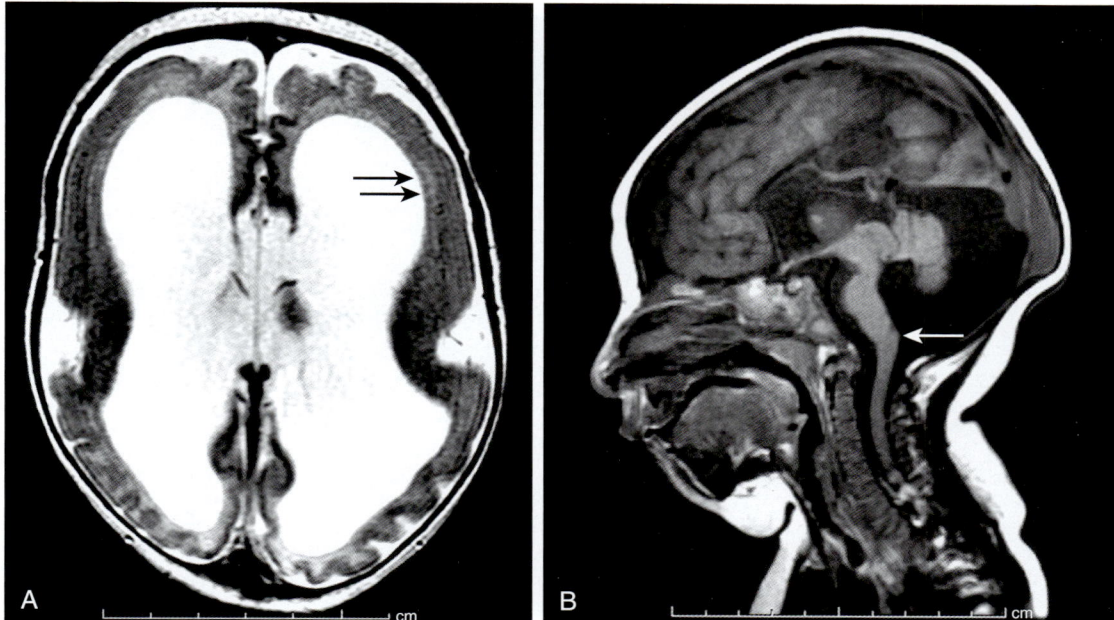

Figure 6.18 Magnetic resonance imaging, type II lissencephaly, Walker-Warburg syndrome. Note in (A) the hydrocephalus, smooth cortical surface anteriorly and pachygyric cortex posteriorly, and, barely observable, the interdigitations of white matter into the cortex with a resulting *cobblestone* appearance *(arrows)*. In (B) note the dysgenetic corpus callosum, cerebellar hypoplasia, and anomalous kinking of the lower brain stem *(arrow)*, all characteristic of Walker-Warburg syndrome. (Courtesy Dr. Omar Khwaja.)

by encoding glycosyl transferases, as shown in Table 6.7.[208,209] The molecular details require further delineation because the precise role of fukutin in glycosylation remains to be clarified, and only 10% to 20% of Walker-Warburg cases exhibit the protein O-mannosyl transferase defect.[202,205] In muscle, correctly glycosylated alpha-dystroglycan is required to interact with extracellular laminin and sarcolemmal beta-dystroglycan, which is bound to dystrophin. In the three disorders, failure of this interaction leads to degeneration of the muscle fiber and *dystrophy* (see Chapter 33). Additional genes implicated in this group of disorders include *POMT2, FKRP, COL4A1, LARGE,* and *POMK*.[210-215]

Polymicrogyria

Anatomical Abnormality. Polymicrogyria is characterized by a great number of small plications in the cortical surface, rendering to the external aspect of the cerebrum the appearance of a wrinkled chestnut (Fig. 6.19). The multitude of small gyri are arranged in complicated festoon-like or glandular formations, appearing to result from fusion of their molecular layers (see Fig. 6.11, lateral convexity).[44,216-218]

Two basic varieties of polymicrogyria, layered and unlayered, can be distinguished from the microscopic appearance (Table 6.10 and Fig. 6.20; see also Fig. 6.11).[a] In the *classic, layered* variety, the cerebral cortex has four distinct layers. Thus a relatively intact outermost molecular layer, a richly cellular second layer consisting of normal superficial cortical neurons, a cell-poor gliotic layer in place of normal deeper cortical neurons, and a fourth layer of relatively preserved neurons arranged in columns are noted (see Fig. 6.20A). The cerebral white

[a]References 20, 44, 93, 137, 219, and 220.

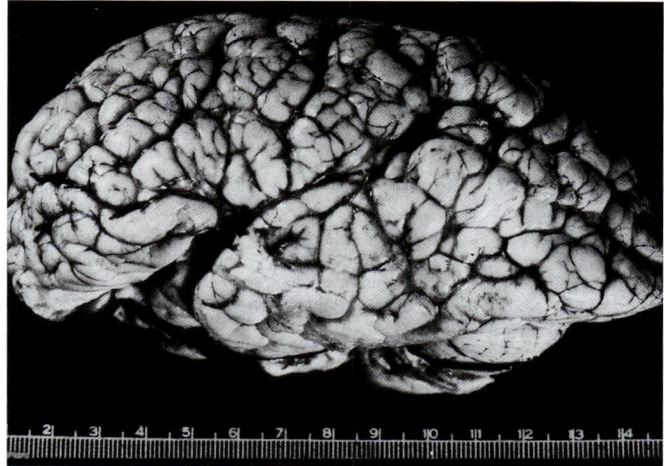

Figure 6.19 Lateral view of the cerebrum from an infant with Zellweger syndrome and polymicrogyria. Note the area of polymicrogyria anterior to the sylvian fissure, involving the convexity of the frontal lobe. (With permission from Volpe JJ, Adams RD. Cerebro-hepato-renal syndrome of Zellweger: an inherited disorder of neuronal migration. *Acta Neuropathol.* 1972;20: 175–198.)

TABLE 6.10   Major Varieties of Polymicrogyria

Layered: *classic* four-layered, probably postmigrational and related to destructive process
Unlayered: *nonclassic,* not four-layered, migrational defect, accompanied by heterotopia and other consequences of migrational disorder

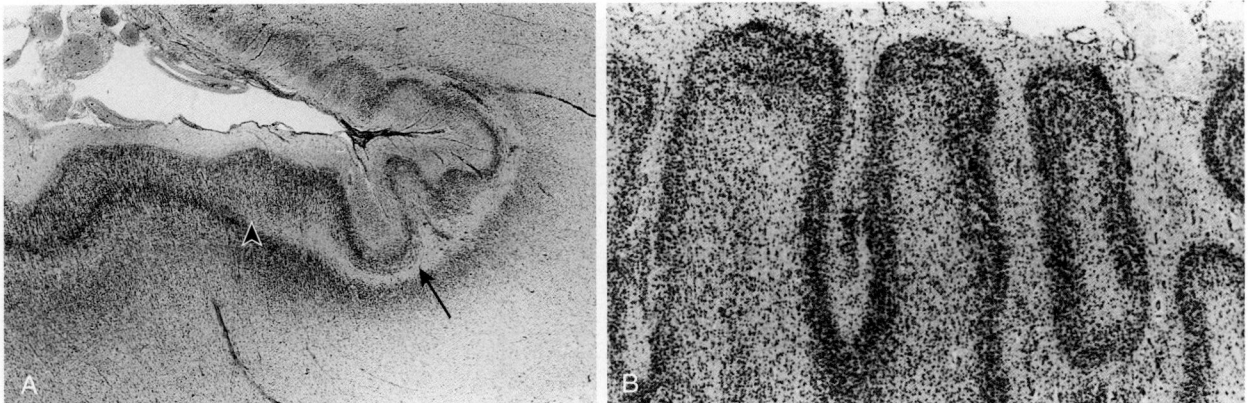

Figure 6.20 Microgyria. (A) *Classic* layered microgyria, with transition between the microgyric and normal cortex. The aneuronal band *(arrow)* of the microgyric segment is continuous with layers III and IV of the normal cortex *(arrowhead)*. Layer II of the microgyric cortex and layer II of the normal cortex are continuous (Nissl stain ×30). (B) Unlayered microgyria in a microencephalic newborn with convulsions and general hypertonia. Note the heterotopic neurons in the subcortical white matter (hematoxylin and eosin, ×87). (A, With permission from Dias MJM, Rijckevorsel GH, Landrieu P, Lyon LG. Prenatal cytomegalovirus disease and cerebral microgyria: evidence for perfusion failure, not disturbance of histogenesis, as the major cause of fetal cytomegalovirus encephalopathy. *Neuropediatrics.* 1984;15:18–24; B, with permission from Barth PG. Disorders of neuronal migration. *Can J Neurol Sci.* 1987;14:1–16.)

matter is much more abundant than in lissencephaly-pachygyria. This type of polymicrogyria often coexists in the margins of more severe ischemic destructive lesions (hydranencephaly) or in association with destructive infectious processes (e.g., toxoplasmosis or CMV infection).[93,137,220-224] In the *nonlayered* variety of polymicrogyria, the neurons destined primarily (although not exclusively) for the outer cortical layers appear to have been impeded in their migrations. The result is a poorly laminated or nonlaminated cortex, which, after the outermost cell-poor molecular layer, consists of an ill-defined zone of larger pyramidal cells (appropriate for deeper cortex) followed by a stream of heterotopic neurons; many of these neurons are smaller pyramidal and granular cells (appropriate for superficial cortical layers) (see Figs. 6.11 and 6.20B). The heterotopic neurons in cerebral white matter are arranged in columns, apparently "glued" to the radial glial fibers.[137] This type of polymicrogyria is characteristic of that seen in Zellweger syndrome (see later discussion).

Timing. The two varieties of polymicrogyria appear to have *differing times of onset.* The nonlayered variety represents a disorder of neuronal migration, and the classic four-layered variety is a postmigrational disorder. The first type includes cases, such as patients with Zellweger syndrome (see Fig. 6.11), with concomitant migrational defects present in the cerebrum as well as in the brain stem or cerebellum. In these instances, the deepest collection of neurons appears to represent heterotopic neurons arrested during migration. Disturbance of neuronal migration as one basic cause of polymicrogyria is supported further by the occurrence of polymicrogyria in index patients and siblings of infants with Miller-Dieker lissencephaly syndrome and in the cerebral hemisphere contralateral to unilateral schizencephaly (see earlier discussion).[225] The time of onset of this nonlayered variety of polymicrogyria appears to be generally no later than the fourth to fifth months of gestation.

The second variety of polymicrogyria includes those cases with evidence of laminar neuronal necrosis in the cortex *after the apparent completion of migration.* Examples of this postmigrational polymicrogyria include those cases associated with carbon monoxide exposure at approximately 20 to 24 weeks[226,227] as well as with other, less well-defined intrauterine insults.[93,222,228-233] In these patients, the sparsely cellular gliotic third layer represents an area of laminar cortical necrosis, and the fourth layer is composed not of heterotopic neurons but of neurons of the deeper layers of previously formed cortex. The *postnatal* evolution of polymicrogyria and periventricular leukomalacia has been documented in a premature infant from 31 weeks' postconceptional age, thereby documenting the postmigrational development of encephaloclastic polymicrogyria.[224] Some examples of polymicrogyria associated with CMV infection, vascular anomalies, ischemic events, or metabolic abnormalities (mitochondrial disorders) could reside in the maldevelopmental categories, encephaloclastic categories, or both.[224,234-238] Indeed, the demonstration of lissencephaly-pachygyria in some infants with CMV infection (see earlier discussion) clearly documents the potential for this viral infection to impair migratory events directly. A few observations suggest that some cases of polymicrogyria are caused by an encephaloclastic process *during* neuronal migration that interfered with the migrational events and produced polymicrogyria, that is, a combination of encephaloclastic and maldevelopmental varieties.[110,218,239,240] An experimental model that supports such a pathogenesis has been described.[241,242]

Clinical Aspects. The best example of a clinically well-defined autosomal recessive disorder of neuronal migration with polymicrogyria and pachygyria is *Zellweger cerebrohepatorenal* syndrome.[137,243-249] The neurological syndrome in these infants is startling and is characterized by marked generalized weakness with severe hypotonia, severe recurrent seizures, and absence or marked impairment of high-level responses to visual, auditory,

TABLE 6.11   Potential Importance of Very Long-Chain Fatty Acids in Neuronal Migration

DISEASE	VERY LONG-CHAIN FATTY ACIDS	PLASMALOGENS	NEURONAL MIGRATION
Zellweger syndrome	↑	↓	Abnormal
Neonatal adrenoleukodystrophy	↑	↓	Abnormal
Bifunctional enzyme	↑	Normal	Abnormal
Rhizomelic chondrodysplasia punctata	Normal	↓	Normal

Data from Moser HW. The peroxisome: nervous system role of a previously underrated organelle. The 1987 Robert Wartenberg lecture. *Neurology.* 1988;38:1617–1627 and Kaufmann WE, Theda C, Naidu S, et al. Neuronal migration abnormality in peroxisomal bifunctional enzyme defect. *Ann Neurol.* 1996;39:268–271.

or somesthetic stimuli. Other features of the syndrome include a distinctive craniofacial appearance, hepatomegaly, multiple renal cortical cysts, and stippled calcification of the patellae. A disturbance of peroxisomal biogenesis is indicated by the demonstration of absence of peroxisomes in the liver and other tissues and certain metabolic abnormalities (e.g., elevated levels of pipecolic acid and very long chain fatty acids and decreased levels of plasmalogens; see Chapter 16). Very long chain fatty acids are important constituents of plasma membranes in the brain; the possibility that the accumulation of these compounds may interfere with normal membrane properties crucial for neuronal migration along radial glial fibers is suggested by the consistent relationship among generalized peroxisomal disorders between this abnormality (rather than others) and abnormal neuronal migration (Table 6.11).[250] This notion is supported further by the occurrence of polymicrogyria in an infant with deficiency of peroxisomal bifunctional enzyme, in which the impairment of peroxisomal function was confined to very long chain fatty acids (and bile acid intermediates).[236,251]

The clinical features of *sporadic cases* of generalized polymicrogyria are not well defined, although seizures are often recorded. In general, a broad range of clinical features has been reported, from severely impaired neurological development and intractable epilepsy to only selective disturbances of neurological function.[44] Unilateral polymicrogyria is a well-documented substrate for congenital hemiplegia.[252] Polymicrogyria may accompany other dysgenetic disorders that have distinctive clinical features (e.g., a form of Joubert syndrome, Aicardi syndrome, Smith-Lemli-Opitz syndrome, periventricular nodular heterotopia; see Chapters 2 and 4).[44,253-255] The postnatal and postmigrational development of bilateral perisylvian polymicrogyria was documented by MRI in a premature infant with periventricular leukomalacia.[224] Focal polymicrogyria is a prominent feature of focal cerebrocortical dysgenesis, the clinical aspects of which are discussed separately later.

Growing numbers of *bilateral symmetrical polymicrogyria syndromes*, some familial, have been recognized (Table 6.12).[192,256-273] The clinical features in most of these disorders appear after the neonatal period. A prominent exception is the bilateral perisylvian polymicrogyric syndromes, many of which are characterized by pseudobulbar palsy with oral-buccal-lingual deficits, feeding disturbances, and facial diparesis as well as seizures from early infancy.

The *radiological diagnosis* of polymicrogyria in the *neonatal period* is often difficult, even with MRI (Fig. 6.21).[124,274] This difficulty relates in part to the lack of myelination and the

TABLE 6.12   Bilateral Symmetrical Polymicrogyria Syndromes

TOPOGRAPHY	GENETICS
Frontal	Sporadic
Frontoparietal	GPR56 (a G protein–coupled receptor)
Perisylvian	Heterogeneous (includes DYNCH1, PI3KCA)
Parasagittal (parieto-occipital)	Sporadic
Temporo-occipital	Heterogeneous (includes FIG4)
Generalized	16q locus

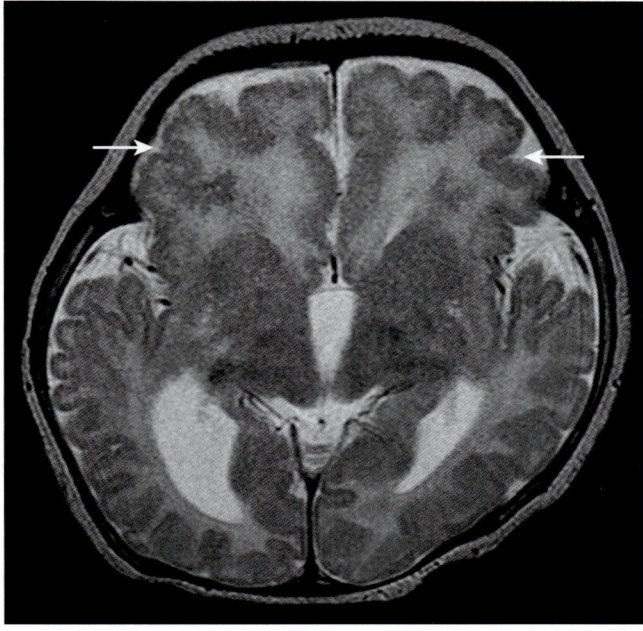

Figure 6.21   Magnetic resonance imaging (MRI), polymicrogyria. This axial T2-weighted MRI scan from an infant with seizures shows bilateral symmetrical frontal polymicrogyria *(arrows)*. Note the multiple but very small sulcal indentations of the cerebral cortex. The cortical surface thus appears somewhat smooth. The distinction from lissencephaly is aided by noting that the cortex is not thick. Also notable are underopercularization of the sylvian fissure and colpocephaly (dilation of occipital horns). (Courtesy Dr. Omar Khwaja.)

TABLE 6.13	Polymicrogyria-Associated Genes According to Head Circumference

CATEGORY	GENES
Microcephaly	ASPM
	COL18A1 (with occipital encephalocele)
	FIG4
	KIF2A
	KIF5C
	RAB3GAP2
	TUBG1
	WDR62
Microcephaly or normal head circumference	DYNC1H1
	GPR56
	TUBA1A
	TUBA8
	TUBB2B
	TUBB3
Macrocephaly	AKT3
	CCND2
	PI3KCA
	PIK3R2

TABLE 6.14	Major Varieties of Cerebral Neuronal Heterotopia

Periventricular (subependymal)
Cerebral white matter
Laminar: subcortical band or double cortex
Nodular: focal or diffuse

less prominent gray-white matter junction in the newborn than at later ages.

Etiology/Genetics: Polymicrogyria. As with schizencephaly, some cases of polymicrogyria have been associated with maternal CMV infection.[275] These cases would be expected to have CMV-associated microcephaly. A number of genetic loci have been associated with polymicrogyria, and the genes for this malformation are beginning to be elucidated. One single-gene cause of polymicrogyria, with associated microcephaly, is recessive mutation of the gene WDR62.[118] Polymicrogyria with occipital encephalocele is another rare syndrome caused by recessive mutations in the gene COL18A1.[276] Some of the genes associated with lissencephaly, including the microtubule protein-encoding genes TUBA1A, TUBA8, TUBB2B, TUBB3, TUB5, and TUBG1, and the kinesin-encoding genes KIF2A and KIF5C,[154,277] DYNC1H1 is yet another cause of genetic polymicrogyria.[192,277] A summary of polymicrogyria-related genes is presented in Table 6.13.

A spectrum of polymicrogyria syndromes associated with megalencephaly has emerged in the past few years. Some patients with hemimegalencephaly have regions of cortex that contain polymicrogyria by MRI, and some with megalencephaly and polymicrogyria have additional symptoms and signs consistent with the syndromes megalencephaly with capillary malformations (MCAP) and megalencephaly with polymicrogyria, polydactyly, and hydrocephalus (MPPH). The genes associated with polymicrogyria and megalencephaly include AKT3, PIK3CA, PIK3R2, and CCND2.[272,278-282] These genes reside in the same pathway as those involved in hemimegalencephaly, discussed in Chapter 5 (see Fig. 5.17). Thus, despite our MRI-based classification of hemimegalencephaly as a disorder of proliferation and polymicrogyria as a disorder of migration or later cortical organization, these disorders share a biological basis in AKT-mTOR pathway mutations that begin to have an effect very early in brain development. It might prove better to consider these disorders to arise during proliferation and to

have subsequent effects on migration and cortical organization. This conundrum of classification speaks to the eventual need for a biological pathway-based classification in the future, to which those who have provided the very useful MRI-based framework have alluded.[2]

Neuronal Heterotopia

Anatomical Abnormality. The least severe of the migrational disturbances, neuronal heterotopia, involves collections of nerve cells in the periventricular region or in subcortical white matter that are apparently arrested during radial migration from the subependymal germinative zones. Such collections are constant accompaniments of the more severe migrational disorders. At the other end of the spectrum, small collections of neurons in cerebral white matter are not unusual as incidental findings on MRI or at autopsy.

Two major varieties of cerebral neuronal heterotopia are recognized (Table 6.14). The heterotopic collections in the periventricular (subependymal) region occur near the site of origin of progenitor cells in the germinative ventricular and subventricular zones (Fig. 6.22A). In the cerebral white matter, heterotopia may occur in a subcortical laminar distribution or as focal or diffuse nodular collections in the white matter. Those in the periventricular region are usually nodular and are termed periventricular nodular heterotopia, periventricular heterotopia, or subependymal heterotopia (see later). Those in the cerebral white matter that occur as a diffuse laminar band below the cerebral cortex are termed band heterotopia or double cortex (see later discussion).

Timing and Clinical Aspects. The onset of neuronal heterotopia is presumed to be no later than the last weeks of major migrational events (i.e., no later than ≈20 weeks of gestation). The clinical features of disorders associated with cerebral neuronal heterotopia were clarified considerably by the advent of MRI scanning.[a] The clinical manifestations of nearly all cases of cerebral neuronal heterotopia begin after the neonatal period. Therefore a detailed discussion is not presented here; however, it should be noted that infants with mutations in FLNA may present with a diffuse lung disease mimicking bronchopulmonary dysplasia before neurological presentation.[313] The characteristic MRI pattern associated with FLNA mutations in females with periventricular heterotopia is shown in Fig. 6.22B. Periventricular heterotopia and band heterotopia (or double cortex) provide insights into mechanisms of neuronal migration and are described briefly. Focal or nodular cerebral white matter heterotopia exhibits clinical features related to the size and location of the heterotopia and are most likely to be encountered in the newborn as a feature of disorders

---

[a]References 34, 35, 72, 93, 166, and 283-312.

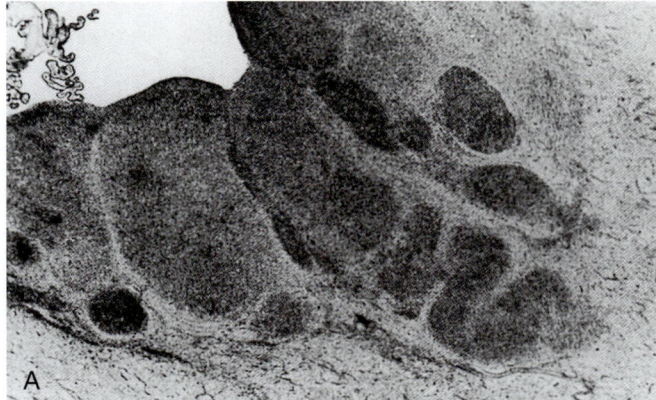
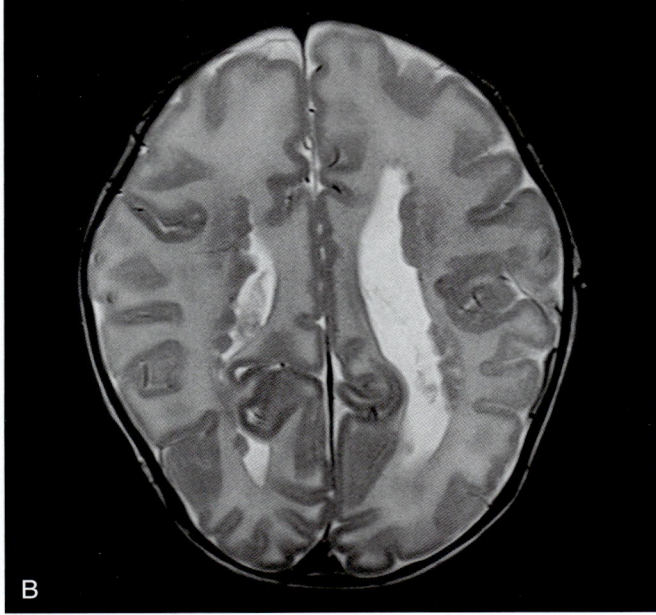

Figure 6.22 Periventricular heterotopia. (A) Nodular masses at the ventricular surface from the brain of a newborn (hematoxylin and eosin, ×12.7). (B) An axial T2-weighted magnetic resonance image of a girl with *FLNA* mutation-positive bilateral periventricular heterotopia. (A, With permission from Barth PG. Disorders of neuronal migration. *Can J Neurol Sci.* 1987;14:1–16.)

TABLE 6.15 Disorders Associated With Neuronal Heterotopia as the Major Manifestation of Migrational Disturbance[a]

Metabolic disorders: neonatal adrenoleukodystrophy, glutaric aciduria type II, nonketotic hyperglycinemia, Leigh disease, Menkes disease, GM_2 gangliosidosis, Hurler disease, Zellweger syndrome, bifunctional enzyme deficiency, carnitine palmitoyltransferase deficiency
Myotonic dystrophy
Neurocutaneous syndromes: neurofibromatosis, tuberous sclerosis, incontinentia pigmenti, Ito hypomelanosis, linear nevus sebaceus, encephalocraniocutaneous lipomatosis, Ehlers-Danlos syndrome
Multiple congenital anomaly syndromes: Smith-Lemli-Opitz, Potter, de Lange, orofacial-digital, Meckel-Gruber, Coffin-Siris
Chromosomal syndromes: trisomy 18, trisomy 13, deletion 4p, trisomy 21
Fetal toxic exposures: carbon monoxide, isotretinoic acid, ethanol, organic mercurial

[a]See text for references. This excludes disorders commonly associated with prominent gyral abnormalities (i.e., schizencephaly, lissencephaly, pachygyria, polymicrogyria). Uncommonly, some of the disorders listed here may also have migrational defects severe enough to have accompanying gyral abnormalities. The genetic disorders summarized in Table 6.15 are not repeated here.

neurons with the mutant gene active do not initiate migration and remain in the periventricular region, whereas neurons with the normal gene active migrate normally. In the autosomal recessive variety of the disorder, related to a mutation of the *ARGEF* gene (ADP ribosylation factor, GEF-2), critical for vesicle trafficking, the mechanism for failure of some neuroblasts to initiate migration is less clear. Importantly, in this disorder, a derangement of neuronal proliferation also occurs, and severe congenital microcephaly results.

In the *double cortex syndrome*, the diffuse laminar heterotopia appears to occur because, as a consequence of random X inactivation, one population of neurons contains only the abnormal gene and thus fails to migrate fully to the cortical plate (see Table 6.16). The characteristic locus of this laminar heterotopia beneath the cerebral cortex is at the site of the critical interface of the intermediate zone and subplate neurons (Fig. 6.23). Presumably the mutated doublecortin is unable to effect the critical interaction between the migrating neurons and the subplate neurons required to penetrate this region and form the cortical plate.[a] As discussed earlier, hemizygous male infants with the doublecortin defect develop lissencephaly, and the fundamental role of doublecortin involves microtubule dynein motor function.

Focal Cerebral Cortical Dysgenesis (Dysplasia)

With the advent of MRI scanning and removal of cortical anomalies for intractable epilepsy, focal disorders of the final stages of neuronal migration to cerebral cortex have been increasingly recognized. The lesions have been described as focal cerebral cortical *dysgeneses* or *dysplasias*.[34,35,287,328-366] The *anatomical descriptions* have not varied appreciably and consist of aberrations of gyral formation (polymicrogyric or pachygyric in

discussed elsewhere in this book.[a] This last diverse group is summarized in Table 6.15.

The two most common heterotopic lesions, periventricular heterotopia and band heterotopia of the double cortex syndrome, are of particular interest (Table 6.15).[b] The most common genetic forms of these two lesions are X-linked. An unusual autosomal recessive type of periventricular heterotopia (with microcephaly) is also recognized (see Table 6.16). In *X-linked periventricular heterotopia*, the anatomical defect is caused by a failure of *initiation of migration*.[41] The gene involved is *filamin*, which encodes filamin-1, an actin-binding protein expressed at high levels in the ventricular zone of the developing cerebrum and crucial for the initial cytoskeletal rearrangement for initiation of migration. Because of random X inactivation,

[a]References 93, 124, 236, 290-295, 297-300, and 314-318.
[b]References 34, 35, 72, 77, 146, 166, 185, 285, 287, 290-303, 307-312, and 319-327.

[a]References 30, 34, 35, 40, 41, 44, and 73.

TABLE 6.16   Major Genetic Syndromes With Cerebral Heterotopia[a]

TYPE OF HETEROTOPIA	SEIZURES	MAJOR COGNITIVE DEFICITS	MODE OF INHERITANCE	MANIFESTATION IN MALES	LOCATION OF GENE	GENE OR GENE PRODUCT
Periventricular heterotopia	Common	Uncommon	X-linked dominant	Lethal(?)[a]	Xq28	Filamin I
Periventricular heterotopia (and microcephaly)	Common	Common	Autosomal recessive	As in females	20q11	ARFGEF2
Double cortex (band or laminar)	Common	Common	X-linked dominant	Lissencephaly	Xq23	Doublecortin

[a]Occasional male patients exhibit periventricular heterotopia.

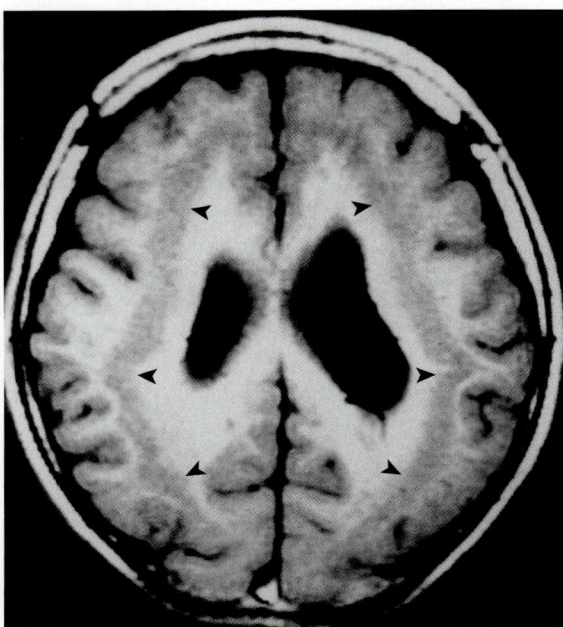

Figure 6.23 Magnetic resonance imaging (MRI), band heterotopia or double cortex syndrome. This T1-weighted MRI scan shows a symmetrical band of heterotopic subcortical gray matter *(arrowheads)* underlying a cerebral cortex with a normal convolutional pattern. (With permission from Miura K, Watanabe K, Maeda N, et al. Magnetic resonance imaging and positron emission tomography of band heterotopia. *Brain Dev.* 1993;15:288–290.)

TABLE 6.17   Major Clinical Syndromes Associated With Focal Cerebral Cortical Dysplasia[a]

SITE OF DYSGENESIS	CLINICAL SYNDROMES
Frontal, temporal, or parietal	Complex or simple partial seizures, hemiparesis (frontal lesions)
Temporal (hippocampus)	Neonatal (subtle) seizures, later multiple seizures, intellectual disability
Left frontotemporal	Developmental dyslexia
Frontal (rolandic)	Focal myoclonus, focal clonic seizures, hemiparesis
Bilateral perisylvian	Facial diplegia, dysarthria-dysphagia, generalized seizures, intellectual disability
Occipital	Congenital hemianopia

[a]See text for references.

appearance), a cerebrocortical plate without normal lamination, and heterotopic neurons in subcortical white matter. The lesions studied most often in specimens obtained at epilepsy surgery may exhibit impaired lamination with normal-appearing neurons or large, dysmorphic (misshapen) neurons. Large cells with immunocytochemical properties of neurons, glia, and multipotent neuroepithelial cells, termed *balloon cells*, may also be present. Those cases with dysmorphic large neurons, with or without the balloon cells, are categorized as *cortical dysplasia of Taylor.*[364] Because MRI has been the basis of the anatomical diagnosis in most cases, and the finding of a *thick* cortical plate with heterotopic gray matter is the prominent feature, it has not been clear whether all the lesions are related more to focal polymicrogyria than to pachygyria. Indeed, the descriptive term *macrogyria* is sometimes used to describe the MRI appearance.

Based on the cytological features, these lesions appear to represent not only disturbances of late neuronal migration but also abnormalities of proliferative and organizational events.

The *clinical syndromes* have been dominated by epilepsy (Table 6.17) and relate in considerable part to the topography of the lesions. The seizures usually begin after the neonatal period. However, in two large series, neonatal seizures occurred in approximately 35% of cases of Taylor-type FCD. Notably, among the 19 patients without balloon cells, approximately 60% had neonatal onset, whereas only 15% of the 15 patients with balloon cells exhibited neonatal seizures.[363,366]

The genetics of FCD now indicate that these disorders primarily affect proliferation, with secondary effects on migration. Thus FCD is covered in more depth in Chapter 5.

Agenesis of the Corpus Callosum, Abnormality of Septum Pellucidum, and Colpocephaly

Agenesis of the corpus callosum is a common accompaniment of the major disorders of neuronal migration, as noted in the previous discussions of the specific disorders. The reasons for the relationship are at least twofold. First, the timing of callosal formation and that of neuronal migration are nearly coincident (see discussion of midline prosencephalic development in Chapter 1). Second, the disturbance of neocortical development caused by the migrational failure is followed by a deficiency in corticocortical fibers destined for the callosum. The first of these reasons may explain the additional frequent accompaniment of neuronal migrational disorder with absence or hypoplasia of the septum pellucidum or persistently wide cavum of the septum pellucidum.

Colpocephaly—the disproportionate enlargement of trigones, occipital horns, and usually temporal horns of the lateral ventricles—is also a frequent accompaniment of neuronal migrational disorders. As mentioned previously (see the discussion of lissencephaly), the enlargement of the trigones and occipital horns stems from failure of development of the splenium of the corpus callosum and the calcarine fissure, and enlargement of the temporal horns results from failure of inversion of the hippocampus, normally provoked by full neocortical development.[124,163,367] Disproportionate enlargement of the trigone and occipital horns of the lateral ventricles can be observed in any destructive disorder with particular involvement of periventricular white matter, such as periventricular leukomalacia, other encephaloclastic processes, or any developmental disorder associated with impairment of myelination (see later discussion of myelination).[368-372] Because the ventricular dilation associated with these diverse processes is also often characterized as *colpocephaly*, the term has lost distinctive meaning.

KEY REFERENCES

1. Barkovich AJ, Kuzniecky RI, Jackson GD, et al. A developmental and genetic classification for malformations of cortical development. *Neurology.* 2005;65:1873-1887.
2. Barkovich AJ, Guerrini R, Kuzniecky RI, et al. A developmental and genetic classification for malformations of cortical development: update 2012. *Brain.* 2012;135:1348-1369.
3. Rakic P. Timing of major ontogenetic events in the visual cortex of the rhesus monkey. In: Buchwald NA, Brazier M, eds. *Brain Mechanisms in Mental Retardation.* New York: Academic Press; 1975:3.
4. Sidman RL, Rakic P. Neuronal migration, with special reference to developing human brain: a review. *Brain Res.* 1973;62:1-35.
7. Rakic P. Defects of neuronal migration and the pathogenesis of cortical malformations. *Prog Brain Res.* 1988;73:15-37.
8. Rakic P. Specification of cerebral cortical areas. *Science.* 1988;241:170-176.
9. Rakic P. Principles of neural cell migration. *Experientia.* 1990;46:882-891.
14. Austin CP, Cepko CL. Cellular migration patterns in the developing mouse cerebral cortex. *Development.* 1990;110:713-732.
15. Walsh C, Cepko CL. Cell lineage and cell migration in the developing cerebral cortex. *Experientia.* 1990;46:940-947.
17. Gray GE, Leber SM, Sanes JR. Migratory patterns of clonally related cells in the developing central nervous system. *Experientia.* 1990;46:929-940.
18. Luskin MB, Pearlman AL, Sanes JR. Cell lineage in the cerebral cortex of the mouse studied in vivo and in vitro with a recombinant retrovirus. *Neuron.* 1988;1:635-647.
22. O'Rourke NA, Dailey ME, Smith SJ, et al. Diverse migratory pathways in the developing cerebral cortex. *Science.* 1992;258:299-302.
25. Komuro H, Rakic P. Selective role of N-type calcium channels in neuronal migration. *Science.* 1992;257:806-809.
26. Komuro H, Rakic P. Modulation of neuronal migration by NMDA receptors. *Science.* 1993;260:95-97.
27. Rakic P. Radial versus tangential migration of neuronal clones in the developing cerebral cortex. *Proc Natl Acad Sci USA.* 1995;92:11323-11327.
28. Leber SM, Sanes JR. Migratory paths of neurons and glia in the embryonic chick spinal cord. *J Neurosci.* 1995;15:1236-1248.
29. O'Rourke NA, Chenn A, McConnell SK. Postmitotic neurons migrate tangentially in the cortical ventricular zone. *Development.* 1997;124:997-1005.
30. Gleeson JG, Walsh CA. New genetic insights into cerebral cortical development. In: Galaburda AM, Christen Y, eds. *Normal and Abnormal Development of Cortex.* Berlin: Springer-Verlag; 1997 [Ch 2].
31. Pearlman AL, Faust PL, Hatten ME, et al. New directions for neuronal migration. *Curr Opin Neurobiol.* 1998;8:45-54.
32. Komuro H, Rakic P. Distinct modes of neuronal migration in different domains of developing cerebellar cortex. *J Neurosci.* 1998;18:1478-1490.
33. Hatten ME. Central nervous system neuronal migration. *Annu Rev Neurosci.* 1999;22:511-539.
34. Walsh CA. Genetic malformations of the human cerebral cortex. *Neuron.* 1999;23:19-29.
35. Walsh CA. Genetics of neuronal migration in the cerebral cortex. *Ment Retard Dev Disabil Res Rev.* 2000;6:34-40.
36. Zecevic N, Rakic P. Development of layer I neurons in the primate cerebral cortex. *J Neurosci.* 2001;21:5607-5619.
37. Rakic P. Elusive radial glial cells: historical and evolutionary perspective. *Glia.* 2003;43:19-32.
39. Rakic P. Developmental and evolutionary adaptations of cortical radial glia. *Cereb Cortex.* 2003;13:541-549.
40. Kato M, Dobyns WB. Lissencephaly and the molecular basis of neuronal migration. *Hum Mol Genet.* 2003;12:R89-R96.
41. Bielas S, Higginbotham H, Koizumi H, et al. Cortical neuronal migration mutants suggest separate but intersecting pathways. *Annu Rev Cell Dev Biol.* 2004;20:593-618.
42. Kriegstein AR, Noctor SC. Patterns of neuronal migration in the embryonic cortex. *Trends Neurosci.* 2004;27:392-399.
44. Guerrini R, Filippi T. Neuronal migration disorders, genetics, and epileptogenesis. *J Child Neurol.* 2005;20:287-299.
45. Noctor SC, Martinez-Cerdeno V, Kriegstein AR. Contribution of intermediate progenitor cells to cortical histogenesis. *Arch Neurol.* 2007;64:639-642.
46. McManus MF, Golden JA. Neuronal migration in developmental disorders. *J Child Neurol.* 2005;20:280-286.
47. Letinic K, Zoncu R, Rakic P. Origin of GABAergic neurons in the human neocortex. *Nature.* 2002;417:645-649.
50. Rakic P. Mode of cell migration to the superficial layers of fetal monkey neocortex. *J Comp Neurol.* 1972;145:61-83.
52. Marin-Padilla M. Cajal-Retzius cells in the development of the neocortex. *Trends Neurosci.* 1998;21:64-71.
53. Reid CB, Tavazoie SF, Walsh CA. Clonal dispersion and evidence for asymmetric cell division in ferret cortex. *Development.* 1997;124:2441-2450.
54. Ware ML, Tavazoie SF, Reid CB, et al. Coexistence of widespread clones and large radial clones in early embryonic ferret cortex. *Cereb Cortex.* 1999;9:636-645.
58. Rakic P, Caviness VS. Cortical development: view from neurological mutants two decades later. *Neuron.* 1995;14:1101-1104.
70. Zheng C, Heintz N, Hatten ME. CNS gene encoding astrotactin, which supports neuronal migration along glial fibers. *Science.* 1996;272:417-419.
71. Gleeson JG, Allen KM, Fox JW, et al. Doublecortin, a brain-specific gene mutated in human x-linked lissencephaly and double cortex syndrome, encodes a putative signaling protein. *Cell.* 1998;92:63-72.
72. Gleeson JG, Minnerath SR, Fox JW, et al. Characterization of mutations in the gene doublecortin in patients with double cortex syndrome. *Ann Neurol.* 1999;45:146-153.
73. Gleeson JG, Lin PT, Flanagan L, et al. Doublecortin is a microtubule-associated protein and is expressed widely by migrating neurons. *Neuron.* 1999;23:257-271.
74. Francis F, Koulakoff A, Boucher D, et al. Doublecortin is a developmentally regulated, microtubule-associated protein expressed in migrating and differentiating neurons. *Neuron.* 1999;23:247-256.
76. Liu JS, Schubert CR, Fu X, et al. Molecular basis for specific regulation of neuronal kinesin-3 motors by doublecortin family proteins. *Mol Cell.* 2012;47:707-721.
77. Fox JW, Lamperti ED, Eksioglu YZ, et al. Mutations in filamin 1 prevent migration of cerebral cortical neurons in human periventricular heterotopia. *Neuron.* 1999;21:1315-1325.

81. Behar TN, Scott CA, Greene CL, et al. Glutamate acting at NMDA receptors stimulates embryonic cortical neuronal migration. *J Neurosci*. 1999;19:4449-4461.

82. Kumada T, Komuro H. Completion of neuronal migration regulated by loss of Ca2+ transients. *Proc Natl Acad Sci U S A*. 2004;101:8479-8484.

87. Welker W. Why does cerebral cortex fissure and fold? A review of determinants of gyri and sulci. In: Jones EG, Peters A, eds. *Cerebral Cortex*. Vol. 8B. New York: Plenum Publishing Corp.; 1990:3-136.

89. Richman DP, Stewart RM, Hutchinson JW. Mechanical model of brain convolutional development. *Science*. 1975;189:18.

90. Van Essen DC. A tension-based theory of morphogenesis and compact wiring in the central nervous system. *Nature*. 1997;385:313-318.

93. Barth PG. Disorders of neuronal migration. *Can J Neurol Sci*. 1987;14:1-16.

96. Denis D, Chateil J-F, Brun M, et al. Schizencephaly: clinical and imaging features in 30 infantile cases. *Brain Dev*. 2000;22:475-483.

97. Granata T, Freri E, Caccia C, et al. Schizencephaly: clinical spectrum, epilepsy, and pathogenesis. *J Child Neurol*. 2005;20:313-318.

105. Bonnemann GC, Meinecke P. Bilateral porencephaly, cerebellar hypoplasia and internal malformations: two siblings representing a probably new autosomal recessive entity. *Am J Med Genet*. 1996;63:428-433.

109. Barkovich AJ, Kjos BO. Schizencephaly: correlation of clinical findings with MR characteristics. *AJNR Am J Neuroradiol*. 1992;13:85-94.

113. Brunelli S, Faiella A, Capra V. Germline mutations in the homeobox gene EMX2 in patients with severe schizencephaly. *Nat Genet*. 1996;12:94-96.

117. Mellado C, Poduri A, Gleason D, et al. Candidate gene sequencing of LHX2, HESX1, and SOX2 in a large schizencephaly cohort. *Am J Med Genet A*. 2010;152A:2736-2742.

118. Yu TW, Mochida GH, Tischfield DJ, et al. Mutations in WDR62, encoding a centrosome-associated protein, cause microcephaly with simplified gyri and abnormal cortical architecture. *Nat Genet*. 2010;42:1015-1020.

119. Yoneda Y, Haginoya K, Kato M, et al. Phenotypic spectrum of COL4A1 mutations: porencephaly to schizencephaly. *Ann Neurol*. 2013;73:48-57.

122. Barkovich AJ, Chuang SH, Norman D. MR of neuronal migration anomalies. *AJNR Am J Neuroradiol*. 1988;8:1009-1017.

131. Dieker H, Edwards RH, Zurhein G. The lissencephaly syndrome. *Birth Defects*. 1969;5:53.

134. Dobyns WB, Stratton RF, Greenberg F. Syndromes with lissencephaly. I: Miller-Dieker and Norman-Roberts syndromes and isolated lissencephaly. *Am J Med Genet*. 1984;18:509-526.

136. Hanaway J, Lee SI, Netsky NG. Pachygyria: relation of findings to modern embryologic concepts. *Neurology*. 1968;18:791-799.

141. Dobyns WB, Andermann E, Andermann F, et al. X-linked malformations of neuronal migration. *Neurology*. 1996;47:331-339.

142. Barkovich AJ, Kuznecky RI, Dopbyns WB, et al. A classification scheme for malformations of cortical development. *Neuropediatrics*. 1996;27:59-63.

145. Ferrie CD, Jackson GD, Giannakodimos S, et al. Posterior agyria-pachygyria with polymicrogyria: evidence for an inherited neuronal migration disorder. *Neurology*. 1995;45:150-153.

146. Fox JW, Walsh CA. Neurogenetics '99—periventricular heterotopia and the genetics of neuronal migration in the cerebral cortex. *J Hum Genet*. 1999;65:19-24.

147. Kato M, Takizawa N, Yamada S, et al. Diffuse pachygria with cerebellar hypoplasia: a milder form of microlissencephaly or a new genetic syndrome? *Ann Neurol*. 1999;46:660-663.

152. Kitamura K, Yanazawa M, Sugiyama N, et al. Mutation of ARX causes abnormal development of forebrain and testes in mice and X-linked lissencephaly with abnormal genitalia in humans. *Nat Genet*. 2002;32:359-369.

154. Bahi-Buisson N, Poirier K, Fourniol F, et al. The wide spectrum of tubulinopathies: what are the key features for the diagnosis? *Brain*. 2014;137:1676-1700.

160. Ledbetter SA, Kuwano A, Dobyns WB, et al. Microdeletions of chromosome 17p13 as a cause of isolated lissencephaly. *Am J Hum Genet*. 1992;50:182-189.

163. Barkovich AJ, Koch TK, Carrol CL. The spectrum of lissencephaly: report of ten patients analyzed by magnetic resonance imaging. *Ann Neurol*. 1991;30:139-146.

164. Dobyns WB. The neurogenetics of lissencephaly. *Neurol Clin*. 1989;7:89-105.

165. Dobyns WB, Elias ER, Newlin AC, et al. Causal heterogeneity in isolated lissencephaly. *Neurology*. 1992;42:1375-1388.

166. Palmini A, Andermann F, de Grissac H, et al. Stages and patterns of centrifugal arrest of diffuse neuronal migration disorders. *Dev Med Child Neurol*. 1993;35:331-339.

169. Pilz DT, Matsumoto N, Minnerath S, et al. LIS1 and XLIS (DCX) mutations cause most classical lissencephaly, but different patterns of malformation. *Hum Mol Genet*. 1998;7:2029-2037.

170. Dobyns WB, Curry CJR, Hoyme HE, et al. Clinical and molecular diagnosis of Miller-Dieker syndrome. *Am J Hum Genet*. 1991; 48:584-594.

171. Toyo-oka K, Shionoya A, Gambello MJ, et al. 14-3-3e is important for neuronal migration by binding to NUDEL: a molecular explanation for Miller-Dieker syndrome. *Nat Genet*. 2003;34:274-285.

173. Bonneau D, Toutain A, Laquerriere A, et al. X-lined lissencephaly with absent corpus callosum and ambiguous genitalia (XLAG): clinical, magnetic resonance imaging, and neuropathological findings. *Ann Neurol*. 2002;51:340-349.

174. Uyanik G, Aigner L, Martin P, et al. ARX mutations in X-linked lissencephaly with abnormal genitalia. *Neurology*. 2003;61:232-235.

176. Kato M, Das S, Petras K, et al. Mutations of ARX are associated with striking pleiotropy and consistent genotype-phenotype correlation. *Hum Mutat*. 2004;23:147-159.

177. Kato M, Dobyns WB. X-linked lissencephaly with abnormal genitalia as a tangential migration disorder causing intractable epilepsy: proposal for a new term, "Interneuronopathy." *J Child Neurol*. 2005;20:392-397.

178. Ross ME, Swanson K, Dobyns WB. Lissencephaly with cerebellar hypoplasia (LCH): a heterogeneous group of cortical malformations. *Neuropediatrics*. 2001;32:256-263.

180. Chang BS, Duzcan F, Kim S, et al. The role of RELN in lissencephaly and neuropsychiatric disease. *Am J Med Genet B Neuropsychiatr Genet*. 2007;144(1):58-63.

181. Bahi-Buisson N, Cavallin M. Tubulinopathies Overview. In: Pagon RA, Adam MP, Ardinger HH, et al., eds. *GeneReviews(R)*. Seattle, WA: University of Washington; 1993.

182. Koizumi H, Tanaka T, Gleeson JG. Doublecortin-like kinase functions with doublecortin to mediate fiber tract decussation and neuronal migration. *Neuron*. 2006;49:55-66.

183. Elias RC, Galera MF, Schnabel B, et al. Deletion of 17p13 and LIS1 gene mutation in isolated lissencephaly sequence. *Pediatr Neurol*. 2006;35:42-46.

184. Sheen VL, Ferland RJ, Harney M, et al. Impaired proliferation and migration in human Miller-Dieker neural precursors. *Ann Neurol*. 2006;60:137-144.

185. Gleeson JG, Luo RF, Grant PE, et al. Genetic and neuroradiological heterogeneity of double cortex syndrome. *Ann Neurol*. 2000;47:265-269.

186. LoTurco J. Doublecortin and a tale of two serines. *Neuron*. 2004;41:175-177.

187. Leventer RJ. Genotype-phenotype correlation in lissencephaly and subcortical band heterotopia: the key questions answered. *J Child Neurol*. 2005;20:307-312.

192. Jamuar SS, Lam AT, Kircher M, et al. Somatic mutations in cerebral cortical malformations. *N Engl J Med*. 2014;371:733-743.

193. Dobyns WB, Pagon RA, Armstrong D, et al. Diagnostic criteria for Walker-Warburg syndrome. *Am J Med Genet*. 1989;32:195-210.

196. Bordarier C, Aicardi J, Goutieres F. Congenital hydrocephalus and eye abnormalities with severe developmental brain defects: Warburg's syndrome. *Ann Neurol*. 1984;16:60-65.

198. Haltia M, Leivo I, Somer H, et al. Muscle-eye-brain disease: a neuropathological study. *Ann Neurol*. 1997;41:173-180.

201. Ross ME. Neurobiology: full circle to cobbled brain. *Nature*. 2002;418:376-377.

204. Vervoort VS, Holden KR, Ukadike KC, et al. POMGnT1 gene alterations in a family with neurological abnormalities. *Ann Neurol*. 2004;56:143-148.

208. Beltran-Valero de Bernabe D, Currier S, Steinbrecher A, et al. Mutations in the O-mannosyltransferase gene POMT1 give

rise to the severe neuronal migration disorder Walker-Warburg syndrome. *Am J Hum Genet.* 2002;71:1033-1043.

209. de Bernabe DB, van Bokhoven H, van Beusekom E, et al. A homozygous nonsense mutation in the fukutin gene causes a Walker-Warburg syndrome phenotype. *J Med Genet.* 2003;40:845-848.

211. Manzini MC, Gleason D, Chang BS, et al. Ethnically diverse causes of Walker-Warburg syndrome (WWS): FCMD mutations are a more common cause of WWS outside of the Middle East. *Hum Mutat.* 2008;29:E231-E241.

231. du Plessis AJ, Kaufmann WE, William MD, et al. Intrauterine-onset myoclonic encephalopathy associated with cerebral cortical dysgenesis. *J Child Neurol.* 1993;8:164-170.

232. Guerrini R, Dubeau F, Dulac O, et al. Bilateral parasagittal parieto-occipital polymicrogyria and epilepsy. *Ann Neurol.* 1997;41:65-73.

235. Kammoun F, Tanguy A, BoesplugTanguy O, et al. Club feet with congenital perisylvian polymicrogyria possibly due to bifocal ischemic damage of the neuraxis in utero. *Am J Med Genet Part A.* 2004;126A:191-196.

243. Volpe JJ, Adams RD. Cerebro-hepato-renal syndrome of Zellweger: An inherited disorder of neuronal migration. *Acta Neuropathol.* 1972;20:175-198.

246. Moser AE, Singh I, Brown FR III, et al. The cerebrohepatorenal (Zellweger) syndrome. Increased levels and impaired degradation of very-long-chain fatty acids and their use in prenatal diagnosis. *N Engl J Med.* 1984;310:1141-1146.

251. Kaufmann WE, Theda C, Naidu S, et al. Neuronal migration abnormality in peroxisomal bifunctional enzyme defect. *Ann Neurol.* 1996;39:268-271.

253. Dixon-Salazar T, Silhavy JL, Marsh SE, et al. Mutations in the AHI1 gene, encoding Jouberin, cause Joubert syndrome with cortical polymicrogyria. *Am J Hum Genet.* 2004;75:979-987.

255. Wieck G, Leventer RJ, Squier WM, et al. Periventricular nodular heterotopia with overlying polymicrogyria. *Brain.* 2005;128:2811-2821.

256. Kuzniecky R, Andermann F, Guerrine R, et al. The epileptic spectrum in the congenital bilateral perisylvian syndrome. *Neurology.* 1994;44:379-385.

258. Gropman AL, Barkovich AJ, Vezina LG, et al. Pediatric congenital bilateral perisylvian syndrome: clinical and MRI features in 12 patients. *Neuropediatrics.* 1997;28:198-203.

260. Barkovich AJ, Hevner R, Guerrini R. Syndromes of bilateral symmetrical polymicrogyria. *AJNR Am J Neuroradiol.* 1999;20:1814-1821.

261. Guerreiro MM, Andermann E, Guerrini R, et al. Familial perisylvian polymicrogyria: a new familial syndrome of cortical maldevelopment. *Ann Neurol.* 2000;48:39-48.

263. Chang BS, Piao X, Bodell A, et al. Bilateral frontoparietal polymicrogyria: clinical and radiological features in 10 families with linkage to chromosome 16. *Ann Neurol.* 2003;53:596-606.

264. Piao X, Basel-Vanagaite L, Straussberg R, et al. An autosomal recessive form of bilateral frontoparietal polymicrogyria maps to chromosome 16q12.2-21. *Am J Hum Genet.* 2002;70:1028-1033.

265. Piao X, Hill RS, Bodell A, et al. G protein-coupled receptor-dependent development of human frontal cortex. *Science.* 2004;303:2033-2036.

266. Chang BS, Piao X, Giannini C, et al. Bilateral generalized polymicrogyria (BGP): A distinct syndrome of cortical malformation. *Neurology.* 2004;62:1722-1728.

270. Piao X, Chang BS, Bodell A, et al. Genotype-phenotype analysis of human frontoparietal polymicrogyria syndromes. *Ann Neurol.* 2005;58:680-687.

271. Baulac S, Lenk GM, Dufresnois B, et al. Role of the phosphoinositide phosphatase FIG4 gene in familial epilepsy with polymicrogyria. *Neurology.* 2014;82:1068-1071.

272. Mirzaa GM, Riviere JB, Dobyns WB. Megalencephaly syndromes and activating mutations in the PI3K-AKT pathway: MPPH and MCAP. *Am J Med Genet C Semin Med Genet.* 2013;163C:122-130.

277. Poirier K, Lebrun N, Broix L, et al. Mutations in TUBG1, DYNC1H1, KIF5C and KIF2A cause malformations of cortical development and microcephaly. *Nat Genet.* 2013;45:639-647.

279. Riviere JB, Mirzaa GM, O'Roak BJ, et al. De novo germline and postzygotic mutations in AKT3, PIK3R2 and PIK3CA cause a spectrum of related megalencephaly syndromes. *Nat Genet.* 2012;44:934-940.

280. Mirzaa GM, Parry DA, Fry AE, et al. De novo CCND2 mutations leading to stabilization of cyclin D2 cause megalencephaly-polymicrogyria-polydactyly-hydrocephalus syndrome. *Nat Genet.* 2014;46:510-515.

281. Mirzaa GM, Conway RL, Gripp KW, et al. Megalencephaly-capillary malformation (MCAP) and megalencephaly-polydactyly-polymicrogyria-hydrocephalus (MPPH) syndromes: two closely related disorders of brain overgrowth and abnormal brain and body morphogenesis. *Am J Med Genet A.* 2012;158A:269-291.

282. Mirzaa GM, Poduri A. Megalencephaly and hemimegalencephaly: breakthroughs in molecular etiology. *Am J Med Genet C Semin Med Genet.* 2014;166:156-172.

289. Huttenlocher PR. Taravath S, Mojtahebi S. Periventricular heterotopia and epilepsy. *Neurology.* 1994;44:51-55.

294. Eksioglu YZ, Scheffer IE, Cardenas P, et al. Periventricular heterotopia: an x-linked dominant epilepsy locus causing aberrant cerebral cortical development. *Neuron.* 1996;16:77-87.

306. Barkovich AJ, Kuzniecky RI. Gray matter heterotopia. *Neurology.* 2000;55:1603-1608.

307. Sheen VL, Dixon PH, Fox JW, et al. Mutations in the X-linked filamin 1 gene cause periventricular nodular heterotopia in males as well as in females. *Hum Mol Genet.* 2001;10:1775-1783.

308. Guerrini R, Mei D, Sisodiya S, et al. Germline and mosaic mutations of FLN1 in men with periventricular heterotopia. *Neurology.* 2004;63:51-56.

309. Sheen VL, Jansen A, Chen MH, et al. Filamin A mutations cause periventricular heterotopia with Ehlers-Danlos syndrome. *Neurology.* 2005;64:254-262.

310. Chang BS, Ly J, Appignani B, et al. Reading impairment in the neuronal migration disorder of periventricular nodular heterotopia. *Neurology.* 2005;64:799-803.

312. Parrini E, Ramazzotti A, Dobyns WB, et al. Periventricular heterotopia: phenotypic heterogeneity and correlation with Filamin A mutations. *Brain.* 2006;129:1892-1906.

325. Sheen VL, Topcu M, Berkovic SF, et al. Autosomal recessive form of periventricular heterotopia. *Neurology.* 2003;60:1108-1112.

326. Sheen VL, Ganesh VS, Topcu M, et al. Mutations in ARFGEF2 implicate vesicle trafficking in neural progenitor proliferation and migration in the human cerebral cortex. *Nat Genet.* 2004;36:69-76.

329. Kuzniecky R, Garcia JH, Faught E, et al. Cortical dysplasia in temporal lobe epilepsy: magnetic resonance imaging correlations. *Ann Neurol.* 1991;29:293-298.

330. Palmini A, Andermann F, Olivier A, et al. Focal neuronal migration disorders and intractable partial epilepsy: results of surgical treatment. *Ann Neurol.* 1991;30:750-757.

331. Palmini A, Andermann F, Olivier A, et al. Focal neuronal migration disorders and intractable partial epilepsy: a study of 30 patients. *Ann Neurol.* 1991;30:741-749.

335. Kuzniecky R, Andermann F, Tampieri D, et al. Bilateral central macrogyria: epilepsy, pseudobulbar palsy, and mental retardation—a recognizable neuronal migration disorder. *Ann Neurol.* 1989;25:547-554.

336. Galaburda AM, Sherman GF, Rosen GD, et al. Developmental dyslexia: four consecutive patients with cortical anomalies. *Ann Neurol.* 1985;18:222-233.

338. Kaufmann WE, Galaburda AM. Cerebrocortical microdysgenesis in neurologically normal subjects: a histopathologic study. *Neurology.* 1989;39:238-244.

343. Berry-Kravis E, Huttenlocher PR, Wollmann RL. Isolated congenital malformation of hippocampal formation as a cause of intractable neonatal seizures [abstract]. *Ann Neurol.* 1989;26:485.

352. Kuzniecky R, Andermann F, Guerrini R. Congenital bilateral perisylvian syndrome—study of 31 patients. *Lancet.* 1993;341:608-612.

355. Kuzniecky R, Morawetz R, Faught E, et al. Frontal and central lobe focal dysplasia: clinical, EEG and imaging features. *Dev Med Child Neurol.* 1995;37:159-166.

356. Barkovich AJ, Kuzniecky RI, Bollen AW, et al. Focal transmantle dysplasia: a specific malformation of cortical development. *Neurology.* 1997;49:1148-1152.

358. Barkovich AJ, Peacock W. Sublobar dysplasia: a new malformation of cortical development. *Neurology.* 1998;50:1383-1387.

359. Spreafico R, Battaglia G, Arcelli P, et al. Cortical dysplasia. An immunocytochemical study of three patients. *Neurology*. 1998; 50:27-36.

361. Casanova MF, Buxhoeveden DP, Cohen M, et al. Minicolumnar pathology in dyslexia. *Ann Neurol*. 2002;52:108-110.

363. Mackay MT, Becker LE, Chuang SH, et al. Malformations of cortical development with balloon cells. Clinical and radiologic correlates. *Neurology*. 2003;60:580-587.

364. Palmini A, Najm I, Avanzini G, et al. Terminology and classification of the cortical dysplasias. *Neurology*. 2004;62:S2-S8.

366. Lawson JA, Birchansky S, Pacheco E, et al. Distinct clinicopathologic subtypes of cortical dysplasia of Taylor. *Neurology*. 2005;64: 55-61.

Full references for this chapter can be found on www.expertconsult .com.

Organizational Events

Hannah C. Kinney ◆ Joseph J. Volpe

NORMAL DEVELOPMENT

Organizational events occur in a peak time period from approximately the fifth month of gestation to several years after birth. However, these complex processes may continue for many more years in human cerebrum. The major developmental features include (1) establishment and differentiation of the subplate neurons; (2) attainment of proper alignment, orientation, and layering (lamination) of cortical neurons; (3) gyral development; (4) elaboration of dendritic and axonal ramifications; (5) establishment of synaptic contacts; (6) cell death and selective elimination of neuronal processes and synapses; and (7) proliferation and differentiation of glia (Table 7.1). These events are of particular importance, because they establish the elaborate circuitry that distinguishes the human brain, and they set the stage for the final developmental event, myelination.

Subplate Neurons

The importance of the subplate neurons in cerebral organizational events was defined by an elegant series of studies both in experimental animals and human brain.[1-22] Cells destined to be subplate neurons are generated in the germinative zones and migrate both radially and tangentially to the primitive marginal zone at approximately 7 weeks of gestation *before* generation and migration of neurons of the cortical plate (Fig. 7.1 and Table 7.2). Initially, these cells are part of the preplate that is split by approximately 10 weeks of gestation by the developing cortical plate into the subplate neurons below and the Cajal-Retzius neurons of the marginal zone above. (The cortical plate neurons give rise to layers II through VI of the cerebral cortex.) Thus the subplate zone contains some of the earliest born neurons of the cerebral cortex, which during this developmental period are more mature than the overlying cortical plate. The subplate neurons rapidly exhibit morphological differentiation and express a variety of receptors for neurotransmitters (gamma-aminobutyric acid [GABA], excitatory amino acids), neuropeptides, and growth factors (nerve growth factor, neuropeptide gamma, somatostatin, calbindin).

The subplate neurons elaborate a dendritic arbor with spines, receive synaptic inputs from ascending afferents from thalamus and distant cortical sites, and extend axonal collaterals to overlying cerebral cortex and to other cortical and subcortical sites (thalamus, other cortical regions, corpus callosum). In addition to the subplate *neurons*, the subplate *zone* contains other tissue components, such as radial glial processes, radially

and tangentially migrating neurons, early developing astrocytes, microglia, and oligodendrocyte precursors, that are also found in other fetal compartments. Yet, this zone is distinguished by an extensive extracellular space that is filled with hydrophilic extracellular matrix (ECM) and heterogeneous contingents of *waiting* cortical afferents and transient synapses.[23] This hydrophilic feature underlies the visibility of the zone in T2-weighted magnetic resonance imaging (MRI) scans of the human fetus from approximately 18 to 26 weeks of gestation (Fig. 7.2).[23,24]

The subplate zone is also molecularly distinct, as determined by the identification of subplate-enriched genes by transcriptome profiling of different fetal layers.[25] Gene expression profiling of the subplate zone in midgestation fetal human brains indicates that the human subplate is functionally enriched for synaptic plasticity[25] and generally shows signs of more advanced maturity compared with the overlying cortical plate. Thus some of the molecular hallmarks of the subplate zone during early development primarily relate to cell maturity, and as subplate cells form, they extend axons and receive synaptic inputs earlier than the cortical plate.[25] Importantly, the subplate is specifically rich in chondroitin sulfate proteoglycans (CSPGs), and the subplate transcriptome is enriched for genes involved in the production of ECM and proteoglycans.[25] CSPGs are known to interact with laminin, fibronectin, tenascin, and collagen, and their differential distribution supports a role in axonal pathfinding and cell migration.

The *functions of the subplate neurons* now appear to be particularly far-reaching (see Table 7.2).[a] Thus they provide a site for synaptic contact for axons ascending from thalamus and other cortical sites, termed *waiting* thalamocortical and corticocortical afferents because their neuronal targets in the cortical plate have not yet arrived or differentiated. These afferents presumably would undergo degeneration if they did not have the subplate neurons as transient targets. Moreover, the subplate neurons have been shown to establish a functional synaptic link between these waiting afferents and their cortical targets. This link could exert a trophic influence on the cortical neuronal targets by the release of neuropeptides or excitatory amino acid neurotransmitter by the subplate axon terminals. There are additional genes with subplate-restricted expression in the cortex that encode secreted proteins, including *Serpini1* (which encodes neuroserpin) and neuronal pentraxin 1 (*Nptx1*). These two proteins are neural specific, with proposed roles

---

[a]References 1-9, 13-15, 17-19, 22, 23, 26, and 27.

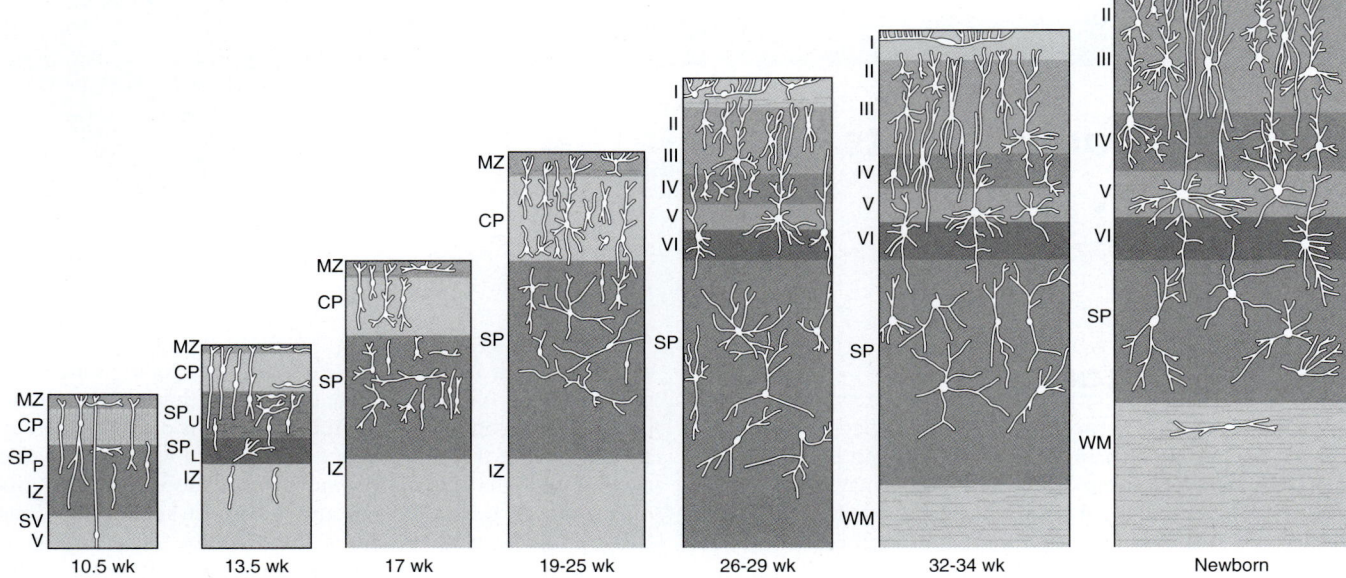

Figure 7.1 Schematic summary of development of human prefrontal cortex. At the earliest age studied (10.5 weeks), the preplate zone has been split by the early-arriving neurons of the cortical plate into neurons of the marginal zone *(MZ)* above and of the subplate zone below. Note the exuberant neuronal development of the subplate zone into the third trimester of gestation. *CP*, Cortical plate; *F*, frontal; *IZ*, intermediate zone; *SP_L*, subplate zone (lower); *SP_P*, subplate-preplate zone; *SP_U*, subplate zone (upper); *SV*, subventricular zone; *V*, ventricular zone; *WM*, white matter. (From Mrzljak L, Uylings HBM, Kostovic I, et al. Prenatal development of neurons in the human prefrontal cortex: I. A qualitative Golgi study. *J Comp Neurol.* 1988;271:355.)

TABLE 7.1   Organization

Peak time period
5 months' gestation—years postnatal
Major events
Subplate neurons—establishment and differentiation
Lamination—alignment, orientation, and layering of cortical plate neurons
Neurite outgrowth—dendritic and axonal ramifications
Synaptogenesis
Cell death and selective elimination of neuronal processes and of synapses
Glial proliferation and differentiation

TABLE 7.2   Importance of Subplate Neurons in Development of Cerebral Cortex

Natural history
SPNs are generated and migrate to beneath the pial surface as part of the preplate *before* generation and migration of neurons of the cortical plate
Early arriving cortical plate neurons split the preplate into the overlying marginal zone and the subplate
SPNs rapidly exhibit morphological differentiation and transiently express a variety of receptors for neurotransmitters and growth factors
SPNs elaborate a dendritic tree, receive synaptic inputs, and extend axonal projections to cortical and subcortical sites
Zone of SPNs is most prominent between approximately 22 and 34 weeks of gestation
About 90% of SPNs undergo programmed cell death postnatally
Functions
Site of synaptic contact for *waiting* thalamocortical and corticocortical afferents before formation of cortical plate
Functional link between *waiting* afferents and cortical targets
Axonal guidance into cerebral cortex for ascending afferents
Involvement in cerebral cortical organization and synaptic development
Pioneering axonal guidance for projections from cortex to subcortical targets

SPNs, Subplate neurons.

---

in synaptic function or maturation. Thus the subplate may additionally influence cortical circuit formation through a transient secretory function. A third function appears to be the guidance by subplate axons entering cerebral cortex of the ascending axons to their targets. Indeed, if the subplate neurons are eliminated, thalamocortical afferents destined for the overlying cortex fail to move superiorly into the cortex at the appropriate site and continue to grow aimlessly in the subcortical region. A fourth function of subplate neurons is involvement in cerebral cortical organization; for example, ocular dominance columns in visual cortex fail to develop if underlying subplate neurons are eliminated during development. Related to this role is the importance for subplate neurons in cortical synaptic development and function. A fifth function appears to be mediated by the descending axon collaterals from the subplate neurons; these collaterals appear to *pioneer* or guide

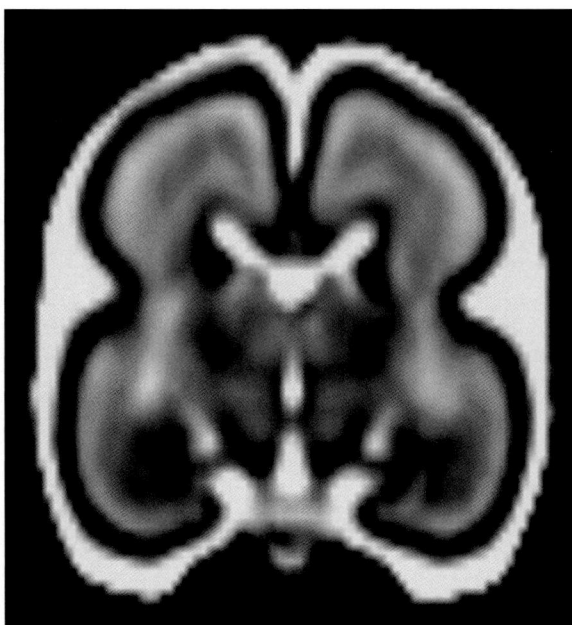

Figure 7.2 Reconstructed T2-weighted MRI image obtained in vivo from a 25-week fetus. Note the high signal intensity in the region of the subplate zone, consistent with its hydrophilic nature. (Courtesy Dr. Caitlin Rollins and Computational Radiology Laboratory, Boston Children's Hospital.)

the initial projections from cerebral cortex toward subcortical targets (e.g., thalamus, corpus callosum, and other cortical sites).

Concomitant studies of subplate neurons of developing *human* cerebral cortex provide a crucial link with the experimental studies (see Fig. 7.3).[13,15-17,19,23,28-31] The subplate neuron layer in human cortex reaches a peak between approximately 24 and 32 weeks of gestation. At this peak time, the width of the subplate zone is approximately four times that of the cortical plate. Programmed cell death (apoptosis) of this layer appears to begin generally late in the third trimester, and approximately 90% of subplate neurons have disappeared after approximately the sixth month of postnatal life.[31] Slightly different time courses for peak development and regression of the subplate neurons exist for somatosensory and visual cortices. In the subplate dissolution stage, which occurs in humans at greater than 35 postconceptional weeks, subplate neurons decline in number and the volume of the subplate zone decreases. The reduction in volume reflects primarily a decrease in extracellular space and fewer axon bundles within the subplate zone. A distinct subplate zone is no longer identifiable by about 6 months post term in humans, but large neurons embedded in white matter are thought to be the remaining subplate cells, which are referred to as interstitial white matter neurons.[31,32]

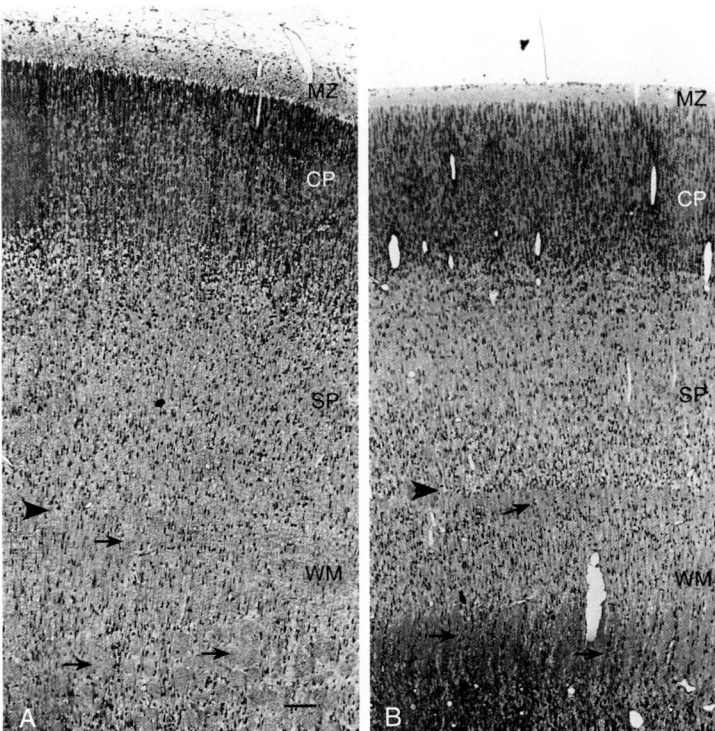

Figure 7.3 Cytoarchitectonics of the subplate zone in the visual area. Shown are A, an 18-week old human and, B, an E78 monkey fetus displayed in plastic 1-μm-thick sections. The subplate zone *(SP)* is characterized by low cell density and presence of mature neurons. The border between the subplate zone and the white matter *(WM)* is relatively sharp because of the presence of well-delineated fiber bundles *(arrows)* in the white matter. External limit of fibers is marked by arrowhead. Note remarkable similarities between the lamination pattern and the cortical plate (CP)-subplate thickness ratio in man and monkey. Bar = 100 μm applies to both illustrations. *MZ,* Marginal zone. (From Kostovic I, Rakic P. Developmental history of the transient subplate zone in the visual and somatosensory cortex of the macaque monkey and human brain. *J Comp Neurol.* 1990;297:441.)

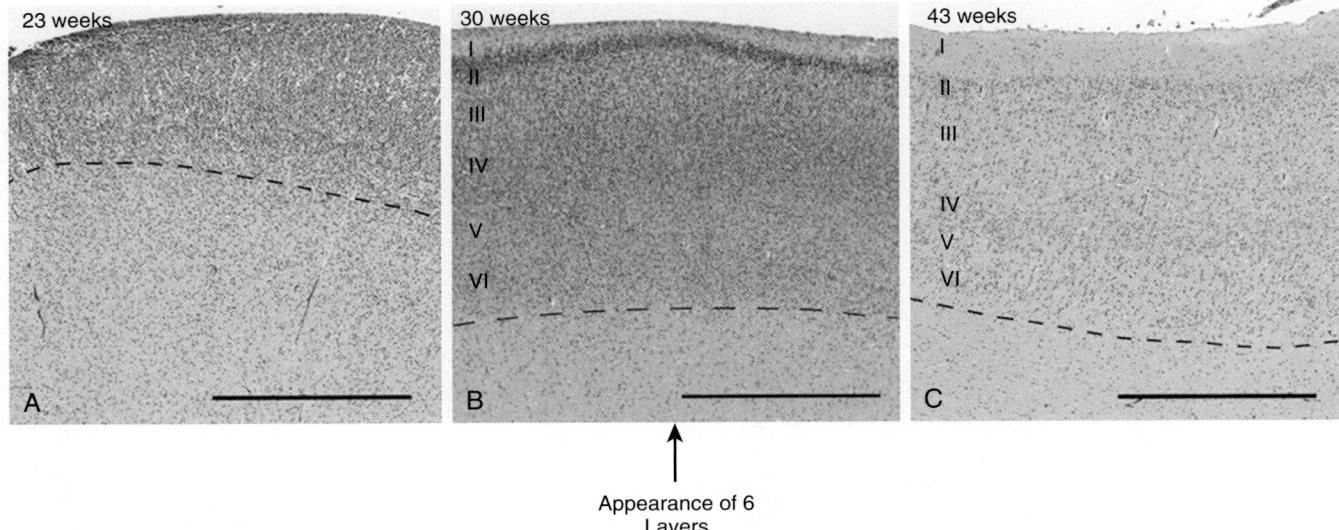

Figure 7.4 Development of human cortical plate in the frontal association cortex. See text for details. The scale bar is one millimeter. (From Andiman SE, et al. The cerebral cortex overlying periventricular leukomalacia: analysis of pyramidal neurons. *Brain Pathol.* 2010;20:803–814, with permission.)

Lamination

Attainment of the proper alignment, orientation, and layering of cortical neurons, defined as lamination, occurs during and following neuronal migration (see Table 7.1). These events are among the earliest in cortical organization.[22,33-36] The microcircuitry of the cerebral cortex underlying cognitive processing is dependent on precise interrelationships between variable numbers of excitatory pyramidal neurons and inhibitory nonpyramidal (granular) neurons in cortical modules. The cortical layers are specialized compartments that contain neurons with unique properties that underlie specific roles in neural circuitry. The normal cerebral cortex is composed of two main classes of neurons: (1) pyramidal neurons, which comprise 75% to 85% of total cortical neurons, are glutamatergic, and project outside the cortex; and (2) nonpyramidal neurons (interneurons), which comprise 15% to 25% of cortical neurons, are GABAergic and project within the cortical layers.[37]

The neocortex begins to transform from an undifferentiated cortical plate to a highly specialized structure at around 30 gestational weeks (Fig. 7.4).[38] At this age, the cortical plate becomes composed of six layers in which each layer is characterized by a specific composite of pyramidal and nonpyramidal neurons. Dramatic changes in lamination, laminar thickness, and pyramidal and nonpyramidal cell differentiation and density in the last half of gestation are consistent with neuroimaging findings of marked increases in cortical thickness and surface area over this same time period (see later). Pyramidal neurons are known to originate from radial progenitors (radial glial cells) in the subventricular zone (SVZ); these early precursors produce neurons destined particularly for the deeper cortical layers and reach the cortex by radial migration before the second half of gestation (see Chapter 6). The early differentiation of pyramidal neurons in layer V is consistent with their early origin and migration. Over the second half of gestation and into infancy, there is a striking increase in the overall thickness of the cortex and in layers I–III, V, and VI. The increase in thickness in layers I–III

in particular over the last half of gestation likely reflects their expansion by late migrating (GABAergic) interneurons, given that the SVZ continues to actively generate mainly GABAergic neurons beyond midgestation (see Chapters 5 and 6).[39,40]

Gyral Development

Gyrification is the process whereby folding patterns of sulci and gyri develop on the surface of the brain. Several of these patterns are asymmetrical between the right and left side of the cerebral hemispheres, and several distinguish the human brain from that of other species. The gyrus is a ridge of cerebral cortex, whereas the sulcus is a depression or furrow on either side of the ridge. *Gyrification results in a dramatic increase in the cortical surface area within the limited and rigid confines of the skull, and thus, in the volume of cortical gray matter.* As discussed later, a striking increase in cerebral cortical volume in the human infant from approximately 28 to 40 weeks after conception has been shown by quantitative MRI measurements of cortical gray matter volumes.[41] Thus a fourfold increase in cerebral cortical gray matter volume could be documented (Fig. 7.5). The changes in cortical gyral development and cortical surface area that accompany and presumably are caused by the increase in cortical volume can be seen by MRI (Fig. 7.6).[42] The formation of gyri and sulci in the brain also allows for compact wiring that promotes and enhances efficient neural processing.[43]

At the time of neural tube closure in the embryonic period, the surface of the brain is smooth, that is, lissencephalic; as development continues, gyri and sulci begin to take shape on the fetal brain surface (Fig. 7.7). The pattern of gyrification follows orderly and defined sequences, such that the brain can be dated to a particular gestational week by its developmental stage of gyrification.[44] Information about these sequences were garnered from 507 brains and serial sections of 207 brains from infants from 10 to 44 gestational weeks of age in the National Perinatal Collaborative Project.[44] The sequential developmental changes of the individual fissures, sulci, and gyri of the cerebral hemispheres throughout the gestational period

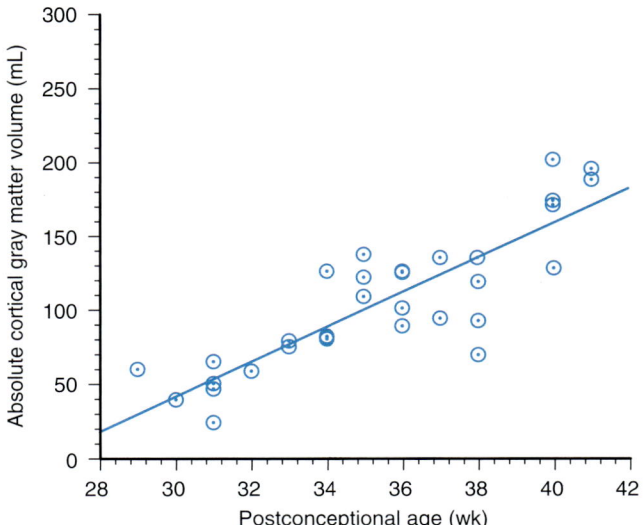

Figure 7.5 Cerebral cortical gray matter volume as a function of postconceptional age. Quantitative volumetric MR determinations of absolute cerebral cortical gray matter volume as a function of postconceptional age in a series (*n* = 35) of preterm and full-term infants. (From Huppi PS, Warfield S, Kikinis R, et al. Quantitative magnetic resonance imaging of brain development in premature and mature newborns. *Ann Neurol.* 1998;43:224–235.)

were tabulated. *The period of greatest development of brain gyrification is during the third trimester of pregnancy*, a period in which the brain undergoes considerable growth.[44] At midgestation, the brain is lissencephalic, except for the presence of the Sylvian fissure and central sulcus[44]; between midgestation and birth, all primary, secondary, and tertiary gyri are formed, an explosive period in gyrification. The *gyrification index (GI),* defined as the ratio between the lengths of coronal outlines for the brain including and excluding the sulcal regions, is a quantitative approach to measure gyrification[45]; brains with higher degrees of cortical folding give higher GI values. This measure was used to quantify the developmental trajectory of gyrification in humans[46] with the major finding that gyrification increases dramatically during the third trimester and then remains relatively constant throughout subsequent development.[46] This anatomical change is readily followed by advanced MRI measures (see later). Little is known about changes in gyrification during childhood and adolescence, although considering the continuing changes in gray matter volume and thickness during this time period, it is conceivable that alterations in the brain surface morphology could also occur during this period of development.[43] Despite the stereotypical development of gyrification, it should be emphasized that there are *structural variations among individuals*, although not apparently between males and females.[44] The central sulcus, for example, varies in location by up to 2 cm between individuals.[43] This variability raises important considerations in analyzing structural and functional brain images in neuroimaging studies.[47] Importantly, there are left-right asymmetries of the transverse temporal gyri, sylvian fissures, and planum temporale.[48] In general, the right cerebral hemisphere shows gyral complexity earlier than the left. Such findings have led to speculations about the significance of left-right asymmetry of the brain as it affects speech and language development.

The *mechanistic basis of cortical folding* is complex and likely involves *multiple interactive factors* (see also Chapters 5 and 6). The following different folding mechanisms have been postulated based mainly on experimental animal data and computer-based modeling: (1) tissue buckling from mechanical stress and external constraints as the brain conforms to the confines of the skull; (2) axonal tethering and local connectivity between developing gyri, or in other words, tension-based morphogenesis;[49] (3) localized cellular proliferation relative to localized cortical surfaces; and (4) radial intercalation of new neurons at the top of the cortical plate that causes the cortical plate to expand tangentially more rapidly than the underlying tissue, and as a result, the cortical plate buckles into a series of folds.[50,51] The size and shape of the lobes of the cerebral hemisphere also involve patterning center(s) of the embryonic forebrain that contains a protomap of the future lobes and involves genetic interactions.[52]

Neurite Outgrowth

Neurite outgrowth refers to the elaboration of dendritic and axonal ramifications of neurons (see Table 7.1). While beginning in the first trimester, it becomes a dominant organizational event in the second half of pregnancy, the neonatal period, and infancy. The most significant early studies of neurite outgrowth in human cerebral cortex were made in 1939 by Conel,[53] whose Golgi-Cox preparations of cerebral cortex from birth to 2 years of age demonstrated progressive enrichment of the dendritic and axonal plexus, with much smaller increases in size and no proportionate increases in the number of individual neurons. The remarkable elaboration of dendritic branching that results can be seen in the cerebrum of a normal child shown in Fig. 7.8. The studies of Mrzljak and co-workers[28] showed similar events in frontal cortex before birth (see Fig. 7.1). Accompanying the elaboration of dendritic and axonal ramifications are the appearance of synaptic elements, the development of neurofibrils, and an increase in size of endoplasmic reticulum within the cytoplasm of cells. The biochemical correlates of these changes are increasing cerebral content of RNA and protein relative to DNA. Immunocytochemical studies document parallel expression of a variety of neurotrophins, neurotransmitters (*N*-methyl-D-aspartate [NMDA], alpha-amino-3-hydroxy-5-methyl-4-isoxazolepropionic acid [AMPA]/kainate, GABA, and glycine receptors), surface glycoconjugates, and cytoskeletal components.[54-67] The maturational changes occur relatively rapidly in the hippocampus, whereas they occur over a more protracted period in the supralimbic region; the latter, of course, is of great significance, because it is the locus of the major association areas. Dendritic development in the human occurs earlier in thalamus and brain stem than in cerebral cortical regions.[68,69] These findings were amplified by studies by Purpura, Huttenlocher, Marin-Padilla, Rakic, and other investigators, who used electron microscopic and immunocytochemical methods as well as Golgi techniques.[28,31,62-66,70-81]

One study of developing human brain demonstrated the strikingly active axonal development in the cerebrum over the last trimester of gestation and in the early postnatal period (Fig. 7.9).[66] Thus immunostaining with GAP-43, a protein expressed on *growing* axons, shows exuberant expression in the cerebral white matter to approximately the subplate region at 20 weeks, to the cortical plate at 27 weeks, within the cortex at 37 weeks, and into the first year of life. This differential pattern

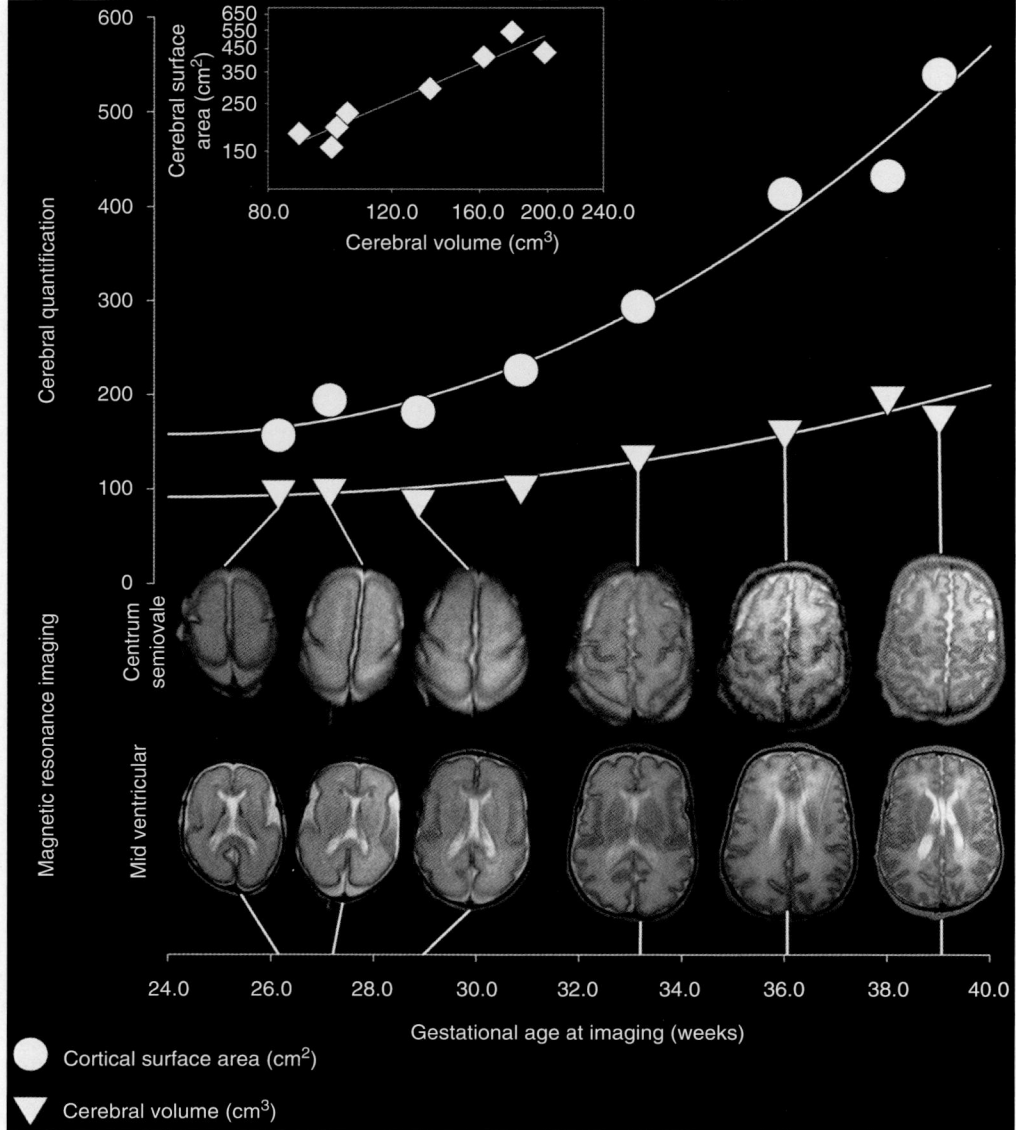

Figure 7.6 Measurements of cortical surface area and volume by advanced magnetic resonance imaging (MRI) *(upper)* and conventional MR images of gyral development *(lower)* during the last 14 weeks of gestation. Data derived from study of 113 preterm infants. (From Kapellou O, Counsell SJ, Kennea NL, Dvet L, et al. Abnormal cortical development after premature birth shown by altered allometric scaling of brain growth. *PLoS Med.* 2006;3:e265.)

may reflect, at 20 weeks, growth of axons from thalamus to subplate neurons, and at 27 weeks, from subplate neurons to cerebral cortex. At 37 weeks, the increase in cerebral cortical expression of GAP-43 may reflect the increase in cortical penetration of thalamic ascending fibers no longer waiting at the subplate layer, in corticocortical fibers, and in descending cortical fibers, initially pioneered by subplate axons (see earlier). These findings are consistent with more recent studies with different techniques by Kostovic and co-workers.[19] Although more data are needed on these issues, it is clear that the *last trimester of human gestation is a period of rapid axonal development.*

The *relationship between neurite outgrowth in cortex and development of functional capacity* can be illustrated in human visual cortex during the third trimester (Fig. 7.10). Most impressive are the appearance and elaboration of basilar dendrites and the tangential spread of apical dendrites. This dendritic development

is accompanied by the appearance of dendritic spines, or in other words, sites of synaptic contact (see the subsequent section on synaptic development). These anatomical expressions of differentiation are paralleled by the neurophysiological expression of maturation of the visual evoked potential (see Fig. 7.10). Such detailed relationships between dendritic structural development and specific details of neurophysiological development have been studied in depth in developing animals.[82]

The *progress of dendritic differentiation depends on the establishment of afferent input and presumably synaptic activity.*[a] In certain developing neural systems, the importance of receiving and making proper connections has been emphasized as highly critical for further organization. At least part of the influence

---

[a]References 28, 54, 60, 61, 70, and 83-89.

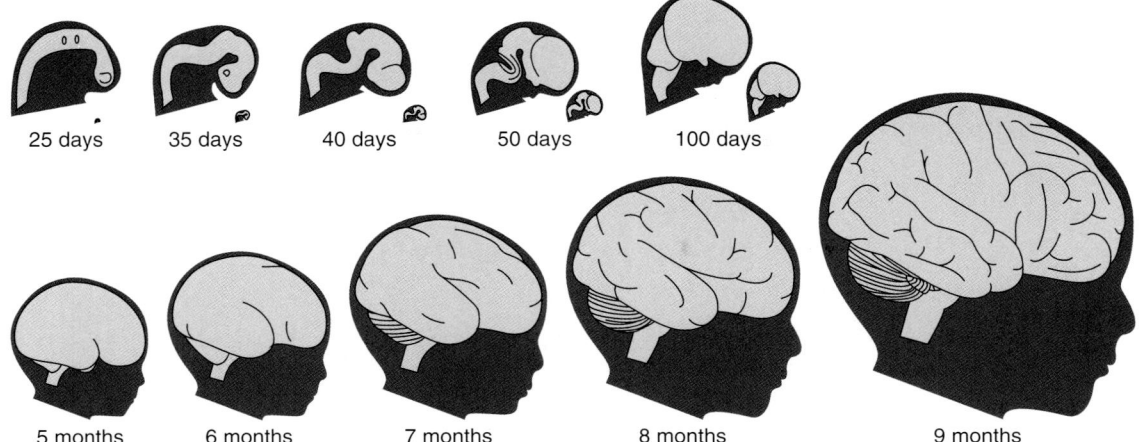

Figure 7.7 Schematic depiction of gyral development in human brain. Note the particularly prominent changes in the last 3 months of gestation. (From Cowan WM. The development of the brain. *Sci Am.* 1979;241:113.)

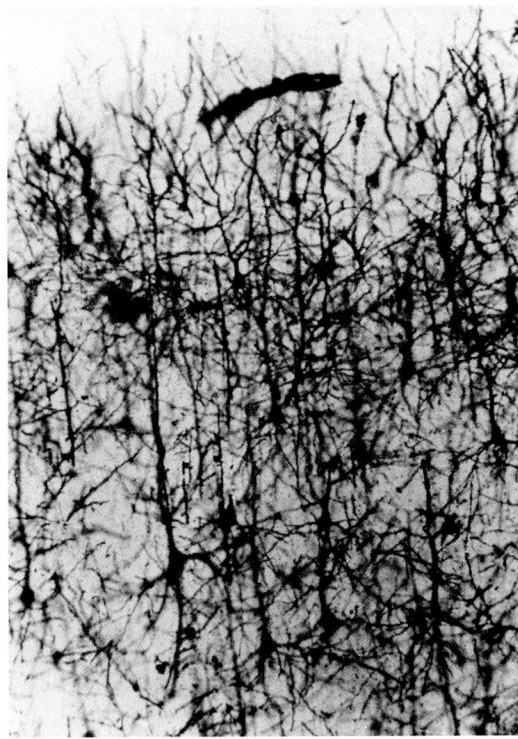

Figure 7.8 Golgi preparation (×80) of middle frontal gyrus from a 6-year-old child without known neurological disease. Note the abundant and complex horizontal and tangential dendritic branches. (From Buchwald NA, Brazier MAB, eds. *Brain Mechanisms in Mental Retardation.* New York: Academic Press; 1975.)

of these connections is mediated by the functional activity generated through them (see earlier discussion of subplate neurons).[90-93] This role of functional activity has implications for the effects of a variety of environmental stimuli on the postnatal progress of organizational development.[54,60] Neuronal activity initiates its effects on dendritic development by inducing calcium influx, both through activation of glutamate receptors, principally the NMDA receptor, but likely also GluR2-deficient AMPA receptors, and by opening of voltage-dependent calcium

channels.[87,88] The calcium-mediated effects include both a direct impact on the actin and microtubular components of the cytoskeleton and on several adhesion molecules and major indirect effects by activating multiple signaling pathways that target nuclear transcription factors and thereby many genes involved in dendritic development. Studies of developing human cerebral cortex show transient exuberant expression of calcium-permeable glutamate receptors in cortical neurons during this perinatal period.[94,95]

The central axon is a smooth, thin process of variable length that extends from the polarized neuronal cell body and propagates action potentials. The *neuronal cytoskeleton of the axon is composed of three different types of filaments: actin microfilaments, microtubules, and intermediate filaments (IFs).*[96] A mechanism for transport down the axon involves a system of both anterograde transport from the cell body to the terminal and retrograde transport from the terminal to the cell body.[96] Once produced in the cell body, membrane-bound organelles, including mitochondria and secretory vesicles, are transported down the length of the axon using microtubules and the motor molecule kinesin, which is thought to *walk* molecules along the microtubule.[97] The growth cone is formed at the tip of the growing axon and is responsible for *sensing* environmental cues, determining the direction of growth, and guiding the growing axon in the proper direction. The *temporal and spatial movement of the axon to its appropriate target is critical to the proper development of neuronal circuits.* This movement is controlled by a number of different environmental cues that direct the axons via interactions with the growth cone receptor. Signals include a number of molecules categorized into three families of ligands—cell adhesion molecules (CAMs), ECM molecules, and ephrins—each of which acts through receptor-mediated interactions on the cell surface of the growth cone.[96] Other signaling factors include the netrins, Slits, and semaphorins.

Advanced diffusion-based MRI imaging known as *tractography* provides further insight into the changes in fiber tract development in the living premature infant (see later).[98] Intracerebral connectivity emerges in a sequential manner, starting from dorsal posterior brain areas, continuing in an anteroventral direction, and ending in inferior temporal and inferior frontal lobes (Fig. 7.11).[99] This observed order follows

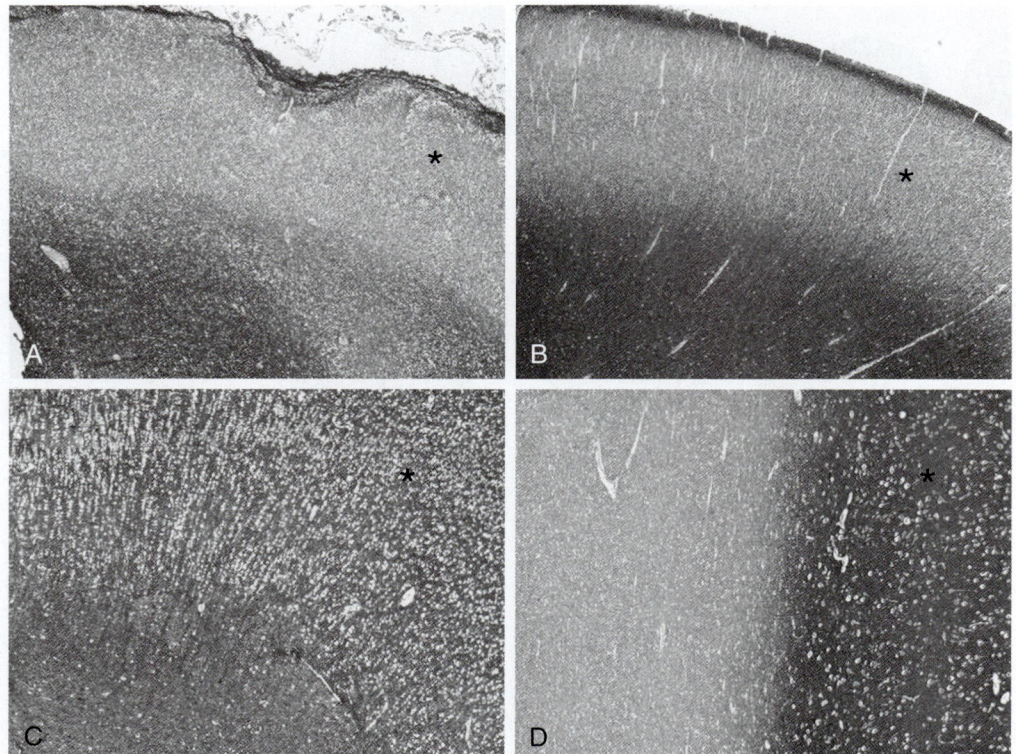

Figure 7.9 GAP-43 expression in developing human parietal white matter and cortex. Cortex is indicated by an asterisk (*). Note at 20 postconceptional (PC) weeks (A), evidence for strong expression in subcortical white matter to a region below the cortical plate, possibly the concentration of subplate neurons. At 27 PC weeks (B), the expression begins to enter the cerebral cortex. By 37 PC weeks (C), diffuse expression in cortex and decreased expression in white matter are apparent. At 144 PC weeks (D), that is, approximately 2 years of age, expression is prominent in cortex but not in white matter. See text for interpretations. Sections are ×40; scale bars are 200 μm. (From Haynes RL, Borenstein NS, DeSilva TM, Folkerth RD, et al. Axonal development in the cerebral white matter of the human fetus and infant. *J Comp Neurol.* 2005;484:156–167.)

the same order of normal gyrification and myelination.[43] Corticocortical association fibers have been found in the cortical plate around 23 to 25 gestational weeks.[19] Decreases in ipsilateral corticocortical connections observed after 22 gestational weeks may be due to axonal loss from failure of final targeting or from pruning after initial exuberant over-connectivity.

Synaptic Development

Synapses are the principal sites for communication between presynaptic and postsynaptic neurons via chemical messengers called neurotransmitters (see Table 7.1). In the human brain, about 10^{15} synaptic contacts interconnect the 10^{10} to 10^{11} neurons.[100] Synaptic formation differs appreciably among brain regions in the human brain. In the brain stem, the number of dendritic spines, the sites of synaptic contacts, in the medullary reticular formation reaches a peak at 34 to 36 weeks of gestation and declines rapidly after birth (see later discussion of disorders of organizational events).[101] In the cerebrum, synapses are observed initially on neurons of the preplate at 4 to 5 gestational weeks and by 10 weeks on neurons in subplate and marginal zones.[22] In the hippocampus, synapses are abundant as early as 15 and 16.5 weeks of gestation (Table 7.3).[102] The earliest synapses in the cerebral cortex are observed around 18 postconceptional weeks and are located on prospective layer V (pyramidal neurons).[31] Shortly after the

TABLE 7.3   Synaptic Formation and Elimination in Human Cerebral Cortex

First synapses involve subplate neurons (e.g., 15–16-week fetal hippocampus)
Synaptogenesis in cortical plate is most active postnatally
Approximately 40% of synapses are eliminated subsequently

pronounced ingrowth of thalamocortical axons to the cortical plate around 21 postconceptional weeks, dendritic spines begin to appear on immature pyramidal neurons and interneurons between 24 and 27 weeks.

With Golgi preparations, Purpura and co-workers[75-78,103] defined the subsequent *progression of dendritic spine development* in the human cortex from the fifth month of gestation (Figs. 7.12 and 7.13). Initially, dendrites appear as thick processes with only a few fine spicules. As development progresses, a great number and variety of dendritic spines appear. In visual cortex, synaptogenesis is fastest between 2 and 4 months after term, a time also critical for the development of function in visual cortex, and maximal synaptic density is attained at 8 months (Fig. 7.14).[78,103] *Synapse elimination* then begins, and by age 11 months, approximately 40% of synapses have been

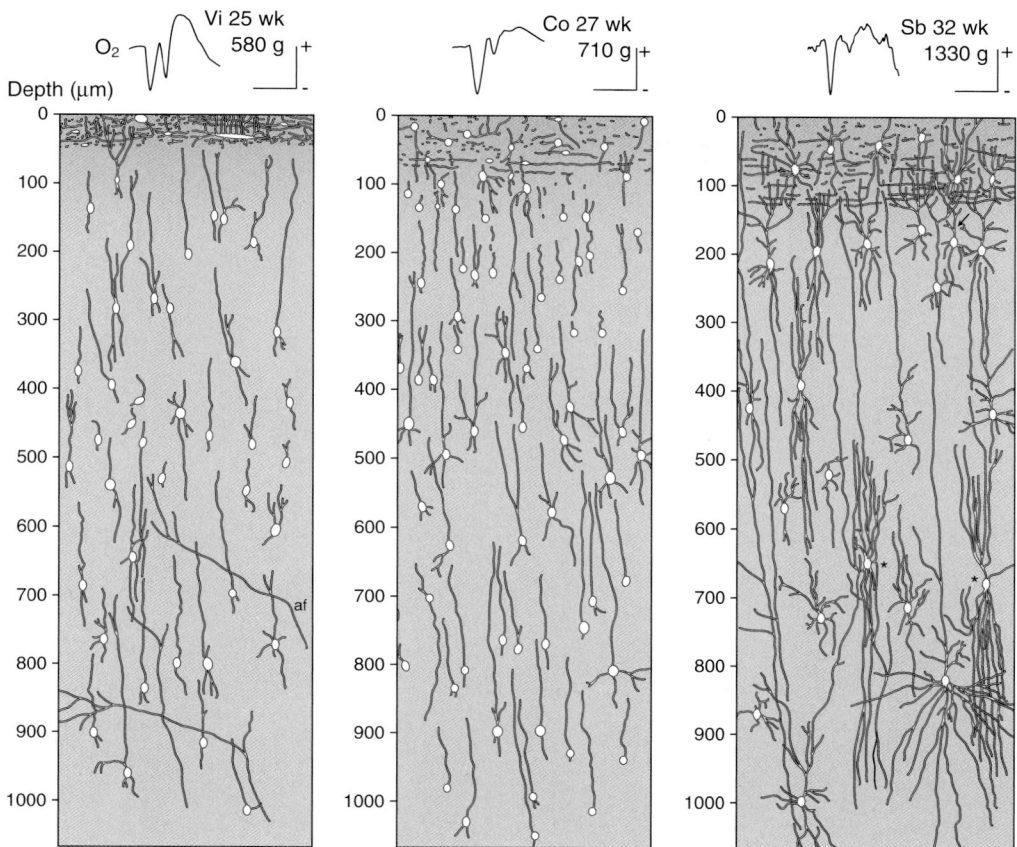

Figure 7.10 Camera lucida composite drawings of neurons in visual (calcarine) cortex of human infants of indicated gestational ages. Note the appearance and elaboration of basilar dendrites and the tangential spread of apical dendrites, as well as the accompanying maturation of the visual evoked response *(top)*. (Courtesy Dr. Dominick Purpura.)

lost. In frontal cortex, the time course of synaptic formation and of elimination differs somewhat from that in visual cortex; maximal synaptic density is reached at approximately 15 to 24 months, and synapse elimination, although reaching the same loss of 40% is more gradual.[103,104] In the prefrontal cortex, synapse elimination extends into midadolescence.[104] Elegant studies in the monkey exhibit more uniformity in the temporal features of synaptogenesis among cortical regions, but the basic principles are formation of earliest synapses in the marginal and subplate zones, an increase in synapses in cortical plate to a peak in excess of the adult number, and a subsequent period of synaptic elimination.[105-108]

Synaptic function results in the development of such neurophysiological measures as cortical evoked responses (see Fig. 7.10). Function is dependent on the action of neurotransmitters. These substances are stored in vesicles and are released from presynaptic nerve terminals at the so-called active zone, a restricted area of the cell membrane situated exactly opposite to the postsynaptic neurotransmitter reception apparatus.[100] At the active zone neurotransmitter, containing synaptic vesicles (SVs) dock, fuse, release their content and are recycled. SV components are initially trafficked to the synapse with members of the kinesin motor family. Exocytoxic function is mediated by a docking/fusion core complex that is regulated by several molecules, including Munc18-1 and syntaxin.[100] Vesicles fuse very quickly

in response to calcium elevations in the cytoplasm; this fusion event is thought to be mediated directly by the SNAREs. Transport proteins are involved in neurotransmitter uptake into the SVs and are composed of proton pumps that generate electrochemical gradients. Vesicular transporters move recycled neurotransmitters from the cells' cytoplasm into the SVs.

The *development of synaptic specificity* begins once a neuron has identified its correct synaptic partner. The initial axodendritic contact is transformed into a functional synapse by the recruitment of presynaptic and postsynaptic components.[109] The factors that stimulate synaptic formation and development in developing brain include initially activity-independent events, (i.e., molecular mechanisms involved in targeting), followed by activity-dependent events occurring after the development of receptors on target neurons and the generation of electrical activity (see previous discussion on neurite outgrowth).[54,60,83,110-113] Many molecules and signaling pathways are involved in dendritic spine development and remodeling. The two principal themes are modulation of the following: (1) ion channels, especially calcium-permeable channels, by neurotransmitters, especially glutamate; and (2) cell surface receptors by a variety of ligands. The intracellular events lead ultimately to effects on actin-binding proteins and the actin cytoskeleton, with resulting changes in spine shape, size, and motility.[113] The importance of synaptogenesis and

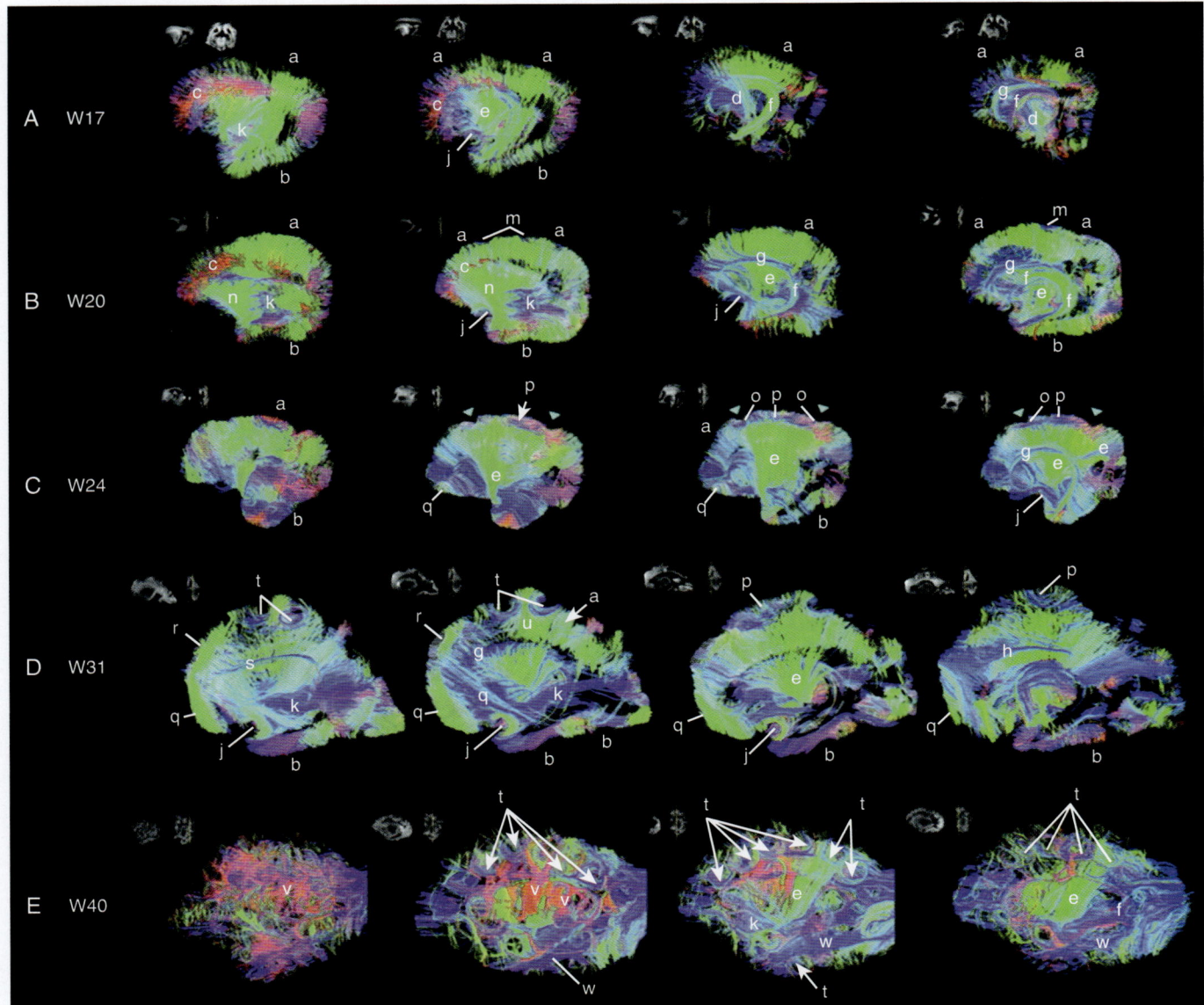

Figure 7.11 Fetal fiber tract development. See text for details. (From Takahashi E, et al. Emerging cerebral connectivity in the human fetal brain: an MR tractography study. *Cereb Cortex.* 2012;22:455–460, with permission.)

synapse elimination in the *plasticity* of the developing nervous system and in the potential effect of experiential factors on developing neural function, including cognitive function, could be enormous.

Cell Death and Selective Elimination of Neuronal Processes and Synapses

Cell death and selective elimination of neuronal processes and synapses, or *regressive events* in brain development, are now recognized to be highly critical (see Table 7.1).[36,78,104,114-130] Results of studies in a variety of developing neuronal systems showed that after formation of neuronal collections by the *progressive* processes of proliferation and migration, cell death occurs.[36,118,122-128,131] Although variable in degree among neuronal regions, typically about half of the neurons in a given collection

die before final maturation. This process of cell death is initiated and sustained by the expression of specific genes and their transcription products that actively kill the neuron.[118,122,125,127] Critical in the final phases of the sequence to cell death is the activation of a family of cysteine proteases known as caspases.[127] The term programmed cell death has been used to emphasize that this is an active developmental process, although more commonly the term apoptosis, a Greek-rooted word referring to the naturally occurring seasonal loss or falling of flowers, is used to refer to this developmentally determined cell death.[36,118,122,125-128,132]

The factors that activate this death system appear to relate to competition of neurons for limited amounts of trophic factors, generated by the target, afferent input, or associated glia. This loss of neurons appears to serve two major functions

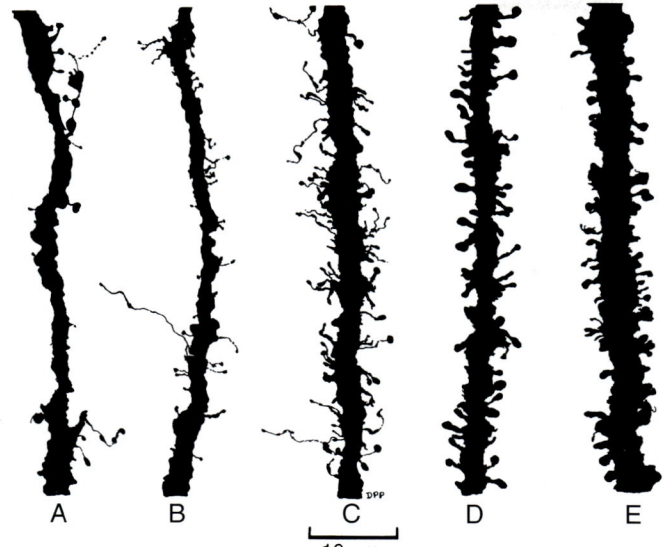

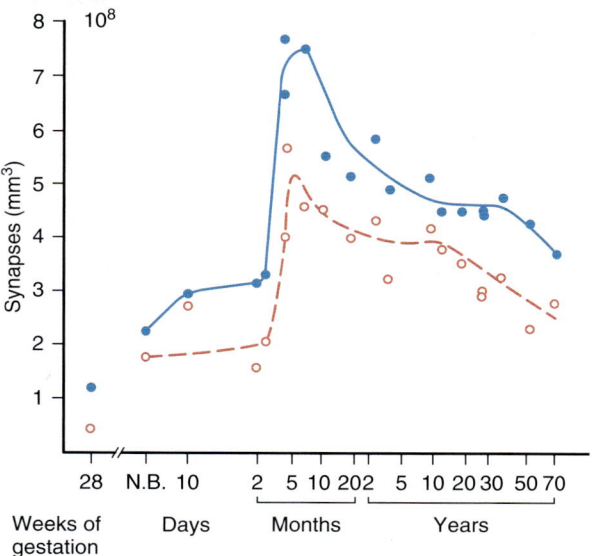

Figure 7.12 Camera lucida drawings of proximal apical dendritic segments of motor cortex pyramidal neurons during development. (A) 18-week-old fetus; (B) 26-week-old fetus; (C) 33-week-old preterm infant; (D) 6-month-old infant; (E) 7-year-old child. Early phase of dendritic spine differentiation in proximal apical segments is associated with the development of long, thin spines and relatively few stubby and mushroom-shaped spines. The latter two types are prominent in the postnatal period and early childhood. (Courtesy Dr. Dominick Purpura.)

Figure 7.14 Synaptic density in layer I and layer II/III of striate cortex. Open circles represent layer I; closed circles represent layer II/III. Note the striking increase in the first postnatal year and the subsequent decline. (From Huttenlocher PR, de Courten C. The development of synapses in striate cortex of man. *Hum Neurobiol.* 1987;6:1.)

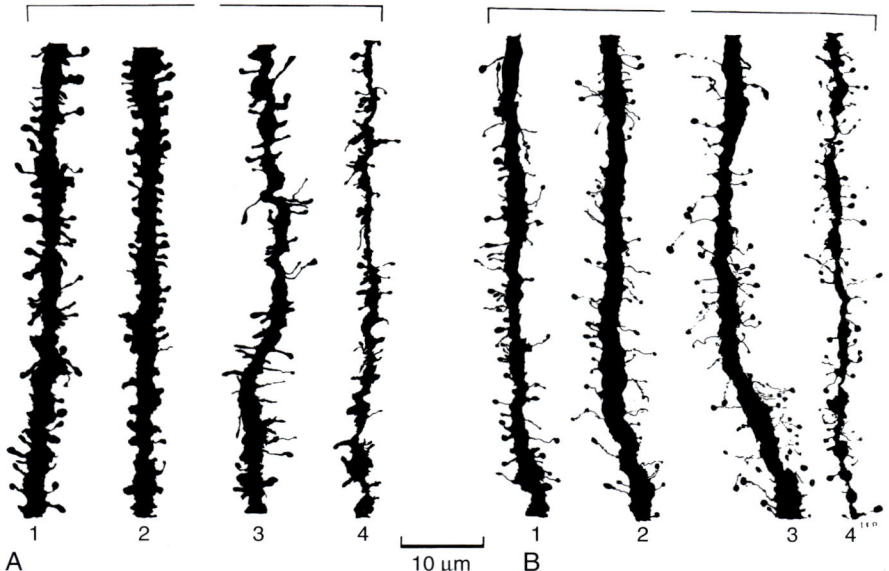

Figure 7.13 Camera lucida drawings of dendritic segments of motor cortex neurons, rapid Golgi preparations, from a normal and a mentally retarded infant. (A) From a normal 6-month-old infant: *1* and *2*, proximal apical dendritic segments with a predominance of stubby and mushroom-shaped spines; *3* and *4*, distal apical dendritic segment and basilar dendritic segment have many more thin spines. (B) From a 10-month-old infant with mental retardation of unknown etiology: *1, 2, 3,* proximal apical and, *4,* basilar dendritic segments. Note the presence in the proximal segments *(1, 2, 3)* of many *long, thin* spines, comparable to the appearance of cortex in normal preterm infants (see Fig. 7.14). (Courtesy Dr. Dominick Purpura.)

in development: quantitative adjustments (numerical matching) of interconnecting populations of neurons and elimination of projections that are aberrant or otherwise incorrect (refinement of synaptic connections or error correction).[a] Failure of cell death or overactivation of this process clearly could have major deleterious implications for brain development and subsequent function.

Neural organization is refined further by a second regressive event, *selective elimination of neuronal processes and synapses*. This event primarily causes the removal of terminal axonal branches and their synapses, although even larger-scale elimination of a total pathway also occurs. Vivid demonstrations of synapse elimination are apparent in developing brain stem and cortex of the human infant (see earlier). The determinants of selective elimination of neuronal processes and synapses are similar to those described for cell death. Activation of the NMDA type of glutamate receptor appears to be an important step in synapse elimination during development.[121] An additional crucial role of the specific region of cerebral cortex in determining the pattern of selective elimination of its terminal axons was shown by studies with cortical transplants in developing rats.[134] Thus cortical neurons transplanted to another region of cortex (as explants) eliminated their distal axon collaterals in the same way as did neurons of the host cortical region (into which they were transplanted), rather than in the way neurons of the donor region eliminated their distal collaterals.

The observations that cell death and elimination of neuronal processes and synapses occur during the organizational period of development have implications for the frequent demonstration that the *plasticity* of developing brain decreases as this period is completed.[114,118,122,123,135-144] It is likely that the regressive events described in this section are modified when the brain is injured and that neuronal processes and synapses destined for elimination can be retained if needed to preserve function. In addition, new projections may develop in response to injury during the period in which the brain has the capacity to perform organizational events. In favor of one or both of these predictions is the demonstration in both human infants and experimental models that, after neonatal cerebral lesions, ipsilateral corticospinal tract projections can be demonstrated and presumably can ameliorate the functional deficit.[139-141,145-158] The demonstration of an ipsilateral corticospinal projection until early childhood in humans suggests that retention of a normally occurring ipsilateral corticospinal tract, which otherwise is eliminated during development, is the crucial event in this form of plasticity.[141,149,159,160] The possible additional role of assumption of motor functions by ipsilateral cerebrum adjacent to the lesion is suggested by other studies.[149,152,161]

Glial Proliferation and Differentiation

Astrocytes, oligodendrocytes, and microglia are the major glial cells of the central nervous system (CNS). Glial proliferation and differentiation are of major importance in developing brain; glial cells clearly outnumber neurons in the CNS. In fact, in human cerebral cortex, glial cells outnumber neurons by approximately 1.25 to 1 and are almost the exclusive cell type in white matter.[162] Astrocytic and oligodendrocytic lineage, proliferation, and differentiation have been the topic of intense

---

TABLE 7.4   Glial Lineage and Differentiation in Forebrain

Astrocytes and oligodendrocytes
Astrocytes are generated primarily *before* oligodendrocytes
Astrocytic and oligodendroglial progenitors are principally subventricular cells and radial glia
Proliferation of these progenitors occurs at their sites of origin and locally (during and after migration)

Microglia
Microglia originate from bone marrow-derived monocytes
Sites of entry from the circulation include the ventricular and subventricular zones
Migration proceeds through the cerebral white matter during mid to late gestation and then to cortex near term

---

investigation in experimental systems in recent years,[163-203] and initial data also are emerging from studies of human brain.[a] The observations are not entirely consistent, but our best attempt at a synthesis is shown in Table 7.4. In general, astrocytes are generated primarily before oligodendrocytes. The progenitors of both astrocytes and oligodendrocytes initially are cells of the SVZ and probably radial glia (see Chapters 5 and 6). Radial glial progenitors may give rise to a glial restricted progenitor that then generates astrocytes or oligodendrocytes. Proliferation of glia, unlike that of neurons, also may occur locally, during and after migration.

Astrocytes

These glial cells are heterogeneous in morphology, function, and regional distribution. *Fibrous astrocytes* populate the white matter where they typically have cylindrical processes, giving the more classic *star-like* appearance, and dense glial filaments that stain with the IF marker glial fibrillary acidic protein (GFAP). *Protoplasmic astrocytes*, on the other hand, populate the gray matter and have more irregular processes and few glial filaments.[219] Protoplasmic astrocytes contact and sheathe synapses by extending thousands of thin processes, with contacts also with blood vessels.[220] Fibrous and protoplasmic astrocytes are developmentally distinct.[221] Markers that can reliably identify subsets of astrocytes are only beginning to be described.

Astrocytes play a variety of *complex nutritive and supportive roles* in relation to neuronal homeostasis and in the reaction to metabolic and structural insults. For example, astrocytes avidly take up glutamate and convert it to glutamine by the action of the astrocyte-specific enzyme glutamine synthetase; this removal of glutamate from the extracellular space is crucial for protection against excitotoxic injury with ischemia, seizures, or hypoglycemia (see Chapters 12, 13, 15, 19, and 25). Other functions include a wide variety of roles in inflammation, immune responses, production of trophic and neuroprotective factors (e.g., antioxidants), and tissue remodeling after injury.[36] In the adult brain, astrocytic endfeet form a sheathing network around the brain vasculature known as the glia limitans, which, together with pericytes and endothelial cells, form a barrier to the passage of molecules, ions, and cells from the bloodstream into the brain parenchyma: the blood-brain barrier (BBB). In

---

this context, astrocytes play an important role in the regulation of cerebral blood flow[222] and in regulating BBB permeability from the bloodstream into the brain parenchyma.

The *last half of human gestation is a crucial time in astrocyte formation in the human cerebral cortex and white matter.* The radial glial cell originates in the ventricular/SVZ and retains connections with the ependyma and pia; it can generate neurons and astrocytes. Its long, thin, and linear processes,, that is, radial glial fibers (RGFs), serve as a guide for migrating neuroblasts and glial cells.[215] Glutamatergic neurons form in the dorsal telencephalic SVZ and migrate along RGFs early in gestation (see Chapters 5 and 6).[223] In the human brain, in contrast to the rodent brain, approximately two-thirds of GABAergic neurons arise from the dorsal telencephalic zone and migrate along RGFs; the remaining one-third originates in the ganglionic eminence and migrates tangentially to the cortex.[224] From 19 to 30 weeks, RGFs are abundant; around 30 to 31 weeks, they begin to transform into fibrous astrocytes in the white matter and from 30 weeks to term gestation (37 to 41 weeks), they progressively disappear as the white matter becomes increasingly populated with transformed astrocytes.[225] By term, RGFs completely disappear, thereby definitively marking the end of radial migration. Fibrous astrocytes in the white matter also form from glial precursors that migrate outward from the ventricular/SVZ independent of RGFs.[225] Reactive gliosis with gemistocytic morphology and GFAP-positive immunostaining begins around midgestation in the human brain.

Oligodendrocytes

Oligodendroglial proliferation and differentiation are crucial for myelination and thus are discussed later in relation to that major developmental event (see Chapter 8).

Microglia

These cells comprise the resident and immune cells of the brain and originate principally if not entirely from bone marrow-derived monocytes.[36] They enter the CNS (especially brain stem and spinal cord) in the first trimester, and in the cerebrum, microglia become apparent in the second trimester within the marginal zone, which is the boundary of the cortical plate and subplate, and the ventricular-SVZs (see Table 7.4).[226-233] A study of developing human cerebrum from 20 weeks of gestation made the striking observation that microglial cells during the second and third trimesters are primarily in the active (ameboid morphology) state and migrate progressively from ventricular-SVZs to cerebral white matter (20 to 35 weeks) and then to cerebral cortex.[234] Migration may occur along white matter tracts, radially oriented vasculature, and residual radial glial cells.[229,234] Although the prevailing notion is that these cells *enter* the ventricular-SVZs via the circulation, whether any of these cells may *originate* in the ventricular-SVZs is unresolved. *The critical point is that the cerebral white matter is heavily populated with activated microglia during a period when developmental events are active and a variety of insults can lead to white matter injury (WMI)* (see Chapters 13 and 15). Microglia, for example, are transiently elevated in the peak window of vulnerability to PVL, well situated to become activated and lead to free radical and cytokine injury to pre-OLs.

Microglial cells play key roles during brain development, involving vascularization,[229] apoptosis,[128] axonal development,[66] and later myelination.[235] In addition to these key beneficial roles,

these cells, when activated by such insults as hypoxia-ischemia or infection-inflammation, can release such substances as cytokines and reactive oxygen and nitrogen species, which could injure *innocent bystanders*, differentiating oligodendrocytes of the premature infant or neurons of the term infant (see Chapters 13 and 15).

Organizational Events Studied In Vivo

Investigation of organizational events in living infants has been based principally on the study of premature infants by advanced MRI methodologies (Table 7.5). Several principal MRI methods have been used and include three structural measures, that is, volumetric MRI, diffusion tensor MRI, and surface-based cerebral cortical measures, as well as functional MRI (fMRI), both task-related (e.g., response to specific sensory input) and resting state (RS) (see Table 7.5). Many excellent reviews of the application of these measures are available[236-240] and are discussed in other relevant chapters in this book (see especially Chapters 10 and 16). *This section focuses on studies relevant to normal development in the fetal and neonatal periods.* Because of the principal application of these measures to preterm infants, the great preponderance of data involves brain development primarily over the period from 28 to 40 postconceptional weeks. These findings are described briefly next.

Volumetric Magnetic Resonance Imaging

Striking increases in total and regional brain volumes are apparent over the last trimester, that is, the last 12 postconceptional weeks (see Table 7.5). An initial report nearly 20 years ago showed a fourfold increase in cerebral cortical gray matter volume from approximately 28 to 40 weeks'

TABLE 7.5 Major Advanced Magnetic Resonance Imaging Measures of Organizational Events in Living Infants

MRI METHOD	MAJOR MEASURES	MAJOR ORGANIZATIONAL EVENT(S) ASSESSED
Volumetric MRI	Total and regional brain volumes	All; specific event(s) depending on region
Diffusion tensor imaging, including tractography	Water diffusion along axons and less commonly, dendrites, and radial fibers; fiber tract mapping	White matter: axonal development and premyelination events Gray matter: axonal and dendritic development
Surface-based cerebral cortical measures	Cortical surface area, cortical thickness, gyral development	Cortical neuronal and subcortical white matter development
Functional MRI, task related or resting state	Neural activity	All, including especially synaptic development

MRI, Magnetic resonance imaging.

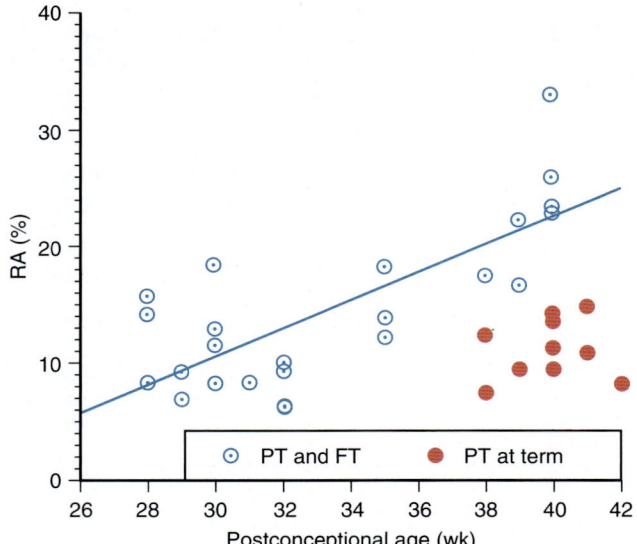

Figure 7.15 Diffusion tensor MR determination of relative anisotropy *(RA)* in cerebral white matter of normal preterm *(PT)* and term *(FT)* infants *(open circles)* as a function of postconceptional age. Note the striking increase in RA, indicative of increasing directionality of diffusion, perhaps related at least in part to oligodendroglial ensheathment of axons, with maturation. The lower values of the preterm infants studied at term *(closed circles)* suggest a deleterious effect of prematurity on this process (see text for details). (From Huppi PA, Maier SE, Peled S, et al. Microstructural development of human newborn cerebral white matter assessed in vivo by diffusion tensor magnetic resonance imaging. *Pediatr Res.* 1998;44:584–590.)

postconceptional age (see Fig. 7.5).[41] Many subsequent studies have confirmed and amplified this initial observation.[236-240] More detailed regional studies have delineated trajectories of increase in specific cortical areas, basal ganglia, thalamus, cerebellum, and other structures. The cellular bases for these increases likely reflect all aspects of the organizational events described earlier, particularly the events involving cortical arrival of late migrating neurons, neuronal differentiation, neurite outgrowth, axonal development, premyelination oligodendroglial events, lamination, and gyrification (see earlier). The multiplicity of effectors of the volumetric increases makes it difficult to delineate the relative importance of each, not only in terms of normal organizational events, but also as causes of impaired volumetric development (see the section on disorders of organizational events).

Diffusion Tensor Magnetic Resonance Imaging

Diffusion tensor imaging (DTI) measures water diffusion along an axis and thereby is *valuable for assessing fiber tracts, especially axons, and less commonly, dendrites* (see Table 7.5).[236,238,239,241] Preferred directionality of water diffusion, measured by DTI as relative or fractional anisotropy (FA), provides information about white matter microstructure and, particularly, the development of white matter fiber tracts. Increases in FA in cerebral white matter was shown in premature infants over the period 28 to 40 weeks' postconception, nearly 20 years ago (Fig. 7.15).[242] Many subsequent studies have confirmed this observation and described important regional differences (see later). The anatomical correlate for this increase in relative

anisotropy (RA) is likely the increase in axonal size and density as development proceeds. However, an additional anatomical determinant, especially later in the third trimester, may reflect axonal ensheathment by premyelinating oligodendrocytes. As noted earlier the latter process is especially active at this time,[213,214] and experimental studies have delineated such a period of *premyelination anisotropy*.[195,243] Differentiation of axial versus radial diffusivity is useful for the distinction of axonal development versus ensheathment by premyelinating oligodendrocytes. Axial diffusivity increases in fiber tracts with axonal development, and radial diffusivity declines in tracts as premyelinating oligodendroglial ensheathment occurs.

Regional differences in development of white matter tracts are reflected by differences in the trajectory of increases in FA.[242,244,245] White matter areas that mature early, such as the posterior limb of the internal capsule and the optic radiations, show a correspondingly early rise in anisotropy.

DTI data also provide information about developing fiber tracts, and such diffusion *tractography* is valuable for visualization of white matter tracts (Figs. 7.16 and 7.17). When combined with fMRI studies, structural connectivity within developing cerebrum can be defined (see later).

Interestingly, in contrast to the increase in FA in developing cerebral *white* matter, *FA declines in developing cerebral cortex*.[246] The higher anisotropy in early developing cortical gray matter may relate to the preponderance of radially oriented fibers, that is, neurons with simple axons and an underdeveloped dendritic tree, RGFs, and the decline over the period from 26 to 40 weeks may reflect the elaboration of the dendritic tree and axonal ramifications and a regression of RGFs (Fig. 7.18).[245,246] A graphical representation of data from Smyser and co-workers[245] shows the simultaneous declines in RA in cerebral cortical areas and increases in RA in corresponding cerebral white matter regions (Fig. 7.19). The crossover point between the maturation lines may reflect the relative rates of white and gray matter development (see Fig. 7.19). The earliest maturing cerebral cortical and white matter areas, that is, primary motor and visual areas, have earlier crossover points than do the later maturing areas, that is, visual association and prefrontal areas (see Fig. 7.19).

Surface-Based, Cerebral Cortical Magnetic Resonance Imaging Measures

Cerebral cortical surface MRI analysis is a relatively recently applied approach to the study of the premature newborn (see Table 7.5). The major foci of this analysis, which uses data from conventional MR images, are *delineation of cortical surface area and folding/gyrification*.[239,240,247-250] Because the last 16 to 20 weeks of gestation is the period of most active cortical folding (see earlier), cortical surface analysis is especially relevant to the premature infant. Cortical surface area increases approximately 12% per week during the premature period.[248] Increases in cortical folding, development of gyri and increases in sulcal depth are similarly dramatic (Fig. 7.20).[240] The anatomical determinants were discussed earlier (see Gyral Development). It is likely that the migration of a full complement of neurons to cortex, including late migrating GABAergic neurons, with expansion especially of superficial cortical layers, followed by elaboration of dendritic and axonal ramifications are critical. However, in addition to the forces generated by development of cerebral cortical surface area, cortical folding likely depends

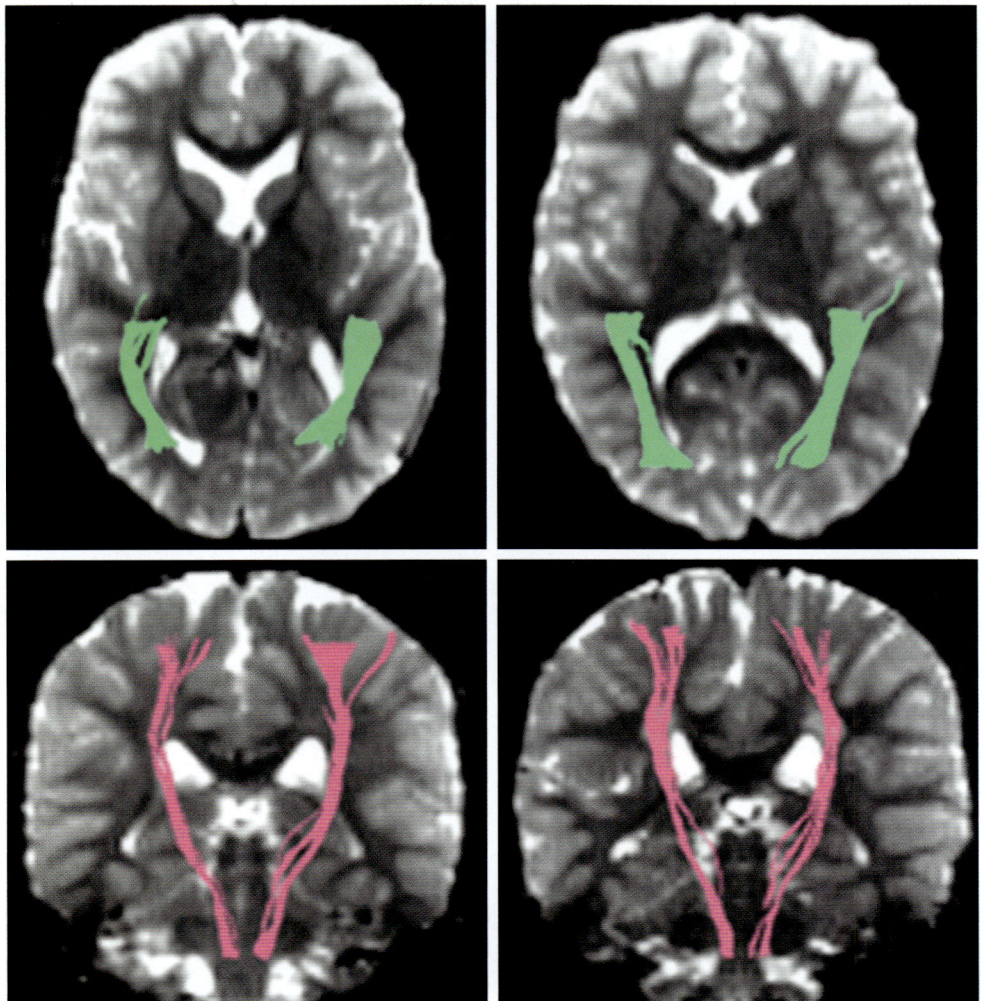

Figure 7.16 Diffusion tractography in two preterm infants studied at term equivalent age. The optic radiations *(green)* and corticospinal tracts *(pink)* are shown. (From Tao JD, Neil JJ. Advanced magnetic resonance imaging techniques in the preterm brain: methods and applications. *Curr Pediatr Rev.* 2014;10:56–64, with permission.)

also on the mechanical tension exerted by axons in rapidly developing subcortical white matter.[49]

Functional Magnetic Resonance Imaging

Whereas the MRI techniques described earlier assess structure, fMRI evaluates neural activity (see Table 7.5). As described in more detail in Chapter 10, the method is based on the fact that neural activation causes local changes in oxyhemoglobin and deoxyhemoglobin levels, changes that result in a detectable MRI signal, and therefore are referred to as the blood oxygenation level dependent (or BOLD) signal. *The neural activity may occur in relation to sensory stimulation (visual, auditory or sensorimotor) or performance of a motor task (active or passive), that is, task-related, or with the infant at rest, that is, RS functional connectivity.*[238,239,251] These methods provide in vivo correlates of functional connectivity in the neonatal brain, and thus are dependent on fiber tract development, neuronal differentiation, synaptic development, and neuronal activity.

Cortical neural activation has been shown by fMRI after visual, auditory, and somatosensory stimulation in the newborn, including the premature newborn.[252-255] A particularly informative report described the maturation of sensorimotor functional responses in the preterm brain.[256] The evolution of the responses induced by passive movement of the wrist is shown in Fig. 7.21. The localized functional activity is seen initially in the contralateral primary sensorimotor cortex at 31 to 32 weeks' postmenstrual age (PMA), then progresses to include the midline supplementary motor area at 33 to 34 weeks, the ipsilateral peri-Rolandic cortex and thalamus at 35 to 36 weeks, and by term equivalent age, an adult-like pattern is seen with activation also of basal ganglia and contralateral opercular cortex/secondary somatosensory cortex. Notably, interhemispheric functional activity increases rapidly during the preterm period to a peak at 36 weeks PMA, but interestingly, then declines at term equivalent age. This decline in functional connectivity could result from increasingly specific functional connectivity.[256]

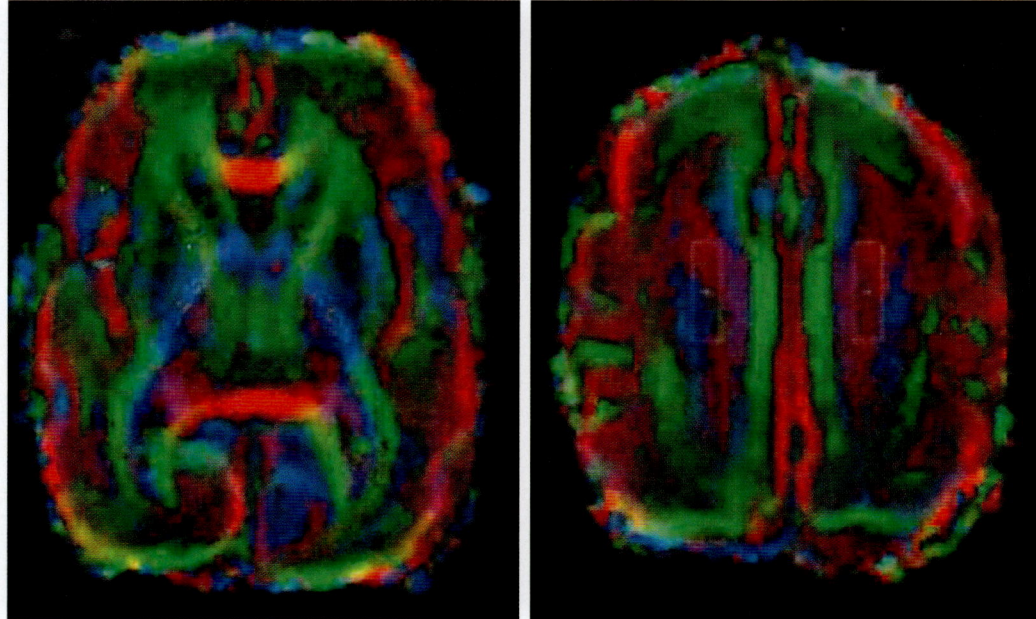

Figure 7.17 Quantitative diffusion tensor imaging. Color anisotropy parameteric maps of a preterm infant brain. The color maps display the direction of individual fibers: right to left *(red)*, anterior to posterior *(green)*, and superior to inferior *(blue)*. (From Tao JD and Neil JJ. Advanced magnetic resonance imaging techniques in the preterm brain: methods and applications. *Curr Pediatr Rev.* 2014;10:56–64, with permission.)

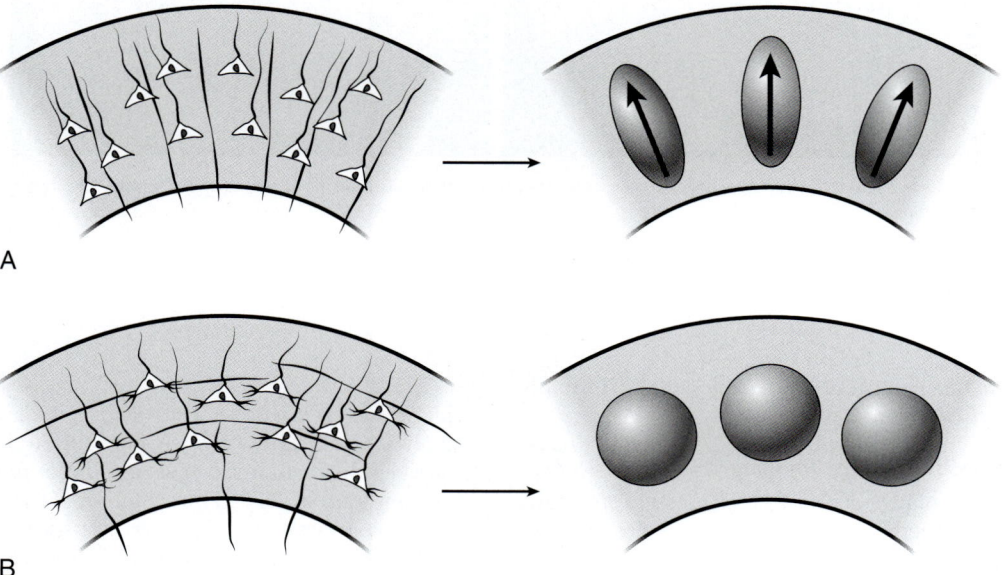

Figure 7.18 Diagram depicting proposed explanation for cortical anisotropy. On the left are representations of cortical microstructure. On the right are the corresponding diffusion ellipsoids at 26 weeks' gestational age (A), radial glial fibers and pyramidal neurons with prominent, radially oriented apical dendrites are shown. This organization has the effect of restricting water displacement parallel to the cortical surface more than displacement orthogonal to it, resulting in diffusion ellipsoids which are nonspherical with their major axes oriented radially *(arrows)*. By 35 weeks' gestational age (B), prominent basal dendrites for the pyramidal cells and thalamocortical afferents have been added. This has the effect of restricting water displacement more uniformly in all directions. As a result, the diffusion ellipsoids are spherical, without a preferred orientation. (From McKinstry RC, et al. Radial organization of developing preterm human cerebral cortex revealed by non-invasive water diffusion anisotropy MRI. *Cereb Cortex.* 2002;12:1237–1243, with permission.)

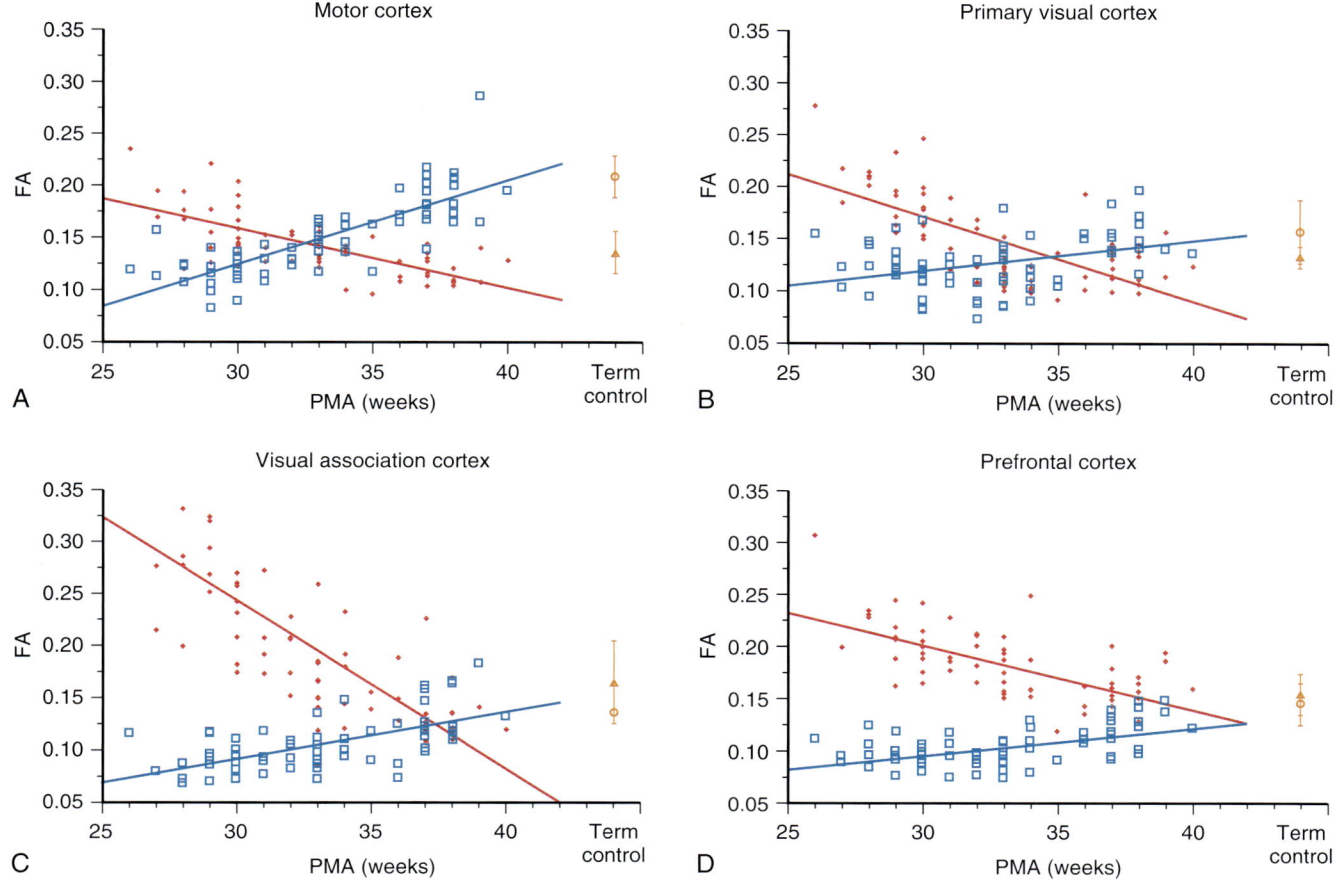

Figure 7.19 Scatter plots demonstrating fractional anisotropy measures versus postmenstrual age in the white *(open squares)* and gray *(red diamonds)* matter of the (A) motor, (B) visual, (C) visual association, and (D) prefrontal areas for very preterm infants. The solid lines depict results from linear regression. Note differences in the crossover point for regression lines for gray and white matter across regions. Values for term-born infants are provided for comparison on far right. (From Smyser TA, et al. Cortical gray and adjacent white matter demonstrate synchronous maturation in very preterm infants. *Cereb Cortex.* 2016;26:3370–3378, with permission.)

A second approach to the investigation of neural connectivity involves *RS connectivity* (see Chapter 10). In this circumstance, the infant is either asleep or resting, and low frequency BOLD signals are studied.[238,239] Temporal correlations within regions and between connected regions are identified. The two principal methods involve either seed correlation analysis (i.e., a specific region of interest, *seed*, is identified and signals from other regions that correlate temporally with the seed region are sought) or independent component analysis (i.e., analysis of signals from the entire brain to identify areas of correlation). Both approaches have been used effectively in the study of premature infants.[251,257-260] Evolution of highly connected cortical regions, that is, *hubs*, especially involving various early maturing cortical areas and thalamus, has been identified from early in the premature period. Short corticocortical connections are apparent initially, and longer corticocortical connections develop toward term. These so-called resting state networks (RSNs) incorporate cortical gray matter regions located initially in primary motor and sensory (somatosensory, visual, and auditory) cortices. The foundations of these networks are identifiable as early as 26 weeks PMA.[251] Thalamocortical connectivity also is especially prominent.[257,261] The rate of development

of the various networks appears to correlate with the rate of development of the regions involved and, presumably therefore, the establishment of connectivity. Thus RSNs involving primary motor and sensory areas are established by term PMA. However, RSNs involving association cortices (e.g., those mediating attentional functions) mature more rapidly after term.[251] These features reflect the development of axons, fiber tracts, myelination, and cortical dendrites. Combining these studies with diffusion tensor tractography provides an insight into the fiber tracts likely involved in interconnecting various components of the developing brain.

DISORDERS OF ORGANIZATIONAL EVENTS

The normative data just reviewed define a critical period in brain development that includes the *perinatal period*. Unfortunately, little is known about disorders of this phase of neural maturation. This ignorance is caused primarily by the inadequacy of standard neuropathologic techniques to evaluate the complex circuitry and synaptic connections of human brain. Earlier, only a few studies using appropriate techniques, such

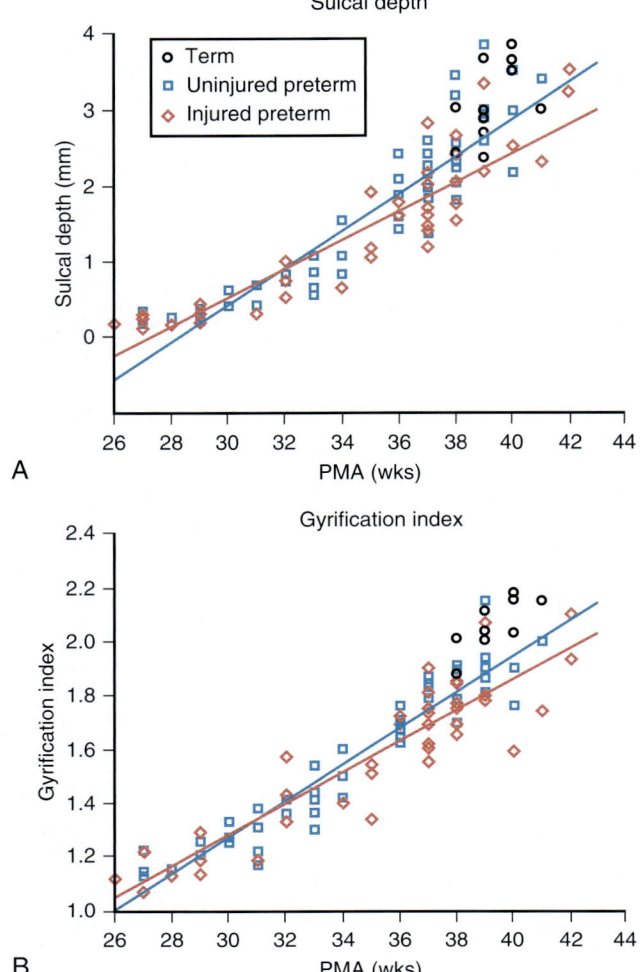

Figure 7.20 Plots of individual mean sucal depth and gyrification index versus postmenstrual age (PMA) for term *(black circles)*, uninjured preterms *(blue squares)*, and injured preterms *(red diamonds)*. Note the striking increase in the preterms (uninjured more than injured) as a function of increasing PMA. (From Shimony JS, et al. Comparison of cortical folding measures for evaluation of developing human brain. *Neuroimage.* 2016;125:180–190, with permission.)

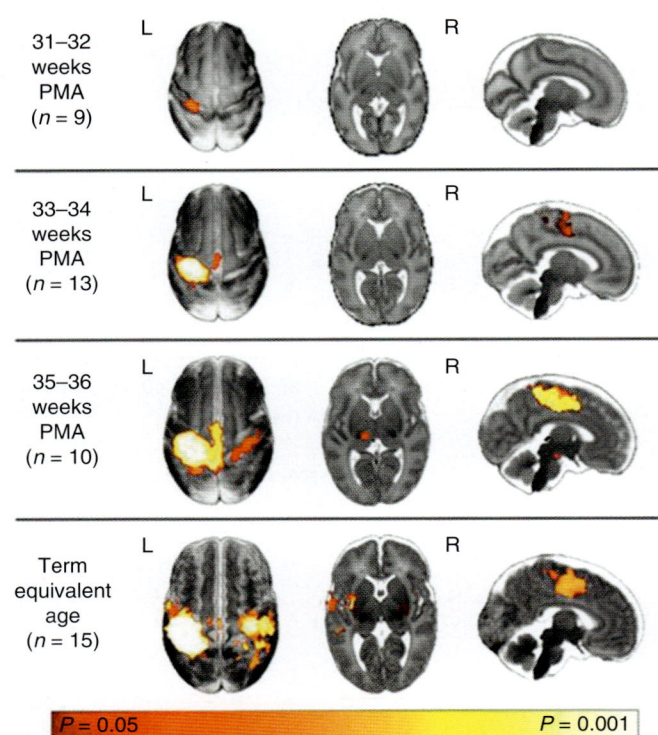

Figure 7.21 Evolution of sensorimotor functional responses induced by passive movement of the right wrist. Following right wrist movement, localized functional activity was identified in all infants in the contralateral *(left)* primary somatosensory cortex. Functional responses can be seen to progress from a contralateral only pattern in the youngest infants at 31 to 32 weeks postmenstrual age (PMA) *(top row, n = 9)*, to include the midline supplementary motor area (SMA) at 33 to 34 weeks *(second row, n = 13)*, and the ipsilateral peri-rolandic cortex and thalamus at 35 to 36 weeks *(third row, n = 10)*. At term equivalent age (37 to 44 weeks; *fourth row, n = 15)*, a mature adultlike activation pattern is seen in the bilateral peri-rolandic regions, basal ganglia, SMA, and contralateral opercular cortex/secondary somatosensory cortex. (From Allievi AG, et al. Maturation of sensori-motor functional responses in the preterm brain. *Cereb Cortex.* 2016;26:402–413, with permission.)

as the Golgi method for staining neuronal processes, were available, and it was often not clear whether the changes observed were primary or secondary, or specific or nonspecific. Although the latter uncertainties often persist, in recent years, the advent of advanced immunocytochemical methodologies, the delineation of molecular genetic defects, and the use of genetically manipulated animals have provided new insights into the identity and the basis of organizational disorders. Moreover, MRI techniques (e.g., quantitative volumetric MRI, diffusion tensor MRI, and fMRI) are clarifying these issues in the living infant (see later discussions and Chapter 10). In Table 7.6, disorders in which prominent deficits involve organizational events are presented as illustrative examples, but the list is not meant to be comprehensive.

Disorders of Subplate Neurons

Clearly, the time periods when the functions of the subplate neurons must be operative in the developing human brain

correspond closely to the times of occurrence of a variety of periventricular hemorrhagic and ischemic lesions (see Chapters 16 and 24). If these lesions disrupt the subplate neurons or their axonal collaterals to subcortical or cortical sites, the functions described earlier would be impaired, and the impact on cortical neuronal development and on a variety of crucial projection systems could be enormous. *Indeed, the major portion of the striking increase in cerebral cortical volume in the last trimester of gestation consists of the extensive elaboration of the afferent fibers, previously "waiting" in contact with subplate neurons, as they enter the cerebral cortex.*[13] As noted later, this increase in cerebral cortical volume is blunted by injury to cerebral white matter in the premature infant. The role of subplate neuronal injury in the encephalopathy of prematurity is discussed in Chapters 14 and 15. In addition, subplate neuronal pathology has been suggested in a variety of other neurological disorders, including epilepsy, autism, and schizophrenia beyond the neonatal period. Drug-resistant epilepsy is often accompanied by severe cortical dysplasias, in which large groups of cells are also abnormally located within the cerebral white matter.[262] It has been postulated that this

TABLE 7.6 Disorders of Organization

Disorders of subplate neurons
    Miscellaneous (see text)
Disorders of lamination
    Miscellaneous (see text)
Disorders of gyrification
    See Chapter 6
Disorders of dendrites and synaptogenesis
    Mental retardation (idiopathic), with or without seizures
    Rett syndrome
    Autism spectrum disorder
    Fragile X syndrome
    Down syndrome
Disorders of axonal outgrowth
    Agenesis of the corticospinal tracts
    Congenital cranial disinnervation disorders
Disorders of glial proliferation and differentiation
    Miscellaneous (see text)
Disorders of multiple organizational events delineated in vivo
    Prematurity-related factors (see Table 7.8)
    Nutritional factors
    Experiential factors

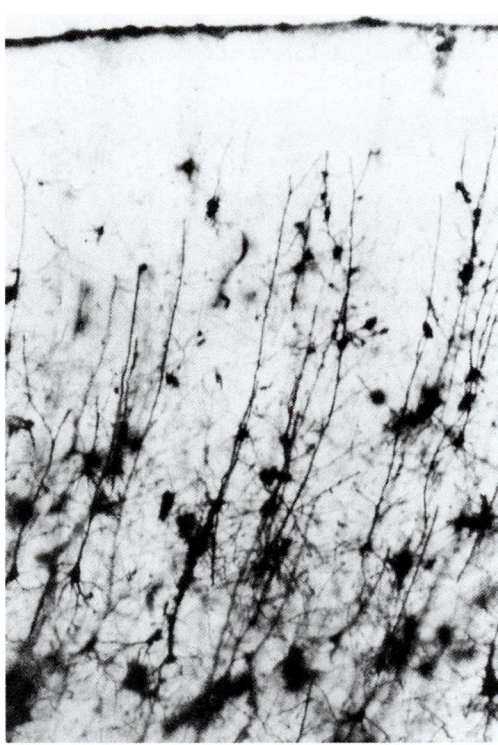

Figure 7.22 Golgi preparation (×80) of middle frontal gyrus from a 10-year-old child with severe mental retardation of unknown origin. Note the relative sparsity of horizontal and tangential dendritic branches (compare with Fig. 7.10). (From Buchwald NA, Brazier MAB, eds. *Brain Mechanisms in Mental Retardation.* New York: Academic Press; 1975.)

excess of interstitial white matter neurons is the result a failure of programmed cell death in subplate cells, although a failure of migration of cortical plate neurons to their final addresses has not been excluded. Excessive numbers of interstitial white matter neurons have been reported in autopsy analyses of the brains of patients with schizophrenia and autism.[263,264] In effect, subplate neurons are the link between developing and mature circuits in the cerebral cortex, and dynamic disorders in their number, position, and molecular and genetic functions can have a major impact on the development of human cognitive and affective processing with far-reaching implications beyond the fetal, premature, and perinatal periods.

Disorders of Lamination

Many malformations of cortical development underlying epilepsy, cerebral palsy, global intellectual disability, and neuropsychiatric disorders include aberrant laminar patterns. These abnormal patterns include focal cortical dysplasia and the *four-layered* types of lissencephaly and polymicrogyria that are discussed in detail in Chapter 6. Layer-specific markers have provided insight into the neurobiology of these patterns. A major goal in developmental neuropathology is to develop a panel of markers to analyze all neuron types and their distribution in the human neocortex to elucidate abnormalities in the position and number of each neuron type in cortical malformations, as well as in metabolic and degenerative diseases that involve selective loss of specific neuron types.[265]

Disorders of Gyrification

Abnormalities in gyrification in the cerebral cortex are associated with various genetic and acquired malformations, including pachygyria, lissencephaly, and polymicrogyria, as reviewed in Chapter 6. Other gyral abnormalities include maldevelopment of individual gyri and/or lobes, resulting, for example, in small superior temporal gyri in Down syndrome.[266]

Disorders of Dendrites and Synaptogenesis

Dendritic pathology occurs in multiple human disorders in early life, of which several major examples are highlighted here for illustration.

Mental Retardation With or Without Seizures

Several studies in which the Golgi technique was used have shown abnormalities of development of dendritic branching and spines in children with idiopathic mental retardation with or without seizures.[74,75,267-271] The children in these studies had no anatomical evidence for destructive disease, metabolic disorder, or other developmental aberration (see Table 7.6). Huttenlocher,[74,270] using the Golgi technique and quantitative estimation of dendritic branching, initially studied 11 brains from individuals with severe mental retardation of unknown cause. In six of these brains, severe defects in the number, length, and spatial arrangement of dendritic branching and in dendritic spines, the sites of synaptic contacts, were demonstrated. The relative sparsity of horizontal and tangential dendritic branches is shown clearly in Fig. 7.22. Four of the six affected children with marked dendritic abnormalities had, in addition to the severe mental retardation, histories of infantile myoclonic seizures and hypsarrhythmic electroencephalograms (EEGs).[74,270,271] Moreover, Purpura[75,267] demonstrated, in a cerebral biopsy specimen of a severely retarded infant, marked abnormalities of dendritic spines, characterized principally by a marked reduction in short, thick-necked spines (see Fig. 7.13). This finding was the only detectable defect in the biopsy specimen and after extensive clinical and laboratory studies yielded negative results.

Insight into a major mechanism in the production of such defects was provided first by the work of Purpura and co-workers.[268,269] Golgi studies of cerebral cortex from five children with mental retardation and seizures (two in one family) demonstrated striking dendritic abnormalities, the most prominent of which was the formation of distinct varicosities along the dendritic processes (Fig. 7.23). Ultrastructural studies showed an aberration of microtubules with loss of the usual parallel array of these structures. These findings indicated that a *disturbance of cytoskeletal structures,* so critical for maintenance of cell shape and for outgrowth of dendrites and axons, can cause a severe dendritic abnormality and marked neurologic disturbance.[269]

More recent work has begun to delineate the molecular bases for at least some of these cases.[113] X-linked genes have been shown to be particularly important, perhaps accounting

in part for the higher incidence of mental retardation in male than in female patients.[272,273] The greatest insight into X-linked mental retardation disorders involves fragile X syndrome and Rett syndrome (discussed subsequently). However, many other genes have recently been identified. Prominent among these are four X-linked genes found mutated in families with mental retardation that encode proteins known as Rho guanine nucleotide exchange factor 6 (ARHGEF6), oligophrenin-1, p21-activated kinase, and guanine dissociation inhibitor 1.[273,274] These proteins are involved in signaling pathways that regulate the actin cytoskeleton, so critical for neurite outgrowth, dendritic spine formation, and morphology and neurotransmitter release. This rapidly evolving field may lead to insights into potential therapies.

Rett Syndrome

Rett syndrome is a complex disorder observed in full form only in females; it constitutes one of the most common causes of mental retardation in girls and women.[275,276] The disorder is characterized clinically by onset of deceleration of rate of head growth in the first months of life, loss of purposeful hand movement near the end of the first year, and development of stereotypical movements with repetitive hand wringing, autism, ataxia, microcephaly, seizures, and global intellectual disabilities before the age of 5 years.[277] Rett syndrome patients also demonstrate a spectrum of sleep disturbances and autonomic and respiratory dysfunction, including erratic breathing while awake with periods of alternating hyperventilation, cyanosis, apnea, abnormal heart rate variability, and sudden death.[278-280] The course is typically progressive until early childhood when it becomes essentially static. The neuropathology consists of a small brain with an apparent disturbance of neuronal development, characterized by dendritic spine abnormalities (decreased spine density, simplified branching) and small, densely packed neurons (Fig. 7.24).[281-283]

The gene involved encodes an X-linked methyl-CpG-binding protein 2 (MeCP2) that selectively binds CpG dinucleotides and mediates transcriptional repression.[276,284-286] MeCP2 regulates the expression of numerous genes, including brain-derived neurotrophic factor (BDNF), and can mediate transcriptional activation, mRNA splicing, and posttranslational procession of microRNAs.[280] Initial data indicate a critical role of MeCP2 in regulation of activity-dependent dendritic growth and

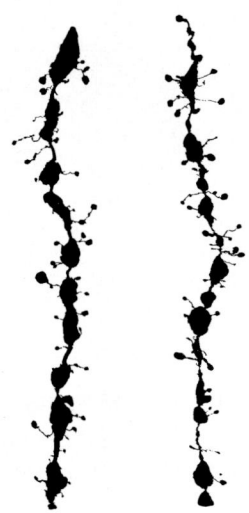

Figure 7.23 Camera lucida drawings of distal dendritic segments from an infant with mental retardation and seizures. Note the irregular varicosities of the dendritic segments. (From Purpura DP, Bodick N, Suzuki K, et al. Microtubule disarray in cortical dendrites and neurobehavioral failure. I. Golgi and electron microscopic studies. *Brain Res.* 1982;281:287–297.)

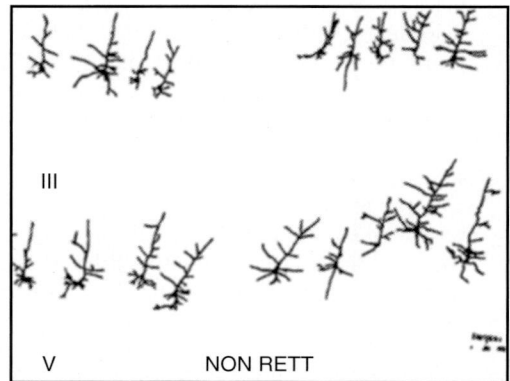
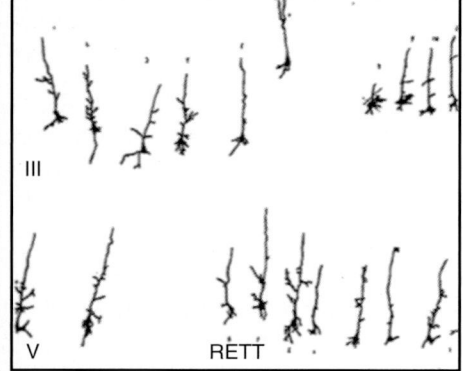

Figure 7.24 Decreased spine density and simplified branching in dendrites of Rett cortical neurons compared to controls using the Golgi method. (From Armstrong D, et al. Selective dendritic alterations in the cortex of Rett syndrome. *J Neuropathol Exp Neurol.* 1995;54:195–201, with permission.)

synaptic maturation.[287] Disturbed synaptogenesis has been identified.[286,288] (A rare male disorder secondary to MeCP2 defects is described in Chapter 29.)

Autism Spectrum Disorder

Autism spectrum disorder (ASD) is a dramatic syndrome characterized by deficits in language and cognitive spheres and by behavioral and repetitive abnormalities. There is a lack of social interaction, with avoidance of eye contact, as well as deficits in verbal and nonverbal communication, emotional control, and understanding the emotions of others.[289] There are also early delays in basic face processing.[290] ASD affects males 2 to 3 times more frequently than females.[289] In the first year of life, infants later diagnosed with ASD are not easily distinguished from normal: by 3 years of age, however, the core symptoms in social communication and restricted/ repetitive behaviors, as well as atypical language trajectories, are clinically expressed.[289]

ASD is not considered a single disorder, but rather, a spectrum of related disorders due to multiple causes resulting from the interaction of genetic and nongenetic risk factors. It can be associated with (caused by) monogenetic disorders, including fragile X syndrome, Rett syndrome (loss of function of MeCP2 protein), and tuberous sclerosis. Recently, there has been an explosion in our understanding of the genetics of ASD risk due to the concentrated efforts of international consortiums that sample thousands of autistic cases compared to controls. Using whole exome sequencing, analysis of rare coding variation in 3871 autism cases and 9937 controls implicated 22 autosomal genes, as well as a set of 107 autosomal genes strongly enriched for those likely to affect risk.[291] The 107 genes incurred loss-of-function mutations in more than 5% of the autistic subjects.[291] Many of the genes encode mainly proteins for synaptic, transcriptional, and chromatin remodeling pathways.

Environmental factors, in addition to genetic factors, are implicated in the pathogenesis of ASD. Prenatal factors related with ASD include exposure to teratogens, such as maternal valproic acid use for seizures,[289] and maternal selective serotonin reuptake inhibitors (SSRIs) use for depression.[289] Perinatal factors include low birth weight, prematurity, and birth asphxia.[289] Studies of survivors of extreme prematurity show an increased prevalence of an atypical social-behavioral profile strongly suggestive of ASD, with abnormalities in cerebellar size and prematurity-related cerebellar injury (infarcts, hemorrhages).[292] A role for cerebellar abnormalities in autism has been postulated in autistic brains.[293,294] The role of the cerebellum in ASD is supported by recognition that this structure is important for social cognition and emotion via extensive cortical interconnections, and not solely involved in sensory-motor control.[295]

Overall, available data suggest *a complex disturbance of neuronal organizational events in brain development*. These organizational events center mainly, but not exclusively, on overall brain growth, synaptogenesis, lamination, and axonal connectivity. The emphasis on synaptogenesis comes primarily from the genetic studies in which there is a convergence of genetic variants in components of synaptic regulation, including receptors, ion channels, neuronal pacemaking proteins, scaffolding proteins, and related transcription and splicing.[291] The emphasis on axonal connectivity is based primarily on neuroimaging studies in living autistic subjects compared to controls.[296] Depending on the experimental paradigm, the major networks implicated in ASD include (1) socioemotional networks, including face processing; (2) corticocerebellar networks[295]; (3) networks involving the interaction between primary sensory networks and subcortical networks (basal ganglia and thalamus)[297]; and (4) higher association frontal networks.[298]

Many neuroimaging studies, mainly involving MRI measures, have provided *neurocorrelates* of the morphological abnormalities.[296] Thus abnormalities have been identified in total and regional brain volumes, sulcal depth, cortical folding, cortical thickness, cortical surface area, regional gyrification, microstructure of white matter tracts, connectivity, and functional networks. Interestingly many of these abnormalities are not apparent in older children and adults with ASD.[299]

Down Syndrome

Down syndrome (trisomy 21) is the most common inherited form of intellectual disability in the United States, affecting 1/700 live births.[300] In early life, the phenotype of Down syndrome is characterized by short stature, abnormal facies, congenital heart disease, developmental delay, global intellectual disability, seizures, and hypotonia that vary in severity from trivial to serious compromise to fatal (inoperable complex congenital heart disease). Still, the survival rate of individuals with Down syndrome has dramatically increased from less than 50% during the mid-1990s to 95% in the early 2000s with a current median life expectancy of 60 years.[301] In their fourth and fifth decades, individuals with Down syndrome develop the cognitive and pathological hallmarks of early-onset Alzheimer disease (AD) with progressive dementia and memory deficits.[302] The brains of individuals with Down syndrome in childhood are about 20% smaller than normally developing brains, even on correction for reduced body size.[303] The brain is brachycephalic with a small cerebellum, simplified gyral appearance, and narrow superior temporal gyrus.[304,305]

Striking abnormalities of dendritic and axonal development have been described in infants with Down syndrome.[75,113,273,306-314] The abnormalities include alterations in cortical lamination, reduced dendritic branching, diminished dendritic spines and synapses, giant spines, and abnormal spine shape.[75,273,306,308-314] Abnormalities are not apparent before 22 weeks of gestation (i.e., before the rapid progression of organizational events). The emergence of lamination, for example, is both delayed and disorganized, notable after 20 to 21 weeks of gestation and over the next 7 to 10 weeks.[266] In the first months of postnatal life, an *excess* in dendritic branching *precedes* the consistent *decrease* observed after approximately 6 months of age. This sequence of excessive initial branching followed by deficits is similar to that seen in certain animal models of impaired dendritic development. Notably, neurons of layers II and IV, which use GABA as neurotransmitter, are deficient in number, and this disturbance would be expected to result in decreased inhibitory activity (i.e., hyperexcitability) in the cerebral cortex in Down syndrome. Two additional factors favor hyperexcitability in the cortex in Down syndrome: the specific nature of the disturbances of ion channels and the shape of dendrite spines. Together with decreased inhibitory activity, these three factors may explain the 5% to 10% incidence of seizures in these patients.[315,316] The demonstration of a defect in antioxidant capacity in Down syndrome neurons, with resulting free radical–mediated cell death, provides another important possible cause for the neuronal disturbance in Down syndrome.[317]

Delayed myelination also has been reported in young children but not in fetuses or newborns with Down syndrome.[318] Brains are affected with delayed myelination in about 23% of individuals with Down syndrome compared to approximately 7% in non-Down syndrome controls.[318] In particular, dysregulation of genes associated with oligodendrocyte differentiation and myelination has been detected in Down syndrome brain and validated via a cross-species comparison to the TS65Dn trisomy mouse model of Down syndrome.[319] Comorbidities of Down syndrome, for example, hypothyroidism, congenital heart disease, and leukemia, contribute to the spectrum of neuropathology in affected individuals. Infants with Down syndrome undergoing cardiac surgery during the first year of life, for example, demonstrate poorer neurodevelopmental outcomes as older infants/toddlers compared to those with Down syndrome without congenital heart disease.[320]

The increased expression of certain genes on Human Chromosome 21 (HC21), alone or in cooperation, is thought to be responsible for the Down syndrome phenotype, including intellectual disability, congenital heart defects, gastrointestinal malformations, immune and endocrine system defects, and early onset of dementia of the Alzheimer type. One such gene encodes a dual specificity tyrosine phosphorylation-regulated kinase 1A (*Dyrk1A*). Dyrk1A is a multifunctional protein kinase with various substrates, such as transcription factors, splicing factors, and synapse-associated proteins.[321] Dyrk1A plays a critical role in neurodevelopment, including neuronal differentiation and synaptic plasticity.[321] The overexpression of the gene for the amyloid precursor protein on HC21 leads to early-onset beta-amyloid plaques in Down syndrome; in addition, affected middle-aged individuals also develop neurofibrillary tangles, neuronal loss, cerebrovascular pathology, white matter alterations, oxidative damage, and neuroinflammation.[322] Information regarding the evolution of AD pathology in Down syndrome has led to a clearer understanding of the temporal and spatial pathogenesis of AD and has suggested a role for amyloid precursor protein both in neurodevelopment in early life and neurodegeneration in early life and neurodegeneration in aging.[323]

Fragile X Syndrome

Fragile X syndrome is a common form of inherited intellectual disability and the leading cause of inherited autism.[324] It is also a disorder mainly of male patients,[325-330] with approximately 1 in 5000 boys affected.[331] The characteristic features of fragile X syndrome other than intellectual disability and autism include language deficits, seizures, sensory hypersensitivity, and hyperarousal. The diagnosis was formerly based on the cytogenetic finding of a fragile site on the X chromosome, which is induced when cells are grown in medium with low folic acid and thymidine. Highly accurate direct DNA diagnostic testing is now widely available for identification of the fragile X syndrome.[328] The molecular defect involves the presence of a large amplification of a trinucleotide repeat sequence in the fragile X gene (*Fmr1*) that causes transcriptional silencing and loss of expression of the fragile X mental retardation protein (FMRP),[332] which is thought to be responsible for the disease signs and symptoms. FMRP is a selective RNA-binding

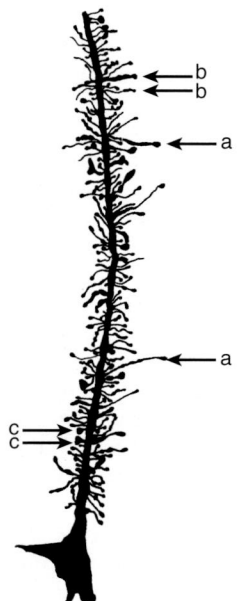

Figure 7.25 Composite camera lucida drawing of Golgi-stained, neocortical, apical dendrite in patients with fragile X syndrome. Note long, tortuous spines with prominent terminal heads *(a)* and irregular dilations *(b)* admixed with apparent decrease of normal short, stubby spines *(c)*. (From Hinton VJ, Brown WT, Wisniewski K, Rudelli RD. Analysis of neocortex in three males with the fragile X syndrome. *Am J Med Genet.* 1991;41:289.)

protein that inhibits the translation of its RNA targets and is most highly expressed in the brain.[331] Many genes bound by FMRP participate in *modulating synaptic plasticity*.[331] Because of the numerous genes affected by the loss of FMRP-regulated translational controls, multiple neuronal signaling pathways involved in local translation are affected, including pathways associated with metabotropic glutamate receptors, ERK, mTOR, GABA receptors, matrix metalloproteinases, and other factors.[324]

The *neuropathology of fragile X syndrome is notable for abnormal dendritic spine morphology* (Fig. 7.25) by Golgi analysis of neocortical neurons.[273,327,329,333,334] The principal findings are an increase in long dendritic spines, fewer short spines, more immature-appearing spines, and fewer mature-appearing spines. That the dendritic abnormality is related to the genetic defect is supported by the finding of similarly abnormal dendritic spines in fragile X gene *(FMR1)* knockout mice.[330,335-337] Thus *these observations may indicate that the crucial morphologic disturbance in this common form of mental retardation involves cortical dendritic development.* The mechanism of this disturbed development appears to relate to the obligatory role played by the FMRP in controlling synaptic plasticity and cytoskeletal organization during neuronal development.[330,338]

Structural MRI studies indicate enlarged gray matter volumes in the caudate and thalamus, as well as in the frontal, cingulate, and fusiform gyri.[324] The basis of this overgrowth is unknown. The most reproducible MRI abnormality is caudate enlargement, implicated in dysfunction in frontostriatal networks in fragile X syndrome. A diffusion tractography study in males with the syndrome also reports an increased density of fiber connections compared to controls, particularly in frontostriatal pathways.[339]

Disorders of Axonal Outgrowth

Impaired axonal development occurs in multiple pediatric disorders of the central and peripheral nervous systems leading to a spectrum of clinical disability. Central disorders in which axonal maldevelopment is primary, selective, or predominant in early life are illustrated here. Axonal injury in the encephalopathy of prematurity is discussed in Chapters 14 to 16, and agenesis of the corpus callosum is discussed in Chapter 2.

Agenesis of the Corticospinal Tracts

This rare condition occurs in relative isolation or in association with diverse disorders, including X-linked congenital aqueductal stenosis, holoprosencephaly, anencephaly, porencephaly, hydranencephaly, Meckel syndrome, Moebius syndrome, agyria, microcephaly with arthrogryposis and renal hypoplasia, schizencephaly, Walker-Warburg syndrome, and hypoxic-ischemic lesions of the cerebral cortex.[340-342] The corticospinal tracts mediate voluntary motor activity, and their absence in early life results in reduced movement and, in some instances, the fetal akinesia deformation sequence.[341] The role of the corticospinal tract in motor dysfunction is underscored by the report of two sibling infants in whom relatively isolated agenesis of the corticospinal tract was associated with delayed motor development, head lag, and spasticity.[343] Agenesis of the corticospinal tract is due to either developmental defects or to destructive lesions rostral to the medulla before its outgrowth and elongation (i.e., in the embryonic period or early part of the second trimester). In anencephaly and holoprosencephaly (i.e., disorders of cortical formation in the embryonic period), for example, agenesis of the corticospinal tract is a constant feature. Destructive lesions to the precentral gyrus due to prenatal hypoxia-ischemia are also found.[340] Yet, this destructive damage likely occurs early in gestation (i.e., the first trimester or early second trimester) to result in anomalous development of the corticospinal tract and not secondary degeneration of axonal fibers, because the histologic hallmarks of acquired damage (i.e., gliosis, macrophagocytic infiltration, and/or wallerian degeneration) are not found. Congenital hemiplegia due to corticospinal tract abnormalities occurs in early life in association with multiple developmental and acquired lesions, including multicystic encephalomalacia, venous infarction, polymicrogyria, and periventricular leukomalacia (PVL),[344,345] and occurs in one-third of patients with the clinical diagnosis of cerebral palsy.[345] The severity of motor dysfunction in such patients correlates with the degree of asymmetry in diffusion measures in the pyramidal tracts, which are defined by diffusion tensor MRI tractography.[345]

Congenital Cranial Disinnervation Disorders

This rare group of genetic disorders is defined by congenital oculomotility syndromes that result from mutations *in genes that are critical to the development and connectivity of cranial motoneurons.*[346] Abnormalities of axonal targeting and anterograde axonal transport have been shown to be important.[346,347]

Other Disorders

Disorders that initial data suggest may be related to a primary disturbance of organizational events were the topic of two reports. Lyon and co-workers[348] described three infants, including two sisters, with a severe congenital encephalopathy manifested by an absent or minimal response to sensory stimuli and profound weakness and hypotonia. At autopsy, the predominant finding was a marked deficiency of cerebral axons with an associated marked decrease in size of corpus callosum and cerebral white matter. Multiple axonal swellings were present in the remaining axons. These authors postulated a primary disorder of axonal development and suggested that "the anomaly may be due to extension of the normal phenomenon of axonal elimination, related to a primary defect of the cytoskeleton." Disorders with somewhat similar findings have been reported.[349,350]

Disorders of Glial Proliferation and Differentiation

Astrocytes and microglia are increasingly recognized to play important roles in the pathogenesis of neurodevelopmental disorders and are not simply *bystanders* to neuronal dysfunction and pathology. Pathological dysfunction of astrocytes and microglia may lead to abnormalities in synapse maturation and function, given the role of these cells in these neural-specific functions. Detailed analyses of neurodevelopmental diseases with known genetic lesions (and their corresponding mouse models) are beginning to reveal that astrocyte dysfunction during development results in disease pathology. These disorders include Rett syndrome, fragile X mental retardation, fetal alcohol spectrum disorders, ASD, Alexander disease, and others. A common finding of many of these studies is that *astrocyte dysfunction has profound non-cell-autonomous effects on surrounding neurons;* thus understanding the mechanisms of astrocyte dysfunction may well be critical to future therapeutic strategies. In *Rett syndrome,* MeCP2-deficient astrocytes may affect normal neuronal development. Conditional reactivation of MeCP2 only in GFAP-positive cells partially rescued defects in MeCP2-deficient mice, including behavioral measures (locomotor activity and respiratory patterns) and neuroanatomical parameters (neuronal soma diameter, hippocampal dendritic branching, and expression of the SV protein vGlut1).[351] The evidence suggests that loss of MeCP2 function in astrocytes contributes to the developmental defects in neurons of MeCP2-deficient mice. *In fragile X syndrome,* immunohistochemical studies demonstrate FMRP expression in developing astrocytes in vitro and possibly in vivo as well. Hippocampal neurons grown on FMR1-deficient astrocytes show abnormal dendritic morphology relative to those grown on wild-type astrocytes,[352] and the intrinsic dendritic defects of FMR1-deficient neurons are significantly rescued when these cells are grown on a monolayer of wild-type astrocytes. *Alexander disease* is currently the only known disease due to a mutation in an astrocyte-specific protein—GFAP (see Chapter 29). The cardinal pathological finding of cytoplasmic GFAP aggregates in astrocytes led to the discovery that gain-of-function point mutations in GFAP are responsible for the disease.[353] The exact mechanism of astrocyte dysfunction is unclear, but the presence of white matter abnormality indicates effects on oligodendrocytes and myelination.

Disorders of Multiple Organizational Events Delineated In Vivo—Related to Prematurity-Related Factors, Nutritional Factors, and Experiential Effects

The application of advanced MRI methodologies to infants in the premature and perinatal periods has provided strong evidence for acquired (nongenetic) disturbances of organizational events

TABLE 7.7 Advanced Magnetic Resonance Imaging Measures of Impaired Organizational Events in Premature Infants

MRI MEASURE	MAJOR FINDINGS
Volumetric MRI	Decreased regional volumes, especially cerebral cortex, white matter, basal ganglia, thalamus, and cerebellum
Diffusion tensor imaging	Decreased fractional anisotropy in white matter, relatively increased radial diffusivity, variably altered axial diffusivity
Surface-based measures	Decreased cerebral cortical surface area and cortical folding/gyrification
Functional MRI	Impaired development of measures of connectivity, including especially thalamocortical connectivity

MRI, Magnetic resonance imaging.

TABLE 7.8 Clinical Correlates in Premature Infants of Advanced Magnetic Resonance Imaging Findings Consistent With Impaired Organizational Events[a]

- Cerebral white matter injury (periventricular leukomalacia spectrum)
- Very low gestational age
- Intrauterine growth retardation
- Postnatal undernutrition/impaired body growth
- Other prematurity-related factors
  - Germinal matrix-intraventricular hemorrhage/periventricular hemorrhagic infarction
- Postnatal systemic infection
  - Dexamethasone administration
  - Pain, stress
  - Morphine administration
  - Patent ductus arteriosus
  - Systemic *illness,* chronic respiratory disease

[a]See text for references.

(see Table 7.6). These disturbances include primarily the variety of deleterious factors associated with *prematurity, nutritional factors*, and *experiential effects*. These three major categories of disturbance are outlined next.

Prematurity—Related Factors

The most common clinical setting associated with disturbances in organizational events is prematurity, especially extreme prematurity. The disturbances are identified, albeit imperfectly, in the living infant primarily by application of the advanced MRI measures described earlier (see Table 7.5). Although the findings are not perfectly consistent, the major changes are measured as follows: by volumetric MRI, decreased total and regional volumes of cerebral cortical regions, cerebral white matter, basal ganglia, thalamus, and cerebellum; by DTI and tractography, lower FA in white matter tracts, impaired development of white matter tracts, involvement of both radial and axial diffusivity, with relatively greater involvement of the former (consistent with involvement of both preoligodendrocyte ensheathment and axons, with perhaps greater involvement of the former); by surface-based measures, diminished cerebral cortical surface area, cortical folding and gyral development; and by fMRI, impaired development of measures of connectivity, especially thalamo-cortical connectivity (Table 7.7).

It should be emphasized that there is considerable variability in the results of the advanced MRI analyses, whether obtained in the neonatal period, usually at term-equivalent age, or subsequently in infancy, childhood, adolescence, and adulthood. The general themes just noted generally persist beyond the neonatal period but often become attenuated or change somewhat in regional characteristics. The effects of such postnatal factors as nutrition, social and parenting factors, educational interventions, and perhaps especially, intrinsic capacity for brain plasticity are important, but not often addressed and difficult to quantify. For this discussion, emphasis is placed on neonatal studies in this context of organizational events of the premature period.

The most prominent clinical correlates of the organizational defects in premature infants defined by advanced MRI are shown in Table 7.8. Although many of the correlates occur in varying combinations, they are discussed separately for convenience.

Cerebral White Matter Injury/Periventricular Leukomalacia Spectrum

Cerebral WMI occurs principally in the context of the PVL spectrum (see Chapters 14 to 16). During the early premature period, this lesion affects at least 50% of infants with varying degrees of severity. As described in detail in Chapter 14, the injury is characterized by varying combinations of two components, that is, focal necrosis deep in cerebral white matter and a more diffuse nonnecrotic white matter lesion characterized by astrogliosis and microgliosis. In modern-day neonatal intensive care facilities, the more diffuse component of the lesion is more prominent, and the focal necrotic component is small (often microscopic) and less prominent. This point is of extreme importance, because such clinical neuroimaging methods as ultrasonography and most clinical MRI scanners are relatively insensitive to the diffuse component, and even the focal lesions are usually microscopic in size and likely below the resolution of current neuroimaging methods, including MRI. In studies of premature infants with the conventional MRI characteristics of WMI, disturbances of advanced MR measures consistent with impaired organizational events are well documented, at term-equivalent age and subsequently.

Volumetric studies at term equivalent age show, as noted in Table 7.7, diminished volumetric development of cerebral cortex, cerebral white matter, thalamus, and basal ganglia.[238,354-359] The progression of the decrement of thalamic volume in premature infants with cystic PVL over the weeks to term equivalent age is shown in Fig. 7.26.

Similarly, *diffusion tensor studies* of infants with WMI studied at term equivalent age or subsequently show altered microstructural organization of multiple cerebral white matter tracts, including corticospinal tracts, cerebral white matter fasciculi, and corpus callosum.[241,242,361-366] Relative changes in the premature period of radial and axial diffusivities are most consistent with a disturbance in ensheathment of preoligodendrocytes, an active process at this time (see earlier), although some evidence also exists for axonal disturbance, either a primary effect or a secondary, trophic effect related to the failure of ensheathment (see Chapter 14).

Cortical folding MR measures also show deficits in infants with WMI.[240] The most distinguishing measures were sulcal depth and GI (Fig. 7.27). These disturbances could relate to decreases in cortical surface area or to white matter disturbance or both (see earlier concerning determinants of cortical folding).

fMRI analyses and therefore measures of connectivity in premature infants with WMI have been accomplished only recently.[251,367] Disturbed development of RS networks has also been shown. The data may reflect a combination of impairments of cerebral white matter, cerebral cortical, and thalamic development (see next).

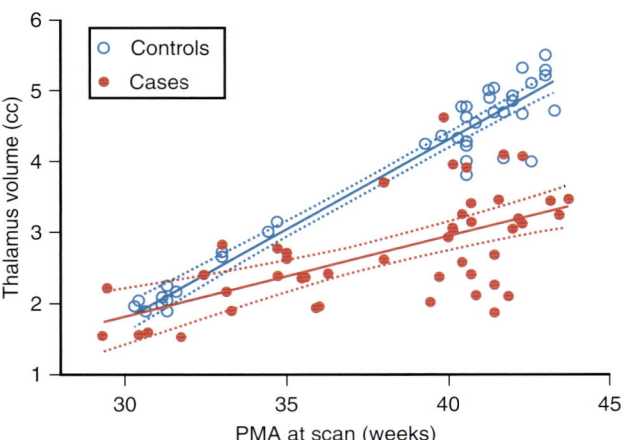

Figure 7.26 Difference in absolute thalamic volumes in preterm infants with cystic periventricular leukomalacia and control infants. (From Kersbergen KJ, et al. Corticospinal tract injury precedes thalamic volume reduction in preterm infants with cystic periventricular leukomalacia. *J Pediatr.* 2015;167:260–268, with permission.)

Potential mechanisms of organizational disturbances with WMI include a complex amalgam of destructive events and developmental disturbances. In cerebral WMI, the primary event is most likely a destructive process (*injury*) and the subsequent trophic/maturational, that is, developmental disturbances are secondary. Fig. 7.28 shows the most probable scenarios of primary injury leading to the secondary developmental organizational deficits defined by the advanced MR measures. It deserves emphasis that the initiating *injury* may reflect the action of an insult on a *specific developmental program* and not necessarily a disruption of cellular or subcellular *structure*. These scenarios and the evidence for each are discussed in detail in Chapters 14 to 16.

Very Low Gestational Age

The degree of immaturity, as reflected in gestational age, is an important and likely independent correlate of MRI measures of impaired organizational events (see Table 7.8). The important caveat, however, is that diffuse, nonnecrotic WMI is often below the resolution capabilities of clinical MR measures; thus WMI may be overlooked. Nonetheless, several important studies have shown subsequent developmental disturbances by advanced MR analyses, in the apparent absence of WMI, with an apparent inverse relation of the severity of the MR abnormalities with gestational age. The abnormalities involve development of cerebral volumes, fiber tracts, cortical surface area, cortical folding, and connectivity. Examples are shown in Figs. 7.29 and 7.30.[242,257-260,368-377] The organizational events likely affected are similar to those just described for cerebral WMI.

Intrauterine Growth Retardation

Intrauterine undernutrition is a principal feature of intrauterine growth retardation (IUGR). Neurodevelopmental impairment after IUGR is well documented, especially in IUGR infants born preterm.[378-380] Although direct injury to the brain, especially ischemic in nature, may occur with IUGR, overt destructive lesions are uncommon. The limited imaging data available

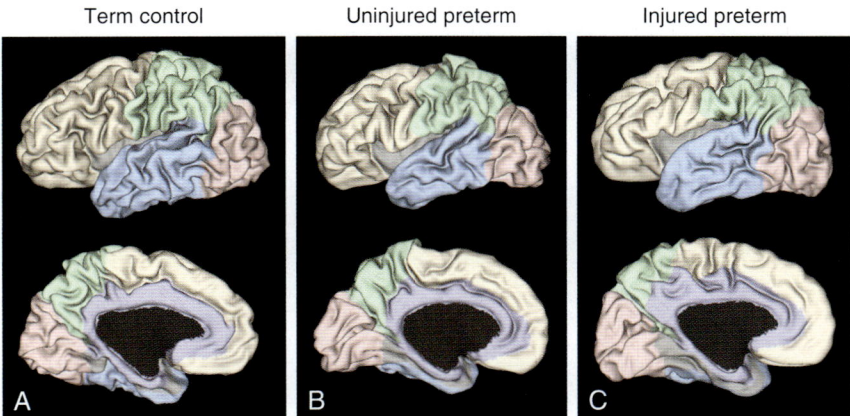

Figure 7.27 Representative left hemispheres at term equivalent PMA from (A) term, (B) uninjured preterm, and (C) injured preterm infants. Note the decrease in sulcal depth and complexity of the temporal index surface from term through injured preterm. Each example was chosen because it provided the result closest to the mean sulcal depth value for each group. The area corresponding to the temporal lobe is shown in light blue, the occipital lobe in rose, the parietal lobe in green, the frontal lobe in yellow, and the limbic area in purple. (From Shimony JS, et al. Comparison of cortical folding measures for evaluation of developing human brain. *Neuroimage.* 2016;125:180–190, with permission.)

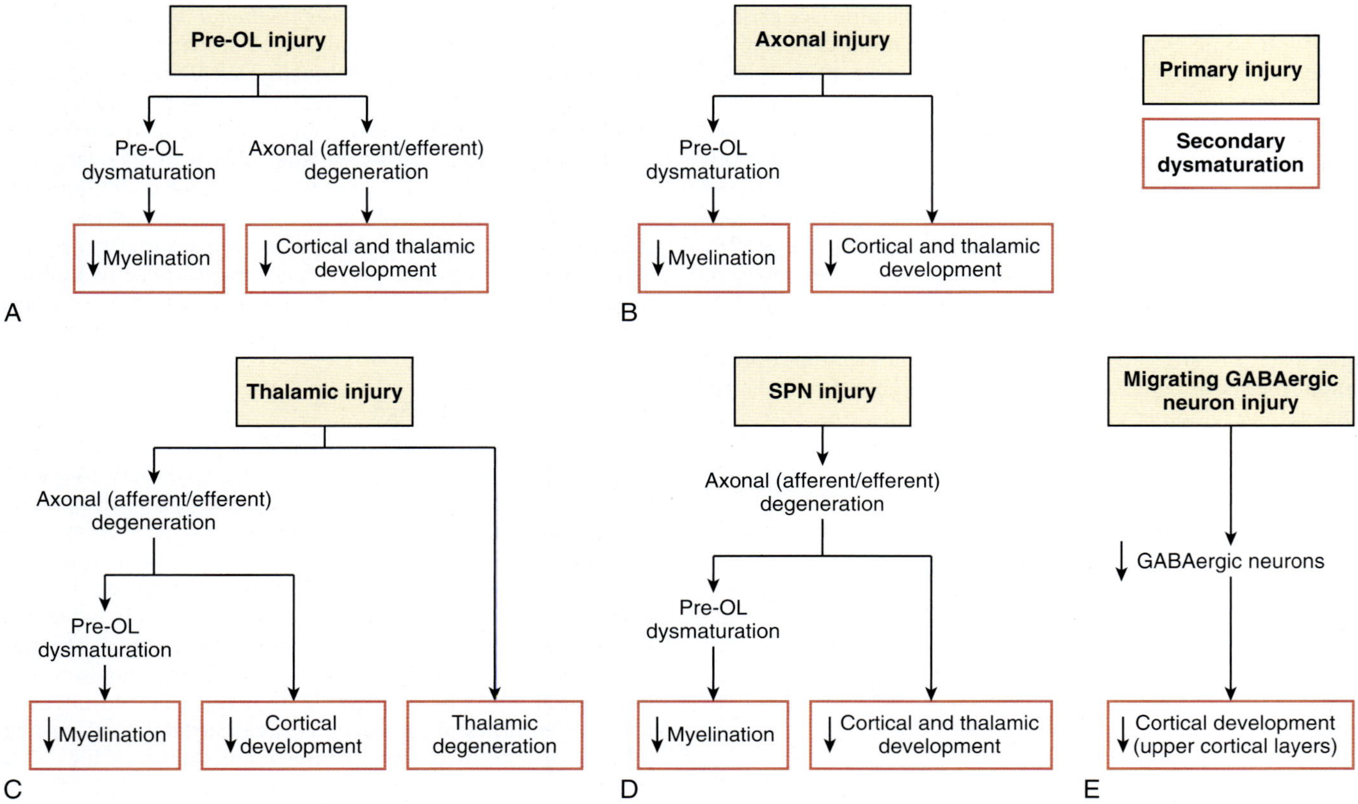

A

Pre-OL injury

Pre-OL dysmaturation

↓Myelination

Axonal (afferent/efferent) degeneration

↓Cortical and thalamic development

B

Axonal injury

Pre-OL dysmaturation

↓Myelination

↓Cortical and thalamic development

Primary injury

Secondary dysmaturation

C

Thalamic injury

Axonal (afferent/efferent) degeneration

Pre-OL dysmaturation

↓Myelination

↓Cortical development

Thalamic degeneration

D

SPN injury

Axonal (afferent/efferent) degeneration

Pre-OL dysmaturation

↓Myelination

↓Cortical and thalamic development

E

Migrating GABAergic neuron injury

↓GABAergic neurons

↓Cortical development (upper cortical layers)

Figure 7.28 Potential sequences of events leading to major brain sequelae observed with periventricular leukomalacia. Potential events are hypomyelination, and impaired cortical and thalamic development (e.g., seen on advanced MR analysis by decreased volume). For each sequence the initiating primary injury is shown, and the subsequent secondary effects are postulated to occur because of maturational/trophic disturbances, as described in the text. *Pre-OL*, Premyelinating oligodendrocyte; *SPN*, subplate neuron. (From Volpe JJ. Brain injury in premature infants: a complex amalgam of destructive and developmental disturbances. *Lancet.* 2009;8:110–124, with permission.)

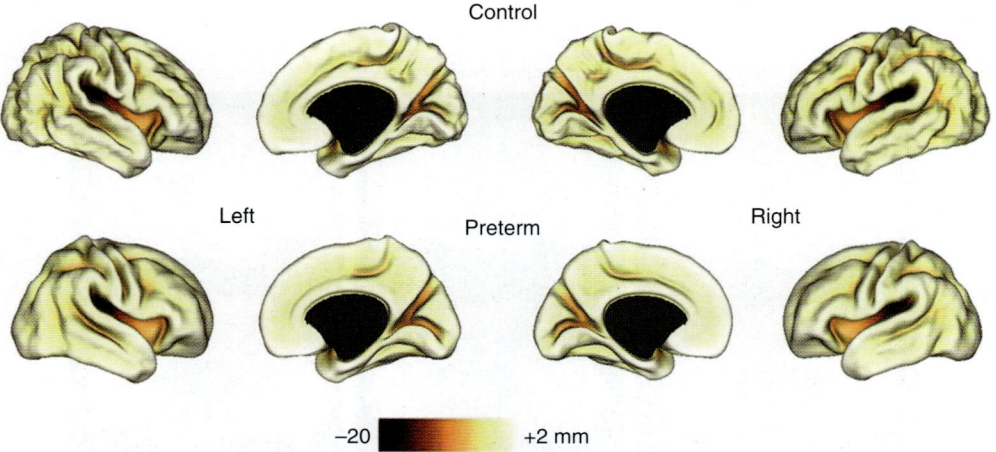

Control

Left   Preterm   Right

−20   +2 mm

Figure 7.29 Decreased gyrification and sulcal depth in preterm infants. Average sulcal depth maps are overlaid. The color bar depicts the scale of sulcal depths in millimeters. Note the decreased gyrification and diminished sulcal depth in the preterms, especially apparent on the lateral views. (From Engelhardt E, et al. Regional impairments of cortical folding in premature infants. *Ann Neurol.* 2015;77:154–162, with permission.)

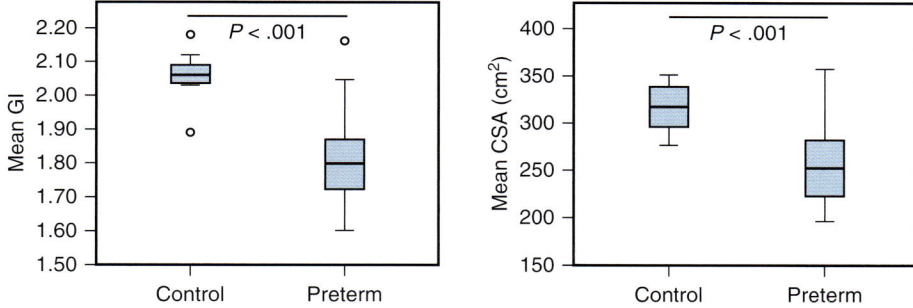

Figure 7.30 Differences in gyrification index (GI) and cortical surface area (CSA) between preterm and control infants. (From Engelhardt E, et al. Regional impairments of cortical folding in premature infants. *Ann Neurol.* 2015;77:154–162, with permission.)

suggest that IUGR, especially in preterms, is associated primarily with impairment of organizational events.

In a seminal report of 28 preterm infants with IUGR and placental insufficiency and studied by volumetric MRI early and at term equivalent age, the preterm infants with IUGR exhibited a 15% lower total brain volume and a 30% lower cerebral cortical gray matter volume than did normally grown preterm control infants.[381] The differences persisted at term equivalent age. No difference in white matter or basal ganglia/thalamus volumes was observed at either age. A subsequent study by the same group showed around birth not only lower cerebral cortical volume, but also reduced cerebral cortical surface area.[382] A later report of preterm infants with and without IUGR and studied at term equivalent age confirmed the reduction in cortical gray matter volume with IUGR and importantly, a 10% reduction in hippocampal volume.[383] The hippocampal effect is noteworthy, because nutritional deprivation during pregnancy is known to increase fetal cortisol levels, and excess corticosteroids have been shown to impair hippocampal growth in subhuman primates.[384] Preterm infants with IUGR studied at 12 months of age showed bilateral reduction in several cortical areas, including the temporal regions.[385] The relative roles of nutritional deficiency, hypoxemia, corticoid exposure in these deleterious effects of IUGR remain to be delineated. In addition, the exact nature of the developmental events involved in these effects at the anatomical level also is unknown.

Presumed Postnatal Undernutrition in Premature Infants

Several lines of evidence suggest that *appropriate nutrition during the premature period* is important for neurodevelopmental outcome and, perhaps therefore, organizational events and that *postnatal undernutrition* is deleterious. Thus multiple studies show that infants with impaired growth during the premature period exhibit poorer neurodevelopmental outcomes than do infants with normal growth.[386-392] Moreover, enhanced nutritional intake, breast feeding, and supplementation with long-chain polyunsaturated fatty acids (e.g., docosahexaenoic acid) enhance both growth and neurodevelopmental outcome in premature infants in most (though not all) studies.[390,393-401]

Insight into a potential effect of postnatal nutrition on organizational events, specifically cerebral cortical development, was provided by a recent serial DTI study of premature infants, scanned first at a median age of 32 weeks' postconception and again at a median age of 40 weeks.[402] Impaired weight, length, and head growth were associated with delayed microstructural development (FA) of cerebral cortical gray matter but not cerebral white matter. As noted earlier, normal maturation of cortex is associated with a decline in FA; presumably secondary to elaboration of neuronal processes consequent to influx of thalamocortical circuitry, late migrating neurons, and influences of subplate neuron connections; and a decline in RGFs. The normal decline in FA in cortex was blunted when body growth was impaired. The changes in FA principally reflected changes in radial diffusion but not axial diffusion, consistent with a delay in neuronal process formation. Notably, the normal increase in FA in cerebral white matter was not disturbed by the slower postnatal growth. These effects were independent of systemic illness, overt brain injury, or necrotizing enterocolitis. Neonatal caloric data were unavailable, but it seems likely that nutritional deficits occurred. The findings suggest that avoiding growth impairment during neonatal care could allow cortical development to proceed normally and perhaps, thereby, prevent subsequent neurodevelopmental disability.[402]

Other Prematurity-Related Factors

A variety of *other factors prevalent in premature infants* have been associated with abnormalities of MR analyses of cerebral volumes, diffusion characteristics of gray or white matter or both, cerebral cortical surface-based measures, and connectivity (see Table 7.8). These factors include germinal matrix-intraventricular hemorrhage, postnatal (systemic) infection, dexamethasone therapy, pain and stress, morphine administration, patent ductus arteriosus, respiratory complications, length of neonatal intensive care unit stay, IUGR, and postnatal nutritional factors/growth failure (see Table 7.8).[a] The imaging and clinical details relating to these factors are reviewed in Chapter 16. The degree to which these factors are accompanied by WMI undetected by conventional imaging (see earlier discussion) is largely unknown. Nevertheless, the findings suggest that the rapidly developing, complex organizational events; especially in the premature period, involving preoligodendroglial proliferation and differentiation, axonal development, subplate neuron structure and function, thalamic development, late migration of interneurons, cerebral cortical differentiation, and synaptic development; are exquisitely vulnerable to primary or secondary perturbation.

---

[a]References 237, 248, 250, 256-260, 368-377, and 402-415.

Experiential Effects

The potential impact of *experiential factors* in regulation of cortical organization was suggested initially by the demonstration that variations in maternal care or related alterations in the environment in experimental animals result in an increase in synaptogenesis.[416-418] Particularly elegant experiments in normal and preterm monkeys showed that premature visual stimulation results in increases in size and proportions of various synapses, presumably by alterations in normal synaptic modification or elimination.[419] Recent study of sensory deprivation in neonatal mice shows pronounced effects on dendritic development in cortex.[420] The likely importance of loss of excitatory input in the genesis of this developmental defect was shown by reproduction of the effect with chronic blockade of NMDA receptors. Studies in human infants suggest that, as in the experimental models, experiential effects are important mediators of certain organizational events. Visual experience of premature infants is associated with an accentuation of the development of visual evoked potentials, a finding consistent with enhancement of dendritic and axonal development and synaptogenesis.[421] In addition, a randomized clinical trial of an individualized developmental care program showed at 9 months' corrected age, improved neurobehavorial function, quantitative EEG evidence of enhanced maturation, and diffusion-tensor MRI evidence of more advanced cerebral white matter fiber tract development.[422] Moreover, a later randomized controlled trial assessed the effectiveness of training parents in reducing stressful experiences in premature infants less than 30-weeks' gestation in the neonatal intensive care unit.[423] The infants of the mothers in the intervention group showed at term equivalent age significantly enhanced maturation and connectivity of cerebral white matter by DTI. The potential role of experiential effects in the neonatal intensive care unit is supported further by a recent report comparing language performance at two years of age in premature infants cared for in a bed space in an active open ward or in a private room in the same hospital.[410] Language scores were higher in the infants cared for in the open ward. More data clearly are needed in these promising areas, especially since the findings have important implications for management.

KEY REFERENCES

1. Luskin MB, Shatz CJ. Studies of the earliest generated cells of the cat's visual cortex: cogeneration of subplate and marginal zones. *J Neurosci.* 1985;5:1062-1075.
2. McConnell SK, Ghosh A, Shatz CJ. Subplate neurons pioneer the first axon pathway from the cerebral cortex. *Science.* 1989;245: 978-982.
4. Friauf E, McConnell SK, Shatz CJ. Functional synaptic circuits in the subplate during fetal and early postnatal development of cat visual cortex. *J Neurosci.* 1990;10:2601-2613.
7. Friauf E, Shatz CJ. Changing patterns of synaptic input to subplate and cortical plate during development of visual cortex. *J Neurophysiol.* 1991;66:2059-2071.
8. Ghosh A, Shatz CJ. Involvement of subplate neurons in the formation of ocular dominance columns. *Science.* 1992;255:1441-1443.
10. Volpe JJ. Subplate neurons—missing link in brain injury of the premature infant? *Pediatrics.* 1996;97:112-113.
11. Marin-Padilla M. Cajal-Retzius cells in the development of the neocortex. *Trends Neurosci.* 1998;21:64-71.

13. Kostovic I, Judas M. Correlation between the sequential ingrowth of afferents and transient patterns of cortical lamination in preterm infants. *Anat Rec.* 2002;267:1-6.
14. Kanold PO, Kara P, Reid RC, et al. Role of subplate neurons in functional maturation of visual cortical columns. *Science.* 2003;301: 521-525.
17. McQuillen PS, Ferriero DM. Perinatal subplate neuron injury: implications for cortical development and plasticity. *Brain Pathol.* 2005;15:250-260.
20. Kostovic I, Judas M. The development of the subplate and thalamocortical connections in the human foetal brain. *Acta Paediatr.* 2010;99:1119-1127.
22. Silbereis JC, Pochareddy S, Zhu Y, et al. The cellular and molecular landscapes of the developing human central nervous system. *Neuron.* 2016;89:248-268.
23. Kostovic I, Kostovic-Srzentic M, Benjak V, et al. Developmental dynamics of radial vulnerability in the cerebral compartments in preterm infants and neonates. *Front Neurol.* 2014;5:1-13.
25. Miller JA, Ding SL, Sunkin SM, et al. Transcriptional landscape of the prenatal human brain. *Nature.* 2014;508:199-206.
26. Bystron I, Blakemore C, Rakic P. Development of the human cerebral cortex: Boulder Committee revisited. *Nat Rev Neurosci.* 2008;9: 110-122.
32. Suarez-Sola ML, Gonzalez-Delgado FJ, Pueyo-Morlans M, et al. Neurons in the white matter of the adult human neocortex. *Front Neuroanat.* 2009;3:7.
35. Marin-Padilla M. Ontogenesis of the pyramidal cell of the mammalian neocortex and developmental cytoarchitectonics: a unifying theory. *J Comp Neurol.* 1992;321:233-240.
36. Kinney HC, Armstrong DL. Perinatal neuropathology. In: Graham DI, Lantos PE, eds. *Greenfield's Neuropathology.* Vol. 1. 7th ed. London: Arnold Publishers; 2002:519-606.
37. Markram H, Toledo-Rodriguez M, Wang Y, et al. Interneurons of the neocortical inhibitory system. *Nat Rev Neurosci.* 2004;5:793-807.
38. Andiman SE, Haynes RL, Trachtenberg FL, et al. The cerebral cortex overlying periventricular leukomalacia: analysis of pyramidal neurons. *Brain Pathol.* 2010;20:803-814.
40. Xu G, Broadbelt KG, Haynes RL, et al. Late development of the GABAergic system in the human cerebral cortex and white matter. *J Neuropathol Exp Neurol.* 2011;70:841-858.
43. White T, Su S, Schmidt M, et al. The development of gyrification in childhood and adolescence. *Brain Cogn.* 2010;72:36-45.
44. Chi JG, Dooling EC, Gilles FH. Gyral development of the human brain. *Ann Neurol.* 1977;1:86-93.
48. Chi JG, Dooling EC, Gilles FH. Left-right asymmetries of the temporal speech areas of the human fetus. *Arch Neurol.* 1977;34:346-348.
50. Striedter GF, Srinivasan S, Monuki ES. Cortical folding: when, where, how, and why? *Annu Rev Neurosci.* 2015;38:291-307.
53. Conel J. *The Postnatal Development of the Human Cerebral Cortex.* Cambridge: Harvard University Press; 1939.
59. Sarnat HB, Nochlin D, Born DE. Neuronal nuclear antigen (NeuN): a marker of neuronal maturation in the early human fetal nervous system. *Brain Dev.* 1998;20:88-94.
63. Hevner RF. Development of connections in the human visual system during fetal mid-gestation: a DiI-tracing study. *J Neuropathol Exp Neurol.* 2000;59:385-392.
65. ten Donkelaar HJ, Lammens M, Wesseling P, et al. Development and malformations of the human pyramidal tract. *J Neurol.* 2004;251:1429-1442.
66. Haynes RL, Borenstein NS, DeSilva TM, et al. Axonal development in the cerebral white matter of the human fetus and infant. *J Comp Neurol.* 2005;484:156-167.
72. Molliver ME, Kostovic I, van der Loos H. The development of synapses in cerebral cortex of the human fetus. *Brain Res.* 1973;50: 403-407.
73. Marin-Padilla M. Abnormal neuronal differentiation (functional maturation) in mental retardation. In: Bergsma D, ed. *Morphogenesis and Malformation of Face and Brain.* New York, NY: Alan R. Liss; 1975:133.
74. Huttenlocher PR. Synaptic and dendritic development and mental defect. In: Buchwald NA, Brazier MAB, eds. *Brain Mechanisms in Mental Retardation.* New York, NY: Academic Press; 1975:123.

75. Purpura DP. Dendritic differentiation in human cerebral cortex: normal and aberrant developmental patterns. In: Kreutzberg GW, ed. *Advances in Neurology*. New York, NY: Raven Press; 1975:91.

78. Huttenlocher PR, de Courten C, Garey LJ, et al. Synaptogenesis in human visual cortex—evidence for synapse elimination during normal development. *Neurosci Lett*. 1982;33:247-252.

81. Becker LE, Armstrong DL, Chan F, et al. Dendritic development in human occipital cortical neurons. *Brain Res*. 1984;315:117-124.

82. Harris KM, Jensen FE, Tsao B. Three-dimensional structure of dendritic spines and synapses in rat hippocampus (CA1) at postnatal day 15 and adult ages: implications for the maturation of synaptic physiology and long-term potentiation. *J Neurosci*. 1992;12:2685-2705.

89. Chen YC, Ghosh A. Regulation of dendritic development by neuronal activity. *J Neurobiol*. 2005;64:4-10.

94. Talos DM, Fishman RE, Park H, et al. Developmental regulation of alpha-amino-3-hydroxy-5-methyl-4-isoxazole-propionic acid receptor subunit expression in forebrain and relationship to regional susceptibility to hypoxic/ischemic injury. I. Rodent cerebral white matter and cortex. *J Comp Neurol*. 2006;497:42-60.

95. Talos DM, Follett PL, Folkerth RD, et al. Developmental regulation of alpha-amino-3-hydroxy-5-methyl-4-isoxazole-propionic acid receptor subunit expression in forebrain and relationship to regional susceptibility to hypoxic/ischemic injury. II. Human cerebral white matter and cortex. *J Comp Neurol*. 2006;497:61-77.

96. Haynes RL, Kinney HC. Central axonal development and pathology in early life. In: *Handbook of Neurochemistry and Molecular Neurobiology*. New York, NY: Springer-Verlag; 2012.

97. Hirokawa N, Takemura R. Kinesin superfamily proteins and their various functions and dynamics. *Exp Cell Res*. 2004;301:50-59.

99. Takahashi E, Folkerth RD, Galaburda AM, et al. Emerging cerebral connectivity in the human fetal brain: an MR tractography study. *Cereb Cortex*. 2012;22:455-464.

101. Takashima S, Mito T. Neuronal development in the medullary reticular formation in sudden infant death syndrome and premature infants. *Neuropediatrics*. 1985;16:76-79.

104. Huttenlocher PR, Dabholkar AS. Regional differences in synaptogenesis in human cerebral cortex. *J Comp Neurol*. 1997;387:167-178.

106. Rakic P, Bourgeois JP, Eckenhoff MF, et al. Concurrent overproduction of synapses in diverse regions of the primate cerebral cortex. *Science*. 1986;232:232-235.

115. Hamburger V, Oppenheim RW. Naturally occurring neuronal death in vertebrates. *Neuroscience*. 1982;1:39.

116. Rakic P, Riley KP. Overproduction and elimination of retinal axons in the fetal rhesus monkey. *Science*. 1983;219:1441-1444.

117. Cowan WM, Fawcett JW, O'Leary DD, et al. Regressive events in neurogenesis. *Science*. 1984;225:1258-1265.

118. Oppenheim RW. Cell death during development of the nervous system. *Annu Rev Neurosci*. 1991;14:453-501.

128. Rakic S, Zecevic N. Programmed cell death in the developing human telencephalon. *Eur J Neurosci*. 2000;12:2721-2734.

135. Kolb B, Whishaw IQ. Plasticity in the neocortex: mechanisms underlying recovery from early brain damage. *Prog Neurobiol*. 1989;32:235-276.

136. Chugani HT, Muller R-A, Chugani DC. Functional brain reorganization in children. *Brain Dev*. 1996;18:347-356.

139. Staudt M, Gerloff C, Grodd W, et al. Reorganization in congenital hemiparesis acquired at different gestational ages. *Ann Neurol*. 2004;56:854-863.

140. Johnston MV. Clinical disorders of brain plasticity. *Brain Dev*. 2004;26:73-80.

148. Farmer SF, Harrison LM, Ingram DA, et al. Plasticity of central motor pathways in children with hemiplegic cerebral palsy. *Neurology*. 1991;41:1505-1510.

153. Maegaki Y, Maeoka Y, Ishii S, et al. Central motor reorganization in cerebral palsy patients with bilateral cerebral lesions. *Pediatr Res*. 1999;45:559-567.

163. Cameron RS, Rakic P. Glial cell lineage in the cerebral cortex: a review and synthesis. *Glia*. 1991;4:124-137.

164. Misson JP, Takahashi T, Caviness VS Jr. Ontogeny of radial and other astroglial cells in murine cerebral cortex. *Glia*. 1991;4:138-148.

165. Knapp PE. Studies of glial lineage and proliferation in vitro using an early marker for committed oligodendrocytes. *J Neurosci Res*. 1991;30:336-345.

169. Luskin MB, Pearlman AL, Sanes JR. Cell lineage in the cerebral cortex of the mouse studied in vivo and in vitro with a recombinant retrovirus. *Neuron*. 1988;1:635-647.

172. Lopes-Cardozo M, Sykes JE, Van der Pal RH, et al. Development of oligodendrocytes. Studies of rat glial cells cultured in chemically-defined medium. *J Dev Physiol*. 1989;12:117-127.

176. Goldman JE, Geier SS, Hirano M. Differentiation of astrocytes and oligodendrocytes from germinal matrix cells in primary culture. *J Neurosci*. 1986;6:52-60.

181. Goldman JE. Regulation of oligodendrocyte differentiation. *Trends Neurosci*. 1992;15:359-362.

183. Barres BA, Hart IK, Coles HSR, et al. Cell death in the oligodendrocyte lineage. *J Neurobiol*. 1992;23:1221-1230.

185. Levison SW, Chuang C, Abramson BJ, et al. The migrational patterns and developmental fates of glial precursors in the rat subventricular zone are temporally regulated. *Development*. 1993;119:611-622.

187. Back SA, Volpe JJ. Cellular and molecular pathogenesis of periventricular white matter injury. *Ment Retard Dev Disabil Res Rev*. 1997;3:96-107.

188. Kinney HC, Back SA. Human oligodendroglial development: relationship to periventricular leukomalacia. *Semin Pediatr Neurol*. 1998;5:180-189.

193. Cai J, Qi YC, Hu XM, et al. Generation of oligodendrocyte precursor cells from mouse dorsal spinal cord independent of Nkx6 regulation and Shh signaling. *Neuron*. 2005;45:41-53.

194. Marshall CAG, Novitch BG, Goldman JE. Olig2 directs astrocyte and oligodendrocyte formation in postnatal subventricular zone cells. *J Neurosci*. 2005;25:7289-7298.

201. Back SA, Rosenberg PA. Pathophysiology of glia in perinatal white matter injury. *Glia*. 2014;62:1790-1815.

208. Armstrong DD. The neuropathology of the Rett syndrome. *Brain Dev*. 1992;14:S89-S98.

209. Marin-Padilla M. Prenatal development of fibrous (white matter), protoplasmic (gray matter), and layer 1 astrocytes in the human cerebral cortex: a Golgi study. *J Comp Neurol*. 1995;357:554-572.

210. Rivkin MJ, Flax J, Mozel R, et al. Oligodendroglial development in human fetal cerebrum. *Ann Neurol*. 1995;38:92-101.

213. Back SA, Luo NL, Borenstein NS, et al. Late oligodendrocyte progenitors coincide with the developmental window of vulnerability for human perinatal white matter injury. *J Neurosci*. 2001;21:1302-1312.

214. Back SA, Luo NL, Borenstein NS, et al. Arrested oligodendrocyte lineage progression during human cerebral white matter development: dissociation between the timing of progenitor differentiation and myelinogenesis. *J Neuropathol Exp Neurol*. 2002;61:197-211.

215. Jakovcevski I, Zecevic N. Sequence of oligodendrocyte development in the human fetal telencephalon. *Glia*. 2005;49:480-491.

216. Rakic S, Zecevic N. Early oligodendrocyte progenitor cells in the human fetal telencephalon. *Glia*. 2003;41:117-127.

218. Volpe JJ, Kinney HC, Jensen FE, et al. The developing oligodendrocyte: key cellular target in brain injury in the premature infant. *Int J Dev Neurosci*. 2011;29:423-440.

221. Marin-Padilla M. *The Human Brain: Prenatal Development and Structure*. Berlin: Springer-Verlag; 2011.

222. Attwell D, Buchan AM, Charpak S, et al. Glial and neuronal control of brain blood flow. *Nature*. 2010;468:232-243.

223. Hodge RD, Kahoud RJ, Hevner RF. Transcriptional control of glutamatergic differentiation during adult neurogenesis. *Cell Mol Life Sci*. 2012;69:2125-2134.

224. Letinic K, Zoncu R, Rakic P. Origin of GABAergic neurons in the human neocortex. *Nature*. 2002;417:645-649.

225. Xu G, Takahashi E, Folkerth RD, et al. Radial coherence of diffusion tractography in the cerebral white matter of the human fetus: neuroanatomic insights. *Cereb Cortex*. 2014;24:579-592.

226. Gould SJ, Howard S. An immunohistological study of macrophages in the human fetal brain. *Neuropathol Appl Neurobiol*. 1991;17:383-390.

228. Rezaie P, Male D. Colonisation of the developing human brain and spinal cord by microglia: a review. *Microsc Res Tech*. 1999;45:359-382.

234. Billiards SS, Haynes RL, Folkerth RD, et al. Development of microglia in the cerebral white matter of the human fetus and infant. *J Comp Neurol.* 2006;497:199-208.

237. Keunen K, Kersbergen KJ, Groenendaal F, et al. Brain tissue volumes in preterm infants: prematurity, perinatal risk factors and neurodevelopmental outcome: a systematic review. *J Matern Fetal Neonatal Med.* 2012;25:89-100.

238. Kwon SH, Vasung L, Ment LR, et al. The role of neuroimaging in predicting neurodevelopmental outcomes of preterm neonates. *Clin Perinatol.* 2014;41:257-283.

239. Tao JD, Neil JJ. Advanced magnetic resonance imaging techniques in the preterm brain: methods and applications. *Curr Pediatr Rev.* 2014;10:56-64.

240. Shimony JS, Smyser CD, Wideman G, et al. Comparison of cortical folding measures for evaluation of developing human brain. *Neuroimage.* 2016;125:780-790.

241. Pandit AS, Ball G, Edwards AD, et al. Diffusion magnetic resonance imaging in preterm brain injury. *Neuroradiology.* 2013;55:65-95.

242. Huppi PS, Maier SE, Peled S, et al. Microstructural development of human newborn cerebral white matter assessed in vivo by diffusion tensor magnetic resonance imaging. *Pediatr Res.* 1998;44:584-590.

246. McKinstry RC, Mathur A, Miller JH, et al. Radial organization of developing preterm human cerebral cortex revealed by non-invasive water diffusion anisotropy MRI. *Cereb Cortex.* 2002;12:1237-1243.

249. Li G, Lin W, Gilmore JH, et al. Spatial patterns, longitudinal development, and hemispheric asymmetries of cortical thickness in infants from birth to 2 years of age. *J Neurosci.* 2015;35:9150-9162.

250. Engelhardt E, Inder TE, Alexopoulos D, et al. Regional impairments of cortical folding in premature infants. *Ann Neurol.* 2015;77:154-162.

253. Seghier ML, Huppi PS. The role of functional magnetic resonance imaging in the study of brain development, injury, and recovery in the newborn. *Semin Perinatol.* 2010;34:79-86.

257. Smyser CD, Inder TE, Shimony JS, et al. Longitudinal analysis of neural network development in preterm infants. *Cereb Cortex.* 2010;20:2852-2862.

258. Ball G, Aljabar P, Zebari S, et al. Rich-club organization of the newborn human brain. *Proc Natl Acad Sci USA.* 2014;111:7456-7461.

259. van den Heuvel MP, Kersbergen KJ, de Reus MA, et al. The neonatal connectome during preterm brain development. *Cereb Cortex.* 2015;25:3000-3013.

266. Golden JA, Hyman BT. Development of the superior temporal neocortex is anomalous in trisomy 21. *J Neuropathol Exp Neurol.* 1994;53:513-520.

267. Purpura DP. Dendritic spine "dysgenesis" and mental retardation. *Science.* 1974;186:1126-1128.

268. Bodick N, Stevens JK, Sasaki S, et al. Microtubular disarray in cortical dendrites and neurobehavioral failure. II. Computer reconstruction of perturbed microtubular arrays. *Brain Res.* 1982;281:299-309.

271. Huttenlocher PR. Dendritic and synaptic pathology in mental retardation. *Pediatr Neurol.* 1991;7:79-85.

275. Amir RE, Van den Veyver IB, Schultz R, et al. Influence of mutation type and X chromosome inactivation on Rett syndrome phenotypes. *Ann Neurol.* 2000;47:670-679.

280. Johnston M, Blue ME, Naidu S. Recent advances in understanding synaptic abnormalities in Rett syndrome. *F1000Res.* 2015;4:F1000 Faculty Rev-1490.

283. Armstrong DD. Can we relate MeCP2 deficiency to the structural and chemical abnormalities in the Rett brain? *Brain Dev.* 2005;27:S72-S76.

285. Van den Veyver IB, Zoghbi HY. Genetic basis of Rett syndrome. *Ment Retard Dev Disabil Res Rev.* 2002;8:82-86.

286. Kaufmann WE, Johnston MV, Blue ME. MeCP2 expression and function during brain development: implications for Rett syndrome's pathogenesis and clinical evolution. *Brain Dev.* 2005;27:S77-S87.

287. Zhou Z, Hong EJ, Cohen S, et al. Brain-specific phosphorylation of MeCP2 regulates activity-dependent Bdnf transcription, dendritic growth, and spine maturation. *Neuron.* 2006;52:255-269.

289. Park HR, Lee JM, Moon HE, et al. A short review on the current understanding of autism spectrum disorders. *Exp Neurobiol.* 2016;25:1-13.

291. De Rubeis S, He X, Goldberg AP, et al. Synaptic, transcriptional and chromatin genes disrupted in autism. *Nature.* 2014;515:209-215.

292. Limperopoulos C. Autism spectrum disorders in survivors of extreme prematurity. *Clin Perinatol.* 2009;36:791-805.

296. Ecker C, Bookheimer SY, Murphy DG. Neuroimaging in autism spectrum disorder: brain structure and function across the lifespan. *Lancet Neurol.* 2015;14:1121-1134.

300. Rachidi M, Lopes C. Mental retardation and associated neurological dysfunctions in Down syndrome: a consequence of dysregulation in critical chromosome 21 genes and associated molecular pathways. *Eur J Paediatr Neurol.* 2008;12:168-182.

305. Wisniewski KE. Down syndrome children often have brain with maturation delay, retardation of growth, and cortical dysgenesis. *Am J Med Genet Suppl.* 1990;7:274-281.

306. Marin-Padilla M. Structural abnormalities of the cerebral cortex in human chromosomal aberrations: a Golgi study. *Brain Res.* 1972;44:625-629.

307. Takashima S, Becker LE, Armstrong DL, et al. Abnormal neuronal development in the visual cortex of the human fetus and infant with Down syndrome. A quantitative and qualitative Golgi study. *Brain Res.* 1981;225:1-21.

310. Becker LE, Armstrong DL, Chan F. Dendritic atrophy in children with Down's syndrome. *Ann Neurol.* 1986;20:520-526.

317. Busciglio J, Yankner BA. Apoptosis and increased generation of reactive oxygen species in Down's syndrome neurons. *Nature.* 1995;378:776-779.

324. Contractor A, Klyachko VA, Portera-Cailliau C. Altered neuronal and circuit excitability in fragile X syndrome. *Neuron.* 2015;87:699-715.

326. Goldson E, Hagerman RJ. The fragile X syndrome. *Dev Med Child Neurol.* 1992;34:826-832.

327. Hinton VJ, Brown WT, Wisniewski K, et al. Analysis of neocortex in three males with the fragile X syndrome. *Am J Med Genet.* 1991;41:289-294.

343. Roessmann U, Horwitz SJ, Kennell JH. Congenital absence of the corticospinal fibers: pathologic and clinical observations. *Neurology.* 1990;40:538-541.

346. Engle EC. Oculomotility disorders arising from disruptions in brainstem motor neuron development. *Arch Neurol.* 2007;64:633-637.

353. Quinlan RA, Brenner M, Goldman JE, et al. GFAP and its role in Alexander disease. *Exp Cell Res.* 2007;313:2077-2087.

354. Panigrahy A, Barnes PD, Robertson RL, et al. Volumetric brain differences in children with periventricular T2-signal hyperintensities: a grouping by gestational age at birth. *AJR Am J Roentgenol.* 2001;177:695-702.

355. Inder TE, Warfield SK, Wang H, et al. Abnormal cerebral structure is present at term in premature infants. *Pediatrics.* 2005;115:286-294.

368. Beauchamp MH, Thompson DK, Howard K, et al. Preterm infant hippocampal volumes correlate with later working memory deficits. *Brain.* 2008;131:2986-2994.

369. Phillips JP, Montague EQ, Aragon M, et al. Prematurity affects cortical maturation in early childhood. *Pediatr Neurol.* 2011;45:213-219.

373. Ball G, Boardman JP, Aljabar P, et al. The influence of preterm birth on the developing thalamocortical connectome. *Cortex.* 2013;49:1711-1721.

382. Dubois J, Benders M, Borradori-Tolsa C, et al. Primary cortical folding in the human newborn: an early marker of later functional development. *Brain.* 2008;131:2028-2041.

388. Ehrenkranz RA, Dusick AM, Vohr BR, et al. Growth in the neonatal intensive care unit influences neurodevelopmental and growth outcomes of extremely low birth weight infants. *Pediatrics.* 2006;117:1253-1261.

398. Deoni SC, Dean DC 3rd, Piryatinsky I, et al. Breastfeeding and early white matter development: a cross-sectional study. *Neuroimage.* 2013;82:77-86.

405. Volpe JJ. Impaired neurodevelopmental outcome after mild germinal matrix-intraventricular hemorrhage. *Pediatrics.* 2015;136:1185-1187.

408. Eikenes L, Lohaugen GC, Brubakk AM, et al. Young adults born preterm with very low birth weight demonstrate widespread white matter alterations on brain DTI. *Neuroimage.* 2011;54:1774-1785.

409. Smith GC, Gutovich J, Smyser C, et al. Neonatal intensive care unit stress is associated with brain development in preterm infants. *Ann Neurol.* 2011;70:541-549.

413. Nosarti C, Nam KW, Walshe M, et al. Preterm birth and structural brain alterations in early adulthood. *Neuroimage Clin.* 2014;6:180-191.

414. Huppi PS, Murphy B, Maier SE, et al. Microstructural brain development after perinatal cerebral white matter injury assessed by diffusion tensor magnetic resonance imaging. *Pediatrics.* 2001;107:455-460.

422. Als H, Duffy FH, McAnulty GB, et al. Early experience alters brain function and structure. *Pediatrics.* 2004;113:846-857.

423. Milgrom J, Newnham C, Anderson PJ, et al. Early sensitivity training for parents of preterm infants: impact on the developing brain. *Pediatr Res.* 2010;67:330-335.

Full references for this chapter can be found on www.expertconsult .com.

Myelination Events

Hannah C. Kinney ◆ *Joseph J. Volpe*

Myelination is characterized by the acquisition of the highly specialized myelin membrane around axons. The time period of myelination in the human is long, beginning mainly in the second trimester of pregnancy and continuing into adult life[1-5] Myelination in the brain begins before birth within the caudal brain stem and progresses rostrally to the forebrain, with the most rapid and dramatic period of human central myelination within the first 2 years of postnatal life. It is during this critical period that myelin is initially laid down in virtually all white matter tracts, with the last site to myelinate intracortical fibers of the cerebral cortex, where myelination extends steadily into the third decade.

NORMAL DEVELOPMENT

The process of myelination begins with proliferation of oligodendroglia, which align along axons (Table 8.1). The plasma membranes of the oligodendroglia become elaborated as the myelin membrane of the central nervous system (CNS).[2,5-9] Thus myelination is considered best in two phases: first, oligodendroglial proliferation and differentiation, and second, myelin deposition around axons.

Oligodendroglial Development

The *progression of the oligodendroglial lineage (OL) proceeds through four basic stages*, beginning with the oligodendroglial progenitor and continuing successively with the preoligodendrocyte, the immature oligodendrocyte, and the mature oligodendrocyte (Fig. 8.1).[7,8,10-17] Oligodendrocytes originate from progenitors in the subventricular zone and also from radial glial progenitors (see Chapter 7). The early phase in oligodendroglial lineage arising from progenitors is a mitotically active migratory cell recognized by the monoclonal antibodies A2B5 and NG2. This cell is generated from midgestation to the early postnatal period.[7,10-14,18] As this cell migrates into the cerebral white matter, oligodendroglial differentiation proceeds to the preoligodendrocyte, a multipolar cell that retains proliferative capacity and is recognized by a monoclonal antibody to sulfatide (O4). The waves of migration of these cells may be the anatomical correlate of the periventricular bands visualized on magnetic resonance imaging (MRI) scans of the premature infant.[19,20] *The O4 positive preoligodendrocyte is the predominant oligodendroglial phase before term and accounts for 90% of the total oligodendroglial population until 28 weeks of gestation* (Fig. 8.2).[13] (The O4 cell differentiates into the postmitotic immature oligodendrocyte, a richly multipolar cell recognized by a monoclonal antibody to galactocerebroside [O1].)[7,10-12] The proportion of O1 cells among the entire oligodendroglial population rises from 5% to 10% before 28 weeks of gestation to 30% to 40% during the premature period and to approximately 50% at term (see Fig. 8.2). In the third trimester of gestation, the O1 cells can be observed to develop striking linear extensions as they wrap around axons in preparation for myelination. This premyelination encasement of axons contributes to an important MRI correlate, the increase in *directionality* of water diffusion measured as increase in relative anisotropy (RA) (see later) (Fig. 8.3).[21-23] This process is followed by differentiation to the mature oligodendrocyte, a strikingly multipolar cell with membrane sheets and recognition by antibodies to myelin basic protein (MBP) and proteolipid protein. This cell becomes the predominant oligodendroglial stage in the months following term and gives rise to myelination.

Human Myelinogenesis Is Stage-Specific and Initiated Only by the O1 Immature Oligodendroglial Lineage

In the well-studied human optic radiation, cell bodies of immature OLs are present by at least 18 gestational weeks, but the first myelin sheaths are not detected until around 30 weeks. During human parietal white matter development, the percentage of immature OLs in the cerebral white matter remains relatively stable until around 30 weeks, at which time the number of immature OLs increases markedly.[13] One explanation for the prolonged *arrest* of human immature OLs in a premyelinating state before 30 weeks may be the lack of appropriate extrinsic factors that switch immature OLs to a myelinating phenotype. *Axon-dependent mechanisms that involve trophic/growth factors appear to play an important role in the timing of the immature OL commitment to myelinogenesis.*[13] The onset of myelination of the optic radiation around 30 weeks coincides with the evolution of the visual evoked response between 32 and 35 weeks to the principal waveforms that closely resemble the mature response that is observed by 39 weeks.[13] Consistent with these observations, there is no apparent contact between immature OLs and axons before the onset of myelinogenesis (Fig. 8.4). The initiation of myelinogenesis around 30 weeks is preceded by the appearance of a subset of specialized OL processes, *pioneer* processes that contact and wrap around axons. These initial contact sites serve to anchor the OL before it initiates the spiral wrapping of myelin along the same or other axon segments (Fig. 8.5).

There is a *transitional phase of myelinogenesis* during which the O4O1 premyelin sheath first forms (see Fig. 8.4), and then later begins to incorporate MBP. Before active myelination, certain MBP isoforms localize to the oligodendroglial cell body and

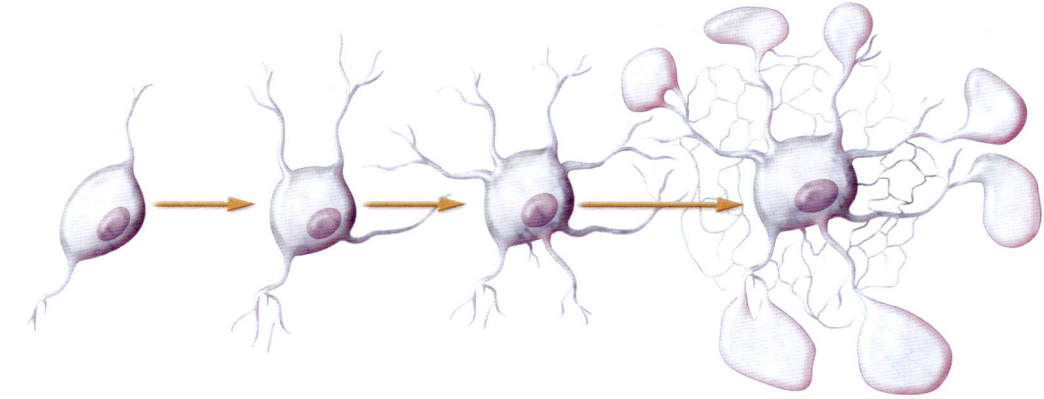

OL Progenitor	Pre-OL	Immature OL	Mature OL
		GalC (O1)	MBP
		Sulfatide (O4)	GalC (O1)
			A2B5
A2B5 NG2	Sulfatide (O4)		

Figure 8.1 **Progression of the oligodendroglial lineage (OL) through the four major stages.** The predominant forms in the premature infant are the O4+ O1− and O4+ O1+ forms. See text for details. (From Back SA, Volpe JJ. Cellular and molecular pathogenesis of periventricular white matter injury. *Ment Retard Dev Disabil Res Rev.* 1997;3:96–107.)

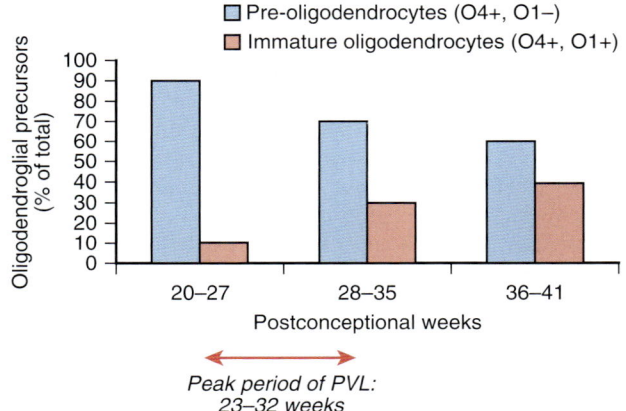

Peak period of PVL: 23–32 weeks

First appearance of MBP ~30 weeks, restricted to periventricular white matter

Figure 8.2 **Timing of the appearance of pre-OLs and immature OLs in the human cerebral white matter (n = 18).** (Data from Back SA, et al. Late oligodendrocyte progenitors coincide with the developmental window of vulnerability for human perinatal white matter injury. *J Neurosci.* 2001;21:1302–1312.)

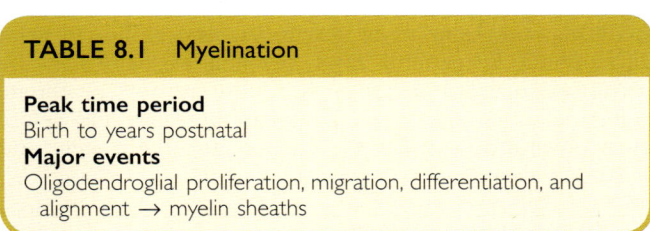

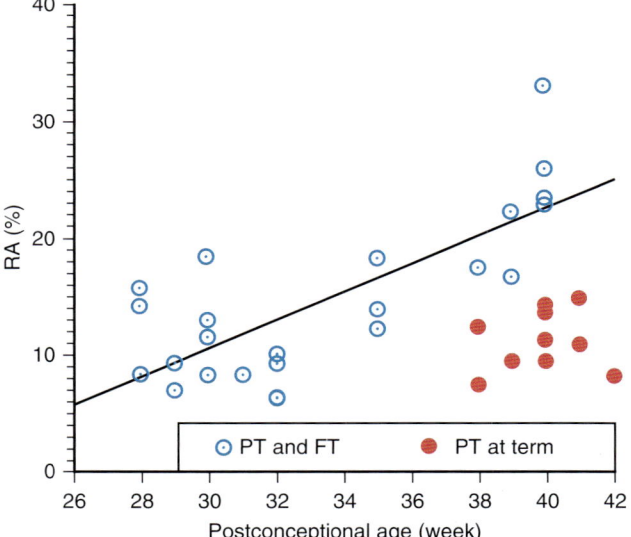

Figure 8.3 **Diffusion tensor MR determination of relative anisotropy (RA) in cerebral white matter of normal preterm (PT) and term (FT) infants (*open circles*) as a function of postconceptional age.** Note the striking increase in RA, indicative of increasing directionality of diffusion, perhaps related at least in part to oligodendroglial ensheathment of axons, with maturation. The lower values of the preterm infants studied at term (*closed circles*) suggest a deleterious effect of prematurity on this process (see text for details). (From Huppi PA, Maier SE, Peled S, et al. Microstructural development of human newborn cerebral white matter assessed in vivo by diffusion tensor magnetic resonance imaging. *Pediatr Res.* 1998;44:584–590.)

TABLE 8.1   Myelination

Peak time period
Birth to years postnatal

Major events
Oligodendroglial proliferation, migration, differentiation, and alignment → myelin sheaths

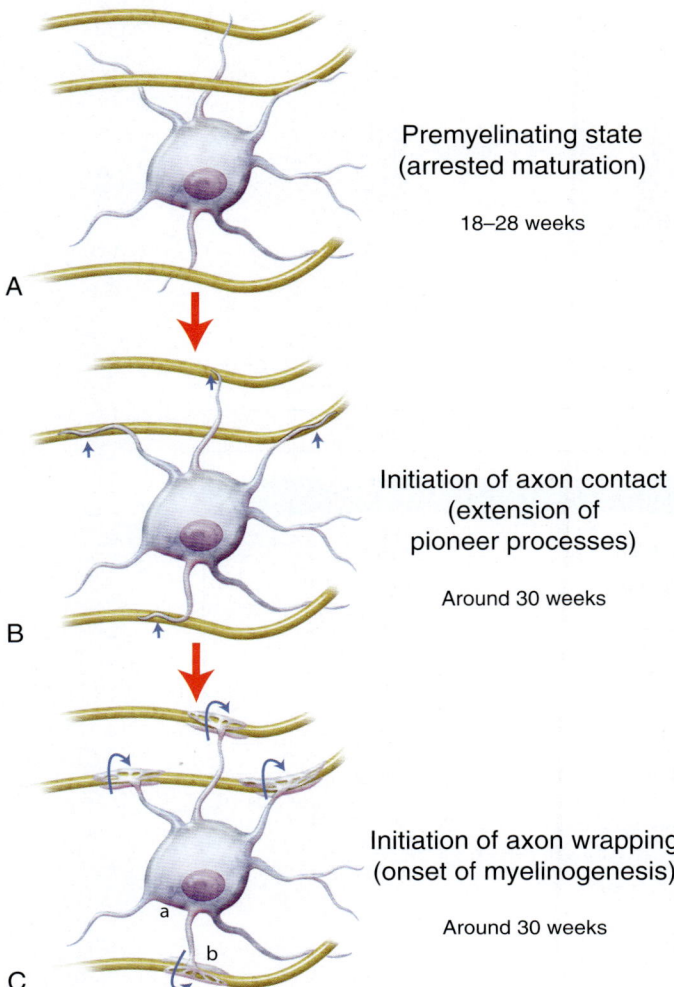

Premyelinating state
(arrested maturation)

18–28 weeks

A

Initiation of axon contact
(extension of
pioneer processes)

Around 30 weeks

B

Initiation of axon wrapping
(onset of myelinogenesis)

Around 30 weeks

a

b

C

Figure 8.4 Cellular sequences of myelin wrapping of axons by oligo-dendrocytes. *a,* Cell body; *b,* wrapping of myelin. (From Back SA, et al. Arrested oligodendrocyte lineage progression during human cerebral white matter development: dissociation between the timing of progenitor differentiation and myelinogenesis. *J Neuropathol Exp Neurol.* 2002;61:197–211.)

TABLE 8.2   Rules of Myelination
• Ontogeny recapitulates phylogeny
• Neuronal maturation before myelin formation
• Caudal to rostral
• Central to poles (occipital > frontal > temporal)
• Posterior to anterior (cerebrum)
• Proximal to distal
• Direction of impulse conduction
• Proximal components faster than distal components
• Components of functional system not simultaneous
• Projection fibers before association fibers

The *molecular determinants of the process of myelination* include a variety of growth factors, hormones, cytokines, surface receptors, and secreted ligands.[a] These molecules include basic fibroblast growth factor, neurotrophin-3, platelet-derived growth factor, insulin-like growth factors, nerve growth factor, transferrin, iron, members of the interleukin-6 family, thyroid hormone, neuregulin, erbB receptors, semaphorins, neuropilin receptors, ephrin, Eph receptors, and Nogo and Nogo receptors. Programmed cell death is an important feature of oligodendroglial development, as it is for neurons (see Chapter 7). Data show that approximately 50% of oligodendroglia will undergo apoptosis during development.[34,35]

Myelination in Human Brain Regions

The most informative of the anatomical descriptions of the *progress of myelination in the human brain* are those by Yakovlev and Lecours[36] and Gilles, Kinney, and co-workers.[3,4,37] Using the Loyez method for staining myelin, Yakovlev and Lecours defined the development of myelin in 25 areas of the human nervous system (Fig. 8.6). Because approximately 7 to 10 myelin lamellae are necessary for resolution by light microscopy, it is not surprising that electron microscopic data demonstrated that the onset of myelination in various brain areas occurs several weeks or more before the onset indicated in Fig. 8.6. Nevertheless, the data of Yakovlev and Lecours[36] provide important information. Several general points can be made on the basis of current knowledge. The process of myelination follows orderly, predictable sequences in which different fiber tracts begin to myelinate before or after birth, and progress at different rates, with tracts that are *fast, intermediate,* and *slow* myelinators relative to each other.[3,4,37]

Myelination Rules

Myelination follows a set of rules, understanding of which helps in the assessment of the status of myelination in different neurological disorders (Table 8.2).[4] The rules are not inviolate, and one rule may supersede another at a particular time or region. Nevertheless, a general understanding of these rules facilitates understanding of the process, and of human brain development in general. First, myelination begins in the peripheral nervous system, where motor roots myelinate before sensory roots. Second, shortly thereafter and before birth, myelin appears in the CNS in the brain stem and

nucleus and later are selectively transported to intracellular regions of myelin compaction.[14] Hence, the mechanism for spatial segregation of MBP mRNAs to the myelin sheath develops, as OLs become mature myelinating cells. MBP is inserted after the generation of a rudimentary premyelin sheath, providing support for the concept that compact myelin is generated after the insertion of MBP into the premyelin sheath.

Recent neuroimaging studies of living newborns between 24 and 40 weeks postconception with *diffusion tensor MRI showed changes in water diffusion that correlate with our morphological* data. Thus, in central white matter, RA, a measure of preferred directionality of water parallel to fiber tracts, increases markedly from 28 to 40 weeks. This increase in anisotropic diffusion occurred in parallel with a decline in overall water diffusion, as measured by the apparent diffusion coefficient. This combination of findings implies restriction of diffusion perpendicular to fiber tracts and could relate to the ensheathment of fibers by OL processes, as shown in our study.

[a]References 7, 8, 10, 11, 15, and 24-33.

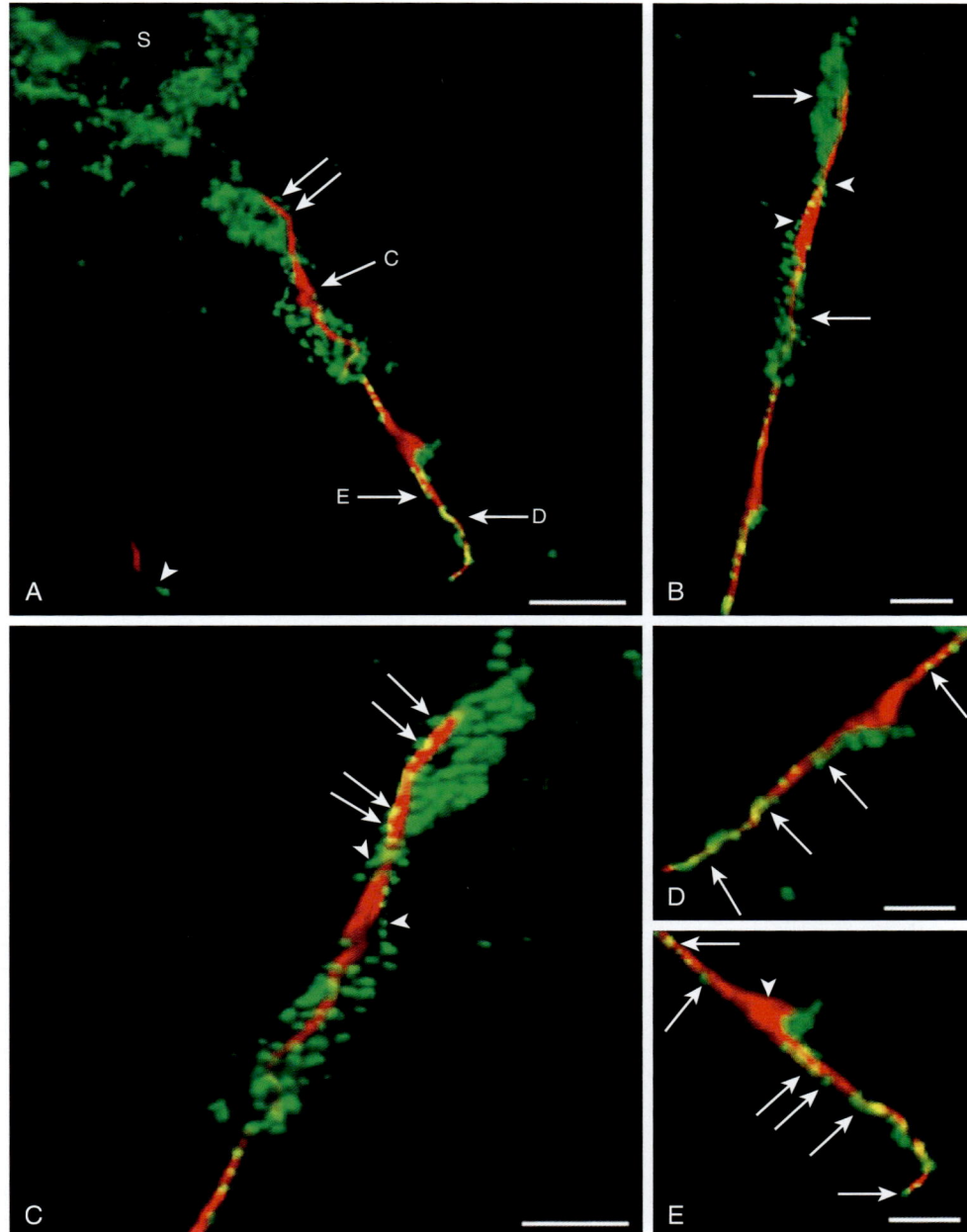

Figure 8.5 Myelin wrapping of axons (*red*, SMI 312) by O4 cells (*green*, O4) in the human optic radiation at 30 gestational weeks. The white arrows indicate the points of contact of O4 with axon. (From Back SA, et al. Arrested oligodendrocyte lineage progression during human cerebral white matter development: dissociation between the timing of progenitor differentiation and myelinogenesis. *J Neuropathol Exp Neurol.* 2002;61:197–211.)

cerebellum in components of some major sensory systems (e.g., medial lemniscus for somesthetic stimuli; lateral lemniscus, trapezoid body, and brachium of the inferior colliculus for auditory stimuli) and in components of some major motor systems (e.g., corticospinal tract in the midbrain and pons and superior cerebellar peduncle). In general, however, and in contrast to the peripheral nervous system, myelination in *central sensory systems tends to precede that in central motor systems.*[36] Third, myelination within the cerebral hemispheres, particularly those regions involved in higher level associative functions and sensory discriminations (e.g., association areas, intracortical

neuropil, and cerebral commissures), occurs well after birth and progresses over decades.

A study of 162 cases at a single children's hospital provided further insight into the progress of myelination from prenatal life through childhood.[3-5] General agreement exists between these data and those obtained by Yakovlev and Lecours,[36] despite the latter's smaller sample size. The median post-term age at which mature myelin was observed in selected brain areas is depicted in Table 8.3. Of the major general rules concerning cerebral myelination in the human, five from the anatomical study of Kinney and co-workers should be emphasized: (1)

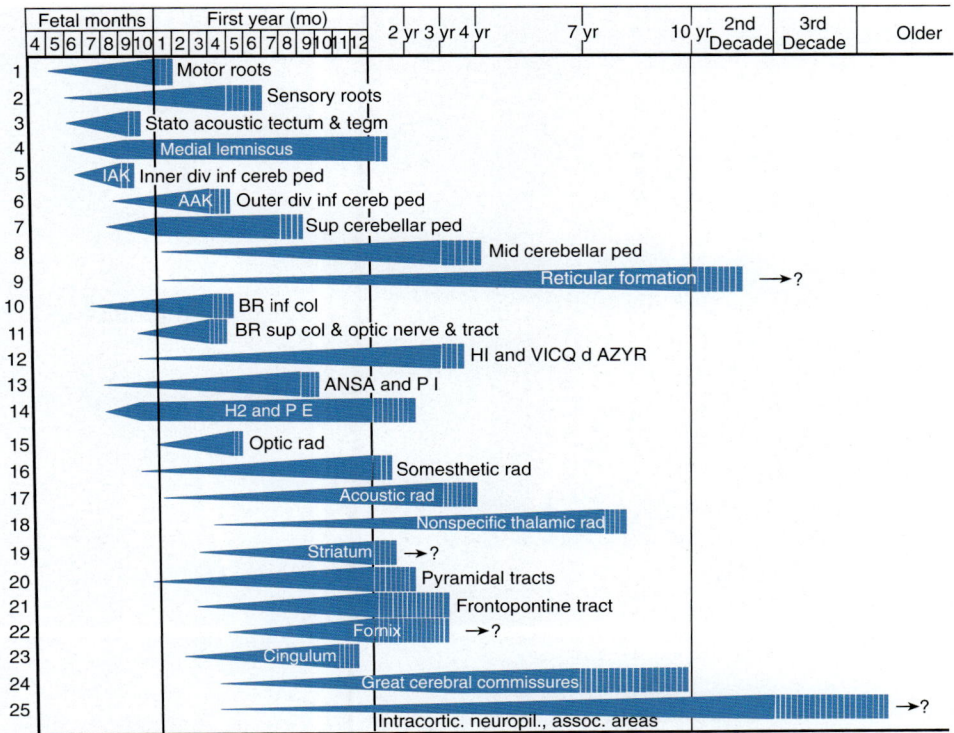

Figure 8.6 Myelogenetic cycles in the human brain. The width and length of the graphs indicate progression in the intensity of staining and the density of myelinated fibers. The vertical strips at the end of graphs indicate the approximate age range of termination of myelination. (Courtesy Dr. Paul Yakovlev.)

TABLE 8.3	Sequences of Myelination: Sites That Begin to Myelinate *Before* Birth			
	≤68 WEEKS	**70–107 WEEKS**	**119–142 WEEKS**	**>144 WEEKS**
Sensory system	Optic tract			
	Optic chiasm			
Auditory			Brachium inferior colliculus	
Other				Tractus solitaries
Pyramidal system	Posterior limb	Pyramid	Cervical CST	
	Midbrain CST		Thoracic CST	
	Pons CST		Lumbar CST	
Extrapyramidal system	Hilus inferior olive	Dentate hilus	Globus pallidus	Central tegmental
	Amiculum inferior	Ansa lenticularis		tract
	Capsule red nucleus	Pontocerebellar fibers		
	Peridentate	Cerebellum lateral		
	Middle-cerebellar	Hemisphere		
	Peduncle			
Central white matter				
Commissures and	Posterior limb			
capsules	Central corona radiate			
Limbic system		Stria medullaris thalami		Anterior commissure
				Outer

CST, Corticospinal tract.

proximal pathways myelinate before distal pathways, (2) sensory pathways myelinate before motor pathways, (3) projection pathways myelinate before cerebral associative pathways, (4) central cerebral sites myelinate before cerebral poles, and (5) occipital poles myelinate before frontotemporal poles.[4,5] The latter two points are illustrated in Fig. 8.7. Overall, the fastest changes in myelination occurred within the first 8 postnatal months.[4] The similarities between the neuroanatomical data and findings made in vivo by MRI (see Chapter 10) are striking, although MRI showed myelin somewhat earlier, especially in the preterm infant (e.g., myelin in the posterior limb of the internal capsule at 36 postceptional weeks versus 44 weeks

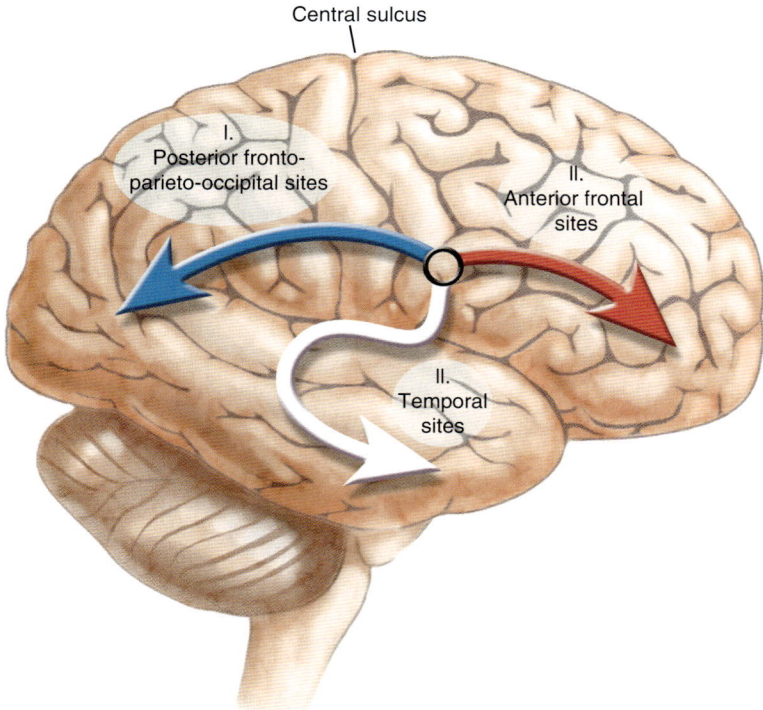

Figure 8.7 Progression of myelination. This drawing of the cerebrum depicts the progression of myelination in telencephalic sites from the central sulcus outward to the poles, with the posterior sites preceding anterior frontotemporal sites. (From Kinney HC, Brody BA, Kloman AS, Gilles FH. Sequence of central nervous system myelination in human infancy. II. Patterns of myelination in autopsied infants. J *Neuropathol Exp Neurol.* 1988;47:217.)

TABLE 8.4   Sequences of Myelination: Sites That Begin to Myelinate *After* Birth

	≤68 WEEKS	70–109 WEEKS	119–142 WEEKS	>144 WEEKS
Sensory system				
Visual	Optic radiation proximal	SAF calcarine cortex		Stripe of Gennari
	Optic radiation distal			
Auditory	Auditory radiation proximal	Heschl's gyrus		
Other			Lateral olfactory stria	
Pyramidal				
Extrapyramidal system		Lateral crus pedunculi	Medial crus pedunculi	
			Putaminal pencils	
Central white matter		Distal radiation to precentral gyrus	Temporal lobe at LGN	
		Posterior frontal	Temporal pole	
		Posterior parietal	Frontal pole	
		Occipital pole	SAF all sites	
Commissures and capsules	Corpus callosum body	Rostrum	Anterior commissure	Extreme capsule
	Splenium	Anterior limb	Inner	
		External capsule		
Limbic system		Cingulum	Mammillothalamic tract	Medial fornix
			Alveus, fimbria	Lateral fornix

LGN, Lateral geniculate nucleus; *SAF,* subcortical association fibers.

in the anatomical study).[38] This difference may relate to the ability of MRI to detect very early myelin wrapping.

In Tables 8.3 and 8.4 the fiber tracts and white matter regions (e.g., temporal pole) are divided into those sites that begin myelination before and after birth, functional systems, for example, sensory systems versus motor versus limbic, and tempo of myelination, that is, fast (within 6 months), ranging to over 8 months (>144 weeks) without attainment of mature staining by the Luxol Fast Blue method. This representation of the process of myelination highlights *fast, intermediate, and slow myelinators.* Moreover, the data help to illustrate the point that disease processes that are acute, if early in the first year of life, can preferentially affect fast myelinators, whereas disease processes that extend over protracted periods are likely to detrimentally affect slow myelinating systems.

DISORDERS

Unequivocal documentation of developmental disturbances of myelin formation in the human has been hindered considerably by the inadequacy of standard neuropathological techniques in quantifying the degree of myelination in brain. Moreover, the most commonly used brain imaging technique in the past, computed tomography (CT), provides little information concerning myelination in the human infant. The advent of MRI provides considerable capability for the monitoring of myelination (see Chapter 10), and MRI is invaluable in defining disturbances of human myelination (see later). Of particular importance are quantitative volumetric MRI determinations and diffusion tensor MRI studies of RA (see later).

Principal Mechanisms of Disordered Myelination

To conceptualize disorders of myelination, three principal mechanisms should be considered: (1) arrested or abnormal development of oligodendrocyte precursors such that mature MBP producing oligodendrocytes are not formed, (2) oligodendroglial dysfunction leads to myelin breakdown, and (3) primary axonal disorders cause aberrant signaling and impaired trophic interactions with developing oligodendrocytes, resulting in impaired myelination or myelin maintenance or both (Fig. 8.8). MRI studies in infants and children have shown apparent impairment in myelination in a wide variety of disorders, including leukodystrophies (see Chapter 29), neuronal degenerations (see Chapter 29), a variety of amino acid and organic acidopathies (see Chapters 27 and 28), mitochondrial and peroxisomal disorders (see Chapter 29), infections (congenital cytomegalovirus and rubella) (see Chapter 34), and neuromuscular disorders (merosin-deficient congenital muscular dystrophy [see Chapter 33]), among others.[38a] For this discussion, we will focus on those entities in which the *impairment of myelination is the dominant neuropathological disturbance* (Table 8.5).

Cerebral White Matter Hypoplasia

Chattha and Richardson[39] reported the clinical and neuropathological features of 12 patients with severe intellectual impairment and spastic quadriparesis that were present from the first weeks of life but nonprogressive. Pregnancy, labor, and delivery were essentially uneventful. Neurological deficits, particularly seizures, were apparent in the neonatal period. Subsequent neurological development was severely impaired. The unifying and outstanding neuropathological feature was a marked deficiency in cerebral white matter, most conspicuous in the centrum ovale (Fig. 8.9). Neurons were normal in appearance, and no gliosis, sign of inflammation, or other indication of a destructive process was present. An inherited developmental aberration in myelin formation was supported by the finding that the series included a set of three affected siblings, and in two other cases a family history of affected siblings was elicited. The biochemical basis of the disorder in myelin formation awaits elucidation. The use of MRI in evaluation of similar patients may lead to further delineation of this disorder. The cases are reminiscent of the murine mutants (e.g., *quaking* and *jimpy* mice) with deficient myelin formation.[40,41] The occurrence of neonatal seizures with this neuropathology raises the possibility of serine synthesis deficiency (see Chapter 29) which was unknown at the time of this report. An autosomal recessive disorder with hypomyelination of the central and peripheral nervous systems, as well as congenital cataract, has also been defined.[42,43] The central nervous system hypomyelination is principally supratentorial. This disorder is

---

TABLE 8.5   Disorders of Myelination

Cerebral white matter hypoplasia
Prematurity-related factors
    Periventricular leukomalacia/cerebral white matter injury
    Other factors (Chapter 7)
Nutritional factors
    Undernutrition
    Breast-feeding
    Iron deficiency
Experiential factors

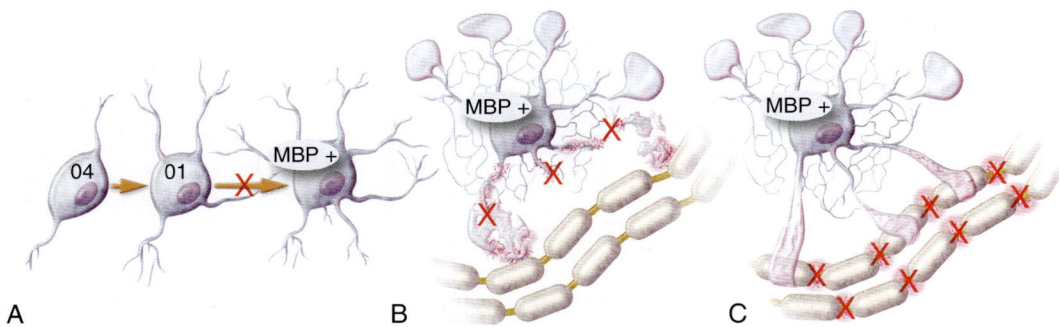

Figure 8.8 Mechanisms of disorders of central myelination. (A) Arrested oligodendroglial lineage (OL) development, (B) OL dysfunction or process loss, and (C) primary axonal injury with abnormal signaling to OLs. *MBP,* Myelin basic protein. (Courtesy Hannah Kinney.)

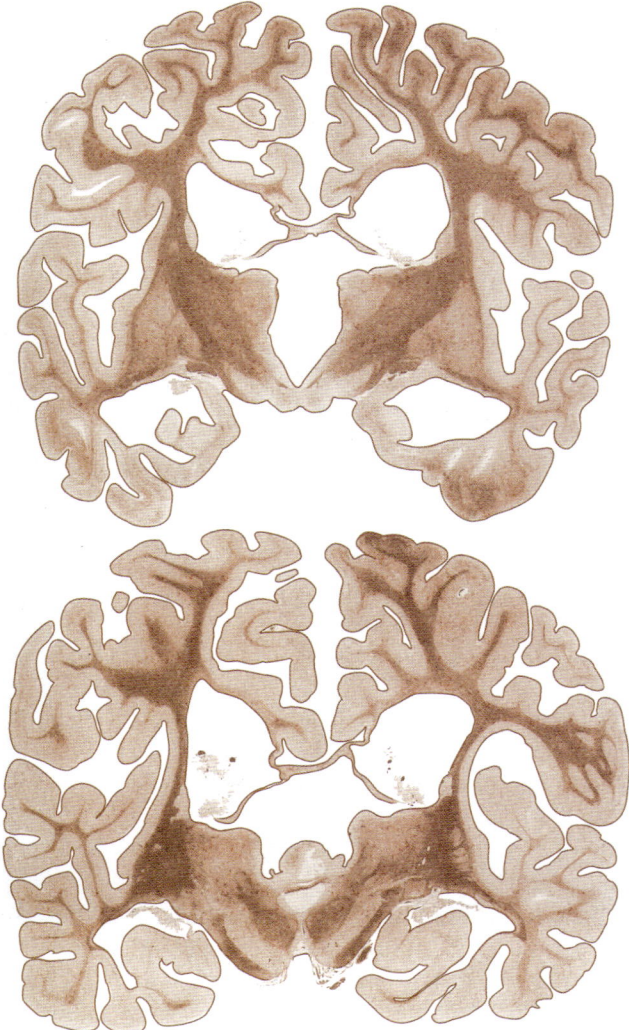

Figure 8.9 Cerebral white matter hypoplasia. Coronal sections of cerebrum, stained for myelin (*dark brown*). Note marked diminution in cerebral myelin, including corpus callosum. As a consequence of the myelin disturbance, ventricular size increases. (From Chattha AS, Richardson EP Jr. Cerebral white-matter hypoplasia. *Arch Neurol.* 1977;34:137.)

TABLE 8.6	Major Neonatal and Subsequent Magnetic Resonance Imaging Findings Consistent With Myelination Failure in Premature Infants[a]

IMAGING MODALITY	PRINCIPAL FINDING(S)
Conventional MRI	Qualitative decrease in cerebral white matter and increased ventricular size
Volumetric MRI	Decreased cerebral white matter volumes, especially periventricular, central corona radiata, and corpus callosum
DTI	Decreased fractional anisotropy in cerebral white matter tracts, relatively increased radial diffusivity
fMRI	Decreased measures of thalamocortical and cortico-cortical connectivity

[a]See text for references.

DTI, Diffusion tensor magnetic resonance imaging; *fMRI*, functional magnetic resonance imaging; *MRI*, magnetic resonance imaging.

caused by a homozygous mutation in the FAM126A gene which encodes the membrane protein, hyccin, critical for myelination.

The decrease in cerebral white matter without evidence of destructive disease in the patients described by Chattha and Richardson[39] is similar to that recorded in the familial disorders of *axonal development* by Lyon and co-workers[44] and others.[45,46] In the latter cases, axonal abnormalities were identifiable, and this finding may be the crucial distinction from the cases of cerebral white matter hypoplasia.

Prematurity-Related Factors

Premature birth and related complications are associated strongly with impaired myelination (see Table 8.5). Cerebral white matter injury is the most common of these complications, but other factors also appear important. The myelination failure in premature infants is difficult to detect at term equivalent age, because the volume of myelinated cerebral white matter accounts for only about 5% of total cerebral white matter at term.[47-55] Because cerebral myelination is principally a *post-term* event, the myelination disturbance becomes more apparent later in infancy and childhood.

The major MRI findings consistent with myelination failure in premature infants are outlined in Table 8.6. Thus, conventional MRI shows a qualitative decrease in cerebral white matter and a corresponding increase in ventricular size, as early as term equivalent age. The advent of volumetric MRI allowed demonstration of quantitative decreases in cerebral white matter, especially involving periventricular and central regions, corona radiata, and corpus callosum. Diffusion tensor MRI (DTI) shows decreased fractional anisotropy in cerebral white matter tracts, consistent with impaired development. Radial diffusivity generally is relatively increased, consistent with a failure of oligodendroglial ensheathment early and of myelin deposition later. Functional MRI studies show decreased measures of connectivity, especially thalamocortical and cortico-cortical, consistent with impaired conduction between sites, a feature dependent on myelin development.

The factors associated with the myelination failure in premature infants and children are multiple, but as noted earlier cerebral white matter injury likely is most important. Examples of the disturbance of myelination in preterm infants studied by conventional MRI and DTI at 7 years of age are shown in Fig. 8.10A and B.[56] The potential mechanisms underlying the myelination failure in the context of white matter injury in the premature infant are discussed in the previous chapter (see Fig. 7.30). Pre-oligodendroglial disturbance, either primary or secondary, with failure of differentiation to myelin-producing cells is critical (see Chapters 14 and 15).

Nutritional Factors

Both experimental and clinical data suggest that nutritional factors are important for myelination. Notably, especially with nutritional factors operating in utero or early postnatal life, it is very difficult to disentangle effects on oligodendroglial

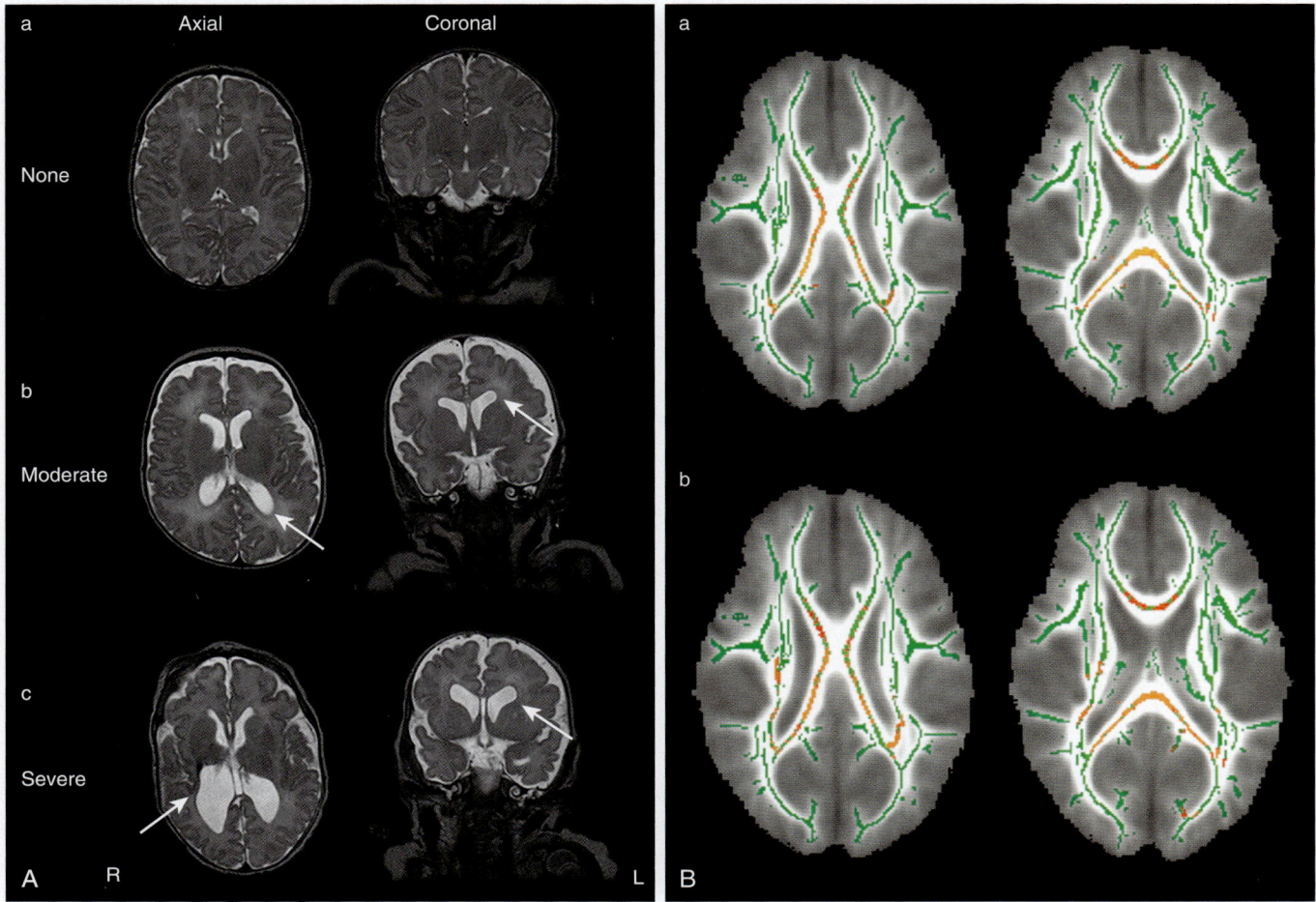

Figure 8.10 (A) White matter abnormality (WMA) in preterm infants scanned at term equivalent postmenstrual age. Axial and coronal T2-weighted MRI illustrating representative example of subjects (a) without WMA, (b) with moderate WMA, and (c) with severe WMA (arrows denote representative areas of WMA). (B) Diffusion tensor MRI at 7 years of age comparing very preterm (VPT) children with and without WMA. Areas of the corpus callosum (CC) differed significantly between VPT children scanned at 7 years of age with and without WMA on neonatal MRI. Results consistent with better myelin development are (a) higher fractional anisotropy (FA) and (b) lower radial diffusivity in the CC in subjects without WMA. Yellow color denotes areas that differ between groups ($P <$ .05). Green color indicates areas with no difference. Results overlaid on averaged FA map. (From Estep ME, et al. *Diffusion tractography and neuromotor outcome in very preterm children with white matter abnormalities. Pediatr Res.* 2014;76:86–92, with permission.)

development (see Chapter 7) from those on myelination per se. Thus, the earlier discussion on nutritional factors and oligodendroglial development should be considered in this context (see Chapter 7). Moreover, direct quantitative information concerning myelin development in *living infants* is modest. Nevertheless, undernutrition, breast-feeding, long-chain polyunsaturated fatty acids (especially docosahexaenoic acid), and iron should be discussed briefly in this context.

Undernutrition. A deleterious effect on myelination of undernutrition in utero or in early infancy seems likely (see Table 8.5). Thus, *intrauterine growth retardation*, especially in preterm infants, is associated with microstructural and volumetric defects in white matter and neurodevelopmental impairment.[57-62] As discussed in detail in Chapter 7 the relative roles of impairment of oligodendroglial differentiation versus impairment of myelination per se is unclear. Undernutrition

in *premature infants* appears to impact principally organizational events, and perhaps preferentially cerebral *cortical* development. In one careful study of premature infants, serial DTI scans showed that growth impairment was followed by delayed microstructural development of cerebral cortex but not of cerebral white matter.[63] More data are needed on this critical issue. Undernutrition *in early infancy* may provide a more suitable clinical setting to investigate nutritional effects specifically on myelin deposition because of the timing of normal myelin development. Relevant data include the demonstration in an older study of a 20% to 30% reduction in cerebrosides and a 15% to 20% reduction in plasmalogens—important myelin lipids—in the cerebral white matter of malnourished infants.[64] The composition of the myelin from these infants was found to be normal, and thus decreased formation of chemically normal myelin was postulated to occur with malnutrition.[65] Results of a later study confirmed these findings.[66] The clinical observation[67] that severe undernutrition to 4 months of age results in a permanent reduction in intelligence quotient (IQ) may also be relevant in this context. Long-term follow-up studies of children undernourished in infancy generally confirm the deleterious effects on intelligence and school performance, although the roles of other factors related to deficient environmental stimulation, *social deprivation*, and confounding deleterious biological factors remain to be defined clearly.[68-79]

Breast-Feeding. As discussed in Chapter 7 regarding nutritional factors and organizational development, breast-feeding has been shown to lead to improved cognitive and behavioral outcomes. A recent report suggests that improved white matter development and specifically, myelination may be critical in mediating these outcomes (see Table 8.5).[80] Thus, a study of 133 healthy term-born children either exclusively breast-fed a minimum of 3 months (mean, 413 days) or exclusively formula fed or fed a mixture of formula and breast milk used advanced magnetic resonance (MR) measures at 10 months to 4 years of age to assess white matter development.[80] The data show that early exclusive breast-feeding was associated with increased development in relatively late maturing white matter regions, including frontal and temporal white matter, peripheral aspects of the internal capsule and corticospinal tracts, superior longitudinal fasciculus, and superior occipitofrontal fasciculus.[80] Notably, these regions are important for specific higher-order cognition domains, in which breast-fed infants have been shown to have improved performance.[80,81] The data amplify earlier volumetric MR studies in adolescents breast-fed as infants who exhibited volumetric increases in total white matter.[82] Moreover, DTI measures in 8-year-old children previously breast-fed also showed better white matter development than in those formula fed, but interestingly, the effect was observed only in boys.[83] The constituents of breast milk important in the beneficial effects on white matter development remain to be determined, but the primary hypothesized constituents are long-chain polyunsaturated fatty acids, especially docosahexaenoic acid and its precursor arachidonic acid (see next section), cholesterol, and, perhaps, growth factors.[79,84] These issues are discussed in more detail in Chapter 16.

Iron Deficiency. Iron deficiency in the neonatal period, a relatively common disorder, is associated with cognitive, motor, and behavioral deficits that may be related to impaired myelination (see Table 8.5). Iron deficiency in this context is usually related to dietary deficiency, but also to breast-feeding and prematurity.[85-87] Indeed as many as 10% of infants 1 to 2 years of age in the United States and 15% of breast-fed Canadian infants exhibit iron deficiency. Because premature birth deprives the infant of the primary period of fetal iron deposition, that is, the third trimester, the risks are still higher in these infants. Although the data are not entirely consistent, most studies show impaired motor, cognitive and behavioral development in iron-deficient infants.[85-93] Although the deleterious effects are generally modest, they may be irreversible if treatment is not prompt. Supportive of an effect on myelination is the finding on studies of auditory and visual evoked potentials of prolonged latencies, without impairment of amplitudes.[88,94-96] The normal maturational decline in latencies relates to acquisition of myelin, whereas changes in amplitude relate more to neuronal development (see

Chapter 10). In one recent study of infants born at ≥35 weeks' gestation, iron deficiency in utero was assessed by cord blood measurements and at least one known intrauterine risk factor for poor iron status (maternal diabetes, pregnancy-induced hypertension, intrauterine growth retardation).[96] Infants with iron deficiency had prolonged interpeak latencies consistent with impaired transmission from the cochlear nuclear complex to the lateral lemniscus, areas undergoing myelination during this period. The findings are consistent with experimental studies indicating that iron deficiency can lead to abnormal or delayed myelination.[97-100] Additionally supportive of an effect on myelination are experimental studies showing the crucial role of iron in the process.[8,85,87,101] Moreover, transferrin concentrations in oligodendrocytes increase during myelination and reach a peak at the height of myelination. Finally, transferrin is involved in the regulation of the transcription of the MBP gene and has a synergistic enhancing effect on myelination with insulin-like growth factor 1.[8] Because iron also plays a critical role in neurotransmitter metabolism, the neural effects of iron deficiency may extend beyond an impairment of myelination.[100] Studies of myelination in living infants by advanced MR measures would be of great interest.

Experiential Factors

Because cerebral myelination is principally a post-term event in human brain, the question of whether experiential effects could alter myelin development is important. Indeed many careful studies show that strong determinants of adverse developmental outcomes in infants and children, even in the absence of overt brain structural disturbances, include such factors as social deprivation, lower socioeconomic status, higher parental job strain, educational and environmental deprivation, and deficient parenting skills.[102] The possibility that such factors could operate to alter myelination is suggested by studies of infants institutionally reared in orphanages under circumstances associated with neglect, including social, emotional, linguistic and cognitive deficiencies. Although disturbances in subsequent behavioral and cognitive functions in such infants are well known, a relation to impaired white matter development has been shown only recently. These recent studies of infants institutionally reared and transferred to foster care, although somewhat limited by small numbers, issues related to selection biases, and other methodological factors, do show significant associations between institutional neglect and microstructural alterations in cerebral white matter.[103-108] A particularly informative large study of Romanian orphans (Bucharest Early Intervention Project) compared infants randomly selected to remain in an institution or to be placed at approximately 2 years of age in supervised foster care. At approximately 8 years of age more than one-half of the children were studied by diffusion tensor MRI.[109] The findings revealed significant associations between neglect in early life and microstructural integrity (fractional anisotropy) of the body of the corpus callosum, tracts involved in limbic circuitry, corona radiata, frontostriatal circuitry, and sensory processing systems. Radial diffusivity, which is sensitive to myelin ensheathment, was particularly affected. (However, the degree to which altered axonal pruning contributed to the white matter findings is difficult to elucidate.) Early intervention (i.e., foster care) promoted more nearly normative white matter development among the previously neglected children. Thus, the data suggest that myelination was affected by early experiential deficiencies associated with neglect and showed capacity for improvement with foster care. The degree to which related effects on myelination occur with less extreme experiential factors is a crucial topic for future research.

REFERENCES

1. Gilles FH, Leviton A, Dooling EC. *The Developing Human Brain: Growth and Epidemiologic Neuropathology*. Boston: John Wright, Inc.; 1983.
2. Bunge RP. Glial cells and the central myelin sheath. *Physiol Rev*. 1968;48:197-251.
3. Brody BA, Kinney HC, Kloman AS, et al. Sequence of central nervous system myelination in human infancy. I. An autopsy study of myelination. *J Neuropathol Exp Neurol*. 1987;46:283-301.
4. Kinney HC, Brody BA, Kloman AS, et al. Sequence of central nervous system myelination in human infancy. II. Patterns of myelination in autopsied infants. *J Neuropathol Exp Neurol*. 1988;47:217-234.
5. Kinney HC, Armstrong DL. Perinatal neuropathology. In: Graham DI, Lantos PE, eds. *Greenfield's Neuropathology*. Vol. 1. 7th ed. London: Arnold Publishers; 2002:519-606.
6. Del Rio-Hortega P. Tercera aportacion al conocimiento morfologico e interpretacion funcional de la oligodendroglia. *Mem Real Soc Espan Hist Nat*. 1928;14:5.
7. Porter B, Tennekoon G. Myelin and disorders that affect the formation and maintenance of this sheath. *Ment Retard Dev Disabil Res Rev*. 2000;6:47-58.
8. de Vellis J, Carpenter E. Development. In: Siegel GJ, Albers RW, Brady ST, et al., eds. *Basic Neurochemistry, Molecular, Cellular, and Medical Aspects*. 7th ed. London: Elsevier; 2006:437-458.
9. Quarles RH, Morell P, McFarland HF. Diseases involving myelin. In: Siegel GJ, Albers RW, Brady ST, et al., eds. *Basic Neurochemistry, Molecular, Cellular, and Medical Aspects*. 7th ed. London: Elsevier; 2006:639-652.
10. Back SA, Volpe JJ. Cellular and molecular pathogenesis of periventricular white matter injury. *Ment Retard Dev Disabil Res Rev*. 1997;3:96-107.
11. Kinney HC, Back SA. Human oligodendroglial development: relationship to periventricular leukomalacia. *Semin Pediatr Neurol*. 1998;5:180-189.
12. Rivkin MJ, Flax J, Mozel R, et al. Oligodendroglial development in human fetal cerebrum. *Ann Neurol*. 1995;38:92-101.
13. Back SA, Luo NL, Borenstein NS, et al. Late oligodendrocyte progenitors coincide with the developmental window of vulnerability for human perinatal white matter injury. *J Neurosci*. 2001;21:1302-1312.
14. Back SA, Luo NL, Borenstein NS, et al. Arrested oligodendrocyte lineage progression during human cerebral white matter development: dissociation between the timing of progenitor differentiation and myelinogenesis. *J Neuropathol Exp Neurol*. 2002;61:197-211.
15. Sherman DL, Brophy PJ. Mechanisms of axon ensheathment and myelin growth. *Nat Rev Neurosci*. 2005;6:683-690.
16. Yue T, Xian K, Hurlock E, et al. A critical role for dorsal progenitors in cortical myelination. *J Neurosci*. 2006;26:1275-1280.
17. Nguyen L, Borgs L, Vandenbosch R, et al. The Yin and Yang of cell cycle progression and differentiation in the oligodendroglial lineage. *Ment Retard Dev Disabil Res Rev*. 2006;12:85-96.
18. Kendler A, Golden JA. Progenitor cell proliferation outside the ventricular and subventricular zones during human brain development. *J Neuropathol Exp Neurol*. 1996;55:1253-1258.
19. Child A-M, Ramenghi LA, Evans DJ, et al. MR features of developing periventricular white matter in preterm infants: evidence of glial cell migration. *AJNR Am J Neuroradiol*. 1998;19:971-976.
20. Battin MR, Maalouf EF, Counsell SJ, et al. Magnetic resonance imaging of the brain in very preterm infants: visualization of the germinal matrix, early myelination, and cortical folding. *Pediatrics*. 1998;101:957-962.
21. Huppi PS, Maier SE, Peled S, et al. Microstructural development of human newborn cerebral white matter assessed *in vivo* by diffusion tensor magnetic resonance imaging. *Pediatr Res*. 1998;44:584-590.
22. Kroenke CD, Bretthorst GL, Inder TE, et al. Diffusion MR imaging characteristics of the developing primate brain. *Neuroimage*. 2005;25:1205-1213.
23. Drobyshevsky A, Song SK, Gamkrelidze G, et al. Developmental changes in diffusion anisotropy coincide with immature oligodendrocyte progression and maturation of compound action potential. *J Neurosci*. 2005;25:5988-5997.
24. Zumkeller W. The effect of insulin-like growth factors on brain myelination and their potential therapeutic application in myelination disorders. *Eur J Paediatr Neurol*. 1997;4:91-101.
25. Ahlgren SC, Wallace H, Bishop J, et al. Effects of thyroid hormone on embryonic oligodendrocyte precursor call development in vivo and in vitro. *Mol Cell Neurosci*. 1997;9:420-432.
26. Vartanian T, Fischbach G, Miller R. Failure of spinal cord oligodendrocyte development in mice lacking neuregulin. *Proc Natl Acad Sci U S A*. 1999;96:731-735.
27. Chan JR, Watkins TA, Cosgaya JM, et al. NGF controls axonal receptivity to myelination by Schwann cells or oligodendrocytes. *Neuron*. 2004;43:183-191.
28. Cohen RI. Visions & reflections: exploring oligodendrocyte guidance: 'to boldly go where no cell has gone before'. *Cell Mol Life Sci*. 2005;62:505-510.
29. Chen S, Velardez MO, Warot X, et al. Neuregulin 1-erbB signaling is necessary for normal myelination and sensory function. *J Neurosci*. 2006;26:3079-3086.
30. Zeger M, Popken G, Zhang J, et al. Insulin-like growth factor type 1 receptor signaling in the cells of oligodendrocyte lineage is required for normal in vivo oligodendrocyte development and myelination. *Glia*. 2007;55:400-411.
31. Taveggia C, Feltri ML, Wrabetz L. Signals to promote myelin formation and repair. *Nat Rev Neurol*. 2010;6:276-287.
32. Kramer AS, Harvey AR, Plant GW, et al. Systematic review of induced pluripotent stem cell technology as a potential clinical therapy for spinal cord injury. *Cell Transplant*. 2013;22:571-617.
33. Franco PG, Pasquini LA, Perez MJ, et al. Paving the way for adequate myelination: the contribution of galectin-3, transferrin and iron. *FEBS Lett*. 2015;589:3388-3395.
34. Barres BA, Hart IK, Coles HSR, et al. Cell death in the oligodendrocyte lineage. *J Neurobiol*. 1992;23:1221-1230.
35. Barres BA, Hart IK, Cotes HSR, et al. Cell death and control of cell survival in the oligodendrocyte lineage. *Cell*. 1992;70:31-46.
36. Yakovlev PI, Lecours AR. The myelogenetic cycles of regional maturation of the brain. In: Minkowski A, ed. *Regional Development of the Brain in Early Life*. Philadelphia: Davis; 1967.
37. Gilles FH. Myelination in the neonatal brain. *Hum Pathol*. 1976;7:244-248.
38. Counsell SJ, Maalouf EF, Fletcher AM, et al. MR imaging assessment of myelination in the very preterm brain. *AJNR Am J Neuroradiol*. 2002;23:872-881.
38a. Schiffmann R, van der Knaap MS. Invited article: an MRI-based approach to the diagnosis of white matter disorders. *Neurology*. 2009;72:750-759.
39. Chattha AS, Richardson EP Jr. Cerebral white-matter hypoplasia. *Arch Neurol*. 1977;34:137-141.
40. Samorajski T, Friede RL, Reimer PR. Hypomyelination in the quaking mouse. A model for the analysis of disturbed myelin formation. *J Neuropathol Exp Neurol*. 1970;29:507-523.
41. Torii J, Adachi M, Volk BW. Histochemical and ultrastructural studies of inherited leukodystrophy in mice. *J Neuropathol Exp Neurol*. 1971;30:278-289.
42. Biancheri R, Zara F, Bruno C, et al. Phenotypic characterization of hypomyelination and congenital cataract. *Ann Neurol*. 2007;62:121-127.
43. Biancheri R, Zara F, Rossi A, et al. Hypomyelination and congenital cataract: broadening the clinical phenotype. *Arch Neurol*. 2011;68:1191-1194.
44. Lyon G, Arita F, Le Galloudec E, et al. A disorder of axonal development, necrotizing myopathy, cardiomyopathy, and cataracts: a new familial disease. *Ann Neurol*. 1990;27:193-199.
45. Lynch BJ, Becich MJ, Torack RM, et al. Arrested maturation of cerebral neurons, axons and myelin: a new familial syndrome of newborns. *Neuropediatrics*. 1992;23:180-187.
46. Curatolo P, Cilio MR, Del Giudice E, et al. Familial white matter hypoplasia, agenesis of the corpus callosum, mental retardation

and growth deficiency: a new distinctive syndrome. *Neuropediatrics*. 1993;24:77-82.

47. Huppi PS, Warfield S, Kikinis R, et al. Quantitative magnetic resonance imaging of brain development in premature and mature newborns. *Ann Neurol*. 1998;43:224-235.

48. Inder TE, Huppi PS, Warfield S, et al. Periventricular white matter injury in the premature infant is associated with a reduction in cerebral cortical gray matter volume at term. *Ann Neurol*. 1999;46:755-760.

49. Thompson DK, Warfield SK, Carlin JB, et al. Perinatal risk factors altering regional brain structure in the preterm infant. *Brain*. 2007; 130:667-677.

50. Eikenes L, Lohaugen GC, Brubakk AM, et al. Young adults born preterm with very low birth weight demonstrate widespread white matter alterations on brain DTI. *Neuroimage*. 2011;54:1774-1785.

51. Panigrahy A, Barnes PD, Robertson RL, et al. Volumetric brain differences in children with periventricular T2-signal hyperintensities: a grouping by gestational age at birth. *AJR Am J Roentgenol*. 2001;177:695-702.

52. Soria-Pastor S, Gimenez M, Narberhaus A, et al. Patterns of cerebral white matter damage and cognitive impairment in adolescents born very preterm. *Int J Dev Neurosci*. 2008;26:647-654.

53. Boardman JP, Craven C, Valappil S, et al. A common neonatal image phenotype predicts adverse neurodevelopmental outcome in children born preterm. *Neuroimage*. 2010;52:409-414.

54. Keunen K, Kersbergen KJ, Groenendaal F, et al. Brain tissue volumes in preterm infants: prematurity, perinatal risk factors and neurodevelopmental outcome: a systematic review. *J Matern Fetal Neonatal Med*. 2012;25:89-100.

55. Kwon SH, Vasung L, Ment LR, et al. The role of neuroimaging in predicting neurodevelopmental outcomes of preterm neonates. *Clin Perinatol*. 2014;41:257-283.

56. Estep ME, Smyser CD, Anderson PJ, et al. Diffusion tractography and neuromotor outcome in very preterm children with white matter abnormalities. *Pediatr Res*. 2014;76:86-92.

57. Padilla N, Falcon C, Sanz-Cortes M, et al. Differential effects of intrauterine growth restriction on brain structure and development in preterm infants: a magnetic resonance imaging study. *Brain Res*. 2011;1382:98-108.

58. Morsing E, Asard M, Ley D, et al. Cognitive function after intrauterine growth restriction and very preterm birth. *Pediatrics*. 2011;127:e874-e882.

59. Eikenes L, Martinussen MP, Lund LK, et al. Being born small for gestational age reduces white matter integrity in adulthood: a prospective cohort study. *Pediatr Res*. 2012;72:649-654.

60. Tanis JC, van der Ree MH, Roze E, et al. Functional outcome of very preterm-born and small-for-gestational-age children at school age. *Pediatr Res*. 2012;72:641-648.

61. Levine TA, Grunau RE, McAuliffe FM, et al. Early childhood neurodevelopment after intrauterine growth restriction: a systematic review. *Pediatrics*. 2015;135:126-141.

62. Guellec I, Marret S, Baud O, et al. Intrauterine growth restriction, head size at birth, and outcome in very preterm infants. *J Pediatr*. 2015;167:975-981.

63. Vinall J, Grunau RE, Brant R, et al. Slower postnatal growth is associated with delayed cerebral cortical maturation in preterm newborns. *Sci Transl Med*. 2013;5:168ra168.

64. Fishman MA, Prensky AL, Dodge PR. Low content of cerebral lipids in infants suffering from malnutrition. *Nature*. 1969;221: 552-553.

65. Fox JH, Fishman MA, Dodge PR, et al. The effect of malnutrition on human central nervous system myelin. *Neurology*. 1972;22:1213-1216.

66. Martinez M. Myelin lipids in the developing cerebrum, cerebellum, and brain stem of normal and undernourished children. *J Neurochem*. 1982;39:1684-1692.

67. Chase HP, Martin HP. Undernutrition and child development. *N Engl J Med*. 1970;282:933-939.

68. Stoch MB, Smythe PM, Moodie AD, et al. Psychosocial outcome and CT findings after gross undernourishment during infancy: a 20-year developmental study. *Dev Med Child Neurol*. 1982;24:419-436.

69. Galler JR, Ramsey F, Solimano G. The influence of early malnutrition on subsequent behavioral development III.

70. Rosso P. Morbidity and mortality in intrauterine growth retardation. In: Senterre J, ed. *Intrauterine Growth Retardation*. New York: Raven Press; 1989:123-142.

71. Ballabriga A. Some aspects of clinical and biochemical changes related to nutrition during brain development in humans. In: Evrard P, Minkowski A, eds. *Developmental Neurobiology*. New York: Raven Press, Ltd.; 1989:271-286.

72. Galler JR, Ramsey FC, Morley DS, et al. The long-term effects of early kwashiorkor compared with marasmus. IV. Performance on the national high school entrance examination. *Pediatr Res*. 1990;28:235-239.

73. Rosso P. Maternal nutrition and fetal growth: implications for subsequent mental competence. In: Rassin DK, Haber B, Drujan BD, eds. *Current Topics in Nutrition and Disease*. Vol. 16. Basic and Clinical Aspects of Nutrition and Brain Development. New York: Alan R. Liss, Inc.; 1987:339-357.

74. Dobbing J. Maternal nutrition in pregnancy and later achievement of offspring: a personal interpretation. *Early Hum Dev*. 1985;12: 1-8.

75. Dobbing J. Infant nutrition and later achievement. *Am J Clin Nutr*. 1985;41:477-484.

76. Stein Z, Susser M. Early nutrition, fetal growth, and mental function: observations in our species. In: Rassin DK, Haber B, Drujan BD, eds. *Current Topics in Nutrition and Disease*. Vol. 16. Basic and Clinical Aspects of Nutrition and Brain Development. New York: Alan R. Liss; 1987:323-338.

77. Gordon N. Some influences on cognition in early life: a short review of recent opinions. *Eur J Paediatr Neurol*. 1998;1: 1-5.

78. Koscik RL, Farrell PM, Kosorok MR, et al. Cognitive function of children with cystic fibrosis: deleterious effect of early malnutrition. *Pediatrics*. 2004;113:1549-1558.

79. Elitt CM, Rosenberg PA. The challenge of understanding cerebral white matter injury in the premature infant. *Neuroscience*. 2014;276:216-238.

80. Deoni SC, Dean DC 3rd, Piryatinsky I, et al. Breastfeeding and early white matter development: a cross-sectional study. *Neuroimage*. 2013;82:77-86.

81. Grossmann T, Johnson MH. The development of the social brain in human infancy. *Eur J Neurosci*. 2007;25:909-919.

82. Isaacs EB, Fischl BR, Quinn BT, et al. Impact of breast milk on intelligence quotient, brain size, and white matter development. *Pediatr Res*. 2010;67:357-362.

83. Ou X, Andres A, Cleves MA, et al. Sex-specific association between infant diet and white matter integrity in 8-y-old children. *Pediatr Res*. 2014;76:535-543.

84. Jensen CL, Voigt RG, Llorente AM, et al. Effects of early maternal docosahexaenoic acid intake on neuropsychological status and visual acuity at five years of age of breast-fed term infants. *J Pediatr*. 2010;157:900-905.

85. Yager JY, Hartfield DS. Neurologic manifestations of iron deficiency in childhood. *Pediatr Neurol*. 2002;27:85-92.

86. Gordon N. Iron deficiency and the intellect. *Brain Dev*. 2003;25: 3-8.

87. Georgieff MK, Innis SM. Controversial nutrients that potentially affect preterm neurodevelopment: essential fatty acids and iron. *Pediatr Res*. 2005;57:99R-103R.

88. Roncagliolo M, Garrido M, Walter T, et al. Evidence of altered central nervous system development in infants with iron deficiency anemia at 6 mo: delayed maturation of auditory brainstem responses. *Am J Clin Nutr*. 1998;68:683-690.

89. Friel JK, Aziz K, Andrews WL, et al. A double-masked randomized control trial of iron supplementation in early infancy in healthy term breast-fed infants. *J Pediatr*. 2003;143:582-586.

90. Lozoff B, De Andraca I, Castillo M, et al. Behavioral and developmental effects of preventing iron-deficiency anemia in health full-term infants. *Pediatrics*. 2003;112:846-854.

91. Kon N, Tanaka K, Sekigawa M, et al. Association between iron status and neurodevelopmental outcomes among VLBW infants. *Brain Dev*. 2010;32:849-854.

92. Lozoff B, Smith JB, Kaciroti N, et al. Functional significance of early-life iron deficiency: outcomes at 25 years. *J Pediatr*. 2013;163:1260-1266.

93. Berglund SK, Westrup B, Hagglof B, et al. Effects of iron supplementation of LBW infants on cognition and behavior at 3 years. *Pediatrics*. 2013;131:47-55.

94. Algarin C, Peirano P, Garrido M, et al. Iron deficiency anemia in infancy: long-lasting effects on auditory and visual system functioning. *Pediatr Res*. 2003;53:217-223.

95. Sarici SU, Serdar MA, Dundaroz MR, et al. Brainstem auditory-evoked potentials in iron-deficiency anemia. *Pediatr Neurol*. 2001;24:205-208.

96. Amin SB, Orlando M, Wang H. Latent iron deficiency in utero is associated with abnormal auditory neural myelination in >/=35 weeks gestational age infants. *J Pediatr*. 2013;163:1267-1271.

97. Ortiz E, Pasquini JM, Thompson K, et al. Effect of manipulation of iron storage, transport, or availability on myelin composition and brain iron content in three different animal models. *J Neurosci Res*. 2004;77:681-689.

98. Beard JL, Wiesinger JA, Connor JR. Pre- and postweaning iron deficiency alters myelination in Sprague-Dawley rats. *Dev Neurosci*. 2003;25:308-315.

99. Connor JR, Menzies SL. Relationship of iron to oligodendrocytes and myelination. *Glia*. 1996;17:83-93.

100. Rao R, Tkac I, Unger EL, et al. Iron supplementation dose for perinatal iron deficiency differentially alters the neurochemistry of the frontal cortex and hippocampus in adult rats. *Pediatr Res*. 2013;73:31-37.

101. Connor JR, Benkovic SA. Iron regulation in the brain: histochemical, biochemical, and molecular considerations. *Ann Neurol*. 1992;32:S51-S61.

102. Pillas D, Marmot M, Naicker K, et al. Social inequalities in early childhood health and development: a European–wide systematic review. *Pediatr Res*. 2014;76:418-424.

103. Eluvathingal TJ, Chugani HT, Behen ME, et al. Abnormal brain connectivity in children after early severe socioemotional deprivation: a diffusion tensor imaging study. *Pediatrics*. 2006;117: 2093-2100.

104. Behen ME, Muzik O, Saporta AS, et al. Abnormal fronto-striatal connectivity in children with histories of early deprivation: a diffusion tensor imaging study. *Brain Imaging Behav*. 2009;3: 292-297.

105. Govindan RM, Behen ME, Helder E, et al. Altered water diffusivity in cortical association tracts in children with early deprivation identified with Tract-Based Spatial Statistics (TBSS). *Cereb Cortex*. 2010;20:561-569.

106. Sheridan MA, Fox NA, Zeanah CH, et al. Variation in neural development as a result of exposure to institutionalization early in childhood. *Proc Natl Acad Sci U S A*. 2012;109:12927-12932.

107. Hanson JL, Adluru N, Chung MK, et al. Early neglect is associated with alterations in white matter integrity and cognitive functioning. *Child Dev*. 2013;84:1566-1578.

108. Kumar A, Behen ME, Singsoonsud P, et al. Microstructural abnormalities in language and limbic pathways in orphanage-reared children: a diffusion tensor imaging study. *J Child Neurol*. 2014;29: 318-325.

109. Bick J, Zhu T, Stamoulis C, et al. Effect of early institutionalization and foster care on long-term white matter development: a randomized clinical trial. *JAMA Pediatr*. 2015;E1-E9.

UNIT II

NEUROLOGICAL EVALUATION

Neurological Examination: Normal and Abnormal Features

Joseph J. Volpe

The neurological evaluation of the newborn comprises, as it does at other ages in pediatric medicine, the history, physical examination, and appropriate specialized studies. Appropriate neurodevelopmental follow-up is the critical next step in the neurological evaluation. The history is discussed best in the context of essentially every chapter of this book and is not repeated in detail here. Appropriate specialized studies (see Chapter 10) and neurodevelopmental follow-up (see Chapter 11) are discussed in separate chapters.

In this chapter, my focus is the neonatal neurological examination because an organized approach to the infant is so critical and, in fact, is the cornerstone of the neurological evaluation. My approach is organized on the framework of the neurological examination of older infants and children but is supplemented and modified significantly for adaptation to the newborn. Too often an organized, systematic approach to the infant is omitted because of the morass of catheters, tubes, monitors, blindfolds, intravenous accoutrements, and the like surrounding the child. It is curiously paradoxical that these outward manifestations of our attempts to provide optimal therapy may interfere significantly with the careful clinical examination that is necessary for rational judgments regarding diagnosis, prognosis, and management. On the other hand, the examiner should remember that the sick newborn, especially the premature infant, often has only tenuous control of such critical functions as respiration and cardiovascular status and that overly vigorous manipulation of the baby may have adverse consequences.

The single most important advice that I can convey concerning the neonatal neurological examination is to stand there and look; do not just do something. Examination of the infant requires patience, a careful eye, and minimal intrusion. Indeed, I am often asked to illustrate how I perform a neurological examination of the infant. The illustration, I fear, has disappointed many who expected that I would perform a series of secret, all-revealing maneuvers. My examination of the infant is dominated by careful observation and very little of the poking, prodding, scratching, and head-dropping maneuvers described in many classical writings. Most of my time is spent watching the infant, with some gentle touches to assess level of consciousness, eye position and movement, facial symmetry and movement, head position, asymmetry of limb positions, onset of spontaneous movement, and so forth. Surely evaluation of tone and reflexes has a role, but most of my examination is performed by watching the infant carefully. It has been somewhat embarrassing for me at times to watch visitors or trainees watch me watch the infant when I felt that they expected to see much more. To repeat, stand there and look; do not just do something.

NORMAL NEUROLOGICAL EXAMINATION

In the following section, the normal features of the neonatal neurological examination are outlined (Table 9.1). Before the formal neurological examination is addressed, brief discussions regarding the determination of gestational age and evaluation of the head are necessary.

Estimation of Gestational Age

Estimation of gestational age is particularly important for several reasons. First, various aspects of the neonatal neurological evaluation change with maturation, and recognition of these changes is critical in assessing the observations. Second, certain disorders are particularly characteristic of infants who are born prematurely but are of average weight for gestational age, those born at term but are small for gestational age, and the like. Third, the same insult (e.g., hypoxia-ischemia) will have a different impact on various regions of the central nervous system, in large part as a function of the gestational age of the infant.

The most helpful information for estimating gestational age is the date of the mother's last menstrual period, particularly in the case of the smallest infants.[1,2] It is unfortunate that often this information is not known precisely. Thus a variety of other measures have been used to estimate gestational age, including anthropometric measurements, such as birth weight and head circumference; certain external characteristics; neurological evaluation; radiological study of bone maturation; certain neurophysiological parameters, especially measurement of motor nerve conduction velocity or the electroencephalogram (EEG); and cranial ultrasonographic determinations of sulcal development. All these approaches have a certain merit as well as significant limitations. Detailed discussion of the aspects of the physical examination useful for the assessment of gestational age is available in multiple sources.[3-13] Of the techniques evaluated, examination of certain external characteristics has been most convenient and generally effective.[2,3,14] I have found four selected external characteristics to be particularly useful: the ear cartilage and its reflection in ear position, the amount of breast tissue, the characteristics of the external genitalia, and the creases of the plantar surface of the foot (Table 9.2).[3,5-7] In the first hours of life, although I routinely assess tone and posture, I do not use these measurements for the principal purpose of assessing gestational age but rather to assess neurological status because in my experience, these measurements are variable and sensitive to exogenous factors, including the process of birth. However, after the first hours of life, some find these evaluations useful for assessing maturation.[2,15,16] These comments are not to deny the value of recognizing the temporal characteristics of neurological maturation, as discussed in detail subsequently, but rather to emphasize that, in my hands, such characteristics are not optimal for the purposes of estimating gestational age, particularly in the immediate neonatal period.

Head: External Characteristics and Rate of Growth

External Characteristics

Skin: Sturge-Weber Syndrome. The external characteristics of the head to be evaluated include the size and shape

---

TABLE 9.1   Neonatal Neurological Examination—Basic Elements

Level of alertness
Cranial nerves
Olfaction (I)
Vision (II)
Optic fundi (II)
Pupils (III)
Extraocular movements (III, IV, VI)
Facial sensation and masticatory power (V)
Facial motility (VII)
Audition (VIII)
Sucking and swallowing (V, VII, IX, X, XII)
Sternocleidomastoid function (XI)
Tongue function (XII)
Taste (VII, IX)
Motor examination
Tone and posture
Motility and power
Tendon reflexes and plantar response
Primary neonatal reflexes
Moro reflex
Palmar grasp
Tonic neck response
Sensory examination

(see later discussion) and the skin. The skin of the head should be examined carefully for the presence of dimples or tracts, subcutaneous masses (e.g., encephalocele, tumor, cephalhematoma, subgaleal hemorrhage), or cutaneous lesions, all generally discussed elsewhere in this book. In this setting I discuss only the significance of *port-wine stains*, congenital vascular abnormalities that are present at birth and persist into adulthood. At birth, these lesions are most often pale-pink macular lesions that subsequently become dark red to purple and often nodular.[17] They are categorized according to their dermatomal distribution (Fig. 9.1). Their importance, apart from the significant cosmetic issue, relates principally to their association with abnormalities of choroidal vessels in the eye, which may result in glaucoma, and of meningeal and superficial cerebral vessels, which may result in cortical lesions with seizures and other neurological deficits (i.e., Sturge-Weber syndrome). The relations between the location of the port-wine stain and the incidence of glaucoma or the intracranial vascular lesion are shown in Table 9.3. In one large series, the intracranial vascular lesion of Sturge-Weber syndrome occurred in 40% to 50% of children with total involvement of V_1.[18,19] Notably, with *partial* involvement of V_1, the risk was markedly lower, and none of the 64 children with involvement of V_2 or V_3 or both (but not V_1) developed either the intracranial lesion or glaucoma.[18,19] The particular prognostic importance of involvement of V_1 (particularly the superior eyelid) has been confirmed in later series.[20-23] The disorder has been shown recently to be caused by a somatic mutation in a gene encoding a guanine nucleotide binding protein (*GNAQ*).[24] The optimal timing of therapy has been the subject of debate. Pulsed dye laser therapy is most effective and best tolerated when used early in infancy.[25,26]

Head Size and Shape. Head circumference is a useful measure of intracranial volume and therefore also of the volume of the brain and cerebrospinal fluid. Less commonly, head circumference is significantly affected by the size of extracerebral spaces, subdural and subarachnoid, or by the intracranial blood volume. Scalp edema, subcutaneous infiltration of fluid from intravenous infusion, and cephalhematomas have obvious effects as well. Nevertheless, measurement of head circumference remains one of the most readily available and useful means for evaluating the status of the central nervous system in the newborn period.

TABLE 9.2   External Characteristics Useful for Estimation of Gestational Age

EXTERNAL CHARACTERISTIC	GESTATIONAL AGE			
	28 WEEKS	**32 WEEKS**	**36 WEEKS**	**40 WEEKS**
Ear cartilage	Pinna soft, remains folded	Pinna slightly harder but remains folded	Pinna harder, springs back	Pinna firm, stands erect from head
Breast tissue	None	None	1–2 mm nodule	6–7 mm nodule
External genitalia: male	Testes undescended, smooth scrotum	Testes in inguinal canal, few scrotal rugae	Testes high in scrotum, more scrotal rugae	Testes descended, pendulous scrotum covered with rugae
External genitalia: female	Prominent clitoris, small, widely separated labia	Prominent clitoris, larger separated labia	Clitoris less prominent, labia majora cover labia minora	Clitoris covered by labia majora
Plantar surface	Smooth	1–2 anterior creases	2–3 anterior creases	Creases cover sole

Adapted from references 3 to 8.

TABLE 9.3 Relation Between Location of Port-Wine Stain and Subsequent Incidence of Glaucoma or Sturge-Weber Syndrome

LOCATION OF PORT-WINE STAIN (DERMATOMAL DISTRIBUTION)	TOTAL NUMBER	INTRACRANIAL VASCULAR LESION ± GLAUCOMA	GLAUCOMA ALONE	PORT-WINE STAIN ONLY
V_1 (total) alone	4	2	1	1
V_1 (total) with other dermatomes	21	9	3	9
V_1 (partial) with or without other dermatomes	17	1	0	16
V_2 alone	29	0	0	29
V_3 alone	13	0	0	13
$V_2 + V_3$ (unilateral or bilateral)	22	0	0	22

Data from Enjolras O, Riche MC, Merland JJ. Facial port-wine stains and Sturge-Weber syndrome. *Pediatrics*. 1985;76:48-51.

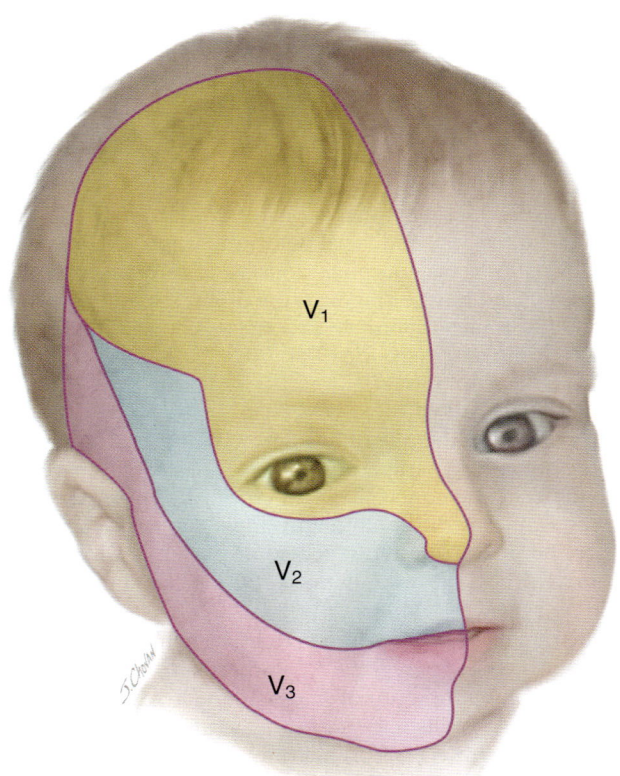

Figure 9.1 Dermatomal distribution of the face. Note the delineation of the three branches of the trigeminal nerve: ophthalmic *(V₁)*, maxillary *(V₂)*, and mandibular *(V₃)*. (From Enjolras O, Riche MC, Merland JJ. Facial port-wine stains and Sturge-Weber syndrome. *Pediatrics.* 1985;76:48-51.)

TABLE 9.4 Distribution of Suture Involvement in Craniosynostosis

SUTURES	PERCENT OF CASES[a] (%)
Sagittal only	56
Coronal only	25
One	13
Both	12
Metopic only	4
Lambdoid only (one or both)	2
Various combinations	13

[a]Total of 519 patients.

Data from Matson D. *Neurosurgery of Infancy and Childhood.* Springfield: Charles C Thomas; 1969.

Longitudinal measurements in particular provide valuable information.

Head circumference is influenced by *head shape*: the more circular the head shape, the smaller the circumference needs be to contain the same area and the same intracranial volume. Infants with relatively large occipital-frontal diameters will have larger measured head circumferences than those with relatively large biparietal diameters. This fact has important implications in evaluating the head circumference of an infant with a skull deformity such as craniosynostosis (see next paragraph). In premature infants, over the first 2 to 3 months of life, there is an impressive change in head shape that is characterized by an increase in occipital-frontal diameter relative to biparietal diameter (Fig. 9.2). Because this alteration occurs over a matter of *weeks*, it usually does not cause major difficulties in the interpretation of head circumference but does remain a fact to be considered, especially in infants with unusually marked dolichocephalic change.

Craniosynostosis, premature closure of cranial suture(s), may affect one or more cranial sutures (Table 9.4).[27,28] Simple sagittal synostosis is most common[27,29] and accounts for 50% to 60% of cases.[30] Coronal synostosis is next most common and accounts for 20% to 30% of cases (see Table 9.4). The diagnosis can be suspected by the shape of the head; with synostosis of a suture, growth of the skull can occur parallel to the affected suture but not at right angles (Fig. 9.3). The "keel-shaped" head of sagittal synostosis is termed *dolichocephaly* or *scaphocephaly*; the wide head of coronal synostosis is called *brachycephaly*; and the tower-shaped head of combined coronal, sagittal, and lambdoid synostosis is known as *acrocephaly*. The initial evaluation has traditionally been skull radiography, although recent work indicates that cranial ultrasonography is as effective as skull radiography except for assessment of the metopic suture and avoids radiation.[31] For infants requiring intervention, three-dimensional (3D) computed

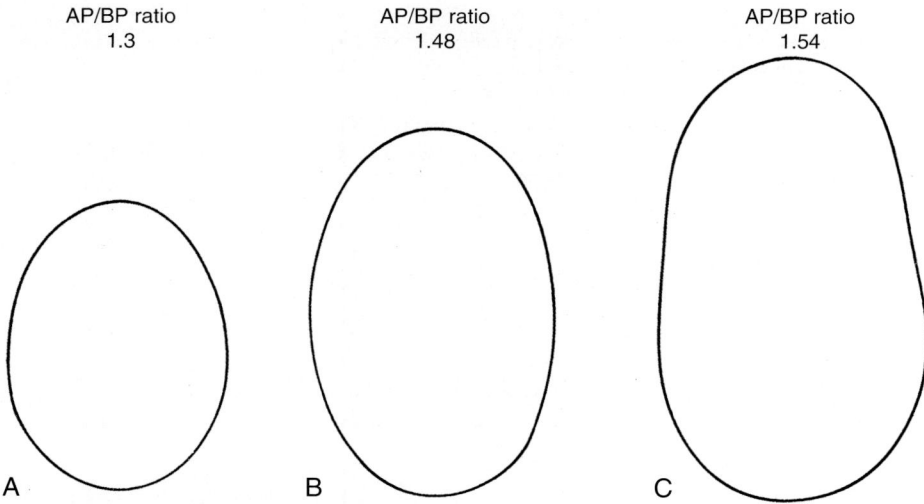

AP/BP ratio
1.3

AP/BP ratio
1.48

AP/BP ratio
1.54

A   B   C

Figure 9.2 Change in head shape in premature infants. Measurements of AP/BP ratio (anterior-posterior [AP] and biparietal [BP] diameters) and drawings of head shape (vertex view) of an infant, born at 28 weeks of gestation, made at (A) 1 week, (B) 5 weeks, and (C) 11½ weeks. (From Baum JD, Searls D. Head shape and size of pre-term low-birthweight infants. *Dev Med Child Neurol.* 1971;13:576.)

tomography (CT) reconstructions are used for surgical planning. Less than 10% of cases of cranial synostosis are familial or represent complex syndromes, the major features, genetics, and neurological outcome of which are summarized in Table 9.5.[28,30,32-38] Most syndromic craniosynostoses are related to mutations in the pathway of the fibroblast growth factor receptor. The outcome in the more common single-suture craniosynostosis is generally favorable, although at least 40% of cases later exhibit learning, behavioral, and other developmental deficits.[30,39,40] Among the subjects with single-suture craniosynostosis, the most neurodevelopmentally vulnerable are those with coronal and lambdoid fusions.[40] The neurological outcome in syndromic craniosynostosis in general is more unfavorable than the outcome in nonsyndromic cases. The importance of early correction of synostosis for optimal cosmetic appearance and other aspects of management are discussed in standard textbooks of neurosurgery. In large series of nonsyndromic cases, outcome has been better for infants operated on early in the first year than later in infancy.[30,41] Surgical approaches have recently been reviewed.[28]

Positional or deformational plagiocephaly has become a frequent clinical issue in recent years. *Plagiocephaly* (*oblique head,* from the Greek) refers to a head appearance in which the occipital region is flattened and the ipsilateral frontal area is prominent, or anteriorly displaced (Fig. 9.4). In positional or deformational plagiocephaly, caused by external molding forces, the ipsilateral ear is also displaced anteriorly and the contralateral face may appear flattened.[28,42,43] Torticollis may be associated and cause a head tilt. Deformation plagiocephaly may be present at *birth*; secondary to *intrauterine* restriction of head movement, as with multiple gestation; abnormal uterine lie or neck abnormality (e.g., torticollis); or may evolve over the *first weeks to months of life,* usually secondary to a *supine sleeping position* as part of the *Back to Sleep* program.[30,42,44,45] Differentiation of deformational plagiocephaly from the rare unilateral lambdoid synostosis, which can also cause occipital flattening, is usually readily made clinically. In the latter the anterior displacement of the frontal area is usually less; the ear is posterior, not anterior, and is displaced inferiorly; and facial deformity is rare. Management of deformational plagiocephaly consists of parental counseling regarding head positioning with the infant supine, supervised time in the prone position, various exercises, and a skull-molding helmet if necessary (see Fig. 9.4).[30,42,46-48]

Rate of Head Growth

Interpretation of the rate of head growth in premature infants is often difficult, in part because *normal postnatal* rates have been difficult to define conclusively (in contrast to normal rates of intrauterine growth, as plotted on most standard charts) and in part because commonly occurring systemic diseases and caloric deprivation in the neonatal period may interfere with brain and head growth.

The rate of head growth in premature infants has been the subject of a variety of reports.[49-65] In the *healthy premature infant,* there is a minimal amount of change in the head circumference in the first days of life; indeed, a small amount of *head shrinkage* with suture overriding has been documented.[51,66] Head shrinkage reaches a peak at approximately 3 days of life, usually averages 2% to 3% of the head circumference at birth, and correlates closely with postnatal weight and urinary sodium losses. In view of these facts and the overriding of sutures, it has been suggested that the head shrinkage relates to water loss from the intracranial compartment.[51]

A longitudinal study of 41 premature infants (of less than 1500 g birth weight) with a favorable neurological outcome at age 2 years (as assessed by neurological examination and the Bayley Mental Developmental Scale) defined the rates of head growth shown in Table 9.6. Thus, after a period of decreasing head circumference in the first week, head growth increased by a mean of approximately 0.50 cm in the second week, 0.75 cm in the third week, and 1.0 cm per week thereafter in the neonatal period. Approximately similar data have been obtained in larger, more recent studies, although rates of 0.75 cm/week were documented in the last 6 to 8 weeks before

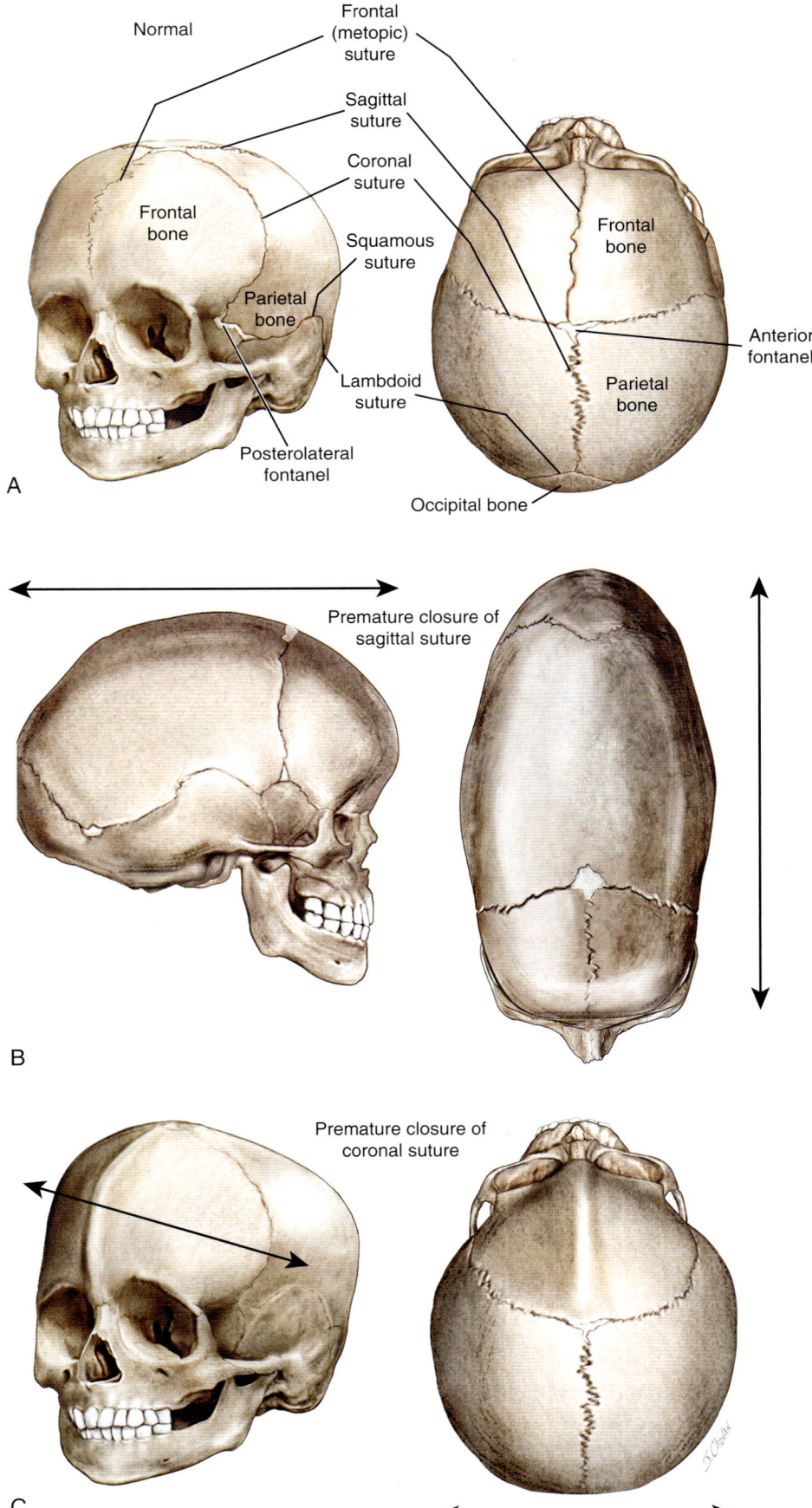

Figure 9.3 Changes related to premature closure of cranial sutures. Schematic diagram of (A) cranial sutures and changes in cranial shape with premature closure of (B) sagittal or (C) coronal sutures.

TABLE 9.5   Craniosynostosis Syndromes

NAME OF SYNDROME	CRANIUM	OTHER MAJOR FEATURES	GENETICS	NEUROLOGICAL OUTCOME
Antley-Bixler	Brachycephaly with multiple synostoses, especially of coronal suture	Maxillary hypoplasia, radiohumeral synostosis, choanal atresia, arthrogryposis	Autosomal recessive	Intelligence probably normal
Apert	Brachycephaly with irregular synostoses, especially of coronal suture	Midfacial hypoplasia, syndactyly of fingers and toes, broad distal phalanx of thumb and big toe	Autosomal dominant (usually new mutation)	Mental retardation or borderline intelligence common
Baller-Gerold	Synostosis of variable sutures, including metopic with trigonocephaly	Radial dysplasia with absent thumbs	Autosomal recessive	Mental retardation common
Carpenter	Acro-brachycephaly with synostosis of coronal, sagittal, and lambdoid sutures	Lateral displacement of inner canthi, polydactyly and syndactyly of feet	Autosomal recessive	Mental retardation common
Crouzon	Acrocephaly (tower-shaped) with synostosis of coronal, sagittal, and lambdoid sutures	Ocular proptosis (shallow orbits) and maxillary hypoplasia	Autosomal dominant (variable expression)	Mental retardation occasional
Greig	High forehead with variable synostosis	Hypertelorism, polydactyly and syndactyly of fingers and toes	Autosomal dominant	Mild mental retardation occasional
Muenke	Brachycephaly with coronal synostosis (unilateral or bilateral), macrocephaly	Mid-face hypoplasia, hypertelorism, hearing loss	Autosomal dominant	Normal intelligence usual
Opitz	Trigonocephaly with synostosis of metopic suture	Upward slant of palpebral fissures, epicanthal folds, narrow palate, anomalies of external ear, loose skin, variable polydactyly or syndactyly of fingers	Autosomal recessive	Mental retardation common
Pfeiffer	Brachycephaly with synostosis of coronal and/or sagittal sutures	Hypertelorism, broad thumbs and toes, partial syndactyly of fingers and toes	Autosomal dominant	Normal intelligence usual
Saethre-Chotzen	Brachycephaly with synostosis of coronal sutures	Prominent ear crus, maxillary hypoplasia, partial syndactyly of fingers and toes	Autosomal dominant (variable expression)	Mental retardation uncommon

term.[63,67] Slower rates of head growth were observed in infants with serious systemic disorders and subsequent neurological impairment.[53] More rapid rates of head growth in the first 6 weeks suggest hydrocephalus (e.g., after intraventricular hemorrhage), as detailed in Chapter 24. It is important to recognize that "sick" preterm infants with systemic disease will often exhibit a "normal" acceleration of head growth (i.e., "catch-up" head growth) after recovery from their illnesses. However, the smallest infants, less than 1000 g birth weight, generally do not exhibit as rapid growth as premature infants greater than 2000 g and do not catch up even by 2 years of age.[57] In addition, preterm infants born small for their gestational age often do not exhibit as rapid head growth or as effective catch-up as infants born average for their gestational age.[60]

The influence of duration of neonatal caloric deprivation (<85 kcal/kg per day) on head growth in the neonatal period was shown initially in a study of 73 preterm infants (mean gestational age, 30 ± 2 weeks) (Fig. 9.5).[68] Three phases of head growth were defined: an initial period of growth arrest or suboptimal head growth, followed by a period of catch-up growth, and terminated by a period of growth along standard curves. The duration of the period of growth arrest or suboptimal growth was directly related to the initial period of caloric deprivation and to the duration of mechanical ventilation, and the period of catch-up growth was directly related to the duration of the preceding caloric deprivation. The rate of head growth along standard curves was between the mean and 1 standard deviation (SD) below the mean for all infants except those calorically deprived the longest (4 to 6 weeks), in whom values were more than 1 SD below the mean. Indeed, such infants calorically deprived for more than 4 weeks had developmental scores below normal ranges at 1 year of corrected age. The deleterious effect of postnatal caloric deprivation is worse for preterm infants born small for their gestational age.[60]

The value of determining neonatal head growth in preterm infants for predicting neurodevelopmental outcome and delineating the relation of such head growth to effective nutrition and body growth has been shown to be particularly effectively in multiple recent studies.[69-73] The overall theme has been a positive relation between better weight gain, linear

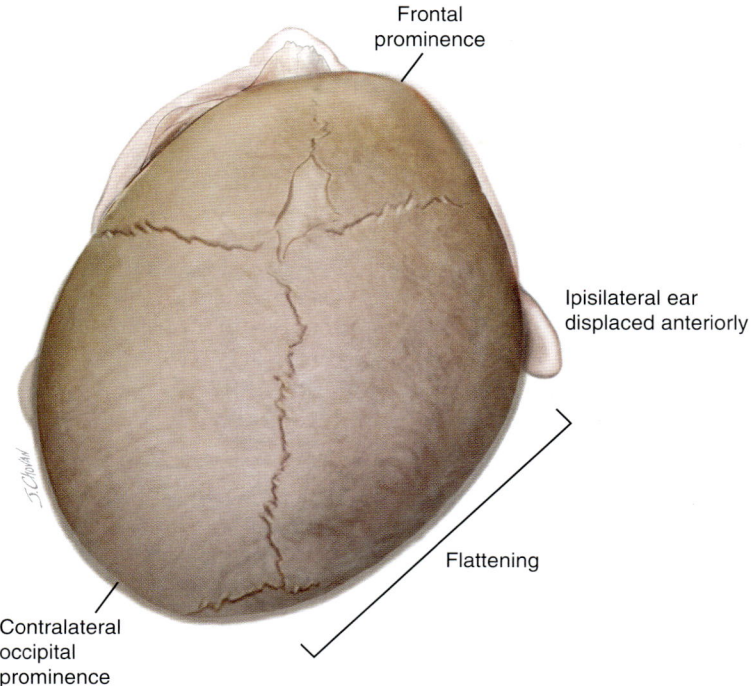

Frontal prominence

Ipisilateral ear displaced anteriorly

Flattening

Contralateral occipital prominence

Figure 9.4 Positional or deformational plagiocephaly. Note the flattening of the right occiput, because the infant is placed primarily in a supine position and the infant's preferred head position is to the right. The other changes are described in the text.

TABLE 9.6	Rates of Head Growth in Premature Infants With Favorable Neurological Outcome
POSTNATAL WEEK	**RATE OF HEAD GROWTH (CM/WEEK)**
First	−0.60
Second	0.50
Third	0.75
After third	1.0

Data from a study of 41 premature infants (<1500 g birth weight) in Gross SJ, Oehler JM, Eckerman CO. Head growth and developmental outcome in very low-birth-weight infants. *Pediatrics.* 1983;71:70-75.

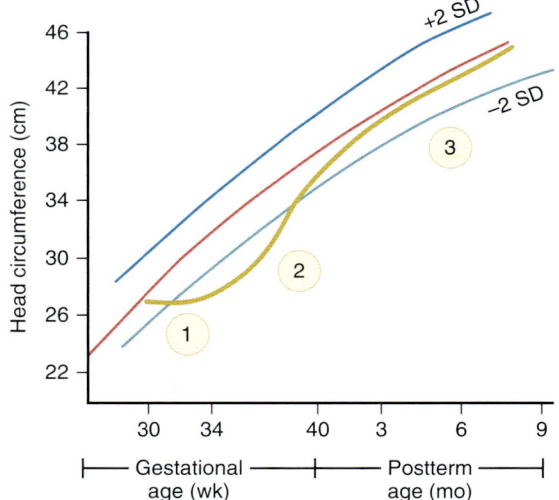

Figure 9.5 Phases of head growth. Phases of head growth derived from data of Georgieff and co-workers and based on a study of 73 premature infants of 30 ± 2 weeks' gestation (mean ± 2 SD). The three phases shown are discussed in the text. (From Georgieff MK, Hoffman JS, Pereira GR, et al. Effect of neonatal caloric deprivation on head growth and 1-year developmental status in preterm infants. *J Pediatr.* 1985;107:581-587.)

growth, head growth, and neurodevelopmental outcome even after control for such confounders as evidence of brain injury. The critical issues regarding the effects of nutrition in the neonatal period and infancy on brain growth and neurological outcome are discussed in more detail in Chapters 7 and 8.

Level of Alertness

The formal neonatal neurological examination should begin with an assessment of the level of alertness. This is perhaps the most sensitive of all neurological functions because it is dependent on the integrity of several levels of the central nervous system (see later). Several different terms have been used to describe this aspect of neurological function, including *state*[74,75] and *vigilance*.[76] It is important to recognize that the level of alertness in the normal infant will vary, depending particularly on time of last feeding, environmental stimuli, recent

experiences (e.g., painful venipuncture), and gestational age.[77-81] Before 28 weeks of gestation, it is difficult to identify periods of wakefulness. Persistent stimulation leads to eye opening and apparent alerting for periods measured principally in seconds. At approximately 28 weeks, however, there is a distinct change in the level of alertness.[76] At that time, a gentle shake will rouse the infant from apparent sleep and will result in alerting for several minutes. Spontaneous alerting also occasionally occurs at this age. Sleep-wake cycles are difficult to observe clinically but can be shown electrophysiologically.[82] By 32 weeks, stimulation is no longer necessary; frequently the eyes remain open, and spontaneous roving eye movements appear. Sleep-wake alternation, as defined by clinical observation, is apparent.[76] By 36 weeks, increased alertness can be observed readily, and vigorous crying appears during wakefulness. By term, the infant exhibits distinct periods of attention to visual and auditory stimuli, and it is possible to study sleep-wake patterns in detail.[78,81,83-87]

Cranial Nerves

Olfaction (I)

Olfaction, a function subserved by the first cranial nerve, is evaluated only rarely in the newborn period. In a study of 100 term and preterm infants, Sarnat observed that all normal infants of more than 32 weeks of gestation responded with sucking, arousal-withdrawal, or both to a cotton pledget soaked with peppermint extract[88]; moreover, 8 of 11 infants of 29 to 32 weeks of gestation, but only 1 of 6 infants of 26 to 28 weeks of gestation also responded. Activation of the orbitofrontal olfactory cortex was detected by near-infrared spectroscopy in full-term newborns exposed to vanilla or maternal colostrum in the first weeks of life.[89]

Olfactory Discriminations. More sophisticated techniques have demonstrated *olfactory discriminations* in newborns.[90,91] Using habituation-dishabituation techniques and recordings of respiration, heart rate, and motor activity, Lipsitt and co-workers demonstrated detection and discrimination among a variety of odorants.[92-94] Mediation of discriminations at a higher level than the periphery was shown by the observation that infants, initially habituated to mixtures of odorants, exhibited dishabituation when presented with the pure components of the mixtures. A particularly interesting demonstration of olfactory discrimination in the infant involved discrimination of the odor of breast pads of the infant's mother from unused pads or those of other nursing mothers.[90,95] Infants consistently adjusted their faces and gazes toward the pads of their own mothers. Later work involving the coupling of stroking with different odorants demonstrated complex associative olfactory learning in the first 48 hours of life.[90,96] That olfactory discrimination develops in utero is suggested by the demonstration of a neonatal preference for the odors of amniotic fluid.[97] Finally, nutrient (breast milk or formula) odor exposure via a pacifier was shown to stimulate nonnutritive sucking during gavage feeding of premature newborns.[98]

Vision (II)

Visual responses, the afferent segment of which is subserved by the second cranial nerve, exhibit distinct changes with maturation in the neonatal period. By 26 weeks, the infant consistently blinks to light.[76,99] By 32 weeks, light provokes eye closure, which persists for as long as the light is present (dazzle reflex of Peiper).[100] A series of behaviors associated with *visual fixation* can be identified by 32 weeks of gestation and can be shown to increase considerably over the next 4 weeks.[101] By 34 weeks, more than 90% of infants will track a fluffy ball of red wool.[102] At 37 weeks, the infant will turn the eyes toward a soft light.[76] By term, visual fixation and

following are well developed.[103-105] For testing of visual fixation and following, I have found most useful as a target a fluffy ball of red yarn. Opticokinetic nystagmus, elicited by a rotating drum, is present in the majority of infants at 36 weeks and is present consistently at term.[100,104,106,107]

The anatomical substrate for visual fixation and following a moving object in the newborn may not be primarily the occipital cortex, as usually thought. Thus, two studies of newborn infants with apparent absence of occipital cortex secondary to maldevelopment (holoprosencephaly) or destructive lesion (congenital hydrocephalus, ischemic injury) suggest that these abilities are mediated at subcortical sites.[108-110] Experimental studies in subhuman primates have defined such a subcortical system involving the retina, optic nerves and tract, pulvinar, and superior colliculus—the "collicular visual system."[111,112] Visual abilities beyond the ability to track a moving object (i.e., visual discriminatory skills; see next paragraphs), however, do require the geniculocalcarine cortical system.

Visual Acuity, Color, and Other Discriminations. Elegant studies have provided important information about neonatal *visual acuity, color perception, contrast sensitivity,* and *visual discrimination.*[105,113-122] Through use of the opticokinetic nystagmus response to striped patterns of varying width, it has been demonstrated that the newborn exhibits at least 20/150 vision.[123] Using a visual fixation technique, Fantz showed that the newborn attended to stripes of ⅛-inch width.[124] Visual acuity in premature infants with birth weights of 1500 to 2500 g studied at approximately 38 weeks' gestational age is similar to that of term infants.[119] Although studies of color perception in the newborn period often have not rigorously distinguished brightness and color, newborn infants will clearly follow a colored object.[125] Color vision is demonstrable by at least as early as 2 months of age.[126,127] Contrast sensitivity increases dramatically between 4 and 9 postnatal weeks.[116]

Discrimination of a rather complex degree has been demonstrated for newborn infants.[105,114,117,118,128-134] Infants as young as 35 weeks of gestation exhibit a distinct visual preference for patterns, particularly those with a greater number of details and larger details. Curved contours are favored over straight lines. Preference for novel patterns becomes apparent at 3 to 5 months.[118] Preference for patterns with facial resemblance develops between approximately 10 and 15 weeks of age[135]; promptly thereafter there is discrimination according to facial features.[136] The degree of contrast has a direct effect on preferences.[137] Binocular vision and appreciation of depth also appear by approximately 3 to 4 postnatal months.[114] Binocular visual acuity increases most rapidly during the same interval.[115] These higher-level visual abilities may reflect a change in the major anatomical substrate from subcortical to cortical structures.[105,112,138] Nevertheless, two functional magnetic resonance imaging (fMRI) studies of infants from the first days of life do show some evidence for activation of the visual cortex with visual stimulation; subcortical structures could not be addressed because of small anatomical size.[139,140] Infants in the first days of life have also been shown to imitate facial gestures (Fig. 9.6).[141,142] In addition, imitation of finger movements, especially involving the left hand, has been demonstrated in healthy term infants.[143] Thus, striking changes in cortically mediated visual function occur in the first weeks and months of postnatal life. It is noteworthy that this is a period for rapid

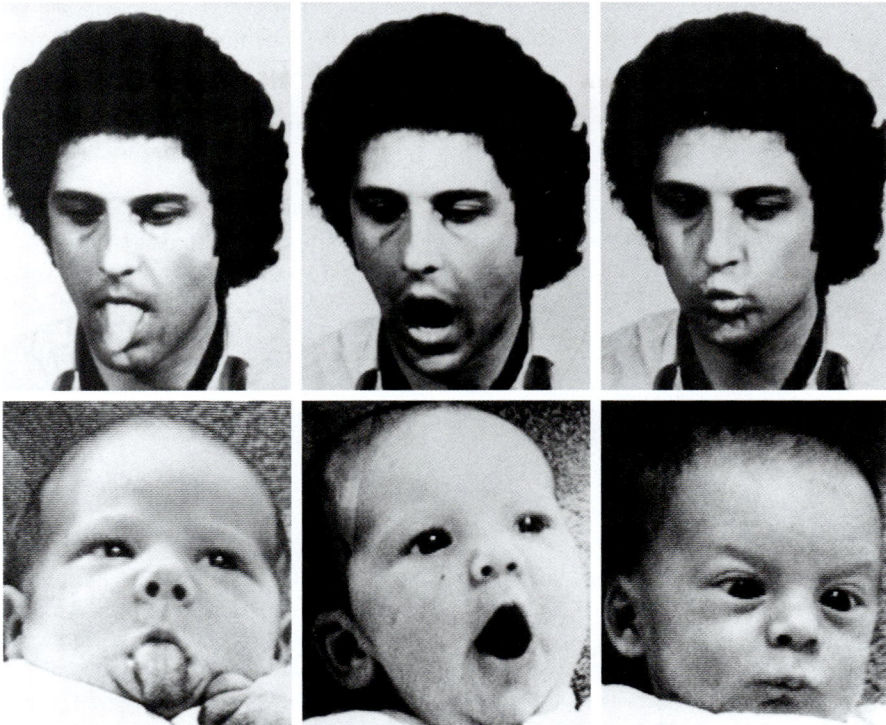

Figure 9.6 Imitation of facial gestures. Sample photographs from videotape recordings of 2- to 3-week-old infants imitating tongue protrusion, mouth opening, and lip protrusion as demonstrated by an adult experimenter. (From Meltzoff AN, Moore MK. Imitation of facial and manual gestures by human neonates. *Science.* 1977;198:75.)

dendritic growth and synaptogenesis in visual cortex and myelination of the optic radiation (see Chapters 7 and 8).

Optic Fundi (II)

The funduscopic examination in the newborn period is facilitated considerably by the aid of a nurse and patience on the part of the examiner. The *optic disc* of the newborn lacks much of the pinkish color observed in the older infant and has a paler, gray-white appearance. This color and the less prominent vascularity of the neonatal optic disc may make distinction from optic atrophy difficult. *Retinal hemorrhages* have been observed in 20% to 40% of all newborn infants, with no association with obvious perinatal difficulties, concomitant central nervous system injury, or neurological sequelae.[100,144-146] A relationship to vaginal delivery is apparent; in one study, 38% of infants delivered vaginally exhibited retinal hemorrhages in contrast to 3% of those delivered by cesarean section (Table 9.7).[145] The hemorrhages generally resolve completely within 7 to 14 days. Consistent with these findings, an evaluation of eight consecutive newborns with retinal hemorrhages by MRI revealed no intracranial abnormalities.[147]

Pupils (III)

The pupils are sometimes difficult to evaluate in the newborn, especially the premature baby, because the eyes are often closed and resist forced opening and the poorly pigmented iris provides poor contrast for visualizing the pupil. The size of the pupils in the premature infant is approximately 3 to 4 mm and is slightly greater in the full-term infant. Reaction to light begins to appear at approximately 30 weeks of gestation, but it is not

TABLE 9.7	Neonatal Retinal Hemorrhage: Influence of Perinatal Factors	
	RETINAL HEMORRHAGES	
PERINATAL FACTOR	**NO. AFFECTED/ TOTAL NO.**	**AFFECTED (%)**
Normal vaginal delivery	48/127	38
Abnormal vaginal delivery	22/69	32
Vaginal delivery		
Spontaneous	61/160	38
Forceps	9/36	25
Cesarean section	1/38	3

Data from Besio R, Caballero C, Meerhoff E, Schwarcz R. Neonatal retinal hemorrhages and influence of perinatal factors. *Am J Ophthalmol.* 1979;87:74-76.

present consistently until approximately 32 to 35 weeks.[99,148] The amplitude of the pupillary response increases markedly between 30 weeks and term (Fig. 9.7).[149] The afferent arc of this reflex leaves the optic tract before the lateral geniculate nucleus and synapses in the pretectal region of midbrain before innervating the Edinger-Westphal nucleus of the oculomotor nerve, the efferent arc of the reflex.

Extraocular Movements (III, IV, VI)

Particular attention should be paid to eye position, spontaneous eye movements, and movements elicited by the *doll's-eyes*

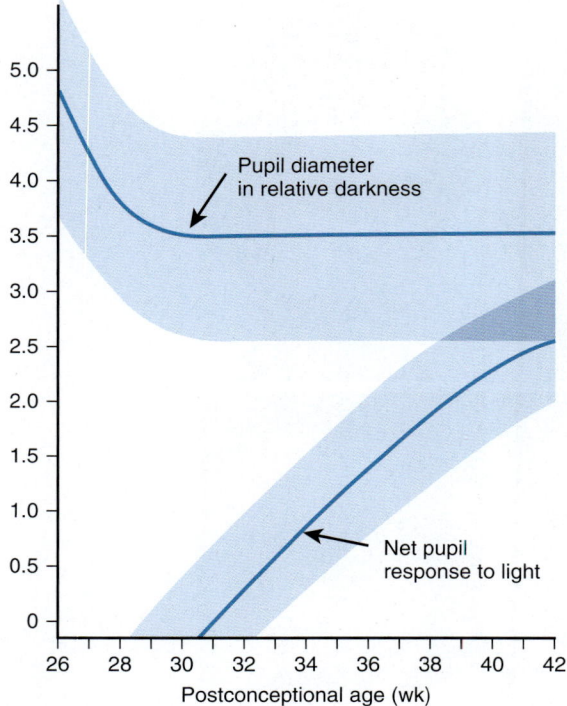

Figure 9.7 Pupil diameter in relation to light. Diameter of pupil in millimeters (mean ± SD) in term and preterm neonates in relative darkness (<10 footcandles) and after light stimulation (600 footcandles). (From Isenberg SJ. Clinical application of the pupil examination in neonates. *J Pediatr.* 1991;118:650.)

maneuver, vertical spin, or caloric stimulation as well as to a variety of abnormal eye movements (see later discussion). These oculomotor functions are subserved by cranial nerves III, IV, and VI and their interconnections within the brain stem. In most premature and some full-term infants, the eyes are slightly dysconjugate at rest, one or the other being 1 to 2 mm out. (This is demonstrated readily by observing the light reflected off each pupil with the light source in the midline at approximately 2 feet from the face.)

As early as 25 weeks of gestation, full ocular movement with the doll's-eyes maneuver can be elicited. Because interfering ocular fixation is not well developed at this stage, elicitation of lateral eye movements with the doll's-eyes maneuver is much easier in the small premature infant than in the full-term infant. Another convenient means of eliciting oculovestibular responses is to spin the baby held upright; the eyes will deviate in a direction opposite to the spin. Rapid maturation of this response with development of nystagmus as well as eye deviation occurs in the first 2 postnatal months.[150] In addition, at 30 weeks of gestation, caloric stimulation with cold water will lead to deviation of the eyes toward the side of the stimulated ear.[151] *Spontaneous* roving eye movements are common at approximately 32 weeks.[152] The tracking movements of full-term and older infants at first are rather jerky and do not become smooth and gliding until approximately the third month of life.[100]

Facial Sensation and Masticatory Power (V)

Subserved by cranial nerve V, the trigeminal nerve, facial sensation is examined best with pinprick. The resulting facial grimace begins on the stimulated side of the face. If the infant has a facial palsy, this response will be impaired and may be mistakenly attributed to involvement of the trigeminal nerve or nucleus. The strength of masseters and pterygoids is also dependent on the motor function of the trigeminal nerve. This strength is assessed by the evaluation of sucking and by allowing the infant to bite down on the examiner's finger.

Facial Motility (VII)

The parameters of interest are the position of the face at rest, the onset of movement, and the amplitude and symmetry of spontaneous and elicited movement. Facial motility is subserved by cranial nerve VII. With the face at rest, attention should be paid to the vertical width of the palpebral fissure, the nasolabial fold, and the position of the corner of the mouth. Examination of the face should never be restricted to observation of elicited movements (e.g., crying) because the quality of *spontaneous* facial movement is of greatest importance in the assessment of cerebral lesions. Subtle lesions at all central levels are best detected by close observation of the *onset* of movement.

Audition (VIII)

The eighth cranial nerve, via its connections in the brain stem and cerebral cortex, subserves auditory function. By 28 weeks, the infant will startle or blink to a sudden, loud noise.[76] As the infant matures, more subtle responses become evident (e.g., cessation of motor activity, change in respiratory pattern, opening of the mouth, and wide opening of the eyes).[100] The relation of such responses to the development of hearing has been the subject of considerable study and controversy, but it is likely that these responses represent the presence of at least some auditory function. Inability to elicit these responses is usually related to the failure to test in quiet surroundings while the baby is alert and not agitated or very hungry and to the failure of ensuring that the ear canals are free of the often copious vernix. In most cases, an infant who does not respond on the initial examination will respond when retested under more favorable conditions. More detailed evaluation of auditory function, including electrophysiological measurements (e.g., brain stem auditory evoked responses; see Chapter 10), certainly is indicated if behavioral responses are consistently absent.

Auditory Acuity, Localization, and Discriminations. More sophisticated studies have provided insight into neonatal *auditory acuity*, *localization*, and *discriminations*. Using the occurrence in the newborn of cardiac acceleration in relation to sound intensity, Steinschneider demonstrated a *threshold* for cardiac acceleration of about 40 dB.[153] *Auditory localization* has been shown by demonstrating loss and recovery of habituation to an auditory stimulus by changing the locus of the stimulus.[154,155] *Auditory-visual coordination* in localization was shown by exposing the infant to his mother speaking before him through a soundproof glass screen, her voice transmitted through a stereo system.[156,157] When the stereo system was in balance (i.e., the voice came from straight ahead), the infant was content, but if the voice appeared to come from a location different from that of the face, the infant became very upset. Maturation of connections between the brain stem auditory nuclei (superior olivary nucleus, nucleus of lateral lemniscus, inferior colliculus), sensory nuclei, and facial nerve nucleus has been studied by measuring the amplitude of the blink response to glabellar tap when the tap is preceded by an auditory tone.[158,159]

TABLE 9.8   Auditory Discriminations in Newborn Infants in First Week of Life[a]

Auditory discriminations based on
   sound intensity, pitch, rhythm
   computer-simulated versus real cry
   phonemic category
   human (preferred) versus nonhuman voice
   mother's voice (preferred) versus other human voice

[a]See text for references.

Through the use of heart rate patterns and a habituation-dishabituation model, it has been possible to demonstrate *auditory discriminations* in 3- to 5-day-old newborn infants on the basis of intensity, pitch, and rhythm (Table 9.8). These findings are of particular interest in view of information suggesting that intensity and pitch discriminations may be mediated at subcortical levels, whereas cortical levels are required for the discrimination of temporal patterns.[160] Discrimination of synthetic speech sounds according to phonemic category and of tonal sounds of different frequencies was demonstrated in newborns in the first days of life.[161-164] Discrimination of real and computer-simulated cries by newborn infants was shown by observing much restlessness and crying in infants stimulated by the real cry and considerably less of such behavior in those stimulated by the computer-simulated cry.[165,166] Moreover, results of other studies indicate a preference of the newborn for the human voice rather than nonhuman sounds[167] and particular preference for the mother's voice rather than another human voice.[168-170] Finally, 2- to 4-week-old infants can learn to recognize a word that their mothers repeat to them over a period of time (2 weeks) and will "remember" the word up to 2 days without intervening presentations.[171]

Studies based on optical topography or fMRI show that newborns in the first days of life respond to normal speech with activation of the temporal regions preferentially in the left hemisphere.[172,173] These interesting observations demonstrate that the newborn brain exhibits the cortical organization to process speech and the regional specification for the left hemisphere for language. Similarly, a magnetoencephalographic study using a paradigm based on sound discrimination and important in auditory cognitive function demonstrated positive responses in newborns shortly after birth.[174]

Sucking and Swallowing (V, VII, IX, X, XII)

Sucking requires the function of cranial nerves V, VII, and XII[100,175]; swallowing, cranial nerves IX and X; and tongue function, cranial nerve XII. The importance of tongue function, particularly the "stripping" action of the medial tongue, has been demonstrated in ultrasonographic and fiberoptic studies of neonatal feeding.[176-179] The act of feeding requires the concerted action of breathing, sucking, and swallowing.[178,180-184] Not surprisingly, the brain stem control centers for these actions, termed *pattern generators*, are closely situated.[184,185] Sucking and swallowing are coordinated sufficiently for oral feeding as early as 28 weeks[152]; this finding is perhaps not surprising because swallowing is observed in utero as early as 11 weeks of gestation.[186] The development of rooting at approximately 28 weeks is a relevant complementing feature. At this early age, however, the synchrony of breathing with sucking and swallowing is not well developed[178]; thus oral feeding is difficult and, in fact, dangerous. By 34 weeks of gestation, however, the normal infant is able to maintain a concerted synchronous action for productive oral feeding.[182,184,187] However, maturation continues rapidly and linkage of breathing, sucking, and swallowing is not achieved fully until 37 weeks of gestation or more.[178,184] Moreover, even in the healthy term infant, the coordination of swallowing and breathing rhythms is not optimal in the first 48 hours of life.[181]

The gag reflex, subserved by cranial nerves IX and X, is an important part of the neurological evaluation in this context. A small tongue blade or a cotton-tipped swab can be used to elicit the reflex. Active contraction of the soft palate, with upward movement of the uvula and of the posterior pharyngeal muscles, should be observed.

Sternocleidomastoid Function (XI)

Function of the sternocleidomastoid muscle is mediated by cranial nerve XI. Because the function of the muscle is to flex and rotate the head to the opposite side, it is difficult to test in the newborn, especially in the premature infant. One useful maneuver with the full-term infant is to gently extend the head over the side of the bed with the child in the supine position. Passive rotation of the head reveals the configuration and bulk of the muscle, and function sometimes can be estimated if the infant attempts to flex the head.

Tongue Function (XII)

Function of the tongue is mediated by cranial nerve XII. The parameters of interest are the size and symmetry of the muscle, the activity at rest, and the movement. Tongue movement is assessed best during the infant's sucking on the examiner's fingertip. The important role of the tongue in oral feeding was discussed in relation to sucking and swallowing.

Taste (VII, IX)

Taste is evaluated only rarely in the neonatal neurological examination. This function is subserved by cranial nerves VII (anterior two thirds of tongue) and IX (posterior one third of tongue). The newborn infant is very responsive to variations in taste and is capable of sharp discriminations. Lipsitt and co-workers used various parameters of sucking behavior, not only to define gustatory discriminations but also to study learning processes in the newborn.[188,189] An apparatus that allows control of the fluid to be obtained by sucking, as well as measurement of duration and frequency of sucking, has been used to demonstrate that, when presented with a sweet fluid (e.g., 15% sucrose), the infant sucks in longer bursts and with fewer rest periods than when presented with water or a salty fluid.[188-190] When the infant is sucking the sweet fluid, the heart rate is increased. It was presumed from these data that the newborn infant "hedonically monitors oral stimuli and signals the pleasantness of such stimuli with the heart rate as an indicator response."[94]

Motor Examination

The major features of the motor examination to be evaluated in the neonatal period are muscle tone and the posture of limbs, motility and muscle power, and the tendon reflexes and plantar response. The infant's postnatal age and level of alertness have an important bearing on essentially all of these features. Unless otherwise indicated, most of the observations to be described next are applicable to an infant more than 24 hours of age and at an optimal level of alertness.

Tone and Posture

Muscle tone is assessed best by passive manipulation of limbs, with the head placed in the midline. Moreover, because the tone of various muscles will in part determine the posture of the limbs at rest, careful observation of posture is valuable for the proper evaluation of tone. Some investigators have devised various maneuvers of passive manipulation of limbs (e.g., approximation of heel to ear, hand to opposite ear [scarf sign], or measurement of angles of certain joints, such as the popliteal angle) to attempt to quantitate tone.[14-16,191] These maneuvers have not been particularly useful for me and are not discussed in detail.

Developmental Aspects. Saint-Anne Dargassies and co-workers have described an approximate caudal-rostral progression in the development of tone, particularly flexor tone, with maturation.[152] At 28 weeks, there is minimal resistance to passive manipulation in all limbs; but by 32 weeks, distinct flexor tone becomes apparent in the lower extremities. By 36 weeks, flexor tone is prominent in the lower extremities and is palpable in the upper extremities. By term, passive manipulation affords appreciation of strong flexor tone in all extremities.

The posture of the infant in repose reflects these changes in tone to some extent. In my experience, these postures are apparent principally when the infant is in a slightly drowsy state. The alert infant at these various gestational ages is more active and motile, and fixed postures or so-called preference postures are difficult to define. This fact has been documented well by Prechtl and co-workers and by others.[193-197] Nevertheless, the quiet infant at 28 weeks often lies with minimally flexed limbs, whereas by 32 weeks, there is distinct flexion of the lower extremities at the knees and hips. By 36 weeks, flexor tone in the lower extremities results in a popliteal angle of 90%, and there is consistent and frequent flexion at the elbows. By term, the infant assumes a flexed posture of all limbs.[76] Fisting, usually bilateral, is the predominant hand posture.[76,198] The evolution of hip and knee flexor tone with maturation is reflected in the developmental increase in pelvic elevation when the infant is in the prone position.[199]

Preference of Head Position. A consistent and interesting aspect of posture in newborn infants is a preference for position of the head toward the right side.[193,200-202] Prechtl and co-workers demonstrated head position toward the right side 79% of the time versus 19% toward the left and 2% toward the midline (Fig. 9.8).[193] In one study, this preference increased with gestational age,[201] whereas in another it decreased.[202] The head orientation preference may be less prominent in the first 24 hours of life.[203] This preference has not been attributable to differences in lighting, nursing practices, or other factors but appears to reflect a normal asymmetry of cerebral function at this age. Notably the left hemisphere, particularly the frontal region, mediates movement of the head to the right. As noted earlier, the left hemisphere appears dominant for speech perception in the newborn.

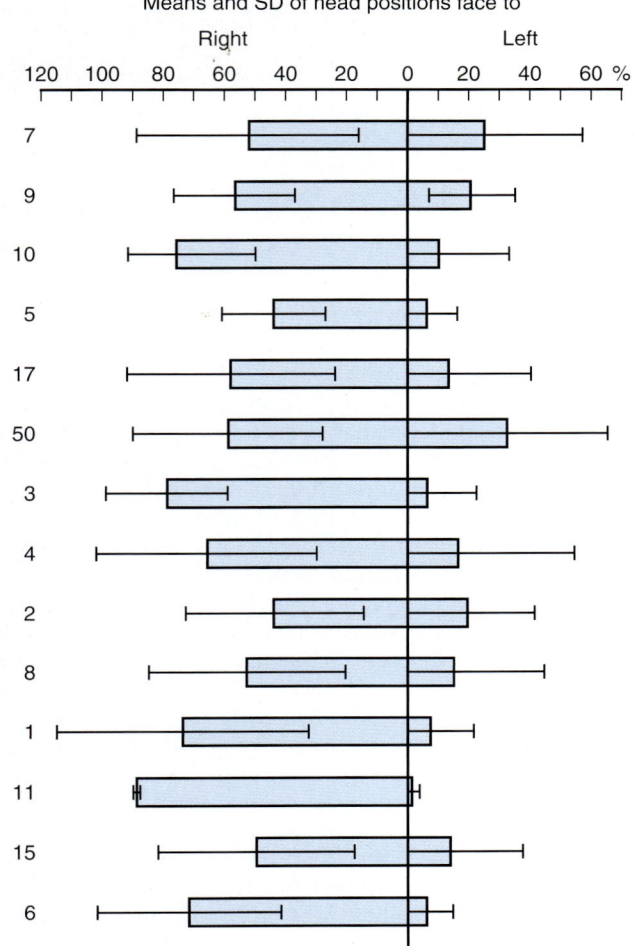

Figure 9.8 Preference of head position. Mean ± SD percentage of minutes from all observations in which each infant (series of 14) had the face to the right or left side. (From Prechtl HF, Fargel JW, Weinmann HM, Bakker HH. Postures, motility and respiration of low-risk pre-term infants. *Dev Med Child Neurol.* 1979;21:3.)

Motility and Power

The quantity, quality, and symmetry of motility and muscle power are the parameters of interest. Prechtl and co-workers[204-206] combined videotape and electrophysiological methods to describe the postnatal development of motor activity in the term infant. In the first 8 weeks, movements with a writhing quality predominate; in the period from 8 to 20 weeks "fidgety" movements are prominent; and after the latter period, rapid large-amplitude antigravity and intentional movements ("swipes and swats") are prominent. In general, preterm infants exhibited similar patterns of motor development when they attained comparable postmenstrual ages, albeit with minor delays in tone and quality of movements.[197,206-208] Prechtl and others[206,209-222] emphasized that the *quality* of *spontaneous* movements in preterm and term infants are of major importance vis à vis the status of the central nervous system.

Saint-Anne Dargassies, using less sophisticated techniques, described the developmental changes in motility in the preterm infant.[76] At 28 weeks, movements tend to involve the entire limb or trunk and may have a slow rotational component or

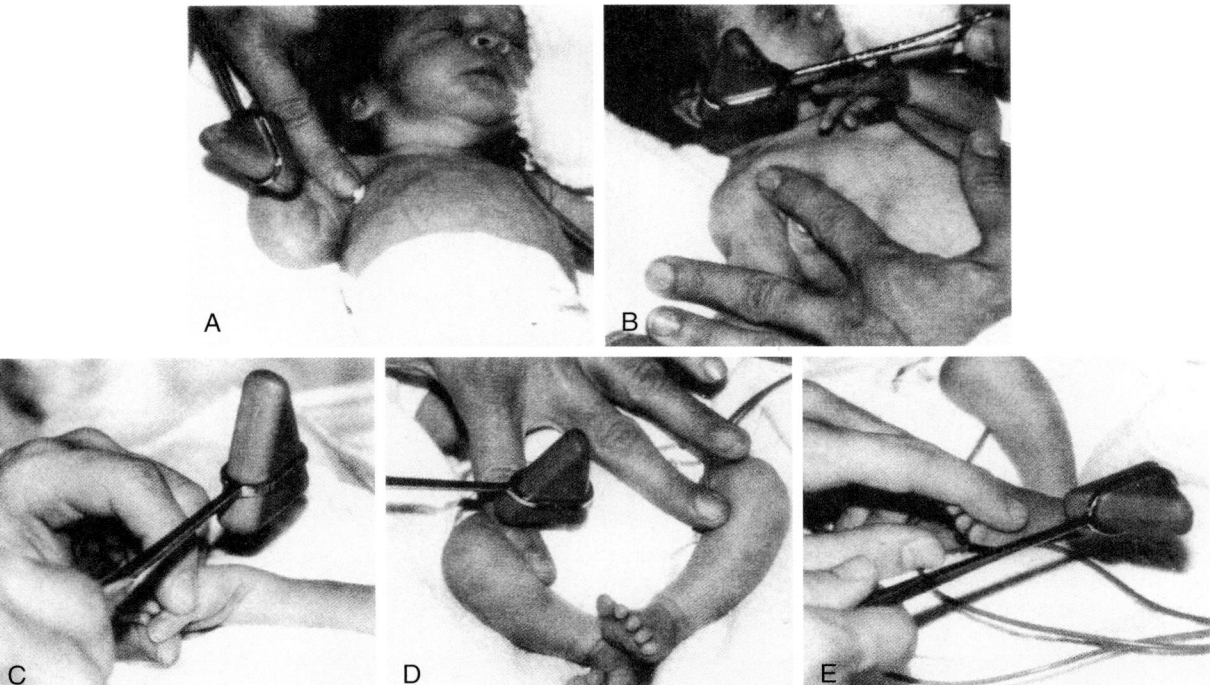

Figure 9.9 **Elicitation of deep tendon reflexes in a premature infant of 32 weeks' gestation.** (A) and (B) Pectoralis major; (C) brachioradialis; (D) thigh adductors and crossed adductors; and (E) Achilles tendon. (From Kuban KC, Skouteli HN, Urion DK, Lawhon GA. Deep tendon reflexes in premature infants. *Pediatr Neurol.* 1986;2:266.)

a fast, large-amplitude characteristic. By 32 weeks of gestation, movements were seen to be predominantly flexor, especially at the hips and knees, often occurring in unison.[76] Although head turning is present, neck flexor and extensor power is negligible, as judged by complete head lag on pull to sit or when the infant is held in the sitting position. By 36 weeks, the active flexor movements of the lower extremities are stronger and often occur in an alternating rather than symmetrical fashion. Flexor movements of the upper extremities are prominent. For the first time, definite neck extensor power can be observed. When the infant is supported in the sitting position, the head is lifted off the chest and remains upright for several seconds. By term, the awake infant is particularly active if stimulated with a gentle shake. Limbs move in an alternating manner, and neck extensor power is still better. Neck flexor power becomes apparent; when the infant is pulled to a sitting position with firm grasp of the proximal upper limbs, the head is held in the same plane as the rest of the body for several seconds.[76]

The importance of a fixed developmental program in motor development is suggested by the similarities in such development in comparing (at the same postmenstrual age) the fetus, the premature infant, and the term infant, albeit with minor exceptions.[a] The similarities outweigh the rather small differences.

Tendon Reflexes and Plantar Response

Tendon Reflexes. Tendon reflexes readily elicited in the term newborn are the pectoralis, biceps, brachioradialis,

knee, adductor, and ankle jerks. I have considerable difficulty obtaining triceps jerks in term infants. Most of these reflexes are elicitable but less active in preterm infants (Figs. 9.9 and 9.10). I prefer a small circular reflex hammer of the "Queen's Square" type. The reflexes are elicited readily by tapping the examiner's finger placed over the tendon of the designated muscle (see Fig. 9.9). An exception is the ankle jerk, which I prefer to elicit by tapping a finger placed over the distal plantar surface of the foot—the tap stretches the Achilles tendon and elicits the reflex. The knee jerk is often accompanied by crossed adductor responses, which should be considered a normal finding in the first months of life (less than 10% of normal infants demonstrate crossed adductor responses after 8 months of age).[225] The adductor jerk is also often accompanied by a crossed adductor response.

Ankle clonus of 5 to 10 beats also should be accepted as a normal finding in the newborn infant if no other abnormal neurological signs are present and the clonus is not distinctly asymmetrical. Ankle clonus usually disappears rapidly, and the existence of more than a few beats beyond 3 months of age is abnormal.

Plantar Response. The plantar response is usually stated to be extensor in the newborn infant.[224,226] This result clearly relates to the manner in which the response is elicited. Using drag of thumbnail along the lateral aspect of the sole, Hogan and Milligan[227] observed bilateral flexion in 93 of 100 newborn infants examined. We[228] observed a similar result in 116 (94%) of 124 infants. In contrast, Ross and associates,[229] using drag of pin or pinprick, observed a predominance of extensor responses, with flexion in only about 5% of patients.

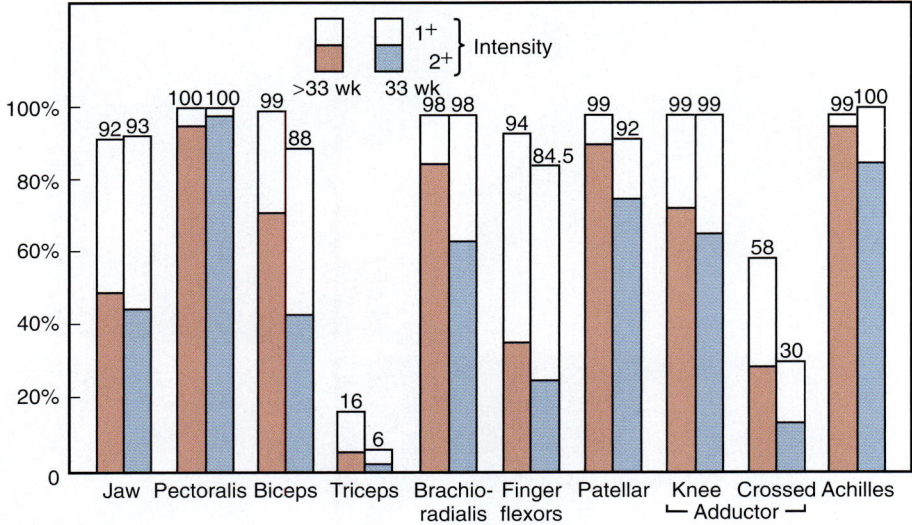

Figure 9.10 Maturity and deep tendon reflexes. Elicitation rate and range of intensity of deep tendon reflexes by maturity (less and greater than 33 weeks' gestation). (From Kuban KC, Skouteli HN, Urion DK, Lawhon GA. Deep tendon reflexes in premature infants. *Pediatr Neurol.* 1986;2:266.)

TABLE 9.9   Evolution of Moro Reflex, Palmar Grasp, and Tonic Neck Response[a]

| NEONATAL REFLEX | AGE (WEEKS OF GESTATION; MONTHS POSTNATAL) | | |
	ONSET (WEEKS)	WELL ESTABLISHED	DISAPPEARS (MONTHS)
Moro reflex	28–32	37 weeks	6
Palmar grasp	28	32 weeks	2
Tonic neck response	35	1 month	6

[a]See text for details.

In the evaluation of the neonatal plantar response, it is necessary to consider at least four competing reflexes leading to movements of the toes. Two reflexes that result in extension are nociceptive withdrawal (often accompanied by triple flexion at hip, knee, and ankle) and contact avoidance (elicited best by stroking the dorsum of the foot, which often occurs inadvertently when the foot is held to elicit the plantar response). Two responses that lead to flexion are plantar grasp and positive supporting reaction (both elicited by pressure on the plantar aspect of the foot). Because of these competing reflexes and the relative inconsistency of responses, I have considered the plantar response to be of limited value in the evaluation of the newborn infant and in the attempt to determine the presence of an upper motor neuron lesion.

Primary Neonatal Reflexes

Many primary neonatal reflexes have been described in the classic writings on the neonatal examination. I have found useful the Moro reflex, the palmar grasp, and the tonic neck response (Table 9.9). In general I find these reflexes to be more valuable in assessment of disorders of the lower motor neuron, nerve, and muscle than of the upper motor neuron.

Moro Reflex

The Moro reflex, elicited best by the sudden dropping of the baby's head in relation to the trunk (the falling head should be caught by the examiner), consists of opening of the hands and extension and abduction of the upper extremities, followed by anterior flexion ("embracing") of the upper extremities and an audible cry. Hand opening is present by 28 weeks of gestation, extension and abduction by 32 weeks, and anterior flexion by 37 weeks.[76] Audible cry appears at 32 weeks. The Moro reflex disappears by 6 months of age in normal infants.[224-226]

Palmar Grasp

Palmar grasp is clearly present at 28 weeks of gestation, is strong at 32 weeks, and is strong enough—and associated with enough extension of upper extremity muscles—to allow the infant to be lifted from the bed at 37 weeks.[76] The palmar grasp becomes less consistent after about 2 months of age, when voluntary grasping begins to develop.

Tonic Neck Response

The tonic neck response, elicited by rotation of the head, consists of extension of the upper extremity on the side to which the face is rotated and flexion of the upper extremity on the side of the occiput (the lower extremities respond similarly but often not as strikingly). The term *fencing posture* is an apt description. The response appears by 35 weeks of gestation[76] but is most prominent about 1 month after term; it disappears by approximately 6 months of age[225,226,230] (although the changes in tone may be palpable for several additional months).[231]

Placing and Stepping

The placing and stepping ("walking") reactions are elicited readily by 37 weeks of gestation.[76] The former is provoked by contacting the dorsum of the foot with the edge of a table. These reflexes are commonly elicited but their significance is not entirely clear.

Sensory Examination

Careful evaluation of sensory function has rarely been a part of the usual neonatal neurological examination. Most often the imprecise term *withdrawal* is used to describe the infant's response. It is noteworthy that the premature infant of just 28 weeks of gestation discriminates touch and pain, the former resulting in alerting and slight motor activity and the latter in withdrawal and cry.[152] The rooting reflex, elicited by tactile stimulation of the perioral region, is well established by 32 weeks of gestation. By approximately 36 weeks, there is rapid turning of the head away from pinprick over the side of the face.

I routinely assess the responses of the infant to multiple (three to five) pinpricks over the medial aspect of the extremities. Responses to be observed are latency, limb movement, facial movement (i.e., grimace), vocalization (i.e., cry), and habituation. A lower-level response is extremely rapid, is stereotyped (e.g., triple flexion at hip, knee, and ankle), and is not accompanied by grimace or cry. There is no clear response decrement with repeated trials (i.e., no habituation). A normal, higher-level response has a recognizable latency and consists usually of an apparently purposeful avoidance maneuver, usually lateral withdrawal, and grimace or cry. The response "dampens" with repeated trials; this characteristic of habituation is an important feature of the normal neonatal response.[232] In a systematic study of 130 healthy newborn infants (124 full term), we observed the higher-level motor response in 94%.[233]

Several careful studies have demonstrated that infants experience pain and that attempts to minimize pain during noxious procedures are beneficial.[234-238] Thus, infants exhibit characteristic behavioral, cardiorespiratory, hormonal, and metabolic responses to pain, retain memory of the pain for a period sufficient to modify subsequent short-term behavior, and respond beneficially to analgesic measures. Careful assessment of the quality of infant cry and facial expressions to pain indicates appreciation of graded levels of pain.[166,234,239] The deleterious effects of painful stimuli on brain growth in preterm infants are described in Chapter 7. Thus the older notion that infants do not experience pain because of their "underdeveloped nervous system" and do not require measures to minimize pain appears finally to have been laid to rest.

ABNORMAL NEUROLOGICAL FEATURES

In the following section, the major *abnormalities* of the neonatal neurological examination are described. Whenever possible, those anatomical loci within the neuraxis that, when deranged, may cause the neurological deficits are identified. In general, such clinicoanatomical correlations in the newborn must be made cautiously. The organization of this discussion is identical to that used to describe the normal neonatal neurological examination.

Abnormalities of Level of Alertness

Abnormalities of the level of alertness are the most common neurological deficits observed in the neonatal period. Detection of such abnormalities, when slight, requires careful observation and consideration of a variety of factors (e.g., time of last feeding, amount of recent sleep interruptions, gestational age, and similar factors).

To ensure consistency and avoid confusion, I use only three terms to characterize the level of alertness: *normal, stupor,* and *coma* (Table 9.10). These characterizations are based principally on three readily determined criteria: (1) the response to arousal maneuvers (i.e., persistent, gentle shaking, pinch, shining of a light, or ringing of a bell) and both (2) the quantity and (3) the quality of motility, both spontaneous and that elicited by pinprick of the medial extremities (see Table 9.10). Infants who are *normally alert* behave in the fashion described in the section on normal neurological findings for gestational age. Infants are considered to be *stuporous* when there is diminished or absent arousal response, and motor responses are diminished. In slight stupor, the infant is awake but "sleepy" or "lethargic," whereas in moderate stupor the infant appears to be asleep; in both states an arousal response, although diminished, is present. In deep stupor, the infant not only appears to be asleep but also cannot be aroused. The distinction between deep stupor and *coma* is based primarily on the quality of the motor responses (i.e., in deep stupor, motor responses are high level in type [nonstereotyped, with definite latency, and habituating], whereas in coma they are low level [stereotyped, rapid in onset, and nonhabituating or totally absent]). Most disorders that affect the neonatal central nervous system disturb the level of alertness at some time, and longitudinal characterization of this level is the

TABLE 9.10	Levels of Alertness in the Neonatal Period			
			MOTOR RESPONSES	
LEVEL OF ALERTNESS	**APPEARANCE OF INFANT**	**AROUSAL RESPONSE**	**QUANTITY**	**QUALITY**
Normal	Awake	Normal	Normal	High level
Stupor				
Slight	"Sleepy"	Diminished (slight)	Diminished (slight)	High level
Moderate	Asleep	Diminished (moderate)	Diminished (moderate)	High level
Deep	Asleep	Absent	Diminished (marked)	High level
Coma	Asleep	Absent	Diminished (marked) or absent	Low level

most sensitive barometer of the newborn infant's neurological status. Use of the terminology described in Table 9.10 enables different examiners to arrive at the same conclusion about an infant's level of alertness and to do so frequently and simply.

Stupor and coma occur in older patients when there is bilateral cerebral disturbance or disturbance of the activating system of reticular gray matter present in the diencephalon (especially thalamus), midbrain, or upper pons.[240,241] Similar correlates may pertain to the newborn infant, but detailed clinicoanatomical correlates of stupor and coma in the newborn period are not yet available.

Abnormalities of Cranial Nerves

Olfaction

Abnormalities of olfaction, detected by the simple bedside technique whereby a cotton pledget soaked with peppermint extract is used, have been demonstrated in infants with absent olfactory bulbs and tracts (i.e., disturbances of prosencephalic development, such as holoprosencephaly).[88] This simple test is recommended also for infants of diabetic mothers, because such infants carry an increased likelihood of olfactory bulb agenesis.[242] The use of olfactory stimuli by Lipsitt and others, as mentioned previously, to demonstrate function probably mediated at the cerebral cortical level (i.e., habituation-dishabituation), suggests the possibility that the study of olfactory responses may provide a means to evaluate higher neurological function in the newborn, at least on a research basis.

Vision

Consistent failure to demonstrate visual following (or optickinetic nystagmus with a rotating drum) in a full-term newborn is a disturbing sign. However, such failure most commonly does not relate to a *primary* disturbance in the optic nerves or tracts but rather is usually part of a constellation of neurological abnormalities indicative of generalized or multifocal disturbance of several levels of the central nervous system. (A less common cause for apparent lack of visual responsiveness is congenital ocular motor apraxia, related usually to cerebellar vermian hypoplasia, but the characteristic head thrusting and inability to initiate saccades usually do not become apparent until head control is achieved at 2 to 3 months of age.[243]) As discussed previously (see the section on normal neurological examination), the earlier notion that visual following of a moving object reflected cerebral function is probably incorrect, and disturbance of such visual following suggests impairment of connections between optic nerves, tract, thalamus, and superior colliculus. Blindness is not a common finding on follow-up examination of the newborn with impaired visual following; visual following usually appears, albeit delayed, in the first weeks of life. However, if pendular "searching" nystagmus, digital manipulation of the globe, and repetitive hand movements before the eyes appear in the first weeks or months of life, congenital blindness is likely, and the locus of the disturbance of optic pathways must be sought in the usual way.

Optic Fundi

A variety of abnormalities of the optic disc and retina may be detected in the neonatal period (Table 9.11).

Optic Disc Hypoplasia or Atrophy. Distinction of optic nerve *hypoplasia-dysplasia* and *optic atrophy* is useful. In *optic*

> **TABLE 9.11 Major Abnormalities of the Optic Fundus in the Neonatal Period**
>
> **Optic disc**
> Hypoplasia-dysplasia
> Atrophy
> **Retina**
> Retinal and preretinal hemorrhages
> Chorioretinitis
> Retinopathy of prematurity
> Retinoblastoma

nerve hypoplasia, the disc is small, one third to one half of the usual size, and occasionally is dysplastic in appearance.[244-247] Other useful findings in diagnosis are a second pigmented ring around the disc and tortuosity or abnormal origin of the vessels originating from the disc. The disorder is bilateral in approximately 85% of cases. This lesion accounts for about 25% of cases of congenital blindness[248] and relates to a disorder during midline prosencephalic development (i.e., second and third months); thus it may be associated with other neurological stigmata of such a disorder (see Chapter 2). Approximately 50% of affected patients subsequently exhibit other signs of cerebral abnormality (i.e., seizures and mental retardation).[245-248] The likelihood of such subsequent neurological deficits varies with the severity of hypoplasia and ranges from approximately 65% with severe bilateral hypoplasia to 40% for milder bilateral or unilateral disease. In one series of *septo-optic dysplasia* (absence of the septum pellucidum with optic hypoplasia-dysplasia), schizencephaly (*porencephaly*) or agenesis of the corpus callosum was associated with 81% of cases with severe bilateral optic disease (see Chapter 2).[247] In septo-optic dysplasia, the lesion is also often associated with hypothalamic-pituitary dysfunction, usually apparent after the neonatal period.[249] Neonatal hypoglycemia with seizures, however, has been reported.[245,246,250] Indeed, in one series selected from an endocrine clinic population, 75% of cases exhibited persistent neonatal hypoglycemia.[251] In approximately 50% of cases of congenital optic nerve hypoplasia with endocrine disturbance, the septum pellucidum is present on neuroimaging. MRI may detect hypothalamic defects in such cases. The endocrine abnormalities are related to impairment in trophic hormone secretions (indicative of hypothalamic maldevelopment), the most common of which involves growth hormone. Impaired growth becomes apparent later in the first or second year of life.[246,251]

In *optic atrophy*, the disc may be normal or nearly normal in size but is poorly vascularized and pale. (Presumably the optic nerve has developed normally and then has been injured or affected by an ongoing metabolic or degenerative process.) Although optic atrophy in the newborn may be associated with other ocular abnormalities (e.g., glaucoma and cataracts), there is no such association in most cases. The etiology is often attributed to injury caused by abnormalities of pregnancy, labor, or delivery, but conclusive data are lacking.

Retinal and Preretinal Hemorrhages. Retinal lesions include *retinal and preretinal hemorrhages*. The former are not of consistent clinical significance, as discussed in the earlier section on normal findings (see Table 9.7). Large preretinal hemorrhages are observed most commonly with major intracranial hemorrhage. These so-called subhyaloid hemorrhages are of ocular venous origin. Consequently increased intracranial pressure is likely to be or to have been present.

Chorioretinitis. Chorioretinitis is observed most commonly with toxoplasmosis, cytomegalovirus, rubella, and herpes simplex infections (see Chapter 34). Chorioretinitis is nearly a constant feature of symptomatic congenital toxoplasmosis, has a predilection for the macular region, and consists of prominent necrotic lesions with striking black pigment as well as yellow scarring. In symptomatic congenital cytomegalovirus infection, retinal lesions occur in about 20% of affected newborns, and although the lesions bear similarities to those in toxoplasmosis, they tend to be less pigmented and more peripheral in location. The chorioretinitis of rubella is readily distinguished from that of toxoplasmosis or cytomegalovirus infection in that it consists of small areas of depigmentation and pigmentation, giving a "salt and pepper" appearance to the retinal surface.

Retinopathy of Prematurity. The earliest vascular changes of retinopathy of prematurity are difficult to detect with certainty by direct ophthalmoscopy.[252,253] Progressive stages of the disease are more readily defined, especially by binocular indirect ophthalmoscopy. These stages include dilation and tortuosity of vessels, neovascularization, hemorrhages, intravitreous proliferation, and, finally, retinal detachment, beginning at the periphery.[253-258] The cornerstone of therapy is confluent diode laser coagulation to arrest progression of the disease.[259]

Retinoblastoma. Although retinoblastoma is only rarely detected in the neonatal period, it is important to recognize it as early as possible to achieve the best possible response to therapy. The usual presenting signs are the so-called white pupil and strabismus.[252] The tumor is bilateral in about one third of cases. In approximately 10% of cases, retinoblastoma is inherited in an autosomal dominant fashion. Thus a family history of an affected sibling should provoke a particularly thorough examination.

Pupils

The size of the pupils relates not only to the parasympathetic constrictor fibers, conveyed by the third cranial nerve, but also to sympathetic dilator fibers from the superior cervical ganglion and to systemic epinephrine from the adrenal medulla. Although afferent connections from the optic pathway may play a role in pupillary size, this part of the reflex arc is rarely the source of pupillary abnormalities in the newborn infant. Abnormal pupillary findings are of great value in clinical neurology in the localization of pathological events that occur in older infants and children. The occurrence and significance of such pupillary findings in the newborn period, however, are still not well defined.

Bilateral Increase in Pupillary Size. A bilateral increase in the size of pupils that are reactive to light is seen commonly during the first hours after perinatal asphyxia in those infants who usually are not seriously affected (Table 9.12) (see Chapter 20). This finding probably relates to systemic epinephrine release in association with asphyxia.[260,261] Late in the course of serious

TABLE 9.12	Major Pupillary Abnormalities and Causes in the Neonatal Period

Bilateral increase in size
Hypoxic-ischemic encephalopathy (reactive early, unreactive late)[a]
Intraventricular hemorrhage (unreactive)
Local anesthetic intoxication (unreactive)
Infantile botulism (unreactive)[b]
Bilateral decrease in size
Hypoxic-ischemic encephalopathy (reactive)
Unilateral decrease in size
Horner syndrome (reactive)
Unilateral increase in size
Convexity subdural hematoma, other unilateral mass (unreactive)
Congenital third-nerve palsy (± unreactive)
Hypoxic-ischemic encephalopathy (± unreactive)

[a]The most common reactivity to light is in parentheses.
[b]Usually midposition and unreactive.

hypoxic-ischemic encephalopathy, especially with other signs of brain stem failure, pupils may be dilated and fixed to light. A similar finding also mediated at the brain stem (midbrain) level is not unusual in massive intraventricular hemorrhage. In local anesthetic intoxication, pupils may be large and unreactive to light because of peripheral parasympatholytic effects (see Chapter 12). In infantile botulism, pupils are usually midposition in size (although they may be dilated) and unreactive to light, also secondary to peripheral synaptic effects (see Chapter 32).

Bilateral Decrease in Pupillary Size. A bilateral decrease in the size of pupils that are reactive to light (although the reaction may be difficult to detect) is seen most often once the first 12 to 24 hours after perinatal asphyxia have passed (see Table 9.12). With hypoxic-ischemic insults that have been well established for hours intrapartum, however, this miosis may be apparent earlier. The pupillary change is usually accompanied by other signs suggestive of parasympathetic discharge (e.g., increased respiratory secretions and gastrointestinal motility and a relative decrease in heart rate). Whether this apparent parasympathetic predominance relates to a central autonomic disturbance or a decrease in systemic catecholamine release is unclear.

Unilateral Decrease in Pupillary Size. A unilateral decrease in size of a pupil that remains reactive to light is seen most often with Horner syndrome (see Table 9.12). In the newborn, this syndrome is almost always associated with a brachial plexus injury, which includes involvement of the eighth cervical root and first thoracic root, destined for the cervical sympathetic ganglion (see Chapter 36).

Unilateral Increase in Pupillary Size. A unilateral increase in the size of a pupil that may be sluggishly reactive or unreactive to light is very unusual in the newborn (unlike older children and adults); this reflects the rarity of the uncal form of transtentorial herniation, which results in compression of the third cranial nerve and its associated parasympathetic fibers. The infrequency of the uncal syndrome is related both to the pliability of the

TABLE 9.13	Transient Abnormalities of Ocular Motility in the Term Newborn	
DISORDER OF OCULAR MOTILITY	**PERCENTAGE OF INFANTS (N = 242) (%)**	**OUTCOME**
Disconjugate gaze (esotropia or exotropia)	9	100% resolved in the neonatal period
Skew deviation	9	77% resolved by 1 month; 23% later developed esctropia
Downward deviation of eyes (while awake)	2	100% resolved by 6 months
Opsoclonus (intermittent)	3	100% resolved by 6 months, most by 1 month

Data from Hoyt CS, Mousel DK, Weber AA. Transient supranuclear disturbances of gaze in healthy neonates. *Am J Ophthalmol.* 1980;89:708-713.

TABLE 9.14	Strabismus in Survivors of Birth Weight Less Than 1500 g[a]
AGE OF TESTING	**PERCENTAGE WITH STRABISMUS (n = 155) (%)**
6 weeks	18
3 months	30
6 months	28[a]
9 months	28
12 months	14

[a]Also at 6 months, 21% of infants with strabismus had neurological abnormalities; 40% of infants with neurological abnormalities had strabismus. Data from van Hof-Van Duin J, Evenhuis-van Leunen A, Mohn G, Baerts W, et al. Effects of very low birth weight (VLBW) on visual development during the first year after term. *Early Hum Dev.* 1989;20:255-266.

neonatal skull and sutures and to the rarity of large *unilateral mass lesions*. In my experience, convexity subdural hematoma is the most common cause of this syndrome in the newborn infant (see Table 9.12 and Chapter 22). However, I have observed unilateral pupillary dilation secondary to transtentorial uncal herniation in neonatal bacterial meningitis.[262]

Unilateral pupillary dilation may be one feature of a congenital third nerve palsy, the other features of which include weakness of medial, superior, and inferior eye movements and ptosis (see Chapter 33). The defects of extraocular movement relate to disturbed innervation of the superior, inferior, and medial rectus and inferior oblique muscles, and the ptosis relates to disturbed innervation of the levator palpebrae.

An unusual acquired cause of unilateral third nerve palsy is neonatal hypoxic-ischemic injury, documented neuropathologically as causing unilateral as well as bilateral nuclear injury in the brain stem, specifically including the third nerve nucleus (see Chapter 18). I have seen this finding in association with the brain stem neuronal injury caused by severe, abrupt, late intrapartum asphyxia (see Chapter 19).

Extraocular Movements

Abnormalities of eye position and eye movement occur in a variety of neonatal neurological states. At least four abnormalities of eye position or eye movement may be observed in *otherwise healthy* term infants examined on the first 3 postnatal days.[263] Their incidence and outcome are summarized in Table 9.13 and noted in the appropriate sections that follow.

Abnormal Eye Position. Abnormalities of eye position occur in either the horizontal plane (dysconjugate) or the vertical plane (skew). Minor degrees of *dysconjugate* eye position at rest or even during spontaneous and elicited movement are not unusual in apparently normal term newborns (see Table 9.13). These disappear in the newborn period. However, in small preterm infants (<1500 g), these abnormalities are more common and may persist (Table 9.14). Indeed, the incidence of *strabismus*

(primarily esotropia) undergoes an interesting developmental increase to a peak at 6 months of age and a nadir at 12 months, which is when approximately 15% of 155 infants in one study exhibited strabismus.[264] Similarly, a recent study of 996 infants born at less than 28 weeks of gestation showed a 14% incidence of strabismus at 2 years of age.[265] A strong relation between the occurrence of strabismus and birth before 26 weeks of gestation or severe fetal growth retardation was noted.[265] In another large study of infants with birth weights below 1500 g, strabismus was associated with evidence of concomitant brain injury. Thus, on follow-up, the incidence varied from approximately 5% in infants with no intraventricular hemorrhage to 16% in those with hemorrhage and to 50% in those with cystic periventricular leukomalacia.[266] In a separate series of preterm infants with later spastic diplegia, 90% had strabismus and all had parieto-occipital white matter injury by MRI.[267] The high incidence of strabismus in preterm infants with white matter injury, principally located in parieto-occipital white matter, is consistent with sophisticated studies in older individuals with infantile onset of strabismus, suggesting that the underlying abnormality is located in the parietal and occipital cortex and the connections thereof.[268]

Skew deviation of the eyes (i.e., vertical disparity in eye position) is not rare in otherwise healthy term infants (see Table 9.13). Interestingly, although most of these cases resolve by 1 month of age, 23% later evolve to esotropia. In older patients, skew deviation is associated with lesions in the brain stem, involving either the region in or around the middle cerebellar peduncle (inferiorly displaced eye) or the medial longitudinal fasciculus (superiorly displaced eye).[269] That a similar correlation may occur in the newborn is supported by our documentation of skew deviation, with right eye down, in an infant with right intracerebellar hemorrhage and associated brain stem compression.[270] Moreover, I have frequently observed skew deviation in association with hypoxic-ischemic encephalopathy and evidence of brain stem neuronal injury as well as with major intraventricular hemorrhage and associated brain stem dysfunction. *Persistent downward deviation of the eyes (tonic downward deviation)* is a rare transient abnormality in otherwise healthy term or preterm infants (see Table 9.12). However, the abnormality may also reflect pretectal disturbance and thereby occur in association with paresis of upward gaze, as in hydrocephalus with a dilated third ventricle or kernicterus (see Chapter 26). With the transient abnormality of the otherwise normal newborn, the doll's-eyes maneuver demonstrates intact vertical gaze, thus indicating dysfunction of unknown cause at supranuclear levels.

Limitation of Eye Movement. Limitations of extraocular movement may occur because of isolated *nerve palsies* (see Chapter 33). Affection of the sixth nerve is the most common of these palsies and causes impaired lateral eye movement with resulting medial deviation.[271-273] This nerve involvement is distinguished from esotropia (strabismus) by the doll's-eyes maneuver, which fails to cause full abduction of the eye in sixth nerve palsy. Most examples of isolated sixth nerve palsy are transient; complete recovery occurs within several weeks.[271] Duane syndrome includes limitation of eye abduction with retraction of the globe and narrowing of the palpebral fissure on adduction of the affected eye (see Chapter 33). Congenital fibrosis of the extraocular muscles is a rare disorder characterized by restrictive paralysis of all extraocular muscles with essentially total ophthalmoplegia with or without ptosis (see Chapter 33).[273,274] Möbius syndrome includes defective eye abduction in approximately 80% of cases; congenital facial diplegia is the hallmark of this disorder (see subsequent discussion and Chapter 33).

Gaze palsies (weakness of conjugate eye movement) in the newborn are most often *horizontal* and may reflect either affection of frontal eye fields for contralateral eye movement or of gaze centers in the pons for ipsilateral eye movement. The former is more common, and both varieties occur most frequently as a feature of hypoxic-ischemic encephalopathy. These two possible anatomical loci for horizontal gaze palsies are distinguished by the doll's-eyes maneuver and by caloric stimulation, which result in movement of the eyes in disturbance of the cerebral eye fields but not in disturbance of the pontine gaze centers. More common in the newborn period is tonic deviation of the eyes to one side as a manifestation of seizure (accompanied often by fine jerking movements of the deviated eyes) or of a postictal state. *Vertical gaze palsies* are rare in the newborn; I have seen only defects of upward gaze with resulting downward deviation, as noted earlier. These abnormalities have occurred on the basis of presumed pretectal involvement by a massively dilated third ventricle (posthemorrhagic hydrocephalus or congenital aqueductal stenosis), major acute intraventricular hemorrhage, kernicterus, posterior fossa hemorrhage, or hypoxic-ischemic encephalopathy.

Abnormal Eye Movements. Abnormal eye movements consist of the horizontal and, occasionally, the vertical jerking movements that are *seizure manifestations, ocular bobbing, paroxysmal downgaze or upgaze, opsoclonus, ocular flutter,* and *nystagmus. Seizures* are discussed in Chapter 12. *Ocular bobbing* is an unusual abnormality of eye movement, described originally by Fisher,[275] and is characterized by intermittent bobbing down and up movements of the eyes that are usually synchronous; ocular bobbing in adults is associated primarily with pontine disturbance. In the newborn, this movement can be difficult to distinguish from seizure; in my experience, ocular bobbing is primarily a rare manifestation of major intraventricular hemorrhage or severe hypoxic-ischemic encephalopathy. *Paroxysmal downgaze* differs from ocular bobbing in its usually benign nature, its

very brief episodic quality, and the lack of bobbing when the eyes return to the meridian. *Episodic (paroxysmal)* downward deviation of the eyes lasting for several seconds may occur in the absence of overt neurological disease and then resolve by 1 to 6 months of age.[276,277] Such episodic deviation may also be a seizure manifestation, and the presence of fine jerking movements of the deviated eyes may help to establish this diagnosis (see Chapter 12). Paroxysmal downward deviation may also occur later in the first year, especially in preterm infants with severe injury (periventricular leukomalacia) of posterior cerebral white matter and, perhaps, connections to the pretectal region.[278] Visual impairment is a frequent accompaniment. *Paroxysmal upgaze*, characterized by episodes of tonic upgaze of 15 to 30 seconds, has been documented as early as the first week of life but usually has its onset at approximately 6 months of age and is later often associated with minor cognitive deficits and ataxia.[279-281] *Opsoclonus* is a dramatic but rare abnormality of eye movement that is characterized by rapid, irregular, multidirectional conjugate jerking of the eyes. Opsoclonus can be a transient abnormality in the term newborn (see Table 9.13). In such cases, resolution usually occurs within a month, invariably by 6 months.[263,282] In older patients, opsoclonus is associated with disturbance primarily of pontine omnipause neurons. The multidirectional nature of the movements is the critical criterion for distinction from seizure. I have observed opsoclonus and *ocular flutter* (jerking similar to that of opsoclonus but confined to the horizontal plane) in infants with maple syrup urine disease, nonketotic and ketotic hyperglycinemia, and posterior fossa hemorrhage.

Nystagmus with onset at birth or the first few days of life should suggest the diagnosis of congenital nystagmus.[283-288] This disorder is characterized by rhythmic, conjugate, horizontal oscillations of both eyes. The horizontal nature of the nystagmus persists with vertical gaze, an important diagnostic point. The disorder may be familial or nonfamilial. The familial variety may be either autosomal dominant, autosomal recessive, or X-linked recessive. The oscillations in an affected family member may be so reduced as to have been overlooked in the past. Visual impairment is present in the minority of patients, and static neurological deficits are present in the majority of nonfamilial (but not familial) cases with visual impairment. Because nystagmus can be observed, albeit uncommonly, in the newborn with severe visual deficit or with diencephalic or brain stem lesions (e.g., congenital tumor), a careful ophthalmological evaluation and an MRI scan should be carried out. A transient, idiopathic nystagmus has been described in early infancy, with disappearance at a mean age of 8 months.[282]

Facial Sensation and Masticatory Power

Abnormality of facial sensation is rarely elicited in the newborn. I have observed several premature infants with a posterior fossa syndrome secondary to an intraventricular hemorrhage (with extension into the fourth ventricle) who had absence or impaired responses to pinprick over the face bilaterally. Careful evaluation of facial sensation, not often performed in the newborn examination, may reveal more deficits than currently recognized.

Disturbance of motor function of the fifth cranial nerve is manifested usually as a defect of sucking and is rarely an isolated finding. Abnormalities of sucking and swallowing are discussed in subsequent sections.

Facial Motility

Abnormalities of facial motility should be sought when the face is at rest, at the onset of movement, during spontaneous facial movement, and during crying or grimacing. Facial weakness secondary to disturbance of the cerebrum is usually more obvious with the baby at rest or during the first movements of spontaneous facial expression and may be completely inapparent during the full movements of crying. Nuclear, cranial nerve, neuromuscular, or muscular lesions, however, are usually more obvious during elicited facial movement, such as a cry or grimace. A simple classification of the types of facial weakness that can occur in the neonatal period is provided, according to the level of the lesion, in Table 9.15. Each of these specific disorders is discussed in more detail in other relevant chapters of this book.

Cerebrum. In facial weakness of cerebral origin, the upper face is spared. Other signs of cerebral deficit are usually present (e.g., hemiparesis [especially of an upper extremity] and seizures). The most common pathological substrate is hypoxic-ischemic encephalopathy, particularly with infarction in the distribution of the middle cerebral artery, and less commonly cerebral contusion (with or without subdural hemorrhage). Cerebral lesions of prenatal onset (e.g., porencephaly) often have relatively less involvement of the face than might be predicted on the basis of the degree of upper extremity weakness and the severity of the lesion on brain imaging. The reason for this apparent facial sparing may relate to the likelihood that, during normal development of the corticobulbar system, there are ipsilateral terminations of each corticobulbar tract that are eliminated postnatally by selective elimination of axonal processes and of synapses (see Chapter 7) but that are retained when the normal contralateral input is lost. Strong support for this notion emanates from the demonstration that the evaluation of older infants and children with hemiparesis revealed facial sparing when lesions occurred prenatally (82% had sparing) but not when lesions occurred beyond the neonatal period.[289] Presumably ipsilateral terminals of the intact corticobulbar tract spared facial function; consistent with this formulation, prenatal lesions did not show facial sparing if they were bilateral (only 8% had sparing).[289] Bilateral facial weakness of cerebral origin may be associated with weakness of sucking, swallowing, and tongue movements as part of a congenital Foix-Chavany-Marie syndrome, secondary either to intrauterine ischemic injury or to cortical dysgenesis involving the perisylvian regions.[290]

Nucleus. Nuclear facial weakness is primarily a manifestation of Möbius syndrome; as such, it is bilateral, involves upper face and lower face (often upper more than lower), and is associated with a variety of other neurological deficits and congenital abnormalities (see Chapter 33). Difficulty with eye closure, flattened nasolabial fold, difficulty sucking, and drooling are prominent features.

In view of the relative frequency of brain stem nuclear injury with perinatal asphyxia, hypoxic-ischemic encephalopathy may be associated with bilateral weakness of both the upper and lower face.

Nerve. Injury to the facial nerve is most often related to intrauterine position during labor with compression of the face against the maternal sacrum (intrauterine position is usually left occiput anterior, and thus most are left facial palsies)[291] or to forceps injury during difficult forceps extractions (see Chapter 36). Rare causes of injury to the facial nerve involve compression from a posterior fossa hematoma, whether intracerebellar or extraparenchymal. In nerve injuries, the upper as well as the lower face is usually affected, and eye closure is notably poor. Because the lesion is unilateral, there is a prominent "pulling" of the lower face toward the normal side during a cry or grimace because of the weakness of muscles on the affected side for lateral movement of the lower face. Occasionally this pulling leads to the impression that the normal side is actually the affected side (Fig. 9.11).

TABLE 9.15	Major Causes of Facial Weakness in the Neonatal Period

Cerebral
Hypoxic-ischemic encephalopathy
Cerebral contusion
Nuclear
Möbius syndrome
Hypoxic-ischemic encephalopathy
Nerve
Traumatic neuropathy
Posterior fossa hematoma
Neuromuscular junction
Myasthenia gravis
Infantile botulism
Muscle
Congenital myotonic dystrophy
Congenital muscular dystrophy
Facioscapulohumeral dystrophy
Nemaline myopathy
Myotubular myopathy
Congenital fiber type disproportion
Mitochondrial disorder: cytochrome *c* oxidase deficiency
Hypoplasia of depressor anguli oris muscle

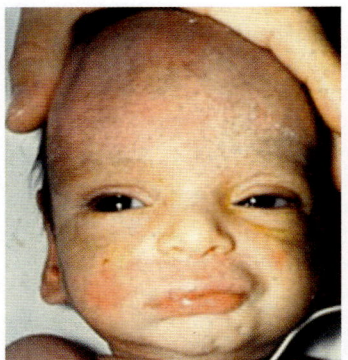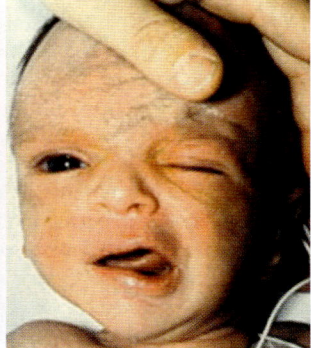

Figure 9.11 Facial paralysis. Facial nerve palsy in a full-term boy at 3 days of age, at rest and on crying. Note, at rest, on the affected side *(right)* the widened palpebral fissure, flattened nasolabial fold, and depressed corner of the mouth. With crying there is "pulling" of the lower face toward the normal *(left)* side because of weakness of muscles on the right for lateral movement of the lower face. (From Renault F, Quijano-Roy S. Congenital and acquired facial palsies. In: Darras BT, Royden Jones H Jr, Ryan MM, DeVivo DC, eds. *Neuromuscular Disorders of Infancy, Childhood, and Adolescence.* 2nd ed. London: Elsevier; 2014:229.)

Neuromuscular Junction. This locus for facial weakness occurs in myasthenia gravis and infantile botulism. Bilateral facial weakness—often with ptosis, dysphagia, and generalized hypotonia—may accompany either the neonatal transient or congenital varieties of myasthenia gravis (see Chapter 32). Diagnosis in the newborn is made best by observing the response to neostigmine or edrophonium. In the former, more common variety of myasthenia gravis, the mother also has the disorder.

In addition to facial diplegia, the infant with infantile botulism exhibits unreactive pupils, dysphagia, peripheral weakness, hypotonia, and constipation.

Muscle. Generalized weakness of the face secondary to myopathic disease is associated most commonly with congenital myotonic dystrophy, congenital muscular dystrophy, facioscapulohumeral dystrophy, nemaline myopathy, myotubular myopathy, congenital fiber-type disproportion, and mitochondrial disorder (cytochrome *c* oxidase deficiency). These disorders often can be distinguished on clinical grounds by recognition of other features (see Chapter 33).

Restricted weakness of the face is characteristic of hypoplasia of the depressor anguli oris muscle (see Chapter 33). In this disorder, the corner of the mouth is unable to retract and to be depressed. This disturbance is especially noticeable during crying. An association with cardiac and other anomalies has been defined.[292]

Audition

Definition of significant hearing loss in the newborn infant by clinical examination is difficult. During the clinical evaluation described in the section on normal neurological findings, it cannot be expected that minor abnormalities in auditory pathways will be detected. However, detection or at least serious suspicion of major hearing deficits is usually possible. In addition to the absence of startle and more subtle responses to sound, a sometimes valuable clue to a serious hearing deficit in the alert young infant is apparent *visual hyperattentiveness* and consistent startle when the examiner approaches the child quickly from the periphery. The use of brain stem auditory evoked potentials is of major value (see Chapter 10). Universal neonatal screening (relative to selected screening) has been shown to lead to the earlier diagnosis of hearing loss and faster intervention.[293] *Close follow-up and repeated examinations are important.* Early diagnosis is critical because language development is benefited by early corrective efforts and impaired by delay in correction (i.e., after 6 months).[293-295] Moreover, hearing loss may be *inapparent* by evoked response audiometry in the neonatal period and appear only as a *progressive* disorder in the first 6 to 8 months of life.[296,297] Thus the identification of the infant at risk for this subsequent hearing loss is crucial.

Serious disturbances of hearing are sometimes categorized under the popular mnemonic *the ABCDs of deafness* (i.e., *A*ffected family, *B*ilirubin injury, *C*ongenital [and neonatal] infection, *D*efect of head or neck, and low birth weight ["small"]) (Table 9.16). Unfortunately this mnemonic neglects the additional category of the term infant subjected to apparent hypoxic-ischemic insults, a category I have added to Table 9.16.

Genetic Deafness. Hereditary forms of deafness are common and account for approximately 50% of all cases of congenital

---

TABLE 9.16   Major Causes of Deafness in the Neonatal Period

Genetic
Isolated: autosomal dominant, autosomal recessive, X-linked recessive
Syndromic: associated with malformations of external ear and ocular, skin, skeletal or systemic disease
Bilirubin and other toxins
Hyperbilirubinemia
Other (e.g., aminoglycosides, furosemide)
Congenital and neonatal infections
Congenital infections: cytomegalovirus, rubella, toxoplasmosis, syphilis, lymphocytic choriomeningitis
Neonatal infection: bacterial meningitis
Defects of the head and neck
Low birth weight
"Hypoxic" injury
Hyperbilirubinemia
Intracranial hemorrhage (?)
Ambient noise (?)
Additive effects (?)
Term infant: hypoxia-ischemia
Perinatal asphyxia
Persistent fetal circulation

---

hearing loss.[298-302] The familial genetic disorders are best categorized as those that are isolated (nonsyndromic) and those that are syndromic (i.e., deficits associated with malformations of the external ear, with eye disease [e.g., cataracts and optic atrophy], with skin disease [e.g., albinism and anhidrosis], with skeletal disease, or with other systemic disorders [e.g., thyroid disease]). Many other hereditary syndromes associated with deafness present later in infancy and childhood. A careful family history is critical. Overall, of the genetic causes, 30% are syndromic (i.e., 15% of total congenital hearing loss, such as those due to Pendred syndrome, Usher syndrome, Waardenberg syndrome, or branchio-oto-renal syndrome). Of these, the first two are autosomal recessive disorders and the latter two are autosomal dominant.[301] The remaining 70% of the genetic causes (i.e., 35% of total congenital hearing loss) are nonsyndromic or isolated. Autosomal dominant, autosomal recessive, X-linked recessive, and mitochondrial inheritances are recognized.[301] The most common disorder involves a gene called *GJB2*, which accounts for approximately half of the cases. The gene encodes a connexin protein involved in gap junctions and perhaps potassium influx for mechanosensory transduction in brain cells.[301]

Bilirubin and Other Toxins. Injury to cochlear nuclei secondary to marked hyperbilirubinemia is an unusual *isolated* cause of severe hearing loss (see Chapter 26).[303-306] More often, other manifestations of bilirubin encephalopathy are present. Results of studies of premature infants suggest that less marked elevations of serum bilirubin level (<20 mg/dL) exert at least an important *additive effect* in the genesis of sensorineural hearing loss.[294,307-310] However, not all studies support this contention.[311]

The toxic effects of *aminoglycosides* are well known, but their overall contribution to serious hearing loss in the newborn period appears to be small.[299,300,303,312-315] However, there is not total agreement on this issue,[316,317] and others have suggested that the combination of aminoglycoside and furosemide is an important factor in neonatal hearing loss.[318] In one study of 35 newborns with sensorineural hearing loss identified by brain stem auditory evoked responses, multivariate analysis identified *furosemide* administration as the only significant factor.[311]

Congenital and Neonatal Infections. The classic *congenital (prenatal)* infection associated with deafness (i.e., rubella) is now a very uncommon cause. Congenital cytomegalovirus infection currently is the most common congenital infection that may result in serious hearing loss (see Table 9.16 and Chapter 34).[319-321] However, toxoplasmosis and congenital syphilis may also cause serious hearing deficits. Lymphocytic choriomeningitis is a fifth, albeit rare prenatal infection associated with hearing loss (see Chapter 34). Bacterial meningitis is the major *neonatal* infection that may result in serious hearing deficits (see Chapter 35).

Defects of Head and Neck. Because the development of the peripheral auditory system is related intimately to the differentiation of the branchial clefts, it is understandable that auditory defects often accompany defects of head and neck. In two large series, 22% and 23% of cases of hearing impairment were related to auriculofacial anomalies.[299,300] Disturbances of the external ear and surrounding structures, some of which are hereditary (e.g., Treacher-Collins mandibulofacial dysostosis), are good examples. Other developmental defects of this type are part of a more generalized dysmorphogenesis (e.g., trisomy 13 to 15).

Low Birth Weight. Premature infants have a distinctly increased incidence of significant hearing loss (see Table 9.16). In an earlier series of 193 surviving preterm infants (gestational age of 28 to 36 weeks), 24 (12%) exhibited definite hearing deficits, particularly of the high-frequency, sensorineural type, on follow-up examination (Fig. 9.12).[322] Other studies indicate incidences of sensorineural hearing loss generally of approximately 5% to 10%.[307-309,314,316,323-326] Although some series report considerably lower incidences,[299-301] a recent nationwide

study in the Netherlands based on excellent screening methods shows that incidence increases with decreasing gestational age (e.g., 1.2% at 31 weeks and 7.5% at 24 weeks).[326]

The etiology of hearing loss with prematurity is probably multifactorial. In an earlier study, a sharp relation with recurrent *cyanotic attacks* was apparent (e.g., 11% of infants of less than 33 weeks of gestation with such attacks were found to be deaf). Later reports also are supportive of a relation in the premature infant between recurrent apneic spells, duration of respiratory therapy, hypoxemia, and subsequent sensorineural hearing loss.[307-309,314,324] One or more of several possible bases for these relationships should be considered. The presumed basis for the relation of hearing deficits to apneic spells, duration of ventilator therapy, or hypoxemia is *hypoxic-ischemic* injury to cochlear nuclei, inferior colliculi, or both in the brain stem (see Chapter 8). Data obtained with brain stem evoked response audiometry suggest that involvement of cochlea may also occur in hypoxic-ischemic disease (see Chapters 10 and 20). Moreover, the demonstration of neonatal *intracranial hemorrhage* involving the auditory nerve and inner ear raises the possibility that hemorrhage also plays a role.[327] A recent study of 1472 surviving preterm infants of 23 to 28 weeks of gestation supports a relation to intraventricular hemorrhage.[325] A third factor, still to be defined further, is the possibility of injury to cochlear hair cells by *excessive acoustic* stimulation provided by incubator or other intensive care unit noises. This notion is supported by circumstantial clinical evidence[328-330] and by the observation that the cochlear hair cells of neonatal animals can be injured by noise levels attained in neonatal incubators.[328,330] Although it is clear that more data are needed,[303] currently a noise level of greater than 45 dB is considered to be of concern in the neonatal intensive care unit.[329] The current recommendation of the American Academy of Pediatrics for noise level limitation is 45 to 55 dB.[331] Notably, the noise levels of various neonatal ventilators have been shown to exceed these levels.[332]

The possibility of the *combined, additive effect of factors* resulting in significant injury, factors that alone are not sufficient to cause injury (e.g., hypoxia, bilirubin, aminoglycosides, furosemide, ambient noise and hemorrhage), must be a major topic for future research. Additive effects of ambient noise

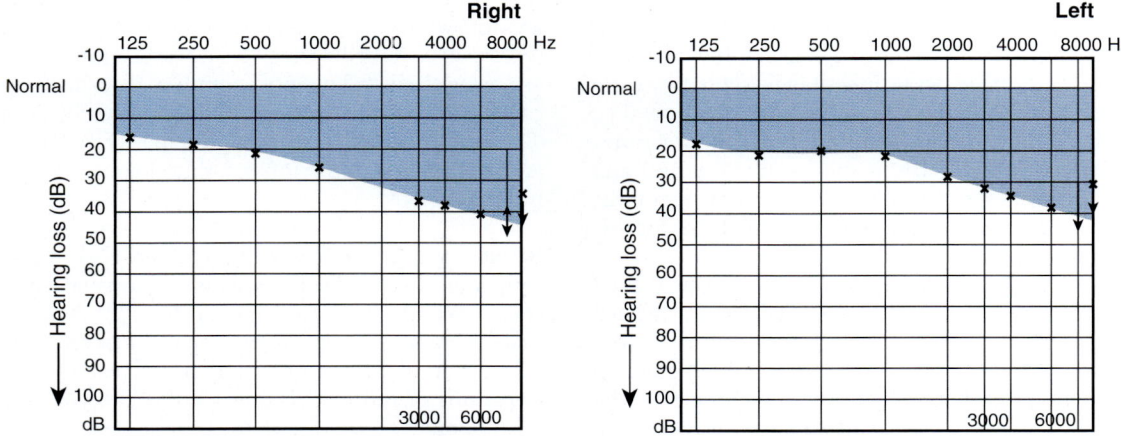

Figure 9.12 Hearing loss in surviving preterm infants. The abnormal audiograms of all 24 children, 8 to 10 years of age, with neurosensory hearing loss were averaged. The deficits (ordinate) were encountered particularly at the high frequencies (abscissa) and were generally symmetric. (From Stennert E, Schulte FJ, Vollrath M, et al. The etiology of neurosensory hearing defects in preterm infants. *Arch Otorhinolaryngol.* 1978;221:171-182.)

and aminoglycosides have been described in experimental animals,[333,334] and disturbances of brain stem auditory evoked responses have been observed in premature infants treated with gentamicin.[314,335] Other observations support additive effects of recurrent apneic spells (and possibly prolonged respirator therapy) and hyperbilirubinemia in the premature infant.[309]

Term Infant, Hypoxia-Ischemia. At least two additional groups of term infants (exclusive of those with kernicterus and congenital or neonatal infection) are at increased risk of sensorineural hearing loss: infants with *perinatal asphyxia* and those with persistent fetal circulation. The incidence of sensorineural hearing loss in infants with hypoxic-ischemic encephalopathy apparently secondary to perinatal asphyxia is variably increased. A recent prospective study of infants treated with hypothermia for perinatal asphyxia ($n = 111$) reported an incidence of bilateral deafness of 4%.[336] This issue is discussed in Chapter 20. The second group of infants, those with persistent fetal circulation, exhibited a 42% incidence of subsequent hearing loss in one series.[296] An increased risk of hearing loss after persistent fetal circulation was also observed in an earlier study.[297] In the later study of Hendricks-Munoz and colleagues, two thirds of the infants with sensorineural hearing loss required hearing aids; interestingly, the hearing deficits appeared after the neonatal period, in the first 6 to 8 months of life. Variables related to the hearing loss included duration of ventilation and, perhaps, use of furosemide. The former factor suggests a possible role for hypoxic-ischemic factors, but values for lowest PaO_2 or arterial blood pressure did not correlate with hearing loss. However, *duration* of hypoxemia was not addressed. More data are needed on these issues.

Sucking and Swallowing

Disturbances of sucking and swallowing very often coexist; even when isolated they can be difficult to distinguish. Disturbances of the gag reflex are very frequent in instances of defective swallowing, but this reflex is usually normal in instances of defective sucking alone. Specific abnormalities of sucking and swallowing in the newborn not uncommonly relate to a nonneurological disturbance (e.g., Pierre Robin anomaly, first arch syndrome, or tracheoesophageal fistula). A framework for formulating the neurological disorders of sucking and swallowing in the newborn is presented in Table 9.17. Each of the specific disorders is discussed in more detail in other relevant chapters of this book. Not listed or discussed here are the multiple malformation syndromes (e.g., first arch, CHARGE [coloboma, heart defects, choanal atresia, retarded growth and development, genital abnormalities, and ear anomalies], orofacial digital) that, in large series, account for more than half of cases of *severe, persistent* sucking and swallowing difficulties at birth and thereafter.[337]

Cerebrum. The most common cause of disturbances of sucking and swallowing in the newborn period is the more generalized depression of central nervous system function associated with most of the encephalopathies discussed in this text. Bilateral cerebral affection with impaired corticobulbar function (of the pyramidal system) is the common denominator. It is likely that a bilateral cerebral white matter disturbance underlies the results of a recent careful study of sucking behavior in 52 premature infants (mean gestational age 29 weeks).[338] Thus

TABLE 9.17	Major Causes of Impaired Sucking and Swallowing in the Neonatal Period[a]

Cerebral
Encephalopathies with bilateral cerebral (pyramidal) involvement: diverse causes
Extrapyramidal-adventitial movements
Congenital isolated pharyngeal dysfunction
Nuclear
Hypoxic-ischemic encephalopathy
Möbius syndrome
Werdnig-Hoffmann disease
Chiari type 2 malformation with myelomeningocele
Nerve
Traumatic facial neuropathy
Posterior fossa hematoma or tumor
Bilateral laryngeal paralysis
Familial dysautonomia (Riley-Day syndrome)
Neuromuscular junction
Myasthenia gravis
Infantile botulism
Muscle
Congenital myotonic dystrophy
Congenital muscular dystrophy
Facioscapulohumeral dystrophy
Nemaline myopathy
Myotubular myopathy
Congenital fiber type disproportion
Mitochondrial myopathy: cytochrome c oxidase deficiency

[a]Malformation syndromes not listed—see text.

specific disturbances of sucking (involving rhythmic jaw and tongue movements; coordination of sucking, swallowing, and respiration; ability to sustain sucking; and persistence of an immature sucking pattern, assessed at 4 to 6 weeks post term and noted in 25% of infants) correlated with abnormal Bayley scores at 2 years of age.

Peculiar adventitial *tongue movements* may occur as unusual findings in the newborn. I have observed tongue thrusting movements as apparent seizure manifestations in association with serious hypoxic-ischemic injury or major intraventricular hemorrhage and as part of the movement disorder in premature infants with severe bronchopulmonary dysplasia (see next discussion). Moreover, the feeding disturbance observed with familial dysautonomia may be accentuated by peculiar tongue rolling (see later discussion in Chapter 32). The pathophysiology of these various tongue movements is unclear, but I suspect that they are mediated centrally at the level of extrapyramidal function. A well-known albeit rare extrapyramidal disorder, recessive GTP (guanosine triphosphate) cyclohydrolase deficiency, also is characterized by neonatal disturbances of sucking and swallowing; some cases have been responsive to treatment with L-dopa.[339]

An interesting syndrome of congenital isolated pharyngeal dysfunction is characterized by total paralysis of the pharyngeal muscles and soft palate, with an inability to swallow or gag and aspiration upon attempts at feeding.[340-343] The lack of abnormality on electromyography (EMG) suggests that this disorder is mediated centrally, above the level of the lower motor neuron. Spontaneous remission has occurred in 50% of cases within the first 6 months of life. The disorder is important to recognize because fatal aspiration has occurred with persistent attempts at oral feeding.

Nuclei. Involvement of the neurons of cranial nerve nuclei V, VII, XI, X, and XII, in various combinations, will disturb sucking and swallowing (see Table 9.17). The three most prominent causes of such involvement are hypoxic-ischemic injury, Möbius syndrome, and Werdnig-Hoffmann disease. Frequently infants with the Chiari type 2 malformation and myelomeningocele have prominent impairment of lower cranial nerve function, including sucking and swallowing, as noted in Chapter 1.[344-352] These deficits presumably relate to deformation of the lower brain stem and dysfunction at the nuclear or root level.

Nerve. Involvement of the facial nerve (see previous discussion and Chapter 33) is very common, and sucking but not swallowing is disturbed. In the rare case of posterior fossa hematoma or tumor, other cranial nerves can be affected, and swallowing may also be disturbed. Bilateral laryngeal paralysis may occur as an isolated abnormality of unknown cause (i.e., unassociated with Chiari type 2 malformation or other neurological defect) or in relation to birth trauma, among other possibilities (see Chapter 36). Stridor is a prominent accompanying sign. Disturbance of autonomic nerve function, as in familial dysautonomia, is a rare cause of swallowing dysfunction in the newborn (see Chapter 32).

Neuromuscular Junction. Both myasthenia gravis and infantile botulism are associated with disturbances of sucking or swallowing or both (see Chapter 32). Congenital myasthenic syndrome with stridor and vocal cord paralysis has been reported.[353]

Muscle Involvement. Of disorders of muscle, congenital myotonic dystrophy is the most common cause of significant impairment of both sucking and swallowing in the newborn. Certain other myopathies can be associated with feeding disturbances, most often because of greater impairment of sucking than of swallowing (see Table 9.17).

Sternocleidomastoid Function

Abnormalities of sternocleidomastoid function result in disturbed flexion and lateral rotation of the head; in the newborn they occur almost exclusively as a feature of congenital torticollis. This disorder is discussed in more detail in Chapter 33. The affected muscle is involved with a contracture that maintains the head in a slightly flexed position, with slight rotation to the opposite side. This posture is most apparent when the infant is viewed from the rear.

Tongue Function

Documented abnormalities of tongue function relate primarily to defects of the neurons of the hypoglossal nucleus and of the muscle itself. The *neuronal disorders* result in atrophy and fasciculations of the tongue. Such fasciculations can be detected reliably only with the tongue at rest, because all infants, especially with crying, have tremulous movements of the tongue that are virtually impossible to distinguish from fasciculations. The latter are most apparent at the periphery of the tongue at rest and, in marked examples, may give the appearance of

a "bag of worms." I have observed fasciculations in newborns with Werdnig-Hoffmann disease and hypoxic-ischemic injury. Atrophy and weakness of the tongue may also occur with Möbius syndrome. A fourth disorder that may affect the twelfth nerve nucleus in early infancy is type II glycogen storage disease (Pompe disease), but fasciculations and weakness usually appear after the neonatal period, and *macroglossia* is common (see Chapter 32).

Involvement of *muscles of the tongue* rarely causes marked weakness. Certain infiltrations, usually resulting in macroglossia, may interfere with tongue function. These disorders include Pompe disease, generalized gangliosidosis, Beckwith syndrome, congenital hypothyroidism, angioma or hamartoma, and isolated macroglossia.

Abnormalities of the Motor Examination

Delineation of motor abnormalities in the newborn is rendered difficult by normal maturational changes in the motility, tone, and character of reflexes (see previous sections). Observation of the posture and ease of passive manipulation of the limbs of infants in quiet repose must always be evaluated as a function of gestational age. Thus a normal infant of 28 weeks of gestation may exhibit relatively little flexor or extensor tone, whereas at 32 weeks of gestation a normal infant may exhibit relatively little flexor tone in the upper extremities but considerable flexor tone in the lower extremities. Moreover, it is critical to emphasize that these conclusions relate to muscle *tone* and not necessarily to muscle power. Pathological hypertonia and hypotonia are detected readily with careful examination. The discussion that follows is based primarily on my experience with a standard clinical approach. Use of more sophisticated techniques (long-term video recordings or quantitative analyses of movement) eventually may lead to better detection of subtle deficits.[204-206,212-216,218-220,222,354-356]

Hypertonia

Hypertonia is not as common a feature of neonatal neurological disease as is hypotonia. When present, hypertonia most often has a plastic quality, which increases with passive manipulation of the limbs and is reminiscent more of gegenhalten or of dystonia in older patients.[269] Only rarely does the increase in tone have the "clasp knife" quality of spasticity. Neonatal hypertonia may be caused by chronic and therefore *intrauterine* injury to the corticospinal tract or extrapyramidal system. Hypoxic-ischemic lesions are the most common cause (see Chapter 19), although markedly increased tone has been described in infants with congenital absence of the pyramidal tracts.[357] *Acute perinatal* causes of hypertonia include *meningeal inflammation* (secondary to bacterial meningitis [see Chapter 35] or to hemorrhage [see Chapters 22 to 24]), *severe bilateral cerebral injury with brain stem release phenomena* (similar to decorticate or decerebrate posturing), *basal ganglia injury* (especially with perinatal hypoxic-ischemic insults [see Chapter 20]), and *brain stem activation* (especially in infants exposed in utero to cocaine or with hyperekplexia [see Chapters 38 and 12, respectively]).

Myogenic causes of hypertonia are myotonia congenita, paramyotonia congenita, or hyperkalemic periodic paralysis (see Chapter 33). Finally, the contractures of arthrogryposis may be *mistaken* for hypertonia, and careful examination is important (see Chapter 31).

Hypotonia and Weakness

Hypotonia is the most common motor abnormality observed in neonatal neurological disorders. It is important to distinguish hypotonia and weakness, but it is unusual to observe hypotonia without at least some weakness in the newborn. Disproportionate involvement occurs but total dissociation is rare. Hypotonia and weakness are discussed in detail in Chapters 30 to 33. Certain *patterns of weakness* are associated with the anatomical loci of disease and are reviewed briefly here.

Focal Cerebral. Focal injury to the cerebrum results in contralateral hemiparesis and a tendency of the eyes to deviate to the side of the lesion. These signs are often not striking in the newborn, but they are definite and, assuredly, detectable, contrary to what is often stated in many standard texts of pediatric neurology and neonatology. Three patterns of lateralized weakness can be defined. Hemiparesis in the term newborn most often affects the upper extremity more prominently than the lower extremity, but in the preterm newborn the opposite occurs (see Chapters 20 and 24). The upper extremity pattern of the term newborn is usually related to an arterial disturbance (primarily affecting the middle cerebral artery), with predominant involvement of the lateral cerebral convexity; the lower extremity pattern is usually related to a unilateral periventricular venous disturbance with predominant involvement of the periventricular white matter. A third variety of focal weakness secondary to focal cerebral injury involves cortical venous infarction, which may occur in either term or preterm infants (especially with bacterial meningitis). The weakness usually involves the superior cerebral convexity and thereby causes either lower extremity monoparesis or, more likely, hemiparesis with greater involvement of the lower than of the upper extremity.

Parasagittal Cerebral. Parasagittal cerebral injury, as occurs after a generalized disturbance in cerebral perfusion in the term newborn, results in weakness of the proximal limbs, upper more than lower, because the lesion resides in the "watershed" region of cerebral convexities (i.e., superomedial aspects; see Chapters 18 and 20).

Periventricular Cerebral (Bilateral). Bilateral cystic periventricular white matter injury, characteristic of the preterm infant, is secondary in largest part to disturbance of cerebral perfusion and results in bilateral, generally symmetric weakness of the lower extremities much more than the upper extremities (see Chapter 16). Before approximately term equivalent, this pattern is difficult to detect in the prematurely born infant. This pattern of weakness can be observed also with the periventricular white matter affection caused by hydrocephalus with dilated lateral ventricles.

Spinal Cord. Involvement of the spinal cord (e.g., cord trauma) usually occurs in the cervical region and initially results in flaccid weakness of all extremities, with *sparing of the face* and the function of other cranial nerves (see Chapter 36). Involvement of sphincters is often prominent, and evolution to spasticity of the lower extremities (and upper extremities if the lesion is in the mid-upper cervical region) usually appears in weeks to months.

Lower Motor Neuron. Involvement of the lower motor neuron (e.g., Werdnig-Hoffmann disease) causes flaccid weakness of all extremities, with initial relative sparing of the face and the function of other cranial nerves (see Chapter 32). Fasciculations may be detectable, particularly in the form of "tremors" of the fingers.

Nerve Roots. Involvement of roots, as with brachial plexus injury, results in discrete and *restricted patterns of focal weakness*, depending on the specific roots involved (see Chapter 36).

Peripheral Nerve. Disease of the peripheral nerves usually results in *generalized* weakness; the newborn only uncommonly exhibits the distal greater than proximal weakness characteristic of neuropathy at later ages (see Chapter 32). Peripheral nerve disease may be *focal* (e.g., in traumatic injury), and such restricted weakness and hypotonia will reflect and suggest this fact (see Chapter 36).

Neuromuscular Junction. Involvement of the *neuromuscular junction* (e.g., in myasthenia gravis and infantile botulism) causes generalized weakness and hypotonia. Accompanying involvement of cranial nerve function, including the face, is common (see Chapter 32).

Muscle. Disease of muscle in the newborn causes generalized weakness and hypotonia, often more prominent in the proximal than the distal limbs. Certain neonatal myopathies also affect face and eye movements and swallowing (see Chapter 33).

Tendon Reflexes and Plantar Response

Abnormalities of *tendon reflexes* are frequent and important accompaniments to disturbances of the motor system in the newborn period. In general, infants with lesions *above the level of the lower motor neuron* (i.e., lesions of the cerebrum or spinal cord) exhibit preserved deep tendon reflexes but do *not* develop the characteristically hyperactive reflexes until weeks or months later (see Chapter 20). When a *lower motor neuron, root,* or *nerve* is involved, deep tendon reflexes are usually *absent* or are barely detectable. Muscle power may be somewhat less affected initially (i.e., there may be modest muscle weakness despite absent reflexes). In disorders of the *neuromuscular junction,* the opposite often occurs (i.e., reflexes may be only slightly affected or unaffected despite striking weakness). In disease of *muscle,* the decrease in deep tendon reflexes parallels the decrease in muscle power.

As indicated in the section on normal neurological findings, the *plantar response* has not been particularly helpful in my evaluation of the neonatal motor system (except in disease of lumbosacral cord or plexus). However, a distinctly asymmetrical response, with one plantar response being extensor, should suggest disease above the level of the lower motor neuron. The most unequivocal extensor responses that I have observed in the newborn infant have accompanied spinal cord injury.

Abnormal Movements

Abnormal movements include myotonia, fasciculations, jitteriness, excessive startles, or more complex adventitial movements. Myotonia and fasciculations are motor abnormalities that have important diagnostic implications and require care for detection. Jitteriness is readily detected but is sometimes confused with other movements (e.g., seizure). The excessive startles of hyperekplexia are closely related (see Chapter 12). A more complex movement disorder occurs particularly with bronchopulmonary dysplasia (see later discussion).

Myotonia. Myotonia is principally observed in myotonic dystrophy; it consists of sustained contraction of a muscle group, usually provoked by percussion. Percussion of the thenar muscles or the mentalis muscle may lead to a persistent "dimple" of the muscle, which is apparent for seconds. This response is very difficult to elicit in the newborn infant (see Chapter 33).

Fasciculation. Fasciculation (i.e., spontaneous contraction of the *group* of muscle fibers that compose a motor unit) is a feature of lower motor neuron disease (e.g., Werdnig-Hoffmann disease). Fasciculations are best observed in the tongue or sometimes in the fingers (if the fingers are observed with the wrist slightly hyperextended).

Jitteriness. Jitteriness is a disorder of movement that is frequently observed in the newborn period; its distinction from seizure is important (see Chapter 12). The movements in jitteriness are generalized and symmetrical, have the qualities primarily of a *coarse* tremor, are exquisitely stimulus-sensitive, and can be diminished effectively by gentle, passive flexion of the limbs. Frequent accompaniments are brisk deep tendon reflexes and an easily elicited Moro reflex. Jitteriness is most frequently related to insults that produce neuronal hyperirritability (e.g., hypoxic-ischemic encephalopathy, hypocalcemia, hypoglycemia, drug withdrawal). However, in many infants, no definable cause is apparent.

Excessive Startles. Startle responses markedly excessive for the stimulation (auditory, somesthetic) that produces them is characteristic of hyperekplexia. As noted earlier, hypertonia is an additional feature. This disorder is discussed in Chapter 12.

Movement Disorder With Bronchopulmonary Dysplasia. Perlman and I defined a striking movement disorder in premature infants with severe bronchopulmonary dysplasia.[358] The clinical features in many ways are similar to extrapyramidal movement disorders of older infants and children. Chronic hypoxemia, hypercarbia, bronchospasm, and inadequate nutrition have been present in all the patients in whom we have observed this disorder. The abnormal movements develop from approximately the third postnatal month and involve the limbs, neck, trunk, and oral-buccal-lingual structures. The limb movements are most prominent distally and consist of rapid, random, jerky movements (similar to chorea) and "restless" movements (similar to akathisia). Similar movements of the neck and face are observed; tongue movements have a "darting quality." The oral-buccal-lingual movements are similar to the dyskinesias of elderly patients. Movements are exacerbated during episodes of respiratory failure and attenuated during sleep. All such infants have exhibited feeding disorders, largely due to the tongue movements. Several infants have exhibited improvement with clonazepam. The natural history has been partial or complete resolution or a static course. Neuropathological findings in the one infant studied were neuronal loss with astrocytosis in caudate, putamen, globus pallidus, and thalamus. Thus these observations defined a previously unrecognized extrapyramidal

disorder of infants with severe bronchopulmonary dysplasia; pathogenesis may be related to chronic hypoxemia.

Abnormalities of Primary Neonatal Reflexes

Moro Reflex

The *Moro reflex* is very sensitive to the infant's level of alertness. The most common cause of a depressed or absent Moro reflex is a generalized disturbance of the central nervous system. Thus, a great variety of disorders may be responsible. An exaggerated, stereotyped, nonhabituating Moro reflex is a common neonatal feature of severe bilateral intrauterine cerebral disturbance (e.g., hydranencephaly and severe micrencephaly vera), perhaps because of release of the brain stem from inhibitory cortical influences. The most useful abnormality of the Moro reflex to elicit is distinct *asymmetry*, which is almost always a feature of root, plexus, or nerve disease. In my experience, focal cerebral injury does not cause a distinct disturbance of the Moro reflex.

Tonic Neck Reflex

As with the Moro reflex, the *tonic neck reflex* normally prominent in the 1-month-old infant may be exaggerated, stereotyped, and nonhabituating with severe fixed bilateral cerebral disturbance. When the tonic neck reflex is "obligatory" (i.e., the full response does not diminish in the normal manner if the head is maintained to the side), other focal cerebral signs (e.g., hemiparesis) are likely to be present or to evolve. Prominent retention of the tonic neck reflex beyond 6 months of age, in my experience, is common in extrapyramidal disorders, such as kernicterus.

Palmar Grasp

Abnormalities of *palmar grasp* are particularly useful if they are asymmetrical, usually reflecting peripheral involvement (i.e., root, plexus, or nerve). As with the Moro reflex, the palmar grasp is exaggerated and nonhabituating in the presence of severe bilateral cerebral disease.[110] Marked retention of the plantar grasp beyond the first 6 months of life is more characteristic of athetoid than spastic cerebral palsy,[230] an observation that suggests an important role for the extrapyramidal motor system in the maturational disappearance of this reflex.

Abnormalities of the Sensory Examination

Abnormalities of sensation are most easily elicited and interpreted in the newborn period in peripheral lesions, especially those involving roots, and in spinal cord injury. The most illustrative of the former is the sensory deficit in infants with *brachial plexus injuries*. In the latter I have observed distinct deficits in response to pinprick in a *segmental distribution* that is usually less extensive than the deficit of motor function (see Chapter 36). Moreover, the finding of sensory deficit in the severely hypotonic infant is strongly suggestive of hypomyelinative polyneuropathy (see Chapter 32).

The major sensory abnormality in *spinal cord injury* relates to the detection of a *sensory level* (i.e., a segmental level below which anesthesia or hypesthesia exists and above which normal sensation occurs). This level corresponds to the approximate segment of cord primarily affected by the injury. (Only occasionally have I been able to detect an area of *hyperesthesia* in a newborn at the segment of the cord injury, as observed in older patients.) Detection of a sensory level is a particularly valuable observation, since it strongly favors the diagnosis of a cord lesion.

Disturbances of sensory function that relate to *lesions of the cerebral hemispheres* are more difficult to document in the newborn period. In my experience, such lesions disturb the so-called higher-level responses described earlier in the discussion of normal neurological findings (i.e., recognizable latency, nonstereotyped movement, accompanying grimace or cry, and habituation). This experience is consistent with the reported observation in an hydranencephalic infant with intact diencephalon but absent parietal lobes of no response decrement to pinprick on any of the administrations of the "five-trial pinprick habituation item"; in fact, the responses "tended to generalize to the whole body and increase in intensity over trials."[110] Thus, the *quality* of the response to pinprick is the critical feature in evaluating sensation vis à vis cerebral lesions.

VALUE OF THE NEONATAL NEUROLOGICAL EXAMINATION

The essential value of the neurological examination in defining the locus and extent of neuropathological involvement and therefore in formulating plans of management is unequivocal in numerous examples of neurological disease. The value of performing a careful neonatal neurological examination, however, is frequently questioned on the basis of two major contentions. The first is that the usual examination permits evaluation of only function of subcortical structures, and the second, related to the first, is that abnormal neurological findings are poor indicators of subsequent deficits of higher neurological function. I consider neither of these contentions to be supported by available data and discuss each briefly in the following sections.

Evaluation of Cerebral Function

The usual support raised for the contention that the neonatal neurological examination permits evaluation of function only of subcortical structures relates to findings of studies of hydranencephalic and anencephalic infants. Such infants often exhibit sleep-wake cycles, blink to light and sound, normal pupillary responses, and reflex extraocular movement.[110,359-361] Facial motility, limb motility, and tendon reflexes exhibit only variable impairment. However, several neurological features are conspicuously disturbed or even absent. Primary neonatal reflexes, although present, are stereotyped, elicited with very brief latencies, and not subject to habituation. Similarly, when occipital and temporal cortices are unequivocally absent, habituation to visual and auditory stimuli is absent. As noted earlier, in one well-studied case in which parietal cortex was apparently absent, habituation to pinprick was absent.[110] Moreover, contrary to the frequently stated misconception, focal cerebral lesions in the newborn result in distinct, although often subtle, focal deficits of limb movement and ocular gaze (see Chapters 16, 20, and 24 on hypoxic-ischemic brain injury and intracranial hemorrhage). Perhaps of greatest importance is the realization that careful clinicoanatomical correlations have only recently begun to be made in neonatal neurology, especially since the advent of MRI. It is to be expected that further significant insight into the impact of cerebral injury on the neonatal neurological examination will be gained from such correlations.

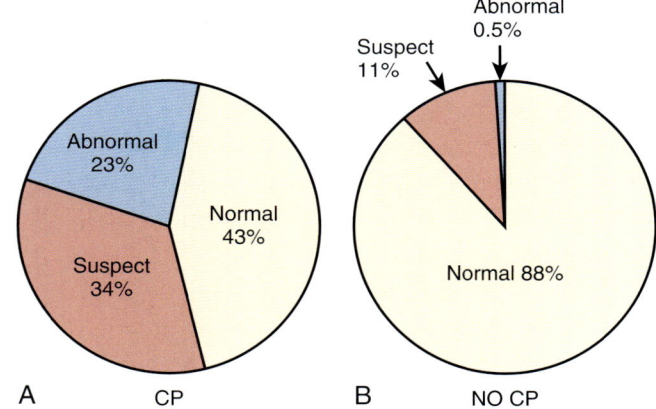

Figure 9.13 Relation of assessment of neonatal neurological status and subsequent outcome. Depicted are overall assessments of neurological status made in the newborn period in (A) infants who later exhibited cerebral palsy (CP) and (B) those who were free of CP. (From Nelson KB, Ellenberg JH. Neonatal signs as predictors of cerebral palsy. *Pediatrics.* 1979;64:225.)

Role in Estimating Prognosis

The contention that the neonatal neurological examination has little predictive value for subsequent neurological abnormality is not supported by a variety of studies.[a] In general, the predictive power of *isolated* neurological signs in the newborn period is not great, but this fact should not detract from the very real predictive value of certain signs or combinations of signs. *Certain neonatal neurological abnormalities* were particularly valuable predictors in the large earlier population studied as part of the Collaborative Perinatal Project of the National Institutes of Health.[362] When infants (predominantly term) who subsequently developed cerebral palsy were compared with those who did not, various abnormalities of limb, neck, or trunk tone carried a 12- to 15-fold enhanced risk; diminished cry for more than 1 day carried a 21-fold enhanced risk; weak or absent sucking a 14-fold enhanced risk; need for gavage or tube feedings a 16- to 22-fold enhanced risk; and diminished activity for more than 1 day carried a 19-fold enhanced risk. Although the actual incidence of infants exhibiting each sign who subsequently developed cerebral palsy was relatively low, usually less than 10%, the predictive power was obviously considerable and alerted the physician to neonatal neurological abnormality. Moreover, I believe that *combinations* of neurological abnormalities greatly increase predictive capacity. This belief, of course, is reasonable in that the occurrence of such combinations in the neonatal period suggests a more severe neurological disturbance. There are data to support this notion.[b] In the aforementioned collaborative project, in which a combination of deficits gave the overall impression of neurological abnormality, 16% of infants later exhibited cerebral palsy. When viewed retrospectively, an overall impression of suspicious or abnormal neurological status was approximately fivefold more likely in infants who later exhibited cerebral palsy than in those who did not (Fig. 9.13). Although the institution in recent years of hypothermia in the management of asphyxiated infants (see Chapter 20) alters the role of neurological assessment during cooling, the

---

[a]References 9, 16, 192, 206, 221, 222, and 362-382.
[b]References 16, 206, 218, 221, 362, 363, 371, 375, 376, 378, 380, and 381.

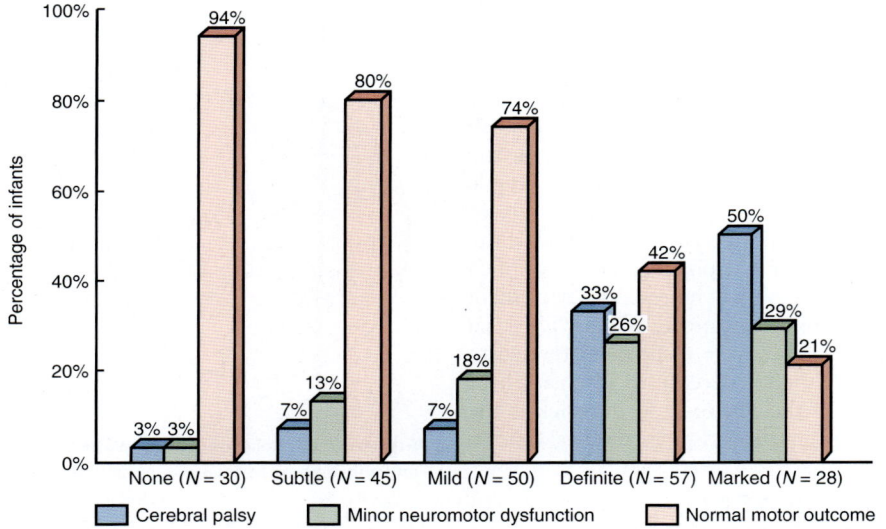

Figure 9.14 **Relationship between number and type of abnormalities observed during neonatal neurodevelopmental examination and later motor development.** Subtle abnormality, one to two minor abnormalities; mild abnormality, three to four minor abnormalities, mild neck extensor tone, or intermittent lower extremity extensor tone; definite abnormality, one major abnormality or at least five minor abnormalities; marked abnormality, at least two major abnormalities or one major and five or more minor abnormalities. (From Allen MC, Capute AJ. Neonatal neurodevelopmental examination as a predictor of neuromotor outcome in premature infants. *Pediatrics.* 1989;83:498.)

value of the examination before onset of cooling and after completion of cooling is still apparent.[9,382]

The value of the neonatal neurological examination in estimating outcome in infants of very low birth weight has also been shown (Fig. 9.14).[370,371] A clear relationship was observed between the severity of the abnormalities at the discharge neurological examination and motor abnormalities at 1 to 5 years of age (see Fig. 9.14).[371] In the latter study, 38% of infants with any abnormality of the neonatal neurological examination at discharge developed cerebral palsy, versus 6% of infants with a normal neonatal neurological examination.[371] Of the infants who developed cerebral palsy, 80% had an abnormal neonatal neurological examination.[371] Other work has emphasized the predictive value of abnormalities of the *quality* of movements in prediction of abnormal neurological outcome.[205,206,219,220-222,383]

The available data thus indicate that the neonatal neurological examination is of major value when carefully and thoughtfully performed. *Serial examinations* are especially useful. It is of critical importance to recognize, however, that *the value of the examination is greatest when it is assessed in the context of the neuropathological disorder* likely to be the cause of the neurological sign or signs. This theme (i.e., correlation of clinical features with the appropriate specialized techniques such as neuroimaging studies) for defining pathology to reach the most meaningful diagnostic and prognostic formulations is recurrent throughout this book.

KEY REFERENCES

1. Sanders M, Allen M, Alexander GR, et al. Gestational age assessment in preterm neonates weighing less than 1500 grams. *Pediatrics.* 1991;88:542-546.
2. Allen MC. Assessment of gestational age and neuromaturation. *Ment Retard Dev Disabil Res Rev.* 2005;11:21-33.
3. Finnstrom O. Studies on maturity in newborn infants. II. External characteristics. *Acta Paediatr Scand.* 1972;61:24-32.
6. Farr V, Kerridge DF, Mitchell RG. The value of some external characteristics in the assessment of gestational age at birth. *Dev Med Child Neurol.* 1966;8:657-660.
7. Dubowitz LM, Dubowitz V, Goldberg C. Clinical assessment of gestational age in the newborn infant. *J Pediatr.* 1970;77:1-10.
8. Ballard JL, Khoury JC, Wedig K, et al. New Ballard score, expanded to include extremely premature infants. *J Pediatr.* 1991;119:417-423.
9. Bonifacio SL, deVries LS, Groenendaal F. Impact of hypothermia on predictors of poor outcome: how do we decide to redirect care? *Semin Fetal Neonatal Med.* 2015;20:122-127.
12. Lissauer T. Physical examination of the newborn. In: Martin RJ, Fanaroff AA, Walsh MC, eds. *Neonatal-Perinatal Medicine. Diseases of the Fetus and Infant.* Vol. 1. 8th ed. Philadelphia: Elsevier; 2006: 513-528.
13. Allan RC, Sayers S, Powers J, et al. The development and evaluation of a simple method of gestational age estimation. *J Paediatr Child Health.* 2009;45:15-19.
15. Dubowitz L, Ricciw D, Mercuri E. The Dubowitz neurological examination of the full-term newborn. *Ment Retard Dev Disabil Res Rev.* 2005;11:52-60.
16. Gosselin J, Gahagan S, Amiel-Tison C. The Amiel-Tison neurological assessment at term: conceptual and methodological continuity in the course of follow-up. *Ment Retard Dev Disabil Res Rev.* 2005;11:34-51.
17. Tallman B, Tan OT, Morelli JG, et al. Location of port-wine stains and the likelihood of ophthalmic and/or central nervous system complications. *Pediatrics.* 1991;87:323-327.
18. Enjolras O, Riche MC, Merland JJ. Facial port-wine stains and Sturge-Weber syndrome. *Pediatrics.* 1985;76:48-51.
19. Enjolras O, Chiron C, Diebler C, et al. New trends for an early diagnosis of the Sturge-Weber syndrome. *Rev Eur Dermatol MST.* 1991;3:21-26. [in French].
20. Pascual-Castroviejo I, Diaz-Gonzalez C, Garcia-Melian RM, et al. Sturge-Weber syndrome: study of 40 patients. *Pediatr Neurol.* 1993;9:283-288.
22. Piram M, Lorette G, Sirinelli D, et al. Sturge-Weber syndrome in patients with facial port-wine stain. *Pediatr Dermatol.* 2012;29: 32-37.
23. Dutkiewicz AS, Ezzedine K, Mazereeuw-Hautier J, et al. A prospective study of risk for Sturge-Weber syndrome in children with upper facial port-wine stain. *J Am Acad Dermatol.* 2015; 72:473-480.

24. Shirley MD, Tang H, Gallione CJ, et al. Sturge-Weber syndrome and port-wine stains caused by somatic mutation in GNAQ. *N Engl J Med.* 2013;368:1971-1979.

25. Nguyen CM, Yohn JJ, Huff C, et al. Facial port wine stains in childhood: prediction of the rate of improvement as a function of the age of the patient, size and location of the port wine stain and the number of treatments with the pulsed dye (585 nm) laser. *Br J Dermatol.* 1998;138:821-825.

26. Chapas AM, Eickhorst K, Geronemus RG. Efficacy of early treatment of facial port wine stains in newborns: a review of 49 cases. *Lasers Surg Med.* 2007;39:563-568.

27. Matson D. *Neurosurgery of Infancy and Childhood.* Springfield: Charles C Thomas; 1969.

28. Governale LS. Minimally invasive pediatric neurosurgery. *Pediatr Neurol.* 2015;52:389-397.

29. Boltshauser E, Ludwig S, Dietrich F, et al. Sagittal craniosynostosis: cognitive development, behaviour, and quality of life in unoperated children. *Neuropediatrics.* 2003;34:293-300.

30. Nagy L, Demke JC. Facial Plast Surg Clin North Am. 2014;22:523-548.

31. Rozovsky K, Udjus K, Wilson N, et al. Cranial ultrasound as a first-line imaging examination for craniosynostosis. *Pediatrics.* 2016;137:e20152230.

32. Jones KL. *Smith's Recognizable Patterns of Human Malformation.* 6th ed. Philadelphia: Elsevier Saunders; 2006.

37. Johnson D, Wilkie AO. Craniosynostosis. *Eur J Hum Genet.* 2011;19: 369-376.

38. Twigg SR, Forecki J, Goos JA, et al. Gain-of-function mutations in ZIC1 are associated with coronal craniosynostosis and learning disability. *Am J Hum Genet.* 2015;97:378-388.

39. Gray KE, Kapp-Simon KA, Starr JR, et al. Predicting developmental delay in a longitudinal cohort of preschool children with single-suture craniosynostosis: is neurobehavioral assessment important? *Dev Med Child Neurol.* 2014;57:456-462.

40. Speltz ML, Collett BR, Wallace ER, et al. Intellectual and academic functioning of school-age children with single-suture craniosynostosis. *Pediatrics.* 2015;135:e615-e623.

41. Patel A, Yang JF, Hashim PW, et al. The impact of age at surgery on long-term neuropsychological outcomes in sagittal craniosynostosis. *Plast Reconstr Surg.* 2014;134:608e-617e.

42. Persing J, James H, Swanson J, et al. Prevention and management of positional skull deformities in infants. *Pediatrics.* 2003;112: 199-202.

43. Maugans TA. The misshapen head. *Pediatrics.* 2002;110:166-167.

44. Littlefield TR, Kelly KM, Pomatto JK, et al. Multiple-birth infants at higher risk for development of deformational plagiocephaly: II. is one twin at greater risk? *Pediatrics.* 2002;109:19-25.

45. Branch LG, Kesty K, Krebs E, et al. Deformational plagiocephaly and craniosynostosis: trends in diagnosis and treatment after the "back to sleep" campaign. *J Craniofac Surg.* 2015;26:147-150.

46. Graham JM Jr, Gomez M, Halberg A, et al. Management of deformational plagiocephaly: repositioning versus orthotic therapy. *J Pediatr.* 2005;146:258-262.

47. Graham JM Jr, Kreutzman J, Earl D, et al. Deformational brachycephaly in supine-sleeping infants. *J Pediatr.* 2005;146:253-257.

48. Bialocerkowski A, Vladusic SL, Howell SM. Conservative interventions for positional plagiocephaly: a systematic review. *Dev Med Child Neurol.* 2005;47:563-570.

57. Sheth RD, Mullett MD, Bodensteiner JB, et al. Longitudinal head growth in developmentally normal preterm infants. *Arch Pediatr Adolesc Med.* 1995;149:1358-1361.

59. Robertson C. Catch-up growth among very-low-birth-weight preterm infants: a historical perspective. *J Pediatr.* 2003;143:145-146.

60. Brandt I, Sticker EJ, Lentze MJ. Catch-up growth of head circumference of very low birth weight, small for gestational age preterm infants and mental development to adulthood. *J Pediatr.* 2003;142:463-468.

61. Latal-Hajnal B, Von Siebenthal K, Kovari H, et al. Postnatal growth in VLBW infants: significant association with neurodevelopmental outcome. *J Pediatr.* 2003;143:163-170.

62. Lofqvist C, Engstrom E, Sigurdsson J, et al. Postnatal head growth deficit among premature infants parallels retinopathy of prematurity and insulin-like growth factor-1 deficit. *Pediatrics.* 2006;117:1930-1938.

63. Ranke MB, Krageloh-Mann I, Vollmer B. Growth, head growth, and neurocognitive outcome in children born very preterm: methodological aspects and selected results. *Dev Med Child Neurol.* 2015;57:23-28.

64. Franz AR, Pohlandt F, Bode H, et al. Intrauterine, early neonatal, and postdischarge growth and neurodevelopmental outcome at 5.4 years in extremely preterm infants after intensive neonatal nutritional support. *Pediatrics.* 2009;123:e101-e109.

65. Villar J, Cheikh Ismail L, Victora CG, et al. International standards for newborn weight, length, and head circumference by gestational age and sex: the Newborn Cross-Sectional Study of the INTERGROWTH-21st Project. *Lancet.* 2014;384: 857-868.

67. Fenton TR. A new growth chart for preterm babies: Babson and Benda's chart updated with recent data and a new format. *BMC Pediatr.* 2003;3:13.

68. Georgieff MD, Hoffman JS, Pereira GR, et al. Effect of neonatal caloric deprivation on head growth and 1-year development status in preterm infants. *J Pediatr.* 1985;107:581-587.

69. Ehrenkranz RA, Dusick AM, Vohr BR, et al. Growth in the neonatal intensive care unit influences neurodevelopmental and growth outcomes of extremely low birth weight infants. *Pediatrics.* 2006;117:1253-1261.

70. Belfort MB, Rifas-Shiman SL, Sullivan T, et al. Infant growth before and after term: effects on neurodevelopment in preterm infants. *Pediatrics.* 2011;128:e899-e906.

71. Vinall J, Grunau RE, Brant R, et al. Slower postnatal growth is associated with delayed cerebral cortical maturation in preterm newborns. *Sci Transl Med.* 2013;5:168ra8.

72. Sammallahti S, Pyhala R, Lahti M, et al. Infant growth after preterm birth and neurocognitive abilities in young adulthood. *J Pediatr.* 2014;165:1109-1115.

73. Pyhala R, Hovi P, Lahti M, et al. Very low birth weight, infant growth, and autism-spectrum traits in adulthood. *Pediatrics.* 2014;134:1075-1083.

74. Prechtl HFR, Beintema D. *The Neurological Examination of the Full Term Newborn Infant.* London: William Heinemann; 1964.

82. Scher MS, Johnson MW, Holditch-Davis D. Cyclicity of neonatal sleep behaviors at 25 to 30 weeks' postconceptional age. *Pediatr Res.* 2005;57:879-882.

88. Sarnat HB. Olfactory reflexes in the newborn infant. *J Pediatr.* 1978;92:624-626.

89. Bartocci M, Winberg J, Ruggiero C, et al. Activation of olfactory cortex in newborn infants after odor stimulation: a functional near-infrared spectroscopy study. *Pediatr Res.* 2000;48:18-23.

97. Varendi H, Christensson K, Porter RH, et al. Soothing effect of amniotic fluid smell in newborn infants. *Early Hum Dev.* 1998;51: 47-55.

98. Bingham PM, Abassi S, Sivieri E. A pilot study of milk odor effect on nonnutritive sucking by premature newborns. *Arch Pediatr Adolesc Med.* 2003;157:72-75.

99. Robinson J, Fielder AR. Pupillary diameter and reaction to light in preterm neonates. *Arch Dis Child.* 1990;65:35-38.

104. Guzzetta A, Cioni G, Cowan F, et al. Visual disorders in children with brain lesions: 1. Maturation of visual function in infants with neonatal brain lesions: correlation with neuroimaging. *Eur J Paediatr Neurol.* 2001;5:107-114.

105. Madan A, Good WV. Visual development in preterm infants. *Dev Med Child Neurol.* 2005;47:276-280.

107. Guzzetta A, Haataja L, Cowan F, et al. Neurological examination in healthy term infants aged 3–10 weeks. *Biol Neonate.* 2005;87: 187-196.

109. Dubowitz LM, Mushin J, De Vries L, et al. Visual function in the newborn infant: is it cortically mediated? *Lancet.* 1986;1: 1139-1141.

110. Aylward GP, Lazzara A, Meyer J. Behavioral and neurological characteristics of a hydranencephalic infant. *Dev Med Child Neurol.* 1978;20:211-217.

111. Jan JE, Wong PK, Groenveld M, et al. Travel vision: "collicular visual system." *Pediatr Neurol.* 1986;2:359-362.

134. Mirabella G, Kjaer PK, Norcia AM, et al. Visual development in very low birth weight infants. *Pediatr Res.* 2006;60:435-439.

137. Farroni T, Johnson MH, Menon E, et al. Newborns' preference for face-relevant stimuli: effects of contrast polarity. *Proc Natl Acad Sci U S A.* 2005;102:17245-17250.

139. Born P, Leth H, Miranda MJ, et al. Visual activation in infants and young children studied by functional magnetic resonance imaging. *Pediatr Res*. 1998;44:578-583.

140. Martin E, Joeri P, Loenneker T, et al. Visual processing in infants and children studied using functional MRI. *Pediatr Res*. 1999;46: 135-140.

141. Meltzoff AN, Moore MK. Imitation of facial and manual gestures by human neonates. *Science*. 1977;198:74-78.

142. Field TM, Woodson R, Greenberg R, et al. Discrimination and imitation of facial expression by neonates. *Science*. 1982;218: 179-181.

143. Nagy E, Compagne H, Orvos H, et al. Index finger movement imitation by human neonates: motivation, learning and left-hand preference. *Pediatr Res*. 2005;58:749-753.

146. Williams MC, Knuppel RA, O'Brien WF, et al. Obstetric correlates of neonatal retinal hemorrhage. *Obstet Gynecol*. 1993;81:688-694.

147. Smith WL, Alexander RC, Judisch GF, et al. Magnetic resonance imaging evaluation of neonates with retinal hemorrhages. *Pediatrics*. 1992;89:332-333.

149. Isenberg SJ. Clinical application of the pupil examination in neonates. *J Pediatr*. 1991;118:650-652.

163. Cheour M, Martynova O, Naatanen R, et al. Speech sounds learned by sleeping newborns. *Nature*. 2002;415:599-600.

164. Carral V, Huotilainen M, Ruusuvirta T, et al. A kind of auditory 'primitive intelligence' already present at birth. *Eur J Neurosci*. 2005;21:3201-3204.

166. Lagasse LL, Neal AR, Lester BM. Assessment of infant cry: acoustic cry analysis and parental perception. *Ment Retard Dev Disabil Res Rev*. 2005;11:83-93.

168. DeCasper AJ, Fifer WP. Of human bonding: newborns prefer their mothers' voices. *Science*. 1980;208:1174-1176.

170. Webb AR, Heller HT, Benson CB, et al. Mother's voice and heartbeat sounds elicit auditory plasticity in the human brain before full gestation. *Proc Natl Acad Sci U S A*. 2015;112:3152-3157.

172. Pena M, Maki A, Kovacic D, et al. Sounds and silence: an optical topography study of language recognition at birth. *Proc Natl Acad Sci U S A*. 2003;100:11702-11705.

173. Dehaene-Lambertz G, Dehaene S, HertzPannier L. Functional neuroimaging of speech perception in infants. *Science*. 2002;298: 2013-2015.

174. Draganova R, Eswaran H, Murphy P, et al. Sound frequency change detection in fetuses and newborns, a magnetoencephalographic study. *Neuroimage*. 2005;28:354-361.

182. Mizuno K, Ueda A. The maturation and coordination of sucking, swallowing and respiration in preterm infants. *J Pediatr*. 2003; 142:36-40.

183. Gewolb I, Bosma J, Reynolds EW, et al. Integration of suck and swallow rhythms during feeding in preterm infants with and without bronchopulmonary dysplasia. *Dev Med Child Neurol*. 2003;45:344-348.

184. Rogers B, Arvedson J. Assessment of infant oral sensorimotor and swallowing function. *Ment Retard Dev Disabil Res Rev*. 2005;11: 74-82.

191. Amiel-Tison C. Neurological evaluation of the maturity of newborn infants. *Arch Dis Child*. 1968;43:89-93.

192. Thorn I. Cerebral symptoms in the newborn. Diagnostic and prognostic significance of symptoms of presumed cerebral origin. *Acta Paediatr Scand*. 1969;(suppl 195):1-8.

198. Faridi MM, Rath S, Aggarwal A. Profile of fisting in term newborns. *Eur J Paediatr Neurol*. 2005;9:67-70.

208. Mercuri E, Guzzetta A, Laroche S, et al. Neurologic examination of preterm infants at term age: comparison with term infants. *J Pediatr*. 2003;142:647-655.

218. Guzzetta A, Mercuri E, Rapisardi G, et al. General movements detect early signs of hemiplegia in term infants with neonatal cerebral infarction. *Neuropediatrics*. 2003;34:61-66.

219. Ferrari F, Cioni G, Einspieler C, et al. Cramped synchronized general movements in preterm infants as an early marker for cerebral palsy. *Arch Pediatr Adolesc Med*. 2002;156:460-467.

220. Groen SE, de Blecourt AC, Postema K, et al. General movements in early infancy predict neuromotor development at 9 to 12 years of age. *Dev Med Child Neurol*. 2005;47:731-738.

221. Paro-Panjan D, Sustersic B, Neubauer D. Comparison of two methods of neurologic assessment in infants. *Pediatr Neurol*. 2005;33:317-324.

222. Stahlmann N, Hartel C, Knopp A, et al. Predictive value of neurodevelopmental assessment versus evaluation of general movements for motor outcome in preterm infants with birth weights <1500 g. *Neuropediatrics*. 2007;38:91-99.

224. Zafeiriou DI. Primitive reflexes and postural reactions in the neurodevelopmental examination. *Pediatr Neurol*. 2004;31:1-8.

225. Paine RS, Brazelton TB, Donovan DE. Evolution of postural reflexes in normal infants and in the presence of chronic brain syndromes. *Neurology*. 1964;14:1036.

228. Rich E, Marshall R, Volpe J. Letter: plantar reflex flexor in normal neonates. *N Engl J Med*. 1973;289:1043.

231. Capute AJ, Palmer FB, Shapiro BK, et al. Primitive reflex profile: a quantitation of primitive reflexes in infancy. *Dev Med Child Neurol*. 1984;26:375-383.

233. Rich EC, Marshall RE, Volpe JJ. The normal neonatal response to pin-prick. *Dev Med Child Neurol*. 1972;16:432.

235. Anand KJS, Hickey PR. Pain and its effects in the human neonate and fetus. *N Engl J Med*. 1987;317:1321-1329.

236. Anand KJ, Carr DB. The neuroanatomy, neurophysiology, and neurochemistry of pain, stress, and analgesia in newborns and children. *Pediatr Clin North Am*. 1989;36:795-822.

241. Posner JB, Saper CB, Schiff ND, et al. *Plum and Posner's Diagnosis of Stupor and Coma*. 4th ed. New York: Oxford University Press; 2007.

244. Walton DS, Robb RM. Optic nerve hypoplasia. A report of 20 cases. *Arch Ophthalmol*. 1970;84:572-578.

245. Margalith D, Jan JE, McCormick AQ, et al. Clinical spectrum of congenital optic nerve hypoplasia: review of 51 patients. *Dev Med Child Neurol*. 1984;26:311-322.

246. Margalith D, Tze WJ, Jan JE. Congenital optic nerve hypoplasia with hypothalamic-pituitary dysplasia. A review of 16 cases. *Am J Dis Child*. 1985;139:361-366.

247. Roberts-Harry J, Green SH, Willshaw HE. Optic nerve hypoplasia: associations and management. *Arch Dis Child*. 1990;65:103-106.

251. Traggiai C, Stanhope R. Endocrinopathies associated with midline cerebral and cranial malformations. *J Pediatr*. 2002;140:252-255.

259. Prepiakova Z, Tomcikova D, Kostolna B, et al. Confluent diode laser coagulation: the gold standard of therapy for retinopathy of prematurity. *J Pediatr Ophthalmol Strabismus*. 2015;52:43-51.

262. Feske SK, Carrazana EJ, Kupsky WJ, et al. Uncal herniation secondary to bacterial meningitis in a newborn. *Pediatr Neurol*. 1992;8:142-144.

263. Hoyt CS, Mousel DK, Weber AA. Transient supranuclear disturbances of gaze in healthy neonates. *Am J Ophthalmol*. 1980;89: 708-713.

267. Seidl Z, Sussova J, Obenberger J, et al. Magnetic resonance imaging in diplegic form of cerebral palsy. *Brain Dev*. 2001;23:46-49.

270. Perlman JM, Nelson JS, McAlister WH, et al. Intracerebellar hemorrhage in a premature newborn: diagnosis by real-time ultrasound and correlation with autopsy findings. *Pediatrics*. 1983;71:159-162.

273. Ryan MM, Engle EC. Disorders of the ocular motor cranial nerves and extraocular muscles. In: Darras BT, Jones HR Jr, Ryan MM, et al., eds. *Neuromuscular Disorders of Infancy, Childhood, and Adolescence. A Clinician's Approach*. 2nd ed. London: Elsevier; 2015:922-957.

281. Ouvrier R, Billson F. Paroxysmal tonic upgaze of childhood—a review. *Brain Dev*. 2005;27:185-188.

282. Morad Y, Benyamini OG, Avni I. Benign opsoclonus in preterm infants. *Pediatr Neurol*. 2004;31:275-278.

288. Ehrt O. Infantile and acquired nystagmus in childhood. *Eur J Paediatr Neurol*. 2012;16:567-572.

289. Lenn NJ, Freinkel AJ. Facial sparing as a feature of prenatal-onset hemiparesis. *Pediatr Neurol*. 1989;5:291-295.

291. Hepner WR. Some observations on facial paresis in the newborn infant: etiology and incidence. *Pediatrics*. 1951;8:494.

301. Smith RJH, Bale JF, White KR. Sensorineural hearing loss in children. *Lancet*. 2005;365:879-890.

302. Lammens F, Verhaert N. Desloovere C. Syndromic disorders in congenital hearing loss. *B-ENT*. 2013;(suppl 21):45-50.

303. Roizen NJ. Nongenetic causes of hearing loss. *Ment Retard Dev Disabil Res Rev*. 2003;9:120-127.

304. Martinez-Cruz CF, Garcia Alonso-Themann P, Poblano A, et al. Hearing and neurological impairment in children with history

of exchange transfusion for neonatal hyperbilirubinemia. *Int J Pediatr.* 2014;2014:605828.

305. Iskander I, Gamaleldin R, El Houchi S, et al. Serum bilirubin and bilirubin/albumin ratio as predictors of bilirubin encephalopathy. *Pediatrics.* 2014;134:e1330-e1339.

306. Corujo-Santana C, Falcon-Gonzalez JC, Borkoski-Barreiro SA, et al. The relationship between neonatal hyperbilirubinemia and sensorineural hearing loss. *Acta Otorrinolaringol Esp.* 2015;66: 326-331.

310. Hulzebos CV, van Dommelen P, Verkerk PH, et al. Evaluation of treatment thresholds for unconjugated hyperbilirubinemia in preterm infants: effects on serum bilirubin and on hearing loss? *PLoS ONE.* 2013;8:e62858.

315. Fjalstad JW, Laukli E, van den Anker JN, et al. High-dose gentamicin in newborn infants: is it safe? *Eur J Pediatr.* 2013;173: 489-495.

317. De Hoog M, van Zanten BA, Hop WC, et al. Newborn hearing screening: tobramycin and vancomycin are not risk factors for hearing loss. *J Pediatr.* 2003;142:41-46.

319. Turner KM, Lee HC, Boppana SB, et al. Incidence and impact of CMV infection in very low birth weight infants. *Pediatrics.* 2014;133:e609-e615.

320. Goderis J, De Leenheer E, Smets K, et al. Hearing loss and congenital CMV infection: a systematic review. *Pediatrics.* 2014;134: 972-982.

321. Toumpas CJ, Clark J, Harris A, et al. Congenital cytomegalovirus infection is a significant cause of moderate to profound sensorineural hearing loss in Queensland children. *J Paediatr Child Health.* 2015;51:541-544.

325. Bolisetty S, Dhawan A, Abdel-Latif M, et al. Intraventricular hemorrhage and neurodevelopmental outcomes in extreme preterm infants. *Pediatrics.* 2014;133:55-62.

326. van Dommelen P, Verkerk PH, van Straaten HL. Hearing loss by week of gestation and birth weight in very preterm neonates. *J Pediatr.* 2015;166:840-843.

329. Etzel RA, Balk SJ, Bearer CF, et al. Noise: a hazard for the fetus and newborn. *Pediatrics.* 1997;100:724-727.

330. Zimmerman E, Lahav A. Ototoxicity in preterm infants: effects of genetics, aminoglycosides, and loud environmental noise. *J Perinatol.* 2013;33:3-8.

331. American Academy of Pediatrics CoEH. Noise: a hazard for the fetus and newborn. American Academy of Pediatrics. Committee on Environmental Health. *Pediatrics.* 1997;100:724-727.

332. Kazemizadeh Gol MA, Black A, Sidman J. Bone conduction noise exposure via ventilators in the neonatal intensive care unit. *Laryngoscope.* 2015;125:2388-2392.

343. Inder TE, Volpe JJ. Recovery of congenital isolated pharyngeal dysfunction: implications for early management. *Pediatr Neurol.* 1998;19:222-224.

346. Cochrane DD, Adderley R, White CP, et al. Apnea in patients with myelomeningocele. *Pediatr Neurosurg.* 1990;16:232-239.

347. Hesz N, Wolraich M. Vocal-cord paralysis and brainstem dysfunction in children with spina bifida. *Dev Med Child Neurol.* 1985;27:528-531.

352. Mizuno K. Neonatal feeding performance as a predictor of neurodevelopmental outcome at 18 months. *Dev Med Child Neurol.* 2005;47:299-304.

353. Al-Shahoumi R, Brady LI, Schwartzentruber J, et al. Two cases of congenital myasthenic syndrome with vocal cord paralysis. *Neurology.* 2015;84:1281-1282.

371. Allen MC, Capute AJ. Neonatal neurodevelopmental examination as a predictor of neuromotor outcome in premature infants. *Pediatrics.* 1989;83:498-506.

376. Dubowitz L, Mercuri E, Dubowitz V. An optimality score for the neurologic examination of the term newborn. *J Pediatr.* 1998;133:406-416.

378. Mercuri E, Guzzetta A, Haataja L, et al. Neonatal neurological examination in infants with hypoxic ischaemic encephalopathy: correlation with MRI findings. *Neuropediatrics.* 1999;30:83-89.

379. Amess PN, Penrice J, Wylezinska M, et al. Early brain proton magnetic resonance spectroscopy and neonatal neurology related to neurodevelopmental outcome at 1 year in term infants after presumed hypoxic-ischaemic brain injury. *Dev Med Child Neurol.* 1999;41:436-445.

381. Als H, Butler S, Kosta S, et al. The Assessment of preterm infants' behavior (APIB): furthering the understanding and measurement of neurodevelopmental competence in preterm and full-term infants. *Ment Retard Dev Disabil Res Rev.* 2005;11:94-102.

382. Sabir H, Cowan FM. Prediction of outcome methods assessing short- and long-term outcome after therapeutic hypothermia. *Semin Fetal Neonatal Med.* 2015;20:115-121.

383. Skiold B, Eriksson C, Eliasson AC, et al. General movements and magnetic resonance imaging in the prediction of neuromotor outcome in children born extremely preterm. *Early Hum Dev.* 2013;89:467-472.

Full references for this chapter can be found on www.expertconsult .com.

Specialized Neurological Studies

Jeffrey J. Neil ◆ *Joseph J. Volpe*

In addition to the neurological examination discussed in Chapter 9, certain specialized studies are critical components of the neurological evaluation of the newborn. Most of these studies are presented in relation to relevant specific disorders throughout this book. However, certain of these specialized aspects, which are not discussed in detail elsewhere and are of definite or potential importance in the neurological evaluation, are reviewed here, including examination of the cerebrospinal fluid (CSF), certain neurophysiological studies (brain stem auditory evoked responses, visual cortical evoked responses, and electroencephalography [EEG]), the major techniques for imaging of brain structure (cranial ultrasound [CUS] and magnetic resonance imaging [MRI]), certain noninvasive continuous monitoring techniques, and methods for physiological brain imaging.

CEREBROSPINAL FLUID EXAMINATION

Examination of the CSF is an important part of the evaluation of a wide variety of neurological disorders, as noted in appropriate chapters throughout this book. In this section, we focus principally on normal CSF in the newborn, particularly the newborn considered at high risk for such neurological disorders.

The principal components of the CSF examination include measurement of intracranial pressure, assessment of the color (e.g., bloody, xanthochromic) and turbidity (e.g., purulent), red blood cell (RBC) and white blood cell (WBC) counts, WBC differential count, and concentrations of protein and glucose. Other, more specialized evaluations (e.g., for microorganisms, various metabolites, and enzymes) are determined by clinical circumstances. In this section, we focus on the WBC and RBC counts and concentrations of protein and glucose.

White Blood Cell, Protein, and Glucose Concentrations

Of the several studies that address normal CSF values in the newborn,[1-13] the studies of Sarff and co-workers[11] and Rodriguez and co-workers[12] are the most informative (although all the data are generally consistent). Sarff and co-workers discussed the CSF findings in 117 high-risk infants (87 term, 30 preterm < 2500 g birth weight; 95 examined in the first week, most with clinical findings indicative of a high risk of infection but without positive cultures for bacteria or other organisms or grossly bloody CSF) (Table 10.1). Mean values for term and preterm infants, respectively, were for WBC counts of 8 and 9/mm³ (60% polymorphonuclear leukocytes), protein concentration 90 and 115 mg/dL, glucose concentrations 52

and 50 mg/dL, and ratio of CSF to blood glucose 81% and 74%. Although the ranges are wide, the values provide a useful framework for evaluating neonatal CSF.

In a subsequent report, Rodriguez and co-workers[12] obtained more detailed data for similarly high-risk infants but of very low birth weight (i.e., <1500 g). When the data were expressed as a function of postconceptional age when the CSF sample was obtained, the values for the more mature infants were similar to the values obtained by Sarff and co-workers (Table 10.2). This similarity could be expected because the infants in the study by Sarff and co-workers were larger and presumably more mature. Notably, however, the least mature infants (26 to 28 weeks of postconceptional age) exhibited values of glucose and protein that were distinctly higher than values observed at later ages. This occurrence, as well as the finding of Sarff and co-workers that preterm infants had relatively high ratios of CSF to blood glucose (see Table 10.1), supports the notion of increased permeability of the blood-brain barrier in the small preterm infant. Moreover, increased permeability for other macromolecules (e.g., immunoglobulin G, alpha-fetoprotein) is suggested by other studies.[14-17] Although the WBC counts in the premature infants studied by Rodriguez and co-workers did not differ as a function of postconceptional age and are similar to those reported by Sarff and co-workers, the percentage of polymorphonuclear leukocytes (7%) is much lower than in the latter study. This discrepancy may be related in part to the error inherent in the study of relatively small numbers of WBCs.

These values for WBC count and protein and glucose concentrations are crucial for the evaluation of the infant with suspected bacterial meningitis or other central nervous system inflammatory processes. Although these issues are discussed in more detail later (see Chapters 34 and 35), combinations of abnormalities are important to recognize, and single values that are questionably abnormal are difficult to interpret conclusively. *Under all circumstances, assessment of the CSF in the context of the clinical setting and the clinical features is most important.*

Red Blood Cell Counts in High-Risk Newborns

Determination of *normal* values for RBCs in neonatal CSF is hindered by the relatively high incidence of germinal matrix–intraventricular hemorrhage, usually clinically silent in the preterm infant (see Chapter 24), and by the likelihood that the process of birth is associated with minor amounts of subarachnoid bleeding. In the study of Sarff and co-workers,[11] the median value for RBC count was 180, with a very wide range (0 to 45,000) (Table 10.3). A similar value was obtained for premature infants in that study. In both the term and preterm infants, the most common value (mode) for RBC count was 0. However, in the report of Rodriguez and co-workers,[12] although a median value of 112 was observed, the mean was 785, and 20% of CSF samples had more than 1000 RBCs/mm^3 (see Table 10.3). These infants were smaller (<1500 g), but ultrasonographic examinations were said to show no evidence of intracranial hemorrhage. However, exclusion of minor subarachnoid hemorrhage by cranial ultrasonography is not reliable.

The aforementioned data indicate that the finding of more than 100 RBCs/mm^3 in the newborn is common and that, in very-low-birth-weight infants, values greater than 1000 occur in a substantial minority in the absence of apparently clinically significant intracranial hemorrhage. Again, the *combination* of findings is important in the evaluation of the CSF for intracranial hemorrhage. Thus the addition of xanthochromia and elevated protein concentration in CSF strongly raises the possibility of a more substantial and, clinically speaking, more important intracranial hemorrhage. This issue is discussed in more detail in Chapter 22.

NEUROPHYSIOLOGICAL STUDIES

Several specialized neurophysiological techniques have been particularly valuable in further defining the neurological maturation of the newborn. Moreover, some of these studies are commonly used in neurological diagnosis. In this section, we cover brain-stem auditory evoked responses, visual evoked responses, and EEG (including amplitude-integrated EEG). The most widely used of these neurophysiological techniques, EEG, is also discussed in relation to seizures in Chapter 12.

Brain-Stem Auditory Evoked Responses

Electrophysiological investigations of the auditory system in the newborn have focused on brain-stem evoked responses. However, cortical auditory evoked responses have been studied, as have visual and somatosensory evoked responses (see later sections), through computer-averaged EEG recordings obtained over the scalp after graded stimuli. Such *cortical responses* have been described in premature and full-term infants,[18-34] demonstrating that peripheral auditory stimuli are transmitted to the primary and secondary auditory cortex of the temporal

---

TABLE 10.1   Cerebrospinal Fluid Findings in High-Risk Newborns

FINDINGS	TERM	PRETERM
White blood cell count per mm^3		
Mean ± standard deviation	8 ± 7	9 ± 6
Range	0–32	0–29
Protein concentration (mg/dL)		
Mean	90	115
Range	20–170	65–150
Glucose concentration (mg/dL)		
Mean	52	50
Range	34–119	24–63
Cerebrospinal fluid/blood glucose (%)		
Mean	81	74
Range	24–248	55–105

Data from Sarff LD, Platt LH, McCracken Jr GH. Cerebrospinal fluid evaluation in neonates: Comparison of high-risk infants with and without meningitis. J Pediatr. 1976;88:473–477; based on 87 term infants and 30 low-birth-weight infants (<2500 g), 95 of whom were examined in the first week of life.

TABLE 10.3   Red Blood Cell Counts (per mm^3) in Cerebrospinal Fluid of High-Risk Newborns

Sarff and co-workers[a]	
Term infants	$n = 87$
	Median: 180
	Range: 0–45,000
Preterm infants (<2500 g)	$n = 30$
	Median: 112
	Range: 0–39,000
Rodriguez and co-workers[b]	
Preterm infants (<1500 g)	$n = 43$
	Mean: 785
	RBCs >1000/mm^3 in 20% of samples

[a]Data from Sarff LD, Platt LH, McCracken Jr GH. Cerebrospinal fluid evaluation in neonates: comparison of high-risk infants with and without meningitis. J Pediatr. 1976;88:473–477.
[b]Data from Rodriguez AF, Kaplan SL, Mason Jr EO. Cerebrospinal fluid values in the very low birth weight infant. J Pediatr. 1990;116:971–974.

TABLE 10.2   Cerebrospinal Fluid Findings in High-Risk Infants of Low Birth Weight (<1500 g)

POSTCONCEPTIONAL AGE (WEEKS)	WHITE BLOOD CELL COUNT (per MM^3 ± SD)	GLUCOSE (MG/DL ± SD)	PROTEIN (MG/DL ± SD)
26–28	6 ± 10	85 ± 39[a]	177 ± 60[a]
29–31	5 ± 4	54 ± 81	144 ± 40
32–34	4 ± 3	55 ± 21	142 ± 49
35–37	6 ± 7	56 ± 21	109 ± 53
38–40	9 ± 9	44 ± 10	117 ± 33

[a]Values for glucose and protein were significantly greater at 26 to 28 weeks than at subsequent postconceptional ages.
SD, Standard deviation.
Data from Rodriguez AF, Kaplan SL, Mason Jr EO. Cerebrospinal fluid values in the very low birth weight infant. J Pediatr. 1990;116:971–974; based on 43 infants, some studied more than once, approximately 80% studied after the first week of life.

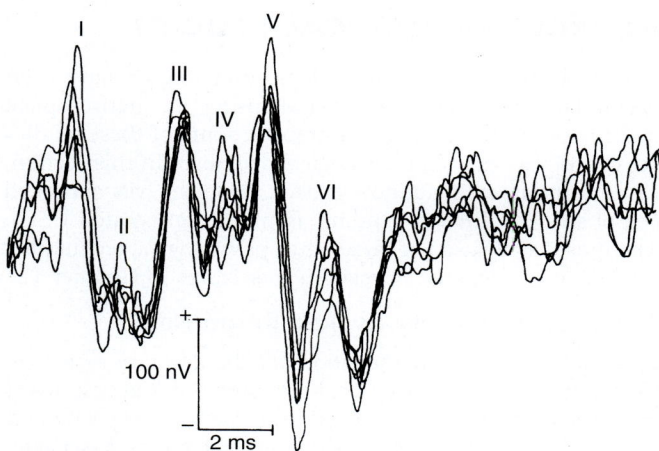

Figure 10.1 Brain-stem auditory evoked response, major waveforms. The responses obtained with several sequential trials were superimposed. The complete response, with the seven definable waves, is not observed in the newborn (see text for details). (From Starr A, Amlie RN, Martin WH, Sanders S. Development of auditory function in newborn infants revealed by auditory brainstem potentials. *Pediatrics.* 1977;60:831–839.)

lobe in the newborn period. Magnetoencephalography has been used to define the maturation of cortical evoked responses from 27 weeks of gestation to term in 18 fetuses.[35,36] This work is noteworthy for the detection of a decrease in latency from 300 ms at 29 weeks of gestation to 150 ms at term. Further, auditory habituation has been demonstrated in fetuses,[37] suggesting that fetal learning is taking place. This novel and noninvasive technique thus not only extends insights into the maturation of auditory cortical areas during the last trimester of human gestation but also demonstrates the applicability of magnetoencephalography to study of the fetus. Nevertheless, measurement of cortical auditory evoked potentials has been difficult to adapt to routine clinical circumstances, in part because the amplitude and latency of the observed responses vary with the infant's level of arousal and in part because of the expense of the technology (magnetoencephalography). In contrast, major attention has been paid to the earlier potentials generated from subcortical structures after auditory stimulation (i.e., the *brain-stem auditory evoked response*).

Major Waveforms and Anatomical Correlates

The brain-stem auditory evoked response reflects the electrical events generated within the auditory pathways from the eighth nerve to the diencephalon and is recorded by electrodes placed usually over the mastoid and vertex. The stimulation is usually a click or pure tone administered at a relatively rapid rate. The latency and amplitude of the components of the response are measured.[24,25,38-44] To avoid movement and other artifacts, the infant is studied preferably during sleep. The complete response consists of seven components, designated consecutively by Roman numerals (Fig. 10.1).[25,38,41] Studies in animals and adult humans indicate that the waves derive from sequential activation of the major components of the auditory pathway.[39,40,45-47] Thus, wave I represents activity of the eighth nerve, wave II the cochlear nucleus, wave III the superior olivary nucleus, wave IV the lateral lemniscus, and wave V the inferior colliculus. The precise origins of waves VI and VII remain to be established, but these waves are probably

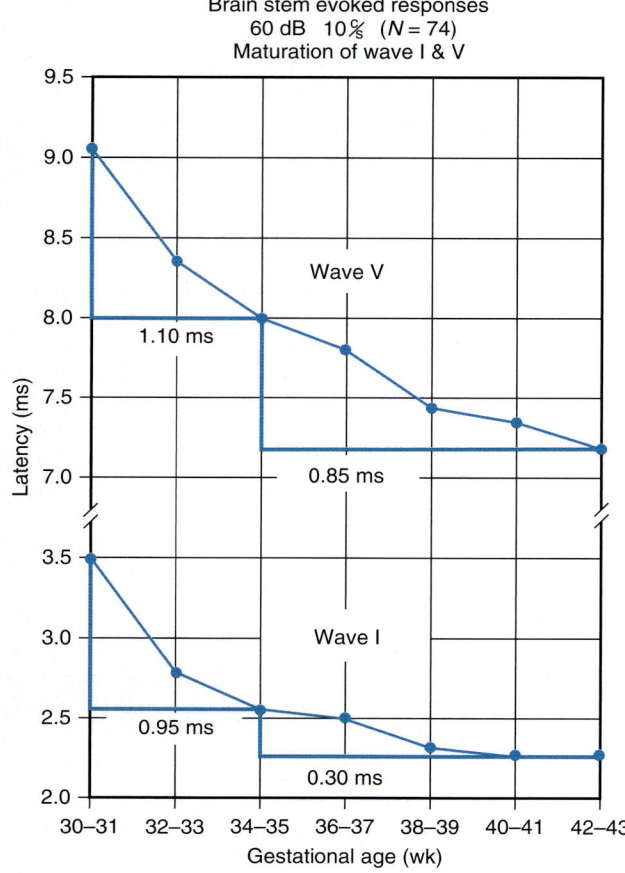

Figure 10.2 Decrease in latencies of major waves of neonatal brain-stem auditory evoked response as a function of gestational age. (From Despland PA, Galambos R. The auditory brainstem response [ABR] is a useful diagnostic tool in the intensive care nursery. *Pediatr Res.* 1980;14:154–158.)

generated in the thalamus and thalamic radiations, respectively. Brain-stem auditory potentials have been well defined in the newborn infant,[24,25,38,41-43,48-63] although all seven components are not observed (see later discussion).

Developmental Changes

Impressive ontogenetic changes in the brain-stem auditory response have been described.[a] The most reproducible and easily definable components are waves I, III, and V; the last is sometimes fused with wave IV. Waves II, VI, and VII have generally been too variable to allow systematic study.[38] The *latencies* of the most prominent components (I, III, IV to V) decrease as a function of gestational age, with a maximal shift occurring in the weeks before 34 weeks of gestation (Fig. 10.2). Moreover, an increase in amplitude and a decrease in threshold of the response occur with increasing gestational age.

Detection of Disorders of the Auditory Pathways

Abundant findings indicate the value of brain-stem auditory evoked response studies in detecting disorders of the auditory pathways in the newborn infant.[b] Definition of such disorders depends on the detection of responses that are abnormal in

---

[a]References 24, 25, 38, 41, 49, 51, 52, 56, 57, and 63-77.
[b]References 24, 25, 38, 41-43, 55, 58-63, and 78-105.

TABLE 10.4   Two Basic Abnormal Patterns of Brain-Stem Auditory Evoked Responses in Neonatal Disease

RESPONSE CHARACTERISTIC	SITE OF DISORDER	
	PERIPHERY	BRAIN STEM
Threshold (wave I)	Elevated	Normal
Wave I latency	Prolonged	Normal
Wave V latency	Prolonged	Prolonged
I–V interval	Normal	Prolonged

TABLE 10.5   Probable or Proven Examples of Neonatal Neurological Disease With Abnormal Brain-Stem Auditory Evoked Responses

NEUROLOGICAL DISORDERS	RELEVANT NEUROPATHOLOGY
Hypoxic-ischemic encephalopathy	Cochlear nuclei, inferior colliculus, cochlea
Hyperbilirubinemia	Cochlear nuclei, inferior colliculus, cochlea, eighth nerve
Bacterial meningitis	Eighth nerve
Congenital viral infection	Cochlea, eighth nerve
Intracranial hemorrhage	Cochlea

threshold sensitivity, conduction time (i.e., latency), amplitude, or conformation. In neonatal studies, deficits in threshold sensitivity and latency have been the most valuable. The general principle is that a lesion at the periphery (middle ear, cochlea, or eighth nerve) results in a heightened threshold and a prolongation of latency of *all* the potentials, including wave I, whereas a lesion in the brain stem causes longer latencies of only those waves originating from structures distal to the lesion, with wave I spared. The essential features of these two basic abnormal patterns of brain-stem auditory evoked responses observed in neonatal patients are depicted in Table 10.4.

Abnormalities of the evoked response in neonatal neurological disease are to be expected, in part because of the known neuropathological involvement of the following: the cochlear nuclei, the inferior colliculus, other brain-stem nuclei, and the cochlea itself by hypoxic-ischemic insult (see Chapter 18); the cochlear nuclei, inferior colliculus, and, perhaps, the cochlea or eighth nerve by hyperbilirubinemia (see Chapter 26); the eighth nerve by bacterial meningitis (see Chapter 35); the cochlea and eighth nerve by congenital viral infections (see Chapter 34); and the cochlea by intracranial hemorrhage (see Chapter 24) (Table 10.5). Indeed, brain-stem evoked response audiometry has been used to describe peripheral and central disturbances in infants with congenital cytomegalovirus infection, hyperbilirubinemia, bacterial meningitis, asphyxia, persistent fetal circulation, aminoglycoside or furosemide administration, trauma to the cochlea or middle ear, and still undefined complications of low birth weight.[a] The particular

importance of *combinations* of these factors in the genesis of permanent deficits has been emphasized. Moreover, neonatal defects may be transient. For example, in one large study (*N* = 92) of term asphyxiated infants, 35% exhibited brain-stem auditory evoked response deficit (increased threshold) in the first 3 days of life, but only 10% had abnormalities at 30 days.[61] Among preterm infants with birth weight less than 1500 g who were studied at term, 14% had evidence of a peripheral impairment (increased threshold), 17% a central impairment (prolonged brain-stem latencies), and 4% a combined impairment, for a total of 27%.[59]

Hearing Screening

Use of the brain-stem auditory evoked response as a screening device for hearing impairment in the neonate has become extremely common, and universal screening is the norm in many countries.[a] The importance of early identification of infants with hearing impairment is based on the realization that acquisition of normal language and of social and learning skills depends on hearing.[b]

The most commonly recommended *screening procedure* for preterm infants consists of testing the infant just before hospital discharge or at least as close to 40 weeks after conception as possible, when he or she is medically stable, and preferably in a room separate from the neonatal unit. Term infants are often tested at any point before discharge.[c] The initial screening procedure has consisted of conventional brain-stem auditory evoked response, automated auditory evoked response, or transient evoked otoacoustic emission. The last detects signals generated by cochlear outer hair cells in response to acoustic stimulation. This technique is faster and less expensive than evoked response audiometry. However, the method does not detect retrocochlear abnormalities (e.g., auditory nerve disease). Infants who fail this test are retested by auditory evoked response study, often an automated study.[107,108,113] The incidence of failure of either screening test at the time of hospital discharge is relatively high, with the actual value depending on the population studied. For low-birth-weight infants tested at term, failure rates as high as 20% to 25% are common.[25,95] Retesting infants after test failure is usually carried out after several weeks or later, often after discharge. With this approach, many infants are lost to follow-up. Because most neonates who fail the first screening procedure exhibit normal responses at the time of the retest,[d] the initial failures are likely transient, reversible disturbances or false-positive results. For example, in one large series of more than 16,000 infants, retesting in the neonatal unit after early test failures resulted in an 80% reduction in failure rate by discharge.[115] In certain high-risk groups, the importance of later testing is emphasized by the report of hearing deficits developing in the first months of life, *after* normal results in the neonatal period (Table 10.6).[82,83,113]

Visual Evoked Responses

Cortical Response

The term *visual evoked response* refers to the electrical response, recorded usually by surface electrodes on the occipital scalp, to

---

[a]References 24, 25, 38, 41-43, 58-63, 77, 78, 80-94, 97, 98, 101, 103, 105, and 106.

[a]References 25, 41, 95, 99, 100, 103, 107, and 108.
[b]References 25, 41, 90, 99-103, 107, and 109-115.
[c]References 25, 99, 100, 107, 111, and 113.
[d]References 25, 41, 51, 54, 55, 95, 99, 100, 107, 111, and 115.

TABLE 10.6   Follow-Up Audiological Diagnostic Evaluation for Infants Who Pass Their Initial Hearing Screening (Adapted From the State of Massachusetts Recommendations)

IMMEDIATELY AFTER DISCHARGE	BY 3 MONTHS OF AGE	AT 6–9 MONTHS OF AGE
CMV	Down syndrome	>10 days mechanical ventilation
Bacterial meningitis	Cleft lip/palate	≤32 weeks gestational age
Parental or medical provider concern	Craniofacial anomalies (microtia/atresia)	<1500 g birth weight
	Syndromes associated with hearing loss (e.g., CHARGE, Treacher Collins, Pierre Robin)	In utero infection associated with hearing loss (e.g., herpes, rubella, syphilis, toxoplasmosis)
	Perinatal asphyxia (therapeutic hypothermia)	Head trauma
	ECMO	Ear pits with preauricular tags
	Hyperbilirubinemia (>20 mg/dL bilirubin)	>7 day course of ototoxic medications including aminoglycosides or in conjunction with loop diuretics
	Permanent childhood hearing loss in immediate family (infant's parents or siblings)	NICU stay for >5 days
		Permanent childhood hearing loss in extended family

CHARGE, Coloboma, heart defects, choanal atresia, retarded growth and development, genital abnormalities, and ear anomalies; CMV, cytomegalovirus; ECMO, extracorporeal membrane oxygenation; NICU, neonatal intensive care unit.

a standardized stimulus, the most common of which is a *light flash* of graded intensity and frequency. Flash visual evoked responses are recorded in response to red light-emitting diodes in goggles placed over the infant's eyes or in an array placed about 6 inches in front of the infant's eyes.[116-118] The fully developed response is complex, but the first two prominent waves consist of first a positive and then a negative deflection. The positive deflection is attributed to postsynaptic activation at the site of the predominant termination of visual afferents, and the negative deflection is attributed to secondary synaptic contacts in the superficial cortical layers.[119] Two features of the response are studied: the quality of the waveform and the latency between stimulus and recorded response. With flash visual evoked responses, variability in latencies can lead to difficulties in interpretation.

An alternative and generally preferable stimulus for visual evoked responses, particularly for study of visual acuity, is a shift (reversal) of a checkerboard pattern (i.e., *pattern-shift or pattern-reversal* visual evoked response).[39,40,116,120-122] This stimulus results in responses with less variable latencies than those obtained with a light-flash stimulus. Although the technique has been used in the newborn,[a] including the preterm newborn,[120,121,124] experience remains limited, in part because obtaining optimal data requires that the newborn *fix* on the visual display. However, reliable data have been obtained, and this technique should prove adaptable to the newborn for wider use.

Developmental Changes

The ontogenetic changes of the visual evoked response in the human newborn have been well established.[116-118,120-122,125-137] A prolonged negative slow wave can be identified as early as 24 weeks of gestation, and this wave ultimately is replaced by the more discrete negative wave noted earlier (Fig. 10.3). The positive wave appears between approximately 32 and 35 weeks of gestation, and by 39 weeks the visual evoked response is

quite well defined. As with the components of the brain-stem auditory evoked response, the latencies of both the positive and negative waves of the visual evoked response decrease in a linear fashion with increasing maturation (Fig. 10.4). This evolution in the quality and latency of the response corresponds well with the behavioral studies of visual function noted in Chapter 9. That this ontogenetic change is principally an inborn program is suggested by the finding that differences between infants born at term and healthy premature infants grown to term are small,[138] and these differences dissipate completely shortly after the time of term.[139] Although the anatomical substrate for the ontogenetic changes is undoubtedly complex, the major maturational changes correspond to the period of rapid dendritic development in the visual cortex and myelination of the optic radiations (see Chapters 7 and 8).

Detection of Disorders of the Visual Pathway

Although neonatal visual evoked responses are not used routinely in clinical practice, premature infants with *serious hypoxemia* secondary to respiratory distress syndrome were shown to lose visual evoked responses during the insult and to regain the responses with restoration of normal blood gas levels.[134,140] Similarly, impairment of the visual evoked response has been demonstrated in the first day after *asphyxia* in term infants, and the severity of the abnormality correlated well with poor neurological outcome.[43,136,141,142] In a study of 36 term infants who experienced *birth asphyxia* and were studied by serial assessment of visual evoked responses, 14 of 16 infants with normal responses in the first week of life were normal on follow-up, and all 20 with abnormal responses persisting beyond the first week died or were *significantly handicapped* at 18 months of age.[142] A related observation in fetal and neonatal lambs indicates the sensitivity of the visual evoked response to asphyxial insult.[143] Abnormalities of the visual evoked response have also been described in infants with *posthemorrhagic hydrocephalus* (see Chapter 24),[116,144,145] a finding probably reflecting the disproportionate dilation of the occipital horns of the lateral ventricles and consequent affection of the geniculocalcarine radiations. Moreover, improvement

---

[a]References 39, 40, 116, 120, 121, and 123.

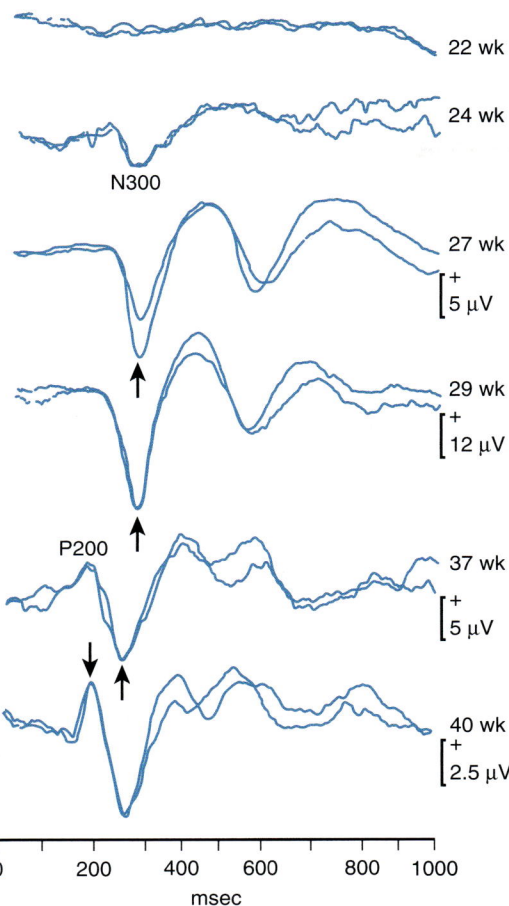

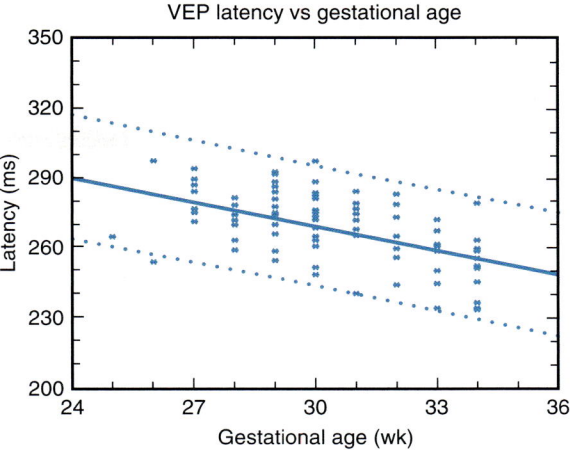

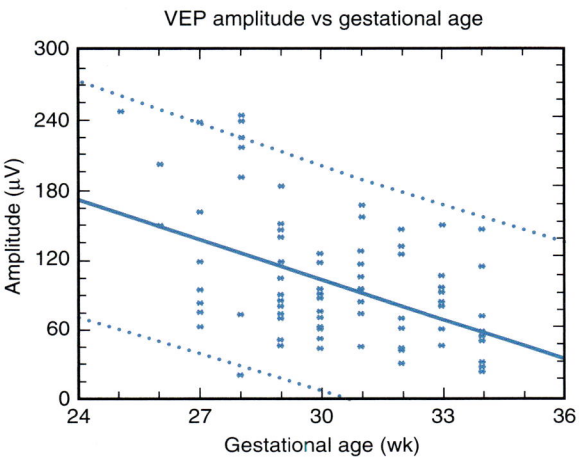

Figure 10.3 Visual evoked potentials to stimulation by light-emitting diode from newborn infants showing no recordable response at 22 weeks of post-conceptional age (PCA), the emergence of N300 at 24 weeks of PCA, the late positivity following the N300 (usually ≈450 ms), which is evident from about 27 weeks onward, and then little change until closer to term. The P200 then emerges and becomes the most prominent wave in the normal term newborn's visual evoked potential. (From Taylor MJ. Visual evoked potentials. In Eyre JA, ed. *The Neurophysiological Examination of the Newborn Infant.* New York: MacKeith Press.)

Figure 10.4 Visual evoked potential latency and amplitude versus gestational age in weeks in 86 preterm infants. The regression line and the 95% confidence interval are indicated. (Latency = 370.7 − 3.4 × ga; amplitude = 440.4 − 11.2 × ga.) (From Pryds O, Trojaborg W, Carlsen J, Jensen J. Determinants of visual evoked potentials in preterm infants. *Early Hum Dev.* 1989;19:117–125.)

in latencies was documented immediately after ventricular tap[145] as well as over a prolonged period after placement of ventriculoperitoneal shunt.[144] The data suggest that the determination of visual evoked responses in the neonatal period provides important information concerning cerebral function, effects of interventions, and outcome.

Electroencephalogram

Normal Development

Maturation of spontaneous EEG recorded activity has been studied in considerable detail in newborn infants, often in combination with studies of sleep states.[139,146-180] With increasing gestational age, impressive elaborations of measurable function occur, characterized principally by more refined organization. Whether infants are born at term or grow to term after uncomplicated premature delivery has little or no effect on these developments. The normal development of EEG patterns in the neonatal period is evaluated best in relation to sleep states. In general, active sleep is the predominant sleep state

in the newborn and consists of greater than 70% of definable sleep time in the smallest premature infants and approximately 50% in term infants. In the following discussion, we review the major changes in EEG over approximately the 12 to 13 weeks before term. Development of EEG is considered best in terms of the continuity of background activity, the synchrony of this activity, and the appearance and disappearance of specific waveforms and patterns (i.e., EEG developmental landmarks) (Table 10.7).[165]

27 to 28 Weeks. Activity at this developmental stage is characteristically discontinuous, with long periods of quiescence (see Table 10.7).[165] The activity that does interrupt the quiescence occurs in generalized rather synchronous bursts (Fig. 10.5). No distinctions between wakefulness and sleep or change in EEG to external stimulus such as loud sound (i.e., reactivity) are apparent.

29 to 30 Weeks. The discontinuity of the EEG continues at this stage, but now the activity is asynchronous (see

TABLE 10.7   Developmental Aspects of Electroencephalographic Activity

POSTCONCEPTIONAL AGE (WEEKS)	CONTINUITY OF BACKGROUND ACTIVITY[a]			SYNCHRONY OF BACKGROUND ACTIVITY[b]			EEG DEVELOPMENTAL LANDMARKS: SPECIFIC WAVEFORMS AND PATTERNS
	AWAKE	QUIET SLEEP	ACTIVE SLEEP	AWAKE	QUIET SLEEP	ACTIVE SLEEP	
27–28	–	D	D	–	++++	++++	—
29–30	D	D	D	0	0	0	1. *Delta brushes* in central regions
—	—	—	—	—	—	—	2. Temporal theta bursts (4–6 Hz)
—	—	—	—	—	—	—	3. Occipital slow activity
31–33	D	D	C	+	+	++	1. *Delta brushes* in occipital–temporal regions
—	—	—	—	—	—	—	2. Temporal alpha bursts replace theta bursts (33 weeks)
—	—	—	—	—	—	—	3. Rhythmic 1.5-Hz activity in frontal leads in transitional sleep
34–35	C	D	C	+++	+	+++	1. Extremely high-voltage beta activity during *delta brushes*
—	—	—	—	—	—	—	2. Temporal alpha bursts disappear
—	—	—	—	—	—	—	3. Frontal sharp-wave transients
36–37	C	D	C	++++	++	++++	1. Central *delta brushes* disappear
—	—	—	—	—	—	—	2. Continuous biooccipital delta activity with superimposed 12–15-Hz activity during active sleep
38–40	C	C	C	++++	+++	++++	1. Occipital *delta brushes* decrease and disappear by 39 weeks
—	—	—	—	—	—	—	2. *Tracé alternant* pattern during quiet sleep

[a]C, Continuous activity; D, discontinuous activity.

[b]0, Total asynchrony; ++++, total synchrony.

EEG, Electroencephalographic.

Adapted from Hrachovy RA, Mizrahi EM, Kellaway P. Electroencephalography of the newborn. In Daly DD, Pedley TA, eds. *Current Practice of Clinical Electroencephalography.* 2nd ed. New York: Raven Press; 1990.

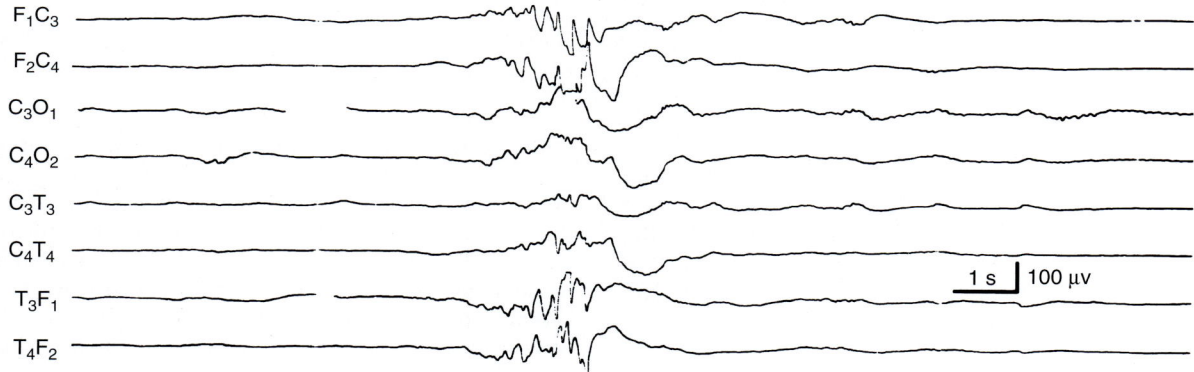

Figure 10.5 Electroencephalogram of a male infant at 27 to 28 weeks of postconceptional age. The bursts of generalized, bilaterally synchronous activity separated by prolonged periods of electrical quiescence are characteristic of this age. Selected sample from a 16-channel recording. (From Hrachovy RA, Mizrahi EM, Kellaway P. Electroencephalography of the newborn. In Daly DD, Pedley TA, eds. *Current Practice of Clinical Electroencephalography.* 2nd ed. New York: Raven Press; 1990.)

Table 10.7 and Fig. 10.6).[165] The principal developmental landmark is the appearance of *delta brushes* (i.e., delta waves of 0.3 to 1.5 Hz with superimposed fast activity in the beta range, usually 18 to 22 Hz), sometimes also called *beta-delta complexes* (Fig. 10.7).[165] These complexes appear in the central regions at this stage. In addition, temporal bursts of theta activity (4 to 6 Hz) are a second developmental landmark of this period (see Fig. 10.7). These bursts occur independently in left and right temporal areas; their sharp configuration has provoked the term *sawtooth pattern.*

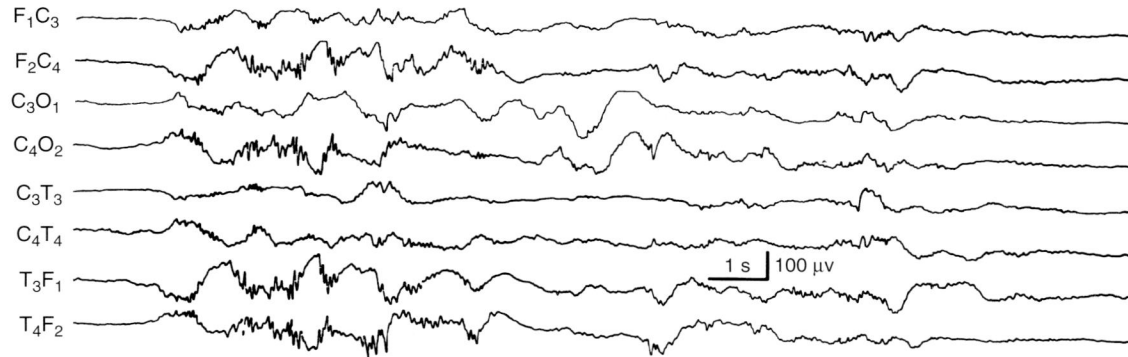

Figure 10.6 *Tracé discontinu* pattern in a male infant with a postconceptional age of 29 to 30 weeks. Selected sample from a 16-channel recording. (From Hrachovy RA, Mizrahi EM, Kellaway P. Electroencephalography of the newborn. In Daly DD, Pedley TA, eds. *Current Practice of Clinical Electroencephalography.* 2nd ed. New York: Raven Press; 1990.)

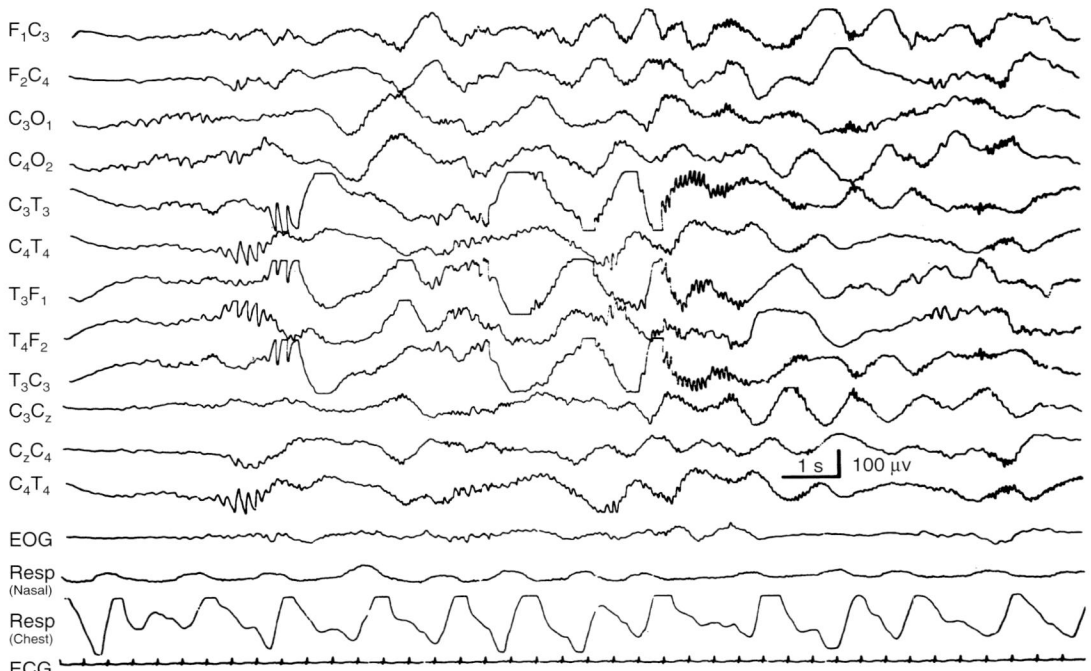

Figure 10.7 Electroencephalogram of a female infant with a postconceptional age of 30 to 32 weeks. *Left,* Brief bursts of 4- to 6-Hz waves of sharp configuration occurring asynchronously in the temporal regions. *Right,* Beta-delta complexes in the central and temporal regions. Selected sample from a 16-channel recording. *ECG,* Electrocardiogram; *EOG,* electro-oculogram. (From Hrachovy RA, Mizrahi EM, Kellaway P. Electroencephalography of the newborn. In Daly DD, Pedley TA, eds. *Current Practice of Clinical Electroencephalography.* 2nd ed. New York: Raven Press; 1990.)

31 to 33 Weeks. At this stage, continuous activity appears during active (or rapid-eye-movement) sleep (see Table 10.7).[165] Moreover, although EEG is generally asynchronous, a degree of synchrony appears in active sleep. The presence of more synchrony in active sleep than in quiet sleep persists throughout the developmental period of the third trimester. The delta brushes now become more prominent in occipital and temporal areas and are apparent particularly in quiet sleep. The temporal theta bursts of earlier stages give way to temporal alpha bursts, still, however, exhibiting the sharp sawtooth pattern (Fig. 10.8).

34 to 35 Weeks. The degree of continuity in the EEG now increases further and is apparent in the awake state as well as in active sleep (see Table 10.7).[165] In concert, the degree of synchrony increases in the awake and active sleep states. Of the developmental EEG landmarks, the delta brushes now exhibit considerably higher-voltage, faster activity. The temporal theta bursts disappear during this phase. Frontal sharp-wave transients (i.e., sharp waves appearing as an abrupt change from background) become apparent (Fig. 10.9) and are characteristic for their diphasic, synchronous, and generally symmetrical

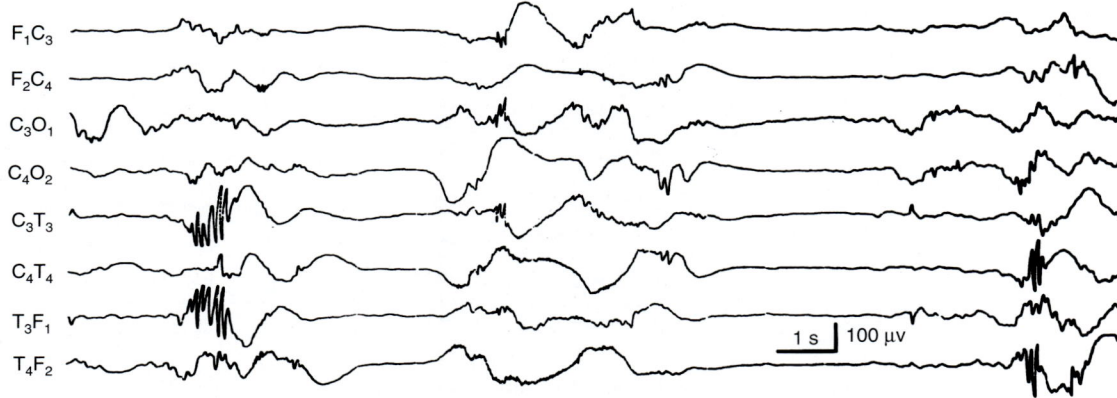

Figure 10.8 Brief bursts of 8- to 9-Hz waves occurring bilaterally in the temporal regions in a female infant with a postconceptional age of 32 to 33 weeks. Selected sample from a 16-channel recording. (From Hrachovy RA, Mizrahi EM, Kellaway P. Electroencephalography of the newborn. In Daly DD, Pedley TA, eds. *Current Practice of Clinical Electroencephalography*. 2nd ed. New York: Raven Press; 1990.)

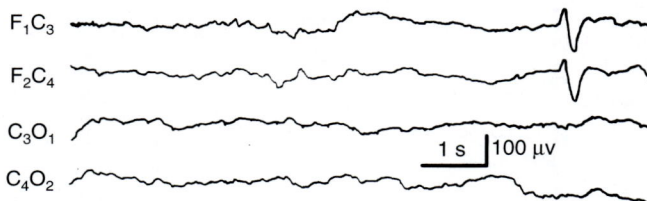

Figure 10.9 Diphasic, bilaterally synchronous, virtually symmetrical frontal sharp waves in transitional sleep in a male infant with a postconceptional age of 36 weeks. Selected sample from a 16-channel recording. (From Hrachovy RA, Mizrahi EM, Kellaway P. Electroencephalography of the newborn. In Daly DD, Pedley TA, eds. *Current Practice of Clinical Electroencephalography*. 2nd ed. New York: Raven Press; 1990.)

TABLE 10.8	Major Electroencephalographic Abnormalities of the Premature and Term Newborn

Disordered development
Depression: lack of differentiation
Excessively discontinuous activity, including burst-suppression pattern
Electrocerebral silence
Unilateral depression of background activity
Periodic discharges
Multifocal sharp waves
Central positive sharp waves
Rhythmic generalized or focal alpha activity
Hypsarrhythmia

Data primarily from Hrachovy RA, Mizrahi EM, Kellaway P. Electroencephalography of the newborn. In Daly DD, Pedley TA, eds. *Current Practice of Clinical Electroencephalography*. 2nd ed. New York: Raven Press; 1990.

configuration. These normal waves should be distinguished from higher-voltage, unilateral, persistently focal, periodic, or semirhythmic sharp waves, which are abnormal and indicative of focal disease (see later discussion). At this stage, the EEG becomes *reactive* to external stimuli. Most commonly, this reactivity consists of a generalized attenuation of the amount and voltage of delta activity, especially apparent in response to sound.

36 to 37 Weeks. The degree of continuity and of synchrony in the awake and active sleep states is still more apparent (see Table 10.7).[165] At this stage, for the first time, the EEG in the awake state differs from that in sleep by the presence of low-voltage activity, with a mixture of activities in the alpha, beta, theta, and delta frequency bands (Fig. 10.10). Of the developmental EEG landmarks, the delta brushes in the central region disappear. These are replaced by similar complexes in the occipital regions (i.e., bioccipital delta with superimposed 12- to 15-Hz activity, which appears during active sleep).

38 to 40 Weeks. At this stage, continuous activity now appears in quiet sleep as well as in active sleep and the awake state (see Table 10.7).[165] A considerable degree of synchrony is present in all states. The occipital delta brushes disappear, and the interesting *tracé alternant* pattern becomes apparent in quiet sleep (Fig. 10.11). This quasiperiodic tracing is characterized by periods of 3 to 15 seconds of generalized voltage attenuation interrupted by higher-voltage, generally synchronous activity. *Tracé alternant* should not be confused with the more ominous burst-suppression pattern (see later discussion).

Clinical Application

The following sections focus on the application of conventional EEG in the clinical arena. The procedure requires skilled technicians and experienced interpreters of the tracing. Definitive assessment of EEG abnormalities in the premature and term newborn requires conventional multichannel EEG. In the following discussion, we review the principal EEG abnormalities of both the premature and term newborn (Table 10.8) except for the EEG correlates of neonatal seizures (see Chapter 12).

Disordered Development. Delineation of abnormalities of EEG maturation clearly requires awareness of the normal developmental changes described in the previous section. Impairment of development level of more than 3 weeks, according to reported gestational age, is clearly abnormal.[165,181] Such disturbances are often but not necessarily associated with

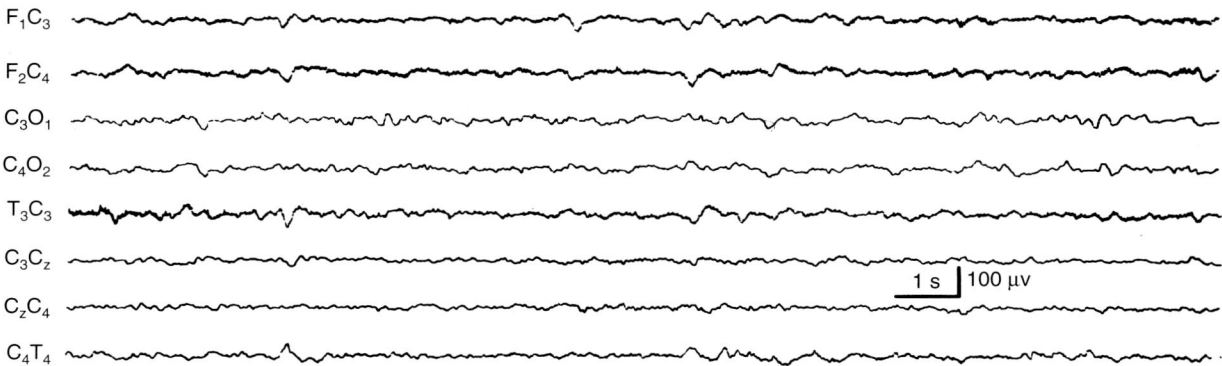

Figure 10.10 Typical awake pattern in a male term infant characterized by a mixture of activities in the alpha, beta, theta, and delta frequency bands. Selected sample from a 16-channel recording. (From Hrachovy RA, Mizrahi EM, Kellaway P. Electroencephalography of the newborn. In Daly DD, Pedley TA, eds. *Current Practice of Clinical Electroencephalography.* 2nd ed. New York: Raven Press; 1990.)

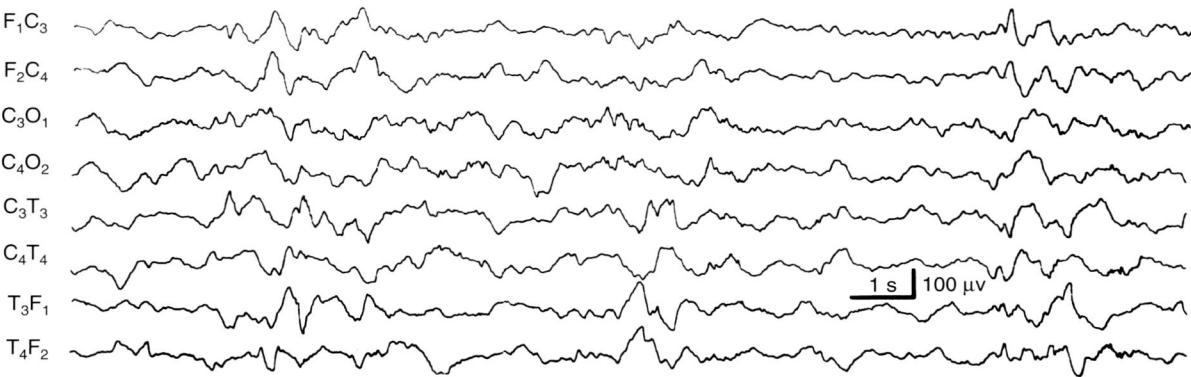

Figure 10.11 *Tracé alternant* pattern in a male term infant. (From Hrachovy RA, Mizrahi EM, Kellaway P. Electroencephalography of the newborn. In Daly DD, Pedley TA, eds. *Current Practice of Clinical Electroencephalography.* 2nd ed. New York: Raven Press; 1990.)

other EEG abnormalities, and the degree of disturbance may differ according to the state of the infant.[181-183] Abnormalities may be apparent only in quiet sleep; thus this sleep state should be included in the EEG evaluation of the newborn.[165] Disturbed development of the EEG does not provide specific information regarding disease process and may reflect either an acute or a chronic disturbance.

Depression and Lack of Differentiation. Depression of background activity, especially of the faster frequencies, often accompanied by lack of differentiation (i.e., disappearance of the normal multiple frequencies), is common after generalized insults, especially hypoxic-ischemic insults (Fig. 10.12).[165,178,181,184,185] Other EEG abnormalities are also often present. In addition to hypoxia and ischemia, other bilateral cerebral insults may produce this EEG pattern, particularly acutely (e.g., bacterial meningitis, encephalitis, and metabolic disorders). Persistence of this EEG pattern is an unfavorable prognostic sign.

Excessively Discontinuous Activity. The development of continuous or intermittent discontinuity of EEG in the term infant is a very common feature of all neonatal encephalopathies. The most extreme of these discontinuous tracings is the *burst-suppression pattern*, which is associated with a very high likelihood of an unfavorable outcome. However, burst-suppression tracings account for the minority of excessively discontinuous neonatal EEGs. Recent data indicate that relatively simple analysis of the latter tracings is highly useful in predicting outcome (see later).

The *burst-suppression pattern* can be considered the most severe of the excessively discontinuous tracings just described. The EEG pattern is characterized by long periods (usually >10 seconds) of marked depression of background activity (voltage <5 μV), alternating with shorter periods of paroxysmal bursts, usually lasting 1 to 10 seconds and characterized by high-voltage (75 to 250 μV) theta and delta activity with intermixed spikes and waves (Fig. 10.13). This EEG pattern should be distinguished from the normal discontinuous tracing of the very immature premature infant and from the *tracé alternant* of quiet sleep of the infant beyond 36 weeks of gestation. Two important distinguishing features of the burst-suppression pattern are persistence of the discontinuous pattern throughout the tracing and nonreactivity (i.e., no change in the EEG with arousal attempts and painful or other stimuli). A burst-suppression pattern that is *reactive* (i.e., is altered by external stimuli) is not as uniformly associated with a poor prognosis as the nonreactive variety described here.[186-191] The poor prognosis

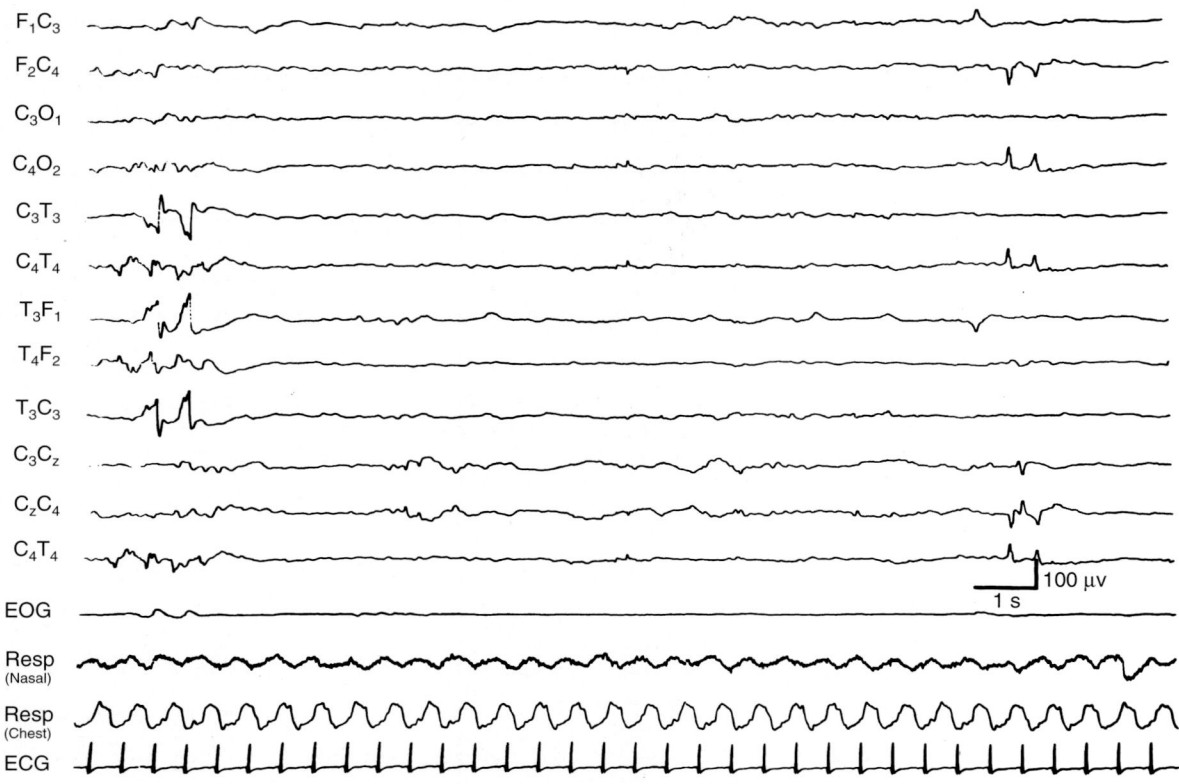

Figure 10.12 Electroencephalogram of a male term infant who had meningitis and hypoxia at birth. Background activity is depressed and undifferentiated, with superimposed abnormal, random sharp waves. Selected sample from a 16-channel recording. *ECG,* Electrocardiogram; *EOG,* electro-oculogram. (From Hrachovy RA, Mizrahi EM, Kellaway P. Electroencephalography of the newborn. In Daly DD, Pedley TA, eds. *Current Practice of Clinical Electroencephalography.* 2nd ed. New York: Raven Press; 1990.)

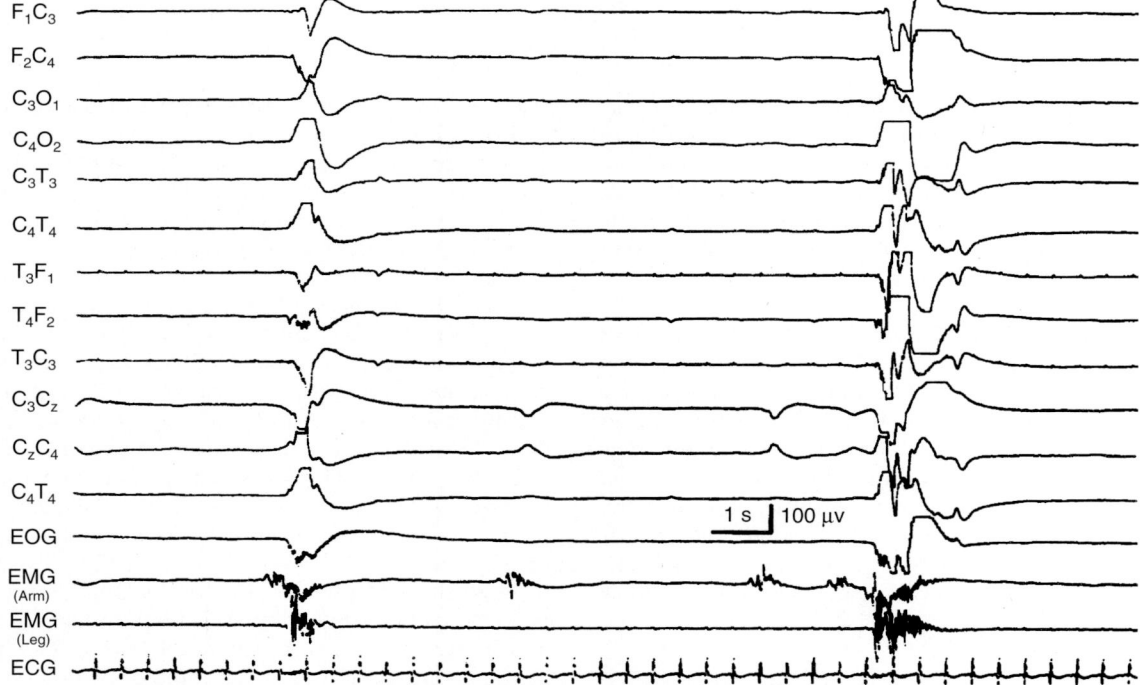

Figure 10.13 Suppression-burst activity in a male term infant with severe neonatal hypoxia. The bursts were associated with myoclonic jerks of the upper and lower extremities (electromyographic channels show myoclonic movement of the arm and leg). This pattern was unremitting during 90 minutes of recording and was nonreactive to intense stimuli. *ECG,* Electrocardiogram; *EMG,* electromyogram; *EOG,* electro-oculogram. (From Hrachovy RA, Mizrahi EM, Kellaway P. Electroencephalography of the newborn. In Daly DD, Pedley TA, eds. *Current Practice of Clinical Electroencephalography.* 2nd ed. New York: Raven Press; 1990.)

TABLE 10.9   Electroencephalography and Prediction of Poor Outcome in Infants With Hypoxic-Ischemic Injury

BACKGROUND PATTERN	SENSITIVITY (95% CI)	SPECIFICITY (95% CI)
Burst suppression	0.87 (0.78–0.92)	0.82 (0.72–0.88)
Low voltage	0.92 (0.72–0.98)	0.99 (0.87–1.0)
Flat trace	0.78 (0.58–0.91)	0.99 (0.88–1.0)

Adapted from Awal MA, Lai MM, Azemi G et al. EEG background features that predict outcome in term neonates with hypoxic ischaemic encephalopathy: a structured review. *Clin Neurophysiol.* 2016;127:285–296.

TABLE 10.10   Duration of Predominant Interburst Interval and Neurological Outcome[a]

PREDOMINANT INTERBURST INTERVAL DURATION[b]	UNFAVORABLE OUTCOME[c]
>30 s	10/10 (100%)
>20 s	12/13 (92%)
>10 s	24/33 (72%)

[a]Data from Menache CC, Bourgeois BFD, Volpe JJ. Prognostic value of neonatal discontinuous EEG. *Pediatr Neurol.* 2002;27:93–101.

[b]Interburst interval duration was obtained by manual measurement with classification into 10-second subintervals (1–10, 11–20, 21–30, >40 seconds); the predominant interval was defined as the interval that accounted for more than 50% of all interburst interval durations.

[c]Death or moderate or severe motor and cognitive deficits were noted on follow-up.

TABLE 10.11   Focal Periodic Electroencephalographic Discharges in the Newborn

	PRETERM	TERM
Characteristics of discharge		
Location	Vertex-central	Temporal
Duration	<1 min	>1 min
Associated electrographic seizures	35%	88%
Origin		
Infarction	15%	88%
Periventricular leukomalacia	27%	0
Other structural abnormalities	27%	0
Unknown	31%	12%
Outcome		
Death	46%	38%
Deficits	27%	50%
Normal	27%	12%

Data from Scher MS, Beggarly M. Clinical significance of focal periodic discharges in neonates. *J Child Neurol.* 1989;4:175–185; *n* = 34 (26 preterm and 8 term).

of various EEG backgrounds, including burst-suppression, for infants with hypoxic-ischemic injury is shown in Table 10.9.[192] Bacterial meningitis is the one disturbance in which I have seen a favorable outcome despite the finding of a burst-suppression EEG during the *acute* disease.[193]

Analysis of the *duration of the predominant interburst interval (IBI)* has proven to be a relatively simple means of *quantitation of excessively discontinuous tracings* in the term infant, and the analysis has major prognostic implications.[194] Thus, of 43 term infants (70% with hypoxic-ischemic encephalopathy) with an excessively discontinuous EEG, 10 parameters regarding the burst and IBIs were quantitated and compared with outcome. One parameter, the IBI duration that accounted for more than 50% of all IBI durations (classified into 10-second blocks), also known as *the predominant IBI duration*, predicted an unfavorable neurological outcome with high specificity (Table 10.10). Thus, IBI durations lasting longer than 30 seconds were invariably associated with an unfavorable outcome, and those with a duration of more than 20 seconds were associated with an unfavorable outcome in 92%. *Of the 43 discontinuous tracings, only 7 (16%) exhibited a burst-suppression pattern*, as defined earlier. Thus, the predominant IBI duration, *readily quantitated at the bedside*, was highly effective and, critically, applicable to the large group of excessively discontinuous tracings in term newborns with encephalopathy.

Electrocerebral Silence. Electrocerebral silence, of course, is the worst end of the continuum from depressed EEG through excessive discontinuity and burst-suppression pattern. Persistence of electrocerebral silence for 72 hours or more is indicative of cerebral death.[195,196] However, electrocerebral silence indicates cerebral cortical death and not necessarily brain-stem death; if clinical evidence of persistent brain-stem failure is not present, survival is possible, although in a persistent vegetative state (see Chapter 9).

Unilateral Depression of Background Activity. A marked voltage asymmetry between hemispheres of background rhythms that persists in all states is clearly different from the normal shifting asymmetries, particularly during quiet sleep (Fig. 10.14). Such persistent unilateral depressions of background activity are indicative usually of a unilateral cerebral lesion that is ischemic, hemorrhagic, or dysgenetic.

Periodic Discharges. Numerous periodic discharges may be seen in neonatal disease states. These complexes may be either strikingly periodic (Fig. 10.15) or only quasiperiodic.[165,178,187,197-200] They can be separated from the normal *transients* noted earlier by their higher voltage, generally longer duration, often polyphasic appearance, and persistent focality. The discharges are located more commonly in the central regions in the premature and in temporal regions in term infants (Table 10.11).[197] Neuropathological substrates are multiple in premature infants, but in the term infant the most common is infarction in the distribution of the middle cerebral artery.

Watanabe and co-workers showed the predictive value of frontal or occipital sharp waves in identifying cystic periventricular leukomalacia (Table 10.12).[200] Thus the presence of one or both of these abnormal sharp waves was superior to the presence of positive rolandic sharp waves (see later) in sensitivity for identifying white matter injury.

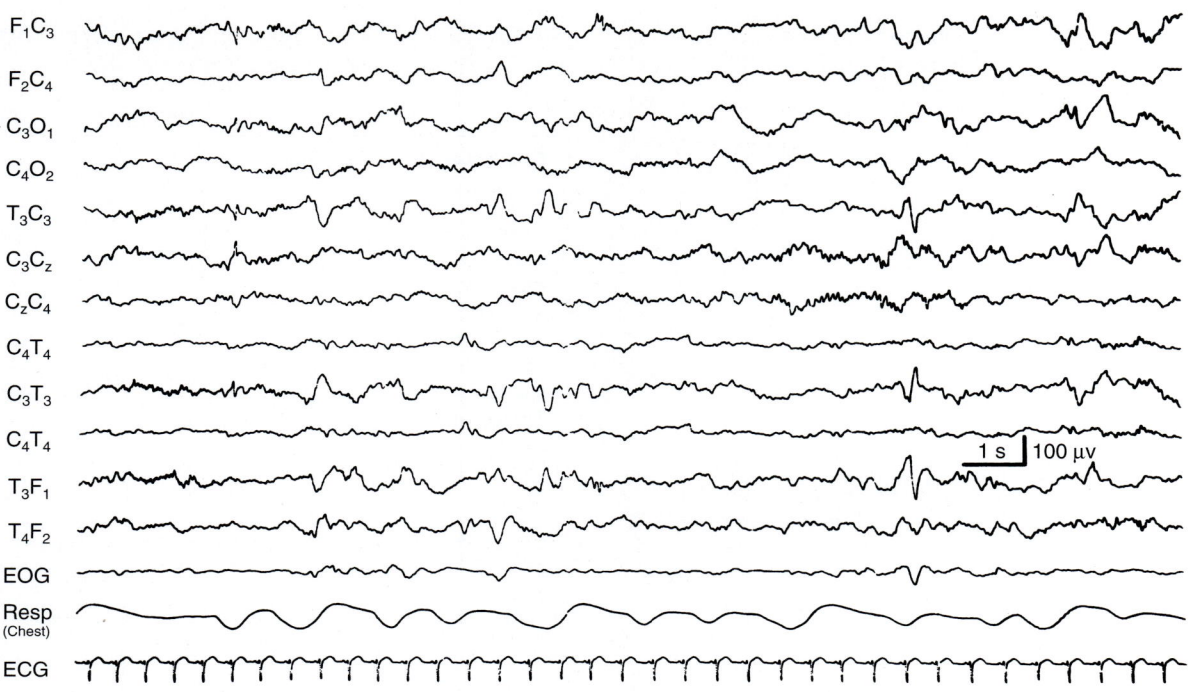

Figure 10.14 Electroencephalogram of a male term infant with a subarachnoid hemorrhage showing suppression of background activity over the right hemisphere. Such unilateral suppressions of background activity are usually associated with an underlying structural lesion. *ECG,* Electrocardiogram; *EOG,* electro-oculogram. (From Hrachovy RA, Mizrahi EM, Kellaway P. Electroencephalography of the newborn. In Daly DD, Pedley TA, eds. *Current Practice of Clinical Electroencephalography.* 2nd ed. New York: Raven Press; 1990.)

TABLE 10.12	Frontal and Occipital Sharp Waves and Positive Rolandic or Vertex (Central) Sharp Waves in Premature Infants

Frontal or occipital sharp waves, or both, present in 100% of cases of severe PVL and in 60%–70% of cases of mild or moderate PVL

PRSs present in 65%–90% of cases of *severe* white matter lesions (i.e., PVL, periventricular hemorrhagic infarction); sensitivity lowest for the most immature infants and for mild or moderate PVL (present in 25% of cases)

PRSs generally apparent when white matter lesions are echodense but not yet cystic by ultrasonography

Lateralization or symmetry of the abnormal waves generally corresponding to lateralization or symmetry of white matter necrosis

Onset of the abnormal waves as early as 2 days, generally peaking between 5 and 14 days; *cystic* PVL noted generally 5–10 days later

PRS, Positive rolandic sharp wave; *PVL,* periventricular leukomalacia.

Multifocal Sharp Waves. *Multifocal sharp waves* are sharp waves of high voltage and relatively long duration occurring in multiple cerebral foci (Fig. 10.16).[165,178] These discharges tend to predominate in temporal regions and are usually accompanied by other EEG abnormalities. The types of underlying pathological features are multiple, and their specific nature determines outcome.

Central Positive Sharp Waves. These distinctive sharp waves, often termed *positive rolandic sharp waves,* are surface positive and occur either unilaterally or bilaterally in central regions (Fig. 10.17). Their particular relation to periventricular white matter injury in the premature infant has been established (see Table 10.12 and Chapter 16).[187,200-209] The apparently superior value of frontal (positive) or occipital (negative) sharp waves regarding sensitivity for white matter injury is discussed earlier (see Table 10.12).[200]

Rhythmic Generalized or Focal Alpha Frequency Activity. This rare discharge may be generalized or focal and consists of periods of rhythmic 8- to 9-Hz activity that is generally synchronous (Fig. 10.18). The activity tends to predominate in the central or temporal regions (an alpha pattern that occurs with seizure is not synchronous). This pattern has been noted with chromosomal abnormalities and inborn errors of metabolism.[165]

Hypsarrhythmia. Although the classical hypsarrhythmic EEG with infantile myoclonic spasms does not usually occur until the second month of life or later, one variety may appear in the newborn (Fig. 10.19). *Hypsarrhythmia* is characterized by periods of marked voltage attenuation interrupted by bursts of asynchronous, high-voltage, slow activity mixed with multifocal spikes and sharp waves.[165] This pattern is differentiated from the burst-suppression pattern described earlier, particularly by the high voltage of the activity during the bursts; in hypsarrhythmia, voltage may reach 1000 μV, whereas in a typical burst-suppression pattern, the voltage of the bursts is usually less than 250 μV.[165]

Value of Serial EEG. The particular value of *serial* EEG in estimating outcome is pronounced.[187,190,204,210] A single EEG, particularly during the acute phase of the disease, may suggest a more ominous outcome than do subsequent EEG studies. The EEG evolves following injury,[211] and the rate of improvement of EEG may be a stronger predictor of outcome than a single EEG in infants with hypoxic-ischemic injury (see Chapter 20).[212,213] This point is illustrated well by the data recorded in Table 10.13, based on a study of 62 infants.[204]

Amplitude-Integrated Electroencephalogram
Methodology and Rationale

Amplitude-integrated EEG (aEEG) is an increasingly used method for the continuous monitoring of cerebral electrical activity in critically ill newborns.[214] It involves either a single-channel recording obtained from one pair of biparietal electrodes or a dual-channel recording from two pairs of electrodes, one pair for each hemisphere.[162,214-222] The EEG signal is band-pass filtered to attenuate activity lower than 2 Hz and higher than 15 Hz (to minimize artifacts).[214,223] The signal is rectified and further processed before being displayed on a modified semilogarithmic scale at a relatively compressed time scale. With many devices, it is possible to select areas of recording and display the corresponding, expanded *raw* EEG trace, which is useful for confirming possible seizure activity.

Among the particular values of this method is ease of application, which means that aEEG leads may be placed by trained personnel in the neonatal intensive care unit (NICU) without necessarily involving a specially trained EEG technologist. Other advantages include the ability to monitor continuously and the capacity to detect seizures, particularly on devices with seizure-detection software. Further, the information provided on background activity can be useful for determining the degree of encephalopathy, effects of drugs, and prognosis. One disadvantage is that the device does not cover the entire brain, thereby potentially missing some focal abnormalities.

Recording

aEEG recordings are evaluated especially for background and seizure activity.[214] The major background patterns identified are termed *continuous normal voltage, discontinuous normal voltage, burst suppression, continuous low voltage,* and *flat trace* (Fig. 10.20). As described later, the last three of these are ominous tracings. Discontinuous normal voltage is considered an intermediate tracing.

Seizure activity on aEEG is characterized in general as a *rapid* rise in both the lower and upper margins of the trace (Fig. 10.21).[214] The experience of the reader is important for detection (see later).

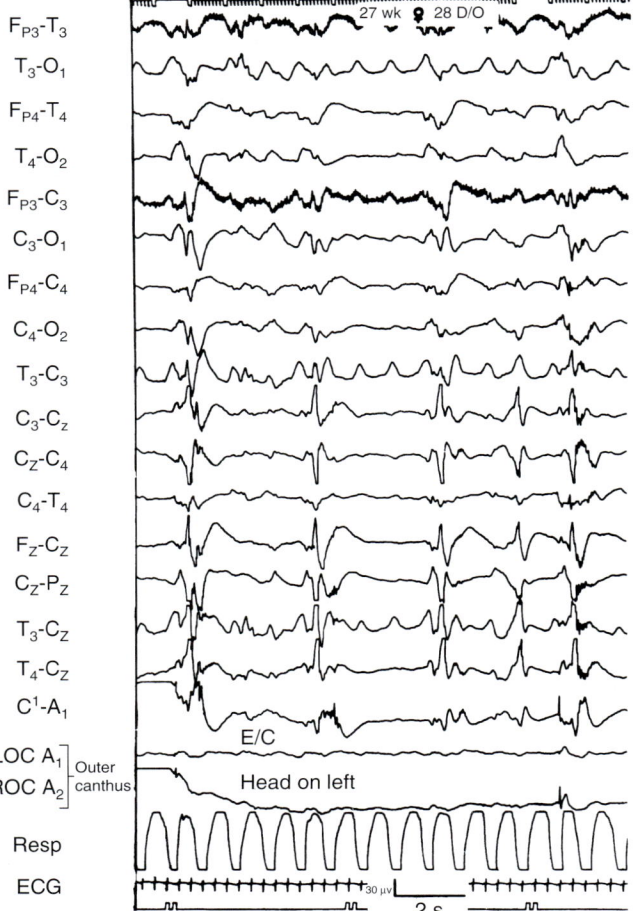

Figure 10.15 Electroencephalogram recording of a 27-week gestation, 28-day-old female infant with periodic lateralizing epileptiform discharges noted at the vertex region with a positive sharp wave morphology. This discharge was also noted with an additional electrode (C¹) referenced to the left ear. *E/C,* Eyes closed; *ECG,* electrocardiogram; *LOC,* left outer canthus; *ROC,* right outer canthus. (From Scher MS, Beggarly M. Clinical significance of focal periodic discharges in neonates. *J Child Neurol.* 1989;4:175–185.)

TABLE 10.13 Serial Electroencephalograms in Preterm Infants (<1200 g) in Relation to Outcome

	OUTCOME			
EEG	**NORMAL**	**SUSPECT**	**ABNORMAL**	**DEATH**
Normal, mildly abnormal, or only one EEG moderately abnormal	76%	13%	4%	7%
Moderately abnormal (≥2 EEGs) or any markedly abnormal	6%	6%	63%	25%

EEG, Electroencephalogram.

Data from Tharp BR, Scher MS, Clancy RR. Serial EEGs in normal and abnormal infants with birth weights less than 1200 grams: a prospective study with long term follow-up. *Neuropediatrics.* 1989;20:64–72; n = 62.

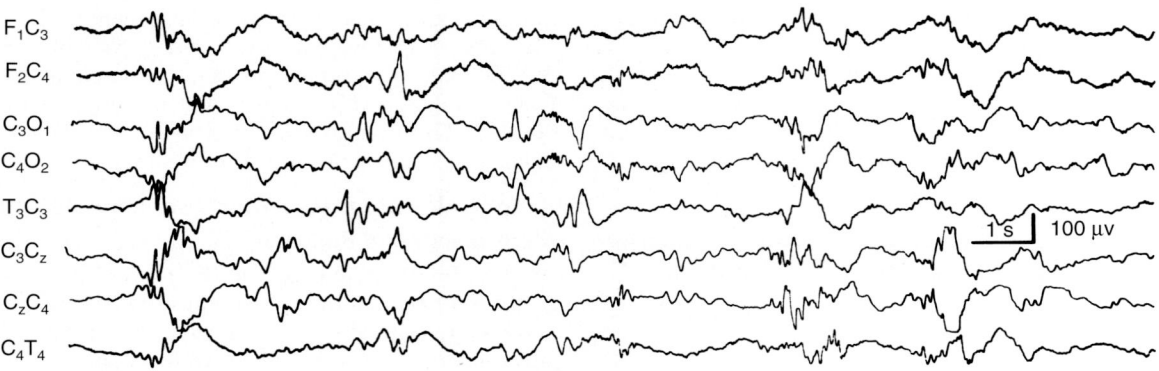

Figure 10.16 Multiple foci of abnormal, high-voltage sharp waves occurring during slow-wave sleep in a male term infant with congenital heart disease, perinatal hypoxia, and respiratory metabolic acidosis. Selected sample from a 16-channel recording. (From Hrachovy RA, Mizrahi EM, Kellaway P. Electroencephalography of the newborn. In Daly DD, Pedley TA, eds. *Current Practice of Clinical Electroencephalography.* 2nd ed. New York: Raven Press; 1990.)

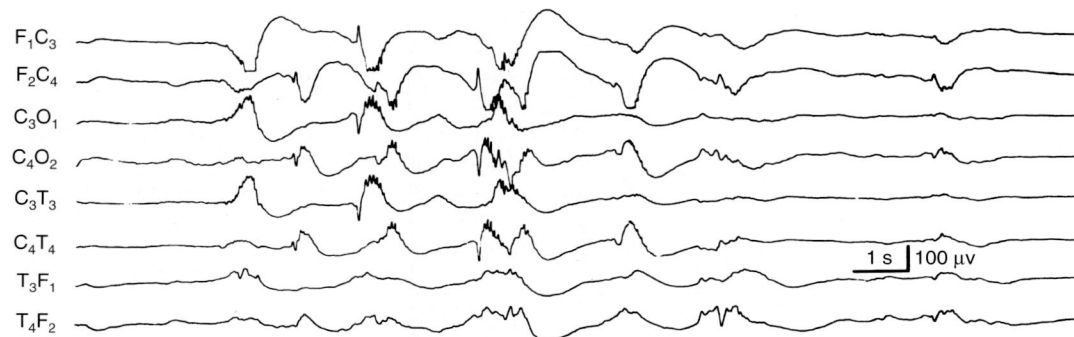

Figure 10.17 Central positive sharp waves in a male infant with an intraventricular hemorrhage; his postconceptional age is 29 to 30 weeks. Selected sample from a 16-channel recording. (From Hrachovy RA, Mizrahi EM, Kellaway P. Electroencephalography of the newborn. In Daly DD, Pedley TA, eds. *Current Practice of Clinical Electroencephalography.* 2nd ed. New York: Raven Press; 1990.)

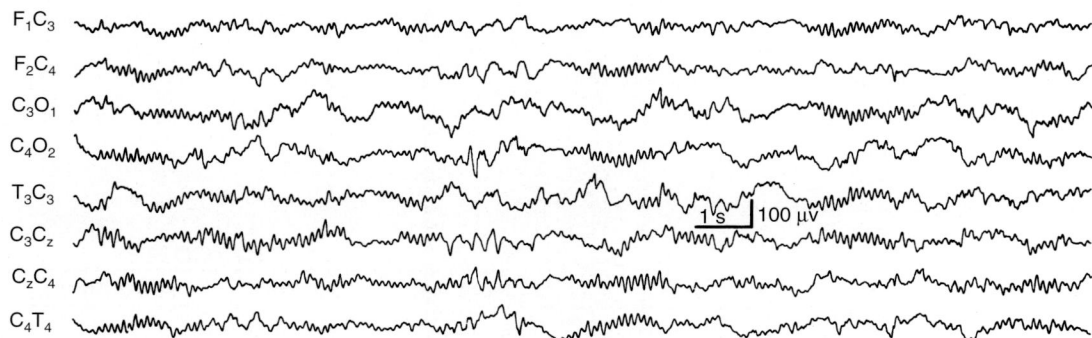

Figure 10.18 Runs of rhythmic 8- to 9-Hz activity occurring synchronously and independently in the left and right central regions in a male term infant with a chromosomal abnormality and multiple congenital anomalies. Such alpha frequency activity may also occur in a generalized fashion. Selected sample from a 16-channel recording. (From Hrachovy RA, Mizrahi EM, Kellaway P. Electroencephalography of the newborn. In Daly DD, Pedley TA, eds. *Current Practice of Clinical Electroencephalography.* 2nd ed. New York: Raven Press; 1990.)

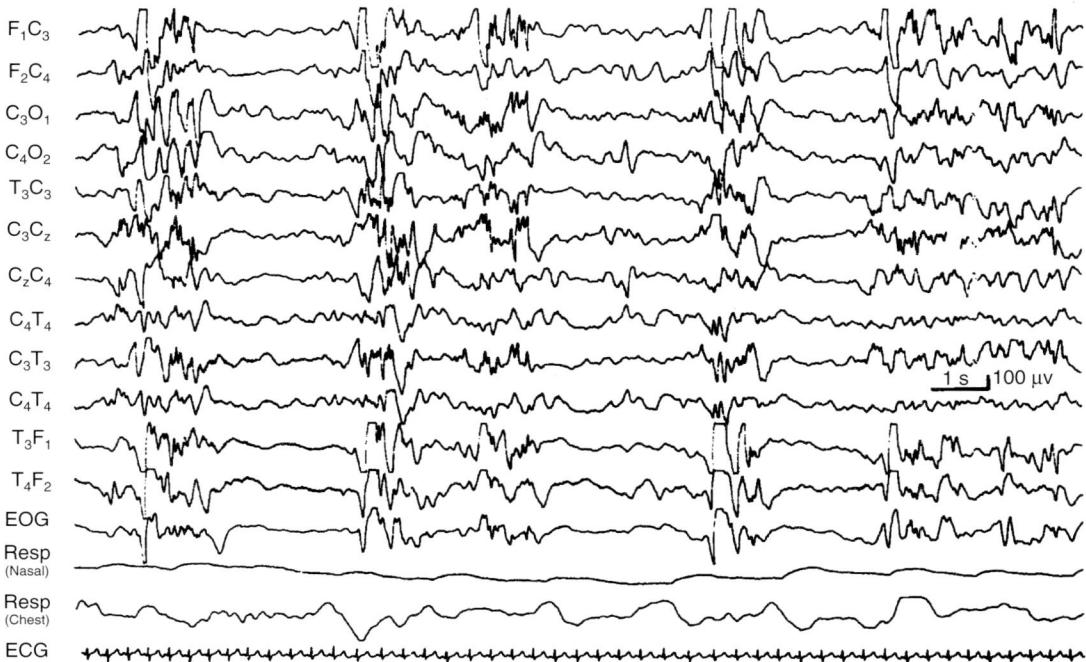

Figure 10.19 Suppression-burst variant of hypsarrhythmia in a 3-week-old male term infant with an inborn error of metabolism, type unknown. The infantile spasms in this patient were accompanied by generalized attenuation episodes in the electroencephalogram. *ECG,* Electrocardiogram; *EOG,* electro-oculogram. (From Hrachovy RA, Mizrahi EM, Kellaway P. Electroencephalography of the newborn. In Daly DD, Pedley TA, eds. *Current Practice of Clinical Electroencephalography.* 2nd ed. New York: Raven Press; 1990.)

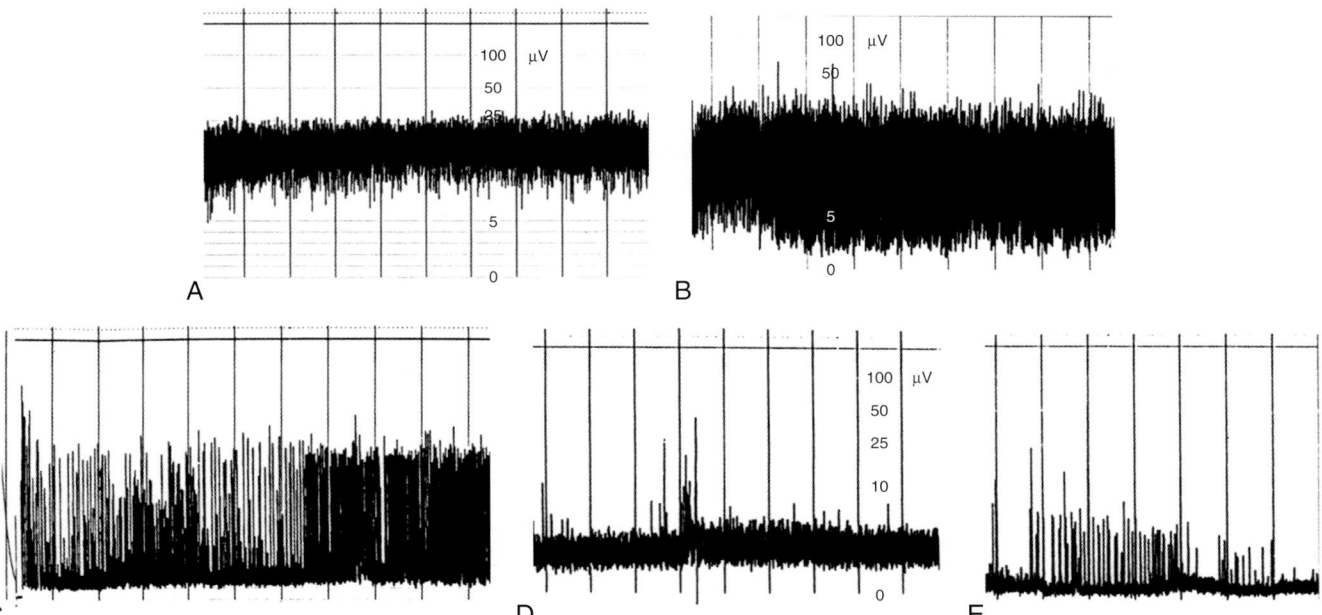

Figure 10.20 Amplitude-integrated electroencephalographic background patterns. Background patterns are (A) continuous normal voltage, (B) discontinuous normal voltage, (C) burst suppression, (D) continuous low voltage, and (E) flat trace. (From de Vries LS, Hellstrom-Westas L. Role of cerebral function monitoring in the newborn. *Arch Dis Child Fetal Neonatal Ed.* 2005;90:F201–F207.)

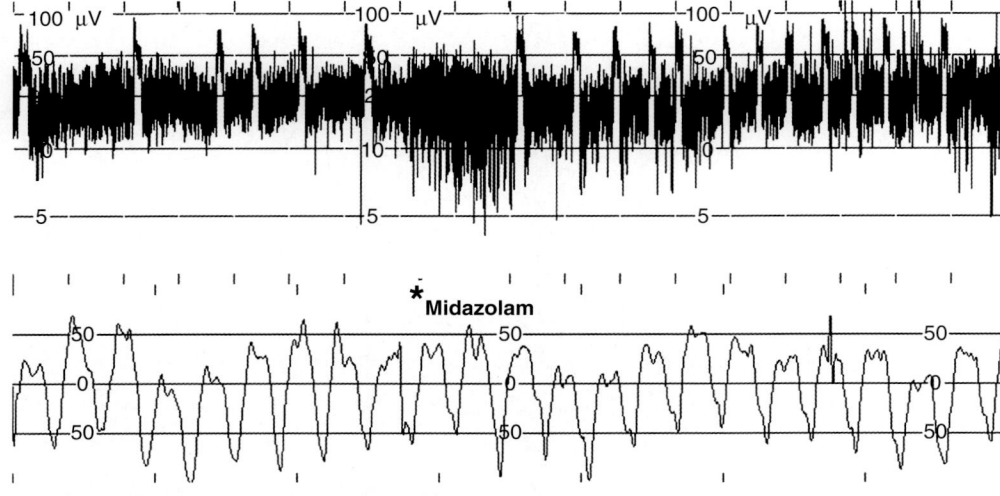

Figure 10.21 Amplitude-integrated electroencephalogram: seizure pattern. Note repetitive discharges on a continuous normal voltage background pattern (*upper trace*). Simultaneous electroencephalogram (*lower trace*), displayed at the asterisk, shows rhythmic epileptic discharges. Midazolam was administered as shown, with no effect on repetitive discharges. (From de Vries LS, Hellstrom-Westas L. Role of cerebral function monitoring in the newborn. *Arch Dis Child Fetal Neonatal Ed.* 2005;90:F201-F207.)

Clinical Applications

As noted earlier, the principal clinical applications of aEEG are assessment of *term infants shortly after perinatal asphyxia* and *detection of seizures*. The value of aEEG in the former instance appears well established, whereas the role in seizure detection requires further clarification.

Assessment of Asphyxiated Term Infants. aEEG has proven very useful in assessment of the asphyxiated term newborn.[214,224-227] A particular goal has been to identify, in the first hours after birth, the likely outcome of the asphyxiated infant. The aEEG *background tracings* have been most useful, particularly the burst-suppression, continuous low-voltage, and flat trace patterns. In one large study, the positive predictive value for unfavorable outcome for aEEG detection of severe abnormalities at 3 hours of life was 78%; at 6 hours, it was 86%.[228] The positive predictive value at 6 hours has been similar in other studies.[221,229] Notably, approximately 10% to 40% of infants with marked background abnormalities may normalize within 24 hours, and more than 50% of this minority group will have a favorable outcome.[225,226] Thus, monitoring the *course of aEEG changes* is useful,[213] although for identification of candidates for neuroprotective therapies, such as therapeutic hypothermia, early detection is crucial (see Chapter 20). Finally, and of additional importance, although aEEG in the first 6 hours was superior to neonatal neurological examination in identifying infants with an unfavorable short-term outcome, the *combination* of aEEG *and* the neurological examination was optimal, with a specificity of 94%.[224]

Detection of Seizures. The value of aEEG in *detection of seizures* has been assessed primarily in asphyxiated term infants.[214,222,230-233] aEEG was not designed as a seizure monitor, although some very experienced users of the method appear skilled at seizure detection. Nevertheless, in one comparative study of aEEG and standard EEG with experienced observers, of 10 infants with ictal activity on EEG, 8 were detected by aEEG, and notably of 16 infants with interictal "multifocal epileptiform activity," only 4 were identified by aEEG.[230] In addition, the experience of the observer is very important in aEEG detection of seizure activity. Thus, in one study involving four neonatologists with no prior experience with aEEG and trained for 3 to 5 hours in seizure detection on the aEEG tracing, only 38% of seizures were detected at the usual paper speed of 6 cm/h.[231] Moreover, focal, low-amplitude, or brief seizures are also readily missed by aEEG.[230,231,233] A more recent study comparing seizure detection by conventional EEG and two-channel aEEG with access to the raw EEG trace and using seizure-detection software showed better aEEG performance; the sensitivity, specificity, positive predictive value, and negative predictive value of aEEG were 75% to 80%.[234] Thus the use of modern equipment is imperative for seizure detection with aEEG.

Other Applications. In initial studies, aEEG has proven useful for a variety of other applications. Thus the method has been used for delineating the effects of anticonvulsant drugs (e.g., midazolam, phenobarbital),[235,236] evaluating sleep-wake cycling in asphyxiated infants,[237] predicting postneonatal epilepsy in asphyxiated infants,[238] defining maturational changes in preterm infants,[239-241] and predicting outcome in premature infants with large intraventricular hemorrhage.[242] Related methods, involving spectral analysis of the EEG and focused more on frequency than on amplitude, are in the developmental stage in the study of the premature infant.[243,244]

Structural Brain Imaging

The three major techniques for demonstrating normal and abnormal brain structure are ultrasonography, computed tomography (CT), and MRI. Ultrasound imaging is the most conveniently performed of these three procedures. CT was the first of the three methods to be used clinically but is now used sparingly, in considerable part because of the radiation exposure. MRI provides the greatest resolution and versatility, and advanced MRI techniques allow evaluation of microstructure and functional networks (see later). Cranial ultrasonography and CT are long-established techniques in the study of the newborn brain; they are noted only briefly here but are illustrated in most chapters of this book. I discuss MRI in more detail, including advanced MRI methods, because this modality has provided important insights into aspects of normal brain development.

Ultrasonography

Ultrasound scanning is one of several techniques that capitalize on the bone-free anterior fontanelle to provide a window into the neonatal brain.[245,246] In addition, use of the posterior fontanelle and of the mastoid fontanelle has markedly improved the value of ultrasonography in the evaluation of posterior fossa structures. The enormous value of the technique in the study of the neonatal brain has been documented in a vast number of original papers and reviews and in several books.[246-254] The specific uses of the technique are documented throughout this book, but it is important simply to emphasize here the value of ultrasound scanning in identification of such diverse intracranial processes as the following: developmental aberrations; hypoxic-ischemic injury; subdural, germinal matrix-intraventricular, and posterior fossa hemorrhage; ventriculitis; tumors; cysts; and vascular anomalies. The basic principles of the technique and the major normal anatomical features, reviewed in previous editions of this book, are summarized in standard writings.[246,255-259] The correspondence between ultrasound imaging planes and brain anatomy is shown in Fig. 10.22.

In addition to structural information, ultrasound also has the capacity to provide measurements related to blood flow. This ability results because the frequency of the ultrasound signal used for imaging undergoes a Doppler shift when it is reflected by a moving structure such as the cells in flowing blood. Thus Doppler ultrasonography has proven useful for evaluating the patency of both arteries and veins. This frequency shift is readily converted to units of velocity (m/s), but deriving a blood flow value (mL/min per g of tissue) from a velocity value is not straightforward, since factors such as the diameter of the vessel, laminar blood flow, and the angle of the ultrasound beam relative to the blood vessel must be taken into account. In practice, the measurement provided is typically the *resistance index (RI) of Pourcelot*,[260,261] given by the formula $RI = (S - D)/S$, where RI is the resistance index and S and D are the peak systolic and end-diastolic velocities of flow, respectively. Notably, RI is not affected by changes in the angle of probe placement. A related index is the so-called *pulsatility index of Gosling*, given by the formula $(S - D)/mean$ velocity. A typical tracing (Fig. 10.23) helps to illustrate these calculations. These measurements are typically taken from the anterior cerebral artery as it wraps around the genu of the corpus callosum or, less commonly, the middle cerebral artery as it turns in a superoinferior direction. These vessels are chosen because the beam from the ultrasound probe, positioned at the anterior fontanel, is parallel to the arteries at these points, providing more consistent measurements.

The average RI tends to decline with age from 0.77 (±0.15) in premature infants to 0.73 (±0.57) in term infants. Overall, an RI between 0.6 and 0.9 can be used as an approximate range to encompass normal values for both term and preterm infants.[262] RI decreases with increases in diastolic flow, such as following acute hypoxic ischemic injury.[263] RI increases with decreases in diastolic flow, such as when hydrocephalus causes an increase in intracranial pressure[264] or with patent ductus arteriosus.[265] It is important to note that in children with cardiac disease, particularly those with left-to-right shunts and extracardiac shunts, RI is unreliable and should not be used.[262]

Computed Tomography

CT scanning is an imaging technique based on the use of ionizing radiation, as in conventional radiography. It is not considered in detail here because it is now a standard radiological procedure and its value is illustrated throughout this book. Nevertheless, in the study of the newborn, a principal disadvantage is the requirement of transport of the infant to the CT scanner. More importantly, the use of ionizing radiation has potential (though not definitively proven) risks of cancer later in life[266-269] and/or neurological impairment.[270,271] Overall, MRI provides superior resolution and richer image contrast. CT is used when MRI is not available, especially in urgent situations.

Magnetic Resonance Imaging

MRI is a mainstay of clinical neuroimaging, and its value became clear over a decade ago.[272-275] Since that time, a rich variety of MRI methods has been developed and is finding its way into clinical practice (Table 10.14). In the following discussion, a brief description of the basic principles of the technique is provided, followed by a description of the various contrast types underlying each method.

In comparison with head ultrasound (HUS), MRI has the disadvantage that infants must be moved from the intensive care unit to the radiology department for study, although this requirement may eventually change as MRI systems suitable for sitting within the NICU are developed. Further, the infant is relatively inaccessible while in the MRI scanner, which becomes problematic in the event of a medical emergency. The major advantage of MRI relative to ultrasonography is that it provides unmatched structural detail and high sensitivity to parenchymal injury.[254,276,277] From an operational standpoint, the imaging of infants requires adaptations of the scanning process. For example, optimal signal-to-noise ratio, and hence better image quality, is achieved when the radiofrequency coil used is size-matched to the infant head, although it remains common practice to use a head coil designed for adult imaging for imaging infants, thereby using a coil that is larger than optimal. In addition, infants are less likely to hold still during the scanning process than are older patients. As a result, it is standard practice in some centers to sedate infants so as to minimize movement. However, a variety of approaches have been developed to mitigate subject motion.[278-286] Thus sedation for scanning should no longer be standard practice, although it may be necessary in some cases.

T1- and T2-Weighted Imaging

Myelination. T1- and T2-weighted images provide mainly structural information (see Table 10.14). Notably, these image types are very sensitive to myelination, with myelinated white matter appearing bright on T1-weighted images and dark on T2-weighted images compared with unmyelinated white matter. This finding provides an opportunity to use MRI to detect

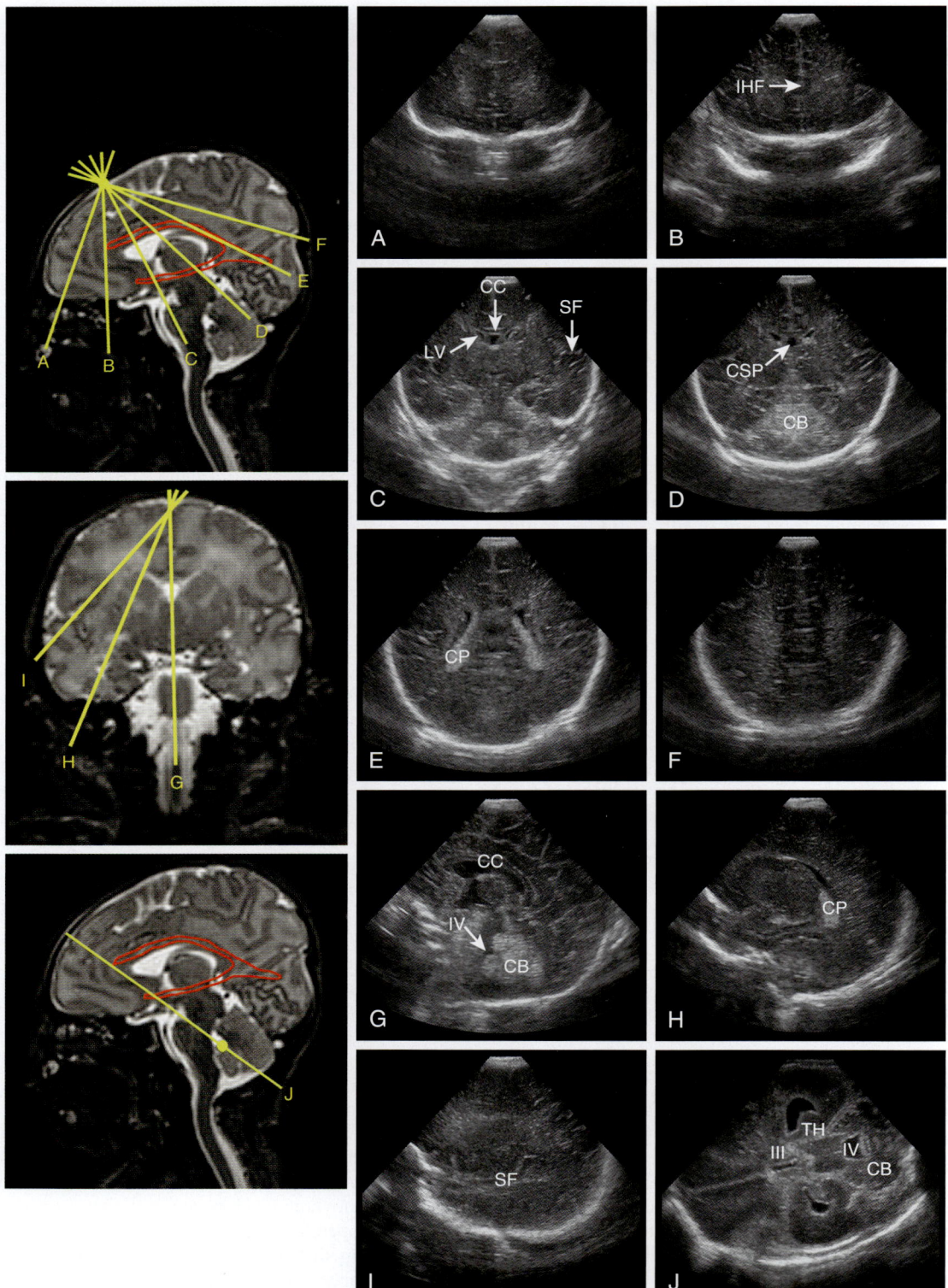

Figure 10.22 Cranial ultrasound images from a term infant. The panels in the left column show magnetic resonance imaging studies on which the outline of the lateral ventricles is drawn in red (note that this infant has mild ventriculomegaly) and the imaging planes are shown in yellow. The letters correspond to the panels in the middle and right columns, which show the matching cranial ultrasound studies. Note that panels (A to I) were obtained through the anterior fontanel. Panel (J) was obtained through the mastoid window. *III*, Third ventricle; *IV*, fourth ventricle; *CB*, cerebellum; *CC*, corpus callosum; *CP*, choroid plexus; *CSP*, cavum septum pellucidum; *IHF*, interhemispheric fissure; *LV*, lateral ventricle; *SF*, sylvian fissure; *TH*, temporal horn of the lateral ventricle.

TABLE 10.14 Magnetic Resonance Imaging Contrast Types

MAGNETIC RESONANCE IMAGING TYPE	CONTRAST MECHANISM	UTILITY
T_1-weighted imaging	Spin-lattice relaxation—sensitive to local chemical environment (CSF, unmyelinated white matter, myelinated white matter, gray matter)	Structural imaging, including gliosis, injury (>48 hours), clotted blood; volumetric measurements, cortical cartography, myelination
T_2-weighted imaging	Spin-spin relaxation—sensitive to local chemical environment	Structural imaging, including gliosis, injury (>48 hours), edema; volumetric measurements, cortical cartography, myelination
Diffusion imaging	Water displacement—can be used to measure water apparent diffusion coefficient and diffusion anisotropy	Acute and subacute injury (apparent diffusion coefficient), integrity of white matter (anisotropy), tractography (anisotropy)
Angiography	Moving *versus* nonmoving water	Stroke, vascular malformation, sinovenous thrombosis
T_2^*-weighted imaging	Magnetic susceptibility—sensitive to deoxyhemoglobin in veins and areas of hemorrhage	Hemorrhage is very conspicuous because of a *bloom* effect related to local magnetic field distortion
Spectroscopy	Signal from MR-detectable nuclei such as ^1H and ^{31}P	^1H spectroscopy can be used to measure lactate and *N*-acetylaspartate levels
Functional MRI	Magnetic susceptibility—sensitive to local changes in blood deoxyhemoglobin levels associated with neuronal activity	Task-based functional MRI is used for detecting areas of activation caused by activity; resting-state functional connectivity MRI is used to detect neural networks
Blood flow	Detection of water in flowing blood	Changes in cerebral blood flow associated with a variety of conditions such as stroke

CSF, Cerebrospinal fluid; *MRI,* magnetic resonance imaging.

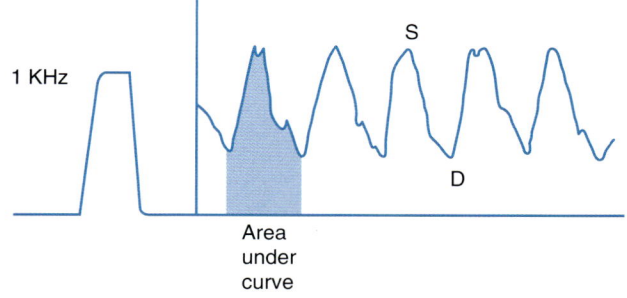

Figure 10.23 Cerebral blood flow velocity tracing obtained at the anterior fontanel from the anterior cerebral artery. The deflection of the electronic internal standard is indicated to the left of the start of the tracing. S refers to peak systolic velocity, D to end diastolic velocity, and the *shaded area* to the area under one velocity waveform. The values for S and D can be used to calculate the resistance index ([S − D]/S); see text for details.

TABLE 10.15 Milestones of Myelination as Shown by Magnetic Resonance Imaging[a]

Birth–1 month
Dorsal midbrain
Cerebellar peduncles
Posterior limb of internal capsule
Lateral thalamus
Paracentral gyri: subcortical white matter
2–4 months
Cerebellar white matter
Anterior limb of internal capsule
Splenium of corpus callosum
Optic radiation
4–6 months
Genu of corpus callosum
Occipital white matter: central
Occipital white matter: peripheral (beginning)
Frontal white matter: central (beginning)
6–9 months
Occipital white matter: peripheral
Frontal white matter: central
Frontal white matter: peripheral

[a]See text for references.

myelination, albeit qualitatively.[287] It also leads to the unusual circumstance in which gray-white image contrast is reversed in newborns compared with older children. As myelination proceeds (Table 10.15), white matter signal intensity gradually changes (Fig. 10.24).[288] Between the ages of 6 and 9 months, white and gray matter signal intensities are similar on both T1- and T2-weighted images, making it difficult to obtain good gray-white image contrast (see Fig. 10.24). Thus, while MRI may still be useful in patients at this age, it is not particularly sensitive for detecting subtle cortical malformations and heterotopias. By the age of 1 year, gray-white contrast is fully reversed and is similar to that of older children and adults.

Volumetry. A valuable use of MRI for the study of normal brain development is quantitative volumetric MRI. Using three-dimensional imaging and tissue segmentation techniques, striking changes in the growth of the brain and of major brain regions with development from 29 to 41 weeks of postmenstrual

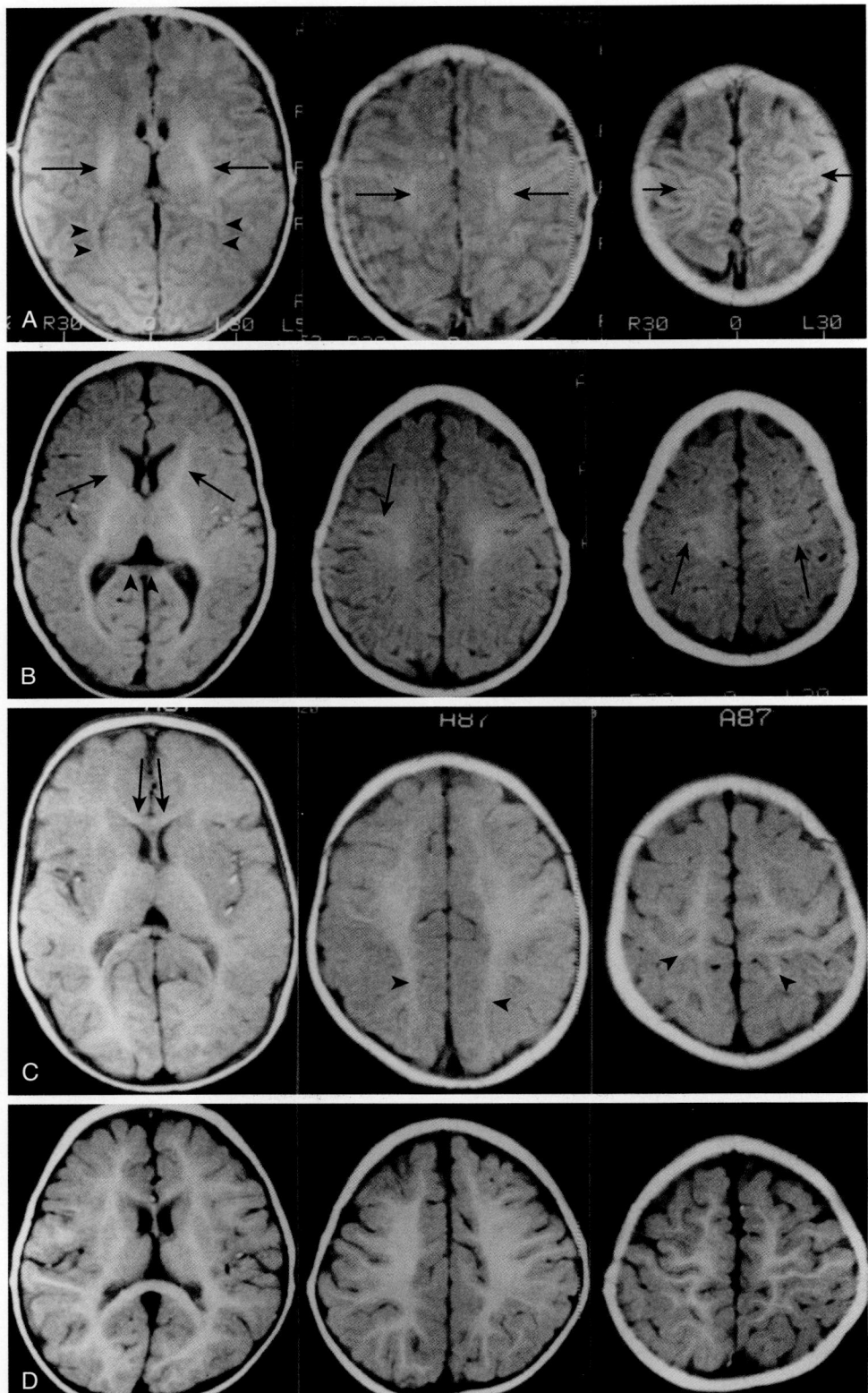

Figure 10.24 T1-weighted magnetic resonance images of brain in healthy **(A)**, 1-month-old **(B)**, 4-month-old **(C)**, 6-month-old, and **(D)**, 8-month-old **infants.** In (A), note increased signal intensity, consistent with myelin, in the posterior limb of the internal capsule *(arrows, left image)*, optic radiations *(arrowheads, left image)*, central corona radiata *(arrows, middle image)*, and paracentral gyri *(arrows, right image)*. In (B), note the addition of increased signal in the anterior limbs of the internal capsule *(arrows, left image)* and splenium of the corpus callosum *(arrowheads, left image)*, as well as intensification of the increased signal in the posterior limb of the internal capsule, optic radiations, and centrum semiovale, with the beginning of arborization of myelin in the paracentral regions *(arrows in middle and right images)*. In (C), note the further progression of myelination with high signal intensity not only in the splenium but also the genu of the corpus callosum *(arrows, left image)* and increased arborization of myelin not only in paracentral regions but also occipital areas *(arrowheads, middle and right images)*. In (D), marked progression of myelination is apparent, with nearly an adult appearance. Arborization of central white matter extends far into subcortical white matter except in the frontal poles. (From Barkovich AJ, Kjos BO, Jackson DE, Norman D. Normal maturation of the neonatal and infant brain: MR imaging at 1.5 T. *Radiology.* 1988;166:173–180.)

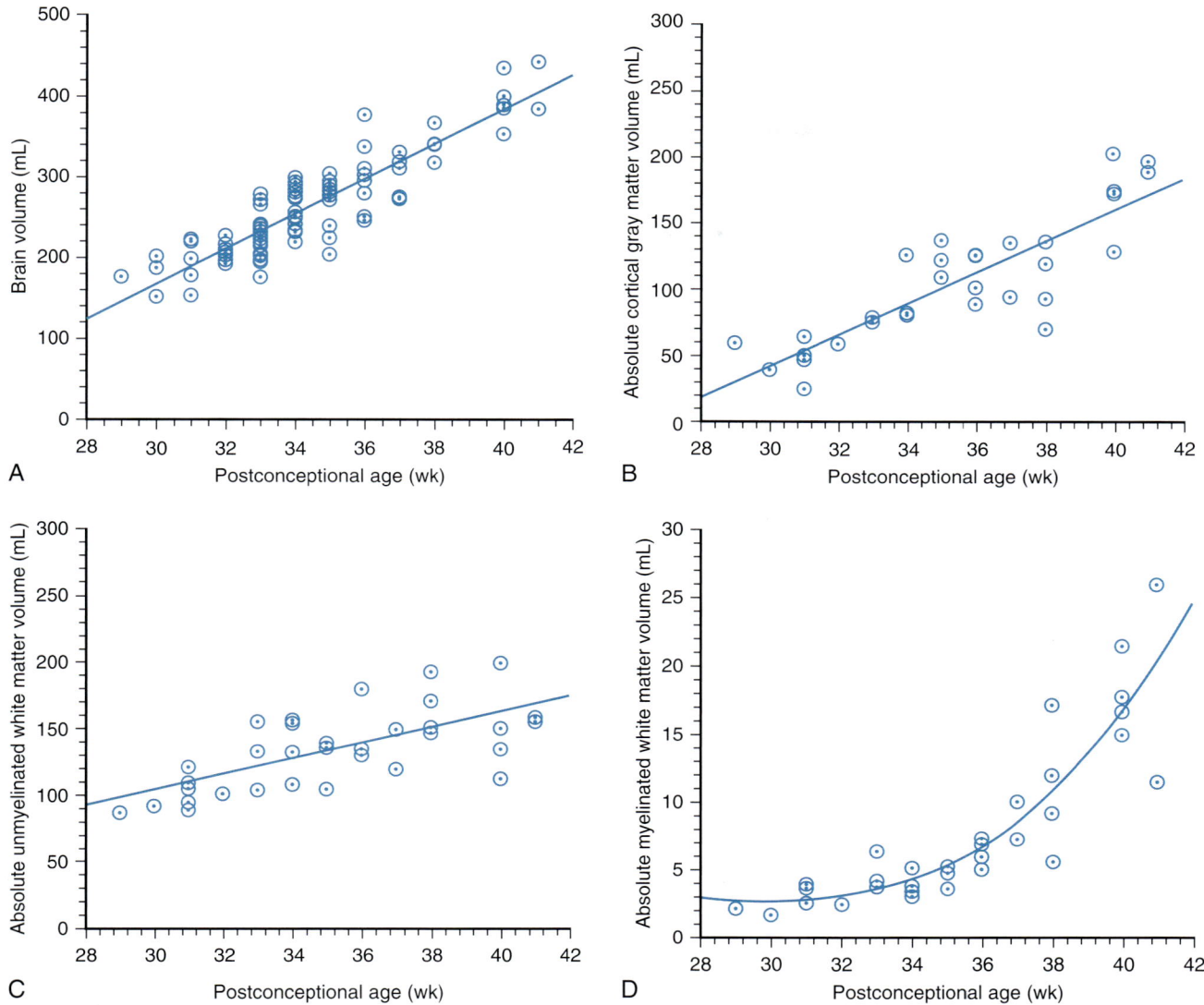

Figure 10.25 Quantitative three-dimensional volumetric magnetic resonance imaging determinations of (A) total brain volume, (B) cortical gray matter volume, (C) unmyelinated white matter volume, and (D) myelinated white matter volume as a function of postconceptional age in 35 premature and full-term infants. (From Huppi PS, Warfield S, Kikinis R, et al. Quantitative magnetic resonance imaging of brain development in premature and mature newborns. *Ann Neurol.* 1998;43:224–235.)

age can be demonstrated (Fig. 10.25).[289] The data show a nearly threefold increase in total brain volume, an approximately fourfold increase in cerebrocortical gray matter volume, an approximately 50% increase in unmyelinated white matter volume, and a dramatic fivefold increase in myelinated white matter volume. The increase in cortical gray matter volume occurs during the time period of rapid growth of cortical neuronal processes and exuberant influx of afferent fibers from subplate neurons and thalamus (see Chapter 7). The fastest increase in cerebral myelin volume occurs between 35 and 41 weeks of postconceptional age and is accompanied by prominent oligodendroglial differentiation (see Chapter 8) and the onset of cerebral myelination. Volumetric studies of children and adults who were born prematurely show decreased volumes of cerebral cortical gray matter and deep nuclear structures, especially thalamus and basal ganglia (see

Chapter 16).[290-298] Moreover, volumetric studies as early as term equivalent have shown decreased cerebral cortical and deep nuclear volumes,[289,299-304] which persist throughout life.[305-310] It is important to bear in mind that cerebral injury leads not only to volume loss but also to signal abnormalities in remaining tissue. Thus, although many MRI scoring systems focus on either volume loss or tissue signal abnormalities, it is preferable to employ a scoring system that takes both into account.[311]

Cartography. *Cartography* involves the analysis of the brain surface, similar to mapping of the earth's surface. The surface to be analyzed is created from T1- and/or T2-weighted images (Fig. 10.26). Once a surface has been generated, a number of summary parameters may be generated to capture features of the cerebral topography. One of the more common of them is *cortical surface area*, which increases dramatically during the immediate

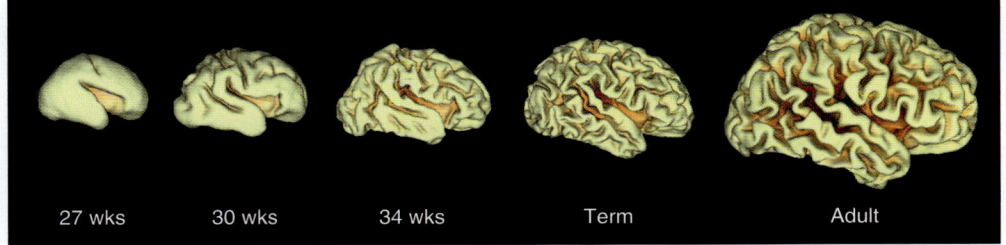

| 27 wks | 30 wks | 34 wks | Term | Adult |

Figure 10.26 Brain surfaces generated from the midcortical thickness of infant brains. Postmenstrual age is shown below each image. Images are shown to scale.

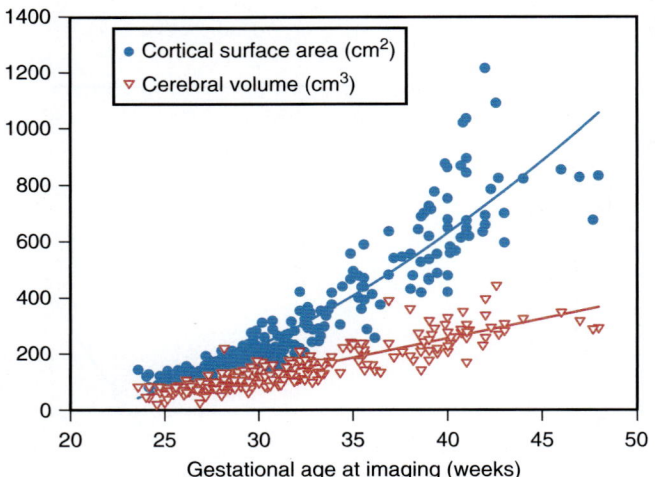

Figure 10.27 Cortical surface area and cerebral volume of preterm infants. A total of 113 preterm infants born between 23 and 30 weeks of gestation were studied by advanced magnetic resonance imaging (see text) to measure cortical surface area and cerebral volume over the period from birth to 48 postconceptional weeks. Note the striking increase in both surface area and volume over the last trimester and the first weeks of postnatal life. (From Kapellou O, Counsell SJ, Kennea NL, et al. Abnormal cortical development after premature birth shown by altered allometric scaling of brain growth. *PLoS Med.* 2006;3:e265.)

postnatal period in preterm infants (Fig. 10.27).[312] The cortex continues to expand between infancy and adulthood, although its areal expansion is nonuniform and bears resemblance to the pattern of human evolutionary expansion.[313] Cortical surface area is also affected by preterm birth and is reduced in preterm infants compared with control infants when evaluated at term-equivalent age (see Chapters 7 and 14).[314,315] A second parameter derived from cartography is the *gyrification index*. This index is a ratio of surface areas; the numerator is the cortical surface area and the denominator is the cerebral hull area, which can be imagined as the area of the surface of the brain as it would be if it were wrapped in cling wrap.[316] For a completely smooth, or lissencephalic, brain, the gyrification index would be 1. As the number and depth of cortical folds increase, the gyrification index increases. As would be expected, the gyrification index increases during normal brain development.[317] As for cortical surface area, the gyrification index is affected by preterm birth and is lower for preterm infants at term-equivalent age compared with control infants in a region-specific fashion (see Chapters 7 and 14).[315] Gyrification index values have also been related to neurodevelopmental outcome.[318] A third index derived

from cortical cartography is *sulcal depth*, which is the distance between the cerebral hull and the bottom of each sulcus.[316] As with the other parameters, sulcal depth increases with brain development.[317,319,320] Sulcal depth measurement has been used to map left-right asymmetries, such as the well-known asymmetry in language areas.[321] Abnormalities of sulcal depth have been described for preterm infants (see Chapters 7 and 14).[315] Finally, disturbances in regional *sulcal patterns* have also been found in preterm infants later in life, particularly of the cingulate sulcus.[322]

Sensitivity to Injury. In contrast to diffusion imaging, which shows injury almost immediately (see later), nonhemorrhagic brain parenchymal injury does not become apparent on T1- and T2-weighted imaging until approximately 48 hours after an ischemic event. Areas of injury then begin to appear hyperintense on T2-weighted images and hypo- or normointense on T1-weighted images.[323] In the case of cortical gray matter injury, the increase in intensity on T2-weighted images can cause the signal intensity of cortex to match that of adjacent white matter, leading to a loss of the *cortical ribbon* on T2-weighted images. From 6 to 10 days after injury, the hyperintensity on T2-weighted imaging evolves to hypointensity, and the injury becomes hyperintense on T1-weighted images.

Diffusion Imaging. The contrast in diffusion imaging is based on water displacements, and a wealth of information is encoded in these displacements. For example, they vary depending on the direction in which they are measured, a property known as *anisotropy*. In white matter, displacements are greater parallel to axons than perpendicular to them. This feature results because water moving parallel to axons can move between myelin layers, thereby not having to cross lipid membranes. Water moving perpendicular to axons must pass through myelin layers or go around them, thereby hindering their motion and reducing their displacements. When diffusion images are obtained, diffusion is measured several times, along different axes, for each slice. For each element, or voxel, in the image, these measurements can be combined to provide a spatial representation of water displacements. This representation can be expressed mathematically as a tensor; hence the name *diffusion tensor imaging*. Although these tensors can be shown as ellipsoids,[324] ellipsoid representations are cumbersome to use in clinical practice. As a result, summary parameters from these ellipsoids are usually shown (Fig. 10.28). The three most important of these parameters are the *apparent diffusion coefficient* (ADC), *diffusion anisotropy*, and the *direction along which water displacements are greatest*. ADC values are typically shown as

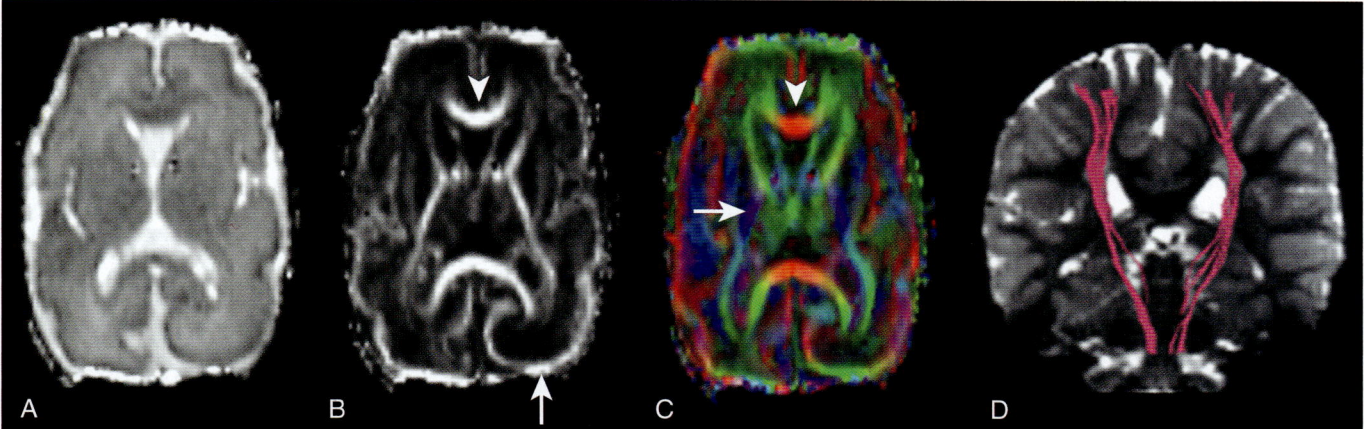

Figure 10.28 Diffusion magnetic resonance imaging data from preterm (panels A–C) and term (panel D) infants. Panel A shows a diffusion map in which image intensity corresponds to water diffusion coefficient. Panel B shows an anisotropy map in which image intensity corresponds to the degree of anisotropy. The arrow indicates an area of the developing cortical plate that has high anisotropy. Panel C is a color map showing the preferred direction of water displacements. Red = mediolateral, green = anteroposterior, blue = superoinferior. Note the mediolateral crossing fibers of the corpus callosum *(arrowhead)* and superoinferior corticospinal fibers of the posterior limb of the internal capsule *(arrow)*. Panel D shows diffusion tractography of the corticospinal tracts *(purple)* in a term infant.

quantitative ADC maps in which image intensity indicates *ADC values* (typically in units of 10^{-3} mm^2/s). In a clinical setting, ADC maps are often shown with inverted contrast, in which areas of low ADC appear bright rather than dark. This depiction is often referred to as the *diffusion-weighted image* as opposed to the *diffusion map* and offers the advantage that areas of low ADC (i.e., areas of subacute injury) appear bright and are thereby more conspicuous than on ADC maps. For diffusion anisotropy maps, areas of high anisotropy (i.e., areas having the greatest directional variation in ADC values) are brighter. Typically areas of white matter have the highest anisotropy, although, during early brain development, the cortical plate also has *high diffusion anisotropy*. The software of many MR scanners also produces a color map representing the *orientation* along which ADC values are highest. For white matter, this orientation is parallel to fiber tracts. In the example shown (see Fig. 10.28), blue represents a superoinferior orientation, red a mediolateral orientation, and green an anteroposterior orientation. Note that the superoinferior fibers of the corticospinal tract in the posterior limb of the internal capsule are blue, the mediolateral fibers of the corpus callosum are red, and the anteroposterior fibers of the anterior limb of the internal capsule are green. In the developing cortical plate, this orientation is *radial*, meaning orthogonal to the cortical surface. This orientation likely is a consequence of the presence of radial glia and the apical dendrites of pyramidal cells[325] and is largely lost by term-equivalent postmenstrual age because of a loss of anisotropy related to growth of dendrites from interneurons, the involution of radial gia, and the elaboration of basal dendrites from pyramidal cells.

Apparent Diffusion Coefficient. ADC values change during development, largely related to a gradual diminution in overall brain water content during development.[326,327] For the developing brain up to term-equivalent age and beyond, ADC values are also higher for white matter than gray matter, leading

to contrast between these two tissue types on ADC maps (see Fig. 10.28). Over time, myelination of white matter and a gradual decrease in brain water content lead to a reduction in ADC values (see Chapters 7 and 8). In adult brain, the values are virtually identical for white and gray matter.

In 1990, it was discovered that ADC values decrease within minutes of acute stroke.[328] Although this phenomenon was initially described for ischemic stroke, it is now known to occur in response to seizure,[329-332] spreading depression,[333-336] excitotoxic injury,[337,338] and trauma[339] as well. The mechanism(s) underlying this phenomenon are not yet fully understood, yet diffusion MRI has become a mainstay of clinical practice because of its unique ability to show injury early. As with virtually all forms of contrast, *the findings on diffusion imaging following injury evolve over time after occurrence of the injury* (see Chapter 20). Further, this evolution is somewhat different for newborns than for adults. For adults with stroke, diffusion abnormalities are present approximately 95% of the time during the acute phase of injury.[340] In infants, this value is closer to 70%. For the other 30%, the ADC values were likely low during the hypoxic-ischemic injury but returned to normal when blood flow and oxygenation were restored (i.e., the infant was delivered). In this case, there is a secondary decline in ADC that takes place over the ensuing 24 to 48 hours.[341] The implication of these findings is that diffusion imaging is most sensitive for detecting ischemic injury in infants between 2 and 4 days after the injury, and diffusion images obtained earlier may not show an injury because of the transient normalization of ADC values. However, earlier imaging is still warranted in infants with severe injury and for whom redirection of care is being considered, since diffusion abnormalities are likely to be present from the time of injury in these patients. From days 6 to 8 after injury, ADC values again change, gradually returning to normal in all infants. Consequently the injury becomes progressively less conspicuous on diffusion imaging in a process known as *pseudonormalization*.[341-344] Wallerian degeneration (degeneration of axons following injury to their associated cell bodies) is an exception to this time course. In this case, the reduction in ADC may emerge more slowly and persist for up to a week after injury.[345,346] The latter time course is most often seen in the corticospinal tracts, optic radiations, and transcallosal tracts. Following pseudonormalization, ADC values often continue to rise and may be higher than normal thereafter. As discussed in Chapter 20, the evolution of ADC values following injury is somewhat slowed by therapeutic hypothermia.

Diffusion Tractography. Tractography is a method that delineates white matter fiber tracts. This involves identifying the orientation along which ADC values are highest for each white matter voxel, which is parallel to the axons in that voxel. Using a white matter seed region as a starting point, this orientation is then used to point the way from one voxel to the next, making it possible to follow tracts from one brain region to another (see Fig. 10.28D). At present, this measure has found little clinical use in neonatology, though it is useful for identifying tracts to be spared in neurosurgical procedures.[347,348] The approach has found use in research studies of infants to define regions of interest for analysis, such as tract-based spatial statistics (TBSS).[349] TBSS involves the alignment of anisotropy maps to a standard-space template followed by projection of individual data onto a representation of major white matter tracts. Analysis is then performed to identify areas where anisotropy values correlate with a parameter of interest, such as neurodevelopmental outcome. For example, using the TBSS approach in a study of preterm infants with follow-up at 2 years, cognitive scores have been correlated with anisotropy values in the corpus callosum, and fine-motor scores were correlated with anisotropy throughout the white matter.[350]

MR Angiography. MR angiography is commonplace in the evaluation of newborns. It is useful for assessing vascular occlusion in perinatal arterial stroke (MR arteriography, Chapter 21)[351] and for detecting sinovenous thrombosis (MR venography, Chapter 21).[352] In patients with suspected venous sinus thrombosis, MR venography should be included as part of the evaluation, and follow-up venography is useful for evaluating the efficacy of therapeutic interventions such as treatment with low-molecular-weight heparin.

Susceptibility-Weighted Imaging. Another form of contrast available in MR images is based on local magnetic susceptibility, sometimes known as T2*-weighted images. These images are extremely sensitive to hemorrhage, which appear as dark areas. Because magnetic field distortions due to susceptibility effects extend beyond the hemorrhage itself, a phenomenon known as the *bloom effect,* small hemorrhages appear as relatively large areas of signal dropout on susceptibility-weighted images, making them very apparent.

Fetal Imaging. Fetal imaging presents a unique set of technical challenges related to movement of the fetus within amniotic fluid and the *filling factor* of the radiofrequency coil used, which must be large enough to include the abdomen of the mother. For technical reasons, typically only T1- and T2-weighted images are obtained, though it will likely be feasible to obtain other image types, particularly diffusion images, in the future. Fetal imaging is done for a variety of indications, such as abnormalities detected on routine fetal ultrasound (often ventriculomegaly), monochorionic twin gestation, maternal infection or major cardiac event, and family history of brain malformation. It is also useful for detecting extracranial anomalies, which may help identify genetic syndromes that have prognostic ramifications.[353]

In cases of ventriculomegaly detected on fetal ultrasound, fetal MRI is effective in identifying associated brain abnormalities that strongly influence prognosis (see Chapter 2). In children with isolated ventriculomegaly, there is a 37% incidence of developmental delay, compared with 84% in children with additional abnormalities.[354] In this population, fetal MRI detects additional CNS abnormalities in 40% to 50% of cases,[355,356] thereby providing important prognostic information. Further, fetal MRI is sensitive on the order of 70% to 100% and specific on the order of 90% to 100% for abnormalities such as cortical brain malformations, posterior fossa anomalies, corpus callosum anomalies, and Chiari malformations/neural tube defects (see Chapters 2 and 31).[357] Other brain abnormalities detectable by fetal MRI are agenesis of the corpus callosum, posterior fossa abnormalities such as Dandy-Walker malformations, and myelomeningocele (see Chapters 2 and 31).[358,359] It is important to obtain postnatal MRI studies on all subjects who have abnormalities on fetal MRI. In part this is because it is possible to obtain images with higher signal-to-noise ratios (and typically better spatial resolution) postnatally. In addition, abnormalities of cortical folding may not be present on early fetal imaging because cortical folding is not yet complete.

MR Spectroscopy. Conventional MRI relies on the detection of the signal from protons (^1H) in water (^1H_2O). The concentration of water ^1H in brain is on the order of 100 M. MR spectroscopy involves the detection of ^1H in brain metabolites, such as lactate, which are present in concentrations on the order of 10 mM. This factor of 10^4 difference in concentration makes MR spectroscopy more challenging than conventional imaging. For example, it is not feasible to obtain a high-resolution image of brain lactate concentration. Instead, an MR spectrum is obtained from a single region of interest (single-voxel spectroscopy), or a grid of spectra is obtained from a thick slice of brain (often known as chemical shift imaging). Through spectral editing, it is possible to obtain MR spectra in such a way as to emphasize the signal from metabolites of interest. However, for typical ^1H spectroscopy in clinical use, the resonance peaks visible are primarily choline, creatine (both creatine and phosphocreatine as a single resonance), N-acetyl-containing compounds (NAA), and lactate (Fig. 10.29). The reasons that these resonances are more conspicuous than others are related to their chemistry and the fact that these metabolites are present in relatively higher concentrations. Choline serves as a component of membranes and is also a constituent of the neurotransmitter acetylcholine. Creatine, when phosphorylated, stores energy in the form of phosphate bonds. (Phosphocreatine levels reflect the cellular energy state, but its detection requires ^{31}P spectroscopy, as creatine and phosphocreatine are indistinguishable using ^1H spectroscopy.) The precise role of NAA in brain metabolism is unclear. It is widely believed that NAA is found primarily in neurons and not glia, but it is probably synthesized in neurons and transported to oligodendrocytes as an acetate source for myelin lipid syntheses (see Chapter 29). Nevertheless, a reduction in NAA level is often taken to reflect a reduction in the number

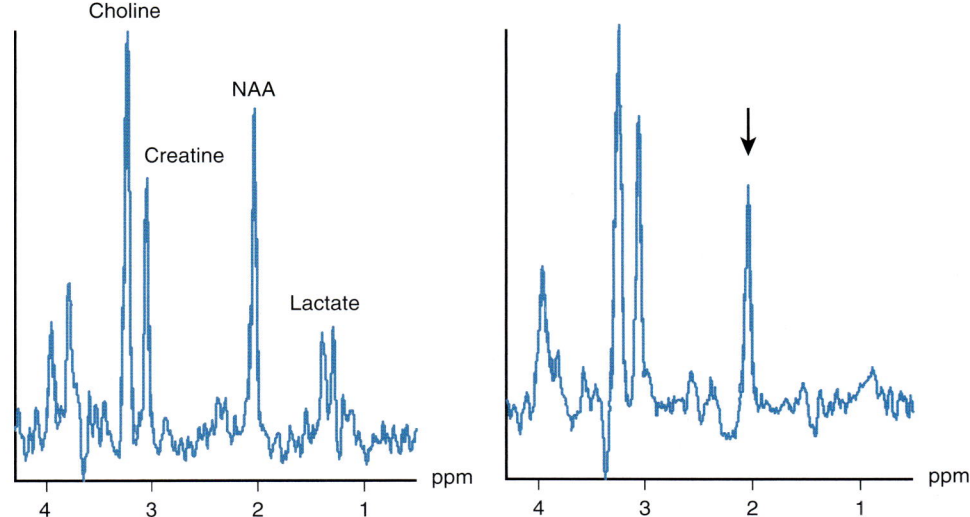

Figure 10.29 ¹H magnetic resonance spectra obtained from a human brain at 3.0 tesla. The spectrum on the left shows a relatively large lactate doublet in an asphyxiated term infant. The spectrum on the right, obtained 9 days later, shows resolution of the lactate doublet and a reduction in the NAA resonance *(arrow)* relative to the choline and creatine resonances due to neuronal loss. *NAA*, N-acetyl aspartate.

of neurons present in a given region, although changes in NAA levels may have multifactorial causes. Lactate is an intermediary of energy metabolism; its levels may be increased under a variety of circumstances, including lack of oxygen and anaerobic glycolysis. Lactate levels may also be increased by the presence of inflammatory cells, which often use anaerobic glycolysis. Note that the ¹H signal from the methyl group of lactate is a doublet (a pair of twin peaks) owing to scalar coupling. In theory, it is possible to quantify metabolite levels (in millimoles [mM]) by comparing resonance amplitudes with the water amplitude in the same brain region. This quantitation is rarely accomplished in clinical practice, though resonance amplitudes are sometimes expressed as ratios. For example, the NAA/choline or NAA/creatine ratio may provide an estimate of the fraction of cells in a given area that are neurons. Finally, nuclei in addition to ¹H are detectable by MR spectroscopy. They include phosphorous (^{31}P), sodium (^{23}Na), an isotope of carbon (^{13}C), and even the other two isotopes of hydrogen (^{2}H and ^{3}H, with ^{3}H being radioactive tritium). Although their detection is certainly of scientific/research interest, particularly detection of hyperpolarized ^{13}C for noninvasive assessment of metabolism, these topics are not covered here because these approaches have not yet found their way into clinical practice.

Studies of ¹H spectroscopy in asphyxiated infants have shown poorer neurodevelopmental outcomes for infants with high lactate and low NAA resonance amplitudes (see Chapter 20).[360] Further, ¹H spectroscopy can be useful for identifying metabolic disorders such as creatine transporter deficiency,[361] Canavan disease,[362] and disorders of energy metabolism (see Chapter 29).[363]

Functional MRI. Functional MRI refers to a form of MRI in which image contrast is based on local neural activity. Neural activation is associated with an increase in local cerebral blood flow with little or no change in local oxyhemoglobin utilization. As a result, neural activation is marked by an increase in local

blood oxygenation levels and a corresponding decrease in local deoxyhemoglobin levels. Deoxyhemoglobin contains reduced iron (Fe^{2+}), which is paramagnetic and affects the local magnetic field. The reduction in local Fe^{2+} associated with neural activation can be detected using a variant of T2*-weighted imaging (see earlier) known as blood oxygenation level–dependent, or BOLD, imaging. In this application, local signal intensity increases in areas of activation because of the reduction in local Fe^{2+} levels. *Task-based functional MRI* involves the observation of areas of activation that appear when the subject carries out a task such as moving a limb. This approach is not particularly useful for infants who, not unexpectedly, are uncooperative at performing tasks, though sleeping or sedated infants do show an activation response to auditory[364] and somatosensory[365,366] stimulation. There is a second form of functional MRI known as *resting-state functional connectivity MRI* (rs-fcMRI). This method is dependent on measuring slow, spontaneous changes in BOLD signal in resting subjects. These fluctuations are physiological, likely representing gradual, spontaneous physiological changes in local neuronal firing rates.[367] As spontaneous activity increases or decreases in one area, areas to which it has excitatory projections have similar changes. (Conversely, areas to which the projection is inhibitory have opposite BOLD signal fluctuations.) Thus areas of cortex that are connected have correlated (or anticorrelated) fluctuations in BOLD signal. Identifying areas for which spontaneous BOLD signal fluctuations are correlated can be used to identify brain networks.[367] This approach is effective even for subjects who are asleep or under anesthesia, though the state of the subject does affect rs-fcMRI data.[368] rs-fcMRI can therefore be applied to infants and used to show the emergence of neural networks (Fig. 10.30). Although rs-fcMRI data from preterm infants have not yet been associated with outcomes, there are methods under development in which these networks can be assessed as a group to provide an indication of the degree of brain maturity (see Chapter 7).[369]

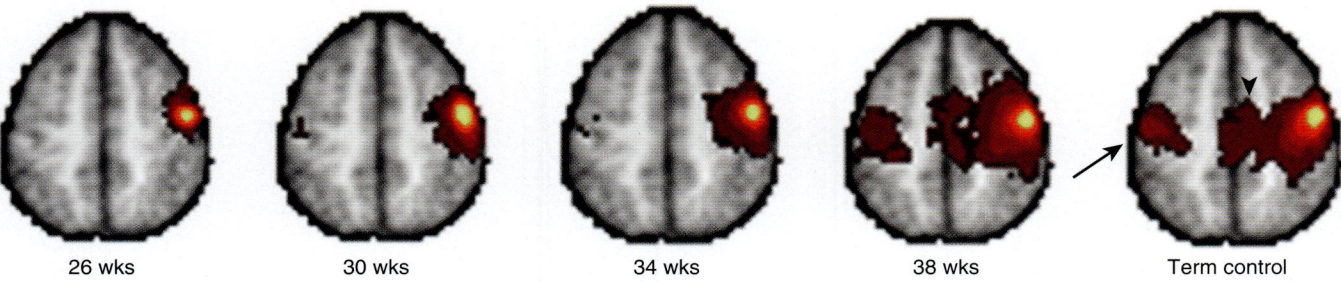

|26 wks|30 wks|34 wks|38 wks|Term control|

Figure 10.30 Resting-state functional connectivity magnetic resonance imaging data from infants at varying postmenstrual ages. The seed region was placed in motor cortex (yellow area in the leftmost panel). Note the emergence of the motor network at 38 weeks' postmenstrual age, including contralateral motor cortex *(arrow)* and supplementary motor cortex *(arrowhead)*.

Near-Infrared Spectroscopy

Near-infrared spectroscopy (NIRS) is an optical technique of potential value in the study of the newborn because the method is capable of noninvasively providing crucial information concerning cerebral hemoglobin oxygen saturation, cerebral blood volume, and cerebral oxygen delivery/metabolism. The method measures a tissue oxygenation index in real time and is most commonly applied to investigate cerebral and renal tissue oxygenation. Although the method has shown great value as a research tool, it is not entrenched as the standard of care in clinical practice. This has been attributed to a variety of causes, including the lack of consensus on calibration standards to improve the validity of the measurements.[370] With the equipment currently available commercially, NIRS is confined to evaluating trends rather than providing quantitative values.[371] As noted in the following, methods currently under development may enable quantitative measures, thereby improving the clinical utility of NIRS.

Basic Principles and Determinations

Applications of NIRS-based techniques to the neonatal population are based on two bio-optical principles.[372-376] First, light in the near-infrared range can easily pass through the thin skin, bone, and other tissues of the infant without significant attenuation of the signal. Second, differential absorption of varying near-infrared wavelengths by oxygenated hemoglobin (HbO_2) and deoxygenated hemoglobin (Hb) allows quantification of changes in HbO_2 and Hb concentrations within the tissue of interest (e.g., brain tissues), based on the modified Beer–Lambert law (Fig. 10.31 and Table 10.16). The method is analogous to the pulse oximetry that is commonly used in clinical practice to monitor arterial oxygen saturation. Both pulse oximetry and NIRS use similar wavelengths of light. For pulse oximetry, the signal is processed to isolate the signal from arterial blood to measure arterial oxygen saturation. Localization is not particularly crucial in this case and is achieved by passing the light through a digit using a pair of optodes. Commercially available NIRS devices work very similarly to pulse oximetry. Since the signal is not usually processed to evaluate arterial blood, NIRS typically provides a relative measure of mixed venous tissue oxygenation. For research applications such as functional activation, localization is a more important consideration and is challenging because of light scatter. When optodes are placed on both sides of the

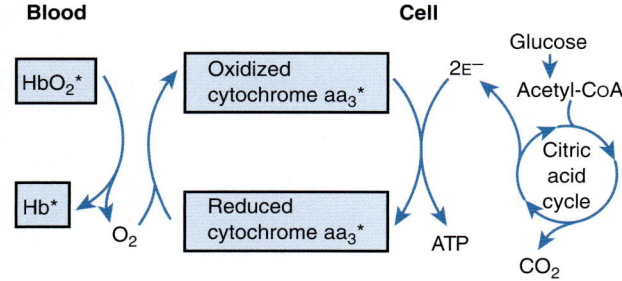

* = Measured by near infrared spectroscopy

Figure 10.31 Schematic of cerebral oxygen delivery by hemoglobin and intracellular oxygen utilization. See text for details. The asterisk denotes values measured by near-infrared spectroscopy. *ATP,* Adenosine triphosphate; *CoA,* coenzyme A; *Hb,* hemoglobin; *HbO₂,* oxygenated hemoglobin.

TABLE 10.16   Near-Infrared Spectroscopy

Principle

By appropriate selection of near-infrared wavelengths, can detect changes in absorbance of HbO_2, Hb, and the oxidation-reduction state of cytochrome aa_3

Determinations

Continuous measurements

Oxygen available in cerebral blood: by measuring HbO_2

Cerebral blood volume: by measuring sum of Hb and HbO_2

Cerebral perfusion: by measuring HbD (see text)

Intracellular oxygen availability or utilization: by measuring relative oxidation-reduction state of cytochrome aa_3

Serial measurements

Cerebral blood flow: by measuring *wash-in* of HbO_2 after brief administration of oxygen

Cerebral venous oxygen saturation: by measuring the change in Hb and HbO_2 after tilting the infant head down

Cerebral function: by measuring the change in Hb and HbO_2 after stimulation

---

Hb, Deoxygenated hemoglobin; *HbD,* difference between oxygenated and deoxygenated hemoglobin (HbD = HbO_2 − Hb); *HbO₂,* oxygenated hemoglobin.

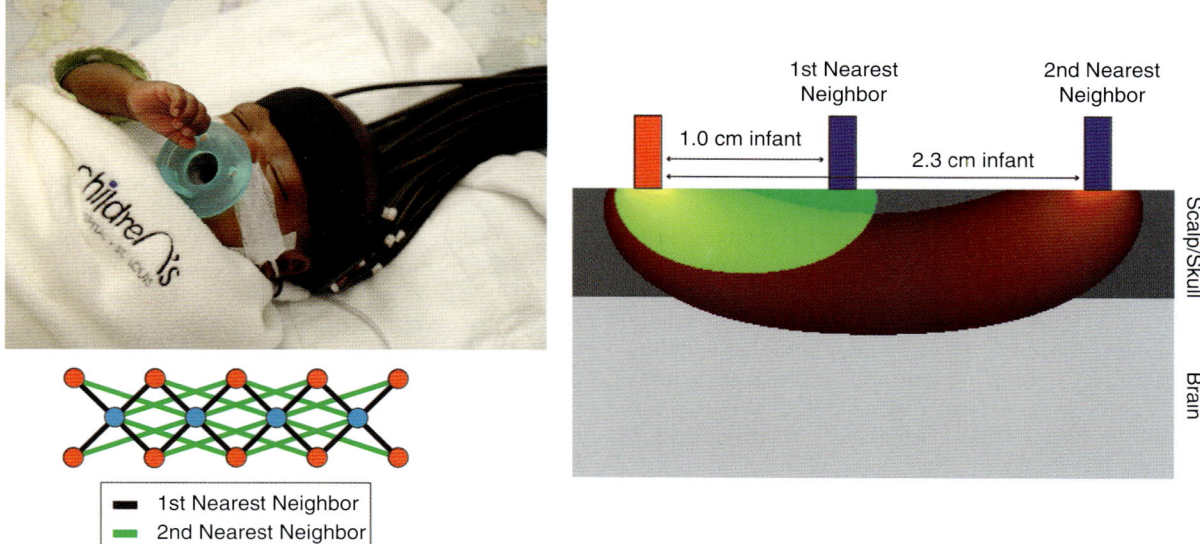

Figure 10.32 Near-infrared spectroscopy. The panel on the upper left shows an infant wearing an optode array. The panel on the lower left shows the optode layout. The panel on the right shows the sensitive volumes for optodes on the grid. The signal shown in green can be subtracted from that in red to reduce contamination from skull and scalp (see text for details). (Courtesy Steve Liao.)

head, the path length of the light that travels between them, due to scatter, is on the order of 5 times the physical distance between them.[377] One means of signal localization involves applying tomographic analysis with a grid of optodes to the scalp (Fig. 10.32) and processing the data to isolate signal from individual optodes.[378,379] It is also possible to improve localization by obtaining a head MRI from which tissue types and configuration can be identified and included in the model for signal analysis.[380,381]

There are also *different forms of NIRS*. The most commonly used and commercially available is *continuous-wave NIRS*. Although this approach provides information on Hb and HbO$_2$, the levels are relative rather than quantitative. Thus data obtained using this form of NIRS would provide information on trends rather than quantitative values. Adaptations, including *frequency-domain*[382,383] and *time-resolved*[384,385] NIRS, in comparison, provide quantitative measures of Hb and HbO$_2$ but require specialized equipment that is not yet routinely available.

The most commonly used parameters available from NIRS are shown in Table 10.17. In addition to these parameters, efforts have been made to measure cerebral blood flow with NIRS. In one approach, an abrupt increase in the inspired O$_2$ concentration was produced and the wash-in of HbO$_2$ was measured as a blood flow tracer, with the arterial input function assessed by conventional pulse oximetry.[386] Unfortunately the signal-to-noise ratio of NIRS data is low and blood oxygen levels are not particularly constant, making accurate measurements challenging. A more fruitful approach has been the use of diffusion correlation spectroscopy, which is based on the optical phase shift caused by the movement of red blood cells in tissue.[387] As with the Doppler flow measurements described earlier, calculating blood flow (mL/min × 100 g tissue) from the optical phase shift requires assumptions about vascular geometry and flow velocities that are difficult to validate. The blood flow parameter calculated is sometimes referred to as a *blood flow index* in recognition of this difficulty. Although an

TABLE 10.17	Parameters Typically Available With Near-Infrared Spectroscopy
PARAMETER	**CALCULATION**
Deoxyhemoglobin (Hb)	Measured directly
Oxyhemoglobin (HbO$_2$)	Measured directly
Total hemoglobin (tHb)	Hb + HbO$_2$
Cerebral blood volume (CBV)	tHb × (molecular weight of Hb/ blood hemoglobin concentration) × (1/brain tissue density)
Cerebral oxygen saturation (ScO$_2$)	HbO$_2$/tHB
Fractional cerebral tissue oxygen extraction	(SaO$_2$ − ScO$_2$)/SaO$_2$ where SaO$_2$ is the arterial oxygen saturation measured by pulse oximetry[a]

[a]Note that ScO$_2$ is weighted toward values from venous blood, which makes up the majority of brain blood. Thus, SaO$_2$ − ScO$_2$ approximates the arteriovenous O$_2$ saturation difference.

CBV, Cerebral blood volume; *Hb*, deoxyhemoglobin; *HbO$_2$*, oxyhemoglobin; *ScO$_2$*, cerebral oxygen saturation; *tHb*, total hemoglobin.

indication of blood flow is valuable in itself, if both cerebral blood flow and oxygen extraction fraction are determined with NIRS, it is possible to obtain an indicator of the cerebral metabolic rate of oxygen consumption.[388,389] Attempts have also been made to measure oxidation-reduction state via NIRS using the absorption of light by oxygenated and deoxygenated cytochrome aa$_3$. Unfortunately the vast majority of infrared light absorbed by the brain is absorbed by hemoglobin, with well under 1% absorbed by cytochrome aa$_3$. This dynamic range problem has hampered efforts to make useful measurements without eliminating the effects of hemoglobin, such as by replacing blood with a perfluorocarbon.[390]

Clinical Application

Application to human infants has provided insights into the value of the NIRS in the assessment of cerebral physiology and metabolism in vivo and into potential mechanisms of brain injury in specific clinical situations. These insights are described briefly next.

Quantitative Determinations of Oxygenated Hemoglobin, Deoxygenated Hemoglobin, and Cerebral Blood Volume in the Newborn.

A large series of studies, particularly by the research group at University College in London, initially provided major insight both into the potential value of NIRS in the study of the newborn brain and into the regulation of cerebral hemodynamics and oxygen delivery. Using the principles and background data described earlier, the British group obtained crucial quantitative data. In an initial report, Wyatt and co-workers[391] showed that cerebral HbO_2 decreases with a modest decrease in arterial oxygen saturation and cerebral blood volume increases, presumably as a result of cerebral vasodilation, with an increase in arterial partial pressure of carbon dioxide ($Paco_2$).

Wyatt and co-workers[392,393] described the use of NIRS to *quantitate cerebral blood volume* and obtained a mean value in premature infants of 2.22 mL/100 g, comparing favorably with the values (2.5 mL/100 g) obtained previously by positron emission tomography (PET).[393] Similar values were obtained by NIRS in a later study.[394] This quantitative approach was used to demonstrate an increase in cerebral blood volume to increases in $Paco_2$ in newborns and an increase in this reactivity of cerebral blood volume to $Paco_2$ with gestational age.[395] Other investigators also showed, using NIRS, that cerebral blood volume increases with increases in $Paco_2$ and simultaneously demonstrated by ^{133}Xe clearance that this increase in blood volume was associated with an increase in cerebral blood flow (CBF) (as expected from the vasodilation caused by increases in $Paco_2$).[396] NIRS parameters also correlate with brain electrical activity. In preterm infants during the first hours of life, both cerebral oxygen saturation and fractional cerebral tissue oxygen extraction correlate positively with spontaneous activity transients and negatively with IBI measured by aEEG, suggesting higher oxygen extraction in preterm infants with higher electrocerebral activity.[397]

Value of NRI in Specific Clinical Situations.

Several studies have documented the value of NIRS in a specific clinical situation. For example, studies of preterm infants with *apnea and bradycardia* suggest that both cerebral oxygen delivery and CBF are impaired during episodes,[398-400] but treatment with increasing the inspired oxygen concentration may lead to hyperoxygenation of the brain.[401] The apparent impairment in CBF with apnea and bradycardia is consistent with the findings of an earlier study of similar infants by Doppler.[402] Similar but less pronounced findings have been observed during the apneic phase of *periodic breathing* in term infants.[403] In a study of *endotracheal suctioning* in preterm infants, the systemic decrease in arterial hemoglobin saturation was accompanied by a decrease in cerebral hemoglobin saturation and an increase in cerebral blood volume.[404] These findings are consistent with the observations during suctioning of elevated central venous pressure and intracranial pressure in the preterm infant.[405,406]

In a study of *gavage feeding* of small preterm infants, decreased cerebral blood volume and HbO_2 were documented.[407] In a study of *asphyxiated infants*, higher cerebral oxygen saturation and lower fractional cerebral tissue oxygen extraction after 24 hours were associated with poor neurodevelopmental outcome, suggesting secondary energy failure in these infants.[408] An investigation of the cerebral hemodynamic effects of *surfactant treatment* of premature infants with respiratory distress syndrome disclosed only small transient perturbations in cerebral HbO_2 concentration and in cerebral blood volume.[409] In the first 3 days of life, infants who later exhibit *severe intraventricular hemorrhage* experience fluctuations in cerebral oxygen extraction as determined by NIRS.[410-412] This finding is consistent with fluctuating CBF, found to be an important pathogenic factor for such hemorrhage (see Chapter 13). *Pressure passive circulation* can be shown with NIRS in preterm infants[411,413-416] and is affected by *deep hypothermic cardiac surgery with cardiopulmonary bypass*[417] during exchange transfusion[418] and with *extracorporeal membrane oxygenation*.[419] NIRS has been used to study the effects of *patent ductus arteriosus*. The majority of the studies show transient or no effect of treatment on cerebral oxygenation parameters,[420-424] though measurement of oxygenation in peripheral tissues such as muscle or kidney may be useful for identifying those infants who would benefit from treatment.[425] One situation in which continuous monitoring for trends in cerebral oxygenation may be particularly useful involves making clinical adjustments, such as changing ventilator settings.[426] NIRS has also been used to compare ventilation strategies.[427,428]

Utilization of NIRS for the study of *cortical activation* has been accomplished by detecting hemodynamic responses to visual, auditory, and olfactory stimulation and to pain.[429-435] The approach appears capable for detecting and generally localizing functional cortical activity in the infant as young as 25 weeks of gestation. Initial research involved the study of the effects of visual activation in the newborn infant.[436] Thus, with visual stimulation, an abrupt increase in cerebral blood volume caused by an increase in both HbO_2 and Hb (findings presumably reflecting an increase in both local CBF and oxygen consumption) was documented by NIRS optodes over the occipital region. More recent studies have involved olfactory, auditory, sensorimotor, and photic stimulation, with the optodes placed on the cranium over the appropriate cortical regions.[379,431,432,434,437-441]

Magnetoencephalography

Magnetoencephalography (MEG) is based on measuring brain electrical activity, similar to EEG. In fact, MEG and EEG are based on the same basic phenomenon—synchronous postsynaptic currents generated in and around neurons. These currents create local field potentials, which are detected by EEG; they also create local magnetic fields, which are again detected by MEG. For both EEG and MEG, brain electrical activity can be modeled as dipolar sources, with EEG being sensitive to both the tangential and radial components of these sources and MEG being sensitive primarily to the tangential components. As a result, MEG is most sensitive to currents in fissural cortex, where pyramidal cells are tangentially oriented with respect to the skull surface. This feature enables MEG to detect activity within sulci, an area from which it can be difficult to record by other means. Another difference between MEG and EEG is the degree of signal distortion that occurs between the current

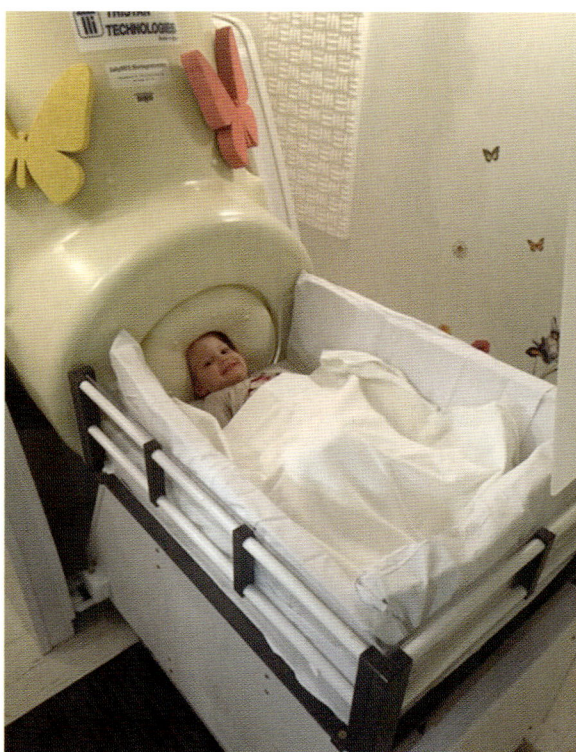

Figure 10.33 A toddler in a magnetoencephalography device.

source and the detector. CSF, skull, and skin have differing conductivities, which causes distortion of electrical fields, but the tissues have similar magnetic permeabilities, thereby causing much less distortion of magnetic fields. Related to this distortion, MEG signals can be measured with millisecond temporal resolution, whereas EEG signals are *temporally smeared* by tissue effects.[442,443]

MEG devices rely on superconducting quantum interference devices (SQUIDs), which allow detection of the brain's magnetic fields without an electric reference. MEG systems may include up to 300 SQUIDs,[444] and some have argued that this may provide higher spatial resolution than EEG, for which little benefit is typically derived from using more than 128 electrodes.[442] The MEG device itself is relatively open (Fig. 10.33), allowing better access to the baby than with MRI, for example. However, the device must be housed in a carefully shielded room. As a result, infants must be taken to the magnetometer rather than evaluated in the intensive care unit, as for EEG.

Setting up a MEG facility is expensive, MEG devices are not commercially available, and the method has yet to find its way into clinical use. Nonetheless, MEG has been used for research studies of infants, mainly involving evaluation of evoked activity. Studies on limited numbers of infants have shown evoked responses in visual, auditory, and somatosensory cortex.[445-447] Preliminary studies also suggest that abnormalities of responses in secondary somatosensory cortex are associated with adverse motor development in very preterm children at age 2 years.[448] Overall, MEG offers a unique opportunity to study higher cortical processing in neonates.

KEY REFERENCES

11. Sarff LD, Platt LH, McCracken GH Jr. Cerebrospinal fluid evaluation in neonates: comparison of high-risk infants with and without meningitis. *J Pediatr.* 1976;88:473-477.
12. Rodriguez AF, Kaplan SL, Mason EO Jr. Cerebrospinal fluid values in the very low birth weight infant. *J Pediatr.* 1990;116:971-974.
13. Wong M, Schlaggar BL, Buller RS, et al. Cerebrospinal fluid protein concentration in pediatric patients: defining clinically relevant reference values. *Arch Pediatr Adolesc Med.* 2000;154:827-831.
16. Adinolfi M, Beck SE, Haddad SA, et al. Permeability of the blood-cerebrospinal fluid barrier to plasma proteins during foetal and perinatal life. *Nature.* 1976;259:140-141.
25. Stapells DR, Kurtzberg D. Evoked potential assessment of auditory system integrity in infants. *Clin Perinatol.* 1991;18:497-518.
33. Fellman V, Kushnerenko E, Mikkola K, et al. Atypical auditory event-related potentials in preterm infants during the first year of life: a possible sign of cognitive dysfunction? *Pediatr Res.* 2004;56: 291-297.
34. Fellman V, Huotilaninen M. Cortical auditory event-related potentials in newborn infants. *Semin Fetal Neonatal Med.* 2006;11: 452-458.
35. Holst M, Eswaran H, Lowery C, et al. Development of auditory evoked fields in human fetuses and newborns: a longitudinal MEG study. *Clin Neurophysiol.* 2005;116:1949-1955.
36. Lowery CL, Eswaran H, Murphy P, et al. Fetal magnetoencephalography. *Semin Fetal Neonatal Med.* 2006;11:430-436.
37. Muenssinger J, Matuz T, Schleger F, et al. Auditory habituation in the fetus and neonate: an fMEG study. *Dev Sci.* 2013;16:287-295.
41. Kennedy CR. The assessment of hearing and brainstem function. In: Eyre JA, ed. *The Neurophysiological Examination of the Newborn Infant.* New York: Mac Keith Press; 1992:79-92.
59. Jiang ZD, Brosi DM, Wilkinson AR. Hearing impairment in preterm very low birthweight babies detected at term by brainstem auditory evoked responses. *Acta Paediatr.* 2001;90:1411-1415.
61. Jiang ZD, Wang J, Brosi DM, et al. One-third of term babies after perinatal hypoxia-ischaemia have transient hearing impairment: dynamic change in hearing threshold during the neonatal period. *Acta Paediatr.* 2004;93:82-87.
95. Robinson RJ. Causes and associations of severe and persistent specific speech and language defects in children. *Dev Med Child Neurol.* 1991;33:943-962.
103. Meyer C, Witte J, Hildmann A, et al. Neonatal screening for hearing disorders in infants at risk: incidence, risk factors, and follow-up. *Pediatrics.* 1999;104:900-904.
105. Jiang ZD, Brosi DM, Li ZH, et al. Brainstem auditory function at term in preterm babies with and without perinatal complications. *Pediatr Res.* 2005;58:1164-1169.
107. Vohr BR, Carty LM, Moore PE, et al. The Rhode Island hearing assessment program: experience with statewide hearing screening (1993–1996). *J Pediatr.* 1998;133:353-357.
108. Johnson JL, White KR, Widen JE, et al. A multicenter evaluation of how many infants with permanent hearing loss pass a two-stage otoacoustic emissions/automated auditory brainstem response newborn hearing screening protocol. *Pediatrics.* 2005;116: 663-672.
112. Joint Committee on Infant Hearing. Year 2000 position statement: principles and guidelines for early hearing detection and intervention programs. *Pediatrics.* 2000;106:798-817.
113. Hayes D. Screening methods: current status. *Ment Retard Dev Disabil Res Rev.* 2003;9:65-72.
115. Shoup AG, Owen KE, Jackson G, et al. The Parkland Memorial Hospital experience in ensuring compliance with Universal Newborn Hearing Screening follow-up. *J Pediatr.* 2005;146:66-72.
116. Taylor MJ. Visual evoked potentials. In: Eyre JA, ed. *The Neurophysiological Examination of the Newborn Infant.* New York: MacKeith Press; 1992:93-111.
120. Roy M-S, Barsoum-Homsy M, Orquin J, et al. Maturation of binocular pattern visual evoked potentials in normal full-term and preterm infants from 1 to 6 months of age. *Pediatr Res.* 1995;37: 140-144.
121. Kos-Pietro S, Towle VL, Cakmur R, et al. Maturation of human visual evoked potentials: 27 weeks conceptional age to 2 years. *Neuropediatrics.* 1997;28:318-323.

138. Engel R. Maturational changes and abnormalities in the newborn electroencephalogram. *Dev Med Child Neurol*. 1965;7:498-506.

139. Parmelee AH. Neurophysiological and behavioral organization of premature infants in the first months of life. *Biol Psychiatry*. 1975;10:501-512.

142. Muttitt SC, Taylor MJ, Kobayashi JS, et al. Serial visual evoked potentials and outcome in term birth asphyxia. *Pediatr Neurol*. 1991;7:86-90.

143. Woods JR Jr, Coppes V, Brooks DE, et al. Birth asphyxia. I. Measurement of visual evoked potential (VEP) in the healthy fetus and newborn lamb. *Pediatr Res*. 1981;15:1429-1432.

145. McSherry JW, Walters CL, Horbar JD. Acute visual evoked potential changes in hydrocephalus. *Electroencephalogr Clin Neurophysiol*. 1982;53:331-333.

146. Dreyfus-Brisac C. The bioelectrical development of the central nervous system during early life. In: Falkner F, ed. *Human Development*. Philadelphia: W. B. Saunders; 1966:286.

153. Guilleminault C, Souquet M. Sleep states and related pathology. In: Korobkin R, Guilleminault C, eds. *Advances in Perinatal Neurology*. New York: Spectrum; 1979:225.

160. Watanabe K. The neonatal electroencephalogram and sleep cycle patterns. In: Eyre JA, ed. *The Neurophysiological Examination of the Newborn Infant*. New York: Mac Keith Press; 1992:11-47.

165. Hrachovy RA, Mizrahi EM, Kellaway P. Electroencephalography of the newborn. In: Daly DD, Pedley TA, eds. *Current Practice of Clinical Electroencephalography*. 2nd ed. New York: Raven Press, Ltd.; 1990:201-241.

178. Mizrahi EM, Hrachovy RA, Kellaway P. *Atlas of Neonatal Electroencephalography*. 3rd ed. Philadelphia: Lippincott Williams & Wilkins; 2004.

192. Awal MA, Lai MM, Azemi G, et al. EEG background features that predict outcome in term neonates with hypoxic ischaemic encephalopathy: a structured review. *Clin Neurophysiol*. 2016;127:285-296.

194. Menache CC, Bourgeois BFD, Volpe JJ. Prognostic value of neonatal discontinuous EEG. *Pediatr Neurol*. 2002;27:93-101.

197. Scher MS, Beggarly M. Clinical significance of focal periodic discharges in neonates. *J Child Neurol*. 1989;4:175-185.

200. Okumura A, Hayakawa F, Kato T, et al. Abnormal sharp transients on electroencephalograms in preterm infants with periventricular leukomalacia. *J Pediatr*. 2003;143:26-30.

204. Tharp BR, Scher MS, Clancy RR. Serial EEGs in normal and abnormal infants with birth weights less than 1200 grams—a prospective study with long term follow-up. *Neuropediatrics*. 1989;20:64-72.

214. deVries LS, Hellström-Westas L. Role of cerebral function monitoring in the newborn. *Arch Dis Child*. 2005;90:F201-F207.

221. Hellström-Westas L, Rosen I, Svenningsen NW. Predictive value of early continuous amplitude integrated EEG recordings on outcome after severe birth asphyxia in full term infants. *Arch Dis Child*. 1995;72:F34-F38.

224. Shalak LF, Laptook AR, Velaphi SC, et al. Amplitude-integrated electroencephalography coupled with an early neurologic examination enhances prediction of term infants at risk for persistent encephalopathy. *Pediatrics*. 2003;111:351-357.

228. Toet MC, Hellström-Westas L, Groenendaal F, et al. Amplitude integrated EEG 3 and 6 hours after birth in full term neonates with hypoxic-ischaemic encephalopathy. *Arch Dis Child Fetal Neonatal Ed*. 1999;81:F19-F23.

229. Eken P, Toet MC, Groenendaal F, et al. Predictive value of early neuroimaging, pulsed Doppler and neurophysiology in full term infants with hypoxic- ischaemic encephalopathy. *Arch Dis Child*. 1995;73:F75-F80.

230. Toet MC, Van der Meij W, de Vries LS, et al. Comparison between simultaneously recorded amplitude integrated electroencephalogram (cerebral function monitor) and standard electroencephalogram in neonates. *Pediatrics*. 2002;109:772-779.

231. Rennie JM, Chorley G, Boylan GB, et al. Non-expert use of the cerebral function monitor for neonatal seizure detection. *Arch Dis Child Fetal Neonatal Ed*. 2004;89:F37-F40.

234. Shah DK, Mackay MT, Lavery S, et al. Accuracy of bedside electroencephalographic monitoring in comparison with simultaneous continuous conventional electroencephalography for seizure detection in term infants. *Pediatrics*. 2008;121:1146-1154.

246. Rennie JM. *Neonatal Cerebral Ultrasound*. Cambridge, UK: Cambridge University Press; 1997.

249. Fawer CL, Calame A. Ultrasound. In: Haddad J, Christmann D, Messer J, eds. *Imaging Techniques of the CNS Of the Neonates*. New York: Springer-Verlag; 1991:79-106.

254. de Vries LS, Volpe JJ. Value of sequential MRI in preterm infants. *Neurology*. 2013;81:2062-2063.

260. Pourcelot L. Diagnostic ultrasound for cerebrovascular disease. In: Donald J, Levi S, eds. *Present and Future Diagnostic Ultrasound*. New York: Wiley; 1976.

262. Lowe LH, Bailey Z. State-of-the-art cranial sonography: part 1, modern techniques and image interpretation. *AJR Am J Roentgenol*. 2011;196:1028-1033.

263. Pinto PS, Tekes A, Singhi S, et al. White-gray matter echogenicity ratio and resistive index: sonographic bedside markers of cerebral hypoxic-ischemic injury/edema? *J Perinatol*. 2012;32:448-453.

264. Nishimaki S, Iwasaki Y, Akamatsu H. Cerebral blood flow velocity before and after cerebrospinal fluid drainage in infants with posthemorrhagic hydrocephalus. *J Ultrasound Med*. 2004;23:1315-1319.

265. Ecury-Goossen GM, Raets MM, Camfferman FA, et al. Resistive indices of cerebral arteries in very preterm infants: values throughout stay in the neonatal intensive care unit and impact of patent ductus arteriosus. *Pediatr Radiol*. 2016;46:1291-1300.

266. Brenner DJ, Doll R, Goodhead DT, et al. Cancer risks attributable to low doses of ionizing radiation: assessing what we really know. *Proc Natl Acad Sci USA*. 2003;100:13761-13766.

267. Karlsson P, Holmberg E, Lundell M, et al. Intracranial tumors after exposure to ionizing radiation during infancy: a pooled analysis of two Swedish cohorts of 28,008 infants with skin hemangioma. *Radiat Res*. 1998;150:357-364.

268. Boice JD Jr. Radiation epidemiology and recent paediatric computed tomography studies. *Ann ICRP*. 2015;44:236-248.

269. Krille L, Dreger S, Schindel R, et al. Risk of cancer incidence before the age of 15 years after exposure to ionising radiation from computed tomography: results from a German cohort study. *Radiat Environ Biophys*. 2015;54:1-12.

270. Hall P, Adami HO, Trichopoulos D, et al. Effect of low doses of ionising radiation in infancy on cognitive function in adulthood: Swedish population based cohort study. *BMJ*. 2004;328:19.

271. Ron E, Modan B, Floro S, et al. Mental function following scalp irradiation during childhood. *Am J Epidemiol*. 1982;116:149-160.

277. Cowan F, Mercuri E, Groenendaal F, et al. Does cranial ultrasound imaging identify arterial cerebral infarction in term neonates? *Arch Dis Child Fetal Neonatal Ed*. 2005;90:F252-F256.

278. Mathur AM, Neil JJ, McKinstry RC, et al. Transport, monitoring, and successful brain MR imaging in unsedated neonates. *Pediatr Radiol*. 2008;38:260-264.

282. Tisdall MD, Hess AT, Reuter M, et al. Volumetric navigators for prospective motion correction and selective reacquisition in neuroanatomical MRI. *Magn Reson Med*. 2012;68:389-399.

283. Gumus K, Keating B, White N, et al. Comparison of optical and MR-based tracking. *Magn Reson Med*. 2015;74:894-902.

285. Ooi MB, Aksoy M, Maclaren J, et al. Prospective motion correction using inductively coupled wireless RF coils. *Magn Reson Med*. 2013;70:639-647.

287. Ganzetti M, Wenderoth N, Mantini D. Whole brain myelin mapping using T1- and T2-weighted MR imaging data. *Front Hum Neurosci*. 2014;8:671.

288. Almli CR, Rivkin MJ, McKinstry RC, et al. The NIH MRI study of normal brain development (Objective-2): newborns, infants, toddlers, and preschoolers. *Neuroimage*. 2007;35:308-325.

289. Huppi PS, Warfield S, Kikinis R, et al. Quantitative magnetic resonance imaging of brain development in premature and mature newborns. *Ann Neurol*. 1998;43:224-235.

293. Abernethy LJ, Cooke RW, Foulder-Hughes L. Caudate and hippocampal volumes, intelligence, and motor impairment in 7-year-old children who were born preterm. *Pediatr Res*. 2004;55:884-893.

294. Reiss AL, Kesler SR, Vohr B, et al. Sex differences in cerebral volumes of 8-year-olds born preterm. *J Pediatr*. 2004;145:242-249.

295. Kesler SR, Ment LR, Vohr B, et al. Volumetric analysis of regional cerebral development in preterm children. *Pediatr Neurol*. 2004;31:318-325.

298. Nosarti C, Giouroukou E, Healy E, et al. Grey and white matter distribution in very preterm adolescents mediates neurodevelopmental outcome. *Brain.* 2008;131:205-217.
304. Thompson DK, Warfield SK, Carlin JB, et al. Perinatal risk factors altering regional brain structure in the preterm infant. *Brain.* 2007;130:667-677.
308. Peterson BS. Brain imaging studies of the anatomical and functional consequences of preterm birth for human brain development. *Ann N Y Acad Sci.* 2003;1008:219-237.
311. Kidokoro H, Neil J, Inder T. A new MRI assessment tool to define brain abnormalities in very preterm infants at term. *AJNR Am J Neuroradiol.* 2013;34:2208-2214.
312. Kapellou O, Counsell SJ, Kennea NL, et al. Abnormal cortical development after premature birth shown by altered allometric scaling of brain growth. *PLoS Med.* 2006;3:e265.
315. Engelhardt E, Inder TE, Alexopoulos D, et al. Regional impairments of cortical folding in premature infants. *Ann Neurol.* 2015;77:154-162.
317. Shimony JS, Smyser CD, Wideman G, et al. Comparison of cortical folding measures for evaluation of developing human brain. *Neuroimage.* 2016;125:780-790.
321. Hill J, Dierker D, Neil J, et al. A surface-based analysis of hemispheric asymmetries and folding of cerebral cortex in term-born human infants. *J Neurosci.* 2010;30:2268-2276.
323. Welch KMA, Windham J, Knight RA, et al. A model to predict the histopathology of human stroke using diffusion and T_2-weighted magnetic resonance imaging. *Stroke.* 1995;26:1983-1989.
326. Huppi PS, Maier SE, Peled S, et al. Microstructural development of human newborn cerebral white matter assessed in vivo by diffusion tensor magnetic resonance imaging. *Pediatr Res.* 1998;44:584-590.
327. Neil JJ, Shiran SI, McKinstry RC, et al. Normal brain in human newborns: apparent diffusion coefficient and diffusion anisotropy measured using diffusion tensor imaging. *Radiology.* 1998;209:57-66.
328. Moseley ME, Kucharczyk J, Mintorovitch J, et al. Diffusion-weighted MR imaging of acute stroke: correlation with T2-weighted and magnetic susceptibility-enhanced MR imaging in cats. *AJNR Am J Neuroradiol.* 1990;11:423-429.
340. Oppenheim C, Stanescu R, Dormont D, et al. False-negative diffusion-weighted MR findings in acute ischemic stroke. *AJNR Am J Neuroradiol.* 2000;21:1434-1440.
341. McKinstry RC, Miller JH, Snyder AZ, et al. A prospective, longitudinal diffusion tensor imaging study of brain injury in newborns. *Neurology.* 2002;59:824-833.
348. Bick AS, Mayer A, Levin N. From research to clinical practice: implementation of functional magnetic imaging and white matter tractography in the clinical environment. *J Neurol Sci.* 2012;312:158-165.
349. Smith SM, Jenkinson M, Johansen-Berg H, et al. Tract-based spatial statistics: voxelwise analysis of multi-subject diffusion data. *Neuroimage.* 2006;31:1487-1505.
350. van Kooij BJ, de Vries LS, Ball G, et al. Neonatal tract-based spatial statistics findings and outcome in preterm infants. *AJNR Am J Neuroradiol.* 2012;33:188-194.
351. Lequin MH, Dudink J, Tong KA, et al. Magnetic resonance imaging in neonatal stroke. *Semin Fetal Neonatal Med.* 2009;14:299-310.
352. Berfelo FJ, Kersbergen KJ, van Ommen CH, et al. Neonatal cerebral sinovenous thrombosis from symptom to outcome. *Stroke.* 2010;41:1382-1388.
353. Saleem SN, Fetal MRI. An approach to practice: a review. *J Adv Res.* 2014;5:507-523.
354. Gupta JK, Bryce FC, Lilford RJ. Management of apparently isolated fetal ventriculomegaly. *Obstet Gynecol Surv.* 1994;49:716-721.
355. Levine D, Barnes PD, Madsen JR, et al. Central nervous system abnormalities assessed with prenatal magnetic resonance imaging. *Obstet Gynecol.* 1999;94:1011-1019.
356. Wagenvoort AM, Bekker MN, Go AT, et al. Ultrafast scan magnetic resonance in prenatal diagnosis. *Fetal Diagn Ther.* 2000;15:364-372.
357. Glenn OA, Cuneo AA, Barkovich AJ, et al. Malformations of cortical development: diagnostic accuracy of fetal MR imaging. *Radiology.* 2012;263:843-855.
358. Glenn OA, Barkovich AJ. Magnetic resonance imaging of the fetal brain and spine: an increasingly important tool in prenatal diagnosis, part 1. *AJNR Am J Neuroradiol.* 2006;27:1604-1611.
359. Glenn OA, Barkovich J. Magnetic resonance imaging of the fetal brain and spine: an increasingly important tool in prenatal diagnosis: part 2. *AJNR Am J Neuroradiol.* 2006;27:1807-1814.
360. Robertson NJ, Thayyil S, Cady EB, et al. Magnetic resonance spectroscopy biomarkers in term perinatal asphyxial encephalopathy: from neuropathological correlates to future clinical applications. *Curr Pediatr Rev.* 2014;10:37-47.
361. Ardon O, Procter M, Mao R, et al. Creatine transporter deficiency: novel mutations and functional studies. *Mol Genet Metab Rep.* 2016;8:20-23.
362. Wittsack HJ, Kugel H, Roth B, et al. Quantitative measurements with localized 1H MR spectroscopy in children with Canavan's disease. *J Magn Reson Imaging.* 1996;6:889-893.
363. Saneto RP, Friedman SD, Shaw DW. Neuroimaging of mitochondrial disease. *Mitochondrion.* 2008;8:396-413.
364. Anderson AW, Marois R, Colson ER, et al. Neonatal auditory activation detected by functional magnetic resonance imaging. *Magn Reson Imaging.* 2001;19:1-5.
365. Arichi T, Moraux A, Melendez A, et al. Somatosensory cortical activation identified by functional MRI in preterm and term infants. *Neuroimage.* 2010;49:2063-2071.
367. Biswal B, Yetkin FZ, Haughton VM, et al. Functional connectivity in the motor cortex of resting human brain using echo-planar MRI. *Magn Reson Med.* 1995;34:537-541.
368. Smyser CD, Snyder AZ, Neil JJ. Functional connectivity MRI in infants: exploration of the functional organization of the developing brain. *Neuroimage.* 2011;56:1437-1452.
369. Smyser CD, Dosenbach NU, Smyser TA, et al. Prediction of brain maturity in infants using machine-learning algorithms. *Neuroimage.* 2016;[epub ahead of print].
371. Liao SM, Culver JP. Near infrared optical technologies to illuminate the status of the neonatal brain. *Curr Pediatr Rev.* 2014;10:73-86.
372. Wyatt JS, Delpy DT. Near infrared spectroscopy. In: Haddad J, Christmann D, Messer J, eds. *Imaging Techniques of the CNS Of the Neonates.* New York: Springer-Verlag; 1991:147-160.
374. du Plessis AJ. Near-infrared spectroscopy for the *in vivo* study of cerebral hemodynamics and oxygenation. *Curr Opin Pediatr.* 1995;7:632-639.
376. Nicklin SE, Hassan IA-A, Wickramasinghe YA, et al. The light still shines, but not that brightly? The current status of perinatal near infrared spectroscopy. *Arch Dis Child.* 2003;88:F263-F268.
378. Gregg NM, White BR, Zeff BW, et al. Brain specificity of diffuse optical imaging: improvements from superficial signal regression and tomography. *Front Neuroenergetics.* 2010;2.
379. Liao SM, Gregg NM, White BR, et al. Neonatal hemodynamic response to visual cortex activity: high-density near-infrared spectroscopy study. *J Biomed Opt.* 2010;15:026010.
383. Franceschini MA, Thaker S, Themelis G, et al. Assessment of infant brain development with frequency-domain near-infrared spectroscopy. *Pediatr Res.* 2007;61:546-551.
385. Hamaoka T, Katsumura T, Murase N, et al. Quantification of ischemic muscle deoxygenation by near infrared time-resolved spectroscopy. *J Biomed Opt.* 2000;5:102-105.
387. Cheung C, Culver JP, Takahashi K, et al. In vivo cerebrovascular measurement combining diffuse near-infrared absorption and correlation spectroscopies. *Phys Med Biol.* 2001;46:2053-2065.
388. Roche-Labarbe N, Carp SA, Surova A, et al. Noninvasive optical measures of CBV, StO(2), CBF index, and rCMRO(2) in human premature neonates' brains in the first six weeks of life. *Hum Brain Mapp.* 2010;31:341-352.
389. Roche-Labarbe N, Fenoglio A, Aggarwal A, et al. Near-infrared spectroscopy assessment of cerebral oxygen metabolism in the developing premature brain. *J Cereb Blood Flow Metab.* 2012;32:481-488.
391. Wyatt JS, Cope M, Delpy DT, et al. Quantification of cerebral oxygenation and haemodynamics in sick newborn infants by near infrared spectrophotometry. *Lancet.* 1986;2:1063-1066.
392. Wyatt JS, Cope M, Delpy DT, et al. Measurement of optical path length for cerebral near-infrared spectroscopy in newborn infants. *Dev Neurosci.* 1990;12:140-144.
393. Altman DI, Perlman JM, Volpe JJ, et al. Cerebral oxygen metabolism in newborn infants measured with positron emission tomography. *J Cerebr Blood Flow Metab.* 1989;9:525.

394. Meek JH, Tyszczuk L, Elwell CE, et al. Cerebral blood flow increases over the first three days of life in extremely preterm neonates. *Arch Dis Child Fetal Neonatal Ed.* 1998;78:F33-F37.

395. Wyatt JS, Edwards AD, Cope M, et al. Response of cerebral blood volume to changes in arterial carbon dioxide tension in preterm and term infants. *Pediatr Res.* 1991;29:553-557.

396. Skov LO, Pryds O, Greisen G. Estimating cerebral blood flow in newborn infants: comparison of near infrared spectroscopy and ^{133}Xe clearance. *Pediatr Res.* 1991;27:445-449.

397. Tataranno ML, Alderliesten T, de Vries LS, et al. Early oxygen-utilization and brain activity in preterm infants. *PLoS ONE.* 2015;10:e0124623.

399. Petrova A, Mehta R. Near-infrared spectroscopy in the detection of regional tissue oxygenation during hypoxic events in preterm infants undergoing critical care. *Pediatr Crit Care Med.* 2006;7:449-454.

401. Baerts W, Lemmers PM, van Bel F. Cerebral oxygenation and oxygen extraction in the preterm infant during desaturation: effects of increasing FiO(2) to assist recovery. *Neonatology.* 2011;99:65-72.

402. Perlman JM, Hersovitch P, Corriveau S, et al. Cerebral blood flow velocity as determined by Doppler is related to regional cerebral blood flow as determined by positron emission tomograpny. *Ann Neurol.* 1985;18:407-408.

403. Urlesberger B, Pichler G, Gradnitzer E, et al. Changes in cerebral blood volume and cerebral oxygenation during periodic breathing in term infants. *Neuropediatrics.* 2000;31:75-81.

404. Shah AR, Kurth CD, Gwiazdowski SG, et al. Fluctuations in cerebral oxygenation and blood volume during endotracheal suctioning in premature infants. *J Pediatr.* 1992;120:769-774.

405. Perlman JM, Volpe JJ. Suctioning in the preterm infant: effects on cerebral blood flow velocity, intracranial pressure, and arterial blood pressure. *Pediatrics.* 1983;72:329-334.

407. van Bel F, Dorrepaal C, Benders M, et al. Changes in cerebral hemodynamics and oxygenation in the first 24 hours following birth asphyxia. *Pediatrics.* 1993;92:365-372.

408. Toet MC, Lemmers PM, van Schelven LJ, et al. Cerebral oxygenation and electrical activity after birth asphyxia: their relation to outcome. *Pediatrics.* 2006;117:333-339.

409. Edwards AD, McCormick DC, Roth SC, et al. Cerebral hemodynamic effects of treatment with modified natural surfactant investigated by near infrared spectroscopy. *Pediatr Res.* 1992;32:532-536.

412. Alderliesten T, Lemmers PM, Smarius JJ, et al. Cerebral oxygenation, extraction, and autoregulation in very preterm infants who develop peri-intraventricular hemorrhage. *J Pediatr.* 2013;162:698-704 e692.

416. Soul JS, Hammer PE, Tsuji M, et al. Fluctuating pressure-passivity is common in the cerebral circulation of sick premature infants. *Pediatr Res.* 2007;61:467-473.

417. Bassan H, Gauvreau K, Newburger JW, et al. Identification of pressure passive cerebral perfusion and its mediators after infant cardiac surgery. *Pediatr Res.* 2005;57:35-41.

418. van de Bor M, Benders MJ, Dorrepaal CA, et al. Cerebral blood volume changes during exchange transfusions in infants born at or near term. *J Pediatr.* 1994;125:617-621.

419. Liem KD, Hopman JCW, Osenburg B, et al. Cerebral oxygenation and hemodynamics during induction of extracorporeal membrane oxygenation as investigated by near infrared spectrophtometry. *Pediatrics.* 1995;95:555-561.

422. van der Laan ME, Roofthooft MT, Fries MW, et al. A hemodynamically significant patent ductus arteriosus does not affect cerebral or renal tissue oxygenation in preterm infants. *Neonatology.* 2016;110:141-147.

425. Underwood MA, Milstein JM, Sherman MP. Near-infrared spectroscopy as a screening tool for patent ductus arteriosus in extremely low birth weight infants. *Neonatology.* 2007;91:134-139.

426. van Bel F, Lemmers P, Naulaers G. Monitoring neonatal regional cerebral oxygen saturation in clinical practice: value and pitfalls. *Neonatology.* 2008;94:237-244.

427. Guerin C, Bailey SM, Mally PV, et al. Randomized control trial comparing physiologic effects in preterm infants during treatment with nasal continuous positive airway pressure (NCPAP) generated by Bubble NCPAP and Ventilator NCPAP: a pilot study. *J Perinat Med.* 2016;44:655-661.

436. Meek JH, Firbank M, Elwell CE, et al. Regional hemodynamic responses to visual stimulation in awake infants. *Pediatr Res.* 1998;43:840-843.

441. White BR, Liao SM, Ferradal SL, et al. Bedside optical imaging of occipital resting-state functional connectivity in neonates. *Neuroimage.* 2012;59:2529-2538.

442. Lopes da Silva F. EEG and MEG: relevance to neuroscience. *Neuron.* 2013;80:1112-1128.

443. Hari R, Parkkonen L. MEG in the study of higher cortical functions. In: Ikeda A, Inoue Y, eds. *Progress in Epileptic Disorders. Event-related Potentials in Patients with Epilepsy: From Current State to Future Prospects.* Vol. 5. Surrey. United Kingdom: John Libbey Eurotext; 2008:103-112.

444. Hari R, Salmelin R. Magnetoencephalography: from SQUIDs to neuroscience. neuroimage 20th anniversary special edition. *Neuroimage.* 2012;61:386-396.

445. Nevalainen P, Lauronen L, Pihko E. Development of human somatosensory cortical functions–what have we learned from magnetoencephalography: a review. *Front Hum Neurosci.* 2014;8:158.

448. Rahkonen P, Nevalainen P, Lauronen L, et al. Cortical somatosensory processing measured by magnetoencephalography predicts neurodevelopment in extremely low-gestational-age infants. *Pediatr Res.* 2013;73:763-771.

Full references for this chapter can be found on www.expertconsult.com.

Neurodevelopmental Follow-Up

Lianne J. Woodward ◆ *Petra S. Hüppi*

Neurodevelopmental follow-up is a critical component of the evaluation of the neurological development and ongoing clinical needs of the high-risk newborn. Such follow-up is important because it has become increasingly clear that a substantial number of infants who exhibit neurological abnormalities or who have other serious conditions in the newborn period will experience later neurological and developmental difficulties that are likely to seriously limit their educational, social, and other life course opportunities. Unfortunately in the neonatal period it is not always possible to accurately predict which infants will experience later neurodevelopmental problems and which will not. Furthermore, children's skills and abilities develop with age and experience, with simpler skills often forming the foundation for the learning of more complex skills. Thus it is often not until a child fails, or is slower to develop a specific skill compared with other children of his or her age, that his or her problem/s become fully apparent. The developmental timing of this will also depend on the function of interest, with neuromotor deficits tending to emerge in the first year of life, while cognitive and behavioral impairment(s) develop more slowly from early childhood to adolescence. Thus it is now widely accepted that high-risk infants require close monitoring and developmental surveillance as part of our ongoing responsibility for care and optimization of their outcomes beyond merely survival and discharge from the neonatal intensive care unit (NICU).[1,2]

Neurodevelopmental follow-up is also important for family support, as well as from a neonatal and public health perspective. First, families want to know if their child is healthy and growing normally, or if problems are likely to be encountered in the future. Such information is valuable for both stress management and family decision-making. It also enables families to proactively plan and advocate for their child's needs. This can be especially relevant at key transition points in a child's life when additional challenges may be encountered by a child, such as starting child care or changing schools. During these times, families are also likely to benefit from extra advice and support.

Second, information about high-risk children's outcomes is crucial for the improvement of existing neonatal services. Specifically, possible positive and negative effects of different medical interventions on neurological and developmental outcomes may not be apparent in the first years of life. Therefore neurodevelopmental follow-up data can provide valuable feedback information about the efficacy and potential risks associated with different clinical care approaches beyond survival and short-term health outcomes. Relatedly, this kind of information can also be extremely useful both for counseling families in the NICU and providing guidance to follow-up and early intervention service providers about the nature of adverse outcomes and when such outcomes may become visible during a child's development.

Finally, from a broader public health perspective, careful follow-up screening on a regular basis helps ensure that child problems are detected early. This is important because targeted interventions can be effective in treating and preventing significant neurodevelopmental problems, which if left untreated may worsen and/or place the child at increased risk of more complex impairments. Thus early screening and intervention serves to not only minimize child and family distress, but also to reduce the burden of long-term care on public health, social, and educational services over the child's life span.

PRINCIPLES AND CONCEPTS OF CHILD DEVELOPMENT

To accurately identify deviations and delays in a child's development, it is essential to have an appreciation of the normative developmental timing of different skills and abilities, and even more importantly, the processes that shape child development. Thus some key principles and concepts of child development are briefly reviewed.

Life Course Development

Child development by definition is recognized to *be dynamic over time and child age*, with both quantitative and qualitative changes in functioning observed from birth to old age.[3] Therefore it is now more common to talk about life course development or *pathways of development* in recognition of the fact that early life experiences can affect an individual's development over his or her life course. Specifically, early perinatal experiences have the potential to both positively or negatively alter an individual's life course trajectory.[4-6] However, in addition, a child's experiences in his or her family, at school, and in his or her community will also mold his or her behavior in unique ways. Thus there is often considerable *inter-* and *intraindividual variability* in observed outcomes for both typically developing and high-risk children. This poses additional challenges for the assessment of delay or impairment in children subject to early neonatal risk, especially at younger ages when this variability is particularly pronounced in the timing of key developmental milestones (e.g., walking and talking). As a result, accurate pediatric diagnosis and prognosis prediction is uniquely challenging because of dynamic changes in children's development with age (Fig. 11.1).

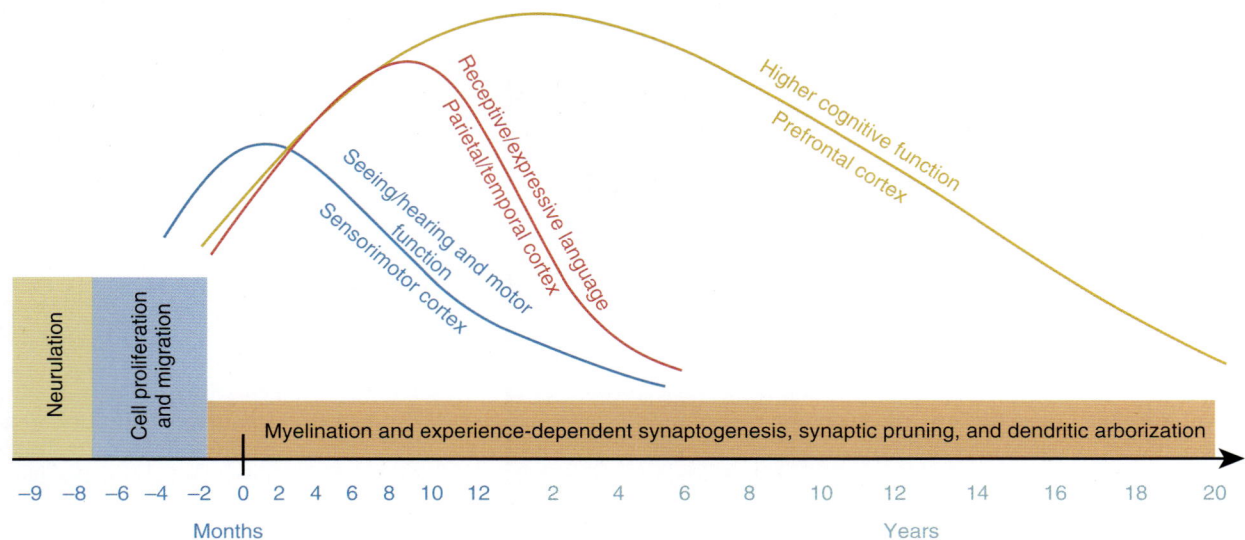

Figure 11.1 Development of key abilities with child age and neurological maturation. (Adapted from Charles A. Nelson, *From Neurons to Neighborhoods*, 2000.)

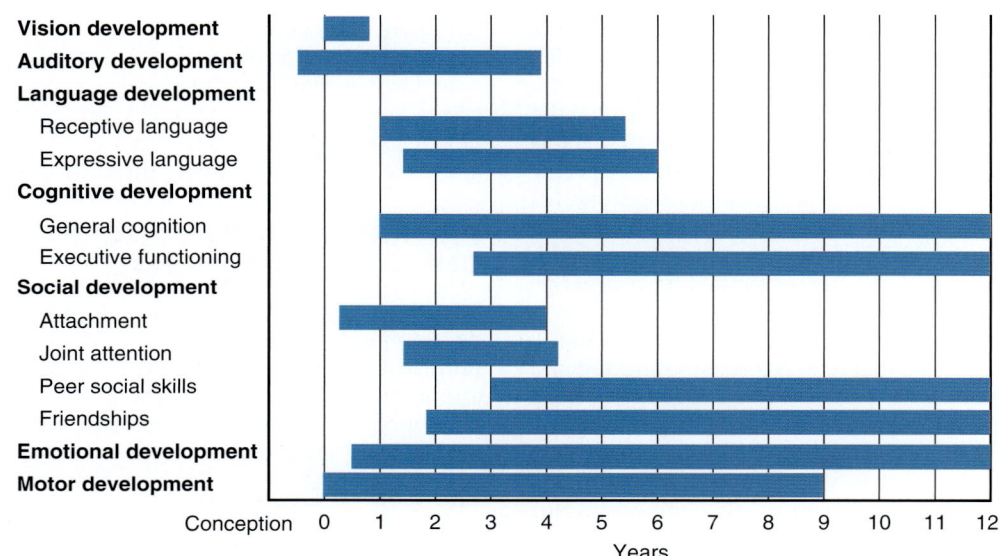

Figure 11.2 Developmental progression of different functional domains.

For this reason, repeated assessments and the collection of information from multiple sources are advised. Longer-term follow-up is also recommended when possible because this will ensure that children are monitored until adaptive functioning in early developing skills, such as emotional and behavioral regulation, is achieved. It also allows for the opportunity to reliably and validly assess more complex abilities that do not come online developmentally until school age and later, but are nonetheless very important for learning and daily life functioning. These include, for example, higher-level cognitive skills such as planning and organization of action, as well as many mental health disorders. Fig. 11.2 provides a broad overview of the approximate developmental progression of functional skills across multiple domains of child development.

Domains of Development

When thinking about child development within this framework, it can be helpful to conceptualize a child's neurodevelopmental functioning as spanning several domains, which include (1) physical health/growth, (2) neuromotor function, (3) language development, (4) cognition and learning, (5) emotional and behavioral well-being or mental health, and (6) social functioning. Although representing somewhat independent skill sets, it is important to note that these domains are also interrelated because functioning in one domain can have an adverse effect on developmental opportunities and functioning in another. Relatedly, early skills acquired during infancy and early childhood form vital building blocks for later competencies not only within the same domain but also across domains. For example, a child with delayed language development may be more prone to develop regulatory and behavior problems because of his or her difficulties in communicating his or her needs to others. Similarly, a child with cerebral palsy (CP) who is unable to participate fully in sport at school may have fewer opportunities to interact and develop friendships with his or her peers, which in turn will limit his or her social learning experiences and long-term social development. These cascading challenges can have adverse cumulative impacts on a child's functioning over time, which is sometimes referred to as the Matthew effect.[7]

Importance of a Child's Postnatal Experiences

Previously a child's functional abilities were viewed as an expression of his or her genetic inheritance and associated brain structural maturational processes. However, a large body of human infant and experimental research now shows that brain development and resulting child functional outcomes are the result of complex interactions between biological and environmental influences.[8-11] Specifically, while an individual's genes provide essential information for establishing basic patterns of neuronal growth and connectivity, it is the interaction of genes and the experiences children have early in life (and the environment in which they have them) that not only shape their developing brain architecture but also how genes are turned on and off, and the way they are expressed (epigenetics). Healthy brain development is optimized when a child is raised in a nurturing environment that is characterized by (1) human interactions that are responsive, emotionally supportive, and developmentally stimulating; (2) adequate nutrition and child health support; (3) protection from threats; and (4) where early learning opportunities are fostered.[12] For the young child, his or her experiences of the world are largely defined by his or her home environment and interactions with parents and other family members. However, unfortunately, not all children experience optimal or even good enough home environments, but rather are exposed to varying degrees of environmental risk, ranging from poverty, social adversity, poor parental mental health, parenting problems, family dysfunction, and neighborhood/community stress or violence. Evidence shows that these adverse experiences, which often co-occur, adversely affect brain development, and, in turn, a child's physical, cognitive, and social development. Often these effects are additive or even interactive, with children exposed to higher levels of family social and economic adversity being at greater risk of neurodevelopmental delay or impairment. Indeed, there is also some suggestion that developmentally vulnerable children may be more sensitive to experiential effects than typically developing children, gaining greater benefit from a nurturing rearing environment and potentially being more severely affected by exposure to an adverse rearing environment.[13,14] The notion that the brain continues to adapt and change in response to experiences throughout childhood and into adulthood is sometimes referred to as *neural plasticity*.[15]

Related to the importance of a child's experiences for brain and behavioral development, it is important to note that the child is not simply a passive recipient of environmental influence, but rather is an active participant in his or her world. This concept was first introduced by Sameroff and Chandler,[16] who argued that the relationship between a child and his or her environment was a transactional one. From this perspective, a child's behavior and neurodevelopmental outcome is the consequence of dynamic, transactional interactions

between genetic, constitutional, neurobiological, biochemical, psychological, and sociological processes. For example, a child who is temperamentally difficult, or is more demanding to care for developmentally, can increase risks of maternal stress/depression as well as marital discord. These parental and family challenges can in turn impede the family's ability to parent and manage difficult child behavior, further exacerbating problems. As highlighted in this example, an implication of the transactional model is not only that environmental factors are important in shaping child outcomes, but also that the child's reciprocal characteristics partially determine the nature of his or her own environment.

WHICH INFANTS NEED FOLLOW-UP?

A child may require specialized neurodevelopmental follow-up for reasons specific to the child and/or his or her family. Table 11.1 provides a list of neonatal medical conditions for which follow-up is recommended based on a more recent multidisciplinary consortium of specialists from Australasia and the United Kingdom.[17] See also those made by the American Academy of Pediatrics [AAP] in 2004.[18] Also listed in Table 11.1 are family factors that may themselves justify child developmental surveillance, but certainly when combined with a clear medical indication reinforce the need for referral because later neurodevelopmental risk is likely to increase as the number of comorbid conditions or risk factors increase. For example, a growth curve analysis of the cognitive trajectories of very preterm (VPT)– and full-term–born children between the ages of 4 and 12 years found that early cerebral white matter abnormalities (WMA) and family social risk contributed additively to children's later cognitive outcome.[11] Cerebral WMA were assessed based on qualitative magnetic resonance imaging (MRI), and social risk consisted of a composite measure of five factors including early motherhood (<21 years), maternal educational underachievement (did not graduate from high school), minority ethnicity, low socioeconomic status (SES), and single parent family. As illustrated in Fig. 11.3, VPT children

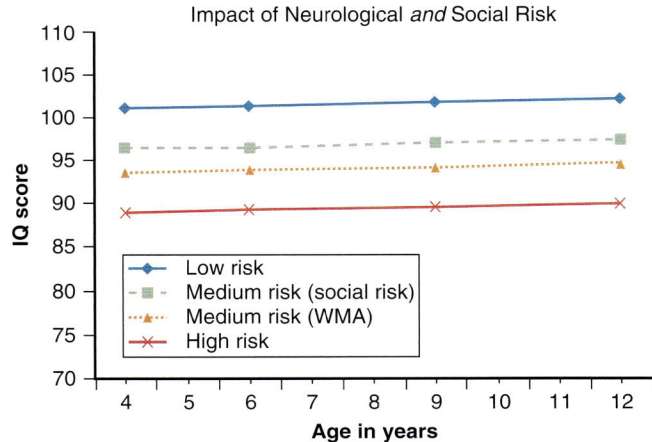

Figure 11.3 Cognitive trajectories of children born prematurely subject to varying degrees of neurological and social risk. *WMA*, White matter abnormalities. (From Mangin, KS, Horwood LJ, Woodward LJ. Cognitive development trajectories of very preterm and typically developing children. *Child Devel.* 2017;88: 282–298.)

TABLE 11.1 Child Health and Family Factors That Indicate the Need for Neurodevelopmental Follow-Up	
CHILD FACTORS	**FAMILY FACTORS**
• VPT: gestational age <32 weeks or very low birth weight (VLBW: <1500 g) • Small for gestational age (SGA: <3rd percentile or <−2 SD weight for gestational age and sex), microcephaly, IUGR with pathological Doppler • Neonatal asphyxia and/or neonatal encephalopathy (including seizure), regardless of cause • Term babies who have received positive pressure ventilation for >24 hours • Congenital brain or heart malformations, genetic syndromes, or inborn errors of metabolism that affect neurodevelopmental outcomes • Congenital infections • NAS • Failed newborn hearing screening • Neonatal central nervous system infections (e.g., meningitis/encephalitis) • Infants requiring major surgery (e.g., brain, cardiac, other thoracic, or abdominal) • Hyperbilirubinemia (bilirubin >400 μmol/L or clinical evidence of bilirubin encephalopathy) • Neurobehavioral abnormalities noted in the newborn period	• High social risk (e.g., interpartner violence, previous child abuse, severe poverty, or homelessness) • Substance abuse by either parent • Major psychiatric history in either parent • Developmental disability in either parent

IUGR, Intrauterine growth restriction; *NAS*, neonatal abstinence syndrome; *SGA*, small for gestational age; *VPT*, very preterm.
From Doyle LW, Anderson PJ, Battin M, et al. Long term follow up of high risk children: who, why and how? *BMC Pediatr.* 2014;14:279.

without moderate to severe WMA on neonatal MRI and no family social risk fared the best, with the highest average cognitive trajectory. The second highest functioning group were those children born VPT who had no observable WMA on term MRI but were raised in family circumstances characterized by high social risk (≥2 social risk factors). These children obtained later IQ scores that were, on average, 4.7 points lower than the lowest risk group, indicating the cognitive risk associated with raising a VPT born child in a socioeconomically disadvantaged family environment. The third best functioning group consisted of those VPT children subject to WMA on neonatal MRI but who were raised in a family environment unaffected by social and economic adversity. These children obtained IQ scores that were on average 7.4 IQ points lower than the lowest risk preterm group. In contrast, when VPT born children were subject to both risk factors (i.e., moderate to severe WMAs and high social risk), the adverse effects on cognitive function were increased, with the average cognitive trajectory for these VPT born children found to be 12 IQ points below that of low-risk (no WMA, low family social risk) VPT born children. These findings demonstrate that the presence of both biological and family social risk have an additive impact on later cognitive function and life course opportunities for children born VPT. They also highlight that it is critically important that every effort be made to ensure that infants being raised in higher social risk families are not lost to follow-up because these children are probably the group that most needs monitoring and support.

MODELS OF NEURODEVELOPMENTAL FOLLOW-UP

Neurodevelopmental follow-up can take several forms depending on the population of concern, the resources available, and the purpose of the visit. The first model consists primarily of *surveillance and monitoring*, which involves observing a child's development and tracking parent concerns over time and across multiple domains of development. Standardized developmental screening measures are typically used to proactively identify children who may have a developmental problem or show early delay in one or more areas of development (e.g., language), which if untreated will place them at increased risk of significant developmental problems in the future. Within this neurodevelopmental screening model, information should also be gathered about possible risk and protective factors in the child's environment that may be assisting or hindering their development, to help inform referral decisions and intervention planning.

A second alternative model or approach consists of in-depth developmental assessment of the child in multiple or specific domains. This may occur at targeted ages to supplement data from routine screening evaluations and is probably most relevant for the highest risk populations of infants. The goal of this approach is to specify the precise nature of the child's developmental problem/s, whether they need intervention, and if so, what approaches would be best.

A third less common approach is a hybrid of the surveillance and assessment models. This approach, which tends to be more common in publicly funded health care systems, seeks to conserve limited resources by providing minimal screening surveillance for all or most at-risk children, with intensive (and expensive) assessment resources limited to those children who fail predetermined screening criteria. Specifically, all children referred for evaluation are monitored regularly using child screening and parent interview measures, with children referred for in-house intensive assessment and ideally treatment on an individual basis. When difficulties resolve, the child would typically be transferred back into the surveillance track where he or she would continue to be monitored.

THE TIMING OF FOLLOW-UP ASSESSMENTS

For high-risk newborn infants, follow-up assessments should be more frequent immediately after discharge, but then become gradually more widely spaced with increasing child age. The goal is to be sure that all expected developmental stages are achieved in the expected time window. The exception to this would be when additional visits were indicated because of the presence of a specific neurodevelopmental problem at the time of discharge from the NICU (e.g., feeding, poor growth), or if new neurodevelopmental problems were detected at a previous follow-up visit. Table 11.2 provides a list of suggested ages based on current recommended standards and relevant child outcomes and family factors to assess. In general, newborns at risk for neurodevelopmental delay should be assessed regularly for early rapid development in the first 2 years (toddlerhood and infancy) at intervals of not more than 6 months apart. After the age of 2 or 3 years, if the child is progressing well, these assessments could be done annually at school entry, with biannual follow-up through middle childhood to test for attention and executive functioning problems, school achievement, and socioemotional adjustment/mental health.

For the child born very or extremely preterm, it is important to note that these ages should be adjusted for the degree of prematurity, especially in a research setting, because data show that without age correction, these children will be unduly disadvantaged on cognitive test measures.[19] This bias is most marked during early childhood but does persist to a lesser degree into school age.[20] In the clinical setting, the overidentification of cognitive delay among children at neurodevelopmental risk may be less of a problem because it may help children access much-needed services. However, for research purposes, when the objective is to assess the extent of a problem and ensure comparability across studies, not correcting for gestational age at birth can be problematic and needs to be a consideration.

DURATION OF FOLLOW-UP

There are usually mandated limits to publicly funded or subsidized neurodevelopmental follow-up, with some programs commonly only receiving health services funding to the age of 3 years, although in some countries this has been extended into the early school years. Data certainly suggest that follow-up until school entry is warranted for several reasons. First, infant and early childhood developmental measures are poor to modest predictors of long-term child outcomes, particularly for cognitive scores.[21-23] Second, some developmental disorders cannot be reliably and accurately assessed at a young age, such as executive function impairments, specific learning problems (e.g., dyscalculia, dyslexia), and common mental health disorders such as attention-deficit/hyperactivity disorder (ADHD) and anxiety disorders. Third, there is growing evidence that a school readiness evaluation can proactively identify children who are at high risk of educational underachievement prior to school entry, assisting in effective utility of limited special needs resources.[24]

NEURODEVELOPMENTAL DOMAINS TO ASSESS

The specific neurodevelopmental outcomes assessed will vary with the child's age and developmental level, but effort should be made to ensure that all the neurodevelopmental domains outlined previously are monitored in some way with age-appropriate tools. Also, as noted previously, different abilities will have particular functional importance at different ages.

Therefore, child and family outcome measures are likely to be influenced by child and family needs/issues at the time of the assessment, or in the near future (e.g., as mothers transition back to work or children transition from kindergarten to school).

The primary focus of the following discussion is to outline relevant areas for assessment from both the child's and the family's perspective, and to indicate how these might vary in importance, depending on the age of the child being seen. Some measurement suggestions are given, but providing detailed advice about specific measures is beyond the scope of this chapter. Where possible we refer the reader to recent reviews in which more detailed information can be found about specific standardized tools, the constructs they measure, child ages for which they are suitable, and a description of their relative psychometric properties.

While assessment with standardized measures will be a central part of the evaluation, we would also echo the advice given in Chapter 9 about the value of direct observation of the child, and also potentially the child's interactions with family members. This can be done informally, or could involve the use of validated global behavior rating scales to provide supplementary information about focused attention, behavioral regulation, joint attention, affect, and so forth. Direct observations should ideally be completed in an independent manner by individual staff interacting with or observing the child in different situations (i.e., during testing or even in the waiting room). These can then be later discussed as a team, with consensus ratings or clinical evaluations made. Attaching an actometer to the child's ankle may also be helpful if ADHD is suspected.

More generally, several other good practice considerations are worth noting before a detailed discussion of neurodevelopmental domains to monitor and/or assess. These are as follows.

Staff Training

The personnel involved will likely vary depending on the number of domain areas to be assessed. However, when assessing children with conditions where multiple functional problems are anticipated, follow-up assessments should involve a multidisciplinary team of health professionals. If straightforward screening measures such as parent report measures are being used, it is often possible for these to be administered by appropriately trained and supervised support staff. But all staff responsible for administering and interpreting specific measures ought to be appropriately qualified and trained to do so. Also, when multiple staff administer the same tool (e.g., Bayley Scales), intertester reliability should be regularly monitored to ensure measurement consistency and avoid problems with tester drift.

Family and Cultural Considerations

Research shows that family engagement is associated with positive outcomes for children.[25,26] In addition, families can provide a perspective on their child that is not readily accessible to the assessment team. They are also the individuals in the child's life that are best placed, and most motivated, to enhance their child's learning experiences and to advocate for their child's needs. As a result, there has been a shift toward the adoption of family-centered care practices worldwide. Key tenets of the family-centered care model include (1) establishing an emotionally and culturally safe/supportive care environment;

TABLE 11.2 Child and Family Outcomes to Be Considered at Different Ages

	AGES AT ASSESSMENT											
	2–6 WEEKS	3–4 MONTHS	8 MONTHS	12 MONTHS	15–18 MONTHS	24 MONTHS	36 MONTHS	4–5 YEARS[a]	6–8 YEARS[b]	12–14 YEARS	TRANSITION TO ADULT	ADULT
Child												
Physical health												
General health	++	++	+++	+++	+++	+++	+++	+++	+++	+++	+++	+++
Growth	++	++	+++	+++	++	+++	+++	+++	+++	+++[c]	++[d]	++[d]
Feeding problems	+++	++	++	++	+	+	+	0	0	0	0	0
Special senses	+++	++	+	+	+	+	+	+	+	+	+	+
Neurological	+++	++	+++	+++	+++	+++	+	+	+++	+	+	+
Motor skills	+	+	+	+++	UR	+/−	+/−	+/−	+++	+++	+++	+++
Blood pressure/ CVS	UR	UR	UR	UR	UR	+/−	+/−	+/−	+	+	++	+++
Respiratory health	+++	++	+++	+++	++	+++	++	+++	+++	+++	+++	+++
Daily functioning	++	++	++	++	++	++	++	++	++	++	++	+++
Learning and cognition												
Development/ cognitive function	+	++	++	++	++	++	++	++	++	++	+	+
Language	+	+	+++[e]	+++[e]	+++[e]	+++[e]	+++	++	++	+	0	0
Preacademic skills	0	0	0	0	0	0	+	0	++	+	0	0
Academic progress	0	0	0	0	0	0	0	0	+++	+++	+	+[f]
Mental health												
Behavior	++	++	+++[e]	+++[e]	+++[e]	+++[e]	+++	+++	+++	+++	+++	+++
Social skills	+	+	+[e]	+[e]	+[e]	+[e]	++[e]	++	++	+	+++	+++
Psychopathology	U	0	0	+[e]	+[e]	+[e]	+[e]	0	0	+++	+++	+++
Risk-taking	0	0	0	0	0	0	0	0	0	++	+++	+[f]
Family												
Parental mental health	++	++	+++	+++	+++	+++	+++	+++	+++	+++	+++	+++
Caregiver-child interaction	+++	+++	+++	+++	+++	+++	+++	+++	+++	+	+	0
Family function	+++	+++	+++	+++	+++	+++	+++	+++	+++	+++	+++	+++
Siblings	++	++	++	++	++	++	++	++	++	++	++	++

[a]Prior to school entry.

[b]1–2 years after starting school.

[c]Growth at 12–14 years includes normal pubertal development.

[d]Overweight/obesity an ongoing issue.

[e]Relevant to early presentation of autism spectrum disorder.

[f]Ongoing life learning.

0, Does not apply; + to +++, reflects relative importance; +/−, of dubious value; CVS, cardiovascular system; UR, unreliable.

Shaded areas represent a suggested minimal checklist for busy clinicians.

From Doyle LW, Anderson PJ, Battin M, et al. Long term follow up of high risk children: who, why and how? *BMC Pediatr.* 2014;1;14:279.

(2) treating families as equal and collaborative partners in all aspects of the follow-up evaluation; (3) providing respectful, compassionate care that is individualized to the child and his or her family; and (4) being culturally and socially responsive to the family's needs and values.[27,28] Strategies for engaging and communicating effectively with families are listed in Table 11.3. Existing staff may require training in these family-centered and culturally sensitive practices.

Choice of Assessment Setting

A major challenge of many follow-up programs is nonattendance and/or high attrition or drop-out over time. The listed family engagement strategies may help reduce this (Table 11.3). However, one of the most concerning aspects of poor attendance is that children from socioeconomically disadvantaged family backgrounds tend to be overrepresented among the "no show" group. Yet, as indicated earlier, there are clear data demonstrating that these children tend to be at greatest developmental risk and

therefore most in need of intervention services.[3,11] To address this problem, some services may choose to offer home visits as an alternative or adjunct to their center-based program. In our experience, even a single home visit during the initial stages of follow-up can help establish a relationship with the family and increase long-term family follow-up compliance. Preliminary data also support this.[29]

Deciding Which Measure to Use

While the choice of measures used for different purposes may vary depending on personnel and regional preferences, several factors should be considered. Measures should have strong psychometric properties, including construct validity and test-retest reliability, as well as inter- and intratester reliability. Preference should also be given to well-standardized measures. That is, they should have good norms that are relevant to the local population. To minimize assessment time, abbreviated measures are sometimes appropriate.

Minimizing Measurement Bias

A final issue to be mindful of is to ensure that measurement bias is minimized. This includes two key forms of bias—tester bias and report source bias. Tester bias results from the evaluator not being blind to the infant's/child's clinical record creating the opportunity for pretesting perceptions of the child's performance to be altered. For example, awareness that the child has severe brain injury on neuroimaging may inadvertently influence a tester's expectations of test performance and possibly their behavior toward the child during testing and scoring, that the child will be a poor performer. This bias is particularly important to eliminate in any research evaluations where the tester should always be blinded to the clinical information of the subject being evaluated.

The second form of bias is that of report source bias. Report source bias occurs when information is obtained from a single informant. This is most relevant for reports of child behavior and is applicable to both the clinical and research setting. Reliance on a single report source such as the primary caregiver can be problematic when his or her perceptions of the child are potentially colored by his or her own mental health difficulties (e.g., depression, anxiety), personal situation, past experiences (in the NICU or with another child), or possibly the quality of his or her own relationship with the child. For example, parents of preterm survivors have been found to report much higher rates of attentional problems than teachers, which may in part reflect either their child's behavior and/or their own understandable, but heightened, anxieties about these possible outcomes based on their earlier NICU experience.[30] Thus, ideally when problems are suspected, it is advisable to obtain the perspectives of multiple significant adults in the child's life.

In line with the developmental framework outlined previously, functional neurodevelopmental domains that should form part of a comprehensive follow-up program include (1) *physical health/growth*, (2) *neuromotor function*, (3) *language development*, (4) *cognition and learning*, (5) *emotional and behavioral well-being or mental health*, and (6) *social functioning*. While all domains are discussed, emphasis is placed on those domains most pertinent to neonatal and neurology follow-up. In addition to child neurodevelopmental domains, relevant family characteristics are also addressed. The overall goal is to highlight relevant child and family variables to assess, and how these may change

---

TABLE 11.3   Strategies to Engage and Work Well With Families

Tips to involve families
- Acknowledge arrival or departure.
  - Share a quick but specific detail about the child's progress.
- Communicate often.
  - Regularly scheduled parent/caregiver meetings.
  - Distribute printed materials (such as a newsletter).
  - Learn from families if communication is efficient and effective.
- Offer home visits when appropriate.
- Notify family of workshops, trainings, and family-child groups.
  - Encourage family peer networking.
- Provide resource materials and ideas for activities that families can do at home and in the community with their children.
- Recognize that family involvement is an ongoing process.
  - Learn from families about prior child evaluation and any new expectations in new settings.
- Acknowledge the perspective of the family on their child's strengths and needs.
- Be sensitive to the diversity in home cultures and how communication may need to be affected.
- Host special family events throughout the year at different times of the day to accommodate a variety of family schedules.
- Be sure families are knowledgeable about provider expectations.

Communication tips
- Be a good listener.
- Communicate strengths first.
- Affirm that families understand the message.
- Describe behaviors rather than use labels or diagnoses.
- Allow time for families to think, process, and respond.
- Be sensitive to the emotional needs of the family.
- Ask for feedback.
- Share resource information.
- Ask questions.
- Wonder with families.

Based on National Infant and Child Care Initiative. Supporting infant/toddler: development, screening and assessment. *Zero to Three*, 2016.

in importance with the age of the child. How comprehensive the follow-up is in terms of the number of domains assessed and depth of measurement will likely vary at each time point depending on the purpose, resources, and time available. The following resources may also be helpful.[27,31]

CHILD CHARACTERISTICS

Physical Health/Growth

This domain includes a number of different areas of potential health concern.

Neurological

A thorough neurological examination, including evaluation of the head, cranial nerves, motor, and sensory system should be completed by a physician who is trained in the neurological examination of the infant and child. This would usually be the pediatrician or child neurologist. The most frequent abnormalities that are found in high-risk infants and children relate to tone, power, and coordination.

Vision and Hearing

Major visual and hearing problems are often diagnosed before discharge home. Hearing screening is often universal for most babies before discharge. Eye examinations are also typically routine for high-risk groups, such as those infants born VPT or less than 1500 g in birth weight. Other high-risk groups who may not have had such assessments before discharge might need specialized follow-up by ophthalmologists or audiologists. Therefore general hearing tests and basic visuomotor assessments should be performed routinely as part of neurodevelopmental follow-up during the first 2 years of life. Infants identified to have abnormal visual (i.e., *strabismus*) or hearing function (*failed hearing screen*) should be referred for assessment. In later childhood, more subtle optical problems such as *refractive errors* and *visual processing* disorders occur more frequently in high-risk groups,[32,33] and these problems can interfere with learning.[34] Similarly, hearing disorders other than deafness, such as *short-term auditory memory problems* or *figure-ground perceptual problems* (difficulty hearing in a noisy background), are common among high-risk infants and can also interfere with learning.[35]

Growth

Assessment of height, weight, and head circumference is relevant at all ages, but especially in early life when growth rates are high, and poor growth can be readily detected with growth charts for child age and sex. This is important because poor growth is common in high-risk infants and may be an indicator of underlying health problems. Better postdischarge linear growth is also associated with better neurodevelopmental outcomes. The WHO Child Growth Standards are available at http://www.who.int/childgrowth/standards/en/index.htm. Specific growth charts also exist for some specific populations, such as children with Down syndrome and Turner syndrome. There are also equations available for estimating total height from knee height, which can be helpful if a child is unable to stand up straight for measurement (e.g., children with CP).[36] In general, growth patterns are more important than single growth measurements in monitoring a child's health and

development. Poor growth is common in VPT infants in the NICU, with human milk–fed infants often more affected.[37] For these children, continued supplementation of energy, protein, and minerals is recommended. Human milk–fed infants may also benefit from partial milk fortification. While many of these infants will catch up in their growth by late infancy, a number will continue to have difficulties through late adolescence, with a minority never catching up. An additional complication for some children as their growth slows with age is overweight and obesity. This is likely to be of greatest concern in developed countries where obesity is a public health problem.

Feeding Problems

Children with neurological problems are at increased risk of feeding problems, and therefore may require prolonged tube feeding after discharge. This can lead to heightened oral sensitivity and delays in adaptive feeding skills that may impede the development of healthy eating skills and physical growth. These difficulties are also highly stressful for families and can create interactional difficulties at mealtimes and more generally. Thus evaluation and support of these problems can require specialized speech pathology therapists with additional radiological evaluations.

Daily Functioning

Skills in daily living, also known as adaptive skills, such as with feeding, dressing, toileting, communication, mobility, socialization, and emotional regulation, appropriate for the age of the child, are all important to consider.

Brain Development. The clinical utility of including an MRI as part of a neurodevelopmental follow-up is highly dependent on the expertise of the person reporting and interpreting the MRI. In particular, in the neonatal period, given the inverted contrasts of white and gray matter compared with adult brain MRI, interpretation can be challenging for the inexperienced reader. However, despite these challenges there have been several features of a neonatal MRI at term that have reasonably good predictive value for later neurodevelopmental outcome, and therefore may be worth considering as part of follow-up. *For the preterm-born infant*, the presence of T1 and T2 characteristics of myelin in the internal capsule and/or asymmetry with absence of myelin on term MRI can be a predictor of high risk of hemiplegia CP in the context of focal cerebral white matter (WM) lesions.[38] Isolated diffuse hyperintense signal on T2-weighted neonatal images, although indicative of a higher water content in these areas and potentially a sign of injury, has in subsequent studies not been able to reliably predict neurodevelopmental outcome.[39,40] Presence of signs of moderate to severe WM injury on term equivalent MRI have also been linked with an increased risk of motor and, to a lesser extent, cognitive impairment assessed with the Bayley Scales in infancy and early childhood.[39,41] In later childhood, these children continued to have neurocognitive impairments across multiple cognitive functions, including executive functions.[42,43] In contrast, VPT children without WM abnormalities on term MRI had generally similar motor and cognitive outcomes as their same-age, full-term peers. These data suggest that a term equivalent MRI with clinical scoring of the conventional T1- and T2-weighted MRI newborns may assist in the identification of infants who are at increased risk of neurodevelopmental problems. Combining MRI at term equivalent with a neurological exam and serial cerebral US data further improves predictability for later neurodevelopmental problems.[44,45] In addition, it will be important to also take other aspects of the child's life into account because a child's developmental progress over the course of childhood will also likely depend on a multitude of contextual factors. Therefore a normal MRI should not be grounds to exclude a child from neurodevelopmental follow-up. Finally, for the preterm child, adding brain biometrics such as biparietal diameter, transcerebellar width, and ventricular size may further improve predictability.[46]

For the *term-born infant with HIE*, brain lesions detected on MRI with and without hypothermia have been shown to have good predictive value for neurodevelopmental outcome.[47-50] For example, the absence of impairment in the signal in the posterior limb of the internal capsule has also been shown to be a powerful predictor of motor disability in the term-born infant with encephalopathy.[51]

Finally, in recent years, the development of image-based analysis with a mathematical and informatics-based approach has been impressive, and these techniques have allowed us to study in more detail the brain structure-function relationships relevant for predicting neurodevelopmental outcomes in high-risk newborns. These techniques include brain volumetry,[52-55] diffusion weighted imaging,[53,56,57] and functional network connectivity analysis.[58,59]

Neuromotor Function

CP and delayed motor development are more prevalent in high-risk populations of children compared with the general population, so repeated neurological assessment is important in the early years. CP represents an umbrella term for conditions that are characterized by a nonprogressive, but not unchanging, motor impairment related to brain disturbances that have occurred early in development.[60-62] Between 1% and 3% of all live-born infants are affected by CP, with this rate increasing to 8% to 40% among high-risk infants, such as those born extremely preterm.[63] It is typical for the severe forms of CP to present earlier in childhood, usually within the first year after birth, with disordered tone and tendon reflexes, along with abnormal motor development. These are categorized into (1) spastic—which can be mono-, di-, or quadriplegic; (2) dystonic; and (3) choreoathetoid forms. Milder CP, however, may not be able to be diagnosed conclusively until later ages, sometimes even after the child has started to walk. Any degree of CP should be graded according to the Gross Motor Function Classification System (GMFCS).[64] A recent systematic review describes the prevalence, type, and distribution of CP according to gestational age.[65] Several reviews have also examined the utility of different tools in predicting CP.[66,67] Findings suggest that assessment of general body movements in the first months of life and MRI at term equivalent can be predictive of CP in high-risk infants.

Apart from CP, many high-risk children have delayed motor development during infancy. Therefore monitoring motor milestones is important. Although some children with initial motor delay will catch up, others will have ongoing problems with motor function and coordination. Yet others may be later diagnosed with developmental co-ordination disorder (DCD).[68] Formal evaluation of milder motor dysfunction is typically done by a physical therapist or an occupational therapist. The pooled prevalence of motor impairment in high-risk preterm children without CP is 19% for moderate impairment and 40% for mild-moderate impairment.[68]

Table 11.4 provides a list of motor scales commonly used in the assessment of infants and children. Several of these infant measures are reviewed by Spittle and colleagues, including Prechtl's General Movements Assessments (birth

TABLE 11.4 Developmental Domains and Measures

DOMAIN	TEST	AGE	SCALE(S)
Motor skills			
	Prechtl's General Movement Assessment	0–20 weeks corrected	Gross movements, writhing movements, fidgety movements
	AIMS	0–18 months	Prone, Supine, Sitting, Standing
	TIMP	34 weeks' gestation to 4 months corrected	Postural and selective control of movement needed for functional motor performance
	NSMDA	1 month–6 years	Gross Motor, Fine Motor, Neurological, Primitive Reflexes, Postural Reactions, Sensorimotor Response
	Bayley Scales of Infant and Toddler Development, 3rd edition	1–42 months	Fine Motor, Gross Motor, Motor (Composite)
	MABC, 2nd edition	3:0–16:11 years	Manual Dexterity, Ball Skills, Static and Dynamic Balance
	BOT-2	4:0–21:11	Fine Motor Precision, Fine Motor Integration, Manual Dexterity, Bilateral Coordination, Balance, Running Speed and Agility, Upper-Limb Coordination, Strength
	GMFCS	<2–18 years	Walks without limitations, walks with limitations, walks using a hand-held mobility device, self-mobility with limitations/may use powered mobility, transported in a manual wheelchair

Continued

TABLE 11.4   Developmental Domains and Measures—cont'd

DOMAIN	TEST	AGE	SCALE(S)
Learning and cognition			
Cognitive function	Bayley Scales of Infant and Toddler Development, 3rd edition	1–42 months	Cognitive Development
	Griffith's Mental Development Scales	0–8 years	Locomotor, Personal-Social, Language, Eye and Hand Coordination, Performance, Practical Reasoning
	WISC-V	6:0–16:11	Verbal Comprehension, Visual Spatial, Working Memory, Fluid Reasoning, Processing Speed, Quantitative Reasoning, Auditory Working Memory, Nonverbal, General Ability, Cognitive Proficiency, Naming Speed, Symbol Translation, Storage and Retrieval
	Stanford-Binet Intelligence Scales	2–85+ years	Fluid Reasoning Knowledge, Quantitative Reasoning, Visual-Spatial Processing, Working Memory
	Differential Ability Scales	2:6–17:11 years	Verbal, nonverbal, and spatial reasoning, Working Memory, Processing Speed, School-Readiness
	Kaufman Assessment Battery for Children	3–18 years	Simultaneous (e.g., face recognition, block counting, conceptual thinking), Sequential (e.g., number recall, word order), Planning (e.g., pattern reasoning, story completion), Learning (e.g., Atlantis, Rebus), Knowledge (e.g., riddles, verbal knowledge)
	A Developmental NEPSY-II	3:0–16:11 years	Executive Function and Attention, Language, Memory & Learning, Sensorimotor, Visuospatial Processing, Social Perception
	TEACh	6:0–15:11 years	Selective Attention, Sustained Attention, Attentional Switching
	Children's Memory Scale	5–16 years	Attention and working memory, Verbal and visual memory, Recall and recognition, Learning characteristics
	D-KEFS	8–89 years	Trail-Making, Verbal Fluency, Design Fluency, Color-Word Interference, Sorting, Twenty Questions, Word Context, Tower, Proverb Tests
	BRIEF	2–90 years	Inhibit, Shift, Emotional Control, Initiate, Working Memory, Plan/Organize, Organization of Materials, Monitor, Behavioral Regulation, Metacognition, Global Executive Composite
	MESL	0–68 months	Gross Motor, Visual Reception, Fine Motor, Expressive Language, Receptive Language
	Willoughby/Pek/Blair Executive Function Assessment Battery	3–5 years	Working Memory Span, Pick the Picture, Silly Sounds Stroop, Spatial Conflict, Spatial Conflict Arrows, Animal Go/No-Go, Something's the Same game
	AWMA	4–22 years	Verbal short-term memory (e.g., nonword recall task), verbal working memory (e.g., listening recall, backward digit recall tasks), visuospatial short-term memory (e.g., dot matrix task), visuospatial working memory (e.g., spatial recall task)
Language	Bayley Scales of Infant and Toddler Development, 3rd edition	1–42 months	Receptive Language, Expressive Language, Language (Composite)
	Rossetti Infant-Toddler Language Scale	0–3 years	Interaction-Attachment, Pragmatics, Gesture, Play, Language Comprehension, Language Expression
	MacArthur-Bates CDI-II	8–37 months	Words and Gestures, Words and Sentences, Expressive Vocabulary and Grammar
	PLS	0–7:11 years	Total Language, Auditory Comprehension, Expressive Communication
	CELF-P	3–6 years	Core Language Score, Receptive Language, Expressive Language, Language Content, Language Structure
	CELF-4	5–21 years	Core Language Score, Receptive Language, Expressive Language, Language Structure, Language Content, Language Memory, Working Memory
	TLC-Expanded	5–18 years	Ambiguous Sentences, Listening Comprehension: Making Inferences, Oral Expression: Recreating Speech Acts, Figurative Language

TABLE 11.4   Developmental Domains and Measures—cont'd

DOMAIN	TEST	AGE	SCALE(S)
	CASL	3–21 years	Lexical/Semantic (Basic Concepts, Antonyms, Synonyms, Sentence Completion, Idiomatic Language), Syntactic (Syntax Construction, Paragraph Comprehension, Grammatical Morphemes, Sentence, Comprehension, Grammaticality Judgment), Supralinguistic (Nonliteral Language, Meaning from Context, Inference, Ambiguous Sentences), Pragmatic (awareness of appropriate language in a situational context and ability to modify as necessary)
	REEL-3	0–3 years	Receptive Language, Expressive Language, Inventory of Vocabulary Words
Pre-academic skills	EMDA	Pre-K–3rd Grade	Math Reasoning, Numerical Operations
	ERDA-II	K–3rd grade	Phonological Awareness, Phonics, Fluency, Vocabulary, Comprehension
	PAL-II	K–6th grade	Phonological Decoding, Morphological Decoding, Silent Reading Fluency, Handwriting, Orthographic Spelling, Narrative Compositional Fluency, Expository Note-Taking and Report-Writing, Orthographic Coding, Phonological Coding, Morphologic/Syntactic Coding, Verbal Working Memory, Rapid Automized Naming/Rapid Alternating Stimulus, Oral Motor Planning, Finger Sense, Numerical Writing, Numeric Coding, Kinesthetic Sense, Working Memory, Sequential Ordering, Basic Arithmetic, Math Operations, Computation Operations, Relationships, Problem-Solving
Academic progress	WIAT	4:0–50:11 years	Oral Reading, Math Fluency, Early Reading Skills, Listening Comprehension, Oral Expression, Written Expression, Reading Comprehension, Sentence Composition
	WRAT4	5–94 years	Word Reading, Reading Comprehension, Spelling, Math Computation, Reading Composite
	WJ IV Tests of ECAD	2:6–7:11 years	General intellectual ability, early academic skills, expressive language skills
Mental health			
Autism	M-CHAT	16–30 months	Autism Spectrum Disorders symptoms
	GARS-3	3–22 years	Restrictive/Repetitive Behaviors, Social Interaction, Social Communication, Emotional Responses, Cognitive Style, Maladaptive Speech
	SCQ	≥4 years	Reciprocal Social Interaction; Communication; Restricted, Repetitive, and Stereotyped Patterns of Behavior
	SRS	4–18 years	Receptive, Cognitive, Expressive, and Motivational aspects of social behavior; Autistic Preoccupations
	ADOS-2	12 months–adulthood	Autism Spectrum Disorders symptoms measured with a series of tasks (e.g., construction, make-believe, joint interaction, conversation and reporting, creating a story, demonstration)
	RITA-T	<3 years	Joint attention, Social awareness, Awareness of human agency, Self-recognition, Fundamental cognitive skill
ADHD	Brown Attention Deficit Disorder Scales for Children and Adolescents	3–18 years	Organizing, Prioritizing and Activating to Work; Focusing, Sustaining and Shifting Attention to Tasks; Regulating Alertness, Sustaining Effort and Processing Speed; Managing Frustration and Modulating Emotions; Utilizing Working Memory and Accessing Recall; Monitoring and Self-Regulating Action
	Conners 3rd edition	6–18 years	Hyperactivity/Impulsivity, Executive Functioning, Learning Problems, Aggression, Peer Relations
Psychopathology	PAPA	2–5 years	Family Structure and Function; Play, Peer, and Sibling Relationships; Daycare/School Experiences; Behaviors/Food Related Behaviors; Sleep Behaviors; Elimination Problems; Somatization; Accidents; Oppositional Defiant Disorder/Conduct Disorder; ADHD; Separation Anxiety; Anxious Affect; Worries; Rituals and Repetitions; Tics; Stereotypes; Reactive Attachment; Depression; Mania; Dysregulation; Life Events; PTSD; Disabilities; Parental Psychopathology; Marital Satisfaction; Socioeconomic Status

Continued

TABLE 11.4   Developmental Domains and Measures—cont'd

DOMAIN	TEST	AGE	SCALE(S)
	DAWBA	5–17 years	Social Aptitudes, Emotion, Hyperactivity, Conduct, Peer, Prosocial
	DICA-IV; DICA-PPYC	6–17 years; 3–7 years	Semistructured diagnostic interview used to assess DSM-IV disorders (e.g., attention-deficit/hyperactivity disorder, major depressive disorder, posttraumatic stress disorder) and risk factors (e.g., conduct disorder, substance use)
	ChIPS	6–18 years	DSM disorders (e.g., ADHD, oppositional defiant disorder, phobias, anxiety disorders, eating disorders, schizophrenia/psychosis)
	SCID	Wide age range	DSM-V disorders
	CBCL	1.5–18 years	Syndrome Scales (Emotionally Reactive, Anxious/Depressed, Somatic Complaints, Withdrawn, Sleep Problems, Attention Problems, Aggressive Behavior), DSM-Oriented Scales (Depressive Problems, Anxiety Problems, Autism Spectrum Problems, Attention Deficit/Hyperactivity Problems, Oppositional Defiant Problems), Internalizing Problems, Externalizing Problems, Total Problems
Risk-taking	HEADSS framework (structured interview)	12–18 years	Home & Environment, Education & Employment, Activities, Drugs, Sexuality, Suicide/Depression
Family			
Parental mental health	GHQ	Wide age range	Screens for common mental disorders and assesses psychiatric well-being generally, including anxiety and depression, social dysfunction, and loss of confidence
	CES-D-R	Wide age range	Depression symptoms (dysphoria, anhedonia, appetite, sleep, thinking/concentration, guilt/worthlessness, fatigue, agitation, suicidal ideation)
	HAM-D, -A	Wide age range	Depression symptoms (sadness, guilt, suicidal ideation, sleep, functionality, psychomotor retardation, agitation, anxiety, somatic and sexual symptoms, weight), depersonalization, paranoia, obsessive/compulsive symptoms; psychic anxiety (mental agitation and psychological distress) and somatic anxiety (physical complaints related to anxiety)
	EPDS	Wide age range	Depression symptoms (anhedonia, self-blame, anxiety, panic, feeling overwhelmed, sleep, sadness, tearfulness, thoughts of self-harm)
	SCID	Wide age range	DSM-V disorders
	STAI	Wide age range	Chronic (trait) and acute (state) anxiety
	IES	Wide age range	Subjective distress caused by traumatic events; yields a total score and Intrusion, Avoidance, and Hyperarousal subscale scores
Caregiver-child interaction	CARE-Index	0–24 months	Maternal sensitivity, control, and unresponsiveness; infant cooperativeness, compulsivity, difficultness, passivity

ADOS-2, Autism Diagnostic Observation Schedule, 2nd edition; *AIMS,* Alberta infant motor scale; *AWMA,* Automated Working Memory Assessment; *BOT-2,* Bruininks-Oseretsky Test of Motor Proficiency, 2nd edition; *BRIEF,* Behavior Rating Inventory of Executive Function; *CASL,* Comprehensive Assessment of Spoken Language; *CBCL,* Child Behavior Checklist; *CDI-II,* Communicative Development Inventories; *CELF-4,* Clinical Evaluation of Language Fundamentals, 4th edition; *CELF-P,* Clinical Evaluation of Language Fundamentals—Preschool; *CES-D-R,* Center for Epidemiologic Studies, Revised; *ChIPS,* Children's Interview for Psychiatric Syndromes; *DAWBA,* Development and Well-Being Assessment; *DICA,* Diagnostic Interview for Children and Adolescents; *DICA-PPYC,* DICA for Parents of Preschool and Young Children; *D-KEFS,* Delis-Kaplan Executive Function System; *ECAD,* Early Cognitive and Academic Development; *EMDA,* Early Math Diagnostic Assessment; *EPDS,* Edinburgh Postpartum Depression Scale; *ERDA-II,* Early Reading Diagnostic Assessment; *GARS-3,* Gilliam Autism Rating Scale, 3rd edition; *GHQ,* General Health Questionnaire; *GMFCS,* Gross Motor Function Classification System; *HAM-D, -A,* Hamilton Scales of Depression/Anxiety; *IES,* Impact of Event Scale; *MABC,* Movement Assessment Battery for Children; *M-CHAT,* Modified Checklist for Autism in Toddlers; *MESL,* Mullen Scales of Early Learning; *NEPSY-II,* NEuroPSYchological Assessment; *NSMDA,* Neuro-Sensory Motor Development Assessment; *PAL-II,* Process Assessment of the Learner; *PAPA,* Preschool Age Psychiatric Assessment; *PLS,* Preschool Language Scales; *REEL-3,* Receptive-Expressive Emergent Language Test—3rd edition; *RITA-T,* Rapid Interactive screening Test for Autism in Toddlers; *SCID,* Structured Clinical Interview for DSM Disorders; *SCID,* Structured Clinical Interview for DSM Disorders; *SCQ,* Social Communication Questionnaire; *SRS,* Social Responsiveness Scale; *STAI,* State-Trait Anxiety Inventory; *TEACh,* Test of Everyday Attention for Children; *TIMP,* Test of Infant Motor Performance; *TLC-Expanded,* Test of Language Competence—Expanded Edition; *WIAT,* Wechsler Individual Achievement Test; *WISC-V,* Wechsler Intelligence Scale for Children, 5th edition; *WJ,* The Woodcock-Johnson; *WRAT4,* Wide Range Achievement Test.

to 20 weeks, corrected for prematurity),[69,70] the Test of Infant Motor Performance (TIMP, 34 weeks to 4 months corrected age),[71-73] Alberta Infant Motor Scale (AIMS, 0 to 18 months),[74] the Neuro-Sensory Motor Development Assessment (NSMDA, 1 month to 6 years),[75] and the motor subscale of the Bayley Scales of Infant and Toddler Development (BTSID, 1 to 42 months).[76] General movements and the TIMP are most useful in the first few months of life, with the AIMS, NSMDA, and Bayley being better from around 4 months upward. In older children, the Movement Assessment Battery for Children

(MABC, 3 to 16 years) tends to be the most widely used motor assessment tool, assessing both fine and gross motor abilities.[77]

Language Development

Language is one of the primary modes by which children communicate and interact with the world. Good language skills provide a vital foundation for social competence,[78] learning,[79,80] and school success.[81] Even relatively small deviations in language development during early childhood can increase children's longer-term educational and social risks. Thus it is essential that early language skills be assessed to ensure early detection of language impairment because earlier treatment has been linked with improved long-term outcomes.[82,83]

Language begins to develop even before birth, with newborn infants already able to recognize their mother's voice. From birth, language development is complex and increases rapidly in a very experience-dependent way. In early childhood, children's language skills are typically divided into *expressive* (what the child says) and *receptive language* skills (what the child can understand). Typically, receptive language skills develop earlier than expressive skills. However, as children grow older, their language abilities become increasingly differentiated and can be classified into semantics, grammar, phonological awareness, discourse, and pragmatics. *Semantics* refers to the meaning of words and sentences. *Grammar* refers to the structure of language, such as the order of words and the use of different tenses. Semantics is usually operationalized as vocabulary or the number of words a child has, and has been shown to predict intelligence.[84] *Phonological awareness* refers to the understanding of speech sounds, which is important for reading. *Discourse* refers to an individual's ability to process and extract the overall message from a conversation or passage of text that requires the integration of information across sentences for a coherent understanding. Finally, *pragmatics* refers to the ability to use language that is appropriate to the conversational or social context. For a review of the language outcomes of children born VPT, see Barre et al.[85] Table 11.4 also provides a summary of infant and child language measures that are available for the assessment of language development at different ages. At early ages, the most commonly used measures include the MacArthur-Bates Communication Development Inventories (CDI-II, 8 to 37 months), the Preschool Language Scales (PLS, birth to 8 years), Receptive-Expressive Emergent Language Test (REEL 3, birth to 3 years), and the language subscale of the BSITD (6 to 42 months).[76] At older ages, the Clinical Evaluation of Language Fundamental preschool (CELF-P, 3 to 6 years) and school age versions (CELF, 5 to 21 years) represent reliable and valid tools.

Cognition and Learning

Cognitive development will be a major component of any clinical or research follow-up assessment because it is one of the most common adverse outcomes experienced by many high-risk infants. It is also relevant at all ages. For example, around a third of infants born VPT will be subject to cognitive delay.[86-89] A number of skills fall within this domain, spanning general cognition or IQ, executive functions, and specific educational abilities such as literacy and numeracy. There is considerable inter- and intraindividual variability in the rate at which children acquire these skills with age. This is especially so in the first 3

to 4 years of life. As a result, it is often difficult to discriminate between mild delays and normal variations in development during this period, whereas there tends to be greater certainty in the detection of cases of severe delay. Mild delay is typically defined as a standardized cognitive or IQ score that is <1 SD below the normative mean but greater than or equal to 2 SDs, whereas severe delay is defined as a standardized cognitive score >2 SD below the normative test mean.

In infancy and toddlerhood, assessment tools tend to focus on general cognitive abilities with the aim of identifying those showing early delay. The most commonly used measures are the BSITD (1 to 42 months) and at earlier ages of the test range, the Griffiths Mental Development Scales, extended revised (birth to 8 years). Sometimes the Mullen Scales of Early Learning (MSEL, birth to 68 months) may be used if a child has limited verbal skills (i.e., a child with Down syndrome or who is on the autistic spectrum). However, this is an older test with somewhat outdated norms and less psychometric data to support its use.

At preschool age and beyond, assessment tools tend to become more specific, reflecting the increased cognitive capabilities of the child. This allows a child's cognitive strengths and vulnerabilities across different cognitive domains to be characterized. Cognitive tests start to be able to differentiate between verbal and spatial cognitive skills, as well as quantify specific cognitive abilities such as memory, attention, executive functioning, and information processing. In terms of global cognitive function, a variety of standardized IQ tests are available, assessing intellectual functioning from about 2.5 years. The most commonly used are the Wechsler scales, which have the advantage of having preschool (4 to 6.5 years), child (6 to 16 years), and adult versions, as well as complementary academic achievement tests (discussed later). Other measures of general intellectual functioning include the Stanford-Binet Intelligence Scales, Differential Ability Scales, and the Kaufman Assessment Battery for Children. For measures such as the Wechsler Scales, abbreviated versions exist, which may be useful for screening and/or research purposes. In addition to these general cognitive measures, there are a number of neuropsychological test batteries and tools for assessing children's risk of memory, executive function, and processing deficits.

Executive functions are a set of interrelated skills that enable an individual to manage, self-regulate, and engage in goal-directed behavior that have been shown to be predictive of educational achievement.[10,90,91] They include inhibitory control, working memory, and cognitive flexibility, as well as more complex planning and organized search abilities that require the integrated coordination of these core components. Until recently, most of these tests were only suitable for school-age children. However, there have been several neuropsychological and/or executive function test batteries developed in recent years. These include the Developmental NEuroPSYchological (NEPSY) assessment (3 to 16:11 years) and a computerized and paper-based executive function battery for preschool children (approximately 3 to 5 years).[92-95] A further measure is the Delis-Kaplan Executive Function System (8 to 89 years).[96] The Test of Everyday Attention (TEACH) is also useful for the assessment of attention from 6 to 15 years,[97] with other approaches reviewed by Mahone and Schneider.[98] Parent completed questionnaire measures are also available, such as the Childhood Executive Functioning Inventory (CHEXI, age range)[99] and the Behavior Rating of Executive

Function scale (BRIEF, with a preschool and school age version, age range 2 to 90 years),[100] although there is some suggestion that these measures may more strongly correlate with child behavior ratings than executive function test performance.[101] In terms of memory measures, one possibility is the Children's Memory Scale (4 to 22 years),[102] which assesses memory and learning in children from 5 to 16 years.

Prior to school entry, an assessment of school readiness is appropriate. The School Readiness Framework recommended by the AAP identifies five key "readiness to learn" domains, spanning physical well-being and motor development, social and emotional development, approaches to learning, communication skills, and general knowledge and cognition.[103] As can be seen, these largely mirror the major domains discussed here. The purpose of a school readiness assessment is *not* to ascertain whether a child should be able to go to school, but rather to determine what resources and supports he or she may need to ensure his or her transition is a successful one. Using this framework, several studies have shown that around 60% of children born VPT will be delayed or impaired in at least one readiness domain, with 44% to 47% subject to difficulties in multiple domains.[24,104] Importantly, the number of readiness domains affected before school entry has been shown to be a strong predictor of later educational risk up to age 9, with two or more affected readiness domains as an effective criterion for referral for educational surveillance and/or additional support during the transition to school.[24] Specifically, over three quarters of VPT children who showed problems in at least two school readiness domains were delayed at school by age 6 and 9 years (OR = 10.6 at age 6 and 7.4 at age 9). These findings clearly demonstrate the importance of a school readiness assessment to enable the early identification of those at high risk of later learning problems who would benefit from closer educational surveillance and/or proactive support. Depending on the resources available, educational referral for VPT children with problems in either one or multiple school readiness domains may be warranted.[24] In addition to assessing a child's developmental needs, it is also important as part of this check-up to consider family and school factors that may also affect his or her educational potential, such as the readiness of the school for the child and the extent of family/community psychosocial adversity.

At school age, numeracy and literacy should be assessed at regular intervals to ensure adequate progress in these areas.[105,106] The extent of this may depend on how much is done and the tools used within the local education system. Examples of academic achievement tests are listed in Table 11.4, with perhaps the most common being the Wechsler Individual Achievement Test (WIAT, >4 years), the Woodcock-Johnson Tests of Achievement (>2 years), and the Wide Range Achievement Test (WRAT4, >5 years). Input from teachers should also be sought, such as through the use of Teacher Assessment of Academic Skills. Children with significant cognitive or learning disorders should receive individualized educational programming so that they can achieve their "personal best," rather than constantly being compared with their peers.

Emotional and Behavioral Well-Being or Mental Health

Infants who are born VPT, who have a neurological abnormality, who have high medical needs, or who have spent a long time in the hospital are particularly prone to these behavioral and mental health disturbances.[107-111] The phenotypic presentation of mental health difficulties varies considerably with child age, but is relevant at all developmental stages. In early life, difficulties tend to manifest as emotional and behavioral regulatory problems, including difficulty soothing, consoling, and settling to sleep; high levels of negative affect in the form of irritability and excessive crying; and disorganized behavior indicated by rapid state changes. Toward the end of the first year and into the second year, some infants may demonstrate signs of delayed language development and social unresponsiveness, which could be an early indication of the presence of autism spectrum disorder. For example, limited interest in interacting with people/objects or exploring the environment, reacting strongly without reason, lack of gestures to communicate (i.e., pointing; joint attention), and appearing fearful or on guard may be a signal for concern. However, accurate assessment and diagnosis tends to be challenging in neurologically at-risk children. There are several reasons for this, including the fact that many of these behaviors are relatively common in very young children, there is considerable interindividual variability within the general population, and also the presence of developmental disability and impairment may confound a mental health diagnosis. Later in life other psychopathologies, such as ADHD, and other externalizing behaviors evolve, along with mood and anxiety, and other internalizing disorders. In the teenage years and later, a small minority may be at risk for major psychiatric disorders.[112] The Diagnostic Classification of Mental Health and Developmental Disorders of Infancy and Early Childhood (DC-05) provides a framework for the prevention, diagnosis, and treatment of mental health problems from 0 to 5 years. At older ages, the DSM-5 is used.

Table 11.4 provides an overview of measures used to assess socioemotional adjustment and/or mental health in infants and children. Several reviews may also be helpful.[113] In terms of a behavioral screening questionnaire that can be completed by significant adults in a child's life, one of the earliest that can be used is the Infant-Toddler Social and Emotional Assessment (ITSEA). This parent-completed scale provides a measure of children's social, emotional, and behavioral problems and competencies and is suitable for use with children between the ages of 12 and 36 months. A short form is also available that provides less information but is very quick to administer. As shown in Table 11.4, other widely used screening measures include the Strengths and Difficulties Questionnaire (SDQ), which has the advantage of being free, brief (and acceptable) to parents, and with good psychometric properties,[114-118] the Child Behavior Checklist,[119] and the Behavioral Assessment System for Children (BASC-2),[120] which have both preschool and child versions.

In addition to these screening measures, several psychiatric interview tools exist for making more in-depth mental health diagnoses, such as anxiety, depression, other internalizing disorders, conduct disorder, major psychiatric illnesses (especially psychosis), autism, ADHD, or obsessive compulsive disorder. These include the Development and Well-Being Assessment (DAWBA: 5 to 17 years),[121] which can be used in conjunction with the SDQ, the Diagnostic Interview for Children and Adolescents (DICA-IV),[122,123] and the Children's Interview for Psychiatric Syndromes (ChIPS: 6 to 18 years).[124] Specific tools for assessing autism risk include the Modified

Checklist for Autism in Toddlers,[125-128] which is useful in screening for autism between 16 and 30 months. For older children, autism screeners include the Gilliam Autism Rating Scale (GARS-2), the Social Communication Questionnaire (SCQ: 4+ years), and the Social Responsiveness Scale (SRS: 4 to 18 years). If concerns are suspected on these screening measures, the next step is usually to administer a diagnostic tool such as the Autism Diagnostic Observation Schedule (ADOS).[129]

Social Development

A related but important aspect of a child's development concerns how he or she gets along with his or her peers and whether he or she is able to form close friendships with other children of the same age. Good social skills are crucial for integration into the peer group. Yet unfortunately for many children with neurodevelopmental problems and their families, this can be an area of anxiety and concern. For example, VPT children often differ physically (e.g., small stature) and psychologically (e.g., shyness, poor attention, lower cognitive abilities) from their peers. This can place them at increased risk of being socially excluded and bullied. These experiences can be extremely distressing, limit social and educational opportunities, and increase their long-term risk.[130] Therefore it is important to include some consideration of the child's experiences and interactions with peers as part of any neurodevelopmental evaluation.

Parental Well-Being and Family Situation

In addition to reviewing a child's developmental progress, it is important to collect information about how the family is coping and any difficulties they may be experiencing, with either the child or other matters that might be affecting the parents' ability to care for their child. This should include information about the family living situation, economic resources, parental mental health, parenting strategies and the quality of parent-child relations, social supports, and family relations in general (e.g., interpartner agreement on child behavior management, child-sibling relations, and family cohesion). This is relevant at all ages, but will be especially helpful soon after birth and discharge home, because this is a time when difficulties are often experienced and parents are most receptive to help. Parental mental well-being is also vital for the establishment of a nurturing and supportive parent-infant relationship.

REFERENCES

1. Aylward GP. Neurodevelopmental outcomes of infants born prematurely. *J Dev Behav Pediatr.* 2014;35:394-407.
2. Marlow N. Outcome following extremely preterm birth. *Curr Paediatr.* 2004;14:275-283.
3. Braveman P, Barclay C. Health disparities beginning in childhood: a life-course perspective. *Pediatrics.* 2009;124:S163-S175.
4. Leve LD, Cicchetti D. Longitudinal transactional models of development and psychopathology. *Dev Psychopathol.* 2016;28:621-622.
5. Cicchetti D, Cannon TD. Neurodevelopmental processes in the ontogenesis and epigenesis of psychopathology. *Dev Psychopathol.* 1999;11:375-393.
6. O'Donnell KJ, Meaney MJ. Fetal Origins of mental health: the developmental origins of health and disease hypothesis. *Am J Psychiatry.* 2017;174:319-328.
7. Seabrook JA, Avison WR. Socioeconomic status and cumulative disadvantage processes across the life course: implications for health outcomes. *Can Rev Sociol.* 2012;49:50-68.
8. Bick J, Nelson CA. Early experience and brain development. *Wiley Interdisc Rev Cogn Sci.* 2017;8:doi:10.1002/wcs.1387.
9. Brown TT, Jernigan TL. Brain development during the preschool years. *Neuropsychol Rev.* 2012;22:313-333.
10. Clark CA, Woodward LJ. Relation of perinatal risk and early parenting to executive control at the transition to school. *Dev Sci.* 2015;18:525-542.
11. Mangin KS, Horwood LJ, Woodward LJ. Cognitive Development Trajectories of Very Preterm and Typically Developing Children. *Child Dev.* 2017;88:282-298.
12. Britto PR, Lye SJ, Proulx K, et al. Nurturing care: promoting early childhood development. *Lancet.* 2017;389:91-102.
13. Forcada-Guex M, Pierrehumbert B, Borghini A, Moessinger A, Muller-Nix C. Early dyadic patterns of mother–infant interactions and outcomes of prematurity at 18 months. *Pediatrics.* 2006;118:e107-e114.
14. Landry SH, Smith KE, Swank PR. Responsive parenting: establishing early foundations for social, communication, and independent problem-solving skills. *Dev Psychol.* 2006;42:627-642.
15. Power JD, Schlaggar BL. Neural plasticity across the lifespan. *Wiley Interdiscip Rev Dev Biol.* 2017;6:doi:10.1002/wdev.216.
16. Sameroff A, Chandler M. Reproductive risk and the continuum of caretaking causality. In: Horowitz F, ed. *Review of Child Development Research.* Vol 4. Chicago: University of Chicago Press; 1975:187-244.
17. Doyle LW, Anderson PJ, Battin M, et al. Long term follow up of high risk children: who, why and how? *BMC Pediatr.* 2014;14:279.
18. American Academy of Pediatrics. Follow-up care of high-risk infants. *Pediatrics.* 2004;114:1377-1397.
19. Anderson PJ, De Luca CR, Hutchinson E, Roberts G, Doyle LW. Underestimation of developmental delay by the new Bayley-III Scale. *Arch Pediatr Adolesc Med.* 2010;164:352-356.
20. Wilson-Ching M, Pascoe L, Doyle LW, Anderson PJ. Effects of correcting for prematurity on cognitive test scores in childhood. *J PaediatrChild Health.* 2014;50:182-188.
21. Wong HS, Santhakumaran S, Cowan FM, Modi N. Developmental assessments in preterm children: a meta-analysis. *Pediatrics.* 2016;138:pii: e20160251.
22. Spencer-Smith MM, Spittle AJ, Lee KJ, Doyle LW, Anderson PJ. Bayley-III Cognitive and Language Scales in Preterm Children. *Pediatrics.* 2015;135:e1258-e1265.
23. Spittle AJ, Spencer-Smith MM, Eeles AL, et al. Does the Bayley-III Motor Scale at 2 years predict motor outcome at 4 years in very preterm children? *Dev Med Child Neurol.* 2013;55:448-452.
24. Pritchard VE, Bora S, Austin NC, Levin KJ, Woodward LJ. Identifying very preterm children at educational risk using a school readiness framework. *Pediatrics.* 2014;134:e825-e832.
25. Williams L. Impact of family-centered care on pediatric and neonatal intensive care outcomes. *AACN Adv Crit Care.* 2016;27:158-161.
26. Brousseau DC, Hoffmann RG, Nattinger AB, Flores G, Zhang Y, Gorelick M. Quality of primary care and subsequent pediatric emergency department utilization. *Pediatrics.* 2007;119:1131-1138.
27. American Academy of Pediatrics. Patient- and family-centered care and the pediatrician's role. *Pediatrics.* 2012;129:394-404.
28. Davidson JE, Aslakson RA, Long AC, et al. Guidelines for family-centered care in the neonatal, pediatric, and adult ICU. *Crit Care Med.* 2017;45:103-128.
29. Vohr B, McGowan E, Keszler L, et al. Impact of a Transition Home Program on Rehospitalization Rates of Preterm Infants. *J Pediatr.* 2017;181:86-92.e81.
30. Bora S, Pritchard VE, Moor S, Austin NC, Woodward LJ. Emotional and behavioural adjustment of children born very preterm at early school age. *J Paediatr Child Health.* 2011;47:863-869.
31. Committee on Practice and Ambulatory Medicine and Bright Futures Periodicity Schedule Workgroup. 2015 Recommendations for Preventive Pediatric Health Care. *Pediatrics.* 2015;136:e727-e729.
32. Molloy CS, Wilson-Ching M, Anderson VA, Roberts G, Anderson PJ, Doyle LW. Visual processing in adolescents born extremely low birth weight and/or extremely preterm. *Pediatrics.* 2013;132:e704-e712.

33. Darlow BA, Clemett RS, Horwood LJ, Mogridge N. Prospective study of New Zealand infants with birth weight less than 1500 g and screened for retinopathy of prematurity: visual outcome at age 7-8 years. *Br J Ophthalmol.* 1997;81:935-940.

34. Molloy CS, Di Battista AM, Anderson VA, et al. The contribution of visual processing to academic achievement in adolescents born extremely preterm or extremely low birth weight. *Child Neuropsychol.* 2017;23:361-379.

35. Davis NM, Doyle LW, Ford GW, et al. Auditory function at 14 years of age of very-low-birthweight. *Dev Med Child Neurol.* 2001;43:191-196.

36. Bell K, Davis P, Boyd R, Stevenson R. Use of segmental lengths for the assessment of growth in children with cerebral palsy. In: *Handbook of Anthropometry: Physical Measures of Human Form in Health and Disease.* New York: Springer; 2012 doi:10.1007/978-1-4419-1788-1_78.

37. Belfort M. Nutritional managment of preterm infants post-discharge. In: Duggan C, Watkins JB, Koletzko B, Walker WA, eds. *Nutrition in Pediatrics.* 5th ed. Hamilton: B.C. Decker; 2016.

38. De Vries L, Groenendaal F, van Haastert IC, Eken P, Rademaker KJ, Meiners LC. Asymmetrical myelination of the posterior limb of the internal capsule in infants with periventricular haemorrhagic infarction: an early predictor of hemiplegia. *Neuropediatrics.* 1999;30:314-319.

39. Kidokoro H, Anderson PJ, Doyle LW, Woodward LJ, Neil JJ, Inder TE. Brain injury and altered brain growth in preterm infants: predictors and prognosis. *Pediatrics.* 2014;134:e444-e453.

40. Leitner Y, Weinstein M, Myers V, et al. Diffuse excessive high signal intensity in low-risk preterm infants at term-equivalent age does not predict outcome at 1 year: a prospective study. *Neuroradiology.* 2014;56:669-678.

41. Woodward LJ, Anderson PJ, Austin NC, Howard K, Inder TE. Neonatal MRI to predict neurodevelopmental outcomes in preterm infants. *N Engl J Med.* 2006;355:685-694.

42. Woodward LJ, Clark CA, Bora S, Inder TE. Neonatal white matter abnormalities an important predictor of neurocognitive outcome for very preterm children. *PLoS ONE.* 2012;7:e51879.

43. Woodward LJ, Clark CA, Pritchard VE, Anderson PJ, Inder TE. Neonatal white matter abnormalities predict global executive function impairment in children born very preterm. *Dev Neuropsychol.* 2011;36:22-41.

44. Leijser LM, de Bruïne FT, van der Grond J, Steggerda SJ, Walther FJ, van Wezel-Meijler G. Is sequential cranial ultrasound reliable for detection of white matter injury in very preterm infants? *Neuroradiology.* 2010;52:397-406.

45. Setänen S, Lahti K, Lehtonen L, et al. Neurological examination combined with brain MRI or cranial US improves prediction of neurological outcome in preterm infants. *Early Hum Dev.* 2014;90:851-856.

46. Melbourne L, Murnick J, Chang T, Glass P, Massaro AN. Regional Brain Biometrics at Term-Equivalent Age and Developmental Outcome in Extremely Low-Birth-Weight Infants. *Am J Perinatol.* 2015;32:1177-1184.

47. de Vries LS, van Haastert IC, Benders MJ, Groenendaal F. Myth: cerebral palsy cannot be predicted by neonatal brain imaging. *Semin Fetal Neonatal Med.* 2011;16:279-287.

48. L'Abee C, de Vries LS, van der Grond J, Groenendaal F. Early diffusion-weighted MRI and 1H-Magnetic Resonance Spectroscopy in asphyxiated full-term neonates. *Biol Neonate.* 2005;88:306-312.

49. Massaro AN. MRI for neurodevelopmental prognostication in the high-risk term infant. *Semin Perinatol.* 2015;39:159-167.

50. Goergen SK, Ang H, Wong F, et al. Early MRI in term infants with perinatal hypoxic-ischaemic brain injury: interobserver agreement and MRI predictors of outcome at 2 years. *Clin Radiol.* 2014;69:72-81.

51. Martinez-Biarge M, Diez-Sebastian J, Wusthoff CJ, et al. Feeding and communication impairments in infants with central grey matter lesions following perinatal hypoxic-ischaemic injury. *Eur J Paediatr Neurol.* 2012;16:688-696.

52. Inder TE, Warfield SK, Wang H, Hüppi PS, Volpe JJ. Abnormal cerebral structure is present at term in premature infants. *Pediatrics.* 2005;115:286-294.

53. Boardman JP, Craven C, Valappil S, et al. A common neonatal image phenotype predicts adverse neurodevelopmental outcome in children born preterm. *Neuroimage.* 2010;52:409-414.

54. Dubois J, Benders M, Borradori-Tolsa C, et al. Primary cortical folding in the human newborn: an early marker of later functional development. *Brain.* 2008;131:2028-2041.

55. Peterson BS. Brain imaging studies of the anatomical and functional consequences of preterm birth for human brain development. *Ann N Y Acad Sci.* 2003;1008:219-237.

56. Drobyshevsky A, Bregman J, Storey P, et al. Serial diffusion tensor imaging detects white matter changes that correlate with motor outcome in premature infants. *Dev Neurosci.* 2007;29:289-301.

57. Kwon SH, Vasung L, Ment LR, Hüppi PS. The role of neuroimaging in predicting neurodevelopmental outcomes of preterm neonates. *Clini Perinatol.* 2014;41:257-283.

58. Muñoz-Moreno E, Fischi-Gomez E, Batalle D, et al. Structural brain network reorganization and social cognition related to adverse perinatal condition from infancy to early adolescence. *Front Neurosci.* 2016;10:560.

59. Smyser CD, Neil JJ. Use of resting-state functional MRI to study brain development and injury in neonates. *Semin Perinatol.* 2015;39:130-140.

60. Bax MC. Terminology and Classification of Cerebral Palsy. *Dev Med Child Neurol.* 1964;6:295-297.

61. Bax MC, Flodmark O, Tydeman C. Definition and classification of cerebral palsy. From syndrome toward disease. *Dev Med Child Neurol Suppl.* 2007;109:39-41.

62. Rosenbaum P, Paneth N, Leviton A, et al. A report: the definition and classification of cerebral palsy April 2006. *Dev Med Child Neurol Suppl.* 2007;109:8-14.

63. Serenius F, Källen K, Blennow M, et al. Neurodevelopmental outcome in extremely preterm infants at 2.5 years after active perinatal care in Sweden. *JAMA.* 2013;309:1810-1820.

64. Palisano R, Rosenbaum P, Walter S, Russell D, Wood E, Galuppi B. Development and reliability of a system to classify gross motor function in children with cerebral palsy. *Dev Med Child Neurol.* 1997;39:214-223.

65. Himpens E, Van den Broeck C, Oostra A, Calders P, Vanhaesebrouck P. Prevalence, type, distribution, and severity of cerebral palsy in relation to gestational age: a meta-analytic review. *Dev Med Child Neurol.* 2008;50:334-340.

66. Bosanquet M, Copeland L, Ware R, Boyd R. A systematic review of tests to predict cerebral palsy in young children. *Dev Med Child Neurol.* 2013;55:418-426.

67. Hadders-Algra M. Early diagnosis and early intervention in cerebral palsy. *Front Neurol.* 2014;5:185.

68. Williams J, Lee KJ, Anderson PJ. Prevalence of motor-skill impairment in preterm children who do not develop cerebral palsy: a systematic review. *Dev Med Child Neurol.* 2010;52:232-237.

69. Einspieler C, Prechtl HF, Ferrari F, Cioni G, Bos AF. The qualitative assessment of general movements in preterm, term and young infants–review of the methodology. *Early Hum Dev.* 1997;50:47-60.

70. Prechtl HF, Einspieler C, Cioni G, Bos AF, Ferrari F, Sontheimer D. An early marker for neurological deficits after perinatal brain lesions. *Lancet.* 1997;349:1361-1363.

71. Campbell SK, Kolobe TH, Osten ET, Lenke M, Girolami GL. Construct validity of the test of infant motor performance. *Phys Ther.* 1995;75:585-596.

72. Campbell SK, Zawacki L, Rankin KM, et al. Concurrent validity of the TIMP and the Bayley III scales at 6 weeks corrected age. *Pediatr Phys Ther.* 2013;25:395-401.

73. Ustad T, Helbostad JL, Campbell SK, et al. Test-retest reliability of the Test of Infant Motor Performance Screening Items in infants at risk for impaired functional motor performance. *Early Hum Dev.* 2016;93:43-46.

74. Piper MC, Darrah J. *Motor Assessment of the Developing Infant.* Philadelphia: WB Saunders; 1994.

75. Burns YR, Ensbey RM, Norrie MA. The neuro-sensory motor developmental assessment part 1: development and administration of the test. *Aust J Physiother.* 1989;35:141-149.

76. Bayley N; 2006. *Bayley Scales of Infant and Toddler Development—Third Edition.* San Antonio: Harcourt Assessment Inc..

77. Schulz J, Henderson SE, Sugden DA, Barnett AL. Structural validity of the movement ABC-2 test: factor structure comparisons across three age groups. *Res Dev Disabil.* 2011;32:1361-1369.

78. Durkin K, Conti-Ramsden G. Language, social behavior, and the quality of friendships in adolescents with and without a history of specific language impairment. *Child Dev.* 2007;78:1441-1457.

79. Koponen T, Mononen R, Räsänen P, Ahonen T. Basic numeracy in children with specific language impairment: heterogeneity and connections to language. *J Speech Lang Hear Res.* 2006;49:58-73.

80. Kelso K, Fletcher J, Lee P. Reading comprehension in children with specific language impairment: an examination of two subgroups. *Int J Lang Commun Disord.* 2007;42:39-57.

81. Bashir AS, Scavuzzo A. Children with language disorders: natural history and academic success. *J Learn Disabil.* 1992;25:53-65, discussion 66-70.

82. Fricke S, Burgoyne K, Bowyer-Crane C, et al. The efficacy of early language intervention in mainstream school settings: a randomized controlled trial. *J Child Psychol Psychiatry.* 2017 May 19;doi:10.1111/jcpp.12737.

83. Fricke S, Bowyer-Crane C, Haley AJ, Hulme C, Snowling MJ. Efficacy of language intervention in the early years. *J Child Psychol Psychiatry.* 2013;54:280-290.

84. Bornstein MH, Haynes OM. Vocabulary competence in early childhood: measurement, latent construct, and predictive validity. *Child Dev.* 1998;69:654-671.

85. Barre N, Morgan A, Doyle LW, Anderson PJ. Language abilities in children who were very preterm and/or very low birth weight: a meta-analysis. *J Pediatr.* 2011;158:766-774.e761.

86. Breeman LD, Jaekel J, Baumann N, Bartmann P, Wolke D. Preterm cognitive function into adulthood. *Pediatrics.* 2015;136:415-423.

87. Woodward LJ, Moor S, Hood KM, et al. Very preterm children show impairments across multiple neurodevelopmental domains by age 4 years. *Arch Dis Child Fetal Neonatal Ed.* 2009;94:F339-F344.

88. Anderson PJ, Doyle LW. Cognitive and educational deficits in children born extremely preterm. *Semin Perinatol.* 2008;32: 51-58.

89. Johnson S. Cognitive and behavioural outcomes following very preterm birth. *Semin Fetal Neonatal Med.* 2007;12:363-373.

90. Blair C, Razza RP. Relating effortful control, executive function, and false belief understanding to emerging math and literacy ability in kindergarten. *Child Dev.* 2007;78:647-663.

91. Clark CA, Pritchard VE, Woodward LJ. Preschool executive functioning abilities predict early mathematics achievement. *Dev Psychol.* 2010;46:1176-1191.

92. Kuhn LJ, Willoughby MT, Blair CB, McKinnon R. Examining an executive function battery for use with preschool children with disabilities. *J Autism Dev Disord.* 2017;47:2586-2594.

93. Willoughby M, Blair C. Test-retest reliability of a new executive function battery for use in early childhood. *Child Neuropsychol.* 2011;17:564-579.

94. Willoughby MT, Pek J, Blair CB. Measuring executive function in early childhood: a focus on maximal reliability and the derivation of short forms. *Psychol Assess.* 2013;25:664-670.

95. Willoughby MT, Wirth RJ, Blair CB. Executive function in early childhood: longitudinal measurement invariance and developmental change. *Psychol Assess.* 2012;24:418-431.

96. Delis DC, Kaplan E, Kramer JH. *Delis Kaplan Executive Function System (D-KEFS).* San Antonio, TX: The Psychological Corporation; 2001.

97. Manly TRI, Anderson V, Nimmo-Smith IT. *TEA-Ch: The Test of Everyday Attention for Children;* 1999. Bury St. Edmunds, England: Thames Valley Test Company Ltd.

98. Mahone EM, Schneider HE. Assessment of attention in preschoolers. *Neuropsychol Rev.* 2012;22:361-383.

99. Thorell LB, Nyberg L. The childhood executive functioning inventory (CHEXI): a new rating instrument for parents and teachers. *Dev Neuropsychol.* 2008;33:536-552.

100. Gioia GIP, Guy S, Kenworthy L. *BRIEF—Behavior Rating Inventory of Executive Function. Professional Manual.* Odessa, FL: Psychological Assessment Resources; 2000.

101. Camerota M, Willoughby MT, Kuhn LJ, Blair CB. The Childhood Executive Functioning Inventory (CHEXI): factor structure, measurement invariance, and correlates in US preschoolers. *Child Neuropsychol.* 2016;13:1-16.

102. Cohen MJ. Children's memory scale. In: Kreutzer JS, Caplan B, DeLuca J, eds. *Encyclopedia of Clinical Neuropsychology.* New York: Springer; 2011:556-559.

103. High PC. School readiness. *Pediatrics.* 2008;121:e1008-e1015.

104. Roberts G, Lim J, Doyle LW, Anderson PJ. High rates of school readiness difficulties at 5 years of age in very preterm infants compared with term controls. *J Dev Behav Pediatr.* 2011;32:117-124.

105. Pritchard VE, Clark CA, Liberty K, Champion PR, Wilson K, Woodward LJ. Early school-based learning difficulties in children born very preterm. *Early Hum Dev.* 2009;85:215-224.

106. Aarnoudse-Moens CS, Weisglas-Kuperus N, van Goudoever JB, Oosterlaan J. Meta-analysis of neurobehavioral outcomes in very preterm and/or very low birth weight children. *Pediatrics.* 2009;124:717-728.

107. Bora S, Pritchard VE, Chen Z, Inder TE, Woodward LJ. Neonatal cerebral morphometry and later risk of persistent inattention/hyperactivity in children born very preterm. *J Child Psychol Psychiatry.* 2014;55:828-838.

108. Lean RE, Melzer TR, Bora S, Watts R, Woodward LJ. Attention and Regional Gray Matter Development in Very Preterm Children at Age 12 Years. *J Int Neuropsychol Soc.* 2017;1-12.

109. Woodward LJ, Lu Z, Morris AR, Healey DM. Preschool self regulation predicts later mental health and educational achievement in very preterm and typically developing children. *Clin Neuropsychol.* 2017;31:404-422.

110. Linsell L, Malouf R, Johnson S, Morris J, Kurinczuk JJ, Marlow N. Prognostic Factors for Behavioral Problems and Psychiatric Disorders in Children Born Very Preterm or Very Low Birth Weight: A Systematic Review. *J Dev Behav Pediatr.* 2016;37: 88-102.

111. Bilgin A, Wolke D. Development of comorbid crying, sleeping, feeding problems across infancy: neurodevelopmental vulnerability and parenting. *Early Hum Dev.* 2017;109:37-43.

112. Johnson S, Wolke D. Behavioural outcomes and psychopathology during adolescence. *Early Hum Dev.* 2013;89:199-207.

113. Brown N, Spittle A. Neurobehavioral evaluation in the preterm and term infant. *Curr Pediatr Rev.* 2014;10:65-72.

114. Van Roy B, Veenstra M, Clench-Aas J. Construct validity of the five-factor Strengths and Difficulties Questionnaire (SDQ) in pre-, early, and late adolescence. *J Child Psychol Psychiatry.* 2008;49:1304-1312.

115. Goodman R, Ford T, Simmons H, Gatward R, Meltzer H. Using the Strengths and Difficulties Questionnaire (SDQ) to screen for child psychiatric disorders in a community sample. *Int Rev Psychiatry.* 2003;15:166-172.

116. Goodman R. Psychometric properties of the strengths and difficulties questionnaire. *J Am Acad Child Adolesc Psychiatry.* 2001;40:1337-1345.

117. Goodman R. The extended version of the Strengths and Difficulties Questionnaire as a guide to child psychiatric caseness and consequent burden. *J Child Psychol Psychiatry.* 1999;40:791-799.

118. Goodman A, Goodman R. Population mean scores predict child mental disorder rates: validating SDQ prevalence estimators in Britain. *J Child Psychol Psychiatry.* 2011;52:100-108.

119. Achenbach TMEC. *Manual for the Child Behavior Checklist and Revised Children Behavior Profile;* 1983. Burlington, VT: Department of Psychiatry, University of Vermont.

120. Reynolds CRKR. *BASC-2 (Behavior Assessment for Children, Second Edition);* 2004. Circle Pines, MN: American Guidance Service.

121. Goodman R, Ford T, Richards H, Gatward R, Meltzer H. The Development and Well-Being Assessment: description and initial validation of an integrated assessment of child and adolescent psychopathology. *J Child Psychol Psychiatry.* 2000;41:645-655.

122. Todd RD, Joyner CA, Heath AC, Neuman RJ, Reich W. Reliability and stability of a semistructured DSM-IV interview designed for family studies. *J Am Acad Child Adolesc Psychiatry.* 2003;42:1460-1468.

123. Herjanic B, Reich W. Development of a structured psychiatric interview for children: agreement between child and parent on individual symptoms. *J Abnorm Child Psychol.* 1997;25:21-31.

124. Weller E, Weller R, Rooney M, Fristad M. *Children's Interview for Psychiatric Syndromes (ChIPS).* Washington, DC: American Psychiatric Press; 1999.

125. Robins DL, Casagrande K, Barton M, Chen CM, Dumont-Mathieu T, Fein D. Validation of the modified checklist for Autism in toddlers, revised with follow-up (M-CHAT-R/F). *Pediatrics*. 2014;133:37-45.

126. Pandey J, Verbalis A, Robins DL, et al. Screening for autism in older and younger toddlers with the Modified Checklist for Autism in Toddlers. *Autism*. 2008;12:513-535.

127. Khowaja MK, Hazzard AP, Robins DL. Sociodemographic barriers to early detection of autism: screening and evaluation using the M-CHAT, M-CHAT-R, and follow-up. *J Autism Dev Disord*. 2015;45:1797-1808.

128. Chlebowski C, Robins DL, Barton ML, Fein D. Large-scale use of the modified checklist for autism in low-risk toddlers. *Pediatrics*. 2013;131:e1121-e1127.

129. Lord C, Rutter M, DiLavore P, Risi S. *Autism Diagnostic Observation Schedule-WPS (ADOS-WPS)*. Los Angeles, CA: Western Psychological Services; 1999.

130. Hack M. Young adult outcomes of very-low-birth-weight children. *Semin Fetal Neonatal Med*. 2006;11:127-137.

UNIT III

NEONATAL SEIZURES

Neonatal Seizures

Nicholas S. Abend ◆ *Frances E. Jensen* ◆ *Terrie E. Inder* ◆ *Joseph J. Volpe*

Seizures in the newborn infant represent the most distinctive frequent manifestations of neurological disease in the neonatal period. The incidence of seizures varies with gestational age and birthweight and is most common in the very low birthweight (VLBW) infant. Estimated incidences are 58/100 live births in the VLBW infant and 1 to 3.5/100 live births in the term infant.[1-4] Compared to seizures at later developmental stages, seizures in the newborn differ in their clinical appearances, electrographic characteristics, etiologies, management, and outcomes. Because most seizures during the newborn period are acute symptomatic seizures due to cerebral injury or dysfunction, they are an important manifestation to alert the clinician to underlying neurological disorders. However, recognition of seizures in the newborn period can be very difficult because of subtle or absent clinical manifestations. To assist in both the accurate identification of seizures in the newborn and the successful treatment with antiepileptic drug therapy, electrophysiological monitoring—either conventional or limited channel monitoring—now plays a critical role within the neonatal intensive care unit. Treatment of neonatal seizures is generally considered necessary because experimental and human evidence suggests seizures may lead to secondary brain injury and are associated with less favorable outcomes. However, antiseizure medications may have associated risks, and there are few data to guide evidence-based management. This chapter reviews the pathophysiology and clinical aspects of neonatal seizures with particular emphasis on the influence of the developmental characteristics of the immature brain.

PATHOPHYSIOLOGY

Mechanisms

A seizure results from an excessive synchronous electrical discharge (i.e., depolarization) of neurons within the central nervous system (CNS).[5-10] Neuronal depolarization is produced by the influx of sodium (Na^+), and repolarization is produced by the efflux of potassium (K^+). Maintenance of the potential across the membrane requires an energy (adenosine triphosphate [ATP])-dependent pump, which extrudes sodium and takes in potassium.

Although the fundamental mechanisms of neonatal seizures are not entirely understood, current data suggest that excessive depolarization may occur because of the imbalance of neural excitation over inhibition for the following reasons (Table 12.1). First, one cause of excessive depolarization may relate to a failure of the ATP-dependent sodium-potassium pump thereby disabling the cell from maintaining a stable membrane potential.

Hypoxemia-ischemia and hypoglycemia, key common processes for neuronal injury in the newborn, can lead to such decreases in cellular energy production. Second, an excess of excitatory neurotransmitters can result in excessive depolarization. This imbalance of excess excitatory neurotransmitters, particularly in relation to the principal excitatory neurotransmitter glutamate, may result from increased synaptic release and/or diminished reuptake in presynaptic nerve endings and glia. Cellular injury, from hypoxic-ischemic neuronal injury, can result in the release of excessive extracellular glutamate.[10,11] Third, a relative deficiency of inhibitory versus excitatory neurotransmitters exists normally in the immature brain and may lead to an excessive rate of depolarization (see later). Developmentally, this enhanced excitation is important for activity-dependent synaptogenesis.[12] However, in the setting of brain injury, this normal enhancement of excitation can be accentuated and lead to excessive depolarization. The brain concentration of gamma-aminobutyric acid (GABA), the major inhibitory neurotransmitter, is lower in the newborn brain than in adulthood. Moreover, these GABA receptors in early life have been shown to be paradoxically excitatory and depolarizing because of a reversal of the chloride gradient in immature neurons compared to the adult.[12-14] This age-specific difference in neurotransmitter receptor function may contribute to the refractoriness of neonatal seizures to conventional antiepileptic drugs mediated via GABA.[12] Fourth, metabolic disturbances occurring in the newborn, such as pyridoxine deficiency, can also lead to seizures. Glutamic acid decarboxylase (GAD), the synthetic enzyme for GABA, requires binding of the critical cofactor of the enzyme, pyridoxine, specifically the active form, pyridoxal-5-phosphate. A state of pyridoxine dependency, in fact, is accompanied by decreased brain and cerebrospinal fluid (CSF) levels of pyridoxal-5-phosphate and GABA.[15-18] The molecular abnormality in this disease involves a defect in lysine degradation leading to an intermediate that forms an adduct with pyridoxal-5 phosphate, thereby preventing its action (see later). Finally, other molecules can influence the membrane's sensitivity to depolarizations such as calcium and magnesium that interact with the neuronal membrane to inhibit Na^+ movement. Thus, hypocalcemia or hypomagnesemia increase the Na^+ influx, resulting in depolarization.

Neuroanatomical and Neurophysiological Substrates

Seizure phenomena in newborns differ considerably from those observed in older humans, and the phenomena in premature infants differ from those in full-term newborns.[7,12,19-34] In the vast majority of neonatal seizures, electrical onset is focal or

TABLE 12.1   Probable Mechanisms of Neonatal Seizures

PROBABLE MECHANISM	DISORDER
Failure of ATP-dependent sodium-potassium pump secondary to decreased adenosine triphosphate	Hypoxemia, ischemia, and hypoglycemia
Excess of excitatory neurotransmitter (i.e., glutamate)	Hypoxemia, ischemia, and hypoglycemia
Deficit of inhibitory neurotransmitter (i.e., GABA)	Pyridoxine dependency
Membrane alteration: increased sodium permeability	Hypocalcemia and hypomagnesemia

ATP, Adenosine triphosphate; *GABA*, gamma-aminobutyric acid.

TABLE 12.2   Perinatal Anatomical and Physiological Features of Importance in Determining Neonatal Seizure Phenomena

Anatomical
- Lamination of cortical neurons
- Neurite outgrowth: dendritic and axonal ramifications
- Synaptogenesis
- Deficient myelination in cortical efferent systems

Physiological
- In limbic and neocortical regions, development of excitatory mechanisms before inhibitory mechanisms
- NMDA receptors overexpressed and exhibit multiple properties that enhance excitation
- AMPA receptors overexpressed and have a subunit composition (deficient GluR2) that enhances excitation
- GABA$_A$ receptors excitatory rather than inhibitory
- Deficient development of substantia nigra system for inhibition of seizures
- Impaired propagation of electrical seizures and resulting lack of correlation of synchronous discharges recorded from surface electroencephalogram with behavioral seizure phenomena

AMPA, α-amino-3-hydroxy-5-methyl-4-isoxazolepropionic acid; *GABA*, gamma-aminobutyric acid; *NMDA*, N-methyl-D-aspartate.

multifocal with the spread of the seizure occurring within one hemisphere[35] and secondary generalization to the contralateral hemisphere only rarely.[35,36] Thus, newborns rarely have well-organized, generalized tonic-clonic seizures, and premature infants have even less well-organized seizures than do term infants. The precise reasons for these differences relate to the status of neuroanatomical and neurophysiological development in the perinatal period.

Neuroanatomical Features

The most critical neuroanatomical developmental processes of relevance to the manifestation of seizure activity in the newborn period are the organizational events (see Chapter 7) (Table 12.2). The relevant events include the attainment of proper cellular orientation, alignment, and layering (i.e., lamination of cortical neurons); the elaboration of axonal and dendritic ramifications; and the establishment of synaptic connections.

Only the first of these processes (lamination) is fully developed by the term equivalent in the human newborn. The latter two events (neurite outgrowth and synaptogenesis) required to provide the cortical connectivity to propagate and sustain a generalized seizure is rudimentary in the term newborn infant. In contrast, in the newborn monkey, the spread of seizure discharges is relatively rapid, and well-organized, synchronous, generalized seizures are readily apparent clinically and electroencephalographically.[37] Such propagation of seizures appears related to the more advanced cortical organization and myelination of cortical efferent systems and interhemispheric commissures present in the newborn monkey.[38,39] The relatively advanced cortical development apparent in limbic structures in the human newborn infant[7,10,40,41] and the connections of these structures to the diencephalon and brain stem may underlie the frequency and dominance of oral-buccal-lingual movements (e.g., sucking, chewing, or drooling), oculomotor movements, and apnea as clinical manifestations of neonatal seizures.

Neurophysiological Features

The relation of excitatory to inhibitory synapses is important in determining the capacity of a focal discharge to both form and then to spread to contiguous and distant brain regions. Strong evidence indicates that the rates of development of the excitatory and inhibitory synaptic activities differ in the newborn cerebral cortex (see Table 12.2). Excitatory activity is mediated by glutamate through two key receptor types, N-methyl-D-aspartate (NMDA) and α-amino-3-hydroxy-5-methyl-4-isoxazolepropionic acid (AMPA). These two excitatory receptors are the predominant neurotransmitter receptors found in the immature brain, with a relative paucity of the principal inhibitory receptors for GABA.[7-11,13,42-58] Indeed, the neonatal period is characterized by levels of excitatory neurotransmitter expression and function that exceed those observed in adult cortical neurons, while inhibition is not yet at adult levels (Fig. 12.1).[12] Moreover, properties of these two glutamate receptors enhance their excitatory function. NMDA receptors in the neonatal period exhibit prolonged duration of the NMDA-mediated excitatory postsynaptic potential, reduced ability of magnesium to block NMDA receptor activity, diminished inhibitory polyamine binding sites, and a greater sensitivity to glycine enhancement.[10,54,55,58-61] Similarly, AMPA receptors in the neonatal period are deficient in the GluR2 subunit responsible for rendering the AMPA channel impermeable to calcium. Thus, these immature AMPA receptors are permeable to calcium and, as a consequence, enhanced excitation.[55-57,62,63] In addition, early in development, the principal inhibitory neurotransmitter, GABA, acts at the major postsynaptic GABA$_A$ receptor (GABA$_A$) to produce excitation rather than inhibition, as occurs later in development.[10,13,54,64] Consistent with these developmental phenomena, it is easier to produce epileptic activity in the immature animal than in the adult (Fig. 12.2).[10,12,65-68]

Insights into the critical developmental relationship between neuronal chloride (Cl⁻) levels and Cl⁻ transport in the perinatal period have major implications for *understanding the basis of GABA excitation, and thus key clinical and therapeutic aspects of neonatal seizures* (Table 12.3). GABA activation of the major postsynaptic GABA$_A$ receptor causes Cl⁻ flux. In the mature neuron, there is Cl⁻ influx down an electrochemical gradient. However, in developing brain, at maturational stages comparable to the human perinatal period, GABA activation causes Cl⁻ efflux,

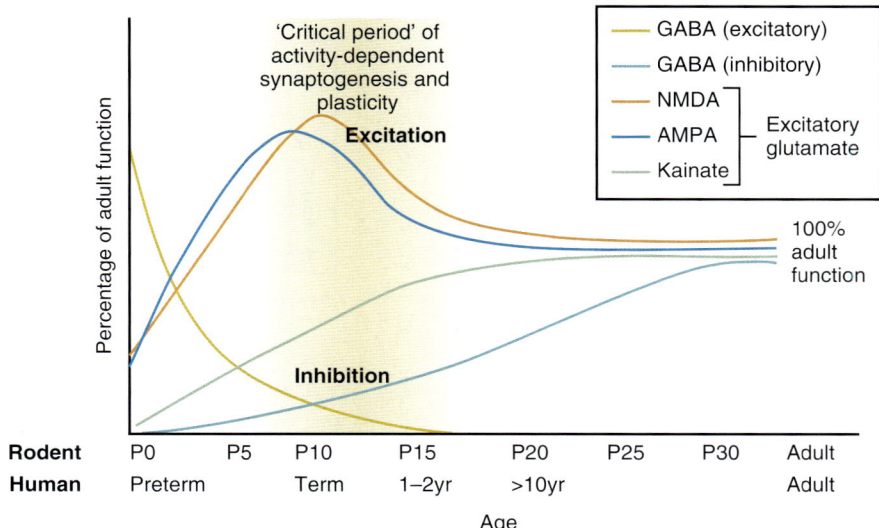

Figure 12.1 Schematic depiction of maturational changes in glutamate and GABA receptor function in the developing brain. Equivalent developmental periods are displayed for rats and humans on the top and bottom axes, respectively. Activation of GABA receptors is depolarizing in rats early in the first postnatal week and in humans up to and including the neonatal period. Functional inhibition, however, is gradually reached overdevelopment in rats and humans. Before full maturation of GABA-mediated inhibition, the NMDA and AMPA subtypes of glutamate receptors peak between the first and second postnatal weeks in rats and in the neonatal period in humans. Kainate receptor binding is initially low and gradually rises to adult levels by the fourth postnatal week. *AMPA*, α-amino-3-hydroxy-5-methyl-4-isoxazole propionate; *GABA*, γ-aminobutyric acid; *NMDA*, N-methyl-D-aspartate; *P*, postnatal day. (From Rakhade SN, Jensen FE. Epileptogenesis in the immature brain: emerging mechanisms. *Nat Rev Med.* 2009;5:380–391, with permission.)

TABLE 12.3   Critical Development Relationships of Neuronal Chloride Levels and Chloride Transport in Excitation of γ-Aminobutyric Acid

GABA is excitatory rather inhibitory in perinatal neurons because of elevated neuronal Cl⁻

GABA_A receptor activation therefore causes Cl⁻ *efflux* and depolarization (excitation) rather than *influx* and hyperpolarization (inhibition)

Elevated neuronal Cl⁻ levels result in the perinatal period because of exuberant development of NKCC1, which mediates Cl⁻ *influx*, in the presence of developmentally low levels of KCC2, which mediates Cl⁻ efflux

With development, NKCC1 declines, KCC2 increases, and thus neuronal Cl⁻ levels decrease; GABA_A receptor activation then results in Cl⁻ influx and hyperpolarization (inhibition)

These developmental changes may explain the imperfect response of neonatal seizures to GABA-agonist antiseizure medications (i.e., phenobarbital, benzodiazepines)

Cl⁻, Chloride; *GABA*, gamma-aminobutyric acid; *KCC2*, potassium-chloride cotransporter; *NKCC1*, sodium-potassium-chloride cotransporter.

---

and GABA activation is therefore excitatory.[13] The basis for this paradoxical effect relates to a *developmental mismatch between the two Cl⁻ transporters that determine neuronal Cl⁻ levels.* Thus, in the perinatal period, in the human cerebral cortex the expression of the Na⁺-K⁺-Cl⁻ cotransporter (NKCC1) responsible for Cl⁻ influx reaches a developmental peak, whereas the expression of the K⁺-Cl⁻ cotransporter (KCC2) responsible for Cl⁻ efflux is relatively low (see Fig. 12.1).[12,13,69-72] The result is a high internal neuronal level of Cl⁻, so when the GABA_A receptor is activated there is efflux (rather than influx) of Cl⁻, resulting in depolarization and excitation. The later developmental upregulation of the KCC2 cotransporter extruding Cl⁻ lowers the internal neuronal Cl⁻ level. Thus, with GABA_A receptor activation there is Cl⁻ influx with hyperpolarization and inhibition.

These findings may explain the therapeutic inconsistency of GABA agonists, such as phenobarbital and benzodiazepines, to be effective anticonvulsants in the newborn infant with seizures. This lack of anticonvulsant pharmacological efficacy is particularly apparent after neonatal hypoxic-ischemic insults, which, in an experimental model, are associated with the up-regulation of NKCC1.[73] *The NKCC1 inhibitor, bumetanide, has potent antiseizure properties by enhancing GABA-mediated inhibition through the blockage of Cl⁻ uptake and the lowering of neuronal Cl⁻ levels* (see later).[13,14] Moreover, because the maturation of the two cotransporters and neuronal Cl⁻ levels occurs in a caudal-rostral direction, spinal cord and brain stem motor neurons would be expected to exhibit GABA-mediated inhibition before the cerebral cortical regions. *This maturational process could explain the frequent occurrence of electroclinical uncoupling/dissociation in which antiseizure medications with GABA agonist mechanisms (i.e., phenobarbital and benzodiazepines) suppress motor manifestations of seizures (by spinal cord and brain stem inhibition) but not cortical electroencephalographic (EEG) manifestations (due to lack of cortex inhibition).*[13,14] The presence of a relative overexpression of NKCC1 versus KCC2 has been documented in postmortem human neonatal brain,[13] and combined with the efficacy in

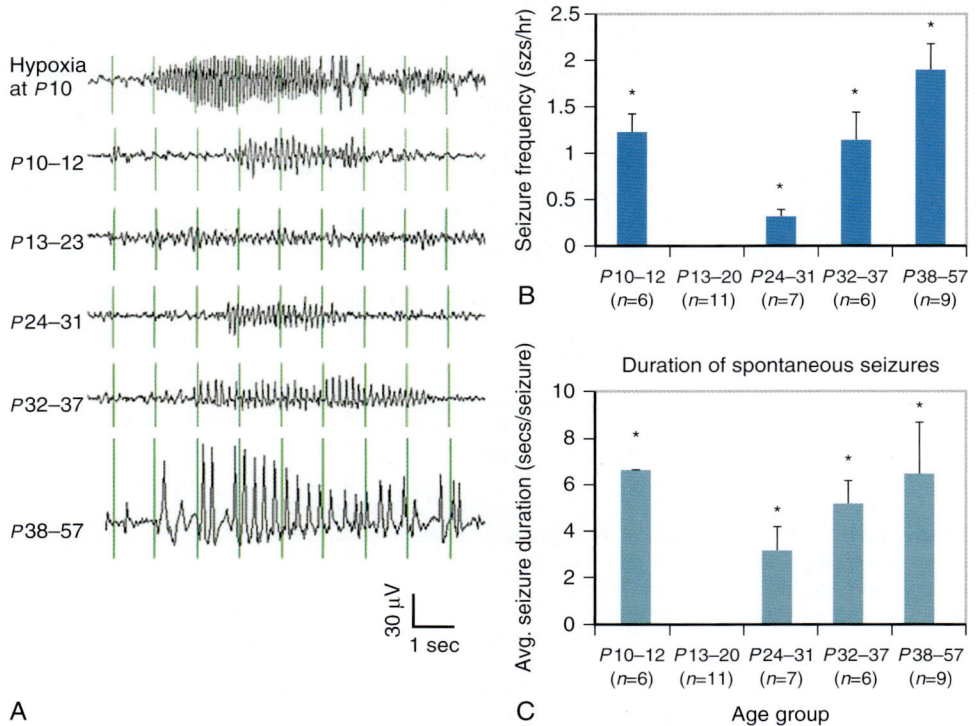

Figure 12.2 Hypoxia-induced seizures in P10 rats and subsequent seizure activity. Electroencephalographic recordings with representations of ictal discharges (A) during hypoxia, 0 to 2 days, 3 to 10 days, 14 to 21 days, 22 to 27 days, and 28 to 47 days following hypoxia. Abnormal activity was classified as seizures when activity was paroxysmal, rhythmic, increasing in amplitude, and greater than 3 seconds in duration. Electrographic seizures associated with abnormal behavioral automatisms were observed within the first 48 hours following hypoxia-induced seizures at P10. There was a decrease in the frequency (B) and duration (C) of the electrographic seizure activity between the ages of P13 and P20. The frequency (B and C) of electrographic seizures associated with abnormal behavior increased again in the animals at P24 to P31 and continued to increase into adulthood. (From Rakhade SN, Jensen FE. Epileptogenesis in the immature brain: emerging mechanisms. *Nat Rev Med.* 2009;5:380–391, with permission.)

rodent neonatal seizure models,[14] a Phase 1 to 2 study has been initiated to examine the safety and pharmacokinetics of the use of bumetanide as a combination anticonvulsant in human infants suffering from acute neonatal seizures.

Energy Metabolism

The most prominent acute biochemical effects of seizures involve energy metabolism (Fig. 12.3).[74-84] Seizures are associated with a greatly increased rate of energy-dependent ion pumping, which is accompanied by a fall in the concentration of ATP and phosphocreatine, the storage form of high-energy phosphate in the brain. The resulting rise in adenosine diphosphate (ADP) has two major effects. First, the rise in ADP leads to the stimulation of glycolysis at the rate-limiting, phosphofructokinase step,[85] which ultimately results in accelerated production of pyruvate (see Fig. 12.3). In the first minutes after the onset of seizure, there is a sharp increase in the rate of glucose utilization.[77,86] In the absence of seizure, a major proportion of the pyruvate formed from glycolysis enters the mitochondrion, is oxidized to carbon dioxide, and is associated with the production of ATP. With seizure activity, however, a considerable proportion of pyruvate is converted in the cytoplasm to lactate in the presence of elevated levels of the reduced form of nicotinamide

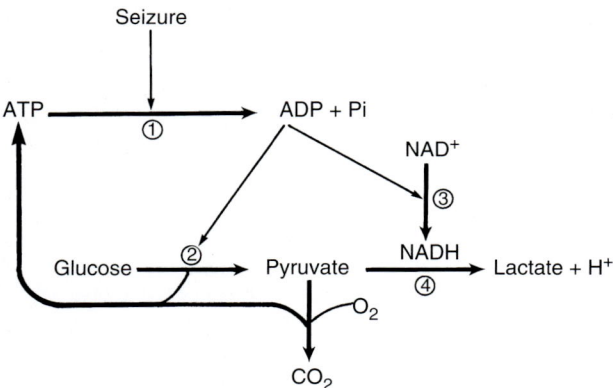

Figure 12.3 Biochemical effects of seizure. The major effects are numbered. *ADP*, Adenosine diphosphate; *ATP*, adenosine triphosphate; *NAD*, nicotinamide adenine dinucleotide; *NADH*, reduced form of nicotinamide adenine dinucleotide; *P_i*, inorganic phosphate.

TABLE 12.4	Seizure-Induced Changes in Brain Energy Metabolites in the Newborn Monkey*	
METABOLITE	CEREBRAL CORTEX (%)	THALAMUS (%)
Glucose utilization	424–598	261–411
Glucose	4	1
Lactate	267–650	308
Phosphocreatine	23–28	28
Adenosine triphosphate	56–77	60

*Values are expressed as a percentage of control. Data from Fujikawa DG, Vannucci RC, Dwyer BE, Wasterlain CG. Generalized seizures deplete brain energy reserves in normoxemic newborn monkeys. *Brain Res.* 1988;454:51–59; and Fujikawa DG, Dwyer BE, Lake RR, Wasterlain CG. Local cerebral glucose utilization during status epilepticus in newborn primates. *Am J Physiol.* 1989;256:C1160–C1167.

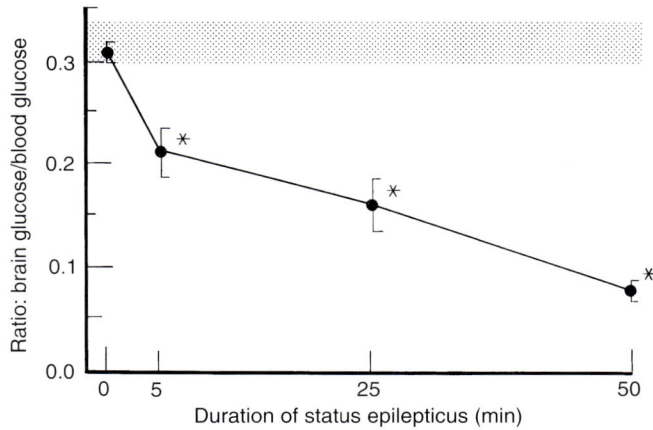

Figure 12.4 Decline in brain glucose concentration with seizure. Ratio of brain glucose to blood glucose levels in convulsing neonatal rats as a function of duration of seizure activity. The *shaded area* represents mean control values ± SE. The *asterisks* indicate difference from controls at $P < .01$. (From Wasterlain CG, Duffy TE. Status epilepticus in immature rats. *Arch Neurol.* 1976;33:821.)

adenine dinucleotide (NADH). Second, the rise in ADP leads to a shift of the redox state in the cytoplasm toward reduction (i.e., NADH; see Fig. 12.3). The excess of lactate, specifically the associated hydrogen ion,[87] has the beneficial effect of causing local vasodilation and a consequent increase in local blood supply and substrate influx.[78,88-90] In addition, seizures are associated with elevated blood pressure, which contributes to increased cerebral blood flow (CBF) and substrate influx.[78,89,91,92] This pressor effect is presumed to be a central autonomic component of the seizure because it can be interrupted by a section of the spinal cord or by administration of sympathetic ganglion-blocking agents.[74] An impairment of cerebrovascular autoregulation with seizure causes the pressor response to result in increased CBF.[89,90,92-94]

Despite these important compensatory factors, in experimental animals neonatal seizures are accompanied by *reductions in brain glucose concentrations*.[75-77,83,88,95-97] In the neonatal rat, rabbit, dog, and monkey, despite normal or slightly elevated blood glucose concentrations, brain glucose concentrations fall dramatically within 5 minutes of onset of seizure to nearly undetectable levels after 30 minutes (Table 12.4 and Fig. 12.4). Concomitant with the fall in brain glucose is a rise in brain lactate, which is used readily as a metabolic fuel in the neonatal brain.[80,84] This fall in brain glucose concentration and rise in brain lactate are directly reminiscent of a hypoxic-ischemic brain insult and presumably relate to the accelerated rate of glucose utilization in an attempt to preserve supplies of phosphocreatine and ATP. Glucose conversion to lactate, which is accelerated with neonatal seizures, results in only two molecules of ATP for each molecule of glucose, as opposed to the 38 molecules of ATP generated when pyruvate enters the mitochondrion and is oxidized to carbon dioxide. Consistently, in vivo studies by magnetic resonance spectroscopy (MRS) of cerebral metabolites in newborn dogs subjected to convulsant-induced seizures demonstrated a prominent decrease in phosphocreatine (with which ATP is in equilibrium) and in intracellular pH.[78,80,81,88] MRS studies by Younkin and colleagues in the human newborns demonstrate the relevance of these experimental data to the clinical situation (Fig. 12.5). Four

newborns had seizures during MRS imaging. The seizures resulted in substantial (~50%) decrease in the phosphocreatine to inorganic phosphate (PCr/Pi) ratio. One newborn's seizures were successfully treated with intravenously administered phenobarbital, which caused an immediate increase in the PCr/Pi ratio. Furthermore, newborns had PCr/Pi ratios of less than 0.8 during seizures and developed long-term neurological sequelae, indicating that neonatal seizures may increase cerebral metabolic demands above energy supply, thereby causing or exacerbating injury.[98] These observations indicate seizures may lead to secondary brain injury in an already injured neonatal brain and therefore have important implications for prognosis and therapy.

Mechanisms of Brain Injury With Seizures

The deleterious effects of seizures may be divided into those related to prolonged seizures (in which the most prominent feature is cell loss) and those related to briefer recurrent seizures (in which the most prominent feature is altered development). While minimal data are available in human newborns (see later discussion), experimental studies are abundant, primarily in developing rodent models. Importantly, although the threshold for seizure generation is lower in the developing brain than in the mature brain, developing neurons are less vulnerable to injury from single prolonged seizures than are mature neurons. This may be due to a lower density of active synapses, lower energy consumption, and immaturity of relevant biochemical cascades to cell death.[99]

Prolonged Seizures

The best-documented mechanisms by which prolonged seizures may cause brain injury are depicted in Fig. 12.6. Seizures may be accompanied by hypoventilation and apnea, which result in hypoxemia and hypercapnia. Hypoxemia may yield cardiovascular dysfunction and ischemic injury to brain, particularly in a newborn whose brain already has been compromised by an insult. Accentuation of the disturbance in cerebral energy metabolism when hypoxemia

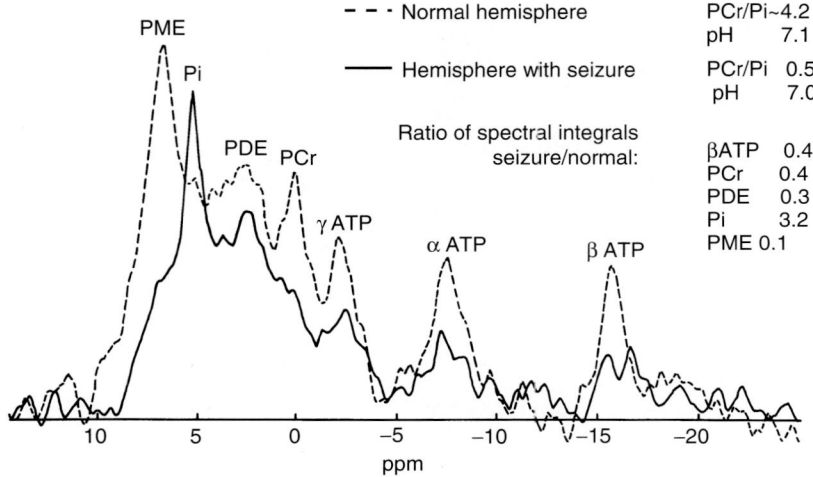

Figure 12.5 Magnetic resonance (phosphorus-31) spectra from a full-term infant during subtle seizure activity (oral-buccal-lingual movements, i.e., lip smacking and chewing). The electroencephalogram demonstrated seizure activity emanating from the left temporal region. The magnetic resonance spectrum from the nonictal hemisphere *(dotted line)* is normal. The spectrum from the ictal hemisphere *(solid line)* exhibits a marked decrease in phosphocreatine (PCr) and adenosine triphosphate (ATP) and a corresponding increase in inorganic phosphate (Pi). *PDE,* Phosphodiesters; *PME,* phosphomonoesters. (Courtesy Dr. Donald Younkin.)

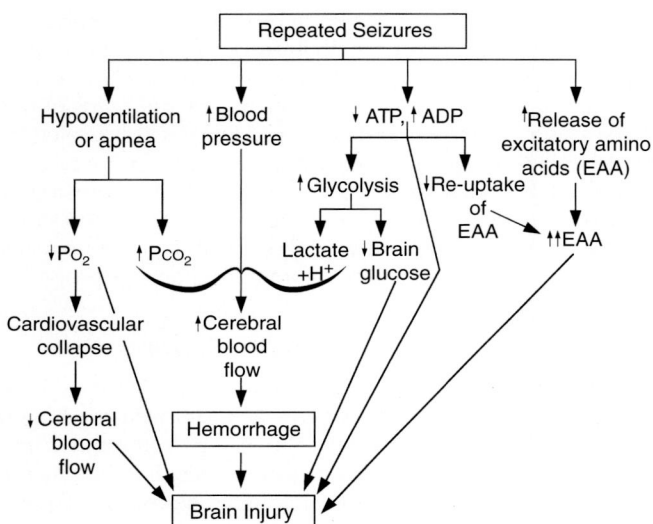

Figure 12.6 Best-documented mechanisms for the occurrence of brain injury consequent to repeated seizures. *ADP,* Adenosine diphosphate; *ATP,* adenosine triphosphate; *EAA,* excitatory amino acids; *PCO₂,* carbon dioxide pressure (especially glutamate); *PO₂,* oxygen pressure.

or hypoxemia-ischemia is combined with seizures has been shown in animal models.[79,81,100-102]

Hypercapnia may combine with seizure-induced adaptive elevations in arterial blood pressure and increased lactate to cause an abrupt increase in CBF in animal models and humans.[a] The importance of this increase in CBF is to maintain substrate supply to the brain and thereby to preserve energy supplies is consistent with the deleterious effect of hypotension when added to seizure, as shown in a neonatal dog model.[79]

[a]References 78, 79, 81, 88-90, 92-94, and 103-112.

Because cardiac dysfunction and diminished cardiac output are late complications of seizures, resulting hypotension, diminished CBF, impaired energy metabolism, and additional brain injury are major threats of repeated prolonged seizures (see Fig. 12.6).[91] Because the impairment of cerebrovascular autoregulation persists into the postictal period, later decreases in blood pressure may also lead to potentially dangerous CBF reductions.[93,94]

Several lines of evidence indicate that *elevations of arterial blood pressure and CBF also occur in the human newborn with seizures,* as described in neonatal animal models. Studies using continuous monitoring of arterial blood pressure demonstrated sharp increases in mean arterial blood pressure during neonatal seizures, including subtle seizures, even in paralyzed patients (Fig. 12.7).[105,113,114] A study of Doppler ultrasound at the anterior fontanelle in 12 newborns demonstrated a sharp increase in CBF velocity during seizures, most of which were subtle in type.[105] Moreover, the likelihood that this increase in CBF velocity is related to an increase in CBF was shown by the direct documentation of an increase in regional CBF by positron emission tomography during a subtle seizure in an infant.[106] In a study of 12 newborns with seizures, ictal measurements of regional CBF by single photon emission computed tomography showed a 50% to 150% increase, and this increase occurred in newborns with subtle seizures and EEG-only seizures.[109] Although the increase in CBF with seizure initially may be an adaptive response to increase substrate supply to the brain at a time of excessive metabolic demand, *this response could become maladaptive in some newborns.* For example, depending on such factors as the gestational age of the newborn or the neuropathological substrate for the seizures, some newborns may have highly vulnerable capillary beds, such as the germinal matrix in premature infants or the margins of ischemic lesions in premature infants or asphyxiated term newborns. Under these circumstances, an increase in CBF could rupture these capillary beds and cause intraventricular hemorrhage, hemorrhagic

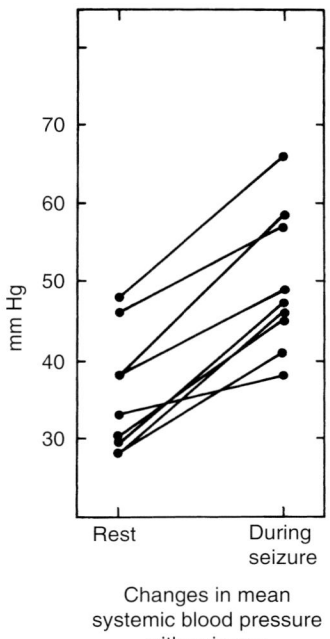

Changes in mean
systemic blood pressure
with seizures

Figure 12.7 Increase in blood pressure with neonatal seizures. Nine infants with subtle seizure phenomena were monitored during ictal episodes. Note the consistent increases in systemic blood pressure. In each infant, a simultaneous increase in cerebral blood flow velocity was documented by the Doppler ultrasound technique at the anterior fontanelle (not shown).

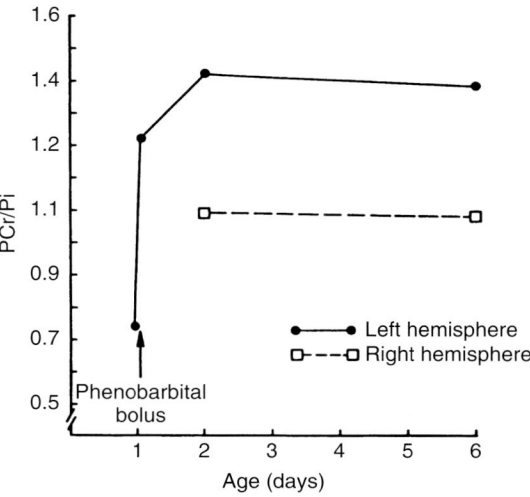

Figure 12.8 Effect of phenobarbital on the depressed ratio of phosphocreatine (PCr) to inorganic phosphorus (Pi) in an infant with seizure emanating from the left hemisphere. Note the immediate and then sustained improvement in cerebral energy state (i.e., increase in PCr/Pi ratio) after treatment with phenobarbital. (Courtesy Dr. Donald Younkin.)

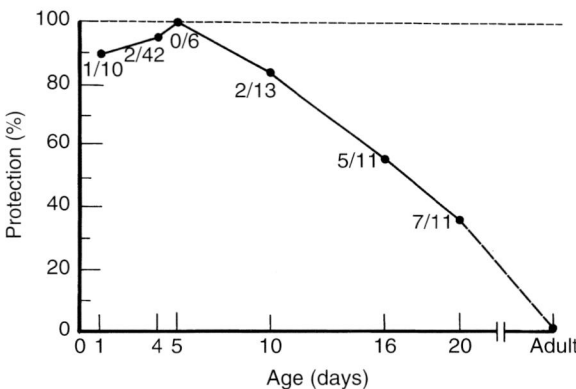

Figure 12.9 Age-dependent protective effect of glucose on mortality from repetitive seizures in the rat. The percentage of protection by glucose equals the number of saline-treated rats minus the number of glucose-treated rats: number of saline treated, dead × 100. (Courtesy Dr. Claude Wasterlain.)

periventricular leukomalacia, or hemorrhagic infarction (see Fig. 12.6).

Repeated prolonged seizures may *be deleterious for the brain, even in the absence of prominent disturbances of ventilation or perfusion* (see Fig. 12.6). The deleterious effects of hypoventilation and apnea can be controlled by prompt and vigorous support of ventilation. However, studies of paralyzed and well-ventilated, primarily adult animals subjected to repeated seizures indicate that eventually adaptive compensatory increases in substrate supply to brain experiencing seizures can no longer adequately compensate for the increase in energy expenditure and the resulting fall in energy reserves. Thus, decreases in brain ATP and phosphocreatine concentrations become progressive and irreparable brain injury may result.[a] *Nevertheless, most studies indicate that the neonatal brain is more resistant to seizure-induced neuronal necrosis than is the adult brain.*[99,125-131] Prevention of the changes in high-energy phosphate levels that appear to be important in the causation of brain injury by pharmacological treatment of seizures was shown by MRS in the neonatal dog.[108] As described previously, changes in high-energy phosphate compounds comparable to those observed in animal models were demonstrated by MRS during subtle seizures in human newborns. Four newborns had seizures during MRS imaging. The seizures resulted in a substantial decrease in the PCr/Pi ratio, and in one newborn whose seizures were successfully treated with intravenously administered phenobarbital, there was an immediate increase in the PCr/Pi ratio (see Figs. 12.5 and 12.8).[98]

Work with newborn animals indicates that *glucose administration* just before seizures prevents the fall in brain glucose level that occurs with status epilepticus and also markedly reduces mortality and brain cell loss.[75,95] This protective effect of glucose was substantially greater in neonatal than in older animals (Fig. 12.9). The precise beneficial effect of the glucose did not seem to relate to brain ATP and phosphocreatine concentrations because neither concentration in the whole brain was altered in these experiments. However, the glucose did appear to serve as a carbon source because DNA, RNA, protein, and cholesterol concentrations were relatively spared in the glucose-treated animals. In a study with potential clinical relevance, glucose administered early during seizures in neonatal rats subjected to hypoxia-ischemia led to decreased mortality but no change in the extent of ischemic brain injury.[97] The potential for important interactions between glucose homeostasis and seizures is raised

[a]References 6, 67, 74, 82, 83, and 115-124.

TABLE 12.5	Evidence Supportive of Major Role of Excitatory Amino Acids as Mediators of Neuronal Death With Prolonged Seizures

Prolonged seizures cause excessive release of glutamate and aspartate at excitatory amino acid synapses
The topography of seizure-related neuronal damage corresponds to the topography of postsynaptic sites innervated by glutamate-aspartate transmitters
Cytopathological features of seizure-related neuronal death are indistinguishable from those of glutamate-induced neuronal death
Specific blockers of glutamate receptors prevent neuronal death with prolonged seizures in vivo, even without preventing seizure activity per se

TABLE 12.6	Major Effects of Recurrent Neonatal Seizures in Experimental Studies

No definite cell loss
Impaired cognitive functions
Synaptic reorganization of axons and terminals in hippocampus (sprouting of mossy fibers)
Decreased neurogenesis in hippocampus
Loss of dendritic spines in hippocampus
Increased susceptibility to later epilepsy because of changes that all favor excitation including: increased NMDA and AMPA receptors and decreased GABA receptors, altered AMPA receptors (decreased GluR2), imbalance of excitatory and inhibitory systems, and altered intrinsic neuronal membrane properties

AMPA, α-amino-3-hydroxy-5-methyl-4-isoxazolepropionic acid; *GABA*, gamma-aminobutyric acid; *NMDA*, N-methyl-D-aspartate.

further by MRS studies of neonatal dogs, which showed that levels of hypoglycemia that do not result in alterations in levels of high-energy phosphates are accompanied by distinct decreases in such levels when seizures occur in addition to hypoglycemia.[78] These data indicate the importance of careful attention to glucose homeostasis in the management of the newborns with seizures, and they raise the possibility that administration of glucose may be a useful adjunct to the therapy of some newborns with seizures.

An *additional mechanism for the genesis of brain injury with severe seizures relates to excitatory amino acids.*[a] Injury to neuronal dendrites and cell bodies, the most prominent acute manifestations of injury from seizures, occurs particularly in limbic structures (e.g., hippocampus) and in distant sites intimately connected with limbic structures (e.g., selected areas of thalamus and cerebellum). The predilection of the limbic system of the newborn for seizure discharges discussed earlier is highly relevant in this regard. The experimental data suggest that the mechanism of neuronal injury in these structures involves *excessive synaptic release of excitatory amino acids*, particularly glutamate, the principal neurotransmitter for the regions that exhibit injury (see Fig. 12.6). When diminution of energy supplies is added, the energy-dependent reuptake systems for excitatory amino acids in presynaptic nerve endings and astrocytes are impaired, and the local accumulation of the neurotransmitters is accentuated (see Fig. 12.6). The result is postsynaptic damage at the axodendritic and axosomatic sites. The evidence that indicates a major role of excitatory amino acids as mediators of neuronal death with prolonged seizures is summarized in Table 12.5. A *particular vulnerability of the developing brain* of the newborn may relate to the rich expression in the developing brain of glutamate receptors, which appear to play an important role in neuronal differentiation and plasticity.[10,11,62,63,137] This rich expression of glutamate receptors, important for normal development, may become a source of overexcitation and neuronal death with repeated or prolonged seizures. Thus, the data suggest that severe seizures can induce a pathological extension of a normal synaptic event and that excitotoxic amino acids may thereby mediate cellular injury,

not only at the site of the epileptic discharge but also at distant sites excited by the epileptic discharge.

Recurrent Seizures

Although most evidence does not suggest serious structural or functional defects from a single neonatal seizure, *recurrent seizures*, even if not prolonged, are associated with long-term functional, morphological, and physiological deficits (Table 12.6).[99,131] The most consistent functional disturbance involves *deficits in cognition.*[99,131,147,148] Visual-spatial memory and learning have been particularly involved, and these deficits are consistent with the locus of the principal structural deficits in the hippocampus. The morphological correlates of the functional disturbances involve *neuronal developmental abnormalities rather than neuronal cell loss.* The most severe disturbances occur in the hippocampus and include dendritic spine loss in CA3 pyramidal cells, and a distinctive pattern of synaptic reorganization of axons and terminals of the dentate granule cells (i.e., mossy fibers).[99,147] The degree of this "sprouting" of mossy fibers correlates with the severity of the cognitive deficits. In addition, dentate granule cell neurogenesis, which, unlike in other cortical areas, persists in the neonatal period, is impaired after recurrent seizures.[149]

Recurrent seizures also lead to *physiological and molecular alterations that favor subsequent neuronal excitability and therefore epileptogenesis*, as well as the occurrence of neuronal injury with subsequent insults.[56-58,99,145,150,151] Alterations include increases in excitatory amino acid receptors (NMDA and AMPA/kainate), decreases in GABA receptors, posttranslational alterations in AMPA receptors (resulting in a decrease in the GluR2 subunit) that render them permeable to calcium, imbalanced excitatory and inhibitory systems, and altered intrinsic neuronal membrane properties—all of which favor excitation.[152-155] Recent data from animal models show that brief episodes of neonatal seizure, produced in particular by hypoxia or hypoxia ischemia, can result in long-term alterations in AMPA receptor subunit composition that can predispose to subsequent spontaneous seizure activity.[154,156-159] Importantly, in a rodent model, the alterations in AMPA receptor subunit composition, and later spontaneous seizures could be reversed by early posttreatment with the AMPA receptor antagonist NBQX.[155,157,158] These data provide evidence that early postseizure treatment may

---
[a]References 6, 10, 11, 55, 56, 67, 82, 83, 116-120, and 132-146.

have clinical potential to mitigate some of the deleterious long-term consequences of neonatal seizures, particularly the later development of epilepsy. Consistent with the deleterious effect of recurrent seizures, an observational study of neonatal electrophysiological monitoring of seizures in term infants with hypoxic-ischemic brain injury targeting anticonvulsants to reduce seizure burden was associated with a lower rate of postneonatal epilepsy.[160]

In addition to the modifications of neurotransmitter expression and function, changes in ion channels and metabolic pathways have been suggested to contribute to *permanent changes in excitability*. KCNQ potassium channels play a very important role in controlling excitation in early-life. The human KCNQ2 and KCNQ3 channel loss-of-function phenotype, benign familial neonatal seizures, suggests these channels are present, active, and important during the neonatal period. A number of medications including flupirtine, a KCNQ channel opener, has been shown to be effective in preventing chemo-convulsant seizures in the neonatal rodent.[161,162]

Recently, an important regulator of protein translation and synthesis, the mTOR (mammalian target of rapamycin) pathway, has been implicated in epileptogenesis in a number of adult seizure models, and overactivation of mTOR is the hallmark defect of the disease tuberous sclerosis (see Chapter 5), which has a high incidence of epilepsy.[163] Similar to adult experimental models, it appears that mTOR upregulation occurs in models of neonatal seizures,[163] and the mTOR inhibitor rapamycin has been shown to prevent acute hypoxia-induced neonatal and convulsant-induced seizures.[164,165]

Taken together, emerging evidence from many experimental models suggests a series of changes that occur in the immature brain in response to early postnatal seizures. First, changes in immediate early genes and posttranslational modifications of existing proteins occur within minutes to hours, whereas transcriptional events and the onset of inflammatory signaling occur within hours to days. Cell death is minimal following seizures in the immature brain compared to the adult. Later changes include gliosis and axonal sprouting, which may contribute to overall network excitability and dysfunction. These changes are outlined in Fig. 12.10, and each represents a separable opportunity to discover novel therapeutic targets that are unique and age-specific to the immature brain.[12]

A critical question, of course, is the extent to which these changes occur in the human newborn who experiences recurrent seizures, and what seizure burden may produce such adverse neurobiological consequences. Although this question remains unanswered, there is mounting evidence that seizures are associated with less favorable neurobehavioral outcomes (see later).

CLINICAL ASPECTS

Historically, most neonatal seizures were identified by direct clinical observation. More recently, many neonatal intensive care units place increased emphasis on EEG monitoring to identify seizures. This monitoring can include principally, conventional EEG, or amplitude-integrated EEG (aEEG), or both.[166-170] An expanded role for EEG monitoring has been advocated by recent guideline and consensus statements (see later discussion).[171-173] However, because this shift toward the use of EEG monitoring is recent, many of the data related to neonatal seizure diagnosis,

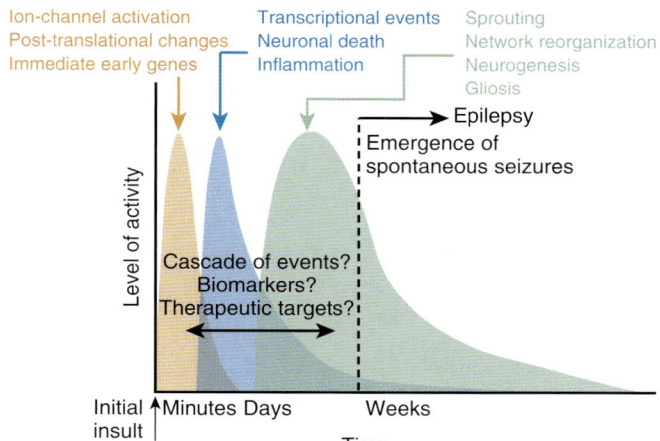

Figure 12.10 Time course of epileptogenesis. An initial insult, such as traumatic brain injury and/or status epilepticus, is followed by a latent period lasting weeks to months or even years before the onset of spontaneous seizures. During this latent period, a cascade of molecular and cellular events occurs that alters the excitability of the neuronal network, ultimately resulting in spontaneous epileptiform activity. The alterations that occur during the latent period might provide a good opportunity for biomarker development and therapeutic intervention. The cascade of events that are presently suggested by experimental evidence can be classified temporally following the initial insult. Early changes, including the induction of immediate early genes and posttranslational modification of receptor and ion-channel related proteins, occur within seconds to minutes. Within hours to days, there can be neuronal death, inflammation, and altered transcriptional regulation of genes, such as those encoding growth factors. A later phase, lasting weeks to months, includes morphological alterations, such as mossy fiber sprouting, gliosis, and neurogenesis. (From Rakhade SN, Jensen FE. Epileptogenesis in the immature brain: emerging mechanisms. *Nat Rev Med.* 2009;5:380–391, with permission.)

management, and outcome are based on studies that relied on clinical identification of seizures. Increasing use of EEG monitoring has raised two important possibilities about data derived from studies of clinically identified seizures. First, some clinically identified motor and behavioral phenomena characterized as seizures do not have a simultaneous EEG seizure correlate; this finding suggests that the occurrence of some neonatal seizures may have been overestimated in the past. Second, many electrographic seizures are not accompanied by clinically observable alterations in neonatal motor or behavioral function; this finding suggests that the occurrence of neonatal seizures may have been underestimated in the past. These observations underscore the importance of EEG data in the identification and management of newborns with seizures.

Seizure Classification

Seizure Types

A *seizure* is defined clinically as a paroxysmal alteration in neurological function (i.e., behavioral, motor, or autonomic function). Such a definition includes clinical phenomena that are associated temporally with seizure activity identifiable on an EEG and, therefore, are clearly epileptic (i.e., related to hypersynchronous electrical discharges that may spread and activate other brain structures). The clinical seizure definition also includes paroxysmal clinical phenomena that are not consistently associated temporally with EEG seizure activity;

TABLE 12.7   Classification of Neonatal Seizures

CLINICAL SEIZURE	ELECTROENCEPHALOGRAPHIC SEIZURE CORRELATE	
	COMMON	UNCOMMON
Subtle	+	
Clonic		
Focal	+	
Multifocal	+	
Tonic		
Focal	+	
Generalized		+
Myoclonic		
Focal, multifocal		+
Generalized	+	

TABLE 12.8   Types of Neonatal Seizures

- Electrographic Seizure: A paroxysmal abnormality in cortical electrical activity that evolves over time and meets criteria in Table 12.9
- Electroclinical Seizure: Electrographic seizure with associated clinical signs
- EEG-Only (subclinical, nonconvulsive, occult) Seizures: Electrographic seizures without clinical signs

EEG, Electroencephalographic.
Adapted with permission from Tsuchida TN, Wusthoff CJ, Shellhaas RA, et al. American Clinical Neurophysiology Society standardized EEG terminology and categorization for the description of continuous EEG monitoring in neonates: report of the American Clinical Neurophysiology Society Critical Care Monitoring Committee. *J Clin Neurophysiol* 2013;30:161–173.

TABLE 12.9   Electrographic Criteria for Neonatal Seizures

- Sudden change in EEG
- Repetitive waveforms that evolve in morphology, frequency, and/or location
- Amplitude: At least 2 μV
- Duration: at least 10 s
- Seizures must be separated by at least 10 s to be considered separate
- Clinical signs may or may not be present

EEG, Electroencephalography.
Adapted from Tsuchida TN, Wusthoff CJ, Shellhaas RA, et al. American Clinical Neurophysiology Society standardized EEG terminology and categorization for the description of continuous EEG monitoring in neonates: report of the American Clinical Neurophysiology Society Critical Care Monitoring Committee. *J Clin Neurophysiol* 2013;30:161–173, with permission.

how many of these clinical phenomena without identifiable EEG correlates are epileptic and just not identifiable on surface-recorded EEG and how many are nonepileptic is not resolved (see later discussion). The classification of neonatal seizures presented here categorizes clinical seizures and designates those clinical seizures likely to be associated with EEG seizure activity.

The classification schemes for neonatal seizures have varied over time (Table 12.7).[174-176] A consensus statement on neonatal EEG terminology by the American Clinical Neurophysiology Society defined three types of neonatal seizures: (1) *clinical-only seizures* in which there is a sudden paroxysm of abnormal clinical change that does not correlate with a simultaneous EEG seizure, (2) *electroclinical seizures* in which there is a clinical seizure coupled with an associated EEG seizure, and (3) *EEG-only seizures* in which there is an EEG seizure that is not associated with any outwardly visible clinical signs. EEG-only seizures are also referred to as *subclinical, nonconvulsive, or occult seizures* (Table 12.8). Neonatal EEG seizures are described as having (1) a sudden EEG change; (2) repetitive waveforms that evolve in morphology, frequency, and/or location; (3) an amplitude of at least 2 μV; and (4) a duration of at least 10 seconds (Table 12.9).[177-179]

Electrographic seizure definitions were provided earlier and are summarized in Table 12.9.[177] It is important to distinguish between electrographic seizures and other related EEG patterns. Although a seizure on EEG is composed of an evolving pattern of epileptiform discharges, not all epileptiform discharges are seizures. *Epileptiform discharges* are brief abnormalities that stand out from the EEG background, usually due to a peaked or sharp appearance. They are sometimes referred to as "sharp waves" or "spikes" because of this EEG appearance. It is normal for newborns to have some sharp waves, and many newborns with epileptiform discharges do not experience seizures. However, epileptiform discharges that occur in runs or are clustered in one brain region are associated with an increased risk of seizure occurrence.[177] In particular, *brief rhythmic discharges* (BRDs) are EEG patterns that meet the criteria for neonatal seizures (sudden, abnormal, evolving) but are shorter in duration than 10 seconds. BRDs have also been referred to as brief intermittent/ictal/interictal rhythmic discharges (BIRDs) or brief electroencephalographic rhythmic discharges (BERDs). BRDs are associated with underlying brain pathology and are associated with the occurrence of seizures, as well as an increased risk of future developmental delay, cerebral palsy, and mortality.[180,181] Further, some BRDs are associated with clinical signs, including focal clonic activity.[180,181] Indicating that the exact separation between seizures and shorter rhythmic discharges may be less distinct. Clearly the 10-second rule is largely arbitrary, and electrographic events with a clinical correlate are generally considered electroclinical seizures even if they last less than 10 seconds.

For those seizures with a clinical correlate, the most recent International League Against Epilepsy seizure classification report classifies neonatal seizures according to the same descriptors as seizures at later ages, rather than as a separate entity as had occurred in prior seizure classification systems.[182-184] However, the *organization of this chapter will retain emphasis of the classification of clinical seizures noted* in Table 12.7.

Despite great efforts to carefully describe the appearance of neonatal seizures, *inter-rater agreement in neonatal seizure identification by clinical observation is suboptimal*. Malone and colleagues presented clinical data and video clips of abnormal neonatal movements from 20 newborns to 137 observers, including 91 physicians from seven neonatal intensive care units. Observers classified the movements as seizure or nonseizure. The average number of correctly classified events was only 50%, compared to the gold standard of EEG classification. Further, interobserver agreement was poor for both physicians and other health care professionals.[185] Similarly, in a study of staff observing high-risk newborns, only 9% of 526 electrographic seizures were identified by clinical observation, indicating that an *underdiagnosis of seizures* occurred. In addition, 78% of 177 nonictal events were incorrectly identified as seizures, indicating that an *overdiagnosis* of seizures occurred.[186] Problematically, the more difficult to diagnose seizure types tend to occur more often than the more readily diagnosed seizure types in newborns. A study of 61 seizures in 24 newborns classified seizures by their most prominent clinical features. Clonic and tonic seizures, which might be more readily identified, only occurred in 20% and 8%, respectively, while orolingual, ocular, and autonomic features, which might be more difficult to identify, were the main features in 55%.[34]

Despite the limitations in clinical recognition of seizures discussed previously, attempts at clinical recognition and classification of neonatal seizures are critical to diagnose seizures and differentiate them from nonictal events. *Four essential clinically evident seizure types* can be recognized: *subtle, clonic, tonic, and myoclonic* (see Table 12.7). Subtle seizures do not have a clear position in the most recent International League Against Epilepsy seizure classification report,[184] but they are very common in newborns and the term is used frequently throughout the literature.[176] Thus, the term is retained as part of the categorization system in this chapter. As discussed further on, a critical fifth seizure type to consider in newborns is seizures with no observable clinical correlate, which have been referred to as *EEG-only seizures, subclinical seizures, nonconvulsive seizures, and occult seizures*. In the terminology used later, *multifocal* refers to clinical activity that involves more than one site, is asynchronous, and, usually, is migratory, whereas *generalized* refers to clinical activity that is diffusely bilateral, synchronous, and nonmigratory.

An important initial distinction in classifying a seizure is whether *it has a generalized or focal mechanism of onset*. Focal seizures have a defined region of onset, and electrical activity initially spreads through neural networks in that region, although the

TABLE 12.10   Manifestations of Subtle Seizures
Ocular phenomena
Tonic horizontal deviation of eyes with or without jerking of eyes[a]
Sustained eye opening with ocular fixation[b]
Oral-buccal-lingual movements
Chewing[b]
Other manifestations
Limb movements
Autonomic phenomena[c]
Apneic episodes[a]

[a]Documented with simultaneous electroencephalographic seizure activity most commonly in term newborns.

[b]Documented with simultaneous electroencephalographic seizure activity most commonly in premature newborns.

[c]Documented with simultaneous electroencephalographic seizure activity as a prominent isolated seizure manifestation most commonly in the premature infants, but autonomic phenomena (e.g., increase in blood pressure) are also common accompaniments of seizures in term newborns.

seizure may spread within the hemisphere or to the contralateral hemisphere with time. Generalized seizures may begin from a specific point, but almost immediately involve bilateral neural networks, such that electrical activity appears on both sides of the brain simultaneously on EEG.[184] *In the vast majority of neonatal seizures, onset is focal or multifocal.* Spread of the seizure within one hemisphere[35] and secondary generalization to the contralateral hemisphere[35,36] are less common in newborns than in older children, presumably because the network connections in the newborn brain are not as fully developed (discussed earlier).

Subtle Seizures. The clinical manifestations of certain neonatal seizures may be overlooked even by skilled observers, and these paroxysmal alterations in neonatal behavior and motor or autonomic function are defined as *subtle seizures* (Table 12.10).[19,174,176] Available information from studies using EEG recording simultaneously with video recording or direct observation suggests that (1) subtle seizures are more common in premature than in full-term infants;[187] and (2) some subtle clinical phenomena in full-term infants are not consistently associated with EEG seizure activity (i.e., clinical-only seizures).[32,33,188-190] Common ictal clinical manifestations, confirmed by simultaneous abnormal EEG discharges, in a group of premature infants of 26 to 32 weeks of gestation, included sustained opening of eyes, ocular movements, chewing, pedaling motions, and a variety of autonomic phenomena.[187] Similar subtle clinical phenomena occur in association with EEG seizure activity in full-term newborns, although slightly less commonly than in preterm newborns.[a] Thus, eye opening, ocular movements (often sustained eye opening with ocular fixation in premature infants and horizontal deviation in term newborns), peculiar extremity movements (e.g., resembling "boxing" or "hooking" movements), mouth movements, and apnea have been documented in association with EEG seizure activity (see Tables 12.10 and 12.11).

---

[a]References 23, 29, 31, 33, 186, and 191-194.

TABLE 12.11	Clinical Manifestations of Electroencephalographic Seizures in Premature Infants
SCHER AND CO-WORKERS[a] (N = 12; MEAN BIRTH WEIGHT, 1358 g)	**RADVANYI-BOUVET AND CO-WORKERS**[b] (N = 21; MEAN BIRTH WEIGHT, 1220 g)
Clonic movements (6)	Sustained eye opening with fixed gaze (15)
Myoclonic movements (2)	Tonic, often with facial "wincing" (8)
Staring (2)	Myoclonic movements (7)
Nystagmus (1)	"Jerks" (1)
Apnea (1)	Pedaling movements (2)
Hiccough (1)	Cry-grimace (3)
Chewing (7)	
Ocular movements (4)	
Apnea (4)	
Tachypnea (3)	
Bradycardia (6)	
Tachycardia (1)	

[a]Data from Scher MS, Painter MJ, Bergman I, Barmada MA, et al. EEG diagnoses of neonatal seizures: clinical correlations and outcome. *Pediatr Neurol.* 1989;5:17–24.
[b]Data from Radvanyi-Bouvet MF, Vallecalle MH, Morel-Kahn F, Relier JP, et al. Seizures and electrical discharges in premature infants. *Neuropediatrics.* 1985;16:143–148.

TABLE 12.12	Clonic Seizures

Focal clonic seizures
Localized clonic jerking
Usually not unconscious
Often associated with EEG seizure
Multifocal clonic seizures
Simultaneous or in sequence clonic jerking from multiple locations
Nonordered (non-Jacksonian) migration
Often associated with EEG seizure
Generalized clonic seizures
Diffusely bilateral, generally symmetrical, and synchronous movements
Rarely, if ever, observed in newborns

EEG, Electroencephalographic.

The frequency with which subtle clinical seizure phenomena are associated with concomitant EEG seizure activity is uncertain. In one study, 22 newborns, approximately 85% of whom were of greater than 36 weeks of gestation, exhibited paroxysms of such ocular abnormalities as eye opening or blinking, oral-buccal-lingual movements, pedaling or stepping movements, or rotary arm movements with an "inconsistent association" with EEG seizure activity. Only tonic horizontal deviation of the eyes was consistently associated with EEG seizure activity.[188] In another report of 44 newborns (28 premature), subtle clinical phenomena, defined as outlined in Table 12.10, accounted for 70% to 75% of all clinical seizures with simultaneous EEG correlates.[29] It is more common for subtle clinical events to have an electrographic correlate (i.e., electroclinical seizures) if the newborn has other types of seizures; these events are somewhat less likely to be seizures when they are the only behavior of clinical concern.[195] However, it is important to recognize that not all epileptic events may be identified by conventional surface EEG recording (see later). Taken together, the data indicate that at least some caution should be used in attributing an epileptic origin to subtle clinical phenomena, particularly when these phenomena are the only seizure manifestation.

The issue of *apnea as a seizure manifestation* deserves special consideration. Although apnea has been demonstrated as a seizure manifestation in premature infants,[23,187,196] most apneic episodes in the premature infants are not epileptic in origin.[187,197-200] However, apnea has been documented with electrical seizure activity, more commonly in the full-term newborns.[31,33,191,201-206] In 14 of the 21 newborns studied by Watanabe and colleagues, the newborns exhibited other subtle phenomena during the apneic seizure (e.g., eye opening, "staring," deviation of the eyes, and mouth movements).[191] Of additional value in clinical identification of apnea as a seizure is the observation that apnea accompanied by EEG seizure activity (i.e., convulsive apnea) is less likely to be associated with bradycardia than is nonconvulsive apnea.[202] However, convulsive apnea that is prolonged may be complicated ultimately by bradycardia.[191,201] Other rarer clinical phenomena observed in newborns with apneic seizures, and occasionally in isolation, include episodic vertical deviation of eyes (usually downward) with or without eye jerking, hyperpnea, vasomotor phenomena, and abnormal cardiac rhythm (usually with bradycardia).[a]

Clonic Seizures. A *clonic seizure* is defined as a seizure characterized by "rhythmic movements of muscle groups in a focal distribution which consist of a rapid phase followed by a slow return movement."[212] Clonic seizures appear as repetitive and rhythmic jerking movements that can affect any part of the body including the face, extremities, and even diaphragmatic or pharyngeal muscles. Clonic seizures represent the clinical seizure type associated most consistently with EEG seizure activity.[32,34,188,213]

Clonic seizures in the newborn are often classified as focal or multifocal (see Tables 12.7 and 12.12). *Focal clonic seizures* involve the face, upper or lower extremities on one side of the body, or axial structures (neck or trunk) on one side of the body. Newborns commonly are not clearly unconscious during or after a focal seizure. The neuropathological condition often is focal (e.g., cerebral infarction), although focal clonic seizures may occur with metabolic encephalopathies. Because focal clonic seizures occur with focal etiologies, it is likely that newborns with only focal clonic seizures have more favorable outcomes than those with other seizures types.[214,215] *Multifocal clonic seizures* involve several body parts, often in a migrating fashion, although the migration most often "marches" in a non-Jacksonian manner (e.g., left arm jerking may be followed by right leg jerking). *Generalized clonic seizures* (i.e., diffusely bilateral, generally symmetrical, and synchronous movements)

[a]References 32, 191, 193, 203, 205, and 207-211.

TABLE 12.13	Tonic Seizures

Focal tonic seizures
Sustained posturing of a limb
Asymmetrical posturing of trunk or neck
Often associated with EEG seizure
Generalized tonic seizures
Tonic extension of upper and lower limbs
Usually not associated with EEG change

EEG, Electroencephalographic.

TABLE 12.14	Relation of Myoclonic Seizures to Electroencephalographic Seizure Discharges

TYPE OF MYOCLONIC SEIZURE	CONSISTENT EEG SEIZURE	INCONSISTENT OR NO EEG SEIZURE
Generalized	35	23
Focal	3	38
Multifocal	0	5

EEG, Electroencephalographic.
Data from Mizrahi EM, Kellaway P. Characterization and classification of neonatal seizures. *Neurology.* 1987;37:1837–1844; *n* = 17.

TABLE 12.15	Myoclonic Seizures

Focal and multifocal myoclonic seizures
Well-localized, single or multiple, migrating jerks, usually of limbs
Usually not accompanied by electroencephalographic seizure discharges
Generalized myoclonic seizures
Single or bilateral synchronous jerks of flexion, more in upper than in lower limbs
May presage infantile spasms with suppression-burst electroencephalographic pattern and hypsarrhythmia
Often associated with EEG seizure

EEG, Electroencephalographic.

are rarely, if ever, observed in newborns. Clonic seizures are often reliably recognized by clinical observation, but they must be distinguished from other repetitive movements, such as jitteriness, tremulousness, and myoclonus (see later). Unlike those nonepileptic movements, the muscle twitches of a clonic seizure cannot be suppressed with gentle pressure and occur spontaneously (see later discussion).

Tonic Seizures. *Tonic seizures* are defined as a "sustained flexion or extension of axial or appendicular muscle groups."[212] Two categories of tonic seizures should be distinguished: focal and generalized tonic seizures (see Tables 12.7 and 12.13). *Focal tonic seizures* consist of sustained posturing of a limb or asymmetrical posturing of trunk or neck. Mizrahi and Kellaway also classified horizontal eye deviation as a focal tonic seizure, although some classify those events as subtle seizures.[188] Focal tonic seizures are associated consistently with EEG seizure discharges.[188] Several nonepileptic conditions may mimic focal tonic seizures. Focal tonic episodes may occur as initial manifestation of *alternating hemiplegia of childhood* in which the EEG is normal, and after the first weeks of life the tonic episodes are followed by the characteristic prolonged periods of hemiparesis.[216,217] *Hemifacial spasm*, a rare disorder in newborns with a posterior fossa lesion (e.g., cerebellar tumor, facial nerve trauma), is not accompanied by abnormal EEG features.[218,219]

Generalized tonic seizures are characterized by tonic extension of both upper and lower extremities (mimicking "decerebrate" posturing) but also by the tonic flexion of upper extremities with the extension of lower extremities (mimicking "decorticate" posturing) (see Table 12.13). The possibility that such clinical seizures represent posturing and are not ictal has been raised because of the frequent association with severe intraventricular hemorrhage and the often poor response to antiseizure medication therapy.[175,220] Approximately 85% of such clinical seizures were not accompanied by electrographic activity or by autonomic phenomena.[33,190] The 15% of generalized tonic seizures that were accompanied by electrographic seizure activity were also accompanied by autonomic phenomena.[33,190] Thus, these generalized tonic events may represent *"brain stem release" phenomena* and uninhibited extensor posturing that appears similar to tonic stiffening in patients with severe brain injury. As an additional mimic to generalized tonic seizures, episodes of generalized hypertonia provoked by minor tactile or other stimuli are characteristic of *hyperekplexia*, which is also known as *startle disease* or *congenital stiff-man syndrome* (see later).[33,190,221-226]

Myoclonic Seizures. Myoclonus is defined as a rapid, isolated jerk which can affect one or multiple muscle groups, can be ictal or nonictal in etiology, and can arise from injury to any level of the nervous system. *Myoclonic seizures* are clinical episodes that are usually not associated with EEG discharges (Table 12.14).[32,188] Myoclonic movements are distinguished from clonic movements by the faster speed of the myoclonic jerk and the predilection for flexor muscle groups. There are three categories of myoclonic seizures: focal, multifocal, and generalized myoclonic seizures (see Tables 12.7 and 12.15). *Focal myoclonic seizures* typically involve flexor muscles of an upper extremity. Of 41 focal myoclonic seizures studied by Mizrahi and Kellaway,[188] only 3 were associated with EEG seizures (see Table 12.14). *Multifocal myoclonic seizures* are characterized by asynchronous twitching of several parts of the body. In five episodes studied by Mizrahi and Kellaway,[188] none had associated EEG seizure discharges (see Table 12.14). *Generalized myoclonic seizures* are characterized by bilateral jerks of flexion of upper and occasionally of lower limbs. These seizures may appear identical to the infantile spasms observed in older infants. Generalized myoclonic seizures are more likely to be associated with EEG seizure discharges than are focal or multifocal myoclonic seizures. Of 58 generalized myoclonic seizures studied by Mizrahi and Kellaway, 35 had associated EEG seizure discharges (see Table 12.13).[188] All three varieties of myoclonic seizures may occur as a feature of severe neonatal epileptic syndromes.

Myoclonic seizures must be distinguished from nonepileptic myoclonus, which can occur with injury to any level of the nervous system and from normal physiological myoclonus,

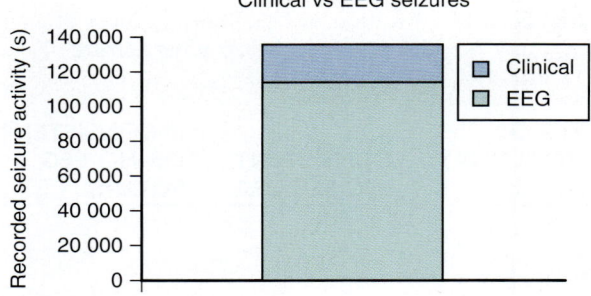

Figure 12.11 Total recorded electrographic seizure activity measured in seconds, versus total clinical seizure manifestations in nine patients with electrographic seizures recorded on continuous video electroencephalography *(EEG)* during the first 72 hours of life. (From Murray DM, Boylan GB, Ali I, Ryan CA, Murphy BP, Connolly S. Defining the gap between electrographic seizure burden, clinical expression and staff recognition of neonatal seizures. *Arch Dis Child Fetal Neonatal Ed.* 2008;93:F187–F191, with permission.)

which occurs in normal newborns. Unlike such other forms of myoclonus, myoclonic seizures are not induced by stimuli and cannot be suppressed by pressure to the affected body part. Furthermore, newborns with myoclonic seizures almost always have abnormal neurological exams, whereas newborns with benign myoclonus are otherwise normal.

Electroencephalographic-Only (Subclinical, Nonconvulsive, Occult) Seizures

A major issue with clinical diagnosis of seizures in newborns is the high incidence of EEG-only seizures in newborns.[a] Numerous studies have indicated that about 80% to 90% of electrographic seizures do not have any associated clinical correlate and therefore would not be identified without continuous EEG monitoring even by the most expert and observant bedside caregivers.[35,186,227,229,237-240] Clancy and colleagues evaluated 41 newborns with seizures happening frequently enough to occur during a routine EEG. Only 21% of 393 seizures identified on EEG were accompanied by clinically evident seizure activity (i.e., electroclinical seizures), while 79% of the seizures identified on EEG were EEG-only seizures. Electroclinical seizures and EEG-only seizures had similar durations, and there were no differences in the degree of encephalopathy. The authors concluded that "unaided visual inspection of infants seriously underestimates true seizure frequency," and that "long-term EEG monitoring may be necessary in many infants to determine their real seizure frequency and to judge the adequacy of antiepileptic drug treatment."[227] In a related study, Murray and colleagues evaluated 51 term newborns with continuous video EEG. Nine newborns experienced a total of 526 electrographic seizures, and only 19% of the electrographic seizure time was accompanied by clinical manifestations (Fig. 12.11). Further, only 9% of electrographic seizures were accompanied by clinical seizure activity that was identified by neonatal staff.[186] These data indicate that the majority of neonatal seizures are EEG-only, that is, identifiable only with EEG monitoring.

In newborns with clinically evident seizures, the administration of antiseizure medications may lead to termination of the clinically evident seizures while electrographic seizures persist, which is an occurrence referred to as electromechanical uncoupling or electromechanical dissociation.[228,229,241] In the study by Clancy and colleagues, 79% of 393 electrical seizures recorded were not accompanied by clinical seizure activity monitored by direct observation; 88% of the total population of patients had been treated with one or more antiseizure medications.[227] Thus, when clinically evident electroclinical seizures terminate following antiseizure medication administration, EEG monitoring may be needed to assess for ongoing EEG-only seizures.

The *reasons for electroclinical dissociation/uncoupling are probably multiple, but data concerning the development of Cl⁻ transporters in perinatal human brain provide a rational explanation.* As discussed earlier, a developmental mismatch occurs between the transporter responsible for Cl⁻ influx (NKCC1) and the transporter responsible for Cl⁻ efflux (KCC2), so that, in the human perinatal brain, neuronal Cl⁻ levels are likely to be high. Thus, GABA activation results in Cl⁻ efflux with resulting depolarization, and thus excitation. Therefore, with treatment with common anticonvulsant medications, such as phenobarbital and benzodiazepines, which are principally GABA agonists, electrographic seizures are not consistently terminated. However, because the maturation of the transporters occurs in a caudal-to-rostral direction,[13,242] neuronal Cl⁻ levels in the brain stem and spinal cord motor systems would be expected to decrease to normal levels before cortical neuronal levels. Thus, GABA activation induced by antiseizure medications would eliminate the motor phenomena of the seizure, but not the cortical electrographic component, resulting in electroclinical dissociation/uncoupling.

The findings described earlier have led to an increased reliance on EEG monitoring with either conventional EEG or aEEG for three main reasons. First, many newborns experience only EEG-only seizures, and EEG-only seizures constitute the majority of neonatal seizures. Second, even in newborns with clinically evident electroclinical seizures, the administration of antiseizure medications may induce electromechanical dissociation/uncoupling with the termination of clinically evident seizures but persisting EEG-only seizures. Third, clinical events may be difficult to distinguish as seizure based on clinical observation, which potentially leads to unnecessary exposure of newborns to antiseizure medications for nonepileptic events. As a result, many neonatal intensive care units place increased importance on EEG monitoring, either using conventional EEG or aEEG, to identify neonatal seizures[166-170]; and, as noted earlier, an expanded role for EEG monitoring has been advocated by recent guidelines, consensus statements, and committee reports (see later discussion).[171-173]

Nonepileptic Movements

Nonepileptic neonatal movements can be difficult to distinguish from seizures by appearance alone, and EEG assessment may be required. Some nonictal movements are benign events while others, although not seizures, are nonetheless abnormal and indicative of underlying brain injury or dysfunction.[243]

Jitteriness. Jitteriness is characterized by movements with qualities primarily of tremulousness but occasionally of clonus. The most consistently defined causes of jitteriness are hypoxic-ischemic encephalopathy, hypocalcemia, hypoglycemia, and drug withdrawal. Five characteristics aid in distinguishing

---

[a]References 22, 23, 29, 31-33, 188, 189, and 227-236.

TABLE 12.16	Distinguishing Between Jitteriness and Seizure	
CLINICAL FEATURE	**JITTERINESS**	**SEIZURE**
Abnormality of gaze or eye movement	0	+
Movements stimulus sensitive	+	0
Predominant movement	Tremor	Clonic jerking
Movements cease with passive flexion	+	0
Associated autonomic changes	0	+

between jitteriness and seizure (Table 12.16). First, jitteriness is not accompanied by ocular phenomena (i.e., eye fixation or deviation); seizures often are associated with ocular phenomena. Second, jitteriness is exquisitely stimulus sensitive; seizures generally are not stimulus sensitive. Third, the dominant movement in jitteriness is tremor (i.e., the alternating movements are rhythmic and of equal rate and amplitude); the dominant movement in seizure is clonic jerking (i.e., movements with a fast and slow component). Fourth, the rhythmic movements of limbs in jitteriness usually can be stopped by gentle passive flexion of the affected limb; seizures do not cease with this maneuver. Finally, jitteriness is not accompanied by autonomic changes (e.g., tachycardia, increase in blood pressure, apnea, cutaneous vasomotor phenomena, pupillary change, salivation, or drooling); seizures may be accompanied by one or more of these autonomic changes. These same distinguishing clinical features are useful in the clinical distinction of episodic movements other than jitteriness that may mimic a seizure.

Tremors. Tremors may be misidentified as clonic seizures because both are characterized by rhythmic oscillatory movements. In tremor, both phases of movement are of the same amplitude and speed, whereas with a clonic seizure there is a fast movement followed by a slower rebound movement. In addition, tremors are generally higher frequency (faster movement) and lower amplitude (smaller and finer movements) than clonic seizures, which are characterized by slower frequency and higher amplitude movements. Finally, tremors are suppressed by subtle pressure or repositioning of the affected body part while seizures persist with pressure or repositioning. Though often spontaneous, tremors may be elicited by stimuli, while seizures arise spontaneously.

Jitteriness and tremors are common and are reported in about half of healthy newborns.[244] A benign tremor is hypothesized to be due to the immaturity of inhibitory neurons[245] or elevated levels of catecholamines.[246] Excessive, pathological tremors can occur with systemic disorders (hypoglycemia, hypocalcemia, infection, drug withdrawal, or thyroid disease) and primary neurological disorders (hypoxic-ischemic encephalopathy or intraventricular hemorrhage). Fine tremors are more likely to be benign or related to electrolyte disturbances while higher-amplitude tremors are more likely to be secondary to brain disorders.[247]

Nonepileptic Myoclonus. Nonepileptic myoclonus may be benign or pathological. Healthy premature infants often demonstrate occasional spontaneous myoclonus. *Benign neonatal myoclonus*, alternately termed benign neonatal sleep myoclonus, can be pronounced, is typically most prominent in sleep, and can last up to several minutes. Benign neonatal myoclonus may be differentiated from pathological myoclonus in that benign myoclonus can be stopped by rousing the infant and typically does not involve the face.[248-255] The episodes usually last for several minutes or more and occur only during sleep, particularly quiet (non-rapid eye movement) sleep. They can be provoked by gentle rocking of the crib mattress in a head-to-toe direction and cease abruptly with arousal. The EEG pattern during the episodes does not show an ictal correlate, and interictal EEG findings are either normal or show minor, nonspecific abnormalities. The episodes can be exacerbated or provoked by treatment with benzodiazepines and resolve within approximately 2 months. The neurological outcome is normal.

Pathological myoclonus is attributed to a brain stem release phenomenon from loss of cortical inhibition of lower circuits. It is frequently seen in infants with severe global brain injury from hypoxia-ischemia, severe intraventricular hemorrhage, and toxic-metabolic disturbances, including drug withdrawal and glycine encephalopathy. These newborns have abnormal neurological exams and abnormal background patterns on EEG.[195,256,257]

Hyperekplexia. Hyperekplexia is also known as *startle disease* or *congenital stiff-man syndrome*.[33,190,221-226,258-264] It is characterized principally by two abnormal forms of response to unexpected auditory, visual, and somesthetic stimuli, which are an exaggerated startle response and sustained tonic spasms.[221-226,258-264] Additional features are generalized hypertonia and prominent nocturnal myoclonus. The "minor" form of hyperekplexia only involves excessive startle, while the "major" form is associated with additional problems, including generalized stiffness while awake, nocturnal myoclonus, and an increased risk of sudden infant death syndrome from central and obstructive apnea.

The hypertonia and exaggerated startle are apparent from the first hours of life, and sudden jerky movements have been noted even in utero. The typical clinical picture is a hyperalert infant who responds to sudden external stimulus, auditory, visual, or somesthetic (simple handling, nose tap, air blow over face) with recurrent startles, increasing rigidity, jittery movements that become rhythmic and mimic seizure, and occasionally apnea. The stiffness may interfere with bathing and diaper changes. Feeding difficulties and spasms can prevent adequate nutrition. Indeed, the tonic spasms may mimic generalized tonic seizures and can be dangerous, because they may lead to apnea. The EEG does not show epileptic discharges associated with the clinical events.

Hyperekplexia may be caused by glycine receptor gene mutations, and clonazepam can be an effective treatment for excessive startle.[195,265] The episodes usually cease spontaneously by the age of approximately 2 years. In some patients, the disorder is inherited in an autosomal dominant fashion, and the responsible gene is on chromosome 5, which is known to encode the α-1 subunit of the glycine receptor. Neurophysiological studies suggest that the primary physiological abnormality is related to increased excitability of reticular neurons in the

TABLE 12.17	Normal Neonatal Motor Activity Commonly Mistaken for Seizure Activity Awake or Drowsy

Roving, sometimes dysconjugate eye movements, with occasional nonsustained nystagmoid jerks at the extremes of horizontal movement (contrast with fixed, tonic horizontal deviation of eyes with or without jerking, characteristic of subtle seizure)
Sucking, puckering movements not accompanied by ocular fixation or deviation
Asleep
Fragmentary myoclonic jerks (may be multiple)
Isolated, generalized myoclonic jerk as infant wakes from sleep

TABLE 12.18	Epileptic Phenomena in the Absence of Surface-Recorded Electroencephalographic Seizure Discharges

Many simple partial seizures in older children and adults have been accompanied by no ictal seizure discharges recorded from surface electrodes
Complex partial seizures in older children and adults emanating from the temporal lobe, particularly the hippocampus, may be undetectable on surface-recorded EEG and even from subdural electrodes; depth electrodes may be required to detect the ictal hippocampal discharges.
Many subtle seizure phenomena in the newborn suggest complex partial seizures; subtle seizures have been documented in congenital maldevelopment of the hippocampus; the hippocampus is a frequent site of neuronal disease in neonatal encephalopathies, especially hypoxic-ischemic encephalopathy
Clinical seizure phenomena can occur in infants with hydranencephaly in the absence of (surface-recorded) EEG discharges
Bilateral, synchronous, and rhythmic myoclonic movements can occur in benign neonatal sleep myoclonus and in benign myoclonus of early infancy, always without seizure discharges from surface-recorded EEG

EEG, Electroencephalographic.

brain stem.[223] The α-1 subunit of the glycine receptor is critical for Cl^- influx and thereby inhibitory interneuron function in spinal cord and brain stem.[225,262,266-268]

Other Normal Motor Activities. Newborns may exhibit additional normal motor activity that could be mistaken for seizures, and these are important to recognize to avoid unnecessarsy diagnostic testing and exposure to antiseizure medications (Table 12.17). Certain unusual but benign paroxysmal neonatal motor phenomena (e.g., paroxysmal downward gaze or upward gaze) also must be distinguished from seizure (see Chapter 9).[269-272]

Does Absence of Electroencephalographic Seizure Activity Indicate That a Clinical Event Is Nonepileptic?

Central to the concept that certain neonatal clinical events are nonepileptic (e.g., brain stem release phenomena) is the lack of a consistent EEG seizure accompaniment. Does the absence of EEG seizure activity rule out an epileptic origin for the clinical activity? Data from older children and adults, as well as in newborns, indicate that *epileptic phenomena can occur in the absence of surface-recorded EEG discharges, and such phenomena can be generated at subcortical (i.e., deep limbic, diencephalic, brain stem) levels* (Table 12.18).[31,249-251,273-283]

Particularly strong support for the notion that neonatal seizures may originate from brain stem structures is provided by rodent studies.[283] Investigators showed that stimulation of the inferior colliculus of the adult rat caused a persistent electrical discharge accompanied by wild running behavior. However, stimulation of this midbrain region in the neonatal rat produced less complex movement such as "forelimb paddling, hind limb treading, and rolling-curling movements of the torso."[283] These may be analogous to the "boxing," "bicycling," and similar movements of the human newborn. Moreover, the sensitivity of the inferior colliculus for the development of the electrical and clinical seizure activity was considerably greater in the newborn than in the older animal. In addition, it is noteworthy that the inferior colliculus of the newborn is particularly sensitive to hypoxic-ischemic brain injury, the most common cause of neonatal seizures.

Several studies of more than 100 newborns with EEG-confirmed seizures have helped to clarify the relationship between subtle seizures and electrographic seizures. First, the proportion of newborns who exhibited subtle clinical seizures was nearly identical among newborns who either did or did not exhibit simultaneous electrographic discharges.[29,33,213] Thus, there was no overrepresentation of subtle seizures in the newborns who did not exhibit an EEG correlate. Second, the groups with and without EEG accompaniments to the subtle seizures were clinically similar and had similar neurological outcomes. Thus, there was no indication that the newborns without consistent EEG correlates to the subtle movements were more likely to have cerebral destruction with resulting "release" phenomena. Third, newborns with subtle seizures sometimes exhibited or did not exhibit concomitant EEG seizures. Finally, the clinical phenomena often began seconds *before* the electrographic discharges. Together, these data indicate that some subtle clinical seizures may originate from subcortical structures and only sometimes propagate to the cortex to produce surface-recorded EEG seizures. This mechanism would account for inconsistent electroclinical correlations and for the fact that the initial EEG change may occur after the initial clinical manifestation.[29,213]

More data are needed regarding the pathophysiology of subtle seizures. Of particular importance is whether such "surface EEG-silent" seizures have the potential to result in brain injury, whether they can be eliminated by conventional antiseizure medication therapy, and whether elimination of the events is associated with more favorable neurobehavioral outcomes.

Seizure Etiology

The majority of neonatal seizures occur in the context of acute neurological disorders. Thus, most neonatal seizures may be considered *acute symptomatic seizures,* which have been defined

TABLE 12.19   Neonatal Seizure Etiologies in Relation to Time of Seizure Onset and Relative Frequency

CAUSE	TIME OF ONSET[a]		RELATIVE FREQUENCY[b]	
	0–3 DAYS	>3 DAYS	PREMATURE	FULL TERM
Hypoxic-ischemic encephalopathy	+		+++	+++
Intracranial hemorrhage[c]	+	+	++	+
Intracranial infection[d]	+	+	++	++
Developmental defects	+	+	++	++
Hypoglycemia	+		+	+
Hypocalcemia[e]	+	+	+	+
Other metabolic[f]	+			+
Epilepsy syndromes[g]	+	+		+

[a]Postnatal age when seizures most commonly begin.

[b]Relative frequency of seizures: +++, most common; ++, less common; +, least common.

[c]Hemorrhages are principally germinal matrix intraventricular, often with periventricular hemorrhagic infarction, in the premature infant and subarachnoid or subdural in the term infant.

[d]Early seizures occur usually with intrauterine nonbacterial infections (e.g., toxoplasmosis, cytomegalovirus infection), and later seizures usually occur with herpes simplex encephalitis or bacterial meningitis.

[e]Two varieties of hypocalcemia (see text).

[f]See text for types.

[g]See text for epilepsy syndromes.

as seizure occurring at the time of a systemic insult or in close temporal association (often 1 week) with a documented brain insult.[284] The current International League Against Epilepsy classifies seizure causes as *genetic, structural metabolic, and unknown*.[285] Within that classification scheme, the majority of neonatal seizures are structural metabolic in etiology.

Determination of the seizure etiology is critical because it affords the opportunity to provide specific treatment and important prognostic information. While there are many causes for neonatal seizures, a relatively limited group of etiologies accounts for the majority of affected newborns. The most common causes and their usual time of onset in premature or full-term infants are shown in Table 12.19. The most common underlying etiologies are hypoxic-ischemic encephalopathy, stroke, intracranial hemorrhage, intracranial infections, and cerebral dysgenesis.[a] Less common but important etiologies include inborn errors of metabolism[288-290] and neonatal epileptic syndromes, such as benign familial neonatal epilepsy (BFNE), benign nonfamilial neonatal seizures ("fifth-day fits"), early myoclonic epilepsy, early infantile epileptic encephalopathy (EIEE), and malignant migrating partial seizures of infancy (see later).[291,292]

The Neonatal Seizure Registry consortium of seven tertiary care pediatric centers in the United States prospectively collected data related to etiology in a cohort of 426 newborns with seizures who underwent continuous EEG (cEEG). The most common seizure etiologies were hypoxic-ischemic encephalopathy in 38%, ischemic stroke in 18%, neonatal onset epilepsy in 13%, intracranial hemorrhage in 11%, neonatal genetic epilepsy syndrome in 6%, congenital cerebral malformation in 4%, and BFNE in 3%. In addition, for all these etiologies, the seizure burden was high, with 59% of subjects having greater than 7 electrographic seizures, and 16% status epilepticus. There was no significant difference in seizure burden between preterm and full-term newborns or among the three most

common causes of seizure (hypoxic-ischemic encephalopathy, ischemic stroke, and intracerebral hemorrhage).[293] These etiologies were similar to those reported in a study by Weeke and colleagues of 378 newborns obtained over a 14-year period with seizures confirmed by EEG or aEEG from a level 3 neonatal intensive care unit. The most common etiologies identified were hypoxic-ischemic encephalopathy (46%), intracranial hemorrhage (12.2%), and perinatal arterial ischemic stroke (10.6%).[294] These etiologies are quite similar to those found in a study by Tekgul and colleagues in which 89 newborns underwent careful etiological evaluation. The most common etiologies were global hypoxic-ischemic encephalopathy in 40%, focal ischemic injury in 38%, intracranial hemorrhage in 17%, cerebral dysgenesis in 5%, transient metabolic disturbance in 3%, infection in 3%, and an inborn error of metabolism in 1%. The etiology remained unknown in 12%.[286] Thus, *in summary three key conditions account for nearly 75% of neonatal seizures*—hypoxic-ischemic brain injury (40% to 50%), arterial stroke (10% to 15%), and intracranial hemorrhage (10% to 20%). The next two most common etiologies are intracranial infection (5%) and cerebral dysgenesis (5%). The remaining less common conditions, accounting for 5% to 10% of all seizures, remain important because of potential therapeutic interventions in transient metabolic disorders and inborn errors of metabolism.

The following discussion briefly discusses common seizure etiologies with an emphasis on seizure characteristics. More detailed discussions of the specific clinical entities may be found in the appropriate chapters of this book.

Hypoxic-Ischemic Encephalopathy

Hypoxic-ischemic encephalopathy is the most common cause of neonatal seizures in both full-term and premature infants accounting for close to one-half of the causes (see Chapters 16 and 18).[a] The seizure burden is often high in

---

[a]References 2, 29, 214, 239, 286, and 287.

[a]References 2, 26, 29, 33, 286, and 293-306.

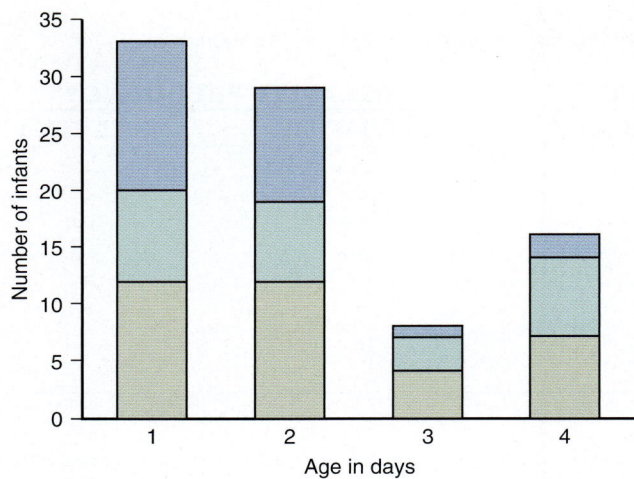

Figure 12.12 Electrographic seizure frequency from day 1 to 4 after birth. Seizure frequency was classified according to sporadic (gray), frequent (light blue), and status epilepticus (dark blue). (From Shah DK, Wusthoff CJ, Clarke P, et al. Electrographic seizures are associated with brain injury in newborns undergoing therapeutic hypothermia. Arch Dis Child Fetal Neonatal Ed. 2014;99:F219–F224, with permission.)

the term newborn with hypoxic-ischemic encephalopathy, and may result in electrographic status epilepticus in between 10% and 15% of cases. A multicenter observational study of 90 newborns treated with therapeutic hypothermia for hypoxic-ischemic encephalopathy and who underwent conventional EEG monitoring identified electrographic seizures in 48%, including 10% with electrographic status epilepticus. Abnormal EEG background features (excessive discontinuity, depressed and undifferentiated patterns, burst suppression, or extremely low voltage) were associated with seizures, but no perinatal variables, including pH less than 6.8, base excess ≤−20, or 10-minute Apgar ≤3, predicted seizure occurrence.[231] Similarly, an earlier single center of 26 consecutive newborns with hypoxic-ischemic encephalopathy undergoing therapeutic hypothermia and continuous conventional EEG monitoring identified electrographic seizures in 65%, which were entirely nonconvulsive in 47% with seizures, and constituted electrographic status epilepticus in 23% with seizures.[233] Regarding the timing of seizures in hypoxic-ischemic encephalopathy (HIE), conventional teaching has been that seizures generally occur in the initial 24 hours of life and become more frequent from 12 to 24 hours after birth. Recent studies using EEG monitoring in consecutive newborns with hypoxic-ischemic encephalopathy confirmed that seizures are most common in the initial 24 hours, but that they can initiate during hypothermia or rewarming, and rarely after a return to normothermia (Fig. 12.12).[232,306,307]

There is some evidence that therapeutic hypothermia may *reduce electrographic seizure exposure in newborns*. However, comparing seizure incidence on studies conducted before and after therapeutic hypothermia utilization may not reflect a reduction in seizures because most studies performed initially relied on clinical observation for seizure identification while most studies performed later used EEG monitoring for seizure identification. Data obtained before the implementation of therapeutic hypothermia as a neuroprotective strategy reported

EEG seizures in 22% to 64% of newborns.[307-309] In newborns with moderate to severe hypoxic-ischemic encephalopathy managed with therapeutic hypothermia, seizures were identified in 30% to 65%.[231,310,311] A single-center study did note a significant reduction in EEG seizure burden in newborns with moderate (but not severe) hypoxic-ischemic encephalopathy who underwent therapeutic hypothermia compared with those who did not receive this treatment, after controlling for degree of magnetic resonance imaging (MRI)–assessed injury, suggesting that therapeutic hypothermia had anticonvulsant therapeutic impact.[312] Similarly, a retrospective study of 107 newborns with hypoxic-ischemic encephalopathy identified seizures in 37 with EEG monitoring. The EEG tracings could be analyzed in 31 newborns, including 15 who received therapeutic hypothermia and 16 who did not receive therapeutic hypothermia. EEG monitoring was initiated earlier in newborns who received therapeutic hypothermia, and despite that group having a longer opportunity for seizure identification with EEG monitoring, the recorded electrographic seizure burden in the cooled group was significantly lower than in the noncooled group (60 vs. 203 minutes). However, this difference was only apparent in those with moderate hypoxic-ischemic encephalopathy.[313]

As described earlier, multiple animal and human studies suggest that seizures exacerbate existing cerebral injury.[149,314-317] Thus, most clinicians aim to identify and manage seizures in these newborns. *A statement from the American Academy of Pediatrics recommends that centers performing therapeutic hypothermia in newborns with hypoxic-ischemic encephalopathy have either aEEG or conventional EEG available for seizure identification.*[172]

Ischemic Stroke

Ischemic stroke is the second most common cause of neonatal seizures in full-term newborns, accounting for between 10% and 20% of cases (see Chapter 21).[286,293,294] The incidence of perinatal arterial stroke is approximately 1 in 1600 to 5000.[318] At least half of neonatal stroke cases are not recognized in the neonatal period, but for those that are diagnosed in the neonatal period, up to 97% present with seizures and 50% have seizures as the only recognized sign.[319] Compared to newborns with more diffuse brain injury, such as hypoxic-ischemic encephalopathy, *those with neonatal stroke as a cause of seizures are more likely to appear active and alert between seizures*. In addition, seizures due to arterial ischemic stroke tend to occur after the first 12 hours of life; that is, somewhat later than those due to hypoxic-ischemic encephalopathy (see Chapter 22). The risk of developing subsequent epilepsy ranges from approximately 10% to 50%, depending on time to follow-up and inclusion criteria.[319-322]

Cerebral sinus venous thrombosis occurs less frequently than arterial stroke in newborns, affecting approximately 1 in 8 to 38,000 children per year; 42% to 78% of these newborns have experienced a venous infarct.[323,324] Seizures are the presenting symptom or a complication of cerebral sinus venous thrombosis in 55% to 80% of the cases, but affected newborns usually also manifest diffuse and focal neurological deficits.

Intracranial Hemorrhage

Intracranial hemorrhage may be difficult to establish conclusively as a cause of seizures distinct from hypoxic-ischemic or traumatic injury because of the frequent association of one or both of these factors with the hemorrhage. Nevertheless, approximately

15% of term infants have intracranial hemorrhage as the primary cause of their seizure, and this incidence is higher in premature infants.[29,306] In the contemporary multicenter neonatal seizure registry study described earlier, intracranial hemorrhage was the etiology in 12% of newborns with seizures,[293] and in the large previously described single-center cohort, 12% had intracranial hemorrhage as the etiology.[294]

Intracerebral hemorrhage often presents with seizures in newborns. In one prospective study of newborns and children with intracerebral hemorrhage, 60% of 20 newborns with intracerebral hemorrhage presented with seizures. In addition, 18 subjects underwent EEG during the acute period, including EEG monitoring in 13, and EEG-only seizures were identified in 25% of the 20 newborns.[325]

Primary subarachnoid hemorrhage, although very common, is usually not of major clinical significance. Nevertheless, seizures can occur secondary to subarachnoid hemorrhage in the full-term infant, and in that context the spells most often have their onset on the second postnatal day.[326] Newborns with subarachnoid hemorrhage in association with hypoxic-ischemic encephalopathy usually exhibit seizures on the first postnatal day, probably as a result of the encephalopathy rather than the hemorrhage. In the interictal period, newborns with seizures secondary to uncomplicated subarachnoid hemorrhage often appear remarkably well.

Germinal matrix-intraventricular hemorrhage, emanating from small blood vessels in the subependymal germinal matrix, is principally a lesion of the premature infants, occurring in the first 3 days of life (see Chapter 24). Seizures in association with this type of hemorrhage usually occur with severe lesions or with accompanying parenchymal involvement or both. In one series of EEG-confirmed seizures, 28 of 62 (45%) of preterm newborns had severe intraventricular hemorrhage with or without periventricular hemorrhagic infarction.[29] More recent studies have documented a high incidence of seizures in the preterm infant in the first 72 hours of life,[327] and these were strongly associated with the presence of intraventricular hemorrhage (IVH). In one study, 95 very preterm infants (<30 weeks gestational age) underwent aEEG monitoring during the first 72 hours of life. The overall incidence of seizures in this sample was 48%. High seizure burden was associated with increased risk of IVH throughout each of the 3 days of monitoring.[234] The seizures observed in this very preterm cohort demonstrated a similar evolution in time line to the seizures of a term infant suffering from HIE with the highest median seizure burden during the 0- to 24-hour period. These observations support the potential role of perinatal asphyxia in the pathway to IVH.

Subdural hemorrhage is often associated with a traumatic event, and it is probably the associated cerebral contusion that results in the convulsive phenomena (see Chapter 22). The most common variety of subdural hemorrhage is the convexity type, and the seizures in this setting are often focal. Historically, in one large series, convulsive phenomena occurred in 50% of newborns with subdural hemorrhage and appeared in the first 48 hours of life.[328] However, in more recent series with less severe hemorrhages, the vast majority of subdural hemorrhages were asymptomatic.[329,330] In most newborns with extra-axial hemorrhage, no neurosurgical intervention is required, and following resolution of the acute symptomatic seizures, the prognosis is excellent.[331]

Intracranial Infection

Intracranial bacterial and nonbacterial infections are not uncommon causes of neonatal seizures (see Chapters 34 and 35). In the contemporary multicenter neonatal seizure registry study described earlier, infection was the etiology in 4% of newborns with seizures.[293] There is an equal incidence in preterm and term infants.[286,331,332] Infections can include congenital infections (such as TORCH [*T*oxoplasmosis, *O*ther, *R*ubella, *C*ytomegalovirus, and *H*erpes infections] infection) or acute CNS infections. Of the bacterial infections, meningitides secondary to *Group B streptococci* and *Escherichia coli* are the most common pathogens. The onset of seizures in these instances is usually in the latter part of the first week and subsequent to that period. The relevant nonbacterial infections include the various neonatal encephalitides: toxoplasmosis, herpes simplex, coxsackievirus B infection, rubella, and cytomegalovirus infection. In intrauterine toxoplasmosis or cytomegalovirus infection that is severe enough to result in neonatal seizures, the episodes occur in the first 3 days of life. Seizures associated with herpes simplex encephalitis tend to occur after 7 days of life. Early-onset disseminated herpes simplex virus (HSV) disease does not usually present with seizures. Seizures are more common in term infants with localized CNS rather than disseminated disease.[333] The infant with this variety of neonatal HSV infection usually has been discharged from the hospital before the illness begins. The usual signs are stupor and irritability, which evolve to seizures (often focal) and, perhaps, coma.

Developmental Defects

Many aberrations of brain development can result in seizures, which begin at any time during the neonatal period. In the contemporary multicenter neonatal seizure registry study described previously, brain malformations were the etiology in 4% of newborns with seizures.[293] Similarly, in prior studies malformations of cortical development accounted for 5% to 9% of neonatal seizures.[286,332] Common malformations include tuberous sclerosis, focal cortical dysplasia, hemimegalencephaly, lissencephaly, subcortical band heterotopia, periventricular nodular heterotopia, schizencephaly, and polymicrogyria (see Chapters 5 and 6). Though these disorders may be the cause of a substantial percent of neonatal seizures, most patients with these malformations do not have seizures in the neonatal period. In tuberous sclerosis, only 5% of children develop seizures in the neonatal period.[334] Outcomes depend primarily on the type and severity of malformation.

Metabolic Disturbances

This category includes abnormalities in the levels of glucose, calcium, magnesium, electrolytes, amino acids, organic acids, blood ammonia, and other metabolites; certain intoxications, especially with local anesthetics; mitochondrial or peroxisomal disturbance; pyridoxine and folinic acid responsive seizures (FARS); and glucose transporter deficiency (Table 12.20). The aberrations in levels of glucose and divalent cations are the most frequent. In the contemporary multicenter neonatal seizure registry study described earlier, the etiology was a transient metabolic disturbance in 4% and an inborn error of metabolism in 3% of newborns with seizures.[293]

TABLE 12.20	Major Metabolic Disturbances Associated With Neonatal Seizures

Hypoglycemia
Hypocalcemia and hypomagnesemia
Local anesthetic intoxication
Hyponatremia
Hypernatremia (especially during correction)
Amino acidopathy (especially nonketotic hyperglycinemia)
Organic acidopathy
Hyperammonemia (often associated with acidopathies)
Mitochondrial disturbance (pyruvate dehydrogenase, cytochrome-c oxidase)
Peroxisomal disturbance (Zellweger syndrome, neonatal adrenoleukodystrophy)
Pyridoxine dependency (also pyridoxal-5-phosphate deficiency)
Folinic acid–responsive seizures
Glucose transporter deficiency
DEND
HI/HA syndrome

HI/HA, Hyperinsulinism/hyperammonemia.

Hypoglycemia. Hypoglycemia is most frequent in small newborns, most of whom are small for their gestational age, and in infants of mothers who are diabetic or prediabetic (see Chapter 25). Hypoglycemia is thought to be responsible for approximately 3% of neonatal seizures, although the incidence has been falling with improved neonatal care.[286] The most critical determinants for the occurrence of neurological symptoms in neonatal hypoglycemia are the *duration of the hypoglycemia and, as a corollary, the amount of time elapsed before treatment is begun.*[335] Neurological symptoms consist most commonly of jitteriness, stupor, hypotonia, apnea, and seizures. In a review of infants who were small for their gestational age and who had hypoglycemia, approximately 80% exhibited neurological symptoms; and more than 50% of symptomatic infants who were small for their gestational age experienced seizures.[336] The onset is usually the second postnatal day. In these newborns, it is often particularly difficult to establish that hypoglycemia is the cause of the neurological syndrome, because perinatal asphyxia, hemorrhage, hypocalcemia, and infection are frequently associated. In an earlier series, although 9% of infants with seizures experienced hypoglycemia, in none was the metabolic defect the only potential etiological factor.[337] In a more recent series, only 3% of neonatal seizures were related to hypoglycemia.[286,295,297] In contrast to the situation with small infants, neurological symptoms, including seizures, are much less frequent in hypoglycemic infants of diabetic mothers (10% to 20%), possibly because the duration of hypoglycemia in the latter infants is relatively brief.[336] Hypoglycemia significant enough to trigger seizures is often associated with adverse neurodevelopmental outcomes.[338]

Hypocalcemia. Hypocalcemia has *two major peaks of incidence in the newborn*. The first peak, which takes place in the *first 2 to 3 days* of life, occurs most often in low-birth-weight newborns, both of average and below-average weight for their gestational age, and in infants of diabetic mothers. In an earlier series, 13% of the infants with seizures exhibited hypocalcemia, but as with hypoglycemia, the metabolic defect was not the only

major etiological possibility.[337] In a later series, hypocalcemia was the cause of 3% of neonatal seizures.[286,295] A therapeutic response to intravenous calcium is of major value in determining whether the low serum calcium is related etiologically to the seizures. Early hypocalcemia may be a condition *associated with* neonatal seizures rather than the cause.[297]

When *hypocalcemia appears later in the neonatal period*, without the complicated associated factors of early-onset hypocalcemia, delineation of hypocalcemia as the major etiological factor in the convulsive phenomena is easier. Classically, these hypocalcemic newborns are large, full-term infants who avidly consume a milk preparation with a suboptimal ratio of phosphorus to calcium and phosphorus to magnesium (e.g., cow's milk or a high-phosphorus synthetic formula). Hypomagnesemia is a frequent accompaniment, or, more rarely, may be present without hypocalcemia.[331,339-341] The neurological syndrome is consistent and distinctive, involving primarily the following: hyperactive tendon reflexes; knee, ankle, and jaw clonus; jitteriness; and seizures. The convulsive phenomena are often focal, both clinically and electroencephalographically.[339,342] Later-onset hypocalcemia of the nutritional type is unusual in the United States. Later-onset hypocalcemic seizures are associated more commonly with endocrinopathy (maternal hyperparathyroidism, neonatal hypoparathyroidism) or with congenital heart disease (with or without DiGeorge syndrome).[343,344] Primary hypomagnesemia—a rare defect of magnesium absorption—may produce a syndrome similar to that just described for late-onset hypocalcemia.[341,345,346] The onset of seizures is most commonly between 2 and 6 weeks of age. Because calcium levels also may be low, the mistaken diagnosis of primary hypocalcemia may be made. Parenteral administration of magnesium prevents the seizures and early infantile death.

Local Anesthetic Intoxication. Seizures are a prominent feature of neonatal intoxication with local anesthetics, which are inadvertently injected, usually into the infant's scalp, at the time of placement of paracervical, pudendal, or epidural block or local anesthesia for episiotomy.[297,347-358] Although direct injection into the fetus is the usual mode of administration, transplacental transmission is possible. Paracervical and pudendal blocks have been the most common forms of maternal analgesia involved in the well-documented cases of fetal injection. *Two distinguishing features of local anesthetic intoxication aid in the differential diagnosis:* (1) pupils fixed to light and often dilated and (2) eye movements fixed to the oculocephalic (doll's eyes) reflex. These latter signs are unusual in hypoxic-ischemic disease in the first 12 hours. The finding that infants with intoxication improve over the first 24 to 48 hours (if properly supported) further distinguishes the disorder from severe hypoxic-ischemic encephalopathy. Clinical signs suggestive of local anesthetic intoxication should alert the physician to a particularly careful inquiry into the obstetrical history and to a search for needle marks on the infant's scalp. Determination of local anesthetic levels in blood and CSF establishes the diagnosis. Management depends on prompt recognition. Vigorous support, especially of ventilation, is essential. The therapy required depends, in part, on the time of recognition of the intoxication; the half-life of the drug in blood is approximately 8 to 10 hours.[359] Removal of the drug is accomplished more effectively by diuresis with acidification of the urine than by exchange transfusion.[359]

Antiseizure medications are of questionable value, and control of seizures is effected best by removal of the local anesthetic. The outcome is good if complications do not occur.

Other Metabolic Disturbances.

Metabolic disturbances other than hypoglycemia and deficiency of divalent cations are uncommon causes of seizures in the newborn (see Table 12.20). Worthy of note are hyponatremia and hypernatremia, hyperammonemia, other amino acid and organic acid abnormalities, mitochondrial disturbances, peroxisomal disorders, pyridoxine dependency, FARS, and glucose transporter deficiency. These metabolic disturbances are all discussed much more extensively in Chapters 27 to 29.

Hyponatremia may result in seizures and often occurs with inappropriate antidiuretic hormone secretion in the context of bacterial meningitis, intracranial hemorrhage, hypoxic-ischemic encephalopathy, or excessive intake of water. The latter may occur in a child with minor gastrointestinal difficulties with inappropriate dilution of formula or excess water (in place of formula) intake.[360] Hypernatremia occurs primarily in severely dehydrated infants or as a complication of overly vigorous use of sodium bicarbonate for the correction of acidosis. Seizures often result during the correction of hypernatremia if markedly hypotonic solutions are used, perhaps secondary to the development of intracellular edema.[361,362] Seizures are most likely to arise in the setting of overly rapid correction with hypotonic fluids.[175,331]

Inborn errors of metabolism may also present with neonatal seizures, and these conditions are discussed in much more detail in Chapters 27 and 28. Disturbances of *amino acid or organic acid metabolism* may result in neonatal seizures, virtually always in the context of other neurological features. The most common of these associated with neonatal seizures are nonketotic hyperglycinemia, sulfite oxidase deficiency, multiple carboxylase deficiency, multiple acyl-coenzyme A dehydrogenase deficiency (glutaric aciduria, type II), and urea cycle defect. Hyperammonemia or acidosis (or both) most commonly accompanies these disturbances. Transient disturbance of the glycine cleavage enzyme may cause neonatal seizures; the diagnosis can be missed if CSF glycine levels are not determined because plasma glycine levels may be normal. The process resolves spontaneously after approximately 6 weeks of age.[363]

Additional unusual causes of neonatal seizures in this context include *mitochondrial or peroxisomal disturbance* (see Chapter 29). Of the former, pyruvate dehydrogenase deficiency and cytochrome *c* oxidase deficiency, with elevated lactate in blood and CSF, are the most common. Although not strictly a "metabolic" disturbance, peroxisomal disease, especially Zellweger syndrome or neonatal adrenoleukodystrophy, associated with elevations of blood levels of very-long-chain fatty acids and other biochemical changes, is associated with severe neonatal seizures, caused by associated cerebral neuronal migrational defects.

Pyridoxine dependency, a disturbance in pyridoxine metabolism, may produce severe seizures that are recalcitrant to usual therapy (see Chapter 29).[15,18,364-391] Onset is usually in the first hours of life, but intrauterine seizures as well as onset after the neonatal period have been observed. Seizures are usually multifocal clonic and recalcitrant to all therapeutic modalities. There is an associated newborn encephalopathy, which may manifest as hyperalertness, tremulousness, or hypothermia.[392] A prodrome of restlessness, irritability, and emesis preceding seizures has been described. A progressive encephalopathy and ultimately death ensue if treatment is not initiated.

Generalized tonic-clonic seizures, a rare form of neonatal seizure, have been described in newborns with pyridoxine dependency. However, the clinical presentation may be varied. Clinical studies also indicate that the disorder may begin after days or weeks; that the seizures may respond initially to anticonvulsant medications; and that doses of pyridoxine greater than 100 mg may be necessary to stop the seizures.[367-371,376,386,393]

Any suspicion of the disorder should lead to a therapeutic trial of pyridoxine (see later). The diagnosis may be suspected from the EEG that usually shows an unusual paroxysmal pattern consisting of generalized bursts of bilaterally synchronous high-voltage 1- to 4-Hz activity with intermixed spikes or sharp waves (Fig. 12.13).[371] Diagnosis is supported by documentation of cessation of seizures and normalization of the EEG findings within minutes after intravenous injection of 50 to 100 mg of pyridoxine. The EEG findings may not normalize for several hours, even when a prompt seizure response is observed. Subsequently complete control of seizures on pyridoxine monotherapy and recurrence on withdrawal established the diagnosis.

Most infants have exhibited subsequent intellectual disability despite therapy from the first days of life. Nevertheless, early therapy may decrease the likelihood or severity, or both, of intellectual deficit; indeed, 8 of the 10 reported infants with normal intellect were identified and treated in the first month of life. However, many infants treated in the first month still exhibit cognitive deficits later. Intrauterine therapy by maternal pyridoxine supplementation may be necessary to prevent fetal brain injury.[386]

The *molecular defect* involves the active form of pyridoxine, pyridoxal-5-phosphate, necessary for the action of GAD, which leads to the synthesis of the inhibitory neurotransmitter GABA.[17,376,377,394,395] This formulation is supported by the finding of low GABA levels as well as elevated glutamate levels in CSF.[18,396-400] The disturbance of pyridoxal-5 phosphate results because of its inactivation by alpha-amino adipic semialdehyde (AASA), an intermediate in the degradation of lysine. AASA accumulates because of a defect in its degradation by AASA dehydrogenase (antiquitin), the result of a mutation in the *ALDH7A1* gene. Elevated urinary AASA is a reliable biomarker for the diagnosis of antiquitin deficiency and, hence, pyridoxine-dependent seizures.[401] The major structural features in pyridoxine-dependent seizures include evidence for both neuronal and white matter injury, with diffuse cortical atrophy, callosal thinning, and impaired cerebral myelination. These findings may relate to the elevation in CSF and brain of glutamate, caused by the molecular defect. Glutamate may lead to neuronal injury by excitotoxic mechanisms and to oligodendroglial injury by free radical mechanisms. *Intrauterine* onset of anatomical disturbance is suggested by the *fetal* imaging finding of partial hypoplasia of the corpus callosum.

Pyridoxamine phosphate oxidase deficiency (PNPO) is a related neonatal epileptic disorder involving synthesis of pyridoxal-5-phosphate.[402] The molecular defect involves PNPO, which is required for synthesis of pyridoxal-5-PO_4. The clinical presentation often includes *fetal* seizures, and infants are often *premature* and exhibit an encephalopathy as well as seizures. The disorder requires treatment with pyridoxal-5 phosphate; pyridoxine, not unexpectedly, is not effective therapy.

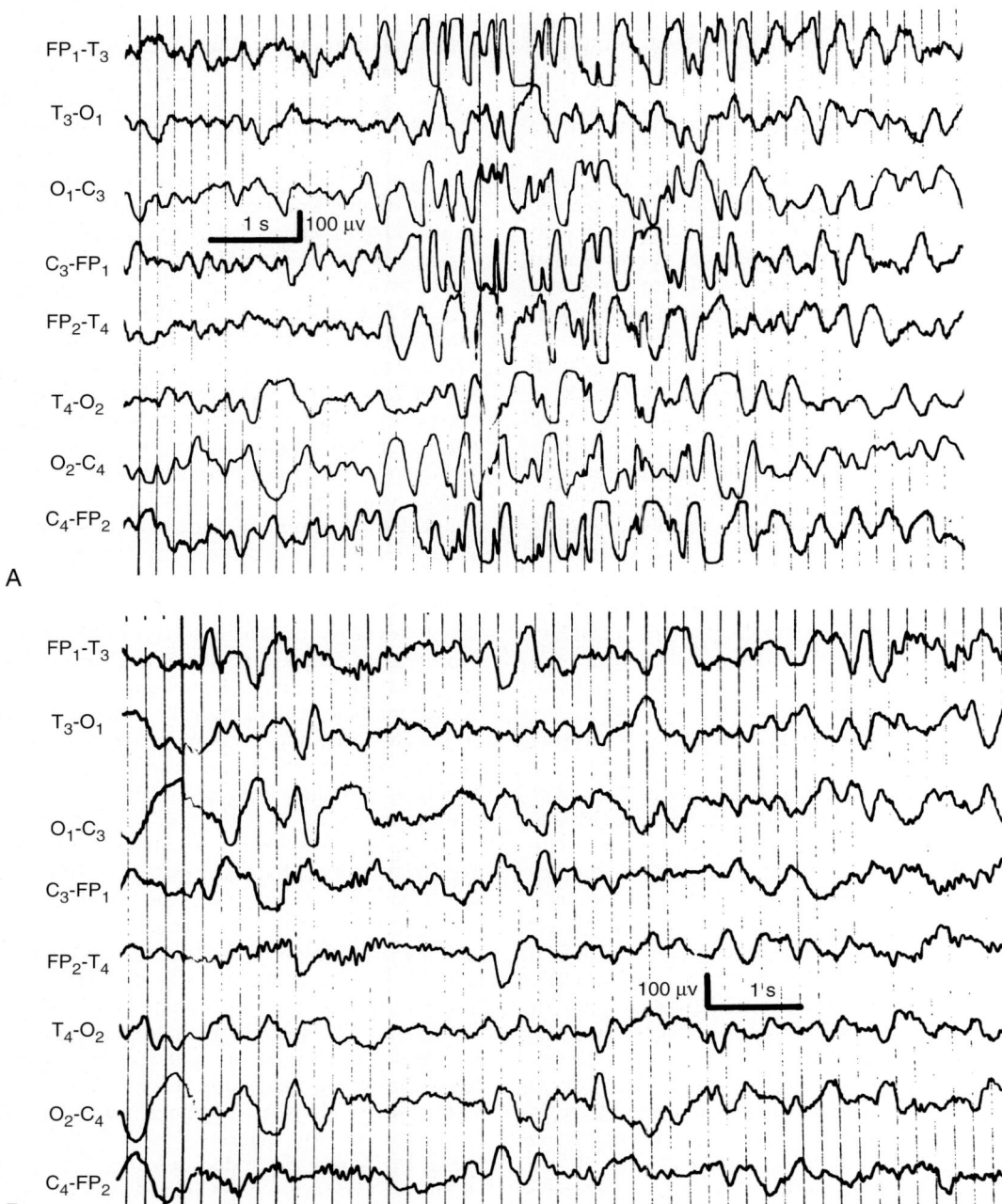

Figure 12.13 Pyridoxine response in an infant with pyridoxine dependency. (A) Before the injection of pyridoxine, the electroencephalogram shows disorganized background with generalized bursts of irregular spikes and sharp–slow wave complexes without clinical accompaniments. Vitamin B_6 was injected 30 seconds later. (B) Ten minutes after vitamin B_6 injection. The discharges have subsided (4 minutes earlier), and the patient shows normal sleep background with early sleep spindles appearing in the tracing. (From Mikati MA, Trevathan E, Krishnamoorthy KS, Lombroso CT. Pyridoxine-dependent epilepsy: EEG investigations and long-term follow-up. *Electroencephalogr Clin Neurophysiol.* 1991;78:215–221.)

Folinic acid-responsive seizures refer to a clinical syndrome of neonatal seizures with onset as early as the first hours of life, responsiveness to oral administration of folinic acid, and the presence on CSF analysis for monoamine neurotransmitters of two unknown metabolic peaks (see Chapter 29).[403-407] The disorder is accompanied by a discontinuous EEG pattern with multifocal sharp waves and progressive cerebral cortical and white matter atrophy. The seizures respond to oral folinic acid at doses ranging from 2 to 20 mg twice daily; the lowest doses have been used in the neonatal period. At least 50% of the infants have had subsequent cognitive deficits. Recent data indicate that FARS and pyridoxine-dependent seizures are syndromes caused by the same genetic defects (see Chapter 29).

A *disorder of glucose transport from blood to brain* is important to recognize because prompt treatment can lead to the cessation of seizures and to improved neurological development.[408-417] This disorder is caused by an autosomal dominant, heterozygous mutation in the GLUT1 transporter (SLC2A1 gene) (see Chapter 29). Approximately 25% of cases have had onset of seizures in the first 2 months of life. The mean age of onset of seizures is 5 months. The striking metabolic findings are low glucose concentrations in CSF with normal blood glucose concentration. The mean ratio of CSF to blood glucose has been 37%. That the hypoglycorrhachia was not the result of increased glycolysis, but rather of impaired glucose transport, is shown by the consistent finding of a low (rather than high) lactate level in CSF. The impaired glucose transport is related to a defect of the glucose transporter (Glut1) responsible for the facilitative diffusion of glucose across the blood-brain endothelial barrier and across the neuronal plasma membrane. Treatment with a ketogenic diet, which supplies usable metabolic fuel for brain energy metabolism not transported by the glucose transporter, is generally effective in leading to seizure control and may blunt the impaired neurological development that is a consistent feature of the disease. However, in general, the beneficial effect of the ketogenic diet is most apparent for seizure control.[395,418,419]

DEND refers to a syndrome characterized by developmental delay, epilepsy, and neonatal diabetes. Characteristic features are a severe neonatal-onset epileptic encephalopathy and diabetes mellitus, associated with a channelopathy involving the endocrine pancreas and the brain.[420] The molecular defect involves an ATP-dependent potassium channel (KATP), responsive to the ratio of intracellular ATP/ADP concentrations. This channel normally closes when the ATP/ADP ratio rises; that is, in association with increased blood glucose. Thus, potassium remains intracellular, and the cell depolarizes. The depolarization leads to Ca^{2+} influx and thereby to physiological insulin release. This mechanism serves to regulate insulin release moment-by-moment in response to blood glucose. In DEND, the channels are unable to close properly. Treatment with insulin is inadequate and does not ameliorate the neurological manifestations. However, sulfonylurea, an oral hypoglycemic agent, binds to the channel, promoting closure and physiological insulin release. Prompt recognition and treatment of this syndrome with oral hypoglycemic agents and not systemic insulin administration are essential for a good neurological outcome.

The *HI/HA syndrome (hyperinsulinism/hyperammonemia syndrome)* also involves regulation of insulin secretion and is associated with neonatal and infantile seizures.[395,418,419] The median age of presentation is 4 to 5 months, although approximately 20% exhibit seizures in the first 72 hours of life in association with hypoglycemia. The hypoglycemia is caused by hyperinsulinism. The molecular defect involves glutamate dehydrogenase (GDH), which generates ATP through the oxidation of glutamate. The rise in ATP to ADP ratio results in closure of K_{ATP} channel and insulin secretion, as discussed re: DEND syndrome. The mutation in the responsible gene (*GLUD1*) impairs its normal inhibition by GTP. Leucine, an endogenous activator of GDH, then operates unopposed to activate GDH and leads to the molecular events described previously for insulin release. Management of the hyperinsulinism in this disorder is accomplished with diazoxide, which promotes the opening of the K_{ATP} channel, thereby inhibiting insulin release. Protein restriction is also useful. The hyperammonemia is mild, is related primarily to upregulated GDH in kidney, and is unrelated to the neurological phenomena. On follow-up, affected infants later exhibit principally atypical absence seizures, learning disabilities, and behavioral problems.

Drug Withdrawal

A rare cause of seizures is passive addiction of the newborn and drug withdrawal. The drugs particularly involved are narcotic-analgesics (e.g., methadone), sedative-hypnotics (e.g., shorter-acting barbiturates), propoxyphene, tricyclic antidepressants, cocaine, and alcohol (see Chapter 38). The usual time of onset of seizures in this setting is the first several days of life.

Neonatal Epilepsy Syndromes

As described earlier, most neonatal seizures represent acute symptomatic (provoked) seizures, but there are rare newborns with epilepsy.[292,421] Several neonatal syndromes are principally distinguished according to their clinical features (see Tables 12.19 and 12.21). The current International League Against Epilepsy classification system defines several electroclinical syndromes with onset in the neonatal and infantile periods. An epilepsy syndrome was defined as "a complex of clinical features, signs, and symptoms that together define a distinctive, recognizable clinical disorder." These distinctive disorders are identifiable on the basis of a typical age of onset, specific EEG characteristics, seizure types, and other factors which, when taken together, permit a specific diagnosis.[184] The classification and terminology used to describe these syndromes have evolved over time.[176,184,243,422] The five major neonatal epilepsy syndromes are discussed next.

Benign Familial Neonatal Epilepsy. This syndrome is an autosomal dominant condition manifesting with seizures in the first week of life.[423-445] Seizure onset is usually on the second or third postnatal day, and in the interictal period the newborn appears well. The seizures most often are focal clonic, focal tonic, or apneic and may occur with a frequency of 10 to 20 per day or higher. The electroclinical characteristics are typical and consist of an initial brief period of EEG flattening, accompanied by apnea and motor activity, followed by a bilateral discharge of spikes and slow waves, accompanied by clonic activity. The disorder is usually self-limited, with cessation of seizures in 1 to 12 months. Neurological development is usually

TABLE 12.21	Major Epilepsy Syndromes With Onset in the Neonatal Period
BFNE
Benign nonfamilial neonatal convulsions (fifth-day fits)
EME
EIEE (Ohtahara syndrome)
Malignant migrating partial seizures

BFNE, Benign familial neonatal epilepsy; *EIEE*, early infantile epileptic encephalopathy; *EME*, early myoclonic encephalopathy.

normal. However, about 10% to 15% of children develop epilepsy later in life.[446] Family histories indicate autosomal dominant inheritance with incomplete penetrance. However, because of the benign course of the disorder, the history of previously affected family members may be overlooked unless specifically sought by direct questioning of parents and sometimes grandparents. Two separate chromosomal loci have been identified (i.e., chromosome 20q13.3 and chromosome 8q24). Both genes encode voltage-gated potassium channels (KCNQ2 on chromosome 20 and KCNQ3 on chromosome 8), which may function in the same heteromeric complex to regulate the threshold for neuronal excitability. BFNE has also been reported in patients with mutations in PRRT2 and genes coding for a sodium channel subunit (SCN2A).[447,448] Mutations in these genes are associated with a spectrum of diseases, including neonatal epileptic encephalopathies.[449] A study of 36 families, which included 33 families with BFNE, found 27 of these families had KCNQ2 mutations, one had a KCNQ3 mutation, and two had SCN2A mutations.[450]

Benign Nonfamilial Neonatal Convulsions. This syndrome is also referred to as "fifth-day fits" or benign idiopathic neonatal seizures. It was initially described in Australia[451-453] and France,[454] and subsequently elsewhere,[297,434,455-458] and is characterized by the onset of seizures in the latter part of the first week of life in apparently healthy full-term infants. The peak time of onset is the fifth day, and approximately 80% to 90% have had their onset between the fourth and sixth days of life. The seizures are usually multifocal clonic, often with apnea. Status epilepticus has occurred in approximately 80% of cases. Despite the abrupt onset and frequent status epilepticus, in most patients seizures cease after 24 hours, and in all patients within 15 days. The patient is normal between seizures; diagnostic testing, including standard laboratory tests and neuroimaging, are normal; and the prognosis is consistently favorable. The interictal EEG is generally normal, although a nonspecific theta pattern referred to as "theta pointu alternant" has been described in some patients. Anticonvulsant medications are often administered acutely in view of status epilepticus, but long-term therapy is generally not needed in view of the self-resolution of seizures in these patients. The demonstration of low zinc levels in the CSF of affected patients[459] raised the possibility of an acute zinc deficiency syndrome,[295] but the origin of the zinc deficiency and confirmation thereof have not been defined. The possibility that some cases of benign nonfamilial neonatal convulsions are related to de novo mutations of KCNQ2, the K+ channel most commonly affected in benign familial neonatal seizures (described earlier), is suggested by a description of four infants.[445]

Early Myoclonic Encephalopathy and Early Infantile Epileptic Encephalopathy (Ohtahara Syndrome). Early myoclonic encephalopathy (EME) and EIEE or Ohtahara syndrome, characteristically present clinically in the first weeks of life (Tables 12.22 and 12.23).[31,384,449,460-482] However, in some patients, these may not present until several weeks or rarely even several months of life. Intrauterine onset has been documented.[468] These disorders are characterized by severe recurrent seizures, principally myoclonic and clonic at the onset in EME and tonic spasms at the onset in EIEE, and a striking suppression-burst EEG pattern. Patients with EME tend to have myoclonic seizures involving any part of the body but may also experience focal motor seizures and tonic spasms. Patients with EIEE tend to have frequent clusters of tonic spasms but may also have focal motor seizures. However, the *characteristics of the suppression-burst EEG pattern differ* (see Table 12.22); in EME, the burst-suppression feature is enhanced by sleep and tends to involve high amplitude bursts followed by brief periods of suppression, whereas in EIEE the pattern is not altered by sleep or waking and is a more typical burst-suppression pattern. Further, the *evolution of the EEG pattern differs*; in EME the burst-suppression pattern persists, whereas in EIEE the pattern evolves to hypsarrhythmia and West syndrome. The *primary etiologies also differ*; in EME the causes are primarily metabolic (especially nonketotic hyperglycinemia but also other amino acid and organic acid disorders), whereas in EIEE the causes are primarily structural (primarily dysgenetic, i.e., migrational defects, microencephaly or hemimegalencephaly, but also encephaloclastic, i.e., hypoxic-ischemic, disorders). Definition of an etiological mechanism is possible in most cases of EIEE, whereas as many as 50% of cases of EME are cryptogenic. Of the structural bases for EIEE, the rare lesion, dentato-olivary dysplasia, is the most difficult to identify in vivo.[466,472,483,484] In addition, while structural malformations are the most common causes of EIEE,[229,291,485] many genetic mutations have been reported to cause EIEE (see Table 12.22).[486]

TABLE 12.22	Early-Onset Epileptic Encephalopathies Characterized by Burst Suppression	
CLINICAL FEATURES	**EME**	**EIEE (OHTAHARA SYNDROME)**
Major clinical seizure types at onset	Myoclonic (also focal motor clonic and tonic)	Tonic spasms (also focal motor clonic)
Electroencephalographic interictal pattern	Suppression burst	Suppression burst
Relation to sleep	Enhanced by sleep	Same asleep and awake
Evolution	Persistent suppression burst	Transition to hypsarrhythmia
Etiology	Metabolic (rarely structural or genetic)	Bilateral structural cerebral lesions (rarely metabolic or genetic)
Outcome	Unfavorable	Unfavorable
Genes	ERBB4, PIGA, SETBP1, SIK1, SLC25A22	STX BP1 in ~30%; KCNQ2 in ~20%; SCN2A in ~10%; AARS, ARX, BRAT1, CACNA2D2, GNAO1, KCNT1, NECAP1, PIGA, PIGQ, SCN8A, SIK1, SLC25A22

EIEE, Early infantile epileptic encephalopathy; *EME*, early myoclonic encephalopathy.

TABLE 12.23   Genes Involved in Early-Onset Epileptic Encephalopathy

GENE	TYPE/INHERITANCE	CLINICAL MANIFESTATION	PROTEIN FUNCTION
ARX	EIEE1/XLR	Ohtahara syndrome	Transcriptional repressor and activator
SLC25A22	EIEE3/X homozygous	Ohtahara syndrome	Glutamate transport into mitochondrion
STXBP	EIEE4/AD	Ohtahara syndrome	Modulator of synaptic vesicle release
SCN1A	EIEE6/X de novo	Dravet syndrome	Subunit of voltage-gated sodium channel
PNKP	EIEE10/AR	Microcephaly, seizures, and developmental delay	Enzyme involved in DNA repair
PLCB1	EIEE12/AR homozygous	Malignant migrating partial seizures in infancy	Phospholipase-C role in intracellular transduction of extracellular signals
KCNT1	EIEE14/sporadic	Malignant migrating partial seizures in infancy	Sodium-activated potassium channel subunit

EIEE, Early infantile epileptic encephalopathy.

Data adapted from Su-Kjeong Hwang SK, Kwon S. Early-onset encephalopathies and the diagnostic approach to underlying causes. *Korean J Pediatr.* 2015;58:407–414.

The predominant genetic defect in EIEE is STXBP1, found in 20% to 30% of patients. STXBP1 promotes the formation of functional vesicle fusion complexes via interaction with two N-terminal domains of syntaxin 1a, and a loss of function mutation impairs this interaction.[487] Patients with STXBP1 encephalopathy present in the neonatal period with severe epilepsy and a suppression-burst pattern on EEG. While refractory seizures are typical, the core of the phenotypic spectrum is the encephalopathy, which is present in the neonatal period.[488]

The second most common genetic defect in EIEE involves KCNQ2 and accounts for 10% of cases. The phenotype is characterized by profound neonatal encephalopathy with severe, frequent, intractable seizures that have been termed KCNQ2 encephalopathy.[489,490] In contrast to BFNE related to KCNQ2 defect (see earlier), the interictal EEG before anticonvulsant administration is multifocal, and there is hypotonia, paucity of spontaneous movements, no visual fixation, and altered reactivity. Whereas mutations that lead to BFNE result in mild reductions in potassium current, the de novo mutations responsible for KCNQ2 encephalopathy represent more profound alterations, in some cases through a dominant negative effect[491,492] or even via gain of function.[493] The best success to date for the management of seizures in KCNQ2 encephalopathy has been with sodium channel blockers and with carbamazepine in particular.[494] Indeed, carbamazepine is emerging as an old drug with a new indication in treating early-onset genetic epilepsies, as relative success has also been reported in treating early epilepsy associated with SCN2A[495] and SCN8A,[496,497] sodium channel gene defects.

Malignant Migrating Partial Seizures of Infancy. This rare neonatal epilepsy syndrome is striking.[477,498-508] Although the usual time of onset of the seizure disorder is at 1 to 3 months, onset in the first days of life has been reported, and approximately one-half of cases have had onset in the first month of life. The seizures are focal clonic at the onset, and over the ensuing weeks become multifocal, extremely frequent, and intractable to antiseizure medications. One report describes a good therapeutic response to levetiracetam.[503] EEG findings show striking multifocal epileptic activity. Detailed metabolic studies and neuroimaging have been reported to be negative for any abnormality. Neuropathological study has shown no abnormality in the neocortex but pronounced hippocampal neuronal loss. Later neurodevelopmental outcome is poor with death or moderate to severe mental retardation in most infants. However, a report of six cases showed mild deficits in two infants.[502] Genetic defects include de novo mutations involving SCN1A (sodium channel) and KCNT1 (potassium channel) and homozygous mutations involving SLC25A22 (glutamate transport into the mitochondrion) and PLC1 (phospholipase C). Recent case reports indicating that KCNQ2 mutations are associated with this epilepsy syndrome suggest benefit from quinidine therapy.[490,494,509]

Diagnosis

Appropriate diagnostic procedures in the newborn infant with seizures can be surmised from the discussion of causes. However, the diagnostic evaluation often is made unnecessarily complicated, and many diagnoses can be strongly suspected by such uncomplicated maneuvers as obtaining a complete prenatal and natal *history* and performing a careful *physical examination.* The first laboratory tests to be performed are directed against the two disorders that are dangerous but readily treated when recognized promptly: hypoglycemia and bacterial meningitis. Thus, blood glucose determination and lumbar puncture should be performed as soon as clinically feasible. In addition, blood should be drawn for determinations of Na^+, K^+, calcium, phosphorus, and magnesium levels. Other imaging and laboratory studies should be directed by specific clinical features. Focal seizures should lead to neuroimaging because of the frequency of focal ischemic cerebral lesions, and MRI is preferred because many focal lesions may not be detected by cranial ultrasound evaluation. As noted earlier, the most common etiologies of neonatal seizures are hypoxic–ischemic encephalopathy, intracranial hemorrhage, and perinatal arterial ischemic stroke. In one study of 354 patients with MRI and ultrasound performed, the diagnosis of important brain lesions would be frequently missed by ultrasound alone. In addition, MRI contributed information beyond ultrasound to the diagnosis in about 40%.[294] Similarly, in a large cohort registry study by the Vermont Oxford Network, the deficiencies of cranial ultrasound and computed tomography scanning compared to MRI for clinically relevant lesions of deep nuclear gray matter injury and focal cortical and white matter injury were highlighted.

Warning signs for inborn errors of metabolism as a cause of neonatal seizures include: (1) seizures beginning in the antepartum period; (2) seizures refractory to anticonvulsant medications; (3) progressive worsening of clinical and EEG abnormalities; (4) EEG showing burst suppression; (5) MRI showing prominent brain atrophy; or (6) findings of hypoxic-ischemic encephalopathy without any obvious hypoxic-ischemic event identified.[288] When laboratory testing is performed, the presence of low CSF glucose (but normal blood glucose) should suggest glucose transporter defect; the presence of elevated CSF glycine despite normal blood amino acids should suggest transient or true nonketotic hyperglycinemia; and the presence of elevated CSF lactate should suggest a mitochondrial disorder. Other CSF abnormalities of diagnostic value in this context are discussed in Chapter 29.

Electroencephalogram and Electroencephalographic Monitoring

EEG provides important diagnostic and prognostic information. Moreover, increasingly, continuous EEG monitoring is performed in neonatal intensive care facilities for several important reasons. EEG data can assist in the determination of whether clinical events are correlated with electrical seizures requiring anticonvulsant medication or with nonepileptic events in which anticonvulsant medication administration can be avoided. As discussed earlier, some seizures have readily identifiable clinical manifestations (i.e., clonic or tonic components), while many seizures have more subtle manifestations (i.e., orolingual, ocular, or autonomic).[34] Thus, clinical diagnosis of seizures may be difficult and unreliable. As described earlier, when compared to the gold standard of EEG data, observers only classify clinical events correctly as seizures about half of the time, and there is poor interobserver agreement.[185] As a result, many nonictal events are classified as seizures, potentially leading to unnecessary exposure to anticonvulsant medications. *Second*, many newborns experience clinically silent seizures, which can only be identified with EEG. In many clinical settings the majority of electrographic seizures are not accompanied by clinically evident seizures,[227] and the majority of time spent having electrographic seizures is not accompanied by clinically evident seizure activity.[186] *Third*, in newborns with clinically evident seizures and administration of anticonvulsant medications, EEG-only seizures may persist (electromechanical uncoupling or dissociation).[228,229,241] Thus, even if management is initiated based on identification of clinically evident seizures, EEG monitoring may be required to fully assess the impact of management on seizure cessation. *Fourth*, assessment of the EEG background may provide important prognostic information (discussed later).

As a result of these data, there is *increasing emphasis on continuous EEG monitoring to aid in management of seizures in newborns*.[510,511] Many neonatal intensive care units report using EEG monitoring, with conventional EEG or aEEG, to identify and manage neonatal seizures.[166-169] In addition, recent guidelines and consensus statements have advocated for EEG monitoring.[171-173] This recommendation has included the need for confirmation of seizures by EEG in specialized settings before therapy[173] and the need for continuous electrophysiological monitoring in the setting of therapeutic hypothermia.[172]

The most comprehensive *guideline on continuous EEG monitoring in the newborn* was produced in 2011 by the American Clinical Neurophysiology Society.[171] The guideline was created to standardize care and define best neuromonitoring practices in the neonatal population, while recognizing that not all recommendations would be feasible or applicable across institutions. The guideline recommendations included that (1) electrodes be placed using the International 10 to 20 system with additional electrocardiogram, respiratory, eye, and electromyography leads; (2) at least 1 hour of recording be assessed to adequately assess cycling through wakefulness and sleep; (3) high-risk newborns be monitored for at least 24 hours to screen for the presence of electrographic seizures; and (4) in newborns with seizures, monitoring occur during seizure management and for an additional 24 hours after the last electrographic seizure.[171] Video EEG recording was recommended for 24 hours rather than a briefer EEG recording because many newborns will not have seizures in the first hour of recording but will experience electrographic seizures within the first day.[311,512,513] Studies in high-risk newborns indicate that the majority of acute seizures occur within 48 hours of the brain insult.[311,327,512-515]

Accurate delineation of seizure phenomena by EEG in the newborn requires experienced electroencephalographers with training in the normal developmental features of EEG in the newborn and skilled EEG technologists for the application of the EEG. A recent report on *Standardized EEG Terminology and Categorization for the Description of Continuous EEG Monitoring in Newborns* was developed by the American Clinical Neurophysiology Society[177] summarizing the many reports of the EEG accompaniments of neonatal seizures.[23,26,27,31-33,516-524] As summarized earlier (see Table 12.9), an electrographic seizure is defined as "a sudden, abnormal electroencephalogram (EEG) event defined by a repetitive and evolving pattern with a minimum 2 microvolt voltage and duration of at least 10 seconds." The major EEG correlates of neonatal seizures thus consist of focal or multifocal spikes or sharp waves or both and focal rhythmic discharges, occurring as a distinct change from background. These discharges may spread to adjacent cortical regions or to homotypic areas of the contralateral hemisphere. Such discharges are distinguished from normal sharp "transients," which are random rather than localized, are not rhythmic, do not spread, and are not followed by voltage suppression. Two general points concerning identification of electrical seizure activity in the newborn should be emphasized. First, neonatal seizures tend to be brief, usually lasting less than 2 minutes (Fig. 12.14).[525] Second, electrographic seizures tend to be focal and well localized, arising most commonly from temporal and central regions, less commonly from occipital regions, and least commonly from frontal regions.

Other specific features of the neonatal EEG that should be evaluated and documented include the behavioral state, EEG background features (symmetry, synchrony, voltage, variability, reactivity, and dysmaturity), the presence or absence of normal elements (delta brushes, rhythmic temporal theta, anterior dysrhythmia), the presence of EEG transient patterns, such as sharp waves and BRDs, and the presence of seizures and status epilepticus.[177]

Amplitude-Integrated EEG

aEEG is in widespread use, especially by neonatologists, as a method to identify electrographic seizures at the bedside (also see Chapter 10). The technique uses a reduced number of electrodes compared to a conventional EEG recording to generate a single channel (two electrodes)[526] or dual-channel (four electrodes) EEG tracing. The EEG signal is modified and compressed using algorithms, which vary slightly between manufacturers,[527] to generate the final display showing several hours of aEEG data on a single screen. Electrographic seizures are characterized by upward arches (Fig. 12.15). The primary advantages of aEEG relate to its relative ease of use. The limited electrode array can be applied by those without specialized training (i.e., not EEG technologists) and the display can be interpreted by bedside caregivers, generally without involvement of electroencephalographers or neurologists.[167] As a result of these advantages and the resource intensity of conventional EEG monitoring, aEEG is widely used in neonatal intensive care units for seizure identification and management.[166,167,169,170]

Some challenges with aEEG have been identified. For example, a survey of neonatologists reported that only 28% felt confident in their aEEG interpretations.[167] In addition, aEEG may underestimate the true incidence of electrographic seizures. In a systematic review of 10 studies of aEEG in newborns for seizure diagnosis,[528] when aEEG was used with the raw EEG tracing available, the median sensitivity was 76% (range 71% to 85%) and the median specificity was 85% (range 39% to 96%). When aEEG was used without the raw EEG tracing the results were worse; the median sensitivity was 39% (range 25% to 80%) and the median specificity was 95% (range 50% to 100%). In addition, seizures that had low amplitude, were brief duration, or occurred distant from the aEEG recording sites, were less likely to be identified. Overall, studies indicate that reliance on aEEG alone might underdiagnose seizures in some newborns.[232,237,526,528-537] The American Clinical Neurophysiology Society's Guidelines on EEG Monitoring in Newborns states that aEEG can be a "useful, initial complementary tool" to EEG monitoring, which remains the gold standard.[171]

Despite the limitations of aEEG, some studies indicate that in comparison to use of clinical signs alone, aEEG may assist in recognition and management of seizures. In a study of 202 newborns, those who underwent aEEG monitoring had greater precision in the diagnosis of neonatal seizures than in contemporary controls with diagnosis by clinical signs alone.[538] Further, more accurate diagnosis of seizures and subsequent management may reduce seizure exposure in newborns. In a

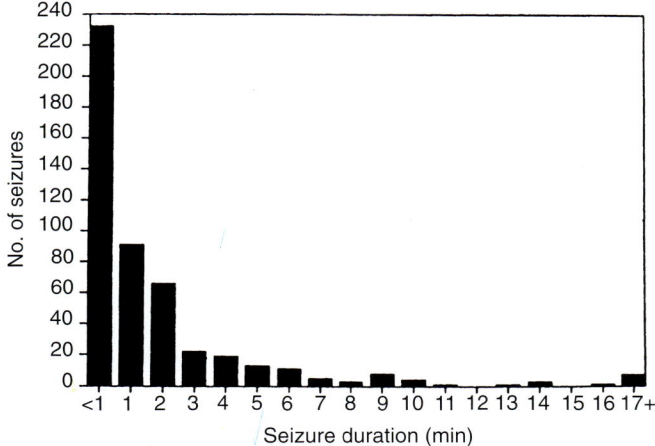

Figure 12.14 Seizure duration. Histogram depicting the distribution of seizure duration among 487 seizures recorded from 42 newborns with seizures. (From Clancy RR, Legido A. The exact ictal and interictal duration of electroencephalographic neonatal seizures. *Epilepsia.* 1987;28:537–541.)

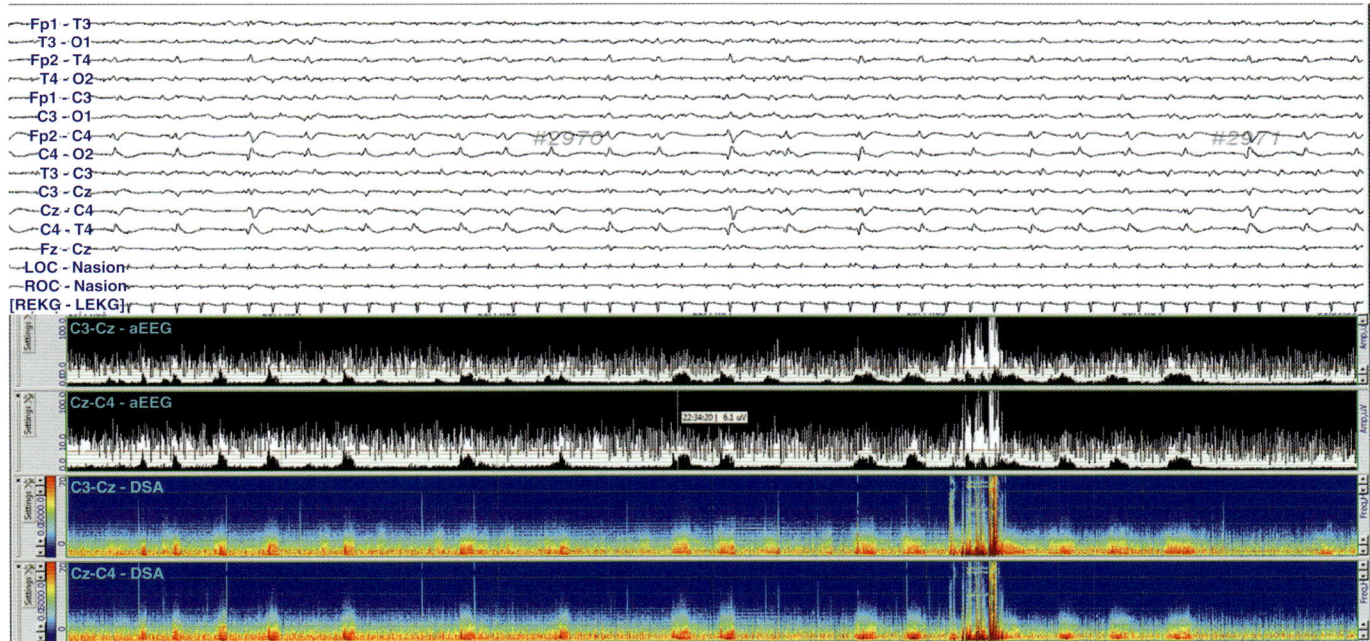

Figure 12.15 Neonatal seizure on conventional electroencephalography (EEG) and amplitude-integrated EEG. *Top.* Conventional EEG with a seizure is evident in the right central (C4) region with about 20 seconds displayed. *Bottom.* Amplitude-integrated EEG with recurrent right hemispheric seizures with about 4 hours displayed. (Personal communication Abend.)

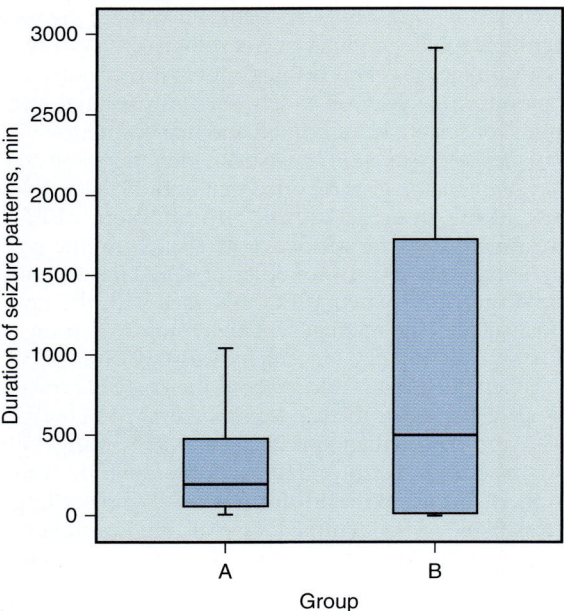

Figure 12.16 Access to amplitude-integrated EEG (aEEG) data led to a trend toward reduced seizure exposure. In a randomized study of 33 infants, neonatologists were allowed to view aEEG in their routine clinical care for 19 patients but were blind to the aEEG data for 14 patients. Among those newborns in whom aEEG was available to neonatologists (Group A), there was a trend toward reduced seizure exposure compared to those newborns in whom neonatologists did not have access to aEEG (Group B). (From van Rooij LG, Toet MC, van Huffelen AC, et al. Effect of treatment of subclinical neonatal seizures detected with aEEG: randomized, controlled trial. *Pediatrics.* 2010;125:e358–e366.)

randomized study of 33 infants, neonatologists were allowed to view aEEG in their routine clinical care for 19 patients but were blind to the aEEG data for 14 patients. Among those newborns in whom aEEG was available to neonatologists, there was a trend toward reduced seizure exposure (Fig. 12.16). Further, patients with lower duration of seizures exhibited less severe brain injury on MRI.[539] Similarly, a prospective single center study assessed 26 newborns who were randomized to have management guided by clinical data only (*n* = 16) or by clinical and EEG data including cEEG and aEEG (*n* = 10). The group with EEG data used for clinical management had a lower seizure burden and more rapid time to treatment completion. In addition, newborns with increasing seizure burden had worse MRI injury scores and lower performance on cognitive, motor, and language composite Bayley scores.[540] More data with larger series will be of great interest, and two large randomized controlled trials of the impact of aEEG monitoring of newborns suspected of having seizures versus standard clinical evaluation are under way in Australia and the Netherlands.

Prognosis
General Outcomes
The major determinant of prognosis in newborn seizures is the neuropathological process that underlies the seizures (see later). However, two other considerations are of importance. The first relates to the fact that the overall prognosis for newborns with seizures has improved over the past several decades. A review of more than 2000 cases of neonatal seizures

in mostly full-term newborns from published reports before and after 1969 demonstrates that mortality has decreased from approximately 40% to 15%.[a] In contrast, the incidence of neurological sequelae (intellectual disability, motor deficits [including cerebral palsy], and epilepsy) in survivors remains high at 20% to 35% with no dramatic change over the past several decades.[176] A recent review of 4538 children with a history of neonatal seizures demonstrated that 18% developed epilepsy, with nearly 70% having onset within the first year. Associated neurological impairments were present in 81% of the children with epilepsy and included 18% with intellectual impairment, 6% with cerebral palsy, and 45% with both cerebral palsy and intellectual impairment.[553]

The second key factor influencing outcome following seizures in the newborn is the gestational age of the infant. Clinical seizures in the preterm infant are commonly associated with severe brain injury and thus, a poor prognosis. In one population-based study of 368 VLBW infants (<1500 g) with clinical seizures, nearly 40% had severe intraventricular hemorrhage and 20% had cystic periventricular leukomalacia.[306] In relation to prognosis, in a study of 82 newborn infants with clinical seizures, all adverse outcomes occurred at twice the frequency in preterm infants than in term-born infants. These outcomes included mortality (42% in preterm infants compared with 16% in term infants); postnatal epilepsy (48% in preterm infants compared with 29% in term infants); cerebral palsy (63% in preterm infants compared with 25% in term infants); and intellectual disability (52% of preterm infants compared with 25% in term infants).[214]

Predicting Outcome in Individual Patients
The overall factors regarding prognosis discussed earlier do not answer the question that is most critical to the physician caring for a newborn with seizures *"How can I predict the outcome in my patient?"* The *two most important factors* in predicting outcome for an individual infant are the infant's underlying neuropathology and the EEG pattern.

Relation of Neurological Disease to Outcome. The *most important determinant of neurological prognosis is the nature of the neuropathological process that underlies* the seizures. The relationship of prognosis with the underlying disease producing the seizures is summarized in Table 12.24.[b] Importantly, nearly all the data are based on follow-up periods that do not extend to school age; thus, the incidence of subtle, but potentially important, intellectual deficits is largely unknown. In addition, in many studies, premature and term infants are considered together. The neurological outcomes related to specific neurological disorders are discussed in other chapters.

Relation of Electroencephalographic to Outcome. Two aspects of the EEG are useful in the assessment of outcome; that is, the *EEG background* and the quantitation of *seizure burden*. A considerable amount of earlier work focused on the *EEG background.*[c] The conclusion that assessment of EEG background

---

[a]References 29, 32, 176, 191, 207, 286, 296, 298, 299, 301-305, 315, 326, 328, 339, 425, and 541-552.
[b]References 32, 191, 207, 220, 239, 286, 296-299, 301, 302, 305, 326, 339, 543, 545, 546, 548-551, and 554.
[c]References 31, 32, 177, 191, 239, 286, 296, 297, 299, 302, 303, 326, 548, 549, 551, and 555-561.

TABLE 12.24 Prognosis of Neonatal Seizures: Relation to Neurological Disease

NEUROLOGICAL DISEASE[a]	NORMAL DEVELOPMENT (%)[b]
Hypoxic-ischemic encephalopathy	50
Intraventricular hemorrhage[c]	10
Primary subarachnoid hemorrhage	90
Hypocalcemia	
Early-onset	50[d]
Later-onset	100[e]
Hypoglycemia	50
Bacterial meningitis	50
Developmental defect	0

[a]Prognosis is for those cases with the stated neurological disease when seizures are a manifestation (thus, value usually differs from overall prognosis for the disease).

[b]Values are rounded off to nearest 5%.

[c]Usually, severe intraventricular hemorrhage is associated with major periventricular hemorrhagic infarction.

[d]Represents primarily the prognosis of complicating illness; prognosis approaches that of later-onset hypocalcemia of the nutritional type if no or only minor neurological illness is present.

[e]Later-onset hypocalcemia of the nutritional type.

TABLE 12.25 Prognosis of Neonatal Seizures: Relation to Electroencephalogram[a]

EEG BACKGROUND	NEUROLOGICAL SEQUELAE (%)
Normal	≤10
Severe abnormalities[b]	≥90
Moderate abnormalities[c]	~50

[a]Based primarily on data (includes both full-term and premature infants) reported in: Lombroso CT. Prognosis in neonatal seizures. *Adv Neurol.* 1983;34:101–113; Rowe JC, Holmes GL, Hafford J, Baboval D, et al. Prognostic value of the electroencephalogram in term and preterm infants following neonatal seizures. *Electroencephalogr Clin Neurophysiol.* 1985;60:183–196; Menache CC, Bourgeois BFD, Volpe JJ. Prognostic value of neonatal discontinuous EEG. *Pediatr Neurol.* 2002;27:93–101.

[b]Burst-suppression pattern, prolonged (>20-second) interburst interval, marked voltage suppression, and electrocerebral silence.

[c]Voltage asymmetries and "immaturity."

EEG, Electroencephalographic.

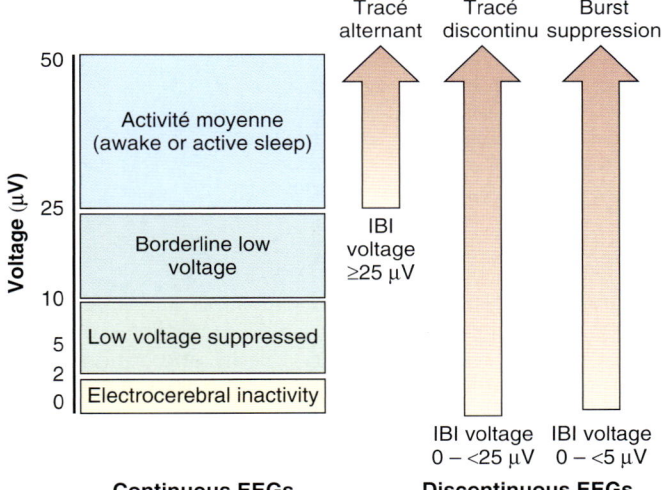

Figure 12.17 Electroencephalographic (EEG) background classification based on the American Clinical Neurophysiology Society standardized EEG recommendations. (From Tsuchida TN, Wusthoff CJ, Shellhaas RA, et al. American Clinical Neurophysiology Society standardized EEG terminology and categorization for the description of continuous EEG monitoring in neonates: report of the American Clinical Neurophysiology Society critical care monitoring committee. *J Clin Neurophysiol.* 2013;30:161–173, with permission.)

infants with seizures (Table 12.25). Most newborns with seizures occurring on a normal EEG background generally have a normal outcome, while 90% of newborns with seizures on an abnormal EEG background (e.g., attenuation in voltage, burst-suppression, or excessive discontinuity) have an abnormal outcome. The burst-suppression pattern (termed *tracé paroxystique* by Monod and Dreyfus-Brisac)[562] is particularly typical of the newborn with severe bilateral cerebral disease and is characterized by relatively long periods of voltage suppression (<5 μV) or by no electrical activity at all in the intervals between the bursts of activity. Moderate background abnormalities, which generally account for approximately 15% to 30% of the tracings,[559] are associated with an intermediate likelihood of sequelae.

The preponderance of data concerning the predictive role of EEG concerns newborns with hypoxic-ischemic encephalopathy. Normal EEG background, particularly in the first day of life, is associated with normal outcomes in 80% to 100% of newborns, burst-suppression background is associated with unfavorable outcomes in 80% to 100% of newborns, and an attenuated EEG background is associated with unfavorable outcomes in 90% to 100% of newborns. Consideration of the impact of sedating medications on the EEG background is important; some newborns with backgrounds that predicted unfavorable outcome yet had favorable outcomes may have had their backgrounds worsened by phenobarbital. In addition, because EEGs may evolve over time, repeat EEG tracings may be useful. *EEGs that remain abnormal are more predictive of unfavorable outcomes.*[177]

Despite the frequently documented relationship between the burst-suppression background pattern or the more common excessively discontinuous tracing with a prolonged (>20-second) interburst interval and poor neurological outcome,[a] some *caution must be used in attributing a grave prognosis to abnormal paroxysmal patterns with long silent periods in premature infants.* This caveat applies especially to premature infants less than 33 to 34 weeks

[a]References 31, 32, 191, 286, 299, 302, 326, 548, 556, 558, 559, 561, and 563-565.

is valuable for *prognostic* estimates must be made with the qualification that evaluations of neonatal EEG findings are sometimes difficult and may vary among interpreters. Recent standardized terminology has been proposed by the American Clinical Neurophysiology Society, and the major EEG background patterns are summarized in Figs. 12.17 and 12.18.[177] In several careful studies, the *background EEG pattern* was found to correlate well with the outcome in both full-term and premature

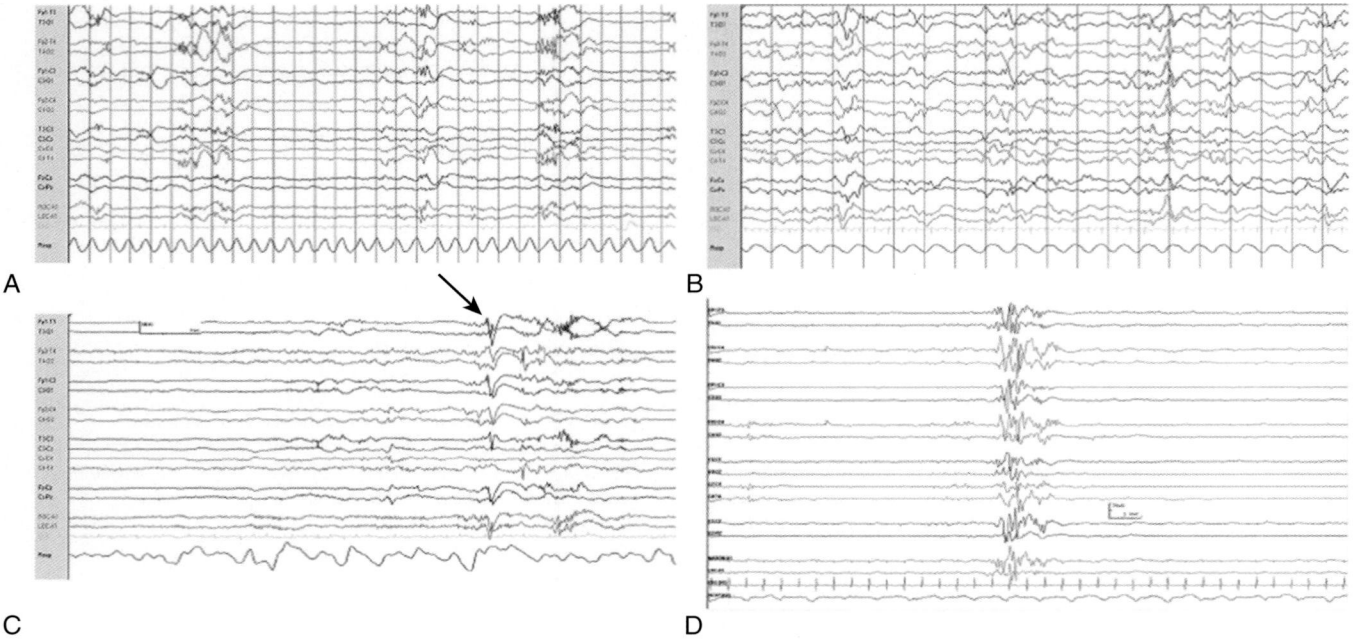

Figure 12.18 Examples illustrating the contrasts between tracé discontinu, tracé alternant, excessive discontinuity, and burst suppression. (A) In tracé discontinu, the bursts are separated by very low voltage, suppressed interburst intervals (IBIs). There are no artifacts from electromyography (EMG) activity or movement, and the respiratory pattern is quite regular. (B) In this example of tracé alternant, however, there is an alternating pattern of high and low voltages but no periods that are consistently suppressed. There are no artifacts from EMG activity or movement, and the respiratory pattern is quite regular. (C) This excessively discontinuous record from a term infant with an acute encephalopathy showing prolonged IBIs, although with some normal features present during bursts, such as the conspicuous encoche frontale seen near its onset *(arrow)*. (D) Burst suppression, in contrast, contains prolonged, extremely suppressed IBIs and bursts composed exclusively of abnormal electrical activity. (From Tsuchida TN, Wusthoff CJ, Shellhaas RA, et al. American clinical neurophysiology society standardized EEG terminology and categorization for the description of continuous EEG monitoring in neonates: report of the American Clinical Neurophysiology Society critical care monitoring committee. *J Clin Neurophysiol.* 2013;30:161–173, with permission.)

of conceptional age, in part because of the normal periodicity and relatively lower interburst voltage in the EEG pattern of the premature infant (see Chapter 10).

The second major value of EEG in assessment of prognosis is *quantitation of seizure burden*. An important question is whether seizures in the newborn lead independently to brain injury and thereby worsen outcome. The answer to this question underlies decisions regarding the importance and aggressiveness of seizure identification and management. Data related to seizures and outcome in experimental animals were discussed in earlier sections. The extent to which seizures produce secondary brain injury versus serving as biomarkers of more severe acute brain injury in human newborns remains uncertain, and the relationship in an individual newborn is likely dependent on the etiology and severity of the acute brain injury, seizure burden, and seizure management strategies. Studies using univariate analyses show associations between seizures and less favorable outcomes, but such studies cannot determine whether the seizures contributed to the worse outcomes (i.e., led to secondary brain injury) or merely served as biomarkers of more severe brain injury and thus predicted worse outcomes (Table 12.26). Studies using multivariate analyses may be more informative as to the impact of seizures on outcome. Several such reports have identified associations between

seizures, particularly high seizure exposures, and unfavorable outcomes in models adjusting for variables reflecting acute brain injury etiology, acute brain injury severity, and critical illness severity. For example, in a study of 63 term-born infants with hypoxic-ischemic encephalopathy who were randomized to treatment of all seizures (clinical + aEEG) compared to treatment of only clinical seizures, a positive correlation was found between seizure duration and MRI injury severity across the entire cohort ($P < .001$) (Fig. 12.19).[539] Of note, this relationship was significant for the newborns treated only for clinical seizures ($P = .001$), but not for those treated for both aEEG and clinical seizures ($P = .292$). In a similar study design of 69 term-born infants with moderate-severe hypoxic-ischemic encephalopathy and clinical seizures randomized to treatment with or without access to EEG data, an association between increasing seizure burden and worsened MRI injury scores ($P < .03$) (Fig. 12.20) was seen.[540] Of greater importance, an association was found between seizure burden and more adverse neurodevelopmental outcomes on Bayley Scales of Infant Development (cognitive composite $R = 0.502$, $P = .03$; motor composite $R = 0.497$, $P = .01$; language composite $R = 0.444$, $P = .03$) (Fig. 12.21). The infants in the aEEG monitored group experienced a lower seizure burden, although neurodevelopmental outcomes were not shown to be statistically different. Larger data sets from

TABLE 12.26   Associations of Seizure Burden With Neurodevelopmental Outcome

STUDY	COHORT	ANALYSIS	KEY FINDINGS
Shah DK, Wusthoff CJ, Clarke P, et al. Electrographic seizures are associated with brain injury in newborns undergoing therapeutic hypothermia. *Arch Dis Child Fetal Neonatal Ed.* 2014;99:F219–F224	85 with moderate-severe HIE managed with TH and monitored with aEEG	Seizure identification: aEEG Multivariate analysis including seizure burden, aEEG background, and Apgar scores. Outcome: MRI injury severity	High electrographic seizure burden associated with a severe pattern of MRI injury (odds ratio 5, 95% confidence interval 1.47–17.05)
Glass HC, Glidden D, Jeremy RJ, et al. Clinical neonatal seizures are independently associated with outcome in infants at risk for hypoxic-ischemic brain injury. *J Pediatr.* 2009;155:318–323	77 with HIE with clinical seizure assessment.	Seizure identification: clinical Multivariate analysis including MRI injury severity. Outcome: Intelligence quotient at 4 years	Every one point increase in the seizure severity scale was associated with a 4.7 point reduction (95% confidence interval −7.2 to −2.2 point reduction) in intelligence quotient at four years. The median intelligence quotients for newborns with no seizures, mild/moderate seizures, and severe seizure burdens were 97, 83, and 67, respectively
Dunne JM, Wertheim D, Clarke P, et al. Automated electroencephalographic discontinuity in cooled newborns predicts cerebral MRI and neurodevelopmental outcome. *Arch Dis Child Fetal Neonatal Ed.* 2017;102:F58–F64	49 with moderate-severe HIE with TH monitored with aEEG	Seizure identification: aEEG Multivariate analysis included seizure burden and aEEG background. Outcome: MRI injury severity	Seizure burden and aEEG discontinuity demonstrated an association between high seizure burden and severe MRI injury (odds ratio 4.2, 95% confidence interval 1.01–17.5). Severe MRI injury was associated with unfavorable neurodevelopmental outcomes assessed with Bayley Scales of Infant Development (Pearson's $R = 0.62$, $P < .001$)
Meyn DF, Jr., Ness J, Ambalavanan N, et al. Prophylactic phenobarbital and whole-body cooling for neonatal hypoxic-ischemic encephalopathy. *J Pediatr.* 2010;157:334–336	42 with HIE treated with phenobarbital prophylactically ($n = 20$) versus only if seizures occurred ($n = 22$)	Seizure identification: aEEG Multivariate analysis with clinical features. Outcome: Neurodevelopmental assessment	Use of prophylactic phenobarbital was associated with a decreased occurrence of seizure in the neonatal period (15% with prophylaxis vs. 82% without prophylaxis, $P < .0001$). Use of prophylactic phenobarbital was associated with improved neurodevelopmental outcomes (odds ratio for moderate to severe neurodevelopmental injury 0.069, $P = .03$)
van Rooij LG, Toet MC, van Huffelen AC, et al. Effect of treatment of subclinical neonatal seizures detected with aEEG: randomized, controlled trial. *Pediatrics.* 2010;125:e358–e366	63 with HIE with aEEG. Randomized to treatment of all seizures (clinical + aEEG) versus treatment of only clinical seizures.	Seizure identification: aEEG + clinical versus clinical. Compared subjects randomized to treatment of clinical + aEEG versus only clinical seizures. Outcome: MRI injury severity and mortality	Nonsignificant trend toward lower seizure exposure with aEEG data. Positive correlation between seizure duration and MRI injury severity across the entire cohort ($P < .001$) and among the newborns treated for only clinical seizures ($P = .001$), but not for the aEEG and clinical group ($P = .292$) (see Fig. 12.22). Newborns who died had experienced a higher seizure duration than those who survived (428 min vs. 164 min)
Srinivasakumar P, Zempel J, Trivedi S, et al. Treating EEG seizures in hypoxic ischemic encephalopathy: a randomized controlled trial. *Pediatrics.* 2015;136:e1302–e1309	69 with moderate-severe HIE or clinical seizures. Excluded newborns with status epilepticus. Randomized to treatment with or without access to EEG data	Seizure identification: Continuous conventional EEG + clinical versus clinical. Compared subjects randomized to treatment with versus without access to EEG data. Outcome: MRI injury severity and neurodevelopmental outcome	Median duration of seizures was lower in the EEG than clinical group. Association between increasing seizure burden and worsened MRI injury scores ($P < .03$) (see Fig. 12.23). Association between seizure burden and lower neurodevelopmental testing on Bayley Scales of Infant Development (cognitive composite $R = 0.502$ $P = .03$; motor composite $R = 0.497$ $P = .01$; language composite $R = 0.444$ $P = .03$) (see Fig. 12.24)
Glass HC, Nash KB, Bonifacio SL, et al. Seizures and magnetic resonance imaging-detected brain injury in newborns cooled for hypoxic-ischemic encephalopathy. *J Pediatr.* 2011;159:731–735.e731	56 with HIE and TH with continuous conventional EEG monitoring.	Seizure identification: Continuous conventional EEG. Univariate Outcome: MRI injury severity	Seizures conferred an increased risk of moderate to severe injury on MRI (relative risk 2.3, $P = .02$)

Continued

TABLE 12.26   Associations of Seizure Burden With Neurodevelopmental Outcome—cont'd

STUDY	COHORT	ANALYSIS	KEY FINDINGS
van Rooij LG, de Vries LS, Handryastuti S, et al. Neurodevelopmental outcome in term infants with status epilepticus detected with amplitude-integrated electroencephalography. *Pediatrics* 2007;120:e354–e363	311 with seizures due to heterogeneous etiologies	Seizure identification: clinical and aEEG. Univariate. Outcome: Neurodevelopmental	Among the newborns with hypoxic-ischemic encephalopathy (but not the full cohort), the duration of status epilepticus was associated with poor outcomes (215 min of seizures in poor outcome vs. 85 min of seizures in good outcome, $P < .05$).
McBride MC, Laroia N, Guillet R. Electrographic seizures in neonates correlate with poor neurodevelopmental outcome. *Neurology.* 2000;55:506–513	68 newborns with heterogeneous etiologies at risk for seizures.	Seizure identification: Continuous conventional EEG. Univariate. Outcome: Mortality, cerebral palsy, microcephaly, and neurodevelopmental.	The presence of seizures was associated with increased risk of death due to neurological causes in the first year of life (relative risk 7, $P < .02$) and cerebral palsy (relative risk 2, $P < .05$). Seizure burden as a categorical variable was associated with microcephaly ($P = .04$), severe cerebral palsy ($P = .03$), and failure to thrive ($P = .03$). Nonsignificant trends in which seizures were associated with increased risks for microcephaly and lower Bayley performance scores. Among asphyxiated newborns, the presence of seizures was associated with increased risk of death from neurological cause ($P = .02$), severe cerebral palsy ($P = .04$), and microcephaly ($P = .05$)
Painter MJ, Sun Q, Scher MS, et al. Neonates with seizures: what predicts development? *J Child Neurol.* 2012;27:1022–1026	52 at risk for seizures	Seizure identification: Continuous conventional EEG. Univariate Outcome: Developmental assessments	Seizure severity predicted outcomes with mild and moderate severity seizures associated with a normal ($P = .002$) or moderate ($P = .007$) outcomes.
Maartens IA, Wassenberg T, Buijs J, et al. Neurodevelopmental outcome in full-term newborns with refractory neonatal seizures. *Acta Paediatr.* 2012;101:e173–e178	46 term with heterogeneous etiologies and seizures refractory to phenobarbital	Seizure identification: Clinical and EEG. Responsiveness to antiseizure medications used as a marker of seizure severity. Univariate Outcome: Infant development at 2 years	Among newborns who had required ≤2 antiseizure medications versus ≥3 antiseizure medications, normal development occurred in 50% versus 5%, moderate disability occurred in 20% versus 27%, and severe disability occurred in 30% versus 68% ($P < .01$)

aEEG, Amplitude-integrated EEG; *EEG,* electroencephalographic; *HIE,* hypoxic-ischemic encephalopathy; *MR,* magnetic resonance imaging; *TH,* therapeutic hypothermia.

current randomized controlled trials with aEEG monitoring that may lower seizure burden in monitored infants across diverse neuropathologies are required to definitely answer the question of the adverse impact of seizures in the newborn infant. However, the current data support that at least in some newborns seizures may cause or accentuate secondary brain injury and subsequent worsening of neurobehavioral outcomes.

Management

Before discussing the usual sequence of therapy in the infant with seizures, it is important to review the selection of the infant to treat and the criteria to determine the adequacy of therapy.

Selection of Whom to Treat

The selection of whom to treat requires the accurate identification of the infant with epileptic seizures. As noted earlier, to accurately recognize a newborn infant with seizures requires continuous electrophysiological monitoring with either gold standard, conventional video EEG, or, if unavailable, limited channel aEEG, because of the very high incidence of clinically silent seizures.

Why *should the infant with seizures be treated with anticonvulsant medication at all*? The answer relates to the potential adverse effects of seizures on ventilatory function, circulation, cerebral metabolism, and subsequent brain development (see earlier). The potential mechanisms of brain injury with repeated seizures include disturbances in CBF, energy metabolism, homeostasis of excitotoxic amino acids, neurogenesis, and subsequent synaptic reorganization (reviewed earlier). Earlier reports, published primarily in the 1980s, showed poorer outcomes in asphyxiated newborns who exhibited seizures than in those who did not (see earlier discussion). The independent effect of seizures, in

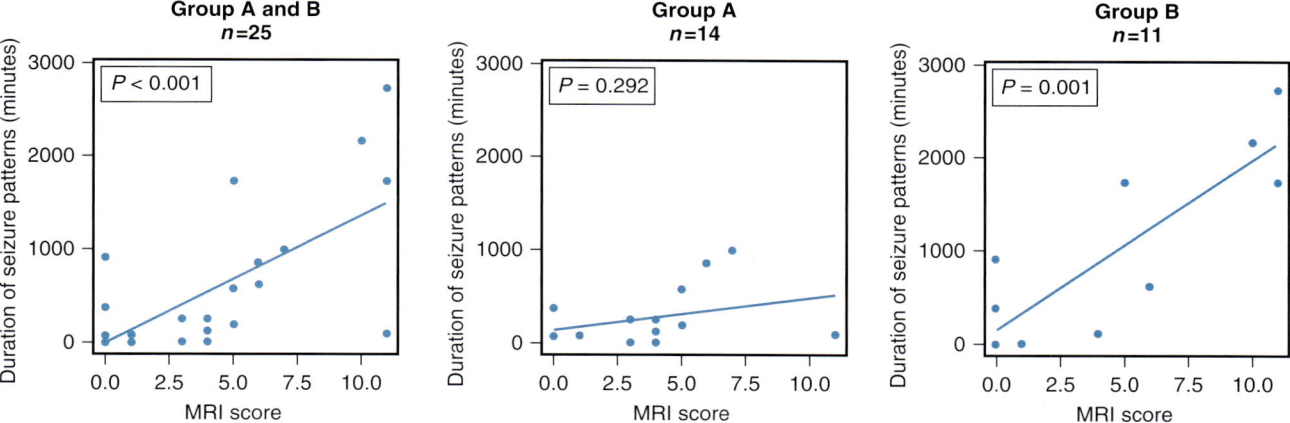

Figure 12.19 **Relationship between seizure duration and MRI scores.** Newborns in Group A were managed based on amplitude-integrated EEG (aEEG) information while newborns in Group B were managed based on only clinical information (e.g., neonatologists were blind to the aEEG data). A significant correlation was found between the duration of seizure patterns and the severity of brain injury in the blinded group, as well as in the whole group. *MRI*, Magnetic resonance imaging. (From van Rooij LG, Toet MC, van Huffelen AC, et al. Effect of treatment of subclinical neonatal seizures detected with aEEG: randomized, controlled trial. *Pediatrics.* 2010;125:e358–e366.)

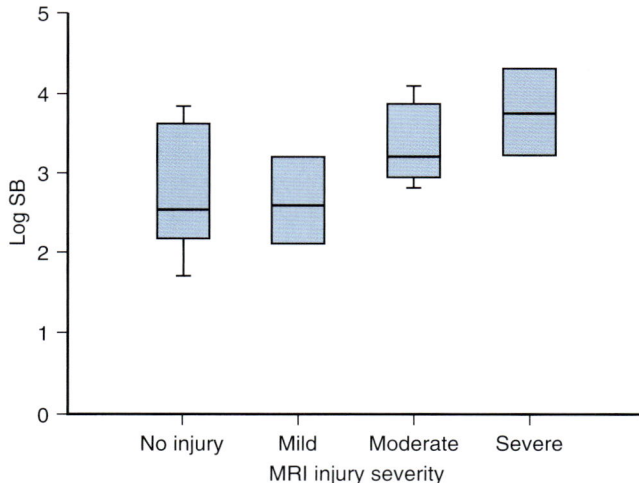

Figure 12.20 Overall trend of electrographic seizure burden (log units) and severity of brain injury on MRI. *MRI*, Magnetic resonance imaging. (From Srinivasakumar P, Zempel J, Trivedi S, et al. Treating EEG seizures in hypoxic ischemic encephalopathy: a randomized controlled trial. *Pediatrics.* 2015;136:e1302–e1309.)

addition to the severity of the pathological features, was not clear from the earlier work. However, more recent reports, characterized by quantitation of electrographic seizures and multivariate analyses adjusting for severity of brain injury suggest that seizures may accentuate brain injury, especially in newborns with hypoxic–ischemic brain injury (see earlier). Although not unequivocally established in the human newborn, *the balance of information indicates that repeated seizures should be stopped because they may induce secondary brain injury and less favorable neurobehavioral outcomes.* While there remains uncertainty as to the extent to which seizures worsen outcomes and in which patients, whether treatment actually improves outcomes, how aggressively to treat seizures, and what medications are

optimal for seizure treatment, the large majority of clinicians treat neonatal seizures.[566] The World Health Organization guideline on neonatal seizures recommends *treatment of all clinical and electrographic seizures.*[173]

The value of implementation of a standardized treatment protocol has been documented in recent studies. One investigation evaluated neonatal status epilepticus management for 6 months before and 12 months after the implementation of a standardized algorithm for therapy in newborn seizures.[567] Adherence of 80% was achieved. After the algorithm, maximum phenobarbital concentrations were decreased (57 vs. 41 μg/mL), fewer patients progressed from seizures to status epilepticus (46% vs. 36%), and hospital length of stay decreased by 10 days in survivors. Although increased attention to neonatal seizure management might lead to concern for overtreatment and elevated exposure to phenobarbital, there is some evidence that early treatment using a coordinated and consistent approach prevents overadministration of anticonvulsant medication. This conclusion is supported by a recent study of 108 newborns with hypoxic-ischemic encephalopathy cared for before and after implementation of a neonatal neurocritical care service. Nearly all newborns (95% to 95%) with seizures received phenobarbital at similar dosing (30 to 33 mg/kg). Although the era after implementation of the service had improved EEG monitoring and improved vigilance for seizures, after adjustment for seizure burden, newborns managed after implementation of the Neonatal Neurocritical Care Service received an average of 30 mg/kg less cumulative phenobarbital and were on maintenance therapy for 5 fewer days.[568] These data indicate that even in the absence of an entirely evidence-based approach to neonatal seizure management, the implementation of a logical and consistent plan may provide benefit. There are many published reviews that summarize clinical approaches to neonatal seizure management.[a]

[a]References 173, 178, 179, 231, 292, 566, and 569-572.

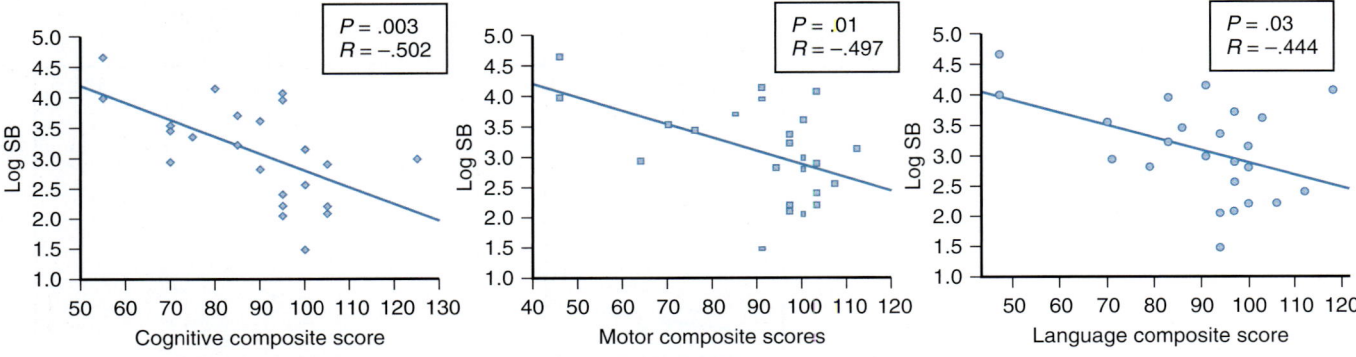

Figure 12.21 Correlation between electrographic seizure burden (log units) and performance scores on Bayley Scales of Infant Development III. (From Srinivasakumar P, Zempel J, Trivedi S, et al. Treating EEG seizures in hypoxic ischemic encephalopathy: a randomized controlled trial. *Pediatrics.* 2015;136:e1302–e1309.)

TABLE 12.27	Survey Results Regarding Monitoring in Preterm and Term Newborns Using Electroencephalographic and Amplitude-Integrated EEG Modalities	
	RESPONDENTS FOR EACH ITEM	
	PRETERM	**TERM**
Method of seizure diagnosis		
Clinical observation only	7%	8%
aEEG	1%	1%
EEG	58%	58%
aEEG or EEG	34%	33%
Continuous monitoring of "at risk" newborns		
Yes with aEEG	22%	24%
Yes with EEG	17%	24%
Yes with aEEG and EEG	15%	19%
No	47%	34%

aEEG, Amplitude-integrated EEG; *EEG,* electroencephalographic.
From Glass HC, Kan J, Bonifacio SL, et al. Neonatal seizures: treatment practices among term and preterm infants. *Pediatr Neurol.* 2012;26:111–115.

Adequacy of Treatment

The decision to initiate seizure therapy and the assessment of the adequacy of treatment rely on the accurate identification of seizures. The *goal of therapy is the elimination of electrical seizure activity,* based on the fact that many seizures in the newborn infant are clinically silent. In addition, the administration of anticonvulsant medications often leads to electromechanical uncoupling/dissociation in which there is cessation of clinical seizures despite the persistence of EEG-only seizures.[227,229,241] Given these difficulties in seizure identification, clinicians must rely on EEG monitoring as the only means for accurate determination of the adequacy of anticonvulsant therapy. A survey of 193 international neurologists, neonatologists, and specialists in neonatal neurology conducted in 2010 reported that the majority of centers used either EEG, aEEG, or a combination for newborns with seizures or at risk for seizures (Table 12.27).[170] Thus, the importance of electrophysiological monitoring to determine accurately the presence of seizure

activity appears essential in determination of the success of anticonvulsant therapy.

As management progresses, the goal of total elimination of electrical seizure activity may have to be adjusted based on individual circumstances. Although the goal of therapy is generally total or near-total elimination of electrographic seizures,[173] in some newborns the doses of anticonvulsant medications required lead to potentially dangerous disturbances of cardiac function, blood pressure, and ventilation. For example, because a newborn with cardiovascular instability may not tolerate multiple anticonvulsant medications, the goal may evolve toward reducing seizure burden as much as possible without worsening cardiovascular function. Similarly, if a diagnosis of brain malformation or other neonatal-onset epileptic encephalopathy is made, the goal might be to reduce seizures as much as possible with an anticonvulsant medication regimen that retains acceptable alertness for long-term use.

Usual Sequence of Therapy

The infant exhibiting repeated seizure activity should be treated promptly. Although there are many knowledge gaps related to neonatal seizure management, a systematic approach to management (as discussed earlier) is valuable. The approach described in previous editions of this book is similar to that recommended by others after systematic literature reviews. However, the lack of extensive, evidence-based information is notable. For example, a 2004 Cochrane Database Systematic Review identified only two randomized, controlled trials related to neonatal seizures, and the authors concluded that there were insufficient data to recommend one anticonvulsant medication over other medications.[573-575] Similarly, a 2013 systematic review identified 571 publications related to neonatal seizure management, but only two randomized controlled trials, and only three additional studies with comparison groups. However, using the available data the authors were able to develop a partially evidence-based treatment algorithm (Fig. 12.22).[570] Similar neonatal management algorithms have been developed by others (Fig. 12.23).[243]

As recommended in previous editions of this book, the World Health Organization recommends phenobarbital as the first agent,[173,576] and, internationally, phenobarbital is the most frequent initial medication administered for neonatal seizures.[170,568,577-580] However, because of the lack of available

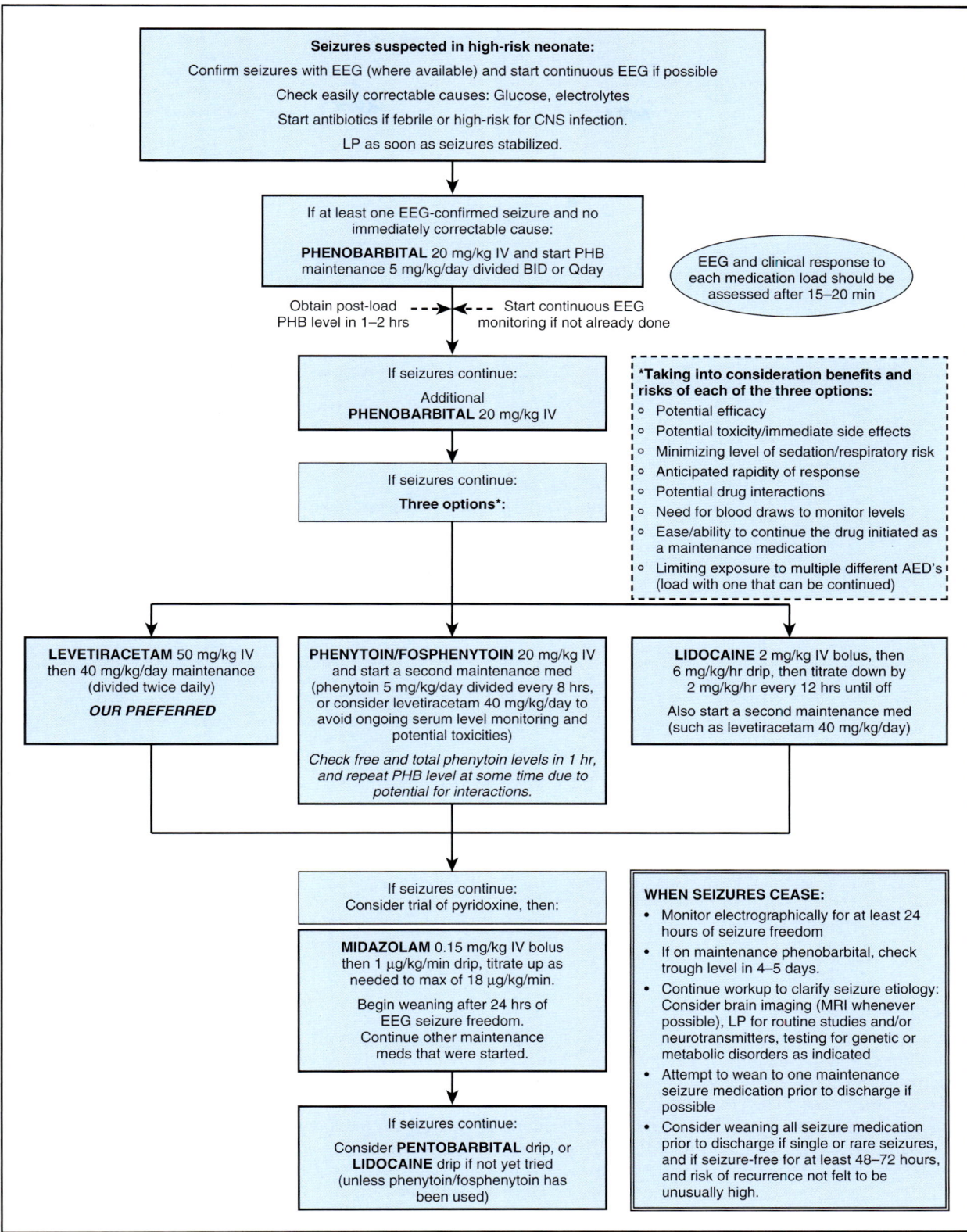

Seizures suspected in high-risk neonate:

Confirm seizures with EEG (where available) and start continuous EEG if possible

Check easily correctable causes: Glucose, electrolytes

Start antibiotics if febrile or high-risk for CNS infection.

LP as soon as seizures stabilized.

If at least one EEG-confirmed seizure and no immediately correctable cause:
PHENOBARBITAL 20 mg/kg IV and start PHB maintenance 5 mg/kg/day divided BID or Qday

Obtain post-load PHB level in 1–2 hrs   Start continuous EEG monitoring if not already done

EEG and clinical response to each medication load should be assessed after 15–20 min

If seizures continue:
Additional **PHENOBARBITAL** 20 mg/kg IV

*Taking into consideration benefits and risks of each of the three options:
- Potential efficacy
- Potential toxicity/immediate side effects
- Minimizing level of sedation/respiratory risk
- Anticipated rapidity of response
- Potential drug interactions
- Need for blood draws to monitor levels
- Ease/ability to continue the drug initiated as a maintenance medication
- Limiting exposure to multiple different AED's (load with one that can be continued)

If seizures continue:
Three options*:

LEVETIRACETAM 50 mg/kg IV then 40 mg/kg/day maintenance (divided twice daily)
OUR PREFERRED

PHENYTOIN/FOSPHENYTOIN 20 mg/kg IV and start a second maintenance med (phenytoin 5 mg/kg/day divided every 8 hrs, or consider levetiracetam 40 mg/kg/day to avoid ongoing serum level monitoring and potential toxicities)
Check free and total phenytoin levels in 1 hr, and repeat PHB level at some time due to potential for interactions.

LIDOCAINE 2 mg/kg IV bolus, then 6 mg/kg/hr drip, then titrate down by 2 mg/kg/hr every 12 hrs until off

Also start a second maintenance med (such as levetiracetam 40 mg/kg/day)

If seizures continue:
Consider trial of pyridoxine, then:

MIDAZOLAM 0.15 mg/kg IV bolus then 1 μg/kg/min drip, titrate up as needed to max of 18 μg/kg/min.

Begin weaning after 24 hrs of EEG seizure freedom. Continue other maintenance meds that were started.

WHEN SEIZURES CEASE:
- Monitor electrographically for at least 24 hours of seizure freedom
- If on maintenance phenobarbital, check trough level in 4–5 days.
- Continue workup to clarify seizure etiology: Consider brain imaging (MRI whenever possible), LP for routine studies and/or neurotransmitters, testing for genetic or metabolic disorders as indicated
- Attempt to wean to one maintenance seizure medication prior to discharge if possible
- Consider weaning all seizure medication prior to discharge if single or rare seizures, and if seizure-free for at least 48–72 hours, and risk of recurrence not felt to be unusually high.

If seizures continue:
Consider **PENTOBARBITAL** drip, or **LIDOCAINE** drip if not yet tried (unless phenytoin/fosphenytoin has been used)

Figure 12.22 An example neonatal seizure management algorithm. *AED,* Antiepileptic drug; *CNS,* central nervous system; *EEG,* electroencephalography; *IV,* intravenous; *LP,* lumbar puncture; *MRI,* magnetic resonance imaging; *PHB,* phenobarbital. (From Slaughter LA, Patel AD, Slaughter JL. Pharmacological treatment of neonatal seizures: a systematic review. *J Child Neurol.* 2013;28:351–364.)

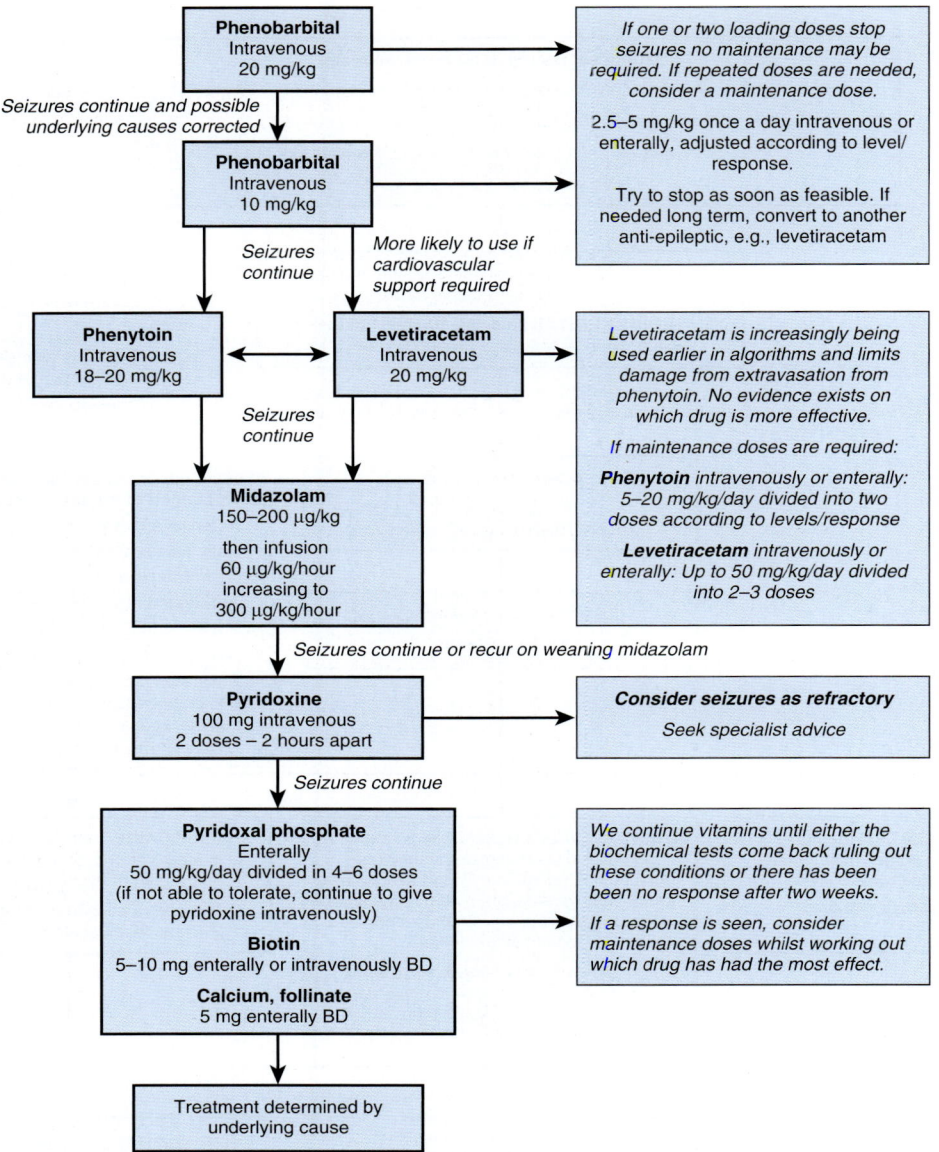

Figure 12.23 An example neonatal seizure management algorithm. (From Hart AR, Pilling EL, Alix JJ. Neonatal seizures—part 2: aetiology of acute symptomatic seizures, treatments and the neonatal epilepsy syndromes. *Arch Dis Child Educ Pract Ed.* 2015;100:226–232, with permission.)

data, there is substantial variability regarding subsequent medication choices and the duration of therapy.[170,577-580] A survey of 193 international neurologists, neonatologists, and specialists in neonatal neurology conducted in 2010 found that the most common first-, second-, and third-line antiseizure medications were phenobarbital, phenytoin, and levetiracetam, respectively (Table 12.28).[170] A typical sequence of therapy is provided in Table 12.29. There is varying familiarity and availability of these medications between institutions and countries, so practice is partially hospital specific.

Before reviewing the individual aspects of the sequence of therapy, it is important to emphasize that before instituting any anticonvulsant therapy, the physician should assess and manage ventilation and perfusion. Moreover, because the administration of certain anticonvulsant medications may impair ventilation, the necessary equipment for support of ventilation should be immediately available, with the expectation that the need for intubation is highly likely. Moreover, the actively convulsing infant should be treated promptly without waiting for implementation of such diagnostic studies as EEG or neuroimaging.

Glucose

If hypoglycemia is present and if the infant is having seizures, then 10% dextrose is given intravenously in a dose of 2 mL/kg (0.2 g/kg), and the newborn is maintained on intravenous dextrose at a rate as high as 0.5 g/kg per hour (8 mg/kg per minute) if necessary (see Chapter 25 for more detail). Although constant infusion of glucose at 8 mg/kg per minute corrects hypoglycemia in less than 10 minutes in most patients,[581]

TABLE 12.28   Survey Results Regarding Choice of Antiseizure Medication for Preterm and Term Newborns

	PRETERM			TERM		
	FIRST	SECOND	THIRD	FIRST	SECOND	THIRD
	n (%)	n (%)	n (%)	n (%)	n (%)	n (%)
Phenobarbital	135 (72.2)	49 (26.2)	2 (1.1)	120 (70.9)	49 (27.2)	3 (1.7)
Lorazepam	41 (21.9)	26 (13.9)	23 (13.1)	42 (23.1)	19 (10.6)	26 (14.9)
Phenytoin	4 (2.1)	76 (40.6)	62 (35.2)	4 (2.2)	77 (42.8)	61 (34.9)
Levetiracetam	2 (1.1)	17 (9.1)	37 (21.0)	2 (1.1)	16 (8.9)	33 (18.9)
Midazolam	5 (2.7)	14 (7.5)	29 (16.5)	5 (2.7)	17 (9.4)	28 (16.0)
Topiramate	0 (0.0)	1 (0.5)	12 (6.8)	0 (0.0)	0 (0.0)	11 (6.3)
Lidocaine	0 (0.0)	4 (2.1)	7 (4.0)	0 (0.0)	2 (1.1)	11 (6.3)
Other	0 (0.0)	0 (0.0)	4 (2.3)	0 (0.0)	0 (0.0)	2 (1.1)

From Glass HC, Kan J, Bonifacio SL, Ferriero DM. Neonatal seizures: treatment practices among term and preterm. *Pediatr Neurol.* 2012;46:111–115.

TABLE 12.29   Acute Therapy of Neonatal Seizures

Phenobarbital: 20 mg/kg, IV (1–2 mg/kg/min)
If necessary:
   Additional phenobarbital: 10 mg/kg IV (to a maximum total
     of 40–50 mg/kg)
    Phenytoin: 20 mg/kg, IV (0.5–1.0 mg/kg/min)
    Fosphenytoin: 20 phenytoin equivalents/kg
    Lorazepam: 0.05–0.10 mg/kg, IV
    Midazolam: 0.2 mg/kg, IV; then, 0.1–0.4 mg/kg/h, IV
Others (as indicated)
Hypoglycemia, glucose, 10% solution: 2 mL/kg, IV
Calcium gluconate, 5% solution: 4 mL/kg, IV
Magnesium sulfate, 50% solution: 0.2 mL/kg, IM
Pyridoxine: 50–100 mg, IV; repeat to maximum of 500 mg if
  needed
Pyridoxal-5-phosphate, 30 mg/kg/day, PO
Folinic acid, 4 mg/kg/day, PO

IM, Intramuscularly; *IV*, intravenously; *PO*, by mouth.

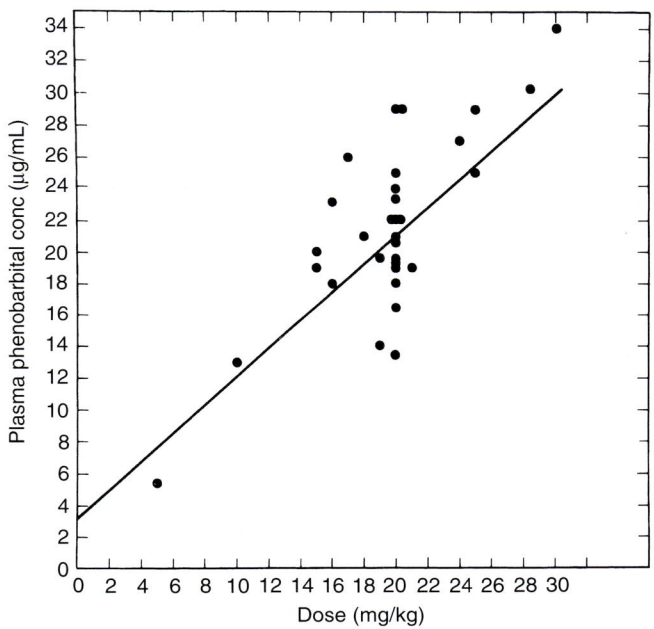

Figure 12.24 Phenobarbital levels after initial bolus. Plasma levels of phenobarbital achieved following the initial intravenous dose in human newborns with seizures. (From Painter MJ, Pippenger C, MacDonald H, Pitlick W. Phenobarbital and diphenylhydantoin levels in neonates with seizures. *J Pediatr.* 1978;92:315–319.)

and is appropriate if the newborn is not having seizures, the faster approach of bolus infusion may be indicated for the newborn experiencing seizures. A second bolus dose can be administered if seizures persist. A topic for future research is the possibility of maintaining supra-normal levels of blood glucose in newborns with frequent seizures, in view of the experimental demonstrations of a decline in brain glucose concentration with seizures and the protective effect of pretreatment with glucose (discussed earlier and in Figs. 12.3 and 12.9).

Anticonvulsant Medications

Phenobarbital. The initial anticonvulsant medication is most often phenobarbital administered intravenously in a loading dose of 20 mg/kg, which is generally delivered over 10 to 15 minutes. Careful surveillance of respiratory effort is important under these circumstances. This dosing is necessary to achieve a blood level of approximately 20 μg/mL (Fig. 12.24), which achieves a clearly measurable anticonvulsant effect in the newborn.[28,582-587] Weight or gestational age does not appear to influence the dose-blood-level relationship appreciably,[582,583,588] although infants less than 30 weeks gestational age may require slightly lower doses to achieve the same blood level.[589] To

achieve the same blood level, the intramuscular dose must be approximately 10% to 15% greater than the intravenous dose.[583] Most clinicians use the intravenous route because of the faster onset of action and the more predictable phenobarbital blood level. If the initial 20 mg/kg dose of phenobarbital is not effective in controlling seizures, many clinicians administer additional doses of 5 to 10 mg/kg each until seizures have ceased, a total dose of 40 mg/kg has been administered, or the patient develops dose-limiting adverse effects (Table 12.30). The goal is to achieve a phenobarbital blood concentration of approximately 40 μg/mL.

Using phenobarbital in this manner, Gilman et al.[586] and Gal et al.[590] attained control of *clinical* seizures in approximately 70% of 71 newborns. Painter and colleagues used approximately

TABLE 12.30   Expected Response of Neonatal Clinical Seizures to Sequence of Therapy

ANTICONVULSANT DRUG[a] (CUMULATIVE DOSE)	CESSATION OF SEIZURES (CUMULATIVE PERCENTAGE) (%)
Phenobarbital, 20 mg/kg	40
Phenobarbital, 40 mg/kg	70
Phenytoin, 20 mg/kg	85
Lorazepam, 0.05–0.10 mg/kg	95–100

[a]All drugs administered intravenously.
Based largely on data of Gilman JT, Gal P, Duchowny MS, Weaver RL, et al. Rapid sequential phenobarbital treatment of neonatal seizures. *Pediatrics.* 1989;83:674–678, and on personal experience.

TABLE 12.31   Response of Neonatal Electrographic Seizures to Phenobarbital and Phenytoin[a]

	EXTENT OF CONTROL	
	COMPLETE (%)	≥80% REDUCTION (%)[a]
Phenobarbital[b] plus	43	
phenytoin	57	80
Phenytoin plus	45	
phenobarbital	62	72

[a]Value includes infants with complete control of seizures and those with 80% or greater reduction (albeit not complete reduction) in seizures.
[b]Blood levels of free phenobarbital were 25 μg/mL and blood levels of free phenytoin were 3 μg/mL. Data from Painter MJ, Scher MS, Stein AD, Armatti S, et al. Phenobarbital compared with phenytoin for the treatment of neonatal seizures. *N Engl J Med.* 1999;341:485–489; the study involved 59 term infants with electrographic seizures, and randomly assigned to receive phenobarbital (n = 30) or phenytoin (n = 29), followed by the two drugs in combination if complete control of electrographic seizures was not attained.

similar doses in a later controlled study of 59 newborns, and the drug completely controlled *electrographic* seizures in only 43% (Table 12.31).[574] An open-label, randomized, controlled trial in India also compared phenobarbital (20 mg/kg) to phenytoin (20 mg/kg) in patients with varied seizure etiologies. Seizures were controlled (defined as a seizure-free period of 24 hours) in significantly more newborns with phenobarbital (72%) than phenytoin (15%). If seizures persisted, newborns crossed-over to the other drug. Overall seizure cessation occurred in significantly more newborns who received phenobarbital first than phenytoin first (91% vs. 80%).[591] A retrospective study of newborns with *electrographically confirmed seizures* (but excluding newborns with status epilepticus) found that of 91 newborns who received phenobarbital, 63% responded completely (cessation of clinical and electrographic seizures), 17% responded partially (reduction but not cessation of electrographic seizures with the first bolus, response to the second bolus), and 21% did not respond.[592] The presence of EEG-only seizures and more abnormal EEG backgrounds predicted a lack of response to phenobarbital.[592]

Even with a favorable initial response to anticonvulsant medication, close observation is required because additional management may be needed. A study using EEG monitoring reviewed by experts calculated electrographic seizure exposure in 19 newborns for 1-hour epochs.[593] The seizure burden was compared in the hour before and subsequent hours after phenobarbitone administration. The seizure burden was reduced by 14 minutes (74% reduction) in the first hour after the administration of phenobarbitone, but the reduction was temporary and not significant within 4 hours. In addition, only phenobarbitone doses of 20 mg/kg resulted in a significant reduction at 1 hour.[593] Total loading doses of phenobarbital in excess of 40 to 50 mg/kg generally do not provide extra benefit. In addition, high levels appreciably sedate the newborn for several days, thereby impairing neurological analysis, and may lead to toxic effects on the cardiovascular system.

Certain *pharmacological properties of phenobarbital are beneficial in the treatment of neonatal seizures.* Thus, the drug enters CSF (and presumably brain) rapidly and with high efficiency (i.e., 30 minutes after an intravenous loading dose was administered, the CSF to blood ratio was 0.58 ± 0.07); the blood level is largely predictable from the dose administered; the agent can be administered intramuscularly as well as intravenously (preferably the latter) for acute therapy; and maintenance therapy is accomplished easily with oral therapy (see later discussion).[584,589] Moreover, experimental data suggest that entrance of phenobarbital into brain is accelerated by the local acidosis associated with seizure.[107] Protein binding is lower in the newborn (33%) than in the older child and adult (41%), and thus free (active) levels of the drug are relatively higher. Because binding may be decreased further by hyperbilirubinemia and apparently other factors still to be defined,[584] routine monitoring of free phenobarbital levels may be optimal for management but is not routinely available.

Despite the concerning adverse profile of phenobarbital on neurons in experimental models, there are some data that phenobarbital-related reduction in seizures might yield more favorable neurobehavioral outcomes. A prospective cohort of 42 newborns with hypoxic–ischemic encephalopathy treated with therapeutic hypothermia were either administered phenobarbital (20 mg/kg) prophylactically (20 newborns) or only if clinical seizures occurred (22 newborns). On univariate analysis, the use of prophylactic phenobarbital was associated with a decreased occurrence of seizure in the neonatal period (15% with prophylaxis vs. 82% without prophylaxis, P < .0001) and decreased occurrence of seizures in the first 24 hours of life (5% with prophylaxis vs. 64% without prophylaxis, P < .0001). On multivariate analysis, which incorporated additional clinical features, such as birth weight and Apgar scores, the use of prophylactic phenobarbital was associated with more favorable neurodevelopmental outcomes.[594]

As discussed earlier, anticonvulsant medications with GABA agonist properties, such as phenobarbital (or benzodiazepines), may not be ideal agents because $GABA_A$ receptors are likely to be excitatory rather than inhibitory in most immature cortical neurons. More rational approaches might convert $GABA_A$ receptors from excitatory to inhibitory and thereby could enhance effectiveness of phenobarbital. Bumetanide inhibits NKCC1, the Cl^- cotransporter responsible for the elevated neuronal Cl^- levels and the depolarizing (excitation) rather than hyperpolarizing (inhibitory) response on $GABA_A$

receptor activation (see earlier). The blockade of NKCC1 decreases neuronal Cl⁻ levels and restores the inhibitory response of GABA$_A$ receptor activation.[13] Bumetanide suppresses epileptiform activity in neonatal rat hippocampal slices in vitro and in neonatal rat brain in vivo.[13] This drug has been used safely as a diuretic in the newborn, and an intravenous preparation is available.[595,596] These features have led to the hypothesis that bumetanide used concurrently with phenobarbital (or benzodiazepines) could be particularly effective, because bumetanide would allow the GABA$_A$ receptor activation produced by phenobarbital to lead to inhibition. A phase 2 feasibility study of combination bumetanide and phenobarbital therapy in newborns with hypoxic–ischemic encephalopathy and electrographic seizures enrolled 14 subjects.[597] Five had seizure reductions, but only two did not need additional rescue therapy. There were no acute adverse effects, but all 11 surviving newborns had hearing impairment. The trial was stopped early because of the concerns over the potential negative auditory adverse effects and limited evidence for efficacy by seizure reduction.[597] A second study of bumetanide for neonatal seizures is currently enrolling subjects.[598]

Phenytoin and Fosphenytoin. In the newborn who continues to experience electrographic or clinical seizures after as much as 40 mg/kg of phenobarbital or in the severely asphyxiated infant in whom less than the full phenobarbital loading dose is deemed appropriate because of cardiopulmonary concerns, phenytoin or fosphenytoin is generally administered as second-line medication.[170] Phenytoin's mechanism involves blocking of sodium channels and, therefore, represents an alternative mechanism to the action of barbiturates (i.e., phenobarbital) and benzodiazepines, which both act on chloride channels. The usual loading dose is 20 mg/kg for phenytoin or 20 phenytoin-equivalents/kg for fosphenytoin. When this approach is used in newborns who continue to exhibit electrographic seizures after 40 mg/kg of phenobarbital, approximately 15% more experience seizure cessation (i.e., to a total of nearly 60%; see Table 12.30). The cumulative response to the combined phenobarbital and phenytoin therapy is similar regardless of which medication is administered first (see Table 12.31). In the study by Painter and colleagues, when phenytoin was used as a first-line medication, 45% had seizure cessation.[574] If clinical seizure is the response end point, nearly 85% of newborns respond (see Table 12.31). However, as noted earlier, clinical seizure is not a suitable parameter for measuring seizure response. If 80% or more reduction of electrographic seizure is considered a favorable response, then the combination of phenobarbital and phenytoin achieves this level of benefit in fully 80% of newborns (see Table 12.31).[574]

The 20 mg/kg loading dose of phenytoin results in a therapeutic blood level of approximately 15 to 20 μg/kg (Fig. 12.25). The dose of phenytoin should be administered at a rate of no more than 1 mg/kg per minute to avoid disturbance of cardiac function, particularly cardiac rhythm. Cardiac rate and rhythm should be monitored during the infusion. Phenytoin should be administered directly into the intravenous line because it is relatively insoluble in aqueous solutions and precipitates in standard dextrose intravenous solutions. The pH of the parenteral solution is 12 and can be irritating to the vein and surrounding tissue; thus, the dose should be followed by a few milliliters of normal saline solution. These

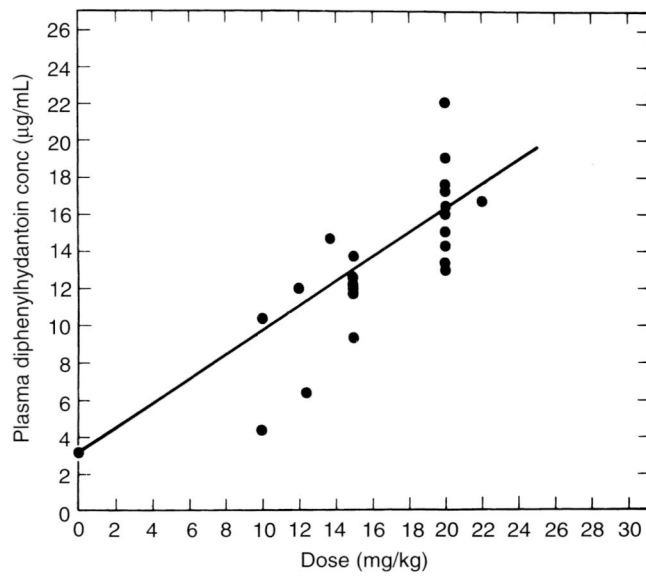

Figure 12.25 **Phenytoin levels after initial bolus.** Plasma levels of phenytoin achieved following the initial intravenous dose in human newborns with seizures. (From Painter MJ, Pippenger C, MacDonald H, Pitlick W. Phenobarbital and diphenylhydantoin levels in neonates with seizures. *J Pediatr.* 1978;92: 315–319.)

characteristics may lead to serious soft tissue injury, and they make fosphenytoin the preferred form for use in the newborn.

Fosphenytoin, a phosphate ester prodrug of phenytoin, has proved to be a major advance in the therapy of status epilepticus and acute seizures.[599-604] The drug's advantages include high water solubility and a pH value closer to neutral, an ease of preparation in standard intravenous solutions, safe intramuscular administration, the absence of tissue injury with intravenous infiltration, and a faster allowable rate of intravenous administration. Fosphenytoin is dosed in *phenytoin equivalents* (1.5 mg of fosphenytoin yields approximately 1 mg of phenytoin), and the effective dose is essentially identical to that described for phenytoin. The drug is converted to phenytoin, primarily by plasma phosphatases, in approximately 8 minutes. The rate of conversion of fosphenytoin to phenytoin appears similar in newborns, infants, and older children.[601,603,604] While fosphenytoin may be associated with fewer potential risks, it is more expensive and not readily available in some hospitals or countries.[566] Nevertheless, it is clearly the preferred form of phenytoin to be used in newborns.

Phenytoin has complicated pharmacokinetics, which makes neonatal use complex. It is highly protein bound, so free levels can be difficult to achieve in newborns with renal or hepatic issues. It also induces hepatic metabolism of many other medications, including phenobarbital, which is often concurrently administered. Thus, levels of hepatically metabolized medications may need to be monitored. Further, maintaining an adequate and stable drug level is difficult, particularly for maintenance administration. Maintenance doses of 5 mg/kg per day divided twice per day (for intravenous formulations) or three times per day (for enteral formulations) are recommended. Drug levels should be followed closely as they can fluctuate substantially.

Benzodiazepines (Lorazepam, Diazepam, Midazolam).
Approximately 20% or more of newborns with electrographic seizures do not respond to the sequential administration of phenobarbital and phenytoin (see Table 12.29). Often lorazepam is administered as a third-line medication, although some clinicians prefer to use lorazepam before phenytoin.[170] Like barbiturates, benzodiazepines act on the GABA receptor and its chloride channel, thus hyperpolarizing the neuron. Thus, benzodiazepines share the mechanistic problems related to GABA activation and chloride levels (see prior discussion) and the adverse effects associated with phenobarbital, including respiratory and, more rarely, cardiovascular depression.

Lorazepam is a benzodiazepine anticonvulsant medication of proven efficacy in older infants and children. Lorazepam enters the brain rapidly and produces a pronounced anticonvulsant effect in less than 5 minutes. Of importance, however, lorazepam is less lipophilic than diazepam, and thus lorazepam does not redistribute from the brain as rapidly as diazepam. The duration of action for lorazepam is generally 6 to 24 hours; that is, longer than diazepam. Moreover, lorazepam appears less likely to produce respiratory depression or hypotension than does diazepam. Lorazepam has been investigated in the newborn in several studies.[605-607] It has been effective in treatment of neonatal clinical seizures, whether as a second drug (after phenobarbital), or as a third drug (after phenobarbital and phenytoin). The onset of effect has been in 2 to 3 minutes, and the duration has extended to 24 hours. The effective dose is 0.05 to 0.10 mg/kg, administered intravenously in 0.05 mg/kg increments over several minutes. The half-life of lorazepam in asphyxiated newborns is approximately 40 hours (i.e., two- to threefold higher values than in the adult).[607] This prolonged half-life could relate to decreased hepatic glucuronidation activity, a normal neonatal finding perhaps accentuated by asphyxial hepatic injury.

Diazepam is an effective anticonvulsant in the newborn but is less used than lorazepam for several reasons. First diazepam is a poor drug for maintenance because of extremely rapid clearance from the brain (minutes after intravenous administration).[608,609] Second, when used with barbiturate, diazepam carries an increased risk of severe circulatory collapse with respiratory failure.[610] Third, the therapeutic dose is variable and is not necessarily less than the toxic dose (doses of 0.30 and 0.36 mg/kg have led to respiratory arrest).[611,612] Fourth, the vehicle for intravenous diazepam, in many preparations, contains sodium benzoate, which is a very effective uncoupler of the bilirubin-albumin complex[613] and theoretically could increase the risk of kernicterus. Results of studies in Gunn rats suggested that the amount of benzoate in the usual diazepam preparation is not high enough to be a serious risk, but the work did not include intravenous administration or measurement of levels of bilirubin in the brain.[614] Although lorazepam shares this potential problem, it appears to be at least as effective, has a longer duration of action, and exhibits less risk of serious side effects (see previous section). Thus, its risk-benefit profile is superior. Despite these limitations, diazepam has been effective as a continuous intravenous infusion. One report described the complete control of seizures in eight term newborns with severe perinatal asphyxia by continuous intravenous infusion of diazepam. Doses of approximately 0.3 mg/kg per hour were required. No patient required assisted ventilation, although stupor and need for gavage feeding were consistently present.[615]

Midazolam is a short-acting benzodiazepine in common use in the treatment of refractory status epilepticus in older infants and children. This drug has the advantage of less respiratory depression and sedation than lorazepam or diazepam.[616] Reports suggest that midazolam is useful in refractory neonatal seizures.[617-619] In a recent study of 13 newborns with electrographic seizures nonresponsive to phenobarbital with or without phenytoin, 8 responded to midazolam administered as a 0.15 mg/kg bolus followed by infusion of 0.4 mg/kg per hour.[618] The remaining 5 nonresponders did respond after an additional bolus and somewhat higher infusion rates (maximum of 1.1 mg/kg per hour). The control of seizures generally was rapid (<2 hours), especially when treatment was begun promptly after the failure of phenobarbital. Midazolam is usually started with a loading dose of 0.05 to 0.2 mg/kg and an infusion of 0.05 to 0.1 mg/kg per hour. If seizures persist, additional loading doses may be administered and the infusion may be increased by 0.05 to 0.1 mg/kg per hour to maximum doses of about 0.5 mg/kg per hour.

Lidocaine. Lidocaine can be used as a second- or third-line agent for refractory neonatal seizures. The medication has good CNS penetration and acts as a depressant, although its mechanism of action as an anticonvulsant medication is uncertain. Lidocaine is used much more frequently in Europe than in North America; one study has shown it to be the third-line agent of choice at multiple major European medical centers.[572] Several reports indicate value for lidocaine as an adjunctive agent in the treatment of neonatal seizures.[575,584,620-622] Data on approximately 100 newborns treated primarily because of the failure of phenobarbital and diazepam indicated cessation of seizures, usually within 10 minutes of the start of intravenous infusion, in approximately 75% of those treated. Dosage schedules varied, but most commonly a starting infusion of approximately 2 to 6 mg/kg per hour, with or without a bolus infusion at the onset, was used. Small studies have found that when added to other anticonvulsant medications, lidocaine has a 70% to 92% response rate.[566] A retrospective study of 319 term and 94 preterm newborns described the response rate to lidocaine for neonatal seizures confirmed by aEEG.[623] Lidocaine had a good (>4 hours with no seizures, no need for rescue medication) or intermediate (0 to 2 hours with no seizures, but rescue medication needed after 2 to 4 hours) effect in 71.4%. Full term newborns had a better response rate than did preterm newborns (76% vs. 55%). In addition, among full-term infants the response to lidocaine was significantly better than to midazolam as second-line antiseizure medication (21% vs. 13%), and there was a trend toward lidocaine superiority as a third-line medication as well (68% vs. 57%).[623]

Because of the cumulative risk of toxicity, lidocaine must be stopped within 36 hours. Furthermore, the dose must be reduced in premature infants or if the newborn is undergoing therapeutic hypothermia, as clearance decreases during hypothermia. Lidocaine can cause arrhythmias and bradycardia. The risk of such side effects can be significantly reduced by carefully following blood levels; the presumed threshold for cardiac and nervous system toxicity is >9 mg/L.[566] It should be avoided in newborns who have congenital heart issues or have received other pro-arrhythmic drugs like phenytoin.[624] In a retrospective study of lidocaine in 368 term and 153 preterm newborns with seizures described earlier,[623] a second analysis assessed cardiac events. These were reported in 11 (2%) of the 521 patients, and in 7 patients a causal relationship was considered plausible. Risk factors for cardiac events were unstable serum potassium levels, cardiac dysfunction, and concurrent phenytoin use. These data indicated that the risk of cardiac events might be lower than previously reported.[625]

Levetiracetam. As a newer anticonvulsant medication, levetiracetam has become a medication used for the treatment of refractory neonatal seizures. In some centers, it is used as a second-line agent before using phenytoin, benzodiazepines, or lidocaine.[170] Levetiracetam likely has a different mechanism of action from other anticonvulsant medications because it prevents neurotransmitter release by binding to a presynaptic vesicle protein, SV2a.[626] Experimental studies have yielded mixed results in terms of the impact of levetiracetam as a neuroprotective strategy, with some data indicating that it may be neuroprotective[627] and other data indicating that in some situations (such as high-dose with hypothermia) the drug is associated with apoptosis.[628]

Although levetiracetam use is increasing, few data are available regarding efficacy. Clinical data consisting of mostly case reports and small series have reported that seizures terminate or decrease in frequency in about 52% to 80% of newborns after receiving levetiracetam.[503,626,629-638] Based on available data, levetiracetam does seem to have a reasonable safety profile with few side effects and without drug-drug interactions, and it is available in an intravenous formulation. Many child neurologists report using levetiracetam off-label for neonatal seizures and often describe a beneficial response.[639] Optimal dosing is unknown, but common dosing involves intravenous loading doses of 30 to 50 mg/kg with escalation to total intravenous loading doses of about 80 to 100 mg/kg if needed. Maintenance doses of 40 to 100 mg/kg per day divided twice or three times per day can be used. Blood levels typically are not followed as they often take several days to return and are not clearly correlated with efficacy. There are ongoing studies of levetiracetam for the treatment of neonatal seizures.[640]

Topiramate. Topiramate is a blocker of the AMPA type of glutamate receptor and was shown in the neonatal rat to have potent anticonvulsant effects versus hypoxia-induced seizures, to have protective properties for neuronal or premyelinating oligodendrocyte injury, and not to exhibit neurotoxicity to developing neurons.[55,58,145,641-644] Unfortunately, although case series describe benefit in some newborns, an intravenous preparation of topiramate is not yet available.[645] Many child neurologists report using topiramate off-label for neonatal seizures, and often describe a beneficial response.[639]

Other Drugs and Treatments. Potential value of *primidone as an antiseizure medication* in the neonatal period is suggested by several reports.[584,616,646,647] In the initial study, primidone was administered orally to 24 infants with neonatal seizures in whom the seizures had recurred despite high levels of phenobarbital (15 to 40 µg/mL) and phenytoin (10 to 20 µg/mL). Seizure control was achieved within 48 hours in 50% of patients, but 34% of infants required up to 9 days for seizure control. The minimum primidone level at which a response occurred was approximately 6 µg/mL. However, marked interpatient variability

was noted in blood levels of primidone, and phenobarbital clearance was prolonged after the addition of primidone. In a second report, 10 infants were treated with oral primidone after discontinuation of previously ineffective anticonvulsant drugs (primarily phenobarbital or phenytoin, or both). Eight patients achieved seizure control within 1 to 5 days of onset of therapy. Blood levels varied between 5 and 16 µg/mL. Because primidone can be administered only orally, it is unlikely to be useful in acute therapy.

Thiopental was reported to be highly effective in the treatment of seizures in nine asphyxiated term newborns who continued to convulse despite mean phenobarbital levels of 28 µg/mL.[648] The dose was 10 mg/kg, administered intravenously over 2 minutes, and response occurred *promptly*. However, a 27% decrease (mean) of arterial blood pressure occurred in six of the nine infants, and each child was treated with pressor agents or volume expansion.

Paraldehyde, administered as an intravenous bolus and then a continuous infusion, was effective as adjunctive therapy in approximately 50% of the infants studied.[584,616,649,650] However, the intravenous form of this drug is no longer available in the United States. Moreover, the potential side effects of respiratory disturbance, secondary to pulmonary excretion of paraldehyde, and of hypotension, make this drug problematic.

Valproic acid, administered orally as adjunctive therapy, led to the control of neonatal seizures recalcitrant to phenobarbital (mean blood level >40 µg/mL) in five of six cases.[651] However, the elevation of blood ammonia required cessation of therapy in three infants. Because of the uncertain risk of valproate hepatotoxicity in this age group, the value of this drug in the treatment of neonatal seizures is uncertain.

Carbamazepine was reported to be effective as an initial agent in the treatment of neonatal seizures in a study of 10 full-term infants with hypoxic-ischemic encephalopathy.[652] All patients showed an *excellent* clinical response. Therapeutic levels were achieved within 2 to 4 hours after a loading dose of 10 mg/kg administered by nasogastric tube. However, variability in blood levels suggests that more data are needed to determine the value of this agent.

There have been case reports of successful use of the *ketogenic* diet for refractory neonatal seizures of unclear etiology.[653] The ketogenic diet is the treatment of choice for patients with glucose transporter defects.

Other medications approved for the treatment of seizures in children or adults are often used in newborns with refractory seizures. These include oxcarbazepine, lamotrigine, felbamate, and vigabatrin. These medications are not available in intravenous formulations and can therefore be more difficult to administer in critically ill newborns. Furthermore, all of these medications are increased slowly over days to weeks, so they are not adequate for the rapid treatment of seizures.[566]

Other Modes of Therapy

Calcium and Magnesium. If hypocalcemia is present, 5% calcium gluconate is given intravenously at a dose of 4 mL/kg (200 mg/kg) (see Table 12.29). The electrocardiogram, or at least cardiac rhythm by auscultation, should be monitored during administration. Phenobarbital can sometimes suppress the seizures of hypocalcemia,[326] and, thus, a decrease in seizures after phenobarbital administration does not rule out hypocalcemia as the cause. If hypomagnesemia is present, magnesium sulfate is given intramuscularly as a 50% solution in a dose of 0.2 mL/kg (see Table 12.29). Approximately half of all newborns with seizures secondary to later-onset hypocalcemia also have hypomagnesemia.[339] The importance of treating these hypocalcemic infants with magnesium is emphasized by the following: (1) the administration of calcium to such infants may increase renal excretion of magnesium, aggravate the hypomagnesemia, and maintain the convulsive state; and (2) the administration of magnesium has been shown to correct both the hypocalcemia and the hypomagnesemia, perhaps by increasing the movement of calcium from bone to plasma.[339] However, magnesium can produce neuromuscular blockade. Transient weakness and hypotonia (without concentrations of plasma magnesium out of the normal range) are often noted in infants who are given magnesium.[339] Maintenance doses of magnesium and calcium should be administered only as long as needed to avoid hypomagnesemia or hypocalcemia.

Metabolic Strategies. Seizures related to other metabolic disturbances or infection require therapeutic approaches that are better discussed in relation to these specific problems (discussed in Chapters 27 to 29).[288] Pearl has developed a useful clinical approach to neonatal or infantile onset epileptic encephalopathy[290] and Ficicioglu and Bearden have described a useful treatment algorithm for neonatal seizures due to some of the most common inborn errors of metabolism (Fig. 12.26).[288]

Recurrent seizures that are not accompanied by any obvious associated findings to aid in diagnosis should raise the possibility of *pyridoxine dependency.* As noted earlier, the molecular defect involves an aldehyde dehydrogenase (antiquitin [ATQ]) in the lysine degradation pathway; the gene involved is *ALDH7A1.* To interrupt seizures a dose of 100 mg of pyridoxine-HCl is

given intravenously accompanied by simultaneous monitoring of the EEG pattern (see Table 12.29), or orally/enterally with 30 mg/kg per day. Infants with pyridoxine dependency may exhibit hypotonia or even apnea after pyridoxine infusion,[371,372] perhaps because of an abrupt increase of synthesis of GABA in the brain and the activation of inhibitory GABA receptors in the brain stem. Therefore, newborns should be monitored closely during and after the infusion. Any uncertainty regarding the response should provoke repeated 100-mg infusions of pyridoxine (to a maximum of 500 mg), a longer trial of oral pyridoxine (15 to 30 mg/kg per day), or both. To ensure that a late and masked response is not missed, treatment with oral/enteral pyridoxine should be continued until the aldehyde dehydrogenase deficiency is excluded by negative biochemical or genetic testing. Long-term treatment dosages vary between 15 and 30 mg/kg per day in infants or up to 200 mg/day in newborns, and 500 mg/day in adults. As described earlier, some infants not responsive to pyridoxine may require pyridoxal-5-phosphate (PLP), the active form of vitamin B₆.[402] In general, a dose of 50 to 100 mg/kg divided 6 times per day is administered for at least a 3- to 5-day trial. PLP is only available in enteral forms and has side effects similar to pyridoxine.[654] In most of the PLP-responsive cases, PNPO deficiency has been identified as the underlying genetic condition (see earlier), but idiopathic PLP response occurs as well.[402,655,656] Because PLP has the potential to treat ATQ deficiency as well as PNPO deficiency, some centers advocate the use of PLP (30 mg/kg per day divided into three dosages), as the first-line vitamin B₆, while other centers advocate the consecutive use when pyridoxine, given over three consecutive days, has failed to control seizures. Finally, pyridoxine-dependent epilepsy is an organic aciduria caused by a deficiency in the catabolic breakdown of lysine;

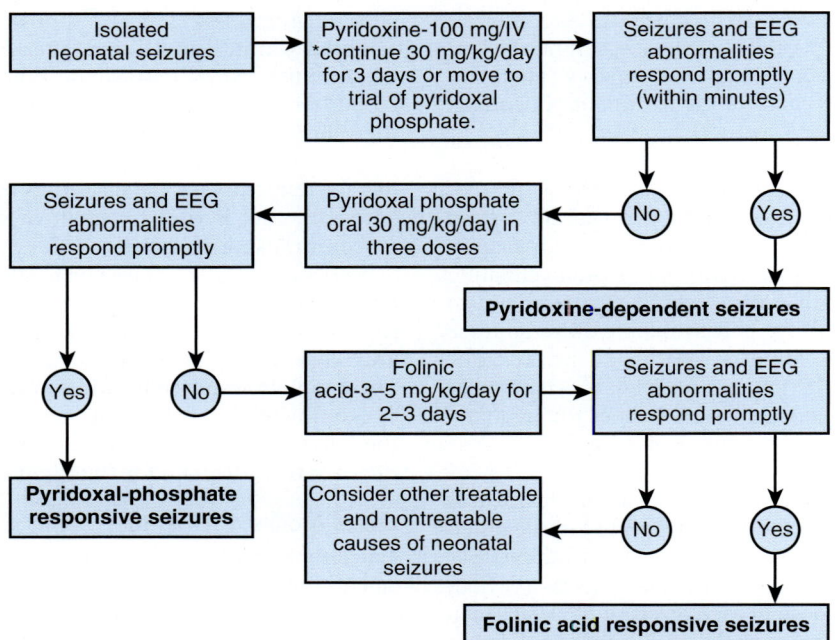

Figure 12.26 Treatment algorithm for neonatal seizures with suspected inborn errors of metabolism. *Some patients may not manifest a clinical or electroencephalographic response to a single intravenous dose of pyridoxine. *EEG,* Electroencephalography; *IV,* intravenous. (From Ficicioglu C, Bearden D. Isolated neonatal seizures: when to suspect inborn errors of metabolism. *Pediatr Neurol.* 2011;45:283–291.)

a lysine-restricted diet may assist in addressing the potential toxicity of accumulating metabolites.

FARS are genetically identical to ATQ deficiency and require specific therapy. FARS were first described in 1995 in patients with intractable seizures and encephalopathy who had two characteristics, but yet unidentified peaks (peak X) in the HPLC chromatogram for CSF monoamine neurotransmitter analysis. Patients showed an improvement of seizures on administration of folinic acid (3 to 5 mg/kg per day). Thus, in refractile epilepsy unresponsive to pyridoxine a trial of *folinic acid (leucovorin)* trial should also be considered, with 3 to 5 mg/kg per day administered for at least 3 to 5 days.

Seizures associated with *biotinidase deficiency* tend to present slightly later, often in the second month of life, and there are often other symptoms, such as an eczematous rash to suggest the diagnosis; in addition, the newborn screen captures at least some of these cases. Because treatment with *biotin 10 mg/day* can lead to favorable neurological outcomes, this disorder should be considered in those newborns with intractable epilepsy of unclear etiology.[657]

The *ketogenic diet* is the optimal treatment for newborns with a *glucose transporter defect* with onset of seizures in the neonatal period (see earlier).

Maintenance Therapy

Typically, maintenance doses are begun 12 hours following administration of the loading dose. These are usually administered in divided doses every 12 hours.

For *phenobarbital,* intravenous, intramuscular, or oral administration is adequate, although the parenteral routes should be used in the seriously ill infant. Drug accumulation results within 5 to 10 days when maintenance doses of *phenobarbital* of 5 mg/kg per day are used (see Fig. 12.26).[582,584] This effect may depress the infant significantly and relates to relatively slow elimination rates in the first 1 to 2 weeks of therapy (Fig. 12.27). These rates are particularly slow in some asphyxiated infants, presumably secondary to hepatic involvement, renal involvement, or both, and lead more readily to drug accumulation than in nonasphyxiated infants.[590,658] However, elimination rates do increase with increasing duration of therapy, and dose requirements may increase.

For *fosphenytoin,* intravenous administration is preferred, although fosphenytoin can be administered intramuscularly. For *phenytoin,* oral administration of phenytoin is less desirable than intravenous, although pharmacokinetic data have modified the prior notion that phenytoin absorption is poor in the newborn.[659-662] Maintenance administration of phenytoin in the newborn is particularly difficult because of its nonlinear kinetics and rapid decrease in elimination rates in the first weeks of life.[659-662] Thus, the apparent half-life of the drug decreases from 57 hours in the first week of life to 20 hours in the fourth week.[659] Careful attention to blood levels is particularly necessary when this drug is used for maintenance.[602]

Two reports suggested that *carbamazepine* may be a useful alternative to phenobarbital or phenytoin in maintenance therapy.[616,652,663] Oral doses of 10 to 15 mg/kg per day were associated with good seizure control.

If medications used to control seizures initially are discontinued quickly (see later discussion) and seizures recur, some clinicians initiate therapy with standard anticonvulsant medications, such as *levetiracetam or oxcarbazepine*, which appear

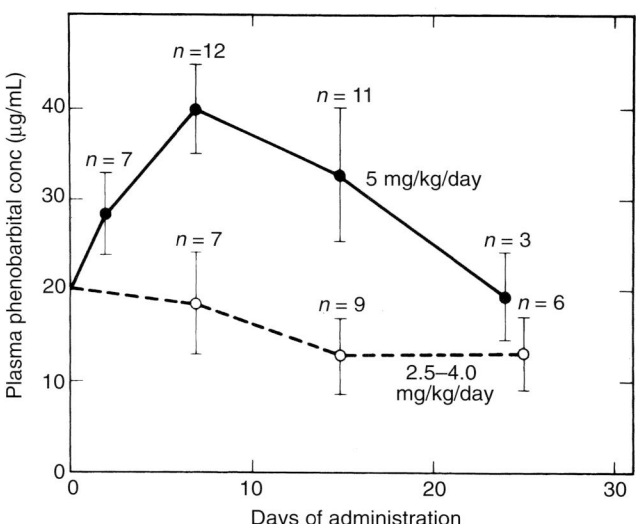

Figure 12.27 Phenobarbital levels achieved on maintenance therapy of 5 mg/kg per day or 2.5 to 4 mg/kg per day as a function of duration of therapy in human newborns. Note the accumulation of drug at the end of the first week of therapy with the higher dose. (From Painter MJ, Pippenger C, MacDonald H, Pitlick W. Phenobarbital and diphenylhydantoin levels in neonates with seizures. *J Pediatr.* 1978;92:315–319.)

to have better tolerability, including less sedation, for long-term use than might occur with re-initiation of phenobarbital. However, more data are needed regarding the role of these newer anticonvulsant medications in young children.

Duration of Therapy

The optimal duration of anticonvulsant therapy for newborns with seizures relates principally to *the likelihood of seizure recurrence if the drugs are discontinued.* What is the risk of subsequent epilepsy in newborns with seizures? The overall incidence of subsequent epilepsy in neonatal seizure survivors has been reported as between approximately 10% and 30%.[a] This range can be refined by considering *three important, readily identified determinants.*[668] The first of these determinants is the neonatal neurological examination. In two studies of asphyxiated infants, the risk of seizure recurrence was approximately 50% when the neurological examination at discharge was abnormal.[191,669] The infants with normal neurological findings did not develop subsequent recurrent seizures. The second determinant is the cause of the neonatal seizures. The risk of subsequent epilepsy after neonatal seizures secondary to perinatal asphyxia is approximately 30% to 50%, and after seizures secondary to cortical dysgenesis, the risk is about 100%. However, simple, late-onset hypocalcemia has essentially no associated risk. Finally, the third determinant is the background EEG pattern (Table 12.32). Of the 54 asphyxiated infants studied by Watanabe and colleagues, none developed subsequent epilepsy when the results of the neonatal interictal EEG tracing were normal or showed only *minimal* or *mild* depression. In contrast, 41% of infants with *marked* depression developed subsequent epilepsy.[191] The value of EEG patterns in determining the risk of subsequent epilepsy has been shown in other studies.[299,667,670]

---

[a]References 29, 31, 191, 239, 286, 299, 302, 304, 548, 561, and 664-667.

TABLE 12.32   Determinants of Duration of Antiseizure Medication

Neonatal neurological examination
Cause of the neonatal seizure
Electroencephalogram

Each of these factors should be assessed carefully to determine the duration of therapy.

Phenobarbital is often maintained for several months because of concern that seizures may recur if the medication is discontinued early.[579] However, there is growing concern about the sedating and potentially neurotoxic effects of anticonvulsant medications, particularly phenobarbital, which have led some clinicians, including ourselves, to attempt discontinuation of anticonvulsant medication as early as possible.[579] *Initial data suggest that early discontinuation of phenobarbital may not impact long-term outcomes.* A study of 146 newborns compared 33 taking phenobarbital and 99 not taking phenobarbital at discharge from the neonatal intensive care unit and found no difference in seizure recurrence or neurological development at 1 to 11 years.[671]

Experimental studies have raised the possibility that phenobarbital may have deleterious long-term effects on the developing brain.[672-678] Initial studies involved rats and cultured cells of neural origin.[679-683] The relation of these data to the human infant is unclear. The time period of the experiments in the rat corresponded to a period in the human from approximately the sixth month of gestation to years postnatally. *Particularly concerning are studies in neonatal rats that showed pronounced apoptotic neurodegeneration within 24 hours after administration of phenobarbital, phenytoin, diazepam, clonazepam, and valproate.*[677,684] *Combinations of drugs produced greater effects.* The doses and blood levels attained were generally comparable to those used in human infants. The neuronal death was associated with reduced expression of neurotrophins and survival-promoting proteins in the brain.

Some human data suggest a possible risk associated with phenobarbital exposure. Studies of children exposed in utero to several antiseizure medications, including phenobarbital and phenytoin have demonstrated an increased risk of cognitive impairments in later childhood.[685-687] A deleterious effect of phenobarbital on cognitive development of infants treated for febrile seizures raised further questions concerning the potential toxicity of phenobarbital.[672,673] However, as just noted, a deleterious effect on neurological development was not noted in infants in whom phenobarbital was discontinued by discharge from the neonatal intensive care unit.[671]

Some of these issues may be slightly less problematic with levetiracetam and topiramate.[644,688] In fact, experimental data suggest that levetiracetam can be antiepileptogenic,[689] and both may be neuroprotective in the setting of hypoxic-ischemic encephalopathy.[690] A study of 280 newborns with comparable seizure etiology and neuroimaging characteristics and which adjusted for the number of electrographic seizures and gestational age found that exposure to increasing doses of phenobarbital and levetiracetam were both associated with worse Bayley Scales of Infant Development scores at 24 months. However, the reductions were more pronounced with phenobarbital. Increased exposure to phenobarbital was associated with worse cognitive and motor scores (8.1- and 9-point decrease per 100 mg/kg; $P = .01$). Increased exposure to levetiracetam also was associated with worse cognitive and motor scores (but to a lesser extent than phenobarbital 2.2- and 2.6-point decrease per 300 mg/kg, $P = .01$). Increasing doses of phenobarbital were also associated with cerebral palsy while levetiracetam was not.[691]

Together, the facts that prolonged exposure to anticonvulsant medications may not provide benefits in long-term neurodevelopment[692-694] or epilepsy and may have associated risks, which suggests that attempts to wean such medications early are appropriate. A review by the World Health Organization recommends the consideration of weaning of anticonvulsant medication after 72 hours of treatment if the neurological examination and/or EEG are normal.[173] The nature of the underlying neuropathology, including the nature and extent of neuroimaging abnormalities, may also assist in determining the risk-benefit of the duration of anticonvulsant therapy, although no formal studies using these guidelines have been undertaken. For those infants who require multiple medications for control, each drug should be weaned individually, with phenobarbital being the last to be discontinued.

KEY REFERENCES

1. Lanska MJ, Lanska DJ, Baumann RJ, et al. A population-based study of neonatal seizures in Fayette County, Kentucky. *Neurology.* 1995;45:724-732.
2. Ronen GM, Penney S, Andrews W. The epidemiology of clinical neonatal seizures in Newfoundland: a population-based study. *J Pediatr.* 1999;134:71-75.
3. Glass HC, Wu YW. Epidemiology of neonatal seizures. *J Pediatr Neurol.* 2009;7:13-17.
7. Moshé SL. Epileptogenesis and the immature brain. *Epilepsia.* 1987;28:S3-S15.
12. Rakhade SN, Jensen FE. Epileptogenesis in the immature brain: emerging mechanisms. *Nat Rev Med.* 2009;5:380-391.
14. Cleary RT, Sun H, Huynh T, et al. Bumetanide enhances phenobarbital efficacy in a rat model of hypoxic neonatal seizures. *PLoS ONE.* 2013;8:e57148.
23. Scher MS, Painter MJ, Bergman I, et al. EEG diagnoses of neonatal seizures: clinical correlations and outcome. *Pediatr Neurol.* 1989;5:17-24.
25. Volpe JJ. Neonatal seizures: current concepts and revised classification. *Pediatrics.* 1989;84:422-428.
28. Painter MJ, Gaus LM. Neonatal seizures: diagnosis and treatment. *J Child Neurol.* 1991;6:101-108.
29. Scher MS, Aso K, Beggarly ME, et al. Electrographic seizures in preterm and full-term neonates: clinical correlates, associated brain lesions, and risk for neurologic sequelae. *Pediatrics.* 1993;91:128-134.
30. Scher MS, Hamid MY, Steppe DA, et al. Ictal and interictal electrographic seizure durations in preterm and term neonates. *Epilepsia.* 1993;34:284-288.
33. Biagioni E, Ferrari F, Boldrini A, et al. Electroclinical correlation in neonatal seizures. *Eur J Paediatr Neurol.* 1998;2:117-125.
34. Nagarajan L, Palumbo L, Ghosh S. Classification of clinical semiology in epileptic seizures in neonates. *Eur J Paediatr Neurol.* 2012;16:118-125.
35. Bye AM, Flanagan D. Spatial and temporal characteristics of neonatal seizures. *Epilepsia.* 1995;36:1009-1016.
36. Clancy RR. The contribution of EEG to the understanding of neonatal seizures. *Epilepsia.* 1996;37:S52-S59.
54. Holmes GL, Ben-Ari Y. The neurobiology and consequences of epilepsy in the developing brain. *Pediatr Res.* 2001;49:320-325.
55. Sanchez RM, Jensen FE. Maturational aspects of epilepsy mechanisms and consequences for the immature brain. *Epilepsia.* 2001;42:577-585.

69. Staley K, Smith R, Schaack J, et al. Alteration of GABAA receptor function following gene transfer of the CLC-2 chloride channel. *Neuron*. 1996;17:543-551.

72. Rivera C, Voipio J, Payne JA, et al. The K⁺/Cl⁻ co-transporter KCC2 renders GABA hyperpolarizing during neuronal maturation. *Nature*. 1999;397:251-255.

76. Fujikawa DG, Vannucci RC, Dwyer BE, et al. Generalized seizures deplete brain energy reserves in normoxemic newborn monkeys. *Brain Res*. 1988;454:51-59.

80. Young RS, Petroff OA, Chen B, et al. Brain energy state and lactate metabolism during status epilepticus in the neonatal dog: in vivo ^{31}P and $_1H$ nuclear magnetic resonance study. *Pediatr Res*. 1991;29:191-195.

83. Wasterlain CG. Recurrent seizures in the developing brain are harmful. *Epilepsia*. 1997;38:728-734.

84. Thoresen M, Hallstrom A, Whitelaw A, et al. Lactate and pyruvate changes in the cerebral gray and white matter during posthypoxic seizures in newborn pigs. *Pediatr Res*. 1998;44:746-754.

88. Young RS, Osbakken MD, Briggs RW, et al. 31P NMR study of cerebral metabolism during prolonged seizures in the neonatal dog. *Ann Neurol*. 1985;18:14-20.

89. Fujikawa DG, Dwyer BE, Wasterlain CG. Preferential blood flow to brainstem during generalized seizures in the newborn marmoset monkey. *Brain Res*. 1986;397:61-72.

97. Cataltepe O, Vannucci RC, Heitjan DF, et al. Effect of status epilepticus on hypoxic-ischemic brain damage in the immature rat. *Pediatr Res*. 1995;38:251-257.

98. Younkin D, Maris JE. The effect of seizures on cerebral metabolites in children. *Pediatr Res*. 1985;19:397.

99. Holmes GL. Effects of seizures on brain development: lessons from the laboratory. *Pediatr Neurol*. 2005;33:1-11.

100. Wirrell EC, Armstrong EA, Osman LD, et al. Prolonged seizures exacerbate perinatal hypoxic-ischemic brain damage. *Pediatr Res*. 2001;50:445-454.

105. Perlman JM, Volpe JJ. Seizures in the preterm infant: effects on cerebral blood flow velocity, intracranial pressure, and arterial blood pressure. *J Pediatr*. 1983;102:288-293.

106. Perlman JM, Herscovitch P, Kreusser KL, et al. Positron emission tomography in the newborn: effect of seizure on regional cerebral blood flow in an asphyxiated infant. *Neurology*. 1985;35:244-247.

109. Borch K, Pryds O, Holm S, et al. Regional cerebral blood flow during seizures in neonates. *J Pediatr*. 1998;132:431-435.

116. Lowenstein DH, Shimosaka S, So YT, et al. The relationship between electrographic seizure activity and neuronal injury. *Epilepsy Res*. 1991;10:49-54.

122. Sankar R, Shin DH, Liu HT, et al. Patterns of status epilepticus-induced neuronal injury during development and long-term consequences. *J Neurosci*. 1998;18:8382-8393.

126. Holmes GL. The long-term effects of seizures on the developing brain: clinical and laboratory issues. *Brain Dev*. 1991;13:393-409.

131. Baram TZ. Long-term neuroplasticity and functional consequences of single versus recurrent early-life seizures. *Ann Neurol*. 2003;54:701-705.

135. Collins RC, Olney JW. Focal cortical seizures cause distant thalamic lesions. *Science*. 1982;218:177-179.

146. Cornejo BJ, Mesches MH, Coultrap S, et al. A single episode of neonatal seizures permanently alters glutamatergic synapses. *Ann Neurol*. 2007;61:411-426.

149. McCabe BK, Silveira DC, Cilio MR, et al. Reduced neurogenesis after neonatal seizures. *J Neurosci*. 2001;21:2094-2103.

154. Rakhade SN, Fitzgerald EF, Klein PM, et al. Glutamate receptor 1 phosphorylation at serine 831 and 845 modulates seizure susceptibility and hippocampal hyperexcitability after early life seizures. *J Neurosci*. 20 12;32:17800-17812.

157. Rakhade SN, Klein PM, Huynh T, et al. Development of later life spontaneous seizures in a rodent model of hypoxia-induced neonatal seizures. *Epilepsia*. 2011;52:753-765.

158. Lippman-Bell JJ, Rakhade SN, Klein PM, et al. AMPA receptor antagonist NBQX attenuates later-life epileptic seizures and autistic-like social deficits following neonatal seizures. *Epilepsia*. 2013;54:1922-1932.

160. de Vries LS, Toet MC. How to assess the aEEG background. *J Pediatr*. 2009;154:625-626.

166. Shah NA, Van Meurs KP, Davis AS. Amplitude-integrated electroencephalography: a survey of practices in the United States. *Am J Perinatol*. 2015;32:755-760.

170. Glass HC, Kan J, Bonifacio SL, et al. Neonatal seizures: treatment practices among term and preterm infants. *Pediatr Neurol*. 2012;46:111-115.

171. Shellhaas RA, Chang T, Tsuchida T, et al. The American Clinical Neurophysiology Society's guideline on continuous electroencephalography monitoring in neonates. *J Clin Neurophysiol*. 2011;28:611-617.

172. Papile LA, Baley JE, Benitz W, et al. Hypothermia and neonatal encephalopathy. *Pediatrics*. 2014;133:1146-1150.

173. World Health Organization. *Guidelines on Neonatal Seizures*. Geneva: World Health Organization; 2011.

177. Tsuchida TN, Wusthoff CJ, Shellhaas RA, et al. American Clinical Neurophysiology Society standardized EEG terminology and categorization for the description of continuous EEG monitoring in neonates: report of the American Clinical Neurophysiology Society Critical Care Monitoring Committee. *J Clin Neurophysiol*. 2013;30:161-173.

179. Abend NS, Wusthoff CJ. Neonatal seizures and status epilepticus. *J Clin Neurophysiol*. 2012;29:441-448.

181. Nagarajan L, Palumbo L, Ghosh S. Brief electroencephalography rhythmic discharges (BERDs) in the neonate with seizures: their significance and prognostic implications. *J Child Neurol*. 2011;26:1529-1533.

185. Malone A, Ryan C, Fitzgerald A, et al. Interobserver agreement in neonatal seizure identification. *Epilepsia*. 2009;50:2097-2101.

186. Murray DM, Boylan GB, Ali I, et al. Defining the gap between electrographic seizure burden, clinical expression and staff recognition of neonatal seizures. *Arch Dis Child Fetal Neonatal Ed*. 2008;93:F187-F191.

188. Mizrahi EM, Kellaway P. Characterization and classification of neonatal seizures. *Neurology*. 1987;37:1837-1844.

189. Mizrahi EM. Neonatal seizures: problems in diagnosis and classification. *Epilepsia*. 1987;28:S46-S55.

213. Weiner SP, Painter MJ, Geva D, et al. Neonatal seizures: electroclinical dissociation. *Pediatr Neurol*. 1991;7:363-368.

214. Ronen GM, Buckley D, Penney S, et al. Long-term prognosis in children with neonatal seizures: a population-based study. *Neurology*. 2007;69:1816-1822.

227. Clancy RR, Legido A, Lewis D. Occult neonatal seizures. *Epilepsia*. 1988;29:256-261.

228. Connell J, Oozeer R, de Vries L, et al. Continuous EEG monitoring of neonatal seizures: diagnostic and prognostic considerations. *Arch Dis Child*. 1989;64:452-458.

229. Scher MS, Alvin J, Gaus L, et al. Uncoupling of EEG-clinical neonatal seizures after antiepileptic drug use. *Pediatr Neurol*. 2003;28:277-280.

230. Shany E, Khvatskin S, Golan A, et al. Amplitude-integrated electroencephalography: a tool for monitoring silent seizures in neonates. *Pediatr Neurol*. 2006;34:194-199.

231. Glass HC, Wusthoff CJ, Shellhaas RA, et al. Risk factors for EEG seizures in neonates treated with hypothermia: a multicenter cohort study. *Neurology*. 2014;82:1239-1244.

232. Shellhaas RA, Soaita AI, Clancy RR. Sensitivity of amplitude-integrated electroencephalography for neonatal seizure detection. *Pediatrics*. 2007;120:770-777.

233. Wusthoff CJ, Dlugos D, Gutierrez-Colina AM, et al. Incidence of electrographic seizures during therapeutic hypothermia for neonatal encephalopathy. *J Child Neurol*. 2011;26:724-728.

235. Wietstock SO, Bonifacio SL, Sullivan JE, et al. Continuous video electroencephalographic (EEG) monitoring for electrographic seizure diagnosis in neonates: a single-center study. *J Child Neurol*. 2016;31:328-332.

236. Nash KB, Bonifacio SL, Glass HC, et al. Video-EEG monitoring in newborns with hypoxic-ischemic encephalopathy treated with hypothermia. *Neurology*. 2011;76:556-562.

238. Clancy RR. Prolonged electroencephalogram monitoring for seizures and their treatment. *Clin Perinatol*. 2006;33:649-665, vi.

239. McBride MC, Laroia N, Guillet R. Electrographic seizures in neonates correlate with poor neurodevelopmental outcome. *Neurology*. 2000;55:506-513.

240. van Rooij LG, de Vries LS, Handryastuti S, et al. Neurodevelopmental outcome in term infants with status epilepticus detected

with amplitude-integrated electroencephalography. *Pediatrics.* 2007;120:e354-e363.

241. Connell J, Oozeer R, de Vries L, et al. Clinical and EEG response to anticonvulsants in neonatal seizures. *Arch Dis Child.* 1989;64:459-464.

286. Tekgul H, Gauvreau K, Soul J, et al. The current etiologic profile and neurodevelopmental outcome of seizures in term newborn infants. *Pediatrics.* 2006;117:1270-1280.

288. Ficicioglu C, Bearden D. Isolated neonatal seizures: when to suspect inborn errors of metabolism. *Pediatr Neurol.* 2011;45:283-291.

289. Pearl PL. New treatment paradigms in neonatal metabolic epilepsies. *J Inherit Metab Dis.* 2009;32:204-213.

290. Pearl PL. Amenable treatable severe pediatric epilepsies. *Semin Pediatr Neurol.* 2016;23:158-166.

293. Glass HC, Shellhaas RA, Wusthoff CJ, et al. Contemporary profile of seizures in neonates: a prospective cohort study. *J Pediatr.* 2016;174:98-103, e1.

302. Bye AME, Cunningham CA, Chee KY, et al. Outcome of neonates with electrographically identified seizures, or at risk of seizures. *Pediatr Neurol.* 1997;16:225-231.

303. Sheth RD. Electroencephalogram confirmatory rate in neonatal seizures. *Pediatr Neurol.* 1999;20:27-30.

305. Garcias Da Silva LF, Nunes ML, Da Costa JC. Risk factors for developing epilepsy after neonatal seizures. *Pediatr Neurol.* 2004;30:271-277.

309. Murray DM, Ryan CA, Boylan GB, et al. Prediction of seizures in asphyxiated neonates: correlation with continuous video-electroencephalographic monitoring. *Pediatrics.* 2006;118:41-46.

310. Glass HC, Nash KB, Bonifacio SL, et al. Seizures and magnetic resonance imaging-detected brain injury in newborns cooled for hypoxic-ischemic encephalopathy. *J Pediatr.* 2011;159:731-735, e731.

311. Wusthoff CJ, Dlugos DJ, Gutierrez-Colina A, et al. Electrographic seizures during therapeutic hypothermia for neonatal hypoxic-ischemic encephalopathy. *J Child Neurol.* 2011;26:724-728.

315. Miller SP, Weiss J, Barnwell A, et al. Seizure-associated brain injury in term newborns with perinatal asphyxia. *Neurology.* 2002;58:542-548.

316. Glass HC, Glidden D, Jeremy RJ, et al. Clinical neonatal seizures are independently associated with outcome in infants at risk for hypoxic-ischemic brain injury. *J Pediatr.* 2009;155:318-323.

322. Wusthoff CJ, Kessler SK, Vossough A, et al. Risk of later seizure after perinatal arterial ischemic stroke: a prospective cohort study. *Pediatrics.* 2011;127:e1550-e1557.

327. Shah DK, Zempel J, Barton T, et al. Electrographic seizures in preterm infants during the first week of life are associated with cerebral injury. *Pediatr Res.* 2010;67:102-106.

396. Gospe SM Jr. Pyridoxine-dependent epilepsy and pyridoxine phosphate oxidase deficiency: unique clinical symptoms and non-specific EEG characteristics. *Dev Med Child Neurol.* 2010;52:602-603.

398. Schmitt B, Baumgartner M, Mills PB, et al. Seizures and paroxysmal events: symptoms pointing to the diagnosis of pyridoxine-dependent epilepsy and pyridoxine phosphate oxidase deficiency. *Dev Med Child Neurol.* 2010;52:e133-e142.

405. Torres OA, Miller VS, Buist NM, et al. Folinic acid-responsive neonatal seizures. *J Child Neurol.* 1999;14:529-532.

413. Gordon N, Newton N. Glucose transporter type 1 (GLUT-2) deficiency. *Brain Dev.* 2003;27:477-480.

414. Leary LD, Wang T, Nordli DR, et al. Seizure characterization and electroencephalographic features in Glut-1 deficiency syndrome. *Epilepsia.* 2003;44:701-707.

415. Wang D, Pascual JM, Yang H, et al. Glut-1 deficiency syndrome: clinical, genetic, and therapeutic aspects. *Ann Neurol.* 2005;57:111-118.

449. Olson HE, Poduri A, Pearl PL. Genetic forms of epilepsies and other paroxysmal disorders. *Semin Neurol.* 2014;34:266-279.

450. Grinton BE, Heron SE, Pelekanos JT, et al. Familial neonatal seizures in 36 families: clinical and genetic features correlate with outcome. *Epilepsia.* 2015;56:1071-1080.

463. Lombroso CT. Early myoclonic encephalopathy, early infantile epileptic encephalopathy, and benign and severe infantile myoclonic epilepsies: a critical review and personal contributions. *J Clin Neurophysiol.* 1990;7:380-408.

464. Ohtahara S, Ohtsuka Y, Yamatogi Y, et al. The early-infantile epileptic encephalopathy with suppression-burst: developmental aspects. *Brain Dev.* 1987;9:371-376.

477. Korff CM, Nordli DR Jr. Epilepsy syndromes in infancy. *Pediatr Neurol.* 2006;34:253-263.

478. Beal JC, Cherian K, Moshe SL. Early-onset epileptic encephalopathies: Ohtahara syndrome and early myoclonic encephalopathy. *Pediatr Neurol.* 2012;47:317-323.

481. Pavone P, Spalice A, Polizzi A, et al. Ohtahara syndrome with emphasis on recent genetic discovery. *Brain Dev.* 2012;34:459-468.

490. Numis AL, Angriman M, Sullivan JE, et al. KCNQ2 encephalopathy: delineation of the electroclinical phenotype and treatment response. *Neurology.* 2014;82:368-370.

491. Miceli F, Soldovieri MV, Ambrosino P, et al. Genotype-phenotype correlations in neonatal epilepsies caused by mutations in the voltage sensor of K(v)7.2 potassium channel subunits. *Proc Natl Acad Sci USA.* 2013;110:4386-4391.

494. Pisano T, Numis AL, Heavin SB, et al. Early and effective treatment of KCNQ2 encephalopathy. *Epilepsia.* 2015;56:685-691.

495. Howell KB, McMahon JM, Carvill GL, et al. SCN2A encephalopathy: a major cause of epilepsy of infancy with migrating focal seizures. *Neurology.* 2015;85:958-966.

498. Coppola G, Plouin P, Chiron C, et al. Migrating partial seizures in infancy: a malignant disorder with developmental arrest. *Epilepsia.* 1995;36:1017-1024.

508. Poduri A, Heinzen EL, Chitsazzadeh V, et al. SLC25A22 is a novel gene for migrating partial seizures in infancy. *Ann Neurol.* 2013;74:873-882.

509. Bearden D, Strong A, Ehnot J, et al. Targeted treatment of migrating partial seizures of infancy with quinidine. *Ann Neurol.* 2014;78:457-561.

511. Shellhaas RA. Continuous long-term electroencephalography: the gold standard for neonatal seizure diagnosis. *Semin Fetal Neonatal Med.* 2015;20:149-153.

512. Lynch NE, Stevenson NJ, Livingstone V, et al. The temporal evolution of electrographic seizure burden in neonatal hypoxic ischemic encephalopathy. *Epilepsia.* 2012;53:549-557.

513. Shah DK, Wusthoff CJ, Clarke P, et al. Electrographic seizures are associated with brain injury in newborns undergoing therapeutic hypothermia. *Arch Dis Child Fetal Neonatal Ed.* 2014;99:F219-F224.

514. Clancy RR, Sharif U, Ichord R, et al. Electrographic neonatal seizures after infant heart surgery. *Epilepsia.* 2005;46:84-90.

515. Naim MY, Gaynor JW, Chen J, et al. Subclinical seizures identified by postoperative electroencephalographic monitoring are common after neonatal cardiac surgery. *J Thorac Cardiovasc Surg.* 2015;150:169-178.

525. Clancy RR, Legido A. The exact ictal and interictal duration of electroencephalographic neonatal seizures. *Epilepsia.* 1987;28:537-541.

526. Shellhaas RA, Clancy RR. Characterization of neonatal seizures by conventional EEG and single-channel EEG. *Clin Neurophysiol.* 2007;118:2156-2161.

528. Rakshasbhuvankar A, Paul S, Nagarajan L, et al. Amplitude-integrated EEG for detection of neonatal seizures: a systematic review. *Seizure.* 2015;33:90-98.

529. Evans E, Koh S, Lerner J, et al. Accuracy of amplitude integrated EEG in a neonatal cohort. *Arch Dis Child Fetal Neonatal Ed.* 2010;95:F169-F173.

533. Wusthoff CJ, Shellhaas RA, Clancy RR. Limitations of single-channel EEG on the forehead for neonatal seizure detection. *J Perinatol.* 2009;29:237-242.

535. van Rooij LG, de Vries LS, van Huffelen AC, et al. Additional value of two-channel amplitude integrated EEG recording in full-term infants with unilateral brain injury. *Arch Dis Child Fetal Neonatal Ed.* 2010;95:F160-F168.

539. van Rooij LG, Toet MC, van Huffelen AC, et al. Effect of treatment of subclinical neonatal seizures detected with aEEG: randomized, controlled trial. *Pediatrics.* 2010;125:e358-e366.

540. Srinivasakumar P, Zempel J, Trivedi S, et al. Treating EEG seizures in hypoxic ischemic encephalopathy: a randomized controlled trial. *Pediatrics.* 2015;136:e1302-e1309.

549. Legido A, Clancy RR, Berman PH. Neurologic outcome after electroencephalographically proven neonatal seizures. *Pediatrics.* 1991;88:583-596.

553. Pisani F, Facini C, Pavlidis E, et al. Epilepsy after neonatal seizures: literature review. *Eur J Paediatr Neurol.* 2015;19:6-14.
560. Boylan GB, Pressier RM, Rennie JM, et al. Outcome of electroclinical, and clinical seizures in the newborn infant. *Dev Med Child Neurol.* 1999;41:819-825.
561. Menache CC, Bourgeois BFD, Volpe JJ. Prognostic value of neonatal discontinuous EEG. *Pediatr Neurol.* 2002;27:93-101.
564. Biagioni E, Bartalena L, Boldrini A, et al. Constantly discontinuous EEG patterns in full-term neonates with hypoxic-ischaemic encephalopathy. *Clin Neurophysiol.* 1999;110:1510-1515.
567. Harris ML, Malloy KM, Lawson SN, et al. Standardized treatment of neonatal status epilepticus improves outcome. *J Child Neurol.* 2016;31:1546-1554.
568. Wietstock SO, Bonifacio SL, McCulloch CE, et al. Neonatal neurocritical care service is associated with decreased administration of seizure medication. *J Child Neurol.* 2015;30:1135-1141.
569. van Rooij LG, van den Broek MP, Rademaker CM, et al. Clinical management of seizures in newborns: diagnosis and treatment. *Paediatr Drugs.* 2013;15:9-18.
574. Painter MJ, Scher MS, Stein AD, et al. Phenobarbital compared with phenytoin for the treatment of neonatal seizures. *N Engl J Med.* 1999;341:485-489.
575. Boylan GB, Rennie JM, Chorley G, et al. Second-line anticonvulsant treatment of neonatal seizures: a video-EEG monitoring study. *Neurology.* 2004;62:486-488.
578. Blume H, Garrison MM, Christakis DA. Neonatal seizures: treatment and treatment variability in 31 United States pediatric hospitals. *J Child Neurol.* 2009;24:148-154.
594. Meyn DF Jr, Ness J, Ambalavanan N, et al. Prophylactic phenobarbital and whole-body cooling for neonatal hypoxic-ischemic encephalopathy. *J Pediatr.* 2010;157:334-336.
595. Sullivan JE, Witte MK, Yamashita TS, et al. Pharmacokinetics of bumetanide in critically ill infants. *Clin Pharmacol Ther.* 1996;60:405-413.
597. Pressler RM, Boylan GB, Marlow N, et al. Bumetanide for the treatment of seizures in newborn babies with hypoxic ischaemic encephalopathy (NEMO): an open-label, dose finding, and feasibility phase 1/2 trial. *Lancet Neurol.* 2015;14:469-477.
610. Prensky AL, Raff MC, Moore MJ, et al. Intravenous diazepam in the treatment of prolonged seizure activity. *N Engl J Med.* 1967;276:779-784.
618. Castro Conde JR, Hernandez Borges AA, Martinez D, et al. Midazolam in neonatal seizures with no response to phenobarbital. *Neurology.* 2005;64:876-879.
620. Hellström-Westas L, Westgren U, Rosén I, et al. Lidocaine for treatment of severe seizures in newborn infants. I. Clinical effects and cerebral electrical activity monitoring. *Acta Paediatr Scand.* 1988;77:79-84.
621. Hellström-Westas L, Svenningsen NW, Westgren U, et al. Lidocaine for treatment of severe seizures in newborn infants. 2. Blood concentrations of lidocaine and metabolites during intravenous infusion. *Acta Paediatr.* 1992;81:35-39.

623. Weeke LC, Toet MC, van Rooij LG, et al. Lidocaine response rate in aEEG-confirmed neonatal seizures: retrospective study of 413 full-term and preterm infants. *Epilepsia.* 2016;57:233-242.
626. Mruk AL, Garlitz KL, Leung NR. Levetiracetam in neonatal seizures: a review. *J Pediatr Pharmacol Ther.* 2015;20:76-89.
632. Abend NS, Gutierrez-Colina AM, Monk HM, et al. Levetiracetam for treatment of neonatal seizures. *J Child Neurol.* 2011;26:465-470.
635. Rakshasbhuvankar A, Rao S, Kohan R, et al. Intravenous levetiracetam for treatment of neonatal seizures. *J Clin Neurosci.* 2013;20:1165-1167.
638. Loiacono G, Masci M, Zaccara G, et al. The treatment of neonatal seizures: focus on Levetiracetam. *J Matern Fetal Neonatal Med.* 2016;29:69-74.
639. Silverstein FS, Ferriero DM. Off-label use of antiepileptic drugs for the treatment of neonatal seizures. *Pediatr Neurol.* 2008;39:77-79.
645. Glass HC, Poulin C, Shevell MI. Topiramate for the treatment of neonatal seizures. *Pediatr Neurol.* 2011;44:439-442.
652. Singh B, Singh P, AlHifzi I, et al. Treatment of neonatal seizures with carbamazepine. *J Child Neurol.* 1996;11:378-382.
653. Cobo NH, Sankar R, Murata KK, et al. The ketogenic diet as broad-spectrum treatment for super-refractory pediatric status epilepticus: challenges in implementation in the pediatric and neonatal intensive care units. *J Child Neurol.* 2015;30:259-266.
654. Pearl PL, Gospe SM. Pyridoxal phosphate dependency, a newly recognized treatable catastrophic epileptic encephalopathy. *J Inherit Metab Dis.* 2007;30:2-4.
655. Wang HS, Kuo MF, Chou ML, et al. Pyridoxal phosphate is better than pyridoxine for controlling idiopathic intractable epilepsy. *Arch Dis Child.* 2005;90:512-515.
667. Toet MC, Groenendaal F, Osredkar D, et al. Postneonatal epilepsy following amplitude-integrated EEG-detected neonatal seizures. *Pediatr Neurol.* 2005;32:241-247.
674. Bromley RL, Leeman BA, Baker GA, et al. Cognitive and neurodevelopmental effects of antiepileptic drugs. *Epilepsy Behav.* 2011;22:9-16.
676. Marsh ED, Brooks-Kayal AR, Porter BE. Seizures and antiepileptic drugs: does exposure alter normal brain development? *Epilepsia.* 2006;47:1999-2010.
684. Bittigau P, Sifringer M, Genz K, et al. Antiepileptic drugs and apoptotic neurodegeneration in the developing brain. *Proc Natl Acad Sci USA.* 2002;99:15089-15094.
691. Maitre NL, Smolinsky C, Slaughter JC, et al. Adverse neurodevelopmental outcomes after exposure to phenobarbital and levetiracetam for the treatment of neonatal seizures. *J Perinatol.* 2013;33:841-846.
694. Maartens IA, Wassenberg T, Buijs J, et al. Neurodevelopmental outcome in full-term newborns with refractory neonatal seizures. *Acta Paediatr.* 2012;101:e173-e178.

Full references for this chapter can be found on www.expertconsult .com.

UNIT IV

HYPOXIC-ISCHEMIC AND RELATED DISORDERS

Pathophysiology: General Principles

Terrie E. Inder ◆ Joseph J. Volpe

Hypoxic-ischemic encephalopathy in the perinatal period is characterized by neuropathological and clinical features that constitute an important portion of neonatal neurology. To understand these features, which are discussed extensively in this unit, it is necessary to be cognizant of the pathophysiological underpinnings, including the physiological and biochemical derangements, that lead to the structural and functional manifestations of this encephalopathy. In this chapter, we first deal with the major modes of cell death in the setting of hypoxic-ischemic injury. We then review the fundamental derangements in cerebral blood flow (CBF) and energy metabolism, on a background of the normal cerebral circulation and biochemistry of the perinatal brain. Much of what we know is based on experimental data, but translational data in humans with neuroimaging supports these concepts (see later). The subsequent effects of these derangements in CBF and energy metabolism, via excitatory, oxidative, and inflammatory pathways, will then be discussed. These insights will form the foundation for reviewing approaches to neuroprotection in the term and premature brain in relation to hypoxic-ischemic injury. The applications of these principles and their related neuropathologies in the setting of the preterm and term infant's brain will be discussed in more detail in the later chapters within this unit.

DEFINITIONS

It seems worthy at the commencement of this chapter and unit to review the key definitions that will be used. *Hypoxemia* refers to deficiency in oxygen within the circulation and at the cellular level. *Ischemia* refers to insufficient perfusion or, more specific to this setting, insufficient CBF. This deficit will usually be associated with concurrent hypoxia at the cellular level. The term *hypoxic-ischemic injury* is often used, due to the intimate nature of these two components in mediating cerebral injury in the newborn infant. Finally, asphyxia refers to an impairment of respiratory gas exchange and therefore a concomitant increased pCO_2 and acidosis combined with hypoxia. *Asphyxia* is usually associated with alterations in CBF, with the increased pCO_2 initially having enhanced CBF via vasodilatory effects. Subsequent impairment of CBF is then usual. Thus central to all mechanisms (hypoxemia, ischemia, and/or asphyxia) is *hypoxia and subsequent substrate deprivation*.

Finally, the terms *neonatal encephalopathy* and *hypoxic-ischemic encephalopathy* should be clarified. *Neonatal encephalopathy* refers to altered behavior in the newborn characteristic of a disturbance in central nervous system functioning. The major etiology of neonatal encephalopathy is hypoxic-ischemic injury, and once identified as the etiology the infant's condition can be more specifically referred to as hypoxic-ischemic encephalopathy, or an encephalopathy resulting from a hypoxic-ischemic insult.[1]

Mode of Cell Death—Necrosis, Apoptosis, and Autophagy

Before defining the underlying *biochemical and physiological principles* that determine cell death in the immature central nervous system, it is important to delineate the *major modes of cell death* and key factors leading to cell death. Two *fundamental modes of cell death* in the nervous system, as in other tissues, are distinguished: *necrosis* and *apoptosis* (Fig. 13.1). It is now clear that hypoxic-ischemic insults may lead to necrosis or apoptosis, or more commonly a continuum, dependent principally on the severity of the insult and the maturational state of the cell. Certain characteristics readily distinguish these two forms of cell death (Table 13.1).[2-14] Thus *necrotic cell death* is characterized by cell swelling, membrane disintegration, cell rupture, release of intracellular contents, and, as a consequence, inflammation and phagocytosis. By contrast, *apoptosis* is characterized by condensation and margination of chromatin, cell shrinkage, relative preservation of cellular membranes, and death without inflammation or alternative.

Apoptotic cell death is difficult to detect in tissue because of the lack of inflammation and the rapid removal of the cell debris. Apoptotic cell death requires activation of specific death genes, adenosine triphosphate (ATP), and new protein synthesis, which result particularly in a series of biochemical changes that include cleavage of DNA at specific sites to result in the characteristic oligonucleosomal fragmentation (see later). Necrotic cell death occurs typically after intense, sometimes relatively brief insults, whereas apoptotic cell death occurs typically after less intense, longer acting insults. Apoptotic cell death appears to be the dominant form of so-called delayed cell death, observable after many hours to several days in various experimental neonatal models and human brain. Important intrinsic properties of the cell itself determine the mode of cell death relating particularly to the developmental stage of the cell. Thus the susceptibility to apoptosis is enhanced in immature versus mature neurons in vitro and in vivo.[7,15-19] Apoptotic cell death was noted to be common in a study of infants who died after intrauterine hypoxic-ischemic insult (see Chapter 18).[12] Moreover, careful studies in the neonatal piglet subjected to hypoxia-ischemia demonstrated in the same paradigm exclusively necrotic cell death in certain neuronal populations,

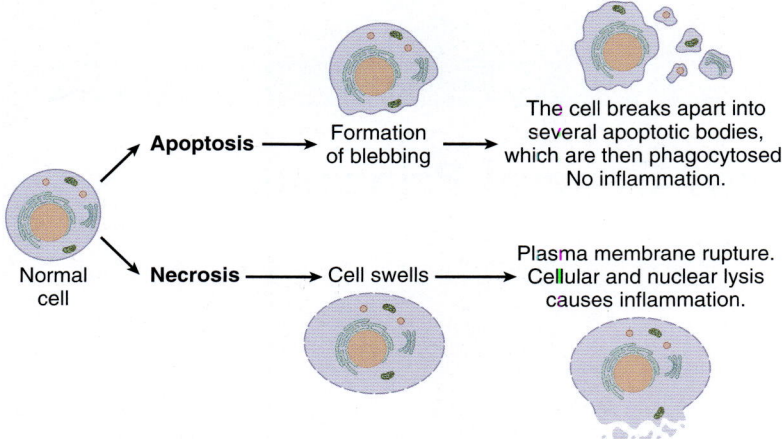

Figure 13.1 Cellular histological images of necrotic and apoptotic cell death.

TABLE 13.1 Necrosis and Apoptosis: Distinguishing Characteristics[a]		
DISTINGUISHING FEATURE	**NECROSIS**	**APOPTOSIS**
Morphology	Cell swelling; dispersed chromatin; membrane fragmentation; inflammatory responses	Cell shrinkage; chromatin condensation; intact membranes; no inflammation
DNA fragmentation	Nonspecific	Specific oligonucleosomal cleavage
Involvement of specific death genes/ enzymes (e.g., Bax, Bid, p53, AIF, PARP, cytochrome c, caspases)	No	Yes
Adenosine triphosphate required	No	Yes
Protein synthesis required	No	Yes
Temporal characteristics	Usually rapid (minutes to hours)	Slow (hours to days)
Insult characteristics	More severe	Less severe

[a]See text for references.

both necrosis and apoptosis in other neuronal populations, but exclusively apoptotic cell death in immature cerebral white matter.[6] Indeed, in many models, electron microscopic study reveals an apoptotic-necrotic continuum in neuronal regions, with clearly apoptotic and necrotic cells present, as well as hybrid cells with "intermediate" characteristics.[20] Often the early cell death appears necrotic and later cell death apoptotic (Fig. 13.2).[21,22]

The *molecular mechanisms involved in apoptosis* associated with *neonatal* hypoxia-ischemia have been clarified considerably, although not completely, in recent years.[14,15,20-29] Although many molecular triggers of apoptosis exist, perhaps most important with hypoxia-ischemia, influx of Ca^{2+} and generation of ROS (see later) are membrane perturbations that involve release of ceramide from sphingomyelin, translocation to the mitochondrion of proapoptotic members of the Bc1-2 family (i.e., Bax, Bid), formation of a mitochondrial permeability pore, release from mitochondrion of cytochrome c and apoptosis-inducing factor, and stimulation of endonucleases by apoptosis-inducing factor and of caspases, especially caspase-3 by cytochrome c. *Both caspase-dependent and caspase-independent mechanisms of apoptotic cell death have been recognized.* Caspases are proteases with cysteine residues in their active sites and catalyze proteolysis at specific aspartate residues—hence the term *caspase.* Caspase-3 is activated within 1 to 3 hours after neonatal

hypoxia-ischemia and is a principal executioner of apoptosis. The substrates attacked by caspases include cytoskeletal and associated proteins, nuclear and DNA-associated proteins, signal transduction proteins, ion channel subunits, and other key molecules. One of the results of the process is DNA cleavage, and poly(ADP ribose) polymerase (PARP), involved in DNA repair, is activated. PARP activation is a prominent feature of the caspase-dependent apoptotic cascade. PARP inactivation occurs by caspase-3–mediated cleavage during the early stages of apoptosis. This inactivation facilitates nuclear disassembly and ensures the completion of the apoptotic process, because PARP activation depletes the cell of ATP, which is essential for apoptosis. The action of apoptosis-inducing factor to cause apoptotic cell death is caspase-*independent* and involves principally translocation to the nucleus and activation of endonucleases. The complex molecular cascades involved in apoptosis occur over many hours and days, thus raising the possibility of interruption of the cascade during a relatively long time window (see later).

More recent attention has been paid to forms of neurodegeneration in the developing brain,[30] which have been termed "pathological apoptosis"[31] and excitotoxic neurodegeneration.[32] Due to the fact that this process rests on a continuum between necrosis and apoptosis, it has also been titled "necroptosis." The important contribution of these

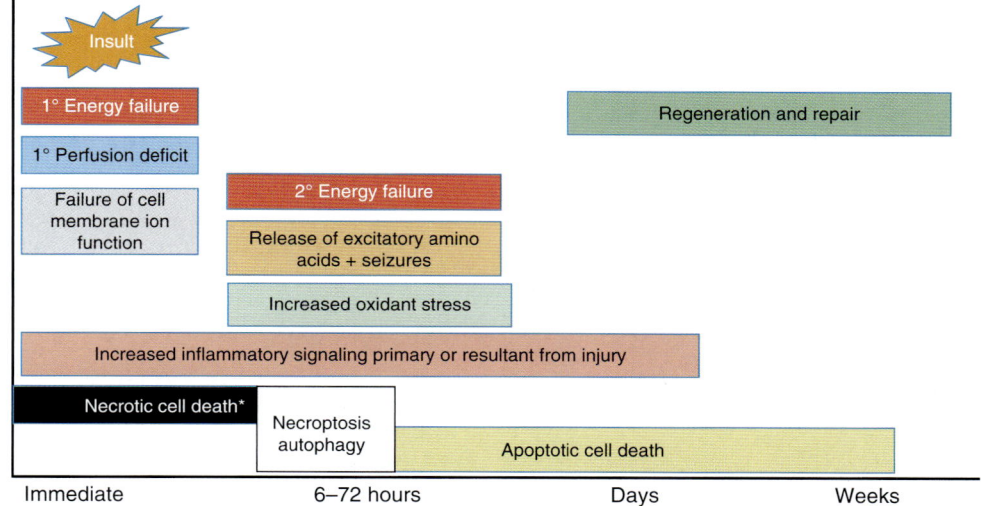

Figure 13.2 The sequence of cellular injury following an acute hypoxic ischemic injury in the immature brain demonstrating the pivotal importance of energy failure with resultant downstream effects.

regulated but morphologically hybrid forms of cell death to hypoxic-ischemic injury in the newborn brain is emerging.[33-35]

These regulated forms of cell death are good examples of molecular switching between apoptotic and necrotic modes of cell death.[36] An additional regulated form of cell death, programmed necrosis, is increasingly recognized as a key form of neurodegeneration and also lies along the apoptosis necrosis continuum.[37] The contribution of these neurodegenerative forms of neuronal cell death in the neonatal brain are still under active investigation.

A final form of cell loss, autophagy, also occurs within the setting of neonatal hypoxic ischemic brain injury.[30,38] Autophagy is an adaptive process through which eukaryotic cells degrade and recycle their own cytoplasm and organelles via lysosomes, in response to unfavorable conditions. Autophagy is considered to be a homeostatic nonlethal stress response protecting the cell from low nutrient supplies.[38] Autophagy is classified as a form of programmed cell death.[39] A histological hallmark of autophagy is the formation of double-membrane autophagosomes derived from the endoplasmic reticulum. These then mature and fuse with lysosomes, followed by degradation or recycling of the autophagosome content.[40] Autophagy is seen in developmental and pathological conditions, and both in vitro and in vivo studies reveal that it has a significant role after neonatal hypoxic-ischemic injury, depending on the severity of the insult, maturation, and cerebral region.[40,41]

Importance of the Reperfusion Period

As discussed in the next section, the cascade of deleterious events that lead to cell death after insults that result in oxygen deprivation and energy failure appears to occur *primarily following the termination of the insult*. Careful studies in animal models and in human patients provide strong support for this notion.[42-51] The phenomena are initiated particularly by energy depletion, accumulation of extracellular excitatory amino acids (particularly glutamate), increase in cytosolic Ca^{2+}, and generation of free radicals. The importance of this "delayed" death of brain in the hours after termination of the insult is related in the largest part to the possibility that intervention during the postinsult

period may be beneficial. Data to support this possibility are now available, with the effectiveness of postnatal neuroprotective approaches, such as therapeutic hypothermia, discussed later.

Initiating Role of Energy Failure

An understanding of the mechanism of cell death in the setting of hypoxic-ischemic injury requires appreciation of the cascade of interrelated cellular events. We will commence with the principal underpinnings of cell death related to energy depletion, which is most commonly the result of *ischemic injury resulting from a failure of adequate CBF*. In earlier years, cell death with oxygen deprivation was explained entirely by reference to the sharply decreased production of high-energy phosphates from anaerobic glycolysis (Figs. 13.3–13.5). The mechanism cited was deficiency of high-energy phosphates that are necessary for synthesis of macromolecules and lipids, and thus maintenance of structural integrity. Several decades of research have made it clear that this explanation is too simple and that cell death does not require energy depletion severe enough to eliminate the synthesis of structural components. However, an initial decrease in high-energy phosphates is capable of *triggering a series of additional mechanisms* that begin with a failure of the ATP-dependent Na^+-K^+ pump. If the insult is very severe, the acute result is Na^+ influx, followed by chloride (Cl^-) and water influx, cell swelling, cell lysis, and thus *early cell death by necrosis* (Fig. 13.6; see also Fig. 13.1).

In the more typical, less severe insult, membrane depolarization occurs and is followed by extracellular accumulation of glutamate, increased cytosolic Ca^{2+}, and a cascade of events leading to a *more delayed cell death*, *principally apoptotic*, although necrosis may also occur by this mechanism. The details are discussed in the ensuing sections. Suffice it to say here that the increased extracellular glutamate results from (1) excessive presynaptic glutamate release (because of membrane depolarization and later increased cytosolic Ca^{2+}) and (2) failure of glutamate uptake mechanisms in presynaptic nerve endings and astrocytes (because of membrane depolarization and failure of high-affinity, Na^+-dependent glutamate transporters). The increase in cytosolic Ca^{2+} is a consequence of (1) *failure of*

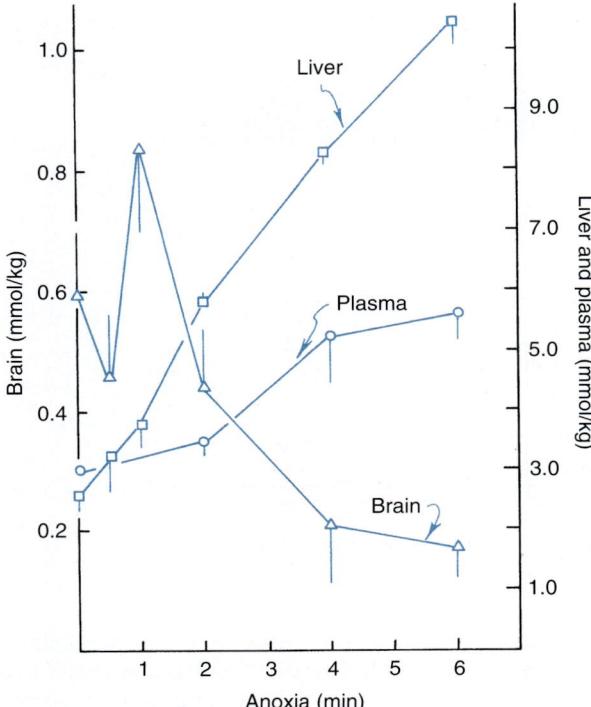

Figure 13.3 **Biochemical effects of hypoxemia.** Concentrations of glucose in brain, liver, and plasma of newborn mice as a function of duration of anoxia (nitrogen breathing). (From Holowach-Thurston J, Hauhart RE, Jones EM. Decrease in brain glucose in anoxia in spite of elevated plasma glucose levels. *Pediatr Res.* 1973;7:691–695.)

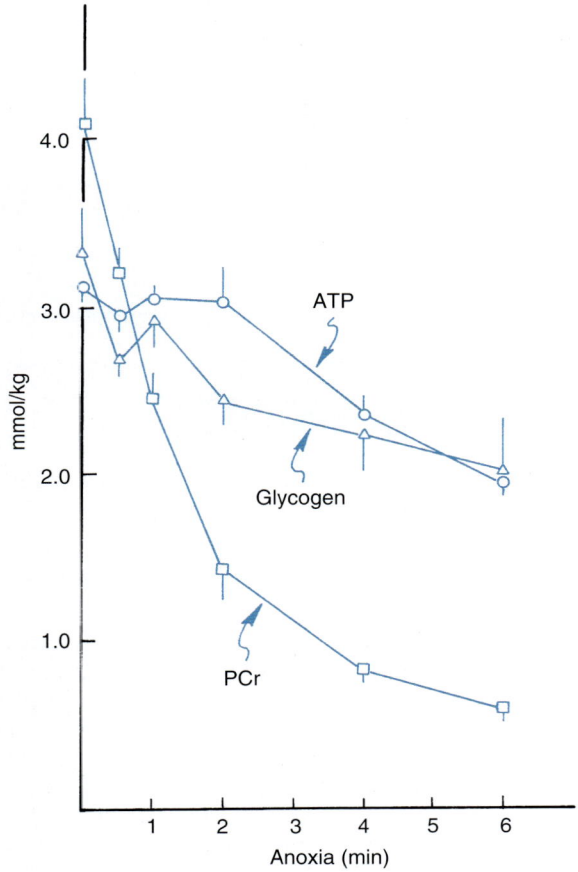

Figure 13.4 **Biochemical effects of hypoxemia.** Concentrations of adenosine triphosphate (ATP), phosphocreatine (PCr), and glycogen in brain of newborn mice as a function of duration of anoxia (nitrogen breathing). (From Holowach-Thurston J, Hauhart RE, Jones EM. Decrease in brain glucose in anoxia in spite of elevated plasma glucose levels. *Pediatr Res.* 1973;7:691–695.)

energy-dependent Ca^{2+}-pumping mechanisms, (2) opening of voltage-dependent Ca^{2+} channels (secondary to membrane depolarization), and probably most important, (3) activation of specific glutamate receptors (see later discussion). The subsequent deleterious events provoked by Ca^{2+} and leading to cell death after these initial events are described later. The pathway to cell death with hypoxic-ischemic insults begins with derangements in CBF, and thus in the following we first discuss CBF and its regulation, and then the biochemical effects of disturbed CBF.

PRIMARY MEDIATORS OF HYPOXIC-ISCHEMIC INJURY IN THE NEWBORN BRAIN—PHYSIOLOGICAL AND BIOCHEMICAL

Major Pathogenetic Themes

The traditional unifying disturbance to neural tissue in hypoxic-ischemic encephalopathy is a deficit in oxygen supply resulting in energy deficit. The perinatal brain can be deprived of oxygen by two major pathogenetic mechanisms: *hypoxemia*, which is a diminished amount of oxygen in the blood supply, and *ischemia*, which is a diminished amount of blood perfusing the brain. The balance of experimental and clinical data leads to the conclusion that *ischemia is the more important of these two forms of oxygen deprivation*. Thus the initial focus of this chapter will be CBF and its perturbation. The conclusion that ischemia is of pivotal importance suggests that

more than deprivation of oxygen is required, supporting that deprivation of *glucose as well as oxygen* is crucial in the genesis of injury. Moreover, the period of *reperfusion* now has been shown clearly to be the time of occurrence of many, if not most, of the deleterious consequences of ischemia on brain metabolism and, ultimately, structure (see later discussion). In most instances, during the perinatal period, hypoxemia or ischemia or both occur as a result of *asphyxia*, which refers to impairment in the exchange of respiratory gases, oxygen, and carbon dioxide. Thus, in asphyxia, the major additional feature is hypercapnia, which results in other metabolic (e.g., additional acidosis) and physiological (e.g., initial increase in CBF) effects. In the following sections, we first discuss CBF in the immature brain and its patterns of perturbation in the preterm and term-born brain. In the next major section, we then discuss the biochemical changes in the brain associated with hypoxemia, ischemia, and asphyxia, initially with an emphasis on carbohydrate and energy metabolism. The manner in which these biochemical changes are affected by other perinatal factors (e.g., the status of carbohydrate metabolism at the time of the insult, the state of brain maturation, and the process of birth) is also described. Subsequent sections synthesize the burgeoning literature on the mechanisms of cell death with oxygen deprivation and focus on the critical importance of

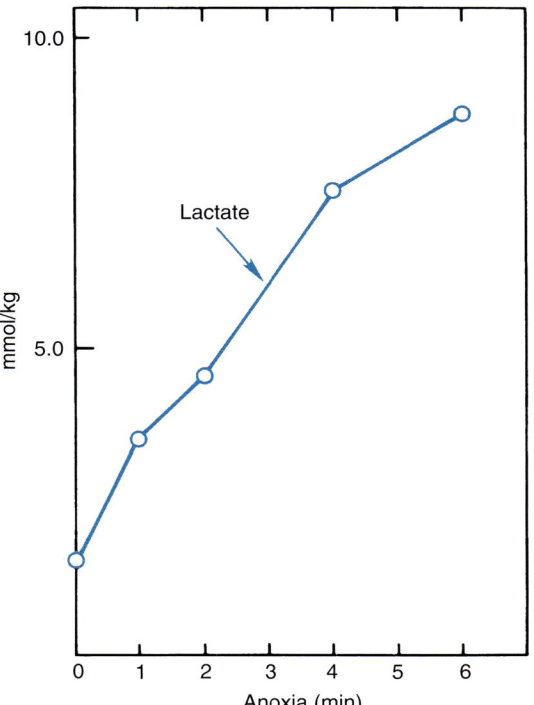

Figure 13.5 Biochemical effects of hypoxemia. Concentrations of lactate in brain of newborn mice as a function of duration of anoxia (nitrogen breathing). (Redrawn from Holowach-Thurston J, Hauhart RE, Jones EM. Decrease in brain glucose in anoxia in spite of elevated plasma glucose levels. *Pediatr Res.* 1973;7:691–695.)

biochemical events beyond glucose and energy metabolism. Particular roles for increase in extracellular glutamate, excessive activation of glutamate receptors (excitotoxicity), increase in cytosolic calcium (Ca^{2+}), and generation of free radicals are emphasized.

PHYSIOLOGICAL MEDIATORS: CEREBRAL BLOOD FLOW

Importance of Cerebral Blood Flow and Regulation

Extensive clinical and neuropathological data emphasize the major role of ischemia in the genesis of brain injury associated with adverse perinatal events. Thus alterations in CBF are of prime importance for understanding the neuropathological and neurological consequences of all varieties of perinatal asphyxial and hypoxic-ischemic insults, as well as the pathogenesis, prevention, and treatment of these consequences. In the following discussion, we review CBF, its regulation, and the changes associated with asphyxia and related hypoxic-ischemic insults. By necessity, the discussion involves studies with experimental animals. However, growing experience with the human newborn, described in the final sections, indicates that the lessons learned from animal research are largely relevant to the perinatal human.

Cerebral Blood Flow: Knowledge From Experimental Studies in Animal Models
Fetal Circulation

The essential features of the fetal circulation, based principally on work with large animals (e.g., sheep, goats, and nonhuman primates), begin with events at the placenta.[52-77] Gas exchange occurs efficiently at the placenta, although oxygen diffusion is somewhat restricted, and fetal arterial oxygen tension values

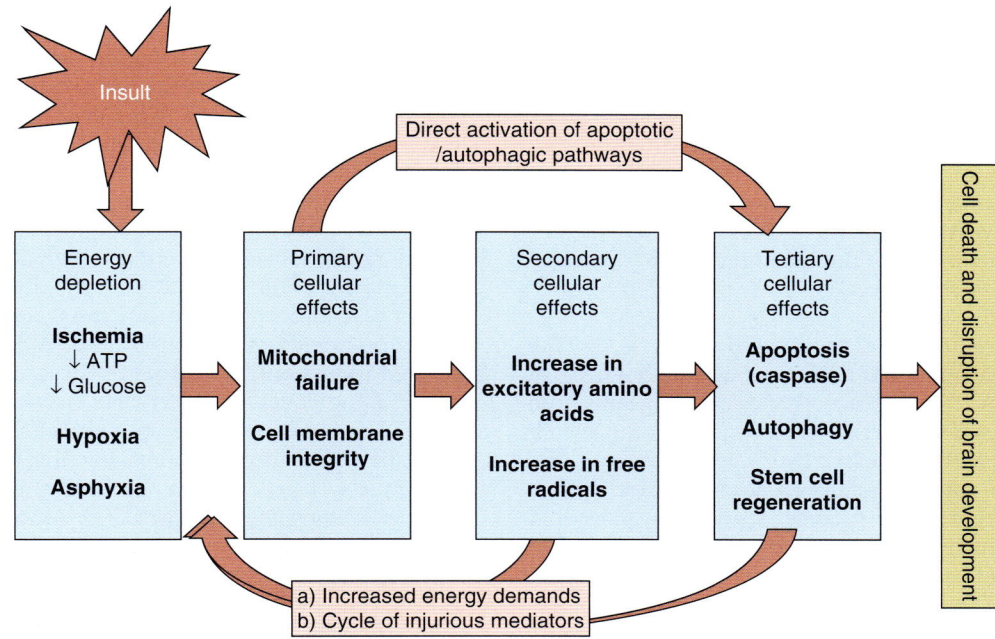

Figure 13.6 Schema of the mechanisms and neuropathologies associated with hypoxic-ischemic brain injury in the newborn infant. *ATP,* Adenosine triphosphate.

TABLE 13.2 Substrate Concentrations in Brain of Hypoxic Puppies (mmol/kg)

TISSUE	PHOSPHOCREATINE	ADENOSINE TRIPHOSPHATE	GLUCOSE	LACTATE
Control				
Parietal cortex	2.74 ± 0.08	2.30 ± 0.08	2.38 ± 0.25	1.08 ± 0.09
Subcortical white matter	1.85 ± 0.22	1.64 ± 0.06	2.14 ± 0.13	1.34 ± 0.07
Hypoxia				
Parietal cortex	2.56 ± 0.06	2.26 ± 0.02	1.64 ± 0.28	12.0 ± 1.4
Subcortical white matter	1.09 ± 0.19	1.40 ± 0.09	0.28 ± 0.04	13.4 ± 1.8

Data from Duffy TE, Cavazzuti M, Cruz NF, Sokoloff L. Local cerebral glucose metabolism in newborn dogs: effects of hypoxia and halothane anesthesia. *Ann Neurol.* 1982;11:233–246.

are considerably lower than maternal values. Compensatory responses to this lower oxygen tension in the fetus include hemoglobin F, with its favorable oxygen affinity curve, polycythemia, and a relatively high cardiac output. Oxygenated blood from the placenta is carried through the umbilical vein, which empties into the inferior vena cava. This well-oxygenated blood enters the right atrium and is preferentially shunted through the patent foramen ovale, ultimately to the aortic arch and then to the coronary and cerebral circulations.[58] Poorly oxygenated blood from the superior vena cava is preferentially shunted into the right ventricle and the pulmonary artery. Because of the high pulmonary vascular resistance, this blood primarily enters the ductus arteriosus and the descending aorta and returns to the placenta through the umbilical arteries.

Regulation of Cerebral Blood Flow: General Principles

CBF in experimental animals has been measured principally by techniques based on the clearance of an inert gas (e.g., xenon and nitrous oxide), carotid artery flow determinations, [^{14}C]antipyrine infusion with autoradiography, and infusion of radioactive microspheres with subsequent tissue sampling. In recent years, near-infrared spectroscopy, sometimes combined with infusion of indocyanine green, and magnetic resonance imaging techniques have been used. Because considerable variability in absolute values of CBF is observed with different techniques, species, modes of anesthesia, preparation of animals, and so forth, we have placed most emphasis in this discussion on the major conclusions of the many studies rather than on the absolute values of CBF recorded. The focus of this section is on the general principles of cerebral hemodynamics, primarily in mature animals; immature animals are discussed subsequently in a separate section.

Autoregulation. *Autoregulation* of CBF refers to the maintenance of a constant CBF over a broad range of perfusion pressures.[59,60,78,79] This constancy of CBF results from arteriolar vasoconstriction with increased perfusion pressure and vasodilation with decreased perfusion pressure.[61,62,78] The mechanisms underlying autoregulation are not entirely understood. Currently the balance of data suggests that autoregulation is mediated primarily by an interplay between endothelial-derived constricting and relaxing factors (see the later discussion of perinatal CBF).[80-82] Autoregulation in the adult human is operative over a range of mean blood pressure between approximately 60 and 150 mm Hg,[78] and the response time is approximately 3 to 15 seconds.[79,83]

Coupling of Cerebral Function, Metabolism, and Blood Flow. Tight coupling of cerebral function, metabolism, and blood flow is well established and can be demonstrated by a variety of correlative physiological, biochemical, and even clinical studies.[59,71,78,84,85] This coupling appears to be mediated by regulation of CBF by one or more local chemical factors that are vasoactive. Vasoactive factors of importance in the brain include H^+, K^+, adenosine, prostaglandins, osmolarity, and Ca^{2+} (Table 13.2). Increase in the perivascular H^+ concentration (i.e., decrease in local pH) is associated with arteriolar vasodilation. Greater neuronal metabolic activity can decrease local pH and therefore increase substrate supply. The effect of perivascular H^+ concentration mediates the vasodilating action of arteriolar carbon dioxide[72-74,78,86] and is important under a variety of other physiological and pathological conditions (see later discussion). This vascular response is well established in the perinatal brain (see later section). K^+ has a vasoactive effect.[75,76,78,87-89] Vasodilation increases linearly with extracellular K^+ levels to 10 mmol/kg (levels >20 mmol/kg induce vasoconstriction). The vasodilation is mediated by a Ca^{2+}-activated K^+ channel on vascular smooth muscle. Because K^+ is released from nerve cells with electrical activity or a variety of insults, including oxygen deprivation (see earlier discussion), this ion may play a role in the regulation of CBF under certain pathological conditions.

Adenosine, administered on the perivascular side of pial arteries, results in a concentration-dependent vasodilation.[78,85,89-91] Changes in adenosine also accompany certain pathological states with changes in CBF, including oxygen deprivation. *Prostaglandins,* particularly prostaglandins E and F$_2$, lead to cerebral vasodilation. The concentrations of these compounds increase in response to cerebral ischemia, and agents that inhibit prostaglandin biosynthesis (e.g., indomethacin) have cerebral vasoconstrictive effects. Prostaglandins appear to be of cerebral hemodynamic importance in immature animals (see later discussion). Increases in perivascular *osmolarity* have a vasodilating effect, and decreases have a vasoconstricting effect.[92] These data may bear on such effects on CBF as the vasodilation associated with infusion of hypertonic solutions.[93] *Ca^{2+}* may also play a role in the control of CBF (e.g., high perivascular concentrations of Ca^{2+} lead to vasoconstriction, and low concentrations lead to dilation of cerebral vessels).[78,94] The ability of Ca^{2+} channel blockers to lead to increases in CBF relates to the prevention of the vasoconstricting effects of Ca^{2+}.[95] Extracellular Ca^{2+} concentrations decline with hypoxia (see earlier discussion) and status epilepticus.[84,96] Other chemical factors (e.g., renin-angiotensin, vasopressin, endogenous opioids,

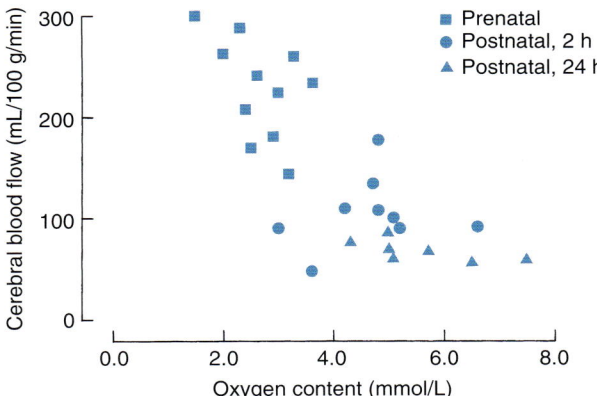

Figure 13.7 Correlation of the perinatal decrease in cerebral blood flow with the increase in arterial oxygen content in the lamb. (From Richardson BS, Carmichael L, Homan J, Tanswell K, Webster AC. Regional blood flow change in the lamb during the perinatal period. *Am J Obstet Gynecol.* 1989;160:919–925.)

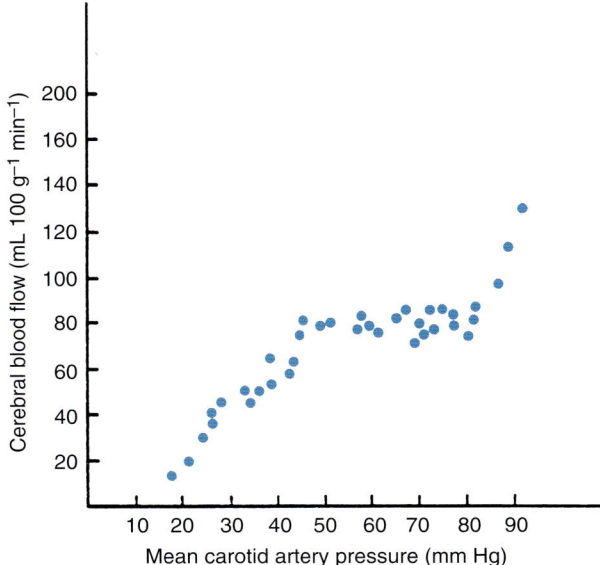

Figure 13.8 Autoregulation of cerebral blood flow in the preterm lamb. See text for details. (From Papile LA, Rudolph AM, Heymann MA. Autoregulation of cerebral blood flow in the preterm fetal lamb. *Pediatr Res.* 1985;19:159–161.)

other neuropeptides, adrenergic compounds, acetylcholine, and endothelium-derived relaxing and constricting factors) may play important roles in the regulation of CBF, but more data are needed on these issues.[80-82,85,97,98] Limited data are available on these agents in immature animals. One report shows that morphine infusions in neonatal piglets result in an upregulation of the vasoconstrictor, endothelin-1, and its receptors.[99]

Cerebral Blood Flow in the Perinatal Period

Ontogenetic Effects. Total and regional CBF changes significantly with maturation. In general, CBF overall increases with postnatal age,[55,100-104] and this increase correlates well with similar increases in cerebral metabolic rates and energy demands, and with neuroanatomical development. Changes in regional CBF with maturation also reflect *coupling with metabolic and anatomical development.* The most dramatic short-term ontogenetic change in CBF occurs around the time of birth. In the lamb, CBF decreases by approximately threefold in the first 24 hours after birth.[105] This decrease correlates well with the postnatal increase in oxygen content (Fig. 13.7), consistent with the importance of oxygen delivery in the regulation of CBF.[104,106]

Regional Effects. Impressive regional differences in CBF are apparent in the perinatal animal, and these differences relate in considerable part to regional differences in metabolic activity. Using the microsphere technique to study regional CBF in term fetal sheep, Ashwal et al.[107] initially noted (1) higher flows in brain stem than in cerebrum and (2) higher values in cortical gray matter than in subcortical white matter.[107] Cavazutti and Duffy[108] amplified these findings in a study of blood flow to 32 brain regions in the newborn dog, confirming the highest CBF in cerebral gray matter, nuclear structures of the brain stem, and diencephalon and lowest in cerebral white matter. Blood flows to the cerebral cortex were approximately 5- to 10-fold of those to subcortical white matter. These regional differences have been confirmed in studies of the perinatal rabbit, lamb, piglet, and puppy.[103,104,109-115] Parallel studies of regional CBF and cerebral glucose metabolism ([2-^{14}C]deoxyglucose method) demonstrated a close correlation with CBF, thus indicating that the *coupling of blood flow and metabolism* is present in the neonatal and adult animal.[116] Finally, studies of blood flow to various

regions of primate cerebrum indicate that the *parasagittal regions,* especially in the posterior aspects of the cerebral hemispheres, have significantly lower flow than other cerebral regions.[117] This finding may have major implications for the distribution of brain injury with perinatal ischemic insults (see the section on parasagittal cerebral injury in Chapter 20).

Cerebral Autoregulation. Cerebral autoregulation appears to be operative over a broad range of arterial blood pressure in the preterm and term fetal lamb, the neonatal lamb, and the neonatal dog.[63-68,85,110,112,118-130] The principal stimulus for the autoregulatory change in vascular diameter appears to be induced largely by the deformation of endothelial cells and generation of endothelial-derived signals that act on the vascular smooth muscle.[124,126,127,131-133] With a decrease in transmural pressure, NO- and Ca^{2+}-activated K^+ channels are important in the vasodilation response, and with an increase in transmural pressure, endothelin-1 is critical in mediation of the vasoconstriction response. The autoregulatory range of blood pressures varies slightly among species and experimental conditions. The curve for the preterm lamb at approximately 80% gestation is shown in Fig. 13.8. The curve for the preterm lamb differs from that for the term or neonatal lamb in two respects.[67] First, the *autoregulatory range in the preterm lamb is narrower,* especially at the upper limit of the curve. Second, and perhaps more strikingly, the *normal arterial blood pressure in the preterm lamb is very near or at the lower autoregulatory limit.* Indeed, in the preterm lamb at 80% of gestation, normal arterial blood pressure is only 5 to 10 mm Hg above the lower limit of the curve, in contrast to the situation in older animals. In a subsequent study that included preterm fetal lambs at approximately 65% gestation (i.e., the onset of the third trimester), the lower autoregulatory limit was *essentially identical* to the normal resting arterial blood pressure.[112] More recent data indicate that the range of blood pressure over which autoregulation is operative decreases with lower gestational age.[129,130] *These data indicate that with decreasing gestational age, resting mean arterial blood pressure (MABP) values approach the lower limit of the autoregulatory plateau, and the range of blood pressure over which CBF remains constant narrows.* Stated in another way, the observations suggest that the margin of safety, at least in the preterm fetus, and to a lesser extent in the term fetus, is small at the lower end of the autoregulatory curve and points to *vulnerability to ischemic brain injury with modest hypotension,* particularly in the preterm animal. *Vulnerability to hypertension* also may result because little change occurs in the upper limit of the autoregulatory range during a brief developmental period (third trimester in the lamb and the human) when normal arterial blood pressure increases markedly.[120] Thus normal arterial blood pressure shifts precariously close to the upper autoregulatory limit and renders capillary beds (e.g., germinal matrix) vulnerable to hemorrhage with modest hypertension.

Autoregulation in the term fetal lamb and in the newborn lamb has been shown to be *sensitive to hypoxia.*[66,68,125,128] Changes in PaO_2 from 20 to 16 mm Hg in the fetal animal and from approximately 70 to 30 mm Hg in the newborn animal abolished autoregulation.[66,68] These decreases in PaO_2 resulted in decreases in arterial oxygen saturation of less than 50%, which can be considered a hypoxic threshold for impairment of cerebrovascular autoregulation. The impairment of autoregulation required only a 20-minute exposure to hypoxia, and autoregulation *did not recover until 7 hours after restoration of normoxia.*[68] Studies in adult animals showed that autoregulation is *abolished in the presence of hypercarbia,*[78,134] and a similar phenomenon was observed in the perinatal animal[135] and in the human preterm newborn.[136] In a single study of the newborn lamb, *systemic acidosis* also was shown to cause a *loss in cerebrovascular autoregulation.*[137]

Regional variation in the decrease in CBF provoked by hypotension to blood pressure values below the lower limit of the autoregulatory plateau has been described in the neonatal piglet, puppy, and lamb.[112,119,120,138-140] In the neonatal piglet, the percentage of reduction in blood flow was least to the brain stem and greatest to the cerebrum.[138,139] In a more detailed regional study in the newborn puppy, the *flow to cerebral white matter was most vulnerable to hypotension.*[119] Similarly, in the preterm lamb, the lower autoregulatory limit with hypotension was lower in the brain stem than in the cerebrum.[112,120] Perhaps even more important, in the preterm lamb at the start of the third trimester, blood flow to cerebral white matter not only was particularly vulnerable to hypotension but also did not recover under conditions of reperfusion that restored blood flow to all other brain regions (Figs. 13.9 and 13.10).[112] The latter observations may have implications for the topography of the injury in the immature human brain with hypoxic-ischemic insults (see the following discussion and Chapters 14 to 16).

Changes in *arterial* PCO_2 (i.e., $PaCO_2$) have marked effects on CBF in perinatal as in adult animals.[108,109,135,141-160] In a study of blood flow to 32 brain regions of the newborn dog, a positive linear correlation was obtained in each structure examined.[108] However, the response to carbon dioxide varied widely among brain regions, ranging from an increase of only 0.15 mL/100 g per minute per mm Hg in PCO_2 in subcortical white matter to an increase of 4.8 in the vestibular and superior olivary nuclei. The *limited vasodilatory response in cerebral white matter* may have implications for the vulnerability of this region to hypoxic-ischemic injury. In general, the higher the blood flow

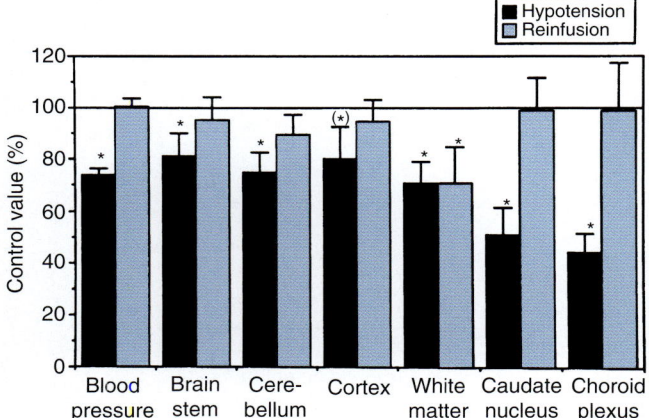

Figure 13.9 **Mean arterial blood pressure and regional cerebral blood flow (CBF; percentage of control values, mean ± SE) after hemorrhagic hypotension and reinfusion in the preterm lamb.** The approximately 25% reduction in blood pressure resulted in significant lowering of CBF in all regions. However, only in cerebral white matter CBF failed to return to baseline levels on reinfusion. (From Szymonowicz W, Walker AM, Yu VY, Stewart ML, Cannata J, Cussen L. Regional cerebral blood flow after hemorrhagic hypotension in the preterm, near-term, and newborn lamb. *Pediatr Res.* 1990;28:361–366.)

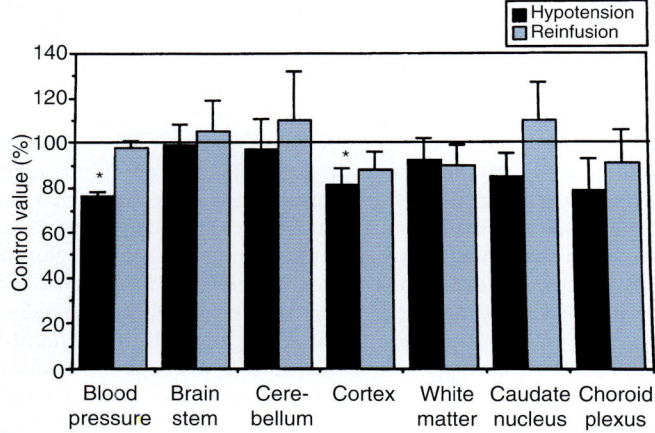

Figure 13.10 **Mean arterial blood pressure and regional cerebral blood flow (CBF; percentage of control values, mean ± SE) after hemorrhagic hypotension and reinfusion in the near-term lamb.** In contrast to the effect on CBF of a similar decrease in blood pressure in the preterm lamb (see Fig. 13.9), during hypotension a significant decline occurred only in cerebral cortex, and on reinfusion all values returned to baseline levels. (From Szymonowicz W, Walker AM, Yu VY, Stewart ML, Cannata J, Cussen L. Regional cerebral blood flow after hemorrhagic hypotension in the preterm, near-term, and newborn lamb. *Pediatr Res.* 1990;28:361–366.)

to a particular structure, the greater the vasodilatory response to increasing PCO_2 (Fig. 13.11).

The effects of profound hypocarbia on CBF are also of importance, as it occurs frequently in sick infants requiring substantial respiratory support. Studies in neonatal lambs indicated an abrupt decrease in CBF with hypocarbia induced by hyperventilation.[109,156,161] The decrease was nonlinear, such that the vasoconstricting effect of hypocarbia declined at lower $PaCO_2$ tensions. Moreover, the decline in CBF became less prominent with time, such that CBF was no longer statistically different in severely hypocarbic animals ($PaCO_2 = 15$ mm Hg)

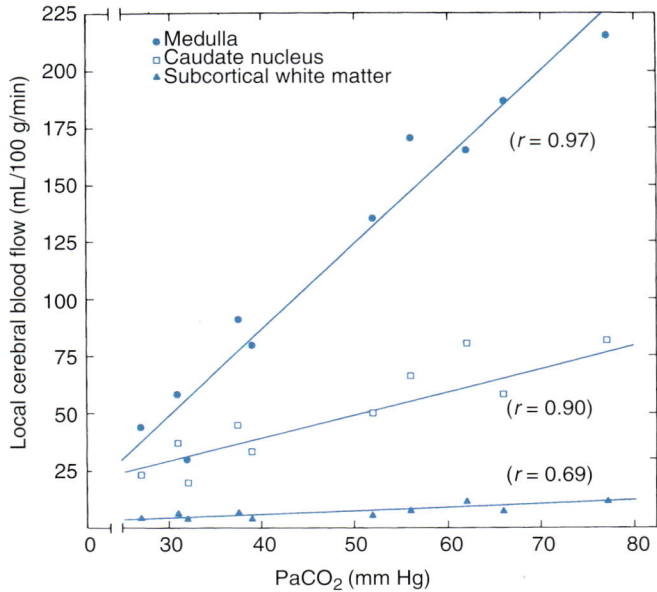

Figure 13.11 Sensitivity of local cerebral blood flow to arterial partial pressure of carbon dioxide (PaCO₂). Note that regions with the higher normocapnic blood flow exhibit the highest sensitivities to PaCO₂. (From Cavazutti M, Duffy TE. Regulation of local cerebral blood flow in normal and hypoxic newborn dogs. *Ann Neurol.* 1982;11:247–257.)

TABLE 13.3 Major Mechanisms for Biochemical Effects of Hypoxemia on Carbohydrate and Energy Metabolism

↑ **Glucose influx to brain**
Link to accelerated glucose utilization
↑ **Glycogenolysis**
Phosphorylase activation (↑ cAMP)
↑ **Glycolysis**
Phosphofructokinase activation (↑ cAMP, ↑ ADP, ↑ P_i, ↓ ATP, ↓ phosphocreatine)
Hexokinase activation (↑ cAMP)
↓ **Brain glucose**
Glucose utilization > glucose influx
↑ **Lactate (and hydrogen ion)**
Anaerobic glycolysis
Impaired utilization of pyruvate (through mitochondrial citric acid cycle–electron transport system)
↓ **Phosphocreatine**
↑ Hydrogen ion production through anaerobic glycolysis
↓ ATP, ↑ ADP
↓ **ATP**
↓ Oxidative phosphorylation

ADP, Adenosine diphosphate; *ATP,* adenosine triphosphate; *cAMP,* cyclic adenosine monophosphate; *P_i,* inorganic phosphate.

---

compared with control animals (PaCO₂ = 36 mm Hg) after 6 hours (Table 13.3). Perhaps most important, the declines in CBF did *not* cause any change in cerebral metabolic rate for oxygen because cerebral oxygen extraction fraction increased. The attenuation of the decline in CBF with increasing duration of hypocarbia probably relates to an increase in perivascular

H⁺ concentration, primarily secondary to an increase in lactate levels. This formulation is supported by *the marked increase in CBF above baseline levels* on restoration of normocarbia.[109]

The effects of *modest hypocarbia* (e.g., PaCO₂ = 26 mm Hg) interact adversely with hypoxic-ischemic insults in the 7-day-old animal.[135,158,160,162] Thus animals exposed to hypoxia-ischemia sustained a greater decline in CBF and a greater degree of brain injury when they were simultaneously rendered modestly hypocarbic, compared with animals who were normocarbic (PaCO₂ = 39 mm Hg) or rendered mildly hypercarbic (PaCO₂ = 54 mm Hg). The latter two groups had better preserved CBF, less severe cerebral metabolic deficits, and less severe brain injury. The modestly hypercarbic animals had the most favorable hemodynamic, biochemical, and neuropathological outcomes. However, more marked hypercarbia accentuated brain injury, because of marked decrease in CBF.[135] The latter effect is presumably related to impaired autoregulation and cardiovascular depression.

Alterations in *arterial* PO₂ (PaO₂) also cause distinct changes in CBF.[a] Decreases in oxygen tension result in increases in blood flow and vice versa. Jones and coworkers[106,164,165] demonstrated that cerebral oxygen delivery is maintained by this increase in CBF over a wide range of arterial oxygen content. In a study of 32 brain regions of the newborn dog, as with *PaCO₂*, the magnitude of the vasodilatory response to hypoxia varied.[108] Hypoxia caused the largest percentage increases in regional blood flow in brain stem structures, moderate increases in cortical and diencephalic structures, and smallest increases in cerebral white matter. These observations again suggest that *cerebral white matter has limited vasodilatory capacity* and thereby has implications for the vulnerability of this region to hypoxic-ischemic injury in the preterm infant (see later discussion and Chapter 15). The *mechanisms* of the increase in CBF with hypoxia are likely to be related to local metabolic factors and to vascular factors per se.[85,166] Thus, with hypoxia, rapid local increases in vasodilatory metabolic factors (e.g., perivascular H⁺, K⁺, adenosine, and prostaglandins) and decreases in vasoconstricting factors (e.g., Ca²⁺) occur. In addition, strikingly rapid decreases in isometric tension generated by the major cerebral arteries isolated from near-term fetal lambs and studied in vitro as isolated segments have been shown with PO₂ lowered to 15 mm Hg.[166] The relaxation was much faster than that observed in adult cerebral arterial segments. Whether this effect is related to local release of NO or another factor remains to be determined. However, the findings indicate that the myogenic properties of the major cerebral vessels themselves must be considered in the evaluation of mechanisms of changes in cerebral hemodynamics. Importance for the large cerebral vessels in regulation of CBF in the preterm human is suggested further by the presence in their vascular wall of a muscularis, in distinct contrast to the absence of a muscularis in the smaller penetrating cerebral arteries and arterioles.[171]

The role of *acidemia* in the regulation of CBF in the perinatal animal requires further study. Whether produced by hypoxemia, lactate infusion, or respiratory means, acidemia caused a sharp increase in CBF in perinatal goats.[172] However, effects were most impressive when acidemia was induced by elevation in PaCO₂, a potent effector of CBF (as described earlier). Moreover, a

---

[a]References 106, 108, 116, 128, 141, 145, and 163-170.

subsequent study of the fetal lamb did not report an alteration in regional CBF over an arterial pH range from 6.9 to 7.5 produced by infusions of lactate or bicarbonate.[145] Studies of newborn dogs and piglets showed inconsistent effects of lactate infusions or other changes in arterial pH on CBF.[173-175]

A role for *adenosine* in regulation of CBF in the immature brain is suggested by observations, primarily in the neonatal piglet.[176,177] Studies correlated CBF with parallel measurements of interstitial concentrations of adenosine and have used specific agonists and antagonists of the A_2 receptor (the adenosine receptor on vascular smooth muscle; the A_1 receptor, the adenosine receptor on neurons, is involved in decreasing glutamate release and Ca^{2+} influx). The data suggest that adenosine has a vasodilatory effect and that it is involved in the cerebrovascular response to decreases in blood pressure and thereby cerebrovascular autoregulation. Recall that brain adenosine concentrations increase with hypoxia and seizures; both conditions require increases in substrate influx to brain. Finally, in addition to its vasodilatory effect, adenosine may influence CBF by inhibitions of platelet aggregation and activation of neutrophils (implicated in endothelial dysfunction), events shown to be important in the postischemic impairment of CBF in adult models.[177,178]

Prostaglandins are important regulators of CBF in the perinatal period.[a] Prostanoids may exhibit vasodilator or vasoconstrictor properties, depending on the specific prostanoid, and they appear to be important in the setting of both the upper and lower limits of autoregulation. However, *in neonatal animals*, prostanoids exert effects that are different from those observed in the adult. In general, these compounds function as cerebral vasodilators and are important in regulation of CBF with decreases in blood pressure within and below the autoregulatory range, with changes in blood PCO_2 and perivascular H^+ concentrations, and following ischemia, asphyxia, and seizures (conditions characterized by increases in cerebral prostaglandin biosynthesis). Prostaglandins also attenuate the vasoconstrictor responses of norepinephrine and are the apparent mediators of the vasodilatory responses of endogenous opiates. As a consequence of these important roles, indomethacin, through its inhibition of cyclooxygenase and thereby prostanoid biosynthesis, may have a variety of important cerebral hemodynamic effects that are vasoconstrictive. Such vasoconstrictor effects may be potentially beneficial (e.g.,

concerning prevention of intraventricular hemorrhage; see Chapter 24), or potentially deleterious (e.g., under conditions requiring maintenance or increase in CBF, as with hypotension, asphyxia, or seizures).

Cerebral Blood Flow During and After Perinatal Asphyxia or Other Hypoxic-Ischemic Insults in Experimental Animal Models

Important cerebral circulatory effects of perinatal asphyxia and related hypoxic-ischemic insults have been defined by studies of a variety of experimental models, some based on techniques that result in impaired gas exchange between the mother and fetus or postnatally, and others based on controlled manipulation of only specific blood gases or of blood pressure.[a] *During asphyxia*, three of these circulatory effects occur initially, and two occur with more prolonged episodes. The effects initially include (1) an alteration in the fetal circulation such that a larger proportion of the cardiac output is distributed to the brain, (2) an increase in total and regional CBF, and (3) a loss of vascular autoregulation, and, later, include (4) a diminution in cardiac output with the occurrence of systemic hypotension, and, largely as a consequence, (5) a decrease in CBF (Table 13.4). *After asphyxia*, critical additional circulatory effects develop, and indeed from the clinical standpoint, these postinsult effects are as important, if not more so, than those occurring during asphyxia (Table 13.5).

Redistribution of Fetal Circulation. Promptly after the onset of asphyxia in the term fetal primate or lamb, cardiac output is

---

[a]References 65, 71, 106-108, 114-116, 119, 128, 129, 139-141, 145, 157, 180, and 196-222.

---

[a]References 85, 113, 114, 126, 127, and 179-195.

TABLE 13.4	Effects of Ischemia on Carbohydrate and Energy Metabolism

↓ Glucose influx to brain
↑ Glycogenolysis
↑ Glycolysis
↓ Brain glucose
↑ Lactate production and tissue acidosis
↓ Phosphocreatine
↓ Adenosine triphosphate

TABLE 13.5   Brain Metabolites in White Matter of Fetal Sheep Made Hypoxic With or Without Hypotension

FETAL CONDITION	WHITE MATTER INJURY	BRAIN METABOLITE*		
		LACTATE	PHOSPHOCREATINE	ADENOSINE TRIPHOSPHATE
Normoxic, normotensive	−	3.2	0.7	0.7
Hypoxic, normotensive	−	9.9[†]	0.5	0.9
Hypoxic, hypotensive	+	19.5[†]	0.3[†]	0.1[†]

*Concentrations are mmol/kg; values are rounded off.
[†]$P < .05$ versus normoxic, normotensive.
Data from Wagner KR, Ting P, Westfall MV, Yamaguchi S, Bacher JD, Myers RE. Brain metabolic correlates of hypoxic-ischemic cerebral necrosis in mid-gestational sheep fetuses: significance of hypotension. *J Cereb Blood Flow Metab.* 1986;6:425-434.

redistributed such that a significantly larger proportion enters the brain, the coronary circulation, and the adrenals, at the expense of blood flow to other regions.[a] Approximately twofold increases in the proportion of cardiac output to brain were noted in studies of term fetal primates. This redistribution of blood flow is reminiscent of the diving reflex observed in aquatic animals and appears designed to protect the most critical and vulnerable organs. The response requires an intact sympathoadrenal system.[52] The important afferent components of the response include particularly the oxygen chemoreceptors.[58,224] Moreover, to be effective, circulation must be maintained—hence the hypertension noted shortly after the onset of fetal asphyxia is particularly important.[52,200,201]

Increase in Cerebral Blood Flow. The major purpose of the circulatory changes as outlined is to maintain CBF in the presence of impending tissue oxygen debt. In experiments with fetal and neonatal lambs, puppies, and primates, CBF in perinatal asphyxia increased generally by 50% to 500%.[b] In severe and prolonged asphyxia, CBF eventually falls as a consequence of decreasing cardiac output (secondary to myocardial failure and hypoxic-induced bradycardia) and the loss of vascular autoregulation.

The *mechanisms* underlying the initial increase in CBF relate in part to cerebral vasodilation, secondary to hypoxemia or hypercapnia, or both, presumably with increased perivascular H^+ concentration.[225,226] Roles for elevated extracellular fluid concentrations of K^+, adenosine, and prostaglandins, all of which increase markedly in brain with hypoxemia and ischemia, are likely.[85,176,177,179,227-231] The particular importance of a rise or at least maintenance of blood pressure in the increase of CBF with asphyxia was indicated by several studies.[200-202] In term fetal sheep subjected to asphyxia by cord compression, the initial increase in MABP persisted for 60 minutes before decreasing to normal values.[200] Carefully controlled experiments with the same animal suggested that fetal blood pressure may be even more critical than local chemical factors, which lead to cerebral vasodilation, in the enhancement of CBF.[201]

Although blood flow to various regions of the brain increases generally in concert with the increase in total CBF, *distinct regional differences* in this increase are apparent. In general, the increase in blood flow is most marked in brain stem structures and is least apparent in cerebral white matter. This general pattern was documented in the fetal lamb, neonatal lamb, and neonatal puppy.[c] This effect has been interpreted as an attempt to maintain the integrity of vital brain stem centers. The mechanism for the heterogeneity in regulation of CBF is unknown; an endogenous opioid-mediated mechanism appears likely.[205,234] Thus administration of naloxone results in an increase in telencephalic blood flow and oxygen metabolism and consequently a decrease in the fraction of CBF to the brain stem. This decrease in the fraction of flow to brain stem may impair the attempt to preserve vital brain stem centers. A likely conclusion from this work is that with hypoxia or asphyxia, the role of endogenous opiates is to suppress the *cerebral* rate of oxygen consumption, with the associated decrease in

telencephalic blood flow serving to preserve the brain stem by an increase in the fraction of total brain blood flow to the brain stem. The burst in release of endogenous opiates with hypoxia and asphyxia and the well-known suppression of cerebral neural activity and oxygen consumption by endogenous opiates support this notion.[235-237] In this context, administration of naloxone during asphyxia may be deleterious to the brain stem.

Loss of Vascular Autoregulation. A serious impairment of cerebral vascular autoregulation develops with perinatal asphyxia with the presence of a pressure-passive CBF.[200] Using the radioactive microsphere technique and producing asphyxia (pH. 6.8 to 7.0) in term fetal sheep by partial occlusion of umbilical vessels, Lou et al.[200] demonstrated a striking pressure-passive CBF. Marked hyperemia, with CBF values up to six times the normal value, occurred when MABP was raised to 60 to 70 mm Hg, whereas CBF declined to close to zero in large cortical areas when MABP was lowered to 30 mm Hg. Vascular autoregulation in these term fetal animals appeared to be very sensitive to asphyxia. The likely mechanism relates most probably to the hypoxemia and hypercapnia that are the hallmarks of perinatal asphyxia. The sensitivity of the autoregulatory system in the fetal and neonatal brain to these alterations in blood gas levels was described earlier (see the section on autoregulation). The implications of these data for ischemic injury to perinatal brain are obvious. In one study of near-term fetal sheep, autoregulation of CBF was lost within 4 minutes of cord occlusion, and overt cerebral injury occurred by 10 minutes secondary to decreased CBF in the presence of hypotension.[128]

Hypotension and Diminished Cerebral Blood Flow. Although the initial response to asphyxia is hypertension, this response is followed by hypotension.[52,128] The rapidity and severity of this occurrence depend on the duration and severity of the asphyxial insult. In large part, this effect is related to a diminution in cardiac output,[100,196] probably secondary to an effect on the myocardium. The consequence for the brain may be devastating, because the impairment of vascular autoregulation leaves CBF at the mercy of perfusion pressure. Deficits in CBF may be marked, with relatively modest changes in MABP. Impressive deficits in CBF (20% to 80%) have been demonstrated, particularly in the parasagittal regions of the cerebral hemispheres and especially posteriorly, in the term fetal monkey subjected to severe and prolonged asphyxia.[117] A similar parasagittal distribution of cerebral cortical injury was demonstrated in near-term fetal sheep subjected to cerebral ischemia.[217,238] The detailed regional study of newborn dogs demonstrated that cerebral white matter also is particularly likely to exhibit diminished blood flow with hypotension.[119] In the preterm sheep (0.65 gestation), cerebral white matter was particularly affected with ischemia, with white matter injury then determined by the topographic distribution within the ischemic regions of vulnerable differentiating oligodendrocytes.[222] These observations correlate well with the neuropathological and clinical observations made by asphyxiated human infants (see Chapters 16 and 20).

A summary of the major relationships between perinatal asphyxia and CBF *during asphyxia* is shown graphically in Fig. 13.12. The initial effects leading to increased CBF are considered best as compensatory, adaptive responses (which could become

---

[a]References 58, 107, 196, 202, 223, and 224.
[b]References 107, 108, 116, 141, 145, 196, 197, 199, 201, 202, and 204-207.
[c]References 65, 108, 114, 116, 145, 201, 204-206, 232, and 233.

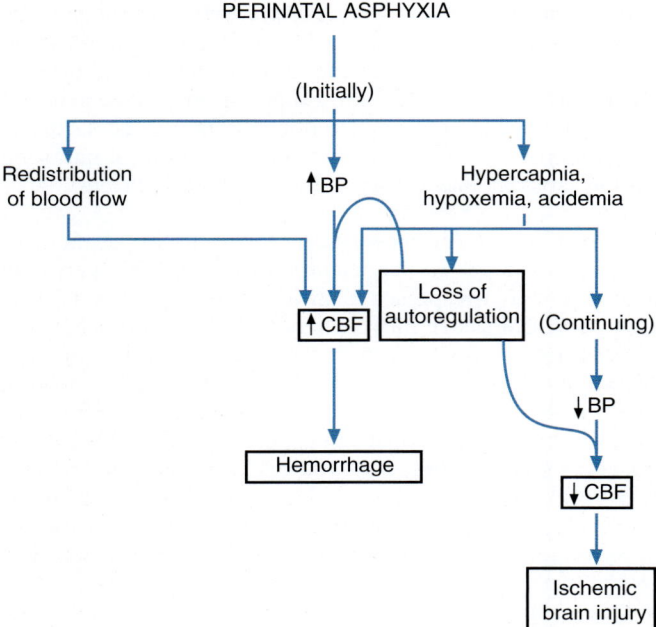

Figure 13.12 Major relationships between perinatal asphyxia and cerebral blood flow (CBF). The major consequences of the changes in cerebral blood flow (i.e., hemorrhage and ischemic brain injury) are shown. *BP*, Blood pressure.

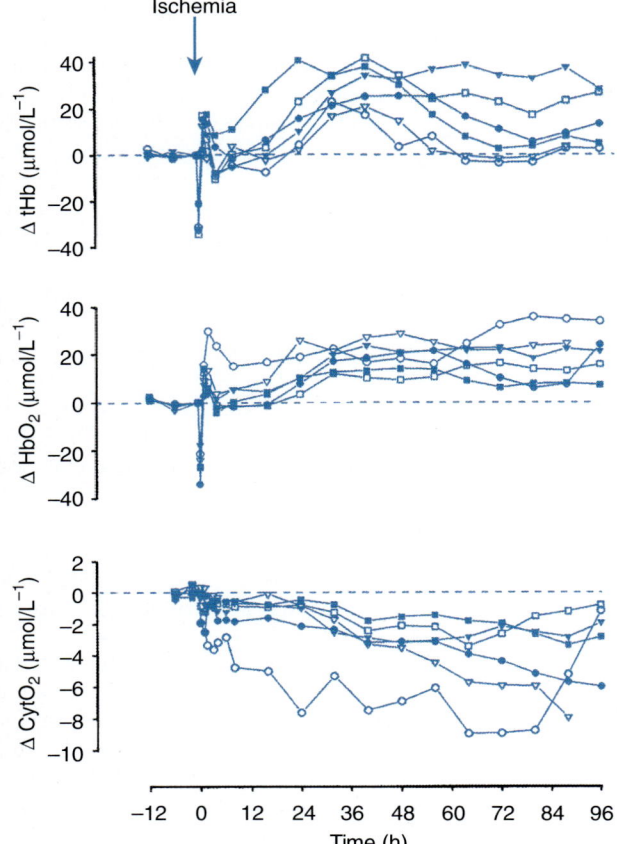

Figure 13.13 Cerebral hemodynamic changes after transient cerebral ischemia in the late-gestation fetal lamb. Changes in total cerebral hemoglobin (tHb), oxygenated hemoglobin (HbO2), and cytochrome oxidase (CytO2) were measured by near-infrared spectroscopy. In each graph, different symbols represent data from separate fetuses. Note the two phases of cerebral vasodilation and increased cerebral blood flow, as assessed by the hemoglobin signals; the early increase occurs in the first 2 to 3 hours after ischemia, and the delayed increase occurs from 12 to 48 hours. The delayed increase in flow is accompanied by a decline in CytO2, consistent with impaired mitochondrial oxygenation. (From Marks KA, Mallard EC, Roberts I, et al. Delayed vasodilation and altered oxygenation after cerebral ischemia in fetal sheep. *Pediatr Res.* 1996;39:48–54.)

maladaptive by leading to hemorrhage in vulnerable capillary beds). The later effects represent a decompensation of these responses and a cascade that leads to diminished CBF and brain injury.

Postasphyxial-Postischemic Effects. The period *after termination of the asphyxial-ischemic insult* is critical because, during this interval, progression to brain injury occurs (see earlier discussion), and in the clinical setting, this time represents a window of opportunity for therapeutic intervention. The principal experimental models used have been near-term fetal sheep and neonatal piglets and rat pups, and the insults have primarily consisted of hypoxia-ischemia and, less commonly, asphyxia.[a] The major circulatory effects identified are summarized in Table 13.5. A consistent observation has been a marked increase in CBF on reperfusion, hyperemia that continues for up to several hours (Fig. 13.13). This *early increase in CBF* is presumably related to the same mechanism operative for the initial increase in CBF during asphyxia noted earlier (i.e., the accumulation of such vasodilating factors as H^+, K^+, adenosine, and prostaglandins). Moreover, superoxide anion, a consequence of reperfusion after asphyxia (see earlier), may lead to a disturbance of cerebrovascular autoregulation through stimulation of vasodilation.[241] This early increase in cerebral perfusion is followed by a decline toward the baseline. In some models, especially if associated with hypotension, CBF declines below normal with the threat of cerebral ischemia.

This postasphyxial cerebral hypoperfusion has not been a consistent feature in all experimental models. It is likely that hypotension could lead to cerebral ischemia in this period, *because autoregulation is not operative* (Fig. 13.14).

Importantly, a second (i.e., "delayed") increase in CBF develops, with onset generally between 12 and 24 hours and with a duration of many hours or a day or more (see Fig. 13.13). This increase is associated with evidence of impaired mitochondrial oxygenation (as assessed by brain levels of oxidized cytochrome c), with the cellular energy failure, and with neuropathological evidence for neuronal and white matter injury. The delayed hyperemia, its association with energy failure, and its correlation with severity of brain injury have also been observed in asphyxiated human infants (Chapters 18 to 20). The mechanisms underlying the vasodilation and hyperemia are not established but may relate in part to NO. Because NO synthesis in endothelial cells (eNOS) is activated after

[a]References 114, 115, 156, 180, 181, 197-199, 207-210, 214-219, 232, and 238-240.

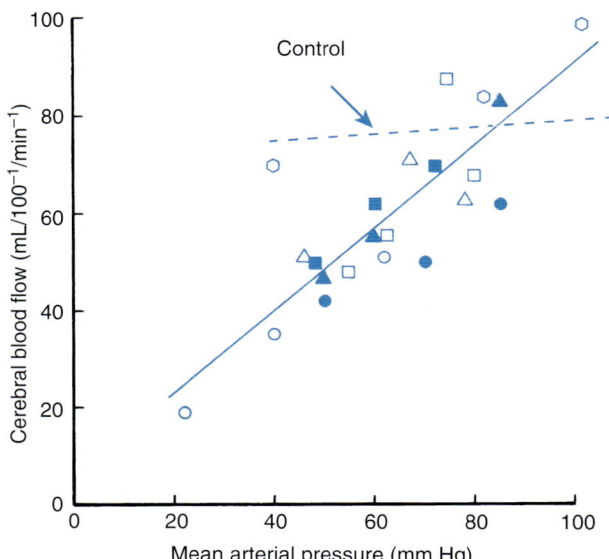

Figure 13.14 Postasphyxial impairment of cerebrovascular autoregulation. Cerebral blood flow versus mean arterial blood pressure following asphyxia. Symbols (n = 7) represent responses to changes in blood pressure in individual asphyxiated lambs (n = 7). The *regression line* is derived from pooled data of all lambs. The *dashed line* represents data from nonasphyxiated (control) lambs. (From Rosenberg AA. Regulation of cerebral blood flow after asphyxia in neonatal lambs. *Stroke.* 1988;19:239–244.)

TABLE 13.6 Effect of Carbohydrate Status on Biochemical Response to Circulatory Arrest (10 Minutes) in Juvenile Monkeys

EXPERIMENTAL CONDITION	BRAIN CONCENTRATION (μmmol/g)	
	ADENOSINE TRIPHOSPHATE	LACTATE
Control	2.2	3.0
Circulatory arrest	0.2	13.0
Circulatory arrest and glucose pretreatment	0.3	33.0

Data from references 269 to 272.

hypoxic-ischemic insults, an attempt to reduce the delayed cerebral hyperemia with an NOS inhibitor was attempted in the fetal sheep model of ischemia.[217,218] The inhibitor did attenuate the delayed hyperemia, but surprisingly, inhibition of NO synthesis *increased* histological injury.[217] This combination of findings suggests that NO synthesis has a protective effect either because of the vasodilatory effect or because of a biochemical effect.

Cerebral Blood Flow in the Human Newborn
Methodology

In approximately the past 25 to 30 years, considerable insight into CBF in the human newborn has been provided by application of one or more of several techniques (Table 13.6). The largest amount of information has been provided by the *xenon-133 clearance technique*.[242-268] The technique uses administration of xenon-133, either by intraarterial or intravenous injection or by inhalation (preferably intravenous injection), and detection of the brain clearance of xenon-133, specifically the gamma radiation thereof, by external detectors. The particular advantage of the xenon-133 clearance technique is the ability to provide quantitative data with relatively low radiation exposure and portable equipment. *Xenon computed tomography* has the advantage of providing regional data, but the technique requires transport to a specialized suite.

Positron emission tomography (PET) has been valuable in demonstration in the premature and term newborn of normal values of regional CBF, coupling with oxygen consumption, increases of flow with seizure, and characteristic changes in premature infants with periventricular hemorrhagic infarction and intraventricular hemorrhage, as well as in term asphyxiated infants with parasagittal cerebral injury. The particular advantage

of PET is the ability to provide not only quantitative data but also regional information. *Single photon emission tomography* also provides regional data but is nonquantitative. *Near-infrared spectroscopy*, a noninvasive optical technique, has the capability to provide serial quantitative measurements of CBF and is discussed in detail in Chapter 10. With *venous occlusion plethysmography*, changes in intracranial volume after brief occlusion of the jugular veins are determined by a strain-gauge instrument placed around the compliant infant skull.[273-277] This technique cannot provide quantitative information and has the disadvantage of causing a transient rise in intracranial pressure. Application of this method is discussed briefly later. The *Doppler ultrasonic technique* for measurement of CBF velocity, a noninvasive method, can provide serial information about cerebrovascular resistance and flow velocity in the insonated cerebral vessels. Determination of changes in volumic flow from the velocity data is complicated by the inability to determine the cross-sectional diameter of the insonated vessel. *Electrical impedance techniques* are noninvasive but have not proven sufficiently sensitive to be consistently useful.[278-280] *MR techniques* for determination of CBF are under intensive study in the human newborn infant, either after administration of a paramagnetic contrast agent (e.g., gadolinium) or by arterial spin labeling (ASL) perfusion-weighted MRI (Fig. 13.15). *ASL perfusion-weighted MRI is the only approach that enables direct and noninvasive measurements of CBF in different brain regions, without the need to inject contrast material or expose the newborn to ionizing radiation.*[281-284] To date, a handful of studies have demonstrated the feasibility of using ASL in newborns.[285-287] In addition, a few recent studies have demonstrated the benefit of combining timely measurements of CBF by ASL-MRI with other modalities, such as near-infrared spectroscopy or MR spectroscopy, to better assess changes in cerebral perfusion, metabolism, and oxygenation in sick newborns.[286-288] The method has been used effectively in studies of CBF with human brain maturation and in several neonatal pathological states (i.e., hypoxic-ischemic encephalopathy, arterial stroke, and congenital heart disease; see Chapters 20 and 21).[289]

Development and Normal Values of Cerebral Blood Flow in the Human Newborn

Changes Immediately After Delivery. A sharp decrease in "apparent" CBF ("apparent" because the plethysmographic

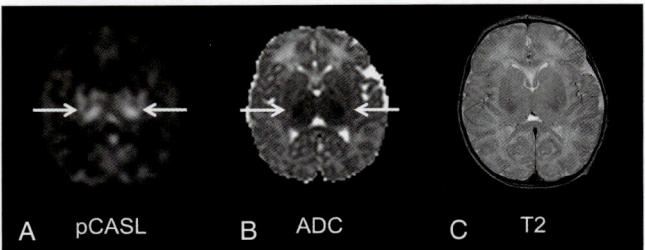

Figure 13.15 An asphyxiated newborn treated with hypothermia showing basal ganglia injury on magnetic resonance imaging (MRI) obtained on day 2 of life. (A) Cerebral blood flow map obtained by pseudocontinuous arterial spin labeling (pCASL), showing higher perfusion *(arrows)* in the bilateral thalami and, to a lesser extent, in the bilateral posterior limb of internal capsule and lentiform nuclei. (B) Apparent diffusion coefficient map showing restricted diffusion *(arrows)* within the same areas. (C) Axial T2-weighted image; changes of T2-weighted images are subtle. (Reprinted with permission from Wintermark P. Injury and repair in perinatal brain injury: insights from non-invasive MR perfusion imaging. *Semin Perinatol.* 2015;39:124–129.)

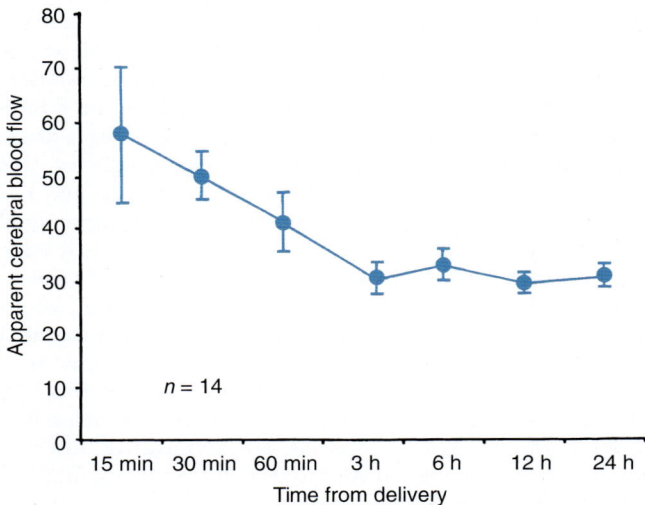

Figure 13.16 Apparent cerebral blood flow in term infants following delivery, as estimated by the jugular venous occlusion plethysmographic technique. Note the decline in the first several hours, followed by stable flow. (From Cooke RW, Rolfe P, Howat P. Apparent cerebral blood-flow in newborns with respiratory disease. *Dev Med Child Neurol.* 1979;21:154.)

method is only semiquantitative) occurs in the term infant in the first hours after delivery (Fig. 13.16).[273] The decrease in the first 3 hours is nearly twofold, and over the ensuing hours, CBF is relatively stable. The reason for the relatively higher value shortly after delivery is not known, although a relationship with higher $PaCO_2$ levels immediately after birth has been suggested. Alternatively, it is possible that a reflex activity, mediated by vagal afferents, is operative because the relatively higher CBF near the time of birth requires intact vagus nerves in the sheep.[141] Both factors may be relevant in the human newborn, when $PaCO_2$ levels may be elevated and vagal activity from lung expansion may be considerable.[273] A third factor may involve arterial oxygen content, because, as noted earlier, a similar sharp decline in CBF after birth has been observed in the lamb and correlates well with the increase

in arterial oxygen content in the newborn versus fetal state. The relatively enhanced CBF in the first minutes to hours after delivery may provide a margin of safety for cerebral metabolic needs in the period of adaptation to birth.

Changes Beyond the Immediate Postpartum Period. Data obtained by PET suggest that CBF is approximately 20% of the adult value in the premature infant of approximately 28 weeks of gestation and approximately 40% of the adult value in the term newborn.[290] Serial studies of CBF in normal preterm infants show an approximately twofold increase in flow over the first 3 days of life, perhaps related to an increase in cardiac output.[291] One study of preterm infants by spatially resolved near-infrared spectroscopy showed a sharp increase in cerebral oxygenation during this period, most consistent with an increase in CBF.[292] Doppler studies of CBF velocity also are consistent with this postnatal increase in CBF (see Chapter 10).[293]

Normal Values. Values for CBF reported in the human premature newborn, studied by xenon clearance and shown in Table 13.7, are generally between 10 and 20 mL/100 g per minute. A similar range is apparent in studies by PET and near-infrared spectroscopy. The correlations with the findings in developing animals described earlier are obvious. Regional values for CBF are notable for higher flows in cerebral gray matter structures than in cerebral white matter.

Regulation in the Human Newborn. The major established regulatory mechanisms for CBF in the human newborn include autoregulation, $PaCO_2$, oxygen delivery, blood glucose, and neuronal activity (e.g., seizure). Certain pharmacological agents also have been shown to exert regulatory effects. These various regulatory factors and their effects on CBF are summarized in Table 13.8 and are reviewed briefly next.

Autoregulation. Autoregulation appears to be operative in both the normal human preterm and full-term infants.[a] *Although the actual limits of the autoregulatory plateau cannot be established with certainty,* the *approximate* autoregulatory range appears to be from 25 to 50 mm Hg MABP. Both the size of this range and its actual upper and lower limits vary according to gestational age (Fig. 13.17) and, likely, postnatal age and multiple other factors. Autoregulation in mature animals and adult humans is rendered inoperative by factors that lead to pronounced vasodilation (e.g., hypercarbia, hypoxia, hypoglycemia, seizure, postasphyxial state, and selected cytokines), and available data suggest that these factors also impair autoregulation in the human infant, particularly the seriously asphyxiated full-term infant and in the sick, mechanically ventilated preterm infant (see Table 13.8).[b]

The problem of a persistent pressure-passive cerebral circulation is particularly important in sick premature infants. Thus initial studies using the invasive technique of radioactive xenon clearance initially showed that certain premature infants, mechanically ventilated and usually clinically unstable, appeared to exhibit pressure-passive cerebral circulation.[200,256] This fundamental initial observation has been confirmed by less invasive methods multiple times.[296-298,301,303] Thus, in such sick

---

[a]References 254, 256, 262, 263, 265-267, and 294-303.
[b]References 256, 260, 265, 267, 268, 296-298, 300, 301, and 304.

TABLE 13.7   Effect of Glucose or Saline Treatment on Brain Adenosine Triphosphate in Hypoxic-Ischemic Rats (Unilateral Carotid Ligation and Hypoxemia)*

EXPERIMENTAL CONDITION	PHOSPHOCREATINE*	ATP*	LACTATE*
Control	3.00	2.41	1.6
Ligation-hypoxemia[†]			
Saline (60 min)	1.00	1.25	11.1
Glucose (60 min)	1.80	2.31	15.2
Saline (120 min)	0.35	0.43	9.4
Glucose (120 min)	1.00	1.80	25.5

*Values are mean concentrations (mmol/kg) in hemisphere ipsilateral to carotid ligation.

[†]All values for ligated-hypoxemic animals different from controls ($P < .05$), and all values for glucose-treated animals different from saline-treated animals ($P < .05$).

ATP, Adenosine triphosphate.

Data from Vannucci RC, Brucklacher RM, Vannucci SJ. The effect of hyperglycemia on cerebral metabolism during hypoxia-ischemia in the immature rat. *J Cereb Blood Flow Metab*. 1996;16:1026–1033.

TABLE 13.8   Tentative Conclusions Concerning Effects of Glucose Administration With Perinatal Hypoxic-Ischemic Insults[a]

Glucose transport into the brain and glucose concentration in the brain are increased. Lactate levels are increased, and intracellular pH values are decreased but recover promptly.

Decrease in the cerebral metabolic rate of oxygen is prevented, perhaps reflecting improved mitochondrial function.

Improvement in high-energy phosphate levels is usual but has not reached statistical significance in all studies.

Neuropathological injury may be prevented, ameliorated, or accentuated, according to the model of hypoxia-ischemia and the species and state of maturation of the animal.

Improved survival occurs and may relate at least partially to improvement in cardiorespiratory function.

Determinations of cerebral lactate and high-energy phosphates, as a function of blood glucose, are needed in asphyxiated human newborns for definitive recommendations concerning glucose supplementation.

[a]See text for references.

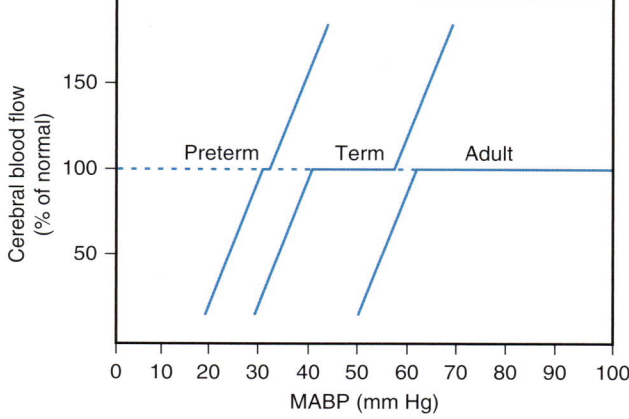

Figure 13.17 An *approximation* of the relationship of cerebral blood flow as a function of mean arterial blood pressure (MABP) with maturation. See text for details.

---

premature infants with pressure-passive cerebral circulation, it would be expected that when blood pressure falls, as occurs commonly in such infants, so would CBF, with the consequence of cerebral ischemia. The presence of arterial end zones and border zones and vulnerable early differentiating oligodendroglia in developing cerebral white matter would render this region especially vulnerable (see Chapter 15). Moreover, the particular danger is compounded by the very low normal blood flow to cerebral white matter in the premature infant, a feature suggesting that a minimal margin of safety may exist. In one serial study of 32 mechanically ventilated premature infants from the first hours, near-infrared spectroscopy was used to demonstrate a pressure-passive cerebral circulation in 53%.[298] The example shown in Fig. 13.18 is typical (i.e., an infant with MABPs that fluctuate gradually over minutes and are accompanied by parallel changes in the cerebral circulation). *The nadirs of blood pressure often are not markedly low and thus may*

be readily overlooked. However, the cumulative effect of many repeated modest declines in CBF is likely to be considerable (see Chapter 15). Importantly, nearly all the cases of PVL (and severe germinal matrix hemorrhage/intraventricular hemorrhage) later identified in the series of 32 infants were in the pressure-passive group.[298] These findings were critical because they suggested that (1) infants with a pressure-passive cerebral circulation could be identified by near-infrared spectroscopy before the occurrence of white matter injury, (2) that the circulatory abnormality is related strongly to the occurrence of white matter injury, and (3) if the pressure-passive state could be corrected, perhaps the white matter injury could be prevented. However, this study involved a relatively small number of infants.

A subsequent study of 90 premature infants used a frequency-based assessment of autoregulation and quantitated the degree and duration of altered autoregulation over the first 5 days of life.[303] *Pressure-passive epochs were documented in 95% of the infants.* The overall mean proportion of the pressure-passive time was 20%, although some infants had a pressure-passive state more than 50% of the time. The likelihood of a pressure-passive state increased with decreasing gestational age and periods of hypotension.

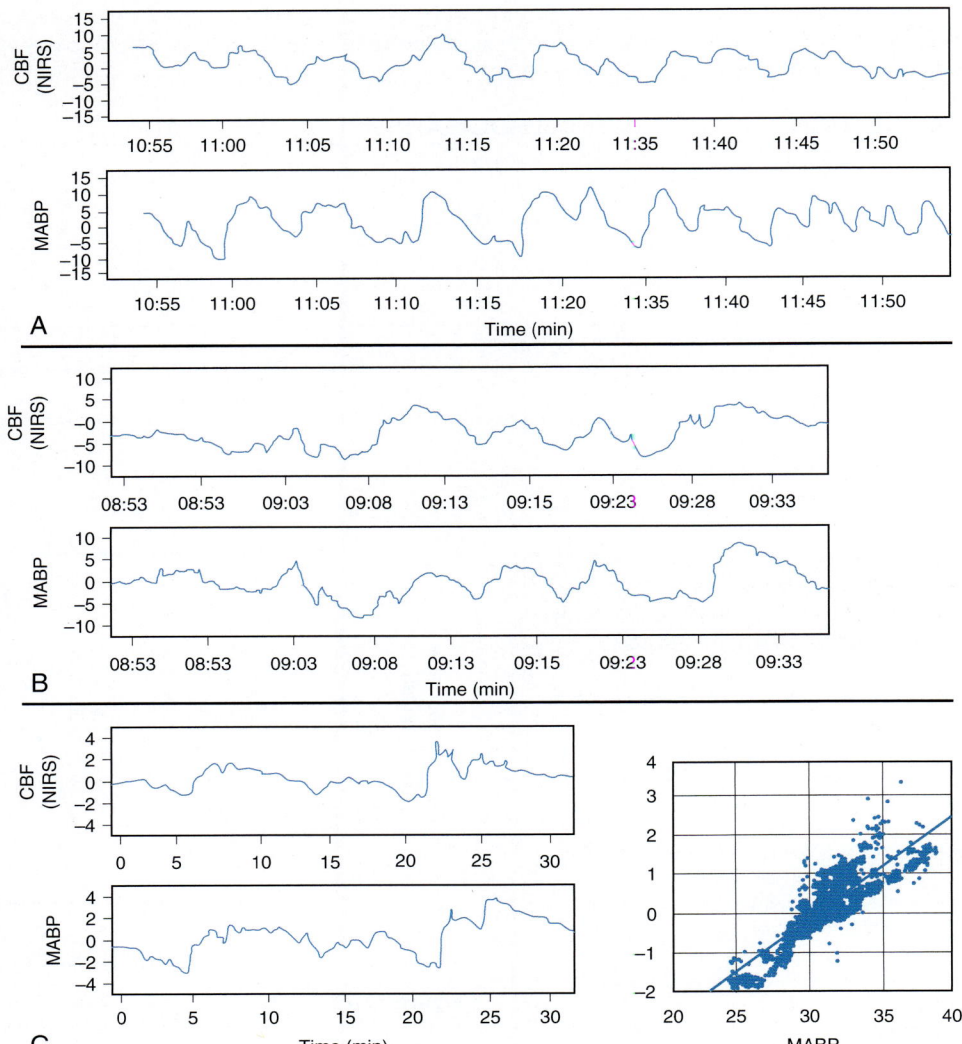

Figure 13.18 Pressure-passive relationship of cerebral blood flow, estimated by near-infrared spectroscopy, and mean arterial blood pressure, in ventilated premature infants. Note the parallel changes in arterial blood pressure and cerebral perfusion (A–C). Note also that the changes in blood pressure are not marked. In (C) all data points are plotted; the linear relationship between blood pressure and cerebral perfusion is apparent. *CBF*, Cerebral blood flow; *MABP*, mean arterial blood pressure. (From Tsuji M, Saul JP, duPlessis A, et al. Cerebral intravascular oxygenation correlates with mean arterial pressure in critically ill premature infants. *Pediatrics.* 2000;106:625–632.)

More recently, using near infrared spectroscopy (NIRS) methodology, high coherence between tissue oxygenation index (TOI) and MABP was also observed with low blood pressure in the sickest infants, suggestive of a narrow window for autoregulation in such sick immature infants.[305] Additional technical analysis with time domain analysis[306] described the cerebral oximetry index (COx) as the moving and linear correlation coefficient between slow waves of MABP and regional cerebral oxygen saturation (rSO$_2$). Researchers observed that lower MABP during the first 3 days of life was associated with impaired autoregulation (COx >0.5) in preterm infants at ≤30 weeks of gestational age. There has been debate regarding whether the two methods are equivalent or one is superior to the other; however, in a series of 60 preterm infants,

time-domain analysis appeared more robust compared with coherence function analysis.[307]

A further index of cerebral vascular reactivity is a correlation coefficient of TOI and MABP (TOx) with HR (tissue oxygenation heart rate, TOHRx), believed to improve the reflection of perfusion with both blood pressure and heart rate.[308] Using this measure in 31 preterm infants at median gestational age of 26 weeks, TOHRx was significantly correlated with gestational age ($R = -0.57$, $P = .007$), birth weight ($R = -0.58$, $P = .006$), and the Clinical Risk Index for Babies II ($R = 0.55$, $P = .0014$)—a prediction score of mortality and morbidity in the preterm infant. Defining "optimal" MABP by the strength of cerebral autoregulation has been studied in adults with traumatic brain injury. By measuring spontaneous fluctuations in cerebral perfusion pressure, it is possible to calculate the range of perfusion pressure where autoregulation is strongest. In one study, patients were more likely to have a favorable outcome when cerebral perfusion pressure was close to "optimal."[309] Recently, continuous monitoring of cerebral vascular reactivity in preterm infants, with TOHRx, has been used to define values of $MABP_{OPT}$ where cerebral vascular reactivity is strongest. Preterm infants who died had a higher mean absolute deviation from $MABP_{OPT}$ than patients who survived. Furthermore, deviation of MABP above the optimal values was observed in infants who had worse germinal matrix-intraventricular hemorrhage grades.[310] (There remain significant technical challenges in obtaining reliable measurements of $MABP_{OPT}$ at the cot side. For example, a minimum of 2 to 4 hours of continuous artifact-free data is necessary to create a reliable U-shaped autoregulatory curve with spontaneous fluctuations in heart rate and TOI. Currently all descriptions of $MABP_{OPT}$ have been undertaken on retrospective analysis of data.)

The *lower limit of the autoregulatory curve in newborns* obviously is of great importance, particularly for management purposes and especially in sick premature infants. The precise lower limit remains unknown, and it is likely that this value varies not only with gestational age but also with postnatal age and with factors that alter the concentration of vasoactive molecules in brain (e.g., blood gases, cytokines, seizures, hypoxia-ischemia). In one report, blood pressure values in the first day of life in infants 24 to 30 weeks of gestation of less than 31 mm Hg were associated with impaired electroencephalogram (EEG) continuity on the EEG, a finding raising the possibility of decreased CBF at such values.[311] Similarly, in a study of extremely low-birth-weight infants (mean birth weight 772 g, mean gestational age 26 weeks) by near-infrared spectroscopy, a pressure-passive cerebral circulation resulted when MABPs were lower than 30 mm Hg.[312,313] However, to what extent, if any, arterial blood pressures lower than 30 mm Hg are clearly dangerous is unclear. Thus a careful study of cerebral electrical activity and cerebral fractional oxygen extraction, presumably a reflection of CBF, in 35 23- to 30-week premature infants showed no electrical abnormality at mean blood pressure levels higher than 23 mm Hg.[313]

Carbon Dioxide. $PaCO_2$ is a potent regulator of CBF in the human newborn.[a] The marked reactivity of CBF to $PaCO_2$ is present in the first hours of life in spontaneously breathing preterm infants but does not appear until the second day in mechanically ventilated preterm infants (Table 13.9).[256,257,263] The reason for the attenuated reactivity of CBF to $PaCO_2$ in the first day of life in mechanically ventilated preterm infants is unclear, although the same phenomenon has been observed in the newborn monkey, rat, dog, and lamb.[144,161,265,314] A state of attenuated or absent reactivity to $PaCO_2$, as with blood pressure, has been observed both in seriously asphyxiated full-term infants and in mechanically ventilated preterm infants before severe intracranial hemorrhage (Table 13.10; see Chapters 14 to 16 and 18 to 20). In general, the loss of reactivity to $PaCO_2$ follows the loss of autoregulation (but precedes loss of reactivity to hypoxemia).[265] In one report, a progressive loss

---

TABLE 13.9 Resistance of High-Energy Phosphate Levels in Perinatal (vs. Adult) Brain to Hypoxic Injury: Probable Mechanisms

Lower rate of energy utilization
Lower rate of accumulation of toxic products (i.e., lactate)
Utilization of lactate and ketone bodies for energy

TABLE 13.10 Effect of Spontaneous Vaginal Delivery on Glycogen, Glycolytic Metabolites, and High-Energy Compounds in Rat Brain

METABOLIC COMPOUND	TIME AFTER DELIVERY (MIN) PERCENTAGE OF TERM FETAL VALUES		
	1	10	60
Glycogen	88	74	90
Lactate	367	408	230
Lactate-pyruvate	425	181	157
Phosphocreatine	38	105	170
Adenosine triphosphate	67	92	96

Data from Vannucci RC, Duffy TE. Influence of birth on carbohydrate and energy metabolism in rat brain. *Am J Physiol.* 1974;226:933–940; and Kohle SJ, Vannucci RC. Glycogen metabolism in fetal and postnatal rat brain: influence of birth. *J Neurochem.* 1977;28:441–443.

---

of cerebrovascular autoregulation was noted with increasing $PaCO_2 \geq 45$ mm Hg.[136]

The *mechanism* for the vasodilating effect of carbon dioxide relates to the increase in *perivascular H^+ concentration*, as observed in experimental models. The observation of a 50% decrease in CBF after sodium bicarbonate administration to term and premature infants with acidosis also supports the important role of perivascular H^+ concentration.[243] The mechanism proposed for a decrease in the latter situation was enhanced movement of bicarbonate across the blood-brain barrier "because of vasodilation caused by the asphyxia" in these infants.[243] The demonstration of a decrease in CBF after sodium bicarbonate administration in acidotic postasphyxial infants may have important implications for management. Sodium bicarbonate is no longer recommended for use in the resuscitation of the term or preterm newborn infant due to its association with an increased mortality and morbidity.[315,316]

Oxygen. Arterial oxygen concentration is an important effector of CBF in the human infant, as it is in the perinatal animal.[a] A vivid demonstration of the vasoconstrictive effect of oxygen is the observation that preterm infants administered 80% oxygen during stabilization at birth had a 23% lower value for CBF

---

[a]References 136, 243, 244, 251, 256, 257, 262, 263, 267, 268, and 313.

[a]References 106, 164, 254, 255, 257, and 317-324.

than infants administered room air during stabilization, when measured by xenon-133 clearance at 2 hours of life.[324] This finding may have implications concerning the use of high concentrations of inspired oxygen at the time of birth. The administration of 100% oxygen for resuscitation of the term newborn infant has been associated with a markedly increased risk for death and has led to the clear recommendation that all term-born infants be resuscitated in room air.[315,325] Arterial oxygen concentration is related not only to PaO_2 but also to hemoglobin concentration and the oxygen affinity of hemoglobin. In preterm infants studied in the first day of life, Pryds and Greisen[257] observed a mean increase in CBF of 11.9% per 1 mmol/kg decrease in hemoglobin concentration. In a separate series of preterm infants studied at a mean postnatal age of 3.7 weeks, a mean increase in CBF of 5% per percentage point of decrease in hematocrit was documented.[254] Oxygen delivery to the brain may be affected not only by hemoglobin concentration but also by the viscosity of blood, at which point the inverse relationship of CBF with hemoglobin concentration becomes more pronounced. However, in general, hematocrit does not alter blood viscosity in the newborn at levels lower than approximately 60% (and perhaps somewhat higher).[267,326,327] Finally, a direct relationship of CBF (determined by xenon-133 clearance) with the relative proportion of fetal hemoglobin has been shown,[320] presumably reflecting the stronger affinity of fetal hemoglobin for oxygen. This conclusion had been suggested by a prior study of CBF velocity.[323]

Glucose. A striking observation by Pryds et al.[253,258] established an important role for glucose in regulation of CBF in the human newborn (see Table 13.8). As discussed in more detail in Chapter 25, an increase in CBF became apparent as blood glucose concentration decreased to less than approximately 30 mg/dL (1.7 mmol/L). Increases in CBF of twofold to threefold then occurred in proportion to the decline in blood glucose. The mechanism for this vasodilatory effect of glucose is not clear, but stimulation of beta-receptors by the increased compensatory secretion of epinephrine is suggested by data in human adults.[265] The clinical significance of this effect of glucose could be appreciable (see Chapter 25).

Neuronal Activity (Seizure). The coupling of neuronal activity to CBF is apparent in at least two situations: sleep states and seizure. A decrease in CBF during *sleep* has been shown by xenon-133 clearance.[328] The effect is not striking. A striking increase (≈50%) in CBF with the excessive neuronal activity of *seizure* has been documented in the human newborn by PET (see Chapter 12).[329] This effect had been suggested by earlier studies of CBF velocity by Doppler.[330]

Pharmacological Agents. Indomethacin and aminophylline are the two pharmacological agents shown to have a clear effect on CBF in the human newborn. *Indomethacin* administration in doses used for closure of the ductus arteriosus led to a 20% to 40% decrease in CBF in the premature infant, as studied by xenon-133 clearance and near-infrared spectroscopy.[194,252,331] Notably, however, no change in CBF, assessed by Doppler, was observed after continuous versus bolus infusion of indomethacin.[332] The vasoconstrictive effect is mediated by the inhibition of synthesis of vasodilatory prostaglandins at the cyclooxygenase step, as shown in experimental models and

studies of isolated neonatal human cerebral artery.[333,334] An increase in cerebrovascular resistance was shown by Doppler studies of very low-birth-weight infants after indomethacin administration.[335] Interestingly, by contrast with indomethacin, *ibuprofen* does not lead to a decline in CBF.[267]

Administration of *aminophylline*, an antagonist of adenosine, led to only a small decrease (10% to 15%) in CBF in the human premature infant within 1 hour of intravenous administration.[264] No alteration of visual evoked potentials accompanied this modest decrease in blood flow. The use of caffeine in the preterm infant has resulted in similar observations of a reduction in CBF. In a study of 40 preterm infants after a loading dose of caffeine using Doppler cerebral sonography, cardiac echocardiography, and cerebral spatially resolved near-infrared spectroscopy, mean anterior cerebral artery peak and time average mean blood flow velocity fell significantly (by 14% and 17.7%, respectively) at 1 hour post-caffeine loading dose. Cerebral TOI fell from predose levels by 9.5% at 1 hour, with partial recovery to 4.9% reduced at 4 hours post dose. There were no significant changes in left or right ventricular output, transcutaneous oxygen saturation, transcutaneous PCO_2, or total vascular resistance.[336] *Dopamine* administered to treat hypotension was reported in two studies to increase CBF as well as arterial blood pressure.[267,312] However, a more recent study of preterm and term piglets showed no increase of CBF with dopamine or dobutamine.[337]

Perinatal Asphyxia, Autoregulation of Cerebral Blood Flow, and Cerebral Hyperemia in the Human Newborn Infant

Impaired Autoregulation. A xenon-133 study of CBF in a group of 19 term and preterm infants first suggested that autoregulation in the human newborn is very sensitive to perinatal asphyxia.[244] Thus 19 infants were examined with the xenon clearance technique "a few hours after birth."[244] Eleven of these infants weighed less than 2000 g. Although most of the infants were considered "distressed," Apgar scores at 5 minutes were less than 7 in only 4 of the 19 infants. At the time of study, pH was less than 7.20 in only 4 infants. For the total group of 19 infants, a linear relationship existed between CBF and systolic blood pressure (Fig. 13.19). This pressure-passive relationship suggests inoperative vascular autoregulation and was seen to a similar degree in the infants less than or more than 2000 g body weight. This apparent impairment of vascular autoregulation is directly reminiscent of the data obtained with fetal and neonatal animals after asphyxia (see the earlier section).

Impaired Vascular Reactivity and Cerebral Hyperemia. Subsequent work clarified the relationship between perinatal asphyxia and the impairment of vascular reactivity—particularly autoregulation. In a systematic study of 19 term infants (mean birth weight, 3200 g) with perinatal asphyxia defined by a 5-minute Apgar score of 5 or lower and umbilical cord pH lower than 7.0, or both, a striking relationship among the severity of brain injury, the absolute value of CBF, and the reactivity to changes in blood pressure and $PaCO_2$ was defined (see Table 13.10).[260] Thus infants with the poorest neurological outcome (isoelectric amplitude-integrated EEG, death) had the highest values for CBF and no autoregulation or carbon dioxide reactivity (see Table 13.9). Infants with a burst-suppression EEG and moderate to severe brain injury had slightly elevated values for CBF and impaired autoregulation but retained reactivity to $PaCO_2$ (see

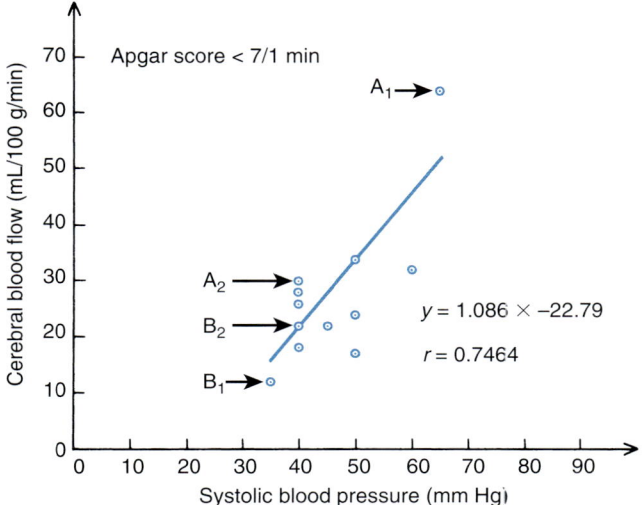

Figure 13.19 Linear relationship between cerebral blood flow and systolic blood pressure in 10 newborns with Apgar scores of less than 7 at 1 minute. Cerebral blood flow (CBF) was measured by the xenon clearance technique. A_1 and A_2 represent measurements of CBF in one patient before and after a spontaneous decrease in blood pressure. B_1 and B_2 represent measurements in another patient before and after a spontaneous increase in blood pressure. (From Lou HC, Lassen NA, Friis-Hansen B. Low cerebral blood flow in hypotensive perinatal distress. *J Pediatr.* 1979;94:118.)

Table 13.10). Infants without evidence of brain injury had normal values for CBF, intact autoregulation, and reactivity to $PaCO_2$. A later study of 16 term infants with hypoxic-ischemic encephalopathy used PET to determine CBF primarily at 1 to 4 days of life and found higher flows in those infants with abnormal neurological outcome (35.6 mL/100 g per minute) than in those with normal neurological outcome (18.3 mL/100 g per minute).[338]

The pronounced, sustained *cerebral hyperemia* observed in the human infant has been shown by less invasive techniques, such as Doppler ultrasound and near-infrared spectroscopy. Thus determinations of CBF velocity in term infants with hypoxic-ischemic encephalopathy from approximately 6 to 130 hours after the insult showed an increase in mean flow velocity with decreased resistance indices (i.e., vasodilation).[339-350] Similarly, studies of asphyxiated human infants on the first day of life by near-infrared spectroscopy are consistent with a loss of vascular reactivity and an increase in cerebral blood volume and CBF, with temporal characteristics similar to those observed in fetal sheep, described earlier.[215,351] The mechanism for this hyperemia is unclear. An increase in neuronal excitability, although documented after hypoxic-ischemic insults, seems unlikely in view of the relation of highest flows to isoelectric EEG. It appears more likely that an accumulation of vasodilatory compounds or vascular injury, or both, occurs and that this accumulation or injury in many ways may be similar in the human newborn and the perinatal animal. Delineation of the mechanisms underlying this vasoparalytic state and cerebral hyperemia after perinatal asphyxia in the human infant will be of major importance and may be able to be further explored with magnetic resonance techniques such as ASL.[285]

The aforementioned data thus define in the postasphyxial human newborn a state of *vasoparalysis* and *cerebral hyperemia* that is correlated with the degree of brain injury and presumably the severity of the asphyxial insult. The altered vascular reactivity, with autoregulation impaired more readily than carbon dioxide reactivity, is similar to observations made in the postasphyxial state in perinatal animal models (see earlier discussion). Presumably, a state of maximal vasodilation exists, related perhaps to the effects of elevated perivascular H^+ concentration, prostaglandins, adenosine, free radicals, or NO, or all these factors. Whether this hyperemic state is caused by the same factors that lead to the brain injury, is an adaptive mechanism to preserve brain tissue, or in some way causes additional brain injury remains to be clarified. It does appear likely that the loss of vascular reactivity renders the infant vulnerable to systemic hypotension and resulting cerebral ischemia.

BIOCHEMICAL MEDIATORS OF HYPOXIC-ISCHEMIC CEREBRAL INJURY—HUMAN NEWBORN AND RELEVANT EXPERIMENTAL MODELS

Normal Carbohydrate and Energy Metabolism

Because glucose and oxygen are the principal driving forces for energy production in brain, the major initial biochemical effects of well-established oxygen deprivation are exerted at the levels of carbohydrate and energy metabolism. A brief review of these areas of metabolism is appropriate here (see also Chapter 25). Detailed discussions are available from other, more specialized sources.[159,352-358]

Glucose Uptake

Glucose from blood is taken up by the brain through a process of carrier-mediated, facilitated diffusion that allows for the transport of glucose faster than would be expected by simple diffusion. Specific glucose transporter proteins are involved (see Chapter 25). The transport process, however, is not energy-dependent and thus differs in that critical fashion from active transport. Glucose transport across the blood-brain barrier uses the heavily glycosylated form of the facilitative glucose transporter protein, GLUT1 (55 kDa). Transport across glial membranes is facilitated by the lower molecular form of GLUT1 (45 kDa), and transport across the neuronal membrane is facilitated by GLUT3. The levels of these proteins are relatively low in the immature brain and are limiting to glucose transport and utilization.[352,353,355-357,359-363] Consistent with the experimental findings, elegant studies of human infants by PET show that the cerebral metabolic rate for glucose in the brain of preterm newborn infants is approximately one-third of that in the brain of adults and that this difference relates to a diminished transport capacity rather than a diminished affinity of the transporters for glucose.[364]

Formation of Glucose-6-Phosphate

Glucose in the brain is phosphorylated to glucose-6-phosphate; the enzyme involved is hexokinase (Fig. 13.20). The activity of hexokinase is linked to glucose uptake by the cell and is inhibited by the product of the reaction, glucose-6-phosphate. The activity of this enzyme is also lower in the neonatal versus adult rat brain.[352,353,356,357,365] Glucose-6-phosphate is a pivotal metabolite in glucose metabolism, with three major fates: (1) glycolysis and, ultimately, energy production; (2) glycogen

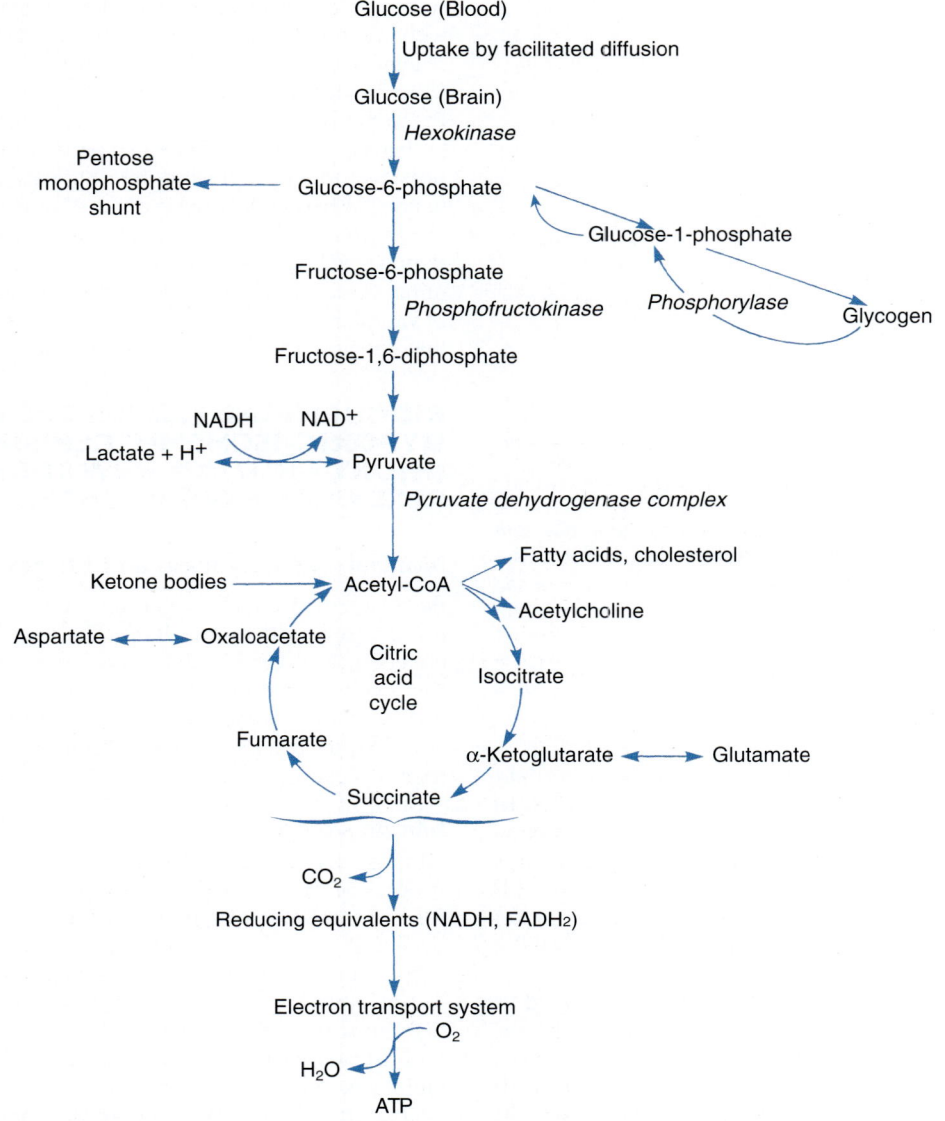

Figure 13.20 Major features of carbohydrate and energy metabolism in brain. See text for details. *ATP*, Adenosine triphosphate; *CoA*, coenzyme A; *FADH₂*, flavin adenine dinucleotide; *NADH*, nicotinamide adenine dinucleotide; *NAD⁺*, oxidized nicotinamide adenine dinucleotide.

synthesis; and (3) the pentose monophosphate shunt for synthesis of lipids (by formation of reduced nicotinamide adenine dinucleotide phosphate [NADPH]) and nucleic acids.

Glycogen Metabolism

Glycogen is found in relatively small concentrations in the brain but represents an important storage form of carbohydrate. Glycogen synthesis and degradation occur primarily in *astrocytes*.[358] Glycogen synthesis proceeds through glucose-1-phosphate and then to glycogen through glycogen synthetase. Glycogen breakdown to glucose-1-phosphate through phosphorylase, and then to glucose-6-phosphate through phosphoglucomutase, is an important mechanism for generating oxidizable substrate by the glycolytic pathway (see Fig. 13.20). Glycogen in astrocytes provides *fuel to neurons* first by conversion to *lactate* and then

transport of lactate by specific monocarboxylate transporters to neurons.[358,366] By a similar mechanism, astrocytes degrade glycogen to *lactate* that is provided to *developing oligodendrocytes*, primarily for lipid biosynthesis.[367] Brain phosphorylase is activated by cyclic adenosine monophosphate (AMP), and levels of cyclic AMP are elevated by certain hormones, such as epinephrine. Epinephrine release is accentuated sharply with hypoxic, ischemic, and asphyxial insults. Although glycogen is broken down in the perinatal brain under certain circumstances, the capacity of the perinatal degradative system, at least in the rodent brain, is considerably less than that in the adult.[368,369]

Glycolysis

The major portion of glucose-6-phosphate enters the glycolytic pathway to result ultimately in the formation of pyruvate. The major control step involves the conversion of fructose-6-phosphate to fructose-1,6-diphosphate; the rate-limiting enzyme involved is phosphofructokinase (see Fig. 13.20). The major mechanism of control of this enzyme is through *allosteric effects*—involving conformational changes of component peptides—and thus it is very rapid in onset. The activity of phosphofructokinase is inhibited by ATP, phosphocreatine (PCr), and low pH and activated by adenosine diphosphate (ADP), inorganic phosphorus (Pi), cyclic AMP, and ammonium ion.

Under *aerobic* conditions, the major product of glycolysis is pyruvate, which enters the mitochondrion and is converted through the pyruvate dehydrogenase complex to acetyl coenzyme A (acetyl-CoA; see Fig. 13.20). This mitochondrial enzyme is inhibited by an increase in the ATP/ADP ratio and is activated by a decrease in this ratio. Acetyl-CoA is used for fatty acid and cholesterol biosynthesis and for acetylcholine synthesis, but particularly for entry into the citric acid cycle for energy production.

Citric Acid Cycle and Electron Transport Chain

Mitochondrial acetyl-CoA enters the citric acid cycle and undergoes oxidation to carbon dioxide (see Fig. 13.20). The rate-limiting step is the conversion of isocitrate to alpha-ketoglutarate, catalyzed by the enzyme isocitrate dehydrogenase. A critical allosteric regulator of this enzyme is the ratio of ATP to ADP; an increase in the ratio causes a decrease in activity of the cycle, and a decrease in the ratio causes an increase in activity of the cycle. The electrons or reducing equivalents (reduced nicotinamide adenine dinucleotide [NADH], flavin adenine dinucleotide [FADH]) generated by the citric acid cycle next enter the electron transport system.

The transport of electrons takes place through a multimember chain of electron carrier proteins and is associated with release of free energy, which is used to generate ATP from ADP and Pi. The free energy, in essence, is "captured" in this high-energy phosphate bond. ATP is generated at three steps in the scheme, and because the final electron acceptor is oxygen, the process is called *oxidative phosphorylation*. Molecular oxygen is reduced, and water is the final product formed. The ATP generated by the citric acid cycle and the electron transport system is transported from the mitochondrion by a specific carrier and ultimately is used in the brain primarily for *transport processes* (especially of ions and neurotransmitters for impulse transmission and for the prevention of dangerous increases thereof; e.g., extracellular glutamate, cytosolic Ca^{2+}) and for *synthetic processes* (especially of neurotransmitters, but also lipids and proteins, particularly in the developing brain). The principal ions involved in ATP consumption are sodium (Na^+), potassium (K^+), and Ca^{2+}; in the adult brain (under normal conditions), approximately 60% to 75% of ATP is used for maintenance of membrane gradients of these three ions, especially Na^+ and K^+.[356,358]

Summary

The concerted action of glycolysis, the citric acid cycle, and the electron transport system, operative under aerobic conditions, results in the formation of 38 molecules of ATP for each molecule of glucose oxidized (Fig. 13.21). The glycolytic portion of the pathway occurs in the cytosol and generates only 2 of the 38 molecules of ATP; the bulk of the ATP is generated in the mitochondrial portion of the pathway, which begins with pyruvate. The ATP generated is transported from

$$Glucose + 2\ NAD^+ + 2\ ADP + 2\ P_i \longrightarrow 2\ Pyruvate + 2\ NADH + 2\ ATP$$

$$2\ Pyruvate + 2\ NADH + 36\ ADP + 36\ P_i + 6\ O_2 \longrightarrow 2\ NAD^+ + 6\ CO_2 + 44\ H_2O + 36\ ATP$$

SUM:
$$Glucose + 38\ ADP + 38\ P_i + 6\ O_2 \longrightarrow 6\ CO_2 + 44\ H_2O + \boxed{38\ ATP}$$

Figure 13.21 Energy production from glucose under aerobic conditions. Contrast with production under anaerobic conditions (see Fig. 13.21). *ADP,* Adenosine diphosphate; *ATP,* adenosine triphosphate; *NADH,* reduced nicotinamide adenine dinucleotide; *NAD⁺,* oxidized nicotinamide adenine dinucleotide; *Pᵢ,* inorganic phosphate.

TABLE 13.11	Effects of Hypoxemia on Carbohydrate and Energy Metabolism
↑ Glucose influx to brain	
↑ Glycogenolysis	
↑ Glycolysis	
↓ Brain glucose	
↑ Lactate production and tissue acidosis	
↓ Phosphocreatine	
↓ Adenosine triphosphate	

the mitochondrion by a specific carrier and is used in the brain for two major purposes: *transport* and *synthetic processes*. Quantitatively, the most important transport processes involve ions in neurons for impulse transmission and maintenance of Ca^{2+} homeostasis. Synthetic processes are important in the developing brain and involve neurotransmitters, structural and functional proteins, and membrane lipids.

Effects of Hypoxemia on Carbohydrate and Energy Metabolism

Major Changes

Hypoxemia is accompanied by numerous effects on carbohydrate and energy metabolism in the brain (Table 13.11),[159,352,353,370,371] effects that are understandable when viewed in the context of the normal metabolism just reviewed. Although it is likely that lack of oxygen is the major pathogenetic factor in these changes, it is difficult to produce hypoxemia experimentally without also causing other major metabolic changes that either accompany the hypoxemic insult or occur as a consequence of the insult (e.g., hypercapnia, acidosis, and hypotension). In most studies, however, these other changes either are prevented or are documented.

The quantitative and temporal aspects of the biochemical changes associated with a severe hypoxemic or anoxic insult (i.e., nitrogen breathing) in the newborn mouse are depicted in Figs. 13.3 to 13.5.[372] The earliest significant changes are a decrease in brain glycogen, an elevation in lactate, and a decrease in PCr. These are followed by a decrease in brain glucose and, finally, ATP. The changes appear to reflect principally the impaired production of high-energy phosphate, secondary to failure of the coupled mitochondrial system of the citric acid cycle and electron transport chain—in turn, a consequence of the lack of the ultimate electron acceptor, oxygen. In response to the anaerobic state, glycolysis becomes the sole source of ATP

$$\text{Glucose} + 2\,\text{ADP} + 2\,P_i \longrightarrow 2\,\text{Lactate}^- + 2\,H^+ + \boxed{2\,\text{ATP}}$$

Figure 13.22 Energy production from glucose under anaerobic conditions. Contrast with production under aerobic conditions (see Fig. 13.20). *ADP,* Adenosine diphosphate; *ATP,* adenosine triphosphate; $P_i,$ inorganic phosphate.

production, and because lactate is the principal product of anaerobic glycolysis, only two molecules of ADP are generated for each molecule of glucose metabolized (Fig. 13.22). This number is clearly a serious difference from the 38 molecules generated under aerobic conditions (see Fig. 13.21). Glycolysis is accelerated 5- to 10-fold, and an attempt to meet this enhanced need for glucose is made by a combination of glycogenolysis and increased net uptake of glucose from blood.[372] (Glycogen contributes approximately one third of the cerebral energy supply under these conditions.[373]) Despite this acceleration, brain energy demands cannot be met, and ATP levels begin to fall after 2 minutes and decrease by 30% after 6 minutes.

The relationship between arterial oxygen delivery and brain PCr levels (expressed as the ratio of PCr to Pi determined by MR spectroscopy) has been clarified in studies of the neonatal dog.[374,375] Thus a crucial threshold decrease in the PCr/Pi ratio of 50% occurred when arterial oxygen pressure decreased to 12 mm Hg (approximate arterial oxygen saturation, 20%).[375] The importance of the 50% decrease in PCr/Pi ratio relates to the finding in the neonatal piglet that at this level, brain lipid peroxidation and impaired Na^+/K^+-ATPase activity occur.[376] The critical value of arterial partial pressure of oxygen (PaO_2) required to lead to the 50% decline in the PCr/Pi ratio in the neonatal dog (12 mm Hg) was higher at 7 to 21 days (17 mm Hg) and higher in the adult (23 mm Hg).[375] This lower threshold value of PaO_2 in the neonatal animal correlated with in vitro data showing more efficient oxygen extraction in the neonatal animals (see later discussion). At any rate, it is clear that *marked hypoxemia* is required to produce serious changes in the brain energy state in the neonatal animal.

Maturational Vulnerability. Studies of the effect of hypoxemia on brain energy metabolism in the immature rat brain have delineated a particular window of vulnerability.[377,378] Thus the most marked declines in PCr and nucleoside triphosphates, defined by MR spectroscopy, occurred in the second postnatal week. This period of heightened vulnerability corresponds with the period of maximal susceptibility to excitotoxic neuronal injury and to epileptogenic effects of hypoxia,[379-381] as well as with the period of maximal expression of specific excitatory amino acid receptors, incomplete maturation of inhibitory transmission, relatively low levels of Ca^{2+} binding proteins, and incomplete maturation of Na^+/K^+-ATPase levels (see later discussion).[382] Taken together, these data suggest that the vulnerability of the immature rat in the second versus the first week of life relates to the increased propensity to develop with hypoxia, a hyperexcitable, hypermetabolic state in neurons, which leads to more marked declines in high-energy phosphates because of increased utilization. These considerations could help explain the greater likelihood of *neuronal* injury with hypoxia in the term brain than in the premature brain of the human.

Regional Vulnerability. Studies in the newborn dog defined the *regional* changes in glucose and high-energy metabolism.[116]

TABLE 13.12	Mechanisms for Increased Cytosolic Calcium in Neurons With Hypoxia-Ischemia
SITE	**MECHANISM**[a]
Plasma membrane	↑ Ca^{2+} influx through voltage-dependent Ca^{2+} channels *(cell depolarization)*
	↑ Ca^{2+} influx through agonist-dependent Ca^{2+} channels *(glutamate action at NMDA and immature AMPA receptors)*[b]
	Activation of phospholipase C and liberation of IP_3 (see below) *(glutamate action at metabotropic receptor)*
	↓ Ca^{2+} efflux through ATP-dependent uniport system *(ATP depletion)*
	↓ Ca^{2+} efflux through Na^+-dependent antiport system *(↓ extracellular Na^+)*
Endoplasmic reticulum	↑ Ca^{2+} release to cytosol through effect of IP_3 (see above)
	↓ Ca^{2+} uptake by ATP-dependent uniport system *(ATP depletion)*
Mitochondrion	↑ Ca^{2+} release to cytosol via Na^+,H^+–dependent antiport system *(↑ cytosolic Na^+,H^+)*

[a]The primary effect of ischemia to cause the indicated change in Ca^{2+} homeostasis is shown in parentheses.
[b]Probably the single most important mechanism.
AMPA, Alpha-amino-3-hydroxy-5-methyl-4-isoxazole-propionic acid; *ATP,* adenosine triphosphate; *Ca^{2+},* calcium; *H^+,* hydrogen; *IP_3,* inositol triphosphate; *Na^+,* sodium; *NMDA,* N-methyl-D-aspartate.

Thus animals subjected to acute hypoxemia (oxygen pressure [PO_2] ≈ 12 mm Hg) and studied by the autoradiographic 2-[^{14}C]deoxyglucose technique exhibited increased glucose utilization in most gray matter structures and every white matter structure. Moreover, the degree of hypoxemia was sufficient to cause the accumulation of lactate in the brain in both gray and white matter, but only in white matter did a decline in energy state occur (Table 13.12). *Thus it appears that anaerobic glycolysis with its accelerated glucose utilization was capable of preserving the energy state in gray matter but not in white matter.* Moreover, the finding that glucose levels declined more drastically in white matter than in gray matter (see Table 13.12) suggests that glucose influx could not meet the increased demands for glucose in white matter. That the rate of glucose metabolism, in fact, was *limited by glucose influx from blood* is supported by the demonstration that local CBF increased insignificantly in relation to white matter but dramatically in relation to gray matter.[108] The apparently limited vasodilatory capacity in white matter is discussed in the section on CBF, but *this imbalance between glucose needs and glucose delivery may contribute to the propensity of neonatal cerebral white matter to hypoxic injury.*

Mechanisms

The mechanisms for the biochemical effects relate to several factors (Table 13.13). ATP levels are preserved initially at the expense of PCr. The *initial* fall in PCr, the principal storage

TABLE 13.13   Deleterious Effects of Calcium in Hypoxia-Ischemia

CALCIUM ACTION	DELETERIOUS EFFECT
Activate phospholipases	Phospholipid hydrolysis and membrane injury Generation of arachidonic acid and ultimately free radicals by cyclooxygenase and lipoxygenase pathways
Activate proteases, disassembly of microtubules	Cytoskeletal disruption (caused by microtubular disruption and proteolysis of neurofilaments) Proteolysis of other cellular proteins
Activate nucleases	Nuclear injury
Activate calcium-ATPase and other energy-dependent calcium extrusion mechanisms	Consumption of ATP at a time of deficient ATP
Enter mitochondrion and uncouple oxidative phosphorylation	Decrease in ATP production
Increase neurotransmitter release (e.g., glutamate, catecholamines)	Activation of glutamate receptors (e.g., calcium influx) Autooxidation of catecholamines with production of free radicals
Activate a protease for transformation of xanthine dehydrogenase to xanthine oxidase	Oxidation of hypoxanthine to xanthine and of xanthine to uric acid with production of free radicals
Activate nitric oxide synthase	Generation of nitric oxide and ultimately peroxynitrite, with toxic effect on neurons

ATP, Adenosine triphosphate.

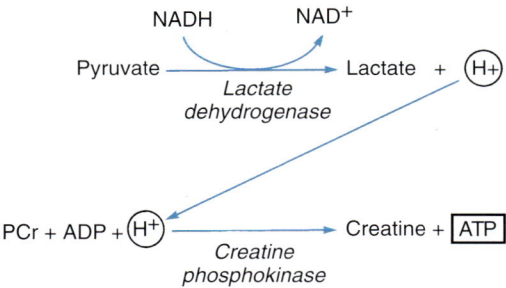

Figure 13.23 **Link between lactate production and hydrolysis of phosphocreatine.** Adenosine triphosphate (ATP) formation is the result. *ADP,* Adenosine diphosphate; *NADH,* reduced nicotinamide adenine dinucleotide; *NAD+,* oxidized nicotinamide adenine dinucleotide; *PCr,* phosphocreatine.

form of high-energy phosphate in brain, relates primarily to the shift in the creatine phosphokinase reaction induced by the hydrogen ion (H^+) generated with lactate formation by anaerobic glycolysis (Fig. 13.23). Later, the creatine phosphokinase reaction is driven by elevated concentrations of both ADP and H^+. The *initial acceleration of glycolysis and the glycogenolysis* may relate to primarily a rise in cyclic AMP levels in the brain, demonstrated to be approximately threefold in the rat after only 30 seconds of nitrogen breathing.[383] Cyclic AMP leads to activation of

phosphorylase for glycogenolysis and of phosphofructokinase (and hexokinase) for glycolysis.[384-386] Further activation of phosphofructokinase and hence glycolysis occurs as ATP levels fall and ADP and Pi levels rise. The fall in brain glucose occurs because the continued excessive utilization of glucose through anaerobic glycolysis, a most inefficient means of generating ATP, outstrips the capacity for glucose delivery from blood. Indeed, after 6 minutes, brain glucose levels had decreased by more than 70%, whereas blood glucose levels had increased by nearly 100% (see Fig. 13.3).[372] *Thus blood glucose level no longer reflected the brain glucose level, an observation of particular clinical relevance.*

The accumulation of lactate and the associated H^+ is worthy of additional emphasis because this accumulation *initially* is a *beneficial* adaptive response to oxygen deprivation, but *later* it can be a serious *deleterious* factor. Thus, initially, the tissue acidosis leads to the generation of ATP from PCr (because of the shift in the creatine phosphokinase reaction) and also to an increase in CBF (because of the local effect of elevated perivascular H^+ concentration on vascular smooth muscle). However, with the progression of lactate formation, severe tissue acidosis develops, and three deleterious effects ensue. The first is an impairment of vascular autoregulation and the potential for ischemic injury to the brain when cerebral perfusion pressure falls (e.g., secondary to the often associated myocardial injury). Second, phosphofructokinase activity is inhibited by low pH, and thus the brain's remaining source of ATP (i.e., glycolysis) is eliminated. Finally, advanced tissue acidosis leads directly to cellular injury and, ultimately, necrosis. A correlation between brain lactate concentration and cellular injury has been demonstrated in the primate brain (see the next section).

Effects of Hypoxia-Ischemia on Carbohydrate and Energy Metabolism

Major Changes

Hypoxic-ischemic insults are accompanied by effects on carbohydrate and energy metabolism in the brain (Table 13.14) that exhibit important similarities to those observed with hypoxemia. Certain differences occur with the addition of ischemia. In earlier years, the most frequently used models with perinatal animals included decapitation, severe hypotension, or occlusion of blood vessels supplying the cranium.[a] The most widely used model in the past 20 years has involved the Vannucci adaptation of the Levine model of unilateral carotid artery ligation, followed by systemic hypoxemia for generally 1 to 3 hours, a procedure that results in hypoxic-ischemic neuronal and white matter injury.[355,393] The combination of hypoxemia and ischemia (i.e., *hypoxic-ischemic insult*) is most relevant to the situation in vivo in the human fetus and newborn. The effects of such an insult on carbohydrate and energy metabolism have been studied in detail in experimental models.[b]

The biochemical features relative to carbohydrate and energy metabolism bear many similarities to those recorded previously for purely hypoxemic insults (see Table 13.14). In the most commonly used model, the hypoxic-ischemic insult is produced in the 7-day-old rat (approximately analogous to a preterm human newborn brain) by a combination of unilateral carotid occlusion and breathing of a low-oxygen (usually 8%) gas

[a]References 100, 239, 240, 355, 357, 368, 369, and 387-392.
[b]References 352, 353, 355, 357, 363, 384, and 392-413.

TABLE 13.14   Free Radicals in Hypoxia-Ischemia

Sources
Mitochondrial electron transport system
Action of cyclooxygenase and lipoxygenase on arachidonic acid
Action of xanthine oxidase on hypoxanthine and xanthine
Autooxidation of catecholamines
Infiltrating reactive microglia
Action of nitric oxide synthase

Endogenous defenses
Major: superoxide dismutase (generates H_2O_2), catalase
(degrades H_2O_2), and glutathione peroxidase (degrades
H_2O_2)
Free radical scavengers: vitamin E (alpha-tocopherol), other
sterols (21-aminosteroids), vitamin C (ascorbic acid),
glutathione, other thiol compounds

Major deleterious effects
Peroxidation of PUFAs of membrane phospholipids (PUFAs
especially abundant in brain membranes)
Damage to DNA and to proteins containing unsaturated or
sulfhydryl groups
Activation of proapoptotic genes

H_2O_2, Hydrogen peroxide; *PUFAs*, polyunsaturated fatty acids.

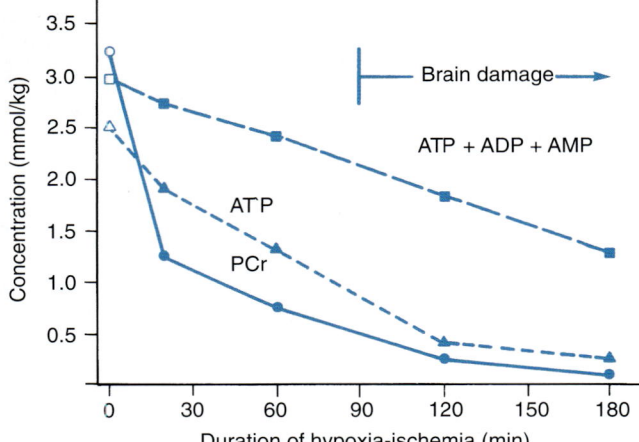

Figure 13.24 Changes in cerebral high-energy phosphate reserves during hypoxia-ischemia in the immature rat. Seven-day-old postnatal rats were subjected to unilateral common carotid artery ligation followed by exposure to hypoxia with 8% oxygen at 37°C. Symbols represent means for adenosine triphosphate (ATP), phosphocreatine (PCr), and total adenine nucleotides (ATP+ADP+AMP). All values are significantly different from control (zero time point). Histological brain damage commences after 90 minutes of hypoxia-ischemia, with increasing severity thereafter. (From Vannucci RC. Experimental biology of cerebral hypoxia-ischemia: relation to perinatal brain damage. *Pediatr Res.* 1990;27:317–326.)

mixture. The *importance of ischemia* in the genesis of the brain injury in this model has been demonstrated by the findings that (1) carotid ligation alone does not lead to a decrease in CBF to the ipsilateral hemisphere, (2) the addition of the hypoxemia leads to marked disturbances in regional blood flow to the ipsilateral hemisphere, and (3) the topography of the injury to this hemisphere correlates closely with the topography of the decreases in regional CBF.[396] Vannucci and colleagues defined the major biochemical changes most clearly.[a] The initial biochemical changes are compatible with accelerated anaerobic glycolysis with lactate accumulation and glycogenolysis. Particular importance for an increased capacity for glucose uptake in the acceleration of glucose utilization has been shown by the demonstration of elevation in the levels of the glucose transporter proteins, GLUT1 (55 kDa) and GLUT3, for transport of glucose across the blood-brain barrier and the neuronal membrane, respectively, in the brain of hypoxic-ischemic 7-day-old rat pups in the first 4 hours after the insult.[363] As with hypoxemia, a role for cyclic AMP in the induction of the glycolysis and glycogenolysis is suggested by marked rises (13-fold) in the levels of this mononucleotide in the first minutes after the onset of ischemia.[414] Nevertheless, brain glucose concentrations fall more severely than with the anoxia of nitrogen breathing; after 2 minutes of ischemia, glucose had decreased markedly, whereas only a modest decrease occurred with nitrogen breathing after this time. Of course, this difference relates to the impairment of CBF and therefore glucose supply with ischemia. An additional difference between ischemia and hypoxemia is the more drastic increase in lactate and tissue acidosis with ischemia, because the circulation is interrupted.[370] The more severe tissue acidosis obtains because the impaired cerebral circulation results in (1) diminished clearance of

accumulated lactate and (2) diminished buffering of tissue carbon dioxide by the bicarbonate buffering system.[370] The increased ratio of lactate to pyruvate in the cytosol is reflected in increased reduction (i.e., decrease) of the $NAD^+/NADH$ ratio. The latter ratio is more oxidized in the mitochondrion because of the limitation in cellular substrate (glucose) supply. (This important limiting role of brain glucose is discussed in more detail later concerning brain carbohydrate status and hypoxic-ischemic injury.) Perhaps most important, high-energy phosphate levels begin to decline within minutes, with the reservoir form, PCr, falling first (Fig. 13.24).[384] Histological evidence of brain injury becomes apparent after approximately 90 minutes.

The particular importance of *ischemia* in the genesis of the deleterious effects of hypoxic-ischemic insults was also shown in the fetal lamb and neonatal piglet.[391,401-403,415,416] In *both animal models, marked hypoxemia did not result in brain injury unless hypotension supervened.* In the piglet, hypotension appeared to be a particular consequence of cardiac dysfunction, and the latter was especially correlated with severe systemic acidosis. In the fetal lamb, pronounced decreases in brain glucose and in high-energy phosphate levels, accompanied by an increase in lactate levels to as high as 16 to 24 mM, were the principal biochemical effects on carbohydrate and energy metabolism. These effects were particularly pronounced in cerebral white matter (Table 13.15). *This regional predilection may be relevant to the propensity of white matter to exhibit injury with hypotension in the premature newborn* (see Chapters 14 to 16).

Secondary Energy Failure

The temporal aspects of the changes in glucose and energy metabolism after hypoxic-ischemic insult in *the living animal*

TABLE 13.15   Glutamate Receptors[a]

TYPE	FUNCTION
Ionotropic	
NMDA	Ca^{2+} entry, Na^+ entry
AMPA	Na^+ entry, Ca^{2+} entry (*immature neurons*)[b]
Kainate	Na^+ entry
Metabotropic	
Ibotenate	Phosphoinositide hydrolysis; protein kinase C activation; Ca^{2+} mobilization from endoplasmic reticulum; multiple downstream effects

[a]The receptors are named according to the glutamate analogue most potent in activation of the individual receptor.

[b]In immature neurons AMPA receptors lack the GluR2 subunit, the subunit which renders the receptor Ca^{2+} impermeable, thus resulting in Ca^{2+}-permeable receptors.

AMPA, Alpha-amino-3-hydroxy-5-methyl-4-isoxazolepropionic acid; *Ca*$^{2+}$, calcium; *Na*$^+$, sodium; *NMDA,* N-methyl-D-aspartate.

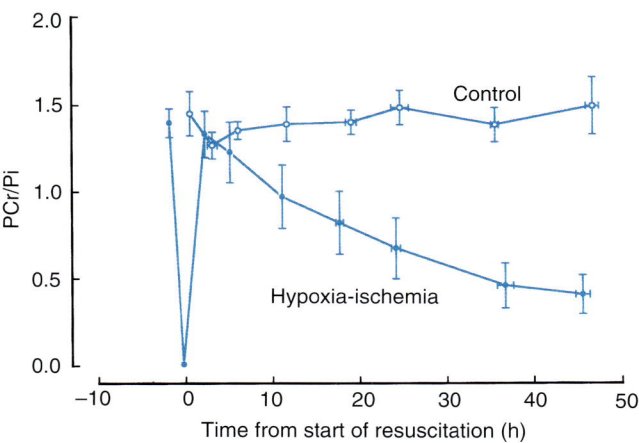

Figure 13.25   High-energy phosphate levels in hypoxia-ischemia in brain of neonatal piglets. Note the sharp decline with the insult, followed by a recovery to baseline in 2 to 3 hours. A few hours later, a second decline ensues and constitutes "secondary energy failure" (see text). PCr, Phosphocreatine; Pi, inorganic phosphate. (From Lorek A, Takei Y, Cady EB, et al. Delayed ("secondary") cerebral energy failure after acute hypoxia-ischemia in the newborn piglet: continuous 48-hour studies by phosphorus magnetic resonance spectroscopy. *Pediatr Res.* 1994;36:699–706.)

have been identified best by studies of the neonatal piglet with phosphorus and proton MR spectroscopy and have defined a delayed, secondary energy failure.[411-413,416] Thus, immediately after the insult, as expected, a marked increase in cerebral lactate levels and a marked decrease in high-energy phosphate levels were documented (i.e., primary energy failure). High-energy phosphate levels *recovered* to baseline levels in 2 to 3 hours (Fig. 13.25); lactate levels improved but did not recover completely. A second decline in high-energy phosphate levels then occurred in the next 24 hours and was especially pronounced at 48 hours (see Fig. 13.25). This *secondary energy failure* and the earlier rise in cerebral lactate levels *have been documented in the human term newborn* subjected to apparent hypoxic-ischemic insult in the context of perinatal asphyxia (see Chapters 18 to 20).[417,418] The onset of the secondary decline in high-energy phosphates varies according to the species and nature of the insult, but in general the onset is clear by 8 to 16 hours and reaches a nadir at 24 to 48 hours. A *major question has been whether the secondary energy decline causes or accentuates brain injury or whether the decline is a consequence of the injury.*

A particularly informative study of the neonatal rat (unilateral carotid ligation and hypoxemia on postnatal day 7) confirmed the occurrence of secondary energy failure, with onset at approximately 18 to 24 hours and a nadir at 48 hours.[419] However, immunocytochemical studies showed that the loss of neuronal proteins became apparent at 6 hours and was very pronounced at 18 hours (i.e., *before* the onset of the secondary energy failure). The temporal characteristics and the additional finding of a loss of total creatine and adenine nucleotides supported the conclusion that the secondary energy depletion is a *consequence* rather than a *cause* of cellular destruction. As discussed earlier, in the hours after the hypoxic-ischemic insult, a cascade of events, including accumulation of excitotoxic amino acids, cytosolic Ca^{2+}, activation of phospholipases, generation of free radicals, and a series of related metabolic events, develops and leads to cell death. The crucial mitochondrial disturbance that precipitates this cascade of deleterious events is responsible for the primary energy failure and *persists* into the period *after* the termination of the insult despite initial recovery of high-energy

phosphates (see later discussion). The particular vulnerability of the mitochondrion during and after ischemia is supported by biochemical and morphological data.[a] Investigators have suggested that the secondary energy failure *initiates* the cascade of events just noted. However, the work just described[419] appears to favor the notion that the secondary energy depletion is a *consequence* of the cascade of events and the resulting cell death.

Effects of Asphyxia on Carbohydrate and Energy Metabolism

Asphyxia, rather than hypoxemia or ischemia or both, is the most common *clinical* insult in the perinatal period that results in the brain injury under discussion. Although hypoxemia and ischemia usually occur concurrently or in sequence with perinatal asphyxia, certain additional metabolic effects, particularly hypercapnia, are prominent. Most experimental studies of perinatal asphyxia have involved lambs and monkeys and have been concerned with changes in CBF and with the neuropathology (see later sections on CBF and Chapters 14, 15, 18, and 19). Some work has provided useful information regarding the biochemical (as well as the physiological) effects in the brain with neonatal asphyxia and is reviewed next.[415,421-427]

Major Changes

Striking changes in biochemical, cardiovascular, cerebrovascular, and electrophysiological parameters were observed in neonatal dogs subjected to ventilatory standstill after paralysis with succinylcholine or curare.[428] *Survival* occurred in all animals after 10 minutes of asphyxia, in two-thirds after 15 minutes of asphyxia, but in only one-fourth after 20 minutes of asphyxia. Changes in *arterial blood gas levels and acid-base status* were dramatic. Thus, after $2\frac{1}{2}$ minutes of respiratory arrest, PaO_2 had fallen to 4 mm Hg, partial pressure of carbon dioxide ($PaCO_2$)

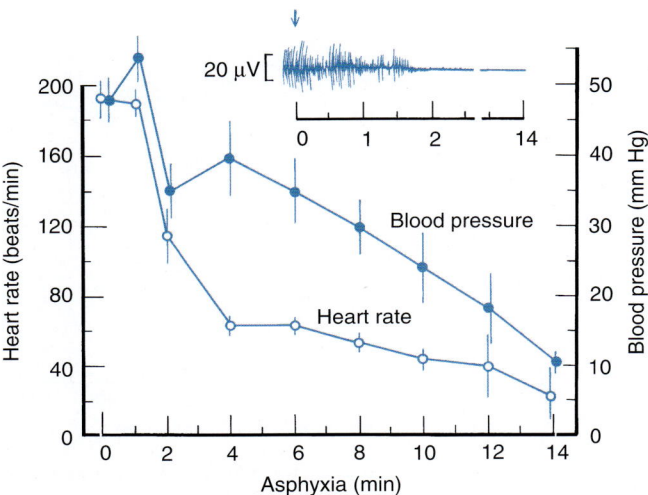

Figure 13.26 Cardiovascular and electroencephalographic effects of asphyxia (respiratory arrest) in newborn dogs. A representative electroencephalogram during 14 minutes of asphyxia is shown in the *upper right*; the *arrow* indicates the onset of respiratory arrest. (From Vannucci RC, Duffy TE. Cerebral metabolism in newborn dogs during reversible asphyxia. *Ann Neurol.* 1977;1:528–534.)

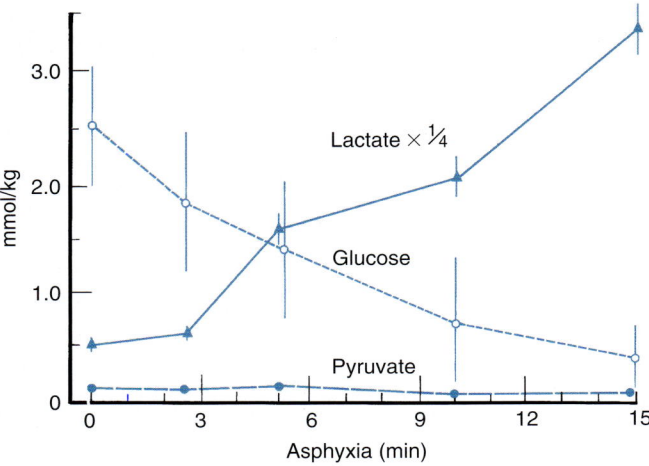

Figure 13.27 Biochemical effects of asphyxia. Concentrations of glucose, pyruvate, and lactate in brain of newborn dogs as a function of duration of asphyxia (respiratory arrest). (From Vannucci RC, Duffy TE. Cerebral metabolism in newborn dogs during reversible asphyxia. *Ann Neurol.* 1977;1:528–534.)

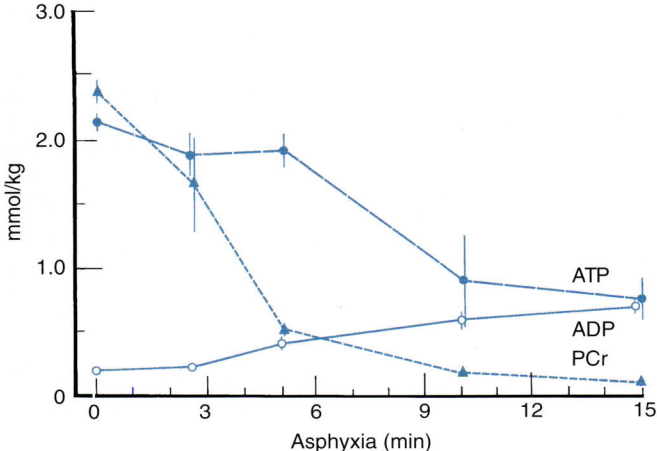

Figure 13.28 Biochemical effects of asphyxia. Concentrations of adenosine triphosphate (ATP), adenosine diphosphate (ADP), and phosphocreatine (PCr) in brain of newborn dogs as a function of duration of asphyxia (respiratory arrest). (From Vannucci RC, Duffy TE. Cerebral metabolism in newborn dogs during reversible asphyxia. *Ann Neurol.* 1977;1:528–534.)

had risen to 51 mm Hg (from control value of 35), and pH had fallen to 7.18 (from control value of 7.38). After 10 minutes, $PaCO_2$ was 100 mm Hg, and pH was 6.79. *Cardiovascular* effects were also marked (Fig. 13.26); MABP declined gradually to a low of 10 mm Hg after 14 minutes, and bradycardia was marked after only 4 minutes. *Cerebral perfusion*, assessed qualitatively by carbon black infusion, overall appeared to decline *pari passu* with MABP, although diminutions were greatest in cerebral cortex and least in brain stem. This more severe affection of *cerebral* flow has been reproduced in other neonatal models of asphyxia (see later discussion). The *EEG* demonstrated rapid deterioration (see Fig. 13.26); between 1 and 2 minutes after the onset of asphyxia, a distinct reduction in the amplitude and frequency occurred, and by $2\frac{1}{2}$ minutes, the EEG was isoelectric. The occurrence of the isoelectric EEG did *not* correlate with any marked change in cerebral perfusion or with any measurable change in brain lactate or ATP levels. In the asphyxiated fetal sheep, this suppression of EEG, initially an energy-conserving protective effect, is mediated by adenosine, an inhibitory neurotransmitter.[427]

Biochemical effects were qualitatively similar to those observed with hypoxemia or ischemia or both (Figs. 13.27 and 13.28). Thus the brain glucose level declined rapidly (despite normal blood glucose level), lactate concentration rose (after a $2\frac{1}{2}$-minute delay), and PCr concentration decreased markedly (to values $\approx 20\%$ of control within 5 minutes). However, ATP levels were maintained for 6 minutes of asphyxia but then declined by 10 minutes. The changes in high-energy phosphates have been documented in the living animal by MR spectroscopy.[421] Thus, after 5 minutes of asphyxia, in which electrocerebral silence occurred after 3 minutes, a 40% decrease in the PCr/Pi ratio and a 30% decrease in the ATP/Pi ratio occurred. Despite these changes, on reinstitution of ventilatory support, cerebral metabolism returned to normal within 20 to 30 minutes. However, studies in neonatal piglets showed that during a similar recovery period after an even less severe asphyxial

insult (2 to 3 minutes), evidence for lipid peroxidation and altered membrane function (depressed Na^+/K^+-ATPase activity) was demonstrable.[423] Production of *intrauterine* asphyxia by impairment of placental blood flow also decreases cerebral high-energy phosphate levels, as measured by MR spectroscopy in the living animal.[429]

Additional Effects of Asphyxia (vs. Solely Hypoxemia or Ischemia or Both)

At least four major factors are added to the constellation of biochemical features controlling the outcome of asphyxia, with its attendant increase in $PaCO_2$. The first three of these factors appear to be beneficial, at least initially, and the fourth of these appears deleterious. *First*, the hypercapnia acts to maintain or even augment CBF through an increase in the perivascular H^+ concentration in the brain, which may be beneficial early in asphyxia. *Second*, the hypercapnia may be associated with a diminution in cerebral metabolic rate. Moderate hypercapnia has been shown to cause a diminution in cerebral metabolic rate in the adult rat brain, adult monkey brain, and developing rat brain.[362,430-432] *Third*, an increase in PaCO$_2$ leads to acidemia, which is accompanied by a shift in the oxygen-hemoglobin dissociation curve such that the affinity of hemoglobin for oxygen is decreased. The result is an increase in the delivery of oxygen to cells. The operation of one or more of these three factors could underlie the protective effect of moderate hypercapnia in immature rats subjected to hypoxia-ischemia.[162,355] The *fourth* important factor relative to hypercapnia and the outcome with asphyxia may be deleterious; intracellular pH falls more drastically for a given amount of lactate formed when the effect of elevated PCO$_2$ is added by asphyxia.[370,422] Thus extreme acidosis and consequent tissue injury could result. Future studies directed at defining the relative roles of these four factors in the genesis of the biochemical and physiological derangements associated with asphyxia in the perinatal animal will be of great interest.

Influence of Carbohydrate Status on Hypoxic-Ischemic Brain Injury

Deleterious Role of Low Brain Glucose in Perinatal Animals

A series of older studies with immature animals suggests a beneficial effect of prior administration of glucose and a deleterious effect of hypoglycemia on the survival response to anoxic insult (i.e., nitrogen breathing).[433-436] The effects of glucose appeared to be exerted on the central nervous system rather than on the heart, because the time to last gasp was altered before cardiac function. This observation is compatible with data indicating the particular resistance of the immature heart to combined hypoxia and hypoglycemia, presumably because of rich carbohydrate stores and high glycogenolytic and glycolytic capacities.[437-439] Later work on the survival and neuropathological response to hypoxia and ischemia of neonatal animals also has demonstrated a beneficial effect of pretreatment with glucose and a deleterious effect of hypoglycemia (Fig. 13.29).[352,353,387,440-443] One study of 185 term human infants who had sustained apparent intrapartum asphyxia (markedly low cord pH) showed a deleterious effect of initial *hypoglycemia* on neurological outcome.[444] Thus, of infants who had initial blood glucose values lower than 40 mg/dL, 56% had an abnormal neurological outcome, versus only 16% among those with initial blood glucose values higher than 40 mg/dL. This apparent deleterious effect of hypoglycemia was also documented in a study focused on the neuroimaging correlates of hypoglycemia in the term-born infant that revealed patterns of brain injury similar to those of hypoxic-ischemic injury.[445] Importantly, in this study the majority of infants had low initial Apgar scores with or without acidemia, suggesting that the hypoglycemia was complicating an underlying asphyxial cerebral insult.

Importance of Endogenous Brain Glucose Reserves. The biochemical mechanisms for the relation between carbohydrate status and resistance to hypoxic-ischemic insult relate to glycolytic capacity. Thus, with hypoxic-ischemic states, the replenishment of brain high-energy phosphate levels depends on anaerobic glycolysis. Because of the 19-fold reduction in ATP production per molecule of glucose when the brain is forced to oxidize glucose anaerobically, the glycolytic rate must

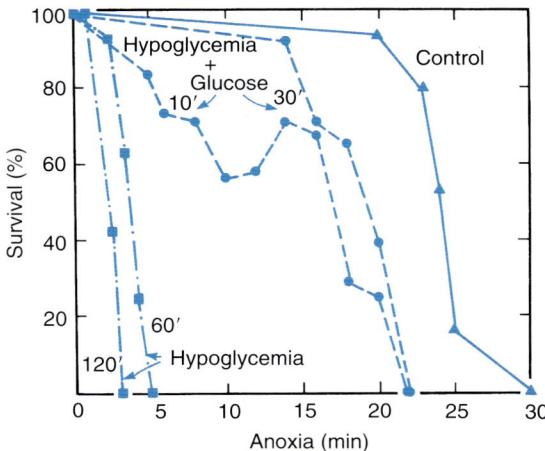

Figure 13.29 **Deleterious effect of hypoglycemia on vulnerability to anoxia (nitrogen breathing).** The percentage of survival of newborn rats was determined as a function of duration of anoxia. Hypoglycemia was produced by insulin injection 1 to 2 hours before onset of anoxia; some hypoglycemic animals were pretreated with glucose (1.8 g/kg subcutaneously) either 10 or 30 minutes before anoxia. (From Vannucci RC, Vannucci SJ. Cerebral carbohydrate metabolism during hypoglycemia and anoxia in newborn rats. *Ann Neurol.* 1978;4:73–79.)

be enhanced greatly. The adaptive mechanisms that come into play for this purpose are summarized in the previous sections. The greatly enhanced glycolytic rate leads to a decline of brain glucose levels.[a] If this decline is prevented (e.g., by prior administration of glucose), the glycolytic rate and hence ATP production are increased, and the biochemical and clinical outcome for animals rendered hypoxic or partially ischemic is improved considerably.[b] Indeed, the careful studies of Vannucci et al.[352,353,442] indicated that the major factor accounting for the difference in outcome between normoglycemic and hypoglycemic animals rendered hypoxic is the amount of *endogenous brain glucose reserves* at the time of the insult. In hypoglycemic animals, a 10- to 20-fold reduction in endogenous brain glucose resulted and correlated best with the impaired glycolytic rate and the decline in high-energy phosphate levels in brain with nitrogen breathing. Brain glycogen levels seemed less important. Thus the capacity for surviving hypoxemia was reduced fivefold in hypoglycemic animals at a time (i.e., 60 minutes after insulin injection) when the brain glycogen level was reduced by only 20%, but brain glucose level was reduced by more than 10-fold (Fig. 13.30). Similarly, reversal of the vulnerability correlated with a rapid normalization of brain glucose levels but no significant change in brain glycogen levels.

Summary. Taken together, these data on immature animals (principally rodents) indicate that carbohydrate status plays an important role in determining the biochemical and clinical responses to hypoxemic and ischemic insults. Hypoglycemia is deleterious, and pretreatment with glucose is beneficial. The mechanism of the effect appears to relate to changes in endogenous, readily mobilized brain glucose reserves, which lead to the enhanced glycolytic rate required to slow the decline

---

[a]References 352, 353, 355, 369, 372, 387, and 428.
[b]References 352, 353, 387, 440, 441, and 446-448.

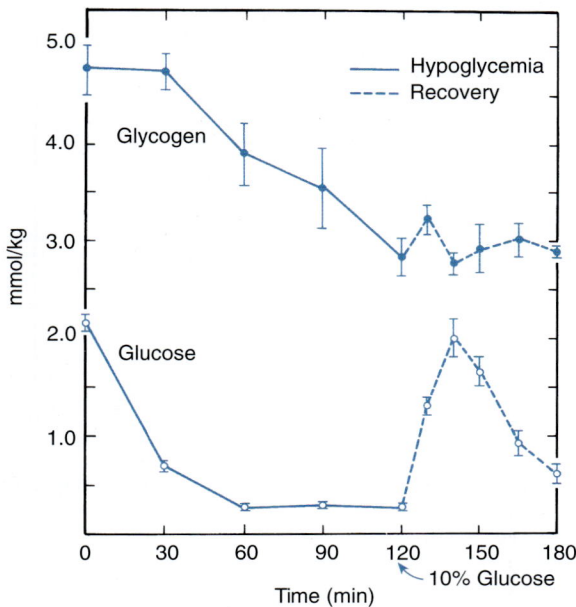

Figure 13.30 Greater importance of brain glucose reserves than glycogen in effects of hypoglycemia on vulnerability to anoxia (nitrogen breathing). Brain glucose and glycogen levels in newborn rats were determined as a function of duration of anoxia. Hypoglycemia was produced by insulin injection at the onset of the experiment. At 60 minutes, survival was fivefold lower in hypoglycemic versus control animals (data not shown). At this 60-minute point, glucose was reduced much more severely than was glycogen. The *arrow* indicates subcutaneous administration of 10% glucose (1.8 g/kg). This resulted in a marked improvement in survival (data not shown) and a normalization of brain glucose but not of glycogen. (From Vannucci RC, Vannucci SJ. Cerebral carbohydrate metabolism during hypoglycemia and anoxia in newborn rats. *Ann Neurol.* 1978;4:73–79.)

of, or even maintain the levels of, high-energy phosphate in the brain.

Deleterious Role of Abundant Brain Glucose in Adult Animals

A potentially deleterious role for abundant brain glucose in the clinical, pathological, and biochemical responses to hypoxemia and ischemia was suggested initially by studies with juvenile rhesus monkeys.[269,270,449,450] In a series of experiments with animals routinely food deprived for 12 to 24 hours before subjection to circulatory arrest, investigators showed that a period of circulatory arrest as long as 14 minutes was compatible with apparently good neurological recovery and "minimal" neuropathological abnormalities, restricted principally to brain stem nuclei, hippocampus, and Purkinje cells.[269] However, animals that were administered an infusion of 1.5 to 3 g/kg of glucose (5% dextrose in saline) that terminated 10 minutes before the 14-minute period of circulatory arrest did very poorly. The clinical course was characterized by seizures, hypertonia, and ultimately decerebrate rigidity, evolving over hours. On sacrifice, in glucose-pretreated monkeys, in contrast to the food-deprived monkeys, the glucose exhibited "changes indicative of widespread injury to tissue…and diffuse cytologic injury" with widespread involvement of the cerebral cortex.[269] In a subsequent study, glucose was administered as a 50% solution in a dose of 2.5 to 5 g/kg 15 minutes before circulatory

TABLE 13.16   Excitation at Glutamate Synapse of *N*-Methyl-D-Aspartate Type

	EFFECT ON EXCITATION	
SITE	**INCREASE**	**DECREASE**
Presynaptic (glutamate release)	Calcium Theophylline	Magnesium Adenosine
Receptor	Glutamate Glycine	APV/CPP Kynurenate
Channel		MK-801/ketamine/ dextromethorphan Magnesium/memantine

APV, 2-amino-5-phosphonovalerate; *CPP*, 3-(2-carboxypiperazine-4-yl)-propyl-1-phosphoric acid.

arrest, and similar clinical and neuropathological consequences were observed.[450]

Importance of Severe Lactic Acidosis in Brain. The biochemical mechanism for the deleterious effect of pretreatment with glucose in the previously mentioned juvenile monkeys may relate to the greater accumulation of lactic acid in the glucose-pretreated than in the food-deprived (control) monkeys (Table 13.16).[271,449] ATP levels declined approximately 10-fold in food-deprived animals subjected to circulatory arrest, and only a minimal difference in the magnitude of that decline was observed in animals pretreated with glucose. However, whereas lactate levels increased approximately fourfold in the food-deprived animals subjected to circulatory arrest, the levels increased more than 10-fold in those pretreated with glucose. The greater increases in brain lactate levels in the glucose-pretreated animals presumably reflected higher endogenous brain glucose reserves and, as a consequence, enhanced lactate production by anaerobic glycolysis. These experiments and related observations with animals rendered severely hypoxemic led Myers and Yamaguchi[272] to suggest that the accumulation of brain lactate to concentrations of approximately 20 mmol/kg or greater leads to tissue destruction and brain edema. This approximate threshold level is supported by the observations that the accumulation of lactate to higher than this level occurs in the brain of monkeys rendered ischemic in those regions that have been shown to be particularly vulnerable to neuronal injury.[271]

Considerable support for the concept of a deleterious effect of abundant glucose and resulting lactic acidosis in brain in the pathogenesis of hypoxic-ischemic brain injury in the adult was provided by further studies in a variety of experimental models in *mature animals*.[272,451-465] A threshold value of lactate of approximately 20 mmol/kg, above which major tissue injury occurs, can be suggested from the data. The apparent mechanism for the principal injury from these high levels of lactate is injury to endothelial cells, and perhaps also to perivascular astrocytes, with resulting disturbance of cerebral perfusion. Direct neuronal injury is likely, but widespread, secondary ischemic injury appears to develop primarily because of the vascular changes.

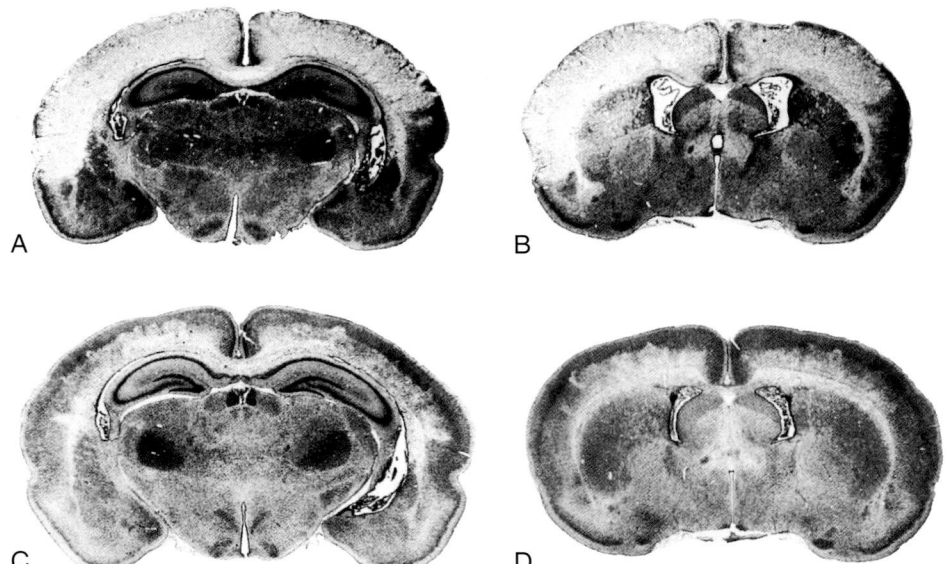

Figure 13.31 Coronal brain sections of rat pups, which had been subjected to bilateral ligation of the carotid arteries followed by exposure to an 8% oxygen atmosphere for 1 hour at the age of 7 days and were sacrificed 72 hours later. Note gross infarction in (A) the neocortex and (B) the lateral part of the striatum in a saline-injected pup. (C and D) Immediate (0 hour) posthypoxic glucose supplement reduced neocortical and striatal infarction. (Hematoxylin and eosin ×2.5 before 52% reduction.) (From Hattori H, Wasterlain CG. Posthypoxic glucose supplement reduces hypoxic-ischemic brain damage in the neonatal rat. *Ann Neurol.* 1990;28:122–128.)

Beneficial(?) Role of Abundant Brain Glucose in Perinatal Animals

In contrast to the deleterious role for glucose in hypoxic-ischemic injury in adult animals, considerable data in the immature rat suggest a beneficial role for abundant glucose administered primarily during or at the termination of the insult.[a] Hattori and Wasterlain,[469] using a model of bilateral carotid occlusion and ventilation with 8% oxygen for 1 hour, showed marked reduction of neuropathological injury in animals treated with supplemental glucose at the termination of the hypoxic breathing (Fig. 13.31). Supplementation 1 hour after termination of the hypoxia had no beneficial effect. In a neonatal lamb model of asphyxia, glucose supplementation prevented the prolonged postasphyxial impairment in cerebral oxygen consumption observed in control (or hypoglycemic) animals (Fig. 13.32).[232] Moreover, neonatal rats breathing 8% oxygen survived twice as long when they were treated with 50% glucose; 50% survival was approximately 4 hours in saline-treated animals versus 8 hours in glucose-treated animals.

The *mechanism* for any beneficial effect of glucose in these perinatal models of hypoxia-ischemia is not conclusively known but probably relates to preservation of mitochondrial energy production. Thus Yager et al.[394] showed that glucose supply becomes limiting in hypoxia-ischemia (unilateral carotid occlusion and 8% oxygen breathing) in the neonatal rat, a conclusion based on the relatively oxidized state of mitochondrial NAD+/NADH. Brain glucose levels clearly increase after glucose supplementation, in several models of hypoxia-ischemia.[353,448] With the model of carotid occlusion and 8% oxygen breathing, brain levels of high-energy phosphates were clearly higher in glucose-treated versus saline-treated animals (Table 13.17).[448] In addition, brain lactate levels in the hypoxic-ischemic neonatal rats were considerably higher in the glucose-treated animals.[448] Indeed, after 2 hours of hyperglycemia, brain lactate levels reached 25.5 mmol/kg. However, no evidence for tissue injury caused by the elevated brain lactate levels was reported, in contrast to the negative effect in the more mature brain.[272,451-465] Moreover, in other perinatal models (in the near-term fetal sheep, the newborn lamb, and the newborn dog), brain lactate levels did not rise to such levels with hypoxia-ischemia or asphyxia.[388-390,471] Increase in brain lactate levels in neonatal brain relative to adult brain is limited by the lower capacity for glucose uptake by the glucose transporter proteins, especially GLUT1 (55 kDa), and by lower hexokinase activity, the rate-limiting enzyme for glucose utilization.[a] Indeed, the possibility should be considered that any increase in lactate that may occur in the glucose-treated animal is used for energy production (by oxidation to pyruvate and entrance into the tricarboxylic acid cycle), because lactate is a preferred fuel in the neonatal brain.[355,448,472-474] Moreover, lactate is transported rapidly across the blood-brain barrier in the immature animal, and at least in the rat, brain pH normalizes by 10 minutes of recovery and tissue lactate levels normalize by 4 hours, unlike the prolonged tissue acidosis that occurs in adult rats subjected to hypoxia-ischemia and glucose treatment.[448] Indeed the combination of rapid utilization of lactate by brain and rapid efflux from brain may explain the lack of serious tissue injury by levels of lactate that lead to injury in the adult brain.

---

[a]References 232, 352, 353, 360, 441, 443, 446, 448, and 466-470.

[a]References 352, 353, 355, 359, 363, and 365.

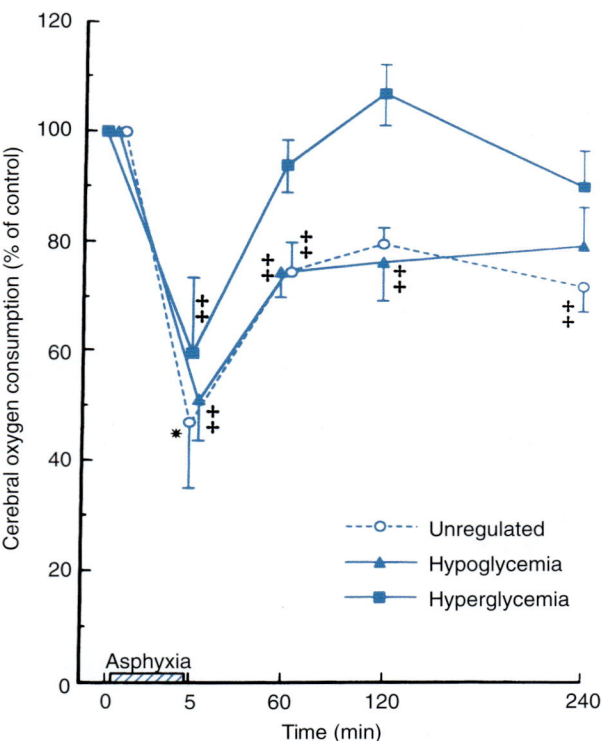

Figure 13.32 Cerebral metabolic rate for oxygen (CMRO₂; percentage of control) over time in the unregulated glucose, hyperglycemic, and hypoglycemic groups of newborn lambs during and after asphyxia. Zero (0) time represents the control measurement that is followed by the 75-minute period of asphyxia. Measurements were then made at 5 minutes and at 1, 2, and 4 hours after asphyxia. All values are means ± SEM. Note the highest CMRO₂ in animals rendered hyperglycemic. $^{++}P < .05$ compared with control; $^{*}P < .005$ compared with control. (From Rosenberg AA, Murdaugh E. The effect of blood glucose concentration on postasphyxia cerebral hemodynamics in newborn lambs. *Pediatr Res.* 1990;27:454–459.)

Enthusiasm for supplementation with glucose during or after hypoxic-ischemic insults in the immature brain must be tempered by the results of four other studies of young animals.[475-477] Thus, in a model of focal ischemia in the 7-day-old rat, glucose administration *after* hypoxia-ischemia led to more severe neuronal injury (although no increase in infarct size) than did saline administration.[475] Moreover, in a model of global hypoxia-ischemia in 1- to 3-day-old piglets, glucose administration *during* the insult led to accentuated neuronal injury.[476] Glucose administration *after* the insult did not ameliorate the injury, as such therapy accomplished in the immature rat (see earlier).[477] Finally, studies of fetal sheep at 80 days of gestation subjected to bilateral carotid occlusion show no effect on the degree of brain injury of prolonged *moderate* hyperglycemia before ischemia and during reperfusion, but a clear detrimental effect when an acute and *marked* increase in plasma glucose concentration (approximately sevenfold greater than control values) was added to the moderate hyperglycemia just before ischemia.[478] Brain lactate levels were not measured. The reasons for the differences in results obtained in the several perinatal models are unclear but may relate to methodological differences.

Summary. Current experimental data allow several tentative conclusions to be made about the effects of glucose administration with perinatal hypoxic-ischemic insults (Table 13.18). On balance, the findings favor maintenance of blood glucose concentrations in the normal range in infants who have sustained hypoxic-ischemic insults or who are at risk for sustaining such insults.

TABLE 13.17   Major Evidence Supporting a Critical Role for Glutamate in Hypoxic-Ischemic Neuronal Death in Developing Brain[a]

In developing neurons in cell culture, excitatory synaptic activity is necessary for hypoxia to lead to neuronal death.
Nonspecific blockade of this synaptic activity prevents hypoxic neuronal death in culture.
Specific glutamate receptor channel blockers also prevent hypoxic neuronal death in culture and in brain slices.
Glutamate accumulates extracellularly in vivo with hypoxic-ischemic insult.
Topography of hypoxic-ischemic neuronal death in vivo is similar to the topography of glutamate synapses.
Increased vulnerability of certain brain structures to hypoxic-ischemic injury during early development correlates, in those structures, with transiently increased concentration of glutamate receptors, which also have molecular characteristics associated with increased calcium influx.
Ontogeny of hypoxic-ischemic neuronal death in vivo is similar to the ontogeny of glutamate-induced neuronal death.
Delayed neuronal death after glutamate exposure in cell culture has a correlate in delayed neuronal death after hypoxia-ischemia in vivo, and both can be prevented by specific glutamate receptor channel blockers, some administered after termination of the insult.

[a]See text for references.

TABLE 13.18   Inflammation in Experimental Models of Perinatal Hypoxic-Ischemic Brain Injury

Microglial activation occurs promptly and briskly after hypoxia-ischemia.
Microglial cells release neurotoxic products (e.g., cytokines and reactive oxygen and nitrogen species).
Cytokines (especially IL-1beta and TNF-alpha) increase promptly in brain after hypoxia-ischemia, and IL-1 receptor antagonists ameliorate hypoxic-ischemic brain injury when they are administered either before or at the termination of hypoxia-ischemia.
Antimicroglial agents (e.g., minocycline) are neuroprotective in several experimental paradigms of perinatal hypoxia-ischemia.
Inflammatory mechanisms provoked by prior exposure to molecular products of infection (e.g., lipopolysaccharide) potentiate subthreshold hypoxic-ischemic insults to lead to severe brain injury.

IL, Interleukin; *TNF,* tumor necrosis factor.

Influence of Maturation on Glucose and Energy Metabolism With Hypoxia-Ischemia

The influence of the maturational state of the brain on the severity and topography of the brain injury caused by hypoxia-ischemia is complex. It is now clear that the long-held general notion that the perinatal brain is more resistant than the adult brain is too simplistic. Evidence indicates that cerebral glucose and energy metabolism are *more resistant* to perturbation by hypoxia-ischemia in the immature than in the adult brain.[a] Some of the mechanisms underlying the resistance of energy metabolism in the immature brain are summarized in Table 13.19. However, neuropathological studies indicate that many critical neuronal groups are *more vulnerable* to hypoxic-ischemic injury in the immature animal.[487-489] This vulnerability of immature neurons relates particularly to enhanced density and function of excitatory amino acid receptors and enhanced vulnerability to attack by reactive oxygen species (ROS) and reactive nitrogen species (RNS), as discussed later. A particular vulnerability of immature oligodendrocytes to hypoxic-ischemic, excitatory amino acid, and free radical injury is discussed later but also is relevant in this context. The various influences of maturation on the regional aspects of hypoxic-ischemic brain injury and on the responses to interventions are highlighted in appropriate subsequent sections of this chapter.

Birth as an Additive or Potentiating Factor in Hypoxic Injury

Perinatal hypoxic-ischemic injury occurs in the setting of a profound alteration of biochemical and physiological homeostasis (i.e., the process of birth). Transient hypoxemia and hypercapnia, variable in severity and duration, are consistent occurrences.[141,490,491] Transient disturbances in CBF may also occur.[196,492] It is appropriate to ask whether the biochemical state of the brain is affected by the major systemic alterations that take place at birth.

Careful studies of the perinatal rat brain indicate that *spontaneous vaginal delivery* is associated with the *signs of hypoxemic or ischemic insult to the brain.*[493,494] Alterations in glycogen, certain glycolytic intermediates, and high-energy compounds after spontaneous vaginal delivery are shown in Table 13.20. Evidence for glycogenolysis, enhanced lactate production, PCr conversion to ATP, and a decline in ATP concentrations is apparent in the first minute after birth. Simultaneous elevation of the concentrations of glucose-6-phosphate and glucose-1-phosphate and decline of the concentration of glycogen are consistent with the occurrence of glycogenolysis.[494] The elevation of lactate level and of the lactate/pyruvate ratio indicates enhanced anaerobic glycolysis. The sharp decline of PCr is not adequate in the first minute to preserve ATP concentrations, and in fact the small persisting deficit in ATP levels 10 minutes after birth is statistically significant.[493] Not shown, but accompanying these changes, is a decline in brain glucose concentrations relative to blood glucose, a finding reflecting further the enhanced glycolysis. By 1 hour after delivery, high-energy phosphate concentrations were no longer depressed, and the ratio of lactate to pyruvate was considerably improved. The latter was normal by 8 hours after delivery.

[a]References 352, 353, 368, 369, 373, 375, 384, 390, 440, 441, and 479-486.

TABLE 13.19 Potentially Valuable Interventions in Prevention or Amelioration of Perinatal Hypoxic-Ischemic Neuronal Injury[a]

Decrease of energy depletion
Hypothermia
Glucose
Sedation
Hypercapnia (mild)
Inhibition of glutamate release
Hypothermia
Calcium channel blockers
Magnesium
Adenosine or adenosine agonists
Free radical scavengers
Anticonvulsants such as lamotrigine, levitaretam
Phenytoin
Cannabinoids
Amelioration of impairment in glutamate uptake
Hypothermia
Blockade of glutamate receptors
NMDA receptor antagonists (MK-801, xenon, memantine, magnesium, ketamine, dextrorphan)
Non-NMDA receptor antagonists (NBQX, CNQX, topiramate)
Blockade of free radical generation
Hypothermia
Inhibitors of cyclooxygenases (e.g., indomethacin)
Inhibitors of lipoxygenases (e.g., AA-861)
Nitric oxide synthase inhibitors (e.g., nitroarginine derivatives, 2-iminobiotin)
Allopurinol
Iron chelators
Fructose-1,6-biphosphate
Removal of free radicals
Free radical scavengers (vitamin E and analogues, edaravone, N-acetylcysteine)
Antioxidant enzyme mimetics
Blockade of downstream effects
Hypothermia
Erythropoietin
Growth factors (insulin-like growth factor-I, brain-derived neurotrophic factor, nerve growth factor)
Caspase inhibitors
Inhibition of inflammatory effects
Hypothermia
Minocycline
Anti–Toll-like receptor agents
Interleukin-1 receptor antagonists
Platelet-activating factor antagonists
Neutropenia

[a]See text for references.
CNQX, 6-cyano-7-nitroquinoxaline-2,3-dione; *NBQX*, 2,3-dihydroxy-6-nitro-7-sulfamoyl-benzo[f]quinoxaline-2,3-dione; *NMDA*, N-methyl-D-aspartate.

Determinations of identical parameters after cesarean section showed very transient and much smaller changes; indeed, no significant change in ATP levels was observed at any time after delivery by cesarean section.[493]

These data indicate that the process of birth through the vaginal route in a neonatal animal model is associated with the biochemical signs of hypoxic insult to brain. The influence of this phenomenon on the impact of hypoxic-ischemic insults

TABLE 13.20   Mild Hypothermia as Neuroprotective Therapy[a]

Principal features
Timing: commence before delayed energy failure and excitatory features such as seizures (i.e., ≈6 h)
Degree: decrease body temperature 3–4°C
Duration: ≈72 h
Mechanisms of benefit
Decrease energy consumption
Decrease accumulation of glutamate
Decrease synthesis of reactive oxygen and nitrogen species
Block downstream molecular cascade to apoptosis
Inhibit inflammatory mechanisms
Synergistic neuroprotective combinations
Hypothermia and xenon
Hypothermia and topiramate
Hypothermia and N-acetylcysteine
Hypothermia and caspase inhibitor

[a]See text for references.

occurring before or immediately after birth is not known. An intuitive conclusion would be that the insult at birth may be additive. However, it is possible that the insult at birth may play a protective role in relation to a subsequent insult. Thus a degree of protection to hypoxic-ischemic neuronal injury has been shown in the immature rat by prior exposure to hypoxia.[495-498] This *hypoxic preconditioning* appears to be related to induction of multiple genes, particularly the transcription factor hypoxia-inducing-factor 1 (HIF1) and its target genes, that blunt the adverse effects of hypoxia-ischemia by induction of vasodilation, glucose transport, glycolysis, and antiexcitotoxic, antioxidant, antiapoptotic, and other mechanisms.

Biochemical Mechanisms of Cellular Injury in Hypoxic-Ischemic Cerebral Injury: Beyond Glucose and Energy Metabolism

The principal biochemical mechanisms of cell death with hypoxia-ischemia and asphyxia are presumably very similar, if not identical, and are initiated by oxygen (and glucose) deprivation and an impairment in energy supplies. Because all the principal, currently considered mechanisms for cell death with oxygen deprivation at least begin with the disturbances of brain glucose and energy metabolism, it is appropriate to synthesize current concepts concerning the mechanisms for cell death immediately after the preceding sections, which emphasize these disturbances. Nevertheless, it is now clear that the mechanisms of cell death with oxygen deprivation are not simply the result of energy failure and, indeed, extend beyond glucose and energy metabolism. An enormous amount of literature attests to the complexity of the mechanisms. In the following section, we attempt to synthesize the essential data and to isolate the most critical mechanisms. The emphasis is on mechanisms of *neuronal death*. Although mechanisms of white matter injury, *especially oligodendroglial death*, bear many similarities, sufficient differences warrant *separate consideration in the next major section*.

As discussed in the next section, the cascade of deleterious events that lead to cell death after insults that result in oxygen deprivation and energy failure appears to occur *primarily following termination of the insult*. Careful studies in animal models and in human patients provide strong support for this notion.[42-50] The phenomena are initiated particularly by energy depletion, accumulation of extracellular excitatory amino acids (particularly glutamate), increase in cytosolic calcium, and generation of free radicals. The importance of this "delayed" death of the brain in the hours after the termination of the insult is related in largest part to the possibility that intervention during the postinsult period could be beneficial. The temporal evolution to cell death is shown in Figs. 13.6 and 13.33.

Role of Accumulation of Cytosolic Calcium

A large body of information indicates a major role for accumulation of cytosolic Ca^{2+} during and after hypoxia-ischemia in the mediation of cell death.[159,384,486,507-519] In perinatal models of hypoxia-ischemia, increased Ca^{2+} uptake into the insulted brain regions, close correlation within brain regions between increased uptake of Ca^{2+} and subsequent neuronal injury, and some protection from subsequent brain injury by pretreatment with voltage-dependent Ca^{2+} channel antagonists have been documented.[a] *Moreover, because a major mechanism of Ca2+ influx into the cytosol is through the* N-methyl-d-aspartate (NMDA) *and* alpha-amino-3-hydroxy-5-methyl-4-isoxazolepropionic acid (AMPA) *types of glutamate receptors, the protection from brain injury afforded by antagonists of these receptors (see later discussion) may be mediated primarily by decreasing the accumulation of cytosolic Ca^{2+}.*

Mechanisms. The mechanisms by which increased cytosolic Ca^{2+} leads to cell death are multiple but are best discussed in the context of normal Ca^{2+} homeostasis (Fig. 13.34).[159,384,507-513,517,525-527] The cellular mechanisms for maintenance of low cytosolic Ca^{2+} concentrations (10^{-7} M) relative to high extracellular Ca^{2+} concentrations (10^{-3} M) are located in the *plasma membrane* (voltage-dependent channels; three agonist-dependent, that is, glutamate-dependent, channels: the NMDA, AMPA [immature, i.e., lacking GluR2 subunit], and metabotropic receptor-activated channels [see later discussion]; an ATP-dependent uniport system, and an Na^+-dependent antiport system), the *endoplasmic reticulum* (an ATP-dependent import system and a release mechanism activated by inositol triphosphate), and the *mitochondrion* (a voltage-dependent channel and an Na^+/H^+-dependent antiport system; see Fig. 13.34).[511-513] The mechanisms for the increased cytosolic Ca^{2+} in neurons subjected to hypoxia-ischemia, and the metabolic and ionic changes caused by ischemia that underlie these mechanisms, are summarized in Table 13.21. *The central roles for ATP depletion, membrane depolarization, and voltage-dependent and glutamate-activated Ca^{2+} channels are apparent.*

The deleterious effects of increased cytosolic Ca^{2+} are multiple and affect the cell in a variety of ways (Table 13.22).[b] These effects include degradation of cellular lipids by activation of phospholipases, of cellular proteins (especially cytoskeletal elements) by activation of proteases, and of cellular DNA by activation of nucleases, as well as crucial indirect mechanisms of destruction mediated by generation of free radicals and nitric oxide (NO; Fig. 13.35). The utilization of ATP by ATP-dependent Ca^{2+}-transport systems, attempting to correct the cytosolic Ca^{2+}

---

[a]References 159, 398, 399, 512, 513, 517, and 520-524.
[b]References 159, 384, 507-513, 517, 519, 522, 526, and 528-533.

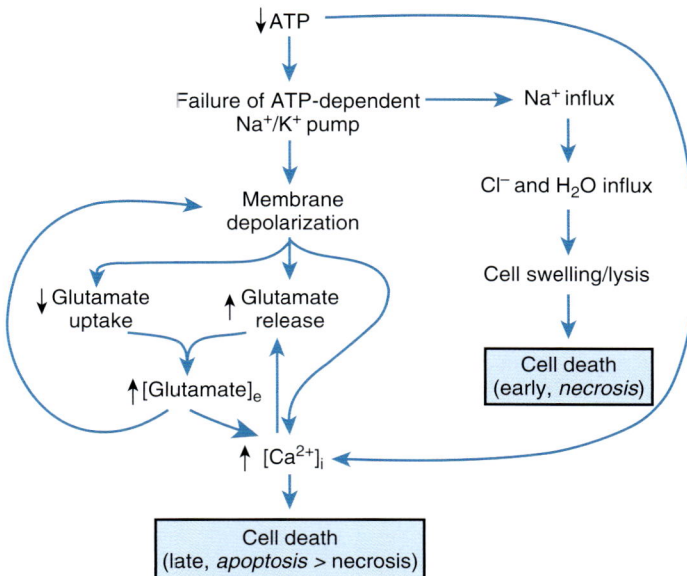

Figure 13.33 Relation between energy depletion and cell death. Early cell death is primarily necrosis, and the more important, later cell death is primarily apoptosis. Concerning the latter, delayed cell death, accumulation of extracellular glutamate with excitotoxicity and elevations of intracellular calcium are important. *ATP,* Adenosine triphosphate; *Ca*$^{2+}$, calcium; *Cl*$^-$, chloride; *K*$^+$, potassium; *Na*$^+$, sodium. See text for details.

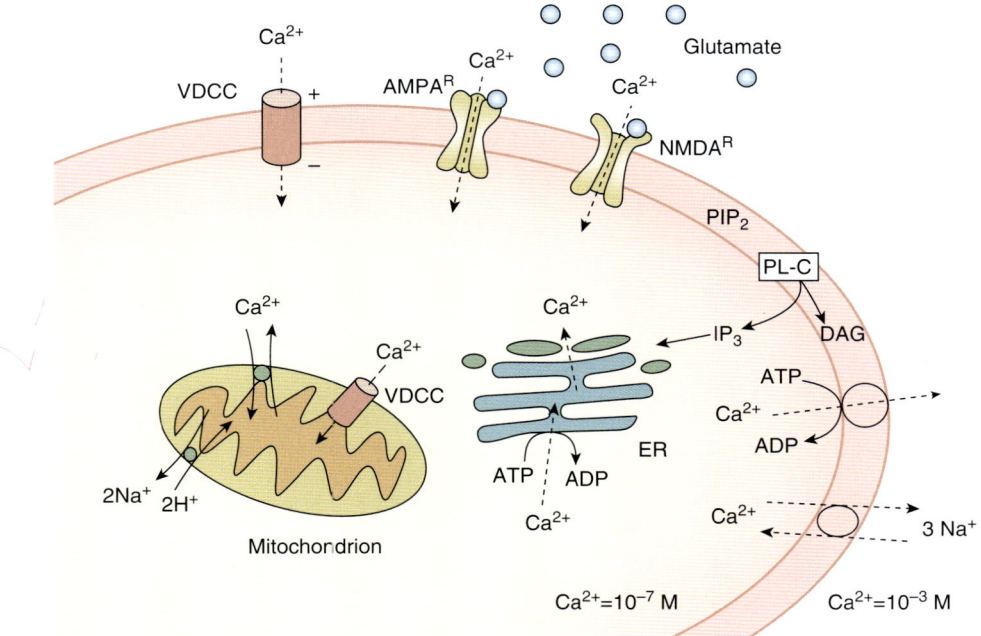

Figure 13.34 Cellular calcium (Ca^{2+}) homeostasis. See text for details. *ADP,* Adenosine diphosphate; *AMPA,* alpha-amino-3-hydroxy-5-methyl-4-isoxazolepropionic acid; *ATP,* adenosine triphosphate; *DAG,* diacylglycerol; *ER,* endoplasmic reticulum; *Na*$^+$, sodium; *NMDA,* N-methyl-D-aspartate; *PIP$_2$,* phosphatidylinositol-4,5-diphosphate; *PL-C,* phospholipase C; *VDCC,* voltage-dependent calcium channel.

accumulation, and the Ca^{2+}-mediated uncoupling of oxidative phosphorylation serve to perpetuate the process (see Fig. 13.35).

Role of Free Radicals: Reactive Oxygen and Nitrogen Species

Free Radicals. The crucial role of free radicals, generated in considerable part by Ca^{2+}-activated processes just described,

in the mediation of cell death with hypoxia-ischemia has been established by the study of a variety of models in vivo, in culture, and in vitro (see later).[13,219,384,519,534-554] The emphasis in these studies has been *neuronal* injury. Discussion of the role of free radicals in *oligodendroglial* injury is contained in a later section. Free radicals are highly reactive compounds with an uneven number of electrons in the outermost orbital. These compounds can react with certain normal cellular components (e.g., unsaturated fatty acids of membrane lipids) and can generate a new free radical and thereby a chain reaction, which results in irreversible biochemical injury (e.g., peroxidation of the unsaturated fatty acids, membrane injury, and cell necrosis). With less intense insults, free radicals can lead to apoptotic cell death by activation of specific death genes.[540,554-557] Free radicals in mammalian cells exist primarily as ROS (e.g., superoxide anion, hydrogen peroxide, hydroxyl radical) or as RNS (e.g., peroxynitrite [$ONOO^-$]; see later discussion). When these reactive species are present in excess, the cell is said to be subjected to oxidative stress or nitrative stress, respectively. Although studies have generally focused on ROS or RNS separately, these species usually exist together (e.g.,

under conditions of hypoxia-ischemia-reperfusion). I discuss the investigations of ROS and RNS in separate sections later.

The principal *sources* of free radicals with hypoxia-ischemia, the endogenous *defenses* against such radicals, and their *major deleterious effects* are summarized in Table 13.23. Of the sources of free radicals with hypoxia-ischemia, the electron transport system is important when oxygen deprivation prevents the complete passage of electrons to cytochrome c oxidase. Free radicals, specifically superoxide anion, are then generated proximal to this terminal enzyme in the electron transport system. The next four sources are directly or indirectly related to cytosolic Ca^{2+} (see Fig. 13.35 and Table 13.22). Arachidonic acid is generated by Ca^{2+}-activated phospholipase A_2, xanthine

TABLE 13.21	Major Neuroprotective Mechanisms of Erythropoietin in Hypoxia-Ischemia

Upstream initiating mechanisms
Antiexcitotoxic (attenuation of glutamate release)
Antioxidant effects
Inhibition of nitric oxide production
Preservation of autoregulation (?)
Downstream mechanisms
Antiapoptotic effects
Survival promoting effects
Stimulation of angiogenesis
Stimulation of neurogenesis
Anti-inflammatory effects (?)

Adapted from Sola A, Wen TC, Hamrick SE, Ferriero DM. Potential for protection and repair following injury to the developing brain: a role for erythropoietin? *Pediatr Res.* 2005;57:110R–117R.

TABLE 13.22	Maturation-Dependent Vulnerability of Differentiating Oligodendrocytes to Excitotoxicity

AMPA receptors (GluR2-deficient) are concentrated on preoligodendrocyte somata, and NMDA receptors are concentrated on preoligodendrocyte processes.
These receptors are overexpressed in cerebral white matter during the peak period of vulnerability to hypoxic-ischemic white matter injury.
Both GluR2-deficient AMPA receptors and NMDA receptors are permeable to calcium.
Ischemia leads to calcium influx through activation of these receptors with either cell death (AMPA activation) or loss of processes (NMDA activation), or both.
Both receptors can be blocked by specific antagonists and lead to protection.

AMPA, Alpha-amino-3-hydroxy-5-methyl-4-isoxazolepropionic acid; *NMDA*, N-methyl-D-aspartate.

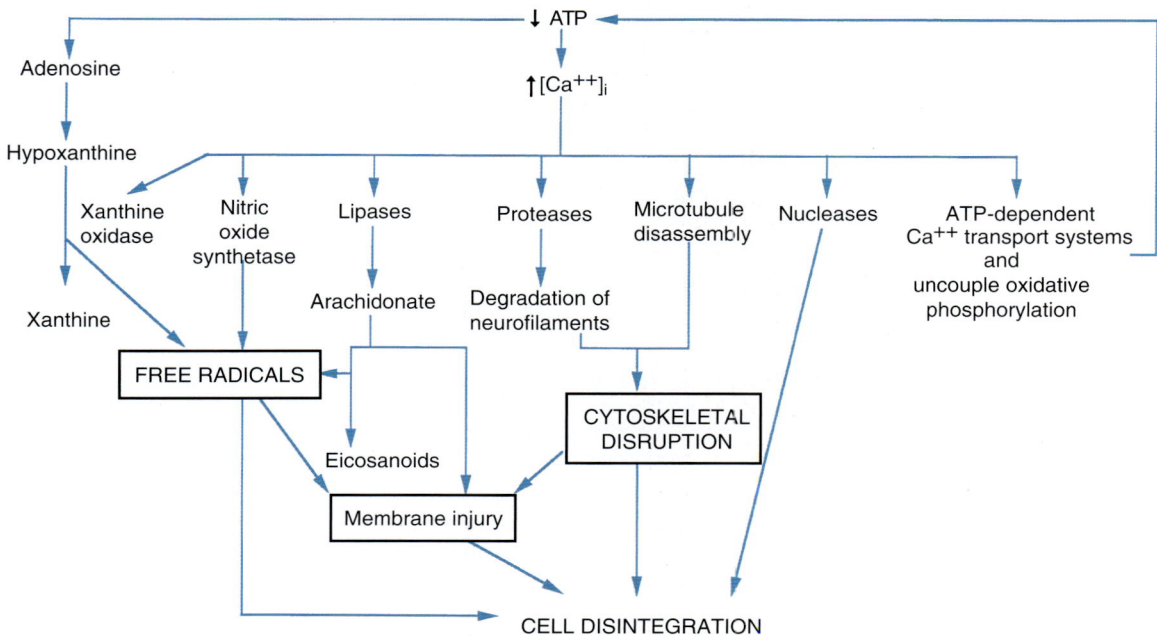

Figure 13.35 Deleterious effects of elevated cytosolic calcium ([Ca^{++}]$_i$). Generation of free radicals is especially important. *ATP*, Adenosine triphosphate. See text for details.

TABLE 13.23   Local Chemical Factors: Change in Brain Extracellular Fluid and Effect on Cerebral Blood Vessels[a]

| LOCAL CHEMICAL FACTOR | CHANGE IN BRAIN EXTRACELLULAR FLUID | | EFFECT ON CEREBRAL VESSELS | |
	HYPOXIA	CORTICAL ACTIVITY[b]	INCREASE	DECREASE
Hydrogen ion	Increase	Increase	Dilate	Constrict
Potassium ion	Increase	Increase	Dilate	Constrict
Adenosine	Increase	Increase	Dilate	Constrict
Prostaglandins	Increase	Increase	Dilate	Constrict
Osmolarity	?	?	Dilate	Constrict
Calcium ion	Decrease	Decrease	Constrict	Dilate

[a]See text for references.
[b]Includes seizures.

oxidase is activated by Ca^{2+}, catecholamine release is stimulated by an increase in cytosolic Ca^{2+}, and NO synthase (NOS; see next section) is activated by Ca^{2+}.[a] Finally, data indicate that early reactive cells at the site of initial insult, especially *microglia*, are potent sources of free radicals (see later discussion).

Reactive Oxygen Species. An important role for ROS in perinatal models of fetal and neonatal hypoxemic, ischemic, hypoxic-ischemic, and asphyxial insults now seems established.[b] After the insults, generation of ROS or elevations of compounds known to lead to generation of ROS have been found. Moreover, studies principally of asphyxia in the newborn lamb and in the neonatal piglet and of hypoxia-ischemia (carotid ligation and low oxygen breathing) in the immature (7-day-old) rat have shown elevations of free radicals, deleterious effects of free radical attack (e.g., evidence for lipid peroxidation), or a neuroprotective effect of treatment (pretreatment, treatment during the insult, or after termination of the insult) with free radical scavengers (e.g., vitamin E analogues, edaravone, or drugs that inhibit free radical formation, such as allopurinol, oxypurinol, indomethacin, superoxide dismutase [SOD], catalase, and iron chelators).[c] The importance of the reperfusion period, rather than the time of the hypoxic-ischemic insult per se, in the generation of the ROS also has been emphasized (Fig. 13.36).

The *major endogenous antioxidant defense system* is illustrated in Fig. 13.37. Thus the most commonly generated initial oxygen free radical, the superoxide anion, is converted to hydrogen peroxide by the enzyme SOD, the three different forms of which are cytosolic copper-zinc SOD, extracellular copper-zinc SOD, and mitochondrial manganese SOD. The hydrogen peroxide generated is detoxified by catalase and glutathione peroxidase. If this step fails or is overloaded, and if iron is available, the Fenton reaction and the production of the deadly hydroxyl radical occur. Studies of animal models and more recent studies of asphyxiated human infants indicate that after hypoxia-ischemia, iron is released and is therefore relatively abundant.[355,539,547,549,605-610] Studies of hypoxia-ischemia in the neonatal mouse indicate that detoxification of hydrogen peroxide is deficient in the immature brain. Thus mice made

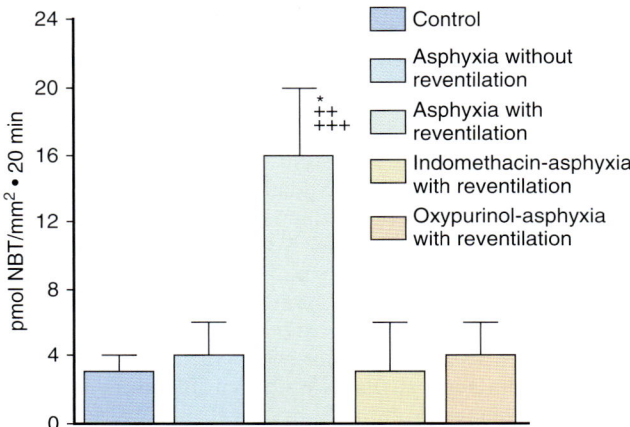

Figure 13.36 Free radical (superoxide anion) production, determined as superoxide dismutase-inhibitable nitroblue tetrazolium (NBT) reduction in control ($n = 7$), asphyxia without reventilation ($n = 9$), asphyxia-reventilation ($n = 11$), asphyxia-reventilation after indomethacin 0.2 mg/kg ($n = 4$), and asphyxia-reventilation after oxypurinol 50.0 mg/kg ($n = 10$) pretreated piglets. Values are mean ± SEM. *$P < .05$ compared with control; ++$P < .05$ compared with asphyxia without reventilation group; +++$P < .05$ compared with indomethacin and oxypurinol pretreatment groups. Note the production of superoxide anion after (with reventilation) but not during (without reventilation) asphyxia and the prevention by administration of indomethacin or oxypurinol. (From Pourcyrous M, Leffler CW, Bada HS, Korones SB, Busija DW. Brain superoxide anion generation in asphyxiated piglets and the effect of indomethacin at therapeutic dose. *Pediatr Res.* 1993;34:366–369.)

transgenic for copper-zinc SOD and therefore overexpressing this enzyme, when subjected to hypoxia-ischemia, exhibit decreased brain injury in the adult but *increased* brain injury in the perinatal period.[548,589] This *exacerbation* of brain injury in the *immature* brain was associated with an accumulation of hydrogen peroxide, because catalase and glutathione peroxidase did not increase in activity in response to the insult (catalase increases after similar hypoxia-ischemia in the adult).[548] Indeed, the levels of glutathione peroxidase decreased after hypoxia-ischemia, and importantly, in the normal animal levels already developmentally low in the perinatal period. Consistent with this, in normally developing rats (P7) rendered hypoxic-ischemic, an accumulation of hydrogen peroxide in the cortex was much greater than occurred with hypoxia-ischemia at later ages (P42).[611] The particular importance of glutathione

[a]References 384, 513, 526, 530-538, 540, 550, and 558-575.
[b]References 13, 179, 405, 538, 539, 548-553, 557, 573, and 576-595.
[c]References 13, 197, 198, 219, 405, 408, 466, 541-553, 557, 577, 584-586, 588, and 590-604.

Superoxide dismutation

$$O_2^{\bullet-} + H^+ \xrightarrow{\text{SOD}} H_2O_2$$

H$_2$O$_2$ detoxification

$$H_2O_2 \xrightarrow[\text{Catalase}]{\text{GSH Peroxidase}} H_2O + O_2$$

Hydroxyl radical formation

$$H_2O_2 + Fe^{++} \xrightarrow[\text{Reaction}]{\text{Fenton}} OH^{\bullet} + OH^- + Fe^{+++}$$

Figure 13.37 Free radical metabolism. The upper two reactions, catalyzed respectively by superoxide dismutases (SOD; both copper-zinc SOD [extracellular and cytosol] and manganese SOD [mitochondrion]) and by GSH peroxidase and catalase, are the major antioxidant defense mechanisms. In the presence of hydrogen peroxide (H$_2$O$_2$) and iron (Fe^{++}), the Fenton reaction (lowest reaction) generates the highly toxic hydroxyl radical. *GSH*, Glutathione; *SOD*, superoxide dismutases.

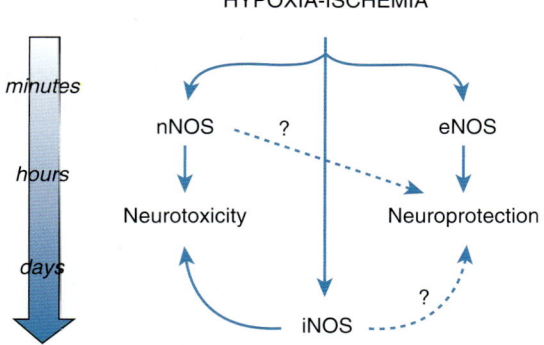

Figure 13.38 Major effects of the various forms of nitric oxide synthase (NOS) after hypoxia-ischemia. Effects in the first minutes to hours and in the hours to days after the insult can be distinguished, although these effects overlap. *Dotted lines* indicate neuroprotective effects that appear plausible under certain circumstances but require more study. See text for details. *eNOS*, Endothelial NOS; *iNOS*, inducible NOS; *nNOS*, neuronal NOS.

peroxidase was shown in two models derived from transgenic mice overexpressing glutathione peroxidase.[612,613] Thus, in cultured neurons exposed to oxidative stress and in a neonatal hypoxic-ischemic model, glutathione peroxidase overexpression led to neuronal protection. Additional importance for glutathione is suggested by the finding in the hypoxic-ischemic 7-day rat that the crucial mitochondrial fraction of glutathione, necessary for glutathione peroxidase function, was markedly decreased after hypoxia-ischemia, with a nadir after 24 hours.[614] Thus the data suggest that the normal immature brain has a limited capacity to detoxify hydrogen peroxide and with hypoxia-ischemia accumulates hydrogen peroxide, both because of this developmental lack and because of failure to respond with an adaptive increase in the antioxidant defense enzymes. With the hypoxia-ischemia–induced increase in iron, generation of the hydroxyl radical and brain injury is the result (see Fig. 13.37).

The *propensity for oxidative neuronal injury* in the immature brain relates not only to the deficient antioxidant defenses just described but also to several *pro-oxidant characteristics*. Thus, at baseline, the developing brain has a relatively high concentration of polyunsaturated fatty acids, especially in neuronal membranes, an excellent target for ROS, and a relatively high concentration of nonprotein-bound iron.[553] Therefore, with exposure to conditions that lead to an increase in ROS (e.g., hypoxia-ischemia-reperfusion) and available iron, the balance strongly favors oxidative injury. Similar considerations apply to the increased oxidative injury observed after hypoxia-ischemia in developing animals or in asphyxiated infants when resuscitation is carried out with 100% oxygen rather than with room air (see Chapter 20).[575,615-622]

Nitric Oxide and Reactive Nitrogen Species. Particular importance for the synthesis of NO by NOS both in normal brain and under conditions of hypoxia-ischemia is now well established.[519,574,623-635] At least three forms of NOS are recognized: a constitutive neuronal form (nNOS), a constitutive endothelial form (eNOS), and an inducible form (iNOS) found in astrocytes and microglia. The constitutive forms are activated by Ca^{2+}, whereas iNOS stimulation appears to be Ca^{2+}

independent and is activated especially well by inflammatory stimuli (e.g., cytokines, lipopolysaccharide [LPS], and oxidative stress). Because NO is a diffusible gas, both its normal functions (i.e., cell signaling and neurotransmission) and its deleterious actions (i.e., neurotoxicity) appear to be mediated by synthesis and then diffusion to intracellular sites and to adjacent cells.

Under *normal* conditions, NO has multiple cellular effects.[635] Many of these, but not all, are initiated by guanylate cyclase activation with the subsequent production of cyclic guanosine monophosphate and protein phosphorylation. This activation occurs when NO binds to the heme group of guanylate cyclase. Other biological effects of NO relate to action of its metabolites. Thus formation of a nitro group (NO$_2$) allows the *nitration* of proteins, especially at tyrosine residues, to form nitrotyrosine. Formation of nitrosonium ion (NO$^+$) allows *nitrosylation* of thiol residues on proteins, especially the cysteine sulfhydryl group. Formation of ONOO$^-$ and other reactive intermediates, including the hydroxyl radical, leads to *oxidation* of multiple amino acid residues, including the formation of nitrotyrosine. The biological effects of these actions of NO include modulation of cell proliferation, apoptosis, mitochondrial energy metabolism, and signal transduction.

Under pathological conditions of *hypoxia-ischemia-reperfusion*, an increase in cytosolic Ca^{2+} is an early event (see earlier). A particularly important effector for the increase in Ca^{2+} is activation of the NMDA receptor (see later). The effects on NO metabolism are multiple and sequential (Fig. 13.38).[519,623-628,634-638] Thus, in the first few minutes, the activity of Ca^{2+}-dependent eNOS in endothelial cells is increased to produce vasodilation and to replenish substrate supply. The activity of Ca^{2+}-dependent nNOS in neurons also is increased, and initially this increase may help improve blood flow because of the presence of nNOS in perivascular nerves.[635] However, the principal effect of induction of nNOS in neurons is the generation of NO that diffuses to adjacent neurons. Under conditions of oxidative stress with abundant superoxide anion (O$_2^{\bullet-}$), NO reacts quickly with O$_2^{\bullet-}$ to form the particularly toxic RNS, ONOO$^-$. Indeed, the affinity of O$_2^{\bullet-}$ for NO to form ONOO$^-$ greatly exceeds the reaction of O$_2^{\bullet-}$ with SOD, and thus ONOO$^-$ formation is greatly favored. This compound leads to neuronal death by multiple

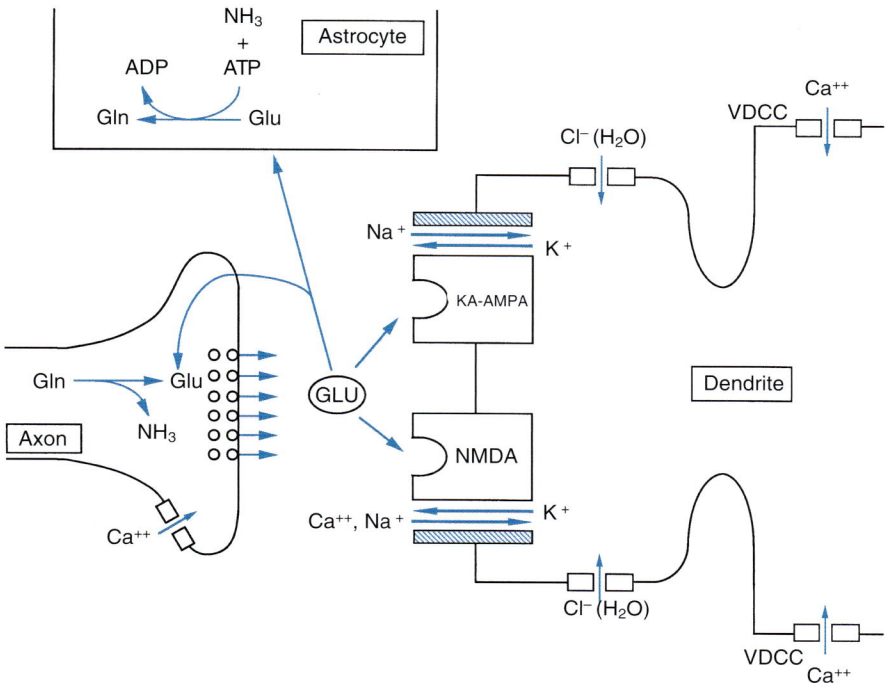

Figure 13.39 Relationships at the glutamate synapse among the presynaptic axonal terminal, the postsynaptic dendrite, and the associated astrocyte. See text for details. In this figure, the non-*N*-methyl-D-aspartate (NMDA; kainate-alpha-amino-3-hydroxy-5-methyl-4-isoxazole-propionic acid [KA-AMPA]) receptors are shown together; see text regarding calcium (Ca⁺⁺) permeability of the AMPA receptor in developing neurons. *ADP,* Adenosine diphosphate; *ATP,* adenosine triphosphate; *Cl⁻,* chloride; *Gln,* glutamine; *Glu,* glutamate; *Na⁺,* sodium; *NH₃,* ammonia; *VDCC,* voltage-dependent calcium channel. (Modified from Siesjö BK. Calcium in the brain under physiological and pathological conditions. *Eur Neurol.* 1990;30:3–9.)

mechanisms, including especially *mitochondrial impairment,* energy depletion, and further failure of Ca²⁺-homeostasis (see earlier).[631-634,639] Glutamate activation of the NMDA receptor is a major cause of the initial increase of cytosolic Ca²⁺ that activates nNOS and leads to this deleterious cascade. Those NMDA receptor–containing neurons that express nNOS are resistant to the deleterious effects of hypoxia-ischemia and excitotoxicity (see later).

A *later result* of hypoxia-ischemia-reperfusion is the *activation of iNOS,* principally in astrocytes and microglia, with a resulting large, sustained increase in NO production, over many hours to days, depending on the experimental model studied (see Fig. 13.38).[634,635] This activation occurs in parallel with inflammatory responses and is based on the activation of specific cell surface receptors for cytokines (tumor necrosis factor-alpha [TNF-alpha], interferon-gamma, and interleukin-1beta [IL-1beta]) and on the intracellular effects of ROS. The deleterious effects of this increase in NO are mediated primarily through formation of ONOO⁻, as discussed earlier. The possibility of a neuroprotective role of NO, mediated by NO⁺, has been raised, because *S*-nitrosylation at critical thiols on the NMDA receptor's redox modulatory site leads to downregulation of channel activity.[637] The biological impact of such a neuroprotective role currently is unclear.

In *perinatal models of asphyxia or hypoxia-ischemia,* evidence for both the neurotoxic effects and the beneficial vascular effects of NO synthesis have been obtained.[a] Evidence for

neurotoxic effects of NOS activation has consisted particularly of demonstration of neuroprotection by specific inhibitors of the synthase (e.g., nitrosoarginine derivatives). Although the data are not completely consistent, on balance the scheme shown in Fig. 13.38 depicts the major effects mediated by stimulation of the several forms of NOS. Particular importance of NO and RNS during development in part is suggested by the observation that the relative resistance of NOS-expressing neurons to NMDA-mediated toxicity is lost after the neonatal period in the developing rat.[553]

Role of Excitatory Amino Acids

A remarkable series of studies over the past several decades has revolutionized the understanding of the role of excitatory amino acids, particularly glutamate, as the mediators of neuronal death under conditions of hypoxia-ischemia. Before discussion of these studies, the normal aspects of glutamate biology at the excitatory synapse are reviewed.

Normal Features. The relationships at the *glutamate synapse* among the presynaptic nerve ending, the postsynaptic dendrite, and the associated astrocyte are shown in Fig. 13.39.[511,512,659-667] Only the ionotropic receptors are shown in Fig. 13.39 (as discussed in the next paragraph). Glutamate release is provoked by the influx of Ca²⁺ into the presynaptic nerve ending. Depolarization of the postsynaptic dendrite is related to Na⁺ entry. The action of glutamate is terminated by potent, high-affinity, Na⁺-dependent reuptake mechanisms in both astrocytes and presynaptic nerve endings. Although the

[a]References 217, 218, 519, 553, 554, 574, 606, 638, and 640-658.

TABLE 13.24   Effect of Hyperventilation and Abrupt Termination Thereof on Cerebral Blood Flow in Newborn Lamb[a]

CONDITION	CEREBRAL BLOOD FLOW[a,b] (PERCENTAGE OF CHANGE)
Hyperventilation	
30 min	−36
6 h	−12[c]
After hyperventilation	
30 min	+210
6 h	+226

[a]No effect on cerebral metabolic rate for oxygen was observed at any time.
[b]Blood flow to cerebral hemispheres and midbrain.
[c]Not significantly different from zero; all other numbers different from control at $P < .05$ level.

Data from Gleason CA, Short BL, Jones MD Jr. Cerebral blood flow and metabolism during and after prolonged hypocapnia in newborn lambs. *J Pediatr.* 1989;115:309–314.

TABLE 13.25   Major Circulatory Effects *During* Perinatal Asphyxia

Initially
Redistribution of cardiac output so larger proportion enters brain
Increase in cerebral blood flow
Loss of cerebral vascular autoregulation
Later
Diminution of cardiac output; hypotension
Decrease in cerebral blood flow

transporters per se are not energy dependent, energy failure, as with hypoxia-ischemia, leads to disruption of Na^+-K^+ ionic gradients across the plasma membrane because of failure of the ATP-dependent Na^+-K^+ pump; the results are *impairment* of the Na^+-dependent glutamate transporters and ultimately *reversal* of transporter function. In the astrocyte, the ATP-dependent enzyme, glutamine synthetase, uses ammonia and glutamate to form glutamine, which diffuses to the presynaptic nerve ending to regenerate glutamate on removal of this second amino group (see Fig. 13.39). ATP depletion also causes this mechanism to fail, and thus clearly ATP depletion results in failure of the major reuptake and removal mechanisms and leads to accumulation of extracellular glutamate and to excitotoxicity (see the following discussion).

These mechanisms of reuptake and removal must be highly efficient, because although the intracellular concentration of glutamate is extraordinarily high (i.e., 5 to 10 mmol/kg), the extracellular concentration is approximately 1000-fold less (i.e., in the low micromolar range or perhaps lower).[660,661,666] The high concentration of glutamate in neurons implies a large release of glutamate into the extracellular space when cell death occurs, an occurrence that is relevant not only to amplification of primary excitotoxic cell death, as occurs with hypoxia-ischemia, but also to the development of secondary excitotoxic cell death from other types of injuries to neurons (e.g., trauma). In addition, release of glutamate from astrocytes may be even more marked than from neurons, under ischemic conditions.[668]

Glutamate acts at both *ionotropic and metabotropic receptors* (Table 13.24).[661,663,665-667,669-683] Three of these are *ionotropic* (i.e., are linked to ion channels). The NMDA receptor is linked to an ion channel for Ca^{2+}, the AMPA receptor is linked to a channel for Na^+ entry, and the kainate receptor is linked to a channel for Na^+ entry. The AMPA receptor is rendered Ca^{2+} impermeable by the presence of one of its four subunits—namely, the GluR2 subunit. This subunit is relatively sparse during early development both in rodent and human neurons, and this feature renders the AMPA receptor in immature neurons Ca^{2+} permeable.[665,666,684-687] This feature may underlie

the involvement of AMPA receptors in the hypoxic-ischemic or glutamate-induced death of immature neurons (see later discussion). Although the NMDA receptor often is considered the most crucial for the excitotoxic effects of glutamate in developing neurons, data suggest comparable importance for the AMPA receptor (see later). Agents that increase or decrease glutamate activation at the synapse mediated by the NMDA receptor-channel complex are shown in Table 13.25. A fourth glutamate receptor type is *metabotropic* (i.e., is coupled through a guanosine triphosphate binding protein [G protein] to an enzyme producing a second messenger, phospholipase C, for phosphoinositide hydrolysis). The resulting products, diacylglycerol and inositol triphosphate, function as second messengers, the former activating protein kinase C, which has many cellular effects, and the latter promoting Ca^{2+} mobilization from the endoplasmic reticulum (see Fig. 13.35).

The normal *ontogeny of glutamate receptors* is relevant to normal brain development and to the vulnerability of immature brain regions to excitotoxic cell death with hypoxia-ischemia. Detailed earlier studies of the development of binding sites for NMDA and non-NMDA receptor agonists in the rat showed a striking increase in the early phases of brain development.[663-665,683,688-694] Later work, largely based on immunocytochemical and in situ hybridization studies, demonstrated the marked developmental increase more clearly, with peak values for the NMDA and AMPA receptors that *exceed* those in the adult brain.[553,685,686] The peak values for NMDA and AMPA receptors were reached at only slightly different ages, with the NMDA peak preceding the AMPA peak. *The timing of these peaks in the rat correlated with the perinatal period for the human brain.* This can be depicted in Fig. 13.40[695] and is discussed with relevance to preterm brain injury (Chapters 14 to 16) and term brain injury (Chapters 18 to 20).

The *molecular characteristics of the NMDA and AMPA receptors* also are developmentally regulated, and the major characteristics of the developing receptors indicate enhanced Ca^{2+} influx.[685,686] Thus, regarding the NMDA receptor, the relative expression of the NR2B subunit compared with that of the NR2A subunit is increased in the immature brain versus that of the adult. *NMDA receptors containing predominantly NR2B exhibit increased duration of NMDA receptor–mediated excitation and increased Ca^{2+} influx.* With regard to the AMPA receptor, in the immature brain the expression of the *GluR2 subunit*, which renders the AMPA receptor Ca^{2+} impermeable, as in the mature brain, is relatively *low. Thus the large numbers of AMPA receptors in developing neurons are largely permeable to Ca^{2+}.*

The transient, dense expressions of these ionotropic glutamate receptors of enhanced functional capabilities have implications not only for their role in normal development

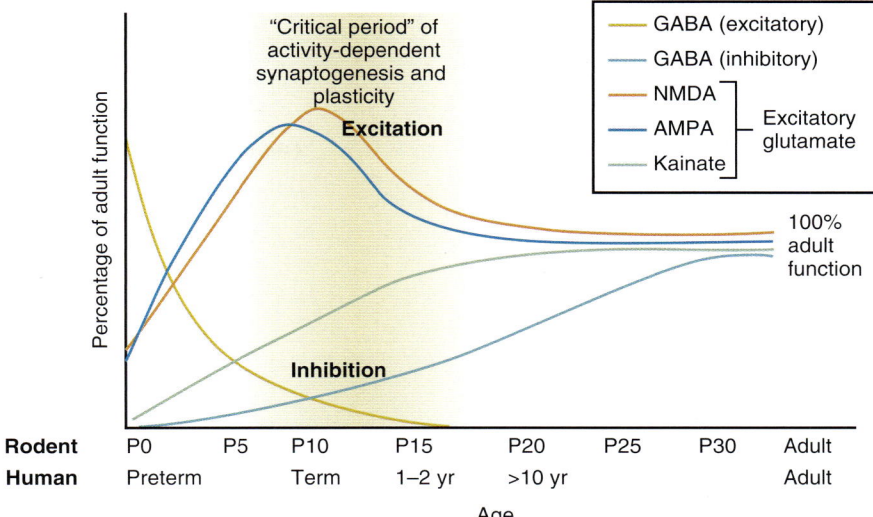

Figure 13.40 Schematic depiction of maturational changes in glutamate and GABA receptor function in the developing brain. Equivalent developmental periods are displayed for rats and humans on the top and bottom axes, respectively. Activation of GABA receptors is depolarizing in rats early in the first postnatal week and in humans up to and including the neonatal period. Functional inhibition, however, is gradually reached over development in rats and humans. Before full maturation of GABA-mediated inhibition, the NMDA and AMPA subtypes of glutamate receptors peak between the first and second postnatal weeks in rats and in the neonatal period in humans. Kainate receptor binding is initially low and gradually rises to adult levels by the fourth postnatal week. *AMPA,* α-amino-3-hydroxy-5-methyl-4-isoxazole propionate; *GABA,* γ-aminobutyric acid; *NMDA,* N-methyl-D-aspartate; *P,* postnatal day. (Reprinted with permission from Rakhade SN, Jensen FE. Epileptogenesis in the immature brain: emerging mechanisms. *Nat Rev Neurol.* 2009;5:380–391.)

but also in determining neuronal death with hypoxia-ischemia (see later). The role of glutamate receptor activation and Ca^{2+} influx relates to such processes as regulation of neurite outgrowth, synapse formation, cell death, selective elimination of neuronal processes, and functional organization of neuronal systems.[663-665,678,685,690,696] *However, in addition, these transient dense expressions of glutamate receptors of enhanced functional capabilities may become the unintended mediators of neuronal death with hypoxia-ischemia* (see later discussion). Moreover, the likelihood that these principles apply to the *developing* human brain is supported by the demonstration of *early overexpression* of glutamate receptors in human hippocampus, cerebral cortex, deep nuclear structures (i.e., basal ganglia and thalamus), and certain brain stem nuclei—regions vulnerable to hypoxic-ischemic injury in the newborn (see Chapters 14 to 20).[663-665,685,687,691,697-701]

Role of Glutamate in Hypoxic-Ischemic Cell Death in Cultured Neurons.

The critical role for glutamate in the mediation of hypoxic-ischemic neuronal death is established by a large body of experimental information, as summarized in Table 13.26.[a] The essential neurotoxicity of glutamate was shown initially in cultured neurons and subsequently in other in vitro and in vivo models (see later).

The crucial initial observation was that cultured hippocampal neurons, obtained from the fetal rat, were *resistant to prolonged anoxia before synapse formation* occurred in the cultures, but they were very sensitive to the same anoxic insult after synaptogenesis was well developed. Thus, such mature cultures markedly

TABLE 13.26	Major Circulatory Effects *Following Perinatal Asphyxia*

Increase in cerebral blood flow beginning within minutes after the insult and lasting for up to several hours
Decline in cerebral blood flow toward baseline or lower, with hypotension, following initial hyperemia
"Delayed" increase in cerebral blood flow ("delayed" hyperemia) beginning between 12 and 24 h and lasting many hours and attenuated by nitric oxide synthase inhibitors
Delayed cerebral hyperemia correlating with impaired mitochondrial oxygenation, "secondary" energy failure, and neuropathological injury

deteriorated in the absence of oxygen.[710] However, when synaptic activity in these mature cultures was blocked by the addition of high concentrations of magnesium, no effect of anoxia on the cultured neurons occurred (Fig. 13.41). Thus the data demonstrated that *synaptic activity resulted in neuronal death* with oxygen deprivation. This protection by synaptic blockage with magnesium was shown later in a hippocampal slice preparation in which neuronal death could be produced in the CA1 region under anoxic conditions.[711]

Because glutamate (as in hippocampus in vivo) was presumed to be the neurotransmitter mediating the synaptic activity in the experiments with the cultured hippocampal neurons and the slice preparation, a nonspecific postsynaptic blocker of glutamate was investigated to prevent the hypoxic neuronal death in culture. This agent protected neurons dramatically from anoxia (Fig. 13.42).[712] The particular role of glutamate

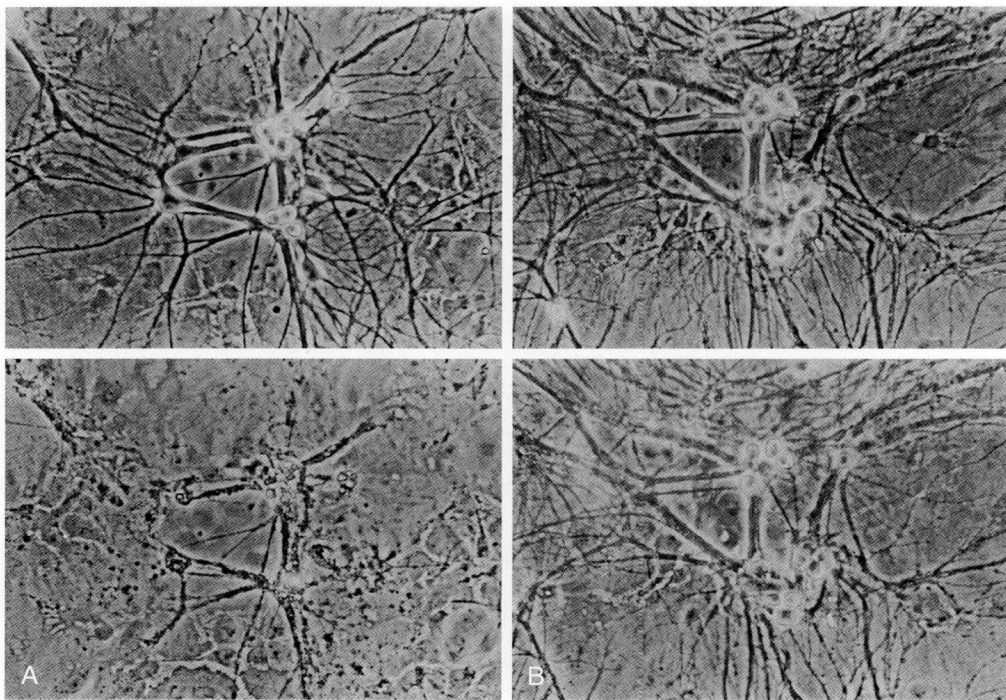

Figure 13.41 Effect of blockade of synaptic activity on anoxic cell death in hippocampal neuronal cultures. (A) Phase contrast micrograph *(top)* shows normoxic culture with abundant neurons; *bottom,* cultures rendered anoxic for 24 hours show extensive neuronal destruction provoked by anoxia. (B) Micrograph shows cultures treated with magnesium chloride to block synaptic activity before *(top)* and after *(bottom)* anoxia. Note the lack of neuronal destruction. (From Rothman SM. Synaptic activity mediates death of hypoxic neurons. *Science.* 1983;220:536–537.)

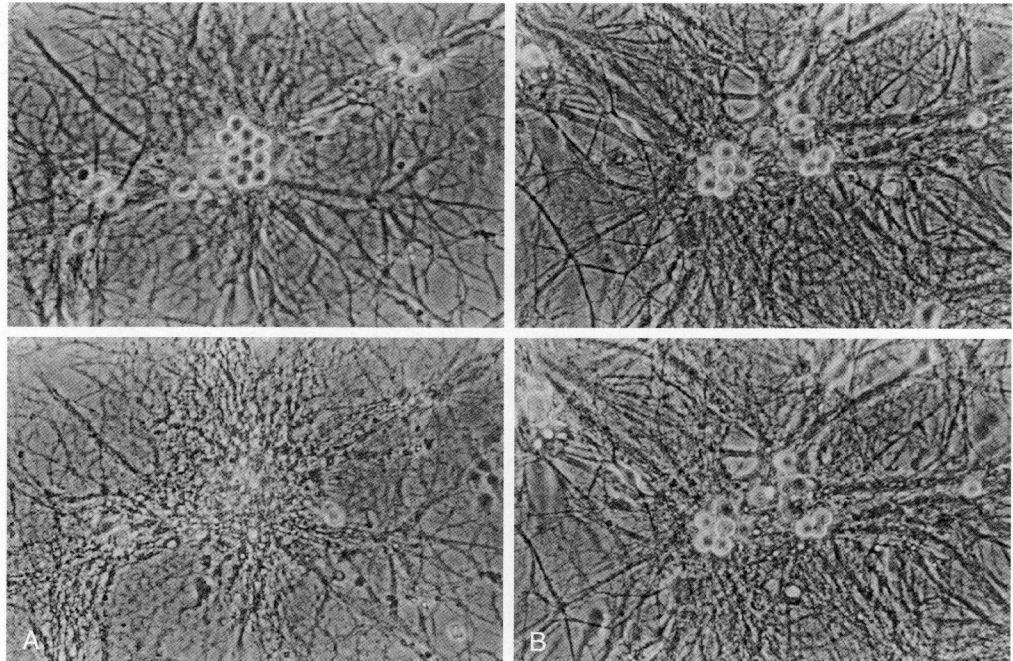

Figure 13.42 Effect of a blocker of the *N*-methyl-D-aspartate (NMDA)-type glutamate receptor on cell death in hippocampal neuronal cultures. (A) Phase contrast micrographs show cultures before *(top)* and 8 hours after *(bottom)* anoxia. Note neuronal destruction after anoxia. (B) Micrographs show cultures treated with the NMDA receptor blocker, gamma-D-glutamylglycine. The appearance before *(top)* and 8 hours after *(bottom)* anoxia are shown. Note the prevention of neuronal destruction in the presence of the blocker. (From Rothman SM. Synaptic release of excitatory amino acid neurotransmitter mediates anoxic neuronal death. *J Neurosci.* 1984;4:1884.)

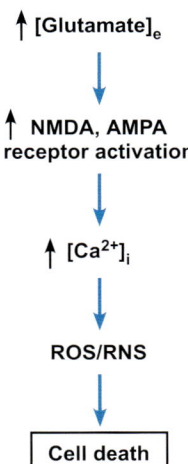

↑ [Glutamate]$_e$

↓

↑ NMDA, AMPA
receptor activation

↓

↑ [Ca^{2+}]$_i$

↓

ROS/RNS

↓

Cell death

Figure 13.43 Mechanisms of glutamate-induced neuronal death. Note the involvement of the N-methyl-D-aspartate (NMDA) and alpha-amino-3-hydroxy-5-methyl-4-isoxazole-propionic acid (AMPA) receptors, the increase in intracellular calcium ([Ca^{2+}]$_i$) the generation of reactive oxygen (ROS) and reactive nitrogen (RNS) species, and the resulting cell death.

synapses in hippocampal neuronal death was supported further shortly thereafter by the demonstration that hypoxic-ischemic neuronal injury could be prevented in vivo by prior section of glutamatergic afferents to the CA1 region.[8,713]

The *mechanisms of glutamate-induced neuronal death* in cultured neurons were elucidated next.[a] Two basic mechanisms were identified. One of these is rapid cell death that occurs in minutes and is initiated by glutamate receptor activation, Na$^+$ entry through all three ionotropic receptors, passive influx of Cl$^-$ down its electrochemical gradient with water following, and ultimately cell swelling and lysis. A second variety, so-called delayed cell death, occurring over many hours, is initiated principally by activation of the NMDA and immature (GluR2-deficient) AMPA receptors, with influx of Ca^{2+} (as well as Na$^+$) and a series of Ca^{2+}-mediated events to cell death (see Table 13.22). *Delayed cell death* appears to be the crucial form of neuronal death in vivo, and the importance of the NMDA and GluR2-deficient AMPA receptors and Ca^{2+} influx is well established by studies of specific blockers of these receptors in cultured cells, brain slices, and in vivo models (see later discussion).[b] The data support the scheme shown in Fig. 13.43. Note the particular involvement of the NMDA and immature GluR2-deficient AMPA receptors. Not shown in the figure is the *accentuation of the increase in cytosolic Ca^{2+}* by Na$^+$ influx through all three ionotropic receptors, membrane depolarization, and opening of voltage-dependent Ca^{2+} channels. Sustained membrane depolarization also leads to *failure of glutamate uptake mechanisms* and to *sustained glutamate release*. Thus cyclical internal amplification with multiple vicious cycles likely becomes operative.

Relevance of Glutamate-Induced Excitotoxicity to Hypoxic-Ischemic Injury in Vivo. The relevance of the *glutamate excitotoxic*

mechanisms to the in vivo situation is now clear.[a] The first body of evidence establishing this relevance showed that *extracellular glutamate concentrations in vivo increase* manifold with hypoxic-ischemic insults.[660] Such increases have been documented in *perinatal* animal models as well as in adults, although glutamate increases tend to be somewhat less in the former models than in the latter.[b] However, studies using microdialysis have documented the accumulation of extracellular glutamate in the brain of asphyxiated fetal sheep and of hypoxic-ischemic immature rats to concentrations of approximately 500 μmmol/L,[739,742,745] concentrations easily sufficient to cause neuronal death in cultured cells. *Moreover, glutamate concentrations in the cerebrospinal fluid of asphyxiated human newborns are markedly greater than concentrations in normal newborns.*[746,747] The reasons for the increase of extracellular glutamate with hypoxic-ischemic insults relate to *impaired uptake of glutamate and to excessive release. The impaired uptake* is related to defective operation of the high-affinity, Na$^+$-dependent glutamate transporters in neurons and astrocytes (because of the failure of the ATP-dependent Na$^+$-K$^+$ pump and loss of the Na$^+$-K$^+$ ionic gradient across the plasma membrane) and to the defective function of the ATP-using glutamine synthetase reaction in astrocytes.[519,666,744,748-751] The transporter function also is disrupted by ROS and RNS and by cytokines (e.g., TNF-alpha), released by activated microglia.[752,753] The *excessive release of glutamate* relates to at least five factors. The first of these is the persistent membrane depolarization resulting from the failure of the ATP-dependent Na$^+$-K$^+$ pump.[754] (The destruction of gamma-aminobutyric acid neurons by hypoxia also may contribute to the excessive excitation and release of glutamate.)[755] The second factor of critical importance is the *reversal* of glutamate transport because of the loss of the Na$^+$-K$^+$ ionic gradient and elevated intracellular Na$^+$ levels. Indeed, this factor may be most important for the sustained release of glutamate into the extracellular space.[756] A third factor is the rapid blockade of inhibitory synaptic transmission with relative preservation of excitatory synaptic transition with anoxia in the immature versus adult animal.[757] A fourth factor promoting the excessive release of glutamate is the acute development of epileptic phenomena after hypoxia in the immature (but not mature) animal.[381] A fifth factor is glutamate release from microglia, a process enhanced in an autocrine manner by TNF-alpha released by microglia with diverse inflammatory stimuli.[758]

The second body of evidence delineating the relevance of glutamate to the in vivo situation is the demonstration in a wide variety of *perinatal models* of hypoxia-ischemia that *glutamate is toxic to neurons in vivo* and that this *toxicity is particularly marked* in the *immature* versus the mature animal.[c] In general, in the immature animal, the most toxic glutamate analogue is NMDA; AMPA is slightly less toxic, and kainate is the least toxic.[d] The approximate time of peak sensitivity in the rat is 6 days for NMDA and 9 to 10 days for AMPA. The particular vulnerability of the brain of the immature animal to hypoxia-ischemia and the importance of the NMDA receptor in this ontogeny of

[a]References 517, 519, 659, 660, 662, 664-666, 678, 680, 682, 690, 691, 693, 702-706, and 714.
[b]References 469, 517, 519, 598, 642, 659, 660, 680, 682, 690, 691, 702-704, 706, and 715-734.

[a]References 517, 519, 642, 659, 660, 678, 680, 682, 684, 685, 690, 691, 693, 708, 723-733, and 735-738.
[b]References 690, 727, 729, 730, 732, and 739-744.
[c]References 379, 519, 553, 662, 664, 665, 685, 690, 706, 709, and 759.
[d]References 642, 662-665, 690, 691, 706, and 760-762.

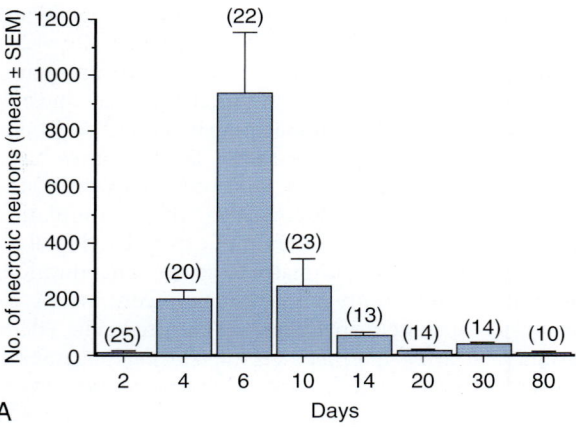

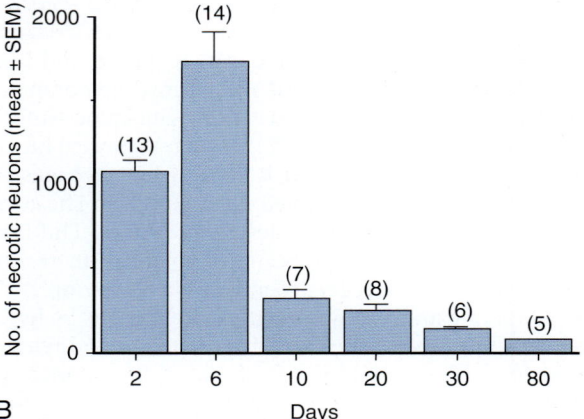

Figure 13.44 Similar developmental profiles of hypoxic-ischemic and N-methyl-D-aspartate (NMDA)-mediated neuronal death. Mean number of neurons destroyed in rat brain under conditions of (A) hypoxia-ischemia, and (B) intrastriatal injection of NMDA (9 nmol). Pups at the age of 6 days show the highest number of necrotic neurons under either condition. The numbers on top of each column represent the number of animals studied for each group. *SEM*, Standard error of the mean. (From Ikonomidou C, Mosinger JL, Salles KS, Labruyere J, Olney JW. Sensitivity of the developing rat brain to hypobaric/ischemic damage parallels sensitivity to N-methyl-aspartate neurotoxicity. *J Neurosci.* 1989;9:2809–2818.)

vulnerability are illustrated by the similar developmental profiles of hypoxic-ischemic neuronal death and NMDA-mediated neuronal death (Fig. 13.44). A similar relationship has been shown for the GluR2-deficient AMPA receptor for the rat.[686] Presumably, these particular vulnerabilities of the immature animal relate at least in part to the transient dense expression of NMDA and GluR2-deficient AMPA receptors during brain development (see earlier discussion).

The third body of evidence linking glutamate to hypoxic-ischemic injury relates to the finding that the topography of glutamate receptors, particularly NMDA and AMPA receptors, corresponds closely to the topography of hypoxic-ischemic neuronal injury observed in vivo.[a] Although more data are needed concerning the perinatal human, the

overwhelming balance of evidence indicates a close relationship between regional neuronal vulnerability to hypoxia-ischemia and regional distribution of glutamate receptors (see Unit I).

Finally, perhaps the strongest evidence of the relevance of the glutamate excitotoxic mechanism to the in vivo situation has been the demonstration of *protection from neuronal death in a variety of perinatal hypoxic-ischemic models by treatment with glutamate receptor blockers*.[a] Most experiments used compounds with effects on the NMDA receptor-channel complex, and in nearly all, benefit was achieved. AMPA antagonists, however, have also been neuroprotective. Benefit was manifested as prevention of morphological, biochemical, or electrophysiological evidence of injury. Although in most studies the antagonists were administered at the onset or during the insult, the most striking has been the marked, though not complete, protection in experiments in which the antagonists were administered *after termination of the insult* (Fig. 13.45). Available data suggest that treatment within 1 to 2 hours is highly effective. This response is compatible with the concepts that delayed cell death is the operative mechanism and that treatment in the clinical situation after termination of the insult ultimately may be beneficial.

Role of Inflammation

The relationship between the brain inflammatory response after hypoxia-ischemia-reperfusion and cell death is discussed in detail later in relation to oligodendroglial injury, as in periventricular leukomalacia (PVL). Similarly, the potentiation of the deleterious effects of hypoxia-ischemia by infection is also emphasized later. Nevertheless, it is important in this context of neuronal death to introduce these concepts, especially in relation to experimental models that focus particularly on gray matter injury rather than white matter injury.

Adult Models of Hypoxic-Ischemic Injury. A series of studies in adult models of hypoxic-ischemic injury, especially models of stroke, initially indicated that inflammatory mechanisms, although important in subsequent reparative processes, are also important in the final common biochemical pathway to hypoxic-ischemic neuronal death.[780-794] The principal sequence of events is the activation of microglia in the first hours after the insult, with the release of a variety of neurotoxic products, including excitatory amino acids, ROS, NO, and certain cytokines. Most important among the cytokines appear to be IL-1beta and TNF-alpha. IL-1beta is particularly important in the activation of endothelial-leukocyte adhesion molecules, especially intercellular adhesion molecule-1 (ICAM-1). The leukocytes involved include not only polymorphonuclear cells but also mononuclear cells, especially of the monocytic-phagocytic series. The leukocytes are important in the release of deleterious compounds, especially ROS and cytokines. The particular importance of activated microglia is supported by the demonstration of neuroprotection by minocycline, a tetracycline analogue that has antimicroglial effects, in several models of hypoxic-ischemic neuronal death.[795-797]

Perinatal Models of Hypoxic-Ischemic Injury. That the sequence of events just explained appears to be operative in *perinatal hypoxia-ischemia* is supported by study of perinatal

---

[a]References 642, 662-665, 683, 685, 686, 690, 693, 694, and 763.

[a]References 699, 723, 724, 728, 731, 733, 735, 736-738, 762, and 764-779.

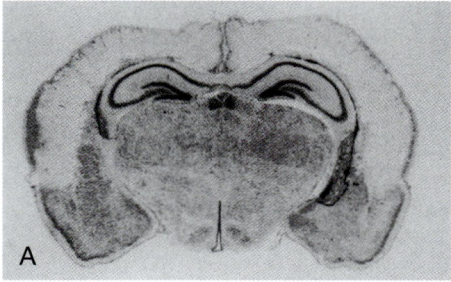
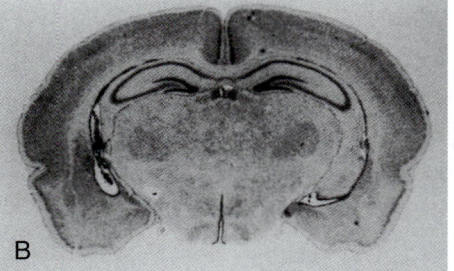
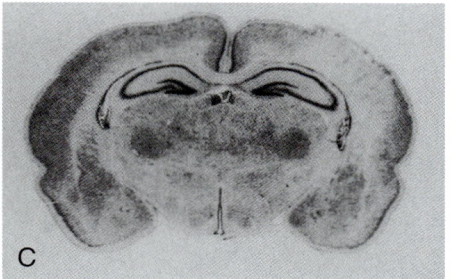
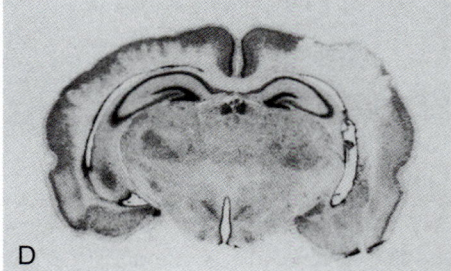
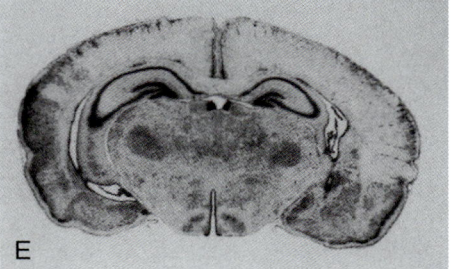

Figure 13.45 Coronal brain sections from rat pups. (A) is from a saline-injected control, and (B) through (E) are from rat pups that were given MK-801 intraperitoneally: (B) 0.5 hour before and (C) immediately, (D) 1 hour, and (E) 4 hours after the hypoxic-ischemic insult. Note the sharply demarcated hypoxic-ischemic infarction in (A). The neuroprotective effects of MK-801 are seen in (B), (C), and (D) in a time-dependent fashion. (Hematoxylin and eosin stain, original magnification ×2.5 before 31% reduction.) (From Hattori H, Morin AM, Schwartz PH, Fujikawa DG, et al. Posthypoxic treatment with MK-801 reduces hypoxic-ischemic damage in the neonatal rat. *Neurology.* 1989;39:713–718.)

TABLE 13.27	Methods for Determination of Cerebral Blood Flow in the Newborn

Xenon-133 clearance techniques (intravenous, intra-arterial, or inhalation administration)

Xenon computed tomography

Positron emission tomography (intravenous administration of $H_2^{15}O$)

Single photon emission computed tomography

Near-infrared spectroscopy (continuous measurement of hemoglobin D [oxyhemoglobin—deoxyhemoglobin] or intermittent inhalation of oxygen)

Doppler ultrasonic techniques

Venous occlusion plethysmography

Electrical impedance techniques

Magnetic resonance techniques[a] (utilization of motion-sensitizing gradient pulses or paramagnetic contrast agent, e.g., gadolinium)

[a]Not yet applied to the newborn.

experimental models (Table 13.27) and human epidemiological data.[787-791,798-808] Thus studies in perinatal rats have shown the *activation of microglia* after hypoxia-ischemia that proceeds more rapidly than in adult animals.[789] Activated microglia begin to accumulate in the first 4 hours after reperfusion and continue to increase over the next 48 hours. *Neutrophil accumulation in brain blood vessels* has been documented on reperfusion after hypoxia-ischemia in the neonatal rat and piglet.[790,799] In the rat model, the accumulation peaked at 4 to 8 hours after reperfusion, although much less infiltration of brain parenchyma

was apparent than that occurring in adult animals.[790,809] However, the neutrophilic accumulation in blood vessels was shown to be important in the genesis of the brain injury by the marked reduction in cerebral edema and subsequent cerebral atrophy in animals made neutropenic before the hypoxic-ischemic insult. Whether the deleterious effect of the neutrophils is related to adherence to endothelium and obstruction of flow or to vascular injury secondary to release of ROS, or to both, remains to be established. Finally, a burst of *cytokine expression*, presumably principally from activated microglia, has been documented in the first 6 hours after cerebral hypoxic-ischemic insult in the immature rat.[787,788,791] Both IL-1beta and TNF-alpha have been shown to increase markedly in the brain in the first 4 to 6 hours after the insult, and notably intracerebral injection of IL-1 receptor antagonist has been shown to ameliorate the brain injury.[788,800] Moreover, pentoxifylline, which inhibits TNF-alpha production, is neuroprotective when administered before hypoxia-ischemia in the 7-day old rat.[801] In addition, the key role of activated microglia in the genesis of neuronal death has been shown by neuroprotection with minocycline in several models of hypoxic-ischemic injury in the neonatal rat, as in adult animals.[810,811] Finally, the potentially deleterious role of the inflammatory cascade is suggested by the partial neuroprotection provided by dexamethasone administered before hypoxia-ischemia in the neonatal rat.[812-814]

Potentiation of Perinatal Hypoxic-Ischemic Brain Injury by Inflammation Provoked by Infection. Potentiation of perinatal hypoxic-ischemic brain injury by inflammation provoked by infection is particularly important in relation to oligodendroglial or white matter injury and is discussed in detail in the next section. However, this situation is likely also important in the

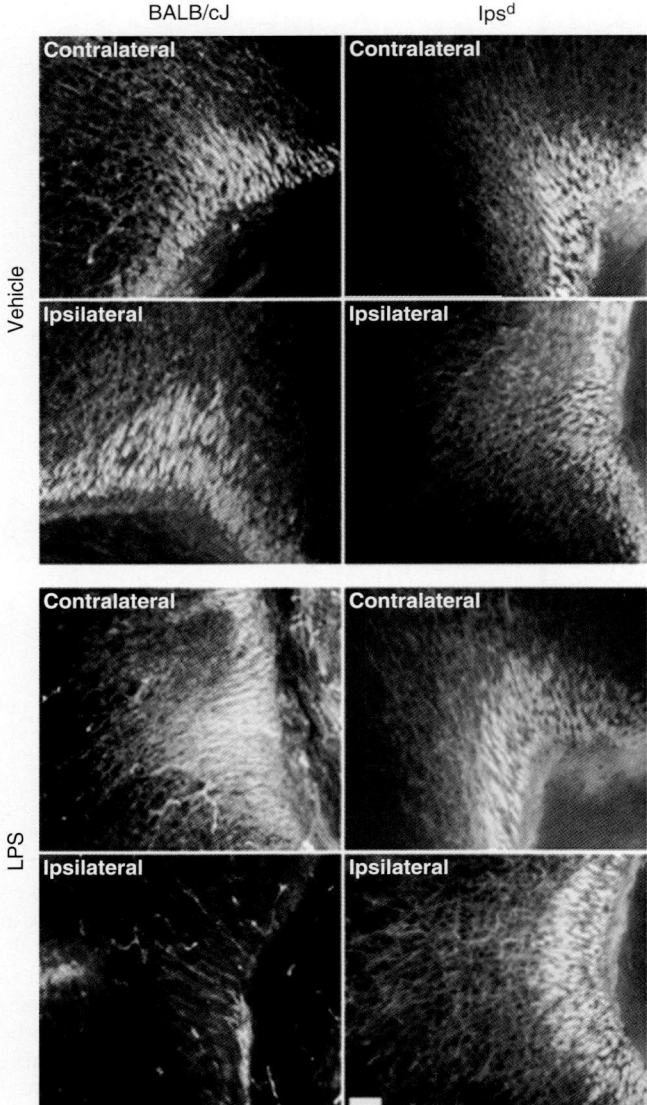

Figure 13.46 Activation of microglia by Toll-like receptor 4 (TLR4) is necessary for the prominent neuronal injury in immature mice treated with lipopolysaccharide (LPS) before a subthreshold hypoxic-ischemic insult. The latter insult was produced by unilateral carotid ligation and hypoxemia in normal (BALB/cJ) and TLR4-lacking (Lps^d) mice. Coronal sections of cerebrum were stained for neurofilament protein. No vehicle-treated animal developed a lesion. By contrast, LPS-pretreated normal animals (BALB/cJ) developed a clear (ipsilateral) hypoxic-ischemic lesion, whereas TLR4-lacking (lps^d) animals did not. (From Lehnardt S, Massillon L, Follett P, et al. Activation of innate immunity in the CNS triggers neurodegeneration through a Toll-like receptor 4-dependent pathway. *Proc Natl Acad Sci U S A.* 2003;100:8514–8519.)

genesis of hypoxic-ischemic neuronal injury. Thus several studies showed a potentiation of hypoxic-ischemic brain injury after pretreatment with LPS.[815-822] The most common paradigm has been the application of a hypoxic-ischemic insult, itself not sufficient to produce brain injury, after short-term (several hours) exposure to LPS, itself not sufficient to produce brain injury. In one report, the effect of LPS was shown to depend on the presence on brain microglia of Toll-like receptor 4 (TLR4), a specific microglial receptor for LPS activation of microglia (see later; Fig. 13.46).[818] The particular involvement

in this combined insult paradigm of an inflammatory cascade, initiated by activated microglia, is suggested by the finding of neuroprotection by pretreatment with dexamethasone.[814] In a related experiment, the use of a glucocorticoid receptor blocker resulted in accentuation of the combined LPS and hypoxic-ischemic injury.[823]

The influence of preceding infection or inflammation on hypoxic-ischemic injury varies according to the timing of the LPS pretreatment. Thus, in the experiments just described, LPS exposure 4 hours before hypoxia-ischemia accentuated injury. A similar potentiation was observed when LPS was administered 72 hours earlier.[824] However, when LPS was administered 24 hours before hypoxia-ischemia, injury was *reduced*. This beneficial effect of LPS preconditioning at 24 hours versus 4 and 72 hours illustrates the potential complexity of the interaction between preceding infection or inflammation and hypoxia-ischemia (see the later discussion on oligodendroglial injury).

Inflammation and Brain Injury in Human Infants. Initial clinical support for a role for inflammation in the genesis of neonatal brain injury emanated especially from epidemiological studies relating *neonatal levels of cytokines in term infants* with brain injury, manifested usually by cerebral palsy defined later in infancy.[825-831] In a minority of these reports, the cytokine evidence of inflammation was a component of an apparent perinatal hypoxic-ischemic insult.[826,829,831] Consistent with these observations is the increased likelihood of later cerebral palsy in newborns who had evidence of chorioamnionitis at birth.[832,833] In the largest case-control study ($N = 231,582$), chorioamnionitis led to a 3.8-fold increased risk for cerebral palsy.[833] The nature of the relationship between perinatal evidence of inflammation and poorer neurological outcome, both in infants with apparent perinatal asphyxial events and in those with no overt hypoxic-ischemic insult, is not entirely clear. The earlier discussion of the potentiating effect of infection or inflammation on subthreshold hypoxic-ischemic insults may be relevant in this context. Further data will be of great interest.

Rationale for Neuroprotective Approaches to Hypoxic-Ischemic Brain Injury Based on Timing and Mechanisms

The fundamental approach to neuroprotection in the human newborn infant is thus based on an understanding of (1) the principal initiating mechanism of injury (hypoxic, ischemic, or asphyxial, or most commonly, some combination); (2) immediate cellular alterations in energy production and impairment in cellular functions, such as membrane potential and structural integrity; (3) subsequent effects of energy failure resulting in excitotoxic and free radical–mediated cellular injury; and (4) delayed apoptotic and autophagic mechanisms of cell death. These mechanisms can have direct cause to effect relationships but also, as important, complex feedback loops that can accelerate energy demands on a dysfunctional metabolic cellular system, thereby propagating ongoing cell death (see Fig. 13.6).

Interventions for Prevention of Neurons From Hypoxic-Ischemic Injury

The insights into the biochemical and cellular mechanisms of neuronal and glial injury with perinatal hypoxic-ischemic-reperfusion insults, as just discussed, provide a rational basis

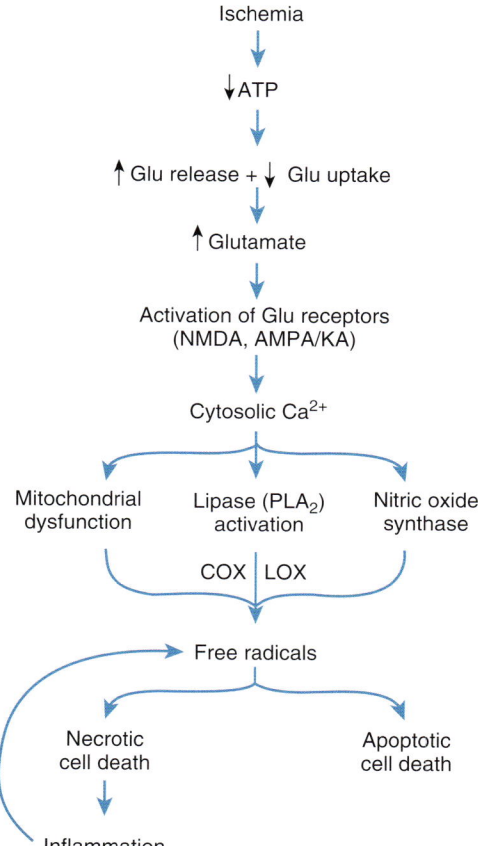

Figure 13.47 General sequence of mechanisms leading to apoptotic and necrotic neuronal death with hypoxia-ischemia. *AMPA*, Alpha-amino-3-hydroxy-5-methyl-4-isoxazole-propionic acid; *ATP*, adenosine triphosphate; *COX*, cyclooxygenase; *Glu*, glutamine; *KA*, kainate; *LOX*, lipoxygenase; *NMDA*, N-methyl-D-aspartate; *PLA₂*, phospholipase A₂. See text for details.

for formulation of interventions to interrupt those mechanisms and thereby prevent or ameliorate the injury. The general sequence of operation of these mechanisms (Fig. 13.47) provides the framework for this discussion of such interventions as outlined in Table 13.28. The following information is derived almost exclusively from data obtained in *perinatal* models of hypoxia-ischemia, *with an emphasis on neuronal injury* (see later for oligodendroglial injury).

Decrease in Energy Depletion. Depletion of high-energy phosphate, not necessarily severe, almost certainly initiates the cascade of events leading to neuronal death (see Fig. 13.47). The most potent and promising intervention to prevent energy depletion is *mild hypothermia* (see Table 13.28; Fig. 13.48).[834-841] In some models, this effect has been correlated with the neuroprotective benefit of this approach. Moreover, mild hypothermia ameliorates the secondary energy failure that follows many hours of reperfusion.[842,843] Nevertheless, the beneficial effects of mild hypothermia occur at *multiple sites* in the cascade to cell death, and the relative importance of each effect remains to be clarified (Table 13.29; see also Table 13.28). A preventive-ameliorative effect of mild hypothermia has been documented in a wide variety of perinatal animal models of hypoxia-ischemia.[834,835,837-842,844-866] In earlier

studies, hypothermia was instituted during hypoxia-ischemia or immediately on reperfusion, or both. In the most recent studies, hypothermia was instituted on reperfusion, to model the usual clinical situation (see Table 13.29). Of particular importance, hypothermia must be commenced before the onset of delayed energy failure and particularly excitatory features, especially seizures. In the experimental models, the onset of the delayed energy failure and seizures is approximately 6 hours after reperfusion. In one especially informative study of ischemic fetal sheep, mild cooling of the cranium *instituted 5.5 hours after the insult* resulted in reduction of injury assessed electrophysiologically and neuropsychologically (Fig. 13.49). (This beneficial effect did not occur in the fetal sheep when hypothermia was instituted at 8.5 hours—just after the occurrence of seizures at 6 to 8 hours.[867]) *Of all the interventions discussed in this section, mild hypothermia has now been proven to be highly effective in reducing neuronal injury and improving short-term and long-term neurodevelopmental outcomes in term born infants with hypoxic-ischemic insults* (see Chapter 20).

The depletion of high-energy phosphates and its initiation of the cascade of events leading to neuronal death can be counteracted in several other ways. The importance of maintenance of glucose at physiological levels was discussed earlier, and data in this regard are summarized in Table 13.18. Sedatives administered in high doses can lead to decreased cerebral metabolic rates and thereby energy preservation.[159] The apparent protective effect of mild hypercapnia, at least in part, may be mediated by decreasing energy utilization.[162] Amiloride, an inhibitor of the Na^+/H^+ transporter, has been shown to be neuroprotective in perinatal hypoxic-ischemic models in vitro and in vivo, and one of the effects of this drug is preservation of energy supplies.[861,868] The Na^+/H^+ transporter is activated with hypoxia-ischemia and leads to sustained intracellular alkalosis, observed in vivo by MR spectroscopy of asphyxiated infants (see Chapter 10). The alkaline pH has multiple effects, including exacerbation of excitotoxicity and impairment of ATP synthesis. Excessive utilization of ATP also can supervene when the increase in intracellular Na^+ concentration leads to activation of the ATP-dependent Na^+/K^+-ATPase.

Inhibition of Glutamate Release. Because glutamate is important in neuronal death, the inhibition of the enhanced glutamate release with hypoxia-ischemia is important (see Fig. 13.47 and Table 13.28). Hypothermia is beneficial at this level both by inhibiting glutamate release and by blunting the disturbance of glutamate transporters that contributes significantly to the accumulation of extracellular glutamate (see earlier).[837,841,869,870] Because Ca^{2+} influx is necessary for glutamate release and because magnesium blocks the former process, part of the beneficial effect of Ca^{2+} channel blockers or of magnesium could occur at this step.[523,871,872] However, Ca^{2+} channel blockers have adverse cardiovascular effects, and magnesium administration in a variety of hypoxic-ischemic models has not been clearly beneficial.[873-875] Adenosine, adenosine agonists, and adenosine antagonists have been studied because activation of the adenosine receptor inhibits glutamate release. Although in some perinatal models adenosine agonists have been beneficial, the available data do not show clearly consistent effects.[876-879]

The neuroprotective effect of free radical scavengers may be exerted partially at the level of glutamate release because

TABLE 13.28 Cerebral Blood Flow in the Newborn as Determined by the Intravenous Xenon-133 Clearance Technique[a]

BIRTH WEIGHT/ GESTATIONAL AGE (MEAN OR RANGE)	NO. OF INFANTS	AGE AT STUDY (MEAN OR RANGE)	CONDITIONS	MEAN CEREBRAL BLOOD FLOW (mL/100 g per min)	REFERENCES (FIRST AUTHOR/ YEAR)
33.4 wk	16	5 days	Stable	29.7	Greisen, 1984[249]
29–34 wk	15	15–17 days	Quiet sleep	17.4	Greisen, 1985[328]
			Active sleep	17.0	
			Wakeful	21.8	
			Unclassified	16.8	
1510 g/31 wk	42	0–5 days	Nonventilatory support	19.8	Greisen, 1986[250]
			Continuous positive airway pressure	21.3	
			Mechanical ventilation (IMV <20)	12.4	
			Mechanical ventilation (IMV >20)	11.0	
			Entire group	15.5	
1340 g/31 wk	15	3.7 wk	Stable	F_1–87.5[b]	Younkin, 1987[254]
				F_2–17.2	
<33 wk	25	1.6 days	Mechanical ventilation	12.3	Greisen, 1987[251]
1420 g/30.9 wk	14	3 h	Glucose ≥1.7 mmol/L	11.8	Pryds, 1988[253]
1210 g/30.5 wk	10	3 h	Glucose ≤1.7 mmol/L	26.0	
1569 g/31.7 wk	21	31 days	Stable	35.4–41.3[b]	Younkin, 1988[255]
1050 g/29.2 wk	18	12.6 h	Stable	13.1	Lipp-Zwahlen, 1989[320]
1540 g/30.4 wk	18	6.4 h	Mechanical ventilation	8.4	Pryds, 1989[256]
1380 g/30.4 wk	8	16.9 h	Mechanical ventilation	10.2	
1470 g/30.3 wk	12	34.3 h	Mechanical ventilation	11.5	
27–33 wk	20	48 h	Mechanical ventilation	10.0	Greisen, 1987[251]
1310 g/29.5 wk	12	2 h	Glucose ≥30 mg/dL	12.0	Pryds, 1990[258]
1500 g/31.2 wk	13	2 h	Glucose ≤30 mg/dL	18.6	
1175 g/29 wk	20	<12 h	Mechanical ventilation	8.7 (total group)	Pryds, 1990[262]
				9.2 (9 infants with normal outcome)	
1300 g/28.0 wk	16	4 days	Before aminophylline	13.2	Pryds, 1991[264]
			After (1 h) aminophylline	10.9	
1060 g/28 wk	10	<36 h	Mechanical ventilation	10.4	Muller, 1997[268]

[a]Excludes studies based on administration of xenon-133 by inhalation or intra-arterial injection and values obtained from infants with documented major brain lesions.
[b]Calculation of cerebral blood flow used partition coefficients derived from studies of adults, which may result in overestimation of cerebral blood flow in the newborn.
IMV, Intermittent mandatory ventilation.

free radicals increase neuronal glutamate release in some models.[880] Moreover, phenytoin has partial neuroprotective effects in cultured neurons and in hypoxic-ischemic models in neonatal rats and fetal guinea pigs, perhaps by blocking Na+ channels and thereby action potential–induced glutamate release.[881-884] The beneficial effect of lamotrigine in an adult model of ischemic neuronal injury probably relates to this anticonvulsant's inhibition of glutamate release.[885] Finally, the recently described neuroprotective effect of cannabinoid agonists in in vitro and in vivo models of neonatal hypoxic-ischemic neuronal injury is mediated in part at the level of glutamate release.[886,887]

Amelioration of Impairment in Glutamate Uptake. As noted earlier, hypothermia may exert some of its neuroprotective effect by decreasing the impairment in astrocytic Na+-dependent, high-affinity glutamate uptake related to ischemia (see Table 13.28). This conclusion is based primarily on studies of neonatal piglets and cultured astrocytes.[870,888]

Blockade of Glutamate Receptors. The neuroprotective effect of NMDA receptor antagonists, especially MK-801 but also xenon, magnesium, ketamine, and dextrorphan, in various models of ischemic neuronal injury, both in culture and in vivo, was discussed earlier concerning glutamate neurotoxicity (see Table 13.26). More often, neuroprotection is achieved when the agents are administered at the termination of the insult or from up to several hours afterward. *Xenon* appears to be particularly efficacious in concentrations likely to be clinically safe.[889,890] Indeed, in one study of hypoxia-ischemia in neonatal rats, *xenon and mild hypothermia acted synergistically to provide neuroprotection* (see Table 13.29). The benefit was greatest when xenon was commenced with the insult, but it was still significant when xenon was used 4 hours after the insult.

Similarly, neuroprotective effects have been apparent in several perinatal models of hypoxia-ischemia by the use of non-NMDA antagonists, especially AMPA antagonists (2,3-dihydroxy-6-nitro-7-sulfamoyl-benzo[f]quinoxaline-2,3-dione

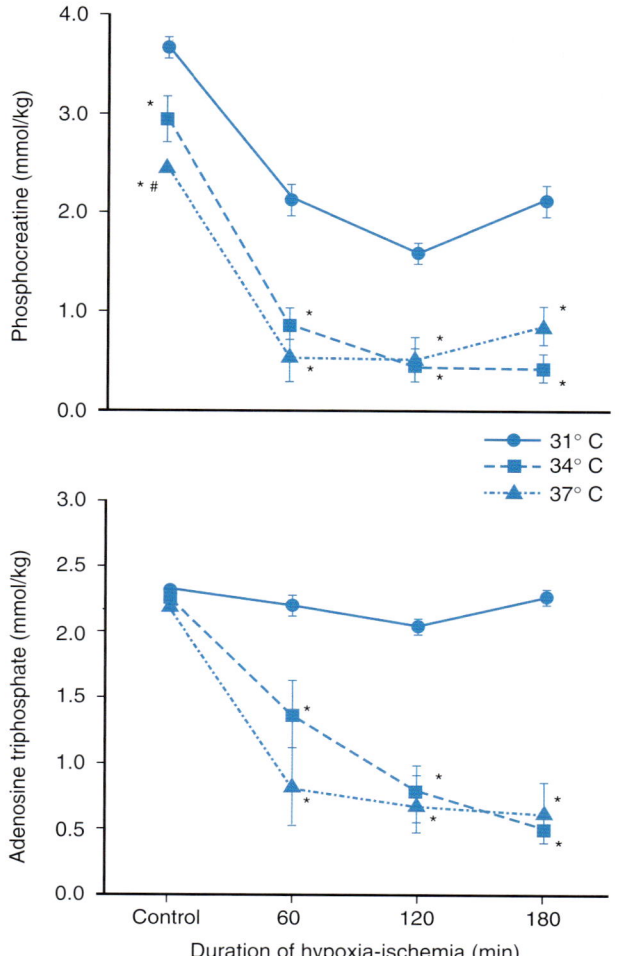

Figure 13.48 Preservation of high-energy phosphate levels in brain of the immature (P7) rat subjected to hypoxia-ischemia at the temperatures shown. With mild hypothermia (31°C), the decline in brain phosphocreatine level was partially prevented, and the decline in ATP levels was completely prevented. (From Yager JY, Asselin J. Effect of mild hypothermia on cerebral energy metabolism during the evolution of hypoxic-ischemic brain damage in the immature rat. *Stroke.* 1996;27:919–926.)

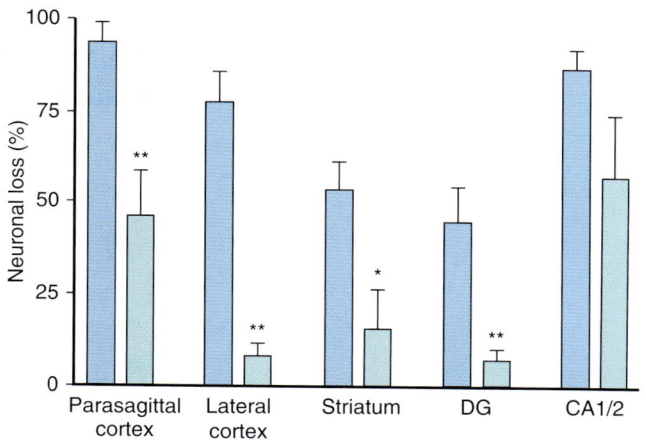

Figure 13.49 Effect of selective cerebral cooling (extradural temperature, 30.4°C) from 6 to 72 hours after ischemia in near-term fetal sheep on neuronal loss in different brain regions 5 days after the ischemia. A significant overall reduction ($P < .001$) in neuronal loss was observed in fetuses treated with selective cerebral cooling (black bars), compared with sham-cooled fetuses (white bars), except in the most severely affected field of the hippocampus (CA1/2). *$P < .05$; **$P < .01$; mean ± SEM. (From Gunn AJ, Gunn TR, Gunning MI, Williams CE, Gluckman PD. Neuroprotection with prolonged head cooling started before postischemic seizures in fetal sheep. *Pediatrics.* 1998;102:1098–1106.)

TABLE 13.29	Regulation of Cerebral Blood Flow in the Human Newborn[a]
INCREASE IN REGULATORY FACTOR	**CHANGE IN CEREBRAL BLOOD FLOW**
BP: normal preterm or term infant	0 (autoregulation)
BP: severely asphyxiated term infant	↑
BP: before severe intracranial hemorrhage or periventricular leukomalacia, or both—in preterm infant	↑
PaCO₂: normal preterm or term infant	↑
PaCO₂: severely asphyxiated term infant	0
PaCO₂: before severe intracranial hemorrhage in preterm infant	0
Total hemoglobin concentration	↓
Proportion of fetal hemoglobin	↑
Glucose (blood)	↓
Seizure	↑
Indomethacin	↓
Ibuprofen	0
Aminophylline	↓

[a]See text for references.

BP, Blood pressure; *PaCO₂*, arterial partial pressure of carbon dioxide in arterial blood.

[NBQX], 6-cyano-7-nitroquinoxaline-2,3-dione [CNQX], topiramate).[736-738,777-779,891,892] Particularly noteworthy is the *synergistic* neuroprotective effect of *topiramate and mild hypothermia* in a perinatal model (P7 rat), in which neither intervention alone produced appreciable benefit (Fig. 13.50). *Topiramate* is of particular interest because postinsult treatment with this drug *also protects developing oligodendrocytes from injury* (see later discussion). Moreover, unlike many other excitatory amino acid antagonists, topiramate, in clinically used doses, does *not* lead to apoptotic neuronal death in the developing brain.[893-895]

Blockade of Free Radical Generation. The downstream intracellular biochemical events leading to cell death include the large series of Ca^{2+}-activated processes, leading to the generation of ROS and RNS, and apoptotic and necrotic cell death (see Table 13.22). *Hypothermia* probably acts at multiple levels in this cascade, but prominent among these effects are reductions in free radical production and NO synthesis (see Tables 13.28

and 13.29).[642,838,839,841,896-899] Inhibitors of free radical production of demonstrated neuroprotective value in various models of hypoxia-ischemia include allopurinol (inhibits xanthine oxidase step), indomethacin (inhibits cyclooxygenase), iron chelation (diminishes hydroxyl radical production by the Fenton reaction), fructose-1,6-biphosphate (preserves intracellular

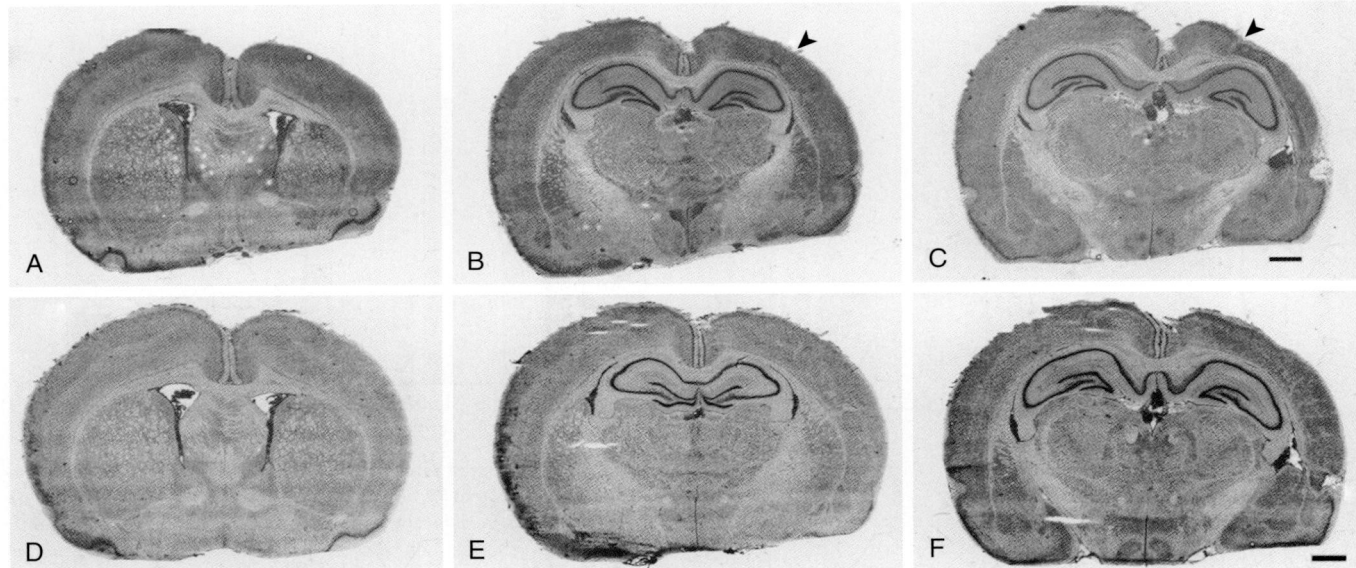

Figure 13.50 Synergistic protective effect of topiramate and mild hypothermia. Comparison of histopathology (coronal sections, cresyl violet) in two P35 rats subjected at P7 to unilateral carotid ligation and hypoxemia, followed by delayed (3 hours) hypothermia with vehicle (A to C) or topiramate (D to F). In the vehicle-treated hypothermic animals, a major lesion *(arrowheads)* is apparent, whereas minimal injury is apparent in the topiramate-treated hypothermic animals. (From Liu Y, Barks JD, Xu G, Silverstein FS. Topiramate extends the therapeutic window for hypothermia-mediated neuroprotection after stroke in neonatal rats. *Stroke.* 2004;25;1460–1465.)

glutathione), and magnesium (inhibits lipid peroxidation; see earlier discussions and references cited herein).[a]

Inhibitors of NO synthesis have been shown to be beneficial in a variety of perinatal models (see earlier discussion). Because of the temporal characteristics of activation of, first, nNOS and, later, iNOS (see Fig. 13.38), specific inhibitors of each isoform have been used in perinatal models.[657,658,903-905] Particularly promising results have been obtained with inhibitors of *both* nNOS and iNOS. Hypothermia also appears to decrease NO generation.[841]

Removal of Free Radicals. A deficiency in antioxidant defenses is an important determinant of neuronal vulnerability in the immature brain (see earlier discussion). Thus accumulation of free radicals occurs, and an important protective intervention involves removal of these injurious components. Two major approaches used have been the administration of free radical scavengers or antioxidant enzyme mimetics. *Free radical scavengers* shown to be effective in perinatal models of hypoxia-ischemia have included vitamin E and its analogues, edaravone and *N*-acetylcysteine (see Fig. 13.36).[b] Of particular interest is the recent demonstration in a hypoxic-ischemic model in the neonatal rat of *synergistic* protection by mild to moderate (30°C) hypothermia (2 hours) and *N*-acetylcysteine (daily), begun following the insult.[906] *N*-acetylcysteine has been shown not only to scavenge free radicals but also to restore intracellular glutathione levels.

Antioxidant enzyme mimetics may prove to be an important advance in the removal of free radicals. Thus these low-molecular-weight, nonpeptidyl molecules mimic the activity of SOD, catalase, or glutathione peroxidase and have the capacity to penetrate the blood-brain barrier.[592,908] Most available data concerning neuroprotective effects have been obtained in adult models, but protection in neonatal hypoxia-ischemia has also been shown.[592]

Blockade of Downstream Effects. Because a substantial proportion of injury to developing neurons with hypoxia-ischemia is apoptotic (see earlier), *inhibitors of apoptotic cell death* have been studied for neuroprotective effects (see Table 13.28). *Hypothermia* has been shown to protect the neonatal rat brain against hypoxia-ischemia by reducing both apoptosis and necrosis (see Table 13.29).[841,864,909,910] The modality may be especially useful against apoptosis, a particularly important mode of neuronal death in neonatal hypoxia-ischemia.[841] Postischemic hypothermia blocks the intense activation of caspase-3, critical for apoptotic cell death after ischemia.[911] Indeed, in the P7 rat model of hypoxia-ischemia, a combination of systemic hypothermia and administration of a pan-caspase inhibitor *synergistically* led to reductions of both caspase-3 activation and neuronal injury in the hippocampus (see Table 13.29).[912]

Erythropoietin (EPO), a glycoprotein originally recognized for its role in erythropoiesis, has been shown to be involved in the adaptive response to perinatal hypoxia-ischemia and to exhibit neuroprotective properties (Table 13.30).[913-919] Thus hypoxia-ischemia leads to an increase in expression of EPO and the EPO receptor, beginning within hours initially in neurons (as well as endothelial cells) and after days, especially in astrocytes.[920-922] The resulting beneficial effects include upstream mechanisms (i.e., antiexcitotoxic effects, attenuation of glutamate release), antioxidant actions (upregulation of glutathione peroxidase, decrease of lipid peroxidation), inhibition of NO production, and downstream mechanisms (i.e., antiapoptotic and

---

[a]References 159, 538, 539, 551, 599, 600, and 900-903.
[b]References 593, 601, 603, 604, 906, and 907.

TABLE 13.30   Relation of Cerebral Blood Flow to Partial Pressure of Carbon Dioxide in Arterial Blood in the Human Preterm Infant in the First 2 Days of Life

AGE	VENTILATION	CHANGE IN CBF (%)/CHANGE IN $PaCO_2$ (mm Hg)
2–3 h	Spontaneously breathing	3.85
2–12 h	Mechanically ventilated	1.50
12–24 h	Mechanically ventilated	1.57
24–48 h	Mechanically ventilated	4.35

CBF, Cerebral blood flow; *$PaCO_2$*, arterial partial pressure of carbon dioxide in arterial blood.

Data for mechanically ventilated infants from Pryds O, Greisen G, Lou H, Friis-Hansen B. Heterogeneity of cerebral vasoreactivity in preterm infants supported by mechanical ventilation. *J Pediatr.* 1989;115:638–645, and derived from 38 preterm infants (mean birth weight 1470 g) with persistently normal neonatal ultrasound scans; data for spontaneously breathing infants from Pryds O, Andersen GE, Friis-Hansen B. Cerebral blood flow reactivity in spontaneously breathing, preterm infants shortly after birth. *Acta Paediatr Scand.* 1990;79:391–396.

survival-promoting effects, as well as stimulation of angiogenesis and neurogenesis; see Table 13.30).[498,913,917,922,923] Although not yet shown in perinatal hypoxia-ischemia, EPO may also serve to preserve cerebrovascular autoregulation and to blunt injurious inflammatory responses.[913] Neuroprotective effects have been shown by treatment *after* as well as before neonatal hypoxia-ischemia. Moreover, although EPO is a 34-kDa glycoprotein, it has been beneficial after *systemic* administration. The principal initiating stimulus for EPO expression is the hypoxia-induced upregulation of hypoxia-inducible factor (HIF1), a transcription factor whose target genes are involved in such key physiological responses as energy metabolism, angiogenesis, and cell proliferation, in addition to EPO expression. Iron is required for degradation of HIF1, and at least part of the neuroprotective benefit of desferrioxamine after hypoxia-ischemia relates to its stabilization of HIF1 and preservation of upregulation of EPO.[922] Upregulation of HIF1 and induction of these adaptive responses underlie the neuroprotection observed in experimental models of *hypoxic-ischemic preconditioning*.[497,498,924-930] EPO produces its key antiapoptotic effects by binding to its receptor, with subsequent activation of the Jak-Stat pathway. The latter involves translocation of Stat-5 to the nucleus, binding to DNA and promoting Bcl-x2 and Bcl2-2 expression, and finally inhibition of caspase-3 activation.[913,917] In addition, NF-kappaB is activated, and the latter ultimately promotes expression of such protective genes as inhibitors of apoptotic protein and SOD. Although *EPO shows great promise as a potential neuroprotective agent*,[913,931] one report indicated *enhanced* neuronal injury when cultured neurons or immature rats were subjected to moderate hypoxia-ischemia *after* treatment with EPO.[932] Clinical situations in which hypoxia-ischemia may occur after treatment with EPO include the asphyxiated fetus or critically ill premature newborn. More data are needed concerning this critical issue.

Because *growth factors and other neurotrophic substances* generally prevent apoptotic cell death, many have been investigated for neuroprotection (see Table 13.28). Those with demonstrated value in various neonatal models of hypoxia-ischemia have included insulin-like growth factor-I (IGF-I), nerve growth factor (NGF), brain-derived neurotrophic factor (BDNF), and growth hormone.[23,910,933-943] Reductions of caspase-3 activation and thus an antiapoptotic effect have been observed after administration of BDNF and IGF-I.[23,941] In addition, IGF-I activates a major pathway mediating neuronal survival involving activation of the serine/threonine kinase AKt.[941] Because in neuronal cultures both BDNF and IGF-I potentiate necrotic cell death with free radical attack, concern exists that, at least under certain circumstances, growth factors may prevent apoptosis but accentuate necrosis.[2] More data are needed.

Inhibition of Inflammatory Effects. As noted earlier, inflammatory mechanisms, initiated after hypoxia-ischemia severe enough to cause tissue necrosis, are important in generating a cascade of deleterious effects that can be cyclical. Thus tissue injury causes inflammation, which in turn causes more tissue injury (see Fig. 13.47). A critical aspect of the inflammatory cascade is the activation of microglia. Other events include release of cytokines and ROS and RNS, accentuation of excitotoxicity, and induction of leukocyte adhesion molecules.

Hypothermia exerts a portion of its neuroprotective effects by suppression of the inflammatory response (see Table 13.28).[841] The responses blunted include microglial activation, generation of free radicals, release of cytokines, and neutrophil accumulation. The first of these effects may be the most important.

Minocycline, a tetracycline derivative, has been shown to be neuroprotective in perinatal models of hypoxia-ischemia, when it is administered either before or immediately after the insult (see Table 13.28; Fig. 13.51).[810,811] The beneficial effects of minocycline have been shown in a variety of other models, including excitotoxicity, oxidative stress, and cytokine attack.[795-797,944-948] The bases for the neuroprotective effects of minocycline are likely multiple, although inhibition of microglial activation appears to be the most important. In one careful experimental study of neonatal hypoxia-ischemia, minocycline *accentuated* neuronal injury.[949] The negative effect was observed in a neonatal mouse model, whereas the beneficial effects have been shown in neonatal rat models. However, a beneficial effect was documented in an adult mouse model of hypoxia-ischemia.[797] Moreover, minocycline was shown to be protective to white matter in perinatal models (see later). Thus this agent, or related antimicroglial agents, shows considerable promise for hypoxic-ischemic neuroprotection (see Table 13.28).

The beneficial effect of *induced neutropenia* before hypoxia-ischemia was discussed earlier.[790] Platelet-activating factor (PAF), the levels of which increase with ischemia-reperfusion, is important in the induction of leukocyte adhesion molecules and thereby subsequent events in the inflammatory cascade. In the immature rat, administration of a *PAF antagonist* has been shown to decrease infarct size with both pretreatment and posttreatment regimens (i.e., begun on reperfusion).[801,950-953] Finally, a critical product of microglia-macrophages is IL-1beta, which, in turn, induces formation of other proinflammatory cytokines, including TNF-alpha. Notably, use of an antagonist of the IL-1 receptor both preinsult and on reperfusion has

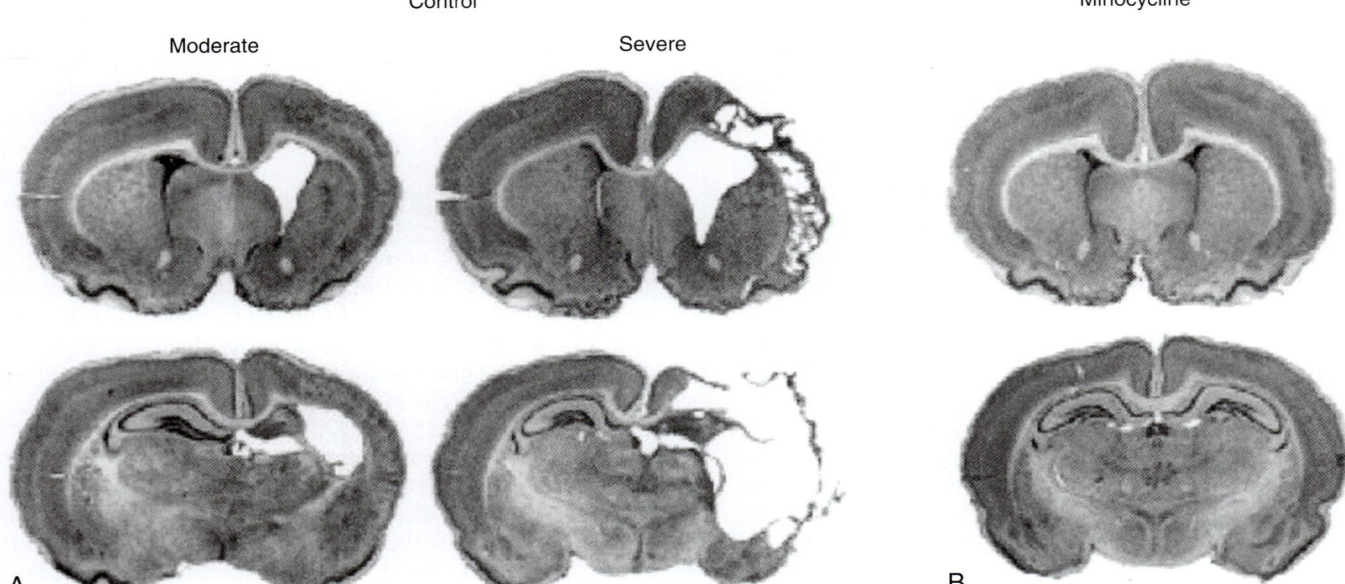

Figure 13.51 Neuroprotective effect of minocycline in hypoxia-ischemia. Representative coronal sections of postnatal day (P) 14 rat brains are shown 1 week after unilateral *(left)* carotid ligation and exposure to hypoxia for 2.5 hours at P7. In a typical example of animals given intraperitoneal injections of minocycline (B) immediately before or after hypoxia, there was little to no damage in almost all brains in comparison with the characteristic moderate or severe injury seen in the hemisphere ipsilateral to carotid ligation in most animals treated with phosphate-buffered saline alone *(control)* (A). (From Arvin KL, Han BH, Du Y, Lin S-Z, Paul SM, Holtzman DM. Minocycline markedly protects the neonatal brain against hypoxic-ischemic injury. *Ann Neurol.* 2002;52;54–61.)

had protective effects in hypoxic-ischemic brain injury in the neonatal rat.[788] These and related issues are discussed further later on, concerning white matter injury.

The Preterm Infant—Biochemical Mechanisms of Oligodendroglial Death With Hypoxia-Ischemia

Intrinsic Vulnerability of Early Differentiating Oligodendroglia to Hypoxic-Ischemic Injury

The principal form of brain injury in the premature infant involves cerebral white matter and, particularly, early differentiating, premyelinating oligodendrocytes (pre-OLs; see Chapters 14 and 15). Pre-OL death is an important characteristic of PVL. As for neuronal death, the most important initiating event is *ischemia* to cerebral white matter (Fig. 13.52). The premature infant has a particular propensity for ischemia to cerebral white matter because of the presence of (1) vascular end zones and border zones in that region and (2) impairment of cerebrovascular autoregulation (see Chapters 14 and 15). The latter leads readily to cerebral ischemia and affection of cerebral white matter vascular border and end zones (see Chapters 14 and 15). The importance of cerebral ischemia in pathogenesis of cerebral white matter injury (i.e., PVL) is illustrated in many models in developing animals (primarily sheep, piglet, rat), in which ischemia has been shown to lead to selective or predominant cerebral white matter injury.[6,222,425,954-983] The principal cellular target has been identified as the preoligodendrocyte (O4+) and the immature oligodendrocyte (O1+), especially the former,[222,959,974,980,984] which together I refer to as pre-OLs. (Recall from Unit 1 that the sequence of oligodendroglial development is the A2B5+ [or NG2+] oligodendrocyte precursor, the O4+ preoligodendrocyte, the O1+ immature oligodendrocyte, and

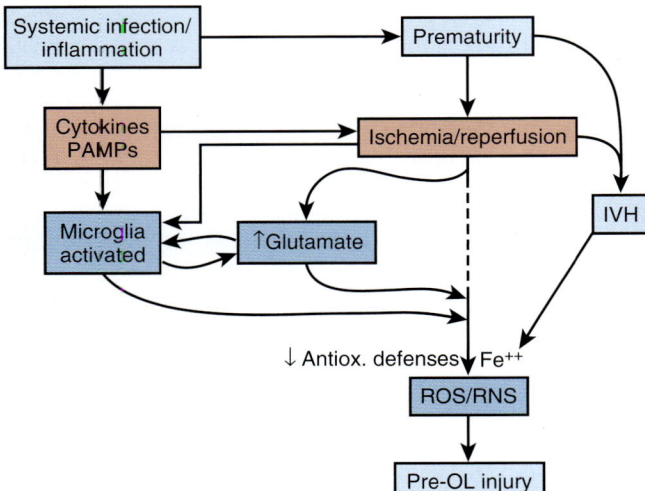

Figure 13.52 Sequence of mechanisms leading to oligodendroglial death. See text for details. The two major upstream mechanisms are ischemia and infection or inflammation *(lighter shading)*, and the two principal downstream mechanisms are excitotoxicity and free radical attack by reactive oxygen species (ROS) and reactive nitrogen species (RNS) *(darker shading)*. IVH, Intraventricular hemorrhage.

the mature, myelin basic protein [MBP+] oligodendrocyte.) Indeed, in one careful study in fetal sheep, under conditions of ischemia, the regional distribution of pre-OLs correlated closely with the regional distribution of the cerebral white matter injury.[222] As discussed in Chapter 15, the pre-OL is the predominant phase of the oligodendroglial lineage observed in human cerebral white matter in the third trimester during the peak period of vulnerability to PVL. In some of the ischemic models, other cellular elements in cerebral white matter (e.g., axons, subplate neurons) or in adjacent neuronal structures (e.g., basal ganglia, cerebral cortex) have been variably affected, but overall the principal cellular target has been the pre-OL.

Infection or Inflammation as an Additional or Potentiating Mechanism

Although ischemia has been the dominant initiating upstream mechanism in the experimental models of white matter injury, infection or inflammation has been shown to lead to injury to pre-OLs in the developing brain (see later). Because a relationship is strongly suspected between maternal intrauterine infection with a systemic fetal inflammatory response and PVL in the human infant, these findings suggest that infection or inflammation is a second important initiating mechanism in cerebral white matter injury (see Fig. 13.52).

Gram-Negative Infection, Endotoxin (Lipopolysaccharide), and White Matter Injury.

A role for maternal/fetal and perhaps neonatal infection in the pathogenesis of PVL was suggested initially by neuropathological studies of human brain and related experimental studies of developing kittens in the 1970s.[985-987] A particular focus on endotoxin (LPS) characterized this earlier work. Subsequent studies have documented varying degrees of white matter injury, including oligodendroglial loss, hypomyelination, ventriculomegaly, and to a lesser extent, cyst formation after systemic or intracerebral injection of LPS to pregnant rats, fetal sheep, and neonatal rats or after induction of gram-negative infection in pregnant rats or pregnant rabbits.[821,822,971,988-1003] Although the neuropathological findings often are not marked and all findings are not consistent among studies, prominent observations, in addition to white matter injury, include infiltration with activated microglia and upregulation of several inflammatory cytokines. These findings are reminiscent of the human lesion (see Chapter 14). Because LPS may cause systemic hypotension, hypoglycemia, a microvascular procoagulant effect, and diminished CBF, cerebral hypoxia-ischemia could complicate these experiments.[1004-1007] However, some studies of LPS-induced white matter injury in fetal sheep do not demonstrate prominent systemic vascular effects.[971]

Because the experimental studies just noted support a relationship between maternal/fetal infection or inflammation and white matter injury, elucidation of the major mechanisms underlying this relation would be critical. Currently data are inconsistent regarding whether LPS, or any related microbial molecular product, may enter the fetus.[1008-1010] Moreover, it is unclear whether LPS can enter the fetal or neonatal brain from the blood (see the next section). However, striking responses in the brain have been well documented after systemic LPS exposure (i.e., upregulation of a variety of cytokines, Fas, NF-kappaB, SOD, ornithine decarboxylase, BDNF, NGF, lipid peroxidation, and of particular importance, the TLRs TLR4 and TLR2, as well as CD14).[1011-1026] In a study using gene microarray techniques, more than a thousand genes were shown to be regulated in the immature rat brain after systemic LPS administration, with a substantial number of cell death–associated genes represented.[1026] *Nearly all the responses involve brain microglia, and at least two of these (i.e., upregulation*

of TLR4 and CD14) are of particular interest because these molecules are the microglial receptors for LPS that mediate innate immunity (see the next section). *Activation of these receptors on microglia results in the death of pre-OLs.*[996]

Innate Immunity and the Relation of Systemic Inflammation to the Brain.

Activation of microglia in the context of infection is postulated to occur in considerable part by way of a relatively small number of specific cell surface receptors (i.e., TLRs) that respond to specific molecular motifs shared by the products of multiple microorganisms (so-called pathogen-associated molecular patterns, or PAMPs).[1025,1027-1033] Because similar molecular motifs are shared by many microbial products, the relatively small number of specific TLRs is the basis for an immediate response to many different organisms (i.e., the mechanism of *innate immunity*). The relevance of this system to the link between maternal/fetal infection and PVL is suggested by the demonstrations that brain microglia contain TLR4, the specific receptor for LPS, the key molecular product of many gram-negative microorganisms, and that when activated by LPS, these microglia secrete diffusible products, perhaps principally NO/ONOO⁻, that are highly toxic to pre-OLs (Fig. 13.53).[996,1034,1035] The mechanisms by which *systemic* LPS produces these responses in the brain are unclear. The possibilities include the following: (1) penetration by LPS of a blood-brain barrier still "immature" in the developing animal or the human premature infant; (2) passage of LPS across a blood-brain barrier compromised by the action of cytokines or by hypoxia-ischemia, or both; (3) passage of LPS into brain across areas devoid of a blood-brain barrier (i.e.,

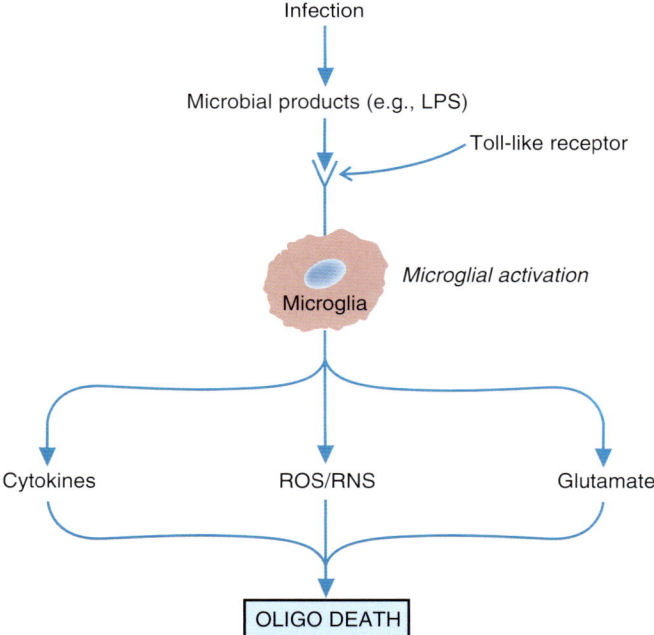

Figure 13.53 **Innate immunity in the pathogenesis of oligodendroglial death.** Activation of specific Toll-like receptors (TLRs) by specific molecular motifs of microbial products (e.g., TLR4 for lipopolysaccharide [LPS] of gram-negative organisms) causes microglial activation and secretion of toxic products, especially reactive oxygen species (ROS) and reactive nitrogen species (RNS). This immediate response to infection (i.e., innate immunity) can cause "innocent bystander" injury to developing oligodendrocytes (OLIGO).

circumventricular organs, with subsequent propagation of immune signals into brain parenchyma); (4) stimulation by LPS of brain endothelial cells with subsequent propagation of immune signals (e.g., cytokines) into brain parenchyma; (5) passage of peripheral LPS-stimulated cytokines across an intact or compromised blood-brain barrier; or (6) penetration of an intact or compromised blood-brain barrier by LPS-stimulated peripheral monocytes.[1018,1022,1025,1028,1036-1046] Experimental data are available to support all these possibilities, although the relevance to the human premature infant remains unclear.

Central Role of Microglia. Although the mechanisms by which maternal/fetal infection and inflammation initiate deleterious molecular and structural events in the brain are not fully understood, *it is clear that microglial cells play a central role.* Moreover, studies in a variety of systems indicate that ROS, RNS, cytokines, and glutamate are important in mediating the actions of these cells (see later). Because mechanisms of ROS/RNS toxicity and excitotoxicity are central to the intrinsic maturation-dependent vulnerability of pre-OLs to both hypoxia-ischemia and infection or inflammation, I further discuss the microglial downstream roles later. However, *it is important here to reemphasize the finding in study of human PVL of the marked microgliosis discovered in the diffuse component of the lesion* (see Chapter 14).[1047] This seminal observation supports their involvement in the human lesion.

The particular involvement of microglia, supported by both human neuropathological observations and by experimental studies, in such an apparently diffuse process as exposure to microbial products or to cytokines, raises the important question of why PVL is confined to the cerebral white matter and spares the overlying cerebral cortex. One potential answer is that hypoxia-ischemia *initiates* the activation of microglia, and the resulting selectivity of cerebral white matter relates to the cerebral hemodynamic and vascular anatomical factors leading to hypoxia-ischemia, as described earlier and in Chapter 15. In addition, however, microglial cells can be identified in the normal human brain very early in development, become abundant in the forebrain from 16 to 22 weeks of gestation, and *notably are concentrated in cerebral white matter, with a deep to superficial gradient.*[1018,1043,1048-1050] Relatively few microglial cells are found in cerebral cortex at this time. *Thus a maturation-dependent population of cells (i.e., microglia) is concentrated in cerebral white matter at the right time and in the right place to contribute to white matter injury when activated.*

Hypoxia-Ischemia and Maternal/Fetal Infection: Potentiating Insults

Deleterious interactions between maternal/fetal infection or inflammation and hypoxia-ischemia could occur at several steps in the pathway to oligodendroglial death (see Fig. 13.52). Thus such potentiation could develop at the level of the major upstream initiating events of hypoxia-ischemia and infection or inflammation, or at the level of the major downstream events of ROS/RNS toxicity and excitotoxicity, or both (see later). Not unexpectedly, most current evidence supporting a potentiating interaction of hypoxia-ischemia and infection or inflammation emanates from experimental studies. However, clinical and neuropathological studies of human PVL also support the notion of a potentiating interaction of these two insults (see Chapters 14 and 15).

Potentiation of Adverse Systemic and Cerebral Circulatory Effects by Combined Infection or Inflammation and Hypoxia-Ischemia. The combination of infection or inflammation and hypoxia-ischemia could result in deleterious circulatory effects, ultimately affecting the cerebral circulation (see Fig. 13.52). Thus, as noted earlier, in some experimental studies, deleterious systemic hemodynamic effects were shown to accompany fetal or neonatal infection or exposure to LPS or cytokines. That a similar interaction could occur in the premature infant is suggested by several reports. Moreover, because several cytokines stimulated by infection, especially TNF-alpha and IL-1beta, exhibit vasoactive properties, it is reasonable to postulate that these inflammatory molecules could contribute to the impaired cerebrovascular autoregulation shown to be important in the pathogenesis of PVL (see Chapter 15).[1051,1052] Under such circumstances, modest decreases in arterial blood pressure could result in decreases in CBF. Indeed, major disturbances in the regulation of CBF and cerebral oxygen delivery have been observed in fetal sheep after relatively low doses of LPS.[1005] Finally, it is well established that hypoxia-ischemia also leads to both systemic and cerebral elevations of vasoactive proinflammatory cytokines (e.g., TNF-alpha and IL-1beta) derived from peripheral monocytes and brain microglia (see earlier).[1053-1056] *Thus the possibility of amplifying or at least additive effects on the systemic and cerebral circulations is considerable in the presence of both infection or inflammation and hypoxia-ischemia.*

Microglia as a Convergence Point in the Potentiation of White Matter Injury by Infection or Inflammation and Hypoxia-Ischemia. Potentiation of the deleterious effects of infection or inflammation and hypoxia-ischemia could also occur downstream of the initiating insults and the effects on the systemic and cerebral circulations (see Fig. 13.52). As discussed earlier concerning neuronal injury, *several studies of immature animals demonstrated that pretreatment with LPS, at doses insufficient alone to cause brain injury, caused a hypoxic-ischemic insult, also insufficient alone to result in appreciable injury, to produce marked degrees of injury, including white matter injury.*[170,815-822] In most of these experimental models, injury to both neurons and differentiating oligodendroglia were observed. Notably, the potentiation of hypoxic-ischemic injury by LPS involved pretreatment in the several hours before hypoxia-ischemia. However, tolerance rather than potentiation was observed when the LPS pretreatment occurred 24 hours before hypoxia-ischemia.[824] The latter effect was shown to be mediated by upregulation of corticosterone after the LPS administration.[823] No benefit was observed when dexamethasone was administered after the hypoxic-ischemic insult. Among the potential beneficial effects of the endogenous glucocorticoids is inhibition of phospholipase A_2 with liberation of arachidonic acid; LPS activates cyclooxygenase 2 expression, involved in arachidonate metabolism, and thereby generation of injurious ROS.[814]

The importance of innate immunity in the genesis of the potentiation of white matter injury by hypoxia-ischemia and infection or inflammation is suggested by the following observations: (1) CD-14, essential for the action of TLR4, the TLR for LPS, was upregulated after LPS treatment,[815] and (2) in parallel experiments with mice lacking TLR4, the combination of LPS and hypoxia-ischemia produced *no* injury.[818] *These data strongly suggest that microglial cells are central to the sensitizing effect of*

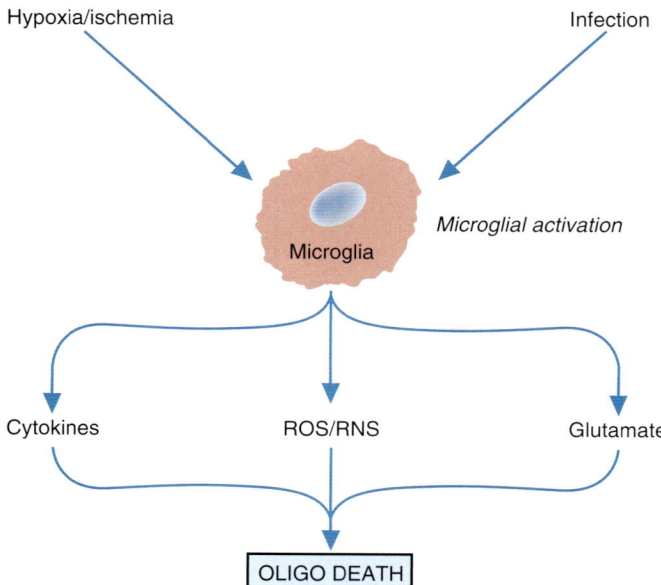

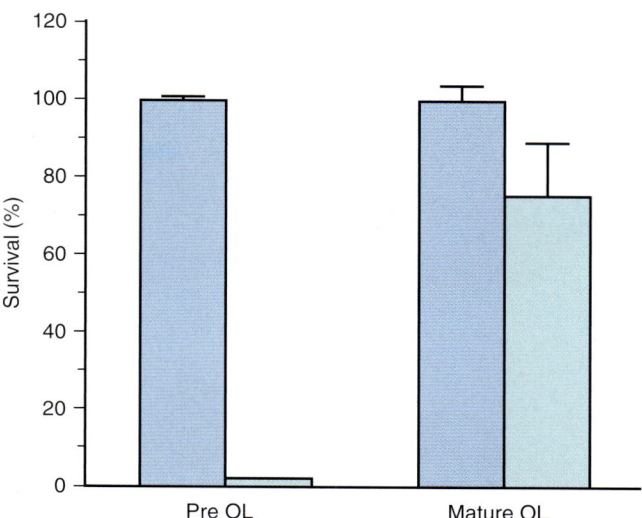

Figure 13.54 Microglia as a central convergence point in the mechanisms of cell death with hypoxia-ischemia and infection. *OLIGO*, Oligodendrocytes; *RNS*, reactive nitrogen species; *ROS*, reactive oxygen species. See text for details.

Figure 13.55 Developing preoligodendrocytes (pre OL) are exquisitely vulnerable to free radical attack (produced by the use of cystine-depleted medium, which leads to decreased intracellular glutathione and oxidative stress), whereas mature oligodendrocytes (mature OL) are resistant. Solid bars are control cells in cystine-containing medium, and hatched bars are cells undergoing free radical attack in cystine-depleted medium. (From Back SA, Gan X, Li Y, Rosenberg PA, Volpe JJ. Maturation-dependent vulnerability of oligodendrocytes to oxidative stress-induced death caused by glutathione depletion. *J Neurosci.* 1998;18:6241–6253.)

LPS and that the two potent activators of microglia, infection (with its associated pathogen-associated molecular patterns; i.e., PAMPs) *and hypoxia-ischemia, may converge on the microglial cell to provoke a deleterious series of effects* (Fig. 13.54). The downstream molecular events involved in the potentiation of hypoxic-ischemic injury by LPS likely involve ROS and, particularly, RNS, cytokines, and glutamate (see Fig. 13.54). These events are discussed next in relation to the maturation-dependent vulnerability of pre-OLs.[54]

Perhaps additional indications of the potentiating interaction of infection or inflammation and hypoxia-ischemia are the demonstrations of the *exacerbation of excitotoxic white matter and gray matter lesions by proinflammatory cytokines*.[802,1057] Excitotoxicity, of course, is a well-established mediator of hypoxic-ischemic death to both pre-OLs and to neurons (see earlier). A central role for *microglia* in this potentiation of excitotoxicity by cytokines is likely because the pretreatment with proinflammatory cytokines increased microglial density in the white matter areas that developed excitotoxic injury.[802] Moreover, TNF-alpha, released from microglia, has been shown to lead, in turn, to the release of glutamate from microglia in an autocrine manner.[758] Also of relevance in this context is the inhibition of glutamate uptake in astrocytes and oligodendrocytes by proinflammatory cytokines (see later discussion).[1058-1061]

Maturation-Dependent Intrinsic Vulnerability of Premyelinating Oligodendrocytes in Cerebral White Matter

An intrinsic vulnerability of pre-OLs in the cerebral white matter of the human premature infant is suggested by experimental studies, by the rarity of the lesion at later ages, by the concentration of these cells in human cerebral white matter during the peak time period for occurrence of PVL, and by their specific involvement in the lesion. To address and clarify the issue of the maturation-dependent vulnerability of oligodendroglial precursors, we and others studied this cell lineage, identified by immunocytochemical criteria (see Unit I), in experimental systems, both in culture and in vivo, and in the human postmortem brain. Within this lineage, as stated earlier, the data indicate that the principal cellular target in PVL is the *pre-OL, a term that includes both the O4+ pre-oligodendrocyte and the O1+ immature oligodendrocyte*. The data indicate that these cells are particularly vulnerable to the *two principal downstream events* in PVL (i.e., *ROS/RNS toxicity* and *excitotoxicity*; see Fig. 13.52), as discussed next.

Reactive Oxygen and Nitrogen Species Toxicity

The most compelling direct evidence that ROS/RNS toxicity is involved in the injury to pre-OLs in PVL emanates from our study of the human lesion reported by Haynes and associates (see Chapter 14).[1047] Thus, using immunocytochemical markers for oxidative (hydroxynonenal) and nitrative (nitrotyrosine) attack, abundant staining was documented in both pre-OLs and reactive astrocytes in PVL. The free radical attack appeared to lead to the death of the former but not the latter. This key discovery of oxidative and nitrative attack in PVL is consistent with experimental data indicative of oxidative and nitrative cellular injury with both hypoxic-ischemic and inflammatory insults to brain (see later), the two likely key upstream mechanisms in PVL (Fig. 13.55). The bases for the maturation-dependent sensitivity of pre-OLs to ROS and RNS toxicity are discussed next.

Reactive Oxygen Species Toxicity. A particular maturation-dependent vulnerability of pre-OLs to both endogenous and exogenous ROS is now well established in both cultured cells and in vivo models (see Fig. 13.55).[980,1062-1067] Thus pre-OLs are killed under conditions of ROS attack that do not harm

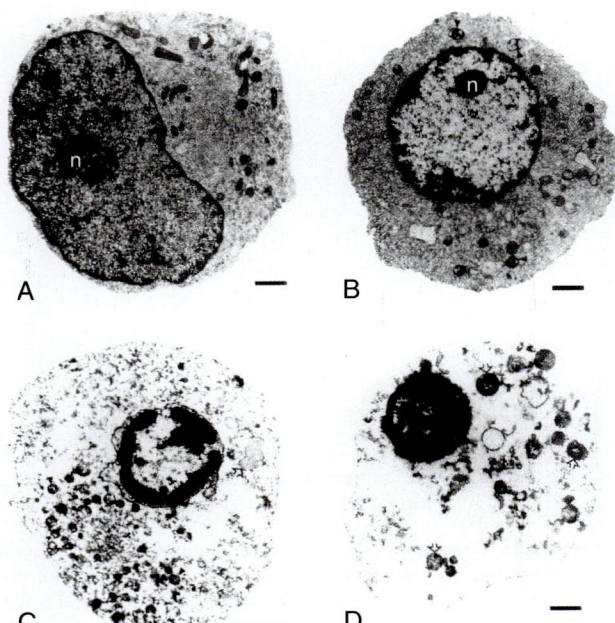

Figure 13.56 Free radical attack causes apoptotic cell death in developing oligodendrocytes. The ultrastructural characteristics of (A), a control cell, and (B) through (D), cells undergoing progressive free radical attack in cystine-depleted medium over 14 hours are shown. Note in (B), the margination and clumping of chromatin; in (C), the condensed marginated chromatin but intact nuclear and plasma membranes; and in (D), the shrunken nucleus with very condensed chromatin but still intact nuclear and plasma membranes. These features are characteristic of apoptosis (see Table 13.1). *n,* Nucleolus. (From Back SA, Gan X, Li Y, Rosenberg PA, Volpe JJ. Maturation-dependent vulnerability of oligodendrocytes to oxidative stress-induced death caused by glutathione depletion. *J Neurosci.* 1998;18:6241–6253.)

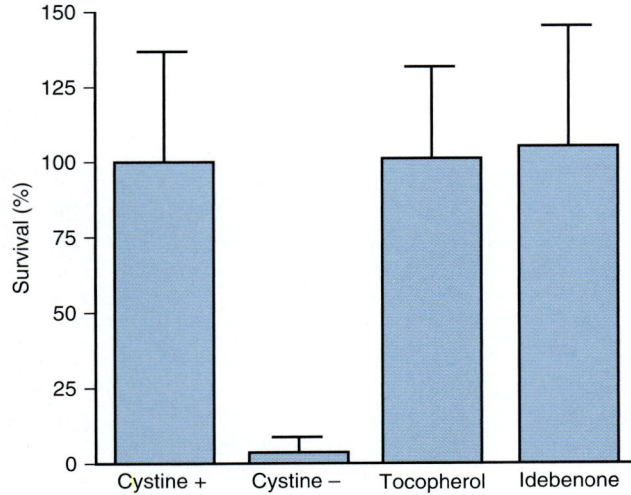

Figure 13.57 Free radical scavengers, alpha-tocopherol and idebenone, protect developing oligodendrocytes in culture from free radical attack. Free radical attack was produced by the use of cystine-depleted medium, which leads to oxidative stress by provoking glutathione depletion, and survival was determined at 24 hours. Note the minimal survival in cystine-depleted medium. When alpha-tocopherol or idebenone was added to the cystine-depleted medium, total protection from free radical–mediated death was observed. The protective effect was observed even when the agents were added as long as 15 hours *after* the onset of cystine depletion. (From Back SA, Gan X, Li Y, Rosenberg PA, Volpe JJ. Maturation-dependent vulnerability of oligodendrocytes to oxidative stress-induced death caused by glutathione depletion. *J Neurosci.* 1998;18:6241–6253.)

mature oligodendrocytes. Moreover, the mechanism of cell death is principally apoptotic (Fig. 13.56). In addition, in cultured pre-OLs, a potent protective effect of clinically safe free radical scavengers (e.g., vitamin E) was shown, even when it was added *after the onset* of ROS attack (Fig. 13.57).[1064] Moreover, vitamin K has been shown to be extraordinarily potent in preventing oxidative injury to developing oligodendrocytes.[1066] The mechanism of the protection by vitamin K was not established, although the vitamin prevented accumulation of ROS in one model of oxidative stress. Moreover, the protective effect occurred even when vitamin K was added hours after the onset of the insult. An important clue to the basis of the particular vulnerability of pre-OLs versus mature cells to ROS toxicity was the discovery that, under conditions of identical exposure to ROS, pre-OLs accumulated ROS, whereas mature cells did not.[1064] The importance of *ROS accumulation in pre-OLs versus mature oligodendrocytes,* despite a similar degree of exposure to ROS, suggested that the intrinsic vulnerability of pre-OLs to oxidation related in part to a *deficit in antioxidant defenses.*

The mechanisms underlying the maturation-dependent vulnerability of developing oligodendrocytes to ROS attack have been addressed in both human brain and in cell culture. The findings in the human brain indicate a delay in the development of enzymes at the SOD and catalase steps (see Chapters 14 and 15), and the findings in cultured pre-OLs show an additional disturbance at the glutathione peroxidase/catalase steps (see

Fig. 13.37).[1068-1070] In addition, the possibility that hydrogen peroxide accumulates and is converted to the hydroxyl radical by the Fenton reaction is suggested by the observations of others of the early appearance of iron in developing human white matter,[1071,1072] as well as by the acquisition of iron by developing oligodendrocytes for differentiation.[1073] In addition, non-protein-bound iron increases prominently in cerebral white matter after hypoxia-ischemia.[1074,1075] Supportive of a relationship between iron and PVL are observations in a mouse model that iron pretreatment increases the amount of white matter injury,[1076] and that for many weeks after human intraventricular hemorrhage, a disorder that sharply increases the risk of PVL,[1077-1079] cerebrospinal fluid levels of nonprotein-bound iron are markedly increased (see Fig. 13.52).[1080] Taken together, the findings indicate a maturation-dependent window of vulnerability to oxidative attack during oligodendroglial development, related principally to the delayed development of antioxidant enzymes and the acquisition of iron for differentiation (see Fig. 13.52).

Multiple reports suggest that the vulnerability to oxidative attack in the premature white matter shares similarities with features in the periphery. Thus studies of plasma of human premature infants indicate a propensity to generate free radicals, including the hydroxyl radical, increases in plasma non-protein-bound iron, accentuated by hypoxia or blood transfusion, and impaired antioxidant defenses.[615,1081-1090]

As for hypoxia-ischemia, experimental studies relevant to maternal/fetal infection and inflammation also indicate a link to oxidative stress. Thus research based primarily on cellular systems indicate that ROS, produced largely by microglia activated by cytokines, LPS, or other factors, are important mediators of oligodendroglial (and neuronal) toxicity in many paradigms.[1091-1100] The critical sequence for the killing of pre-OLs by LPS-activated microglia is LPS activation of the TLR-4 receptor, generation of superoxide anion, nitric oxide, and then peroxynitrite, the final mediator of pre-OL death.[996,1034]

Reactive Nitrogen Species Toxicity.

As with oxidative stress, experimental studies in a variety of models demonstrated the importance of RNS in the cascade to cell death induced by hypoxia-ischemia-reperfusion (see earlier). The presence of NOS in neurons (including subplate neurons), astrocytes, activated microglia, endothelial cells, and perhaps pre-OLs (see later) provides abundant sources for NO. NO toxicity to oligodendrocytes was shown in primary cultures, oligodendroglial-derived cell lines, and isolated rat optic nerves.[633,1101-1107] The work of my colleagues and I showed that NO toxicity to oligodendrocytes is maturation dependent, with pre-OLs much more vulnerable than mature MBP-expressing oligodendrocytes.[1101] The mechanisms of the NO toxicity to pre-OLs are likely multiple. Thus, in the presence of activated microglia, formation of superoxide anion and NO and then $ONOO^-$ is important.[1034] However, NO can lead to pre-OL death directly and without formation of $ONOO^-$. Thus, in the latter instance, NO acts as a mitochondrial poison, with subsequent translocation of apoptosis-inducing factor from mitochondria to nuclei and caspase-independent cell death.[1101] *Relevance of these mechanisms to human PVL is indicated* by the finding of a significant increase in the number of iNOS-positive astrocytes in the diffuse component of PVL (see Chapter 14). The data suggest that a key source of NO in the human lesion, potentially leading to a major portion of the nitrative stress identified previously in diffuse PVL,[1047] is the reactive astrocyte (see Chapter 15).

As for hypoxia-ischemia, experimental studies relevant to maternal/fetal infection and inflammation also indicate a link to RNS toxicity. Thus research based primarily on cellular systems indicate that RNS, produced largely by microglia activated by cytokines, LPS, or other factors, but also probably produced by astrocytes, are important mediators of oligodendroglial (and neuronal) toxicity in a variety of models.[1034,1108-1112] Interferon-gamma is of particular importance in this context for several reasons. First, induction of iNOS, particularly in microglia but also in astrocytes, appears to be the principal mode of killing induced by this cytokine.[1034,1108-1114] Second, of proinflammatory cytokines thus far studied, interferon-gamma appears to be the most toxic to oligodendrocytes, and particularly developing oligodendrocytes.[1115-1118] Third, although data are not entirely consistent concerning toxicity of TNF-alpha to oligodendrocytes,[1104,1118-1126] it is clear that TNF-alpha potentiates the oligodendroglial toxicity of interferon-gamma.[1115,1119,1127] Moreover, in one careful study of the entire oligodendroglial lineage, the toxicity of TNF-alpha decreased as maturation progressed.[1128] Fourth, interferon-gamma levels increase in the neonatal piglet brain after systemic LPS treatment.[1054] Fifth, mice made transgenic for cerebral expression of interferon-gamma exhibit marked hypomyelination and impaired remyelination.[1129,1130] Finally, our studies of human PVL showed in the diffuse component of the lesion abundant interferon-gamma expression in astrocytes and interferon-gamma receptor expression in pre-OLs (see Chapter 4).[1131] Taken together, the data suggest that RNS toxicity is involved in cell death with infection or inflammation, and that interferon-gamma especially, through induction of iNOS and thereby NO production, may be a critical mediator of pre-OL death in PVL. TNF-alpha likely plays a critical role as well.

Excitotoxicity

An intrinsic maturation-dependent vulnerability of pre-OLs to excitotoxicity was shown by experimental studies and by related observations of developing human brain (see Chapter 15). Indeed, with free radical toxicity, excitotoxicity may be considered one of the two major downstream mechanisms in the cascade to oligodendroglial death (see Fig. 13.52). Glutamate is capable of inducing maturation-dependent death of pre-OLs by nonreceptor and receptor-mediated mechanisms. The *nonreceptor-mediated mechanism* involves glutamate competition for the cystine transporter and promotion of cystine efflux under conditions of high extracellular levels of glutamate.[1062] The results are depletion of intracellular glutathione (which requires cysteine for biosynthesis) and cell death by oxidative stress.[1062-1064] However, the substantial levels (millimolar) of glutamate required for this effect suggest that this mechanism may operate in vivo only under extreme pathological conditions.

By contrast, the *receptor-mediated mechanism*, which requires micromolar levels of glutamate, is more likely to occur in vivo, as shown directly in animal models by us and others (see later). In the following discussion, I review evidence for glutamate elevations in white matter in vivo, the sources of glutamate, the receptors involved, and the interaction of excitotoxicity and ROS/RNS toxicity.

Elevated Glutamate Levels in Vivo.

Although the elevation of brain glutamate levels in vivo with hypoxia-ischemia and inflammation has been recognized in cerebral neuronal structures,[744] only recently have such elevations been documented in cerebral white matter.[1132] Thus, in an established model of cerebral white matter injury produced by umbilical cord occlusion in near-term fetal sheep, marked increases in extracellular glutamate were detected in white matter by microdialysis in the hours after occlusion. The extent of the increase in extracellular glutamate correlated directly with the ultimate extent of white matter injury. The *delayed* increase in glutamate over the *hours* after the insult was much greater than the increase during the insult and is considered to be the more important increase in the genesis of the injury. This delayed and large increase has been observed in other models in which an effect on glutamate transport systems occurs (see the next section).

Sources of Glutamate.

The sources of glutamate in cerebral white matter after hypoxia-ischemia appear to be principally glutamate transporters.[1133,1134] Glutamate levels in white matter are regulated by high-affinity, Na^+-dependent glutamate transporters on oligodendroglia, astrocytes, axons, and probably microglia.[1133,1134] The two principal transporters, GLAST and GLT-1, are involved. When ATP levels fall and the energy-dependent Na^+-K^+ cellular gradient is lost, the glutamate transporters fail and operate in reverse. This fact may underlie the potentiation of pre-OL excitotoxicity by impaired mitochondrial function.[1135] Oligodendrocytes are quantitatively important cells for glutamate transport in white matter, and *both pre-OLs and axons appear to be the major sources for extracellular glutamate with hypoxia-ischemia, oxygen-glucose deprivation, or inflammation.*[984,1059,1133,1134,1136-1139] Recently described vesicular release from axons also could be involved.[1140,1141] With ischemia, astrocytes also are important sources.[1142,1143] Although a portion of this latter effect is reversal of transport, another mechanism involves ischemic activation of the $Na^+/K^+/Cl^-$ cotransporter, with Cl^- and water import, astrocyte swelling, and ultimately lysis, with the release of intracellular glutamate. Microglial cells, activated by inflammatory stimuli, also release glutamate by varied mechanisms that may include the reversal of an Na^+-dependent transporter, operation of the cystine-glutamate antiporter, and vesicular release.[758,1134,1144-1148] Additional links of altered glutamate homeostasis to inflammation include the potent inhibition of glutamate transport in oligodendrocytes by TNF-alpha and in astrocytes by IL-1beta.[1058-1061]

Relevance of this work on glutamate transport and thereby excitotoxicity to the other major downstream mechanism of pre-OL death initiated by hypoxia-ischemia or inflammation (see Fig. 13.52; i.e., ROS/RNS toxicity) is suggested by the demonstration that ROS disrupts glutamate transport in astrocytes.[752] Because excitotoxicity to pre-OLs is mediated in considerable part by the generation of ROS (see later), the possibilities of amplification of the two downstream mechanisms of excitotoxicity and ROS/RNS attack through effects on glutamate transport are real.

Involvement of glutamate transport in the maturation-dependence of pre-OL toxicity and in the genesis of human PVL is suggested by the demonstration of overexpression of glutamate transporters in cerebral white matter in the fetal sheep and in the human infant during the time period of peak vulnerability to PVL (see Chapter 15).[1149,1150] Our studies of the human brain also demonstrate that the glutamate transporter is overexpressed in the pre-OL.[1149]

Glutamate Receptors. Only in the past decade has it become clear that oligodendrocytes contain glutamate receptors, which, when excessively activated, can lead to cell injury. The most widely studied type of glutamate receptor, the AMPA/KA type, concentrated in cell somata, leads to cell death when excessively activated (see later). The more recently discovered type, the NMDA receptor, concentrated in oligodendroglial processes, leads to the loss of cell processes when excessively activated. I discuss each of these in sequence next.

Oligodendrocytes express *AMPA/kainate (AMPA/KA)-type glutamate receptors*, the activation of which results in cell death.[1067,1133,1135,1151-1159] Our study of excitotoxicity to the major phases of the oligodendroglial lineage showed that the toxicity is maturation dependent and that both functional activity and subunit expression of AMPA/KA receptors are downregulated in mature oligodendrocytes versus pre-OLs.[1160] The relevance of these findings to hypoxia-ischemia was suggested by the demonstration in culture by others and by us that receptor-mediated excitotoxicity was the principal mechanism for pre-OL death with oxygen-glucose deprivation.[1067,1136,1153,1158,1161-1163] Relevance to hypoxia-ischemia in vivo was shown after the development of a rodent model of hypoxia-ischemia–induced PVL (P7 rat subjected to unilateral carotid ligation and hypoxemia).[1164] This white matter injury could be prevented by *systemic* administration, beginning immediately *after* insult, of NBQX, an AMPA/KA antagonist (Fig. 13.58).[1164] Because NBQX may not be clinically safe, in

subsequent work, topiramate, a clinically safe anticonvulsant drug with AMPA blocking properties, was shown to also have a similar protective effect.[1165] Additionally supportive of a relationship among hypoxia-ischemia, excitotoxicity, and PVL is the observation that AMPA receptors are overexpressed (relative to the mature brain) in the white matter of developing rats during the peak period of vulnerability of this species for selective hypoxic-ischemic white matter injury (see earlier).[686]

The mechanism of the receptor-mediated toxicity appears to involve Ca^{2+} influx.[a] The basis for the Ca^{2+} influx relates to the expression in developing versus mature oligodendrocytes of AMPA receptors that lack the GluR2 subunit, the subunit that renders the receptor Ca^{2+} impermeable.[1067,1151,1165] *Relevance of these observations to PVL is suggested by the demonstration that pre-OL killing induced by oxygen-glucose deprivation occurs by Joro spider toxin–sensitive Ca^{2+} permeable AMPA/KA receptors.*[1067] Moreover, of potential clinical relevance is the additional finding that *sublethal oxygen-glucose deprivation resulted in enhanced toxicity to subsequent exposure to oxygen-glucose deprivation (or to kainate)* because of downregulation of the GluR2 subunit and an increase in Ca^{2+} influx.[1067] Studies of cerebral hemodynamics in the premature infant suggest that infants with a pressure-passive cerebral circulation experience *multiple*, but usually not severe, declines in CBF (see later discussion). Finally, and perhaps most important, in developing white matter of the rat brain and, critically, the *human brain*, not only are AMPA receptors *overexpressed* during the peak period of vulnerability to PVL, but also these receptors are relatively deficient in the GluR2 subunit and are thereby Ca^{2+} permeable.[686,687,1165]

A major advance in the understanding of oligodendroglial excitotoxicity was the recent discovery of *NMDA receptors on processes of oligodendrocytes*, from the developing to the mature, myelin-producing stages.[1159,1168-1171] When activated by ischemic conditions or exposure to agonists, loss of processes occurs. Moreover, NMDA receptors are permeable to Ca^{2+}, and it is likely that the downstream mechanisms related to Ca^{2+} influx, generation of ROS/RNS, account for the deleterious effects. Because axons can release glutamate, the findings suggest that the presence of NMDA receptors on oligodendrocytes provides a mechanism of axonal-oligodendroglial signaling important for myelination. However, with excessive glutamate, as occurs with ischemia, this normal mechanism becomes pathological. The data suggest an additional site for protection of pre-OLs from ischemic injury. Indeed, in preliminary data, we showed a potent protective effective of memantine, a specific NMDA antagonist, in a neonatal rat model of hypoxic-ischemic white matter injury. Moreover, preliminary studies of human brain showed, analogous to the findings with AMPA receptors, a marked expression of NMDA receptors in pre-OLs in human cerebral white matter during the peak period of vulnerability to PVL. The findings of NMDA receptors on pre-OLs may help explain the white matter injury produced in developing mice and rabbits by intracerebral injection of ibotenic acid and NMDA, both agonists of the NMDA receptor.[802,1172-1174] However, because NMDA receptors are also present on microglia and astrocytes, secondary effects involving pre-OLs could account for some of the white matter injury in these models. At any rate, the findings of an overexpression of both Ca^{2+}-permeable AMPA receptors and NMDA receptors on pre-OLs suggest a

---

[a]References 686, 1067, 1136, 1151, 1158, 1160, 1166, and 1167.

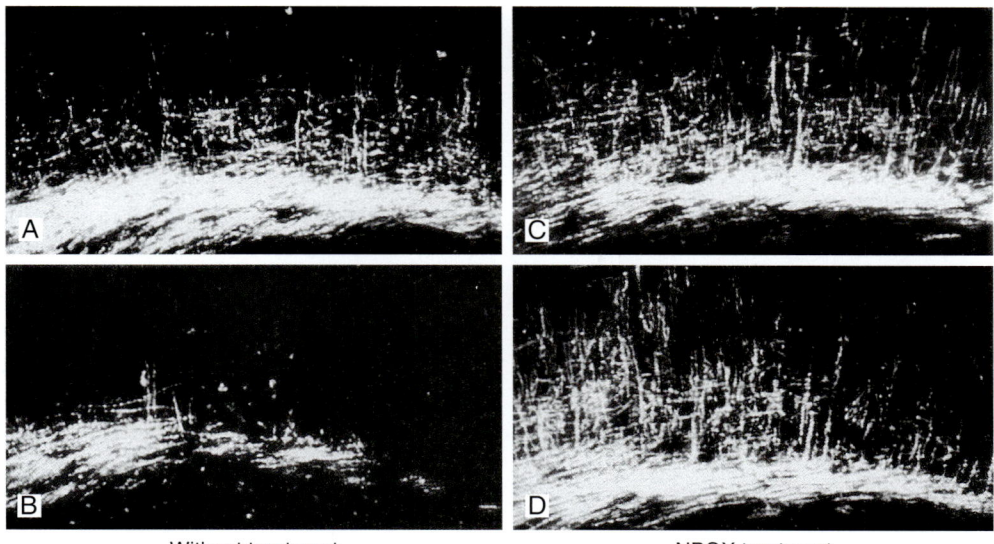

Without treatment   NBQX treatment

Figure 13.58 Protection from hypoxic-ischemic cerebral white matter injury in the immature (P7) rat by systemic administration of the non-N-methyl-D-aspartate (NMDA) receptor blocker, 2,3-dihydroxy-6-nitro-7-sulfamoyl-benzo[f]quinoxaline-2,3-dione (NBQX), after the termination of the insult. (A) through (D) show myelin basic protein (MBP) staining in cerebral white matter at P11, 4 days after cerebral hypoxia-ischemia produced by unilateral carotid ligation and hypoxemia at P7. Developing oligodendrocytes at P7 normally differentiate into MBP-positive oligodendrocytes by P11. At the termination of the insult on P7, animals received either injection of (A and B) vehicle or (C and D) NBQX, the non-NMDA receptor blocker. (A) and (C) show MBP staining contralateral to the ligation, and (B) and (D) show staining ipsilateral to the ligation. Note the marked disturbance in the hypoxic-ischemic (ipsilateral) hemisphere in the nontreated animal (B compared with A) and the protection afforded by NBQX in the hypoxic-ischemic hemisphere in the treated animal (D compared with C). Rights were not granted to include this figure in electronic media. Please refer to the printed book. (From Follett P, Rosenberg PA, Volpe JJ, Jensen FE. NBQX attenuates excitotoxic injury in developing white matter. *J Neurosci.* 2000;20:9235–9241.)

TABLE 13.31	Relation of Outcome in Term Infants to Mean Cerebral Blood Flow in the First 12 Hours After Asphyxia[a]			
CLINICAL GROUP	**NEUROLOGICAL OUTCOME**	**MEAN CBF (mL/100 g per min)**	**MABP REACTIVITY**[b]	**CARBON DIOXIDE REACTIVITY**[c]
Asphyxiated	Death or severe brain injury	30.6	−	−
Asphyxiated	Moderate to severe brain injury	15.1	−	+
Asphyxiated	Normal	9.2	+	+
Nonasphyxiated	Normal	11.9	+	+

[a]CBF determined in three groups of asphyxiated infants at mean age of 9 hours and in a group of nonasphyxiated infants at the age of 1–5 days.

[b]MABP reactivity: −, CBF fluctuates directly with MABP (i.e., autoregulation not operating); +, CBF does not change with MABP (i.e., autoregulation normal).

[c]Carbon dioxide reactivity: −, CBF does not change directly with changes in $PaCO_2$ (i.e., lack of normal reactivity of CBF); +, CBF changes directly with changes in $PaCO_2$ (i.e., normal reactivity of CBF).

CBF, Cerebral blood flow; *MABP*, mean arterial blood pressure; *PaCO_2*, arterial partial pressure of carbon dioxide.

Data from Pryds O, Greisen G, Lou H, Friis-Hansen B. Vasoparalysis associated with brain damage in asphyxiated term infants. *J Pediatr.* 1990;117:119–125.

particularly maturation-dependent vulnerability of these cells to excitotoxicity (Table 13.31).

The findings concerning AMPA and NMDA receptors on pre-OL cell bodies and processes, respectively, suggest the possibility of differential effects and temporal aspects of excessive activation of these receptors (Fig. 13.59). Thus activation of the NMDA receptor, which can flux Ca^{2+} more readily and more vigorously than even GluR2-deficient AMPA receptors, would lead initially to the loss of oligodendroglial processes but not cell death. By contrast, more pronounced or prolonged exposure to glutamate may be required to activate the AMPA receptors to lead to cell death. The consequence of both could be subsequent hypomyelination, although perhaps the possibilities of recovery would be greater if only cell processes were lost and the cell body was spared. Additionally possible are secondary axonal disturbances, caused by a failure of both ensheathment by pre-OLs and subsequent myelination (see Fig. 13.59).

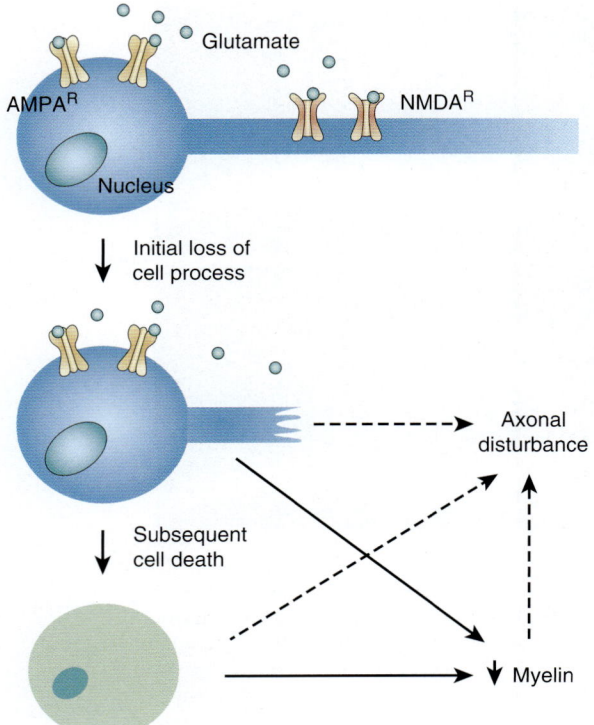

Figure 13.59 Potential differential effects and temporal aspects of excitotoxicity to developing oligodendrocytes. The intact cell *(top)* has alpha-amino-3-hydroxy-5-methyl-4-isoxazole-propionic acid (AMPA) receptors primarily on the cell soma and N-methyl-D-aspartate (NMDA) receptors primarily on the cell processes. Initially with excess extracellular glutamate, activation of NMDA receptors could lead to loss of cell processes, and if excitotoxicity continues, to activation of AMPA receptors and cell death. Either event could lead to impaired myelination *(solid arrows)* and potentially also to axonal disturbance *(dotted lines)*.

Relation of Excitotoxicity to Reactive Oxygen Species/Reactive Nitrogen Species Toxicity. A direct relationship between the two downstream mechanisms leading to death of pre-OLs (i.e., excitotoxicity and ROS/RNS toxicity; see Fig. 13.52) is suggested by the demonstrations that AMPA/KA receptor toxicity to oligodendroglial precursors is accompanied by the generation of ROS and RNS.[1158,1167,1175] The occurrence of nitrotyrosine immunoreactivity in pre-OLs suggested that, under these conditions, $ONOO^-$ is the key RNS. This deadly compound is likely formed from NO, produced by Ca^{2+}-activated iNOS in the oligodendrocytes and superoxide anion, produced by one or more of several Ca^{2+}-inducible enzymes resulting in ROS formation.[1175] The oxidative stress associated with AMPA receptor activation in oligodendrocytes is greater than that associated with activation in neurons.[714] The use of an SOD/catalase mimetic, Euk, protected pre-OLs from excitotoxicity.[1158] This nonpeptidyl molecule has neuroprotective properties in vivo (see the earlier discussion on neuronal death). Thus the data indicate how multiple maturation-dependent characteristics of pre-OLs interact in an amplifying manner to produce a highly vulnerable cell, with the upstream mechanisms (hypoxia-ischemia and inflammation) converging on two interacting downstream mechanisms (excitotoxicity and free radical attack; see Fig. 13.52).

Interventions for Prevention of Oligodendrocytes From Hypoxic-Ischemic and Inflammatory Injury

As for the earlier discussion of neuronal death, the insights into the biochemical and cellular mechanisms of injury to differentiating oligodendrocytes by hypoxia-ischemia and inflammation, as just discussed, provide a rational basis for the formulation of mechanisms to interrupt those mechanisms and thereby to prevent or ameliorate the injury. The sequence just described and the best candidates for intervention are shown in Fig. 13.60. Some of the interventions have been shown to be effective against neuronal death (see earlier) and thus will be particularly promising as an approach to dual neuronal-oligodendroglial protection, a feature of some perinatal human hypoxic-ischemic lesions.

Prevention of Hypoxia-Ischemia. Prevention of hypoxia-ischemia is discussed in detail in Chapters 16, 17, and 20. Prevention requires detection of the infant with impaired cerebrovascular autoregulation, and this requirement may be possible with *near-infrared spectroscopy*, with subsequent correction of the cerebrovascular disturbance. Progress in these areas has been accomplished in recent years.

Prevention of Infection or Inflammation. Prevention of the infection or inflammation upstream mechanism appears most promising at the level of interventions to *blunt or prevent microglial activation, cytokine action, or related inflammatory cascades* (see Fig. 13.60). In experimental models, the use of *minocycline* has been most promising (see the earlier discussion regarding neuronal protection).[1176-1180] Melatonin may exert some of its white matter protection at this level.[1181] Thus these agents or related antimicroglial compounds could be useful against both gray matter (neuronal) and white matter (oligodendroglial) injury.

The antenatal administration of corticosteroids is associated with a decreased incidence of cerebral white matter injury in the premature newborn (see Chapter 16). Whether this effect relates to the well-documented anti-inflammatory properties of the drug is unclear. Whether other targets (e.g., TLRs or their downstream molecules) would be suitable for interventions remains unclear. Such approaches are in the early phases of development.[1182]

Prevention of Excitotoxicity. Concerning the two major downstream mechanisms, excitotoxicity and free radical attack, *blockade of non-NMDA, particularly AMPA receptors*, appears very promising to prevent pre-OL death (see earlier discussion; see Fig. 13.60).[1164,1165] The apparently clinically safe agent, *topiramate*, is very effective in a well-characterized animal model.[893,1165]

The *blockade of NMDA receptors* appears similarly promising to prevent the loss of pre-OL processes (see Fig. 13.60; see earlier). *Memantine* may be the most clinically safe NMDA receptor antagonist in this setting.[1183] More data are needed. The potentially beneficial effect of *melatonin* on white matter injury in an animal model involving direct injection of an NMDA agonist may occur in part at this level.[1184]

Combination therapy with non-NMDA and NMDA antagonists could be particularly useful in two ways. This approach may provide optimal protection for pre-OLs and may also combine an important neuronal protective effect (see the discussion on neuronal protection).

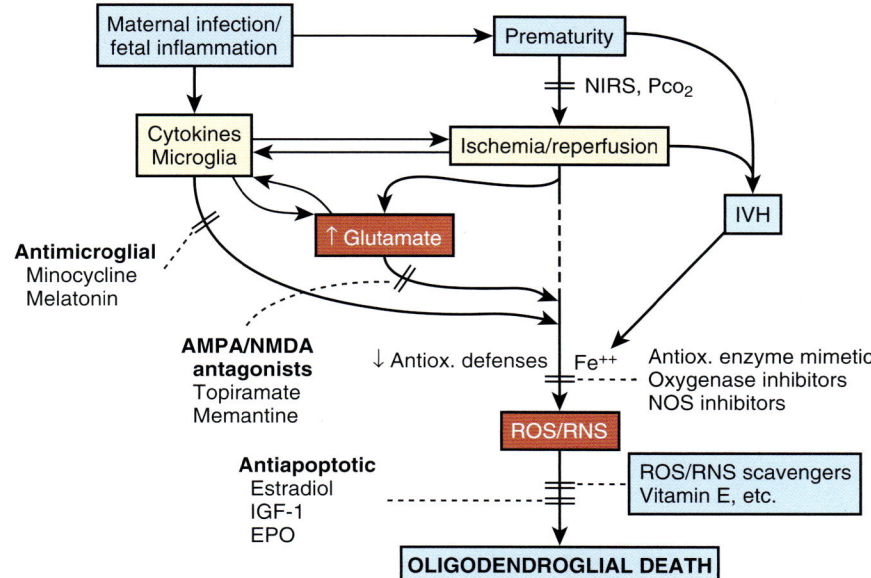

Figure 13.60 Interventions for prevention of injury to developing oligodendrocytes resulting from hypoxic-ischemic and inflammatory insults. *AMPA*, Alpha-amino-3-hydroxy-5-methyl-4-isoxazole-propionic acid; *Fe⁺⁺*, iron; *IVH*, intraventricular hemorrhage; *NIRS*, near-infrared spectroscopy; *NMDA*, N-methyl-D-aspartate; *NOS*, nitric oxide synthase; *RNS*, reactive nitrogen species; *ROS*, reactive oxygen species. See text for details.

Prevention of Free Radical Generation. *ROS* and *RNS attack* is a critical area because the deleterious effects of both upstream mechanisms *and* the major portion of excitotoxicity occur through the actions of ROS/RNS (see Fig. 13.60). *Counteraction of the impaired antioxidant defenses in pre-OLs* and thereby prevention of free radical accumulation by the use of mimetics of antioxidant enzymes may be of particular value,[1158] because nonpeptidyl agents can enter the brain. The *prevention of free radical generation* by vitamin K may be a particularly powerful approach because available data indicate high potency for this intervention and effectiveness even hours after the onset of free radical accumulation (see earlier).[1066] This agent should be safe in premature infants, because vitamin K is administered routinely in newborns for blood coagulation in vivo and is protective in vitro in very low concentrations. The *inhibition of enzymes that are crucial in the genesis of oxygen free radicals* (e.g., oxygenase inhibitors, especially 12-lipoxygenase) by specific agents may also be valuable, based on published data.[1185] Whether these agents are useful in vivo remains to be determined. Because of the important role of nitrative mechanisms, the use of *inhibitors of NO synthesis* may be particularly valuable (see earlier). More data are needed.

Scavenging of Free Radicals. Scavengers of ROS/RNS may be particularly useful against pre-OL death, because these agents also would be useful against neuronal death (see earlier; Fig. 13.60). Vitamin E and related scavengers have been effective, especially in cultured models.[907,1064] One *free radical scavenging* agent, the spin-trapping agent alpha-phenyl-*N*-tert-butyl-nitrone (PBN), administered systemically after the hypoxic-ischemic insult, attenuated white matter injury in the immature rat.[1186]

Blockade of Downstream Effects. The principal downstream effects in the cascade to pre-OL cell death involve progression to apoptosis. Thus studies of pre-OLs undergoing free radical attack,[1064] hypoxic-ischemic white matter injury in the neonatal piglet,[6] and human neuropathology (see Chapters 14 and 15) indicate that apoptosis is the principal mechanism of pre-OL death in PVL. Thus, antiapoptotic interventions, as discussed for neuronal protection (see earlier), are relevant in this context.

Of the agents that block apoptotic mechanisms and are shown to be protective to neurons (see earlier), *several growth factors* have been most effective versus pre-OL death. Thus *IGF-I* has been shown to be protective to pre-OLs in the hypoxic-ischemic neonatal rat[1187] and in near-term fetal sheep.[1188] In both paradigms, IGF-I suppressed apoptotic death and promoted oligodendroglial precursor proliferation. The antiapoptotic effect involves activation of Akt and prevention of both mitochondrial cytochrome c release and caspase activation.[1188-1190] Administration of the peptide was by the intracerebral or intraventricular route, and thus clinical application could be problematic. However, a report in hypoxic-ischemic *adult* rats suggested appreciable neuroprotection after intravenous administration of the N-terminal tripeptide of IGF-I.[1191]

Other growth factors may also be protective against pre-OL death. In separate animal models involving excitotoxic or inflammatory mechanisms, BDNF and ciliary neurotrophic factor (CNTF) have shown benefit.[942,1192] Finally, the recently described protective effect of *estradiol* in neonatal white matter injury appears to be primarily antiapoptotic.[1193]

Among other interventions discussed in relation to neuronal protection, *mild hypothermia* was shown to decrease postischemic white matter injury sharply in the near-term fetal sheep.[1194,1195] Protection was associated with reduced caspase-3 activation. However, hypothermia was not effective when it was delayed until 5.5 hours after reperfusion. Moreover, because, unlike in hypoxic-ischemic *neuronal* injury, the insults that lead to white matter injury in the human infant are likely to be mild, multiple, and protracted, hypothermia does not appear to be an ideal intervention.

EPO, discussed earlier as particularly promising with regard to neuronal protection, may be predicted to be promising against white matter injury as well, in view of several of its molecular effects (e.g., antiapoptotic, antioxidant, antiexcitotoxic). Several randomized controlled trials using EPO in the preterm infant have now been undertaken, with some preliminary supportive results. The Swiss trial dosing used 3000 IU/kg within 3 hours, at 12 to 18 and at 36 to 42 hours after birth, a regimen closely following experimental data arguing for very early initiation as well as a high dose of rhEPO to achieve therapeutic levels in the brain within the most vulnerable, early postnatal period. A subset of patients were examined at term-corrected age by cranial MRI, which showed significantly lower white and gray matter injury scores after rhEPO treatment.[1196] However, the 2-year outcomes with Bayley scales of infant development were not improved, both in that subset and in the entire study population.[1197] A more recent study included 800 infants of ≤32 weeks' gestational age and within 72 hours after birth. The infants were randomly assigned to receive rhEPO (500 IU/kg; $n = 366$) or placebo ($n = 377$) intravenously within 72 hours after birth and then once every other day for 2 weeks. Death and moderate/severe neurological disability occurred in 91 of 338 very preterm infants (26.9%) in the placebo group and in 43 of 330 very preterm infants (13.0%) in the rhEPO treatment group (relative risk [RR] = 0.40, 95% confidence interval [CI] = 0.27 to 0.59, $P < .001$) at 18 months of corrected age. The rate of moderate/severe neurological disability in the rhEPO group (22 of 309, 7.1%) was significantly lower compared with that in the placebo group (57 of 304, 18.8%; RR = 0.32, 95% CI = 0.19 to 0.55, $P < .001$), and no excess adverse events were observed.[1198] Such findings await replication in current ongoing trials before the more widespread initiation of EPO as a neuroprotective agent in the preterm infant.

KEY REFERENCES

1. Volpe JJ. Neonatal encephalopathy: an inadequate term for hypoxic-ischemic encephalopathy. *Ann Neurol.* 2012;72:156-166.
14. Mattson MP, Bazan NG. Apoptosis and necrosis. In: Siegel GJ, Albers RW, Brady ST, et al., eds. *Basic Neurochemistry. Molecular, Cellular and Medical Aspects.* 7th ed. New York: Elsevier; 2006:603-615.
15. Zhu CL, Xu FL, Wang XY, et al. Different apoptotic mechanisms are activated in male and female brains after neonatal hypoxia-ischaemia. *J Neurochem.* 2006;96:1016-1027.
18. Liu CL, Siesjo BK, Hu BR. Pathogenesis of hippocampal neuronal death after hypoxia-ischemia changes during brain development. *Neuroscience.* 2004;127:113-123.
19. Zhu C, Wang X, Xu F, et al. The influence of age on apoptotic and other mechanisms of cell death after cerebral hypoxia-ischemia. *Cell Death Differ.* 2005;12:162-176.
23. Han BH, D'Costa A, Back SA, et al. BDNF blocks caspase-3 activation in neonatal hypoxia-ischemia. *Neurobiol Dis.* 2000;7:38-53.
24. Manabat C, Han BH, Wendland M, et al. Reperfusion differentially induces caspase-3 activation in ischemic core and penumbra after stroke in immature brain. *Stroke.* 2003;34:207-213.

25. Aito H, Aalto KT, Raivio KO. Biphasic ATP depletion caused by transient oxidative exposure is associated with apoptotic cell death in rat embryonal cortical neurons. *Pediatr Res.* 2002;52:40-45.
26. Joly L-M, Benjelloun N, Plotkine M, et al. Distribution of poly-(ADP-ribosyl)ation and cell death after cerebral ischemia in the neonatal rat. *Pediatr Res.* 2003;53:776-782.
28. Daval JL, Pourie G, Grojean S, et al. Neonatal hypoxia triggers transient apoptosis followed by neurogenesis in the rat CA1 hippocampus. *Pediatr Res.* 2004;55:561-567.
29. Malagelada C, Xifro X, Minano A, et al. Contribution of caspase-mediated apoptosis to the cell death caused by oxygen-glucose deprivation in cortical cell cultures. *Neurobiol Dis.* 2005;20:27-37.
30. Northington FJ, Chavez-Valdez R, Martin LJ. Neuronal cell death in neonatal hypoxia-ischemia. *Ann Neurol.* 2011;69:743-758.
33. Northington FJ, Zelaya ME, O'Riordan DP, et al. Failure to complete apoptosis following neonatal hypoxia-ischemia manifests as "continuum" phenotype of cell death and occurs with multiple manifestations of mitochondrial dysfunction in rodent forebrain. *Neuroscience.* 2007;149:822-833.
34. Northington FJ, Chavez-Valdez R, Graham EM. Necrostatin decreases oxidative damage, inflammation, and injury after neonatal HI. *J Cereb Blood Flow Metab.* 2011;31:178-189.
35. Verghese PB, Sasaki Y, Yang D. Nicotinamide mononucleotide adenylyl transferase 1 protects against acute neurodegeneration in developing CNS by inhibiting excitotoxic-necrotic cell death. *Proc Natl Acad Sci USA.* 2011;108:19054-19059.
37. Nagley P, Higgins GC, Atkin JD, et al. Multifaceted deaths orchestrated by mitochondria in neurones. *Biochim Biophys Acta.* 2010;1802:167-185.
38. He C, Klionsky DJ. Regulation mechanisms and signaling pathways of autophagy. *Annu Rev Genet.* 2009;43:67-93.
39. Bursch W. The autophagosomal-lysosomal compartment in programmed cell death. *Cell Death Differ.* 2001;8:569-581.
40. Descloux C, Ginet V, Clarke PG, et al. Neuronal death after perinatal cerebral hypoxia-ischemia: focus on autophagy-mediated cell death. *Int J Dev Neurosci.* 2015;45:75-85.
41. Ginet V, Pittet MP, Rummel C, et al. Dying neurons in thalamus of asphyxiated term newborns and rats are autophagic. *Ann Neurol.* 2014;76:695-711.
91. O'Regan M. Adenosine and the regulation of cerebral blood flow. *Neurol Res.* 2005;27:175-181.
99. Van Woerkom R, Beharry KDA, Modanlou HD, et al. Influence of morphine and naloxone on endothelin and its receptors in newborn piglet brain vascular endothelial cells: clinical implications in neonatal care. *Pediatr Res.* 2004;55:147-151.
129. van Os S, Liem D, Hopman J, et al. Cerebral O2 supply thresholds for the preservation of electrocortical brain activity during hypotension in near-term-born lambs. *Pediatr Res.* 2005;57:358-362.
130. van Os S, Klaessens J, Hopman J, et al. Cerebral oxygen supply during hypotension in near-term lambs: a near-infrared spectroscopy study. *Brain Dev.* 2006;28:115-121.
140. Hilario E, Rey-Santano MC, Goni-de-Cerio F, et al. Cerebral blood flow and morphological changes after hypoxic-ischaemic injury in preterm lambs. *Acta Paediatr.* 2005;94:903-911.
160. Greisen G, Vannucci RC. Is periventricular leucomalacia a result of hypoxic-ischaemic injury? Hypocapnia and the preterm brain. *Biol Neonate.* 2001;79:194-200.
169. Fumagalli M, Mosca F, Knudsen GM, et al. Transient hyperoxia and residual cerebrovascular effects in the newborn rat. *Pediatr Res.* 2004;55:380-384.
171. Kuban KC, Gilles FH. Human telencephalic angiogenesis. *Ann Neurol.* 1985;17:539-548.
193. Pourcyrous M, Busija DW, Shibata M, et al. Cebrovascular responses to therapeutic dose of indomethacin in newborn pigs. *Pediatr Res.* 1999;45:582-587.
194. Patel J, Roberts I, Azzopardi D, et al. Randomized double-blind controlled trial comparing the effects of ibuprofen with indomethacin on cerebral hemodynamics in preterm infants with patent ductuc arteriosus. *Pediatr Res.* 2000;47:36-42.
195. Brown DW, Lee D, Kumaran VS, et al. Age-dependent cerebral hemodynamic effects of indomethacin in the newborn piglet. *J Appl Physiol.* 2004;97:1880-1887.

220. Giussani DA, Thakor AS, Frulio R, et al. Acute hypoxia increases S100beta protein in association with blood flow redistribution away from peripheral circulations in fetal sheep. *Pediatr Res.* 2005;58:179-184.

221. van Os S, van den Tweel E, Egberts H, et al. Cerebral cortical tissue damage after hemorrhagic hypotension in near-term born lambs. *Pediatr Res.* 2006;59:221-226.

222. Riddle A, Luo NL, Manese M, et al. Spatial heterogeneity in oligodendrocyte lineage maturation and not cerebral blood flow predicts fetal ovine periventricular white matter injury. *J Neurosci.* 2006;26:3045-3055.

255. Younkin D, Delivoria-Papadopoulos M, Reivich M, et al. Regional variations in human newborn cerebral blood flow. *J Pediatr.* 1988;112:104-108.

260. Pryds O, Greisen G, Lou H, et al. Vasoparalysis associated with brain damage in asphyxiated term infants. *J Pediatr.* 1990;117:119-125.

265. Pryds O. Control of cerebral circulation in the high-risk neonate. *Ann Neurol.* 1991;30:321-329.

270. Myers RE. Brain damage due to asphyxia: mechanism of causation. *J Perinat Med.* 1981;9:78-86.

281. Biagi L, Abbruzzese A, Bianchi MC, et al. Age dependence of cerebral perfusion assessed by magnetic resonance continuous arterial spin labeling. *J Magn Reson Imaging.* 2007;25:696-702.

283. Wang J, Licht DJ. Pediatric perfusion MR imaging using arterial spin labeling. *Neuroimaging Clin N Am.* 2006;16:149-167, ix.

285. De Vis JB, Hendrikse J, Petersen ET, et al. Arterial spin-labelling perfusion MRI and outcome in neonates with hypoxic-ischemic encephalopathy. *Eur Radiol.* 2015;25:113-121.

288. Wintermark P, Hansen A, Warfield SK, et al. Near-infrared spectroscopy versus magnetic resonance imaging to study brain perfusion in newborns with hypoxic-ischemic encephalopathy treated with hypothermia. *Neuroimage.* 2014;85:287-293.

289. De Vis JB, Alderliesten T, Hendrikse J, et al. Magnetic resonance imaging based noninvasive measurements of brain hemodynamics in neonates: a review. *Pediatr Res.* 2016;80:641-650.

293. Fukuda S, Kato T, Kakita H, et al. Hemodynamics of the cerebral arteries of infants with periventricular leukomalacia. *Pediatrics.* 2006;117:1-8.

303. Soul JS, Hammer PE, Tsuji M, et al. Fluctuating pressure-passivity is common in the cerebral circulation of sick premature infants. *Pediatr Res.* 2007;61:467-473.

305. Wong FY, Silas R, Hew S, et al. Cerebral oxygenation is highly sensitive to blood pressure variability in sick preterm infants. *PLoS ONE.* 2012;7:e43165.

306. Gilmore MM, Stone BS, Shepard JA, et al. Relationship between cerebrovascular dysautoregulation and arterial blood pressure in the premature infant. *J Perinatol.* 2011;31:722-729.

307. Eriksen VR, Hahn GH, Greisen G. Cerebral autoregulation in the preterm newborn using near-infrared spectroscopy: a comparison of time-domain and frequency-domain analyses. *J Biomed Opt.* 2015;20:037009.

308. Mitra S, Czosnyka M, Smielewski P, et al. Heart rate passivity of cerebral tissue oxygenation is associated with predictors of poor outcome in preterm infants. *Acta Paediatr.* 2014;103:e374-e382.

309. Aries MJ, Czosnyka M, Budohoski KP, et al. Continuous determination of optimal cerebral perfusion pressure in traumatic brain injury. *Crit Care Med.* 2012;40:2456-2463.

310. da Costa CS, Czosnyka M, Smielewski P, et al. Monitoring of cerebrovascular reactivity for determination of optimal blood pressure in preterm infants. *J Pediatr.* 2015;167:86-91.

315. Perlman JM, Wyllie J, Kattwinkel J, et al. Part 7: Neonatal resuscitation: 2015 international consensus on cardiopulmonary resuscitation and emergency cardiovascular care science with treatment recommendations. *Circulation.* 2015;132:S204-S241.

350. Ilves P, Lintrop M, Metsvaht T, et al. Cerebral blood-flow velocities in predicting outcome of asphyxiated newborn infants. *Acta Paediatr.* 2004;93:523-528.

356. Erecinska M, Cherian S, Silver IA. Energy metabolism in mammalian brian during development. *Prog Neurobiol.* 2004;73:397-445.

357. Vannucci RC, Brucklacher RM, Vannucci SJ. Glycolysis and perinatal hypoxic-ischemic brain damage. *Dev Neurosci.* 2005;27:185-190.

393. Vannucci RC, Vannucci SJ. Perinatal hypoxic-ischemic brain damage: evolution of an animal model. *Dev Neurosci.* 2005;27:81-86.

419. Vannucci RC, Towfighi J, Vannucci SJ. Secondary energy failure after cerebral hypoxia-ischemia in the immature rat. *J Cereb Blood Flow Metab.* 2004;24:1090-1097.

427. Hunter CJ, Bennet L, Power GG, et al. Key neuroprotective role for endogenous adenosine A(1) receptor activation during asphyxia in the fetal sheep. *Stroke.* 2003;34:2240-2245.

444. Salhab WA, Wyckoff MH, Laptook AR, et al. Initial hypoglycemia and neonatal brain injury in term infants with severe fetal acidemia. *Pediatrics.* 2004;114:361-366.

445. Burns CM, Rutherford MA, Boardman JP, et al. Patterns of cerebral injury and neurodevelopmental outcomes after symptomatic neonatal hypoglycemia. *Pediatrics.* 2008;122: 65-74.

470. Callahan DJ, Engle MJ, Volpe JJ. Hypoxic injury to developing glial cells: protective effect of high glucose. *Pediatr Res.* 1990;27:186-190.

475. Sheldon RA, Partridge JC, Ferriero DM. Postischemic hyperglycemia is not protective to the neonatal rat brain. *Pediatr Res.* 1992;32:489-493.

498. Gidday JM. Cerebral preconditioning and ischaemic tolerance. *Nat Rev Neurosci.* 2006;7:437-448.

527. Annunziato L, Cataldi M, Pignataro G, et al. Glutamate-independent calcium toxicity: introduction. *Stroke.* 2007;38: 661-664.

552. Tan S, Zhou F, Nielsen VG, et al. Increased injury following intermittent fetal hypoxia-reoxygenation is associated with increased free radical production in fetal rabbit brain. *J Neuropathol Exp Neurol.* 1999;58:972-981.

574. Murphy S. Production of nitric oxide by glial cells: regulation and potential roles in the CNS. *Glia.* 2000;29:1-14.

575. Saugstad OD. Oxidative stress in the newborn—a 30-year perspective. *Biol Neonate.* 2005;88:228-236.

591. Ortega-Gutierrez S, Garcia JJ, MartinezBallarin E, et al. Melatonin improves deferoxamine antioxidant activity in protecting against lipid peroxidation caused by hydrogen peroxide in rat brain homogenates. *Neurosci Lett.* 2002;323:55-59.

592. Shimizu K, Rajapakse N, Horiguchi T, et al. Neuroprotection against hypoxia-ischemia in neonatal rat brain by novel superoxide dismutase mimetics. *Neurosci Lett.* 2003;346: 41-44.

594. Sanchez-Alvarez R, Almeida A, Medina JM. Oxidative stress in preterm rat brain is due to mitochondrial dysfunction. *Pediatr Res.* 2002;51:34-39.

595. Calamandrei G, Venerosi A, Valazano A, et al. Increased brain levels of F2-isoprostane are an early marker of behavioral sequels in a rat model of global perinatal asphyxia. *Pediatr Res.* 2004;55:85-92.

611. Lafemina MJ, Sheldon RA, Ferriero DM. Acute hypoxia-ischemia results in hydrogen peroxide accumulation in neonatal but not adult mouse brain. *Pediatr Res.* 2006;59:680-683.

612. Sheldon RA, Jiang X, Francisco C, et al. Manipulation of antioxidant pathways in neonatal murine brain. *Pediatr Res.* 2004;56:656-662.

613. McLean CW, Mirochnitchenko O, Claus CP, et al. Overexpression of glutathione peroxidase protects immature murine neurons from oxidative stress. *Dev Neurosci.* 2005;27:169-175.

618. Maniscalco WM, Watkins RH, Roper JM, et al. Hyperoxic ventilated premature baboons have increased p53, xxidant DNA damage and decreased VEGF expression. *Pediatr Res.* 2005;58:549-556.

619. Dohlen G, Carlsen H, Blomhoff R, et al. Reoxygenation of hypoxic mice with 100% oxygen induces brain nuclear factor-kappa B. *Pediatr Res.* 2005;58:941-945.

620. Shimabuku R, Ota A, Pereyra S, et al. Hyperoxia with 100% oxygen following hypoxia-ischemia increases brain damage in newborn rats. *Biol Neonate.* 2005;88:168-171.

631. Kindler DD, Thiffault C, Solenski NJ, et al. Neurotoxic nitric oxide rapidly depolarizes and permeabilizes mitochondria by dynamically opening the mitochondrial transition pore. *Mol Cell Neurosci.* 2003;23:559-573.

632. Waxman SG. Nitric oxide and the axonal death cascade. *Ann Neurol.* 2003;53:150-153.

639. Araujo IM, Verdasca MJ, Ambrosio AF, et al. Nitric oxide inhibits complex I following AMPA receptor activation via peroxynitrite. *Neuroreport.* 2004;15:2007-2011.

687. Talos DM, Follett PL, Folkerth RD, et al. Developmental regulation of alpha-amino-3-hydroxy-5-methyl-4-isoxazole-propionic acid receptor subunit expression in forebrain and relationship to regional susceptibility to hypoxic/ischemic injury. II. Human cerebral white matter and cortex. *J Comp Neurol.* 2006;497:61-77.

700. Ritter LM, Unis AS, Meador-Woodruff JH. Ontogeny of ionotropic glutamate receptor expression in human fetal brain. *Brain Res Dev Brain Res.* 2001;127:123-133.

701. Panigrahy A, Rosenberg PS, Assmann S, et al. Differential expression of glutamate receptor subtypes in human brainstem sites involved in perinatal hypoxia-ischemia. *J Comp Neurol.* 2001;437:196-208.

734. Poulsen CF, Simeone TA, Maar TE, et al. Modulation by topiramate of AMPA and kainate mediated calcium influx in cultured cortical, hippocampal and cerebellar neurons. *Neurochem Res.* 2004;29:275-282.

737. Koh S, Tibayan FD, Simpson JN, et al. NBQX or topiramate treatment after perinatal hypoxia-induced seizures prevents later increases in seizure-induced neuronal injury. *Epilepsia.* 2004;45:569-575.

744. Hagberg H, Peebles D, Mallard C. Models of white matter injury: comparison of infectious, hypoxic-ischemic, and excitotoxic insults. *Ment Retard Dev Disabil Res Rev.* 2002;8: 30-38.

752. Rao SD, Yin HZ, Weiss JH. Disruption of glial glutamate transport by ractive oxygen species produced in motor neurons. *J Neurosci.* 2003;23:2627-2633.

778. Sfaello I, Baud O, Arzimanoglou A, et al. Topiramate prevents excitotoxic damage in the newborn rodent brain. *Neurobiol Dis.* 2005;20:837-848.

779. Noh MR, Kim SK, Sun W, et al. Neuroprotective effect of topiramate on hypoxic ischemic brain injury in neonatal rats. *Exp Neurol.* 2006;201:470-478.

796. Lee SM, Yune TY, Kim SJ, et al. Minocycline inhibits apoptotic cell death via attenuation of TNF-alpha expression following iNOS/NO induction by lipopolysaccharide in neuron/glia co-cultures. *J Neurochem.* 2004;91:568-578.

797. Morimoto N, Shimazawa M, Yamashima T, et al. Minocycline inhibits oxidative stress and decreases in vitro and in vivo ischemic neuronal damage. *Brain Res.* 2005;1044:8-15.

801. Eun B-L, Liu X-H, Barks JDE. Pentoxifylline attenuates hypoxic-ischemic brain injury in immature rats. *Pediatr Res.* 2000;47:73-78.

802. Dommergues M-A, Patkai J, Renauld J-C, et al. Proinflammatory cytokines and interleukin-9 exacerbate excitotoxic lesions of the newborn murine neopallium. *Ann Neurol.* 2000;47: 54-63.

814. Ikeda T, Mishima K, Aoo N, et al. Dexamethasone prevents long-lasting learning impairment following a combination of lipopolysaccharide and hypoxia-ischemia in neonatal rats. *Am J Obstet Gynecol.* 2005;192:719-726.

820. Larouche A, Roy M, Kadhim H, et al. Neuronal injuries induced by perinatal hypoxic-ischemic insults are potentiated by prenatal exposure to lipopolysaccharide: animal model for perinatally acquired encephalopathy. *Dev Neurosci.* 2005;27:134-142.

821. Wang X, Hagberg H, Zhu C, et al. Effects of intrauterine inflammation on the developing mouse brain. *Brain Res.* 2007;1144:180-185.

822. Wang X, Hagberg H, Nie C, et al. Dual role of intrauterine immune challenge on neonatal and adult brain vulnerability to hypoxia-ischemia. *J Neuropathol Exp Neurol.* 2007;66: 552-561.

823. Ikeda T, Yang L, Ikenoue T, et al. Endotoxin-induced hypoxic-ischemic tolerance is mediated by up-regulation of corticosterone in neonatal rat. *Pediatr Res.* 2006;59:56-60.

829. Foster-Barber A, Dickens B, Ferriero DM. Human perinatal asphyxia: correlation of neonatal cytokines with MRI and outcome. *Dev Neurosci.* 2002;23:213-218.

831. Bartha AI, Foster-Barber A, Miller SP, et al. Neonatal encephalopathy: association of cytokines with MR spectroscopy and outcome. *Pediatr Res.* 2004;56:960-966.

833. Wu YW, Escobar GJ, Grether JK, et al. Chorioamnionitis and cerebral palsy in term and near-term infants. *JAMA.* 2003;290:2677-2684.

840. Thoresen M, Whitelaw A. Therapeutic hypothermia for hypoxic-ischaemic encephalopathy in the newborn infant. *Curr Opin Neurol.* 2005;18:111-116.

841. Gunn AJ, Thoresen M. Hypothermic neuroprotection. *NeuroRx.* 2006;3:154-169.

861. Robertson NJ, Bhakoo K, Puri BK, et al. Hypothermia and amiloride preserve energetics in a neonatal brain slice model. *Pediatr Res.* 2005;58:288-296.

863. Tooley JR, Eagle RC, Satas S, et al. Significant head cooling can be achieved while maintaining normothermia in the newborn piglet. *Arch Dis Child.* 2005;90:F262-F266.

864. Zhu C. Wang X, Xu F, et al. Intraischemic mild hypothermia prevents neuronal cell death and tissue loss after neonatal cerebral hypoxia-ischemia. *Eur J Neurosci.* 2006;23: 387-393.

865. George S, Scotter J, Dean JM, et al. Induced cerebral hypothermia reduces post-hypoxic loss of phenotypic striatal neurons in preterm fetal sheep. *Exp Neurol.* 2007;203:137-147.

872. Zhu HD, Meloni BP, Bojarski C, et al. Post-ischemic modest hypothermia (35 degrees C) combined with intravenous magnesium is more effective at reducing CA1 neuronal death than either treatment alone following global cerebral ischemia in rats. *Exp Neurol.* 2005;193:361-368.

886. Fernandez-Lopez D, Martinez-Orgado J, Nunez E, et al. Characterization of the neuroprotective effect of the cannabinoid agonist WIN-55212 in an in vitro model of hypoxic-ischemic brain damage in newborn rats. *Pediatr Res.* 2006;60:169-173.

889. Ma D, Hossain M, Chow A, et al. Xenon and hypothermia combine to provide neuroprotection from neonatal asphyxia. *Ann Neurol.* 2005;58:182-193.

890. Dingley J, Tooley J, Porter H, et al. Xenon provides short-term neuroprotection in neonatal rats when administered after hypoxia-ischemia. *Stroke.* 2006;37:501-506.

891. Liu Y, Barks JD, Xu G, et al. Topiramate extends the therapeutic window for hypothermia-mediated neuroprotection after stroke in neonatal rats. *Stroke.* 2004;35:1460-1465.

894. Bittigau P, Sifringer M, Genz K, et al. Antiepileptic drugs and apoptotic neurodegeneration in the developing brain. *Proc Natl Acad Sci USA.* 2002;99:15089-15094.

899. McManus T, Sadgrove M, Pringle AK, et al. Intraischaemic hypothermia reduces free radical production and protects against ischaemic insults in cultured hippocampal slices. *J Neurochem.* 2004;91:327-336.

905. van den Tweel ERW, van Bel F, Kavelaars A, et al. Long-term neuroprotection with 2-iminobiotin, an inhibitor of neuronal and inducible nitric oxide synthase, after cerebral hypoxia-ischemia in neonatal rats. *J Cereb Blood Flow Metab.* 2005;25:67-74.

913. Sola A, Wen TC, Hamrick SE, et al. Potential for protection and repair following injury to the developing brain: a role for erythropoietin? *Pediatr Res.* 2005;57:110R-117R.

919. Statler PA, McPherson RJ, Bauer LA, et al. Pharmacokinetics of high-dose recombinant erythropoietin in plasma and brain of neonatal rats. *Pediatr Res.* 2007;61:671-675.

923. Kumral A, Gonenc S, Acikgoz O, et al. Erythropoietin increases glutathione peroxidase enzyme activity and decreases lipid peroxidation levels in hypoxic-ischemic brain injury in neonatal rats. *Biol Neonate.* 2005;87:15-18.

928. Hagberg H, Dammann O, Mallard C, et al. Preconditioning and the developing brain. *Semin Perinatol.* 2004;28:388-395.

931. Strunk T, Hartel C, Schultz C. Does erythropoietin protect the preterm brain? *Arch Dis Child.* 2004;89:F364-F366.

941. Brywe KG, Mallard C, Gustavsson M, et al. IGF-I neuroprotection in the immature brain after hypoxia-ischemia, involvement of Akt and GSK3beta? *Eur J Neurosci.* 2005;21:1489-1502.

942. Husson I, Rangon CM, Lelievre V, et al. BDNF-induced white matter neuroprotection and stage-dependent neuronal survival following a neonatal excitotoxic challenge. *Cereb Cortex.* 2005;15:250-261.

943. Bemelmans AP, Husson I, Jaquet M, et al. Lentiviral-mediated gene transfer of brain-derived neurotrophic factor is neuroprotective in a mouse model of neonatal excitotoxic challenge. *J Neurosci Res.* 2006;83:50-60.

959. Follett P, Rosenberg P, Volpe JJ, Jensen FE. NBQX attenuates excitotoxic injury in developing white matter. *J Neurosci.* 2000;20:9235-9241.

962. Duncan JR, Cock ML, Harding R, et al. Relation between damage to the placenta and the fetal brain after late-gestation placental embolization and fetal growth restriction in sheep. *Am J Obstet Gynecol.* 2000;183:1013-1022.

964. Skoff RP, Bessert DA, Barks JDE, et al. Hypoxic-ischemic injury results in acute disruption of myelin gene expression and death of oligodendroglial precursors in neonatal mice. *Int J Dev Neurosci.* 2001;19:197-208.

966. Ness JK, Romanko MJR, Rothstein RP, Wood TL, et al. Perinatal hypoxia-ischemia induces apoptotic and excitotoxic death of periventricular white matter oligodendrocyte progenitors. *Dev Neurosci.* 2001;23:203-208.

971. Mallard C, Welin A-K, Peebles D, et al. White matter injury following systemic endotoxemia or asphyxia in the fetal sheep. *Neurochem Res.* 2003;28:215-223.

975. McQuillen PS, Sheldon RA, Shatz CJ, et al. Selective vulnerability of subplate neurons after early neonatal hypoxia-ischemia. *J Neurosci.* 2003;23:3308-3315.

976. Zaidi AU, Bessert DA, Ong JE, et al. New oligodendrocytes are generated after neonatal hypoxic-ischemic brain injury in rodents. *Glia.* 2004;46:380-390.

977. Baud O, Daire JL, Dalmaz Y, et al. Gestational hypoxia induces white matter damage in neonatal rats: a new model of periventricular leukomalacia. *Brain Pathol.* 2004;14:1-10.

978. Robinson S, Petelenz K, Li Q, et al. Developmental changes induced by graded prenatal systemic hypoxic-ischemic insults in rats. *Neurobiol Dis.* 2005;18:568-581.

980. Back SA, Luo NL, Mallinson RA, et al. Selective vulnerability of preterm white matter to oxidative damage defined by F(2)-isoprostanes. *Ann Neurol.* 2005;58:108-120.

984. Back SA, Craig AS, Kayton R, et al. Hypoxia-ischemia preferentially triggers glutamate depletion from oligodendroglia and axons in perinatal cerebral white matter. *J Cereb Blood Flow Metab.* 2007;27:334-347.

998. Paintlia MK, Paintlia AS, Barbosa E, et al. N-acetylcysteine prevents endotoxin-induced degeneration of oligodendrocyte progenitors and hypomyelination in developing rat brain. *J Neurosci Res.* 2004;78:347-361.

999. Rodts-Palenik S, WyattAshmead J, Pang Y, et al. Maternal infection-induced white matter injury is reduced by treatment with interleukin-10. *Am J Obstet Gynecol.* 2004;191:1387-1392.

1003. Rousset CI, Chalon S, Cantagrel S, et al. Maternal exposure to LPS induces hypomyelination in the internal capsule and programmed cell death in the deep gray matter in newborn rats. *Pediatr Res.* 2006;59:428-433.

1022. Hagberg H, Mallard C. Effect of inflammation on central nervous system development and vulnerability. *Curr Opin Neurol.* 2005;18:117-123.

1026. Eklind S, Hagberg H, Wang X, et al. Effect of lipopolysaccharide on global gene expression in the immature rat brain. *Pediatr Res.* 2006;60:161-168.

1030. Abreu MT, Arditi M. Innate immunity and toll-like receptors: clinical implications of basic science research. *J Pediatr.* 2004;144:421-429.

1034. Li J, Baud O, Vartanian T, et al. Peroxynitrite generated by inducible nitric oxide synthase and NADPH oxidase mediates microglial toxicity to oligodendrocytes. *Proc Natl Acad Sci USA.* 2005;102:9936-9941.

1035. Barger SW, Goodwin ME, Porter MM, et al. Glutamate release from activated microglia requires the oxidative burst and lipid peroxidation. *J Neurochem.* 2007;101:1205-1213.

1041. Monje ML, Toda H, Palmer TD. Inflammatory blockde restores adult hippocampal neurogenesis. *Science.* 2003;302:1760-1765.

1042. Pachter JS, De Vries HE, Fabry Z. The blood-brain barrier and its role in immune privilege in the central nervous system. *J Neuropathol Exp Neurol.* 2003;62:593-604.

1059. Pitt D, Nagelmeier IE, Wilson HC, et al. Glutamate uptake by oligodendrocytes. Implications for excitotoxicity in multiple sclerosis. *Neurology.* 2003;61:1113-1120.

1065. Fragoso G, Martinez Bermudez AK, Liu HN, et al. Developmental differences in H2O2-induced oligodendrocyte cell death: role of glutathione, mitogen-activated protein kinases and caspase 3. *J Neurochem.* 2004;90:392-404.

1067. Deng W, Rosenberg PA, Volpe JJ, et al. Calcium-permeable AMPA/kainate receptors mediate toxicity and preconditioning by oxygen-glucose deprivation in oligodendrocyte precursors. *Proc Natl Acad Sci USA.* 2003;100:6801-6806.

1069. Baud O, Haynes RF, Wang H, et al. Developmental up-regulation of MnSOD in rat oligodendrocytes confers protection against oxidative injury. *Eur J Neurosci.* 2004;20:29-40.

1099. Godbout JP, Berg BM, Kelley KW, et al. alpha-Tocopherol reduces lipopolysaccharide-induced peroxide radical formation and interleukin-6 secretion in primary murine microglia and in brain. *J Neuroimmunol.* 2004;149:101-109.

1100. Block ML, Hong JS. Microglia and inflammation-mediated neurodegeneration: Multiple triggers with a common mechanism. *Prog Neurobiol.* 2005;76:77-98.

1101. Baud O, Li J, Zhang Y, et al. Nitric oxide-induced cell death in developing oligodendrocytes is associated with mitochondrial dysfunction and apoptosis-inducing factor translocation. *Eur J Neurosci.* 2004;20:1713-1726.

1130. Lin W, Kemper A, Dupree JL, et al. Interferon-gamma inhibits central nervous system remyelination through a process modulated by endoplasmic reticulum stress. *Brain.* 2006;129:1306-1318.

1131. Folkerth RD, Keefe RJ, Haynes RL, et al. Interferon-gamma expression in periventricular leukomalacia in the human brain. *Brain Pathol.* 2004;14:265-274.

1139. Domercq M, Etxebarria E, Perez-Samartin A, et al. Excitotoxic oligodendrocyte death and axonal damage induced by glutamate transporter inhibition. *Glia.* 2005;52:36-46.

1142. Wilke SR, Thomas R, Allcock N, et al. Mechanism of acute ischemic injury of oligodendroglia in early myelinating white matter: the importance of astrocyte injury and glutamate release. *J Neuropathol Exp Neurol.* 2004;63:872-881.

1143. Thomas R, Salter MG, Wilke S, et al. Acute ischemic injury of astrocytes is mediated by Na-K-Cl cotransport and not Ca2+ influx at a key point in white matter development. *J Neuropathol Exp Neurol.* 2004;63:856-871.

1144. Barger SW, Basile AS. Activation of microglia by secreted amyloid precursor protein evokes release of glutamate by cystine exchange and attenuates synaptic function. *J Neurochem.* 2001;76:846-854.

1160. Jensen FE. Role of glutamate receptors in periventricular leukomalacia. *J Child Neurol.* 2005;20:950-959.

1161. Tekkok SB, Goldberg MP. AMPA/kainate receptor activation mediates hypoxic oligodendrocyte death and axonal injury in cerebral white matter. *J Neurosci.* 2001;21:4237-4248.

1168. Salter MG, Fern R. NMDA receptors are expressed in developing oligodendrocyte processes and mediate injury. *Nature.* 2005;438:1167-1171.

1169. Karadottir R, Cavelier P, Bergersen LH, et al. NMDA receptors are expressed in oligodendrocytes and activated in ischaemia. *Nature.* 2005;438:1162-1166.

1171. Matute C. Oligodendrocyte NMDA receptors: a novel therapeutic target. *Trends Mol Med.* 2006;12:289-292.

1174. Sfaello I, Daire JL, Husson I, et al. Patterns of excitotoxin-induced brain lesions in the newborn rabbit: a neuropathological and MRI correlation. *Dev Neurosci.* 2005;27:160-168.

1183. Manning SM, Talos DM, Zhou C, et al. NMDA receptor blockade with memantine attenuates white matter injury in a rat model of periventricular leukomalacia. *J Neurosci.* 2008;28:6670-6678.

1184. Husson I, Mesples B, Bac P, et al. Melatoninergic neuroprotection of the murine periventricular white matter againstneonatal excitotoxic challenge. *Ann Neurol.* 2002;51:82-92.

1186. Lin S, Cox HJ, Rhodes PG, et al. Neuroprotection of alpha-phenyl-n-tert-butyl-nitrone on the neonatal white matter is associated with anti-inflammation. *Neurosci Lett.* 2006;405:52-56.

1187. Lin SY, Fan LW, Pang Y, et al. IGF-1 protects oligodendrocyte progenitor cells and improves neurological functions following cerebral hypoxia-ischemia in the neonatal rat. *Brain Res.* 2005;1063:15-26.

1190. Ness JK, Scaduto RC, Wood TL. IGF-I prevents glutamate-mediated Bax translocation and cytochrome C release in O4(+) oligodendrocyte progenitors. *Glia.* 2004;46:183-194.

1191. Guan J, Thomas GB, Lin H, et al. Neuroprotective effects of the N-terminal tripeptide of insulin-like growth factor-1, glycine-proline-glutamate (GPE) following intravenous infusion in hypoxic-ischemic adult rats. *Neuropharmacology*. 2004;47:892-903.

1195. Bennet L, Roelfsema V, George S, et al. The effect of cerebral hypothermia on white and grey matter injury induced by severe hypoxia in preterm fetal sheep. *J Physiol*. 2007;578:491-506.

1196. Leuchter RH, Gui L, Poncet A, et al. Association between early administration of high-dose erythropoietin in preterm infants and brain MRI abnormality at term-equivalent age. *JAMA*. 2014;312:817-824.

1197. Natalucci G, Latal B, Koller B, et al. Effect of early prophylactic high-dose recombinant human erythropoietin in very preterm enfants on neurodevelopmental outcome at 2 years: a randomized clinical trial. *JAMA*. 2016;315:2079-2085.

1198. Song J, Sun H, Xu F, et al. Recombinant human erythropoietin improves neurological outcomes in very preterm infants. *Ann Neurol*. 2016;80:24-34.

Full references for this chapter can be found on www.expertconsult.com.

Encephalopathy of Prematurity: Neuropathology

Hannah C. Kinney ◆ Joseph J. Volpe

The major neuropathological substrate of human preterm brain injury is the *encephalopathy of prematurity*, a term coined to characterize the multifaceted gray and white matter lesions in the preterm brain that reflect acquired and developmental factors in combination (Table 14.1).[1] The encephalopathy of prematurity is also associated with hemorrhages, notably in the germinal matrix of the ganglionic eminence (GE) (see Chapter 24) and cerebellum (see Chapter 23) and with focal micro- or macroinfarcts. Because the responsible insults occur at a time of rapid brain growth, a host of developmental programs may be affected, resulting in maturational defects that compound the acquired lesion (e.g., hypoxic-ischemic injury leading to loss of preoligodendrocytes [pre-OLs] and subsequent impaired maturation and, as a consequence, impaired myelination). The cause of the encephalopathy of prematurity is multifactorial and includes cerebral hypoxia-ischemia and systemic infection/inflammation, which results in glutamate, free radical, and/or cytokine toxicity to pre-OLs, axons, and neurons (see Chapter 15). Contributory roles for impaired nutrition, pain, stress, drugs and other factors associated with neonatal intensive care seem likely but remain to be clarified (see Chapters 15 and 16). Given the heterogeneity and diverse combinations of the lesions that comprise the encephalopathy of prematurity, it is not surprising that the spectrum of neurodevelopmental abnormalities in preterm survivors is wide and includes, often in combination, a variety of cognitive, behavioral, socialization, attentional, and motor deficits (see Chapter 16). The patterns and mechanisms of injury are highly dependent upon the specific maturational stages of OLs, neurons, and axons over the last half of gestation (i.e., the time frame of occurrence of the encephalopathy).

NEUROPATHOLOGICAL FEATURES OF THE ENCEPHALOPATHY OF PREMATURITY

Periventricular Leukomalacia

The central feature of the encephalopathy of prematurity is periventricular leukomalacia (PVL). This lesion is the major white matter component of the encephalopathy and is defined as focal periventricular necrosis associated with more diffuse reactive gliosis and microglial activation in the surrounding cerebral white matter.[2] Thus PVL has two components, focal and diffuse. The seminal publication of Banker and Larroche in 1962[3] characterized this lesion in detail and related it to adverse cardiorespiratory events and cerebral ischemia in the affected infants, with the focal lesion apparently occurring in deep arterial border zones and end zones in the periventricular white matter (Fig. 14.1).

The *necrotic foci likely represent a core infarct with destruction of all cellular elements,*[2] while the astrocytic and microglial response in the surrounding white matter represents less severe and potentially reversible ischemic injury.[2] The necrotic foci progress from coagulative necrosis (characteristic of the histology of tissue ischemia in all tissues, with hypereosinophilia, nuclear pyknosis, and axonal spheroids) to organizing necrosis with reactive gliosis, macrophagocytic infiltration, and tissue disintegration and then end-stage cystic formation and gliosis (Fig. 14.2).[4] This latter variety of PVL (i.e., with focal cysts, the more severe end of a spectrum) is termed *cystic PVL* in the neuroimaging literature (see the section on neuropathology in living infants, later).

Importantly, *the necrotic foci are not always apparent upon macroscopic examination.* In autopsy studies in our hospital from the modern era of intensive care, 46% to 82% of PVL cases, depending upon the data set, have only microscopic necrotic foci (with macrophagocytic infiltration) that measure less than 2 mm in diameter (Fig. 14.3).[5] These punctate white matter lesions are now the most common focal manifestation of PVL at autopsy.

Nevertheless, visually obvious foci of necrosis, or "white spots," as well as cysts greater than 2 mm in diameter are still detected at autopsy (Fig. 14.4).[5] The small necrotic foci do not result in cysts but rather focal areas of gliosis. In the neuroimaging literature, this variety of PVL is often termed *noncystic PVL*. The small foci of gliosis may account for the focal punctate lesions seen by magnetic resonance imaging (MRI) (see the section on neuropathology in living infants, later, and Chapter 16), although careful anatomical imaging correlations are lacking.

Diffuse white matter gliosis without periventricular necrotic foci occurs frequently in preterm brains,[5] but its relationship to PVL is uncertain (e.g., whether or not it represents the least severe end of a spectrum of ischemic injury to the premyelinated white matter, with PVL at the most severe end). Reactive gliosis and activated microglia are the two major inflammatory components of PVL (Fig. 14.5).[2] Presumed to be initially protective against pre-OL cell damage, these cells carry the potential for compounding tissue injury when the insult is prolonged and/or severe. Reactive gliosis in PVL is preferentially located in the deep as opposed the intragyral white matter and thereby may define injury in the vascular distal fields of the cerebral white matter. Activated microglia likewise conform to

TABLE 14.1   Neuropathological Features of the Encephalopathy of Prematurity

I. White matter lesions
   A. Periventricular leukomalacia
      1. Focal white matter necrosis
      2. Diffuse white matter gliosis and activation of microglia
   B. Acute loss of pre-oligodendrocytes (pre-OLs)
   C. Expression of markers of oxidative and nitrative stress in pre-OLs.
   D. Replenishment of pre-OLs
   E. Arrested maturation of pre-OLs
   F. Hypo- and/or delayed myelination
   G. Increased EAAT—immunopositive astrocytes
   H. Increased inducible nitric oxide synthase—immunopositive astrocytes and microglia
II. Gray matter lesions
   A. Neuronal loss and/or gliosis in gray matter sites in variable combinations
      1. Thalamus, basal ganglia, hippocampus, cerebellar dentate nucleus
      2. Deficit of interstitial neurons in cerebral white matter
      3. Decrease of GABAergic neurons in cerebral white matter
   B. Diffuse and focal periventricular axonal injury

EAAT, Excitatory amino acid transporter.

this regional distribution, while macrophages are prominent in the organizing necrotic foci of the periventricular regions. Both astrocytes and microglia/macrophages produce inflammatory cytokines, and immunocytochemical studies in PVL demonstrate increased cytokine expression within them as a distinctive feature of the histopathology. Notably, reactive astrocytes in PVL express interferon-γ and thus are a potential source for this toxic cytokine, particularly to pre-OLs compared with mature OLs.[6] Reactive astrocytes and microglia/macrophages also help to protect pre-OLs from excitotoxic injury by the upregulation of the glutamate transporter excitatory amino acid transporter (EAAT) and uptake of excessive extracellular glutamate, as suggested by the finding that the percentage of EAAT2-immunopositive astrocytes is increased in PVL as compared with control white matter; moreover, macrophages in the necrotic foci express EAAT2.[7] Yet reactive astrocytes and microglia may contribute to free radical injury in PVL, as indicated by intense expression of inducible nitric oxide synthase (iNOS), a marker of nitrative stress, in reactive astrocytes in the acute through chronic stages of PVL, and in activated microglia primarily in the acute stage, this last observation suggesting an early role for microglial iNOS in the pathogenesis of PVL.[8,9] In addition, the density of iNOS-immunopositive cells is significantly increased in the diffuse component in cerebral white matter.[8]

The *cellular evolution of PVL* involves acute loss of pre-OLs[8]; some OL cell bodies appear to survive with loss of cell processes, others with morphological dysfunction in myelin formation as well as subsequent hypomyelination.[10] Immunocytochemical analysis using an antibody to Olig2, a pan-OL lineage marker, indicates no significant difference in Olig2 cell density in the periventricular or intragyral white matter between PVL cases

and controls.[10] Moreover, early lineage markers suggest that there is an attempt at replenishment of pre-OLs by proliferation of progenitors, but these pre-OLs fail to mature. The cellular result is dominance of pre-OLs over mature OLs (see further on and Chapter 15).[11] Consistent with a maturational disturbance of pre-OLs, qualitative abnormalities of myelin basic protein (MBP) staining in both the diffuse and necrotic components of PVL occur despite preserved Olig2 cell density. These include excessive MBP immunostaining in enlarged OL perikarya that presumably reflects a functional derangement in MBP transport from its site of production in the OL cell body to the OL processes.[10]

Free radical injury to pre-OLs in PVL is indicated by early immunocytochemical evidence for protein nitration and lipid peroxidation of pre-OLs in the diffusely gliotic component of PVL (Fig. 14.6).[8] In addition, F(2)-isoprostanes, an arachidinate metabolite/lipid peroxidation marker of oxidative damage, is significantly increased in the white matter of early PVL cases.[12] The end stage of PVL is delayed myelination or hypomyelination of the cerebral white matter and compensatory ventricular enlargement

Gray Matter Lesions in Encephalopathy of Prematurity

Neuronal loss and/or gliosis are the histopathological hallmarks of gray matter injury in the encephalopathy of prematurity and occur in virtually all gray matter sites, albeit in variable combinations (Fig. 14.7). Over one-third of PVL cases demonstrate overt gray matter lesions characterized by neuronal loss and/or gliosis[5]; microglial activation is often striking. Of note, more refined techniques, such as analysis of dendritic and spine number and morphology, may ultimately detect neuronal deficits at the subcellular (and molecular) levels (see Chapter 15). The incidence of neuronal loss, as assessed semiquantitatively in tissue sections, is 38% in the thalamus, 33% in the globus pallidus and hippocampus, and 29% in the cerebellar dentate nucleus.[5] Gliosis without obvious neuronal loss is more common than combined neuronal loss and gliosis, occurring in the thalamus (56% of PVL cases), globus pallidus (60%), hippocampus (47%), basis pontis (100%), inferior olive (92%), and brain-stem tegmentum (43%).[5] In a histopathological survey of brain injury in infants with very low birth weights, the frequency of neuronal loss (sites unspecified) is reportedly less than that of cerebral white matter abnormalities.[13] Because detection of neuronal loss and gliosis is a somewhat crude measure of neuronal disturbance, the possibility of even more frequent neuronal disturbance is likely. Moreover, neuronal loss and gliosis may not reflect primary injury but rather secondary dysmaturational effects caused by trophic and retrograde and anterograde disturbances (see later).

Thalamus

Thalamic injury associated with PVL may be heterogeneous and occur in different patterns, reflecting different types of insults. Four different patterns of thalamic injury have been recognized: (1) diffuse gliosis with or without neuronal loss; (2) microinfarcts with focal neuronal loss; (3) macroinfarcts in the distribution of the posterior cerebral artery; and (4) status marmoratus.[14] These different patterns likely reflect separate pathogenetic mechanisms, including diffuse hypoxia-ischemia and focal arterial embolism, as well as potentially different

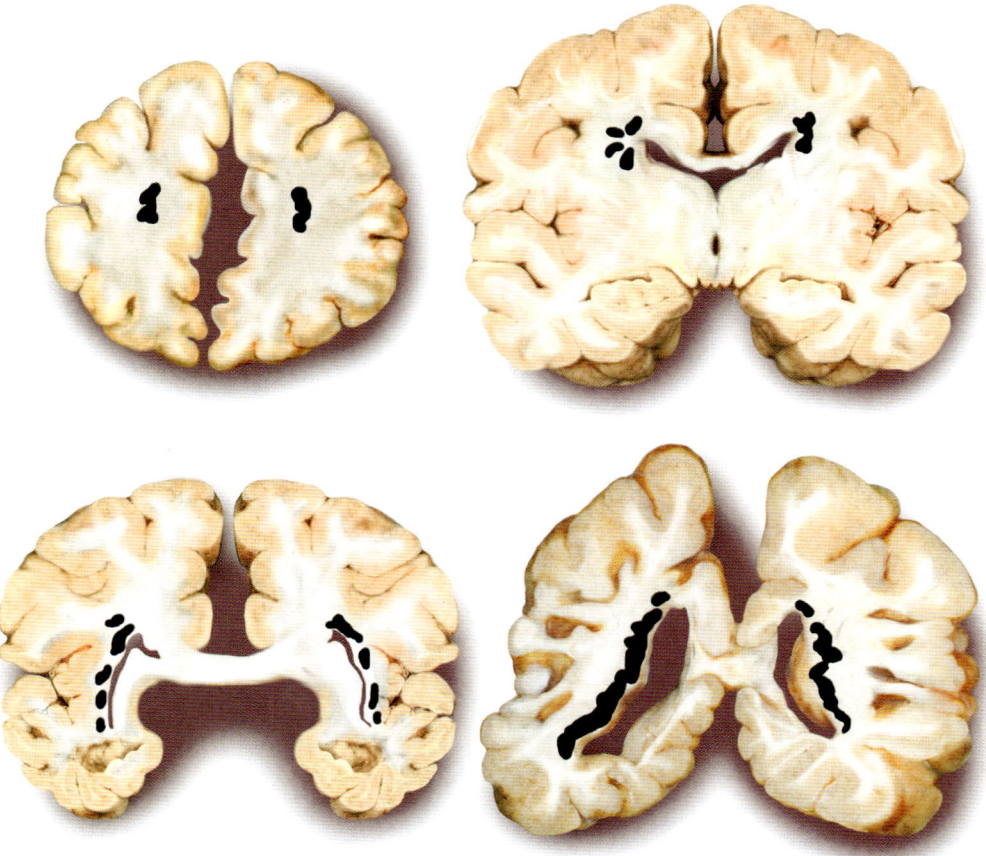

Figure 14.1 **Topographical occurrence of periventricular leukomalacia.** The seminal publication of Banker and Larroche in 1962 characterized this lesion in detail and related it to adverse cardiorespiratory events and cerebral ischemia in affected infants, with the lesion occurring in deep arterial border zones in the periventricular white matter *(solid black ovals)*. (From Banker BQ, Larroche JC. Periventricular leukomalacia of infancy. A form of neonatal anoxic encephalopathy. *Arch Neurol.* 1962; 7:386–410, with permission.)

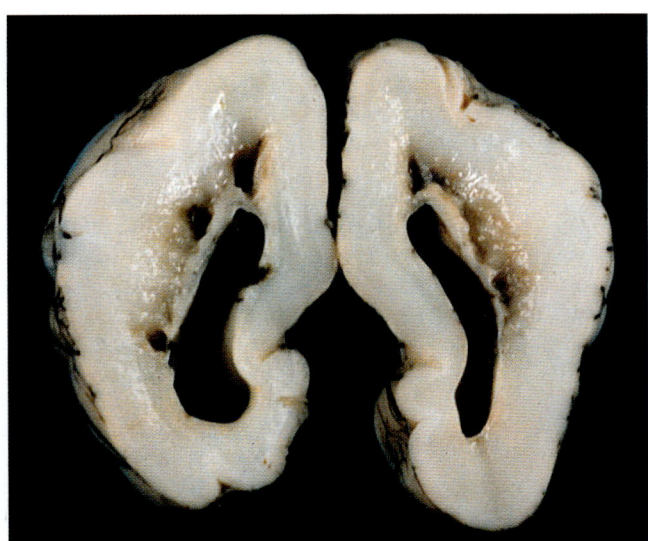

Figure 14.2 Cavitating periventricular leukomalacia in a 4-week-old newborn delivered at 24 gestational weeks. (Courtesy Hannah Kinney.)

temporal characteristics of the responsible insults. Diffuse diminutions in thalamic volume are seen in older children with PVL (Fig. 14.8).[15] The thalamic volumetric disturbances could reflect either direct injury or secondary anterograde and retrograde effects related to axonal and subplate neuron disturbance (see later).

Cerebral Cortex

During the last half of gestation, the neocortex transforms from an undifferentiated cortical plate to a highly specialized structure (see Chapter 7). Around 30 gestational weeks, the cortical plate comprises six layers, each of which is characterized by a specific composite of differentiating pyramidal and nonpyramidal neurons.[16] The cortex increases in thickness because of striking increases in the neuropil (e.g., neuronal cell size, dendritic arborization, spine formation, and arrival of preterminal afferents) (see Chapter 7). Relative to excitotoxicity, the excitatory amino acid receptor GluR2 is low in the pyramidal and nonpyramidal neurons in the cerebral cortex during the preterm period.[17,18] In a study of PVL cases compared to controls adjusted for postconceptional age, there was a marked reduction

Focal necrosis (<2 mm) in periventricular white matter

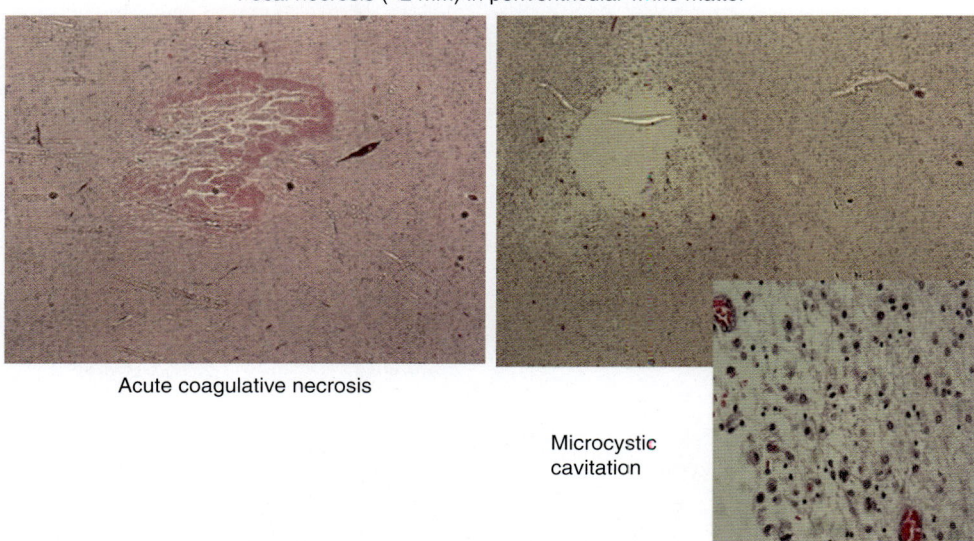

Acute coagulative necrosis

Microcystic cavitation

Figure 14.3 Microscopic stages of periventricular leukomalacia from acute coagulative necrosis to microcystic cavitation (<2 mm in diameter). The inset shows macrophages associated with the cavitation.

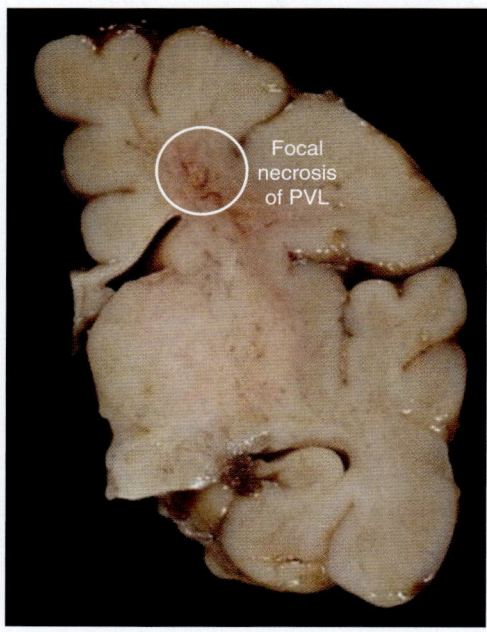

Focal necrosis of PVL

Figure 14.4 Foci of necrosis in deep white matter appear as the typical "white spots" *(within circle)* of organizing periventricular leukomalacia **(PVL).** Histologically, the white spot is composed of lipid-laden macrophages.

(38%) in the density of layer V neurons in all areas sampled in the PVL cases ($n = 17$) compared with controls ($n = 12$) adjusted for postconceptional age at or greater than 30 weeks, when the six-layer cortex is visually distinct ($P < .024$). This reduction may reflect a dying-back loss of somata secondary to transection of layer V axons projecting through the necrosis in the underlying white matter. This study underscores the role of secondary cortical effects in the encephalopathy of prematurity.

Late Migrating GABAergic Neurons

A defining feature of cortical development in the human preterm period is the late development of the GABAergic interneurons that play a key role in cortical specification, output, and synaptic plasticity (see Chapter 7).[19,20] At least 20% of GABAergic neurons migrate through the white matter to the cerebral cortex over late gestation.[19] This migration peaks around term and then declines and ends within the first 6 postnatal months; in parallel, the GABAergic neuronal density increases in the cortex over late gestation, peaks at term, and declines thereafter.[21] One report has shown a deficit in GABAergic neurons in cerebral white matter in infants with PVL.[21]

Subplate Neurons

Deficit of Neurons in the Subplate Zone and White Matter in the Encephalopathy of Prematurity. There is damage to neurons not only in gray matter sites but also to those located in the cerebral white matter and subplate region. The density of granular neurons is significantly reduced in the periventricular and central white matter and the subplate region in PVL.[22] These neurons are likely late-migrating GABAergic neurons and/or non-GABAergic constituents of the subplate region and interstitial white matter.[22] In regard to the former possibility, a reduction in the density of GAD67-immunopositive neurons and neurons expressing the $GABA_A\alpha1$ receptor has been reported in human perinatal white matter lesions (with and without focal necrosis).[19] Notably, in contrast to granular neurons, there is not a consistent deficit in unipolar, bipolar, multipolar, or inverted pyramidal neurons in the white matter or subplate region in PVL.[22] The finding of reduced density of white matter neurons in the necrotic foci in PVL is not unexpected, since necrosis involves destruction of all cellular elements. *On the other hand, the deficit in the granular neurons distant from the focally necrotic lesions (i.e., in the subplate region), presumably in areas with less severe insult, is of major interest.* The preferential damage to granular neurons, including those distant from the necrotic foci, suggests that this particular subtype is

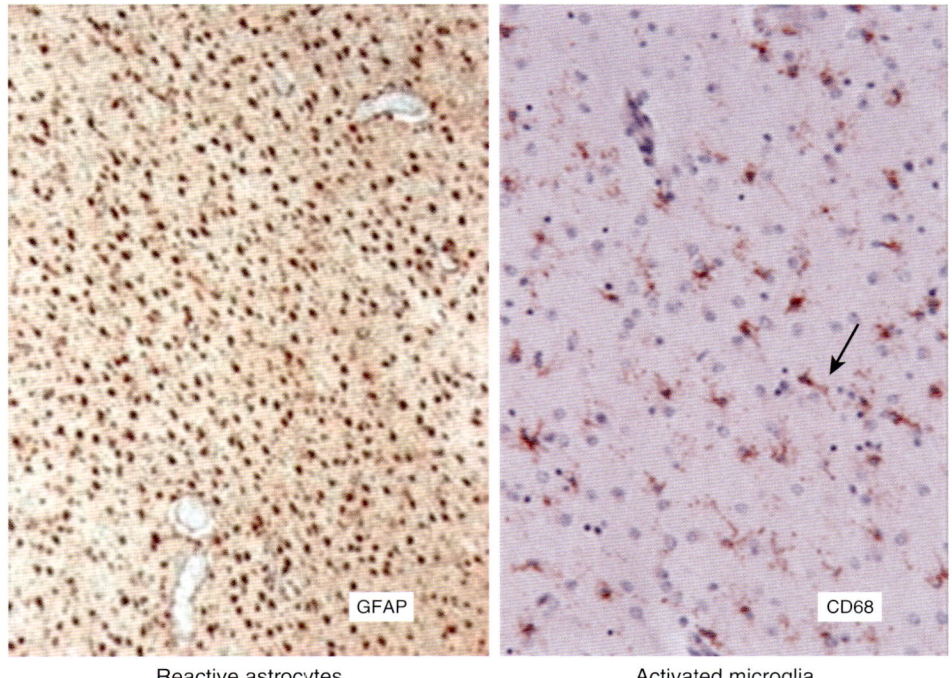

Reactive astrocytes   Activated microglia

Figure 14.5 Diffuse astrogliosis (GFAP) and diffuse activation of microglia (CD68) in the cerebral white matter surrounding necrotic periventricular foci.

TABLE 14.2	Radial Glial Pathology in Periventricular Leukomalacia

I. Development
   A. 19–30 weeks: radial glial fibers abundant
   B. 30–31 weeks: onset of transformation of radial glial fibers into fibrous astrocytes
   C. 30 weeks–term: progressive disappearance of radial glial fibers as white matter is increasingly populated with transformed astrocytes
   D. 40 weeks: end of major radial glial-mediated neuronal migration
II. Pathology in periventricular leukomalacia
   A. Loss of radial glial fibers in periventricular necrotic foci
   B. Potential deficit of fibrous astrocytes in cerebral white matter

exquisitely sensitive to hypoxia-ischemia. Because of the critical roles of subplate neurons in cerebral cortical development, such injury could have important secondary deleterious effects in cortex (see later).

Radial Glial Fibers

Development of Radial Glial Fibers and Astrocytes in the Cerebral White Matter in the Preterm Period. The last half of human gestation is a crucial time in astrocyte formation in the cerebral cortex and white matter. The radial glial cell originates in the ventricular zone/subventricular zone (SVZ), retains connections with the ependyma and pia, and is capable of generating neurons and astrocytes (Table 14.2).[23] Early in development these cells are important neuronal progenitors (see Chapter 5). Radial glial cells have long, thin, linear processes

(i.e., radial glial fibers [RGFs]), which serve as a guide for migrating neuroblasts and glial cells.[24] Glutamatergic neurons form in the dorsal telencephalic pallium and migrate along RGFs early in gestation (see Chapter 6).[20] In the human brain, in contrast to the rodent brain, approximately two thirds of GABAergic neurons arise from the dorsal telencephalic zone and migrate along RGFs; the remaining one third originate in the GE and migrate tangentially to the cortex (see Chapter 5).[25] From 19 to 30 weeks, RGFs are abundant; around 30 to 31 weeks, they begin to transform into fibrous astrocytes in the white matter; and from 30 weeks to term, they progressively disappear as the white matter becomes increasingly populated with transformed astrocytes (see Table 14.2).[26-28] By term, RGFs completely disappear, thereby definitively marking the end of radial migration. Fibrous astrocytes in the white matter also form from glial precursors that migrate outward from the ventricular zone/SVZ independent of RGFs.[29] Reactive gliosis with gemistocytic morphology and immunostaining positive for glial fibrillary acidic protein (GFAP) begins around midgestation in the human brain.[2] There is presumed loss and fragmentation of RGFs transected by focal periventricular necrosis (see Table 14.2). RGF damage could adversely affect radial neuronal migration with secondary maldevelopment of the vertical columns of the cerebral cortex. This idea of diffuse loss of RGFs has not been rigorously tested, however, in the preterm brain with the necessary tissue methods to define quantitative derangements in cortical mini- and macrocolumn formation. Damage to RGFs may also potentially impair astrocytic development, as fibrous astrocytes in the white matter develop from the transformation of RGFs, and protoplasmic astrocytes in the cortex transform from layer I astrocytes following RGF migration.[29] A deficit in fibrous and/or protoplasmic astrocytes in the encephalopathy of prematurity may potentially be

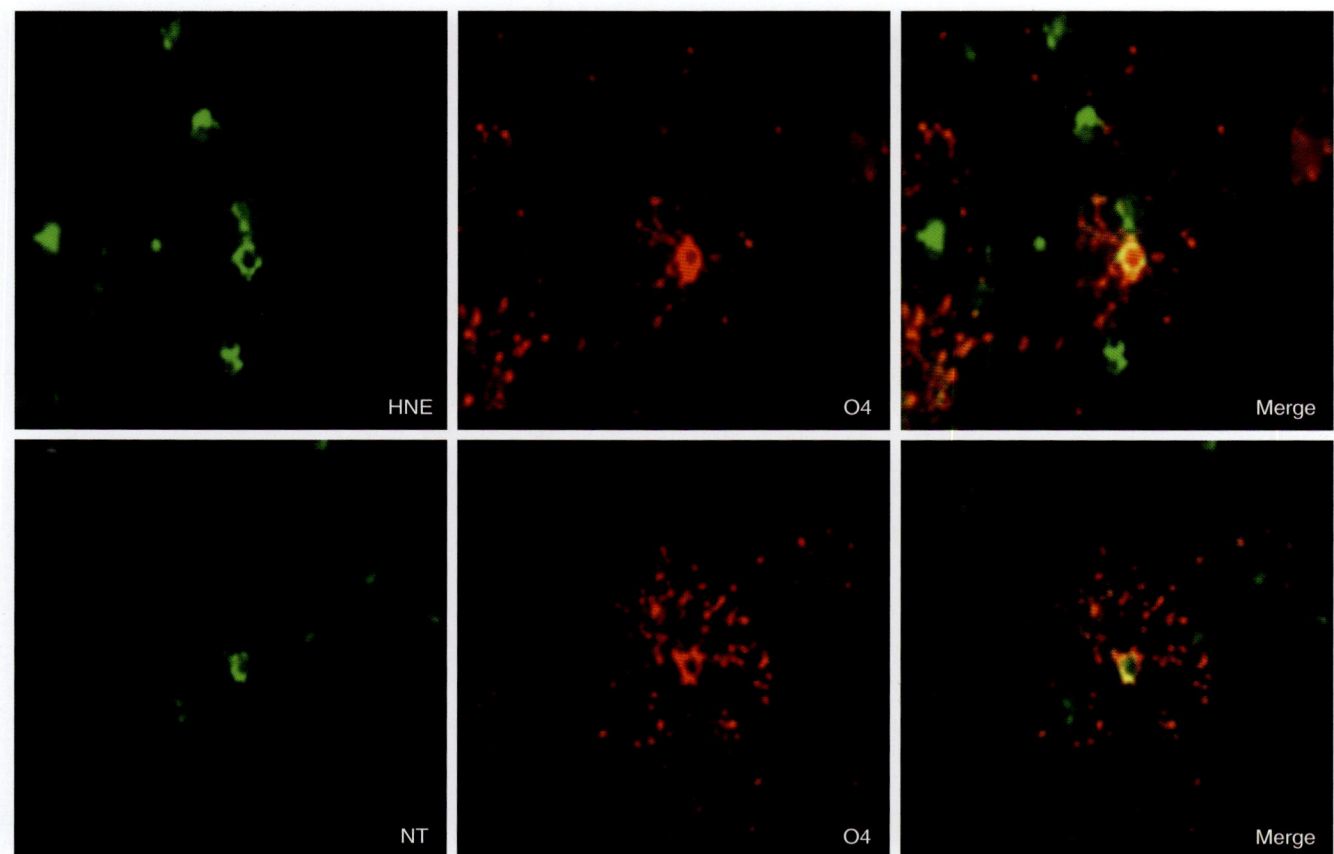

Figure 14.6 Oxidative and nitrative injury in developing oligodendrocytes (OLs) in periventricular leukomalacia. The O4 marker identifies the pre-OL that has sustained oxidative (HNE) and nitrative (NT) injury. *HNE,* 4-Hydroxy-2-nonenal (marker of lipid peroxidation); *NT,* nitrotyrosine (marker of free radical-induced protein nitration). (From Haynes, et al. Nitrosative and oxidative injury to premyelinating oligodendrocytes in periventricular leukomalacia. *J Neuropathol Exp Neurol.* 2003;62:441–450, with permission.)

masked by gliosis, as there are no quantitative criteria for an *adequate* astrocytic response. Nevertheless, reactive astrocytes in the encephalopathy of prematurity demonstrate evidence of oxidative and nitrative stress, which is potentially primary and could lead to an *inadequate* glial response.[8,9] Indeed, "acutely damaged glia" in PVL may represent astrocytes undergoing cell death. Given the role of astrocytes in protecting against ischemic injury via glutamate uptake and in orchestrating cytokine responses, damage to them secondary to potential RGF injury in the encephalopathy of prematurity could be especially deleterious. The delineation of RGF pathology in the encephalopathy of prematurity is an important direction for future research.

White Matter Axons

Diffuse Axonal Injury in the Cerebral White Matter in the Encephalopathy of Prematurity. With β-amyloid precursor protein, axonal spheroids are detected within the necrotic lesions of PVL, whether focal or large (Fig. 14.9).[30,31] This finding is not unexpected in view of the injury to all cellular elements in the focal areas of necrosis. *However, surprisingly perhaps, in the more diffuse nonnecrotic component of PVL, evidence for axonal injury has recently been gathered.* With the apoptotic marker fractin,

diffuse axonal injury is detected in the white matter distant from acute or organizing necrotic foci, suggesting a widespread axonopathy in PVL (Fig. 14.10).[30,31] This diffuse axonal damage could reflect secondary degeneration of thalamocortical afferents complicating primary thalamic neuronal loss. Alternatively, hypoxic-ischemic or inflammatory injury directly to the axon, with secondary impairments in axonal-OL interactions in the initiation and maintenance of myelination, seems possible (see later). Irrespective of its pathogenesis, widespread axonal damage likely contributes to the reduced white matter volume and callosal thinning in end-stage PVL. Axonal injury throughout the diffuse and focal components of PVL may also lead to architectonic changes in the overlying cerebral cortex.[32]

Neural Repair

Evidence is mounting that tissue repair is under way in the encephalopathy of prematurity within the neonatal period (Table 14.3). In this regard, as noted earlier, Olig2 cell density at the necrotic foci is *increased* in PVL cases compared with that in sites distant from these foci, suggesting that OLs are migrating to the ischemic core to replenish OL cell number.[10] In PVL, the stem cell immunomarker nestin, demonstrates increased expression in glia and neurons, attributed to nestin

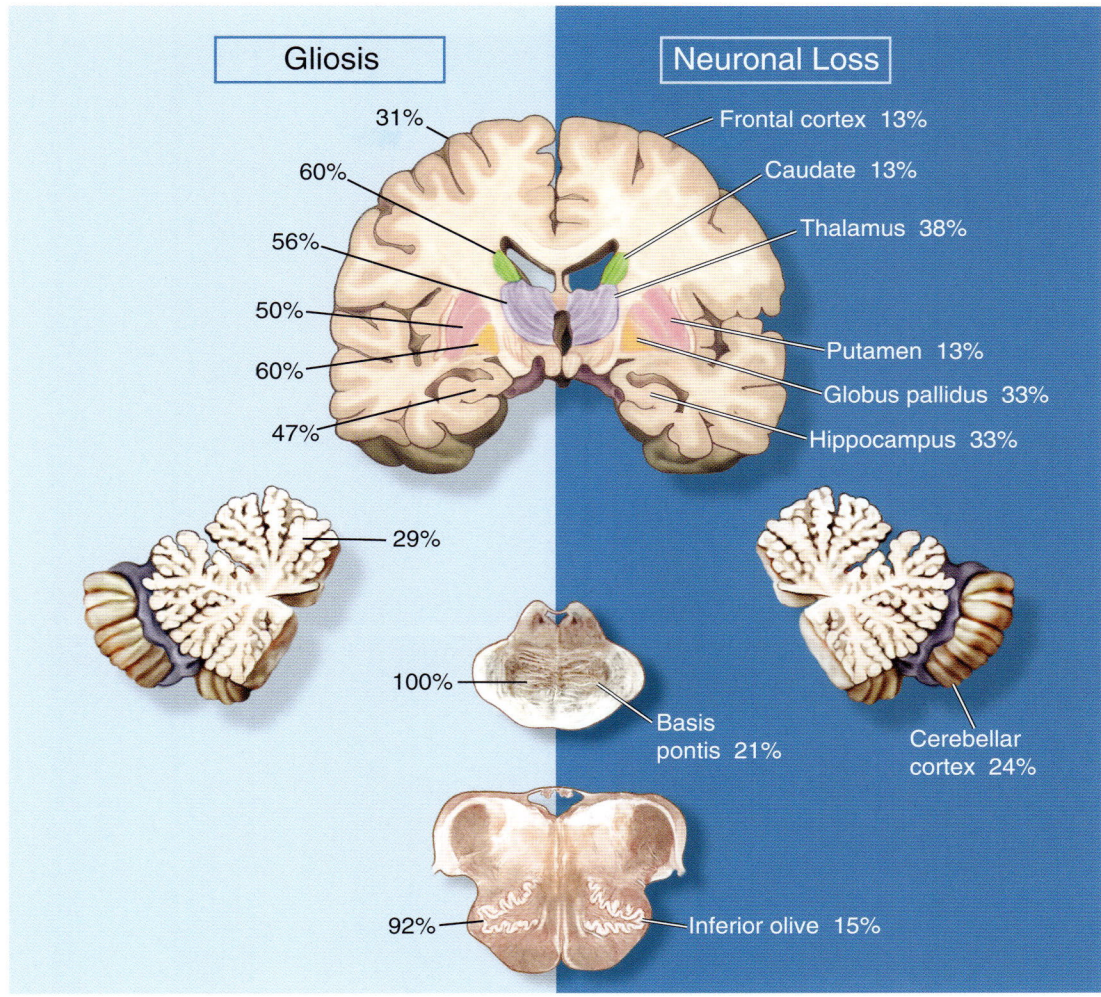

Gliosis

31%
60%
56%
50%
60%
47%

29%

100%

92%

Neuronal Loss

Frontal cortex 13%
Caudate 13%
Thalamus 38%
Putamen 13%
Globus pallidus 33%
Hippocampus 33%

Basis pontis 21%

Cerebellar cortex 24%

Inferior olive 15%

Figure 14.7 Gray matter lesions associated with periventricular leukomalacia. Percentages give proportion of cases in study (*n* = 41) with gray matter site involvements. (From Pierson CR, et al. Gray matter injury associated with periventricular leukomalacia in the premature infant. *Acta Neuropathol.* 2007;114:619–631, with permission.)

TABLE 14.3   Repair and Plasticity of Encephalopathy of Prematurity

I. White matter changes
   A. Increased expression of stem cell immunomarker, nestin
   B. Increased Olig2 cell density at periventricular necrotic foci
   C. Increased density of cells immunopositive for doublecortin, immunomarker of migrating neurons
II. Cerebral cortex changes
   A. Leptomeningeal heterotopia complicating subpial hemorrhage
   B. Transformation of pyramidal neurons with amputated dendrites into star cells
   C. Transformation of projection pyramidal neurons with transected axons into intracortical short axon cells
   D. Diminution in number of pyramidal neurons in layer V overlying periventricular leukomalacia lesion

Olig2, Oligodendrocyte transcription factor.

upregulation in response to injury rather than regeneration of new cells.[33] Using doublecortin (DCX) immunopositivity as a marker of postmitotic migrating neurons, we found significantly increased densities of DCX-immunopositive cells in PVL cases compared with controls in the SVZ, necrotic foci, and subcortical white matter in the perinatal time window (i.e., 35–42 postconceptional weeks). These increased DCX-immunopositive neurons may be *en route* to replenish the loss of white matter neurons. Their increased density in the SVZ suggests that the regenerative capacity originates in this germinal site.[34] Successful incorporation of the DCX-immunopositive cells into the neuronal circuitry of the white matter in PVL will ultimately depend upon timing and extent of injury as well as the availability of neurotropic factors necessary for cellular differentiation and the formation of functional circuits.

Plasticity of the Neocortex Following Hemorrhagic and Hypoxic-Ischemic Encephalopathies. The cerebral cortex has been studied in children who survived days, weeks, months, and even years after sustaining hemorrhagic and hypoxic-ischemic

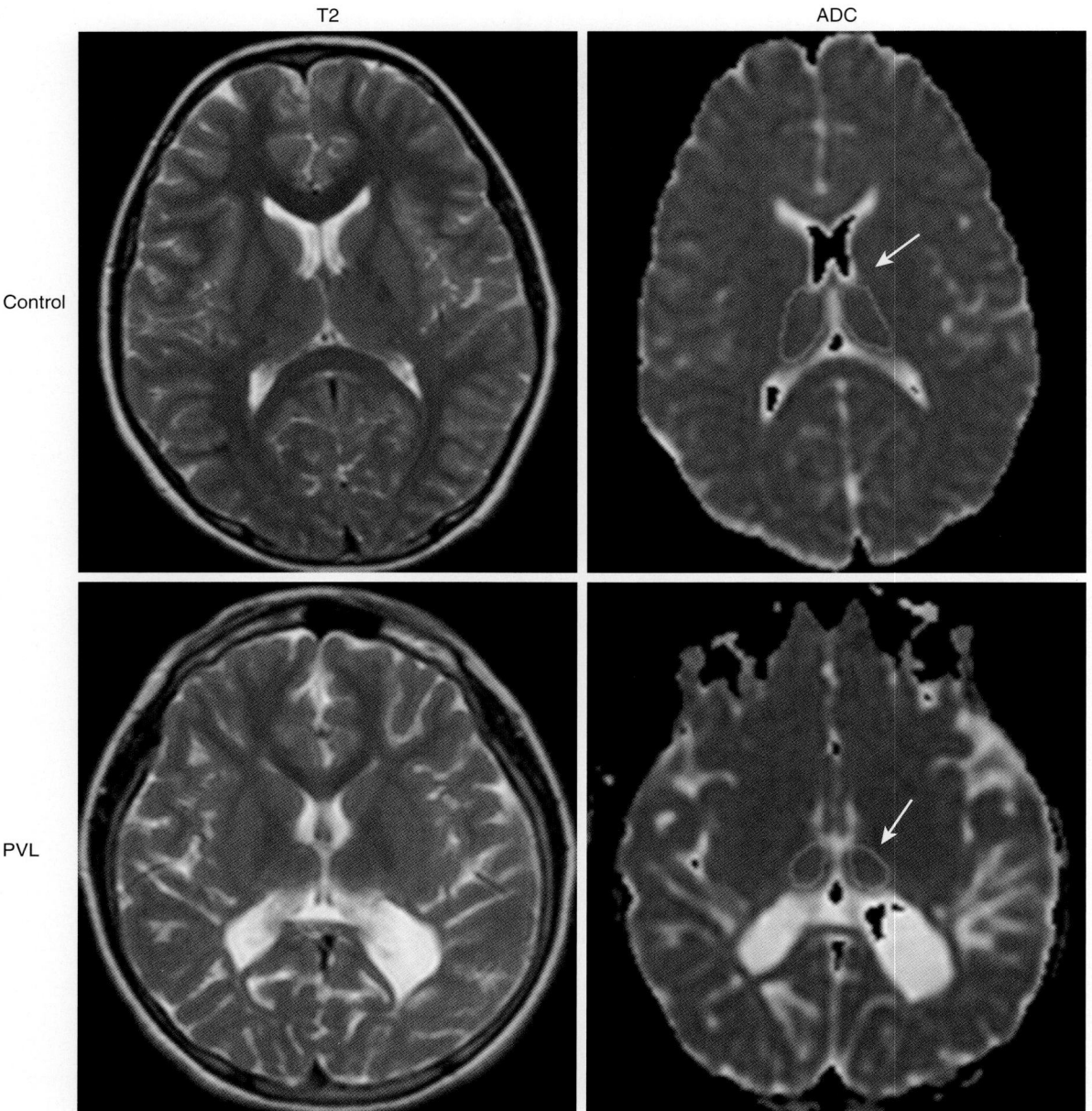

Figure 14.8 Thalamic damage in children with periventricular leukomalacia (PVL). The arrows in the right panels show size of the thalamus in controls (*n* = 74) compared with atrophy of the thalamus (*n* = 17) associated with PVL. (From Nagasunder AC, et al. Abnormal microstructure of the atrophic thalamus in preterm survivors with periventricular leukomalacia, *AJNR Am J Neuroradiol.* 2011;32:185–191, with permission.)

lesions to the cerebral cortex and/or underlying white matter.[32] Such studies reveal changes in the subsequent development of the cortex that could be responsible for clinical epilepsy, cerebral palsy, and intellectual impairment.[32] The postnatal development of the gray matter adjacent to these lesions is altered in a specific manner (see Table 14.3). The postnatal resolution (scarring) of subpial hemorrhage, for example, causes structural changes in the superficial layers of the cortex and permanent leptomeningeal heterotopia. The pyramidal cells of layers II and III, whose apical dendrites had been partially amputated by hemorrhage, can become star cells.

The postnatal development of the cerebral cortex overlying white matter infarcts (partly deprived of sensory information because of the destruction of afferent fibers and contact loss from them) is adversely affected. Projection pyramidal cells (long axon) axotomized by the subjacent lesion survive the insult and are transformed into intracortical short-axon cells. The intrinsic neuropil of the gray matter (partially isolated) increases in an irregular manner, which can be seen using immunohistochemical techniques and Golgi's method: areas with a great increase in fibers alternate with areas with few fibers. The presence of large neurons (Golgi method) with long

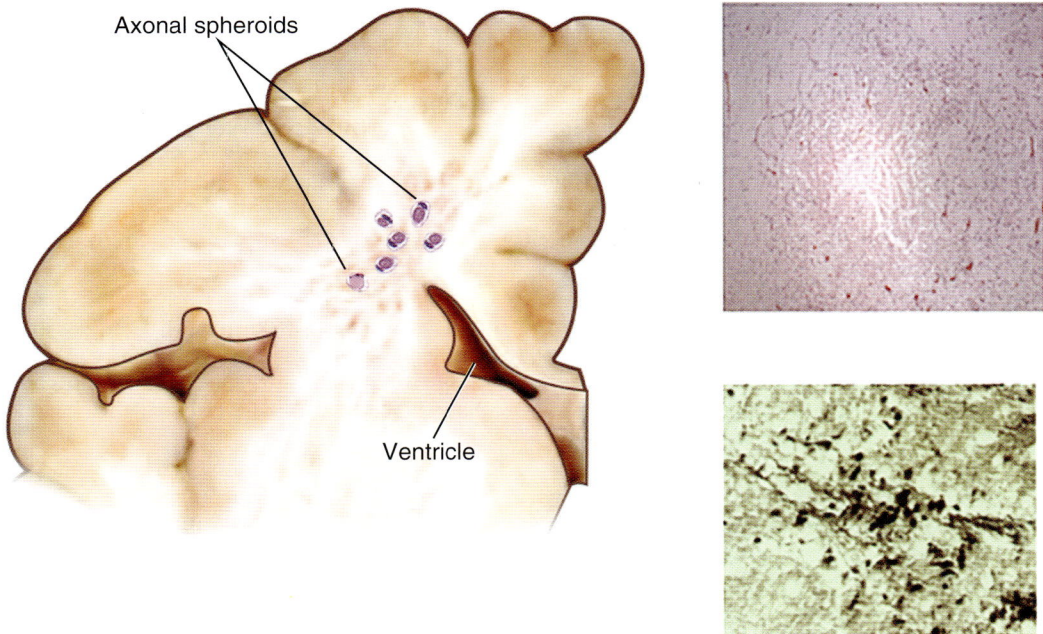

Figure 14.9 Focal periventricular necrosis with axonal damage. The immunomarker to β-amyloid demonstrates acute axonal (transected) spheroids in organizing foci of necrosis.

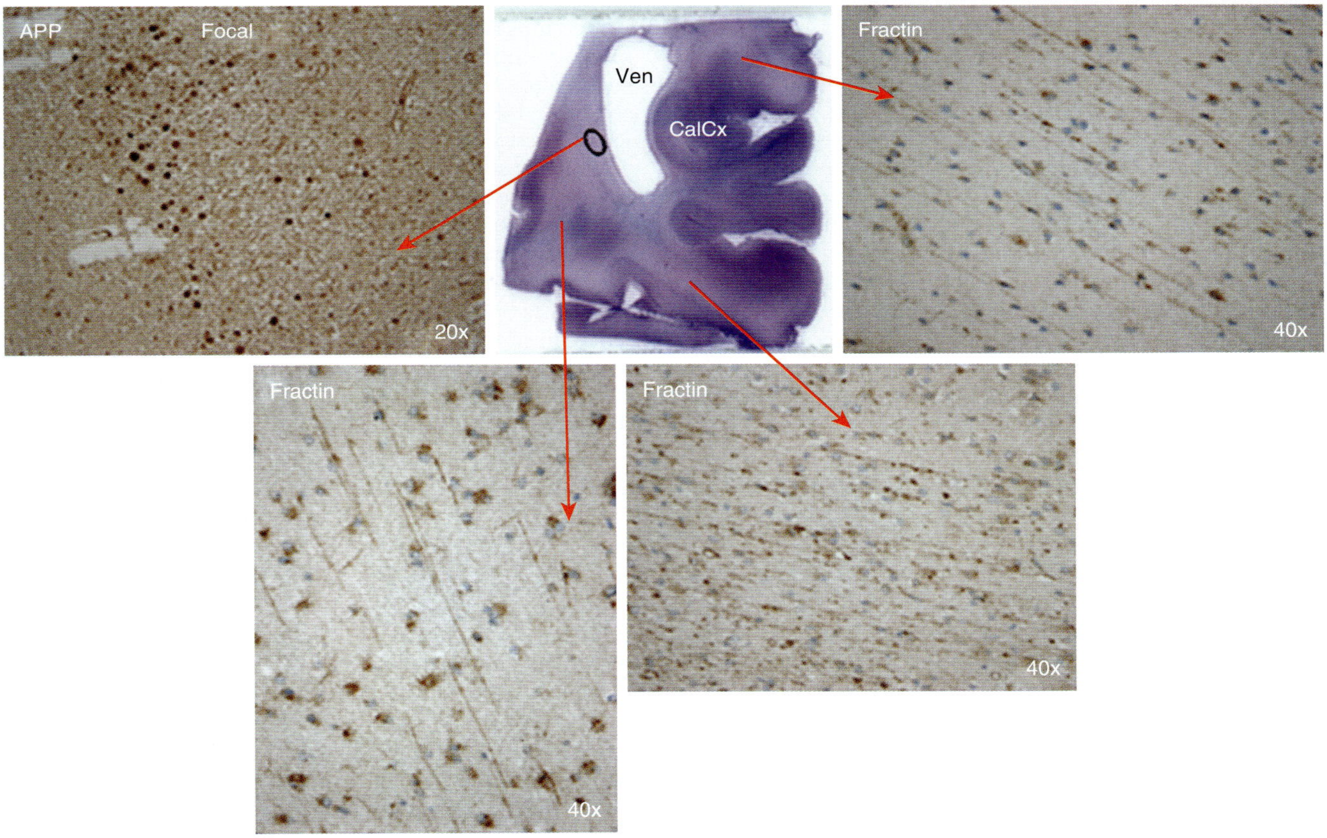

Figure 14.10 Diffuse and focal (periventricular) axonal injury in periventricular leukomalacia. The diffuse injury is visualized by the apoptotic marker fractin. Note the linear areas of fractin-positivity, reflecting axonal degeneration. *APP*, Amyloid precursor protein; *CalCx*, Calcarine cortex; *Ven*, ventricle. (From Haynes RL, et al. Diffuse axonal injury in periventricular leukomalacia as determined by apoptotic marker fractin. *Pediatr Res.* 2008;63: 656–661.)

dendrites covered with spines (acquired neuronal hypertrophy) is frequent. To what extent these remarkable changes occur in premature infants with major parenchymal lesions remains to be established.

Cerebellum

The cerebellum in the preterm infant demonstrates bilateral, symmetrical deficits in hemispheric volume without overt parenchymal hemorrhage or infarction.[35,36] This reduced volume is commonly associated with intraventricular or subarachnoid hemorrhage.[37] Moreover, impaired cerebellar development is associated with supratentorial lesions, especially PVL and periventricular hemorrhagic venous infarction (see Chapter 24), suggesting the possibility of transsynaptic mechanisms in its pathogenesis via corticopontocerebellar pathways.[35,36] Yet neuroimaging studies also indicate a gradual deficit in cerebellar volume in preterm infants, associated in the majority of cases with infratentorial hemosiderin deposition.[37] Thus it has been postulated that blood products (hemosiderin/nonheme iron) in the cerebrospinal fluid lead to cerebellar underdevelopment owing to their toxic effects upon the proliferating granule precursor cells of the external granular layer, which are located directly at the interface with the subarachnoid space and which later migrate inward to form the internal granular layer.[37] Nevertheless, this idea, based upon neuroimaging studies, has not been verified anatomically by quantitative analysis of the cell number of the internal granular layer.

Direct injury to other cerebellar neurons also seems likely. Indeed, semiquantitative analysis of the cerebellum has revealed moderate loss of cortical neurons in 24% of cases with PVL (see Fig. 14.7) and moderate loss of dentate neurons in 29% of cases,[5] in association with reactive astrocytes. Thus the neuropathological features (notably gliosis) suggest an acquired insult rather than underdevelopment. Yet the distinction between atrophy and underdevelopment is difficult in the developing cerebellum, in which migration from the external to the internal granular layer is protracted over the last half of gestation into infancy. That is, a particular insult may lead simultaneously to *atrophy* with dropout of cells already at their proper address (inciting gliosis) *and underdevelopment* due to disruption of proliferating or migrating cells, or both, and with both mechanisms resulting in an incomplete complement of neurons. Indeed, the pathology of the cerebellum epitomizes the "complex amalgam" of the encephalopathy of prematurity, where developmental and destructive processes intersect.[1] Similarly, regarding the cerebellar relay nuclei, it is uncertain if the neuronal loss in the basis pontis and inferior olive, the major cerebellar relay nuclei, which is seen

in 21% of PVL cases,[5] is primary or secondary to transsynaptic degeneration.

ENCEPHALOPATHY OF PREMATURITY—NEUROPATHOLOGY IN LIVING INFANTS

The neuropathology of the encephalopathy of prematurity, as just described from neuropathological studies, involves predominantly cerebral white matter and multiple neuronal/axonal structures. The neuronal/axonal disease in the encephalopathy is apparent in cerebral cortex, cerebral white matter, thalamus, basal ganglia, brain stem, and cerebellum. Detection of the white and gray matter lesions in living infants by neuroimaging is discussed and illustrated in detail in Chapters 7 and 16. A very brief consideration is presented here.

Cerebral White Matter Injury

Cerebral white matter injury represents a spectrum of disease by neuropathological study, with "focal necrotic/cystic" PVL the most striking and diffuse "nonnecrotic/noncystic disease" the least striking. The diffuse component of PVL may underlie the finding of diffuse excessive high signal intensity (DEHSI) detectable by MRI. The principal MRI features of PVL, their relative frequency in living premature infants and the postulated neuropathological correlates are shown in Table 14.4. (The MRI features are discussed in detail in Chapter 16.) In *focal necrotic/cystic disease* the focal necrotic lesions are large and evolve to cysts readily identified by cranial ultrasonography (Fig. 14.11). Such lesions are now apparent in less than 5% of very preterm infants in modern neonatal intensive care units. MRI, unlike cranial ultrasonography, also readily detects such cystic lesions (see Table 14.4). However, MRI also demonstrates small focal necrotic lesions that do not evolve to cysts (likely the small gliotic scars seen by neuropathology) (see Table 14.4 and Fig. 14.12). These focal punctate lesions, which can be termed *focal necrotic/noncystic*, are observed in approximately 15% to 20% of very preterm infants (see Chapter 16). *Nonnecrotic/noncystic* cerebral white matter injury, a more diffuse abnormality, in which cysts or focal necrotic lesions are either not present or are minute in size and below the level of resolution of conventional neuroimaging, accounts for the majority of the white matter disease in modern neonatal intensive care units (see Table 14.4). MRI is the most effective imaging modality for detection of this milder form of cerebral white matter disease and shows DEHSI in cerebral white matter, possibly reflecting diffuse gliosis (see Figs. 14.11 and 14.12).[38] The subsequent disturbance of white matter *development* associated with cerebral white matter disease becomes apparent by term-equivalent age and beyond (e.g.,

TABLE 14.4 Major Neuropathological Varieties of Cerebral White Matter Injury/Periventricular Leukomalacia Spectrum in Premature Infants and Postulated Magnetic Resonance Imaging Features

| NEUROPATHOLOGY | | MRI FINDINGS | | |
FOCAL	DIFFUSE	FOCAL	DIFFUSE	RELATIVE FREQUENCY (MRI)
Necrosis/cysts	Gliosis	"Cysts"	DEHSI	≤5%
Necrosis/gliotic scars	Gliosis	PWMLs	DEHSI	15%–20%
Necrosis microscopic or absent	Gliosis	Absent	DEHSI	≥50% (?)

DEHSI, Diffuse excessive high signal intensity; *MRI*, magnetic resonance imaging; *PVL*, periventricular leukomalacia; *PWMLs*, punctate white matter lesions.

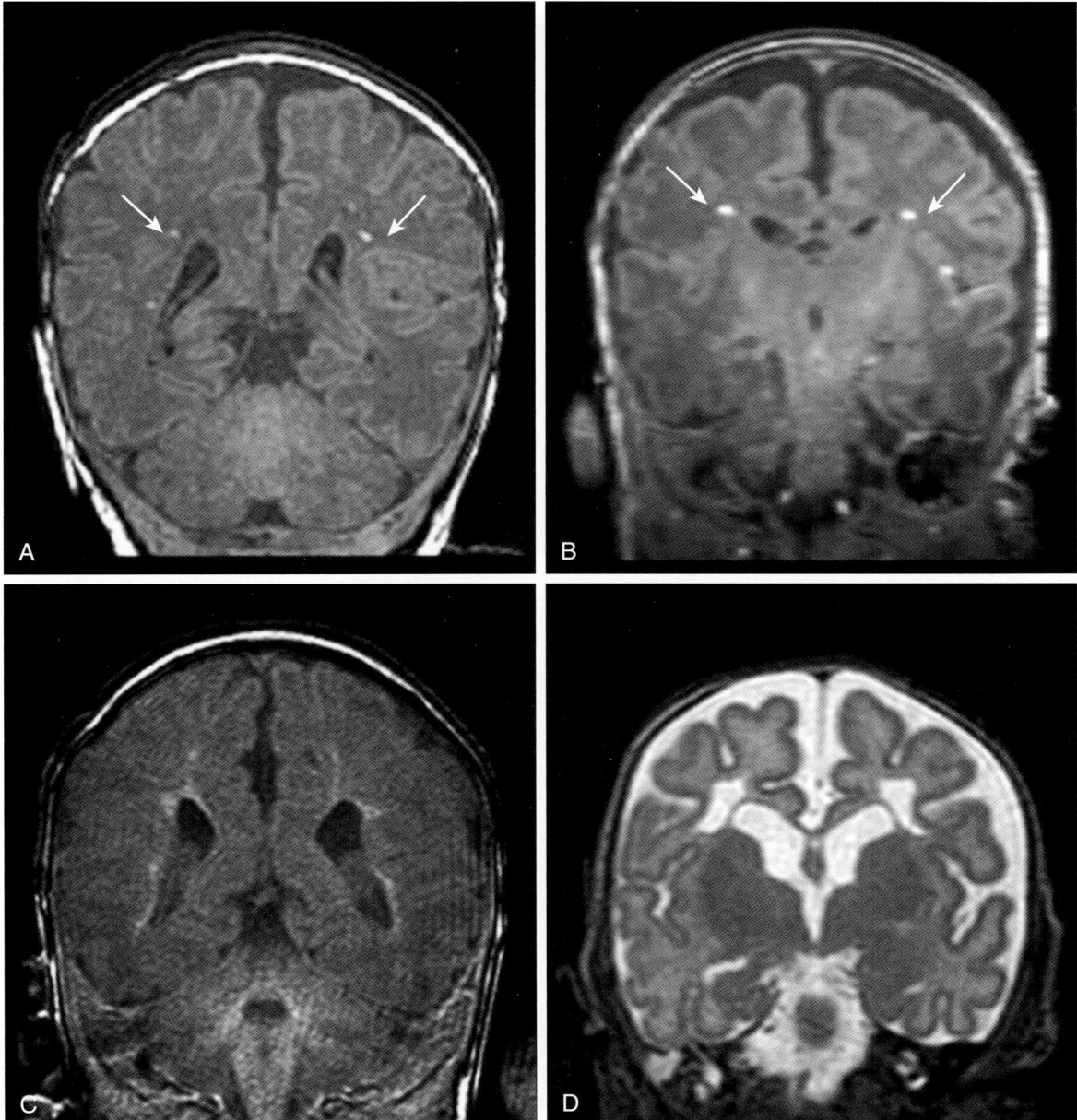

Figure 14.11 Magnetic resonance imaging of "focal necrotic/noncystic" and "focal necrotic/cystic" cerebral white matter injury in premature infants studied at term-equivalent age. Note, in A to C, the increase in size of punctate periventricular white matter lesions, presumed to be focal necrotic lesions. In D, overt cystic lesions are apparent. (From Kidokoro H, Anderson PJ, Doyle LW, et al. Brain injury and altered brain growth in preterm infants: predictors and prognosis. *Pediatrics*. 2014;134:e444–e453, with permission.)

as ventricular dilation by cranial ultrasonography). MRI-based techniques best identify the subsequent impairment of cerebral myelination, principally a postterm event (see Chapter 8).

Neuronal-Axonal Abnormalities

Many of the disturbances in cerebral white matter and in the various neuronal/axonal structures described earlier can be detected in living infants by advanced MRI methods (Table 14.5).[39-56] Because these findings reflect principally impairment of *organizational developmental* events, they are discussed and illustrated in Chapter 7 (see also Chapter 16).

Potential Sequences of Events in the Encephalopathy of Prematurity

The *potential sequences of events leading to the major brain sequelae identified in very preterm infants by MRI are shown in* Fig. 14.13. As discussed previously,[1] these mechanisms include a complex amalgam of destructive and developmental disturbances. In cerebral white matter injury the *primary* event is most likely a destructive process (*injury*) and the subsequent trophic/maturational events (i.e., developmental disturbances) are *secondary* (see Fig. 14.13). Of the six potential scenarios

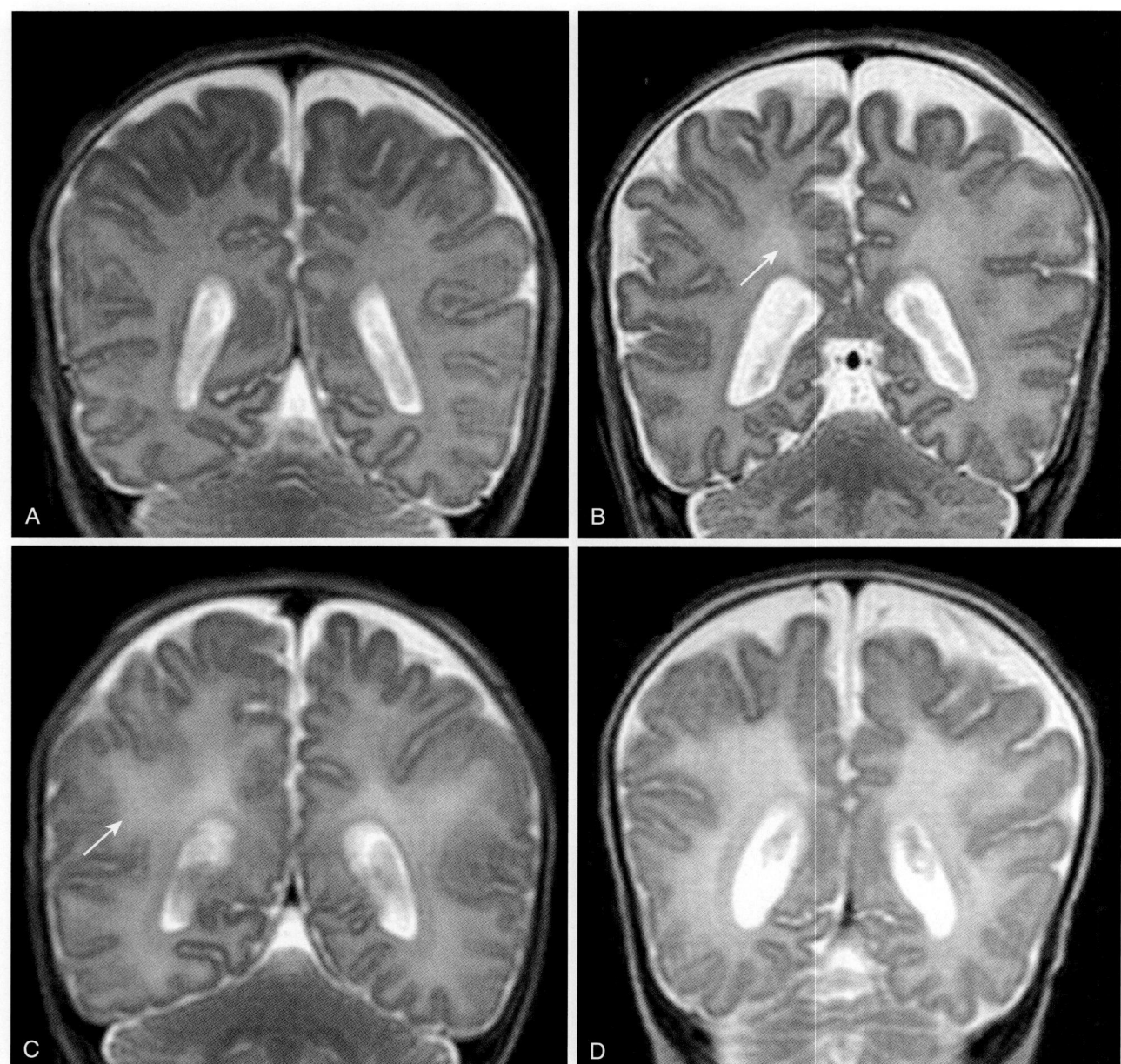

Figure 14.12 Magnetic resonance imaging (MRI) scans (T-2 weighted) of "nonnecrotic/noncystic" cerebral white matter injury in preterm infants. (A) A normal scan for comparison. (B–D) Increasing degrees of abnormally increased signal in periventricular regions only (B) or more extensively in cerebral white matter (C and D) (diffuse excessive high signal intensity, or DEHSI). (From Kidokoro, et al. High signal intensity on T2-weighted MR imaging at term-equivalent age in preterm infants does not predict 2-year neurodevelopmental outcomes. *AJNR Am J Neuroradiol.* 2011;32:2005–2010, with permission.)

concerning the primary and secondary events, the first is the best supported by available data. However, importantly, rigorous studies of the other scenarios in human infants are sparse, and it is quite possible that all scenarios are operative to varying degrees. The degree to which one or the other predominates may relate to a variety of associated factors (see later).

Preoligodendrocyte Injury, Primary

Pre-OL injury leading to impaired pre-OL maturation, a central feature of cerebral white matter disease, would lead to an impairment of myelination, the hallmark of PVL (see Fig. 14.13A). In addition, however, pre-OL injury could also lead to a failure of axonal development and ultimately axonal degeneration. The important trophic role of OLs for axonal development, survival, and function has been established in experimental models.[57-68] As noted earlier and in Chapter 7, accompanying the ensheathment of axons by pre-OLs, axonal growth in the cerebral white matter is markedly exuberant during the premature period; thus a particular need for trophic support is apparent. Diffusion-based MRI studies of cerebral white matter in premature infants show abnormalities consistent with axonal deficiency, which could reflect impaired axonal development, axonal degeneration, or both.[39,48,49,69-75] The consequences of the axonal deficiency would be diminished volumes of cerebral cortex and thalamus/basal ganglia, secondary to retrograde and anterograde (transsynaptic) effects

(i.e., projection fibers to and from cortex, thalamus, and basal ganglia, and commissural and association fibers to and from cortex) (see Fig. 14.13A).[1]

Axonal Injury, Primary

Axonal injury could be a primary event with PVL (see Fig. 14.13B). As noted earlier axonal disruption occurs in the areas of focal necrosis. Perhaps more importantly, in the wider spread, diffuse component of PVL axonal degeneration, detected by the apoptotic marker fractin, has been discovered.[30] This observation is consistent with the finding of axonal injury in experimental models of hypoxic-ischemic injury analogous to PVL.[76-80] The active axonal development in cerebral white matter in premature infants (see earlier and Chapter 7) could make these fibers especially vulnerable. Although it is unclear whether the axonal degeneration in diffuse PVL is a primary injury or secondary effect, if the former did occur, the expected secondary developmental effects would be both the hypomyelination (due to failure of axonal ensheathment by pre-OLs and thereby loss of trophic axonal/oligodendroglial interactions) and the decreased cortical and thalamic/basal ganglia volumes (via anterograde and retrograde effects) observed in surviving premature infants (see Fig. 14.13B).

Thalamic Injury, Primary

The possibility of *thalamic injury* as a primary event is suggested by experimental observations in a developing animal model of hypoxic-ischemic injury[81] and, as noted earlier, neuropathological

---

TABLE 14.5   Major Advanced MRI Findings in Premature Infants With Cerebral White Matter Injury[a]

MRI MEASURE	MAJOR FINDINGS
Volumetric MRI	Decreased regional volumes of cerebral cortex, cerebral white matter, basal ganglia, and thalamus
DTI	Decreased fractional anisotropy in cerebral white matter, relatively increased radial diffusivity, variably altered axial diffusivity
Surface-based measures	Decreased cerebral cortical surface area and cortical folding/gyrification
Functional MRI	Impaired development of measures of connectivity, including especially thalamocortical connectivity

[a]See text for references and Chapter 7.
DTI, Diffusion tensor imaging; *MRI,* magnetic resonance imaging.

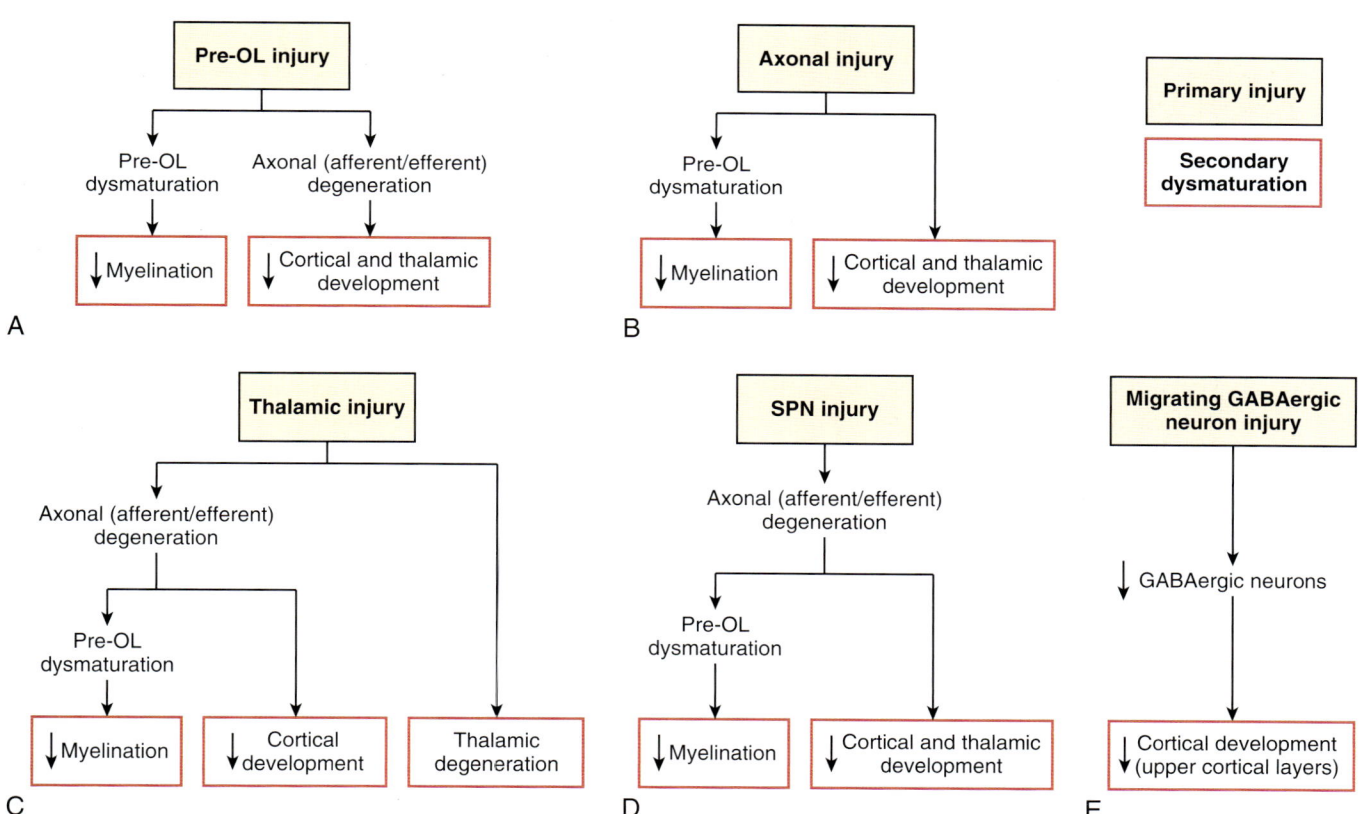

Figure 14.13 Potential sequences of events in the encephalopathy of prematurity (see text). Each sequence illustrates the progression from primary injury *(shown in yellow)* to secondary dysmaturational events, resulting in the major findings observed by magnetic resonance imaging *(red-outlined boxes).*

study of human infants with PVL shows thalamic neuronal/axonal abnormalities in approximately 60%.[5,14] However, the principal findings (i.e., neuronal loss, gliosis, axonal degeneration) do not allow distinction of primary injury from secondary trophic/developmental effects. If primary thalamic neuronal injury does occur, expected secondary effects would involve white matter axons and ensheathing pre-OLs, with subsequent hypomyelination as well as impaired development of both cerebral cortex and thalamus, as noted by advanced MRI studies (see Fig. 14.13C).[1]

Subplate Neuronal Injury, Primary

Injury to subplate neurons could have major secondary trophic/maturational disturbances affecting both cerebral cortex and thalamus in view of the key role of this transient neuronal population in the development of thalamocortical and corticocortical circuits (see earlier and Chapter 7). Considerable experimental data support this contention.[1,82-91] A brief earlier report showed increased apoptosis in the subplate of infants with PVL.[21] A more detailed recent report has shown a prominent decrease in subcortical white matter neurons, presumably subplate neurons, in infants with PVL.[22] If these observations reflect a primary neuronal injury, secondary anterograde effects would involve cerebral cortical targets and retrograde effects would impact afferent white matter axons and their originating neurons in thalamus and distant cortical regions (see Fig. 14.13D). Axonal degeneration would lead to subsequent hypomyelination, as discussed earlier, for pre-OL and axonal injury. Notably, selective subplate neuronal death was identified in a neonatal rat model of hypoxic-ischemic injury akin to PVL.[92]

Late Migrating GABAergic Neuronal Injury, Primary

Because the diffuse component of PVL includes the migrating path of the *late generated GABAergic neurons* from the SVZ and GE, the possibility of direct injury to these critical cells is real (see earlier). An earlier report showed a deficit in GABAergic neurons in central white matter in infants with PVL.[21] As noted earlier, a larger recent study also showed a pronounced deficit in central white matter neurons in such infants.[22] Whether these findings reflect direct injury or decreased generation from an impaired SVZ is unclear. An earlier report suggests that precursor cells in the dorsal telencephalic SVZ, the source of 65% of the GABAergic neurons destined for human cortex, are vulnerable to hypoxia-ischemia.[93] On balance, it appears that there is a deficit in late-migrating GABAergic neurons in human PVL, but the mechanism is unclear. Because these GABAergic neurons contribute importantly to the thickness of upper cortical layers, a blunting or diminution of this migration could have important structural and functional consequences.[1] Moreover, such a defect could explain, at least in part, the disturbances in cerebral cortical volumes, thickness, and surface area defined by advanced MRI methods (see Fig. 14.13E and Chapters 7 and 16).

Cerebral Cortical Neuronal Injury, Primary

A sixth scenario centered on the cerebral cortical neuron is suggested by recent experiments in an excellent fetal sheep model of PVL.[94] Thus, induction of cerebral ischemia in fetal sheep at the equivalent of 26 to 28 weeks of human gestation, sufficient to produce diffuse white matter changes comparable to human PVL, led to impaired cortical neuronal development detectable 4 weeks later. The measures of cortical dendritic development consistent with deficits in dendritic arbor formation included quantitative analysis of dendritic arbors in Golgi-Cox preparations and diffusion tensor imaging (DTI) measures of fractional anisotropy (FA) of cerebral cortex.[94] The normal decline in FA in cortex with development, caused by elaboration of neuronal dendritic arbors (see Chapter 7), failed to occur in the animals with white matter injury, and direct analysis of such arbors by the Golgi studies confirmed the defect. The impaired dendritic development was associated with a blunting of the normal increase in cerebral cortical volume during this interval. There was no loss of cortical neurons per se. The data suggest that the ischemic insult irreversibly altered the *development program* for dendritic development, *without causing a direct loss of the neurons.* Thalamic volumes and subsequent myelination were not studied, although it could be postulated that afferent and efferent axonal degeneration could occur, with subsequent maturational/trophic effects on myelination and thalamus, as described in the other five scenarios. *No comparable neuropathological studies of dendritic development in cortex of premature human infants are available but are clearly needed.* A recent study of very preterm infants by DTI also showed a failure in the decline of FA in cerebral cortex[95] and thus may represent the human equivalent of the fetal sheep study. In the human study, a relation to cerebral white matter injury could not be shown, although overt white matter injury was uncommon in the cohort, perhaps reflecting the fact that diffuse, noncystic white matter disease is likely below the resolution of conventional MRI.

Conclusion

To conclude, it is unclear which of the six potential scenarios is most important in the encephalopathy of prematurity. It seems likely that more than one and perhaps all the scenarios shown in Fig. 14.13 operate to a varying extent. Determinants of the relative importance of each scenario could relate to such factors as the gestational age of the infant, the timing and nature of the insult or insults, such critical associated factors as disturbed nutritional state, exposure to glucocorticoids or other drugs, and many parameters yet to be defined. The most important lesson is that the encephalopathy of prematurity is a *complex amalgam of destructive and developmental disturbances;* its full understanding will require deeper insight into the extraordinary spectrum of developmental events and neuropathological consequences of the impairment thereof occurring in the gestational period and beyond.

REFERENCES

1. Volpe JJ. Brain injury in premature infants: a complex amalgam of destructive and developmental disturbances. *Lancet Neurol.* 2009;8:110-124.
2. Folkerth RD, Kinney HC. Perinatal neuropathology. In: Louis DN, Love S, Ellison DW, eds. *Greenfield's Neuropathology.* Vol. 1. 8th ed. London: Arnold; 2009.
3. Banker BQ, Larroche JC. Periventricular leukomalacia of infancy. A form of neonatal anoxic encephalopathy. *Arch Neurol.* 1962;7:386-410.
4. Kinney HC, Volpe JJ. Perinatal panencephalopathy in premature infants: is it due to hypoxia-ischemia? In: Haddah GG, Yu SP, eds. *Brain Hypoxia and Ischemia With Special Emphasis on Development.* New York: Humana Press; 2009:153-186.

5. Pierson CR, Folkerth RD, Billards SS, et al. Gray matter injury associated with periventricular leukomalacia in the premature infant. *Acta Neuropathol.* 2007;114:619-631.

6. Folkerth RD, Keefe RJ, Haynes RL, et al. Interferon-gamma expression in periventricular leukomalacia in the human brain. *Brain Pathol.* 2004;14:265-274.

7. DeSilva TM, Kinney HC, Borenstein NS, et al. The glutamate transporter is transiently expressed in developing human cerebral white matter. *J Comp Neurol.* 2007;501:879-890.

8. Haynes RL, Folkerth RD, Keefe R, et al. Nitrosative and oxidative injury to premyelinating oligodendrocytes is accompanied by microglial activation in periventricular leukomalacia in the human premature infant. *J Neuropathol Exp Neurol.* 2003;62:441-450.

9. Haynes RL, Folkerth RD, Trachtenberg FL, et al. Nitrosative stress and inducible nitric oxide synthase expression in periventricular leukomalacia. *Acta Neuropathol.* 2009;118:391-399.

10. Billiards SS, Haynes RL, Folkerth RD, et al. Myelin abnormalities without oligodendrocyte loss in periventricular leukomalacia. *Brain Pathol.* 2008;18:153-163.

11. Buser JR, Maire J, Riddle A, et al. Arrested preoligodendrocyte maturation contributes to myelination failure in premature infants. *Ann Neurol.* 2012;71:93-109.

12. Back SA, Luo NL, Mallinson RA, et al. Selective vulnerability of preterm white matter to oxidative damage defined by F(2)-isoprostanes. *Ann Neurol.* 2005;58:108-120.

13. Golden JA, Gilles FH, Rudewlli R, et al. Frequency of neuropathological abnormalities in very low birth weight infants. *J Neuropathol Exp Neurol.* 1997;56:472-478.

14. Ligam P, Haynes RL, Folkerth RD, et al. Thalamic damage in periventricular leukomalacia: novel pathologic observations relevant to cognitive deficits in survivors of prematurity. *Pediatr Res.* 2009;65:524-529.

15. Nagasunder AC, Kinney HC, Bluml S, et al. Abnormal microstructure of the atrophic thalamus in preterm survivors with periventricular leukomalacia. *AJNR Am J Neuroradiol.* 2011;32:185-191.

16. Andiman SE, Haynes RL, Trachtenberg FL, et al. The cerebral cortex overlying periventricular leukomalacia: analysis of pyramidal neurons. *Brain Pathol.* 2010;20:803-814.

17. Talos DM, Fishman RE, Park H, et al. Developmental regulation of alpha-amino-3-hydroxy-5-methyl-4-isoxazole-propionic acid receptor subunit expression in forebrain and relationship to regional susceptibility to hypoxic/ischemic injury. I. Rodent cerebral white matter and cortex. *J Comp Neurol.* 2006;497:42-60.

18. Talos DM, Follett PL, Folkerth RD, et al. Developmental regulation of alpha-amino-3-hydroxy-5-methyl-4-isoxazole-propionic acid receptor subunit expression in forebrain and relationship to regional susceptibility to hypoxic/ischemic injury. II. Human cerebral white matter and cortex. *J Comp Neurol.* 2006;497:61-77.

19. Xu G, Broadbelt KG, Haynes RL, et al. Late development of the GABAergic system in the human cerebral cortex and white matter. *J Neuropathol Exp Neurol.* 2011;70:841-858.

20. Rubenstein JL. Annual research review: development of the cerebral cortex: implications for neurodevelopmental disorders. *J Child Psychol Psychiatry.* 2011;52:339-355.

21. Robinson S, Li Q, Dechant A, et al. Neonatal loss of gamma-aminobutyric acid pathway expression after human perinatal brain injury. *J Neurosurg.* 2006;104:396-408.

22. Kinney HC, Haynes RL, Xu G, et al. Neuron deficit in the white matter and subplate in periventricular leukomalacia. *Ann Neurol.* 2012;71:397-406.

23. Gray GE, Sanes JR. Lineage of radial glia in the chicken optic tectum. *Development.* 1992;114:271-283.

24. Sidman RL, Rakic P. Development of the human nervous system. In: Adams RD, Haymaker W, eds. *Cytology and Cellular Neuropathology.* 2nd ed. Springfield, IL: Charles C Thomas; 1973.

25. Letinic K, Rakic P. Telencephalic origin of human thalamic GABAergic neurons. *Nat Neurosci.* 2001;4:931-936.

26. deAzevedo LC, Fallet C, Moura-Neto V, et al. Cortical radial glial cells in human fetuses: depth-correlated transformation into astrocytes. *J Neurobiol.* 2003;55:288-298.

27. Kadhim HJ, Gadisseux JF, Evrard P. Topographical and cytological evolution of the glial phase during prenatal development of the human brain: histochemical and electron microscopic study. *J Neuropathol Exp Neurol.* 1988;47:166-188.

28. Choi BH, Lapham LW. Radial glia in the human fetal cerebrum: a combined Golgi, immunofluorescent and electron microscopic study. *Brain Res.* 1978;148:295-311.

29. Marin-Padilla M. *The Human Brain: Prenatal Development and Structure.* Berlin: Springer-Verlag; 2011.

30. Haynes RL, Billiards SS, Borenstein NS, et al. Diffuse axonal injury in periventricular leukomalacia as determined by apoptotic marker fractin. *Pediatr Res.* 2008;63:656-661.

31. Deguchi K, Oguchi K, Matsuura N, et al. Periventricular leukomalacia: relation to gestational age and axonal injury. *Pediatr Neurol.* 1999;20:370-374.

32. Marin-Padilla M. Developmental neuropathology and impact of perinatal brain damage. 2. White matter lesions of the neocortex. *J Neuropathol Exp Neurol.* 1997;56:219-235.

33. Okoshi Y, Mizuguchi M, Itoh M, et al. Altered nestin expression in the cerebrum with periventricular leukomalacia. *Pediatr Neurol.* 2007;36:170-174.

34. Haynes RL, Xu G, Folkerth RD, et al. Potential neuronal repair in cerebral white matter injury in the human neonate. *Pediatr Res.* 2011;69:62-67.

35. Limperopoulos C, Benson CB, Bassan H, et al. Cerebellar hemorrhage in the preterm infant: ultrasonographic findings and risk factors. *Pediatrics.* 2005;116:717-724.

36. Limperopoulos C, Soul JS, Haidar H, et al. Impaired trophic interactions between the cerebellum and the cerebrum among preterm infants. *Pediatrics.* 2005;116:844-850.

37. Volpe JJ. Cerebellum of the premature infant—rapidly developing, vulnerable, clinically important. *J Child Neurol.* 2009;24:1085-1104.

38. Kidokoro H, Anderson PJ, Doyle LW, et al. Brain injury and altered brain growth in preterm infants: predictors and prognosis. *Pediatrics.* 2014;134:e444-e453.

39. Huppi PS, Maier SE, Peled S, et al. Microstructural development of human newborn cerebral white matter assessed in vivo by diffusion tensor magnetic resonance imaging. *Pediatr Res.* 1998;44:584-590.

40. Panigrahy A, Barnes PD, Robertson RL, et al. Volumetric brain differences in children with periventricular T2-signal hyperintensities: a grouping by gestational age at birth. *AJR Am J Roentgenol.* 2001;177:695-702.

41. Inder TE, Warfield SK, Wang H, et al. Abnormal cerebral structure is present at term in premature infants. *Pediatrics.* 2005;115:286-294.

42. Thompson DK, Warfield SK, Carlin JB, et al. Perinatal risk factors altering regional brain structure in the preterm infant. *Brain.* 2007;130:667-677.

43. Boardman JP, Craven C, Valappil S, et al. A common neonatal image phenotype predicts adverse neurodevelopmental outcome in children born preterm. *Neuroimage.* 2010;52:409-414.

44. Zubiaurre-Elorza L, Soria-Pastor S, Junque C, et al. Gray matter volume decrements in preterm children with periventricular leukomalacia. *Pediatr Res.* 2011;69:554-560.

45. Kwon SH, Vasung L, Ment LR, et al. The role of neuroimaging in predicting neurodevelopmental outcomes of preterm neonates. *Clin Perinatol.* 2014;41:257-283.

46. Kersbergen KJ, de Vries LS, Groenendaal F, et al. Corticospinal tract injury precedes thalamic volume reduction in preterm infants with cystic periventricular leukomalacia. *J Pediatr.* 2015;167:260-268, e3.

47. Counsell S, Shen Y, Boardman JP, et al. Axial and radial diffusivity in preterm infants who have diffuse white matter changes on MRI at term equivalent age. *Pediatrics.* 2006;117:376-386.

48. Skranes J, Vangberg TR, Kulseng S, et al. Clinical findings and white matter abnormalities seen on diffusion tensor imaging in adolescents with very low birth weight. *Brain.* 2007;130(Pt 3):654-666.

49. Cheong JL, Thompson DK, Wang HX, et al. Abnormal white matter signal on MR imaging is related to abnormal tissue microstructure. *AJNR Am J Neuroradiol.* 2009;30:623-628.

50. Bassi L, Chew A, Merchant N, et al. Diffusion tensor imaging in preterm infants with punctate white matter lesions. *Pediatr Res.* 2011;69:561-566.

51. van Pul C, van Kooij BJ, de Vries LS, et al. Quantitative fiber tracking in the corpus callosum and internal capsule reveals microstructural abnormalities in preterm infants at term-equivalent age. *AJNR Am J Neuroradiol.* 2012;33:678-684.

52. Pandit AS, Ball G, Edwards AD, et al. Diffusion magnetic resonance imaging in preterm brain injury. *Neuroradiology.* 2013;55(suppl 2):65-95.

53. Estep ME, Smyser CD, Anderson PJ, et al. Diffusion tractography and neuromotor outcome in very preterm children with white matter abnormalities. *Pediatr Res.* 2014;76:86-92.

54. Shimony JS, Smyser CD, Wideman G, et al. Comparison of cortical folding measures for evaluation of developing human brain. *Neuroimage.* 2016;125:780-790.

55. Smyser CD, Neil JJ. Use of resting-state functional MRI to study brain development and injury in neonates. *Semin Perinatol.* 2015;39:130-140.

56. Smyser CD, Snyder AZ, Shimony JS, et al. Effects of white matter injury on resting state fMRI measures in prematurely born infants. *PLoS ONE.* 2013;8:e68098.

57. Bjartmar C, Yin X, Trapp BD. Axonal pathology in myelin disorders. *J Neurocytol.* 1999;28:383-395.

58. Biffiger K, Bartsch S, Montag D, et al. Severe hypomyelination of the murine CNS in the absence of myelin-associated glycoprotein and fyn tyrosine kinase. *J Neurosci.* 2000;20:7430-7437.

59. Gotow T, Leterrier JF, Ohsawa Y, et al. Abnormal expression of neurofilament proteins in dysmyelinating axons located in the central nervous system of jimpy mutant mice. *Eur J Neurosci.* 1999;11:3893-3903.

60. Lappe-Siefke C, Goebbels S, Gravel M, et al. Disruption of *Cnp1* uncouples oligodendroglial functions in axonal support and myelination. *Nat Genet.* 2003;33:366-374.

61. Rasband MN, Tayler R, Kaga Y, et al. CNP is required for maintenance of axon-glia interactions at nodes of Ranvier in the CNS. *Glia.* 2005;50:86-90.

62. Dutta R, Trapp BD. Pathogenesis of axonal and neuronal damage in multiple sclerosis. *Neurology.* 2007;68:S22-S31.

63. Roy K, Murtie JC, El-Khodor BF, et al. Loss of erbB signaling in oligodendrocytes alters myelin and dopaminergic function, a potential mechanism for neuropsychiatric disorders. *Proc Natl Acad Sci U S A.* 2007;104:8131-8136.

64. Nakazawa T, Nakazawa C, Matsubara A, et al. Tumor necrosis factor-alpha mediates oligodendrocyte death and delayed retinal ganglion cell loss in a mouse model of glaucoma. *J Neurosci.* 2006;26:12633-12641.

65. Drobyshevsky A, Song SK, Gamkrelidze G, et al. Developmental changes in diffusion anisotropy coincide with immature oligodendrocyte progression and maturation of compound action potential. *J Neurosci.* 2005;25:5988-5997.

66. Wilkins A, Majed H, Layfield R, et al. Oligodendrocytes promote neuronal survival and axonal length by distinct intracellular mechanisms: a novel role for oligodendrocyte-derived glial cell line-derived neurotrophic factor. *J Neurosci.* 2003;23:4967-4974.

67. Dai X, Lercher LD, Clinton PM, et al. The trophic role of oligodendrocytes in the basal forebrain. *J Neurosci.* 2003;23:5846-5853.

68. Du YZ, Dreyfus CF. Oligodendrocytes as providers of growth factors. *J Neurosci.* 2002;68:647-654.

69. Counsell SJ, Allsop JM, Harrison MC, et al. Diffusion weighted imaging of the brain in preterm infants with focal and diffuse white matter abnormality. *Pediatrics.* 2003;112:1-7.

70. Miller SP, Vigneron DB, Henry RG, et al. Serial quantitative diffusion tensor MRI of the premature brain: development in newborns with and without injury. *J Magn Reson Imaging.* 2002;16:621-632.

71. Huppi PS, Murphy B, Maier SE, et al. Microstructural brain development after perinatal cerebral white matter injury assessed by diffusion tensor magnetic resonance imaging. *Pediatrics.* 2001;107:455-460.

72. Martinussen M, Fischl B, Larsson HB, et al. Cerebral cortex thickness in 15-year-old adolescents with low birth weight measured by an automated MRI-based method. *Brain.* 2005;128:2588-2596.

73. Vangberg TR, Skranes J, Dale AM, et al. Changes in white matter diffusion anisotropy in adolescents born prematurely. *Neuroimage.* 2006;32:1538-1548.

74. Anjari M, Srinivasan L, Allsop JM, et al. Diffusion tensor imaging with tract-based spatial statistics reveals local white matter abnormalities in preterm infants. *Neuroimage.* 2007;35:1021-1027.

75. Counsell SJ, Dyet LE, Larkman DJ, et al. Thalamo-cortical connectivity in children born preterm mapped using probabilistic magnetic resonance tractography. *Neuroimage.* 2007;34:896-904.

76. Sizonenko SV, Sirimanne E, Mayall Y, et al. Selective cortical alteration after hypoxic-ischemic injury in the very immature rat brain. *Pediatr Res.* 2003;54:263-269.

77. McCarran WJ, Goldberg MP. White matter axon vulnerability to AMPA/kainate receptor-mediated ischemic injury is developmentally regulated. *J Neurosci.* 2007;27:4220-4229.

78. Tekkok SB, Goldberg MP. AMPA/kainate receptor activation mediates hypoxic oligodendrocyte death and axonal injury in cerebral white matter. *J Neurosci.* 2001;21:4237-4248.

79. Wakita H, Tomimoto H, Akiguchi I, et al. Axonal damage and demyelination in the white matter after chronic cerebral hypoperfusion in the rat. *Brain Res.* 2002;924:63-70.

80. Alix JJ, Zammit C, Riddle A, et al. Central axons preparing to myelinate are highly sensitivity to ischemic injury. *Ann Neurol.* 2012;72:936-951.

81. Northington FJ, Ferriero DM, Flock DL, et al. Delayed neurodegeneration in neonatal rat thalamus after hypoxia-ischemia is apoptosis. *J Neurosci.* 2001;21:1931-1938.

82. Volpe JJ. *Neurology of the Newborn.* 5th ed. Philadelphia: Elsevier; 2008.

83. Volpe JJ. Subplate neurons—missing link in brain injury of the premature infant? *Pediatrics.* 1996;97:112-113.

84. McConnell SK, Ghosh A, Shatz CJ. Subplate neurons pioneer the first axon pathway from the cerebral cortex. *Science.* 1989;245:978-982.

85. Ghosh A, Antonini A, McConnell SK, et al. Requirement for subplate neurons in the formation of thalamocortical connections. *Nature.* 1990;347:179-181.

86. Ghosh A, Shatz CJ. Involvement of subplate neurons in the formation of ocular dominance columns. *Science.* 1992;255:1441-1443.

87. Ghosh A, Shatz CJ. A role for subplate neurons in the patterning of connections from thalamus to neocortex. *Development.* 1993;117:1031-1047.

88. Kostovic I, Judas M. Correlation between the sequential ingrowth of afferents and transient patterns of cortical lamination in preterm infants. *Anat Rec.* 2002;267:1-6.

89. Kanold PO, Kara P, Reid RC, et al. Role of subplate neurons in functional maturation of visual cortical columns. *Science.* 2003;301:521-525.

90. Kanold PO. Transient microcircuits formed by subplate neurons and their role in functional development of thalamocortical connections. *Neuroreport.* 2004;15:2149-2153.

91. Bystron I, Molnar Z, Otellin V, et al. Tangential networks of precocious neurons and early axonal outgrowth in the embryonic human forebrain. *J Neurosci.* 2005;25:2781-2792.

92. McQuillen PS, Sheldon RA, Shatz CJ, et al. Selective vulnerability of subplate neurons after early neonatal hypoxia-ischemia. *J Neurosci.* 2003;23:3308-3315.

93. Romanko MJ, Rothstein RP, Levison SW. Neural stem cells in the subventricular zone are resilient to hypoxia/ischemia whereas progenitors are vulnerable. *J Cereb Blood Flow Metab.* 2004;24:814-825.

94. Dean JM, McClendon E, Hansen K, et al. Prenatal cerebral ischemia disrupts MRI-defined cortical microstructure through disturbances in neuronal arborization. *Sci Transl Med.* 2013;5:168ra167.

95. Vinall J, Grunau RE, Brant R, et al. Slower postnatal growth is associated with delayed cerebral cortical maturation in preterm newborns. *Sci Transl Med.* 2013;5:168ra168.

Encephalopathy of Prematurity: Pathophysiology

Stephen A. Back ◆ *Joseph J. Volpe*

OVERVIEW OF PATHOGENESIS

The preterm white matter is susceptible to a broad spectrum of injury severity that ranges from diffuse nondestructive lesions to the severe necrotic lesions of periventricular leukomalacia (PVL). The factors that contribute to the spectrum of severity remain incompletely defined, but a number of fundamental physiological factors related to cerebral blood flow (CBF), including cerebral oxygenation, hypercarbia, levels of glucose and its metabolites, as well as a variety of inflammatory factors, likely influence the severity of white matter injury (WMI). The propensity to injury is initiated by two major *upstream mechanisms*, primarily *ischemia* but also *infection/inflammation* (Box 15.1 and Fig. 15.1). These mechanisms may operate in concert to potentiate each other. The critical *downstream mechanisms* involve at least three successive distinct injury responses that disrupt preterm white matter maturation at a critical period in development (Fig. 15.2). The first coincides with early WMI and involves a confluence of maturation-dependent pathogenetic factors that selectively trigger the degeneration of late oligodendrocyte progenitors (preOLs) through hypoxia-ischemia and potentially other factors that include infection and inflammation. In response to preOL loss, early OL progenitors display remarkable plasticity, which is inherent to neuroglia. During this second subacute phase of WMI, early OL progenitors undergo a robust proliferative response that regenerates the preOLs required for OL differentiation and myelination. During the third and chronic phase of WMI, preOL differentiation is disrupted by the chronic injury environment, which coincides with disturbances in the normal progression of myelination.

Ischemia

Premature infants have a propensity for the development of global cerebral ischemia that particularly injures the white matter. Because of the limitations of current approaches to measure preterm human CBF, it has not been feasible to directly quantify human cerebral white matter flow to related disturbances in flow to WMI. Nevertheless, a role for ischemia is supported by a diverse array of clinical observations as well as experimental studies. Collectively, these findings support that moderately severe ischemia is necessary but not sufficient to generate WMI. The topography of WMI is related to a complex constellation of vascular anatomical, physiological, cellular maturational, and metabolic factors that define the timing of appearance and distribution of WMI.

Periventricular Vascular Anatomical and Physiological Factors

The development of the vasculature that supplies the preterm human cerebral white matter is significant for arterial end and border zones. Considerable study previously focused on the hypothesis that more severe *focal necrotic white matter lesions* coincide with regions of greater ischemia generated within these *arterial end zones*.[1-8] (The earlier concept that the deep periventricular region also contained arterial border zones involving so-called ventriculofugal arteries[1,3] is not supported by later studies as reviewed by Gilles and co-workers.[9,10]) The periventricular arterial end zones originate from vessels penetrating the cerebral wall from the pial surface. These long penetrating arteries are derived from the middle cerebral artery, and, to a lesser extent, the anterior or posterior cerebral artery, and they terminate in the deep periventricular white matter (Fig. 15.3). The end zones that result are essentially *distal fields in the periventricular white matter* that are hypothesized to be more susceptible to a fall in perfusion pressure and CBF.

The penetrating cerebral arteries can be further divided into the long penetrators that terminate deep in periventricular white matter and the short penetrators that extend only into subcortical white matter (see Fig. 15.3).[6] At 24 to 28 weeks of gestation, the long penetrators have relatively few side branches and infrequent intraparenchymal anastomoses with each other and with the short penetrators, which also are relatively sparse. Thus, end zones and border zones may exist at this time in the cerebral white matter relatively distant from the periventricular region. From 32 weeks to term, maturation of the short penetrators and the anastomoses between the long and short penetrators occurs and may promote CBF more similar to the term infant.

The susceptibility to hypoperfusion may also be influenced by the rate at which the vascular supply matures in the white matter. The last 16 weeks of human gestation is a period of active maturation of the periventricular vasculature.[4-6,11,12] Indeed, this development could be used as an index of cerebrovascular maturity.[4] Detailed analysis of the development of the vascular supply to the periventricular preterm white matter defined an avascular area at the common site of WMI. This avascular area may represent an area of vascular immaturity or an area of particular predilection to significant vascular necrosis that occurred in association with more severe WMI (Fig. 15.4).

Consistent with the immaturity of the vascular supply of the preterm brain are human and experimental studies that

BOX 15.1   Cerebral White Matter Injury: Pathogenesis[a]

Periventricular Vascular Anatomical and Physiological Factors
Potential arterial end zones and border zones
Very low physiological blood flow to cerebral white matter under basal
    conditions

**Cerebral Ischemia, Impaired Cerebrovascular Autoregulation,
and Pressure-Passive Cerebral Circulation**
Danger of systemic hypotension
Danger of marked hypocarbia

Infection and Inflammation
Propensity for maternal/intrauterine infection and for fetal systemic
    inflammatory response
Propensity for postnatal infection
Presence of Toll-like receptors on microglia capable of producing
    pre-OL death on activation by release of ROS, RNS, and cytokines
Maturation-dependent concentration of microglia in cerebral white
    matter during the peak period of vulnerability to PVL
TNF-α in cerebrospinal fluid and brain in PVL
Interferon-gamma toxicity potentiated by TNF-α and greater to
    preOLs than to mature cells

Potentiating Relationship of Infection/Inflammation and Ischemia
Infection/inflammation leading to impaired cerebral perfusion
Microglia as a convergence point for both infection/inflammation and
    ischemia

**Intrinsic Vulnerability of Cerebral White Matter of Premature
Newborn**
Vulnerability of preOLs to free radical attack
    Production of both ROS and RNS
    Deficient antioxidant defenses
    Acquisition of iron
Vulnerability of preOLs to excitotoxicity
    Exuberant expression of glutamate transporter
    Exuberant expression of AMPA receptors, which also are deficient
        in the GluR2 subunit and therefore calcium permeable
    Exuberant expression of NMDA receptors, which are calcium
        permeable
Presence of other potentially vulnerable, rapidly differentiating cellular
    elements
Axons
Maturation arrest of preOLs in chronic phase of white matter injury
    Pronounced early proliferative response of oligodendrocyte
        progenitors precedes an increase in preOLs
    Diffuse activation of microglia and astrocytes
    Disruption of extracellular matrix signaling in lesions enriched in
        reactive astrocytes
    Disturbances in normal progression of oligodendrocyte maturation
        and myelination

*AMPA, Alpha-amino-3-hydroxy-5-methyl-4-isoxazolepropionic acid; NMDA,
N-methyl-D-aspartate; pre-OLs, premyelinating oligodendrocytes; PVL,
periventricular leukomalacia; RNS, reactive nitrogen species; ROS, reactive
oxygen species; TNF, tumor necrosis factor.*
[a]Includes those factors shown in human premature brain (see Chapter 13 for
additional factors based on experimental studies).

have demonstrated *the significantly lower basal blood flow to preterm cerebral white matter.* Low basal white matter flow was suggested initially by xenon clearance studies that documented mean global CBF values in ventilated human premature infants of only ~10 to 12 mL/100 g/min.[13] Subsequent xenon studies confirmed these very low mean global values (see Chapter 13).[14-20] Importantly, studies of *regional* CBF by positron emission tomography confirmed the low global values and further documented that surviving preterm infants with normal or nearly normal neurological outcome had basal flow that ranged from only 1.6 to 3.0 mL/100 g per minute.[21] These very low values in white matter were approximately 25% of those in cortical gray matter, a regional difference confirmed in a study using single photon emission tomography.[21,22] These basal flow values of less than 5.0 mL/100 g per minute are markedly less than the threshold value for viability in adult human brain of 10 mL/100 g per minute (*normal* CBF in the adult is ≈50 mL/100 g per minute).[23] *The very low values of volemic flow in cerebral white matter in the human premature infant suggest a minimal margin of safety for blood flow to cerebral white matter in such infants and suggests that the susceptibility of the preterm infant to WMI is related to a heightened propensity for ischemia.*

Cerebral Ischemia, Impaired Cerebrovascular Autoregulation, and Pressure-Passive Cerebral Circulation

An apparent impairment of cerebrovascular regulation in sick premature infants may render cerebral white matter more vulnerable to injury from ischemia (see Box 15.1). *Clinically stable premature infants* seem less likely to exhibit this apparent lack of cerebrovascular autoregulation.[13,14,24-26] Early radioactive xenon clearance studies showed that certain premature infants, mechanically ventilated and often clinically unstable, appeared to exhibit pressure-passive cerebral circulation (Fig. 15.5).[16,26-28] This fundamental observation has been confirmed by less invasive methods multiple times.[29-38] Thus, in such sick premature infants with a pressure-passive cerebral circulation, it would be expected that when blood pressure falls, as occurs commonly in such infants, so would CBF, with consequent cerebral ischemia. With intact cerebrovascular autoregulation, CBF is not pressure passive but rather remains constant over a wide range of blood pressure because of arteriolar dilation with decreases in blood pressure and arteriolar constriction with increases in blood pressure (see the curve for the mature *child* in Fig. 15.6). *The propensity to a pressure-passive abnormality in premature infants* may relate in part to an absent muscularis around penetrating cerebral arteries and arterioles in the third trimester in the human brain.[9,10,39]

The proportion of infants with a pressure-passive cerebral circulation and the duration of the abnormality appear to be substantial (see Chapter 13). In a serial study of 32 mechanically ventilated premature infants from the first hours of life, near-infrared spectroscopy (NIRS) was used to demonstrate a pressure-passive cerebral circulation in 53% (see Chapter 13).[31] The nadirs of blood pressure often are not markedly low and thus could be readily overlooked with routine monitoring. Importantly, nearly all the cases of WMI (and severe intraventricular hemorrhage) were in the pressure-passive group.[31]

In a later, more detailed study of a larger number of infants (*N* = 90), pressure-passive periods were identified in 95% of the infants, and the overall mean proportion of the pressure-passive time was 20%.[33] Some infants had a pressure-passive circulation more than 50% of the time. The likelihood of a pressure-passive state increased with decreasing gestational age and periods of hypotension.

Although the numbers were small, these studies suggest that (1) infants with impaired cerebrovascular autoregulation and a pressure-passive cerebral circulation could be identified

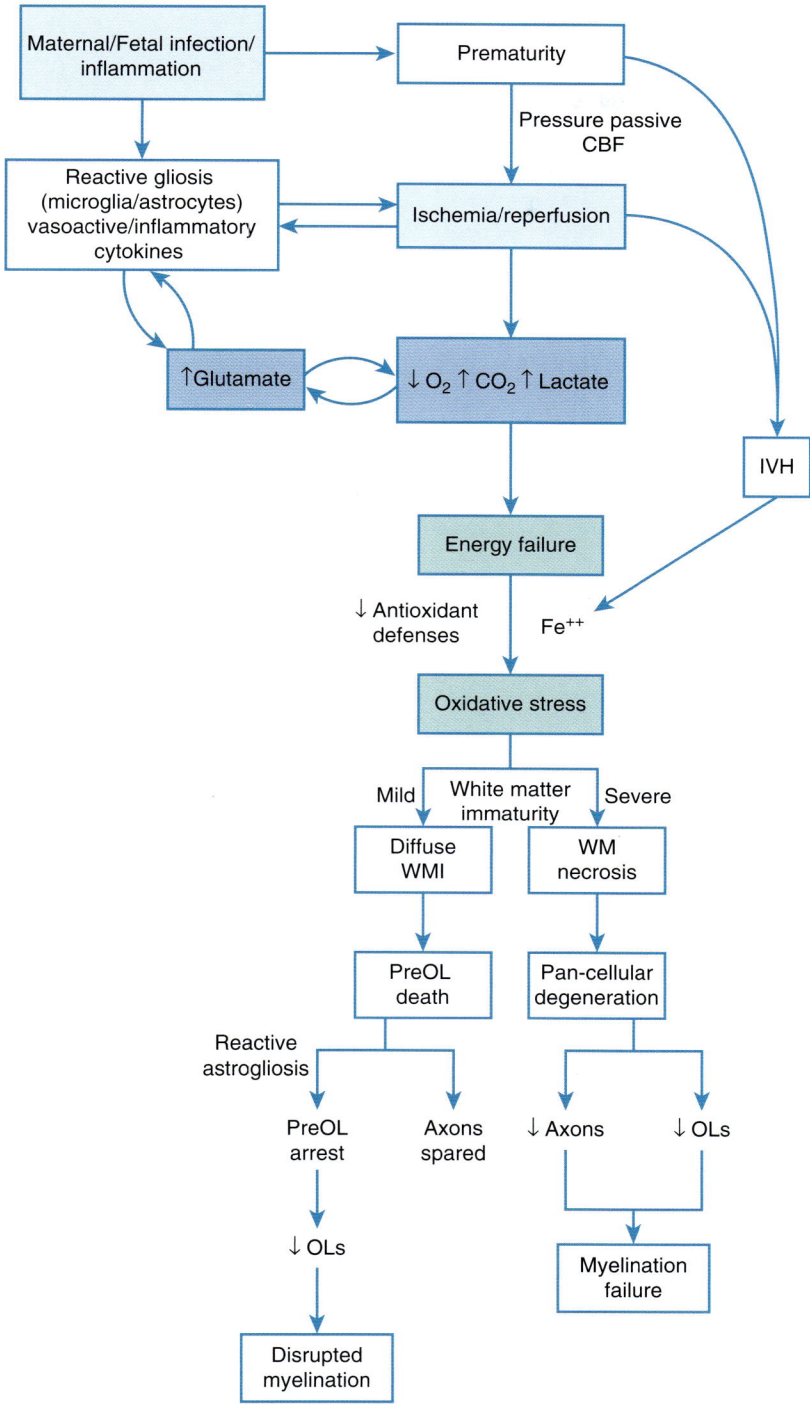

Figure 15.1 Pathogenesis of cerebral white matter injury. The two major upstream mechanisms are ischemia and infection/inflammation *(color 1)*. The two major downstream mechanisms are disturbances in glutamate homeostasis, which results in excitotoxicity, and disrupted energy metabolism *(color 2)* that together contribute to energy failure and oxidative stress *(color 3)*. The magnitude of oxidative stress contributes to the propensity for less severe diffuse WMI, which selectively targets preOLs or more severe cystic white matter necrosis that results in loss of all cellular elements. Downstream of oxidative stress-induced cell death, chronic WMI progressive along two distinct pathways. Disruption of the normal progression of myelination *(left pathway)* occurs downstream of a series of dysmaturation events that result in regeneration of preOLs that fail to differentiate to myelinating oligodendrocytes. Myelination failure in focal or more diffuse regions of necrosis *(right pathway)* occurs due to a loss of axons and oligodendrocytes that together are required for myelination. *CBF*, Cerebral blood flow; *Fe^{++}*, ferrous iron; *Glc*, glucose; *IVH*, intraventricular hemorrhage; *PreOL*, pre-oligodendrocyte; *OL*, oligodendrocyte; *WM*, white matter. (See Chapter 13 for details.)

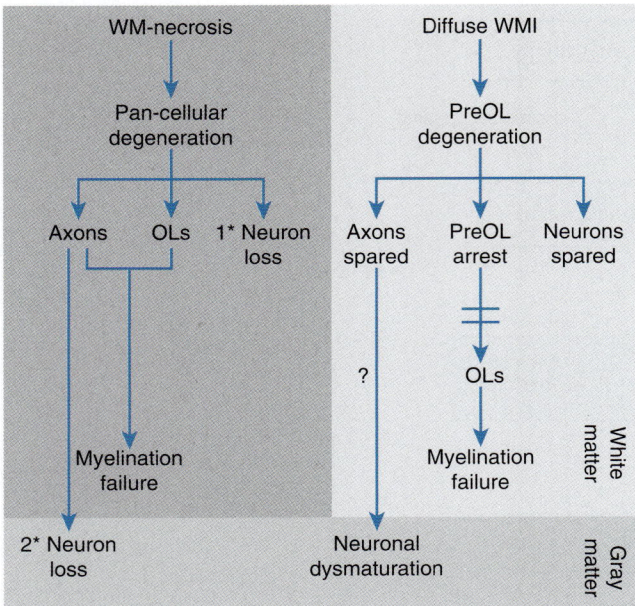

Figure 15.2 In premyelinated white matter (WM), the cellular mechanisms and extent of neuroaxonal degeneration and myelination failure are distinct for necrotic and diffuse WM injury (WMI). WM necrosis (cystic periventricular leukomalacia/microcysts; left panel) is characterized by loss of all cellular elements in necrotic foci (glia, axons, and interstitial neurons). Degeneration of axons and oligodendrocytes (OLs) both contribute to myelination failure. Retrograde degeneration of axons in necrotic foci contributes to neuronal loss in cerebral gray matter. Diffuse WMI (right panel) involves selective degeneration of OL progenitors (preOLs) with sparing of premyelinating axons and interstitial neurons. Note that recent experimental data support a role for selective vulnerability of larger caliber early myelinating axons that appear later in white matter development as myelination progresses.[302] Myelination failure is related to a failure of preOL differentiation (preOL arrest) to OLs. The mechanism of neuronal dysmaturation is unclear and may involve a direct effect of gray matter ischemia on maturation of dendrites and spines as well as axonal factors related to chronic white matter inflammation. (Reprinted with permission from Back SA, Miller SP. Brain injury in premature neonates: a primary cerebral dysmaturation disorder? *Ann Neurol.* 2014;75:469–486.)

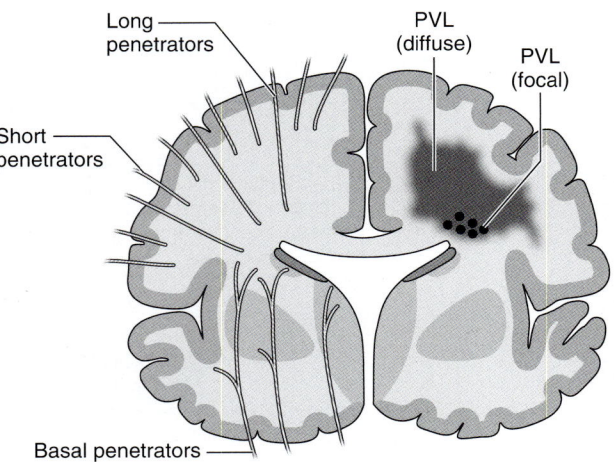

Figure 15.3 Coronal section of cerebrum (schematic) depicting the vascular supply in one hemisphere and the two components (focal and diffuse) of periventricular leukomalacia (PVL) in the other. See text for details. (Vessels redrawn from Rorke LB. Anatomical features of the developing brain implicated in pathogenesis of hypoxic-ischemic injury. *Brain Pathol.* 1992;2:211–221.)

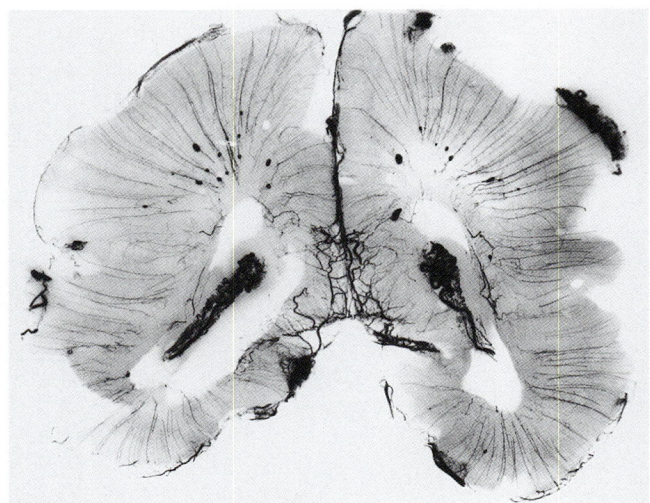

Figure 15.4 Microangiography of the occipital region in a premature infant with periventricular leukomalacia. Note the apparent avascular areas at the sites of leukomalacia, which may be due to a region of vascular degeneration related to hypoxia-ischemia. (From Takashima S, Tanaka K. Development of cerebrovascular architecture and its relationship to periventricular leukomalacia. *Arch Neurol.* 1978;35:11–16.)

by NIRS before the occurrence of WMI, (2) the circulatory abnormality was related to the occurrence of such injury, and (3) if the pressure-passive state could be corrected, the WMI could be prevented. A limitation of these studies is a lack of *regional* estimates of *white matter flow*. NIRS is limited to measurements of CBF at the cortical surface that may not reflect white matter flow during a suspected ischemic event. It would be particularly informative to measure temporal changes in white matter flow under basal conditions as well as during ischemia and reperfusion, as is feasible experimentally (see later).[40,41]

Factors That Predispose to a Pressure Passive Circulation

A number of metabolic abnormalities that influence vascular reactivity are likely to promote the pressure passive state. Both hypocarbia ($PCO_2 < 30$ mm Hg) and hypercarbia ($PCO_2 > 55$ mm Hg) can significantly perturb CBF.[24,42-46] Hypocarbia may promote hypotension and an increased risk for intraventricular hemorrhage and WMI[47,48] through disturbances in CBF.[49] The pronounced reduction in more severe cystic WMI appeared

to be related to a decrease in days of mechanical ventilation,[50] possibly related to reduced hypocarbic alkalosis, which can promote hypotension. Early studies identified that hypocarbia is a potential risk factor for more severe WMI.[51-54] Analysis of the cumulative exposure to hypocarbia demonstrated an increased risk for more severe WMI[55] that was confirmed in a large study of nearly 800 infants studied in the first 7 days of life and found to have a strong association with WMI identified as echolucencies on cranial ultrasonography (Fig. 15.7).[56] Infants with the highest quartile of cumulative exposure to hypocarbia had more than a fivefold increased risk

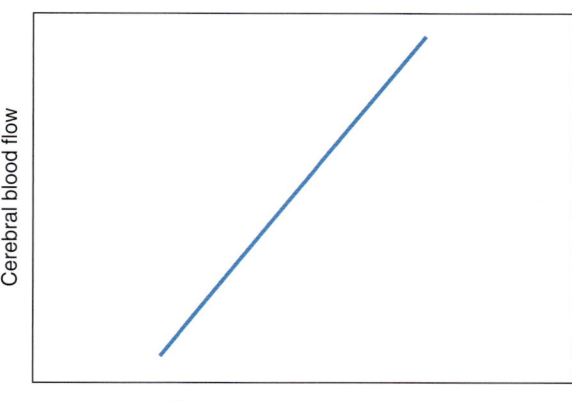

Figure 15.5 Pressure-passive relationship of cerebral blood flow and mean arterial blood pressure. (See text for details.)

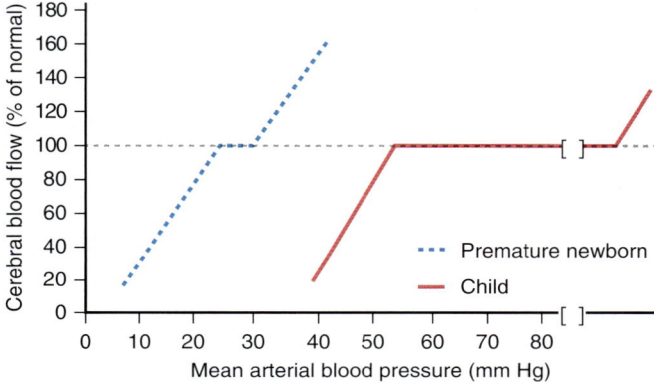

Figure 15.6 Probable relationships between cerebral blood flow and mean arterial blood pressure in the healthy premature newborn and the mature child. (See text for details.)

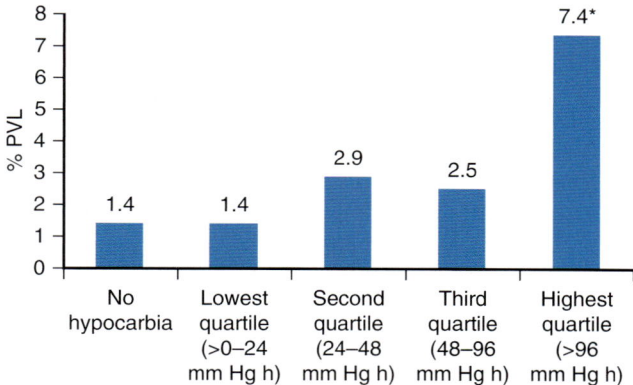

Figure 15.7 Cumulative index of hypocarbia in the first week of life and the occurrence of periventricular leukomalacia (PVL). The study involved 925 infants with a range of birth weights of 501 to 1249 g. PVL was identified by the occurrence of echolucencies on cranial ultrasonography at approximately 28 days of age. Hypocarbia was defined as an arterial partial pressure of carbon dioxide ($PaCO_2$) lower than 35 mm Hg, and the cumulative index of exposure to hypocarbia was calculated as ($35 - PaCO_2$) multiplied by the time interval in hours for each 6-hour block in a 24-hour day. The frequency of PVL in the highest quartile of the cumulative index of exposure differed from that with no hypocarbia ($P < .03$). (From Shankaran S, Langer JC, Kazzi SN, Laptook AR, et al. Cumulative index of exposure to hypocarbia and hyperoxia as risk factors for periventricular leukomalacia in low birth weight infants. *Pediatrics.* 2006;118:1654–1659.)

may account for the demonstrated relationships between marked hypocarbia or hypotension and WMI.[14,53-56,67-70]

Factors That Influence the Timing and Distribution of White Matter Injury

A complex interplay of factors appears to define the enhanced propensity of the preterm human white matter to injury. As discussed earlier, these include an immature vascular supply and disturbances in cerebrovascular autoregulation that can particularly render CBF pressure passive in the setting of critical illness. Central unresolved questions are the factors that define the distribution of WMI and the developmental window of heightened vulnerability. Moreover, is a greater magnitude of ischemia necessary and sufficient to render certain regions more susceptible to more severe necrotic WMI? Often, but not exclusively, the focal necrotic lesions that affect all cellular elements localize to deep cerebral white matter in a periventricular distribution. These lesions frequently coincide with more superficial diffuse cerebral WMI that principally targets oligodendroglial precursor cells (preOLs). Is selective preOL death and the relative sparing of other cellular elements perhaps related to less severe ischemia sustained by diffuse WMI?

Multiple studies in preterm fetal sheep have confirmed that, as observed in humans, the cerebral white matter has an intrinsically lower basal CBF than other gray matter regions[40,71,72] and also displays a pressure passive circulation relative to term and adult animals.[73-75] We achieved spatially resolved quantitative measurements of fetal CBF in utero that were co-registered with histologically defined analyses of WMI. Flow in periventricular white matter was 60% to 70% lower than that observed in cerebral cortex.[40] However, under conditions of moderately severe global cerebral ischemia, the nadir of ischemic CBF was

of WMI when compared with infants in the lowest quartile.[56] The contribution of hypercarbia to WMI is less well defined. Although trials of permissive hypercapnia found no evidence of cystic WMI by cranial ultrasound evaluation,[57,58] abnormal white matter microstructure was identified when extremely low birth weight (ELBW) infants were evaluated at term by diffusion tensor magnetic resonance imaging (MRI).[59]

Similarly unclear is the role of hypoxemia in promoting WMI through disturbances in cerebral autoregulation. Isolated acute hypoxemia has not been directly demonstrated to promote WMI independently of ischemia.[60] Although transient hypoxemia caused inconsistent white and gray matter injury in the midgestation or near-term sheep,[61-63] WMI was notably more severe when significant hypotension was observed.[64]

Additional potential reasons for a pressure-passive cerebral circulation include the mechanical trauma of labor or vaginal delivery to the easily deformed cranium of the premature infant[26,29-32,65,66] A combination of these factors or other factors (e.g., cytokine-mediated vascular effects) could be operative. Finally, *even in the presence of intact cerebrovascular autoregulation*, marked cerebral vasoconstriction or severe systemic hypotension could lead to sufficiently impaired CBF to vascular end zones and border zones to result in cerebral WMI. This explanation

BOX 15.2 Factors Supporting That Global Cerebral Ischemia Is Necessary but Not Sufficient to Define the Spatial Distribution of White Matter Injury in Preterm Fetal Sheep

Basal flow was ~60%–70% lower in cerebral white matter than adjacent gray matter structures such as cerebral cortex and basal ganglia

During moderately severe ischemia, CBF decreased proportionally to ~10%–15% of basal flow in both white and gray matter

No measurable gradients of CBF between superficial cerebral cortex and deep cerebral white matter

Vulnerable white matter regions did not sustain greater reductions in CBF and blood flow was not greater in regions that lacked white matter injury

In regions with similar ischemic flow, the distribution of white matter injury was defined by the density of susceptible preOLs

_____

CBF, Cerebral blood flow; *preOL*, pre-oligodendrocyte.
ªSee references 40 and 41.

similar in multiple cerebral gray matter regions relative to the white matter. After 30 minutes of ischemia, both cortical and white matter flows decreased proportionally to ~10% to 15% of basal flows. Later studies confirmed these observations and found that there were no pathologically significant gradients of flow between fetal cerebral cortex and deep cerebral white matter during either ischemia or reperfusion. Moreover, histologically confirmed WMI did not localize to regions susceptible to greater ischemia, nor did less vulnerable regions of white matter have greater blood flow during ischemia. *These findings supported that ischemia is necessary but not sufficient to generate WMI* (Box 15.2). Even under conditions of moderately severe uniform ischemia, some regions of white matter were relatively spared, whereas other neighboring regions sustained significantly more cell death.

To address this paradox, in a series of studies in preterm fetal sheep we identified that *in regions that sustained similar ischemic CBF, the distribution of WMI was explained by the distribution of one particular cell type, the preOLs* (see Chapters 13 and 14). Human preOLs are markedly more susceptible to hypoxia-ischemia and oxidative stress than other neural cell types.[76,77] In regions that contained more differentiated oligodendrocytes, the susceptibility to WMI was significantly reduced.[40,41] The timing of appearance of preOLs during white matter development also significantly influences the magnitude and distribution of WMI. In preterm fetal rabbits, we identified a window in preterm white matter development (embryonic day 25) when the white matter is populated by a less mature population of early oligodendrocyte progenitors. These early progenitors give rise to preOLs and are much more resistant to hypoxia-ischemia than are the preOLs.[78] Importantly, *these early progenitors rapidly respond to injury by mounting a robust proliferative response that initiates repair of WMI by regenerating preOLs* (see later).[79] Consistent with these observations, the rabbit E25 white matter was highly resistant to pronounced cerebral ischemia in contrast to the E27 white matter when preOLs are diffusely present.[80] *Hence, both the timing of appearance and the distribution of preOLs define the location of susceptible regions of white matter under conditions of moderately severe ischemia.*

It is also clinically important to identify the factors that define the pathogenesis of more severe WMI. The *duration* of cerebral ischemia is a critical factor that defines the burden of white matter necrosis. In preterm fetal sheep, graded WMI is generated that is related to the duration of ischemia.[40] As discussed earlier, it is also likely that the magnitude of a number of systemic factors (e.g., hypotension) and metabolic factors (e.g., hypoxemia, hypocapnia, hypoglycemia, lactic acidosis) interact to determine the severity of ischemic WMI. Given how low basal CBF is in human preterm white matter, regional blood flow and metabolism may be equivalently low and matched for metabolic requirements. Ischemia may be relatively well tolerated unless there is pronounced energy failure that shifts the balance toward focal or more diffuse necrotic cell death. *Hence, ischemia appears to be necessary but not sufficient to cause WMI, and cellular maturational and metabolic factors likely influence the severity of the WMI response.*

It is also currently unclear if recurrent hypoxia-ischemia predisposes to more severe WMI. In preterm-equivalent neonatal rats, a pronounced increase in cell death was observed in chronic WMI after recurrent hypoxia-ischemia.[79] However, in preterm fetal sheep that develop WMI that more closely resembles human, recurrent hypoxia-ischemia did not trigger more pronounced WMI. This suggests that recurrent hypoxia-ischemia may confer protection against more severe WMI through an ischemic tolerance-like mechanism.[81] This is an important direction for future study.

Clinical Factors Supporting a Role for Hypoxia-Ischemia in the Pathogenesis of White Matter Injury

Additional clinical evidence supportive of a relationship between impaired CBF and the occurrence of WMI includes the association of the injury with markers of hypoxic-ischemic events (e.g., neonatal acidosis, elevations of plasma uric acid on the first day of life), episodes of mean arterial blood pressure less than 30 mm Hg, hypovolemia, oliguria, abrupt decreases in blood pressure in chronically hypertensive premature newborns (in whom cerebrovascular autoregulation may be present but with the curve shifted to the right), patent ductus arteriosus, congenital heart disease, and severely ill infants treated with extracorporeal membrane oxygenation (ECMO) or cardiac surgery.[66,82-98] The adverse effect of patent ductus arteriosus on the cerebral circulation, documented by earlier studies,[99-101] as well as subsequently,[88,102-104] supports a direct link between cerebral ischemia and WMI. Thus, infants with the most severe derangement of CBF (i.e., retrograde flow in diastole) had a 36% incidence of PVL (ultrasonographic criteria) versus a 15% incidence in those infants with no retrograde flow.[88] Escalating doses of indomethacin were not shown to reduce the incidence of WMI or intraventricular hemorrhage.[105] The high frequency of the lesion in the hypoxemic and hypotensive infants treated with ECMO also demonstrates a striking relationship with apparent cerebral ischemia (Table 15.1).[106] Other pathological evidence for generalized ischemic insults (e.g., selective neuronal necrosis) also was present in these infants (see Table 15.1).

A relationship of cerebral ischemia with WMI may be operative in infants with apneic spells. A relationship of apnea and bradycardia with WMI has been suspected for many years because earlier work, performed before the era of cranial ultrasonography, showed an association between spastic diplegia and apneic-bradycardic episodes.[107] Studies of CBF

TABLE 15.1 Prominence at Autopsy of Periventricular White Matter Injury Among Hypoxic-Ischemic Lesions in Infants Treated With Extracorporeal Membrane Oxygenation[a]

LESION	NO. (PERCENTAGE OF TOTAL)[b]
Periventricular leukomalacia	18 (78%)
Diffuse white matter injury	8 (35%)
Selective neuronal necrosis	
Thalamus	9 (39%)
Inferior olivary nucleus	8 (35%)
Cerebral infarction[c]	7 (30%)

[a]Derived from 23 infants (born at 35 to 41 weeks of gestation) treated with extracorporeal membrane oxygenation at Boston Children's Hospital from 1984 to 1991 (Kupsky W, personal communication, 1992). Nine infants (39%) also sustained subdural, subarachnoid, or intraparenchymal hemorrhage (see Chapter 22).

[b]Infants often had more than one lesion; thus, percentages exceed 100%.

[c]Four infarcts were hemorrhagic.

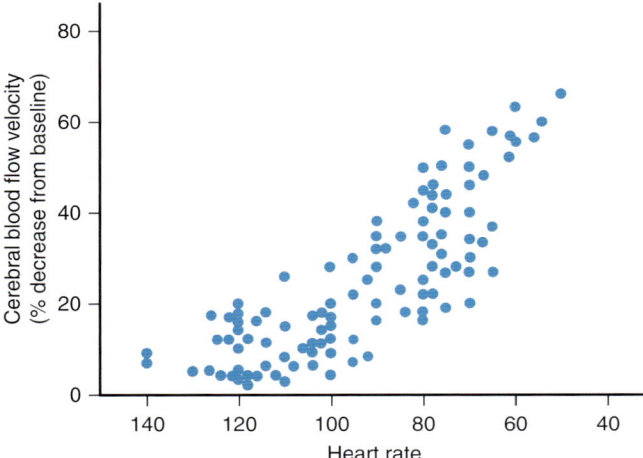

Figure 15.8 Effect of apnea and bradycardia on cerebral blood flow velocity. Cerebral blood flow velocity, quantitated as area under the velocity curve, is shown as a function of heart rate with apnea in premature infants. Individual values for 101 separate episodes of apnea and bradycardia are shown. (From Perlman JM, Volpe JJ. Episodes of apnea and bradycardia in the preterm newborn: Impact on cerebral circulation. *Pediatrics.* 1985;76:333–338.)

velocity by Doppler showed an impairment in cerebral flow velocity with mild to moderate bradycardia (80 to 100 beats/min) and a marked impairment with severe bradycardia (<80 beats/min) (Fig. 15.8).[108] Studies with NIRS documented a sharp decrease in cerebral oxygenated hemoglobin and cerebral blood volume in association with apneic spells with bradycardia,[109-112] and findings were consistent with the likelihood of a decrease in CBF with such spells. Chronic hypoxemia in rodents generates transient maturational disturbances in white matter myelination.[60] Preclinical studies found that resolution of this dysmyelination was promoted by caffeine.[113] Since caffeine therapy is an effective treatment for apnea of prematurity,[114,115] its potential benefits to reduce WMI and related motor deficits were evaluated in several large clinical studies. However, longer-term outcome studies have not demonstrated reduced neurological morbidity related to caffeine therapy.[116,117]

Several neuroimaging and postmortem studies have identified that near-term and term infants with congenital heart disease have reduced brain volumes associated with a high risk for WMI and that the WMI often precedes surgical interventions.[118-120] In a large autopsy series of infants dying after cardiac surgery, WMI was the dominant lesion (nearly 80% of cases).[95] Although WMI was originally thought to be related to perioperative hypoxia-ischemia during cardiac repair,[121] more recent studies found that infants with congenital heart disease have low preoperative CBF that is associated with an increased risk for WMI.[122] Reduced cerebral flow is associated with reduced cerebral oxygen delivery and reduced brain volumes.[123,124] Survivors of cyanotic congenital heart lesions, particularly those with transpositions of the great arteries or hypoplastic left heart syndrome, are now surviving with significant motor and neurobehavioral disabilities that point to widely distributed white matter and gray matter disturbances that disrupt brain connectivity.[125,126] The similarities between the pathogenesis of these conditions and preterm survivors are striking and support that disturbances in CBF and metabolism are linked to the spectrum of white matter and gray matter pathology in both disorders.

It should finally be emphasized that preterm infants and infants with congenital heart disease are also commonly at risk for *exposure to hypoxemia or hyperoxia*. The extent to which either insult *independently* contributes to WMI is currently unclear. Although exposure to both hypoxemia and hyperoxia is common in critically ill neonates, *these infants are at risk for concomitant hypoxia-ischemia and other causes of WMI*. It has thus been difficult in human studies to identify infants with relatively isolated exposure to hyperoxia. Similarly, there are no well-defined human neuropathological features that characterize the cerebral response to isolated chronic hypoxemia, because preterm survivors with chronic lung disease often sustain other forms of WMI related to hypoxia-ischemia, hyperoxia, or intraventricular hemorrhagic infarction. There are thus *no human pathological studies that have defined the features of cerebral injury related to hyperoxia or hypoxemia, alone.*

As recently reviewed and summarized in Box 15.3, experimental findings from animal models have, in fact, identified that *exposure to hypoxia-ischemia, hypoxia, and hyperoxia results in strikingly different forms of WMI.*[60] Global cerebral hypoxia-ischemia models in preterm fetal sheep, for example, display disturbances in cerebral autoregulation and regional white matter blood flow. These models generate graded cerebral WMI that closely resembles the spectrum of human preterm WMI that ranges from diffuse WMI to focal cystic necrotic lesions (see earlier discussion).[127] In addition, acute WMI selectively triggers the necrotic and apoptotic degeneration of preOLs and results in chronic persistent reactive astrogliosis and microgliosis. By contrast, chronic hypoxia in neonatal rodents spares preOLs but causes delayed apoptosis of mature oligodendrocytes. Chronic hyperoxia similarly spares preOLs but causes apoptosis of early oligodendrocytes, which are the precursors to preOLs.[128]

Although *neither hypoxemia nor hyperoxia generates a spectrum of pathology that resembles human WMI,* improved animal models are clearly needed to further define how hypoxemia or hyperoxia modifies the response to hypoxia-ischemic to disrupt cerebral white or gray matter maturation. Isolated chronic hypoxia, for example, disrupts EGF receptor-mediated mechanisms that are required for the survival and generation of new oligodendrocytes[129,130] and thus may have significant consequences for white matter regeneration and repair processes. Moreover, chronic hypoxia disrupts preOL maturation and myelination through dysregulation of Wnt activity.[131-133] Oxygen tension via hypoxia-inducible factor also influences Wnt activation to promote preOL maturation arrest and disrupts white matter angiogenesis, which is required for axon integrity[134] as well as maintenance of neural stem cell niches for neurogenesis.[135,136]

Infection/Inflammation

Infection/inflammation is the second major upstream event in pathogenesis (see Box 15.1 and Fig. 15.1). Thus, an important series of clinical/epidemiological, neuropathological, and experimental studies suggest that maternal intrauterine infection and fetal systemic inflammation are involved in the pathogenesis of a proportion of cases of WMI. Postnatal infections were also significantly associated with increased risk for WMI. The magnitude of the role of infection/inflammation and especially the potential mechanisms thereof are still unresolved issues. Several fundamental questions remain to be resolved. First, rigorous outcome measures to identify and quantify antecedent maternal-fetal infections were frequently lacking. Confirmation of infection by placental pathology was not consistently used in most studies. Second, many studies relied on relatively insensitive neuroimaging modalities to detect WMI, and often, imaging was not obtained in close temporal proximity to the suspected time of infection. Third, although infections were expected to render the white matter more susceptible to injury, there has been little experimental exploration of potential mechanisms of infection-mediated tolerance in preterm white matter. Studies in near-term animals support that the timing of an inflammatory challenge is critical in rendering the brain susceptible or resistant to hypoxia-ischemia. As demonstrated in neonatal rodents,[137,138] in some settings, a low-grade antecedent infection may *protect* against more severe injury from a subsequent more severe insult such as hypoxia-ischemia.[139]

Clinical/Epidemiological Observations

Clinical and epidemiological studies suggest a link between maternal and fetal infection, inflammation, and the occurrence of WMI (see Chapters 13 and 16).[140,141] The most commonly held view is that maternal intrauterine infection causes a fetal systemic inflammatory response that results in injury to cerebral white matter. There are several potential mechanisms by which WMI may occur. A fetal systemic inflammatory response may disrupt CBF via cardiovascular insufficiency and secondary cerebral hypoperfusion, as demonstrated in experimental models.[142] As discussed later, inflammation may disrupt cerebral vascular reactivity, as in the setting of chorioamnionitis. For example, inflammation may also potentially trigger direct degeneration of cells in the white matter through mechanisms involving cytotoxic cytokines.

The fetal systemic inflammatory response, recognized for many years, is defined in considerable part by detection of proinflammatory cytokines in blood. A relationship with WMI or associated cerebral palsy in premature infants is suggested by the finding of increased incidence of these outcomes in the presence of (1) evidence for maternal and fetal infection/inflammation (e.g., chorioamnionitis, funisitis, premature rupture of membranes);[140,141,143-153] (2) elevated levels of proinflammatory cytokines, especially interleukin-6 (IL-6) and IL-1β, in amniotic fluid[154] or umbilical cord blood;[140,152,155-157] and (3) evidence for intrauterine T-cell activation.[155] However, nearly all these studies used for the diagnosis of WMI the ultrasonographic finding of echolucencies (i.e., apparent *cystic* WMI). As noted earlier, cystic WMI now is recognized to account for less than 5% of WMI. Cranial ultrasonography also has poor sensitivity and specificity to detect multifocal noncystic WMI, which comprises the majority of cases (see Chapter 14). The potential mis-classification of noncystic WMI as *controls* makes the interpretation of these data difficult. Moreover, two studies of former preterm infants showed no significant relationship between levels of proinflammatory cytokines in early neonatal blood and the later diagnosis of cerebral palsy.[158,159]

The role of chorioamnionitis in the pathogenesis of WMI has received considerable attention but remains unresolved because of several important limitations.[160] The majority of early studies used cranial ultrasonography to detect WMI and relied on clinical rather than histopathological criteria. One study of 126 infants showed no correlation between clinical chorioamnionitis and ultrasonographically demonstrated WMI.[161] Some studies used cerebral palsy as an outcome measure rather than assessment of WMI by neuroimaging. Two large meta-analysis studies found a significantly increased risk for cerebral palsy in studies that diagnosed chorioamnionitis by clinical (OR 2.42) or histopathological (OR 1.83) criteria. However, these studies did not evaluate the spectrum of WMI, including more severe cystic WMI, as well as other forms of cerebral pathology that may have contributed to cerebral palsy. Moreover, chorioamnionitis may increase the risk for adverse outcomes related to postnatal infections,[162-164] necrotizing enterocolitis,[163,165,166] or symptomatic hypotension.[167] Greater attention to these postnatal risk factors would strengthen the analysis of the independent contribution of prenatal chorioamnionitis to WMI or cerebral palsy. Few studies have combined MRI-defined WMI with rigorous evaluation of maternal and fetal inflammatory responses by placental pathology to confirm exposure to chorioamnionitis. In a study of 100 consecutive premature infants studied by MRI at term, no significant relationship was noted between the occurrence of chorioamnionitis or prolonged rupture of membranes and moderate to severe WMI.[168] Several additional prospective MRI-based studies similarly failed to find an association between histopathologically confirmed chorioamnionitis and disturbances in brain maturation or injury.[169-172]

Since as many as 25% of all infants who weigh less than 1500 g at birth experience neonatal sepsis,[173-176] a role for *postnatal* infection/inflammation in WMI has been studied. In the aforementioned MRI study of 100 premature infants, a weak relationship was noted between neonatal sepsis and WMI identified at term.[177] Other reports have shown an increased rate of WMI, cerebral palsy, or other neurodevelopmental disabilities in preterm infants after neonatal sepsis.[98,162,164,178] This relationship is particularly apparent among infants of ELBW (401 to 1000 g), of whom 65% exhibit at least one infection during the postnatal period.[164] In a key study of 92 premature infants, postnatal infections and hypotension, but not histologically defined chorioamnionitis, were associated with increased risk for MRI-defined WMI.[170] Despite the lack of strong associations between prenatal chorioamnionitis and adverse neurodevelopmental outcomes, chorioamnionitis may indirectly increase the risk for postnatal infections and hypotension as independent risk factors for cerebral ischemia and WMI.

Potential Role of Proinflammatory Cytokines in White Matter Injury

A potential role for inflammation and, specifically, cytokines in the pathogenesis of WMI has been proposed from human and experimental studies that have detected proinflammatory cytokines in early or advanced stages of WMI.[179-184] Experimental studies in fetal sheep found that circulating IL1-β and IL-6 cross the blood-brain barrier to access the central nervous system (CNS).[185] Moreover, ischemia-related disruptions in blood-brain barrier permeability were attenuated with neutralizing antibodies directed against either of these cytokines.[186,187] Perhaps related to these findings are the demonstrations in living premature infants of a relationship between elevated levels of interferon-gamma (IFN-γ) in blood or cerebrospinal fluid (CSF) and ultrasonographically defined WMI[188,189] or tumor necrosis factor-α (TNF-α) in CSF and MRI-defined WMI.[190] In preterm infants with WMI studied postmortem, IFN-γ was highly expressed in white matter lesions.[184] An additional source of proinflammatory cytokines within the CNS are microglia or astrocytes that are resident in the white matter. In chronic human diffuse WMI, activated microglial are abundantly present.[191]

In experimental models, several microglial-derived inflammatory cytokines have been shown to cause early WMI through peroxynitrite-mediated toxicity to the OL lineage.[192-196] Bacterial endotoxin exposure similarly may exacerbate WMI via peroxisomal dysfunction and related oxidative stress.[197,198] Experimental and clinical studies have found that proinflammatory cytokines are detected in association with WMI[157,180,184,190,199-203] and can disrupt white matter development in neonatal animal models.[204,205] The principal cytokines observed in human WMI are TNF-α, IL-1β and IFN-γ. The toxicity of these cytokines to preOLs has been proposed as a potential mechanism for *early* WMI. Support for this hypothesis is weakened by the lack of several critical observations. Human pathology studies have relied heavily on cytokine staining in *chronic* WMI samples, but detection of cytokines has not been done in *early* WMI when the majority of preOL degeneration occurs. Immunohistochemical detection of cytokines in human tissue sections is also a relatively insensitive means to detect differences in cytokine levels. Cytokine detection in human chronic WMI has also been largely restricted to lesions with *cystic* WMI, whereas the majority of contemporary patients sustain mostly multifocal noncystic WMI. Hence, a role for proinflammatory cytokines in the pathogenesis of the major form of early human WMI remains unresolved.

Delineation of the insult leading to the brain cytokine response in WMI would be of major value in the understanding of pathogenesis. A potential interacting role for systemic infection/inflammation with hypoxia-ischemia has been suggested from experimental studies in which endotoxin exposure was shown to either dampen or potentiate the severity of cerebral injury depending on the timing of exposure.[139] Identification of the initiating insult is difficult in neuropathological studies, but available data *suggest a role both for hypoxia-ischemia and systemic infection/inflammation*. In the neuropathological series of Kadhim and associates,[182] the 19 cases with WMI and cytokine staining in the lesions had *asphyxia* in the background, although cases complicated by systemic infection had the greatest staining. Thus, the degree to which hypoxia-ischemia contributed to the inflammatory response in these cases of human WMI is unclear and important to consider. It is well established in animal models of WMI that ischemia/reperfusion is associated with a brisk inflammatory response, characterized by activation of microglial cells, secretion of cytokines, mobilization, adhesion and migration of macrophages and inflammatory cells, and reactive astrocytosis.[206-221] Persistence of this response, with activated microglia and astrocytes, for many *weeks* following the insult has been documented in hypoxic-ischemic models in immature animals and in human stroke.[206,216,221] As discussed later, activated microglial cells also secrete toxic diffusible products (e.g., reactive oxygen species [ROS] and reactive nitrogen species [RNS]) that may be more injurious than cytokines in the genesis of WMI.

Cellular Mediators of Inflammation

Although the mechanisms by which maternal and fetal infection/inflammation initiate deleterious molecular and structural events in the brain are not fully understood, *microglia are present during the early and advanced stages of WMI* (see Fig. 15.1 and Chapter 13). During normal brain development, microglia have key roles in clearance of apoptotic cells arising from programmed cell death and in synaptic pruning. Microglia are broadly classified in two major phenotypes that are biased toward proinflammatory or antiinflammatory actions.[222-225] During the immediate early phase of WMI, microglia may initiate or potentiate cell death via ROS and RNS and perhaps glutamate.[226] The mechanisms of ROS/RNS toxicity and excitotoxicity have the potential to contribute to the intrinsic maturation-dependent vulnerability of preOLs to both hypoxia-ischemia and infection/inflammation (see also Chapter 13). During the more chronic stages of WMI, the activation state of human microglia has not been defined. It has been proposed that during the progressive remodeling of the white matter after injury, microglia may assume a more antiinflammatory role that could contribute to repair processes to promote oligodendrocyte maturation and myelination in neonatal WMI[227] and multiple sclerosis.[228] This topic is an important direction for future study.

Microglial cells can be identified in normal human brain very early in development, become abundant in forebrain from 16 to 22 weeks of gestation, and *are concentrated in cerebral white matter, with a deep-to-superficial gradient.*[229-238] Relatively fewer microglial cells are found in cerebral cortex at this time. In one longitudinal study of human postmortem brain, the density of microglia reached a peak during the period of greatest vulnerability to WMI (third trimester of gestation) and declined markedly in white matter after 37 weeks of gestation.[233] As density declined in cerebral white matter, it increased in cerebral cortex. This observation suggests that a wave of migrating microglia is apparent in cerebral white matter at the optimum time for activation by hypoxia-ischemia or infection or both. *Thus, although more data on these developmental features are needed, a maturation-dependent population of cells (i.e., microglia) may be concentrated in cerebral white matter at the right time and location to contribute to WMI when activated.*

Infection and Hypoxia-Ischemia-Potentiating Insults

Deleterious interactions between prenatal (maternal or fetal) and postnatal infection/inflammation and hypoxia-ischemia could occur at several steps in the pathway to WMI (see Box 15.1 and Fig. 15.1). Thus, such potentiation could develop at the level of the major upstream initiating events of hypoxia-ischemia and infection/inflammation or at the level of the major downstream events of oxidative stress and excitotoxicity. Not unexpectedly, most current evidence supporting a potentiating interaction of infection/inflammation and hypoxia-ischemia emanates from experimental studies (see Chapter 13). However, clinical and neuropathological studies of human PVL also support the notion of a potentiating interaction.

Inflammation-Induced Sensitization of White Matter Injury

Both experimental and clinical studies provide support for potential interactions between distinct injurious factors that may potentiate or reduce the severity of WMI. Although most of the experimental studies have focused on sensitization of the term infant brain, they provide an important new direction to define the impact of multifactorial events on the progression of WMI during the early phase of cell death and the later stages of regeneration and repair. Of particular importance to the pathogenesis of early WMI is the *notion that infection/inflammation may potentiate or mitigate WMI arising from cerebral hypoxia-ischemia.*

As discussed earlier, antenatal or postnatal infection/sepsis may have adverse systemic and cerebral circulatory effects that contribute to WMI. Major disturbances in the regulation of CBF and cerebral oxygen delivery have been observed in fetal sheep after relatively low doses of lipopolysaccharide.[239,240] Significant episodes of chorioamnionitis are associated with funisitis, fetal and postnatal hemodynamic instability, and signs of persistent inflammatory states.[241-243] For example, in one study of 61 consecutively born preterm infants (<32 weeks of gestation), the risk of WMI, identified by MRI and ultrasonography, was enhanced with a history of histological chorioamnionitis *only in the presence* of *concurrent* placental vascular disturbances consistent with a placental perfusion defect.[172] Whether the latter was caused by intrauterine infection was not clear, although such a relationship has been shown.[244] Histological chorioamnionitis *without placental perfusion defect* was *not* associated with white matter disease.

Because several cytokines stimulated by infection, especially TNF-α and IL-1β, exhibit vasoactive properties, it is reasonable to postulate that these inflammatory molecules could contribute to impaired cerebrovascular autoregulation, likely important in the pathogenesis of WMI (see earlier discussion).[182,245-247] Hypoxia-ischemia (*without infection*) also leads to both systemic and cerebral elevations of vasoactive proinflammatory cytokines (e.g., TNF-α and IL-1β) derived from peripheral monocytes and brain microglia.[248-251] A resident population of microglia is concentrated in human preterm cerebral white matter with the potential to be activated and become injurious during the early phase of WMI (see earlier).[233] *Thus, activated microgliosis is a consistent and prominent feature of early and chronic white matter lesions*[76,191,236-238] *with the potential to exert vasoactive effects that may promote or amplify the extent of WMI due to hypoxia-ischemia.*

It is also important to consider the potential impact of subclinical factors that in isolation would not be injurious but in combination may synergize to potentiate WMI. The combination of infection/inflammation and hypoxia-ischemia could result in deleterious systemic circulatory effects that ultimately affect the cerebral circulation (see Fig. 15.1). Many other maternal or iatrogenic factors may also induce fetal stress and alter the susceptibility to hypoxia-ischemia.[252]

Although in some experimental studies, deleterious systemic hemodynamic effects have been shown to accompany fetal or neonatal infection or exposure to lipopolysaccharide or cytokines, equally important to consider is the *concept of inflammation/infection mediated tolerance to a hypoxic-ischemic event, which may reduce the severity of WMI.* Mechanisms of ischemic tolerance/preconditioning have been extensively described in neonatal hypoxia-ischemia.[253-257] Studies in neonatal rodents have demonstrated that the *timing* of an inflammatory challenge relative to subsequent hypoxia-ischemia defines the severity of cerebral injury, which may be *attenuated or enhanced.*[137,138,258-265]

Thus, taken together, a growing body of experimental, neuropathological, and clinical evidence suggests that infection/inflammation and hypoxia-ischemia may interact to influence the magnitude of WMI. The identification of mechanisms of sensitization would have major implications concerning the means of surveillance of infants at risk and the approaches to prevention and are critical for future research.

Intrinsic Vulnerability of the Premature Newborn to Acute Cerebral White Matter Injury

The cerebral white matter of the premature infant is intrinsically susceptible to a broad spectrum of injury (see Box 15.1). At the more severe end are the now relatively rare severe destructive lesions that result in microscopic or macroscopic cystic white matter necrosis and the nonselective degeneration of all cell types within these lesions. In addition to glia, migrating and interstitial white matter neurons, subplate neurons, and axons may degenerate in necrotic lesions, as supported by both human and experimental studies.[40,266-269] Neuroimaging studies support that the majority of infants sustain focal or diffuse non-necrotic white matter lesions. Neuropathology studies support that these nondestructive lesions involve a maturation-dependent *intrinsic* vulnerability of the cerebral white matter that targets the oligodendrocyte lineage. This intrinsic vulnerability is supported by experimental studies (see Chapter 13), by the decline in incidence of relatively restricted WMI later in gestation, by the concentration of vulnerable preOLs during the peak time period of occurrence of the lesion,[270] and by the selective degeneration of preOLs in the early lesions.[77] The intrinsic vulnerability relates principally to the two major downstream mechanisms of WMI (i.e., free radical attack by ROS and RNS and excitotoxicity; see Box 15.1). The details of the intrinsic vulnerabilities, as derived from experimental studies, are described in Chapter 13. Here are emphasized studies performed on human premature brain that have defined a role for preOL death as a key initiating event in the pathogenesis of chronic WMI as discussed later.

Vulnerability to Free Radical Attack

Both experimental and human pathology studies support that preOLs selectively degenerate during the early phase of WMI. A role for oxidative stress in preOL degeneration is supported by in vitro, experimental, and human neuropathology studies (Box 15.4). The fetal cerebral white matter is rich in membrane lipids that are readily oxidized.[271-273] The developing white matter may be more vulnerable to oxidative damage due to a delay in the expression of the antioxidant enzymes, superoxide dismutases-1 and -2, catalase, and glutathione peroxidase,[274-276] but expression data in rat and human have not been confirmed with enzyme activity data. Although controversy exists regarding the role of RNS in the pathogenesis of early WMI, human preterm white matter is especially prone to lipid peroxidation-mediated injury.[76,77] Both the biochemical and immunohistochemical detection of protein, lipid, and DNA adducts generated by reaction oxygen and nitrogen species (e.g., protein carbonyls, 4-hydroxynonenal and 8-oxo-deoxyguanosine) are unreliable in human preterm WMI.[77] Sensitive detection of the aldehydes formed from lipid hydroperoxides is specifically achieved in glia by measurement of F_2-isoprostanes, which are stable adducts in postmortem human tissue.[277] F_2-isoprostanes were significantly elevated in histopathologically confirmed cases

---

> **BOX 15.4** Findings Supporting a Role for Oxidative Injury to Preterm Human Cerebral White Matter
>
> ◆ Detectable levels of staining for the iron binding protein ferritin in preterm human white matter suggest the possibility of iron-mediated generation of reactive oxygen species during hypoxia-ischemia.
> ◆ Reduced staining for antioxidant enzymes (superoxide dismutase 1 and 2, catalase, and glutathione peroxidase) in preterm human white matter suggests reduced antioxidant defenses.
> ◆ Preterm human early WMI displays elevated levels of markers of lipid peroxidation by staining and by biochemical detection of F_2-isoprostanes.
> ◆ Preterm human cerebral cortex and adjacent regions of early WMI display low levels of F4-neuroprostanes, a marker of oxidative damage to neurons and axons.
>
> *WMI, White matter injury.*

---

of early WMI[77] and coincided with the levels detected in the cerebral cortex where severe perinatal asphyxia was confirmed. This oxidative damage was accompanied by a pronounced increase in degenerating cells in the periventricular white matter, which were shown to be preOLs (Fig. 15.9). F_4-neuroprostanes, a specific marker of oxidative injury to *neuronal* elements, were not detected in white matter or cerebral cortex, consistent with the notion that neurons and axons were spared (Fig. 15.10). *Hence, oxidative damage selectively targeted the preterm white matter, and the degree of oxidative damage sustained in the early phases of WMI is considerable and comparable to that sustained in severe perinatal asphyxia from hypoxic-ischemia.*

The mechanisms underlying the maturation-dependent vulnerability of developing white matter to ROS attack has been extensively studied in an attempt to design protective strategies against WMI (see also Chapter 13). Definition of the timing of ROS generation requires animal studies. Studies in a mid-gestation fetal sheep asphyxial model of preterm WMI found that the peak of free radical generation was delayed and not detected until several hours after the insult.[278] This timing likely reflected a delayed wave of ROS generation that occurs during the peak of cell death. Studies in a preterm fetal rabbit model of placental insufficiency detected increased superoxide production during the immediate ischemia-reperfusion period. Early delivery of a superoxide dismutase mimic or antioxidants significantly reduced hypertonia in this model of mixed cerebral palsy.[226] Early superoxide generation is consistent with the delay in expression of copper-zinc superoxide dismutase, manganese superoxide dismutase, and catalase in preterm human white matter.[274] The possibility that superoxide generation promotes the accumulation of hydrogen peroxide and its conversion to the hydroxyl radical by the Fenton reaction is suggested by the early appearance of iron in developing human white matter,[279,280] as well as by the acquisition of iron by developing oligodendrocytes for differentiation.[281] Supportive of a relationship between iron and WMI is the observation that, for many weeks after human intraventricular hemorrhage, a disorder that sharply increases the risk of WMI,[282-284] CSF levels of non–protein-bound iron are markedly increased.[285] In addition, several reports suggest that the vulnerability to oxidative attack in the premature white matter shares similarities with systemic features. Studies of

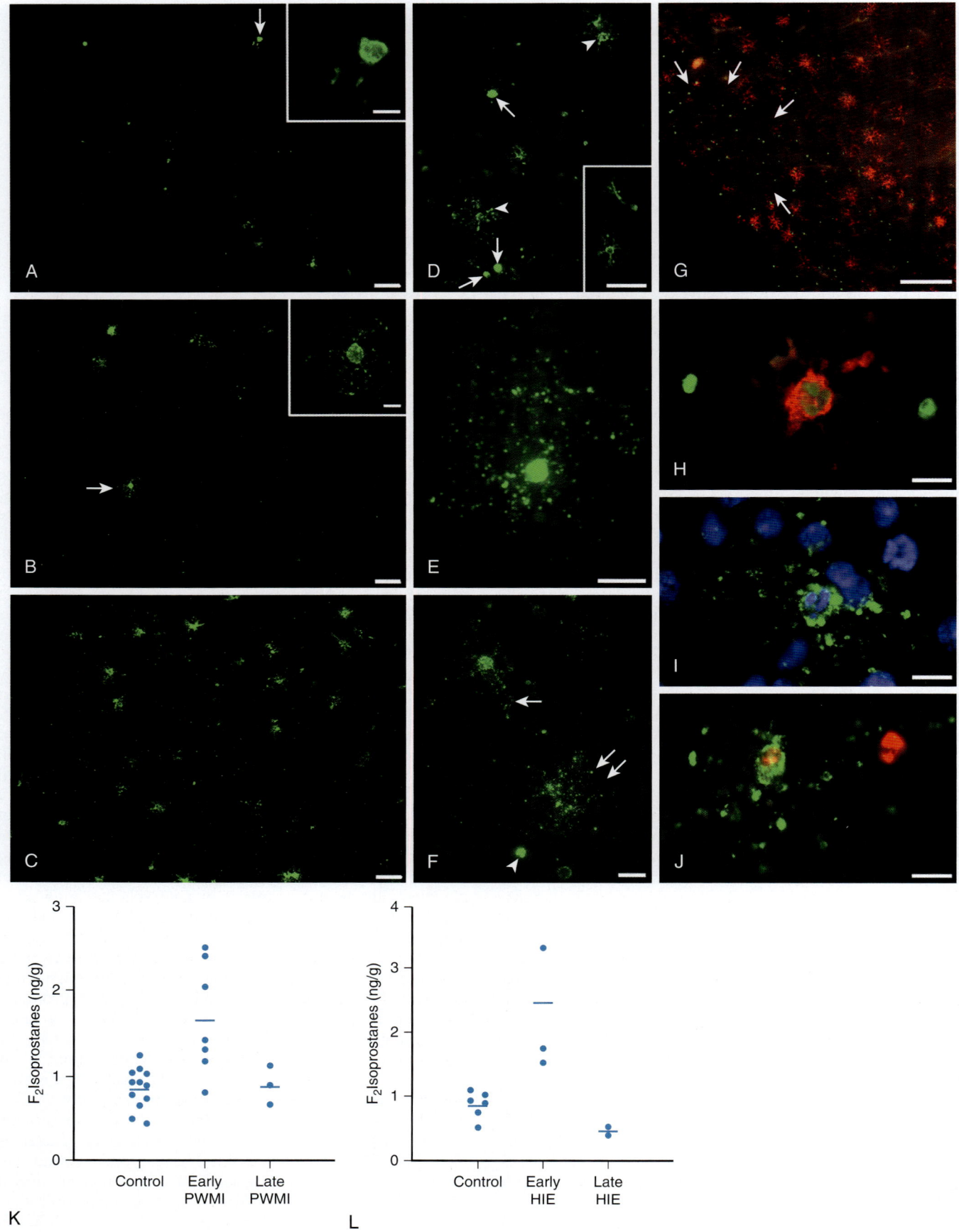

Figure 15.9 Oxidative stress selectively causes preOL degeneration in early human preterm diffuse white matter injury (WMI). (A to C) Typical example of a gradient of early WMI that preferentially localized to deeper areas of cerebral white matter in A and B with more normal appearing white matter in C. Note the severely damaged cell remnants in A (arrow; detail in inset) and the paucity of normal appearing preOLs in B (arrow; detail in inset). (D) Typical appearance of shrunken degenerating preOLs (arrows) scattered among more normal-appearing cells (arrowheads), also shown in the inset. (E and F) Typical morphology of degenerating preOLs. (G) PreOLs (red) also are vulnerable in the subventricular zone deep to the periventricular white matter where a focal lesion is seen (arrows) that contains many degenerating cells (green). (H to J) Examples of apoptotic preOLs with a typical fragmented condensed nucleus. (K) F_2-isoprostanes, a sensitive and specific marker of oxidative injury in human autopsy tissue, were significantly elevated in the periventricular white matter from cases of early preterm WMI (PWMI) relative to age-matched control cases or those diagnosed with more chronic PWMI. (L) The levels of oxidative damage in early WMI in K were similar in magnitude to that measured in cortical gray matter lesions from autopsy cases with early term hypoxic-ischemic encephalopathy (HIE). Note that the F_2-isoprostanes were significantly elevated in the early late HIE cases relative to controls or those diagnosed with more chronic HIE. Scale bars: A to C, 50 μm; Inset in A and B, 10 μm; D and inset in D, 50 μm; E, 10 μm; F, 20 μm; G, 200 μm; H to J, 10 μm. (Adapted with permission from Back SA, Luo NL, Mallinson RA, et al. Selective vulnerability of preterm white matter to oxidative damage defined by F2-isoprostanes. *Ann Neurol.* 2005;58:108–120.)

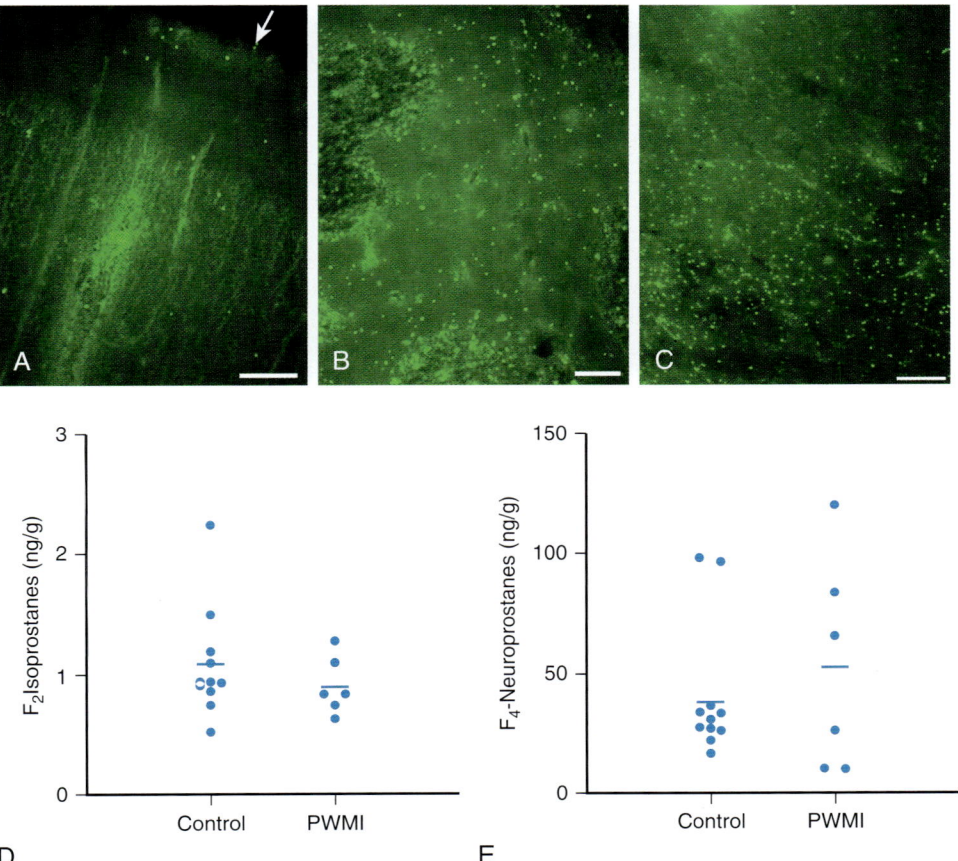

Figure 15.10 In contrast to preOLs, neurons and axons are markedly more resistant to oxidative injury in gray and white matter. (A and B) Typical paucity of neuronal death in the overlying cerebral cortex (A) from a preterm infant with diffuse white matter injury (WMI) at autopsy that showed extensive preOL degeneration (B and C). The individual degenerating cells appear as bright green dots. The arrow in A marks the pial surface. (D and E). When compared to controls, no significant oxidative injury to the cerebral cortex was observed in autopsy brains where significant preterm WMI (PWMI) was observed. F_2Isoprostanes are a general marker of oxidative injury to cells, and F_4-Neuroprostanes specifically detect injury to neurons and axons. Scale bars: A, 200 μm; B, 100 μm; C, 200 μm. (Adapted with permission from Back SA, Luo NL, Mallinson RA, et al. Selective vulnerability of preterm white matter to oxidative damage defined by F2-isoprostanes. *Ann Neurol.* 2005;58:108–120.)

plasma of human premature infants indicated a propensity to generate free radicals, including the hydroxyl radical; increases in plasma non–protein-bound iron, accentuated by hypoxia or blood transfusion; and impaired antioxidant defenses.[286-293] *Taken together, the findings support a maturation-dependent window of vulnerability to oxidative attack during the period in preterm white* *matter development when preOLs predominate in the white matter* (see Chapter 13 and Box 15.1).

Vulnerability to Excitotoxicity

As detailed in Chapter 13, glutamate is capable of inducing maturation-dependent death of preOLs by non–receptor-mediated and receptor-mediated mechanisms. The *non–receptor-mediated mechanism* involves glutamate competition for the cystine transporter and promotion of cystine efflux under conditions of high extracellular levels of glutamate.[294-296] Depletion of intracellular glutathione (which requires cysteine for biosynthesis) is accompanied by cell death by oxidative stress. However, the substantial levels (millimolar) of glutamate required for this effect suggest that this mechanism may not operate in vivo under most pathological conditions. By contrast, the *receptor-mediated mechanism*, which requires micromolar levels of glutamate, is more likely to occur in vivo, as shown directly in animal models (see Chapter 13). Both α-amino-3-hydroxy-5-methyl-4-isoxazolepropionic acid (AMPA) and *N*-methyl-D-aspartate (NMDA) receptors appear to be involved.

The *principal sources of elevated extracellular glutamate* in cerebral white matter with hypoxia-ischemia are glutamate transporters (see Chapter 13). Glutamate transporters constitute a family of 5 human genes, EAAT1-5.[297] The important transporters in the forebrain are EAAT1-3. All three transporters are detected in developing white matter, but expression in preOLs has not been specifically defined.[298,299]

Failure of glutamate uptake and actual reversal of transport occur in the setting of energy failure because of the failure of the high-affinity sodium-potassium ion pump. Experimental in vitro studies support the concept of a fatal feedback loop in developing OLs whereby in the setting of energy failure, reverse glutamate transport occurs to provide a source of extracellular glutamate.[300-302] When activated, glutamate receptors expressed on the same cells mediate excessive influx of calcium, which triggers excitotoxic injury and cell death. This model of excitotoxic injury in the immature brain contrasts with that in the mature brain and may be a cell-autonomous process in which certain populations of cells provide both the source and the target for pathological accumulations of glutamate.

Excessive glutamate receptor activation during ischemia requires an elevation in extracellular glutamate and a concomitant glutamate loss from at least one cellular compartment. The *potential sources of glutamate release to cerebral white matter* include astrocytes, OLs, axons and cells of the choroid plexus. In experimental perinatal hypoxia-ischemia studies, depletion of glutamate in vivo was most pronounced in axons and premyelinating stages of the OL lineage, which suggested that re-uptake mechanisms may be immature in the perinatal brain or dysfunctional during hypoxia-ischemia.[303]

The critical initiators of excitotoxic cell death are *glutamate receptors*. Focal expression of NMDA receptors on the processes of OL progenitors and mature OLs in vivo mediates a rapid, Ca^{2+}-dependent, disintegration of OL processes under in vitro conditions that mimic ischemia, and NMDA receptors have been found on premyelinating oligodendrocytes in developing human white matter.[304-308] As described in Chapter 13, glutamate toxicity to preOLs in vitro is also mediated by ionotropic glutamate receptors (iGluRs) of the AMPA/kainate type.[309-319] Although these in vitro studies suggest that calcium-permeable AMPA receptors on preOLs might be important in WMI, there remains uncertainty about whether preOLs in vivo express this type of receptor. Cells deficient in the GluR2 subunit render them Ca^{2+} permeable and thereby capable of toxicity. Increased expression of the GluR4 subunit occurs between 23 and 32 weeks of gestation in human parietal white matter and

P7 rat corpus callosum.[320] The timing of calcium permeable AMPA type glutamate receptor expression and NMDA receptor expression during human and rat white matter development thus appears to coincide with the window of heightened susceptibility to WMI,[306,321,322] but there remains uncertainty about whether human preOLs in vivo express these types of receptors during the peak period for WMI during preterm white matter development. Further in vivo studies are needed to verify the direct toxicity of glutamate to preOLs, other OL lineage stages, and astrocytes.[308,323-325] NMDA and AMPA/kainate receptor antagonists prevented myelin loss after perinatal hypoxia-ischemia in the term equivalent rat.[320,326,327] However, the efficacy of glutamate receptor antagonists to directly block degeneration of preOLs and axons in vivo remains largely unstudied.

Other Potentially Vulnerable White Matter–Associated Cellular Elements

Preterm cerebral white matter contains numerous neurons that include transient populations (e.g., migrating neuronal progenitors and subplate neurons) as well as interstitial neurons that appear to reside permanently in the white matter. *Axons* are in a state of very active development in cerebral white matter of the human premature infant.[328,329] The confluence of developing ascending and descending projection fibers, commissural fibers, and sagittal corticocortical association fibers in the peritrigonal region is particularly prominent at this time and may also degenerate in more severe WMI.[330]

Data from experimental studies found that immature neurons in preterm white and gray matter are surprisingly resistant to moderately severe hypoxia-ischemia that is of sufficient magnitude to cause diffuse WMI and selective preOL degeneration.[331,332] Not unexpectedly, both neurons and axons nonselectively undergo necrotic degeneration in more severe destructive lesions that diffusely target glia as well. *Subplate neurons* were initially proposed to be selectively vulnerable to hypoxia-ischemia in neonatal rats,[333] but subsequent extensive studies found that this transient population degenerates primarily in severe lesions in association with other populations of cortical neurons.[269] In more severe WMI, preterm human subplate neurons degenerate in lesions where other populations of neurons also degenerate.[266,267] In chronic diffuse noncystic WMI, the subplate and adjacent regions display evidence of sustained inflammatory responses.[334] Studies in preterm fetal sheep found that diffuse WMI was not accompanied by acute or delayed degeneration of migrating neurons destined to become GABAergic interneurons.[332] A single small neuropathological study found a decrease in GABAergic neurons in the white matter of infants with severe necrotic WMI, but other classes of neurons that typically degenerate in such lesions were not studied.[335] More data are needed on this issue.

Axonal degeneration is a prominent feature of WMI when necrosis is identified.[336,337] For example, axonal injury has been observed in regions of chronic human diffuse WMI that are adjacent to regions of necrosis,[337] but these dystrophic axons are likely to be structurally continuous with the degenerating axons in necrotic foci. Necrotic lesions are a minor component of WMI in both recent human studies[191] and experimental models[338] and comprise only about 5% of the total burden of WMI. During the *acute* phase of diffuse WMI in preterm fetal sheep, axonal injury was rarely observed,[40] and in chronic

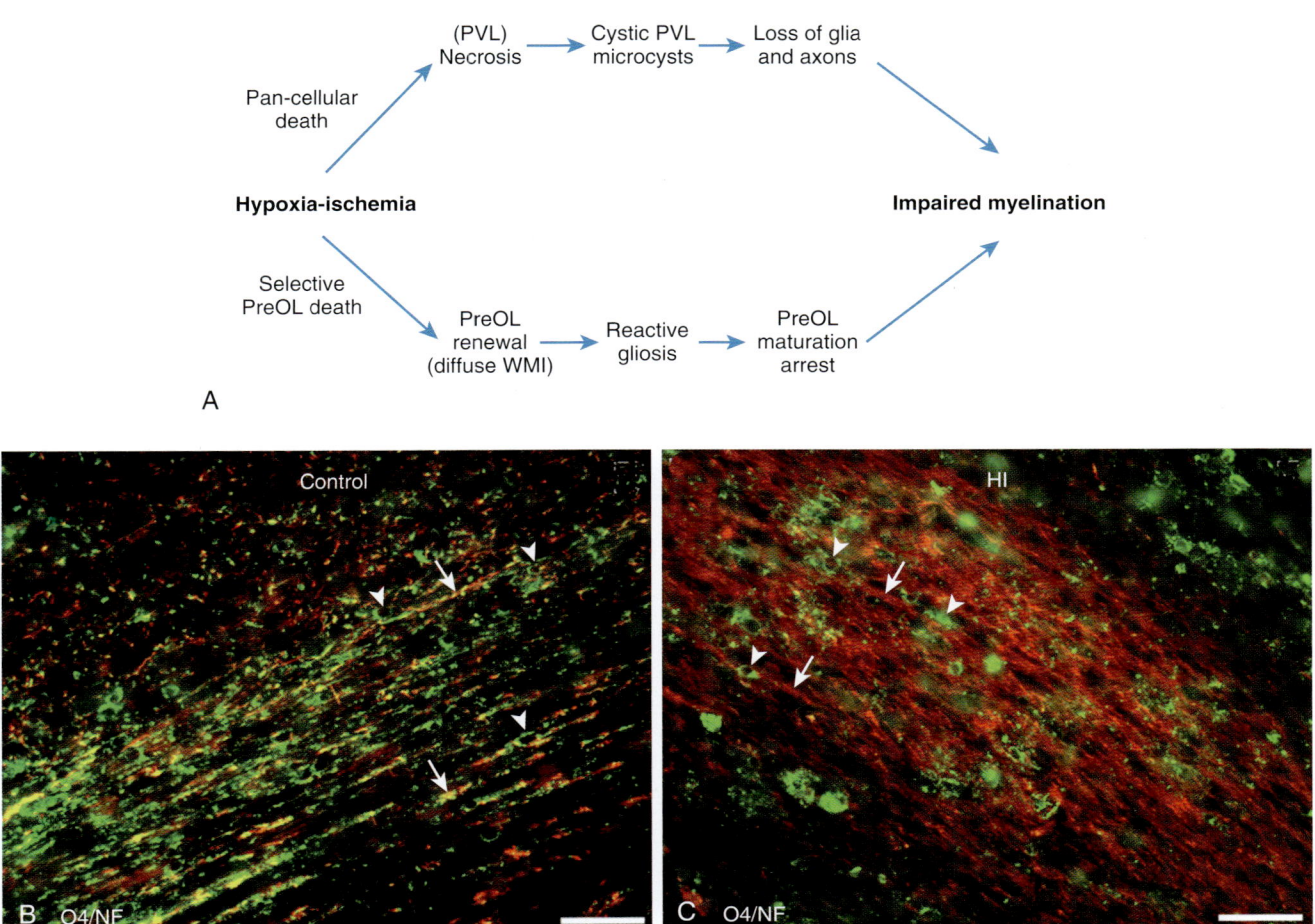

Figure 15.11 Pathogenesis of myelination failure in chronic diffuse white matter injury (WMI). (A) Distinctly different pathogenetic mechanisms mediate abnormal myelination in focal necrotic lesions (periventricular leukomalacia [PVL]; upper pathway) versus lesions with diffuse WMI (lower pathway). When more severe, hypoxia-ischemia (HI) triggers white matter necrosis (upper pathway) with pancellular degeneration that depletes the white matter of glia and axons. Severe necrosis results in cystic PVL, whereas milder necrosis results in microcysts. Milder HI (lower pathway) selectively triggers early preOL death, but preOLs are rapidly regenerated in chronic lesions enriched in reactive astrocytes that contribute to a block in preOL differentiation to myelinating oligodendrocytes. Myelination failure in diffuse WMI thus results from preOL arrest rather than axonal degeneration, as occurs with white matter necrosis. The lower pathway is the dominant one for many contemporary preterm survivors, whereas the minor upper pathway reflects the declining burden of white matter necrosis. (B) Typical appearance of normal early myelination in neonatal rodents. Axons are visualized in red, and early myelination of axons is in green. (C) Arrested maturation of preOLs in a chronic white matter lesion where numerous preOLs (*green*) are seen, but the axons (*red*) are diffusely unmyelinated. Scale bars = 100 μm. (Reprinted with permission from Back SA, Miller SP. Brain injury in premature neonates: a primary cerebral dysmaturation disorder? *Ann Neurol.* 2014;75:469–486.)

diffuse WMI, no significant axonal degeneration, axonal loss, or shift in the distribution of axon calibers was observed by quantitative electron microscopy studies.[339] Hence, the major sites of axonal degeneration are necrotic lesions, and axons appear to be structurally intact in diffuse WMI. The *functional integrity* of axons in diffuse lesions is difficult to study and is an important direction for future study.

Factors Related to the Progression of Chronic White Matter Injury

As discussed earlier, focal necrotic WMI results in myelination failure, which is likely to be permanent, because it is typically accompanied by loss of all glial cells, including preOLs and

astrocytes, as well as loss of axons that are required for myelination (Fig. 15.11). The pathogenesis of focal necrotic WMI is distinct from the processes that lead to non-necrotic diffuse WMI (Box 15.5). The evolution of diffuse WMI comprises two major overlapping events that contribute to a process of disrupted regeneration and repair of chronic lesions with disturbances in the normal progression of oligodendrocyte lineage maturation and myelination (see Fig. 15.11). The first event involves an *early cell proliferative response* to WMI in which early oligodendrocyte progenitor cells increase in subacute lesions. This plasticity response results in regeneration of preOLs that have degenerated during acute WMI. The second overlapping event occurs over days to weeks and involves a *disruption in the normal maturational processes* by which preOLs differentiate to myelinating oligodendrocytes. Hence, despite the pronounced selective degeneration of preOLs in early diffuse WMI, disturbances in myelination in chronic lesions do not appear to arise from a loss of myelinating cells but rather from newly generated oligodendrocyte progenitor cells (OPCs) that fail to fully mature (see earlier).

Glial Cell Proliferative Responses

Although it was initially hypothesized that abnormal myelination arises from a persistent loss of preOLs,[340] several later experimental studies found that surviving preOLs in preterm-equivalent rats rapidly increased in number to regenerate depleted preOLs.[79,341,342] Although preOLs are a mitotically active population of cells, expansion of the preOL pool appears to be driven mostly by a large reservoir of early OL progenitors that proliferate locally in white matter lesions. A potential alternative source is the neural stem cell–rich subventricular zone, where less robust generation of OL lineage cells has been observed.[343-345] Several human studies similarly have found that preOLs are not depleted in chronic lesions.[191,346] Despite a pronounced loss of preOLs during the acute phase of WMI,[77] rigorous quantitative studies identified a significant diffuse *increase* in the total pool of oligodendrocyte lineage cells in chronic lesions from subjects that survived for about 2 to 3 weeks after birth.[191] This increase in oligodendrocyte lineage cells was related to a significant increase in preOLs. The expansion in the pool of human preOLs was associated with diffuse activation of microglia and astrocytes. This diffuse inflammatory response thus accompanies the robust proliferative response of early OL progenitors and points to a generalized activation of multiple glial cell populations in response to WMI.

Disrupted preOL Maturation in Chronic Lesions

A major consequence of the chronic glial inflammatory response in advanced white matter lesions is a *disruption of the normal progression of oligodendrocyte lineage maturation and myelination.* Although a large pool of preOLs are regenerated and survive in chronic WMI, these cells fail to normally differentiate. In preterm equivalent rodents and preterm fetal sheep, chronic hypoxic-ischemic lesions display disrupted maturation of preOLs that fail to normally progress to myelinating oligodendrocytes. In diffuse WMI in preterm sheep, an approximate doubling in the density of preOLs in lesions coincided with approximately a 50% reduction in oligodendrocytes.[338] In human chronic diffuse WMI, an increase in preOLs similarly coincided with a decline in the total percentage of oligodendrocytes.[191] It is important to note that this arrested maturation of preOLs was significantly associated with the magnitude of astrogliosis both in preterm fetal sheep and humans.[191,338] As discussed later, several astrocyte-derived factors have been linked to arrested preOL maturation and myelination failure.

Since preOLs do not differentiate along their normal developmental time course, disturbances in myelination occur despite the presence of numerous intact axons within the chronic lesions. In chronic diffuse WMI in preterm fetal sheep, for example,[40] no significant axonal degeneration, axonal loss, or shift in the distribution of axon sizes was identified by light or quantitative electron microscopy studies.[338,339] The *long-term functional integrity of axons* in chronic WMI is important to define, since viable OLs and myelination are critical for axon survival.[347]

The impact of preOL arrest on the severity of recurrent WMI is unclear from experimental studies. Preterm-equivalent rodents displayed a pronounced increase in cell death in chronic WMI after recurrent hypoxia-ischemia.[79] However, in preterm fetal sheep, whose lesions more closely resemble humans, recurrent hypoxia-ischemia did not trigger enhanced WMI, which suggested that preOL maturation arrest may confer protection against recurrent WMI.[81] An important future direction would be a detailed cellular and molecular analysis of mechanisms of ischemic tolerance in chronic preterm WMI.

Molecular Mechanisms of Arrested Maturation of preOLs and Myelination Disturbances

Recognition that a sizeable pool of preOLs persists in chronic white matter lesions suggests the potential to promote repair of WMI through strategies that promote preOL differentiation. Disrupted maturation of oligodendrocyte progenitors in chronic white matter lesions has been extensively studied in experimental models of adult myelination failure related to multiple sclerosis and vascular dementias. From such studies a complex array of intrinsic, extrinsic, and epigenetic factors have been shown to regulate the cell cycle, maturation, and myelination of oligodendrocyte lineage cells.[348-352] Numerous genes are activated by oxidative stress, which regulates OL maturation, and oxidative stress promotes global histone acetylation, which can block OL differentiation.[353-357] Post-transcriptional control by microRNAs regulates OL differentiation and OL progenitors that lack mature microRNAs display arrested maturation.[358,359]

Disruption of the extracellular matrix is a prominent feature of chronic WMI and is linked to diffuse reactive astrogliosis. In diffuse preterm human WMI, the extracellular matrix (ECM) is a *rich source of hyaluronic acid (HA) and one of its receptors, CD44.*[191] *CD44-positive reactive astrocytes* are significantly associated with the magnitude of WMI. Reactive astrocytes synthesize high-molecular-weight forms of hyaluronic acid that accumulates in lesions.[360] Arrest of preOL maturation is stimulated both in vitro and in vivo by high-molecular-weight forms of hyaluronic acid that are digested to bioactive forms by CNS enriched hyaluronidases that orient to the extracellular matrix.[81,361-363] Pharmacological inhibition of hyaluronidases promotes OL maturation in vitro and myelination in vivo, which is accompanied by enhanced nerve conduction.[363]

Reactive astrocytes display enhanced expression of *bone morphogenetic proteins* that inhibit OL progenitor differentiation and promote astrocyte differentiation.[364] The *Notch ligand Jagged1* is elevated on reactive astrocytes in demyelinating lesions and activates Notch signaling on OL progenitors, preventing their maturation.[365] Dysregulation of *WNT-beta catenin signaling* in OL progenitors promotes preOL arrest, delays normal myelination, and disrupts remyelination.[131,133,366-369] Constitutive expression of the *epidermal growth factor receptor* (EGFR) in neonatal white matter promotes proliferation of OL progenitors,[370] and enhanced EGFR signaling stimulates adult CNS myelination and remyelination.[371] EGFR activation via an intranasally administered form of EGF reduced OL death from chronic neonatal hypoxia, promoted OL maturation and myelination, and led to functional improvement.[130]

Since multiple signaling pathways appear to be involved in the pathogenesis of chronic WMI and myelination failure, one potential therapeutic strategy is to target multiple signaling pathways via the pleiotropic growth factor, erythropoietin (EPO), which has demonstrated actions to promote angiogenesis, neurogenesis, and gliogenesis during normal brain maturation.[306,372-377] A randomized trial of intravenously administered recombinant high-dose EPO to preterm infants in the first 2 days of life was safe and associated with enhanced MRI-defined white matter maturation,[378,379] but 2-year neurodevelopmental outcomes were not improved.[380] A recent double-blinded, placebo-controlled trial of EPO administered with therapeutic hypothermia showed potential benefit for neonatal encephalopathy in term infants. MRI-defined brain injury in the perinatal period was significantly reduced, as well as improved motor function at 1 year of age.[381]

An important future direction will be to define the evolution of cerebral white matter lesions over months to years to identify the relative contributions of dysmyelination and axonal dysfunction to functional disabilities in preterm survivors. Such information is of critical importance to define the period over which chronic WMI may be repaired and to better identify mechanisms to promote additional regeneration and repair of WMI.

KEY REFERENCES

2. De Reuck JL. Cerebral angioarchitecture and perinatal brain lesions in premature and full-term infants. *Acta Neurol Scand.* 1984;70:391-395.
3. De Reuck J, Chattha AS, Richardson EP Jr. Pathogenesis and evolution of periventricular leukomalacia in infancy. *Arch Neurol.* 1972;27:229-236.
4. Takashima S, Tanaka K. Development of cerebrovascular architecture and its relationship to periventricular leukomalacia. *Arch Neurol.* 1978;35:11-16.
7. Larroche JC. *Developmental Pathology of the Neonate.* New York: Excerpta Medica; 1977.
8. Inage YW, Itoh M, Takashima S. Correlation between cerebrovascular maturity and periventricular leukomalacia. *Pediatr Neurol.* 2000;22:204-208.
10. Nelson MD, Gonzalez-Gomez I, Gilles FH. The search for human telencephalic ventriculofugal arteries. *AJNR Am J Neuroradiol.* 1991;12:215-222.
12. Ballabh P, Braun A, Nedergaard M. Anatomic analysis of blood vessels in germinal matrix, cerebral cortex, and white matter in developing infants. *Pediatr Res.* 2004;56:117-124.
21. Altman DI, Powers WJ, Perlman JM, et al. Cerebral blood flow requirement for brain viability in newborn infants is lower than in adults. *Ann Neurol.* 1988;24:218-226.
23. Powers WJ, Grubb RL, Darriet D, et al. Cerebral blood flow and cerebral metabolic rate of oxygen requirements for cerebral function and viability in humans. *J Cereb Blood Flow Metab.* 1985;5:600-608.
24. Pryds O. Control of cerebral circulation in the high-risk neonate. *Ann Neurol.* 1991;30:321-329.
25. Younkin DP, Reivich M, Jaggi JL, et al. The effect of hematocrit and systolic blood pressure on cerebral blood flow in newborn infants. *J Cereb Blood Flow Metab.* 1987;7:295-299.
28. Muller AM, Morales C, Briner J, et al. Loss of CO_2 reactivity of cerebral blood flow is associated with severe brain damage in mechanically ventilated very low birth weight infants. *Eur J Paediatr Neurol.* 1997;5:157-163.
30. von Siebenthal K, Beran J, Wolf M, et al. Cyclical fluctuations in blood pressure, heart rate and cerebral blood volume in preterm infants. *Brain Dev.* 1999;21:529-534.
31. Tsuji M, Saul JP, du Plessis A, et al. Cerebral intravascular oxygenation correlates with mean arterial pressure in critically ill premature infants. *Pediatrics.* 2000;106:625-632.
32. Lemmers PM, Toet M, van Schelven LJ, et al. Cerebral oxygenation and cerebral oxygen extraction in the preterm infant: the impact of respiratory distress syndrome. *Exp Brain Res.* 2006;173:458-467.
33. Soul JS, Hammer PE, Tsuji M, et al. Fluctuating pressure-passivity is common in the cerebral circulation of sick premature infants. *Pediatr Res.* 2007;61:467-473.
35. Rhee CJ, Fraser CD, Kibler K, et al. The ontogeny of cerebrovascular pressure autoregulation in premature infants. *Acta Neurochir Suppl.* 2016;122:151-155.
36. O'Leary H, Gregas MC, Limperopoulos C, et al. Elevated cerebral pressure passivity is associated with prematurity-related intracranial hemorrhage. *Pediatrics.* 2009;124:302-309.
37. Wong FY, Silas R, Hew S, et al. Cerebral oxygenation is highly sensitive to blood pressure variability in sick preterm infants. *PLoS ONE.* 2012;7:e43165.
38. da Costa CS, Czosnyka M, Smielewski P, et al. Monitoring of cerebrovascular reactivity for determination of optimal blood pressure in preterm infants. *J Pediatr.* 2015;167:86-91.
39. Iadecola C, Nedergaard M. Glial regulation of the cerebral microvasculature. *Nat Neurosci.* 2007;10:1369-1376.
40. Riddle A, Luo NL, Manese M, et al. Spatial heterogeneity in oligodendrocyte lineage maturation and not cerebral blood flow predicts fetal ovine periventricular white matter injury. *J Neurosci.* 2006;26:3045-3055.
41. McClure MM, Riddle A, Manese M, et al. Cerebral blood flow heterogeneity in preterm sheep: lack of physiologic support for vascular boundary zones in fetal cerebral white matter. *J Cereb Blood Flow Metab.* 2008;28:995-1008.
46. Gleason CA, Short BL, Jones MD Jr. Cerebral blood flow and metabolism during and after prolonged hypocapnia in newborn lambs. *J Pediatr.* 1989;115:309-314.
48. Erickson SJ, Grauaug A, Gurrin L, et al. Hypocarbia in the ventilated preterm infant and its effect on intraventricular haemorrhage and bronchopulmonary dysplasia. *J Paediatr Child Health.* 2002;38:560-562.
49. Greisen G, Vannucci RC. Is periventricular leucomalacia a result of hypoxic-ischaemic injury? Hypocapnia and the preterm brain. *Biol Neonate.* 2001;79:194-200.
50. Hamrick SE, Miller SP, Leonard C, et al. Trends in severe brain injury and neurodevelopmental outcome in premature newborn infants: the role of cystic periventricular leukomalacia. *J Pediatr.* 2004;145:593-599.

53. Okumura A, Hayakawa F, Kato T, et al. Hypocarbia in preterm infants with periventricular leukomalacia: the relation between hypocarbia and mechanical ventilation. *Pediatrics*. 2001;107: 469-475.

55. Wiswell TE, Graziani LJ, Kornhauser MS, et al. Effects of hypocarbia on the development of cystic periventricular leukomalacia in premature infants treated with high-frequency jet ventilation. *Pediatrics*. 1996;98:918-924.

56. Shankaran S, Langer JC, Kazzi SN, et al. Cumulative index of exposure to hypocarbia and hyperoxia as risk factors for periventricular leukomalacia in low birth weight infants. *Pediatrics*. 2006;118:1654-1659.

59. Ou X, Glasier CM, Ramakrishnaiah RH, et al. Diffusion tensor imaging in extremely low birth weight infants managed with hypercapnic vs. normocapnic ventilation. *Pediatr Radiol*. 2014;44:980-986.

66. Bassan H, Gauvreau K, Newburger JW, et al. Identification of pressure passive cerebral perfusion and its mediators after infant cardiac surgery. *Pediatr Res*. 2005;57:35-41.

72. Gleason CA, Hamm C, Jones MD Jr. Cerebral blood flow, oxygenation, and carbohydrate metabolism in immature fetal sheep in utero. *Am J Physiol*. 1989;256:R1264-R1268.

74. Papile LA, Rudolph AM, Heymann MA. Autoregulation of cerebral blood flow in the preterm fetal lamb. *Pediatr Res*. 1985;19:159-161.

76. Haynes RL, Folkerth RD, Keefe RJ, et al. Nitrosative and oxidative injury to premyelinating oligodendrocytes in periventricular leukomalacia. *J Neuropathol Exp Neurol*. 2003;62:441-450.

77. Back SA, Luo NL, Mallinson RA, et al. Selective vulnerability of preterm white matter to oxidative damage defined by F_2-isoprostanes. *Ann Neurol*. 2005;58:108-120.

78. Back SA, Han BH, Luo NL, et al. Selective vulnerability of late oligodendrocyte progenitors to hypoxia-ischemia. *J Neurosci*. 2002;22:455-463.

79. Segovia K, McClure M, Moravec M, et al. Arrested oligodendrocyte lineage maturation in chronic perinatal white matter injury. *Ann Neurol*. 2008;63:517-526.

80. Buser JR, Segovia KN, Dean JM, et al. Timing of appearance of late oligodendrocyte progenitors coincides with enhanced susceptibility of preterm rabbit cerebral white matter to hypoxia-ischemia. *J Cereb Blood Flow Metab*. 2010;30:1053-1065.

81. Hagen MW, Riddle A, McClendon E, et al. Role of recurrent hypoxia-ischemia in preterm white matter injury severity. *PLoS ONE*. 2014;9:e112800.

82. Low JA, Froese AF, Galbraith RS, et al. The association of fetal and newborn metabolic acidosis with severe periventricular leukomalacia in the preterm newborn. *Am J Obstet Gynecol*. 1990; 162:977-981.

88. Shortland DB, Gibson NA, Levene MI, et al. Patent ductus arteriosus and cerebral circulation in preterm infants. *Dev Med Child Neurol*. 1990;32:386-393.

95. Kinney HC, Panigrahy A, Newburger JW, et al. Hypoxic-ischemic brain injury in infants with congenital heart disease dying after cardiac surgery. *Acta Neuropathol (Berl)*. 2005;110:563-578.

96. Hammers AL, Sanchez-Ramos L, Kaunitz AM. Antenatal exposure to indomethacin increases the risk of severe intraventricular hemorrhage, necrotizing enterocolitis, and periventricular leukomalacia: a systematic review with metaanalysis. *Am J Obstet Gynecol*. 2015;212:505.e1-505.e3.

97. Morgan JL, Nelson DB, Casey BM, et al. Impact of metabolic acidemia at birth on neonatal outcomes in infants born before 34 weeks' gestation. *J Matern Fetal Neonatal Med*. 2016;1-4.

98. Tsimis ME, Johnson CT, Raghunathan RS, et al. Risk factors for periventricular white matter injury in very low birthweight neonates. *Am J Obstet Gynecol*. 2016;214:380.e1-380.e6.

99. Perlman JM, Hill A, Volpe JJ. The effect of patent ductus arteriosus on flow velocity in the anterior cerebral arteries: ductal steal in the premature newborn infant. *J Pediatr*. 1981;99:767-771.

100. Lipman B, Serwer GA, Brazy JE. Abnormal cerebral hemodynamics in preterm infants with patent ductus arteriosus. *Pediatrics*. 1982;69: 778-781.

105. Sperandio M, Beedgen B, Feneberg R, et al. Effectiveness and side effects of an escalating, stepwise approach to indomethacin treatment for symptomatic patent ductus arteriosus in premature infants below 33 weeks of gestation. *Pediatrics*. 2005;116:1361-1366.

108. Perlman JM, Volpe JJ. Episodes of apnea and bradycardia in the preterm newborn: impact on cerebral circulation. *Pediatrics*. 1985;76:333-338.

110. Urlesberger B, Kaspirek A, Pichler G, et al. Apnea of prematurity and changes in cerebral oxygenation and cerebral blood volume. *Neuropediatrics*. 1999;30:29-33.

111. Payer C, Urlesberger B, Pauger M, et al. Apnea associated with hypoxia in preterm infants: impact on cerebral blood volume. *Brain Dev*. 2003;25:25-31.

113. Back SA, Craig A, Ling Luo N, et al. Protective effects of caffeine on chronic hypoxia-induced perinatal white matter injury. *Ann Neurol*. 2006;60:696-705.

114. Schmidt B, Roberts RS, Davis P, et al. Caffeine therapy for apnea of prematurity. *N Engl J Med*. 2006;354:2112-2121.

115. Henderson-Smart DJ, De Paoli AG. Methylxanthine treatment for apnoea in preterm infants. *Cochrane Database Syst Rev*. 2010;(12):CD000140.

116. Schmidt B, Anderson PJ, Doyle LW, et al. Survival without disability to age 5 years after neonatal caffeine therapy for apnea of prematurity. *JAMA*. 2012;307:275-282.

117. Lodha A, Seshia M, McMillan DD, et al. Association of early caffeine administration and neonatal outcomes in very preterm neonates. *JAMA Pediatr*. 2015;169:33-38.

119. Miller SP, McQuillen PS, Hamrick SE, et al. Abnormal brain development in newborns with congenital heart disease. *N Engl J Med*. 2007;357:1928-1938.

120. Licht DJ, Shera DM, Clancy RR, et al. Brain maturation is delayed in infants with complex congenital heart defects. *J Thorac Cardiovasc Surg*. 2009;137:529-536, discussion 536-537.

121. du Plessis AJ, Newburger J, Jonas RA, et al. Cerebral oxygen supply and utilization during infant cardiac surgery. *Ann Neurol*. 1995;37:488-497.

123. Jain V, Buckley EM, Licht DJ, et al. Cerebral oxygen metabolism in neonates with congenital heart disease quantified by MRI and optics. *J Cereb Blood Flow Metab*. 2014;34:380-388.

124. Sun L, Macgowan CK, Sled JG, et al. Reduced fetal cerebral oxygen consumption is associated with smaller brain size in fetuses with congenital heart disease. *Circulation*. 2015;131:1313-1323.

125. Volpe JJ. Encephalopathy of congenital heart disease—destructive and developmental effects intertwined. *J Pediatr*. 2014;164:962-965.

128. Wellmann S, Buhrer C, Schmitz T. Focal necrosis and disturbed myelination in the white matter of newborn infants: a tale of too much or too little oxygen. *Front Pediatr*. 2014;2:143.

130. Scafidi J, Hammond TR, Scafidi S, et al. Intranasal epidermal growth factor treatment rescues neonatal brain injury. *Nature*. 2014;506:230-234.

131. Fancy SP, Baranzini SE, Zhao C, et al. Dysregulation of the Wnt pathway inhibits timely myelination and remyelination in the mammalian CNS. *Genes Dev*. 2009;23:1571-1585.

132. Fancy SP, Harrington EP, Baranzini SE, et al. Parallel states of pathological Wnt signaling in neonatal brain injury and colon cancer. *Nat Neurosci*. 2014;17:506-512.

133. Fancy SP, Harrington EP, Yuen TJ, et al. Axin2 as regulatory and therapeutic target in newborn brain injury and remyelination. *Nat Neurosci*. 2011;14:1009-1016.

135. Licht T, Dor-Wollman T, Ben-Zvi A, et al. Vessel maturation schedule determines vulnerability to neuronal injuries of prematurity. *J Clin Invest*. 2015;125:1319-1328.

137. Eklind S, Mallard C, Arvidsson P, et al. Lipopolysaccharide induces both a primary and a secondary phase of sensitization in the developing rat brain. *Pediatr Res*. 2005;58:112-116.

138. Eklind S, Mallard C, Leverin A, et al. Bacterial endotoxin sensitizes the immature brain to hypoxic—ischaemic injury. *Eur J Neurosci*. 2001;13:1101-1106.

139. Mallard C, Hagberg H. Inflammation-induced preconditioning in the immature brain. *Semin Fetal Neonatal Med*. 2007;12:280-286.

147. Mittendorf R, Montag AG, MacMillan W, et al. Components of the systemic fetal inflammatory response syndrome as predictors of impaired neurologic outcomes in children. *Am J Obstet Gynecol*. 2003;188:1438-1444, discussion 1444-1436.

150. Resch B, Vollaard E, Maurer U, et al. Risk factors and determinants of neurodevelopmental outcome in cystic periventricular leucomalacia. *Eur J Pediatr*. 2000;159:663-670.

151. Wu YW, Colford JM. Chorioamnionitis as a risk factor for cerebral palsy. A meta-analysis. *JAMA*. 2000;284:1417-1424.

152. Yoon BH, Romero R, Park JS, et al. Fetal exposure to an intra-amniotic inflammation and the development of cerebral palsy at the age of three years. *Am J Obstet Gynecol*. 2000;182:675-681.

155. Duggan PJ, Maalouf EF, Watts TL, et al. Intrauterine T-cell activation and increased proinflammatory cytokine concentrations in preterm infants with cerebral lesions. *Lancet*. 2001;358: 1699-1700.

157. Yoon BH, Romero R, Yang SH, et al. Interleukin-6 concentrations in umbilical cord plasma are elevated in neonates with white matter lesions associated with periventricular leukomalacia. *Am J Obstet Gynecol*. 1996;174:1433-1440.

158. Nelson KB, Grether JK, Dambrosia JM, et al. Neonatal cytokines and cerebral palsy in very preterm infants. *Pediatr Res*. 2003;53:600-607.

160. Chau V, McFadden DE, Poskitt KJ, et al. Chorioamnionitis in the pathogenesis of brain injury in preterm infants. *Clin Perinatol*. 2014;41:83-103.

161. Locatelli A, Vergani P, Ghidini A, et al. Duration of labor and risk of cerebral white-matter damage in very preterm infants who are delivered with intrauterine infection. *Am J Obstet Gynecol*. 2005;193:928-932.

162. Chau V, Brant R, Poskitt KJ, et al. Postnatal infection is associated with widespread abnormalities of brain development in premature newborns. *Pediatr Res*. 2012;71:274-279.

163. Shah DK, Doyle LW, Anderson PJ, et al. Adverse neurodevelopment in preterm infants with postnatal sepsis or necrotizing enterocolitis is mediated by white matter abnormalities on magnetic resonance imaging at term. *J Pediatr*. 2008;153:170-175, 175.e1.

164. Stoll BJ, Hansen NI, AdamsChapman I, et al. Neurodevelopmental and growth impairment among extremely low-birth-weight infants with neonatal infection. *JAMA*. 2004;292:2357-2365.

165. Martin CR, Dammann O, Allred EN, et al. Neurodevelopment of extremely preterm infants who had necrotizing enterocolitis with or without late bacteremia. *J Pediatr*. 2010;157:751-756.e1.

166. Schulzke SM, Deshpande GC, Patole SK. Neurodevelopmental outcomes of very low-birth-weight infants with necrotizing enterocolitis: a systematic review of observational studies. *Arch Pediatr Adolesc Med*. 2007;161:583-590.

167. Lee SY, Ng DK, Fung GP, et al. Chorioamnionitis with or without funisitis increases the risk of hypotension in very low birthweight infants on the first postnatal day but not later. *Arch Dis Child Fetal Neonatal Ed*. 2006;91:F346-F348.

168. Inder TE, Warfield SK, Wang H, et al. Abnormal cerebral structure is present at term in premature infants. *Pediatrics*. 2005;115: 286-294.

169. Reiman M, Kujari H, Maunu J, et al. Does placental inflammation relate to brain lesions and volume in preterm infants? *J Pediatr*. 2008;152:642-647, 647.e1-647.e2.

170. Chau V, Poskitt KJ, McFadden DE, et al. Effect of chorioamnionitis on brain development and injury in premature newborns. *Ann Neurol*. 2009;66:155-164.

171. Sato M, Nishimaki S, Yokota S, et al. Severity of chorioamnionitis and neonatal outcome. *J Obstet Gynaecol Res*. 2011;37:1313-1319.

172. Kaukola T, Herva R, Perhomaa M, et al. Population cohort associating chorioamnionitis, cord inflammatory cytokines and neurologic outcome in very preterm, extremely low birth weight infants. *Pediatr Res*. 2006;59:478-483.

173. Stoll BJ, Hansen N, Fanaroff AA, et al. Late-onset sepsis in very low birth weight neonates: the experience of the NICHD neonatal research network. *Pediatrics*. 2002;110:285-291.

175. Makhoul IR, Sujov P, Smolkin T, et al. Pathogen-specific early mortality in very low birth weight infants with late-onset sepsis: a national survey. *Clin Infect Dis*. 2005;40:218-224.

177. Inder TE, Wells SJ, Mogridge N, et al. Defining the nature of the cerebral abnormalities in the premature infant—a qualitative magnetic resonance imaging study. *J Pediatr*. 2003;143:171-179.

182. Kadhim HJ, Tabarki B, Verellen G, et al. Inflammatory cytokines in the pathogenesis of periventricular leukomalacia. *Neurology*. 2001;56:1278-1284.

183. Kadhim HJ, Tabarki B, De Prez C, et al. Interleukin-2 in the pathogenesis of perinatal white matter damage. *Neurology*. 2002;58: 1125-1128.

184. Folkerth RD, Keefe RJ, Haynes RL, et al. Interferon-gamma expression in periventricular leukomalacia in the human brain. *Brain Pathol*. 2004;14:265-274.

185. Threlkeld SW, Lynch JL, Lynch KM, et al. Ovine proinflammatory cytokines cross the murine blood-brain barrier by a common saturable transport mechanism. *Neuroimmunomodulation*. 2010;17: 405-410.

187. Chen X, Sadowska GB, Zhang J, et al. Neutralizing anti-interleukin-1beta antibodies modulate fetal blood-brain barrier function after ischemia. *Neurobiol Dis*. 2015;73:118-129.

189. Schmitz T, Heep A, Groenendaal F, et al. Interleukin-1beta, interleukin-18, and interferon-gamma expression in the cerebrospinal fluid of premature infants with posthemorrhagic hydrocephalus-markers of white matter damage? *Pediatr Res*. 2007;61: 722-726.

190. Ellison VJ, Mocatta TJ, Winterbourn CC, et al. The relationship of CSF and plasma cytokine levels to cerebral white matter injury in the premature newborn. *Pediatr Res*. 2005;57:282-286.

191. Buser J, Maire J, Riddle A, et al. Arrested pre-oligodendrocyte maturation contributes to myelination failure in premature infants. *Ann Neurol*. 2012;71:93-109.

193. Li J, Baud O, Vartanian T, et al. Peroxynitrite generated by inducible nitric oxide synthase and NADPH oxidase mediates microglial toxicity to oligodendrocytes. *Proc Natl Acad Sci USA*. 2005;102: 9936-9941.

200. Lin CY, Chang YC, Wang ST, et al. Altered inflammatory responses in preterm children with cerebral palsy. *Ann Neurol*. 2010;68: 204-212.

205. Favrais G, van de Looij Y, Fleiss B, et al. Systemic inflammation disrupts the developmental program of white matter. *Ann Neurol*. 2011;70:550-565.

223. Hu X, Leak RK, Shi Y, et al. Microglial and macrophage polarization-new prospects for brain repair. *Nat Rev Neurol*. 2015;11: 56-64.

226. Drobyshevsky A, Luo K, Derrick M, et al. Motor deficits are triggered by reperfusion-reoxygenation injury as diagnosed by MRI and by a mechanism involving oxidants. *J Neurosci*. 2012;32: 5500-5509.

228. Miron VE, Boyd A, Zhao JW, et al. M2 microglia and macrophages drive oligodendrocyte differentiation during CNS remyelination. *Nat Neurosci*. 2013;16:1211-1218.

230. Rezaie P, Cairns NJ, Male DK. Expression of adhesion molecules on human fetal cerebral vessels: relationship to microglial colonisation during development. *Brain Res Dev Brain Res*. 1997;104: 175-189.

233. Billiards SS, Haynes RL, Folkerth RD, et al. Development of microglia in the cerebral white matter of the human fetus and infant. *J Comp Neurol*. 2006;497:199-208.

234. Monier A, Evrard P, Gressens P, et al. Distribution and differentiation of microglia in the human encephalon during the first two trimesters of gestation. *J Comp Neurol*. 2006;499:565-582.

237. Verney C, Pogledic I, Biran V, et al. Microglial reaction in axonal crossroads is a hallmark of noncystic periventricular white matter injury in very preterm infants. *J Neuropathol Exp Neurol*. 2012;71: 251-264.

238. Supramaniam V, Vontell R, Srinivasan L, et al. Microglia activation in the extremely preterm human brain. *Pediatr Res*. 2013;73:301-309.

241. Yanowitz TD, Jordan JA, Gilmour CH, et al. Hemodynamic disturbances in premature infants born after chorioamnionitis: association with cord blood cytokine concentrations. *Pediatr Res*. 2002;51:310-316.

243. Yanowitz TD, Baker RW, Roberts JM, et al. Low blood pressure among very-low-birth-weight infants with fetal vessel inflammation. *J Perinatol*. 2004;24:299-304.

261. Wang X, Stridh L, Li W, et al. Lipopolysaccharide sensitizes neonatal hypoxic-ischemic brain injury in a MyD88-dependent manner. *J Immunol*. 2009;183:7471-7477.

266. Kinney H, Haynes R, Xu G, et al. Neuron deficit in the white matter and subplate in periventricular leukomalacia. *Ann Neurol*. 2012;71:397-406.

267. Andiman SE, Haynes RL, Trachtenberg FL, et al. The cerebral cortex overlying periventricular leukomalacia: analysis of pyramidal neurons. *Brain Pathol*. 2010;20:803-814.

268. Pierson CR, Folkerth RD, Billiards SS, et al. Gray matter injury associated with periventricular leukomalacia in the premature infant. *Acta Neuropathol*. 2007;114:619-631.

270. Back SA, Luo NL, Borenstein NS, et al. Late oligodendrocyte progenitors coincide with the developmental window of vulnerability for human perinatal white matter injury. *J Neurosci.* 2001;21:1302-1312.

274. Folkerth R, Haynes R, Borenstein NS, et al. Developmental lag in superoxide dismutases relative to other antioxidant enzymes in premyelinated human telencephalic white matter. *J Neuropathol Exp Neurol.* 2004;63:990-999.

275. Baud O, Haynes R, Wang H, et al. Developmental up-regulation of MnSOD in rat oligodendrocytes confers protection against oxidative injury. *Eur J Neurosci.* 2004;19:2669-2681.

276. Baud O, Greene A, Li J, et al. Glutathione peroxidase-catalase cooperativity is required for resistance to hydrogen peroxide by mature rat oligodendrocytes. *J Neurosci.* 2004;24:1531-1540.

279. Iida K, Takashima S, Ueda K. Immunohistochemical study of myelination and oligodendrocyte in infants with periventricular leukomalacia. *Pediatr Neurol.* 1995;13:296-304.

285. Savman K, Nilsson UA, Blennow M, et al. Non-protein-bound iron is elevated in cerebrospinal fluid from preterm infants with posthemorrhagic ventricular dilation. *Pediatr Res.* 2001;49:208-212.

291. Hirano K, Morinobu T, Kim H, et al. Blood transfusion increases radical promoting non-transferrin bound iron in preterm infants. *Arch Dis Child Fetal Neonatal Ed.* 2001;84:F188-F193.

294. Oka A, Belliveau MJ, Rosenberg PA, et al. Vulnerability of oligodendroglia to glutamate: pharmacology, mechanisms and prevention. *J Neurosci.* 1993;13:1441-1453.

298. Desilva TM, Kinney HC, Borenstein NS, et al. The glutamate transporter EAAT2 is transiently expressed in developing human cerebral white matter. *J Comp Neurol.* 2007;501:879-890.

300. Fern R, Moller T. Rapid ischemic cell death in immature oligodendrocytes: a fatal glutamate release feedback loop. *J Neurosci.* 2000;20:34-42.

301. Alix JJ, Fern R. Glutamate receptor-mediated ischemic injury of premyelinated central axons. *Ann Neurol.* 2009;66:682-693.

302. Alix JJ, Zammit C, Riddle A, et al. Central axons preparing to myelinate are highly sensitivity to ischemic injury. *Ann Neurol.* 2012;72:936-951.

306. Jantzie LL, Miller RH, Robinson S. Erythropoietin signaling promotes oligodendrocyte development following prenatal systemic hypoxic-ischemic brain injury. *Pediatr Res.* 2013;74:658-667.

308. Salter MG, Fern R. NMDA receptors are expressed in developing oligodendrocyte processes and mediate injury. *Nature.* 2005;438:1167-1171.

315. Rosenberg PA, Dai W, Gan XD, et al. Mature myelin basic protein expressing oligodendrocytes are insensitive to kainate toxicity. *J Neurosci Res.* 2003;71:237-245.

321. Talos DM, Follett PL, Folkerth RD, et al. Developmental regulation of alpha-amino-3-hydroxy-5-methyl-4-isoxazole-propionic acid receptor subunit expression in forebrain and relationship to

regional susceptibility to hypoxic/ischemic injury. II. Human cerebral white matter and cortex. *J Comp Neurol.* 2006;497:61-77.

328. Judas M, Rados M, JovanovMilosevic N, et al. Structural, immunocytochemical, and MR imaging properties of periventricular crossroads of growing cortical pathways in preterm infants. *AJNR Am J Neuroadiol.* 2005;26:2671-2684.

329. Haynes RL, Borenstein NS, DeSilva TM, et al. Axonal development in the cerebral white matter of the human fetus and infant. *J Comp Neurol.* 2005;484:156-167.

331. Dean J, McClendon E, Hansen K, et al. Prenatal cerebral ischemia disrupts MRI-defined cortical microstructure through disturbances in neuronal arborization. *Sci Transl Med.* 2013;5:101-111.

332. McClendon E, Chen K, Gong X, et al. Prenatal cerebral ischemia triggers dysmaturation of caudate projection neurons. *Ann Neurol.* 2014.

337. Haynes RL, Billiards SS, Borenstein NS, et al. Diffuse axonal injury in periventricular leukomalacia as determined by apoptotic marker fractin. *Pediatr Res.* 2008;63:656-661.

338. Riddle A, Dean J, Buser J, et al. Histopathological correlates of MRI-defined chronic perinatal white matter injury. *Ann Neurol.* 2011;70:493-507.

339. Riddle A, Maire J, Gong X, et al. Differential susceptibility to axonopathy in necrotic and non-necrotic perinatal white matter injury. *Stroke.* 2012;43:178-184.

349. Emery B, Agalliu D, Cahoy JD, et al. Myelin gene regulatory factor is a critical transcriptional regulator required for CNS myelination. *Cell.* 2009;138:172-185.

363. Preston M, Gong X, Su W, et al. Digestion products of the PH20 hyaluronidase inhibit remyelination. *Ann Neurol.* 2013;73:266-280.

371. Aguirre A, Dupree JL, Mangin JM, et al. A functional role for EGFR signaling in myelination and remyelination. *Nat Neurosci.* 2007;10:990-1002.

374. Juul SE, Mayock DE, Comstock BA, et al. Neuroprotective potential of erythropoietin in neonates; design of a randomized trial. *Matern Health Neonatol Perinatal.* 2015;1:27.

379. O'Gorman RL, Bucher HU, Held U, et al. Tract-based spatial statistics to assess the neuroprotective effect of early erythropoietin on white matter development in preterm infants. *Brain.* 2015;138(Pt 2):388-397.

380. Natalucci G, Latal B, Koller B, et al. Effect of early prophylactic high-dose recombinant human erythropoietin in very preterm infants on neurodevelopmental outcome at 2 years: a randomized clinical trial. *JAMA.* 2016;315:2079-2085.

381. Wu YW, Mathur AM, Chang T, et al. High-dose erythropoietin and hypothermia for hypoxic-ischemic encephalopathy: a phase II trial. *Pediatrics.* 2016;137.

Full references for this chapter can be found on www.expertconsult .com.

Encephalopathy of Prematurity: Clinical-Neurological Features, Diagnosis, Imaging, Prognosis, Therapy

Jeffrey J. Neil ◆ *Joseph J. Volpe*

This chapter addresses the clinical aspects of the encephalopathy of prematurity, a term coined to characterize the multifaceted, nonhemorrhagic white and gray matter lesions in the premature brain that reflect a combination of destructive and dysmaturational effects (see Chapter 14).[1] The central pathology is cerebral white matter injury (WMI)/periventricular leukomalacia (PVL), with a variety of associated neuronal/axonal deficits. The latter affect principally cerebral cortex and deep gray matter structures, especially thalamus (see Chapter 14). Other lesions also often present in preterm infants include germinal matrix-intraventricular hemorrhage (IVH) (see Chapter 24) and cerebellar disturbances (see Chapters 4 and 23), which are discussed elsewhere in this book. The pathophysiology of the encephalopathy of prematurity is multifactorial, but principally involves molecular events initiated by hypoxia-ischemia and systemic inflammation (see Chapter 15). The prevailing underlying theme is *initial primary injury leading to secondary dysmaturation* (see Chapter 14). Because the encephalopathy is diverse regionally, the spectrum of neurodevelopmental impairments is broad and includes, often in combination, a variety of cognitive, behavioral, socialization, attentional, and motor deficits (see later).

CLINICAL SETTINGS

The rate of preterm birth (<37 weeks' gestation) remains slightly higher than 10% worldwide, with rates varying from 5% to 18% across 184 countries studied (http://www.who.int/mediacentre/factsheets/fs363/en/). This relatively high frequency translates into more than 15 million preterm births worldwide in 2010. In the United States, the preterm birthrate has shown a slow and steady decline over the past decade,[2] reaching 9.6% for the period 2012 to 2014 (March of Dimes Premature Birth Report Card; http://www.marchofdimes.org/mission/prematurity-reportcard.aspx), corresponding to nearly 400,000 newborns born preterm per year.[3] Preterm birth is a leading cause of long-term neurological disabilities in children[4] and has been estimated to have cost the US health care system more than $26 billion in 2005.[5] A disproportionate fraction of these costs originates from very preterm infants (VPT, <32 weeks' gestation), who account for more than 2/3 of the costs associated with preterm birth despite representing just 20% of the preterm population.[5] A particularly vulnerable subgroup is the very low birthweight (VLBW) infant (<1500 g at birth). In 2014, this group comprised 1.4% of total births (approximately 4,000,000), corresponding to approximately 55,000 infants per year in the United States.[6] In addition, the survival of preterm infants has improved over the past decades, particularly for those born extremely preterm (<28 weeks' gestation). For example, survival of infants born at 22 to 28 weeks' gestation increased from 70% in 1993 to 79% in 2012.[7] While these advances are encouraging, the morbidity associated with preterm birth—including impairments in development, learning, behavior, and social interaction—remains high.[7-10] In a study examining data from the year 2012, survival without morbidity ranged from 9% for infants born at 24 weeks' gestation to 59% for those born at 28 weeks' gestation.[7] Finally, the incidence of late preterm births (34 to 36 weeks' gestation) has remained steady at approximately 6.8%, corresponding to 270,000 births per year in the United States.[6] While late preterm infants tend to be less severely affected than infants from other preterm groups, neuropathological studies show that the spectrum of brain injury is similar to that found in early preterm infants, although the injury is generally less severe.[11]

The *principal clinical settings* for the encephalopathy of prematurity include especially those for PVL, the unifying pathology (Table 16.1). As discussed in Chapter 15, the major pathogenetic themes are cerebral ischemia and systemic infection/inflammation (maternal infection/fetal systemic inflammation or neonatal infection/systemic inflammation). The propensity to ischemia relates especially to the high frequency of a pressure-passive cerebral circulation, particularly in the sick, ventilated infant, a variety of cardiorespiratory events leading to periods of decreased blood pressure, and respiratory complications associated with hypocarbia or hypoxemia (see Chapter 15). The relation to maternal intrauterine or neonatal infection and fetal or neonatal systemic inflammation indicates importance for clinical settings indicative of placental inflammation, documented early neonatal infection, and noninfectious disorders with severe systemic inflammation, especially necrotizing enterocolitis (see Chapter 15). Thus in view of the central importance of PVL, the encephalopathy of prematurity involves an interplay between *two major initiating insults, hypoxia-ischemia and systemic infection/inflammation.*[12-21] Experimental studies provide strong evidence that these two insults can potentiate one another.[22-31] Antenatal factors associated with adverse outcome for preterm infants include maternal diabetes, inadequate prenatal care, malnutrition, and maternal infection. Often in the latter studies, the distinction between antenatal factors that promote premature birth and

TABLE 16.1	Principal Clinical Settings for the Encephalopathy of Prematurity

Primarily Hypoxia-Ischemia[a]
Fetal metabolic acidosis
Respiratory insufficiency secondary to severe RDS
Cardiac insufficiency or hypotension or both
- Severe respiratory disease
- Recurrent apneic spells
- Large PDA
- Congenital heart disease
- Sepsis

Primarily Systemic Inflammation[a]
Maternal intrauterine infection
Neonatal sepsis
Necrotizing enterocolitis

[a]Hypoxia-ischemia and inflammation can be additive or potentiating, and the former is associated with a brisk inflammatory response.
See text for references. *PDA*, Patent ductus arteriosus; *RDS*, respiratory distress syndrome.

TABLE 16.2	Clinical Correlates of Periventricular Leukomalacia and the Encephalopathy of Prematurity

TOPOGRAPHY OF THE MAJOR INJURY	NEONATAL PERIOD	LONG-TERM SEQUELAE
Periventricular white matter, including descending motor fibers, optic radiations, and association fibers; and associated deficits of cerebral cortex, basal ganglia, thalamus, and cerebellum	Probable lower limb weakness	Spastic diplegia Motor deficits (without spastic diplegia) Cognitive deficits Visual deficits Behavioral/ attentional/ socialization deficits

those that lead directly or indirectly to cerebral injury is very difficult. Thus, *overall, perinatal factors associated with increased risk of PVL* include: (1) fetal metabolic acidosis; (2) systemic fetal inflammation; (3) respiratory insufficiency secondary to severe respiratory distress syndrome or recurrent apneic spells; (4) cardiac insufficiency secondary to severe respiratory disease, recurrent apneic spells, large patent ductus arteriosus, severe congenital cardiac disease, or vascular collapse (e.g., in association with sepsis); and/or (5) conditions that lead to elevated concentrations of inflammation-related proteins in the circulation, such as necrotizing enterocolitis (see Table 16.1; see later).

NEUROLOGICAL SYNDROME

The *acute neurological correlates* of PVL, those that are present while the infant is in the neonatal intensive care unit (NICU), have been difficult to establish. This difficulty relates principally to the problems of carrying out a careful neurological examination in the sick, labile, premature infant and the frequent association of other neurological manifestations related to complicating hemorrhagic and neuronal injury. The ability to identify the focal component of this lesion in the neonatal period by ultrasonography has facilitated identification of some neonatal neurological correlates. In previous years, when large cystic PVL lesions were seen commonly in premature infants, we saw a substantial number of infants with weakness of lower limbs in the first weeks of life associated with focal periventricular white matter injury documented by ultrasound scan (Table 16.2). In general, the weakness in the neonatal period is not marked, even in the presence of relatively large lesions. However, in recent years with the marked predominance of noncystic PVL, such specific motor deficits have been very unusual to identify. The frequent affection of optic radiations[32-38] is consistent with electrophysiological studies that indicate a high incidence of disturbance of visual-evoked potentials, but impairments in visual perception and visual fields[38-63] are not typically detectable until later in life (see Table 16.2).

Recognition of a distinct *neonatal* neurological syndrome associated with PVL and other anatomical features of the encephalopathy of prematurity also has been very difficult because of the rapidly changing *normal* neurological characteristics of the premature infant (see Chapter 9). For example, the normal infant of 28 weeks' gestation requires stimulation for arousal from sleep. At 32 weeks' gestation, spontaneous arousal occurs, but vigorous crying during wakefulness is unusual. Only at 40 weeks' gestation should the observer expect to see discrete periods of attention to visual and auditory stimuli. Similarly, periodic breathing in a full-term newborn is much more likely to be an abnormal finding than in a premature infant at 32 weeks' gestation. Further, absent pupillary reaction to light is usual at 28 weeks but is unusual at 32 to 34 weeks. However, full extraocular movements with oculocephalic (doll's eyes) maneuver are present in the youngest normal infants (i.e., 28 weeks' gestation or even younger). In addition, hypotonia in the upper extremities is usual at 28 or 32 weeks' gestation but is abnormal at term. Finally, spontaneous movements also exhibit a progression from lower to upper extremities from 28 weeks' gestation to term, so that *weakness* of upper extremities must be defined with caution in the premature infant.

The issue of *neonatal seizures* in the context of the sick preterm infant is critical to address (Table 16.3). While neonatal seizures are characteristic of moderate to severe hypoxic-ischemic encephalopathy in the term infant (see Chapter 18), recent electrophysiological studies show that they also are common in VPT infants.[64] However, only the minority of electrical seizures have an obvious clinical correlate in preterm (as well as term) infants (see Chapter 12). A recent study of 95 VPT infants evaluated by amplitude-integrated encephalography (aEEG) from the first day of life showed that fully 48% exhibited seizures in the first 72 hours of life.[64] The presence of seizures on the second postnatal day was associated with white matter injury (detected by magnetic resonance imaging [MRI] at term equivalent age) (relative risk, 3.0 [1.3 to 6.6]). Only 7% of the infants with electrographic seizures had clinically detected seizures. Importantly, seizures were associated with poorer early language development. The data suggest that the clinical assessment of the very preterm infant should include

TABLE 16.3	**Frequency and Importance of Neonatal Seizures in the Sick Preterm Infant**

Amplitude-integrated EEG (aEEG) detected electrographic seizures in 48% of sick very preterm infants in the first 72 hours of life.

Only 7% of the infants with electrographic seizures had clinically detected seizures.

Seizures on postnatal day 2 were associated with cerebral white matter injury detected by magnetic resonance imaging at term equivalent age.

Seizures were associated with poorer language development.

Data from Vesoulis ZA, Inder TE, Woodward LJ, et al. Early electrographic seizures, brain injury, and neurodevelopmental risk in the very preterm infant. *Pediatr Res.* 2014;75:564–569.

TABLE 16.4	**Value of EEG in Detection of Cerebral White Matter Injury in Premature Infants**

"Acute-stage abnormalities"—decreased continuity, lower background amplitude, or both—observed on days 1–4 of life (and rarely thereafter) with subsequently proven PVL (ultrasonography)

Abnormal sharp waves of value are positive rolandic or vertex (central), positive frontal, and negative occipital

Positive rolandic sharp waves (>0.1/minute) present in 65%–90% of cases of severe PVL and 25% of mild or moderate PVL

Frontal positive or occipital negative sharp waves or both present in 100% of cases of severe PVL and in 60%–90% of mild or moderate PVL

Abnormal sharp waves accompany echodense lesions and precede the development of echolucent, presumed cystic change by ultrasonography

Peak period of occurrence of sharp waves 5–14 days

See text for references. *PVL*, Periventricular leukomalacia.

diligent attempts at recognition of subtle seizures and liberal use of aEEG (see section on diagnosis). The findings also have implications regarding the apparent perinatal timing of insults leading to PVL, as they suggest that injury sufficient to cause seizures occurs within the first days after birth (see later).

DIAGNOSIS

Unlike the term infant with hypoxic-ischemic encephalopathy, the value of the neurological examination and metabolic biomarkers in diagnosis of the encephalopathy of prematurity is limited. EEG has not been used extensively, although the potential value of conventional EEG and aEEG deserves exploration (see earlier and next section). Neuroimaging is of major diagnostic importance, and cranial ultrasonography and MRI are the key imaging methodologies.

Electroencephalogram

Because the encephalopathy of prematurity includes cerebral cortical and thalamic abnormalities (see Chapter 14), it is reasonable to expect that conventional or aEEG would provide important diagnostic information (Table 16.4). Concerning *conventional EEG,* serial EEG studies have been shown of value in identifying preterm infants with PVL and presumed neuronal disease. Thus, in one important study, EEG findings referred to as *acute-stage abnormalities* (*decreased continuity, lower background amplitude, or both*) were observed mainly on days 1 to 4 of life in infants with subsequent ultrasonographically identified PVL. Later, *chronic-stage abnormalities* (*deformed slow activity and abnormal sharp waves*) were observed, mainly on days 5 to 14 and resolving within 1 to 2 months. Chronic-stage EEG abnormalities were more severe and persisted longer in patients with extensive cystic PVL compared with patients with milder PVL, suggesting that EEG findings correlate with PVL severity.[65] Another EEG abnormality, *positive rolandic sharp waves,* has been identified as a specific, though not particularly sensitive, marker for overt PVL.[66] The presence of additional abnormalities—occipital sharp waves (negative polarity) and frontal sharp waves (positive polarity)—increases sensitivity for cystic PVL.[67] These EEG findings also are of prognostic value, as the presence of positive rolandic sharp waves has been associated with adverse motor outcome.[68] Although brain injury

such as grade III/IV IVH or cystic PVL detected by cranial ultrasound or MRI during the neonatal period is the most significant marker for predicting adverse outcomes (see later), EEG provides prognostic value independent of neuroimaging findings and clinical risk factors.[69,70] In addition to abnormalities of EEG background, approximately 30% of patients with PVL presented with seizures and 65% with episodes of apnea.[71,72]

The findings described earlier regarding early detection of seizures by aEEG are relevant here (see Neurological Syndrome). Notably, the onset of aEEG seizures in the first days of life is consistent with the conventional EEG findings just described, suggesting that the timing of the insult(s) leading to the encephalopathy of prematurity involves early perinatal and neonatal events, at least initially.

Neuroimaging

Neuroimaging of Cerebral White Matter in the Encephalopathy of Prematurity

Relevant Neuropathology. The *hallmark of the encephalopathy of prematurity* is cerebral white matter injury or PVL (see Chapter 14). To understand the value and the challenges of neuroimaging of the encephalopathy in the neonatal period, we should review briefly the neuropathology of PVL and related cerebral white matter injury. PVL consists of two distinct components: *focal necrosis*, with loss of all cellular elements, dorsal and lateral to the lateral ventricles, and a more cell-specific *diffuse injury* involving pre-oligodendrocytes (pre-OLs) in cerebral white matter and marked by astrogliosis and microgliosis. A spectrum of severity is recognized[15] and *in living infants* is based on neuroimaging (principally MRI). Thus PVL can be categorized into three subtypes (Table 16.5). The most severe form involves focal necroses that are macroscopic in size, that is, relatively large, more than several millimeters, and evolve to tissue dissolution and cystic change over a period of weeks. This *focal necrotic/cystic form* is often simply termed *cystic PVL* (Fig. 16.1) and is readily detected by cranial ultrasonography or MRI (see later). Cystic PVL is now uncommon and has an overall incidence in living

TABLE 16.5   The Spectrum of Periventricular Leukomalacia in Premature Infants

FORM OF PVL	FOCAL PERIVENTRICULAR INJURY	DEGREE OF DIFFUSE WHITE MATTER INJURY[a]	IMAGING CORRELATE[a]	APPROXIMATE INCIDENCE (%)
Severe ("cystic")	Large areas of macroscopic necrosis, evolving to cysts	Severe	Periventricular cysts	5
Moderate ("noncystic")	Smaller areas of macroscopic necrosis, evolving to gliotic scarring	Intermediate	Periventricular signal abnormality on CUS and punctate white matter lesions on MRI	25
Mild	Microscopic areas of necrosis	Mild	No periventricular signal abnormality	? 25–35

[a]The diffuse component of white matter injury is manifest on MRI as diffuse signal abnormality on T_2-weighted imaging or as diffuse abnormalities on diffusion imaging.
CUS, Cranial ultrasonography; MRI, magnetic resonance imaging; PVL, periventricular leukomalacia.

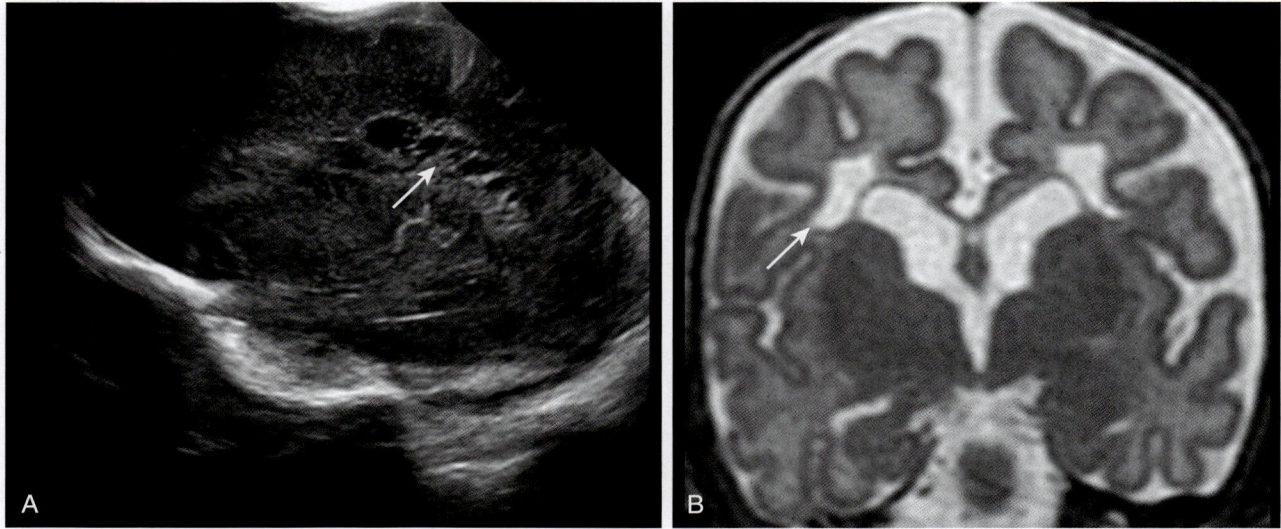

Figure 16.1 Images of severe cystic periventricular leukomalacia. (A) A parasaggital ultrasound image showing numerous large cysts superolateral to the lateral ventricle *(arrow)*. (B) A coronal T_2-weighted image in which cysts are present superolateral to the lateral ventricles *(arrow)*.

VLBW infants of 5% or less.[7,73] In the largest neuropathological series of preterm infants ($n = 41$), approximately 40% exhibited PVL with focal necroses, but *macroscopic* necroses were observed in only 18% of these PVL cases (only 7% of the total of autopsied preterm infants).[74] A moderate form of PVL involves focal necrotic lesions that are 1 to 2 mm in size and, on tissue dissolution, evolve not to cysts but rather to focal glial scars, sometimes visible as punctate areas of increased signal intensity on T_1-weighted MRI (Fig. 16.2). This form, often termed *noncystic PVL*, occurs in approximately 25% of living infants. Finally, the least severe form of PVL involves a focal necrotic component less than 1 mm in size, that is, microscopic and so small as to be invisible to neuroimaging. This mild form, like all forms of PVL, exhibits the diffuse gliosis described in Chapter 14. The degree of the diffuse abnormality generally correlates with the severity of PVL (see Table 16.5). The MRI correlate of the diffuse gliosis likely is the diffuse signal change described later. The mild form of PVL is likely present in a substantial minority of premature infants (see later). In the

neuropathological series just noted, fully 82% of PVL cases (34% of the total series of autopsied premature infants) had focal necrotic lesions that were less than 1 mm and therefore likely below the detection of conventional clinical MRI scanners. Such cases would be classified (mistakenly) as *nonnecrotic* by MRI. All three subtypes of PVL include the diffuse component, characterized by astrogliosis/microgliosis, and, after the initial pre-OL cell death, an excess of oligodendroglial progenitors. These oligodendroglial progenitors, however, fail to differentiate into myelin-producing cells (see Chapters 14 and 15). The severity of the diffuse component appears to parallel the severity of the PVL.

A *form of cerebral white matter injury with no necroses and only the diffuse white matter gliosis must be considered*. It is noteworthy that in the total group of 41 autopsied premature infants by Pierson et al.,[74] approximately 40% had *only* diffuse gliosis, with *no* focal necroses. In strict terminology, these cases without any necroses should not be termed *PVL*. This diffuse-lesion-only may be the least severe form of cerebral white matter injury,

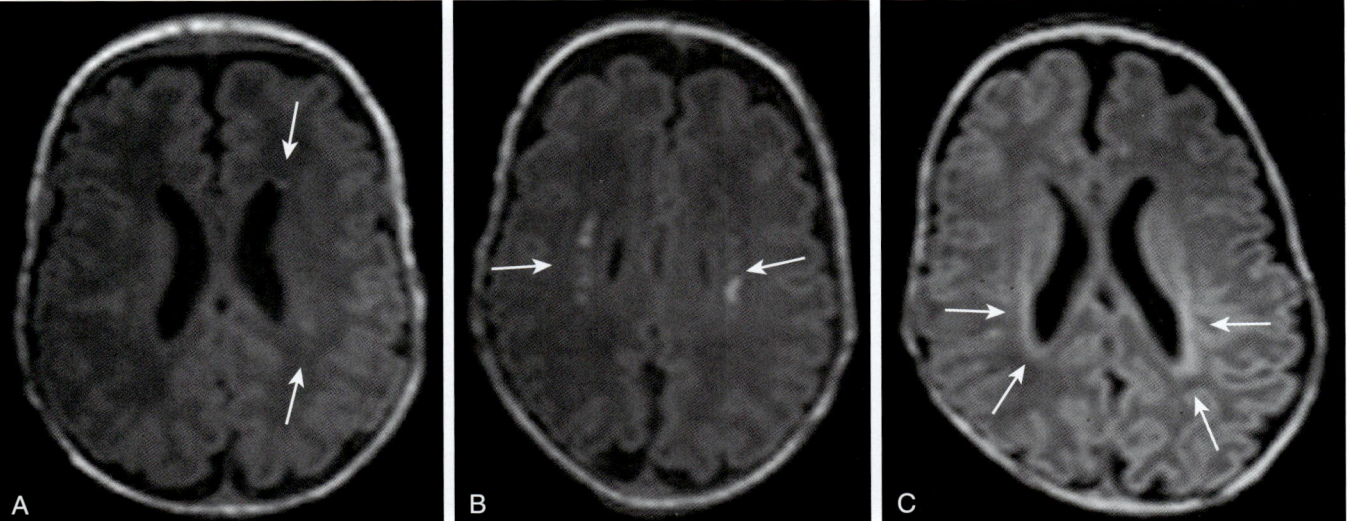

Figure 16.2 Axial T₁-weighted images showing examples of noncystic PVL visible as areas of increased signal intensity in the periventricular areas *(arrows)*. The severity of injury increases from panels A to B to C.

TABLE 16.6   Ultrasonographic Diagnosis of Periventricular Leukomalacia—Appearance, Temporal Features, and Pathological Correlation

ULTRASONOGRAPHIC APPEARANCE	TEMPORAL FEATURES	NEUROPATHOLOGICAL CORRELATION
Echogenic foci, bilateral, posterior > anterior	First week	Necrosis with congestion and/or hemorrhage, (size > 1 cm)
Echolucent foci ("cysts")	1–3 weeks	Cyst formation secondary to tissue dissolution (size > 3 mm)
Ventricular enlargement, often with disappearance of "cysts"	≥2–3 months	Deficient myelin formation; gliosis, often with collapse of cyst

Derived from the studies of "cystic PVL" by Nwaesei et al.,[530] Fawer et al.,[531] Hope et al.,[532] de Vries et al.,[32] Rodriguez et al.,[533] Carson et al.,[35] Paneth et al.,[34] and personal unpublished material, with permission.

but *because its MRI appearance is likely identical to the least severe form of PVL, that is, with microscopic necroses, distinction in vivo is not currently possible.* Whether these infants consistently exhibit diffuse signal abnormality on MRI is unknown. Moreover, whether infants with the diffuse gliotic component without any necrotic component subsequently exhibit the neuronal/axonal dysmaturational effects of the encephalopathy of prematurity also is not known. The particular potential importance of diffuse white matter gliosis without focal necroses relates not only to its high frequency in neuropathological studies of premature infants, but also to the recent observations of Buser et al.,[75] who not only confirmed the high frequency but who *also showed in cerebral white matter the characteristic excess of pre-OLs and their maturational arrest,* as observed in the diffuse component of PVL. These findings suggest that such infants in vivo could develop the impairment of myelination and perhaps also the secondary dysmaturational effects on neuronal/axonal structures consequent to disrupted myelination (see Chapter 14). The important point in this context is that accurate identification of the *diffuse white matter cellular abnormalities in vivo in the neonatal period currently is not clearly possible.* Experimental data based on imaging at 11.7T suggest potential for identifying and quantifying white matter gliosis (as well as microscopic necrosis).[76] However, the imaging was carried out *ex vivo,* and

the safety of imaging human preterm brain at 11.7T has not been established.

Cranial Ultrasonography. Cranial ultrasonography is of great value in diagnosis (Tables 16.6–16.8). The cysts of cystic PVL are readily visible by cranial ultrasonography (see Table 16.6; Figs. 16.3–16.5). They are located primarily just lateral to the atria of the lateral ventricles, and extend anteriorly, and to some extent posteriorly, with increasing severity (Fig. 16.6). They are sometimes only visible for a few weeks and may have fully resolved by term equivalent, but their presence is predictive of subsequent cerebral palsy.[77] Their *resolution* is likely due to development of a gliotic scar with collapse of the cyst (see Chapter 14; Fig. 16.7). As a result, their manifestation at term equivalent may be subtle, consisting of mild to moderate ventricular dilatation and an irregularly contoured ventricular wall.

The ultrasonographic imaging correlates of noncystic PVL are generally not obvious (see Tables 16.7 and 16.8).[78] Some data suggest that cerebral white matter echodensity at least as echogenic as the choroid plexus and persisting for at least 7 days is significant. Further, the presence of white matter inhomogeneity or a *patchy* appearance on ultrasonography should also alert the clinician to potential white matter

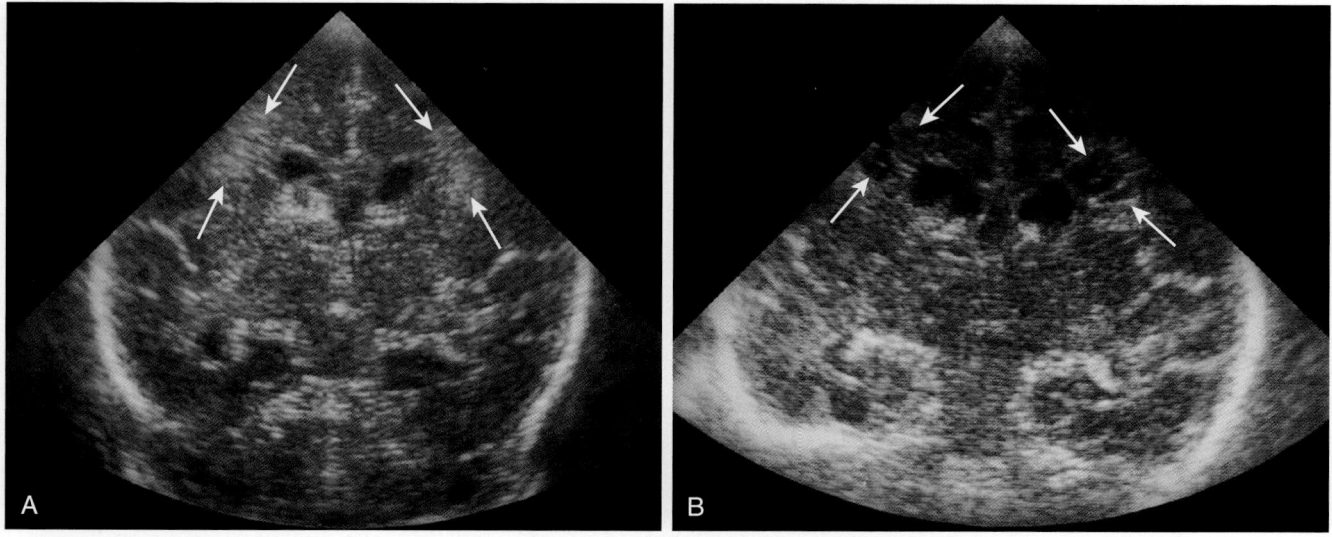

Figure 16.3 Coronal ultrasound scans of periventricular leukomalacia in a premature infant on postnatal days (A) 5 and (B) 24. Note in A, the periventricular echodensities *(arrows)* and in B, the small echolucent foci, consistent with cysts, in the same areas *(arrows)*.

TABLE 16.7   Cranial Ultrasonography Not Highly Predictive of Noncystic Periventricular Leukomalacia Identified by Magnetic Resonance Imaging

| | **MRI FINDING AT TERM** | | |
CRANIAL ULTRASOUND FINDING	NORMAL	WHITE MATTER SIGNAL ABNORMALITY	CYSTIC CHANGE
Normal or transient echodensity (n = 74)	48	25	1
Prolonged echodensity (n = 19)	10	9	0
Echolucencies (n = 3)	0	0	3

MRI, Magnetic resonance imaging.

Data adapted from Inder TE, Anderson NJ, Spencer C, Wells S, Volpe JJ. White matter injury in the premature infant: a comparison between serial cranial sonographic and MR findings at term. *AJNR Am J Neuroradiol.* 2003;24:805–809.

TABLE 16.8   Cranial Ultrasonography and the Diagnosis of Periventricular Leukomalacia

Echolucencies on US are sensitive and specific for focal cystic lesions

Echodensities on US may be transient (<7 days), prolonged >7 days, or evolve to lucencies

Transient echodensities are generally not predictive of WM abnormality on MRI at term

Echodensities that are prolonged (>7 days) or severe or apparent after the first week of life are variably predictive of WM abnormality on MRI at term

Mild or moderate WM signal abnormalities on MRI at term are poorly predicted by cranial ultrasonography; approximately 70% of noncystic white matter abnormality on MRI at term is not detected by cranial ultrasonography

See text for references.

MRI, Magnetic resonance imaging; *US,* ultrasonography; *WM,* white matter.

abnormalities (Fig. 16.8).[79] This patchy appearance can sometimes be hemorrhagic in origin, and a combination of diffusion- and susceptibility-weighted MRI can help identify a hemorrhagic component.[80] Although PVL is principally a nonhemorrhagic lesion, occasionally secondary hemorrhage can be dramatic (Fig. 16.9).

Magnetic Resonance Imaging. The focal necrotic/cystic component of PVL, observed well on cranial ultrasound, is readily demonstrated by MRI as well (see Table 16.5). However, the much more common moderate (noncystic) forms of PVL often also are detected by MRI and generally not by cranial ultrasonography (see Table 16.7). Indeed, the high frequencies of noncystic cerebral white matter abnormality, manifested either as focal punctate white matter lesions or, even more commonly, of the mildest form of PVL (with microscopic necroses), manifested only as diffuse MRI signal change, were unexpected until the application of MRI (see Table 16.5).[78,81-91] The *frequency of the diffuse abnormality on MRI increases as a function of postnatal age.* In one series with serial MRI scans,

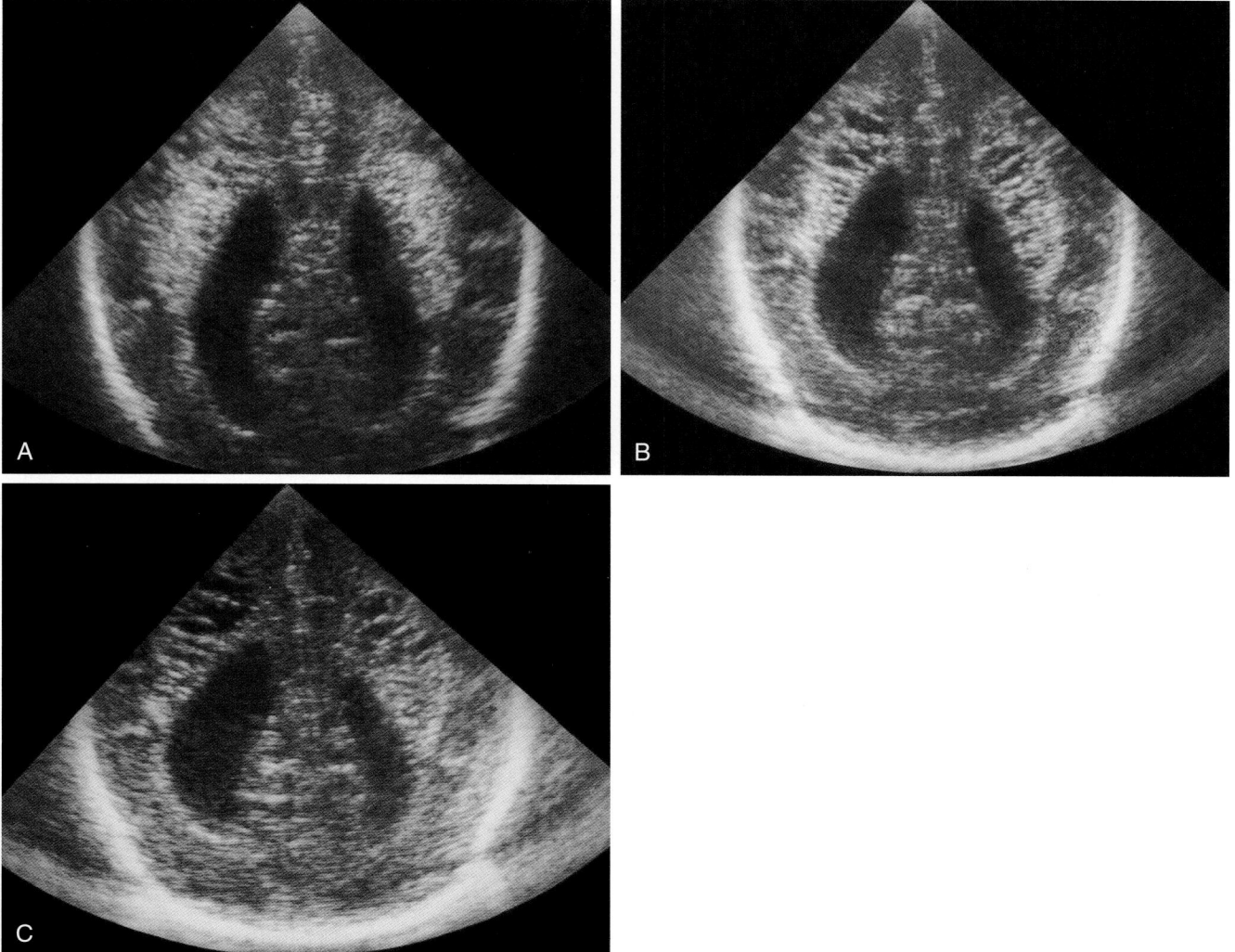

Figure 16.4 Coronal ultrasound scans angled slightly posteriorly to image the peritrigonal regions in periventricular leukomalacia. The scans were obtained in a premature infant at (A) 10, (B) 17, and (C) 25 days of age. Note the evolution from echodensities to multiple small echolucencies in the periventricular white matter.

the finding of diffuse MRI signal abnormality in premature infants with a median gestational age of 27 weeks increased from 21% in the first postnatal week, to 53% over the next several weeks, to 79% at term equivalent.[82] In a later prospective study of 100 premature infants, 64 exhibited white matter signal abnormality at term.[83]

The neuropathological correlates of the diffuse white matter signal abnormality, known as diffuse excessive high signal intensity (DEHSI), are unclear. A reasonable speculation is that the abnormality reflects the diffuse gliotic (astrogliosis and microgliosis) component of PVL. It is seen best on T_2-weighted images at term equivalent age[84] and is a common finding (see earlier).[90] While these white matter signal intensity changes are associated with increased water diffusion coefficient values on diffusion imaging, the qualitative identification of signal changes on T_2-weighted images is subjective. Further, recent studies have failed to identify a relationship between these signal changes and outcome at either 18 or 30 months of age.[92,93]

However, the absence of a later clinical correlate to DEHSI does not necessarily mean that a degree of white matter injury isn't present. Indeed, in the neuropathological series referred to earlier,[74] the focal necrotic component was less than 1 mm in most cases and likely below the resolution of clinical MRI scanners. Moreover, as noted earlier, in 42% of the entire series of autopsied premature infants diffuse gliosis *without* focal necrosis was present. Whether the subsequent neuronal/axonal abnormalities observed in the encephalopathy of prematurity and likely important for long-term outcome were present is unknown. Moreover, the lack of later clinical abnormalities also could reflect the beneficial effects of plasticity.

Other potential MRI correlates of diffuse cerebral white matter injury in the neonatal period include disturbances of white matter structure detected *via* diffusion anisotropy maps (Fig. 16.10) and abnormalities of ^1H spectroscopy, with both involving areas of white matter that may appear normal on conventional, T_1- and T_2-weighted, imaging.[94]

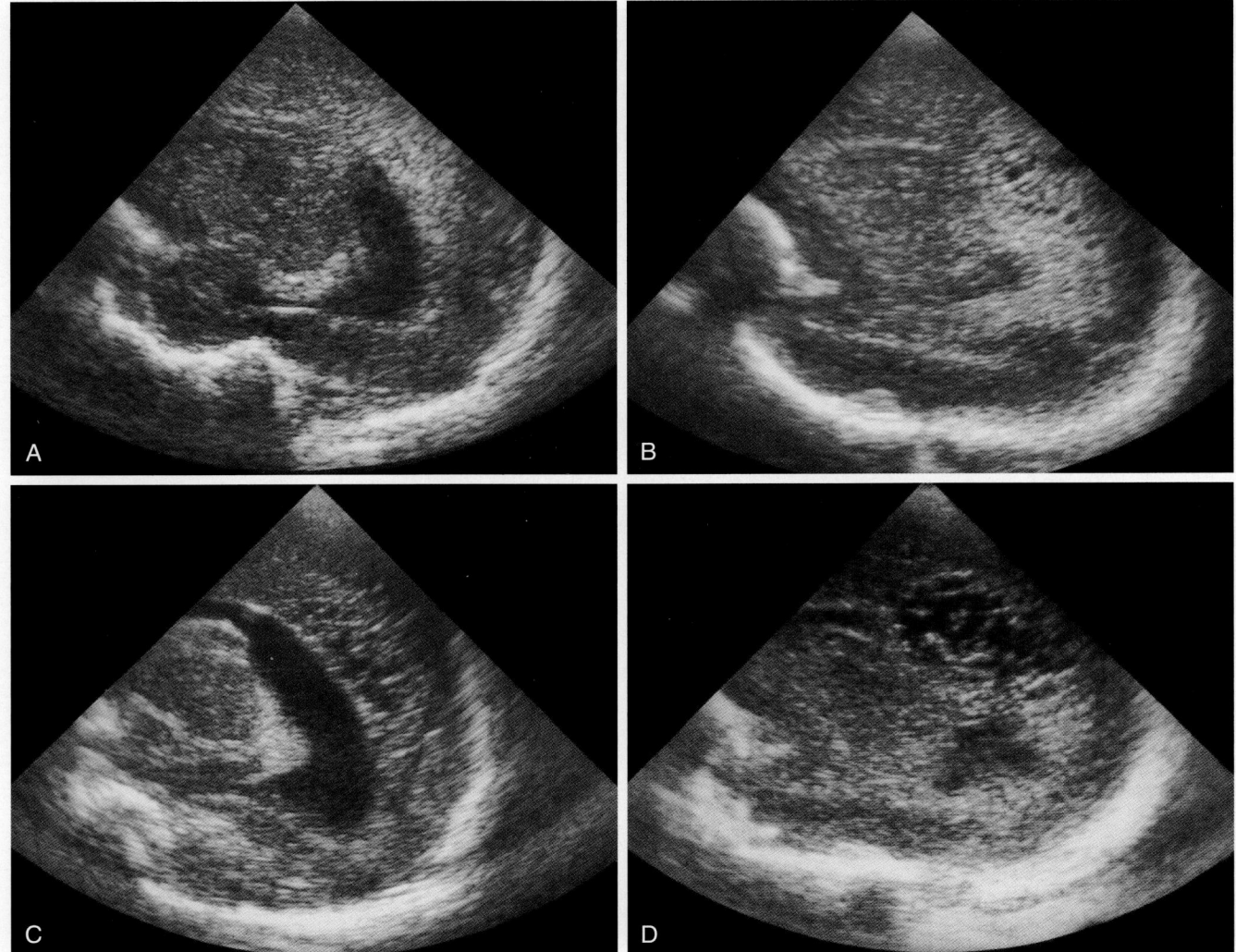

Figure 16.5 Parasagittal ultrasound scans of periventricular leukomalacia obtained from a premature infant at (A) 2, (B) 13, (C) 17, and (D) 26 days of age. Note the evolution from echodensity to multiple small echolucencies in the periventricular white matter adjacent to the trigone of the lateral ventricles.

Neuroimaging of Neuronal/Axonal Components in the Encephalopathy of Prematurity

The *neuronal/axonal* components of the encephalopathy of prematurity are difficult to visualize by neuroimaging in the acute period. However, over the ensuing weeks such abnormalities become prominent and are detectable by advanced MRI methods (see later).

PROGNOSIS AND CLINICOPATHOLOGICAL CORRELATIONS

Difficulties of Delineating Prognosis and Clinicopathological Correlations in Premature Infants

Delineation of prognosis and, in particular, clinicopathological correlations attributable to the encephalopathy of prematurity is hindered by (1) in vivo identification of the encephalopathy, (2)

the concurrence of brain abnormality secondary to a variety of deleterious postnatal events unrelated to the encephalopathy of prematurity, and (3) definition of the specific regions affected—especially those involved in dysmaturation subsequent to the initial destructive effects. Concerning *the in vivo identification of the encephalopathy*, the central feature is cerebral white matter injury (see earlier and Chapter 14). At present, *identification of the white matter lesion of the encephalopathy of prematurity in vivo is accomplished most definitively by detection of the focal necrotic component of PVL*. Unfortunately, the difficulty of such detection is related to the relatively small proportion of cases in which the focal necrotic component of PVL would be expected to be detectable by clinically available conventional MRI scanners (Table 16.9). As noted earlier, in the neuropathological series cited,[74] 41% ($n = 17$) had PVL, and among this PVL group, fully 82% ($n = 14$) had focal necrotic lesions that were smaller than 1 mm and visible only by microscopy.[74] Thus only 3 of the 17 infants (8%) with PVL had focal necrotic lesions likely readily detected by MRI. The remaining 14 infants (92%) with PVL had microscopic

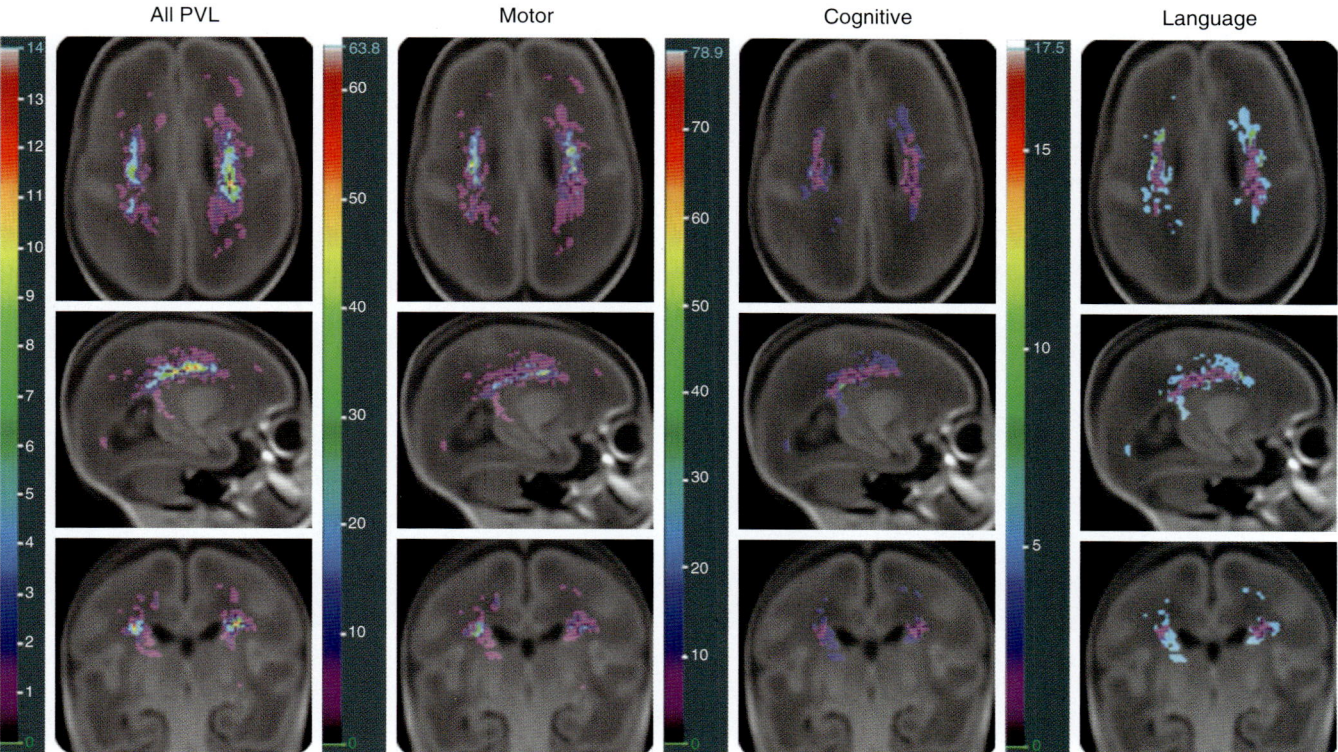

Figure 16.6 Odds ratio maps of noncystic periventricular leukomalacia (PVL) for motor *(second column),* cognitive *(third column),* and language *(fourth column)* outcomes overlaid on a T₁-weighted neonatal brain template. The first column shows the spatial cumulative map including all noncystic signal abnormalities seen in any of 58 very preterm neonates. Note that the signal intensity abnormalities most commonly involve the white matter adjacent to the trigone and posterior body of the lateral ventricles. Note also that they also tend to involve the left hemisphere more than the right. The maximum odds ratio values on the motor, cognitive, and language odds ratio maps are 63.8, 78.9, and 17.5, respectively. (From Guo T, Duerden EG, Adams E, et al. Quantitative assessment of white matter injury in preterm neonates: association with outcomes. *Neurology.* 2017;88:614–622.)

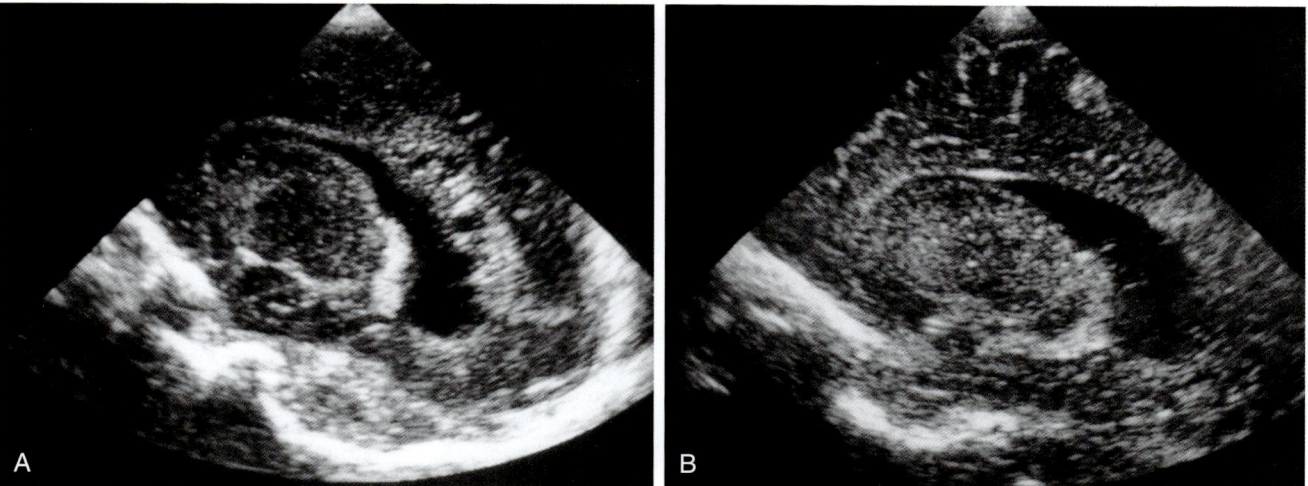

Figure 16.7 Parasagittal ultrasound scans obtained from a premature infant at (A) 24 and (B) 93 days of age. Note that the echolucent cysts apparent at 24 days have disappeared by 93 days of age. The trigonal region of the lateral ventricle at 93 days is dilated because of loss of periventricular white matter and failure of early myelination.

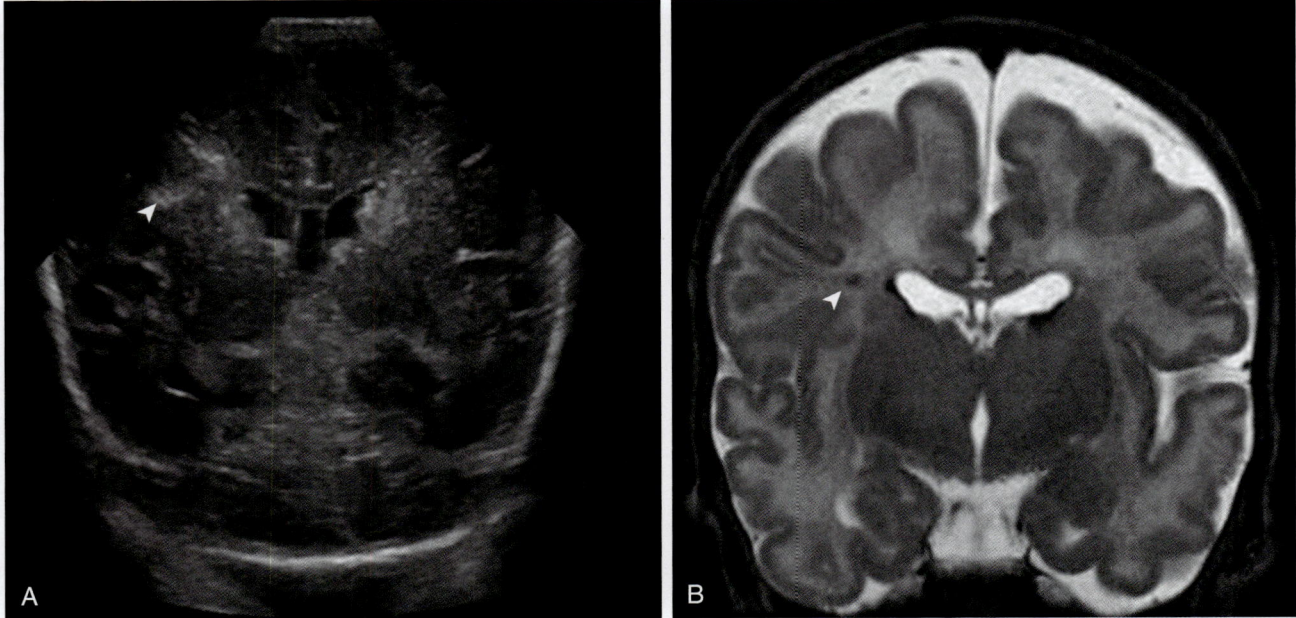

Figure 16.8 Coronal ultrasound scan in a 28-week preterm infant on day of life 5 shows periventricular white matter echodensity (A). Note the corresponding lesion that appears dark on the T₂-weighted image (*arrowhead,* B) obtained at term equivalent age.

TABLE 16.9	Major Difficulties in Delineating Prognosis and Clinicopathological Correlations in Encephalopathy of Prematurity

In vivo identification of the cerebral white matter injury—microscopic areas of necrosis are very frequent and are invisible to conventional MRI

Common indicators of white matter injury detectable by MRI, for example, punctate white matter lesions, may be apparent early in the neonatal course but disappear by term equivalent age

In vivo identification of neuronal/axonal deficits are very difficult in the acute/subacute period and, later, require advanced MRI methods for detection

Many other concurrent factors, related to drugs, pain, stress, nutrition, experiential events, independently may have deleterious effects on the developing premature brain

MRI, Magnetic resonance imaging.

lesions predicted to be below the detection of clinically used MRI scanners. However, it is possible that such lesions could exhibit surrounding inflammatory changes that allow them to be detectable, at least *early and transiently*. For example, in a recent report of 112 premature infants with punctate white matter lesions on MRI, approximately one-third were only visible on an early scan and were no longer apparent at term (see Table 16.9).[95] Similarly, in a recent study in which 54 infants underwent MRI studies at 32 weeks' postmenstrual age and at term equivalent, the white matter injury (consisting of cysts or increased focal signal intensity in the periventricular area on T₁-weighted imaging) appeared less severe on the MRI study at term equivalent age in 24 infants. *These findings suggest that*

a portion of the injury apparent at 32 weeks was no longer detectable by MRI at term equivalent in nearly half the infants.[96] In two recent large studies of premature infants (<33 weeks' gestational age and <28 weeks' gestational age) MRI at term equivalent age did detect moderate/severe WMI in nearly 20%.[97,98] Nevertheless many studies based on conventional MRI likely underestimate infants with white matter injury as well as the neuronal/axonal defects of the encephalopathy of prematurity (see Chapter 14). This concern can be allayed partially by detection of white matter microstructural impairment by diffusion-based MRI at term equivalent age or later (see Fig. 16.10 and see later). Currently, the availability of such advanced magnetic resonance (MR) methodologies is limited.

Concerning the *concurrence of brain abnormality secondary to other deleterious postnatal factors*, many studies do not systematically address the effects of such factors. The latter may include specific drugs (e.g., glucocorticoids, narcotics, sedatives), pain, stress, nutrition, experiential factors, infection, etc.

Concerning *definition of the specific brain regions affected*, particularly cerebral cortex and other gray matter structures, the principal difficulties relate to the dysmaturational nature of the brain abnormalities (relating to impaired organizational developmental events—see Chapter 7), their later occurrence, and the advanced MRI techniques required for detection (e.g., volumetric MRI, diffusion tractography, cerebral cortical surface-based measures, functional MRI; see Table 16.9). Many follow-up studies do not include such measures either in the neonatal period or later.

Thus, in the sections to follow, although we emphasize outcomes in premature infants with clearly defined white matter injury with evidence for focal necroses or, in some studies, evidence for microstructural white matter injury, and presumably therefore the encephalopathy of prematurity, we also discuss other large-scale studies of premature infants without

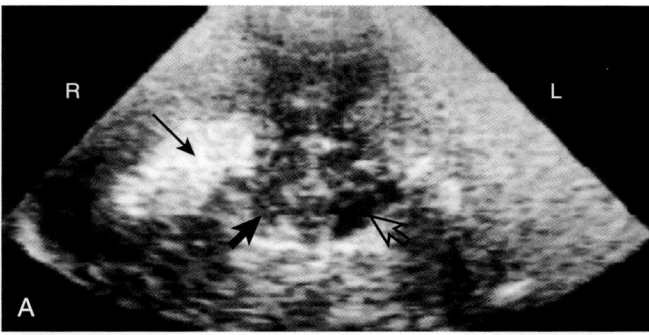

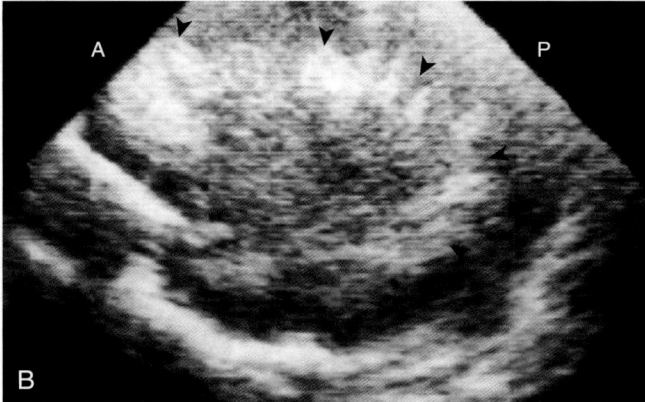

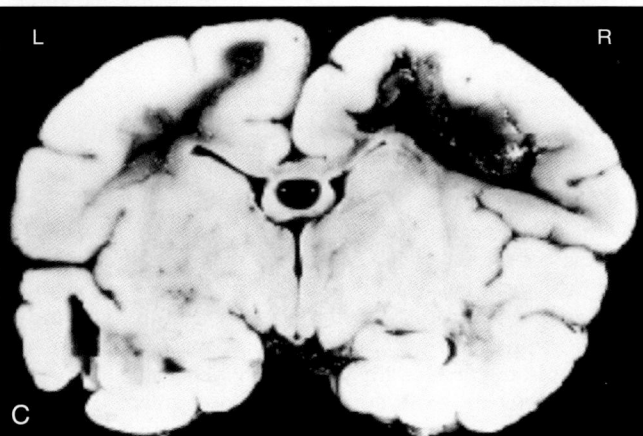

Figure 16.9 Ultrasound scan of hemorrhagic periventricular leukomalacia from an infant of 33 weeks of gestation who experienced cardiorespiratory arrest at 20 days of age. (A) Coronal section shows ovoid echodense area in right periventricular region *(long arrow)*; a smaller periventricular echodense area is present on the left. The lateral ventricles are marked by short arrows. (B) Right parasagittal scan shows extensive anteroposterior region of periventricular echodensity *(arrowheads)*. (C) Coronal section of cerebrum from the same infant, who died several days later, shows massive hemorrhagic periventricular leukomalacia on the right and a smaller area on the left.

imaging evidence of overt injury with focal necroses, with the presumption, based in part on the neuropathological studies, that the encephalopathy is present and invisible to the imaging modalities used. Relatively strong correlations can be found between some outcomes, the degree of brain injury, and its location in connections to and from primary motor or sensory cortices (see sections on spastic diplegia and visual impairment). These correlations result because the involved cerebral regions include areas of *eloquent* cortex with clearly defined afferent

and efferent pathways and functional correlates. In contrast, the imaging correlates of cognitive and behavioral impairment, which are common in preterm children, are not so discrete, likely because these functions are anatomically more widely distributed. Consequently, as described below, these correlates often reflect an overall burden of injury rather than injury to a specific brain area. Such outcomes may be related to abnormality in more than one type of brain tissue (white matter, cortex, deep nuclear gray matter). In some instances, an overall *global abnormality score* derived from assessment of the entire brain shows the strongest relation to outcome, although such scores may not provide precise clinicopathological, correlative information.

Clinicopathological Correlates

The *major long-term correlates* of the encephalopathy of prematurity include motor deficits—spastic diplegia and less severe motor deficits—and a variety of cognitive, behavioral, attentional and socialization defects (see Table 16.2). These neurological disturbances relate in varying degrees to the cerebral white matter injury and to the associated deficits of cerebral cortex, thalamus, basal ganglia, and cerebellum, as outlined next.

Motor Deficits

Motor deficits observed later in premature infants are common, but over the past decades these deficits have declined, particularly in severity. The motor deficits consist of the major spastic motor deficits, often categorized as *cerebral palsy*, and relatively minor motor deficits involving coordination and other more subtle aspects of motor function, sometimes referred to as *developmental coordination disorder*. We discuss the major and minor motor deficits next.

Spastic Diplegia. Premature infants may exhibit a variety of major motor deficits related to PVL, severe IVH (see Chapter 24), and stroke (see Chapter 21), among other pathologies. In the context of this chapter on the encephalopathy of prematurity, the principal major motor deficit is *spastic diplegia*. This motor disturbance has as its central feature spastic paresis of the extremities with affection of lower more than upper limbs. The incidence of this motor deficit has declined markedly in the past two decades and is generally approximately 2% to 3%,[97,99] although in the extremely preterm infant the incidence can be as high as 10%.[100]

Two major lines of evidence indicate that the focal necroses of PVL result in spastic diplegia and its variants. First, the topography of the focal lesions includes the region of cerebral white matter traversed by descending fibers from motor cortex, and those subserving function of lower extremities are more likely to be affected by the periventricular locus of the necrosis (Fig. 16.11). More severe lesions, with lateral extension into the centrum semiovale and corona radiata, would be expected to affect upper extremities and intellectual functions as well. Indeed, patients with spastic diplegia with significant involvement of upper extremities exhibit other manifestations of more severe cerebral disturbance, including intellectual deficits (Table 16.10).[101-104]

A second line of evidence linking spastic diplegia and focal PVL, related to the first, is that the ultrasonographic and MRI correlates of the focal necrotic component of PVL, especially

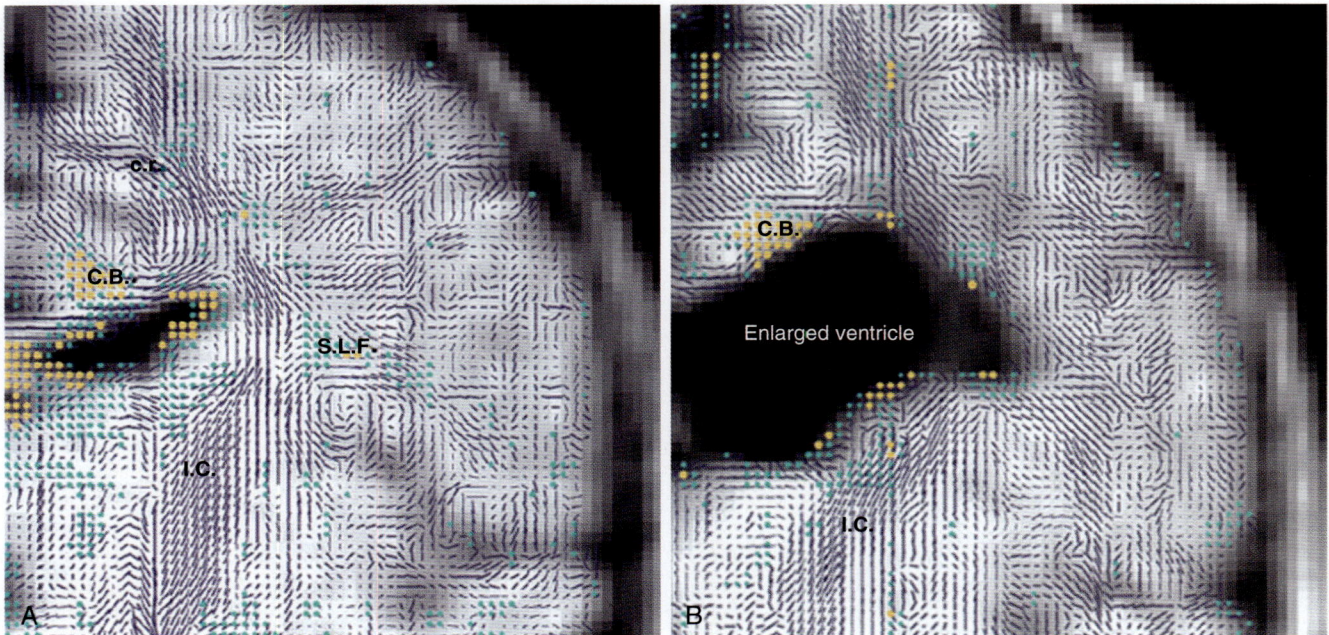

Figure 16.10 Diffusion vector maps overlaid on coronal diffusion weighted images for a premature infant at term with no white matter injury (A) and a premature infant at term with perinatal white matter injury (B). The posterior limb of the internal capsule (*I.C.*) in (A) shows more homologous directed vectors that are longer and more densely packed than in the internal capsule of (B). Anteroposterior-oriented white matter fibers in the area of the superior longitudinal fasciculus (*S.L.F.*; yellow and green dots with yellow representing higher anisotropy than green) in (A) indicate the presence of fiber bundles that are missing or are less prominent in (B). The only discrete anteroposterior fiber bundles that definitely are present in (B) are the cingulate bundle (*C.B.*). Fibers of the corona radiata appear less well-organized in (B) than (A). (From Huppi PS, Murphy B, Maier SE, et al. Microstructural brain development after perinatal cerebral white matter injury assessed by diffusion tensor magnetic resonance imaging. *Pediatrics.* 2001;107:455–460.)

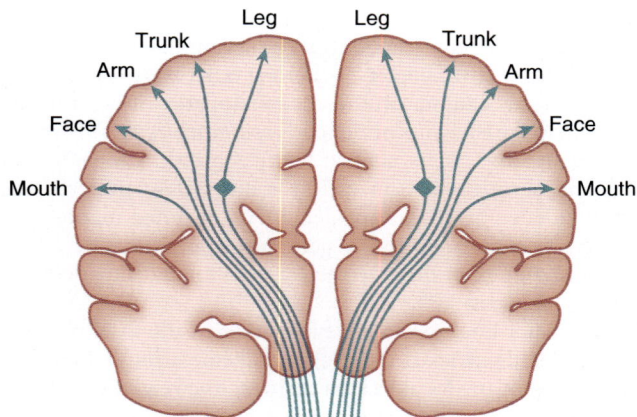

Figure 16.11 Schematic diagram of corticospinal tracts from their origin in the motor cortex, with descent past the periventricular region and into the internal capsule. The locus of periventricular leukomalacia (*marked square areas*) would be expected to affect, particularly, descending fibers for lower extremity more than the laterally placed fibers for upper extremity and face.

cystic PVL, are associated with spastic diplegia.[33,34,38,40,105-122] The severity and extent of injury, as manifested by cystic change or ventricular dilation or both, are correlated with more severe involvement of lower limbs, prominent involvement of upper limbs, and impairment of cognitive function. Further, in a study in which the location of cysts and/or signal abnormality on MR was compared with motor outcome, cysts located more anteriorly, near the corticospinal tracts, were most strongly associated with motor deficits (see Fig. 16.6).[96] The motor deficits in premature infants with mild spastic diplegia may disappear in the first several years of life, especially if the white matter lesions are noncystic by ultrasonography.[39]

In addition to the evidence cited above indicating that spastic diplegia is caused by periventricular injury to descending corticospinal tracts, injury to thalamocortical sensory afferents may also play a role in the motor deficits associated with PVL. Several studies using diffusion tensor imaging with diffusion anisotropy measures (see Chapter 10) to evaluate white matter integrity found correlations between the degree of white matter abnormality in thalamocortical tracts and motor deficits in older children who had been born prematurely.[123-126] Thus it has been hypothesized that disruption of sensorimotor loops involved in motor control plays an important role in the motor deficits associated with PVL. Nevertheless, in a recent report in which both corticospinal and thalamocortical tracts were assessed, correlation of motor dysfunction in spastic diplegia was greater for impairment of the former than the latter.[127]

Other Motor Disturbances. At least one-half of preterm infants exhibit motor disturbances despite the absence of cerebral palsy (Table 16.11).[128] These include difficulties in gross and/or fine motor skills, involving especially balance, visual motor

TABLE 16.10   Intellectual Function in Preterm Infants With Spastic Diplegia and Spastic Quadriplegia

INTELLECTUAL FUNCTION	SPASTIC DIPLEGIA[a] (n = 81) (%)	SPASTIC QUADRIPLEGIA[a] (n = 56) (%)
Normal or IQ ≥70	68	14
Moderate mental retardation	15	21
Severe mental retardation	17	54

[a]Spastic diplegia—lower extremities affected more than upper extremities; spastic quadriplegia—lower and upper extremities equally affected.

Data from Pharoah PO, Cooke T, Rosenbloom L, Cooke RW. Effects of birth weight, gestational age, and maternal obstetric history on birth prevalence of cerebral palsy. *Arch Dis Child.* 1987;62:1035–1040.

TABLE 16.11   Beyond Cerebral Palsy— Common Motor Disturbances in Premature Infants

Early difficulties in:
- gross and/or fine motor skills
- balance
- visual-motor integration
- hand-eye coordination
- manual dexterity

Later difficulties in:
- running
- drawing
- ball skills
- coordination

TABLE 16.12   Spectrum of Neurodevelopmental (Nonmotor) Deficits in Premature Infants

Cognitive
   Overall intellectual disability
   Executive dysfunction
   Language impairment
Behavior
   Attentional dysfunction
Socialization
   Autistic phenomena
Visual
   Cerebral visual impairment

integration, hand-eye coordination, manual dexterity, and related motor impairments. These disturbances are manifest in infancy as delayed motor milestones; at school age with impairment in activities ranging from running, ball skills, and drawing; and in adolescence and adulthood with clumsiness and dyscoordination. Although these deficits are minor in comparison to cerebral palsy, they are much more common and may affect quality of life.

The *clinicopathological correlates* of these disturbances are likely multiple. In keeping with a relation to the white matter injury of the encephalopathy of prematurity, long-term follow-up studies of preterm infants with white matter signal abnormalities detected on conventional (T_1- and T_2-weighted) MRI at term equivalent were strongly predictive of motor impairment at ages 2 and 5 years.[89,129] Further, diffusion abnormalities of white matter, including the internal capsule and corticospinal tracts, have been associated with similarly abnormal motor outcomes.[130-134] Whether gray matter structures involved in the encephalopathy of prematurity, for example, basal ganglia and thalamus, are involved seems likely, but has not been studied specifically. Recent work suggests importance also for cerebellar impairment.[98,128,135-137] More data are needed on this important issue.

Neurodevelopmental (Nonmotor) Deficits

Neurodevelopmental, nonmotor deficits now dominate the long-term neurological correlates of the encephalopathy of prematurity. These can be considered in terms of cognitive, behavioral, socialization, and visual deficits (Table 16.12).

Cognitive Deficits. Cognitive performance involves a complex series of functions that can be parsed in many ways. In this section, we review overall intelligence quotient (IQ) measures (often from younger populations) followed by outcome measures involving more specific cognitive functions, including language and executive function (EF) (Table 16.13).

Concerning *overall cognitive performance*, fully 30% to 50% of very preterm survivors exhibit cognitive deficits, and as a group, preterm infants have lower developmental quotients than their term-born counterparts. In a meta-analysis published in 2002,[138] the weighted mean difference in cognitive scores of preterm and term-born control infants was 10.9 (95% CI 9.2 to 12.5). This difference was directly proportional to gestational age or weight at birth, with values ranging as high as 22.7 (95% CI 16.3 to 29.1) for infants born weighing less than 750 g.[139] A 10-point reduction in IQ has significant meaning for an individual child, but also has meaning at a group level. For example, if one assumes, as an approximation, that the standard deviation of IQ values is similar between term and preterm children, a 10-point reduction in the mean value (from 100 to 90) corresponds to an increase in the fraction of children with IQ below 85 from 16% to 37%, and an increase in the fraction with IQ below 70 from 2.5% to 9%. This shift in distribution has social consequences, and it is well known that preterm children require a disproportionate amount of follow-up resources.[140]

Concerning the *clinicopathological correlates of the cognitive deficits* in premature infants, consistent with the concept of the encephalopathy of prematurity, *white matter injury* appears central. A relation of severe cognitive deficits to white matter involvement is apparent in infants with cystic PVL and

TABLE 16.13   Relation of Cerebral White Matter Abnormalities Identified by Magnetic Resonance Imaging at Term Equivalent to Outcome in Premature Infants at 2 Years of Age

OUTCOME MEASURE	WHITE MATTER ABNORMALITY AT TERM[a]				P
	NONE (n = 47)	MILD (n = 85)	MODERATE (n = 29)	SEVERE (n = 6)	
MDI cognitive score	92	85	80	70	<.001
PDI psychomotor score	95	91	80	56	.008
Severe motor delay (%)	4	5	26	67	<.001
Cerebral palsy (%)	2	6	24	67	<.001
Neurosensory impairment (%)	4	9	21	50	.003

[a]Severity of white matter abnormality graded according to a numerical scale based on nature and extent of white matter signal abnormality, white matter volume loss, cystic abnormalities, ventricular dilation, and thinning of the corpus callosum.

MDI, Mental Development Index; PDI, Psychomotor Development Index.

Adapted from Woodward LJ, Anderson PJ, Austin NC, Howard K, Inder TE. Neonatal MRI to predict neurodevelopmental outcomes in preterm infants. *N Engl J Med.* 2006;355:685–694.

spastic involvement of both upper and lower extremities, as described earlier (see Table 16.10). Notably, most infants with noncystic PVL exhibit only minor motor deficits, but prominent cognitive disturbance. Involvement of cerebral white matter fibers subserving visual, auditory, somesthetic, and associative functions may be crucial in this context. Indeed, the peritrigonal region, a site of predilection of PVL, is a region containing a high concentration of interhemispheric callosal commissural fibers, intrahemispheric associative fibers, and ascending (thalamocortical) and descending (cortical to deep nuclear structures and to brain stem/cord) projection fibers.[141,142] In an assessment of the relationship between the amount of white matter involved with PVL and cognitive outcome, the involvement of frontal white matter particularly predicted adverse cognitive and motor outcomes (see Fig. 16.6).[96] However, this regional distinction is not dramatic and has not been emphasized by others.[143,144]

The *importance of white matter injury in relation to cognitive outcome* was suggested by a series of studies that reported an association of impaired neurodevelopment in premature infants studied in *later infancy, childhood, and adolescence* in whom neuroimaging during the neonatal period showed white matter signal abnormality, ventricular dilation, and qualitative measures of diminished white matter volume.[145] The largest well-characterized study to date (n = 167) of VPT (<30 weeks' gestation) showed clearly the relationship between the frequency and severity of these neonatal MRI measures (obtained at term equivalent age) and subsequent cognitive motor deficits (see Table 16.13).[89] The increasing severity of white matter injury was accompanied by such abnormalities of gray matter as increased size of the subarachnoid space and impaired gyral maturation. The likely relation of the latter dysmaturation to primary injury to white matter was detailed in Chapters 7 and 14. Since the seminal work just described, there have been a large number of studies principally confirming the earlier observation.[91,146-148] White matter abnormality can also be quantified with diffusion imaging, particularly through measures of diffusion anisotropy (see Chapter 10).[134,149-151] For example, in a study of preterm children with follow up at 2 years, cognitive scores were correlated with anisotropy values in the corpus callosum.[152]

Consistent with the concept that primary cerebral white matter injury is related to the *secondary developmental disturbances of cerebral cortex, thalamus, and basal ganglia* seen in premature infants (see Chapter 14), a particularly detailed MRI study defined a *common neonatal image phenotype* that appeared to predict adverse neurodevelopmental outcome in children born preterm.[144] Based on a study of 80 preterm infants (mean gestational age 29 weeks) by MRI at term equivalent age, Boardman and collaborators delineated the common image phenotype as diffuse white matter injury and tissue volume reduction in the thalamus, globus pallidus, periventricular white matter, corona radiata, and central region of the centrum semiovale. The abnormal image phenotype was associated with reduced median DQ (DQ = 92) at 2 years compared with control infants (DQ = 112). In a similar study of adolescent children, Soria-Pastor et al. also found that lower white matter volume was associated with IQ and processing speed.[143]

Because our current concept of the encephalopathy of prematurity involves primary white matter injury leading to secondary dysmaturation of gray matter structures (see Chapter 14), it would be predicted that imaging studies of preterm infants later in life would show evidence of such developmental disturbances. Gray matter tissue signal abnormalities in preterm infants are less common *in the neonatal period* than are white matter signal abnormalities, perhaps consistent with the uncommon occurrence of acute neuronal injury. Gray matter abnormality is more typically manifest near term equivalent age as *alterations of cortical folding and/or enlarged extracerebral spaces*. As discussed in Chapter 7, dramatic changes in cortical folding take place during the third trimester of gestation. This process can be disrupted in preterm infants. For reasons that have not been fully elucidated, these cortical folding abnormalities most commonly involve the temporal and inferior frontal areas as well as the cingulate sulcus.[153] In a study of 167 VPT, gray matter abnormalities were found in half of the infants and consisted of abnormal/immature cortical folding patterns and/or enlarged subarachnoid space.[89] These abnormalities were associated with an increased risk of severe cognitive delay, psychomotor delay, and cerebral palsy at age 2 years, but the association was less robust than that with white matter abnormalities in the same study.[89] The *potential links between*

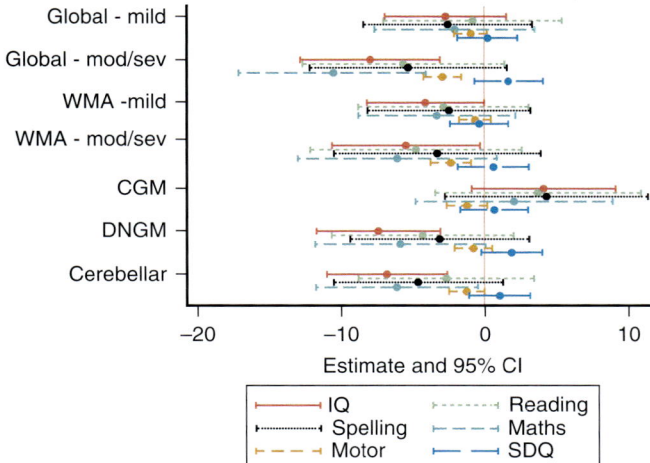

Figure 16.12 A plot showing the relationship of magnetic resonance imaging findings at term equivalent age for 186 preterm children and neurodevelopmental outcome at age 7 years. Full scale IQ was measured using the Wechsler Abbreviated Scale of Intelligence. Word, reading, spelling, and math computational skills were assessed with the *Wide Range Achievement Test* —Fourth edition. Motor skills were assessed using the Movement Assessment Battery for Children. Parents rated their child's behavior using the Strengths and Difficulties Questionnaire (SDQ) (note that for this test, higher scores indicate worse outcome). *CGM*, Cortical gray matter; *DNGM*, deep nuclear gray matter; *WMA*, white matter abnormality. (From Anderson PJ, Treyvaud K, Neil JJ, et al. Associations of newborn brain magnetic resonance imaging with long-term neurodevelopmental impairments in very preterm children. *J Pediatr.* 2017;187:58-65 e51.)

cerebral white matter injury and cortical folding abnormalities were discussed in Chapter 7, but may involve impairment of late migrating GABAergic neurons to superficial layers of cerebral cortex or of tension generated by underlying developing white matter. Perhaps more promising markers of cerebral cortical maturational impairment and subsequent outcome will include the cortical folding measures outlined recently by Shimony et al. (see Chapter 7).[154] In a study of neurodevelopmental outcomes in preterm children in which correlations were sought between abnormalities on MRI at term equivalent age and outcome at age 7 years,[155] T_1- and T_2-weighted MRI studies were scored for signal abnormality and/or volume loss in white matter, cortex, deep nuclear gray matter, and cerebellum. Higher global, deep gray matter and cerebellar as well as white matter abnormality scores were related to poorer IQ and motor function (Fig. 16.12).[155] Notably, abnormalities of the area of basal ganglia showed a strong relation to cognitive outcome. While area reduction could be related to direct injury to deep nuclear gray matter, it is more likely that basal ganglia area reduction reflects a disruption of reciprocal connections between basal ganglia and cortex as a consequence of white matter injury or cortical dysmaturation or both (see Chapter 14).

In addition to findings on conventional MRI, MR volumetry (see Chapter 10) has also been applied to evaluate preterm children and outcomes. *Widespread alterations in cerebral volumes* have been described for preterm infants imaged at term equivalent age,[156] and a number of studies have related volume changes with neurodevelopmental outcome. At short-term follow-up (<2 years), neurodevelopmental disability was associated with volumetric reductions in cerebral white matter, cerebral cortex, deep nuclear gray matter,[157-159] hippocampus, total cerebral tissue,[88,160,161] and cerebellum.[162]

EF is a broad term that refers to coordination of many interrelated processes and involves purposeful, goal-directed behavior that is instrumental in cognitive, behavioral, emotional, and social functions. While there is not yet consensus on the exact components of EF, it may be considered to include cognitive flexibility, goal setting, attentional control, and information processing.[163] Executive dysfunction, then, is not a unitary disorder, but reflects a range of impairment phenotypes.

One of the functional implications of executive dysfunction is poor academic performance (which may also be caused by low IQ), and a number of studies have shown poorer academic performance for preterm children on standardized testing.[164-167] Deficits in academic performance may also be manifest as learning disability. In a study of 75 children weighing less than 800 g at birth who had a verbal or performance IQ ≥85, 65% of preterm children met criteria for learning disability, as compared with 13% of the control group.[168] Findings on subtests were consistent with the large body of evidence showing that academic underachievement arises, at least in part, from executive dysfunction.

Concerning clinicopathological correlations, the association between imaging findings and executive/academic dysfunction in preterm children has been evaluated in multiple studies. In the study noted earlier with outcomes at age 7 years (see Fig. 16.12),[155] higher cerebral white matter, deep gray matter, and global abnormality scores were related to spelling and math computation. Studies focused on white matter injury have also noted associated impairments in executive functioning,[169,170] verbal and visuospatial working memory,[88,171] and learning.[173] *Overall the frequent concurrence of cerebral white matter abnormality with disturbances of gray matter structures is consistent with the central concept of the encephalopathy of prematurity.*

Language delay is common in preterm children (see Table 16.12).[174-178] The language and communication problems are often attributed to delayed development with the expectation of later catch-up. However, meta-analysis indicates that language deficits persist in preterm children with a severity comparable to that documented in other cognitive domains.[174,177,178] The language deficits affect quality of life, including friendship quality, reading skills, and overall academic achievement.[179-181] Language function can be divided into simple (vocabulary words and short phrases) and complex (wording, meaning of concepts, use of verbs, relational terms, and complex sentences). In a meta-analysis,[175] preterm children were found to lag behind term control children in both simple (0.5 SD, 95% CI 0.3 to 0.6) and complex (0.6 SD, 95% CI 0.4 to 0.8) language measures.

When considering the imaging correlates of language dysfunction, current concepts indicate that the anatomical substrate of language function involves widely distributed areas. Functional MRI studies show that language networks are detectable in preterm infants, despite the fact that the infants will not have any fluent speech for more than a year.[182-184] The imaging correlates of language impairment in preterm children are likely multiple, but white matter disturbance is identified commonly. For example, white matter injury has been associated with impaired language skills.[185,186] Cerebellar lesions in the absence of overt cerebral lesions have also been associated with abnormalities of receptive and expressive language.[187] Recall, however, that most cerebral white matter injury in premature infants may be below the resolution of conventional MRI (see earlier). Further, reduced corpus callosum volumes, consistent with white matter injury, have been related to impaired verbal fluency.[188]

Behavioral Disturbances. Especially common sequelae in premature infants involve behavioral issues, especially *attention-deficit/hyperactivity disorder* (*ADHD*). ADHD is relatively common among preterm children, with prevalence rates of 10% to 20%.[189] In a recent meta-analysis, preterm children had a relative risk of 2.64 compared with term-born children.[138] The prevalence also varies with degree of prematurity, and in one study was 17% for infants born weighing less than 750 g as compared with 6% in infants weighing 750 to 1499 g at birth.[139] ADHD has been associated with such neonatal medical factors as chronic lung disease, sepsis, and necrotizing enterocolitis, as well as intracranial hemorrhage and white matter injury.[134] It has also been suggested that reduction of perinatal systemic inflammation could reduce the incidence of ADHD.[190] Notably, systemic inflammation is an important precipitant of cerebral white matter injury (see Chapter 15). There are relatively few studies linking imaging abnormalities with attentional difficulties in preterm children, but one study comparing MRI at term equivalent age with outcome at age 7 years found that the strongest link with attention difficulties was abnormalities in deep nuclear gray matter.[191] The latter are commonly associated with cerebral white matter injury in the encephalopathy of prematurity.

Socialization Deficits—Autism Spectrum Disorders. Approximately 20% of preterm toddlers have abnormalities on early screening tests for autism spectrum disorder (ASD), such as the Modified Checklist for Autism in Toddlers (MCHAT), suggesting that they are at high risk for ASD.[134] Major motor, cognitive, visual, and hearing impairments may lead to false-positive screening tests, and these impairments may account for more than half of the positive MCHAT screens in extremely low gestational age newborns.[192-194] Nevertheless, even after those with such impairments are eliminated, 10% of children—nearly double the expected rate—screen positive. The perinatal clinical correlates of ASD and other social/behavioral issues in preterm infants are not yet fully delineated.[195] However, the risk of ASD does increase with the degree of prematurity, either with or without intellectual disability.[196,197] From a neuroimaging standpoint, ASD has been associated with cystic white matter lesions and cerebellar abnormalities during the perinatal period, although in studies with relatively small numbers of subjects.[198-200]

Visual Deficits. A number of injuries can lead to visual impairment in preterm children, ranging from retinopathy of prematurity (ROP) through injury to white matter visual pathways, thalamus, and cerebral cortex. In this section, we focus primarily on visual impairment caused by brain injury. Much of the visual impairment found in preterm children can be classified as cortical or cerebral visual impairment (CVI), which is defined as bilateral impairment of visual acuity due to damage to cerebral visual areas.[201] In a study of 105 preterm infants and 67 control infants, 24% of the preterm children met criteria for CVI, compared to 7% of controls (OR 3.86, 95% CI: 1.40 to 10.70). Several studies have evaluated the association between brain injury and visual impairment. Perhaps not surprisingly, PVL has a strong association with visual impairment,[202,203]

as the primary area of injury includes the optic radiations (geniculocalcarine tracts) and visual association fibers. More severe PVL correlates with poorer future vision,[58,204] and lesions of the peritrigonal white matter and optic radiations, as well as of the occipital cortex, have been associated with abnormality of visual acuity and function.[39,58]

CVI, though defined on the basis of visual acuity, is also associated with impaired visual perception and visual-motor integration. Geldof et al. have proposed that these impairments are related to injury involving occipital-parietal-frontal neural circuitries.[207] These circuitries are mediated by cerebral white matter regions particularly likely to be affected in cerebral white matter injury in premature infants. Consistent with the importance of cerebral white matter injury in recovery is the finding that only 42% of children with PVL and CVI show improvement in visual function, a proportion considerably lower than the 78% of a heterogeneous group of infants with primarily striate cortical injury.[208]

A number of studies have evaluated the relationship between the quality of MRI diffusion parameters of the geniculocalcarine tract (usually fractional anisotropy, see Chapter 10) and visual function.[209-211] In general, higher anisotropy values corresponded to better visual function. In one study of 142 preterm children and 32 control children who were evaluated at age 7 years, diffusion abnormalities were also found in association with white matter injury on conventional MRI and with ROP.[212] The association of abnormalities of the geniculocalcarine tract with ROP suggests that cerebral white matter changes not only can cause visual impairment, but can be caused by other abnormalities. In the case of ROP, it has been postulated that the abnormalities of the geniculocalcarine tract are a consequence of trans-synaptic effects. Other studies concerning structure function relationships include a volumetric study in which reduced occipital regional volumes were associated with impaired visual function.[212]

MANAGEMENT

Management of the encephalopathy of prematurity focuses especially on the central and initial neuropathological feature, that is, cerebral white matter injury. Prevention of the diverse dysmaturational events that occur in the weeks to months subsequent to the initiating white matter injury and during the remarkable series of complex developmental events normally occurring in brain (see Chapter 7) remains largely unknown and will only be discussed later in this section (see section on neurorestorative interventions). Thus the focus in this discussion of management will be prevention and treatment of cerebral white matter injury in the premature infant. As discussed in detail in Chapters 13 and 15, the two principal upstream mechanisms leading to this injury are *hypoxia-ischemia* and *infection-inflammation*. Thus the major emphases of management relate to these two mechanisms. The basic elements of management are outlined in Table 16.14.

Antenatal Interventions
Prevention of Premature Birth

Prevention of premature birth would be the most decisive way to prevent cerebral white matter injury of prematurity (Table 16.14). Attempts at prevention have emphasized (1) identification of the woman at high risk for premature delivery, (2) management

---

TABLE 16.14   Basic Elements of the Management of the Encephalopathy of Prematurity

Antenatal
Prevention of prematurity
Antenatal magnesium
Antenatal steroids
Antenatal antibiotics and other antiinflammatory agents
Optimal management of labor and delivery
Delayed cord clamping/umbilical cord milking (?)
Newborn resuscitation
Ventilation
Oxygen
Carbon dioxide
Perfusion
Glucose
Seizures
Indomethacin (?)
Neuroprotective interventions
Neurorestorative interventions

---

of such a woman with a combination of approaches, and (3) early treatment of premature labor, primarily with tocolytic agents (see Chapter 24). Overall, results thus far have not been dramatically beneficial.

Antenatal Magnesium

Magnesium sulfate has been used for many years in obstetrics as a tocolytic agent for preterm labor and as therapy for preeclampsia. The evidence of its effectiveness for the latter purpose is stronger than that concerning its role as a tocolytic (see Chapter 24). Particular interest for the maternal use of magnesium sulfate in the prevention of neurological deficits in infants born prematurely began with a report that only 7.1% of VLBW infants with later cerebral palsy were exposed to maternal magnesium sulfate versus 36% of a control group.[213] In a subsequent study of approximately 1000 premature infants, those whose mothers received magnesium sulfate had a lower prevalence of cerebral palsy (0.9%) than those whose mothers did not receive this agent (7.7%).[214] However, subsequent evidence regarding benefit for magnesium sulfate for prevention of cerebral palsy or associated brain lesions or both has not been consistently positive.[215-231] Meta-analyses have shown that antenatal magnesium sulfate administered for neuroprotection in preterm infants is associated with a reduction of cerebral palsy at a corrected age of 18 to 24 months,[232-234] but studies of longer-term outcomes have failed to show benefit.[235,236]

Experimental studies concerning a beneficial role for magnesium in prevention or amelioration of hypoxic-ischemic death also have yielded conflicting results. Thus, in perinatal hypoxic-ischemic models in the rat, piglet, and fetal lamb, magnesium sulfate treatment either during or immediately following the insult did not ameliorate adverse biochemical, neurophysiological, or neuropathological effects.[237-239] Nevertheless, other experimental work supported the potential value of magnesium by several mechanisms (i.e., antiexcitatory amino acid [impairs release, blocks the N-methyl-D-aspartate (NMDA) receptor], antioxidant [essential for glutathione biosynthesis], anticytokine [decreases levels of inflammatory

cytokines], and antiplatelet [decreases platelet aggregation] effects).[240-246] Perhaps the most likely beneficial effect of magnesium relates to its strong vasodilatory properties, which can lead to an increase in uteroplacental blood flow and perhaps also to improved fetal perfusion.[247-251] Such effects also could decrease the likelihood that the infant postnatally would experience a pressure-passive cerebral circulation and thereby cerebral ischemia and periventricular white matter injury (see Chapter 13).

A recent large randomized trial suggests that the gestational age of the infant may be critical in determining whether antenatal magnesium sulfate is beneficial.[252] Thus, in infants born at less than 32 weeks of gestation, 82% of the preterm infants in the study, magnesium sulfate was associated with a reduction in occurrence of echolucency or echodensity. Moreover, a reduced risk of cerebral palsy at 2 years of age (OR 0.63, 95%, CI 0.42 to 0.95) was observed and could be partially accounted for by the ultrasonographic findings. More data are needed on these issues.

Antenatal Steroids

Antenatal administration of glucocorticoids may be useful in prevention of cerebral white matter injury in premature infants (see Table 16.14). Several studies using cranial ultrasonography for detection of largely cystic PVL have shown a beneficial effect.[253-258] Antenatal steroids also have a clear benefit in reducing the incidence of germinal matrix-intraventricular hemorrhage. The beneficial effects of steroids occur after a complete course and preferably, with betamethasone. Perhaps related to these effects, a recent review noted that a single course of antenatal steroids was associated with a reduced risk of cerebral palsy (RR 0.83, CI 0.74 to 0.93), psychomotor development index less than 70 (RR 0.79, CI 0.73 to 0.85), and less overall severe disability (RR 0.79, CI 0.73 to 0.85).[259]

The basis for the beneficial effect of antenatal steroids likely relates at least in part to the long-established enhancement of pulmonary maturation and the consequent decrease in respiratory distress syndrome.[260] Treated infants have improved cardiovascular stability, with less hypotension postnatally and less need for blood pressure support.[257,261-263] This beneficial postnatal hemodynamic effect could relate to less likelihood of impaired cerebrovascular autoregulation because of improved placental blood flow (see Chapter 24). The possibility also exists that glucocorticoids have a beneficial effect on brain maturation, especially the periventricular vasculature (see Chapter 24).

Not all infant populations are benefitted similarly by antenatal glucocorticoids. For example, a recent study showed no difference in respiratory distress syndrome or IVH after antenatal corticosteroids.[264] Moreover, certain steroid preparations, for example, dexamethasone, have been associated with adverse effects on brain development especially when used for prolonged periods postnatally (see Chapters 4 and 7).

Antenatal Antibiotics and Other Antiinflammatory Agents

Antibiotics. In a subset of infants, maternal intrauterine infection and fetal systemic inflammation appear important in pathogenesis of cerebral white matter injury (see Table 16.14; see Chapter 15). Moreover, maternal intrauterine infection is a major cause of spontaneous preterm labor. A study of over 4000 women in spontaneous preterm labor compared administration of erythromycin and/or amoxicillin-clavulanate with that of placebo.[265] At age 7 years the children administered either antibiotic regimen showed *no benefit in functional attainment*, those administered erythromycin showed an *increase* in functional impairment, and those administered either antibiotic regimen showed an *increase in risk of cerebral palsy*.[265] Thus the *routine* use of antibiotics is not of apparent benefit in mothers in spontaneous labor. In a separate study, the use of erythromycin in preterm labor with premature rupture of membranes led to a small reduction in adverse short-term neonatal outcome, but the adverse effect of erythromycin in the study just described raises questions about the merit of this practice.[266] Note that these data do not address the antibiotic treatment of overt chorioamnionitis in mothers with premature rupture of membranes or mothers with positive Group B streptococcal cultures (see Chapter 35).

N-Acetylcysteine. Another antenatal attempt to combat the effects of intrauterine infection/systemic inflammation involves the use of *N*-acetylcysteine (NAC; see Table 16.14).[267,268] NAC is a free radical scavenger that, in experimental models of chorioamnionitis, has been shown to cross the blood-brain barrier, decrease oxidative stress, and exhibit multiple antiinflammatory effects. In a recent study of mothers with chorioamnionitis, 22 were randomized to receive either intravenous NAC or saline before delivery and for 2.5 days past delivery.[268] In saline-treated infants cerebrovascular autoregulation was impaired, but in NAC-treated infants this critical parameter, a potential precursor to hypoxic-ischemic injury, was preserved. Whether this apparent beneficial effect will lead to prevention of brain injury or dysfunction will require a larger study. Nevertheless, the data are of interest.

Optimal Management of Labor and Delivery

Potentially deleterious effects of labor and delivery relate in considerable part to the easily deformed, particularly compliant skull of the premature infant (see Table 16.14). Such deformations could lead to such cerebral hemodynamic disturbances as increases in venous pressure and perhaps an impairment of cerebrovascular autoregulation (see Chapter 13). Prolonged labor and breech delivery potentially could lead to such hemodynamic effects (see Chapter 24). The relation of cerebral white matter injury to such clinical markers as fetal metabolic acidosis (see earlier) supports the notion that labor and delivery are important periods for careful management to prevent hypoxic-ischemic insults or the development of cerebrovascular autoregulatory dysfunction that might lead to hypoxia-ischemia subsequently. Such issues as the role of elective cesarean section or the timing of the latter in relation to duration of labor are relevant in this context (see Chapter 24).

Delayed Cord Clamping/Umbilical Cord Milking

These mechanisms of placental transfusion, currently under intensive study, theoretically could lead to such favorable consequences as improved hemodynamics (see Table 16.14; see Chapter 24). Whether either approach is beneficial in prevention of hypoxic-ischemic insults and cerebral white matter injury is unknown. Currently infants who require resuscitation are not candidates for these approaches (see Chapter 24).

Newborn Resuscitation

The importance of prompt temperature stabilization and establishment of adequate ventilation and perfusion in the newly born premature infant is paramount. Hypoxemia and hypercarbia should be avoided because these two conditions can result in a pressure-passive circulation (see Chapter 13). Because of a structurally immature myocardium, the VLBW infant has limited capacity to adapt to the pronounced changes in pre- and afterload occurring around the time of birth.[269] This transient phenomenon may lead to reduced systemic and cerebral blood flow (CBF).[270] A recent small study showed that impaired perfusion on day one correlates with an adverse outcome (IVH and PVL).[270] Thus the findings define "*a vulnerable phase of the circulation during adaptation*" and indicate the importance of extra vigilance in management of the circulation at this time.

Concern for *potential deleterious effects of hyperoxia* (e.g., oxidative stress, vasoconstriction, organ injury—including retina and brain) led in the first decade of this century to a major change in practice from the use in resuscitation of 100% oxygen to much lower levels. A survey in 2015 of 25 countries found that only 4 used 100% oxygen and greater than 70% used ≤40% oxygen.[271] In addition, the 2015 guidelines released by an International Consensus group, including the American Heart Association, recommended that resuscitation of preterm newborns less than 35 weeks' gestation be initiated with relatively low oxygen levels, 21% to 30%.[272] However, the largest randomized controlled trial to date recently showed that resuscitation of infants less than 28 weeks' gestation with room air versus 100% oxygen resulted in higher hospital mortality (22% vs. 6%).[273] Similarly, a large retrospective Canadian study showed that after a change of resuscitation guidelines from 100% to room air, severe neurological injury increased (OR 1.36, CI 1.11 to 1.66).[274] More data are needed concerning this important issue.

Ventilation

Maintenance of adequate ventilation is a central aspect of postnatal *supportive care*, an imprecise term that refers to the maintenance also of temperature, perfusion, and metabolic status. The importance of these various postnatal aspects of management cannot be overemphasized; disturbances of ventilation and perfusion particularly may play an important role in determining the ultimate severity of neurological injury.

Oxygen

In the following discussion we will review the deleterious effects of overt hypoxemia and hyperoxemia. The issue of the optimal range of oxygen saturation in premature infants has been the topic of considerable research in recent years.[275-281] The principal comparisons have been between groups with oxygen saturation targets of 85% to 89% versus 91% to 95%. No dramatic differences in outcomes were observed, although in the most recent study the lower oxygen saturation group had nonsignificantly higher rates of death or disability at 2 years but significantly increased risks of this combined outcome and of death alone in post hoc combined analyses.[281] In general, the neurodevelopmental outcomes and rates of serious ROP were similar between the two groups, although necrotizing enterocolitis, a major risk factor for cerebral white matter injury (see earlier), occurred less frequently in the higher oxygen group.

TABLE 16.15	Deleterious Consequences of Disturbed Oxygenation

Hypoxia
Pressure-passive cerebral circulation
White matter (and potentially neuronal) injury
Impaired pre-oligodendrocyte differentiation
Hyperoxia
Increased oxidative stress
Cerebral vasoconstriction
Impaired periventricular angiogenesis
Retinopathy of prematurity
Pontosubicular neuronal necrosis

TABLE 16.16	Common Causes of Hypoxemia in Low-Birth-Weight Infants

Feeding procedures
Overfeeding with abdominal distention, neck flexion, and
   hand-under-jaw feeding
Crying
Airway manipulations
Suctioning, neck flexion, neck hyperextension, and poorly
   placed nasal mask or endotracheal tube
Diagnostic procedures
Painful procedures and abdominal examination with
   compression
Seizures
Apneic episodes
Other
Handling, excessive noise, active sleep, and ambient
   temperature out of infant's thermoneutral zone

The most reasonable current conclusion is that "targeting an oxygen saturation of 91% to 95% is safer than targeting an oxygen saturation of 85% to 89%."[281]

Hypoxemia. Avoidance of oxygen deprivation is a cornerstone of supportive therapy. Hypoxemia may lead to a disturbance of cerebrovascular autoregulation and, as a consequence, a *pressure-passive circulation* (Table 16.15; see Chapter 13). Under such circumstances, the infant is vulnerable to ischemic cerebral white matter injury with only moderate decreases in arterial blood pressure (see Chapter 15). Indeed, this hemodynamic mechanism may be the most important by which hypoxemia leads to parenchymal injury. The propensity for white matter injury presumably relates in part to the limited vasodilatory capacity in neonatal cerebral white matter in the presence of anaerobic glycolysis, increased substrate demand and a cellular population, pre-OLs, exquisitely vulnerable to hypoxia-ischemia and resulting oxidative attack (see Chapter 15).

Concerning *detection and causes of hypoxemia*, very diligent surveillance is critical. The use of pulse oximetry and transcutaneous oxygen monitoring has demonstrated that among infants in neonatal intensive care facilities, especially low-birth-weight infants, episodes of hypoxemia are more frequent than often thought and are readily overlooked by *periodic* sampling of arterial blood. Thus *continuous* transcutaneous oxygen or pulse oximetry monitoring in sick, low-birth-weight infants has detected some very frequent and, in some cases, previously unsuspected causes of hypoxemia (Table 16.16).[282-299]

Continuous transcutaneous oxygenation measurement *via* pulse oximetry has become standard practice, but it would be more relevant to measure *cerebral* oxygenation *via* near infrared spectroscopy (NIRS; Chapter 10). For example, NIRS has been used to show that hypoxemia with apnea results in *cerebral deoxygenation*.[300] In a multicenter, phase II, randomized trial of 166 infants born at less than 28 weeks' gestation, continuous NIRS monitoring was used during the first 72 hours of life with a standardized approach to maintaining cerebral oxygenation. This regimen was associated with a significant reduction of time spent with cerebral oxygenation below 55%,[301] but serial cranial ultrasound studies and MRI at term equivalent age did not show any difference in severity of injury in monitored and control infants.[302] However, it has been suggested that the incidence of intermittent hypoxia in extremely low-birth-weight infants progressively increases over the first 4 weeks of postnatal life, with a subsequent plateau followed by a slow decline beginning at weeks 6 to 8,[303] raising the possibility that longer-term cerebral

monitoring may be useful. *This timing is interesting because some clinical, imaging, and neuropathological data suggest that the first days and weeks of life are critical, concerning the timing of cerebral white matter injury (see earlier).* Overall, while the use of continuous NIRS monitoring of cerebral oxygenation is promising, there is not yet sufficient evidence from outcome-based clinical trials to recommend its routine use.

Hyperoxia. Although hypoxemia is serious and requires prompt reaction, overreaction also may be deleterious if *hyperoxia* is produced (see Table 16.15). The latter may lead to *white matter or neuronal injury*. Experimental studies also show that hyperoxia can lead to cerebral white matter injury similar to PVL (see Chapter 15 and later). Moreover, the neuropathological data reviewed in Chapter 14 suggest a role for hyperoxia in the genesis of a specific pattern of neuronal injury, pontosubicular necrosis. In addition, the possibility that hyperoxia may contribute to neuronal and white matter injury by causing a reduction in CBF must be considered. Reductions of CBF of 20% to 30% were shown with hyperoxia in newborn puppies, although the arterial oxygen tensions (PaO_2) of approximately 350 mm Hg used were very high.[304] Notably, in human premature infants, CBF measured by xenon clearance 2 hours after birth was 23% lower in infants who were resuscitated with 80% oxygen versus infants resuscitated with room air.[305] In view of the critical role of cerebral ischemia in the genesis of cerebral white matter injury, this apparent effect of hyperoxia requires further study, especially in view of the recent studies concerning oxygen levels in resuscitation (see earlier).

Finally, although the cause of *ROP* is now recognized to be complex, hyperoxia remains an important factor.[306,307] Nevertheless, the use of lower oxygen levels in preterm infants to reduce the risk of retinopathy of maturity remains an area of active research. In a recent meta-analysis, lower oxygen saturation targets did reduce the risk of ROP, but were also associated with higher mortality.[308] The issue of recommended oxygen saturation target range was discussed earlier.

Is the Optimal Oxygen Saturation in Premature Infants Age-Dependent? *Recent experimental studies* raise the question of whether the identification of optimal oxygen tension for premature infants depends not only on the absolute value but also the postnatal age of the infant. Thus at birth the transition from intrauterine placental to postnatal pulmonary oxygenation results in a drastic increase in brain oxygenation.[309] This abrupt increase in oxygenation leads in experimental models to a diminution in brain expression of the hypoxia-inducible factor, HIF 1α/HIF 2α genes. Among the results of the latter is an increase in Wnt signaling and a decrease in VEGF expression, unlike the normal physiological situation with lower oxygen tension in fetal brain during pregnancy.[310-312] These molecular events result in a *diminution in angiogenesis*, particularly in periventricular vessels, which are the last to mature in developing white matter. The anatomical consequences are periventricular vascular underdevelopment and local hypoxia-ischemia with the propensity to development *of focal periventricular necrosis and cyst formation*, that is, typical *cystic* PVL. (Note that this mechanism does not involve oxidative stress which, as described in Chapter 15, appears to be important in a neonatal rodent model of hyperoxia-induced PVL.)[313] Later, under conditions of hypoxia, as can occur in the postnatal period because of pulmonary, cardiac, and other neonatal complications, there is upregulation of HIF 1α/HIF 2α and Wnt signaling that leads to *arrest of pre-OL maturation diffusely in cerebral white matter*. The result of the pre-OL maturation failure, of course, would be hypomyelination, the hallmark of the diffuse component of PVL, as observed in both clinical and experimental studies (see earlier and Chapter 14). Accompanying upregulation of VEGF leads to enhancement of angiogenesis and thereby a decline in propensity to periventricular cystic lesions. (The similarities of this pathophysiology to ROP are apparent, wherein the initial relative hyperoxia leads to diminished retinal angiogenesis and, as a result, retinal hypoxia-ischemia, with the latter then resulting in retinal injury and excessive angiogenesis.) The implications for management of the premature infant are that hyperoxia should be avoided, especially in the early postnatal period. Indeed, it has been postulated that "restraint in using high Fi0₂ with careful monitoring of arterial oxygen saturation by pulse oximetry might have contributed to the decline of cystic PVL observed over the last decades."[309] Whether a graded postnatal increase in Fi0₂ levels from early to later in the postnatal period would be appropriate management for the sick premature infant is an important question, based on the experimental data just described. More data are needed on these critical issues.

Carbon Dioxide

Because $PaCO_2$ may have serious metabolic and vascular effects, careful control thereof is critical (see Table 16.14). As with oxygen determinations, periodic sampling of arterial blood is not an optimal means to monitor $PaCO_2$ serially. Experience with continuous transcutaneous monitoring of PCO_2 or serial measurements of end-tidal carbon dioxide pressure indicates that events as frequent as, and often similar to, those recorded in Table 16.16 result in marked changes in $PaCO_2$.[289,292,314-316] However, the use of end-tidal CO_2 is somewhat problematic in premature infants for such technical issues as leakage around uncuffed endotracheal tubes and other factors. Sampling breath close to the carina by measuring distal end-tidal CO_2 is less susceptible to such factors. A recent small study showed that the latter approach improved ability to maintain infant CO_2

TABLE 16.17	Deleterious Consequences of Disturbed Carbon Dioxide Levels

Hypercarbia (marked)
Vascular
Pressure-passive cerebral circulation
Cerebral vasodilation with hemorrhagic complications (e.g., intraventricular hemorrhage)
Metabolic
Cerebral acidosis
Hypocarbia
Vascular
Diminished cerebral blood flow: ischemic injury

levels in a predetermined *safe* range (PCO_2 30 to 60 mm Hg) and led to a decline in incidence of IVH and PVL.[317]

Hypercarbia. Marked elevations of $PaCO_2$ are particularly dangerous in such infants because of the resulting increase in tissue PCO_2 and consequent worsening of intracellular acidosis in brain (Table 16.17). Perhaps more important than the *metabolic* effects and worsening of tissue acidosis are the *vascular* effects of hypercarbia. Thus hypercarbia results in an impairment of cerebrovascular autoregulation and, as a consequence, a pressure-passive circulation (see Chapter 13). In one study of 43 ventilated preterm infants in the first week of life, a progressive loss of vascular autoregulation was observed with $PaCO_2$ values of 45 mm Hg or greater.[318] As noted previously concerning hypoxemia, with hypercarbia the infant becomes especially vulnerable to ischemic cerebral injury with decreases in arterial blood pressure. Moreover, because of the potent vasodilatory effect of hypercarbia, CBF may increase and may cause a risk of hemorrhage in vulnerable capillary beds (e.g., germinal matrix and thereby intraventricular hemorrhage). These adverse effects with marked hypercarbia should be contrasted with the apparent *beneficial* effects of *mild* hypercarbia during hypoxia-ischemia (see later).

Hypocarbia. The effect of *hypocarbia* on CBF is pronounced (see Table 16.17). Although marked diminutions have been documented in adult humans and animals,[319-321] the findings in neonatal animals have not been entirely consistent.[322-332] Differences in results appear to relate in part to species and methodological differences. The following conclusions seem warranted. With hypocarbia to approximately 20 mm Hg, little change in CBF occurs. With lower levels (mean, 17 mm Hg), a definite decline in regional CBF occurs in the puppy.[327] However, in the piglet, extreme hypocarbia (<15 mm Hg) is necessary to produce statistically significant decreases in CBF.[326] Perhaps the most consistent observation in the several animal models is that the linear relationship between $PaCO_2$ and CBF becomes curvilinear at tensions lower than 20 to 25 mm Hg[319,324,326]; the decrease in CBF for a given decrease in $PaCO_2$ becomes *considerably less* than it is above this lower range of $PaCO_2$. In addition, adaptation occurs such that in the newborn lamb, CBF after 6 hours of $PaCO_2$ of 15 mm Hg is not statistically different from that in control animals.[330] Perhaps of greatest importance despite the decreases in CBF in newborn animals, no change in cerebral metabolic rate for oxygen occurs, primarily because of an increase in oxygen extraction.[328,330] Thus mild hypocarbia may be of little or no danger, *although data in the human newborn concerning hypocarbia are of concern (see later).*

Perhaps relevant in this context is the demonstration that *mild hypocarbia (PaCO$_2$ of 26 mm Hg) interacted adversely with hypoxic-ischemic insults in the immature rat.*[333-335] Thus animals exposed to hypoxia-ischemia during mild hypocarbia sustained a larger decline in CBF, a greater degree of cerebral glucose and energy depletion, and more neuropathological evidence of brain injury than did animals exposed to the same insult but with normocarbia (PaCO$_2$ of 39 mm Hg) or mild hypercarbia (PaCO$_2$ of 54 mm Hg). The latter two groups had better preserved CBF, less severe cerebral biochemical deficits, and less severe brain injury. The mildly hypercarbic animals had the most favorable hemodynamic, biochemical, and neuropathological outcomes.

CBF in the human infant is responsive to changes in PaCO$_2$, except under conditions of maximal vasodilation in the mechanically ventilated preterm infant (in the first days of life).[318,336-342] *Concern for impaired CBF with vasoconstriction caused by hypocarbia seems warranted.* Thus, in one study of 32 ventilated premature infants on the first day of life, values of PaCO$_2$ lower than 25 mm Hg were associated with slowing of the EEG tracing and increased cerebral fractional oxygen extraction, likely related to decreased cerebral oxygen delivery induced by hypocarbia.[342] Moreover, an increased risk for cystic PVL was shown after cumulative time periods of PaCO$_2$ lower than 25 mm Hg.[343-345] An earlier study also suggested a threshold value of 25 mm Hg.[346] Moreover, in another report, 21 of 56 ventilated preterm infants (37%) who were exposed to a maximally low PaCO$_2$ value of less than 20 mm Hg at least once during the first 3 days of life developed large periventricular cysts or cerebral palsy, or both.[347] Although the potency of the relationship between hypocarbia and PVL or cerebral palsy, or both, varied somewhat among earlier studies, the relationship has received considerable support.[346,348-354] Indeed, a report of 778 premature infants (birth weight, 501 to 1249 g) measured a *cumulative index of hypocarbia (PaCO$_2$ ≤ 35 mm Hg) over the first 7 days of life and found a strong association with the occurrence of cystic PVL, identified as echolucencies on cranial ultrasonography* (Fig. 16.13).[354] As noted in Chapter 24, extremes of PaCO$_2$ are also associated with intraventricular hemorrhage.[355,356]

Perfusion

The maintenance of adequate perfusion to brain is a critical aspect of supportive care (see Table 16.14) and important for prevention of additional ischemic cerebral white matter injury. The basic elements of maintenance of adequate perfusion are summarized in Table 16.18 and in the following discussion.

Recognition of Pressure-Passive Cerebral Circulation

The problem of impaired cerebrovascular autoregulation and a *pressure-passive cerebral circulation is particularly severe in the sick premature infant.* Numerous studies using invasive and noninvasive methods have shown the pressure-passive state.[336,357-365] In one series (N = 32) of ventilated premature infants studied by NIRS from the first hours of life, 53% were found to have extended periods of a pressure-passive state (Fig. 16.14; see Chapter 13).[360] *Moreover, the nadirs of blood pressure were often not markedly low* and thus could be readily overlooked. A later study of 90 premature infants used a more sophisticated frequency-based assessment by NIRS and found that fully 95% of the infants had pressure-passive epochs in the first days of

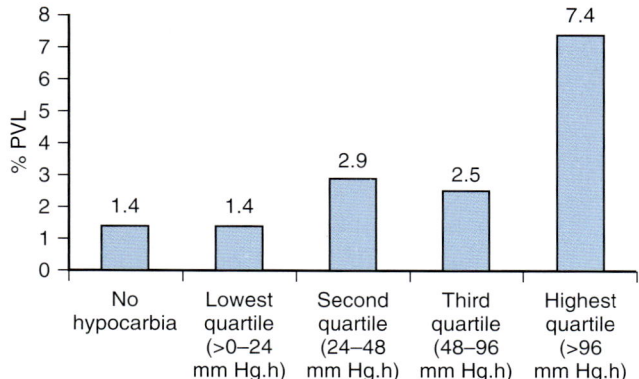

Figure 16.13 Cumulative index of hypocarbia in the first week of life and the occurrence of periventricular leukomalacia (PVL). Study involved 778 infants with range of birth weights of 501 to 1249 g. PVL was identified by the occurrence of echolucencies on cranial ultrasonography at approximately 28 days of age. Hypocarbia was defined as PaCO$_2$ less than 35 mm Hg, and the cumulative index of exposure (CIE) to hypocarbia was calculated as (35 − PaCO$_2$) multiplied by the time interval in hours for each 6-hour block in a 24-hour day. The frequency of PVL in the highest quartile of CIE differed from that with no hypocarbia (P <.03). (From Shankaran S, Langer JC, Kazzi SN, et al. Cumulative index of exposure to hypocarbia and hyperoxia as risk factors for periventricular leukomalacia in low birth weight infants. *Pediatrics*. 2006;118:1654–1659.)

TABLE 16.18 Maintenance of Adequate Perfusion
Recognition of pressure-passive cerebral circulation
Recognition of "normal" arterial blood pressure level
Avoidance of systemic hypotension (may cause ischemic injury)
Avoidance of systemic hypertension (may cause hemorrhagic complications)
Avoidance of hyperviscosity

life.[363] The overall mean proportion of pressure-passive time was 20%, although some of the smallest infants were in a pressure-passive state more than 50% of the time. Hypotension (see later) also was a common finding, and the likelihood of a pressure-passive state increased with both decreasing gestational age and hypotension. However, the pressure-passive state fluctuated over time and occurred commonly without low blood pressures. Hypoxia and hypercarbia, as with severe respiratory disease, are known precipitants of a pressure-passive cerebral circulation. Necrotizing enterocolitis, a strong risk factor for cerebral white matter injury (see earlier), also is associated with impaired cerebrovascular autoregulation.[366] Thus continuous monitoring of cerebral hemodynamics by a methodology such as NIRS would be valuable to determine whether an infant is in a pressure-passive state at any given blood pressure. Further insights into the causes of the cerebrovascular regulatory abnormality could lead to correction of the abnormality and perhaps prevention of ischemic brain injury in these infants. Recent studies have shown promise for techniques based on NIRS, Doppler measurements of CBF velocity, plethysmographic analysis of pulse oximetry signal, and echocardiography/Doppler-derived superior vena cava flow.[18,270,366-370] Further data will be of great interest.

The lower limit of the autoregulatory curve in newborns, especially preterm newborns, obviously is of great importance

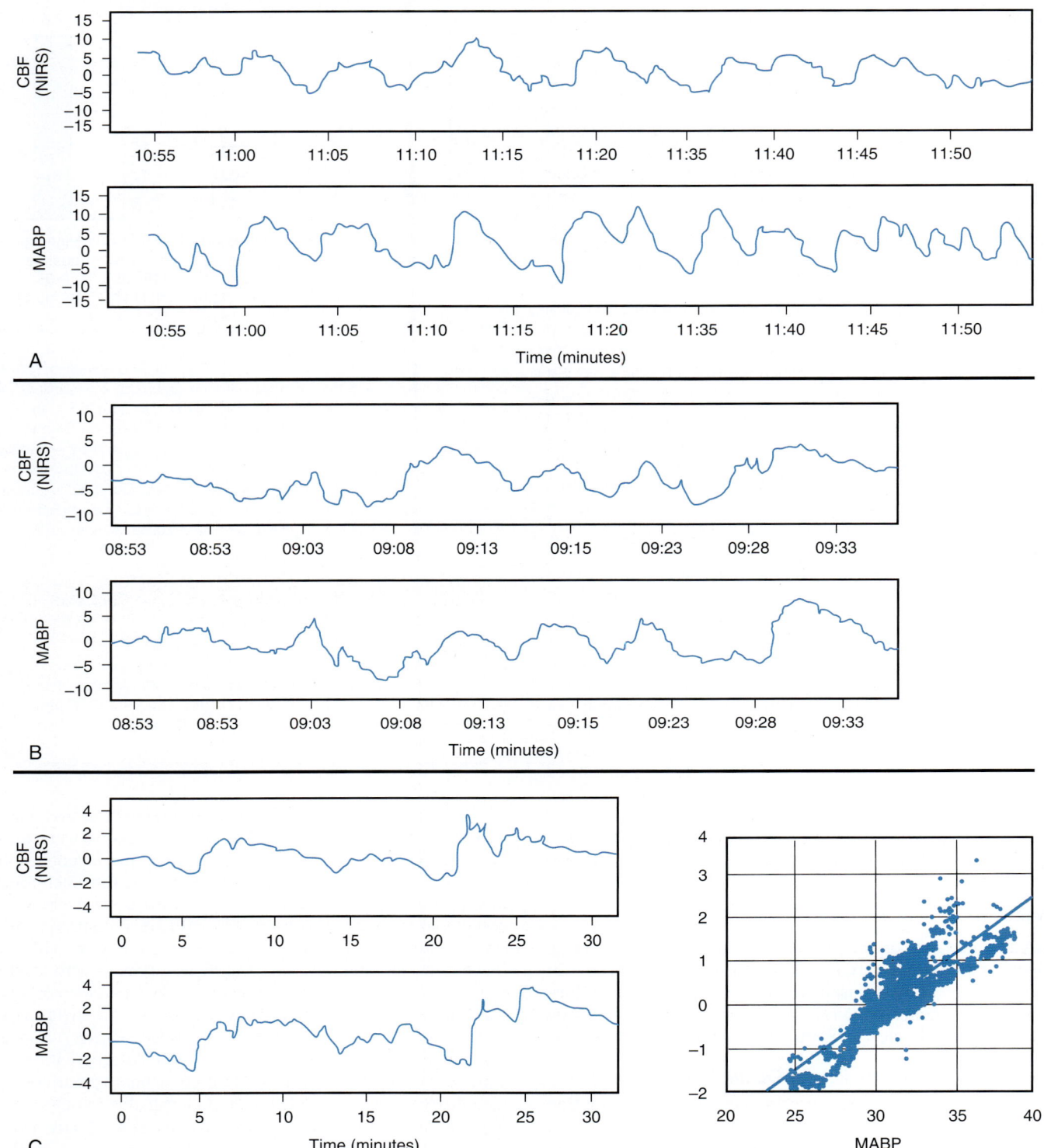

Figure 16.14 Pressure-passive relationship of cerebral blood flow, estimated by near-infrared spectroscopy (see Chapter 10), and mean arterial blood pressure in ventilated premature infants. Note the parallel changes in arterial blood pressure and cerebral perfusion (A–C). Note also that the changes in blood pressure are not marked. In (C) all data points are plotted; the linear relationship between blood pressure and cerebral perfusion is apparent. *CBF,* Cerebral blood flow; *MABP,* mean arterial blood pressure; *NIRS,* near infrared spectroscopy. (From Tsuji M, Saul JP, du Plessis A, et al. Cerebral intravascular oxygenation correlates with mean arterial pressure in critically ill premature infants. *Pediatrics.* 2000;106:625–632.)

for management purposes. The precise lower limit is unknown and likely fluctuates for a given infant. Critical determining factors, in addition to gestational age, likely include such vasoactive factors as blood gases, seizures, hypoxia-ischemia, and cytokines. Several reports provide insight into the lower limit of the autoregulatory curve.[361,364,365] Thus, in a study of infants of 24 to 30 weeks of gestation on the first day of life, mean blood pressure values lower than 31 mm Hg were associated with impaired EEG continuity, perhaps related to decreased CBF at such values.[364] Similarly, in a study of extremely low-birth-weight infants (mean birth weight, 772 g; mean gestational age, 26 weeks) by NIRS, a pressure-passive cerebral circulation resulted when mean arterial blood pressures were less than 30 mm Hg (Fig. 16.15).[361] However, to what extent, if any, arterial blood pressures lower than 30 mm Hg are dangerous is unclear. Thus a study of cerebral electrical activity and cerebral fractional oxygen extraction, presumably a reflection in part of the adequacy of CBF, in 35 23- to 30-week premature infants showed no electrical abnormality at mean blood pressures higher than 23 mm Hg.[365] Clearly, more data combining cerebral hemodynamic and functional parameters are needed.

Recognition of Normal Arterial Blood Pressure Levels in the Newborn

A series of studies has investigated normal values for arterial blood pressure in the newborn.[371-391] In the first 12 hours of life, an inverse relationship between birth weight and blood pressure was shown (Table 16.19 and Fig. 16.16). Although this relationship continued over the next 2 days, a postnatal increase in mean blood pressure also was apparent. In a study of 131 premature infants in a neonatal intensive care unit, mean blood pressure over the first 96 hours was described by a linear function (mean blood pressure in mm Hg = 31.6 + (0.1 × hours age) + (0.0057 × birth weight in g)).[384] In a study of 147 infants born at 28 to 36 weeks' gestation, blood pressure

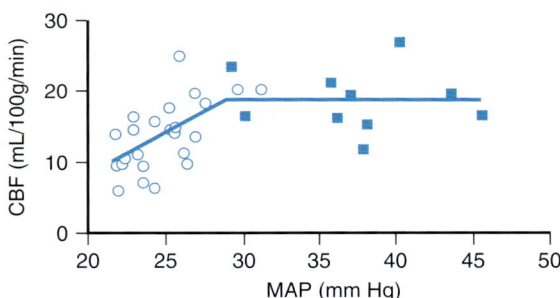

Figure 16.15 Analysis of cerebral autoregulation in extremely low-birth-weight infants (mean, 772 g). Infants studied were either clinically normotensive (*closed squares*) or were clinically hypotensive and studied just before treatment with dopamine (*open circles*). A breakpoint in the autoregulation curve relating cerebral blood flow (CBF), determined by near-infrared spectroscopy, to mean arterial blood pressure (MAP) was identified at MAP = 29 mm Hg. (From Munro MJ, Walker AM, Barfield CP. Hypotensive extremely low birth weight infants have reduced cerebral blood flow. *Pediatrics.* 2004;114:1591–1596.)

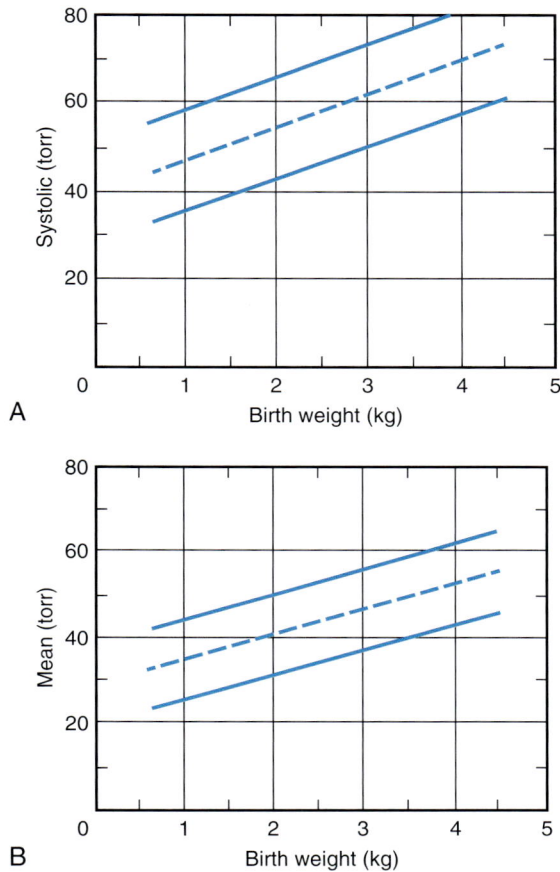

Figure 16.16 Blood pressure as a function of birth weight. (A) Systolic and, (B) mean arterial blood pressure (in the first 12 hours of life) as a function of birth weight. (From Versmold HT, Kitterman JA, Phibbs RH, Gregory GA, Tooley WH. Aortic blood pressure during the first 12 hours of life in infants with birth weight 610 to 4,220 grams. *Pediatrics.* 1981;67:607.)

BIRTH WEIGHT (g)	POSTNATAL AGE (HOURS)					
	3	12	24	48	72	96
500	35(23)[a]	36(24)	37(25)	39(28)	42(30)	44(33)
1000	38(26)	39(27)	40(28)	42(31)	45(33)	47(35)
1500	40(29)	43(30)	43(31)	45(33)	48(36)	50(38)

TABLE 16.19 Mean Arterial Blood Pressure as a Function of Birth Weight and Postnatal Age

[a]Values are for mean blood pressure and, *in parentheses, the 10th percentile for the birth weight and postnatal age.*
Data condensed from Watkins AM, West CR, Cooke RW. Blood pressure and cerebral haemorrhage and ischaemia in very low birthweight infants. *Early Hum Dev.* 1989;19:103–110.

rose during the first 2 weeks of life and stabilized thereafter at levels close to those of term-born infants.[390] It is clear that awareness of these dynamically changing normal values is important for management.

Avoidance of Systemic Hypotension

In view of the aforementioned considerations concerning pressure-passive cerebral circulation and neonatal blood pressure data, it is clear that systemic hypotension must be avoided because of the danger of cerebral hypoperfusion (see Table 16.18). Moreover, because *normal* arterial blood pressure values in the newborn are relatively low and may be dangerously close to the downslope of even an intact autoregulatory curve, the *margin of safety* for arterial blood pressure sufficient to maintain adequate cerebral perfusion is likely to be small. As noted in Chapter 13 concerning pathogenesis, brain regions that are particularly vulnerable include the cerebral white matter in the premature newborn. The particular importance of *duration* as well as severity of hypotension in the genesis of brain injury in the premature newborn was shown clearly by a study of 98 infants.[392] Thus the cumulative effects of hypotension should be watched for and avoided. As noted earlier, the unresolved question, especially in the premature infant, is the definition of hypotension. *Common definitions include values of mean arterial blood pressure lower than the 10th percentile for birth weight and postnatal age (see Table 16.19), lower than the infant's gestational age, or less than 30 mm Hg.* The relatively high frequency of low blood pressures is highlighted in two recent studies. Thus, in the study depicted in Table 16.19, 43% of the group had mean blood pressures lower than the 10th percentile for weight and postnatal age for 2 consecutive hours at some time during the first 96 hours of life.[384] In a recent study of 90 infants who weighed less than 1500 g at birth, hypotension, defined in this way, was particularly common in the smallest infants, with periods of hypotension exceeding 80% of the epochs studied on days 3 to 5.[363] The most important definition of hypotension, of course, is the blood pressure below which functional or structural injury is likely. This value is generally unknown and likely varies according to multiple associated clinical factors in a given infant.

An important cause of serious systemic hypotension is *cardiogenic*. The structural immaturity of the myocardium is an important starting substrate. The adaptive challenges at birth were discussed earlier. In one study of 86 premature infants (<2000 g) with some evidence of asphyxia (i.e., Apgar scores <3 at 1 minute and <6 at 5 minutes), minimum systolic and diastolic blood pressures were significantly lower postnatally than in infants with normal Apgar scores, and infants with the low Apgar scores who died had lower pressures than those who survived.[383] Cardiogenic shock associated with perinatal asphyxia in the preterm infant was shown to respond to inotropic agents.[393,394] However, the mode and the timing of interventions for low blood pressures and the potential adverse effects of these interventions are controversial.[386,389,391,395-399] The relative roles of volume expansion, dopamine, dobutamine, phosphodiesterase III inhibitors (e.g., milrinone), and corticosteroids are currently under active study.[361,395-397,400,402] Detailed discussion is beyond the scope of this book.

Other important causes of systemic hypotension and apparent impairment of CBF with implications for management include, particularly, patent ductus arteriosus and recurrent apneic spells.

In *patent ductus arteriosus*, use of the transcutaneous Doppler ultrasound technique at the anterior fontanelle has shown a marked decrease in CBF velocity during patency of the ductus and an increase after spontaneous, medical (indomethacin), or surgical closure.[403-411] In many infants, retrograde flow can be documented during diastole. The changes in the cerebral circulation are apparently caused by diminutions in systemic blood pressure, diastolic more than systolic, and by diastolic *runoff* through the ductus. The findings led us to postulate the possibility of *ductal steal* in the premature infant.[403] The demonstration of a markedly higher incidence of PVL (ultrasonographic criteria) among infants with patent ductus arteriosus when retrograde flow in diastole is present supports this notion.[408] However, a recent study showed that cerebral oxygenation and oxygen extraction may remain unchanged in the presence of hemodynamically significant patent ductus arteriosus.[412] Nevertheless, it is reasonable to consider whether patent ductus arteriosus, under certain circumstances, may *contribute* to the occurrence of ischemic brain injury in the infant.[413,414] Whether the apparent value of indomethacin in prevention of intraventricular hemorrhage and improvement of cognitive outcome in male infants[415,416] is relevant in this context is possible but not established (see Chapter 24). Indomethacin may have a beneficial effect in decreasing cerebral white matter injury, even in the absence of patent ductus arteriosus (see later).[417] More data are needed on these issues.

Of additional implications for management are data suggesting that serious impairments in cerebral perfusion occur during *apneic spells* and may result from the impaired cardiac function with these spells.[299,300,418-420] In a study of 101 apneic episodes in preterm infants, we observed a striking relationship between decreases in CBF velocity and severity of bradycardia during the apneic episodes (Fig. 16.17).[421] With bradycardia of 100 beats/minute or less, a prominent decrease in CBF velocity became obvious, and with bradycardia of 80 beats/minute or less, the decrease was marked. The decreases in heart rate were accompanied by decreases in blood pressure, and the latter appeared to cause the changes in the cerebral

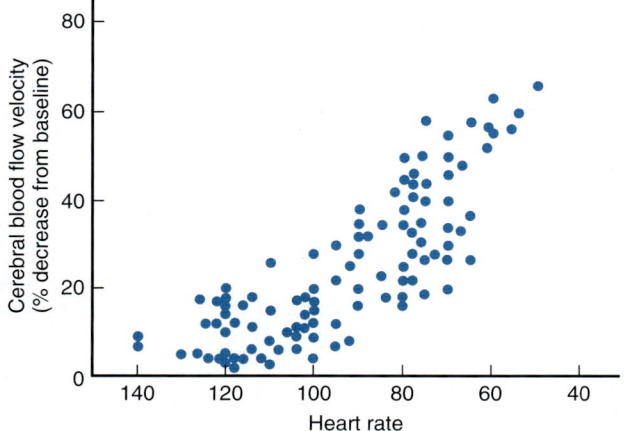

Figure 16.17 Effect of apnea and bradycardia on cerebral blood flow velocity. Cerebral blood flow velocity, quantitated as area under the velocity curve, is shown as a function of heart rate with apnea in 15 premature infants. Individual values for 101 separate episodes of apnea and bradycardia are shown. (From Perlman JM, Volpe JJ. Episodes of apnea and bradycardia in the preterm newborn: impact on cerebral circulation. *Pediatrics*. 1985;76:333–338.)

circulation. Several studies of preterm infants during apnea and bradycardia by near-infrared spectroscopy confirmed the decrease in apparent CBF.[300,418-420,422,423] When the disturbance in CBF is coupled with the hypoxemia that has been shown to accompany the spells, the dangers to the brain are obvious. In addition, earlier clinical data showed that the incidence of spastic diplegia is increased in infants with apnea and severe bradycardia.[101] In view of the observations reviewed earlier that correlate spastic diplegia with PVL, the major ischemic lesion of the preterm infant (see the section on clinicopathological correlation), the possibility that apneic episodes with severe bradycardia contribute to ischemic brain injury becomes strong. The implication for therapy is obvious: intervention appears to be needed urgently for episodes with bradycardia of 80 beats/minute or less, and in view of the data recorded in Fig. 16.17, urgent intervention may be indicated for episodes with bradycardia of 80 to 100 beats/minute.

Avoidance of Systemic Hypertension

The other side of the coin regarding the issue of cerebral ischemia just discussed is cerebral overperfusion. Because of the pressure-passive cerebral circulation, increases in systemic blood pressure, especially abrupt increases, could lead to rupture of certain vulnerable capillaries and thereby to hemorrhagic complications (see Table 16.18). The causes of such elevations in blood pressure, discussed in more detail in Chapter 24, range from apparently innocuous events, such as simple handling of the infant, to more obvious events such as overly exuberant administration of volume expanders or pressor agents, seizures, pneumothorax, or abrupt closure of patent ductus arteriosus. In the premature infant, vulnerable capillaries in the germinal matrix could rupture and result in intraventricular hemorrhage, or those in the region of PVL could burst and produce massive hemorrhagic lesions in cerebral white matter (see Chapter 24). The essential point is that arterial blood pressure must be monitored carefully, and events that lead to abrupt increases in arterial blood pressure must be prevented or corrected promptly.

An additional problem of systemic hypertension in this context is the possibility of occurrence of *ischemic* injury in association with treatment of *chronic* hypertension. The latter is not uncommon in premature infants with bronchopulmonary dysplasia.[421,424] In one series of nine infants with chronic hypertension, when previously effective antihypertensive therapy unexpectedly decreased blood pressure markedly and for a mean duration of 17 hours in four patients, oliguria and neurological abnormalities, particularly seizures but also infarction in one case, developed.[425] The blood pressure, although sharply decreased with the episodes, was not outside the normal range. The data suggest that the cerebrovascular autoregulatory curve was shifted to the right with chronic hypertension, as described in experimental models and in human adults with hypertension,[426-429] and rendered the infant vulnerable to decreases in blood pressure not necessarily out of the normal range. Thus caution is necessary in the treatment of chronic hypertension in the newborn to avoid ischemic complications.[430]

Glucose

Maintenance of adequate glucose levels is of major importance in premature infants because glucose supply to cerebral white matter is especially important for its viability (see Table 16.14).

This notion relates in part to the very low values for cerebral oxygen consumption in cerebral white matter of the human preterm infant (see Chapters 13 and 25). The observation raises the possibility that, to some extent, cerebral white matter energy needs are met by anaerobic glycolysis, which generates 19-fold less adenosine triphosphate (ATP) than does aerobic glycolysis (see Chapter 13). In addition, endogenous glucose reserves are limited in premature infants (see Chapter 13), and thus hypoglycemia is produced readily. This propensity is accentuated by perinatal hypoxia-ischemia, a common precursor to cerebral white matter injury in premature infants (see Pathogenesis earlier and Chapter 15). Management of glucose homeostasis and hypoglycemia in the premature infant is discussed in Chapter 25.

Seizures

Seizures in premature infants present a difficult problem in management. Firstly, as discussed earlier (see the section on clinical settings), electrographic seizures occur in approximately 50% of premature infants in the first 72 hours of life; only the minority of these have a clear clinical correlate.[64] Thus detection of the seizures requires aEEG or conventional EEG monitoring. Secondly, seizures increase cerebral metabolic demands, and it is of interest in this regard that the presence of seizures on the second postnatal day was associated with white matter injury detected at term by MRI.[64] Whether seizures contribute to causation of the injury or reflect the presence of injury is unclear. Thirdly, experimental studies indicate that neonatal seizures have deleterious effects on brain structure (especially regarding axonal and synaptic development [see Chapter 12]). Taken together, the data suggest that more diligent attempts to detect electrographic seizures in premature infants are indicated, and appropriate therapeutic interventions should be implemented (see Chapter 12).

Indomethacin

A potential role for indomethacin in the prevention of cerebral white matter injury was shown by a study published in 2006.[417] Thus indomethacin was administered either for a prolonged course of treatment (≥4 days) or a short course (≤3 days). In this prospective study of 57 infants who were treated with indomethacin to prevent the development of a hemodynamically significant, symptomatic patent ductus arteriosus, a prolonged course of treatment was used when the short course was not effective in closure of the ductus. White matter injury was identified by MRI. Infants who received a short course of indomethacin had a 38% incidence of moderate to severe white matter injury versus only 4% in those who received a prolonged course (Table 16.20). A more recent study confirms apparent benefit from a prolonged course of indomethacin.[97] Other studies, addressed to the use of indomethacin to prevent intraventricular hemorrhage (see Chapter 24), showed no difference in development of ultrasonographically detected PVL or of cerebral palsy at 36 months of age.[431,432] Of additional relevance, an analysis of 27 observational studies of *antenatal* indomethacin used for tocolysis in preterm labor showed an increased risk of PVL (largely ultrasonographically identified) and of necrotizing enterocolitis, a risk factor for cerebral white matter injury.[433] Thus currently the value of prophylactic *postnatal* use of indomethacin in prevention of cerebral white matter injury is uncertain. More data clearly are needed.

TABLE 16.20	Preventative Effect of Indomethacin on Cerebral White Matter Injury in Premature Infants

INDOMETHACIN TREATMENT	MODERATE-SEVERE WHITE MATTER INJURY NO./TOTAL (%)
Short course	11/29 (38%)
Prolonged course	1/24 (4%)

Infants were born after 24 to 28 weeks' gestation. White matter injury was determined by MRI (see text). Short course, ≤3 days; prolonged course, ≥4 days.

Data from Miller SP, Mayer EE, Clyman RI, et al. Prolonged indomethacin exposure is associated with decreased white matter injury detected with magnetic resonance imaging in premature newborns at 24 to 28 weeks' gestation at birth. *Pediatrics*. 2006;117:1626–1631.

TABLE 16.21	Neuroprotective Interventions in the Encephalopathy of Prematurity

LIKELY TARGET	MAJOR AGENT(S)
Microglial Activation/ Inflammation	Minocycline
	Melatonin
Excitotoxicity	Memantine
	Topiramate
Antioxidant Defenses/Free Radical Generation	Oxygenase inhibitors
	NOS inhibitors
	Antioxidative enzyme mimetics
Free Radical Scavengers	Free radical scavengers— N-acetylcysteine, vitamin E, vitamin K
Multiple Mechanisms	Erythropoietin[a]
	IGF-1[b]
	EGF[b]
	Hypothermia (?)
	Estradiol

[a]Studied in human preterm infants (see text).
[b]Exhibits neuroprotective properties and promotes differentiation.
Based principally on experimental studies.

Whether an alternative cyclo-oxygenase inhibitor would be valuable prophylactically also awaits further study.

The basis for any beneficial effect of indomethacin is not known. Patent ductus arteriosus closure did not appear to account for the beneficial effect because benefit for prolonged indomethacin course was noted even in the absence of patent ductus.[417] Possible relevant effects of indomethacin include widening of the range of cerebral vascular autoregulation, prevention of generation of free radicals at the cyclooxygenase step, or antiinflammatory effects (see Chapter 13).

Neuroprotective Interventions

In this section we use the term *neuroprotective* for those agents that act principally by preventing direct pre-OL injury or death. In a subsequent section, we use the term *neurorestorative* for those interventions that act later to counteract the secondary dysmaturational effects of the encephalopathy of prematurity.

Neuroprotective interventions have focused on the prevention of pre-OL injury or death. Many excellent neonatal experimental models of hypoxic-ischemic or inflammatory white matter injury, similar to PVL, have identified a considerable number of effective neuroprotective agents. The likely mechanistic targets of these agents are shown in Table 16.21. The mechanisms of pre-OL injury and the effects of these agents are described in Chapters 13 and 15. Of these, only erythropoietin (EPO) has been studied in detail in human premature infants and will be emphasized in the following.

Erythropoietin

EPO has been considered as a neuroprotective strategy for a variety of conditions for both term and preterm infants; the focus here will be on preterm infants. As of this writing, many studies of EPO in preterm infants are ongoing.[434] One randomized, masked, multicenter trial (29 subjects treated with EPO, 27 with darbepoetin, and 24 with placebo, Bayley-III scores measured at 18 to 22 months) showed higher cognitive scores among darbepoetin (96.2 ± 7.3; mean ± SD) and EPO recipients (97.9 ± 14.3) compared with placebo recipients (88.7 ± 13.5; *P* = .01). No EPO/darbepoetin recipients had cerebral palsy, compared with 5 in the placebo group (*P* <.001). Later follow-up (3.5 to 4 years of age) showed better cognitive

outcomes and less neurodevelopmental impairment in the treated group.[435] In a more recent study of recombinant human EPO (rhEPO), 228 preterm infants were randomized to rhEPO and 220 to placebo; both conventional and diffusion tensor MRI studied at term equivalent age showed less white matter injury and better white matter development in the rhEPO-treated infants.[436,437] However, at 2 years there were no statistically significant differences in neurodevelopmental outcomes.[438,439] Whether follow-up at school age, when cognitive testing can be more detailed and reliable, will show benefit suggested by the early MRI data awaits further study. Notably the timing of EPO administration differed between the two reported cohorts. In the former,[438] the medication was administered 3×/week through 35 weeks' postmenstrual age. In the latter,[439] it was administered at less than 3 hours, at 12 to 18 hours, and at 36 to 42 hours after birth. Thus, in the former instance rhEPO may have functioned both as a neuroprotective *and* neurorestorative intervention, whereas in the latter cohort rhEPO may have functioned only as a neuroprotective agent. Perhaps consistent with this notion, the largest study to date randomized 800 infants of less than 32 weeks' gestation to placebo or rhEPO administered intravenously within 72 hours after birth and then once every other day for 2 weeks.[440] The rate of moderate/severe neurological disability at 18 months' corrected age was significantly lower in the rhEPO group (7.1%) versus the placebo group (18.8%; RR = 0.32, CI 0.19 to 0.55, *P* <.001).

The mechanisms of action of EPO are likely multiple (see Chapter 13), as the agent has antiinflammatory, antiexcitotoxic, antioxidant, and antiapoptotic effects.[441] EPO has been shown to prevent/mitigate white matter injury in experimental models.[442,443] Moreover, EPO promotes oligodendrocyte *development* after hypoxic-ischemic insults and thus has restorative properties.[444,445] In vivo, EPO is probably generated primarily from astrocytes,[446] which are abundant in the diffuse component of PVL (see Chapter 14 and earlier). Interestingly, EPO also promotes *cerebral cortical development* after hypoxia-ischemia,[447] again, consistent with its multifaceted restorative effects on cellular development in brain. These multiple effects on development, as well as its potential neuroprotective effects, make EPO an excellent candidate for benefit, with reference to *both the primary injury and secondary dysmaturational effects* that are the foundation of the encephalopathy of prematurity.

Epidermal Growth Factor, Insulin-Like Growth Factor

Although not yet studied in human preterm infants, *both epidermal growth factor (EGF) and insulin-like growth factor (IGF-1)* have beneficial effects in experimental models of preterm white matter injury (see Table 16.21). Using an established mouse model of very preterm white matter injury, Scafidi et al. showed that either selective overexpression of human EGF receptor in oligodendroglial lineage cells or the intranasal administration of EGF immediately after injury led to decreased oligodendroglial death, enhanced generation of new oligodendroglia from progenitor cells, and promotion of functional recovery.[448] More data are needed.

IGF-1 has shown protective effects versus white matter injury in studies of neonatal animal models (hypoxia-ischemia, lipopolysaccharide-induced inflammation) and cultured pre-OLs.[449-453] Two issues limit enthusiasm for this agent: First, the peptide must be administered intraventricularly, and second, the beneficial effect is dose-related, with lower doses effective and higher doses toxic. Nevertheless, IGF-1 is useful when given *after* the insult, rescues pre-OLs in immature white matter, and promotes myelination following hypoxia-ischemia. Further data would be of interest.

Hypothermia

Therapeutic hypothermia is effective for treating brain injury in term infants, and its neuroprotective benefit involves multiple mechanisms in the cascade to cell death (see Table 16.21; Chapter 20). However, its potential value in preterm infants has not been carefully studied. In 2014, the Committee on the Fetus and Newborn of the American Academy of Pediatrics concluded that information regarding the safety and efficacy of cooling treatment of encephalopathic infants born at less than 35 weeks of gestational age is lacking.[454] Experimental studies suggest potential value after *acute* hypoxic-ischemic insults. Thus, in a study of preterm fetal sheep (0.7 gestation) exposed to umbilical cord occlusion followed 90 minutes later by 70 hours of intrauterine cranial hypothermia, hypothermia was associated with a significant overall reduction in loss of immature oligodendrocytes in the periventricular white matter and neuronal loss in the hippocampus and basal ganglia. There was also evidence of suppression of apoptosis and inflammation.[455] These findings raise the possibility that therapeutic hypothermia could be effective in preterm infants with an *acute* insult (as opposed to the more common, sustained insults underlying the encephalopathy of prematurity [see earlier]).[456] The safety of hypothermia in preterm infants, especially VPT, has not yet been demonstrated.

Neurorestorative Interventions

Because, in the encephalopathy of prematurity, a variety of dysmaturational events occur subsequent to the primary injury, the possibility of later interventions to counteract these events is raised. We will term these interventions *neurorestorative*. The

---

TABLE 16.22   Neurorestorative Interventions in the Encephalopathy of Prematurity

Pharmacologic agents
  Erythropoietin
  ?EGF, IGF-1
Nutritional factors
  Quality and source of milk
  Components of milk
  Breastfeeding
Experiential factors
  Visual
  Auditory
  Pain, stress
Individualized care
Early intervention programs
Stem cells
Parenting/educational/social factors

EGF, Epidermal growth factor; *IGF-1*, insulin-like growth factor.

---

best-established and perhaps most important of the *failures of maturation* involves pre-OLs and the resulting hypomyelination (see Chapter 14). Disturbances of development of neuronal/axonal structures accompany the pre-OL maturational failure and may occur, at least in part, as *a consequence* of this failure (see Chapter 14). A number of restorative pharmacological interventions have been addressed in experimental models (Table 16.22). Of these, only EPO has been studied in human preterm infants (see earlier concerning neuroprotection). In addition, a number of other interventions, related to neonatal and later postnatal care and involving nutritional, experiential, care-giving, and parenting factors, may also be involved in restorative effects and will be described briefly next (see Table 16.22).

Nutrition

A large corpus of clinical, epidemiological, and experimental studies show that *appropriate nutrition during the premature period* is important for neurodevelopmental outcome and that *postnatal undernutrition* is deleterious.[457-459] Overall, the data raise the possibility that optimal nutrition, both in the neonatal period and the subsequent posthospitalization period, could be a restorative intervention in the infant with the encephalopathy of prematurity. The potential high prevalence of impaired nutrition in premature infants is illustrated by observations that 50% of VLBW preterm infants had a discharge weight less than the 10th percentile for postmenstrual age, and 27% had a discharge weight less than the 3rd percentile.[460,461]

Several lines of evidence suggest that nutritional factors are important for neurodevelopmental outcome and perhaps, therefore, the critical organizational events occurring during the postnatal time period in premature infants. First, many studies have shown that infants with impaired growth (somatic and cranial) during the premature period exhibit poorer developmental outcomes than do infants with normal growth.[459,462-472] A study of 95 preterm infants showed that infants with slower postnatal growth had diffusion tensor MRI data showing delayed microstructural development of cerebral cortex.[473] Recall that normal maturation of the cerebral cortex is related to the influx of thalamocortical circuitry, late migrating

GABAergic neurons, and influences of subplate neurons (see Chapter 7), all processes that appear to be adversely affected in the encephalopathy of prematurity (see Chapter 14).

The *quality of the milk provided to the infant*, perhaps not unexpectedly, is important in relation to neurological outcome. Thus available data indicate particular value concerning outcome for fortified preterm versus term formula, for human milk versus formula, and for fortified human milk versus no fortification.[459,474-480] *Breast-feeding* is of particular value, and several MRI volumetric and diffusion tensor MRI studies have shown better white matter maturation in such infants.[457,475,478,479] Breast milk also is associated with lower risk for necrotizing enterocolitis, a known risk factor for white matter injury.

Specific components of milk likely also are critical. Although beyond the scope of this chapter, particular value for *long-chain polyunsaturated fatty acids* is suggested by available data. Concerning supplementation with the former, although not all findings are consistent, favorable effects on visual function and cognitive function have been reported.[459,481,482] Supplementation to the *lactating mother* who is breast-feeding has been most effective. A recent study of preterm infants in which polyunsaturated fatty acid levels in red blood cells were measured noted a correlation of these levels with microstructural maturation of cerebral white matter as measured by diffusion MRI.[483]

Experiential

The potential impact of *experiential factors* in regulation of cortical organization was discussed in Chapter 7. Although emphasis is often placed on the deleterious effects of altered experience in the neonatal period in the premature infant, the *potential benefit of experiential factors as restorative therapies is important to consider* (see Table 16.22). The most relevant in this context relate to visual and auditory input and to the nature of the care of the infant in the neonatal care unit. These factors are discussed next.

Visual. As discussed earlier, central visual impairment is a common feature of the encephalopathy of prematurity. Whether optimal visual experience in premature infants could counteract these deleterious central visual effects, that is, have restorative properties, is important to consider. Elegant experiments in normal and preterm monkeys showed that premature visual stimulation results in increases in size and proportions of synapses in visual cortex, presumably by alterations in normal synaptic modification or elimination.[484] Moreover, visual deprivation has the opposite effect. Studies in human infants suggest that as in the experimental models, experiential effects are important mediators of certain organizational events. Visual experience of premature infants is associated with accentuation of the development of the visual evoked potential, a finding consistent with enhancement of dendritic and axonal development and synaptogenesis.[485] More data are needed on these issues and how visual experience could enhance development of the cerebral visual system.

Auditory. Recent work suggests that modification of the auditory environment may have a beneficial effect on cortical development in premature infants. Thus, as discussed in Chapter 9, sound levels in many open neonatal intensive units, incubators, and ventilators can exceed current recommendations

of the American Academy of Pediatrics.[486-490] In part because of these observations, many neonatal intensive care units are designed to minimize ambient noise, often by maintaining infants in single rooms. Recent data suggest that this approach may have an adverse effect on language outcome in premature infants.[491,492] Thus, in a study of 136 preterm infants assigned to either open ward or single room bedspaces, infants kept in single patient rooms had lower language scores at age 2 years, as well as abnormalities of cortical folding in the superior temporal area, after controlling for potential confounders.[491] This finding was attributed to the auditory environment of the NICU bedspaces, with infants in the open wards exposed to more language, often *overhearing* discussions among medical personnel during the course of a typical day. In comparison, babies in single patient rooms had less speech exposure. In a subsequent study,[492] neurodevelopmental outcome was assessed for infants from both private room and open ward bedspaces while taking into account maternal involvement in NICU care. Infants with high maternal involvement from both single patient and open ward bedspaces had higher cognitive and language scores on the Bayley Scales of Infant Development-III at age 18 months than did infants with low maternal involvement. The effect size was greater for children from single rooms. This second study suggests that the level of language exposure depends on a variety of factors, of which room type is only one. Other influences, such as maternal characteristics (e.g., socioeconomic status, availability of maternity leave, time spent with the baby) and the NICU culture (e.g., encouraging family members to read to babies), are also relevant (see later).

The pathophysiology underlying these effects is likely related to the relationship between sensory input and auditory network maturation.[493,494] There is a striking development of the auditory system from preterm birth to term equivalent age. The connections between the cochlea and the brain stem are established by 24 to 25 weeks and between the temporal lobe and the auditory cortex by as early as 30 to 31 weeks.[495,496] Auditory evoked potentials are detectable by the 28th week of gestation, and from 28 weeks' until 34 weeks' gestation there is a marked reduction in response latency as neural pathways mature. Before full-term birth, infants demonstrate auditory responses, and it is believed that the pitch, intensity, and pattern of *in utero* auditory exposures activate the system and stimulate association between the cortex and the cochlea. For preterm infants, it is biologically plausible that an important factor in their subsequent language impairment relates to disruption of this developmental sequence caused by a lack of language exposure. Consistent with this hypothesis, functional connectivity MRI (Chapter 10) data show that disruption of brain networks detected at term equivalent persists into childhood.[497] Overall, these studies emphasize the importance of the NICU auditory environment. *In the infant with the encephalopathy of prematurity and its associated disturbances in development of multiple neural networks, the data suggest the possibility of promoting normal development by optimizing the auditory environment.* While the ideal NICU auditory environment is not yet known, it appears important that NICU policies and design take into account the auditory environment to optimize language exposure.

Pain, Stress. Pain and stress in the neonatal intensive care unit, common experiences for the preterm infant, have been shown to have adverse effects on neurodevelopmental, behavioral, and cognitive outcomes.[498-501] Recent studies suggest that these effects are associated with abnormalities of brain development, similar in many respects to the encephalopathy of prematurity (see later). The findings suggest that reduction of pain and stress in these infants could serve as a restorative intervention, as discussed in this overall section (see Table 16.22).

Two particularly informative studies addressed the effects on brain development at term equivalent age in preterm infants as a function of number of stressful events[502] or of numbers of painful procedures.[503] The findings were consistent with impaired white matter and cortical development. In the study of Smith et al.[502] a disturbance of interhemispheric connectivity between the temporal lobes was identified. This observation suggests involvement of commissural interconnections, also frequently a site of cerebral white matter injury in the encephalopathy of prematurity. Additional evidence of a relation of stress to cerebral white matter development emanates from a later randomized controlled clinical trial that assessed the effectiveness of training parents in reducing stressful experiences in premature infants less than 30 weeks' gestation in the neonatal intensive care unit.[504] The infants of the mothers in the intervention group showed at term equivalent age significantly enhanced maturation and connectivity of cerebral white matter by advanced MRI techniques. These and related data caused the American Academy of Pediatrics to emphasize the need in neonatal intensive care facilities for "a pain-prevention program that includes strategies for minimizing the number of painful procedures performed."[505] Reduction of pain and stress by pharmacological means is difficult because of potentially deleterious effects of commonly used analgesics (see Chapter 38).

Individualized Care

In the last several decades, a variety of approaches to individualized care have been developed in an attempt to minimize the stresses described above and to maximize comfort (see Table 16.22).[506] The possible *neurorestorative* role of this approach was suggested by a randomized clinical trial of the Als individualized developmental care program, which showed, at 9 months' corrected age, improved neurobehavioral function, quantitative EEG evidence of enhanced maturation, and diffusion-tensor MRI evidence of more advanced cerebral white matter fiber tract development.[507] Benefits were still present at 8 years of age.[508] A variety of approaches to such *developmental care* have been taken. Many elements of developmental care have been identified, including patient positioning, light, sound, handling, approaches to feeding, and inclusion of parents in care.[509-511] Perhaps as a consequence of this richness of approaches, many of which have been used in various combinations, the literature relating developmental care with outcome is somewhat fragmented with respect to the elements used and the findings somewhat inconsistent regarding neurodevelopmental outcome. A comprehensive review of this literature is beyond the scope of this chapter. Nevertheless, the initial findings regarding beneficial effects on brain organizational events suggest that at least some of the approaches could lead to mitigation and recovery of the dysmaturational features of the encephalopathy of prematurity.

Early Intervention Programs

Because organizational events in brain development (see Chapter 7) are active for at least several years postnatal, many interventions, especially infant behavioral and developmental intervention programs, have attempted to harness those brain developmental capabilities to improve motor and cognitive outcomes after the neonatal period (see Table 16.22). Infants with features of the encephalopathy of prematurity are especially targeted. The results have been mixed, but most consistently, short-term benefits have been demonstrated.[512-514] Detailed consideration of the specific early intervention programs and their impact is beyond the scope of this presentation (see also Chapter 11).

Parenting/Educational/Social Factors

Although the anatomical substrate remains essentially unknown, many studies in recent years have shown that factors relating to parenting, education, and social context beyond the neonatal period are critical determinants of ultimate outcome (see Table 16.22). The biological bases for these effects are unclear and likely diverse. Detailed discussion is beyond the scope of this chapter (see also Chapter 11). Nevertheless, importance is established for parental (especially maternal) education, parenting skills, maternal-infant feeding interactions, social class, and economic status (especially overt poverty).[515-519] Delineation of the effects of these factors on brain organizational events awaits further study.

Stem Cells

Experimental studies of brain injury in preterm animals suggest that stem cell therapies may be effective for neurorestoration (see Table 16.22).[520-522] The major types of cells used thus far include neural, embryonic, mesenchymal, umbilical cord, and induced pluripotent stem cells. A variety of routes of stem cell administration have been explored, and *intranasal* administration may be the most efficient and least invasive. Stem cells administered intranasally appear to target the injury site after entering the brain via olfactory neural processes traversing the cribriform plate.[523] Studies of rodent models of preterm brain injury have shown that this route can be effective for mitigating injury to myelin[524] and improving behavioral outcome.[525] In addition, direct injection of stem cells into a lateral ventricle has been shown to reduce myelin loss following a variety of insults, suggesting that stem cells adapt their response to the nature of the injury.[526] The precise neuroprotective factors released by stem cells are not known with certainty, but the effects on oligodendroglial and myelin development and on behavioral outcome also can be achieved with administration of extracellular vesicles derived from stem cells in lieu of stem cells per se.[527]

Perhaps of most relevance to cerebral white matter injury in the premature infant is a recent study of such injury produced by hypoxia-ischemia in the 3-day-old rat.[528] Oligodendrocyte progenitor cells produced from embryonic stem cells were transplanted into the injured cerebrum. The transplanted cells survived, underwent differentiation, formed myelin sheaths, and stimulated proliferation of endogenous neural stem cells. Functional benefit was shown after 6 weeks.

The most relevant human study in this context is the transplantation of human neural stem cells into the brains of four patients with connatal Pelizaeus-Merzbacher disease (see Chapter 29).[529] After 1 year, diffusion tensor imaging suggested myelin ensheathment of axons. Although more data are needed, the findings are promising regarding stem cell therapy in cerebral white matter disease, such as the central neuropathology in the encephalopathy of prematurity.

KEY REFERENCES

1. Volpe JJ. Brain injury in premature infants: a complex amalgam of destructive and developmental disturbances. *Lancet Neurol.* 2009;8: 110-124.
7. Stoll BJ, Hansen NI, Bell EF, et al. Trends in care practices, morbidity, and mortality of extremely preterm neonates, 1993-2012. *JAMA.* 2015;314:1039-1051.
11. Haynes RL, Sleeper LA, Volpe JJ, et al. Neuropathologic studies of the encephalopathy of prematurity in the late preterm infant. *Clin Perinatol.* 2013;40:707-722.
12. Dammann O, Leviton A. Intermittent or sustained systemic inflammation and the preterm brain. *Pediatr Res.* 2014;75:376-380.
15. Volpe JJ, Kinney HC, Jensen FE, et al. The developing oligodendrocyte: key cellular target in brain injury in the premature infant. *Int J Dev Neurosci.* 2011;29:423-440.
17. Tsimis ME, Johnson CT, Raghunathan RS, et al. Risk factors for periventricular white matter injury in very low birthweight neonates. *Am J Obstet Gynecol.* 2016;214:380.e381-e386.
23. Favrais G, van de Looij Y, Fleiss B, et al. Systemic inflammation disrupts the developmental program of white matter. *Ann Neurol.* 2011;70:550-565.
27. Wang LW, Chang YC, Lin CY, et al. Low-dose lipopolysaccharide selectively sensitizes hypoxic ischemia-induced white matter injury in the immature brain. *Pediatr Res.* 2010;68:41-47.
28. Wang X, Hagberg H, Nie C, et al. Dual role of intrauterine immune challenge on neonatal and adult brain vulnerability to hypoxia-ischemia. *J Neuropathol Exp Neurol.* 2007;66:552-561.
63. Guzzetta A, Mazzotti S, Tinelli F, et al. Early assessment of visual information processing and neurological outcome in preterm infants. *Neuropediatrics.* 2006;37:278-285.
64. Vesoulis ZA, Inder TE, Woodward LJ, et al. Early electrographic seizures, brain injury, and neurodevelopmental risk in the very preterm infant. *Pediatr Res.* 2014;75:564-569.
65. Kidokoro H, Okumura A, Hayakawa F, et al. Chronologic changes in neonatal EEG findings in periventricular leukomalacia. *Pediatrics.* 2009;124:e468-e475.
70. Hayashi-Kurahashi N, Kidokoro H, Kubota T, et al. EEG for predicting early neurodevelopment in preterm infants: an observational cohort study. *Pediatrics.* 2012;130:e891-e897.
72. Resch B, Resch E, Maurer-Fellbaum U, et al. The whole spectrum of cystic periventricular leukomalacia of the preterm infant: results from a large consecutive case series. *Childs Nerv Syst.* 2015;31:1527-1532.
74. Pierson CR, Folkerth RD, Billiards SS, et al. Gray matter injury associated with periventricular leukomalacia in the premature infant. *Acta Neuropathol.* 2007;114:619-631.
75. Buser JR, Maire J, Riddle A, et al. Arrested preoligodendrocyte maturation contributes to myelination failure in premature infants. *Ann Neurol.* 2012;71:93-109.
79. van Wezel-Meijler G, De Bruine FT, Steggerda SJ, et al. Ultrasound detection of white matter injury in very preterm infants: practical implications. *Dev Med Child Neurol.* 2011;53:29-34.
80. Niwa T, de Vries LS, Benders MJ, et al. Punctate white matter lesions in infants: new insights using susceptibility-weighted imaging. *Neuroradiology.* 2011;53:669-679.
88. Woodward LJ, Edgin JO, Thompson D, et al. Object working memory deficits predicted by early brain injury and development in the preterm infant. *Brain.* 2005;128:2578-2587.
89. Woodward LJ, Anderson PJ, Austin NC, et al. Neonatal MRI to predict neurodevelopmental outcomes in preterm infants. *N Engl J Med.* 2006;355:685-694.
92. Skiold B, Vollmer B, Bohm B, et al. Neonatal magnetic resonance imaging and outcome at age 30 months in extremely preterm infants. *J Pediatr.* 2012;160:559-566.e551.
94. Chau V, Synnes A, Grunau RE, et al. Abnormal brain maturation in preterm neonates associated with adverse developmental outcomes. *Neurology.* 2013;81:2082-2089.
95. Kersbergen KJ, Benders MJ, Groenendaal F, et al. Different patterns of punctate white matter lesions in serially scanned preterm infants. *PLoS ONE.* 2014;9:e108904.
96. Guo T, Duerden EG, Adams E, et al. Quantitative assessment of white matter injury in preterm neonates: association with outcomes. *Neurology.* 2017;88:614-622.
97. Gano D, Andersen SK, Partridge JC, et al. Diminished white matter injury over time in a cohort of premature newborns. *J Pediatr.* 2015;166:39-43.
99. van Haastert IC, Groenendaal F, Uiterwaal CS, et al. Decreasing incidence and severity of cerebral palsy in prematurely born children. *J Pediatr.* 2011;159:86-91, e81.
100. Serenius F, Ewald U, Farooqi A, et al. Neurodevelopmental outcomes among extremely preterm infants 6.5 years after active perinatal care in Sweden. *JAMA Pediatr.* 2016;170:954-963.
121. Ohgi S, Akiyama T, Fukuda M. Neurobehavioural profile of low-birthweight infants with cystic periventricular leukomalacia. *Dev Med Child Neurol.* 2005;47:221-228.
122. Tang-Wai R, Webster RI, Shevell MI. A clinical and etiologic profile of spastic diplegia. *Pediatr Neurol.* 2006;34:212-218.
126. Trivedi R, Agarwal S, Shah V, et al. Correlation of quantitative sensorimotor tractography with clinical grade of cerebral palsy. *Neuroradiology.* 2010;52:759-765.
127. Lee JD, Park HJ, Park ES, et al. Motor pathway injury in patients with periventricular leukomalacia and spastic diplegia. *Brain.* 2011;134:1199-1210.
128. Spittle AJ, Orton J. Cerebral palsy and developmental coordination disorder in children born preterm. *Semin Fetal Neonatal Med.* 2014;19:84-89.
129. Spittle AJ, Cheong J, Doyle LW, et al. Neonatal white matter abnormality predicts childhood motor impairment in very preterm children. *Dev Med Child Neurol.* 2011;53:1000-1006.
133. De Bruine FT, Van Wezel-Meijler G, Leijser LM, et al. Tractography of white-matter tracts in very preterm infants: a 2-year follow-up study. *Dev Med Child Neurol.* 2013;55:427-433.
134. Rogers CE, Smyser T, Smyser CD, et al. Regional white matter development in very preterm infants: perinatal predictors and early developmental outcomes. *Pediatr Res.* 2016;79:87-95.
135. Rose J, Cahill-Rowley K, Vassar R, et al. Neonatal brain microstructure correlates of neurodevelopment and gait in preterm children 18-22 mo of age: an MRI and DTI study. *Pediatr Res.* 2015;78:700-708.
137. Wang S, Fan GG, Xu K, et al. Altered microstructural connectivity of the superior and middle cerebellar peduncles are related to motor dysfunction in children with diffuse periventricular leucomalacia born preterm: a DTI tractography study. *Eur J Radiol.* 2014;83:997-1004.
141. Judas M, Rados M, Jovanov-Milosevic N, et al. Structural, immunocytochemical, and MR imaging properties of periventricular crossroads of growing cortical pathways in preterm infants. *Am J Neuroadiol.* 2005;26:2671-2684.
142. Kostovic I, Judas M. Prolonged coexistence of transient and permanent circuitry elements in the developing cerebral cortex of fetuses and preterm infants. *Dev Med Child Neurol.* 2006;48:388-393.
143. Soria-Pastor S, Gimenez M, Narberhaus A, et al. Patterns of cerebral white matter damage and cognitive impairment in adolescents born very preterm. *Int J Dev Neurosci.* 2008;26:647-654.
144. Boardman JP, Craven C, Valappil S, et al. A common neonatal image phenotype predicts adverse neurodevelopmental outcome in children born preterm. *Neuroimage.* 2010;52:409-414.
147. de Bruine FT, van den Berg-Huysmans AA, Leijser LM, et al. Clinical implications of MR imaging findings in the white matter in very preterm infants: a 2-year follow-up study. *Radiology.* 2011;261:899-906.
152. van Kooij BJ, de Vries LS, Ball G, et al. Neonatal tract-based spatial statistics findings and outcome in preterm infants. *AJNR Am J Neuroradiol.* 2012;33:188-194.
155. Anderson PJ, Treyvaud K, Neil JJ, Cheong JLY, et al. Associations of newborn brain magnetic resonance imaging with long-term neurodevelopmental impairments in very preterm children. *J Pediatr.* 2017;187:58-65 e51.
158. Young J, Powell T, Morgan BR, et al. Deep grey matter growth predicts neurodevelopmental outcomes in very preterm children. *Neuroimage.* 2015;111:360-368.
162. Van Kooij BJ, Benders MJ, Anbeek P, et al. Cerebellar volume and proton magnetic resonance spectroscopy at term, and neurodevelopment at 2 years of age in preterm infants. *Dev Med Child Neurol.* 2012;54:260-266.

163. Burnett AC, Scratch SE, Anderson PJ. Executive function outcome in preterm adolescents. *Early Hum Dev.* 2013;89:215-220.
166. Litt JS, Gerry Taylor H, Margevicius S, et al. Academic achievement of adolescents born with extremely low birth weight. *Acta Paediatr.* 2012;101:1240-1245.
167. Hutchinson EA, De Luca CR, Doyle LW, et al. School-age outcomes of extremely preterm or extremely low birth weight children. *Pediatrics.* 2013;131:e1053-e1061.
169. Edgin JO, Inder TE, Anderson PJ, et al. Executive functioning in preschool children born very preterm: relationship with early white matter pathology. *J Int Neuropsychol Soc.* 2008;14:90-101.
171. Clark CA, Woodward LJ. Neonatal cerebral abnormalities and later verbal and visuospatial working memory abilities of children born very preterm. *Dev Neuropsychol.* 2010;35:622-642.
173. Omizzolo C, Scratch SE, Stargatt R, et al. Neonatal brain abnormalities and memory and learning outcomes at 7 years in children born very preterm. *Memory.* 2014;22:605-615.
176. Vohr B. Speech and language outcomes of very preterm infants. *Semin Fetal Neonatal Med.* 2014;19:78-83.
177. Carter FA, Msall ME. Language abilities as a framework for understanding emerging cognition and social competencies after late, moderate, and very preterm birth. *J Pediatr.* 2017;181:8-9.
180. Durkin K, Conti-Ramsden G. Language, social behavior, and the quality of friendships in adolescents with and without a history of specific language impairment. *Child Dev.* 2007;78:1441-1457.
181. Conti-Ramsden G, Durkin K, Simkin Z, et al. Specific language impairment and school outcomes. I: identifying and explaining variability at the end of compulsory education. *Int J Lang Commun Disord.* 2009;44:15-35.
184. Smyser CD, Inder TE, Shimony JS, et al. Longitudinal analysis of neural network development in preterm infants. *Cereb Cortex.* 2010;20:2852-2862.
186. Reidy N, Morgan A, Thompson DK, et al. Impaired language abilities and white matter abnormalities in children born very preterm and/or very low birth weight. *J Pediatr.* 2013;162:719-724.
187. Limperopoulos C, Bassan H, Gauvreau K, et al. Does cerebellar injury in premature infants contribute to the high prevalence of long-term cognitive, learning, and behavioral disability in survivors? *Pediatrics.* 2007;120:584-593.
189. Johnson S, Marlow N. Preterm birth and childhood psychiatric disorders. *Pediatr Res.* 2011;69:11R-18R.
190. O'Shea TM, Downey LC, Kuban KK. Extreme prematurity and attention deficit: epidemiology and prevention. *Front Hum Neurosci.* 2013;7:528.
191. Murray AL, Scratch SE, Thompson DK, et al. Neonatal brain pathology predicts adverse attention and processing speed outcomes in very preterm and/or very low birth weight children. *Neuropsychology.* 2014;28:552-562.
193. Kuban KC, O'Shea TM, Allred EN, et al. Positive screening on the Modified Checklist for Autism in Toddlers (M-CHAT) in extremely low gestational age newborns. *J Pediatr.* 2009;154:535-540.e531.
195. Linsell L, Malouf R, Johnson S, et al. Prognostic factors for behavioral problems and psychiatric disorders in children born very preterm or very low birth weight: a systematic review. *J Dev Behav Pediatr.* 2016;37:88-102.
197. Schieve LA, Clayton HB, Durkin MS, et al. Comparison of perinatal risk factors associated with autism spectrum disorder (ASD), intellectual disability (ID), and co-occurring ASD and ID. *J Autism Dev Disord.* 2015;45:2361-2372.
198. Brossard-Racine M, du Plessis AJ, Limperopoulos C. Developmental cerebellar cognitive affective syndrome in ex-preterm survivors following cerebellar injury. *Cerebellum.* 2015;14:151-164.
207. Geldof CJ, van Wassenaer AG, de Kieviet JF, et al. Visual perception and visual-motor integration in very preterm and/or very low birth weight children: a meta-analysis. *Res Dev Disabil.* 2012;33:726-736.
211. Groppo M, Ricci D, Bassi L, et al. Development of the optic radiations and visual function after premature birth. *Cortex.* 2014;56:30-37.
212. Thompson DK, Thai D, Kelly CE, et al. Alterations in the optic radiations of very preterm children-Perinatal predictors and relationships with visual outcomes. *NeuroImage Clin.* 2014;4:145-153.
232. Conde-Agudelo A, Romero R. Antenatal magnesium sulfate for the prevention of cerebral palsy in preterm infants less than 34 weeks' gestation: a systematic review and metaanalysis. *Am J Obstet Gynecol.* 2009;200:595-609.
233. Doyle LW, Crowther CA, Middleton P, et al. Magnesium sulphate for women at risk of preterm birth for neuroprotection of the fetus (Review). *Cochrane Database Syst Rev.* 2009;(1):CD004661.
235. Chollat C, Enser M, Houivet E, et al. School-age outcomes following a randomized controlled trial of magnesium sulfate for neuroprotection of preterm infants. *J Pediatr.* 2014;165:398-400. e393.
236. Doyle LW, Anderson PJ, Haslam R, et al. School-age outcomes of very preterm infants after antenatal treatment with magnesium sulfate vs placebo. *JAMA.* 2014;312:1105-1113.
252. Hirtz DG, Weiner SJ, Bulas D, et al. Antenatal magnesium and cerebral palsy in preterm infants. *J Pediatr.* 2015;167:834-839. e3.
258. Chawla S, Natarajan G, Shankaran S, et al. Association of neurodevelopmental outcomes and neonatal morbidities of extremely premature infants with differential exposure to antenatal steroids. *JAMA Pediatr.* 2016;170:1164-1172.
259. Sotiriadis A, Tsiami A, Papatheodorou S, et al. Neurodevelopmental outcome after a single course of antenatal steroids in children born preterm: a systematic review and meta-analysis. *Obstet Gynecol.* 2015;125:1385-1396.
260. Crowther CA, McKinlay CJ, Middleton P, et al. Repeat doses of prenatal corticosteroids for women at risk of preterm birth for improving neonatal health outcomes. *Cochrane Database Syst Rev.* 2015;(7):CD003935.
265. Kenyon S, Pike K, Jones D, et al. Childhood outcomes after prescription of antibiotics to pregnant women with preterm rupture of the membranes: 7-year follow-up of the ORACLE I trial. *Lancet.* 2008;372:1310-1318.
266. Bedford Russell AR, Steer PJ. Antibiotics in preterm labour—the ORACLE speaks. *Lancet.* 2008;372:1276-1278.
268. Jenkins DD, Wiest DB, Mulvihill DM, et al. Fetal and neonatal effects of n-acetylcysteine when used for neuroprotection in maternal chorioamnionitis. *J Pediatr.* 2016;168:67-76.e66.
270. Van Laere D, O'Toole JM, Voeten M, et al. Decreased variability and low values of perfusion index on day one are associated with adverse outcome in extremely preterm infants. *J Pediatr.* 2016;178:119-124.
272. Copublishing of the pediatric and neonatal portions of the 2015 International Consensus on cardiopulmonary resuscitation and emergency cardiovascular core science with treatment recommendations and the 2015 American Heart Association Guidelines update for cardiopulmonary resuscitation and emergency cardiovascular care. *Pediatrics.* 2015;136:S83-S87.
273. Oei JL, Saugstad OD, Lui K, et al. Targeted oxygen in the resuscitation of preterm infants, a randomized clinical trial. *Pediatrics.* 2017;139:e20161452.
279. Synnes A, Miller SP. Oxygen therapy for preterm neonates: the elusive optimal target. *JAMA Pediatr.* 2015;169:311-313.
281. Tarnow-Mordi W, Stenson B, Kirby A, et al. Outcomes of two trials of oxygen-saturation targets in preterm infants. *N Engl J Med.* 2016;374:749-760.
299. Poets CF, Roberts RS, Schmidt B, et al. Association between intermittent hypoxemia or bradycardia and late death or disability in extremely preterm infants. *JAMA.* 2015;314:595-603.
301. Hyttel-Sorensen S, Pellicer A, Alderliesten T, et al. Cerebral near infrared spectroscopy oximetry in extremely preterm infants: phase II randomised clinical trial. *BMJ.* 2015;350:7635.
302. Plomgaard AM, Hagmann C, Alderliesten T, et al. Brain injury in the international multicenter randomized SafeBoosC phase II feasibility trial: cranial ultrasound and magnetic resonance imaging assessments. *Pediatr Res.* 2016;79:466-472.
303. Martin RJ, Wang K, Koroglu O, et al. Intermittent hypoxic episodes in preterm infants: do they matter? *Neonatology.* 2011;100:303-310.
308. Fang JL, Sorita A, Carey WA, et al. Interventions to prevent retinopathy of prematurity: a meta-analysis. *Pediatrics.* 2016;137: e20153387.
309. Wellmann S, Buhrer C, Schmitz T. Focal necrosis and disturbed myelination in the white matter of newborn infants: a tale of too much or too little oxygen. *Front Pediatr.* 2014;2:1-4.
312. Guo F, Lang J, Sohn J, et al. Canonical Wnt signaling in the oligodendroglial lineage-puzzles remain. *Glia.* 2015;63:1671-1693.

313. Gerstner B, DeSilva TM, Genz K, et al. Hyperoxia causes maturation-dependent cell death in the developing white matter. *J Neurosci.* 2008;28:1236-1245.

317. Kugelman A, Golan A, Riskin A, et al. Impact of continuous capnography in ventilated neonates: a randomized, multicenter study. *J Pediatr.* 2016;168:56-61.e2.

318. Kaiser JR, Gauss CH, Williams DK. The effects of hypercapnia on cerebral autoregulation in ventilated very low birth weight infants. *Pediatr Res.* 2005;58:931-935.

321. Davis SM, Ackerman RH, Correia JA, et al. Cerebral blood flow and cerebrovascular CO_2 reactivity in stroke-age normal controls. *Neurology.* 1983;33:391-399.

342. Victor S, Appleton RE, Beirne M, et al. Effect of carbon dioxide on background cerebral electrical activity and fractional oxygen extraction in very low birth weight infants just after birth. *Pediatr Res.* 2005;58:579-585.

345. Murase M, Ishida A. Early hypocarbia of preterm infants: its relationship to periventricular leukomalacia and cerebral palsy, and its perinatal risk factors. *Acta Paediatr.* 2005;94:85-91.

354. Shankaran S, Langer JC, Kazzi SN, et al. Cumulative index of exposure to hypocarbia and hyperoxia as risk factors for periventricular leukomalacia in low birth weight infants. *Pediatrics.* 2006;118:1654-1659.

355. Fabres J, Carlo WA, Phillips V, et al. Both extremes of arterial carbon dioxide pressure and the magnitude of fluctuations in arterial carbon dioxide pressure are associated with severe intraventricular hemorrhage in preterm infants. *Pediatrics.* 2007;119:299-305.

356. Altaany D, Natarajan G, Gupta D, et al. Severe intraventricular hemorrhage in extremely premature infants: are high carbon dioxide pressure or fluctuations the culprit? *Am J Perinatol.* 2015;32(9):839-844.

362. Lemmers PM, Toet M, van Schelven LJ, et al. Cerebral oxygenation and cerebral oxygen extraction in the preterm infant: the impact of respiratory distress syndrome. *Exp Brain Res.* 2006;173:458-467.

363. Soul JS, Hammer PE, Tsuji M, et al. Fluctuating pressure-passivity is common in the cerebral circulation of sick premature infants. *Pediatr Res.* 2007;61:467-473.

365. Victor S, Marson AG, Appleton RE, et al. Relationship between blood pressure, cerebral electrical activity, cerebral fractional oxygen extraction, and peripheral blood flow in very low birth weight newborn infants. *Pediatr Res.* 2006;59:314-319.

366. Schat TE, van der Laan ME, Schurink M, et al. Assessing cerebrovascular autoregulation in infants with necrotizing enterocolitis using near-infrared spectroscopy. *Pediatr Res.* 2016;79:76-80.

369. Rhee CJ, Fraser CD 3rd, Kibler K, et al. Ontogeny of cerebrovascular critical closing pressure. *Pediatr Res.* 2015;78:71-75.

370. Kenosi M, Naulaers G, Ryan CA, et al. Current research suggests that the future looks brighter for cerebral oxygenation monitoring in preterm infants. *Acta Paediatr.* 2015;104:225-231.

389. Fernandez E, Watterberg KL, Faix RG, et al. Incidence, management, and outcomes of cardiovascular insufficiency in critically ill term and late preterm newborn infants. *Am J Perinatol.* 2014;31:947-956.

391. Batton B, Li L, Newman NS, et al. Evolving blood pressure dynamics for extremely preterm infants. *J Perinatol.* 2014;34:301-305.

395. Weindling AM, Bentham J. Commentary on "blood pressure in the neonate.". *Acta Paediatr.* 2005;94:138-140.

397. Barrington KJ, Dempsey EM. Cardiovascular support in the preterm: treatments in search of indications. *J Pediatr.* 2006;148:289-291.

398. Osborn DA, Evans N, Kluckow M. Left ventricular contractility in extremely premature infants in the first day and response to inotropes. *Pediatr Res.* 2007;61:335-340.

413. Dix L, Molenschot M, Breur J, et al. Cerebral oxygenation and echocardiographic parameters in preterm neonates with a patent ductus arteriosus: an observational study. *Arch Dis Child Fetal Neonatal Ed.* 2016.

417. Miller SP, Mayer EE, Clyman RI, et al. Prolonged indomethacin exposure is associated with decreased white matter injury detected with magnetic resonance imaging in premature newborns at 24 to 28 weeks' gestation at birth. *Pediatrics.* 2006;117:1626-1631.

423. Schmid MB, Hopfner RJ, Lenhof S, et al. Cerebral oxygenation during intermittent hypoxemia and bradycardia in preterm infants. *Neonatology.* 2015;107:137-146.

430. Dionne JM, Abitbol CL, Flynn JT. Hypertension in infancy: diagnosis, management and outcome. *Pediatr Nephrol.* 2012;27:17-32.

433. Hammers AL, Sanchez-Ramos L, Kaunitz AM. Antenatal exposure to indomethacin increases the risk of severe intraventricular hemorrhage, necrotizing enterocolitis, and periventricular leukomalacia: a systematic review with metannalysis. *Am J Obstet Gynecol.* 2015;12:505.e501-e513.

434. Juul SE, Pet GC. Erythropoietin and neonatal neuroprotection. *Clin Perinatol.* 2015;42:469-481.

435. Ohls RK, Cannon DC, Phillips J, et al. Preschool assessment of preterm infants treated with darbepoetin and erythropoietin. *Pediatrics.* 2016;137:1-9.

437. O'Gorman RL, Bucher HU, Held U, et al. Tract-based spatial statistics to assess the neuroprotective effect of early erythropoietin on white matter development in preterm infants. *Brain.* 2015;138:388-397.

438. Ohls RK, Kamath-Rayne BD, Christensen RD, et al. Cognitive outcomes of preterm infants randomized to darbepoetin, erythropoietin, or placebo. *Pediatrics.* 2014;133:1023-1030.

441. Rangarajan V, Juul SE. Erythropoietin: emerging role of erythropoietin in neonatal neuroprotection. *Pediatr Neurol.* 2014;51:481-488.

447. Jantzie LL, Corbett CJ, Firl DJ, et al. Postnatal erythropoietin mitigates impaired cerebral cortical development following subplate loss from prenatal hypoxia-ischemia. *Cereb Cortex.* 2015;25:2683-2695.

448. Scafidi J, Hammond TR, Scafidi S, et al. Intranasal epidermal growth factor treatment rescues neonatal brain injury. *Nature.* 2014;506:230-234.

454. Committee on F Newborn, Papile LA, et al. Hypothermia and neonatal encephalopathy. *Pediatrics.* 2014;133:1146-1150.

456. Laptook AR. Birth asphyxia and hypoxic-ischemic brain injury in the preterm infant. *Clin Perinatol.* 2016;43:529-545.

458. Cusick SE, Georgieff MK. The role of nutrition in brain development: the golden opportunity of the "first 1000 days". *J Pediatr.* 2016;175:16-21.

459. Belfort MB, Ehrenkranz RA. Neurodevelopmental outcomes and nutritional strategies in very low birth weight infants. *Semin Fetal Neonatal Med.* 2017;22:42-48.

461. Griffin IJ, Tancredi DJ, Bertino E, et al. Postnatal growth failure in very low birthweight infants born between 2005 and 2012. *Arch Dis Child Fetal Neonatal Ed.* 2016;101:F50-F55.

464. Ehrenkranz RA, Dusick AM, Vohr BR, et al. Growth in the neonatal intensive care unit influences neurodevelopmental and growth outcomes of extremely low birth weight infants. *Pediatrics.* 2006;117:1253-1261.

465. Lira PIC, Eickmann SE, Lima MC, et al. Early head growth: relation with IQ at 8 years and determinants in term infants of low and appropriate birthweight. *Dev Med Child Neurol.* 2010;52:40-46.

467. Neubauer V, Griesmaier E, Pehbock-Walser N, et al. Poor postnatal head growth in very preterm infants is associated with impaired neurodevelopment outcome. *Acta Paediatr.* 2013;102:883-888.

470. Leppanen M, Lapinleimu H, Lind A, et al. Antenatal and postnatal growth and 5-year cognitive outcome in very preterm infants. *Pediatrics.* 2014;133:63-70.

472. Sammallahti S, Pyhala R, Lahti M, et al. Infant growth after preterm birth and neurocognitive abilities in young adulthood. *J Pediatr.* 2014;165:1109-1115.

477. Bernard JY, De Agostini M, Forhan A, et al. Breastfeeding duration and cognitive development at 2 and 3 years of age in the EDEN mother-child cohort. *J Pediatr.* 2013;163:36-42.e31.

478. Deoni SC, Dean DC 3rd, Piryatinsky I, et al. Breastfeeding and early white matter development: a cross-sectional study. *Neuroimage.* 2013;82:77-86.

480. Gibertoni D, Corvaglia L, Vandini S, et al. Positive effect of human milk feeding during NICU hospitalization on 24 month neurodevelopment of very low birth weight infants: an italian cohort study. *PLoS ONE.* 2015;10:e0116552.

483. Tam EW, Chau V, Barkovich AJ, et al. Early postnatal docosahexaenoic acid levels and improved preterm brain development. *Pediatr Res.* 2016;79:723-730.

491. Pineda RG, Neil J, Dierker D, et al. Alterations in brain structure and neurodevelopmental outcome in preterm infants hospitalized in different neonatal intensive care unit environments. *J Pediatr.* 2014;164:52-60.

492. Lester BM, Salisbury AL, Hawes K, et al. 18-month follow-up of infants cared for in a single-family room neonatal intensive care unit. *J Pediatr.* 2016;177:84-89.

497. Kwon SH, Scheinost D, Vohr B, et al. Functional magnetic resonance connectivity studies in infants born preterm: suggestions of proximate and long-lasting changes in language organization. *Dev Med Child Neurol.* 2016;58:28-34.

505. Committee on Fetus and Newborn and Section on Anesthesiology and Pain Medicine. Prevention and management of procedural pain in the neonate: an update. *Pediatrics.* 2016;137:e20154271.

508. McAnulty GB, Duffy FH, Butler SC, et al. Effects of the newborn individualized developmental care and assessment program (NIDCAP) at age 8 years: preliminary data. *Clin Pediatr (Phila).* 2010;49: 258-270.

511. Pineda R, Guth R, Herring A, et al. Enhancing sensory experiences for very preterm infants in the NICU: an integrative review. *J Perinatol.* 2017;37:323-332.

512. Orton J, Spittle A, Doyle L, et al. Do early intervention programmes improve cognitive and motor outcomes for preterm infants after discharge? A systematic review. *Dev Med Child Neurol.* 2009;51:851-859.

514. Spittle A, Orton J, Anderson PJ, et al. Early developmental intervention programmes provided post hospital discharge to prevent motor and cognitive impairment in preterm infants (Review). *Cochrane Database Syst Rev.* 2015;(11):CD005495.

517. Doyle LW, Cheong JL, Burnett A, et al. Biological and social influences on outcomes of extreme-preterm/low-birth weight adolescents. *Pediatrics.* 2015;136:e1513-e1520.

518. Linsell L, Malouf R, Morris J, et al. Prognostic factors for poor cognitive development in children born very preterm or with very low birth weight: a systematic review. *JAMA Pediatr.* 2015;169: 1162-1172.

520. Titomanlio L, Kavelaars A, Dalous J, et al. Stem cell therapy for neonatal brain injury: perspectives and challenges. *Ann Neurol.* 2011;70:698-712.

521. Fleiss B, Guillot PV, Titomanlio L, et al. Stem cell therapy for neonatal brain injury. *Clin Perinatol.* 2014;41:133-148.

528. Chen LX, Ma SM, Zhang P, et al. Neuroprotective effects of oligodendrocyte progenitor cell transplantation in premature rat brain following hypoxic-ischemic injury. *PLoS ONE.* 2015;10: e0115997.

529. Osorio MJ, Rowitch DH, Tesar P, et al. Concise review: stem cell-based treatment of Pelizaeus-Merzbacher disease. *Stem Cells.* 2017;35: 311-315.

Full references for this chapter can be found on www.expertconsult .com.

Intrauterine, Intrapartum Assessments in the Term Infant

Terrie E. Inder ◆ *Joseph J. Volpe*

The focus in this chapter is the assessment of fetal well-being, particularly as a means for recognition of the infant that may be at risk of hypoxic-ischemic cerebral injury. The identification of an intrauterine disturbance in gas exchange between the human fetus and mother (i.e., asphyxia), or the likelihood that such a disturbance will occur during labor or delivery is critical in view of the large body of data that intrauterine asphyxia occurs in a large proportion of infants with hypoxic-ischemic encephalopathy. Moreover, attempts at prevention of the brain injury caused by intrauterine asphyxia—antepartum and intrapartum—demand precise awareness of when such injury is imminent. Although the most definitive information concerning detection of hypoxic-ischemic insult to the fetus still applies primarily to the intrapartum period, major advances in antepartum assessment have been made. This chapter reviews the major current means of antepartum assessment of the fetus and the approach to intrapartum assessment. In addition, we will briefly summarize novel fetal and placental imaging techniques using magnetic resonance imaging (MRI). Issues related to genetic disorders and cerebral genesis (Unit 1) and fetal cerebral metabolic disorders (Chapters 27, 28 and 29) are reviewed in other sections of the book.[1-10]

ANTEPARTUM ASSESSMENT

Although the nature, timing, and frequency are not entirely established, it is clear that some hypoxic-ischemic insults affect the brain before labor and delivery (i.e., during the antepartum period). The search for means of assessing such disturbances, acute or chronic, has been the subject of a vast amount of obstetrical research. Antepartum surveillance regimens were developed principally to prevent stillbirth. Thus, the evaluation of antepartum techniques of monitoring for a reduction in hypoxic-ischemic injury has not been specifically studied. However, with the expansion of monitoring, the impact of monitoring on Apgar scores and neonatal intensive care admission has allowed some insights (see later). In this section, a brief review of the current means of fetus evaluation during the antepartum period is provided. The techniques are described as those based on measurement of fetal movement, fetal heart rate, a combination of factors that include fetal movement and heart rate (biophysical profile), fetal growth, and blood flow velocity in uterine and fetal blood vessels (Table 17.1). All of these techniques are usually applied with greater frequency to women who are deemed to be at greater risk for pregnancy and neonatal complications. Thus, identifying the fetus at risk for cerebral injury may allow timely detection of impending fetal jeopardy allowing intervention or delivery to reduce the risk of possible cerebral injury. Pregnancy conditions that have been associated with increased risk of short-term and long-term neurological sequelae[11] for which antenatal testing may be appropriate are outlined in Table 17.2.

A common theme found in relation to all the techniques outlined later is that the presence of normal results is associated with good fetal and neonatal outcomes. Thus, *the absence of any abnormality can be reassuring.* However, abnormal tests have low positive predictive values for abnormal outcomes, making their utility as diagnostic tests for fetal vulnerability poor. Finally, many studies have not included outcomes of greatest relevance, including neonatal morbidity and neurodevelopmental outcomes.

Fetal Movement and Behavioral States

Fetal movement is a useful indicator of fetal health.[12-23] Techniques for monitoring fetal movement have included systematic maternal recording of perceived activity (the most convenient and widely used), electromechanical devices (tocodynamometry, primarily an investigative tool), and real-time ultrasonography (see Table 17.1). Real-time ultrasonography has received increasingly wide clinical and investigational use because of the diversity of information that it can provide.

Fetal movements are one aspect of the determination of fetal behavioral states. Fetal behavioral states are defined according to the quantitative and qualitative aspects of fetal body movements, eye movements, and fetal heart rate.[20,23-30] Distinct fetal states are definable by 36 to 38 weeks of gestation and recognizable behavioral states at that time are summarized in Table 17.3. These states approximate *neonatal* behavioral states, that is, quiet sleep (1F), REM sleep (2F), quiet waking (3F), and active waking (4F). Active sleep (2F) is the most frequently observed, followed by quiet sleep (1F).[23] The waking states are either infrequent (4F) or rare (3F).

Maturational Changes

Distinct maturational changes in fetal movement can be identified (Fig. 17.1).[13,22,23] Although with ultrasonography it is possible to detect movement as early as the second month of gestation,[31-33] maternal perception of movement (*quickening*) occurs at approximately 16 weeks. Thereafter, the movements increase in strength and reach a plateau from 26 to 32 weeks of gestation. An abrupt fall to a second plateau occurs between 32 and 36 weeks. No appreciable change occurs thereafter until delivery.

Prechtl and others[16,18,21,34-38] emphasized the quality of fetal movements and the striking maturational changes in the variety and complexity of these movements. Certain fetal movements increase in incidence gradually with advancing gestation (e.g., breathing, sucking, and swallowing), other movements increase in incidence to a plateau (e.g., general movements, isolated arm movements), and still others increase in incidence and then decrease (e.g., startles, hiccups).

Relation to Fetal Well-Being

The relation of quantity and quality of fetal movement to fetal well-being is illustrated by the study summarized in Fig. 17.2. Decreased fetal movements perceived by the mother over the 7 days before delivery can be documented in a series of pregnancies with "unfavorable perinatal outcome" (i.e., abnormal intrapartum fetal heart rate patterns, depressed Apgar scores, and antepartum or intrapartum stillbirth).[13] The most common denominator of fetal inactivity was *chronic uteroplacental insufficiency.* A report that suggests the value for prompt detection and evaluation of decreased fetal movement involved pregnant women who were instructed to report to the delivery unit if 2 hours elapsed without 10 fetal movements perceived. Further evaluations and any indicated interventions for fetal compromise were performed.[18] During the study period, fetal mortality among women with such decreased fetal movement was 10 per 1000; in the control period immediately before onset of the study, fetal mortality with such decreased fetal movement was 44 per 1000.

A recent Cochrane review of the efficacy of fetal movement counting for the assessment of fetal well-being included five studies with 71,458 women.[39] All included women with uncomplicated pregnancies, except one study which included high-risk women as participants. Two studies compared fetal

---

TABLE 17.1 Major Means of Antepartum Assessment of the Human Fetus

Fetal movement
Detection by maternal perception or by real-time ultrasonography
Fetal heart rate
Nonstress test: response of fetal heart rate to movement
Contraction stress test: response of fetal heart rate to stimulated (oxytocin and nipple stimulation) or spontaneous uterine contraction
Fetal biophysical profile
Combination of fetal breathing, movement, tone, heart rate reactivity, and amniotic fluid volume
Fetal growth
Detection of intrauterine growth retardation
Fetal blood flow velocity
Detection by the Doppler technique of flow velocity in umbilical and fetal systemic and cerebral vessels

---

TABLE 17.2 Pregnancy Conditions to Consider Heightened Antepartum Assessment of the Human Fetus Due to Risk for Fetal Loss or Cerebral Injury

Maternal conditions
Maternal thyroid disease
Maternal hypertension—essential or preeclampsia
Maternal diabetes—preexisting or gestational
Maternal immune disorders—isoimmunization, antiphospholipid disorder
Maternal chronic medical conditions—SLE, renal disease
Maternal drug or infectious exposure
Fetoplacental conditions
Fetal growth restriction
Fetal anatomical anomaly
Abnormality of amniotic volume—oligohydramnios or polyhydramnios
Multiple gestation—particularly monochorionic
Previous fetal demise
Other
Environmental risk—ionizing radiation, lead, mercury

SLE, Systemic lupus erythematosus.

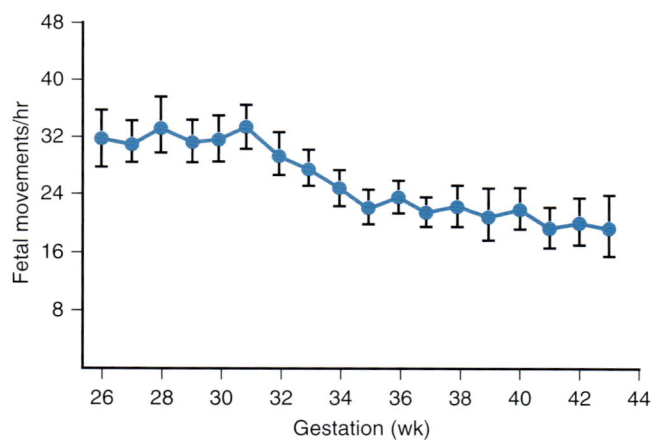

Figure 17.1 Relation of quantity of fetal movement to gestational age. Movements were quantitated by maternal perception. (From Rayburn WF. Antepartum fetal assessment: monitoring fetal activity. *Clin Perinatol.* 1982;9: 231–240.)

TABLE 17.3 Fetal Behavioral States at 38 Weeks of Gestation

STATE[a]	BODY MOVEMENTS	EYE MOVEMENTS	FETAL HEART RATE PATTERN
1F	Absent (occasional startle)	Absent	Narrow variability, isolated acceleration
2F	Present (frequent bursts)	Present	Wide variability, acceleration with movement
3F	Absent	Present	Wide variability, no accelerations
4F	Present (almost continuous)	Present (continuous)	Long accelerations or sustained tachycardia

See text for references.
[a]These fetal states approximate neonatal behavioral states, that is, quiet sleep (1F), active sleep (2F), quiet waking (3F), and active waking (4F).

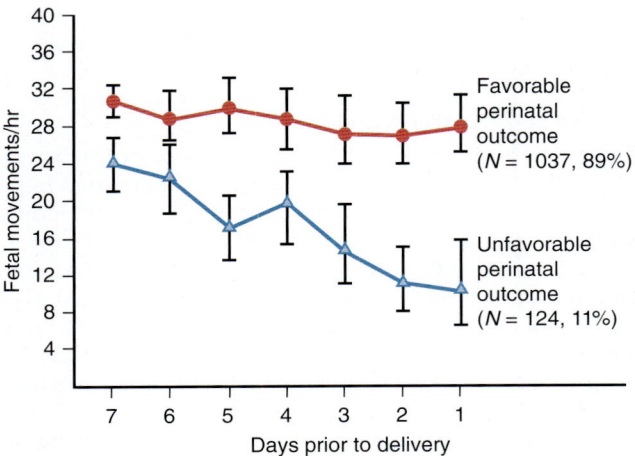

Figure 17.2 Relation of decrease in quantity of fetal movement over 7 days before delivery to unfavorable perinatal outcome. See text for details. (From Rayburn WF. Antepartum fetal assessment: monitoring fetal activity. *Clin Perinatol.* 1982;9:231–240.)

movement counting with standard care, as defined by trial author.[40,41] Two studies compared two types of fetal movement counting:[42,43] comparing once-a-day (Cardiff count-to-10) with more than once-a-day fetal movement counting methods. One study compared fetal movement counting with hormone assessment evaluated with an average of five determinations of serum total estriol and human placental lactogen.[44]

The first comparison of fetal movement monitoring compared with standard care showed no difference in mean stillbirth rates (standard mean difference [SMD] 0.23, 95% CI –0.61 to 1.07) or fetal deaths. There was no difference in cesarean section rate between groups within any of these three comparisons of fetal movement monitoring. There were no data on perinatal mortality or severe morbidities.

The conclusions of the Cochrane review were that sufficient evidence did not exist to influence clinical practice. In particular, only two studies compared the counting of fetal movements with standard antenatal care.[40,41] It is noteworthy that the larger cluster randomized controlled trial (RCT)[40] comparing routine fetal movement counting with *normal care*, which included fetal movement counting at the discretion of the caregiver (8.9% in a subset of *control* participants), demonstrated a strong trend to a reduction in stillbirth. However, this did not translate to reduced perinatal mortality or morbidity across all studies, including this RCT.

Fetal Neurological Examination

The observations described in the preceding sections are reminiscent of those made during the neonatal neurological examination. The utilization of fetal movements as part of a detailed analysis of fetal behavior by real-time ultrasonography led to the identification of *distinct behavioral states*, as noted earlier. These analyses include assessment of a variety of specific body movements (e.g., yawning, stretching, and startle), as well as fetal eye movements, posture, breathing, and heart rate. The analogy of these phenomena to those observed after birth in the premature infant (see Chapter 9) is obvious, and, to a major extent, one can consider these observations *a kind of fetal neurological examination*. When amplified by such assessments as habituation of the

fetus to vibrotactile stimuli or response to acoustical stimuli, the analogy to neurological assessment becomes even more impressive.[22,23,45-52] Detailed analysis of the *quantity and quality of fetal breathing* can provide still further information about the fetal nervous system.[a] With the wide use of real-time ultrasonography, standardization of observable neurological phenomena, and, importantly, the correlation of aberrations with the topography of neuropathology, highly valuable evaluation of the fetal central nervous system and dysfunction should be possible. The design of appropriate interventions for disturbances then would be an appropriate next step.

Fetal Heart Rate: Nonstress and Stress Tests

The evaluation of fetal well-being by *antepartum* fetal heart rate testing is a standard obstetrical practice in high-risk pregnancies. The two commonly used techniques determine fetal heart rate changes with either stimulated (or spontaneous) uterine contractions (contraction stress test) or spontaneous fetal events (e.g., fetal movement test, or nonstress test) (see Table 17.1).

Nonstress Test

Of the two techniques, the *nonstress test* is the approach used as an initial evaluation.[55-58] In general, the particular value of the technique is the determination of a healthy fetus[55,56,58-60] based on demonstration of at least two accelerations of fetal heart rate during the period of observation (usually ≈40 minutes), generally in association with fetal movement or vibroacoustical stimulation. The accelerations must exceed 15 beats/min and last at least 15 seconds; the normal result is called a *reactive* nonstress test. A *nonreactive* test is characterized by the failure to note such accelerations over the observation period. The demonstration of accelerations of fetal heart rate with acoustical stimulation and the correlation of a reactive acoustical stimulation test with the conventional nonstress test have led to use of such stimulation as part of the nonstress test in many centers.[22,51,56-58]

In *the predictive value* of nonstress testing, the incidence of fetal distress leading to cesarean delivery increases from about 1% to 20% when antepartum reactive and nonreactive patterns are compared.[51,55,56] It is clear, however, that most *abnormal* or nonreactive tests are not followed by difficulties with labor and delivery. A normal, reactive nonstress test is highly predictive of fetal well-being. *Thus, as with most other modes of fetal evaluation including antepartum and intrapartum, the prediction of a normal fetus and the relative lack of need for intervention are the greatest values of the test.* However, the test does not detect such important maternal-fetal problems as oligohydramnios, umbilical cord or placental abnormalities, growth disorders, and twin demise. When suspicion or concern for such problems exists, another approach using ultrasonography, as in fetal biophysical profile, is essential.[58] Despite the rational approach to these measures of fetal behavior and well-being, several randomized prospective trials that have used weekly nonstress surveillance tests have shown no benefit to the fetus or infant.[52,61-63]

Contraction Stress Test

The *contraction stress test* was most commonly used in the past as a follow-up evaluation after a nonreactive stress test. Experimental data suggest that the occurrence of late decelerations with contractions, the basis for a *positive* (abnormal) *stress test*, is

---
[a]References 16, 22, 35, 37, 53, 54.

an early warning sign of uteroplacental insufficiency.[58-60,64] The established clinical and experimental premise of the stress test is that chronic uteroplacental insufficiency results in late decelerations of the fetal heart rate, a sign of fetal hypoxia (see following discussion) in response to uterine contractions; these can be stimulated by breast stimulation or oxytocin infusion.[58,65-68] In approximately 10% of women, spontaneous uterine contractions obviate the need to stimulate uterine contractions. A *positive* (abnormal) *result* is indicated by persistent late decelerations over several or more contractions; these positive tests can be subdivided further as *reactive*, when accompanied by accelerations at some time during the test, or *nonreactive*, when not accompanied by accelerations. An *equivocal result* refers to the occurrence of nonpersistent *late decelerations*. A *negative stress test* is defined as absence of any late decelerations with the contractions.

As with nonstress testing and other fetal assessments, a negative stress test is a reliable indicator of fetal well-being. The predictive value of a positive stress test was demonstrated in one multi-institutional study of high-risk pregnancies. A negative test was followed by perinatal death in less than 1% of cases versus 5% to 20% of infants with positive contraction tests. The lower value was for infants with reactive positive tests; the higher value was for those with nonreactive positive tests.[66-68] Similarly, an Australian study showed that among 72 patients with nonreactive positive spontaneous contraction stress test results, there was a 28% perinatal mortality rate. Of the 52 infants who survived the neonatal period, 42 were assessed with 27% having neurological handicap.[60]

Currently, the contraction stress test is no longer the principal method for follow-up in most centers.[58] This change relates to logistical and interpretive difficulties and relatively low positive-predictive values. The fetal biophysical profile is now favored as the primary means of fetal surveillance for high-risk pregnancies, identified by a nonreactive nonstress test or other evidence.[58]

Fetal Biophysical Profile

In view of the relatively high incidence of false-positive assessments with the tests of fetal heart rate just described, *a series of fetal measures*, termed a *composite biophysical profile*, has been used to refine antepartum evaluation.[57,58,69-77] These measures include quantitation *not only of fetal heart rate reactivity* (see the earlier discussion of the nonstress test), but also of *fetal breathing movements, gross body movements, fetal tone* (as assessed by posture and flexor-extensor movements), and *amniotic fluid volume* (see Table 17.1). Each item is graded, usually on a score of 0 to 2. The use of *real-time ultrasonography* has made such an assessment possible, and the relative ease of this methodology in modern obstetrical centers has led to widespread use. The rationale of using such a profile is entirely reasonable (i.e., the various measures reflect activity of several levels of the central nervous system, including cerebrum, diencephalon, and brain stem). The predictive value of the score is demonstrated by the data in Fig. 17.3, which illustrate the relation of the fetal biophysical score to umbilical venous pH determined by cordocentesis.[78] Similar correlations are available regarding incidence of meconium passage during labor, signs of intrapartum fetal distress, and perinatal mortality.[58,72] Of particular importance, the degree of abnormality of the fetal biophysical score has been shown to correlate with cerebral palsy (Fig. 17.4) and predicted perinatal

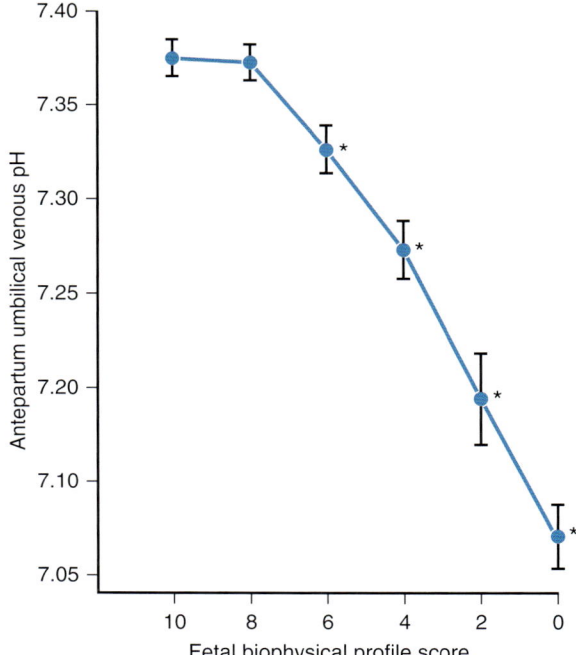

Figure 17.3 Relation of fetal biophysical profile score to mean umbilical vein pH (±2 SD) in fetal blood obtained by cordocentesis. A progressive and highly significant direct linear relationship exists between abnormal biophysical profile (BPP) scores (≤6) and umbilical vein pH (P <.01). Asterisks denote a significantly lower mean pH compared with the value recorded for the immediately higher BPP score. (From Manning FA. Fetal assessment by evaluation of biophysical variables. In Creasy RK, Resnik R, eds. *Maternal-Fetal Medicine*. 4th ed. Philadelphia: WB Saunders; 1999.)

mortality (Table 17.4).[58,77] Data from a single center suggested that alterations in obstetrical management provoked by the results of the score could lead to a threefold to fourfold decline in cerebral palsy rates.[77] Despite these positive results, a recent Cochrane review found no significant difference in outcomes between those high-risk pregnancies monitored with biophysical profile as compared with other forms of fetal assessment, mainly fetal heart rate monitoring.[79] This supports the challenge in the widespread implementation of these evaluative tools of fetal well-being in randomized controlled trials, despite strong and rational observational data. The apparent lack of benefit may relate to subject selection, application of the testing, and/or limitations in the outcome measures.

Fetal Growth

As with other antepartum assessments, advances in ultrasound technology have provided the capability of accurate quantitative assessment of fetal growth.[7,80] The particular value of this assessment is in the detection of intrauterine growth retardation (see Table 17.1), although other aberrations of growth (e.g., large body size and large head) have important implications for management of labor, delivery, and the neonatal period, as discussed elsewhere in this book. Detection of intrauterine growth retardation is important, principally because significant management decisions follow. Most such fetuses are "constitutionally small," are not at increased perinatal risk, and do not require aggressive intervention.[7] However, some such infants (≈5% to 10%) exhibit a major developmental anomaly,

TABLE 17.4   Fetal Biophysical Score: Relation to Outcome and Recommended Management

BIOPHYSICAL PROFILE SCORE[a]	INTERPRETATION	PREDICTED PERINATAL MORTALITY	RECOMMENDED MANAGEMENT
0/10	Severe acute asphyxia	60/100	Immediate delivery by cesarean section
2/10	Acute fetal asphyxia, most likely with chronic decompensation	125/100	Delivery for fetal indications (usually cesarean section)
4/10	Acute fetal asphyxia likely; if oligohydramnios present, chronic asphyxia also very likely	9.1/100	Delivery by obstetrically appropriate method with continuous monitoring
10/10	No evidence of fetal asphyxia	<0.1/100	No acute intervention

[a]Values intermediate between 4/10 and 10/10 not shown.
Adapted from Harman CR. Assessment of fetal health. In Creasy RK, Resnik R, Iams JD, eds. *Maternal-Fetal Medicine: Principles and Practice.* 5th ed. Philadelphia: WB Saunders; 2004, with permission.

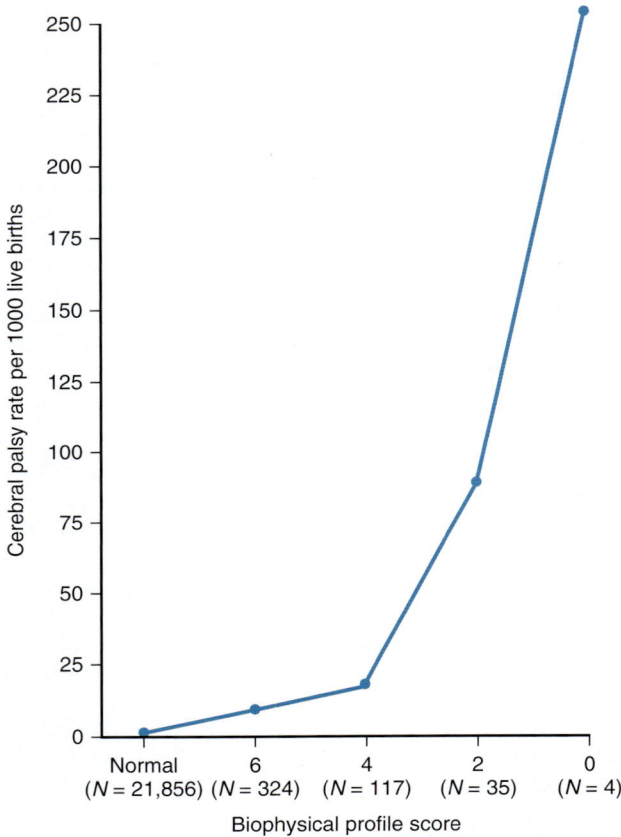

Figure 17.4 Relationship between last fetal biophysical profile score and incidence of cerebral palsy. An inverse, exponential, and highly significant relationship is apparent (P <.001). (From Harman CR. Assessment of fetal health. In Creasy RK, Resnik R, Iams JD, eds. *Maternal-Fetal Medicine: Principles and Practice.* 5th ed. Philadelphia: WB Saunders; 2004.)

including chromosomal aberration, that may require further intrauterine assessment (e.g., amniocentesis and chromosomal or other genetic analyses). Of greatest importance, particularly in this context, is that approximately 10% to 15% of infants with intrauterine growth retardation are growth retarded because of uteroplacental failure and are *at risk for intrapartum asphyxia.*[7,81-87] In one series from a single high-risk service, 35%

of growth-retarded fetuses exhibited intrapartum fetal heart rate abnormalities indicative of fetal distress.[82] A significant increase in fetal asphyxia, as judged by cord acid-base studies, was apparent even when growth-retarded infants were compared with other high-risk groups.[83] Moreover, growth-retarded infants with intrapartum fetal heart decelerations demonstrate considerably higher umbilical artery lactate levels than do normally grown infants with similar decelerations.[84] Hence, growth-retarded infants tolerate labor less well than do normally grown infants, perhaps in part due to deficient stores of glycogen in liver, heart, and, possibly, in the brain. Therefore, antepartum detection of such infants is important in formulating rational decisions concerning further assessment of the fetus (e.g., fetal biophysical profile, Doppler blood flow velocity studies) and optimal management of labor and delivery (see next section).

Doppler Measurements of Blood Flow Velocity in Maternal Umbilical and Fetal Cerebral and Ductus Venosus Vessels

Doppler velocimetry is now a well-described technique used to assess fetal status (Table 17.5). Several vessels have been interrogated, including the (maternal) uterine artery, fetal middle cerebral artery (MCA), umbilical artery, umbilical vein, and ductus venosus (DV). The most commonly examined and clinically useful vessel is the fetal umbilical artery. The waveform in normally growing fetuses is characterized by high-velocity diastolic flow; the commonly measured indices include systolic/diastolic ratio, resistance index, and pulsatility index (PI) (see Chapter 10).[88] Marked abnormality in the waveform is characterized by absent or reversed diastolic flow. These waveforms correlate histopathologically with small artery obliteration in placental tertiary villi, and functionally with fetal hypoxia, acidosis, and prenatal morbidity and mortality.[89] These studies have been undertaken predominantly in women who have a fetal diagnosis of intrauterine growth retardation.

Umbilical Artery

Most studies based on the use of Doppler in pregnancy have focused on the umbilical artery.[a] The principal quantitative parameters of the Doppler waveform used have been the *pulsatility index of Gosling* (peak systolic velocity [S] − end diastolic

---

[a]References 19, 58, 81, 85, 86, 90-105.

TABLE 17.5	Doppler Measurements of Blood Flow Velocity to Assess Fetal Status		
METHOD	**MEASURES**	**INDICATIONS**	**VALUE**
Umbilical cord artery	Pulsatility index Resistive index Diastolic flow—absent or reversed	High-risk fetus, particularly IUGR	Reduction in fetal mortality and in obstetrical interventions
Fetal middle cerebral artery	Cerebral blood flow velocity Resistive index Pulsatility index	High-risk fetus, particularly IUGR	Abnormal MCA PI was associated with greater perinatal morbidity
Fetal ductus venosus	a-Wave characteristics Diastolic flow measures	IUGR—particularly useful between 20 and 32 weeks gestation	Determination of delivery by DV. measures resulted in slight increase in mortality but reduction in morbidity

DV, Ductus venosus; IUGR, intra-uterine growth restriction; MCA, middle cerebral artery; MCR, middle cerebral artery.

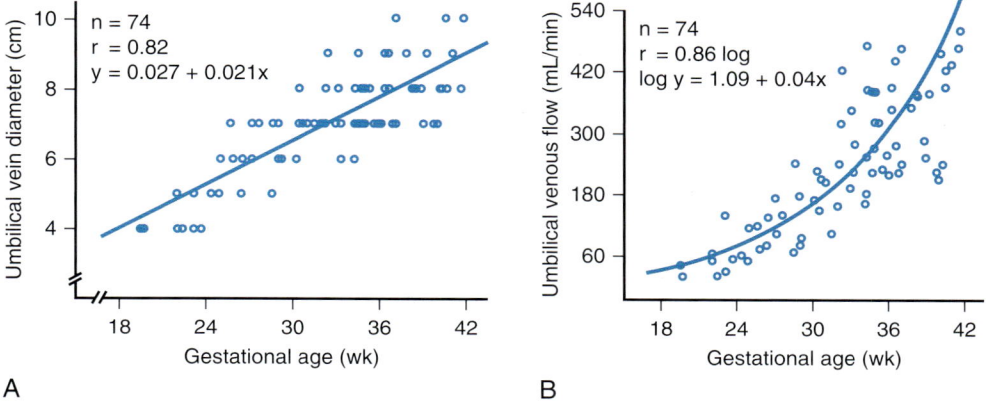

Figure 17.5 Relationship between umbilical vein diameter and umbilical venous flow in human pregnancy **(n = 74).** (A) Umbilical vein diameter. (B) Umbilical venous flow. Note the linear increase in venous diameter and the exponential increase in blood flow. (From Sutton MS, Theard MA, Bhatia SJ, et al. Changes in placental blood flow in the normal human fetus with gestational age. *Pediatr Res.* 1990;28:383–387.)

velocity [D]/mean velocity), the *resistance index of Pourcelot* (S – D/S), and the *S/D ratio*. The values of these ratios, in general, are not affected by the angle of insonation, which is clearly difficult to maintain as a constant in the clinical situation. The pulsatility index and the resistance index reflect vascular resistance, in large part. The principal change in umbilical artery blood flow velocity with progression of *normal pregnancy* is a decline in the resistance parameters.[58,91,93,99,106] Although the decline is gradual, a more pronounced decrease occurs after 30 weeks of gestation. This decrease is considered secondary to a decrease in placental vascular resistance, related particularly to increased numbers of small vessels. A similar phenomenon was documented in the fetal lamb.[107] The decrease in placental vascular resistance with advancing pregnancy is accompanied by an increase in volemic placental blood flow, calculated in human fetuses by simultaneous measurements of the blood flow velocity in the umbilical vein and the cross-sectional area of that vessel by combined Doppler and imaging ultrasonography (Fig. 17.5).[108]

The major application of Doppler studies of blood flow velocity in the umbilical artery has been in the investigation of the high-risk fetus.[a] In intrauterine growth retardation, the principal finding is an increase in the resistance measures.[a] With progression of this disturbance in resistance measures in the umbilical artery, marked impairment of the end diastolic flow or even loss or reversal of diastolic flow (an ominous sign) may occur (Fig. 17.6).

In one study, the changes in resistance indices *preceded* antepartum late heart-rate decelerations in more than 90% of fetuses who developed such decelerations, and the median duration of the interval between the severe abnormality of resistance measure and decelerations was 17 days.[115] The importance of the rising placental vascular resistance to the fetus is shown by the striking curvilinear relationship between the pulsatility index in the umbilical artery and the lactate concentration in fetal blood, a measure of fetal hypoxia (Fig. 17.7).[116] The clinical predictive value of the diastolic flow in the umbilical artery was apparent in a study of 459 high-risk pregnancies.[106] Thus, the rate of fetal or neonatal death in the presence of end diastolic flow was 4%, increased to 41% with absence of flow, and increased to 75% with reversal of flow. With further prompt and detailed fetal assessments and appropriate interventions, an unfavorable outlook with absence of diastolic flow has not been so evident.[58,119] However, reversal of flow is

[a]References 19, 58, 81, 85, 86, 90-92, 94, 95, 97-99, 101-106, 109-119.

[a]References 19, 81, 85, 86, 91, 92, 98, 99, 101-106, 109, 111, 118.

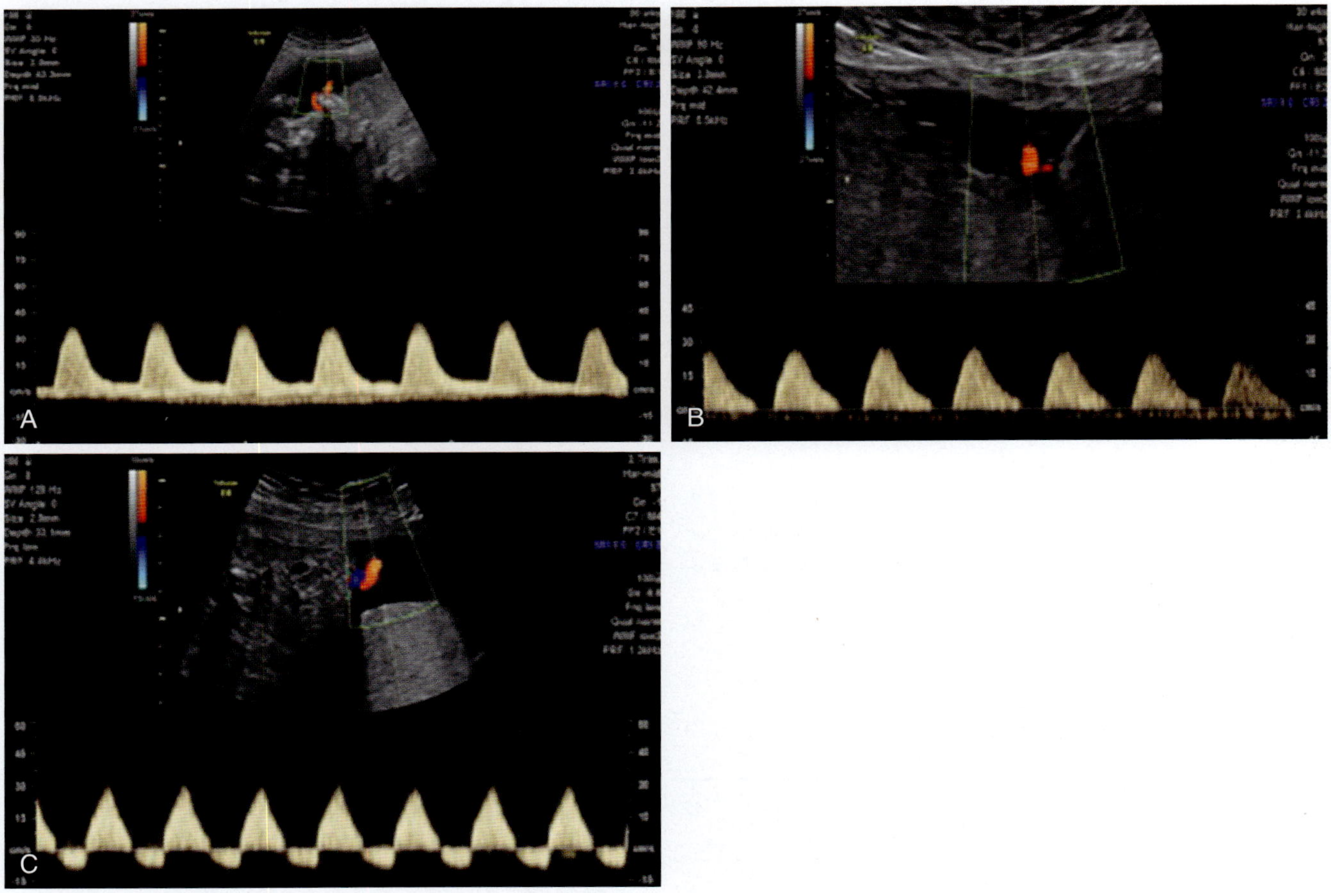

Figure 17.6 Changes in umbilical artery waveforms. (A) Normal with positive end-diastolic flow (EDF). (B) Abnormal with absent EDF. (C) Abnormal with reversed EDF. (Reprinted with permission from Everett TR, Peebles DM. Antenatal tests of fetal wellbeing. *Sem Fetal Neonatal Med.* 2015;20(3):138–143.)

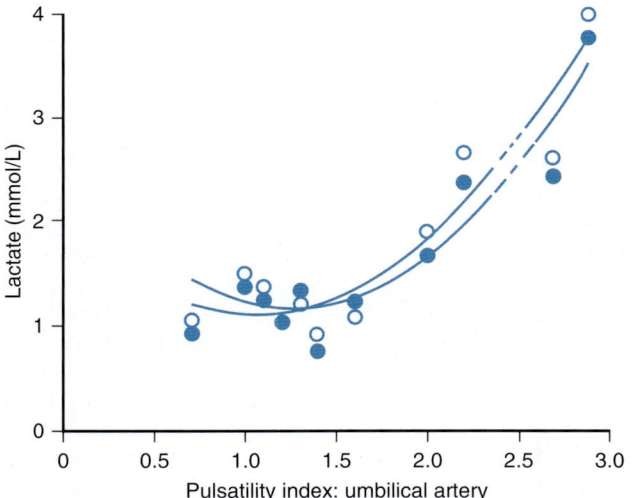

Figure 17.7 Relationship between lactate concentration of fetal blood (sampled from the umbilical vein *[solid circles]* or artery *[open circles]* at the time of cesarean section) and pulsatility index obtained from the umbilical artery before delivery. Note the marked increase in fetal blood lactate with increasing pulsatility index (i.e., increasing placental vascular resistance). (From Ferrazzi E, Pardi G, Bauscaglia M, et al. The correlation of biochemical monitoring versus umbilical flow velocity measurements of the human fetus. *Am J Obstet Gynecol.* 1988;159: 1081–1087.)

associated with a considerable risk of fetal compromise, perinatal mortality, neonatal neurological disturbances, and subsequent neurodevelopmental disability, with the risk magnitude varying considerably with the selection of the population studied.

The use of Doppler assessment of the umbilical artery flow in fetuses with growth restriction or those at risk (e.g., hypertensive pregnancies) has been shown to lead to a reduction in perinatal mortality and reduced unnecessary obstetrical intervention.[120] Further meta-analyses, comparing the use of umbilical Doppler in high-risk groups, have confirmed this conclusion. A recent Cochrane review with 18 studies and >10,000 pregnancies demonstrated that women with Doppler assessment had a significantly lower perinatal mortality (1.2%) compared with those without Doppler studies (1.7%) (RR: 0.67; 95% CI: 0.46, 0.96). Although the data for secondary outcomes showed that there were fewer adverse outcomes in the Doppler group, this finding did not reach statistical significance.[121] Interestingly, there was a reduction in interventions such as induction of labor and cesarean delivery in the Doppler group. Importantly, though, there is a lack of data on long-term neurological development on the infants in either group, and whereas the quality of data is described as low, the most recent study suitable for inclusion is more than a decade old.

The central abnormality in the growth-retarded fetus leading to the increase in placental vascular resistance is a disturbance in placental vessels.[122] The major features include loss of small blood vessels, decreased vascular diameter because of media and intima thickening, and thrombosis. Placental vascular obstruction produced by a variety of experimental techniques in pregnant sheep reproduced the changes in the resistance measures observed in the human fetus.[123] Indeed, elevated umbilical artery resistance measures have been observed in a variety of pathological conditions of the placenta, including partial abruption, placental scarring from intervillous thrombosis, and inflammatory villitis secondary to bacterial or viral infection.[58] Accordingly, the value of this technique in the evaluation of a wide variety of high-risk pregnancies is very high.

The utility of Doppler umbilical arterial evaluation was recently recognized by the Society for Maternal-Fetal Medicine, which published a clinical guideline concerning Doppler assessment in intrauterine growth restriction (IUGR).[124] The recommendations included: (1) Doppler examination of any vessel is not recommended as a screening tool for identifying pregnancies that will subsequently be complicated by IUGR; (2) antepartum surveillance of a viable fetus with suspected IUGR should include Doppler examination of the umbilical artery, as its use is associated with a significant decrease in perinatal mortality; (3) once IUGR is suspected, umbilical artery Doppler studies should be performed usually every 1 to 2 weeks to assess for deterioriation, and, if normal, they can be extended to less frequent intervals; (4) Doppler assessment of additional fetal vessels has not been sufficiently evaluated in randomized trials to recommend its routine use in clinical practice in fetuses with suspected IUGR; (5) antenatal corticosteroids should be administered if absent or reversed end-diastolic flow is noted before 34 weeks in a pregnancy with suspected IUGR; (6) as long as fetal surveillance remains reassuring, women with suspected IUGR and absent umbilical artery end-diastolic flow may be managed expectantly until delivery at 34 weeks; and (7) as long as fetal surveillance remains reassuring, women with suspected IUGR and reversed umbilical artery end-diastolic flow may be managed expectantly until delivery at 32 weeks.

In contrast, Doppler measurement of umbilical artery flow has been shown repeatedly not to be useful in a low-risk or unselected population.[125,126] A recent Cochrane review, including >14,000 women from 20 studies, compared the outcomes of low-risk pregnancies with either routine ultrasound or no Doppler ultrasound. This comparison failed to demonstrate a reduction in perinatal death or serious neonatal morbidity in the Doppler group, nor were there differences in the secondary outcomes, including prematurity, mode of delivery, neonatal resuscitation, or a 5-minute Apgar score <7.[121]

Fetal Cerebral Vessels

Soon after the initial applications of Doppler for study of umbilical blood flow velocity followed the successful study of blood flow velocity in fetal cerebral vessels, particularly the MCA. This now widely used methodology allows monitoring during pregnancy of cerebral hemodynamics, perhaps the most crucial physiological process with regard to fetal brain injury.

During normal pregnancy, in contrast to the decreasing values for resistance measures defined in the umbilical circulation, values in the cerebral circulation change little until approximately the last 5 weeks, when a distinct decline is apparent (Fig. 17.8).[58,99,106,127-132] In addition, mean cerebral

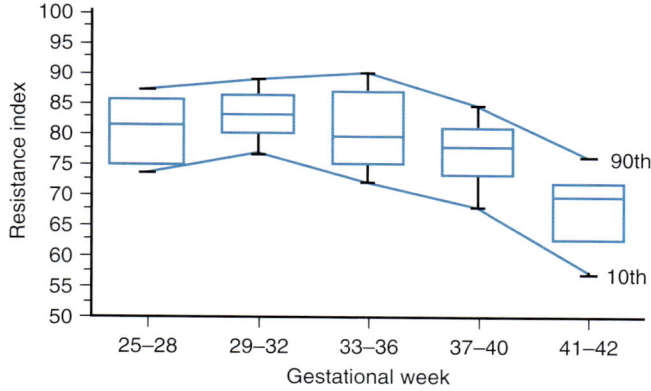

Figure 17.8 Resistance index values of fetal intracranial arterial velocity waveforms in normal pregnancies. The framed areas represent the values between the 25th and 75th percentiles for each gestational age period. The medians (*horizontal lines within the framed areas*) and the 10th and 90th percentiles are indicated. Note the sharp decline in the last month of pregnancy. (From Kirkinen P, Müller R, Huch R, Huch A. Blood flow velocity waveforms in human fetal intracranial arteries. *Obstet Gynecol.* 1987;70:617–621.)

blood flow velocity has been shown to increase during the same period that resistance appears to decrease.[128] This combination of findings suggests an increase in cerebral blood flow during the last trimester of pregnancy, perhaps related to cerebral vasodilation, or development of vascular beds, or both. A particular role for development of cerebrovascular reactivity to relatively low oxygen tension in the fetus is suggested by the findings that cerebral resistance indices in the fetus have been shown to be more responsive to blood oxygen tension than to carbon dioxide tension, and that in the immediate postnatal period, when blood oxygen tensions rise dramatically, cerebral mean flow velocity transiently declines markedly (consistent with an increase in cerebrovascular resistance).[128,133]

As with Doppler studies of the umbilical vessels, study of cerebral blood flow velocity has been routinely directed at the growth-retarded fetus. The dominant abnormality has been a diminished value of cerebral resistance indices, in contrast to the elevated value in the umbilical artery (Fig. 17.9).[a] This apparent vasodilation in the cerebrum at a time of decreasing umbilical flow has been interpreted as an adaptive response, perhaps mediated by hypoxia, and has been termed *fetal brain sparing*. It seems reasonable to suggest that, with severe impairment of umbilical flow and hypoxia, such an adaptive response could become insufficient. Indeed, the decline in cerebral resistance indices and the increase in umbilical resistance indices have been quantitatively combined as a cerebral-to-umbilical ratio. This ratio has been predictive of such subsequent disturbances as fetal distress requiring cesarean section, fetal acidosis, and early neonatal complications (Table 17.6).[141]

The value of MCA Doppler in the prediction of adverse fetal outcome and fetal assessment has been inconsistent. Some studies have suggested that the MCA Doppler measures are useful, whereas others have found poor predictive value.[142-145]

Recently, a meta-analysis of 35 eligible studies including 4025 fetuses was performed.[146] It is worth noting that within the included studies the definition of IUGR varied, the timing

---

[a]References 58, 81, 102, 104-106, 127, 131, 134-140.

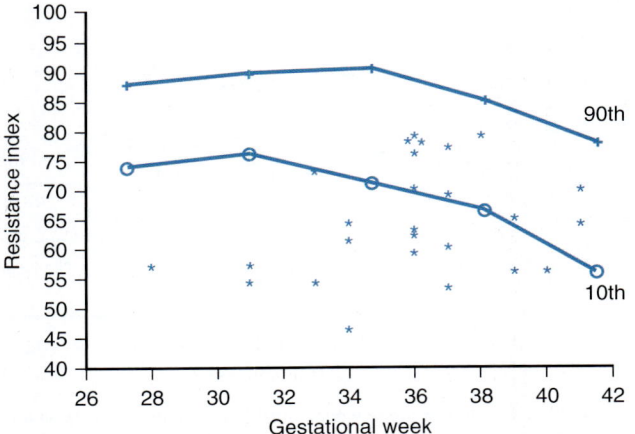

Figure 17.9 Resistance index values in fetal intracranial arteries of small-for-dates newborns (*asterisks*). The 10th and 90th percentiles for normal pregnancy are indicated by the lines. Note the lower resistance values in the small-for-dates newborns. (From Kirkinen P, Müller R, Huch R, Huch A. Blood flow velocity waveforms in human fetal intracranial arteries. *Obstet Gynecol.* 1987;70: 617–621.)

TABLE 17.6   Neonatal Outcome as a Function of Ratio of Cerebral-Umbilical Pulsatility Index

	RATIO <1.08 (n = 18)[a]	RATIO >1.08 (n = 72)[a]
Small for gestational age	100%	38%
Cesarean section (for fetal distress)	89%	12%
Umbilical vein pH (mean)	7.25	7.33
Five-minute Apgar score <7	17%	3%
Neonatal complications[b]	33%	1%

[a]Ratio of pulsatility index from cerebral circulation to index from umbilical artery; normal mean value is approximately 2.0.
[b]Intracerebral hemorrhage, seizures, respiratory distress syndrome.
Data from Gramellini D, Folli MC, Raboni S, et al. Cerebral-umbilical Doppler ratio as a predictor of adverse perinatal outcome. *Obstet Gynecol.* 1992;79:416–420, with permission.

of MCA recordings in relation to outcomes differed, and the definition of abnormal MCA also varied, though most used PI < 2 SD or PI < fifth centile. This meta-analysis found that low MCA PI appears to be predictive of impaired fetal well-being assessed either by acidosis (pH < 7.20) at birth or by higher likelihood of 5-minute Apgar score <7 (positive LR: 1.65 [1.07, 2.52]), and increased admission to a NICU (positive LR: 4.00 [2.16, 7.50], negative LR: 0.62 [0.47, 0.82]). Abnormal MCA recording was also predictive of an overall composite measure of adverse perinatal outcome (positive LR: 2.77 [1.93, 3.96], negative LR 0.58 [0.44, 0.69]) and perinatal mortality (positive LR: 1.36 [1.10, 1.67], negative LR: 0.51 [0.29, 0.89]). Although these findings suggest that there is an association between abnormal MCA recordings and adverse outcomes, the association is weak.

Finally, the potential value of Doppler study of the cerebral circulation in other fetal states is suggested by the demonstration of increased values for pulsatility index in the presence of hydrocephalus.[127,147] This observation is identical to that made postnatally with posthemorrhagic hydrocephalus (see Chapters 10 and 24), and it raises the possibility of the use of Doppler in determination of the need for intervention in fetal hydrocephalus. Changes in cerebral blood flow velocity also have been documented with changes in fetal behavioral states and after administration of indomethacin to the mother.[136,148]

Ductus Venosus

The DV is a fetal vessel connecting the abdominal umbilical vein to the left portion of the inferior vena cava just below the diaphragm. The function of the DV is to shunt the substrate-rich blood coming from the placenta via the umbilical vein to the heart. The DV diverts 25% of the blood, with the remainder being distributed to the liver and joining the circulation via the hepatic portal system.

The DV waveform can be detected by Doppler and is sensitive to cardiac function, which in turn is adversely affected by chronic severe decrease in substrate/oxygen availability. In response to hypoxia, the DV becomes more dilated and there is reduced flow during ventricular diastole, resulting in increased DV pulsatility index for veins (PIV), followed by increasingly retrograde flow during atrial systole, seen as absent or reversed a-wave (Fig. 17.10).

The utility of the DV waveform is primarily in the very premature fetus with IUGR, or in the preterm fetus with abnormal UA waveforms. Reversal or absence of the DV a-wave (see Fig. 17.10), particularly in combination with umbilical vein pulsations, has been shown to be closely associated with an umbilical cord pH < 7.20 at delivery (65% sensitivity and 95% specificity).[149] Similarly, these DV Doppler changes are associated with an 11-fold increase in major adverse neonatal outcomes and a doubling in neonatal mortality.[150]

A recent study (TRUFFLE) used DV Doppler measures to assist in determining timing of delivery in preterm infants with IUGR. In cases where delivery was determined by increased DV pulsatility index or absent DV a-wave, perinatal mortality was 6% in control and 10% in the DV Doppler measures group. However, neurological impairment at 2 years of age was reduced in the measures group from 9% to 5%, respectively. In those for whom delivery timing was based on reduced and more complex measures of heart rate variability from the Doppler, perinatal mortality and abnormal 2-year outcomes were reduced at 7% compared to 15%, respectively. Although the outcomes were not significantly different between groups, the study suggests that delivery based on Doppler changes may provide better long-term outcomes, possibly at the expense of a small increase in perinatal mortality.[151]

Sequence of Changes in Doppler Parameters in the Fetus With Intrauterine Growth Restriction

The traditional view of the changes in Doppler parameters was that as placental function deteriorated, there would be a clearly defined sequence of changes in Doppler findings with an initial increase in umbilical artery impedance (followed by changes in the waveform: absent end-diastolic flow [EDF] and then reversed EDF). As placental function deteriorated further, the reduction in oxygen and substrate to the fetus would result in a brain-sparing effect with a measurable reduction in the MCA impedance. Changes in the DV, initially with increased

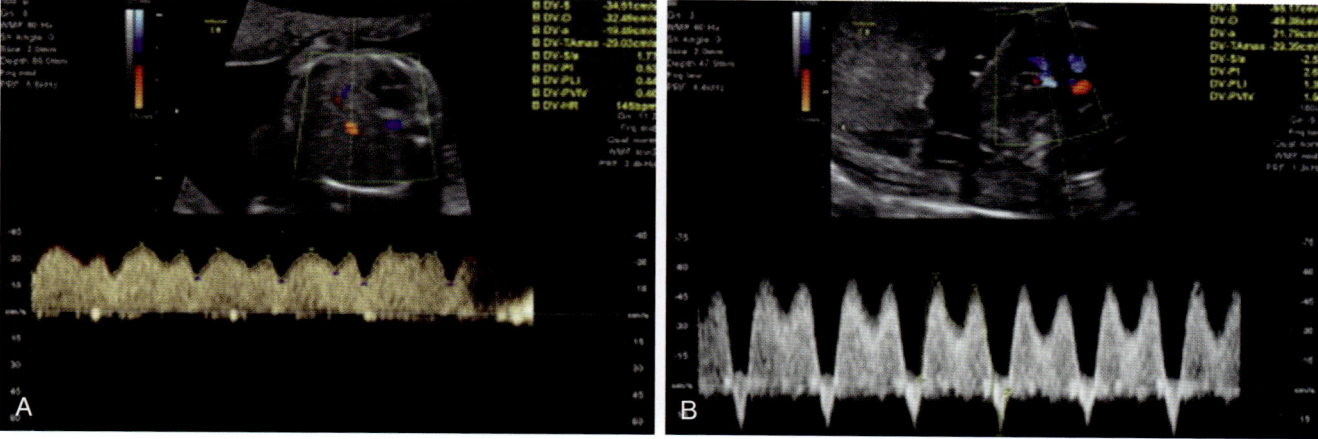

Figure 17.10 Ductus venosus Doppler. Changes in ductus venosus waveforms. (A) Normal with positive a-wave. (B) Abnormal with a-wave reversal. (Reprinted with permission from Everett TR, Peebles DM. Antenatal tests of fetal wellbeing. *Sem Fetal Neonatal Med.* 2015;20(3):138–143.)

pulsatility index and then reversal of the a-wave, would be later signs, as the fetal myocardium became increasingly hypoxic and functioned suboptimally.[152]

The recent PORTO study[153] has challenged this viewpoint. This prospective study of 1116 fetuses with estimated fetal weight <10th centile demonstrated there is no single predominant pattern of Doppler changes. Nearly half (46%) of fetuses showed changes initially in the umbilical artery with pulsatility index >95th centile or absent or reversed EDF, 27% had MCA pulsatility index <5th centile, and 11% had abnormal DV measures (either pulsatility index >95th centile, or absent, or reversed a-wave.)

The pattern of adverse outcomes, such as intraventricular hemorrhage, periventricular leukomalacia, hypoxic ischemic encephalopathy, necrotizing enterocolitis, bronchopulmonary dysplasia, sepsis, and death, is also of interest. Eighty-six percent of fetuses with abnormal umbilical artery Doppler measures had adverse outcomes, compared to 51% with abnormal MCA and only 25% with abnormal DV Doppler measures. In contrast to the TRUFFLE study, this study included late preterm gestations, up to 36⁶ weeks' gestation. These findings demonstrate that the pattern of Doppler changes in a fetus with IUGR may vary significantly and that a combined set of measures from the umbilical cord, MCA, and the DV may provide complementary information from each of the measures that may assist the clinician in evaluating fetal risk.

INTRAPARTUM ASSESSMENT

The occurrence of injury to brain during the birth process has been the focus of clinical research for more than a century. Considerable work has shown that brain injury in the intrapartum period does occur and affects a large absolute number of infants worldwide. It is obscure in most cases in terms of exact timing and precise mechanisms, awaits more sophisticated means of detection in utero, and represents potentially preventable neurological morbidity.[154] Among the many adverse consequences of the increase in obstetrical litigation has been a tendency in some quarters of the medical profession to deny the importance, or even the existence, of intrapartum brain injury. This tendency is

TABLE 17.7	Major Means of Intrapartum Assessment of the Fetus

Meconium passage
Fetal heart rate
Fetal acid-base status
Other techniques
  Transcutaneous monitoring of blood gases and pH
  Near-infrared spectroscopy
  Doppler measurements of fetal blood flow velocity
  Fetal electroencephalogram

particularly unfortunate in that it is clear that true obstetrical malpractice is a rare occurrence and that the obstetrician is called on to deal with perhaps the most dangerous period in an individual's life with inadequate methods. Recognition from experimental studies shows that a considerable proportion of hypoxic-ischemic brain injury evolves *after* cessation of the insult and can be interrupted to a considerable extent by several approaches (see Chapters 13 and 18 to 20). Therefore the ultimate possibility of intervention both in utero and in the early postnatal period is strongly suggested. Denial that intrapartum injury occurs may impair development and application of such brain-saving intervention.

Determination of the nature and timing of cerebral injury is challenging to determine. The most commonly cited marker of hypoxic-ischemic cerebral injury is the pattern of fetal heart rate. The alterations in fetal heart rate that occur with disturbances to fetal well-being have been defined in great detail in the past several decades with the widespread use of electronic fetal monitoring, usually supplemented with fetal blood sampling to assess acid-base status. The passage of meconium in utero is an often-cited but far less useful indicator of serious fetal distress (see later). In the following sections, we will review the basic elements of intrapartum assessment of the human fetus (Table 17.7), namely, the implications of meconium passage in utero, the important fetal heart rate patterns, and the relation of fetal heart rate alterations to fetal acidosis and to neurological morbidity in the newborn period. Finally, we will briefly discuss

TABLE 17.8	Relationship Between Intrapartum Asphyxia and Cerebral Palsy: Term Infants	
COUNTRY	**YEARS OF INFANTS' BIRTHS**	**PERCENTAGE RELATED TO ASPHYXIA**
United States	1959–1966	12%
Australia	1975–1980	17%
Finland	1978–1982	24%
Ireland	1981–1983	23%
England	1984–1987	17%
Sweden	1987–1990	17%
Sweden	1991–1994	24%

See text for references.

certain other measures of fetal surveillance. In the first section that follows, the relationship between intrapartum asphyxia and cerebral palsy is reviewed.

Relationship Between Intrapartum Asphyxia and Cerebral Palsy

Numerous epidemiological studies have shown that most cases of cerebral palsy observed in children are *not* related to intrapartum asphyxia.[155-164] Related clinical epidemiological data also support this conclusion.[77,164-176]

The epidemiological data have been derived from studies of many thousands of infants born over the past 3 to 4 decades, including the era of modern perinatology and neonatology (Table 17.8). Thus, if one excludes premature infants in whom the overwhelming balance of data shows that timing of injury is primarily postnatal (see Chapters 14 to 16), approximately 12% to 24% of cases of cerebral palsy can be related to intrapartum asphyxia. Indeed, if one considers the six large-scale studies of term infants born in the last 3 decades, the data are remarkably consistent in showing that 17% to 24% of cases of cerebral palsy are related to intrapartum asphyxia. A careful MRI study of 40 individuals with cerebral palsy also led to the conclusion that 17% to 24% of term infants sustained their injury from *perinatal* events.[177,178]

Although the data just described indicate that the majority of children examined later with the diagnosis of cerebral palsy did not sustain intrapartum asphyxia, the findings have been interpreted by some clinicians to mean that intrapartum brain injury is rare or nonexistent and therefore unimportant. As noted in the introduction to this section, such a conclusion is incorrect. A sizable body of clinical and brain imaging data shows that brain injury occurs intrapartum in a large absolute number of infants (see Chapter 20). In view of the relatively high prevalence of cerebral palsy, in most countries, generally 2 to 3 cases per 1000 children born, even a relatively small percentage of cases caused by intrapartum events translates into a very large absolute number. (Consider the approximately 4 million live births and the 8000 to 9000 new cases of cerebral palsy in the United States yearly.) These points were stated eloquently in an exchange of communications in *The Lancet* (Table 17.9).[177,178]

The tasks for the future are to devise technologies that can aid in definition of the exact timing and mechanisms of this intrapartum

TABLE 17.9	Interesting Exchanges Published in *The Lancet* Concerning Intrapartum Events and Cerebral Palsy

Editorial (Anonymous), November 25, 1989
"In light of the evidence reviewed above, the continued willingness of doctors to reinforce the fable that intrapartum care is an important determinant of cerebral palsy can only be regarded as shooting the specialty of obstetrics in the foot."

Letter to *The Lancet*[a]
"However medicolegally comforting the new epidemiological orthodoxy you espouse may be, most of us will continue to believe that severe hypoxia/ischemia is deleterious to the brain, that the longer it goes on the worse the effect, and that delayed, inefficient, or inappropriate treatment can be disastrous. It is no longer a matter for conjecture whether asphyxia and cerebral damage are causally related, or merely occur in the same antenatally imperfect individual. Ultrasonography, and many other objective tests of cerebral structure and function allow us to follow the time course of evolving neuronal damage in the postnatal period following severe asphyxia."

"You suggest that by accepting '...the fable that intrapartum care is an important determinant of cerebral palsy,' the specialty of obstetrics is shooting itself in the foot, and that it is time to look elsewhere. We are concerned that by ignoring the 23% of cerebral palsy that *is* related to intrapartum asphyxia, obstetricians and their colleagues will take the advice too literally and shoot themselves somewhere else."

[a]From Hope PL, Moorcraft J. Cerebral palsy in infants born during trial of intrapartum monitoring. *Lancet*. 1990;335:238, with permission.

brain injury and to develop interventions both during and after the insult that will prevent brain injury in the affected infants.

Meconium Passage in Utero

Fetal hypoxia may lead to meconium passage in utero secondary to increased intestinal peristalsis and, perhaps, also to relaxation of the anal sphincter. However, the increased vagal tone associated with fetal maturation may lead to meconium passage; approximately 10% to 20% of apparently normal pregnancies at term and 25% to 50% of postdate pregnancies are accompanied by meconium-stained amniotic fluid. Thus, although the presence of meconium-stained amniotic fluid during labor is a potentially ominous sign concerning fetal well-being, controversy exists over the relative importance of this sign.[179-196] The discrepancy in conclusions may relate in part to the failure to assess *the timing and quantity of meconium passed*. In a prospective study of 2923 pregnancies, Meis and co-workers[188] observed the presence of meconium-stained amniotic fluid in 646 (22%) of cases. Meconium passage was classified as either early (light or heavy) or late. *Early* passage referred to meconium noted on rupture of the fetal membranes before or during the active phase of labor; *light* or *heavy* designations were made on the basis of quantity (and color). *Late* passage referred to meconium-stained amniotic fluid passed in the second stage of labor, after clear fluid had been noted previously. Patients with *early-light* meconium-stained amniotic fluid constituted approximately 54% of the total group with stained fluid and were no more likely to be depressed at birth than were control patients. Patients with *late* passage of

TABLE 17.10	Timing of Meconium Passage Before Birth

CLINICOPATHOLOGICAL FEATURE	PROBABLE DURATION BEFORE BIRTH
Pigment-laden macrophages in amnion	>1 hour
Pigment-laden macrophages in chorion	>3 hour
Meconium-stained fetal nails	>4–6 hour

Data from Miller PW, Coen RW, Benirschke K. Dating the time interval from meconium passage to birth. *Obstet Gynecol.* 1985;66:459–462, with permission.

TABLE 17.11	Fetal Heart Rate Patterns: Major Causes and Usual Significance	

FETAL HEART RATE PATTERN	MAJOR CAUSE	USUAL SIGNIFICANCE
Loss of beat-to-beat variability	Multiple	Variable
Early decelerations	Head compression	Benign
Late decelerations	Uteroplacental insufficiency	Ominous
Variable decelerations	Umbilical cord compression	Variable

meconium constituted approximately 21% of the total group with stained fluid and exhibited 1- and 5-minute Apgar scores lower than 7 two to three times more often than did control patients, but this difference was not statistically significant. (In a subsequent study, the same investigators demonstrated that the presence of *both late* passage of meconium *and* certain intrapartum fetal heart rate abnormalities, i.e., loss of beat-to-beat variability and variable decelerations [see next section], sharply increased the likelihood of depressed Apgar scores.[190]) Finally, however, patients with *early-heavy* meconium-stained amniotic fluid, which constituted 25% of the total group, had a sharply increased likelihood of neonatal depression as well as intrapartum and neonatal death. Significantly, of this group 33% exhibited Apgar scores lower than 7 at 1 minute, and 6.3% had scores lower than 7 at 5 minutes. Early-heavy meconium-stained amniotic fluid was also associated with other signs of fetal distress (e.g., *fetal heart rate abnormalities*) and with antecedent obstetrical conditions that lead to neonatal morbidity. Thus, the data suggest that the timing and quantity of meconium passage are critical variables in attempting to assess the significance of this occurrence for fetal well-being. Presumably, these two aspects of meconium passage correlate with the duration and severity of the intrauterine insult. Clinical estimation of the timing of meconium passage in utero is aided by examination of placental membranes or of the newborn (Table 17.10).[197] In general, *in most cases*, the finding of meconium-stained amniotic fluid is not of serious import concerning intrauterine asphyxia. Moreover, in view of the high rate of meconium passage without serious perinatal complications, the most prevalent current view is that "the presence of meconium per se does not imply fetal distress during labor until other parameters, e.g., fetal heart rate abnormalities, support such a contention."[196] However, a recent study continues to confirm the association of thick meconium with acute hypoxic-ischemic cerebral injury. In this study of 405 infants >35 weeks gestation with early encephalopathy, clinical markers, and neuroimaging consistent with hypoxic-ischemic injury, 29% had thick meconium at delivery versus 7% of controls. On multivariable analysis, thick meconium was one of seven intrapartum factors that was independently associated with hypoxic-ischemic injury.[198]

Fetal Heart Rate Alterations

In most medical centers, the central means of the intrapartum assessment of fetal well-being is electronic fetal monitoring.[191,195,199-216] Evaluation of fetal heart rate, particularly in relation to uterine contractions, is the most widely used form of electronic fetal monitoring. Although the necessity and relative merits of electronic fetal heart rate monitoring have been the subjects of disagreement,[a] utilization of such monitoring during labor has been standard obstetrical practice in the United States. The bases for the major controversy concerning the value of electronic monitoring of the fetal heart rate are that (1) the abnormalities are detected in labor in a large number of infants who are normal at birth and on follow-up, and (2) the increase in operative deliveries provoked by the finding of such abnormalities has had little or no impact on adverse neurological outcome, particularly cerebral palsy. It is beyond the scope of this book to discuss in detail the relative merits of the use of electronic fetal monitoring in all pregnancies versus use in high-risk pregnancies only. It is perhaps worthy of emphasis only that in the so-called Dublin trial of nearly 13,000 women, a study generally acknowledged to be among the best designed of all trials, the use of electronic fetal monitoring was followed by a decrease in the incidence of neonatal seizures, and the presence of certain heart rate patterns (see subsequent discussion) was an important predictor of abnormal neonatal neurological examinations.[163,224] A decrease in neonatal seizures was documented in a meta-analysis of 12 studies involving 59,324 infants.[213] In another well-designed study, 27% of the 78 patients with cerebral palsy who had intrapartum fetal monitoring exhibited multiple late decelerations or decreased beat-to-beat variability of the heart rate.[214] In a further study of 405 infants with proven neonatal hypoxic-ischemic injury, abnormal fetal heart rate tracing was observed in 77% and was independently associated with disease with an odds ratio of 12.75.[198]

The major aspects of the fetal heart rate pattern evaluated are divided into *baseline features* (i.e., rate and beat-to-beat variability) and *periodic features* (i.e., accelerations or decelerations), usually in relation to uterine contractions (Fig. 17.11 and Table 17.11). The significance of these aspects of the fetal heart rate is discussed in detail in standard writings on maternal-fetal medicine. A brief overview is provided next.

Rate

Assessment of the fetal heart rate begins with the finding that the normal heart rate (± 2 standard deviations) is 120 to 160 beats/minute (see Fig. 17.11).[191,231] Abnormalities of baseline fetal heart rate are suspicious, but in the absence of disturbances of beat-to-beat variability or decelerations (see later discussions), these abnormalities usually do not reflect an ominous event,

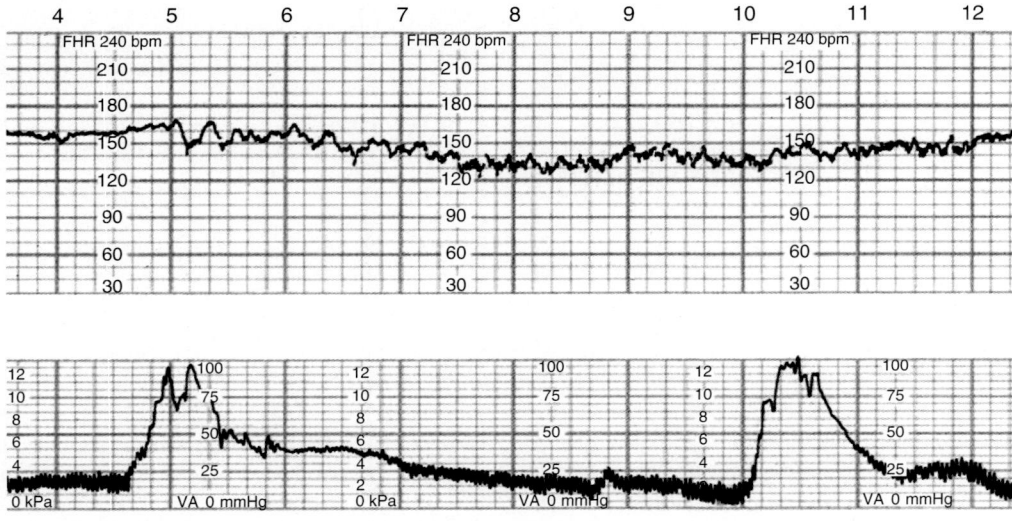

Figure 17.11 Fetal heart rate tracing, normal pattern. The *upper trace* represents the fetal heart rate, and the *lower trace* represents uterine activity. The fetal heart rate ranges generally between 130 and 150 beats/minute, with normal beat-to-beat variability of approximately 10 to 15 beats/minute. The uterine contractions shown are approximately 5 minutes apart. *bpm,* Beats per minute; *FHR,* fetal heart rate. (Courtesy Dr. Barry Schifrin.)

such as severe fetal hypoxia.[191,216] The most common cause of baseline tachycardia in the fetus is maternal fever secondary to amnionitis. Maternal fever can also occur following maternal epidural administration,[232] particularly as many as >75% of women in labor in developed countries will receive epidural for pain relief. Other causes include fetal infection, certain drugs (e.g., atropine and beta-sympathomimetics), arrhythmia, and maternal anxiety. Fixed tachycardia with loss of beat-to-beat variability, especially in relation to patterns of deceleration, may be observed with fetal hypoxia and has been observed in infants before intrapartum or early neonatal death.[233] In these instances, the tachycardia may reflect a fetal response to massive blood loss, since this is the best compensatory mechanism to maintain cardiac output given the limitations on stroke volume (Fig. 17.12).[234]

Baseline bradycardia with average beat-to-beat variability and no sign of fetal compromise is observed most commonly in the postmature fetus.[191] Bradycardia may be observed with fetal heart block, as a drug effect and with hypothermia. Baseline bradycardia as a feature of fetal hypoxia is accompanied by loss of beat-to-beat variability and decelerations.

Beat-to-Beat Variability

Normal fetal heart rate exhibits fluctuations of approximately 6 to 25 beats/minute (see Fig. 17.11).[216,235,236] This beat-to-beat variability reflects the modulation of heart rate by autonomic, particularly parasympathetic, input and especially depends on inputs from cerebral cortex, diencephalon, and upper brain stem to the cardiac centers in the medulla and then to the vagus nerve.[191,200,216,237-239] Of the autonomic input, parasympathetic influences are more important than sympathetic influences.[216,240-242] *The presence of normal beat-to-beat variability is considered the best single assessment of fetal well-being.*[191,216,231,239] Indeed, the presence of normal variability is a reassuring finding in the presence of the mild variable decelerations common in the second stage of labor.[191] Loss of or diminished beat-to-beat variability may be observed not only with significant

fetal hypoxia but also with prematurity, fetal sleep, drugs (e.g., sedative-hypnotics, narcotic-analgesics, benzodiazepines, atropine, and local anesthetics), congenital malformations (e.g., anencephaly), and intrauterine, antepartum cerebral destruction.[a] *The loss of beat-to-beat variability coupled with variable or late decelerations (see subsequent sections) significantly enhances the likelihood that the fetus is undergoing significant hypoxia.*[191,200,216,231,239] The importance of careful longitudinal assessment of heart rate variability has been suggested.[234] Ample documentation has shown the association between decreased fetal heart rate variability and decelerations, fetal acidosis, intrauterine fetal death, and low Apgar scores.[191,216,239,240]

Accelerations

Increases or decreases in fetal heart rate associated particularly with contractions are designated *accelerations* or *decelerations* and constitute the periodic features of the fetal heart rate. Accelerations during the uterine contractions of labor, as in the case of antepartum contractions (see previous discussion) or with fetal movement, are not of concern and in fact are generally considered a sign of fetal well-being.[191,246,247] Uncommonly, heart rate accelerations may be an early sign of compression of the umbilical vein.[191,248] Maintenance of fetal heart rate variability is a reassuring sign of fetal well-being in the presence of such accelerations.

Decelerations

Decelerations are of three major types: early, late, and variable (Figs. 17.13–17.15; see Table 17.11). These decreases in heart rate associated with uterine contraction have significantly different mechanisms and implications for outcome.

Early Type. An *early deceleration* is one that begins with the onset of a contraction, reaches its peak with the peak of the contraction, and then returns to normal baseline levels as

---

[a]References 191, 200, 216, 231, 239, 243-245.

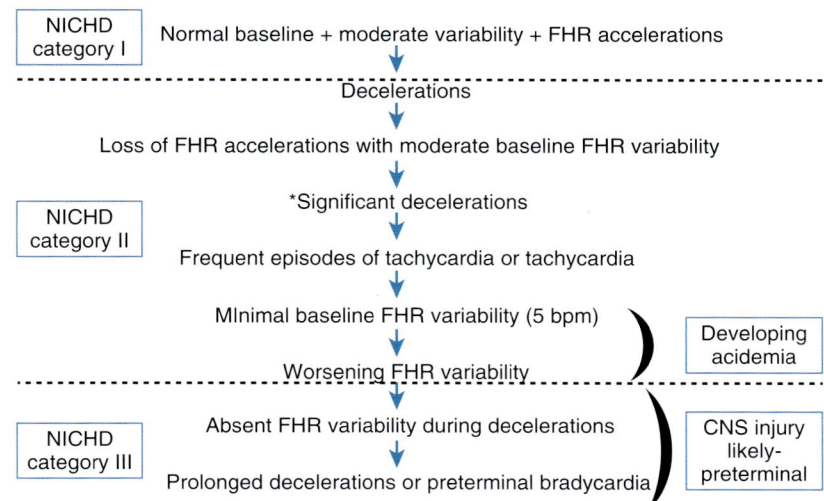

Figure 17.12 Progression of fetal heart rate pattern of deteriorating fetus. Progressive fetal heart rate (FHR) changes. *Significant decelerations include: (A) variables lasting >60 seconds and reaching nadir <60 beats per minute (bpm) below baseline; (B) variables lasting >60 seconds and reaching nadir <60 bpm regardless of baseline; (C) lates of any depth; (D) prolonged deceleration (>2 to <10 min); and (E) decelerations accompanied by compensatory tachycardia. *CNS,* Central nervous system; *NICHD,* Eunice Kennedy Shriver National Institute of Child Health and Human Development. (Reprinted with permission from Vintzileos AM, Smulian JC. Decelerations, tachycardia, and decreased variability: have we overlooked significance of longitudinal fetal heart rate changes for detecting intrapartum fetal hypoxia? *Am J Obstet Gynecol.* 2016;215(3):261–264).

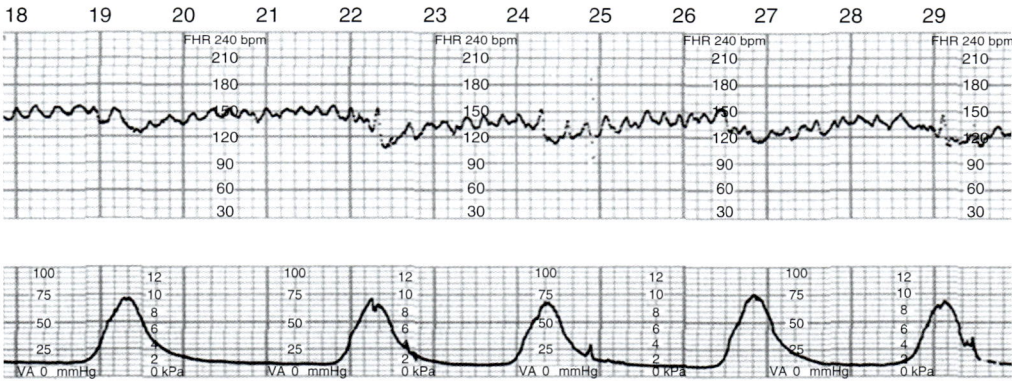

Figure 17.13 Fetal heart rate tracing, early deceleration. Note the typical early deceleration (i.e., the deceleration begins with the onset of the contraction, reaches its peak with the peak of the contraction, and returns to a normal baseline as the contraction ends). Variability is preserved. *bpm,* Beats per minute; *FHR,* fetal heart rate. (Courtesy Dr. Barry Schifrin.)

the contraction ends (see Fig. 17.13).[191,216,249,250] These decelerations appear to be related to compression of the fetal head and are mediated by vagal input to the heart.[251-253] The mechanism of this effect of head compression may relate to a transient increase in intracranial pressure with secondary hypertension and bradycardia through the Cushing reflex. Early decelerations are not associated with fetal hypoxia, as reflected in fetal acid-base measurements or in neonatal depression.[191,224,254]

Late Type. A *late deceleration* is one that begins after a contraction starts, but reaches a peak well after the peak of contraction is reached and does not return to baseline until 30 to 60 seconds after the contraction is completed (see Fig. 17.14).[191,216,230,255] These decelerations are related primarily

to *uteroplacental insufficiency* (e.g., placental disorder, uterine hyperactivity, and maternal hypotension) and are mediated by fetal hypoxia (see Table 17.11).[a] Such decelerations are unusual with fetal scalp pressure of oxygen (PO$_2$) greater than 20 mm Hg, but appear in more than 50% of infants with fetal scalp PO$_2$ less than 10 mm Hg.[262] It is understandable that fetal hypoxia occurs after the onset of a uterine contraction when uteroplacental insufficiency is present, because uterine contractions normally reduce uterine blood flow and thereby oxygen delivery to the fetus.[208,263] Fetal hypoxia causes bradycardia by a multifactorial mechanism that primarily includes a chemoreceptor-mediated vagal response initially and then a direct effect on myocardial function.[208,260,261,264]

---

[a]References 191, 208, 216, 230, 239, 256-261.

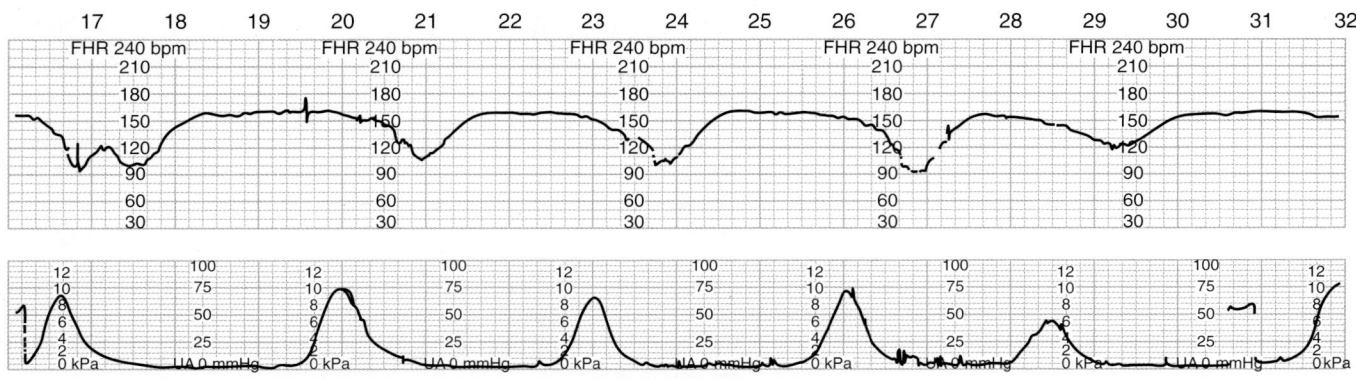

Figure 17.14 Fetal heart rate tracing, late deceleration. Note the late decelerations (i.e., the peak of the deceleration is reached well after the peak of the contraction). The absent variability is consistent with decreased cerebral oxygenation. *bpm*, Beats per minute; *FHR*, fetal heart rate. (Courtesy Dr. Barry Schifrin.)

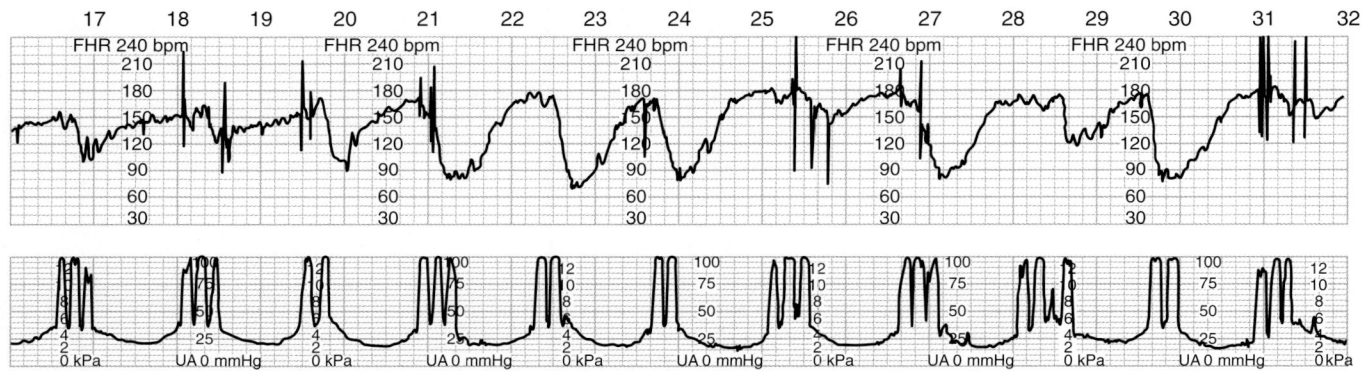

Figure 17.15 Fetal heart rate tracing, variable deceleration. Note the recurrent variable decelerations, as described in the text, associated here with maternal pushing, evidenced by the spikes in uterine activity (*lower trace*). The decreasing variability is concerning for recurrent ischemia and fetal compromise. *bpm*, Beats per minute; *FHR*, fetal heart rate. (Courtesy Dr. Barry Schifrin.)

The initial reflex vagally mediated response is accompanied by normal fetal heart rate variability and thus "normal CNS integrity," whereas the nonreflex myocardial late deceleration is observed without heart rate variability and thus "inadequate fetal cerebral and myocardial oxygenation."[216]

The *causal relationship* between fetal hypoxia and late decelerations has been shown in several ways. First, as just noted, the decelerations have been correlated temporally with fetal hypoxia, identified with fetal capillary blood sampling and tissue oxygen electrodes.[256,262] Second, when fetal oxygenation is improved by the administration of 100% oxygen to the normotensive mother or of intravenous fluids and pressors to the hypotensive mother, the bradycardia may cease. Third, a strong correlation exists between the occurrence of late decelerations and alterations in fetal acid-base status secondary to fetal hypoxia.[258]

The possibility that the *late decelerations* may have *secondary deleterious effects* was suggested by studies in subhuman primates that showed that late decelerations are accompanied not only by fetal hypoxia and acidosis but also by hypotension. The bradycardia per se appeared to cause the hypotension.[257] Moreover, studies with fetal sheep documented decreased cardiac output with bradycardia, particularly at rates lower than 60 beats/min.[51,261,265,266] Data on cerebral blood flow are lacking, however.

The *duration of asphyxia* with late decelerations required to produce brain injury is not entirely clear, although experiments with fetal monkeys suggested that time periods less than 1 hour are not generally sufficient.[267] Studies of human infants also suggested that a time period of less than 1 hour is not likely to be harmful.[268,269] However, *this conclusion must be made very cautiously* because the *severity of the insult* is critical and has not been studied systematically with regard to the timing required to produce fetal brain injury. Indeed, in the case of severe, abrupt, terminal insults (i.e., acute *total* asphyxia just before delivery), brain injury appears to occur after insults of less than 1 hour.[270,271]

Variable Type. The most commonly observed fetal heart rate deceleration is *variable deceleration*,[191,231] which occurs in a substantial minority of all fetuses (see Fig. 17.15).[209,272] This characteristically abrupt slowing of the fetal heart rate may begin before, with, or after the onset of the uterine contraction and is variable in duration. The deceleration pattern is principally the result of varying degrees of umbilical cord compression (see Table 17.11).[51,191,200,250,258] Thus, this periodic pattern is more common with nuchal, short, or prolapsed umbilical cord or decreased amniotic fluid volume (oligohydramnios, ruptured membranes). The *mechanism* of the bradycardia is considered to be an increase in peripheral resistance, which leads to fetal hypertension that, in turn, causes baroreceptor-stimulated, vagally mediated bradycardia.[273] Occasionally, the umbilical cord compression with each contraction can be prevented by alteration of maternal position. Distinction of early from late cord compression can be made on the basis of determinations of fetal carbon dioxide pressure (PCO_2) and base excess; thus, respiratory acidosis reflects early umbilical cord compression with impaired umbilical blood flow, and metabolic acidosis indicates late cord compression with fetal tissue hypoxia.[274] When variable decelerations are accompanied by or evolve into late decelerations, or *when beat-to-beat variability is diminished or lost* (even without late decelerations), the likelihood of significant fetal hypoxia is markedly enhanced.[191,216,228,258,272]

Taxonomy of Fetal Heart Rate Patterns

The currently accepted taxonomy, endorsed by the American College of Obstetricians and Gynecologists (ACOG),[275] divides all patterns of EFM into 3 categories: category I (normal), category II (indeterminate), and category III (abnormal) (see Fig. 17.12, Table 17.12), based on the ability to predict acid-base status at the time. The ACOG recommendations concerning the timing of monitoring do not provide instructions regarding longitudinal fetal heart rate assessments. Some investigators consider careful longitudinal assessment during labor, especially considering the evolution of category II patterns, critical for early detection of the deteriorating fetus.[234]

Relation of Fetal Heart Rate Abnormalities to Neonatal Neurological Course and Subsequent Outcome

A distinct relationship has been demonstrated between intrapartum abnormalities of fetal heart rate, sometimes with documented fetal acidosis, and neurological morbidity in the neonatal period and after 1 year of follow-up.[a] In a prospective study, 50 infants of high-risk mothers who were provided intrauterine fetal heart rate monitoring during labor were examined by a pediatric neurologist in the neonatal period and then were subsequently evaluated periodically (Table 17.13).[216,276,278-280] Thirty-eight of the infants exhibited *clearly abnormal fetal heart rate patterns*. These were categorized as *moderate to severe variable decelerations* (defined as decelerations to 70 to 80 beats/minute for >60 seconds with three contractions or to a rate of <70 beats/minute for 30 to 60 seconds), *severe variable decelerations* (decelerations to a rate of <70 beats/minute for ≥60 seconds), and *late decelerations* (a uniform deceleration of the

[a]References 216, 224, 230, 268, 269, 276-280.

TABLE 17.12 Three-Tier Nomenclature of the Fetal Heart Tracing

Category I
Category I FHR tracings include all of the following
- Baseline rate: 110–160 beats per minute
- Baseline FHR variability: moderate
- Late or variable decelerations: absent
- Early decelerations: present or absent
- Accelerations: present or absent

Category II
Category II FHR tracings include all FHR tracings not categorized as Category I or Category III. Category II tracings may represent an appreciable fraction of those encountered in clinical care. Examples of Category II FHR tracings include any of the following:

Baseline rate
- Bradycardia not accompanied by absent baseline variability
- Tachycardia

Baseline FHR variability
- Minimal baseline variability
- Absent baseline variability with no recurrent decelerations
- Marked baseline variability

Accelerations
- Absence of induced accelerations after fetal stimulation

Periodic or episodic decelerations
- Recurrent variable decelerations accompanied by minimal or moderate baseline variability
- Prolonged deceleration more than 2 minutes but less than 10 minutes
- Recurrent late decelerations with moderate baseline variability
- Variable decelerations with other characteristics such as slow return to baseline, overshoots, or *shoulders*

Category III
Category III FHR tracings include either:
- Absent baseline FHR variability and any of the following
  - Recurrent late decelerations
  - Recurrent variable decelerations
  - Bradycardia
- Sinusoidal pattern

FHR, Fetal heart rate.

Reprinted with permission from Macones GA, Hankins GD, Spong CY, Hauth J, Moore T. The 2008 National Institute of Child Health and Human Development workshop report on electronic fetal monitoring: update on definitions, interpretation, and research guidelines. *Obstet Gynecol.* 2008;112(3):661–666.

TABLE 17.13 Neonatal Neurological Course and Subsequent Development in Electronically Monitored Infants

	FETAL HEART RATE PATTERNS[a]		
TIME OF EVALUATION	**NORMAL**	**MODERATE TO SEVERE VARIABLE DECELERATIONS**	**SEVERE VARIABLE AND/OR LATE DECELERATIONS**
Neonatal (48–72 hour)	16%[a]	63%	73%
1 year	0%	6%	27%
6–9 year	0%	0%	10%

[a]Percentage of patients with fetal heart rate pattern and abnormal neurological evaluation.

fetal heart rate of any magnitude that occurred consistently in the late phase of each contraction). A striking relationship of these patterns with the occurrence of neonatal neurological signs was apparent (see Table 17.13). The most consistent sign was hypotonia. By 1 year of age, many fewer abnormalities were apparent, although approximately 25% of the infants with severe variable decelerations or late decelerations, or both, exhibited neurological disturbances (see Table 17.13). Of the abnormal infants at 1 year of age, approximately 30% exhibited severe deficits. Only 10% of the group with abnormal fetal heart rate patterns had abnormal neurological evaluations at 6 to 9 years of age.[278] These data demonstrate that certain abnormal intrapartum fetal heart rate patterns alone can be valuable indicators of intrauterine insults, presumably hypoxic-ischemic, that result in neurological injury. Further support for this notion is provided by the demonstration of markedly elevated levels of brain-specific creatine phosphokinase in umbilical cord blood of infants with similarly ominous fetal heart rate alterations.[281] In the latter study, approximately 29% of this group exhibited poor neurological outcome. However, the disappearance of a large portion of the neurological disturbance by 6 to 9 years of age, as shown by Painter and co-workers,[278,279] suggests that the plasticity of the developing human brain is capable of overcoming much of the injury apparent earlier in life, if that injury is not severe. Finally, as noted earlier concerning a study of 405 infants with MRI proven acute hypoxic-ischemic injury, abnormal fetal heart rate results were observed in 77% and were independently associated with brain injury with an odds ratio of 12.75.[198]

With regard to the three-tier classifications of the fetal heart rate tracings, category I patterns are considered normal and do not require intervention. However, ongoing assessment is important because patterns can change over time. Moderate variability and presence of accelerations,[282,283] features of category I patterns, have both been associated with normal neonatal umbilical cord blood pH (>7.20).

The majority of intrapartum fetal heart rate tracings are category II.[284,285] There are, however, specific elements of category II patterns, such as tachycardia, bradycardia, absent or minimal variability, absence of accelerations, and late or prolonged decelerations, which have been associated with acidemia, as noted earlier (see Fig. 17.13 and Table 17.12). Despite certain category II features being associated with acidemia, as with category III patterns, these elements of category II tracings have a generally low-positive predictive value for acidemia or adverse outcomes.[285]

Elements of category III patterns,[275] including absent variability with recurrent late or variable fetal heart rate decelerations, or bradycardia, or a sinusoidal pattern, have been associated with abnormal arterial pH, encephalopathy, and cerebral palsy.[284-286] Although category III patterns are not highly predictive of adverse outcomes,[287] their association necessitates intervention.

Fetal Electrocardiogram

The possibility that analysis of the fetal electrocardiogram could add appreciably to the identification of fetal compromise secondary to intrapartum hypoxia was suggested by studies in the United Kingdom and Sweden.[288-292] The parameters of greatest apparent value are elevation of the ST segment and shortening of the QT interval, which become progressively worse with fetal hypoxia.

The mediator of these effects on the myocardium appears to be the surge in catecholamines provoked by hypoxia.[292] Clearly, such information about myocardial insufficiency is relevant to the central nervous system because, ultimately, with asphyxia myocardial insufficiency results in the ischemia that causes brain injury. In a multicenter randomized trial in Sweden involving 4966 women with term fetuses, women were monitored either with fetal heart rate monitoring alone or with fetal heart rate monitoring in addition to evaluation of the electrocardiogram (for elevated ST segment).[290,291] In those women managed according to fetal heart rate monitoring in addition to evaluation of the electrocardiogram, the investigators noted less umbilical cord metabolic acidosis, fewer 1-minute Apgar scores lower than 4, less neonatal encephalopathy, and no neonatal seizures. Subsequent work suggests that in the distressed acidotic fetus, the QT interval is shortened irrespective of changes in heart rate.[292] Thus, this approach appeared initially to add significantly to the information gained from assessment of the fetal heart rate. However, the method requires *placement of a fetal scalp electrode* and thereby is more invasive than fetal heart rate monitoring. Moreover, a recent randomized multicenter trial of 11,108 women attempting vaginal delivery at >36 weeks of gestation showed that fetal ECG ST-segment analysis used as an adjunct to conventional intrapartum electronic fetal heart rate monitoring did not improve perinatal outcomes or decrease operative delivery rates.[293]

Fetal Acid-Base Status

As alluded to in the previous section, certain fetal heart rate patterns are indicative of (or ultimately productive of) fetal hypoxia and the biochemical correlate of tissue oxygen debt, fetal acidosis. Fetal acidemia may occur as a consequence of accumulation of (1) carbon dioxide and thereby carbonic acid; (2) *metabolic* acids, particularly lactate but also ketone bodies; or (3) both the carbonic and noncarbonic acids. Carbon dioxide, which is highly diffusible and thereby subject to rapid changes, can lead to alterations in fetal pH that occur and resolve quickly. By contrast, metabolic acids, which accumulate usually as a consequence of oxygen deprivation and thus anaerobic glycolysis (or incomplete oxidation of fatty acids), increase in tissue and blood more slowly and thus cause slower and more sustained alterations in fetal pH. More detailed consideration of the relevant biochemical aspects is presented in Chapter 13.

Although most studies of *fetal acidosis* are assessed by measurements from the umbilical artery at delivery, the intrapartum use of fetal scalp blood samples provides more nearly real-time information. However, the need for fetal scalp access prevents this approach from being widely used.[294] *Indeed, more commonly used than scalp sampling as an adjunct to fetal heart rate monitoring is assessment of acceleration of fetal heart rate to vibroacoustical (or tactile) stimulation; the presence of acceleration is a reliable indicator of fetal pH higher than 7.2 (normal fetal scalp pH is greater than 7.25; values lower than 7.20 are considered to be of concern).*[294]

Normal values for fetal blood gas and acid-base measures, obtained from umbilical artery at delivery, are shown in Table 17.14.[269,295,296] In one large series, the 2.5th percentile values for umbilical artery pH and base deficit were 7.10 and 11, respectively.[296] The value of fetal acid-base measurements as an *adjunct* to fetal heart rate monitoring in the assessment of fetal well-being is well established, although the extent of that value is not without controversy.[195,223,269,294,297-319] Results of several studies showed a strong correlation between the duration and severity of fetal heart rate deceleration patterns of the variable and late types and the occurrence of fetal acidosis or acidosis at delivery.[a]

Alterations in Fetal Acid-Base Measurements and Neonatal Outcome

Alterations in fetal acid-base measurements, particularly when combined with fetal heart rate assessment, are effective predictors of the *condition of the infant at birth*. An early, careful study of 587 high-risk pregnancies, in which fetal heart rate patterns and fetal acid-base data were combined, showed a strong correlation between biochemically documented fetal asphyxia and subnormal Apgar scores at 1 and 5 minutes and abnormal neurological signs in the first hour.[a] A later study showed the particular predictive value of the measurement of base deficit in umbilical arterial blood (Table 17.15).[311] Thus, *deficits less than 12 mmol/L very rarely resulted in moderate or severe neurological signs.* Fully 41% of infants with umbilical artery base deficits in excess of 16 mmol/L exhibited such signs. The particular importance of the *base deficit* may relate to the measure's reflection of the accumulation of metabolic acids and thereby not only the severity but also the *duration* of the hypoxic-ischemic insult (see earlier). The severity of fetal acidosis at delivery has been studied most commonly in relation to umbilical artery pH, and although valuable data have been obtained, a relatively high incidence of neonatal neurological complications after presumed prolonged partial asphyxia is not observed until markedly low pH values are obtained (see next section). This difficulty may relate in part to the finding that umbilical artery pH may decline rapidly and may recover promptly with transient changes in PCO_2.

As just noted, the relation of neonatal neurological features to the *severity of fetal acidosis*, as manifested by umbilical arterial pH values at delivery, was delineated in several large-scale studies.[b] Thus, in a study of 129 term, singleton infants with umbilical pH less than 7.00,[306] a distinct relationship between severity of the acidosis and neonatal neurological and systemic manifestations of presumed hypoxic-ischemic insult was observed (Table 17.16). As stated earlier, despite the high incidence of neonatal neurological

---

[a]References 181, 208, 209, 269, 294, 300, 311, 314, 320-326.

---

[a]References 181, 208, 209, 269, 294, 300, 311, 314, 320-326.
[b]References 294, 306, 309, 310, 312-317, 319.

TABLE 17.14 Mean Fetal Blood Gas and Acid-Base Data as Measured in Umbilical Artery at Delivery

VARIABLE	MEAN VALUE
pH	7.26
Partial pressure of oxygen	15 mm Hg
Oxygen saturation	25%
Partial pressure of carbon dioxide	48 mm Hg
Base deficit[a]	5 mmol/L

[a]Base deficit is concentration of bicarbonate lower than normal. When the term base excess is used, the concentration value is expressed as a negative number.

Data from Low JA. Fetal acid-base status and outcome. In Hill A, Volpe JJ, eds. *Fetal Neurology.* New York: Raven Press; 1989, with permission.

TABLE 17.15 Relation Between Fetal Acidemia and Neonatal Encephalopathy

NEONATAL ENCEPHALOPATHY[a]	UMBILICAL ARTERY BASE DEFICIT		
	4–12 mmol/L (n = 116)	12–16 mmol/L (n = 58)	>16 mmol/L (n = 59)
None	89%	72%	39%
Minor	10%	19%	20%
Moderate	1%	7%	29%
Severe	0%	2%	12%

[a]Minor encephalopathy, "irritability or jitteriness"; moderate, "profound lethargy or abnormal tone"; severe, "coma or abnormal tone and seizures."

Data from Low JA, Lindsay BG, Derrick EJ. Threshold of metabolic acidosis associated with newborn complications. *Am J Obstet Gynecol.* 1997;177:1391–1394, with permission.

TABLE 17.16 Relation Between Severity of Fetal Acidosis and Neonatal Neurological and Systemic Features

CLINICAL DYSFUNCTION	UMBILICAL ARTERY pH			
	6.61–6.70	6.71–6.79	6.80–6.89	6.90–6.99
Hypoxic-ischemic encephalopathy[a]	80%	60%	33%	12%
Renal dysfunction	60%	53%	26%	16%
Cardiac dysfunction	60%	60%	30%	18%
Pulmonary dysfunction	80%	47%	30%	12%
None	20%	40%	48%	75%

[a]Manifested as seizures and hypotonia in 76%, seizures only in 6%, and hypotonia only in 18%.

Data from Goodwin TM, Belai I, Hernandez P, Durand M, et al. Asphyxial complications in the term newborn with severe umbilical acidemia. *Am J Obstet Gynecol.* 1992;167:1506–1512, with permission, derived from study of 129 term infants with umbilical arterial pH < 7.00.

TABLE 17.17 Relationship Between Fetal Asphyxia (Defined by Fetal Acidemia) in Term Infants and Neurological Outcome at 1 Year of Age

	NEUROLOGICAL OUTCOME		
	NORMAL	MINOR DEFICIT	MAJOR DEFICIT
Control (n = 76)	93%	6%	1%
Fetal asphyxia (n = 37)	61%	25%	14%

Data from Low JA, Galbraith RS, Muir DW, Killen HL, et al. Motor and cognitive deficits after intrapartum asphyxia in the mature fetus. *Am J Obstet Gynecol.* 1988;158:356–361.

TABLE 17.18 Umbilical Artery pH and Neonatal Outcome

	PERINATAL MORTALITY (ODDS RATIO)	PERINATAL MORBIDITY (ODDS RATIO)	CEREBRAL PALSY (ODDS RATIO)
pH < 7.00	6.1 (0.9–41.6)	12.5 (6.1–25.6)	
pH < 7.10	7.1 (3.3–15.3)	2.4 (1.3–4.2)	
pH < 7.20	4.3 (2.2–8.7)	2.2 (1.3–3.7)	2.3 (1.3–4.2)[a]

[a]Seven reports with 1117 cases and controls with pH threshold 7.00–7.20
Data from Malin G, Morris RK, Khan KS. Strength of association between umbilical cord pH and perinatal and long term outcomes: systematic review and meta-analysis. *BMJ.* 2010;340:c1471. doi: 10.1136/bmj.c1471, with permission.

phenomena, overall, 78% of the infants with umbilical pH less than 7.00 were normal on follow-up examinations. In a later report, 62% of term infants with pH of or less than 7.00 had no neonatal clinical abnormalities.[315]

Alterations in Fetal Acid-Base Measurements and Later Neurological Outcome

The relationship between fetal acidemia and later neurological outcome was studied particularly well by Low and co-workers.[301] These investigators defined the *neurological outcome* at 1 year of age of 37 term infants identified prospectively by detection of fetal asphyxia in term infants derived from a high-risk obstetrical population (Table 17.17). Fourteen percent of the infants with fetal asphyxia had major deficits at 1 year, and a relationship between outcome and severity of acidosis in the asphyxiated group was apparent. However, approximately 85% of the asphyxiated infants either were normal or exhibited only minor deficits at 1 year of age (see Table 17.17). In the relatively uncommon circumstance of severe, abrupt, terminal insults (i.e., acute *total* asphyxia), umbilical cord blood pH most often is *not* markedly depressed; in one large series (N = 47), 60% of such infants (who later exhibited major neurological deficits) had umbilical cord pH higher than 7.00, and in this and other series, cord pH in the normal range was documented.[270,271]

A recent systematic review was undertaken of 51 studies of 481,753 term infants correlating neonatal mortality, clinical evidence of hypoxic-ischemic insult, and cerebral palsy with umbilical cord gases with various thresholds (<7.00, <7.10, and <7.20). A graded increase in the risk of perinatal mortality and morbidity with increasing acidemia status at birth was documented (Table 17.18). The correlation with cerebral palsy was much weaker than that of neonatal mortality and morbidity with seven studies showing nonsignificant increase in risk at various degrees of acidosis. However, when subjected to meta-analysis for the 1117 cases and controls, the odds ratio became significant at 2.3 (95% CI 1.3 to 4.2).[327] It is also important to note that additional neurological outcomes are not well documented in these studies, with cerebral palsy being a severe and crude marker for adverse motor outcome. Thus, more detailed neurological outcomes would be necessary to truly define the relationship between acidemia and outcome.

Supporting the value of fetal acid-base assessment *in conjunction with* fetal heart rate monitoring was a study of

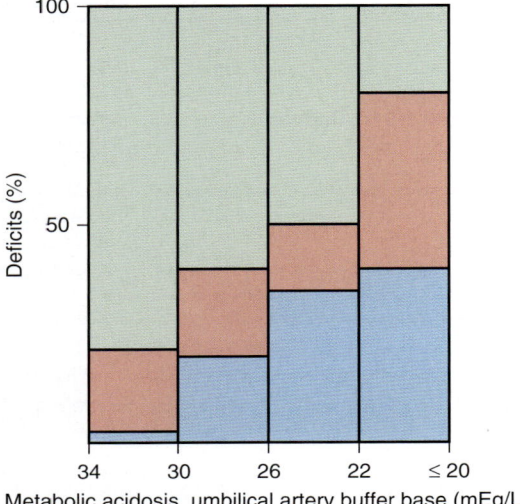

Figure 17.16 Relation of intrapartum fetal hypoxia to neurological outcome, derived from a study of 60 infants, 42 of whom were full term. Intrapartum fetal hypoxia is expressed as the degree of acidosis, assessed by umbilical artery buffer base values. *Significant* metabolic acidosis in this laboratory is considered to be a buffer base level of less than 34 mEq/L (base deficit >12 mmol/L). Major *(blue)* and minor *(red)* deficits are motor or cognitive (or both) in type. See text for details. (From Low JA, Galbraith RS, Muir DW, Killen HL, et al. Factors associated with motor and cognitive deficits in children after intrapartum fetal hypoxia. *Am J Obstet Gynecol.* 1984;148:533–539.)

60 children with intrapartum fetal hypoxia documented by fetal acid-base studies after detection of fetal heart rate abnormalities.[268] Of the 60 infants, 29% exhibited neurological deficits at age 1 year; the deficits included motor abnormalities in approximately one third. Of the infants with deficits, approximately one half were marked. The severity of deficits correlated closely with the severity of the intrapartum hypoxia as judged by the associated acidosis (Fig. 17.16). Moreover, analysis of the intrapartum obstetrical and biochemical data in the usual case of prolonged partial asphyxia suggested that *the likelihood of neurological deficits correlated with duration of the insult and that approximately 1 hour was a critical time period.* In infants without deficits, the data indicated that metabolic acidosis developed

during the hour before delivery. In children with minor deficits, the data indicated that acidosis had been developing at least over the hour before delivery. In children with major deficits, the data indicated that acidosis had developed over a period "in excess of one hour."[268] The results of a later study by the same group also were consistent with the duration of 1 hour as an important threshold.[195] As noted earlier, the circumstance of severe, abrupt, terminal asphyxia may lead to brain injury with durations of less than 1 hour.[270,271]

Thus, current observations demonstrate the predictive value of intrapartum monitoring of fetal acid-base status. Moreover, the observations provide major insight into the importance not only of *severity* but also of a critical threshold of *duration* of the hypoxic insult. The latter observations are compatible with experimental data obtained with the fetal monkey that suggest that several hours of *partial asphyxia* result in serious neurological deficits.[328]

Other Techniques for Monitoring Fetal Well-Being Intrapartum

Fetal Pulse Oximetry

Although intermittent measurements of fetal pH, PO_2, and PCO_2 by sampling of fetal scalp blood have provided useful information, *continuous* intrauterine assessment would be of great value. As noted earlier with regard to the fetal heart rate assessments, longitudinal evaluations appear best for the prompt detection of the deteriorating fetus. Also, as noted earlier, the role of fetal scalp blood sampling is limited by difficulties with access, safety, and accuracy of information.[216] With pulse oximetry, continuous measurements of arterial oxygen saturation can be achieved by application of the oximeter sensor on the infant's cheek. The principle of oximetry relates to the differential absorption of red-infrared (735 nm) and near-infrared (890 nm) by oxyhemoglobin and deoxyhemoglobin. Oximeters in newborns placed on the fingers or toes are based on transmission of light through an emitting optode and reception of light after absorption by the two chromophores by a receiving optode. In fetal oximetry, the optode on the fetal cheek both emits the light and receives the reflected light after absorption.

Initial studies showed that the method is feasible and capable of reproducibly monitoring oxygen saturation.[329-333] Large-scale studies showed that an arterial oxygen saturation of 30% is an apparent threshold for detection of fetal acidosis, as demonstrated by simultaneous fetal scalp blood sampling or umbilical artery blood sampling at delivery. In one study, the use of fetal pulse oximetry in conjunction with fetal heart rate monitoring of high-risk pregnancies led to a 50% reduction in operative deliveries.[333] However, in a randomized trial of more than 5000 women, the use of fetal pulse oximetry and knowledge of intrapartum fetal oxygen saturation had no significant effect on the rates of cesarean delivery overall or specifically for the indication of nonreassuring fetal heart rate.[334] Thus, to what extent this promising methodology will serve as an adjunct to fetal heart rate monitoring remains to be established.

Fetal Electroencephalogram

Although the value of monitoring fetal heart rate and fetal acid-base status is apparent from the data available, a more direct means of assessing the status of the central nervous system in utero obviously would be preferred. One attempt in this direction was the earlier study of the *fetal electroencephalogram (EEG)* during labor by Rosen and co-workers.[335-342] By correlating the fetal patterns on the EEG with fetal heart rate tracings, neonatal assessment, and neurological evaluation at age 1 year, these investigators were able to demonstrate that brain injury is incurred in utero during labor in selected high-risk patients. Late decelerations of the fetal heart rate and traction of the head with forceps were among the factors shown to be associated with voltage suppression on the EEG.[336] Prolonged voltage suppression and persistent sharp waves were shown to be associated with neurological abnormality in the neonatal period and at 1 year of age.[341-343] The relevant abnormalities on the EEG were adapted to a system of computer interpretation, and investigators showed that the fetal EEG accurately predicted 63% of infants found to be abnormal (primarily delayed neurological development) at 1 year of age.[341-343] When data related to fetal heart rate, Apgar scores, and neonatal neurological examination were considered in addition to the findings on the fetal EEG, the accuracy of prediction increased to 80%. These observations, with a physiological measure of central nervous system function during labor, indicated that brain injury occurring in utero often can be detected at that time. The possibility of identifying such patients has major implications for interventions at the time of or immediately following the injurious insult in utero as well as shortly after birth.

Because of methodological difficulties, use of fetal EEG has not reached the level of clinical applicability, despite attempts to develop electrodes more easily used in clinical obstetrics.[344,345] Certainly, evaluation of fetal cerebral electrical activity has provided insight into timing of disturbance to the fetal central nervous system during labor, but technological advances are required before application to clinical practice is feasible. One potential solution is a more simplified system based on real-time spectral analysis of the fetal EEG obtained from two leads embedded in a single probe that can be applied to the fetal scalp by suction cups.[346] The spectral analysis of the signal on the fetal EEG determines frequency and amplitude of the signal. The most useful measure is the spectral edge frequency: the frequency lower than which 90% of the power of the power spectrum resides. Changes in spectral edge frequency correlate with changes in behavioral state, and during episodes of variable decelerations, a decrease in spectral edge frequency has been observed. Whether this limited measure of the fetal EEG will prove clinically useful remains to be established.

Doppler Measurements of Blood Flow Velocity

The value of measurements of blood flow velocity in the umbilical and fetal cerebral arteries in antepartum monitoring was described earlier. The feasibility of measurements of umbilical arterial blood flow velocity intrapartum has been demonstrated.[347-351] Although application of the technique has provided useful pathophysiological information, the method has not proven applicable for widespread clinical use.

Measurement of uterine blood flow velocity has been correlated with uterine contractions during labor (Table 17.19).[350] A linear decrease in velocity was shown with the increase in intrauterine pressure with contractions.

Of particular interest has been the determination of blood flow velocity during labor in the fetal anterior and middle

TABLE 17.19	Decrease in Uterine Blood Flow Velocity as a Function of Increase in Intrauterine Pressure With Contractions
PRESSURE INCREASE (mm Hg)	**VELOCITY DECREASE (MEDIAN)**
10	8%
20	23%
30	30%
40	44%
50	65%
60	60%

Data from Janbu T, Nesheim BI. Uterine artery blood velocities during contractions in pregnancy and labour related to intrauterine pressure. *Br J Obstet Gynaecol.* 1987;94:1150–1155, with permission.

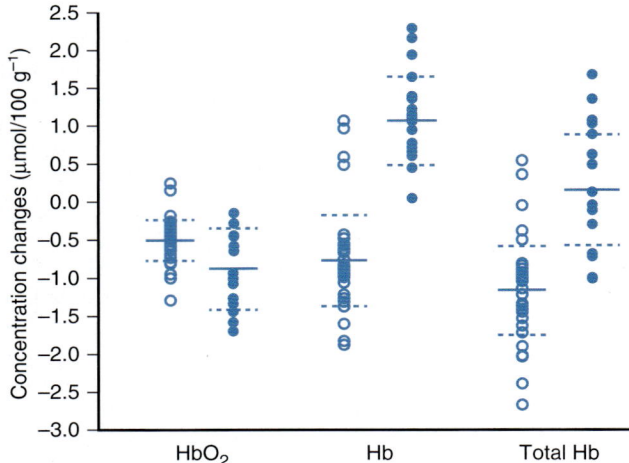

Figure 17.17 Near-infrared spectroscopic findings obtained from human fetuses during normal uterine concentrations (*left: open circles*) and those accompanied by fetal heart rate decelerations (*right: solid circles*). Mean values ± standard deviations are indicated. Note the lower oxyhemoglobin (HbO₂) and higher deoxyhemoglobin (Hb), indicative of cerebral hemoglobin oxygen desaturation, in contractions complicated by fetal heart rate decelerations. (From Peebles DM, Edwards AD, Wyatt JS, Bishop AP, et al. Changes in human fetal cerebral hemoglobin concentration and oxygenation during labor measured by near-infrared spectroscopy. *Am J Obstet Gynecol.* 1992;166:1369–1373.)

cerebral arteries, insonated either through the anterior fontanelle by transvaginal Doppler ultrasound or through the transabdominal approach with duplex Doppler.[352,353] An approximately 40% decrease in resistance index in the MCA was observed between contractions during active labor in one study.[353] One of several explanations for this observation is the occurrence of vasodilation caused by accumulation of vasoactive molecules (e.g., hydrogen ion, adenosine, prostaglandins) provoked by intermittent ischemia. Further studies would be of interest, although technical difficulties in obtaining reproducible measurements have proved substantial.

Near-Infrared Spectroscopy

An approach to intrapartum fetal monitoring of potential value involves the use of near-infrared spectroscopy for the study of *fetal cerebral hemodynamics and oxygenation.* As described in Chapter 10, application of a near-infrared light source and a photon-counting device to the cranium of the newborn and appropriate selection of light wavelengths can obtain information about intracranial concentrations of oxygenated and deoxygenated hemoglobin. With such data, information concerning cerebral hemoglobin oxygen saturation, cerebral oxygen delivery, and cerebral blood volume can be determined. This method, like intrapartum Doppler study, has provided useful pathophysiological information, but the method has not proven applicable for widespread clinical use.

Peebles and co-workers[354-358] designed a rubber probe that incorporates two fiberoptic bundles containing the near-infrared light source and the photon counter, separated by approximately 3 to 4 cm. This probe can be attached to the fetal head after membranes have ruptured and when cervical dilation is sufficient to attach the probe. Initial studies showed that with normal uterine contractions, cerebral content of both oxygenated and deoxygenated hemoglobin, and thereby total hemoglobin, decreased. The data suggested a decline in cerebral blood volume with contractions. With late fetal heart rate decelerations, a different pattern emerged. Oxygenated hemoglobin declined, whereas deoxygenated hemoglobin increased, a finding indicating cerebral hemoglobin oxygen desaturation (Fig. 17.17). This observation suggests a decrease in cerebral oxygen delivery with the decelerations. One possible

reason for this decrease would be a reduction in cerebral blood flow. Another study of 14 women under epidural analgesia during uncomplicated labor at term showed that the supine position was associated with a decline in mean cerebral oxygenated hemoglobin concentration sufficient to produce an 8.3% decrease in mean cerebral oxygen saturation.[357] This finding may reflect a decrease in uterine blood flow, secondary to maternal aortocaval obstruction by the gravid uterus, resulting in fetal hypoxemia. Further studies would be of interest, but the expense of the instrumentation and technical difficulties in obtaining reproducible measurements in the clinical setting have proved substantial.

Techniques Evaluating Fetal Brain Development and Placental Development

To date, the techniques discussed in this chapter have focused on an identification of deteriorations in fetal assessments that may indicate that a fetus is undergoing hypoxic or ischemic injury. Thus, such evaluations reflect concurrent cerebral injury, whether from severe placental dysfunction, such as intrauterine growth restriction, or during labor. A more effective method of fetal assessment for the future would include a thorough evaluation incorporating placental functioning, brain development, and any deviations from typical brain development. These profiles may allow the clinician to evaluate vulnerability to injury, rather than concurrent injury. This may alter clinician decision-making, including the timing and method of delivery, such as cesarean section, to avoid labor.

Placental Evaluation

MRI has been performed in pregnancy for >30 years,[359] mainly as a second-line imaging modality of the fetus used in combination with ultrasound examination. MRI is more expensive and not as widely available as ultrasound examination, but benefits from a larger field of view and from multiplanar capabilities, including acceptable spatial and temporal resolutions of high-contrast images. MRI is now being used increasingly more often in pregnancy, especially at advanced gestational age or in obese women. MRI of the placenta has been developed primarily to improve the diagnosis of placenta accreta.

MRI can be used with traditional structural imaging to determine shape, size, placement, and other abnormalities. Placental size is expressed in terms of thickness in the midportion of the organ and should be between 2 and 4 cm. Placental thinning has been described in systemic vascular and hematological diseases that result in micro-infarctions. Thicker placentas (>4 cm) are seen in fetal hydrops, antepartum infections, maternal diabetes, and maternal anemia.[360] MRI has been very useful in the evaluation of and planning for surgical intervention in placental implantation disorders, such as accreta. In addition, MRI can define the nature and extent of abruption or any scarred placental tissues (Fig. 17.18).

In addition, MRI in pregnancy benefits from the experience of functional MRI (fMRI) that has been gained in other specialties; specific sequences have provided a promising insight into fetal brain and placental function in vivo. Techniques of fMRI allow the assessment of several functional aspects of tissue being studied, which includes microvascular parameters, oxygenation, and metabolism (Table 17.20). Dynamic contrast-enhanced (DCE) MRI and arterial spin labeling (ASL) MRI can study tissue perfusion. Blood oxygen level–dependent (BOLD) MRI and oxygen-enhanced (OE) MRI can assess tissue oxygenation. Diffusion-weighted (DW) studies provide information on diffusion within tissues, and perfusion can be approximated using intravoxel incoherent motion (IVIM) MRI. These techniques have been applied in the human setting (see Table 17.20).

If these techniques can assist in the early identification of placental dysfunction and/or identify placenta that may be challenged during labor and delivery, such measures may have the *best capability* to identify risk before any cerebral injury.

Fetal Cerebral Evaluation

The techniques that are used in the evaluation of the structural and functional development of the immature brain (fully outlined in Chapter 10) can also be applied to the fetal brain, as demonstrated in Unit 1 (see Chapters 7 and 8). However, imaging of the fetal brain is more challenging, due to imaging a small brain at a considerable distance from the coil on the abdomen, thereby reducing signal to noise, and fetal motion. Nevertheless, recent work has demonstrated the applicability to the fetus of advanced MRI of structure (conventional imaging, diffusion tractography), biochemistry (spectroscopy), and function (resting state fMRI and activation f MRI) (Fig. 17.19). These MRI techniques build on a baseline of structural imaging to expanded functional insights, all of which are likely to render details that are of great relevance to the later neurodevelopmental outcome of the fetus.

TABLE 17.20 Magnetic Resonance Imaging Measures of Placental Function

MRI TECHNIQUE	PARAMETERS	APPLICATIONS	REFERENCES
Dynamic contrast enhanced	Gradient echo SI and PS	Altered perfusion throughout the placenta in normal placenta and IUGR	Gowland P. Placental MRI. *Semin Fetal Neonatal Med* 2005;10:485–490. Francis ST, Duncan KR, Moore RJ
Arterial spin labeling	Single spin echo EPI flow (Delta SI) Perfusion (F)	Altered perfusion	Baker PN, Johnson IR, Gowland PA. Noninvasive mapping of placental perfusion. *Lancet.* 1998;351:1397–1399.
Blood oxygen level dependent analysis	T2-weighted EPI with T2ª-weighted multi-echo signal including monoexponential decay fit	Increased signal intensity throughout the placenta	Huen I, Morris DM, Wright C, et al. R1 and R2* changes in the human placenta in response to maternal oxygen challenge. *Magn Reson Med.* 2012;70:1427–1433. Derwig I, Barker GJ, Poon L, et al. Association of placental T2 relaxation times and uterine artery Doppler ultrasound measures of placental blood flow. *Placenta.* 2013;34:474–479.
Diffusion weighted	Diffusion-weighted imaging with signal intensity for variable b-values	ADC	Moore RJ, Strachan BK, Tyler DJ, et al. In utero perfusing fraction maps in normal and growth restricted pregnancy measured using IVIM echo-planar MRI. *Placenta.* 2000;21:726–732.
Intravoxel incoherent motion	Exponential fit of the signal relative to B values (SI) and BI exponential fit	Altered perfusion measures	Nieto F, Wikstrom AK, Wikstrom J. Placental perfusion in normal pregnancy and early and late preeclampsia: a magnetic resonance imaging study. *Placenta.* 2014;35:202–206.
Magnetic resonance spectroscopy	Chemical shift imaging for phosphate of ATP, phosphocreatine	Altered energy markers	Weindling AM, Griffiths RD, Garden AS, Martin PA, Edwards RH. Phosphorus metabolites in the human placenta estimated in vivo by magnetic resonance spectroscopy. *Arch Child.* 1991;66:780–782.

ADC, Altered apparent diffusion coefficient; *ATP,* adenosine triphosphate; *EPI,* echo-planar imaging; *IUGR,* intrauterine growth restriction; *MRI,* magnetic resonance imaging; *PS,* permeability surface area; *SI,* signal intensity.

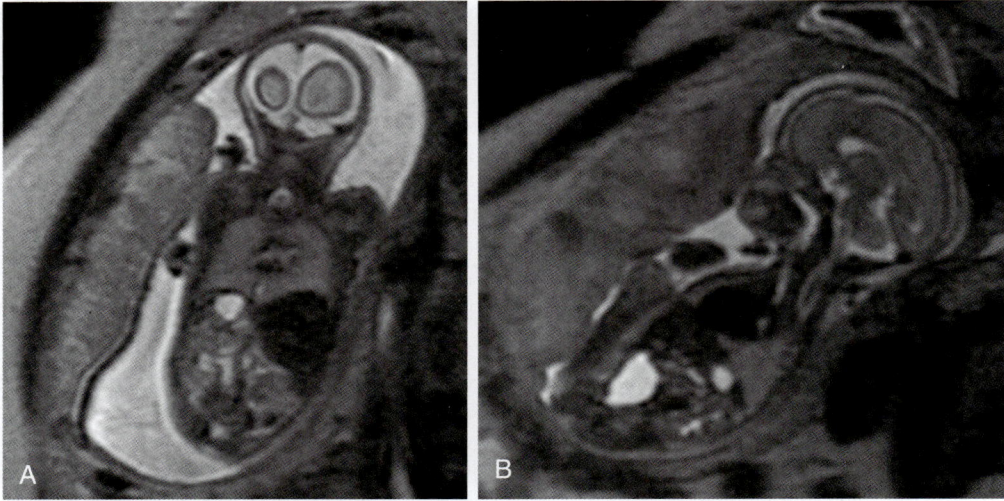

Figure 17.18 Placental magnetic resonance imaging. (A) T2-weighted image of a 26-week healthy placenta. Note the homogeneous high-signal intensity throughout the organ. (B) T2-weighted image of a 26-week placenta from a growth-restricted fetus. Note the heterogeneity in signal intensity, thought to correlate with areas of infarction, necrosis, or fibrosis. (Reprinted with permission from Andescavage NN, du Plessis AJ, Limperopoulos C. Advanced magnetic resonance imaging of the placenta: exploring the in utero placenta-brain connection. *Semin Perinatol.* 2015;39(2):113–123.)

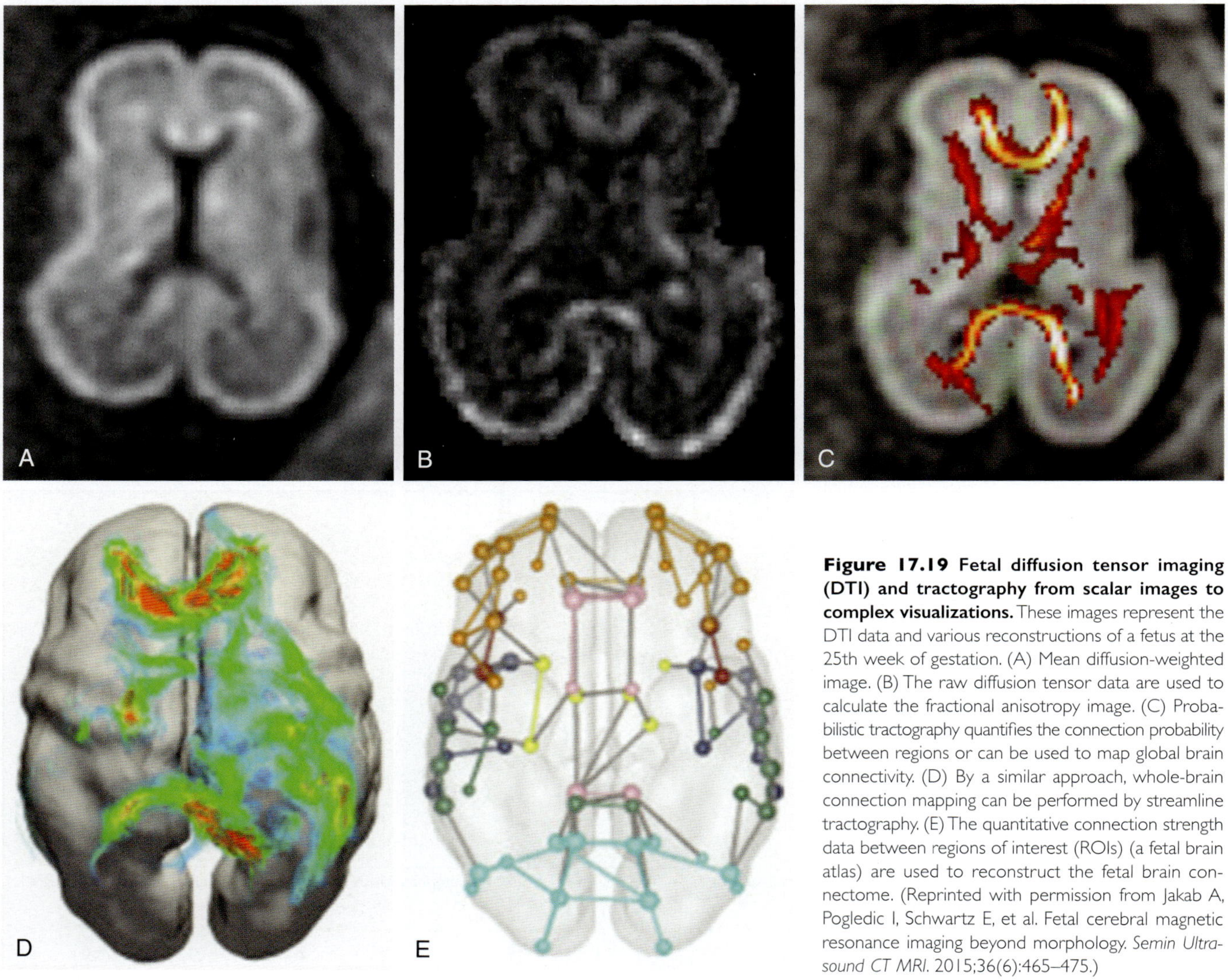

Figure 17.19 Fetal diffusion tensor imaging (DTI) and tractography from scalar images to complex visualizations. These images represent the DTI data and various reconstructions of a fetus at the 25th week of gestation. (A) Mean diffusion-weighted image. (B) The raw diffusion tensor data are used to calculate the fractional anisotropy image. (C) Probabilistic tractography quantifies the connection probability between regions or can be used to map global brain connectivity. (D) By a similar approach, whole-brain connection mapping can be performed by streamline tractography. (E) The quantitative connection strength data between regions of interest (ROIs) (a fetal brain atlas) are used to reconstruct the fetal brain connectome. (Reprinted with permission from Jakab A, Pogledic I, Schwartz E, et al. Fetal cerebral magnetic resonance imaging beyond morphology. *Semin Ultrasound CT MRI.* 2015;36(6):465–475.)

KEY REFERENCES

1. Kok RD, vandenBergh AJ, Heerschap A, et al. Metabolic information from the human fetal brain obtained with proton magnetic resonance spectroscopy. *Am J Obstet Gynceol.* 2001;185:1011-1015.

2. Levine D, Barnes PD, Robertson RR, et al. Fast MR imaging of fetal central nervous system abnormalities. *Radiology.* 2003;229: 51-61.

3. Eswaran H, Wilson JD, Preissl H, et al. Magnetoencephalographic recordings of visual evoked brain activity in the human fetus. *Lancet.* 2002;360:779-780.

5. Righini A, Bianchini E, Parazzini C, et al. Apparent diffusion coefficient determination in normal fetal brain: a prenatal MR imaging study. *AJNR Am J Neuroradiol.* 2003;24:799-804.

6. Gowland P, Fulford J. Initial experiences of performing fetal fMRI. *Exp Neurol.* 2004;190:S22-S27.

9. Roelants-van Rijn AM, Groenendaal F, Stoutenbeek P, et al. Lactate in the foetal brain: detection and implications. *Acta Paediatr.* 2004;93:937-940.

10. Bijma HH, Schoonderwaldt EM, vanderHeide A, et al. Ultrasound diagnosis of fetal anomalies: an analysis of perinatal management of 318 consecutive pregnancies in a multidisciplinary setting. *Prenat Diagn.* 2004;24:890-895.

13. Rayburn WF. Antepartum fetal assessment—monitoring fetal activity. *Clin Perinatol.* 1982;9:231.

14. Neldam S. Fetal movements as an indicator of fetal well-being. *Dan Med Bull.* 1983;30:274-278.

18. Moore TR, Piacquadio K. A prospective evaluation of fetal movement screening to reduce the incidence of antepartum fetal death. *Am J Obstet Gynecol.* 1989;160:1075-1080.

21. Prechtl HFR. State of the art of a new functional assessment of the young nervous system. An early predictor of cerebral palsy. *Early Hum Dev.* 1997;50:1-11.

27. Drogtrop AP, Ubels R, Nijhuis JG. The association between fetal body movements, eye movements and heart rate patterns in pregnancies between 25 and 30 weeks of gestation. *Early Hum Dev.* 1990;23:67-73.

31. Birnholz JC, Farrell EE. Ultrasound images of human fetal development. *Am Sci.* 1984;72:608.

32. Birnholz JC, Stephens JC, Faria M. Fetal movement patterns: a possible means of defining neurologic developmental milestones in utero. *AJR Am J Roentgenol.* 1978;130:537-540.

39. Mangesi L, Hofmeyr GJ, Smith V, et al. Fetal movement counting for assessment of fetal wellbeing. *Cochrane Database Syst Rev.* 2015;(10):CD004909.

40. Grant A, Elbourne D, Valentin L, et al. Routine formal fetal movement counting and risk of antepartum late death in normally formed singletons. *Lancet.* 1989;2:345-349.

41. Saastad E, Israel P, Ahlborg T, et al. Fetal movement counting—effects on maternal-fetal attachment: a multicenter randomized controlled trial. *Birth.* 2011;38:282-293.

49. Kisilevsky BS, Muir DW, Low JA. Human fetal responses to sound as a function of stimulus intensity. *Obstet Gynecol.* 1989;73:971-976.

50. Parkes MJ, Moore PJ, Moore DR, et al. Behavioral changes in fetal sheep caused by vibroacoustic stimulation: the effects of cochlear ablation. *Am J Obstet Gynecol.* 1991;164:1336-1343.

57. Platt LD, Paul RH, Phelan J, et al. Fifteen years of experience with antepartum fetal testing. *Am J Obstet Gynecol.* 1987;156:1509-1515.

61. Kidd LC, Patel NB, Smith R. Non-stress antenatal cardiotocography—a prospective randomized clinical trial. *Br J Obstet Gynecol.* 1985;92:1156-1159.

62. Lumley J, Lester A, Anderson I, et al. A randomized trial of weekly cardiotocography in high-risk obstetric patients. *Br J Obstet Gynaecol.* 1983;90:1018-1026.

63. Flynn AM, Kelly J, Mansfield H, et al. A randomized controlled trial of non-stress antepartum cardiotocography. *Br J Obstet Gynaecol.* 1982;89:427-433.

73. Vintzileos AM, Gaffney SE, Salinger LM, et al. The relationships among the fetal biophysical profile, umbilical cord pH, and Apgar scores. *Am J Obstet Gynecol.* 1987;157:627-631.

74. Vintzileos AM, Campbell WA, Nochimson DJ, et al. The use and misuse of the fetal biophysical profile. *Am J Obstet Gynecol.* 1987;156:527-533.

75. Johnson JM, Harman CR, Lange IR, et al. Biophysical profile scoring in the management of the postterm pregnancy: an analysis of 307 patients. *Am J Obstet Gynecol.* 1986;154:269-273.

78. Manning FA. Fetal assessment by evaluation of biophysical variables. In: Creasy RK, Resnik R, eds. *Maternal-Fetal Medicine.* 4th ed. Philadelphia: WB Saunders; 1999:319-330.

79. Lalor JG, Fawole B, Alfirevic Z, et al. Biophysical profile for fetal assessment in high risk pregnancies. *Cochrane Database Syst Rev.* 2008;(23):CD000038.

83. Low JA, Boston RW, Panchan SR. Fetal asphyxia during the intrapartum period in intrauterine growth retarded infants. *Am J Obstet Gynecol.* 1972;113:351.

84. Lin CC, Moawad AH, Rosenow PJ, et al. Acid-base characteristics of fetuses with intrauterine growth retardation during labor and delivery. *Am J Obstet Gynecol.* 1980;137:553-559.

86. Steiner H, Staudach A, Spitzer D, et al. Growth deficient fetuses with absent or reversed umbilical artery end-diastolic flow are metabolically compromised. *Early Hum Dev.* 1995;41:1-9.

87. Resnik R, Creasy RK. Intrauterine growth restriction. In: Creasy RK, Resnik R, Iams JD, eds. *Maternal-Fetal Medicine, Principles and Practice.* 5th ed. Philadelphia: WB Saunders; 2004:495-512.

90. Schulman H. The clinical implications of Doppler ultrasound analysis of the uterine and umbilical arteries. *Am J Obstet Gynecol.* 1987;156:889-893.

93. Hendricks SK, Sorensen TK, Wang KY, et al. Doppler umbilical artery waveform indices—normal values from fourteen to forty-two weeks. *Am J Obstet Gynecol.* 1989;161:761-765.

94. McParland P, Pearce JM. Doppler blood flow in pregnancy. *Placenta.* 1988;9:427-450.

95. Carroll BA. Duplex Doppler systems in obstetric ultrasound. *Radiol Clin North Am.* 1990;28:189-203.

96. Newnham JP, Patterson LL, James IR, et al. An evaluation of the efficacy of Doppler flow velocity waveform analysis as a screening test in pregnancy. *Am J Obstet Gynecol.* 1990;162:403-410.

97. Ritchie JW. Use of Doppler technology in assessing fetal health. *J Dev Physiol.* 1991;15:121-123.

103. Adiotomre PNA, Johnstone FD, Laing IA. Effect of absent end diastolic flow velocity in the fetal umbilical artery on subsequent outcome. *Arch Dis Child.* 1997;76:F35-F38.

104. Dubiel M, Sudmundsson S, Gunnarsson G, et al. Middle cerebral artery velocimetry as a predictor of hypoxemia in fetuses with increased resistance to blood flow in the umbilical artery. *Early Hum Dev.* 1997;47:177-184.

105. Harrington K, Thompson MO, Carpenter RG, et al. Doppler fetal circulation in pregnancies complicated by pre-eclampsia or delivery of a small for gestational age baby: 2. Longitudinal analysis. *Br J Obstet Gynaecol.* 1999;106:453-466.

118. Hawdon JM, Ward Platt MP, McPhail S, et al. Prediction of impaired metabolic adaptation by antenatal Doppler studies in small for gestational age fetuses. *Arch Dis Child.* 1992;67:789-792.

119. Schreuder AM, McDonnell M, Gaffney G, et al. Outcome at school age following antenatal detection of absent or reversed end diastolic flow velocity in the umbilical artery. *Arch Dis Child.* 2002;86:108-114.

120. Westergaard HB, Langhoff-Roos J, Lingman G, et al. A critical appraisal of the use of umbilical artery Doppler ultrasound in high-risk pregnancies: use of meta-analyses in evidence-based obstetrics. *Ultrasound Obstet Gynecol.* 2001;17:466-476.

121. Alfirevic Z, Stampalija T, Gyte GM. Fetal and umbilical Doppler ultrasound in high-risk pregnancies. *Cochrane Database Syst Rev.* 2013;(11):CD007529.

124. Society for Maternal-Fetal Medicine Publications Committee, Berkley E, Chauhan SP, et al. Doppler assessment of the fetus with intrauterine growth restriction. *Am J Obstet Gynecol.* 2012;206:300-308.

126. Goffinet F, Paris-Llado J, Nisand I, et al. Umbilical artery Doppler velocimetry in unselected and low risk pregnancies: a review of randomised controlled trials. *Br J Obstet Gynaecol.* 1997; 104:425-430.

131. Chandran R, Serraserra V, Sellers SM, et al. Fetal cerebral Doppler in the recognition of fetal compromise. *Br J Obstet Gynaecol.* 1993;100:139-144.

132. Veille JC, Hanson R, Tatum K. Longitudinal quantitation of middle cerebral artery blood flow in normal human fetuses. *Am J Obstet Gynecol.* 1993;169:1393-1398.

143. Fieni S, Gramellini D, Piantelli G. Lack of normalization of middle cerebral artery flow velocity prior to fetal death before the 30th week of gestation: a report of three cases. *Ultrasound Obstet Gynecol.* 2004;24:474-476.

144. Oros D, Figueras F, Cruz-Martinez R, et al. Longitudinal changes in uterine, umbilical and fetal cerebral Doppler indices in late-onset small-for-gestational age fetuses. *Ultrasound Obstet Gynecol.* 2011;37:191-195.

145. Severi FM, Bocchi C, Visentin A, et al. Uterine and fetal cerebral Doppler predict the outcome of third-trimester small-for-gestational age fetuses with normal umbilical artery Doppler. *Ultrasound Obstet Gynecol.* 2002;19:225-228.

146. Morris RK, Say R, Robson SC, et al. Systematic review and meta-analysis of middle cerebral artery Doppler to predict perinatal wellbeing. *Eur J Obstet Gynecol Reprod Biol.* 2012;165:141-155.

149. Baschat AA, Gembruch U, Weiner CP, et al. Qualitative venous Doppler waveform analysis improves prediction of critical perinatal outcomes in premature growth-restricted fetuses. *Ultrasound Obstet Gynecol.* 2003;22:240-245.

150. Bilardo CM, Wolf H, Stigter RH, et al. Relationship between monitoring parameters and perinatal outcome in severe, early intrauterine growth restriction. *Ultrasound Obstet Gynecol.* 2004;23:119-125.

151. Lees CC, Marlow N, van Wassenaer-Leemhuis A, et al. 2 year neurodevelopmental and intermediate perinatal outcomes in infants with very preterm fetal growth restriction (TRUFFLE): a randomised trial. *Lancet.* 2015;385:2162-2172.

153. Unterscheider J, Daly S, Geary MP, et al. Predictable progressive Doppler deterioration in IUGR: does it really exist? *Am J Obstet Gynecol.* 2013;209:539.e1-539.e7.

154. Volpe JJ. Neonatal encephalopathy: an inadequate term for hypoxic-ischemic encephalopathy. *Ann Neurol.* 2012;72:156-166.

158. Hagberg B, Hagberg G, Olow I. The changing panorama of cerebral palsy in Sweden. 6. Prevalence and origin during the birth year period 1983-1986. *Acta Paediatr.* 1993;82:387-393.

164. Kuban KCK, Leviton A. The epidemiology of cerebral palsy. *N Engl J Med.* 1994;330:188-195.

165. Nelson KB. What proportion of cerebral palsy is related to birth asphyxia? [editorial]. *J Pediatr.* 1988;112:572-574.

169. Melone PJ, Ernest JM, O'Shea MD Jr, et al. Appropriateness of intrapartum fetal heart rate management and risk of cerebral palsy. *Am J Obstet Gynecol.* 1991;165:272-276.

170. Nelson KB, Leviton A. How much of neonatal encephalopathy is due to birth asphyxia? *Am J Dis Child.* 1991;145:1325-1331.

171. Stanley FJ, Blair E. Why have we failed to reduce the frequency of cerebral palsy? *Med J Aust.* 1991;154:623-626.

173. Hagberg B, Hagberg G, Olow I, et al. The changing panorama of cerebral palsy in Sweden. 7. Prevalence and origin in the birth year period 1987-90. *Acta Paediatr.* 1996;85:954-960.

175. Hagberg B, Hagberg G, Beckung E, et al. Changing panorama of cerebral palsy in Sweden. VIII. Prevalence and origin in the birth year period 1991-94. *Acta Paediatr.* 2001;90:271-277.

176. Clark SL, Hankins GDV. Temporal and demographic trends in cerebral palsy—fact and fiction. *Am J Obstet Gynecol.* 2003;188:628-633.

177. Truwit CL, Barkovich AJ, Koch TK, et al. Cerebral palsy: MR findings in 40 patients. *AJNR Am J Neuroradiol.* 1992;13:67-78.

178. Volpe JJ. Value of MR in definition of the neuropathology of cerebral palsy in vivo. *AJNR Am J Neuroradiol.* 1992;13:79-83.

193. Spinillo A, Capuzzo E, Orcesi S, et al. Antenatal and delivery risk factors simultaneously associated with neonatal death and cerebral palsy in preterm infants. *Early Hum Dev.* 1997;48:81-91.

194. Glantz JC, Woods JR. Significance of amniotic fluid meconium. In: Creasy RK, Resnik R, eds. *Maternal-Fetal Medicine.* 4th ed. Philadelphia: WB Saunders; 1999:393-403.

195. Low JA, Victory R, Derrick EJ. Predictive value of electronic fetal monitoring for intrapartum fetal asphyxia with metabolic acidosis. *Obstet Gynecol.* 1999;93:285-291.

198. Martinez-Biarge M, Diez-Sebastian J, Wusthoff CJ, et al. Antepartum and intrapartum factors preceding neonatal hypoxic-ischemic encephalopathy. *Pediatrics.* 2013;132:e952-e959.

203. Zuspan FP, Quilligan EJ, Iams JD, et al. NICHD Consensus Development Task Force report: predictors of intrapartum fetal distress—the role of electronic fetal monitoring. *J Pediatr.* 1979;95:1026-1030.

204. Krebs HB, Petres RE, Dunn LJ, et al. Intrapartum fetal heart rate monitoring. I. Classification and prognosis of fetal heart rate patterns. *Am J Obstet Gynecol.* 1979;133:762-772.

213. Thacker SB, Stroup DF, Peterson HB. Efficacy and safety of intrapartum electronic fetal monitoring: an update. *Obstet Gynecol.* 1995;86:613-620.

214. Nelson KB, Dambrosia JM, Ting TY, et al. Uncertain value of electronic fetal monitoring in predicting cerebral palsy. *N Engl J Med.* 1996;334:613-618.

215. MacDonald D. Cerebral palsy and intrapartum fetal monitoring. *N Engl J Med.* 1996;334:659-660.

216. Parer JT, Nageotte MP. Intrapartum fetal surveillance. In: Creasy RK, Resnik R, Iams JD, eds. *Maternal-Fetal Medicine, Principles and Practice.* 5th ed. Philadelphia: WB Saunders; 2004:403-427.

217. Thacker SB. The efficacy of intrapartum electronic fetal monitoring. *Am J Obstet Gynecol.* 1987;156:24-30.

221. Shy KK, Luthy DA, Bennett FC, et al. Effects of electronic fetal-heart-rate monitoring, as compared with periodic auscultation, on the neurologic development of premature infants. *N Engl J Med.* 1990;322:588-593.

222. Freeman R. Intrapartum fetal monitoring—a disappointing story. *N Engl J Med.* 1990;322:624-626.

225. Morrison JC, Chez BF, Davis ID, et al. Intrapartum fetal heart rate assessment—Monitoring by auscultation or electronic means. *Am J Obstet Gynecol.* 1993;168:63-66.

226. Vintzileos AM, Antsaklis A, Varvarigos I, et al. A randomized trial of intrapartum electronic fetal heart rate monitoring versus intermittent auscultation. *Obstet Gynecol.* 1993;81:899-907.

228. Williams KP, Galerneau F. Intrapartum fetal heart rate patterns in the prediction of neonatal acidemia. *Am J Obstet Gynecol.* 2003;188:820-823.

229. Althuse JE, Petersen SM, Fox HE, et al. Can electronic fetal monitoring identify preterm neonates with cerebral white matter injury? *Obstet Gynecol.* 2005;105:458-465.

232. Riley LE, Celi AC, Onderdonk AB, et al. Association of epidural-related fever and noninfectious inflammation in term labor. *Obstet Gynecol.* 2011;117:588-595.

234. Vintzileos AM, Smulian JC. Decelerations, tachycardia, and decreased variability: have we overlooked the significance of longitudinal fetal heart rate changes for detecting intrapartum fetal hypoxia? *Am J Obstet Gynecol.* 2016;215:261-264.

235. Paul RH, Suidan AK, Yeh S, et al. Clinical fetal monitoring. VII. The evaluation and significance of intrapartum baseline FHR variability. *Am J Obstet Gynecol.* 1975;123:206-210.

246. Powell OH, Melville A, MacKenna J. Fetal heart rate acceleration in labor: excellent prognostic indicator. *Am J Obstet Gynecol.* 1979;134:36-38.

247. Krebs HB, Petres RE, Dunn LJ, et al. Intrapartum fetal heart rate monitoring. VI. Prognostic significance of accelerations. *Am J Obstet Gynecol.* 1982;142:297-305.

248. James LS, Yeh MN, Morishima HO, et al. Umbilical vein occlusion and transient acceleration of the fetal heart rate. Experimental observations in subhuman primates. *Am J Obstet Gynecol.* 1976;126:276-283.

256. Althabe O Jr, Schwarcz RL, Pose SV, et al. Effects on fetal heart rate and fetal pO₂ of oxygen administration to the mother. *Am J Obstet Gynecol.* 1967;98:858-870.

257. James LS, Morishima HO, Daniel SS, et al. Mechanism of late deceleration of the fetal heart rate. *Am J Obstet Gynecol.* 1972;113:578-582.

258. Cibils LA. Clinical significance of fetal heart rate patterns during labor. V. Variable decelerations. *Am J Obstet Gynecol.* 1978;132:791-805.

259. Mueller-Heubach E, Myers RE, Adamsons K. Fetal heart rate and blood pressure during prolonged partial asphyxia in the rhesus monkey. *Am J Obstet Gynecol.* 1980;137:48-52.

262. Aarnoudse JG, Huisjes HJ, Gordon H, et al. Fetal subcutaneous scalp PO₂ and abnormal heart rate during labor. *Am J Obstet Gynecol.* 1985;153:565-566.

263. Greiss FC. A clinical concept of uterine blood flow during pregnancy. *Obstet Gynecol.* 1967;40:595.

269. Low JA. Fetal acid-base status and outcome. In: Hill A, Volpe JJ, eds. *Fetal Neurology.* New York: Raven Press; 1989:195-214.

270. Pasternak JF, Gorey MT. The syndrome of acute near-total intrauterine asphyxia in the term infant. *Pediatr Neurol.* 1998;18:391-398.

271. Korst LM, Phelan JP, Wang YM, et al. Acute fetal asphyxia and permanent brain injury: a retrospective analysis of current indicators. *J Matern Fetal Med.* 1999;8:101-106.

272. Krebs HB, Petres RE, Dunn LJ. Intrapartum fetal heart rate monitoring. VIII. Atypical variable decelerations. *Am J Obstet Gynecol.* 1983;145:297-305.

273. Goodlin RC, Haesslein HC. Fetal reacting bradycardia. *Am J Obstet Gynecol.* 1977;129:845-856.

275. American College of Obstetricians and Gynecologists. ACOG Practice Bulletin No. 106: Intrapartum fetal heart rate monitoring: nomenclature, interpretation, and general management principles. *Obstet Gynecol.* 2009;114:192-202.

280. Low JA, Killen H, Derrick EJ. The prediction and prevention of intrapartum fetal asphyxia in preterm pregnancies. *Am J Obstet Gynecol.* 2002;186:279-282.

284. Larma JD, Silva AM, Holcroft CJ, et al. Intrapartum electronic fetal heart rate monitoring and the identification of metabolic acidosis and hypoxic-ischemic encephalopathy. *Am J Obstet Gynecol.* 2007;197:e301-e308.

285. Cahill AG, Roehl KA, Odibo AO, et al. Association and prediction of neonatal acidemia. *Am J Obstet Gynecol.* 2012;207:206.e1-206.e8.

286. Sameshima H, Ikenoue T. Predictive value of late decelerations for fetal acidemia in unselective low-risk pregnancies. *Am J Perinatol.* 2005;22:19-23.

287. Cahill AG, Spain J. Intrapartum fetal monitoring. *Clin Obstet Gynecol.* 2015;58:263-268.

289. Rosen KG. Fetal electrocardiogram waveform analysis in labour. *Curr Opin Obstet Gynecol.* 2001;13:137-140.

290. Amer-Wahlin I, Hellsten C, Noren H, et al. Cardiotocography only versus cardiotocography plus ST analysis of fetal electrocardiogram for intrapartum fetal monitoring: a Swedish randomised controlled trial. *Lancet.* 2001;358:534-538.

293. Belfort MA, Saade GR, Thom E, et al. A randomized trial of intrapartum fetal ECG ST segment analysis. *N Engl J Med.* 2015;373:632-641.

296. Helwig JT, Parer JT, Kilpatrick SJ, et al. Umbilical cord blood acid-base state: what is normal? *Am J Obstet Gynecol.* 1996;174:1807-1814.

297. Gilstrap LD, Leveno KJ, Burris J, et al. Diagnosis of birth asphyxia on the basis of fetal pH, Apgar score, and newborn cerebral dysfunction. *Am J Obstet Gynecol.* 1989;161:825-830.

299. Ruth VJ, Raivio KO. Perinatal brain damage: predictive value of metabolic acidosis and the Apgar score. *BMJ.* 1988;297:24-27.

300. Low JA. The role of blood gas and acid-base assessment in the diagnosis of intrapartum fetal asphyxia. *Am J Obstet Gynecol.* 1988;159:1235-1240.

301. Low JA, Galbraith RS, Muir DW, et al. Motor and cognitive deficits after intrapartum asphyxia in the mature fetus. *Am J Obstet Gynecol.* 1988;158:356-361.

303. Low JA, Muir DW, Pater EA, et al. The association of intrapartum asphyxia in the mature fetus with newborn behavior. *Am J Obstet Gynecol.* 1990;163:1131-1135.

306. Goodwin TM, Belai I, Hernandez P, et al. Asphyxial complications in the term newborn with severe umbilical acidemia. *Am J Obstet Gynecol.* 1992;167:1506-1512.

309. van den Berg PP, Nelen WLDM, Jongsma HW, et al. Neonatal complications in newborns with an umbilical artery pH<7.00. *Am J Obstet Gynecol.* 1996;175:1152-1157.

310. Belai YI, Goodwin TM, Durand M, et al. Umbilical arteriovenous PO2 and PCO2 differences and neonatal morbidity in term infants with severe acidosis. *Am J Obstet Gynecol.* 1998;178:13-19.

311. Low JA, Lindsay BG, Derrick EJ. Threshold of metabolic acidosis associated with newborn complications. *Am J Obstet Gynecol.* 1997;177:1391-1394.

313. Shankaran S. Identification of term infants at risk for neonatal morbidity. *J Pediatr.* 1998;132:571-572.

314. Carter BS, McNabb F, Merenstein GB. Prospective validation of a scoring system for predicting neonatal morbidity after acute perinatal asphyxia. *J Pediatr.* 1998;132:619-623.

316. daSilva S, Hennebert N, Denis R, et al. Clinical value of a single postnatal lactate measurement after intrapartum asphyxia. *Acta Paediatr.* 2000;89:320-323.

317. Toh VC. Early predictors of adverse outcome in term infants with post-asphyxial hypoxic ischaemic encephalopathy. *Acta Paediatr.* 2000;89:343-347.

318. Williams KP, Singh A. The correlation of seizures in newborn infants with significant acidosis at birth with umbilical artery cord gas values. *Obstet Gynecol.* 2002;100:557-560.

319. Ross MG, Gala R. Use of umbilical artery base excess: algorithm for the timing of hypoxic injury. *Am J Obstetr Gynecol.* 2002;187:1-9.

321. Hon EH, Khazin AF. Observations on fetal heart rate and fetal biochemistry. I. Base deficit. *Obstet Gynecol.* 1969;105:721.

322. Kubli FW, Hon EH, Khazin AF, et al. Observations on heart rate and pH in the human fetus during labor. *Am J Obstet Gynecol.* 1969;104:1190-1206.

327. Malin GL, Morris RK, Khan KS. Strength of association between umbilical cord pH and perinatal and long term outcomes: systematic review and meta-analysis. *BMJ.* 2010;340:c1471.

330. Kuhnert M, Seelbach-Goebel B, Butterwegge M. Predictive agreement between the fetal arterial oxygen saturation and fetal scalp pH: results of the German multicenter study. *Am J Obstet Gynecol.* 1998;178:330-335.

331. Seelbach-Gobel B, Heupel M, Kuhnert M, et al. The prediction of fetal acidosis by means of intrapartum fetal pulse oximetry. *Am J Obstet Gynecol.* 1999;180:73-81.

332. Garite TJ, Dildy GA, McNamara H, et al. A multicenter controlled trial of fetal pulse oximetry in the intrapartum management of nonreassuring fetal heart rate patterns. *Am J Obstet Gynecol.* 2000;183:1049-1058.

333. Kuhnert M, Schmidt S. Intrapartum management of nonreassuring fetal heart rate patterns: a randomized controlled trial of fetal pulse oximetry. *Am J Obstet Gynecol.* 2004;191:1989-1995.

334. Bloom SL, Spong CY, Thom E, et al. Fetal pulse oximetry and cesarean delivery. *N Engl J Med.* 2006;355:2195-2202.

336. Rosen MG, Scibetta JJ, Hochberg CJ. Fetal electroencephalography. IV. The FEEG during spontaneous and forceps births. *Obstet Gynecol.* 1973;42:283-289.

337. Rosen MG, Scibetta J, Chik L, et al. An approach to the study of brain damage. The principles of fetal electroencephalography. *Am J Obstet Gynecol.* 1973;115:37-47.

343. Sokol RJ, Rosen MG, Chik L. Fetal electroencephalographic monitoring related to infant outcome. *Am J Obstet Gynecol.* 1977;127:329-330.

346. Thaler I, Boldes R, Timor-Tritsch I. Real-time spectral analysis of the fetal EEG: a new approach to monitoring sleep states and fetal condition during labor. *Pediatr Res.* 2000;48:340-345.

348. Sarno AP Jr, Ahn MO, Brar HS, et al. Intrapartum Doppler velocimetry, amniotic fluid volume, and fetal heart rate as predictors of subsequent fetal distress. I. An initial report. *Am J Obstet Gynecol.* 1989;161:1508-1514.

349. Mansouri H, Gagnon R, Hunse C. Relationship between fetal heart rate and umbilical blood flow velocity in term human fetuses during labor. *Am J Obstet Gynecol.* 1989;160:1007-1012.

353. Yagel S, Anteby E, Lavy Y, et al. Fetal middle cerebral artery blood flow during normal active labour and in labour with variable decelerations. *Br J Obstet Gynaecol.* 1992;99:483-485.

355. Peebles DM, Spencer JA, Edwards AD, et al. Relation between frequency of uterine contractions and human fetal cerebraloxygen saturation studied during labour by near infrared spectroscopy. *Br J Obstet Gynaecol.* 1994;101:44-48.

359. Smith FW, Adam AH, Phillips WD. NMR imaging in pregnancy. *Lancet.* 1983;1:61-62.

360. Masselli G, Gualdi G. MR imaging of the placenta: what a radiologist should know. *Abdom Imaging.* 2013;38:573-587.

Full references for this chapter can be found on www.expertconsult .com

Hypoxic-Ischemic Injury in the Term Infant: Neuropathology

Hannah C. Kinney ◆ Joseph J. Volpe

Hypoxic-ischemic brain injury is a very important neurological problem of the perinatal period. This importance relates to the general gravity of the lesions and to the relatively large number of affected infants. In the premature infant this encephalopathy is often accompanied by intraventricular hemorrhage and its concomitants, which contribute to the neurological morbidity (see Chapter 24). Thus it is apparent that a basic understanding of hypoxic-ischemic brain injury provides insight into a major portion of neonatal neurology. The subsequent neurological deficits of concern are principally a variety of motor deficits, especially spasticity, but also choreoathetosis, dystonia, and ataxia, often grouped together as *cerebral palsy*, with or without accompanying cognitive deficits and seizures.

In this chapter, we review the neuropathology and pathogenesis of neonatal hypoxic-ischemic encephalopathy. The major lesions are discussed separately, although commonly there is overlap in the occurrence of each lesion. In Chapters 19 and 20, we review the pathogenesis and clinical features of neonatal hypoxic-ischemic encephalopathy, using the same framework of neuropathological lesions discussed in this chapter.

NEUROPATHOLOGY

The neuropathological features of neonatal hypoxic-ischemic encephalopathy vary considerably with the gestational age of the infant, the nature of the insult, the types of interventions, and other factors, most still to be defined. Nevertheless, certain basic lesions can be recognized, and recognition of these lesions provides a useful framework for the discussion of clinical aspects. The major neuropathological varieties are shown in Table 18.1. In the context of generalized hypoxemia-ischemia, the focus of this chapter, the first three varieties are most common and discussed next. Stroke occurs in the context of multiple etiologies and is discussed separately in Chapter 21.

Brain Swelling and Brain Necrosis

Brain swelling is discussed separately from the recognized neuropathological disorders associated with perinatal hypoxic-ischemic insults because some workers have suggested that brain swelling is a separate and dominant lesion that may lead to additional brain injury. This view is derived principally from experience with adult patients and from experimental data (see later discussion). Indeed, it is well known in standard neuropathological writings concerning adult patients that severe hypoxic-ischemic insults are associated with a major degree of brain swelling and increased intracranial pressure and that

the latter may accentuate neurological morbidity. Extrapolation of such data to the neonatal brain cannot be made a priori. Earlier work with neonatal kittens and rats indicated a relative resistance of immature brain to the development of prominent edema produced by hypoxic-ischemic or cold-induced injury; similar insults regularly produce pronounced brain edema in adult animals.[1,2] Therefore it is reasonable to ask whether brain swelling with hypoxic-ischemic injury is a consistent feature in the human newborn with perinatal asphyxia.

Pathological Aspects in Human Infants

Pathological studies of neonatal hypoxic-ischemic encephalopathy do not provide decisive support for the occurrence of brain swelling as a separate and dominant lesion without comparable degrees of tissue necrosis.[3-8] Several older reports do emphasize brain swelling in asphyxiated newborn infants.[9-12] However, often the definition of swelling is not precise, the degree of associated brain injury is not clearly quantitated, the length of time spent on ventilatory and circulatory support before death is not defined, and the type of management after the insult is not described. These factors have major bearing on the questions of whether edema, in fact, was present, and if so, whether it was simply the *consequence* of brain necrosis or was a predominant lesion per se. Moreover, because fetal and neonatal human brain contains more water than myelinated, mature brain and the immature brain swells considerably during fixation, Gilles et al.[13] suggested that "much of what has been called edema in the fixed brain may well reflect the initial high water content of this tissue plus the water accumulated during fixation." The absence of external signs of swelling and of necrosis caused by transtentorial (hippocampal) or transmagnal (cerebellar) herniation in the huge autopsy population of the National Collaborative Perinatal Project has been emphasized.[13]

Several clinical studies also indicated that primary brain swelling (i.e., in the absence of marked brain necrosis) is not a prominent feature of hypoxic-ischemic encephalopathy in the human newborn.[14-18] In one study, clearly increased intracranial pressure (i.e., >10 mm Hg) was observed in only 22% of 32 asphyxiated term newborns; it did not compromise cerebral perfusion pressure, it reached a maximum at 36 to 72 hours, and it correlated with computed tomography (CT) evidence for early brain necrosis.[17] In a second systematic study, intracranial pressure reached a maximum at a mean age of 29 hours and was not correlated with clinical or electroencephalographic evidence for neurological deterioration.[16] Changes in cerebral perfusion pressure most often reflected decreases in arterial

TABLE 18.1	Major Neuropathological Varieties of Neonatal Hypoxic-Ischemic Encephalopathy

Selective neuronal necrosis
Parasagittal cerebral injury
Periventricular leukomalacia
Focal (and multifocal) ischemic brain necrosis—stroke

TABLE 18.2	Evidence Against Early Brain Edema as a Causative Factor in Hypoxic-Ischemic Brain Injury[a]

Intracranial pressure (ICP) >10 mm Hg is uncommon in asphyxiated term infants
When ICP >10 mm Hg occurs, timing is relatively late (i.e., 24–72 h)
Marked decreases in cerebral perfusion pressure (CPP) are uncommon, and decreases in CPP that do occur are usually caused by decreases in blood pressure rather than by increases in ICP

[a]See text for references.

blood pressure rather than increases in intracranial pressure.[16] Moreover, administration of mannitol in a single dose to asphyxiated infants in a controlled study had no beneficial clinical effect.[18] These observations support the conclusion that early brain edema is a *consequence rather than a causative factor of* hypoxic-ischemic brain injury (Table 18.2).[14-18]

Experimental Aspects in Perinatal Animals

Intrauterine Partial Asphyxia in the Fetal Monkey. The notion that brain swelling is an important *early* feature with perinatal hypoxic-ischemic insults and the *cause* of subsequent tissue necrosis is based on studies with term fetal monkeys by Myers and co-workers.[19-25] In these experiments, in association with "prolonged partial asphyxia" of the term fetal monkey (produced by a variety of procedures that impair placental gas exchange, such as maternal hypotension, maternal hypoxemia, and umbilical cord compression), a pattern of cerebral injury characterized by necrosis and edema was observed. The topography of the necrosis was typical of the parasagittal cerebral injury observed in the asphyxiated human term infant (see later discussion).

Associated with the cerebral injury in the monkeys was *brain swelling*, defined primarily by gyral flattening. The edema was considered to be intracellular on the basis of electron microscopic observations in related experiments.[25] In similar experiments, statistically significant changes in brain water content could not be demonstrated.[24] On balance, the brain swelling in these experiments appears most likely to be secondary to the pronounced tissue injury (with cytotoxic edema) rather than a primary event leading to the injury. This possibility would be compatible with conclusions derived from human pathological material (see earlier discussion).

Intrauterine Partial Asphyxia in the Fetal Lamb. Studies of the fetal lamb subjected to intrauterine partial asphyxia do not support the notion of brain edema, at least of the vasogenic variety, as an important consequence of acute hypoxic-ischemic brain injury in this model.[26,27] Extravascular plasma volume was quantitated by the iodine-125-labeled albumin method with asphyxia and was found not to be significantly increased in cerebrum, brain stem, or cerebellum.[26] Moreover, the postasphyxial delayed cerebral hypoperfusion observed in this model occurred in the absence of brain edema.[27] In later studies of near-term fetal lambs subjected to hypoxia-ischemia, findings indicative of *cytotoxic* edema correlated with documented neuronal injury were obtained—a correlation consistent with the observations in human infants (see earlier).[28]

Hypoxic-Ischemic Insult in the Neonatal Rat and Piglet. Careful morphological, physiological, and biochemical studies of the neonatal rat and piglet subjected to a combination of ischemia (carotid ligation) and hypoxemia also failed to support the notion of brain edema as a primary or injury-causing result of hypoxic-ischemic insult.[29-38] In the studies of neonatal rats, although the water content of brain increased, a close correlation was defined between the degree of tissue necrosis and the increase in brain water. No sign of transtentorial or cerebellar herniation was observed, *unlike the case in adult animals similarly studied.* No inverse correlation of cerebral blood flow (CBF) and brain water content could be identified over the 6 days following the hypoxic-ischemic insult. Moreover, administration of four doses of mannitol over 2 days following the insult did not ameliorate the incidence, distribution, or severity of the extensive tissue injury, despite reduction in the increase in brain water content in the hypoxic-ischemic hemisphere.[30] In addition, the spatial relationships between this increase in brain volume and the tissue injury did not suggest that the apparent edema caused or contributed to the cerebral injury.[33] The conclusion is that the brain *edema* is a "consequence rather than a cause of major ischemic damage in the immature animal."[29-31,33-35,37]

Selective Neuronal Necrosis: Patterns of Injury

Selective neuronal necrosis is the most common variety of injury observed in neonatal hypoxic-ischemic encephalopathy. The term refers to necrosis of neurons in a characteristic although often widespread distribution. Neuronal necrosis often coexists with other distinctive manifestations of neonatal hypoxic-ischemic encephalopathy (see later sections), and in fact it is very unusual to observe one of the other varieties of neonatal hypoxic-ischemic encephalopathy without some degree of selective neuronal injury as well. The topography of the neuronal injury depends in considerable part on the severity and temporal characteristics of the insult and on the gestational age of the infant. Three basic patterns derived primarily from correlative clinical and brain imaging findings and observed best in term infants can be distinguished (Table 18.3). *Diffuse neuronal injury* occurs with very severe and very prolonged insults in both term and premature infants. A *cerebrocortical–deep nuclear* neuronal predominance occurs in primarily term infants with moderate to severe, relatively prolonged insults. The deep nuclear involvement includes basal ganglia (especially putamen) and thalamus. *Deep nuclear–brain-stem* neuronal predominance occurs in primarily term infants with severe, relatively abrupt insults. Two additional patterns, *pontosubicular* neuronal injury

TABLE 18.3 Major Patterns of Selective Neuronal Injury and Characteristics of Usual Insult in Term Newborns

PATTERN[a]	USUAL INSULT
Diffuse	Very severe, very prolonged
Cerebral cortex–deep nuclear[b]	Moderate to severe, prolonged
Deep nuclear[b]–brain stem	Severe, abrupt

[a]The patterns reflect areas of *predominant* neuronal injury; considerable overlap is common. Note that two additional patterns of selective neuronal necrosis (i.e., *pontosubicular* and *cerebellar*) that occur predominantly in premature newborns (see text) are not listed here because the temporal characteristics of the insults are unknown.

[b]Deep nuclear: basal ganglia (especially putamen) and thalamus.

and *cerebellar* injury, occur particularly in premature infants with a still-to-be-defined temporal pattern of insult (see later discussion), but these patterns are usually accompanied by other features of selective neuronal injury and are discussed in this overall context. In the discussion that follows, we review the cellular aspects of selective neuronal injury, the regions of predilection, and the current concepts of pathogenesis. Because autopsied newborns have complex clinical problems, it is not possible at postmortem examination to determine with absolute certainty which of the many insults, alone or in combination, are responsible for the neuropathological findings. Indeed, hypoxia-ischemia, hypoglycemia, and hyperbilirubinemia are all characterized by acute neuronal necrosis, neuronal loss, or gliosis, albeit in different topographic distributions, and all share common mechanisms of cell injury, particularly glutamate toxicity.

Cellular Aspects

As the name selective *neuronal* necrosis implies, the neuron is the primary site of injury.[4-6,8] Experimental studies indicate that the first observable change in the neuron is cytoplasmic vacuolation, caused by mitochondrial swelling, occurring within 5 to 30 minutes after the onset of hypoxia.[39-42] In contrast to the rapid onset of *neuronal* changes in tissue cultures of neonatal mouse cerebellum exposed to hypoxia, no structural alteration was observed in astrocytes.[42] However, as discussed later, studies of a variety of developing models suggest that differentiating oligodendrocytes exhibit approximately the same sensitivity to glucose and oxygen deprivation as do neurons. On balance, the data suggest that in the immature and mature brain, the order of vulnerability is neuron → oligodendroglia → astrocyte → microglia. In the context of the present discussion, the neuron is the cellular element most vulnerable to hypoxia-ischemia.

The *temporal features* of neuronal and related changes in neonatal human brain have been well documented.[3-8,43,44] The major changes to be seen by classic light microscopy occur after 24 to 36 hours and are characterized by marked eosinophilia of neuronal cytoplasm, loss of Nissl substance (endoplasmic reticulum), condensation (pyknosis) or fragmentation (karyorrhexis) of nuclei, and breakdown of nuclear and plasma membranes, often with observable cell swelling (Fig. 18.1). Two factors alter the ability to identify such neuronal changes early

after perinatal asphyxia: (1) the gestational age of the infant and (2) the nature of the survival period. Thus recognition of neuronal changes in premature infants is difficult because of the close packing of immature cortical neurons and their relative lack of Nissl substance. Moreover, the brain of any infant who has been maintained on a respirator for several days, with compromised ventilation or perfusion, may have undergone enough autolysis to obscure early cellular changes. When these factors are not taken into account, the presence and magnitude of neuronal injury may be misjudged and may lead to spurious conclusions about the nature of the neuropathology.

The early neuronal changes are followed in several days by overt signs of cell necrosis (Fig. 18.2). Associated with this is the appearance of microglia and, by 3 to 5 days after the insult, hypertrophic astrocytes. Foamy macrophages consume the necrotic debris, and a glial mat forms over the next several weeks. Severe lesions may result in cavity formation, especially in the cerebral cortex.[3,5-8]

Apoptotic as well as *necrotic* cell death is observed in hypoxic-ischemic disease in human infants, as in neonatal animal models.[8,43,45-52] In one study of neuronal injury after *birth asphyxia*, the mean fractions of apoptotic and necrotic cells in cerebral cortex were 8.3% and 20.8%, respectively.[43] In a study of the neonatal piglet subjected to hypoxia-ischemia, apoptotic neuronal death predominated among immature neurons and necrotic cell death among mature neurons.[45] A similar susceptibility of immature neurons to apoptosis has been shown in *N*-methyl-D-aspartate (NMDA)–treated neurons in culture.[50] In one specific form of human neonatal injury, pontosubicular necrosis (see later), the predominant form of cell death appears to be apoptosis.[47,53]

Regional Aspects (Autopsied Infants)

As noted earlier, three major regional patterns of selective neuronal necrosis can be delineated in the human newborn, especially the term infant (see Table 18.3). In *diffuse* disease, certain neurons at essentially all levels of the neuraxis are affected. In predominantly *cerebral–deep nuclear* disease, the prominent involvement is of cerebral neocortex, hippocampus, and basal ganglia–thalamus. In predominantly *deep nuclear–brain stem* disease, *basal ganglia–thalamus–brain stem* is the topography. A fourth pattern, more commonly observed in the preterm infant, *pontosubicular necrosis,* is characterized by involvement of neurons of the base of the pons and the subiculum of the hippocampus (see later). A fifth pattern, observed particularly in the small premature infant but to a different degree in the term infant, involves the *cerebellum* (see later). Given that *overlap among these groups is the rule rather than the exception,* we discuss diffuse disease first, since all the vulnerable groups are involved.

Diffuse Neuronal Injury. The major sites of predilection for diffuse neuronal necrosis in the term and preterm newborn infant are shown in Table 18.4.[2-6,8,43,47,54-75]

Cerebral Cortex. Neurons of the cerebral cortex in the term infant are particularly vulnerable, most notably the hippocampus (pyramidal cells) among the cerebral cortical regions. Sommer's sector (and contiguous areas) in the term newborn and the subiculum of the hippocampus in the premature newborn (see later discussion) are especially prone to injury (see Table 18.4). With more severe injury in the term infant, the better

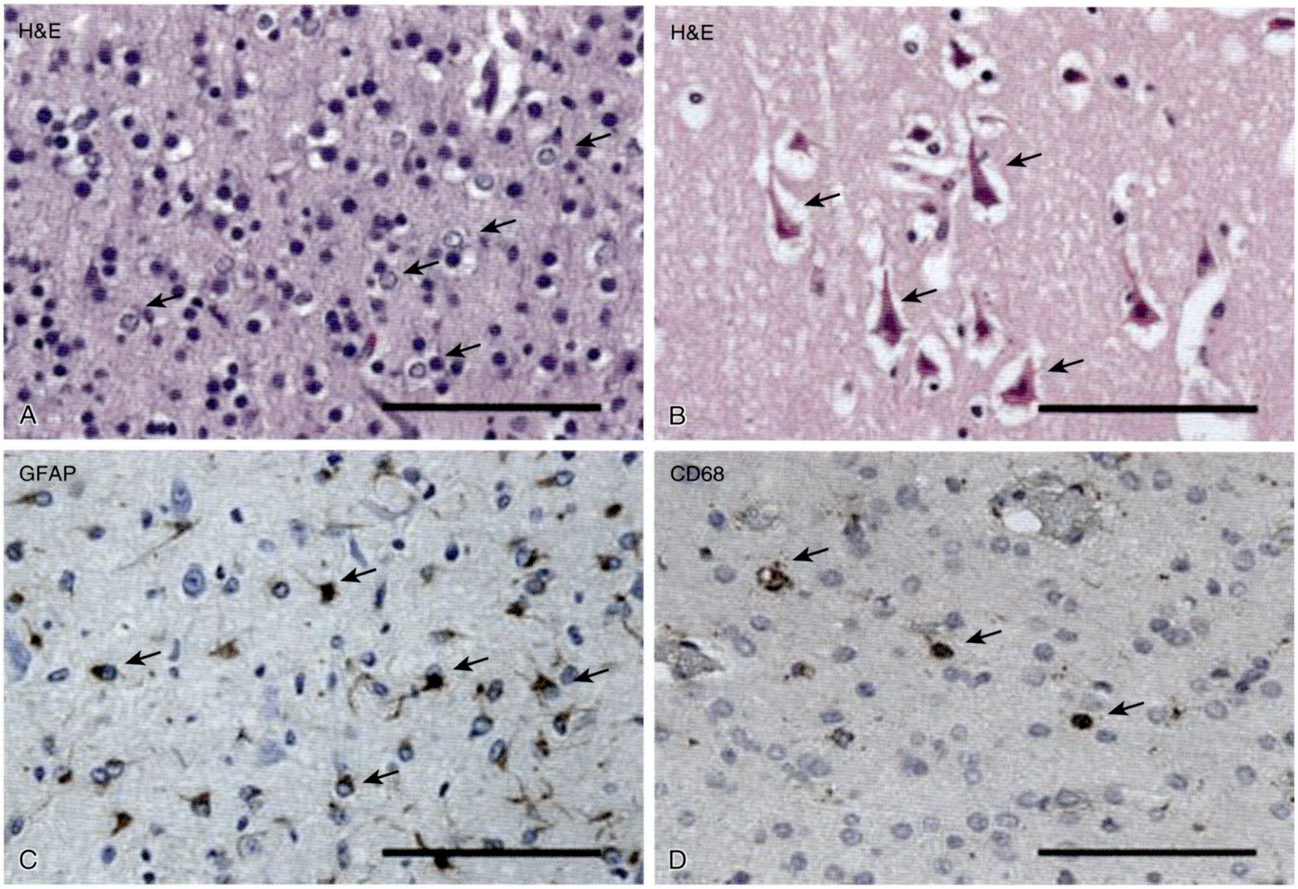

Figure 18.1 Ischemic neuronal injury *(arrowheads)* within the neonatal cerebral cortex. Note the characteristic features of (A) astrogliosis characterized by "naked" glial nuclei *(arrows)* (hematoxylin and eosin [H&E] stain); (B) acutely necrotic, hyper-eosinophilic neurons *(arrows)* (the classic *red dead* neurons of ischemic injury) (H&E); (C) reactive astrocytes stained for glial fibrillary acid protein *(arrows)* (GFAP); and (D) diffusely activated microglia stained for CD68 *(arrows)*. (With permission from Andiman SE, Haynes RL, Trachtenberg FL, et al. The cerebral cortex overlying periventricular leukomalacia: analysis of pyramidal neurons. *Brain Pathol*. 2010;20:803–814.)

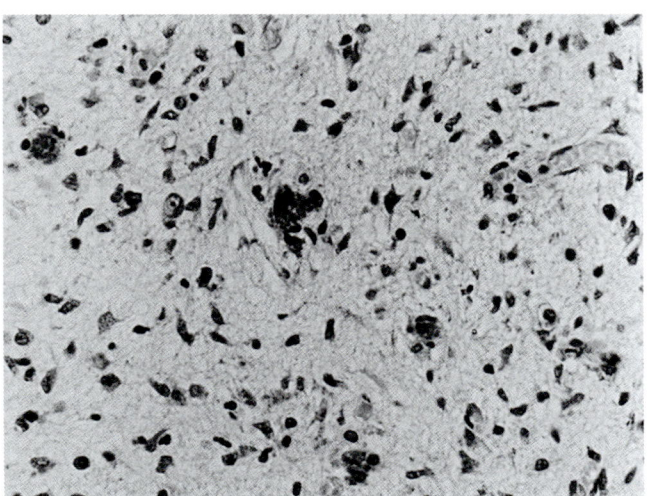

Figure 18.2 Selective neuronal necrosis. Note the *encrusted* necrotic neuron in the center of the figure. Most of the other cells in this brain-stem nucleus are reactive astrocytes and microglia. (Courtesy Dr. Margaret G. Norman.)

differentiated neurons of the calcarine (visual) cortex and of the precentral and postcentral cortices (i.e., perirolandic cortex) may be injured. In very severe injury, diffuse involvement of cerebral cortex occurs. Neurons in deeper cortical layers and particularly in the depths of sulci are especially affected. A role for patterns of blood flow in the determination of the topography is apparent from the more severe neuronal injury consistently observed in border zones between the major cerebral arteries, especially in the posterior cerebrum, and in the depths of sulci. Perhaps reflecting the relative immaturity of cerebral cortical neurons in premature infants, involvement of cerebral cortex is uncommon,[75] particularly in comparison with neurons of deep nuclear structures and brain stem (see later). However, sophisticated brain imaging studies of *premature infants at term-equivalent age and later in childhood show impressive abnormalities of cerebral cortex* (see Chapters 7, 14, and 16). Thus diminutions of cerebral cortical volumes and gyral development have been documented. The disturbances may reflect abnormalities of cerebral cortical *development* and may be related to concomitant cerebral white matter injury (see Chapter 14). The important point in this context is that the

TABLE 18.4 Sites of Predilection for the Diffuse Form of Hypoxic-Ischemic Selective Neuronal Injury in Premature and Term Newborns[a]

BRAIN REGION	PREMATURE	TERM NEWBORN
Cerebral neocortex		+
Hippocampus		
Sommer's sector		+
Subiculum	+	
Deep nuclear structures		
Caudate-putamen	+	+
Globus pallidus	+	+
Thalamus	+	+
Brain stem		
Cranial nerve nuclei	+	+
Pons (ventral)	+	+
Inferior olivary nuclei	+	+
Cerebellum		
Purkinje cells		+
Granule cells (internal, external)	±	±
Spinal cord		
Anterior horn cells (alone)		±
Anterior horn cells and contiguous cells (? infarction)	±	

+, Common; ±, less common.
[a]See text for references.

abnormalities of cerebral cortex may not reflect direct cortical neuronal necrosis, at least as evidenced by histological criteria.

Deep Nuclear Structures. Involvement of deep nuclear structures, *principally thalamus and basal ganglia,* is particularly characteristic of hypoxic-ischemic neuronal injury in both preterm and term newborns. With diffuse disease, *thalamus* is particularly vulnerable. As discussed later, a particular pattern of injury in term newborns involves a combination of affection of neurons of thalamus, basal ganglia, and brain stem, with relative sparing of cerebral cortical neurons. Hypothalamic neurons and those of the lateral geniculate nuclei (thalamus) are also especially vulnerable. In preterm newborns, involvement of deep nuclear structures is a major form of gray matter injury.[75] Injury to thalamus and basal ganglia was apparent in 40% to 50% of one series of 41 premature infants studied at autopsy (see later).[75] Of the *basal ganglia,* neurons of the caudate, putamen, and globus pallidus are often injured in both term and premature newborns (see Table 18.4). Neurons of the putamen (and head of the caudate nucleus) are somewhat more likely to be affected in the term infant, whereas neurons of the globus pallidus are more likely to be affected in the premature infant.[5,6] This distinction is subtle, however. Neuronal injury to basal ganglia is usually accompanied by thalamic neuronal injury. Indeed, in my experience, the combination of putaminal and thalamic neuronal injury is typical of neonatal hypoxic-ischemic disease, especially in the term infant.

Brain Stem. Particularly characteristic of hypoxic-ischemic encephalopathy in the newborn is involvement of the brain stem.[4,6-8,54-67,69-72,74-88] In general, hypoxic-ischemic injury to brain stem in the term newborn tends to be more or less restricted to neurons. With premature infants, although neurons are involved primarily, injury may be so marked as to result in cystic necrosis.[65] As discussed later, involvement of neurons of brain stem may occur in combination with basal ganglia and thalamic involvement.

In *midbrain,* the inferior colliculus stands out in terms of vulnerability. This is in keeping with the studies of Ranck, Windle, and Faro[89,90] of asphyxiated fetal monkeys, particularly with total asphyxia. Neuronal injury is also found frequently in the neurons of the oculomotor and trochlear nuclei, substantia nigra, and reticular formation.

In *pons,* particularly frequently involved are the motor nuclei of the fifth and seventh cranial nerves, the reticular formation, the dorsal cochlear nuclei, and the pontine nuclei. Striking involvement of the nuclei in ventral pons and of the neurons of the subicular portion of the hippocampus in some cases led Friede[6] to the term *pontosubicular neuronal necrosis.* This pattern of injury is discussed later.

In *medulla,* particularly vulnerable are the dorsal nuclei of the vagus, nucleus ambiguus (ninth and tenth cranial nerves), inferior olivary nuclei, and the cuneate and gracilis nuclei. Involvement of neurons of the inferior olivary nuclei is the single most common brain-stem neuronal lesion in both term and preterm infants.[8,72,75] In one series of 41 premature infants studied at autopsy, fully 90% had evidence of inferior olivary injury.[75] Important clinical correlates of many of these brain stem lesions are discussed in Chapter 20.

Cerebellum. The cerebellum is especially vulnerable to hypoxic-ischemic neuronal injury, and the Purkinje cells in the term infant and the granule cell neurons (of both the internal and external granule cell layers) in both the term and premature infant are the most vulnerable cerebellar neurons (see Table 18.4). Neurons of the vermis may be especially easily injured in the term infant.[91,92] Neurons of the dentate nucleus (and other roof nuclei) are also somewhat susceptible to injury, more so in the preterm newborn than at later ages. In the term infant, a subsequent disturbance of cerebellar growth, especially involving the vermis, has been observed by magnetic resonance imaging (MRI).[91,92] In this setting, frequent concomitant injury to thalamus and basal ganglia also raises the possibility of transsynaptic effects.[91-93] Involvement of the cerebellum, especially the cerebellar hemispheres, and subsequently impaired cerebellar growth are particular features of very premature infants and are sufficiently distinctive to be discussed as a separate form of selective neuronal necrosis (see later).

Spinal Cord. Affection of anterior horn cells by hypoxic-ischemic injury has been identified.[5,94,95] This involvement is accompanied clinically by hypotonia and weakness and electrophysiologically by signs of anterior horn cell disturbance; it may underlie at least some cases of so-called atonic cerebral palsy (see Chapter 20). The neuronal injury occurs in typical form in the term infant and is similar cytopathologically to that observed in other regions. When present in the premature infant, the lesion, as with hypoxic-ischemic injury to brain stem, often also involves contiguous cellular elements, which may have the histological appearance of infarction and may be accompanied by hemorrhage.[94]

Cerebral–Deep Nuclear Neuronal Injury. Although systematic data are difficult to gather, MRI studies of *asphyxiated* term infants suggest that approximately 35% to 85% exhibit predominantly cerebral–deep nuclear neuronal involvement.[96-102] Among neurons of cerebral cortex, those in the parasagittal areas of perirolandic cortex are especially likely to be affected. Involvement of hippocampus and other neocortical areas was described earlier. The most common additional neuronal lesion affects basal ganglia, especially putamen, and thalamus. The pathogenesis appears usually to involve a *moderate or moderate-to-severe insult that evolves in a gradual manner* (i.e., a "prolonged, partial" insult; see the section on pathogenesis in Chapter 19).

Deep Nuclear–Brain-Stem Neuronal Injury. Although involvement of neurons of basal ganglia and thalamus occurs in approximately two thirds of *asphyxiated* term infants, in approximately 15% to 20% of infants with hypoxic-ischemic disease, involvement of deep nuclear structures (i.e., basal ganglia, thalamus, and tegmentum of brain stem) is the *predominant* lesion.[6,70,71,79,85,103-105] Until the advent of MRI, detection of this deep gray matter predominance in the living infant had not been accomplished readily; thus the relative frequency of this pattern of neuronal injury was not recognized. However, studies based on MRI and careful clinical-pathological correlations have delineated this pattern as a distinct entity.[70,71,85] The topography of the neuropathology is illustrated in Fig. 18.3.

At least some cases of this predominantly deep gray matter form of selective neuronal injury may evolve to *status marmoratus,* a disorder of basal ganglia and thalamus not seen in its complete form until the latter part of the first year of life, despite the perinatal timing of the insult. The basic initiating role of hypoxia-ischemia is demonstrated not only by clinical data in human infants (see later discussion) but also by the reproduction of the lesion in the newborn rat subjected to hypoxic-ischemic insult[106,107] as well as in the term fetal monkey subjected to intrauterine asphyxia.[19]

Status marmoratus has three major features: neuronal loss, gliosis, and hypermyelination.[5-7,108] *Hypermyelination* is the characteristic feature of the lesion; this term refers to an apparent increase in amount and an abnormal distribution of myelinated fibers within the affected nuclear structures, especially the putamen (Fig. 18.4). The hypermyelination has been noted at as early as 8 months of life.[6] The abnormal myelin pattern gives a *marbled appearance* to the basal ganglia, hence the term *status marmoratus* or *état marbré.* Previous observations by light microscopy had led to the suggestion that the many myelinated fibers in status marmoratus were axons, and the idea that such apparent overgrowth was a result of aberrant myelination of nerve fibers was accepted for many years. However, electron microscopic techniques were used to show that the abnormal myelinated fibers, at least in part, are astrocytic processes.[109] It appears that the very young brain, at the time of normal myelination, may myelinate fibers that are not axonal in origin. Thus this distinctive response to injury appears to depend on the *time of occurrence* of the insult as well as the locus of the injury. Nevertheless, the proportion of infants with hypoxic-ischemic involvement of basal ganglia and thalamus who develop status marmoratus and the determinants for the occurrence of this relatively specific pathological response to injury versus that of only gliosis and atrophy remain to be determined. Concerning the sequela of gliosis

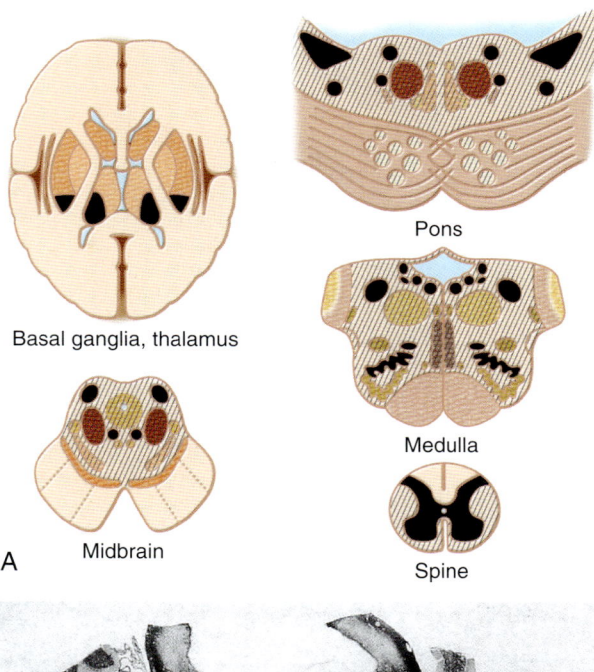

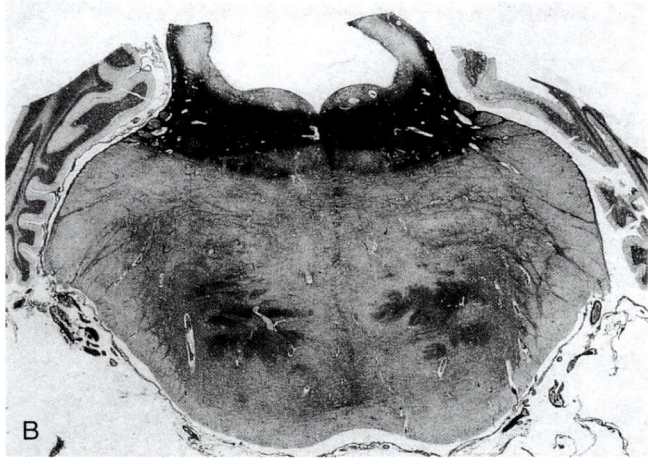

Figure 18.3 Neuropathology of the deep nuclear–brain-stem form of selective neuronal necrosis. (A) Schematic depiction of the topography of the lesions in a typical case of a term newborn subjected to severe, terminal asphyxia. Dark areas indicate nuclei with neuronal loss, and the diagonally striped areas indicate regions of marked gliosis. (B) Holzer stain of the pons for gliosis in a typical case. The tegmentum is atrophied and deeply stained because of gliosis; the base of the pons is nearly normal. (With permission from Natsume J, Watanabe K, Kuno K, Hayakawa F, Hashizume Y. Clinical, neurophysiologic, and neuropathological features of an infant with brain damage of total asphyxia type (Myers). *Pediatr Neurol.* 1995;13:61–64.)

and atrophy alone, a reasonable speculation is that an injury so severe as to eliminate oligodendrocytes as well as neurons may prevent the occurrence of the typical hypermyelination of status marmoratus. As discussed later (see the section on pathogenesis in Chapter 19), the hypoxic-ischemic insult associated with the occurrence of predominant involvement of deep gray matter structures typically is *severe* and *abrupt* in evolution (i.e., an "acute, total" insult).

Pontosubicular Neuronal Necrosis. Pontosubicular neuronal necrosis is a fourth type of selective neuronal injury with predominant involvement of neurons of the basis pontis (i.e.,

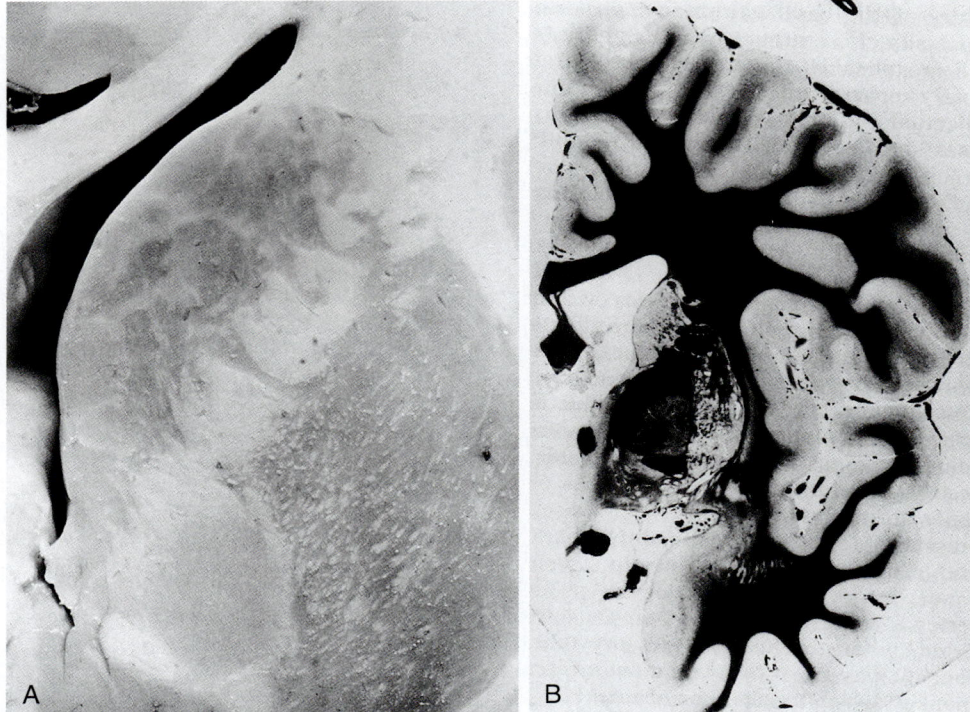

Figure 18.4 Status marmoratus. Coronal sections of cerebrum from two infants who died several years after the perinatal insult. (A) Formalin-fixed and unstained; note the marbled appearance of the caudate nucleus and putamen. (B) Stained for myelin; note the black-staining myelin, particularly in the putamen. (Courtesy Dr. EP Richardson Jr.)

TABLE 18.5	Pontosubicular Neuronal Necrosis in the Premature Newborn[a]

Pons and subiculum are common sites of neuronal injury in the premature newborn
Strong association with periventricular leukomalacia
Clinically associated with hypoxia-ischemia, hypocarbia, and hyperoxia (reproducible in newborn rat by hyperoxia alone)

[a]See text for references.

TABLE 18.6	Cerebellar Injury in the Premature Newborn

Cerebellar injury, especially involving cerebellar hemispheres, generally bilateral and symmetrical, especially in very small premature infants
Microscopic features include cerebellar neuronal injury (including neuronal precursors of external granule cell layer), cerebellar white matter necrosis/gliosis, and neuronal injury to brain stem relay nuclei to cerebellum
Diminished cerebellar volume is the most common structural sequela
Often associated with supratentorial injury, especially intraventricular hemorrhage and cerebral white matter injury, and with injury to relay nuclei in brain stem, all principally hypoxic-ischemic in nature
Etiology may reflect a combination of transsynaptic trophic disturbances and direct neuronal injury.

---

not the tegmentum, as described earlier) and the subiculum of hippocampus.[47,66,67,74,78,80-83,110-112] Among all types of selective neuronal injuries, pontosubicular neuronal necrosis is by far the least common. The lesion is characteristic of the premature infant but occurs in infants up to 1 to 2 months beyond term (Table 18.5).[66,67,78,80-83,110,113] A strong association exists with periventricular leukomalacia (PVL). Although the disorder is characterized principally by affection of neurons of ventral pons and of subiculum of hippocampus, neuronal death in the fascia dentata of hippocampus was observed in 60% of cases in one series.[67] In several neuropathological studies that included electron microscopy, labeling of oligonucleosomal fragments, and detection of Fas receptor and activated caspase-3, the neuronal death in pontosubicular neuronal necrosis appeared to be predominantly apoptotic.[47,53,111,112,114]

Cerebellar Injury. *Cerebellar injury is particularly characteristic of premature infants, especially those of extremely low birth weight,*

and is sufficiently distinctive to be considered a fifth type of selective neuronal necrosis (Table 18.6). This injury has occurred primarily in premature infants with serious respiratory disease, although single major hypoxic-ischemic insults typical of asphyxiated term infants have not been present. Cerebellar disturbance has been identified most often by the finding by MRI of bilateral, generally symmetrical decreases of cerebellar hemispheric volumes at term-equivalent age or later in infancy or childhood.[115-127] Although a few cases have been focal and asymmetrical, suggestive of infarction, nearly all abnormalities

TABLE 18.7	Predominant MRI Patterns of Injury and Approximate Frequency in Presumed Neonatal Hypoxic-Ischemic Encephalopathy[a]
PREDOMINANT BRAIN STRUCTURE(S) INVOLVED	**APPROXIMATE PERCENT OF TOTAL[b]**
Selective neuronal injury	—
Diffuse (*global*)	5%–10%
Deep nuclear—cerebral cortex	40%–80%
Deep nuclear—brain stem	10%–20%
Parasagittal cerebral injury	40%–60%
Cerebral white matter injury	15%

[a]Data from references cited in the text, involving primarily term newborns with perinatal asphyxia (fetal heart rate abnormalities, acute sentinel event, cord blood acidosis, low Apgar scores, neonatal encephalopathy, and presumed hypoxia-ischemia) (see Chapters 19 and 20 for clinical details).
[b]Lesions often overlap; thus numbers do not add up to 100%. Table does not include asphyxiated infants with normal MRI (15% to 30%) or stroke pattern (5% to 10%).

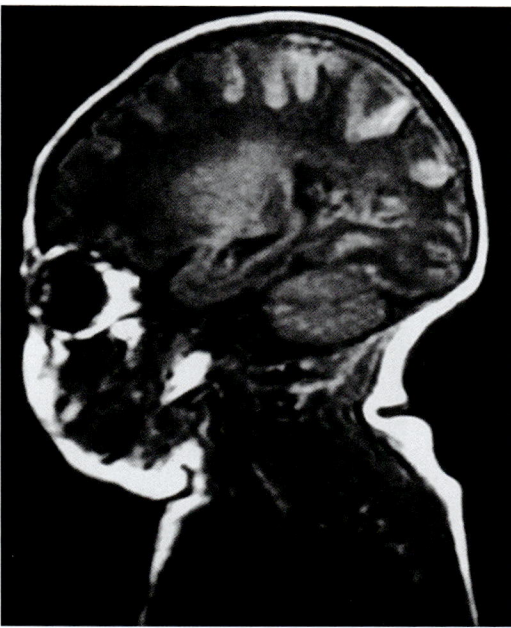

Figure 18.5 Magnetic resonance imaging scan of cortical neuronal injury. Infant had severe apnea on the first day of life, and scan was performed on the third postnatal day. On this parasagittal fluid-attenuated inversion recovery image, note the striking cortical highlighting, especially marked in depths of sulci.

have consisted of bilateral and symmetrical diminutions in size. The possibility that the proliferating neuronal precursor cells of the external granule cell layer are injured, especially by hemosiderin from intraventricular hemorrhage, is suggested by recent MRI studies (see Chapters 14 and 23). The additional possibility of a trophic disturbance, perhaps related to supratentorial white matter injury, is suggested by a strong association with *cerebral* white matter injury (see Chapters 14 and 23).[123,125,126] Moreover, the high frequency of injury to neurons of brain-stem cerebellar relay nuclei (see earlier) also raises the possibility of impaired trophic interactions at the transsynaptic level.

Regional Aspects (Living Infants)

The regional features of *selective neuronal injury* have been identified in living infants by neuroimaging, especially MRI.[70,71,73,85,128-142] The *three major patterns* include diffuse neuronal injury (involving cerebral cortex, deep nuclear structures [basal ganglia and thalamus], and brain stem), deep nuclear–cerebral cortex injury, and deep nuclear–brain-stem injury (Table 18.7). The most common temporal characteristics of the insults leading to these three major regional patterns were noted earlier (see Table 18.3). Pontosubicular neuronal necrosis and most cerebellar neuronal injuries, identified neuropathologically (see earlier), are not readily visualized in vivo.

The major regional patterns of selective neuronal injury very often occur in combination, although, despite the overlap, a single *predominant pattern* can frequently be identified. The cerebral cortical involvement is most prominent in perirolandic cortex and in depths of sulci. The deep nuclear involvement is most prominent in thalamus and putamen, and the intervening posterior limb of the internal capsule is affected in moderate or severe thalamoputaminal injury. The affection of the posterior limb has important prognostic implications (see Chapter 20).[136,143] The brain-stem involvement is most apparent in dorsal tegmental areas. Examples of these patterns are shown in Figs. 18.5 to 18.8 and discussed in greater detail

in Chapters 19 and 20. The relative distribution of the three predominant neuronal patterns defined by MRI in primarily full-term infants with the clinical characteristics of perinatal asphyxia is shown in Table 18.7.

Parasagittal Cerebral Injury

Cellular and Regional Aspects (Autopsied Infants)

Parasagittal cerebral injury refers to a lesion of the cerebral cortex and subcortical white matter with a characteristic distribution (i.e., parasagittal and superomedial aspects of the cerebral convexities) (Figs. 18.9 and 18.10). The injury is bilateral and, although usually symmetrical, may be more striking in one hemisphere than the other. The posterior aspect of the cerebral hemispheres, especially the parieto-occipital regions, is more impressively affected than the anterior aspect. The term *watershed infarct* has been used to describe the lesion and to emphasize its ischemic nature (see later discussion). We prefer the more descriptive term *parasagittal cerebral injury*.

Parasagittal cerebral injury is characterized by necrosis of the cortex and the immediately subjacent white matter; neuronal elements are most severely affected. The areas of infarction may be hemorrhagic, although more usually they are not. In particularly severe cases, the necrosis extends to a large proportion of the lateral cerebral convexity (see Fig. 18.10B), especially in the parieto-occipital regions, the most vulnerable regions of the cerebrum. The precise pathological evolution of parasagittal cerebral injury in the newborn is not known, but atrophic gyri, ulegyria, or both are the chronic neuropathological correlates. Parasagittal cerebral injury is characteristic of the full-term infant with perinatal asphyxia; it is unlikely, in fact, that cerebral necrosis in the parasagittal distribution occurs in the premature infant to a major degree, for reasons outlined in the section on periventricular leukomalacia.

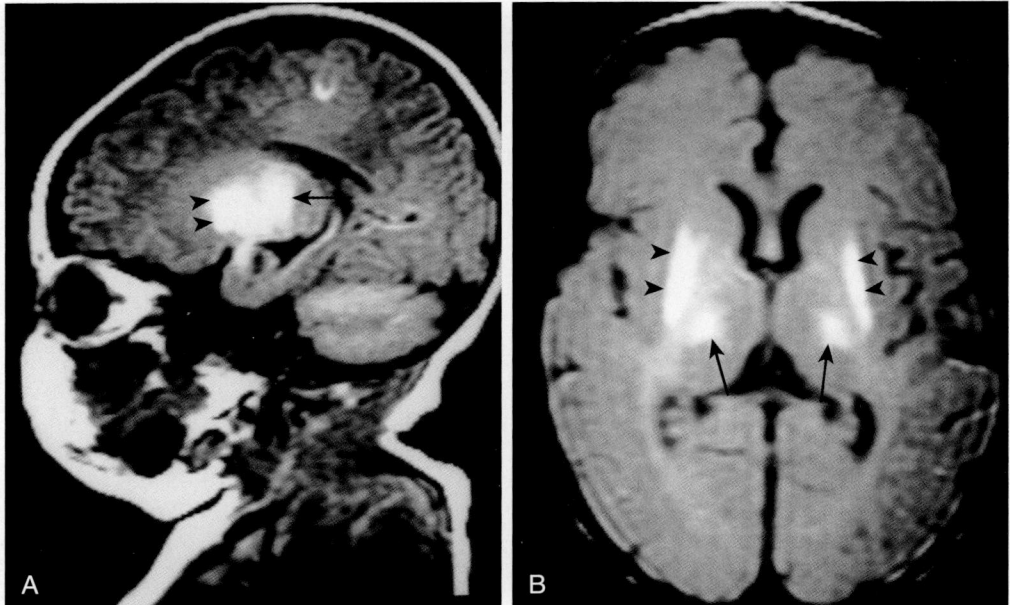

Figure 18.6 **Magnetic resonance imaging scans of hypoxic-ischemic injury to basal ganglia and thalamus.** Scans obtained from a 5-day-old infant who experienced severe perinatal asphyxia. (A) Note, in the parasagittal T1-weighted image, markedly increased signal in basal ganglia, especially in putamen *(arrowheads)*, and thalamus *(arrow)*. (B) The axial proton density image also demonstrates the injury well in the same distribution. (Courtesy Dr. Patrick Barnes.)

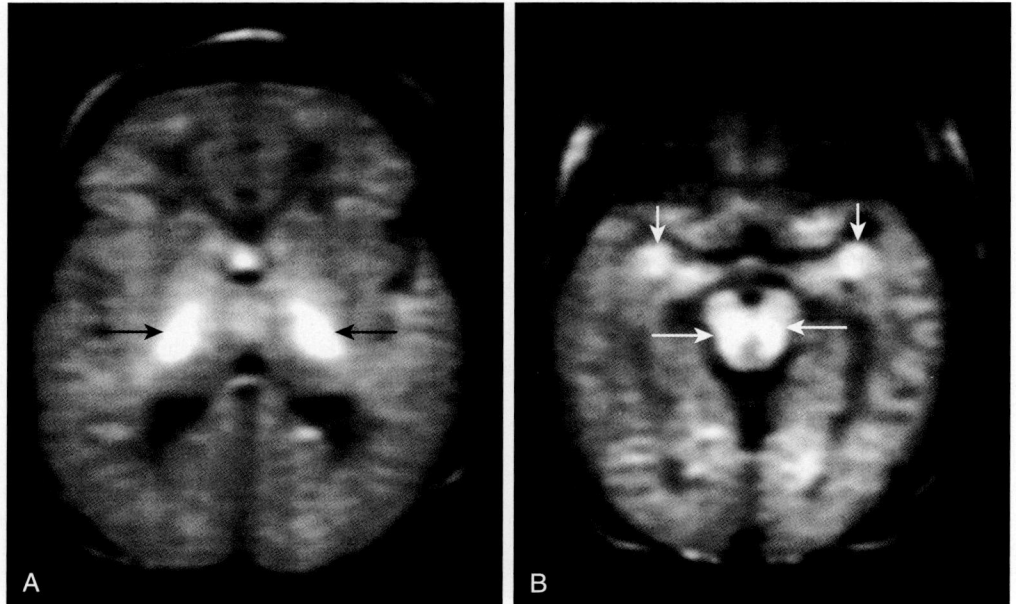

Figure 18.7 **Diffusion-weighted magnetic resonance image (DWI) of deep nuclear and brain-stem injury.** This full-term infant experienced a severe late intrapartum asphyxial insult. Magnetic resonance imaging (MRI) and DWI scans were carried out late on the first postnatal day. No definite abnormality was discerned by conventional MRI (not shown). However, DWI shows striking decreased diffusion (increased signal) in basal ganglia–thalamus *(arrows* in A), hippocampus *(short arrows* in B), and midbrain tegmentum *(long arrows* in B).

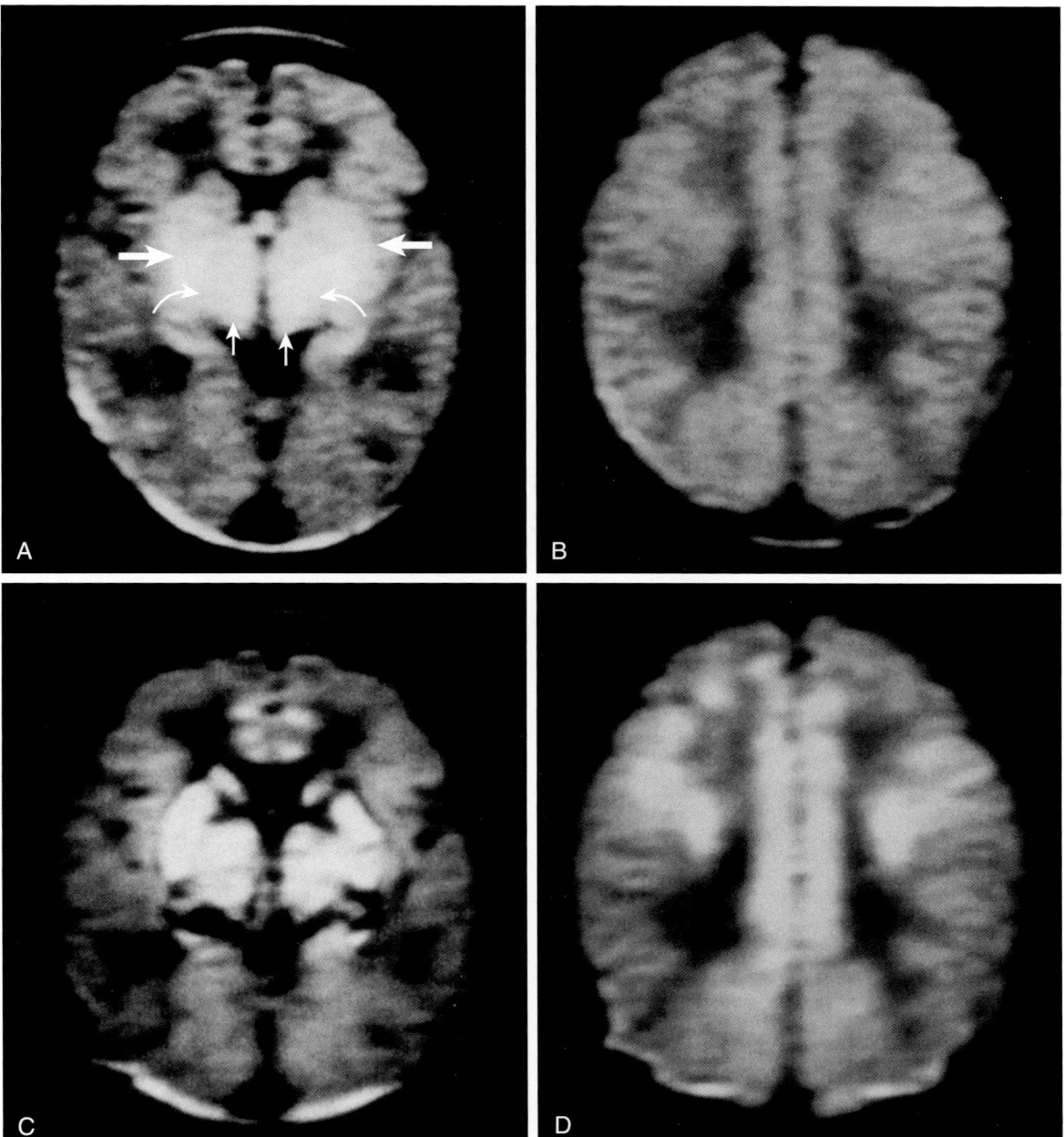

Figure 18.8 Differential regional decreases in diffusion after neonatal hypoxia-ischemia. Diffusion-weighted magnetic resonance images (A and B) obtained 6 hours after cardiorespiratory arrest show bright signal—that is, decreased diffusion—in basal ganglia *(thick arrows)*, thalami *(curved arrows)*, and dorsal brain stem *(thin arrows)*. There is no decrease in diffusion in cerebral cortex. Diffusion-weighted images (C and D) obtained 32 hours after cardiorespiratory arrest show persistence of the decreased diffusion in deep nuclear structures (A) but also bright signal (decreased diffusion) in cerebral cortex. Conventional magnetic resonance imaging (not shown) at 6 hours was normal but clearly abnormal at 32 hours. (With permission from Soul JS, Robertson RL, Tzika AA, du Plessis AJ, Volpe JJ. Time course of changes in diffusion-weighted magnetic resonance imaging in a case of neonatal encephalopathy with defined onset and duration of hypoxic-ischemic insult. *Pediatrics.* 2001;108:1211–1214.)

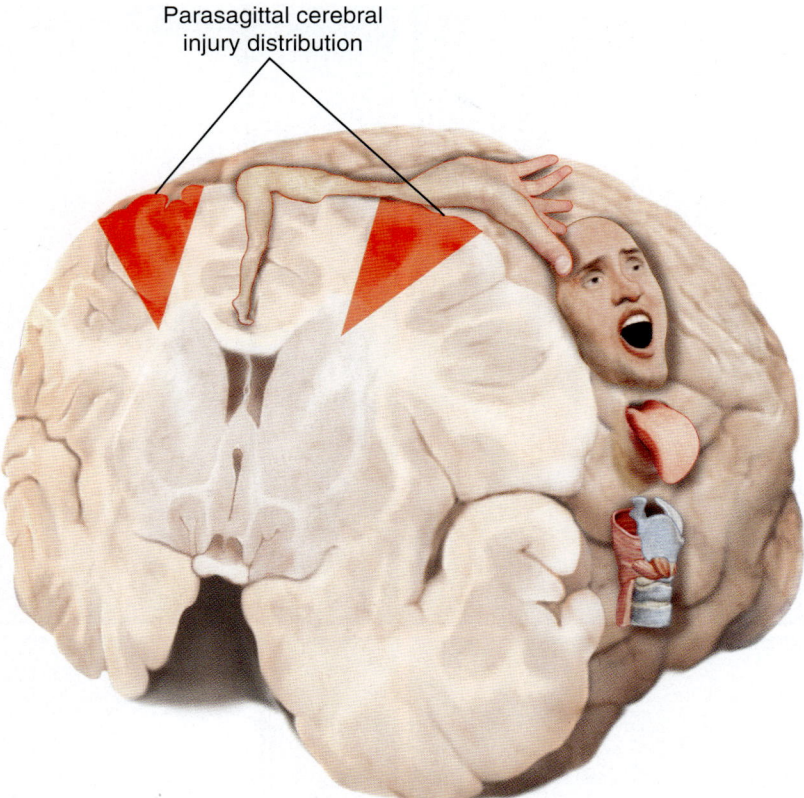

Parasagittal cerebral
injury distribution

Figure 18.9 Parasagittal cerebral injury, coronal view. Schematic diagram of the distribution of the injury, which is indicated by symmetrical red areas in superomedial aspects of cerebrum.

Parasagittal cerebral injury has been well documented in classic neuropathological writings (e.g., the work of Friede,[144] Courville,[145] and Norman et al.[146]), particularly those concerned with older survivors with cerebral palsy. However, the lesion has been more difficult to define as *an isolated entity* in neuropathological studies of infants dying in the neonatal period, although examples are apparent (see Fig. 18.10). We believe that the difficulty in pathological identification of the discrete lesion in the neonatal period relates to the severe nature of the cases in *newborns who die.* Thus the neuropathological findings are most often diffuse and severe, very frequently complicated by autolytic changes related to survival for many hours or days on life support. These diffuse changes obscure elemental lesions, such as parasagittal cerebral injury, which, however, are identifiable in those less severely affected infants who *survive.* In keeping with this explanation is the observation of a high frequency in asphyxiated term newborns (≈90% of whom survive) of parasagittal cerebral injury identifiable by radionuclide brain scanning,[147,148] positron emission tomography,[149] and especially MRI[99,131,150] (see section on diagnosis in Chapter 20). Indeed, in a recent MRI study of 173 term infants with neonatal encephalopathy, fully 45% (*n* = 78) were found to have watershed injury as the predominant lesion.[131] The computed tomography scan, still often used in evaluation of such infants, is not particularly sensitive for the detection of this lesion because the axial images frequently fail to detect the superficial corticosubcortical lesions of parasagittal injury. The advent of MRI scanning, with coronal and lateral views, has proved more effective in identification of parasagittal

cerebral injury in vivo and has provided further documentation of its frequency (see Chapter 20).

The pathogenesis of parasagittal cerebral injury relates principally to a disturbance in cerebral perfusion. The two factors underlying the propensity of the parasagittal region to ischemic injury relate to parasagittal vascular anatomical factors and cerebral ischemia with a pressure-passive state of the cerebral circulation, as mentioned in the discussion of pathogenesis in Chapter 19.

Regional Aspects (Living Infants)

Parasagittal cerebral injury, often characterized as a "watershed" injury, has been identified in approximately 40% to 60% of asphyxiated newborns (see Table 18.7).[70,71,73,85,128-143,151,152] MRI is the best neuroimaging modality for identifying the lesion (Figs. 18.11 and 18.12 and Chapter 19).

Cerebral White Matter Injury

Regional Aspects (Autopsied Infants)

Cerebral white matter injury is a common neuropathological accompaniment of hypoxic-ischemic encephalopathy in the term infant. The features are reminiscent of those described in detail in Chapter 14 concerning the premature infant; they are not reiterated here.

Regional Aspects (Living Infants)

MRI studies of term infants with hypoxic-ischemic encephalopathy indicate that the predominant lesion may involve *primarily cerebral white matter.*[130,133,153,154] Approximately

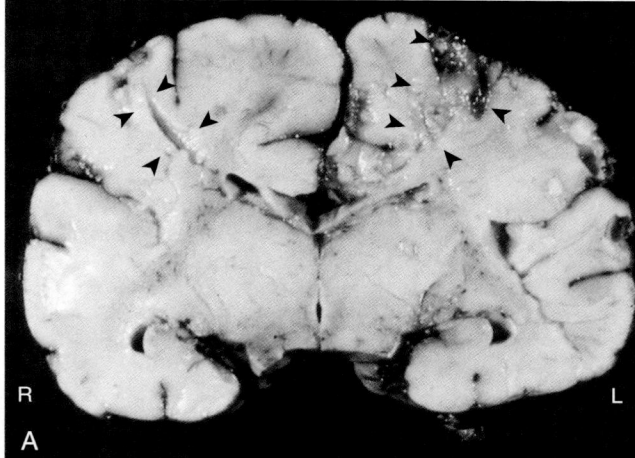

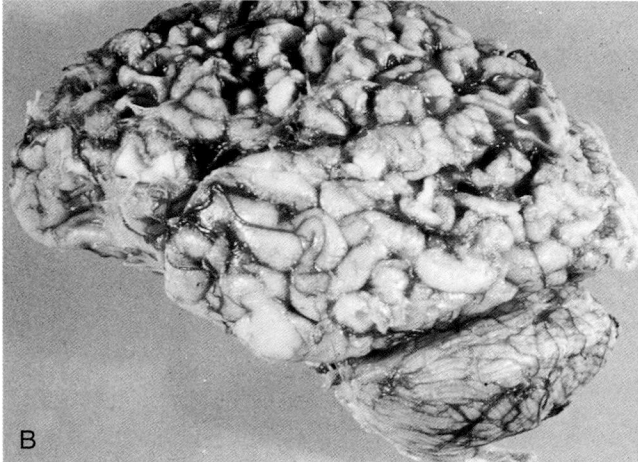

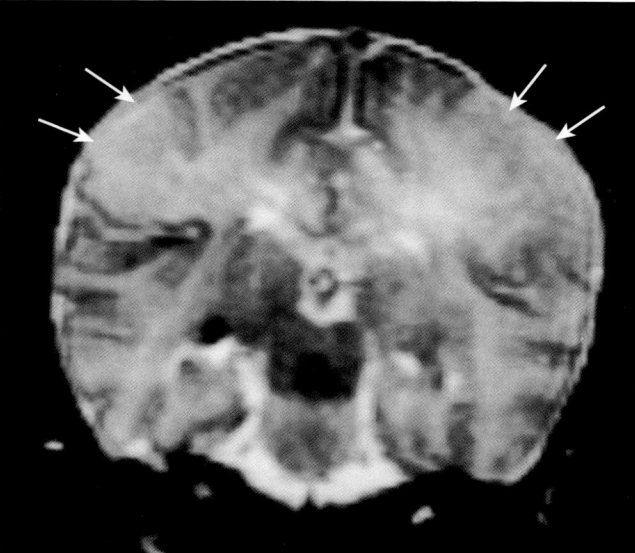

Figure 18.11 Magnetic resonance imaging (MRI) of parasagittal cerebral injury. Coronal T2-weighted MRI scan obtained on postnatal day 4 from an infant with perinatal asphyxia and neonatal seizures. Note the striking abnormality in parasagittal areas bilaterally *(arrows)*. Computerized tomography performed one day earlier produced equivocal findings (not shown). (Courtesy Dr. Patrick Barnes.)

Figure 18.10 **Parasagittal cerebral injury.** (A) Coronal section of cerebrum in an asphyxiated, full-term infant who died on the third postnatal day. Areas of necrosis of cerebral cortex and subcortical white matter in the parasagittal regions are marked by arrowheads. (B) Lateral view of cerebral convexity in a 6-month-old infant who had experienced severe perinatal asphyxia. Note the cortical atrophy in parasagittal distribution (compare with Fig. 18.8). (B, Courtesy Dr. Alan Hill.)

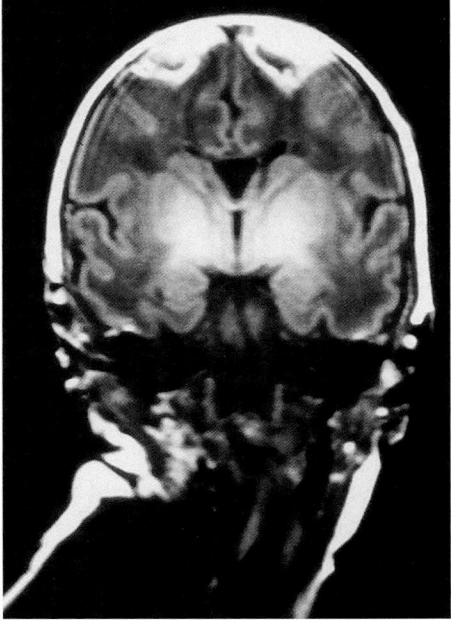

Figure 18.12 Magnetic resonance imaging (MRI) of parasagittal cerebral injury. Coronal T1-weighted MRI, obtained on the fifth postnatal day in an asphyxiated term infant, shows striking triangular lesions in the parasagittal areas bilaterally. Increased signal is also apparent in basal ganglia and thalamus bilaterally. (Courtesy Dr. Alan Hill.)

15% of infants exhibit this pattern of injury as the dominant abnormality (see Table 18.7). The involvement, detected by MRI (Fig. 18.13), is usually more prominent posteriorly than anteriorly and affects periventricular and central white matter. The similarities with cerebral white matter injury (or periventricular leukomalacia) of very premature infants are apparent (see Chapter 16 for details). Important contributing pathogenetic factors for predominant cerebral white matter injury in infants with hypoxic-ischemic encephalopathy are late preterm gestational age, neonatal hypoglycemia, and often chronic hemodynamic instability. The last of these is supported by the observation that the majority of term infants with congenital heart disease dying days after cardiac surgery exhibit, at autopsy, periventricular leukomalacia as a prominent lesion.[72] Involvement of cerebral white matter is also the dominant neuroimaging feature of infants with complex congenital heart disease both before and after cardiac surgery.[155]

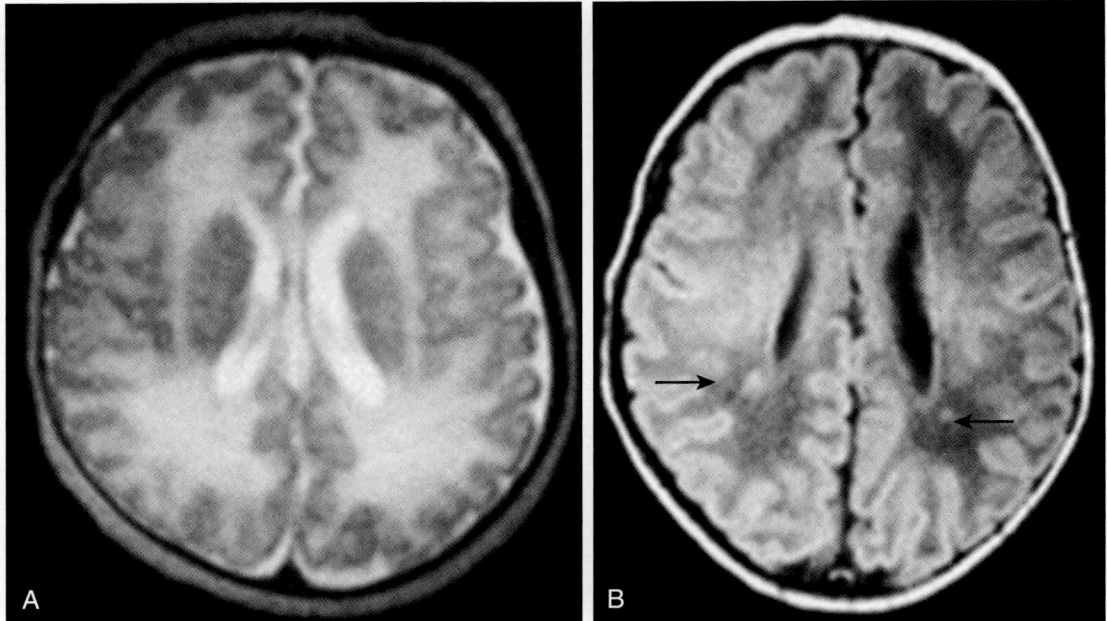

Figure 18.13 Magnetic resonance imaging (MRI) scan of cerebral white matter injury in postasphyxial term newborns. Note in (A), the T2-weighted image, abnormally increased signal in the posterior cerebral white matter. In a separate case (B), the T1-weighted image shows abnormally decreased signal in posterior cerebral white matter and focal punctate lesions *(arrows)*. (With permission from Martinez-Biarge, Bregant T, Wusthoff CJ, et al. White matter and cortical injury in hypoxic-ischemic encephalopathy: antecedent factors and 2-year outcome. *J Pediatr*. 2012;161(5):799–807.)

REFERENCES

1. Spector RG. Water content of the immature rat brain following cerebral anoxia and ischaemia. *Br J Exp Pathol*. 1962;43:472.
2. Streicher E, Wisniewski H, Klatzo I. Resistance of immature brain to experimental cerebral edema. *Neurology*. 1965;15:833.
3. Larroche JC. *Developmental Pathology of the Neonate*. New York: Excerpta Medica; 1977.
4. Norman MG. Perinatal brain damage. In: Rosenberg HS, Boilande RP, eds. *Perspectives in Pediatric Pathology*. Vol. 4. Chicago: Mosby; 1978:41-92.
5. Rorke LB. *Pathology of Perinatal Brain Injury*. New York: Raven Press; 1982.
6. Friede RL. *Developmental Neuropathology*. 2nd ed. New York: Springer-Verlag; 1989.
7. Rorke LB. Anatomical features of the developing brain implicated in pathogenesis of hypoxic-ischemic injury. *Brain Pathol*. 1992; 2(3):211-221.
8. Folkerth RD, Kinney HC. Disorders of the perinatal period. In: Love S, Louis DN, Ellison D, eds. *Greenfield's Neuropathology*. Vol. 1. 8th ed. London: Hodder Arnold; 2008:241-334.
9. Clifford SH. The effects of asphyxia on the newborn infant. *J Pediatr*. 1941;18:567.
10. Thorn K. Cerebral symptoms in the newborn. *Acta Paediatr Scand*. 1969;195(suppl):1-8.
11. Pryse-Davies J, Beard RW. A necropsy study of brain swelling in the newborn with special reference to cerebellar herniation. *J Pathol*. 1972;109:51.
12. Anderson JM, Belton NR. Water and electrolyte abnormalities in the human brain after severe intrapartum asphyxia. *J Neurol Neurosurg Psychiatry*. 1974;37(5):514-520.
13. Gilles FH, Leviton A, Dooling EC. *The Developing Human Brain: Growth and Epidemiologic Neuropathology*. Boston: John Wright, Inc.; 1983.
14. Levene MI, Evans DH. Medical management of raised intracranial pressure after severe birth asphyxia. *Arch Dis Child*. 1985;60(1):12-16.
15. Levene MI, Evans DH, Forde A, Archer LNJ. Value of intracranial pressure monitoring of asphyxiated newborn infants. *Dev Med Child Neurol*. 1987;29(3):311-319.
16. Clancy R, Legido A, Newell R, Bruce D, Baumgart S, Fox WW. Continuous intracranial pressure monitoring and serial electroencephalographic recordings in severely asphyxiated term neonates. *Am J Dis Child*. 1988;142(7):740-747.
17. Lupton BA, Hill A, Roland EH, Whitfield MF, Flodmark O. Brain swelling in the asphyxiated term newborn: pathogenesis and outcome. *Pediatrics*. 1988;82(2):139-146.
18. Adhikari M, Moodley M, Desai PK. Mannitol in neonatal cerebral oedema. *Brain Dev*. 1990;12(3):349-351.
19. Myers RE. Four patterns of perinatal brain damage and their conditions of occurrence in primates. *Adv Neurol*. 1975;10(1):223-234.
20. Brann AW Jr, Myers RE. Central nervous system findings in the newborn monkey following severe in utero partial asphyxia. *Neurology*. 1975;25(4):327-338.
21. Myers RE. Two patterns of perinatal brain damage and their conditions of occurrence. *Am J Obstet Gynecol*. 1972;112(2):246-276.
22. Myers RE. Fetal asphyxia due to umbilical cord compression. Metabolic and brain pathologic consequences. *Biol Neonate*. 1975; 26(1):21-43.
23. Myers RE. Two classes of dysergic brain abnormality and their conditions of occurrence. *Arch Neurol*. 1973;29(6):394-399.
24. Selzer ME, Myers RE, Holstein SB. Prolonged partial asphyxia: effects on fetal brain water and electrolytes. *Neurology*. 1972; 22(7):732-737.
25. Bondareff W, Myers RE, Brann AW. Brain extracellular space in monkey fetuses subjected to prolonged partial asphyxia. *Exp Neurol*. 1970;28(1):167-178.
26. Tweed WA, Pash M, Doig G. Cerebrovascular mechanisms in perinatal asphyxia: the role of vasogenic brain edema. *Pediatr Res*. 1981;15(1):44-46.
27. Rosenberg AA. Regulation of cerebral blood flow after asphyxia in neonatal lambs. *Stroke*. 1988;19(2):239-244.

28. De Haan HH, Gunn AJ, Williams CE, Gluckman PD. Brief repeated umbilical cord occlusions cause sustained cytotoxic cerebral edema and focal infarcts in near-term fetal lambs. *Pediatr Res.* 1997;41:96-104.

29. Rice JE III, Vannucci RC, Brierley JB. The influence of immaturity on hypoxic-ischemic brain damage in the rat. *Ann Neurol.* 1981;9(2):131-141.

30. Mujsce DJ, Christensen MA, Vannucci RC. Cerebral blood flow and edema in perinatal hypoxic-ischemic brain damage. *Pediatr Res.* 1990;27(5):450-453.

31. Mujsce DJ, Towfighi J, Stern D, Vannucci RC. Mannitol therapy in perinatal hypoxic-ischemic brain damage in rats. *Stroke.* 1990;21(8):1210-1214.

32. Stonestreet BS, Burgess GH, Cserr HF. Blood-brain barrier integrity and brain water and electrolytes during hypoxia/hypercapnia and hypotension in newborn piglets. *Brain Res.* 1992;590:263-270.

33. Vannucci RC, Christensen MA, Yager JY. Nature, time-course, and extent of cerebral edema in perinatal hypoxic-ischemic brain damage. *Pediatr Neurol.* 1993;9(1):29-34.

34. Vannucci RC, Christensen MA, Yager JY. Cerebral edema and perinatal hypoxic-ischemic (H-1) brain damage. *Pediatr Res.* 1993;355A.

35. Rose VC, Shaffner DH, Gleason CA, Koehler RC, Traystman RJ. Somatosensory evoked potential and brain water content in post-asphyxic immature piglets. *Pediatr Res.* 1995;37:661-666.

36. Rumpel H, Buchli R, Gehrmann J, Aguzzi A, Illi O, Martin E. Magnetic resonance imaging of brain edema in the neonatal rat: a comparison of short and long term hypoxia-ischemia. *Pediatr Res.* 1995;38:113-118.

37. Nedelcu J, Klein MA, Aguzzi A, Boesiger P, Martin E. Biphasic edema after hypoxic-ischemic brain injury in neonatal rats reflects early neuronal and late glial damage. *Pediatr Res.* 1999;46:297-304.

38. Dijkhuizen RM, deGraaf RA, Tulleken KAF, Nicolay K. Changes in the diffusion of water and intracellular metabolites after excitotoxic injury and global ischemia in neonatal rat brain. *J Cereb Blood Flow Metab.* 1999;19(3):341-349.

39. Levy DE, Brierley JB, Silverman DG, Plum F. Brief hypoxia-ischemia initially damages cerebral neurons. *Arch Neurol.* 1975;32(7):450-456.

40. Brown AW, Brierley JB. The earliest alterations in rat neurones and astrocytes after anoxia-ischaemia. *Acta Neuropathol.* 1973;23(1):9-22.

41. Salford LG, Plum F, Brierley JB. Graded hypoxia-oligemia in rat brain. II. Neuropathological alterations and their implications. *Arch Neurol.* 1973;29(4):234-238.

42. Kim SU. Brain hypoxia studied in mouse central nervous system cultures. I. Sequential cellular changes. *Lab Invest.* 1975;33(6):658-669.

43. Edwards AD, Yue X, Cox P, et al. Apoptosis in the brains of infants suffering intrauterine cerebral injury. *Pediatr Res.* 1997;42:684-689.

44. Becher JC, Bell JE, Keeling JW, McIntosh N, Wyatt B. The Scottish perinatal neuropathology study: clinicopathological correlation in early neonatal deaths. *Arch Dis Child Fetal Neonatal Ed.* 2004;89:F399-F407.

45. Yue X, Mehmet H, Penrice J, et al. Apoptosis and necrosis in the newborn piglet brain following transient cerebral hypoxia-ischemia. *Neuropathol Appl Neurobiol.* 1997;23(1):16-25.

46. Edwards AD, Mehmet H. Apoptosis in perinatal hypoxic-ischaemic cerebral damage. *Neuropathol Appl Neurobiol.* 1996;22:482-503.

47. Bruck Y, Bruck W, Kretzschmar HA, Lassmann H. Evidence for neuronal apoptosis in pontosubicular neuron necrosis. *Neuropathol Appl Neurobiol.* 1996;22(1):23-29.

48. Mazarakis ND, Edwards AD, Mehmet H. Apoptosis in neural development and disease. *Arch Dis Child.* 1997;77(3):F165-F170.

49. Pulera MR, Adams LM, Liu HT, et al. Apoptosis in a neonatal rat model of cerebral hypoxia-ischemia. *Stroke.* 1998;29(12):2622-2629.

50. McDonald JW, Behrens MI, Chung C, Bhattacharyya T, Choi DW. Susceptibility to apoptosis is enhanced in immature cortical neurons. *Brain Res.* 1997;759(2):228-232.

51. Taylor DL, Edwards AD, Mehmet H. Oxidative metabolism, apoptosis and perinatal brain injury. *Brain Pathol.* 1999;9(1):93-117.

52. Bossenmeyer-Pourie C, Koziel V, Daval J-L. Effects of hypothermia on hypoxia-induced apoptosis in cultured neurons from developing rat forebrain: comparison with preconditioning. *Pediatr Res.* 2000;47:385-391.

53. Van Landeghem FKH, Felderhoff-Mueser U, Moysich A, et al. Fas (CD95/Apo-1)/Fas ligand expression in neonates with pontosubicular neuron necrosis. *Pediatr Res.* 2002;51:129-135.

54. Leech RW, Alvord EC Jr. Anoxic-ischemic encephalopathy in the human neonatal period. The significance of brain stem involvement. *Arch Neurol.* 1977;34(2):109-113.

55. Norman MG. Unilateral encephalomalacia in cranial nerve nuclei in neonates: report of two cases. *Neurology.* 1974;24(5):424-427.

56. Norman MG. Antenatal neuronal loss and gliosis of the reticular formation, thalamus, and hypothalamus. A report of three cases. *Neurology.* 1972;22(9):910-916.

57. Schneider H, Ballowitz L, Schachinger H, Hanefeld F, Dröszus JU. Anoxic encephalopathy with predominant involvement of basal ganglia, brain stem and spinal cord in the perinatal period. Report on seven newborns. *Acta Neuropathol.* 1975;32(4):287-298.

58. Griffiths AD, Laurence KM. The effect of hypoxia and hypoglycaemia on the brain of the newborn human infant. *Dev Med Child Neurol.* 1974;16(3):308-319.

59. Grunnet ML, Curless RG, Bray PF, Jung AL. Brain changes in newborns from an intensive care unit. *Dev Med Child Neurol.* 1974;16(3):320-328.

60. Schneck SA, Neubuerger KT. Lesions of the brain in hyaline membrane disease of infants. *Acta Neuropathol.* 1962;2:11.

61. Buckingham S, Sommers SC, Sherwin RP. Lesions of the dorsal vagal nucleus in the respiratory distress syndrome. *Am J Clin Pathol.* 1967;48(3):269-276.

62. Hall JG. A histological investigation of the auditory pathways in neonatal asphyxia. *Acta Otolaryngol.* 1962;45:369.

63. Hall JG. On the neuropathological changes in the central nervous system following neonatal asphyxia. *Acta Otolaryngol.* 1963;188(suppl):331.

64. Leech RW, Brumback RA. Massive brain stem necrosis in the human neonate: presentation of three cases with review of the literature. *J Child Neurol.* 1988;3(4):258-262.

65. Pindur J, Capin DM, Johnson MI, Rance NE. Cystic brain stem necrosis in a premature infant after prolonged bradycardia. *Acta Neuropathol.* 1992;83(6):667-669.

66. Hashimoto K, Takeuchi Y, Takashima S. Hypocarbia as a pathogenic factor in pontosubicular necrosis. *Brain Dev.* 1991;13(3):155-157.

67. Torvik A, Skullerud K, Andersen SN, Hurum J, Maehlen J. Affection of the hippocampal granule cells in pontosubicular neuron necrosis. *Acta Neuropathol.* 1992;83(5):535-537.

68. Galloway PG, Roessmann U. Neuronal karyorrhexis in Sommer's sector in a 22-week stillborn. *Acta Neuropathol.* 1986;70(3):343-344.

69. Becker LE, Takashima S. Chronic hypoventilation and development of brain stem gliosis. *Neuropediatrics.* 1985;16(1):19-23.

70. Natsume J, Watanabe K, Kuno F, Hayakawa F, Hashizume Y. Clinical, neurophysiologic, and neuropathological features of an infant with brain damage of total asphyxia type (Myers). *Pediatr Neurol.* 1995;13:61-64.

71. Roland EH, Poskitt K, Rodriguez E, Lupton BA, Hill A. Perinatal hypoxic-ischemic thalamic injury: clinical features and neuroimaging. *Ann Neurol.* 1998;44:161-166.

72. Kinney HC, Panigrahy A, Newburger JW, Jonas RA, Sleeper LA. Hypoxic-ischemic brain injury in infants with congenital heart disease dying after cardiac surgery. *Acta Neuropathol.* 2005;110(6):563-578.

73. Cowan F, Rutherford M, Groenendaal F, et al. Origin and timing of brain lesions in term infants with neonatal encephalopathy. *Lancet.* 2003;361(9359):736-742.

74. Bell JE, Becher JC, Wyatt B, Keeling JW, McIntosh N. Brain damage and axonal injury in a Scottish cohort of neonatal deaths. *Brain.* 2005;128:1070-1081.

75. Pierson CR, Folkerth RD, Billards SS, et al. Gray matter injury associated with periventricular leukomalacia in the premature infant. *Acta Neuropathol.* 2007;114:619-631.

76. Roland EH, Hill A, Norman MG, Flodmark O, MacNab AJ. Selective brainstem injury in an asphyxiated newborn. *Ann Neurol.* 1988;23(1):89-92.

77. Takashima S. Olivocerebellar lesions in infants born prematurely. *Brain Dev.* 1982;4(5):361-366.

78. Takashima S, Mito T, Houdou S, Ando Y. Relationship between periventricular hemorrhage, leukomalacia and brainstem lesions in prematurely born infants. *Brain Dev.* 1989;11(2):121-124.

79. Kreusser KL, Schmidt RE, Shackelford GD, Volpe JJ. Value of ultrasound for identification of acute hemorrhagic necrosis of thalamus and basal ganglia in an asphyxiated term infant. *Ann Neurol.* 1984;16(3):361-363.

80. Skullerud K, Westre B. Frequency and prognostic significance of germinal matrix hemorrhage, periventricular leukomalacia, and pontosubicular necrosis in preterm neonates. *Acta Neuropathol.* 1986;70(3):257-261.

81. Skullerud K, Skjaeraasen J. Clinicopathological study of germinal matrix hemorrhage, pontosubicular necrosis, and periventricular leukomalacia in stillborn. *Childs Nerv Syst.* 1988;4(2):88-91.

82. Armstrong DL, Sauls CD, Goddard-Finegold J. Neuropathologic findings in short-term survivors of intraventricular hemorrhage. *Am J Dis Child.* 1987;141:617-621.

83. Scher MS, Painter MJ. Electroencephalographic diagnosis of neonatal seizures: issues of diagnostic accuracy, clinical correlation, and survival. In: Wasterlain CG, Vert P, eds. *Neonatal Seizures.* New York, NY: Raven Press; 1990:15-26.

84. Gilles FH. Hypotensive brain stem necrosis. Selective symmetrical necrosis of tegmental neuronal aggregates following cardiac arrest. *Arch Pathol.* 1969;88:32-41.

85. Pasternak JF, Gorey MT. The syndrome of acute near-total intrauterine asphyxia in the term infant. *Pediatr Neurol.* 1998;18:391-398.

86. Sugama S, Ariga M, Hoashi E, Eto Y. Brainstem cranial-nerve lesions in an infant with hypoxic cerebral injury. *Pediatr Neurol.* 2003;29:256-259.

87. Sugama S, Eto Y. Brainstem lesions in children with perinatal brain injury. *Pediatr Neurol.* 2003;28:212-215.

88. Sarnat HB. Watershed infarcts in the fetal and neonatal brainstem. An aetiology of central hypoventilation, dysphagia, Mobius syndrome and micrognathia. *Eur J Paediatr Neurol.* 2004;8:71-87.

89. Ranck JB, Windle WF. Brain damage in the monkey, maccaca mulatta, by asphyxia neonatorum. *Exp Neurol.* 1959;1:130.

90. Faro MD, Windle WF. Transneuronal degeneration in brains of monkeys asphyxiated at birth. *Exp Neurol.* 1969;24(1):38-53.

91. Sargent MA, Poskitt KJ, Roland EH, Hill A, Hendson G. Cerebellar vermian atrophy after neonatal hypoxic-ischemic encephalopathy. *AJNR Am J Neuroradiol.* 2004;25:1008-1015.

92. Connolly DJ, Widjaja E, Griffiths PD. Involvement of the anterior lobe of the cerebellar vermis in perinatal profound hypoxia. *AJNR Am J Neuroradiol.* 2007;28(1):16-19.

93. LeStrange E, Saeed N, Cowan FM, Edwards AD, Rutherford MA. MR imaging quantification of cerebellar growth following hypoxic-ischemic injury to the neonatal brain. *AJNR Am J Neuroradiol.* 2004;25:463-468.

94. Sladky JT, Rorke LB. Perinatal hypoxic-ischemic spinal cord injury. *Pediatr Pathol.* 1986;6(1):87-101.

95. Clancy RR, Sladky JT, Rorke LB. Hypoxic-ischemic spinal cord injury following perinatal asphyxia. *Ann Neurol.* 1989;25(2):185-189.

96. Martin E, Barkovich AJ. Magnetic resonance imaging in perinatal asphyxia. *Arch Dis Child.* 1995;72:F62-F70.

97. Barkovich AJ, Hallam D. Neuroimaging in perinatal hypoxic-ischemic injury. *Ment Retard Dev Disabil Res Rev.* 1997;3:1-14.

98. Rutherford M, Pennock J, Schwieso J, Cowan F, Dubowitz L. Hypoxic-ischaemic encephalopathy: early and late magnetic resonance imaging findings in relation to outcome. *Arch Dis Child Fetal Neonatal Ed.* 1996;75:F145-F151.

99. Kuenzle C, Baenziger O, Martin E, et al. Prognostic value of early MR imaging in term infants with severe perinatal asphyxia. *Neuropediatrics.* 1994;25:191-200.

100. Rutherford MA, Pennock JM, Schwieso JE, Cowan FM, Dubowitz LM. Hypoxic ischaemic encephalopathy: early magnetic resonance imaging fundings and their evolution. *Neuropediatrics.* 1995;26:183-191.

101. Mercuri E, Ricci D, Cowan FM, et al. Head growth in infants with hypoxic-isehmic encephalopathy: correlation with neonatal magnetic resonance imaging. *Pediatrics.* 2000;106:235-243.

102. Rutherford MA, Azzopardi D, Whitelaw A, et al. Mild hypothermia and the distribution of cerebral lesions in neonates with hypoxic-ischemic encephalopathy. *Pediatrics.* 2005;116:1001-1006.

103. Wilson ER, Mirra SS, Schwartz JF. Congenital diencephalic and brain stem damage: neuropathologic study of three cases. *Acta Neuropathol.* 1982;57(1):70-74.

104. Parisi JE, Collins GH, Kim RC, Crosley CJ. Prenatal symmetrical thalamic degeneration with flexion spasticity at birth. *Ann Neurol.* 1983;13(1):94-97.

105. Cohen M, Roessmann U. In utero brain damage: relationship of gestational age to pathological consequences. *Dev Med Child Neurol.* 1994;36:263-270.

106. Johnston MV. Neurotransmitter alterations in a model of perinatal hypoxic-ischemic brain injury. *Ann Neurol.* 1983;13(5):511-518.

107. McDonald JW, Johnston MV. Physiological and pathophysiological roles of excitatory amino acids during central nervous system development. *Brain Res Brain Res Rev.* 1990;15(1):41-70.

108. Malamud N. Status marmoratus: a form of cerebral palsy following either birth injury or inflammation of the central nervous system. *J Pediatr.* 1950;37:610.

109. Borit A, Herndon RM. The fine structure of plaques fibromyeliniques in ulegyria and in status marmoratus. *Acta Neuropathol.* 1970;14(4):304-311.

110. Mito T, Kamei A, Takashima S, Becker LE. Clinicopathological study of pontosubicular necrosis. *Neuropediatrics.* 1993;24:204-207.

111. Stadelmann C, Mews I, Srinivasan A, Deckwerth TL, Lassmann H, Brück W. Expression of cell death-associated proteins in neuronal apoptosis associated with pontosubicular neuron necrosis. *Brain Pathol.* 2001;11(3):273-281.

112. Rossiter JP, Anderson LI, Yang F, Cole GM. Caspase-3 activation and caspase-like proteolytic activity in human perinatal hypoxic-ischemic brain injury. *Acta Neuropathol.* 2002;103:66-73.

113. Ahdab-Barmada M, Moossy J, Nemoto EM, Lin MR. Hyperoxia produces neuronal necrosis in the rat. *J Neuropathol Exp Neurol.* 1986;45(3):233-246.

114. Takizawa Y, Takashima S, Itoh M. A histopathological study of premature and mature infants with pontosubicular neuron necrosis: neuronal cell death in perinatal brain damage. *Brain Res.* 2006;1095(1):200-206.

115. Allin M, Matsumoto H, Santhouse AM, et al. Cognitive and motor function and the size of the cerebellum in adolescents born very pre-term. *Brain.* 2001;124(Pt 1):60-66.

116. Johnsen SD, Tarby TJ, Lewis KS, Bird R, Prenger E. Cerebellar infarction: an unrecognized complication of very low birthweight. *J Child Neurol.* 2002;17:320-324.

117. Peterson BS, Vohr B, Staib LH, et al. Regional brain volume abnormalities and long-term cognitive outcome in preterm infants. *JAMA.* 2000;284:1939-1947.

118. Mercuri E, Atkinson J, Braddick O, et al. Visual function in full-term infants with hypoxic-ischaemic encephalopathy. *Neuropediatrics.* 1997;28:155-161.

119. Argyropoulou MI, Xydis V, Drougia A, et al. MRI measurements of the pons and cerebellum in children born preterm; associations with the severity of periventricular leukomalacia and perinatal risk factors. *Neuroradiology.* 2003;45(10):730-734.

120. Bodensteiner JB, Johnsen SD. Cerebellar injury in the extremely premature infant: newly recognized but relatively common outcome. *J Child Neurol.* 2005;20:139-142.

121. Johnsen SD, Bodensteiner JB, Lotze TE. Frequency and nature of cerebellar injury in the extremely premature survivor with cerebral palsy. *J Child Neurol.* 2005;20:60-64.

122. Limperopoulos C, Soul JS, Gauvreau K, et al. Late gestation cerebellar growth is rapid and impeded by premature birth. *Pediatrics.* 2005;115:688-695.

123. Limperopoulos C, Soul JS, Haidar H, et al. Impaired trophic interactions between the cerebellum and the cerebrum among preterm infants. *Pediatrics.* 2005;116:844-850.

124. Miall LS, Cornette LG, Tanner SF, Arthur RJ, Levene MI. Posterior fossa abnormalities seen on magnetic resonance brain imaging in a cohort of newborn infants. *J Perinatol.* 2003;23:396-403.

125. Srinivasan L, Allsop J, Counsell SJ, et al. Smaller cerebellar volumes in very preterm infants at term-equivalent age are associated with the presence of supratentorial lesions. *AJNR Am J Neuroradiol.* 2006;27(3):573-579.

126. Shah DK, Anderson PJ, Carlin JB, et al. Reduction in cerebellar volumes in preterm infants: relationship to white matter injury and neurodevelopment at two years of age. *Pediatr Res.* 2006;60:97-102.

127. Bodensteiner JB, Johnsen SD. Magnetic resonance imaging (MRI) findings in children surviving extremely premature delivery and extremely low birthweight with cerebral palsy. *J Child Neurol.* 2006;21(9):743-747.

128. Barkovich AJ, Westmark K, Partridge C, Sola A, Ferriero DM. Perinatal asphyxia: MR findings in the first 10 days. *AJNR Am J Neuroradiol.* 1995;16:427-438.

129. Kaufman SA, Miller SP, Ferriero DM, Glidden DH, Barkovich AJ, Partridge JC. Encephalopathy as a predictor of magnetic resonance imaging abnormalities in asphyxiated newborns. *Pediatr Neurol.* 2003;28:342-346.

130. Rutherford M, Counsell S, Allsop J, et al. Diffusion-weighted magnetic resonance imaging in term perinatal brain injury: a comparison with site of lesion and time from birth. *Pediatrics.* 2004;114:1004-1014.

131. Miller SP, Ramaswamy V, Michelson D, et al. Patterns of brain injury in term neonatal encephalopathy. *J Pediatr.* 2005;146:453-460.

132. Okereafor A, Allsop J, Counsell SJ, et al. Patterns of brain injury in neonates exposed to perinatal sentinel events. *Pediatrics.* 2008;101:906-914.

133. Li AM, Chau V, Poskitt KJ, et al. White matter injury in term newborns with neonatal encephalopathy. *Pediatr Res.* 2009; 65(1):85-89.

134. Chau V, Poskitt KJ, Sargent MA, et al. Comparison of computer tomography and magnetic resonance imaging scans on the third day of life in term newborns with neonatal encephalopathy. *Pediatrics.* 2009;123:319-326.

135. Steinman KJ, Gorno-Tempini ML, Glidden DV, et al. Neonatal watershed brain injury on magnetic resonance imaging correlates with verbal IQ at 4 years. *Pediatrics.* 2009;123(3):1025-1030.

136. Martinez-Biarge M, Diez-Sebastian J, Kapellou O, et al. Predicting motor outcome and death in term hypoxic-ischemic encephalopathy. *Neurology.* 2011;76(24):2055-2061.

137. Martinez-Biarge M, Diez-Sebastian J, Rutherford MA, Cowan FM. Outcomes after central grey matter injury in term perinatal hypoxic-ischaemic encephalopathy. *Early Hum Dev.* 2010;86(11):675-682.

138. Bednarek N, Mathur A, Inder T, Wilkinson J, Neil J, Shimony J. Impact of therapeutic hypothermia on MRI diffusion changes in neonatal encephalopathy. *Neurology.* 2012;78(18):1420-1427.

139. Cheong JL, Coleman L, Hunt RW, et al. Prognostic utility of magnetic resonance imaging in neonatal hypoxic-ischemic encephalopathy: substudy of a randomized trial. *Arch Pediatr Adolesc Med.* 2012;166(7):634-640.

140. Harteman JC, Groenendaal F, Toet MC, et al. Diffusion-weighted imaging changes in cerebral watershed distribution following neonatal encephalopathy are not invariably associated with an adverse outcome. *Dev Med Child Neurol.* 2013;55(7):642-653.

141. Harteman JC, Nikkels PG, Benders MJ, Kwee A, Groenendaal F, de Vries LS. Placental pathology in full-term infants with hypoxic-ischemic neonatal encephalopathy and association with magnetic resonance imaging pattern of brain injury. *J Pediatr.* 2013;163(4):968-975, e962.

142. Shankaran S, McDonald SA, Laptook AR, et al. Neonatal magnetic resonance imaging pattern of brain injury as a biomarker of childhood outcomes following a trial of hypothermia for neonatal hypoxic-ischemic encephalopathy. *J Pediatr.* 2015;167:987-993.

143. Volpe JJ. Neonatal encephalopathy: an inadequate term for hypoxic-ischemic encephalopathy. *Ann Neurol.* 2012;72(2):156-166.

144. Friede RL. *Developmental Neuropathology.* New York: Springer-Verlag; 1975.

145. Courville CB. *Birth and Brain Damage.* Pasadena: M. F. Courville; 1971.

146. Norman RM, Urich H, McMenemey WH. Vascular mechanisms of birth injury. *Brain.* 1957;80:49.

147. Volpe JJ, Pasternak JF. Parasagittal cerebral injury in neonatal hypoxic-ischemic encephalopathy: clinical and neuroradiologic features. *J Pediatr.* 1977;91(3):472-476.

148. O'Brien MJ, Ash JM, Gilday DL. Radionuclide brain-scanning in perinatal hypoxia/ischemia. *Dev Med Child Neurol.* 1979;21:161.

149. Volpe JJ, Herscovitch P, Perlman JM, Kreusser KL, Raichle ME. Positron emission tomography in the asphyxiated term newborn: parasagittal impairment of cerebral blood flow. *Ann Neurol.* 1985;17(3):287-296.

150. Yokochi K, Fujimoto S. Magnetic resonance imaging in children with neonatal asphyxia: correlation with developmental sequelae. *Acta Paediatr.* 1996;85:88-95.

151. Perez A, Ritter S, Brotschi B, et al. Long-term neurodevelopmental outcome with hypoxic-ischemic encephalopathy. *J Pediatr.* 2013;163(2):454-459, e451.

152. Harteman JC, Groenendaal F, Benders MJ, Huisman A, Blom HJ, de Vries LS. Role of thrombophilic factors in full-term infants with neonatal encephalopathy. *Pediatr Res.* 2013;73(1):80-86.

153. Logitharajah P, Rutherford MA, Cowan FM. Hypoxic-ischemic encephalopathy in preterm infants: antecedent factors, brain imaging, and outcome. *Pediatr Res.* 2009;66(2):222-229.

154. Martinez-Biarge M, Bregant T, Wusthoff CJ, et al. White matter and cortical injury in hypoxic-ischemic encephalopathy: antecedent factors and 2-year outcome. *J Pediatr.* 2012;161(5):799-807.

155. Volpe JJ. Encephalopathy of congenital heart disease-destructive and developmental effects intertwined. *J Pediatr.* 2014;164(5):962-965.

Hypoxic-Ischemic Injury in the Term Infant: Pathophysiology

Joseph J. Volpe

This chapter addresses the pathophysiology of hypoxic-ischemic injury. The neuropathology of this injury, just discussed in detail in Chapter 18, includes three principal lesions, that is, *selective neuronal necrosis, parasagittal cerebral injury,* and *cerebral white matter injury*. I will discuss each of these lesions separately, because in the infant with hypoxic-ischemic disease one or the other tends to predominate. However, magnetic resonance imaging (MRI) studies of such infants do show considerable overlap in the occurrence of the lesions (see Chapter 18). Additionally, although we will discuss pathophysiology for these three categories of injury separately, *several pathogenetic themes recur*. These themes include initiating factors, principally ischemia, impinging on specific anatomical and metabolic cellular and regional characteristics that underlie a maturation-dependent vulnerability. Ischemia is linked to a variety of deleterious perinatal events (see Chapter 17) and to impaired cerebrovascular autoregulation. Regional patterns of ischemic injury occur especially in vascular border zones and end zones. At the cellular level, ischemia leads to cell death, both neuronal and oligodendroglial, via a cascade of events that particularly includes excitotoxicity. The pathophysiological events and the cascade to cell death most often occur over relatively protracted temporal periods and thereby afford opportunities for preventative/ameliorative interventions (see Chapter 20).

SELECTIVE NEURONAL NECROSIS

Selective neuronal necrosis is the most common variety of injury observed in neonatal hypoxic-ischemic encephalopathy and refers to necrosis of neurons in a characteristic, although often widespread, distribution (see Chapter 18). MRI studies show an overall incidence of approximately 80% in infants with hypoxic-ischemic disease (see Chapter 18). Neuronal necrosis often coexists with other distinctive manifestations of neonatal hypoxic-ischemic encephalopathy (see later sections), and in fact it is very unusual to observe one of the other varieties of neonatal hypoxic-ischemic encephalopathy without some degree of selective neuronal injury as well. The topography of the neuronal injury depends in considerable part on the severity and temporal characteristics of the insult and on the gestational age of the infant. *Three basic patterns* derived primarily from correlative clinical and brain imaging findings, and observed best in term infants, can be distinguished (Table 19.1). *Diffuse* neuronal injury *(cerebral cortical, deep nuclear, brain stem)* occurs with very severe, relatively prolonged insults in

both term and premature infants; a *cerebral cortical–deep nuclear* neuronal predominance occurs in primarily term infants with moderate to severe, relatively prolonged insults. The deep nuclear involvement includes basal ganglia (especially putamen) and thalamus. *Deep nuclear–brain stem* neuronal predominance occurs in primarily term infants with severe, relatively abrupt insults. Two other patterns, *pontosubicular* neuronal injury and *cerebellar* injury, are uncommon and will be noted only briefly in the following discussion.

Pathogenesis
Cerebral Ischemia, Impaired Cerebrovascular Autoregulation, and Pressure-Passive Cerebral Circulation

Cerebral ischemia, with deprivation of oxygen and glucose, followed by reperfusion and the cascade of metabolic events described in Chapter 13, is the likely pathogenetic sequence in selective neuronal necrosis (Box 19.1). Although the causative relation between cerebral ischemia and both selective neuronal necrosis and parasagittal cerebral injury (see later) has been established in several excellent perinatal animal models (see previous section), studies in *human infants* also provide excellent support for the role of diminished cerebral blood flow (CBF) secondary to systemic hypotension. Thus, as discussed in detail in Chapter 13, because of the *impaired vascular autoregulation* in asphyxiated infants, CBF becomes passively related to arterial blood pressure (Fig. 19.1 and see Box 19.1). The impaired vascular autoregulation has been documented in the hours to days after the insult and, by extrapolation from experimental data (see Chapter 13), is presumed to begin during the insult, when hypotension is most pronounced. This situation makes the infant exquisitely vulnerable to the diminutions in blood pressure characteristic of severe asphyxia, and those regions most vulnerable are in the distribution of selective neuronal necrosis as well as the watershed, that is, parasagittal, distributions of the cerebrum (see later). The data of Pryds and co-workers[1,2] show clearly that those asphyxiated term infants with impaired autoregulation have the poorest neurological outcome (see Fig. 19.1).

The *causes of the pressure-passive circulation* in the asphyxiated newborn could relate to such factors as (1) the hypoxemia or hypercarbia or both of the primary asphyxial insult, (2) the postasphyxial impairment in vascular reactivity observed in experimental models of perinatal asphyxia and presumably related to the effect of one or more of the vasodilatory compounds that accumulate secondary to ischemia-reperfusion (see Chapter 13), (3) an "immature" autoregulatory system with

TABLE 19.1 Major Patterns of Selective Neuronal Injury and Characteristics of Usual Insult in Term Newborns

PATTERN[a]	SEVERITY AND TIMING OF USUAL INSULT[b]
Diffuse (cerebral cortex, deep nuclear, brain stem)	Severe, prolonged
Cerebral cortex–deep nuclear[b]	Moderate, prolonged
Deep nuclear[c]–brain stem	Severe, abrupt

[a]The patterns reflect areas of *predominant* neuronal injury; considerable overlap is common.

[b]Severity and timing of insult are estimates, based on clinical and experimental studies (see text).

[c]Deep nuclear: basal ganglia (especially putamen) and thalamus.

BOX 19.1 Selective Neuronal Necrosis: Pathogenesis

Cerebral ischemia
  Impaired cerebrovascular autoregulation with pressure-passive
    cerebral circulation
  Systemic hypotension
Regional vascular factors
Regional metabolic factors
Regional distribution of excitatory (glutamate) receptors on neurons[a]
Factors related to the hypoxic-ischemic insult
  Severity and temporal characteristics
  Preceding/concomitant infection/inflammation

[a]Single most important factor for determining regional distribution of selective neuronal necrosis.

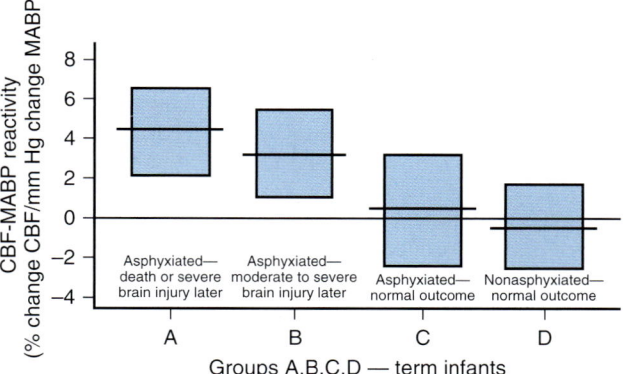

Figure 19.1 Cerebrovascular autoregulation, expressed as reactivity of cerebral blood flow to changes in mean arterial blood pressure, in a group of 19 asphyxiated term newborns and 12 control infants. Note the normal reactivity in the control infants (D) and the loss of reactivity in the infants with the poorest outcomes (A and B). *CBF,* Cerebral blood flow. (Data from Pryds O, Greisen G, Lou H, Friis-Hansen B. Vasoparalysis associated with brain damage in asphyxiated term infants. *J Pediatr.* 1990;117:119–125.)

limited capacity for reactivity because of the deficient arteriolar muscular lining of penetrating cerebral arteries and arterioles in the third trimester,[3,4] (4) an autoregulatory system with a lower limit so close to the range of *normal* blood pressure that even slight hypotension places CBF on the down slope of the curve (see Chapter 15), or (5) a combination of these factors. Whatever the mechanisms, the clinical implications are enormous. Falls in arterial blood pressure lead to decreases in CBF and injury to certain vulnerable brain *cells*, that is, neurons in the distribution of selective neuronal necrosis, and *regions*, that is, parasagittal cerebrum (see later).

Regional Vascular Factors

The reasons for the *selective vulnerability* of neuronal groups in the central nervous system have become increasingly clear in recent years. *Regional vascular factors* certainly can play a role because neuronal injury is more marked in vascular border zones and end zones (see Box 19.1). The vulnerable vascular zones include, for depths of cortical sulci, end zones of short penetrating vessels; for basal ganglia and thalamus (including posterior limb of the internal capsule), end zones of lenticulostriate, Heubner and posterior cerebral arteries; and for brain stem, end zones and border zones in the vertebrobasilar system.[5-7] The predilection of cerebral cortical neuronal injury for parasagittal regions likely relates to their occurrence within the border zones of all three major cerebral vessels (see later).

The role of vascular factors in pathogenesis of pontosubicular necrosis is likely complex. Thus, the documented relationship of the lesion to hypocarbia and to hyperoxemia suggests a role for cerebral vasoconstriction.[8-10] However, possibly additionally important, the rapid neuronal maturation in the pons and subiculum during the time of occurrence of this lesion suggests that vulnerability of this region may relate in part to the simultaneous occurrence of neuronal differentiation and a propensity of these neurons to undergo apoptosis.[10a-10d]

Regional Metabolic Factors

Regional metabolic factors could play a central role (see Box 19.1). Those factors that lead to hypoxic cell death in experimental systems (see Chapter 13) raise the possibilities of regional differences in anaerobic glycolytic capacity, energy requirements, lactate accumulation, mitochondrial function, calcium influx, nitric oxide synthesis, and free radical formation and scavenging capacity. For example, the high metabolic rate and energy utilization of deep gray matter may contribute to the especial vulnerability of these neurons to the severe, abrupt ischemic insults that lead to particular injury to these neuronal structures (see later). Although relatively little is known about these regional metabolic issues in *human brain*, recent data suggest a role for impaired antioxidant defenses (see Chapters 14 and 18).

Regional Distribution of Excitatory (Glutamate) Receptors

The *regional distribution of glutamate receptors, particularly of the N-methyl-D-aspartate (NMDA) and alpha-amino-3-hydroxy-5-methyl-4-isoxazole propionic acid (AMPA) types,* now appears to be the *single most important determinant of the distribution of selective neuronal injury* (see Box 19.1). As discussed in detail in Chapter 13, the topography of hypoxic-ischemic neuronal death in vivo is similar to the topography of glutamate synapses; the particular vulnerability of certain neuronal groups in the perinatal period correlates with a transient, maturation-dependent density of glutamate receptors; extracellular glutamate increases dramatically at such receptors with hypoxia-ischemia; and hypoxic-ischemic neuronal death in vivo can be prevented by administration of blockers of the NMDA receptor-channel complex and, to a considerable extent also, of non-NMDA receptors, especially Ca^{2+}-permeable AMPA receptors (see Chapter 13). The demonstration that the molecular mechanisms by which activation of the glutamate receptors leads to cell death operate over hours *after termination of the insult* and that prevention or amelioration of such excitotoxic injury can be effected by glutamate receptor blockers administered also after termination of the insult has profound and obvious clinical implications (see Chapters 13 and 20).

The importance of the regional distribution of glutamate receptors in the determination of regional selectivity of neuronal injury is particularly apparent in basal ganglia and thalamus. Thus, first, it is clear that there is a transient, dense glutamatergic innervation of the basal ganglia and thalamus in the perinatal period, both in experimental models (see Chapter 13) and in the human.[11-15] Second, the development of vulnerability of striatum and thalamus to hypoxic-ischemic injury parallels the expression of glutamate receptors and the vulnerability to direct injections of glutamate (see Chapter 13). Third, extracellular glutamate levels have been shown to rise in perinatal models of hypoxic-ischemic striatal injury (see Chapter 13). Fourth, a highly effective blocker of perinatal hypoxic-ischemic deep nuclear is MK-801, a specific blocker of the NMDA receptor-channel complex (see Chapter 13). Fifth, there is a specific hierarchy of potency of glutamate receptor agonists for production of striatal injury, and this potency parallels the expression of receptor subtypes and the inhibitory capabilities of specific receptor antagonists (see Chapter 13).

As noted earlier, neuronal injury in brain stem often accompanies such injury in basal ganglia and thalamus. Notably, studies of the developmental profiles of glutamate receptor subtype binding in the human brain stem have shown transient elevations in inferior olive and basis pontis of NMDA and kainate receptors in early infancy.[16,17] The likely importance of the development of glutamate receptor expression in vulnerable brain stem nuclei is also discussed in Chapter 18.

Perhaps related to the role of glutamate receptors of the NMDA type in pathogenesis of selective striatal neuronal injury is a *relative sparing of nicotinamide adenine dinucleotide phosphate (NADPH)–diaphorase neurons* in hypoxia-ischemia.[18,19] *NADPH diaphorase* has been shown to be identical to nitric oxide synthase, and generation of nitric oxide has been shown to be one mechanism whereby activation of NMDA receptors (which contact NADPH-diaphorase neurons) leads to striatal neuronal death (see also Chapter 13). Since nitric oxide synthase is activated by Ca^{2+}, and Ca^{2+} influx follows activation of the NMDA receptor (see Chapter 13), the data suggest a sequence of NMDA receptor activation, activation of nitric oxide synthase, generation of nitric oxide, and diffusion of nitric oxide (a highly reactive molecule that can generate free radicals) to adjacent neurons, and free radical–mediated cell death. It is noteworthy that the peak period of vulnerability of striatal neurons in the immature rat corresponds to the peak periods of sparing of NADPH-diaphorase neurons and of hypoxic-ischemic vulnerability.[18,19] The reason for the relative sparing of NADPH-diaphorase neurons remains unclear, but this sparing may contribute importantly to perinatal striatal neuronal death. Currently, it is not known whether a similar sparing of nitric oxide–synthesizing neurons contributes to selective neuronal injury in cerebral cortical and other areas vulnerable

in hypoxia-ischemia in the neonatal human. However, potential importance for neuronal nitric oxide synthase in mediation of such hypoxic-ischemic neuronal injury is suggested by the results of a study of the development of neuronal expression of the enzyme in human brain.[20] The striking findings were a higher density of nitric oxide synthase–positive neurons in late fetal human brain than in adult brain and a concentration of such neurons in areas known to be injured in selective neuronal necrosis, that is, deeper layers of cerebral cortex, striatum, and brain stem tegmentum.

Recent studies of glutamate receptors in developing *human* cerebral cortex suggest that a transient expression of Ca^{2+}-permeable AMPA receptors and NMDA receptors occurs around the time of term birth (Fig. 19.2).[21,22] Thus, the theme is similar to that for basal ganglia and brain stem, that is, a maturation-dependent exuberant expression of Ca^{2+}-permeable glutamate receptors becomes lethal to neurons with excessive activation, as occurs with cerebral ischemia.

Factors Related to the Hypoxic-Ischemic Insult

Severity and Temporal Characteristics. Factors related to the *severity and the temporal characteristics* of the insult appear to be of particular importance in determining the major pattern of selective neuronal injury in the newborn (see Table 19.1).[5,23] Severe and prolonged insults result in diffuse and marked neuronal necrosis, involving the many levels of the neuraxis described earlier as the *diffuse* pattern of injury. The *cerebral–deep nuclear* pattern of neuronal injury appears to be related to insults that are less severe and prolonged, often termed *partial, prolonged asphyxia*. The *deep nuclear–brain stem* pattern of injury to basal ganglia–thalamus–brain stem has been described in human infants with a severe, abrupt event, often termed *total asphyxia*. It is postulated that the severe, abrupt event prevents the operation of major adaptive mechanisms normally operative with asphyxial events (see Chapter 13). The most important of these may be the diversion of blood from the cerebral hemispheres to the *vital* deep nuclear structures. Because the latter have high rates of energy utilization and also a high content of glutamate receptors, these nuclei are particularly likely to be injured. In the more prolonged and less severe insults, the diversion of blood to deep nuclear structures occurs at least to a degree, and thus the cerebral regions are more likely to be affected. Studies in the near-term fetal lamb indicate that the severe terminal insult that results in injury to deep nuclear structures especially may be likely to occur after brief, repeated hypoxic-ischemic insults *first* cause a cumulative deleterious effect on cardiovascular function that presumably *then* can result in a severe late insult.[23-27]

Difficulty of Determining Timing and Duration of Insult(s). In the clinical setting available methods are not ideal for determining timing and duration of hypoxic-ischemic insults.[5] As delineated in Chapter 17, the large majority of insults occur in the late intrauterine/intrapartum period. In the living infant MRI studies can be valuable in delineating approximate timing, albeit not with extreme accuracy (see Chapter 20).

Classic studies with term fetal monkeys by Myers and co-workers provide insight into the relation of timing and duration of hypoxic-ischemic insults to certain patterns of injury. For example, the deep nuclear-brain stem pattern was produced by *total asphyxia* in the term fetal monkey.[28,29] The sequence

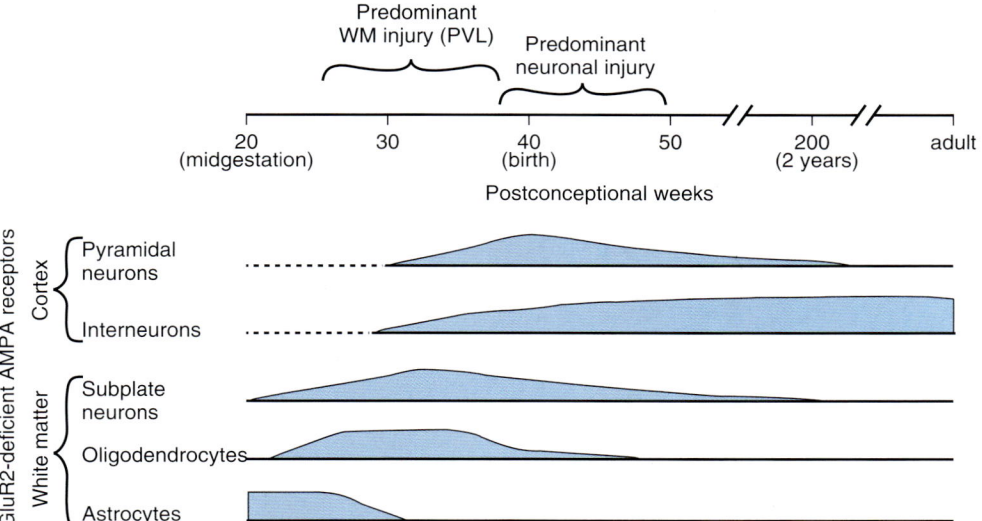

Figure 19.2 Transient expression of Ca^{2+}-permeable (GluR2-deficient) alpha-amino-3-hydroxy-5-methyl-4-isoxazole propionic acid (AMPA) receptors in cerebral cortex and cerebral white matter (WM) in developing human brain. Note the transient dense expression of GluR2-deficient AMPA receptors in cortical pyramidal neurons around the time of term. N-methyl-D-aspartate receptors show a similar time course (data not shown). The changes in cerebral WM are discussed in Chapter 15 in relation to periventricular leukomalacia (PVL). (From Talos DM, Follett PL, Folkerth RD, Fishman RE, et al. Developmental regulation of alpha-amino-3-hydroxy-5-methyl-4-isoxazole-propionic acid receptor subunit expression in forebrain and relationship to regional susceptibility to hypoxic/ischemic injury. II. Human cerebral white matter and cortex. J Comp Neurol. 2006;497:61–77.)

of events was rapidly progressive fetal hypoxia, hypercarbia, acidosis, hypotension, and brain injury within approximately 10 to 15 minutes. The topography of the neuropathology is markedly similar to that in the human fetus subjected to apparent total asphyxia, for example, with cord prolapse or uterine rupture. In one carefully documented human study, this neuropathology was identified by neuroimaging after such sentinel events occurring generally from 10 to 46 minutes before delivery.[30]

Term fetal monkeys subjected to a partial rather than total interference with respiratory gas exchange (produced by halothane-induced hypotension) developed physiological derangements over longer periods), so-called prolonged partial asphyxia.[31,32] The maternal event resulted in more slowly evolving hypoxia and acidosis, followed by late decelerations of the fetal heart rate, diminished cardiac output, hypotension, and evidence for cerebral ischemia. Brain injury became apparent after several hours, and the topography involved cerebral cortex (especially in paracentral areas), basal ganglia, and thalamus, as in human infants (see Table 19.1) If the insults were especially severe and prolonged, brain stem was also involved, as in the diffuse pattern noted in Table 19.1.

As noted earlier, determination of timing and severity of insult in the perinatal clinical setting is hindered by the lack of available methods, whether they be real-time fetal monitoring or retrospective estimates by various magnetic resonance determinations. Indeed, in the 80% to 90% of cases of infants with hypoxic-ischemic disease, in which an overt fetal sentinel event is not present, the uncertainty in timing is often measured in hours, often many hours or more, and not minutes. These issues are discussed in detail in Chapter 17.

Preceding or Concomitant Infection/Inflammation. As discussed in Chapter 13, experimental data demonstrate the *potentiation of hypoxic-ischemic insults by preceding or concomitant infection/inflammation.* Thus, hypoxic-ischemic insults not severe enough to cause injury alone can be rendered seriously injurious if the fetus or infant is exposed to inflammatory factors associated with intrauterine or postnatal infection. This phenomenon could underlie, at least in part, the accentuated risk of apparent hypoxic-ischemic brain injury observed in infants who sustain their insults in association with chorioamnionitis and/or who have elevated levels of cytokines in blood or cerebrospinal fluid.[33-44] However, it should be emphasized that the vast majority of term infants exposed to chorioamnionitis have an uncomplicated neonatal course and neurologic outcome, and overall, histologic chorioamnionitis does not appear to increase the risk of adverse outcome even in infants with hypoxic-ischemic encephalopathy.[45] Nevertheless, in the subset of infants with histologic chorioamnionitis *and* evidence of a fetal placental response, for example, villitis, adverse outcome is increased.[44] The presence or absence of a *fetal inflammatory response* may be most critical, perhaps both by local placental vascular obliterative/blood flow effects and by potentiation of hypoxic-ischemic effects, as described in Chapter 13.

PARASAGITTAL CEREBRAL INJURY

Parasagittal cerebral injury refers to a lesion of the cerebral cortex and subcortical white matter with a characteristic distribution, that is, parasagittal, superomedial aspects of the cerebral convexities (Figs. 19.3 and 19.4; see Chapter 18). The injury is bilateral and, although usually symmetrical,

Parasagittal cerebral
injury distribution

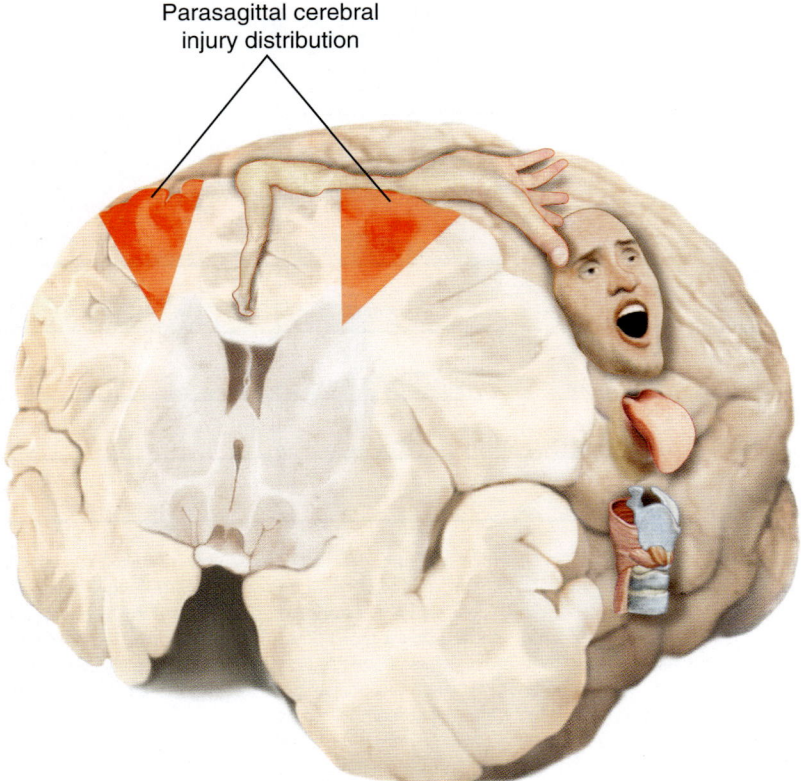

Figure 19.3 Parasagittal cerebral injury, coronal view. Schematic diagram of the distribution of the injury, which is indicated by symmetrical red areas in superomedial aspects of cerebrum.

Parasagittal cerebral
injury distribution

Branches of posterior
cerebral artery

Branches of anterior
cerebral artery

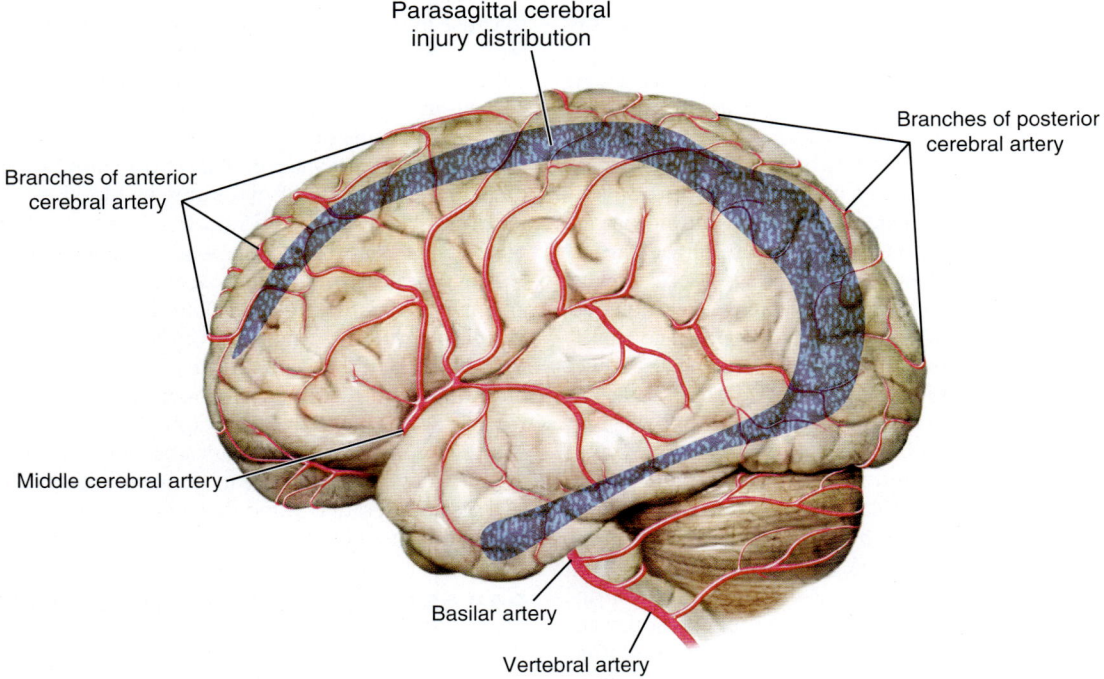

Middle cerebral artery

Basilar artery

Vertebral artery

Figure 19.4 Parasagittal cerebral injury, lateral view. Schematic diagram of cerebral convexity, lateral view, showing distribution of major cerebral arteries. Distribution of injury, shown by line-marked area, is in border zones and end fields of these arteries.

may be more striking in one hemisphere than the other. The posterior aspect of the cerebral hemispheres, especially the parietal-occipital regions, is more impressively affected than the anterior aspect. The terms *watershed infarct* and *watershed injury* have been used to describe the lesion and to emphasize its ischemic nature (see later discussion). I prefer the more descriptive term *parasagittal cerebral injury*. As detailed in Chapter 18, parasagittal cerebral injury has been identified by neuroimaging in approximately 40% to 60% of asphyxiated term newborns. At the cellular level, parasagittal cerebral injury is characterized by necrosis of the cortex and the immediately subjacent white matter; neuronal elements are most severely affected, but premyelinating oligodendrocytes of subcortical white matter are also involved.

Pathogenesis

The pathogenesis of parasagittal cerebral injury relates principally to a disturbance in cerebral perfusion. The two factors underlying the propensity of the parasagittal region to ischemic injury relate to parasagittal vascular anatomical factors and cerebral ischemia, often associated with a pressure-passive state of the cerebral circulation (Box 19.2). The reasons that one infant with ischemia may develop primarily parasagittal cerebral injury and another, the various patterns of selective neuronal necrosis, are not entirely clear. As discussed in the section on selective neuronal necrosis, the *severity* and the *temporal characteristics of the insult* are likely to be very important (see later). Indeed, some degree of concomitant selective neuronal injury, particularly involving basal ganglia and thalamus, is common in my experience and documented by multiple MRI studies (see Chapter 18).

Cerebral Ischemia, Impaired Cerebrovascular Autoregulation, Pressure-Passive Cerebral Circulation

The importance of the asphyxial/post-asphyxial impairment of cerebrovascular autoregulation (see Chapter 13) in the genesis of cerebral ischemia with associated systemic circulatory failure is apparent for parasagittal cerebral injury, as described earlier for selective neuronal necrosis (see earlier discussion). Nevertheless, it is important to recognize that even in the presence of intact autoregulation, severe hypotension, below the lower limit of the autoregulatory curve, will result in cerebral ischemia.

Parasagittal Vascular Anatomical Factors

The likely areas of greatest ischemia relate to parasagittal vascular anatomic factors (see Box 19.2). Thus, the areas of necrosis in parasagittal cerebral injury are in the *border zones* between the end fields of the major cerebral arteries (see Fig.

19.4).[46,47] These border zones are the brain regions most susceptible to a fall in cerebral perfusion pressure. Meyer,[46] who defined the characteristic topography of the cerebral lesions in 30 infants more than 50 years ago, related the injury to systemic hypotension. This watershed concept is based on the analogy with an irrigation system supplying a series of fields with water and emphasizes the vulnerability of the *last fields* when the head of pressure falls.[48,49] Experimental support for this concept initially was provided in the monkey by Brierley and co-workers,[50,51] who produced rapid, profound systemic hypotension and prevented hypoxemia when respiratory failure developed. Typical watershed lesions were produced in the cerebral cortex (and cerebellum) and were ascribed to the sharply reduced CBF. As we[52,53] observed in asphyxiated human infants, more marked injury was demonstrated in the *posterior* cerebrum in the experimental animals, as well as in the adult human.[47,50,51] The more marked injury in posterior cerebrum presumably relates to the fact that this region represents the watershed of all three major cerebral vessels (see Fig. 19.4).

The border zone concept has received ample additional experimental support in several developing animal models. Parasagittal cerebral cortical-subcortical injury has been documented in the perinatal monkey, sheep, rabbit, and mouse subjected to a variety of insults complicated by hypotension and presumed or documented cerebral ischemia.[5,23,27,31,54-59] The studies of the near-term sheep fetus showed particularly well the greater vulnerability of the parasagittal regions versus more laterally placed cerebrum with less than maximal insults (Fig. 19.5). Moreover, the cellular pattern of laminar necrosis of cortical pyramidal neurons was similar to the pattern observed in the asphyxiated human infant.[60] Interestingly, although parasagittal cerebral cortex was most vulnerable, with prolonged ischemia (e.g., 40 minutes) many other regions become affected

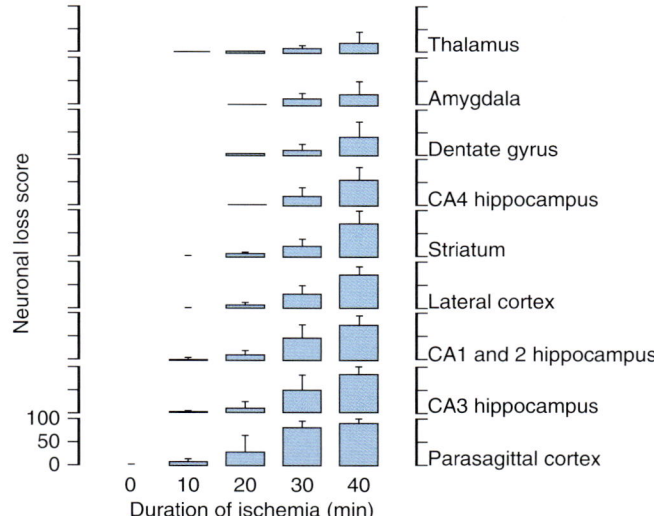

Figure 19.5 Neuronal damage in nine brain regions following increasing durations of ischemia. These regions are ranked in inverse order of total damage scores: the parasagittal cortex was the most severely and earliest damaged *(bottom)*, whereas the thalamus *(top)* showed the least damage. The damage scores are on a linearized scale. *0* to *100, 0*, no neuronal loss; *100*, total necrosis. (From Williams CE, Gunn AJ, Mallard C, et al. Outcome after ischemia in the developing sheep brain: an electroencephalographic and histological study. *Ann Neurol.* 1992;31:14–21.)

BOX 19.2   Selective Neuronal Necrosis: Pathogenesis

Cerebral ischemia
  Impaired cerebrovascular autoregulation with pressure-passive
    cerebral circulation
  Systemic hypotension
Parasagittal vascular factors
  Arterial border zones and end zones
**Excitatory (glutamate) receptors on neurons and premyelinating
  oligodendrocytes**

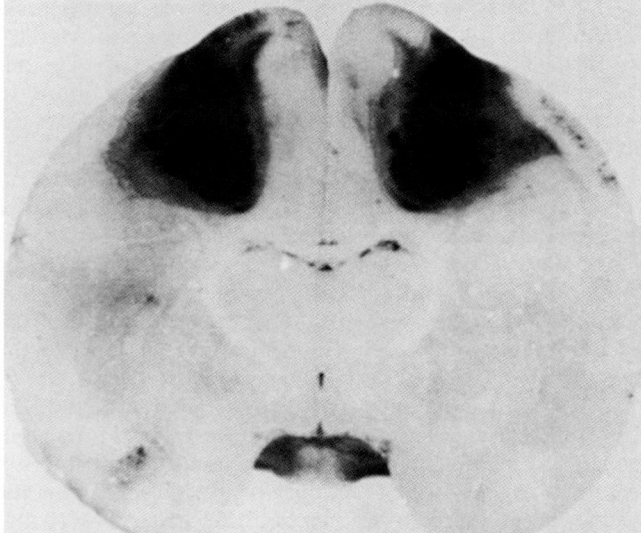

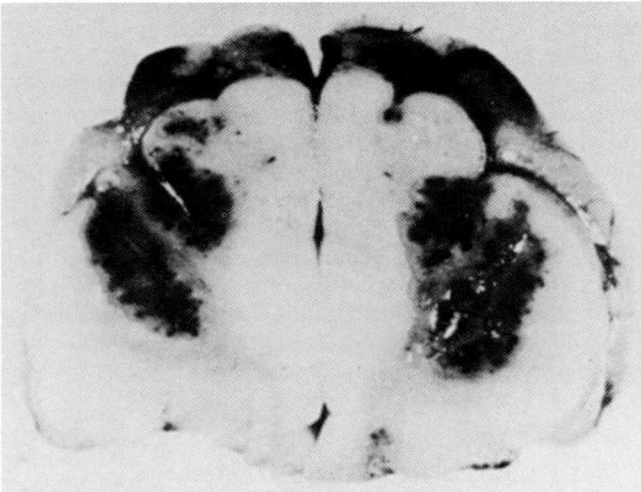

Figure 19.6 Cerebral lesions after prolonged partial asphyxia of the term fetal monkey. Coronal sections of cerebrum. Note the symmetrical, parasagittal distribution of necrosis and observe the similarity to the topography of the injury in asphyxiated infants (see Chapter 18). (From Brann AW Jr, Myers RE. Central nervous system findings in the newborn monkey following severe in utero partial asphyxia. *Neurology.* 1975;25:327.)

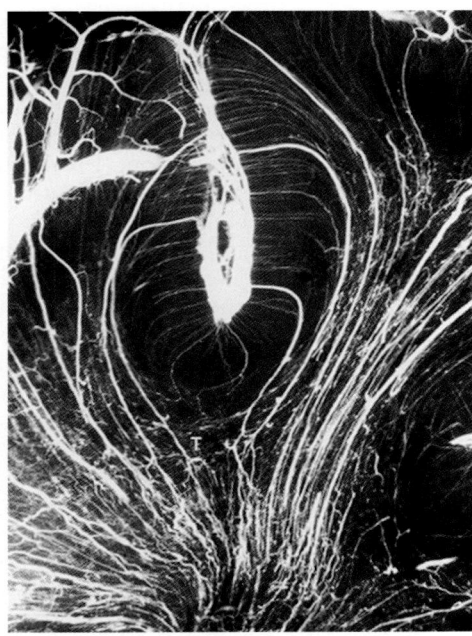

Figure 19.7 Vascular supply to depth of sulcus in full-term newborn. Postmortem microarteriography demonstrates the relatively avascular, triangular area (T) at the depth of the sulcus. (From Takashima S, Armstrong DL, Becker LE. Subcortical leukomalacia. Relationship to development of the cerebral sulcus and its vascular supply. *Arch Neurol.* 1978;35:470.)

and the parasagittal predilection is less apparent (see Fig. 19.5). The latter situation is reminiscent of findings with severely asphyxiated human infants who die. A vivid example of the occurrence of parasagittal cerebral injury in a *primate model* of intrauterine asphyxia and fetal cerebral ischemia is provided by elegant studies of the term fetal monkey (Fig. 19.6).[31]

It should be noted that although vascular border zones are the most vulnerable to drops in perfusion pressure, *other "distal fields,"* not necessarily border zones, for example, posterior occipital regions, are particularly vulnerable and are especially affected by systemic hypotension. Moreover, certain border zones supplied by larger *proximal* branches of cerebral vessels (e.g., temporal region between middle and posterior cerebral arteries) would be expected to be less vulnerable and, indeed, tend to be relatively less affected in parasagittal cerebral injury,

whether in the asphyxiated infant, hypotensive adult human, or monkey (see Chapter 18).[50,51]

In addition to the recognized vascular border zones and end zones just described, a factor related to *vascular development* appears to predispose the human newborn to ischemic injury of cortex and subcortical white matter. Takashima and co-workers[61] have shown that as sulci form and deepen near term in the human brain, the penetrating vessels from the meningeal arteries are forced to bend acutely at the cortical–white matter junction. This bending results in a triangular area at the depth of the sulcus (the site of particular predilection for ischemic cerebral injury), which represents a border zone of relative avascularity between the penetrating vessels (Fig. 19.7). This relatively avascular region presumably is even more vulnerable to a fall in perfusion pressure within the border zone regions between the major cerebral vessels. Thus we are dealing with a border zone within a border zone, which results during a specific phase of gyral and vascular development in human brain. These observations may explain why the cerebral injury in the parasagittal vascular border zones is more severe in the depths of sulci and why there is the subsequent characteristic "mushroom" appearance of the atrophic gyri (Fig. 19.8).[62-74] In the living infant, more severe affection of depths of sulci in parasagittal cerebral injury are apparent by MRI (see Chapter 20), and in some cases the unusual appearance of "subcortical leukomalacia" in parasagittal areas may be identified by brain imaging.[75-77]

Excitatory (Glutamate) Receptors on Neurons and Premyelinating-Oligodendrocytes. The final pathway to cell death occurs both in neurons of cerebral cortex and premyelinating oligodendrocytes (pre-OLs) of subcortical

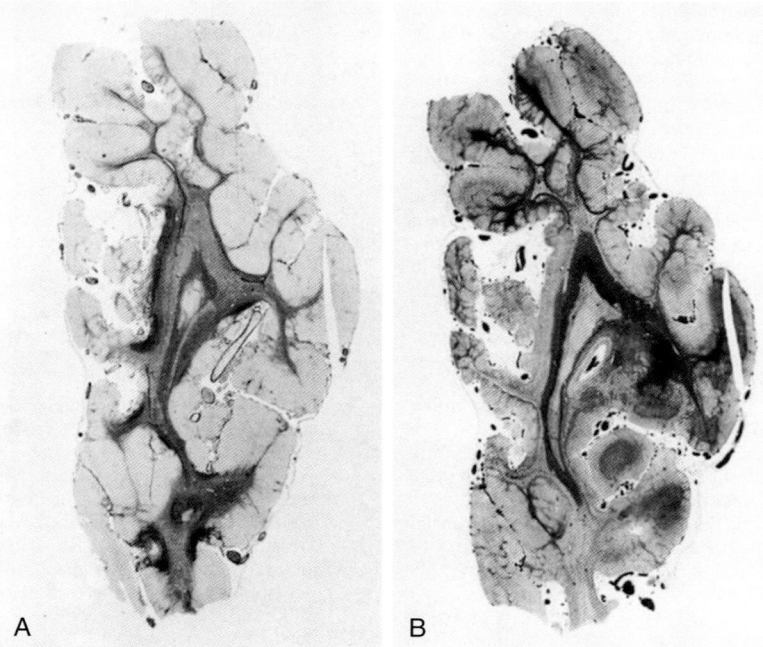

Figure 19.8 Ulegyria. Coronal section of cerebrum, stained for (A) glial fibers and (B) myelin. Note the mushroom-shaped gyri, especially in parasagittal areas. (From Norman MG. Perinatal brain damage. In: Rosenberg HS, Bolande RP, eds. *Perspectives in Pediatric Pathology.* Chicago: Mosby; 1978.)

white matter involved in the parasagittal lesions (see Box 19.2). The pathogenetic mechanisms operative in both neurons and pre-OLs involve principally excitatory (glutamate) receptors. The details for neurons were noted earlier concerning selective neuronal necrosis and for pre-OLs in Chapter 15.[78]

CEREBRAL WHITE MATTER INJURY/ PERIVENTRICULAR LEUKOMALACIA

In a minority of term infants with hypoxic-ischemic encephalopathy the predominant lesion involves primarily cerebral white matter (see Chapter 18). Approximately 15% of infants exhibit this pattern of injury as the dominant abnormality on neuroimaging (see Chapter 18). Periventricular and central cerebral white matter are involved, and the appearance is similar to "noncystic periventricular leukomalacia," as described for premature infants in Chapter 14. The principal cellular target is likely the pre-OL, as in the typical white matter injury of premature infants. Indeed, this oligodendroglial sub-type is the most abundant stage of the oligodendroglial lineage even at term in the human brain.[78]

Pathogenesis

The pathogenesis of cerebral white matter injury of the term infant with hypoxic-ischemic disease likely is similar to that described for the premature infant (see Chapter 15). As with the premature infant, the pathogenetic cascade likely includes the presence in cerebral white matter of vulnerable pre-OLs, the initiating injurious mechanism of ischemia, with energy deprivation, leading to excitotoxicity, microglial activation, Ca²⁺ influx, and free radical attack.[78] The associations of predominant white matter injury identified by MRI in term infants with hypoxic-ischemic encephalopathy with chronic hemodynamic

instability, hypoglycemia, and congenital heart disease (before and after cardiac surgery) support this formulation.[5,79-83] A potentiating role for systemic inflammation, with or without infection, also is apparent. These and related issues have been described in depth in Chapter 15.

REFERENCES

1. Pryds O, Greisen G, Lou H, et al. Vasoparalysis associated with brain damage in asphyxiated term infants. *J Pediatr.* 1990;117:119-125.
2. Greisen G. Effect of cerebral blood flow and cerebrovascular autoregulation on the distribution, type and extent of cerebral injury. *Brain Pathol.* 1992;2:223-228.
3. Kuban KC, Gilles FH. Human telencephalic angiogenesis. *Ann Neurol.* 1985;17:539-548.
4. Nelson MD, Gonzalez-Gomez I, Gilles FH. The search for human telencephalic ventriculofugal arteries. *AJNR Am J Neuroradiol.* 1991;12:215-222.
5. Volpe JJ. Neonatal encephalopathy: an inadequate term for hypoxic-ischemic encephalopathy. *Ann Neurol.* 2012;72:156-166.
6. Rorke LB. *Pathology of Perinatal Brain Injury.* New York: Raven Press; 1982.
7. Gilles FH. Hypotensive brain stem necrosis. Selective symmetrical necrosis of tegmental neuronal aggregates following cardiac arrest. *Arch Pathol.* 1969;88:32-41.
8. Ahdab-Barmada M, Moossy J, Nemoto EM, et al. Hyperoxia produces neuronal necrosis in the rat. *J Neuropathol Exp Neurol.* 1986;45:233-246.
9. Hashimoto K, Takeuchi Y, Takashima S. Hypocarbia as a pathogenic factor in pontosubicular necrosis. *Brain Dev.* 1991;13:155-157.
10. Friede RL. *Developmental Neuropathology.* 2nd ed. New York: Springer-Verlag; 1989.
10a. Mito T, Kamei A, Takashima S, et al. Clinicopathological study of pontosubicular necrosis. *Neuropediatrics.* 1993;24:204-207.
10b. Bruck Y, Bruck W, Kretzschmar HA, et al. Evidence for neuronal apoptosis in pontosubicular neuron necrosis. *Neuropathol Appl Neurobiol.* 1996;22:23-29.

10c. Stadelman C, Mews I, Srinivasan A, et al. Expression of cell death-associated proteins in neuronal apoptosis associated with pontosubicular neuron necrosis. *Brain Pathol.* 2001;11:273-281.

10d. Rossiter JP, Anderson LI, Yang F, et al. Caspase-3 activation and caspase-like proteolytic activity in human perinatal hypoxic-ischemic brain injury. *Acta Neuropathol.* 2002;103:66-73.

11. Barks JD, Silverstein FS, Sims K, et al. Glutamate recognition sites in human fetal brain. *Neurosci Lett.* 1988;84:131-136.

12. McDonald JW, Trescher WH, Johnston MV. The selective ionotropic-type quisqualate receptor agonist AMPA is a potent neurotoxin in immature rat brain. *Brain Res.* 1990;526:165-168.

13. Lee HS, Choi BH. Density and distribution of excitatory amino acid receptors in the developing human fetal brain—a quantitative autoradiographic study. *Exp Neurol.* 1992;118:284-290.

14. Piggott MA, Perry EK, Perry RH, et al. N-methyl-D-aspartate (NMDA) and non-NMDA binding sites in developing human frontal cortex. *Neurosci Res Commun.* 1993;12:9-16.

15. Johnston MV. Neurotransmitters and vulnerability of the developing brain. *Brain Dev.* 1995;17:301-306.

16. Kinney HC, Panigrahy A, Newburger JW, et al. Hypoxic-ischemic brain injury in infants with congenital heart disease dying after cardiac surgery. *Acta Neuropathol (Berl).* 2005;110:563-578.

17. Panigrahy A, Rosenberg PS, Assmann S, et al. Differential expression of glutamate receptor subtypes in human brainstem sites involved in perinatal hypoxia-ischemia. *J Comp Neurol.* 2001;437:196-208.

18. Ferriero DM, Arcavi LJ, Sagar SM, et al. Selective sparing of NADPH-diaphorase neurons in neonatal hypoxia-ischemia. *Ann Neurol.* 1988;24:670-676.

19. Ferriero DM, Arcavi LJ, Simon RP. Ontogeny of excitotoxic injury to nicotinamide adenine dinucleotide phosphate diaphorase reactive neurons in the neonatal rat striatum. *Neuroscience.* 1990;36:417-424.

20. Downen M, Zhao ML, Lee P, et al. Neuronal nitric oxide synthase expression in developing and adult human CNS. *J Neuropathol Exp Neurol.* 1999;58:12-21.

21. Talos DM, Follett PL, Folkerth RD, et al. Developmental regulation of alpha-amino-3-hydroxy-5-methyl-4-isoxazole-propionic acid receptor subunit expression in forebrain and relationship to regional susceptibility to hypoxic/ischemic injury. II. Human cerebral white matter and cortex. *J Comp Neurol.* 2006;497:61-77.

22. Jantzie LL, Talos DM, Jackson MC, et al. Developmental expression of N-methyl-D-aspartate (NMDA) receptor subunits in human white and gray matter: potential mechanism of increased vulnerability in the immature brain. *Cereb Cortex.* 2015;25:482-495.

23. Yager JY, Ashwal S. Animal models of perinatal hypoxic-ischemic brain damage. *Pediatr Neurol.* 2009;40:156-167.

24. Mallard EC, Williams CE, Gunn AJ, et al. Frequent episodes of brief ischemia sensitize the fetal sheep brain to neuronal loss and induce striatal injury. *Pediatr Res.* 1993;33:61-65.

25. Mallard EC, Waldvogel HJ, Williams CE, et al. Repeated asphyxia causes loss of striatal projection neurons in the fetal sheep brain. *Neuroscience.* 1995;65:827-836.

26. Mallard EC, Williams CE, Johnston BM, et al. Repeated episodes of umbilical cord occlusion in fetal sheep lead to preferential damage to the striatum and sensitize the heart to further insults. *Pediatr Res.* 1995;37:707-713.

27. De Haan HH, Gunn AJ, Williams CE, et al. Brief repeated umbilical cord occlusions cause sustained cytotoxic cerebral edema and focal infarcts in near-term fetal lambs. *Pediatr Res.* 1997;41:96-104.

28. Myers RE. Four patterns of perinatal brain damage and their conditions of occurrence. *Adv Neurol.* 1975;10:223-234.

29. Myers RE. Two patterns of perinatal brain damage and their conditions of occurrence. *Am J Obstet Gynecol.* 1972;112:246-276.

30. Pasternak JF, Gorey MT. The syndrome of acute near-total intrauterine asphyxia in the term infant. *Pediatr Neurol.* 1998;18:391-398.

31. Brann AW Jr, Myers RE. Central nervous system findings in the newborn monkey following severe in utero partial asphyxia. *Neurology.* 1975;25:327-338.

32. Leung AS, Leung EK, Paul RH. Uterine rupture after previous cesarean delivery: maternal and fetal consequences. *Am J Obstet Gynecol.* 1993;169:945-950.

33. Martin-Ancel A, Carcia-Alix A, Pascual-Salcedo D, et al. Interleukin-6 in the cerebrospinal fluid after perinatal asphyxia is related to early and late neurological manifestations. *Pediatrics.* 1997;100:789-794.

34. Grether JK, Nelson KB. Maternal infection and cerebral palsy in infants of normal birth weight. *J Am Med Assoc.* 1997;287:207-211.

35. Nelson KB, Dambrosia JM, Grether JK, et al. Neonatal cytokines and coagulation factors in children with cerebral palsy. *Ann Neurol.* 1998;44:665-675.

36. Grether JK, Nelson KB, Dambrosia JM, et al. Interferons and cerebral palsy. *J Pediatr.* 1999;134:324-332.

37. Foster-Barber A, Dickens B, Ferriero DM. Human perinatal asphyxia: correlation of neonatal cytokines with MRI and outcome. *Dev Neurosci.* 2002;23:213-218.

38. Shalak LF, Perlman JM. Infection markers and early signs of neonatal encephalopathy in the term infant. *Ment Retard Dev Disabil Res Rev.* 2002;8:14-19.

39. Shalak LF, Laptook AR, Jafri HS, et al. Clinical chorioamnionitis, elevated cytokines, and brain injury in term infants. *Pediatrics.* 2002;110:673-680.

40. Wu YW, Escobar GJ, Grether JK, et al. Chorioamnionitis and cerebral palsy in term and near-term infants. *J Am Med Assoc.* 2003;290:2677-2684.

41. Silveira RC, Procianoy RS. Interleukin-6 and tumor necrosis factor-α levels in plasma and cerebrospinal fluid of term newborn infants with hypoxic-ischemic encephalopathy. *J Pediatr.* 2003;143:625-629.

42. Bartha AI, Foster-Barber A, Miller SP, et al. Neonatal encephalopathy: association of cytokines with MR spectroscopy and outcome. *Pediatr Res.* 2004;56:960-966.

43. Rouse DJ, Landon M, Leveno KJ, et al. The Maternal-fetal medicine units cesarean registry: chorioamnionitis at term and its duration-relationship to outcomes. *Am J Obstet Gynecol.* 2004;191:211-216.

44. Mir IN, Johnson-Welch SF, Nelson DB, et al. Placental pathology is associated with severity of neonatal encephalopathy and adverse developmental outcomes following hypothermia. *Am J Obstet Gynecol.* 2015;213:849.e1-e7.

45. Shalak L, Johnson-Welch S, Perlman JM. Chorioamnionitis and neonatal encephalopathy in term infants with fetal acidemia: histopathologic correlations. *Pediatr Neurol.* 2005;33:162-165.

46. Meyer JE. Über die lokalisation fruhkindlicher hirschaden in arteriellen grenzgebieten. *Arch Psychiatr Nervenchr.* 1953;190:328.

47. Adams JH, Brierley JB, Connor RC, et al. The effects of systemic hypotension upon the human brain. Clinical and neuropathological observations in 11 cases. *Brain.* 1966;89:235-268.

48. Zulch KJ. Die pathogenese von massenblutung und erweichung unter besonderer berucksichtigung klinischer gesichtspunkte. *Acta Neurochir.* 1961;7:51.

49. Torvik A. The pathogenesis of watershed infarcts in the brain. *Stroke.* 1984;15:221-223.

50. Brierley JB, Excell BJ. The effects of profound systemic hypotension upon the brain of *M. rhesus*: physiological and pathological observations. *Brain.* 1966;89:269-298.

51. Brierley JB, Brown AW, Excell BJ, et al. Brain damage in the rhesus monkey resulting from profound arterial hypotension. I. Its nature, distribution and general physiological correlates. *Brain Res.* 1969;13:68-100.

52. Volpe JJ, Pasternak JF. Parasagittal cerebral injury in neonatal hypoxic-ischemic encephalopathy: clinical and neuroradiologic features. *J Pediatr.* 1977;91:472-476.

53. Volpe JJ, Herscovitch P, Perlman JM, et al. Positron emission tomography in the asphyxiated term newborn: parasagittal impairment of cerebral blood flow. *Ann Neurol.* 1985;17:287-296.

54. Takashima S, Ando Y, Takeshita K. Hypoxic-ischemic brain damage and cerebral blood flow changes in young rabbits. *Brain Dev.* 1986;8:274-277.

55. Yoshioka H, Iino S, Sato N, et al. New model of hemorrhagic hypoxic-ischemic encephalopathy in newborn mice. *Pediatr Neurol.* 1989;5:221-225.

56. Williams CE, Gunn AJ, Synek B, et al. Delayed seizures occurring with hypoxic-ischemic encephalopathy in the fetal sheep. *Pediatr Res.* 1990;27:561-565.

57. Williams CE, Gunn AJ, Mallard C, et al. Outcome after ischemia in the developing sheep brain: an electroencephalographic and histological study. *Ann Neurol.* 1992;31:14-21.

58. Gunn AJ, Parer JT, Mallard EC, et al. Cerebral histologic and electrocorticographic changes after asphyxia in fetal sheep. *Pediatr Res.* 1992;31:486-491.

59. Marks KA, Mallard CE, Roberts I, et al. Nitric oxide synthase inhibition attenuates delayed vasodilation and increases injury after cerebral ischemia in fetal sheep. *Pediatr Res.* 1996;40:185-191.

60. Larroche JC. *Developmental Pathology of the Neonate.* New York: Excerpta Medica; 1977.

61. Takashima S, Armstrong DL, Becker LE. Subcortical leukomalacia. Relationship to development of the cerebral sulcus and its vascular supply. *Arch Neurol.* 1978;35:470-472.

62. Kuenzle C, Baenziger O, Martin E, et al. Prognostic value of early MR imaging in term infants with severe perinatal asphyxia. *Neuropediatrics.* 1994;25:191-200.

63. Rutherford MA, Pennock JM, Dubowitz L. Cranial ultrasound and magnetic resonance imaging in hypoxic-ischaemic encephalopathy: a comparison with outcome. *Dev Med Child Neurol.* 1994;36:813-825.

64. Rollins NK, Morriss MC, Evans D, et al. The role of early MR in the evaluation of the term infant with seizures. *AJNR Am J Neuroradiol.* 1994;15:239-248.

65. Mercuri E, Rutherford M, Cowan F, et al. Early prognostic indicators of outcome in infants with neonatal cerebral infarction: a clinical, electroencephalogram, and magnetic resonance imaging study. *Pediatrics.* 1999;103:103-139.

66. de Vries LS, Groenendaal F, Eken P, et al. Infarcts in the vascular distribution of the middle cerebral artery in preterm and fullterm infants. *Neuropediatrics.* 1997;28:88-96.

67. Trauner DA, Mannino FL. Neurodevelopmental outcome after neonatal cerebrovascular accident. *J Pediatr.* 1986;108:459-461.

68. Bode H, Strassburg HM, Pringsheim W, et al. Cerebral infarction in term neonates: diagnosis by cerebral ultrasound. *Childs Nerv Syst.* 1986;2:195-199.

69. Filipek PA, Krishnamoorthy KS, Davis KR, et al. Focal cerebral infarction in the newborn: a distinct entity. *Pediatr Neurol.* 1987;3:141-147.

70. Coker SB, Beltran RS, Myers TF, et al. Neonatal stroke: description of patients and investigation into pathogenesis. *Pediatr Neurol.* 1988;4:219-223.

71. Hernanz-Schulman M, Cohen W, Genieser NB. Sonography of cerebral infarction in infancy. *AJR Am J Roentgenol.* 1988;150:897-902.

72. Roodhooft AM, Parizel PM, Van Acker KJ, et al. Idiopathic cerebral arterial infarction with paucity of symptoms in the full-term neonate. *Pediatrics.* 1987;80:381-385.

73. Sran SK, Baumann RJ. Outcome of neonatal strokes. *Am J Dis Child.* 1988;142:1086-1088.

74. Fujimoto S, Yokochi K, Togari H, et al. Neonatal cerebral infarction: symptoms, CT findings and prognosis. *Brain Dev.* 1992;14:48-52.

75. Trounce JQ, Levene MI. Diagnosis and outcome of subcortical cystic leucomalacia. *Arch Dis Child.* 1985;60:1041-1044.

76. Houdou S, Takashima S, Takeshita K, et al. Infantile subcortical leukohypodensity demonstrated by computed tomography. *Pediatr Neurol.* 1988;4:165-167.

77. Yokochi K. Clinical profiles of subjects with subcortical leukomalacia and border-zone infarction revealed by MR. *Acta Paediatr.* 1998;87:879-883.

78. Volpe JJ, Kinney HC, Jensen FE, et al. The developing oligodendrocyte: key cellular target in brain injury in the premature infant. *Int J Dev Neurosci.* 2011;29:423-440.

79. Rutherford M, Counsell S, Allsop J, et al. Diffusion-weighted magnetic resonance imaging in term perinatal brain injury: a comparison with site of lesion and time from birth. *Pediatrics.* 2004;114:1004-1014.

80. Li AM, Chau V, Poskitt KJ, et al. White matter injury in term newborns with neonatal encephalopathy. *Pediatr Res.* 2009;65:85-89.

81. Logitharajah P, Rutherford MA, Cowan FM. Hypoxic-ischemic encephalopathy in preterm infants: antecedent factors, brain imaging, and outcome. *Pediatr Res.* 2009;66:222-229.

82. Martinez-Biarge M, Bregant T, Wusthoff CJ, et al. White matter and cortical injury in hypoxic-ischemic encephalopathy: antecedent factors and 2-year outcome. *J Pediatr.* 2012;161:799-807.

83. Volpe JJ. Encephalopathy of congenital heart disease—destructive and developmental effects intertwined. *J Pediatr.* 2014;164:962-965.

Hypoxic-Ischemic Injury in the Term Infant: Clinical-Neurological Features, Diagnosis, Imaging, Prognosis, Therapy

Terrie E. Inder ◆ Joseph J. Volpe

The clinical aspects of neonatal hypoxic-ischemic encephalopathy (HIE) are appropriately discussed following the neuropathology (see Chapter 18) and pathophysiology (see Chapter 19), because understanding of the clinical phenomena is facilitated greatly by an awareness of the underlying pathological substrates. Moreover, choice of appropriate diagnostic modalities, formulation of rational prognostic statements, and development of appropriate plans of management are based, in many ways, on awareness of the probable neuropathologies. In this chapter, we discuss the clinical settings for neonatal HIE, the clinical syndrome, diagnostic studies, clinical correlations, prognosis, and management.

CLINICAL SETTINGS

The importance of the early recognition of the clinical risk factors for hypoxic-ischemic cerebral injury in the term born infant has escalated significantly in the last decade with the implementation of successful neuroprotection with therapeutic hypothermia (see later sections). To initiate such therapy requires a recognition of the infant who may have suffered hypoxic-ischemic cerebral injury—predominantly in the peripartum period. *The peripartum period is defined as the period shortly before, during, and immediately after birth.* The clinical settings for neonatal HIE are dominated by the ultimate occurrence of ischemia (i.e., diminished blood supply to brain), usually, but not necessarily, preceded or accompanied by hypoxemia (i.e., a diminished amount of oxygen in the blood supply). Hypoxemia leads to brain injury principally by causing myocardial disturbance and loss of cerebrovascular autoregulation, with ischemia the major consequence. The temporal characteristics and the severity of the hypoxemia and ischemia, as well as the gestational age of the infant, are the principal determinants of the type of resulting neuropathology (see Chapters 18 and 19).

The major causes of serious hypoxemia in the peripartum period are: (1) hypoxia-ischemia with intrauterine disturbance of gas exchange across the placenta (i.e., asphyxia) or with failure to establish independent respiration at the time of birth or both; (2) postnatal respiratory insufficiency secondary to severe respiratory disease; and (3) severe right-to-left shunt secondary to persistent fetal circulation or cardiac disease. The major causes of serious ischemia are: (1) intrauterine asphyxia (i.e., hypoxemia, hypercarbia, and acidosis) with cardiac insufficiency and loss of cerebrovascular autoregulation both in

utero and at the time of birth; (2) postnatal cardiac insufficiency secondary to severe hypoxemia or congenital heart disease; and (3) postnatal (postcardiac) circulatory insufficiency secondary to patent ductus arteriosus (with "ductal steal") or vascular collapse (e.g., with sepsis).

In this chapter, we will focus on the encephalopathic syndrome in the term infant *and* the presence of evidence for peripartum hypoxic-ischemic injury. We prefer the term "peripartum" hypoxic-ischemic injury as it acknowledges the potential presence of (1) fetal or maternal prepartum conditions that may accentuate propensity to intrapartum hypoxic-ischemic injury; (2) intrapartum hypoxic–ischemic injury per se; and (3) the often associated protracted postpartum resuscitative efforts for such infants, with no or low heart rate for several minutes. Although the postnatal cardiac compromise is not the primary etiology of the poor birth transition, it may contribute to the extent of the ultimate hypoxic-ischemic cerebral injury in the infant. However, there is also evidence that even with prolonged resuscitation, in the era of therapeutic hypothermia there can be better outcomes than might be expected (see the section on prognosis).[1]

It is important to recognize that not all neonatal encephalopathies are related to hypoxic-ischemic disease. Antepartum and postpartum disorders (e.g., infectious, metabolic, dysgenetic) may lead to neonatal encephalopathies,[2,3] as discussed throughout this book. In one large population-based observational study, the prevalence of moderate to severe encephalopathy was 1.64 per 1000 live term births, and the prevalence of "birth asphyxia" was 0.86 per 1000 live term births.[4] Fully 56% of all cases of newborn encephalopathy were related to hypoxic-ischemic injury that occurred during the intrapartum period. These findings are consistent with a more recent large cohort study of 4165 singleton term infants with any one of the following: seizures, stupor, coma, Apgar score at 5 minutes less than 3 and/or receiving hypothermia therapy.[5] In this study, 15% of the infants experienced a clinically recognized sentinel event, such as antenatal hemorrhage (presumably, often placental abruption), uterine rupture, or cord prolapse, all of which are capable of compromising oxygen supply. Almost one half of the infants displayed umbilical cord blood gas acidemia and/or fetal bradycardia. Of note, signs of inflammation were also not uncommon with 27% of mothers displaying elevated maternal temperature in labor and 11% clinical chorioamnionitis. However, the contributing role of chorioamnionitis is not consistently supported.[6] Although intrapartum sentinel events provide clear evidence of a hypoxic-ischemic insult, in three studies of neonatal encephalopathy, sentinel intrapartum events were only identified in 8% to 25% of infants.[7-9] In a referral sample of 500 term infants with neonatal encephalopathy evaluated for therapeutic hypothermia, 48 (9%) had a sentinel birth event.[10] Thus, it can be challenging to confirm an hypoxic-ischemic etiology for the infant with neonatal encephalopathy and/or the need for resuscitation as only 10% to 20% of such infants may have a clinical history of a major risk factor, whereas approximately 50% or more may have a constellation of risk factors including maternal history, cord acidemia, and the need for resuscitation that supports this as the most likely etiology for their neurological syndrome.

In addition, although obvious, hypoxic-ischemic injury may affect the infant's brain during the antepartum and postnatal periods, *albeit much less commonly than the intrapartum period*. On the basis of earlier work,[11-27] approximately 20% of hypoxic-ischemic injury recognized in the newborn period was said to be related primarily to antepartum insults. These data should be interpreted with the awareness that assessment of timing of insults to the fetus in these reports generally was based on imprecise methods, and the variability of findings is considerable. Moreover, more recent studies with consistent use of magnetic resonance imaging (MRI) suggest that the large majority of hypoxic-ischemic injury occurs during the intrapartum period.

The best data indicate that most infants with neonatal HIE and intrapartum evidence of hypoxic-ischemic insult exhibit, on MRI, evidence only of injury from the immediate peripartum period with no clear evidence of long-standing antenatal hypoxic-ischemic disease (Table 20.1).[28,29]

In one study of 245 term infants with neonatal encephalopathy and evidence of intrauterine asphyxia, fully 80% had evidence of acute lesions (within the period immediately before or during labor and delivery) consistent with hypoxic-ischemic disease, 16% had normal MRI scans, and only 4% had concomitant evidence of chronic antenatal injury (see Table 20.1).[28] In another MRI study of 173 term newborns with encephalopathy and signs of intrauterine asphyxia, only acute injury was observed.[29] Related clinical and epidemiological data also support a marked preponderance of intrapartum events in the origin of neonatal HIE, especially in the term infant.[30-32]

The principal *intrapartum events* leading to hypoxic-ischemic fetal insults include acute placental or umbilical cord disturbances, such as abruptio placentae or cord prolapse, prolonged labor with transverse arrest, difficult forceps extractions, or rotational maneuvers (see Chapters 17 to 19). *Postpartum events* alone (e.g., severe persistent fetal circulation, severe recurrent apneic spells, cardiac failure secondary to large patent ductus arteriosus or other congenital heart disease, severe pulmonary disease) may lead to HIE and may account for approximately 5% to 10% of cases.[30] Most of these and related *postnatal* factors are much more important in the pathogenesis of hypoxic-ischemic brain injury in the *premature infant* than in the term infant (see Chapters 14 to 16). Although hypoxic-ischemic injury certainly can occur in the antepartum period (e.g., secondary to maternal trauma, maternal hypotension, uterine hemorrhage), this injury cumulatively accounts for between 5% and 20% of neonatal HIE (as noted earlier). However, antepartum factors appear to be of some importance in the risk for neonatal encephalopathy related to peripartum events. Such factors may indeed *predispose* to intrapartum hypoxia-ischemia during the stresses of labor and delivery, especially through threats to placental flow. Such factors include maternal diabetes, preeclampsia, placental vasculopathy, intrauterine growth restriction, and twin gestation that may compromise fetal cerebral perfusion (Table 20.2; see Chapter 13). In one series, such factors were present in approximately one third of cases of intrapartum asphyxia.[30] Indeed, "perinatal asphyxia" was identified in 27% of infants of diabetic mothers, and its occurrence correlated closely with diabetic vasculopathy (nephropathy) and presumed placental vascular insufficiency.[33] In a more recent cohort of infants that received therapeutic

---

TABLE 20.1   Timing of Insults Leading to Hypoxic-Ischemic Encephalopathy

Of 245 infants who had an MRI scan after neonatal neurological signs ("neonatal encephalopathy"), and evidence of intrapartum perinatal asphyxia:
  197 (80%) had MRI evidence of *acute peripartum* lesions consistent with hypoxic-ischemic insult; only 8 (4%) also had MRI evidence of antenatal injury
  40 (16%) had normal MRI scans
  8 (4%) had other disorders (e.g., neuromuscular or metabolic diseases)

MRI, Magnetic resonance imaging.
Data from Cowan F, Rutherford M, Groenendaal F, et al. Origin and timing of brain lesions in term infants with neonatal encephalopathy. *Lancet*. 2003;361:736–742.

TABLE 20.2   Antepartum/Maternal Clinical Factors Associated With Neonatal Encephalopathy

		FREQUENCY IN GENERAL POPULATION (%)	FREQUENCY IN HIE POPULATION (%)
Antepartum/Maternal	Hypothyroidism	0.5[713]	3
	Obesity	10–25[714]	15–50[a]
	Diabetes (particularly pregestational)	0.5–2[715]	5–20[a]
	Fetal growth restriction <5%	5	10–15
	Hypertension	3–5[716]	5–15
	Clinical chorioamnionitis	1–4[717]	5–10

[a]Dependent on geographical cohort.
HIE, Hypoxic-ischemic encephalopathy.

hypothermia (*n* = 98), the frequency of pregestational diabetes and preeclampsia were significantly higher (threefold to fivefold) in women with infants requiring cooling.[9]

Regarding intrauterine growth restriction, in the largest North American series of neonatal encephalopathy, collected by the Vermont Oxford Registry, 16% of infants were defined as less than the 10th% for weight.[5] In a major controlled study of neonatal encephalopathy, 16% of infants with neonatal encephalopathy were growth-restricted compared to only 1.2% of term infants without encephalopathy. Growth restriction was the strongest predictor of neonatal encephalopathy examined, associated with a 30-fold increase in risk.[26] In a regional study of moderate or severe neonatal encephalopathy in term infants, 17% were small for their gestational age.[8] The additional stress of labor would be expected to compromise placental blood flow. Similarly, impaired placental function and an increased risk of perinatal asphyxia in *the infant with intrauterine growth restriction* are recognized and appear to account for some of the increased risk of subsequent neurological disability in such infants.[34-41] In the most recent series of infants receiving hypothermia, infant birthweight below the 5th percentile for gestational age was significantly associated with the need for therapeutic hypothermia.[9] Other factors (e.g., dysmorphic syndromes, severe undernutrition, infection) may also lead to increased risk of neurological disability in intrauterine growth restriction.[38,42-46] Moreover, studies in fetal and neonatal animals suggest that the mechanisms for the increased vulnerability of the growth-restricted fetus relate not only to placental insufficiency but also to diminished glucose reserves in the heart, liver, and brain, and to impaired capability to increase substrate supply to the brain with the hypoxic stress of vaginal delivery.[47,48]

Other less characterized maternal factors have been recognized as important risk factors for neonatal encephalopathy, although pathogenetic mechanisms remain unclear. One such factor is maternal hypothyroidism. In four prospective studies, an elevated risk of up to 10-fold was found for maternal hypothyroidism in infants with neonatal encephalopathy (see Table 20.2).[5,7,26,49] Further, maternal drug use can impair the transition of infants after delivery, and infants can display abnormal neurological signs that can mimic neonatal encephalopathy. The details of these agents are outlined in Chapter 38.

Although the particular importance of intrauterine hypoxic-ischemic injury, especially intrapartum asphyxia with or without antepartum predisposing factors, in the genesis of the clinical syndrome of neonatal HIE is apparent, most infants who experience intrapartum hypoxic-ischemic insults do *not* exhibit overt neonatal neurological features *or* subsequent neurological evidence of brain injury.[a] The severity and duration of the hypoxic-ischemic insult is obviously critical. The elegant studies of Low[16,17,50] and others[51,52] demonstrate a striking relationship among the severity and duration of intrapartum hypoxia, assessed by the use of fetal acid-base studies (see Chapter 17), the subsequent occurrence of a neonatal neurological syndrome, and later neurological deficits. Current data suggest that approximately 10% of all term deliveries require some resuscitation with 1% requiring extensive resuscitation,[56,57] Of the latter. only 1 to 3 per 1000 will develop signs of evolving encephalopathy consistent with HIE.[31,55,58,59]

---

[a]References 2, 11, 12, 23, 25, 27, and 50-55.

NEUROLOGICAL SYNDROME

The neurological syndrome that accompanies serious peripartum hypoxic-ischemic cerebral injury is the prototype for neonatal HIE. *In considering the nature and timing of hypoxia-ischemia as the etiology of neonatal HIE,* we consider three features to be important: (1) evidence of fetal distress and/or fetal risk for hypoxia-ischemia (e.g., fetal heart rate (FHR) abnormalities, sentinel event, fetal acidemia); (2) the need for resuscitation and/or low Apgar scores; and (3) an overt neonatal neurological syndrome in the first hours or day of life.

Although not discussed here in depth, important *systemic abnormalities,* presumably related to ischemia, often accompany the neonatal neurological syndrome. The relative frequencies of manifestations of organ injury in term infants with evidence of asphyxia have been investigated in several studies.[53,54,60-64] The findings varied as a function of the severity of asphyxia and the definitions of organ dysfunction. In combined data from two reports (Table 20.3),[54,60] approximately 20% of infants with apparent fetal asphyxia had no evidence of organ injury. Evidence of involvement of the central nervous system occurred in 62% of infants. Indeed, in 16% of infants, involvement of only the nervous system was apparent. The order of frequency of systemic organ involvement overall has been hepatic > pulmonary > renal > cardiac. In an autopsy series, cardiac involvement was the most common among affection of systemic organs.[65] With careful electrocardiographic and enzymatic studies of living infants after perinatal asphyxia, evidence of myocardial ischemia has been commonly observed.[66] Representative data from a well-studied series of 144 infants with moderate-severe encephalopathy, found that all infants displayed some form of organ dysfunction, with pulmonary and hepatic approximately 85%, renal 70%, and cardiac 60%.[64] These frequencies may relate, in part, to the nature of the diagnostic categories for these abnormalities, but confirm that multiorgan dysfunction is very common in the setting

---

TABLE 20.3   Manifestations of Organ Injury in Term Asphyxiated Infants[a]

ORGAN	PERCENTAGE OF TOTAL
None	0–36
CNS only	0–36
CNS and one or more other organs	46–100
Renal & cardiac approx. 65%: Pulmonary & liver approx. 85%	
Other organ(s), no CNS	10–20

[a]Cumulative total of 107 term infants; definition of asphyxia in both series included umbilical cord arterial pH < 7.2.

CNS, Central nervous system.

Data from Perlman JM, Tack ED, Martin T, et al. Acute systemic organ injury in term infants after asphyxia. *Am J Dis Child.* 1989;143:617–620; Martin-Ancel A, Garcia-Alix A, Gaya F, et al. Multiple organ involvement in perinatal asphyxia. *J Pediatr.* 1995;127:786–793; Shah P, Riphagen S, Beyene J, Perlman M. Multiorgan dysfunction in infants with post-asphyxial hypoxic-ischaemic encephalopathy. *Arch Dis Child Fetal Neonatal Ed.* 2004;89(2):F152–F155; Phelan JP, Ahn MO, Korst L, Martin GI, Wang YM. Intrapartum fetal asphyxial brain injury with absent multiorgan system dysfunction. *J Matern Fetal Med.* 1998;7(1):19–22.

TABLE 20.4 Standardized Scoring Systems for Neonatal Encephalopathy

SCORING SYSTEM	PURPOSE/UTILITY	NUMBER OF ELEMENTS	ELEMENTS	EEG NECESSARY
Sarnat	Prognosis applied in first 7 days	14	Alertness, tone, posture, reflexes, myocolonus, suck, Moro, oculovestibular, tonic neck, pupils, heart rate, secretions, GI motility, seizures, EEG	Yes
Modified Sarnat	Prognosis applied in first 7 days	5	Alertness, tone, suck, Moro, seizures	No
Thompson	Prognosis applied in first 7 days	6	Alertness, tone, respiratory status, reflexes, seizure, feeding method	No
NICHD	Selection in first 6 h of life of moderate-severe NE for hypothermia	9	Alertness, spontaneous activity, posture, tone, suck, Moro, pupils, heart rate, respirations	No
SIBEN	Defining mild, moderate, and severe NE in first 6 h of life	10	Alertness, spontaneous activity, posture, tone, suck, Moro, pupils, heart rate, respirations, seizures	No

EEG, Electroencephalography; *GI*, gastrointestinal; *NE*, neonatal encephalopathy; *NICHD*, National Institute of Child Health and Human Development; *SIBEN*, Score of the Iberoamerican Society of Neonatology.

of moderate-severe peripartum HIE and should be sought by appropriate diagnostic studies.

Defining the neurological syndrome of HIE by clinical evaluation is important. Central to this definition is awareness of the characteristics of the normal neurological examination (see Chapter 9). The abnormal features of the examination in infants with HIE were discussed in previous editions of this book and in Chapter 9. To improve interobserver reliability, standardized scores have been developed, and have proven useful in large-scale clinical research studies (see later) (Table 20.4)[67-69]

The initial neurological examination classification systems developed evaluated infants over the first week of life to define the severity of their encephalopathy for prognostication. The first of these scoring systems was that developed by Sarnat, which was based on serial examinations of 21 term-born infants over the first few weeks of life.[70] Three clinical stages of "postanoxic encephalopathy" were described. Stage 1 lasted less than 24 hours and was characterized by hyperalertness, uninhibited Moro and stretch reflexes, sympathetic effects, and a normal electroencephalogram. Stage 2 was marked by obtundation, hypotonia, strong distal flexion, and multifocal seizures. The electroencephalography (EEG) showed a periodic pattern sometimes preceded by continuous delta activity. Infants in stage 3 were stuporous, flaccid, and their brain stem and autonomic functions were suppressed. The EEG was isopotential or had infrequent periodic discharges. Infants who did not enter stage 3 and who had signs of stage 2 for less than 5 days appeared normal in later infancy. Persistence of stage 2 for more than 7 days, or failure of the EEG to revert to normal, was associated with later neurologic impairment or death. This classification system was then further simplified, to be known as the Modified Sarnat score (see Table 20.4).

The next scoring system developed for prognostication in neonatal encephalopathy was the Thompson Encephalopathy Score, developed in 1997 (see Table 20.4).[68] This scoring system was simpler to apply and did not require EEG to increase its widespread applicability. The initial evaluation showed a good

correlation between the maximal score in the first 7 days of life and neurodevelopmental outcome at 18 months in 44 infants with neonatal HIE.

It is important to note that both the Sarnat and the Thompson scoring systems aimed to define neonatal neurological signs *during the first week of life* to improve the prediction of subsequent neurological deficits. However, as the era of neuroprotection emerged, it became apparent that a standardized neonatal neurological examination tool to be applied *in the first few hours of life* would be necessary to define eligibility for randomized controlled trials, such as therapeutic hypothermia. For some of the latter trials, the modified Sarnat and Thompson scales were used. For the largest North American study, a new scoring system was developed: the NICHD (National Institute of Child Health and Human Development) Neonatal Encephalopathy Scoring System (see Table 20.4).[71] The aim of this scoring system was to identify infants with moderate-severe encephalopathy who were eligible for entry into the trial within the first 6 hours of life. There was recognition that the examination could evolve over the first day of life, as described by Sarnat and Thompson (see temporal evolution of the neurological syndrome later).

To further refine the NICHD scoring system by the addition of a *mild encephalopathy* grouping, the HIE Score of the Iberoamerican Society of Neonatology (SIBEN) was developed in 2016 and involved the assessment of 10 clinical aspects that could be undertaken from immediately after delivery room resuscitation (see Tables 20.4 and 20.5).[72] The recognition of mild encephalopathy is of great relevance as it is recognized that at least 40% of hypoxic-ischemic cerebral injury presents as mild disease (see later).[59] To classify HIE as mild, moderate, or severe, each item evaluated varies according to the degree of severity (see Table 20.5). With this scoring system, a point is given to every item that corresponds to a level in the SIBEN score, with the diagnosis of HIE considered in the presence of three points or more. This scoring system has been evaluated in clinical practice in Brazil, but it remains under ongoing investigation for its utility in application to the evaluation of all infants requiring resuscitation who may benefit from therapeutic hypothermia. It remains the only current published

TABLE 20.5   SIBEN Neurological Score

		MILD	MODERATE	SEVERE
Level of consiousness		Hyperalert	Lethargy	Stupor/Coma
Spontaneous activity		Normal	Decreased	Not present
Posture		Mild distal flexion	Marked distal flexion	Decerebrate
Tone		Normal	Hypotonia	Flaccidity
Suck		Weak	Weak or absent	Not present
Moro		Strong	Weak	Not present
Pupils		Mydriasis	Miosis	Diverted/nonreactive
Heart rate (HR)		Tachycardia	Bradycardia	Lack of HR variability
Breathing		Spontaneous	Periodic	Apnea
Seizures		Absent	Present—Frequent	Present—infrequent

SIBEN, Score of the Iberoamerican Society of Neonatology.

TABLE 20.6   Clinical Features of Severe HIE: Birth to 12 Hours

Depressed level of consciousness: usually deep stupor or coma
Ventilatory disturbance: "periodic" breathing or respiratory failure
Intact pupillary responses
Intact oculomotor responses
Hypotonia, minimal movement > hypertonia
Seizures

HIE, Hypoxic-ischemic encephalopathy.

scoring system to include the evaluation of all three grades of neonatal encephalopathy in the first 6 hours of life.

Temporal Evolution of the Neurological Syndrome

The temporal evolution of the neurological syndrome in the era before therapeutic hypothermia has been outlined in detail in previous editions of this book. This evolution is most readily apparent in severely affected infants. With less severe forms of HIE changes in the clinical syndrome may be less stereotyped, and thus careful serial clinical evaluation every hour over the first 6 to 12 hours of life may be more sensitive to the evolution.

With regard to the most severe form of neonatal encephalopathy, occurring in 20% of HIE,[59] a clear evolution has been documented. Although the temporal evolution of the neurological syndrome is more complex in the infant undergoing therapeutic hypothermia because of sedation and response to hypothermia, the principles remain unchanged.

In the first hours after the insult, signs of presumed bilateral cerebral hemispheral disturbance predominate (Table 20.6).[73,74]

The severely affected infant is either deeply stuporous or in coma (i.e., not arousable and minimal, or no response to sensory input). Periodic breathing, or respiratory irregularity akin to this pattern, is prominent, which may be considered as a form of respiratory disturbance as a neonatal counterpart of Cheyne-Stokes respiration, which is observed in older children and adults with bilateral hemispheral disease. In one series, approximately 80% of infants with severe neonatal encephalopathy had abnormal breathing patterns, particularly periodic breathing.[75] Those most severely affected may exhibit

marked hypoventilation or apnea. Pupillary responses to light are intact, spontaneous eye movements are present, and eye movements with the oculocephalic response (doll's eyes maneuver) are usually full. (Pupillary size is variable, although dilated reactive pupils tend to predominate in the less affected infants, and constricted reactive pupils are common in the more severely affected infants.[70]) Commonly, disconjugate eye movements are apparent. However, only in a few babies are eye signs of major brain stem disturbance seen. Fixed, midposition, or dilated pupils and eye movements fixed to the doll's eyes maneuver and to cold caloric stimulation are unusual at this stage. If either of these signs is evident at this time, especially in the full-term infant, injury to the brain stem is likely. Most infants at this stage are markedly and diffusely hypotonic with minimal spontaneous or elicited movement. Less severely affected infants have a preserved tone. Others exhibit an increased tone, especially with prominent involvement of the basal ganglia.

Clinical seizure-like activity often occurs by 6 to 12 hours after birth in approximately 50% to 60% of the infants who ultimately have seizures.[24,55,76] (This early onset of seizures is unlike the later onset, 19 to 28 hours, in infants with neonatal arterial ischemic stroke [see Chapter 21].) A major challenge occurs in the correct clinical recognition of seizures. In one recent study of staff observing high-risk newborns, only 9% of 526 electrographic seizures were identified by clinical observation, indicating an *underdiagnosis of seizures*. In addition, 78% of 177 nonictal events were incorrectly identified as seizures, indicating an *overdiagnosis* of seizures.[77] Problematically, the more difficult to diagnose seizure types tend to occur more often than the more readily diagnosed seizure types in newborns. A study of 61 seizures in 24 newborns classified seizures by their most prominent clinical features. Clonic and tonic seizures, which might be more readily identified, only occurred in 20% and 8%, respectively, while orolingual, ocular, and autonomic features, which might be more difficult to identify, were the main features in 55%.[78] These clinical features contrast with the high frequency of focal clonic seizures in infants with neonatal arterial ischemic stroke (see Chapter 21).

Thus, neonatal seizures in the setting of HIE are frequently subtle or clinically invisible. More recent studies using EEG in the assessment of infants with moderate-severe HIE and undergoing therapeutic hypothermia identified the median timing of onset of EEG seizure activity at 13 hours (interquartile

TABLE 20.7 Clinical Features of Severe HIE: 12–24 Hours

Variable change in level of alertness
More seizures
Apneic spells
Jitteriness
Weakness
    Proximal limbs, upper > lower (full term)
    Hemiparesis (full term)
    Lower limbs (premature)

HIE, Hypoxic-ischemic encephalopathy.

TABLE 20.8 Clinical Features of Severe HIE: 24–72 Hours

Stupor or coma
Respiratory arrest
Brain stem oculomotor and pupillary disturbances

HIE, Hypoxic-ischemic encephalopathy.

TABLE 20.9 Clinical Features of Severe HIE: After 72 Hours

Persistent, yet diminishing stupor
Disturbed sucking, swallowing, gag, and tongue movements
Hypotonia > hypertonia
Weakness
Proximal limbs, upper > lower
Hemiparesis

HIE, Hypoxic-ischemic encephalopathy.

range [IQR]: 11 to 22 hours), with maximal seizure burden at a median of 19 hours (IQR: 12 to 29 hours).[79]

From approximately 12 to 24 hours, the infant's level of consciousness changes in a variable manner (Table 20.7).

Infants with severe disease remain deeply stuporous or in a coma. Infants with less severe disease may often begin to exhibit some degree of improvement in alertness. A recent report from Biselele et al. serially examined 21 infants with evidence of hypoxic-ischemic insult and found that in the first hour 70% of the infants that displayed neurological signs scored greater than 7 on the Thompson scale (see earlier), thereby permitting entry into therapeutic hypothermia; while at 6 hours only 20% of infants scored at this level.[80] The authors warn that this "apparent" improvement may prevent infants that need to receive therapeutic hypothermia from being eligible, if their examination is delayed to close to 6 hours of life. Thus, it is regarded that in many of these infants, this *improvement is more apparent than real*, because the appearance of alertness may not be accompanied by visual fixation or following, habituation to sensory stimulation, or other signs of cerebral function. The notion of apparent rather than real improvement in such cases is supported further by the occurrence at this time of seizures (as noted earlier, median occurrence at 13 hours), apneic spells, jitteriness, and weakness. Apneic spells appear in approximately 50% of infants (65% in one series).[11,12,75] Jitteriness develops in about one-fourth of infants and may be so marked that the movements are mistaken for seizures. Distinction can usually be made at the bedside (see Chapter 9). Infants with involvement of basal ganglia may exhibit an increase in their hypertonia, especially in response to handling. Many infants manifest definite, albeit not marked, weakness (see Table 20.7). Although precise correlation is often difficult, these infants appear from the clinical circumstances surrounding their insult to have sustained particularly marked *ischemic* insults. Full-term infants most often exhibit weakness in the hip–shoulder distribution, with more impressive involvement usually of the proximal extremities. Distinct asymmetry of these latter motor findings is unusual to elicit at this time, although a few full-term infants do exhibit weakness that is confined to or is clearly more severe on one side than on the other.

Between approximately **24 and 72 hours**, the severely affected infant's level of consciousness often deteriorates further, and deep stupor or coma may ensue (Table 20.8).

Respiratory arrest may occur, often after a period of irregularly irregular ("ataxic") respirations. Brain stem oculomotor disturbances are now more common. These usually consist of skew deviation and loss of responsiveness of the eyes to the doll's eyes maneuver and to cold caloric stimulation. (Rarely, ocular bobbing may appear.) Pupils may become fixed to light in the mid or dilated position. Reactive but constricted pupils are more common in less severely affected infants. Babies who die with HIE most often do so at this time, particularly if the criterion is "brain death."[81] In one large series of infants who died after perinatal asphyxia and HIE, the median age of death was 2 days.[65] The cause for the apparent delay in progression to brain death until this period is not known definitely, but delayed cell death has been documented in in vivo models and in neurons in culture (see Chapters 13, 18, and 19). The importance of excitatory amino acids, calcium-mediated deleterious metabolic events, and free radical production has been detailed in Chapter 13. Indeed, studies by MR spectroscopy in the asphyxiated human infant (see later) have documented a delayed deterioration of cerebral energy state. However, although delayed cell death most probably accounts for this clinical deterioration, consideration should also be given to the occurrence of frequent subclinical electrical seizures as the reason for the deterioration. Although EEG is required for this determination, the potential effectiveness of anticonvulsant therapy warrants the procedure.

Infants who survive to greater than 72 hours will at this point usually improve over the next several days to weeks; however, certain neurological features persist (Table 20.9).

Although the level of consciousness improves, often dramatically, mild to moderate stupor continues. Disturbances of feeding are extremely common and relate to abnormalities of sucking, swallowing, and tongue movements. The power and coordination of the muscles involved (innervated by cranial nerves V, VII, IX, X, and XII) are deranged. A few infants require tube feedings for weeks to months, particularly those with involvement of deep nuclear gray matter and brain stem (see Prognosis). In the large series studied by Brown and co-workers,[11,12] 80% of infants required early tube feedings because of feeding difficulty. Generalized hypotonia of limbs is common, although hypertonia, particularly with the passive manipulation of limbs, is frequent on careful examination, especially among infants with prominent involvement of basal ganglia. The patterns of weakness discussed in the previous section become more readily elicited, although the weakness is rarely marked.

DIAGNOSIS

The recognition of neonatal HIE depends principally on information gained from a careful history and a thorough neurological examination. The contributing role of certain metabolic derangements requires evaluation. Determination of the site or sites and extent of the injury is made by the history, neurological examination, EEG, and neuroimaging studies (ultrasonography, MRI).

History

Recognition of neonatal HIE requires awareness of those intrauterine situations that account for most cases. Thus, information should be sought regarding maternal disorders with an increased risk for peripartum HIE (see Table 20.2) and that could lead to uteroplacental insufficiency and disturbances of labor or delivery that could impair placental respiratory gas exchange or fetal blood flow. The value of fetal evaluation including electronic fetal monitoring, particularly when supplemented by fetal blood sampling to determine acid-base status, is discussed in Chapter 17.

Neurological Examination

Recognition of the neurological signs outlined previously provides critical information concerning the presence, site, and extent of hypoxic-ischemic injury in the newborn infant. The neurological examination plays two critical roles. First, the systematic neurological examination in the first 6 hours of life may allow recognition by the clinician of the presence and severity of any neonatal HIE. This is essential to allow that infant to be eligible for potentially neuroprotective strategies, such as therapeutic hypothermia. Second, the regular and systematic neurological examination of the infant with encephalopathy over the first week of life carries very important information for establishing a prognosis (see the section on prognosis).

Metabolic Parameters

Certain metabolic derangements may contribute significantly to the severity and qualitative aspects of the neurological syndrome, and the diagnostic evaluation should include evaluation of such derangements. Hypoglycemia, hyperammonemia, hypocalcemia, hyponatremia (inappropriate secretion of antidiuretic hormone [ADH]), hypoxemia, and acidosis are among the metabolic complications that may occur, often because of associated disorders, and that may exacerbate certain neurological features or add new ones.

Of particular interest in this context is the occurrence of *hypoglycemia* and its potential role in the accentuation of brain injury. In a detailed study of 185 infants with evidence of intrauterine asphyxia (cord pH < 7.00), fully 15% exhibited blood glucose concentrations lower than 40 mg/dL in the first 30 minutes of life.[82] The hypoglycemia may relate, in large part, to enhanced anaerobic glycolysis and, therefore, glucose use, in

an attempt to preserve cellular energy levels (see Chapter 13). By multivariate analysis, the odds ratio (OR) for an abnormal neurological outcome was 18.5 when infants with blood glucose levels lower than 40 mg/dL were compared with those with levels higher than 40 mg/dL. These data may have important implications for management (see later).

Hyperammonemia may occur in newborns with severe perinatal asphyxia.[83] Although very uncommon, levels of approximately 300 to 900 μg/mL have been detected in the first 24 hours of life and are usually accompanied by elevated serum glutamic oxaloacetic transaminase levels. Clinical correlates may be difficult to distinguish from those secondary to HIE, although hyperthermia and hypertension have been frequent additions in patients with hyperammonemia. Clinical improvement is coincident with falling blood ammonia levels. The pathogenesis of the hyperammonemia is unclear, although a combination of increased protein catabolism, secondary to hypoxic "stress,"[84] and impaired liver function, and therefore hepatic urea synthesis, is a good possibility (see Chapter 27). Recall that hepatic disturbance is a common feature of the systemic multiorgan dysfunction observed with intrauterine asphyxia (see earlier).

Other metabolic parameters have been studied and some may hold promise as measures of severity of the hypoxic-ischemic insult (Table 20.10), although currently the precise sensitivity and specificity of these determinations require further study before general use is warranted. The metabolites and markers are best considered in terms of their relevance to energy metabolism, excitatory amino acids, free radical metabolism, inflammation, brain-specific proteins, and compounds from other organ systems that may have sustained hypoxic-ischemic injury (see Table 20.10). Thus, the early clinical detection of blood or cerebrospinal fluid (CSF) biomarkers might allow an earlier diagnosis compared with neuroimaging. This identification would allow the earlier initiation of intervention measures to improve neonatal survival and reduce the degree of brain injury. In summary, such biomarkers could be important for diagnosis of neonatal HIE, selection of intervention, determination of efficacy, as well as assessment of the severity of illness and the estimation of prognosis.

Concerning *energy metabolism*, perinatal asphyxia has been associated with hypoglycemia, elevated lactate in blood and CSF, elevated lactate/creatinine (L/C) ratio in urine, and elevated lactate and hydroxybutyrate dehydrogenases in CSF.[82,85-88] Of these, the value of detection of early hypoglycemia was discussed earlier. Of particular interest is the ratio of L/C in urine. In a study of 40 infants with evidence of intrapartum asphyxia, the mean (±SD) ratio within 6 hours of life was 16.8 ± 27.4 in the asphyxiated infants who subsequently developed the clinical features of HIE versus 0.2 ± 0.1 in those who did not develop encephalopathy, and 0.09 ± 0.02 in normal infants.[87] Moreover, the ratio was significantly higher in the infants who had neurological sequelae at 1 year (25.4 ± 32.0) than in those with favorable outcomes (0.6 ± 1.5). The degree of elevation of lactate in blood at 30 minutes of life also may be a useful predictor of the severity of perinatal asphyxia.[88] A more recent study of L/C in urine by proton nuclear MR spectroscopy within 6 and 24 hours after birth in 50 normal infants and 50 infants with asphyxia who developed HIE showed that the L/C ratio was elevated among asphyxiated neonates in the first 6 hours after birth to 11-fold greater than in normal

TABLE 20.10	Potential Adjunctive Determinations in Blood, Urine, or Cerebrospinal Fluid in Assessment of Perinatal Asphyxia[a]
DETERMINATION	**BODY FLUID**
Energy metabolism	
Glucose	Blood
Lactate	Blood, CSF
Lactate/creatinine ratio	Urine
Lactate dehydrogenase	CSF
Excitatory amino acids	
Glutamate	CSF
Aspartate	CSF
Glycine	CSF
Free radical metabolism	
Hypoxanthine	Blood, urine
Uric acid	Blood, urine
Nonprotein-bound iron	Blood
Protein carbonyls	CSF
Isoprostanes	CSF
Ascorbic acid	CSF
Arachidonate metabolites	CSF
Nitric oxide	Blood, CSF
Antioxidant enzymes	CSF
Inflammatory markers	
Interleukin-6	Blood, CSF
Interleukin-10	CSF
Interleukin-1 beta	Blood
Tumor necrosis factor-alpha	Blood, CSF
Brain-specific proteins	
Neuron-specific enolase	Blood, CSF
Neurofilament protein	CSF
Protein S-100	Blood, urine, CSF
Glial fibrillary acidic protein	Blood, CSF
Creatine kinase-BB	Blood, CSF
Other	
Erythropoietin	Blood
Nerve growth factor	CSF
Cyclic adenosine monophosphate	CSF

[a]See text for references.

CSF, Cerebrospinal fluid.

neonates (P = .0001).[89] This ratio decreased to 1.5 ± 0.55 for asphyxiated cases over the first 24 hours after birth, fivefold greater than in the control group (P = .0001). The severity of asphyxia correlated with the greater L/C ratio among cases (P = .0007). The sensitivity and specificity of the L/C ratio were 96.1% and 100%, respectively. This measure is not yet used in routine clinical practice for the detection or confirmation of HIE.

Concerning *excitatory amino acids*, elevations of the excitotoxic amino acids glutamate, aspartate, and glycine (through the *N*-methyl-D-aspartate [NMDA] receptor) have been observed in CSF in the first day of life (see Table 20.10).[90-94] Correlations with severity of HIE have been shown. Clinical observation showed increased levels of serum glutamate after neonatal HIE insult.[95,96] Within 24 hours, the increase of glutamate was significant, and reached a peak at day 3 of postnatal life. At day 7 (recovery period) the levels returned to normal, and serum glutamic acid concentrations were closely related to the severity of HIE.[97]

Concerning *free radical metabolism*, many studies support the involvement of reactive oxygen and nitrogen species in the final common pathway to cell death with neonatal HIE (see Table 20.10).[98-115] These studies have shown elevations in sources of free radicals (e.g., hypoxanthine, non-protein-bound iron, arachidonate metabolites), indicators of lipid peroxidation (e.g., isoprostanes) or oxidized proteins (e.g., protein carbonyls), and markers of free radical use (e.g., ascorbic acid, antioxidant enzymes). Of particular note in clinical studies is superoxide dismutase (SOD), an antioxidant enzyme that removes the oxygen free radical, superoxide, to protect cells from free radical damage (see Chapter 13). Its activity level reflects the oxygen free radical scavenging capacity. Glutathione peroxidase, a second key antioxidant enzyme, detoxifies hydrogen peroxide, the product of action of SOD. In addition, also frequently studied is the lipid peroxidation product of free radical activity, malondialdehyde (MDA), which reflects the extent of oxidative damage to cells. Thus, excess free radicals consume SOD, produce a large amount of MDA, promote the release of inflammatory factors in brain tissue, induce nerve cell apoptosis, and increase permeability of the blood-brain barrier in neonatal HIE.[116] A study of 50 cases of asphyxiated full-term newborns found that serious asphyxia resulting in the death of newborns with HIE was associated with concentrations of MDA and glutathione peroxidase in plasma and CSF that were significantly higher than in infants who survived.[117] In neonatal HIE with epilepsy, serum MDA concentrations were significantly higher than in HIE without seizures.[118] Moreover, serum MDA concentrations were increased with the degree of brain injury, which was confirmed by imaging analysis.[119] Clinical studies found that in the acute stage of HIE, serum SOD concentrations were significantly decreased compared to those of a healthy control group, and MDA concentrations were significantly increased.[120]

Concerning *inflammatory markers*, related potentially to hypoxic-ischemic or intrauterine infection or both, elevations of certain cytokines (interleukin [IL]-6, IL-10, IL-1beta, IL-18, ICAM-1, P-selectin, and tumor necrosis factor-alpha) have been documented in blood and CSF in both term and preterm infants (see Table 20.10).[121-127] The degree to which the elevations in cytokines are primary or secondary is unclear (see Chapter 13). A recent review of the role of inflammation in the exacerbation and recovery from hypoxic-ischemic injury outlines the key mediators.[128]

Concerning *brain-specific proteins*, specific components of neurons (neuron-specific enolase, neurofilament protein, creatine kinase-BB [CK-BB]) and astrocytes (S-100, glial fibrillary acidic protein, CK-BB) have been studied in blood and CSF to detect evidence of neuronal and glial injury.[127,129-154] In general, elevations of these markers in blood or CSF in the first hours of life after perinatal asphyxia have correlated approximately with the severity of clinical and brain imaging findings. However, the value of studies of blood is tempered somewhat by the finding of S-100 and neuron-specific enolase (NSE) in placenta; this suggests that these molecules are not entirely brain specific.[148] A recent study of infants receiving hypothermia treatment for neonatal HIE demonstrated abnormal changes in blood NSE that correlated with brain injury on neuroimaging.[155] However, findings in relation to the severity of the injury remain variable.

Available data suggest that the determination of CK-BB is a very sensitive indicator of brain disturbance.[132,134-140,145,150,151]

However, the extreme sensitivity of the indicator in blood impairs the specificity of the measure because variable but appreciable proportions of infants with elevated concentrations of CK-BB in cord blood or neonatal blood samples have no evidence of irreversible brain injury and have a normal neurological outcome. However, two studies of the concentrations of CK-BB in *CSF* suggested greater specificity as well as sensitivity concerning identification of hypoxic-ischemic brain injury than with determination of blood CK-BB concentrations (see Table 20.10).[140,145]

Concerning *other markers*, elevations of erythropoietin in blood and nerve growth factor and cyclic adenosine monophosphate in CSF have been documented after perinatal asphyxia (see Table 20.10).[156-159] The value of these markers and the significance of their elevations remain to be established.

Currently, none of the markers has been established to be of sufficiently high sensitivity and specificity to be appropriate for general clinical use. However, several appear to be promising (see Review.)[127]

Lumbar Puncture

A lumbar puncture should be performed on any infant with HIE in whom the diagnosis is unclear. It is particularly important to rule out other potentially treatable intracranial disorders (e.g., early-onset meningitis) that may mimic the clinical features of HIE.

Electroencephalogram

The EEG changes in HIE may provide valuable information concerning the severity of the injury.[70,160-189] Although a considerable variety of tracings may be observed, the most common evolution of EEG changes in severe HIE is depicted in Fig. 20.1.

The initial alteration is voltage suppression and a decrease in the frequency (i.e., slowing) into the delta and low theta ranges. Within approximately 1 day, and often less, an excessively discontinuous pattern appears, characterized by periods of greater voltage suppression interspersed with bursts, usually asynchronous, of sharp and slow waves. Some infants exhibit multifocal or focal sharp waves or spikes at this time, often with

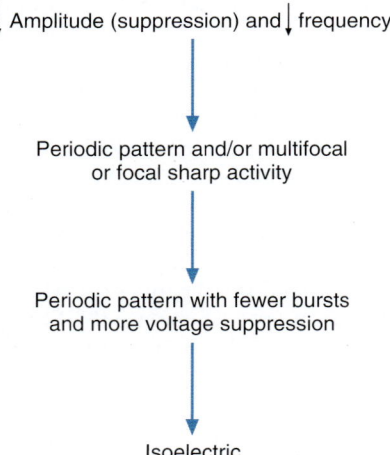

Figure 20.1 Evolution of the electroencephalographic changes in severe hypoxic-ischemic encephalopathy. See text for temporal aspects.

a degree of periodicity. Over the next day or so, the excessively discontinuous pattern may become very prominent, with more severe voltage suppression and fewer bursts, now characterized by spikes and slow waves. This *burst-suppression pattern* is of ominous significance, especially in the full-term infant (see Chapter 10). However, it is critical to recognize that excessively discontinuous patterns with prolonged interburst intervals (IBIs), which are not as severe as classic burst-suppression patterns, nevertheless also are associated with an unfavorable outcome (see the later section on prognosis and Chapter 10). Indeed, in one large series of infants, only 16% of excessively discontinuous tracings (in patients with a generally unfavorable outcome) exhibited burst-suppression patterns by classic definition.[190] Notably, however, as many as 50% of asphyxiated term infants with a burst-suppression pattern identified by amplitude-integrated EEG (aEEG) *in the first hours of life* develop normal or nearly normal tracings within 24 hours (see later).[191] In the severely affected infant, the excessively discontinuous EEG may then evolve into an isoelectric tracing and a hopeless prognosis. Caution in the interpretation of apparent isoelectric tracings in the newborn not undergoing hypothermia therapy, *especially in the first 10 hours of life*, is indicated by the findings of Pezzani and co-workers,[169] which showed that of 17 asphyxiated newborns with isoelectric or "minimal" background activity in the first 10 hours, one was normal and one exhibited only epilepsy on follow-up (15 of the 17 died in the neonatal period). In general, those asphyxiated infants whose EEG tracings revert to normal within approximately 1 week have favorable outcomes.[70,191]

aEEG is a commonly applied method for continuous monitoring of electrical activity in the newborn (see Chapter 10)[192] and has considerable value in the assessment of the encephalopathic term newborn (Fig. 20.2).[191-197] This approach has been crucial in the selection of infants for treatment with mild hypothermia (see later). The most useful tracings for detection of severe encephalopathy have been continuous low-voltage, flat, and burst-suppression tracings. Positive predictive values (PPVs) for an unfavorable outcome with such tracings in the first hours of life are 80% to 90% (see the later section on prognosis). Of infants with these marked background abnormalities, 10% to 50% may normalize within 24 hours. Rapid recovery is associated with a favorable outcome in 60% of cases.

Although the aEEG acquired within the first 6 hours of age has been considered one of the best predictors of neurological outcome at 18 months in infants with neonatal HIE who did not receive hypothermia therapy,[198] since the widespread use of hypothermia therapy, the predictive value of early aEEG has changed, and infants have been shown to have a normal neurological outcome if the aEEG background voltage activity recovers by 48 hours.[199-201] In a recent meta-analysis of nine studies with 520 infants treated with therapeutic hypothermia for moderate or severe HIE, the predictive value of an abnormal tracing on aEEG, acquired at 6, 24, 48, and 72 hours of age, was examined.[202] The authors found that (1) a persistent, severely abnormal aEEG background at 48 hours of age or beyond predicted an adverse outcome (PPV value 85% and diagnostic OR 67 at 48 hours); and (2) at 6 hours of age, the aEEG background in hypothermia-treated infants had a good sensitivity at 96% (95% confidence interval [CI], 89% to 97%) but low specificity at 39% (95% CI, 32% to 45%).

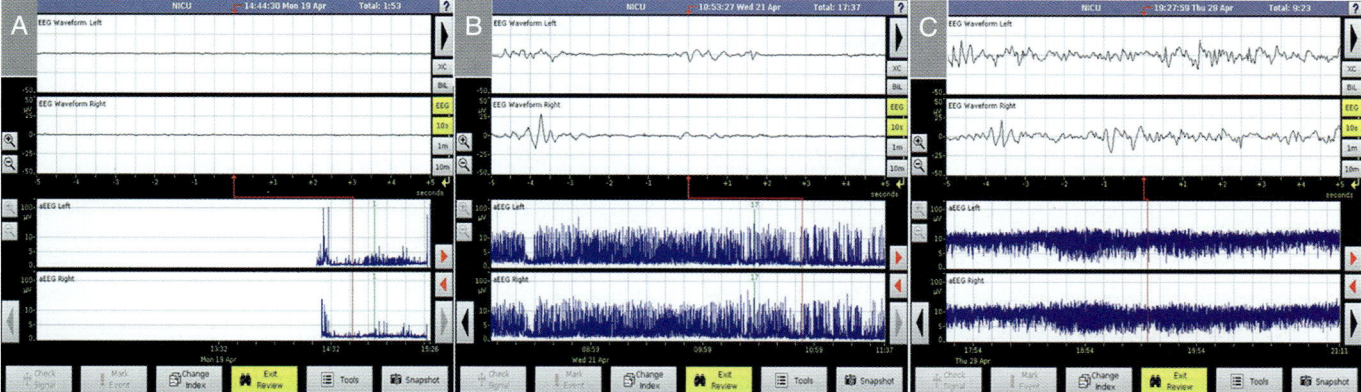

Figure 20.2 Term infant born via emergency cesarean section for fetal bradycardia with Apgar scores 1,[1] 4,[5] and 4.[10] Seizures began at 3 hours of age. Received therapeutic hypothermia from 3 hours of life. aEEG studies at 3 hours of life (A), day 3 (B), and day 7 (C) present the evolution from a suppressed flat tracing to burst suppression by day 3 and normal amplitude with cyclicity on day 7.

Continuous monitoring of conventional EEG with portable equipment has been found to be particularly useful in the identification of *seizure activity* (see Chapter 12).[171,203] Early detection of the seizures and the evaluation of response to anticonvulsant therapy are facilitated by modern portable monitoring systems. EEG data can assist in the determination of whether clinical events are correlated with electrical seizures requiring anticonvulsant medication or with nonepileptic events in which anticonvulsant medication administration can be avoided. As discussed earlier, some seizures have readily identifiable clinical manifestations (i.e., clonic or tonic components), while many seizures have more subtle manifestations (i.e., orolingual, ocular, or autonomic).[78] The most comprehensive *guideline on continuous EEG monitoring in the newborn* was produced in 2011 by the American Clinical Neurophysiology Society.[204] The guideline was created to standardize care and define the best neuromonitoring practices in the neonatal population, while recognizing that not all recommendations would be feasible or applicable across institutions. The guideline recommendations included that (1) electrodes be placed using the International 10 to 20 system with additional electrocardiogram, respiratory, eye, and electromyography leads; (2) at least 1 hour of recording be assessed to adequately assess cycling through wakefulness and sleep; (3) high-risk newborns be monitored for at least 24 hours to screen for the presence of electrographic seizures; and (4) in newborns with seizures, monitoring occur during seizure management and for an additional 24 hours after the last electrographic seizure.[204] Video EEG recording was recommended for 24 hours rather than a briefer EEG recording because many newborns will not have seizures in the first hour of recording but will experience electrographic seizures within the first day.[205,206] A statement from the American Academy of Pediatrics recommends that centers performing therapeutic hypothermia in newborns with HIE have either aEEG or conventional EEG available for seizure identification.[207] This approach provides insight not only into potentially treatable conditions (frequent, clinically silent seizures) but also into the status of the cerebral hemispheres in an infant who is heavily sedated or therapeutically paralyzed.

TABLE 20.11	Most Frequent Correlations of Electroencephalographic Patterns and Table: Topography of Neonatal Hypoxic-Ischemic Brain Injury[a]
EEG PATTERN	**TYPE OF HYPOXIC-ISCHEMIC BRAIN INJURY**
Excessive discontinuity, burst suppression, persistent marked voltage suppression, isoelectric EEG pattern	Diffuse cortical and thalamic neuronal necrosis
Excessive sharp waves: positive vertex or rolandic, positive frontal, and negative occipital sharp waves	Periventricular leukomalacia (also periventricular hemorrhagic infarction; see Chapters 16 and 24)
Focal periodic lateralized epileptiform discharges	Focal cerebral ischemic necrosis (infarction)

[a]See text for references.

EEG, Electroencephalographic.

The *type of EEG abnormality* may indicate a specific pathological variety of hypoxic-ischemic brain injury (Table 20.11).

Diffuse and severe abnormalities (excessive discontinuity with prolonged IBI, burst suppression, marked voltage suppression, isoelectric EEG) are observed most commonly with diffuse cortical neuronal necrosis. Involvement of thalamus may also be important (see Chapter 10).[a]

The particular value of *serial EEG* in assessment of the asphyxiated infant is pronounced.[185,187,209] A single EEG study, particularly during the acute phase of the disease, may suggest a more ominous outcome than do subsequent EEG studies (see Chapter 10).[210] Focal periodic epileptiform discharges are

---

[a]References 162, 164-167, 171, 179, 183-188, and 208.

characteristic of focal cerebral infarction[211,212]; in one series, approximately 90% of infants with such discharges had infarctions (see Chapter 21).[211]

The role of the EEG in the *assessment of brain death* in the asphyxiated newborn has not been delineated decisively.[81,213-222] Thus, an isoelectric EEG can be observed in infants with *cerebral neuronal necrosis but not death of the entire brain* (i.e., brain death). Conversely, persistent EEG activity for many days has been documented in infants with clinical and radionuclide evidence of brain death.[81,217,218,223] Currently, the guidelines of the Task Force for the Determination of Brain Death in infants between the ages of 7 days and 2 months requires two clinical examinations indicative of loss of all cerebral and brain stem function and two isoelectric EEG tracings carried out according to standardized techniques separated by 48 hours.[224] Although data are limited,[217,218] a 72-hour observation period for term infants less than 7 days of age appears warranted in most cases and only when the cause of the coma is unequivocally established.

Neuroimaging Evaluation

Neuroimaging is used to identify the key neuropathologies, as outlined in Chapter 18. These include: (1) selective neuronal necrosis, including three basic patterns, that is, diffuse injury, cerebral cortex-deep nuclear injury, and deep nuclear-brain stem injury; (2) parasagittal cerebral injury; (3) periventricular leukomalacia (see Chapter 16); and (4) focal ischemic necrosis and stroke (see Chapter 21). The accurate diagnostic application of neuroimaging modalities in the newborn infant with HIE is related to the level of radiological expertise for the acquisition and interpretation of the studies, regardless of the neuroimaging method. The methods of acquisition and level of experience in the interpretation of neuroimaging studies in the newborn can vary greatly between institutions. Integration of neonatal, neuroradiological, and radiological physicians by joint conference and review of case materials on a regular basis (e.g., weekly) will assist in improved communication and the application of modern neuroimaging methods. In addition, expert interpretation at a center of excellence in perinatal and neonatal neurology should be requested.

Cranial Ultrasound

Cranial ultrasound remains the most commonly used neuroimaging modality in the neonatal intensive care unit (NICU) setting, and is commonly applied to the term infant with neonatal encephalopathy. In the Vermont Oxford Neonatal Encephalopathy Registry, cranial ultrasound was acquired in nearly 40% of all infants with neonatal encephalopathy on a median of day 4 of life.[225] Cranial ultrasound may be the only imaging modality possible if an infant is too clinically unstable to transport from the neonatal intensive care unit. Cranial ultrasound is sensitive for parenchymal hemorrhage, ventricular size, gross brain malformations, and cystic changes in the brain parenchyma (see Chapter 10). It is less sensitive for smaller and more subtle abnormalities within the brain, including cerebral cortical or brain stem neuronal disease, noncystic white-matter abnormalities, and minor cerebral dysgenesis. It is a very useful screening evaluation in the term infant, with encephalopathy; cerebral dysgenesis has been identified in approximately 2% to 4% of infants who had been diagnosed with hypoxic-ischemic injury (Table 20.12). Cranial ultrasound is often used to assess the presence of slit-like ventricles, or sulcal effacement related to cerebral edema, and hemispheric or basal ganglia echodensity. Cranial ultrasound also can detect severe deep nuclear gray matter injury (Figs. 20.3 and 20.4). However, cranial ultrasound lacks sensitivity in defining the full extent of the cerebral lesions, even in severe encephalopathy, and particularly in the first 24 hours of life.[226,227] Because of the delay in the evolution of cranial ultrasound abnormalities by a minimum of 48 hours, detection of pronounced abnormalities on the first day of life may assist in identifying established severe HIE originating before the onset of labor.[228]

Computed Tomography

Computed tomography (CT), in medical centers without ready access to MRI, has some value in the initial evaluation of the

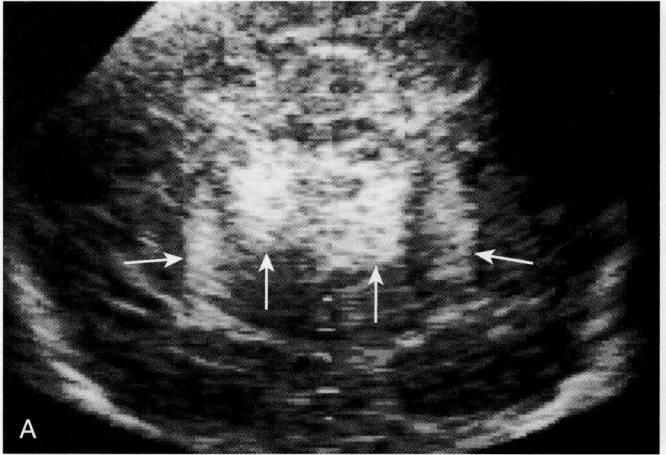
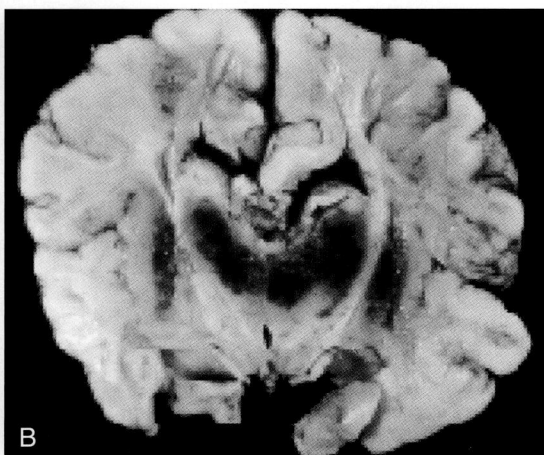

Figure 20.3 Hypoxic-ischemic injury to basal ganglia in a 24-hour-old full-term infant who experienced severe perinatal asphyxia. (A) Coronal ultrasound scan shows marked bilateral echodensities in the region of basal ganglia and thalamus *(arrows)*. The ventricles are not visible. (B) Coronal section of the cerebrum from the same infant, who died at 80 hours of age. Note the bilateral areas of hemorrhagic necrosis, involving the putamen, globus pallidus, and thalamus.

TABLE 20.12 Neuroimaging Characteristics on Magnetic Resonance Imaging in Term Encephalopathy

STUDY	COWAN 2003[28]	MILLER 2005[29]	OKEREAFOR 2008[10]	CHAU 2009[229]	STEINMAN 2009[274]	RUTHERFORD 2010[476]	VERMONT OXFORD 2014[225]	CHEONG 2012[477]	MARTINEZ-BIARGE 2010 2011[275,276]
Inclusion criteria	Either fetal heart rate monitoring abnormalities or cord pH <7.1 or delayed respiration or 5-min Apgar <7 or Multiorgan failure	One of: Apgar score ≤5 at 5 min, pH <7.1, BD >10	Acute sentinel event; umbilical cord prolapsed (19%), uterine rupture (23%), placental abruption (46%)	Neonatal encephalopathy and one of "fetal distress" cord acidemia, 5-min Apgar ≤5, or both	One of: Apgar score ≤5 at 5 min, pH <7.0, BD >10	Neonatal encephalopathy and abnormal EEG and cord pH <7.0 or delayed respiration or 10-min Apgar <5, or both	Seizures or stupor Coma or hypothermia or Apgar at 5 min <3	Two of: Apgar score ≤5 Need for mechanical ventilation at 10 min pH <7.0, BD >12	Term neonatal encephalopathy and MRI in first 6 weeks Apgar score ≤5 at 5 min or pH <7.1, or both "fetal distress"
Number of infants	245	173	48	48	64	67 no hypothermia	1,074	61 no hypothermia	425
Day of MRI scan (range)	14 days of birth	6 days (1–24)	10 days	72 h	14 days	8 days (2–30)	7 days	6 days (3–8)	10 days (2–42)
No abnormality	16%	30%		33%	40%	20%	18%	13%	See cortical injury
Basal ganglia/thalamus	80%	25%	75% any 65% moderate-severe	31%	33%	80% any 58% moderate-severe	30%	36% moderate-severe	41%
Cortical injury	10%	45%	58%	36%	45%	63%	15%	28%	44% (n = 186) normal or white matter/cortical
White-matter injury	5%	Not recorded	Not recorded	21%	15%	84% any 13% severe	25%	23%	See cortical injury
Other diagnosis	4%	None noted	None noted	Arterial infarction in 10%	4%	4%	2%	See cortical injury	11% from total of 555

EEG, Electroencephalographic; MRI, magnetic resonance imaging.
From Inder T. Role of Neuroimaging, Chapter 10. In: Neonatal Encephalopathy and Neurologic Outcome, Second Edition. Washington DC, 2014, American College of Obstetrics & Gynecology.

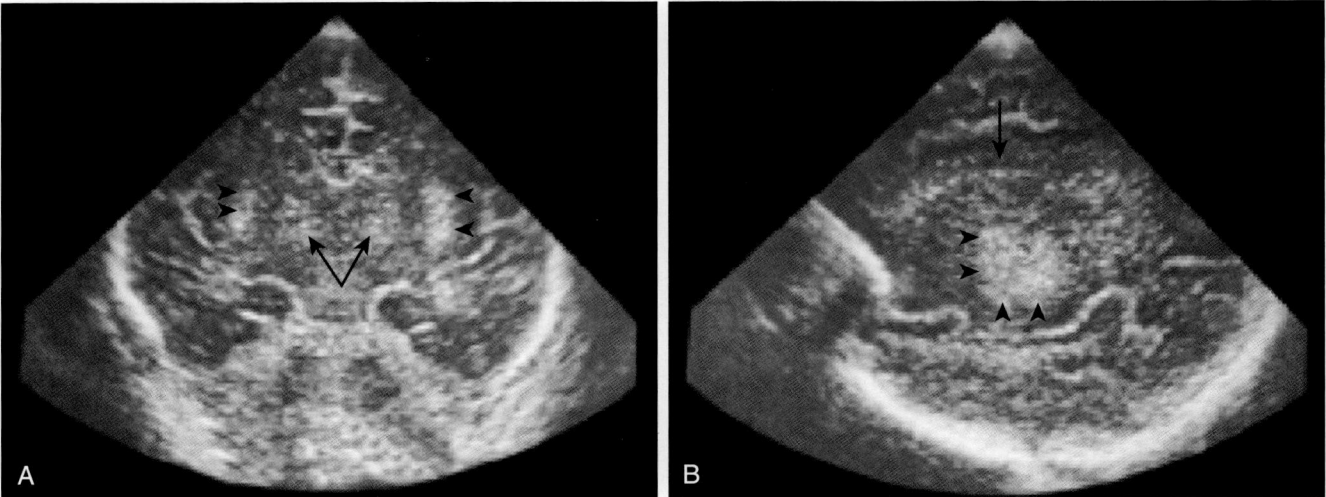

Figure 20.4 Perinatal asphyxia. (A) Coronal and (B) parasagittal ultrasound scans in a 1-day-old full-term infant who experienced perinatal asphyxia. In A, note the increased echogenicity in the basal ganglia (putamen) *(arrowheads)* and the thalamus *(arrows)*. In B, note the increased echogenicity in the region of the thalamus and basal ganglia *(arrowheads)*; the slit-like lateral ventricle is indicated by the arrow for orientation. A computed tomography scan on day 6 (not shown) demonstrated decreased attenuation in the echogenic areas.

TABLE 20.13   Neuroimaging Results

	ULTRASOUND	CT	MRI
Number of infants	2006/4111 (48.8)	933/4107 (22.7)	2690/4109 (65.5)
Day of life at first scan, median (interquartile range)	2 (1–3); N = 2001	2 (2–3); N = 928	6 (4–8); N = 2682
Any reported abnormality	642/1985 (32.3)	552/930 (59.4)	1798/2676 (67.2)
Intraventricular hemorrhage	171/2001 (8.5)	110/930 (11.8)	220/2686 (8.2)
Extraaxial hemorrhage	59/2003 (2.9)	321/927 (34.6)	487/2686 (18.1)
Parenchymal hemorrhage	90/2001 (4.5)	125/929 (13.5)	292/2687 (10.9)
Deep nuclear gray matter abnormality	140/1994 (7.0)	65/926 (7.0)	603/2671 (22.6)
Cystic white matter injury	43/1997 (2.2)	24/928 (2.6)	131/2677 (4.9)
Diffuse white matter injury	—	—	628/2674 (23.5)
Venous or arterial occlusion	22/1980 (1.1)	54/925 (5.8)	183/2657 (6.9)
Ventriculomegaly	84/2004 (4.2)	39/929 (4.2)	92/2687 (3.4)
Cerebellar injury	21/1986 (1.1)	29/929 (3.1)	137/2677 (5.1)
Brain stem injury	—	7/927 (0.8)	126/2677 (4.7)
Diffuse cortical signal abnormality	—	—	572/2673 (21.4)
Parasagittal watershed injury	—	—	285/2665 (10.7)
Absent posterior limb of the internal capsule	—	—	114/2659 (4.3)
Other abnormality	329/2000 (16.5)	190/931 (20.4)	588/2686 (21.9)

Data presented as n/N (%) unless noted otherwise.

CT, Computed tomography; *MRI,* magnetic resonance imaging.

Courtesy Barnette AR, Horbar JD, Soll RF, et al. Neuroimaging in the evaluation of neonatal encephalopathy. *Pediatrics.* 2014;133(6):e1508–e1517.

infant with HIE. As we discuss later, MRI is far preferable. CT does have several useful characteristics, including high sensitivity for the detection of acute hemorrhage and bone abnormalities, a short examination time, and wide availability. These features are useful in the evaluation of acute brain pathology, particularly in the setting of traumatic brain injury. However, in the setting of HIE, MRI is more sensitive, particularly for injury to the cerebral cortex, deep nuclear gray matter, and cerebral white matter. These characteristics are demonstrated by the results from neuroimaging of 1421 term infants with neonatal encephalopathy in the Vermont Oxford Neonatal Encephalopathy Registry from 2006 to 2008 (Table 20.13).

The advantage of MRI, relative to CT, was further demonstrated by a comparison of the same infants undergoing direct imaging comparisons on the same day in this cohort (Table 20.14). Particularly apparent is the superiority of MRI in the diagnosis of deep gray matter injury and cerebral parenchymal injury. These data are consistent with another report comparing CT scans with MRI on day 3 of life in the setting of acute neonatal encephalopathy (Fig. 20.5). In this study of 48 term born infants with HIE, it was noted that the

TABLE 20.14	Neuroimaging Findings in Infants With 2 Types of Imaging on the Same Day					
	ULTRASOUND VERSUS CT		**ULTRASOUND VERSUS MRI**		**CT VERSUS MRI**	
	ULTRASOUND	CT	ULTRASOUND	MRI	CT	MRI
Intraventricular hemorrhage	2/43 (5)	4/43 (9)	3/47 (6)	5/47 (11)	8/70 (11)	9/70 (13)
Extraaxial hemorrhage	2/42 (5)	10/43 (23)	1/46 (2)	11/47 (23)	17/69 (25)	14/70 (20)
Parenchymal hemorrhage	5/42 (12)	7/43 (16)	3/46 (7)	6/47 (13)	10/69 (14)	13/70 (19)
Subependymal hemorrhage	1/42 (2)	2/43 (5)	1/46 (2)	2/47 (4)	0/69 (0)	1/70 (1)
Deep nuclear gray matter abnormality	1/42 (2)	4/42 (10)	4/46 (9)	11/47 (23)	8/69 (12)	18/70 (26)
Cystic white matter injury	0/42 (0)	2/42 (5)	0/46 (0)	4/47 (9)	1/69 (1)	2/70 (3)
Venous or arterial occlusion	0/42 (0)	1/42 (2)	0/46 (0)	2/47 (4)	12/69 (17)	13/70 (19)
Cerebellar injury	1/42 (2)	3/43 (7)	0/46 (0)	4/47 (9)	1/69 (1)	5/70 (7)
Brain stem injury					6/69 (9)	6/70 (9)

Data presented as *n/N* (%).

CT, Computed tomography; *MRI*, magnetic resonance imaging.

Courtesy Barnette AR, Horbar JD, Soll RF, et al. Neuroimaging in the evaluation of neonatal encephalopathy. *Pediatrics.* 2014;133(6):e1508–e1517.

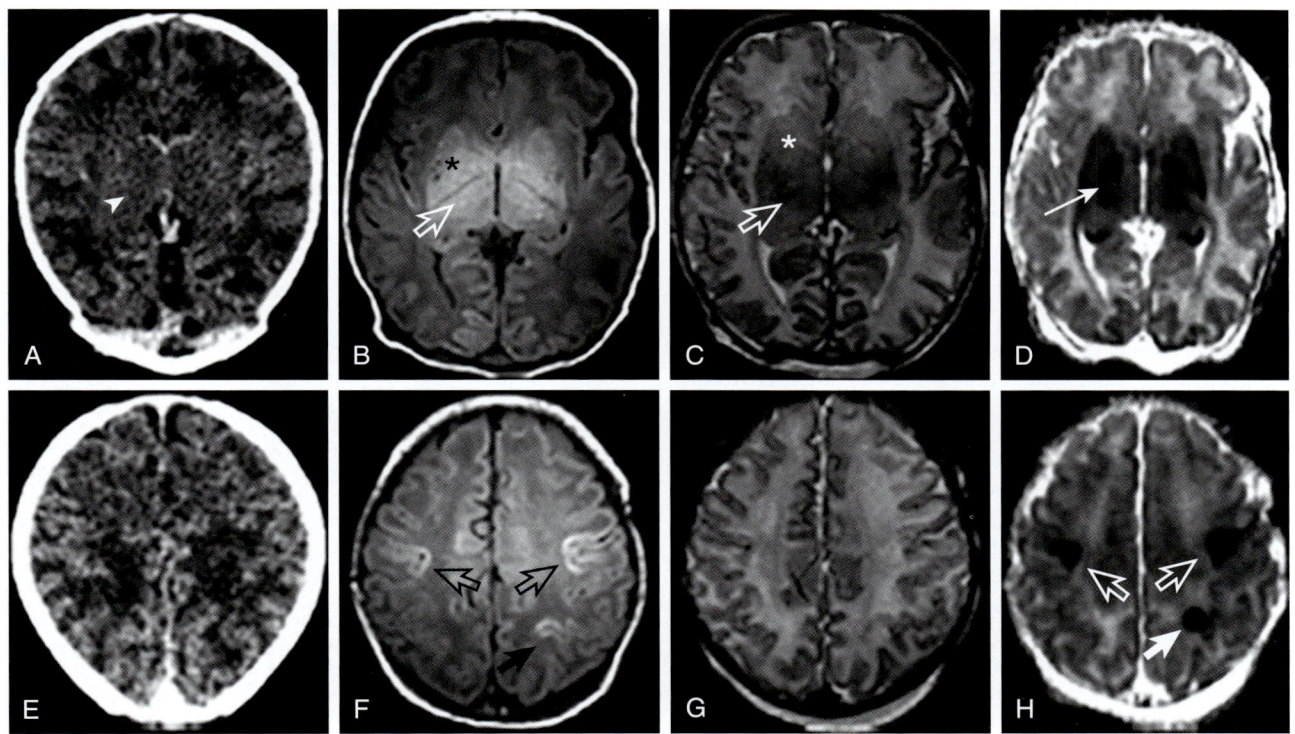

Figure 20.5 **Comparison of computed tomography (CT) versus magnetic resonance imaging (MRI) at day 3 of life in hypoxic-ischemic encephalopathy.** CT identifies BN-predominant pattern but not cortical injury. This newborn has the BN-predominant pattern (A to D). The injury in the BN is apparent on CT, MRI, and the apparent diffusion coefficient (ADC) map. Superiorly, a focal stroke *(white arrow)* in the left parietal lobe, and cortical injury in the paracentral gyri bilaterally *(empty white arrows)* can be seen on the ADC map (H) as restricted diffusion areas, but are not evident on CT (E). On MRI, these lesions are most readily seen as hyperintensities on T1-weighted imaging *(black and empty arrows, F)*. (Courtesy Chau V, Poskitt KJ, Sargent MA, et al. Comparison of computer tomography and magnetic resonance imaging scans on the third day of life in term newborns with neonatal encephalopathy. *Pediatrics.* 2009;123:319–326.)

extent of cortical injury and focal-multifocal lesions, such as strokes and white matter injury, was less apparent on CT than MRI, particularly diffusion-weighted MRI (DWI).[229] Of particular importance, in addition to its limited diagnostic role, there are increasing concerns regarding the impact of radiation exposure from CT on the developing brain (i.e., the risk of future malignancy and later cognitive impairments). These concerns are outlined in Chapter 10. Until further data are available, this neuroimaging technique should be restricted to select settings in which the information obtained from the imaging

TABLE 20.15 Major Techniques for Diagnosis of Specific Neuropathological Types of Neonatal HIE

	DIAGNOSTIC TECHNIQUE		
NEUROPATHOLOGICAL TYPE	MRI	CT	ULTRASOUND
Selective neuronal necrosis: cerebral cortical	++	+	−
Selective neuronal necrosis: basal ganglia and thalamus	++	+	+
Selective neuronal necrosis: brain stem	++	±	−
Parasagittal cerebral injury	++	+	−
Focal and multifocal ischemic brain injury	++	++	+
Periventricular leukomalacia	++	+	++[a]

[a]Very useful for detection of focal component; not useful for detection of diffuse component or "noncystic periventricular leukomalacia" (see text).

++, Very useful; +, useful; ±, questionably useful; −, not useful.

CT, Computed tomography; *HIE*, hypoxic-ischemic encephalopathy; *MRI*, magnetic resonance imaging.

study is clearly of benefit to the patient and cannot be readily obtained with some other modality. Examples would include infants with severe head trauma at risk for major epidural bleeding and those who require more definitive imaging in a very brief period because of severe clinical instability.

Magnetic Resonance Imaging

MRI provides the highest sensitivity for both anatomical and functional detail and also offers an array of imaging options that can be tailored to the specific clinical question (see later). MRI, however, does have some drawbacks compared with other imaging modalities, particularly in the neonatal period. Unlike cranial ultrasound, patients must typically be transported to a radiology suite from the neonatal intensive care unit for MRI, which may pose some risk to those infants who are unstable. Safely imaging encephalopathic neonates is a unique challenge. Studies have shown that at least 20% of term-born infants with severe HIE cannot be safely transported to the MRI scanning suite because of the severity of their illness.[230] Further information on MRI in infants and the techniques applied in MRI are detailed in Chapter 10.

MRI has been used in a large number of studies of neonatal HIE.[28,29,226,231-272] The entire spectrum of hypoxic-ischemic brain injury has been demonstrated (Table 20.15). The major findings by MRI are outlined in Table 20.16.

Conventional MRI shows the abnormalities in the first 3 to 4 days, but generally not on the first day. However, DWI, based on the molecular diffusion of water, is not only more sensitive than conventional MRI, but also shows abnormalities earlier, often in the first 24 to 48 hours after birth (see later discussion, Fig. 20.6). The correlates of the MRI findings with the neuropathological states described in Chapter 18 are apparent (Figs. 20.7 to 20.14). Thus, *selective cerebral cortical neuronal injury* is manifested by loss of the cerebral gray-white matter differentiation and by cortical high signal (highlighting) on T1-weighted (T1W) or fluid-attenuated inversion recovery (FLAIR) images at the sites of particular predilection, the parasagittal perirolandic cortex, and the depths of sulci (see Fig. 20.7).

Decreased diffusion (increased signal) is seen on DWI (see Fig. 20.8).

Selective cerebral cortical neuronal injury is usually accompanied by involvement of *basal ganglia (especially dorsal putamen) and thalamus (especially lateral thalamus*; see Fig. 20.9).

TABLE 20.16 Major Aspects of Magnetic Resonance Imaging in the Diagnosis of HIE in the Term Infant[a]

Major conventional MRI findings in first week

Cerebral cortical gray-white differentiation lost (on T1W or T2W)

Cerebral cortical high signal (T1W and FLAIR), especially in parasagittal perirolandic cortex

Basal ganglia/thalamus, high signal (T1W and FLAIR, usually associated with the cerebral cortical changes but possibly alone with increased signal in brain stem tegmentum in cases of acute severe insults; see Chapter 18)

Parasagittal cerebral cortex, subcortical white matter, high signal (T1W and FLAIR)

Periventricular white matter, decreased signal (T1W) or increased signal (T2W)

Posterior limb of internal capsule, decreased signal (T1W or FLAIR)

Cerebrum in a vascular distribution, decreased signal (T1W), but much better visualized as decreased diffusion (increased signal) on diffusion-weighted MRI

Diffusion-weighted MRI more sensitive than conventional MRI, especially in first days after birth, when former shows decreased diffusion (increased signal) in injured areas

[a]See text for references and more details concerning timing of findings.

FLAIR, Fluid-attenuated inversion recovery; *MRI*, magnetic resonance imaging; *T1W and T2W*, T1- and T2-weighted images.

In the unusual cases of principally deep nuclear and brain stem involvement, as with severe, acute asphyxial insults, high signal (T1W or FLAIR) is seen in the brain stem tegmentum as well as in the basal ganglia. DWI is more sensitive for detection of cerebral cortical and deep nuclear involvement (see Fig. 20.10).

In one series of 173 encephalopathic term newborns, predominant involvement of perirolandic cortex and basal ganglia/thalamus was observed in 44 (25%) and in an additional 24 (14%) in association with predominant involvement of parasagittal regions.[273] *Parasagittal cerebral injury* is seen readily as areas of increased signal (T1W and FLAIR) in the parasagittal cerebral cortex and subcortical white matter (see Figs. 20.11 and 20.12).

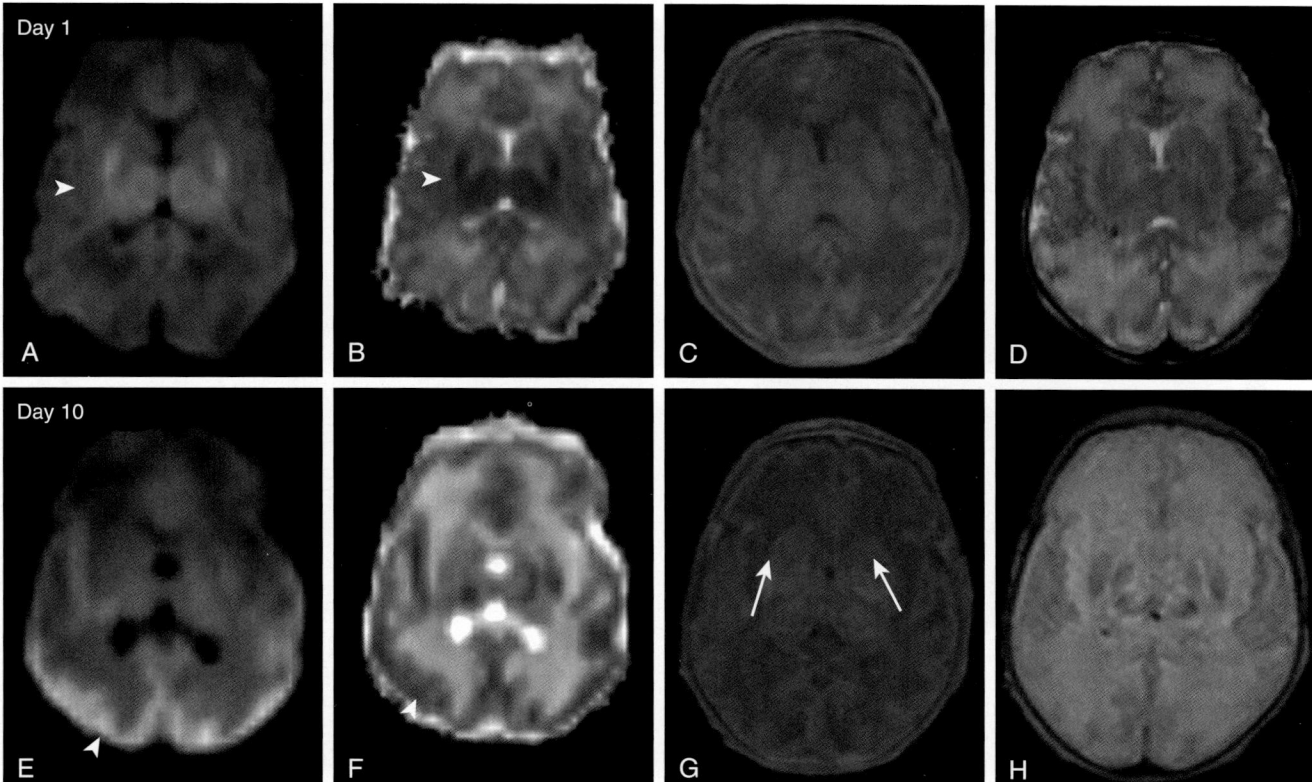

Figure 20.6 Deep nuclear-cortical selective neuronal injury. An infant at 35 weeks of gestation with a history of placental abruption for several hours before hospital admission. Apgars 1 (at 1 minute), 3 (at 5 minutes), and 7 (at 10 minutes). No hypothermia therapy was commenced. Magnetic resonance imaging of axial imaging on the first day of life for diffusion-weighted imaging (A), apparent diffusion coefficient map imaging (B), T1-weighted imaging (C), and T2-weighted imaging (D) reveal isolated thalamic and deep nuclear gray-matter injury that is most apparent on the diffusion imaging *(thick arrowheads)*. At day 10 there is now evolution, with more prominent T1- and T2-weighted signal changes in the deep nuclear gray matter and the thalamus, and prominent restriction in the cortical ribbon on diffusion-weighted (E) and apparent diffusion coefficient map (F, *thick arrowheads*) imaging, suggesting a secondary neuronal degeneration. The extent of the conventional injury in the deep gray matter is apparent (G and H). (Images were prepared by Dr Joshua Shimony, neuroradiologist at Washington University in St. Louis and are courtesy of ACOG.)

The relative distribution of the abnormalities among many large-scale MRI studies has varied somewhat because of different schemes for analysis (see Table 20.12).[a] In general, approximately 15% to 30% of MRI scans have been normal. Lesions in basal ganglia/thalamus, either predominantly or more commonly accompanying other areas of involvement, are present in approximately 40% to 80% of cases. Because the lesions in basal ganglia and thalamus often are microscopic in size, some instances of involvement likely may not be detected by MRI. Abnormalities of parasagittal (watershed) white matter and cortex are present in approximately 40% to 60%. The involvement of cortex in the watershed lesions also is likely an underestimate, because the cortical involvement typically is laminar (especially layers 3 and 5), and the entire cortical thickness in the human newborn is only approximately 2 mm.[283] In more severe cases the classic watershed parasagittal cerebral injury involving cortex and subcortical/central white matter is readily apparent. Involvement of basal ganglia *and* brain stem preferentially occurs in approximately 10% to 20% of

cases, usually following a catastrophic sentinel event (see later). Preferential involvement of periventricular/central white matter, similar to periventricular leukomalacia of premature infants, is noted as a dominant feature in only approximately 15% of cases, and occurs especially in infants of somewhat lower gestational age (late preterms),[279,280,284] or in the context of hypoglycemia or prolonged cardiovascular instability (e.g., congenital heart disease).[285]

Although many of the lesions just discussed are visualized well by conventional MRI, they are visualized better and, importantly, earlier by *DWI* (see Fig. 20.14). Increased signal on DWI, indicative of decreased water diffusion, has been shown in experimental models of focal cerebral ischemia and in adult stroke in the first 1 to 2 hours after the insult.[286-292] Many studies of newborns with hypoxic-ischemic disease have demonstrated the superior sensitivity of DWI versus conventional MRI in delineating the site and extent of tissue injury early in the neonatal period.[a] The DWI signal in neonatal HIE is influenced greatly by the timing of the scan and the

[a]References 10, 28, 29, 229, 264, 270, 272, and 274-282.

[a]References 242, 243, 253, 254, 271, 279, and 293-301.

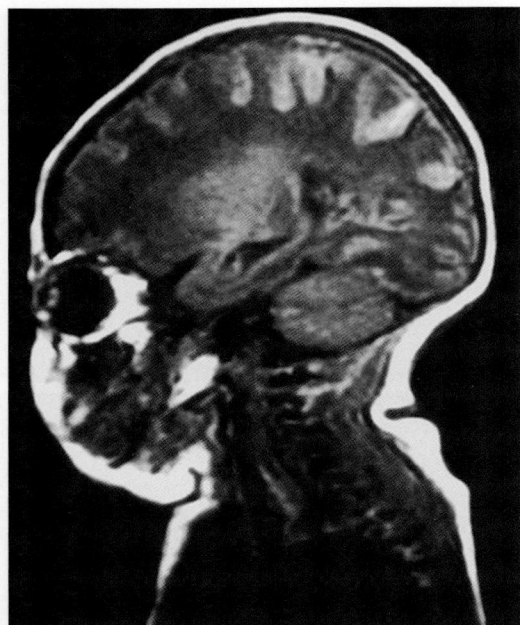

Figure 20.7 Magnetic resonance imaging scan of cortical neuronal injury. The infant had severe apnea on the first day of life, and the scan was performed on the third postnatal day. On this parasagittal fluid-attenuated inversion recovery image, note the striking cortical highlighting, especially marked in the depths of sulci.

region studied.[261,263-267,269,270] The *timing* of DWI abnormality in asphyxiated term infants with presumed selective neuronal necrosis or parasagittal cerebral injury, or both, is shown in Fig. 20.15.[298]

Thus, although some infants exhibit abnormality on the first day, injury is generally underestimated at that time. The nadir for diffusion occurs between the second and third days. By 7 to 8 days, pseudonormalization is apparent and is probably related to recovery processes that ultimately lead to angiogenesis and other factors causing increased diffusion. *Thus, the optimal time for detection of DWI abnormality in the most common varieties of hypoxic-ischemic disease in the term newborn is approximately 2 to 3 days* (see Fig. 20.15). In *adult human stroke* (i.e., permanent occlusion), diffusion is decreased *in the first hours after the insult and remains low* until pseudonormalization occurs at 7 to 9 days.[302] This time course is similar to that observed in animal models of permanent vascular occlusion. By contrast, in newborns, the insult usually is *transient* and is followed by reperfusion. In animal models of transient occlusion, during the occlusion diffusion decreases, whereas on reperfusion, diffusion recovers before a secondary decline many hours later, as in the usual asphyxiated human infant (see Fig. 20.15). The *evolution of these diffusion changes appears to be altered by the commencement of therapeutic hypothermia,* which is associated with a more protracted pseudonormalization of the diffusion coefficient, with full normalization requiring greater than 10 days.[303] This more protracted course may reflect a slower evolution to cell death and thereby provide a longer window for a second neuroprotective agent. Further studies are needed to confirm this evolution of the diffusion findings in the setting of therapeutic hypothermia.

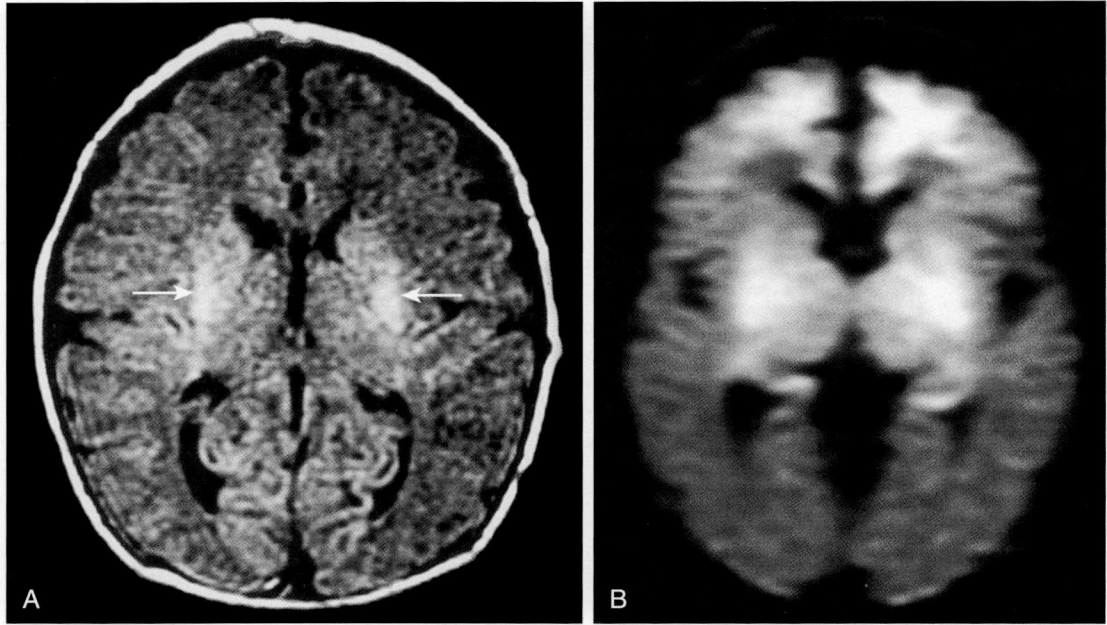

Figure 20.8 Magnetic resonance imaging (MRI) scans of selective neuronal injury. The infant experienced intrapartum asphyxia and had seizures on the first postnatal day. Scans were performed on the fifth postnatal day. (A) The axial fluid-attenuated inversion recovery image shows increased signal in putamen bilaterally *(arrows)* but no definite abnormality in the cerebral cortex. (B) By contrast, diffusion-weighted MRI (DWI) shows striking increased signal (i.e., decreased diffusion) in the frontal cortex (in addition to more pronounced basal ganglia abnormality).

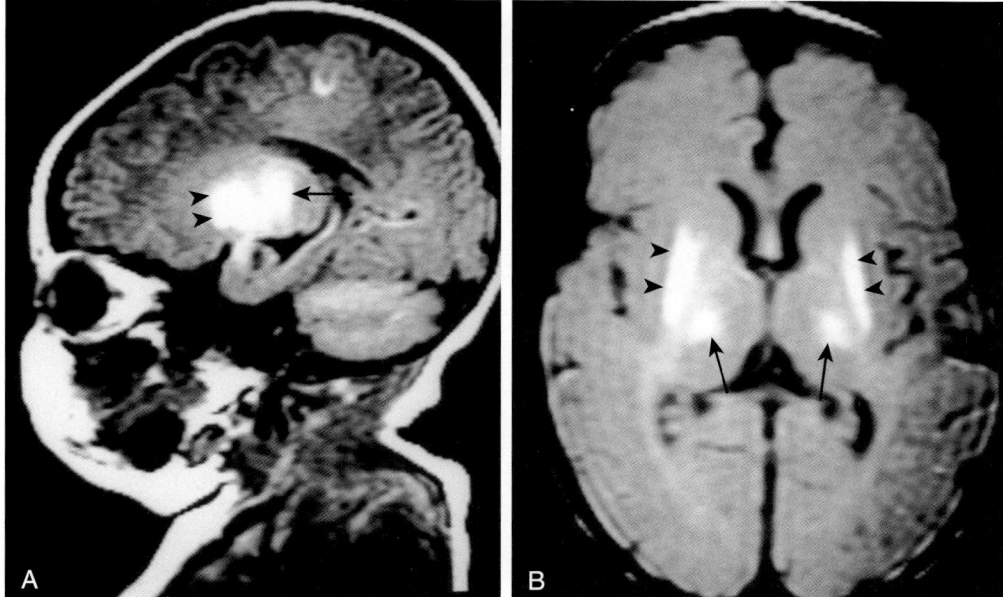

Figure 20.9 Magnetic resonance imaging scans of hypoxic-ischemic injury to basal ganglia and thalamus. Scans were obtained from a 5-day-old infant who experienced severe perinatal asphyxia. (A) Note in the parasagittal T1-weighted image markedly increased signal in the basal ganglia, especially the putamen *(arrowheads)*, and in the thalamus *(arrow)*. (B) The axial proton density image also demonstrates the injury well in the same distribution. (Courtesy Dr. Patrick Barnes.)

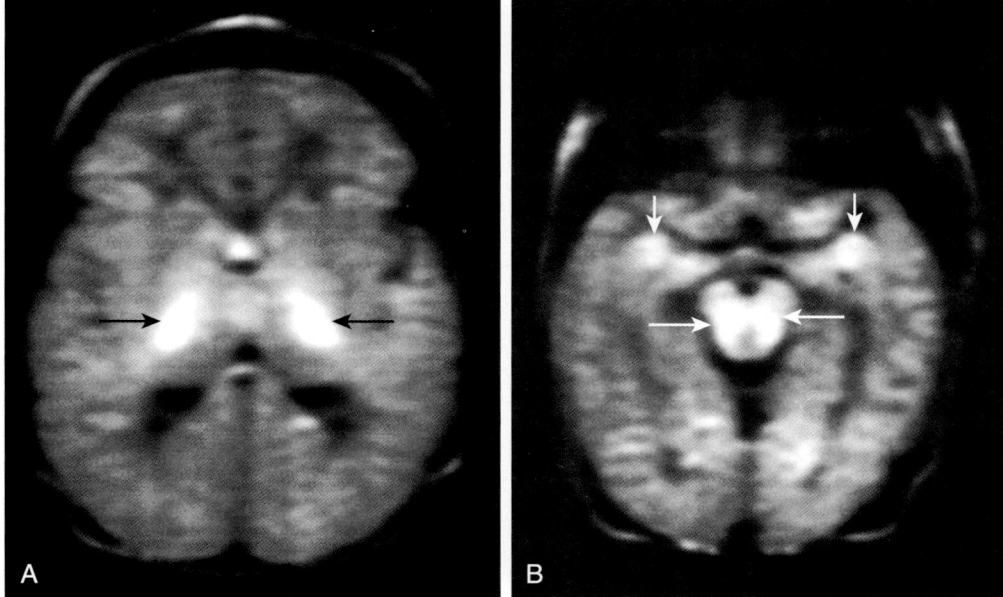

Figure 20.10 Diffusion-weighted magnetic resonance imaging (DWI) of deep nuclear and brain stem injury. This full-term infant experienced a severe late intrapartum asphyxial insult. MRI and DWI scans were carried out late on the first postnatal day. No definite abnormality was discerned by conventional MRI (not shown). However, DWI shows striking decreased diffusion (increased signal) in the basal ganglia–thalamus *(arrows* in A), the hippocampus *(short arrows* in B), and the midbrain tegmentum *(long arrows* in B).

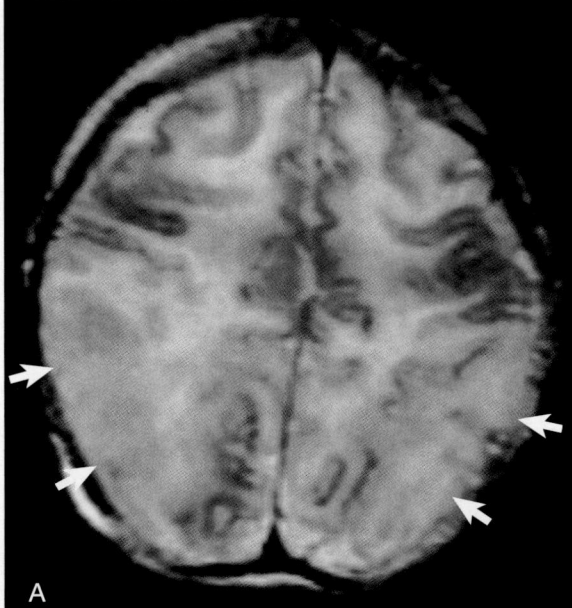

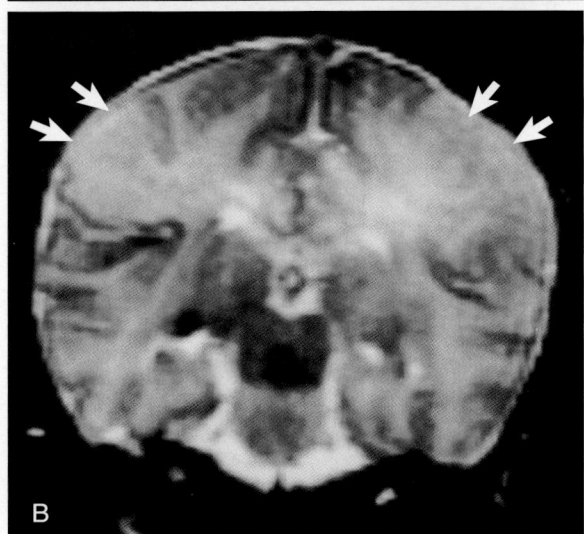

Figure 20.11 Magnetic resonance imaging (MRI) scan of parasagittal cerebral injury. (A) Axial T2-weighted MRI scan obtained on postnatal day 5 from an infant with perinatal asphyxia and neonatal seizures shows a striking loss of normal cerebral gray–white matter signals symmetrically in parasagittal regions, especially posteriorly *(arrows)*. A computed tomography (CT) scan obtained 2 days earlier (not shown) showed much less well-localized decreased attenuation. (B) Coronal T2-weighted MRI scan obtained on postnatal day 4 from an infant with perinatal asphyxia and neonatal seizures. Note the striking abnormality in parasagittal areas bilaterally *(arrows)*. A CT scan performed 1 day before showed equivocal findings (not shown). (Courtesy Dr. Patrick Barnes.)

The importance of the *region injured* in the evolution of changes in diffusion is illustrated by the scans shown in Fig. 20.16.[295] Thus, in this unusual example of precise knowledge of the timing of the insult (postnatal cardiac arrest), decreased diffusion in basal ganglia and thalamus was apparent at 6 hours of age, but decreased diffusion did not appear in the cerebral cortex until 32 hours. Other investigators showed that although severe white matter injury is associated with early decreased diffusion, with more moderate white matter injury

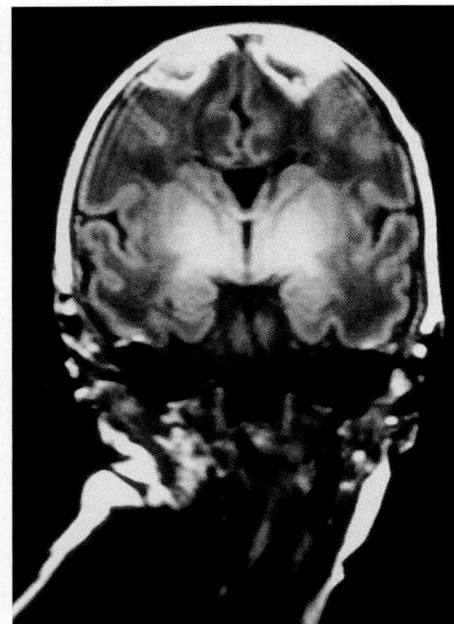

Figure 20.12 Magnetic resonance imaging (MRI) scan of parasagittal cerebral injury. Coronal T1-weighted MRI, obtained on the fifth postnatal day in an asphyxiated term infant, shows striking, triangular lesions in the parasagittal areas bilaterally. The increased signal is also apparent in the basal ganglia and the thalamus bilaterally. (Courtesy Dr. Alan Hill.)

diffusion is normal or slightly increased early and increases in the ensuing days (Fig. 20.17).[279] A similar increase in white matter diffusion was observed in cerebral hypoxia–ischemia in the neonatal rat.[304]

To *summarize*, MRI clearly provides superior imaging resolution for delineation of all hypoxic-ischemic lesions, both in the neonatal period and on follow-up (see Tables 20.15 and 20.16). DWI provides the capability for identification of injury by 24 to 48 hours after asphyxia in the term infant to assist in the early delineation of the nature and severity of cerebral injury.

Cerebral Metabolic-Hemodynamic Neurodiagnostic Studies

Neurodiagnostic studies that address changes in metabolism and physiology after perinatal hypoxic-ischemic insults include MR spectroscopy, positron emission tomography (PET), near-infrared spectroscopy, and other measures of the cerebral circulation (see Chapter 10). Of these, *MR spectroscopy* has proven most useful for diagnostic assessment and is emphasized here.

Magnetic Resonance Spectroscopy

MR spectroscopy has proven to be a diagnostic modality of particular importance in the evaluation of the infant with perinatal hypoxic-ischemic brain injury. Both phosphorus and proton MR spectroscopy are useful, although currently the more readily available proton MR spectroscopy is used most widely. Indeed, over the past few years at our institution, proton MR spectroscopy has joined DWI as part of the standard evaluation of infants evaluated by MR techniques for hypoxic-ischemic disease. The basic principles of phosphorus and proton MR spectroscopy and the normative data obtainable are described

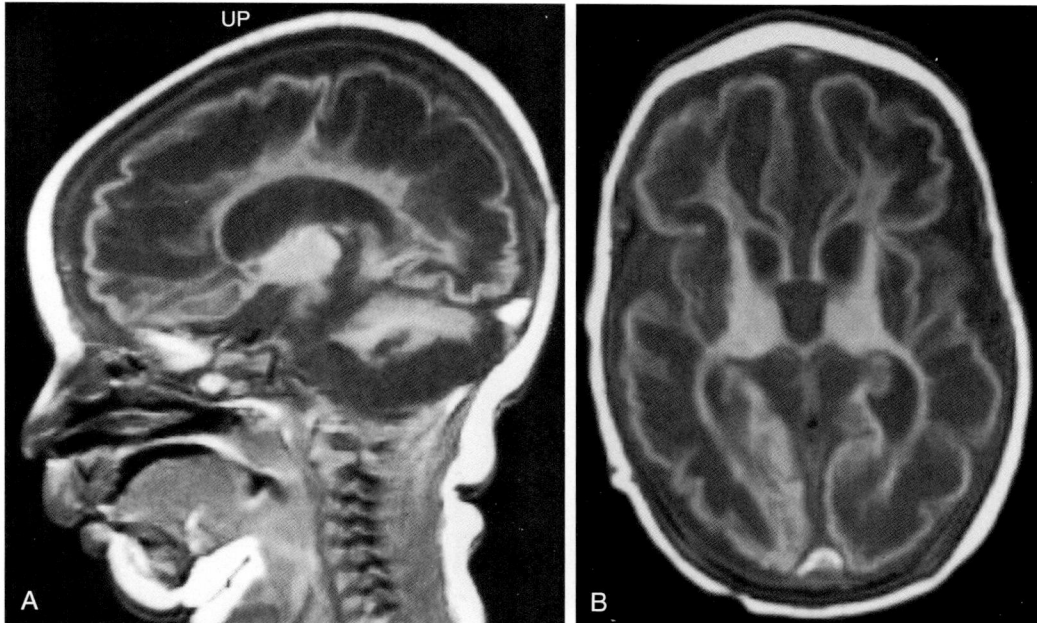

Figure 20.13 Magnetic resonance imaging scan of multifocal ischemic brain necrosis. The scan was obtained at 6 weeks of age in an infant who had severe perinatal asphyxia. T1-weighted images in the (A) sagittal and (B) axial planes show striking changes consistent with multicystic encephalomalacia.

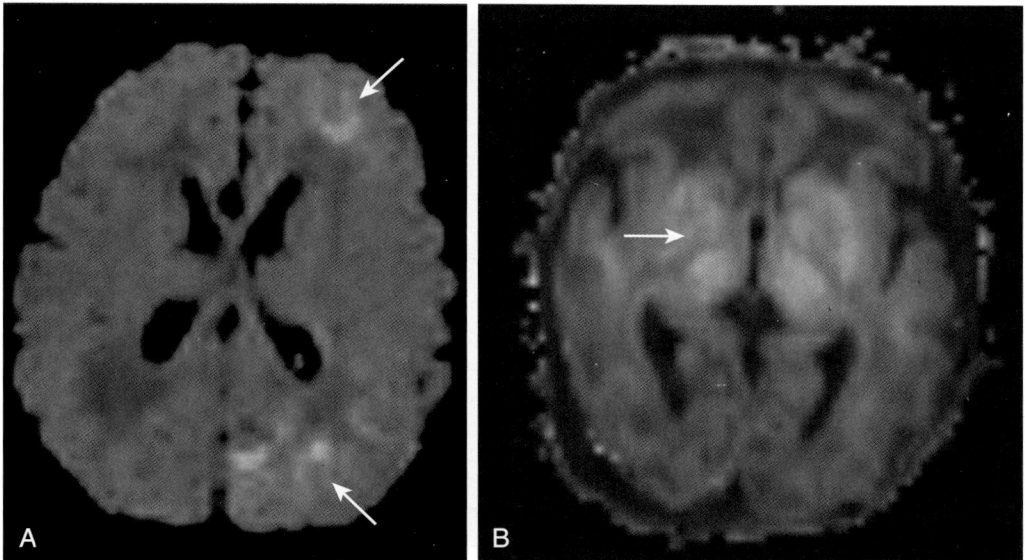

Figure 20.14 Common patterns of cerebral injury represented by diffusion-weighted images at days 2 to 3 after birth. The areas of injury appear bright. Panel A shows watershed injury, predominantly in the anterior and posterior watershed areas of the left hemisphere. Panel B shows the basal ganglia/thalamic injury.

in Chapter 10. The value of these techniques in the assessment of HIE in the term infant is summarized in Table 20.17.

Phosphorus Magnetic Resonance Spectroscopy. Multiple studies of infants who sustained perinatal asphyxia, especially intrapartum, have focused on phosphorus-31 (^{31}P) spectra.[305-314] The sequence of findings has been initially normal spectra (concentrations of phosphocreatine [PCr], inorganic phosphate [P_i],[315] and adenosine triphosphate [ATP]) in the first hours after birth, followed by a decline in concentration of PCr and a rise in that of P_i (and thus a decline in the PCr/P_i ratio) over approximately the next 24 to 72 hours (Fig. 20.18; see Table 20.17). In the most severely affected infants, ATP concentrations also decline at this time. Subsequently, spectra return to normal over the ensuing weeks, although the total ^{31}P signal may be reduced when marked loss of brain tissue has occurred.[308] *This sequence of events is directly reminiscent of the progression of the "delayed energy failure"* described in Chapter 13. This secondary energy failure correlates directly with the ultimate degree of cell death. Consistent with the experimental data, the severity of

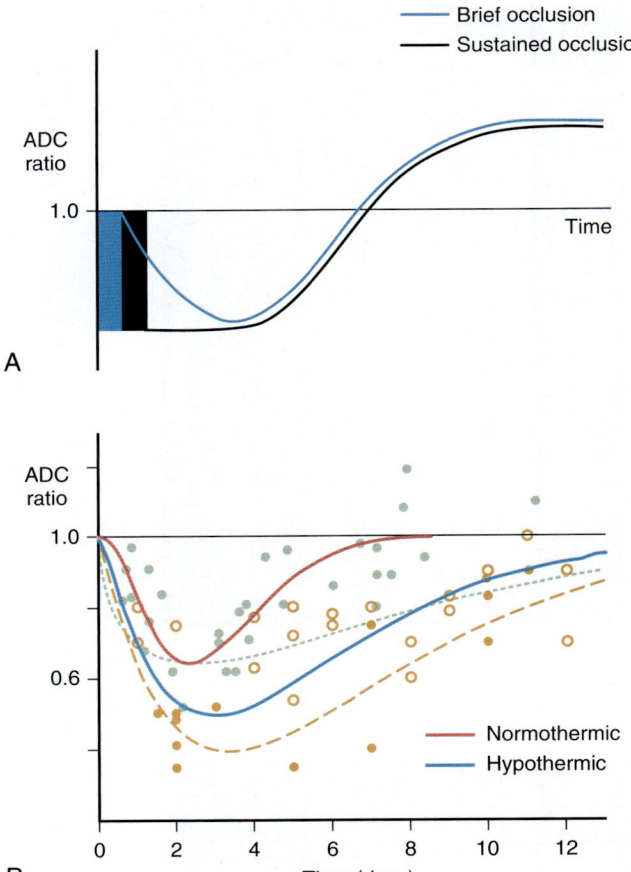

Figure 20.15 (Panel A) The time course of apparent diffusion coefficient (ADC) change following brain injury. Blue represents a 30-minute occlusion. Black represents a 90-minute occlusion. The data are a composite from animal studies. (Panel B) The time course of ADC change following brain injury in term-born human infants. Red represents normothermic infants. Blue shows infants treated with therapeutic hypothermia. ADC ratios rather than absolute ADC values are used in the ordinate of both panels because ADC values vary regionally in infants and the areas of injury vary infant to infant. The ratio represents injured tissue over normal tissue, so values < 1 indicate a reduction in ADC values. (A, adapted from McKinstry RC, Miller JH, Snyder AZ, et al. A prospective, longitudinal diffusion tensor imaging study of brain injury in newborns. *Neurology.* 2002;59(6):824–833; and B, adapted from Bednarek N, Mathur A, Inder T, et al. Impact of therapeutic hypothermia on MRI diffusion changes in neonatal encephalopathy. *Neurology.* 2012;78:1420–1427.)

---

this delayed energy failure in human infants correlates closely with the severity of the neonatal neurological syndrome (Fig. 20.19) and with the subsequent occurrence of neurological deficits (see later).[311,312,314] The findings not only demonstrate the value of phosphorus MR spectroscopy in the early delineation of impairments of energy metabolism in the asphyxiated infant but also provide important prognostic information (see the section on prognosis).

Phosphorus MR spectroscopy also is valuable in detection of a paradoxical postischemic increase in intracellular pH (pH$_i$).[314] The evolution of this increase in the days to weeks after hypoxia-ischemia correlates with the degree of brain injury. This *postischemic alkalinization* may lead to cellular injury and appears related, in considerable part, to postischemic activation of the neuronal and glial sodium-hydrogen transporter. Consistent with

---

TABLE 20.17   Value of Magnetic Resonance Spectroscopy in Assessment of HIE in the Term Infant[a]

Phosphorus magnetic resonance spectroscopy

Detects high-energy phosphates (PCr, ATP), inorganic phosphate, and pH$_i$; in first few hours after insult PCr, ATP, and pH$_i$ are often normal.

After approximately 8 h, with development of secondary energy failure, PCr (and later ATP) declines, and pH$_i$ increases.

In first 1–2 weeks, the severity of decline in PCr and the increase in pH$_i$ correlate with the severity of brain injury.

Proton magnetic resonance spectroscopy

Detects multiple compounds, especially lactate, N-acetylaspartate, choline, creatine, and glutamate.

Lactate is elevated as early as a few hours after the insult, and it appears to be an earlier indicator of brain injury than is diffusion-weighted magnetic resonance imaging.

In the first days after insult, elevations of lactate (and perhaps glutamate) and declines in N-acetylaspartate are identified, and the severity of changes correlates with the severity of brain injury.

[a]See text for references.

ATP, Adenosine triphosphate; *HIE,* hypoxic-ischemic encephalopathy; *PCr,* phosphocreatine; *pH$_i$,* intracellular pH.

---

this formulation, experimental data indicate a neuroprotective role for amiloride, a sodium-hydrogen exchange blocker, when administered after ischemia (see Chapter 13 and later).

Proton Magnetic Resonance Spectroscopy. Proton MR spectroscopy (see Chapter 10) has been applied extensively to the study of infants with HIE.[272,295,313,316-344] Although not all the reported observations are entirely consistent, important and consistent findings can be recognized (see Table 20.17). First, in the acute period, as early as a few hours after birth, *elevation in cerebral lactate*, often expressed as the ratio of lactate to N-acetylaspartate (NAA), creatine, or choline, can be detected (see Fig. 20.10A). Indeed, detection of lactate by proton MR spectroscopy is a more consistent indicator of brain injury than is DWI (or other imaging modality) in the first hours after hypoxic-ischemic injury.[330] *Currently, MR spectroscopy may be considered as the most sensitive modality for detection of neonatal brain disturbance in the acute period.* More data regarding sensitivity and specificity for structural injury are needed. During this early period, ratios of NAA to choline or creatine have been either unchanged or only slightly decreased. The elevated lactate is most pronounced in deep nuclear structures, especially basal ganglia and thalamus, with their high metabolic rate and propensity for hypoxic-ischemic injury. The acutely elevated lactate correlates with the severity of the neonatal neurological syndrome, the subsequent delayed energy failure (Fig. 20.20B), and the neurological deficits on follow-up (see the section on prognosis). Lactate levels may remain elevated for weeks, perhaps in part because of enhanced glycolysis and lactate production by astrocytes. Second, after days to weeks, ratios of NAA to choline or creatine decline and reflect tissue injury. Recall from Chapter 10 that NAA is contained in neurons (and presumably axons) and in

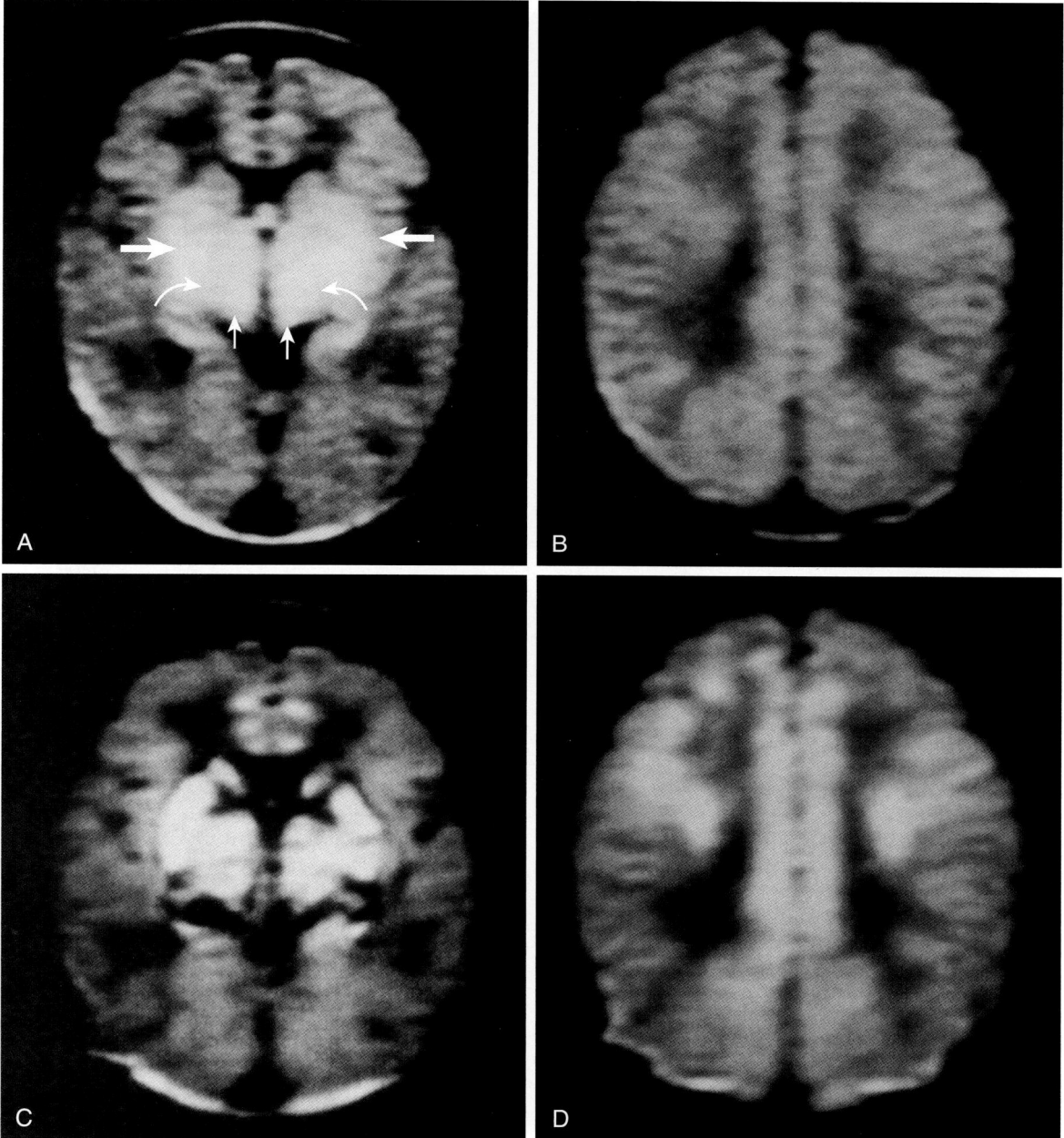

Figure 20.16 Differential regional decreases in diffusion after neonatal hypoxia-ischemia. Diffusion-weighted magnetic resonance imaging (DWI) images A and B, obtained 6 hours after cardiorespiratory arrest, show a bright signal (i.e., decreased diffusion) in the basal ganglia *(thick arrows)*, the thalami *(curved arrows)*, and the dorsal brain stem *(thin arrows)*. There is no decrease in diffusion in the cerebral cortex. DWI images C and D, obtained 32 hours after cardiorespiratory arrest, show persistence of the decreased diffusion in deep nuclear structures and a bright signal (decreased diffusion) in the cerebral cortex. Conventional magnetic resonance imaging (not shown) at 6 hours was normal, but at 32 hours it was clearly abnormal. (From Soul JS, Robertson RL, Tzika AA, du Plessis AJ, et al. Time course of changes in diffusion-weighted magnetic resonance imaging in a case of neonatal encephalopathy with defined onset and duration of hypoxic-ischemic insult. *Pediatrics.* 2001;108:1211–1214.)

oligodendroglial precursors. Thus, the declines in NAA in both gray and white matter are not surprising. The severity of the decline in NAA correlates with the severity of subsequent neurological deficits. Glutamate levels also have been shown to be elevated in the first days of life in infants with severe HIE.[329] This determination is more difficult than that for lactate or NAA and may not be as useful.

Positron Emission Tomography

Although PET is not a routine diagnostic procedure (for the reasons described in Chapter 10), the technique has provided major insight into the frequency, basic nature, and probable pathogenesis of the cerebral injury observed in asphyxiated *term* infants.[345] Because experience with adult patients had indicated that measurements of regional cerebral blood flow

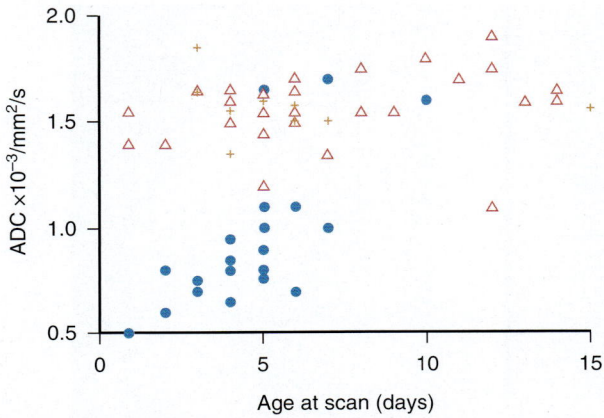

Figure 20.17 Diffusion abnormalities in cerebral white matter after apparent neonatal hypoxia-ischemia. The infants were born at term and were control (+), with severe white abnormalities on conventional magnetic resonance imaging (MRI) (●), or with moderate white matter abnormalities (△) on conventional MRI. Note in the infants with severe white matter abnormalities, diffusion was clearly decreased in the first week, whereas in the infants with moderate abnormalities, diffusion was not decreased. A nonsignificant increase in diffusion was noted in the latter infants after the first week. (Based on Rutherford M, Counsell S, Allsop J, et al. Diffusion-weighted magnetic resonance imaging in term perinatal brain injury: a comparison with site of lesion and time from birth. *Pediatrics.* 2004;114:1004–1014.)

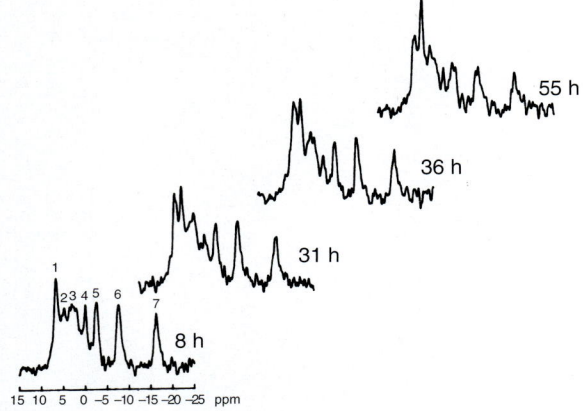

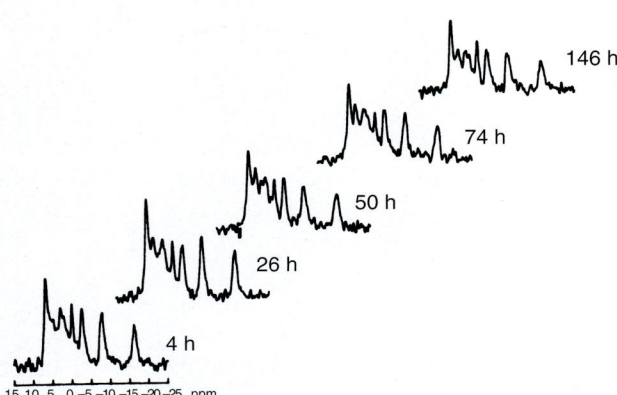

Figure 20.18 Phosphorus (P)-31 magnetic resonance spectra from two asphyxiated infants born at 37 and 36 weeks of gestation. Postnatal ages at the time of study are indicated. *(Top)* Peak assignments (numbers *1* to *7*) are as follows: *1,* phosphomonoester (PME); *2,* inorganic P (P_i); *3,* phosphodiester (PDE); *4,* phosphocreatine (PCr); *5, 6,* and *7,* gamma, alpha, and beta nucleotide triphosphate (mainly adenosine triphosphate [ATP]). At 8 hours, spectra were within normal limits (i.e., PCr/P_i was 0.99, ATP/total P was .09, and intracellular pH [pH_i] was 7.06; pH_i rose to a maximum of 7.28 at 36 hours). Minimum value for PCr/P_i was 0.32 at 55 hours, when ATP/total P was only .04 and pH_i was 6.99. The infant died at age 60 hours. *(Bottom)* At 4 hours, PCr/P_i and ATP/total P were normal at .97 and .09, respectively, and pH_i was 7.08 (pH_i rose to a maximum of 7.23 at 26 hours). The minimum value for PCr/P_i was 0.65 at 50 hours, but by 146 hours it was normal. ATP/total P never fell below normal. However, the infant died at age 27 days with cerebral atrophy. (From Azzopardi D, Wyatt JS, Cady EB, et al. Prognosis of newborn infants with hypoxic–ischemic brain injury assessed by phosphorus magnetic resonance spectroscopy. *Pediatr Res.* 1989;25:445–451.)

(CBF) provided critical information concerning the topography of hypoxic-ischemic cerebral injury, PET was studied in a series of 17 asphyxiated term infants with the $H_2^{15}O$ technique to measure regional CBF.[345] The infants had experienced primarily intrapartum asphyxia, exhibited the clinical syndrome described earlier, including proximal limb weakness, and were evaluated by PET during the acute period of their illness (i.e., the first week). The *disturbance of regional CBF in the asphyxiated infants* constituted a continuum of deviation from the normal (or nearly normal) pattern. The consistent and apparently unifying abnormality was a relative decrease in CBF to parasagittal regions, generally symmetrical and more marked posteriorly than anteriorly. The extent of the relative decreases in parasagittal CBF correlated directly with the severity of clinical manifestations.[345]

The *structural correlates* of the decrease in CBF in parasagittal regions were elucidated in four infants by technetium brain scan and by neuropathology and consisted of parasagittal cerebral injury. Thus, our CBF findings by PET indicated that *parasagittal cerebral injury* is a *common* feature in neonatal HIE, at least in patients who survive the perinatal insult.[345] This observation has been confirmed and amplified by subsequent studies with MRI (see earlier discussion).

CLINICOPATHOLOGICAL CORRELATIONS

The neurological correlates of HIE, as observed in the neonatal period and subsequently, are understood when one recalls the topography of the neuropathological lesions. Considerably more is known about the long-term neurological correlates of the several lesions than about the correlates in the newborn period. Indeed, in the latter instance, correlates must be made with some reservation. The reasons for the difficulty in establishing

correlations relate primarily to the large degree of overlap in the occurrence of the basic lesions and to the heretofore imperfect definition of topography by available imaging studies. Although the overlap of the various lesions will be a persistent confounder, improvements in imaging, especially the use of MRI, have allowed better definition of the topography of the brain injury in the neonatal period. The latter now has allowed certain probable correlations to be made. In the following discussion, we review the major neuropathological lesions in terms of the neurological correlates in the newborn period and subsequent periods (i.e., neurological sequelae).

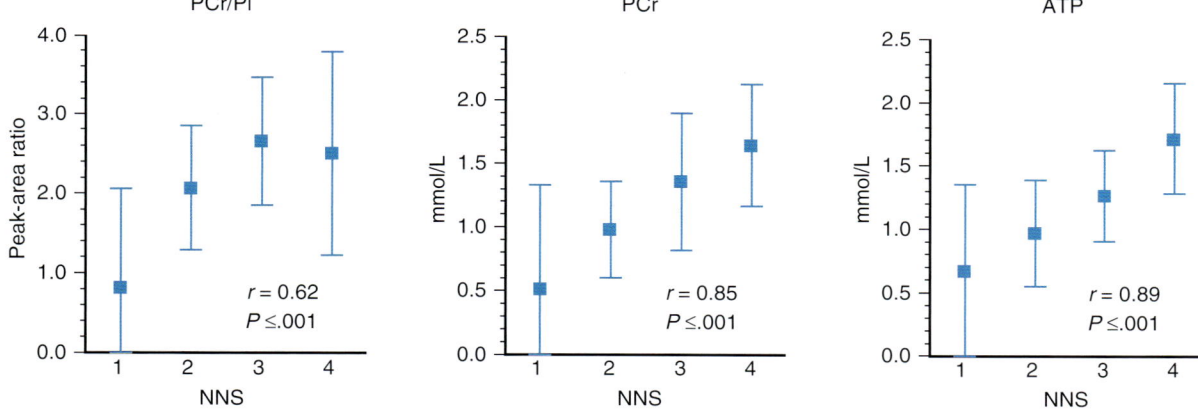

Figure 20.19 Relationship between cerebral levels of high-energy metabolites (mean ± SD), determined by phosphorus magnetic resonance spectroscopy, and the severity of the neonatal neurological syndrome (NNS) in 23 asphyxiated term newborns. The numerical scoring was as follows: NNS1, severe; NNS2, moderate; NNS3, mild; and NNS4, normal neurological examination in healthy control infants. *ATP*, adenosine triphosphate; *PCr*, phosphocreatine; *Pi*, inorganic phosphate. (From Martin E, Buchli R, Ritter S, et al. Diagnostic and prognostic value of cerebral ³¹P magnetic resonance spectroscopy in neonates with perinatal asphyxia. *Pediatr Res.* 1996;40: 749–758.)

TABLE 20.18   Clinical Correlates of Selective Neuronal Necrosis[a]

| | **NEUROLOGICAL FEATURES[b]** | |
TOPOGRAPHY OF THE MAJOR INJURY	NEONATAL PERIOD	LONG-TERM SEQUELAE
Cerebral cortex; basal ganglia; thalamus; reticular formation; brain stem nuclei, including inferior colliculus, cochlear nuclei, and motor nuclei of cranial nerves; cerebellum; anterior horn cells	Stupor and coma Seizures Hypotonia Hypertonia-dystonia[c] Oculomotor disturbances[d] Disturbed sucking, swallowing, and tongue movements[d]	Cognitive deficits[c] Spastic quadriparesis Choreoathetosis[c] Dystonia[c] Seizure disorder Ataxia Bulbar and pseudobulbar palsy[d]

[a]As discussed in the text, three major forms of selective neuronal necrosis should be recognized: diffuse, cerebral cortical–deep nuclear, and deep nuclear–brain stem.

[b]All the neurological features may be seen to varying degrees in the diffuse form of selective neuronal necrosis.

[c]Common abnormalities in those infants with involvement of basal ganglia and thalamus.

[d]Common additional abnormalities in those infants with involvement of brain stem tegmentum (and usually associated with deep nuclear involvement).

Selective Neuronal Necrosis

Neonatal Correlates

The neurological correlates in the *neonatal period* are diverse, as is the topography of the major neuronal injury (Table 20.18).

Of the major varieties of selective neuronal necrosis (diffuse, cerebral cortical–deep nuclear, deep nuclear–brain stem, and pontosubicular necrosis [see Chapter 18]), tentative clinical correlates can be established for the first three. In the *diffuse variety of selective neuronal necrosis*, associated with very severe and prolonged insults, all levels of the neuraxis are affected. With this variety, we have attributed the derangement of the level of consciousness to the involvement of the bilateral cerebral hemispheres or the reticular activating system in the upper brain stem and diencephalon, including the thalamus. Indeed, in one careful series studied by MRI, the involvement of basal ganglia and thalamus was associated strongly with severe encephalopathy, including a decreased level of alertness.[278] Seizures appear to relate to cerebral cortical injury, although some of the seizure phenomena, especially some of the tonic phenomena, may emanate from subcortical nuclear structures in basal ganglia, thalamus, or midbrain. The uncommon but dramatic occurrence of the syndrome of inappropriate ADH secretion or diabetes insipidus presumably relates to hypothalamic neuronal involvement. The hypotonia could relate to cerebral cortical or anterior horn cell disturbances or combinations of both. Electrophysiological evidence (e.g., fibrillations), as well as clinical data (hypotonia, absent deep tendon reflexes, weakness), support a role for anterior horn cell involvement, especially in severe, diffuse disease.[346,347] The oculomotor abnormalities presumably relate primarily to the disturbance of cranial nerve nuclei (III, IV, and VI). The impairments of sucking (V), swallowing (IX and X), and tongue movements (XII) also are probably largely the basis of brain stem cranial nerve nuclear involvement. However, a contribution of corticobulbar disturbance to these deficits is possible. The facial appearance of an infant with striking brain stem involvement, proven neuropathologically, is shown in Fig. 20.21.

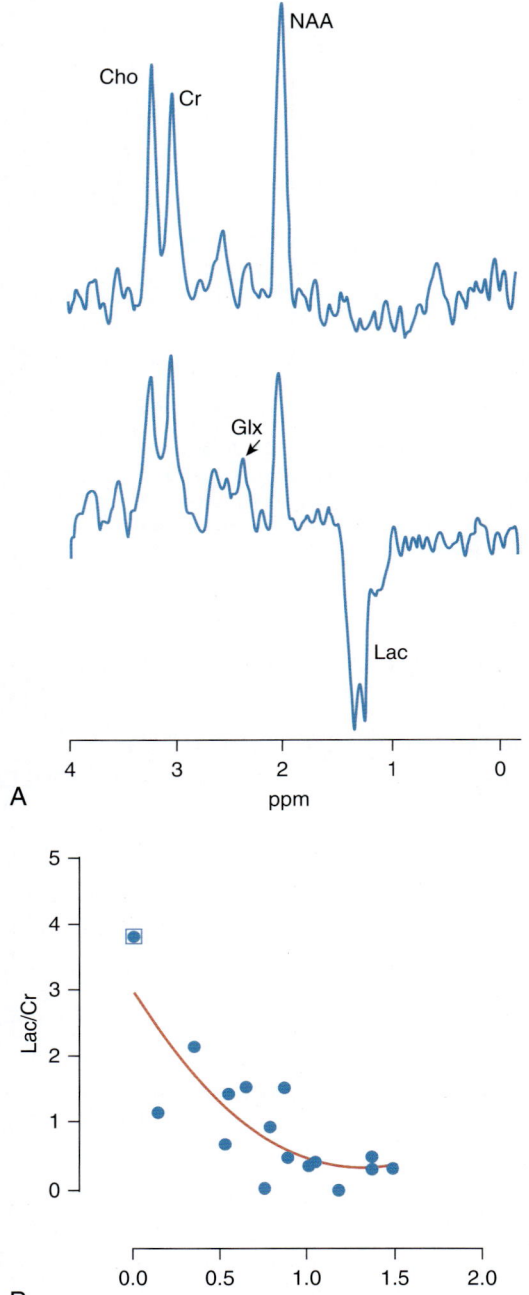

A

B

Figure 20.20 Proton magnetic resonance (MR) spectroscopy from basal ganglia in 16 asphyxiated term newborns. (A) Spectra from a control infant *(upper tracing)* and from a severely asphyxiated infant *(lower tracing)*, both obtained at 14 hours of age. Note the striking lactate peak in the asphyxiated infant. (B) Relationship between lactate/creatine (Lac/Cr) measured by proton MR spectroscopy at 4 to 18 hours of age and phosphocreatine/inorganic phosphate (PCr/Pi) measured by phosphorus MR spectroscopy at 33 to 106 hours. Note the correlation between the severity of the early increase in lactate and the degree of secondary energy failure as manifested by the decreased PCr/Pi ratio. *Cho,* choline; *Glx,* glutamic acid; *NAA,* N-acetylaspartate. (From Hanrahan JD, Sargentoni J, Azzopardi D, et al. Cerebral metabolism within 18 hours of birth asphyxia: a proton magnetic resonance spectroscopy study. *Pediatr Res.* 1996;39:584–590.)

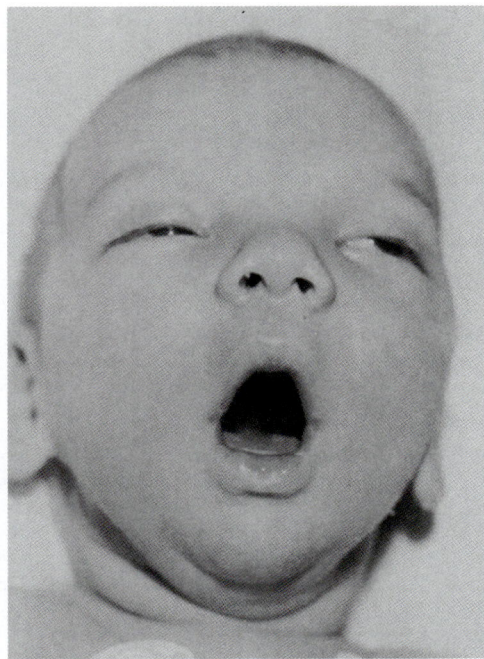

Figure 20.21 Facial appearance at age 1 month in an infant who experienced perinatal asphyxia. Note the disconjugate gaze, ptosis, marked facial weakness, and wide-open mouth. The infant also exhibited fasciculations of the tongue on physical examination. (From Roland EH, Hill A, Norman MG, et al. Selective brainstem injury in an asphyxiated newborn. *Ann Neurol.* 1988;23:89–92.)

With the *cerebral cortical–deep nuclear variety of selective neuronal necrosis,* associated with moderate to severe and relatively prolonged insults, the involvement of the cerebral cortex, the basal ganglia (especially the putamen), and the thalamus predominates (see Chapter 18). The major clinical difference from the syndrome just described is the occurrence of *increased tone* in many such affected infants. The hypertonia often increases with stimulation, especially manipulation, and has characteristics of dystonia. We have attributed this finding to extrapyramidal involvement, perhaps unmasked by the less severe injury to the pyramidal system that occurs with the diffuse variety of selective neuronal injury.

With the *deep nuclear–brain stem variety of selective neuronal necrosis,* associated with severe and abrupt insults, the involvement of the basal ganglia, thalamus, and brain stem tegmental neurons occurs, with relative sparing of the cerebral cortex. The major additional clinical correlates relate to brain stem injury and include ptosis, oculomotor disturbances, facial diparesis, ventilatory disturbances, and impaired sucking and swallowing.[61,348,349]

Long-Term Correlates

The *long-term neurological sequelae* depend on the topography of the neuronal injury. With the *diffuse variety of selective neuronal necrosis,* intellectual retardation is nearly uniform and is the consequence principally of cerebral cortical injury (see Table 20.18). However, injury to the basal ganglia,[350,351] thalamus, and cerebellum (see later) could play a role. (The possibility of impairment of subsequent cortical neuronal differentiation is raised by experimental data,[352,353] but studies of human infants are lacking.) The spastic motor deficits could relate to cortical injury, although the relative roles of concomitant ischemic parasagittal cerebral injury and cerebral white matter injury/ periventricular leukomalacia have not been elucidated. Seizure disorders, which develop in approximately 10% to 30% of infants with HIE (see Chapter 12), probably relate to cerebral cortical injury. Impairment of cortical visual functions occurs in severely affected infants, and cerebral cortical atrophy was reported to be the principal finding on CT in approximately 60% of such patients.[354-357] MRI studies have emphasized the association of basal ganglia or thalamic lesions and cerebral white matter injury with impaired visual function in such infants.[358-360] (The improvement of vision in as many as 50% of such infants over the first 2 years of life may reflect the operation of cortical organizational events, i.e., brain plasticity, as outlined in Unit I.) Disturbances of hypothalamic neurons presumably underlie the early sexual maturation that occurs in 10% of term asphyxiated infants with other signs of neurological disturbance.[361] Impairments of sucking, swallowing, and facial movement may relate to nuclear injury (i.e., bulbar palsy), although some infants also exhibit the features of upper motor neuron injury (i.e., pseudobulbar palsy), probably cerebral in origin, such as "all-or-none smile" and fixed facial expression with drooling.[362,363] Hyperactivity and impaired attentive capacities, particularly observable (unmasked?) in less affected patients, may relate to involvement of neurons of the reticular activating system, the basal ganglia, or the cerebellum.[364-366] The substantial minority of infants with hearing deficits presumably may have involvement of dorsal cochlear nuclei (which subserve perception of higher frequency sounds) or of cochlea, or both. The involvement of the superior olivary nucleus and the inferior colliculus may contribute. Finally, the involvement of anterior horn cells may explain the characteristic persistence of hypotonia in the first months of life, and when it is severe, this topography of involvement may explain the unusual persistence into childhood of hypotonia and weakness (i.e., atonic quadriparesis or "atonic cerebral palsy").

With the *cerebral cortical–deep nuclear variety of selective neuronal necrosis*, the major clinical features include not only the deficits attributable to cerebral cortical neuronal injury but also those related to the involvement of the basal ganglia and the thalamus, which are discussed separately later. With the *deep nuclear–brain stem variety of selective neuronal necrosis*, the additional clinical features relate not only to the basal ganglia–thalamic involvement, discussed separately later, but also to the brain stem injury. All surviving infants with this injury have prolonged difficulties with feeding, usually for many months and often requiring tube feeding.[61,348,367,368] Approximately 20% to 30% require gastrostomy for feeding (see the later section on prognosis). However, because of the relative sparing of cerebral cortex with this variety of selective neuronal injury, up to 50% of these patients have been found to exhibit normal cognition.[61]

With *involvement of basal ganglia and thalamus*, whether as a component of the cerebral–deep nuclear variety of selective neuronal necrosis or the deep nuclear syndrome with brain stem involvement, subsequent extrapyramidal abnormalities are not uncommon. The neurodevelopmental, motor, and feeding outcomes of a large series of infants with basal ganglia and thalamic injury on MRI have been recently reviewed (see Prognosis).[275,276,369] Unknown numbers of such infants develop

the neuropathological lesion *status marmoratus* (see Chapter 18), but the fundamental clinicoanatomical correlate is neuronal loss in the putamen and the thalamus, whether or not the final pathological appearance is that of status marmoratus.[370,371] The essential anatomical combination for choreoathetosis and dystonia appears to be *bilateral* involvement of the basal ganglia and *intact* pyramidal tracts because, in one neuropathological series, the several patients without choreoathetosis had unilateral or bilateral sparing of the basal ganglia or degeneration of the pyramidal tracts.[372] The thalamoputaminal involvement is different from the subthalamic nucleus and globus pallidus distribution in bilirubin encephalopathy, the other major neonatal disorder with subsequent choreoathetosis (see Chapter 26). Careful studies using MRI in infants with "dyskinetic" or "athetoid" cerebral palsy demonstrated the thalamoputaminal predilection in hypoxic-ischemic disease.[373,374] Indeed, the thalamus was affected without putaminal involvement as often as with putaminal involvement, and more often than with the involvement of the putamen alone.[373] Of particular interest and not readily explicable is the finding that the onset of the extrapyramidal abnormalities is not clearly apparent until after 6 to 12 months and often much later. Thus, most such infants develop overt choreoathetosis or dystonia, or both, between 1 and 4 years of age.[375-377] Abnormal motor development and hypertonia commonly are obvious before this time (i.e., as early as 6 months of life).[360]

An important percentage of children will not develop abnormal movements until as late as 7 to 14 years of age (see Table 20.19).[377-381] In the largest reported series of the *delayed-onset syndrome*, the mean age of onset of choreoathetosis and dystonia was 12.9 years, and the mean duration of progression was 7 years (Table 20.19).[381] Four of the 10 patients studied had attained early developmental milestones at ages within the normal range. Although the children ultimately had mild to moderate motor disability, all were ambulatory. The only class of drugs with clear benefit was anticholinergic medication, perhaps reflecting that the relatively spared cholinergic neurons were responsible for the development of the extrapyramidal clinical phenomena.[381]

Intellectual function often is *relatively* preserved in those infants with choreoathetosis. Thus, in the older literature, intellectual function in infants with "athetoid cerebral palsy," presumably many or most of whom had putaminothalamic

TABLE 20.19	Delayed-Onset Dystonia After Perinatal Asphyxia

The mean age of onset of dystonia, often with choreoathetosis, is 12.9 years.

Nearly 50% of patients have a history of normal neurological development.

Approximately 80% have other neurological signs, but fewer than 50% have overt "cerebral palsy."

Intellect is in normal range in approximately 80%.

Progression of dystonia continues for a mean of 7 years to moderate disability (not wheelchair bound).

Treatment with anticholinergic agents may be beneficial.

Data from Saint-Hilaire MH, Burke RE, Bressman SB, et al. Delayed-onset dystonia due to perinatal or early childhood asphyxia. *Neurology.* 1991;41:216–222.

injury to a varying degree, was not noted to be markedly affected consistently.[382-385] In the largest reported series of the delayed-onset extrapyramidal syndrome, 8 of 10 individuals had a normal intelligence quotient.[381] The pathological substrate for the intellectual failure with injury to the basal ganglia and the thalamus presumably relates, in considerable part, to any associated hypoxic-ischemic cerebral cortical neuronal injury; indeed, in the large neuropathological series of Malamud,[372] approximately 50% of patients with severe involvement (i.e., the pathological features of status marmoratus) exhibited neuropathological signs of cerebral cortical injury. However, these latter patients also manifested thalamic injury, and approximately one-third of patients with pathologically proven status marmoratus, and with impaired intellect, exhibited thalamic injury *without* significant involvement of the cerebral cortex.[372] This finding suggests that the thalamic injury can play an important role in causing the intellectual deficits. MRI data support this contention (see the section on prognosis).[29,386] These observations have major implications for the *role of the thalamus in the development of intellectual function.*

The clinical correlates of the *cerebellar vermian atrophy/ hypoplasia* that is a common sequela in term infants with hypoxic-ischemic disease (see Chapter 18) remain to be defined. This abnormality may contribute to varying degrees of motor incoordination, occasionally including overt ataxia. Cognitive and behavioral deficits also could be correlates of the cerebellar involvement (see later).

Parasagittal Cerebral Injury

Neonatal Correlates

The neurological correlates in the *neonatal period* include particularly weakness of proximal limbs, which is consistently more prominent in the upper rather than the lower extremities (Table 20.20).

This pattern of weakness is readily predicted from the topography of the lesion (Fig. 20.22). The topographical

TABLE 20.20   Clinical Correlates of Parasagittal Cerebral Injury

TOPOGRAPHY OF THE MAJOR INJURY	NEUROLOGICAL FEATURES	
	NEONATAL PERIOD	LONG-TERM SEQUELAE
Cerebral cortex and subcortical white matter, superomedial (parasagittal) convexities, and posterior > anterior cerebrum	Proximal limb weakness upper > lower	Spastic quadriparesis Intellectual deficits (often "specific")

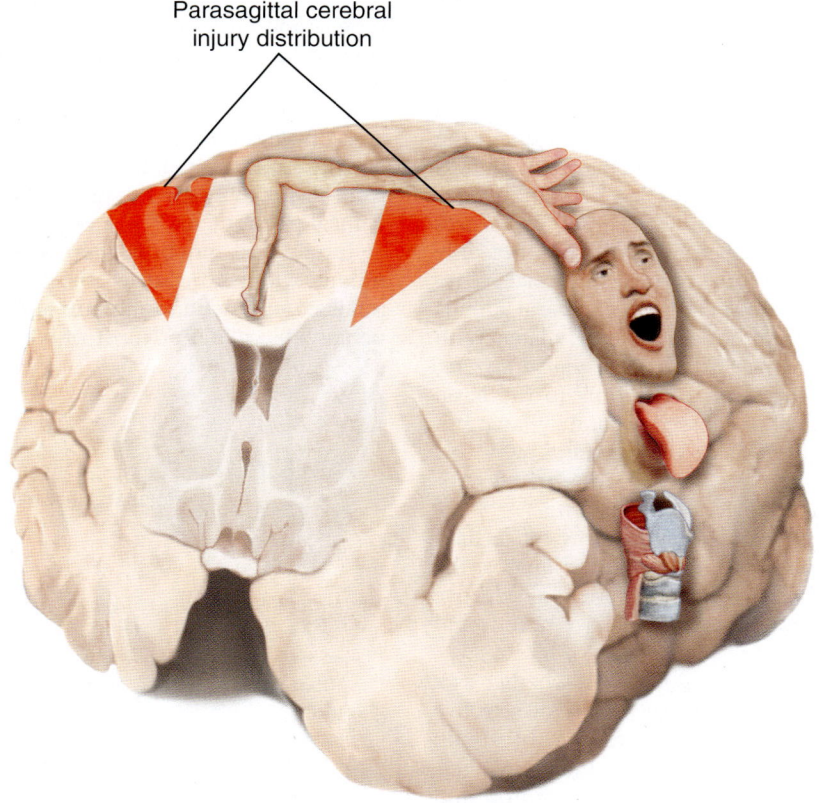

Parasagittal cerebral injury distribution

Figure 20.22 Schematic diagram of representation of the homunculus on the motor cortex and the sites of parasagittal cerebral injury *(red triangular areas bilaterally).* Note that the proximal extremities, upper more than lower, are most likely to be affected.

representation of the homunculus on the motor cortex indicates that the proximal extremities, upper more than lower, lie within the distribution of the necrosis of the cerebral cortical neurons and their descending corticospinal tract fibers in subcortical white matter. Other deficits referable to parasagittal cerebral injury are likely, but ready detection of such deficits in the newborn requires specialized clinical techniques. For example, careful analysis of "cortical" somesthetic-visual-auditory associations, functions residing within the areas of posterior cerebrum especially affected in parasagittal necrosis, has not been accomplished in the newborn. This topic is clearly important for future clinical research. The advances in electrophysiological, behavioral, and functional MR techniques for assessing such associative functions in the newborn (see Chapters 9 and 10) could be used effectively in this clinical setting. Indeed, the disturbances of visual- and somatosensory-evoked responses observed in asphyxiated infants appear to correlate with cerebral injury in the parasagittal cerebral distributions, affecting parieto-occipital regions in the former instance (visual-evoked responses) and parietal regions in the latter instance.[354,387]

Long-Term Correlates

The *long-term sequelae* of parasagittal cerebral injury relate primarily to motor and cognitive function, particularly the latter.[29,274,281,388,389] However, in general, subsequent deficits are less common than in infants who also exhibit deep nuclear injury (see the section on prognosis later).[29] The motor deficits, when present, include particular involvement of proximal limbs, upper more than lower, as in the neonatal period (see Table 20.20). Although severely affected infants exhibit multiple cognitive deficits, many infants have exhibited "specific" intellectual deficits, such as disproportionate disturbances in the development of language or of visual-spatial abilities, or both.[388,390-393] We believe these discrete intellectual deficits to relate particularly to the larger, posteriorly located lesions (i.e., in posterior parietal-occipital-temporal regions) that reside within areas of critical importance for many associative functions, especially those relating to auditory and visual input and output, and to a variety of visual–motor phenomena.

PROGNOSIS

Precise determination of the prognosis in the term newborn who sustains a hypoxic-ischemic insult is hindered by the difficulties in determining the severity of the insult. As indicated earlier, most of the primary insults occur in utero, and the difficulties of determining the degree of hypoxemia and ischemia in the fetus are obvious. The value of *electronic fetal monitoring* and associated fetal blood sampling may be appreciable, but further advances in monitoring the status of the fetal brain clearly are needed (see Chapter 17). Because significant intrauterine (particularly intrapartum) hypoxic-ischemic insult is usually associated with depressed Apgar scores, correlation of outcome with the *Apgar score* also has been used for assessing the prognosis. The presence of a *neonatal neurological syndrome* is a crucial indicator of a perinatal insult with the potential to cause neurological injury. Moreover, certain *specific aspects of the neurological syndrome* (e.g., seizures and duration of abnormalities) are useful in estimating outcome. Finally, selected neurodiagnostic studies, such as *EEG, evoked potentials, ultrasound, CT,* and *MRI,* are also of proven prognostic value. Value for *MR spectroscopy* is also

indicated by more recent data. In the following discussion, the relative value of each of these factors in estimating outcome is evaluated.

An important general question to consider is the spectrum of neurological deficits observed subsequently, and specifically, whether impairment of cognitive functions can occur in *the absence of prominent motor deficits (i.e., cerebral palsy)*. Large-scale studies show that cognitive impairment without overt cerebral palsy is not uncommon after neonatal HIE.[386,388,394-396] In the largest available series, among survivors of HIE, 9% of children without cerebral palsy had an IQ at 6 to 7 years of less than 70 and fully 31% had scores ranging from 70 to 84.[396] Children with cerebral palsy did have a poorer cognitive outcome (i.e., 96% had an IQ < 70). Overall, 14% of infants treated with hypothermia developed cerebral palsy, versus 28% of those not treated with hypothermia, and the rates of occurrence of cognitive impairment without cerebral palsy were approximately similar in the two treatment groups.

Apgar Scores, Fetal Acidosis, and Neonatal Resuscitation

Because hypoxic-ischemic injury is one cause of *depressed Apgar scores,* and because depressed Apgar scores imply the possibility of an ongoing hypoxic-ischemic insult, correlation of outcome with such scores has been attempted for many years. This approach is fraught with hazards for several reasons. First, precise quantitation of the Apgar score varies among observers, sometimes considerably. Second, each of the five factors that make up the score is given equal weight, and clearly the importance of each for central nervous system integrity differs greatly. Third, causes of the depressed scores, other than hypoxic-ischemic insult,[397-404] include laryngeal inhibition (e.g., caused by aspiration of a small amount of amniotic fluid or by oronasopharyngeal–laryngeal stimulation from suction catheters), maternal medications or anesthesia, and prematurity, and are associated with generally favorable prognoses unless additional postnatal insults occur. In a population-based cohort study of 235,165 term infants, of the 292 with a 5-minute Apgar score of 0 to 3, only 16, or 6.8%, later exhibited cerebral palsy.[405] Similarly, in another series of 1200 consecutive deliveries, only 20% of infants with a 5-minute Apgar score of less than 7 had acidosis with a pH of 7.10 or less (umbilical artery).[406] This tenuous relationship between apparent fetal asphyxia and low Apgar scores has been confirmed.[53,400,407-412]

The value of the "extended" Apgar score (i.e., the score after 5 minutes) was demonstrated initially by data from the Collaborative Perinatal Project of the National Institutes of Health and was published over 35 years ago (Table 20.21).[413] The likelihood of cerebral palsy in infants weighing 2500 g or more increased dramatically with the increasing duration of Apgar scores of 3 or less, especially after 15 minutes. Infants with such scores experienced a progressive increase in mortality rate, so that almost 60% of those with Apgar scores of 0 to 3 after 20 minutes subsequently died. Similarly, premature infants also exhibited a distinctly worsening prognosis with low "extended" Apgar scores. It is likely that the major determinant of the poor outcome with longer duration of a low Apgar score in both premature and full-term infants was, in the largest part, the severity of the initial intrauterine insult. However, even though low Apgar scores for as long as 15 minutes are associated with high mortality rates, the majority of *survivors* escaped *major*

TABLE 20.21	Relation of Apgar Score to Mortality and Cerebral Palsy[a]	
APGAR SCORE OF 0–3	**DEATH IN FIRST YEAR (%)**	**CEREBRAL PALSY IN SURVIVORS (WITH KNOWN OUTCOME) (%)[b]**
1 min	3	1
5 min	8	1
10 min	18	5
15 min	48	9
20 min	59	57

[a]For infants ≥2501 g.

[b]Neurological sequelae less pronounced than cerebral palsy were not quantitated.

Adapted from Nelson KB, Ellenberg JH. Apgar scores as predictors of chronic neurologic disability. *Pediatrics*. 1981;68:36–44.

TABLE 20.22   New Expanded and Traditional Apgar Score for Evaluation of the Newborn Infant

Expanded Apgar

C	Continuous positive airway pressure[a]
O	Oxygen
M-B	Mask and bag ventilation[b]
I	Intubation and ventilation
N	Neonatal chest compression
E	Exogenous surfactant
D	Drugs

Scoring each item of expanded Apgar:

0 = intervention was performed; 1 = no intervention was performed

[a]: score 0 if "mask and bag" or "intubation and ventilation" is scored 0

[b]: score 0 if "intubation and ventilation" is scored 0

Traditional Apgar

A	Appearance (skin color)	
	2 = completely pink	
	1 = centrally pink with acrocyanosis	
	0 = centrally blue or pale	
P	Pulse (HR)	
	2 = > 100 beats per minute	
	1 = < 100 beats per minute	
	0 = no heart beat	
G	Grimacing (reflex)	
	2 = Appropriate for gestational age	
	1 = Reduced for gestational age	
	0 = No reflex response	
A	Activity (muscle tone)	
	2 = Appropriate for gestational age	
	1 = Reduced for gestational age	
	0 = No reflex response	
R	Respiration (chest movement)	
	2 = Regular chest movement	
	1 = Small or irregular chest movement	
	0 = No chest movement	

HR, Heart rate.

neurological injury (see Table 20.21). It is important to note that neurological sequelae less severe than cerebral palsy were not quantitated in this earlier study.[53,404,414-416] Even with the worst of Apgar scores at 1 minute of age (i.e., 0 or apparent stillbirth), in a large series (*n* = 93), of the 40% of infants who survived, approximately 60% had a normal outcome.[416] However, of the 58 infants whose Apgar score still was 0 at 10 minutes of age, 57 died, and the sole survivor had an abnormal neurological outcome.

More recent data in the era of hypothermia treatment suggest value for the 10-minute Apgar score. Thus, in a substudy of 174 infants in the NICHD randomized, controlled trial of therapeutic hypothermia, 64/85 (75%) of those with a 10-minute Apgar score of 0 to 3 had death/disability compared with 40/89 (45%) of those with scores greater than 3. Each point increase in the 10-minute Apgar scores was associated with a significantly lower adjusted risk of death/disability, death, death/IQ < 70, death/cerebral palsy (CP), and disability/IQ < 70 and CP among survivors (all *P* < 0.05). Among the 24 children with a 10-minute Apgar score of 0, five (21%) survived without disability. The risk-adjusted probabilities of death/disability were significantly lower in cooled infants with Apgar scores of 0 to 3. The authors concluded that although the low 10-minute Apgar scores were associated with poorer school-age outcomes, approximately 20% of infants with a 10-minute Apgar score of 0 survived without disability to school age.[417]

Finally, a novel method of adapting the original Apgar score to provide a combined score[418] that includes elements of respiratory management, chest compressions and the administration of drugs, in addition to the elements of the traditional Apgar score, has been shown to improve the short-term predictive power of this resuscitative evaluation (Table 20.22). Future data may show that this combined score better correlates with outcomes.

The severity of *fetal acidosis*, as determined by the measurement of umbilical arterial pH and base deficit, is a useful reflection of the severity and duration of intrauterine hypoxia–ischemia. The relationship between the severity of fetal acidosis and neonatal neurological features as well as neurological outcome is reviewed in Chapter 17.

Certain aspects of the *neonatal resuscitation*, and particularly the need for positive pressure ventilation and more intensive cardiopulmonary resuscitation efforts (e.g., chest compressions), are predictive of an unfavorable outcome. Hence, as outlined earlier the Combined Apgar score uses this information in addition to the parameters of the traditional Apgar score for prognostication (see Table 20.22). In one careful study, when the need for cardiopulmonary resuscitation was associated with evidence of fetal acidemia (pH < 7.00), five of five infants either died in the neonatal period or exhibited neonatal seizures, whereas of 10 infants requiring such resuscitation measures, but without evidence of an appreciable intrauterine insult (cord pH normal), all 10 had a normal outcome.[419] In a later study, the requirement for intubation in full-term infants with severe fetal acidemia (i.e., umbilical arterial pH ≤ 7.0) was associated with a 6.4-fold increase in abnormal neurological outcome.[82] The importance of the duration of delayed onset of breathing, also presumably reflecting the severity of the intrauterine insult, was emphasized by a study of 165 infants who exhibited "postasphyxial encephalopathy."[420] Thus, the

TABLE 20.23 Relation of Three Key Early Neonatal Variables to Risk of Severe Adverse Outcome With Neonatal Hypoxic-Ischemic Encephalopathy

VARIABLES	PROBABILITY OF SEVERE OUTCOME[a]	
	PERCENTAGE OF TOTAL	95% CONFIDENCE INTERVAL
None	46	33–58
One variable		
CC	69	NA
Resp.	67	NA
BD	6	NA
Overall	64	54–73
Two variables		
CC and Resp.	67	NA
CC and BD	77	NA
BD and Resp.	81	NA
Overall	77	66–85
Three variables		
CC and Resp. and BD	93	81–99

[a]Severe adverse outcome was defined as death or severe neurological disability; total N = 302.

BD, Base deficit ≥16; CC, chest compression for >1 minute; NA, not applicable; Resp., age at onset of respiration ≥30 minutes.

Data from Shah PS, Beyene J, To T, et al. Postasphyxial hypoxic–ischemic encephalopathy in neonates: outcome prediction rule within 4 hours of birth. Arch Pediatr Adolesc Med. 2006;160:729–736.

rate of death or subsequent neurological deficits was 42% with delayed onset of breathing for 1 to 9 minutes, 56% for 10 to 19 minutes, and 88% for more than 20 minutes. An additional prognostic feature of the first 30 minutes of life in asphyxiated term infants with severe fetal acidemia (umbilical arterial pH ≤ 7.0) is the occurrence of hypoglycemia.[82] Thus, the 15% of acidemic infants in this study with an initial blood glucose of 40 mg/dL or lower had an 18.5-fold increased risk for death or moderate to severe encephalopathy than those with a glucose concentration higher than 40 mg/dL.

A recent study of more than 300 term infants with apparent intrapartum asphyxia and HIE identified three key variables that together provided a strong prediction of a serious adverse outcome (death or severe neurological sequelae) (Table 20.23).[421] The data suggested that the combination of need for chest compressions for more than 1 minute, a base deficit of 16 or greater, and age at onset of respiration at 30 minutes or greater was associated with a 93% risk of serious adverse outcome. The findings could be useful not only for early prognostication but also perhaps for decision-making concerning neuroprotective therapies. The additions of pH and arterial carbon dioxide pressure (PCO_2) of cord blood gas measurements also provide predictive accuracy.[422]

Neonatal Neurological Syndrome

The occurrence of a recognizable neonatal neurological syndrome after signs of intrauterine asphyxia (see earlier) is the single most useful indicator that a significant hypoxic-ischemic insult to the brain has occurred. Studies completed since the 1970s, but before the era of hypothermia treatment, support this contention and suggest the occurrence of improvements in overall outcome.[a] In an excellent representative earlier series of 93 patients (most term infants) reported by Brown and co-workers[11] in 1974, perinatal asphyxia was manifested by such features as meconium-stained amniotic fluid, fetal bradycardia, the need for endotracheal intubation, assisted ventilation at birth, and Apgar scores of less than 3 at 1 minute, or less than 5 at 5 minutes, *in addition to neurological signs*, such as feeding difficulties, apnea, seizures, and hypotonia. Approximately 20% of the infants died in the neonatal period, approximately 40% subsequently exhibited neurological sequelae, and approximately 40% were found to be normal. In later series, although direct comparisons are hindered by differences in selection criteria, the outcome was somewhat better. Among term infants, only approximately 10% died in the neonatal period, and approximately 75% (i.e., nearly 85% of survivors) were normal on follow-up.

The likelihood of neurological sequelae in infants after hypoxic-ischemic insult *without* a neonatal neurological syndrome is not known absolutely. The regionalization of *both* perinatal and pediatric care in the area served by Brown and co-workers[11] allowed these investigators to conclude that such an occurrence was very unlikely. A similar conclusion can be drawn from a later study.[55] Although more data are needed on this issue, the available information suggests that the occurrence of neonatal neurological features provides the best indicator of infants at risk for subsequent significant neurological deficits. However, these issues will require systematic reconsideration in the current era of hypothermia treatment.

Specific Aspects

Certain aspects of the neonatal neurological syndrome particularly useful in estimating the prognosis include the *severity of the syndrome*, the *presence of seizures*, and the *duration of the abnormalities*.

Before discussing these specific neurological aspects, it is important to recognize that certain aspects of the *non-neurological evaluation* may provide prognostic information. Thus, in a study of asphyxiated infants (defined by depressed Apgar scores or fetal acidosis or both), of the 22 term infants with normal urine output, the mortality rate was approximately 5%, and neurological sequelae occurred in only 10% of survivors, whereas, with oliguria persisting beyond 24 hours of life, the mortality rate was 33%, and neurological sequelae occurred in 67% of survivors.[426] A similar relationship between the severity of renal injury and an unfavorable neurological outcome was shown in the preterm infants. However, as also observed by others, neurological abnormalities in the neonatal period and on follow-up can occur in the absence of apparent renal injury (see the earlier section on neurological syndrome).[53,425,426]

The *severity* of the neonatal neurological syndrome is of major value. Thus, when systematically quantitated, the severity correlated directly with the incidence of neurological sequelae.[b] The studies of Finer and co-workers,[20,394,431] which involved 226 full-term infants with HIE, and of Thornberg and co-workers,

---

[a]References 11, 14-17, 20, 23, 25, 29, 55, 70, 250, 278, 327, 394, 402, 419, 420, and 423-444.
[b]References 17, 23, 29, 55, 84, 250, 278, 327, 394, 419, 420, 424, 427, 428, 430-432, 437, 439-442, 444, and 445.

TABLE 20.24   Outcome of Term Infants With HIE as a Function of Severity of Neonatal Neurological Syndrome[a]

SEVERITY OF NEONATAL SYNDROME[b]	NO. OF PATIENTS	PERCENTAGE OF TOTAL		
		DEATHS[c] (%)	NEUROLOGICAL SEQUELAE (%)[d]	NORMAL (%)
Mild	115	0	0	100
Moderate	136	5	24	71
Severe	40	8	20	0
All	291	13	14	73

[a]Derived from 291 full-term infants with HIE.

[b]Mild, "hyperalert, hyperexcitable; normal muscle tone, no seizures"; moderate, "hypotonia, decreased movements, and often seizures"; severe, "stuporous, flaccid, and absent primitive reflexes."

[c]Includes in-hospital and postdischarge deaths.

[d]Principally spastic motor deficits and cognitive disturbances.

HIE, Hypoxic-ischemic encephalopathy.

Data from Robertson C, Finer N. Term infants with HIE: outcome at 3.5 years. *Dev Med Child Neurol.* 1985;27:473–484; and Thornberg E, Thiringer K, Odeback A, Milsom I. Birth asphyxia: incidence, clinical course and outcome in a Swedish population. *Acta Paediatr.* 1995;84:927–932.

TABLE 20.25   Seizures as an Unfavorable Prognostic Sign in Neonatal Hypoxic-Ischemic Encephalopathy in Term Infants[a]

Seizures increase the risk of neurological sequelae by as much as 40-fold

Seizures persistently recalcitrant to anticonvulsant treatment are nearly uniformly associated with death or subsequent neurological deficits

Early onset of seizures increases the risk of adverse outcome, and the risk is approximately 75% with onset in the first 4 h

[a]See text for references.

which involved 65 such infants, demonstrated this point clearly (Table 20.24).[55] Although the overall incidence of death or neurological sequelae was 27%, infants with a mild neonatal syndrome had *no* subsequent deficits, whereas those with a severe syndrome uniformly either died (80%) or exhibited sequelae (20%). Prolonged follow-up is important; in one report of teenage outcome among term infants with moderate neonatal encephalopathy and considered normal on earlier assessment (*n* = 28), the majority exhibited some learning problems or behavioral disturbances, or both, at the later evaluation.[444] Later neurodevelopmental follow-up has also identified some disability in infants that had mild neonatal encephalopathy. In one population of infants with mild HIE (*n* = 34), followed to 9 years, lower mean IQ (98.6 vs. 109 [*P* = 0.21]), increased thought problems (*P* = 0.001), and impaired motor assessment and manual dexterity (*P* = 0.002) were observed.[446-448]

The presence of *seizures* as part of the neonatal neurological syndrome increases the risk for neurological sequelae (Table 20.25).[a] The incidence of neurological sequelae in infants with seizures is as much as 40-fold greater than the incidence in

those without seizures. Thus, in one series of 27 infants with HIE complicated by seizures, death, or subsequent neurological deficits occurred in 67%.[55] Moreover, neurological sequelae are more likely if seizures occur in the first 12 hours or are difficult to control. For example, in one series of 45 infants, 76% with seizure onset at 4 hours of age or less died or exhibited neurological sequelae.[420] In another study of 68 term newborns with apparent HIE, the *combination* of a neonatal neurological syndrome and seizures on the first day of life predicted abnormal outcome with 94% specificity and 72% sensitivity.[442] The degree to which the seizures per se *contribute* to the poorer outcome in certain cases (see Chapter 12) or simply reflect a more serious insult is unresolved.

The *duration* of neonatal neurological abnormalities is useful in identifying the infant at greatest risk for sequelae.[a] In two large series, essentially all infants who exhibited no neurological abnormalities after about 1 week of life (or on "discharge from the hospital") were normal on follow-up.[20,70] In a more recent series of 84 infants, approximately 90% of those with a normal examination at 7 days were normal on follow-up, and 10% had only mild abnormalities.[439] In another careful study of 23 severely asphyxiated infants, all 17 infants who were normal on follow-up exhibited neurological signs for less than 2 weeks.[70] Our experience is similar. Thus, the duration of neurological abnormalities is a good indicator of the severity of hypoxic-ischemic injury, and the disappearance of abnormalities by 1 or 2 weeks is an excellent prognostic sign. However, such analyses do not include systematic evaluation at school age; therefore, the possibility of learning disturbances cannot be conclusively ruled out.

Results of Neurodiagnostic Techniques

Because outcome clearly relates to the severity of the neuropathology, any specialized technique that defines the extent of brain injury in the newborn period should provide valuable information regarding prognosis. Such techniques include electrophysiological measures, especially EEG, but also

[a]References 14, 15, 20, 29, 53, 55, 70, 419, 420, 425, 430, 432, 435, 439, 440, 442, and 449-453.

[a]References 20, 70, 414, 432, 433, and 439.

TABLE 20.26   Electroencephalographic Patterns of Prognostic Significance in Asphyxiated Term Infants[a]

Associated with favorable outcome
Mild depression (or less) on day 1
Normal background by day 7
Associated with unfavorable outcome
Predominant interburst interval >20 s on any day
Burst-suppression pattern on any day
Isoelectric tracing on any day
Mild (or greater) depression after day 12

[a]See text for references. Associations with favorable or unfavorable outcome are generally 90% or greater, but the clinical context must be considered.

TABLE 20.27   Predominant Interburst Interval Duration in Prediction of Outcome[a]

Predominant interburst interval duration is obtained readily by manual measurement of the predominant interval accounting for more than 50% of all interburst interval durations
A predominant interburst interval duration of more than 30 s is associated with an unfavorable outcome in 100% of cases, a duration of more than 20 s is associated with an unfavorable outcome in 92% of cases, and an interval lasting longer than 10 s is associated with an unfavorable outcome in 72% of cases
The predominant interburst interval duration is more useful than the burst-suppression periodic pattern because the latter accounts for a small minority of discontinuous tracings

[a]See text for details and Chapter 4.

evoked potentials, brain imaging methods, and methods to evaluate cerebral hemodynamics and metabolism.

Electroencephalography and Evoked Potentials

As discussed in the diagnosis section, *specific EEG patterns* are indicative of particular types of hypoxic-ischemic brain injury (see Table 20.11). Such information, especially when coupled with imaging data, is valuable for prognostic assessment (see earlier).

The *severity* of EEG abnormalities and their *duration* in the asphyxiated infant also are of prognostic importance (Table 20.26).[a] Regarding *severity*, in the term infant the most common feature is a continuous or intermittent discontinuity of EEG (see Chapters 10 and 12). The most extreme of these discontinuous tracings is the *burst-suppression pattern*, which is associated with a very high likelihood of an unfavorable outcome, especially when the tracing is non-reactive (see Chapter 10). However, burst-suppression tracings account for a *minority* of excessively discontinuous neonatal EEG tracings. We have found that a relatively simple means of quantitation of excessively discontinuous tracings in the term infant (i.e., analysis of the duration, in 10-second blocks, of the predominant IBI) has major prognostic value (Table 20.27).[190] Predominant IBI durations of more than 30 seconds were invariably associated with an unfavorable outcome, and durations of more than 20 seconds were associated with an unfavorable outcome in 92%. Notably, predominant IBI durations of more than 10 seconds still predicted abnormal outcome in 72%. Of the 43 discontinuous tracings studied, only 7 (16%) exhibited a burst-suppression pattern, as defined classically (see Table 20.27 and Chapter 10). Thus, the predominant IBI duration, readily quantitated at the bedside, was highly effective and, critically, applicable to *most* excessively discontinuous tracings in the term newborn with encephalopathy.

Regarding the *duration* of EEG abnormalities, as with the neonatal neurological syndrome, recovery of normal EEG background by day 7 is associated with a favorable outcome (see Table 20.26). In one large series of 77 term infants with apparent HIE and studied at 7 days of age, of 52 with a normal EEG tracing, 83% were later (at 1 year of age) found to be normal, 17% had mild abnormalities, and none had severe abnormalities.[439]

TABLE 20.28   Value of Amplitude-Integrated Electroencephalography in Assessment of Asphyxiated Term Infants[a]

Detection of severe abnormalities (i.e., CLV, FT, BSP) in the first hours of life has a positive predictive value of an unfavorable outcome of 80%–90%
Severe abnormalities may improve within 24 h (≈50% of BSP and 10% of CLV/FT)
Rapid recovery of severe abnormalities is associated with a favorable outcome in 60% of cases
The *combination* of early neonatal neurological examination and early aEEG enhances the positive predictive value and specificity

[a]See text for references.
aEEG, amplitude-integrated encephalography; *BSP*, burst-suppression pattern; *CLV*, continuous low voltage; *FT*, flat trace.

Consistent with earlier work, studies in the era of therapeutic hypothermia show that the early return of sleep-wake cycling and the normalization of background EEG abnormalities are good prognostic indicators.[192,456] The link between timing of this evolution and prognostic ability can be altered by therapeutic hypothermia, so that delayed recovery may still be associated with a normal outcome.[201] A normal EEG recorded soon after birth is highly associated with a normal outcome at 2 years.[457] However, an abnormal EEG soon after birth may recover over subsequent days, but if it remains abnormal at 48 hours a poor prognosis is highly likely.[457]

aEEG has been of considerable value in the estimation of prognosis in the asphyxiated term newborn (Table 20.28).[191-196,198,227,454,458] As described earlier in Chapters 10 and 12, the most useful tracings for detection of severe encephalopathy have been continuous low-voltage, flat, and burst-suppression patterns. Because PPVs for such tracings in the first hours of life are 80% to 90%, aEEG has been valuable for early selection of infants for neuroprotective therapies (e.g., hypothermia; see later). Notably, 10% to 15% of infants with these marked background abnormalities may normalize within

[a]References 70, 160, 169, 170, 173, 175, 176, 178, 180-184, 187, 190, 439, and 453-455.

TABLE 20.29   Prognostic Value of Visual- and Somatosensory-Evoked Potentials in Term Infants With Hypoxic-Ischemic Encephalopathy (<6 Hours of Age)

RESULT OF EVOKED POTENTIALS	TOTAL NO.	OUTCOME		
		NORMAL	SEQUELAE	DEATH
Somatosensory				
Normal	12	11	0	1
Delayed	8	4	2	2
No response	14	0	0	14
Visual				
Normal	12	10	2	0
Delayed	14	5	0	9
No response	8	0	0	8

Data from Eken P, Toet MC, Groenendaal F, De Vries LS. Predictive value of early neuroimaging, pulsed Doppler and neurophysiology in full-term infants with hypoxic-ischaemic encephalopathy. *Arch Dis Child Fetal Neonatal Ed.* 1995;73:F75–F80.

24 hours. Rapid recovery is associated with a favorable outcome in 60% (see Table 20.28). Importantly, although aEEG in the first 6 hours is slightly superior to the neonatal neurological examination in identifying infants with an unfavorable outcome, the *combination* of aEEG *and* the neurological examination is more nearly optimal, with a specificity of 94%.[194] The positive predictive value of a severely abnormal aEEG for death or disability at 6 hours is approximately 0.60, and this value declines slightly, but not significantly, in cooled infants.[457,459]

Serial *visual-evoked potentials* carried out in term asphyxiated infants have been shown to provide valuable prognostic information.[356,460,461] In one study of 34 full-term infants with HIE who were studied *within 6 hours of delivery*, the finding of normal visual-evoked potentials was associated with a normal neurological outcome in 10 of 12 infants, whereas no response to visual input was followed by death in 8 of 8 infants (Table 20.29).[227] However, the 14 infants with delayed latencies had an intermediate outcome.

Serial *somatosensory-evoked potentials* also have been shown to provide valuable prognostic information in assessment of the asphyxiated infant.[227,462–467] In 20 survivors of asphyxia at term, all 13 infants with normal outcome had normal somatosensory-evoked response by 4 days of age, whereas the 7 infants with subsequent deficits had abnormal or absent responses beyond 4 days.[464] One study of 34 term infants with HIE who were evaluated *within 6 hours of delivery* showed striking predictive value for favorable or unfavorable outcomes with normal potentials or no response, respectively (see Table 20.29).[227] Moreover, compared with the results with visual-evoked potentials, fewer infants had intermediate abnormalities on somatosensory-evoked potential testing (see Table 20.29).[227] Thus, the data suggest that somatosensory-evoked potentials could be useful for early prognostic formulations.

Ultrasound

In the *term infant*, as discussed earlier (see the section on diagnosis), major injury to basal ganglia and thalamus and focal and multifocal ischemic parenchymal lesions have been identified and have contributed to prediction of outcomes. However, most scans do not show such discrete lesions.[468,469] In one careful study of 40 term infants with HIE and cranial ultrasonography in the first week, 13 of 14 infants (93%),

with either a normal scan or with isolated germinal matrix or intraventricular or subarachnoid hemorrhage, were normal on follow-up.[226] Of the remaining infants, the ultrasonographic findings nearly consistently associated with subsequent neurological deficits were *bilateral* abnormalities of basal ganglia in 9 infants, focal parenchymal echodensities or apparent stroke in 8, or a featureless appearance with patchy echodensities in 7. Periventricular echodensities may occur in the asphyxiated term infant, as in the preterm infant, but they are generally observed uncommonly. Confusion sometimes exists concerning the finding in the asphyxiated term infant of small ventricles or those that cannot be visualized. Whereas this observation has been said to be indicative of major brain edema,[469] in another study this finding was present in 62% of control subjects in the first week of life and could not be clearly related to structural disease.[468] In the latter study, the finding of a normal ultrasound scan in 9 of the 32 term infants with HIE was followed by a normal outcome in 8 of the 9 infants.[468]

Magnetic Resonance Imaging

Because the likelihood, nature, and severity of subsequent neurological deficits in the infant with HIE are related most decisively to the extent and specific topography of the lesions, MRI should prove to be the best imaging modality for determining prognosis. Studies of *term infants* support this prediction.[a] Particularly vivid examples of the value of neonatal MRI in establishing prognosis were discussed earlier and include those infants with evidence of selective neuronal necrosis of the major varieties defined in Chapter 18 (i.e., the diffuse type, the cerebral–deep nuclear type, and the deep nuclear–brain stem type). Of all imaging modalities currently applied to the newborn, only MRI provides consistent delineation, particularly of involvement of specific areas of the cerebral cortex, basal ganglia, thalamus, and brain stem, as well as the cerebral white matter.

The relation of motor and cognitive outcomes to topography of injury delineated by neonatal MRI can be summarized generally as follows. Infants with *normal MRI findings* generally do not exhibit *major* motor or cognitive deficits.[28,29,282]

---

[a]References 29, 61, 226, 236, 237, 240, 241, 245, 247-250, 253, 256, 258, 296, 348, 362, 386, and 470-472.

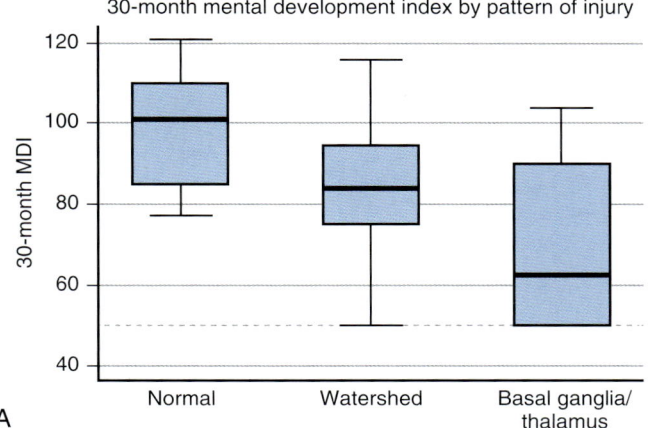

30-month mental development index by pattern of injury

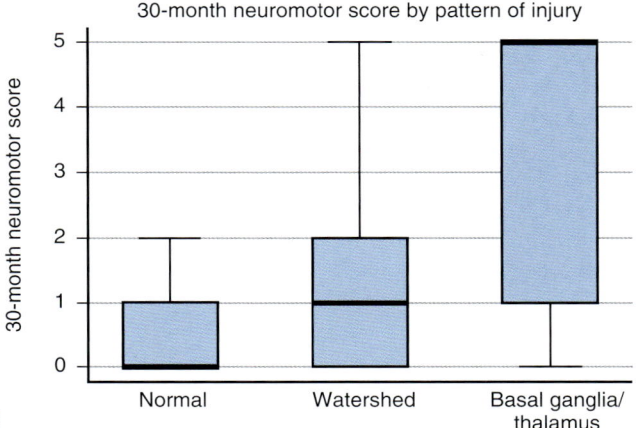

30-month neuromotor score by pattern of injury

Figure 20.23 Relationship between predominant regions injured and neurological outcome. Predominant regional patterns were obtained by magnetic resonance imaging (MRI) in 173 term infants with encephalopathy, most probably resulting from hypoxia–ischemia. The relative distribution of MRI patterns was "parasagittal watershed" (n = 78), "basal ganglia/thalamus" (n = 44), or "normal" (n = 51). (A) Box plot of the 30-month Mental Development Index (MDI) by the pattern of injury. The MDI was lowest in the infants with the basal ganglia/thalamus predominant pattern, with intermediate scores in infants with the watershed pattern (P = .0007). The *thick line* represents the median, with the 25th and 75th percentiles as the lower and upper limits of the box; whiskers indicate the 5th and 95th percentiles. The *dashed line* indicates the lowest attainable MDI score. (B) Box plot of the 30-month neuromotor score by the pattern of injury. Neuromotor impairments were most severe in the infants with the basal ganglia/thalamus pattern (P = .0001). (From Miller SP, Ramaswamy V, Michelson D, et al. Patterns of brain injury in term neonatal encephalopathy. *J Pediatr.* 2005;146:453–460.)

Infants with *prominent basal ganglia/thalamic (BG/T)* lesions have the poorest motor and cognitive outcomes. A particularly useful predictor of prominent subsequent motor deficits (i.e., cerebral palsy) is MRI evidence of severe BG/T injury and abnormal signal in the posterior limb of the internal capsule (PLIC) (Fig. 20.23).[248,275,276,296,473-475]

In a well-studied series of 175 infants with neonatal HIE and BG/T lesions, a striking relationship was apparent between the severity of the lesions, the presence of an abnormal PLIC signal, and cerebral palsy in survivors (Fig. 20.23 from Volpe). With mild lesions (n = 28), the PLIC signal was abnormal in none,

equivocal in 4, and normal in 24; only 3 of the 24 infants (12%) developed cerebral palsy. However, with severe BG/T lesions (n = 63), the PLIC signal was abnormal in 62—all of whom developed cerebral palsy. The severity of BG/T lesions also provides information regarding other neurological outcomes (Figs. 20.24 to 20.27).

Infants with *predominant parasagittal watershed lesions* have more prominent cognitive than motor deficits (see earlier). In this group especially, cognitive deficits may occur without appreciable motor deficits.[a]

Infants with the quantitatively unusual but distinctive pattern of *injury to BG/T and brain stem tegmentum*, which is common after severe sentinel events, have the highest likelihood of death. Mortality rates are as high as 35%.[276,282,348]

Infants with *predominantly cerebral white matter injury*, present in only approximately 15% of term infants with HIE, exhibit cognitive deficits more than motor deficits. Important contributing factors in pathogenesis include late preterm gestational age, neonatal hypoglycemia, and chronic hemodynamic instability, similar to congenital heart disease.[282,285]

Combining the findings of BG/T injury and abnormalities in the PLIC, Martinez-Biarge and co-workers developed algorithms for outcomes.[275] The severity of the BG/T and PLIC lesions is shown in Fig. 20.24. The algorithms for outcomes of mild (see Fig. 20.25), moderate (see Fig. 20.26), and severe injury (see Fig. 20.27) are shown.

A large meta-analysis evaluated 32 studies of MRI in 860 non-cooled infants with neonatal encephalopathy.[341] Conventional MRI, mostly using scoring systems based on T1- and T2-weighted imaging, had a pooled sensitivity of 0.91 and specificity of 0.51 to predict adverse outcome (death and/or moderate/severe disability, depending on the individual study) at 12 or more months of age. Late MRI (defined as MRI between day 8 and 30 of life) had higher sensitivity but lower specificity than early MRI (performed between day 1 and 7 of life). However, there was significant statistical heterogeneity between studies.

Hypothermia does not appear to alter the prognostic value of MRI, although two studies showed that it *may alter the timing of changes seen on MRI* (see Fig. 20.15).[303] Another prospective study using serial MRI found that the T1/T2 changes appeared later (by day 3 of life in noncooled infants, but not until the MRI on day 10 of life in 2 of the cooled infants).[261] Despite these limitations, recent analyses showed that predictive values of MRI do not seem to be affected by therapeutic hypothermia. Rutherford and colleagues studied 131 infants from the TOBY (TOtal Body hYpothermia) cooling trial[476] and found that in the infants treated with therapeutic hypothermia, fewer BG/T lesions and fewer abnormalities in the PLIC were identified in comparison to noncooled infants. Infants who were cooled were more likely to have normal scans. The ability of major MRI abnormalities to predict death or major disability at 18 months was almost identical in both groups (cooled infants, sensitivity 0.88, specificity 0.82, PPV 0.76, and negative predictive value (NPV) 0.91; non-cooled group, sensitivity 0.94, specificity 0.68, PPV 0.74, and NPV 0.92). In the Infant Cooling Evaluation (ICE) trial, fewer newborns in the hypothermia group had moderate/severe white matter or gray matter abnormalities

---

[a]References 29, 274, 281, 282, 388, and 389.

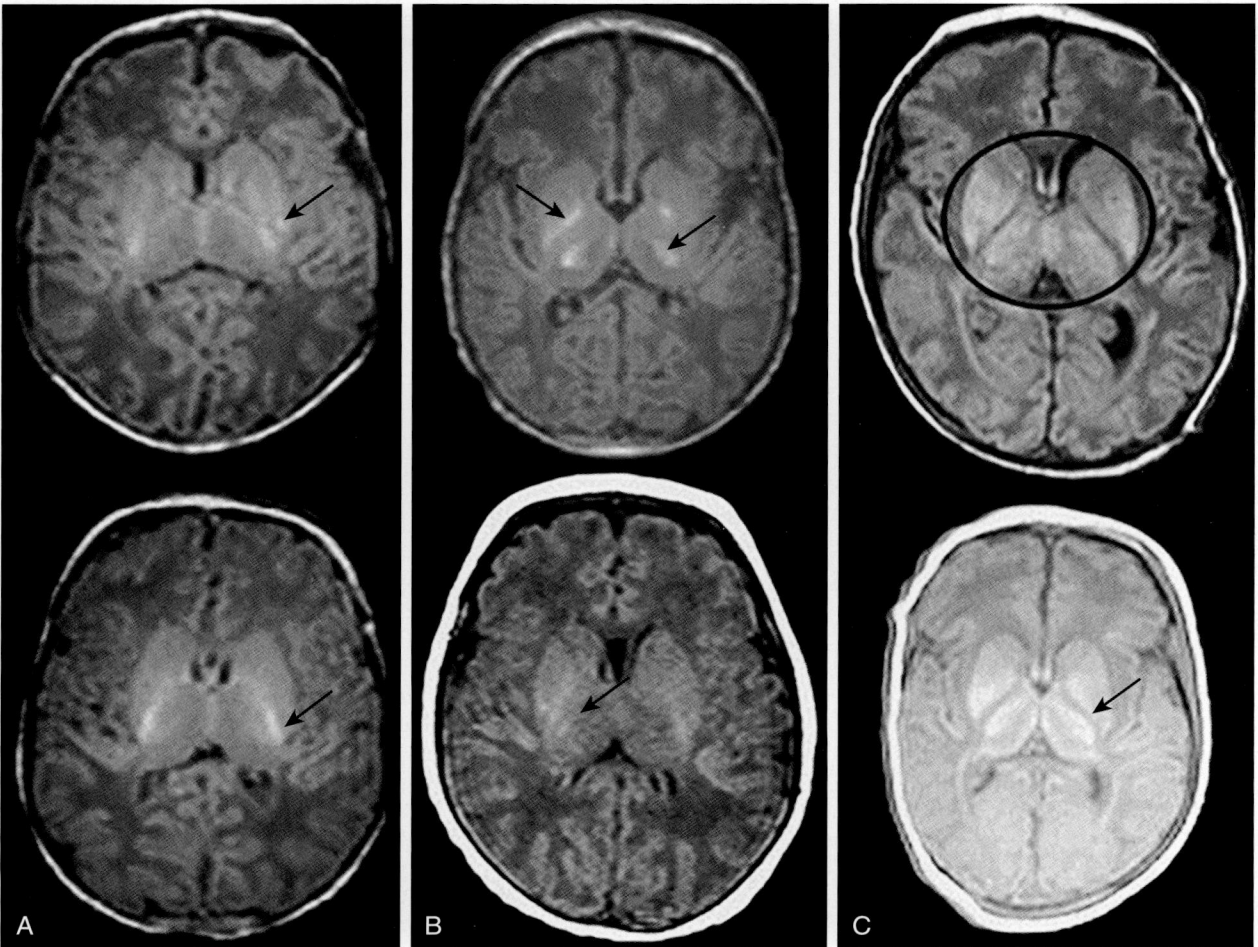

Figure 20.24 Top row: Axial T1-weighted images showing: (A) mild basal ganglia/thalamic (BG/T) lesions *(arrow)*; (B) moderate BG/T injury *(arrows)*; (C) severe BG/T abnormalities *(circled)*. Bottom row: Axial T1-weighted images showing: (A) normal signal intensity (SI) in the posterior limb of the internal capsule (PLIC) *(arrow)*; (B) equivocal, asymmetrical and slightly reduced SI in the PLIC *(arrow)*; and (C) abnormal, absent SI in the PLIC *(arrow)*. (Courtesy of Martinez-Biarge M, Diez-Sebastian J, Rutherford MA, Cowan FM. Outcomes after central grey matter injury in term perinatal hypoxic-ischaemic encephalopathy. *Early Hum Dev.* 2010;86:675–682.)

on T1/T2-weighted scans as compared with infants in the normothermia group; but abnormal MRI findings were still predictive of outcome in both the normothermia and the hypothermia groups.[477] The sensitivity of T1/T2 and diffusion abnormalities to predict adverse outcome was low (0.27 to 0.60) but specificity was high (0.92 to 0.95). In the National Institute of Child Health and Human Development cooling trial, the sensitivity, specificity, PPV, and NPV of moderate/severe brain injury on neonatal MRI to predict death or IQ less than 70 at 6 to 7 years of age were similar between the hypothermia group (0.77, 0.85, 0.71, and 0.89, respectively), and the control group (0.85, 0.66, 0.69, and 0.83, respectively).[396] Death or IQ less than 70 occurred in 4 of 50 children with normal MRI in the neonatal period. A recent systematic review[478] has analyzed MRI studies in detail and determined the pooled sensitivity, specificity, PPV, and NPV as follows: *DWI:* ≤1 wk: sensitivity 0.58 and specificity of 0.89; *apparent diffusion coefficient (ADC) at ≤1 wk:* sensitivity 0.79 and specificity 0.85; *T1/T2:* ≤1 wk: sensitivity 0.84 and specificity 0.90, ≤2 wk: sensitivity 0.98 and specificity 0.76, ≤6 wk: sensitivity 0.83 and specificity 0.53.

Thus, MRI remains a very powerful tool in the prognosis of an infant with HIE with or without therapeutic hypothermia.

Magnetic Resonance Spectroscopy

MR spectroscopy of both the proton and phosphorus types has been useful in determination of outcome in neonatal hypoxic-ischemic disease in the term newborn. The data should be interpreted in the context of the findings in experimental models of an early increase in cerebral lactate, detectable by proton MR spectroscopy, preceding a "secondary delayed energy failure," characterized by a decline in high-energy phosphate compounds, detectable by phosphorus MR spectroscopy (see Chapter 10). (The primary, initial energy failure occurs close to the time of the initial insult, usually in utero and before any measurements can be made.)

Studies by *proton MR spectroscopy* performed in the first several days of life showed distinctly elevated cerebral lactate in asphyxiated human infants.[a] The elevation in lactate is apparent

---

[a]References 313, 318-321, 323, 326-328, 330-339, and 475.

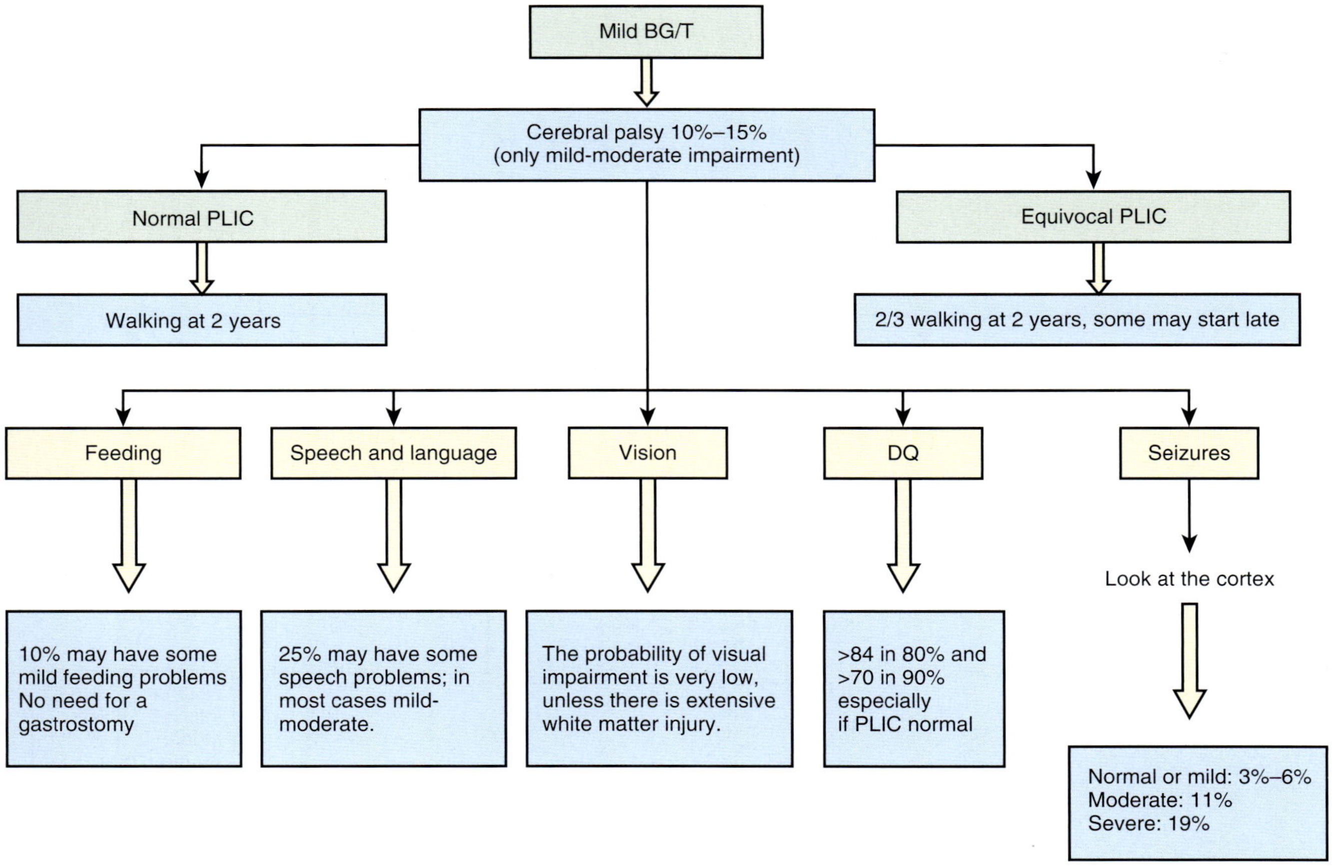

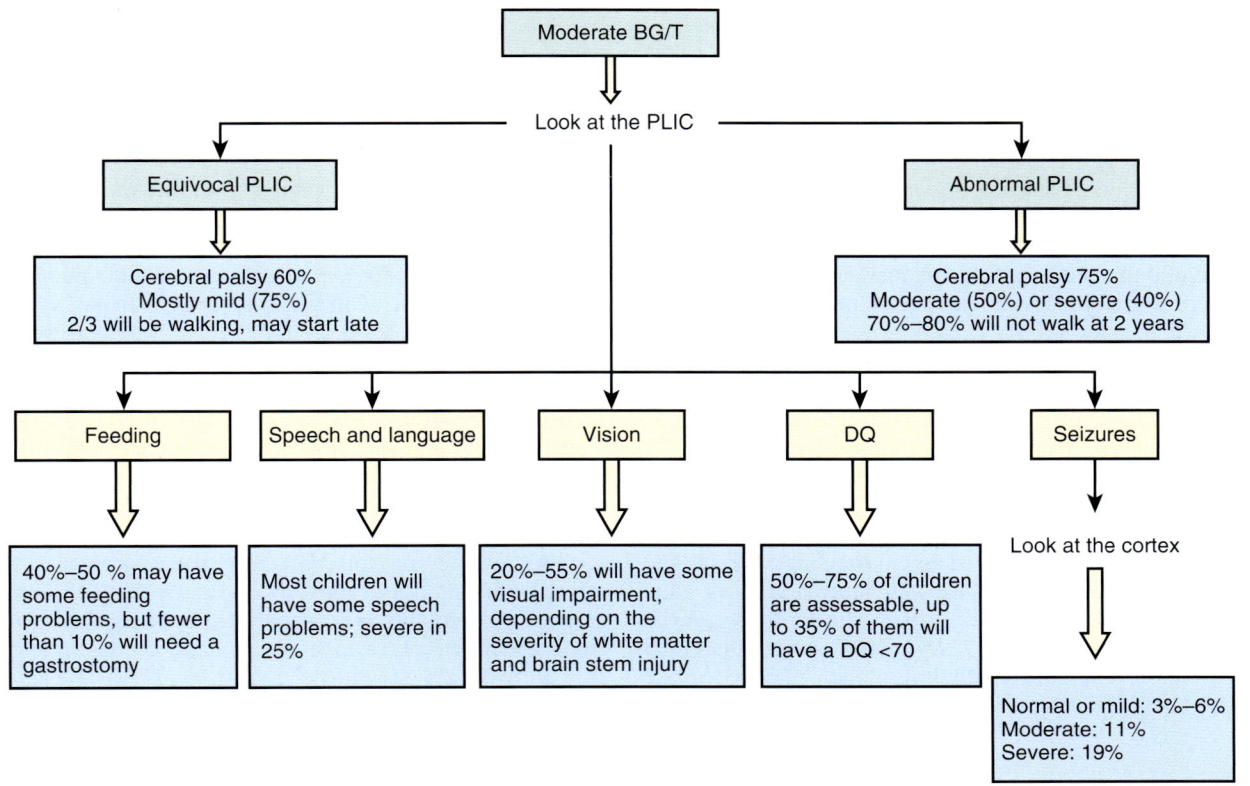

Figure 20.25 Flow chart showing patterns of outcome with mild basal ganglia/thalamic (BG/T) injury. *DQ*, developmental quotient; *PLIC*, posterior limb of the internal capsule. (Courtesy of Martinez-Biarge M, Diez-Sebastian J, Rutherford MA, Cowan FM. Outcomes after central grey matter injury in term perinatal hypoxic-ischaemic encephalopathy. *Early Hum Dev.* 2010;86:675–682.)

Figure 20.26 Flow chart showing patterns of outcome with moderate basal ganglia/thalamic (BG/T) injury. *DQ*, developmental quotient; *PLIC*, posterior limb of the internal capsule. (Courtesy Martinez-Biarge M, Diez-Sebastian J, Rutherford MA, Cowan FM. Outcomes after central grey matter injury in term perinatal hypoxic-ischaemic encephalopathy. *Early Hum Dev.* 2010;86:675–682.)

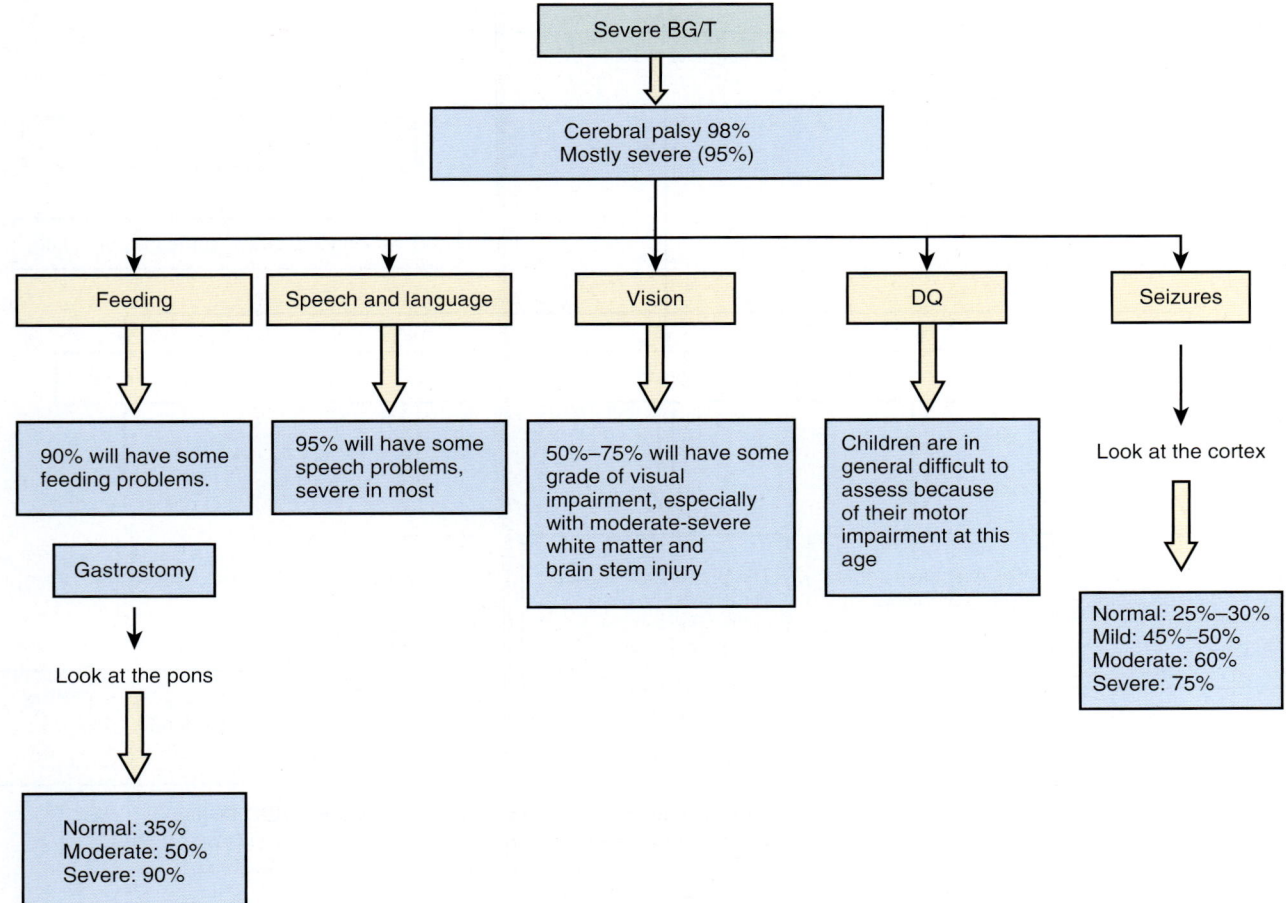

Figure 20.27 Flow chart showing patterns of outcome with severe basal ganglia/thalamic (BG/T) injury. *DQ,* developmental quotient. (Courtesy Martinez-Biarge M, Diez-Sebastian J, Rutherford MA, Cowan FM. Outcomes after central grey matter injury in term perinatal hypoxic-ischaemic encephalopathy. *Early Hum Dev.* 2010;86:675–682.)

in the first 18 hours of life and, importantly, correlates with the severity of the delayed secondary energy failure observed on subsequent days (see Fig. 20.20B), the neonatal neurological syndrome, and the neurological outcome (Fig. 20.28).[318,326-328,339] Infants with the poorest outcomes have persistently elevated lactate levels (i.e., for several weeks or more),[313,314,324] whereas those with favorable outcomes had resolution of lactate elevations during this interval.

NAA, a marker of the neuronal-axonal unit as well as oligodendroglial precursors and immature oligodendrocytes,[479,480] is usually only variably affected during these early phases.[a] However, a decline in NAA does become apparent after many days to weeks as tissue loss becomes established.

Thayyil and colleagues pooled 10 studies that evaluated the Lac/NAA ratio in the basal ganglia, with a median cut-off value between normal and abnormal of 0.29.[341] The pooled sensitivity was 0.82 and specificity was 0.95 for a value greater than 0.29 to predict a poor outcome (death or disability measured at ≥12 months). These investigators considered the Lac/NAA ratio

in the deep nuclear gray matter to be the most accurate MR spectroscopy biomarker for prediction of outcome.

MR spectroscopy also appears to be valuable in prognostication in the hypothermia era. Corbo and colleagues evaluated 38 infants with birth asphyxia,[482] half of whom were cooled. There were lower levels of Lac in the infants treated with hypothermia, but the NAA ratios were not different between the two groups. Ancora and colleagues[483] followed to 2 years of age, 20 newborns who were treated for HIE with selective head cooling and had MRI in the neonatal period. NAA/Cr in the basal ganglia (value ≤0.67) had a PPV of 1.0 and NPV of 0.93 to predict poor outcomes (death or severe cerebral palsy at 2 years of age).

Studies by *phosphorus MR spectroscopy* performed in the first week of life show a delayed secondary decline in high-energy phosphate compounds in asphyxiated human infants.[308,309,311,312] This decline becomes apparent generally on the second day of life and reaches a nadir at 2 to 4 days of life. The severity of this delayed secondary energy failure correlates with the severity of both the neonatal neurological syndrome (see Fig. 20.19) and the subsequent neurological deficits (Fig. 20.29).[311,312] As noted earlier, the sustained alkaline intracellular pH identified

---

[a]References 320, 322, 325, 327-329, 332-334, 336, 338, 475, and 481.

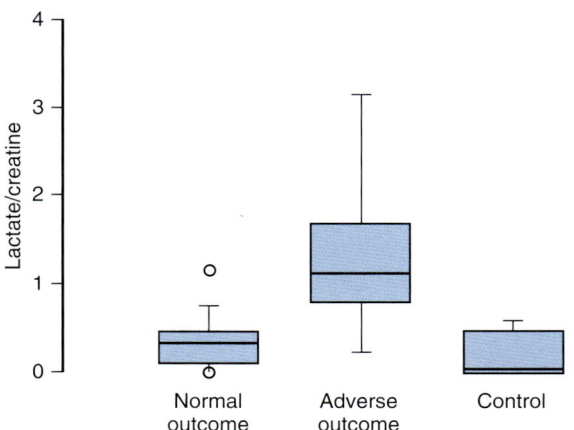

Figure 20.28 Relation between the lactate/creatine ratio obtained by proton magnetic resonance spectroscopy in the first 18 hours of life, and the neurological outcome. Median, interquartile ranges, and upper and lower adjacent values of the ratios in infants with normal outcome, infants with abnormal outcome, and control infants are shown. The value for infants with adverse outcome was significantly different from the values for both infants with normal outcome and control infants. (From Hanrahan JD, Cox IJ, Azzopardi D, et al. Relation between proton magnetic resonance spectroscopy within 18 hours of birth asphyxia and neurodevelopment at 1 year of age. *Dev Med Child Neurol.* 1999;41:76–82.)

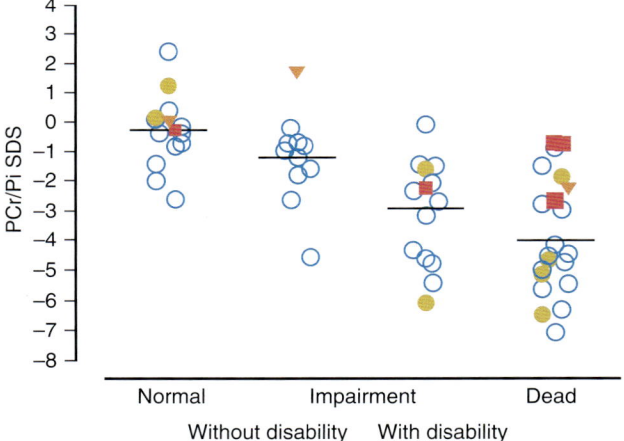

Figure 20.29 Relation between phosphocreatine/inorganic phosphate (PCr/Pi) standard deviation score (SDS), determined by phosphorus magnetic resonance spectroscopy (during the period of secondary energy failure) as a number of standard deviations from the mean of control values, and neurodevelopmental outcome, determined by evaluation at 4 years in 62 asphyxiated infants. *Open circles* represent term average for gestational age (AGA) infants, *closed circles* represent term small for gestational age (SGA) infants, *closed triangles* represent preterm AGA infants, and *closed squares* represent preterm SGA infants. (From Roth SC, Baudin J, Cady E, et al. Relation of deranged neonatal cerebral oxidative metabolism with neurodevelopmental outcome and head circumference at 4 years. *Dev Med Child Neurol.* 1997;39:718–725.)

by phosphorus MR spectroscopy also correlates with poor neurodevelopmental outcome.[314]

Currently, proton MR spectroscopy is used much more widely than phosphorus MR spectroscopy in the evaluation of newborn infants, because this approach, unlike phosphorus

MR spectroscopy, is adapted readily to clinically used MR instruments. Thus, although the data obtained by phosphorus MR spectroscopy have provided important information, it is likely that future work will continue to be carried out primarily with proton MR spectroscopy.

Computed Tomography

Although MRI has the greatest predictive capability and is the preferred imaging modality, historically, CT in the neonatal period has provided adjunctive information of prognostic value. As noted in the section on diagnosis, in infants with major injury to the basal ganglia and thalamus, to a considerable extent CT defines the site and extent of the lesion and allows estimation of the neurological sequelae outlined in the section on clinicopathological correlations. More often, however, the CT appearance in the infant with HIE cannot be so neatly categorized.

In the *term infant*, several earlier series categorized the CT findings as normal or showing variable degrees of hypoattenuation or hemorrhage, or both.[423,484-488] At the extremes of injury, CT scans can be of some assistance. Infants with normal CT scans will rarely exhibit severe neurological deficits on follow-up, and infants with scans demonstrating severe abnormalities, such as marked diffuse hypodensity, rarely are normal on follow-up. Moreover, those unusual infants with major degrees of intracerebral hemorrhage, usually indicative of hemorrhagic infarction, almost always exhibit neurological deficits on follow-up. However, in several reported series, as many as one-third of infants with less severe degrees of hypoattenuation had no intraparenchymal hemorrhage; in this group, the outcome is variable and not readily predicted. Nevertheless, it is apparent that in more than one-half of term infants with HIE, the CT scan provides some useful prognostic information. This proportion may be increased by a follow-up CT study at 2 to 6 weeks of age, when initially ambiguous findings may evolve to either a normal or an overtly abnormal scan.[486]

Measurement of Cerebral Blood Flow Velocity, Cerebral Blood Volume, or Cerebral Blood Flow

Although not commonly used for the assessment of brain injury and the estimation of outcome in neonatal HIE, measurements of CBF velocity, cerebral blood volume and CBF have provided useful prognostic information. A series of studies has established that the postasphyxial human newborn exhibits a state of vasoparalysis and cerebral hyperemia, which is detectable as increased CBF velocity and decreased cerebrovascular resistance by Doppler studies, as increased cerebral blood volume by near-infrared spectroscopy, and as increased CBF by xenon-133 clearance or PET (see Chapter 13). These changes are correlated with the degree of brain injury, as discussed next.

Measurements of *CBF velocity by the Doppler technique* at the anterior fontanelle have provided useful prognostic information in full-term asphyxiated infants studied in the first days of life. Determination of CBF velocity in such infants generally, from approximately 1 to 6 days after the insult, showed an increase in mean flow velocity with decreased resistance indices (i.e., cerebral vasodilation).[489-498] One large study involved 39 term asphyxiated infants with "postasphyxial encephalopathy" in whom Doppler measurements from the anterior cerebral artery from the first hour delineated distinct abnormalities at a median age of 26 hours (i.e., increased CBF velocity and decreased Pourcelot resistance index).[494] This constellation suggested a state of cerebral hyperemia with vasodilation, leading to both decreased resistance and increased flow. The mechanism underlying this "delayed hyperemia" is unclear (see Chapter 13). The cerebral hyperemia could account in part for the increase in intracranial pressure (ICP) sometimes observed at this time in severely asphyxiated infants (see Chapter 19). An important point for this discussion is that the changes were correlated with unfavorable outcome. Thus, no infant with CBF velocity greater than 3 standard deviations above the mean survived without severe neurological impairment.[494] One report showed that the increased CBF velocity in infants with an unfavorable outcome is not apparent until 12 to 24 hours of age, and thus earlier measurements do not have appreciable prognostic value.[498] Similar measurements on infants subjected to therapeutic hypothermia have not been reported.

That the Doppler measurements reflected cerebral vasodilation, at least in part, was shown in studies of similar infants by *near-infrared spectroscopy*.[499-501] Such studies of asphyxiated human infants on the first day of life suggested an increase in both cerebral blood volume and CBF. Moreover, other work with near-infrared spectroscopy showed that the state of cerebral hyperemia is accompanied by evidence of diminished oxygen extraction and elevated cerebral venous oxygen saturation, perhaps reflecting tissue injury.[502] Several investigators have attempted to use near-infrared spectroscopy measurements for both short- and long-term outcomes in infants after birth asphyxia with limited success to date. One study showed that infants with HIE ($n = 12$) who had a poor outcome (death, cerebral palsy, or global delays at 12 months) had a higher level of cerebral oxygenation, measured as tissue oxygenation index at 12 hours of age, than infants with a normal outcome.[503] A related study reported similar findings in 22 term infants with HIE in which in the first day of life the tissue oxygenation index was 80% in infants with abnormal outcomes at 1 year versus 75% in infants with normal 1-year outcomes ($P = .04$). A larger study ($n = 39$) in the era of therapeutic hypothermia again demonstrated that cerebral oxygenation was higher in newborns with an adverse outcome.[504] Whether the use of near-infrared spectroscopy could provide valuable information for long-term prognostic estimation is not established by these short-term studies, but it seems possible.

Decisive demonstration of both the prognostic value of direct measurement of CBF and of the likelihood that the studies using Doppler ultrasound and near-infrared spectroscopy reflected cerebral hyperemia was accomplished by direct measurements in asphyxiated infants *by xenon-133 clearance and by PET*.[505,506] In the large series of infants studied by xenon clearance, infants with the poorest outcome had the highest values for CBF in the first day of life (see Chapter 13). Asphyxiated infants who died or had severe brain injury had mean CBF of 30.6 mL/100 g per minute; those who had moderate to severe brain injury had CBF of 15.1 mL/100 g per minute; and those with normal outcome had CBF of 9.2 mL/100 g/min. That the low Pourcelot resistance index shown by Doppler reflected cerebral vasodilation, presumably secondary to vasoparalysis, also was shown by Pryds and co-workers,[505] who demonstrated no reactivity of flow to arterial blood pressure or arterial carbon dioxide tension ($PaCO_2$) in the group with poorest outcome,

no reactivity to blood pressure (although retained reactivity to carbon dioxide) in the group with intermediate outcome, and retained reactivity to both pressure and carbon dioxide in the group with normal outcome. A later study of 16 term infants with HIE used PET to determine CBF primarily at 1 to 4 days of life and found higher flows in those infants with abnormal neurological outcome (35.6 mL/100 g/min) than in those with normal neurological outcome (18.3 mL/100 g/min).[506]

That these measures of cerebral hyperemia are *not* related to increased cerebral metabolic rate was shown by a study of 20 infants with HIE with PET measurements of cerebral metabolic rate for glucose.[507] Thus, the total cerebral metabolic rate for glucose was *inversely* correlated with severity of the encephalopathy and the degree of neurological deficits. Those infants with the most severe deficits later had the lowest neonatal values of cerebral metabolic rate for glucose.

Conclusion

No neurodiagnostic technique is capable of diminishing the importance of the clinical evaluation of the infant in assessment of outcome, although MRI appears to have the strongest prognostic capability of all the complementary technologies. In clinical practice, a combination of clinical history and examination, electrophysiology, and neuroimaging with MRI constitutes the best complete evaluation to enable the most accurate prognostication for the term infant with HIE.

MANAGEMENT

Management of the term-born infant with HIE requires attention to the involvement of multiple systems. Although we will emphasize the neurological aspects of therapy, it is the rule rather than the exception that infants with HIE have disturbances of pulmonary, cardiovascular, hepatic, and renal functions as well.[54,60,63-65,426,508] The emphasis on management is in terms of the following: *prevention* of peripartum hypoxic-ischemic insult; *recognition* of peripartum hypoxic-ischemic insult; *stabilization* of systemic physiology, including respiratory, cardiovascular and metabolic; *control of seizures*; commencement of *neuroprotective therapy*; (therapeutic hypothermia), if indicated; and consideration of other potential neuroprotective intervention therapies (Table 20.30). Concerning all of these, it is important to note that the major portion of

---

TABLE 20.30   Basic Elements of the Management of Neonatal Hypoxic-Ischemic Encephalopathy

Prevention of peripartum hypoxic-ischemic injury
Recognition of peripartum hypoxic-ischemic injury
Stabilization of systemic physiology, including respiratory, cardiovascular, and metabolic
- maintenance of adequate ventilation
- maintenance of adequate perfusion
- maintenance of adequate glucose levels

Control of seizures
Commencement of *therapeutic hypothermia, if indicated*
Consideration of *other potential neuroprotective intervention therapies*

neuronal death following hypoxic-ischemic insult evolves *after* termination of the insult (i.e., often during the time that the therapeutic maneuvers to be reviewed next are applied).

Prevention of Peripartum Hypoxic-Ischemic Insult

A critical aspect of management is prevention of the hypoxic-ischemic insult, and because most infants appear to experience the primary insult in utero, prevention of intrauterine asphyxia is paramount (see Table 20.30). Detailed discussion of the management of pregnancy, labor, and delivery is beyond the scope of this book, but the basic elements of this aspect of management are summarized in Table 20.31 and are based on the considerations discussed in Chapter 17.

The first goal is identification of the fetus being subjected to or likely to experience hypoxic-ischemic insults with labor and delivery. Thus, antepartum assessment (see Chapter 17) with identification of the high-risk pregnancy is central. The fetus should be monitored during the intrapartum period primarily by the electronic techniques described in Chapter 17, supplemented, when necessary, by fetal blood sampling to determine pH and blood gas values. The need for better methods to assess *fetal neurological status*, particularly fetal cerebral hemodynamics and metabolism, and placental functioning, was emphasized earlier. The particular mode of intervention for the fetus threatened by hypoxic-ischemic insult depends on a variety of factors related to the fetus and the mother, but often cesarean section is a critical intervention in the prevention of the degree of asphyxia that leads to brain injury.

Recognition of Peripartum Hypoxic-Ischemic Injury

The recognition of the risk factors for peripartum hypoxic-ischemic injury and the associated neurological syndrome associated with HIE can be challenging, as discussed earlier (see Tables 20.2 to 20.6). Thus, clinical suspicion must be high at all at-risk settings to fully evaluate the infant. This evaluation is accomplished best as part of a clinical practice guideline to standardize the approach of the clinical team to such infants and should consider inclusion of the following:

1. Evaluation for metabolic acidemia with cord blood gas measurement or infant blood gas measurement within 60 minutes of birth.
2. Optimal resuscitation and stabilization of the infant, as discussed later.
3. Avoidance of hyperthermia by the removal of external heat sources, such as overhead heating devices in the resuscitation room, until a clinical decision about the need for neuroprotective therapy is made.
4. Systematic serial neurological examination of the infant with a standardized neurological scoring system over the first few hours of life to define the presence and severity of any encephalopathy.

5. Consideration of electrophysiological monitoring to assess background cerebral activity during the first few hours of life. This assessment is accomplished readily with aEEG.

Stabilization of Systemic Physiology

This aspect of management relates to respiratory, cardiovascular, and metabolic status (see Table 20.30).

Maintenance of Adequate Ventilation

Maintenance of adequate ventilation is a central aspect of *supportive care*, an imprecise term that refers to the maintenance also of temperature, perfusion, and metabolic status. The importance of these various postnatal aspects of management cannot be overemphasized, although a significant intrauterine insult has occurred in most asphyxiated infants, postnatal disturbances of ventilation and perfusion particularly may play an important role in determining the ultimate severity of neurological injury. In this section, we discuss the particular importance of maintenance of adequate arterial concentrations of oxygen and carbon dioxide.

Oxygen

Hypoxemia. The avoidance of oxygen deprivation clearly is a cornerstone of supportive therapy. Hypoxemia may lead to a disturbance of cerebrovascular autoregulation and, as a consequence, a *pressure-passive circulation* (Table 20.32; see Chapter 13). Under such circumstances, the infant is vulnerable to superimposed ischemic cerebral injury with only moderate decreases in arterial blood pressure. Indeed, this mechanism may be the most important by which hypoxemia leads to parenchymal injury. Provision of adequate oxygen also is necessary to prevent additional *neuronal and white matter injury* (see Table 20.32).

The *most common cause of serious persistent hypoxemia* in the *term* infant, persistent pulmonary hypertension of the newborn, can be complex to manage. The risk for this condition may be elevated in the setting of therapeutic hypothermia.[509,510] It has also been suggested that the presence of this severe respiratory complication may further compromise the well-being of infants receiving hypothermia by leading to greater cerebral hypoxemia.[511] The management of persistent pulmonary hypertension of the newborn is discussed in standard writings on neonatology. Suffice it to say here that the principal therapeutic modalities range from oxygen and assisted ventilation to the administration of pulmonary vasodilator drugs (e.g., nitric oxide), passive hyperventilation, and high-frequency ventilation.

TABLE 20.31	Prevention of Peripartum Hypoxic-Ischemic Injury

Antepartum assessment and identification of the high-risk pregnancy
Electronic fetal monitoring
Fetal blood sampling
Appropriate interventions (e.g., cesarean section)

TABLE 20.32	Deleterious Neurological Consequences of Disturbed Oxygenation

Hypoxemia
Pressure-passive cerebral circulation
Neuronal and white matter injury
Hyperoxia
Cerebral vasoconstriction
Increased oxidative stress
Neuronal and white matter injury
Increased mortality

Extracorporeal membrane oxygenation has been used for the most severe cases, although the advent of nitric oxide therapy decreased the need for this invasive approach considerably.

Hyperoxia. Although hypoxemia is serious and requires prompt reaction, overreaction also may be deleterious if *hyperoxia* is produced (see Table 20.32). Hyperoxia may lead to cerebral vasoconstriction or increased oxidative stress or both (see Chapters 13 and 16). The result may be *neuronal or white matter injury, or both.* Experimental and neuropathological data support this conclusion (see Chapter 19). For example, the neuropathological data reviewed in Chapter 18 suggest a role for hyperoxia in the genesis of a specific pattern of neuronal injury, pontosubicular necrosis, which is most common in the premature infant. In addition, the possibility that hyperoxia may contribute to neuronal injury by causing a reduction in CBF must be considered. Reductions of CBF of 20% to 30% were shown with hyperoxia in newborn puppies, although the arterial oxygen tensions (PaO_2) of approximately 350 mm Hg used were very high.[512] In one study of 218 term infants with "postasphyxial HIE," infants who experienced severe hyperoxia ($PaO_2 > 200$ mm Hg) in the first hours of life had an increased risk on multivariate analysis of adverse neurological outcome (OR 3.85; 95% CI, 1.67 to 8.86; *P* = .002).[513] This deleterious effect was accentuated if severe hypocarbia also occurred (see later). A more recent report shows that infants with perinatal acidemia and an initial $PaO_2 > 100$ mm Hg had higher incidences of HIE and of abnormal MRI findings.[514]

Concern about deleterious effects of hyperoxia has led, in recent years, to a reconsideration of previous recommendations to use 100% oxygen in resuscitation.[515-520] Resuscitation with room air versus 100% oxygen has been associated with reduced neonatal mortality. Resuscitation with 100% oxygen also appears to increase oxidative stress.[521] A recent meta-analysis compared 100% oxygen resuscitation to room air resuscitation of depressed term newborn infants.[522] The data showed a lower mortality both in the first week of life (OR 0.70; 95% CI, 0.50 to 0.98) and at 1 month and beyond (OR 0.63; 95% CI, 0.42 to 0.94) in the room air resuscitation group. Importantly, the incidence of severe HIE (stage II and stage III) was similar between the two groups. Whether the higher levels of oxygen administered contribute to increased oxidative stress in brain, deleterious for both neurons and differentiating oligodendrocytes (see Chapters 13, 14, 15, 17, and 18), is not yet known, although experimental data support this possibility (see Chapter 16).[523] The International Liaison Committee on Resuscitation (ILCOR) recommendations for neonatal resuscitation in the term-born infant requiring resuscitation include initiation of oxygen with room air or oxygen concentrations between 21% (room air) and 40%, with increasing oxygen to be used if the response is poor.[524]

Carbon Dioxide

Because $PaCO_2$ may have serious metabolic and vascular effects, careful control thereof is critical (Table 20.33). A consistent body of evidence appears to indicate deleterious effects of alterations in $PaCO_2$ on outcomes following cerebral injury.[525] These effects may relate to hypocarbia, hypercarbia, or the degree of variability in $PaCO_2$ levels.[526] As with oxygen determinations, periodic sampling of arterial blood is not an optimal means to monitor serially and to maintain $PaCO_2$. Experience with continuous

TABLE 20.33   Deleterious Consequences of Disturbed Carbon Dioxide Levels

Hypercarbia (marked)
Metabolic
    Cerebral acidosis
Vascular
    Pressure-passive cerebral circulation
    Cerebral vasodilation with hemorrhagic complications (e.g., hemorrhagic infarction)
    Intracranial "steal"
Hypocarbia
Vascular
    Diminished cerebral blood flow: ischemic injury

transcutaneous monitoring of PCO_2 or serial measurements of end-tidal carbon dioxide pressure indicates that frequent clinical events result in marked changes in $PaCO_2$.[527-531]

Hypercarbia. Marked elevations of $PaCO_2$ are particularly dangerous in infants with HIE because of the resulting increase in tissue PCO_2 and consequent worsening of intracellular acidosis in brain (see Table 20.33). Perhaps more important than the *metabolic* effects and worsening of tissue acidosis are the *vascular* effects of hypercarbia. Thus, hypercarbia results in an impairment of cerebrovascular autoregulation and, as a consequence, a pressure-passive circulation (see Chapter 13). In one careful study of 43 ventilated preterm infants in the first week of life, a progressive loss of vascular autoregulation was observed with $PaCO_2$ values of 45 mm Hg or greater.[532] As noted previously, with hypercarbia resulting in potent vasodilatory effects, CBF may increase and may cause a risk of hemorrhage in vulnerable capillary beds (e.g., margins of an infarct and thereby hemorrhagic infarct in the term infant with HIE). Finally, the cerebral vasodilation in uninjured areas may lead to "steal" of blood from those reversibly injured areas in need of maximal substrate supply. (This risk, shown in adult experimental models, has not been studied in a newborn model.)

Hypocarbia. The effect of *hypocarbia* on CBF is pronounced. Although marked diminutions have been documented in adult humans and animals,[533-535] the findings in neonatal animals have not been entirely consistent.[536-546] Differences in results appear to relate in part to species and methodological differences. The following conclusions seem warranted. With hypocarbia to approximately 20 mm Hg, little change in CBF occurs. With lower levels (mean, 17 mm Hg), a definite decline in regional CBF occurs in the puppy,[541] more marked (30% to 60%) in regions with highest basal levels of blood flow and, therefore, highest sensitivity to carbon dioxide (see Chapter 13) (i.e., brain stem and diencephalon). However, in the piglet, extreme hypocarbia (<15 mm Hg) is necessary to produce statistically significant decreases in blood flow, and in this animal, the cerebrum and not the brain stem or diencephalon is affected.[540] Perhaps the most consistent observation in the several animal models is that the linear relationship between $PaCO_2$ and CBF becomes curvilinear at tensions lower than 20 to 25 mm Hg[533,538,540]; the decrease in CBF for a given decrease in $PaCO_2$ becomes *considerably less* than it is above this lower range of $PaCO_2$. In addition, adaptation occurs such that in the newborn lamb, CBF after 6 hours of $PaCO_2$ of 15 mm Hg is not statistically different from that in control animals.[544] Perhaps of greatest importance despite the decreases in CBF in newborn animals, no change in cerebral metabolic rate for oxygen occurs, primarily because of an increase in oxygen extraction.[542,544] Thus, mild hypocarbia may be of little or no danger, although data in the human newborn concerning hypocarbia are of concern (see later).

Perhaps relevant in this context is the demonstration that mild hypocarbia ($PaCO_2$ of 26 mm Hg) interacted adversely with hypoxic-ischemic insults in the immature rat.[547-549] Thus, animals exposed to hypoxia-ischemia during mild hypocarbia sustained a larger decline in CBF, a greater degree of cerebral glucose and energy depletion, and more neuropathological evidence of brain injury than did animals exposed to the same insult but with normocarbia ($PaCO_2$ of 39 mm Hg) or mild hypercarbia ($PaCO_2$ of 54 mm Hg). The latter two groups had better preserved CBF, less severe cerebral biochemical deficits, and less severe brain injury. The mildly hypercarbic animals had the most favorable hemodynamic, biochemical, and neuropathological outcomes.

CBF in the human infant is responsive to changes in $PaCO_2$, except under conditions of maximal vasodilation in the mechanically ventilated preterm infant (in the first days of life) and in the asphyxiated term infant.[505,532,550-555] *Concern for impaired CBF with vasoconstriction caused by hypocarbia seems warranted.* One study of 217 term infants with HIE showed, on multivariate analysis, an association between adverse neurological outcome and $PaCO_2$ lower than 20 mm Hg in the first hours of life (OR 2.34; 95% CI, 1.02 to 5.37; $P = .04$).[513] The risk was accentuated (OR 4.56) when severe hyperoxia also was present. The investigators postulated that aggressive early management and resuscitation may be contributory.

In the largest study to date of the impact of $PaCO_2$ in infants receiving therapeutic hypothermia, 202 infants in the NICHD randomized controlled trial of systemic therapeutic hypothermia had multiple blood gases recorded prospectively: prerandomization, randomization, 4, 8, and 12 hours of intervention.[556] Subsequent blood gases were obtained as per clinical care and were recorded once daily during study intervention. Hypocarbia was common. A total of 181 newborns had at least one $PaCO_2$ concentration below 35 mm Hg, and 100 infants had at least one $PaCO_2$ concentration below 25 mm Hg from birth to 12 hours of intervention (~16.9 hours of age [mean]). Importantly, 95% of these infants were intubated in the delivery room with the median duration of intubation 6 days. Thus, many infants received significant ventilatory support, which has been shown to increase the risk for hypocarbia in the setting of HIE.[557] In relation to neurodevelopmental outcome at 18 to 22 months, infants with poor outcome had significantly lower minimum $PaCO_2$ concentrations (median 22 vs. 26 mm Hg), greater fluctuations in $PaCO_2$ concentrations (difference in maximum and minimum $PaCO_2$, SD of $PaCO_2$) and cumulative $PCO_2 < 35$ mm Hg. The study did not find any relationship to hypercarbia exposure but the early period of observation in the first 16 hours of life may have limited the observation of hypercarbia. Thus, hypocarbia and fluctuations in $PaCO_2$, particularly in ventilated infants, are critical to avoid to optimize subsequent neurodevelopmental outcomes in infants with HIE, irrespective of additional neuroprotective approaches.

TABLE 20.34 Maintenance of Adequate Perfusion

Recognition of pressure-passive cerebral circulation
Recognition of "normal" arterial blood pressure level
Avoidance of systemic hypotension (may cause ischemic injury)
Avoidance of systemic hypertension (may cause hemorrhagic complications)

Maintenance of Adequate Perfusion

The maintenance of adequate perfusion to brain is a critical aspect of supportive care (Table 20.34). Prevention of additional ischemic injury is important. The basic elements of maintenance of adequate perfusion are summarized in Table 20.34 and in the following discussion.

Recognition of Pressure-Passive Cerebral Circulation

As discussed in Chapter 19 (concerning pathogenesis) and Chapter 13, the cerebral circulation of the infant with HIE appears to be pressure passive. This occurrence may relate to a disturbance of autoregulation by complicating hypoxemia or hypercarbia, or both; a postasphyxial impairment of vascular reactivity as observed in experimental models of perinatal asphyxia; an "immature" autoregulatory system with blunted capacity for reactivity because of the deficient arterial muscularis of penetrating cerebral vessels in the third trimester; an intact or partially intact autoregulatory mechanism but with "normal" neonatal blood pressure dangerously close to the downslope of the autoregulatory curve; or a combination of these factors (see Chapters 13 and 18). The important point is that the physician must be aware of the pressure-passive state, must monitor blood pressure continuously and diligently, and must maintain blood pressure at adequate levels to avoid cerebral ischemia or overperfusion. Studies of CBF in human infants with xenon-clearance techniques have documented a *pressure-passive state of the cerebral circulation* in seriously *asphyxiated term infants* (see Chapter 13 and earlier discussion).

Recognition of Normal Arterial Blood Pressure Levels in the Newborn

A series of studies has investigated normal values for arterial blood pressure in the newborn.[558-574] In the largest, most recent series of 406 healthy term-born infants, day 1 median (5th percentile) values for systolic, diastolic, and mean arterial pressure were 65 mm Hg (55 mm Hg), 45 mm Hg (30 mm Hg), and 48 mm Hg (40 mm Hg), respectively. On day 4, these values had increased to 70 mm Hg, 46 mm Hg, and 54 mm Hg, respectively. In clinical practice, we aim to maintain mean arterial blood pressure (monitored by arterial catheter) at greater than 45 mm Hg and to avoid systolic blood pressures greater than 75 mm Hg, principally by maintaining adequate comfort measures, including sedation.

Avoidance of Systemic Hypotension

In view of the aforementioned considerations concerning a pressure-passive cerebral circulation and neonatal blood pressure data, it is clear that systemic hypotension must be avoided because of the danger of cerebral hypoperfusion (see Table 20.34). Moreover, because "normal" arterial blood pressure values in the newborn are relatively low and may be dangerously

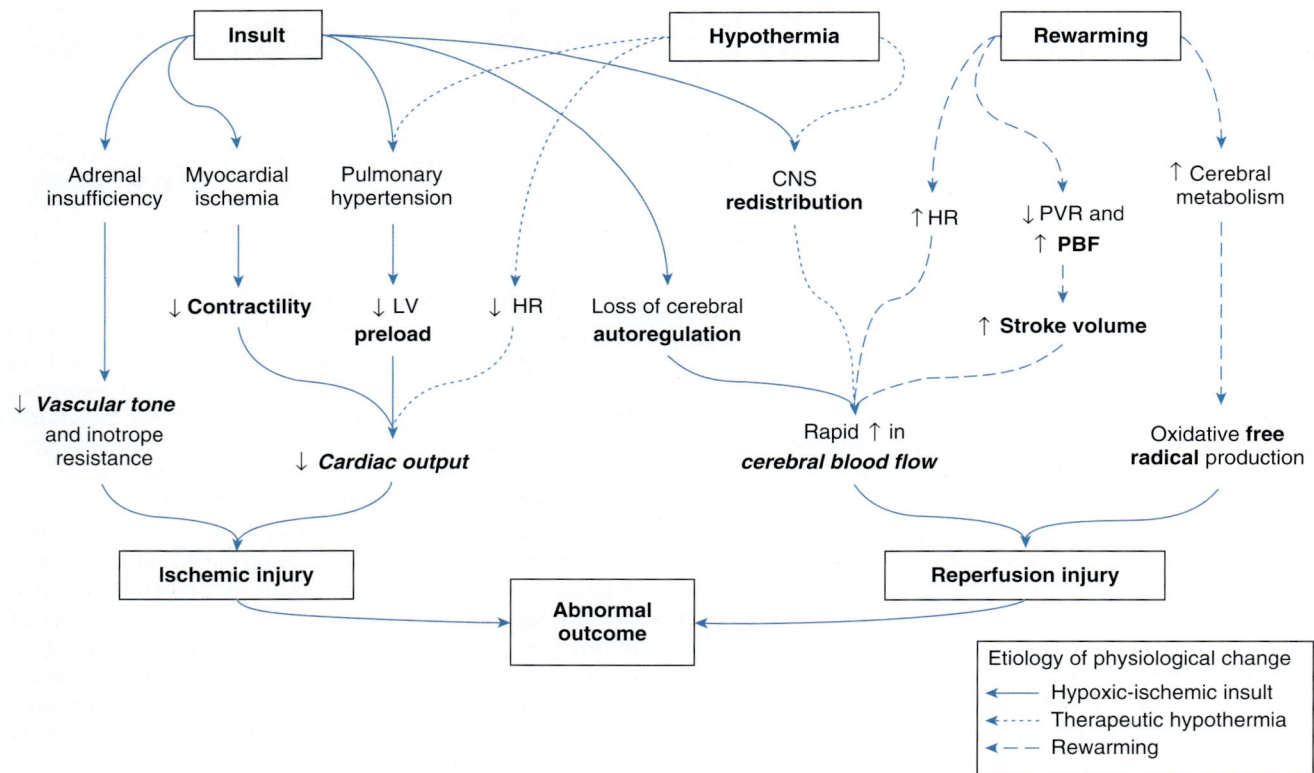

Figure 20.30 Interrelationship between contributors to ischemic injury resulting from initial insult, TH, and reperfusion injury on rewarming. Both ischemia and reperfusion injury may contribute to the degree of brain injury via modification of cardiovascular factors. Resumption of cellular activity after transient suppression is a putative source of potentially damaging oxidative radicals. *HR*, Heart rate; *LV*, left ventricle; *PBF*, pulmonary blood flow; *PVR*, pulmonary vascular resistance; *RV*, right ventricle. (From Giesinger RE, Bailey LJ, Deshpande P, McNamara PJ. Hypoxic–ischemic encephalopathy and therapeutic hypothermia: the hemodynamic perspective. *J Pediatr.* 2017;180:22–30.)

close to the downslope of even an intact autoregulatory curve, the margin of safety for arterial blood pressure sufficient to maintain adequate cerebral perfusion is likely to be small. As noted in Chapter 13 concerning pathogenesis, brain regions that are particularly vulnerable include neuronal-rich areas (cerebral cortex, basal ganglia, thalamus) and regions with vascular border zones and end zones (the parasagittal cerebral areas in the term newborn and to a lesser extent, the periventricular white matter).

The principal *causes* of serious systemic hypotension in the asphyxiated infant are *cardiogenic*. Evidence of ischemia to papillary muscle, subendocardial region, and myocardium more diffusely has been demonstrated in asphyxiated infants.[575-583] In a study of 20 asphyxiated term infants, 8 exhibited myocardial dysfunction in the first 2 postnatal days, and this dysfunction was associated with both reduced cardiac output and lower mean CBF velocity than observed on recovery at 3 days.[583] With the introduction of therapeutic hypothermia as standard of care in the infant with moderate-severe HIE, cardiovascular evaluation and management has become more challenging. The impact of therapeutic hypothermia on the cardiovascular system has been extensively reviewed recently and is outlined in Fig. 20.30.[584]

The evaluation of the cardiovascular system is more challenging in the infant receiving therapeutic hypothermia, due to bradycardia with resulting decreased cardiac output,

peripheral vasoconstriction with hypothermia, and persisting lactic acidemia from the initial ischemic insult. Thus, targeted echocardiography has been recommended to better define the nature of contributing cardiovascular factors, such as cardiac output, superior vena caval flow, and pulmonary hypertension (see review).[584] The relative roles of volume expansion, dopamine, dobutamine, phosphodiesterase III inhibitors (e.g., milrinone), and corticosteroids are currently under active study and relate in part to the underlying pathophysiology (as outlined in Fig. 20.30).[585-590] Detailed discussion is beyond the scope of this book.

Avoidance of Systemic Hypertension

The other side of the coin regarding the issue of cerebral ischemia just discussed is cerebral overperfusion. Because of a pressure-passive cerebral circulation, increases in systemic blood pressure, especially abrupt increases, could lead to rupture of certain vulnerable capillaries and thereby to hemorrhagic complications (see Table 20.34; Fig. 20.30). The causes of such elevations in blood pressure can range from apparently innocuous events, such as simple handling of the infant, to more obvious events, such as overly exuberant administration of volume expanders or pressor agents, seizures, pneumothorax, or abrupt closure of patent ductus arteriosus. Concern for the role of cerebral overperfusion is prominent in the era of therapeutic hypothermia. In one study of a series of 24 term-born infants receiving therapeutic hypothermia, normal brain MRI was associated with lower cerebral blood flow, which further declined in those undergoing hypothermia therapy, compared with infants with poor radiologic outcome who had a higher baseline and a progressive rise in cerebral blood flow despite therapeutic hypothermia.[591] Because cerebral hyperfusion may occur following cerebral injury (see Chapter 13), the apparent hyperperfusion in the infants with abnormal MRI may reflect a consequence rather than a cause of injury. More data are needed to resolve this issue.

One of the vulnerable periods for cerebral overperfusion in the term infant receiving therapeutic hypothermia is the period of rewarming, which occurs 72 hours after hypothermia has been commenced. In the full-term infant, vulnerable capillaries include those at the margins of cerebral infarcts or in residual germinal matrix, and thus hemorrhagic infarction or intraventricular hemorrhage may occur. In a cohort of 160 asphyxiated neonates, of whom 9% developed intraventricular hemorrhage, hemorrhage at the time of rewarming was associated with a greater degree of hemodynamic instability.[592] The essential point is that arterial blood pressure must be monitored carefully, and events that lead to abrupt increases in arterial blood pressure must be prevented or corrected promptly.

Maintenance of Adequate Glucose Levels

The roles for endogenous glucose stores, particularly *at the time* of the asphyxial insult, and for the addition of exogenous glucose after the insult, remain to be established clearly for the human infant. In Chapter 13, the available information based on experiments in immature and mature animals was reviewed. The former experiments suggest, although not uniformly, a generally beneficial effect of glucose, and the latter experiments suggest a deleterious effect. These experiments are relevant particularly to the treatment of the asphyxiated human *fetus* and, thus, the management of labor and delivery, detailed consideration of which is not within the province of this book.

The precise role of glucose in the management of the infant who *already has experienced an asphyxial insult* needs to be defined further. As described in detail in Chapter 13, studies in perinatal models of hypoxic-ischemic insults indicate that the effects of glucose administration vary considerably, perhaps because of species and other methodological differences. Neuropathological injury has been reported to be prevented, ameliorated, or accentuated in different models. Improved survival with glucose administration is generally consistent and may relate at least partially to improvement in cardiorespiratory function.

In human studies, intrapartum hypoxia-ischemia disturbs the typical metabolic transition and increases the likelihood of low blood glucose concentrations through several mechanisms. There is prolonged duration of anaerobic glycolysis, leading to a rapid depletion of glycogen stores. Infants with HIE have significantly lower blood glucose concentrations in the delivery room (before intravenous glucose has been given) than do matched healthy infants (1.95 [SD 0.63 mmol/L] vs. 3.16 [SD 0.31 mmol/L]).[593] In addition to depleted stores, the infant with HIE may have increased peripheral glucose utilization, which can be compounded by transient hyperinsulinism,[594] and impaired counter-regulatory hormone and enzyme responses. These factors may account for the high prevalence (25%) of infants with moderate to severe HIE with blood glucose values

of less than 2.6 mmol/L, as reported to the UK TOBY cooling register.[595] Several clinical observational studies have suggested a *potentiating impact of hypoglycemia on cerebral injury in the infant with HIE.* One report involved 185 term-born infants with acidemia (pH < 7.0) admitted to a NICU, and found that those with an initial blood glucose concentration of 2.22 mmol/L (45 mg/dL) or less were at a higher risk of abnormal neurological outcome than infants whose first blood glucose measurement was more than 2.22 mmol/L (56% vs. 16%). In a multivariate logistic analysis that included severity of acidosis and other measures of illness severity at birth, the OR for low blood glucose and poor outcome was 18.5 (95% CI, 3.1 to 111.9).[82] In a smaller study of 52 infants with HIE, blood glucose values of less than 2.6 mmol/L, 0 to 6 hours following birth, were associated with poor neurodevelopmental outcome at 24 months, but the association was insignificant after adjustment for severity of HIE.[596] These authors concluded that hypoglycemia may be a marker of the duration and severity of the ischemic insult rather than an independent injurious factor. In a more recent study of infants with HIE (defined as umbilical artery pH values of <7.1, umbilical artery base deficits of >10 mmol/L, or 5 minutes Apgar scores of ≤5), the presence of hypoglycemia (any blood glucose concentration <2.6 mmol/L within 24 hours of birth) predicted corticospinal tract injury (OR 3.72; 95% CI, 1.02 to 13.57) and poor neurodevelopmental outcomes at 12 months in multivariate regression analyses that controlled for clinical markers of the degree of hypoxia–ischemia.[597] The authors hypothesized that the ischemic cerebral insult may have increased the vulnerability of the brain at levels of blood glucose that are tolerated, in the absence of HIE, by a healthy, breast-fed infant. These conclusions were shared in a recent editorial related to the impact of hypoglycemia on patterns of cerebral injury on MRI in the term-born infant.[598]

There are insufficient data concerning the blood glucose level that will provide optimal glucose delivery to the brain, as outlined in a recent review of this topic.[599] By definition, an infant with moderate to severe HIE displays abnormal neurological signs and should therefore have blood glucose levels maintained above 2.5 mmol/L. However, infants with HIE may require higher concentrations of glucose,[600] as suggested by animal data and human studies described earlier.

Regarding *hyperglycemia,* early hyperglycemia (>150 mg/dL, >8.3 mmol/L) has been associated with greater risk of neurodevelopmental disability (adjusted OR 6.2 and 2.7, respectively) 18 months in term infants with HIE.[601,602] In a further secondary analysis of the NICHD Cool Cap study of 194 term-born infants with HIE, in the first 12 hours, 9% (18/194) of infants had ≥1 episode of hypoglycemia, 45% (87/194) had ≥1 episode of hyperglycemia, and 46% (89/194) were normoglycemic.[603,604] In this study, in the hyperglycemic infants it was apparent that hypothermia therapy conferred a lower risk of adverse outcome (adjusted risk ratio [aRR] 0.80; 95% CI, 0.66 to 0.99), whereas there was no reduction in risk of adverse outcome associated with hypothermia therapy in the normoglycemic (aRR 0.95; 95% CI, 0.70 to 1.27) or hypoglycemic infants (aRR 1.03; 95% CI, 0.52 to 2.00). A further small study examined the extent by which glucose variability influenced outcomes in term-born infants with hypoxic-ischemic injury. The neurodevelopmental outcomes from 8 of 23 patients were considered severe, and this group demonstrated a significant increase of mean absolute glucose

TABLE 20.35	Maintenance of Adequate Blood Glucose Levels

Maintain a blood glucose concentration of approximately 50–100 mg/dL

Avoid hypoglycemia because it may cause neuronal injury

Avoid marked hyperglycemia because it may provoke hemorrhage (through a hyperosmolar effect) or may worsen cerebral lactic acidosis

change from birth (95% CI, –0.28 to –0.03; RR = 0.1; P = 0.03). There were no differences between outcome groups with regard to the number of patients with hyperglycemia (mean), and/or one or multiple hypo- or hyperglycemic measurement(s). There were also no differences between groups for mean glucose.[603]

Given the evidence presented, it has been postulated that glucose may be a marker of the timing and severity of brain injury. Thus, hypoglycemia may be a marker of a more severe and prolonged hypoxic-ischemic insult, compared with hyperglycemia, which may represent an acute insult. The latter may demonstrate greater benefit from hypothermia therapy. In addition, major fluxes in blood glucose also may be injurious. Thus, in collaboration with guidelines from broader arenas of knowledge/research/academic discovery, we currently recommend that glucose supplementation be adjusted to maintain a blood glucose level between approximately 50 and 100 mg/dL (Table 20.35) and that fluxes be minimized.

Control of Seizures

Therapy for seizures begins with careful serial observations to detect clinical seizure activity (see Chapter 12). Seizures, an accompaniment of the majority of cases of serious HIE, may cause further injury to the brain. For example, in one detailed study of 90 term infants with perinatal asphyxia, each increase in seizure severity score was independently associated with an increase in lactate and a decrease in NAA, which was assessed by MR spectroscopy (see Chapter 12)[335] Later clinical studies support the conclusion that greater frequency and severity of seizures in infants with HIE are associated with a greater degree of brain injury and poorer neurodevelopmental outcome.[605-609] Seizures are associated with a *markedly accelerated cerebral metabolic rate*, and if, as indicated earlier, cerebral metabolism is not operating at optimal aerobic capacity (e.g., because of mitochondrial injury), this acceleration may lead to a rapid fall in brain glucose, an increase in lactate, and a decrease in high-energy phosphate compounds. Moreover, the excessive synaptic release of certain excitotoxic amino acids (e.g., glutamate) also may lead to cellular injury. In addition, seizures are associated frequently with hypoventilation and apnea with consequent *hypoxemia and hypercarbia*, the dangers of which have been discussed. Studies with transcutaneous tissue electrodes suggest that these latter changes may occur with seizures that are so subtle that they are readily missed clinically. In addition, neonatal seizures are associated with *abrupt elevations in arterial blood pressure* (see Chapter 12), and hence the possibility of inducing hemorrhage, as discussed earlier. Moreover, studies of ischemia in the term fetal lamb indicate that epileptiform activity is a prominent feature in the hours following the insult (maximum at 10 hours, duration

of 72 hours) and that cortical neuronal necrosis occurs in the same cortical areas and to a degree that correlates with the extent of epileptiform activity.[610] Moreover, infants with poorly controlled seizures have more frequent and severe neurological sequelae than infants whose seizures are well controlled.[20,335,611,612] Obviously, this difference may relate to the severity of the initial injury rather than to additional injury from repetitive seizures. Indeed, studies in neonatal rats subjected to hypoxia-ischemia and subsequent chemically induced seizures at 2, 6, and 12 hours of recovery showed no accentuation of brain damage compared with histopathological findings in rats subjected to hypoxia–ischemia without induced seizures.[613-615] However, the convulsing animals developed hypoglycemia and a mortality rate of 53%, both of which could be improved by glucose supplementation.[613] Nevertheless, on balance, the data do raise the possibility of a deleterious effect of multiple seizures in the infant with HIE. Careful attention to glucose homeostasis clearly is critical in this context.

Phenobarbital remains the preferred drug for the treatment of seizures in neonatal HIE; details of the administration of this drug are described in Chapter 12. The *timing* of treatment has been somewhat controversial. *Pretreatment* with barbiturates (i.e., before the onset of seizures) has been considered because of studies in adult animals that barbiturates in high doses are beneficial in ischemia (by causing reduction of cerebral metabolic rate, cerebral vasoconstriction, reduction of brain edema, or removal of harmful free radicals)[616-621] and studies in *perinatal animals* that suggest a beneficial effect in several nonprimate species and in term fetal monkeys.[549,622-629] In the study of the fetal monkey by Cockburn and co-workers,[628] anesthetic doses of pentobarbital that were administered to the mothers produced *anesthesia* in the fetuses, which were then delivered and asphyxiated experimentally. When compared with animals delivered under local anesthesia before asphyxia, the barbiturate-treated animals had prolongation of time to last gasp, accelerated establishment of rhythmic breathing after resuscitation, and less histological evidence of neuronal injury. In the only study of *neonatal monkeys* treated with barbiturates *after birth* but before asphyxia, no beneficial effect on time to last gasp, survival, or CBF could be detected.[630] In this study, a 20-mg/kg dose of phenobarbital was administered in the 18 hours before asphyxia, and animals were *sedated but not anesthetized*, a potentially important difference from the study of Cockburn and co-workers.[628] No experimental studies have been reported in which barbiturates have been administered *after* a perinatal asphyxial insult.

Studies of pretreatment of asphyxiated term infants with barbiturates (i.e., before the occurrence of seizures) have shown interesting but not entirely consistent results.[631,632] In one randomized, controlled trial of 32 severely asphyxiated term infants, thiopental was administered initially at a mean age of 2.3 hours and then by constant infusion over 24 hours.[632] Seizures occurred in approximately 75% of both treated and control infants. Moreover, the mortality rate and neurological outcome were similar in the two groups. Of concern is that hypotension occurred in nearly 90% of the treated group and required pressor agents in 30%.

An earlier study, which used a slightly smaller number of severely asphyxiated infants, suggested benefit for relatively high doses of phenobarbital administered shortly after birth.[633] A total of 14 infants were treated within 60 minutes of delivery with phenobarbital (10 mg/kg, followed in 4 hours by 10 mg/kg per day), in addition to assisted ventilation, glucocorticoid, and fresh frozen plasma. (Another group of 16 infants did not receive glucocorticoid or fresh frozen plasma therapy and were given phenobarbital only if seizures did not respond to diazepam.) Plasma levels of phenobarbital in the early-treated infants were approximately 25 μg/mL on the first day and rose to a peak of 40 to 70 μg/mL on the second and third days. Respiratory "insufficiency" was noted at levels higher than approximately 40 μg/mL, and phenobarbital administration "may have prolonged ventilator treatment in some infants."[633] When compared with infants not treated early with phenobarbital, the early phenobarbital-treated infants had lower mortality rates (14% vs. 50%) and a more frequent normal outcome in survivors (83% vs. 50%). Obviously, the numbers are small, the groups were not comparably treated with respect to factors other than phenobarbital, and the side effects are disturbing.

A later study evaluated the effect of administration of 40 mg/kg of phenobarbital to term infants with "severe asphyxia" (initial arterial pH ≤ 7.0 and base deficit of 15 mEq/L or more, Apgar score ≤3 at 5 minutes of age, or failure to initiate spontaneous respirations by 10 minutes of age) at a mean age of 6 hours and before the onset of clinical seizures.[634] Seizures occurred in 9 of 15 treated infants versus 14 of 16 "control" infants ($P = .11$). At 3 years of age, normal outcome was noted in 11 of 15 treated infants versus only 3 of 16 control infants ($P = .003$). Thus, although early onset of high-dose phenobarbital therapy was not associated with a statistically significant reduction in the occurrence of seizures, a beneficial effect on neurological outcome was suggested.

The potential value of prophylactic phenobarbital (40 mg/kg given at the time of onset of cooling) was studied in 42 infants with HIE.[635] A decrease in the frequency of neurodevelopmental impairment in the prophylactic phenobarbital group (23%) versus the nonprophylactic group (45%) was not statistically significant. There were fewer clinical seizures in the prophylactic group than in the cooled infants not given prophylactic phenobarbital (15% vs. 82%; $P < .0001$). More data will be of interest.

Currently, we do not administer phenobarbital routinely before the onset of clinical or electrographic seizures. However, we use the EEG tracing to identify seizures and to provoke prompt treatment. Phenobarbital sometimes is not optimally effective in the severely asphyxiated infant. This situation results most probably because (1) phenobarbital is a gamma-aminobutyric acid (GABA) agonist; (2) GABA receptors tend to be excitatory in the newborn brain because of high intracellular chloride levels; and (3) the expression of the NKCC1 transporter for chloride influx is activated after hypoxia-ischemia (see Chapter 12).[636] However, trials of newer additive agents, such as bumetanide, a diuretic and inhibitor of NKCC1, and levetiracetam, are currently underway. The largest published study to date is an open-label, dose finding, and feasibility phase 1/2 trial, with recruitment of full-term infants less than 48 hours of age with HIE and electrographic seizures not responding to a loading dose of phenobarbital (NCT01434225). The authors reported on 14 infants (10 males) with bumetanide dose allocation: 0.05 mg/kg, $n = 4$; 0.1 mg/kg, $n = 3$; 0.2 mg/kg, $n = 6$; 0.3 mg/kg, $n = 1$.[637] All infants received at least one dose of bumetanide with the second dose of phenobarbital; three were withdrawn for reasons unrelated

to bumetanide, and one because of dehydration. All but one infant also received aminoglycosides. Five infants met EEG criteria for seizure reduction (1 on 0.05 mg/kg, 1 on 0.1 mg/kg and 3 on 0.2 mg/kg), and only 2 of the 14 did not need rescue antiepileptic drugs (i.e., met rescue criteria; 1 on 0.05 mg/kg and 1 on 0.3 mg/kg). Three of 11 surviving infants had hearing impairment confirmed on auditory testing between 17 and 108 days of age. The most common nonserious adverse reactions were moderate dehydration in 1, mild hypotension in 7, and mild to moderate electrolyte disturbances in 12 infants. The trial was stopped early because of serious adverse reactions and limited evidence for seizure reduction. The authors concluded that bumetanide as an add-on to phenobarbital did not improve seizure control in newborn infants who have HIE, and might increase the risk of hearing loss, which highlighted the risks associated with the off-label use of drugs in newborn infants. A further randomized, controlled trial (NCT00830531) is currently being undertaken in the United States with phenobarbital combined with either 0.1 mg/kg, 0.2 mg/kg, or 0.3 mg/kg of bumetanide as determined by the status of the dose escalation design.

Topiramate, an anticonvulsant agent, which potentiates the neuroprotective effect of hypothermia (see later and Chapter 13), is also a candidate for further study in the context of HIE. Further data are required before implementation of these agents as standard clinical practice.

Neuroprotective Interventions

As described in detail in Chapters 13 and 19, the principal mechanisms of neuronal death in HIE operate after termination of the insult, are initiated by the activation of glutamate receptors, occur over hours, and involve the accumulation of cytosolic calcium and the activation of a variety of calcium-mediated deleterious events, including especially the generation of free radicals, such as superoxide anion, hydroxyl radical, and nitric oxide derivatives. Free radical-mediated cell death also appears to be the final common pathway for cell death (see Chapters 13 and 19). *The exciting implication concerning management is that interruption of this deleterious cascade, even after termination of the insult, could prevent or ameliorate the brain injury in perinatal hypoxic-ischemic disease.* In Chapter 13, potential neuroprotective interventions shown to be of value in a variety of experimental models of hypoxia-ischemia are discussed. In this section, we discuss primarily those agents studied in human newborns (Table 20.36).

The approaches that have been studied in human infants and considered here are therapeutic hypothermia, anticonvulsant therapy, xenon, antioxidants, melatonin, erythropoietin, magnesium, calcium channel blockers, and stem cell transplantation (see Table 20.36). Several other promising pharmacologic agents, still in a preclinical stage, are also noted briefly.

Hypothermia

Although for many decades, deep hypothermia to body temperatures less than 20°C has been shown to be valuable for neuroprotection during cardiac surgery with circulatory bypass or circulatory arrest, in recent years, after numerous experimental studies in a variety of models of perinatal hypoxia-ischemia, it has shown a pronounced beneficial effect with induced hypothermia of only a few degrees (i.e., "mild" hypothermia; see Chapter 13) has been shown. This approach has been studied in human infants with HIE and is now adopted worldwide. The *principal determinants of neuroprotective benefit* for mild hypothermia have related to *timing* (onset of hypothermia before delayed energy failure and excitatory features, such as seizures [i.e., ≈6 hours]), *degree* (decrease of body temperature by 3°C to 4°C), and *duration* (≈72 hours). The *mechanisms of benefit* appear to include a decrease in energy consumption, a decrease in the accumulation of extracellular glutamate, a decrease in the generation of reactive oxygen and nitrogen species, inhibition of inflammatory mechanisms, and the interruption of downstream molecular cascades to apoptosis (see Chapter 13). On the background of the promising results of mild hypothermia in experimental models, multicenter, randomized, clinical trials in term infants with HIE were initiated with consistent findings of benefit.[71,476,601,638-655]

Two principal approaches have been used: selective head cooling (by a water-circulating cap, "Cool Cap") or whole body cooling (by water-circulating blankets) (Fig. 20.31). The first large-scale multicenter study reported involved *selective head cooling*.[601]

In this landmark study, 218 infants with moderate to severe encephalopathy and abnormal aEEG were randomized

to cooling therapy that began before 5.5 hours of age and continued for 72 hours. In a minority of infants (*n* = 46) who had *severe* aEEG abnormalities, no effect on death or severe disability at 18 months was observed. However, in a majority of infants who had *moderate* aEEG abnormalities (*n* = 172), a significantly lower rate of this unfavorable outcome was observed in the hypothermic group versus the control group (48% vs. 66%, *P* = .02).

Similarly, early promising results were obtained from the multicenter trial of *whole body cooling*.[71] The total group included 208 infants with moderate or severe encephalopathy; aEEG was not used in this study. Cooling was begun at a mean age of 4.3 hours to an esophageal temperature of 33.5°C and was continued for 72 hours. Death or moderate or severe disability occurred in 44% of the hypothermic infants versus 62% of the control infants (*P* = .01).

In the most recent meta-analysis of 11 randomized controlled trials of 1505 term and late preterm infants with moderate/severe encephalopathy and evidence of intrapartum asphyxia,[510] therapeutic hypothermia resulted in a significant and clinically important reduction in the combined outcome of mortality or major neurodevelopmental disability to 18 months of age (typical RR 0.75 [95% CI, 0.68 to 0.83]; typical risk differences [RD] −0.15, [95% CI, −0.20 to −0.10]); number needed to treat for an additional beneficial outcome (NNTB) 7 (95% CI, 5 to 10) (8 studies, 1344 infants) (Fig. 20.32). Cooling also resulted in statistically significant reductions in mortality (typical RR 0.75 [95% CI, 0.64 to 0.88]; typical RD −0.09 [95% CI, −0.13 to −0.04]); NNTB 11 (95% CI, 8 to 25 [11 studies, 1468 infants]) and in neurodevelopmental disability in survivors (typical RR 0.77 [95% CI, 0.63 to 0.94]; typical RD −0.13 [95% CI, −0.19 to −0.07]); NNTB 8 (95% CI, 5 to 14; [8 studies, 917 infants]).

The selection of infants that may benefit from hypothermia therapy has been investigated and the following indications for the initiation of hypothermia endorsed by the American Academy of Pediatrics[207]:

1. More than 35 weeks gestational age
2. Less than 6 hours of age
3. "Evidence of asphyxia," as defined by the presence of at least 1 to 2 of the following:

TABLE 20.36	Neuroprotective Interventions in the Human Fetus and Newborn[a]

Mild hypothermia
Anticonvulsant drugs
Xenon
Antioxidants—*N*-Acetylcysteine, allopurinol
Melatonin
Erythropoietin
Magnesium
Calcium channel blockers
Stem cell transplantation
Other pharmacologic agents

[a]See text for details.

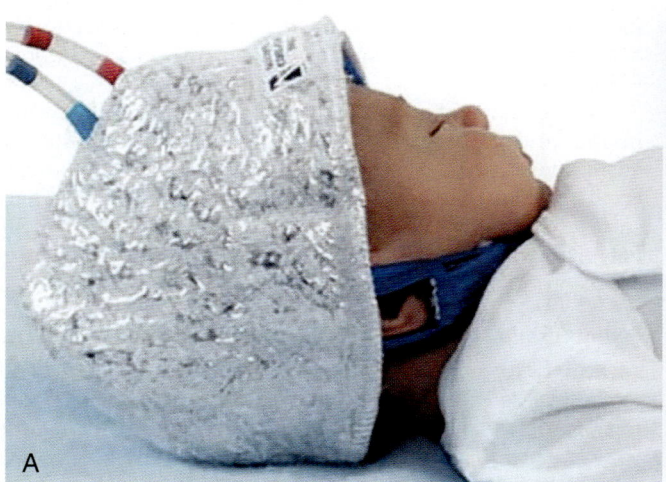
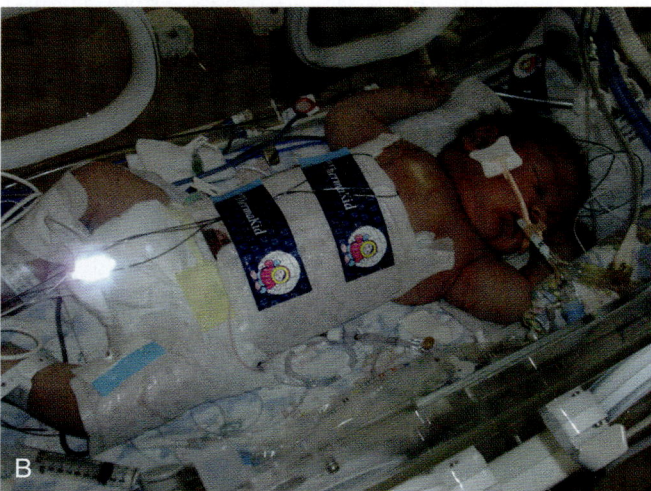

Figure 20.31 Two approaches to hypothermia. (A) Selective head cooling with head wrap and chin straps. (B) Infant receiving whole body therapeutic hypothermia via body wrap.

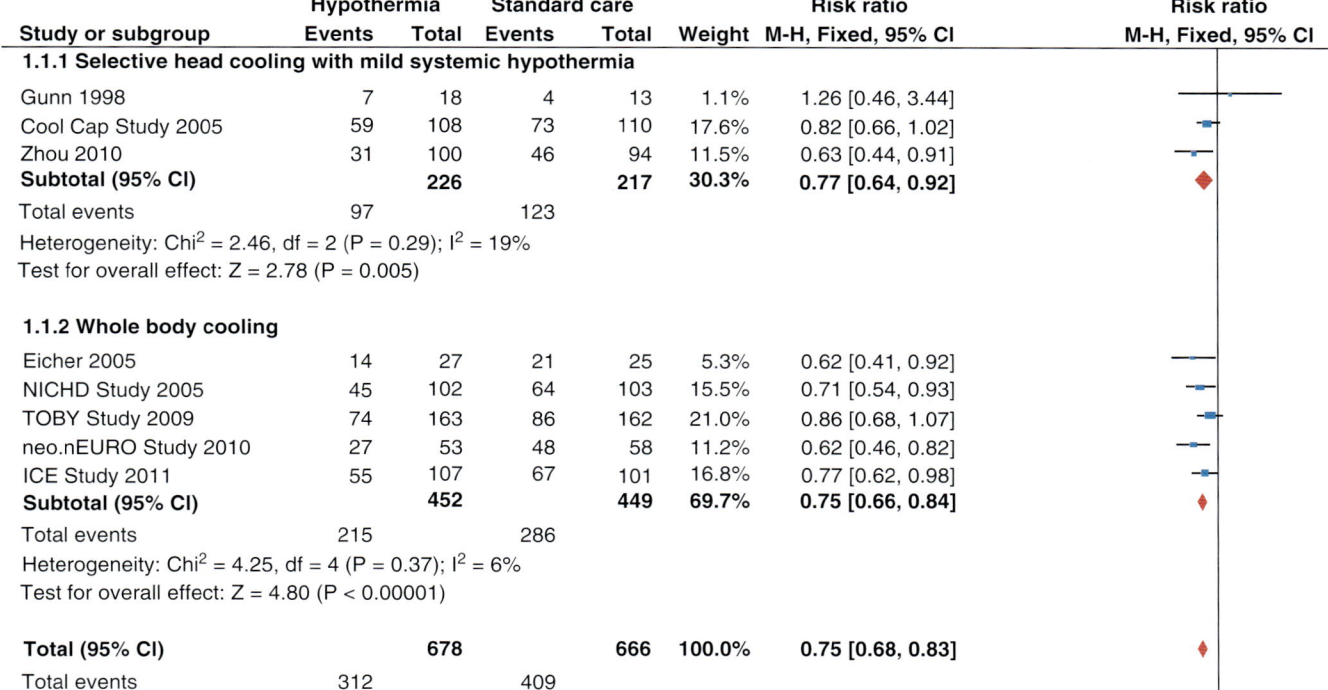

A

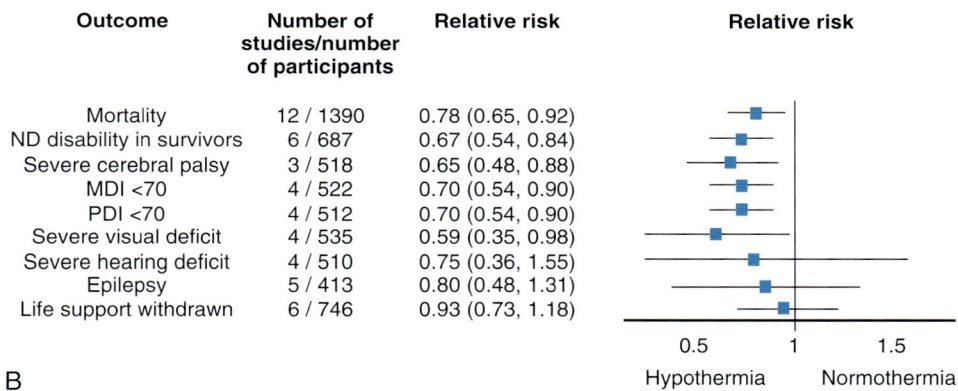

B

Figure 20.32 **Therapeutic hypothermia outcomes.** (A) Primary outcomes in randomized controlled trials of therapeutic hypothermia. (B) Outcomes from therapeutic hypothermia in neonatal hypoxic-ischemic encephalopathy.

- Apgar score less than 6 at 10 minutes or continued need for resuscitation with positive pressure ventilation or chest compressions at 10 minutes
- Any acute perinatal sentinel event that may result in HIE (e.g., abruptio placentae, cord prolapse, severe FHR abnormality)
- Cord pH < 7.0 or base excess of −16 mmol/L or less
- If cord pH is not available, arterial pH < 7.0 or base excess less than −16 mmol/L within 60 minutes of birth
4. Presence of moderate/severe neonatal encephalopathy on clinical examination

The issue of initiation of therapeutic hypothermia in mildly encephalopathic infants is currently under active investigation. Although infants with milder degrees of clinical encephalopathy were not eligible in any of the RCTs, a small number of mildly

encephalopathic infants were enrolled in two trials (total *n* = 79).[651,656] This inclusion of milder cases may reflect the difficulty of firmly assigning the severity of NE within the first hours of life and is consistent with the common clinical situation.[595,657,658] Zhou et al. randomized 39 infants with mild NE, 21 to treatment with hypothermia, and 18 controls.[656] No infant with mild NE met the primary outcome of death or severe disability. However, 33% (13/39) of those with mild NE were found to have a moderately abnormal outcome (a developmental quotient between one to two standard deviations below the mean at 18 months of age, with the Gesell Child Development Age Scale). Stratification by treatment group showed that 29% (6/21) who received hypothermia versus 39% (7/18) of control infants had a moderately abnormal outcome (*P* = 0.3). In the ICE trial, Jacobs et al. randomized 40 infants with mild neonatal encephalopathy, 16 to treatment with hypothermia, and 24 controls.[651] A total of 30% (12/40) of infants with mild NE met the composite primary outcome of death or severe disability at 2 years of age. Severe disability was defined as any one of: cerebral palsy, a Psychomotor Development Index score on the Bayley-II of greater than two standard deviations below the mean, a Motor Composite Scale score on the Bayley-III of greater than two standard deviations below the mean, or a disability level on the Gross Motor Function Classification System of two to five. Stratification by treatment group showed that 25% (4/16) who received therapeutic hypothermia versus 33% (8/24) of control infants met the primary outcome (RR 0.53; 95% CI, 0.17 to 1.66). Thus, both of these demonstrated a trend toward improved outcome among the hypothermia group, with an RR reduction with hypothermia treatment of 26% in the study of Zhou et al., and 24% in the ICE trial. These reductions in the risk of adverse outcomes are similar to those reported for death or disability for therapeutic hypothermia in the setting of moderate–severe neonatal encephalopathy, but are very underpowered for definition. Finally, it is noteworthy that the rates of adverse outcome for infants with mild NE after therapeutic hypothermia reported in both trials are almost identical to the frequency of moderate-severely abnormal MRIs (23%) among infants with mild NE reported in other studies.[658-660] Thus, the inclusion of such infants with mild disease for treatment in clinical practice continues to expand without any randomized trial.[595,657,658] Further data are needed on the efficacy of this neuroprotective therapy in this group.[656]

Thus, to conclude, it is clear from available clinical and preclinical evidence that moderate therapeutic hypothermia should be implemented as soon as possible, before the onset of secondary injury and continued until this period of secondary energy failure has resolved.[661] Infants cooled within 3 hours of birth appear to have better neurodevelopmental outcomes compared with infants whose cooling commences between 3 hours and 6 hours.[662] Following 72 hours of cooling, infants should be *slowly* rewarmed (0.5°/hour). This rate is based on animal data showing increased seizures[663] and increased cortical apoptosis with[664] rapid rewarming. Longer periods of cooling (>72 hours) or deeper cooling to less than 33.5°C has not been shown to be of benefit, and is harmful.[665-668] The risk factors associated with therapeutic hypothermia appear to be relatively minor compared to the potential benefit from the therapy.[510]

To conclude, it is now clear that early implementation of therapeutic hypothermia to at-risk infants for HIE reduces the extent of cerebral injury on MRI, reduces mortality, and improves neurodevelopmental outcomes. Further research is required to determine the extent to which mild HIE is an indication for the implementation of this approach.

Other Neuroprotective Agents

As discussed in Chapter 13, experimental studies suggest that some neuroprotective agents appear to have synergistic or, at least, strong additive effects with hypothermia in models of neonatal hypoxia–ischemia. The principal agents studied have been anticonvulsant drugs, including phenobarbital, topiramate, and levetiracetam; xenon, antioxidants, including *N*-acetylcysteine and allopurinol; and agents with multiple effects, including erythropoietin and IGF-1. Other neuroprotective interventions for neonatal HIE not studied in relation to hypothermia also will be noted briefly later.

Anticonvulsant Drugs

Anticonvulsant drugs may play a neuroprotective role in addition to their anticonvulsant action (see Table 20.36). The potential role for phenobarbital administered prophylactically in infants treated with hypothermia was discussed in the section on control of seizures. A potential role for topiramate in this context, discussed in Chapter 13, and for levetiracetam was noted earlier. This potential is based on studies of experimental models of neonatal HIE, in conjunction with hypothermia, particularly by Silverstein and colleagues.[669] Topiramate is not available in parenteral form. Levetiracetam is of particular interest because the agent does not cause neuronal apoptosis in the neonatal animal; it is used for treatment of seizures in the human newborn and is available in parenteral form.

Xenon

Xenon is a potent anesthetic with a low gas partition coefficient. It crosses the blood-brain barrier easily and leads to rapid induction of anesthesia. Neuroprotective effects of xenon have been demonstrated in combination with hypothermia (see Table 20.36).[670,671] Xenon was reported to be safe for use with hypothermia in a phase II randomized study of outcomes after demonstration of similar results as cooling therapy alone.[672] An open-label randomized controlled trial of 92 infants (46 assigned to hypothermia alone, and 46 to hypothermia and xenon therapy) showed no significant differences in lactate/NAA ratio in the thalamus or fractional anisotropy in the posterior limb of the internal capsule.[673] The investigators concluded that administration of xenon "is unlikely to enhance the neuroprotective effect of cooling after birth asphyxia."[673]

Antioxidants—N-Acetylcysteine, Allopurinol

Because oxidative stress is an important mechanism of neonatal hypoxic-ischemic brain injury (see Chapters 13 and 19), agents with antioxidant properties might be anticipated to be useful in neuroprotection. Experimental studies of hypoxia-ischemia in the neonatal rat support this possibility.[674] N-*acetylcysteine* in combination with hypothermia was particularly beneficial. Potential value for *N*-acetylcysteine is supported by its ability to cross the blood-brain barrier and relative safety. Data in human infants treated with hypothermia would be of interest.

Allopurinol, a xanthine oxidase inhibitor and free radical scavenger, has neuroprotective properties. Data from one report suggested a beneficial effect of allopurinol therapy on free radical formation (measured by the assay of markers in plasma), cerebral hemodynamics (measured by near-infrared spectroscopy), and electrical brain activity (measured by a cerebral function monitor). Short-term outcome (death, neurological abnormalities at discharge) tended to be more favorable in the treated infants, but the difference did not achieve statistical significance.[675] A later study also suggested the benefit for allopurinol in asphyxiated term infants.[676] In 2014, a large trial of *maternal treatment* with allopurinol during fetal hypoxia did not significantly lower neuronal damage markers in umbilical cord blood. However, post hoc analysis revealed a potential benefit in the treatment of females (NCT00189007).[677] Several underpowered clinical trials suggest modest benefit of allopurinol in neonatal HIE.[675,678,679] Whether allopurinol could enhance the benefit of hypothermia is unknown but perhaps worthy of study.

Melatonin

Melatonin (*N*-acetyl-5-methoxytryptamine) is an endogenous indolamine that has shown promising effects in the treatment of HIE. It has antioxidant, antiinflammatory, and antiapoptotic properties.[680] Melatonin freely crosses the blood-brain barrier. In an animal model of neonatal asphyxia melatonin has been shown to protect the brain independently[681] or in concert with therapeutic hypothermia.[682] Aly and colleagues demonstrated in a small pilot study of infants with moderate to severe HIE that the combination of melatonin and therapeutic hypothermia was efficacious in reducing oxidative stress and improved survival with favorable neurodevelopmental outcome at 6 months of age.[683] Optimal dose, route, and duration of administration still need to be delineated.

Erythropoietin

Erythropoietin (EPO) has been investigated as a neuroprotective strategy for both term and preterm infants. EPO is a glycoprotein shown to be involved in the adaptive response to perinatal hypoxia-ischemia and to exhibit neuroprotective properties.[684-686] The principal sequence of adaptive events is the induction by hypoxia of a hypoxia-inducible factor, a transcription factor, that then leads to increased expression of EPO and its receptor in neurons, astrocytes, oligodendroglia, microglia, and endothelial cells. The principal neuroprotective mechanisms involve antiexcitotoxic, antioxidant, antiinflammatory, and antiapoptotic effects (see Chapter 13). Numerous experimental studies of neonatal hypoxia-ischemia have shown reductions in brain injury with administration of EPO.[687,688] Neuroprotective effects in animal models have been shown by treatment *after* as well as before the hypoxic-ischemic insult. Moreover, although EPO is a 34-kDa glycoprotein, it has been beneficial after *systemic* administration. Two clinical trials in human infants with HIE, before the era of hypothermia treatment, suggested a beneficial effect of EPO treatment (for 5 days or 14 days) on neurological outcome.[689,690]

The possibility that EPO might have an added or even synergistic neuroprotective effect when combined with hypothermia is suggested in part by the broad spectrum of deleterious mechanisms blunted by these two modalities. Initial studies in experimental models provided inconsistent results.[691,692] However, a small phase 1 trial (*n* = 24) suggested benefit for the addition of EPO to hypothermia for HIE.[693] Moreover, a later phase II trial (*n* = 50) of EPO administered in the first week in combination with hypothermia treatment appeared to result in less MRI brain injury and improved 1 year motor function.[694] The potential of more prolonged EPO treatment with a longer dosing interval is suggested by a recent safety trial of darbopoietin, an EPO-derived molecule with an extended circulating half-life.[695]

Currently there are two active clinical trials (NCT01913340 and NCT01732146) examining EPO in combination with hypothermia in infants with HIE. The "Neonatal Erythropoietin and Therapeutic Hypothermia Outcomes in Newborn Brain Injury" study (NCT01913340) assesses an EPO dose of 1000 U/kg per dose IV × 5 doses, while the "Efficacy of Erythropoietin to Improve Survival and Neurological Outcome in Hypoxic Ischemic Encephalopathy" study (NCT01732146) evaluates

intravenous erythropoietin at 1000 to 1500 U/kg per dose three times every 24 hours with the first dose within 12 hours of delivery. The outcomes of these trials are awaited before incorporation of this neuroprotective approach as complementary to therapeutic hypothermia.

The possibility should be considered that prolonged EPO therapy could be effective in *reparative, restorative* mechanisms after the initial hypoxic-ischemic injury. Thus, EPO not only has neuroprotective properties but also promotes neurogenesis, oligodendroglial development and angiogenesis (see Chapters 13 and 16). Prolonged EPO treatment perhaps could be useful for recovery/restoration after neuronal and white matter injury. The availability of an agent like darbopoietin (see earlier) with a prolonged circulatory half-life and longer dosing intervals could be valuable in this context.

Magnesium

Magnesium sulfate has been used for many years in obstetrics as a tocolytic agent for preterm labor and as therapy for preeclampsia. The evidence of its effectiveness for the latter purpose is stronger than that for its role as a tocolytic. Although magnesium has been shown to be neuroprotective in some animal models of neonatal HIE, the data are inconsistent.[696] Similarly, data are not consistent for a beneficial role for antenatal magnesium in prevention of preterm brain injury. Tagin and colleagues in a recent meta-analysis of all available trial data demonstrated that there is insufficient evidence to determine if magnesium therapy given shortly after birth to newborns with HIE reduces death or moderate-to-severe disability.[697] Currently, an ongoing phase III clinical trial (NCT01646619) is assessing whether the addition of magnesium sulfate to therapeutic hypothermia for infants who are asphyxiated at birth provides additional benefit to survival and outcomes compared to cooling alone.

Calcium Channel Blockers

Because a central mediator of the cascade to neuronal death is elevated cytosolic calcium, caused in part by enhanced calcium influx, the possibility of a protective effect of calcium channel blockers has been investigated. Experimental studies show some benefit (see Chapter 13). However, a single small study of a calcium channel blocker in the treatment of severely asphyxiated infants indicated that further understanding of the toxicity of these agents is necessary before a beneficial effect can be expected.[698] We are unaware of any current studies of the use of calcium channel blockers in asphyxiated human infants.

Stem Cell Therapy

A potential role for stem cell therapy for neuroprotection and neurorestoration in neonatal HIE is suggested by recent experimental observations (see Table 20.36). Such a role in the treatment of cerebral white matter injury in premature infants and in term infants with neonatal arterial ischemic stroke is discussed in Chapters 16 and 21. In the context of neonatal HIE the principal agents studied in experimental models have been human cord blood, multipotent stem cells and progenitor cells, and neural stem cells.[699] Although results are not entirely consistent, generally beneficial effects have been documented. Cord blood is an excellent source of stem and progenitor cells. Experimental studies show that infusion of human cord blood in the first 24 hours after hypoxia–ischemia or at 7 days has led to variable benefit, most often functional.[700-704] The benefit likely relates not to the major engraftment of cells but rather to antiapoptotic and antiinflammatory effects and perhaps trophic effects on endogenous cells. The administration of autologous, volume- and red-blood-cell-reduced human cord blood to human infants appears to be safe and feasible[699] and has been proposed for use in conjunction with hypothermia treatment. Although multiple issues require resolution (e.g., timing, dose, and duration), this avenue of therapy should be explored in carefully designed, controlled trials. An initial trial by Cotten and co-workers of autologous cord blood infusion in term infants with HIE is underway (NCT00593242).[705]

Other Pharmacological Agents

Experimental studies suggest potential neuroprotective roles in neonatal HIE for a variety of other agents, including caspase inhibitors, IGF-1, cannabinoids, and osteopontin (see Table 20.36).[706-712] No trials in human infants are available.

Conclusions

The prospective studies of the *individual* agents and interventions discussed in the preceding sections and those likely to be evaluated in the future based on experimental data are necessary and appropriate. However, it seems likely that *combinations* of agents, including those that affect different levels of the cascade to cell death described in Chapter 13, will prove optimal. Moreover, such combinations may include *sequential* administration, beginning intrapartum and continuing postnatally. Approaches that are likely to affect common initiating mechanisms (e.g., cerebrovascular autoregulation, cerebral ischemia), as well as common downstream mechanisms (e.g., excitotoxicity, free radical attack, inflammation, apoptosis, especially at multiple sites), will have particular value because both neuronal and oligodendroglial injury could be ameliorated. *Mild hypothermia* is now an established approach. Agents that potentiate the effect of hypothermia remain crucial topics for future research. Subsequent to or concomitant with the initial phase of neuroprotection, the institution of neurorestorative therapies (e.g., erythropoietin, human cord blood transplantation) may be critical for reparative and regenerative processes.

KEY REFERENCES

1. Shah P, Anvekar A, McMichael J, et al. Outcomes of infants with Apgar score of zero at 10 min: the West Australian experience. *Arch Dis Child Fetal Neonatal Ed.* 2015;100:F492-F494.
2. Nelson KB, Leviton A. How much of neonatal encephalopathy is due to birth asphyxia? *Am J Dis Child.* 1991;145:1325-1331.
3. Edwards AD, Nelson KB. Neonatal encephalopathies. Time to reconsider the cause of encephalopathies. *BMJ.* 1998;317:1537-1538.
4. Pierrat V, Haouari N, Liska A, et al. Prevalence, causes, and outcome at 2 years of age of newborn encephalopathy: population based study. *Arch Dis Child.* 2005;90:F257-F261.
5. Nelson KB, Bingham P, Edwards EM, et al. Antecedents of neonatal encephalopathy in the Vermont Oxford Network Encephalopathy Registry. *Pediatrics.* 2012;130:878-886.
6. Jenster M, Bonifacio SL, Ruel T, et al. Maternal or neonatal infection: association with neonatal encephalopathy outcomes. *Pediatr Res.* 2014;76:93-99.
7. Adamson SJ, Alessandri LM, Badawi N, et al. Predictors of neonatal encephalopathy in full-term infants. *BMJ.* 1995;311:598-602.
9. Nelson DB, Lucke AM, McIntire DD, et al. Obstetric antecedents to body-cooling treatment of the newborn infant. *Am J Obstet Gynecol.* 2014;211:155. e151-e156.
10. Okereafor A, Allsop J, Counsell SJ, et al. Patterns of brain injury in neonates exposed to perinatal sentinel events. *Pediatrics.* 2008;101:906-914.
51. Nelson KB, Ellenberg JH. Obstetric complications as risk factors for cerebral palsy or seizure disorders. *JAMA.* 1984;251:1843-1848.
57. Wyckoff MH, Aziz K, Escobedo MB, et al. Part 13: neonatal resuscitation: 2015 American Heart Association guidelines update for cardiopulmonary resuscitation and emergency cardiovascular care. *Circulation.* 2015;132:S543-S560.
58. Wu YW, Backstrand KH, Zhao S, et al. Declining diagnosis of birth asphyxia in California: 1991-2000. *Pediatrics.* 2004;114:1584-1590.
59. Lee AC, Kozuki N, Blencowe H, et al. Intrapartum-related neonatal encephalopathy incidence and impairment at regional and global levels for 2010 with trends from 1990. *Pediatr Res.* 2013;74(suppl 1):50-72.
64. Shah P, Riphagen S, Beyene J, et al. Multiorgan dysfunction in infants with post-asphyxial hypoxic-ischaemic encephalopathy. *Arch Dis Child.* 2004;89:152-155.
67. Amiel-Tison C. A method for neurological evaluation within the first year of life: experience with full-term newborn infants with birth injury. *Ciba Found Symp.* 1978;59:107-137.
68. Thompson CM, Puterman AS, Linley LL, et al. The value of a scoring system for hypoxic ischaemic encephalopathy in predicting neurodevelopmental outcome. *Acta Paediatr.* 1997;86:757-761.
69. Dubowitz L, Ricci WD, Mercuri E. The Dubowitz neurological examination of the full-term newborn. *Ment Retard Dev Disabil Res Rev.* 2005;11:52-60.
70. Sarnat HB, Sarnat MS. Neonatal encephalopathy following fetal distress. A clinical and electroencephalographic study. *Arch Neurol.* 1976;33:696-705.
72. Perez JM, Golombek SG, Sola A. Clinical hypoxic–ischemic encephalopathy Score of the Iberoamerican Society of Neonatology (SIBEN): a new proposal for diagnosis and management. *Rev Assoc Med Bras.* 2017;63:64-69.
78. Nagarajan L, Palumbo L, Ghosh S. Classification of clinical semiology in epileptic seizures in neonates. *Eur J Paediatr Neurol.* 2012;16:118-125.
80. Biselele T, Naulaers G, Tady B. Evolution of the Thompson score during the first 6 h in infants with perinatal asphyxia. *Acta Paediatr.* 2014;103:145-148.
116. Kumar A, Mittal R, Khanna HD, et al. Free radical injury and blood-brain barrier permeability in hypoxic–ischemic encephalopathy. *Pediatrics.* 2008;122:e722-e727.
155. Roka A, Kelen D, Halasz J, et al. Serum S100B and neuron-specific enolase levels in normothermic and hypothermic infants after perinatal asphyxia. *Acta Paediatr.* 2012;101:319-323.
192. de Vries LS, Hellstrom-Westas L. Role of cerebral function monitoring in the newborn. *Arch Dis Child.* 2005;90:F201-F207.
196. Shany E, Goldstein E, Khvatskin S, et al. Predictive value of amplitude-integrated electroencephalography pattern and voltage in asphyxiated term infants. *Pediatr Neurol.* 2006;35:335-342.
200. Hallberg B, Grossmann K, Bartocci M, et al. The prognostic value of early aEEG in asphyxiated infants undergoing systemic hypothermia treatment. *Acta Paediatr.* 2010;99:531-536.
201. Azzopardi D, Toby Study Group. Predictive value of the amplitude integrated EEG in infants with hypoxic ischaemic encephalopathy: data from a randomised trial of therapeutic hypothermia. *Arch Dis Child Fetal Neonatal Ed.* 2014;99:F80-F82.
204. Shellhaas RA, Chang T, Tsuchida T, et al. The American Clinical Neurophysiology Society's Guideline on continuous electroencephalography monitoring in neonates. *J Clin Neurophysiol.* 2011;28:611-617.
205. Lynch NE, Stevenson NJ, Livingstone V, et al. The temporal evolution of electrographic seizure burden in neonatal hypoxic ischemic encephalopathy. *Epilepsia.* 2012;53:549-557.
207. Committee on Fetus and Newborn, Papile LA, Baley JE, et al. Hypothermia and neonatal encephalopathy. *Pediatrics.* 2014;133:1146-1150.
225. Barnette AR, Horbar JD, Soll RF, et al. Neuroimaging in the evaluation of neonatal encephalopathy. *Pediatrics.* 2014;133:e1508-e1517.

229. Chau V, Poskitt KJ, Sargent MA, et al. Comparison of computer tomography and magnetic resonance imaging scans on the third day of life in term newborns with neonatal encephalopathy. *Pediatrics.* 2009;123:319-326.

230. Glass HC, Bonifacio SL, Shimotake T, et al. Neurocritical care for neonates. *Curr Treat Options Neurol.* 2011;13:574-589.

241. Rutherford M, Pennock J, Schwieso J, et al. Hypoxic-ischaemic encephalopathy: early and late magnetic resonance imaging findings in relation to outcome. *Arch Dis Child.* 1996;75:F145-F151.

242. Mercuri E, Cowan F, Rutherford M, et al. Ischaemic and haemorrhagic brain lesions in newborns with seizures and normal Apgar scores. *Arch Dis Child.* 1995;73:F67-F74.

251. Rutherford M. *MRI of the Neonatal Brain.* Philadelphia: WB Saunders; 2002.

259. Barkovich AJ. *Pediatric Neuroimaging.* 4th ed. Philadelphia: Lippincott Williams & Wilkins; 2005.

261. Gano D, Chau V, Poskitt KJ, et al. Evolution of pattern of injury and quantitative MRI on days 1 and 3 in term newborns with hypoxic–ischemic encephalopathy. *Pediatr Res.* 2013;74:82-87.

262. Srinivasakumar P, Zempel J, Wallendorf M, et al. Therapeutic hypothermia in neonatal hypoxic ischemic encephalopathy: electrographic seizures and magnetic resonance imaging evidence of injury. *J Pediatr.* 2013;163:465-470.

263. Cavalleri F, Lugli L, Pugliese M, et al. Prognostic value of diffusion-weighted imaging summation scores or apparent diffusion coefficient maps in newborns with hypoxic–ischemic encephalopathy. *Pediatr Radiol.* 2014;44:1141-1154.

264. Agut T, Leon M, Rebollo M, et al. Early identification of brain injury in infants with hypoxic ischemic encephalopathy at high risk for severe impairments: accuracy of MRI performed in the first days of life. *BMC Pediatr.* 2014;14:177.

265. Chalak LF, Sanchez PJ, Adams-Huet B, et al. Biomarkers for severity of neonatal hypoxic–ischemic encephalopathy and outcomes in newborns receiving hypothermia therapy. *J Pediatr.* 2014;164:468-474. e461.

267. Ryan ME. MRI predicts outcome after HIE treated with hypothermia. *Pediatr Neurol Briefs.* 2015;29:11.

272. Groenendaal F, de Vries LS. Fifty years of brain imaging in neonatal encephalopathy following perinatal asphyxia. *Pediatr Res.* 2017;81:150-155.

275. Martinez-Biarge M, Diez-Sebastian J, Rutherford MA, et al. Outcomes after central grey matter injury in term perinatal hypoxic-ischaemic encephalopathy. *Early Hum Dev.* 2010;86:675-682.

276. Martinez-Biarge M, Diez-Sebastian J, Kapellou O, et al. Predicting motor outcome and death in term hypoxic–ischemic encephalopathy. *Neurology.* 2011;76:2055-2061.

277. Barkovich AJ, Westmark K, Partridge C, et al. Perinatal asphyxia: MR findings in the first 10 days. *AJNR Am J Neuroradiol.* 1995;16:427-438.

279. Rutherford M, Counsell S, Allsop J, et al. Diffusion-weighted magnetic resonance imaging in term perinatal brain injury: a comparison with site of lesion and time from birth. *Pediatrics.* 2004;114:1004-1014.

281. de Vries LS, Cowan FM. Evolving understanding of hypoxic-ischemic encephalopathy in the term infant. *Semin Pediatr Neurol.* 2009;16:216-225.

282. Volpe JJ. Neonatal encephalopathy: an inadequate term for hypoxic–ischemic encephalopathy. *Ann Neurol.* 2012;72:156-166.

298. McKinstry RC, Miller JH, Snyder AZ, et al. A prospective, longitudinal diffusion tensor imaging study of brain injury in newborns. *Neurology.* 2002;59:824-833.

299. De Vries LS, Van der Grond J, Van Haastert IC, et al. Prediction of outcome in new-born infants with arterial ischaemic stroke using diffusion-weighted magnetic resonance imaging. *Neuropediatrics.* 2005;36:12-20.

300. Miller SP. Newborn brain injury: looking back to the fetus. *Ann Neurol.* 2007;61:285-287.

303. Bednarek N, Mathur A, Inder T, et al. Impact of therapeutic hypothermia on MRI diffusion changes in neonatal encephalopathy. *Neurology.* 2012;78:1420-1427.

305. Hope PL, Costello AM, Cady EB, et al. Cerebral energy metabolism studied with phosphorus NMR spectroscopy in normal and birth-asphyxiated infants. *Lancet.* 1984;2:366-370.

328. Barkovich AJ, Baranski K, Vigneron D, et al. Proton MR spectroscopy for the evaluation of brain injury in asphyxiated, term neonates. *AJNR Am J Neuroradiol.* 1999;20:1399-1405.

329. Groenendaal F, RoelantsvanRijn AM, vanderGrond J, et al. Glutamate in cerebral tissue of asphyxiated neonates during the first week of life demonstrated in vivo using proton magnetic resonance spectroscopy. *Biol Neonate.* 2001;79:254-257.

332. Roelants-Van Rijn AM, Van Der Grond J, De Vries LS, et al. Value of ^{1}H-MRS using different echo times in neonates with cerebral hypoxia-ischemia. *Pediatr Res.* 2001;49:356-362.

333. Miller SP, Newton N, Ferriero DM, et al. Predictors of 30-month outcome after perinatal depression: role of proton MRS and socioeconomic factors. *Pediatr Res.* 2002;52:71-77.

334. Bartha AI, Foster-Barber A, Miller SP, et al. Neonatal encephalopathy: association of cytokines with MR spectroscopy and outcome. *Pediatr Res.* 2004;56:960-966.

335. Miller SP, Weiss J, Barnwell A, et al. Seizure-associated brain injury in term newborns with perinatal asphyxia. *Neurology.* 2002;58:542-548.

340. Zhu W, Zhong W, Qi J, et al. Proton magnetic resonance spectroscopy in neonates with hypoxic-ischemic injury and its prognostic value. *Transl Res.* 2008;152:225-232.

343. Degraeuwe P, Jaspers GJ, Robertson NJ, et al. Magnetic resonance spectroscopy as a prognostic marker in neonatal hypoxic–ischemic encephalopathy: a study protocol for an individual patient data meta-analysis. *Syst Rev.* 2013;2:96.

344. Wisnowski JL, Wu TW, Reitman AJ, et al. The effects of therapeutic hypothermia on cerebral metabolism in neonates with hypoxic–ischemic encephalopathy: an in vivo 1H-MR spectroscopy study. *J Cereb Blood Flow Metab.* 2016;36:1075-1086.

366. Lou HC, Rosa P, Pryds O, et al. ADHD: increased dopamine receptor availability linked to attention deficit and low neonatal cerebral blood flow. *Dev Med Child Neurol.* 2004;46:179-183.

367. Sugama S, Ariga M, Hoashi E, et al. Brainstem cranial-nerve lesions in an infant with hypoxic cerebral injury. *Pediatr Neurol.* 2003;29:256-259.

383. Hagberg B, Hagberg G, Olow I. The changing panorama of cerebral palsy in Sweden 1954-1970. I. Analysis of the general changes. *Acta Paediatr Scand.* 1975;64:187-192.

385. Rosenbloom L. Dyskinetic cerebral palsy and birth asphyxia. *Dev Med Child Neurol.* 1994;36:285-289.

386. Barnett A, Mercuri E, Rutherford M, et al. Neurological and perceptual-motor outcome at 5–6 years of age in children with neonatal encephalopathy: relationship with neonatal brain MRI. *Neuropediatrics.* 2002;33:242-248.

387. de Vries LS, Pierrat V, Eken P, et al. Prognostic value of early somatosensory evoked potentials for adverse outcome in full-term infants with birth asphyxia. *Brain Dev.* 1991;13:320-325.

428. Amiel-Tison C, Ellison P. Birth asphyxia in the fullterm newborn: early assessment and outcome. *Dev Med Child Neurol.* 1986;28:671-682.

429. Nelson KB, Ellenberg JH. The asymptomatic newborn and risk of cerebral palsy. *Am J Dis Child.* 1987;141:1333-1335.

430. Ellenberg JH, Nelson KB. Cluster of perinatal events identifying infants at high risk for death or disability. *J Pediatr.* 1988;113:546-552.

432. Ishikawa T, Ogawa Y, Kanayama M, et al. Long-term prognosis of asphyxiated full-term neonates with CNS complications. *Brain Dev.* 1987;9:48-53.

439. Caravale B, Allemand F, Libenson MH. Factors predictive of seizures and neurologic outcome in perinatal depression. *Pediatr Neurol.* 2003;29:18-25.

441. Badawi N, Felix JF, Kurinezuk JF, et al. Cerebral palsy following term newborn encephalopathy: a population-based study. *Dev Med Child Neurol.* 2005;47:293-298.

442. Miller SP, Latal B, Clark H, et al. Clinical signs predict 30-month neurodevelopmental outcome after neonatal encephalopathy. *Am J Obstet Gynecol.* 2004;190:93-99.

443. Miller SP, Ferriero DM, Leonard C, et al. Early brain injury in premature newborns detected with magnetic resonance imaging is associated with adverse early neurodevelopmental outcome. *J Pediatr.* 2005;147:609-616.

446. Van Kooij BJ, Van Handel M, Uiterwaal CS, et al. Corpus callosum size in relation to motor performance in 9- to 10-year-old

children with neonatal encephalopathy. *Pediatr Res.* 2008;63:103-108.

448. van Handel M, de Sonneville L, de Vries LS, et al. Specific memory impairment following neonatal encephalopathy in term-born children. *Dev Neuropsychol.* 2012;37:30-50.

457. Murray DM, Boylan GB, Ryan CA, et al. Early EEG findings in hypoxic–ischemic encephalopathy predict outcomes at 2 years. *Pediatrics.* 2009;124:e459-e467.

458. Hellstrom-Westas L, Rosen I. Continuous brain-function monitoring: state of the art in clinical practice. *Semin Fetal Neonatal Med.* 2006;11:503-511.

459. Hellstrom-Westas L. Monitoring brain function with aEEG in term asphyxiated infants before and during cooling. *Acta Paediatr.* 2013;102:678-679.

473. Vermeulen RJ, van Schie PE, Hendrikx L, et al. Diffusion-weighted and conventional MR imaging in neonatal hypoxic ischemia: two-year follow-up study. *Radiology.* 2008;249:631-639.

474. Rutherford M, Malamateniou C, McGuinness A, et al. Magnetic resonance imaging in hypoxic-ischaemic encephalopathy. *Early Hum Dev.* 2010;86:351-360.

475. Alderliesten T, de Vries LS, Benders MJ, et al. MR imaging and outcome of term neonates with perinatal asphyxia: value of diffusion-weighted MR imaging and (1)H MR spectroscopy. *Radiology.* 2011;261:235-242.

476. Rutherford M, Ramenghi LA, Edwards AD, et al. Assessment of brain tissue injury after moderate hypothermia in neonates with hypoxic-ischaemic encephalopathy: a nested substudy of a randomised controlled trial. *Lancet Neurol.* 2010;9:39-45.

477. Cheong JL, Coleman L, Hunt RW, et al. Prognostic utility of magnetic resonance imaging in neonatal hypoxic–ischemic encephalopathy: substudy of a randomized trial. *Arch Pediatr Adolesc Med.* 2012;166:634-640.

482. Corbo ET, Bartnik-Olson BL, Machado S, et al. The effect of whole-body cooling on brain metabolism following perinatal hypoxic–ischemic injury. *Pediatr Res.* 2012;71:85-92.

483. Ancora G, Testa C, Grandi S, et al. Prognostic value of brain proton MR spectroscopy and diffusion tensor imaging in newborns with hypoxic–ischemic encephalopathy treated by brain cooling. *Neuroradiology.* 2013;55:1017-1025.

484. Flodmark O, Becker LE, Harwood-Nash DC, et al. Correlation between computed tomography and autopsy in premature and full-term neonates that have suffered perinatal asphyxia. *Radiology.* 1980;137:93-103.

497. Jongeling BR, Badawi N, Kurinczuk JJ, et al. Cranial ultrasound as a predictor of outcome in term newborn encephalopathy. *Pediatr Neurol.* 2002;26:37-42.

503. Ancora G, Maranella E, Grandi S, et al. Early predictors of short term neurodevelopmental outcome in asphyxiated cooled infants. A combined brain amplitude integrated electroencephalography and near infrared spectroscopy study. *Brain Dev.* 2013;35:26-31.

504. Lemmers PM, Zwanenburg RJ, Benders MJ, et al. Cerebral oxygenation and brain activity after perinatal asphyxia: does hypothermia change their prognostic value? *Pediatr Res.* 2013;74:180-185.

514. Kapadia VS, Chalak LF, Dupont TL, et al. Perinatal asphyxia with hyperoxemia within the first hour of life is associated with moderate to severe hypoxic–ischemic encephalopathy. *J Pediatr.* 2013;163:949-954.

515. Saugstad OD, Ramji S, Irani SF, et al. Resuscitation of newborn infants with 21% or 100% oxygen: follow-up at 18 to 24 months. *Pediatrics.* 2003;112:296-300.

516. Vento M, Asensi M, Sastre J, et al. Resuscitation with room air instead of 100% oxygen prevents oxidative stress in moderately asphyxiated term neonates. *Pediatrics.* 2001;107:642-647.

522. Rabi Y, Rabi D, Yee W. Room air resuscitation of the depressed newborn: a systematic review and meta-analysis. *Resuscitation.* 2007;72:353-363.

523. Solberg R, Longini M, Proietti F, et al. Resuscitation with supplementary oxygen induces oxidative injury in the cerebral cortex. *Free Radic Biol Med.* 2012;53:1061-1067.

524. Perlman JM, Wyllie J, Kattwinkel J, et al. Part 7: Neonatal Resuscitation: 2015 International Consensus on Cardiopulmonary Resuscitation and Emergency Cardiovascular Care Science With Treatment Recommendations. *Circulation.* 2015;132:S204-S241.

525. Roberts BW, Karagiannis P, Coletta M, et al. Effects of $PaCO_2$ derangements on clinical outcomes after cerebral injury: a systematic review. *Resuscitation.* 2015;91:32-41.

532. Kaiser JR, Gauss CH, Williams DK. The effects of hypercapnia on cerebral autoregulation in ventilated very low birth weight infants. *Pediatr Res.* 2005;58:931-935.

535. Davis SM, Ackerman RH, Correia JA, et al. Cerebral blood flow and cerebrovascular CO_2 reactivity in stroke-age normal controls. *Neurology.* 1983;33:391-399.

546. Kamei A, Ozaki T, Takashima S. Monitoring of the intracranial hemodynamics and oxygenation during and after hyperventilation in newborn rabbits with near-infrared spectroscopy. *Pediatr Res.* 1994;35:334-338.

548. Vannucci RC, Brucklacher RM, Vannucci SJ. Effect of carbon dioxide on cerebral metabolism during hypoxia-ischemia in the immature rat. *Pediatr Res.* 1997;42:24-29.

551. Pryds O, Greisen G. Effect of P_aCO_2 and haemoglobin concentration on day to day variation of CBF in preterm neonates. *Acta Paediatr Scand Suppl.* 1989;360:33-36.

554. Pryds O, Edwards AD. Cerebral blood flow in the newborn infant. *Arch Dis Child.* 1996;74:F63-F69.

556. Pappas A, Shankaran S, Laptook AR, et al. Hypocarbia and adverse outcome in neonatal hypoxic–ischemic encephalopathy. *J Pediatr.* 2011;158:752-758 e751.

557. Nadeem M, Murray D, Boylan G, et al. Blood carbon dioxide levels and adverse outcome in neonatal hypoxic–ischemic encephalopathy. *Am J Perinatol.* 2010;27:361-365.

570. Hegyi T, Anwar M, Carbone MT, et al. Blood pressure ranges in premature infants: II. The first week of life. *Pediatrics.* 1996;97:336-342.

571. Watkins AM, West CR, Cooke RW. Blood pressure and cerebral haemorrhage and ischaemia in very low birthweight infants. *Early Hum Dev.* 1989;19:103-110.

572. Laughon M, Bose C, Allred E, et al. Factors associated with treatment for hypotension in extremely low gestational age newborns during the first postnatal week. *Pediatrics.* 2007;119:273-280.

584. Giesinger RE, Bailey LJ, Deshpande P, et al. Hypoxic–ischemic encephalopathy and therapeutic hypothermia: the hemodynamic perspective. *J Pediatr.* 2017;180:22-30.e22.

585. Weindling AM, Bentham J. Commentary on "blood pressure in the neonate". *Acta Paediatr.* 2005;94:138-140.

588. Paradisis M, Evans N, Kuckow M, et al. Pilot study of milrinone for low systemic blood flow in very preterm infants. *J Pediatr.* 2006;148:306-313.

592. Al Yazidi G, Boudes E, Tan X, et al. Intraventricular hemorrhage in asphyxiated newborns treated with hypothermia: a look into incidence, timing and risk factors. *BMC Pediatr.* 2015;15:106.

593. Basu P, Som S, Choudhuri N, et al. Contribution of the blood glucose level in perinatal asphyxia. *Eur J Pediatr.* 2009;168:833-838.

596. Nadeem M, Murray DM, Boylan GB, et al. Early blood glucose profile and neurodevelopmental outcome at two years in neonatal hypoxic-ischaemic encephalopathy. *BMC Pediatr.* 2011;11:10.

597. Tam EW, Haeusslein LA, Bonifacio SL, et al. Hypoglycemia is associated with increased risk for brain injury and adverse neurodevelopmental outcome in neonates at risk for encephalopathy. *J Pediatr.* 2012;161:88-93.

598. Inder T. How low can I go? The impact of hypoglycemia on the immature brain. *Pediatrics.* 2008;122:440-441.

599. Boardman JP, Hawdon JM. Hypoglycaemia and hypoxic-ischaemic encephalopathy. *Dev Med Child Neurol.* 2015;57(suppl 3):29-33.

601. Gluckman PD, Wyatt JS, Azzopardi D, et al. Selective head cooling with mild systemic hypothermia after neonatal encephalopathy: multicentre randomised trial. *Lancet.* 2005;365:663-670.

607. Glass HC, Hong KJ, Rogers EE, et al. Risk factors for epilepsy in children with neonatal encephalopathy. *Pediatr Res.* 2011;70:535-540.

608. Glass HC, Nash KB, Bonifacio SL, et al. Seizures and magnetic resonance imaging-detected brain injury in newborns cooled for hypoxic–ischemic encephalopathy. *J Pediatr.* 2011;159:731-735.e731.

612. McBride MC, Laroia N, Guillet R. Electrographic seizures in neonates correlate with poor neurodevelopmental outcome. *Neurology.* 2000;55:506-513.

637. Pressler RM, Boylan GB, Marlow N, et al. Bumetanide for the treatment of seizures in newborn babies with hypoxic ischaemic encephalopathy (NEMO): an open-label, dose finding, and feasibility phase 1/2 trial. *Lancet Neurol.* 2015;14:469-477.

638. Gunn AJ, Gluckman PD, Gunn TR. Selective head cooling in newborn infants after perinatal asphyxia: a safety study. *Pediatrics.* 1998;102:885-892.

639. Azzopardi D, Robertson NJ, Cowan FM, et al. Pilot study of treatment with whole body hypothermia for neonatal encephalopathy. *Pediatrics.* 2000;106:684-694.

640. Battin MR, Dezoete A, Gunn TR, et al. Neurodevelopmental outcome of infants treated with head cooling and mild hypothermia after perinatal asphyxia. *Pediatrics.* 2001;107:480-484.

641. Battin MR, Penrice J, Gunn TR, et al. Treatment of term infants with head cooling and mild systemic hypothermia (34.5°C) after perinatal asphyxia. *Pediatrics.* 2003;111:244-251.

642. Eicher DJ, Wagner CL, Katikaneni LP, et al. Moderate hypothermia in neonatal encephalopathy: efficacy outcomes. *Pediatr Neurol.* 2005;32:11-17.

644. Higgins RD, Raju TN, Perlman J, et al. Hypothermia and perinatal asphyxia: executive summary of the National Institute of Child Health and Human Development workshop. *J Pediatr.* 2006;148:170-175.

645. Edwards AD, Azzopardi DV. Therapeutic hypothermia following perinatal asphyxia. *Arch Dis Child Fetal Neonatal Ed.* 2006;91: F127-F131.

646. Wyatt JS, Gluckman PD, Liu PY, et al. Determinants of outcomes after head cooling for neonatal encephalopathy. *Pediatrics.* 2007; 119:912-921.

647. Azzopardi DV, Strohm B, Edwards AD, et al. Moderate hypothermia to treat perinatal asphyxial encephalopathy. *N Engl J Med.* 2009;361:1349-1358.

648. Laptook AR. The neo.nEURO.network hypothermia randomized controlled trial. *Pediatrics.* 2010;126:e965-e966.

650. Edwards AD, Brocklehurst P, Gunn AJ, et al. Neurological outcomes at 18 months of age after moderate hypothermia for perinatal hypoxic ischaemic encephalopathy: synthesis and meta-analysis of trial data. *BMJ.* 2010;340:c363.

651. Jacobs SE, Morley CJ, Inder TE, et al. Whole-body hypothermia for term and near-term newborns with hypoxic–ischemic encephalopathy: a randomized controlled trial. *Arch Pediatr Adolesc Med.* 2011;165:692-700.

652. Thoresen M. Hypothermia after perinatal asphyxia: selection for treatment and cooling protocol. *J Pediatr.* 2011;158:e45-e49.

653. Tagin MA, Woolcott CG, Vincer MJ, et al. Hypothermia for neonatal hypoxic ischemic encephalopathy: an updated systematic review and meta-analysis. *Arch Pediatr Adolesc Med.* 2012;166:558-566.

655. Azzopardi D, Strohm B, Marlow N, et al. Effects of hypothermia for perinatal asphyxia on childhood outcomes. *N Engl J Med.* 2014;371:140-149.

656. Zhou WH, Cheng GQ, Shao XM, et al. Selective head cooling with mild systemic hypothermia after neonatal hypoxic–ischemic encephalopathy: a multicenter randomized controlled trial in China. *J Pediatr.* 2010;157:367-372, 372 e361-e363.

659. Dupont TL, Chalak LF, Morriss MC, et al. Short-term outcomes of newborns with perinatal acidemia who are not eligible for systemic hypothermia therapy. *J Pediatr.* 2013;162:35-41.

672. Dingley J, Tooley J, Liu X, et al. Xenon ventilation during therapeutic hypothermia in neonatal encephalopathy: a feasibility study. *Pediatrics.* 2014;133:809-818.

679. Kaandorp JJ, van Bel F, Veen S, et al. Long-term neuroprotective effects of allopurinol after moderate perinatal asphyxia: follow-up of two randomised controlled trials. *Arch Dis Child Fetal Neonatal Ed.* 2012;97:F162-F166.

685. Xiong T, Qu Y, Mu D, et al. Erythropoietin for neonatal brain injury: opportunity and challenge. *Int J Dev Neurosci.* 2011;29:583-591.

693. Rogers EE, Bonifacio SL, Glass HC, et al. Erythropoietin and hypothermia for hypoxic–ischemic encephalopathy. *Pediatr Neurol.* 2014;51:657-662.

694. Wu YW, Mathur AM, Chang T, et al. High-dose erythropoietin and hypothermia for hypoxic–ischemic encephalopathy: a phase II trial. *Pediatrics.* 2016;137:E20160191.

695. Baserga MC, Beachy JC, Roberts JK, et al. Darbepoetin administration to neonates undergoing cooling for encephalopathy: a safety and pharmacokinetic trial. *Pediatr Res.* 2015;78:315-322.

696. Galinsky R, Bennet L, Groenendaal F, et al. Magnesium is not consistently neuroprotective for perinatal hypoxia-ischemia in term-equivalent models in preclinical studies: a systematic review. *Dev Neurosci.* 2014;36:73-82.

707. Nijboer CH, Heijnen CJ, van der Kooij MA, et al. Targeting the p53 pathway to protect the neonatal ischemic brain. *Ann Neurol.* 2011;70:255-264.

711. Bolouri H, Savman K, Wang W, et al. Innate defense regulator peptide 1018 protects against perinatal brain injury. *Ann Neurol.* 2014;75:395-410.

Full references for this chapter can be found on www.expertconsult .com.

Stroke in the Newborn

Terrie E. Inder ◆ Joseph J. Volpe

The presentation and etiologies of stroke in the newborn differ from those of children and adults and, in many cases, remain unrecognized. Perinatal ischemic stroke has been defined as "*a group of heterogeneous conditions in which there is a focal disruption of cerebral blood flow secondary to arterial or cerebral venous thrombosis or embolization, between 20 weeks of fetal life through twenty-eighth postnatal day confirmed by neuroimaging or neuropathologic studies.*"[1] Thus the clinical entity of ischemic perinatal stroke includes focal or multifocal ischemic injury to the central nervous system of either arterial or venous etiology that can occur during the prenatal, intrapartum, or postnatal periods. The perinatal period carries the highest risk of stroke in the pediatric age range. Stroke affects about 1 in 1600 to 4000 births, including 1 in 140 preterm births (at or before 34 weeks' gestation).[2-6] Approximately 80% of neonatal strokes are ischemic and 20% are cerebral sinovenous thrombosis (CSVT) or hemorrhage. Ischemic strokes may be arterial or venous, and arterial strokes may be due to thromboembolism or in situ thrombosis, as in older children.

CLASSIFICATION-NOMENCLATURE

Multiple subclassifications of perinatal stroke have been proposed and relate to three key factors, that is, the type of vessel affected, the timing, and the clinical presentation.[6] We will use the classification outlined in Table 21.1. Thus perinatal ischemic strokes are divided into those that are arterial or venous in origin. The former are more common and can be divided according to their time of occurrence. Prenatal/fetal arterial ischemic stroke (AIS) includes intrauterine events from approximately 20 weeks of gestation to the time of delivery. Neonatal AIS includes those exhibiting overt clinical phenomena (usually seizures) in the neonatal period (<28 days), and *presumed* perinatal AIS includes those that present clinically (usually a focal neurological deficit) at >28 days of life and with an infarct on neuroimaging consistent with a perinatal origin. In the following we discuss in sequence the Neuropathology, Pathogenesis, Clinical Features, Diagnosis, Prognosis and Management, first of Prenatal and Neonatal AIS, and then of CSVT. Presumed perinatal AIS, which presents clinically after the neonatal period, is not discussed further.

PERINATAL ARTERIAL ISCHEMIC STROKE

Neuropathology

For perinatal AIS, we include the localized areas of necrosis that occur *within the distribution of single (or multiple) major cerebral vessel or vessels*. Involvement of *specific vascular distributions* thus is the distinguishing hallmark of this lesion.

Frequency at Autopsy, Cellular Aspects, Topography

The *relative frequency* of these ischemic lesions *at autopsy* was emphasized by a neuropathological review of 592 infants examined over a 4-year period.[7] Cerebral infarcts with arterial occlusion were seen in 5.4% of infants. The incidence as a function of gestational age was 0% for infants less than 28 weeks, approximately 5% for those between 28 and 32 weeks, 10% for those between 32 and 37 weeks, and 15% for those between 37 and 40 weeks. Involvement of the middle cerebral artery (MCA) occurred in approximately one half of the affected infants (Fig. 21.1). Multiple smaller vessels were the sites of occlusion in the remaining cases. The predominance of the MCA distribution has been more marked in infants identified in vivo by brain imaging modalities (see later discussion).

The *cellular aspects of the neuropathology* of these lesions are dominated by necrosis of all cellular elements within specific arterial distributions (i.e., an infarction). The cellular features relate primarily to the time after the insult.[8-13] After 18 to 24 hours, anoxic neuronal change is apparent by light microscopy; earlier, no change may be detectable. Shortly thereafter, activated cells of the monocyte-macrophage type migrate from vessels and enter the lesion as elongated and pleomorphic microglial cells. These cells become foamy macrophages by 36 to 48 hours. Astrocytic hypertrophy, with the characteristically large, eosinophilic, sail-like cytoplasm of the gemistocytic astrocyte, becomes apparent by 3 to 5 days. Astrocytic proliferation, with prominent staining of glial acidic protein in astrocytic fibers, then forms a dense mat of glial fibrillary processes. This process occurs over weeks to months. Mineralization of neurons, sometimes with more diffuse calcification, may occur. Cavity formation is common and is discussed later.

The *topography of infarction in arterial distribution*, occurring in the perinatal period and identified in the newborn by brain imaging, is distinctive (Table 21.2).[2,14-38] Approximately 75% of lesions are unilateral, and nearly all the unilateral lesions involve the MCA. Of all *unilateral* MCA infarcts, approximately 65% involve the distribution of the left artery.

When these focal and multifocal necroses of brain of the prenatal and early postnatal periods are associated with dissolution of tissue and cavity formation, the terms *porencephaly, hydranencephaly*, and *multicystic encephalomalacia* are used to describe the lesions.[13,39-41] In this discussion, we use the term *porencephaly* to refer to a single unilateral cavity within the cerebral hemisphere that may or may not communicate with the lateral ventricle (Fig. 21.2).[42] When related to ischemia (rather than intracerebral hemorrhage or

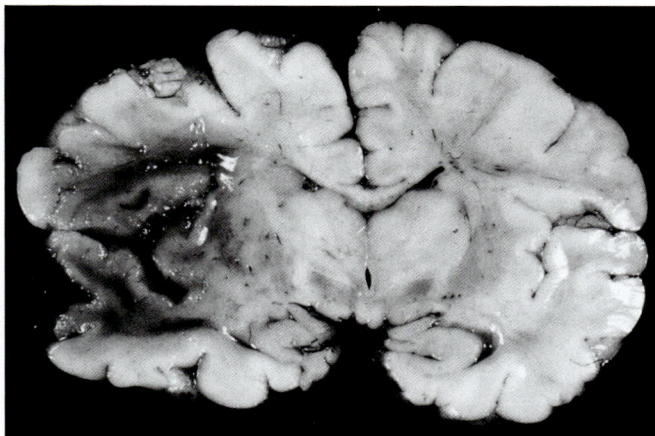

Figure 21.1 Focal ischemic brain injury. Coronal section of the cerebrum from a full-term infant with thrombosis of the left middle cerebral artery and a large ischemic infarct. The infant died 2 days after birth complicated by meconium aspiration. (From Barmada MA, Moossy J, Shuman RM. Cerebral infarcts with arterial occlusion in neonates. *Ann Neurol.* 1979;6:495–502.)

TABLE 21.1	Classification of Perinatal Ischemic Stroke

Perinatal Arterial Ischemic Stroke (AIS)
Prenatal/fetal AIS[a]
Neonatal AIS (NAIS)[a]
   Preterm
   Term
Presumed perinatal AIS
Perinatal Cerebral Sinovenous Thrombosis (CSVT)[a]

[a]Discussed in this chapter.

TABLE 21.2	Perinatal Arterial Ischemic Stroke: Topography of Infarction

TOPOGRAPHY OF INFARCTION	PERCENTAGE OF TOTAL (%)
Laterality	
Unilateral	75
Bilateral	25
Vascular distribution	
Left MCA	55
Right MCA	30
Bilateral MCA	10
Other arteries	5

MCA, Middle cerebral artery.
Data derived from 244 infants (90% full term) studied primarily by magnetic resonance imaging (see references in text); 45 are personal cases. Numbers are rounded off.

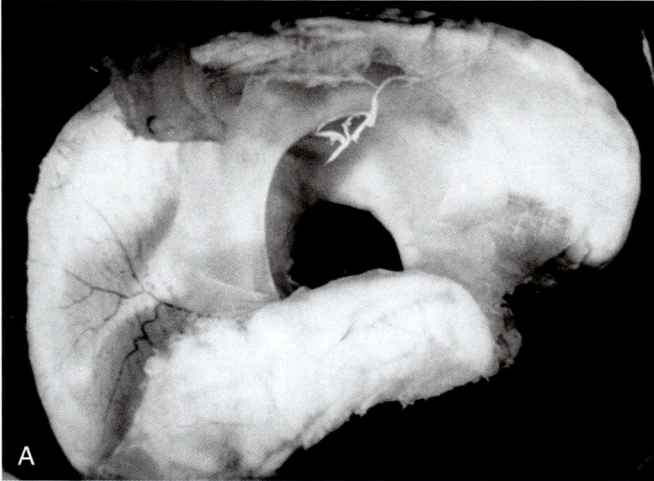

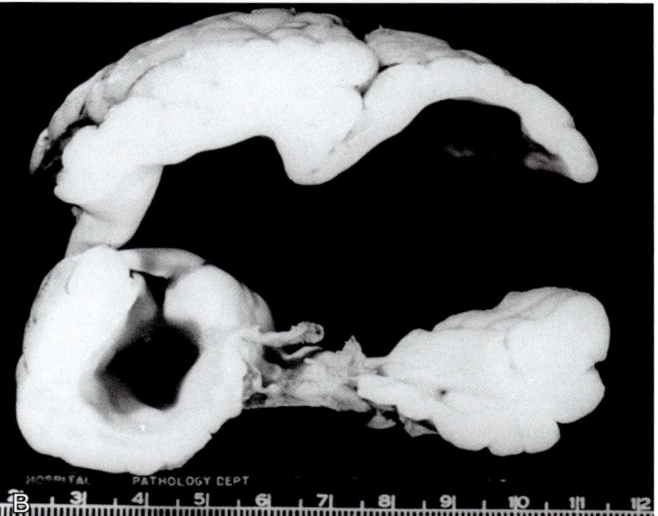

Figure 21.2 Focal ischemic brain injury with porencephaly. The infant, who died after 2 months, also exhibited a large head. (A) Lateral view of cerebrum floating in water. (B) Coronal section of cerebrum. Note the destruction in the distribution of the right middle cerebral artery; no lesion of the right internal carotid or middle cerebral artery could be demonstrated. Associated hydrocephalus was related to aqueductal obstruction; the cause was unknown. (From Norman MG. Perinatal brain damage. In: Rosenberg HS, Bolande RP, eds. *Perspectives in Pediatric Pathology.* Chicago: Mosby; 1978.)

infection), porencephaly is the sequela of an infarction with involvement of both cortex and cerebral white matter in the distribution of a single major cerebral vessel. *Hydranencephaly* refers to massive bilateral lesions, in which most or all of both hemispheres are reduced to cerebrospinal fluid (CSF)-filled sacs.

When related to ischemia, hydranencephaly most commonly is the sequela of bilateral cerebral infarction, with involvement of both cortex and cerebral white matter in the distribution of both internal carotid arteries (i.e., the anterior circulation). Because the posterior cerebral artery may have its origin from the anterior circulation in nearly 25% of newborns, the posterior cerebral artery distribution may also be affected.[43] *Multicystic encephalomalacia* refers to *multiple* cavitated foci of cerebral necrosis, usually bilateral in distribution. Most examples of these serious and relatively unusual lesions, when related to ischemia, are the sequelae of predominantly cerebral white matter destruction caused by generalized ischemia (i.e., more analogous to severe periventricular leukomalacia than to affection of single or several vessels).

TABLE 21.3	Factors Determining the Propensity of Immature Cerebrum to Undergo Dissolution

High content of water
Relative paucity of tightly packed, myelinated fiber bundles
Deficient astroglial response

Factors Determining the Propensity to Cavitation

The time period involved in the propensity to cavitation is from approximately the second trimester of gestation to the first postnatal weeks or months. The major factors determining the propensity of human brain to undergo dissolution and cavitation with necrosis during this time are primarily threefold (Table 21.3). The relatively *high water content* is characteristic of unmyelinated tissue and approaches 90% of wet weight in fetal brain. In contrast, myelinated white matter in the mature human brain is composed of approximately 70% water.[44] The deposition of myelin lipids occurs principally postnatally pari passu with the diminution of water content and the development of tightly packed fiber bundles. This axonal fiber development is reflected in the increasing anisotropic diffusion demonstrated in human brain of 28 to 40 postconceptional weeks by diffusion tensor magnetic resonance imaging (MRI).[45] Thus the first two factors, high water content and relative paucity of tightly packed myelinated fibers, are complementary and result in a tissue that is quite different from the relatively dense, mature cerebrum. Therefore dissolution of tissue is prone to occur with ischemic or other types of necrosis. The additional evolution from dissolution to cavitation relates importantly to the deficient astroglial response to injury.[11] This deficient response is both quantitative and qualitative. As discussed in Chapter 7, rapid proliferation of glia in human cerebrum does not begin until the last half of gestation and continues for many months postnatally; therefore the number of astrocytes to respond to injury may be relatively less than at later ages. In addition, some deficiency in the astrocytic response per se (i.e., the proliferation and hypertrophy of the cell and the development of glial fibers important for the formation of a tight glial scar) does appear to occur. As a consequence, areas of necrosis become areas of cavitation with deficient glial lining. The glial components in multicystic encephalomalacia are more obvious than in most cases of porencephaly and hydranencephaly, at least in part because of the less complete destruction of entire regions of brain and relative sparing of some glial cells in the former lesion, as opposed to the latter two lesions.

The importance of *timing* of ischemic injury in the development of porencephaly and hydranencephaly is well demonstrated by experiments with fetal monkeys.[46,47] Animals whose carotid arteries were ligated in the second trimester of gestation (latter part of the second trimester) developed cavitated areas of necrosis, similar to those in hydranencephaly or porencephaly and observable at term. Hydranencephaly resulted especially with early second trimester ligation, and porencephaly resulted from late second trimester ligations. An example of porencephaly produced experimentally in the fetal monkey by unilateral carotid ligation in the latter part of the second trimester is shown in Fig. 21.3. Vascular ligation before

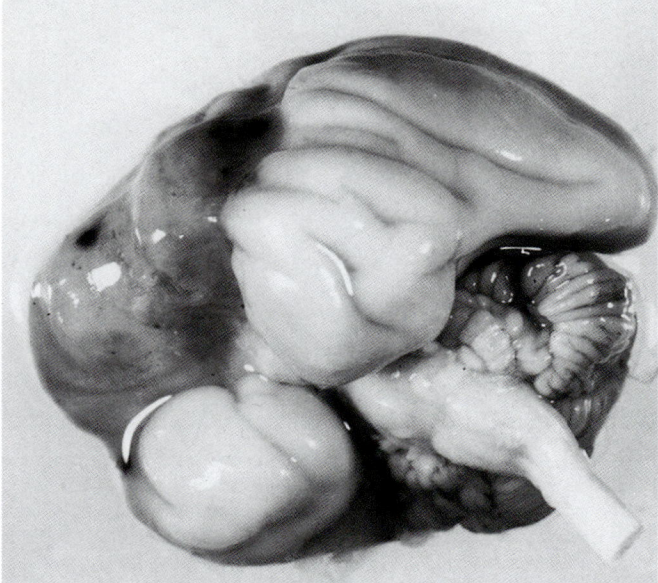

Figure 21.3 Porencephaly produced experimentally by vascular occlusion in the fetal monkey. At 90 days of gestation (term is ~160 days), the fetus was exposed surgically, and the carotid artery was ligated in the neck. The pregnancy was allowed to continue until term, when the fetus was delivered by cesarean section. This right lateral view demonstrates a sharply circumscribed area of infarction with a membrane-covered cyst. (Courtesy Dr. Philip R. Dodge.)

the early to middle second trimester of gestation resulted in cerebral *dysgenesis*, characterized by gyral abnormalities that were not further defined.[47,48] A combination of destructive and dysgenetic features occurred with middle second trimester ligations in the monkey. The analogy in the human is the finding of polymicrogyria in the margins of porencephalies of prenatal origin in the human fetus.[12,49]

Prenatal ultrasonographic studies followed by postnatal imaging and neuropathology clearly demonstrated the human correlates of the studies with monkeys concerning the importance of timing of the insult for the occurrence of cavitation.[11,12,50-59] Porencephaly and hydranencephaly have been documented to develop after insults as early as 20 to 27 weeks, and multicystic encephalomalacia has occurred after insults as early as 30 weeks. Causes of the fetal ischemia in these well-studied cases have included severe maternal hypotension secondary to cardiac failure, anaphylaxis, attempted maternal suicide with butane gas, maternal abdominal trauma, placental and umbilical cord catastrophes, and death of one twin (see later discussion).

Pathogenesis

Although the pathogenetic factors of perinatal stroke related to arterial or venous origin differ in many respects, there is considerable overlap among these two categories. Moreover, in both perinatal arterial and venous stroke, *multiple* coexisting pathogenetic factors are often involved. Although there is considerable overlap in causes of *prenatal* and *neonatal* AIS, we will discuss each entity separately. The principal causes are outlined in Table 21.4 according to the major pathogenetic mechanism.

TABLE 21.4	Major Causes of Perinatal Arterial Ischemic Stroke

Focal and multifocal cerebrovascular occlusion-insufficiency
Vascular abnormality (prenatal)
Vascular maldevelopment
Vasculopathy
Familial, proliferative
Collagen IV A 1 mutation
Isoimmune thrombocytopenia
Vasospasm
Cocaine
Vascular distortion

Embolus (prenatal or neonatal)
Placental thromboses or tissue fragments, detritus (twin pregnancy with dead co-twin)
Involuting fetal vessels (thrombi)
Catheterized vessels (thrombi or air)
Cardiac: congenital heart disease with right-to-left shunt, patent foramen ovale, atrial myxoma, rhabdomyoma (tuberous sclerosis),

Thrombus (arterial or venous) (prenatal or neonatal)
Meningitis with arteritis or phlebitis
Trauma
Dissection
Fibromuscular dysplasia
Vascular ligation-manipulation: extracorporeal membrane oxygenation (ECMO)
Disseminated intravascular coagulation (e.g., sepsis, twin pregnancy with dead co-twin)
Prothrombotic/hypercoagulable, endogenous factors: factor V Leiden mutation, protein C deficiency, protein S deficiency, prothrombin mutation, antithrombin III deficiency, antiphospholipid antibodies, *MTHFR* mutation, elevated lipoprotein α, elevated factor VIIIc
Hypernatremia-dehydration
Polycythemia
Generalized systemic circulatory insufficiency
Prenatal
Maternal hypotension or cardiac arrest
Maternal trauma (?)

Neonatal
Perinatal asphyxia
Systemic hypotension or cardiac arrest
Congenital heart disease with cardiac failure (exclusive of thromboembolic phenomena)

MTHFR, Methylene tetrahydrofolate reductase.

Prenatal Arterial Ischemic Stroke

Vascular Abnormalities. *Prenatal stroke* has been increasingly identified in utero with advances in fetal imaging. Many of these disorders are related to *vascular abnormalities* (see Table 21.4). A particularly well-documented case of a prenatal focal parenchymal defect with porencephaly, secondary to *vascular maldevelopment* (see Table 21.4), involved the lenticulostriate branches of the MCA and the anterior choroidal arteries.[60] Of additional interest in this case was the occurrence of polymicrogyric cortex in the margins of the porencephalic defect, compatible with a destructive process in the sixth month of gestation. The similarity to the experiments involving second trimester carotid occlusion in fetal monkeys discussed earlier is interesting.

Intrauterine focal or multifocal *ischemic injury secondary to vasculopathy* (see Table 21.4) has been shown in several disorders. A multifocal vascular disorder in association with hydranencephaly in utero was observed in association with a proliferative vasculopathy.[8,61-64] The likelihood of a genetic disorder was supported by the occurrence of multiple affected siblings in three families. In two cases, a mitochondrial disorder was suspected because of the finding of low levels of complexes III and IV of the electron transport chain.[63,64] Microangiopathy related to a *mutation in collagen IV A1* appeared to underlie another familial disorder with congenital porencephaly.[65,66] In a second disorder, *neonatal isoimmune thrombocytopenia,* intrauterine multifocal cystic lesions have been described and are generally considered to represent a sequela of intracerebral hemorrhage.[67-72] However, the apparent relation to vascular territories suggests an ischemic lesion (perhaps with secondary hemorrhage).[68,69,73] Endothelial injury and even thrombosis have been observed in other types of immune thrombocytopenia.[74-76]

Vasospasm may underlie the focal cerebral infarctions observed with intrauterine exposure to cocaine (see Chapter 38).[77-79] The vasospasm is postulated to occur secondary to transplacentally acquired cocaine as well as to the surge of catecholamines caused by the systemic and local cerebral effects of cocaine, as detailed in Chapter 38.

Emboli. *Sources of emboli* (see Table 21.4) may include placental fragments or clots (e.g., with placental infarcts), or thrombi in fetal vessels. The *placenta* has been recognized increasingly as a potential source of emboli and cerebral infarction.[80-84] The principal placental lesions have involved fetal vessels (fetal thrombotic vasculopathy, or fetal vasculitis) and have been associated with intrauterine infection with chorioamnionitis and maternal and, perhaps, fetal coagulopathies. Related placental lesions could underlie in part the increased risk of perinatal stroke with preeclampsia, ovarian-hyperstimulating treatments in women with a history of infertility, and severe intrauterine growth retardation.[35,80,85] Emboli from the fetal venous circulation could enter the arterial circulation by passage across the foramen ovale.

Twin-Twin Transfusion Syndrome. The most dramatic example of prenatal AIS occurs as a component of the twin-twin transfusion syndrome (TTTS). *Twin gestation* deserves special consideration as a cause of focal and multifocal ischemic brain injury, often related to *thromboembolic* phenomena (Tables 21.4 and 21.5).[7,11,38,78,86-127] As discussed later, *generalized as well as focal disturbance of cerebral blood flow* is involved in the origin of the neuropathology. Most of the clinically significant brain injury observed with twin gestation occurs in monozygotic *monochorionic* (i.e., a single placenta) twin gestations. Approximately 65% of twin gestations are dizygotic, diamniotic, dichorionic, and generally not associated with brain injury (except for a modest risk related to prematurity or the rare occurrence of stroke). Approximately 35% of twin gestations are monozygotic. Of the latter, approximately 30% are diamniotic, dichorionic (if the zygote splits early before blastocyst formation). However, approximately 70% of monozygotic twin gestations are diamniotic but *monochorionic* (when the zygote splits after blastocyst formation). In the latter group, in which each

TABLE 21.5   Brain Injury in Monochorionic Twins[a]

General features
Incidence of brain injury overall ≈30%, before modern day treatment
Occurrence of brain injury associated with placental vascular anastomoses, particularly artery to vein, with *twin-twin transfusion syndrome*; incidence of death or brain injury in untreated severe twin-twin transfusion syndrome >80%
Intrauterine death of one twin commonly associated with brain injury in the surviving twin, but most twin gestations with brain injury in one or both twins *not* complicated by fetal death

Neuropathology
Injury in first half of pregnancy
Porencephaly-microcephaly
Polymicrogyria
Rarely, anencephaly, exencephaly, encephalocele

Injury in second half of pregnancy
Isolated or multiple infarcts
Porencephaly with or without polymicrogyria
Hydranencephaly
Multicystic encephalomalacia
Periventricular leukomalacia
Rarely, venous thrombosis with hemorrhagic infarct
Pathogenesis

With death of co-twin
Severe hypotension with cerebral ischemia (hemorrhage into dead fetus)
Disseminated intravascular coagulation (thromboplastin material from dead fetus)
Thromboembolic (placental material, detritus from dead fetus)

With or without death of co-twin
Fetofetal transfusion leading to, in *the donor*, hypovolemia, hypotension, severe anemia, resulting in oligohydramnios ("stuck twin"), and cerebral hypoxic-ischemic injury, and in *the recipient*, hypervolemia, polycythemia, hyperviscosity, cardiac failure, resulting in polyhydramnios, premature delivery, and cerebral hypoxic-ischemic injury
Mechanical factors: transient disturbance of umbilical blood flow by compression or distortion, placental circulatory stasis with thromboembolism

[a]See text for references.

fetus shares the single placenta, the risk of brain injury is considerable (see Table 21.5). In this context occur *placental vascular anastomoses*, especially arteriovenous connections, in which placental tissue perfused by an artery from one fetus is drained by a vein from the other.[128] These vascular connections involve one or more arteries or veins from one fetus inserting into a common placental cotyledon of the other fetus and, thereby, allow for potential abnormal volume distribution between the fetuses.[129] In most situations, the anastomoses are balanced, but in 10% to 20%, they are unbalanced, and the TTTS results. The TTTS is the setting for most of the brain injury associated with twin gestations. Although this brain injury may occur consequent to the fetal death of a co-twin, most such injury occurs without such fetal death.

The *neuropathology* of brain injury associated with twin gestations relates particularly to the timing of the injury, as outlined in Table 21.5. Disturbances in early brain development (e.g., anencephaly and encephalocele) occur only rarely, and such early lesions are considered to be caused by vascular insufficiency. Also of presumed vascular basis are the somewhat more common occurrences of microcephaly with multiple porencephalies and of polymicrogyria. The polymicrogyria may contain features both of a disorder of neuronal migration (nonlayered cortex, heterotopias) and of a postmigrational encephaloclastic process (cortical laminar necrosis). The *most characteristic lesions are associated with insults in the second trimester and later* and consist of the full range of focal, multifocal, and generalized ischemic lesions (i.e., isolated infarction, porencephaly, hydranencephaly, multicystic encephalomalacia, and periventricular leukomalacia). Concerning the most serious of the ischemic lesions (i.e., hydranencephaly and severe porencephaly), twin gestations accounted for 11% of all cases in one series.[91] In most such cases, a deceased co-twin is identified.[91,123,125] (The incidence of deceased co-twin in these most severe cases could be higher because the remnants of such a co-twin are easily missed without careful examination of the placenta. In addition, the prenatal mortality in twins is high [i.e., approximately 20% to 80% of twins detected in the first trimester of gestation were singletons by the time of birth].)[110,130,131]

Pathogeneses of the brain injuries in monochorionic twin gestations are best divided into those associated with *a dead co-twin* and those associated with *severe TTTS*, but not necessarily fetal demise. Pathogenesis in cases with *death of a co-twin* includes the following: (1) now considered most common, fetal exsanguination from the surviving to the dead fetus through placental anastomoses, resulting in severe hypotension and cerebral ischemia; (2) thrombosis caused primarily by transfer of thromboplastin material from the dead twin, with disseminated intravascular coagulation resulting; and (3) embolus from the placenta or the dead fetus through the fetal vascular anastomoses (see Table 21.5).[101] Pathogenesis in the more common situation of *severe TTTS* relates principally to the cerebral hemodynamic consequences of TTTS (see Table 21.5). Thus the donor fetus experiences hypovolemia, hypotension, and severe anemia, with diminished cerebral blood flow and cerebral hypoxic-ischemic injury the consequence. Because of decreased renal blood flow, oliguria leads to oligohydramnios with the additional potential for umbilical cord disturbance or placental compression. The recipient fetus experiences hypervolemia, polycythemia, hyperviscosity, and cardiac failure and thereby risks generalized and focal (thrombotic) cerebral circulatory insufficiency. Polyhydramnios and resulting premature delivery may contribute to risk. These hemodynamic factors may be complicated by or conceivably superseded by mechanical factors (e.g., disturbances by compression or distortion of umbilical blood flow or of placental flow, with risk of thrombosis; see Table 21.5).

Therapy has been directed toward the pregnancies complicated by severe TTTS (Table 21.6). Two fundamental approaches (i.e., serial amnioreduction and fetoscopic laser occlusion of the vascular anastomoses) have been used.[129,132-137] Diagnosis of severe TTTS in the second trimester of gestation and institution of therapy shortly thereafter have comprised the usual protocol. The benefit of laser therapy relates to the reduction of the vascular anastomoses (a single amnioreduction to reduce polyhydramnios is carried out at the time of the laser surgery; see Table 21.6). In 2004, following the publication of

TABLE 21.6   Survival and Neurological Outcome in Severe Twin-Twin Transfusion Syndrome as a Function of Treatment

	NONE	AMNIOREDUCTION	LASER
Survival at 28 days	20%–30%	55%	75%
Normal neurological outcome	20%–30%[a]	50%–60%	85%
Brain injury	20%–30%	15%	5%

[a]Long-term follow-up data are limited.

Data for amnioreduction and intrauterine laser surgery, Senat MV, Deprest J, Boulvain M, Paupe A, Winer N, Ville Y. Endoscopic laser surgery versus serial amnioreduction for severe twin-to-twin transfusion syndrome. *N Engl J Med.* 2004;351:136–144; Graef C, Ellenrieder B, Hecher K, et al. Long-term neurodevelopmental outcome of 167 children after intrauterine laser treatment for severe twin-twin transfusion syndrome. *Am J Obstet Gynecol.* 2006;194:303–308; and from Behrendt N, Galan HL. Twin-twin transfusion and laser therapy. *Curr Opin Obstet Gynecol.* 2016;28(2):79–85, with permission. See text for references for no treatment.

the Eurofetus randomized control trial, laser therapy became the treatment of choice and indeed standard of care for this condition.[132] Combining subsequent published series, perinatal survival of at least one twin after laser therapy was reported in the region of 81% to 88%, and survival of both twins, in 52% to 54% of pregnancies.[138] Most recent directions in the management of TTTS have involved refinements in the prediction of the disease, clarification of the optimum frequency of surveillance, technique of laser ablation, prediction of adverse outcome after treatment, and development of other vascular ablative techniques. Improvements in intrauterine monitoring, including fetal echocardiography and advanced Doppler studies, have guided earlier treatment, which now includes more advanced methods of selective fetoscopic laser photocoagulation with laser photocoagulation of the surface of the placenta.[129] In the largest and most recent follow-up study comparing the standard fetoscopic laser surgery approach to the Solomon technique of more extensive laser photocoagulation, no differences were observed in fetal deaths (16% to 18%), neonatal deaths (4%), and survival with neurodevelopmental impairment (9% to 11%).[137] The Solomon technique is now favored because of the reduction in short-term complications, that is, twin anemia–polycythemia sequence or recurrent TTS.

Vascular Distortion. *Vascular distortion* is a potential cause of intrauterine stroke (see Table 21.4). We raise this possibility because extremes of neck extension or rotation have the potential to produce impairment of blood flow in the vertebrobasilar system or in the carotid system, respectively. Precedent for such occurrences in older patients is available.[139-145] The vertebrobasilar system may be particularly vulnerable in the fetus and newborn because of poorly developed ligamentous structures of the upper cervical spine that allow sliding and slipping movements between the atlantooccipital and atlantoaxial articulations.[13,146,147] Hyperextension of the head may cause inversion of the atlas through the foramen magnum and impair flow coursing through the vertebral arteries.[148] In a careful postmortem study, cerebral artery compression was shown in three of five infants with neck extension and in three of nine cases of neck rotation.[147]

Intrauterine Trauma. *Intrauterine trauma*, secondary to blunt trauma to the maternal abdomen, has resulted in prenatal stroke (see Table 21.4). The mechanism of this effect is not clear.[71,72,149]

TABLE 21.7   Major Risk Factors for Neonatal Arterial Ischemic Stroke

SOURCE OF RISK FACTOR	RISK FACTOR
Maternal (prepartum)	Primiparous
	Infertility
	Smoking
	Intrauterine growth retardation
	Preeclampsia
	Thrombophilia
Maternal (peripartum)	Maternal fever
	Maternal infection
	Prolonged rupture of membranes
	Intrapartum complications
Neonatal	Male
	Apgar score <7 (5 min)
	Prolonged resuscitation
	Hypoglycemia
	Early-onset sepsis/meningitis
	Congenital heart disease
	Vascular abnormality
	Thrombophilia
Placenta	Cord complication
	Chorioamnionitis
	Chronic villitis with obliterative fetal vasculopathy, thrombotic vasculopathy, small placenta

Derived from references 36, 152, 154-156,158-160.

Neonatal Arterial Ischemic Stroke

Pathogenesis of NAIS. Neonatal arterial ischemic stroke (NAIS) includes those examples of perinatal stroke that *present clinically in the neonatal period*, usually with seizures (see later). Before discussing the major causes of NAIS, that is, thrombosis or embolus, it should be emphasized that (1) the cause most often is unclear, and (2) *multiple* maternal, neonatal, and placental risk factors are often present. Some of the more common of these risk factors are shown in Table 21.7.

Maternal risk factors include primiparous pregnancy, infertility, maternal smoking, intrauterine growth retardation, thrombophilia, and signs of an intrauterine inflammatory state, for example, maternal fever (intrapartum), maternal infection, prolonged rupture of membranes, chorioamnionitis, and placental inflammatory features (see later; Table 21.7).[35,36,85,150-160]

Neonatal risk factors include male gender, early-onset sepsis-meningitis, thrombophilia, congenital heart disease, hypoglycemia, and signs of intrapartum hypoxic-ischemic events (depressed Apgar score, need for resuscitation).[153] In one large study (International Pediatric Stroke Study), among newborns with stroke, 30% received resuscitation, 23% had systemic infection, and less than 20% exhibited prothrombotic or cardiac abnormalities.[153]

Placental factors include chorioamnionitis and, particularly, chronic villitis with obliterative fetal vasculopathy and fetal thrombotic vasculopathy.

The *principal pathogenetic mediators* of NAIS in these settings are arterial occlusion by thrombosis or embolus or generalized circulatory insufficiency with particular affection of a single vessel (see Table 21.4). Some specific examples of these mechanisms follow.

Thrombus, Embolus. *Arterial occlusion by embolus or thrombus* (see Table 21.4) is a well-documented neonatal cause of focal and multifocal parenchymal defects.[a] Often it has been difficult by clinical imaging or even pathological criteria to distinguish between a thrombotic and embolic process. As noted earlier, the lesions have been observed principally in the regions of the middle (and sometimes anterior) cerebral arteries (see Figs. 21.1 and 21.2).

Emboli. *Sources of emboli* (see Table 21.4) may be similar to those in some cases of prenatal stroke (see earlier) and include placental fragments or clots, for example, with placental infarcts; thrombi in involuting fetal vessels, for example, umbilical vein, portal vein, or ductus arteriosus; and thrombi or air in punctured or catheterized vessels. As noted earlier, the *placenta* has been recognized increasingly as a potential source of emboli and occurrence of cerebral infarction (see earlier).[80-83,152,158] Emboli from the fetal or neonatal venous circulation could enter the arterial circulation by passage across the foramen ovale. In 50% to 90% of normal newborns at rest interatrial left to right shunting is documented readily, and in approximately 60% of healthy newborns studied at 24 hours of age, right-to-left blood flow could be demonstrated across the foramen ovale.[180,181]

Other sources of emboli include thrombi in the internal carotid artery, portal vein, central venous catheter (thrombus or air), and the heart.[182-184] Cardiac sources of emboli are relatively uncommon in the newborn period, although infants with *congenital heart disease, especially with right to left shunts*, may exhibit thromboembolic phenomena of cerebral arteries.[170,185-191] Stroke with congenital heart disease can occur in the preoperative, intraoperative, or postoperative periods.[158] The characteristics of the cardiac lesion and the management thereof are important determinants for stroke, with strongest associations with an intracardiac right-to-left shunt, preoperative balloon atrial septostomy, transposition of the great arteries, or single ventricle physiology.[158] In addition, such operative features as duration of bypass, age at surgical correction, and need for reoperation increase the likelihood of occurrence of stroke with congenital heart disease. Diagnostic procedures, including cardiac catheterization and the more recent use of ventricular assist devices as a bridge from extracorporeal membrane oxygenation (ECMO) have been associated with AIS.[186,189,190] Rarer causes of cardiac emboli include single cases of atrial myxoma and rhabdomyoma (infant with tuberous sclerosis) that we have seen.

Our suspicion has been that emboli may be more common causes of NAIS than currently recognized. It is noteworthy that cerebral emboli at later ages more commonly affect the left hemisphere (perhaps because of the direct route from the aorta of the left common carotid artery), and the left hemisphere predominance in neonatal MCA stroke is striking (see Table 21.2). In addition, transient right-to-left shunting through the ductus arteriosus also might favor the occurrence of left hemispheral emboli. Further support for a relative frequency of embolic infarction in NAIS is the finding by serial Doppler studies of four infants with focal MCA strokes of an ipsilateral decrease in cerebral blood flow velocity at the time of diagnosis of the infarct and a reemergence of blood flow in the ensuing days, consistent with embolic occlusion with subsequent fragmentation and distal migration of embolic fragments.[79]

Thrombi. *Thrombosis* may involve arteries or veins (see Table 21.4). The most common cause of NAIS related to an abnormality of the artery or vein per se is the vasculitis associated with *bacterial meningitis* (see Chapter 35). Cases of apparent occlusion caused by extremes of *neck movement* or *cranial trauma* may relate to vascular injury and resulting thrombosis (see earlier discussion of vascular distortion, concerning prenatal AIS).[a] Neonatal stroke has also been described in relation to carotid artery *dissection* and to *fibromuscular dysplasia* affecting multiple intracranial vessels.[194,195]

ECMO may lead to focal cerebral infarction by several mechanisms, including thrombus (see Table 21.4 and Chapter 22). In one series of 180 infants subjected to serial brain imaging studies, 16 (9%) exhibited a major brain lesion, 6 of the 16 infants exhibited focal ischemic lesions, and 10 exhibited hemorrhagic lesions.[196] Of the 6 ischemic lesions, 5 were in the right hemisphere, that is, ipsilateral to the carotid artery ligation. Of the 10 hemorrhagic lesions, 7 were in the left hemisphere and only 3 in the right hemisphere; the origin of the hemorrhages in the infants treated with ECMO is discussed in Chapter 22. A preponderance of right hemispheric *ischemic* phenomena has been observed by others.[197-199] The mechanisms for the right hemispheral infarcts include the following: (1) prior ischemic injury, secondary to persistent pulmonary hypertension and the associated systemic hypotension and impaired cerebrovascular autoregulation (secondary to hypoxemia or hypercarbia or both), partially compensated by cerebral vasodilation before institution of carotid ligation and ECMO; (2) ischemia caused by the carotid artery ligation because of insufficient collateral circulation through the circle of Willis; (3) ischemia caused by impaired cerebrovascular autoregulation during ECMO with disproportionate decrease in cerebral blood flow with hypotension in the right hemisphere because of the ligated carotid artery; and (4) thrombosis propagated into the anterior cerebral circulation from the ligated carotid.[196-198,200] The occurrence of ischemic lesions in the left hemisphere could

---

relate to emboli emanating from the ECMO circuit or to a *steal* phenomenon caused by the strong collateral flow from the left cerebral circulation to the right.[201,202]

Abnormalities of blood volume and coagulability account for most of the remaining cases of thrombosis in NAIS. *Hypernatremia-dehydration,* which leads to thrombosis probably by a combination of vascular and hypovolemic causes, is among the unusual causes of neonatal thrombosis, affecting either arteries or veins, most commonly veins (see Table 21.4). *Disseminated intravascular coagulation* in association with sepsis is among the most commonly documented causes for thrombosis in many *neuropathological series.* For example, in the study of 29 newborns with cerebral infarcts and arterial occlusions by Barmada and co-workers,[7] disseminated intravascular coagulation, usually with sepsis, was present in approximately two thirds. *Polycythemia* rarely has been associated with neonatal ischemic lesions, often complicated by hemorrhage.[203-205] Polycythemia may lead to arterial or venous thrombosis, and the nature of the pathology in neonatal cases is rarely clear. Impaired cognitive outcome, possibly related to ischemic cerebral phenomena, has been documented in infants with polycythemia and hyperviscosity.[206-208] Increased cerebrovascular resistance and diminished cerebral blood flow velocity, determined by Doppler studies, also have been observed in polycythemic infants with hyperviscosity,[208-211] and decreased cerebral blood flow and oxygen delivery have been shown directly by studies of neonatal piglets with hyperviscosity produced by infusion of cryoprecipitate.[212] The hemodynamic factors are probably important in genesis of the overt ischemic lesions associated with polycythemia, but it is necessary to recognize that such lesions are very unusual even among polycythemic infants with neurological symptoms.

Prothrombotic/hypercoagulable endogenous factors and other genetic factors are recognized to be of importance in the genesis of perinatal NAIS (Tables 21.4 and 21.8).[158,169,175-177,213-224] Similarly, these factors are frequent contributing factors in sinovenous thrombosis in newborns (see later).[225-230] The most commonly implicated factors in NAIS have been the factor V Leiden mutation, prothrombin mutation, methylene tetrahydrofolate reductase (MTHFR) deficiency (with resulting hyperhomocysteinemia), protein C deficiency, antithrombin III deficiency, and elevated lipoprotein *a.* Although present in 30% to 70% of cases of neonatal stroke, *these factors are usually combined*

TABLE 21.8   Prothrombotic Factors in Neonatal Arterial Stroke[a]

Prothrombotic factors associated with neonatal arterial stroke in 30%–70% of cases
Most common factors: factor V Leiden mutation, prothrombin mutation, *MTHFR* mutation, protein C deficiency, protein S deficiency, antithrombin III deficiency, antiphospholipid antibodies, elevated lipoprotein *a,* elevated factor VIIIc
Usually (50%–80%) associated with other pathogenetic factors (i.e., preeclampsia, gestational diabetes, placental vasculopathy, chorioamnionitis, signs of "perinatal asphyxia," sepsis, congenital heart disease)

[a]See text for references.
MTHFR, Methylene tetrahydrofolate reductase.

---

with other pathogenetic factors that favor thrombosis or embolus, that is, preeclampsia, placental vasculopathy, chorioamnionitis, signs of *perinatal asphyxia,* sepsis, and congenital heart disease (see later). Indeed, although we classify these disorders here under *thrombosis,* the likely mechanism of cerebral stroke in these disorders may relate less to thrombosis in situ in cerebral vessels but rather to embolus from thrombi in other sites, such as placenta, involuting fetal vessels, or the heart.

The potential importance of the inherited deficiencies was suggested initially by the detection of a syndrome of multiple thromboses, primarily venous, and particularly associated with hemorrhagic, ischemic skin lesions termed *purpura fulminans* in newborns with inherited deficiencies principally of protein C or protein S.[73,231-238] In general, in these two disorders thromboses were predominantly systemic, although cerebral ischemic lesions in arterial distributions were observed. Several newborns with isolated cerebral ischemic lesions have been described.[172,239,240] The mechanism is related to failure of the protein C regulatory system to limit coagulation and augment fibrinolysis. This system is composed of protein C, the pivotal regulatory vitamin K–dependent protein, protein S, a cofactor of activated protein C, and two additional proteins. Of particular interest, protein C and protein S levels are low in the neonatal period, although the activity of protein S is less impaired than that of protein C because of low levels also of a protein that inactivates protein S.[241,242] Indeed, protein C activity is extremely low in approximately 30% of preterm twin gestations and in approximately 35% of preterm infants with respiratory distress syndrome.[238,241]

One of the most important of the prothrombotic factors is the factor V Leiden mutation or so-called resistance to activated protein C.[3,177,178,217] In this disorder there is a defect in factor V, a procoagulant molecule, such that the factor cannot be inactivated by activated protein C. This so-called factor V Leiden mutation thus causes a *resistance* to the normal inactivating property of activated protein C. The result is an excess of the procoagulant, factor V. The newborn may have a particular propensity for thrombosis with the factor V Leiden mutation because, unlike the relatively low levels of protein C in the newborn, factor V levels are similar to adult values. Therefore the capacity of protein C to inactivate the factor V, even without the Leiden mutation, is diminished.[243] This defect has been described in association with neonatal cerebral infarction in many infants.[a] Careful examination of the placenta has led to detection of placental thromboses,[173,217] a finding suggesting that one mechanism of stroke in this setting is embolus originating in the placenta and reaching the fetal cerebral circulation via the foramen ovale. (Approximately 60% of fetal cardiac output enters brain from this right-to-left shunt.) In approximately 50% of cases, other risk factors, for example, perinatal complications, infection, cardiac disease, or presence of another endogenous prothrombotic factor, were present.

Generalized Systemic Circulatory Insufficiency. An apparently *generalized* disturbance of systemic circulation with impaired perfusion of brain in the past has been considered to account for a considerable proportion of ischemic cerebral lesions, occurring especially in the peripartum period (see Table 21.4). Indeed

---

[a]References 33, 35, 171, 173, 174, 177, 217, 222, 223, 243-247.

TABLE 21.9   Risk of Perinatal Arterial Stroke as a Function of Risk Factors Present Before Delivery

A. RISK FACTORS	ODDS RATIO (95% CONFIDENCE INTERVAL)	P VALUE
Preeclampsia	5.3 (1.3–22.0)	.02
Oligohydramnios	5.4 (0.9–31.3)	.06
Cord abnormality	3.6 (1.0–12.7)	.05
Primiparity	2.5 (1.0–6.4)	.05
Prolonged rupture of membranes	3.8 (1.1–12.8)	.03
Chorioamnionitis	3.4 (1.1–10.5)	.03

B. NUMBERS OF RISK FACTORS[a]	PERCENTAGE OF CASES (N = 37)	ODDS RATIO (95% CONFIDENCE INTERVAL)
≥1	86%	4.2 (1.4–14.8)
≥2	69%	6.5 (2.6–16.5)
≥3	60%	25.3 (7.9–87.1)
≥4	31%	24.1 (4.7–230.0)

[a]Includes risk factors shown in A, and in addition, decreased fetal movement, prolonged second stage of labor, fetal heart rate abnormalities, and history of infertility (treated with ovarian-stimulating drugs, which are prothrombotic).

Data from Lee J, Croen LA, Backstrand KH, et al. Maternal and infant characteristics associated with perinatal arterial stroke in the infant. *JAMA.* 2005;293:723–729, with permission.

the frequent occurrence of "prolonged second stage of labor," "fetal heart rate abnormalities," "signs of perinatal asphyxia," placental and cord "complications" and related features have suggested that a generalized circulatory insufficiency could *contribute* to the pathogenesis of neonatal stroke.[a] However, it is unclear how the strikingly unilateral predominance, in the distribution often of only a single vessel, could occur in the presence of an *apparently* generalized disturbance of perfusion. The phenomenon has been observed in the fetal and neonatal monkey.[249] Possible explanations include variations in the *development of the cerebral vessels or their responses to regulatory effectors.* It is noteworthy that the vessels of the anterior circulation, unlike those of the vertebrobasilar circulation, have a dense sympathetic innervation.[250] Thus asphyxia, a potent sympathetic stimulator, may be particularly likely to induce vasoconstriction in the anterior circulation and thereby favor the preponderance of focal cerebral ischemic lesions in the distribution of the MCA. A speculation would be that this innervation may exhibit asymmetries during development and that this developmental feature might explain some of the unilateral lesions seen with this apparently generalized insult. A second major possibility involves the *potential of emboli (clot and/or debris) from the involuting placenta to the brain.*[154] Thus in fetal sheep rendered hypoxic, the ductus venosus dilates and leads to a marked increase in flow through this vessel.[251] This vascular structure bypasses the liver and provides a direct pathway from the placenta to the brain via the foramen ovale. Whether this phenomenon occurs in the hypoxic human fetus is unknown, although the enhanced flow through the ductus venosus has been shown in human infants with intrauterine growth retardation, placental compromise, and hypoxia.[252]

Importance of Multiple Risk Factors. The importance of multiple risk factors and the nature of these factors in the genesis of perinatal arterial stroke is illustrated by the data shown earlier

in Table 21.9.[85] In this careful study of 37 cases, although data on endogenous prothrombotic factors were not available, the importance of such factors as preeclampsia, chorioamnionitis, prolonged rupture of membranes, and cord abnormality (tight nuchal cord, umbilical cord knot, body cord) is shown (see Table 21.9). Moreover, the markedly increased risk related to *multiple* rather than single risk factors is apparent. The data further illustrate that the pathogenesis of perinatal arterial stroke is very often multifactorial.

Clinical Features of NAIS

The clinical hallmark of NAIS in term infants is *seizure, especially focal seizure,* with *onset after 12 hours* of life.[158,160,253] This timing of seizures is different than in hypoxic-ischemic encephalopathy when seizures occur most often in the first 12 hours. In one careful study, the mean time of seizure onset in NAIS was 27.8 hours versus 5.1 hours in hypoxic-ischemic encephalopathy.[253] In a larger cohort (n = 79) median postnatal age of seizure onset was 19 hours.[160] Notably, again in contrast to hypoxic-ischemic disease, among infants with stroke only 10% (n = 8) exhibited encephalopathy, and of these most (n = 6) had mild encephalopathy.[160]

The clinical presentation of NAIS in *preterm infants* differs from that in term infants.[158] Indeed, commonly the former infants are asymptomatic and NAIS is identified on routine cranial ultrasonography.[37] This observation raises the question of whether NAIS is more common in premature infants than currently thought because cranial ultrasonography is not as sensitive for detection of NAIS as is MRI (see Chapter 10). In a carefully studied series, most preterm infants with NAIS presented with respiratory difficulties or apnea (83%) whereas only 30% presented with seizure.[254]

Diagnosis of NAIS

Diagnosis of NAIS is best considered in terms of the initial assessment and more definitive diagnosis. The latter is accomplished with neuroimaging.

---

[a]References 36, 38, 85, 150, 154, 155, 160, 178, 248.

Initial Evaluation

As noted earlier, the most common initial clinical sign of NAIS is a seizure, usually focal, occurring in the first 24 hours of life in an infant without other overt neurological signs. As in any other infant with seizures, laboratory studies should be carried out to rule out seizure etiologies requiring prompt and often specific intervention, such as hypoglycemia, infection, electrolyte or metabolic abnormalities (see Chapter 12). Electroencephalography (EEG) is of particular value because focal findings can aid in identification of the location of the stroke. In one large series of infants with stroke or with hypoxic-ischemic encephalopathy, 75% of infants with focal seizures were shown to have stroke.[253]

Neuroimaging

After the initial evaluation suggests NAIS, neuroimaging is performed. The initial assessment often is cranial ultrasonography. MRI is the definitive approach. Computed tomography (CT), formerly used in diagnosis, is not recommended because it is less effective than MRI and subjects the infants to radiation exposure (see later).

Cranial Ultrasonography. *Cranial ultrasonography* commonly is used initially. The evolution of the ultrasonographic appearance of acute infarction may consist in the hours after onset of symptoms of no definite abnormality. However, over the ensuing days the evolution of the ultrasonographic appearance of acute infarction consists of echodensity in a vascular distribution, usually that of the MCA (Fig. 21.4). Over the ensuing weeks the echodensity evolves to echolucency, often passing through a stage of heterogeneous appearance termed checkerboard.[255] Nevertheless, the *sensitivity* of ultrasound for detection of stroke is not optimal and is time-dependent. In two large studies the sensitivity of early ultrasound scan (1 to 3 days) for detection of MRI-proven arterial infarction was 30% to 70%, although scans later (4 to 14 days) detected abnormality in 86%.[256,257] Nevertheless, because the distribution of the MCA is affected in most cases and the region of the Sylvian fissure is visualized well on coronal ultrasound scans, careful cranial ultrasonography can be useful. Unfortunately, detection of smaller strokes, especially those involving superficial cortical branches, can be problematic with cranial ultrasonography.[258]

Computed Tomography. *Cranial computed tomography* (cranial CT) offers higher image resolution than ultrasound but exposes the infant to irradiation. The demonstration by CT of the uncommon occurrence of hemorrhagic transformation of a MCA stroke is shown in Fig. 21.5. Unfortunately, CT may underestimate the presence and size of the stroke (Fig. 21.6).[259]

Magnetic Resonance Imaging. MRI not only is the most sensitive technique for detection of neonatal stroke, but the modality provides the best available anatomic resolution (Figs. 21.7 and 21.8; see also Fig. 21.6).[259,260] The specific magnetic resonance (MR) modalities and their value have been effectively reviewed by Lehman and Rivkin.[158] Thus the specific sequences include diffusion-weighted imaging (DWI), T1- and T2-weighted imaging (T1W and T2W), and susceptibility weighted imaging (SWI). Magnetic resonance angiography (MRA) of the head and neck for assessment of craniocervical arteriopathy is useful because MRA can be added readily to the initial MRI evaluation. Vascular imaging has not been studied as much in neonatal stroke as it has in older children and adults. Several reports illustrate the ability of MRA to detect cervicocephalic arterial dissection and asymmetry of cerebrovascular trees in newborn infants with NAIS.[261-263] MRI is also important because the clinical presentations of neonatal arterial ischemic and sinovenous strokes overlap.

The several MRI sequences outlined above are important not only for careful anatomical identification of NAIS but also for timing and evolution of the injury.[158] DWI is useful for detection of cytotoxic edema and thus is sensitive within hours of the initial stroke. Unlike ischemia/reperfusion injury, as in hypoxic-ischemic encephalopathy, when cytotoxic edema is slow to evolve and is detectable by DWI after 48 hours, in neonatal stroke (as in adult stroke) vascular occlusion leads to cytotoxic edema within hours (Fig. 21.9; see Chapters 10 and 20). The DWI abnormality is very prominent at 2 to 4 days after the initial injury.[264,265] In a detailed study of the evolution of changes on T1W and T2W, Dudink et al. showed that in the first postnatal week, T2W images showed high signal intensity in affected cortical gray matter and white matter and T1W images showed low signal intensity in the involved cortical gray matter.[264] In the ensuing several weeks, cortical gray matter signal intensity was high on T1W imaging and low on T2W imaging. After 1 to 2 months with tissue dissolution, the infarcted area evolved into areas of tissue loss and cysts (Figs. 21.10–21.12).[158]

MRI studies of NAIS confirm the geographic features described earlier (see the section on neuropathology). Thus the large majority are unilateral, involve the left hemisphere, and the MCA distribution.[35,37] Interestingly, however, the location of AIS *within the MCA territory* varies in term and preterm neonates. *Term neonates* usually show *cortical branch strokes* (59%) within the MCA territory while *lenticulostriate branch infarcts* are commonly observed in *preterms* (39%).[156,266]

Main branch MCA strokes occur with approximately equal frequency in term and preterm infants. Notably, as reviewed by Lehman and Rivkin,[158] the arterial involvement in the preterm infant was shown to differ with gestational age. Among infants of <28 to 32 weeks of gestational age, most had lenticulostriate involvement, whereas in older (32 to 36 weeks of gestational age) preterm infants, cortical branch infarcts represented a majority. These findings are consistent with the conclusion that most of the term neonatal MCA strokes reflect cortical branch involvement.[156,266]

Newer Magnetic Resonance Imaging Techniques. *Newer MRI techniques* have provided further delineation of focal ischemic lesions (Fig. 21.13). Thus *diffusion tensor imaging with or without tractography* helps in identification of an asymmetry of the corticospinal tracts and can predict hemiplegia, as has been shown in preterm infants.[267] In addition, as noted earlier, *vascular imaging* with MRA of the head and neck can assess the possibility of craniocervical arteriopathy, such as dissection.[158] Such studies could be especially useful in the infant with abnormal neck position in utero or during delivery. In addition, detection of an intracranial arteriopathy or an unusual vascular lesion, such as aneurysm or arteriovenous malformation, all of which may mimic AIS, would lead to specific therapeutic considerations (see Chapter 37).

Text continued on p. 578

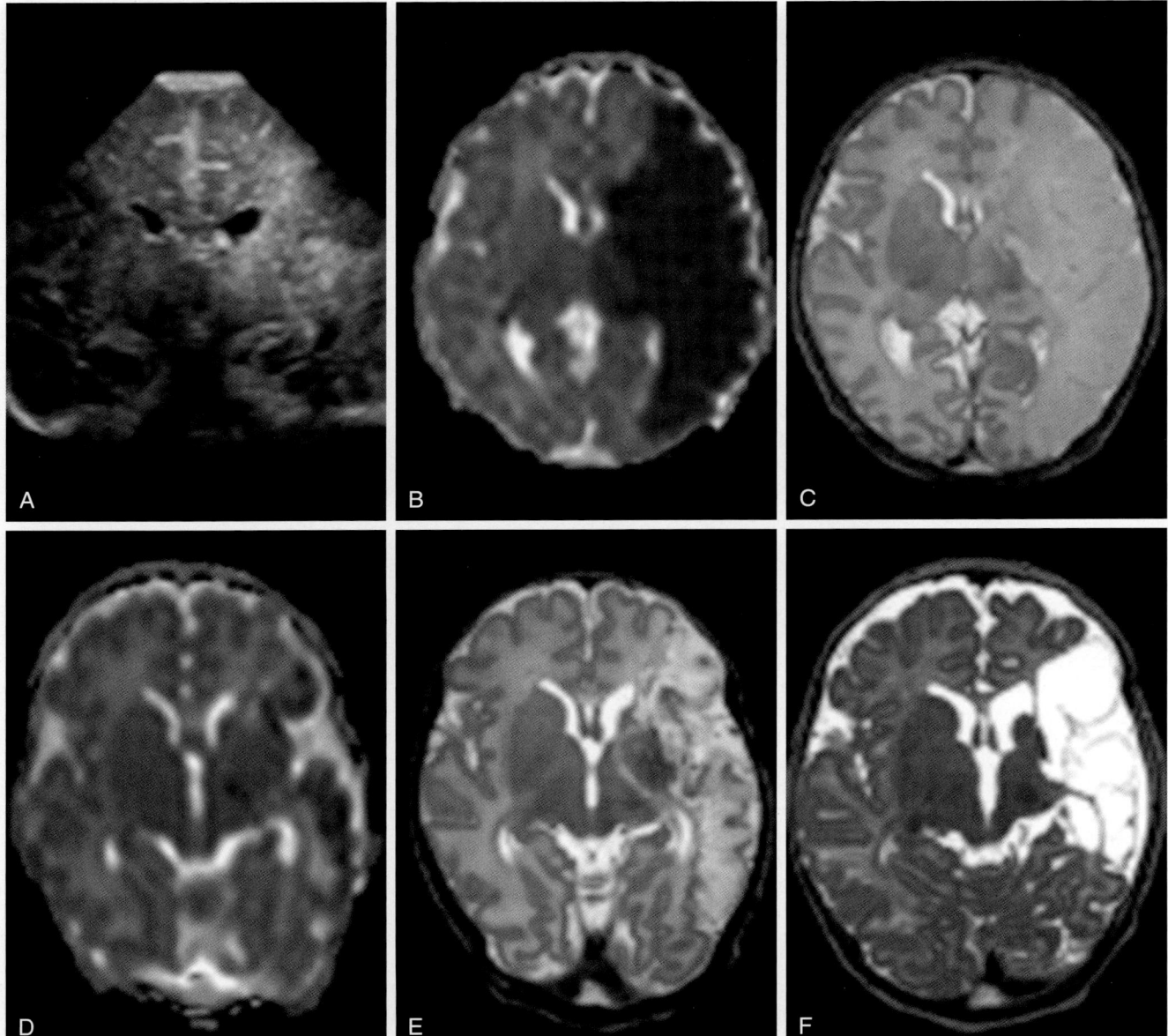

Figure 21.4 Cranial ultrasound and magnetic resonance imaging. Findings of a full-term infant with a perinatal arterial ischemic stroke. Cranial ultrasound on day 5 shows an area of increased echogenicity in the territory of the left middle cerebral artery, including involvement of the thalamus (A). A magnetic resonance image (MRI), including T2-weighted imaging (C) and diffusion-weighted imaging (ADC map) (B), was obtained on the same day and showed a main branch middle cerebral artery stroke. A second MRI, acquired at the age of 10 days, showed pseudonormalization of the diffusion abnormalities (D), but cystic evolution of the white matter (E). At 3 months of age, multicystic encephalomalacia can be seen in the former stroke area (F). Because of the extent of the injury, this infant was closely followed, and the development of unilateral spastic cerebral palsy, hemianopia, and postnatal epilepsy was observed in the first 6 months after birth. (From van der Aa NE, Benders MJ, Groenendaal F, de Vries LS. Neonatal stroke: a review of the current evidence on epidemiology, pathogenesis, diagnostics and therapeutic options. *Acta Paediatr.* 2014;103(4):356–364.)

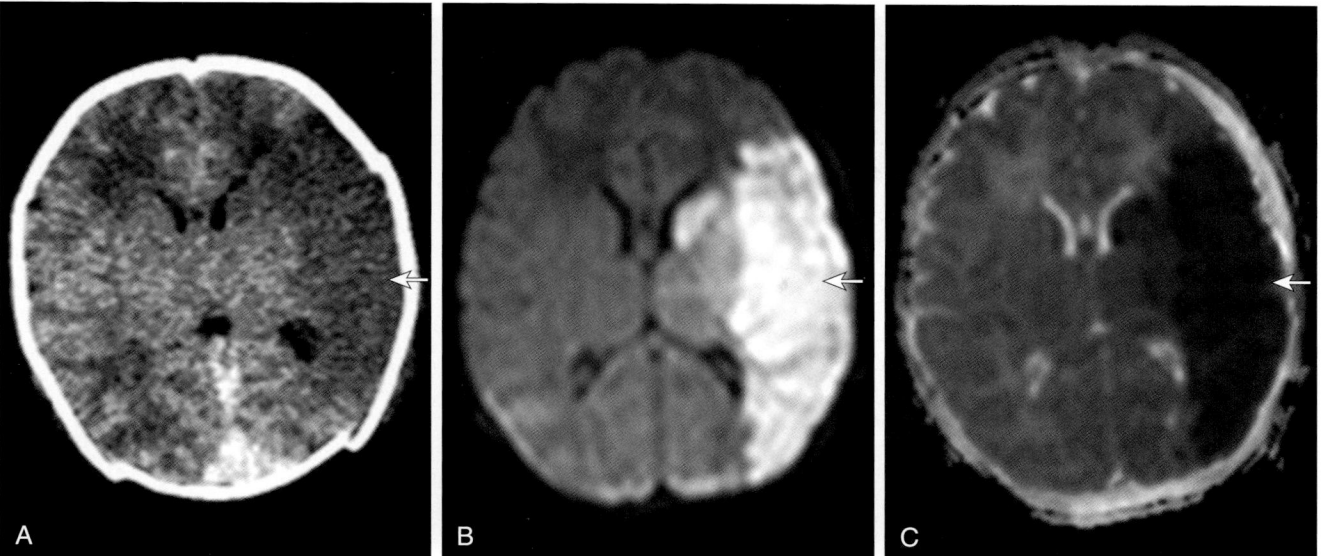

Figure 21.5 Comparison of computed tomography with magnetic resonance imaging. Comparison of cranial computed tomography (CCT) and brain magnetic resonance imaging (MRI) for demonstration of neonatal arterial ischemic stroke in a 1-day-old term infant who presented with a right focal seizure. (A) An axial CCT image reveals hypodensity *(white arrow)* in the left middle cerebral artery (MCA) territory consistent with acute infarction. (B) Axial MRI diffusion-weighted trace image of the same patient in A reveals clearly demarcated area of infarct as a region of hyperintensity *(white arrow)* in the left MCA territory. (C) Diffusion-weighted image apparent diffusion coefficient map reveals region of signal hypointensity and restricted diffusion *(white arrow)* to match area of signal hyperintensity observed in B. (From Lehman LL, Rivkin MJ. Perinatal arterial ischemic stroke: presentation, risk factors, evaluation, and outcome. *Pediatr Neurol.* 2014;51(6):760–768.)

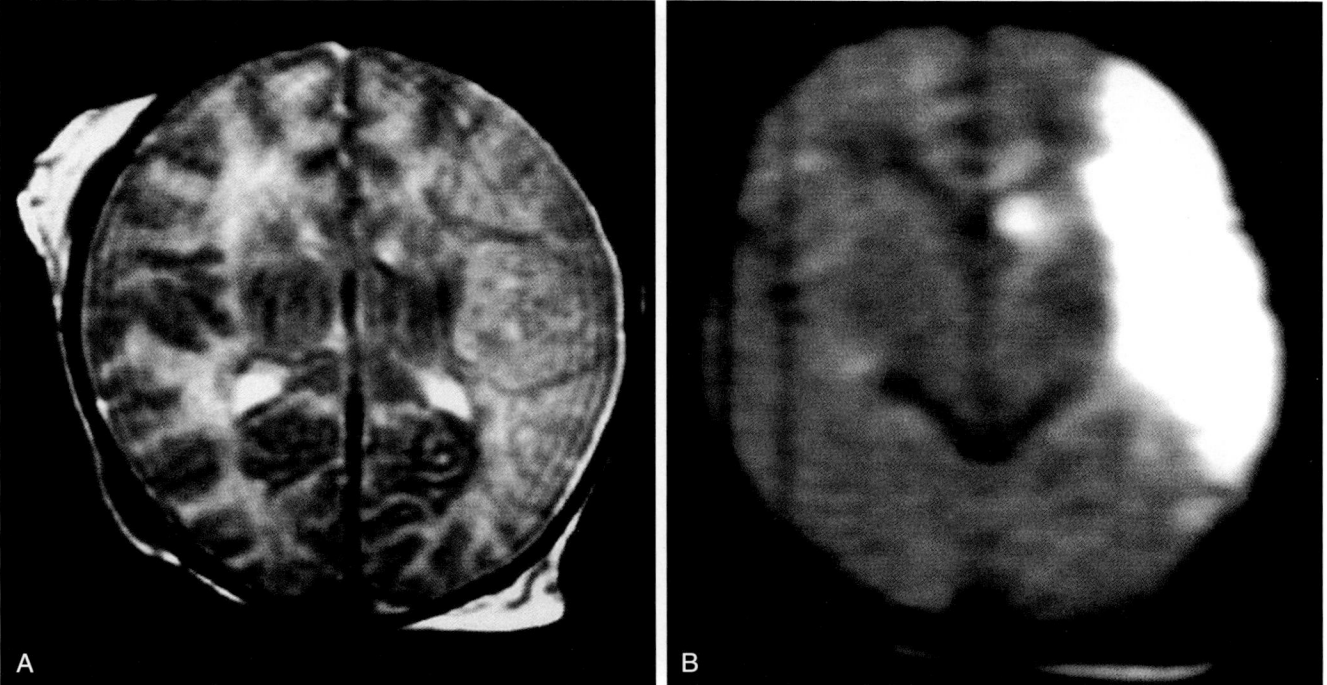

Figure 21.6 Magnetic resonance imaging (MRI) scans of focal ischemic cerebral injury. Scans were performed on the third postnatal day. (A) Axial T2W MRI scan shows a lesion in the distribution of the main branch of the left middle cerebral artery. (B) The diffusion-weighted imaging scan demonstrates the lesion more strikingly.

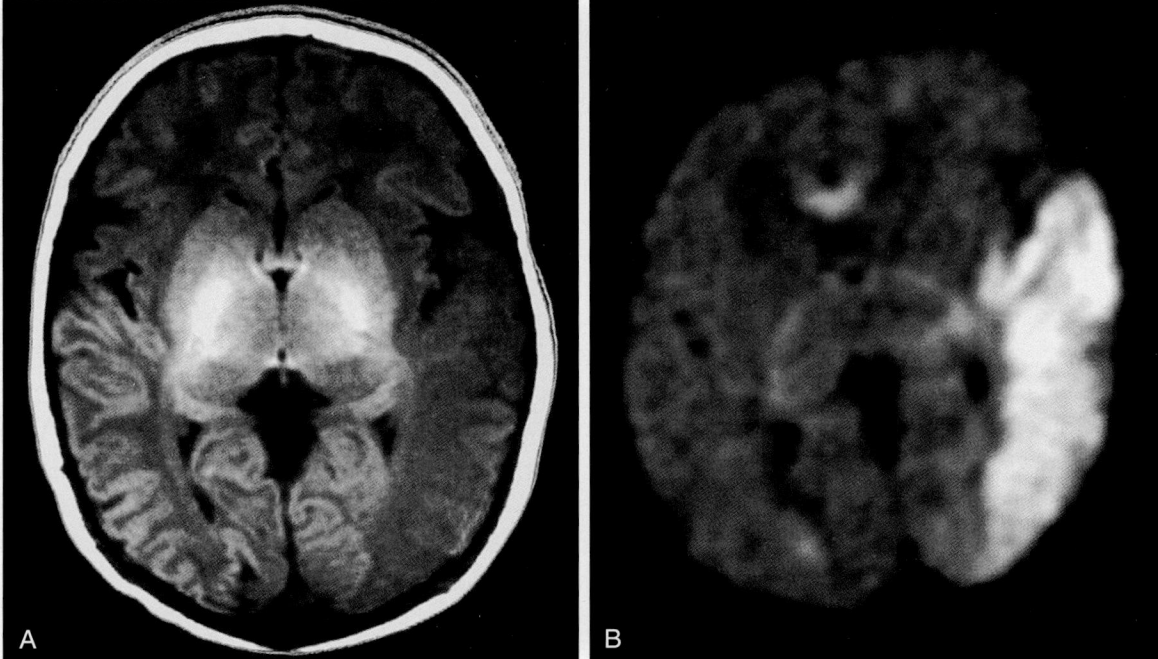

Figure 21.7 Magnetic resonance imaging (MRI) scans of focal ischemic cerebral injury. Scans were formed on the third postnatal day. (A) Axial T1W MRI scan shows an area of decreased signal in the distribution of the posterior division of the left middle cerebral artery. (The normal increased signal bilaterally in the posterior limb of the internal capsule also is apparent.) (B) The diffusion-weighted imaging scan demonstrates the apparent infarction more strikingly.

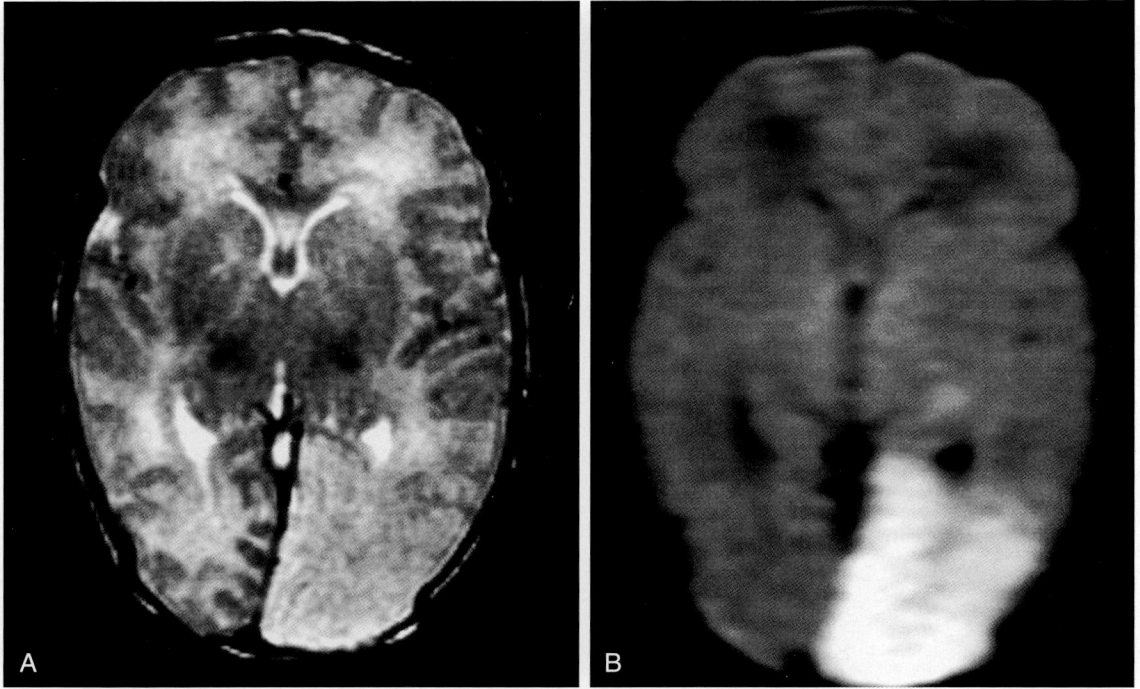

Figure 21.8 Magnetic resonance imaging scans of focal ischemic cerebral injury. Scans were performed on the fifth postnatal day. (A) Axial T2W magnetic resonance imaging shows increased signal in the distribution of the left posterior cerebral artery. (B) The diffusion-weighted imaging scan demonstrates the apparent infarction more strikingly.

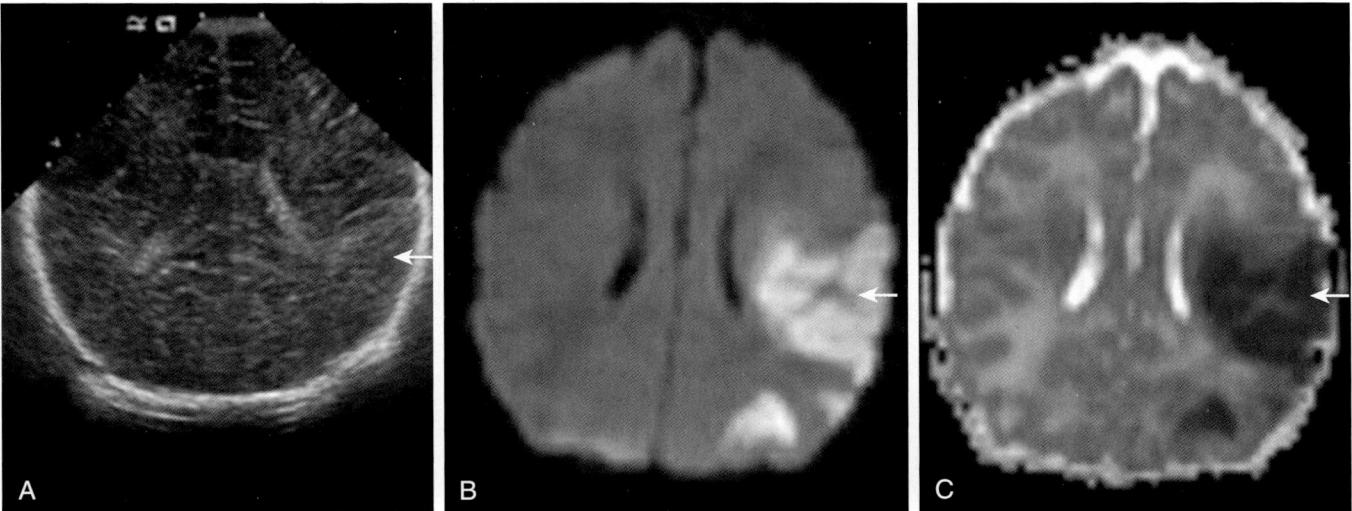

Figure 21.9 Comparison of head ultrasound and brain. Magnetic resonance imaging (MRI) of neonatal arterial ischemic stroke in a 1-day-old term infant who presented with a right focal seizure. (A) Head ultrasound reveals hyperechogenicity in the left cerebral hemisphere (indicated by *white arrow*) concerning ischemic injury. (B) Axial MRI diffusion-weighted trace image of the same patient observed in A reveals well-defined hyperintensity (indicated by *white arrow*) in the left middle cerebral artery (MCA) territory. (C) Diffusion-weighted image of apparent diffusion coefficient map of matching slice observed in B reveals corresponding hypointensity (indicated by white arrow) in the left MCA territory. (From Lehman LL, Rivkin MJ. Perinatal arterial ischemic stroke: presentation, risk factors, evaluation, and outcome. *Pediatr Neurol.* 2014;51(6):760–768.)

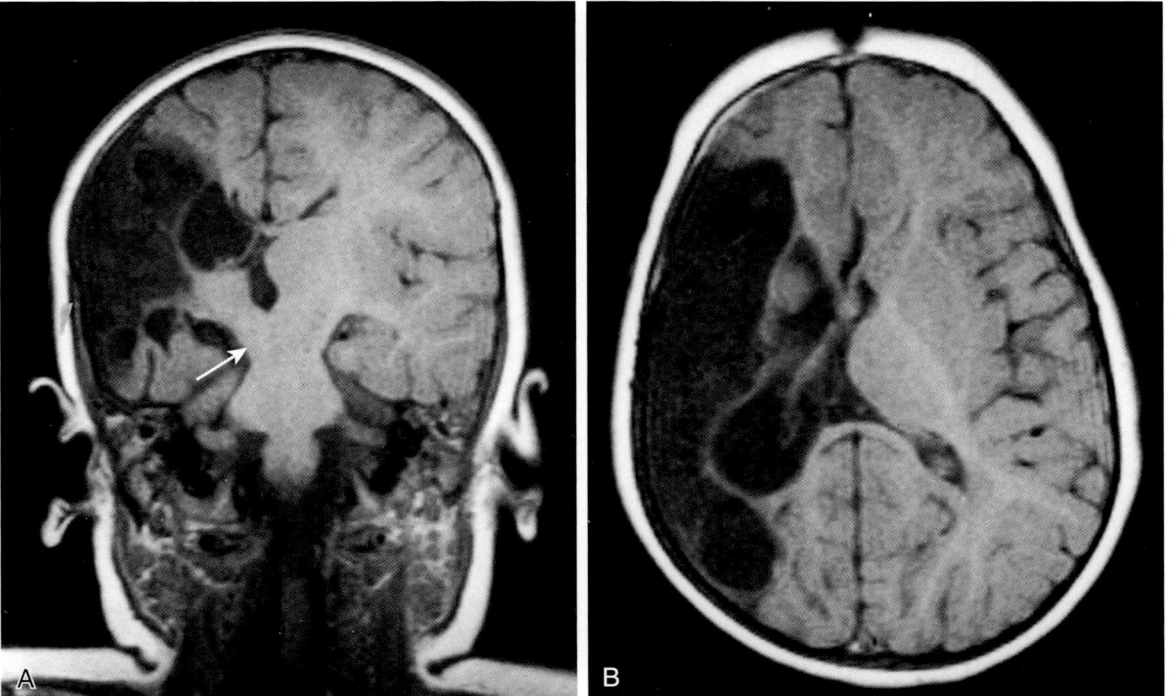

Figure 21.10 Magnetic resonance imaging scans of focal cerebral infarction. Scan was obtained at 6 months of age in a full-term infant who experienced an infarction in the distribution of the right middle cerebral artery, shown by computed tomography scan, in the neonatal period. Note on these T1-weighted images in the (A) coronal and (B) axial planes the distinct area of decreased signal in the territory of the right middle cerebral artery and the compensatory dilation of the right lateral ventricle. Note also the smaller cerebral peduncle on the right *(arrow)* in (A) consistent with wallerian degeneration of corticospinal tract fibers.

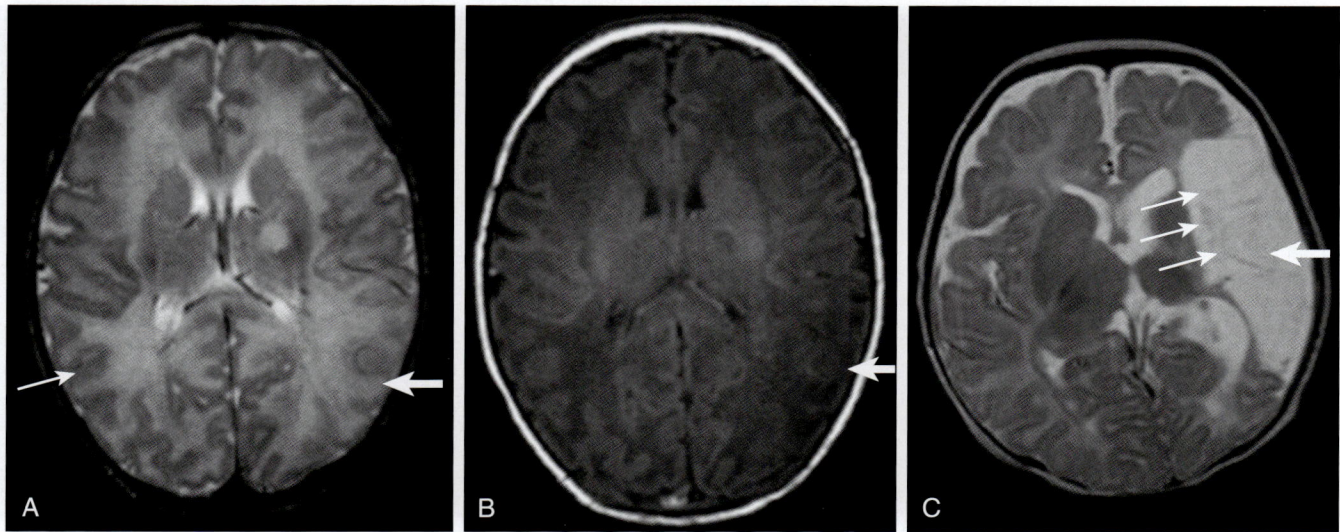

Figure 21.11 Comparison of magnetic resonance imaging (MRI) appearance of a patient with acute neonatal arterial ischemic stroke (AIS) compared with MRI of a patient with presumed perinatal AIS. (A) T2-weighted (T2-W) axial image obtained in a 1-day-old term infant who presented with seizure reveals hyperintensity *(thick arrow)* in gray matter cortex and underlying white matter with loss of gray and/or white matter differentiation in the left middle cerebral artery territory *(thick arrow)*, consistent with acute infarction compared with the normal right side with dark cortex *(thin arrow)* and normal differentiation of the white and gray matter. (B) T1-weighted axial image, obtained in the same patient at the same time as image in A, reveals signal hypointensity in cortical gray matter *(thick arrow)* matching the area of hyperintensity observed in A consistent with a diagnosis of acute neonatal AIS. (C) T2-W image obtained in a 3-month-old infant with an unremarkable neonatal history who presented at 3 months of age with a prematurely appearing right-hand preference reveals an area of hyperintensity and cystic change *(thick arrow)* with cystic septations *(thin arrows)* typically of chronic infarction. (From Lehman LL, Rivkin MJ. Perinatal arterial ischemic stroke: presentation, risk factors, evaluation, and outcome. *Pediatr Neurol.* 2014;51(6):760–768.)

TABLE 21.10	Thrombophilia Studies in Neonatal Arterial Ischemic Stroke

Protein C functional assay[a]
Protein S functional assay[a]
Factor V Leiden functional assay or factor V Leiden gene mutation
Prothrombin gene mutation on (20210)
Antithrombin functional assay
Serum homocysteine level
Serum lipoprotein (a)
Serum lupus anticoagulant[b]
Anti-cardiolipin antibodies[b]
Anti-B2 glycoprotein antibodies[b]

---

[a]Proteins C and S reach adult levels at 6 to 12 months of life. If levels are only slightly low in the newborn, a repeat level should be obtained later in the first year.

[b]Antiphospholipid antibodies—can be tested in mother or infant.

TABLE 21.11	Long-Term Neurological Outcome in Term Infants With Neonatal Arterial Ischemic Stroke

Magnetic resonance imaging is valuable in estimation of prognosis by determining both the extent of the unilateral lesion and the presence of milder injury of the contralateral hemisphere.

Hemiparesis occurs in approximately 25%–35% of survivors.

Hemiparesis occurs in nearly 100% if the lesion involves the distribution of the *stem* of the middle cerebral artery (cerebral cortex—white matter—basal ganglia—posterior limb of the internal capsule).

The presence of concomitant, albeit milder injury to the contralateral hemisphere sharply increases the likelihood of hemiparesis.

Cognitive deficits occur approximately in 50%–70% of survivors when studied at *school age.*

Epilepsy occurs in approximately 15%–40% of survivors

Prothrombotic/Thrombophilia Studies

The potential role of *prothrombotic abnormalities* in pathogenesis of NAIS was discussed earlier (see the section on pathogenesis). The diagnostic approach suggested by Lehman and Rivkin[158] is appropriate (Table 21.10).

Prognosis of NAIS

The *long-term neurological sequelae* of lesions identified by MRI in the neonatal period have included principally motor deficits,

cognitive/behavioral disorders, and epilepsy (Table 21.11).[a] The principal findings and conclusions are shown in Table 21.11.

Hemiparesis

Hemiparesis occurs subsequently in 25% to 35% of surviving term infants with apparent unilateral cerebral infarction (see Table 21.11). When hemiparesis occurs, the motor disturbance

---

[a]References 2, 3, 31, 32, 34, 35, 37, 158, 175, 177, 268–284.

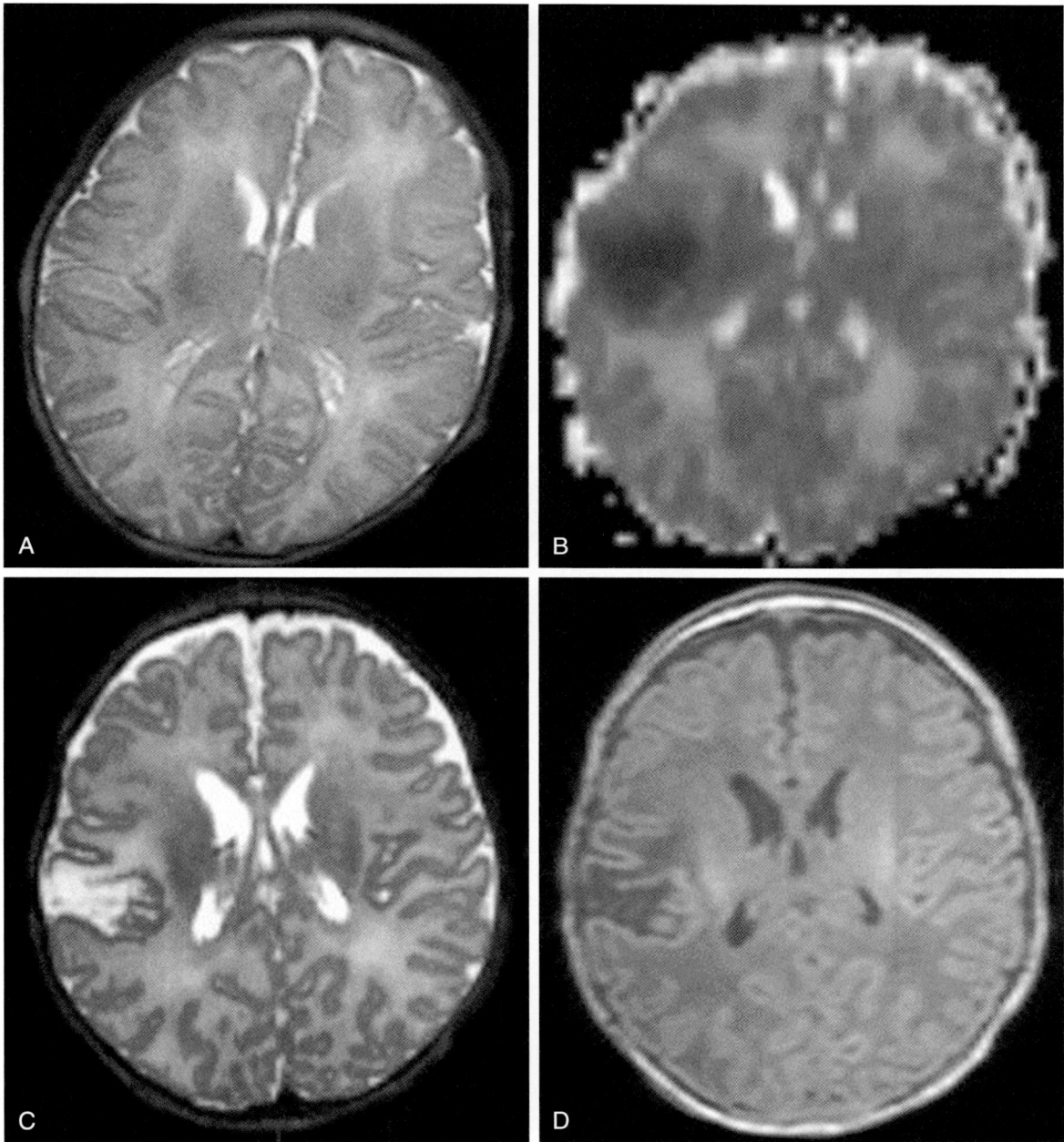

Figure 21.12 At 4 days of life (A), the T2-weighted image and (B) the apparent diffusion coefficient map display restricted diffusion in the right middle cerebral artery distribution. At 19 days of life, established injury is seen in both (C) T1- and (D) T2-weighted imaging. (From Barnette A, Inder T. Evaluation and management of stroke in the neonate. *Clin Perinatol.* 2009;36(1):125–136.)

becomes overt after approximately 6 months of age. The distribution of weakness involves contralateral face and upper extremity more than lower extremity, because of the anatomical distribution of the MCA (Fig. 21.14). *The likelihood of hemiparesis depends on the extent of the lesion or on the presence of involvement, albeit not severe, of the contralateral hemisphere or both.* Thus the likelihood of hemiparesis is nearly 100% if the distribution of the stem of the MCA is affected, that is, cerebral cortex, white matter, basal ganglia, and posterior limb of the internal capsule. If the distributions of a cortical branch or only the lenticulostriate vessels are affected, the likelihood of hemiparesis

is less than 10%. For example, hemiparesis is rare if the internal capsule is involved together with *either* basal ganglia *or* cerebral cortical involvement. When the hemisphere contralateral to the infarction is affected, even if not severely, the likelihood of hemiparesis approaches 100%. This occurrence presumably relates to an inability of the opposite hemisphere to reestablish its earlier developed ipsilateral corticospinal tract innervation, the presence of which has been demonstrated in older hemiplegic patients by a variety of functional studies.[285-287] This plasticity may require many months to evolve. For example, in one study, both infants with *moderate* hemiparesis at 6 to 8 months of age

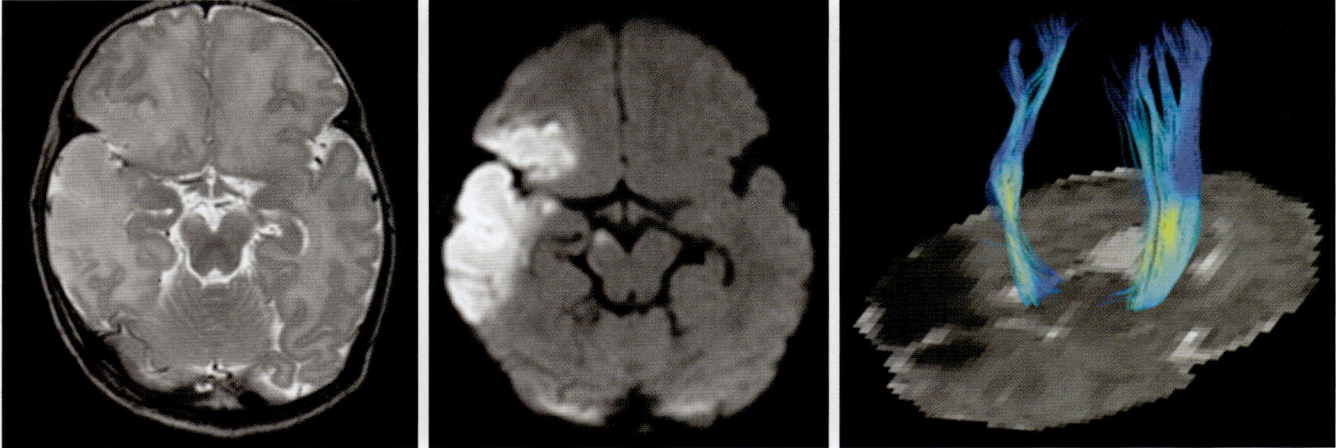

Figure 21.13 Axial T2-weighted magnetic resonance imaging (MRI; *left*), diffusion weighted imaging (DWI; *middle*), and tractography *(right)* on day 3 in an infant with a middle cerebral artery infarct and involvement of the ipsilateral corticospinal tract after mild perinatal asphyxia. An area of increased signal intensity with loss of gray white matter differentiation and increased signal intensity in the ipsilateral cerebral peduncle is seen on T2-weighted MRI. This is seen as restricted diffusion with DWI. Tractography demonstrates a clear asymmetry between the ipsilateral and contralateral corticospinal tracts. (From Groenendaal F, de Vries LS. Fifty years of brain imaging in neonatal encephalopathy following perinatal asphyxia. *Pediatr Res.* 2017;81(1–2):150–155.)

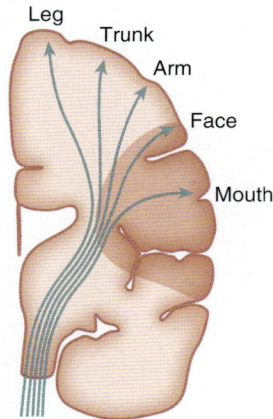

Figure 21.14 Schematic diagram of origin and descent of corticospinal tract fibers and location of the usual infarction in the distribution of the middle cerebral artery *(marked area)*. Note that face and upper extremity are more likely to be affected than lower extremity.

had no hemiparesis on follow-up at 2 years of age, and three of nine infants with severe hemiparesis early had only moderate weakness later.[288] When DWI shows extensive *involvement* of the corticospinal tract, that is, extending from the posterior limb of the internal capsule to the ipsilateral cerebral peduncle, nearly all such infants developed hemiplegia.[281] The predictive importance of involvement of the descending corticospinal tract was shown also by Kirton et al.[289]

Cognitive Function

Cognitive function is impaired after *unilateral* infarctions in approximately 25% to 50% of infants (see Table 21.11). In general, the likely involvement of language versus nonlanguage functions bears no consistent relation to location of the injury on the right side or left side, although one study observed spatial deficits more commonly with right hemispheral lesions and language deficits more with left hemispheral lesions.[271,273,288,290,291]

In one recent large study, infants with NAIS studied at 7 years of age exhibited rates of *impaired language and low academic skills* of 49% and 28% respectively.[282] Of particular note, Westmacott et al., showed a *late emergence of cognitive deficits after unilateral neonatal stroke.*[292,293] Thus as preschoolers, the patients' performance did not differ from a normative sample for Full Scale IQ, Verbal IQ, or Performance IQ. However, at school age, Full Scale IQ was lower, with 69% of the children showing emerging deficits in nonverbal reasoning, working memory, and processing speed. In addition, the *particular vulnerability of the developing neonatal brain* is suggested by the demonstration that later cognitive function is worse among children whose stroke occurred in the neonatal period vs. occurrence later in infancy and childhood.[292,293] Often accompanying the cognitive deficits are a variety of behavioral abnormalities, such as hyperactivity, and attentional and related problems.[37]

Seizure Disorders

Subsequent epilepsy occurs in approximately 15% to 40% of infants on follow-up after unilateral infarctions (see Table 21.11). The seizures are often focal and are variably responsive to therapy. In one recent series of 55 infants, 16% developed epilepsy at a mean age of 4 years and 2 months.[294] The major risk factor was infarction in the territory of the right MCA infarction or in multiple territories. In another study, size of the infarct was a key risk factor.[295] In the most recent large series, of 40 infants with NAIS heralded by a neonatal seizure, 15 (38%) had active epilepsy at follow-up.[283]

Management of NAIS

The management of the infant with NAIS should begin with careful attention to fluid and electrolyte status and supportive measures related to cardiorespiratory function. Thrombolytic therapy is not a practical consideration because the timing of the initiating lesion is generally not known and is generally many hours before diagnosis.

Acute Therapy

The *principal acute therapy from the neurological perspective is treatment of the seizures* that herald most cases of NAIS. Prompt treatment of seizures is supported by data in adult stroke that seizures are related to poorer outcome and in animal models that seizures increase lesion volume.[158] Perhaps most important, as reviewed in Chapter 12, both experimental and clinical data indicate that neonatal seizures can lead to or enhance brain injury.

Supportive therapies include management of comorbidities. Careful attention to blood glucose homeostasis is important. The unusual occurrence of hemorrhagic transformation should be avoided by assurance of vitamin K administration and prevention of thrombocytopenia.

Anticoagulant/Antiplatelet Therapy

The *issue of use of anticoagulant/antiplatelet therapy is controversial.* The purpose of such therapy would be to prevent propagation or recurrence of thrombus, as in a prothrombotic state or meningitis, to prevent embolism, as in cardiac disease, or to combat both of these possibilities, as in complex congenital heart disease. Thus guidelines from the American Heart Association and the American College of Chest Physicians (CHEST) recommend anticoagulation for infants with stroke who have a prothrombotic state, a documented source of cardioembolism, or congenital heart disease.[158] The most commonly used agent is low-molecular-weight heparin. In the absence of a genetic defect of coagulation or a rare arteriopathy, *long-term anticoagulation therapy is not recommended in NAIS* because the recurrence risk in large series is only approximately 1% to 2%.[296]

Hypothermia

A possible role for *hypothermia* in management of neonatal stroke is suggested by observations in a group of infants with hypoxic-ischemic encephalopathy treated with this modality, as described in Chapter 20.[297] Of the 15 infants with stroke, 5 had been treated with hypothermia and had no seizures, whereas 7 of the 10 with stroke but not treated with hypothermia had neonatal seizures. Whether seizure absence will correlate with more favorable outcome will be of great interest. The findings do raise the question of whether therapeutic hypothermia should be instituted more broadly in NAIS.

Erythropoietin

Erythropoietin, an agent with neuroprotective and neurorestorative properties (see Chapters 13, 16, and 20), has been shown in experimental models of neonatal stroke to lead to a reduction in infarct volumes and improvement of neurological function, even after delayed treatment.[298-303] A recent feasibility and safety study of erythropoietin for neuroprotection after NAIS showed no adverse effects. The study was too small to assess neuroprotective effect, but in the small group investigated ($n = 10$) no apparent differences in residual infarct volume or neurodevelopmental outcome (compared to historical controls) were apparent.[304]

Stem Cells

A potential restorative therapy involves the use of *stem cells*.[305-308] Several stem and progenitor cells have shown promise when administered hours to days after onset of injury in experimental models of neonatal stroke. The principal agents used have included induced pluripotent stem cells, neural stem cells, and mesenchymal cells. The latter can be derived from extra-embryonic tissues, such as placenta, umbilical cord, and Wharton jelly. The mechanisms of benefit vary somewhat with the stem cell used, but experimental studies suggest reduction of apoptosis, anti-inflammatory effects, stimulation of local neurotrophic factors, promotion of endogenous cell proliferation, stimulation of maturation of neuronal and oligodendroglial precursors, and enhancement of functional recovery. Importantly, delayed *intranasal administration* of mesenchymal stem cells after experimental neonatal stroke significantly enhanced somatosensory function 14, 21 and 28 days after stroke, reduced tissue loss, and improved motor function 28 days after stroke.[305-309] Autologous umbilical cord blood–derived cells, which have a number of obvious advantages from ethical and safety standpoints, have reached the stage of phase 1 clinical trials following NAIS (ClinicalTrials.gov reference NCT 01700166). Whether such cells, with or without added genetic modifications, will be useful in human infants with NAIS remains to be established, but future work will be of great interest.

Later Therapies

Therapies beyond the neonatal period are beyond the scope of this chapter. Early implementation of physical, occupational, and speech therapy is likely important for maximizing outcome.[158] The most recent addition in trial design for early rehabilitation for perinatal stroke has involved including parents in the development of the Early Therapy in Perinatal Stroke (eTIPS) program—a parent-delivered, home-based complex intervention addressing a current gap in practice for infants in the first 6 months of life after unilateral perinatal stroke and with the aim of improving motor outcome. This trial will commence in 2017.[310] Additional measures include constraint-induced movement therapy and extensive gait training. Of particular interest have been reports of implementation of *noninvasive neuromodulation* in children with hemiparesis after NAIS. These noninvasive approaches include inhibitory repetitive transcranial magnetic stimulation and transcranial direct current stimulation.[311,312] Future work will be of great interest.

CEREBRAL SINOVENOUS THROMBOSIS

Venous thrombosis, recognized best in the neonatal period by MRI, is more common than previously expected in the era before MRI.[a] CSVT has a lower reported incidence than NAIS, with incidences ranging from 0.6 to 12 per 100,000 live births.[227,324] This wide range in incidence may reflect differences in frequency of performance of neuroimaging (especially MRI) and the MRI sequences used. Moreover, it is generally assumed that CSVT remains somewhat overlooked because of relative lack of awareness among clinicians, the often nonspecific clinical presentation, and the relative difficulty of radiological diagnosis.

---

[a]References 179, 227, 229, 230, 245, 313-323.

TABLE 21.12   Neonatal Cerebral Sinovenous Thrombosis[a]

Superior sagittal sinus involvement in ≈65% of patients; thrombosis of lateral sinus in ≈50% or deep venous system in ≈50%; multiple site involvement in ≈50%

Infarction present in 40%–80% and hemorrhagic in most; intraventricular hemorrhage present in 35%–55%; hemorrhage in caudate and thalamus less common

Seizures initial presentation in 60%–70% of cases

Diagnosis best made by MRI/MRV

Pathogenesis often involving *multiple* factors, most often preeclampsia, maternal diabetes, perinatal "distress," congenital cardiac disease, ECMO, sepsis, dehydration, or prothrombotic coagulation defect

[a]See text for references; also includes unpublished personal experience.
ECMO, Extracorporeal membrane oxygenation; *MRI/MRV,* magnetic resonance imaging/magnetic resonance venography.

A higher incidence, of up to 4%, has been reported in preterm infants, but this may reflect the routine use of careful cranial ultrasound in these infants.[324,325]

Neuropathology of CVST

Approximately 65% of the thromboses affect the superior sagittal sinus, especially the posterior portion, and the remainder involve the lateral sinus (50%) or deep veins (e.g., straight sinus and Galenic system [50%]; Table 21.12). Infarction is present in 40% to 60% of cases; brain edema is the principal finding in those without infarction. The infarcts characteristically are hemorrhagic. MRI often demonstrates hemorrhagic infarction in the parasagittal regions bilaterally with sagittal sinus thrombosis and hemorrhagic infarction in the region of the striatum and internal capsule with deep venous thrombosis (involving internal cerebral and terminal veins). Intraventricular hemorrhage is present in 35% to 55% of cases and is often associated with infarction involving the thalamus and internal capsule.

Pathogenesis of CVST

The pathogenesis of CSVT exhibits similarities to that for NAIS. However, the distribution of risk factors differs to a considerable degree.

Risk Factors

As with NAIS, pathogenesis of CSVT is often multifactorial. However, in one large cohort study, a single risk factor was present in 48% of cases and multiple risk factors could be identified in 39%.[326] Preeclampsia, which involves a hypercoagulable state, is a common *maternal* risk factor. Other common maternal factors include gestational diabetes,[323,324,327] maternal fever, and chorioamnionitis. *Peripartum complications* (presence of meconium, hypoxia, acidosis, newborn resuscitation) were present in 70% of a large series.[328] Congenital heart disease was a dominant factor in 22% of the same series. Another large series identified congenital heart disease in only 2%.[324] Other common factors included dehydration (20%) and sepsis/meningitis.[328] In a report of 52 well-studied newborns with CSVT from the Netherlands, fully 60% experienced a complicated delivery, including vacuum or forceps delivery, a

finding that raises the possibility that cranial molding leading to venous sinus obstruction could be particularly important.[324]

The role of *prothrombotic factors* is not entirely clear.[324] Such abnormalities have been described in 15% to 20%, but the abnormalities often are considered *minor* and occur in the context of other risk factors.[328,329]

Clinical Features of CVST

Neonatal CSVT presents with seizures in 60% to 70% of cases.[a] Onset is most often in the first 48 hours after birth.[323,324] Importantly however, seizures are often preceded or accompanied by altered consciousness (*lethargy;* 65%)[328,329] and, only somewhat less frequently, by poor feeding, apnea, respiratory distress, irritability, or hypotonia. At least 70% of infants have in their background such peripartum risk factors as presence of meconium, hypoxia, sepsis/meningitis, acidosis, and newborn resuscitation.[328] Moreover, other associated disorders include dehydration and congenital heart disease.

Progression of clinical signs may occur, especially with development of major hemorrhage into the infarction, intraventricular hemorrhage, or thrombus propagation. Major degrees of hemorrhagic infarction occur in approximately 60% of cases.[328] Thrombus propagation occurs over the first week in approximately 25% of untreated patients.[330]

Diagnosis of CVST

Initial Evaluation

The initial diagnostic evaluation of the infant with suspected CSVT is similar to that outlined for NAIS. The emphasis of this section is diagnosis by neuroimaging.

Neuroimaging

Neuroimaging plays a key role in the diagnosis of CSVT.[227] The primary goal of neuroimaging is (1) to visualize and characterize the thrombus, (2) to identify the degree of impaired flow within the affected venous system, and (3) to define secondary consequences, such as infarction or hemorrhage, or both. Different techniques have been applied in the diagnostic workup of CSVT: cranial ultrasonography (especially with color Doppler studies), CT with or without venography (CTV), MRI with or without venography (MRV), and conventional angiography (Fig. 21.15).[227,331,332] MRI is the diagnostic modality of choice in CSVT and combines both conventional and advanced sequences, such as diffusion-weighted/tensor imaging (DWI/DTI) and SWI. Neuroimaging findings in CSVT may be subtle, and a number of potential pitfalls, such as anatomical variants of the cerebral venous system, make diagnosis challenging.[333] In addition, the MRI signal characteristics of a venous thrombus may vary depending upon its age and the MR sequence used. A high index of suspicion as well as familiarity with the neuroimaging findings is important for an early, sensitive, and specific diagnosis of CSVT in the newborn infant.

Cranial Ultrasonography. *Cranial ultrasonography,* used as a screening procedure, may provide clues of the presence of CSVT. The features most likely to be detected are intraventricular hemorrhage, often with ipsilateral thalamic hemorrhage or centrally located hemorrhagic venous infarction. As noted

[a]References 227, 229, 230, 245, 313, 315, 317-320, 322-324.

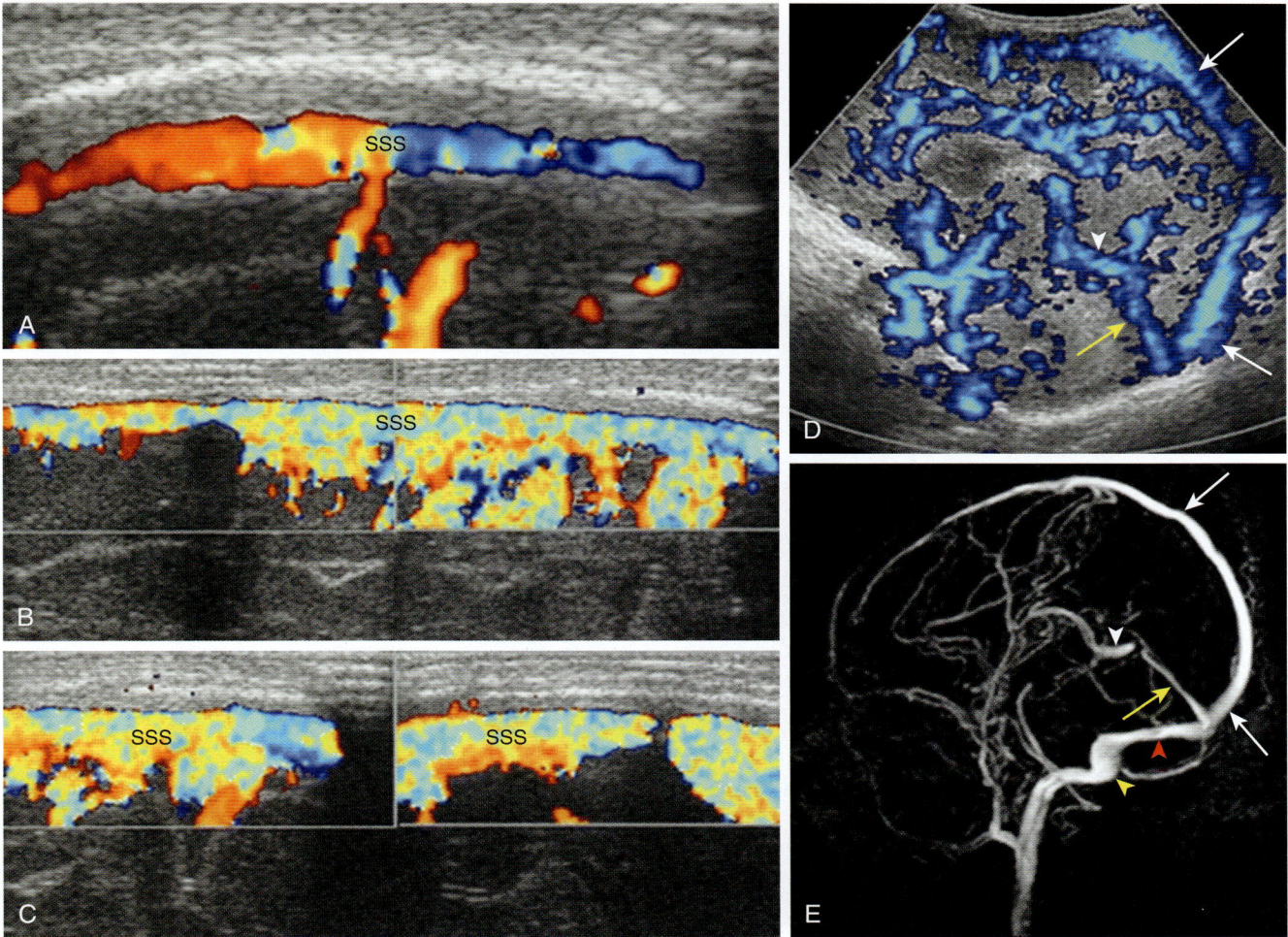

Figure 21.15 Normal superior sagittal sinus (SSS) in a 40-week gestational age newborn. Sagittal color Doppler ultrasound images of the (A) anterior, (B) middle, and (C) posterior SSS obtained through the anterior fontanelle, sagittal suture, and posterior fontanelle, respectively. Comparison to (D) power Doppler sagittal image acquired from the anterior fontanelle including the majority of the SSS *(white arrows)*, vein of Galen *(arrowhead)* and straight sinus *(yellow arrow)*. (E) Time-of-flight (TOF) magnetic resonance venography demonstrates patency of the cerebral venous sinuses: SSS *(white arrows)*, vein of Galen *(white arrowhead)*, straight sinus *(yellow arrow)*, transverse sinuses *(red arrowhead)*, and sigmoid sinuses *(yellow arrowhead)*. Inferior sagittal sinus was not seen on the reformat or source images (From Miller E, Daneman A, Doria AS, et al. Color Doppler US of normal cerebral venous sinuses in neonates: a comparison with MR venography. *Pediatr Radiol.* 2012;42(9):1070–1079.)

earlier, hemorrhagic infarction is apparent in approximately 50% to 60% of infants with CSVT, and intraventricular hemorrhage is noted in approximately 33% of infants with deep cerebral venous sinuses and hemorrhagic infarction in thalamus and/or caudate.[230,329]

Cranial ultrasound with color Doppler is a useful complementary ultrasonographic technique. A recent study evaluated 50 consecutive infants (30 males [60%]; 25 to 41 weeks old; mean, 37 weeks) with cranial ultrasonography with color Doppler and compared results with evaluation by MRI/MRV.[334] Excellent US-MRI agreement was noted for visualization of superior sagittal sinus, cerebral veins, straight sinus, torcular Herophili, sigmoid sinus, superior jugular veins (94% to 98%), and transverse sinuses (82% to 86%; see Fig. 21.15). In 10 cases (20%), MRV showed flow gaps whereas normal flow was demonstrated with US. Visualization of the inferior sagittal sinus was limited with both imaging techniques.

Computed Tomography. *CT*, although no longer a preferred technique, can identify major CSVT. The classic features include the *dense triangle* or the *cord sign*, depicting increased density over the major venous sinus on plain CT and the *empty triangle* or *empty delta* sign in a contrast-enhanced CT.[329] CT may lead to false positive results in newborns because of increased hematocrit and slower venous flow and involves radiation exposure. Thus we do not recommend this approach unless MRI is unavailable.

Magnetic Resonance Imaging/Magnetic Resonance Venography. MRI with MRV is clearly the most definitive diagnostic neuroimaging approach.[323,324,327-329,335] MRI is especially useful for detection of infarction (Figs. 21.16 and 21.17; see Chapters 10 and 20). With DWI the parenchymal lesions are apparent within minutes-hours of the injury. Coupled with time-of-flight MRV, the cerebral venous sinuses and deep venous system can be imaged without contrast. Some caution in interpretation is needed, however, as lower venous flow, a smaller caliber venous sinus, and skin molding can also cause the appearance of a flow gap in the venous sinuses. These findings

should, therefore, be interpreted in the context of the additional MR findings just noted and the clinical condition of the infant.

Associated lesions like thalamic hemorrhage, intraventricular hemorrhage, or parenchymal hemorrhagic infarction are commonly seen (see Figs. 21.16 and 21.17; see the section on neuropathology). In the largest series with CSVT (*n* = 52), thalamic hemorrhage, intraventricular hemorrhage, or parenchymal hemorrhagic infarction was observed in 25

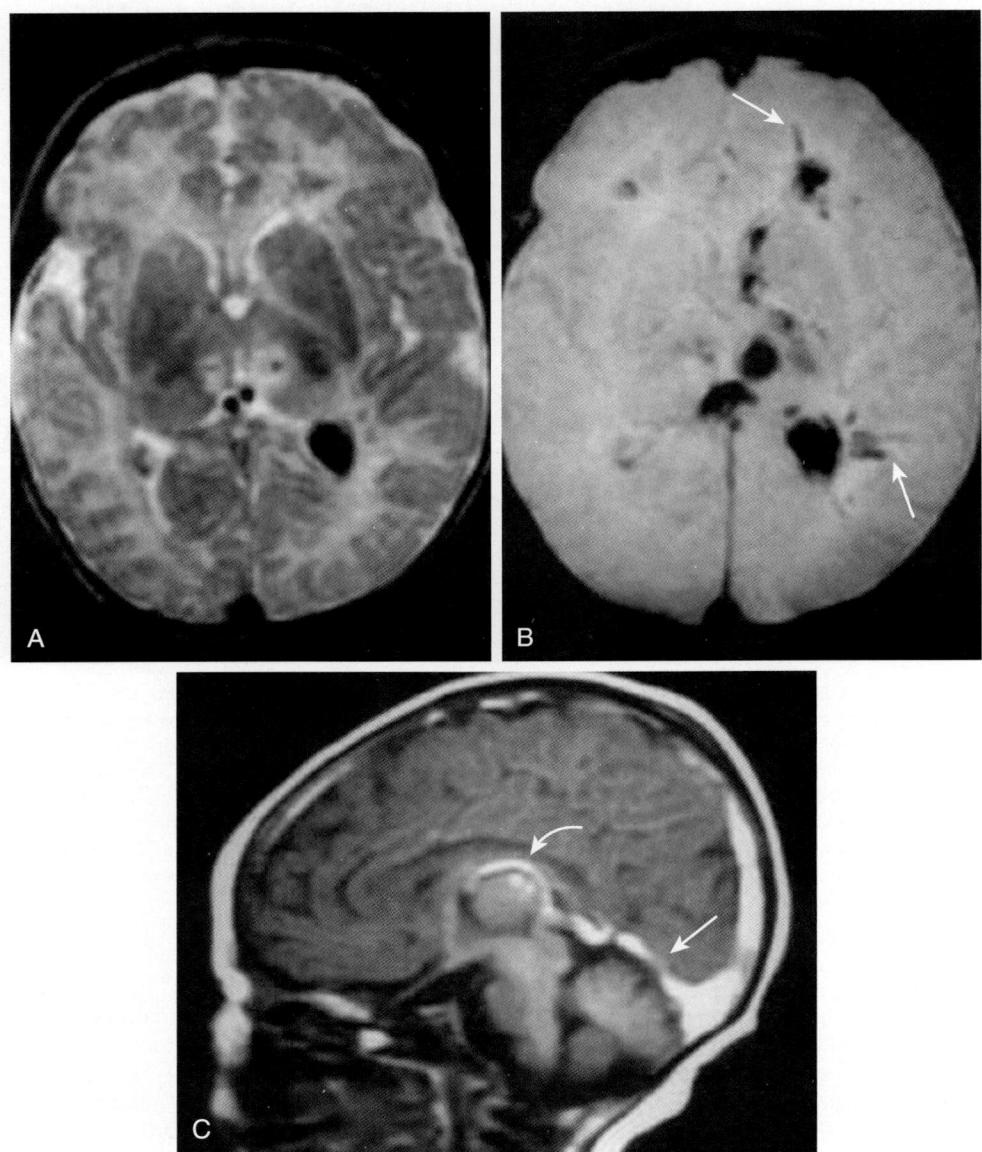

Figure 21.16 Conventional magnetic resonance imaging of cerebral sinovenous thrombosis in the newborn. Combined deep and superficial venous thrombosis with hemorrhage in a neonate. An 11-day-old girl presented with drowsiness and pyrexia. (A) Axial T2-weighted MR image demonstrates bilateral thalamic T2 hyperintensity and low signal hemorrhage within the periventricular white matter, left capsular white matter, and deep gray matter, more marked on the left. The hypointensity is much more conspicuous on the equivalent (B) axial T2-weighted MR image. The low signal within the superior sagittal sinus and internal cerebral veins represents early thrombus rather than evidence of flow. The linear hypointensities within deep white matter probably represent thrombus within medullary veins (*arrows*). (C) Sagittal T1-weighted MR image reveals high signal thrombus within the superior sagittal sinus, straight sinus (*arrow*), and internal cerebral veins (*curved arrow*). (From Connor SE, Jarosz JM. Magnetic resonance imaging of cerebral venous sinus thrombosis. *Clin Radiol.* 2002;57(6):449–461.)

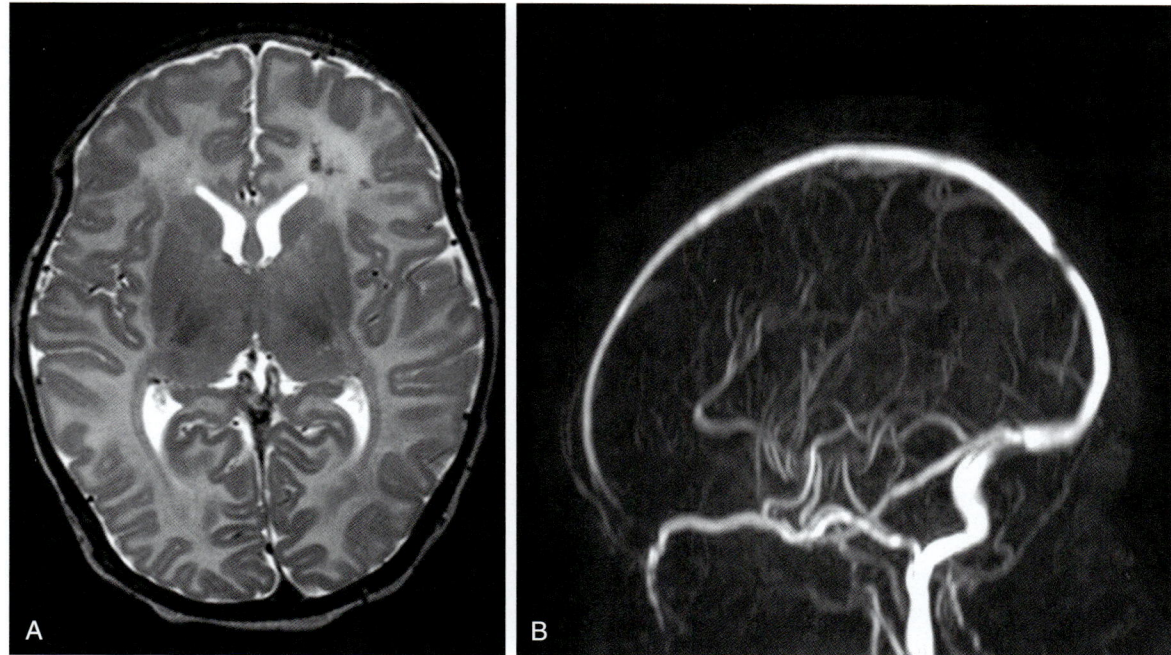

Figure 21.17 (A) Axial T2-weighted spin echo (T2SE) image showing predominantly left-sided punctate white matter lesions. (B) Time-of-flight magnetic resonance venography image showing absent flow in the straight sinus. (From Berfelo FJ, Kersbergen KJ, van Ommen CH, et al. Neonatal cerebral sinovenous thrombosis from symptom to outcome. *Stroke.* 2010;41:1382–1388.)

(48%), 29 (56%), and 41 (79%) of the infants, respectively.[324] Straight sinus thrombosis or complex multiple-sinus thrombosis was associated most frequently with severe hemorrhagic infarction of basal ganglia and/or thalamus. In infants with multiple-sinus thrombosis without associated cerebral lesions (3 of 26), the straight sinus was not involved. Multiple-sinus thrombosis was present in 9 of the 10 newborns who died.

Prognosis

The outcome of CSVT differs in several respects from that just described for NAIS. Thus *neonatal death* with NAIS is rare, less than 1%. With CSVT mortality rates vary, but the largest series report rates of 10% to 20%.[227,323,324,328,329] The higher mortality rates in CSVT may reflect in considerable part the accompanying disorders leading to CSVT, as well as the associated cerebral parenchymal lesions, especially when multiple sinuses are involved.

Long-term neurological sequelae with CSVT include motor deficits, cognitive impairment, and epilepsy (Table 21.13). Motor impairment occurs in approximately 50% of survivors and is most often bilateral, unlike the nearly uniform hemiparesis in NAIS.[a] The rates of cognitive impairment vary in part according to the duration of follow-up but range from 10% to 60%.[227,323,324,328,329] Epilepsy is reported in 20% to 40% of survivors.[227,324,329] In general, the neurological deficits occur in

TABLE 21.13	Neonatal and Long-Term Neurological Correlates of Neonatal Cerebral Sinovenous Thrombosis[a]
NEUROLOGICAL CORRELATES	**AFFECTED (%)**
Motor impairment, usually bilateral	50
Cognitive deficits	10–60
Seizures	29–40

[a]See text for references. Includes unpublished personal cases.

those infants with parenchymal lesions, especially hemorrhagic infarction.

Management

Acute Therapy

The acute therapy of CSVT is similar to that noted for NAIS: management of comorbidities and seizures. In CSVT such comorbidities as sepsis, meningitis, and dehydration require especially prompt treatment. Considerations for treatment of seizures are as noted for NAIS and as discussed in detail in Chapter 12.

Anticoagulant Therapy

No worldwide consensus in the management of neonatal CSVT has evolved, but a *distinct tendency toward increased use*

---

[a]References 227, 323, 324, 328, 329, 336-339.

of anticoagulation has developed in recent years.[340] However, this tendency varies remarkably by region. In one large study, treatment with anticoagulation was recorded in 25% of cases in the United States, 68% of cases in Canada, and 80% of cases in Europe.[328] Prevention of clot propagation is the principal reason for therapy. Propagation occurs in 25% to 30% of cases, most often in the first week after the primary insult. Initiation of anticoagulation treatment reduces the rate to about 3%.[329] No apparent increased risk of bleeding has been observed. In general, anticoagulation is recommended in infants with CSVT without hemorrhage, and many centers also use anticoagulation with CSVT with thalamic hemorrhage.[340,341] Low-molecular-weight heparin is used most commonly and such therapy requires close monitoring to ensure adequate dosing. Follow-up imaging studies should include assessment after 6 weeks to evaluate recanalization. If recanalization is complete, therapy can be discontinued. If recanalization is not complete, therapy for 6 additional weeks is carried out.[329]

Other Interventions

Supportive care strategies are also under investigation in perinatal CSVT. Tan et al.[342] have demonstrated that the occipital bone compression seen in supine newborn infants can be associated with CSVT, presumably because of increased venous stasis. Later work by this group revealed that a pillow alleviating occipital decompression can increase blood flow in the sigmoid sinus and superior sagittal sinus, thus representing a possible noninvasive intervention for the treatment of CSVT or even a prevention strategy in high-risk infants.[343]

KEY REFERENCES

1. Raju TN, Nelson KB, Ferriero D, et al. Ischemic perinatal stroke: summary of a workshop sponsored by the National Institute of Child Health and Human Development and the National Institute of Neurological Disorders and Stroke. *Pediatrics.* 2007;120(3):609-616.
3. Nelson KB, Lynch JK. Stroke in newborn infants. *Lancet.* 2004;3:150-158.
4. Schneider AT, Kissela B, Woo D, et al. Ischemic stroke subtypes: a population-based study of incidence rates among blacks and whites. *Stroke.* 2004;35(7):1552-1556.
5. Schulzke S, Weber P, Luetschg J, et al. Incidence and diagnosis of unilateral arterial cerebral infarction in newborn infants. *J Perinat Med.* 2005;33(2):170-175.
6. Kirton A, Deveber G. Perinatal ischemic stroke. *Stroke Rev.* 2006;10:38-47.
14. Mannino FL, Trauner DA. Stroke in neonates. *J Pediatr.* 1983;102(4):605-610.
15. Ment LR, Duncan CC, Ehrenkranz RA. Perinatal cerebral infarction. *Ann Neurol.* 1984;16(5):559-568.
16. Trauner DA, Mannino FL. Neurodevelopmental outcome after neonatal cerebrovascular accident. *J Pediatr.* 1986;108(3): 459-461.
18. Filipek PA, Krishnamoorthy KS, Davis KR, et al. Focal cerebral infarction in the newborn: a distinct entity. *Pediatr Neurol.* 1987;3(3):141-147.
24. Sran SK, Baumann RJ. Outcome of neonatal strokes. *Am J Dis Child.* 1988;142(10):1086-1088.
31. de Vries LS, Groenendaal F, Eken P, et al. Infarcts in the vascular distribution of the middle cerebral artery in preterm and fullterm infants. *Neuropediatrics.* 1997;28:88-96.
32. Mercuri E, Rutherford M, Cowan F, et al. Early prognostic indicators of outcome in infants with neonatal cerebral infarction: a clinical, electroencephalogram, and magnetic resonance imaging study. *Pediatrics.* 1999;103:103-139.
33. Govaert P, Matthys E, Zecic A, et al. Perinatal cortical infarction within middle cerebral artery trunks. *Arch Dis Child.* 2000;82(1):F59-F63.
34. Sreenan C, Bhargava R, Robertson CMT. Cerebral infarction in the term newborn: clinical presentation and long-term outcome. *J Pediatr.* 2000;137:351-355.
35. Golomb MR, MacGregor DL, Domi T, et al. Presumed pre- or perinatal arterial ischemic stroke: risk factors and outcomes. *Ann Neurol.* 2001;50:163-168.
36. Ramaswamy V, Miller SP, Barkovich AJ, et al. Perinatal stroke in term infants with neonatal encephalopathy. *Neurology.* 2004;62:2088-2091.
37. Lee J, Croen LA, Lindan C, et al. Predictors of outcome in perinatal arterial stroke: a population-based study. *Ann Neurol.* 2005;58(2):303-308.
38. Benders MJNL, Groenendaal F, Uiterwaal CSPM, et al. Maternal and infant characteristics associated with perinatal arterial stroke in the preterm infant. *Stroke.* 2007;38:1759-1765.
56. Amato M, Huppi P, Herschkowitz N, et al. Prenatal stroke suggested by intrauterine ultrasound and confirmed by magnetic resonance imaging. *Neuropediatrics.* 1991;22(2):100-102.
63. Castro-Gago M, Alonso A, Pintos-Martinez E, et al. Congenital hydranencephalic-hydrocephalic syndrome associated with mitochondrial dysfunction. *J Child Neurol.* 1999;14:131-135.
72. Ozduman K, Pober BR, Barnes P, et al. Fetal stroke. *Pediatr Neurol.* 2004;30(3):151-162.
73. Smith CD, Baumann RJ. Clinical features and magnetic resonance imaging in congenital and childhood stroke. *J Child Neurol.* 1991;6(3):263-272.
77. Chasnoff IJ, Bussey ME, Savich R, et al. Perinatal cerebral infarction and maternal cocaine use. *J Pediatr.* 1986;108(3):456-459.
79. Perlman JM, Rollins NK, Evans D. Neonatal stroke: clinical characteristics and cerebral blood flow velocity measurements. *Pediatr Neurol.* 1994;11:281-284.
80. Burke CJ, Tannenberg AE, Payton DJ. Ischemic cerebral injury, intrauterine growth retardation, and placental infarction. *Dev Med Child Neurol.* 1997;39:726-730.
81. Kraus FT, Acheen VI. Fetal thrombotic vasculopathy in the placenta: cerebral thrombi and infarcts, coagulopathies, and cerebral palsy. *Hum Pathol.* 1999;30:759-769.
82. Kraus FT. Cerebral palsy and thrombi in placental vessels of the fetus: insights from litigation. *Hum Pathol.* 2003;28:246-248.
83. Redline RW. Severe fetal placental vascular lesions in term infants with neurologic impairment. *Am J Obstet Gynecol.* 2005;192:452-457.
84. Curry CJ, Bhullar S, Holmes J, et al. Risk factors for perinatal arterial stroke: a study of 60 mother-child pairs. *Pediatr Neurol.* 2007;37(2):99-107.
85. Lee J, Croen LA, Backstrand KH, et al. Maternal and infant characteristics associated with perinatal arterial stroke in the infant. *JAMA.* 2005;293:723-729.
87. Manterola A, Towbin A, Yakovlev PI. Cerebral infarction in the human fetus near term. *J Neuropathol Exp Neurol.* 1966;25(3):479-488.
105. Weig SG, Marshall PC, Abroms IF, et al. Patterns of cerebral injury and clinical presentation in the vascular disruptive syndrome of monozygotic twins. *Pediatr Neurol.* 1995;13:279-285.
106. Van Bogaert P, Donner C, David P, et al. Congenital bilateral perisylvian syndrome in a monozygotic twin with intrauterine death of the co-twin. *Dev Med Child Neurol.* 1996;38:166-171.
108. Maier RF, Bialobrzeski B, Gross A, et al. Acute and chronic fetal hypoxia in monochorionic and dichorionic twins. *Obstet Gynecol.* 1996;86:973-977.
114. Pharoah POD, Adi Y. Consequences of in-utero death in a twin pregnancy. *Lancet.* 2000;355(9215):1597-1602.
115. Pharoah POD. Cerebral palsy in the surviving twin associated with infant death of the co-twin. *Arch Dis Child Fetal Neonatal Ed.* 2001;84:F111-F116.
116. Seng YC, Rajadurai VS. Twin-twin transfusion syndrome: a five year review. *Arch Dis Child Fetal Neonatal Ed.* 2000;83(3):F168-F170.
117. Scher AI, Petterson B, Blair E, et al. The risk of mortality or cerebral palsy in twins: a collaborative population-based study. *Pediatr Res.* 2002;52:671-681.

118. Duncombe GJ, Dickinson JE, Evans SF. Perinatal characteristics and outcomes of pregnancies complicated by twin-twin transfusion syndrome. *Obstet Gynecol*. 2003;101(6):1190-1196.

119. Buldini B, Drigo P, Via LD, et al. Symmetrical thalamic calcifications in a monozygotic twin: case report and literature review. *Brain Dev*. 2005;27:66-69.

120. Mari G, Roberts A, Detti L, et al. Perinatal morbidity and mortality rates in severe twin-twin transfusion syndrome: results of the International Amnioreduction Registry. *Am J Obstet Gynecol*. 2001;185:708-715.

121. Lopriore E, Nagel HTC, Vandenbussche FPHA, et al. Long-term neurodevelopmental outcome in twin-to-twin transfusion syndrome. *Am J Obstet Gynecol*. 2003;189(5):1314-1319.

122. Chiswick M. Assessing outcomes in twin-twin transfusion syndrome. *Arch Dis Child Fetal Neonatal Ed*. 2000;83(3):F165-F167.

123. Hahn JS, Lewis AJ, Barries P. Hydranencephaly owing to twin-twin transfusion: serial fetal ultrasonography and magnetic resonance imaging findings. *J Child Neurol*. 2003;18:367-370.

124. Glinianaia SV, Pharoah POD, Wright C, et al. Fetal or infant death in twin pregnancy: neurodevelopmental consequence for the survivor. *Arch Dis Child*. 2002;86(1):F9-F15.

125. Zankl A, Brooks D, Boltshauser E, et al. Natural history of twin disruption sequence. *Am J Med Genet A*. 2004;127A(2):133-138.

126. Dickinson JE, Duncombe GJ, Evans SF, et al. The long term neurologic outcome of children from pregnancies complicated by twin-twin transfusion syndrome. *BJOG*. 2005;112(1):63-68.

127. Golomb MR, Williams LS, Garg BP. Perinatal stroke in twins without co-twin demise. *Pediatr Neurol*. 2006;35(1):75-77.

128. Redline RW. Nonidentical twins with a single placenta—disproving dogma in perinatal pathology. *N Engl J Med*. 2003;349(2):111-114.

129. Behrendt N, Galan HL. Twin-twin transfusion and laser therapy. *Curr Opin Obstet Gynecol*. 2016;28(2):79-85.

132. Senat MV, Deprest J, Boulvain M, et al. Endoscopic laser surgery versus serial amnioreduction for severe twin-to-twin transfusion syndrome. *N Engl J Med*. 2004;351:136-144.

133. Lopriore E, Sueters M, Middeldorp JM, et al. Neonatal outcome in twin-to-twin transfusion syndrome treated with fetoscopic laser occlusion of vascular anastomoses. *J Pediatr*. 2005;147:597-602.

134. Graef C, Ellenrieder B, Hecher K, et al. Long-term neurodevelopmental outcome of 167 children after intrauterine laser treatment for severe twin-twin transfusion syndrome. *Obstet Gynecol*. 2006;194:303-308.

135. Lopriore E, van Wezel-Meijler G, Middeldorp JM, et al. Incidence, origin, and character of cerebral injury in twin-to-twin transfusion syndrome treated with fetoscopic laser surgery. *Am J Obstet Gynecol*. 2006;194(5):1215-1220.

136. Norton ME. Evaluation and management of twin-twin transfussion syndrome: still a challenge. *Am J Obstet Gynecol*. 2007;196:419-420.

137. van Klink JM, Slaghekke F, Balestriero MA, et al. Neurodevelopmental outcome at 2 years in twin-twin transfusion syndrome survivors randomized for the Solomon trial. *Am J Obstet Gynecol*. 2016;214(1):113 e111-e117.

138. Akkermans J, Peeters SH, Klumper FJ, et al. Twenty-five years of fetoscopic laser coagulation in twin-twin transfusion syndrome: a systematic review. *Fetal Diagn Ther*. 2015;38(4):241-253.

145. Choi KD, Shin HY, Kim JS, et al. Rotational vertebral artery syndrome: oculographic analysis of nystagmus. *Neurology*. 2005;65:1287-1290.

146. Pamphlett R, Murray N. Vulnerability of the infant brain stem to ischemia: a possible cause of sudden infant death syndrome. *J Child Neurol*. 1996;11:181-184.

149. Hayes B, Ryan S, Stephenson JBP, et al. Cerebral palsy after maternal trauma in pregnancy. *Dev Med Child Neurol*. 2007;49:700-706.

150. Wu YW, March WM, Croen LA, et al. Perinatal stroke in children with motor impairment: a population-based study. *Pediatrics*. 2004;114(3):612-619.

151. Simchen MJ, Goldstein G, Lubetsky A, et al. Factor v Leiden and antiphospholipid antibodies in either mothers or infants increase the risk for perinatal arterial ischemic stroke. *Stroke*. 2009;40(1):65-70.

152. Elbers J, Viero S, MacGregor D, et al. Placental pathology in neonatal stroke. *Pediatrics*. 2011;127(3):e722-e729.

153. Kirton A, Armstrong-Wells J, Chang T, et al. Symptomatic neonatal arterial ischemic stroke: the International Pediatric Stroke Study. *Pediatrics*. 2011;128(6):e1402-e1410.

154. Michoulas A, Basheer SN, Roland EH, et al. The role of hypoxia-ischemia in term newborns with arterial stroke. *Pediatr Neurol*. 2011;44(4):254-258.

155. Tuckuviene R, Christensen AL, Helgested J, et al. Infant, obstetrical and maternal characteristics associated with thromboembolism in infancy: a nationwide population-based case-control study. *Arch Dis Child Fetal Neonatal Ed*. 2012;97(6):F417-F422.

156. Harteman JC, Groenendaal F, Kwee A, et al. Risk factors for perinatal arterial ischaemic stroke in full-term infants: a case-control study. *Arch Dis Child Fetal Neonatal Ed*. 2012;97(6):F411-F416.

157. Darmency-Stamboul V, Chantegret C, Ferdynus C, et al. Antenatal factors associated with perinatal arterial ischemic stroke. *Stroke*. 2012;43(9):2307-2312.

158. Lehman LL, Rivkin MJ. Perinatal arterial ischemic stroke: presentation, risk factors, evaluation, and outcome. *Pediatr Neurol*. 2014;51(6):760-768.

159. Tibussek D, Sinclair A, Yau I, et al. Late-onset group B streptococcal meningitis has cerebrovascular complications. *J Pediatr*. 2015;166(5):1187-1192 e1181.

160. Martinez-Biarge M, Cheong JLY, Diez-Sebastian J, et al. Risk factors for neonatal arterial ischemic stroke: the importance of the intrapartum period. *J Pediatr*. 2016;173:62-68.

175. Gunther G, Junker R, Strater R, et al. Symptomatic ischemic stroke in full-term neonates: role of acquired and genetic prothrombotic risk factors. *Stroke*. 2000;31:2437-2441.

176. Hogeveen M, Blom HJ, van Amerogen M, et al. Hyperhomocysteinemia as risk factor for ischemic and hemorrhagic stroke in newborn infants. *J Pediatr*. 2002;141:429-431.

177. Mercuri E, Cowan F, Gupte G, et al. Prothrombotic disorders and abnormal neurodevelopmental outcome in infants with neonatal cerebral infarction. *Pediatrics*. 2001;107:1400-1404.

178. Lynch JK, Hirtz DG, De Veber G, et al. Report of the National Institute of neurological disorders and stroke workshop on perinatal and childhood stroke. *Pediatrics*. 2002;109:116-123.

179. Golomb MR, Dick PT, MacGregor DL, et al. Neonatal arterial ischemic stroke and cerebral sinovenous thrombosis are more commonly diagnosed in boys. *J Child Neurol*. 2004;19: 493-497.

182. Alfonso I, Prieto G, Vasconcellos E, et al. Internal carotid artery thrombus: an underdiagnosed source of brain emboli in neonates? *J Child Neurol*. 2001;16:446-447.

186. Liu XY, Wong V, Leung M. Neurologic complications due to catheterization. *Pediatr Neurol*. 2001;24(4):270-275.

187. Domi T, Edgell DS, McCrindle BW, et al. Frequency, predictors, and neurologic outcomes of vaso-occlusive strokes associated with cardiac surgery in children. *Pediatrics*. 2008;122(6):1292-1298.

188. Chen J, Zimmerman RA, Jarvik GP, et al. Perioperative stroke in infants undergoing open heart operations for congenital heart disease. *Ann Thorac Surg*. 2009;88(3):823-829.

189. Morales DL, Almond CS, Jaquiss RD, et al. Bridging children of all sizes to cardiac transplantation: the initial multicenter North American experience with the Berlin Heart EXCOR ventricular assist device. *J Heart Lung Transplant*. 2011;30(1):1-8.

190. Almond CS, Morales DL, Blackstone EH, et al. Berlin Heart EXCOR pediatric ventricular assist device for bridge to heart transplantation in US children. *Circulation*. 2013;127(16): 1702-1711.

191. Sinclair AJ, Fox CK, Ichord RN, et al. Stroke in children with cardiac disease: report from the International Pediatric Stroke Study Group Symposium. *Pediatr Neurol*. 2015;52(1):5-15.

194. Lequin MH, Peeters EA, Holscher HC, et al. Arterial infarction caused by carotid artery dissection in the neonate. *Eur J Paediatr Neurol*. 2004;8:155-160.

195. Kaneko K, Someya T, Ohtaki R, et al. Congenital fibromuscular dysplasia involving multivessels in an infant with fatal outcome. *Eur J Pediatr*. 2004;163:241-244.

215. Chow G, Mellor D. Neonatal cerebral ischaemia with elevated maternal and infant anticardiolipin antibodies. *Dev Med Child Neurol*. 2000;42:412-413.

216. Smith RA, Skelton M, Howard M, et al. Is thrombophilia a factor in the development of hemiplegic cerebral palsy? *Dev Med Child Neurol*. 2001;43:724-730.

217. Lynch JK, Nelson KB, Curry CJ, et al. Cerebrovascular disorders in children with the factor V Leiden mutation. *J Child Neurol*. 2001;16(10):735-744.

218. Aronis S, Bouza H, Pergantou H, et al. Prothrombotic factors in neonates with cerebral thrombosis and intraventricular hemorrhage. *Acta Paediatr.* 2002;91:87-91.

219. Ebeling F, Petaja J, Alanko S, et al. Infant stroke and beta-2-glycoprotein 1 antibodies: six cases. *Eur J Pediatr.* 2003;162(10):678-681.

220. Cowan F, Rutherford M, Groenendaal F, et al. Origin and timing of brain lesions in term infants with neonatal encephalopathy. *Lancet.* 2003;361(9359):736-742.

221. Verdu A, Cazorla MR, Moreno JC, et al. Prenatal stroke in a neonate heterozygous for factor V Leiden mutation. *Brain Dev.* 2005;27:451-454.

222. De Haan TR, Van Wezel-Meijler G, Beersma MF, et al. Fetal stroke and congenital parvovirus B19 infection complicated by activated protein C resistance. *Acta Paediatr.* 2006;95:863-867.

223. Reid S, Halliday J, Ditchfield M, et al. Factor V Leiden mutation: a contributory factor for cerebral palsy? *Dev Med Child Neurol.* 2006;48(1):14-19.

224. Gelfand AA, Croen LA, Torres AR, et al. Genetic risk factors for perinatal arterial ischemic stroke. *Pediatr Neurol.* 2013;48(1):36-41.

225. Baud O, Picard V, Durand P, et al. Intracerebral hemorrhage associated with a novel antithrombin gene mutation in a neonate. *J Pediatr.* 2001;139:741-743.

226. Friese S, Muller-Hansen I, Schoning M, et al. Isolated internal cerebral venous thrombosis in a neonate with increased lipoprotein (a) level: diagnostic and therapeutic considerations. *Neuropediatrics.* 2003;34:36-39.

227. deVeber G, Andrew M, Adams C, et al. Cerebral sinovenous thrombosis in children. *N Engl J Med.* 2001;345(6):417-423.

228. Abrantes M, Lacerda AF, Abreu CR, et al. Cerebral venous sinus thrombosis in a neonate due to factor V Leiden deficiency. *Acta Paediatr.* 2002;91(2):243-245.

229. Hunt RW, Badawi N, Laing S, et al. Pre-eclampsia: a predisposing factor for neonatal venous sinus thrombosis? *Pediatr Neurol.* 2001;25:242-246.

230. Wu TW, Miller SP, Chin K, et al. Multiple risk factors in neonatal sinovenous thrombosis. *Neurology.* 2002;59:438-440.

231. Mahasandana C, Suvatte V, Chuansumrit A, et al. Homozygous protein S deficiency in an infant with purpura fulminans. *J Pediatr.* 1990;117(5):750-753.

247. Debus OM, Kosch A, Strater R, et al. The factor V G1691A mutation is a risk for porencephaly: a case-control study. *Ann Neurol.* 2004;56:287-290.

248. Steinlin M, Pfister I, Pavlovic J, et al. The first three years of the Swiss Neuropaediatric Stroke Registry (SNPSR): a population-based study of incidence, symptoms and risk factors. *Neuropediatrics.* 2005;36:90-97.

251. Kiserud T, Ozaki T, Nishina H, et al. Effect of NO, phenylephrine, and hypoxemia on ductus venosus diameter in fetal sheep. *Am J Physiol Heart Circ Physiol.* 2000;279(3):H1166-H1171.

252. Kiserud T, Kessler J, Ebbing C, et al. Ductus venosus shunting in growth-restricted fetuses and the effect of umbilical circulatory compromise. *Ultrasound Obstet Gynecol.* 2006;28(2):143-149.

253. Rafay MF, Cortez MA, de Veber GA, et al. Predictive value of clinical and EEG features in the diagnosis of stroke and hypoxic ischemic encephalopathy in neonates with seizures. *Stroke.* 2009;40(7):2402-2407.

254. Golomb MR, Garg BP, Edwards-Brown M, et al. Very early arterial ischemic stroke in premature infants. *Pediatr Neurol.* 2008;38(5):329-334.

257. Cowan F, Mercuri E, Groenendaal F, et al. Does cranial ultrasound imaging identify arterial cerebral infarction in term neonates? *Arch Dis Child Fetal Neonatal Ed.* 2005;90:F252-F256.

258. van der Aa NE, Dudink J, Benders MJ, et al. Neonatal posterior cerebral artery stroke: clinical presentation, MRI findings, and outcome. *Dev Med Child Neurol.* 2013;55(3):283-290.

259. Barnette AR, Horbar JD, Soll RF, et al. Neuroimaging in the evaluation of neonatal encephalopathy. *Pediatrics.* 2014;133(6):e1508-e1517.

260. Robertson RL, Robson CD, Zurakowski D, et al. CT versus MR in neonatal brain imaging at term. *Pediatr Radiol.* 2003;33(7):442-449.

261. Koelfen W, Wentz U, Freund M, et al. Magnetic resonance angiography in 140 neuropediatric patients. *Pediatr Neurol.* 1995;12:31-38.

262. Kuker W, Mohrle S, Mader I, et al. MRI for the management of neonatal cerebral infarctions: importance of timing. *Childs Nerv Syst.* 2004;20(10):742-748.

263. Lequin MH, Dudink J, Tong KA, et al. Magnetic resonance imaging in neonatal stroke. *Semin Fetal Neonatal Med.* 2009;14(5):299-310.

264. Dudink J, Mercuri E, Al-Nakib L, et al. Evolution of unilateral perinatal arterial ischemic stroke on conventional and diffusion-weighted MR imaging. *AJNR Am J Neuroradiol.* 2009;30(5):998-1004.

265. Groenendaal F, de Vries LS. Fifty years of brain imaging in neonatal encephalopathy following perinatal asphyxia. *Pediatr Res.* 2017;81(1-2):150-155.

266. Benders MJ, Groenendaal F, Uiterwaal CS, et al. Maternal and infant characteristics associated with perinatal arterial stroke in the preterm infant. *Stroke.* 2007;38(6):1759-1765.

267. Roze E, Benders MJ, Kersbergen KJ, et al. Neonatal DTI early after birth predicts motor outcome in preterm infants with periventricular hemorrhagic infarction. *Pediatr Res.* 2015;78(3):298-303.

278. Mercuri E, Barnett A, Rutherford M, et al. Neonatal cerebral infarction and neuromotor outcome at school age. *Pediatrics.* 2004;113:95-100.

279. Boardman JP, Ganesan V, Rutherford M, et al. Magnetic resonance image correlates of hemiparesis after neonatal and childhood middle cerebral artery stroke. *Pedaitrics.* 2005;115:321-326.

280. Bax M, Tydeman C, Flodmark O. Clinical and MRI correlates of cerebral palsy: the European Cerebral Palsy Study. *JAMA.* 2006;296(13):1602-1608.

281. Husson B, Hertz-Pannier L, Renaud C, et al. Motor outcomes after neonatal arterial ischemic stroke related to early MRI data in a prospective study. *Pediatrics.* 2010;126(4):912-918.

282. Chabrier S, Peyric E, Drutel L, et al. Multimodal outcome at 7 years of age after neonatal arterial ischemic stroke. *J Pediatr.* 2016;172:156-161 e153.

283. Fox CK, Glass HC, Sidney S, et al. Neonatal seizures triple the risk of a remote seizure after perinatal ischemic stroke. *Neurology.* 2016;86(23):2179-2186.

284. van der Aa NE, Northington FJ, Stone BS, et al. Quantification of white matter injury following neonatal stroke with serial DTI. *Pediatr Res.* 2013;73(6):756-762.

289. Kirton A, Shroff M, Visvanathan T, et al. Quantified corticospinal tract diffusion restriction predicts neonatal stroke outcome. *Stroke.* 2007;38(3):974-980.

291. Kolk A, Talvik T. Cerebral lateralization and cognitive deficits after congenital hemiparesis. *Pediatr Neurol.* 2002;27:356-362.

292. Westmacott R, MacGregor D, Askalan R, et al. Late emergence of cognitive deficits after unilateral neonatal stroke. *Stroke.* 2009;40(6):2012-2019.

293. Westmacott R, Askalan R, MacGregor D, et al. Cognitive outcome following unilateral arterial ischaemic stroke in childhood: effects of age at stroke and lesion location. *Dev Med Child Neurol.* 2010;52(4):386-393.

294. Suppiej A, Mastrangelo M, Mastella L, et al. Pediatric epilepsy following neonatal seizures symptomatic of stroke. *Brain Dev.* 2016;38(1):27-31.

295. Wusthoff CJ, Kessler SK, Vossough A, et al. Risk of later seizure after perinatal arterial ischemic stroke: a prospective cohort study. *Pediatrics.* 2011;127(6):e1550-e1557.

296. Fullerton HJ, Wu YW, Sidney S, et al. Risk of recurrent childhood arterial ischemic stroke in a population-based cohort: the importance of cerebrovascular imaging. *Pediatrics.* 2007;119(3):495-501.

297. Harbert MJ, Tam EW, Glass HC, et al. Hypothermia is correlated with seizure absence in perinatal stroke. *J Child Neurol.* 2011;26(9):1126-1130.

298. Sun Y, Calvert JW, Zhang JH. Neonatal hypoxia/ischemia is associated with decreased inflammatory mediators after erythropoietin administration. *Stroke.* 2005;36(8):1672-1678.

299. Sola A, Rogido M, Lee BH, et al. Erythropoietin after focal cerebral ischemia activates the Janus Kinase-signal transducer and activator of transcription signaling pathway and improves brain injury in postnatal day 7 rats. *Pediatr Res.* 2005;57:481-487.

301. Gonzalez FF, Abel R, Almli CR, et al. Erythropoietin sustains cognitive function and brain volume after neonatal stroke. *Dev Neurosci.* 2009;31(5):403-411.

303. Ehrenreich H, Hasselblatt M, Dembowski C, et al. Erythropoietin therapy for acute stroke is both safe and beneficial. *Mol Med.* 2002;8(8):495-505.

304. Benders MJ, van der Aa NE, Roks M, et al. Feasibility and safety of erythropoietin for neuroprotection after perinatal arterial ischemic stroke. *J Pediatr.* 2014;164(3):481-486.

305. van Velthoven CT, Gonzalez F, Vexler ZS, et al. Stem cells for neonatal stroke—the future is here. *Front Cell Neurosci.* 2014;8:207.

306. Chau MJ, Deveau TC, Song M, et al. iPSC Transplantation increases regeneration and functional recovery after ischemic stroke in neonatal rats. *Stem Cells.* 2014;32(12):3075-3087.

309. van Velthoven CT, Sheldon RA, Kavelaars A, et al. Mesenchymal stem cell transplantation attenuates brain injury after neonatal stroke. *Stroke.* 2013;44(5):1426-1432.

310. Basu AP, Pearse JE, Baggaley J, et al. Participatory design in the development of an early therapy intervention for perinatal stroke. *BMC Pediatr.* 2017;17(1):33.

311. Kirton A. Filling a lacune in perinatal stroke outcomes. *Dev Med Child Neurol.* 2016;58(1):8-9.

312. Kirton A, Ciechanski P, Zewdie E, et al. Transcranial direct current stimulation for children with perinatal stroke and hemiparesis. *Neurology.* 2017;88(3):259-267.

323. Fitzgerald KC, Williams LS, Garg BP, et al. Cerebral sinovenous thrombosis in the neonate. *Arch Neurol.* 2006;63:405-409.

324. Berfelo FJ, Kersbergen KJ, van Ommen CH, et al. Neonatal cerebral sinovenous thrombosis from symptom to outcome. *Stroke.* 2010;41(7):1382-1388.

325. Raets MM, Sol JJ, Govaert P, et al. Serial cranial US for detection of cerebral sinovenous thrombosis in preterm infants. *Radiology.* 2013;269(3):879-886.

326. Moharir MD, Shroff M, Pontigon AM, et al. A prospective outcome study of neonatal cerebral sinovenous thrombosis. *J Child Neurol.* 2011;26(9):1137-1144.

328. Jordan LC, Rafay MF, Smith SE, et al. Antithrombotic treatment in neonatal cerebral sinovenous thrombosis: results of the International Pediatric Stroke Study. *J Pediatr.* 2010;156(5):704-710, 710.e1-710.e2.

329. Yang JY, Chan AK, Callen DJ, et al. Neonatal cerebral sinovenous thrombosis: sifting the evidence for a diagnostic plan and treatment strategy. *Pediatrics.* 2010;126(3):e693-e700.

331. Wagner MW, Bosemani T, Oshmyansky A, et al. Neuroimaging findings in pediatric cerebral sinovenous thrombosis. *Childs Nerv Syst.* 2015;31(5):705-712.

332. Carducci C, Colafati GS, Figa-Talamanca L, et al. Cerebral sinovenous thrombosis (CSVT) in children: what the pediatric radiologists need to know. *Radiol Med.* 2016;121(5):329-341.

333. Bracken J, Barnacle A, Ditchfield M. Potential pitfalls in imaging of paediatric cerebral sinovenous thrombosis. *Pediatr Radiol.* 2013;43(2):219-231.

334. Miller E, Daneman A, Doria AS, et al. Color Doppler US of normal cerebral venous sinuses in neonates: a comparison with MR venography. *Pediatr Radiol.* 2012;42(9):1070-1079.

339. Saxonhouse MA, Burchfield DJ. The evaluation and management of postnatal thromboses. *J Perinatol.* 2009;29(7):467-478.

340. Kirton A, deVeber G. Paediatric stroke: pressing issues and promising directions. *Lancet Neurol.* 2015;14(1):92-102.

341. van der Aa NE, Benders MJ, Groenendaal F, et al. Neonatal stroke: a review of the current evidence on epidemiology, pathogenesis, diagnostics and therapeutic options. *Acta Paediatr.* 2014;103(4):356-364.

342. Tan M, Deveber G, Shroff M, et al. Sagittal sinus compression is associated with neonatal cerebral sinovenous thrombosis. *Pediatrics.* 2011;128(2):e429-e435.

343. Tan MA, Miller E, Shroff MM, et al. Alleviation of neonatal sinovenous compression to enhance cerebral venous blood flow. *J Child Neurol.* 2013;28(5):583-588.

Full references for this chapter can be found on www.expertconsult.com.

UNIT V

INTRACRANIAL HEMORRHAGE

Intracranial Hemorrhage: Subdural, Subarachnoid, Intraventricular (Term Infant), Miscellaneous

Terrie E. Inder ◆ Jeffrey M. Perlman ◆ Joseph J. Volpe

Intracranial hemorrhage in the neonatal period is an important clinical problem. Its importance relates to a relatively high frequency of occurrence, accompanied at times by serious neurological sequelae or even death. Over the last decade there have been changes in the relative frequency of intracranial hemorrhage owing to changes in obstetrical practice, such as increased vacuum-assisted delivery and reduced rotational forceps as well as the improved survival of preterm infants with complex intracranial hemorrhagic lesions. Moreover, systematic neuroimaging studies in otherwise asymptomatic term infants have led to a new awareness of the incidence of more clinically benign forms of intracranial hemorrhage.

In this chapter, an overview of neonatal intracranial hemorrhage and the basic elements of recognition are presented. Detailed discussion is devoted to subdural hemorrhage, primary subarachnoid hemorrhage, intraventricular hemorrhage of the *full-term infant*, and certain unusual, miscellaneous examples of neonatal intracranial hemorrhage. The critical problem of germinal matrix–intraventricular hemorrhage of *the premature infant* is discussed in Chapter 24, and cerebellar hemorrhage, in Chapter 23. Various traumatic extracranial and intracranial hemorrhages, now generally unusual, are considered in Chapter 36.

OVERVIEW

Classification

The major clinically important types of neonatal intracranial hemorrhages are (1) epidural hemorrhage; (2) subdural hemorrhage, including posterior fossa subdural hemorrhage; (3) primary subarachnoid hemorrhage; (4) cerebellar hemorrhage; (5) intraventricular hemorrhage; and (6) other forms of intraparenchymal hemorrhage (other than cerebellar). The approximate incidence, anatomical site of blood, relative frequency in premature versus term infants, and the usual clinical gravity are noted in Table 22.1.

The *incidence of intracranial hemorrhage* has been challenging to define, because most studies have focused on symptomatic newborns. In one small study of symptomatic infants, the estimated incidence was 4.9 per 10,000 live births.[1] The largest epidemiological data relate to the Californian Perinatal Database, with maternal and neonatal hospital discharge records on 600,000 infants (2500 to 4000 g) born to nulliparous women. These data demonstrate the following: incidences of symptomatic intracranial hemorrhage associated with spontaneous delivery (1 per 1900 births), vacuum extraction delivery (1 per 860 births), and forceps delivery (per 664 births).[2] In contrast, more recent studies using neuroimaging, such as magnetic resonance imaging (MRI), in *asymptomatic* newborn infants in the first month of life have revealed a much higher frequency of intracranial hemorrhage.[3] A large prospective MRI (0.2T) study of asymptomatic term newborns found an 8% prevalence of subdural hemorrhage.[3,4] A second study of 88 asymptomatic neonates born via vaginal delivery who underwent cranial MRI (3T) between the ages of 1 and 5 weeks demonstrated 17 term infants with intracranial hemorrhage, for a study prevalence of 26%.[5] Such findings suggest that asymptomatic intracranial hemorrhage in term newborns is much more frequent than had previously been thought.

With these limitations regarding the incidence of intracranial hemorrhage in mind, Table 22.1 provides a summary of the location, incidence, and usual clinical gravity of the main types of hemorrhages. In summary, *subdural hemorrhage* is more frequent in the full-term than in the premature infant and is frequently asymptomatic; if large, however, it can be clinically serious. *Primary subarachnoid hemorrhage*, more frequent in the premature than in the full-term infant, is, in general, common but is almost always clinically benign. *Cerebellar hemorrhage*, more frequent in the premature than in the full-term infant, can be serious when large. *Intraventricular hemorrhage*, almost exclusively a lesion of the premature infant, is, in contrast to the other three types of hemorrhages, both common and usually serious. Intraventricular hemorrhage has recently been more commonly recognized in the term infant, particularly related to sinovenous thrombosis and/or hypoxic-ischemic cerebral injury. Other forms of *intraparenchymal hemorrhage*, more frequent in the full-term than in the premature infant, are uncommon and are of variable clinical gravity.

Recognition of Hemorrhage
Three Major Steps

Three major steps must be taken to ensure recognition of neonatal intracranial hemorrhage. First, *predisposing factors* should be identified. As outlined in more detail in subsequent sections, these factors include the gestational history, the details of labor and delivery, the maturation of the baby, the occurrence of *hypoxic* events, the modes of resuscitation, and so forth. Second, definition of *abnormal clinical features* must be made early in the neonatal course. Particular attention should be given to subtle

TABLE 22.1   Major Sites of Neonatal Intracranial Hemorrhage

TYPE OF HEMORRHAGE	INCIDENCE	ANATOMICAL SITE OF BLOOD	MATURATION OF INFANT	USUAL CLINICAL GRAVITY
Extradural (epidural) (see Chapter 36)	Very rare	Between skull and outside of dura	FT > PT	Variable
Subdural	5%–25%	Between dura and arachnoid	FT > PT	Benign
Subarachnoid	1%–2% FT 10% PT	Between arachnoid and pia	PT > FT	Benign
Cerebellar (see Chapter 23)	0.1% FT 5% PT	Cerebellar hemispheres and/or vermis	PT > FT	Serious
Intraventricular (see Chapter 24)	0.2% FT 15% PT	Within ventricles or including periventricular hemorrhagic infarction	PT > FT	Serious
Parenchymal	0.1% FT 2%–4% PT	Cerebral parenchyma	FT > PT	Variable

FT, Full-term; *PT*, preterm (<32 weeks).

Note that, additionally, subgaleal cephalohematoma and other traumatic forms of hemorrhage are reviewed in Chapter 36.

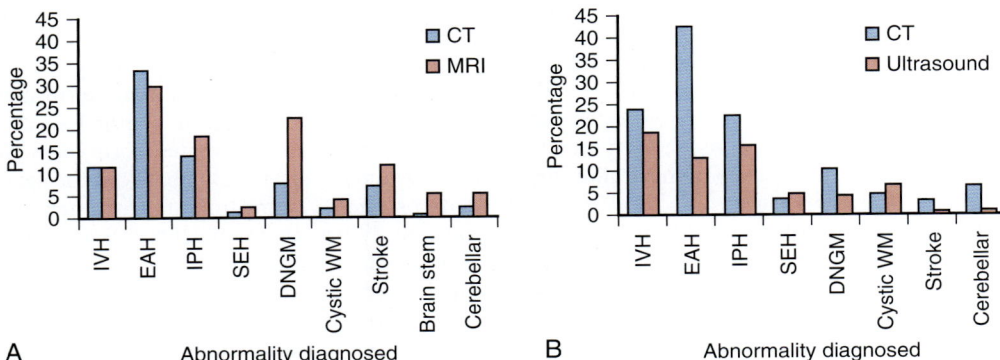

Figure 22.1 Comparison of results of infants imaged with (A) both MRI and CT (*N* = 651) and (B) both cranial ultrasound and CT (*N* = 245). *CT*, Computed tomography; *Cystic WM*, cystic white matter injury; *DNGM*, deep nuclear gray matter abnormality; *EAH*, extra-axial hemorrhage; *IPH*, intraparenchymal hemorrhage; *IVH*, intraventricular hemorrhage; *SHE*, subependymal hemorrhage. (Reprinted with permission from Barnette AR, Horbar JD, Soll RF, et al. Neuroimaging in the evaluation of neonatal encephalopathy. *Pediatrics.* 2014;133:e1508–e1517.)

neurological signs, as outlined later. Third, visualization of the site and extent of the hemorrhage should be implemented by an *imaging technique*, often initially by ultrasound scan and then more definitively by MRI or computed tomography (CT) (indicated only if needed emergently). Intracranial hemorrhage may first be suspected because a lumbar puncture, often carried out to rule out sepsis, reveals *cerebrospinal fluid (CSF)* consistent with hemorrhage. In view of this role of the CSF examination, interpretation of the CSF findings is also discussed further on. However, lumbar puncture is not the diagnostic test of choice for intracranial hemorrhage and may potentially pose a risk to the infant if a large posterior fossa hemorrhage is present.

Neuroimaging in the Recognition of Intracranial Hemorrhage

Three key methods of neuroimaging are applied in the recognition of intracranial hemorrhage. Cranial ultrasound is portable and easily accessible in the preterm and sick term infant, making it a common choice for investigating brain injury in the encephalopathic infant. Unfortunately there is a lack of sensitivity for intracranial hemorrhage and brain injury. In a

recent study analyzing 4098 term infants born between 2006 and 2010 from 95 centers,[6] imaging was performed for 2006 with cranial ultrasound, 933 with CT, and 2690 with MRI. The number of patients with no, one, two, and all three types of imaging were 678 (16.5%), 1405 (34.3%), 1845 (45.0%), and 170 (4.1%), respectively (*N* = 4098 patients). Although cranial ultrasound identified intraventricular hemorrhage well, it lacked the sensitivity of MRI and CT for identifying other types of hemorrhages and intracranial injuries. Of particular note, cranial ultrasound was particularly limited in detecting all forms of extra-axial hemorrhage (subdural, subarachnoid, and extradural) (Fig. 22.1 and Table 22.2).[7]

CT use was recommended by the 2002 American Academy of Neurology practice parameters for infants with birth trauma and a low hematocrit or coagulopathy[8] on the basis of data from two small studies reporting on CT diagnoses of intracranial hemorrhages leading to interventions.[9,10] However, there were no comparisons with cranial ultrasound for these 31 infants. In the patients in the Barnette series, the largest published to date in term infants with encephalopathy who were examined with two imaging modalities, CT was superior to ultrasound

TABLE 22.2   Neuroimaging Findings of Infants With Two Types of Imaging on the Same Day[a]

	ULTRASOUND VERSUS CT		ULTRASOUND VERSUS MRI		CT VERSUS MRI	
	ULTRASOUND	CT	ULTRASOUND	MRI	CT	MRI
Intraventricular hemorrhage	2/43 (5)	4/43 (9)	3/47 (6)	5/47 (11)	8/70 (11)	9/70 (13)
Extra-axial hemorrhage	2/42 (5)	10/43 (23)	1/46 (2)	11/47 (23)	17/69 (25)	14/70 (20)
Parenchymal hemorrhage	5/42 (12)	7/43 (16)	3/46 (7)	6/47 (13)	10/69 (14)	13/70 (19)
Subependymal hemorrhage	1/42 (2)	2/43 (5)	1/46 (2)	2/47 (4)	0/69 (0)	1/70 (1)
Deep nuclear gray matter abnormality	1/42 (2)	4/42 (10)	4/46 (9)	11/47 (23)	8/69 (12)	18/70 (26)
Cystic white matter injury	0/42 (0)	2/42 (5)	0/46 (0)	4/47 (9)	1/69 (1)	2/70 (3)
Venous or arterial occlusions	0/42 (0)	1/42 (2)	0/46 (0)	2/47 (4)	12/69 (17)	13/70 (19)
Cerebellar injury	1/42 (2)	3/43 (7)	0/46 (0)	4/47 (9)	1/69 (1)	5/70 (7)
Brain stem injury					6/69 (9)	6/70 (9)

[a]Data presented as n/N (%) unless otherwise noted.

CT, Computed tomography; MRI, magnetic resonance imaging.

From Barnette AR, Horbar JD, Soll RF, et al. Neuroimaging in the evaluation of neonatal encephalopathy. *Pediatrics.* 2014;133:e1508–e1517.

for the detection of hemorrhage. Although the authors were unable to determine the impact of the imaging findings of the infants who needed surgical intervention, only 9 of 933 infants with CT examinations underwent any central nervous system surgery. In addition, this study documented that CT performed relatively poorly for the delineation of the common patterns of brain injury in neonatal encephalopathy, including deep nuclear gray matter and white matter injury. In comparison with MRI, CT detected less than one third of deep nuclear gray matter injuries and few brain-stem or cerebellar lesions. These findings are consistent with previous publications showing that MRI detects brain injuries and malformations in infants that are missed by CT.[11-13]

Because CT scanning has inherent risks, alternative neuroimaging modalities should be considered. Major national and international organizations agree that there is probably no amount of radiation that can be considered absolutely safe.[14] Recent data from irradiated children demonstrate small but significant increases in cancer risk, even at levels of radiation (25 to 50 milligray; 1.8 to 3.8 millisievert) comparable with those produced by neonatal and pediatric CT scans.[15,16] In addition, radiation may also have harmful cognitive effects. In immature animal models, the cerebellum and cerebral cortical migration appeared to be sensitive to damage from radiation.[17,18] The Image Gently campaign promotes reducing the frequency of CT imaging and minimizing medical radiation exposure.

The diagnostic accuracy of MRI is similar to that of CT in scanning for intracranial hemorrhage (see Fig. 22.1 and Table 22.2), with improved sensitivity for clinically important forms of cerebral parenchymal injury in both the preterm and term infant. The development of more rapid MRI sequences to allow for brief diagnostic scans for cerebral hemorrhage will enhance physician comfort with this as a first-line technique.

Cerebrospinal Fluid in the Recognition of Intracranial Hemorrhage

Traumatic Lumbar Puncture. The finding of bloody cerebrospinal fluid (CSF) in a newborn is common (occurring in >⅓ of all CSF samples within a neonatal intensive care unit); it is often attributed to *traumatic* lumbar puncture.[19] This conclusion primarily relates to the relative difficulty of performing the

TABLE 22.3   Computed Tomography Scan Correlates of Bloody Cerebrospinal Fluid in 76 Infants Weighing Less Than 2000 g

BLOOD ON SCAN	NO. OF PATIENTS	PERCENTAGE OF TOTAL GROUP
None	6	8%
Subarachnoid	22	29%
Germinal matrix— intraventricular	48	63%

puncture in the newborn but also to the relative frequency of finding bloody CSF in infants without overt neurological signs. It is, however, likely that traumatic lumbar puncture in the newborn is much less common than is generally thought. For example, in a study in which lumbar punctures were performed on the third postnatal day in all premature infants of less than 2000 g, the 76 infants who had *grossly* bloody CSF with elevated protein content were evaluated by CT (Table 22.3). Only 6 (8%) had no increased attenuation consistent with blood. Subarachnoid blood was detectable in 22 (29%), and intraventricular hemorrhage was noted in 48 (63%). Few studies have attempted to correlate the findings of red cells on CSF with the nature and extent of intracranial hemorrhage in either the preterm or term infant.

Cerebrospinal Fluid Findings of Intracranial Hemorrhage. CSF findings that indicate intracranial hemorrhage are, primarily, xanthochromia of the centrifuged fluid and elevations of the number of red blood cells (RBCs) as well as the protein content. Particular emphasis should be placed on the occurrence of *combinations* of findings rather than on a single, isolated abnormality.

Xanthochromia of the CSF develops within several hours after hemorrhage in older children and adults. In one particularly large study of adults with subarachnoid hemorrhage, nearly 90% exhibited xanthochromia within 12 hours of the ictus.[20] The evolution of xanthochromia in newborns has not been studied systematically, although our impression is that it appears to occur more slowly than in older patients. This slower evolution may relate to a delay in the induction of the enzyme heme oxygenase, which is located in the arachnoid and is responsible for the conversion of heme to bilirubin, the major pigment accounting for xanthochromia of the CSF.[21] In adult rats, the activity of heme oxygenase reaches peak values 6 to 12 hours after injection of heme into the subarachnoid space.[21] These data are closely comparable with the clinical observations of adult patients cited. Determination of the significance of xanthochromia in newborns is occasionally difficult in the presence of elevated serum bilirubin levels.

The number of *RBCs* that should be considered significant is difficult to state conclusively, in part because of the remarkably wide range of values considered normal (see Chapter 10).[22-30] In studies of infants in neonatal intensive care units, median values of 100 to 200 RBC/μL have been observed. A more recent study reported even higher values for mean RBCs when the lumbar puncture was undertaken by a resident. In a study of 184 cases, 64% of infants had RBC counts below 100,000.[31] In the only report with ultrasonographic correlates, among 43 infants of less than 1500 g birth weight, the median value was 112, but the mean value was 785, and 20% of CSF samples had more than 1000 RBCs/mm.[29] These infants did not exhibit ultrasonographic evidence of intracranial hemorrhage. However, exclusion of minor subarachnoid hemorrhage by cranial ultrasonography is not reliable. Thus, the data indicate that findings of more than 100 RBCs/mm in the newborn are common, and in the very low-birth-weight infants, values greater than 1000 occur in a substantial minority in the absence of apparently clinically significant intracranial hemorrhage. Again, the *combination* of findings is important in the evaluation.

Values for CSF *protein* are higher in newborns in an intensive care unit than in older children. In the series of Sarff and co-workers,[28] an average protein content in CSF of 90 mg/dL was observed for term infants and a content of 115 mg/dL for preterm infants. We have obtained similar data.[27] In general, values for CSF protein are higher in the most premature infants; in one series, the mean value at 26 to 28 weeks of postconceptional age was 177 mg/dL; at 35 to 37 weeks, it was 109 mg/dL.[29] Values in intracranial hemorrhage are usually severalfold higher than these. A recent study found that CSF protein concentrations increased by approximately 2 mg/dL for every 1000 CSF RBCs.[32]

Finally, determination of the CSF *glucose* level may be helpful in the diagnosis. In term and preterm infants evaluated in a neonatal intensive care unit and free of intracranial infection, the ratios of CSF to blood glucose levels are relatively high (i.e., 0.81 and 0.74, respectively).[28] As with CSF protein levels, values for CSF glucose tend to be higher in the most premature infants; in one series, the mean value at 26 to 28 weeks was 85 mg/dL; at 38 to 40 weeks, it was 44 mg/dL.[29] After neonatal intracranial hemorrhage, the CSF glucose level is frequently low (Table 22.4).[33-37] Indeed, in one study in which serial lumbar punctures were performed (for therapeutic purposes) on 13 infants with intraventricular hemorrhage, the CSF glucose concentration decreased on subsequent measurements in *all* the infants.[37] Of the 13 infants, 11 had CSF glucose values lower than 30 mg/dL at some point subsequent to the hemorrhage, and values of 10 mg/dL or less were common. The low values occurred as early as 1 day after the hemorrhage but usually became apparent between approximately 5 and 15 days after

TABLE 22.4	Major Features of Hypoglycorrhachia After Neonatal Intracranial Hemorrhage

- Nearly uniform occurrence after major hemorrhage
- Onset usually 5–15 days after hemorrhage
- Duration of weeks to months
- Accompanied by concomitant decrease in cerebrospinal fluid lactate level

Mechanism not proved but probably related to impaired glucose transport

the hemorrhage. The depressed CSF glucose values persist for weeks and have been noted as long as 3 months after the hemorrhage.[33,34,36]

The basis of hypoglycorrhachia is probably related to an impairment of the mechanisms of glucose transport into the CSF. This impairment may occur at the level of the plasma membrane glucose transporter.[38] Other proposed pathogeneses have included glucose use by RBCs or by contiguous brain. The former is ruled out by the lack of correlation between RBC number and CSF glucose level and by the negligible rates of glucose consumption observed when the cellular CSF is incubated in vitro. The possibility of excessive anaerobic use of glucose by contiguous brain rendered hypoxic-ischemic by hemorrhage, ventricular dilation, or other insult[39] appears unlikely in view of simultaneous serial determinations of CSF glucose and lactate.[37] Thus, in 13 infants described with CSF hypoglycorrhachia, CSF glucose and lactate concentrations decreased pari passu; if anaerobic use of glucose had been operative, a concomitant increase in CSF lactate would have been expected. These observations favor the notion of a defect in glucose transport mechanisms.

An important practical problem arises when the low CSF glucose level is accompanied by pleocytosis and elevated protein content. This not uncommon occurrence is related presumably to meningeal inflammation from blood products and raises the question of bacterial meningitis. Although appropriate cultures are always indicated and even initiation of antimicrobial therapy may be necessary (until results of cultures are known), the CSF formula of pleocytosis, depressed glucose, and elevated protein content is not infrequent after neonatal intracranial hemorrhage.

The *optimal imaging procedure for diagnosis* becomes apparent in the following discussions of the respective lesions. The relative value of cranial ultrasonography, CT, and MRI in diagnosis is reviewed in Chapter 10. Suffice it to say here that cranial ultrasonography is often used as a screening procedure, MRI is the most effective methodology, and CT is used for a more rapid emergent approach. The features of MRI signal change over the days and weeks after neonatal parenchymal hemorrhage and are reviewed in Table 22.5. The MRI changes relate primarily to changes in hemoglobin state, which proceed from predominantly intracellular deoxyhemoglobin to intracellular methemoglobin to extracellular methemoglobin and finally to hemosiderin.

SUBDURAL HEMORRHAGE

The incidence of subdural hemorrhage has been underestimated because many such hemorrhages appear to be asymptomatic. Whitby et al.[4] studied 111 term infants with a 0.2T MRI scanner

TABLE 22.5	Predominant Changes in Magnetic Resonance Imaging Signal After Parenchymal Hemorrhage	
	SIGNAL CHANGES	
AGE OF HEMORRHAGE	**T1-WEIGHTED**	**T2-WEIGHTED**
1–3 days	Isointense	Low
3–10 days	High	Low
10–21 days	High	High
3–6 weeks	High	High
6 weeks–10 months	Isointense	Low

Adapted from Rutherford M. *MRI of the Neonatal Brain*. Philadelphia: WB Saunders; 2002 and from personal experience.

TABLE 22.6	Neuropathology of Subdural Hemorrhage
SOURCE OF BLEEDING	**LOCATION OF HEMATOMA**
Tentorial laceration	Infratentorial (posterior fossa), supratentorial
Straight sinus, vein of Galen, transverse sinus, and infratentorial veins	—
Occipital osteodiastasis	Infratentorial (posterior fossa)
Occipital sinus	—
Falx laceration	Longitudinal cerebral fissure
Inferior sagittal sinus	—
Superficial cerebral veins	Surface of cerebral convexity

and documented an 8% prevalence of subdural hemorrhage in newborns. He found that subdural hemorrhage was associated with vaginal delivery. All subdural hemorrhages resolved at follow-up imaging 4 weeks later. In both asymptomatic and symptomatic subdural hemorrhages, the supratentorial component was in a posterior location over the occipital or parietal lobes. No subdural hemorrhages were located over the frontal lobes. Of the nine infants with asymptomatic subdural hemorrhages, one had isolated supratentorial hematomas, six had isolated infratentorial hematomas, and two had subdural hemorrhages in both compartments. There were no subdural hemorrhages in the infants delivered by cesarean section. In a second study, Looney et al.[5] studied 88 asymptomatic term infants with a 3T MRI scanner within the first month of life and identified 17 intracranial hemorrhages, of which 16 were subdural. There were nine isolated subdural hemorrhages that were mostly infratentorial or associated with occipital lobe subdural hemorrhage. The infants with subdural hemorrhages were all born by vaginal delivery. There was no proven association with instrumental delivery. The long-term outcome associated with these subdural hemorrhages remains unknown.

It is important to note that the pattern of subdural hemorrhage in asymptomatic term infants is different from that found in infants with nonaccidental head injuries. Nonaccidental head injuries typically cause subdural hematomas that are generally located in the interhemispheric fissure or over the cerebral convexities; these hematomas are often but not always of differing ages.

In contrast, symptomatic subdural hemorrhage in the newborn infant is very uncommon. However, if symptomatic, recognition of the disorder is important because therapeutic intervention can be lifesaving in patients with large hemorrhages.

Neuropathology
Anatomy of Major Veins and Sinuses
The neuropathology of neonatal subdural hemorrhage is readily understood after a brief review of the major anatomical features of the veins and sinuses involved in the production of such hemorrhage (Fig. 22.2). The deep venous drainage of the cerebrum empties into the great cerebral vein of Galen at the junction of the tentorium and falx. The confluence of the vein of Galen and the inferior sagittal sinus, the latter located in the inferior margin of the falx, forms the straight sinus.

This sinus proceeds directly posteriorly and joins the superior sagittal sinus, located in the superior margin of the falx, to form the transverse sinus. Blood in the transverse sinuses, located in the lateral margins of the tentorium, proceeds eventually to the jugular vein. Blood in the posterior fossa in part drains into the occipital sinus, which empties into the torcular. The superficial portion of the cerebrum is drained by the superficial, bridging cerebral veins, which empty into the superior sagittal sinus. Tears of these several veins or venous sinuses, occurring secondary to forces to be described and often accompanying laceration of the dura, result in subdural hemorrhage.

Major Varieties of Subdural Hemorrhage
The four major varieties of neonatal subdural hemorrhage include the following (Table 22.6): tentorial laceration with rupture principally of the straight sinus, transverse sinus, vein of Galen, or smaller infratentorial veins; occipital osteodiastasis with rupture of the occipital sinus; falx laceration with rupture of the inferior sagittal sinus; and rupture of bridging superficial cerebral veins.

Tentorial Laceration. With *major, lethal tears* of the tentorium, hemorrhage is most often infratentorial.[40-47] This finding is the case particularly with rupture of the vein of Galen or straight sinus or with severe involvement of the transverse sinus. The clots extend into the posterior fossa and, when large, very rapidly result in lethal compression of the brain stem.[40,41,46-51] A massive infratentorial hemorrhage from a rupture of the vein of Galen also may occur without visible tear of the tentorium.

Lesser degrees of tentorial injury, with the advent of modern brain imaging techniques, are recognized now to be more common than the major lethal lacerations just described and probably are much more common than previously suspected. Thus several series, the largest and most recent described earlier, have documented a spectrum of intracranial hemorrhage, primarily subdural, associated with apparent or presumed tentorial injury.[a] This spectrum, summarized in Table 22.7, includes both *infratentorial* (usually retrocerebellar) subdural hemorrhage (Fig. 22.3), secondary to inferior extension, and *supratentorial* subdural hemorrhage, secondary to superior

---

[a]References 1, 4, 5, 10, 40, 42-47, 50, 52-58.

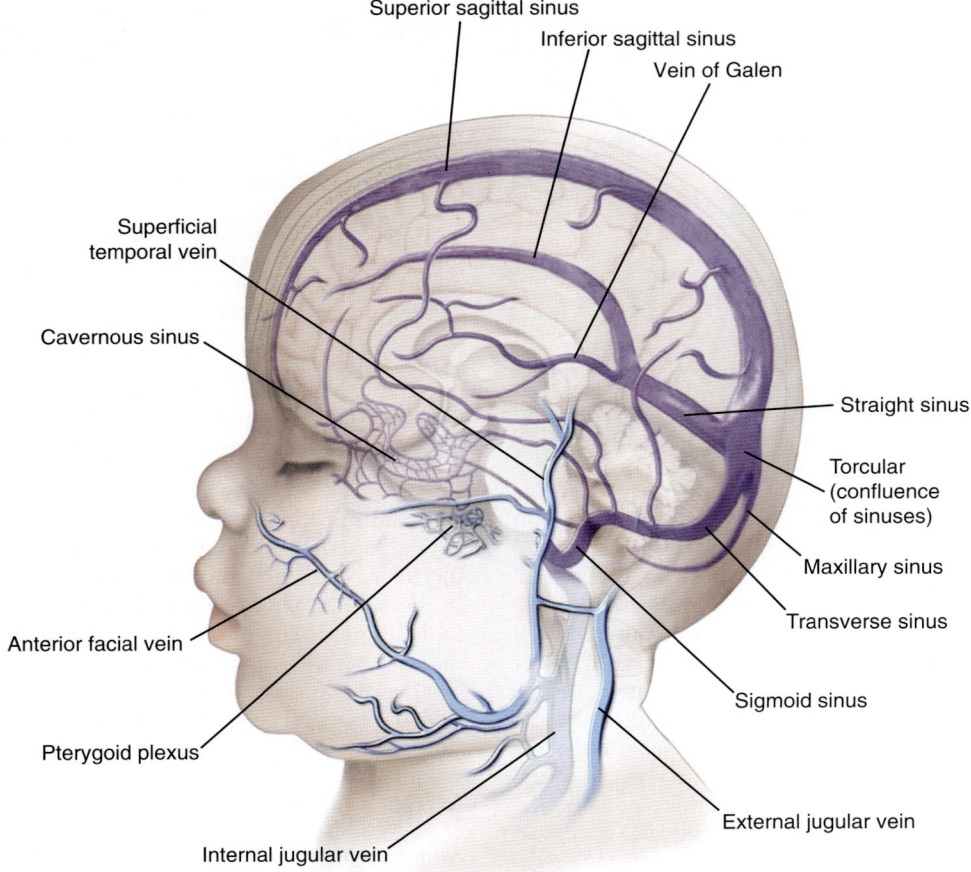

Figure 22.2 Major cranial veins and dural sinuses. The ventricular system is also outlined. The superior sagittal sinus runs in the superior border of the falx; the inferior sagittal and straight sinuses run in the inferior border; and the transverse sinus runs in the outer border of the tentorium. The occipital sinus (shown but not labeled) runs in the midline of the posterior fossa and empties into the torcular.

TABLE 22.7   Spectrum of Tentorial Hemorrhage[a]

Anterior extension
- Excrescence (on free edge of tentorium)
- Velum interpositum
- Intraventricular
- Subarachnoid

Superior extension
- Supratentorial subdural
- Cerebral parenchymal hemorrhage[b]

Inferior extension
- Infratentorial (posterior fossa) subdural
- Cerebellar parenchymal hemorrhage[b]

---
[a]See text for references.
[b]Often associated hemorrhage rather than true extension.

---

extension. It is important to note that the infratentorial posterior fossa subdural hemorrhages may relate also to tears of cerebellar bridging veins, with or without accompanying overt tears of the tentorium. In addition to infratentorial or supratentorial extension, the hemorrhage of a tentorial tear may remain *confined*

to the free edge of the tentorium, most often near the junction of the tentorium and falx (Fig. 22.4; see also Fig. 22.3), or it may extend *anteriorly* further into the subarachnoid space, velum interpositum, or ventricular system (see Table 22.6). Very minor varieties of this spectrum may account for the relatively high RBC counts in CSF in *normal* newborns (see earlier discussion).

Occipital Osteodiastasis. A prominent traumatic lesion in some infants who die after breech delivery is occipital diastasis with posterior fossa subdural hemorrhage and laceration of the cerebellum (see Table 22.6 and Chapter 36).[10,59-61] The diastasis lesion consists of traumatic separation of the cartilaginous joint between the squamous and lateral portions of the occipital bone.[59,62] In its most severe form, the dura and occipital sinuses are torn, resulting in massive subdural hemorrhage in the posterior fossa and cerebellar laceration. The bony lesion may be more common than has generally been recognized because it is easily missed at postmortem examination.

Falx Laceration. Laceration of the falx alone is distinctly less common than laceration of the tentorium and usually occurs at a point near the junction of the falx with the tentorium.

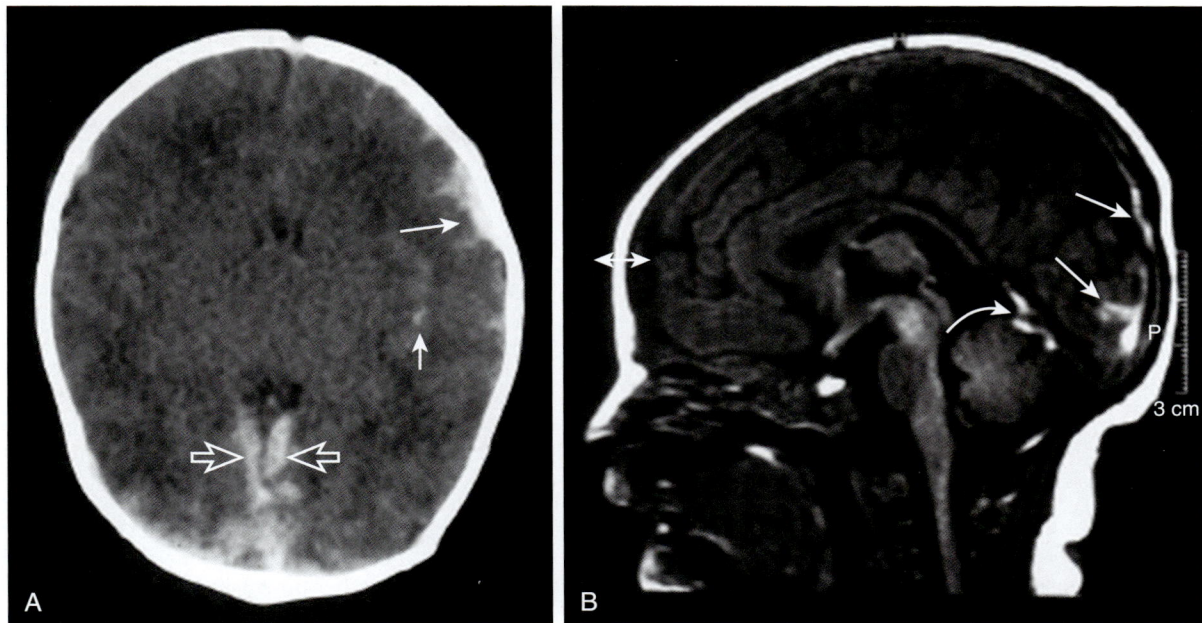

Figure 22.3 Tentorial subdural hemorrhage at the junction of the falx and tentorium. (A) Computed tomography reveals a subdural hematoma along the tentorium *(open arrows)*, a small subdural hematoma underlying the coronal suture *(long arrow)*, and subarachnoid blood in the sylvian fissure *(short arrow)*. (B) Sagittal T1 image (TR = 500 ms). (Reprinted with permission from Chamnanvanakij S, Rollins N, Perlman JM. Subdural hematoma in term infants. *Pediatr Neurol.* 2002;26:301–304.)

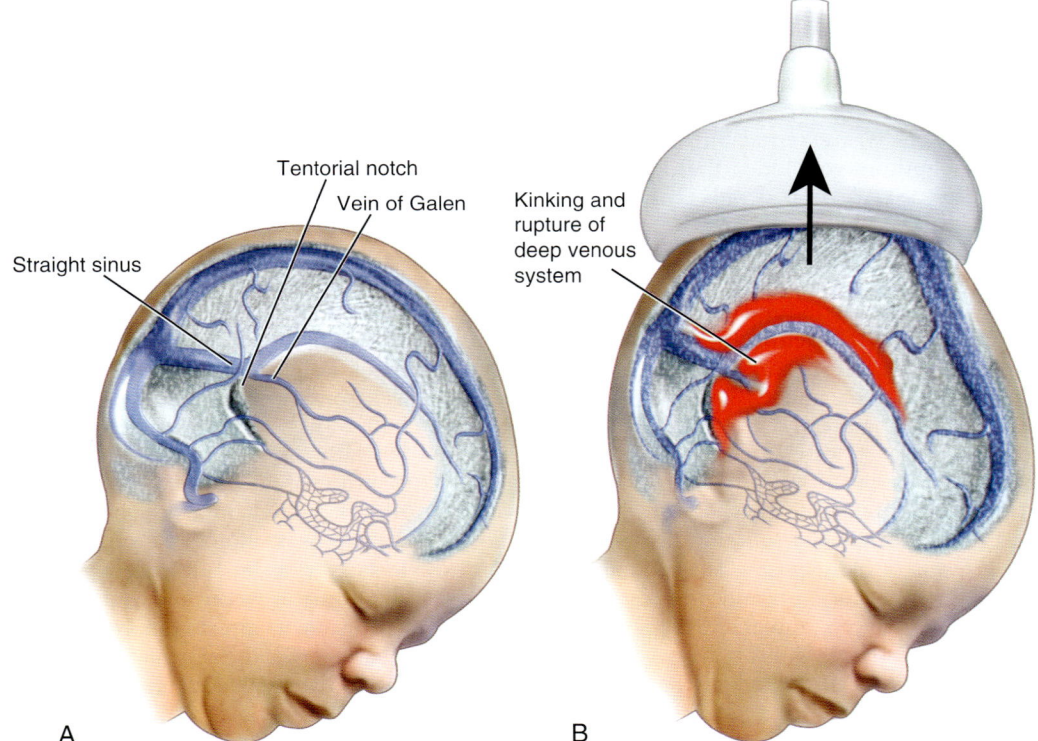

Figure 22.4 The likely mechanism of tentorial hemorrhage after vacuum extraction. (A) The vein of Galen joins the straight sinus and tributaries from the deep venous system at the tentorial notch. (B) Traction in the occipitofrontal direction produces stress on the vertical axis of the falx and tentorium with kinking of the deep venous system. Engorgement and venous rupture lead to hemorrhage into the surrounding subdural space. (From Hanigan WC, Morgan AM, Stahlberg LK, Hiller JL. Tentorial hemorrhage associated with vacuum extraction. *Pediatrics.* 1990;85:534–539.)

The source of bleeding is usually the inferior sagittal sinus, and the clot is located in the cerebral fissure over the corpus callosum (see Table 22.6).

Superficial Cerebral Vein Rupture. Rupture of the bridging superficial cerebral veins results in hemorrhage over the cerebral convexity, the well-known convexity subdural hematoma (see Table 22.6). The hematoma is usually more extensive over the lateral aspect of the convexity than near the superior sagittal sinus. Although convexity subdural hemorrhage is usually unilateral, bilateral lesions are not uncommon.[a] Subarachnoid blood is a typical accompaniment. Convexity subdural hemorrhage is not a rare event, and, indeed, in small amounts, it is a frequent incidental finding at autopsy of the term infant.[51,58] The trauma that leads to the hemorrhage may result also in *cerebral contusion*, which, in fact, may dominate the clinical picture.

Pathogenesis

Subdural hemorrhage in the neonatal period is most commonly a traumatic lesion, especially *when the lesion is large*.[b] Most such cases have involved full-term infants. Many of these series reported symptomatic infants. In asymptomatic infants, subdural hemorrhages are associated with vaginal delivery and not cesarean section, supporting that vaginal delivery may be associated with greater risk for trauma. However, in asymptomatic term infants with subdural hemorrhages, neither assisted vaginal delivery nor clinical evidence of neonatal birth trauma could be used to predict the presence of hemorrhage. Most (13 of 17, or 76%) of the cases were in the setting of nonassisted vaginal birth. This is in agreement with the findings of Whitby et al.,[4] who described nine neonates with asymptomatic hemorrhage; in only two of the nine neonates with subdural hemorrhages was external birth trauma an associated finding. The authors concluded that a subdural hematoma was not necessarily associated with obvious birth trauma. Holden et al.[56] identified 4 of 11 neonates with clinically silent intracranial hemorrhage by cranial ultrasound; in all, vaginal delivery was uneventful.

With regard to symptomatic subdural hemorrhages, as the incidence of grossly traumatic deliveries has decreased, the relative proportion of premature infants with subdural hemorrhage has increased as well. Indeed, in some surveys, the proportion of cases in premature and full-term infants has been approximately similar.[59,67] However, most modern reports still indicate a predominance of full-term infants, especially with cerebral convexity subdural hemorrhages.[c]

The pathogenesis of *major* neonatal subdural hemorrhage is best considered in terms of predisposing factors referable to the mother, the infant, the duration and progression of labor, and the manner of delivery (Table 22.8). Thus large symptomatic subdural hemorrhage is most likely to occur under the circumstances where the head of the infant is subjected to unusual or rapid deforming stresses such as compression, molding, or stresses on extraction. This can include circumstances such as (1) when the infant's head is relatively large and/or the birth canal is relatively small;

TABLE 22.8	Pathogenesis of Neonatal Subdural Hemorrhage
AT RISK	**PREDISPOSING FACTORS**
Mother	Primipara
	Older multipara
	Small birth canal
Infant	Large, full term
	Premature
Labor	Precipitous
	Prolonged
Delivery	Breech extraction
	Foot, face, or brow presentation
	Difficult forceps or vacuum extraction
	Difficult rotation

(2) when the skull is unusually compliant, as in a premature infant; (3) when the pelvic structures are unusually rigid, as in a primiparous or older multiparous mother; (4) when the duration of labor is either unusually brief, not allowing enough time for dilation of the pelvic structures, or unusually long, subjecting the head to prolonged compression and molding; (5) atypical presentations, such breech (with poor adaptation of the birth canal), face, or brow presentation; or (6) difficult vacuum extraction or challenging forceps or rotational maneuvers.

Under the circumstances just described, excessive vertical molding and fronto-occipital elongation or oblique expansion of the head may occur (see Fig. 22.4). These effects can result in stretching of both the falx and one or both leaves of the tentorium, with a tendency for tearing of the tentorium, particularly near its junction with the falx, or, less commonly, tearing of the falx itself. Even if a laceration does not occur, the sinuses into which the vein of Galen drains can be stretched, and the result may be a tear of the vein of Galen or its immediate tributaries. Similarly, rupture of cerebellar bridging veins may occur in this context.[47] Tear of the falx occurs particularly with *extreme* fronto-occipital elongation, especially that associated with face or brow presentation. Extreme vertical molding appears to underlie many tears of superficial cerebral veins and the formation of a convexity subdural hematoma. In the special case of occipital osteodiastasis with breech delivery, the injury results from suboccipital pressure, which most commonly occurs if the fetus is forcibly hyperextended with the head trapped beneath the symphysis.[10,59] The lower edge of the squamous portion of the occipital bone is displaced in a forward direction, thus lacerating dura, occipital sinus, or cerebellum. (A roughly analogous situation in the supratentorial compartment probably occurs with difficult forceps extractions, which may result in skull fracture, convexity subdural hemorrhage, and cerebral contusion by direct compressive effects.)

Fortunately many of the aforementioned pathogenetic factors have been eliminated by vastly improved obstetrical practices in most medical centers. Indeed, subdural hemorrhage is not invariably due to trauma alone and can result from other contributing risk factors. For example, coagulation disturbances (e.g., maternal aspirin ingestion, early vitamin K deficiency secondary to maternal phenobarbital administration) may play at least a contributing role in some infants.[1,10,70,71] Moreover, with the advent of intrauterine brain imaging, subdural hematoma has been identified in the fetus before intrapartum events could

---

[a]References 1, 10, 47, 55, 57, 63–65.
[b]References 1, 10, 40–47, 49, 54, 55, 64, 66.
[c]References 1, 10, 42–46, 54, 68, 69.

be responsible.[71-76] In one report, maternal abuse with blunt abdominal trauma was documented in an infant with bilateral subdural hematomas identified in the first day of life.[64] In other intrauterine cases, other forms of external abdominal pressure or coagulopathy have been important.[71]

Clinical Features

In contrast to the considerable amount of medical writings relative to the neuropathological and radiological aspects of subdural hemorrhage, surprisingly few clinical neurological data are available. However, some important conclusions can be drawn from our own observations and from those recorded by other investigators.[a]

Tentorial Laceration, Occipital Diastasis, and Syndromes Associated With Posterior Fossa Subdural Hematoma

Rapidly Lethal Syndromes. Tentorial laceration with *massive* infratentorial hemorrhage, an extremely rare disorder in the modern obstetrical era, is associated with neurological disturbance from the time of birth.[42,49] The majority of the most severely affected infants weigh more than 4000 g at birth. Initially, the baby demonstrates signs of midbrain–upper pons compression (i.e., stupor or coma, skew deviation of eyes with lateral deviation that is not altered by the "doll's eyes" maneuver, and unequal pupils, with some disturbance of response to light). With such infratentorial hemorrhage, nuchal rigidity with retrocollis or opisthotonos may also be a helpful early sign.[46,89] When these features are associated with bradycardia,[40] a large infratentorial clot with brain-stem compression should be suspected. Over minutes to hours, as the clot becomes larger, stupor progresses to coma, pupils may become fixed and dilated, and signs of lower brain-stem compression appear. Ocular bobbing and ataxic respirations may occur; finally, respiratory arrest ensues.

The severe clinical syndrome associated with *occipital osteodiastasis* resembles that described for major tentorial laceration. With occipital osteodiastasis, delivery is characteristically breech. A depressed Apgar score at 1 minute is common, and the course is one of rapid deterioration. In the six infants described by Wigglesworth and Husemeyer,[59] the age at the time of death ranged from 7 to 45 hours.

Less Malignant Syndromes Associated With Posterior Fossa Subdural Hematoma. Less severe clinical syndromes accompany most examples of *posterior fossa subdural hematoma* currently encountered on obstetrical and neonatal services.[b] These syndromes appear to result from smaller tears of the tentorium than those just noted, from rupture of bridging veins from superior cerebellum without tentorial tear, or perhaps from lesser degrees of occipital diastasis. The clinical syndrome consists of three phases. First, no neurological signs are apparent for a period that varies from several hours after birth (usually a difficult vacuum, forceps, or breech extraction or all three) to as much as 3 or 4 days of age. Most commonly, the interval is less than 24 hours. Presumably, this period is associated with slow enlargement of the hematoma. Second, various signs develop referable to increased intracranial pressure (e.g., full fontanelle, irritability, *lethargy*). Most of these signs appear

to relate to the evolution of hydrocephalus secondary to a block of CSF flow in the posterior fossa. Third, signs referable to disturbance of brain stem develop, including respiratory abnormalities, apnea, bradycardia, oculomotor abnormalities, skew deviation of eyes, and facial paresis. These deficits relate to direct compressive effects of the posterior fossa hematoma. In addition to brain-stem signs, seizures occur in the majority of infants, perhaps because of accompanying subarachnoid blood. In infants who clearly worsen over hours or a day or more, as do approximately half, lethal brain-stem compression may develop.

In more recent years, more common lesions of *particularly small* posterior fossa subdural hemorrhages have been identified by CT or MRI during the investigation of more subtle neurological abnormalities in term infants. In one carefully studied series of 26 small subdural hemorrhages detected by CT, 19 were infratentorial; the leading clinical features were respiratory abnormalities (apnea, *dusky episodes*) in approximately 60% and neurological features (subtle seizures, hypotonia, apnea) in approximately 40%.[10,57] None of the infants developed progressive neurological signs. In addition, two recent case reports describe the finding of vocal cord paralysis in infants who presented with stridor and respiratory distress and exhibited subdural hemorrhages diagnosed on subsequent MRI.[90-92] Finally, as noted earlier, the most common presentation of subdural hemorrhage in the term infant is to be completely asymptomatic to the clinical providers.[3-5]

Falx Laceration

No careful description of the clinical course of falx tears with major subdural hemorrhage is available. Yet in view of the locus of the hematoma, it is likely that initially bilateral cerebral signs will appear. However, striking neurological findings probably do not develop until the clot has extended infratentorially; the resulting syndrome is then similar to that described for tentorial laceration and posterior fossa subdural hematoma.

Cerebral Convexity Subdural Hemorrhage

Subdural hemorrhage over the cerebral convexities is associated with at least three neurological syndromes (Table 22.9). First and probably most commonly, minor degrees of hemorrhage occur, and *minimal* or *no clinical signs* are apparent. Irritability, a *hyperalert* appearance, unexplained apneic episodes, or no signs have been noted.[4,10,40,57]

Second, *signs of focal cerebral disturbance* may occur, with the most common time of onset being the second or third day of life. With this syndrome, seizures, often focal, are common and are frequently accompanied by other focal cerebral signs (e.g., hemiparesis, deviation of eyes to the side contralateral to the hemiparesis; however, the eyes move by doll's eyes

TABLE 22.9	Neurological Syndromes Associated With Subdural Hemorrhage of Cerebral Convexity

Minimal or no clinical signs
Focal cerebral syndrome: hemiparesis, deviation of eyes to side of lesion, focal seizures, homolateral pupillary abnormality
Chronic subdural effusion

---

[a]References 1, 10, 40-48, 53, 55, 57, 60, 69, 77-90.
[b]References 1, 10, 42-44, 46, 53, 57, 61, 69, 90.

maneuver, because this is a cerebral lesion). These focal cerebral signs are definitive, *although usually not striking*. The most distinctive neurological sign with major convexity subdural hemorrhage is dysfunction of the third cranial nerve on the side of the hematoma; this dysfunction is usually manifested by a nonreactive or poorly reactive, dilated pupil.[40,79,84-86] The latter occurs secondary to compression of the third nerve by herniation of the temporal lobe through the tentorial notch. An excellent example of such a neurological syndrome associated with subdural hematoma was a newborn with hemophilia that we studied.[84]

A third clinical presentation may be the occurrence of subdural hemorrhage in the neonatal period with few clinical signs and then the development over the next several months of a *chronic subdural effusion*. It is certainly well known that many infants presenting in the first 6 months of life with an enlarging head, increased transillumination, and chronic subdural effusions have no known cause for the lesion and that subdural hemorrhage can evolve into subdural effusion.[93-95] However, the timing of the subdural hemorrhage as perinatal or postnatal may be unknown and must raise concerns for the occurrence of nonaccidental injury in the neonatal period.[96]

Diagnosis

The diagnosis of major neonatal subdural hemorrhage depends principally on recognition of the clinical syndrome, with subsequent definitive demonstration by a brain imaging study.

Clinical Syndromes

The clinical syndromes previously reviewed are often sufficiently distinctive to raise the suspicion of a large subdural hemorrhage as well as the specific variety thereof. Neurological signs primarily referable to the brain stem should suggest infratentorial hematoma. Neurological signs primarily referable to the cerebrum should suggest convexity subdural hematoma. These signs should provoke more definitive and prompt diagnostic studies because the clinical course may deteriorate very rapidly. Lumbar puncture is *not* a good choice for diagnostic study in this setting because of the possibility of provoking herniation, either of cerebellar tonsils into the foramen magnum in the presence of a posterior fossa subdural hematoma or of the temporal lobe into the tentorial notch in the presence of a large unilateral convexity subdural hematoma.

Computed Tomography, Magnetic Resonance Imaging, and Ultrasound Scans

Although *CT* is a definitive means of demonstrating the site and extent of neonatal subdural hemorrhage, MRI is superior and currently recommended. When MRI is not available soon enough, CT is particularly useful for a rapid diagnosis and defining the location and extent of the lesions. Examples of the CT demonstration of the varieties of subdural hemorrhage just discussed are shown in Fig. 22.4. MRI is more effective than CT in the delineation of posterior fossa subdural hemorrhage (Figs. 22.5 to 22.7).[1,45,97-99] This particular superiority of MRI in the evaluation of posterior fossa hemorrhage also applies to other types of lesions in this location (see Chapter 10). Detection of subdural hematoma by *ultrasound scanning* (Fig. 22.8), although reported, is generally difficult.[43,46,64,100] Moreover, even when these hematomas are detected, the extent and distribution of supratentorial lesions are usually demonstrated far better by MRI or CT and of infratentorial lesions by MRI. In addition,

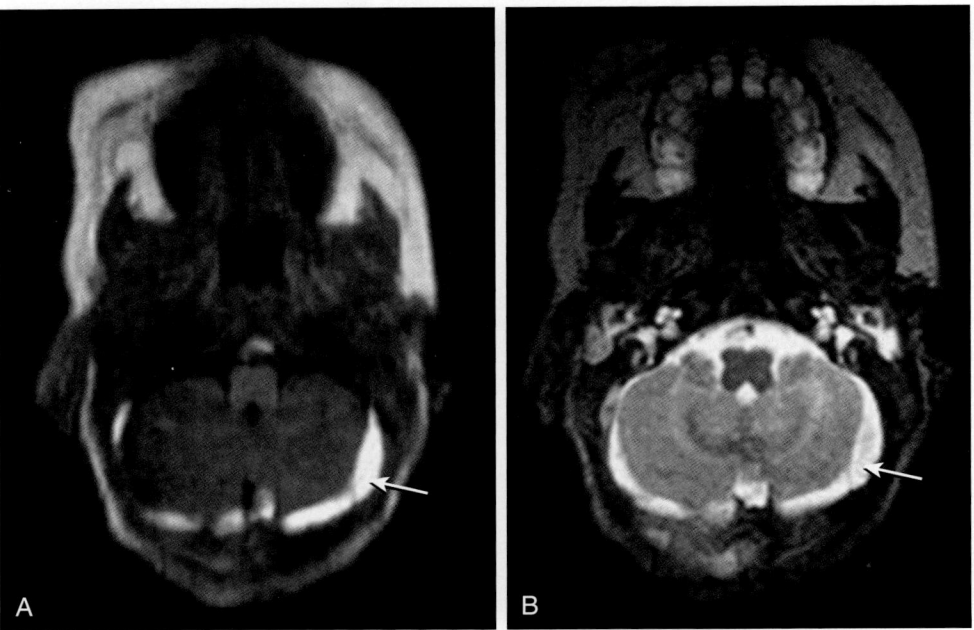

Figure 22.5 Subdural hemorrhage with retrocerebellar hemorrhage. This term infant was delivered by vacuum extraction. Apgar scores were 3 at 1 minute and 7 at 5 minutes. He developed convulsions on day 1 and was imaged at 14 days. (A) T1-weighted (spin echo [SE] 860/20) sequence. There is high signal in the posterior fossa, consistent with subdural hemorrhage *(arrow)*. (B) T2-weighted (2700/120) sequence. The hemorrhage has high signal intensity, consistent with a perinatal lesion. Differentiation from transverse sinus thrombosis may be difficult. (From Rutherford M. Part 4: Disorders in the newborn infant. Hemorrhagic lesions of the newborn brain. Chapter 9 in: MRI of the Neonatal Brain. http://www.mrineonatalbrain.com.)

the vast majority of subdural hematomas are infratentorial, where ultrasound has even greater challenges in accurate diagnosis. The major difficulty of ultrasound scanning relates to acoustical interference by bone and to near-field transducer artifacts.

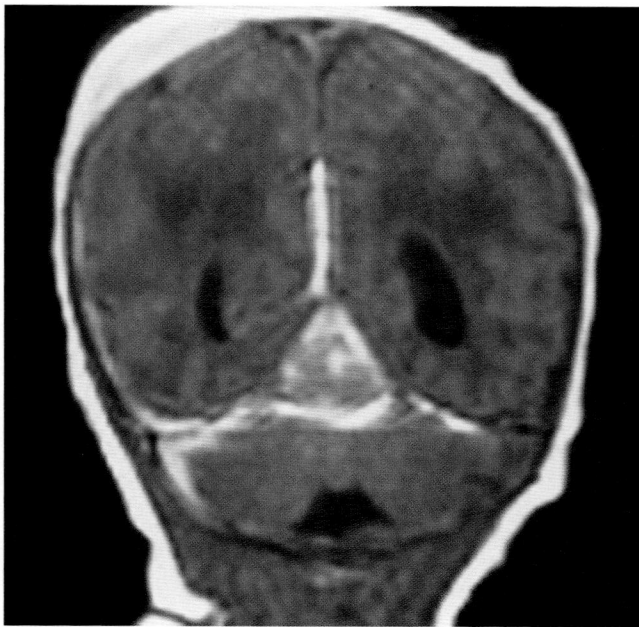

Figure 22.6 Posterior fossa subdural hemorrhage, magnetic resonance imaging. Coronal T1-weighted image shows the central tentorial hematoma and layered blood along both leaves of the tentorium and the posterior falx. A small subdural hematoma in the right posterior fossa is seen. The blood in the right parietal region is due to a cephalhematoma (better seen on axial images). (Adapted with permission from Castillo M, Fordham, LA. MR of Neurologically symptomatic newborns after vacuum extraction delivery. *AJNR Am J Neuroradiol.* 1995;16:816–818.)

Skull Radiographs

Occipital osteodiastasis may be demonstrated by skull radiographs. The lateral view shows the lesion (Fig. 22.9).

Prognosis

Infants with major symptomatic *lacerations of the tentorium and falx* and massive degrees of subdural hemorrhage have a very poor prognosis. Nearly all die; the rare survivor is left with hydrocephalus secondary to obstruction of CSF flow at the tentorial notch or over the convexities. Similarly, severe *occipital diastasis* and its complications have been associated with a poor

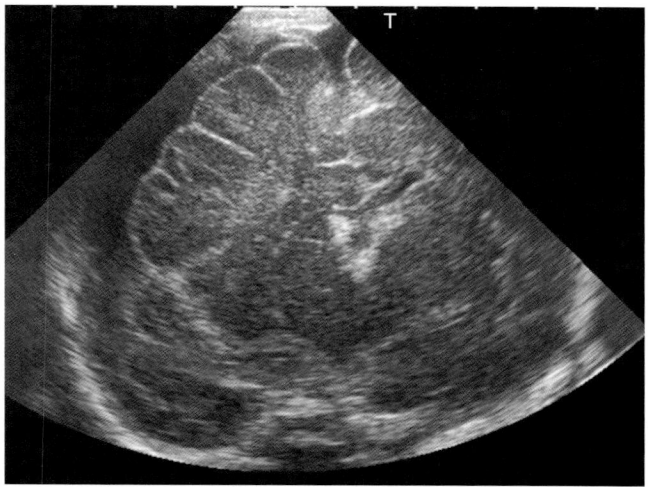

Figure 22.8 Subdural hemorrhage. A full-term infant with difficult delivery who required resuscitation and displayed neonatal encephalopathy. Cranial ultrasound scan on admission to the neonatal intensive care unit displayed a very large subdural hemorrhage. (Image courtesy Linda de Vries, MD, University Medical Center, Utrecht, The Netherlands.)

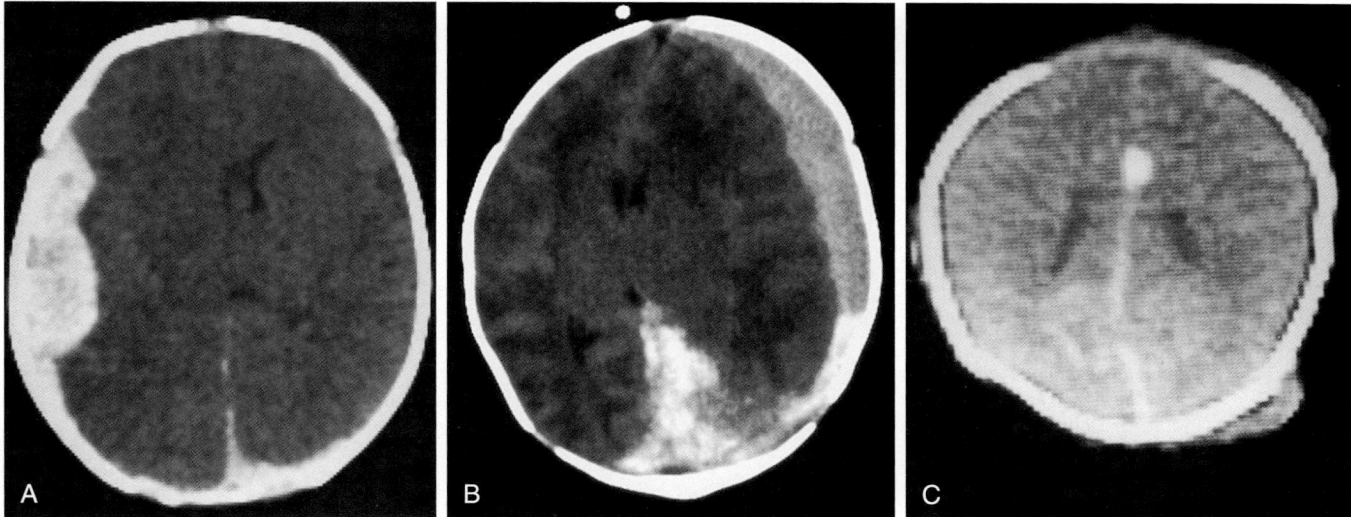

Figure 22.7 Subdural hemorrhage, computed tomography scans. (A) Convexity subdural hematoma in a newborn with severe hemophilia. Note the area of increased attenuation on the right, representing the hematoma, and the shift of ventricles to the left. (B) Convexity subdural hematoma on the left in a 1-day-old infant delivered by forceps because of head entrapment. The infant's pupil was dilated on the side of the lesion. Note also deviation of midline structures to the right and probable tentorial tear, with associated hemorrhage. (C) Probable falx tear in a newborn of 4780 g delivered by a difficult breech extraction. Note the small circular area of increased attenuation in the midline, representing hemorrhage in the inferior margin of the falx.

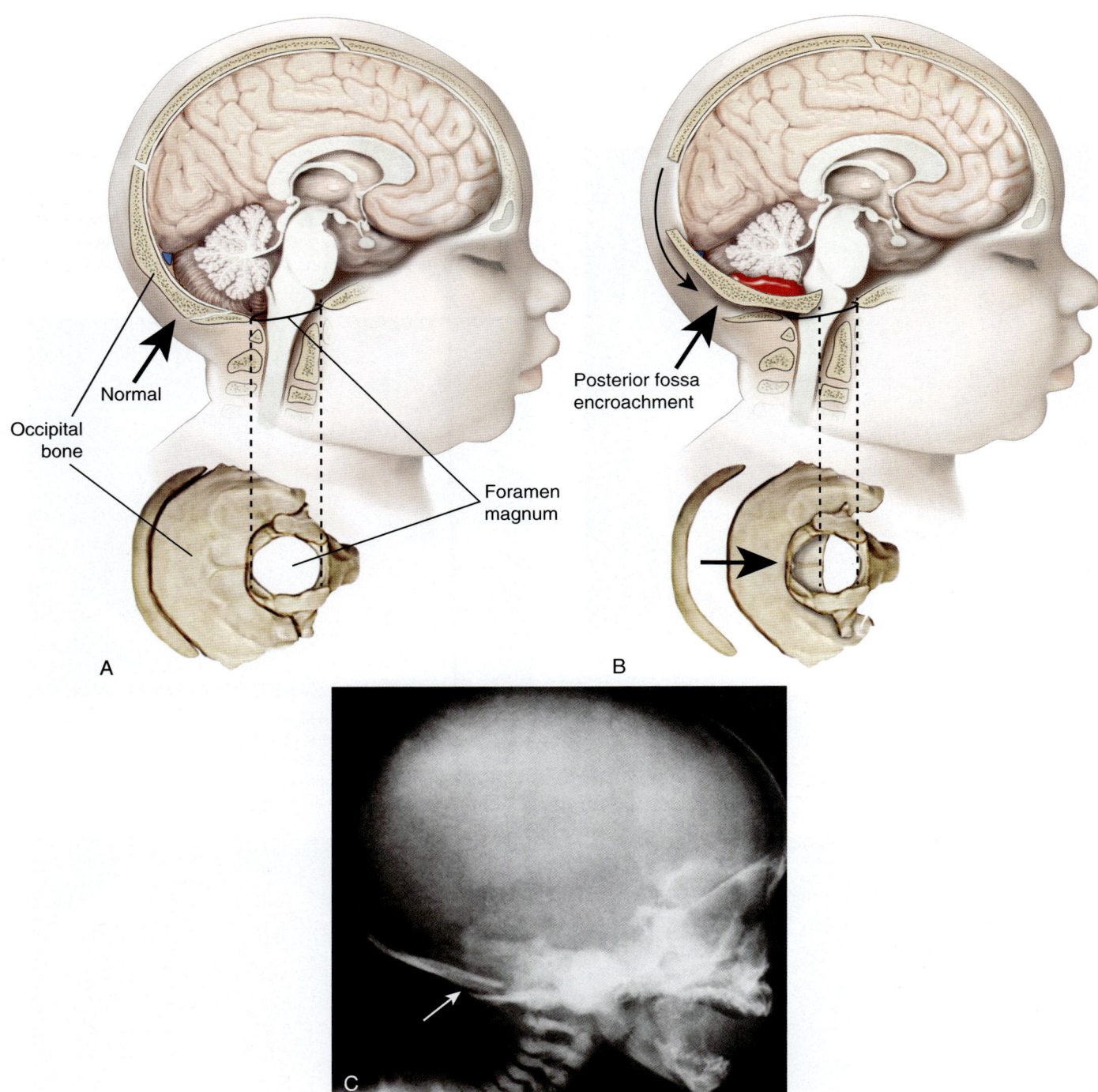

Figure 22.9 Occipital osteodiastasis. Schematic diagram of the cranium illustrating (A) the normal state *(arrow)* and (B) occipital osteodiastasis with posterior fossa encroachment *(arrow)*. (C) Lateral radiograph of the skull demonstrating occipital osteodiastasis in an autopsy case *(arrow)*. (From Pape KE, Wigglesworth JS. *Hemorrhage, Ischemia, and the Perinatal Brain*. Philadelphia: JB Lippincott; 1979.)

TABLE 22.10	Outcome With Subdural Hemorrhage of Posterior Fossa[a]		
SURGICAL EVACUATION (N = 81)	OUTCOME		
	GOOD TO EXCELLENT	MAJOR SEQUELAE	DEATHS
Yes (46)	85%	10%	5%
No (35)	88%	7%	5%

[a]See text for references; also includes unpublished personal cases. Lesions have been of moderate or large size.

outcome. Nevertheless it is possible that early diagnosis could lead to beneficial intervention.

Although they are often serious lesions, *moderate posterior fossa subdural hematomas*, frequently recognized in recent years primarily by CT and MRI, are associated with an outcome that is variable but dependent on size, rapidity of diagnosis, and, when necessary, intervention (Table 22.10).[a] Thus of 30 surgically treated infants, 80% either were normal or exhibited minor neurological deficits on follow-up. Approximately 15% of surgically treated patients developed communicating hydrocephalus that required shunt placement. Of 40 nonsurgically treated infants, nearly 90% had a favorable outcome (see Table 22.10). In earlier reports, as many as 40% to 50% of infants who did not undergo operations died, probably because of rapidly progressive lesions, the gravity of which escaped prompt detection. The *small* posterior fossa subdural hemorrhages described in hospital-based series are associated with no major sequelae or death.[4,5,57]

The prognosis of patients with moderate or large *convexity subdural hemorrhage* is relatively good; from 50% to 90% of affected infants are well on follow-up.[b] The remainder are left with focal cerebral signs and, occasionally, hydrocephalus. The deficits appear to relate to associated parenchymal lesions. The small subdural hemorrhages detected by widespread imaging in recent years have a generally favorable short-term outcome,[4,5,57] although the longer-term prognosis remains unknown at this stage.

Management

Tentorial and Falx Lacerations, Occipital Osteodiastasis, and Posterior Fossa Subdural Hematoma

The severity of the initial trauma and the rapid progression to brain-stem compromise have rendered effective treatment nearly impossible in *major* tears of the tentorium and falx and in overt occipital osteodiastasis with *severe* subdural hemorrhage. Theoretically, rapid surgical evacuation may provide some hope for salvage of the affected baby. Some support for this suggestion is obtained by the experience just reviewed with less severe posterior fossa subdural hematomas (see Table 22.10). Rapid detection and prompt surgical evacuation in the presence of progression of neurological signs have been of value in the management of these lesions. However, a normal outcome has been documented in posterior fossa subdural hematoma *without* surgical intervention (see Table 22.10). In

summing up the available literature, several key points are apparent: *Close surveillance alone* is appropriate *in the absence of* major neurological signs, particularly brain-stem signs, or worsening neurological status. Surgery should not be delayed if clear neurological deterioration becomes apparent. With small lesions, close surveillance is almost always followed by a favorable outcome.

Cerebral Convexity Subdural Hematoma

Effective management of the infant with an acute convexity subdural hematoma requires careful sequential clinical observation. Surgery is not mandatory if the infant is stable neurologically.[43] The need for surgery is based on large size of the lesion, signs of increased intracranial pressure, and neurological deficits, particularly if findings suggest incipient transtentorial herniation. If a stable subdural hemorrhage evolves to subdural effusion, subdural taps can be used to reduce signs of increased intracranial pressure and to prevent the development of craniocerebral disproportion, the latter serving only to perpetuate subdural bleeding.[93] Repeated subdural taps should not be performed if the infant is asymptomatic and the head is not growing rapidly. The development of constricting *subdural membranes* was overestimated in the past. The smaller convexity subdural hemorrhages detected by imaging in recent years rarely require intervention.

PRIMARY SUBARACHNOID HEMORRHAGE

Primary subarachnoid hemorrhage is hemorrhage within the subarachnoid space that is not secondary to extension from subdural, intraventricular, or cerebellar hemorrhage. Moreover, also excluded from this category are cases in which subarachnoid blood is secondary to extension from intracerebral hematoma, a structural vascular lesion (e.g., aneurysm or arteriovenous malformation), tumor, hemorrhagic infarction, or major coagulation disturbance (see later discussion of miscellaneous causes of intracranial hemorrhage). Primary subarachnoid hemorrhage, defined in this way, is a very frequent variety of neonatal intracranial hemorrhage, mostly because the category includes the many newborn infants, particularly premature infants, with a few hundred RBCs per cubic millimeter in the CSF. The frequency of *clinically significant* primary subarachnoid hemorrhage was overestimated in the past, particularly in the premature infant but also in the full-term infant, mostly because of the lack of brain imaging data to identify intraventricular hemorrhage. As reviewed in Table 22.3, in our own series of infants weighing less than 2000 g with grossly bloody CSF, only 29% exhibited subarachnoid hemorrhage alone, and 63% exhibited intraventricular hemorrhage (although with blood also in the subarachnoid space). Moreover, even many term infants with bloody CSF who, in the past, would have been considered to have primary subarachnoid hemorrhage on clinical grounds, have now been shown by more detailed neuroimaging studies—including ultrasound, CT, or MRI scans—to have intraventricular hemorrhage. Finally, a localized variant of subarachnoid hemorrhage, involving the subpial space and superficial cerebral cortex, should also be recognized in this context; this lesion often occurs with subarachnoid hemorrhage and, on brain imaging, may be difficult to distinguish from typical primary subarachnoid hemorrhage (see later).

[a]References 1, 10, 43, 44, 46, 53, 61, 69, 90.
[b]References 1, 10, 43, 55, 79, 101.

Neuropathology

Blood is usually located most prominently in the pia-arachnoid space over the cerebral convexities, especially posteriorly, and in the posterior fossa.[67,102,103] Small amounts of subarachnoid blood are not infrequently found at postmortem examinations of newborns not suspected clinically of having sustained intracranial hemorrhage.[51,67] Less commonly, large amounts of blood are observed. The source of the bleeding in primary subarachnoid hemorrhage is presumed to be small vascular channels derived from the involuting anastomoses between leptomeningeal arteries present during brain development.[104] Origin from bridging veins within the subarachnoid space is also possible.[47,60] At any rate, primary subarachnoid hemorrhage in newborn patients is unlike the dramatic large vessel, arterial hemorrhage in older patients.

Neuropathological complications of neonatal primary subarachnoid hemorrhage are very unusual. Even in major degrees of hemorrhage, significantly increased intracranial pressure with brain-stem compression is rare. The only significant, albeit very uncommon, sequela clearly related to the hemorrhage is hydrocephalus. The latter is secondary either to adhesions around the outflow of the fourth ventricle or around the tentorial notch—which result in obstruction to CSF flow—or to adhesions over the cerebral convexities, which result in impaired CSF flow or absorption.

The *variant of subarachnoid hemorrhage* noted earlier involves localized bleeding in the *subpial* region, with involvement of the most superficial aspect of cerebral cortex.[84,90,105,106] Although this hemorrhage often occurs together with subarachnoid hemorrhage, in subpial hemorrhage, the blood is found beneath the pia and is contiguous with bleeding in the most superficial, largely glial-populated region of cerebral cortex. The usual location for this type of hemorrhage is in the region of the anterior temporal lobe, near the pterion (a point at the junction of the coronal, squamous sphenosquamous, and sphenofrontal sutures) or in localized cerebral regions beneath cranial sutures.

Pathogenesis

The pathogenesis of neonatal primary subarachnoid hemorrhage is not entirely understood, but most of the *major* hemorrhages appear to relate, on clinical grounds, to trauma or to circulatory events related to prematurity. The relationships of trauma to the genesis of major subarachnoid hemorrhage are similar in many respects to those described earlier for subdural hemorrhage. The relationships to prematurity are similar to those described in Chapter 24 for germinal matrix–intraventricular hemorrhage of the premature infant. Common to both pathogenetic themes is the substrate of maturation-dependent involution of leptomeningeal anastomotic channels.[104] The pathogenesis of the common smaller subarachnoid hemorrhages is unclear because most of these hemorrhages occur without any apparent traumatic or circulatory abnormality.

The interesting *subpial hemorrhages* may relate to local trauma with resulting disruption of small veins because the lesions occur at sites in proximity to cranial sutures and to likely movement of bone during normal delivery.[106] Thus, in one series of seven cases, four occurred in proximity to the pterion and the remainder occurred beneath the coronal or squamosal sutures.[106]

TABLE 22.11	Neurological Syndromes Associated With Primary Subarachnoid Hemorrhage

Minimal or no clinical signs
Seizures in full-term infant; considered *well* during interictal period
Catastrophic deterioration

Clinical Features

Three major syndromes with primary subarachnoid hemorrhage can be distinguished (Table 22.11). First, and *undoubtedly most commonly*, minor degrees of hemorrhage occur, and minimal or no signs develop. Second, primary subarachnoid hemorrhage can result in *seizures*, especially in full-term infants (see Chapter 12). The seizures usually have their onset on the second postnatal day. In the interictal period, these babies usually appear remarkably well, and the description "well baby with seizures" often seems appropriate. In the subpial variant, the seizures are often focal, reflecting the localized nature of these lesions.

A third and rare syndrome is massive subarachnoid hemorrhage with *catastrophic deterioration* and a rapidly fatal course. The infants have usually sustained severe perinatal asphyxia, sometimes with an element of trauma at the time of birth.[40,49] The neurological syndrome is similar to the catastrophic deterioration described in Chapter 24 for some patients with large intraventricular hemorrhage.

Diagnosis

The diagnosis of primary subarachnoid hemorrhage is usually made by MRI or CT; on rare occasions it is made by ultrasound (see earlier discussion of neuroimaging).[7] On CT, distinction from the normal, slightly increased attenuation in the region of the falx and major venous sinuses in the newborn may be difficult. Sometimes the possibility of primary subarachnoid hemorrhage is raised initially by the findings of an elevated number of RBCs and an elevated protein content in the CSF, usually obtained for another purpose (e.g., to rule out meningitis). Exclusion of another cause of blood in the subarachnoid space (e.g., extension from subdural, cerebellar, or intraventricular hemorrhage) or from certain unusual sources (e.g., tumor, vascular lesions) is made best by MRI or CT.[7] The localized subpial hemorrhages, often with superficial cortical hemorrhage, are observable both by MRI or CT (Fig. 22.10).

Ultrasonography is insensitive in detecting subarachnoid hemorrhage per se because of the normal increase in echogenicity around the periphery of the brain.[107] A large subarachnoid hemorrhage occasionally distends the sylvian fissure and thus becomes detectable, but care must be taken not to confuse a sylvian fissure distended with blood from the wide fissure seen consistently in premature infants and resulting from the normal separation of the frontal operculum and superior temporal region until late in gestation (Fig. 22.11).[108]

Prognosis

In general the prognosis for infants with primary subarachnoid hemorrhage without serious traumatic or hypoxic injury is

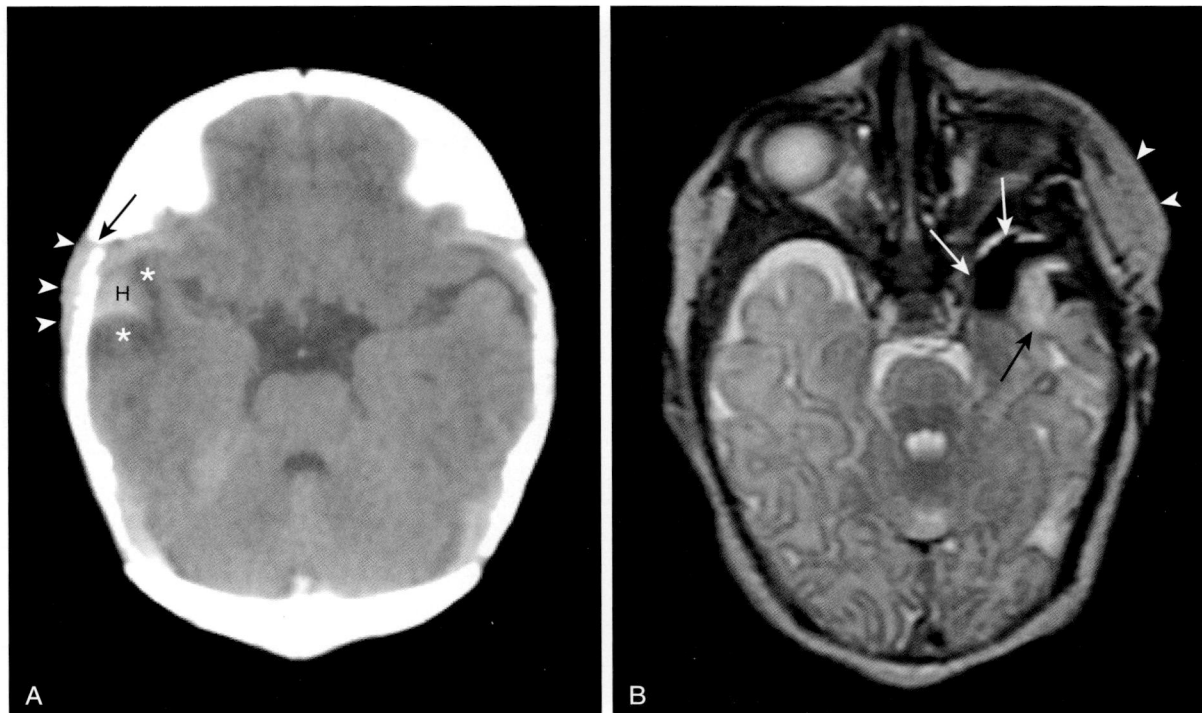

Figure 22.10 Subpial hemorrhage. (A) Computed tomography scan performed at 8 hours of life in a term infant with apnea; note the hemorrhage *(H)*, which tracks the subpial space and adjacent low-attenuation edema *(asterisks)*. Note also the pterion *(arrow)* and associated soft tissue swelling *(arrowheads)*. (B) T2-weighted magnetic resonance imaging scan, performed on the second postnatal day in an infant with apnea and seizures at 24 hours of life, shows subpial hemorrhage *(white arrows)*, which is of low signal in the acute period, in the region of the anterior temporal lobe, near the pterion (see text), a site of predilection for this type of hemorrhage. Parenchymal edema *(black arrow)* and soft tissue swelling *(white arrowheads)* are also apparent. (From Huang AH, Robertson RL. Spontaneous superficial parenchymal and leptomeningeal hemorrhage in term neonates. *AJNR Am J Neuroradiol.* 2004;25:469–475.)

good. The specific outcome correlates reliably with the neonatal clinical syndrome. Thus, the many infants with minimal signs in the neonatal period and documentation of subarachnoid blood do well virtually uniformly. Those few full-term infants with seizures as the primary manifestation of the hemorrhage are normal on follow-up in at least 90% of cases (see Chapter 12). The rare patient with a catastrophic course with massive subarachnoid hemorrhage of unknown origin either suffers serious neurological residua or dies. The principal sequela, albeit unusual, after major subarachnoid hemorrhage is hydrocephalus.

Management

The management is essentially that of posthemorrhagic hydrocephalus and is discussed in detail in Chapter 24 in relation to intraventricular hemorrhage of the premature infant.

INTRAVENTRICULAR HEMORRHAGE OF THE TERM INFANT

Although intraventricular hemorrhage is predominantly a lesion of the premature infant, this variety of hemorrhage has been documented repeatedly by ultrasound, MRI, or CT scans as well as by postmortem study of term infants.[1,67,89,108-134] A few of these hemorrhages are caused by intraventricular extension of blood

from large hemorrhagic infarctions, ruptured vascular lesions (e.g., arteriovenous malformations, aneurysms), or tumors, which are discussed separately (see the later section on miscellaneous examples of neonatal intracranial hemorrhage). In this section, we consider those cases in which intraventricular hemorrhage per se is the dominant lesion in a *term infant*. Moreover, we emphasize here intraventricular hemorrhages of appreciable size, because minor degrees of intraventricular hemorrhage with or without subependymal or choroid plexus hemorrhage are not rare in asymptomatic full-term infants.[5,123,124,128,129] For example, in one ultrasonographic study of 1000 consecutive healthy term newborns, intracranial hemorrhage was detected in 3.5%, with a subependymal locus in 2.0%, a choroid plexus locus in 1.1%, and a parenchymal locus in 0.4%.[129] In a large study of encephalopathic term infants, intraventricular hemorrhage was identified in approximately 2%, although the site of origin was not defined.[7,128,129]

Neuropathology

The neuropathology of major intraventricular hemorrhage of the term infant differs from that of the premature infant (see Chapter 24), primarily in relation to the principal sites of origin of the hemorrhage (Table 22.12). In term infants, *neuropathological studies* have indicated that most intraventricular hemorrhages encountered in the early neonatal period emanate from bleeding

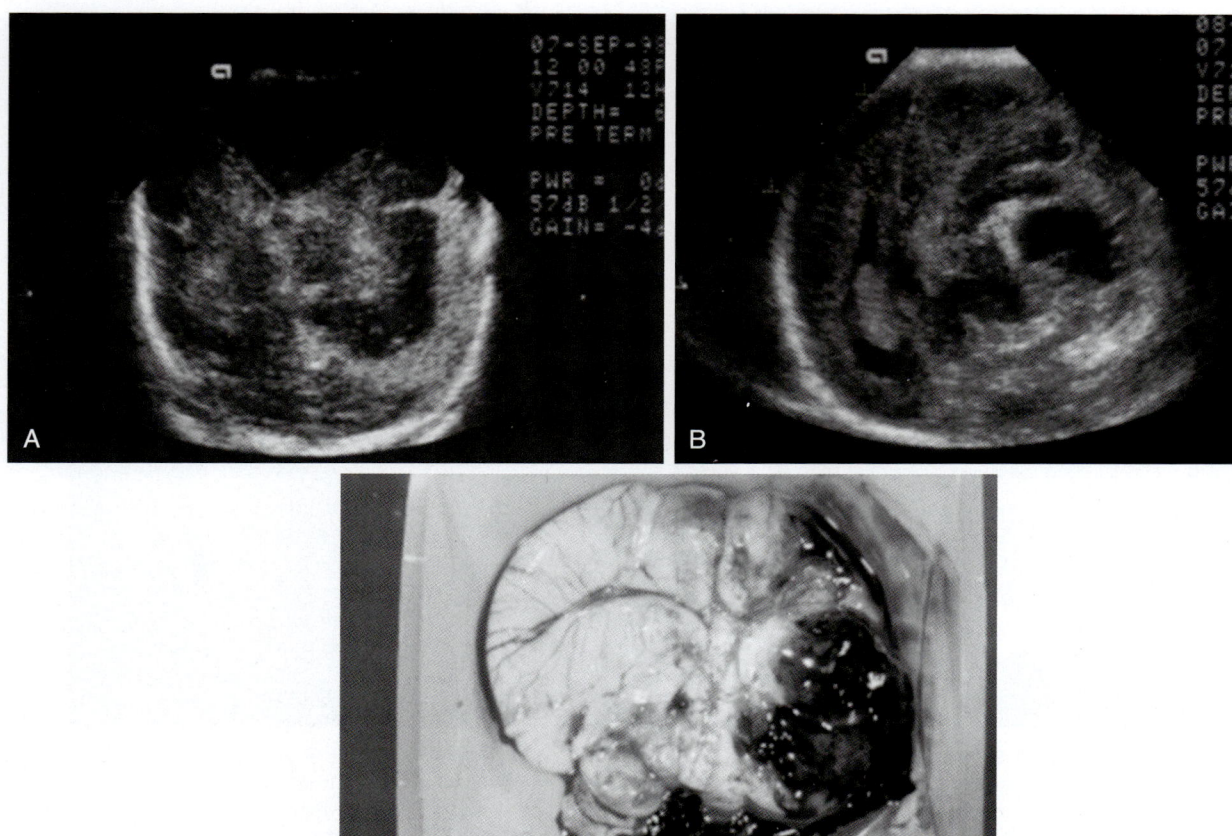

Figure 22.11 Extensive subarachnoid hemorrhage detected by cranial ultrasound scan (A) Cranial ultrasound scan obtained on postnatal day 9. Observe the increased echogenicity extending inferiorly from within the left sylvian fissure. (B) Coronal ultrasound scan obtained 24 hours later. Observe the larger-appearing lesion with areas of hyperechogenicity interspersed with areas of hypoechogenicity. A midline shift is also present. (C) Brain specimen from the postmortem examination. Observe the large organized hematoma involving the left posterior parietal cortex. The hematoma was confined to the subarachnoid space. (Reprinted with permission from Chamnanvanakij S, Perlman JM. Extensive late-onset primary subarachnoid hemorrhage in a preterm infant. *Pediatr Neurol.* 1999;21:735–738.)

TABLE 22.12   Sites of Origin of Intraventricular Hemorrhage of the Term Infant[a]

Choroid plexus (35%)
Thalamus (24%)
Subependymal germinal matrix, caudate (17%)
Periventricular cerebral parenchyma (14%)
Source unclear (10%)

[a]Data derived from brain imaging of 29 full-term infants with intraventricular hemorrhage.
Data from Wu YW, Hamrick SEG, Miller SP, Haward MF, et al. Intraventricular hemorrhage in term neonates caused by sinovenous thrombosis. *Ann Neurol.* 2003;54:123–126.

---

in the choroid plexus.[a] Particularly common sites within the choroid are the posterior tufts in the region of the atrium of the lateral ventricle.[67] In somewhat fewer term infants with intraventricular hemorrhage studied neuropathologically, the site of origin was the subependymal germinal matrix, particularly the region of the thalamocaudate groove (slightly posterior to the region overlying the head of the caudate nucleus as in the premature newborn), which is the last area of matrix to dissipate in the human newborn. Large-scale *ultrasonographic studies* of healthy term newborns examined in the first days of life suggest, however, that the subependymal germinal matrix may be a more common site of intraventricular hemorrhage in the term infant than previously suspected.[123,124,128,129] For example, in the study of 1000 term newborns of Heibel and coworkers,[128,129] of 20 infants with intraventricular blood (albeit generally small amounts in these *asymptomatic* infants), 9 had

---

[a]References 60, 67, 123, 130, 133, 134.

choroid plexus hemorrhage and 11 had subependymal germinal matrix hemorrhage.

The conclusions just mentioned concerning site of origin must be interpreted in the context of the two largest studies of *major* intraventricular hemorrhages in *living term infants*, identified by CT scan ($n = 19$)[125,126] or by CT and MRI scan ($n = 29$).[133,134] In the larger of these two studies (see Table 22.12), the choroid plexus (35%) and thalamus (24%) were the sites of origin in the majority of cases (see Table 22.12).[133,134] The thalamus was a more common site than the choroid plexus in the earlier study based entirely on CT.[125,126] Thalamic origin of hemorrhage is associated more prominently than is choroid plexus origin with moderate to severe intraventricular hemorrhage and with venous thrombosis (see later). Subependymal germinal matrix overlying the caudate is often difficult to distinguish from an apparent caudate origin and accounts for nearly 20% of cases. Intraventricular extension from periventricular hemorrhagic infarction accounts for a small minority of cases (see Table 22.12). With imaging that includes MRI, a site of origin of hemorrhage is obscure in only approximately 10% of cases.[125,126,134] The neuropathological sequelae of intraventricular hemorrhage (e.g., posthemorrhagic hydrocephalus) are similar in the term and premature infant (see Chapter 24).

Pathogenesis

The principal pathogenetic themes are often multiple, but *apparent disturbances in cerebral blood flow, venous pressure, coagulation, and vascular integrity*, as well as mechanical *trauma*, are prominent.[a] Many of the pathogenetic factors relative to these themes, discussed in relation to intraventricular hemorrhage of the premature infant, are relevant here (see Chapter 24). However, two aspects of pathogenesis are somewhat different in the term infant compared with the premature infant. First, the role of *trauma* may be somewhat more important in the term infant. Among those cases with adequate perinatal data, an appreciable minority experienced difficult deliveries because of forceps rotations, vacuum-assisted delivery, and breech extractions. The specific relationships between the trauma and the occurrence of intraventricular hemorrhage are not entirely clear, but presumably some of the factors described earlier for cerebellar hemorrhage (see the pathogenesis section) that lead to increases in cerebral venous pressure are important. A second aspect of pathogenesis in the term infant that appears different from that in the preterm infant is the *more prominent role of coagulation disturbance*. Thus, in the largest reported series, 40% of infants tested had coagulation factor abnormalities consistent with a hypercoagulable state, had disseminated intravascular coagulation, or were receiving extracorporeal membrane oxygenation (ECMO).[134] Consistent with the importance of a hypercoagulable state,[133,134] recent data strongly indicate an important role for *cerebral sinovenous thrombosis* in the final cascade to intraventricular hemorrhage in the term infant. An earlier report based on CT scanning suggested that thalamic venous hemorrhagic infarction was important in pathogenesis.[125,126] A later study using MRI demonstrated thrombosis in the vein of Galen or major venous sinuses in approximately 30% of cases of intraventricular hemorrhage and showed parenchymal findings (hemorrhagic

infarct) consistent with thrombosis in an additional 25%.[133,134] Venous thrombosis was associated with nearly all the thalamic infarcts.[134] Sinovenous thrombosis is more extensively reviewed in Chapter 21.[133]

Clinical Features

The onset of the neurological syndrome varies with the cause. Infants with perinatal complications usually exhibit distinct abnormalities from the first day or two of life, whereas infants with no clear cause of the syndrome often present later, sometimes as late as the second to fourth *weeks* of life. The neurological syndrome is characterized by irritability, stupor, apnea, and particularly seizures.[a] The seizures are usually focal or multifocal and occur in approximately 50% to 65% of cases. Other features include fever, jitteriness, and signs of increased intracranial pressure (e.g., full fontanelle, vomiting). Approximately 50% of infants with large hemorrhages develop hydrocephalus that requires placement of a ventriculoperitoneal shunt. An additional 20% of infants develop ventricular dilation that ceases to progress without therapy. Approximately half of the infants recover totally within 2 to 3 weeks; the remainder improve but continue to exhibit neurological abnormalities and subsequently neurological deficits.

Diagnosis

The diagnosis of the intraventricular hemorrhage is readily made by neuroimaging techniques, as outlined earlier. The thalamic source of origin and any associated venous thromboses are determined best by MRI scan (Figs. 22.12 and 22.13). MRI also demonstrates parenchymal involvement better than ultrasound or CT and clearly is the preferred imaging modality. In addition, magnetic resonance venography can evaluate the patency of the cerebral veins. Because of the unusual occurrence of choroid plexus arteriovenous malformation—a lesion that raises serious therapeutic questions—some investigators have suggested angiography in infants with apparent choroid plexus origin of hemorrhage and no apparent causative factors.[133]

Prognosis

At first glance, the overall outcome of intraventricular hemorrhage for the term infant appears to be somewhat worse than that for the premature infant (Table 22.13).[b] This apparent difference relates in part to the finding that smaller lesions, without parenchymal involvement, make up a greater proportion of the hemorrhages identified in premature infants. For example, in one series of 15 term infants, 67% of hemorrhages were classified as "grade III or IV."[126,128] In a later series of nine infants, all four of the infants with an unfavorable outcome had "grade III or IV" hemorrhage.[1] In the largest reported series ($n = 29$), 45% of lesions were *moderate* or "severe."[134] The specific outcome in term infants relates in part to the cause. Those infants with major perinatal complications in the background or on ECMO exhibit neurological deficits in most instances, whereas infants with no etiological factors recognized are usually normal on follow-up examinations.[c] The relative frequency of accompanying parenchymal injury appears to underlie the differences in outcome. Infants who

---

[a]References 1, 64, 89, 110, 111, 114, 118-122, 125-128, 133, 134.

[a]References 1, 64, 89, 110, 111, 114, 118-122, 125-128, 131-134.
[b]References 64, 89, 110, 111, 114, 118-121, 125, 126, 128.
[c]References 64, 89, 110, 111, 114, 118-121, 125, 126, 128, 129.

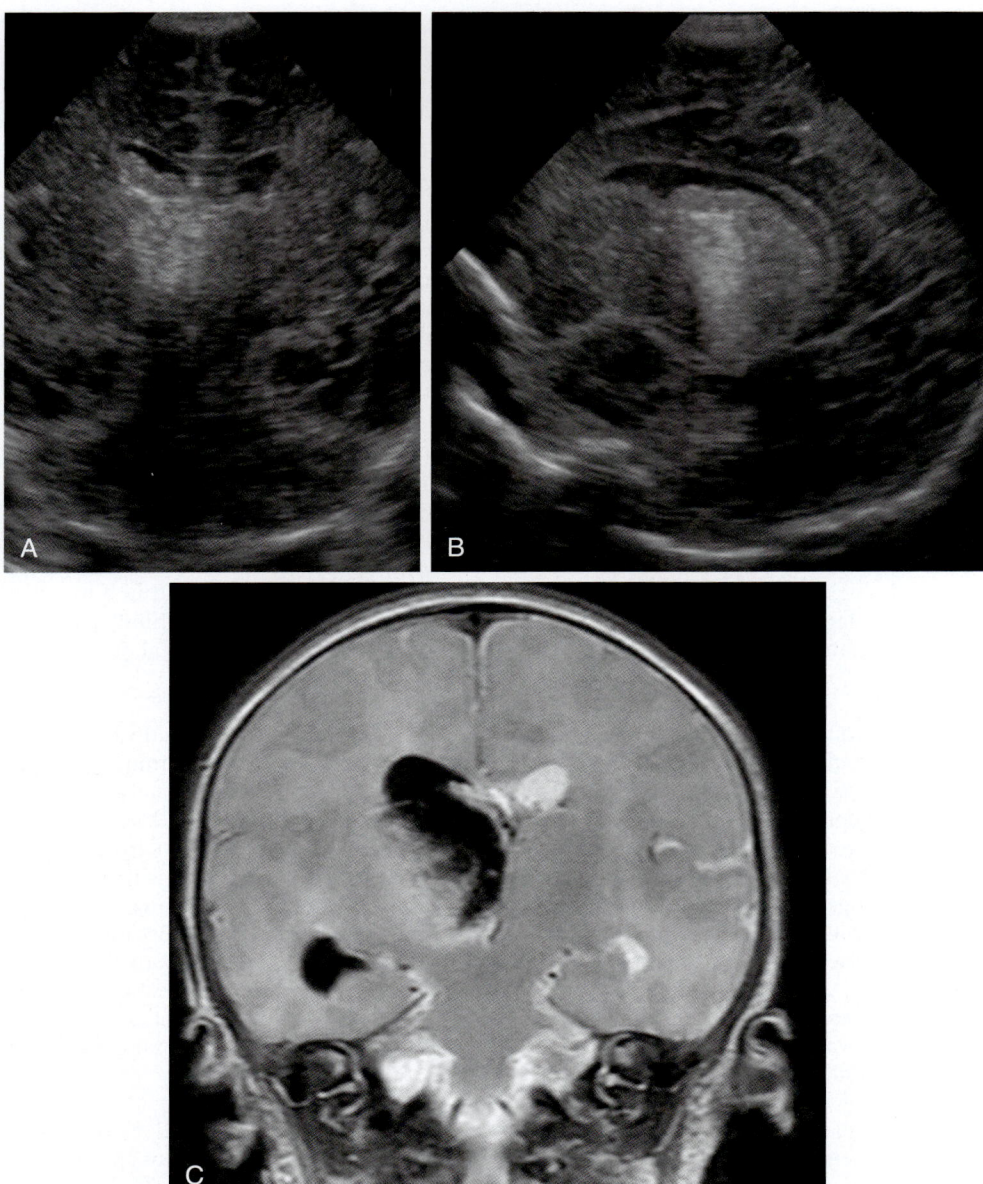

Figure 22.12 Cranial ultrasound and magnetic resonance imaging (MRI) scans of intraventricular hemorrhage (IVH) originating in the thalamus. A 2-day-old premature infant born after 33 weeks of gestation and delivered vaginally with Apgar scores of 9 and 9 at 1 and 5 minutes, respectively. She presented with seizures on the first postnatal day. (A) Cranial ultrasound demonstrated increased echogenicity within the right thalamus on the coronal view and (B) associated intraventricular hemorrhage on the sagittal view. (C) The MRI coronal T2 scan demonstrates a large right thalamic hemorrhage that dissects into the right lateral ventricle.

TABLE 22.13	Outcome of Intraventricular Hemorrhage of the Term Infant[a]	
Outcome	**Total**
Normal	55%
Neurological deficits (major)	40%
Hydrocephalus (shunted)	50%
Dead	5%

[a]Derived from data on 84 infants reported in references listed in text and unpublished personal cases.

develop intraventricular hemorrhage as a consequence of thalamic hemorrhagic infarction have a less favorable outlook than those who do not have thalamic involvement.[a] In the large series of infants with thalamic hemorrhagic lesions with intraventricular hemorrhage ($n = 12$) reported by Roland and co-workers,[125,126] 83% had cerebral palsy (usually hemiparesis), whereas only 29% of the term infants with intraventricular hemorrhage without thalamic involvement had cerebral palsy.

[a]References 111, 114, 125, 126, 134, 135.

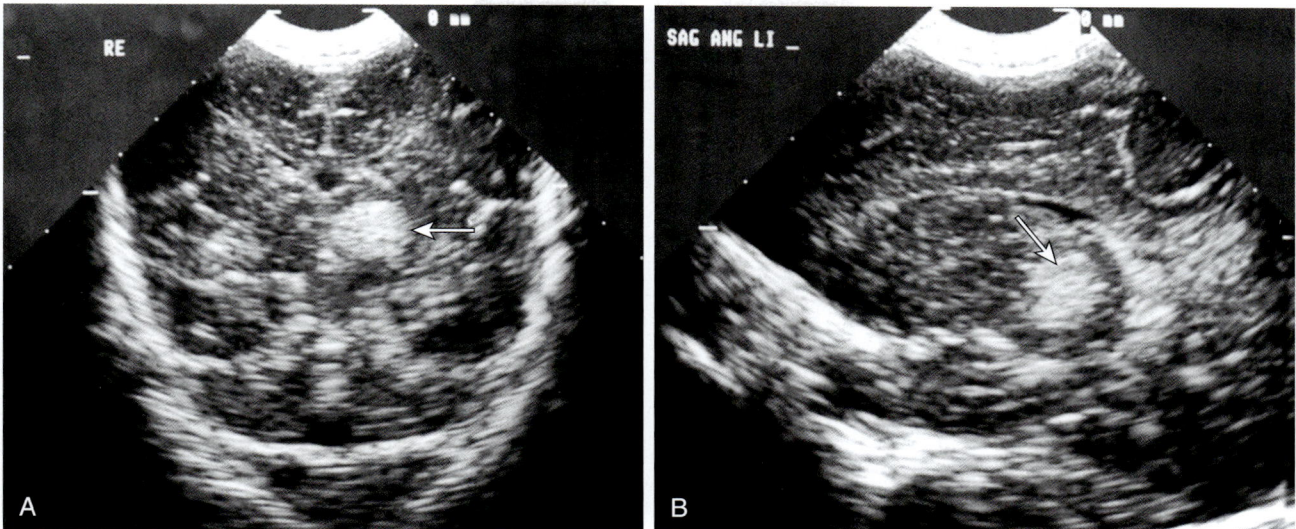

Figure 22.13 Ultrasound scan of unilateral thalamic *hemorrhage.* (A) Coronal and (B) sagittal scans obtained on day 3 in an infant weighing 2120 g with persistent fetal circulation. Note the circular area of echodensity in the region of the thalamus *(arrow in each).* (From de Vries LS, Smet M, Goemans N, Wilms G, et al. Unilateral thalamic haemorrhage in the pre-term and full-term newborn. *Neuropediatrics.* 1992;23:153–156.)

Management

Management of intraventricular hemorrhage for term infants is similar to that described in detail in Chapter 24 for premature infants. In addition, the timing and choices of intervention for any posthemorrhagic hydrocephalus that develops are also similar.

MISCELLANEOUS EXAMPLES OF NEONATAL INTRACRANIAL HEMORRHAGE

The major unusual and miscellaneous examples of intracranial hemorrhage are associated with trauma, hemorrhagic infarction, coagulation disturbance, vascular defect, cerebral tumor, and unknown factors (Table 22.14). These examples are reviewed briefly in the following subsections.

Trauma

Although trauma usually results in subdural hemorrhage or primary subarachnoid hemorrhage (see previous sections), epidural, intraventricular, or intracerebral hemorrhage may also be observed. Epidural hemorrhage is discussed in Chapter 36. Intraventricular hemorrhage of the traumatic variety is discussed in earlier sections. Traumatic intracerebral hemorrhage is rare, but when it occurs it is almost always an accompaniment of major extracerebral hemorrhage.[136] Trauma severe enough to produce major hemorrhage most often results in injury to scalp and skull (see Chapter 36). The precise site and extent of intracranial involvement are best determined by MRI or CT.

Hemorrhagic Infarction

Hemorrhagic infarction results when the injured although functional capillaries in an ischemic infarct are ruptured by release of an arterial obstruction (e.g., embolus), by an increase in venous pressure, or when small amounts of bleeding from injured capillaries are not controlled by an intact clotting

TABLE 22.14	Miscellaneous Examples of Neonatal Intracranial Hemorrhage

Trauma
Epidural hemorrhage
Intracerebral hemorrhage
Hemorrhagic infarction
Embolus
Venous thrombosis
Arterial thrombosis
Coagulation disturbance
Thrombocytopenia
Deficiency of coagulation factors
Vascular defect
Aneurysm
Arteriovenous malformation
Coarctation of the aorta
Cerebral tumor
Unknown cause
Extracorporeal membrane oxygenation

system. Thus hemorrhagic infarction is observed in the newborn primarily with (1) embolic arterial occlusion because of distal movement of the embolus, (2) venous thrombosis because of the increase in venous pressure proximally, and (3) arterial thrombosis (or perhaps vasospasm) that is partial (or intermittent) or accompanied by a disturbance of coagulation (see Table 22.14). The specific causes, incidence, diagnosis, and outcomes are discussed in Chapter 21 under Stroke of the Newborn.

Unilateral thalamic hemorrhagic lesions may represent a specific variety of hemorrhagic infarction.[135,137,138] This type of lesion has been observed in both premature and term infants, particularly after perinatal asphyxia, persistent fetal circulation with hypotension, and sinovenous thrombosis. Identification is

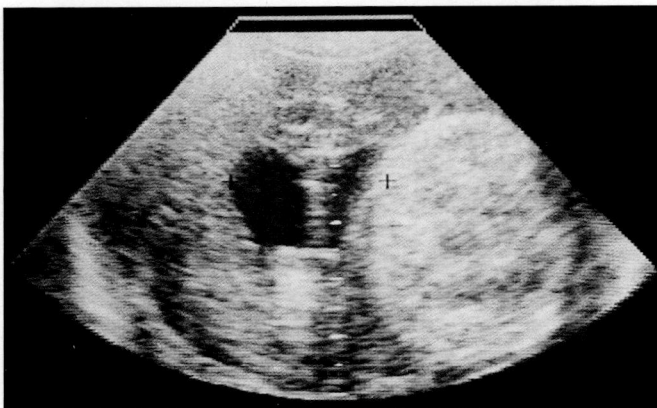

Figure 22.14 Ultrasound scan of hemorrhage into basal ganglia from an infant with congenital fibrinogen deficiency. Note the large circular echodense lesion in the region of the left putamen. (Courtesy Dr. Gary Shackelford.)

readily made by cranial ultrasonography, CT, and MRI (see Figs. 22.12 and 22.13). The relationship of this unilateral hemorrhagic lesion with the bilateral hemorrhagic necrosis observed in thalamus and basal ganglia of asphyxiated term infants (see Chapter 20) and with the syndrome of intraventricular hemorrhage with apparent thalamic hemorrhagic infarction[126,134] is not clear. The outcomes vary, related in part to the extent of the lesion, presence of other cerebral lesions, and involvement of the posterior limb of the internal capsule. In general the outcomes have been more favorable in infants with unilateral thalamic *hemorrhage*, unlike the unfavorable outcome in the thalamic hemorrhagic lesion associated with intraventricular hemorrhage.

Coagulation Defect

The most common coagulation disturbances *primarily* responsible for neonatal intracranial hemorrhage are thrombocytopenia and defects of a coagulation factor or factors (see Table 22.14 and Fig. 22.14).

Thrombocytopenia

Thrombocytopenia of a severe degree may lead to neonatal intracranial hemorrhage. However, the major causes of neonatal thrombocytopenia (i.e., immune disorders, congenital and neonatal infections, maternal drugs, organic acidopathies, and congenital bone marrow hypoplasias) often dominate the clinical picture through extraneural manifestations, including bleeding at various sites. Indeed, except for isoimmune thrombocytopenia, thrombocytopenia is only very uncommonly associated with serious neonatal intracranial hemorrhage.[138,139]

Neonatal Isoimmune Thrombocytopenia. *Neonatal isoimmune thrombocytopenia* is an unusual but important cause of intrauterine hemorrhagic lesions.[a] This fetal hematological disorder occurs in 0.2 per 1000 live births and is related to passive transfer from mother to fetus of antibodies against a fetal platelet antigen inherited from the father and absent in the mother. In approximately 85% of all cases in white infants,

the antigen is the so-called HPA-1a antigen (human platelet antigen 1a). In Japanese infants, the antigen usually is HPA-4a.[147] Other platelet antigens, implicated in the minority of cases, are HPA-3a and HPA-5b.[146,149] Major intrauterine intracranial lesions have been described as a consequence of neonatal isoimmune thrombocytopenia.[a] Although the lesions are usually characterized as *intracerebral hemorrhage*, their frequent location in an apparent vascular distribution, evolution to porencephalic cyst, and reported association with vascular thrombi suggest that at least some are fundamentally ischemic, perhaps with hemorrhage as a secondary event (see also Chapters 20 and 21). Moreover, the finding that antibodies to HPA-1a also react with an endothelial cell surface antigen further supports the notion of an ischemic basis for at least a portion of the intrauterine cystic lesions. Optic nerve atrophy or hypoplasia is a common accompaniment of the severe porencephalic lesions.[144,145] Prevention of the intrauterine lesions is difficult because of their frequently early intrauterine occurrence (possible in the second trimester, although usually in the third trimester). Because the risk of recurrence of intracranial hemorrhage in subsequent pregnancies is 80% to 90%, fetal management is critical.

Current management is somewhat controversial. Fetal genotyping by amniocentesis coupled with genotyping of the father will indicate whether the fetus contains the offending antigen and thus is at risk. If the previous affected pregnancy involved fetal intracranial hemorrhage, intravenous immunoglobulin G is administered weekly, beginning in the second trimester, preferably several weeks before the occurrence of hemorrhage in the previous pregnancy.[146,151-153] This approach leads to elevations of the fetal platelet count and a sharp reduction in the risk of fetal intracranial hemorrhage.[153,154] This has been redefined to include a management algorithm based on risk stratification.[153] Intracranial hemorrhage with isoimmune thrombocytopenia may also occur in apparent relation to labor and delivery and consist of subdural hemorrhage, subarachnoid hemorrhage, and intracerebral hemorrhage, often in combination. Management postnatally consists of transfusion of compatible antigen-negative platelets and administration of intravenous immunoglobulin.[146,155-157]

Deficiency of Coagulation Factors

Deficits of coagulation factors may also result in neonatal intracranial hemorrhage (see Table 22.14). The deficits may occur secondary to a congenital deficiency (e.g., hemophilia A), severe liver disease, disseminated intravascular coagulation, or vitamin K deficiency. Except for the first of these examples, evidence of extraneural bleeding is almost always present. Moreover, with severe liver disease, the clinical picture is usually dominated by systemic disturbances related to hepatic failure. Disseminated intravascular coagulation can lead to all varieties of intracranial hemorrhage and to extramedullary hematoma of the spinal cord as well.[158] Congenital deficiency of coagulation factors, especially hemophilia, and vitamin K deficiency are briefly reviewed next.

Congenital Deficiency of Coagulation Factors. The most common congenital deficiency of a coagulation factor that

---

[a]References 1, 89, 128, 137, 140-150.

[a]References 1, 89, 128, 140-146, 148-150.

results in neonatal intracranial hemorrhage is hemophilia. Thus, deficiencies of factor VIII (hemophilia A) or of factor IX (hemophilia B) have been associated with neonatal intracranial hemorrhage.[84,159-163] In a recent systematic review, newborns with hemophilia, compared with the general population, were found to be 44 times (95% CI: 34.7 to 57.1, P <.01) more likely to experience a symptomatic intracranial hemorrhage and 8 times (95% CI: 5.38 to 12.6, P <.01) more likely to experience extracranial hemorrhage at birth.[163] In newborns with hemophilia, the odds ratio of experiencing intracranial hemorrhage, was 4.4 (95% CI: 1.46 to 13.7, P = .008) following an assisted vaginal delivery and 0.34 (95% CI: 0.14 to 0.83, P = .018), or less likely, following cesarean section compared with vaginal delivery.[163] The lesions described have been predominantly subdural, although intracerebral, cerebellar, and epidural hemorrhages have been observed, often also in association with subdural hemorrhage. Neurological sequelae have occurred in the majority of patients. It is crucial to consider such a coagulation disturbance in unexplained neonatal intracranial hemorrhage, especially subdural hemorrhage in a term infant, so as to institute appropriate replacement therapy promptly.

Other coagulation defects rarely associated with neonatal intracranial hemorrhage include acquired deficiency of factor VIII (secondary transplacental transfer of an inhibitory antibody),[164] congenital factor X deficiency,[165-167] and congenital fibrinogen deficiency (see Fig. 22.14). Fatal intracerebral hemorrhage secondary to bleeding from a hemorrhagic infarct caused by venous thrombosis in the setting of a defect in the antithrombin gene is a rare example of lethal hemorrhage resulting from a defect in a procoagulant factor.[168]

Vitamin K Deficiency. Three neonatal syndromes of vitamin K deficiency are recognized: early hemorrhagic disease, with onset in the first 24 hours; classic hemorrhagic disease, with onset between 1 and 7 days; and late hemorrhagic disease, with onset usually in the second month of life. *Early hemorrhagic disease* may be accompanied by intracranial as well as systemic hemorrhage and is usually associated with maternal anticonvulsant therapy, which increases degradation of vitamin K. *Classic hemorrhagic disease* is characterized by systemic and, only rarely, intracranial bleeding and is associated with lack of neonatal administration of vitamin K and unknown additional factors.[169]

Late hemorrhagic disease, the major subject of this section, is characterized *particularly by intracranial bleeding*, and the principal cause for the vitamin K deficiency appears to be a combination of low vitamin K content of breast milk (lower than cow's milk and conventional formula) and lack of administration of vitamin K at birth (to augment the *physiologically* lower levels of vitamin K that occur in the newborn).[65,169-182] More recently, refusal or omission of vitamin K prophylaxis has been increasing and places newborn infants at risk for life-threatening bleeding. Over an 8-month period, seven infants were encountered with confirmed vitamin K deficiency and five developed vitamin K–deficiency bleeding. The mean age of the seven infants was 10.3 weeks (range, 7 to 20 weeks). None of the infants had received vitamin K at birth, and all were found to have profoundly deranged coagulation parameters, which corrected rapidly with administration of vitamin K in intravenous or intramuscular form. Of the seven infants, four had intracranial

hemorrhage; two of these infants required urgent neurosurgical intervention.[183] A commentary accompanying this report from Tennessee by Volpe[184] identified that the reasons for parental decline of vitamin K included concern about an increased risk of leukemia related to vitamin K administration (a notion not supported by the most recent findings),[185] an impression that the injection was unnecessary, and a desire to avoid exposure of the infant to vaccines containing *toxins*.[186] Analogous data are available from Great Britain, Ireland, and Israel.[187,188] The Israeli study was particularly notable: although 63% of expecting parents held academic degrees, 60% to 70% did not know that providing vitamin K to a newborn can prevent serious bleeding and 68% had not yet decided whether they intended to provide their newborn with vitamin K.[188] Volpe concluded that the need for repeated parental education of the purpose, value, and safety of vitamin K administration, preferably by the intramuscular route as recommended by the American Academy of Pediatrics, was critical. Finally, a further report from New Zealand noted similar findings, with four cases of late intracranial hemorrhage noted in infants who had not received vitamin K prophylaxis at birth.[189] The effect on the clotting system is the failure of vitamin K to carboxylate and thereby render functional the clotting factors II (prothrombin), VII, IX, and X, with a resulting prolongation of both the prothrombin time and the partial thromboplastin time.[190] The disorder is more common in Asia but has been observed in the United States, Great Britain, and many other countries.[65,69,172-183,189-191]

The onset is usually not apparent for several weeks, although easy bruising is frequently recorded in the first weeks. In one series, the median age of onset of intracranial hemorrhage was 56 days.[65,69] The major presenting features are seizures, depressed level of consciousness, and signs of increased intracranial pressure (e.g., tense fontanelle, vomiting). The varieties of hemorrhage have included primarily intracerebral hemorrhage and accompanying subarachnoid hemorrhage, although subdural and intraventricular hemorrhages have also been reported in a substantial minority.[65,69,191] The diagnosis of the site and extent of hemorrhage is readily made by MRI or CT (Fig. 22.15). Most affected infants with major intracranial hemorrhage involving cerebral parenchyma and not solely the subarachnoid space have been left with serious neurological deficits. Only 10% to 30% of infants with late hemorrhagic disease and intracranial hemorrhage have been normal on follow-up. The clotting defects are correctable in a matter of hours by vitamin K administration, and the disorder is preventable by prophylactic administration of vitamin K at birth, either intramuscular or oral.[a] Using a sensitive assay of vitamin K deficiency (i.e., detection of protein induced by vitamin K absence [PIVKA-II]), Hathaway and co-workers showed, in a study in Thailand, that a single oral dose at birth reduced the incidence of vitamin K deficiency at 1 month in breast-fed infants to 18% compared with 60% in untreated infants; the incidence was reduced to 6% in infants who were given vitamin K intramuscularly.[177]

Vascular Defect

The two major intracranial vascular defects that may cause neonatal intracranial hemorrhage are congenital arterial

---

[a]References 65, 69, 176, 177, 179-183, 189.

TABLE 22.15   Aneurysms With Presentation in the First 3 Months of Life[a]

Clinical presentation
Subarachnoid hemorrhage, massive, with full or bulging anterior fontanelle and catastrophic neurological deterioration
Seizures, usually focal
Focal neurological signs, nature depending on location of aneurysm or associated intracerebral hematoma
Diagnosis
Computed tomography demonstrates large subarachnoid hemorrhage, intraparenchymal hematoma, or both
Magnetic resonance imaging may demonstrate the aneurysm
Cerebral angiography, computed tomography angiography, or magnetic resonance angiography needed to demonstrate exact site of lesion in vasculature
Outcome
Rapid diagnosis and surgical therapy associated with good outcome

[a]See text for references.

TABLE 22.16   Arteriovenous Malformations (Not Involving Vein of Galen) With Presentation in the First 3 Months of Life[a]

Location
Cerebral hemisphere
Thalamus–third ventricle
Choroid plexus
Posterior fossa
Spinal cord
Common presentations
- Intracranial hemorrhage (with signs of increased intracranial pressure):
- Intracerebral hemorrhage ± IVH
- IVH alone
- Posterior fossa hemorrhage
- Seizures, often focal
- Congestive heart failure with cranial bruit
- Hydrocephalus
- Opisthotonos, brain-stem signs (especially posterior fossa lesions)
- Paraplegia (spinal cord lesions)

IVH, Intraventricular hemorrhage.
[a]See text for references.

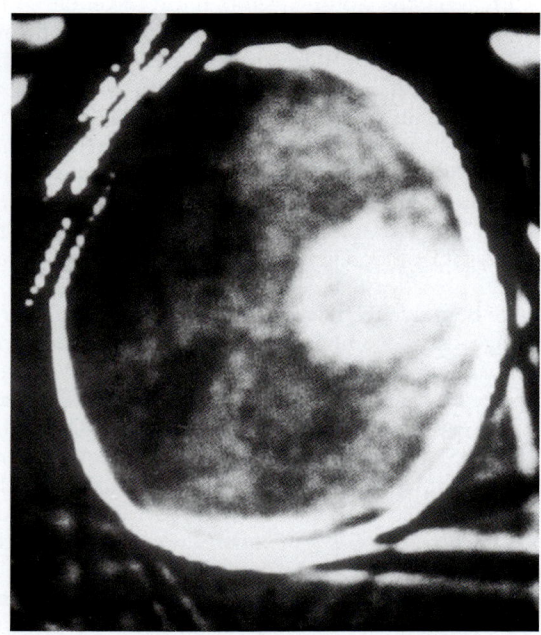

Figure 22.15 Computed tomography scan of intracerebral hemorrhage secondary to vitamin K deficiency. Note the large hematoma in the left cerebral hemisphere.

aneurysm and arteriovenous malformation (see Table 22.16). The former is more likely to result in presentation with intracranial hemorrhage than the latter, although both are rare occurrences. A systemic vascular lesion, coarctation of the aorta, is also associated with neonatal intracranial hemorrhage.

Aneurysm

Congenital arterial aneurysm with rupture has been recorded in more than 20 infants in the first 3 months of life (Table 22.15).[192-214] The onset of the neurological deterioration is generally abrupt and occurs as early as the first days of life.

The *clinical presentation* is dominated by acute major subarachnoid hemorrhage with signs of increased intracranial pressure (full or bulging anterior fontanelle) and rapid neurological deterioration (Table 22.16). Seizures, often focal, also occur in approximately half of the cases. Focal neurological signs are present in a similar proportion; their nature relates to the site of the aneurysm (e.g., hemiparesis with middle cerebral artery aneurysm and brain-stem signs with aneurysms of the vertebrobasilar circulation). *Sites of the lesions* have consisted of the middle cerebral artery (11 cases), anterior cerebral artery (5 cases), internal carotid artery near its bifurcation into anterior and middle cerebral arteries (2 cases), circle of Willis near the junction of the posterior communicating and posterior cerebral arteries (2 cases), and vertebrobasilar circulation (5 cases). The lesions are usually large. The *anatomical defect* involves the internal elastic lamina and muscularis, which are thinned, fragmented, or absent. The *diagnosis* usually made with neuroimaging, notably by MRI or CT, which shows subarachnoid hemorrhage, parenchymal hemorrhage, or both. MRI may demonstrate the aneurysm (Fig. 22.16). Cerebral angiography is usually required to define the anatomical features of the vascular lesion, especially concerning the presence of features (e.g., neck) important for surgical intervention. MR angiography or CT angiography may provide similar information in a less invasive manner. The *outcome* relates in considerable part to the size and location of the lesion. Surgical clipping and cure are often possible except for so-called *giant aneurysms* or lesions located in vessels that are inaccessible or that cannot be clipped, as with basilar aneurysms. In one report, coil embolization was effective.[210-214]

Arteriovenous Malformation

Arteriovenous malformation is a rare cause of neonatal intracranial hemorrhage but an important one to recognize

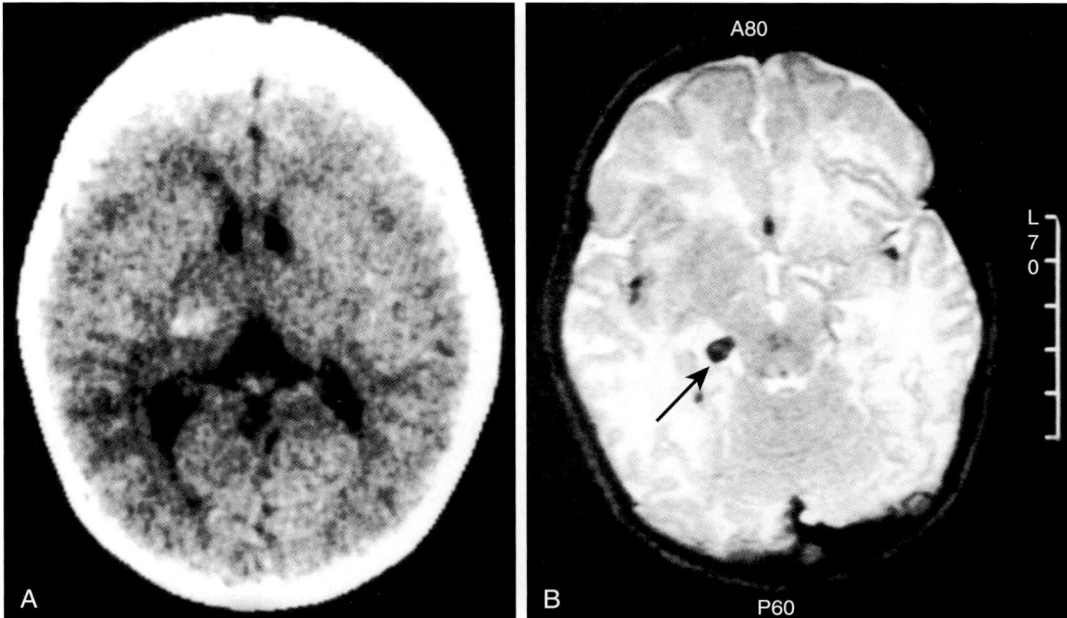

Figure 22.16 Congenital aneurysm in a 7-week-old infant with a 2-week history of left focal seizures. (A) Computed tomography (CT) shows only a small hemorrhagic lesion in the right posterior thalamus. (B) Magnetic resonance imaging obtained shortly after the CT scan demonstrates flow void in the perimesencephalic cistern *(arrow)*, consistent with an aneurysm (later proven by cerebral angiography). (From Putty TK, Luerssen TG, Campbell RL, Boaz JC, et al. Magnetic resonance imaging diagnosis of a cerebral aneurysm in an infant: case report and review of the literature. *Pediatr Neurosurg.* 1990–1991;16:48–51.)

and treat appropriately.[133,215-233] Of all neonatal arteriovenous malformations, those that involve the vein of Galen are most common. However, vein of Galen malformations rarely manifest clinically as intracranial hemorrhage and are discussed with brain tumors in Chapter 37. Arteriovenous malformations not involving the vein of Galen but manifesting clinically in the first 3 months of life, the subject of this section, commonly herald their presence by *intracranial hemorrhage* (see Table 22.16). (Notably, however, approximately half of such cases presenting in the neonatal period are found to have cardiac manifestations, especially congestive heart failure.) Most commonly, the intracranial hemorrhage is intracerebral, intraventricular, or both. This propensity to produce hemorrhage at these loci relates to the most common sites for the vascular malformations (i.e., cerebral hemispheres, thalamus–third ventricle, and choroid plexus, which together account for 70% of all reported lesions; see Table 22.16). *Other clinical presentations*, sometimes occurring with hemorrhage, include seizures, congestive heart failure (secondary to high cardiac output), hydrocephalus (secondary to increased venous pressure or obstruction of CSF pathways), opisthotonos with other brain-stem signs (posterior fossa lesions), or paraplegia, either congenital or of abrupt onset in the neonatal period (spinal cord lesions). The *diagnosis* is suspected by the occurrence of unexplained intracranial hemorrhage or one or more of the other clinical features noted in Table 22.16. Color Doppler ultrasonography is an effective means of assessing the site of the lesion.[223,231]

Angiography (conventional, MR, or both) is required to identify the anatomical details of the malformation and its vascular feeders. Treatment consists of surgical extirpation and has been curative except with very large lesions or those in

loci that preclude surgical attack. Embolic therapy, as in the management of vein of Galen malformations (see Chapter 37), is an alternative therapeutic modality.

Coarctation of the Aorta

A major *systemic* vascular defect, coarctation of the aorta, has been associated rarely with the occurrence of intracranial hemorrhage in the newborn.[216,234-236] The hemorrhages documented in the 6 patients included subarachnoid, intraventricular, and intracerebral lesions.[216,235,236] The cause of the hemorrhage in newborns was thought to be systemic hypertension, which, in four of the five infants reported, was only moderate (90 to 110 mm Hg systolic).[216] Cerebral hemorrhage complicates coarctation of the aorta in older patients in as many as 10% of cases and has been attributed in some cases not only to brachiocephalic hypertension but also to frequently associated cerebral aneurysms. In neonatal patients, no cerebral aneurysms have been found on angiography or on postmortem examination, but small aneurysms cannot be excluded. The important points are that infants with coarctation of the aorta must be considered at risk for the occurrence of serious intracranial hemorrhage and that systemic hypertension perhaps need not be dramatic to provoke this complication. Perhaps related to this association is the demonstration of multiple cerebral arteriovenous malformations (although without hemorrhage) in an infant with coarctation of the aorta.[217,227]

Cerebral Tumor

Hemorrhage associated with brain tumor has been observed in the newborn period. More commonly, the clinical presentation is that of signs of increased intracranial pressure, hydrocephalus, macrocephaly, and focal neurological signs (see Chapter 37).

Unknown Cause

Infants, almost exclusively full term, occasionally exhibit focal parenchymal hemorrhage, usually into cerebral white matter but also into thalamus, basal ganglia, brain stem, or spinal cord without definable cause.[a] The cerebral lesions become manifest most often on the first day or so of life with seizures, frequently focal. Motor deficits are common and are generally predictable by the topography of the lesion. Cerebral lesions may be accompanied by hemiparesis. An infant with a medullary hemorrhage exhibited bilateral diaphragmatic paralysis, impaired sucking and swallowing, and tongue fasciculations.[239] Another infant with a spinal cord hemorrhage exhibited an abrupt onset of quadriplegia.[240] Subsequent motor deficits may occur, but full recovery is not unusual. Hydrocephalus has appeared secondary to extension of parenchymal hemorrhage to the lateral ventricles or subarachnoid space. One potential cause for this group of lesions is an arteriovenous malformation that is too small to be detected by conventional imaging techniques or is obliterated by the hemorrhage. Some may represent hemorrhagic infarctions not clearly demonstrated by ultrasonography, CT, or MRI.

Extracorporeal Membrane Oxygenation

ECMO is a technique of cardiopulmonary bypass used for term and near-term infants with pulmonary failure that is potentially reversible but has not been responsive to trials of conventional or high-frequency ventilation or inhaled nitric oxide. Infants subjected to ECMO have exhibited a variety of intracranial hemorrhagic and ischemic phenomena. The hemorrhagic phenomena are discussed in this context.

Patient Selection and Technique

Infants chosen for ECMO therapy have had intractable respiratory failure secondary to a variety of disorders that have in common a high intrinsic mortality rate (>50%) and a potential for reversibility, either spontaneously or by surgery. The disease states that have led to ECMO therapy in major series have been, in general order of frequency, meconium aspiration syndrome, congenital diaphragmatic hernia, persistent pulmonary hypertension, sepsis, and respiratory distress syndrome.[242-262] The short-term benefit of ECMO is apparent from data collected from 200 centers in North America and elsewhere on more than 3500 newborns; these data show an overall survival rate of 83% in infants with a predicted mortality rate in excess of 80%.[245] These findings are supported by a single-center experience spanning 37 years (1973–2010), where the overall survival to hospital discharge was 84%.[262] The success in recent years of other modalities (e.g., high-frequency oscillatory ventilation, inhaled nitric oxide) has changed the composition of populations treated with ECMO to a somewhat more severe spectrum of disease.

ECMO is carried out by the venoarterial or venovenous technique. The largest reported experience is with the former. In venoarterial ECMO, the right internal jugular vein is cannulated, the catheter is passed into the right atrium, the cranial opening

[a]References 1, 64, 89, 90, 110, 111, 114, 118-121, 128, 141, 148, 216, 235, 237-243.

TABLE 22.17	Hemorrhagic Lesions in Infants Treated With Extracorporeal Membrane Oxygenation
LOCATION	**NO. OF INFANTS**
Cerebral	—
Frontal	12
Parietal	3
Temporal	4
Occipital	6
Periventricular white matter	4
Germinal matrix	17
Intraventricular	6
Basal ganglia	2
Posterior fossa	—
Cerebellar	9
Mesencephalon	1
Subarachnoid	4
Total	68

Data from Taylor GA, Fitz CR, Kapur S, Short BL. Cerebrovascular accidents in neonates treated with extracorporeal membrane oxygenation: sonographic-pathologic correlation. *AJR Am J Roentgenol.* 1989;153:355–361.

of the jugular vein is permanently ligated, and venous blood from the atrium is drained to the extracorporeal membrane oxygenator. After the addition of oxygen and removal of carbon dioxide by the membrane oxygenator, the blood is warmed and pumped by nonpulsatile flow to the infant through a catheter placed in the right common carotid artery and is directed into the right aortic arch. As with the jugular vein, the cranial opening of the common carotid artery is ligated. (In recent years, reconstruction of the right common carotid artery following termination of ECMO has commonly been carried out.) Anticoagulation therapy with heparin is administered systemically for the duration of the bypass procedure to prevent clotting in the ECMO circuit. With venovenous ECMO, the right common carotid artery is not cannulated and blood is returned to the central venous circulation. A recent single-center report suggests that this approach is associated with fewer neurological complications, including intracranial hemorrhage.[263]

Intracranial Hemorrhage

Intracranial hemorrhage and ischemic lesions of brain have been documented in infants treated with ECMO.[a] In most series, with findings based on brain imaging studies, 20% to 50% of such infants exhibit intracranial abnormalities. Approximately 40% of these abnormalities (i.e., those in 10% to 20% of infants) are of major severity. Approximately 40% of the intracranial abnormalities are purely hemorrhagic lesions, approximately 20% are hemorrhagic complicating apparent ischemic lesions, and approximately 40% are nonhemorrhagic ischemic lesions. Ischemic lesions consist primarily of periventricular leukomalacia, cerebral infarction (hemorrhagic in ≈50% of cases), and selective neuronal necrosis.

Hemorrhagic lesions observed in infants treated with ECMO are varied (see Table 22.17). In one large series ($n = 68$),

[a]References 134, 242, 244, 246, 248, 250, 251, 255, 256, 259, 263-277.

although 34% of lesions were relatively minor germinal matrix or intraventricular hemorrhages, particularly the former, 37% were cerebral parenchymal hemorrhages. Of the cerebral hemorrhages, 40% or more have been observed in unusual locations (i.e., beyond the confines of the anterior circulation and in the temporal or occipital lobes).[246,268] In addition, 15% of the hemorrhages, usually serious, have been in the posterior fossa, primarily involving cerebellum (see Table 22.17).[244,250,261] In a recent report from the Netherlands spanning 21 years, involving a total of 677 infants, and using cranial ultrasound imaging, brain injury was identified in 17.3%, with primary hemorrhage (8%) the most frequent. Stroke was identified in 5% of cases and was notably left-sided, as was lobar hematoma noted in 2%.[261] The *laterality* of hemorrhagic and ischemic lesions in infants treated with ECMO has been the subject of controversy. In one study, major hemorrhagic cerebral lesions occurred predominantly on the left (seven of nine cases), whereas major ischemic cerebral lesions occurred predominantly on the right (five of six cases).[246] Other reports have not described the left-sided preponderance of hemorrhagic cerebral lesions.[244,250,261,268,276]

The right hemispheric predominance of ischemic lesions has been observed by others.[250,261,275] For example, in a separate study, 8 of 36 infants exhibited evidence of ischemic lesions, with 5 of the 8 in the right hemisphere, 1 in the left, and 2 bilateral.[250,261] Moreover, although some reports described a nearly equal distribution of ischemic lesions, the distributions did *not* conform to the left hemispheric predominance characteristic of strokes of other causes in newborns (see Chapter 21). Thus, on balance, the data suggest that focal cerebral infarcts in infants treated with ECMO preferentially affect the right hemisphere.

The hemorrhagic lesions in infants treated with ECMO are identified most readily by ultrasonography during ECMO and by MRI when the infant is not receiving ECMO. Because some of the hemorrhages may be slow to clot as a result of systemic heparinization, some variability in echogenicity on ultrasound scan or in attenuation on CT may be observed, especially acutely (Fig. 22.17). For similar reasons, blood-fluid levels and rapidly expanding hematomas may be observed in affected infants.

Mechanisms of Hemorrhagic and Ischemic Brain Injury With Extracorporeal Membrane Oxygenation

The mechanisms underlying hemorrhagic and ischemic brain injury in infants subjected to ECMO are undoubtedly multifactorial. Before discussing the likely mechanisms, we briefly review the cerebral hemodynamic effects as defined primarily by Doppler ultrasonic studies of cerebral blood flow velocity.

Cerebral Hemodynamics in Infants Treated With Extracorporeal Membrane Oxygenation. The *cerebral hemodynamic effects* of ligation of the common carotid artery and jugular vein in infants subjected to ECMO have been evaluated by Doppler ultrasonic measurements of cerebral blood flow velocity and by near-infrared spectroscopy.[260,275,276,278-286] The principal findings shortly after common carotid ligation are (1) an abrupt initial 50% decrease in systolic flow velocity in the right middle cerebral artery at the time of ligation with a return to 70% of baseline within 5 minutes and (2) a corresponding decline in resistance index and an increase in diastolic flow velocity.

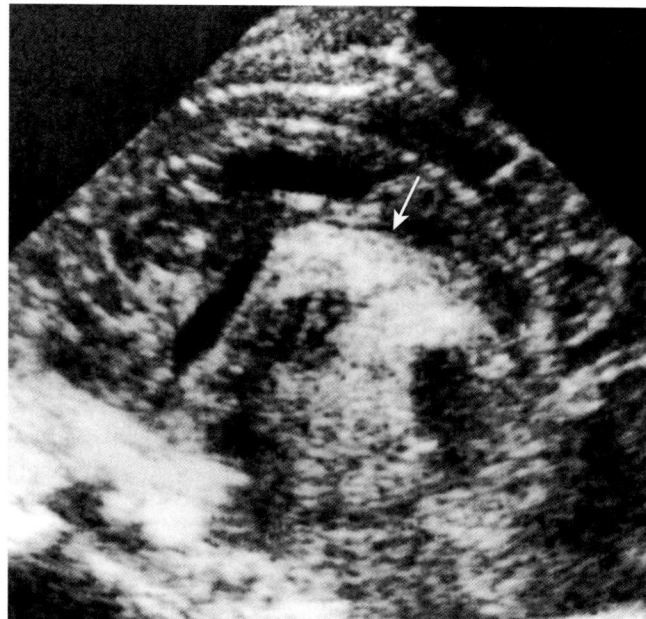

Figure 22.17 **Ultrasound scan of intracranial hemorrhage in association with extracorporeal membrane oxygenation (ECMO).** Sagittal scan from an infant of 35 weeks' gestation with a congenital diaphragmatic hernia, treated with ECMO; the ultrasound scan was normal before ECMO. The scan shows a large posterior fossa hemorrhage with characteristically heterogeneous echogenicity. Blood is also present in the third ventricle *(arrow).* Hemorrhage in the cerebellar parenchyma and in the subarachnoid space cannot readily be distinguished. (From Taylor GA, Fitz CR, Kapur S, Short BL. Cerebrovascular accidents in neonates treated with extracorporeal membrane oxygenation: sonographic-pathologic correlation. *AJR Am J Roentgenol.* 1989;153:355–361.)

Taken together, these data suggest that an initial important hemodynamic effect of ECMO is a decline in right cerebral perfusion followed by vasodilation with a compensatory increase in perfusion. However, measurements of volemic blood flow are not available, and the difficulties of drawing conclusions concerning volemic flow based solely on measurements of blood flow velocity are described in Chapter 10. Nevertheless, the possibility of ischemic injury to the right hemisphere acutely must be considered. However, an acute decline in perfusion to *both* cerebral hemispheres is supported by the findings with near-infrared spectroscopy of an acute decline in oxyhemoglobin concentration and a corresponding increase in deoxyhemoglobin concentration.[260] A decline in perfusion to the left as well as the right hemisphere may reflect an inability of the left internal carotid to supply *both* hemispheres acutely. Despite the decrease in flow velocity and oxyhemoglobin concentrations, prompt relative compensation for the common carotid ligation by collateral vessels occurs. Collateral circulation to the right cerebral hemisphere has been shown in the Doppler studies to emanate from (1) the left anterior circulation (i.e., from the anterior communicating artery), (2) the left posterior circulation (i.e., from the posterior communicating artery through the circle of Willis), and (3) from the right external carotid artery to the right internal carotid artery. The action of the collaterals emanating from the left anterior circulation may account for the approximately 50% increase in mean flow velocity in the left internal carotid artery during ECMO and the increase in oxyhemoglobin and decline in deoxyhemoglobin within 60 minutes of onset of ECMO.[260,284]

A second notable hemodynamic effect of ECMO involves the posterior circulation. Thus, *in addition to* potential compromise of the arterial supply to the right anterior circulation, a disturbance of arterial supply to the *posterior circulation* is suggested by Doppler studies. In one study of 40 infants during ECMO, retrograde flow in the right vertebral artery, consistent with vertebral steal, was observed in 30%.[284,285] The demonstrations of impaired brachial flow velocity after cannulation and both improvement of brachial flow velocity and reinstitution of anterograde vertebral flow after removal of the arterial cannula suggested that the vertebral artery flow abnormality was related to partial obstruction of the origin of the right subclavian artery by the cannula (from the common carotid artery) in the innominate artery.[284,285] Whether ischemia in the distribution of the posterior circulation may occur consequent to vertebral steal remains unclear (see later discussion).

A third notable hemodynamic effect of ECMO relates to the effects of ligation of the jugular vein. In a study of 23 consecutive infants subjected to ECMO, Taylor and Walker demonstrated reduction in blood flow velocity in the superior sagittal sinus in 10 (43%).[287] In 9 of these 10 infants, the disturbance in venous flow persisted for over 48 hours and, notably, was followed by the appearance of a variety of hemorrhagic or ischemic lesions. These observations raise the possibility that jugular venous occlusion may be an important pathogenetic factor for the occurrence of brain injury with ECMO (see later discussion). This finding may be relevant to the frequent occurrence of venous thrombosis in infants on ECMO.[277,287]

Studies of cerebral blood flow by positron emission tomography and of cerebral vessels by MR angiography suggest that in the weeks *following* ECMO, no major hemodynamic effects are apparent.[288,289] Moreover, the symmetry of cerebral blood flow shown by positron emission tomography was present, whether or not the previously ligated common carotid artery was reanastomosed.[289]

Pathogenesis of Intracranial Hemorrhage With Extracorporeal Membrane Oxygenation. The pathogenesis of intracranial hemorrhage with ECMO may relate to one or more of four major factors (Table 22.18). Infants subjected to ECMO may have intractable pulmonary failure, commonly complicated by

cardiac insufficiency and hypotension. In one series of infants with persistent pulmonary hypertension, a common cause of the need for ECMO, approximately 50% of those not treated with ECMO sustained cerebral infarction.[290] Such infarcts, with their injured microvasculature, would have a high likelihood of becoming hemorrhagic on reperfusion with ECMO, especially when coupled with other factors that encourage hemorrhage. Venous infarction has been well documented in infants who received ECMO, and extension of hemorrhage into the lateral ventricles is an important cause of intraventricular hemorrhage in these infants.[134,277] The possibility that ischemia predisposes to the occurrence of intracranial hemorrhage with ECMO is also supported by the demonstration of elevated blood lactate levels before ECMO in infants who later developed intracranial hemorrhage relative to lactate levels in infants who did not develop hemorrhage.[291] Other factors of potential importance include heparinization and an abrupt increase in cerebral blood flow with the institution of ECMO. The increase in cerebral blood flow could be related to one or more of three factors. The first of these is the correction of the hypocarbia induced by the hyperventilation used as therapy before institution of ECMO. The hyperemic effect of correcting hypocarbia was clearly shown in an animal model.[292] The second factor is the restoration of the circulation by ECMO in infants who typically are hypotensive before onset of ECMO; the occurrence of impaired cerebrovascular autoregulation, shown in newborn lambs subjected to ECMO,[292,293] accentuates this factor. Third, cerebral blood flow may increase, particularly in the left hemisphere, as suggested by Doppler studies of the internal carotid artery (see earlier discussion), because the right hemisphere becomes perfused by collaterals (anterior and posterior communicating arteries) emanating from the left hemisphere. Left hemispheric hyperperfusion would be consistent with the suggestion from studies in human infants of left hemispheric predominance for hemorrhagic cerebral lesions in infants with ECMO (see earlier discussion).

Increased venous pressure, suggested by Doppler studies of venous blood flow velocity in the superior sagittal sinus,[287] may also contribute to the pathogenesis of intracranial hemorrhage (see Table 22.18). Moreover, the venous factor may be particularly important in the pathogenesis of the posterior fossa hemorrhages, which occur with unusually high frequency in infants treated with ECMO (see earlier discussion).

Outcome in Infants Treated With Extracorporeal Membrane Oxygenation. Conclusions concerning outcome in infants treated with ECMO are based on data obtained from a large number of informative studies.[241-243,247-250,252-259,294-309] Data are best evaluated as a function of the birth weight of the infants (Table 22.19). In general, premature infants do less well than heavier and more mature infants.[247,255,259] Thus overall mortality rates are markedly higher in smaller versus larger infants (see Table 22.19). In one large study of 1524 premature infants treated with ECMO, the mortality rate was 39%.[259] Of this cohort, the 185 infants with intracranial hemorrhage had a 57% mortality rate. Similarly, major neuroimaging abnormalities, particularly hemorrhagic, are twice as common in smaller infants. Indeed, major intracranial hemorrhage is a primary cause of the higher mortality in smaller infants.[247,255] Major developmental delay (developmental quotient <70) is present in 10% to 20% of all infants treated with ECMO, but again,

---

TABLE 22.18   Pathogenesis of Hemorrhagic Brain Lesions in Infants Treated With Extracorporeal Membrane Oxygenation

Prior infarction
Secondary hemorrhage during extracorporeal membrane oxygenation
Heparinization
Increase in cerebral blood flow
Increase in arterial carbon dioxide tension after hypocarbia
Increase in blood pressure with impaired cerebrovascular autoregulation
Collateral circulation: left greater than right hemisphere
Increased central venous pressure
Jugular vein ligation

TABLE 22.19   Outcome in Infants Treated With Extracorporeal Membrane Oxygenation[a]

OUTCOME	PERCENTAGE OF INFANTS		
	2000–2500 g	>2500 g	TOTAL
Mortality rate (%)	34	11	14
Neuroimaging abnormality (major) (%)	41	21	27
Major intracranial hemorrhage (%)	28	11	13
Developmental quotient <70 (%)	38	8	12

[a]n = 29 for infants with birth weight 2000–2500 g; n = 235 for infants with birth weight >2500 g.

Data from Revenis ME, Glass P, Short BL. Mortality and morbidity rates among lower birth weight infants (2000–2500 g) treated with extracorporeal membrane oxygenation. *J Pediatr.* 1992;121:452–458, and Ljsselstijn H, van Heljst AF. Long-term outcome of children treated with neonatal extracorporeal membrane oxygenation: increasing problems with increasing age. *Semin Perinatol.* 2014;38(2):114–21.

TABLE 22.20   New Overview of Long-Term Outcomes Following Neonatal ECMO

	INFANCY (<2 YEARS)	PRESCHOOL AGE (2–5 YEARS)	SCHOOL AGE (6–12 YEARS)	ADOLESCENCE (>12 YEARS)
Medical outcome				
Lung function	Airflow obstruction,[7,8] normal lung volume,[7,8] and hyperinflation in CDH[9]	—	Airflow obstruction,[10,11,13] air trapping[10,13]; problems mainly in CDH patients[13]	Airflow obstruction and air trapping[10]
Exercise capacity	—	Decreased[14]	Decreased[11,14] to normal[10]	Normal[10]
Growth	Normal[5,7] to slightly decreased weight[8] especially in CDH[9]	Normal[14]	Normal,[12,14] decreased height and weight in CDH[12]	—
SNHL	Prevalence ranging from 3% to 26%, in different studies over time[17-22,33]			
Chronic kidney disease	Abnormal urine protein/creatinine ratio or estimated glomerular filtration rate in 11%[31]			
(Neuro)developmental outcome				
Motor function	Normal in 84%[32]	Normal in 64%–73%[16,36]	Normal in 43%[39] and normal in 71% of CDH patients[36]	—
Cognition	Normal in 92%[32]	Normal average scores[15,33,38,45]	Normal in 68%[39] and normal average scores[43]	—
Neuropsychological tests	—	Decreased scores at verbal, reasoning, and spatial abilities,[22] and neuropsychological deficit at ≥1 domain in 11%[38]	Spatial ability scores below 10th percentile in 26%,[39] visual-motor integration below average in 20%,[43] memory problems in 26%–48%,[39] decreased working speed in 70%,[43] and decreased accuracy in 39%[43]	Memory problems in 46%–57%[36]
School performance	—	—	Special education 9%–20%[39,43]; extra support 20%–39%[39,43]	—
Behavior	—	Normal in 48.5%–65%,[45,47] more problems compared with controls in social, attention, and hyperactivity domains[38]	Clinical total problems 18%, social problems 5%, and attention problems 6%[43]	Self-reported externalizing problems 6%[36]

CDH, Congenital diaphragmatic hernia; *ECMO,* extracorporeal membrane oxygenation; *SNHL,* sensorineural hearing loss.

Data from Ljsselstijn H, van Heljst AF. Long-term outcome of children treated with neonatal extracorporeal membrane oxygenation: increasing problems with increasing age. *Semin Perinatol.* 2014;38(2):114–121.

the rate is considerably higher in smaller (38%) versus larger (8%) infants (see Table 22.19). Major neurological defects occur in approximately 10% to 20% of infants treated with ECMO (Table 22.20). Sensorineural hearing loss was observed in 12% and 15% of two well-studied series of infants,[301,305] but the rate was 4% in other series.[241,303] Not unexpectedly, adverse neurological and cognitive outcomes are approximately twice as common in infants who exhibit major hemorrhagic and

nonhemorrhagic neuroimaging abnormalities or seizures (or both) in the neonatal period than in infants who do not exhibit such evidence of parenchymal injury.[a] The number of infants followed to school age has been relatively small. Further data will be of major interest.

---

[a]References 242, 244, 248, 250, 254, 258, 276, 302, 308, 309.

KEY REFERENCES

1. Hanigan WC, Powell FC, Miller TC, et al. Symptomatic intracranial hemorrhage in full-term infants. *Childs Nerv Syst.* 1995;11:698-707.
2. Towner D, Castro MA, Eby-Wilkens E, et al. Effect of mode of delivery in nulliparous women on neonatal intracranial injury. *N Engl J Med.* 1999;341:1709-1714.
3. Rooks VJ, Eaton JP, Ruess L, et al. Prevalence and evolution of intracranial hemorrhage in asymptomatic term infants. *AJNR Am J Neuroradiol.* 2008;29:1082-1089.
4. Whitby EH, Griffiths PD, Rutter S, et al. Frequency and natural history of subdural haemorrhages in babies and relation to obstetric factors. *Lancet.* 2004;363:846-851.
5. Looney CB, Smith JK, Merck LH, et al. Intracranial hemorrhage in asymptomatic neonates: prevalence on MR images and relationship to obstetric and neonatal risk factors. *Radiology.* 2007;242:535-541.
6. Pfister RH, Bingham P, Edwards EM, et al. The Vermont Oxford Neonatal Encephalopathy Registry: rationale, methods, and initial results. *BMC Pediatr.* 2012;12:1-11.
7. Barnette AR, Horbar JD, Soll RF, et al. Neuroimaging in the evaluation of neonatal encephalopathy. *Pediatrics.* 2014;133:e1508-e1517.
8. Ment LR, Bada HS, Barnes P, et al. Practice parameter: neuroimaging of the neonate: report of the Quality Standards Subcommittee of the American Academy of Neurology and the Practice Committee of the Child Neurology Society. *Neurology.* 2002;58:1726-1738.
9. Odita JC, Hebi S. CT and MRI characteristics of intracranial hemorrhage complicating breech and vacuum delivery. *Pediatr Radiol.* 1996;26:782-785.
10. Perrin RG, Rutka JT, Drake JM, et al. Management and outcomes of posterior fossa subdural hematomas in neonates. *Neurosurgery.* 1997;40:1190-1199, discussion 1199-1200.
11. Chau V, Poskitt KJ, Sargent MA, et al. Comparison of computer tomography and magnetic resonance imaging scans on the third day of life in term newborns with neonatal encephalopathy. *Pediatrics.* 2009;123:319-326.
12. Miller SP, Cozzio CC, Goldstein RB, et al. Comparing the diagnosis of white matter injury in premature newborns with serial MR imaging and transfontanel ultrasonography findings. *AJNR Am J Neuroradiol.* 2003;24:1661-1669.
13. Miller SP, Ferriero DM. From selective vulnerability to connectivity: insights from newborn brain imaging. *Trends Neurosci.* 2009;32:496-505.
14. American Academy of Pediatrics. Committee on Environmental Health. Risk of ionizing radiation exposure to children: a subject review. *Pediatrics.* 1998;101:717-719.
15. Hall EJ, Brenner DJ. Cancer risks from diagnostic radiology. *Br J Radiol.* 2008;81:362-378.
16. Pearce MS, Salotti JA, Little MP, et al. Radiation exposure from CT scans in childhood and subsequent risk of leukaemia and brain tumours: a retrospective cohort study. *Lancet.* 2012;380:499-505.
17. Cui L, Pierce D, Light KE, et al. Sublethal total body irradiation leads to early cerebellar damage and oxidative stress. *Curr Neurovasc Res.* 2010;7:125-135.
18. Schull WJ. Brain damage among individuals exposed prenatally to ionizing radiation: a 1993 review. *Stem Cells.* 1997;15:129-133.
19. Srinivasan L, Shah SS, Abbasi S, et al. Traumatic lumbar punctures in infants hospitalized in the neonatal intensive care unit. *Pediatr Infect Dis J.* 2013;32:1150-1152.
20. Walton JN. *Subarachnoid Haemorrhage.* Edinburgh: Livingstone; 1956.
27. Escobedo M, Barton L, Volpe J. Cerebrospinal fluid studies in an intensive care nursery. *J Perinat Med.* 1975;3:204-210.
29. Rodriguez AF, Kaplan SL, Mason EO Jr. Cerebrospinal fluid values in the very low birth weight infant. *J Pediatr.* 1990;116:971-974.
31. Shafer S, Rooney D, Schumacher RE, et al. Lumbar punctures at an academic level 4 NICU: indication for a new curriculum. *Teach Learn Med.* 2015;27:205-207.
32. Hines EM, Nigrovic LE, Neuman MI, et al. Adjustment of cerebrospinal fluid protein for red blood cells in neonates and young infants. *J Hosp Med.* 2012;7:325-328.

36. Nelson RM, Bucciarelli RL, Nagel JW, et al. Hypoglycorrhachia associated with intracranial hemorrhage in newborn infants. *J Pediatr.* 1979;94:800-803.
40. Craig WS. Intracranial haemorrhage in the new-born: a study of diagnosis and differential diagnosis based upon pathological and clinical findings in 126 cases. *Arch Dis Child.* 1938;13:89-124.
43. Hayashi T, Hashimoto T, Fukuda S, et al. Neonatal subdural-hematoma secondary to birth injury—clinical analysis of 48 survivors. *Childs Nerv Syst.* 1987;3:23-29.
44. Tanaka Y, Sakamoto K, Kobayashi S, et al. Biphasic ventricular dilatation following posterior fossa subdural hematoma in the full-term neonate. *J Neurosurg.* 1988;68:211-216.
45. Hanigan WC, Morgan AM, Stahlberg LK, et al. Tentorial hemorrhage associated with vacuum extraction. *Pediatrics.* 1990;85:534-539.
46. Huang CC, Shen EY. Tentorial subdural hemorrhage in term newborns - ultrasonographic diagnosis and clinical correlates. *Pediatr Neurol.* 1991;7:171-177.
47. Squier W, Mack J. The neuropathology of infant subdural haemorrhage. *Forensic Sci Int.* 2009;187:6-13.
52. Blank NK, Strand R, Gilles FH, et al. Posterior fossa subdural hematomas in neonates. *Arch Neurol.* 1978;35:108-111.
53. Koch TK, Jahnke SE, Edwards MS, et al. Posterior fossa hemorrhage in term newborns. *Pediatr Neurol.* 1985;1:96-99.
56. Holden KR, Titus MO, Van tassel P. Cranial magnetic resonance imaging examination of normal term neonates: a pilot study. *J Child Neurol.* 1999;14:708-710.
57. Chamnanvanakij S, Rollins N, Perlman JM. Subdural hematoma in term infants. *Pediatr Neurol.* 2002;26:301-304.
59. Wigglesworth JS, Husemeyer RP. Intracranial birth trauma in vaginal breech delivery: the continued importance of injury to the occipital bone. *Br J Obstet Gynaecol.* 1977;84:684-691.
60. Pape KE, Wigglesworth JS. *Haemorrhage, Ischaemia and the Perinatal Brain.* Philadelphia: JB Lippincott; 1979.
65. Aydinli N, Citak A, Caliskan M, et al. Vitamin K deficiency—late onset intracranial haemorrhage. *Eur J Paediatr Neurol.* 1998;2:199-203.
68. Flodmark O, Fitz CR, Harwood-Nash DC. CT diagnosis and short-term prognosis of intracranial hemorrhage and hypoxic/ischemic brain damage in neonates. *J Comput Assist Tomogr.* 1980;4:775-787.
70. Renzulli P, Tuchschmid P, Eich G, et al. Early vitamin K deficiency bleeding after maternal phenobarbital intake: management of massive intracranial haemorrhage by minimal surgical intervention. *Eur J Pediatr.* 1998;157:663-665.
71. Akman CI, Cracco J. Intrauterine subdural hemorrhage. *Dev Med Child Neurol.* 2000;42:843-846.
75. Rotmensch S, Grannum PA, Nores JA, et al. In utero diagnosis and management of fetal subdural hematoma. *Am J Obstet Gynecol.* 1991;164:1246-1248.
76. Piastra M, Pietrini D, Massimi L, et al. Severe subdural hemorrhage due to minimal prenatal trauma. *J Neurosurg Pediatr.* 2009;4:543-546.
82. Gilles FH, Shillito J Jr. Infantile hydrocephalus. Retrocerebellar subdural hematoma. *J Pediatr.* 1970;76:529-537.
84. Volpe JJ, Manica JP, Land VJ, et al. Neonatal subdural hematoma associated with severe hemophilia A. *J Pediatr.* 1976;88:1023-1025.
85. Deonna T, Calame A, van Melle G, et al. Hypoglycorrhachia in neonatal intracranial hemorrhage. Relationship to posthemorrhagic hydrocephalus. *Helv Paediatr Acta.* 1977;32(4–5):351-361.
87. Ravenel SD. Posterior fossa hemorrhage in the term newborn: report of two cases. *Pediatrics.* 1979;64:39-42.
88. Serfontein GL, Rom S, Stein S. Posterior fossa subdural hemorrhage in the newborn. *Pediatrics.* 1980;65:40-43.
89. Scher MS, Wright FS, Lockman LA, et al. Intraventricular hemorrhage in the full-term neonate. *Arch Neurol.* 1982;39:769-772.
90. Hernansanz J, Munoz F, Rodriguez D, et al. Subdural hematomas of the posterior fossa in normal-weight newborns. Report of two cases. *J Neurosurg.* 1984;61:972-974.
91. Forbes E, Patel N, Kasem K. Unilateral vocal cord paralysis associated with subdural haemorrhage in a newborn infant. *J Perinatol.* 2010;30:563-565.
92. Alshammari J, Monnier Y, Monnier P. Clinically silent subdural hemorrhage causes bilateral vocal fold paralysis in newborn infant. *Int J Pediatr Otorhinolaryngol.* 2012;76:1533-1534.

96. Minns RA. Subdural haemorrhages, haematomas, and effusions in infancy. *Arch Dis Child.* 2005;90:883-884.

98. Barkovich AJ. *Pediatric Neuroimaging.* 4th ed. Philadelphia: Lippincott Williams & Wilkins; 2005.

99. Rutherford MA. *MRI of the Neonatal Brain.* London; New York: W.B. Saunders; 2002.

100. Levene MI, Williams JL, Fawer CL. *Ultrasound of the Infant Brain.* London: Blackwell Scientific Publications, Ltd.; 1985.

102. Dooling EC, Leviton A, Gilles FH. *The Developing Human Brain: Growth and Epidemiologic Neuropathology.* Boston: J. Wright-PSG; 1983.

106. Huang AH, Robertson RL. Spontaneous superficial parenchymal and leptomeningeal hemorrhage in term neonates. *AJNR Am J Neuroradiol.* 2004;25:469-475.

107. Shackelford GD, Volpe JJ. Cranial ultrasonography in the evaluation of neonatal intracranial hemorrhage and its complications. *J Perinat Med.* 1985;13:293-304.

108. Chamnanvanakij S, Perlman JM. Extensive late-onset primary subarachnoid hemorrhage in a preterm infant. *Pediatr Neurol.* 1999;21:735-738.

109. Donat JF, Okazaki H, Kleinberg F. Intraventricular hemorrhage in full-term and premature infants. *Mayo Clin Proc.* 1978;53:437.

111. Palma PA, Miner ME, Morriss FH Jr, et al. Intraventricular hemorrhage in the neonate born at term. *Am J Dis Child.* 1979;133: 941-944.

112. Ludwig B, Brand M, Brockerhoft P. Post-partum CT examination of the heads of full-term infants. *Neuroradiology.* 1980;20:145.

113. LeBlanc R, O'Gorman AM. Neonatal intracranial hemorrhage: a clinical and serial computerized tomographic study. *J Neurosurg.* 1980;53:642.

114. Mitchell W, O'Tuama L. Cerebral intraventricular hemorrhages in infants: a widening age spectrum. *Pediatrics.* 1980;65:35-39.

116. Levene MI, Wigglesworth JS, Dubowitz V. Cerebral structure and intraventricular haemorrhage in the neonate: a real-time ultrasound study. *Arch Dis Child.* 1981;56:416-424.

117. Flodmark O, Scott G, Harwood-Nash DC. Clinical significance of ventriculomegaly in children who suffered perinatal asphyxia with or without intracranial hemorrhage: an 18 month follow-up study. *J Comput Assist Tomogr.* 1981;5:663.

124. Hayden CK Jr, Shattuck KE, Richardson CJ, et al. Subependymal germinal matrix hemorrhage in full-term neonates. *Pediatrics.* 1985;75:714-718.

125. Zorzi C, Angonese I, Nardelli GB, et al. Spontaneous intraventricular haemorrhage in utero. *Eur J Pediatr.* 1988;148:83-85.

126. Roland EH, Flodmark O, Hill A. Thalamic hemorrhage with intraventricular hemorrhage in the full-term newborn. *Pediatrics.* 1990;85:737-742.

128. Jocelyn LJ, Casiro OG. Neurodevelopmental outcome of term infants with intraventricular hemorrhage. *Am J Dis Child.* 1992;146: 194-197.

132. Monteiro JP, Roulet-Perez E, Davidoff V, et al. Primary neonatal thalamic haemorrhage and epilepsy with continuous spike-wave during sleep: a longitudinal follow-up of a possible significant relation. *Eur J Paediatr Neurol.* 2001;5:41-47.

133. Heck DV, Gailloud P, Cohen HL, et al. Choroid plexus arteriovenous malformation presenting with intraventricular hemorrhage. *J Pediatr.* 2002;141:710-711.

134. Wu YW, Hamrick SE, Miller SP, et al. Intraventricular hemorrhage in term neonates caused by sinovenous thrombosis. *Ann Neurol.* 2003;54:123-126.

138. De Vries LS, Smet M, Goemans N, et al. Unilateral thalamic haemorrhage in the pre-term and full-term newborn. *Neuropediatrics.* 1992;23:153-156.

148. Hanigan WC, Powell FC, Palagallo G, et al. Lobar hemorrhages in full-term neonates. *Childs Nerv Syst.* 1995;11:276-280.

150. Kanhai HH, Brand A. Fetal thrombocytopenia. In: James DK, Steer PJ, Weiner CP, eds. *High Risk Pregnancy Management Options.* 3rd ed. Philadelphia: Elsevier; 2006.

151. Radder CM, Brand A, Kanhai HH. A less invasive treatment strategy to prevent intracranial hemorrhage in fetal and neonatal alloimmune thrombocytopenia. *Am J Obstet Gynecol.* 2001;185:683-688.

152. Radder CM, Roelen DL, van de Meer-Prins EM, et al. The immunologic profile of infants born after maternal immunoglobulin treatment and intrauterine platelet transfusions

for fetal/neonatal alloimmune thrombocytopenia. *Am J Obstet Gynecol.* 2004;191:815-820.

154. Bussel J, Berkowitz R, McFarland J, et al. In-utero platelet transfusion for alloimmune thrombocytopenia. *Lancet.* 1988;2: 1307-1308.

153. Pacheco LD, Berkowitz RL, Moise KJ Jr, et al. Fetal and neonatal alloimmune thrombocytopenia: a management algorithm based on risk stratification. *Obstet Gynecol.* 2011;118:1157-1163.

155. Delbos F, Bertrand G, Croisille L, et al. Fetal and neonatal alloimmune thrombocytopenia: predictive factors of intracranial hemorrhage. *Transfusion.* 2016;56:59-66.

161. Bray GL, Luban NL. Hemophilia presenting with intracranial hemorrhage. An approach to the infant with intracranial bleeding and coagulopathy. *Am J Dis Child.* 1987;141:1215-1217.

162. Yoffe G, Buchanan GR. Intracranial hemorrhage in newborn and young infants with hemophilia. *J Pediatr.* 1988;113:333-336.

165. Sumer T, Ahmad M, Sumer NK, et al. Severe congenital factor X deficiency with intracranial haemorrhage. *Eur J Pediatr.* 1986;145: 119-120.

166. Ermis B, Ors R, Tastekin A, et al. Severe congenital factor X deficiency with intracranial bleeding in two siblings. *Brain Dev.* 2004;26:137-138.

167. Herrmann FH, Navarette M, Salazar-Sanchez L, et al. Homozygous Factor X gene mutations Gly380Arg and Tyr163delAT are associated with perinatal intracranial hemorrhage. *J Pediatr.* 2005;146:128-130.

172. Lane PA, Hathaway WE, Githens JH, et al. Fatal intracranial hemorrhage in a normal infant secondary to vitamin K deficiency. *Pediatrics.* 1983;72:562-564.

173. McNinch AW, Orme RL, Tripp JH. Haemorrhagic disease of the newborn returns. *Lancet.* 1983;1:1089-1090.

180. Von Kries R, Gobel U. Vitamin K prophylaxis and vitamin K deficiency bleeding (VKDB) in early infancy. *Acta Paediatr.* 1992;81:655-657.

181. Vitamin KAHTF, Merenstein GB, Hathaway WE, et al. Controversies concerning vitamin K and the newborn. *Pediatrics.* 1993;91:1001-1003.

182. von Kries R, Hachmeister A, Gobel U. Oral mixed micellar vitamin K for prevention of late vitamin K deficiency bleeding. *Arch Dis Child Fetal Neonatal Ed.* 2003;88:F109-F112.

183. Schulte R, Jordan LC, Morad A, et al. Rise in late onset vitamin K deficiency bleeding in young infants because of omission or refusal of prophylaxis at birth. *Pediatr Neurol.* 2014;50:564-568.

184. Volpe JJ. Intracranial hemorrhage in early infancy—renewed importance of vitamin K deficiency. *Pediatr Neurol.* 2014;50:545-546.

185. Shearer MJ. Vitamin K deficiency bleeding (VKDB) in early infancy. *Blood Rev.* 2009;23:49-59.

186. Warren M, Miller A, Traylor J, et al. Late vitamin K deficiency bleeding in infants whose parents declined vitamin K prophylaxis. *MMWR Morb Mortal Wkly Rep.* 2013;62:901-902.

189. Darlow BA, Phillips AA, Dickson NP. New Zealand surveillance of neonatal vitamin K deficiency bleeding (VKDB): 1998–2008. *J Paediatr Child Health.* 2011;47:460-464.

193. Jones RK, Shearburn EW. Intracranial aneurysm in a four-week-old infant. Diagnosis by angiography and successful operation. *J Neurosurg.* 1961;18:122-124.

197. Lee YJ, Kandall SR, Ghali VS. Intracerebral arterial aneurysm in a newborn. *Arch Neurol.* 1978;35:171-172.

198. Grode ML, Saunders M, Carton CA. Subarachnoid hemorrhage secondary to ruptured aneurysms in infants. Report of two cases. *J Neurosurg.* 1978;49:898-902.

205. Boop FA, Chadduck WM, Sawyer J, et al. Congenital aneurysmal hemorrhage and astrocytoma in an infant. *Pediatr Neurosurg.* 1991;17:44-47.

206. Piatt JH Jr, Clunie DA. Intracranial arterial aneurysm due to birth trauma. Case report. *J Neurosurg.* 1992;77:799-803.

209. Pollo C, Meagher-Villmure K, Bernath MA, et al. Ruptured cerebral aneurysm in the early stage of life—a congenital origin? *Neuropediatrics.* 2004;35:230-233.

210. Song JK, Niimi Y, Brisman JL, et al. Multiple cerebral aneurysms in a neonate: occlusion and rupture. *J Neurosurg.* 2005;102:81-85.

213. Ko A, Filardi T, Giussani C, et al. An intracranial aneurysm and dural arteriovenous fistula in a newborn. *Pediatr Neurosurg.* 2010;46:450-456.

214. Tai YP, Chou IC, Yang MS, et al. Neonatal intracranial aneurysm rupture treated by endovascular management: a case report. *Pediatr Neonatol.* 2010;51:249-251.

222. Godersky JC, Menezes AH. Intracranial arteriovenous anomalies of infancy: modern concepts. *Pediatr Neurosci.* 1987;13:242-250.

224. Wakai S, Andoh Y, Nagai M, et al. Choroid plexus arteriovenous malformation in a full-term neonate. Case report. *J Neurosurg.* 1990;72:127-129.

229. Rodesch G, Malherbe V, Alvarez H, et al. Nongalenic cerebral arteriovenous malformations in neonates and infants. Review of 26 consecutive cases (1982–1992). *Childs Nerv Syst.* 1995;11:231-241.

231. Hayashi T, Ichiyama T, Nishikawa M, et al. A case of large neonatal arteriovenous malformation with heart failure. Color Doppler sonography, MRI and MR angiography as early non-invasive diagnostic procedures. *Brain Dev.* 1996;18:236-238.

232. Nakayama H, Suzuki S, Hikino S, et al. Multiple cerebral arteriovenous fistulas and malformations in the neonate. *Pediatr Neurol.* 2001;25:236-238.

233. Kraneburg UM, Nga VD, Ting EY, et al. Intracranial pial arteriovenous fistula in infancy: a case report and literature review. *Childs Nerv Syst.* 2014;30:365-369.

235. Mehwald PS, Dittrich S, Grohmann J, et al. Coarctation of the aorta presenting as cerebral hemorrhage. *J Pediatr.* 2005;146:293.

236. Bagdure D, Bartakian S, Kaufman J. Coarctation of aorta and vein of Galen aneurysmal malformation in a neonate. *Curr Opin Pediatr.* 2011;23:249-252.

241. Schumacher RE, Palmer TW, Roloff DW, et al. Follow-up of infants treated with extracorporeal membrane oxygenation for newborn respiratory failure. *Pediatrics.* 1991;87:451-457.

242. Korinthenberg R, Kachel W, Koelfen W, et al. Neurological findings in newborn infants after extracorporeal membrane oxygenation, with special reference to the EEG. *Dev Med Child Neurol.* 1993;35:249-257.

243. Glass P, Bulas DI, Wagner AE, et al. Severity of brain injury following neonatal extracorporeal membrane oxygenation and outcome at age 5 years. *Dev Med Child Neurol.* 1997;39:441-448.

246. Mendoza JC, Shearer LL, Cook LN. Lateralization of brain lesions following extracorporeal membrane oxygenation. *Pediatrics.* 1991;88:1004-1009.

247. Revenis ME, Glass P, Short BL. Mortality and morbidity rates among lower birth weight infants (2000 to 2500 grams) treated with extracorporeal membrane oxygenation. *J Pediatr.* 1992;121:452-458.

254. Vaucher YE, Dudell GG, Bejar R, et al. Predictors of early childhood outcome in candidates for extracorporeal membrane oxygenation. *J Pediatr.* 1996;128:109-117.

255. Hardart GE, Fackler JC. Predictors of intracranial hemorrhage during neonatal extracorporeal membrane oxygenation. *J Pediatr.* 1999;134:156-159.

256. Desai SA, Stanley C, Gringlas M, et al. Five-year follow-up of neonates with reconstructed right common carotid arteries after extracorporeal membrane oxygenation. *J Pediatr.* 1999;134:428-433.

257. Davis PJ, Firmin RK, Manktelow B, et al. Long-term outcome following extracorporeal membrane oxygenation for congenital diaphragmatic hernia: the UK experience. *J Pediatr.* 2004;144:309-315.

258. Parish AP, Bunyapen C, Cohen MJ, et al. Seizures as a predictor of long-term neurodevelopmental outcome in survivors of neonatal extracorporeal membrane oxygenation (ECMO). *J Child Neurol.* 2004;19:930-934.

259. Hardart GE, Hardart MK, Arnold JH. Intracranial hemorrhage in premature neonates treated with extracorporeal membrane oxygenation correlates with conceptional age. *J Pediatr.* 2004;145:184-189.

262. Gray BW, Haft JW, Hirsch JC, et al. Extracorporeal life support: experience with 2,000 patients. *ASAIO J.* 2015;61:2-7.

263. Roberts J, Keene S, Heard M, et al. Successful primary use of VVDL+V ECMO with cephalic drain in neonatal respiratory failure. *J Perinatol.* 2016;36:126-131.

268. Taylor GA, Fitz CR, Kapur S, et al. Cerebrovascular accidents in neonates treated with extracorporeal membrane oxygenation: sonographic-pathologic correlation. *AJR Am J Roentgenol.* 1989;153:355-361.

270. Wiznitzer M, Masaryk TJ, Lewin J, et al. Parenchymal and vascular magnetic resonance imaging of the brain after extracorporeal membrane oxygenation. *Am J Dis Child.* 1990;144:1323-1326.

271. Bulas DI, Taylor GA, Fitz CR, et al. Posterior fossa intracranial hemorrhage in infants treated with extracorporeal membrane oxygenation: sonographic findings. *AJR Am J Roentgenol.* 1991;156:571-575.

272. Jarjour IT, Ahdab-Barmada M. Cerebrovascular lesions in infants and children dying after extracorporeal membrane oxygenation. *Pediatr Neurol.* 1994;10:13-19.

273. Evans MJ, McKeever PA, Pearson GA, et al. Pathological complications of non-survivors of newborn extracorporeal membrane oxygenation. *Arch Dis Child.* 1994;71:F88-F92.

274. Van Meurs KP, Nguyen HT, Rhine WD, et al. Intracranial abnormalities and neurodevelopmental status after venovenous extracorporeal membrane oxygenation. *J Pediatr.* 1994;125:304-307.

277. Wu YW, Miller SP, Chin K, et al. Multiple risk factors in neonatal sinovenous thrombosis. *Neurology.* 2002;59:438-440.

278. Taylor GA, Catena LM, Garin DB, et al. Intracranial flow patterns in infants undergoing extracorporeal membrane oxygenation: preliminary observations with Doppler US. *Radiology.* 1987;165:671-674.

279. Mitchell DG, Merton D, Desai H, et al. Neonatal brain: color Doppler imaging. Part II. Altered flow patterns from extracorporeal membrane oxygenation. *Radiology.* 1988;167:307-310.

280. Taylor GA, Short BL, Glass P, et al. Cerebral hemodynamics in infants undergoing extracorporeal membrane oxygenation: further observations. *Radiology.* 1988;168:163-167.

281. Raju TN, Kim SY, Meller JL, et al. Circle of Willis blood velocity and flow direction after common carotid artery ligation for neonatal extracorporeal membrane oxygenation. *Pediatrics.* 1989;83:343-347.

287. Taylor GA, Walker LK. Intracranial venous system in newborns treated with extracorporeal membrane oxygenation: Doppler US evaluation after ligation of the right jugular vein. *Radiology.* 1992;183:453-456.

290. Klesh KW, Murphy TF, Scher MS, et al. Cerebral infarction in persistent pulmonary hypertension of the newborn. *Am J Dis Child.* 1987;141:852-857.

291. Grayck EN, Meliones JN, Kern FH, et al. Elevated serum lactate correlates with intracranial hemorrhage in neonates treated with extracorporeal life support. *Pediatrics.* 1995;96:914-917.

292. Gleason CA, Short BL, Jones MD Jr. Cerebral blood flow and metabolism during and after prolonged hypocapnia in newborn lambs. *J Pediatr.* 1989;115:309-314.

293. Short BL, Walker LK, Bender KS, et al. Impairment of cerebral autoregulation during extracorporeal membrane oxygenation in newborn lambs. *Pediatr Res.* 1993;33:289-294.

298. Dworetz AR, Moya FR, Sabo B, et al. Survival of infants with persistent pulmonary hypertension without extracorporeal membrane oxygenation. *Pediatrics.* 1989;84:1-6.

299. Glass P, Miller M, Short B. Morbidity for survivors of extracorporeal membrane oxygenation: neurodevelopmental outcome at 1 year of age. *Pediatrics.* 1989;83:72-78.

301. Hofkosh D, Thompson AE, Nozza RJ, et al. Ten years of extracorporeal membrane oxygenation: neurodevelopmental outcome. *Pediatrics.* 1991;87:549-555.

306. Kornhauser MS, Baumgart S, Desai SA, et al. Adverse neurodevelopmental outcome after extracorporeal membrane oxygenation among neonates with bronchopulmonary dysplasia. *J Pediatr.* 1998;132:307-311.

307. Nield TA, Langenbacher D, Poulsen MK, et al. Neurodevelopmental outcome at 3.5 years of age in children treated with extracorporeal life support: relationship to primary diagnosis. *J Pediatr.* 2000;136:338-344.

308. Goodman M, Gringlas M, Baumgart S, et al. Neonatal electroencephalogram does not predict cognitive and academic achievement scores at early school age in survivors of neonatal extracorporeal membrane oxygenation. *J Child Neurol.* 2001;16:745-750.

309. Amigoni A, Pettenazzo A, Biban P, et al. Neurologic outcome in children after extracorporeal membrane oxygenation: prognostic value of diagnostic tests. *Pediatr Neurol.* 2005;32:173-179.

Full references for this chapter can be found on www.expertconsult.com.

Cerebellar Hemorrhage

Catherine Limperopoulos ◆ *Adré J. du Plessis* ◆ *Joseph J. Volpe*

Cerebellar hemorrhage has been increasingly detected in both preterm and full-term newborns in recent years. Currently, our understanding of cerebellar hemorrhagic injury and its long-term neurological sequelae has significantly changed, in large part due to increasing survival of critically ill infants and the greater availability and application of magnetic resonance imaging (MRI). Early studies reported a prevalence of cerebellar hemorrhage as high as 25% in premature infants at autopsy, usually associated with complicated births and a striking clinical presentation.[1-7] Given the relative insensitivity to posterior fossa structures of cranial ultrasonography (US) through the anterior fontanel approach, it was not until the advent of focused mastoid foramen views[8-12] that an unexpectedly high incidence of cerebellar lesions was noted in living premature infants (see later).

CEREBELLAR HEMORRHAGE: PRETERM INFANTS

Prevalence

Cerebellar hemorrhage is now recognized as an important complication of premature birth and is more common among premature than term infants. Older neuropathological series reported an incidence among premature infants less than 32 weeks of gestation or less than 1500 g birth weight, or both, ranging from 15% to 25%.[1,3,4,6,13] In contrast to these neuropathological reports, some large studies of living premature infants by computed tomography (CT) did not demonstrate cerebellar hemorrhage.[14,15] The reason for the discrepancy may not relate simply to differences between dead and living populations. Flodmark et al.[4] observed 15 cases of cerebellar hemorrhage at autopsy (all in premature infants) from 79 infants studied by CT for perinatal asphyxia. Among these 15 autopsy-proven cases, the hemorrhage was identified by CT in only one. (Ten of the lesions were considered to be "probably below the resolving power of the CT scanner.") Similarly, in infants evaluated by US through the anterior fontanel, the identification of cerebellar hemorrhage is unusual.[9,16,17] The advent of imaging through the mastoid fontanel, the thinnest region of the temporal bone at the junction of the squamosal, lambdoidal, and occipital sutures, has greatly facilitated accurate imaging of the posterior fossa in the newborn (Figs. 23.1 and 23.2).[8,9,12,18,19] Recent studies using this *mastoid window* report a high incidence of cerebellar hemorrhage in preterm infants. The largest reported study to date, based on use of this *mastoid window* in the evaluation of 1242 infants weighing less than

1500 g, showed an overall incidence of cerebellar hemorrhage of approximately 3% (Table 23.1).[8] However, the incidence varied markedly as a function of birth weight. *Infants of less than 750 g of birth weight had the highest incidence (i.e., 8.7% overall, and notably, 17% in the last 2 years of the 5-year study).* Infants between 750 and 1499 g exhibited an overall incidence of approximately 2.7%. Indeed, in this large cohort, nearly 60% of all cerebellar hemorrhages were in the infants who weighed less than 750 g. Thus, cerebellar hemorrhage is particularly a lesion of the most immature infants. More recent data suggest that cerebellar hemorrhage in the preterm infant is even more prevalent, described in up to 19% of preterm infants of less than 32 weeks' gestation.[10,21-23] The addition of the mastoid fontanel window in cranial US improved the detection of cerebellar hemorrhage compared to detection by the anterior and posterior fontanel US views alone.[10,21-23] With the mastoid view, abnormalities in the posterior fossa were detected in 71% of preterm infants but were missed using the anterior or posterior fontanel views.[10] Notably, approximately half of small hemorrhagic cerebellar lesions (e.g., punctate hemorrhages) were undetected, even when the mastoid fontanel approach was used.[10,22] When MRI is routinely performed in very preterm infants (<32 weeks gestational age), the incidence of cerebellar hemorrhage is still higher, ranging from 15% to 24%,[10,22-25] but may be underdiagnosed if specific MRI sequences (e.g., susceptibility-weighted imaging) are not performed.[26] With the latter approach and 3T-MRI, 37% of preterm newborns less than 33 weeks of gestation had cerebellar hemorrhage identified (Table 23.2).[27]

Neuropathology

Four major categories of lesions have been described in infants with cerebellar hemorrhage (Table 23.3). Primary cerebellar hemorrhage likely accounts for most cases of cerebellar hemorrhage in the preterm infant.

Primary cerebellar hemorrhage is the best studied of the destructive cerebellar lesions in premature infants. There is a broad spectrum in the severity of cerebellar hemorrhages reported, ranging from mild punctate lesions, focal unilateral lesions, to the less common and more extensive bihemispheric and vermian hemorrhages (Figs. 23.3 to 23.5). The more extensive lesions range from partial inferomedial hemorrhage to near-total destruction of the cerebellum and may be associated with pontine hypoplasia on subsequent MRI (Fig. 23.6).[28,29] Recently, a cerebellar hemorrhage grading scheme was proposed (Table 23.4).[22] The hemorrhages are followed by cerebellar atrophy, detectable about 2 months later in 37%. Atrophy

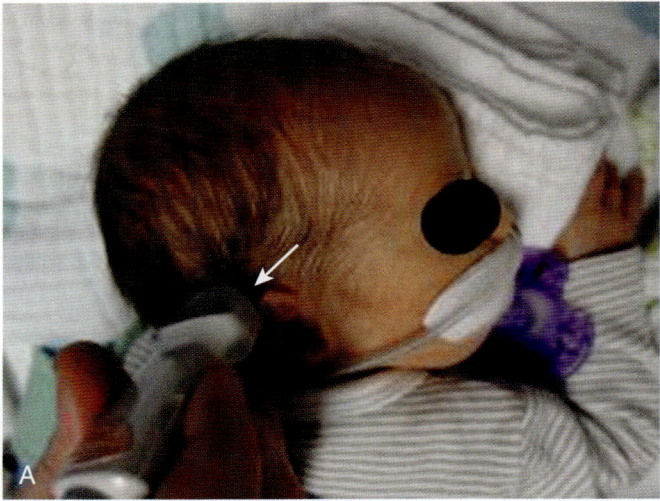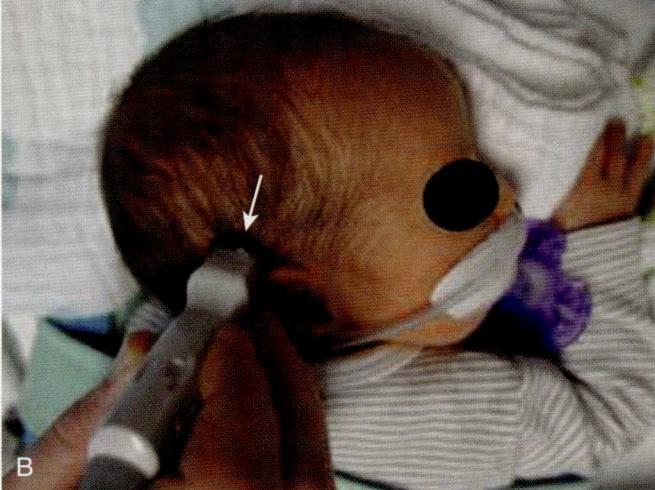

Figure 23.1 Probe positioning for mastoid fontanel cranial ultrasonography, axial (A) and coronal (B) views. (From Steggerda SJ, van Wezel-Meijler G. Cranial ultrasonography of the immature cerebellum: role and limitations. *Semin Fetal Neonatal Med.* 2016;21:295–304.)

TABLE 23.1	Incidence of Cerebellar Hemorrhage in Premature Infants by Birth Weight
BIRTH WEIGHT	**INCIDENCE[a]**
<750 g	20/230 (8.7%)[b]
750–999 g	4/602 (0.7%)
1000–1499 g	11/410 (2.7%)
Total	35/1242 (2.8%)

[a]Incidence is expressed as *n/N* (%).
[b]Incidence in the last 2 years of the 5-year study period was 17%.
Data from Limperopoulos C, Benson CB, Bassan H, et al. Cerebellar hemorrhage in the preterm infant: ultrasonographic findings and risk factors. *Pediatrics.* 2005;116:717–724.

TABLE 23.2	Incidence of Cerebellar Hemorrhage in Premature Infants Less Than 32 Weeks Gestation by Imaging Modality
Cranial ultrasound (with mastoid view)	3%–9%[a]
Magnetic resonance imaging (MRI)	15%–37%[a,b]
Sensitivity/specificity of routine CUS relative to MRI	18%/100%[c]
Positive/negative predictive value of routine cranial ultrasound	100%/84%[c]
Sensitivity/specificity of additional cranial ultrasound views relative to MRI	45%/100%[c]
Positive/negative predictive value of additional cranial ultrasound views	100%/89%

[a]Data from Staggerda SJ, van Wezel-Meijler G. Cranial ultrasonography of the immature cerebellum: role and limitations. *Semin Fetal Neonatal Med.* 2016;21:295–304.
[b]Data from Gano D, Ho ML, Partridge JC, et al. Antenatal exposure to magnesium sulfate is associated with reduced cerebellar hemorrhage in preterm newborns. *J Pediatr.* 2016;178:68–74.
[c]Data from Staggerda SJ, Leijser LM, Wiggers-de Bruïne FT, van der Grond J, Walther FJ, van Wezel-Meijler G. Cerebellar injury in preterm infants: incidence and findings on US and MR imaging. *Radiology.* 2009;252:190–199.

is focal in the unilateral lesions and more generalized in the bilateral lesions. Notably, reductions in contralateral *cerebral* volumes have been defined and likely reflect impaired remote transsynaptic trophic effects.[30]

A recent neuropathologic study[31] reported that the principal locus of cerebellar hemorrhage was the ventral aspect of the posterior lobe of the cerebellum and vermis. The cerebellar hemorrhages tended to be bilateral and involved the vermis (74%). Microscopically, the hemorrhages were located in the white matter or in the cerebellar cortex near the junction of the white matter and the internal granule cell layer and were associated with germinal matrix hemorrhage (95%) and pontosubicular necrosis (69%). More than half also had neuronal loss/gliosis in the inferior olivary nucleus and the dentate, which likely represents a transsynaptic degenerative process (Fig. 23.7).

Cerebellar infarction is a recognized complication of extreme preterm birth.[28,29,32] Distinction of hemorrhagic venous infarction from primary cerebellar hemorrhage can be very difficult, even at microscopic examination. Cerebellar infarcts typically involve the bilateral inferior parts of the cerebellar

TABLE 23.3	Neuropathology of Neonatal "Cerebellar Hemorrhage"

Primary cerebellar hemorrhage
Venous (hemorrhagic) infarction
Extension into cerebellum of intraventricular or subarachnoid blood or both
Traumatic laceration of cerebellum or rupture of major veins or occipital sinus (with or without occipital diastasis)

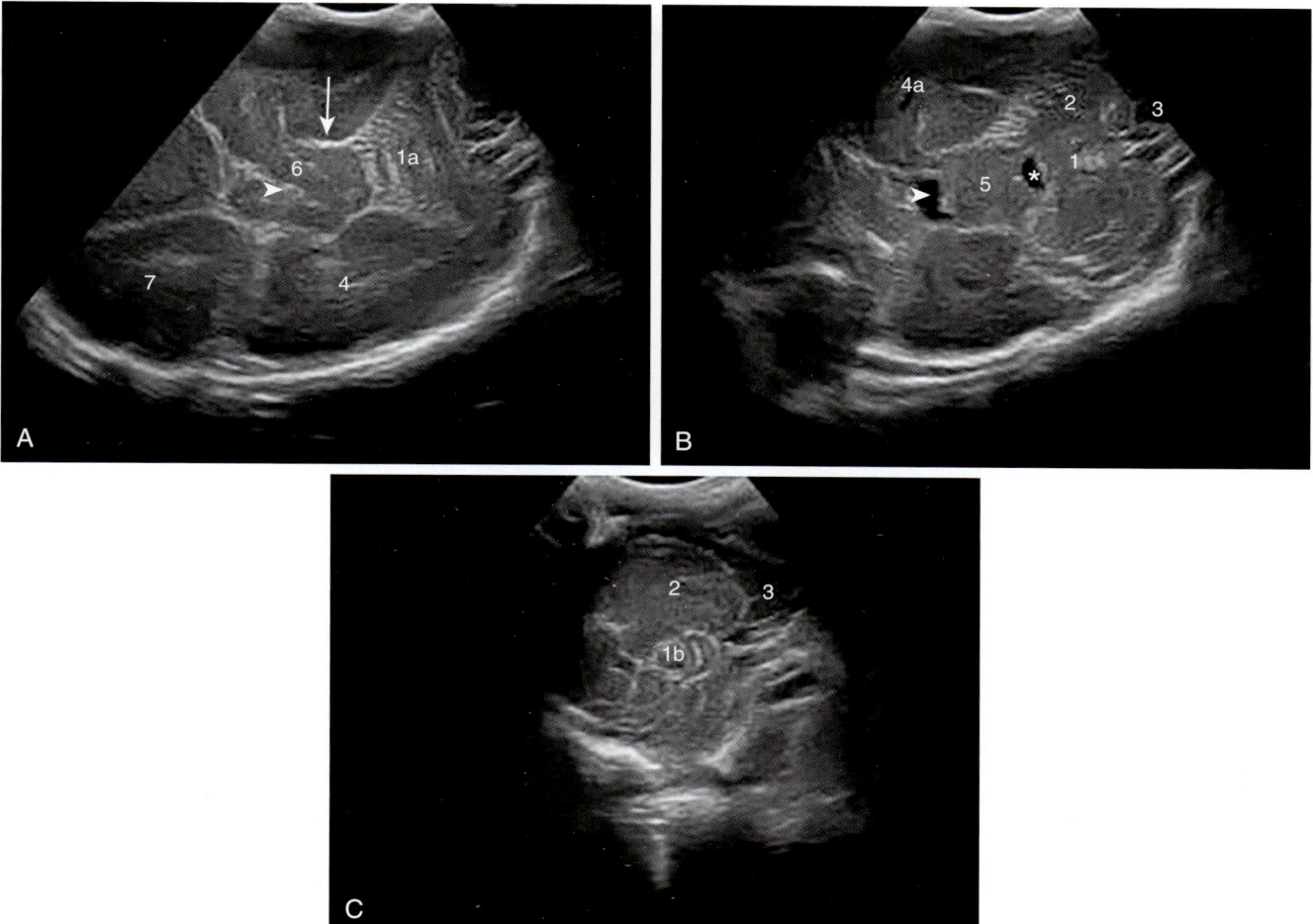

Figure 23.2 Normal superior (A), middle (B), and inferior (C) axial views using the mastoid fontanel as an acoustic window in a preterm infant (gestational age 28 weeks), showing cerebellar vermis (1) with superior (1a) and inferior (1b) part, cerebellar hemisphere (2), cisterna magna (3), temporal lobe (4), temporal horn (4a), pons (5), cerebral peduncle (6), frontal lobe (7), fourth ventricle (asterisk), perimesencephalic cistern (arrow), interpedunclar fossa (short arrow), and prepontine cistern (arrowhead). (From Steggerda SJ, van Wezel-Meijler G. Cranial ultrasonography of the immature cerebellum: role and limitations. Semin Fetal Neonatal Med. 2016;21:295–304.)

TABLE 23.4	Grading Scheme for Cerebellar Hemorrhage

Grade 1: Unilateral small punctate lesions (≤3 mm)
Grade 2: Bilateral small punctate lesions (≤3 mm)
Grade 3: Extensive unilateral lesions (>3 mm)
Grade 4: Bilateral extensive lesions (>3 mm)

Data from Kidokoro H, Anderson PJ, Doyle LW, Woodward LJ, Neil JJ, Inder TE. Brain injury and altered brain growth in preterm infants: predictors and prognosis. *Pediatrics*. 2014;134:e444–e453.

hemispheres, suggesting a vascular distribution in the territory of the posterior inferior cerebellar arteries,[28] and often occur in combination with supratentorial white matter injury, suggesting a more generalized hypoxic-ischemic insult.

The extension of blood from intraventricular or subarachnoid spaces has been suggested as a cause of cerebellar hemorrhage. This notion was raised particularly by the studies of Donat et al.[2] In 10 of their 20 cases of cerebellar hemorrhage, secondary dissection of blood into the cerebellum appeared to occur either from the fourth ventricle into the vermis or, less frequently, from the subarachnoid space into the cerebellar hemispheres. In these cases, massive hemorrhage into the lateral ventricles was the original source of the blood. This notion is supported by observations of a strong association of cerebellar hemorrhage with cerebral intraventricular hemorrhage (IVH).[6,13] (Indeed, in the aforementioned study of 1242 premature infants who were less than 1500 g of birth weight and studied in vivo by US, about two-thirds of cases were associated with IVH.)[8,17] Similarly, neuropathological studies also report that cerebellar hemorrhage is accompanied by IVH in 95% of cases.[31] Hemosiderin deposition on the cerebellar surface from extraaxial blood can have toxic effects and result in injury to underlying structures (e.g., the external granule cell layer) and may impair the immature and rapidly developing cerebellum (Chapter 4). However, a recent neuropathology report found no evidence for dissection of blood from the fourth ventricle or from the subarachnoid space that originates from IVH.[31]

Similarly, in a study of 73 preterm newborns with cerebellar hemorrhages, 70% (51/73) had no IVH and only 10% (7/73) had severe IVH.[27]

The fourth potential mechanism of cerebellar hemorrhage, *traumatic injury*, with laceration of cerebellum or with rupture of cerebellar bridging veins or occipital sinus, often occurring with occipital osteodiastasis, was discussed in Chapter 22 (see the section on subdural hemorrhage). This category may be important to some *term* infants with hemorrhage.[33-35] In the preterm infant, the ventral posterior loci of cerebellar hemorrhage is in a distribution that corresponds to the posterior inferior veins that drain the inferior cerebellar hemispheres into the transverse sinus, and the inferior vermis into the confluens.[31] The compliant skull of the preterm infant would render it vulnerable to compression of the occipital region by external forces, displacing the squamous portion of the occipital bone and distorting the venous sinuses at the confluens, thereby increasing venous pressure, and preferentially affecting the ventral cerebellum. This mechanism of injury raises the possibility that cerebellar hemorrhage can arise from a venous source.[31]

The neuroimaging of the loci of the hemorrhages within the cerebellum in the *small premature infant* includes both the hemisphere and the vermis. The lesions tend to be focal and localized. Approximately 70% of the lesions are localized to one cerebellar hemisphere, and 20% are localized to the vermis (Table 23.5).[8] Smaller lesions have included both subpial and subependymal locations, which are the sites of the germinal matrices in the external granule cell layer and subependymal zones, respectively. More recently, very small or punctate cerebellar hemorrhagic lesions have been reported on MRI (Figs. 23.8 and 23.9).[20,22,36] The more widespread use of MRI and the newer MRI techniques, such as susceptibility-weighted imaging, have increased the detection of these punctate lesions, which are difficult to detect by cranial US.[20,22] In large lesions, the cerebellar cortex and underlying white matter are destroyed. Notably, the neuropathological study by Haines et al.[31] showed that cerebellar hemorrhage was mulitfocal with lesions of

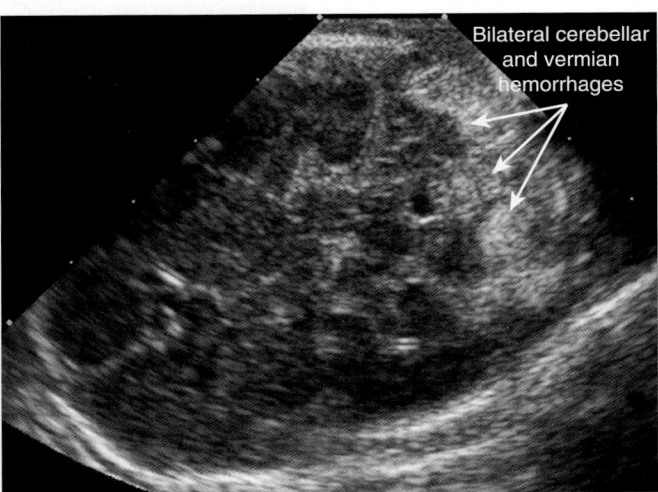

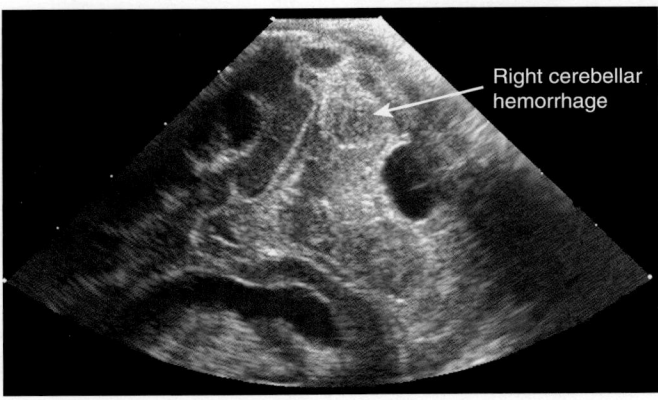

Figure 23.3 Ultrasonography image of the posterior fossa obtained through the mastoid fontanelle depicts a right cerebellar hemorrhage. (From Limperopoulos C, Benson CB, Bassan H, et al. Cerebellar hemorrhage in the preterm infant: ultrasonographic findings and risk factors. *Pediatrics.* 2005;116:717–724.)

Figure 23.4 Ultrasonography image of the posterior fossa obtained through the mastoid fontanelle depicts a bilateral cerebellar hemispheric and vermian hemorrhage. (From Limperopoulos C, Benson CB, Bassan H, et al. Cerebellar hemorrhage in the preterm infant: ultrasonographic findings and risk factors. *Pediatrics.* 2005;116:717–724.)

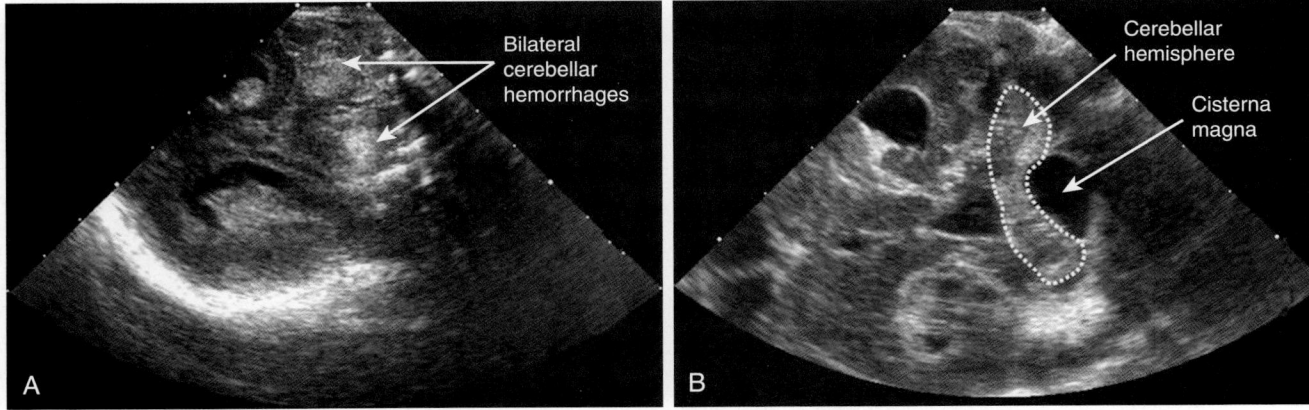

Figure 23.5 Ultrasonography images of the posterior fossa obtained through the mastoid fontanelle depict bilateral cerebellar hemispheric hemorrhage (A) and bilateral CBH resulting in cerebellar atrophy (B). (From Limperopoulos C, Benson CB, Bassan H, et al. Cerebellar hemorrhage in the preterm infant: ultrasonographic findings and risk factors. *Pediatrics.* 2005;116:717–724.)

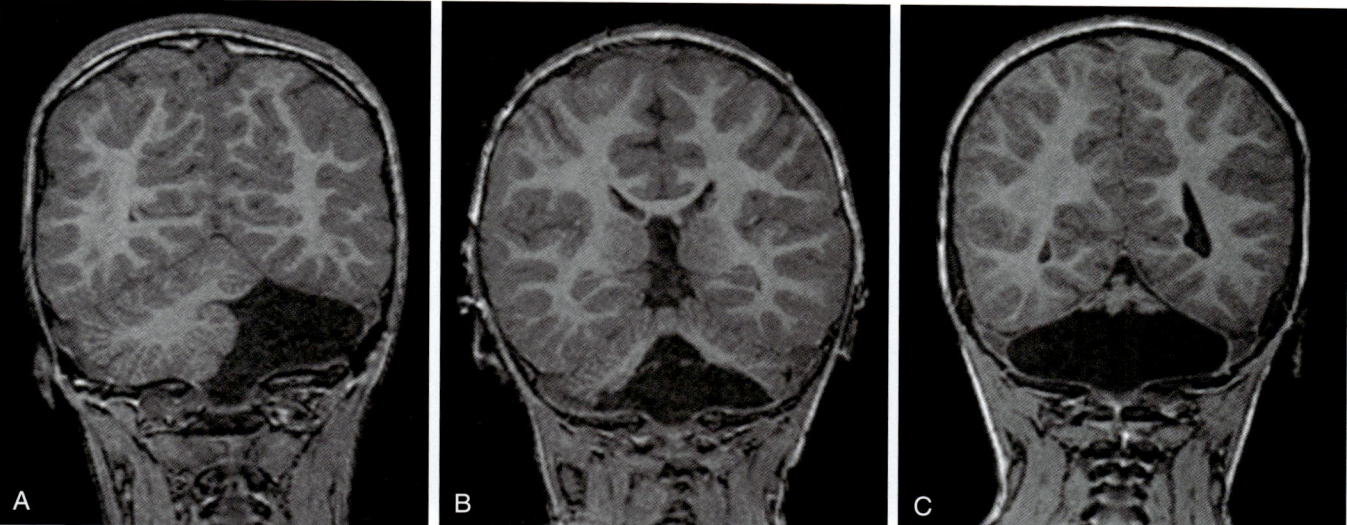

Figure 23.6 Follow-up brain magnetic resonance imaging (coronal spoiled gradient recalled T1-weighted) of infants with isolated cerebellar hemorrhagic injury on neonatal cranial ultrasound. (A) Complete absence of the left cerebellar hemisphere with preservation of the right cerebellar hemisphere and vermis. (B) Absence of the inferior cerebellar vermis and inferior portions of both cerebellar hemispheres. (C) Near-total cerebellar destruction with only a small amount of superior cerebellar vermis present. (From Limperopoulos C, Bassan H, Gauvreau K, et al. Does cerebellar injury in premature infants contribute to the high prevalence of long-term cognitive, learning, and behavioral disability in survivors? *Pediatrics.* 2007;120:584–593.)

TABLE 23.5	Loci of Cerebellar Hemorrhage by Ultrasonography in Premature Infants
LOCUS	**OCCURRENCE (%)**
Unilateral hemisphere	71
Vermis	20
Both hemispheres and vermis	9
Isolated[a]	23

[a]No supratentorial hemorrhage.

Data from Limperopoulos C, Benson CB, Bassan H, et al: Cerebellar hemorrhage in the preterm infant: ultrasonographic findings and risk factors. *Pediatrics.* 2005;116:717–724.

TABLE 23.6	Loci of Cerebellar Hemorrhage by Magnetic Resonance Imaging in the Full-Term Infant
LOCUS	**OCCURRENCE (N = 20) NO. (%)**
Cerebellar hemorrhage	17 (85)
Bilateral	7 (41)
Bilateral + vermis	3 (18)
Unilateral right,	3 (18)
Unilateral right + vermis	1 (6)
Unilateral left	3 (18)
Cerebellar nonhemorrhagic infarction	3 (15)
Associated supratentorial abnormalities	12 (60)

Data from Limperopoulos C, Robertson RL, Sullivan NR, Bassan H, du Plessis AJ. Cerebellar injury in term infants: clinical characteristics, MRI findings, and outcome. *Pediatr Neurol.* 2009;41:14–18.

variable size and histopathological age, suggesting that cerebellar hemorrhage may develop as a series of recurrent hemorrhagic episodes occurring over a period of time.

CEREBELLAR HEMORRHAGE: TERM INFANT

The topography of cerebellar hemorrhage in the *term* infant can be divided into two broad categories. In recent reports, the most common pattern consists of small hemorrhages deep within the cerebellum, which are usually bilateral and involve the vermis in approximately one-quarter of cases. About half of these small lesions are tiny punctate lesions.[35,37] The second category of cerebellar injury are large hemispheric and vermian hemorrhages, primarily medial and superior in location (Fig. 23.10). These large cerebellar lesions are frequently associated with subsequent cerebellar hemispheric and vermis atrophy (Table 23.6).[35,37]

Pathogenesis

The pathogenesis of cerebellar hemorrhage is undoubtedly multifactorial, but particular importance can be attributed to respiratory and circulatory events related to prematurity, and, in selected instances, traumatic delivery (breech or forceps extractions, or both).[a] In the premature infant, the pathogenesis bears similarities to that of IVH (Chapter 24). In the term infant, the pathogenesis appears to relate principally to hypoxic-ischemic and traumatic events. The pathogenesis

[a]References 1, 3, 6, 8, 13 and 38-41.

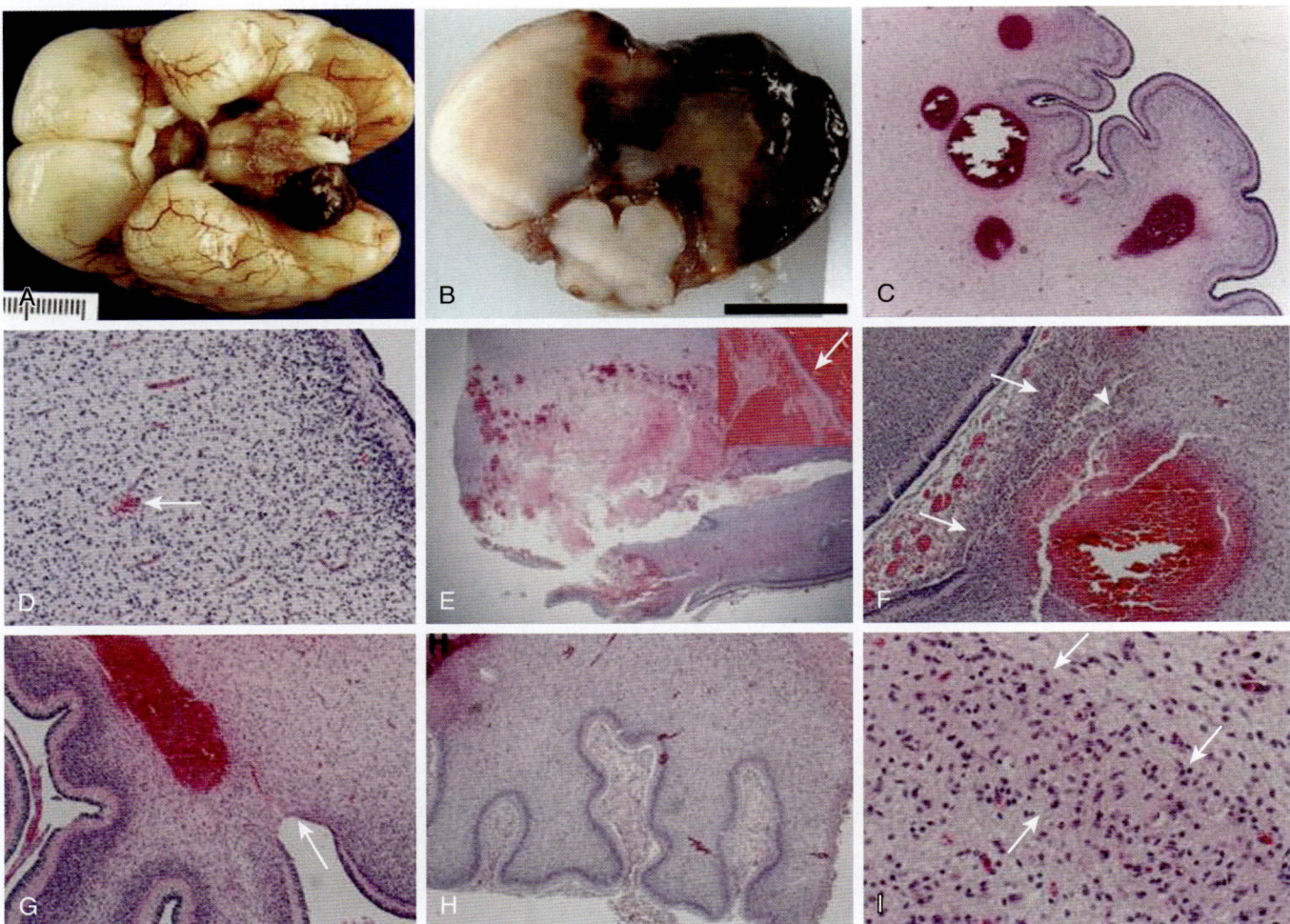

Figure 23.7 Neuropathology of cerebellar hemorrhage. (A) Gross photograph of a 25-week-gestation infant with a large cerebellar hemorrhage involving the ventral surface. (B) Horizontal section through the cerebellum and rostral medulla of (A) showing multiple hemorrhages destroying cerebellar parenchyma. (C) Low-powered photomicrograph showing multiple recent hemorrhages at the interface of the emerging internal granule layer and the white matter. (D) Often small, relatively inconspicuous hemorrhages are noted near, or at a distance, from a large hemorrhage *(arrow)*. (E) Low-powered photomicrographs from a 28-week-gestation infant showing a large destructive hemorrhage. Inset photomicrograph of the hemorrhage at high power showing the remnants of the cortex *(arrow)*. Small hemorrhages (B to D) may enlarge and become confluent resulting in these large destructive lesions. Hemorrhage may extend into and disrupt the cortex (F) *(arrows)*, or there may be focal cerebellar cortical loss *(arrow)* associated with a nearby hemorrhage, suggesting that hemorrhages are associated with hypoxic–ischemic processes (G) *(arrow)*. Cerebellar hemorrhages frequently show a mixture of recent hemorrhages with more subacute changes, such as hemosiderin-laden macrophages *(arrowhead)* (F), suggesting that some larger lesions may be due to repeated bouts of hemorrhage. With longer survival periods, cerebellar hemorrhage is associated with cortical atrophy (H) as seen in this photomicrograph from a 1-month-old infant, born at 27 weeks. (I) High-powered photomicrograph of the cerebellar dentate *(arrows)* from the same case in (C) showing marked neuronal loss and gliosis. Bar = 1 cm in (B). (From Pierson CR, Al Sufiani F. Preterm birth and cerebellar neuropathology. *Semin Fetal Neonatal Med.* 2016;21:305–311.)

of cerebellar hemorrhage is best considered in terms of intravascular, vascular, and extravascular factors (Table 23.7).

Intravascular Factors

Pressure-Passive Cerebellar Circulation. As discussed in Chapters 13 and 15, the cerebral circulation of the newborn, especially the sick preterm newborn, is pressure passive. If the pressure-passive state of the cerebral circulation also affects the cerebellar circulation, which is likely, then vulnerable

capillaries (see vascular factors later) can be exposed to bursts of arterial pressure flow, caused by hypertensive spikes, infusions of colloid, and so forth (see also Chapter 24). Rupture is a potential result. Notably, the autoregulatory capacity of the cerebellum is even narrower than that of the cerebrum, and ischemia may develop.[42] In one large series, several pathogenetic factors that are potentially consistent with the occurrence of ischemia included a relation to fetal distress, the need for an emergency cesarean section, the requirement of pressor

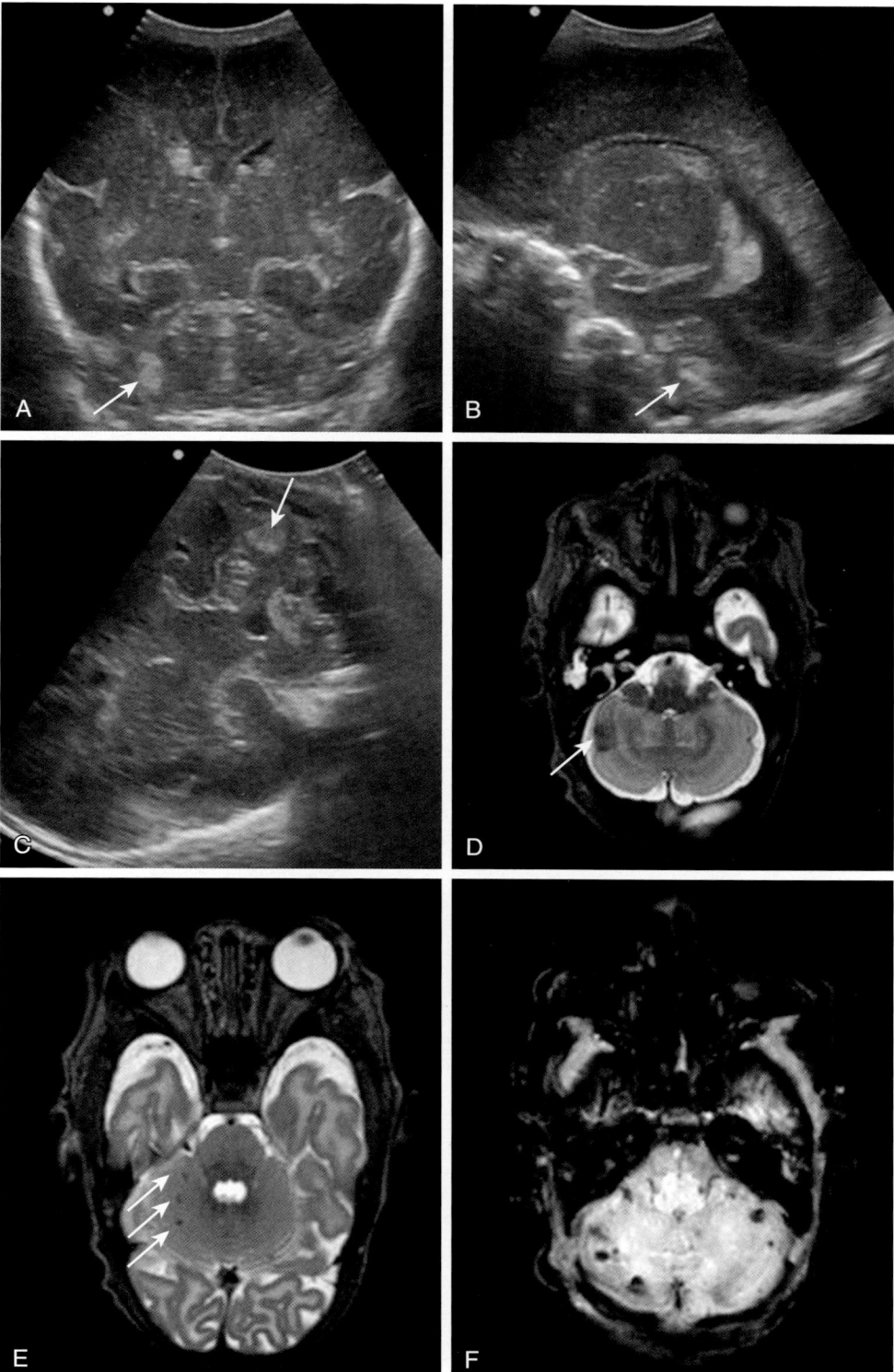

Figure 23.8 Preterm infant (gestational age 26 weeks), cranial ultrasound performed at fourth postnatal day. (A) Coronal view through anterior fontanel shows bilateral intraventricular hemorrhage and echogenicity in the right cerebellar hemisphere *(arrow)*. (B) Parasagittal view shows the small intraventricular hemorrhage and echogenicity within the right cerebellar hemisphere *(arrow)*. (C) Coronal view through the right mastoid fontanel clearly demonstrates the small convexity lesion in the right cerebellar hemisphere *(arrow)*. (D) Magnetic resonance imaging (MRI) in the same infant, obtained at term age *(arrow)*. (E) T2-weighted MRI shows convexity hemorrhage in the right cerebellar hemisphere and punctate hemorrhages in the right hemisphere not detected by ultrasound *(arrows)*. (F) Susceptibility-weighted image demonstrates multiple bilateral cerebellar hemorrhages. (From Steggerda SJ, van Wezel-Meijler G. Cranial ultrasonography of the immature cerebellum: role and limitations. *Semin Fetal Neonatal Med.* 2016;21: 295–304.)

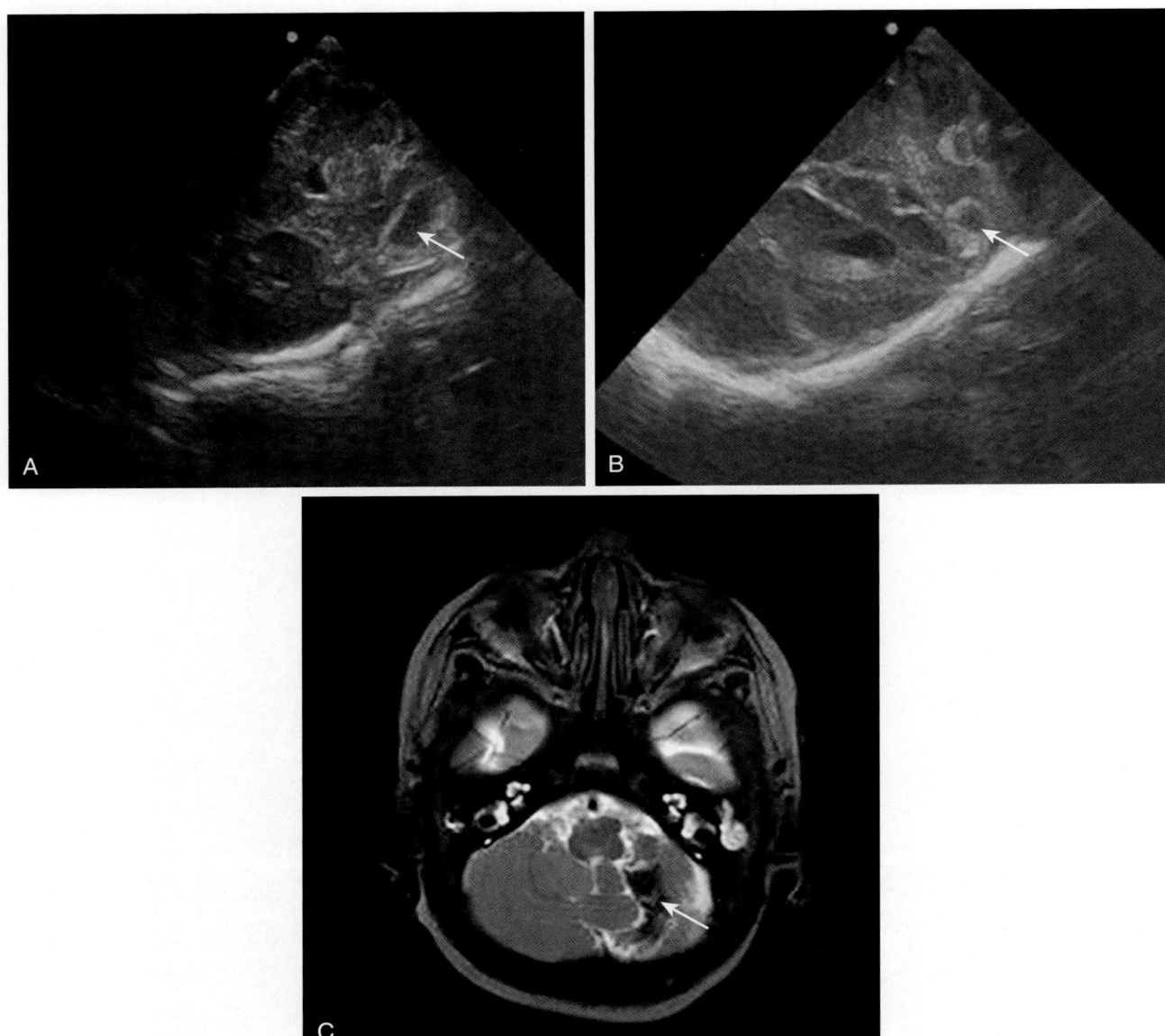

Figure 23.9 Preterm infant (gestational age 25 weeks) who was readmitted after surgery for gastric perforation and patent ductus arteriosus. No previous mastoid fontanel scan was performed. Axial (A) *(arrow)* and coronal (B) *(arrow)* views obtained through right mastoid fontanel on 28th postnatal day show increased echogenicity with central echolucency in the left cerebellar hemisphere, which is suspect for subacute cerebellar hemorrhage. (C) Magnetic resonance imaging at term age shows residual hemorrhage in the slightly smaller left cerebellar hemisphere *(arrow)*. (From Steggerda SJ, van Wezel-Meijler G. Cranial ultrasonography of the immature cerebellum: role and limitations. *Semin Fetal Neonatal Med.* 2016;21:295–304.)

support, patent ductus arteriosus (PDA), and low pH in the early neonatal period (relative to matched controls without cerebellar hemorrhage).[8] More recent studies have identified similar risk factors, including fetal heart rate abnormalities, intubation at birth, high-frequency oscillation ventilation, mechanical ventilation greater than or equal to 7 days, hypotension, the need for volume expanders, high-dose caffeine, sepsis, PDA, and grade 3 to 4 IVH.[17,22,27,43,44]

Increased Venous Pressure, Compliant Skull. A potentially important factor, in the premature newborn only somewhat more than the term infant, is the *compliant skull.* External pressure, which causes occipital compression, results in forward movement of the upper part of the squamous portion of the occipital bone under the parietal bones, thus distorting the venous sinuses at the torcular and increasing venous pressure. This phenomenon has been demonstrated radiographically and at postmortem examination.[34,45,46] Moreover, forward movement of the lower portion of the squamous bone, as discussed with occipital diastasis, could distort the occipital sinus and its tributaries with a similar effect on venous pressure. These bony distortions would be expected with breech extractions and

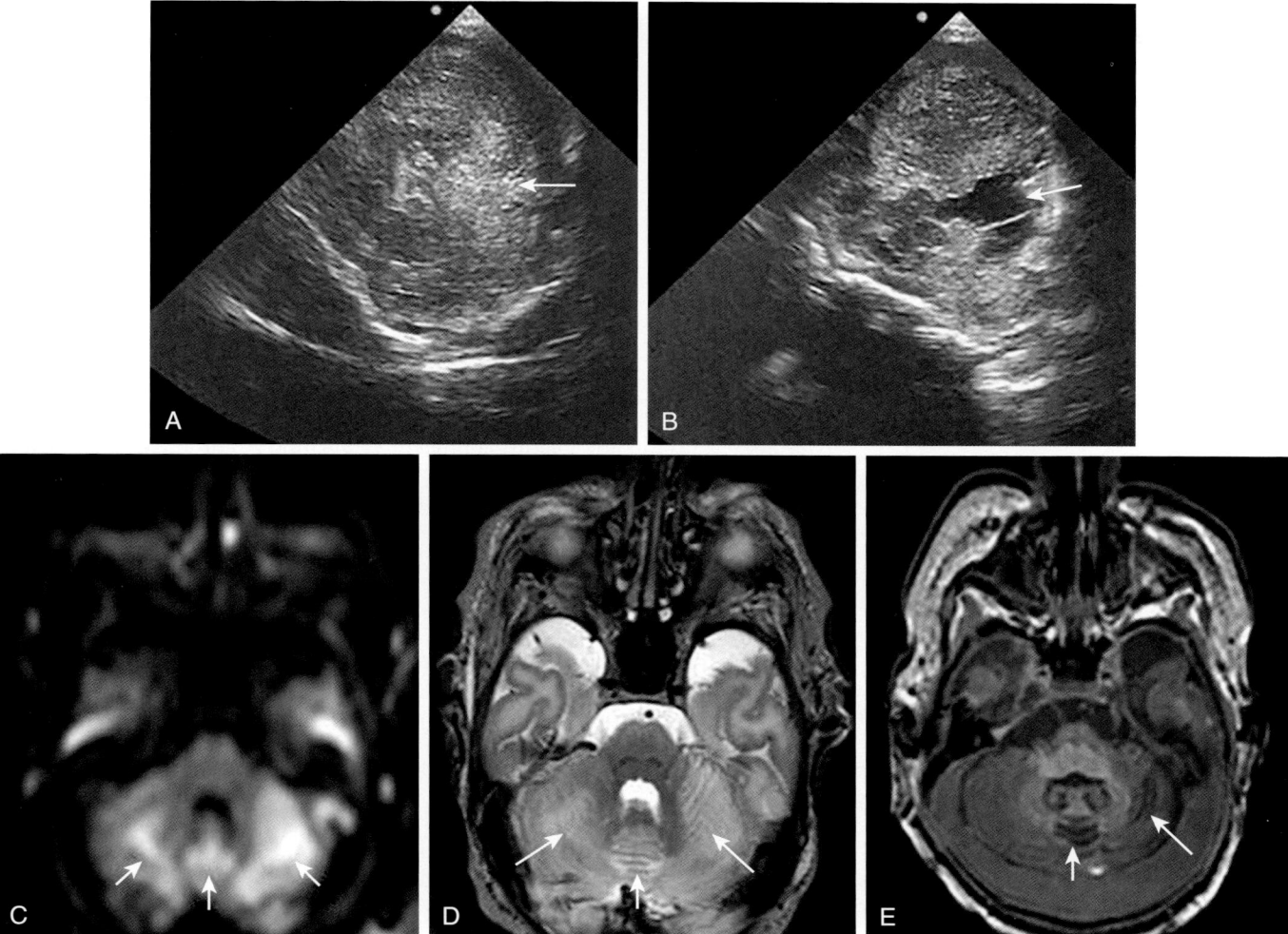

Figure 23.10 Axial ultrasound scan in full-term neonate (gestational age 40 weeks, Group B streptococcus meningitis) using the right mastoid fontanelle as an acoustic window. (A) On the fourth day of life, demonstrating abnormal echogenicity of cerebellar vermis and hemispheres *(arrow)*. (B) Follow-up ultrasound scan on 11th day of life, demonstrating loss of parenchymal tissue of cerebellar vermis and left cerebellar hemisphere, and loss of normal structure and anatomical landmarks. The fourth ventricle is widened and irregularly shaped *(arrow)*. Magnetic resonance imaging (MRI) in the same neonate on the fifth day of life. (C) Diffusion-weighted image showing abnormal signal intensity in the cerebellar vermis *(short arrow)* and both hemispheres *(arrows)*. (D) T2-weighted MR image showing abnormal high signal in corresponding areas *(arrows)*. (E) T1-weighted MR image on the 12th day of life showing destructive lesions of the cerebellar vermis *(short arrow)* and the left hemisphere *(arrow)*. (From Steggerda SJ, de Bruïne FT, Smits-Wintjens VE, Walther FJ, van Wezel-Meijler G. Ultrasound detection of posterior fossa abnormalities in full-term neonates. *Early Hum Dev.* 2012;88:233–239.)

difficult forceps extractions. In one series of term infants with cerebellar hemorrhage, such intrapartum events were present in the majority of cases.[41] More recent data show that 30% of term cerebellar hemorrhages were associated with assisted vaginal deliveries (forceps or vacuum).[35]

The possibility that such phenomena could occur *postnatally* was emphasized in a series of patients with cerebellar hemorrhage who had received positive-pressure ventilation by means of a face mask attached by a band across the occiput.[6] The band caused occipital molding and compression of the type just described, which resulted in distortion and obstruction of major venous sinuses. However, use of the face mask is by no means an essential factor because in most other large

series of pathologically proven cerebellar hemorrhage in the premature infant, the lesion did not occur in such a clinical setting.[1-3,8,13,16] Nevertheless, occipital compression can occur readily in the small infant by such maneuvers as fixation of the head in the supine position for nursing, bag and mask resuscitation, placement of the endotracheal tube, and puncture of the scalp vein.[45]

Disturbed Coagulation. Although not common, disturbed coagulation may contribute to pathogenesis. Cerebellar hemorrhage has been described in association with vitamin K deficiency[47] and thrombocytopenia.[37] The latter was present in single cases of cerebellar hemorrhage with methylmalonic

TABLE 23.7   Pathogenesis of Cerebellar Hemorrhage

Intravascular factors
Pressure-passive cerebellar circulation/ischemia
Increased venous pressure (compliant skull)
Disturbed coagulation
Vascular factors
Tenuous vascular integrity
Involuting vessels: subependymal and subpial germinal matrices
Vessels in the internal granule cell layer
Hypoxia-ischemia
Extravascular factors
Direct external effects on cerebellar parenchyma and vessels
  (compliant skull)
Poor vascular support: subependymal and subpial germinal
  matrices
Extension from intraventricular hemorrhage

acidemia and with propionic acidemia.[48] An infant with cerebellar hemorrhage associated with isovaleric acidemia—a metabolic disorder frequently complicated by thrombocytopenia—had a blood dyscrasia that was not characterized in detail.[49] (Other pathogenetic factors also were present in these patients with organic acidopathies; e.g., infusion of hypertonic solutions, cardiac failure, and cerebellar edema with upward herniation.) Maternal conditions, including deficiency of factor V Leiden, have also been associated with cerebellar hemorrhage in the term infant.[35]

Vascular Factors

Tenuous Vascular Integrity. An intrinsic vulnerability of certain cerebellar capillaries was suggested by Wigglesworth and Husemeyer.[50] Thus, the rich capillary beds of the subpial region and the core of the cerebellar folia are in "a continual process of remodeling," especially in the premature infant. These vessels may be expected to be vulnerable to rupture.

Subependymal and Subpial Germinal Matrix Vessels. Germinal matrices—richly vascularized structures—are present in the cerebellum. In the premature infant, they occur in the subependymal region around the fourth ventricle, and in both the premature and term infant, they are present in the subpial, external granule layer. The latter layer is especially prominent in the premature infant (see Chapter 4). In the perinatal period, the subependymal region provides glial precursors for migration to cerebellar white matter, and the external granule layer provides neuronal precursors for migration to the internal granule cell layer. These structures and their capillaries are in various stages of involution and, presumably, may be more vulnerable to rupture.

Internal Granule Cell Layer. The internal granule cell layer is one of the most highly vascularized areas of the brain and one of the major regions where cerebellar hemorrhages appear to originate in premature infants.[31] Vessels at the white matter-internal granule cell layer interface are immature during this vulnerable developmental period due to the rapid angiogenesis that is occurring to support the rapidly expanding internal granule cell population.

Hypoxia-Ischemia. As discussed in Chapter 24 (the section on IVH), hypoxic-ischemic brain insults may predispose to secondary parenchymal hemorrhage. There are a number of potential pathways through which this could occur, including reperfusion injury to the vasculature, loss of cerebral pressure-flow autoregulation, and disturbances in the coagulation cascade. In a recent study of severe hypoxic-ischemic encephalopathy in term infants, hemorrhagic cerebellar injury (by susceptibility-weighted MRI) was present in 18% of cases.[37] Other studies have also reported cerebellar hemorrhage[16,35] in hypoxic-ischemic encephalopathy with extensive cerebellar and vermis injury.

Extravascular Factors

Tear of Cerebellar Parenchyma and Vessels: Compliant Skull. The distortion of vessels discussed earlier concerning the infant's compliant skull could result in rupture by direct effects, rather than, or in addition to, the effects on venous pressure. Similarly, these compressive forces could cause upward cerebellar herniation, particularly of the superior vermis into the tentorial notch, with resulting contusion or laceration. The cerebellar vermis is an important site of the origin of cerebellar hemorrhage in the term infant.

Poor Vascular Support: Subependymal and Subpial Germinal Matrix Regions. The subependymal and subpial germinal matrices described earlier are gelatinous regions that provide poor support for the small vessels that course through them. Presumably, this deficiency of extravascular support encourages rupture.

Extension From Intraventricular Hemorrhage. The reasons for the apparent capacity of blood within the fourth ventricle and subarachnoid space of the posterior fossa to dissect into the cerebellum in certain cases are unclear (see earlier). Moreover, the precise frequency of this cause of *cerebellar* hemorrhage is not known; the 50% frequency suggested by Donat et al.[2] is probably too high. In a large ultrasonographic series, although 77% of cerebellar hemorrhages in premature infants were associated with IVH, the hemorrhages were relatively small in about one-half of these.[8] More recent reports of cerebellar hemorrhage detected by conventional MRI corroborate the high prevalence of concomitant IVH (in ~2/3 cases) described in previous studies.[10,22] Conversely, Gano et al.[27] reported that cerebellar hemorrhage occurred primarily in the absence of IVH. Nevertheless, in those cases of cerebellar hemorrhage with large IVH, the three factors of potential importance in permitting the extension of blood into the cerebellum relate to (1) the state of development of the cerebellum (e.g., incomplete myelination of cerebellar white matter and the presence of the external granule cell layer), (2) a large quantity of blood associated with the IVH, and (3) increased intracranial pressure, especially within the fourth ventricle and subarachnoid space of the posterior fossa.

Clinical Features

The clinical syndrome varies considerably according to the size of the lesion and the gestational age of the infant.[a] In

---

[a]References 1, 5, 8, 13, 16, 33, 34, 38-40, 50, and 51.

term infants with major degrees of hemorrhage, onset of clinical symptoms in the first 24 hours has been most common. The neurological syndrome is composed most consistently of signs of brain stem compression, especially apnea or respiratory irregularities (within 12 hours of birth), sometimes with bradycardia, and of obstruction to cerebrospinal fluid (CSF) flow, especially full fontanelle, separated sutures, and moderately dilated ventricles on CT/MRI or ultrasound scan. The need for neurosurgical intervention (e.g., hematoma evacuation, ventriculoperitoneal shunt placement) has been described.[35] Careful examination has also revealed specific additional signs of brain stem dysfunction (e.g., skew deviation of eyes, facial paresis, intermittent tonic extension of limbs, opisthotonos, and degrees of quadriparesis).[5,35,39-41] Seizures may occur within the first 36 hours of life. Neonatal mortality is as high as 10% in these infants.[35]

The most rapid progression of signs has occurred *with large lesions in small premature infants* who soon died, most within 36 hours of the onset of deterioration.[1,3,6,13] However, in recent years, with detection of the many *smaller lesions in premature infants*, clinical signs referable to the brain stem are subtle or nonexistent, and cerebellar hemorrhage tends to be clinically silent and detected primarily by US and/or MRI.[8,12] Clinical seizures[52] and unexplained motor agitation have been described in a subset of premature infants in the days preceding the diagnosis of cerebellar hemorrhage.[53]

Diagnosis

The essential issue in the recognition of cerebellar hemorrhage is a high index of suspicion. Clinical signs referable to brain stem dysfunction or increased intracranial pressure or both (see the section on clinical features) should provoke careful *ultrasound scan* through the *mastoid window*. With this approach, larger lesions are readily detected. However, smaller lesions may be missed and false positive diagnoses may occur (see Figs. 23.8 and 23.9). The sensitivity and specificity of cranial ultrasound compared with MRI for posterior fossa findings are 18% and 100%, respectively. When incorporating the mastoid view, the sensitivity of ultrasound increased to 45% while specificity was 100% (see Table 23.2).[54] The cerebellum, especially the vermis, is normally quite echogenic; careful attention to any lack of symmetry in echogenicity is important in the diagnosis of hemorrhage. (Posterior fossa subdural hemorrhage may be difficult to distinguish from intrinsic cerebellar hemorrhage by ultrasound scan,[55] although multiple parasagittal views or imaging through the posterior fontanelle are useful.) Early detection of cerebellar hemorrhage is clinically important, as infants are at increased risk of developing posthemorrhagic ventricular dilatation, requiring serial US examinations and neurosurgical intervention.[37,56]

An *MRI scan* is necessary to define the extent and distribution of the lesion most decisively. MRI is especially valuable for assessment of the anatomy of both the posterior fossa and the supratentorial structures. Its increased sensitivity in detecting smaller cerebellar hemorrhages in preterm and full-term infants has led to its increasing use.[10,22,35,37,54]

Prognosis

The outcome in *premature infants* with the largest lesions was initially reported to be poor. The earlier series of cases reported were identified at postmortem examination.[1,3,6,13] Subsequently,

six premature infants with cerebellar hemorrhage were identified during life, either by CT[38] or by ultrasound scan,[5,52,57] and all died, often with complicating systemic illness. However, with the detection of the more typical smaller hemorrhages by US through the mastoid window in the small premature infant, it has become clear that the outcome is not dire. In more recent series, the mortality rate ranged from 14% to 50%, although the survivors demonstrated greater neonatal morbidities, including longer requirements for supplemental oxygen, mechanical ventilation, and days in the neonatal intensive care unit, as well as a high incidence of gastrointestinal perforation and retinopathy of prematurity ≥stage III.[8,17,50,58] Some of the latter outcomes, of course, are not related directly to the cerebellar hemorrhage.

In studies of premature infants with longer follow-up and probably somewhat larger lesions, neurological deficits ranged from 30% to 100% and included gross and fine motor delays, cerebral palsy, and movement disorders.[32,50,58-62] Children with more extensive cerebellar hemorrhages had significantly worse neurological outcomes. In view of the growing awareness of cerebellum in cognitive and social-behavioral functions, it is of great interest that recent data show that affected small premature infants exhibit cognitive deficits, (40% to 100%) and language impairments (40% to 77%).[29,61] Moreover, approximately 35% have behavioral problems and autism spectrum disorders. It is noteworthy that socialization difficulties and a positive autism screening (42%) were almost exclusively associated with injury to the vermis in one careful study.[61] *Collectively, these studies point to a prevalent developmental form of the cerebellar cognitive affective*[63] *syndrome similar to that previously described in adults.*[64] Schmahmann and Sherman[65] provided the first comprehensive description of the "cerebellar cognitive-affective syndrome," a syndrome of "higher-order" dysfunction following cerebellar injury in adults with discrete cerebellar injury; this syndrome included executive, visual-spatial, and linguistic dysfunction, as well as impaired attention.[65] In fact, a functional topography of the cerebellum has been proposed based on its widespread anatomical connections with the cerebral cortex and recent neuroimaging investigations (Fig. 23.11).[66-76] Supporting this concept, these functional subregions of the cerebellum at a hemispheric, lobular, and nuclear level[77-79] provide a framework for understanding the *role of the developing cerebellum in motor, cognitive, language, and social-affective skills.* Notably, these developmental consequences include *cerebellar connections to the cerebrum.* In premature infants, recent studies have demonstrated that isolated, discrete cerebellar hemorrhage is associated with subsequent impairment of regional and remote neocortical circuits in the cerebrum. Specifically, when compared with the cerebral hemisphere ipsilateral to the injured cerebellar hemisphere, cerebral cortical gray matter, dorsolateral prefrontal, premotor, sensorimotor, midtemporal, and inferior occipital volumes are reduced.[80] These remote regional effects also predicted domain-specific functional deficits in these children. A study by Limperopoulos et al.[30] in premature infants with cerebellar hemorrhage showed a significant association between early signs of autism spectrum disorders and dorsolateral prefrontal volume, between gross motor scores and sensorimotor volumes, and between cognitive and language scores, and premotor and midtemporal volumes. Each unit increase in the corresponding regional cerebral volume was associated with lower odds of an abnormal outcome score, adjusted for age at

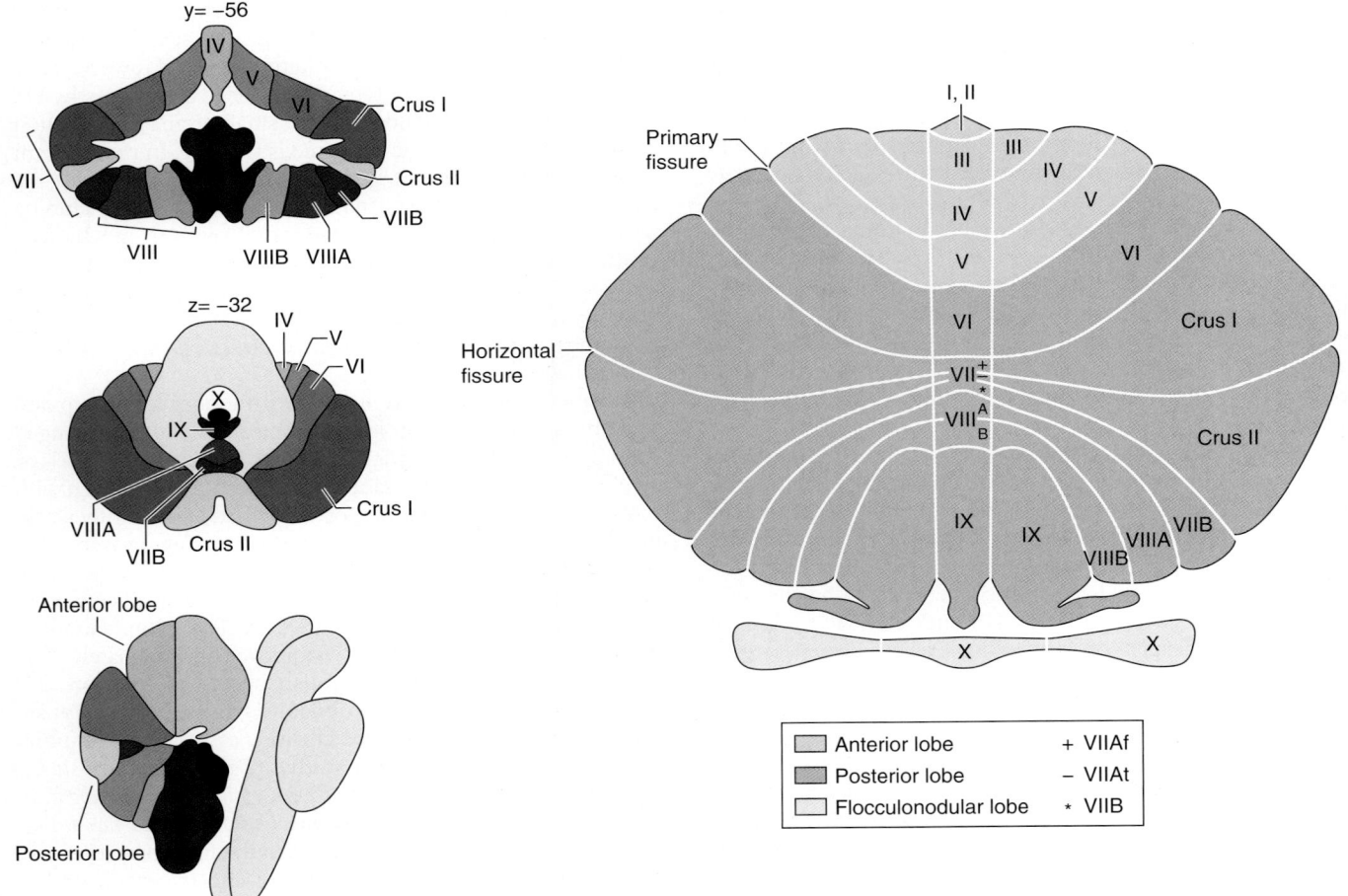

Figure 23.11 Cerebellar anatomy. *(Upper)* Cerebellar lobules shown in coronal, axial, and sagittal slices from the Spatially Unbiased Infra-tentorial Template (SUIT) cerebellar atlas; individual lobules are labeled and color-coded. *(Lower)* Flattened cerebellum showing lobules I–X, including the subdivisions of lobule VII (Crus I, Crus II, VIIB) and lobule VIII (VIIIA and VIIIB); the anterior (lobules I–V), posterior (lobules VI–IX), and flocculonodular (lobule X) lobes of the cerebellum are shown. (From Stoodley CJ, Limperopoulos C. Structure–function relationships in the developing cerebellum: evidence from early-life cerebellar injury and neurodevelopmental disorders. *Semin Fetal Neonatal Med.* 2016;21:356–364.)

MRI and contralateral cerebellar volume. This phenomenon of changes in cerebral volumes in the presence of cerebellar injury has been termed *developmental diaschisis*, which is likely related to the interruption of transsynaptic trophic interactions between the cerebellum and cerebrum, which are normally maintained by appropriate activation through afferent neural pathways. *These studies suggest that preterm cerebellar hemorrhage results in the disruption of selective supratentorial neural systems with a loss of neuronal activation, which is critical for development.*

The outcome in *term infants* in general has been characterized by a high likelihood of subsequent neurological deficits. In two earlier series, of the 10 infants identified during life by CT,[38-41] all survived. All four infants were treated surgically in one series,[38] and none of six was treated surgically in the other series.[39-41] Of the 10 infants, all have subsequent neurological deficits, especially motor, with consistent but variable involvement of intellect. Approximately one-half of both surgically treated and nontreated infants developed hydrocephalus, which required ventriculoperitoneal shunts. In a later series of 10 infants, neurological deficits were present

in the majority of survivors.[16] In one carefully studied group of six term infants evaluated at a mean age of 32 months, five had prominent deficits relative to cerebellar disturbance, including intention tremor, dysmetria, truncal ataxia, and hypotonia.[41] Such deficits were confirmed in a later series.[34,35] A large, more recent study reported wide-ranging disabilities including expressive language delays (44%), behavioral difficulties (~40%), and cognitive deficits (~30%).[35] Children with larger cerebellar hemorrhages that resulted in cerebellar hemispheric and vermian atrophy or both, have significantly greater motor, cognitive, behavioral, and expressive language deficits, compared to those with small cerebellar lesions. Undoubtedly, these clinical phenomena relate to the destruction of cerebellar tissue, and perhaps to subsequent aberrations of cerebellar development. Recall that inward migration of external granule cells to the internal granule cell layer is active in the neonatal period and subsequently in early infancy. Other neurological deficits observed (e.g., cerebral palsy) may relate to the frequently associated supratentorial lesions (see earlier discussion).

Management

Early detection by ultrasound scan, CT, or MRI is critical. A high index of suspicion is important. The most difficult issue relates to the decision concerning surgical intervention. Important determining factors include size and location of the hemorrhage, rapidity of neurological deterioration, and seriousness of pulmonary or other systemic disorders that could preclude anesthesia and major surgery. Numerous reports document survival after surgical evacuation by posterior fossa craniotomy in *full-term infants*.[34,38,81-83] However, Fishman et al.[39-41] documented survival with no worse neurological sequelae in six full-term infants who were treated with medical support alone. Thus, surgery is not obligatory and, in fact, is probably not indicated unless the infant's neurological status fails to stabilize. Placement of a ventriculoperitoneal shunt is necessary in nearly one-half of affected infants, with or without surgical evacuation. Even during the neonatal period, temporary ventriculostomy may be necessary for infants with acute hydrocephalus that occurs before resolution of the obstructing cerebellar hematoma.[39-41]

The appropriate therapeutic approach to the *premature infant* is not fully established. Preventative interventions relate to the management of labor, delivery, and the sick, ventilated infant, as described in Chapter 24, for intraventricular hemorrhage. Infants with large lesions should be followed for progression as noted for term infants. However, surgery is particularly problematic in very small infants, who, unfortunately, are also the most likely to exhibit cerebellar hemorrhage. Most lesions currently identified in premature infants have not required surgical intervention. A recent report showed that antenatal magnesium sulfate exposure in preterm infants of less than 33 weeks' gestation was associated with decreased MRI-detected cerebellar hemorrhage but not with other types of preterm brain injuries.[27] These data suggest that magnesium sulfate promotes some degree of neuroprotection. Further studies are needed to confirm these initial findings and identify other modifiable risk factors for cerebellar hemorrhage in the preterm infant.

REFERENCES

1. Grunnet ML, Shields WD. Cerebellar hemorrhage in the premature infant. *J Pediatr.* 1976;88:605-608.
2. Donat JF, Okazaki H, Kleinberg F. Cerebellar hemorrhages in newborn infants. *Am J Dis Child.* 1979;133:441.
3. Martin R, Roessmann U, Fanaroff A. Massive intracerebellar hemorrhage in low-birth-weight infants. *J Pediatr.* 1976;89:290-293.
4. Flodmark O, Becker LE, Harwood-Nash DC, et al. Correlation between computed tomography and autopsy in premature and full-term neonates that have suffered perinatal asphyxia. *Radiology.* 1980;137:93-103.
5. Perlman JM, Nelson JS, McAlister WH, et al. Intracerebellar hemorrhage in a premature newborn: diagnosis by real-time ultrasound and correlation with autopsy findings. *Pediatrics.* 1983;71:159-162.
6. Pape KE, Armstrong DL, Fitzhardinge PM. Central nervous system pathology associated with mask ventilation in the very low birthweight infant: a new etiology for intracerebellar hemorrhages. *Pediatrics.* 1976;58:473-483.
7. Bejar R, Coen RW, Ekpoudia I, et al. Real time ultrasound diagnosis of hemorrhagic pathological conditions in the posterior fossa of preterm neonates. *Neurosurgery.* 1985;16:281-289.
8. Limperopoulos C, Benson C, Bassan H, et al. Cerebellar hemorrhage in the preterm infant; ultrasonographic characteristics and risk factors. *Pediatrics.* 2005;116:717-724.
9. Merrill JD, Piecuch RE, Fell SC, et al. A new pattern of cerebellar hemorrhages in preterm infants. *Pediatrics.* 1998;102:E62.
10. Steggerda SJ, Leijser LM, Wiggers-de Bruine FT, et al. Cerebellar injury in preterm infants: incidence and findings on US and MR images. *Radiology.* 2009;252:190-199.
11. Di Salvo DN. A new view of the neonatal brain: clinical utility of supplemental neurologic US imaging windows. *Radiographics.* 2001;21:943-955.
12. Steggerda S, van Wezel-Meijler G. Cranial ultrasonography of the immature cerebellum: role and limitations. *Semin Fetal Neonatal Med.* 2016;21:295-304.
13. Shuman RM, Oliver TK. Face masks defended. *Pediatrics.* 1976;58:621.
14. Papile LA, Burstein J, Burstein R, et al. Incidence and evolution of subependymal and intraventricular hemorrhage: a study of infants with birth weights less than 1,500 gm. *J Pediatr.* 1978;92:529-534.
15. Ahmann PA, Lazzara A, Dykes FD, et al. Intraventricular hemorrhage in the high-risk preterm infant: incidence and outcome. *Ann Neurol.* 1980;7:118-124.
16. Miall LS, Cornette LG, Tanner SF, et al. Posterior fossa abnormalities seen on magnetic resonance brain imaging in a cohort of newborn infants. *J Perinatol.* 2003;23:396-403.
17. Steggerda S, De Bruine F, van den Berg-Huysmans A, et al. Small cerebellar hemorrhage in preterm infants: perinatal and postnatal factors and outcome. *Cerebellum.* 2013;12:794-801.
18. Correa F, Enriquez G, Rossello J, et al. Posterior fontanelle sonography: an acoustic window into the neonatal brain. *AJNR Am J Neuroradiol.* 2004;25:1274-1282.
19. Barkovich AJ. *Pediatric Neuroimaging.* 4th ed. Philadelphia: Lippincott Williams & Wilkins; 2005.
20. Deleted in review.
21. Soudack M, Jacobson J, Raviv-Zilka L, et al. Cerebellar hemorrhage in very low birth weight premature infants: the advantage of the posterolateral fontanelle view. *J Clin Ultrasound.* 2013;41:395-401.
22. Neubauer V, Djurdjevic T, Griesmaier E, et al. Routine magnetic resonance imaging at term-equivalent age detects brain injury in 25% of a contemporary cohort of very preterm infants. *PLoS ONE.* 2017;12:e0169442.
23. Parodi A, Morana G, Severino M, et al. Low-grade interaventricular hemorrhage: is ultrasound good enough? *J Matern Fetal Neonatal Med.* 2015;28:2261-2264.
24. Van Kooij B, Benders M, Anbeek P, et al. Cerebellar volume and proton magnetic resonance spectroscopy at term, and neurodevelopment at 2 years of age in preterm infants. *Dev Med Child Neurol.* 2012;54:260-266.
25. Kidokoro H, Anderson P, Doyle L, et al. Brain injury and altered brain growth in preterm infants: predictors and prognosis. *Pediatrics.* 2014;134:e444-e453.
26. Kim H, Gano D, Ho M, et al. Hindbrain regional growth in preterm newborns and its impairment in relation to brain injury. *Hum Brain Mapp.* 2016;37:678-688.
27. Gano D, Ho ML, Partridge JC, Glass HC, et al. Antenatal exposure to magnesium sulfate is associated with reduced cerebellar hemorrhage in preterm infants. *J Pediatr.* 2016;178:68-74.
28. Bodensteiner JB, Johnsen SD. Cerebellar injury in the extremely premature infant: newly recognized but relatively common outcome. *J Child Neurol.* 2005;20:139-142.
29. Johnsen SD, Bodensteiner JB, Lotze TE. Frequency and nature of cerebellar injury in the extremely premature survivor with cerebral palsy. *J Child Neurol.* 2005;20:60-64.
30. Limperopoulos C, Chilingaryan G, Sullivan N, et al. Injury to the premature cerebellum: outcome is related to remote cortical development. *Cereb Cortex.* 2014;24:728-736.
31. Haines K, Wang W, Pierson C. Cerebellar hemorrhagic injury in premature infants occurs during a vulnerable developmental period and is associated with wider neuropathology. *Acta Neuropathol Commun.* 2013;1:69.
32. Mercuri E, He J, Curati W, et al. Cerebellar infarction and atrophy in infants and children with a history of premature birth. *Pediatr Radiol.* 1997;27:139-143.
33. Hanigan WC, Powell FC, Miller TC, et al. Symptomatic intracranial hemorrhage in full-term infants. *Childs Nerv Syst.* 1995;11:698-707.
34. Perrin RG, Rutka JT, Drake JM, et al. Management and outcomes of posterior fossa subdural hematomas in neonates. *Neurosurgery.* 1997;40:1190-1199.

35. Limperopoulos C, Robertson R, Sullivan N, et al. Cerebellar injury in term infants: clinical characteristics, magnetic resonance imaging findings, and outcome. *Pediatr Neurol.* 2009;41:1-8.

36. Melbourne L, Chang T, Murnick J, et al. Clinical impact of term-equivalent magnetic resonance imaging in extremely low-birth-weight infants at a regional NICU. *J Perinatol.* 2016;36:985-989.

37. Steggerda S, de Bruine F, Smits-Wintjens V, et al. Posterior fossa abnormalities in high-risk term infants: comparison of ultrasound and MRI. *Eur Radiol.* 2015;25:2575-2583.

38. Scotti G, Flodmark O, Harwood-Nash D, et al. Posterior fossa hemorrhages in the newborn. *J Comput Assist Tomogr.* 1981;5:68.

39. Fishman MA, Percy AK, Cheek WR, et al. Successful conservative management of cerebellar hematomas in term neonates. *J Pediatr.* 1981;98:466.

40. Cheek WR, Fishman MA, Speer ME. Cerebellar hemorrhage in the term neonate. *Pediatr Neurosurg.* 1985;5:48.

41. Williamson WD, Percy AK, Fishman MA. Cerebellar hemorrhage in the term neonate: developmental and neurologic outcome. *Pediatr Neurol.* 1985;1:356-360.

42. Calkins H, Shyr Y, Frumin H, et al. The value of the clinical history in the differentiation of syncope due to ventriculr tachycardia, atrioventricular block, and neurocardiogenic syncope. *Am J Med.* 1995;98:365-373.

43. McPherson C, Neil J, Tjoeng T, et al. A pilot randomized trial of high-dose caffeine therapy in preterm infants. *Pediatr Res.* 2015;78:198-204.

44. Sehgal A, El-Naggar W, Glanc P, et al. Risk factors and ultrasonographic profile of posterior fossa haemorrhages in preterm infants. *J Paediatr Child Health.* 2009;45:215-218.

45. Pape KE, Wigglesworth JS. *Haemorrhage, Ischaemia and the Perinatal Brain.* Philadelphia: JB Lippincott; 1979.

46. Newton TH, Gooding CA. Compression of superior sagittal sinus by neonatal calvarial molding. *Radiology.* 1975;115:635-640.

47. Chaou WT, Chou ML, Eitzman DV. Intracranial hemorrhage and vitamin K deficiency in early infancy. *J Pediatr.* 1984;105:880.

48. Dave P, Curless RG, Steinman L. Cerebellar hemorrhage complicating methylmalonic and proprionic acidemia. *Arch Neurol.* 1984;41:298.

49. Fischer AQ, Challa VR, Burton BK, et al. Cerebellar hemorrhage complicating isovaleric acidemia: a case report. *Neurology.* 1981;31:746.

50. Zayek M, Benjamin J, Maertens P, et al. Cerebellar hemorrhage: a major morbidity in extremely preterm infants. *J Perinatol.* 2012;32:699-704.

51. Fishman M. Personal communication; 1993 (oral).

52. McCarthy L, Donoghue V, Murphy J. Ultrasonically detectable cerebellar haemorrhage in preterm infants. *Arch Dis Child Fetal Neonatal Ed.* 2011;96:F281-F295.

53. Ecury-Goossen G, Dudink J, Lequin M, et al. The clinical presentation of preterm cerebellar haemorrhage. *Eur J Pediatr.* 2010;169:1249-1253.

54. Steggerda S, De Bruine F, Smits-Wintjens V, et al. Ultrasound detection of posterior fossa abnormalities in full-term neonates. *Early Hum Dev.* 2012;88:233-239.

55. Grant EG, Schellinger D, Richardson JD. Real-time ultrasonography of the posterior fossa. *J Ultrasound Med.* 1983;2:73.

56. Limperopoulos C, Folkerth R, Barnewolt CE, et al. Posthemorrhagic cerebellar disruption mimicking Dandy-Walker malformation: fetal imaging and neuropathology findings. *Semin Pediatr Neurol.* 2010;17:75-81.

57. Reeder JD, Setzer ES, Kaude JV. Ultrasonographic detection of perinatal intracerebellar hemorrhage. *Pediatrics.* 1982;70:385.

58. Bednarek N, Akhavi A, Pietrement C, et al. Outcome of cerebellar injury in very low birth-weight infants: 6 case reports. *J Child Neurol.* 2008;23:906-911.

59. Messerschmidt A, Fuiko R, Prayer D, et al. Disrupted cerebellar development in preterm infants is associated with impaired neurodevelopmental outcome. *Eur J Pediatr.* 2008;167:1141-1147.

60. Tam E, Miller S, Studholme C, et al. Differential effects of intraventricular hemorrhage and white matter injury on preterm cerebellar growth. *J Pediatr.* 2011;158:366-371.

61. Limperopoulos C, Bassan H, Gauvreau K, et al. Does cerebellar injury in premature infants contribute to the high prevalence of long-term cognitive, learning, and behavioral disability in survivors? *Pediatrics.* 2007;120:584-593.

62. Dyet L, Kennea N, Counsel S, et al. Natural history of brain lesions in extremely preterm infants studied with serial magnetic resonance imaging from birth and neurodevelopmental assessment. *Pediatrics.* 2006;118:536-548.

63. Brossard-Racine M, du Plessis A, Limperopoulos C. Developmental cerebellar cognitive affective syndrome in ex-preterm survivors following cerebellar injury. *Cerebellum.* 2015;14:151-164.

64. Schmahmann J, Sherman J. The cerebellar cognitive affective syndrome. *Brain.* 1998;121:561-579.

65. Schmahmann J, Sherman J. Cerebellar cognitive affective syndrome. *Int Rev Neurobiol.* 1997;41:433-440.

66. Ramnani N. The primate cortico-cerebellar system: anatomy and function. *Nat Rev Neurosci.* 2006;7:511-522.

67. Wedeen V, Hagmann P, Tseng W, et al. Mapping complex tissue architecture with diffusion spectrum magnetic resonance imaging. *Magn Reson Med.* 2005;54:1377-1386.

68. Rorden C, Karnath H, Bonilha L. Improving lesion-symptom mapping. *J Cogn Neurosci.* 2007;19:1081-1088.

69. Adams W, Sheslow D. *The Wide Range Assessment of Visual-Motor Abilities.* Wilmington: Wide Range, Inc.; 1995.

70. Gioia G, Espy K, Isquith P. *The Behavior Rating Inventory of Executive Function-Preschool Version (BRIEF-P).* Odessa: Psychological Assessment Resource; 2003.

71. Dimitrova A, Weber J, Redies C, et al. MRI atlas of the human cerebellar nuclei. *Neuroimage.* 2002;17:240-255.

72. Mori S, Van Zijl P. Fiber tracking: principles and strategies—a technical review. *NMR Biomed.* 2002;15:468-480.

73. Wakana S, Jiang H, Nagae-Poetscher L, et al. Fiber tract-based atlas of human white matter anatomy. *Radiology.* 2004;230:77-87.

74. Mamata H, Mamata Y, Westin C, et al. High-resolution line scan diffusion tensor MR imaging of white matter fiber tract anatomy. *AJNR Am J Neuroradiol.* 2002;23:67-75.

75. Counsell S, Dyet L, Larkman D, et al. Thalamo-cortical connectivity in children born preterm mapped using probabilistic magnetic resonance tractography. *Neuroimage.* 2007;34:896-904.

76. Stoodley C, Limperopoulos C. Structure-function relationships in the developing cerebellum: evidence from early-life cerebellar injury and neurodevelopmental disorders. *Semin Fetal Neonatal Med.* 2016;21:356-364.

77. Clausi S, Bozzali M, Leggio M, et al. Quanitification of gray matter changes in the cerebral cortex after isolated cerebellar damage: a voxel-based morphometry study. *Neuroscience.* 2009;162:827-835.

78. Kim S, Ugurbil K, Strick P. Activation of a cerebellar output nucleus during cognitive processing. *Science.* 1994;265:949-951.

79. Deistung A, Stefanescu M, Ernst T, et al. Structural and functional magnetic resonance imaging of the cerebellum: considerations for assessing cerebellar ataxias. *Cerebellum.* 2016;15:21-25.

80. Limperopoulos C, Chilingaryan G, Guizard N, et al. Cerebellar injury in the premature infant is associated with impaired growth of specific cerebral regions. *Pediatr Res.* 2010;68:145-150.

81. Odeku EL, Adcock KJ. Neonatal hydrocephalus due to intracerebellar hematoma. *Int Surg.* 1969;51:302.

82. Schreiber MS. Posterior fossa (cerebellar) haematoma in the newborn. *Med J Aust.* 1963;2:713.

83. Rom S, Serfontein GL, Humphreys RP. Intracerebellar hematoma in the neonate. *J Pediatr.* 1978;93:486.

Preterm Intraventricular Hemorrhage/ Posthemorrhagic Hydrocephalus

Terrie E. Inder ◆ Jeffrey M. Perlman ◆ Joseph J. Volpe

Germinal matrix hemorrhage–intraventricular hemorrhage (GMH-IVH) is the most common variety of neonatal intracranial hemorrhage and is characteristic of the premature infant.[1] The importance of the lesion relates not only to its high incidence but also to the essential gravity of the larger forms of IVH and their attendant complications. Moreover, the major forms of brain injury of the premature infant occur most commonly in the context of IVH, either as an apparent consequence of the IVH or as an associated finding.

The *magnitude of the problem* of IVH in the premature infant relates to the relatively high and unchanging incidence of prematurity, the relatively high survival rates of premature infants, and the relatively high incidence of IVH. Thus, in the approximately four decades from the 1970s to the present in the United States, the proportion of live births born as very low birthweight (VLBW), weighing less than 1500 g increased from 1.17% to 1.45%.[2-5] In the last decade since 2006, a modest reduction in the incidence of preterm birth has been predominantly due to a reduction in late preterm births (infants between 34 and 36 weeks' gestation), with no reduction in the incidence of VLBW infants.[6] In 2012, 11.55% of infants were born preterm (gestational age at birth <37 weeks), with nearly 8% weighing less than 2500 g (defined as low birthweight—LBW), 1.42% weighing less than 1500 g (VLBW), and 0.7% weighing less than 1000 g (defined as extremely low birthweight—ELBW).

In view of the approximately 4 million live births each year in the United States, approximately 55,000 VLBW infants, of which nearly one-half are ELBW infants, will be born each year in this country alone. This number of VLBW and ELBW infants born each year over the last two decades has not changed.[6] However, there has been a continual decline in mortality rates,[7-18] such that approximately 90% of infants between 500 and 1500 g birthweight survive the neonatal period.[19] Indeed, even among infants of birthweights 500 to 1000 g, current survival rates are approximately 70%,[19-22] although there is variation noted internationally.[19] The greatest improvements in survival over the last decade have been among those infants born at less than 28 weeks' gestation, notably those also at high risk for IVH. Between 1993 and 2013 within the United States, the survival for infants at 25 to 28 weeks' gestation increased approximately 2% at each gestational age per year.[23] The increased survival was accompanied by an increased use of antenatal corticosteroids and delivery by cesarean section for infants less than 28 weeks' gestation.[18,24] With *increasing survival in these most immature infants at greatest risk for IVH, the absolute number of infants affected by IVH within the United States alone is close to 10,000 infants each year.*

The *incidence* of IVH in premature infants, although lower than it was two decades ago, is high (Table 24.1). In six well-studied series of premature infants (total of ≈1200) subjected to routine computed tomography (CT) or ultrasound scans and studied in the late 1970s and early 1980s, the incidence generally ranged from 40% to 50%.[25-30] Among this group, a local series of 460 infants (birthweight <2250 g) had an incidence of IVH of 39%.[29] However, subsequently, the incidence of IVH in the mid-1980s in the same unit for infants less than 2000 g birthweight was 29%.[31] Incidences derived from infants studied in the late 1980s were approximately 20%.[32-36] In the mid-1990s values generally were less than 20% and often approximately 15%.[1,37-40] However, over the 2000s, the incidence of IVH has remained unchanged, with an overall incidence for all IVH of 25% (Fig. 24.1).[13,15,17,41,42]

IVH has most frequently been graded as grades I–IV. The grading system most commonly used for IVH in the infant was first reported by Papile and colleagues[30] and is based on the presence of blood in the amount of blood in the germinal matrix and the lateral ventricles. Initially this classification was developed for CT scanning but is now commonly used for any form of neuroimaging (Fig. 24.2).

Grade I represents hemorrhage confined to the subependymal germinal matrix, grade II has hemorrhage within the lateral ventricles without ventricular dilatation, grade III IVH has hemorrhage with distention resulting in ventricular dilatation and/or hemorrhage occupying more than 50% of the ventricle, and grade IV IVH has parenchymal hemorrhage. Although grade IV IVH is a periventricular hemorrhagic infarction (see later) rather than an extension of IVH per se, most reports continue to classify the cranial ultrasound findings according to the earlier (Papile) classification system and use the term *grade IV IVH* for this severe lesion. Because the pathogenesis of grade IV IVH relates to the severity of the IVH per se (see later), the term has some merit. However, this term can also limit the understanding of the pathogenesis and outcomes of this lesion and is not preferred by us (see later).

In one of the largest reported series, 247,392 VLBW infants were observed between 2009 and 2013 from 917 neonatal intensive care units (NICUs) as part of the Vermont-Oxford Database (data provided from 2009 to 2013 from Vermont Oxford Network Database; see Figs. 24.1 and 24.3). Thus the incidence of all grades of IVH remained static over this 5-year period at 24% to 26%, with the incidence of the most

TABLE 24.1   High Incidence of Intraventricular Hemorrhage in Premature Infants[a]

YEARS OF STUDY	CRITERIA FOR INCLUSION	INCIDENCE (%)
Late 1970s–1980s	Premature: several different birthweights and gestational ages	40–50
Late 1980s	<1500 g	20
Late 1990s	<1500 g	15–20
Present	<1500 g	20–25

[a]See text for references; values for incidence are rounded off.

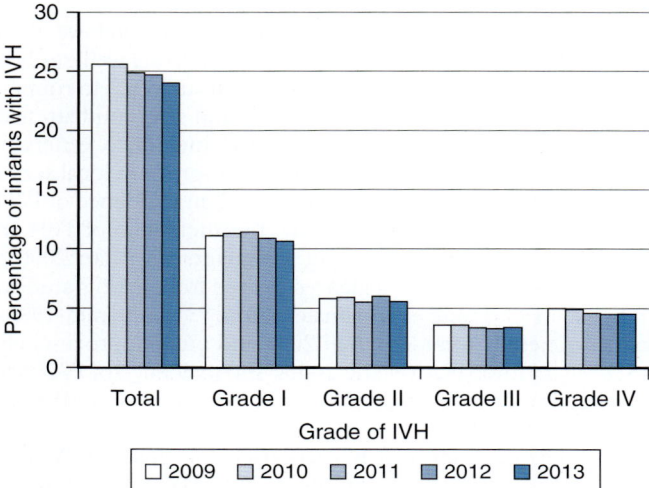

Figure 24.1 The percentage of very preterm infants with birthweight less than 1500 g with intraventricular hemorrhage (IVH) by year from 2009 to 2013. Data were collected from the Vermont-Oxford Network assessing approximately 55,000 very low-birthweight infants every year. Note that the percentage of infants with IVH has not significantly changed, although there is a small trend toward a reduction in 2012–13.

severe forms of IVH (grade III and IV) approximately 5%. It has been hypothesized that a true decline in the incidence of IVH may be hidden because of the fact that over the past 5 to 10 years there has been a greater number of extremely immature infants, with a higher risk of IVH, being resuscitated and surviving. However, the data from the Vermont-Oxford Database from 2009 to 2013 demonstrate that the percentage of preterm infants less than 750 g across this 5-year period was stable at 18%.

More recent data suggest that there may be a small decline in the risk of high-grade IVH for infants with gestational ages 26 to 28 weeks, with no change in the most immature infants of 22 to 25 weeks' gestation (Fig. 24.4).[23] This decline may be related to greater use of antenatal steroids, prophylactic indomethacin, and/or mode of delivery (see later). It has long been known that there is an increased risk for all forms of IVH in the most immature preterm infants (see Fig. 24.3).[31,37,40,43,44] For infants less than 750 g, the risk of *any* IVH is approximately threefold higher than for a preterm infant over 1250 g (42%

vs. 14%). The most immature infants also carry the greatest risk for the more severe forms of IVH, with a 10-fold higher risk of grade III–IV IVH (20% vs. 2.1%; see Fig. 24.3).[22] For an infant less than 750 g, an approximately equal risk exists for grades I through IV at about 10% (see Fig. 24.3).

In this chapter, the neuropathology, pathogenesis, clinical features, diagnosis, prognosis, and management of IVH and its complications will be reviewed. The prominent position of this lesion in neonatal medicine has been accompanied by a large increase in work from several disciplines. This chapter attempts to integrate this information in a meaningful way without oversimplifying a clearly complex problem.

NEUROPATHOLOGY

The neuropathology of IVH is best considered in terms of the site of origin (primarily the germinal matrix), the spread of the hemorrhage throughout the ventricular system, the neuropathological consequences of the hemorrhage, and the neuropathological accompaniments not necessarily related directly to the IVH.

The basic lesion in germinal matrix hemorrhage–IVH is bleeding into the subependymal germinal matrix. This region is represented by the ventricular-subventricular zone described in Chapter 6. Over the final 12 to 16 weeks of gestation, this matrix becomes less and less prominent and is essentially exhausted by term (see later discussion). This region is highly cellular, gelatinous in texture, and as would be expected for a structure with active cellular proliferation, richly vascularized. To understand the nature of IVH, it is useful to review first the arterial and venous supply to the germinal matrix.

Arterial Supply to Subependymal Germinal Matrix

The arterial supply to the subependymal germinal matrix is derived particularly from the anterior cerebral artery (through Heubner artery), the middle cerebral artery (primarily through the deep lateral striate branches but also through penetrating branches from surface meningeal branches), and the internal carotid artery (through the anterior choroidal artery; Fig. 24.5).[45,46] The relative importance of these arteries in the vascular supply to the capillaries of the matrix is not entirely clear; different studies have attributed particular importance to the Heubner artery[45,47] and to the lateral striate arteries.[48] However, it is likely that the terminal branches of this arterial supply constitute a vascular end zone and thus a vulnerability to ischemic injury.

Capillary Network

The rich arterial supply just described feeds an elaborate *capillary bed* in the germinal matrix.[45,47-52] This bed generally is composed of relatively large, irregular endothelial-lined vessels that do not exhibit the characteristics of arterioles or venules and are classified as capillaries or channels, or both. Pape and Wigglesworth[47] characterized the anatomical appearance as "a persisting immature vascular rete in the subependymal matrix which is only remodeled into a definite capillary bed when the germinal matrix disappears." As term approaches, some of the larger endothelial-lined vessels acquire a collagenous adventitial sheath[48] and can be categorized appropriately as veins,[51] as also described in the matrix of the monkey.[53] The nature of the endothelial-lined vessels in this microvascular

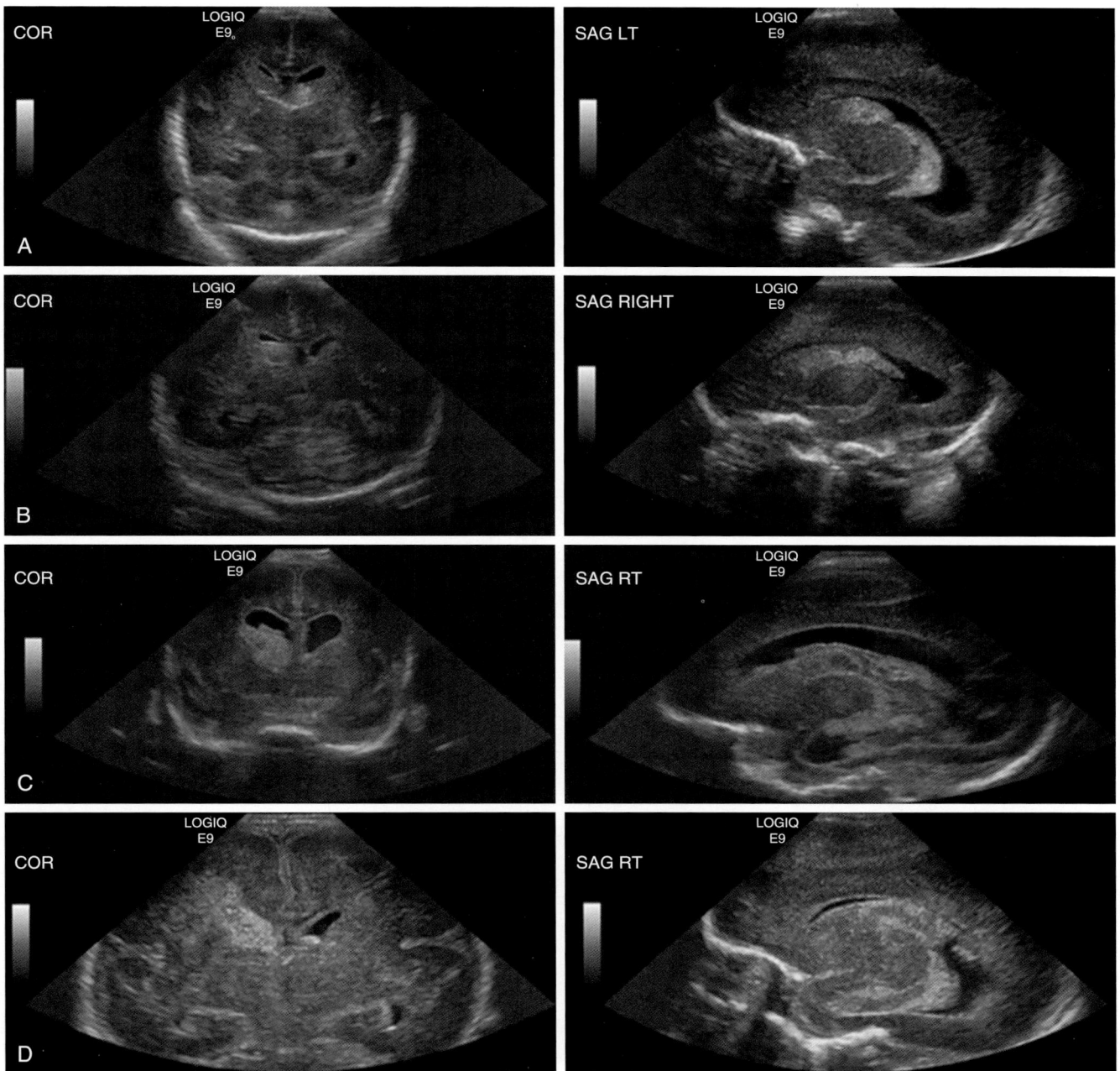

Figure 24.2 Grading of the severity of germinal maxtrix–intraventricular hemorrhage (IVH): coronal (COR) and parasagittal (SAG) ultrasound scans. (A) Germinal matrix hemorrhage—grade I; (B) intraventricular hemorrhage (note is filling less than 50% of the ventricular area)—grade II; (C) intraventricular hemorrhage with ventricular dilatation—grade III; (D) large intraventricular hemorrhage with associated parenchymal echogenicity (hemorrhagic infarct)—grade IV.

bed may be of pathogenetic importance concerning germinal matrix hemorrhage.

These germinal matrix vessels exhibit a variety of unique characteristics that may underlie the fragility and propensity to hemorrhage. These characteristics include exuberant angiogenesis, related to high vascular endothelial growth factor (VEGF) and angiopoietin levels, discontinuous glial endfeet of the blood-brain barrier, relative lack of pericytes, immature basal lamina characteristics, and developmentally regulated

expression of vascular wall characteristics, including molecules such as alkaline phosphatase, and high morphometric ratio of diameter to wall thickness.[54-58]

Venous Drainage of Subependymal Germinal Matrix

The rich microvascular network just described is continuous with a well-developed deep venous system. This venous drainage eventually terminates in the great cerebral vein of Galen

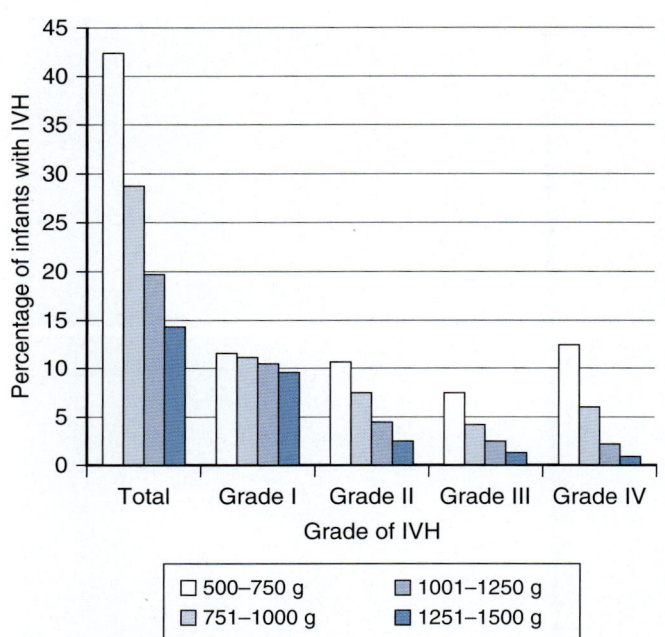

Figure 24.3 The percentage of very preterm infants with birthweight less than 1500 g with intraventricular hemorrhage (IVH) by birthweight groupings for 2013. Data were collected from the Vermont-Oxford Network, assessing approximately 55,000 very low birthweight infants every year.

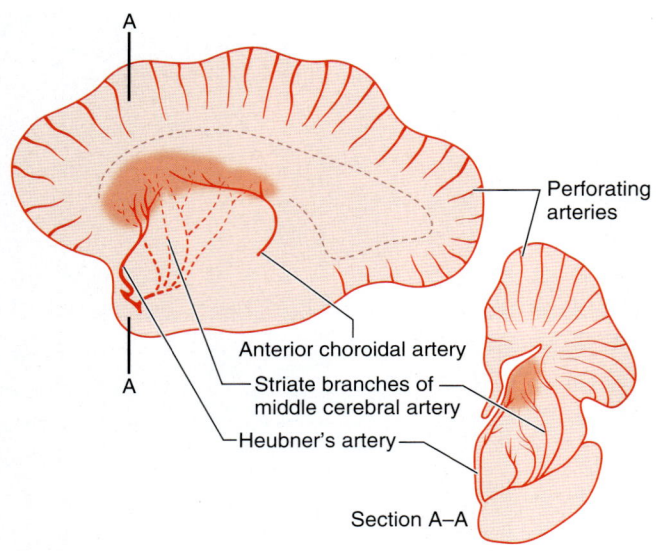

Figure 24.5 Arterial supply. Arterial supply to the subependymal germinal matrix at 29 weeks of gestation. (From Hambleton G, Wigglesworth JS. Origin of intraventricular haemorrhage in the preterm infant. *Arch Dis Child.* 1976;51: 651–659.)

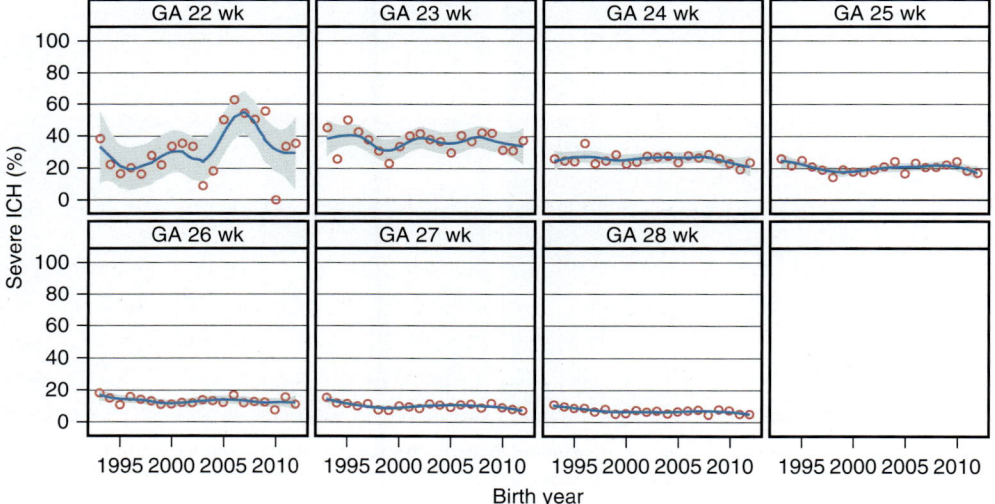

Figure 24.4 Severe intracranial hemorrhage (ICH) by birth year and gestational age (GA) for infants born at GA 22 to 28 weeks in Neonatal Research Network centers 1993–2012. In each graph, circles show the percent of infants born each year who were evaluated by cranial sonogram and diagnosed with grade 3 to 4 ICH, a smoothed curve shows the trend, and shading indicates a 95% CI for the curve. The year-GA interaction was significant, $P = .03$. Relative risks for the change per year were adjusted for study center, maternal race/ethnicity, infant GA, SGA, and sex. (From Stoll BJ, Hansen NI, Bell EF, Walsh MC, Carlo WA, Shankaran S, Laptook AR, Sánchez PJ, Van Meurs KP, Wyckoff M, Das A, Hale EC, Ball MB, Newman NS, Schibler K, Poindexter BB, Kennedy KA, Cotten CM, Watterberg KL, D'Angio CT, DeMauro SB, Truog WE, Devaskar U, Higgins RD; Eunice Kennedy Shriver National Institute of Child Health and Human Development Neonatal Research Network. Trends in care practices, morbidity, and mortality of extremely preterm neonates, 1993–2012. *JAMA.* 2015;314:1039–1051.)

(Fig. 24.6).[59] In addition to the matrix region, this venous system drains blood from the cerebral white matter, choroid plexus, striatum, and thalamus through the medullary, choroidal, thalamostriate, and terminal veins. Indeed, the terminal vein, which runs essentially within the germinal matrix, is the principal terminus of the medullary, choroidal, and thalamostriate veins. The latter three vessels course primarily *anteriorly* to a point of confluence at the level of the head of the caudate nucleus to form the terminal veins, which empty into the internal cerebral vein that courses directly *posteriorly* to join the vein of Galen. Thus at the usual site of germinal matrix hemorrhage,

the direction of blood flow changes in a peculiar U-turn. This feature may have pathogenetic implications (see later section). This venous anatomy is also relevant to the occurrence of periventricular hemorrhagic infarction (see later discussion).

Site of Origin and Spread of Intraventricular Hemorrhage

Site of Origin

The site of origin of IVH characteristically is the *subependymal germinal matrix* (Fig. 24.7). This cellular region immediately ventrolateral to the lateral ventricle serves as the source of cerebral excitatory neuronal precursors between approximately 10 to 20 weeks of gestation and in the second half of gestation provides neuroglial precursors that become cerebral oligodendroglia and astrocytes and late migrating GABAergic neurons destined for the cerebral cortex and, especially, the thalamus (see Unit I).[60-65] Indeed, elegant studies of Del Bigio showed exuberant proliferation of precursor cells in the germinal matrix until 28 weeks of gestation, with a rapid decline thereafter.[66] For reasons discussed earlier, the many thin-walled vessels in the matrix are a ready source of bleeding. The matrix undergoes progressive decrease in size, from a width of 2.5 mm at 23 to 24 weeks, to 1.4 mm at 32 weeks, to nearly complete involution by approximately 36 weeks.[43] The matrix from 28 to 32 weeks is most prominent in the thalamostriate groove at the level of the head of the caudate nucleus at the site of or slightly posterior to the foramen of Monro,[45,66-71] and this site is the most common for germinal matrix hemorrhage. Before 28 weeks, hemorrhage in persisting matrix over the body of the caudate nucleus may also be found. Hemorrhage from choroid plexus occurs in nearly 50% of infants with germinal matrix hemorrhage and IVH,[72] and in more mature infants especially, it may be the major site of origin of IVH (see Chapters 20 to 22).

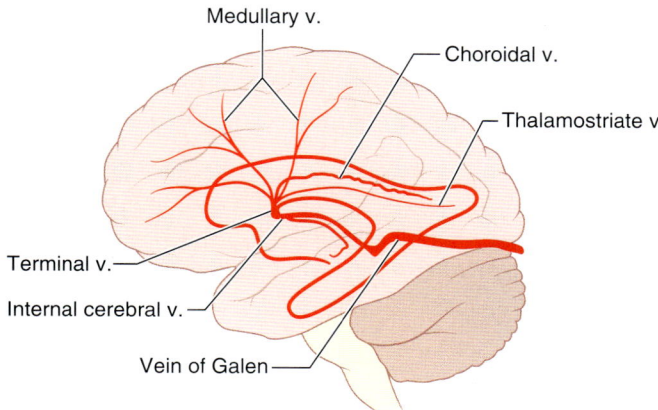

Figure 24.6 Veins of the Galenic system, midsagittal view. Note that the medullary, choroidal, and thalamostriate veins come to a point of confluence to form the terminal vein. The terminal vein, which courses through the germinal matrix, empties into the internal cerebral vein, and the major flow of blood changes direction sharply at that junction.

Labels in figure: Medullary v.; Choroidal v.; Thalamostriate v.; Terminal v.; Internal cerebral v.; Vein of Galen

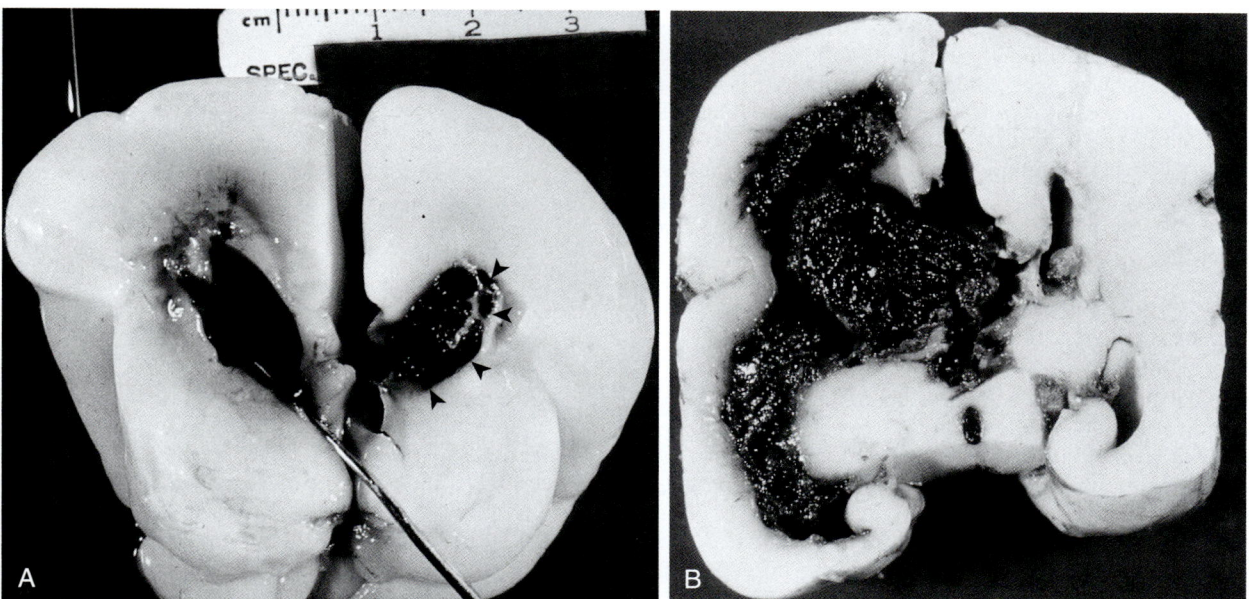

Figure 24.7 Germinal matrix–intraventricular hemorrhage. Coronal sections of cerebrum. (A) Germinal matrix hemorrhage *(arrowheads)* at the level of the head of the caudate nucleus and foramen of Monro (see probe), with rupture into the lateral ventricles. (B) Massive intraventricular hemorrhage. Obstruction at the foramen of Monro has caused severe, unilateral ventricular dilation.

The vascular *site of origin* of germinal matrix hemorrhage within the microcirculation of this region appears most commonly to be the prominent endothelial-lined vessels described earlier, not clearly arterial or venous.[45,51,67,71,73-75] Particular importance for vessels in free communication with the venous circulation (e.g., capillary-venule junction or small venules) is suggested by the emergence of solution into germinal matrix hemorrhage from postmortem injection into the jugular veins but not from injection into the carotid artery.[73] Histochemical studies of germinal matrix vessels at the site of hemorrhage also are consistent with an origin at the capillary-venule or small venule level.[75] Multiple microcirculatory sites involving small vessels lined only by endothelium may be involved, depending on the clinical circumstances.

Spread of Intraventricular Hemorrhage

In the approximately 80% of cases with germinal matrix hemorrhage in which blood enters the lateral ventricles, spread occurs throughout the ventricular system (Fig. 24.8).[45,70,71] Blood proceeds through the foramina of Magendie and Luschka and tends to collect in the basilar cisterns in the posterior fossa; with substantial collections, the blood may incite an obliterative arachnoiditis over days to weeks with obstruction to cerebrospinal fluid (CSF) flow. Other sites at which particulate blood clot may lead to impaired CSF dynamics are the aqueduct of Sylvius and the arachnoid villi (see later discussion of hydrocephalus).

Neuropathological Consequences of Intraventricular Hemorrhage

Several neuropathological states occur as apparent consequences of IVH, including germinal matrix destruction, cerebral white matter injury/dysmaturation, cerebral gray matter dysmaturation, cerebellar dysmaturation, periventricular hemorrhagic infarction, and posthemorrhagic hydrocephalus.

Germinal Matrix Destruction

Destruction of germinal matrix and, importantly, its precursor cells for glia, especially oligodendroglial precursor cells (OPCs) and late migrating GABAergic neurons, is a consistent and expected feature of germinal matrix hemorrhage (see Fig. 24.9).[66,67,71] The hematoma is frequently replaced by a cyst, the walls of which include hemosiderin-laden macrophages and reactive astrocytes. The destruction of glial precursor cells may have a deleterious influence on subsequent brain development, as outlined next (see Fig. 24.9).

Cerebral White Matter Injury/Dysmaturation

As described earlier and in Unit I, the germinal matrix (ganglionic eminence during the developmental period of major occurrence of GMH-IVH; i.e., 24 to 32 weeks' gestation) is a principal source of proliferation of OPCs, which later in the third trimester migrate into the cerebral white matter, differentiate, and after term equivalency produce cerebral myelin.[60,61] Loss of these myelin-producing cells could lead to impaired cerebral development. Importantly, studies of postmortem human brains with GMH-IVH, as well as experimental models of GMH, have shown impairment of proliferation of OPCs and their subsequent migration and differentiation.[66,76,77] Experimental studies suggest that these deleterious effects on OPCs are mediated by blood products, inflammatory compounds,

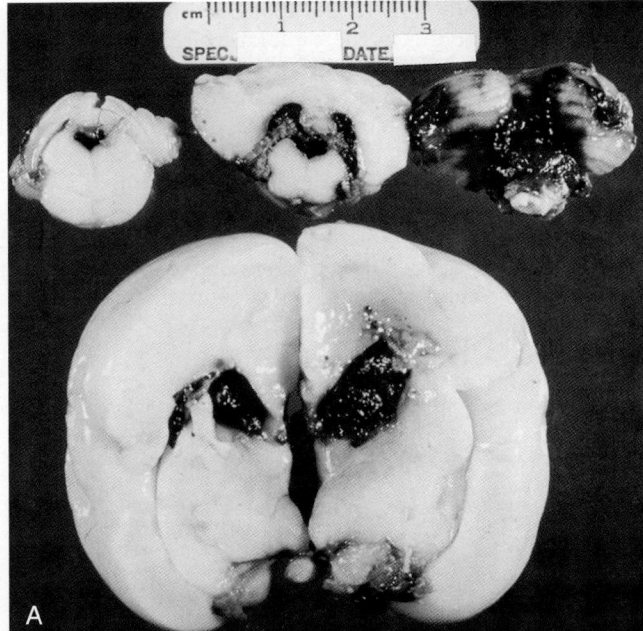

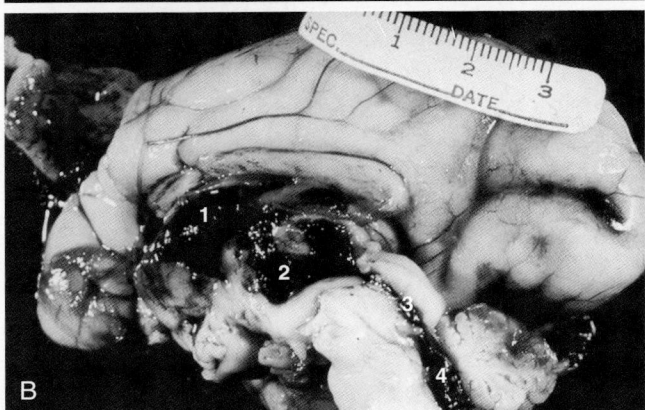

Figure 24.8 Spread of intraventricular hemorrhage. (A) Coronal and (B) sagittal views. In A, note blood in the lateral ventricles, aqueduct of Sylvius, the fourth ventricle, and the subarachnoid space around the cerebellum and lower brain stem. In B, note blood throughout the ventricular system (the numbers *1* to *4* refer to lateral ventricle, third ventricle, aqueduct, and fourth ventricle, respectively).

and microglia. Indeed microglial activation in the germinal matrix and periventricular white matter has been shown in the postmortem human brain with GMH ± IVH.[66,78] The role of microglia in the mediation of cerebral white matter injury/dysmaturation is discussed in more detail in Chapter 15 concerning the pathophysiology of periventricular leukomalacia.

A related possibility for a deleterious effect of GMH-IVH on cerebral white matter involves free-radical mediated effects on differentiating oligodendrocytes (OLs) and perhaps also on rapidly growing axons in the cerebral white matter (see Chapter 15), related in part to the release of nonheme iron from the hemorrhage.[79]

Cerebral Gray Matter Dysmaturation

A deleterious effect of mild GMH-IVH on cerebral cortical and thalamic volumetric development is suggested by recent

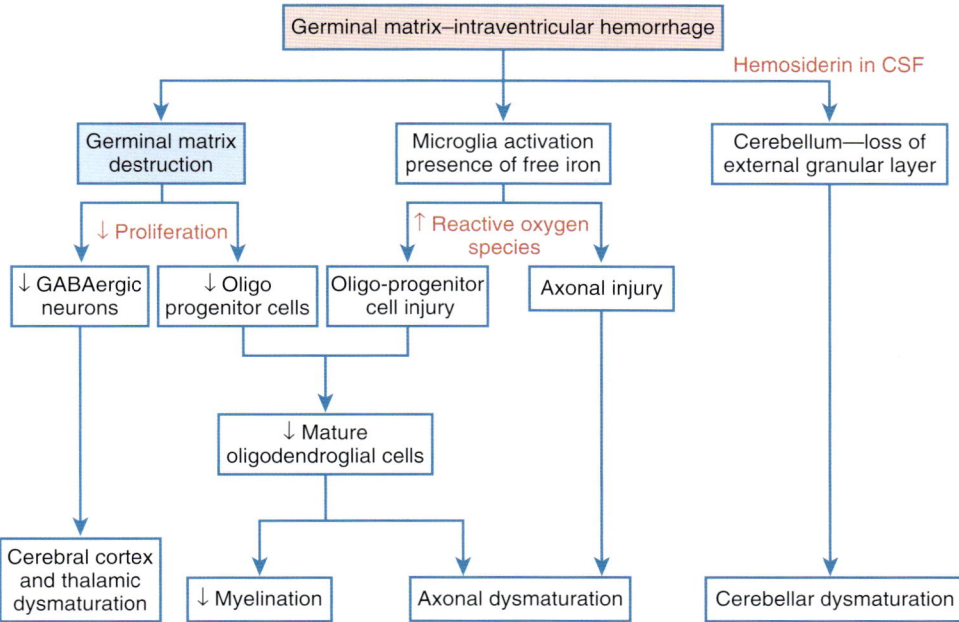

Figure 24.9 Neuropathologic consequences of germinal matrix–intraventricular hemorrhage on cerebral white and gray matter, and cerebellum.

magnetic resonance imaging (MRI) studies (see later). However, data are limited, and careful neuropathological analysis is lacking. If initial findings are corroborated, a role for germinal matrix destruction should be considered (see Fig. 24.9). As noted earlier, during the developmental period of the peak occurrence of GMH-IVH, the germinal matrix contributes to the generation and later migration of GABAergic neurons for cerebral cortex but especially also for association nuclei in the thalamus, both critical for high-level cognitive functioning.[62-65]

Cerebellar Dysmaturation

Cerebellar dysmaturation, principally in the form of diminished cerebellar volumetric growth, in the absence of overt parenchymal destructive disease, is the most common cerebellar abnormality of the premature infant.[80] Although multiple pathogenetic factors likely operate, strong evidence supports an important role for IVH and associated extraaxial blood.

The possibility that the cerebellar underdevelopment in premature infants may be related to adverse effects of blood products has been raised principally by the observations of Messerschmidt and co-workers, who have described the severe end of the spectrum of the acquired cerebellar growth failure.[81-83] In their series of 35 infants (mean gestational age, 27 weeks; mean birthweight, 900 g), after an initially normal cerebellar ultrasonographic examination in the first week of life, subsequent ultrasound and then MRI scans identified a gradual deficit in volume, without any apparent injury pattern, over the ensuing weeks. The pons and medulla also were found to be small subsequently. Using MRI sequences optimal for detection of hemosiderin, they identified infratentorial hemosiderin deposition in 70% of infants.[83] The deposition was particularly prominent on the cerebellar surface but was also noted on the surface of the brain stem and in the fourth ventricular region (Fig. 24.10). Hemosiderin in the posterior

fossa conveyed a sensitivity of 0.70 (95% confidence interval [CI], 0.48 to 0.86) and a specificity of 0.95 (CI, 0.84 to 0.99), with a positive predictive value of 0.88 and a negative predictive value of 0.87, for cerebellar underdevelopment.[83] Nearly all infants had experienced IVH, and 69% had posthemorrhagic hydrocephalus. A later study of 172 preterm infants identified a linear relationship between IVH and decreased cerebellar volumes with advancing postnatal age.[84] A recent report of 72 preterm infants confirmed these observations, even in the presence of grade II IVH.[85] Consistent with the possibility of a direct relationship between extraaxial blood and impaired cerebellar development is a recent report that showed by MRI a significant relationship between the presence of extraaxial blood and diminished cerebellar volumetric growth with advancing postnatal age, equivalent to the third trimester.[86,87] As discussed in Chapter 4, this developmental period is characterized by maximal proliferative activity in the external granular layer located on the surface of the cerebellum and crucial for cerebellar growth.[88]

Thus the data raise the strong possibility that the key targets for the adverse effects of blood over the surface of the cerebellum of the small premature infant are the *granule precursor cells of the external granular layer*.[88] The proliferating cells of the external granular layer are located directly at the interface with the subarachnoid space. Impairment of the survival or proliferation, or both, of these cells could result in the cerebellar underdevelopment, as evidenced by MRI. The effect on the external granular layer would result not only in deficient generation of internal granule cells but also in disturbance of the granular excitatory input to Purkinje cells and other cells of the molecular layer. The result would be deficient development of the full spectrum of cerebellar circuitry.

The mechanisms of disturbance to the external granular layer in the context of hemosiderin deposition almost certainly would relate to the *generation of free radicals, especially reactive*

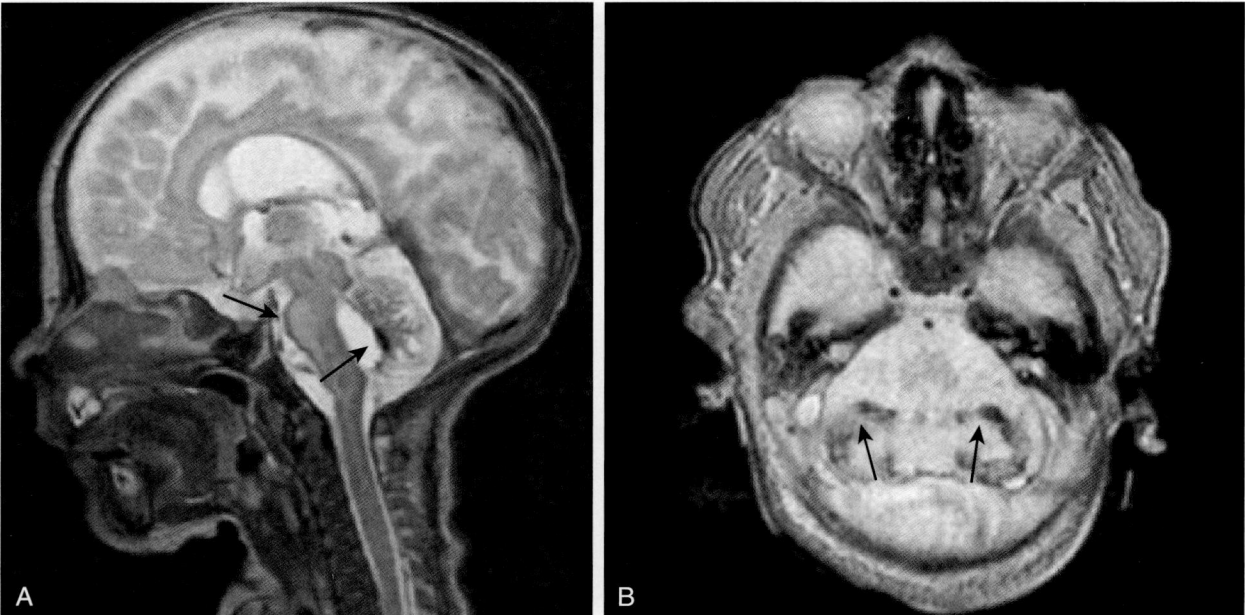

Figure 24.10 Cerebellar underdevelopment and hemosiderin deposition by magnetic resonance imaging (MRI) in a newborn at term equivalent age. Sagittal T2-weighted MRI (A) from a 13-week-old infant born at 26 weeks' gestation shows small vermis, enlarged fourth ventricle, reduced dimensions of the brain stem, and inclined tentorium; hemosiderin deposition is apparent on the surface of the pons and the lining of the fourth ventricle (*black arrows*). Horizontal MRI (B) shows reduced volume of cerebellar hemispheres with hemosiderin deposition in both hemispheres (*black arrows*). (Reproduced with permission from Messerschmidt A, Prayer D, Brugger PC, Boltshauser E, Zoder G, Sterniste W, Pollak A, Weber M, Birnbacher R. Preterm birth and disruptive cerebellar development: assessment of perinatal risk factors. *Eur J Paediatr Neurol.* 2008;12:455–460.)

oxygen species (Fig. 24.11). Hemosiderin is derived from blood by the following sequential steps: hemolysis of red blood cells, formation of heme, conversion of heme to free iron (and biliverdin, carbon monoxide) by heme oxygenase, and formation of ferritin and then hemosiderin.[89] Free iron is toxic because it leads to the generation of reactive oxygen species, especially the hydroxyl radical by the Fenton reaction. In one adult study of brain with hemosiderin deposits, free iron was increased 2.5-fold in the cerebellar cortex and 14.5-fold in the medulla. In experimental models, intracortical injections of free iron lead to lipid peroxidation products and epileptogenic necrotic foci.[90] In addition, hemosiderin, although a storage form of iron, may also release iron from its protein matrix.[91-93] The central nervous system has limited ability to discharge iron, and thus the accumulated iron can produce a chronic deleterious effect.[90] Notably, studies of CSF of infants with posthemorrhagic hydrocephalus show persistence of copious amounts of nonprotein-bound iron for weeks after IVH.[94]

Periventricular Hemorrhagic Infarction

Approximately 10% to 15% of VLBW infants with IVH also exhibit a characteristic parenchymal lesion (i.e., a relatively large region of hemorrhagic necrosis in the periventricular white matter), just dorsal and lateral to the external angle of the lateral ventricle (Fig. 24.12).[14,17,42] The incidence of the lesion increases with decreasing gestational age, such that in infants of less than 750 g, periventricular hemorrhagic infarction accounts for nearly 15% of all cases with IVH (see

later).[a] The distribution of high-grade IVH (grades 3 and 4 IVH) for each gestational age from 1993 to 2013 shows the very high incidence of severe IVH in the most immature infants (see Fig. 24.4).[23]

Large-scale ultrasonographic studies have defined the *topographic characteristics of periventricular hemorrhagic infarction.* The parenchymal hemorrhagic necrosis is strikingly asymmetrical; in the largest early series reported,[96] 67% of such lesions were exclusively unilateral, and in virtually all the remaining cases, lesions were grossly asymmetrical, although bilateral. Approximately one-half of the lesions were extensive and involved the periventricular white matter from frontal to parieto-occipital regions (Fig. 24.13); the remainder were more localized. Approximately 80% of cases were associated with large IVH. Commonly (and mistakenly), the parenchymal hemorrhagic lesion is described as an *extension* of IVH. Several neuropathological studies have shown that simple extension of blood into cerebral white matter from the germinal matrix or lateral ventricle does *not* account for the periventricular hemorrhagic necrosis.[29,72,95-101] In a later ultrasonographic report of 58 infants, findings were similar: the lesion was unilateral in 74%, extensive (involving two or more lobar territories) in 67%, and associated with large IVH in 88%.[102] The lobar distribution indicates that the majority of lesions involved the frontal and parietal regions. Approximately 50% of the cases exhibited a

---

[a]References 10, 14, 17, 22, 42, and 95.

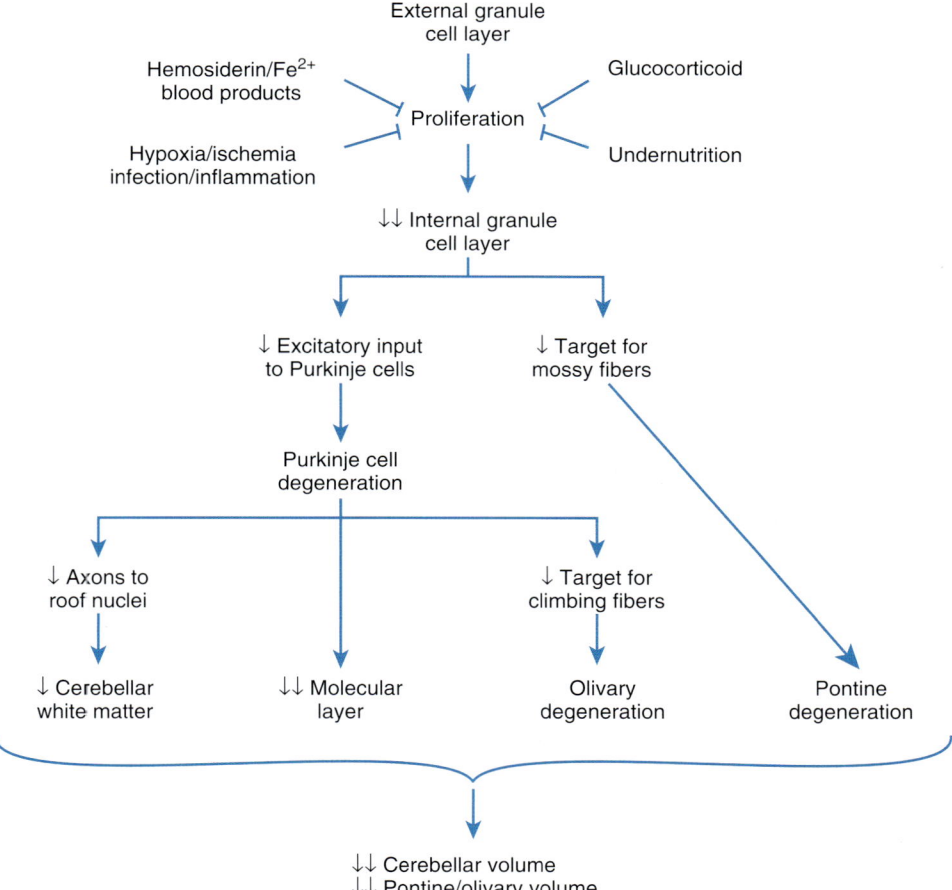

Figure 24.11 Likely mechanisms by which direct adverse effects on the external granule cell layer lead to diminished volumetric development of cerebellum and pontine and olivary nuclei. (From Volpe JJ. Cerebellum of the premature infant: rapidly developing, vulnerable, clinically important. *J Child Neurol.* 2009;24:1085–1104.)

midline shift of cerebral structures, consistent with the severity of the lesions. A more recent report of somewhat more localized lesions showed that a majority of the lesions were predominantly parietal with fewer in the frontal and temporal regions.[103] This lobar predominance has implications for outcome (see later).

Microscopic study of the periventricular hemorrhagic necrosis just described indicates that the lesion is a *hemorrhagic infarction.*[29,96-101,104] The careful studies of Gould and co-workers[98] and Takashima and co-workers[104] emphasized that (1) the hemorrhagic component consists usually of perivascular hemorrhages that follow closely the fan-shaped distribution of the medullary veins in periventricular cerebral white matter (Fig. 24.14A and B), and (2) the hemorrhagic component tends to be most concentrated near the ventricular angle where these veins become confluent and ultimately join the terminal vein in the subependymal region. Thus the periventricular hemorrhagic necrosis occurring in association with large IVH is, in fact, a *venous infarction.* The *most common neuropathological sequela* of periventricular hemorrhagic infarction is a large *porencephalic cyst* at the site of the lesion, either alone (66%) or in combination with smaller cysts (23%).[102] The large cyst communicates often, although not invariably, with the lateral ventricle.

Periventricular hemorrhagic infarction is distinguishable neuropathologically from secondary hemorrhage into periventricular leukomalacia, which is the ischemic, usually nonhemorrhagic, and symmetrical lesion of periventricular white matter of the premature infant (see later discussion). Distinction of these two lesions in vivo, however, is sometimes difficult. Indeed, because the pathogeneses of periventricular hemorrhagic infarction and periventricular leukomalacia overlap (see later discussion), it is to be expected that the lesions often coexist, thereby sometimes causing confusion in interpretation of cranial ultrasound scans.[1] In Table 24.2, the basic features of these two periventricular white matter lesions of the premature infant are compared.

The *pathogenesis* of periventricular hemorrhagic infarction appears to be related causally to the GMH-IVH. A direct relation to the latter lesion seems likely on the basis of three fundamental findings.[96,102] First, 80% to 90% of the reported parenchymal lesions are observed in association with large (and almost invariably) asymmetrical GMH-IVH. Second, the parenchymal lesions invariably occurred *on the same side* as the larger amount of germinal matrix and intraventricular blood (Table 24.3). Third, in some cases, the lesions were shown to develop and progress after the occurrence of the GMH-IVH. More than one-half of the lesions were detected after the second postnatal day, when approximately 75% of cases of IVH have already occurred (see the section on

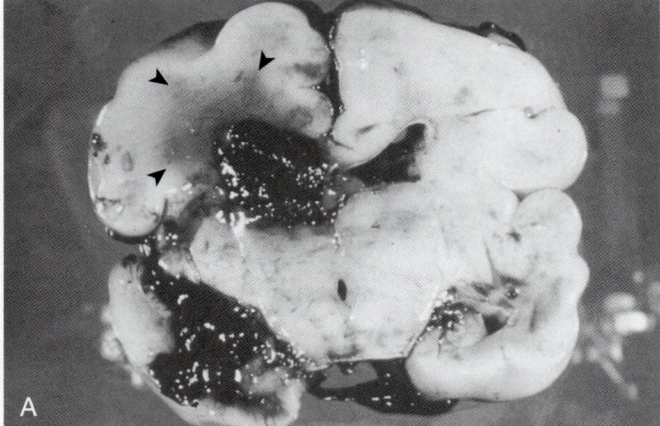

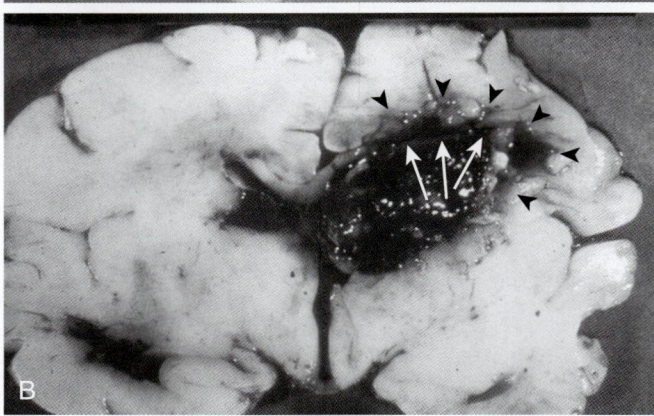

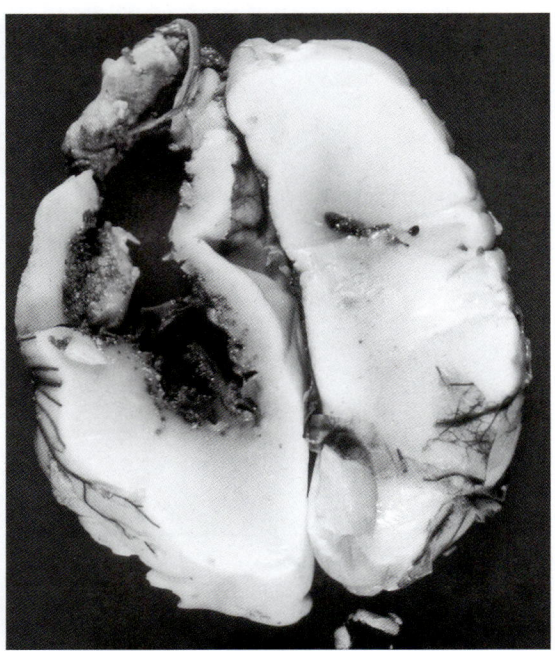

Figure 24.13 **Periventricular hemorrhagic infarction, neuropathology.** Horizontal section of cerebrum above the level of lateral ventricles from a premature infant who died on the sixth postnatal day, 3 days after severe intraventricular hemorrhage. Hemorrhagic necrosis in left cerebral white matter separated from the brain section during fixation and revealed a shaggy margin of the hemorrhagic infarction. See text for details.

Figure 24.12 **Periventricular hemorrhagic infarction with intraventricular hemorrhage; coronal sections of cerebrum.** (A) Early lesion; note evolving hemorrhagic infarction *(arrowheads)* on the same side as larger intraventricular hemorrhage. (B) More advanced lesion; note hemorrhagic necrosis with liquefaction in periventricular white matter *(arrowheads)* on the same side as larger intraventricular hemorrhage. The ependymal lining is marked by white arrows.

TABLE 24.2	Periventricular White Matter Lesions in the Premature Infant With Intraventricular Hemorrhage		
	LESION		
	PERIVENTRICULAR HEMORRHAGIC INFARCTION		**PERIVENTRICULAR LEUKOMALACIA**
Likely site of circulatory disturbance	Venous		Arterial
Grossly hemorrhagic	Invariable		Uncommon
Markedly asymmetrical	Nearly invariable		Uncommon
Evolution	Single large cyst		Multiple small cysts

TABLE 24.3	Laterality of Apparent Periventricular Hemorrhagic Infarction and Concurrent Asymmetrical Intraventricular Hemorrhage	
SEVERITY OF INTRAVENTRICULAR HEMORRHAGE	**PERIVENTRICULAR HEMORRHAGIC INFARCTION HOMOLATERAL**	**PERIVENTRICULAR HEMORRHAGIC INFARCTION CONTRALATERAL**
Grade III	47	0
Grades I–II	5	4

Data from Guzzetta F, Shackelford GD, Volpe S, Perlman JM, Volpe JJ. Periventricular intraparenchymal echodensities in the premature newborn: critical determinant of neurologic outcome. *Pediatrics.* 1986;78:995–1006.

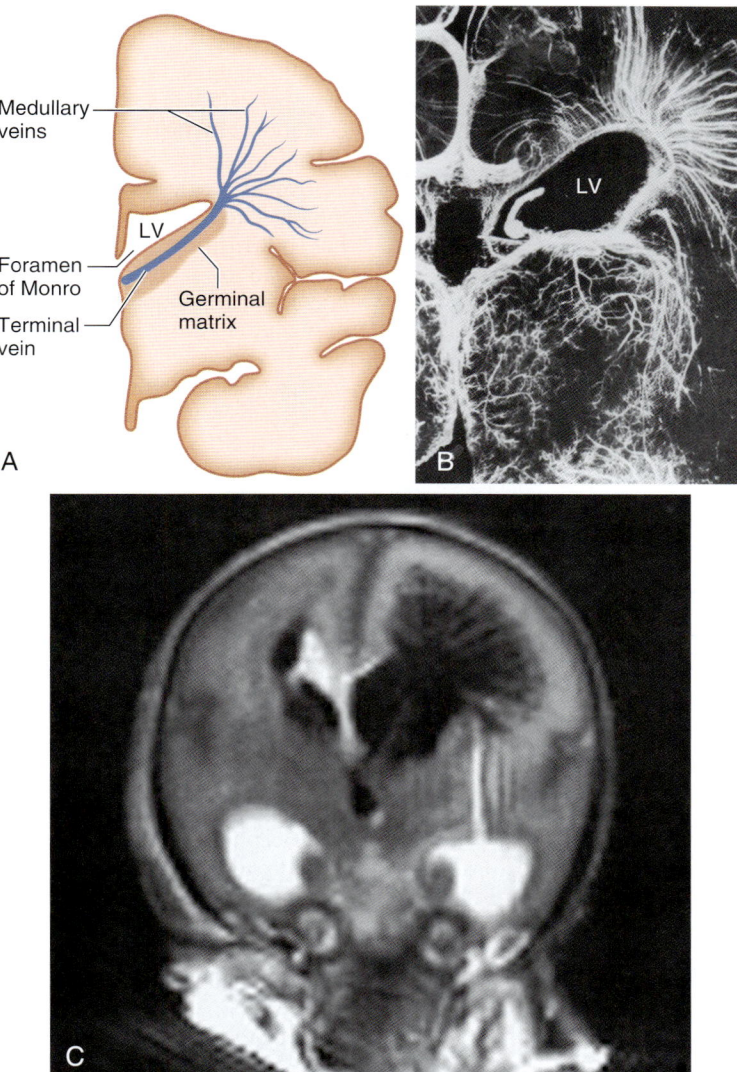

Figure 24.14 Venous drainage of cerebral white matter in schematic and actual appearances.
(A) Schematic diagram shows that the medullary veins, arranged in a fan-shaped distribution, drain blood from the cerebral white matter into the terminal vein, which courses through the germinal matrix. (B) Postmortem venogram obtained from a human newborn shows the actual appearance of the vessels. (C) Periventricular hemorrhagic infarction: coronal magnetic resonance imaging scan (fast spin-echo image) demonstrating bilateral germinal matrix–intraventricular hemorrhages, with an apparent periventricular hemorrhagic infarction on the side of the larger amount of germinal matrix and intraventricular blood (reader's right). Note the fan-shaped linear distribution of increased signal in the parenchymal lesion (reader's right), consistent with a combination of intravascular thrombi and perivascular hemorrhage along the course of the medullary veins. *LV,* Lateral ventricle. (B From Takashima S, Mito T, Ando Y. Pathogenesis of periventricular white matter hemorrhages in preterm infants. *Brain Dev.* 1986;8:25–30. C From Counsell SJ, Maalouf EF, Rutherford MA, Edwards AD. Periventricular haemorrhagic infarct in a preterm neonate. *Eur J Paediatr Neurol.* 1999;3:25–28.)

diagnosis). The association of large asymmetrical GMH-IVH with progression to ipsilateral periventricular hemorrhagic infarction has been confirmed.[102,105-108] These data suggest that the IVH or its associated germinal matrix hemorrhage leads to obstruction of the terminal veins and thus impaired blood flow in the medullary veins with the occurrence of hemorrhagic venous infarction. A similar conclusion was suggested from a neuropathological study.[98] The timing of this progression to infarction is often very rapid because, in most cases, the severe IVH and the periventricular hemorrhagic infarction are detected simultaneously.

This pathogenetic formulation received strong support from Doppler determinations of blood flow velocity in the terminal vein during the evolution of the infarction in the living premature infant; obstruction of flow in the terminal vein by the ipsilateral GMH-IVH was shown clearly.[109,110] Moreover, the finding of elevated lactate in structures adjacent to the GMH, in the distribution of tributaries of the terminal

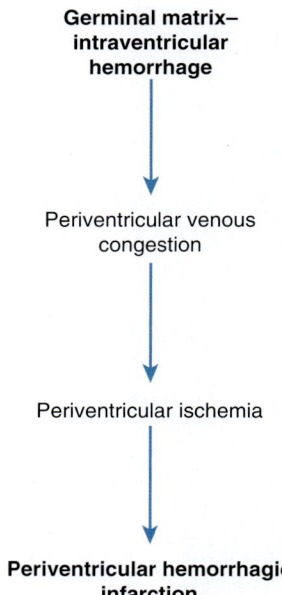

Figure 24.15 Pathogenesis of periventricular hemorrhagic infarction. The formulation indicates a central role for germinal matrix–intraventricular hemorrhage in causation of the periventricular venous infarction.

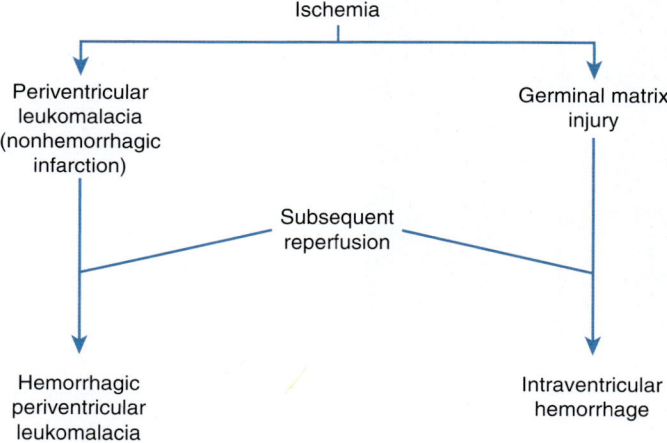

Figure 24.16 Pathogenesis of hemorrhagic periventricular leukomalacia.

vein, further supports the occurrence of ischemia secondary to venous obstruction by the matrix hemorrhage.[111] Finally, an MRI study of acute periventricular hemorrhagic infarction has shown an appearance consistent with a combination of intravascular thrombi and perivascular hemorrhage along the course of the medullary veins within the area of infarction (see Fig. 24.14C).[112]

The pathogenetic scheme that is considered to account for most examples of periventricular hemorrhagic infarction is shown in Fig. 24.15. This scheme should be distinguished from that operative for hemorrhagic periventricular leukomalacia (Fig. 24.16), although the lesions could coexist. The frequency of coexistence of the two lesions is not known. In addition, the two pathogenetic schemes could operate in sequence; that is, periventricular leukomalacia could become secondarily

hemorrhagic (and perhaps a larger area of injury) when GMH or IVH subsequently causes venous obstruction.

The deleterious neurological effects of periventricular hemorrhagic infarction may relate not only to destruction of cerebral white matter per se but also to the effects of the white matter injury on cerebral cortical development. Thus careful neuropathological study of cerebral cortical organization in infants who died with major hemorrhagic white matter lesions has shown striking alterations in neuronal axonal and dendritic ramifications in areas overlying the white matter destruction.[113] Moreover, in unpublished work from our group, cerebral cortical gray matter volume was shown by three-dimensional MRI to be reduced at term in premature infants with periventricular hemorrhagic infarction.[114] These abnormalities are postulated to be secondary to disturbances of afferent input to and efferent input from the areas of cortex by disruption of the respective white matter axons. Another potential cause of the cortical abnormalities could be the destruction of subplate neurons by the white matter infarction.[115] These neurons are critical for cerebral cortical organization and are abundant in subcortical white matter in the human premature infant (see Unit 1). Whatever the mechanism, these *cerebral cortical* abnormalities with periventricular hemorrhagic infarction could be very important in determining subsequent cognitive deficits and seizure disorders.

Hydrocephalus

An additional neuropathological consequence of IVH is progressive posthemorrhagic ventricular dilation (i.e., hydrocephalus). The likelihood and the rapidity of evolution of hydrocephalus after IVH are related directly to the quantity of intraventricular blood. Thus, with large IVH, hydrocephalus may evolve over days (*acute* hydrocephalus), and with smaller IVH, the process evolves usually over weeks (*subacute-chronic* hydrocephalus; see later discussion).

Acute hydrocephalus is accompanied by particulate blood clot, readily demonstrated in life by ultrasound scan (see later discussion). The particulate clot may impair CSF absorption by obstruction of the arachnoid villi. This mechanism may be particularly likely in the newborn, in whom only microscopic arachnoid villi (and not larger, later appearing arachnoid granulations) are present.[116-118] The possibility that endogenous fibrinolytic mechanisms mediated by plasminogen activation are deficient in the CSF of the premature infant is suggested by the findings that plasminogen levels are extremely low in the CSF of such infants,[119] whereas in infants with recent IVH, the levels of plasminogen activator inhibitor are relatively high.[120,121] This combination of findings may limit the infant's capacity to mediate clot lysis after IVH.

Subacute-chronic hydrocephalus relates most commonly either to an obliterative arachnoiditis in the posterior fossa (which results in either obstruction of fourth ventricular outflow or flow through the tentorial notch) or to aqueductal obstruction by blood clot, disrupted ependyma, and reactive gliosis.[47,67,122-124] The obliterative arachnoiditis is probably most important. Two molecules important in fibroproliferative responses have been shown to be upregulated in infants with posthemorrhagic hydrocephalus.[125-128] Transforming growth factor-beta 1, derived in this setting from platelets, is a cytokine chemotactic for fibroblasts and important in the upregulation of genes encoding collagen, fibronectin, and other extracellular matrix proteins.[125,127,128] Procollagen 1C-peptide, involved in collagen fiber formation and tissue deposition, also has been shown to be elevated in CSF of infants with posthemorrhagic hydrocephalus.[126]

The *deleterious effects of hydrocephalus on cerebral white matter* are discussed later (see section on progressive posthemorrhagic ventricular dilatation). Prominent affection of white matter axons and microcirculation is emphasized.

Neuropathological Accompaniments of Intraventricular Hemorrhage

Several neuropathological states are common accompaniments of IVH, but, in contrast to the states just described, these are generally not caused by the IVH. The two most common accompaniments are periventricular leukomalacia and selective neuronal necrosis.

Periventricular Leukomalacia

Periventricular leukomalacia, the generally symmetrical, nonhemorrhagic, and apparently ischemic white matter injury of the premature infant (see Chapters 14 to 16), was observed to some degree in 75% of one series of infants who died with IVH.[72] The frequent association of classic necrotic/cystic periventricular leukomalacia and IVH also was emphasized in three other neuropathological reports,[99,104,129] as well as in two large ultrasonographic studies.[17,42] Although it has been reported that approximately 25% of examples of periventricular leukomalacia become hemorrhagic,[72,130] especially when associated coagulopathy is present, this figure includes examples that have been accompanied by large IVH and that probably represent the venous infarction discussed earlier as periventricular hemorrhagic infarction. Takashima and co-workers[104] suggested that the two lesions (i.e., periventricular hemorrhagic infarction and hemorrhagic periventricular leukomalacia) may be distinguishable in part on the basis of topography. Thus hemorrhagic periventricular leukomalacia has a predilection for periventricular arterial border zones, particularly in the region near the trigone of the lateral ventricles. Venous infarction, especially its most hemorrhagic component, is particularly prominent more anteriorly; that is, the lesion radiates from the periventricular region at the site of confluence of the medullary and terminal veins and assumes a roughly triangular, fan-shaped appearance in periventricular white matter.

IVH *also may contribute to the occurrence of periventricular leukomalacia.* The possibility of periventricular white matter injury caused by blood products is raised both by experimental studies and by the demonstration that the presence of IVH is associated with a sharply increased risk of ultrasonographic correlates (e.g., echolucencies) of white matter injury.[38,42] In one such study, cystic periventricular leukomalacia by ultrasonography was accompanied by IVH in 67% of cases versus only 17% in infants without the cystic injury.[42] A later correlate of white matter injury, nonprogressive ventriculomegaly, is also associated especially with impaired cognitive function in infants with IVH (see Chapter 16).[131,132] Moreover, the neurodevelopmental outcome of preterm infants with later ventricular dilation was worse in those who had associated IVH versus those who did not.[133] Finally, infants with only mild degrees of IVH exhibit a poorer neurodevelopmental outcome than infants with no IVH.[134] The most likely mechanism of white matter

injury with intraventricular or (parenchymal blood) involves *increased free radical formation*, provoked perhaps in part by ischemia-reperfusion but also particularly by local release of iron from the blood.[94,135,136] Supportive of this suggestion is the demonstration that non-protein-bound iron was found in the CSF of 75% of preterm infants with posthemorrhagic ventriculomegaly for many *weeks* after the IVH.[94] Of particular importance in this context are the recent observations of the crucial role of free radicals in the pathogenesis of cerebral white matter injury in the premature infant (see Chapter 15).

Selective Neuronal Necrosis

Selective neuronal necrosis, secondary to hypoxia-ischemia in the premature infant, particularly involves the pons, deep nuclear structures, especially the thalamus and basal ganglia, and hippocampus (see Chapter 14). Although each of these lesions is more commonly encountered in association with IVH, the relationship is particularly notable for pontine neuronal necrosis. In two carefully studied neuropathological series,[72,129] 46% and 71% of infants with IVH exhibited pontine neuronal necrosis. Accompanying neuronal necrosis in the subiculum of the hippocampus is common but not invariable.[a] All the infants with IVH accompanied by pontine neuronal necrosis in the series of Armstrong and co-workers[72] died of respiratory failure; previous investigations had suggested that the pontine lesion is related to hypoxic-ischemic insult, hyperoxia, and hypocarbia.[117,139] Involvement of the inferior olivary nucleus often accompanies the pontine disturbance, and thus cerebellar afferent systems are often affected. This involvement could contribute to the decreased volume of cerebellum observed by volumetric MRI in infants after severe IVH.[114]

PATHOGENESIS

The pathogenesis of IVH is considered best in terms of intravascular, vascular, and extravascular factors. Clearly, the pathogenesis of IVH is multifactorial, and to some extent different combinations of these factors are operative in different patients. Nevertheless, several of the factors are important in every patient, as discussed in the following sections.

Intravascular Factors

Intravascular factors are those that relate primarily to the regulation of blood flow, pressure, and volume in the microvascular bed of the germinal matrix (Table 24.4). Factors that relate to platelet-capillary function and to blood clotting capability may play a contributory pathogenetic role in certain patients.

Fluctuating Cerebral Blood Flow

The major importance of fluctuating cerebral blood flow in the pathogenesis of IVH was shown in a study by Perlman and co-workers[140] of ventilated preterm infants with respiratory distress syndrome. Using the Doppler technique at the anterior fontanelle to insonate the pericallosal branch of the anterior cerebral artery (the latter an important source of blood supply to the germinal matrix), we asked whether alterations in cerebral

---

[a]References 28, 47, 117, 129, 137, and 138.

TABLE 24.4   Pathogenesis of Germinal Matrix–Intraventricular Hemorrhage: Intravascular Factors

Fluctuating cerebral blood flow
Ventilated preterm infant with respiratory distress syndrome
Increase in cerebral blood flow
Systemic hypertension: importance of pressure-passive
    circulation
Rapid volume expansion
Hypercarbia
Decreased hematocrit
Decreased blood glucose
Increase in cerebral venous pressure
Venous anatomy: U-turn in direction of venous flow
Labor and vaginal delivery
Respiratory disturbances
Decrease in cerebral blood flow (followed by reperfusion)
Systemic hypotension: importance of pressure-passive
    circulation
Platelet and coagulation disturbance

TABLE 24.5   Relation of Fluctuating Cerebral Blood Flow Velocity to Subsequent Development of Intraventricular Hemorrhage

CEREBRAL BLOOD FLOW VELOCITY PATTERN	SUBSEQUENT IVH	NO IVH
Fluctuating	21	2
Stable	7[a]	20

[a]Other provocative factors (e.g., pneumothorax) present in four patients.
IVH, Intraventricular hemorrhage.

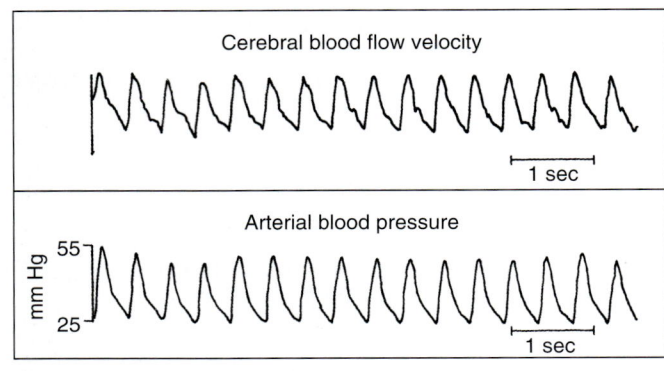

A

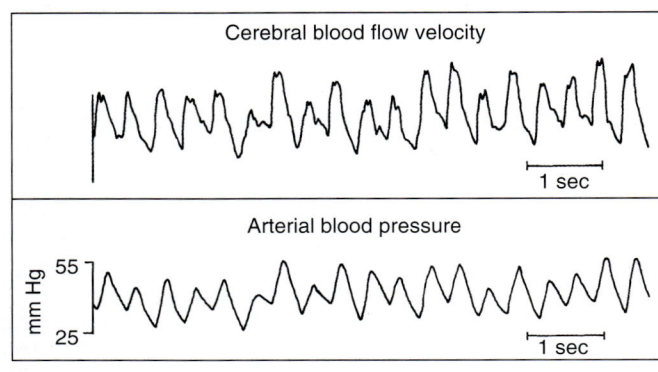

B

Figure 24.17 Cerebral blood flow velocity in ventilated premature infant with respiratory distress syndrome. The upper trace of each pair is the cerebral blood flow velocity, obtained at the anterior fontanelle, and the lower trace is the simultaneous blood pressure obtained with an umbilical artery catheter. (A) Stable pattern and (B) fluctuating pattern. See text for description.

blood flow velocity in the first hours and days of life could be identified and related to the subsequent development of IVH. The findings were decisive. Two patterns of cerebral blood flow velocity were noted on the first day of life: a stable pattern and a fluctuating pattern (Fig. 24.17). The *stable pattern* was characterized by equal peaks and troughs of systolic and diastolic flow velocity (see Fig. 24.17A). In contrast, the *fluctuating pattern* was characterized by marked, *continuous alterations* in both systolic and diastolic flow velocities (see Fig. 24.17B); blood flow velocity tracings closely reflected similar patterns of arterial blood pressure, simultaneously obtained from the abdominal aorta through an umbilical artery catheter (see Fig. 24.17). A striking relationship of the fluctuating pattern of cerebral blood flow velocity to the subsequent occurrence of IVH was defined when the infants were studied by serial cranial ultrasound scans (Table 24.5).

The aforementioned observations were important for two reasons: First, they identified a subset of infants with respiratory distress syndrome at extreme risk for the subsequent occurrence of IVH and therefore prime candidates for preventive

interventions (see later discussion). Second, they suggested a rational pathogenetic mechanism for the development of IVH with the respiratory distress syndrome (i.e., continuous fluctuations of blood flow in the vulnerable matrix microvessels, leading to rupture of these vessels). The relationship of the fluctuating phenomena to the hypoperfusion-reperfusion cycles discussed later is striking. The relationship between fluctuating cerebral blood flow velocity and occurrence of major IVH was later confirmed.[141] Two studies[142,143] in which fluctuations in flow velocity were less than 10% (coefficient of variation) did not show a correlation of fluctuations with the occurrence of IVH, consistent with the earlier observation of Perlman and co-workers[140] that fluctuations of this small degree do not lead to IVH.

The cause of the fluctuations in both the systemic and cerebral circulations is related to the mechanics of ventilation[144-148] and to primary and secondary cardiovascular effects, including lowered cardiac stroke volume and cardiac output, often combining effects on both systemic and cerebral blood flows from cardiovascular and ventilatory management (Fig. 24.18).[149,150] Thus hypercarbia, hypovolemia, hypotension, *restlessness*, patent ductus arteriosus, and relatively high inspired oxygen concentrations have all correlated with the occurrence of fluctuations in cerebral blood flow velocity.[141,147,148,151-153]

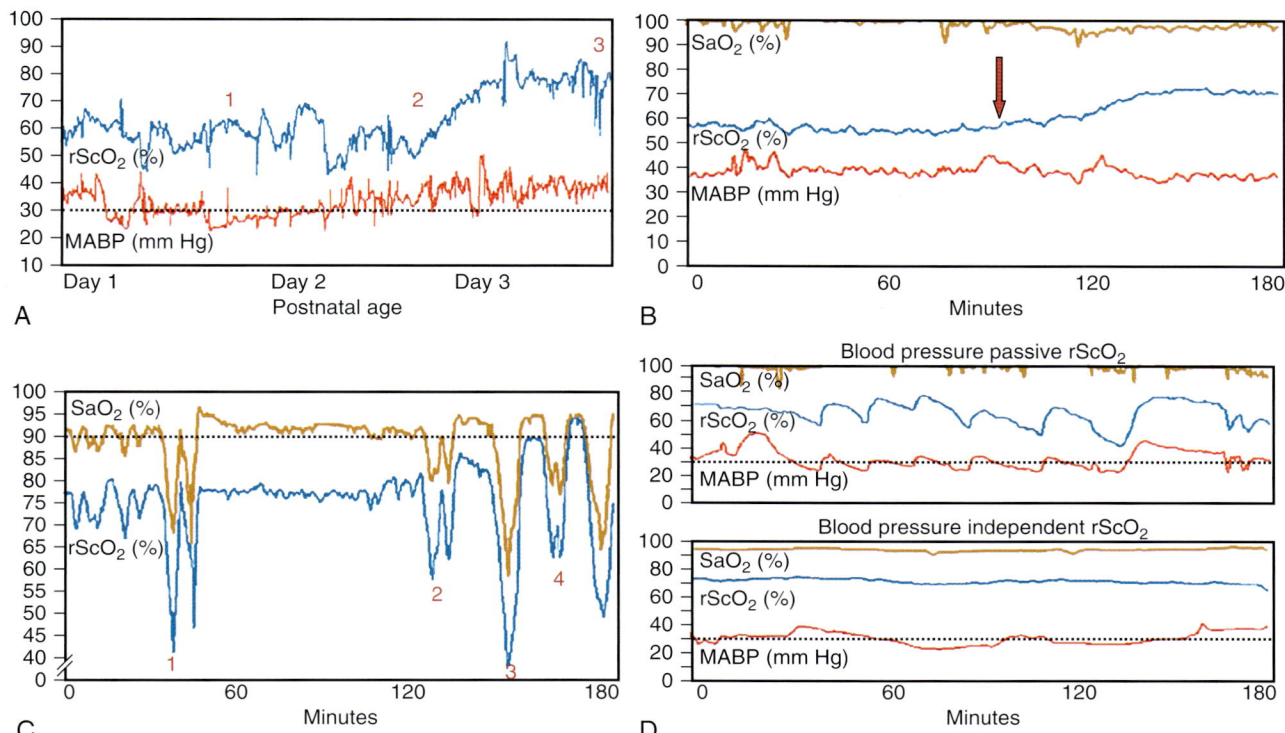

Figure 24.18 Patterns of regional cerebral saturation (rScO$_2$) and near arterial blood pressure during neonatal illness and procedures. (A) Patterns of rScO$_2$ and near arterial blood pressure during and after closure of a hemodynamically important patent ductus arteriosus (PDA) in a 28-week-old preterm neonate. Note the sometimes unusually low rScO$_2$ during PDA (1), the increase of rScO$_2$ after the start of indomethacin treatment (2), and the "normalization" of rScO$_2$ values after ductal closure (3). (B) Pattern of rScO$_2$ during high-frequency oscillation with high mean airway pressures (MAP: 18 cm H$_2$O) and subsequent lowering *(red arrow)* to 14 cm H$_2$O. Note the rather low rScO$_2$ values (53%) and its increase to reference values after adjustment (lowering) of the MAP. (C) Simultaneous patterns of SaO$_2$ and rScO$_2$ before, during, and after recurrent apneas in an unstable preterm neonate. Note the quick recovery of rScO$_2$ after the first apnea is treated with extra oxygen (1, 2) and the subsequent apnea is treated with extra oxygen (3, 4), showing extremely high rScO$_2$ levels, up to 94%. (D) Patterns of rScO$_2$ and mean arterial blood pressure (MABP). Note the similar patterns of rScO$_2$ and MABP in the upper part (blood pressure passive cerebral oxygenation) and the stable rScO$_2$, despite large swings in MABP from 24 to 40 mm Hg, in the lower part (blood pressure–independent cerebral circulation). (From van Bel F, Lemmers P, Naulaers G. Monitoring neonatal regional cerebral oxygen saturation in clinical practice: value and pitfalls. *Neonatology.* 2008;94:237–244.)

Increases in Cerebral Blood Flow: Importance of Pressure-Passive Circulation

The close temporal correlation between the occurrence of IVH and abrupt increases in arterial blood pressure, apparent cerebral blood flow (jugular venous occlusion plethysmography), and cerebral blood flow velocity[145,154-159] has supported the earlier suggestion[45] that increases in cerebral blood flow play an important pathogenetic role in IVH. A *particularly likely cause of the premature infant's apparent propensity for dangerous elevations of cerebral blood flow is a pressure-passive state of the cerebral circulation.*[114,160-169] As discussed in Chapters 13 and 15, severely impaired cerebrovascular autoregulation was identified in approximately 50% of ventilated very low birthweight infants studied by near-infrared spectroscopy in the first several days of life.[169] Using a more sophisticated approach with the same methodology, Soul and co-workers[114] showed that *fully 87 of 90 infants studied in the first 5 days of life had pressure-passive periods, and for the total group, these periods accounted for a mean of 20% of*

the time. Indeed, some infants exhibited the pressure-passive state more than 50% of the time. In addition, hypercarbia and perhaps decreased hematocrit or decreased blood glucose may contribute to severe enough elevations in cerebral blood flow in the premature infant to provoke IVH (see later discussion).

A more complex interaction of the cardiovascular system—both systemic and cerebral—has recently been explored by simultaneous study of neonatal echocardiography and near infrared spectroscopy. In a prospective study of 22 preterm infants between 23 and 27 weeks studied in the first 3 days of life, different patterns of changes in hemodynamics were found in very preterm neonates who developed high-grade IVH compared with those who did not.[149] Importantly, in the infants of the grade IV IVH group, the changes in systemic and cerebral hemodynamics *preceded* the occurrence of the bleeding and revealed a pattern consistent with a hypoperfusion-reperfusion cycle. More specifically, the infants in the grade IV IVH group had lower cardiac stroke volume and mean blood pressure on study entry at around 6 hours of life. In addition, they also

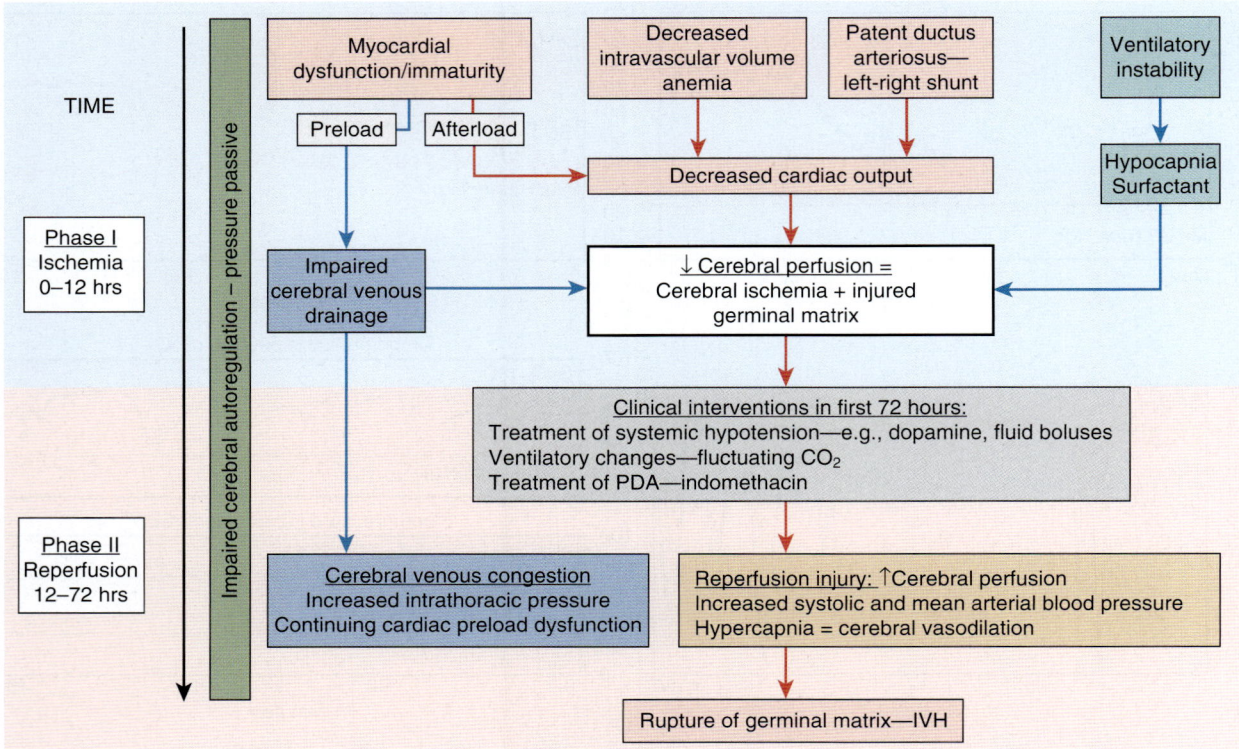

Figure 24.19 Mechanisms of cerebral ischemia and reperfusion in the pathogenesis of germinal matrix–intraventricular hemorrhage (IVH). *PDA,* Patent ductus arteriosus.

had lower cerebral rSO₂ and higher cerebral functional oxygen extraction during the first 12 hours of monitoring, suggestive of initial low cerebral blood flow in patients. *Importantly, this period of hypoperfusion was followed by increased cardiac stroke volume and evidence of cerebral reperfusion,* all of which preceded the radiological recognition of IVH. The high concordance in timing and measures of systemic and cerebral vascular changes are consistent with systemic and cerebral hypoperfusion-reperfusion cycles, apparently important in the causative pathway to high-grade IVH.

The importance of cerebral hypoperfusion-reperfusion cycles is also emphasized in a study using superior vena cava (SVC) flow as a surrogate for systemic blood flow and showing that most cases of high-grade IVH were first noted after low SVC flow normalized. A recent case-control study using NIRS also found higher cerebral rSO₂ and lower cerebral oxygen extraction values before the occurrence of high-grade IVH.[150,170] However, this study did not document the initial cerebral ischemic period and did not monitor systemic hemodynamics. As the systemic and cerebral ischemic period is transient, and because in the study just cited the cranial ultrasound studies were performed on average only every 21 hours, it is conceivable that the period of cerebral ischemia was missed. The underlying primary cause or causes of the cerebral ischemia leading to predisposition to the development of high-grade IVH is/are not known. Myocardial immaturity, with an increased sensitivity to afterload, has been postulated as *one of the primary etiological factors* of the decreased cardiac output and resultant low cerebral blood flow in the very early hours following delivery of the very preterm newborn. Such findings require further confirmation to propose rational consideration of interventions to prevent a primary

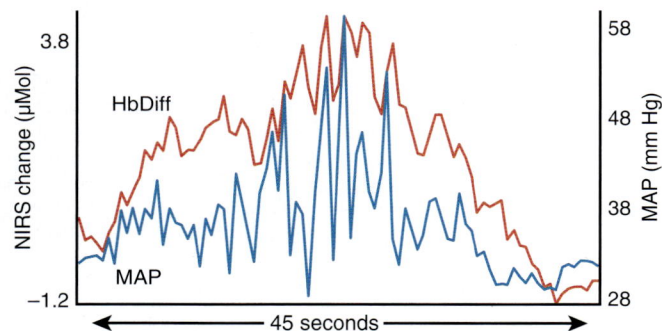

Figure 24.20 **Changes in blood pressure (mean arterial pressure [MAP]) and cerebral perfusion (hemoglobin difference [HbDiff]) during a diaper change.** Simultaneous tracings were obtained from a premature infant (30 weeks of gestational age). Note the marked, parallel increase in cerebral perfusion, determined by near-infrared spectroscopy (NIRS), and in arterial blood pressure, obtained from an umbilical artery catheter. (Courtesy Dr. Adre du Plessis.)

and important period of cerebral hypoperfusion. The potential sequence of cardiovascular changes is outlined in Fig. 24.19.

Elevations of Arterial Blood Pressure and Pressure-Passive Cerebral Circulation. Concerning the role of elevations in arterial blood pressure, the presence of a pressure-passive cerebral circulation would be expected to lead to an increase in cerebral blood flow in association with increases in blood pressure, with the potential consequence being rupture of vulnerable germinal matrix vessels. The striking increase in cerebral blood flow associated with increases in blood pressure can be shown in real time by near-infrared spectroscopy (Fig. 24.20). A decisive

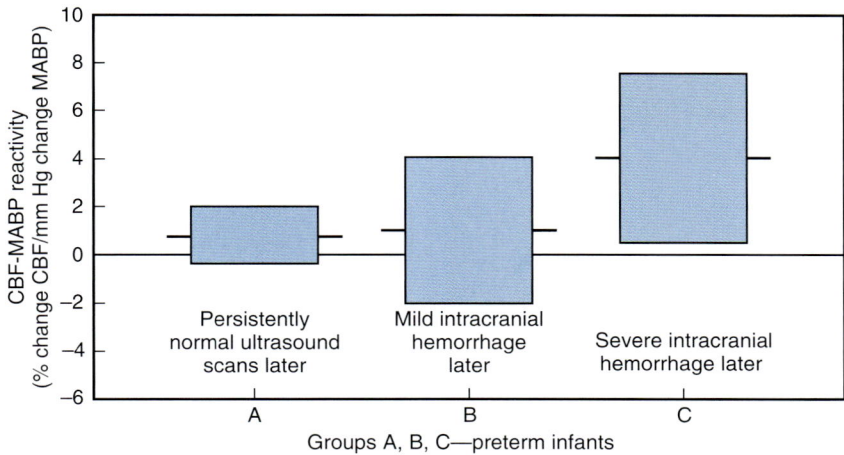

Figure 24.21 Cerebral blood flow *(CBF)*—mean arterial blood pressure *(MABP)* reactivities (percentage of change in CBF per millimeter of mercury change in MABP) in premature infants before intracranial hemorrhage. CBF-MABP reactivities were obtained in the first 2 days of life (primarily in the first 24 hours) in 57 mechanically ventilated preterm infants who had normal ultrasound scans at the time of the reactivity measurements and who were followed subsequently by ultrasonography. Groups A, B, and C were determined by the results of the subsequent scans. The average reactivity and 95% confidence limits for each group are shown. Intact autoregulation (i.e., zero value for CBF-MABP reactivity) was present in those infants who had subsequent scans that were normal or showed only mild hemorrhage. Infants who later developed severe hemorrhage had a pressure-passive cerebral circulation. (Redrawn from Pryds O, Greisen G, Lou H, Friis-Hansen B. Heterogeneity of cerebral vasoreactivity in preterm infants supported by mechanical ventilation. *J Pediatr.* 1989;115:638–645.)

demonstration of the relation between pressure-passive cerebral circulation and the occurrence of IVH was obtained from a classic study of 57 preterm infants supported by mechanical ventilation during at least the first 48 hours of life (Fig. 24.21). Infants in whom ultrasonographic signs of severe IVH developed had prior evidence of a pressure-passive cerebral circulation, whereas those with intact cerebrovascular autoregulation developed either no hemorrhage or only mild hemorrhage (see Fig. 24.21).[161,162] The work of Tsuji and co-workers showed that 47% of infants with impaired cerebrovascular autoregulation developed IVH (or periventricular leukomalacia, or both), whereas only 13% of those with intact autoregulation developed these lesions.[169] Consistent with a potential role for arterial hypertension in this setting is the demonstration of a relationship between maximum systolic blood pressure above a threshold value and subsequent occurrence of IVH.[171] The limit for the highest tolerable peak systolic blood pressure was markedly lower for the smaller infants.[171] A particular role for minute-to-minute alterations in blood pressure has also been demonstrated.[172]

A more recent study continued to suggest the importance of elevations in cerebral perfusion being associated with high-grade IVH.[173] Thus cranial Doppler studies for middle cerebral artery cerebral blood flow velocity in 185 preterm infants who were receiving mechanical ventilation showed that severe IVH (grades 3 to 4) was associated with an elevation in diastolic closing margin—a measure of cerebral perfusion in diastole that exceeds "cerebral closing margin." The measures were a complex combination of assumptions based on Doppler-based estimations of cerebrovascular resistance and compliance. This modeling requires replication, but the findings suggest that high-grade IVH was associated with excessive cerebral perfusion. The timing of this elevation in relation to the timing of the IVH was not delineated within the study.

Moreover, as discussed in Chapter 13, the upper limit of the normal autoregulatory range in the infant is dangerously close to the upper limit of the range of normal blood pressure. Studies in developing animals indicate that the receptor number for specific vasoconstricting prostaglandins, which are important in setting the upper limit of the autoregulatory range in the adult, are low early in maturation and thereby impair protection of the cerebral circulation from increases in blood pressure.[174]

Whether the pressure-passive cerebral circulatory state relates to dysfunctional autoregulation per se, to maximal vasodilation caused by hypercarbia or hypoxemia (or both), to the cranial trauma of even a *normal* vaginal delivery, to dopamine therapy for hypotension, or to *normal* arterial blood pressures in the premature infant that are dangerously close to the upslope of a normal autoregulatory curve remains unclear. Experimental support for these several possibilities is available (see Chapter 13).[45,145,163,174–181] Whatever the mechanism, however, the balance of current data imparts particular importance to events that cause elevations in arterial blood pressure, especially abrupt elevations, in the small premature infant.

Causes of Increased Arterial Blood Pressure in the Human Newborn. The causes of abrupt elevations in arterial blood pressure sometimes shown to be accompanied by increased cerebral blood flow velocity by the Doppler technique, or increased cerebral blood volume by near-infrared spectroscopy in the premature infant, are clearly important to detect (and to prevent, whenever possible; Table 24.6). These causes include the following: such *physiological* events as rapid eye movement (REM) sleep and the first minutes and hours after birth; such *caretaking* concomitants as inadvertent noxious stimulation, abdominal examination, handling (see Figs. 24.10 and 24.22), instillation of mydriatics, and tracheal suctioning (Fig. 24.23);

TABLE 24.6   Major Causes of Increased Blood Pressure or Cerebral Blood Flow in the Premature Infant[a]

Related to "physiological" events
Postpartum status
Rapid eye movement sleep
Related to caretaking procedures
Noxious stimulation
Motor activity: spontaneous or with handling
Tracheal suctioning
Instillation of mydriatics
Related to systemic complications
Pneumothorax
Rapid volume expansion: exchange transfusion, other rapid colloid infusion
Ligation of patent ductus arteriosus
Related to neurological complications
Seizure

[a]See text for references.

systemic complications such as pneumothorax and rapid infusion of colloid; and neurological complications such as seizures.[154,155,158,182-209]

Although the degree to which these events contribute to the pathogenesis of IVH requires further quantitation and probably depends on concomitant clinical circumstances, particular importance can be attributed to *pneumothorax*.[142,155,210-214] In one earlier study of nine infants, pneumothorax was accompanied consistently by abrupt elevations of systemic blood pressure and cerebral blood flow velocity, and these circulatory changes were followed within hours by IVH.[155] Studies in newborn dogs documented abrupt increases in arterial blood pressure on rapid evacuation of pneumothorax.[211] Thus both clinical and experimental data emphasize the potentially deleterious circulatory effects of neonatal pneumothorax.

The complexity of interaction between respiratory and cardiovascular factors in the pathway to IVH is also notable with regard to pneumothorax. A major reduction in the risk of pneumothorax occurred following the administration of exogenous surfactant therapy. Indeed, the administration of surfactant reduced the risk of pneumothoraxes by almost 50% (RR 0.63; 95% CI, 0.53 to 0.75). However, despite this reduction in pneumothorax with surfactant administration, there has been no reduction in the incidence of IVH. One possible explanation for this lack of reduction in IVH may relate

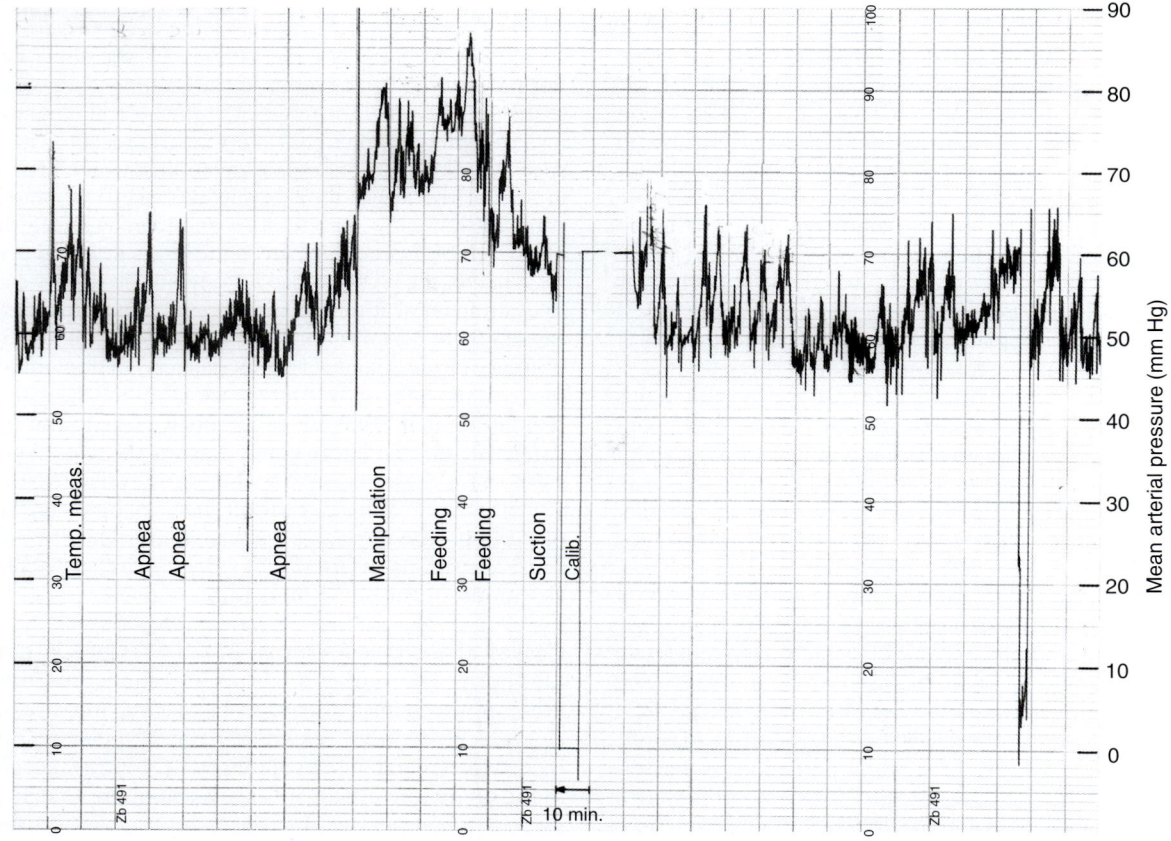

Figure 24.22 Increases of arterial blood pressure in the small premature infant. Continuous recording of mean aortic pressure in a 20-hour-old premature infant weighing 880 g. Note the marked and sustained increase with manipulation. The infant subsequently developed an intraventricular hemorrhage. (From Lou HC, Lassen NA, Friis-Hansen B. Is arterial hypertension crucial for the development of cerebral haemorrhage in premature infants? *Lancet.* 1979;1:1215–1217.)

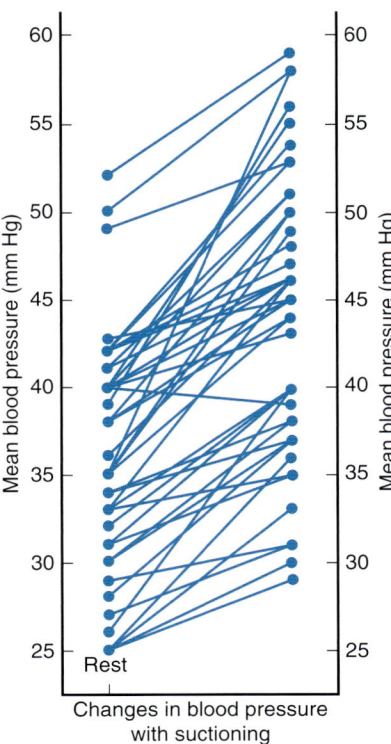

Figure 24.23 Changes in blood pressure with tracheal suctioning in premature infants. Note the increase in blood pressure that accompanied suctioning in all but one infant.

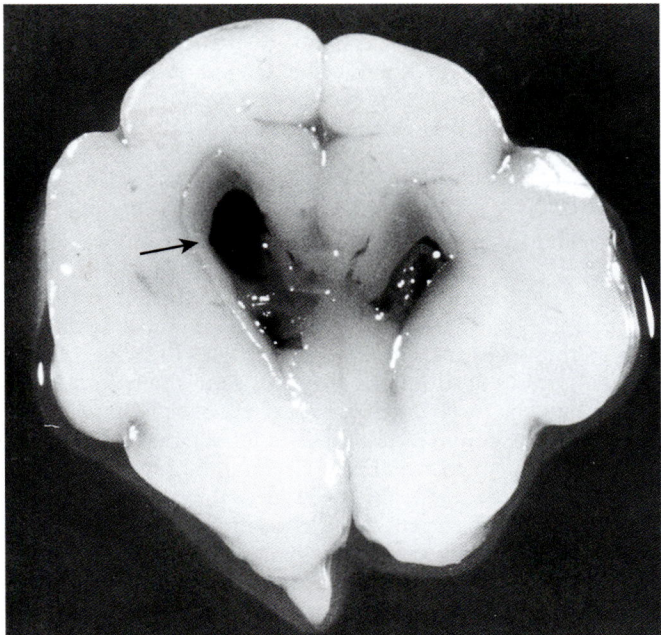

Figure 24.24 Intraventricular hemorrhage in the newborn beagle puppy. Gross intraventricular hemorrhage with dilation of the lateral ventricle *(arrow)* in cerebrum of a 24-hour-old puppy subjected to hypertension. (From Goddard J, Lewis RM, Armstrong DL, Zeller RS. Moderate, rapidly induced hypertension as a cause of intraventricular hemorrhage in the newborn beagle model. *J Pediatr.* 1980;96:1057–1060.)

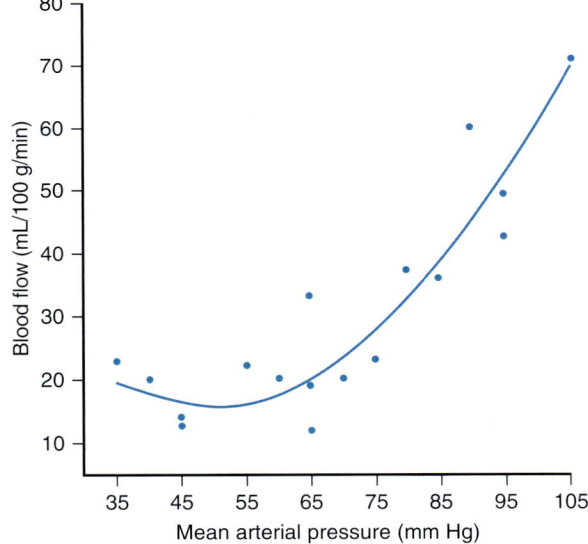

Figure 24.25 Increase in blood flow to germinal matrix with increase in arterial blood pressure in the newborn dog. Blood pressure was elevated by infusion of phenylephrine. Blood flow to the germinal matrix was measured by ^{14}C-iodoantipyrine autoradiography. (From Pasternak JF, Groothuis DR. Autoregulation of cerebral blood flow in the newborn beagle puppy. *Biol Neonate.* 1985;48:100–109.)

to changes in cardiovascular and respiratory stability during surfactant administration. As early as 1992, it was noted that during surfactant administration adverse changes in systemic and cerebral oxygenation could be seen. This has been replicated with less severe impact in recent years, with 62% of premature infants displaying reductions in cerebral electrophysiological activity with intubation and surfactant administration.[215] Thus surfactant administration may have a *double-edge* effect with a positive impact, with reduction of pneumothorax being offset by a potential negative effect of reduced cerebral perfusion during its administration. To determine the impact of therapies during this period of physiological instability in the preterm infant, monitoring of cerebral perfusion can provide much-needed guidance.

Relevant Experimental Studies: Role of Hypertension. The particular importance of abrupt increases in systemic blood pressure, and cerebral blood flow in pathogenesis has been demonstrated conclusively in elegant *experimental* studies in the newborn beagle puppy[178,216-224] and in the preterm sheep fetus.[225] The newborn puppy, which has been studied most extensively, has a subependymal germinal matrix approximately comparable to that of the human premature infant of 30 to 32 weeks of gestation.[226] Germinal matrix hemorrhage–IVH is produced most readily in this animal by a sequence of hypotension and hypertension produced by blood removal and volume reinfusion (Fig. 24.24). The marked increase in germinal matrix flow provoked by hypertension has been demonstrated strikingly by autoradiography (Fig. 24.25).[178]

Rapid Volume Expansion. The role of *rapid volume expansion* (see Table 24.4) involves not only the administration of blood or other colloid, as described in relation to systemic hypertension, but also the administration of hyperosmolar materials, such as hypertonic sodium bicarbonate. Pressure-passive cerebral circulation may not be the sole or even the principal means by which such infusions may lead to IVH, particularly in the case of *sodium bicarbonate*. Although the dangers of rapid infusion of hyperosmolar solutions had been noted for many years, an association of IVH in the premature infant administered sodium bicarbonate was emphasized initially by Simmons and co-workers[227] from study of an autopsy population. The association was later confirmed in a CT study of premature infants, and the importance of rapidity of infusion was made apparent.[228] Conflicting reports on the pathogenetic role of sodium bicarbonate[212,229-236] relate in part to the failure to take into account such factors as rapidity of administration and also to the problems of extrapolating data to living infants from studies of dead infants, particularly in the case of IVH. At any rate, the mechanism for the effect of rapid infusion of hyperosmolar sodium bicarbonate on intracranial hemorrhage may relate in part to the abrupt elevation of arterial pressure of carbon dioxide ($PaCO_2$) that results in the poorly ventilated or nonventilated patient from the buffering effect of the bicarbonate. The elevated $PaCO_2$ would then act on cerebral arterioles, by causing an increase in perivascular hydrogen ion (H^+) concentration, to increase cerebral perfusion as outlined next.

Hypercarbia. The role of *hypercarbia* in causing increases in cerebral blood flow of pathogenetic importance for IVH may be appreciable in selected infants. Hypercarbia, a common accompaniment of respiratory distress syndrome, respiratory complications, apneic episodes, and so forth, has been demonstrated conclusively to be a potent means for increasing cerebral blood flow in experimental studies (see Chapter 13). Indeed, careful studies of mechanically ventilated preterm infants show a pronounced reactivity of cerebral blood flow to changes in $PaCO_2$ ($\approx$30% increase in cerebral blood flow per kilopascal [kPa] increase in $PaCO_2$) after the first 24 hours of life.[162,163,166,237-240] Notably, in the first 24 hours of life, this normal reactivity was attenuated markedly ($\approx$10% increase in cerebral blood flow per kPa increase in $PaCO_2$) in mechanically ventilated infants with normal subsequent ultrasonograms, but it was actually *absent* in infants with subsequent severe IVH.[161] This observation suggested that, in the first day of life at least, hypercarbia of at least a moderate degree may not be a major pathogenetic factor for severe IVH in mechanically ventilated infants. A similar lack of correlation between hypercarbia and IVH is apparent in several other studies.[213,235,241] An increased risk for IVH after hypercarbia, however, is suggested in several other reports,[106,142,242-244] including three that used multivariate analysis.[214,244,245] In a particularly large study (n = 463), hypercarbia (defined as $PaCO_2$ >60 mm Hg) showed a positive relation with IVH.[214,243,247] In a later study of *permissive hypercapnia* to 45 to 55 mm Hg (vs. 35 to 45 mm Hg in the control group) in ventilated premature infants, no statistically significant difference in IVH was noted between the groups, although the incidence of severe IVH was 29% in the permissive hypercapnia group versus 20% in the control group (not statistically significant).[248] Thus a role for hypercarbia in the pathogenesis of IVH may require particularly marked elevations of $PaCO_2$. Consistent with this speculation is the demonstration that hypercapnia leads to clearly impaired autoregulation at $PaCO_2$ levels above 45 mm Hg (Fig. 24.26).[208] Such levels were shown to be significantly associated with the occurrence of

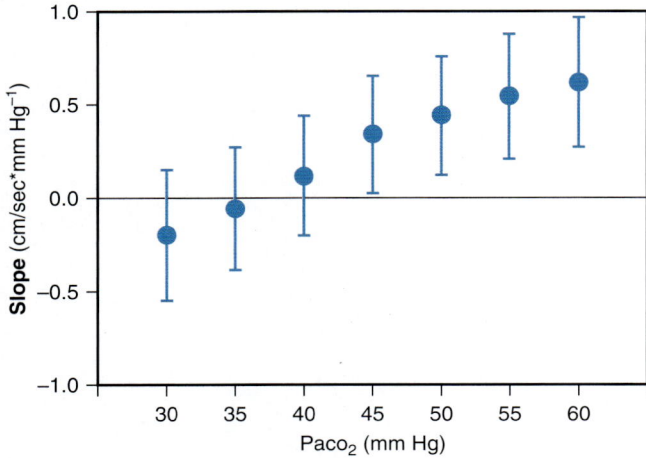

Figure 24.26 Impaired autoregulation with hypercapnia. Estimated mean slopes and 95% confidence intervals of the autoregulatory plateau for arterial carbon dioxide tension ($PaCO_2$) values 30, 35, 40, 45, 50, 55, and 60 mm Hg for 43 very low birthweight infants. Bars indicate 95% confidence intervals for the mean slopes of the autoregulatory plateaus for $PaCO_2$ 30 (n = 82), 35 (n = 94), 40 (n = 100), 45 (n = 103), 50 (n = 100), 55 (n = 90), and 60 mm Hg (n = 83). The horizontal line at slope 0 indicates intact autoregulation. The estimated means of the slope of the autoregulatory plateau (cm/sec* mm Hg^{-1}) increased as $PaCO_2$ increased (P = .004). (From Kaiser JR, Gauss CH, Williams DK. The effects of hypercapnia on cerebral autoregulation in ventilated very low birthweight infants. *Pediatr Res.* 2005;58:931–935.)

severe IVH and periventricular hemorrhagic infarction in a study of 58 infants.[249]

Decreased Hemoglobin. The role of *decreased hematocrit* in causing increases in cerebral blood flow of pathogenetic importance for IVH may be greater than was previously suspected. Thus, as described in Chapter 13, an inverse correlation exists in the human infant between hemoglobin concentration and cerebral blood flow, as well as between the concentration of adult versus fetal hemoglobin (higher hemoglobin oxygen affinity) and cerebral blood flow.[162,163,250-253] In one study of premature infants in the first days of life, cerebral blood flow increased by 12% per 1-mM decrease in hemoglobin.[162,250] The inverse relationship between hematocrit and cerebral blood flow described previously in experimental studies has been suggested to result from changes in arterial oxygen content or blood viscosity. Because alterations in newborn hematocrit to less than 60% have little influence on blood viscosity, the major factor in the studies of human infants is considered to be related to arterial oxygen content and thereby cerebral oxygen delivery. Cerebral blood flow presumably increases to maintain cerebral oxygen delivery at a constant level. Consistent with this possibility, apparently *stable* premature infants with low hematocrits (<21%) had clinically unsuspected high cardiac output.[254] The adaptive response of increased cerebral blood flow may become maladaptive if certain vulnerable capillary beds (e.g., in the germinal matrix) are exposed to the elevated cerebral blood flow. When one considers that iatrogenic blood loss, owing to repeated blood sampling, and low initial blood volume are common in sick premature infants, especially during the periods of highest risk for occurrence of IVH, the role of decreased hematocrit as a cause of IVH could be considerable.

Potentially consistent with supporting the role of anemia in the risk for IVH, a recent study demonstrated an increased risk of severe IVH among VLBW infants following a red cell transfusion within the first 72 hours of birth. This finding remained significant after controlling for confounding variables (RR, 2.02 [95% CI, 1.54 to 3.33]).[255] The authors were unable to determine the underlying mechanism, given the retrospective nature of the review, but one possibility for the increased risk is concomitant anemia requiring transfusion, rather than the transfusion itself. However, the infants developing IVH may have been sicker and thus at greater risk. Indeed, although there was no difference in coagulation measures, the infants with IVH received more frozen plasma and platelet transfusions and had longer ampicillin courses, higher nucleated RBC counts, more vasopressor use, and a higher mortality rate.

Relevant in this context are results of studies of the timing of cord clamping. Delayed cord clamping (DCC; 30 seconds), compared with immediate cord clamping (6 to 7 seconds), is associated with a slightly higher baseline hematocrit (49% vs. 46%), higher mean blood pressure (33.8 vs. 31.9 mm Hg), increased superior vena caval flow, and a significantly reduced risk for IVH (14% vs. 36%).[256,257] This reduction in IVH with DCC is supported by a meta-analysis of the randomized trials in preterm infants, although it is noteworthy that the largest studies included involve larger preterm infants with birthweights greater than 1500 g.[258] Because of these benefits in preterm infants and the advantages of increasing iron stores in healthy term-born infants, the American College of Obstetricians and Gynecologists recommended a delay in umbilical cord clamping in vigorous term and preterm infants for at least 30 to 60 seconds after birth.[259]

Blood Glucose. *Decreased blood glucose* now should be considered in the evaluation of pathogenetic factors for IVH in view of the observation that cerebral blood flow increases twofold to threefold when blood glucose declines to levels lower than 1.7 mM in the premature infant.[162,238,260] Blood glucose levels lower than 1.7 mM in premature infants are not unusual in the first days of life in many NICUs (see Chapter 25).

Increased blood glucose has also been evaluated as a potential risk factor for IVH. In a recent case-control study of high-grade IVH (n = 70) compared with no IVH (n = 108), infants with IVH had significantly more hyperglycemic events (2.9 ± 1.7 vs. 2.4 ± 1.8 events, P < .05) with longer duration (22.2 ± 14.2 vs. 14.1 ± 12.5 hours, P < .001) and a higher hyperglycemic index (1.0 ± 0.9 vs. 1.4 ± 1.0, P = .003). Respiratory distress syndrome, hypotension, and thrombocytopenia increased the adjusted OR for IVH. Hypoglycemia was not independently associated with IVH. Conversely, the increase in hyperglycemic duration most prominently increased the aOR for severe IVH (OR = 10.33; 95% CI, 10.0 to 10.6; P = .033). To avoid hyperglycemia, insulin therapy is often initiated. However, an important randomized controlled trial of *tight* glycemic control with insulin versus standard care documented a nonsignificant trend toward an increase in the incidence of grade III/IV IVH in the insulin-treated group (insulin 6/38 infants, 14%, vs. standard care 3/43, 7%, P = .35).[261] The insulin-treated group did have more episodes of hypoglycemia. Thus avoidance of protracted hyperglycemia and hypoglycemia may be most prudent as further data are collected on this clinical factor.

Finally, it has been suggested that alterations in the osmotic gradient may occur with hyperglycemia and other metabolic derangements, such as hypernatremia, leading to an increase in the intravascular pressure relative to the surrounding extravascular tissue that may predispose to IVH.[262] Several cohort studies have shown that those states associated with an alteration in the osmotic balance, such as hyperglycemia and hypernatremia (even high sodium intake in the absence of hypernatremia), are associated with an increased risk for IVH.[263-266] However, the retrospective nature of these studies cannot delineate the underlying mechanism for this increased risk.

Increases in Cerebral Venous Pressure

Elevations of cerebral venous pressure may contribute to the occurrence of IVH. Indeed, the potential importance of venous factors is suggested by the demonstration that with postmortem injection of carotid artery or jugular vein in infants with germinal matrix hemorrhage, the injected material entered the hemorrhage only through venous injections.[73] Moreover, careful anatomical studies also are consistent with an origin at the level of the capillary-venule junction or the small venule.[75] The *most important causes* for such increases are labor and delivery, asphyxia, and respiratory complications (see later discussion).

Importance of Venous Anatomy. The particular importance of increased venous pressure in the pathogenesis of IVH relates in part to the *venous anatomy* in the region of the germinal matrix (see Fig. 24.6). Thus the direction of deep venous flow takes a peculiar U-turn in the subependymal region at the level of the foramen of Monro (i.e., the most common site of germinal matrix hemorrhage). Also at this site is the point of confluence of the medullary, thalamostriate, and choroidal veins to form, in sequence, the terminal vein and then the internal cerebral vein, which ultimately empties into the vein of Galen.

Labor and Delivery. Concerning labor and delivery, marked increases in cerebral venous pressure must be common accompaniments. Indeed, in one study of 46 infants, when measurement of "fetal head compression pressure" was determined by a compression transducer positioned between the fetal head and the wall of the uterus,[267] the overall mean pressure was 158 mm Hg. *Deformations of the particularly compliant premature skull* are likely to accentuate the increases in venous pressure caused by normal labor. Indeed, the deleterious effects of labor (see later discussion) appear to be most pronounced in the most premature infants.[34,106,236,268,269] The skull deformations can lead to obstruction of major venous sinuses and presumably increased venous pressure.[47,270] Support for this notion has been provided by studies of blood flow velocity in the sagittal sinus, cerebral blood volume, and intracranial pressure during such manipulations as external pressure on the skull or rotation of the neck.[271,272] These effects may be expected to be greater with breech delivery. Available data are somewhat inconsistent concerning a relationship between such factors as presence or absence of labor, duration of labor, mode of delivery, and the occurrence of IVH, although in general the studies were not designed to address these issues specifically and were retrospective.[212,233,273-287] The inconsistency of the data, however, does not rule out a *contributory role* of intrapartum

TABLE 24.7   Occurrence of Germinal Matrix Hemorrhage as a Function of Route of Delivery and Duration of Labor

LABOR	ROUTE OF DELIVERY	
	VAGINAL	**ABDOMINAL**
None	—	6.1% (8/131)
<6 h	23.2% (19/82)	14.7% (12/129)
6–12 h	22.5% (9/40)	18.5% (5/27)
>12 h	32.1% (9/28)	25.0% (3/12)

Data from Leviton A, Fenton T, Kuban KC, Pagano M. Labor and delivery characteristics and the risk of germinal matrix hemorrhage in low birth weight infants. *J Child Neurol.* 1991;6:35–40.

events in causation of IVH in certain infants. Thus, in a study that addressed the role of presence or absence of labor, duration of labor, mode of labor, and potential confounders in a multivariate analysis, Leviton and co-workers[34] showed that infants delivered vaginally were more likely to develop IVH than those delivered abdominally, that labor longer than 12 hours increased risk of IVH regardless of the mode of delivery, and that the occurrence of labor before abdominal delivery increased the incidence of IVH by 2 to 4 times, depending on the duration of labor (Table 24.7). In a separate study of 201 VLBW infants, multivariate analysis also indicated an increased risk (2.2-fold) of IVH for infants delivered vaginally, a very low risk (7%) for infants delivered abdominally with no labor, and an increased risk among infants delivered abdominally for labor greater than 10 hours in duration (40%).[288] Subsequent investigations of 229 and 254 infants, respectively, show an increased risk of IVH occurring in the first 3 to 12 hours of life as a function of active labor and vaginal delivery.[106,107,287] Finally, a multicenter study of 4795 infants of less than 1500 g birthweight showed an incidence of *grade III and IV IVH* in 19% of vaginally delivered infants and 11% of those delivered by cesarean section without labor.[269] On balance, these data suggest that labor and delivery influence the risk of IVH in premature infants and have implications concerning a potential role for cesarean section in prevention (see later discussion).

The most recent studies of mode of delivery relative to IVH have continued to demonstrate conflicting results, with several finding no association with method of delivery.[289-292] A recent study of 158 infants born at less than 1500 g found that there was an increased risk of mild IVH among infants with vaginal delivery versus cesarean section before the second stage of labor.[293] The studies that did not report an association between mode of delivery and IVH did not comment on the duration of labor or the stage during which the cesarean section was performed, possibly explaining the discrepancies in the literature. Of note, it has been recently shown that head position, both before delivery and in the neonatal nursery, may also alter cerebral venous drainage. One study with near-infrared spectroscopy showed that cerebral venous drainage may be impaired in prone or side positions.[272]

Hypoxic-Ischemic Injury. With perinatal asphyxial events, circulatory collapse may lead to hypoxic-ischemic cardiac failure and, as a consequence, increased cerebral venous pressure. The cardiac disturbance is caused by injury of papillary muscle, subendocardial tissue, and myocardium.[294-303] The importance of increased venous pressure in association with asphyxia in the causation of IVH was shown in experimental studies of preterm fetal sheep.[225] Thus it seems likely that increased venous pressure could contribute to the propensity to IVH observed after serious asphyxia. Consistent with this notion are the strong relationships among such factors as severe umbilical cord acidemia, low Apgar scores, the need for neonatal resuscitation, and the occurrence of severe IVH (see later).[249,304] Other factors associated with asphyxia, such as ischemic injury to the germinal matrix and hypercarbia, are also likely important.

Respiratory Disturbances. Concerning *respiratory disturbances*, available data suggest that such factors as positive-pressure ventilation with relatively high peak inflation pressure, tracheal suctioning, abnormalities of the mechanics of respiration, and pneumothorax may be major causes of increased cerebral venous pressure in the premature infant.[303,305-311] Thus, extending earlier observations,[307,310,312] Cowan and Thoresen[305] used Doppler measurements of blood flow velocity in the superior sagittal sinus to demonstrate a striking sensitivity of the venous circulation to the level of peak inflation pressure; the smallest infants exhibited the most marked effects.

The possibility of a particular importance for venous abnormalities in causation of IVH was raised by a study of intubated preterm infants with respiratory distress syndrome under conditions in which dangerous alterations in arterial blood pressure occur (i.e., elevations with tracheal suctioning[189] and fluctuations with breathing out of synchrony with the ventilator[144]). The effects on the venous circulation were dramatic.[309] With elevations in arterial blood pressure produced by tracheal suctioning, pronounced changes in venous pressure also occurred (Fig. 24.27A). Moreover, because the magnitude and the direction of the changes in venous pressure often were not similar to those in arterial pressure, striking changes in perfusion pressure resulted (see Fig. 24.27B). Similarly, because fluctuations in arterial blood pressure were associated with noncoordinated fluctuations in venous pressure (Fig. 24.28A), pronounced and continuous alterations in perfusion pressure resulted (see Fig. 24.28B). Thus, under both circumstances, *decreases* in perfusion pressure by as much as 10 to 20 mm Hg were followed in seconds by abrupt, similar *increases* in perfusion pressure. Because these changes occur essentially on a beat-to-beat basis, it is unlikely that autoregulation, even if functional, could protect critical capillary beds by causing the changes in arteriolar diameter necessary to maintain constant cerebral blood flow under such circumstances. Thus the previously established role for disturbed mechanics of respiration with fluctuations in arterial blood pressure in the causation of IVH (see Table 24.5)[140] may be mediated as much by alterations on the venous side of the cerebral circulation as by alterations on the arterial side. A similar conclusion can be drawn for the previously established role[155] in the causation of IVH of abruptly increased arterial blood pressure with pneumothorax, because this respiratory complication has been shown to cause abruptly increased venous pressure as well.[211,303,313,314] A study of 58 cases of severe IVH with periventricular hemorrhagic infarction showed a significant relationship of pneumothorax with the occurrence of the lesion.[249]

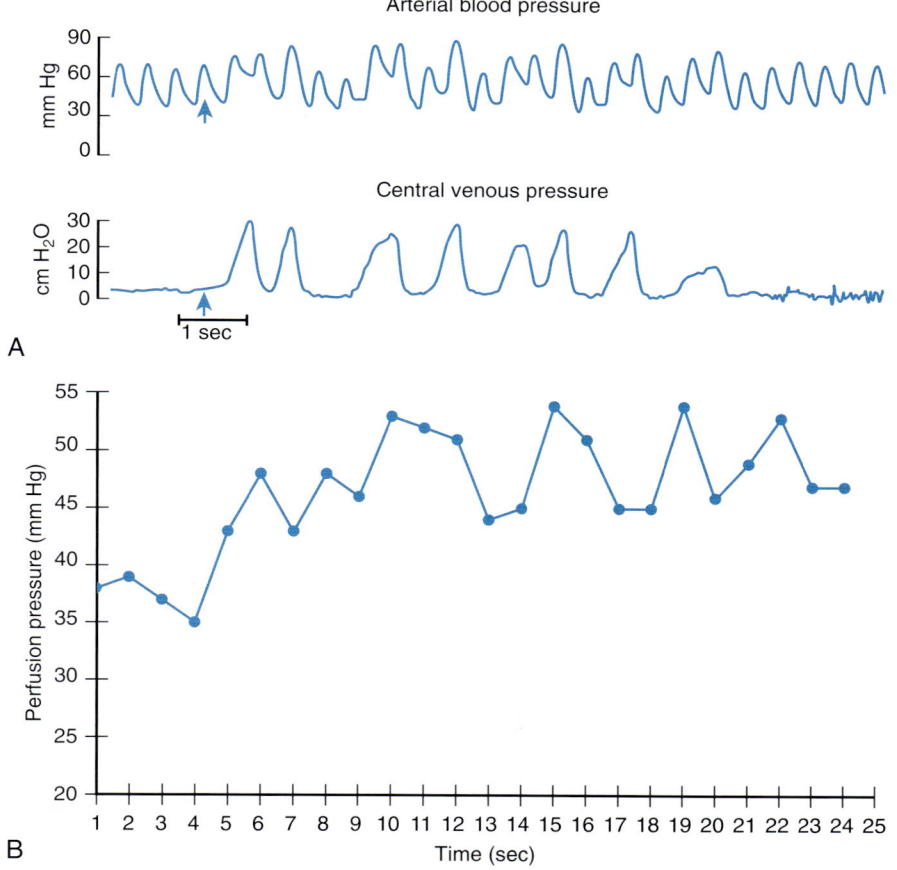

Figure 24.27 Venous pressure response to suctioning. (A) Simultaneous venous pressure and arterial blood pressure tracings from a premature infant during tracheal suctioning *(arrowhead)*. Note the pronounced increases in venous pressure after onset of suctioning. (B) Graphic plot of calculated changes in perfusion pressure during the same suctioning episode. (Adapted from Perlman JM, Volpe JJ. Are venous circulatory abnormalities important in the pathogenesis of hemorrhagic and/or ischemic cerebral injury? *Pediatrics.* 1987;80:705–711.)

Decreases in Cerebral Blood Flow

Importance of Pressure-Passive Cerebral Circulation. Decreases in cerebral blood flow, occurring either prenatally (perhaps primarily intrapartum) or postnatally, may play an important role in pathogenesis of IVH in certain infants. The principal consequence of the decreased cerebral blood flow is injury of germinal matrix vessels, which rupture subsequently on reperfusion. The importance of vascular border zones and end zones in the matrix, as well as the intrinsic vulnerability of the matrix vessels to oxygen deprivation, is emphasized later (see the section on vascular factors). As indicated earlier, hemorrhagic hypotension preceding volume reexpansion is the optimal means to produce IVH experimentally in the newborn beagle puppy. In the premature infant, decreases in cerebral blood flow are most likely with perinatal hypoxia-ischemia and with various postnatal events that result in systemic hypotension. Because of the pressure-passive cerebral circulation in sick premature infants, this hypotension can lead to a decrease in cerebral blood flow. Recall that a detailed study of 90 premature infants in the first 5 days of life showed that more than 95% had pressure-passive periods, with a mean total time of pressure-passivity of 20%.[114]

Perinatal Hypoxic-Ischemic Events. Although it is not an obligatory event for development of IVH, the infant with prior perinatal asphyxia clearly has an increased likelihood of developing IVH, and, in our experience, the hemorrhage in such infants tends to be relatively large. Indeed, a study of 58 infants with periventricular hemorrhagic infarction found a strong association of the lesion with fetal distress and the need for emergency cesarean section, low Apgar scores, and the need for respiratory resuscitation.[249] Perinatal hypoxic-ischemic events presumably explain, at least in part, the relation between low Apgar scores, early acidosis, early use of bicarbonate or pressors, hypocarbia, and the subsequent overall occurrence of IVH, particularly lesions that develop in the first 12 hours.[a] The mechanism for provocation of IVH with perinatal asphyxia is complex and includes increases in cerebral blood flow associated with impaired vascular autoregulation, increases in cerebral venous pressure, and decreases in cerebral blood flow associated with hypotension, with resulting injury to matrix capillaries. Release of endogenous vasodilators (e.g., adrenomedullin) in the

[a]References 212, 244, 249, 287, 304, and 315-317.

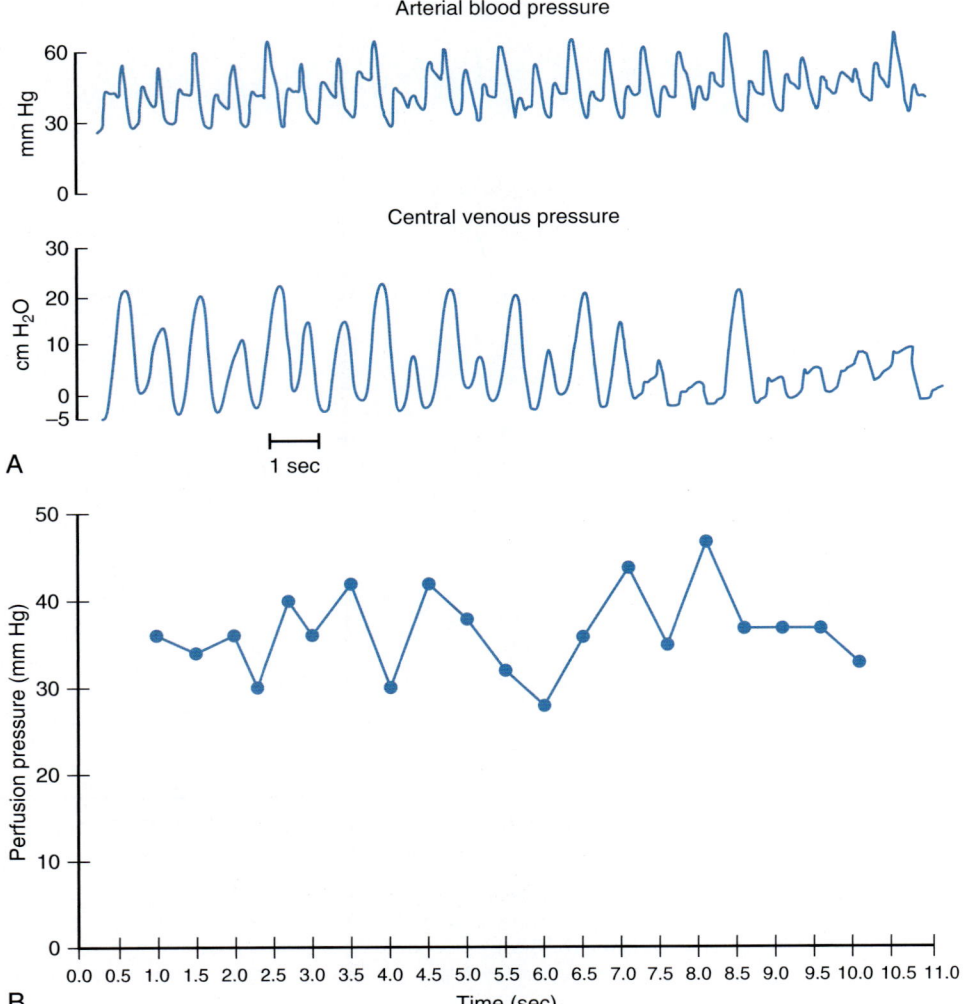

Figure 24.28 Correlation of fluctuations in arterial and venous pressure. (A) Simultaneous venous pressure and arterial blood pressure tracings from an infant with fluctuating blood pressure. Note that the marked fluctuations in arterial pressure are associated with marked fluctuations in venous pressure. (B) Graphic plot of calculated changes in perfusion pressure in the same infant. (Adapted from Perlman JM, Volpe JJ. Are venous circulatory abnormalities important in the pathogenesis of hemorrhagic and/or ischemic cerebral injury? *Pediatrics.* 1987;80:705–711.)

first hours after birth may also play a role in this situation.[318] Studies of the concentrations of brain-specific creatine kinase isoenzymes in cord blood or blood samples obtained early in the postnatal period or of the hypoxanthine metabolite, uric acid, in blood samples obtained on the first postnatal day, in preterm infants who later developed IVH, support the notion that late intrauterine injury (perhaps asphyxia) may be involved in at least some cases of IVH.[319-321] In one study, those infants who developed IVH had cord blood levels of brain-specific creatine kinase (CK-BB) that were 6 times greater than those in the infants who did not develop IVH.[319] Moreover, the possibility of a perinatal hypoxic-ischemic insult to brain as a predecessor to IVH is suggested also by the finding of depressed amplitude-integrated electroencephalographic activity before the occurrence of the hemorrhage in 4 of 10 carefully studied preterm infants.[322] In a separate study, early continuous electroencephalographic monitoring detected such

abnormalities as excessive discontinuity before the occurrence of IVH.[323] These abnormalities are similar to those produced by hypoxic-ischemic insults (see Chapter 10).

More recent studies have documented a high incidence of seizures in the preterm infant in the first 72 hours of life,[324] accompanied by a strong association with the presence of IVH. In one study, 95 VPT infants underwent aEEG monitoring during the first 72 hours of life. The overall incidence of seizures in this sample was 48%. High seizure burden was associated with increased risk of IVH throughout each of the 3 days of monitoring.[325] The seizures observed in this very preterm cohort demonstrated a similar evolution in the timeline to the seizures of a term infant suffering from hypoxic-ischemic encephalopathy (HIE) with the highest median seizure burden during the 0- to 24-hour period. These observations support a potential role of perinatal asphyxia in the pathway to IVH.

Postnatal Ischemic Events. The importance of *postnatal decreases in cerebral blood flow* in the pathogenesis of IVH has been shown by studies using a combination of noninvasive methods to evaluate the cerebral circulation.[170,287,326-328] Notably, however, a relationship with decreases in *mean arterial blood pressure*, when infants who developed IVH were compared with infants who did not develop IVH, was not uniformly shown. *Thus the changes in cerebral hemodynamics could occur without pronounced disturbances of mean arterial blood pressure.* These findings of a lack of association between mean arterial blood pressure and IVH were recently replicated. Rhee and co-workers documented no relationship between systemic blood pressure and risk for IVH but did document a relationship between measures of cerebral blood flow with IVH.[173] This finding continues to emphasize the inability of systemic measures of blood pressure to define the adequacy of cerebral perfusion. Because impaired autoregulation and fluctuations in blood pressure are both frequent but not necessarily constant in the sick preterm infant,[114] intermittent declines in cerebral blood flow could occur without pronounced changes in mean blood pressure. Thus *continuous measurements of the cerebral circulation are critical in determining changes in cerebral blood flow in the sick, ventilated infant.*

Nevertheless the importance of postnatal decreases in arterial blood pressure in the pathogenesis of IVH is suggested by several studies in which arterial blood pressure was monitored continuously from birth or the first hours of life. In a study of approximately 25,000 VLBW infants, severe IVH was 3 times more common in those infants requiring cardiopulmonary resuscitation (15.3%) at delivery than in those not requiring resuscitation (4.9%).[329] A relationship between arterial hypotension and subsequent occurrence of IVH has been documented frequently.[172,212,330-332] Although the possibility of ischemic insult to germinal matrix in the postnatal period is obvious in association with such occurrences as severe apnea, myocardial failure, sepsis, and so forth, sharp decreases in blood pressure have also been shown to precede the more widely recognized increases provoked by ordinary caretaking procedures.[188] By continuous monitoring of arterial blood pressure during such procedures as auscultation of the chest, taking of temperature, and suctioning, the increases in blood pressure previously noted were shown to be preceded by a decrease in blood pressure. The decreases were most pronounced in the infants requiring the most intensive ventilatory support. The biphasic response of decrease and then increase in blood pressure is qualitatively similar to the sequence required to produce IVH in the beagle puppy (see earlier). The rebound elevation of cerebral blood flow velocity observed after apnea and bradycardia is relevant in this context.[333]

Of particular importance concerning a role for postnatal ischemia is the demonstration by near-infrared spectroscopy in 24 preterm infants in the first 24 hours of life that cerebral blood flow was significantly lower in infants with subsequent demonstration of IVH (median, 7.0 mL/100 g/min) than in those without IVH (median, 12.2 mL/100 g/min).[334] In addition supportive of a relationship between postnatal ischemic events and the occurrence of IVH is the demonstration of decreased cardiac output in the first 36 hours of life in infants who developed the lesion, especially with severe IVH.[335] Similarly, the occurrence of periventricular hemorrhagic infarction with severe IVH was strongly associated with metabolic acidosis in the first days of life and a need

for pressor support and volume expanders.[249] Finally, the beneficial effect of delayed versus immediate clamping of the umbilical cord on the incidence of IVH is considered to be likely caused in considerable part by stabilization of cerebral blood flow and prevention of ischemia.[256,336] However, as mentioned earlier, the interrelationships between cerebral hypoperfusion and IVH appear complex, with an early ischemic period potentially increasing the vulnerability for reperfusion injury to the germinal matrix. These evolutions can only be evaluated with the presence of *monitoring of both systemic and cerebral hemodynamics simultaneously.*

The contributory role of *maternal intrauterine infection and fetal systemic inflammation* in the pathogenesis of IVH likely is mediated by effects on the cerebral circulation. Although data are not entirely consistent concerning a relationship between chorioamnionitis and the occurrence of IVH, several reports indicate an association with IVH of elevated levels of specific cytokines, especially interleukin-6 (IL-6), in cord or early neonatal blood.[337-344] Infants with chorioamnionitis *and* fetal cord vasculitis had higher IL-6 levels and likelihood of IVH than those with fetal vasculitis alone.[339] The findings suggest that maternal intrauterine infection that leads to a systemic fetal inflammatory response is critical. Indeed, a recent large study of periventricular hemorrhagic infarction (*n* = 58) found no association with maternal fever, maternal infection, or pathologically confirmed chorioamnionitis.[249] The principal mechanism of the fetal/neonatal cytokine effect is likely circulatory disturbance. Thus decreased arterial blood pressure, often requiring pressor support, has been shown in the infants with elevated IL-6.[339,342] IL-6, like several other cytokines, has vasodilator properties that likely lead to the decreased blood pressure and presumably cerebral blood flow (Fig. 24.29). Whether IL-6 or related cytokines impair cerebrovascular autoregulation is plausible but not yet shown.

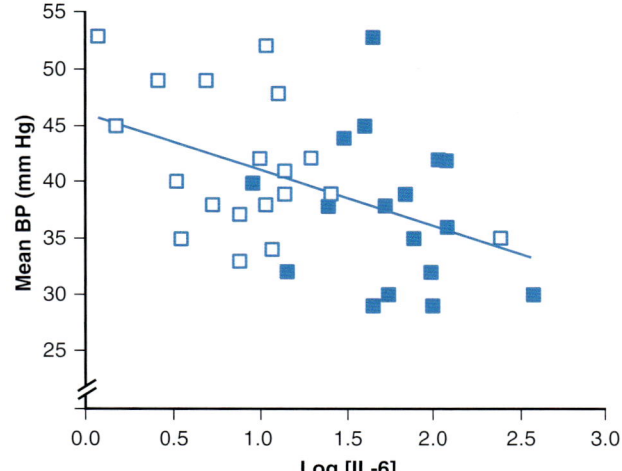

Figure 24.29 Relationship between mean arterial blood pressure (BP) and interleukin-6 (IL-6) concentration. Mean BP was inversely correlated (R^2 = 0.21, P < .01) with log IL-6. Solid square, chorioamnionitis; open square, no chorioamnionitis. (From Yanowitz TD, Jordan JA, Gilmour CH, Towbin R, et al. Hemodynamic disturbances in premature infants born after chorioamnionitis: association with cord blood cytokine concentrations. *Pediatr Res.* 2002;51:310–316.)

Platelet and Coagulation Disturbances

Disturbances of platelet-capillary function and coagulation may contribute to the pathogenesis of IVH (see Table 24.4). The lack of uniformity in results of studies designed to investigate the pathogenetic role of such disturbances, however, emphasizes that the role is likely to be contributory or important only in certain patients.

Platelet-Capillary Function. Regarding platelet-capillary function, an earlier prospective study is of particular interest.[345] Forty percent of infants of less than 1500 g birthweight exhibited platelet counts less than 100,000/mm³,[319] and most of these thrombocytopenic infants had abnormal bleeding times. The incidences of IVH in thrombocytopenic versus nonthrombocytopenic infants were 78% versus 48% for those weighing less than 1000 g. Additional analysis for other factors potentially important for causation of IVH suggested that the presence of thrombocytopenia was an independent pathogenetic factor. Subsequent work has both confirmed and refuted a role for thrombocytopenia in the pathogenesis of IVH.[346-348]

While subsequent work has both confirmed and refuted a role for thrombocytopenia in the pathogenesis of IVH,[346,347,349] the most recent studies have tended to support an association. The largest of these evaluated 655 infants born at less than 32 weeks' gestational age, 44% of whom had thrombocytopenia. Within this cohort there was a 30% (85/286) incidence of IVH in those with thrombocytopenia versus 14% (53/369) in those with a normal platelet count.[347] Interestingly there was no correlation between the severity of thrombocytopenia and the incidence of IVH; rather the relationship was dichotomous.[346,347] Similarly no protective effect was demonstrated with increased platelet transfusion, as might be expected if there was a linear correlation with platelet count.[350] In an alternate cohort of 251 neonates, Rastogi and colleagues found no significant difference in severe IVH with or without thrombocytopenia in isolation, but the odds of a severe IVH were increased fourfold if there was a sudden drop in the platelet count. The odds increased to 14 times the baseline if this sudden decline occurred from a baseline of thrombocytopenia.[349] The exact mechanism between IVH and thrombocytopenia has not yet been elucidated. Some evidence suggests that premature infants demonstrate elevated levels of prostacyclin before the occurrence of IVH.[351] Because prostaglandins have an impact not only on platelet function but also on such factors as cerebral blood flow and free radical production that also may be important in pathogenesis of IVH, it is not clear to what extent effects on platelet-capillary function were independently related to causation of IVH.

Perhaps relevant to the possibility of disturbed platelet *function* (rather than platelet count) in some infants before the occurrence of IVH is the study by Rennie and co-workers[351] of circulating levels of the principal metabolite of prostacyclin in preterm infants. Prostacyclin is a potent perturbant of platelet-capillary function and is produced in elevated amounts, probably by lung, in respiratory distress syndrome and with mechanical ventilation. Evidence was obtained for elevated levels of prostacyclin before the occurrence of IVH. Because prostaglandins additionally have an impact on such factors as cerebral blood flow and free radical production that also may be important in the pathogenesis of IVH, it is not clear to what extent effects on platelet-capillary function were independently

related to causation of IVH. More data are needed on these issues.

Coagulation. Disagreement exists concerning the role of coagulopathy in causation of IVH.[212,274,346,348,352-362] It could be postulated that prothrombotic disturbances (e.g., factor V Leiden mutation, prothrombin mutation) would increase IVH by provoking deep venous thrombosis or would decrease IVH by preventing extension of small hemorrhages. Because disturbances of coagulation are not uncommon in preterm infants with other provocative factors for IVH (e.g., serious respiratory distress syndrome, asphyxia) or may occur *secondary* to major hemorrhage, an independent pathogenetic role for such disturbances has been difficult to establish. Although administration of fresh frozen plasma was shown in one study to decrease the incidence of IVH,[352] no effect on coagulation measures accompanied the apparent beneficial effect. Moreover, a later investigation failed to show a beneficial effect of prophylactic early fresh frozen plasma in premature infants.[356,363] Administrative of antithrombin III, known to be low in premature infants, did not alter the incidence of IVH in a randomized study.[361]

Recent reports have examined the potential role of mutations in coagulation proteins as possible risk modifiers for IVH. Several common mutations in coagulation proteins are associated with increased tendency to thrombotic events. Those that have been investigated most included factor XIII Val34Leu mutation, factor V Leiden, factor II (prothrombin) G20210A, and MTHFR C677T. Factor XIII stabilizes the fibrin clot, and thus it is hypothesized that low levels of factor XIII may predispose to IVH. Low factor XIII levels in preterm infants may contribute to the relatively higher fibrinolytic activity documented in preterm infants.[364] Two recent studies, however, failed to find any association between factor XIII-Val34Leu mutation and IVH.[365,366] Factor V Leiden is a common mutation in the white population and is associated with thrombotic events, with decreased inactivation of factor V leading to increased thrombin generation. The role of factor V Leiden in risk of IVH is unclear. Results have been conflicting with some studies suggesting a significant role for factor V Leiden in the risk of IVH,[359,362,367] while others suggest no role,[359,362,367,368] or a mixed pattern, whereby the mutation is associated with low-grade IVH (grade I or II), but a reduced risk of severe IVH.[360,366]

There have been similarly conflicting findings for prothrombin G20210A mutations and the development of IVH.[365,367] Two mutations (C677T and A1298C) in the 5,10-methylene tetrahydrofolate reductase (MTHFR) gene lead to hyperhomocysteinemia under conditions of decreased folate or B$_{12}$ concentrations and an increased risk of thrombosis. Although no consistent association has been found with this mutation and IVH,[360,364] a recent report by Ment and co-workers did find a significantly increased association of this polymorphism among preterm infants, specifically with grade II–IV IVH.[369]

Potential Role of Drugs. The possibility that *maternal ingestion of certain drugs*, such as aspirin, can result in impaired neonatal hemostasis and provoke IVH was suggested by two earlier reports.[370,371] It is not likely, however, that such factors play a major independent role.[354] Similarly, retrospective data suggest that the use of heparin as an intravascular flush to maintain

TABLE 24.8	Pathogenesis of Germinal Matrix–Intraventricular Hemorrhage: Vascular Factors

Tenuous capillary integrity
Involuting, remodeling capillary bed
Deficient vascular lining
Large vascular and luminal area
Vulnerability of matrix capillaries to hypoxic-ischemic injury
Vascular border zones
High requirements for oxidative metabolism

patency of umbilical artery catheters increases the risk of IVH by fourfold.[372] Whether this effect is related to a disturbance of coagulation or to selection bias because of the use of heparin in sick premature infants who develop IVH for other reasons is unclear. A subsequent report also suggested an increasing risk for IVH in premature infants as a function of the daily dose of heparin.[373] More data are needed.

Vascular Factors

Vascular factors are those referable to the blood vessels of the germinal matrix (Table 24.8). As discussed earlier (see the section on neuropathology), the vascular site of origin likely involves the rich microcirculation of the germinal matrix and, specifically, endothelial-lined vessels not readily characterized as arterial or venous. Thus vascular factors are best grouped in two categories—those suggesting (1) that the integrity of small matrix vessels is tenuous and (2) that these vessels are particularly vulnerable to hypoxic-ischemic injury (see Table 24.8).

Tenuous Vascular Integrity

Three lines of anatomical evidence suggest that the integrity of the microvasculature is tenuous in the germinal matrix (see Table 24.8). First, these vessels, like the germinal matrix itself, are in a process of involution. Pape and Wigglesworth[47] characterized the elaborate capillary bed of the germinal matrix as "a persisting immature vascular rete," an immature microvascular network that is remodeled into a mature capillary bed when the matrix disappears. In keeping with this notion, transmission electron microscopic studies of the matrix reveal many small vessels with the absence of a complete basal lamina, a fenestrated lining, and other features characteristic of immature vessels.[374] This involuting remodeling capillary bed may be expected to be more susceptible to rupture than would more mature vessels.

Second, many studies emphasized that the matrix microcirculation is composed of simple endothelial-lined vessels, often of a larger size than capillaries but not readily categorized as arterioles or venules because of absence of muscle and collagen.[47-50,52,67-70,75,375] Particularly careful studies have documented in detail the absence of muscle[48] and of type VI collagen.[375] Investigators have postulated that such vessels are likely to be more susceptible to rupture. In favor of this postulate is the demonstration in the newborn beagle puppy of matrix vessels that are similar to those just described (i.e., relatively large size and thin walls[376]); these vessels are the sites of hemorrhage in this animal model of germinal matrix hemorrhage–IVH. Recent work emphasized the high vascular

density of the germinal matrix and the abundance of small veins, the walls of which are lined only by endothelial cells.[51,377]

Third, an electron microscopic study of cortical and germinal matrix vessels showed a twofold to fourfold greater diameter of both the vessels and the lumina of the vessels of the germinal matrix versus those of the cortical plate in infants of 25 to 33 weeks of gestation.[378] At 37 weeks of gestation, this difference had disappeared and, notably, the diameters of the matrix vessels and their lumina were twofold to threefold smaller than at 25 to 33 weeks. Thus, in the age range of greatest propensity for occurrence of IVH, the diameters are unusually large, a finding of potential pathogenetic importance because of the Laplace law, which states that the larger the vessel diameter, the greater the total force on the wall at any given pressure.

Fourth, as noted earlier, additional potential characteristics leading to fragility of the vasculature include discontinuous glial endfeet, relative lack of pericytes, and immature basal lamina components, among other features. Exuberant angiogenesis, postulated to be related partially to relative hypoxia of the richly cellular matrix and manifested by high VEGF and angiopoietin-2 levels, may lead to fragility and relative ease of rupture (see the earlier section on the site of origin).

The possibility should be considered that the effects of these maturational deficiencies of germinal matrix vessels underlie the interesting observation that women with a diagnosis of preeclampsia exhibit a lower risk for an infant with IVH (2.5%) than women without this diagnosis (17%).[35] This lower risk for IVH has been confirmed.[379,380] Infants born to preeclamptic mothers exhibit a variety of features suggestive of accelerated maturation of the brain and other organs.[212,381-383]

Vulnerability to Hypoxic-Ischemic Injury

Two features suggest a particular vulnerability of matrix capillaries to hypoxic-ischemic injury (see Table 24.8). First, as shown by Takashima and Tanaka,[46] at the usual site for matrix hemorrhage a vascular border zone exists between the end fields of the striate and thalamic arteries (Fig. 24.30). The demonstration of heterogeneity of blood flow within the matrix of the beagle puppy may represent the physiological correlate of the anatomical data.[222] Studies of hypotension in the fetal rat also demonstrate a vulnerability of the matrix to ischemia.[384] Thus it can be postulated that the matrix vessels could be readily injured by ischemia, and on reperfusion of these injured vessels, hemorrhage could occur. As indicated earlier, this notion is supported by the finding in the beagle puppy model of IVH that the free radical scavenger superoxide dismutase prevents hemorrhage caused by the usual hypotension-reperfusion sequence. Similarly, certain older studies in human infants (see later discussion) suggest that vitamin E, a free radical scavenger, has a preventive effect on IVH.

Second, matrix capillaries, like other brain capillaries, appear to have a high requirement for oxidative metabolism. Thus brain endothelial cells have been shown to contain 3 to 5 times more mitochondria than systemic capillary endothelial cells.[385,386] This intense oxidative activity would complement the presence of a vascular border zone in the matrix in enhancing the vulnerability of matrix vessels to ischemic insults.

Extravascular Factors

Extravascular factors are those referable to the space surrounding the germinal matrix capillaries (Table 24.9). These factors are

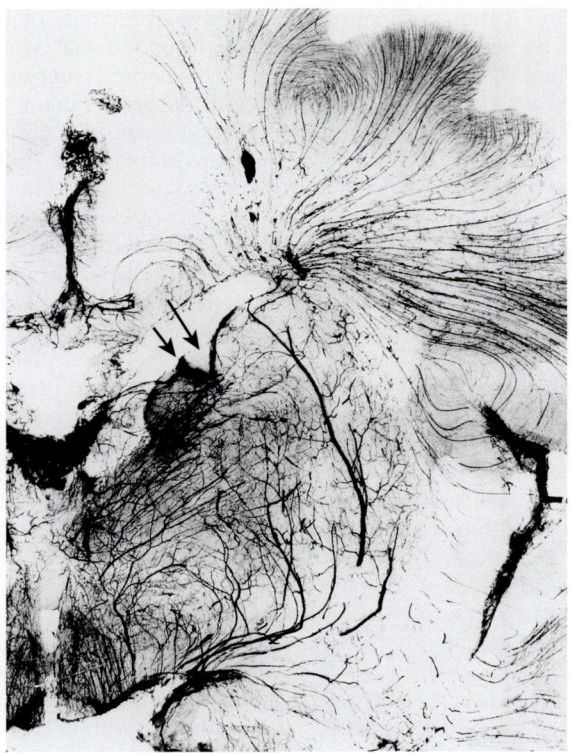

Figure 24.30 Vascular border zone and end zone at the site of germinal matrix hemorrhage. Postmortem arteriography of cerebral hemisphere (coronal section) of a premature infant of 32 weeks of gestational age. Note the triangular avascular area *(large arrow)* at the border zone between the end fields of the thalamostriate and medullary arteries at the site of a small subependymal hemorrhage *(small arrow)*. (From Takashima S, Tanaka K. Microangiography and vascular permeability of the subependymal matrix in the premature infant. *Can J Neurol Sci.* 1978;5:45–50.)

**TABLE 24.9   Pathogenesis of Germinal Matrix–
Intraventricular Hemorrhage:
Extravascular Factors**

Deficient vascular support
Fibrinolytic activity
Postnatal decrease in extravascular tissue pressure (?)

grouped best into the following three categories: deficient vascular support, fibrinolytic activity, and postnatal decrease in extravascular tissue pressure.

Deficient Vascular Support

The germinal matrix can be seen by gross examination to be a gelatinous, friable structure, and by microscopic examination to be deficient in supporting mesenchymal and glial elements.[45,67,387] Thus investigators have suggested that the extravascular space provides poor support for the large, endothelial-lined capillaries that course through it and that are the site of the hemorrhage. This formulation received experimental support from studies of the germinal matrix of the beagle puppy, which showed that large portions of the capillary walls lacked any direct contact with perivascular structures (unlike the capillaries in the

cerebral cortex or caudate nucleus).[376] Decisive demonstration of the potential importance of deficient vascular support in the human infant is derived from the work of Gould and Howard.[387] Thus, assessing astrocytic fibrillary development by immunocytochemical staining for glial fibrillary acidic protein (GFAP), these investigators showed minimal astrocytic development as late as 27 weeks of gestation and prominent GFAP staining, not until 31 weeks. A later detailed study also showed deficient GFAP and astrocytic endfeet overlying the germinal matrix vasculature during the gestational period of 23 to 34 weeks.[388] Because of the role of glial fibers in capillary stabilization, these data suggest an important role for deficient astrocytic development in pathogenesis of IVH in the premature infant. Lastly, immunomicroscopy of neuropathology specimens have shown that staining for tight junction proteins (ZO-1, claudin, and occludin) in the germinal matrix vessels at 24 weeks revealed reduced and immature staining patterns. Immature tight junctions between endothelial cells would affect the functionality of the blood-brain barrier and could predispose the vessels to hemorrhagic rupture.[389]

Fibrinolytic Activity

An excessive amount of fibrinolytic activity has been defined in the periventricular, germinal matrix region of the human premature infant (see Table 24.9).[390,391] Although the source of this activity is not established conclusively, it is likely that the fibrinolytic activity reflects the proteolytic action of the plasmin-generating system. This extracellular proteolytic system is composed of plasminogen activator, plasminogen, and plasmin.[392,393] Plasminogen activator, a protease secreted from cells, activates plasminogen to generate the protease plasmin, which, in turn, can degrade a wide variety of extracellular proteins. This system is involved in many developing, remodeling tissues as a normal maturational process. Fibrinolysis is only one action of this proteolytic system. In developing chick spinal cord, this system is most active during glial proliferation. Moreover, studies in cell culture show that the immature astrocyte (not the mature astrocyte) is the principal source for plasminogen activator and the action of this proteolytic system. Glial proliferation is very active in the germinal matrix at the usual time of occurrence of germinal matrix hemorrhage. It is reasonable to suspect that this fibrinolytic activity, an epiphenomenon of the proteolytic system required for remodeling of the germinal matrix, allows the small capillary hemorrhages of the matrix to become the large lesions characteristic of IVH.

Postnatal Decrease in Extravascular Tissue Pressure

The possibility that a postnatal decrease in extravascular tissue pressure causes an increase in the transmural intravascular-extravascular pressure gradient sufficient to provoke hemorrhage was raised by studies of the beagle puppy.[394,395] Administration of prolactin was shown to decrease the incidence and severity of hemorrhage in that animal model. The relevance to hemorrhage in the human premature infant, however, is unclear because the timing of the apparent postnatal decrease in extracellular volume in the premature infant[262,396-398] (i.e., 2 to 3 days of life) occurs *after* the peak time of occurrence of IVH. As noted earlier, it has been suggested that alterations in the osmotic gradient may occur with hyperglycemia and other metabolic derangements, such as hypernatremia, leading to an increase in the intravascular pressure relative to the surrounding

TABLE 24.10	Catastrophic Clinical Syndrome With Germinal Matrix–Intraventricular Hemorrhage

Inexorable evolution in minutes to hours
Neurological features
   Stupor → coma
   Respiratory disturbance → apnea
   Generalized tonic seizures
   "Decerebrate" posturing
   Pupils fixed to light
   Eyes fixed to vestibular stimulation
   Flaccid quadriparesis

TABLE 24.11	Saltatory Clinical Syndrome With Germinal Matrix–Intraventricular Hemorrhage

Stuttering evolution: hours to days
Neurological features
Altered level of consciousness
Altered motility (usually decreased)
Hypotonia
Abnormally tight popliteal angle
Abnormal eye position or movement or both
Respiratory disturbance

tissue that may predispose to IVH.[262] Several cohort studies have shown that these states associated with an alteration in the osmotic balance, such as hyperglycemia and hypernatremia (even high sodium intake in the absence of hypernatremia), are associated with an increased risk for IVH.[263-266] However, the retrospective nature of these studies cannot delineate the underlying mechanism for this increased risk.

Interaction of Pathogenetic Factors

As indicated throughout the preceding discussion, not *all* the pathogenetic factors operate in every case. *Clinical circumstances dictate which factors are most critical in the individual infant.* Perhaps the best example of the interaction of the most important pathogenetic factors is provided by the clinical situation of the premature infant who is mechanically ventilated for serious respiratory distress syndrome (see Fig. 24.19), the clinical setting for the largest proportion of all cases of IVH.

CLINICAL FEATURES

The principal clinical setting for IVH is a premature infant with respiratory distress syndrome severe enough to require mechanical ventilation. The *time of onset of hemorrhage*, defined most clearly by serial cranial ultrasonography (see the section on diagnosis), is the first day of life in at least 50% of affected infants, and by 72 hours, approximately 90% of the lesions can be identified. The timing of the initial clinical features, as expected, is similar.

Three Basic Syndromes

Three basic clinical syndromes accompany IVH: (1) a *catastrophic* deterioration (Table 24.10), (2) a *saltatory* deterioration (Table 24.11), and (3) a *clinically silent* syndrome. The least common but most dramatic of these is the catastrophic deterioration, which occurs in infants with the most severe hemorrhages. More common is the saltatory deterioration, and *most common of all is the clinically silent syndrome.* The latter two syndromes occur most often, although not exclusively, in infants with smaller lesions.

Catastrophic Syndrome

The catastrophic syndrome is dramatic in presentation (see Table 24.10). The deterioration evolves in minutes to hours and consists of deep stupor or coma, respiratory abnormalities (arrhythmias, hypoventilation, and apnea), generalized tonic seizures, decerebrate posturing, pupils fixed to light, eyes fixed

to vestibular stimulation, and flaccid quadriparesis. The clinical distinction between tonic seizures and *decerebrate* posturing is very difficult in this setting. Indeed, generalized tonic seizures in this setting most often do represent posturing rather than an epileptic phenomenon (see Chapter 12). The wide range of frequencies of seizure phenomena recorded with IVH (≈15% to 35%)[202,399-403] in part reflects this difficulty. In my experience, seizures occurring with IVH early in the neonatal course usually are associated with periventricular hemorrhagic infarction.

This impressive neurological syndrome is associated with numerous other features—for example, falling hematocrit, bulging anterior fontanelle, hypotension, bradycardia, temperature derangements, metabolic acidosis, and abnormalities of glucose and water homeostasis.[401,404-407] The latter include, particularly, inappropriate antidiuretic hormone secretion and, less commonly, diabetes insipidus.[404,407]

This catastrophic neurological syndrome most likely reflects the movement of blood through the ventricular system, with sequential affection of the diencephalon, midbrain, pons, and medulla. The signs of increased intracranial pressure reflect acute hydrocephalus. The outcome, often poor, reflects the severity of the hemorrhage and, particularly, the extent of complicating parenchymal involvement (see the section on prognosis).

Saltatory Syndrome

The saltatory syndrome is much more subtle in presentation (see Table 24.11).[408,409] The most common presenting signs are (1) an alteration in the level of consciousness, (2) a change (usually a decrease) in the quantity and quality of spontaneous and elicited motility, (3) hypotonia, and (4) subtle aberrations of eye position and movement (e.g., skew deviation, vertical drift, usually down, and incomplete horizontal movement with the doll's eyes maneuver). In some patients, disturbances of respiratory function appear to be concomitants, but more data are needed on this issue. In one careful study of serial clinical evaluations and ultrasonographic examinations, an abnormal popliteal angle was found to be a particularly useful diagnostic sign.[403] Eighty-four percent of premature infants with IVH (vs. 10% of infants without hemorrhage) exhibited an abnormally tight angle, perhaps secondary to meningeal irritation. The signs of the saltatory syndrome evolve over many hours, and the deterioration often ceases, only to begin anew after several more hours. This stuttering course may continue for a day or more. The outcome, most often favorable, again relates to the ultimate severity of the hemorrhage and any accompanying parenchymal involvement (see the section on prognosis).

Clinically Silent Syndrome

The neurological signs of the saltatory syndrome may be so subtle that they are overlooked. Indeed, in a prospective study of infants subjected to clinical assessment and CT scan in the first week of life, only approximately 50% of cases of IVH were correctly predicted to have the lesion on the basis of clinical criteria.[402] The most valuable sign was an unexplained fall in hematocrit or a failure of hematocrit to rise after transfusion. In the serial study of Dubowitz and co-workers,[403] approximately 75% of cases had three or more of the abnormal neurological signs of the saltatory syndrome. Thus, in 25% to 50% of infants with IVH, even careful, serial clinical assessments may fail to reveal a distinct constellation of signs indicative of the lesion.

DIAGNOSIS

Initial Approach

The two essential steps in establishing the diagnosis of IVH are recognition of the *clinical setting* and use of a suitable *screening procedure.* In view of the high incidence of the hemorrhage, any very premature infant in a neonatal intensive care facility can be at risk. Thus such infants should be subjected to a suitable screening procedure.

Although *the screening procedure of choice is portable cranial ultrasonography* (see the section on ultrasound scan later), *lumbar puncture (LP),* usually obtained for such purposes as evaluation for meningitis, has provided useful information. The characteristic CSF profile of intracranial hemorrhage consists initially of many red blood cells and elevated protein content, followed shortly by xanthochromia and depressed glucose content (see Chapter 22). The first two of these CSF abnormalities are the most critical in early recognition. The degree of elevation of CSF protein correlates approximately with the severity of the hemorrhage. For example, in one study of 48 cases of CT-proven IVH, the mean CSF protein in the small lesions (subependymal hemorrhage or less than 10% of ventricular area filled with blood) was 254 mg/dL; in the moderate lesions (10% to 50% of the ventricular area filled with blood), it was 746 mg/dL; and in the largest lesions (more than 50% of the ventricular area filled with blood), it was 1668 mg/dL.[410] However, the dispersion of the mean values was so large that the CSF protein content could be used only as an approximation of severity of hemorrhage.

In the following sections, the principal means of visualizing germinal matrix hemorrhage–IVH (i.e., ultrasonography, MRI) will be reviewed.

Ultrasound Scan

Ultrasound scan of the neonatal cranium is the procedure of choice in the diagnosis of germinal matrix hemorrhage–IVH. The basic principles of the technique, the features of the instruments used, and the normal anatomical features visualized are described in Chapter 10. Since the initial reports of the value of the technique in diagnosis of IVH,[411-417] a vast experience has demonstrated the reliability and versatility of the procedure in this clinical setting.[a] High-resolution imaging, portable instrumentation, lack of ionizing radiation,

---

[a]References 16, 17, 27, 38, 48, 108, 245, 249, and 418-442.

and relative affordability have been the major advantages. In the following subsections, we illustrate the value of cranial ultrasound scanning in identification of hemorrhage and in determination of timing, severity, and progression of the lesion.

Identification of the Hemorrhage

Ultrasound scan is effective in identification of all degrees of severity of IVH from isolated germinal matrix hemorrhage to major degrees, with or without periventricular hemorrhagic infarction. The physical basis of the dense echoes that correlate with the hemorrhage is probably the formation of fibrin mesh within the clot.[436]

The major elemental lesion, of course, is *hemorrhage within the germinal matrix* (see Fig. 24.2A). *Intraventricular bleeding* results in echogenic material that fills a portion or all of the lateral ventricular system (see Fig. 24.2B and C). *Periventricular hemorrhagic infarction* complicating major IVH is a striking echogenic lesion, globular, crescentic, or fan shaped in configuration, usually unilateral, and located on the side of the largest amount of germinal matrix or intraventricular blood or both (Fig. 24.31). The echogenic portion of the lesion is located most commonly in the frontal and parietal regions. The subsequent finding of porencephalic cyst at the site of such a hemorrhagic intracerebral lesion (see Figs. 24.31 and 24.32) reflects the essential ischemic nature of the lesion (see the section on mechanisms of brain injury later). The *single, large, unilateral,* or *asymmetrical* porencephalic cyst that occurs as a consequence of periventricular hemorrhagic infarction differs from the *multiple, small, symmetrical* cysts observed as a consequence of periventricular leukomalacia (see Chapter 14). The evolution of the typical unilateral or grossly asymmetrical periventricular hemorrhagic infarction after ipsilateral germinal matrix or IVH, or both, has been well documented.[105,249] *Posthemorrhagic ventricular dilation* is demonstrated very well by cranial ultrasound scan. This disorder and its management are discussed in detail later (see the section on management).

Grading the Severity of Hemorrhage

The grading system that we have used is based on the presence and amount of blood in the germinal matrix and lateral ventricles (Table 24.12); determination of the presence of blood in the matrix is best made on the coronal scan, and determination of the amount of blood in the lateral ventricles

TABLE 24.12	Grading of Severity of Germinal Matrix–Intraventricular Hemorrhage by Ultrasound Scan
SEVERITY	**DESCRIPTION**
Grade I	Germinal matrix hemorrhage with no or minimal intraventricular hemorrhage (<10% of ventricular area on parasagittal view)
Grade II	Intraventricular hemorrhage (10%–50% of ventricular area on parasagittal view)
Grade III	Intraventricular hemorrhage (>50% of ventricular area on parasagittal view; usually distends lateral ventricle)
Separate notation	Periventricular echodensity (location and extent)

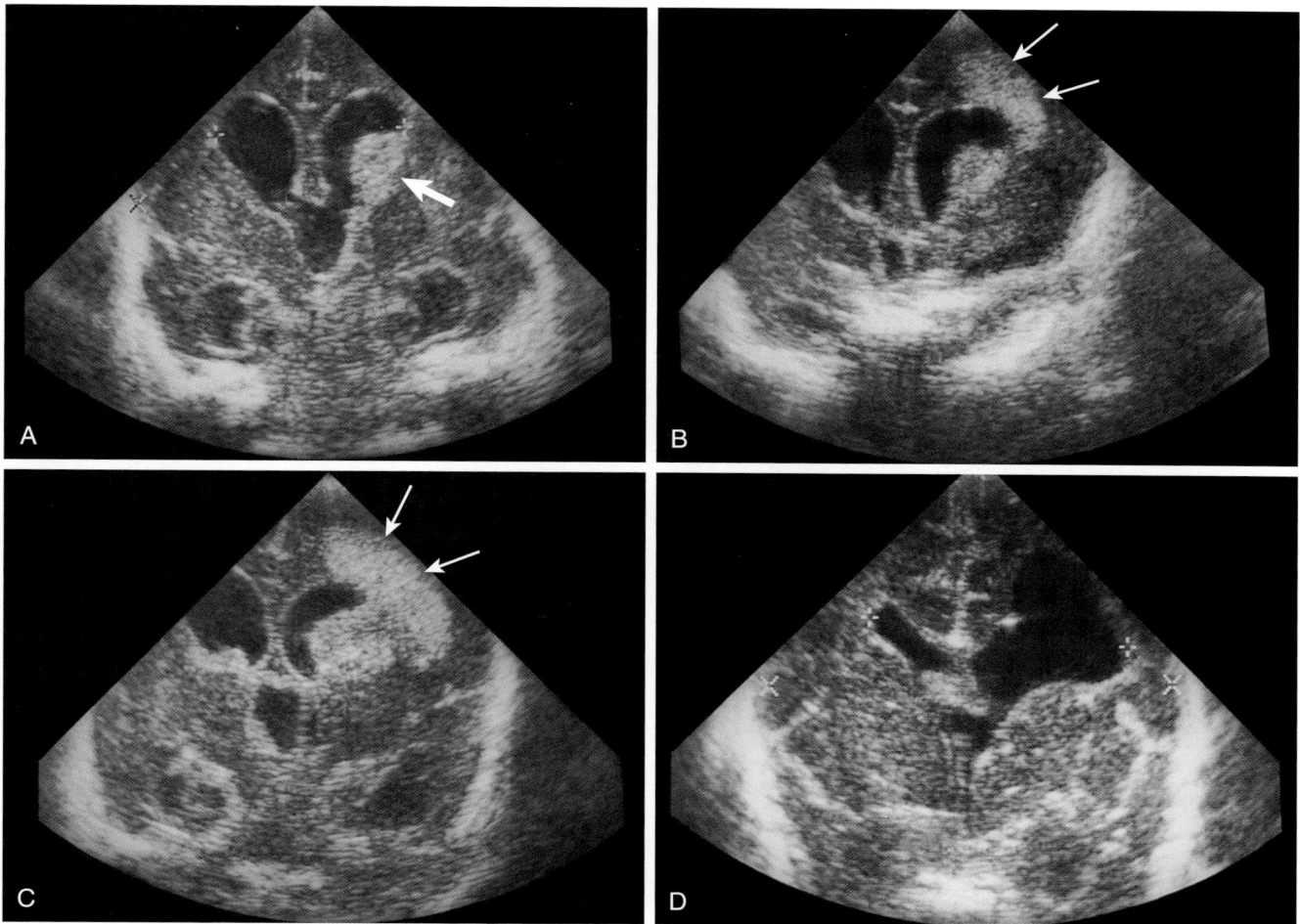

Figure 24.31 Ultrasound scans of evolution of periventricular hemorrhagic infarction. Coronal scans obtained from a premature infant of 30 weeks of gestation on (A–C) day 7 and, D, day 60. The three coronal scans obtained on day 7 were separated by minutes to several hours and show a bulging germinal matrix hemorrhage (*arrow* in A) that increases in size (B and C); with the increasing size, a crescentic periventricular echodensity (*arrows*) consistent with periventricular hemorrhagic infarction develops. Note in C the midline shift to the right. (D) Two months later, a large single porencephalic cyst is observed at the site of the infarction.

is best made on the parasagittal scan. In this classification, the presence of periventricular hemorrhagic infarction or of other parenchymal lesions is noted separately because these abnormalities generally are not caused simply by *extension* of matrix hemorrhage or IVH into normal brain parenchyma (see earlier discussion).

Timing of Hemorrhage

Serial ultrasound scans of premature infants have provided invaluable information concerning the *time of onset of hemorrhage*, and this information, of course, is critical for deciding when to screen for the presence of hemorrhage. In a cumulative series of 105 infants with IVH studied by real-time ultrasonography from the first hours of life, approximately 50% had onset of hemorrhage on the first postnatal day, an additional 25% on the second day, and an additional 15% on the third day (Table 24.13).[a] In a single study of 1105 infants weighing 2000 g or less at birth, approximately 40% of the 265 who developed IVH did so within the first 5 hours of life.[36] The likelihood of onset of hemorrhage on the first postnatal day varies inversely with birthweight; in one series, 62% of hemorrhages in infants between 500 and 700 g birthweight occurred in the first 18 hours.[44] In general, if screening were to be confined to a single postnatal day in the first days of life, a scan on the fourth postnatal day would be expected to detect approximately 90% of all hemorrhages. However, *progression* of the lesions occurs in approximately 20% to 40% of the affected infants, with maximal extent of the lesion attained usually within 3 to 5 days of the initial diagnosis.[a] Thus a second scan after approximately 5 days is necessary to identify the maximal extent of hemorrhage in the many infants who exhibit progression. I prefer a regimen of two scans in the first week, with timing of subsequent scans determined by the initial findings and clinical events (see later).

---

[a]References 44, 107, 241, 315, 425, 427, and 430.

[a]References 44, 419, 425, 430, 432, and 437.

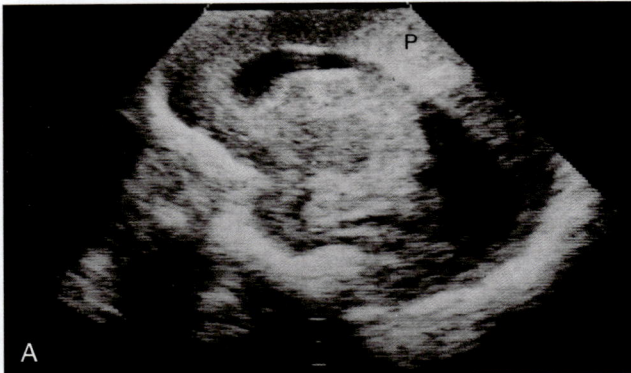

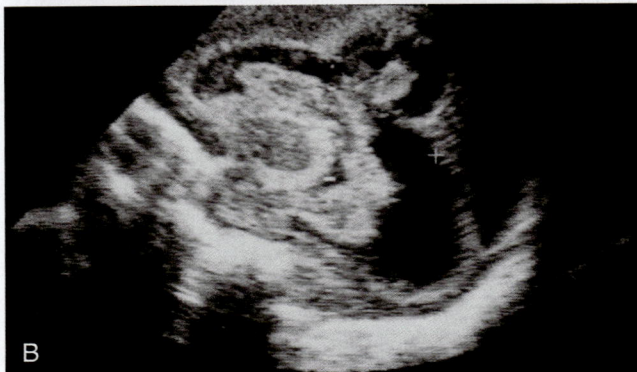

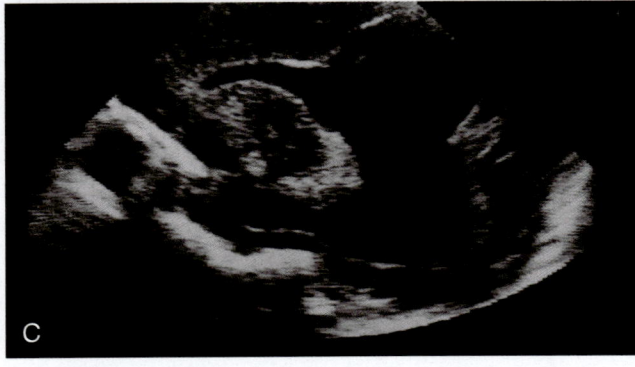

Figure 24.32 Periventricular hemorrhagic infarction with evolution to porencephalic cyst, ultrasound scans. (A) At 9 days of age, the intraparenchymal lesion *(p)* and ventricular dilation are visible on parasagittal ultrasound scan. Remaining intraventricular clot is also apparent. (B) At 3 weeks of age, the cystic cavity becomes apparent, as necrotic tissue and clot retract. (C) At 2 months of age, a large porencephalic cyst has evolved pari passu with increased ventricular dilation.

Severity of Hemorrhage

The relative distribution of the severity of IVH has been elucidated more effectively with ultrasound scan than was possible with CT scan, because the *single* CT scan usually obtained could not be expected to identify the maximal severity of hemorrhage in many of the cases. With serial ultrasound scans, this problem is obviated. However, large-scale ultrasonographic studies have used different grading systems and inclusion criteria and have often grouped together infants with grade III IVH and periventricular hemorrhagic infarction. The relative distribution of severity of IVH in infants of less than 1500 g birthweight, based on our unpublished data and that

TABLE 24.13	Approximate Time of Occurrence of Germinal Matrix–Intraventricular Hemorrhage Identified by Ultrasound Scan
POSTNATAL DAY	**PERCENTAGE OF INFANTS WITH GERMINAL MATRIX–INTRAVENTRICULAR HEMORRHAGE[a] (%)**
1	50
2	25
3	15
≥4	10

[a]Approximately 20%–40% of these infants exhibit progression of hemorrhage over 3–5 days.

TABLE 24.14	Severity of Germinal Matrix–Intraventricular Hemorrhage Identified by Ultrasound Scan
SEVERITY[a]	**PERCENTAGE OF INFANTS WITH GERMINAL MATRIX–INTRAVENTRICULAR HEMORRHAGE (%)**
Grade I	40
Grade II	25
Grade III	20
Intraventricular hemorrhage and apparent periventricular hemorrhagic infarction	15[b]

[a]See Table 24.13 for grading system.
[b]In approximately 90%, the accompanying intraventricular hemorrhage was grade III in severity.
From unpublished personal data from approximately 400 premature infants with germinal matrix–intraventricular hemorrhage.

in the literature, is shown in Table 24.14, Fig. 24.1.[13–17,22,41,42,443] Approximately 20% of the hemorrhages were large (i.e., grade III), with blood usually filling and dilating the lateral ventricles on parasagittal scan (see Table 24.12 for grading system). Approximately 15% of all the infants with hemorrhage had, in addition, large periventricular echodensity consistent with periventricular hemorrhagic infarction. In these infants, the severity of the IVH was grade III in approximately 90%.

Particular emphasis should be placed on large IVH with periventricular hemorrhagic infarction, because this lesion accounts for most of the morbidity attributable to IVH per se. This striking lesion is particularly characteristic of the most immature infants (see earlier). Thus, in one series of 2667 infants, IVH with periventricular hemorrhagic infarction accounted for 20% to 30% of all IVH in infants born at 24 to 26 weeks of gestation but less than 5% of all IVH at 30 to 32 weeks of gestation (see Fig. 24.3).[17] It is also important to note that the incidence of high-grade IVH (grade III and IV) has not changed markedly overall in the last 20 years in all premature infants less than

TABLE 24.15 Short-Term Outcome of Germinal Matrix–Intraventricular Hemorrhage as a Function of Severity of Hemorrhage and Birthweight[a]

SEVERITY OF HEMORRHAGE[b]	DEATHS IN FIRST 14 DAYS[c]		PVD (SURVIVORS >14 DAYS)[c]	
	<750 g (n = 75)	751–1500 g (n = 173)	<750 g (n = 56)	751–1500 g (n = 165)
Grade I	3/24 (12)	0/80 (0)	1/21 (5)	3/80 (4)
Grade II	5/21 (24)	1/44 (2)	1/16 (6)	6/43 (14)
Grade III	6/19 (32)	2/26 (8)	10/13 (77)	18/24 (75)
Grade III and apparent PHI	5/11 (45)	5/23 (22)	5/6 (83)	12/18 (66)

[a]Values are n (%).

[b]For grading system, see Table 24.12.

[c]Deaths occurring later in the neonatal period are not shown; the total mortality rates (early and late deaths) are approximately 50%–100% greater for each grade of hemorrhage and birthweight than those shown in the table for early deaths alone.

PHI, Periventricular hemorrhagic infarction; PVD, progressive ventricular dilation.

Data from Murphy BP, Inder TE, Rooks V, Taylor GA, et al. Posthemorrhagic ventricular dilatation in the premature infant: natural history and predictors of outcome. *Arch Dis Child Fetal Neonatal Ed.* 2002;87:F37–F41.

28 weeks (see Fig. 24.4). However, there has been some decline in infants born at 26 weeks (19% to 11%, $P = .03$), 27 weeks 15% to 7%, $P = .02$), and 28 weeks (11% to 5%, $P < .01$), but not for infants born at 22 to 25 weeks (Fig. 24.4).

Computed Tomography Scan

The CT scan demonstrates the site and extent of IVH very effectively.[25,30,401,444-450] Indeed, in the first edition of this book, it was stated that "the CT scan is the most definitive means to define the site(s) and extent of periventricular-intraventricular hemorrhage (PIVH)."[145] Ultrasound scan has displaced CT as the principal diagnostic technique, not only because of equivalent resolution for identification of the hemorrhage but also because CT has the disadvantages of requiring the sick premature infant to be transported and of exposing the brain and eyes to ionizing radiation. If MRI is unavailable, CT retains some value, however, for identification of complicating hemorrhagic lesions, such as subdural hemorrhage, hemorrhagic posterior fossa lesions, and certain cerebral parenchymal hemorrhagic abnormalities (see Chapter 10).

Magnetic Resonance Imaging Scan

MRI has been shown to provide excellent images of IVH, especially after the first few days of the hemorrhage.[108,451-456] However, MRI currently cannot supplant ultrasonography in the evaluation of IVH, because the former technique requires transport to the scanner, has a relatively long data acquisition time, precludes the use of metallic materials still often found on neonatal monitoring and support equipment, and is expensive. The effectiveness of MRI in demonstration of the parenchymal details of periventricular hemorrhagic infarction with germinal matrix hemorrhage–IVH was illustrated earlier (see Figs. 24.12 and 24.14).[112]

PROGNOSIS

Prognosis is best considered in terms of the short-term outcome (mortality rate and development of progressive ventricular dilation) and the long-term outcome (neurological sequelae). We will emphasize the relationship of outcome with the severity of hemorrhage and parenchymal abnormalities identifiable on neonatal brain imaging studies—especially the most widely used modality, cranial ultrasonography.

Short-Term Outcome: Mortality Rates and Progressive Ventricular Dilation

The *short-term outcome* relates clearly to the severity of the hemorrhage and to the degree of prematurity. The mortality rates and incidences of progressive posthemorrhagic ventricular dilation (i.e., hydrocephalus) are shown in Table 24.15 as a function of the severity of the hemorrhage, documented primarily by ultrasound scan, and the infant's birthweight.[443] Although the data are derived from a single study of 248 infants, findings of other reports are more or less similar.[a] Thus, with small lesions, confined to the germinal matrix or accompanied by small amounts of intraventricular blood (grade I), mortality rates are low, comparable to those of small premature infants without hemorrhage, and the frequency of progressive ventricular dilation in survivors is very uncommon. With moderate (grade II) lesions, mortality rates are higher only in the smallest infants (<750 g), and approximately 5% to 15% of survivors develop progressive ventricular dilation. With severe (grade III) lesions (i.e., blood filling the ventricles), mortality rates are approximately 30% in the infants weighing less than 750 g at birth but still less than 10% in the infants with a birthweight of 751 to 1500 g; approximately 75% of survivors exhibit progressive ventricular dilation in both groups. For those infants who, in addition to severe IVH, also exhibit apparent periventricular hemorrhagic infarction, mortality rates approach 50% in the infants weighing less than 750 g at birth and are approximately 20% in those with a birthweight of 751 to 1500 g, and the incidences of subsequent hydrocephalus are still higher. Indeed, for the now prominent population of infants of less than 750 g birthweight, survival without progressive ventricular dilation is very unusual with these severe lesions. A recent review of changes in a geographical cohort in Nova Scotia[476] revealed that although overall mortality in very preterm infants had significantly decreased over time, from 17.4% during 1993–97 to 7.7% during 2008–10 ($P < .001$), mortality in very preterm infants with grade IV IVH (risk 47%)

[a]References 15, 16, 22, 25, 29, 38, 39, 42, 131, 426, and 457-475.

had not changed significantly over time (P = .152). In addition, the rate of withdrawal of care in IVH was 15.1% for all infants with IVH. This rate had not significantly changed over time (P = .287). The rate of withdrawal of care in grade IV IVH was 39% for all infants with grade IV IVH and 83% for infants with grade IV IVH who died. These two rates had not significantly changed over time (P = .475 and P = .275, respectively).

The progressive ventricular dilation that occurs in survivors does not necessarily require a procedure to divert CSF from the lateral ventricles (i.e., ventriculostomy or ventriculoperitoneal shunt). Indeed, many infants, especially with less severe IVH, exhibit cessation of progression, with or without resolution, with no therapy. The natural history of posthemorrhagic ventricular dilation is discussed in more detail in the subsequent section, along with outcomes.

Long-Term Outcome: Neurological Sequelae

The *long-term neurodevelopmental outcome* of the infant with IVH depends on two key factors: the immaturity of the infant and the degree of parenchymal injury. The latter ranges from germinal matrix destruction to periventricular hemorrhagic infarction (see Fig. 24.9). Associated concurrent neuropathologies (see earlier) also may contribute importantly to long-term outcome. There are several limitations to our ability to define the full consequences of IVH in the immature brain, including the inability to assess fully the presence of microstructural brain injury, the impact on subsequent developmental processes, and related factors. Thus, most literature has focused on associations between cranial ultrasound findings and outcome, with only an approximate relationship existing between the quantity of intraventricular blood and the neurologic outcome (see Table 24.14).[a] Although the incidence of major neurological sequelae (spastic motor deficits, major cognitive deficits) after minor degrees of hemorrhage is slightly higher than that in infants without hemorrhage and increases to approximately 50% in infants with severe hemorrhage, a *clearly higher* incidence occurs in infants with IVH complicated by periventricular hemorrhagic infarction or cystic periventricular leukomalacia, or both. *Prognostic estimates* can thus be refined considerably by assessment of the presence and the degree of parenchymal injury by detailed imaging. It is highly likely that such estimates could also be considerably improved by more sophisticated understanding of the full impact of GMH-IVH on subsequent cerebral development.

A recent meta-analysis summarized nine cohort studies to compare neurodevelopmental outcomes in three groups—no IVH, mild (grade I–II) IVH, and severe (grade III–IV) IVH.[517] (In the analysis, the authors used the term *periventricular* IVH, and therefore PIVH, rather than GMH-IVH, as in this chapter.) The analysis documented that mild PIVH (two studies,[518,519] 3508 subjects, unadjusted OR 1.48; 95% CI, 1.26 to 1.73; I^2 = 79%) and severe PIVH (8830 subjects, unadjusted OR 4.72; 95% CI, 4.21 to 5.31; I^2 = 97%) were both associated with higher odds of the primary outcome of death or moderate-severe neurodevelopmental impairment (NDI) at 18 to 24 months of life when compared with infants without IVH. The analysis also evaluated the secondary outcome of moderate-severe NDI, defined as moderate to severe cerebral palsy; moderate

to severe cognitive delay; severe visual impairment, defined as visual acuity less than 6/60 (metric scale) in the better eye; or severe hearing impairment, defined as requirement of unilateral/bilateral hearing aids or cochlear implants, distinct from mortality. Mild PIVH was associated with higher odds of moderate-severe NDI compared with no IVH among those who survived to discharge (3032 subjects, unadjusted OR 1.75; 95% CI, 1.40 to 2.20; I^2 = 76%; adjusted OR 1.39; 95% CI, 1.09 to 1.77, I^2 = 70%). Severe IVH was also associated with higher odds of the outcome compared with no IVH (13,691 subjects, unadjusted OR 3.36; 95% CI, 3.06 to 3.68; I^2 = 39%; 2670 subjects, adjusted OR 2.44; 95% CI, 1.73 to 3.42; I^2 = 82%). Finally, severe IVH was associated with higher odds of moderate-severe NDI when compared with mild IVH among survivors (880 subjects, unadjusted OR 2.62; 95% CI, 1.83 to 3.74; I^2 = 0%; 1686 subjects, adjusted OR 2.16; 95% CI, 1.36 to 3.43; I^2 = 0%). This study is informative in two ways: First, and importantly, it highlights the presence of increased risk for NDI in the preterm infant with grade I–II IVH. Second, however, the odds ratio (OR) estimates for each of these outcomes is still relatively low and thus renders individual prognostication challenging.[520] As discussed later, it may be possible to improve prognostications with more advanced neuroimaging techniques.

One of the largest studies contributing to our understanding of the neurodevelopmental consequences of IVH has been the EPIPAGE study that enrolled 1954 infants less than 32 weeks' gestation[521] and described a clear relationship between greater severity of IVH and an increased risk of adverse neurological outcome. Even in isolated grade I–II IVH the rates of cerebral palsy increased substantially from a baseline of 5.5% to 8.1% for grade I IVH (n = 229) and 12.2% for grade II IVH (n = 168). Notably, cerebral palsy rates with isolated grade I–III IVH also rose with immaturity from 5% in infants born at 31 to 32 weeks to 10% to 15% in those born at 27 to 30 weeks and 33% in those born at 24 to 26 weeks. Patra and colleagues also[134] reported that grade I–II IVH was associated with a twofold increase in the risk of lower cognitive performance (Mental Developmental Index) and a 2.6-fold increase in the risk of neuromotor abnormalities (cerebral palsy and tone) after controlling for social and neonatal factors (gender, bronchopulmonary dysplasia, sepsis, necrotizing enterocolitis, maternal marital status, race, and education). Two recent additional studies also showed that grade I–II IVH was associated with worse Mental Developmental Index (MDI) and Psychomotor Developmental Index (PDI) scores,[134,522,523] but that this outcome was dependent on gestational age, being significant only at less than 28 to 29 weeks' gestation. For school-aged outcomes, Sherlock and colleagues examined 298 preterm infants less than 1000 g at age 8 years to determine the impact of IVH in relation to neuromotor and cognitive outcomes.[524] They documented that no IVH was associated with cerebral palsy rates of 6.7%, with no rise in association with grade I IVH (6.4%), but a marked elevation with grade II IVH to 24%.

Despite these large data sets, there continues to be disagreement about the significance of low-grade IVH, with two recent studies having directly conflicting results. Payne and colleagues enrolled 1472 infants, all less than 27 weeks' gestation. Comparing infants with no IVH and low-grade IVH, they found no difference in rates of cerebral palsy (8% vs. 9%), or NDI (10% vs. 10%), with similarly no increased

---

[a]References 16, 29, 39, 96, 99–101, 105, 131, 133, 134, 426, 460, 462–466, 468, 469, 471, and 477–516.

risk on multivariate analysis.[525] Contrary to this, Bolisetty and colleagues enrolled an alternate cohort also of 1472 infants less than 29 weeks' gestation and found a consistent association between low grades of IVH and both cerebral palsy (no IVH vs. I–II IVH; 6.5% vs. 10.4%) and moderate-severe neurosensory impairment (no IVH vs. I–II IVH; 12% vs. 22%). On multivariate analysis there remained a one-and-a-half-times increased risk of moderate to severe neurosensory impairment with low-grade IVH, when controlling for gestation, gender, SGA, chronic lung disease, ROP, and PVL.[526] The notable differences between these two studies is that Payne and colleagues had a 1- to 2-week lower mean gestational age for all subgroups, with slightly worse outcomes among infants without IVH, and had fewer infants with a low-grade IVH (270 vs. 336). All of the studies have been limited by the necessity to combine grades I and II IVH into a composite for statistical purposes and by the inability to distinguish the key neuropathologies that may be leading to the subsequent impairment in neurodevelopmental outcome. Cranial ultrasound has been demonstrated to have poor diagnostic utility for diffuse white matter injury, which has been shown to occur in up to 75% of preterm infants (see Chapters 10 and 16). Concomitant cerebral white matter injury is also an important determinant of outcome with IVH, as described earlier. Thus low-grade IVH could be a visible marker on cranial ultrasound for the more important neuropathology of cerebral white matter injury, which on MR imaging has been shown to be highly predictive of both motor and cognitive deficits.[527]

Of note, the elevation of risk for poor outcomes with low-grade IVH with increasing immaturity may also suggest an independent role for the loss of the glial and neuronal precursors from the immature germinal matrix.[520] This concept of disturbed cerebral development following low-grade IVH is supported by the work of Vasileiadis and co-workers,[528] who analyzed cerebral volumes on MRI at term equivalent in 12 infants with IVH (seven infants had grade I IVH, four infants had grade II IVH, and one infant had grade III IVH, with no persistent ventriculomegaly; the IVH was bilateral for eight infants). The volumes were compared with 11 preterm infants without IVH. The volume of cortical gray matter on MRI was significantly reduced by 16% in the IVH group (no-IVH group: 122 ± 12.9 mL; IVH group: 102 ± 14.6 mL; $F = 13.218$). There was no difference in the volumes of subcortical gray matter, white matter, and CSF.

Periventricular Hemorrhagic Infarction—Major Determinant of Long-Term Outcome

Clearly, major determinants of outcome in the premature infant are the presence and severity of associated periventricular hemorrhagic infarction. Although many studies have addressed the outcome in this group, quantitative conclusions are difficult to draw because the selection criteria differ, the numbers of infants are often relatively small, the lesion usually is not quantitated, and the mortality rates vary, in part because of differences in policies of termination of life support in the severely affected infant. Nevertheless, more recent studies[a] provide useful data and complement the largest single study reported earlier ($n = 75$).[96] In the latter study, the *degree* of

---

[a]References 16, 102, 103, 476, 516, and 529.

TABLE 24.16 Long-Term Outcome: Neurological Sequelae in Survivors With Germinal Matrix–Intraventricular Hemorrhage as a Function of Severity of Hemorrhage[a]

SEVERITY OF HEMORRHAGE[b]	INCIDENCE OF DEFINITE NEUROLOGICAL SEQUELAE[c] (%)
Grade I	15
Grade II	25
Grade III	50
Grade III and apparent periventricular hemorrhagic infarction	75

[a]See text for references. Data are derived from reports published since 2002 and include personal published and unpublished cases.

[b]For grading system, see Table 24.12.

[c]Mean values (to nearest 5%); considerable variability among studies was apparent, especially for the severe lesions. Definite neurological sequelae included principally cerebral palsy or mental retardation, or both.

---

parenchymal injury was quantitated after identification on ultrasound scan as a large intraparenchymal echodensity (i.e., >1 cm), presumed to represent periventricular hemorrhagic infarction.[96] Among the 75 infants studied, the mortality rate was 59%. This finding should be contrasted with a mortality rate of 8% in the same neonatal unit at the same time for infants with the severest grade of IVH (i.e., grade III IVH but no associated periventricular hemorrhagic infarction). Among the 22 survivors who could be examined on follow-up, 87% exhibited major motor deficits, and 68% had cognitive function less than 80% of normal. The motor deficits correlated with the topography of the parenchymal lesions and thus consisted of either spastic hemiparesis or asymmetrical spastic quadriparesis. In more recent reports, the incidence of major motor deficits has been lower (i.e., ≈50% in 36 surviving infants <32 weeks of gestational age,[16] and 60% in 30 surviving infants <2500 g birthweight[249]).

Prognostic estimation can be refined by considering the severity of the periventricular hemorrhagic infarction (Tables 24.16 and 24.17). Thus, among infants with extensive lesions (i.e., echodensity that included frontoparieto-occipital regions (Figs. 24.32 and 24.33), 30 of 38 (81%) died, and of the eight survivors, seven had subsequent motor deficits.[96] *However, caution is necessary in extrapolating these small numbers to all infants; careful consideration of associated lesions (e.g., periventricular leukomalacia) and other clinical aspects is necessary.* Among infants with *localized* lesions (i.e., echodensity confined to frontal, parietal, temporal, or occipital regions (Fig. 24.34), the outcome was more favorable than after extensive echodensity for both unilateral and bilateral lesions. Thus major spastic motor deficits occurred in only 50% with unilateral localized lesions, and major cognitive deficits appeared in only 12% of these infants. Even with bilateral localized disease, major cognitive deficits occurred in only 50%. In a recent study,[102,516] only 4 of 12 (33%) infants with unilateral localized lesions had an abnormal motor examination at 2 years of age. Consistent with this *more favorable outcome for localized lesions*, a study of unilateral periventricular echodensities that evolved to porencephalic cyst reported a developmental

TABLE 24.17   Outcome of Intraventricular Hemorrhage as a Function of the Severity of Associated Periventricular Intraparenchymal Echodensity

| | SEVERITY OF IPE[a] | | | |
OUTCOME	UNILATERAL EXTENSIVE	LOCALIZED	BILATERAL EXTENSIVE	LOCALIZED
Mortality rate	21/27 (78%)	8/23 (35%)	9/11 (82%)	6/14 (43%)
Major motor deficits[b]	5/6 (83%)	4/8 (50%)	2/2 (100%)	5/6 (83%)
Cognitive <75%[c]	5/6 (83%)	1/8 (12%)	2/2 (100%)	3/6 (50%)

[a]See text for definitions of "extensive" and "localized."
[b]Includes only overt spastic motor deficits.
[c]Age range at testing generally 1 to 4 years; tests included varying combinations of Bayley, Stanford-Binet, Vineland, Wechsler, and Verbal Language Development Scales.
IPE, Intraparenchymal echodensity.

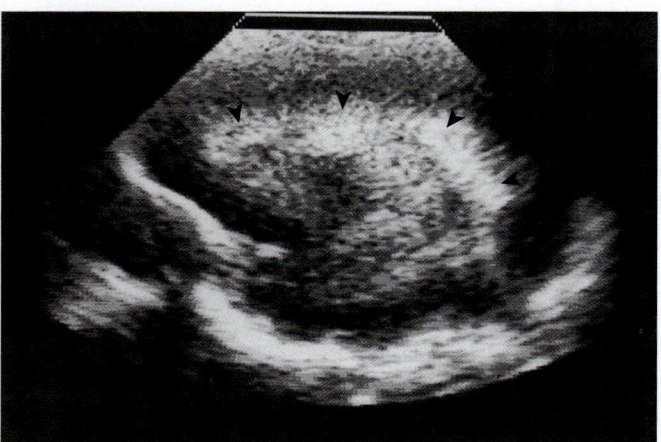

Figure 24.33 Ultrasound scan of periventricular intraparenchymal echodensity, extensive. Note that the lesion *(arrowheads)* extends from frontal to occipital regions.

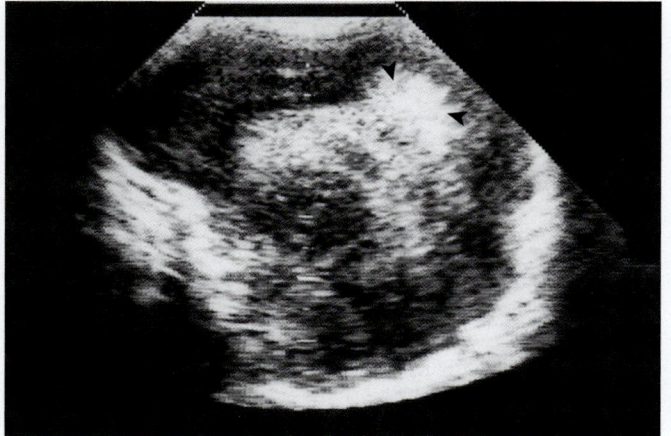

Figure 24.34 Ultrasound scan of periventricular intraparenchymal echodensity, localized. Note that the lesion *(arrowheads)* is confined to the posterior parietal region.

quotient less than 80 in five of nine localized lesions, versus six of seven diffuse lesions; spastic motor deficits occurred in four of nine localized lesions versus seven of seven diffuse lesions.[530] The relationship of the superior–inferior involvement of the motor tracts is represented on the cerebral topography of the

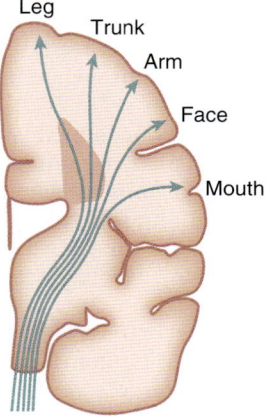

Figure 24.35 Schematic diagram of the location of periventricular hemorrhagic infarction and descending corticospinal tract motor fibers. Note that the topography of the lesion accounts for the subsequent spastic hemiparesis with prominent involvement of lower as well as upper extremity.

major motor tracts in Fig. 24.35. The relationship between the anterior-posterior distribution of periventricular hemorrhagic infarction and outcome is controversial. The discrepancies could relate in part to differing definitions of anterior and posterior. An earlier report indicated that motor deficits were more likely with posterior than anterior lesions,[530] whereas more recent work found more motor deficits with anterior than posterior lesions.[249,516] Posterior (peritrigonal) lesions have been noted to be especially closely associated with subsequent cognitive deficits[530] and microcephaly.[249,516]

The largest recent series further refine neurodevelopmental outcomes in relation to the regional position of the parenchymal hemorrhage.[103] In the setting of the commonest lesion in the parietal region, cerebral palsy occurred in one-half of infants, with the majority being unilateral spastic in nature. However, an important subgroup of infants with temporal lobe hemorrhages were noted to have a very high risk of behavioral and cognitive challenges (Fig. 24.36).

MANAGEMENT

Management of neonatal germinal matrix hemorrhage–IVH is considered best in terms of (1) prevention, (2) initial or acute measures, and (3) treatment of posthemorrhagic ventricular

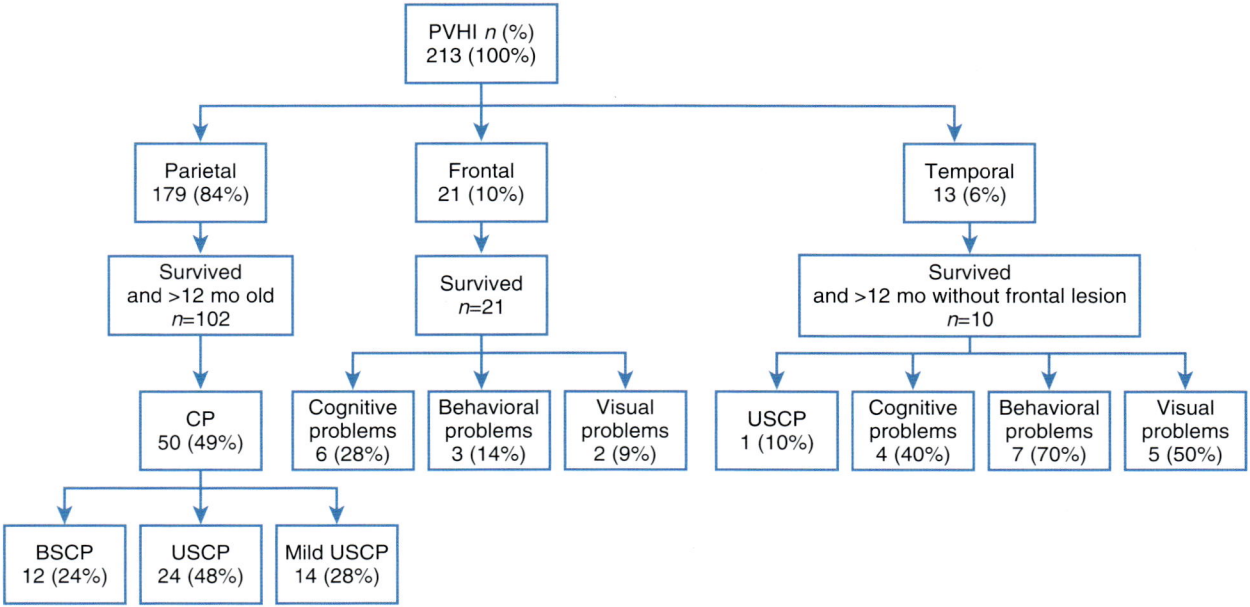

Figure 24.36 Flowchart of overall review of children with periventricular hemorrhagic infarction (PVHI) treated in a single unit from 1999 to 2012. Only survivors older than 12 months corrected age were included in the analysis of features of neurodevelopmental outcome. Children with temporal PVHI and bilateral frontal cystic periventricular leukomalacia were excluded. *BSCP*, Bilateral spastic cerebral palsy; *CP*, cerebral palsy; *USCP*, unilateral spastic cerebral palsy. (From Soltirovska Salamon A, Groenendaal F, van Haastert IC, Rademaker KJ, Benders MJ, Koopman C, de Vries LS. Neuroimaging and neurodevelopmental outcome of preterm infants with a periventricular haemorrhagic infarction. *Dev Med Child Neurol.* 2014;56:547–555.)

TABLE 24.18	Prevention of Germinal Matrix–Intraventricular Hemorrhage: Perinatal Interventions

Prevention of preterm birth
Transportation in utero
Prenatal pharmacological interventions
   Glucocorticoids
   Phenobarbital
   Vitamin K
   Magnesium sulfate
Optimal management of labor and delivery
Delayed umbilical cord clamping
Umbilical cord milking
Temperature stability
Newborn resuscitation

dilation. In the following discussion, we consider these three aspects and conclude with a rational sequence of management.

Prevention

As with many neonatal neurological disorders, the primary goal in management of IVH is prevention. Rational attempts at prevention require an understanding of pathogenesis (see earlier discussion). The relevant prenatal (Table 24.18) and postnatal interventions are discussed next in the context of current concepts of pathogenesis discussed earlier.

Perinatal Interventions

Prevention of Premature Birth. The most decisive way to prevent IVH would be to prevent premature birth. Those

pathogenetic factors referable to the regulation of cerebral blood flow and the microvascular network of the germinal matrix of the premature brain obviously cannot be altered after birth. Indeed, the magnitude of the problem of IVH relates directly to the fact that annually more than 300,000 premature infants (birthweight <2500 g) are born in the United States (≈8% of the 4,000,000 births yearly), and more important, approximately 60,000 of these infants weigh less than 1500 g at birth.[3-6,531,532] Notably, in the United States, the rate of very low birthweight (i.e., <1500 g) infants has actually increased from 1.17% to 1.42% in the past 30 years.[2,4,5,531,533-536]

Attempts at prevention of premature birth have been based on three major approaches, operating in sequence: (1) identification of the woman at high *risk* for premature delivery; (2) management of such a woman with a combination of patient education, treatment of infection, comprehensive health care, and early detection of premature labor; and (3) early treatment of premature labor, primarily with tocolytic agents.[2,531,533,534,537-561] Despite comprehensive prevention programs and aggressive use of tocolytic agents, or both, results have not shown consistent benefit.[a]

Of particular interest has been the beneficial effect of progesterone or 17-alpha-hydroxyprogesterone caproate (17P) in reduction of preterm delivery.[562,563] In one large multicenter, randomized clinical trial of 17P begun at 16 to 20 weeks of gestation in women with a history of previous preterm delivery, the rate of preterm delivery in the 17P-treated group was 36% versus 55% in the placebo group.[562] Notably, the incidence of IVH in these infants who weighed less than 2500 g at

---

[a]References 531, 533, 534, 537-552, 554-557, and 559-561.

TABLE 24.19   Antenatal Steroids and Prevention of Intraventricular Hemorrhage

Single most effective antenatal pharmacological intervention for prevention of intraventricular hemorrhage
Reduced incidence of both total and severe intraventricular hemorrhage
Reduced incidence of cystic periventricular leukomalacia
Betamethasone preferred over dexamethasone
Mechanism of beneficial effects not established: improved cerebral hemodynamics and maturational benefits most likely

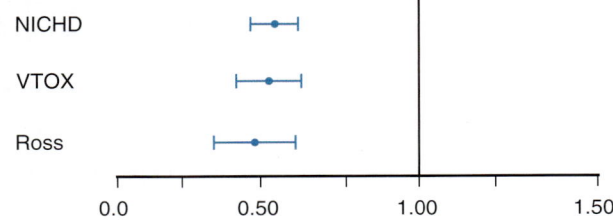

Figure 24.37 **Intraventricular hemorrhage and antenatal steroids.** Unadjusted odds ratio and 95% confidence intervals for the occurrence of severe intraventricular hemorrhage after antenatal steroid treatment (vs. no treatment) in three separate studies of infants of less than 1500 g birthweight (the National Institute of Child Health and Human Development Neonatal Research Network [NICHD], the Vermont-Oxford Trials Network [VTOX], and the database of Ross Laboratories [Ross]). The total number of infants was approximately 18,000. (Data from Wright LL, Horbar JD, Gunkel H, Verter J, et al: Evidence from multicenter networks on the current use and effectiveness of antenatal corticosteroids in low birth weight infants. *Am J Obstet Gynecol.* 1995;173:263–269.)

birth was 1.3% in the 17P-treated group versus 5.2% in the placebo group. A more recent study of 45 singleton pregnancies randomized after successful tocolysis and arrest of preterm labor included 22 women who received 17 P and 23 placebo.[564] The mean gestational age at delivery ($P = .07$) and the interval from treatment to delivery ($P = .2$) were not affected by 17 P. However, significantly fewer women in the 17 P group delivered at less than 34 weeks (14 vs. 21, $P = .03$). There was also a significant reduction in the risk of neonatal sepsis ($P = .04$) and grade III/IV IVH ($P = .02$) in the 17 P group.

Transportation in Utero. If premature labor and delivery cannot be prevented, then the pregnant woman should be transported to a perinatal center specializing in high-risk deliveries.[565-567] Infants thus transported in utero have a considerably lower incidence of IVH than apparently similar infants transported after delivery.[145] Whether this difference relates to inherently lower risk in pregnant women who are transported compared with those who are not transported, the type of management of labor and delivery, neonatal resuscitation factors, complications during transport, or a combination of these factors is not yet clear.

Prenatal Pharmacological Interventions. Because of the possibility that factors related to labor and delivery or to the immediate postnatal period may play a role in the pathogenesis of IVH, a preventive intervention that could be instituted in the presence of impending premature delivery has been sought. Antenatal administration of *glucocorticoids*, usually betamethasone or dexamethasone, currently is the most clearly beneficial antenatal intervention to decrease the incidence of all varieties of IVH (Table 24.19). The beneficial effect was observed initially in studies of the use of antenatal glucocorticoids to promote fetal lung maturation.[568] An early brief report suggested that this therapy resulted in a decreased incidence of IVH postnatally.[569] In a subsequent careful study, the incidence of germinal matrix hemorrhage–IVH was twofold to threefold lower in infants whose mothers received a complete course of steroids antenatally, compared with infants whose mothers received no steroids or an incomplete course.[570] Similar beneficial effects of glucocorticoid have been well documented.[288] Multivariate analysis suggested that the effect was *not* related to a lower incidence of complications of respiratory distress syndrome, although the severity of the respiratory disease was less in the treated infants.[570,571] A large amount of subsequent work demonstrated the beneficial effect of antenatal glucocorticoids

(Fig. 24.37).[269,317,572-585] The beneficial effect has been observed most decisively after a *complete* course of treatment (maternal receipt of two or more doses of glucocorticoid within a week of delivery with an interval of 12 hours from the last dose [or 24 hours from the first dose] to delivery) but also has been observed with a *partial* course (less than two doses in the week before delivery).[a] Two issues of importance relate to the benefits and hazards of (1) different corticosteroid preparations and (2) repeated courses of antenatal steroids. Concerning the former, *betamethasone* is preferred over dexamethasone because of more favorable pharmacokinetics, better pulmonary maturation enhancement, and less toxicity.[581,586-590] However, some investigators consider the two agents similar in terms of risks and benefits.[591]

Repeated antenatal glucocorticoid courses have not been recommended as routine clinical practice because of adverse effects on fetal growth and cerebral cortical maturation documented in animals[592] and humans.[581,593-598] However, one randomized clinical trial ($n = 982$) showed benefit of repeat doses for respiratory outcome but no additional benefit concerning incidence of IVH.[599] Another, smaller trial ($n = 249$) of mothers who received a course of betamethasone followed by a single booster dose of betamethasone just before preterm birth showed a trend for worse survival and increased respiratory disease but no effect on incidence of IVH for those receiving the booster dose of betamethasone versus placebo.[600]

The most recent Cochrane review of single versus repeated course of antenatal corticosteroids included 10 trials, with a total of 4733 women and 5700 infants.[601] The comparison was between treatment of women who remain at risk of preterm birth seven or more days after an initial course of prenatal corticosteroids with repeat dose(s), compared with no repeat corticosteroid treatment. Repeated corticosteroid reduced the risk of respiratory distress syndrome (RR 0.83; 95% CI, to 0.91). There was no effect on the incidence of IVH. Treatment with repeat dose(s) of corticosteroid was associated with a reduction in mean birthweight (mean difference [MD] −75.79 g; 95% CI,

---

[a]References 269, 317, 571, 573, 575, and 581.

−117.63 to −33.96; nine trials, 5626 infants). At early childhood follow-up, no statistically significant differences were seen for infants exposed to repeat prenatal corticosteroids compared with unexposed infants for the primary outcomes (total deaths; survival free of any disability or major disability; disability; or serious outcome) or in the secondary outcome growth assessments. Finally, twin gestations may not show the same beneficial effects of antenatal corticosteroids, with a recent study showing no difference in respiratory distress syndrome or other neonatal morbidities, including IVH.[602]

The basis for the beneficial effect of antenatal steroids may relate to the improved cardiovascular stability in the treated infants. Thus antenatal steroid therapy is associated with less need for blood pressure support and less hypotension postnatally.[573,581,603,604] That this beneficial postnatal hemodynamic effect could be related to improved placental blood flow (and thereby less likelihood of impairment of the infant's cerebrovascular autoregulation) seems possible because antenatal betamethasone has been shown to lead to a decrease in placental vascular resistance.[605] Perhaps relevant in this context is the observation that antenatal steroid administration is associated with a reduced incidence of cystic periventricular leukomalacia postnatally.[509,510,533-535] The possibility also exists that the therapy leads to the beneficial effect on IVH in part by stimulation of maturation of brain structures (e.g., germinal matrix).[570,573,606]

In conclusion, antenatal corticosteroids reduce the risk for IVH in singleton preterm infants, particularly when a completed course is given and betamethasone is the agent administered. The biological basis for this benefit remains unclear. Optimal preparations, dosing, and timing to delivery remain worthy of investigation, particularly in the setting of multiple births.

Antenatal administration of *phenobarbital* led to interesting results in five studies.[607-618] Initial studies raised the possibility that antenatal phenobarbital may have a small protective effect against IVH. However, later work failed to show a significant protective effect. Currently this approach appears not to be beneficial for the prevention of IVH.

Because the function of vitamin K–dependent coagulation factors in preterm infants is approximately 30% to 60% of the function in adults, *vitamin K* was administered intramuscularly to women in premature labor at least 4 hours before delivery in an attempt to prevent IVH.[619] The incidence of IVH in the prenatally treated infants was 5%, compared with 33% in the control infants. Although the infants treated prenatally with vitamin K had normal prothrombin activity (compared with 67% of normal in control infants), no statistically significant relationship existed between prothrombin activity and the occurrence of IVH. In a subsequent larger study (*n* = 100), antenatal administration of vitamin K resulted in a lower incidence of total IVH (16% vs. 36% in control infants) and of severe IVH (0% vs. 11% in control infants).[620] However, uncertainty concerning the role of vitamin K per se persists, despite these interesting data. Moreover, two later studies of antenatal vitamin K administration, combined in one of the studies with antenatal phenobarbital administration, showed no significant beneficial effect on hemostasis or incidence and severity of IVH.[611,621-623] Thus, on balance, it does not appear that antenatal vitamin K is useful for the prevention of IVH.

As described in Chapter 16, some data, although not consistent, indicate that the use of *antenatal magnesium sulfate* (principally for tocolysis) is followed by a lower incidence of cerebral palsy in the premature infants so treated. Although one preliminary report suggested that antenatal magnesium sulfate therapy results in a lower incidence of "grade III or IV IVH," most data do not show a beneficial effect on IVH or cerebral palsy, or both.[379,380,578,624-630] More concerning, some reports noted an increase in perinatal and postnatal mortality after antenatal magnesium administration.[631,632] Other studies did not show this increased mortality.[628,630,633] A more recent report showed a decreased incidence of IVH after the combination of antenatal magnesium and aminophylline, but the population was not randomized, and the numbers of infants with IVH were small (1 of 78 in the treated group and 7 of 68 in the control group).[634] A review of the nine best trials concluded that antenatal magnesium sulfate has no beneficial effect on "the risk of neonatal morbidity."[635]

Optimal Management of Labor and Delivery—Delivery Mode. As discussed earlier concerning pathogenesis, potentially deleterious effects of labor and delivery relate principally to the easily deformed, particularly compliant skull of the premature infant. Such deformations presumably could lead to dangerous elevations of venous pressure and perhaps to an impairment of cerebrovascular autoregulation (analogous to that observed in adult patients with head trauma).[636] Prolonged labor and breech delivery would be considered most likely to lead to such hemodynamic effects, and some, but not all, work supports this contention.[a] In one large prospective study that used multivariate analysis (see Table 24.7), abdominal delivery appeared to be protective concerning germinal matrix hemorrhage, and longer duration of labor was deleterious. In a later study, cesarean section before the active phase of labor resulted in a lower frequency of progression to severe IVH but did not affect total incidence of IVH.[638] Another study identified a twofold lower incidence of grade III/IV IVH in infants delivered by cesarean section without labor versus section delivery with labor, but the difference disappeared after logistic regression analysis.[285] Thus the potential value for cesarean section in selected preterm infants for the prevention of IVH is suggested by some, but not all, work; more data are needed to define the specific clinical circumstances that should lead to a recommendation for abdominal delivery.

Delayed Cord Clamping. DCC by 30 to 120 seconds rather than immediate clamping has been reported to be associated with less need for transfusion and lower rate of IVH. In December 2012, the American College of Obstetricians and Gynecologists recommended a delay of 30 to 60 seconds in umbilical cord clamping for all preterm deliveries.[641] Most recently in January 2017, the American College of Obstetricians and Gynecologists recommended a delay in umbilical cord clamping in vigorous term and preterm infants who do not require resuscitation for at least 30 to 60 seconds after birth.[259]

Although DCC has been associated with a decrease in the overall incidence of IVH, it has not been shown to have a beneficial effect on severe IVH, and thus its clinical application has not been uniformly embraced.[642] It is also worthy of note that both the ACOG and ILCOR recommendations are in

---

[a]References 27, 34, 45, 49, 70, 72, 106, 140, 185, 191, 212, 214, 233, 269, 280-285, 288, 313, 371, 376, 396, and 637-640.

vigorous preterm infants. There are no data on DCC in the premature infant in need of resuscitation.

With regard to subsequent outcomes, a recent randomized controlled trial reported the effects of placental transfusion on neonatal and 18-month outcomes in preterm infants with singleton fetuses (*n* = 208) between 24 weeks of gestation and 32 weeks of gestation.[643] There were no differences in the number of infants who received phototherapy, days of phototherapy, delivery room resuscitation, Neonatal Acute Physiology scores at 12 hours of age, and the rates of IVH or late-onset sepsis between the groups. However, at 18 to 22 months, DCC was found to be protective against motor scores less than 85 on the Bayley Scales of Infant Development. The authors concluded that although DCC did not alter the incidence of IVH or late-onset sepsis in preterm infants, it improved motor function at 18 to 22 months' corrected age.

Umbilical Cord Milking. An alternative to DCC is umbilical cord milking (UCM), a procedure that can be performed in 20 seconds. UCM is performed by holding the infant at or 20 cm below the level of the placenta.[257] The cord is pinched as close to the placenta as possible and milked toward the infant for 2 seconds. The cord is then released and allowed to refill with blood for 1 to 2 seconds between each milking motion, a process repeated a total of 4 times. After completion, the cord is clamped and the newborn handed to the resuscitation team. Milking the cord 4 times provides a similar amount of placental-fetal blood as with DCC for 30 seconds.[644]

A recent meta-analysis of UCM, including seven randomized clinical trials involving 501 infants delivered at less than 33 weeks, demonstrated that infants who underwent UCM had a higher hemoglobin level and lower risk of oxygen requirement at 36 weeks and IVH of all grades compared with those who underwent immediate cord clamping.[645] A recent pilot study of 75 extremely premature neonates (born at a gestational age <29 weeks) randomly assigned to receive UCM or immediate cord clamping also demonstrated a 50% reduction in total IVH[646] with UCM. Moreover, in another recent retrospective study of 318 infants born at less than 30 weeks, UCM was associated with reductions in IVH, necrotizing enterocolitis, and death before hospital discharge.[647] Concerning the mechanism of benefit from UCM, a further study that enrolled 197 infants (mean gestational age 28 ± 2 weeks) reported a higher hemoglobin level at birth, improved hemodynamics (higher blood flow and improved blood pressure), and improved urine output with UCM compared with DCC in preterm infants delivered by cesarean section.[648] The authors also noted SVC flow and higher right ventricular output in infants treated with UCM.

A concern has been raised over UCM relating to the rapidity of the delivery of the bolus of blood. Rapid changes in venous pressure during UCM were addressed in an early trial that demonstrated no greater increase in venous pressures with UCM compared with uterine contractions or a newborn cry during intact placental circulation.[649] A recent meta-analysis evaluating the safety and efficacy of UCM at birth concluded that there was a lower risk of oxygen requirement at 36 weeks and IVH of all grades.[645]

The potential for developing hyperbilirubinemia is another issue of concern with UCM. A Cochrane review found that none of the infants with elevated bilirubin levels required phototherapy treatment or exchange transfusions.[641] However,

in populations more susceptible to neonatal hyperbilirubinemia, especially those of Asian ethnicity, careful monitoring of the serum bilirubin level is warranted.

According to the 2010 International Consensus on Cardiopulmonary Resuscitation and Emergency Cardiovascular Care Science With Treatment Recommendations[650] and subsequent review of both DCC and cord milking in preterm newborns in the 2015 Umbilical Cord Management in the International Liaison Committee on Resuscitation (ILCOR) systematic review,[651,652] DCC for longer than 30 seconds was proposed as reasonable for both term and preterm infants who do not require resuscitation at birth. However, it was felt that there was insufficient evidence to recommend "delayed" cord clamping for infants who required resuscitation at birth, and more randomized trials involving such infants were needed. ILCOR also suggested that cord milking should not be routinely used for infants born at less than 29 weeks of gestation outside of a research setting because of concerns over rapid volume changes. Further studies are warranted to elucidate this issue, because cord milking may improve the initial mean blood pressure, hematologic indices, and reduce intracranial hemorrhage. However, there is currently no evidence with regard to improvements in long-term outcomes.

Temperature Stabilization. Unless significant preventative efforts are made, periviable newborns will quickly lose heat in the delivery room by evaporation of amniotic fluid from the baby's body, by conduction of heat from the body touching cooler surfaces, by convection to cooler surrounding air, and by radiation to cooler objects in the vicinity. For every 1°C below 36°C on admission temperature, mortality increases by 28%. The periviable infant should be placed in a high diathermancy food-grade polyethylene bag or wrap without initial drying up to the level of the shoulders.[653,654] Multiple studies have shown that plastic bags and wraps improve temperature on admission to the NICU, but as of yet there are no studies powered for important clinical outcomes, such as mortality or IVH.

Although normothermia may reduce *cold stress*, there are few studies to support an association of admission temperature or admission hypothermia to an increased risk for IVH. A single observational study of 271 VLBW infants showed that after correction for confounders by multivariate logistic regression analysis admission hypothermia (at ≤35.5 and at ≤35°C) was not associated with IVH.[655]

Newborn Resuscitation. Consideration of the intravascular pathogenetic factors makes it clear that certain practices in newborn resuscitation may increase the likelihood of IVH in the premature infant (Table 24.20). In particular, overly rapid infusion of volume expanders or of hypertonic solutions, such as sodium bicarbonate, should be avoided.

Concerning cerebrovascular autoregulation, the most important admonition in neonatal resuscitation is to establish adequate ventilation promptly to prevent hypoxemia and hypercarbia, two alterations that result readily in pressure-passive cerebral circulation.[145,162] Because of the latter facts and because hyperventilation in animals[175] and humans[656] sufficient to decrease $PaCO_2$ to approximately 25 mm Hg restores autoregulation after hypoxia, two retrospective studies of hyperventilation in the first 2 hours of life and the subsequent occurrence of IVH were conducted.[657,658] The data in the initial

TABLE 24.20	Progressive Ventricular Dilation After Intraventricular Hemorrhage

Etiology: acute, particulate blood clot; chronic, obliterative arachnoiditis in posterior fossa; aqueductal obstruction less commonly

Temporal features: usual onset of progression 1–3 weeks after hemorrhage; rapidity of evolution directly related to severity of hemorrhage

Rapid head growth or signs of increased intracranial pressure or both **following** ventricular dilation by days to weeks

Posterior horns of lateral ventricles dilating before, and more severely than, anterior horns

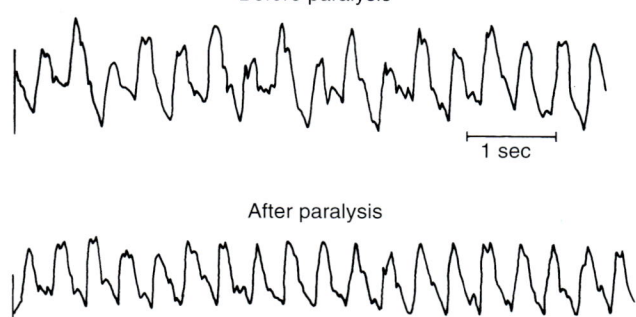

Figure 24.38 **Effect of muscle paralysis on fluctuating cerebral blood flow velocity from a ventilated, preterm infant with respiratory distress syndrome.** Before paralysis, the constantly fluctuating peak systolic and end-diastolic flow velocities are apparent. After paralysis was induced by pancuronium, the fluctuating pattern was eliminated.

study suggested that $PaCO_2$ values less than 35 mm Hg led to a decrease in incidence of subsequent IVH,[658] but a subsequent study failed to confirm this observation.[657] Currently, it seems prudent to recommend that adequate ventilation be established promptly in the resuscitation of the newborn infant, and that hypoxemia and hypercarbia be avoided. However, this goal does not require systematic early intubation of all ELBW infants (≤1000 g) at the slightest signs of respiratory distress.[659] An individualized approach to intubation is important. It is also important that if continuous positive airway pressure (CPAP) is to be used as the principal mode of ventilator support, an adequate but not excessive end expiratory pressure must be provided, with the goal of avoiding overdistention or elevated intrathoracic pressures.

Postnatal Interventions

Postnatal interventions aimed at reducing the risk for IVH have principally focused on cardiorespiratory management to reduce fluctuations in cerebral perfusion and pharmacological approaches to enhance cerebral blood flow and improve vascular stability.

Correction of Fluctuating Cerebral Blood Flow Velocity. The nearly invariable relationship between fluctuating cerebral blood flow velocity in the ventilated premature infant with respiratory distress syndrome and the subsequent occurrence of IVH (see Table 24.5) led to a search for interventions that could prevent this hemodynamic disturbance. Muscle paralysis with pancuronium bromide was found to be highly effective for the rapid conversion of the fluctuating pattern to a stable velocity (Fig. 24.38).[140] Moreover, muscle paralysis eliminated the fluctuations in venous pressure that accompany the cerebral arterial fluctuations (see earlier discussion).[309] Thus a prospective, randomized study of muscle paralysis from the first day of life to 72 hours of age in ventilated premature infants with the fluctuating hemodynamic disturbance was undertaken.[660] *All* the control infants (i.e., nonparalyzed) developed IVH, consistent with previous observations.[140] After completion of the controlled study,[660] a second study in 72 ventilated premature infants with the fluctuating circulatory abnormality for the first 72 hours of life showed a prominent reduction in IVH, including especially severe IVH.

Importantly, the fluctuations were related to the infant breathing out of synchrony with the ventilator, inducing a *pulses paradoxus*–like effect. Paralysis eliminated the infant's own breathing activity with immediate stabilization of the blood pressure and fluctuating cerebral blood flow velocity patterns. Over the last 10 years, several clinical and therapeutic factors have reduced the occurrence of this potential deleterious relationship. First, the near-universal use of antenatal glucocorticoids has reduced the severity of respiratory distress syndrome and improved the stability of the infant's blood pressure. Consequently, there has been a lesser requirement for volume expanders and/or inotrope use. Second, the early use of surfactant replacement therapy for infants with evidence of respiratory distress syndrome has facilitated the earlier extubation of infants, reducing the severity of their respiratory instability and the length of time that the infant is ventilated. Third, modern ventilators now have sophisticated feedback strategies that facilitate the infant's breathing in synchrony with the ventilator. In this regard, in a report in 2015 of 47,816 VLBW infants in the Vermont Oxford Network, only 50% of these infants ever received any positive pressure ventilation. Sixty percent of infants were ventilated for less than 24 hours, and 80% for less than 7 days. Thus it is the most immature and sick infants (<20% of VLBW infants) who may remain ventilator dependent during the first few critical days when the risk for IVH is highest and reducing fluctuations in systemic and cerebral perfusion are most often considered.

For those infants who may appear *irritable*, the use of sedatives is a clinical option. In our own experience and that of the more recent published literature, the *need* for muscle paralysis now is rare.[661] Of note, however, the use of opiates and benzodiazepines has increased dramatically over the past two decades in some centers (Fig. 24.39). The factors responsible for this increase in use are unclear, but it has not been driven by clear data indicating that such practice reduces the risk for IVH.

In view of the increased use of sedation rather than paralysis, it is plausible that the use of such sedatives may reduce the tendency for fluctuating cerebral blood flow associated with handling, painful procedures, and/or mechanical *fighting* of the ventilator, thereby leading to lower rates of IVH. Nevertheless, the impact of opioids on acute brain injury and long-term neurodevelopment in mechanically ventilated preterm neonates

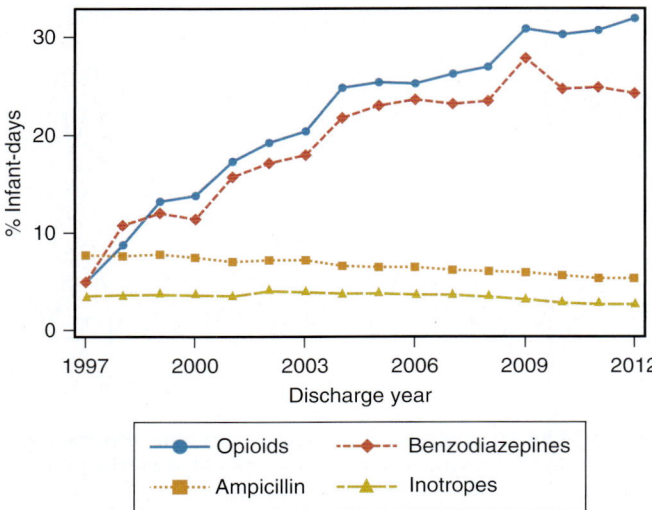

Figure 24.39 Opioid and benzodiazepine administration compared with ampicillin and inotrope administration over time. (From Zimmerman KO, Smith PB, Benjamin DK, Laughon M, Clark R, Traube C, Sturmer T. Hornik CP. Sedation, analgesia, and paralysis during mechanical ventilation of preterm infants. *J Pediatr.* 2017;180:99–104, figure 2.)

has been examined in two large randomized controlled trials, where no *difference in the composite outcome of severe IVH, PVL, or death was detected.* It is worthy of note that infants that required additional boluses of morphine in the morphine group demonstrated an increased risk for IVH.[582] However, long-term follow-up was also concerning, as it revealed conflicting results regarding the neurodevelopmental impact of early morphine exposure in preterm neonates. Even though the randomized Neurologic Outcomes and Preemptive Analgesia in Neonates study (NEOPAIN)[582] showed no difference in overall intelligence between groups, morphine exposure was associated with a smaller head circumference, impaired short-term memory, and social problems at 5 to 7 years of age compared with the placebo group. An understanding of how to best target sedation and/or paralysis is limited in these studies because of a lack of knowledge of cerebral perfusion and autoregulation. If accurate monitoring of cerebral perfusion were achievable, then a more rational targeted approach would identify which infant might benefit from sedation/paralysis to minimize any fluctuations in cerebral blood flow.

Correction or Prevention of Other Major Hemodynamic Disturbances. As indicated in the earlier discussion of pathogenesis, increases and decreases in cerebral arterial blood flow and increases in cerebral venous pressure can be involved in the pathogenesis of IVH. Thus care must be taken to prevent sharp elevations in blood pressure and cerebral blood flow with excessive handling, tracheal suctioning, rapid infusions of blood or other colloid, exchange transfusions, apneic spells, seizures, pneumothorax, and hypercarbia. As noted earlier, the use of antenatal corticosteroids, coupled with targeted surfactant replacement therapy, has reduced many of these events, particularly pneumothorax. Fluctuating $PaCO_2$ or hypocarbia also should be avoided.[246] Several smaller retrospective studies suggested that alterations in various monitoring and caretaking procedures, resulting in *minimal stimulation,* led to a decrease in

incidence of IVH.[662-664] However, out of necessity, the use of historic controls made it difficult to specify the most important alterations. A subsequent prospective study in which infants were randomly assigned to a carefully quantitated *reduced manipulation* protocol ($n = 62$) or to standard care ($n = 94$) did not show a significant difference in incidence of IVH (30% in study infants, 37% in control infants).[332]

In an attempt to avoid (rapid) fluctuations in CBF during routine care, several nursing interventions have been proposed. These nursing interventions are especially important during the first 72 hours after birth because most GMH-IVH develops during this time frame. The first of these interventions consists of positioning the head of the infant in a neutral (i.e., midline) position, enabling optimal cerebral venous drainage through the internal jugular veins.[665-667] As a consequence, hampered venous drainage and ultimately bleeding is believed to be prevented.[272,668,669] Low-quality evidence obtained in very small studies indicates that there is no significant effect on *cerebral oxygenation* by head rotation and/or head tilting in preterm infants.[670,671] One study performed by Liao and co-workers[672] revealed a small, statistically significant, one-sided decrease in $rScO_2$ after head rotation to the left. However, this decline of only 1% is unlikely to be of clinical significance. The second proposed intervention consists of elevating the head of the incubator 15 to 30 degrees upward (i.e., tilting) to facilitate venous outflow from the brain by promoting hydrostatic cerebral venous drainage.[673]

Finally, elevations in venous pressure must be avoided by prompt treatment of myocardial impairment (e.g., in the asphyxiated infant) and factors that may increase intrathoracic pressure and thereby cerebral venous pressure, such as pneumothorax and vigorous tracheal suctioning. A more extensive evaluation of myocardial function by functional echocardiography may assist in the decision to reduce cardiovascular afterload or manage preload. Management that is limited to evaluation of a single mean arterial blood pressure will likely result in inadequate or inappropriate therapy.

The role of *surfactant* per se in prevention of the hemodynamic disturbances associated with mechanical ventilation of infants with respiratory distress syndrome and thereby IVH is not entirely clear. Thus a series of earlier studies using one of at least seven different preparations of surfactant in *prophylactic* or *rescue* trials resulted in findings that were not entirely uniform.[674-693] In general, however, neonatal mortality rates, severity of respiratory distress, and air-block complications (e.g., pneumothorax) were reduced. The incidence and severity of IVH most often were either unchanged or reduced. The occurrence, albeit unusual, of increased incidence of IVH in surfactant-treated infants and the failure of a consistent decrease in incidence of IVH (despite a decrease in respiratory disease) in such infants led to the suspicion that surfactant treatment may have deleterious cerebral hemodynamic effects. Available data suggest that surfactant therapy may cause a transient increase in cerebral blood flow velocity and cerebral blood volume and electroencephalographic depression, but the effects are generally not marked.[694-700] Moreover, no clinical or biochemical evidence of deleterious effects (e.g., serum CK-BB levels) has been demonstrated.[701] In addition, the combined use of antenatal glucocorticoids and postnatal surfactant has added benefits concerning the prevention of IVH.[692,702,703]

Alternative methods of mechanical ventilation (i.e., high-frequency oscillatory ventilation or high-frequency jet ventilation) are not clearly superior to conventional ventilation regarding the incidence of IVH.[704-710] Indeed, in initial work, the incidence of severe IVH was higher in infants treated with high-frequency oscillatory ventilation (26%) than in infants treated with conventional mechanical ventilation (18%), and the neurological outcome was poorer in the former group of infants.[707,708] A subsequent multicenter study showed a similarly higher incidence of IVH (36% vs. 20%),[709] but four later studies showed no increase in incidence of IVH in infants treated with high-frequency oscillatory ventilation.[710-713] A significantly deleterious effect concerning IVH also was not observed in two studies of high-frequency jet ventilation,[706,714] although an increase in the incidence of cystic periventricular leukomalacia was documented in one report.[714] More data are needed on these issues. Most frequently, early nasal CPAP is being used in the delivery room or early in the neonatal course. A meta-analysis of 2364 infants comparing CPAP with mechanical ventilation, CPAP resulted in a small but clinically significant reduction in the incidence of BPD at 36 weeks (typical RR 0.89; 95% CI, 0.79 to 0.99) and death or BPD (typical RR 0.89; 95% CI, 0.81 to 0.97).[715] There was no difference in the rates of IVH. Early CPAP did appear to be associated with a higher risk for pneumothorax if surfactant therapy was not administered.

The use of *inhaled nitric oxide* for premature infants with severe respiratory failure, related most often to severe respiratory distress syndrome, currently is under active investigation.[716-724] The gas is used for pulmonary benefits related to its strong pulmonary vasodilator properties. Thus far, no consistent significant differences in the rate of IVH in infants treated with nitric oxide have been reported. One controlled study of 793 infants 34 weeks of gestational age or younger described a decline in *grade 3 or 4* hemorrhage in infants treated with nitric oxide from the first days of life but only in infants of birthweight 750 to 999 g.[721] Another report described improved neurodevelopmental outcome in infants treated with inhaled nitric oxide, but the neuropathological basis for the improvement was not clear.[716]

Correction of Abnormalities of Coagulation. Although in selected infants abnormalities of coagulation (or of platelet-capillary interactions) may play a role in the pathogenesis of IVH, it is unclear whether interventions to correct or prevent such abnormalities are indicated for all premature infants. Thus in one controlled study of the administration of fresh frozen plasma (10 mL/kg) to premature infants on admission to the nursery and again at 24 hours of life, treated infants exhibited a decrease in the overall incidence of IVH (14% vs. 41% in untreated infants).[352] However, no difference in incidence of severe IVH was noted, and no clear effect on coagulation variables could be demonstrated. The possibility was raised that the fresh frozen plasma exerted its benefit by "stabilizing the circulation" rather than by an effect on coagulation. Two later studies of administration of fresh frozen plasma showed no benefit regarding prevention or extension of IVH or on neurological outcome at 2 years.[355,356,363] Thus, at present, no clear indication exists for the routine administration of fresh frozen plasma postnatally to premature infants for prevention of IVH.

Pharmacological Interventions

Indomethacin. In the last edition of this book, we reviewed 19 controlled studies of indomethacin as a means to prevent IVH.[725-740] The drug was studied particularly for prophylaxis, rather than treatment, of patent ductus arteriosus, and it was generally administered initially before 12 hours of age. A summary of the pooled results showed that indomethacin administration led to a decrease in the incidence of overall IVH (RR, 0.88; 95% CI, 0.80 to 0.96) and of severe IVH (RR, 0.66; 95% CI, 0.53 to 0.82).[736,741] In the largest early series ($n = 431$), Ment and co-workers[742] observed a decrease in the incidence of total IVH (18% to 12%) and *grade IV* IVH (4.5% to 0.5%). However, in this study, early-onset IVH was excluded, and the marked preponderance of *grade IV* IVH relative to *grade III* IVH (10:1) in the control population was unusual and raised the possibility of an undefined unusual characteristic of the control population.[743] Indeed, in centers where the incidence of grades III and IV IVH in the control population was greater than 10%, indomethacin administration was shown to lead to a significant reduction in these severe hemorrhages (OR, 0.54; 95% CI, 0.36 to 0.82; $P < .005$), whereas in centers where the incidence was less than 10%, indomethacin did not lead to a significant reduction (OR, 0.72; 95% CI, 0.39 to 1.33; $P < .3$).[733]

An interesting development in this area was the repeat analysis of the data from the earlier study of Ment and co-workers ($n = 431$; Table 24.21).[737] Thus the beneficial effect of indomethacin on IVH was shown in *male* but not female patients. A repeat analysis of the later larger study of prophylactic indomethacin ($n = 1202$) showed a weak differential effect of indomethacin by sex; for severe IVH, the incidences in indomethacin-treated versus placebo groups were 9.8% versus 11.7% (OR, 0.46 to 1.44) for female patients but 8.6% versus 14.7% (OR, 0.31 to 0.94) for male patients.[738] *Thus, on balance, in the total experience with indomethacin, a generally favorable preventive effect of the drug on IVH seems apparent, particularly or exclusively in male patients.* Follow-up of the large series of infants studied by Ment and co-workers showed no difference in the development of ultrasonographically demonstrated cystic periventricular leukomalacia or in incidences of cerebral palsy or of cognitive impairment at 36 months of age.[39,744] Other investigators also have shown no beneficial long-term neurodevelopmental effects.[736,740,741] However, again, when male and female patients are analyzed separately, a clear cognitive benefit is apparent in male but not female patients (Table 24.22).

The complexity of the issues of indomethacin prophylaxis (IP) regarding prevention of IVH and the role of the patent ductus arteriosus in this context is illustrated in more recent work. Thus a retrospective study during the period 2003–10[745] involved 13,754 infants with a birthweight ≤1000 g admitted to the participating centers with IP given to 4255 eligible infants. The first prophylactic dose of indomethacin was given at ≤6 hours of age in 2340 infants and at greater than 6 to 24 hours of age in 1915 infants. Bivariate analyses indicated lower incidences of IVH or death and severe IVH or death in the group receiving IP at ≤6 hours of age compared with those administered IP at greater than 6 to 24 hours of age. However, after multivariate correction, statistically significant associations did not persist. The primary outcomes of indomethacin timing and unadjusted risk for IVH and patent ductus arteriosus (PDA) are shown in Table 24.23. Thus this study confirmed

TABLE 24.21   Effect of Prophylactic Indomethacin Administration on Incidence and Severity of Intraventricular Hemorrhage: Effect of Gender[a]

	FEMALE PATIENTS (n = 196)		MALE PATIENTS (n = 235)	
	SALINE	INDOMETHACIN	SALINE	INDOMETHACIN
No IVH	89 (86%)	78 (84%)	93 (78%)	106 (91%)
IVH	14 (14%)	15 (16%)	26 (22%)	10 (9%)
Grade I			5	4
Grade II			12	6
Grade III			1	0
Grade IV			8	0

[a]Breslow-Day test for homogeneity (female vs. male), $P = .013$ for IVH/no IVH.

IVH, Intraventricular hemorrhage.

Data from Ment LR, Vohr BR, Makuch RW, et al. Prevention of intraventricular hemorrhage by indomethacin in male preterm infants. *J Pediatr.* 2004;145:832–834.

TABLE 24.22   Effect of Prophylactic Indomethacin Administration on Neurodevelopment: Effect of Gender[a]

	AGE AT FOLLOW-UP		
	3 YEARS	6 YEARS	8 YEARS
Female patients			
Saline	88.5 ± 17.3	92.0 ± 21.7	92.6 ± 22.3
Indomethacin	83.5 ± 22.0	93.2 ± 25.2	90.8 ± 24.8
Male patients			
Saline	77.8 ± 25.1	86.8 ± 29.8	89.9 ± 30.0
Indomethacin	87.4 ± 20.6	96.6 ± 19.6	95.4 ± 23.4

[a]Scores are based on the Peabody Picture Vocabulary Test-R. For male patients, saline versus indomethacin, $P = .017$.

Data from Ment LR, Vohr BR, Makuch RW, Westerveld M, et al. Prevention of intraventricular hemorrhage by indomethacin in male preterm infants. *J Pediatr.* 2004;145:832–834.

that IP before 6 hours of age does not decrease the incidence of IVH or death compared with later administration up to 24 hours of age. Similar findings were reported by Yanowitz and co-workers.[746] In this large cohort, there was no impact on the incidence of any IVH-related outcomes relative to the timing of IP, including analysis by any sex or gestational grouping. The authors concluded that administration of prophylactic indomethacin at ≤6 hours of age was not associated with a lower incidence of IVH or death in ELBW infants. However, medical treatment or surgical ligation of PDA or death was significantly less frequent among the infants who received IP ≤6 hours of age compared with later administration.

On balance, although the overall data are interesting and provocative, the findings do not appear sufficiently conclusive to recommend routine IP for the prevention of IVH. Many academic centers have taken a *risk-based* approach, administering prophylactic indomethacin to treat PDA and reduce the risk for IVH in the highest risk infants—those most immature who have not received antenatal corticosteroids and have significant cardiorespiratory instability. This tentative conclusion, however, will need reassessment in the context of the recent finding that prolonged indomethacin prophylactic exposure in premature newborns of 24 to 28 weeks of gestation is associated with decreased white matter injury detected by MRI (see Chapter 16).[747]

The mechanisms of a beneficial effect of indomethacin may relate to the circulatory and metabolic consequences of the drug. First, indomethacin was shown in the beagle puppy model of IVH to decrease baseline cerebral blood flow and to diminish the occurrence of IVH after hemorrhagic hypotension and volume reexpansion.[748] The decrease in cerebral blood flow after indomethacin was replicated in several animal models.[749-757] The circulatory effects are presumed to be secondary to the drug's inhibition of prostaglandin biosynthesis. Indeed, studies in newborn piglets showed that indomethacin not only decreased baseline cerebral blood flow by approximately 20% to 30% but also, perhaps more important, attenuated the cerebral hyperemia induced by asphyxia (combined hypoxia-hypercarbia).[758,759]

Studies of human preterm infants suggest that the increase in cerebrovascular resistance and decline in cerebral blood flow observed in perinatal animals may also occur in the infant. Thus a decrease in cerebral blood flow velocity and an increase in resistance indices were documented by the Doppler technique after administration of indomethacin to human infants.[760-766] Indeed, a *decrease in cerebral blood flow after administration of indomethacin* was shown clearly by Pryds and co-workers,[767] who used the xenon clearance method to define in six premature infants a mean decrease in cerebral blood flow of 24%. The effect of indomethacin began within minutes and continued for at least an hour. Studies with near-infrared spectroscopy also clearly documented a decline in cerebral blood volume, flow, and oxygen delivery after administration of indomethacin to human infants.[768-772] Finally, *ibuprofen*, shown to be effective in prophylaxis for patent ductus arteriosus, is not associated with the unfavorable cerebral hemodynamic effects of indomethacin.[773-777] However, prophylactic ibuprofen does not have a preventive effect for IVH.[775,776]

A second aspect of the indomethacin action that may be of benefit in prevention of IVH relates to the inhibition of the formation of free radicals generated by the cyclooxygenase portion of the pathway of prostaglandin biosynthesis (the portion affected by indomethacin).[778] *This mechanism may be of relevance concerning the male versus female effects noted earlier.* Thus, male cells have been shown to be more susceptible

TABLE 24.23 Indomethacin Timing and Unadjusted Risk for Intraventricular Hemorrhage and Patent Ductus Arteriosus

	TIME OF INDOMETHACIN		
PRIMARY OUTCOME	**≤6 h (n = 2340)**	**>6–24 h (n = 1915)**	**P**
Total IVH (any grade)	747 (32%)	630 (33%)	.39
Total IVH or death	976 (42%)	871 (45%)	.01
Severe IVH (grade 3/4)	413 (17%)	347 (18%)	.60
Severe IVH or death	711 (30%)	647 (34%)	.02
PDA	778 (33%)	688 (36%)	.07
PDA or death	1088 (46.5%)	984 (51.5%)	<.001
PDA receiving treatment	500 (22%)	564 (30%)	<.001
PDA receiving treatment or death	858 (37.1%)	900 (47.2%)	<.001

IVH, Intraventricular hemorrhage; *PDA*, patent ductus arteriosus.

From Mirza H, Laptook AR, Oh W, Vohr BR, Stoll BJ, Kandefer S, Stonestreet BS, and Generic Database Subcommittee of the NICHD Neonatal Research Network. Effects of indomethacin prophylaxis timing on IVH and PDA in extremely low birth weight (ELBW) infants. *Arch Dis Child Fetal Neonatal Ed.* 2016;101:F418–F422.

to free radical–mediated cell death because of a deficiency in antioxidant defenses at the glutathione peroxidase step.[779]

A third potentially beneficial effect of indomethacin is an acceleration of maturation of microvessels in the germinal matrix. Thus indomethacin administration to the newborn beagle puppy led to increased laminin deposition in basement membranes of matrix microvessels.[780] This effect was apparent on the second postnatal day, 1 day after the first injection of the drug.

Other Pharmacological Approaches

Several previous drugs have been studied historically to reduce the risk of IVH but are currently not in routine clinical use. These include etamsylate, phenobarbital, and vitamin E. For historic relevance, they are briefly summarized here.

Etamsylate. Etamsylate (formerly ethamsylate) was initially evaluated in five smaller RCTs that all documented benefit with a reduction in IVH in treated infants.[760,781-783] However, enthusiasm for etamsylate was dampened by the results of an international, multicenter randomized trial that involved 334 infants of less than 32 weeks of gestation.[784] Thus no difference was seen between the treated and control groups in incidence of all IVH (35% vs. 37%) or of severe IVH or *major* ultrasonographic lesions (13% vs. 12%). Etamsylate in this trial was administered *within 4 hours of birth* (i.e., later than the *1 hour* in two large trials that demonstrated a protective effect of etamsylate).[782,783] However, still more discouraging, long-term follow-up of the earlier cohorts showed no decrease in rates of cerebral palsy in the etamsylate-treated group.[785]

Phenobarbital. Phenobarbital was evaluated in nine controlled studies as a means to prevent IVH.[212,213,419,786-793] The results were not consistent. Although the studies had small methodological differences, the essential similarities in methods were more prominent; that is, phenobarbital was administered generally from the first hours of life, and phenobarbital levels attained were usually 20 to 25 µg/mL. The largest reported study[213] was composed of 280 intubated premature infants. The data showed a higher overall incidence of IVH in the phenobarbital-treated infants than in the controls.[213]

Vitamin E. Vitamin E was evaluated as a means to prevent IVH in several studies that showed a reduction in IVH, most notably severe IVH.[212,794-799] Nevertheless, enthusiasm for the use of vitamin E for prevention of IVH was tempered by the largest study, that of Phelps and co-workers.[795] This investigation of 287 premature infants was designed to evaluate the efficacy of vitamin E in the prevention of retinopathy of prematurity. Vitamin E was administered *intravenously* initially and later by the oral route. The data showed not only that vitamin E did not prevent retinopathy of prematurity but also that the treated infants exhibited a *higher* incidence of severe IVH (25% in treated infants, 15% in control infants). This effect was most marked in infants less than 1000 g (36% in treated infants, 11% in control infants). A later report concerning vitamin E focused on the smallest infants (<1000 g), those with the highest risk of the most severe hemorrhages, and reported a beneficial effect of vitamin E in the smaller group of infants (501 to 750 g), with a 50% decrease in incidence of total IVH (60% vs. 32%, *P* = .045) and an even more marked decrease in incidence of IVH of severe variety (29% vs. 4%, *P* = .023).[798] No increase in mortality rate, sepsis, or necrotizing enterocolitis (previously suggested, potential deleterious effects of vitamin E)[800] was observed in the vitamin E–treated infants. However, a review of 26 randomized clinical trials of relevance to the role of vitamin E concluded that, in preterm infants, vitamin E supplementation reduced the risk of IVH when administered by routes other than intravenous and at serum tocopherol levels that did not exceed 3.5 mg/dL.[799] In current clinical neonatal practice, intravenous vitamin E is not readily available and is not routinely administered for the prevention of IVH.

Conclusions

The advances in understanding the pathogenesis of germinal matrix hemorrhage–IVH, as discussed earlier, led to the formulation of rational interventions to prevent hemorrhages. Both perinatal and postnatal interventions show considerable promise. Perinatal interventions include prevention of premature birth (currently a focus of the March of Dimes Foundation in the United States), transportation of the premature infant to a tertiary facility in utero rather than after birth (an

TABLE 24.24	Acute Management of Germinal Matrix–Intraventricular Hemorrhage

Maintenance of cerebral perfusion
    Cautious control of blood pressure
    Lowering of increased intracranial pressure: rarely indicated
Prevention of cerebral hemodynamic disturbances
    Avoidance of fluctuating or increased arterial blood
        pressure, hypercarbia, hypoxemia, acidosis, hyperosmolar
        solutions, rapid volume expansion, pneumothorax, and
        seizures
Other supportive care
Serial ultrasound scans
Management of posthemorrhagic hydrocephalus

approach of proven value), *prenatal administration especially of glucocorticoid*, and optimal management of labor and delivery with DCC or UCM, prevention of hypo- or hyperthermia, and high-quality respiratory care. Postnatal interventions include avoidance of fluctuating cerebral blood flow velocity, correction or prevention of other major hemodynamic disturbances, and correction of abnormalities of coagulation. Postnatal pharmacological interventions that have been studied in detail include phenobarbital, indomethacin, etamsylate, and vitamin E. No single agent among this group has been shown to consistently lead to a decrease in the incidence *and* severity of IVH. However, a high-risk very preterm infant without perinatal exposure to maternal antenatal corticosteroids with cardiorespiratory instability after birth may selectively benefit from the administration of prophylactic indomethacin.

Acute Management of Intraventricular Hemorrhage

Most often, the physician has been unable to prevent IVH and is faced with the task of managing the infant who has sustained this potentially serious intracranial event. The basic elements of acute management are shown in Table 24.24.

Maintenance of Cerebral Perfusion

The critical initial task is to maintain cerebral perfusion. As discussed previously, cerebral perfusion pressure is related to the mean arterial blood pressure minus the intracranial pressure. With *major* IVH, because of the potential for decreased arterial blood pressure and very occasionally elevated intracranial pressure, cerebral perfusion may be compromised.

Arterial blood pressure must be maintained at adequate levels, although this control of blood pressure must be carried out cautiously because of the likely presence of pressure-passive cerebral circulation. Overly exuberant therapeutic responses may contribute to the conversion of a moderate lesion to a severe one.

Intracranial pressure should not be allowed to remain excessive, although major elevations are *extremely* rare with IVH. Moreover, direct measurements of intracranial pressure in all cases of IVH are *not practical*. Selection of those rare patients with large lesions and clinical signs of increased intracranial pressure (e.g., full anterior fontanelle) is important and may be worthy of review with neurosurgery colleagues for consideration of an acute decompression, if feasible and appropriate.

Prevention of Cerebral Hemodynamic Disturbances

The other side of the coin concerning cerebral perfusion is avoidance of abrupt increases in cerebral blood flow and the other hemodynamic disturbances important in the pathogenesis of hemorrhage. Such disturbances may lead to progression of hemorrhage. Thus, the factors previously discussed concerning prevention of hemorrhage must be considered: avoidance of fluctuating or increased arterial blood pressure, hypercarbia, hypoxemia, acidosis, hyperosmolar solutions, rapid volume expansion, and pneumothorax. Because seizures appear to be much more common than previously recognized in VPT infants and may provoke cerebral hyperfusion by an effect on arterial blood pressure, as well as by local factors in brain, overt seizures should be treated vigorously in the setting of major IVH (see Chapter 12). More recent studies have documented that close to one-half of very preterm infants experience seizures in the first 72 hours of life.[324] High seizure burden has been associated with increased risk of IVH.[325]

Serial Ultrasound Scans

If the infant survives the acute period, serial assessments of ventricular size by ultrasound scan should be conducted. Serial assessment is necessary because, as discussed later, the classic signs of evolving hydrocephalus (i.e., rapid head growth, full anterior fontanelle, and separated cranial sutures) do not appear for days to weeks *after* ventricular dilation has already commenced. We have recommended a minimum frequency of twice a week for cranial ultrasounds for monitoring for the development of progressive ventricular dilatation in the setting of IVH. Posthemorrhagic ventricular dilatation and its management are described in the following sections.

Posthemorrhagic Hydrocephalus
Incidence and Definition

Hydrocephalus, which is progressive ventricular dilation secondary to a disturbance in CSF dynamics, is a not uncommon sequela of IVH (see Table 24.20).[a] As might be expected, the incidence of posthemorrhagic progressive ventricular dilation is related closely to the severity of the initial hemorrhage (see later). However, because ventricular dilation may occur after IVH as a result of periventricular leukomalacia or periventricular hemorrhagic infarction, or both, posthemorrhagic ventriculomegaly should not be equated with hydrocephalus. The most important aspect of this differentiation relates to the timing of the ventriculomegaly. If there has been a large grade III or IV IVH, and one is following serial cranial ultrasound scans every 3 to 4 days, then it is possible to better delineate the etiology of the ventriculomegaly relating to hydrocephalus (posthemorrhagic) or ex vacuo loss of white matter volume. Another manner in which one can delineate such evolution is to consider the extraaxial space. If there is an increase in the extraaxial space that accompanies the ventriculomegaly, then it is likely that this represents an ex vacuo phenomenon rather than hydrocephalus, which tends to produce diminution of the extraaxial space.

Indeed, clinical distinction between ventriculomegaly secondary to periventricular cerebral atrophy and ventriculomegaly

---

[a]References 25, 27, 127, 128, 245, 426, 430, 435, 443, 458, 460–463, 466, 467, 469–471, 484, 485, and 801–814.

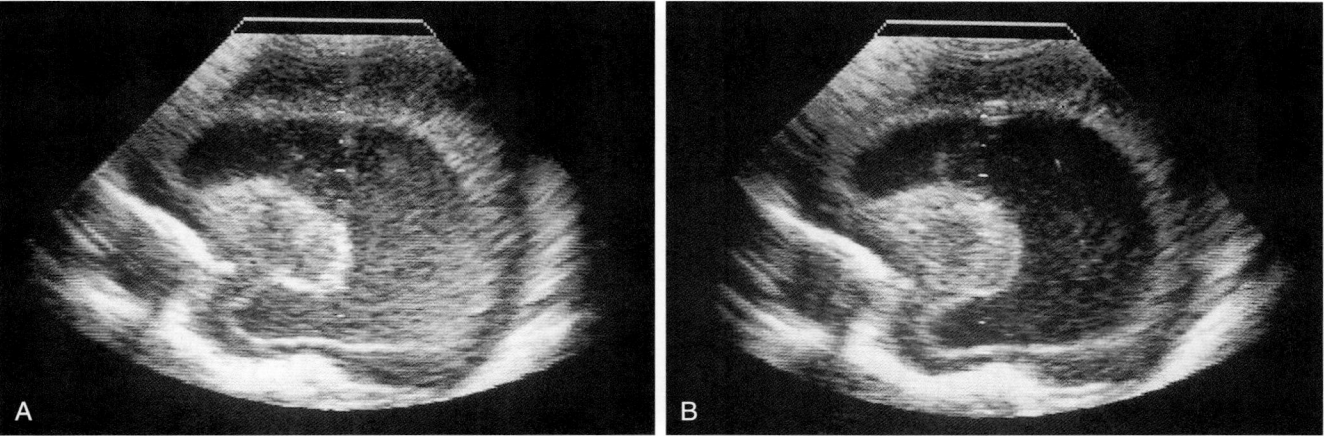

Figure 24.40 Acute hydrocephalus with intraventricular hemorrhage: pathogenesis. Parasagittal ultrasound scans were performed (A) immediately after the examiner turned the patient's head from right to left and (B) after 10 minutes. In moderately to markedly dilated lateral ventricles, echogenic particulate matter is prominent immediately after (A) turning of head and disappears (B) over the next 10 minutes.

secondary to hydrocephalus with attendant impairment of CSF dynamics is critical for formulation of appropriate management decisions. Close surveillance and neuroimaging usually provide the necessary information to make the distinction.

Ventricular size and shape can be affected by the original parenchymal injury in addition to white matter volume loss/underdevelopment associated with the encephalopathy of prematurity (see Chapter 16).

Pathogenesis

The pathogenesis of posthemorrhagic hydrocephalus can be considered in terms of either the acute process, apparent within days (particularly after severe IVH), or the subacute-chronic process, apparent within weeks. *Acute* hydrocephalus appears to be secondary to an impairment of CSF absorption caused by particulate blood clot and demonstrable by ultrasound scan (Fig. 24.40).[815] The important role of *the combination of deficient fibrinolytic properties and enhanced fibroproliferative characteristics* of the CSF of infants with posthemorrhagic hydrocephalus includes the deficient fibrinolytic properties with low plasminogen and high plasminogen activator inhibitor levels in CSF of premature infants after IVH.[119-121] The enhanced fibroproliferative properties appear to relate to the upregulation after IVH of CSF levels of transforming growth factor-beta 1 and procollagen 1C-peptide.[125-128] The impairment of CSF flow is usually distal to the outflow of the fourth ventricle, because most examples of posthemorrhagic hydrocephalus are of the communicating type. The latter has been demonstrated by radionuclide lumbar cisternography and by ultrasonographic demonstration of a decrease in ventricular size immediately after removal of CSF from the lumbar space.[466,484,811,816,817] Obstruction at the level of the aqueduct by blood clot, debris, and subependymal scarring still occurs, with some important frequency.

Evolution

The ventricular dilation may begin essentially with the hemorrhage, especially with larger IVH. More often, definite ventricular dilation and particularly the progression thereof

begin within 1 to 3 weeks of the hemorrhage. Unfortunately, the traditional clinical criteria of evolving hydrocephalus (i.e., rapid head growth, full anterior fontanelle, and separated cranial sutures) do not appear for days to weeks *after* ventricular dilation has already been present. This phenomenon was surmised on the basis of neuropathological[785] and clinical data.[818] The availability of serial ultrasound studies has allowed repeated observation of this occurrence. As discussed in more detail in the management section, the rapidity of progression of posthemorrhagic ventricular dilation relates principally to the severity of the hemorrhage.

To quantitate the extent of ventricular dilation, standard ventricular measurements have been developed.[819] These measures focus on the anterior horn width (AHW), thalamo-occipital diameter, and ventricular index (VI).[819] Development of normal values for postmenstrual age allows the clinician to plot the evolution of ventricular enlargement over time following IVH.

To diagnose and evaluate PHVD, measurements of ventricular size on cranial ultrasound are superior to any subjective assessments of elevated ICP, like a tense fontanel, sunset phenomena of the eyes, or measurements of head circumference.[820-823] In clinical practice, the VI of the lateral ventricles, as measured on cranial ultrasound (Fig. 24.41), is most frequently used for monitoring ventricular size following GMH-IVH. In some studies,[412,824,825] measurements of the VI are expressed as a ratio to the hemispheric width (HW). Although a rise in ICP may be accompanied by an increase in VI, often the VI only starts to enlarge in more severe hydrocephalus and consequently may fail to identify neonates with mild dilation.[826,827] The first sign of an increase in ICP is more frequently a change in ventricular shape with rounding of the frontal horns and an increase in AHW (see Fig. 24.41). Hence the AHW has been suggested to be a more sensitive marker for early or mild ventricular enlargement than the VI. The depth of the occipital horn of the lateral ventricle (thalamo-occipital distance [TOD]; see Fig. 24.41) has also been recommended as a valuable addition for the evaluation of ventricular size following GMH-IVH. Occipital horn enlargement is often visible before

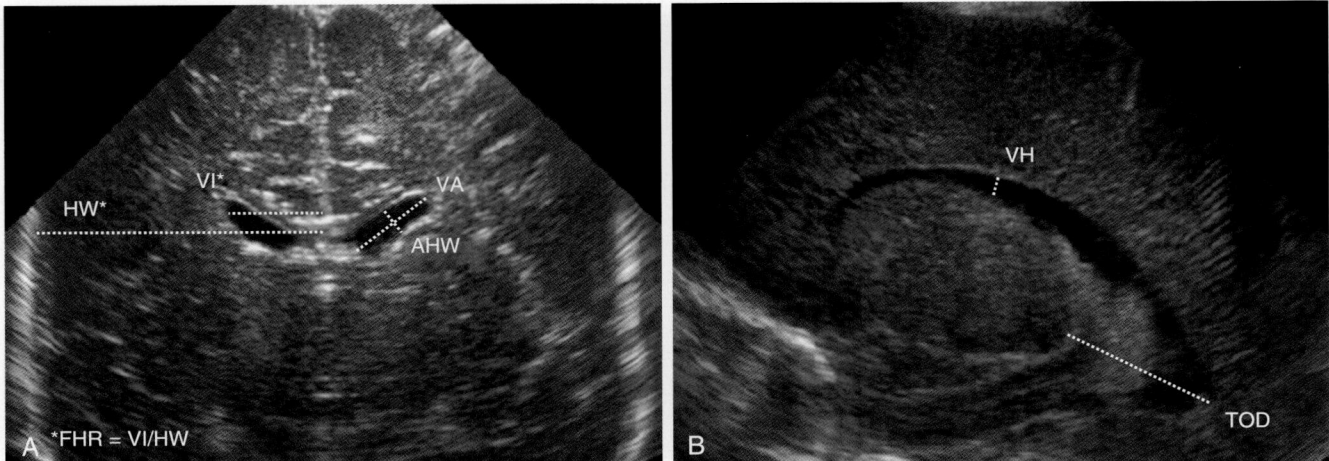

Figure 24.41 Ventricular parameters measured in the (A) coronal and (B) sagittal planes by cranial ultrasonography. *AHW*, Anterior horn width; *FHR*, frontal horn ratio; *HW*, hemispheric width; *TOD*, thalamo-occipital distance; *VA*, ventricular axis; *VH*, ventricular height; *VI*, ventricular index. (From Brouwer MJ, de Vries LS, Pistorius L, Rademaker KJ, Groenendaal F, Benders MJ. Ultrasound measurements of the lateral ventricles in neonates: why, how and when? A systematic review. *Acta Paediatr.* 2010;99:1298–1306.)

any increase in frontal horn dimensions. The occipital horns are usually dilated to a greater extent than the frontal horns and may represent the only site of ventricular dilation.[416,421,828] Although the data from several cross-sectional studies have been summarized (Fig. 24.42),[819] important questions remain as to which measure on cranial ultrasound is most indicative of raised intracranial pressure that would necessitate or guide the need for decompression of PHVD.

Reasons for Ventricular Dilation Before Rapid Head Growth

The reasons for the impressive ventricular dilation before the development of rapid head growth and signs of increased intracranial pressure must relate to the developmental state of the cerebrum in the premature infant. The three most relevant features are (1) the paucity of cerebral myelin, (2) the relative excess of water in the centrum semiovale, and (3) the relatively large subarachnoid space. In experimental and human hydrocephalus, the cerebral white matter is encroached on, and central gray structures are relatively spared.[829] The paucity of myelin and the relative excess of water in the cerebral white matter of the premature infant would serve to accentuate this general feature of hydrocephalus. It can be postulated that less force is required to compress this immature cerebral white matter than to overcome the restrictions of the dura and skull. This notion is supported by the disproportionate dilation of the occipital versus frontal horns with posthemorrhagic hydrocephalus. The third factor (i.e., the relatively large subarachnoid space in the premature infant, reflected by the enhanced cranial transillumination in the normal premature infant) may have an important contributory effect, because this space could be encroached on even after ventricular dilation but before separation of sutures (Figs. 24.43 and 24.44).

Relation of Ventricular Dilation to Brain Injury

The precise relation of progressive posthemorrhagic ventricular dilation to brain injury is unclear. This issue is considered best in terms of experimental and clinical studies.

Experimental Studies. The pathogenesis of brain injury in hydrocephalus is multifactorial. Deleterious effects of hydrocephalus on the brain include disturbances of cerebral white matter, cerebral blood vessels, and cerebral cortex.[830] Concerning cerebral white matter, the earliest changes (1 week after induction of experimental hydrocephalus) involve OLs and myelin, with a decrease in myelin-associated enzymes (e.g., ceramide galactosyltransferase) and structural proteins (e.g., myelin basic protein). Later, after several weeks, axonal loss and impaired myelination are apparent. Investigators reported that shunting at 1 week, but not at 4 weeks, when axonal loss had occurred, allowed recovery of myelination.[831,832] In later stages of maturation, hydrocephalus can delay myelination, which may recover to some extent after shunting.[831,833,834] The late occurrence of axonal loss with hydrocephalus was noted in earlier studies.[835-842] Thus if this stage is not reached, therapy appears to be beneficial in preventing permanent structural deficits.

A role for *cerebral vascular changes and ischemia* in the genesis of the white matter injury in experimental hydrocephalus is demonstrated by morphological studies that show an attenuation of the caliber of major cerebral vessels and a decrease in the secondary and tertiary vessels in cerebral white matter.[830,839,843] These changes may underlie, at least in part, the decrease in volemic cerebral blood flow and alterations in energy metabolism in hydrocephalic animal models.[830,844-846] Also supportive of cerebral ischemia are the findings in cerebral white matter of increased cerebral rates of glucose metabolism (presumably anaerobic glycolysis), elevated lactate, decreased high-energy phosphates, and elevated free radicals.[834,847-850] In addition, evidence for a brisk inflammatory response in cerebral white matter suggest another source for free radical–mediated white matter injury (see Chapters 13 and 15).[851] These mechanisms, leading to free radical production, are particularly relevant in view of the data demonstrating the particular vulnerability of differentiating oligodendroglia to free radical attack (see Chapter 13).[852] These biochemical changes and neurochemical signs of axonal loss could be prevented by early shunting

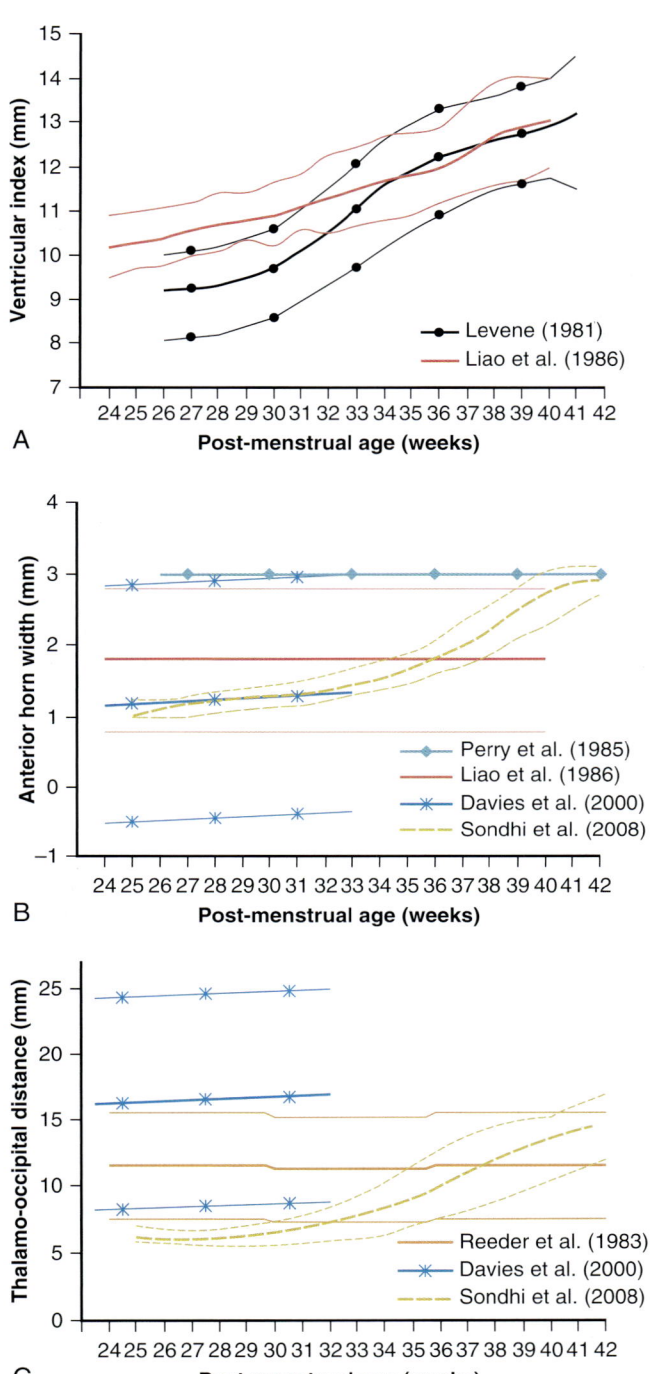

A

B

C

Figure 24.42 Overview of the reference curves for the (A) ventricular index, (B) anterior horn width, and (C) thalamo-occipital distance according to Davies et al. (regression line with 95% confidence interval), Levene, Liao et al. (mean ± 2 SD), Perry et al., Reeder et al. (mean ± 2 SD), and Sondhi et al. (Adapted from Davies et al., Levene, Liao et al., and Sondhi et al. From Brouwer MJ, de Vries LS, Pistorius L, Rademaker KJ, Groenendaal F, Benders MJ. Ultrasound measurements of the lateral ventricles in neonates: why, how and when? A systematic review. *Acta Paediatr.* 2010;99:1298–1306.)

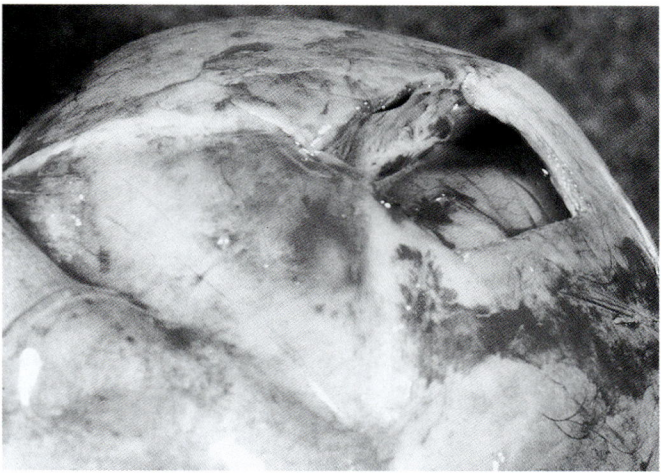

Figure 24.43 Prominent subarachnoid space in the premature infant. Bone has been removed from the left parietal region of an infant of 29 weeks of gestation. Note the large subarachnoid space. (Courtesy Dr. James Rohrbaugh.)

in the various experimental models.[830,846,847,853] Moreover, the vascular attenuation may represent the anatomical substrate for the increase in cerebrovascular resistance and decrease in volemic cerebral blood flow and flow velocity in human infants with hydrocephalus (see later discussion).

Of particular additional interest are alterations in *cerebral cortical neurons* in hydrocephalic animal models. Thus disturbances in catecholaminergic and serotonergic neurotransmitter development and in synaptogenesis and evidence for neuronal degeneration have been delineated.[830,854-864] Animal studies also show that the hydrocephalus can particularly disturb brain development during the phase of cell proliferation.[865,866] These effects could reflect, in part, disturbance to the ascending and descending axons in the cerebral white matter with secondary anterograde and retrograde effects on the organizational development of the cerebral cortex. When specifically addressed in the various experimental studies, the deleterious effects were shown to be reversible when the hydrocephalic state was corrected early. The specific roles of duration of dilation, severity thereof, and presence and degree of intracranial hypertension in determining reversibility remain to be defined clearly.

Human Studies. Data from studies of infants concerning the deleterious effect of progressive posthemorrhagic ventricular dilation relate to cerebral hemodynamics, neurophysiological function, morphological disturbances, biochemical indicators of hypoxia, and clinical outcome (Table 24.25). The data are sometimes difficult to interpret conclusively, because such details as rate of progression, degree and duration of ventriculomegaly, intracranial pressure, preceding parenchymal injury, and neurological outcome are often not provided. Nevertheless, the findings suggest at least transient disturbances.

Concerning *cerebral hemodynamics*, a systematic study of nine infants with posthemorrhagic hydrocephalus initially demonstrated *impaired blood flow velocity* in the anterior cerebral arteries that was reversed with therapy to correct the hydrocephalic state.[155] The disturbance of cerebral blood flow velocity appeared to correlate more closely with ventriculomegaly than with increased intracranial pressure.

Extracerebral cerebrospinal fluid

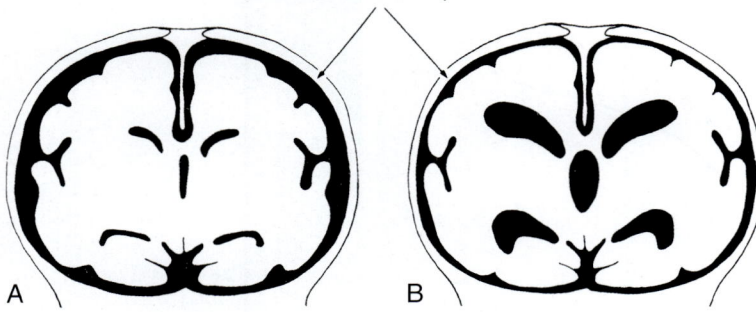

Figure 24.44 Postulated contributory mechanism for development of posthemorrhagic ventricular dilation before rapid head growth. (A) Normal premature brain. (B) Evolving posthemorrhagic hydrocephalus encroaching on subarachnoid space. (From Pape KE, Wigglesworth JS. *Haemorrhage, Ischaemia, and the Perinatal Brain.* Philadelphia: JB Lippincott; 1979.)

TABLE 24.25   Cerebral Hemodynamic, Neurophysiological, and Biochemical Evidence of at Least Transient Disturbance With Posthemorrhagic Ventricular Dilation in Human Infants[a]

Cerebral hemodynamics
Decreased cerebral blood flow velocity–increased cerebrovascular resistance–decreased cerebral compliance (Doppler)
Decreased cerebral blood flow (positron emission tomography)
Decreased cerebral oxygenated hemoglobin, blood volume, and indicator of cerebral blood flow (near-infrared spectroscopy)

Neurophysiological function
Abnormal visual evoked responses
Abnormal brain stem auditory evoked responses
Abnormal somatosensory evoked responses

Biochemical parameters
Increased cerebrospinal fluid hypoxanthine
Increased cerebrospinal fluid nonprotein-bound iron
Decreased oxidized cytochrome aa$_3$ in brain (near-infrared spectroscopy)

[a]See text for references.

Subsequent studies of cerebral blood flow velocity confirmed the fundamental observation.[867-883] The principal finding with posthemorrhagic hydrocephalus is evidence for increased cerebrovascular resistance, by means of resistance indices, and for diminished mean cerebral blood flow velocity. Removal of CSF by LP or ventricular drainage led to improvement in both parameters, except in infants with ventriculomegaly secondary to periventricular white matter atrophy. Data from studies of infants concerning the deleterious effect of progressive posthemorrhagic ventricular dilation relate to cerebral hemodynamics, neurophysiological function, morphological disturbances, biochemical indicators of hypoxia, and clinical outcome (see Table 24.25). The data are sometimes difficult to interpret conclusively because such details as rate of progression, degree and duration of ventriculomegaly, intracranial pressure, preceding parenchymal injury, and neurological outcome are often not provided. Nevertheless, the findings suggest at least transient disturbances.

With gradual increases in intracranial pressure and volume, cerebral compliance is sufficient to prevent alterations in cerebral hemodynamics, perhaps in part by obliteration of the subarachnoid space and encroachment of the infant's cerebral white matter (see earlier discussion). However, available data suggest that (1) a critical point of altered cerebral compliance is reached when further increases will elevate cerebrovascular resistance, and (2) this critical point can be detected by Doppler measurements of the resistive index (RI) before and after a small increase in intracranial pressure induced by external compression of the anterior fontanelle by the ultrasonic transducer.[881,882] Thus Taylor and co-workers[814,881,882] showed the following: (1) a close correlation between the (percentage) change in resistive index (ΔRI) before and after compression ([RI after compression – RI before compression]/RI before compression; Fig. 24.45A) and the intracranial pressure; and, importantly, (2) a clear distinction between ΔRI in infants with posthemorrhagic hydrocephalus who required a shunt versus the ΔRI in infants who had arrest of their posthemorrhagic hydrocephalus (see Fig. 24.45B).[882] Because of the challenges in measurement of RI clinically, this measure is not routinely used in clinical evaluation of the preterm infant with PHVD.

Additional studies suggest that the changes in cerebral blood flow velocity parameters reflect lower volemic cerebral blood flow.[884] Thus PET scanning (H$_2$^{15}O technique) has shown an increase in regional cerebral blood flow in five infants with posthemorrhagic hydrocephalus immediately after removal of CSF by LP (unpublished). Moreover, near-infrared spectroscopy has shown evidence for an increase in cerebral blood flow after CSF removal in 16 infants with posthemorrhagic hydrocephalus.[884]

Concerning *neurophysiological function, visual evoked potentials* have been shown to be altered by posthemorrhagic ventricular dilation. The measurement may be expected to be a sensitive indicator of neurological dysfunction with posthemorrhagic hydrocephalus, because, as noted earlier, the ventricular dilation characteristically affects posterior horns disproportionately. Two studies initially demonstrated prolonged latencies of visual evoked potentials with posthemorrhagic hydrocephalus in the premature infant.[885,886] Improvement in latencies was demonstrated 1 to 2 weeks after placement of a ventriculoperitoneal shunt and within minutes after direct

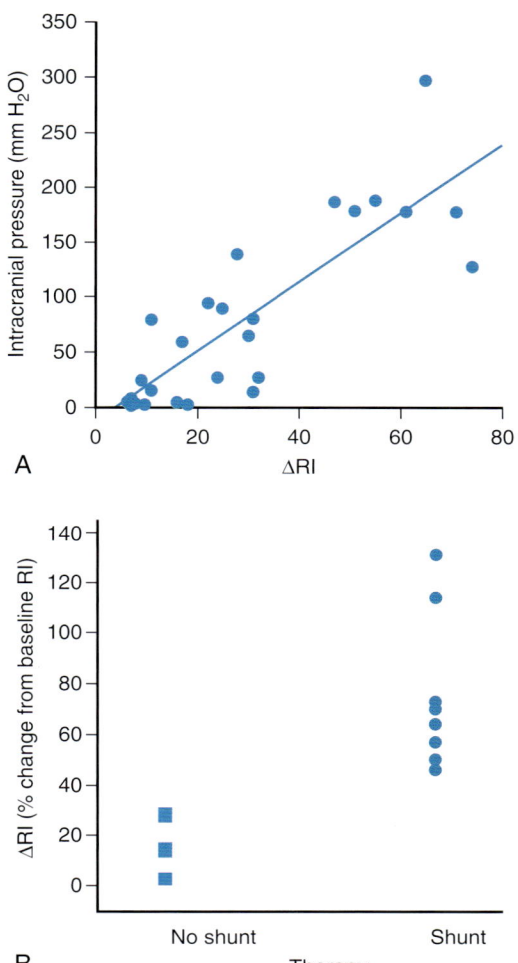

Figure 24.45 Resistive index (RI) in relation to intracranial pressure or shunt indication. Relationship of the RI, obtained by Doppler from the pericallosal artery in a series of infants with posthemorrhagic hydrocephalus, as a function of (A) intracranial pressure or (B) subsequent need for shunt placement. ΔRI is the percentage of change in RI before and after compression of the fontanelle ([RI after compression − RI before compression]/RI before compression). See text for details. (From Taylor GA, Madsen JR. Neonatal hydrocephalus: Hemodynamic response to fontanelle compression: correlation with intracranial pressure and need for shunt placement. *Radiology.* 1996;201: 685–689.)

combined parameters in nine preterm infants: nine with cranial ultrasound scan data, eight with NIRS data, seven with aEEG data, and four with VEPs. The resistive index was stable and remained unchanged after decompression in all patients. Before decompression, the mean rcSO$_2$ value was 42.6 ± 12.9% and increased to 55 ± 12.2% after decompression. With increasing ventricular width, FTOE showed a mean value of 0.51 ± 0.05 and decreased to a mean of 0.39 ± 0.12 after decompression. Amplitude-integrated electroencephalography showed a more continuous pattern, and VEPs showed delayed latencies in all patients before intervention, improving afterward. These findings all support the improvement in cerebral hemodynamics and function following therapy.[889]

Concerning *morphological evidence for brain injury* with posthemorrhagic ventricular dilation, data from autopsy studies of human infants who did not have markedly advanced disease are few. Studies of biopsies taken at the time of shunt placement have shown four major findings: (1) disruption of ependyma, (2) direct evidence for axonal injury (*axonal ballooning*), (3) lipid-laden microglia, and (4) diminished number of myelinated axons.[830,832,836,890-894] A potential biochemical correlate of this injury is the elevation of CSF levels of such brain-specific proteins as GFAP, neurofilament protein, and S-100 protein in CSF of infants with posthemorrhagic ventricular dilation.[895] These findings are reminiscent of the more carefully controlled observations made in experimental models of hydrocephalus. However, the relation of these changes to the rate of progression and severity of ventriculomegaly, intracranial hypertension, and neurological outcome is unclear.

Biochemical evidence of free radical–mediated injury is suggested by several lines of evidence. Thus a study of 12 infants with posthemorrhagic hydrocephalus demonstrated *markedly elevated CSF levels of hypoxanthine*, a marker for hypoxic tissue and free radical generation, before treatment.[896] Successful treatment of the ventriculomegaly by LP or ventriculoperitoneal shunt led to marked decreases of CSF hypoxanthine levels in all but one infant.[896] Although the morphological effects of hydrocephalus on cerebral vessels and the resulting deleterious cerebral hemodynamic effects appear to be the most probable explanation for tissue hypoxia, the possibility that elevated levels of vasoconstricting eicosanoids (e.g., thromboxanes) or edema-producing eicosanoids (e.g., leukotrienes) are important should be considered. Such eicosanoids have been shown to be elevated in the CSF of infants with posthemorrhagic hydrocephalus.[897] In addition, elevated levels of non-protein-bound iron have been observed in CSF of premature infants for weeks after IVH.[94] Free iron can lead to generation of the highly injurious hydroxyl radical (see Chapters 13 and 15). Additional biochemical evidence for oxygen deficiency at the mitochondrial level is the demonstration by near-infrared spectroscopy of an increase in *brain levels* of *oxidized cytochrome aa$_3$* after LP in infants with posthemorrhagic hydrocephalus, accompanied by increased intracranial pressure.[811,898]

Prevention

Because blood products and protein in the CSF presumably lead to the impaired fibrinolysis and the arachnoiditis that causes subsequent hydrocephalus in infants with IVH, serial LPs to remove blood products and administration of fibrinolytic agents to dissolve blood clot have been used to attempt to prevent the development of posthemorrhagic hydrocephalus. The rationale

removal of ventricular fluid.[885,886] These data suggest that an axonal disturbance is caused by distention of occipital horns and that this disturbance can be reversed by effective therapy. A second parameter of neurophysiological function, *brain stem auditory evoked potentials*, also has been shown to be altered by posthemorrhagic ventricular dilation and corrected by CSF removal.[887] A third parameter of neurophysiological function, *somatosensory evoked responses*, also has been shown to be altered by posthemorrhagic ventricular dilation and to be corrected by either spontaneous arrest of ventricular growth or shunt placement.[888] The effect on latency was most marked in infants with increased intracranial pressure. The mechanism of the effect could relate in part to affection of ascending thalamocortical fibers that course around the dilated body of the lateral ventricle. A recent study examined

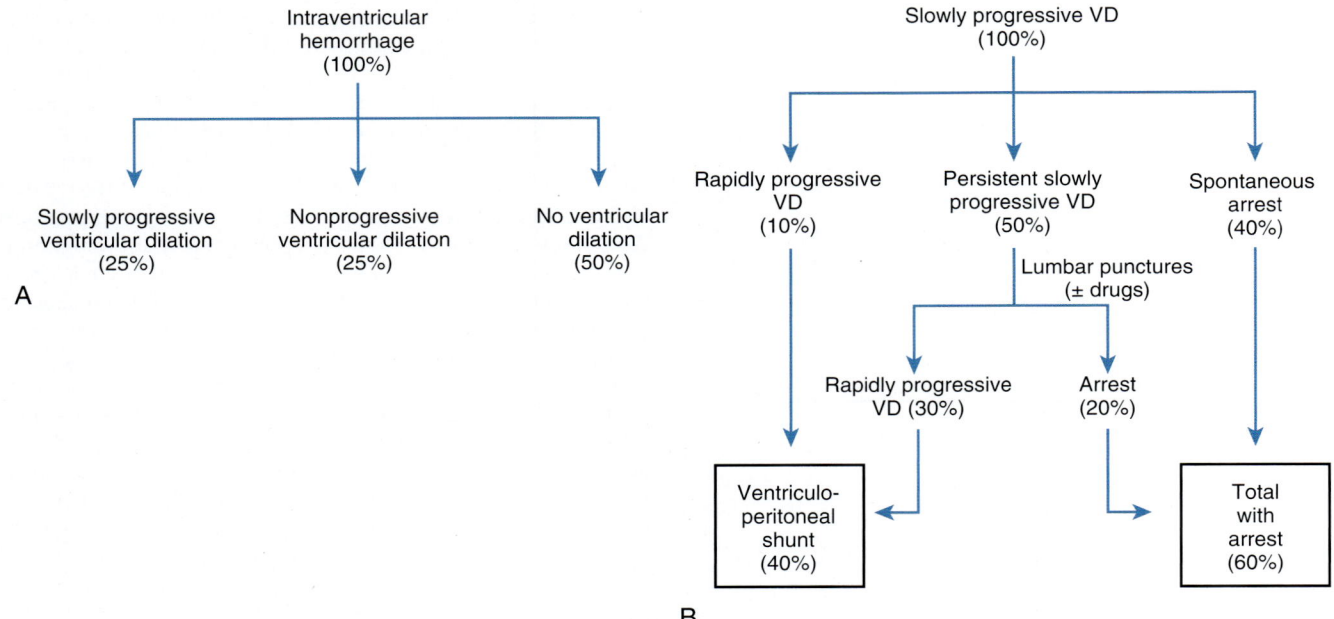

Figure 24.46 (A) Likelihood of progressive ventricular dilation after intraventricular hemorrhage. The schema begins with all infants with intraventricular hemorrhage (*not* germinal matrix hemorrhage alone). Data are derived from 221 infants studied by Murphy et al.; numbers are rounded off. (B) Outcome of infants with slowly progressive ventricular dilation (VD). The starting population of infants (100%) is the 25% of infants with intraventricular hemorrhage, shown in (A), who developed slowly progressive ventricular dilation. The starting population of slowly progressive ventricular dilation includes only infants of less than 1500 g birthweight, 31% of whom had birthweights lower than 750 g and 81% of whom had grade III or grade IV intraventricular hemorrhage; the population does not include 15% of infants who died (principally of systemic complications of prematurity). (Data from Murphy BP, Inder TE, Rooks V, Taylor GA, et al. Posthemorrhagic ventricular dilatation in the premature infant: natural history and predictors of outcome. *Arch Dis Child Fetal Neonatal Ed.* 2002;87:F37–F41.)

was that repeated LPs would accelerate removal of blood and protein from the CSF and would thereby lessen the chance for the development of hydrocephalus. Thirty-eight infants with moderate or severe IVH identified by CT were randomized to receive serial LPs or no punctures from the time of diagnosis of the hemorrhage. The data showed no difference in the development of hydrocephalus, despite punctures performed until CSF was clear and colorless, with protein content less than 180 mg/dL. A later study of 47 infants with grade III or IV IVH, in whom LPs were commenced at mean postnatal age of 11 days and continued for 20 days, also failed to show a difference in the incidence of subsequent hydrocephalus requiring placement of a ventriculoperitoneal shunt (39% in control group, 42% in treated group).[899] In this study, a mean total of 67 ± 101 mL of CSF was removed, with 16 ± 12 LPs.

A second approach to prevention of severe posthemorrhagic hydrocephalus involves the use of intraventricular *fibrinolytic* therapy. This approach was stimulated by the observation of successful dissolution of intraventricular blood clots and improved outcome in adults with IVH treated with intraventricular infusion of urokinase.[900,901] Moreover, endogenous fibrinolytic activity was shown to be absent in the CSF of premature infants until at least 17 days after the occurrence of IVH.[902] The impaired endogenous fibrinolytic activity may relate to a combination of low levels of plasminogen in CSF after IVH and of high levels of plasminogen activator inhibitor in the posthemorrhagic CSF.[119,120] In an initial encouraging report, Whitelaw and co-workers[903] treated nine

infants with evolving posthemorrhagic hydrocephalus at 8 to 27 days of age, with intraventricular infusion of streptokinase for 12 to 72 hours.[904] Only one of the nine infants in the initial report ultimately required ventriculoperitoneal shunt, and based on parallel studies in a multicenter trial,[466] approximately 60% of this group would have been expected to develop hydrocephalus requiring shunt placement. A subsequent study of four infants with urokinase resulted in favorable results (i.e., none required a ventriculoperitoneal shunt).[905] A later investigation of 22 preterm infants with progressive posthemorrhagic ventricular dilation treated with intraventricular instillation of recombinant tissue plasminogen activator resulted in the need for shunt placement in 45% versus 71% in historic controls.[906] These favorable results were followed by two later studies that recorded no benefit from intraventricular urokinase or streptokinase.[907,908] A Cochrane review "found no good evidence" that streptokinase is useful in this context.[909] It is possible that the usual timing of the onset of therapy, generally after the first week of life, is too late to prevent the progressive changes provoked by the initial blood clots. Early therapy, however, carries the theoretical risk that hemorrhage could be precipitated by the fibrinolytic therapy.

Management of Progressive Posthemorrhagic Ventricular Dilation

Natural History. Management of progressive posthemorrhagic ventricular dilation must begin with the recognition of the natural history of the disorder (Fig. 24.46). Although definitions

TABLE 24.26 Progressive Ventricular Dilation, Ventriculoperitoneal Shunt and Mortality as a Function of Severity of Intraventricular Hemorrhage

SEVERITY OF IVH[a]	PVD IN SURVIVORS >14 DAYS OLD	VPS IN SURVIVORS[b] PVD	VPS IN SURVIVORS[b] TOTAL	LATE MORTALITY[c]
Grade I/II	11/160 (7%)	1/11 (9%)	1/160 (0.6%)	14/160 (9%)
Grade III	28/37 (76%)	10/28 (36%)	10/37 (27%)	6/37 (16%)
Grade IV	17/24 (71%)	8/17 (47%)	8/24 (33%)	7/24 (29%)

[a]Grading as described in Table 24.12, except the combination of IVH and apparent periventricular hemorrhagic infarction is termed grade IV.

[b]VPS in infants with PVD and in the total group of infants surviving >14 days.

[c]Late mortality is death after 14 days; most deaths are related to systemic complications of prematurity.

IVH, Intraventricular hemorrhage; *PVD*, progressive ventricular dilation; *VPS*, ventriculoperitoneal shunt.

Data from Murphy BP, Inder TE, Rooks V, Taylor GA, et al. Posthemorrhagic ventricular dilatation in the premature infant: natural history and predictors of outcome. *Arch Dis Child Fetal Neonatal Ed.* 2002;87:F37–F41.

of progressive ventricular dilation and descriptions of evolution, management, and outcome vary considerably among studies, the data shown in Fig. 24.46, based on our personal published and unpublished observations, bear similarities to those reported by others.[a] Currently, approximately 50% of infants with grade II–IV IVH exhibit no or minimally nonprogressive ventricular dilation. Of those with grade II–IV IVH, approximately 65% will exhibit ventricular dilation. For 35% this is not progressive and, at least in part, may reflect cerebral white matter injury, such as periventricular leukomalacia (see Chapter 16). The remaining 40% to 50% of infants with IVH develop slowly progressive ventricular dilation (see Fig. 24.46). These infants usually have moderate degrees of ventricular dilation and intracranial pressure measurements that are generally stable and normal or nearly normal. In our experience, mean values for intracranial pressure (anterior fontanelle sensor) in this group are approximately 50 to 80 mm H_2O, near or just above the upper limit of normal, and the rate of head growth is appropriate for gestational development.

Currently, we use serial measurements of (1) rate and severity of progression of ventricular dilation (ultrasonography), (2) rate of head growth, and (3) clinical signs of increased intracranial pressure to follow infants with posthemorrhagic ventricular dilation. On the basis of this experience, summarized in Fig. 24.46, three groups of infants who have grade II–IV IVH who are evaluated can be categorized for management: group I, those with the onset of slowly progressive ventricular dilation who spontaneously arrest; group II, those with *persistent* slowly progressive ventricular dilation who may either arrest after LP or need placement of a subgaleal shunt or ventricular access device (VAD); and group III, those with rapidly progressive ventricular dilation.

Approximately 65% of those infants with progressive posthemorrhagic ventricular dilation will exhibit arrest, most often within 4 weeks, usually with partial or total resolution of the ventricular dilation (see Fig. 24.46). Of the remaining infants with slowly progressive ventricular dilation, most continue to progress for more than 4 weeks (persistent slowly progressive ventricular dilation) and, if not treated, develop severe ventricular dilation. A smaller proportion of the starting group (≈15%) develop this rapid progression even before 4 weeks (see Fig. 24.46). In these infants, intracranial pressure increases rapidly, usually within days of onset of rapid progression, and is followed closely and consistently by rapid head growth and often by such clinical signs as full anterior fontanelle and separated cranial sutures. Rates of head growth greater than 2 cm/week usually signal the rapid progression,[805,806] although rates greater than 1.5 cm/week are considered indicative of this phase by others.[823] In our experience, values for intracranial pressure in this group may increase rapidly to greater than 150 mm H_2O. These infants rarely resolve and often require acute surgical intervention with a subgaleal shunt or VAD.

The severity of the initial IVH is the most critical determinant of not only the likelihood of progressive ventricular dilation (see Table 24.16) but also the temporal evolution and course. Thus, with moderate hemorrhages, the onset of the slowly progressive ventricular dilation is usually after 10 to 14 days, and spontaneous arrest is more likely. With severe hemorrhages, the onset of the ventricular dilation may be within several days, the phase of slow progression may be very brief, and the likelihood of spontaneous resolution may be relatively low. Indeed, in most series, the vast majority of infants who develop rapidly progressive hydrocephalus, either initially or later, had experienced severe IVH, with or without periventricular hemorrhagic infarction. In a study of 221 infants with IVH and survival after the acute neonatal period (>14 days), only 7% of infants with grades I/II IVH developed progressive ventricular dilation, whereas approximately 75% of infants with grades III and IV IVH, respectively, did so (Table 24.26).[443] In addition, among the group with grade I/II IVH, less than 1% eventually required a ventriculoperitoneal shunt, whereas 25% to 35% of infants with grades III and IV IVH required a ventriculoperitoneal shunt.

Basic Groups for Management

For the purposes of formulating management, as noted in the previous section, three basic groups can be gleaned from the data. These are summarized in Table 24.27.

Rapidly Progressive Ventricular Dilation

The major treatment choices for this treatment group are outlined in Table 24.28. In this clinical setting, close surveillance

[a]References 25, 27, 245, 426, 430, 435, 443, 458, 461-463, 466, 467, 469-471, 484, 485, 801, 803, 805, 807, 813, and 910-912.

TABLE 24.27   Management Groups for Posthemorrhagic Hydrocephalus

I.	Slowly progressive ventricular dilation: moderate dilation, appropriate rate of head growth, stable RI/ΔRI; <2 weeks
II.	Persistent slowly progressive ventricular dilation: similar to I, except that duration is >2 weeks and rate of head growth and RI/ΔRI may begin to increase
III.	Rapidly progressive ventricular dilation: moderate to severe dilation, clearly excessive rate of head growth, RI/ΔRI clearly increased
IV.	Arrested progression: spontaneous arrest of ventricular dilation or arrest following lumbar puncture

ΔRI, Change in resistive index; *RI,* resistive index.

TABLE 24.28   Management of Posthemorrhagic Hydrocephalus: Group I

Slowly progressive ventricular dilation: moderate dilation, appropriate rate of head growth (and RI and ΔRI), duration <2 weeks
1. Close surveillance

ΔRI, Change in resistive index; *RI,* resistive index.

TABLE 24.29   Management of Posthemorrhagic Hydrocephalus: Group II (Predominant)

Progressive ventricular dilation: moderate to severe dilation
1. Serial lumbar punctures 2–3 only maximal (consider for temporization)
2. Ventricular drainage
   a. Direct external ventricular drain
   b. Tunneled external ventricular drain
   c. Subcutaneous ventricular catheter to reservoir or to subgaleal or supraclavicular spaces
3. Ventriculoperitoneal shunt or external third ventriculostomy and choroid plexus ablation

alone certainly is no longer appropriate, because an infant with rapidly progressive ventricular dilation can develop severe ventricular dilation (measures I cranial ultrasound measures >97th%) within days. The specific criteria used to define this stage are based on progression of dilation that is measured in days, rate of head growth in excess of 2.0 cm/week, ventricular size (superior to inferior borders) that increases excessively for the AHW, VI, or thalamo-occipital diameter.[466,484,805,807,823] The treatment choices include neurosurgical intervention with an appropriate CSF drainage device. The devices that are most commonly used are internal ventricular drains tunneled to a subcutaneous ventricular reservoir device that is drained on a daily basis, or to a surgically established subcutaneous supraclavicular pouch, or to the subgaleal space.

Slowly Progressive Ventricular Dilation

Infants who exhibit persistent slowly progressive ventricular dilation in the first 4 weeks of life following IVH (Table 24.29) have been the subject of controversy regarding management. Because spontaneous arrest, if it will occur, usually does so within 4 weeks, close surveillance for a minimum of 4 weeks following IVH is appropriate. We recommend surveillance with cranial ultrasound measures of ventricular size every 2 to 4 days to monitor increases in ventricular dimensions, with reduction to 1 to 2 times per week after 2 weeks of stable measures. If ventricular dilation continues to progress, the principal treatment choices are serial LPs or ventricular drainage interventions.

Serial Lumbar Punctures. Cessation of posthemorrhagic ventricular dilation in association with serial LPs has been well documented.[a] However, no consensus exists on whether this therapeutic modality is consistently beneficial in arresting progression or improving outcome.[918] Nevertheless, the technique is useful for at least temporary improvement (i.e., arrest of progression and intermittent decrease in ventricular size) if two criteria are met. The first criterion is to establish the presence of communication between the lateral ventricles and lumbar subarachnoid space, and the second is to remove an adequate quantity (usually a relatively large volume) of CSF.[817] A substantial volume of CSF must be removed to effect arrest of progression of the hydrocephalic process and intermittent decreases in ventricular size.[b] Although quantitative data for premature newborns with hydrocephalus are lacking, our observations indicate that, on average, volumes of approximately 10 to 15 mL/kg are most often necessary. The critical volume must be determined for each infant, and cranial ultrasonography before and after CSF removal is important in this regard. Thus clinical recommendations are for two to three lumbar punctures to determine whether the progressive ventricular dilatation can be arrested before consideration of neurosurgical intervention.

The *timing of onset of LP therapy* appears to be important. Thus, in a study of 95 infants with hydrocephalus after grade III IVH, de Vries and co-workers showed that intervention with serial LPs after the VI (see Fig. 24.41)[917] *exceeded the 97th percentile but before the ventricular size had increased 4 mm higher than that percentile (i.e., "early intervention"),* ventriculoperitoneal shunt was required in only 16%.[473,917] Those not treated with LPs until after the VI had increased to more than 4 mm above the 97th percentile line ultimately required shunt placement in 62% of cases. Serial LPs represent the least invasive of the therapeutic modalities noted in Table 24.30 and may lead to temporary or even permanent arrest of the hydrocephalic process. However, timing of therapy appears critical (Fig. 24.47).[918]

Complications of LP therapy include rare events such as meningitis, epidural abscess, vertebral osteomyelitis, and late occurrence of intraspinal epidermoid tumor.[919,920] When large volumes of CSF are removed, attention to fluid status is important to avoid hyponatremia. The risk of complicating meningitis has been unusually high in some small series (e.g., 27%).[921] The use of unstyletted needles has been associated with the rare examples of late epidermoid tumors.[920] Such needles should be avoided.

---

[a]References 25, 426, 443, 466, 467, 473, 484, 807, 813, 817, and 913-917.
[b]References 426, 443, 466, 467, 473, 484, 817, and 910.

TABLE 24.30 Management of Posthemorrhagic Hydrocephalus: Group III

Rapidly progressive ventricular dilation: moderate to severe dilation, excessive rate of head growth, and RI/ΔRI clearly increased
1. Serial lumbar punctures (consider for temporization)
2. Ventricular drainage
   a. Direct external ventricular drain
   b. Tunneled external ventricular drain
   c. Subcutaneous ventricular catheter to reservoir or to subgaleal or supraclavicular spaces
3. Ventriculoperitoneal shunt

ΔRI, Change in resistive index; *RI,* resistive index.

Drugs That Decrease Cerebrospinal Fluid Production. In previous years, carbonic anhydrase inhibitors were used to control hydrocephalus by causing a reduction in CSF production. Acetazolamide leads to a 50% reduction in CSF production.[922] The effect of acetazolamide on CSF production has been shown in human infants.[923] However, two large studies of the use of acetazolamide and furosemide in the treatment of posthemorrhagic hydrocephalus resulted in the conclusion that the combination "cannot be recommended."[472,812,924] In conclusion, the combined and long-term use of acetazolamide (100 mg/kg/day) and furosemide (1 mg/kg/day) does not appear to have clear benefit in therapy and may be associated with risk. Although the use of acetazolamide *alone* has not been studied in a controlled fashion as a complement to LPs, currently we do not recommend the use of either of these agents in the management of posthemorrhagic hydrocephalus.

Ventricular Drainage. Ventricular drainage is indicated for infants who have not responded adequately to LP and who

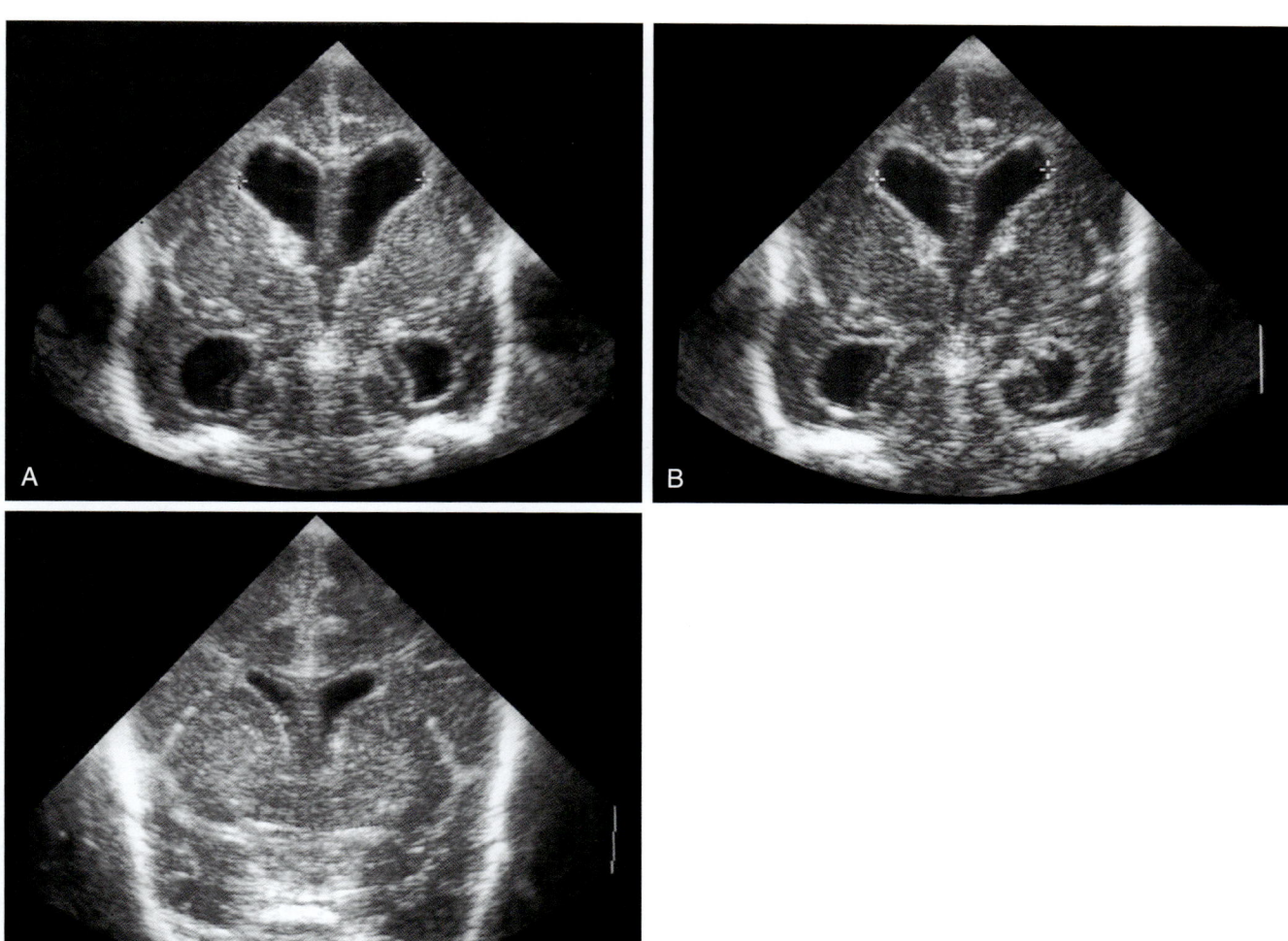

Figure 24.47 Beneficial response of slowly progressive ventricular dilation to lumbar puncture and removal of cerebrospinal fluid (CSF). Coronal ultrasound scans were obtained, (A) immediately before lumbar puncture and (B) immediately after removal of 10 mL/kg (body weight) of CSF in a 5-week-old premature infant with progressive posthemorrhagic ventricular dilation. Note the decrease in size of the lateral ventricles after the tap. (C) Obtained 2 weeks after a 3-week course of serial lumbar punctures. No further therapy was required.

TABLE 24.31   Effect of Drainage, Irrigation, and Fibrinolytic Therapy on the Distribution of Bayley Developmental Indices

| | TREATMENT | | SEVERE DISABILITY (<55) | | | |
	DRIFT (N = 35/34), n (%)	Standard (N = 32), n (%)	OR (95% CI)	P	OR (95% CI) Adjusted for Gender, Birthweight, and Grade of IVH	P
MDI						
≥85	8 (23)	9 (28)	0.31 (0.11–0.86)	.024	0.17 (0.05–0.57)	.004
70–84	9 (26)	3 (9)				
55–69	7 (20)	1 (3)				
<55	11 (31)	19 (59)				
PDI						
≥85	4 (12)	5 (16)	0.54 (CI 0.20–1.45)	.22	0.21 (0.05–0.85)	.028
70–84	5 (15)	5 (16)				
55–69	11 (32)	4 (13)				
<55	14 (41)	18 (56)				

DRIFT, Drainage, irrigation, and fibrinolytic therapy; *IVH*, intraventricular hemorrhage; *OR*, odds ratio.
From Whitelaw A, Jary S, Kmita G, et al. Randomized trial of drainage, irrigation and fibrinolytic therapy for premature infants with posthemorrhagic ventricular dilatation: developmental outcome at 2 years. *Pediatrics.* 2010;125:e852–e858.

are not good candidates for placement of a ventriculoperitoneal shunt. Reasons for the latter situation are, first, an infant who is too small or too ill to tolerate the surgical procedure and, second, an infant who has bloody or highly proteinaceous CSF that may lead to shunt obstruction. Essentially, the goal of ventricular drainage is temporization, although in a minority of infants, the time gained also allows reopening of pathways of CSF flow and absorption (see later discussion). The *value* of external ventricular drainage in the treatment of ventricular dilation in premature infants has been documented in several studies.[a] Four basic approaches have been used: (1) a novel procedure of ventricular drainage, irrigation, and fibrinolytic therapy ("DRIFT"); (2) a direct external ventricular drain (EVD); (3) an EVD tunneled subcutaneously to an external drip chamber; and (4) a completely internal ventricular drain tunneled to a subcutaneous reservoir, to a surgically established subcutaneous supraclavicular pouch, or to the subgaleal space.

DRIFT. A novel approach of ventricular *d*rainage, *i*rrigation, and *f*ibrinolytic *t*herapy was shown in a pilot study to be of benefit in the management of rapidly progressive posthemorrhagic hydrocephalus.[128,936] The goals of the procedure are to remove deleterious blood products, antifibrinolytic and fibroproliferative molecules (see earlier), and toxic compounds (free radicals, non-protein-bound iron), to provide the antifibrinolytic agent tissue-type plasminogen activator, and to control intracranial pressure. Two ventricular catheters are placed, one in the frontal horn and one in the occipital horn, tissue-type plasminogen activator is administered intraventricularly, and after 8 hours, irrigation with artificial CSF is commenced and is carried out for 72 hours. In the initial study of 24 infants (median birthweight, 1150 g) with grade III IVH, 16 with parenchymal lesions, only 26% required a ventriculoperitoneal shunt.[936] Outcome was better than in historic controls; in infants with parenchymal

lesions, 70% were free of major cognitive deficits and 40% had no major motor deficits, and in infants without parenchymal lesions, all were normal. Subsequently, a multicenter randomized trial (n = 70) comparing DRIFT with conventional therapy found no difference in the primary outcomes of death or need for shunt.[937] Moreover, 35% of the infants in the DRIFT group developed secondary IVH, usually in the 24 hours after onset of therapy, whereas only 8% of the conventionally treated infants developed such hemorrhage. However, on follow-up, infants in the DRIFT intervention arm, despite an increased risk of cerebral hemorrhage, had better neurodevelopmental outcomes (Table 24.31).[938] Of 39 infants assigned to DRIFT, 21 (54%) died or were severely disabled versus 27 of 38 (71%) in the standard group (adjusted OR, 0.25 [95% CI, 0.08 to 0.82]). Among the survivors, 11 of 35 (31%) in the DRIFT group had severe cognitive disability versus 19 of 32 (59%) in the standard group. Despite these promising neurodevelopmental outcomes, DRIFT currently is not a recommended intervention for posthemorrhagic hydrocephalus.[939]

Direct External Ventricular Drains. Direct EVDs have been in use for many years, although less so in recent years. Some investigators have suggested performance of the tap under ultrasonic guidance.[940,941] The catheter is maintained in a closed system with a reservoir, the height of which can be adjusted to determine intracranial pressure and to regulate rate of drainage. In general, the rate of CSF drainage is approximately 10 to 15 mL/kg body weight per day. This fluid should be calculated in determining daily fluid requirements. Duration of drainage is generally approximately 5 to 7 days.

Tunneled External Ventricular Drains. The more common approach to external ventricular drainage for neonatal posthemorrhagic hydrocephalus involves not a direct route from the skin surface to the ventricle but rather a *tunneled ventricular catheter* (see Table 24.30). With this approach, a subcutaneous tunnel is established from the point of entry

---

[a]References 443, 461, 471, 805, 810, and 925-935.

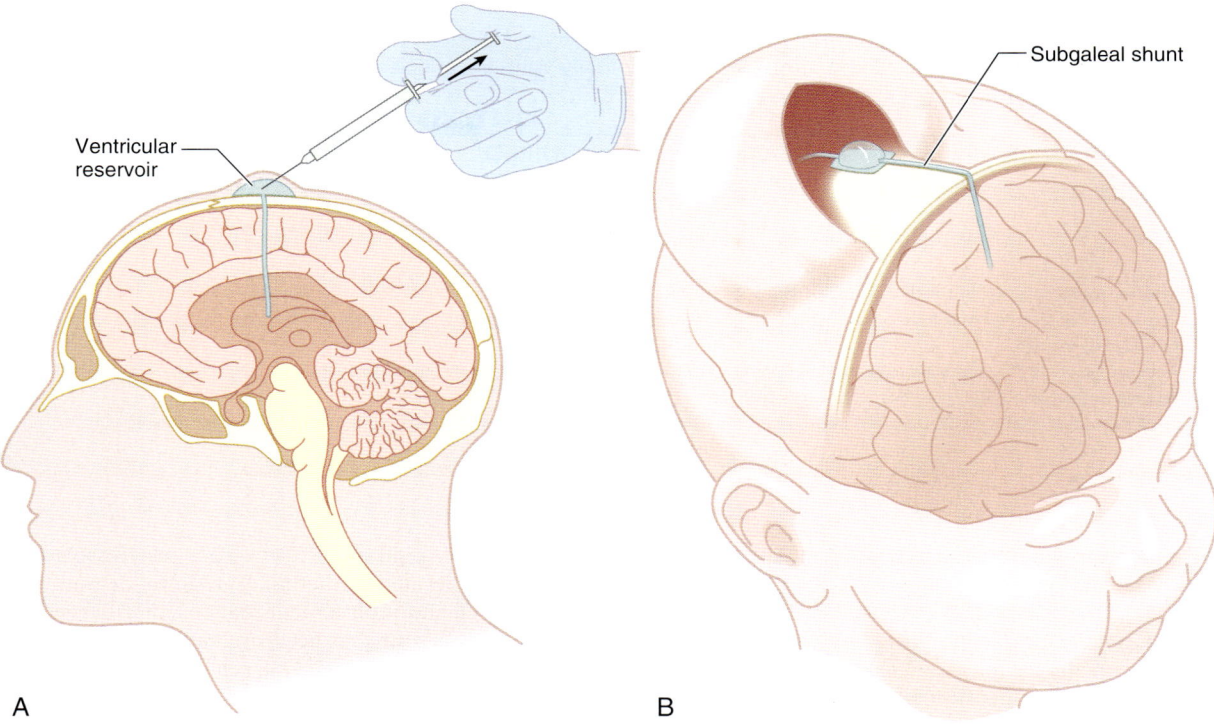

Figure 24.48 Illustration of the ventricular reservoir (A) and subgaleal shunt (B) devices.

at the skin surface to the point of penetration of the skull and ultimately the cerebral wall. The use of a subcutaneous tunnel decreases the risk of infection and thereby allows a longer duration for the drainage (i.e., several weeks vs. 5 to 7 days with direct external ventricular drainage). As with direct EVDs, the rate of CSF removal can be modulated by alteration of the height of the external drip chamber. The ultimate need for shunt placement depends on severity of the initial IVH but generally was approximately 50% to 70%.[810,927,930,932]

Subcutaneous Ventricular Catheter With a Reservoir. A third major approach to temporizing ventricular drainage, and now perhaps the most commonly used, involves a tunneled ventricular catheter that is connected to a subcutaneous reservoir, which can be tapped several times daily for CSF removal (see Table 24.30) ("VAD"),[471,473,928,933-935,942] or to a surgically prepared subcutaneous pouch in the supraclavicular region or to the subgaleal space (Fig. 24.48).[929,931]

de Vries and co-workers studied the use of a subcutaneous reservoir after either early or late LPs for hydrocephalus after grade III IVH.[473,917] Approximately one-third of infants who continued to progress after early LPs and were treated with a subcutaneous reservoir required a ventriculoperitoneal shunt. By contrast, approximately 80% of infants who had *more severe* hydrocephalus and were treated with a reservoir immediately or after LPs required ventriculoperitoneal shunts. Overall, 66% of infants treated with a reservoir required a ventriculoperitoneal shunt. *Thus the possibility that a ventricular drain to a subcutaneous reservoir will be curative and not merely temporization decreases with more severe hydrocephalus.* This has now led to the establishment

of a randomized controlled trial that is still in progress (ELVIS trial).[943]

A recent systematic review of the therapy for PHVD,[939] including the surgical management, concluded that VADs, EVDs, ventriculosubgaleal (VSG) shunts, or LPs are treatment options in the management of PHH, with clinical judgment necessary for determining best therapy in the individual patient. The summarized evidence supported the conclusion that VADs led to reduced morbidity and mortality when compared with EVDs. Moreover, 10 studies supported the safety and efficacy of VADs, or Ommaya reservoirs, for the aspiration of CSF, ventricular decompression, and lowering of intracranial pressure.[944-951]

Subcutaneous Ventricular Cather With a Subgaleal Pouch (Ventricular-Subgaleal Shunt). The particular value of *placement of a VSG shunt to reduce the need for permanent shunt placement* has been the focus of several recent reports. Thus a large prospective study reported a statistically significant decreased need for permanent CSF diversion in infants treated with VSG shunts.[952] Sixty-six percent of infants (20 of 30) treated with VSG shunts required VP shunts and 33% (10 of 30) remained shunt free; this finding was compared with a group of infants treated with VADs, in which 75% (49 of 65) required VP shunts and 25% of infants (16 of 65) remained shunt-free.[952,953]

Finally, the risks of the drainage devices, particularly infection, are important considerations. Lam and Heilman demonstrated that VSG shunting significantly reduced the need for daily CSF aspiration, which may decrease the risk of introducing a de novo CSF infection.[954] A chi square test performed on their data indicated that a VSG shunt reduced the need for

TABLE 24.32 Outcome of Premature Infants Referred to a Neurosurgical Service With Rapidly Progressive Posthemorrhagic Hydrocephalus Treated Initially With Ventricular Drainage[a]

SEVERITY OF HEMORRHAGE[b]	NO.	OUTCOME			
		DEATH (%)	REQUIRED SHUNT (%)	MOTOR DEFICITS (%)	ABNORMAL DQ[c] (%)
Grade III	24	4	78	54	8
Grade IV	48	62	94	100	78

[a]Rapidly progressive posthemorrhagic hydrocephalus was identified by "progressive and marked ventriculomegaly despite serial lumbar punctures." The ventricular catheter was tunneled to a subcutaneous reservoir, from which "5–20 mL of CSF" was removed daily. Outcome data are rounded off. Note that this selected population of infants was particularly severely affected.
[b]Severity of hemorrhage: grade III is equivalent to grade III in Table 11.13; grade IV includes parenchymal hemorrhagic lesions.
[c]Abnormal development quotient (DQ): more than 2 SD below the mean.
Data from Levy ML, Masri LS, McComb JG. Outcome for preterm infants with germinal matrix hemorrhage and progressive hydrocephalus. *Neurosurgery.* 1997;41:1111–1117.

daily CSF aspiration when compared with a VAD ($\chi^2 = 19.2$, df = 1, $P = .000016$, $P < .05$).[954]

Conclusion Concerning Temporizing Ventricular Drainage Procedures. In conclusion, the essential point is that ventricular catheterization, which drains CSF either into a subcutaneous reservoir *that can be tapped percutaneously or into a subgaleal or supraclavicular pouch, is effective temporization* for treatment of rapidly progressive posthemorrhagic hydrocephalus. A substantial minority of infants so treated will escape ultimate VP shunt placement, but more important, the majority who ultimately will require a shunt will be better able to tolerate the procedure and more likely to have CSF free enough of blood products to avoid frequent shunt obstruction. Finally, the impact of such removal of CSF on later neurodevelopmental outcomes will await results from current randomized controlled trials of early versus later drainage.

Ventriculoperitoneal Shunt. Placement of a shunt system that diverts CSF from the lateral ventricles to the peritoneal cavity (definitive therapy for hydrocephalus; see Table 24.30) has been associated with variable success in reports from many medical centers.[a] Shunt placement in small premature infants carries a considerable morbidity, secondary to various shunt-related complications, such as ulceration of scalp, ventriculitis, sepsis, and need for frequent revisions. Indeed, poor outcome is related in part to the occurrence of shunt infection. Thus the value of procedures for temporization (i.e., VADs) is considerable. Systematic data for brain injury caused by posthemorrhagic hydrocephalus *alone* are difficult to obtain, because major parenchymal lesions play a dominant role in causing subsequent neurological deficits in these infants.[b] This fact is demonstrated clearly by the data recorded in Table 24.32. The principal determinant of unfavorable outcome appears to relate to the occurrence of parenchymal injury consequent to the IVH (periventricular hemorrhagic infarction) or to preceding ischemic insults (periventricular leukomalacia). However, the brain already injured by hemorrhage or ischemia may be more

vulnerable to additional injury from progressive ventricular dilation or elevated intracranial pressure, or both. The exact timing of VP shunt placement remains controversial. A weight of 1500 g frequently has been used as a criterion for VP shunt placement.[947] Evaluation of CSF cell count, protein, and glucose levels was not found to be related to the occurrence of shunt failure or infection in the one large study population.[971] Based on these findings, the authors recommended that the placement of the shunt be performed when the infant's age, weight, and overall stability allow.

Endoscopic Third Ventriculostomy. Endoscopic third ventriculostomy (ETV) for the treatment of hydrocephalus in infants and children is a relatively new procedure that has not been fully evaluated in the treatment of PHVD. In a review of 52 consecutive ETV procedures in 49 infants with hydrocephalus, most infants (31 patients) had aqueductal stenosis.[939] Of the seven infants with preterm PHVD, six required a shunt after ETV. Thus infants with PHVD from premature birth did not appear to benefit from ETV.[972] In another single-institution retrospective case series, 18 preterm infants with PHVD were treated initially with Ommaya reservoir placement: one infant died, five received a VP shunt, and nine underwent ETV.[973] Three patients did not require any further intervention. While overall 59% were shunt-free at the last follow-up, five of the nine patients who were treated with ETV had to undergo repeated surgery for VP shunt placement. The authors recommended combining placement of an Ommaya reservoir with ETV to reduce shunt dependency for preterm infants with PHVD. Finally, a large (101 patients) multicenter, retrospective study evaluated the success rate of ETV in patients with hydrocephalus from subarachnoid hemorrhage, IVH, and/or CSF infection; a minority of the patients (25% [25 of 101]) had PHVD of prematurity.[974] Overall, ETV was successful in 52% of the premature infants with PHVD. Similar data were obtained in a multi-institutional review.[975] ETV was especially useful in 100% (13 of 13) of children with preterm PHVD, who had been initially treated with a shunt. ETV was unsuccessful in 12 of 12 infants treated with ETV as the first-line treatment. Thus, although further investigation is warranted, currently there appear to be limitations to ETV as a *first-line surgical treatment in PHVD in premature infants.*

---

[a]References 469, 471, 473, 485, 807, 913, 925, 946, and 955-969.
[b]References 469, 471, 485, 807, 913, 925, 946, 959, 961-966, and 968-970.

KEY REFERENCES

5. Martin JA, Kochanek KD, Strobino DM, et al. Annual summary of vital statistics—2003. *Pediatrics*. 2005;115:619-634.
6. Osterman MJ, Kochanek KD, MacDorman MF, et al. Annual summary of vital statistics: 2012–2013. *Pediatrics*. 2015;135:1115-1125.
13. Davis JM, Parad RB, Michele T, et al. Pulmonary outcome at 1 year corrected age in premature infants treated at birth with recombinant human CuZn superoxide dismutase. *Pediatrics*. 2003;111:469-476.
14. Darlow BA, Cust AE, Donoghue DA. Improved outcomes for very low birthweight infants: evidence from New Zealand national population based data. *Arch Dis Child*. 2003;88:23-28.
18. Manuck TA, Rice MM, Bailit JL, et al. Preterm neonatal morbidity and mortality by gestational age: a contemporary cohort. *Am J Obstet Gynecol*. 2016;215:103.e101-103.e114.
19. Shah PS, Lui K, Sjors G, et al. Neonatal outcomes of very low birth weight and very preterm neonates: an international comparison. *J Pediatr*. 2016;177:144-152.e146.
20. MacDonald H, Committee on Fetus and Newborn. Perinatal care at the threshold of viability. *Pediatrics*. 2002;110:1024-1027.
23. Stoll BJ, Hansen NI, Bell EF, et al. Trends in care practices, morbidity, and mortality of extremely preterm neonates, 1993–2012. *JAMA*. 2015;314:1039-1051.
24. Ancel PY, Goffinet F, Kuhn P, et al. Survival and morbidity of preterm children born at 22 through 34 weeks' gestation in France in 2011: results of the EPIPAGE-2 cohort study. *JAMA Pediatr*. 2015;169:230-238.
38. Kuban K, Sanocka U, Leviton A, et al. White matter disorders of prematurity: association with intraventricular hemorrhage and ventriculomegaly. *J Pediatr*. 1999;134:539-546.
39. Ment LR, Vohr B, Oh W, et al. Neurodevelopmental outcome at 36 months' corrected age of preterm infants in the multicenter indomethacin intraventricular hemorrhage prevention trial. *Pediatrics*. 1996;98:714-718.
44. Perlman JM, Volpe JJ. Intraventricular hemorrhage in extremely small premature infants. *Am J Dis Child*. 1986;140:1122-1124.
52. Ballabh P, Hu FB, Kumarasiri M, et al. Development of tight junction molecules in blood vessels of germinal matrix, cerebral cortex, and white matter. *Pediatr Res*. 2005;58:791-798.
55. Dummula K, Vinukonda G, Xu H, et al. Development of integrins in the vasculature of germinal matrix, cerebral cortex, and white matter of fetuses and premature infants. *J Neurosci Res*. 2010;88:1193-1204.
62. Bystron I, Blakemore C, Rakic P. Development of the human cerebral cortex: Boulder Committee revisited. *Nat Rev Neurosci*. 2008;9:110-122.
66. Del Bigio MR. Cell proliferation in human ganglionic eminence and suppression after prematurity-associated haemorrhage. *Brain*. 2011;134:1344-1361.
76. Vinukonda G, Csiszar A, Hu F, et al. Neuroprotection in a rabbit model of intraventricular haemorrhage by cyclooxygenase-2, prostanoid receptor-1 or tumour necrosis factor-alpha inhibition. *Brain*. 2010;133:2264-2280.
78. Supramaniam V, Vontell R, Srinivasan L, et al. Microglia activation in the extremely preterm human brain. *Pediatr Res*. 2013;73:301-309.
79. Volpe JJ, Kinney HC, Jensen FE, et al. The developing oligodendrocyte: key cellular target in brain injury in the premature infant. *Int J Dev Neurosci*. 2011;29:423-440.
84. Tam EW, Miller SP, Studholme C, et al. Differential effects of intraventricular hemorrhage and white matter injury on preterm cerebellar growth. *J Pediatr*. 2011;158:366-371.
85. Jeong HJ, Shim SY, Cho HJ, et al. Cerebellar development in preterm infants at term-equivalent age is impaired after low-grade intraventricular hemorrhage. *J Pediatr*. 2016;175:86-92.e82.
88. Volpe JJ. Cerebellum of the premature infant—rapidly developing, vulnerable, clinically important. *J Child Neurol*. 2009;24:1085-1104.
102. Bassan H, Benson CB, Limperopoulos C, et al. Ultrasonographic features and severity scoring of periventricular hemorrhagic infarction in relation to risk factors and outcome. *Pediatrics*. 2006;117:2111-2118.
103. Soltirovska Salamon A, Groenendaal F, van Haastert IC, et al. Neuroimaging and neurodevelopmental outcome of preterm infants with a periventricular haemorrhagic infarction located in the temporal or frontal lobe. *Dev Med Child Neurol*. 2014;56:547-555.
132. Miller SP, Ferriero DM, Leonard C, et al. Early brain injury in premature newborns detected with magnetic resonance imaging is associated with adverse early neurodevelopmental outcome. *J Pediatr*. 2005;147:609-616.
133. Vollmer B, Roth S, Riley K, et al. Neurodevelopmental outcome of preterm infants with ventricular dilatation with and without associated haemorrhage. *Dev Med Child Neurol*. 2006;48:348-352.
134. Patra K, Wilson-Costello D, Taylor HG, et al. Grades I–II intraventricular hemorrhage in extremely low birth weight infants: effects on neurodevelopment. *J Pediatr*. 2006;149:169-173.
149. Noori S, McCoy M, Anderson MP, et al. Changes in cardiac function and cerebral blood flow in relation to peri/intraventricular hemorrhage in extremely preterm infants. *J Pediatr*. 2014;164:264-270.e261-263.
150. Alderliesten T, Lemmers PM, Smarius JJ, et al. Cerebral oxygenation, extraction, and autoregulation in very preterm infants who develop peri-intraventricular hemorrhage. *J Pediatr*. 2013;162:698-704.e692.
167. Boylan GB, Young K, Panerai RB, et al. Dynamic cerebral autoregulation in sick newborn infants. *Pediatr Res*. 2000;48:12-17.
169. Tsuji M, Saul JP, du Plessis A, et al. Cerebral intravascular oxygenation correlates with mean arterial pressure in critically ill premature infants. *Pediatrics*. 2000;106:625-632.
173. Rhee CJ, Kaiser JR, Rios DR, et al. Elevated diastolic closing margin is associated with intraventricular hemorrhage in premature infants. *J Pediatr*. 2016;174:52-56.
185. Lou HC, Lassen NA, Friis-Hansen B. Is arterial hypertension crucial for the development of cerebral haemorrhage in premature infants? *Lancet*. 1979;1:1215-1217.
190. Perlman JM, Volpe JJ. Seizures in the preterm infant: effects on cerebral blood flow velocity, intracranial pressure, and arterial blood pressure. *J Pediatr*. 1983;102:288-293.
201. Porter FL, Miller JP, Cole FS, et al. A controlled clinical trial of local anesthesia for lumbar punctures in newborns. *Pediatrics*. 1991;88:663-669.
209. van Bel F, Lemmers P, Naulaers G. Monitoring neonatal regional cerebral oxygen saturation in clinical practice: value and pitfalls. *Neonatology*. 2008;94:237-244.
215. Shangle CE, Haas RH, Vaida F, et al. Effects of endotracheal intubation and surfactant on a 3-channel neonatal electroencephalogram. *J Pediatr*. 2012;161:252-257.
217. Goddard J, Lewis RM, Armstrong DL, et al. Moderate, rapidly induced hypertension as a cause of intraventricular hemorrhage in the newborn beagle model. *J Pediatr*. 1980;96:1057-1060.
218. Goddard-Finegold J, Armstrong D, Zeller RS. Intraventricular hemorrhage following volume expansion after hypovolemic hypotension in the newborn beagle. *J Pediatr*. 1982;100:796-799.
244. Fabres J, Carlo WA, Phillips V, et al. Both extremes of arterial carbon dioxide pressure and the magnitude of fluctuations in arterial carbon dioxide pressure are associated with severe intraventricular hemorrhage in preterm infants. *Pediatrics*. 2007;119:299-305.
255. Baer VL, Lambert DK, Henry E, et al. Among very-low-birth-weight neonates is red blood cell transfusion an independent risk factor for subsequently developing a severe intraventricular hemorrhage? *Transfusion*. 2011;51:1170-1178.
257. Katheria AC, Leone TA, Woelkers D, et al. The effects of umbilical cord milking on hemodynamics and neonatal outcomes in premature neonates. *J Pediatr*. 2014;164:1045-1050.e1041.
258. Rabe H, Diaz-Rossello JL, Duley L, et al. Effect of timing of umbilical cord clamping and other strategies to influence placental transfusion at preterm birth on maternal and infant outcomes. *Cochrane Database Syst Rev*. 2012;(8):CD003248.
259. Committee on Obstetric Practice American College of Obstetricians and Gynecologists, Committee Opinion Number 684. Delayed umbilical cord clamping after birth. *Obstet Gynecol*. 2017;129:e5-e10.
263. Auerbach A, Eventov-Friedman S, Arad I, et al. Long duration of hyperglycemia in the first 96 hours of life is associated with

severe intraventricular hemorrhage in preterm infants. *J Pediatr.* 2013;163:388-393.

266. Barnette AR, Myers BJ, Berg CS, et al. Sodium intake and intraventricular hemorrhage in the preterm infant. *Ann Neurol.* 2010;67:817-823.

284. Hansen A, Leviton A. Labor and delivery characteristics and risks of cranial ultrasonographic abnormalities among very-low-birth-weight infants. *Am J Obstet Gynecol.* 1999;181:997-1006.

292. Haque KN, Hayes AM, Ahmed Z, et al. Caesarean or vaginal delivery for preterm very-low-birth weight (< or = 1,250 g) infant: experience from a district general hospital in UK. *Arch Gynecol Obstet.* 2008;277:207-212.

293. Gawade PL, Whitcomb BW, Chasan-Taber L, et al. Second stage of labor and intraventricular hemorrhage in early preterm infants in the vertex presentation. *J Matern Fetal Neonatal Med.* 2013;26:1292-1298.

304. Lavrijsen SW, Uiterwaal CSPM, Stigter RH, et al. Severe umbilical cord acidemia and neurological outcome in preterm and full-term neonates. *Biol Neonate.* 2005;88:27-34.

317. Heuchan AM, Evans N, Smart DJH, et al. Perinatal risk factors for major intraventricular haemorrhage in the Australian and New Zealand Neonatal Network, 1995–97. *Arch Dis Child.* 2002;86:F86-F90.

324. Shah DK, Zempel J, Barton T, et al. Electrographic seizures in preterm infants during the first week of life are associated with cerebral injury. *Pediatr Res.* 2010;67:102-106.

327. Kissack CM, Garr R, Wardle SP, et al. Postnatal changes in cerebral oxygen extraction in the preterm infant are associated with intraventricular hemorrhage and hemorrhagic parenchymal infarction but not periventricular leukomalacia. *Pediatr Res.* 2004;56:111-116.

328. Osborn DA, Evans N, Kluckow M, et al. Low superior vena cava flow and effect of inotropes on neurodevelopment to 3 years in preterm infants. *Pediatrics.* 2007;120:372-380.

336. Baenziger O, Stolkin F, Keel M, et al. The influence of the timing of cord clamping on postnatal cerebral oxygenation in preterm neonates: a randomized, controlled trial. *Pediatrics.* 2007;119:455-459.

341. Kassal R, Anwar M, Kashlan F, et al. Umbilical vein interleukin-6 levels in very low birth weight infants developing intraventricular hemorrhage. *Brain Dev.* 2005;27:483-487.

343. Krediet TG, Kavelaars A, Vreman HJ, et al. Respiratory distress syndrome-associated inflammation is related to early but not late peri/intraventricular hemorrhage in preterm infants. *J Pediatr.* 2006;148:740-746.

349. Baer VL, Lambert DK, Henry E, et al. Severe thrombocytopenia in the NICU. *Pediatrics.* 2009;124:e1095-e1100.

350. Von Lindern JS, Hulzebos CV, Bos A, et al. Thrombocytopaenia and intraventricular haemorrhage in very premature infants: a tale of two cities. *Arch Dis Child Fetal Neonatal Ed.* 2012;97:F348-F352.

357. Ramenghi LA, Gill BJ, Tanner SF, et al. Cerebral venous thrombosis, intraventricular haemorrhage and white matter lesions in a preterm newborn with Factor V (Leiden) mutation. *Neuropediatrics.* 2002;33:97-99.

364. Baier RJ. Genetics of perinatal brain injury in the preterm infant. *Front Biosci.* 2006;11:1371-1387.

365. Hartel C, Konig I, Koster S, et al. Genetic polymorphisms of hemostasis genes and primary outcome of very low birth weight infants. *Pediatrics.* 2006;118:683-689.

367. Ramenghi LA, Fumagalli M, Groppo M, et al. Germinal matrix hemorrhage: intraventricular hemorrhage in very-low-birth-weight infants: the independent role of inherited thrombophilia. *Stroke.* 2011;42:1889-1893.

377. Ballabh P, Braun A, Nedergaard M. Anatomic analysis of blood vessels in germinal matrix, cerebral cortex, and white matter in developing infants. *Pediatr Res.* 2004;56:117-124.

408. Volpe JJ. Neonatal periventricular hemorrhage: past, present, and future [editorial]. *J Pediatr.* 1978;92:693-696.

409. Volpe JJ. Intracranial hemorrhage in the newborn: current understanding and dilemmas. *Neurology.* 1979;29:632-635.

437. Volpe JJ. Intraventricular hemorrhage and brain injury in the premature infant. Diagnosis, prognosis, and prevention. *Clin Perinatol.* 1989;16:387-411.

443. Murphy BP, Inder TE, Rooks V, et al. Posthemorrhagic ventricular dilatation in the premature infant—natural history and predictors of outcome. *Arch Dis Child.* 2002;87:F37-F41.

446. Volpe JJ. Neonatal intracranial hemorrhage. Pathophysiology, neuropathology, and clinical features. *Clin Perinatol.* 1977;4:77-102.

456. Barkovich AJ, Raybaud C, eds. *Pediatric Neuroimaging.* 5th ed. Philadelphia: Lippincott Williams & Wilkins; 2012.

472. Kennedy CR, Ayers S, Campbell MJ, et al. Randomized, controlled trial of acetazolamide and furosemide in posthemorrhagic ventricular dilation in infancy: follow-up at 1 year. *Pediatrics.* 2001;597-607.

473. de Vries LS, Liem KD, vanDijk K, et al. Early versus late treatment of posthaemorrhagic ventricular dilatation: results of a retrospective study from five neonatal intensive care units in The Netherlands. *Acta Paediatr.* 2002;91:212-217.

474. Futagi Y, Suzuki Y, Toribe Y, et al. Neurodevelopmental outcome in children with posthemorrhagic hydrocephalus. *Pediatr Neurol.* 2005;33:26-32.

475. Ment LR, Allan WC, Makuch RW, et al. Grade 3 to 4 intraventricular hemorrhage and Bayley scores predict outcome. *Pediatrics.* 2005;116:1597-1598, author reply 1598.

476. Radic JA, Vincer M, McNeely PD. Outcomes of intraventricular hemorrhage and posthemorrhagic hydrocephalus in a population-based cohort of very preterm infants born to residents of Nova Scotia from 1993 to 2010. *J Neurosurg Pediatr.* 2015;15:580-588.

500. Vohr B, Garcia-Coll C, Flanagan P, et al. Effects of intraventricular hemorrhage and socioeconomic status on perceptual, cognitive, and neurologic status of low birth weight infants at 5 years of age. *J Pediatr.* 1992;121:280-285.

511. de Vries LS, Radenmaker KJ, Groenendaal F, et al. Correlation between neonatal cranial ultrasound, MRI in infancy and neurodevelopmental outcome in infants with a large intraventricular haemorrhage with or without unilateral parenchymal involvement. *Neuropediatrics.* 1998;29:180-188.

515. Futagi Y, Toribe Y, Ogawa K, et al. Neurodevelopmental outcome in children with intraventricular hemorrhage. *Pediatr Neurol.* 2006;34:219-224.

516. Bassan H, Limperopoulos C, Visconti K, et al. Neurodevelopmental outcome in survivors of periventricular hemorrhagic infarction. *Pediatrics.* 2007;120:785-792.

517. Mukerji A, Shah V, Shah PS. Periventricular/intraventricular hemorrhage and neurodevelopmental outcome: a meta-analysis. *Pediatrics.* 2015;136:1132-1143.

519. Goldstein RF, Cotten CM, Shankaran S, et al. Influence of gestational age on death and neurodevelopmental outcome in premature infants with severe intracranial hemorrhage. *J Perinatol.* 2013;33:25-32.

520. Volpe JJ. Impaired neurodevelomental outcome after mild germinal matrix-intraventricular hemorrhage. *Pediatrics.* 2015;136:1185-1187.

524. Sherlock RL, Anderson PJ, Doyle LW. Neurodevelopmental sequelae of intraventricular haemorrhage at 8 years of age in a regional cohort of ELBW/very preterm infants. *Early Hum Dev.* 2005;81:909-916.

525. Payne AH, Hintz SR, Hibbs AM, et al. Neurodevelopmental outcomes of extremely low-gestational-age neonates with low-grade periventricular-intraventricular hemorrhage. *JAMA Pediatr.* 2013;167:451-459.

526. Bolisetty S, Dhawan A, Abdel-Latif M, et al. Intraventricular hemorrhage and neurodevelopmental outcomes in extreme preterm infants. *Pediatrics.* 2014;133:55-62.

527. Woodward LJ, Anderson PJ, Austin NC, et al. Neonatal MRI to predict neurodevelopmental outcomes in preterm infants. *N Engl J Med.* 2006;355:685-694.

529. Calisici E, Eras Z, Oncel MY, et al. Neurodevelopmental outcomes of premature infants with severe intraventricular hemorrhage. *J Matern Fetal Neonatal Med.* 2015;28:2115-2120.

558. Hall RT. Prevention of premature birth: do pediatricians have a role? *Pediatrics.* 2000;105:1137-1140.

562. Meis PJ, Klebanoff M, Thom E, et al. Prevention of recurrent preterm delivery by 17 alpha-hydroxyprogesterone caproate. *N Engl J Med.* 2003;348:2379-2385.

564. Briery CM, Klauser CK, Martin RW, et al. The use of 17-hydroxy progesterone in women with arrested preterm labor: a randomized clinical trial. *J Matern Fetal Neonatal Med.* 2014;27:1892-1896.

576. Shankaran S, Bauer CR, Bain R, et al. Relationship between antenatal steroid administration and grades III and IV intracranial hemorrhage in low birth weight infants. *Am J Obstet Gynecol.* 1995;173:305-312.

577. Horbar JD. Antenatal corticosteroid treatment and neonatal outcomes for infants 501 to 1500 gm in the Vermont-Oxford Trials Network. *Am J Obstet Gynecol.* 1995;173:275-281.

585. Blickstein I, Reichman B, Lusky A, et al. Plurality-dependent risk of severe intraventricular hemorrhage among very low birth weight infants and antepartum corticosteroid treatment. *Am J Obstet Gynecol.* 2006;194:1329-1333.

587. Volpe JJ. Encephalopathy of prematurity includes neuronal abnormalities. *Pediatrics.* 2005;116:221-225.

590. Parikh N, Lasky RE, Kennedy KA, et al. Postnatal dexamethasone therapy and cerebral tissue volumes in extremely low birth weight infants. *Pediatrics.* 2007;119:265-272.

601. Crowther CA, McKinlay CJ, Middleton P, et al. Repeat doses of prenatal corticosteroids for women at risk of preterm birth for improving neonatal health outcomes. *Cochrane Database Syst Rev.* 2015;(7):CD003935.

602. Viteri OA, Blackwell SC, Chauhan SP, et al. Antenatal corticosteroids for the prevention of respiratory distress syndrome in premature twins. *Obstet Gynecol.* 2016;128:583-591.

616. Crowther C, Henderson-Smart D. Prenatal phenobarbital before very-preterm birth and neurodevelopmental outcome. *Lancet.* 2003;360:1529-1530.

628. Crowther CA, Hiller JE, Doyle LW, et al. Effect of magnesium sulfate given for neuroprotection before preterm birth—a randomized controlled trial. *JAMA.* 2003;290:2669-2676.

629. Mittendorf R, Dammann O, Lee KS. Brain lesions in newborns exposed to high-dose magnesium sulfate during preterm labor. *J Perinatol.* 2006;26:57-63.

642. Committee on Obstetric Practice, American College of Obstetricians and Gynecologists, Committee opinion no. 543. Timing of umbilical cord clamping after birth. *Obstet Gynecol.* 2012;120:1522-1526.

648. Katheria AC, Truong G, Cousins L, et al. Umbilical cord milking versus delayed cord clamping in preterm infants. *Pediatrics.* 2015;136:61-69.

651. Perlman JM, Wyllie J, Kattwinkel J, et al. Part 7: neonatal resuscitation: 2015 international consensus on cardiopulmonary resuscitation and emergency cardiovascular care science with treatment recommendations. *Circulation.* 2015;132:S204-S241.

652. Wyllie J, Perlman JM, Kattwinkel J, et al. Part 7: neonatal resuscitation: 2015 international consensus on cardiopulmonary resuscitation and emergency cardiovascular care science with treatment recommendations. *Resuscitation.* 2015;95:e169-e201.

655. Audeh S, Smolkin T, Bental Y, et al. Does admission hypothermia predispose to intraventricular hemorrhage in very-low-birth-weight infants? *Neonatology.* 2011;100:373-379.

672. Liao SM, Rao R, Mathur AM. Head position change is not associated with acute changes in bilateral cerebral oxygenation in stable preterm infants during the first 3 days of life. *Am J Perinatol.* 2015;32:645-652.

684. Horbar JD, Soll RF, Sutherland JM, et al. A multicenter randomized, placebo-controlled trial of surfactant therapy for respiratory distress syndrome. *N Engl J Med.* 1989;320:959-965.

697. Hellström-Westas L, Bell AH, Skov L, et al. Cerebroelectrical depression following surfactant treatment in preterm neonates. *Pediatrics.* 1992;89:643-647.

700. Roll C, Knief J, Horsch S, et al. Effect of surfactant administration on cerebral haemodynamics and oxygenation in premature infants—a near infrared spectroscopy study. *Neuropediatrics.* 2000;31:16-23.

715. Subramaniam P, Henderson-Smart DJ, Davis PG. Prophylactic nasal continuous positive airways pressure for preventing morbidity and mortality in very preterm infants. *Cochrane Database Syst Rev.* 2005;(3):CD001243.

716. Mestan KKL, Marks JD, Hecox K, et al. Neurodevelopmental outcomes of premature infants treated with inhaled nitric oxide. *N Engl J Med.* 2005;353:23-32.

723. Kinsella JP, Abman SH. Inhaled nitric oxide in the premature newborn. *J Pediatr.* 2007;151:10-15.

724. Hintz SR, Van Meurs KP, Perritt R, et al. Neurodevelopmental outcomes of premature infants with severe respiratory failure enrolled in a randomized controlled trial of inhaled nitric oxide. *J Pediatr.* 2007;151:16-22, 22.e11-e13.

726. Ment LR, Duncan CC, Ehrenkranz RA, et al. Randomized low-dose indomethacin trial for prevention of intraventricular hemorrhage in very low birth weight neonates. *J Pediatr.* 1988;112:948-955.

734. Schmidt B, Davis P, Moddemann D, et al. Long-term effects of indomethacin prophylaxis in extremely-low-birth-weight infants. *N Engl J Med.* 2001;344:1966-1972.

738. Ohlsson A, Roberts RS, Schmidt B, et al. Male/female differences in indomethacin effects in preterm infants. *J Pediatr.* 2005;147:860-862.

739. Clyman RI, Saha S, Jobe A, et al. Indomethacin prophylaxis for preterm infants: the impact of 2 multicentered randomized controlled trials on clinical practice. *J Pediatr.* 2007;150:46-50. e42.

740. Clyman RI, Chorne N. Patent ductus arteriosus: evidence for and against treatment. *J Pediatr.* 2007;150:216-219.

741. Fowlie PW, Davis PG. Prophylactic intravenous idomethacin for preventing mortality and morbidity in preterm infants. *Cochrane Database Syst Rev.* 2005.

745. Mirza H, Laptook AR, Oh W, et al. Effects of indomethacin prophylaxis timing on intraventricular haemorrhage and patent ductus arteriosus in extremely low birth weight infants. *Arch Dis Child Fetal Neonatal Ed.* 2016;101:F418-F422.

784. The EC Ethamsylate Trial Group. The EC randomised controlled trial of prophylactic ethamsylate for very preterm neonates: early mortality and morbidity. *Arch Dis Child.* 1994;70:F201-F205.

799. Brion LP, Bell EF, Raghuveer TS. Vitamin E supplementation for prevention of morbidity and mortality in preterm infants. *Cochrane Database Syst Rev.* 2005;(3).

814. Taylor GA. Sonographic assessment of posthemorrhagic ventricular dilatation. *Radiologic Clin North Am.* 2001;39:541-551.

819. Brouwer MJ, de Vries LS, Pistorius L, et al. Ultrasound measurements of the lateral ventricles in neonates: why, how and when? A systematic review. *Acta Paediatr.* 2010;99:1298-1306.

825. Sondhi V, Gupta G, Gupta PK, et al. Establishment of nomograms and reference ranges for intra-cranial ventricular dimensions and ventriculo-hemispheric ratio in newborns by ultrasonography. *Acta Paediatr.* 2008;97:738-744.

832. Del Bigio MR, Wilson MJ, Enno T. Chronic hydrocephalus in rats and humans: white matter loss and behavior changes. *Ann Neurol.* 2003;53:337-346.

850. Del Bigio MR, Khan OH, da Silva Lopes L, et al. Cerebral white matter oxidation and nitrosylation in young rodents with kaolin-induced hydrocephalus. *J Neuropathol Exp Neurol.* 2012;71:274-288.

866. Owen-Lynch PJ, Draper CE, Mashayekhi F, et al. Defective cell cycle control underlies abnormal cortical development in the hydrocephalic Texas rat. *Brain.* 2003;126:623-631.

883. Maertzdorf WJ, Vles JSH, Beuls E, et al. Intracranial pressure and cerebral blood flow velocity in preterm infants with posthaemorrhagic ventricular dilatation. *Arch Dis Child.* 2002;87:185-188.

884. Soul J, Eichewald E, Walter G, et al. CSF removal in infantile posthemorrhagic hydrocephalus results in significant improvement in cerebral hemodynamics. *Pediatr Res.* 2004;55:872-876.

889. Norooz F, Urlesberger B, Giordano V, et al. Decompressing posthaemorrhagic ventricular dilatation significantly improves regional cerebral oxygen saturation in preterm infants. *Acta Paediatr.* 2015;104:663-669.

895. Whitelaw A, Rosengren L, Blennow M. Brain specific proteins in posthaemorrhagic ventricular dilatation. *Arch Dis Child Fetal Neonatal Ed.* 2001;84:F90-F91.

909. Whitelaw A. Intraventricular streptokinase after intraventricular hemorrhage in newborn infants. *Cochrane Database Syst Rev.* 2005.

917. de Vries LS, Benders M, Groenendaal F. *Improved outcome in preterm infants with a large intraventricular hemorrhage: a relationship with*

earlier intervention? Pediatric Academic Societies 2006: Annual Meeting, Abstract #3590.3369.

918. Whitelaw A. Repeated lumbar or ventricular punctures in newborns with intraventricular hemorrhage. *Cochrane Database Syst Rev*. 2005.

923. Carrion E, Hertzog JH, Medlock MD, et al. Use of acetazolamide to decrease cerebrospinal fluid production in chronically ventilated patients with ventriculopleural shunts. *Arch Dis Child*. 2001;83:68-71.

924. Whitelaw A. Diuretic therapy for newborn infants with posthemorrhagic ventricular dilatation. *Cochrane Database Syst Rev*. 2005.

937. Whitelaw A, Evans DA, Carter M, et al. Randomised clinical trial of prevention of hydrocephalus after intraventricular hemorrhage in premature infants: brain-washing versus tapping fluid. *Pediatrics*. 2007;119:e1071-e1078.

938. Whitelaw A, Jary S, Kmita G, et al. Randomized trial of drainage, irrigation and fibrinolytic therapy for premature infants with posthemorrhagic ventricular dilatation: developmental outcome at 2 years. *Pediatrics*. 2010;125:e852-e858.

939. Mazzola CA, Choudhri AF, Auguste KI, et al. Pediatric hydrocephalus: systematic literature review and evidence-based guidelines. Part 2: Management of posthemorrhagic hydrocephalus in premature infants. *J Neurosurg Pediatr*. 2014;14:8-23.

943. de Vries LS, Brouwer AJ, Groenendaal F. Posthaemorrhagic ventricular dilatation: when should we intervene? *Arch Dis Child Fetal Neonatal Ed*. 2013;98:F284-F285.

951. Kormanik K, Praca J, Garton HJ, et al. Repeated tapping of ventricular reservoir in preterm infants with post-hemorrhagic ventricular dilatation does not increase the risk of reservoir infection. *J Perinatol*. 2010;30:218-221.

954. Lam HP, Heilman CB. Ventricular access device versus ventriculosubgaleal shunt in post hemorrhagic hydrocephalus associated with prematurity. *J Matern Fetal Neonatal Med*. 2009;22:1097-1101.

971. Fulkerson DH, Sivaganesan A, Hill JD, et al. Progression of cerebrospinal fluid cell count and differential over a treatment course of shunt infection. *J Neurosurg Pediatr*. 2011;8:613-619.

972. Elgamal EA, El-Dawlatly AA, Murshid WR, et al. Endoscopic third ventriculostomy for hydrocephalus in children younger than 1 year of age. *Childs Nerv Syst*. 2011;27:111-116.

973. Peretta P, Ragazzi P, Carlino CF, et al. The role of Ommaya reservoir and endoscopic third ventriculostomy in the management of post-hemorrhagic hydrocephalus of prematurity. *Childs Nerv Syst*. 2007;23:765-771.

974. Siomin V, Cinalli G, Grotenhuis A, et al. Endoscopic third ventriculostomy in patients with cerebrospinal fluid infection and/or hemorrhage. *J Neurosurg*. 2002;97:519-524.

975. Kulkarni AV, Drake JM, Mallucci CL, et al. Endoscopic third ventriculostomy in the treatment of childhood hydrocephalus. *J Pediatr*. 2009;155:254-259.e251.

Full references for this chapter can be found on www.expertconsult .com.

METABOLIC ENCEPHALOPATHIES

Glucose

Jeffrey M. Perlman ◆ *Joseph J. Volpe*

Glucose, like oxygen, is of essential and fundamental importance for brain metabolism. Indeed, because oxygen consumption is relatively low in the neonatal human brain and minimal in such areas as cerebral white matter (see Chapter 13), glucose supply to the brain may be even more important. The major source of brain glucose is the blood supply; thus it is readily understood that serious encephalopathy may ensue when the glucose content of blood becomes deficient.

In this chapter, the normal aspects of glucose metabolism in the brain are discussed, followed by a review of the biochemical derangements that occur with hypoglycemia. The neuropathology of hypoglycemia is described next and, on the background of the biochemical and neuropathological derangements, the clinical aspects are reviewed. To begin the discussion, an attempt to define hypoglycemia is presented with an explanation of why this attempt is so difficult.

DEFINITION

Definition of a blood glucose level that should be considered too low is difficult, in part because the newborn does not have the neural capacity to demonstrate when the critical lower limit has been passed, consistently and by overt symptoms. Thus the critical limit of blood glucose level for the maintenance of neonatal neuronal integrity in various clinical circumstances is unknown. Relevant clinical circumstances include those with (1) reduced availability of glucose or alternative fuels (ketone bodies, lactate), because of deficient glycogen and fat stores or impaired hepatic gluconeogenesis or both (e.g., intrauterine growth restriction, prematurity); (2) increased systemic glucose utilization (e.g., infant of a diabetic mother, hyperinsulinism, cold stress, sepsis); (3) increased cerebral glucose utilization (e.g., hypoxic-ischemic states, seizures); or (4) decreased cerebral utilization (e.g., hypotension). Moreover, and perhaps most important, the lower limits of blood glucose are likely higher when there are also concomitant insults that increase cerebral demand for glucose and that are deleterious to the brain (e.g., hypoxemia, ischemia, repetitive seizures). Indeed, the concept of an additive and potentiating role of hypoglycemia in the production of brain injury in the sick newborn infant is a critical neurological aspect of neonatal hypoglycemia.

Definition of a blood glucose level below which hypoglycemia should be designated is complex and cannot be based on a single number that can be uniformly applied to all infants. Attempts at such definitions have been based on *statistical* thresholds derived from the study of serial changes of blood glucose in *normal* infants; on *operational* thresholds based on

blood glucose levels and the presence or absence of symptoms or risk factors; on *neurophysiological* thresholds based on changes in brain stem auditory evoked responses (BSAERs), cerebral blood flow (CBF), or cerebral glucose metabolism; and on neurological outcome thresholds based on neurodevelopmental outcome as a function of different blood glucose levels (see next). The results of seven large-scale studies concerning the incidence of *hypoglycemia* in various neonatal populations are shown in Table 25.1[1-7] and noted in relevant sections that follow.

Postnatal Changes

During the first 2 hours of postnatal life, plasma glucose levels decline to a nadir followed by a rise, reaching a steady-state glucose concentration by 3 to 4 hours after birth. Glucose levels then increase to higher and relatively more stable concentrations, generally above 60 mg/dL by 12 hours after birth (Fig. 25.1).[1,2,4,8] This adaptation is associated in part with the hepatic release of glucose at the rate of 4 to 6 mg/min per kg (see later).[8] These neonatal glucose levels are less than those in the adult and rise slowly to achieve the latter levels by the third or fourth day.[1,2,4]

Statistical Thresholds

Historically, the designation of hypoglycemia has usually been based on statistical measures (i.e., marked deviation from *normal* blood glucose levels). Previous determinations of such blood glucose levels in the newborn were derived from infants generally not fed in the first hours of life.[9] Such determinations led to the definition of *significant hypoglycemia* in the newborn as a whole blood glucose concentration lower than 30 mg/dL in the term infant and lower than 20 mg/dL in the preterm infant. Subsequent reports in healthy infants, initially breast-fed within the first 3 hours,[1,4,8,10] show that blood glucose concentrations as low as 30 mg/dL are observed in some infants within 1 to 2 hours after birth and are usually transient, asymptomatic, and considered to be part of normal adaptation to postnatal life.[11]

Operational Thresholds

Cornblath and co-workers suggested that the term *hypoglycemia* is not readily defined for individual patients and that *operational thresholds* (i.e., "a concentration of blood or plasma glucose at which clinicians should consider intervention") should be established.[8] An *operational threshold* by itself is an indication for action and is not diagnostic of disease or predictive of adverse neurological sequelae. These thresholds were defined as less than 45 mg/dL (2.5 mmol/L) for "the infant with abnormal clinical signs" and less than 36 mg/dL (2.0 mmol/L) for the

TABLE 25.1   Incidence of Hypoglycemia According to Blood/Plasma Glucose Levels at Varying Postnatal Age

REFERENCE	GLUCOSE CONCENTRATION (mg/dL)	INCIDENCE (%)	HOURS FOLLOWING DELIVERY
Srinivasan and colleagues[a]	<40 (plasma)	13	3
Heck and Erenberg[b]	<30 (plasma)	8	48
Hawdon[a]	<47 (blood)	12	96
Hoseth et al[a]	<47 (blood)	14	96
	<40 (blood)	4	
	<30 (blood)	0.4	
Lucas et al[c]	<45 (blood)	66	120
	<30 (blood)	28	
	<10 (blood)	10	
Harris et al[d]	<47 (blood)	51	≤48
	<40 (blood)	19	
Kaiser et al[e]	<45 (plasma)	19.3	3
	<30 (plasma)	10.3	
	<10 (plasma)	6.4	

[a]Healthy, appropriate for gestational age babies.
[b]Healthy, small or large for gestational age, term babies.
[c]Infants <1850 g birthweight (mean, 1337 g).
[d]>35 Weeks, high-risk infants (small or large for gestational age, infant of diabetic mothers, late preterm).
[e]Infants 23 to 42 weeks.

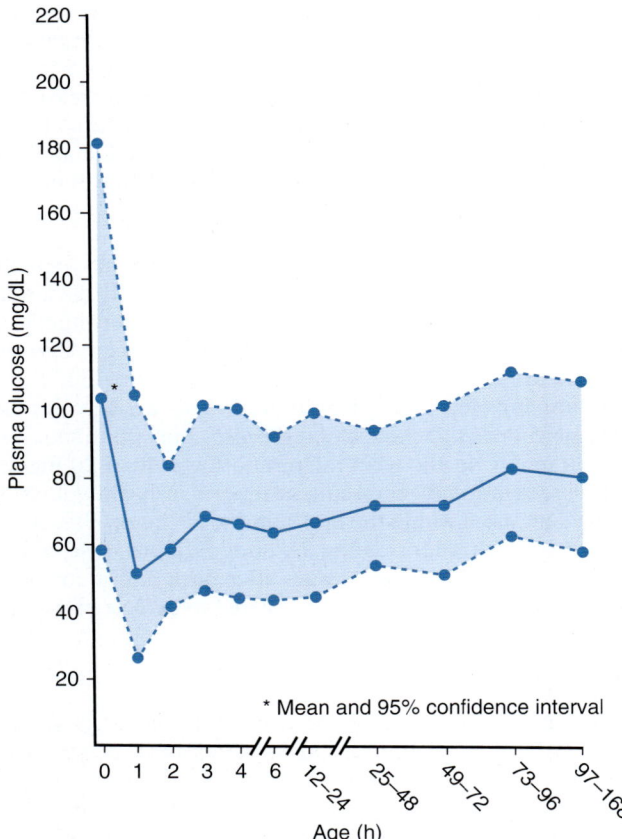

Figure 25.1 Neonatal glucose values. Plasma glucose values during the first week of life in healthy term newborns appropriate for gestational age. (Adapted from Srinivasan G, Pildes RS, Cattamanchi G, et al. Clinical and laboratory observations: plasma glucose values in normal neonates—a new look. *J Pediatr.* 1986;109:114–117.)

asymptomatic infant and the infant "at risk for hypoglycemia" (without regard to other influencing factors mentioned previously). Using this threshold, Harris and colleagues recently studied infants above 35 weeks of gestational age (GA) and noted hypoglycemia (blood sugar < 47 mg/dL [2.6 mmol/dL]) in 51% of high-risk infants (small or large for GA infants, infants of diabetic mothers, or late preterm infants) and in 19% of infants with a blood sugar below 36 mg/dL (2 mmol/L) (see Table 25.1).[6] Clearly the incidence of hypoglycemia will vary substantially depending on the applied operational threshold (see later; also see Table 25.1). The operational threshold still focuses, however, on individual glucose concentrations and does not address whether the threshold level of blood glucose represents the threshold level for neuronal injury. Hawdon makes the plausible argument that hypoglycemia should perhaps be defined as a persistently low blood glucose level in a baby at risk for impaired metabolic adaptation but with no abnormal clinical signs or a single low blood glucose level in a baby presenting with abnormal clinical signs.[3]

Neurophysiological Threshold

The complexity of defining hypoglycemia is further illustrated by the lack of consistency in a particular threshold value and outcome (see next). Thus determinations of BSAERs in a small series of term infants showed prolonged latencies at levels lower than approximately 47 mg/dL (Fig. 25.2) (see later discussion).[12] A later report of a single infant did not detect prolongation of latency to wave V until blood glucose fell to 25 mg/dL.[13]

Other relevant physiological measures include CBF and cerebral glucose metabolism. Thus two studies of human infants showed that CBF increases at glucose values lower than 30 mg/dL and that transport becomes limiting for cerebral glucose utilization at a glucose level lower than approximately 54 mg/dL. In addition, the level of blood glucose required for brain homeostasis is different in the infant with *impaired CBF*, as

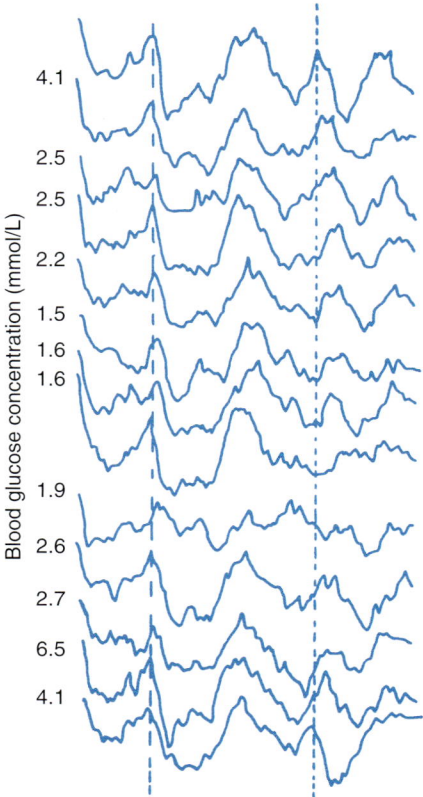

Figure 25.2 Serial brain stem auditory evoked potentials recorded in a 2-day-old infant in relation to his blood glucose concentration. The vertical lines indicate the latency between wave I and wave V in the initial recording during normoglycemia. Note the prolongation of latency when blood glucose values decreased to 2.5 mmol/L and lower. (From Koh TH, Aynsley-Green A, Tarbit M, Eyre JA. Neural dysfunction during hypoglycaemia. *Arch Dis Child.* 1988;63:1353–1358.)

with hypotension, or with *increased cerebral glucose utilization*, as with seizures, or with the anaerobic glycolytic metabolism of hypoxia-ischemia or asphyxia (see later discussion). Moreover, the ability to compensate for low cerebral fuel availability during hypoglycemia includes the capacity to use nonglucose cerebral fuels such as lactate and ketones.[14] However, regarding the latter, recent evidence suggests that neonatal hypoglycemia within the first 48 hours evolves in the context of a hypoketotic state, with varying levels of lactate and detectable insulin levels in many infants.[15,16]

Because the rate of ketone utilization by the brain is directly proportional to plasma concentrations, the contribution of ketones to neonatal brain metabolism is less than one tenth that of older children with similar degrees of hypoglycemia.

Neurological Outcome Thresholds

A careful epidemiological study suggested a deleterious effect on subsequent cognitive development in infants whose plasma glucose levels were less than approximately 47 mg/dL on at least one occasion on 3 or more separate days (see Table 25.1 and Fig. 25.3).[5] Abnormalities in arithmetic and motor scores persisted at 7.5 to 8 years.[17] Conversely, in a subsequent study that attempted to duplicate these findings,[18] 47 of 566 infants of

GA below 32 weeks with a blood glucose level below 47 mg/dL on at least 3 days were matched with hypoglycemia-free infants and followed up through 15 years. The investigators found no difference in physical disability or developmental progress at 2 years or in psychometric assessment at 15 years.[18] In a recent retrospective review of 1943 infants (23 to 42 weeks GA), early transient newborn hypoglycemia was noted in 19.3% using a value of 45 mg/dL (<2.6 mmol/L), 10.3% using a value of 40 mg/dL (<2.3 mmol/L), and in 6.4% using a value of <35 mg/dL (<2.0 mmol/L) (see Table 25.1).[7] In this study, in assessing for multiple confounding variables, transient hypoglycemia was associated with a decreased probability of proficiency on literacy and mathematics fourth-grade achievement tests at 8-year testing (see later).[7] As will be discussed, the preponderance of evidence suggests that *duration* and *degree* of depression of blood glucose are both important.

In summary, defining hypoglycemia is highly complex and must be individualized according to the infant's clinical situation. The definition requires consideration of factors that influence the vulnerability of specific cells and regions in the brain, the status of brain energy reserves, hepatic glycogen reserves, and gluconeogenic capacity, such as the GA of the infant, status of intrauterine nutrition, prior or concomitant hypoxic-ischemic insults, and seizures, among others. These and related issues are discussed subsequently.

NORMAL METABOLIC ASPECTS

Brain as the Primary Determinant of Glucose Production

The pathophysiology of neonatal hypoglycemic encephalopathy has as its basis the importance of glucose as the primary metabolic fuel for the brain. Glucose for normal brain metabolism is derived from the blood, and glucose production in mammals is primarily a function of the liver. The postnatal induction of hepatic glycogenolysis and gluconeogenesis and the interplay of insulin, glucagon, catecholamines, corticosteroids, and other hormones in the regulation of hepatic glucose metabolism have been reviewed in detail by others.[19-23] It need only be emphasized here that the brain appears to be the major determinant of (hepatic) glucose production.[24] Thus glucose production was measured in a series of infants and children from 1 to 25 kg in body weight by a continuous 3- to 4-hour infusion of the nonradioactive tracer, 6,6-dideuteroglucose. Glucose production on a body-weight basis was found to be twofold to threefold greater in newborns than in older patients. The infants clearly had disproportionately higher rates of glucose production as compared with adult subjects. This observation becomes understandable when glucose production is plotted as a function of estimated brain weight (Fig. 25.4). The linear relationship suggests that the disproportionately high rates of glucose production in the neonatal period relate to the disproportionately large neonatal brain. Because central nervous system consumption of glucose accounts for 30% or more of total hepatic glucose output, at least in the premature infant, this relationship between glucose production rate and brain weight seems reasonable.[25]

The mechanisms by which utilization of glucose by the brain may regulate hepatic glucose output are unknown. It is possible that the effect is mediated by subtle changes in blood glucose levels acting directly on pancreatic insulin secretion or

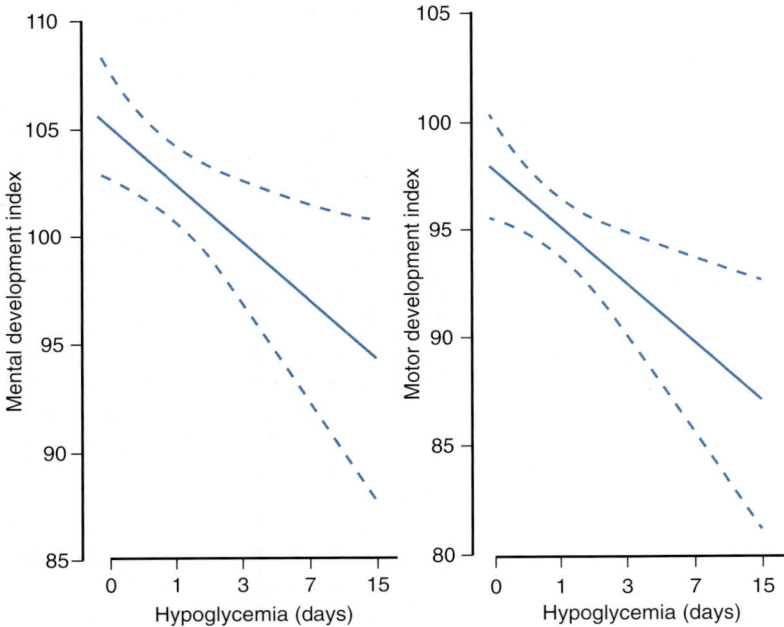

Figure 25.3 Logarithm of days of recorded hypoglycemia lower than 2.6 mmol/L related to the Bayley Mental Development Index and Bayley Psychomotor Development Index at 18 months (corrected age) in a series of 433 premature infants. Regression slopes and 95% confidence intervals (*dashed lines*) are shown adjusted for days of ventilation, gender, social class, birthweight, and fetal growth retardation. Data shown are for both genders and all social classes combined and for no ventilation. For infants ventilated for 1 to 6, 7 to 14, or more than 14 days, subtract 5, 10, or 15 points, respectively, for mental development index and 4.5, 9.0, or 13.5 points, respectively, for psychomotor development index. (From Lucas A, Morley R, Cole TJ. Adverse neurodevelopment outcome of moderate neonatal hypoglycaemia. *Br Med J.* 1988;297:1304–1308.)

on hepatic glucose output. More provocative is the possibility that the brain mediates control over hepatic glucose production by neural or hormonal effectors originating within the central nervous system.[26] This possibility leads to the interesting logical extension that disturbances of the brain may *lead to* disturbances in glucose output by the liver and *result in* hypoglycemia or hyperglycemia (see later discussion). Moreover, the size of the brain per se may also possibly lead to disturbances in glucose output secondary to changes in glucose utilization. At any rate, in the normal human, from the newborn period to adulthood, it is now clear that a very close relationship exists between brain mass and glucose production.

Glucose Metabolism in the Brain

Glucose metabolism in the brain is depicted in a simplified fashion in Fig. 25.5. Those aspects particularly relevant to this chapter are shown; a further review of cerebral glucose and energy metabolism is contained in Chapter 13.[26-29]

Glucose Uptake

Glucose uptake from the blood into the brain occurs by a process that is not energy-dependent but that proceeds faster than expected by simple diffusion (i.e., carrier-mediated facilitated diffusion). The transport is mediated by a specific protein, a glucose transporter.[29-34]

The brain glucose transporter is concentrated in the capillaries and the concentration of the transporter increases with development. In the rat, the lower apparent blood-brain glucose permeability in the newborn (≈25% of adult values) is related to a lower concentration of the glucose transporter (not to a lower affinity of the transporter for glucose). Studies of human premature infants also suggest that the number of available endothelial transporters is approximately one third to one half the value for the adult human brain.[25] The importance of the transporter for brain function and structure is illustrated by the occurrence of seizures and developmental delay in infants with partial deficiency of the transporter (see Chapters 12 and 29).[31,32] The glucose concentration normally present in blood in the newborn rat is approximately one fourth that required for glucose uptake to proceed at maximal velocity.[28] *Studies of the human premature infant by positron emission tomography (PET) indicate that at a plasma glucose level of approximately 3 µmol/mL (i.e., ≈54 mg/dL), transport becomes limiting for cerebral glucose utilization.*[25] *Thus uptake is one potential site for regulation of glucose metabolism in the brain, and this regulation is particularly dependent on changes in blood glucose concentrations.*

Hexokinase

The initial step in glucose utilization in the brain is phosphorylation to glucose-6-phosphate by *hexokinase* (see Fig. 25.5). This enzyme is inhibited not only by its product but also by adenosine triphosphate (ATP). Under certain circumstances, hexokinase is an important control point in glycolysis.[31,35]

Major Fates of Glucose-6-Phosphate

The product of the hexokinase reaction, glucose-6-phosphate, is at an important branch point in glucose metabolism (see Fig. 25.5). From glucose-6-phosphate originate pathways to the

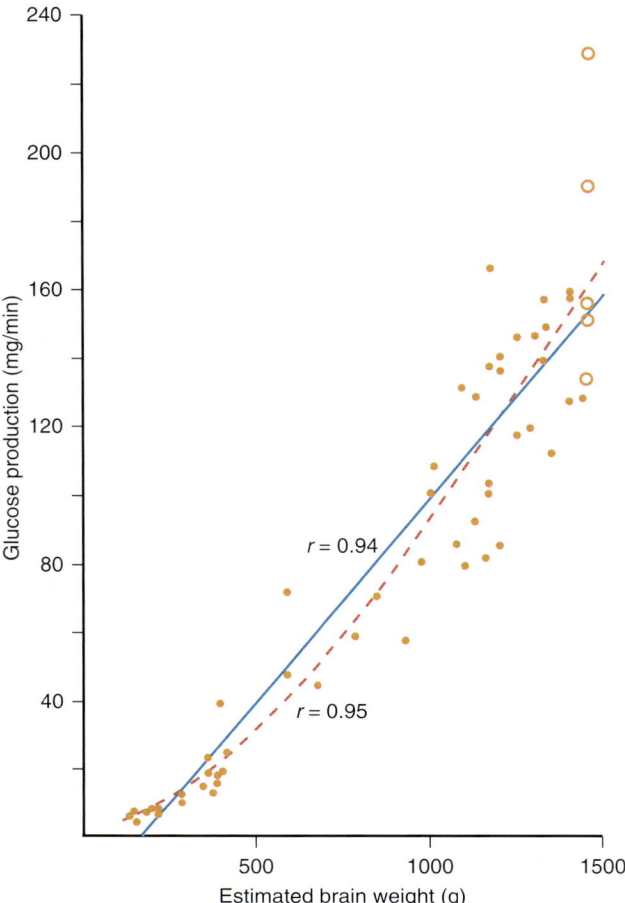

Figure 25.4 Linear relationship between glucose production and (estimated) brain weight in subjects ranging from premature infants of approximately 1000 g to adults. Glucose production was measured by continuous infusion of 6,6-dideuteroglucose. The linear and quadratic functions are depicted by solid and dashed lines, respectively. (From Bier DM, Leake RD, Haymond MW. Measurement of true glucose production rates in infancy and childhood with 6,6-dideuteroglucose. *Diabetes.* 1977;26:1016–1023.)

formation of glycogen, to the pentose monophosphate shunt, and through glycolysis to pyruvate. *Glycogen* is important as a readily available store of glucose in the brain; glycogenolysis is an actively regulated process that is called into play during periods of glucose lack (i.e., hypoglycemia) or accelerated glucose utilization (e.g., oxygen deprivation [with associated anaerobic glycolysis] or seizures). Glycogen is concentrated in astrocytes, and with low brain glucose, astrocytic glycogenolysis is activated to produce glucose-6-phosphate. The latter is converted to lactate, which then enters the neuron for use as an energy source (see later).[36] The *pentose monophosphate shunt* provides reducing equivalents, important for lipid synthesis, and ribose units, important for nucleic acid synthesis. These two synthetic processes are of particular importance in the developing brain. The generation of reducing equivalents is also critical for the generation of reduced glutathione, which is crucial for defense against free radicals and thereby hypoglycemic cellular injury (see later discussion).

The major fate of glucose-6-phosphate in the brain is entrance into the *glycolytic pathway*, principally for the

ultimate production of *chemical energy* in the form of high-energy phosphate bonds (i.e., ATP and its storage form, phosphocreatine). When oxidized aerobically, each molecule of glucose generates 38 molecules of high-energy phosphate compounds. The next several sections describe the utilization of glucose for energy production.

Phosphofructokinase

The most critical step in the glycolytic pathway is the conversion of fructose-6-phosphate to fructose-1,6-diphosphate; the enzyme involved, phosphofructokinase, is a major regulatory, rate-limiting step in glycolysis (see Fig. 25.5). The enzyme is inhibited by ATP and is activated by adenosine diphosphate (ADP). The ammonium ion (NH_4^+), generated by amino acid transamination, is also a potent activator of this complex.

Pyruvate

The glycolytic pathway ultimately results in the formation of pyruvate, most of which enters the mitochondrion and is converted to acetyl-coenzyme A (acetyl-CoA) (see Fig. 25.5). However, pyruvate can also result in the formation of lactate when the cytosolic redox state is shifted toward reduction. Conversely, under the conditions of hypoglycemia (i.e., [1] available lactate and deficient pyruvate, [2] a cytosolic redox state that is normal or shifted toward oxidation, and [3] the action of lactate dehydrogenase), lactate can lead to formation of pyruvate and can become an energy source (see later discussion). Finally, alanine may be converted to pyruvate by transamination and can therefore become a source of glucose or acetyl-CoA.

Acetyl-Coenzyme A

The formation of acetyl-CoA by pyruvate dehydrogenase is the major starting point for the citric acid cycle (see Fig. 25.5). This step is an important rate-limiting process in glucose utilization in the neonatal brain.[28] Acetyl-CoA is also the major starting point for the synthesis of brain lipids and acetylcholine. Moreover, ketone bodies are converted to acetyl-CoA to become an energy source.

Citric Acid Cycle

The citric acid cycle (with the linked electron transport system) ultimately results in the complete oxidation of the carbon of glucose to carbon dioxide and the generation of nearly all the ATP derived from this sugar (Fig. 25.6). Transamination reactions interface this segment of glucose utilization with certain amino acids, which thereby can be used for energy production.

Glucose as the Primary Metabolic Fuel for Brain

The role of glucose as the primary fuel for the production of chemical energy and the maintenance of normal function in the *mature brain* are supported by three main facts.[26,28,37,38] First, the respiratory quotient (i.e., carbon dioxide output/oxygen uptake) of the brain is approximately 1, a finding indicating that carbohydrate is the major substrate oxidized by neural tissue. Glucose is the only carbohydrate extracted by the brain in any significant quantity. Second, cerebral glucose uptake is almost completely accounted for by cerebral oxygen uptake. Third, central nervous system function is rapidly and seriously disturbed by hypoglycemia.

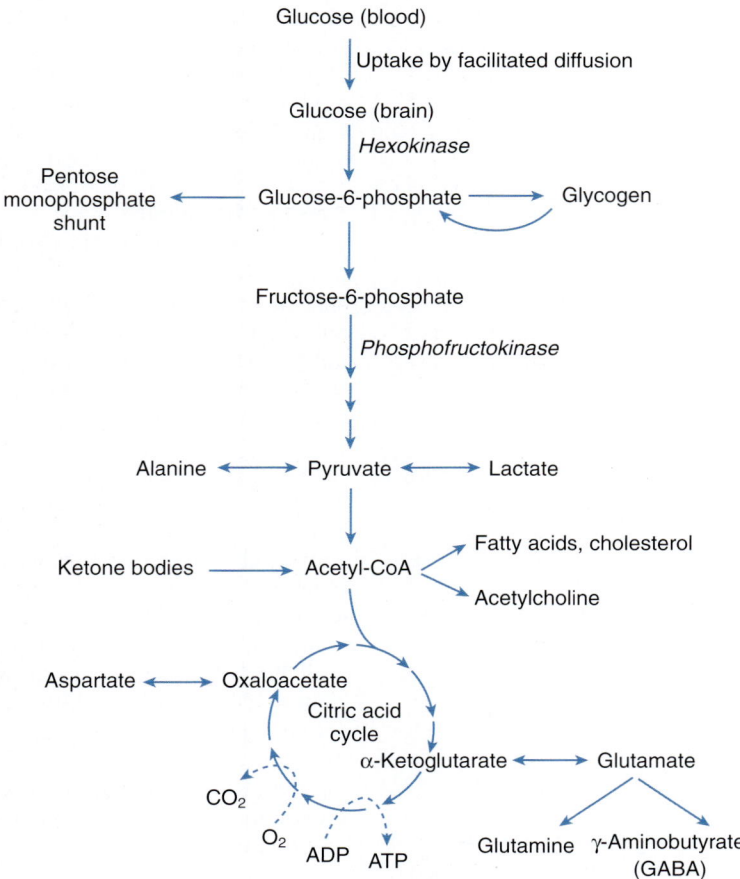

Figure 25.5 Glucose metabolism in the brain. See text for details. *ADP,* Adenosine diphosphate; *ATP,* adenosine triphosphate; *CoA,* coenzyme A.

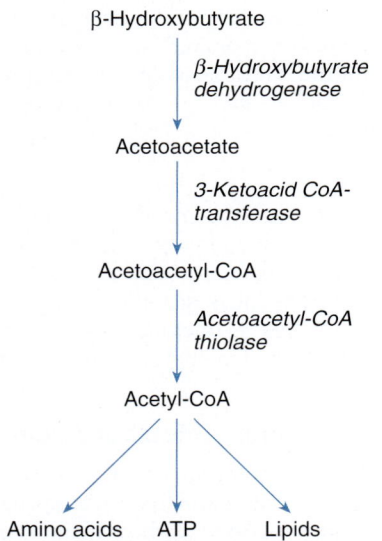

Figure 25.6 Ketone body use in brain. See text for details. *ATP,* Adenosine triphosphate; *CoA,* coenzyme A.

Current data support a similar preeminence for glucose in the *immature brain.*[26,29] Thus studies in the newborn dog indicate that glucose consumption in the brain accounts for 95% of cerebral energy supply.[39] Moreover, studies in term fetal sheep demonstrated that, under aerobic conditions, glucose

is the main substrate metabolized for energy production.[40] Glucose/oxygen quotients of approximately 1.1 were obtained in two different laboratories.[40-42] The glucose/oxygen quotient is equivalent to the arteriovenous difference of glucose (×6) divided by the arteriovenous difference of oxygen and represents the fraction of cerebral oxygen consumption required for the aerobic metabolism of cerebral glucose. Although the data demonstrate that glucose is the primary substrate metabolized by the brain, the finding that the values for glucose/oxygen quotients are slightly but consistently in excess of 1 suggests that a portion of the glucose is used for purposes other than complete oxidation to generate high-energy phosphate bonds. Other data, based on the fate of labeled glucose in the brain, indicate that glucose is also used for the synthesis of other materials (e.g., amino acids via transaminations and lipids via appropriate biosynthetic pathways; see Fig. 25.5).[37] Syntheses of membrane lipids and proteins, of course, are critical events in the developing brain and probably account for a relatively larger proportion of cerebral glucose utilization than in the mature brain.

Important *regional* and *developmental* changes in cerebral glucose utilization have been defined primarily in animals but also in human infants.[a] Thus, early in development, regional differences are relatively few, and brain stem structures

[a]References 25, 26, 28, 29, and 43-46.

generally exhibit the highest rates of glucose utilization. With development, increases in cerebral glucose utilization are most prominent, particularly in cerebral cortical regions. In the human infant, the developmental progression in the first year of life occurs first in the sensorimotor cortex and thalamus, next in the parietal, temporal, and occipital cortices, and last in the frontal cortex and association areas.[44,45] Careful studies in animals, focused primarily on electrophysiological maturation of the brain stem and diencephalic structures, showed a close correlation between increases in rates of glucose utilization and the acquisition of neuronal function.[28]

Additional compelling evidence for the obligatory role of glucose in the developing brain emanates from studies of human newborns by PET. Thus values for cerebral metabolic rate for oxygen in the brain of premature and term infants are only 3% and 28%, respectively, of the adult values.[47] One reasonable conclusion from these data is that glucose is critical for energy production in the brain, especially in the premature infant. The data raise the possibility that anaerobic glucose utilization is important in the neonatal brain, and because energy production is markedly less with anaerobic versus aerobic metabolism (see Chapter 13), glucose *delivery* to the brain is critical for energy production in the neonatal brain, especially in the premature infant.

Alternative Substrates for Glucose in Brain Metabolism

Overview

Although glucose is the primary metabolic fuel for the brain, it is apparent that certain other substrates can also be used for energy production and other metabolic purposes. Under normal circumstances, such alternative substrates are probably not of major importance for energy production. However, under conditions in which glucose is limited (e.g., hypoglycemia), alternative substrates may spare brain function and structure. Substances such as lactate, pyruvate, free fatty acids, glycerol, a variety of ketoacids (i.e., ketone bodies), and certain amino acids have been shown to be capable of partially or wholly supporting respiration of *brain tissue slices* and related in vitro systems.[a] Certain of these substrates are produced *in the brain* during hypoglycemia (e.g., amino acids from the degradation of protein and fatty acids from the degradation of phospholipid) and are potentially utilizable as alternative energy sources (see later discussion). Clearly, however, these latter alternative substrates are not optimal because their sources (i.e., proteins and phospholipids) are largely structural components, and conservation of energy production at the cost of brain structure is not a desirable adaptive response. Moreover, because most of the systemically produced alternative substrates noted either do not appear in appreciable quantities in blood or are not capable of crossing the blood-brain barrier to a major extent, they can contribute relatively little to brain energy levels in hypoglycemia. The two substrates most often considered to be useful as primarily blood-borne, alternative sources of brain energy with hypoglycemia are ketone bodies and lactate; considerable data show evidence of their value for the support of oxidative metabolism in the neonatal brain.[3,26-29,50-56]

[a]References 6, 15, 27, 28, 48, and 49.

Ketone Bodies

Appreciable data have accumulated to suggest that ketone bodies may be used as alternative substrates for brain metabolism in the neonatal period. Ketone bodies are taken up by the brain by a carrier-mediated transport system and are subsequently used according to the reactions outlined in Fig. 25.6.[28,57,58]

Energy Production. Studies of *newborn infants* have demonstrated that the cerebral extraction of ketone bodies from blood is markedly greater in the newborn than it is in older infants and adults.[28,59] Associated with this finding is an enhanced rate of ketone body utilization in the newborn brain. Thus it was shown that ketone bodies account for approximately 12% of total cerebral oxygen consumption in newborns subjected to 6-hour fasts. An enhanced capacity to use ketone bodies was also demonstrated in the *human fetal brain*.[60] These data indicate relevance for animal studies that demonstrate relatively high activities for the enzymes involved in ketone body utilization in the immature versus the mature brain.[61,62] These enzymatic activities have also been demonstrated in the human fetal brain.[62]

Thus the newborn brain, at least under conditions of brief fasting, normally satisfies a small portion of its energy demands by the conversion of ketone bodies to acetyl-CoA, which then proceeds through the citric acid cycle (see Fig. 25.5). Whether ketone bodies satisfy a greater portion of cerebral energy demands when glucose is deficient is a separate issue and not so readily demonstrated (see later). As noted previously, recent evidence suggests that neonatal hypoglycemia within the first 48 hours appears to be a hypoketotic state, with varying levels of lactate and detectable insulin levels in many infants. This suggests that during this early time frame lactate may be more important than ketones as alternative energy source to glucose.[3] Moreover, experimental data in the newborn dog do not support an important role for ketone bodies in this context (see later discussion).[26,39]

Limitations of Hepatic Ketone Synthesis. Utilization of ketone bodies as alternative substrates for glucose in brain energy production under conditions of glucose deprivation depends on the capacity of the liver to deliver these compounds to the blood. Data obtained in human newborn infants suggest that hepatic ketone synthesis is restricted during the early neonatal period.[14] The findings demonstrate (1) low levels of ketone bodies, (2) failure of ketone bodies to rise with fasting (in contrast to fasting in older children), and (3) failure of ketone bodies to rise with hypoglycemia (Table 25.2). In a subsequent study, relatively low plasma concentrations of ketone bodies were also documented with formula feeding.[63] Because cerebral utilization of ketone bodies linearly depends on plasma concentrations,[63] these data from studies of human infants suggest that *limitations of hepatic ketone synthesis* prevent a major role for these materials as alternative metabolic substrates in the brains of human infants with hypoglycemia. *However, these data do not rule out the possibility that exogenous administration of ketone bodies or of exogenous sources of ketone bodies (e.g., fatty acids) could serve as alternative metabolic substrates.* One report demonstrated cerebral uptake of exogenously administered beta-hydroxybutyrate for the management of hypoglycemic infants in the first year of life.[64]

TABLE 25.2 Failure of Ketone Bodies to Increase in Blood With Hypoglycemia

INFANTS	KETONE BODIES (mmol/L)	
	BETA-HYDROXYBUTYRATE	ACETOACETATE
Normoglycemic, term, AGA	0.31 ± 0.04	0.06 ± 0.01
Hypoglycemic, term, AGA	0.16 ± 0.03	0.02 ± 0.01
Hypoglycemic, SGA	0.24 ± 0.07	0.03 ± 0.01

AGA, Appropriate for gestational age; *SGA*, small for gestational age.
Data from Stanley CA, Anday EK, Baker L, Delivoria-Papadopoulos M. Metabolic fuel and hormone responses to fasting in newborn infants. *Pediatrics.* 1979;64:613–619.

TABLE 25.3 Lactate as Important Alternative Substrate for Brain Energy Production With Hypoglycemia in the Newborn Dog

BLOOD GLUCOSE[a]	SOURCE OF CEREBRAL ENERGY REQUIREMENTS		
	GLUCOSE	LACTATE	BETA-HYDROXYBUTYRATE
Normoglycemia	95%	4%	<1%
Hypoglycemia (13 mg/dL)	48%	52%	<1%
Hypoglycemia (5 mg/dL)	42%	56%	2%

[a]Two hours after injection of insulin (or placebo).
Data from Hernandez MJ, Vannucci RC, Salcedo A, Brennan RW. Cerebral blood flow and metabolism during hypoglycemia in newborn dogs. *J Neurochem.* 1980;35:622–628.

Lactate

Lactate as an important energy source in neonatal hypoglycemia was suggested by elegant experiments in the newborn dog.[a] Thus determinations of cerebral metabolic rates for oxygen, glucose, lactate, and beta-hydroxybutyrate were accomplished by measurements of CBF and cerebral arteriovenous differences of these compounds.[39] These data were then used to determine the relative proportions of cerebral energy requirements derived from glucose, lactate, and beta-hydroxybutyrate under conditions of normoglycemia and insulin-induced hypoglycemia (Table 25.3). During normoglycemia, the newborn dog obtained 95% of its cerebral energy requirements from glucose and only a small fraction from lactate (4%) and beta-hydroxybutyrate (<1%).[39] With hypoglycemia, in concert with the expected decline in cerebral utilization of glucose, a striking increase in lactate use was observed (see Table 25.3). (No appreciable change in the contribution of ketone body utilization was noted.) In subsequent experiments, no significant decrease in brain high-energy phosphate levels occurred under these conditions.[65,67] *Thus the data indicate that increased utilization of lactate spared brain energy levels under conditions of severe hypoglycemia.*

The *mechanisms* by which blood lactate leads to energy production in the brain probably include enhanced lactate uptake by the brain from blood and active oxidation to pyruvate by lactate dehydrogenase (see Fig. 25.5). Indeed, available data indicate that lactate uptake in newborn dogs occurs at a rate that exceeds that of adult dogs, even when arterial lactate concentrations are within or near the physiological range.[b] Concerning conversion of lactate to pyruvate, the activity of

lactate dehydrogenase in the brain of the perinatal animal has been shown to be relatively high.[28,69-71] Moreover, other data suggest that the neonatal brain may have a particular ability to use lactate as a brain energy source as an adaptation to the relative lactic acidemia in the first hours and days after birth.[39,72] Lactic acidemia related to the hypoxic stress of *normal* vaginal delivery has been documented in newborn rats and lambs.[26,28,73,74] These data also bear on the relative resistance of the neonatal versus the adult brain to hypoglycemic injury (see later). The sparing role of lactate in neonatal hypoglycemia requires further elucidation, but the data from studies of the newborn dog suggest that this role is considerable.

BIOCHEMICAL ASPECTS OF HYPOGLYCEMIA

The *pathophysiological aspects* of the encephalopathy caused by hypoglycemia are best considered in terms of the *initial* biochemical effects on brain metabolism, the *later* effects, and the *combined* effects of hypoglycemia with hypoxemia, ischemia, or seizures. These combined effects may be of major clinical relevance because hypoglycemia rarely occurs as an isolated neonatal event and also because hypoglycemia not severe enough to cause brain injury alone may attain that capacity when combined with certain other deleterious insults to brain metabolism.

Major Initial Biochemical Effects of Hypoglycemia on Brain Metabolism
Major Biochemical Changes

At the outset, it is crucial to recognize that *no* biochemical effects of hypoglycemia occur as long as the initial physiological response of *increased CBF* supplies sufficient glucose to the

---

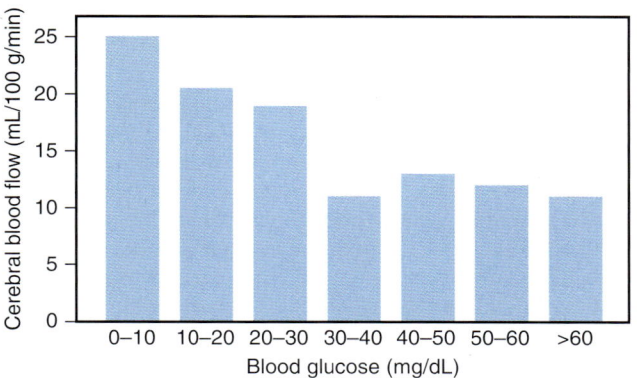

Figure 25.7 Cerebral blood flow as a function of blood glucose measured 2 hours after birth in 25 premature newborns. Cerebral blood flow was determined by xenon clearance. Note the increase in cerebral blood flow that begins with blood glucose lower than 30 mg/dL. (Values are means calculated and redrawn from data from Pryds O, Christensen NJ, Friis HB. Increased cerebral blood flow and plasma epinephrine in hypoglycemic, preterm neonates. *Pediatrics.* 1990;85:172–176.)

TABLE 25.4	Major Initial Biochemical Effects of Hypoglycemia on Brain Metabolism

- $\downarrow\downarrow$ Brain glucose
- $\uparrow$ Glycogen $\rightarrow$ glucose
- $\downarrow\downarrow$ CMR glucose
- $\pm\downarrow$ CMR oxygen
- $\pm\downarrow$ ATP, phosphocreatine
- $\uparrow$ CMR lactate
- $\downarrow$ Amino acids, $\uparrow$ ammonia
- ?$\uparrow$ Ketone body utilization
- $\downarrow$ Synthesis of acetylcholine

$\downarrow$, Decreased; $\downarrow\downarrow$, moderately decreased; $\uparrow$, increased; $\rightarrow$, conversion to; $\pm$, with or without; *ATP*, adenosine triphosphate; *CMR*, cerebral metabolic rate.

brain. This initial hyperemic response, first described in adult models of hypoglycemia,[27] was documented in neonatal animal models[74,76] and human infants.[18,77-79] The marked increase in CBF begins in the human infant when blood glucose declines to less than approximately 30 mg/dL (Fig. 25.7). Studies of changes in cerebral blood volume, measured continuously in preterm infants by near-infrared spectroscopy (see Chapter 11), suggested that previously unperfused capillaries are recruited to maintain glucose levels in the brain with hypoglycemia.[79] However, clearly with marked decreases in cerebral glucose delivery (e.g., because of marked decreases in blood glucose or impaired CBF, or both) or with marked increases in cerebral glucose utilization (e.g., because of seizure), biochemical derangements begin.

The major *initial* biochemical effects of hypoglycemia on brain metabolism are summarized in Table 25.4.[a] The principal consequences involve cerebral glucose metabolism and the metabolic attempts to preserve cerebral energy status by use of alternatives to glucose. Sharp falls in brain glucose

concentrations are expected. Glycogenolysis responds in an attempt to restore some of the brain's supply of glucose. Nevertheless, the result is a sharp decrease in the cerebral metabolic rate for glucose. However, an important feature of hypoglycemia, noted in 1948 in humans[88] and subsequently studied in more detail in experimental animals,[26,81,85] is a disproportionately smaller disturbance of the cerebral metabolic rate for oxygen. Indeed, in neonatal animals, cerebral metabolic rates of oxygen tend to be unchanged.[26,39] This discrepancy between the cerebral utilization of glucose and that of oxygen implies that the brain's energy needs are being met by alternative substrates to glucose (see next paragraph). Indeed, except in very severe hypoglycemia, significant declines in high-energy phosphate levels in the brain are not consistent initial features.

The preservation of oxidative metabolism and high-energy phosphate levels in the brain despite the decrease in cerebral glucose metabolic rate presumably relates to the use of alternative substrates (see Table 25.4). The major substrates considered are lactate, ketone bodies, and amino acids. As noted previously, *lactate* is the most likely candidate as the *major* alternative substrate for maintenance of the brain's oxidative metabolism during hypoglycemia, and the increase in its rate of utilization in the newborn dog with hypoglycemia is sufficient to account for preservation of the cerebral metabolic rate for oxygen and of tissue levels of high-energy phosphate compounds (see Table 25.3). The possibility of increased *ketone body* utilization as an additional alternative energy source is suggested by data in adult and young (not newborn) animals.[85,89] However, as described earlier, direct measurements of ketone body utilization in the hypoglycemic newborn dog did not suggest that ketone bodies are important alternative substrates, at least in that insulin-induced model.[26,28,39] Other alternative substrates for glucose or energy production or both are *amino acids*. Indeed, a sharp decrease in brain concentrations of most, although not all, amino acids occurs, with a consequent increase in brain ammonia levels (through transamination and deamination reactions; see Table 25.4 and subsequent discussion).

Dissociation of Impaired Brain Function and Energy Metabolism

Changes in brain energy metabolism do not clearly explain the striking changes in clinical signs and the electroencephalographic (EEG) activity of the brain during the initial phases of hypoglycemia. Thus, although findings differ qualitatively if newborn or adult animals are studied, in general the evolution with hypoglycemia of clinical changes from an alert state to a depressed level of consciousness (and even to seizures) and of EEG changes from normal activity to slowing (and even to burst-suppression patterns and seizure discharges) occurs *with no definite change in ATP levels* in the whole brain or the cerebral cortex and several other brain regions.[a] In many respects, this dissociative phenomenon is similar to that observed in the initial phases of hypoxic–ischemic insults (see Chapter 13). It is unclear whether this occurrence is an adaptive phenomenon (i.e., when faced with an imminent power failure, the brain curtails neuronal activity), perhaps to conserve energy stores.

The *mechanism* by which the dissociation of functional and electrical activity of the brain from brain energy levels

[a]References 26, 27, 29, 37, 39, 56, 65, and 80-87.

[a]References 26, 27, 29, 37, 39, 56, 80-82, and 85-87.

occurs may relate to certain of the metabolic concomitants of hypoglycemia (see Table 25.4). Such concomitants could include alterations in relative amounts of excitatory and inhibitory amino acids, in tissue levels of ammonia, or in neurotransmitter metabolism. Indeed, the degradation of amino acids described earlier results in an increase in levels of *brain ammonia* that are considered potentially sufficient to produce stupor in adult hypoglycemic animals.[85] Whether such levels are generated in newborn animals is unknown. Data in mature rats rendered hypoglycemic demonstrated that *impaired synthesis of acetylcholine* (see Table 25.4) occurs in the first minutes after onset of hypoglycemia.[90] Indeed, only modest decreases in plasma glucose levels caused 20% to 45% decreases in concentrations of acetylcholine and 40% to 60% decreases in the synthesis of this neurotransmitter in the cortex and striatum.[90] The likely mechanism of this disturbance relates to a decrease in synthesis of acetyl-CoA because of the drastic decrease in brain glucose and, as a consequence, glycolysis. Even with modest hypoglycemia, pyruvate concentrations in the brain decrease by 50% in minutes.[85] Data concerning acetylcholine synthesis in hypoglycemic *newborn animals* are lacking, but similar sharp decreases in brain glucose and pyruvate[65] levels suggest that the same impairment of acetylcholine synthesis is likely.

Major Later Biochemical Effects of Hypoglycemia on Brain Metabolism

Glucose and Energy Metabolism

The major *later* biochemical effects of hypoglycemia are summarized in Table 25.5. Because most of the available data have been derived from studies of mature animals and the limited data in newborn animals suggest some differences (although also many similarities) compared with mature animals, in the following discussion I review the major effects on the mature and immature nervous systems separately.

Biochemical Changes in the Mature Animal

Glucose and Energy Metabolism. The biochemical effects of severe or prolonged hypoglycemia include an accentuation of the changes described in the previous section as well as the addition of other effects (see Table 25.5). Thus the decreases in brain glucose level become very marked, the cerebral metabolic rate of glucose falls drastically, and a distinct decrease in cerebral

oxidative metabolism and in the synthesis of high-energy phosphate compounds becomes apparent.[a]

Metabolic Responses to Preserve Brain Energy Levels. To preserve brain energy levels, the use of endogenous amino acids—derived from protein degradation, glycolytic intermediates, and lactate—continues as described earlier for initial biochemical effects (glycogen is essentially exhausted by this time). Indeed, as a consequence of the use of amino acids, ammonia levels in the brain increase markedly (i.e., 10- to 15-fold). An additional metabolic response (i.e., phospholipid degradation with the generation of free fatty acids) becomes apparent. The free fatty acids become an energy source in severe hypoglycemia. However, the responses are insufficient in severe and prolonged hypoglycemia to prevent the onset of declines in levels of high-energy phosphate compounds in the brain and the occurrences of coma and an isoelectric EEG pattern.[27,85] At this point, an additional series of events develops.

Intracellular Calcium and Cell Injury With Hypoglycemia. At approximately the time of onset of EEG isoelectricity, striking changes in intracellular calcium (Ca^{2+}) and extracellular potassium (K^+) occur and appear to initiate a series of events that result in cell death.[27,29,83,93] Thus at this time the capacity of the neuron to maintain normal energy-dependent ionic gradients is lost, extracellular Ca^{2+} levels decrease abruptly by approximately 6-fold, and extracellular K^+ levels increase by approximately 14-fold. Movements of Ca^{2+} into the cell and of K^+ out of the cell account for these observations. The initiating event is probably failure of the energy-dependent sodium-K^+ (Na^+/K^+) pump, which extrudes Na^+ and retains K^+. With failure of this system, sodium accumulates intracellularly, K^+ is extruded, and sustained membrane depolarization occurs; the intracellular increase of Na^+ then leads to activation of the Na^+/Ca^{2+} exchange system and movement of Ca^{2+} intracellularly in exchange for Na^+. Additional crucial effects of this membrane depolarization are excessive release of excitatory amino acids from synaptic nerve endings and reduced reuptake secondary to failure of glutamate transport; the resulting extracellular accumulation of these excitatory neurotransmitters and consequent activation of glutamate receptors result in a variety of deleterious effects, including influx of Ca^{2+} (see later). Ca^{2+} also may accumulate intracellularly because of failure of energy-dependent Ca^{2+} transport mechanisms designed to maintain low cytosolic Ca^{2+} levels (see Chapter 13). The metabolic consequences of these ionic changes appear to be similar to those described in Chapter 13 concerning the mechanisms of cell death with oxygen deprivation. The importance of cytosolic Ca^{2+}-induced phospholipase activation (see Chapter 13) is emphasized by the observation of an abrupt decline in phospholipid concentration in the brain and a further elevation in free fatty acid concentration. The deleterious effects of arachidonate (e.g., generation of free radicals and harmful vasoactive compounds) are summarized in Chapter 13. Thus the final common pathway to neuronal injury in hypoglycemia may be very similar to that in oxygen deprivation and relates especially to the accumulation of cytosolic Ca^{2+}. Moreover, in hypoglycemia as in hypoxia-ischemia, *massive* depletion of

---

TABLE 25.5   Major Later Biochemical Effects of Hypoglycemia on Brain Metabolism

- ↓↓↓ Brain glucose
- ↓↓↓ CMR glucose
- ↓ CMR oxygen
- ↓ ATP, phosphocreatine
- ↑ CMR lactate
- ↓↓ Amino acids (except glutamate and aspartate), ↑ ammonia
- ↓ Phospholipids, ↑ free fatty acids
- ↑ Intracellular calcium, ↑ extracellular potassium
- ↑ Extracellular glutamate
- ↓ Glutathione, ↑ oxidative stress

↓, Decreased; ↓↓, moderately decreased; ↓↓↓, severely decreased; ↑, increased; *ATP*, adenosine triphosphate; *CMR*, cerebral metabolic rate.

---

[a]References 27, 29, 81, 83-85, 91, and 92.

TABLE 25.6 Cerebral Glucose, Pyruvate, Lactate, and High-Energy Phosphates With Hypoglycemia in the Newborn Dog

BLOOD GLUCOSE (mg/dL)[b]	CEREBRAL METABOLITE (PERCENTAGE OF CONTROL)[a]				
	GLUCOSE (%)	PYRUVATE (%)	LACTATE (%)	PHOSPHOCREATINE (%)	ATP (%)
20–30	9	86	69	91	93
10–20	1	35	45	98	100
<10	1	36	26	91	97

[a]All values for glucose, pyruvate, and lactate, but none for phosphocreatine and ATP, were statistically significant from control values.

[b]Two hours after insulin injection.

ATP, Adenosine triphosphate.

Data from Vannucci RC, Nardis EE, Vannucci SJ, Campbell PA. Cerebral carbohydrate and energy metabolism during hypoglycemia in newborn dogs. *Am J Physiol.* 1981;240:R192–R199.

high-energy phosphate compounds does not appear to be an obligatory event in producing cell death.

Role of Excitotoxic Amino Acids in Hypoglycemic Neuronal Death.

As discussed in Chapter 13, considerable data indicate that the mechanism of cell death with hypoxia-ischemia is mediated by the extracellular accumulation of excitatory amino acids, which are toxic in high concentrations. *It now appears likely that excitatory amino acids play a major role in the mediation of neuronal death with hypoglycemia.* Evidence in support of this conclusion includes the demonstration of a rise in extracellular concentrations of excitatory amino acids (aspartate and glutamate) in advanced hypoglycemia and an attenuation of neuronal injury by simultaneous administration of antagonists of the *N*-methyl-D-aspartate (NMDA) type of glutamate receptor, both in in vivo models in cultured neurons.[27,29,91,93-100] These observations suggest that the Ca^{2+} accumulation and Ca^{2+}-mediated deleterious events, noted in the previous section and described in detail in Chapter 13, including especially the generation of reactive oxygen and nitrogen species, are intertwined with and provoked in considerable part by activation of the NMDA receptor, with the resulting influx of Ca^{2+} through the NMDA channel (as well as through voltage-dependent Ca^{2+} channels). The free radicals generated result in DNA damage and, as a consequence, the DNA repair enzyme poly(ADP-ribose) polymerase-1 (PARP). With excessive activation of PARP and, as a consequence, adenosine depletion, energy failure and activation of apoptosis occur.[100] PARP inhibitors have been shown to protect neurons from hypoglycemia in in vitro and in vivo experimental models.[100] Thus the data concerning excitotoxicity and the prevention thereof raise interesting new therapeutic possibilities for the prevention or amelioration of hypoglycemic neuronal death—possibilities that exhibit analogies with potential therapies for ischemic neuronal death (see Chapter 13).

Biochemical Changes in the Newborn Animal

Similarities and Differences in Changes in the Newborn and Adult Brain. Many of the biochemical effects of hypoglycemia described earlier in the adult brain can be documented in the neonatal brain, such as sharp decreases in levels of glucose, diminished cerebral utilization of glucose, and diminished concentrations of glycolytic intermediates (see

Table 25.5).[a] However, *certain metabolic differences* from the changes observed in the adult brain are prominent (e.g., preservation of phosphocreatine and ATP levels despite severe decreases in glucose levels and markedly greater utilization of lactate as an alternative substrate for energy metabolism). The data contained in Table 25.6 show that hypoglycemia severe enough to deplete brain of glucose almost entirely is accompanied by some preservation of such glycolytic intermediates as pyruvate and lactate and, most strikingly, by complete preservation of phosphocreatine and ATP levels. Indeed, hypoglycemia of comparable severity in the adult animal causes marked reductions in the levels of phosphocreatine and ATP in the brain.[84,85]

The relative preservation of the energy status of a brain with severe hypoglycemia in the newborn animal is accompanied by a similar *preservation of neurological function and electrical activity.* Thus, in the adult rat, insulin-induced hypoglycemia to plasma glucose values of approximately 35 mg/dL resulted in prominent slowing on the EEG tracing, and plasma glucose values of approximately 30 mg/dL resulted in lethargy and markedly slow activity on the EEG tracing.[84,85] Prolongation of this degree of hypoglycemia for approximately 1 hour resulted in coma and an isoelectric EEG pattern.[84,85] These latter states were attained in less time in the adult animals when plasma glucose levels were reduced to 10 to 15 mg/dL.[84] In contrast, in the newborn rat rendered hypoglycemic to a plasma glucose level of approximately 15 mg/dL, no change in neurological function could be observed over 2 hours.[82] In the newborn dog, prominent slow activity on the EEG tracing was observed only at plasma glucose levels lower than approximately 20 mg/dL. Moreover, at plasma glucose values of approximately 10 to 15 mg/dL (i.e., levels sufficient to cause an isoelectric EEG pattern in the adult dog), considerable electrical activity, albeit slow, was apparent in the newborn dog.[65] Indeed, at this level, seizure discharges often became apparent, and the accompanying respiratory failure and cardiovascular collapse could result in death of the animal.[65]

Reasons for the Relative Resistance of the Newborn Brain to Hypoglycemia. The data reviewed demonstrate clearly a

---

[a]References 26, 29, 39, 65, 82, and 99.

TABLE 25.7   Major Reasons for the Relative Resistance of the Newborn Animal to Hypoglycemia

- Diminished cerebral energy utilization
- Increased cerebral blood flow with even moderate hypoglycemia
- Increased cerebral uptake and utilization of lactate
- Resistance of the heart to hypoglycemia

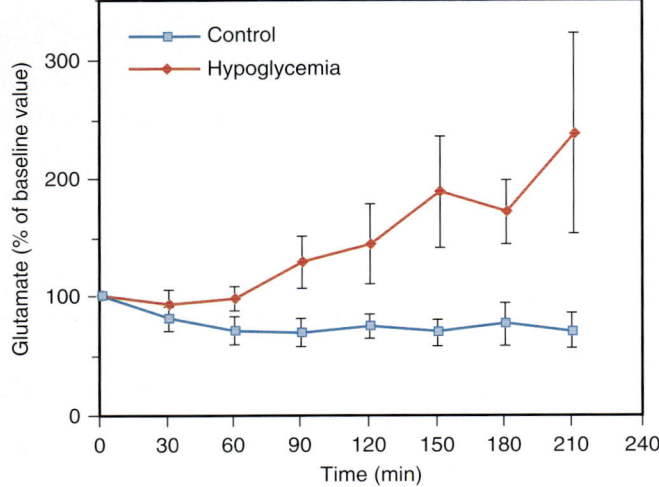

Figure 25.8 Increase in extracellular glutamate with hypoglycemia in the immature rat. The striatal glutamate efflux (i.e., extracellular glutamate) in control ($n = 6$) and hypoglycemic ($n = 6$) postnatal day 7 rats was determined by microdialysis. Hypoglycemia was produced by insulin injection. In hypoglycemic animals, the striatal glutamate efflux increased gradually and peaked at 240% of control values. (From Silverstein FS, Simpson J, Gordon KE. Hypoglycemia alters striatal amino acid efflux in perinatal rats: an in vivo microdialysis study. *Ann Neurol.* 1990;28:516–521.)

relative resistance of the newborn versus the adult animal to the deleterious effects of hypoglycemia. The major reasons for this relative resistance are shown in Table 25.7. Of particular importance is the lower cerebral energy requirement in the immature brain with the consequently *lower rate of energy utilization*. This situation, discussed in Chapter 13 concerning the relative resistance of the perinatal brain to hypoxic injury, presumably relates first to the less developed dendritic-axonal ramifications and synaptic connections and, as a consequence, energy-dependent ion pumping and neurotransmitter synthesis. However, the relatively advanced dendritic development and synaptogenesis in the occipital cortex of the human newborn may explain the predominance of occipital involvement observed on magnetic resonance imaging (MRI) of hypoglycemic newborns (see later). The second reason for the relative resistance of the newborn animal and human to hypoglycemia relates to the *marked increase in CBF* provoked by even moderate hypoglycemia. As noted earlier, blood glucose levels lower than 30 mg/dL in the human newborn are associated with prominent increases in CBF. In mature animals, severe hypoglycemia is required to lead to increases in CBF. The third reason for the relative resistance to hypoglycemia presumably relates to an *increased capacity for both cerebral uptake and utilization of lactate for brain energy production* (see previous discussion of alternative substrates).[26,28,39,67] Fourth, severe hypoglycemia does not have as profound an effect on cardiovascular function in the newborn as in the adult animal.[65] The *relative resistance of the immature heart* relates to its rich endogenous carbohydrate stores (glucose and glycogen), which can be mobilized for energy during hypoglycemia, and the capacity of the immature heart to use fuels other than glucose for energy.[101,102] Thus, although it is clear that more data are needed concerning the impact of hypoglycemia on the neonatal brain, current information suggests that cerebral and myocardial metabolic capacities provide remarkable degrees of resistance.

Role for Excitotoxic Amino Acids in Hypoglycemic Neuronal Death.

A possible role for excitatory amino acids in hypoglycemic neuronal death with severe hypoglycemia in neonatal animals, as in mature animals (see earlier discussion), is suggested by studies of severe insulin-induced hypoglycemia in 7-day-old rats.[103] Thus insulin-induced hypoglycemia caused an increase in striatal extracellular glutamate, measured by microdialysis, with the onset of the increase at blood glucose levels of 20 mg/dL (Fig. 25.8). After $3\frac{1}{2}$ hours of hypoglycemia (terminal glucose level of < 5 mg/dL), striatal glutamate was approximately 2.4-fold higher than baseline levels. The increased extracellular glutamate may be caused by failure of high-affinity glutamate uptake mechanisms or by increased release (secondary to synaptic release provoked by membrane depolarization [resulting from Na^+ or Ca^{2+} influx] or by reversal of the Na^+-dependent glutamate transport system [resulting from increased intracellular Na^+], or by both mechanisms). The potential consequence would be excitotoxic neuronal death by the mechanisms described in Chapter 13. Prevention of neuronal death in organotypic hippocampal cultures derived from newborn rat brains and maintained in the absence of glucose by the NMDA receptor antagonist MK-801 also illustrates the importance of excitotoxic mechanisms in hypoglycemic neuronal death.[97] The prevention of neuronal death by addition of the antagonist 30 minutes *after* the insult may have important therapeutic implications. The increase in apparent affinity of the NMDA receptor observed in the hypoglycemic piglet suggests that the excitotoxic potential of glutamate may be enhanced by hypoglycemia.[99]

Glutathione Depletion and Oxidative Stress.

A role for oxidative stress in hypoglycemic cell death was suggested by studies of cultured neural cells and a newborn piglet model.[104,105] In cultured cells, glucose deprivation caused a decrease in glutathione levels and then cell death. Glucose is involved in the production of reduced glutathione by generating reducing equivalents and providing a carbon source required for biosynthesis of this critical antioxidant. That the cell death in the studies of cultured glial cells was mediated by oxidative stress and free radical attack was shown by the demonstration of protection by free radical scavengers. Because Ca^{2+} influx and glutamate receptor activation in neurons may lead to the generation of free radicals (see Chapter 13), the deleterious effect of reduced glutathione levels could be critical in the final common pathway to cell death with hypoglycemia. Studies of the hypoglycemic newborn piglet showed markedly elevated mitochondrial production of reactive oxygen species.[104] The demonstration that brain-derived neurotrophic factor (BDNF)

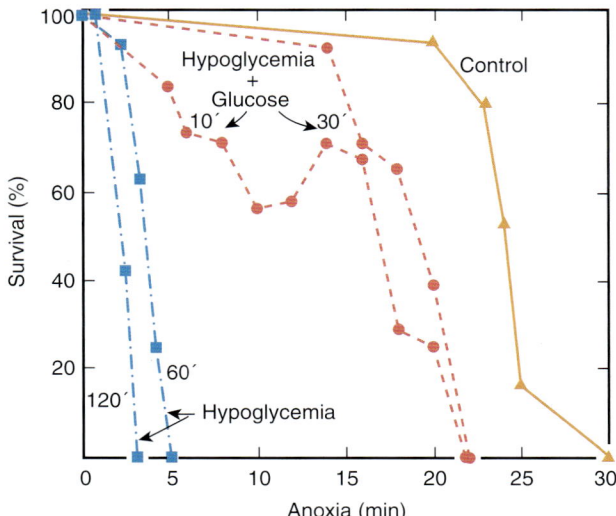

Figure 25.9 Deleterious effect of hypoglycemia on vulnerability to anoxia (nitrogen breathing). The percentage of survival of newborn rats was determined as a function of duration of anoxia. Hypoglycemia was produced by insulin injection 1 to 2 hours before the onset of anoxia; some hypoglycemic animals were pretreated with glucose (1.8 g/kg, subcutaneously) either 10 or 30 minutes before anoxia. (From Vannucci RC, Vannucci SJ. Cerebral carbohydrate metabolism during hypoglycemia and anoxia in newborn rats. *Ann Neurol.* 1978;4:73–79.)

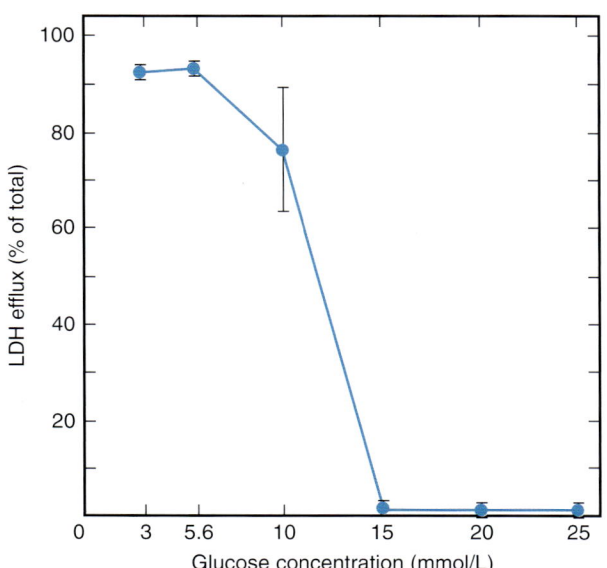

Figure 25.10 Beneficial effect of glucose on hypoxia-induced cellular injury in differentiating glial cells, primarily astrocytes. Cellular injury was determined by measurement of efflux of lactate dehydrogenase (LDH) from the damaged cells. Primary glial cell cultures were grown for 18 days, when differentiation was active, and subjected to hypoxia, with the indicated concentrations of glucose in the culture medium. (From Callahan DJ, Engle MJ, Volpe JJ. Hypoxic injury to developing glial cells: protective effect of high glucose. *Pediatr Res.* 1990;27:186–190.)

protected cultured neurons from hypoglycemic injury further suggests a role for oxidative stress because BDNF induces antioxidant systems.[106]

Hypoglycemia and Hypoxemia or Asphyxia

Hypoglycemia and Hypoxemia

The vulnerability of the immature brain to hypoxemic injury is enhanced by concomitant hypoglycemia, an observation first made in 1942.[107] Studies of cerebral carbohydrate metabolism during hypoxemia and hypoglycemia in newborn rats have provided further insight into the mechanism of this effect.[26,82] Thus newborn rats subjected to hypoxemia by breathing 100% nitrogen exhibited greater mortality rates when they were also subjected to insulin-induced hypoglycemia (Fig. 25.9). Indeed, animals rendered hypoglycemic for 1 hour experienced a fivefold reduction in survival ability, and those hypoglycemic for 2 hours did even worse. Supplementation of hypoglycemic animals with glucose before anoxia improved outcome (see Fig. 25.9). Animals rendered hypoglycemic as well as hypoxemic exhibited less accumulation of lactate in the brain and a faster decline in cerebral energy reserves (ATP and phosphocreatine) than those rendered hypoxemic alone. Moreover, glucose supplementation ameliorated the adverse metabolic effects. The mechanism for the enhanced deleterious effect of hypoxemia when hypoglycemia was associated appeared to relate to a diminution in brain glucose reserves and thus retarded glycolytic flux. The improvement with glucose supplementation supports this notion.

Studies of cultured immature glial cells are relevant to the adverse effect of the combination of hypoxemia and hypoglycemia. Thus not only are immature astrocytes more vulnerable to glucose deprivation than are mature glial cells[108] but also, of special interest in this context, glucose deprivation

markedly accentuates the vulnerability of differentiating glial cells to oxygen deprivation (Fig. 25.10).[109] This effect of glucose deprivation on immature glial cells is apparent in both differentiating astrocytes and oligodendroglia.[109]

Hypoglycemia and Asphyxia

Study of the newborn dog has demonstrated the deleterious effect of hypoglycemia when combined with asphyxia.[26,67] Thus, to approximate clinical circumstances more closely (than the nitrogen breathing of the experiments just described), neonatal dogs were asphyxiated with and without prior induction of hypoglycemia to plasma glucose levels of approximately 20 mg/dL. The data showed striking worsening of the cerebral metabolic effects of asphyxia in animals rendered hypoglycemic versus those that were normoglycemic. Thus, whereas in normoglycemic animals levels of glycolytic substrates subsequent to the phosphofructokinase step increased secondary to the expected acceleration of anaerobic glycolysis, in hypoglycemic animals no such increase occurred, in keeping with a failure of enhancement of anaerobic glycolysis. Moreover, whereas hypoglycemia alone resulted in little or no alteration in levels of high-energy phosphate compounds, when combined with asphyxia a drastic reduction in these compounds resulted. ATP levels declined with asphyxia by 61% in the hypoglycemic animals compared with only 13% in the normoglycemic animals. Thus the data extended the findings described earlier with the combination of hypoglycemia and hypoxemia and indicated that hypoglycemia combined with asphyxia leads to greater cerebral metabolic derangements than those observed with asphyxia alone.

A deleterious effect of hypoglycemia in the *postasphyxial* period was shown by studies of newborn lambs.[110] Here cerebral fractional oxygen extraction remained depressed relative to values in control or hyperglycemic animals for as long as 4 hours following termination of asphyxia (the last time point studied).

A study of 185 term infants with severe fetal acidemia (umbilical arterial pH < 7.00) suggested an important role for postasphyxial postnatal hypoglycemia in the genesis of brain injury.[111] Thus 27 (14.5%) of the 185 infants had an initial blood glucose level of 40 mg/dL or lower. Of these 27 infants, 56% (15) had an abnormal neurological outcome, whereas only 16% (26) of the 158 infants with a blood glucose level higher than 40 mg/dL had an abnormal outcome. Infants with abnormal outcomes and a blood glucose level of 40 mg/dL or lower did not appear to have sustained a more pronounced asphyxial insult because they had a higher cord pH (6.86 vs. 6.75) and lower base deficit (−19 vs. −23.8). By multivariate logistic analysis, initial blood glucose was significantly associated with abnormal outcome (odds ratio 18.5; 95% confidence interval [CI], 3.1 to 111.9). Consistent with these observations, recent MRI studies of infants with postasphyxial hypoxic-ischemic encephalopathy show more frequent and more severe brain injury in infants who had complicating hypoglycemia postnatally than in those who did not.[112-114]

Summary

Taken together, these observations demonstrate that hypoglycemia potentiates the deleterious effects of hypoxemia or asphyxia on the newborn mammalian brain, including the human brain, and that such deleterious effects are potentiated also in the postasphyxial period by hypoglycemia. These findings may have major clinical relevance (see later). Indeed, these insults frequently occur together in the clinical arena (see later discussion), and they raise the possibility that degrees of hypoxemia or asphyxia or both *and* hypoglycemia, which alone would not cause brain injury, may do so when acting in concert.

Hypoglycemia and Ischemia
Enhanced Vulnerability of the Hypoglycemic Brain to Ischemic Insult

The vulnerability of the brains of *mature animals* to ischemic insult is enhanced by concomitant hypoglycemia.[115] Increases of mortality, acute neurological phenomena (e.g., seizures), and neurological deficits in survivors were apparent in the hypoglycemic versus normoglycemic animals. The mechanism of this effect presumably was similar to that just described; that is, diminished glucose reserves in the hypoglycemic brain were unable to maintain the accelerated glycolytic flux necessary to maintain cerebral energy reserves under anaerobic (ischemic) conditions. (Recall the 19-fold difference in ATP production from glucose metabolism under anaerobic versus aerobic conditions; see Chapter 13.)

The *degree of ischemia* is important in the enhancement of vulnerability of hypoglycemic brain to ischemia. Thus, with only moderate hypotension in the mature rat (blood pressure reduced to 60 mm Hg), although energy failure was enhanced in hypoglycemic brain, neuronal necrosis was not accentuated.[116]

Data relative to *neonatal animals* also suggest a crucial role for blood glucose in the determination of ischemic brain injury. Thus studies of 7-day-old rats subjected to hypoxic-ischemic insult showed an increase in mitochondrial oxidation in contrast to the decrease observed in the adult brain. This observation indicates a disturbance in the immature brain of glucose influx and utilization, the major source of mitochondrial reducing equivalents.[117] Hypoglycemia presumably would accentuate this disturbance. Direct demonstration of the deleterious additional effect of hypoglycemia in neonatal hypoxia-ischemia was shown in the 7-day-old rat pup.[118] Thus Yager and co-workers subjected the pups to hypoglycemia by fasting or insulin injection before inducing hypoxia-ischemia. Although the hypoglycemia was relatively mild (i.e., 5.4, 4.3, and 3.4 mmol/L for control, insulin-injected, and fasting animals, respectively), the brain injury was accentuated in the insulin-injected animals. The fasted animals had the least damage, apparently because of enhanced ketogenesis exhibited by this group. Finally, studies in an excellent ischemic model of cerebral white matter injury in a preterm fetal sheep model showed a striking inverse relation between blood glucose level and degree of ischemic injury.[119]

Observations relative to the *neonatal human* that suggest an enhanced vulnerability to ischemic injury with hypoglycemia are derived from studies of infants with hypoplastic left heart syndrome.[120] Thus periventricular leukomalacia, an ischemic lesion (see Chapter 14), occurred particularly in infants with decreased blood glucose as well as with the presumed ischemia associated with this severe cardiac lesion. In the previously noted MRI studies of asphyxiated human newborns, cerebral white matter injury is also a prominent feature.[112-114] In the immature rat with hypoglycemia, of all brain regions, cerebral white matter showed the poorest compensatory increase in blood flow and the greatest reduction in cerebral metabolic rate for glucose.[75]

Impaired Vascular Autoregulation and the Likelihood of Ischemic Insult in Hypoglycemia

The enhanced vulnerability of the hypoglycemic brain to major ischemic insult, as just described, is particularly important because of the likelihood of ischemia to certain brain regions during hypoglycemia with only moderate hypotension. This likelihood relates to the impairment of vascular autoregulation that has been documented with hypoglycemia in experimental studies.[26,27,75,121,122] A tissue autoradiographic technique was used initially to measure regional CBF in 25 brain structures in the hypoglycemic rat. Siesjo and co-workers[122] observed diminutions in CBF with only moderate hypotension (mean arterial blood pressure of 80 mm Hg; i.e., impaired autoregulation) in several brain regions. The latter included the cerebral cortex, hippocampus, and thalamus, each of which exhibits particular vulnerability to hypoglycemic neuronal injury. The regional decreases in blood flow were to values as low as 10% of control values. In separate experiments, diminutions in CBF with hypoglycemia and moderate hypotension were shown to enhance the deterioration of cerebral energy state and, as a consequence, to enhance K^+ release from cerebral cortical cells.[123,124] The mechanism of the effect of hypoglycemia on autoregulation remains to be defined. (A disturbance in the synthesis of a neurotransmitter [acetylcholine?] involved in the regulation of local cerebrovascular tone seems possible.) The effect of hypoglycemia in the mature animal on cerebrovascular reactivity is not confined to autoregulation and indeed includes reactivity to arterial carbon dioxide pressure and a variety of pharmacological vasodilators and vasoconstrictors.[125]

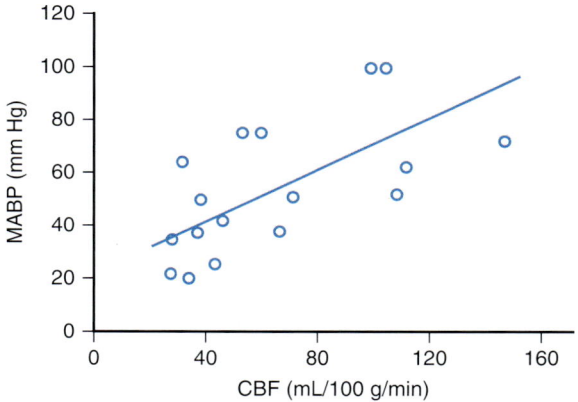

120
100
80
60
40
20
0

MABP (mm Hg)

0   40   80   120   160
CBF (mL/100 g/min)

Figure 25.11 Correlation of cerebral blood flow (CBF) with mean arterial blood pressure (MABP). A pressure-passive relationship exists between CBF and MABP in the newborn dog during hypoglycemia. (From Anwar M, Vannucci RC. Autoradiographic determination of regional cerebral blood flow during hypoglycemia in newborn dogs. *Pediatr Res.* 1988;24:41–45.)

A decisive demonstration of the impairment of cerebrovascular autoregulation with hypoglycemia was made in the newborn dog (Fig. 25.11).[81] The mechanism of this effect in the neonate, as in the adult animal, is unclear.[125]

Summary

The observations reviewed indicate that the cerebral metabolic and vascular derangements caused by hypoglycemia render the brain more susceptible to ischemic insults. Thus major brain ischemia would be expected to result in greater brain injury with hypoglycemia than with normoglycemia. Perhaps more important, the data indicate that ischemia to certain brain regions is particularly likely to occur with even *moderate* hypotension because of the impairment in cerebrovascular autoregulation. The observations emphasize the importance of controlling both circulatory function in hypoglycemic infants and glucose homeostasis in infants experiencing or at risk for ischemic insults to the brain. Moreover, as with hypoxemia and asphyxia, the data suggest the clinically important possibility that degrees of ischemia and hypoglycemia that alone would not cause brain injury might do so when acting together.

Hypoglycemia and Seizures

Consideration of the effects of seizures on cerebral glucose and energy metabolism (see Chapter 12) leads to the prediction that hypoglycemia would be deleterious in the presence of seizures. Thus seizures are associated with accelerated energy utilization (secondary to the increased neuronal activity and energy-dependent ion pumping), which leads to a severalfold increase in the rate of glucose utilization. The resulting increased demand for glucose produces a diminution in brain glucose concentrations despite the maintenance of normal blood glucose concentrations. Therefore, if supplies of glucose in the brain during seizures decrease further because of hypoglycemia, a serious deficit of cerebral energy reserves may be expected to occur particularly rapidly. Earlier studies of paralyzed, ventilated mature rats subjected to bicuculline-induced seizures and concomitant hypoglycemia by starvation demonstrated this deficit.[126] *An additional abnormality* in the hypoglycemic convulsing animals was *a decrease in CBF*, in contrast to an increase in CBF in the convulsing, normoglycemic animals. This decrease in CBF is obviously particularly serious in a situation such as repetitive seizures, in which the supply of exogenous substrate is already limiting for cerebral metabolism. The cause of the decrease in CBF was unclear, although a combination of myocardial dysfunction and impairment of autoregulation could be important (see earlier discussion).

Studies in *newborn monkeys and puppies* also indicated a deleterious effect of the combination of hypoglycemia and seizures.[127-129] Thus, in the newborn puppy, more severe decreases in cerebral high-energy phosphate compounds occurred with the combination of seizures and hypoglycemia than with hypoglycemia, as just described. Indeed, decreases in blood glucose levels not sufficient to lead to a decrease in phosphocreatine levels resulted in significant decreases when seizures were added.[127] In the newborn monkey, repeated seizures resulted in virtual total depletion of brain glucose and marked depletion of high-energy phosphate levels, and glucose supplementation was required to prevent these changes.[128,129]

The aforementioned data underscore the *importance of controlling seizures in infants with accompanying hypoglycemia.* Moreover, they emphasize the necessity of monitoring glucose homeostasis in any infant exhibiting seizures and again raise the possibility that degrees of hypoglycemia and seizure activity, which alone would not cause brain injury, may do so when acting in concert.

NEUROPATHOLOGY

Definition of the neuropathology of neonatal hypoglycemia has been made particularly difficult by the almost invariable association of other insults, especially hypoxia-ischemia, that also cause brain injury. Nevertheless, data from studies of animals, including subhuman primates as well as from the few reports of affected human newborns, lead to several conclusions. *First*, hypoglycemia, if severe or prolonged, results in injury to neurons primarily but also to glia. *Second*, the topography of the injury is somewhat different from that observed with hypoxic-ischemic injury. *Third*, when associated with other insults to the brain (e.g., hypoxia-ischemia), hypoglycemia of a degree not sufficient to cause brain injury alone can probably play an important contributory role in the genesis of neuronal injury.

Experimental Observations

A distinct correlation between the severity and duration of hypoglycemia and the occurrence of brain injury was demonstrated in studies of monkeys subjected to insulin-induced hypoglycemia with carefully maintained ventilation, perfusion, and temperature.[130,131] Thus the brain of the adolescent monkey subjected to blood glucose levels of less than 20 mg/dL for more than 2 hours usually exhibited neuropathological aberrations. Of 10 such animals, 6 exhibited cerebral cortical injury, whereas of 4 animals subjected to this degree of hypoglycemia for less than 2 hours, only 1 exhibited cerebral cortical injury. The brain injury involved neurons particularly, and the areas especially vulnerable were *cerebral cortex, mainly the parieto-occipital region.* Less commonly involved were neurons of the hippocampus, the caudate nucleus, and the putamen. Detailed studies in the mature rat indicated that the neuronal injury with hypoglycemia is particularly pronounced

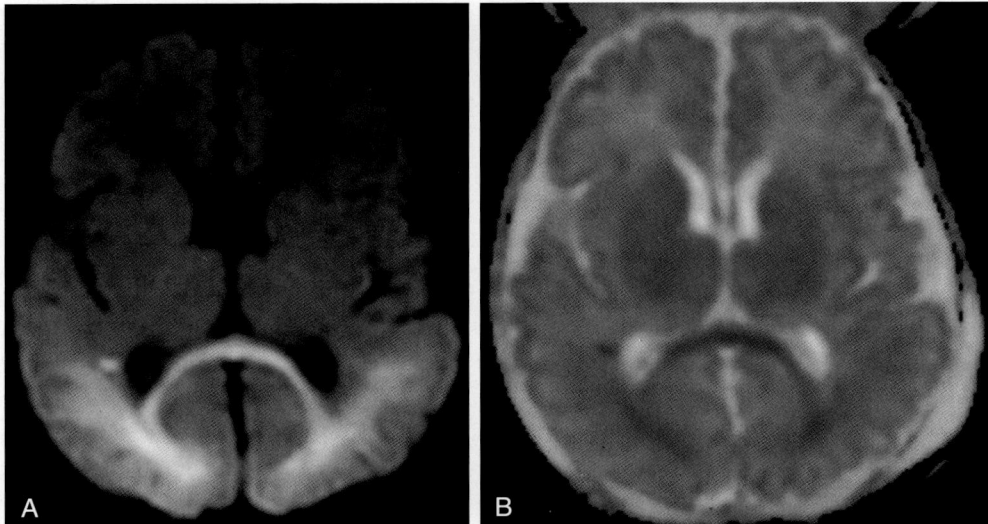

Figure 25.12 Structural changes with neonatal hypoglycemia, studied by computed tomography and magnetic resonance imaging (MRI) in a term infant. A MRI scan from a term infant with Apgar scores of 9 and 9 at 1 and 5 minutes who was found unresponsive at 36 hours, with hypothermia and hypoglycemia (blood sugar 17 mg/dL). B, The diffusion-weighted image (DWI) shows restricted diffusion predominantly involving the occipital lobe and noted on the corresponding apparent diffusion coefficient (ADC) map.

in regions contiguous to cerebrospinal fluid, such as superficial cerebral cortical layers.[27,116,132-134] This observation suggested that the agent causing the neuronal death is derived from the extracellular space, and the evidence, described earlier, that excitotoxic amino acids are involved in the neuronal death is relevant in this context. Moreover, the neuropathological demonstration that the early lesion in hypoglycemic neuronal injury involves dendrites also is consistent with an excitotoxic mechanism.

Limited data are available concerning the potentiating deleterious effects of hypoglycemia and ischemia. However, a single well-studied monkey that experienced a degree of hypoglycemia (no time when blood glucose level fell to < 20 mg/dL) and of moderate hypotension, either of which alone not sufficient to cause brain injury, demonstrated striking neuronal injury in the border zone distribution between the middle cerebral and anterior cerebral arteries.[130,131] This pattern of injury is characteristic of marked falls in cerebral perfusion pressure (see Chapter 19) and demonstrates the potentiating deleterious effect of hypoglycemia with ischemia. This observation corroborates the experimental observations (see earlier discussion) indicating a potentiation of ischemic injury by hypoglycemia.

Human Observations
Neonatal Neuropathology

The limited observations in human newborns suggest that the lessons learned from the animal studies are relevant. Thus a correlation between the severity and duration of hypoglycemia and the degree of neuronal injury is apparent.[135,136] In one series of 17 largely premature infants who experienced *transient hypoglycemia* (blood glucose level < 20 mg/dL) and *hypoxia* confined to the first day of life, no increase in brain injury could be discerned over and above that expected with the concomitant *hypoxia*.[136] In another series, marked and diffuse

neuronal injury was apparent in 2- and 3-day-old premature infants whose hypoglycemia was not effectively treated before death.[135] In these *untreated and inadequately treated* patients, the neuronal injury involved essentially every level of the nervous system, including the anterior horn cells of the spinal cord, but with a particular predilection for the *posterior cerebrum*, as in the monkey experiments (see earlier discussion). This posterior cerebral predilection has been demonstrated in the hypoglycemic newborn by computed tomography, MRI, and single photon emission computed tomography (SPECT) blood flow scans (Fig. 25.12; see later).[137-144] The reasons for the posterior parieto-occipital predominance in human infants is not entirely clear but could relate in considerable part to the active state of neuronal development, both dendritic arborization and synaptogenesis, in the posterior cerebral cortex relative to other cortical areas (see Chapter 7). This active development is likely accompanied by higher energy needs, development of excitatory amino acid receptors, and related changes that would increase the likelihood of neuronal injury with glucose deprivation.[145-148] The lesions in the neuropathological study did not exhibit selective involvement of border zones, or Purkinje cells, as in hypoxic-ischemic injury. Moreover, involvement of upper cortical neuronal layers occurred with neonatal hypoglycemia, a finding, as described earlier, suggestive of an agent (excitatory amino acid?) borne in cerebrospinal fluid. This cortical topography is different from that observed with ischemia (i.e., selective involvement of intermediate and deeper cortical layers).[149,150]

Although neuronal injury dominates the neuropathological picture in neonatal hypoglycemia, concomitant injury to glia is also detectable.[135] Indeed, the classic neuropathological studies of Larroche[150] showed that hypoglycemia is a precedent of periventricular leukomalacia. Moreover, decreased blood glucose was an important pathogenetic factor in careful studies of infants with hypoplastic left heart syndrome, in whom periventricular leukomalacia is a prominent sequela.[120] Studies of oligodendrocyte precursor cells and cerebellar slice cultures showed that hypoglycemia induces apoptotic cell death and inhibits differentiation and myelination.[151] Moreover, the experimental observations of vulnerability of differentiating glial cells to glucose deprivation and to excitatory amino acids (see earlier discussion and Chapter 13) are clearly relevant in this context. The posterior cerebral predilection may relate to the relatively high concentration of oligodendroglial precursor cells in this region of neonatal white matter; these cells are particularly vulnerable to energy deprivation (see Chapters 14 and 15). These findings may account for the subsequent disturbance of myelination noted in animal studies and in surviving human infants (see later discussion).[150,152]

Neuropathological Sequelae

The neuropathological *sequelae* of severe neonatal hypoglycemic encephalopathy reflect injury particularly to the cerebral cortex but also to subcortical white matter, especially posteriorly (see Fig. 25.12).[137,138,140-143,153] These include microcephaly and widened sulci, with atrophic gyri, as well as diminution in myelinated cerebral white matter, with dilated lateral ventricles. The effect on myelination may be a consequence of the glial injury.

Unresolved Issues

Despite the informative aforementioned data, the anatomical correlates of *marginal* hypoglycemia in combination with other insults (e.g., hypoxemia, ischemia, and seizures) remain to be defined. Precedent from experimental studies, biochemical and neuropathological in design (see earlier discussions), lead one to speculate that these combined insults, which are quite prevalent, may result in brain injury that was not recognized in the past. However, this notion remains to be proven conclusively in the human newborn. Moreover, the impact of these combined insults on *development* of the nervous system, particularly the organizational aspects thereof, is totally unexplored. The application of newer techniques for assessing dendritic and synaptic development (see Chapter 2) in the brains of affected infants is a critical topic for future research.

CLINICAL ASPECTS

The clinical aspects of neonatal hypoglycemia encompass a wide variety of disorders and pathogeneses, with the common denominator being the decrease in blood glucose concentration. Consequently and not surprisingly, considerable heterogeneities in incidence, occurrence of symptoms, and prognosis are apparent. Nevertheless, certain unifying characteristics can be recognized and are emphasized in the following discussion.

Incidence

The incidence of neonatal hypoglycemia in a given population varies considerably, depending on the following: the relative number of preterm and term infants; the degree of risk of the population; the time of screening; the time and type of feeding; the control of temperature, ventilation, and circulation; and, above all, the definition of hypoglycemia (see Table 25.1). Moreover recent evidence indicates that the use of continuous interstitial glucose monitoring identifies low glucose concentrations in a substantial number of infants

TABLE 25.8   Incidence and Duration of Hypoglycemia in Preterm Infants[a]

	PLASMA GLUCOSE (mmol/L)		
	<0.06	<1.6	<2.6
Total occurrences	10%	28%	66%
Duration (no. of days concentration recorded)			
1	8%	20%	32%
2	1%	4%	18%
≥3	1%	4%	16%

[a]The population comprised 661 preterm infants (<1850 g at birth) who survived for more than 48 hours. <0.06 mmol/L = 1 mg/dL glucose, 1.6 mmol/L = 28 mg/dL glucose, <2.6 mmol/L = 47 mg/dL glucose.
Data from Lucas A, Morley R, Cole TJ. Adverse neurodevelopment outcome of moderate neonatal hypoglycaemia. *Br Med J.* 1988;297:1304–1308.

(25%) that were not detected with intermittent glucose testing and, in some cases, that persisted for up to 5 hours.[154] In one study of 232 *low-risk* infants in a level 1 nursery, the onset of hypoglycemia occurred at a mean age of 3.4 hours, with incidences of 8% when the definitions were blood glucose levels lower than 30 mg/dL in the full-sized term infant and lower than 20 mg/dL in the low-birthweight infant and 21% when the definition was a blood glucose level lower than 40 mg/dL in all infants.[155] In a large multicenter study of 661 preterm infants with birthweight of less than 1850 g who were subjected to "broadly similar early feeding practices," fully 10% had at least one value of blood glucose less than approximately 10 mg/dL (0.06 mmol/L), 28% at least one value less than approximately 30 mg/dL (1.6 mmol/L), and 66% at least one value less than 45 mg/dL (2.6 mmol/L) (Table 25.8).[5] The proportions were 1%, 4%, and 16% of infants with values less than 10, 30, and 45 mg/dL, respectively, *on 3 or more days* (see later discussion).[5] Among healthy breast-fed term infants, median values were 2.8 to 3.1 mmol/L (50 to 56 mg/dL); in two large studies[4,156] values did not vary appreciably between 3 and 72 hours of age. Notably, approximately 17% had values of plasma glucose lower than 2.16 mmol/L (<40 mg/dL) at 3 hours of age and 10% had such values at 72 hours.[156] Approximately 5% had values lower than 1.6 mmol/L (<29 mg/dL) at 3 and 72 hours.[156] The incidence of hypoglycemia is highest for certain *high-risk* infants. Harris and colleagues evaluated 514 high-risk infants ≥ 35 weeks (i.e., large for GA, infants of diabetic mothers, small for GA, and later preterms) and reported that 51% became hypoglycemic (<2.6 mM) (<47 mg/dL) and 19% had severe hypoglycemia (<2.0 mM) (<36 mg/dL).[6] Most (81%) episodes occurred in the first 24 hours. Of the 260 infants with hypoglycemia, 79% had no clinical symptoms, 15% were too sleepy to feed, and 7% were jittery (Table 25.9). Importantly, 37% exhibited hypoglycemia after three normal blood sugar levels (see Table 25.9). Thus, although the largest proportion of infants identified as hypoglycemic in the early neonatal period exhibit only transient depression of blood glucose levels, large absolute numbers of infants do exhibit levels considered low by generally accepted definitions. Thus we are dealing with a very common abnormality.

TABLE 25.9   Characteristics of Hypoglycemia in a High-Risk Population (n = 260)[a]

BLOOD GLUCOSE CHARACTERISTICS	PERCENTAGE/DURATION
Blood glucose <47 mg/dL (2.6 mmol/L)	~51%
Blood glucose <36 mg/dL (2.0 mmol/L)	~19%
Evolved in first 6 h	48%
Evolved in first 24 h	81%
Hypoglycemia evolved after three normal values	37%
Median duration of an episode	1.4 h

[a]The patient population comprised 514 infants identified at high risk for hypoglycemia; (51%) developed hypoglycemia. High-risk infants—small or large infants, infants of diabetic mothers, late preterm infants.

Adapted from Harris DL, Weston PJ, Harding JE. Incidence of neonatal hypoglycemia in babies identified as at risk. *J Pediatr.* 2012;161:787–779.

Clinical Categorization of Neonatal Hypoglycemia

A classification of neonatal hypoglycemia should incorporate the clinical setting, timing, and duration and severity of hypoglycemia.[6,8,10,157] A reasonable classification, as outlined next, includes early transitional-adaptive hypoglycemia, hypoglycemia associated with impaired metabolic adaptation, hypoglycemia associated with intrauterine growth restriction, and severe recurrent hypoglycemia. Albeit overlapping, the classification provides a useful framework for discussion. *Early transitional-adaptive hypoglycemia* usually occurs in the first 3 to 12 hours after sudden withdrawal of maternally derived substrate at birth. These infants fail to make the appropriate adaptive metabolic adjustments during the transition from intrauterine to extrauterine life. *Hypoglycemia associated with impaired metabolic adaptation* occurs principally as an associated finding in infants with a variety of disorders, particularly involvement of the central nervous system. In many respects, this group could be considered a subtype of early transitional–adaptive hypoglycemia. Hypoglycemia associated with intrauterine growth restriction is an extension of an intrauterine disturbance, often undernutrition, that may affect glycogen and lipid stores, gluconeogenic capacity, and ketone production.[16] *Severe recurrent hypoglycemia* is secondary to specific primary enzymatic or metabolic–endocrine abnormalities involving glucose homeostasis.

Early Transitional-Adaptive Hypoglycemia

Early transitional-adaptive hypoglycemia is a relatively common variety of neonatal hypoglycemia. The pathophysiology involves failure of one or more of the early adaptive responses to birth, such as the upregulation of glycogenolysis and gluconeogenesis. Thus, included in this somewhat heterogeneous hypoglycemic group are infants whose mothers received excessive glucose intrapartum (resulting in the downregulation of glycogenolysis and gluconeogenesis and increased insulin secretion); large-for-GA infants of diabetic, gestational diabetic, or nondiabetic mothers (resulting in excessive insulin); hypothermic infants (resulting in excessive glucose utilization for heat production and factors still to be defined); or asphyxiated infants (resulting in excessive anaerobic metabolism of glucose, glycogen

TABLE 25.10   Major Causes of Neonatal Hypoglycemia[a]

Early transient hypoglycemia
- Prematurity
- Perinatal hypoxia-ischemia
- Intrauterine growth restriction
- Sepsis
- Hypothermia
- Polycythemia
- Congenital heart disease

Hypoglycemia associated with impaired metabolic adaptation
- Infant of diabetic mother
- Preterm infants
- Large for gestational age infant
- Intrauterine growth restriction
- Perinatal hypoxia-ischemia

Hypoglycemia associated with intrauterine growth restriction

Severe, recurrent hypoglycemia
- Hyperinsulinism
  - Potassium-ATP (K_{ATP}) channel hyperinsulinism
  - Glucokinase hyperinsulinism
  - Short chain L-3-hydroxyacyl-coenzyme dehydrogenase deficiency
  - Beckwith-Wiedemann syndrome
  - Infant of a diabetic mother (poorly controlled)
- Endocrine deficiencies
  - Panhypopituitarism
  - Isolated growth hormone deficiency
  - Cortisol deficiency
  - Hypothyroidism
- Hereditary metabolic defects
  - Carbohydrate metabolism
    - Galactosemia
    - Glucose 6 phosphate deficiency
    - Phosphoenolpyruvate carboxykinase deficiency
    - Fructose 1,6 diphosphatase deficiency
  - Organic acid metabolism
    - Pyruvate carboxylase deficiency
    - Propionic acidemia
    - Methymalonic acidemia
    - Mitochondrial disorders
    - Fatty acid oxidation disorders

[a]See text for references.

depletion, and hyperinsulinism of unknown causes [see later] [Table 25. 10]). *Preterm* asphyxiated infants are particularly at risk because of diminished glycogen stores (most hepatic glycogen accumulation occurs in the third trimester of pregnancy). *Onset of hypoglycemia* in this category is characteristically *very early*, duration is relatively brief, degree is relatively mild, and response to glucose administration is prompt. Relatively few of these patients exhibit symptoms clearly referable to hypoglycemia.[8-11,16,157-160] Prognosis depends to a large extent on any accompanying disorder; however, the contributory role of the hypoglycemia remains to be clarified. For example, in a study of 185 term infants with severe fetal acidemia and presumed asphyxia, 14% exhibited a blood glucose in the first 30 minutes of 40 mg/dL or lower; of these infants, 56% had an abnormal short-term neurological outcome versus 16% of those with a blood glucose greater than 40 mg/dL.[111]

Hypoglycemia Associated With Impaired Metabolic Adaptation

Hypoglycemia associated with impaired metabolic adaptation is also relatively common in neonates (see Table 25.10). The pathophysiology is considered to represent a hypoketotic form of hypoglycemia, which, in infants or children, appears to be caused by a lower glucose threshold for the suppression of insulin secretion than would be normal and results in impaired glucose and ketone production.[16,161] Included in this group are appropriate-for-GA term and preterm infants, although small-for-GA infants are overrepresented. These infants may have been subjected to a variety of *associated illnesses*, which include disorders of the central nervous system, especially interruption of placental flow (asphyxia) resulting in perinatal hypoxia-ischemia, intracranial hemorrhage, and such systemic disorders as congenital heart disease (with decreased perfusion to the liver). The overlap with early transitional adaptive hypoglycemia is apparent. The association of this category with central nervous system disturbances is of particular pathogenetic interest because of data demonstrating a close relationship between hepatic glucose production and brain mass (see earlier discussion). Thus the brain disturbance may have an adverse impact on the regulation of hepatic glucose production. Additional pathogenetic factors potentially operative with cerebral disturbance, especially asphyxia, are (1) enhanced cerebral utilization of glucose secondary to anaerobic glycolysis, (2) glycogen depletion secondary to intrapartum stress-induced catecholamine release, and (3) hypersecretion of insulin.[a] This form of hypoglycemia usually has its onset on the first day of life (although usually later than in the early transitional group), duration is variable, degree is relatively mild, and response to glucose therapy is prompt. (In the *severely "asphyxiated" infant*, onset is earlier, degree is marked, and, if complicated by relative hyperinsulinism, response to glucose therapy may not be prompt.) Approximately 50% (or more) of the infants in this category exhibit neurological symptoms, although—in view of the associated disorders—the relation of such symptoms to hypoglycemia is difficult to determine decisively. The outlook depends particularly on the associated disorders, but, again, the contributory role of the hypoglycemia remains to be defined.

Neonatal Hypoglycemia Associated With Intrauterine Growth Restriction

Intrauterine undernutrition is a dominant feature of the disorder. Pathogenesis includes the following: (1) inadequate production of glucose and energy because of both diminished glycogen and lipid stores and defective gluconeogenesis and (2) excessive glucose utilization because of both the relatively large brain (major consumer) compared with the liver (major producer) and, in some infants at least, relative hyperinsulinism.[b] Regarding the latter, in a recent paper of 27 small-for-GA infants, plasma insulin levels were inappropriately elevated during hypoglycemia in 22, and the remaining 5 infants had inappropriately low β-hydroxybutyrate and nonesterified fatty acids during hypoglycemia as supportive biochemical evidence of hypoglycemic hyperinsulinism.[163] All infants required a glucose infusion rate of at least 8 mg/kg per minute to maintain normoglycemia (median 15.6 mg/kg per minute). No correlation was found between maximum glucose infusion rate to maintain normoglycemia and plasma insulin level during hypoglycemia. Clinical signs are common, and this group represents the best category for evaluating the relation between clinical signs and blood glucose levels. The onset of hypoglycemia occurs in the latter part of the first day. The degree of hypoglycemia may be moderate to severe, duration can be prolonged, and response to glucose administration requires relatively large amounts. The outlook depends in largest part on the duration and severity of hypoglycemia and, as a corollary, the time before the onset of adequate therapy.

Severe Recurrent Hypoglycemia

Severe recurrent hypoglycemia is the least common variety of neonatal hypoglycemia. The single feature that distinguishes this group from those just described is the persistence and the recurrence of the hypoglycemia. Included in this category are principally term-appropriate or large-for-GA infants with primary disorders of glucose homeostasis. The major causes are detailed in Table 25.10.[a] The onset of hypoglycemia in these disorders varies with the specific entity, but degree is usually severe, duration is prolonged, and symptoms are almost invariable. The outlook depends primarily on detection of the disorder, institution of specific therapy when possible, and, particularly, rapid and adequate maintenance of blood glucose levels.

The most common causes of persistent hypoglycemia in the newborn are *hyperinsulinemic hypoglycemia of infancy* and *congenital hyperinsulinism*. These inherited disorders relate to abnormalities of the mechanisms of insulin secretion by the pancreatic beta cell. The final stage of insulin secretion is regulated by the action of a receptor-channel complex composed of the sulfonylurea receptor (SUR1) and inwardly rectifying K^+ channel (Kir6.2). The channel is closed when the ATP/ADP ratio rises in the beta cell. Closure results in an increase in intracellular K^+, membrane depolarization, Ca^{2+} influx, and insulin release.[168,169] Glucose entry through the GLUT2 transporter upregulates insulin secretion by glucose metabolism, generation of ATP, and closure of the Kir6.2 channel. Another regulator of insulin secretion is the action of glutamate dehydrogenase and generation of ATP from glutamate, with resulting closure of the channel. Glutamate dehydrogenase is allosterically activated by leucine. The most common genetic causes of congenital hyperinsulinism are inactivating mutations of the ABCC8 and KCNJ11 genes coding for the two subunits of the ATP-sensitive K(+) (KATP) channel in the beta cell of the pancreas.[172] As noted earlier, the related proteins are respectively the high-affinity SUR1 and the Kir6.2 channels.[173] Histologically, two types of congenital hyperinsulinism have been mainly described, focal and diffuse. The focal form, localized to one region of the pancreas, has been associated with paternal isodisomy for a KATP mutation in beta cells, whereas the diffuse form is associated with autosomal recessive and dominant mutations in the ABCC8 and KCNJ11 genes.[173] The focal form, related

---

[a]References 9, 10, 14, 16, 157, 161, and 162.
[b]References 8-10, 16, 157, 162, and 163.

[a]References 8, 10, 16, 157, and 164-171.

TABLE 25.11   Major Neurological Features in Small for Gestational Age Infants With Hypoglycemia

CLINICAL FEATURES

- Changes in level of consciousness
  Irritability
  Lethargy
  Stupor
- Jitteriness/tremor
- Seizures
- Apnea and other respiratory abnormalities
- Feeding poorly
- Hypotonia

Data from Cornblath M, Hawdon JM, Williams AF, et al. Controversies regarding definition of neonatal hypoglycemia: suggested operational thresholds. *Pediatrics.* 2000;105:1141–1145.

TABLE 25.12   Brain Imaging Abnormalities (and Neurological Outcome) in Severe Neonatal Hypoglycemia[a]

Neonatal blood glucose levels
  ≤20 mg/dL: 74%
  ≤25 mg/dL: 90%
  ≤30 mg/dL: 95%
Major imaging findings
Occipital with or without parietal lesions (75%)
Corticospinal tract involvement (15%)
Watershed pattern (10%)
Neurological sequelae
Total: 84%
Developmental delay/mental retardation: 84%
Seizures: 66%
Visual impairment: 37%[b]
Microcephaly: 32%

[a]See text for references.
[b]Testing inconsistent; likely an underestimate.

to an area of beta-cell adenomatosis, is potentially curable by surgery.

Neurological Features

The neurological features of neonatal hypoglycemia are best considered in terms of their relative frequency, severity, and nature. These aspects of the clinical syndrome vary as a function of the clinical circumstances (e.g., infant of diabetic mother, infant with *asphyxia*) as well as of the duration and severity of the hypoglycemia, particularly the length of time before adequate therapy is instituted (see the later section "Seizures: Importance of Duration of Hypoglycemia"). The neurological features that are concomitants of any associated disorders may obscure or accentuate those related to hypoglycemia.

Major Neurological Features

The most representative group of infants to define the neurology of neonatal hypoglycemia is the classic transient group (i.e., small-for-GA infants with classic transient hypoglycemia; Table 25.11).[8,10,174] The clinical hallmark of this disorder is the combination of stupor and jitteriness. In standard writings, stupor either is not commented on or is categorized in an imprecise manner (e.g., *lethargy* and *somnolence*). In a recent report by Harris and colleagues involving 260 infants with a blood glucose below 47 mg/dL, 79% of infants with hypoglycemia were asymptomatic, 15% were too sleepy to feed (likely a marker of altered level of consciousness), and 7% were jittery.[6] It is rare to see a symptomatic hypoglycemic small-for-GA infant with a normal level of alertness. Jitteriness occurs in at least 80% of symptomatic infants and seizures occur in more than 50%. Respiratory disturbances and hypotonia are also relatively common. Hypotonia is present in the majority of the affected infants, although the precise frequency is difficult to define from reported cases and therefore is probably underestimated. Further delineation of the relative frequency of the neurological features of neonatal hypoglycemia is now difficult because of close surveillance and prompt treatment of infants at risk.

Seizures: Importance of Duration of Hypoglycemia

The incidence of seizures with hypoglycemia remains unclear. In one older study, late diagnosis, onset of therapy, and control of hypoglycemia were common in infants who experienced seizures.[175] Similar data have been obtained by other investigators.[176] However, the incidence and frequency of seizures with hypoglycemia may be underestimated because seizures may be subclinical and require continuous EEG monitoring for detection. The relatively high frequency of subclinical seizures requiring continuous monitoring for detection is well documented for other neonatal neurological disorders, especially hypoxic-ischemic encephalopathy (see Chapters 12 and 20).

Brain Imaging in Neonatal Hypoglycemia

A series of reports have identified, by brain imaging, a specific pattern of cerebral abnormality involving principally the parieto-occipital regions (Table 25.12).[114,177-182] Consistent with the reported neuropathology (see earlier), the dominant finding has been abnormal signal intensity by MRI in the parieto-occipital region (Figs. 25.13 and 25.14). The involved areas exhibit restricted diffusion on diffusion-weighted MRI (DWI) (see Figs. 25.13 and 25.14). The topography is seen better in the acute stage by DWI than by conventional MRI. Magnetic resonance spectroscopy shows no or mild elevations of lactate with advanced lesions. The findings of no or mild elevations of lactate indicate that the lesion is not ischemic in basic nature but rather is related to glucose deprivation. Although 10% to 15% of the lesions resolve, most are followed in subsequent weeks and months by loss of cerebral cortex and white matter, often with ventricular dilation. A more diffuse pattern of cerebral cortical injury may occur with very severe hypoglycemia.[113,183] In general the posterior cerebral involvement includes both cortex and underlying white matter, seen best acutely by DWI imaging (see Table 25.12). Conventional MRI sequences often show predominantly white matter involvement. Other lesions (see Table 25.12) are seen in a minority of infants and are often related to associated insults.[112,113,183]

Prognosis

Mortality and neurological outcome in neonatal hypoglycemic states relate to the rapidity of onset of adequate therapy and

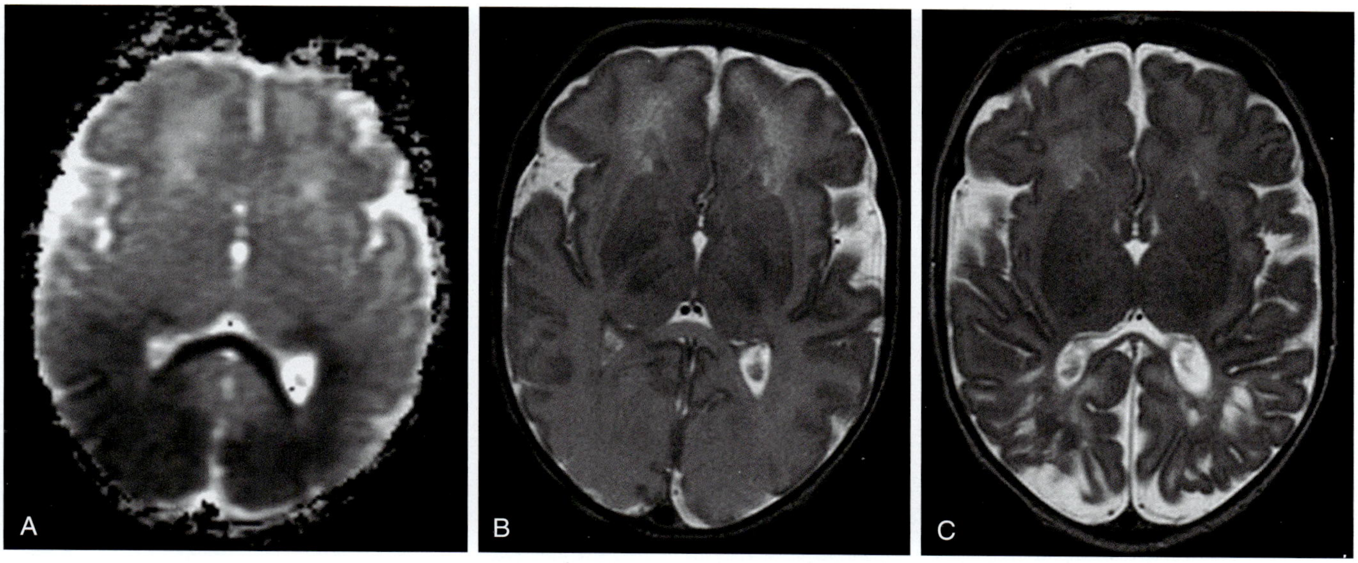

Figure 25.13 Conventional magnetic resonance imaging (MRI) and diffusion-weighted MRI (DWI) in neonatal hypoglycemia. A, ADC map (DWI), B, T-2 weighted (T2W) MRI on day 6, and, C, T2W MRI on day 44, from a term infant with a minimum blood glucose of 1.1 mmol/L at 92 hours of age. Note in A the area of decreased diffusion (dark in the ADC map) in the parieto-occipital cortex, subcortical white matter, and splenium of the corpus callosum and in B the loss of gray-white matter differentiation in the parieto-occipital cortex and white matter on the T2W MRI. In C, atrophy of the parieto-occipital region and splenium is apparent on the T2W image at 44 days. (From Filan PM, Inder TE, Cameron FJ, Kean MJ, et al. Neonatal hypoglycemia and occipital cerebral injury. *J Pediatr.* 2006;148:552–555.)

TABLE 25.13 Neurological Outcome After Neonatal Hypoglycemia as a Function of Neonatal Neurological Features

NEONATAL CLINICAL SYNDROME	NEUROLOGICAL OUTCOME[a] NORMAL (%)	TRANSIENT ABNORMALITY (%)	ABNORMAL (%)
Neurological features: seizures	38	12	50
Neurological features: no seizures	76	12	12
No neurological features	80	14	6

[a]Follow-up examination was at 1 to 4 years of age.

Adapted from Koivisto M, Blanco SM, Krause U. Neonatal symptomatic and asymptomatic hypoglycaemia: a follow-up study of 151 children. *Dev Med Child Neurol.* 1972;14:603–614.

to the associated disorders. Mortality because of untreated hypoglycemia is now rare. Sequelae include particularly disturbances of neurological development and intellectual function; visual disturbances; motor deficits, especially spasticity and ataxia; seizure disorders; and microcephaly.[a] As one may predict from the topography of the neuropathological lesions, disturbances of neurological development and subsequent intellectual function and visual disturbances are the most common deficits, presumably reflecting the cerebral cortical neuronal and white matter (glial) injury. Prognosis is best considered in relation to neonatal neurological brain imaging and degree of duration of moderate hypoglycemia, as discussed next.

Relation of Neurological Outcome to Neonatal Neurological Features

A distinct correlation exists between neurological outcome and neonatal clinical features (Table 25.13). This is particularly true when *series exclude those infants with secondary associated hypoglycemia*, in whom neonatal clinical features and neurological sequelae secondary to the associated disorders are difficult to distinguish from those secondary to the hypoglycemia. In one series of 151 infants with neonatal hypoglycemia followed for 1 to 4 years, the occurrence of seizures as part of the neonatal neurological syndrome was associated with a clearly abnormal outcome in 50% and with transient neurological abnormalities that were no longer apparent in an additional 12%.[175] In contrast, infants with no neonatal neurological features (i.e., asymptomatic infants) were clearly abnormal on follow-up examination in only 6% of cases. Infants with neurological features but *not* seizures did nearly as well as those without any

[a]References 7, 8, 10, 15, 112, 113, 158, 174, 175, and 183-185.

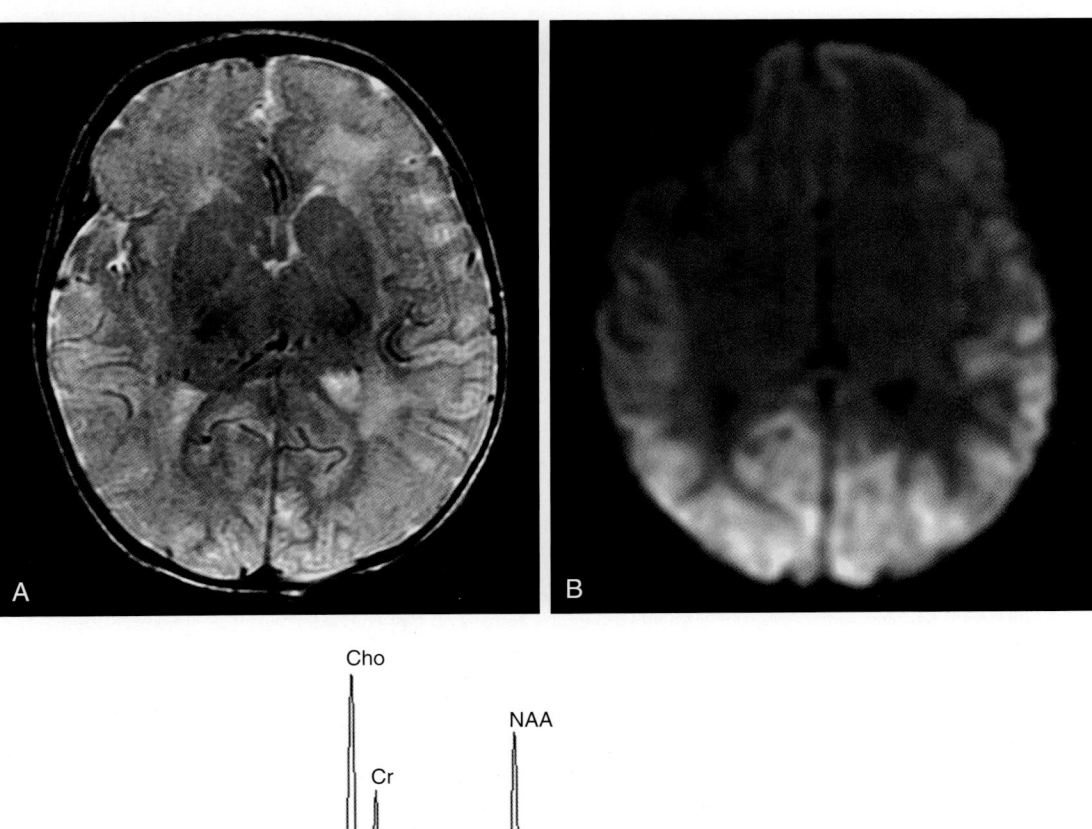

Figure 25.14 Proton magnetic resonance spectroscopy (MRS) and diffusion-weighted magnetic resonance imaging (DWI) in neonatal hypoglycemia. Images are from a term infant with a minimum blood glucose of 5 mg/dL on day 2. On day 6, A, axial T2-weighted MRI shows a subtle loss of gray-white differentiation in parieto-occipital areas. However, in B, DWI shows markedly decreased diffusion (high signal) in these regions, and in C, MRS demonstrates only a slight elevation of lactate. *Cho,* Choline; *Cr,* creatine; *NAA, N*-acetylaspartate. (Courtesy Dr. Omar Khwaja.)

neurological features (see Table 25.13). However, the relatively brief follow-up period in this study is noteworthy.

In a study with a longer follow-up period of 39 hypoglycemic infants, most of whom were small for GA, the prognostic importance of neonatal symptoms was reaffirmed.[184] Although mean intelligence quotient (IQ) scores were not significantly different between the total hypoglycemic group and the matched control group, a significantly larger number of the hypoglycemic children (13 of 25) had IQ scores less than 86 than did the control children (6 of 27) at 5 to 7 years of age. The lower scores were attributed to poor verbal skills (likely expressive language delay). Children who did most poorly had *seizures* as part of their neonatal neurological syndrome.

Relation of Brain Imaging to Outcome

Although duration of hypoglycemia is difficult to determine from the published reports, the degree of hypoglycemia in infants with pronounced imaging findings, especially generally, has been marked (see Table 25.12). Thus 70% of cases had glucose levels of 20 mg/dL or lower and only 5% had levels of 30 mg/dL or higher. The rate of neurological sequelae is variable but generally is greater than 50%. Severity is also variable, but the majority of infants exhibit mild or moderate deficits. Visual impairment, including blindness, occurs in approximately one third of infants. However, testing is inconsistent, and it is possible that disturbed higher visual function and visual associations are more common consistent with the locus of the disease. Indeed,

TABLE 25.14 Neurological Outcome in Preterm Infants With Moderate Hypoglycemia[a,b]

DURATION OF HYPOGLYCEMIA (DAYS)	PERCENTAGE OF ALL INFANTS STUDIED (%)	PERCENTAGE WITH NEURODEVELOPMENTAL IMPAIRMENT (%)[a]
≥3	15	29
≥5	6	42
≥7	3	40

[a]Neurodevelopmental impairment consisted of cerebral palsy (≈40%) or developmental delay (i.e., Bayley mental or motor score of ≥ 70 [≈60%]). The population consisted of 661 preterm infants (<1850 g at birth) who survived for more than 48 hours. Moderate hypoglycemia consisted of at least one daily value of plasma glucose lower than 2.6 mmol/L (≈47 mg/dL).
[b]See text for references.
Data from Lucas A, Morley R, Cole TJ. Adverse neurodevelopment outcome of moderate neonatal hypoglycaemia. *Br Med J.* 1988;297:1304–1308.

involvement of the parieto-occipital cortex with long-term sequelae has been described in a well-delineated neurological syndrome of cortical visual loss, occipital localization-related epilepsy, and psychomotor retardation.[141,186] It will be of great interest to determine whether milder degrees of hypoglycemia have milder and transient abnormalities, detectable perhaps by DWI. These observations raise the possibility that neurological features, such as impaired higher visual functions, may have been undetected in previous follow-up studies, indicating that a focus on such functions will be important in future work.

Neurocognitive Outcome in Infants With Moderate Hypoglycemia (Blood Sugar < 47 mg/dL)

Although study design and populations have varied and data are not entirely consistent, neurological outcome does appear to be influenced by moderate hypoglycemia, including both its *duration* and *degree*. Thus findings from a multicenter prospective study of preterm infants suggest that even *moderate hypoglycemia* (at least one daily value of plasma glucose < 2.6 mmol/L, or ≈47 mg/dL) may be deleterious if it is present for 3 or more days (Table 25.14).[5] The data shown in Table 25.14 indicate an approximately 30% incidence of neurodevelopmental sequelae when moderate hypoglycemia was present for 3 days or more and approximately 40% when it was present for 5 days or more. Notably, relatively large proportions of all infants studied were affected (see Table 25.14). These findings emphasize the importance of *duration* of hypoglycemia, even if moderate, in the determination of prognosis. Follow-up of this population showed persistence of abnormalities in arithmetic and motor scores at 7.5 to 8 years.[5] However, a second group attempting to replicate the findings of this study[18] more recently followed 47 of 566 infants of less than 32 weeks' GA who presented with a blood glucose level below 47 mg/dL on at least 3 days and who were matched with nonhypoglycemic infants. These investigators found no difference in physical disability or developmental progress at 2 years or in psychometric assessment at 15 years.[18]

An added impact of intrauterine growth retardation is suggested by a study of 62 small-for-GA preterm infants with neonatal hypoglycemia defined as values lower than 2.6 mmol/L or 47 mg/dL.[172] The data showed a strong correlation with persistent neurodevelopmental deficits and reduced head circumference, *especially in infants with recurrent episodes of moderate hypoglycemia* (compared with infants with a single episode of more pronounced hypoglycemia).[174]

The degree of *moderate hypoglycemia* is also important. Thus in a recent retrospective review of 1943 infants (23 to 42 weeks' GA), early transient neonatal hypoglycemia was noted in 19.3% using a value of 45 mg/dL (<2.6 mm/L), 10.3% using a value of 40 mg /dL (<2.3 mm/L) and 6.4% using a value of less than 35 mg/dL (<2.0 mm/L).[7] In confounding for multiple variables in this study, this transient hypoglycemia was associated with a decreased probability of proficiency on literacy and mathematics fourth-grade achievement tests at 8-year testing. For the 3 hypoglycemia cutoffs, the adjusted odds ratios (95% confidence intervals) for literacy were 0.62 (0.45–0.85), 0.43 (0.28–0.67), and 0.49 (0.28–0.83), respectively, and the adjusted odds ratios (95% CIs) for mathematics were 0.78 (0.57–1.08), 0.51 (0.34–0.78), and 0.49 (0.29–0.82), respectively.[7] An additional retrospective study of 832 *moderately preterm* infants (32 to 35⁵⁄₇ weeks' GA) showed a graded association between hypoglycemic thresholds of less than 40 mg/dL (2.2 mmol/L) and neurodevelopmental impairment at 4-year follow-up.[185] Specifically, a documented glucose value of 1.7 mmol/L (30 mg/dL) was relatively common (8.1%) and increased the risk of developmental delay from 9.1% to approximately 20% (odds ratio 2.4 [95% CI, 1.23–4.77]).[185] These observations reemphasize the importance of moderate hypoglycemia in the genesis of brain injury.

In recent years, infants at risk for hypoglycemia have been *screened from the first hours of life*, and low glucose levels have been treated promptly. In general, the results have shown a relation between transient, relatively brief, mild hypoglycemia (<2.2 mmol/L, <40 mg/dL) and a favorable neurological outcome.[160,187] A recent prospective cohort study involving 528 high-risk neonates with a GA of at least 35 weeks, all of whom were treated early to maintain a blood glucose concentration of at least 47 mg/dL (2.6 mmol/L), was undertaken to evaluate the impact of treatment on outcome. In addition, interstitial glucose concentrations were continuously monitored. When infants with neonatal hypoglycemia were treated to maintain a blood glucose concentration of at least 47 mg/dL, the hypoglycemia was not associated with an increased risk of a primary outcome of neurosensory impairment and processing difficulty at 2-year follow-up (risk ratio, 0.95; 95% CI, 0.75 to 1.20; *P* = .67) as compared with infants without hypoglycemia. Interestingly, continuous interstitial glucose monitoring indicated that

TABLE 25.15   Neurocognitive Outcome in Infants With Moderate Hypoglycemia (Blood Sugar <47 mg/dL)

- Duration of hypoglycemia is an important determinant of outcome
  - Small for gestational age preterm infants with recurrent episodes of moderate hypoglycemia are at increased risk for neurodevelopmental deficits
- Transient hypoglycemia at cutoff values <45 mg/dL, <40 mg/dL, and < 35 mg/dL is associated with a decreased probability of proficiency in literacy and mathematics on a fourth-grade proficiency test
- Moderate hypoglycemia *treated promptly* is not followed by increased risk for neurodevelopmental deficits at 2 years.

episodes of low glucose concentrations were common (25%) even in infants with intermittent normal blood glucose concentrations while receiving treatment for hypoglycemia (Table 25.15).[154]

Management

Management of the infant with neonatal hypoglycemia is considered best in terms of *prevention and therapy.* Major advances in both these aspects of management have been made in the past 20 years.

Prevention

Prevention of neonatal hypoglycemia must involve factors related to pregnancy, labor, delivery, and the early neonatal period. These factors are discussed most appropriately in standard texts of perinatology and neonatology. During pregnancy, importance can be attributed to control of maternal diabetes, nutrition, intrauterine growth restriction, and other factors that cause prematurity. Prevention and control of perinatal *asphyxia* are clearly of major significance. Of particular relevance *after delivery* are (1) identification of the high-risk infant, (2) minimization of excessive caloric expenditures by maintenance of temperature in the normal range, (3) implementation of oral feedings (breast-feeds when possible) as soon as possible after birth, (4) careful surveillance for clinical symptoms, and (5) determination of blood glucose level before the first feeding and subsequently according to the clinical setting. Early discharge of preterm infants before the firm establishment of oral feedings should be avoided to prevent the postdischarge evolution of hypoglycemia.[11,188]

Simple preventive guidelines in *asymptomatic infants* can be summarized as follows.[11,157] In the *healthy appropriately grown term infant,* facilitating normal feeding is sufficient. In *preterm infants* of less than 32 to 34 weeks' GA or those with respiratory distress, establishment of enteral feedings is relatively slow and intravenous glucose, generally commencing at 4 to 6 mg glucose/kg per minute, is needed. Because breast-fed neonates do not receive full caloric intake for several days after birth, it has been suggested that they are able to compensate for low glucose by the generation of ketones as an alternative fuel for the brain. However, ketones are low in breast-fed babies during the first 1 to 2 days after birth and then rise modestly over 2 to 3 days after birth (0.7 to 1.4 mmol/L) before falling to very low levels as breast milk production matures.[189] The

low levels of ketones and free fatty acids appear to be explained by incomplete suppression of insulin release in the face of low plasma glucose concentrations. Importantly, without specific measurements of plasma ketone concentrations, it cannot be assumed that ketones are available as an alternative fuel to support brain metabolism when normal neonates develop hypoglycemia or that breast-fed babies are protected against potential adverse effects of hypoglycemia by ketones if their postnatal fasting period becomes too long.[14]

For clearly *intrauterine growth–restricted infants,* management depends in part on the initial glucose values but usually includes early introduction of enteral feedings plus or minus intravenous glucose infusions. Such infants may require from 6 to 8 mg/kg per minute and on occasions even higher glucose infusion rates particularly with relative hyperinsulinism. For *infants of diabetic mothers,* early glucose screening (highest incidence of hypoglycemia is at ~2 to 4 hours of age), early enteral feeding and regular prefeed glucose monitoring are crucial. Excessive rapid intravenous glucose infusion should be avoided to prevent overstimulation of the infant's pancreas, already primed to produce hyperinsulinism.

A recent approach adopted by Harris and colleagues is to treat infants with a blood glucose less than 47 mg/dL (2.6 mmol/L) using 40% dextrose gel.[190,191] This approach is based on a randomized double-blind placebo-controlled trial of infants of 35 to 42 weeks' GA, less than 48 hours of age, and at risk of hypoglycemia (infant of a diabetic mother [gestational, type 1, or type 2], late preterm [35 or 36 weeks' gestation], small [birthweight <10th centile or <2500 g], or large [birthweight >90th centile or >4500 g] who received either 40% dextrose gel 200 mg/kg or placebo gel and feeds). The gel is massaged into the buccal mucosa and the baby is encouraged to feed. Of the 237 infants treated, there were 118 (50%) in the dextrose group and 119 (50%) in the placebo group. Dextrose gel reduced the frequency of treatment failure compared with placebo (16 [14%] vs. 29 [24%]; relative risk 0.57, 95% CI 0.33 to 0.98; $P = .04$). No serious adverse events were noted. This treatment approach has not yet been widely adopted in the United States.

Therapy

When to Treat. The major issues in therapy relate to when and how to treat. Detection of hypoglycemia at the bedside, previously dependent on Dextrostix determinations, has been facilitated in many units by portable reflectance meters, electrochemical glucose meters, and related instruments.[192] Confirmation of low values with laboratory determinations is important. The difficult issue in this context, of course, is the definition of hypoglycemia. Moreover, treatment depends on whether the infant is symptomatic or not. The American Academy of Pediatrics (AAP) has recently published guidelines for screening and management of postnatal glucose homeostasis in late-preterm (34 to 36 6/7 weeks' GA), term small-for-GA infants, and infants who were born to mothers with diabetes/large-for-GA infants (Fig. 25.15).[11] These guidelines suggest that late-preterm and small-for-GA infants be screened at 0 to 24 hours and infants of diabetic mothers and large-for-GA infants (i.e., ≥34 weeks' GA) at 0 to 12 hours. In the *asymptomatic infant,* the AAP suggests for values less than 25 mg/dL (birth to 4 hours), or less than 35 mg/dL (4 to 24 hours of age), that the infant be fed and rechecked in an hour; if the blood glucose

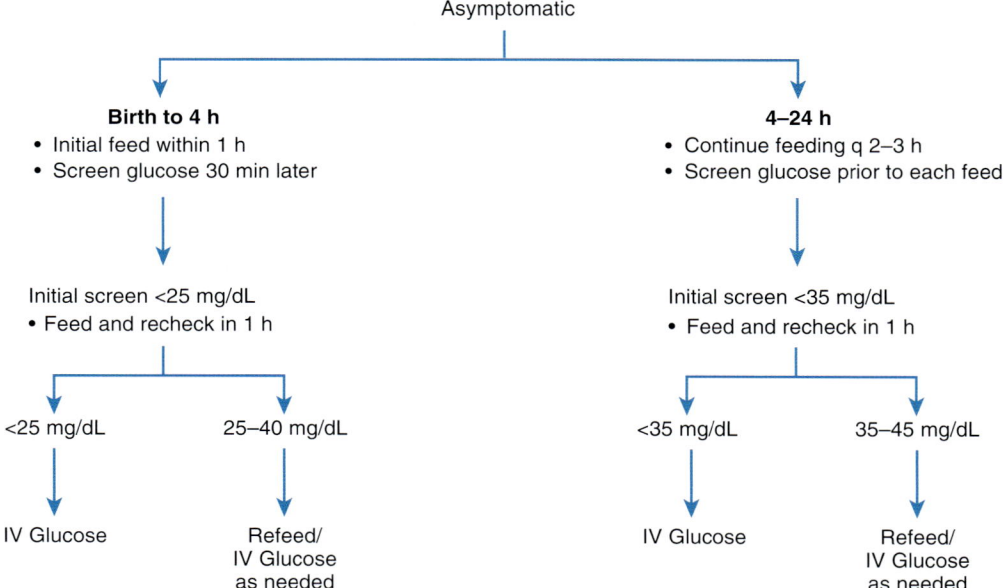

Asymptomatic

Birth to 4 h
- Initial feed within 1 h
- Screen glucose 30 min later

Initial screen <25 mg/dL
- Feed and recheck in 1 h

<25 mg/dL → IV Glucose

25–40 mg/dL → Refeed/ IV Glucose as needed

4–24 h
- Continue feeding q 2–3 h
- Screen glucose prior to each feed

Initial screen <35 mg/dL
- Feed and recheck in 1 h

<35 mg/dL → IV Glucose

35–45 mg/dL → Refeed/ IV Glucose as needed

Target glucose screen 45 mg/dL prior to routine feeds
Glucose dose = dextrose 10% at 2 mL/kg (200 mg/kg) and/or IV glucose infusion at 5–8 mg/kg per min (80–100 mL/kg per day)
Achieve plasma glucose level of 40–50 mg/dL

Figure 25.15 Algorithm depicting a scheme for the screening and management of postnatal glucose homeostasis in asymptomatic late preterm and term infants, small for gestational age infants, large for gestational age infants, and infants of diabetic mothers. *IV,* Intravenous. (Adapted from Adamkin DH, Committee on Fetus and Newborn. Clinical report—postnatal glucose homeostasis in late-preterm and term infants. *Pediatrics.* 2011;127:575.)

remains below 25 mg/dL or below 35 mg/dL, intravenous glucose should be administered. For symptomatic babies and a glucose level below 40 mg/dL, intravenous glucose is recommended (see Fig. 25.15).[11] However, we favor the following approach: intravenous glucose should be considered in any infant with a persistently low blood glucose level who is at risk for impaired metabolic adaptation (e.g., small-for-GA infant, infant of a diabetic mother, or the infant with concomitant hypoxic–ischemic insult), even with no abnormal clinical signs, or a single low blood glucose level in an infant presenting with abnormal clinical signs.[3] We suggest this approach based on (1) neurophysiological,[12] epidemiological,[5,17,18] and clinical[174] observations that levels less than 50 mg/dL can be associated with evidence for neurophysiological or neurodevelopmental dysfunction; (2) the PET observation that cerebral glucose utilization in the premature infant may be limited by glucose transport at levels of plasma glucose less than approximately 54 mg/dL; (3) the likelihood that degrees of hypoglycemia not sufficient to cause brain injury alone may do so when combined with other factors deleterious to the central nervous system; (4) the lack of precise information regarding the level of blood glucose below which neuronal injury is likely to occur; (5) the realization that the parieto-occipital region and higher visual functions are most sensitive to hypoglycemia and that such cortical functions have not been carefully studied in most previous follow-up reports; and (6) the ample experimental evidence that blood glucose levels are not accurate predictors of brain glucose levels, particularly in states such as asphyxia or seizures. It is essential that the physician consider the status of

both *cerebral glucose delivery* (i.e., CBF) as well as blood glucose content and *cerebral glucose utilization.*

How to Treat. If a decision is made to treat an infant, the next issue is the manner of therapy. A small group of infants requires specific therapies for hormonal or enzymatic aberrations; these therapies are discussed in detail elsewhere.[10,11,16,157,170] For the large group of infants in whom glucose alone is the mainstay of therapy, it is prudent to avoid the relatively large bolus infusion, particularly in the premature infant. Lilien and co-workers[193] demonstrated particular effectiveness and safety of a *minibolus infusion* of 200 mg/kg (2 mL of 10% glucose injected over 1 minute), immediately followed by a continuous glucose infusion of 5 to 8 mg/kg per minute.[11,184] The minibolus infusion results in rapid correction of blood glucose level (usually within 1 minute), and a relative stability of values between approximately 70 and 80 mg/dL occurs thereafter with the continuous infusion of 5 to 8 mg/kg per minute, approximately the maximum usable dose of glucose in the newborn (Fig. 25.16).[8,157,193,194] *Careful assessment of the initial clinical response after the minibolus infusion is essential,* especially if the indication for the infusion was seizure, because of variability in the response to blood glucose level; a second minibolus infusion may be necessary. *Continued careful monitoring of clinical response and blood glucose level* also is important because certain infants (e.g., those with hyperinsulinism) may require higher maintenance doses of glucose, whereas some infants require lower maintenance doses to avoid hyperglycemia.[10,11,157,192] In general, after blood glucose levels are stable at 70 to 100 mg/dL,

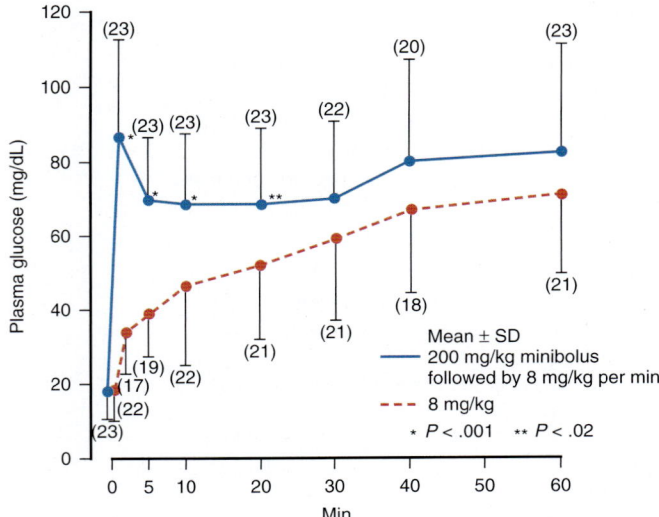

Figure 25.16 **Response to minibolus therapy in hypoglycemia.** Composite of blood glucose response to 200 mg/kg glucose minibolus followed by 8 mg/kg per minute constant glucose infusion in 23 hypoglycemic newborn infants and composite of blood glucose response to 8 mg/kg per minute constant glucose infusion without minibolus in 22 previously studied hypoglycemic infants. (From Lilien LD, Pildes RS, Srinivasan G. Treatment of neonatal hypoglycemia with minibolus and intravenous glucose infusion. *J Pediatr.* 1980;97:295–298.)

the dextrose concentration in the infusion may be decreased by 1 to 2 mg/kg per minute every 6 to 12 hours.[157] Glucose levels are monitored closely and should be maintained at more than 50 mg/dL. It is important not only to correct hypoglycemia but also to avoid hyperglycemia (see later). For infants whose glucose levels do not increase adequately despite higher infusion rates of at least 10 to 12 mg/kg per minute or who require infusion rates of more than 12 mg/kg per minute or if hypoglycemia recurs, hyperinsulinism should be considered. Treatment for the latter condition includes diazoxide or octreotide (both of which suppress insulin secretion) or pancreatic surgery.[169] Less likely causes include specific hormonal defects (e.g., hypopituitarism) or a metabolic disorder (see earlier), each of which requires specific therapy. Hydrocortisone, previously used in this context at 5 mg/kg every 12 hours, has benefit by increasing gluconeogenesis (from protein sources) and decreasing peripheral glucose utilization. This agent has been used less in recent years; if administered, it should be discontinued as soon as feasible.

Recent findings indicate that the rate of glucose infusion to correct hypoglycemia is not clear cut. Thus, in a study of infants (≤35 weeks GA) with hypoglycemia treated to maintain a blood glucose concentration of at least 47 mg/dL (2.6 mmol/L), a surprising finding was the association of neurosensory impairment, especially cognitive delay, with higher glucose concentrations and less glucose stability, indicated by a larger proportion of time outside a central range of 54 to 72 mg/dL in the first 48 hours.[154] Of concern is the observation that rapid correction of hypoglycemia to higher blood glucose concentrations may be associated with an adverse outcome. This unanticipated finding must be interpreted with caution, since the study was observational. Furthermore, the association was seen only in tests of general development and not in

tests of processing ability.[154] Hyperglycemia (blood glucose concentration of >180 mg/dL [10.0 mmol/L]) has been shown previously to be associated with increased mortality and neurodevelopmental impairment in very preterm infants,[195-198] but an association has not previously been reported in more mature infants, especially at glucose concentrations typically regarded as being within the normal range.

Conclusions

The definition of hypoglycemia and the level below which the risk for neurocognitive injury is increased remain unclear. This definition may differ for infants with transient adaptive hypoglycemia as opposed to those infants with congenital hyperinsulinism. These differences may in part explain the differences in treatment thresholds put forth by the American Academy of Pediatrics[11] and the Pediatric Endocrine Society.[199] Moreover, the observations that with interstitial monitoring up to 25% of periods of hypoglycemia go undetected, coupled with the observation that rapid correction of hypoglycemia may be associated with neurosensory issues, creates the clinical dilemma of whom to screen and when and how to treat. Future research is clearly of paramount importance.

KEY REFERENCES

1. Srinivasan G, Pildes RS, Cattamanchi G, et al. Clinical and laboratory observations. Plasma glucose values in normal neonates: a new look. *J Pediatr.* 1986;109:114-117.
2. Heck LJ, Erenberg A. Serum glucose levels in term neonates during the first 48 hours of life. *J Pediatr.* 1987;110:119-122.
3. Hawdon JM. Definition of neonatal hypoglycaemia: time for a rethink? *Arch Dis Child Fetal Neonatal Ed.* 2013;98:F382-F383.
4. Hoseth E, Joergensen A, Ebbesen F, et al. Blood glucose levels in a population of healthy, breast fed, term infants of appropriate size for gestational age. *Arch Dis Child Fetal Neonatal Ed.* 2000;83:F117-F119.
5. Lucas A, Morley R, Cole TJ. Adverse neurodevelopmental outcome of moderate neonatal hypoglycaemia. *Br Med J.* 1988; 297:1304-1308.
6. Harris DL, Weston PJ, Harding JE. Incidence of neonatal hypoglycemia in babies identified as at risk. *J Pediatr.* 2012;161: 787-791.
7. Kaiser JR, Bai S, Gibson N, et al. Association between transient newborn hypoglycemia and fourth-grade achievement test proficiency: a population-based study. *JAMA Pediatr.* 2015;169:913-921.
8. Cornblath M, Hawdon JM, Williams AF, et al. Controversies regarding definition of neonatal hypoglycemia: suggested operational thresholds. *Pediatrics.* 2000;105:1141-1145.
9. Cowett RM. Hypoglycemia and hyperglycemia in the newborn. In: Polin RA, Fox WW, eds. *Fetal and Neonatal Physiology.* Vol. 1. 2nd ed. Philadelphia: WB Saunders; 1998:596-608.
10. Rozance PJ, Hay WW. Hypoglycemia in newborn infants: features associated with adverse outcomes. *Biol Neonate.* 2006;90:74-86.
11. Adamkin DH. Clinical report—postnatal glucose homeostasis in late-preterm and term infants. *Pediatrics.* 2011;127:575-579.
12. Koh TH, Aynsley-Green A, Tarbit M, et al. Neural dysfunction during hypoglycaemia. *Arch Dis Child.* 1988;63:1353-1358.
13. Cowett RM, Howard GM, Johnson J, et al. Brain stem auditory-evoked response in relation to neonatal glucose metabolism. *Biol Neonate.* 1997;71:31-36.
15. Harris DL, Weston PJ, Harding JE. Lactate, rather than ketones, may provide alternative cerebral fuel in hypoglycaemic newborns. *Arch Dis Child Fetal Neonatal Ed.* 2015;100:F161-F164.
16. Stanley CA, Rozance PJ, Thornton PS, et al. Re-evaluating "transitional neonatal hypoglycemia": mechanism and implications for management. *J Pediatr.* 2015;166:1520-1525 e1521.
17. Lucas A, Morley R. Outcome of neonatal hypoglycaemia [Letter to the Editor]. *Br Med J.* 1999;318:194.

18. Tin W, Brunskill G, Kelly T, et al. 15-year follow-up of recurrent "hypoglycemia" in preterm infants. *Pediatrics*. 2012;130:e1497-e1503.
19. Hawdon JM, Aynsley-Green A, Alberti KG, et al. The role of pancreatic insulin secretion in neonatal glucoregulation. I. Healthy term and preterm infants. *Arch Dis Child*. 1993;68:274-279.
20. Hawdon JM, Ward Platt MP. Metabolic adaptation in small for gestational age infants. *Arch Dis Child*. 1993;68:262-268.
21. Hawdon JM, Weddell A, Aynsley-Green A, et al. Hormonal and metabolic response to hypoglycaemia in small for gestational age infants. *Arch Dis Child*. 1993;68:269-273.
22. Hawdon JM, Aynsley-Green A, Ward Platt MP. Neonatal blood glucose concentrations: metabolic effects of intravenous glucagon and intragastric medium chain triglyceride. *Arch Dis Child*. 1993;68:255-261.
23. Hawdon JM, Aynsley-Green A, Bartlett K, et al. The role of pancreatic insulin secretion in neonatal glucoregulation. II. Infants with disordered blood glucose homeostasis. *Arch Dis Child*. 1993;68:280-285.
24. Bier DM, Leake RD, Haymond MW, et al. Measurement of "true" glucose production rates in infancy and childhood with 6,6-dideuteroglucose. *Diabetes*. 1977;26:1016-1023.
25. Powers WJ, Rosenbaum JL, Dence CS, et al. Cerebral glucose transport and metabolism in preterm human infants. *J Cereb Blood Flow Metab*. 1998;18:632-638.
26. Vannucci RC. Cerebral carbohydrate and energy metabolism in perinatal hypoxic-ischemic brain damage. *Brain Pathol*. 1992;2:229-234.
28. Nehlig A, Pereira de Vasconcelos A. Glucose and ketone body utilization by the brain of neonatal rats. *Prog Neurobiol*. 1993; 40:163-221.
29. Yager JY. Hypoglycemic injury to the immature brain. *Clin Perinatol*. 2002;29:651-674.
31. DeVivo DC, Trifiletti RR, Jacobson RI, et al. Defective glucose transport across the blood-brain barrier as a cause of persistent hypoglycorrhachia, seizures, and developmental delay. *N Engl J Med*. 1991;325:703-709.
32. Fishman RA. The glucose-transporter protein and glucopenic brain injury. *N Engl J Med*. 1991;325:731-732.
33. Vannucci SJ. Developmental expression of GLUT1 and GLUT3 glucose transporters in rat brain. *J Neurochem*. 1994;62:240-246.
36. Brown AM, Ransom BR. Astrocyte glycogen and brain energy metabolism. *Glia*. 2007;55:1263-1271.
39. Hernandez MJ, Vannucci RC, Salcedo A, et al. Cerebral blood flow and metabolism during hypoglycemia in newborn dogs. *J Neurochem*. 1980;35:622-628.
44. Chugani HT, Phelps ME. Maturational changes in cerebral function in infants determined by [18]FDG positron emission tomography. *Science*. 1986;231:840-843.
46. Chugani HT, Phelps ME, Mazziotta JC. Positron emission tomography study of human brain functional development. *Ann Neurol*. 1987;22:487-497.
47. Altman DI, Powers WJ, Perlman JM, et al. Cerebral blood flow requirement for brain viability in newborn infants is lower than in adults. *Ann Neurol*. 1988;24:218-226.
50. Dombrowski GJ Jr, Swiatek KR, Chao KL. Lactate, 3-hydroxybutyrate, and glucose as substrates for the early postnatal rat brain. *Neurochem Res*. 1989;14:667-675.
51. Young RS, Petroff OA, Chen B, et al. Preferential utilization of lactate in neonatal dog brain: in vivo and in vitro proton NMR study. *Biol Neonate*. 1991;59:46-53.
54. Thurston JH, Hauhart RE, Schiro J. β-Hydroxybutyrate reverses insulin-induced hypoglycemic coma in suckling-weaning mice despite low blood and brain glucose levels. *Metab Brain Dis*. 1986;1:63-81.
56. Lin C-H, Gelardi NL, Cha C-J, et al. Cerebral metabolic response to hypoglycemia in severe intrauterine growth-retarded rat pups. *Early Hum Dev*. 1998;52:1-11.
60. Adam PAJ, Raiha N, Rahiala E, et al. Oxidation of glucose and D-beta-OH-butyrate by the early human fetal brain. *Acta Paediatr Scand*. 1975;64:17.
62. Page MA, Williamson DH. Enzymes of ketone-body utilization in human brain. *Lancet*. 1971;2:6.
63. Anday EK, Stanley CA, Baker L, et al. Plasma ketones in newborn infants: absence of suckling ketosis. *J Pediatr*. 1981;98:628.
64. Plecko B, Stoeckler-Ipsiroglu S, Schober E, et al. Oral beta-hydroxybutyrate supplementation in two patients with hyperinsulinemic hypoglycemia: monitoring of beta-hydroxybutyrate levels in blood and cerebrospinal fluid, and in the brain by in vivo magnetic resonance spectroscopy. *Pediatr Res*. 2002;52:301-306.
66. Young RS, Petroff OA, Chen B, et al. Brain energy state and lactate metabolism during status epilepticus in the neonatal dog: in vivo ^{31}P and ^{1}H nuclear magnetic resonance study. *Pediatr Res*. 1991;29:191-195.
69. Kuhlman RE, Lowry OH. Quantitative histochemical changes during the development of the rat cerebral cortex. *J Neurochem*. 1956;1:173.
75. Anwar M, Vannucci RC. Autoradiographic determination of regional cerebral blood flow during hypoglycemia in newborn dogs. *Pediatr Res*. 1988;24:41-45.
76. Mujsce DJ, Christensen MA, Vannucci RC. Regional cerebral blood flow and glucose utilization during hypoglycemia in newborn dogs. *Am J Physiol*. 1989;256:H1659-H1666.
77. Pryds O, Christensen NJ, Friis HB. Increased cerebral blood flow and plasma epinephrine in hypoglycemic, preterm neonates. *Pediatrics*. 1990;85:172-176.
78. Pryds O. Control of cerebral circulation in the high-risk neonate. *Ann Neurol*. 1991;30:321-329.
79. Skov L, Pryds O. Capillary recruitment for preservation of cerebral glucose influx in hypoglycemic, preterm newborns: evidence for a glucose sensor? *Pediatrics*. 1992;90:193-195.
82. Vannucci RC, Vannucci SJ. Cerebral carbohydrate metabolism during hypoglycemia and anoxia in newborn rats. *Ann Neurol*. 1978;4:74.
84. Ratcheson RA, Blank AC, Ferrendelli JA. Regionally selective metabolic effects of hypoglycemia in brain. *J Neurochem*. 1981;36:1952.
85. Ghajar JBG, Plum F, Duffy TE. Cerebral oxidative metabolism and blood flow during acute hypoglycemia and recovery in unanesthetized rats. *J Neurochem*. 1982;38:397.
86. Petroff OAC, Young RSK, Cowan BE. [1]H nuclear magnetic resonance spectroscopy study of neonatal hypoglycemia. *Pediatr Neurol*. 1988;4:31-34.
87. Brown AM. Brain glycogen re-awakened. *J Neurochem*. 2004; 89:537-552.
90. Ghajar JBG, Gibson GE, Duffy TE. Regional acetylcholine metabolism in brain during acute hypoglycemia and recovery. *J Neurochem*. 1985;44:94.
91. Behar KL, Hollander JA, Petroff OAC. Effect of hypoglycemic encephalopathy upon amino acids high-energy phosphates, and pHi in the rat brain in vivo, detection by sequential ^{1}H and ^{31}P NMR spectroscopy. *J Neurochem*. 1985;44:1045.
92. Wieloch T, Harris RJ, Symon L, et al. Influence of severe hypoglycemia on brain extracellular calcium and potassium activities, energy, and phospholipid metabolism. *J Neurochem*. 1984;43:160-168.
93. Wieloch T. Hypoglycemia-induced neuronal damage prevented by an N-methyl-D-aspartate antagonist. *Science*. 1985;230:681-683.
94. Sandberg M, Butcher SP, Hagberg M. Extracellular overflow of neuroactive amino acids during severe insulin induced hypoglycemia in vivo dialysis of the rat hippocampus. *J Neurochem*. 1986;47:178-184.
95. Facci L, Leon A, Skaper SD. Hypoglycemic neurotoxicity in vitro: involvement of excititory amino acid receptors and attenuation by monosialoganglioside GM1. *Neuroscience*. 1990;37:709-716.
96. Papagapiou MP, Auer RN. Regional neuroprotective effects of the NMDA receptor antagonist MK-801 (Dizocilpine) in hypoglycemic brain damage. *J Cereb Blood Flow Metab*. 1990;10:270-276.
97. Tasker RC, Coyle JT, Vornov JJ. The regional vulnerability to hypoglycemia-induced neurotoxicity in organotypic hippocampal culture—protection by early tetrodotoxin or delayed MK-801. *J Neurosci*. 1992;12:4298-4308.
98. Simon RP, Schmidley JW, Meldrum BS, et al. Excitotoxic mechanisms in hypoglycaemic hippocampal injury. *Neuropathol Appl Neurobiol*. 1986;12:567-576.
99. McGowan JE, Hayneslaing AG, Mishra OP, et al. The effect of acute hypoglycemia on the cerebral NMDA receptor in newborn piglets. *Brain Res*. 1995;670:283-288.

100. Suh SW, Aoyama K, Chen YM, et al. Hypoglycemic neuronal death and cognitive impairment are prevented by poly(ADP-ribose) polymerase inhibitors administered after hypoglycemia. *J Neurosci.* 2003;23:10681-10690.

101. Shelley HJ. Glycogen reserves and their changes at birth and in anoxia. *Br Med J.* 1961;17:137.

102. Dawes GS, Mott JC, Shelley HJ. The importance of cardiac glycogen for the maintenance of life in fetal lambs and newborn animals during anoxia. *J Physiol.* 1960;152:271.

103. Silverstein FS, Simpson J, Gordon KE. Hypoglycemia alters striatal amino acid efflux in perinatal rats: an in vivo microdialysis study. *Ann Neurol.* 1990;28:516-521.

104. McGowan JE, Chen L, Gao D, et al. Increased mitochondrial reactive oxygen species production in newborn brain during hypoglycemia. *Neurosci Lett.* 2006;399:111-114.

105. Suh SW, Gum ET, Hamby AM, et al. Hypoglycemic neuronal death is triggered by glucose reperfusion and activation of neuronal NADPH oxidase. *J Clin Invest.* 2007;117:910-918.

107. Himwich HE, Bernstein AO, Herlich H. Mechanisms for the maintenance of life in the newborn during anoxia. *Am J Physiol.* 1942;135:387.

108. Juurlink BHJ, Hertz L, Yager JY. Astrocyte maturation and susceptibility to ischaemia or substrate deprivation. *Dev Neurosci.* 1992;3:1135-1137.

109. Callahan DJ, Engle MJ, Volpe JJ. Hypoxic injury to developing glial cells: protective effect of high glucose. *Pediatr Res.* 1990;27:186-190.

110. Rosenberg AA, Murdaugh E. The effect of blood glucose concentration on postasphyxia cerebral hemodynamics in newborn lambs. *Pediatr Res.* 1990;27:454-459.

111. Salhab WA, Wyckoff MH, Laptook AR, et al. Initial hypoglycemia and neonatal brain injury in term infants with severe fetal acidemia. *Pediatrics.* 2004;114:361-366.

112. Wong DS, Poskitt KJ, Chau V, et al. Brain injury patterns in hypoglycemia in neonatal encephalopathy. *AJNR Am J Neuroradiol.* 2013;34:1456-1461.

113. Tam EW, Haeusslein LA, Bonifacio SL, et al. Hypoglycemia is associated with increased risk for brain injury and adverse neurodevelopmental outcome in neonates at risk for encephalopathy. *J Pediatr.* 2012;161:88-93.

114. Harteman JC, Groenendaal F, Benders MJ, et al. Role of thrombophilic factors in full-term infants with neonatal encephalopathy. *Pediatr Res.* 2013;73:80-86.

117. Yager JY, Brucklacher RM, Vannucci RC. Cerebral oxidative metabolism and redox state during hypoxia-ischemia and early recovery in immature rats. *Am J Physiol.* 1991;261:H1102-H1108.

118. Yager JY, Heitjan DF, Towfighi J, et al. Effect of insulin-induced and fasting hypoglycemia on perinatal hypoxic-ischemic brain damage. *Pediatr Res.* 1992;31:138-142.

119. Riddle A, Maire J, Cai V, et al. Hemodynamic and metabolic correlates of perinatal white matter injury severity. *PLoS ONE.* 2013;8:e82940.

120. Glauser TA, Rorke LB, Weinberg PM, et al. Acquired neuropathologic lesions associated with the hypoplastic left heart syndrome. *Pediatrics.* 1990;85:991-1000.

125. Gomez B, Garcia-Villallon AL, Frank A, et al. Effects of hypoglycemia on the cerebral circulation in awake goats. *Neurology.* 1992;42:909-916.

127. Young RS, Cowan BE, Petroff OA, et al. In vivo ^{31}P and in vitro ^{1}H nuclear magnetic resonance study of hypoglycemia during neonatal seizure. *Ann Neurol.* 1987;22:622-628.

128. Dwyer BE, Wasterlain CG. Neonatal seizures in monkeys and rabbits: brain glucose depletion in the face of normoglycemia, prevention by glucose loads. *Pediatr Res.* 1985;19:992-995.

129. Fujikawa DG, Vannucci RC, Dwyer BE, et al. Generalized seizures deplete brain energy reserves in normoxemic newborn monkeys. *Brain Res.* 1988;454:51-59.

133. Auer RN, Kalimo H, Olsson Y, et al. The temporal evolution of hypoglycemic brain damage. I. Light- and electron-microscopic findings in the rat cerebral cortex. *Acta Neuropathol.* 1985;67:13-24.

134. Auer RN, Wieloch T, Olsson Y, et al. The distribution of hypoglycemic brain damage. *Acta Neuropathol.* 1984;64:177-191.

135. Anderson JM, Milner RD, Strich SJ. Effects of neonatal hypoglycaemia on the nervous system: a pathological study. *J Neurol Neurosurg Psychiatry.* 1967;30:295-310.

136. Griffiths AD, Laurence KM. The effect of hypoxia and hypoglycaemia on the brain of the newborn human infant. *Dev Med Child Neurol.* 1974;16:308-319.

137. Spar JA, Lewine JD, Orrison WW Jr. Neonatal hypoglycemia: CT and MR findings. *AJNR Am J Neuroradiol.* 1994;15:1477-1478.

138. Barkovich AJ, Ali FA, Rowley HA, et al. Imaging patterns of neonatal hypoglycemia. *AJNR Am J Neuroradiol.* 1998;19:523-528.

139. Chiu NT, Huang CC, Chang YC, et al. Technetium-99m-HMPAO brain SPECT in neonates with hypoglycemic encephalopathy. *J Nucl Med.* 1998;39:1711-1713.

140. Kinnala A, Rikalainen H, Lapinleimu H, et al. Cerebral magnetic resonance imaging and ultrasonography findings after neonatal hypoglycemia. *Pediatrics.* 1999;103:724-729.

141. Caraballo RH, Sakr D, Mozzi M, et al. Symptomatic occipital lobe epilepsy following neonatal hypoglycemia. *Pediatr Neurol.* 2004;31:24-29.

142. Alkalay AL, Flores-Sarnat L, Sarnat HB, et al. Brain imaging findings in neonatal hypoglycemia: case report and review of 23 cases. *Clin Pediatr (Phila).* 2005;44:783-790.

143. Murakami Y, Yamashita Y, Matsuishi T, et al. Cranial MRI of neurologically impaired children suffering from neonatal hypoglycaemia. *Pediatr Radiol.* 1999;29:23-27.

144. Filan PM, Inder TE, Cameron FJ, et al. Neonatal hypoglycemia and occipital cerebral injury. *J Pediatr.* 2006;148:552-555.

145. Huttenlocher PR, Dabholkar AS. Regional differences in synaptogenesis in human cerebral cortex. *J Comp Neurol.* 1997;387:167-178.

146. Huttenlocher PR, de Courten C. The development of synapses in striate cortex of man. *Hum Neurobiol.* 1987;6:1-9.

147. Purpura DP. Dendritic differentiation in human cerebral cortex: normal and aberrant developmental patterns. *Adv Neurol.* 1975;12:91-134.

148. Takashima S, Chan F, Becker LE, et al. Morphology of the developing visual cortex of the human infant: a quantitative and qualitative Golgi study. *J Neuropathol Exp Neurol.* 1980;39:487-501.

149. Friede RL. *Developmental Neuropathology.* 2nd ed. New York: Springer-Verlag; 1989.

150. Larroche JC. *Developmental Pathology of the Neonate.* New York: Excerpta Medica; 1977.

151. Yan H, Rivkees SA. Hypoglycemia influences oligodendrocyte development and myelin formation. *Neuroreport.* 2006;17:55-59.

153. Banker BQ. The neuropathological effects of anoxia and hypoglycemia in the newborn. *Dev Med Child Neurol.* 1967;9:544-550.

154. McKinlay CJ, Alsweiler JM, Ansell JM, et al. Neonatal glycemia and neurodevelopmental outcomes at 2 years. *N Engl J Med.* 2015;373:1507-1518.

156. Diwakar KK, Sasidhar MV. Plasma glucose levels in term infants who are appropriate size for gestation and exclusively breast fed. *Arch Dis Child Fetal Neonatal Ed.* 2002;87:F46-F48.

157. Rozance PJ, Hay WW Jr. Describing hypoglycemia—definition or operational threshold? *Early Hum Dev.* 2010;86:275-280.

158. Stenninger E, Flink R, Eriksson B, et al. Long term, neurological dysfunction and neonatal hypoglycaemia after diabetic pregnancy. *Arch Dis Child.* 1998;79:F174-F179.

159. Schaefer-Graf UM, Rossi R, Buhrer C, et al. Rate and risk factors of hypoglycemia in large-for-gestational-age newborn infants of nondiabetic mothers. *Am J Obstet Gynecol.* 2002;187:913-917.

160. Brand PL, Molenaar NL, Kaaijk C, et al. Neurodevelopmental outcome of hypoglycaemia in healthy, large for gestational age, term newborns. *Arch Dis Child.* 2005;90:78-81.

161. Hawdon JM. Postnatal metabolic adaptation and neonatal hypoglycaemia. *Paediatr. Child Health.* 2016;26:135-139.

163. Arya VB, Flanagan SE, Kumaran A, et al. Clinical and molecular characterisation of hyperinsulinaemic hypoglycaemia in infants born small-for-gestational age. *Arch Dis Child Fetal Neonatal Ed.* 2013;98:F356-F358.

164. Sovik O. Inborn errors of amino acid and fatty acid metabolism with hypoglycemia as a major clinical manifestation. *Acta Paediatr Scand.* 1989;78:161-170.

165. Perelmuter B, Goodman SI, McCabe ER. Galactosaemia with fatal cerebral oedema. *J Inherit Metab Dis.* 1989;12:489-490.

166. Zeller J, Bougneres P. Hypoglycemia in infants. *Trends Endocrinol Metab.* 1992;3:366-370.

167. Bell JJ, August GP, Blethen SL, et al. Neonatal hypoglycemia in a growth hormone registry: incidence and pathogenesis. *J Pediatr Endocrinol Metab*. 2004;17:629-635.

168. Sperling MA, Menon RK. Differential diagnosis and management of neonatal hypoglycemia. *Pediatr Clin North Am*. 2004;51:703-723.

169. Hussain K. Congenital hyperinsulinism. *Semin Fetal Neonatal Med*. 2005;10:369-376.

170. Hussain K, Aynsley-Green A. Hyperinsulinaemic hypoglycaemia in preterm neonates. *Arch Dis Child Fetal Neonatal Ed*. 2004;89:F65-F67.

171. Menni F, de Lonlay P, Sevin C, et al. Neurologic outcomes of 90 neonates and infants with persistent hyperinsulinemic hypoglycemia. *Pediatrics*. 2001;107:476-479.

172. Faletra F, Snider K, Shyng SL, et al. Co-inheritance of two ABCC8 mutations causing an unresponsive congenital hyperinsulinism: clinical and functional characterization of two novel ABCC8 mutations. *Gene*. 2013;516:122-125.

173. Saint-Martin C, Arnoux JB, de Lonlay P, et al. KATP channel mutations in congenital hyperinsulinism. *Semin Pediatr Surg*. 2011;20:18-22.

174. Duvanel CB, Fawer CL, Cotting J, et al. Long-term effects of neonatal hypoglycemia on brain growth and psychomotor development in small-for-gestational-age preterm infants. *J Pediatr*. 1999;134:492-498.

175. Koivisto M, Blanco-Sequeiros M, Krause U. Neonatal symptomatic and asymptomatic hypoglycaemia: a follow-up study of 151 children. *Dev Med Child Neurol*. 1972;14:603-614.

177. Montassir H, Maegaki Y, Ogura K, et al. Associated factors in neonatal hypoglycemic brain injury. *Brain Dev*. 2009;31:649-656.

178. Tam EW, Widjaja E, Blaser SI, et al. Occipital lobe injury and cortical visual outcomes after neonatal hypoglycemia. *Pediatrics*. 2008;122:507-512.

179. Musson RE, Batty R, Mordekar SR, et al. Diffusion-weighted imaging and magnetic resonance spectroscopy findings in a case of neonatal hypoglycaemia. *Dev Med Child Neurol*. 2009;51:653-654.

180. Montassir H, Maegaki Y, Ohno K, et al. Long term prognosis of symptomatic occipital lobe epilepsy secondary to neonatal hypoglycemia. *Epilepsy Res*. 2010;88:93-99.

181. Caksen H, Guven AS, Yilmaz C, et al. Clinical outcome and magnetic resonance imaging findings in infants with hypoglycemia. *J Child Neurol*. 2011;26:25-30.

182. Gataullina S, De Lonlay P, Dellatolas G, et al. Topography of brain damage in metabolic hypoglycaemia is determined by age at which hypoglycaemia occurred. *Dev Med Child Neurol*. 2013;55:162-166.

183. Burns CM, Rutherford MA, Boardman JP, et al. Patterns of cerebral injury and neurodevelopmental outcomes after symptomatic neonatal hypoglycemia. *Pediatrics*. 2008;122:65-74.

184. Pildes RS, Cornblath M, Warren I, et al. A prospective controlled study of neonatal hypoglycemia. *Pediatrics*. 1974;54:5-14.

185. Kerstjens JM, Bocca-Tjeertes IF, de Winter AF, et al. Neonatal morbidities and developmental delay in moderately preterm-born children. *Pediatrics*. 2012;130:e265-e272.

186. Karimzadeh P, Tabarestani S, Ghofrani M. Hypoglycemia-occipital syndrome: a specific neurologic syndrome following neonatal hypoglycemia? *J Child Neurol*. 2011;26:152-159.

187. Dalgic N, Ergenekon E, Soysal S, et al. Transient neonatal hypoglycemia—long-term effects on neurodevelopmental outcome. *J Pediatr Endocrinol Metab*. 2002;15:319-324.

188. Hume R, McGeechan A, Burchell A. Failure to detect preterm infants at risk of hypoglycemia before discharge. *J Pediatr*. 1999;134:499-502.

189. Hawdon JM, Ward Platt MP, Aynsley-Green A. Patterns of metabolic adaptation for preterm and term infants in the first neonatal week. *Arch Dis Child*. 1992;67:357-365.

190. Harris DL, Weston PJ, Signal M, et al. Dextrose gel for neonatal hypoglycaemia (the Sugar Babies Study): a randomised, double-blind, placebo-controlled trial. *Lancet*. 2013;382:2077-2083.

191. Brown LD, Rozance PJ. A sweet addition for the treatment of neonatal hypoglycemia. *J Pediatr*. 2016;170:10-12.

192. Michel A, Kuster H, Krebs A, et al. Evaluation of the Glucometer Elite XL device for screening for neonatal hypoglycaemia. *Eur J Pediatr*. 2005;164:660-664.

193. Lilien LD, Pildes RS, Srinivasan G. Treatment of neonatal hypoglycemia with minibolus and intravenous glucose infusion. *J Pediatr*. 1980;97:295.

194. Bier DM, Leake RD, Arnold KJ. Glucose production rates in infancy and childhood. *Pediatr Res*. 1976;10:405.

195. Hays SP, Smith EO, Sunehag AL. Hyperglycemia is a risk factor for early death and morbidity in extremely low birth-weight infants. *Pediatrics*. 2006;118:1811-1818.

196. van der Lugt NM, Smits-Wintjens VE, van Zwieten PH, et al. Short and long term outcome of neonatal hyperglycemia in very preterm infants: a retrospective follow-up study. *BMC Pediatr*. 2010;10:52.

197. Alexandrou G, Skiold B, Karlen J, et al. Early hyperglycemia is a risk factor for death and white matter reduction in preterm infants. *Pediatrics*. 2010;125:e584-e591.

198. Stensvold HJ, Strommen K, Lang AM, et al. Early enhanced parenteral nutrition, hyperglycemia, and death among extremely low-birth-weight infants. *JAMA Pediatr*. 2015;169:1003-1010.

199. Thornton PS, Stanley CA, De Leon DD, et al. Recommendations from the pediatric endocrine society for evaluation and management of persistent hypoglycemia in neonates, infants, and children. *J Pediatr*. 2015;167:238-245.

Full references for this chapter can be found at www.expertconsult.com.

Bilirubin

Jeffrey M. Perlman ◆ *Joseph J. Volpe*

An important relationship between bilirubin and injury to the neonatal central nervous system has been recognized for many years. The first comprehensive description of the most overt form of bilirubin encephalopathy (i.e., kernicterus) was provided by Schmorl in 1903.[1] The development of therapeutic measures, such as exchange transfusion, and of preventive measures, such as the use of anti-Rh immune globulin to prevent maternal sensitization, resulted in a marked decrease in this overt form of bilirubin encephalopathy. Subsequently implementation of predischarge universal screening coupled with the appropriate use of phototherapy and post–hospital discharge follow-up has been shown to be an extremely important strategy in the prevention of severe neonatal hyperbilirubinemia.[2-4] The total impact of these strategies on hospital readmissions in the first 1 to 2 weeks of life remains to be defined.[2-5]

In this chapter, normal bilirubin structure and metabolism, the pathophysiology of hyperbilirubinemia and bilirubin neurotoxicity, and the neuropathological and clinical aspects of bilirubin injury to the neonatal central nervous system are reviewed.

NORMAL BILIRUBIN STRUCTURE AND METABOLISM

Central to an understanding of the relation of bilirubin to neonatal brain injury is an awareness of the normal aspects of bilirubin structure, properties, and metabolism in the newborn. Thus, before the pathophysiology of bilirubin encephalopathies is discussed, certain highly relevant aspects of the chemical structure and solubility of bilirubin, as well as normal bilirubin metabolism, are briefly reviewed.

Bilirubin Structure and Properties

Bilirubin is a catabolic product of the porphyrin ring, derived from heme (see subsequent discussion). This compound can exist in plasma as bilirubin anion (monoanion or dianion form) (Fig. 26.1A) or as bilirubin acid (see Fig. 26.1B). Bilirubin dianion binds actively to albumin. The dianion is not highly soluble in lipid or nonpolar solvents,[6,7] but in view of the two polar carboxyl groups and oxidipyrryl (lactam) groups, it is not surprising that the anionic forms of bilirubin are relatively soluble in polar solvents. Although the anionic forms were considered previously to be the principal free bilirubin species in plasma, more recent work showed that at physiological pH the acceptance of two hydrogen ions results in bilirubin diacid (see Fig. 26.1B). The diacid has a rigid folded structure, maintained by six internal hydrogen bonds involving all the polar groups,

thereby rendering the molecule poorly soluble in aqueous solutions.[8] However, the compound does passively diffuse across plasma membranes of cells (see later). When the concentration of free bilirubin diacid exceeds its limit of aqueous solubility (≈70 nM at physiological pH), the compound exists as soluble oligomers and metastable microaggregates. Moreover, at very high concentrations of the diacid, insoluble precipitates form that may result in major injury to membranes. At *physiological pH*, the species of free bilirubin are approximately 82% diacid, 16% monoanion, and 2% dianion.[8] These chemical properties of bilirubin are important in understanding the neurotoxicity of bilirubin (see later discussion).

Bilirubin Metabolism

Normal bilirubin metabolism is considered best in terms of the following sequential events: (1) production, (2) transport, (3) hepatic uptake, (4) conjugation, (5) excretion, and (6) enterohepatic circulation (Fig. 26.2).[9-11]

Production

Bilirubin is the end product of the catabolism of heme, the major source of which is circulating hemoglobin (see Fig. 26.2). In the newborn infant, the normal destruction of circulating red blood cells in the reticuloendothelial system accounts for approximately 75% of the daily production of bilirubin. The conversion of the heme moiety to bilirubin requires the sequential action of two enzymes, heme oxygenase (to form biliverdin) and a reduced nicotinamide adenine dinucleotide phosphate (NADPH)–dependent biliverdin reductase (to form bilirubin). Approximately 25% of the daily production of bilirubin in the newborn is derived from sources other than senescent red blood cells. This *other* fraction has two major components: a nonerythropoietic component, resulting from turnover of nonhemoglobin sources of heme (e.g., cytochromes, catalase, peroxidase, and myoglobin), and an erythropoietic component, resulting from the destruction of products of ineffective erythropoiesis.

Transport

Bilirubin leaves the site of production in the reticuloendothelial system and is transported in plasma bound to albumin (see Fig. 26.2). Human albumin has a single, tight, high-affinity (or primary) binding site for bilirubin and one or more (probably two) weaker, lower-affinity binding sites.[10,12-14] The capacity of serum albumin to bind bilirubin is known as the *binding capacity*, and the strength of the bilirubin-albumin bond is referred to as the *binding affinity*. The amount of *free bilirubin*

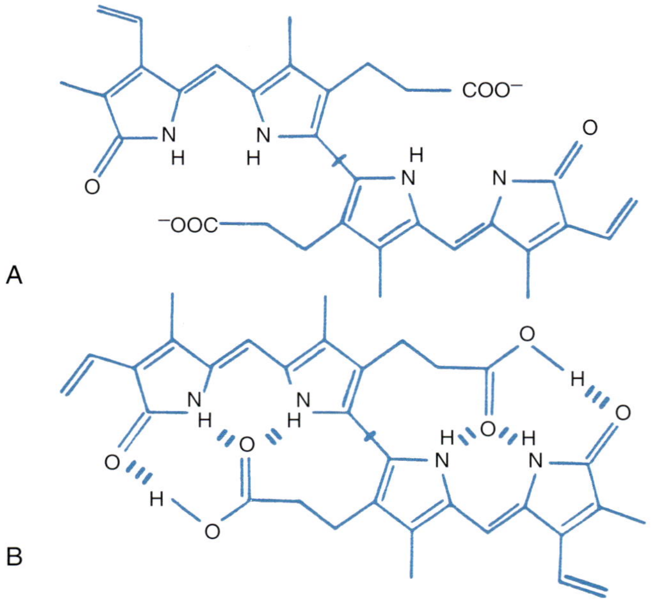

Figure 26.1 Chemical structures of bilirubin. (A) Bilirubin dianion, with two free carboxyl groups; bilirubin monoanion has one free carboxyl group. (B) Bilirubin diacid, the predominant form of free bilirubin in plasma at physiological pH. See text for details. (From Brodersen R. Bilirubin transport in the newborn infant, reviewed in relation to kernicterus. *J Pediatr.* 1980;96:349–356.)

TABLE 26.1 Major Causes of Neonatal Unconjugated Hyperbilirubinemia

Increased production
Hemolytic disease
Immune-mediated: Rh or ABO incompatibility
Inherited red blood cell defects: red blood cell membranes (e.g., spherocytosis), hemoglobin (e.g., thalassemias), or red blood cell metabolism (e.g., glucose-6-phosphate dehydrogenase deficiency[a])
Other
Hematoma, including cerebral, or other extravasation of blood
Polycythemia
Sepsis[a]
Infant of diabetic mother
Increased enterohepatic circulation
Breast-milk feeding
Bowel obstruction
Decreased conjugation
Prematurity
Glucose-6-phosphase dehydrogenase deficiency
Uridine glucuronyl transferase deficiency (e.g., Crigler-Najjar, Gilbert syndrome)
Hypothyroidism

[a]Decreased conjugation/clearance also involved.
Adapted from Maisels MJ. Jaundice. In: MacDonald MG, Mullett MD, Seshia MMK, eds. *Avery's Neonatology Pathophysiology and Management of the Newborn.* 6th ed. Philadelphia: Lippincott Williams & Wilkins; 2005.

(i.e., bilirubin not bound to albumin) is very low at physiological pH. These last three characteristics of a given serum-binding capacity, binding affinity, and amount of free bilirubin can be estimated by in vitro measurements[15] and provide a measure, albeit only approximate, of the amount of bilirubin that may be available to cause neuronal injury (see later discussion).

Hepatic Uptake

Hepatocytes have a selective and highly efficient system for removing unconjugated bilirubin from plasma. This mechanism requires several different organic anion transport proteins.[4,10] Variants of one of these, organic anion transporter 2 (OATP2), may be important in determining the elevated risk of severe hyperbilirubinemia in Asian infants.[16] In the hepatocyte, the transported bilirubin is bound to ligandin, a cytosolic protein, that facilitates transfer to the endoplasmic reticulum, the site of bilirubin conjugation.[10]

Conjugation

Conversion of bilirubin to excretable monoconjugates and diconjugates is carried out primarily by the microsomal enzyme uridine-diphosphate (UDP)–glucuronyl transferase (A1 isoform). The protein is encoded by the *UGT1A1* gene.[17] Variants of the *UGT1A1* gene appear to be important in determining the elevated risk of severe hyperbilirubinemia in Asian infants.[18-20] The disconjugate accounts for approximately 90% of total bilirubin glucuronide conjugates.[10,21]

Excretion

The conjugated bilirubin is excreted into the bile. Because this event occurs across a concentration gradient, an energy-dependent active transport system is involved.[4,10] The conjugated bilirubin is then transported to the small intestine, where it is primarily further degraded by intestinal bacteria and excreted in the stool.

Enterohepatic Circulation

Enterohepatic circulation also occurs. Intestinal beta-glucuronidase hydrolyzes the conjugated bilirubin, thus releasing free bilirubin, which is then reabsorbed and transported by the portal circulation to the liver (see Fig. 26.2).

PATHOPHYSIOLOGY

Hyperbilirubinemia

Although the relationship between serum levels of unconjugated bilirubin and neurotoxicity is not simple (see subsequent sections), a general link can be discerned between neonatal hyperbilirubinemia and the risk of neural injury. The major causes of neonatal hyperbilirubinemia, including the universal (*physiological*) elevation of bilirubin in the newborn, are reviewed next.

Major Causes

In the newborn period, numerous disorders may lead to elevated concentrations of unconjugated bilirubin (Table 26.1).[21] These include the following: disorders with *increased production*, principally hemolytic disease, secondary to blood group incompatibility; intrinsic defects of red blood cells or hemoglobin; degradation of extravascular blood (i.e., hemorrhage); polycythemia; sepsis; disorders with disturbed gastrointestinal transit and therefore *increased enterohepatic circulation; disorders of bilirubin conjugation,* including inherited

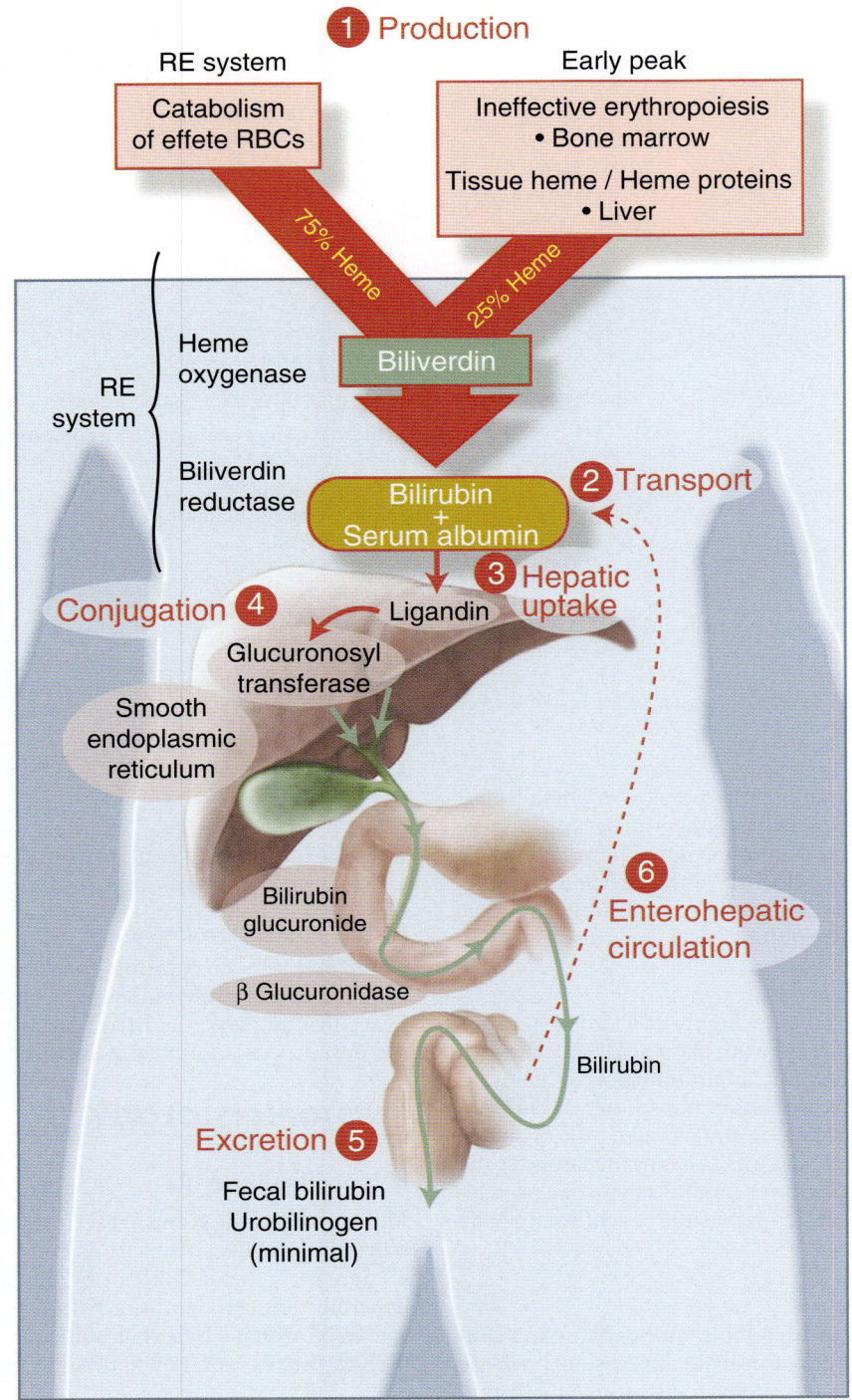

Figure 26.2 Bilirubin metabolism. See text for details. *RBCs*, Red blood cells; *RE system*, reticuloendothelial system.

and acquired defects (e.g., prematurity); and hormonal disturbances (e.g., hypothyroidism).[21] Central to the frequency of hyperbilirubinemia in the newborn is the development of hyperbilirubinemia that occurs normally and onto which these other causes are grafted. This *physiological jaundice of the newborn* may be better termed *developmental hyperbilirubinemia* because it is very difficult to define precisely when this neonatal process is physiological and when it is pathological.[21]

Physiological Hyperbilirubinemia

Definition. *Physiological hyperbilirubinemia* refers to the elevation of serum bilirubin values that occur in essentially every newborn infant in the first week of life. In classic earlier studies of formula-fed white and African American full-term infants, the serum bilirubin level rose gradually to a mean peak of approximately 6 mg/dL by 48 to 72 hours of life and then declined relatively rapidly to a slightly elevated level, approximately 3 mg/dL, at approximately 5 days of life. After the peak bilirubin level was reached, little change occurred for several days; then a second, gradual decline occurred, with normal levels reached by approximately 2 weeks.[22] Thus, two phases could be identified in the human, and the mechanisms underlying these were studied in detail in the neonatal monkey, in which the biphasic course is also apparent.[22] With the current increase in breast-feeding in the United States and elsewhere, peak values for bilirubin clearly are greater than in the earlier studies. Thus, in predominantly breast-fed white and African American term infants, the normal peak value is 8 to 9 mg/dL, and the decline is slower.[21] In Asian newborns (predominantly breast-fed), the peak values, 10 to 14 mg/dL, are still higher than those in white and African American infants.[2,20] In the premature infant, the peak serum bilirubin concentration occurs slightly later than in the full-term infant (i.e., approximately the fourth to fifth day) and is higher (i.e., mean: 10 to 12 mg/dL); normal levels may not be reached until 3 to 4 weeks of age.[2] More importantly, the term *physiological hyperbilirubinemia* in the *premature infant* is misleading because such values are potentially dangerous (see later).[21] Indeed, in infants of very low birth weight, phototherapy is recommended well before values reach 10 to 12 mg/dL (see later).

The *late preterm infant* (i.e., 35 to 37 weeks of gestation) presents a situation intermediate between the clearly premature infant and the full-term infant (38 to 42 weeks of gestation). Thus, several studies showed that such infants have a severalfold higher risk of significant hyperbilirubinemia in the first week of life.[23-25] In a careful study through the first 7 days of life, near-term infants exhibited a later and higher peak value of bilirubin than did term infants. Moreover, the higher values declined more slowly in the near-term infants. Overall, 10% of the full-term infants had significant hyperbilirubinemia requiring phototherapy, versus 25% in the near-term group.[26] These data highlight the importance of particularly close follow-up of near-term infants after hospital discharge (see later).

Mechanisms. The mechanisms considered important in the genesis of physiological hyperbilirubinemia are shown in Table 26.2. Although evidence has been mustered for all these factors, studies of the newborn monkey provided considerable insight into their relative importance.[22] Thus, the *first phase* of hyperbilirubinemia (see previous section) has been shown to relate to the combined effects of (1) increased bilirubin load to the liver and (2) decreased bilirubin-conjugating capacity. The source of the increased bilirubin load to the liver includes both hemoglobin and nonhemoglobin sources as well as the enterohepatic circulation[27]; the latter is increased in the newborn because of deficient bacterial degradation of bilirubin and increased activity of intestinal beta-glucuronidase.[28] The defective bilirubin conjugating capacity is related to a diminished activity of hepatic UDP-glucuronyl transferase, which undergoes a rapid developmental change from negligible levels at birth to adult levels after several days.[22] Prematurity results in more severe neonatal hyperbilirubinemia, principally because of a delayed maturation of the hepatic UDP-glucuronyl

TABLE 26.2	Probable Mechanisms Involved in Physiological Hyperbilirubinemia[a]

Increased bilirubin production
  ↑ Red blood cell volume
  ↓ Red blood cell survival
  ↑ "Other" sources
Increased enterohepatic circulation
Decreased hepatic uptake of bilirubin from plasma
  ↓ Membrane transport
  ↓ Ligandin
Defective bilirubin conjugation
  ↓ Uridine-diphosphate-glucuronyl transferase

[a]See text for references.
↑, Increased; ↓, decreased.

transferase.[10,22] More recent studies in human infants have refined the earlier observations. Thus the possibility of impaired transport of bilirubin into the hepatocyte because of genetic variants of organic anion transporters (see earlier) is likely important, perhaps especially in Asian infants.[20] The diminished levels of ligandin in hepatic cytosol are likely less important. Genetic variants of the *UGT1A1* gene as well as the long-recognized developmental deficiency of the glucuronyl transferase may also be important. Increase in the enterohepatic circulation is likely important in *jaundice associated with breast milk feedings* because breast milk contains beta-glucuronidase, which can degrade conjugated bilirubin in the small intestine.[21,29] In addition, lipoprotein lipase activity in breast milk has been suggested to lead to the increased release of free fatty acids (anions) from triglycerides and thereby to a disturbance of hepatic uptake. Pregnanediol in breast milk may also inhibit bilirubin conjugation. Finally, the common *delay in adequate caloric intake* with breast-feeding is considered of most importance in jaundice associated with breast-feeding; the mechanism of the deleterious effect of caloric deprivation on bilirubin homeostasis remains unclear.[21]

Important Determinants of Neuronal Injury by Bilirubin

The critical event in the genesis of brain injury caused by bilirubin is entrance of bilirubin into brain and exposure to neurons.[11,21,30-32] The predominance of available data indicates that bilirubin per se and more specifically the bilirubin no longer bound to albumin, that is, *unbound or "free" bilirubin*, is the form that ultimately leads to neuronal injury (see later discussion).[11]

Interrelationships of Bilirubin, Albumin, and Hydrogen Ion

To derive the important determinants of neuronal injury by bilirubin, it is necessary to recognize the critical reactions shown in Fig. 26.3. As noted earlier, at physiological pH, the predominant species of unbound bilirubin in plasma is bilirubin acid. Consideration of these equilibria makes it clear that the potential means for increasing the exposure of neurons to bilirubin acid would include increasing the quantity of [bilirubin anion]-albumin (i.e., *unconjugated bilirubin*) and especially thereby unbound or free bilirubin, disturbing the binding of bilirubin anion to albumin, decreasing the quantity of albumin that is free

1.   [Bilirubin anion]-Albumin $\rightleftharpoons$ [Bilirubin anion] + Albumin

2.   [Bilirubin anion]+ 2H$^+$ $\rightleftharpoons$ [Bilirubin acid]

Sum: [Bilirubin anion]-Albumin + 2H$^+$ $\rightleftharpoons$ [Bilirubin acid] + Albumin

Figure 26.3 Relationships among bilirubin anion, either bound to albumin or *free*, hydrogen ion, albumin, and bilirubin acid. See text for details.

TABLE 26.3   Important Determinants of Neuronal Injury by Bilirubin

- Concentration of serum unconjugated and free (unbound) bilirubin
- Concentration of serum albumin
- Bilirubin binding by albumin
- Concentration of hydrogen ions (pH)
- Blood-brain barrier
- Neuronal susceptibility

TABLE 26.4   Relationship Between Maximum Serum Bilirubin Concentration and Kernicterus in Newborns With Hemolytic Disease[a]

MAXIMUM BILIRUBIN CONCENTRATION (mg/dL)	TOTAL NO. OF CASES	NO. WITH KERNICTERUS
30–40	11	8 (73%)
25–29	12	4 (33%)
19–24	13	1 (8%)
10–18	24	0

[a]See text for references.

---

to bind bilirubin, and increasing the quantity of hydrogen ions (i.e., lowering pH) (Table 26.3). Additional factors that interrelate closely with those just enumerated include the status of the blood-brain barrier and the susceptibility of target neurons to bilirubin injury; these factors are considered separately in later sections. In the following discussion of the determinants of bilirubin neurotoxicity, it becomes clear that the importance of each factor must vary with the clinical circumstances (see Table 26.3).[11]

Concentration of Serum Unconjugated and Free Bilirubin

Unconjugated Bilirubin. Although it is generally recognized that serum levels of unconjugated bilirubin must be elevated to cause neurotoxicity, the relationship between such elevations and brain injury is not simple. In the *full-term infant with marked hyperbilirubinemia* secondary to *hemolytic disease*, a clear correlation can be discerned between the occurrence of kernicterus and the maximal recorded level of serum bilirubin (Table 26.4).[11,21,33,34] In a review of 52 infants with hemolytic disease (33 Rh incompatibility, 19 ABO incompatibility) and comorbid factors, approximately 95% of whom developed kernicterus, the peak total serum bilirubin in both groups was *approximately 32 mg/dL*, with an *approximate range of 18 to 51 mg/dL*.[34]

The neural risk of marked hyperbilirubinemia in *full-term infants without hemolysis* is less clear. Indeed, an earlier analysis of available studies by Newman and Maisels[35] suggested that the risk for neurological sequelae is distinctly less for hyperbilirubinemic infants without hemolytic disease compared with the risk for infants with hemolytic disease. Subsequent observations supported this contention, including a study by Newman and associates of 140 treated infants (phototherapy $n = 136$) and exchange transfusion ($n = 5$) with peak serum bilirubin levels largely between 25 and 29.9 mg/dL.[36] There were no cases of kernicterus. However, multiple reports describe the occurrence of kernicterus, identified by neuropathological, neuroradiological, or clinical criteria, after apparent nonhemolytic hyperbilirubinemia.[32,34,37-40] Furthermore, in a review of 35 selected infants with nonhemolytic, *idiopathic* hyperbilirubinemia and documented acute or chronic bilirubin encephalopathy, all infants had peak total serum bilirubin levels greater than 20 mg/dL (Fig. 26.4).[34] Indeed, more than 90% of the infants with kernicterus had peak levels higher than 25 mg/dL. Notably, however, fully 25% had peak levels lower than 30 mg/dL.[34] Nevertheless, current observations suggest that hemolytic conditions are often overlooked in the absence of a detailed search for immune-mediated mechanisms by advanced techniques.[41] It seems reasonable to conclude that hyperbilirubinemia, in most cases, is a necessary but usually not sufficient condition to explain kernicterus. Factors acting in concert with bilirubin, including duration of exposure to bilirubin or albumin binding of bilirubin, must be evaluated to seek a satisfactory explanation for the risk of developing kernicterus (see later).[2,34] These issues are discussed in detail later (see the section on the relationship of neurological sequelae in term infants to degree of hyperbilirubinemia). The relationships between neonatal bilirubin values and neurological outcome in *premature infants* are probably different from those in full-term infants. Indeed, kernicterus has been demonstrated repeatedly in the *premature infant without marked hyperbilirubinemia* (see later discussion).[21,40,42-44] These infants have usually exhibited a variety of complicating illnesses (e.g., acidosis, hyperbilirubinemia, sepsis, asphyxia, hypothermia, intraventricular hemorrhage). In one often-cited, relatively large collection of premature infants with kernicterus ($n = 6$), peak total serum bilirubin levels were in excess of 20 mg/dL (range, 22 to 26 mg/dL).[45] However, in this report, the gestational age of the six infants ranged from 34 to 36 weeks. Studies of bilirubin-induced auditory disturbances in smaller premature infants (28 to 32 weeks of gestational age) document neurological dysfunction at much lower bilirubin levels.[46,47] The critical issue of the premature infant is discussed later (see the section on clinical features).

Free Bilirubin. Because of the recognition that the fraction of bilirubin not bound to albumin is the critical component involved in bilirubin's entry into the brain and in neurotoxicity

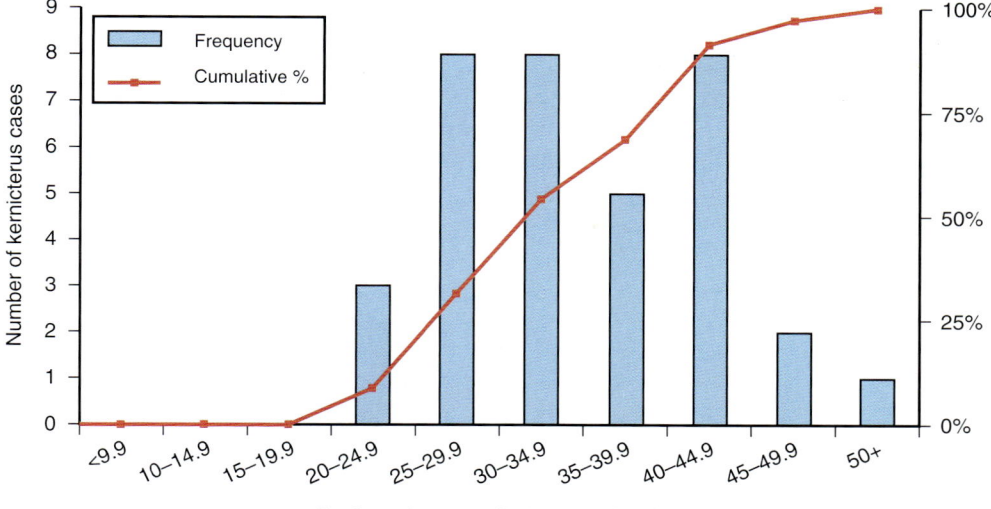

Figure 26.4 **Distribution of peak total serum bilirubin level in term and near-term newborns with idiopathic jaundice who developed kernicterus (*n* = 35).** The bars refer to frequency, that is, number of cases (left Y-axis) and the line to cumulative percentage (right Y-axis). Rights were not granted to include this figure in electronic media. Please refer to the printed book. (From Ip S, Chung M, Kulig J, O'Brien R, et al. An evidence-based review of important issues concerning neonatal hyperbilirubinemia. *Pediatrics.* 2004;114:e130–e153.)

(see later) and because of the demonstration of kernicterus in premature infants without markedly elevated levels of unconjugated bilirubin, intensive investigation has been directed toward measurement of the quantity of that fraction of unconjugated serum bilirubin, namely, unbound (i.e., *free*) bilirubin.[a] In general, premature infants with higher levels of free bilirubin exhibit kernicterus at postmortem examination more often than those with lower levels. In a recent study of 1100 infants of extremely low birth weight in whom total and unbound bilirubin levels were measured at 5 days, irrespective of the clinical status, an increasing level of unbound bilirubin was associated with higher rates of death, neurodevelopmental impairment, or hearing loss at 18- to 22-month follow-up.[51]

Disturbances of the brain stem auditory evoked response (BSAER) are observed at lower levels of free bilirubin in premature versus full-term infants (see later).[46,47] Measuring the total bilirubin/albumin molar ratio (BAMR) was initially considered to be more clinically relevant and had been shown to be highly correlated with unbound bilirubin when the latter serum concentrations are less than but not greater than 0.6 μg/dL.[52] However, in a recent randomized study in preterm infants of ≤32 weeks' gestation with hyperbilirubinemia, no significant effect of the additional use of the bilirubin–albumin ratio compared with total serum bilirubin (TSB)–based treatment on the neurodevelopmental outcome at 18 to 24 months corrected age was observed.[53] Thus it is clear that free bilirubin levels *alone* do not clearly distinguish premature infants who will develop kernicterus from those who will not. Moreover the use of phototherapy may in addition affect this relationship. Thus photoisomers, which account for up to 25% of the total bilirubin produced during phototherapy, may affect bilirubin–albumin binding, altering the level of unbound circulating bilirubin.[15,54,55] The important point is that other determinants (e.g., concerning

albumin-bilirubin binding, status of the blood-brain barrier, and neuronal susceptibility; see Table 26.3) are also often present in the sick premature infant and contribute to the likelihood of bilirubin injury (see subsequent sections). Experimental studies support a relationship between free or unbound bilirubin and neuronal injury.[11,49,56]

Concentration of Serum Albumin

Consideration of the equilibria among albumin-bound bilirubin anion, albumin, hydrogen ion, and bilirubin acid (see Fig. 26.3) makes it apparent that the concentration of serum albumin is important in determining the neurotoxicity of bilirubin (see Table 26.3). At lower concentrations of serum albumin, the overall reaction favors the formation of unbound bilirubin anion and, ultimately, bilirubin acid. Indeed, in experimental systems, the toxic effects of bilirubin on enzymatic systems or on cultured cells of neural origin can be reversed by the addition of albumin.[7,11,57] Moreover, evidence indicates that infants at the greatest risk for kernicterus in the absence of marked hyperbilirubinemia (i.e., sick premature infants) usually exhibit concentrations of serum albumin that are lower than those in healthy premature and full-term infants.[21,58,59] Indeed, in one study of 27 premature infants with kernicterus, serum albumin levels were statistically significantly lower than in a comparable control group.[59] However, the latter observation has not been entirely consistent, in keeping with the importance of such other factors as the bilirubin binding affinity and binding capacity of albumin (see following discussion).

Bilirubin Binding by Albumin

The capacity of serum albumin to bind bilirubin depends on such factors as the affinity of the albumin for bilirubin and the competition between bilirubin and other endogenous and exogenous anions for albumin binding sites.[7,11,21,46,60-63] The clinical importance of the ability of albumin to bind bilirubin

---

[a]References 11, 13, 21, 32, 46, and 48-50.

TABLE 26.5 Factors of Potential Importance in Enhancing Bilirubin Neurotoxicity With Asphyxia[a]

- Impaired bilirubin–albumin binding and increased proportion of free bilirubin (endogenous anions)
- Increased proportion of bilirubin as bilirubin acid (acidosis)
- Increased blood-brain transport of bilirubin (hypercarbia, increased bilirubin acid, and potentially impaired adenosine triphosphate–dependent transporters)
- Enhanced susceptibility of neurons to bilirubin injury (hypoxia-ischemia)
- Enhanced susceptibility of neurons to hypoxic-ischemic excitotoxic injury (free bilirubin)

[a]Probable mechanisms are in parentheses; see text for references.

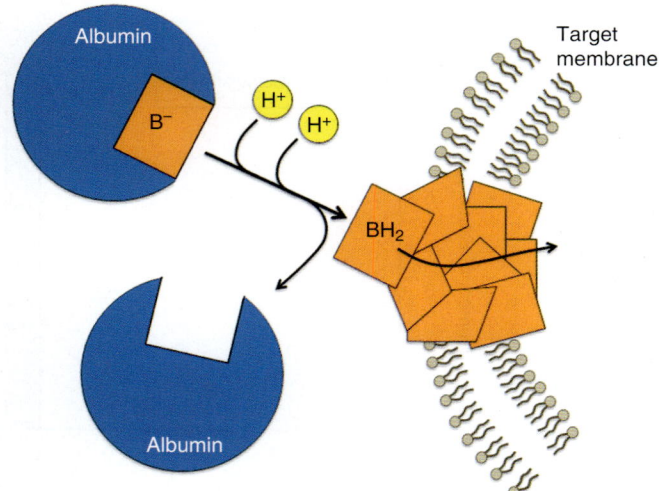

Figure 26.5 Proposed mechanism of advanced bilirubin acid deposition in the lipid bilayer of cellular membranes. See text for details. B^-, Bilirubin anion; BH_2, bilirubin acid. (Adapted from Brodersen R. Binding of bilirubin to albumin and tissues. In: Stern L, ed. *Physiological and Biochemical Basis for Perinatal Medicine.* Basel: Karger; 1981.)

is emphasized by the demonstrations that premature infants who develop kernicterus without marked hyperbilirubinemia may have disturbances of the affinity or capacity, or both, of albumin to bind bilirubin.[7,58,59] Similarly, a relationship between bilirubin–albumin binding and the subsequent cognitive outcome of premature infants who required neonatal intensive care further supports the clinical importance of this binding.[64]

Affinity of Newborn Albumin for Bilirubin. The affinity of albumin for bilirubin is less in the newborn than in the older infant.[7,11,63,65] Adult levels of binding affinity are not reached until as late as 5 months of age. Moreover, binding affinity is lower in the premature infant than in the term infant and is lower in sick infants than in well infants. The explanation for the lower binding affinity of neonatal albumin is not entirely clear. The search for competing anions or for compositional differences in the protein as the unifying explanation has not been fruitful. The leading possibility is that a difference in *conformation* of the albumin is responsible.[11] Moreover, it is likely that the conformational difference relates to the humoral environment of the neonatal albumin because adult serum albumin infused into newborns loses its superior binding affinity over 24 hours.[66]

Endogenous Anions. Endogenous anions that may compete with bilirubin for albumin binding sites include nonesterified fatty acids and other organic anions.[a] *Nonesterified fatty acids* are anions at physiological pH and are present in high concentrations with hypothermia, hypoxemia, hypoglycemia, sepsis, starvation, the administration of heparinized blood (through heparin's activation of triglyceride lipase), and intravenous alimentation with lipid.[67,68] A recent report describes the uncoupling of unbound from total bilibulin as a result of unbound free fatty acids in premature infants treated with intralipids.[67] Studies of *asphyxiated infants with metabolic acidosis* demonstrated impaired bilirubin binding to albumin that could not be attributed to the low pH per se.[69] Rather, the data indicated the presence of *organic anions* in the plasma of asphyxiated, acidotic infants that compete with bilirubin for albumin binding sites. This finding may represent one of several mechanisms of potential importance in enhancing bilirubin neurotoxicity with asphyxia (Table 26.5).

Exogenous Anions. Many exogenous anions may compete with bilirubin for albumin binding sites.[a] However, the largest proportion of such substances has been shown to displace bilirubin from albumin in vitro and in relatively high concentrations. Agents that appear to be particularly potent competitors for bilirubin binding sites include sulfonamides (especially sulfisoxazole), ibuprofen, and various penicillins (especially ceftriaxone). Indeed, ceftriaxone is a more potent bilirubin displacer than sulfisoxazole.[61]

Concentration of Hydrogen Ions: Acidosis

Results of experimental and clinical studies indicate that acidosis facilitates the neurotoxicity of bilirubin.[7,59,69,70] Experimental data suggest that the principal deleterious effect of acidosis occurs at the level of cellular binding, at the uptake of bilirubin, or both.[7,71] Thus enhanced binding and uptake of bilirubin in the presence of acidosis have been demonstrated with cells in tissue culture, liposomes, red blood cell membranes, rat brain slices, and rat brain in vivo.[7,71,72] It is likely that the striking increase in brain bilirubin levels in neonatal rat brain observed during and shortly after anoxia[73] also relates to acidosis. Moreover, the acidosis associated with asphyxia may be similarly important in enhancing the bilirubin neurotoxicity of that insult (see Table 26.5). The mechanism by which acidosis leads to increased neuronal binding, brain uptake of bilirubin, or both, presumably relates to the conversion of bilirubin anion to bilirubin acid (see Fig. 26.3) on acceptance of two hydrogen ions. Bilirubin anion binds to cellular surface membrane components, primarily phospholipids, but also gangliosides and sphingomyelin, and this binding is increased by decreased pH.[74] This electrostatic interaction of the bilirubin anion and the cationic membrane lipid moieties is followed rapidly by the formation of bilirubin acid in the membrane, aggregation of bilirubin acid, irreversible binding to the membrane, and membrane injury, uptake, or both (see later discussion) (Fig. 26.5). This effect of acidosis, when

---

[a]References 7, 20, 60, 61, 66, and 67.

[a]References 7, 20, 46, 60, 61, 66, 69, and 70.

exerted at the level of the endothelial cells of the blood-brain barrier, perhaps could lead to increased transport of bilirubin across the barrier into the brain, in addition to the effect exerted at the level of the neuron (i.e., bilirubin acid binding, neuronal uptake, and neuronal death; see later sections concerning the blood-brain barrier and mechanisms of neurotoxicity).

Blood-Brain Barrier

The entry of bilirubin into the central nervous system can potentially occur across the blood-brain or blood (choroid plexus)–cerebrospinal fluid barrier. It is likely, although not established, that transport across the blood-brain barrier is the more important of these two mechanisms. The blood-brain barrier is composed of the brain capillary endothelial cells with characteristic tight intercellular junctions. The choroid plexus does not contain such tight junctions. Export of bilirubin from the neurons and glia to the extracellular space and hence to the blood by capillary endothelial cells of the blood-brain barrier includes transport-mediated efflux across the blood-brain barrier. A similar process extrudes bilirubin from cerebrospinal fluid to blood through the cells of the choroid plexus.[11] There are at least two types of transporters: ATP-binding cassette transporter B1 (ABCB1) P-glycoprotein, which is localized to the luminal (blood side) face of capillary endothelial cells of the blood-brain barrier, and ATP-binding cassette transporter C1 (ABCC1) multidrug resistance–associated protein 1 (MRP1), which is localized to the basolateral face of the choroid plexus epithelium of the blood–cerebrospinal fluid barrier.[11,30,75-77] These transporters are upregulated with hyperbilirubinemia. However, disturbance in their function (e.g., genetic variants and possibly energy depletion) can render the brain in a given infant highly susceptible to the accumulation of bilirubin within neurons and glia, with resulting neurotoxicity.[11] These transport mechanisms are summarized in Table 26.6.

In this context, it is most reasonable to consider bilirubin entry into the brain across either an intact or a disrupted blood-brain barrier (Table 26.7). The clinical circumstances largely determine the status of the blood-brain barrier (see Table 26.7).

Bilirubin Transport Across an Intact Blood-Brain Barrier. The likelihood of the passage of bilirubin across an *intact blood-brain barrier* is suggested by the finding that free bilirubin binds to phospholipid (e.g., plasma membrane phospholipid of capillary endothelial cells). Such bilirubin-phospholipid complexes are very lipophilic[6,8,30]; thus they would be expected to move bilirubin across the blood-brain barrier readily (Fig. 26.6). Therefore the aforementioned factors that lead to elevations of bilirubin no longer bound to albumin (i.e., *free* bilirubin) would be expected to enhance the movement of bilirubin across the blood-brain barrier. Studies in animals have demonstrated such movement across the intact blood-brain barrier, particularly in the younger as opposed to the more mature animal,[78,79] and the occurrence of kernicterus in older children with apparently intact blood-brain barriers further supports this concept.[80] As noted earlier, the predominant species of unbound bilirubin in plasma is the diacid, with the minority as the monoanion or dianion. These species readily diffuse across cell membranes.[8] When free bilirubin is only moderately higher than its aqueous saturation ($\approx$70 nM), soluble oligomers and metabolic microaggregates of the diacid form

---

TABLE 26.6   Brain Transport Mechanisms and Prevention of High Cellular Bilirubin[a]

- Bilirubin entry into the CNS potentially can occur across the blood-brain barrier and blood (choroid plexus)–CSF barrier.
- Prevention of high cellular (and CSF) bilirubin levels depends on the action of two large families of ABC efflux transporters (ACCB1 P-glycoprotein is localized to the luminal face of the capillary endothelial cells of the blood-brain barrier and ABCC1 multidrug resistance–associated protein [MRP1] is localized to the basolateral aspect of the blood–cerebrospinal fluid barrier).
- The function of the transporters is to export bilirubin from brain cells to the extracellular space and then across capillary endothelial cells to blood (similar transport from CSF to blood by the choroid plexus transporters also occurs).
- Disturbances in action of these transporters, because of genetic variants or perhaps ATP depletion, could play a major role in determining neuronal susceptibility to bilirubin injury.

[a]See text for references.

ABC, Adenosine triphosphate–binding cassettes; *ABCC1,* ATP-binding cassette transporter C1; *ACCB1,* ATP-binding cassette transporter B1; *ATP,* adenosine triphosphate; *CNS,* central nervous system; *CSF,* cerebrospinal fluid; *MDR/PGP,* multidrug-resistance P-glycoprotein; *MRP,* multidrug-resistant protein.

TABLE 26.7   Bilirubin Transport and the Blood-Brain Barrier

Bilirubin transport across intact blood-brain barrier
- Unbound (free) bilirubin: passive diffusion
- Increased cerebral blood flow (hypercarbia, seizure)

Bilirubin transport across disrupted blood-brain barrier
- Hyperosmolar load (hyperosmolar solutions, exchange transfusion)
- Hypercarbia with acidosis
- Asphyxia
- Acidosis (?)[a]
- Vasculitis (meningitis)
- Abrupt increases in arterial blood pressure and/or venous pressure (?)[a]

[a]Question marks indicate experimental data that are suggestive but not yet conclusive.

---

and bind to the outer leaflet of the plasma membrane. The result is a modest perturbation of membrane structure that may enhance the further uptake of bilirubin (see Fig. 26.5). These occurrences merge with the mechanism of bilirubin transport across a disrupted blood-brain barrier (see following section). Conditions such as acidosis that favor the formation of bilirubin acid (see Fig. 26.3) may be expected to provoke this series of events.[81]

Studies of isolated brain capillary cells support this notion of toxicity of bilirubin to endothelia, with an associated effect on membrane transport.[81]

A role for *increased cerebral blood flow* in the enhanced transport of bilirubin across an intact blood-brain barrier may

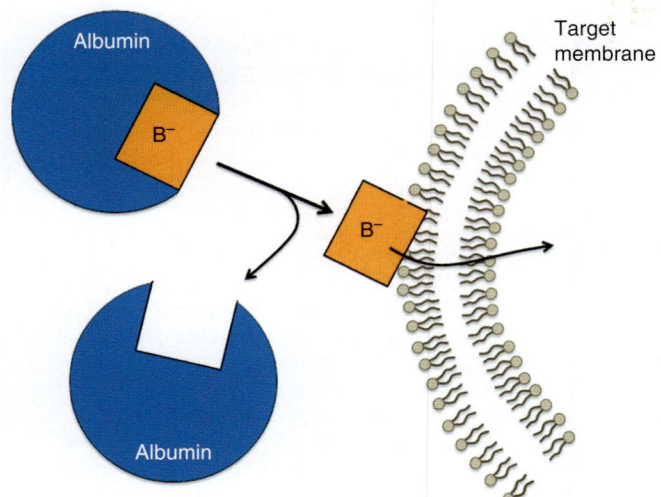

Figure 26.6 Proposed mechanism of bilirubin entry into cells and passage across an intact blood-brain barrier. Bilirubin anion (B⁻) (or bilirubin acid [BH₂]) binds to membrane phospholipid of the target plasma membrane (e.g., brain endothelial cell, neuronal or glial cell) and is transported across the membrane as a lipid-soluble, bilirubin-phospholipid complex.

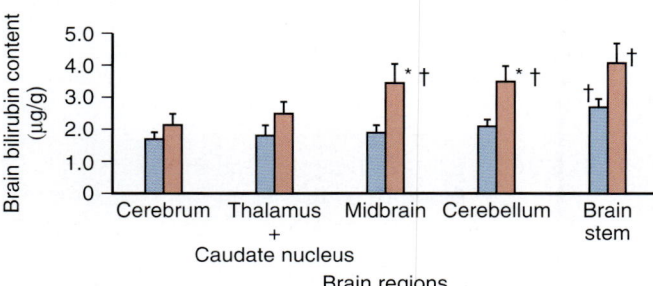

Figure 26.7 Increase in brain bilirubin content with hypercarbia (arterial carbon dioxide pressure, ≈70 mm Hg) and consequent increased cerebral blood flow in the neonatal piglet. *Blue bars* show regional brain bilirubin content in the control group (n = 14); *pink bars* show regional brain bilirubin content in the hypercarbia group (n = 10). Note the increase in brain bilirubin in several brain regions with hypercarbia. Mean ± SEM; *, $P < .05$ as compared with control; †, $P < .05$ as compared with cerebral value within the same group. (From Burgess GH, Oh W, Bratlid D, Brubakk AM, et al. The effects of brain blood flow on brain bilirubin deposition in newborn piglets. *Pediatr Res.* 1985;19:691–696.)

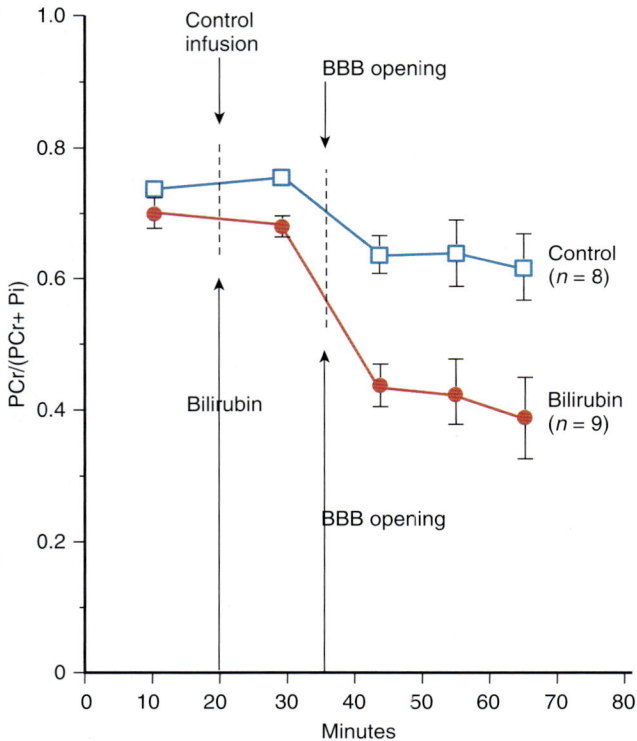

Figure 26.8 Changes in phosphocreatine (PCr)/(PCr + inorganic phosphorus [Pi]) with bilirubin and control infusions before and after hyperosmolar opening of the blood-brain barrier. Results expressed as mean ± SD; values were obtained by magnetic resonance spectroscopy. *BBB,* Blood-brain barrier. (From Ives NK, Bolas NM, Gardiner RM. The effects of bilirubin on brain energy metabolism during hyperosmolar opening of the blood-brain barrier: an in vivo study using ³¹P nuclear magnetic resonance spectroscopy. *Pediatr Res.* 1989;26:356–361.)

be predicted if, as just discussed, bilirubin can be transported across an intact blood-brain barrier. Direct demonstration of an increase in bilirubin transport by an increase in cerebral blood flow was made in studies of neonatal piglets subjected to moderate hypercarbia (Fig. 26.7).[82] No increase in albumin uptake occurred; thus the blood-brain barrier remained intact under these conditions. The implications of this observation are considerable, because abrupt increases in cerebral blood flow are not uncommon in the premature infant, particularly the sick infant, with impaired cerebrovascular autoregulation (see Chapters 13, 15, 16, and 24).

Bilirubin Transport Across a Disrupted Blood-Brain Barrier. The likelihood of the passage of bilirubin, even still bound to albumin, across a *disrupted blood-brain barrier*, caused by

exposure to *hyperosmolar materials*, is suggested by the results of experimental studies, primarily in the rat (see Table 26.7).[83,84] Thus, unilateral kernicterus was produced in the rat by the infusion of bilirubin-albumin after reversible opening of the blood-brain barrier was accomplished on the same side by the infusion of hypertonic arabinose. The infusion of hyperosmolar materials is a well-established means for disturbing endothelial tight junctions and thereby the blood-brain barrier.[85] That it was indeed the bilirubin-albumin complex that entered the brain was shown by demonstrating an increase in brain concentration of albumin as well as bilirubin in the affected hemisphere. Subsequent studies confirmed the increase in brain bilirubin concentration under these conditions.[83,84,86] An approximate similarity of the topography of the bilirubin deposition to that of kernicterus was reported in the initial work, but the critical question concerning whether the brain bilirubin deposition was followed by neuronal injury was not answered. However, subsequent studies did demonstrate alterations in electroencephalography and in brain energy metabolism parallel to the uptake of bilirubin (Fig. 26.8).[83,87] These data raise the possibility that sudden or sustained increases in serum osmolality (e.g., in the sick premature infant administered hypertonic glucose or sodium bicarbonate, in association with hypothalamic disturbance after asphyxia or intraventricular hemorrhage, or following an exchange transfusion) could lead to abrupt increases in brain bilirubin levels even in the absence of marked hyperbilirubinemia.[88]

A second potential means of disrupting the blood-brain barrier in the newborn is *hypercarbia* (see Table 26.7). Thus experimental data suggest that hypercarbia can disturb the blood-brain barrier and induce kernicterus in puppies.[89] A careful study of the rat demonstrated that marked hypercarbia (carbon dioxide pressure [PCO_2], 100 mm Hg), independent of acidosis, caused a more than twofold increase in brain bilirubin concentration as well as in the brain albumin level.[90] The mechanism of the effect of hypercarbia could involve the impact of maximal vasodilation and an abrupt increase in cerebral blood flow on the integrity of the blood-brain barrier. These data raise the possibility that hypercarbia in the sick premature infant could contribute to the transport of bilirubin into the brain of the infant without marked hyperbilirubinemia.

Asphyxia may lead to disruption of the blood-brain barrier, at least in mature animals (see Table 26.7). Moreover, kernicterus has been produced readily in the asphyxiated but not in the nonasphyxiated monkey or rabbit.[91] In addition, in the Gunn rat, it leads to hearing impairment at levels of bilirubin otherwise insufficient to lead to injury.[92] It is tempting to suggest that the association of kernicterus and asphyxia in the human infant could stem, at least in part, on a disturbance in the blood-brain barrier. However, the only direct measurement of albumin transport across the blood-brain barrier in an asphyxiated perinatal animal involved the fetal lamb, and no significant increase in transport could be demonstrated. The possibility that asphyxia, by way of the associated acidosis, could lead to the enhanced formation of bilirubin acid at the endothelial cell surface, injury to the blood-brain barrier, and the transport of *bilirubin acid* (see previous section) remains to be determined. Moreover, the marked hypercarbia associated with asphyxia could lead to increased brain uptake of bilirubin through both an intact blood-brain barrier, as described earlier, and a disrupted blood-brain barrier, as just described. Finally, the ATP-dependent transporters on brain endothelial cells (see Table 26.6) perhaps could be impaired by the energy depletion of asphyxia. This issue requires further study, but it may add to the mechanisms of potentiation of bilirubin neurotoxicity with asphyxia (see Table 26.5).

Intracranial infection, particularly meningitis, is associated with *vasculitis* and a clearly compromised blood-brain barrier (see Table 26.7). A possible role for this mechanism in the genesis of kernicterus is suggested by clinical data.[93] Thus, in two affiliated neonatal facilities, four infants with kernicterus were observed at postmortem examination over 5 years; of these four babies, all exhibited sepsis and two had meningitis. Whether the effect of sepsis-meningitis was at the level of the blood-brain barrier, enhanced neuronal susceptibility to bilirubin injury because of concomitant neuronal injury (see later discussion), or a combination of these factors requires further study. In a more recent report, the presence of sepsis (odds ratio [OR] = 20.6) greatly increased the risk of acute bilirubin encephalopathy.[94]

Finally, the possibility that the blood-brain barrier can be disrupted transiently by abrupt *increases in blood pressure, especially in the infant with impaired autoregulation, or by increased venous pressure*, with an associated increase in transport of bilirubin into brain, is suggested by several lines of evidence (see Table 26.7). First, as noted earlier, circumstances that cause an increase in cerebral blood flow, such as hypercarbia, are associated with the increased transport of bilirubin into brain. An *abrupt increase in blood pressure* in the sick infant with a pressure-passive cerebral circulation would be expected to cause an abrupt increase in cerebral blood flow (see Chapters 13 and 24). Seizure, which causes an abrupt increase in blood pressure and cerebral blood flow in the newborn (see Chapter 12), may also lead to transient disruption of the blood-brain barrier. Such a disruption was documented shortly after a seizure in the human adult and was delineated carefully in animal models. *Abrupt increases in venous pressure* are common in sick premature infants, particularly in relation to respiratory disturbances (see Chapter 24). More data are needed concerning the possibility that transient disruptions in the blood-brain barrier are an important means for the entry of bilirubin into the neonatal brain.

Neuronal Susceptibility

The distinctive regional topography of brain injury with kernicterus (see subsequent discussion) and the predilection for involvement of neurons indicate a selective susceptibility of specific neurons to bilirubin injury. The mechanisms accounting for this selective susceptibility are unclear and cannot be explained solely by bilirubin transport across the blood-brain barrier, particularly the disrupted barrier, or with patterns of highest regional cerebral blood flow or metabolic rate.[11,83]

The predilection of bilirubin injury for *neurons* rather than glia (see later discussion of neuropathology) was reproduced in cultured cells.[95,96] This predilection may relate to aspects of neuronal surface membranes (e.g., abundance of gangliosides) that lead more readily to binding of bilirubin and to the initial steps leading to membrane injury (see later discussion of mechanisms of neurotoxicity). This speculation is only one of many possible explanations, however.

Perhaps of particular clinical importance, available data suggest that *concomitant injury to neurons* enhances the likelihood of bilirubin encephalopathy. The potentiating role of asphyxia may be a good example of this effect (see Table 26.5). Thus, in this circumstance, concomitant injury to neurons may render the cell more susceptible to uptake of and injury by bilirubin, and, as will be discussed regarding mechanisms of neurotoxicity, exposure of neurons to bilirubin may enhance the susceptibility to hypoxic-ischemic excitotoxic neuronal injury. As noted earlier, these factors related to neuronal susceptibility are among several other factors that may underlie the increased likelihood of bilirubin encephalopathy with asphyxia (see Table 26.5). Nevertheless, it also must be considered that other insults to neurons by such factors as hypoglycemia, metabolic aberrations, intracranial hemorrhage, infection, trauma, or exposure to toxic agents may have critical additive effects with bilirubin by producing concomitant injury to neurons. The role of such factors in enhancing neuronal susceptibility to injury could be very important and requires further study. The demonstrations that bilirubin toxicity to cultured cells is enhanced by otherwise nontoxic concentrations of tumor necrosis factor-alpha (TNF-α) and endotoxin (lipopolysaccharide) suggest a mechanism whereby sepsis-meningitis could enhance neuronal susceptibility to bilirubin injury.[11,97] The role of inflammatory mechanisms in bilirubin-induced excitotoxicity is also relevant to this issue (see later).[97,98] Finally, the observation that immature rat brain is rich in heme oxygenase,[99] which could lead ultimately to

TABLE 26.8   Potential Mechanisms for Bilirubin Neurotoxicity[a]

Impairment of
- Glucose utilization
- Oxidative phosphorylation, adenosine triphosphate levels
- DNA synthesis
- Protein synthesis
- Activity of many enzymes
- Protein phosphorylation
- Neurotransmitter synthesis
- Ion transport
- Synaptic transmission
- Excitatory amino acid homeostasis
- Cytosolic calcium concentration
- Free radical homeostasis
- Inflammatory homeostasis
- Apoptotic/survival balance

[a]Based on numerous studies performed in vivo and in vitro (cultured cells, tissue extracts); see text for references.

TABLE 26.9   Brain Energy Metabolites 15 Minutes After Intracarotid Infusion of Osmotic Agent (Arabinose) and Bilirubin in the Rat[a]

METABOLITE	CONTROL	BILIRUBIN
Phosphocreatine	4.93	2.04
Adenosine triphosphate	2.83	1.72
Glycogen	2.82	1.20
Glucose	2.95	1.02
Lactate	2.27	10.55

[a]Values are mmol/kg brain tissue; all differences are significant at the $P < .05$ level.

Data from Wennberg RP, Johansson BB, Folbergrova J, Siesjo BK. Bilirubin-induced changes in brain energy metabolism after osmotic opening of the blood-brain barrier. *Pediatr Res.* 1991;30:473–478.

the formation of bilirubin from local heme sources, raises the possibility that certain neurons could be exposed to particularly high local concentrations of bilirubin. Further information concerning the factors that could activate heme oxygenase, increase availability of its substrate, or both would be of interest concerning neuronal susceptibility to bilirubin injury.

Nonneuronal cells, including especially astrocytes and microglia, also show sensitivity to unconjugated bilirubin, and their responses may play a role in modulating the toxicity of bilirubin to neurons.[11] The interactions of these cells are described later (see potential sequence for bilirubin neurotoxicity). Bilirubin toxicity to other cellular structures including unmyelinated axons and differentiating oligodendrocytes is suggested by several experimental studies.[100-102] Relevance to the human neuropathology (see later) remains to be clarified.

Mechanisms of Bilirubin Neurotoxicity

Spectrum of Effects of Bilirubin on Cellular Functions

The mechanism of injury of neurons by bilirubin is not entirely resolved, but recent work has provided important insights (see later). Previous work indicated that bilirubin exerts a deleterious effect on a wide variety of cellular events. Various in vitro and in vivo studies, primarily with animals, including Gunn rats, and more recently a genetically engineered mouse model created by introducing a premature stop codon in the *Ugt1a1* gene and resulting in an inactive glucuronyl transferase,[103] have demonstrated disturbances in glucose utilization, oxidative phosphorylation, glycogen synthesis, citric acid cycle function, cyclic adenosine monophosphate synthesis, amino acid and protein metabolism, DNA synthesis, lipid metabolism, myelination, synthesis and transport of neurotransmitters, ion transport, synaptic transmission, excitatory amino acid homeostasis, cytosolic calcium levels, nitric oxide release, free radical homeostasis including glutathione content,[104,105] inflammatory homeostasis, and apoptotic/survival balance (Table 26.8).[a] A recent case report of a 32-week 1600-g

[a]References 11, 31, 57, 87, 97, and 104-107.

premature infant with total serum bilirubin levels of 13.1, 28.8, and 21.4 mg/dL on the first, second, and fourth postnatal days and who died on the fourth day may add further insight into the cellular and molecular changes contributing to bilirubin-induced neuropathology.[108] Compared with age-matched controls, increased blood vessel density with ill-defined luminal structures was observed in mesencephalon, pons, medulla corpus striatum, and hippocampus. The last two regions exhibited increased expression of vascular endothelial growth factor (VEGF) and vascular endothelial growth factor receptor-2 (VEGFR-2) as well as albumin extravasation into brain parenchyma.[109]

A particular importance for *disturbance of mitochondrial function and thereby energy metabolism* has been suggested by several studies using biochemical measurements and magnetic resonance (MR) spectroscopy to analyze energy metabolites, including high-energy phosphate levels.[31,110] Thus a rapid decline in high-energy phosphate levels was observed in brain 15 minutes after the entrance of bilirubin by disruption of the blood-brain barrier (Table 26.9).[110] The findings were indicative of a disturbance in oxidative phosphorylation, with the depletion of glucose and glycogen and accumulation of lactate indicative of an increase in glycolytic rates in an attempt to restore energy potential. Moreover, similar experiments, also using MR spectroscopy, documented in vivo the disturbance in high-energy phosphate levels (see Fig. 26.8).[87] The importance of hypoxia in potentiating the effect of bilirubin on energy metabolism was also shown by MR spectroscopy in a similar model (Fig. 26.9).[111] In addition, brief exposure of immature primary cortical neurons to bilirubin rapidly and selectively inhibited the mitochondrial respiratory chain at the level of the cytochrome *c* oxidase complex.[112] This effect resulted in an impairment in oxygen consumption, inner mitochondrial membrane energy failure, and apoptosis. In addition, there was an increase in free radicals—that is, oxidized glutathione and superoxide anion. The antioxidant glycoursodeoxycholic acid blocked the inhibitory effects on cytochrome *c* activity with prevention of oxidative stress, metabolic alterations, and cellular death.[112]

Involvement of excitotoxic mechanisms in bilirubin-induced injury emanated initially from the demonstrations in the Gunn rat

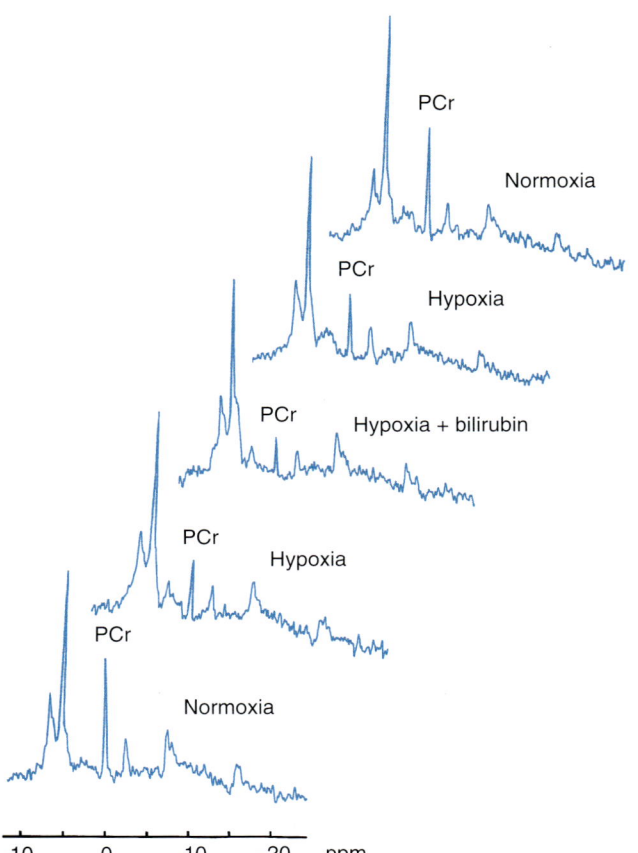

Figure 26.9 Deleterious effect of bilirubin in the presence of hypoxia in brain slices. A representative sequence of spectra collected hourly over a 5-hour experimental period is shown. Alterations in the superfusate are as labeled, with progression from bottom left to top right. Bilirubin at a concentration of 40 µmol/L (bilirubin–albumin molar ratio, 5:1) in combination with hypoxia was associated with a reversible fall in phosphocreatine (PCr) to less than the steady-state reduction observed during hypoxia (tracing immediately above). (From Ives NK, Cox DWG, Gardiner RM, Bachelard HS. The effects of bilirubin on brain energy metabolism during normoxia and hypoxia: an in vitro study using ^{31}P nuclear magnetic resonance spectroscopy. *Pediatr Res*. 1988;23: 569–573.)

that (1) bilirubin-induced neuronal injury could be blocked by administration of the *N*-methyl-D-aspartate (NMDA) receptor antagonist MK-801 and (2) excitotoxic neuronal injury induced by injection of NMDA into striatum is accentuated by bilirubin entry into the region. These observations suggested that excitotoxic mechanisms could contribute to the neuronal injury caused by bilirubin.[97] Recent experimental evidence suggests that as in hypoxia-induced excitotoxicity, the final common pathway to cell death involves the generation of reactive oxygen and nitrogen species (see Chapter 13). Thus, using rat cortical neurons, the role of nitric oxide (NO) and NMDA glutamate receptors in bilirubin neurotoxicity was evaluated. Bilirubin increased the expression of neuronal nitric oxide synthase (nNOS), as well as the production of nitrites and cyclic guanosine monophosphate (GMP), which was accompanied by protein oxidation and cell demise, whereas the major cellular antioxidant defense system, provided by glutathione, was impaired. Moreover, bilirubin-induced neuronal oxidative

injury was prevented by NO synthesis inhibition as well as by blockade of the NMDA receptor channel with MK-801. These findings point to NO as a key mediator of bilirubin-induced neuronal oxidative injury and suggests that the upregulation of nNOS and neurotoxicity occur through the NMDA receptor.[104] The sequence of events then could be similar to that described in hypoxia-ischemia (see Chapter 13) and in hypoglycemia (see Chapter 25), whereby a disturbance in high-energy phosphate levels leads to impairment of energy-dependent glutamate uptake mechanisms in both nerve terminals and astrocytes, a resulting accumulation of extracellular glutamate, and neuronal death initiated by activation of glutamate receptors, particularly the NMDA receptor. The demonstration of an impairment of glutamate uptake mechanisms by synaptic vesicles treated with bilirubin[107] suggested that bilirubin itself could cause or accentuate the increase in extracellular glutamate. These considerations provided an additional reason for a link between hypoxic-ischemic insults and bilirubin neuronal injury (see Table 26.5).[96] Moreover, the finding that the *combination* of lipopolysaccharide and bilirubin exacerbated excitotoxic neuronal injury induced by bilirubin suggests a mechanism whereby sepsis could increase the risk of kernicterus.[97]

The involvement of inflammatory mechanisms in bilirubin-induced injury is based primarily on studies of experimental models. The pivotal roles of microglia and astrocytes are apparent. Thus microglia exposed to unconjugated bilirubin become activated and secrete multiple inflammatory cytokines, potentially injurious to neurons. A neuroprotective effect of the antimicroglial agent minocycline in Gunn rats supports a deleterious role of such an inflammatory mechanism. An important role for astrocytes in inducing the inflammatory response is suggested by the demonstration that astrocytes exposed to bilirubin release multiple inflammatory cytokines.[98] Immature astrocytes release more TNF-α than more mature cells. These glia-mediated inflammatory mechanisms would be expected to contribute importantly to bilirubin-induced neurotoxicity both by accentuating excitotoxicity and generating free radicals (see Chapter 14).

Potential Sequence for Bilirubin Neurotoxicity

The observations of bilirubin-induced energy depletion, excitotoxicity, and free radical attack just reviewed should be viewed in the context of a broader cellular and molecular scheme (Fig. 26.10).[8,30,113] Since the early 2000s, studies based on concentrations of free bilirubin more relevant to the clinical setting suggest that the principal subcellular compartments affected are the *plasma membrane* and the *mitochondrion* and that the major cell types involved are the *neuron* and the *astrocyte* (see earlier).

Plasma Membrane and Excitotoxicity. Although bilirubin dianion and its rapidly formed diacid can bind to phospholipids and diffuse passively across the plasma membrane, disturbance of the plasma membrane can also occur. The results are accentuation of bilirubin uptake and disturbance of certain plasma membrane functions (e.g., glutamate transport). Impairment of glutamate transport in neurons and *especially astrocytes* causes an increase in extracellular glutamate (see earlier).[97] The result is excessive activation of neuronal NMDA receptors with an increase in cytosolic calcium, the generation of free radicals, and neuronal necrosis, apoptosis, or both as

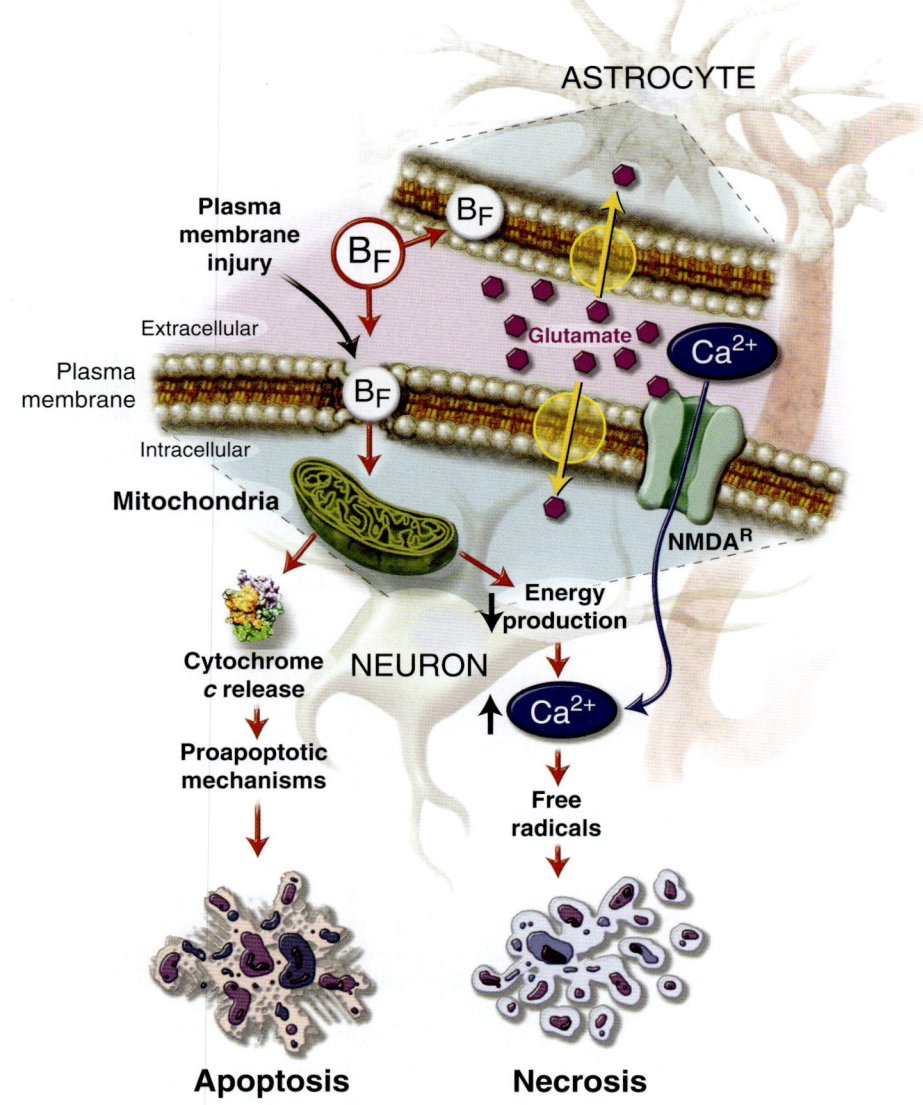

Figure 26.10 Potential sequence for bilirubin neurotoxicity. See text for details. Note the particular importance of mitochondrial disturbance and impaired glutamate homeostasis with increased extracellular glutamate and resulting excitotoxicity. B_F, Free bilirubin; Ca^{2+}, calcium; *NMDA*, N-methyl-D-aspartate.

described for hypoxia-ischemia in Chapter 13. Prevention of bilirubin-induced injury by specific inhibitors of the NMDA receptor (e.g., MK-801) supports this formulation.[11,114]

Astrocytes also sustain injury from unconjugated bilirubin, although their vulnerability to cell death is less than that for neurons.[97,105] Bilirubin induces a rapid increase in extracellular glutamate content,[98] predominantly via immature astrocytes,[97] that appears to result from several factors. First, impairment of *glutamate transport* is greater in astrocytes than in neurons; thus the accumulation of extracellular glutamate attributable to astrocytic dysfunction is greater than that for neurons (see Fig. 26.10). Second, astrocytes exposed to bilirubin release cytokines such as TNF-α and interleukin-1beta, which also

impair glutamate transport; therefore the action of these cytokines may add to the accumulation of extracellular glutamate (see Fig. 26.10).[98] Immature astrocytes also release more TNF as compared with the more differentiated cells. In addition, bilirubin-induced activation of NF-kappa B has an age-dependent profile, an effect that can be related to the greater amount of cytokine secretion by these cells. Third, because high-affinity sodium-dependent glutamate transport is impaired secondary to energy depletion and the resulting disturbance of ionic gradients (see Chapter 13), the energy depletion associated with bilirubin mitochondrial toxicity (see later) adds to the transport failure (or even reversal of transport) and accumulation of extracellular glutamate.

TABLE 26.10   Potential Novel Interventions Versus Bilirubin Neurotoxicity[a]

N-methyl-D-aspartate receptor blockers (e.g., memantine, dextromethorphan, magnesium, MK-801)
Antioxidant therapies (free radical scavengers, antioxidant enzyme mimetics)
Antiinflammatory, antimicroglial agents (e.g., minocycline)
Antiapoptotic agents
Combinations of interventions

[a]Based on experimental studies (see text for references).

TABLE 26.11   Neuropathological States With Bilirubin Staining of Brain Nuclei

Acute bilirubin encephalopathy, or kernicterus, of the full-term (or premature) infant *with* marked hyperbilirubinemia
Acute bilirubin encephalopathy, or kernicterus, of the premature infant *without* marked hyperbilirubinemia
Secondary bilirubin staining of brain nuclei of the premature infant (*without* marked hyperbilirubinemia)

Importance of the Mitochondrion. In addition to the plasma membrane and excitotoxic effects, bilirubin exposure in clinically relevant concentrations has important effects on *mitochondria* (see Fig. 26.10).[8,11,31] What results is not only diminished energy production but also permeabilization of mitochondrial membranes and release of cytochrome *c*.[31] The latter then leads to apoptotic neuronal death by binding to apoptosis protease activating factor-1, activation of caspases, and execution of the cell death program (see earlier).

Final Common Pathway to Cell Death. The final common pathway for both the plasma membrane effects with excitotoxicity and the mitochondrial disturbances includes an increase in cytosolic calcium and the generation of free radicals (see Fig. 26.10) (see Chapter 13).[105,113] The result is apoptotic cell death, necrotic cell death, or both. Both neurons and astrocytes can be affected, although neurons are more vulnerable. The intensity and duration of the stimulus determine whether neuronal death will be apoptotic or necrotic (see Chapter 13). High bilirubin concentrations, longer exposures, or both result in necrosis and lower concentrations or shorter exposures result in apoptosis.[11,102] A particular although not exclusive importance for apoptotic cell death with bilirubin toxicity was suggested by the observation that inhibition of the proapoptotic enzyme p38 MAP kinase by minocycline prevented cerebellar neuronal cell death with bilirubin exposure.[115] (This effect was likely independent of the antimicroglial effects of minocycline, as discussed in Chapter 13.) Moreover, minocycline administered to the newborn Gunn rat prevented the marked apoptotic cell death that resulted in cerebellar hypoplasia in that animal.[115] *Combination* of *antiapoptotic* (caspase inhibitor) and *antiexcitotic* (MK-801) agents may exhibit *synergy* in neuronal protection from bilirubin toxicity.[114]

Implications for Therapy

The sequence outlined in Fig. 26.10 and the supporting experimental data suggest several potential sites for therapeutic intervention (Table 26.10). Thus blockade of NMDA receptors has been shown to be highly effective, depending on the experimental model. MK-801 is the most effective NMDA inhibitor but unfortunately is not clinically safe (see Chapters 13 and 20). However, memantine, magnesium, or dextromethorphan would be potentially more useful. Scavenging of free radicals with such agents as vitamin E or related compounds or enhancing antioxidant defenses with antioxidant enzyme mimetics may be of potential value. Antiapoptotic interventions

may also be beneficial (see Chapter 20), and the beneficial effects of minocycline in two rat models are relevant in this context. *Combinations* of interventions may have *synergistic* effects, as noted earlier for antiapoptotic (caspase inhibitor) and antiexcitoxic (MK-801) agents. At any rate, insights into the mechanisms of bilirubin neurotoxicity raise important new possibilities for prevention of this injury. Nonetheless the most important therapeutic intervention is the rapid lowering of the bilirubin level with either phototherapy and/or exchange transfusion (see later).

NEUROPATHOLOGY

The classic neuropathology of acute bilirubin encephalopathy consists of two essential features: bilirubin staining of specific nuclear groups *and* neuronal necrosis.[116-119] The former is the earliest and most dramatic finding of bilirubin encephalopathy and the latter is a later occurrence (in subsequent days), presumably in large part a consequence of the bilirubin uptake. Although the bilirubin staining of nuclei gives rise to the term *kernicterus*, to avoid later confusion I use this term for encephalopathy that includes *both* the staining *and* evidence for neuronal injury.

Three neuropathological states should be recognized in association with bilirubin staining of brain nuclei in the newborn (Table 26.11). The first two states (acute bilirubin encephalopathy, or kernicterus by my definition) occur in the full-term (or premature) infant with marked hyperbilirubinemia or in the premature infant *without* marked hyperbilirubinemia. The third variety, bilirubin staining *without* related neuronal injury, also occurs in the premature infant without marked hyperbilirubinemia.[118,119]

In the following discussion, the neuropathology of acute bilirubin encephalopathy or kernicterus is reviewed in detail as the essential variety of bilirubin injury to the central nervous system. Because the pathological features of the disorder in the full-term (or premature) infant with marked hyperbilirubinemia and in the premature infant *without* marked hyperbilirubinemia are similar, these disorders are discussed together. (Indeed, these two neuropathological states appear to differ principally only in pathogenesis.) Finally, briefer note is made of the third variety of bilirubin staining of brain, the apparently secondary staining of brain nuclei by bilirubin (see Table 26.11).

Acute Bilirubin Encephalopathy-Kernicterus

The essential hallmarks of acute bilirubin encephalopathy, or kernicterus, are bilirubin staining of neurons and neuronal necrosis. These characteristics are discussed separately next, although they are inextricably intertwined.

Bilirubin Staining

Bilirubin staining is most apparent in fresh specimens or in frozen sections, especially in infants surviving only several days, and it occurs in a characteristic topography (Fig. 26.11; Table 26.12).[39,71,108,116-120] Those regions most commonly affected are as follows: basal ganglia, particularly the globus pallidus and subthalamic nucleus; hippocampus, specifically, the so-called sectors CA2,3; substantia nigra; various cranial nerve nuclei, particularly the oculomotor, vestibular, auditory (especially cochlear nuclei but also superior olivary complex, nuclei of lateral lemniscus, inferior colliculi) and facial nerve nuclei; various other brain stem nuclei, particularly the reticular formation of pons and the inferior olivary nuclei; certain cerebellar nuclei, particularly the dentate; and anterior horn cells of the spinal cord. Similarities in the topography in full-term (or premature) infants with marked hyperbilirubinemia, premature infants *without* marked hyperbilirubinemia, the homozygous Gunn rat, and a genetically engineered mouse model (created by introducing a premature stop codon in the *Ugt1a1* gene which results in an inactive enzyme) are striking (see Table

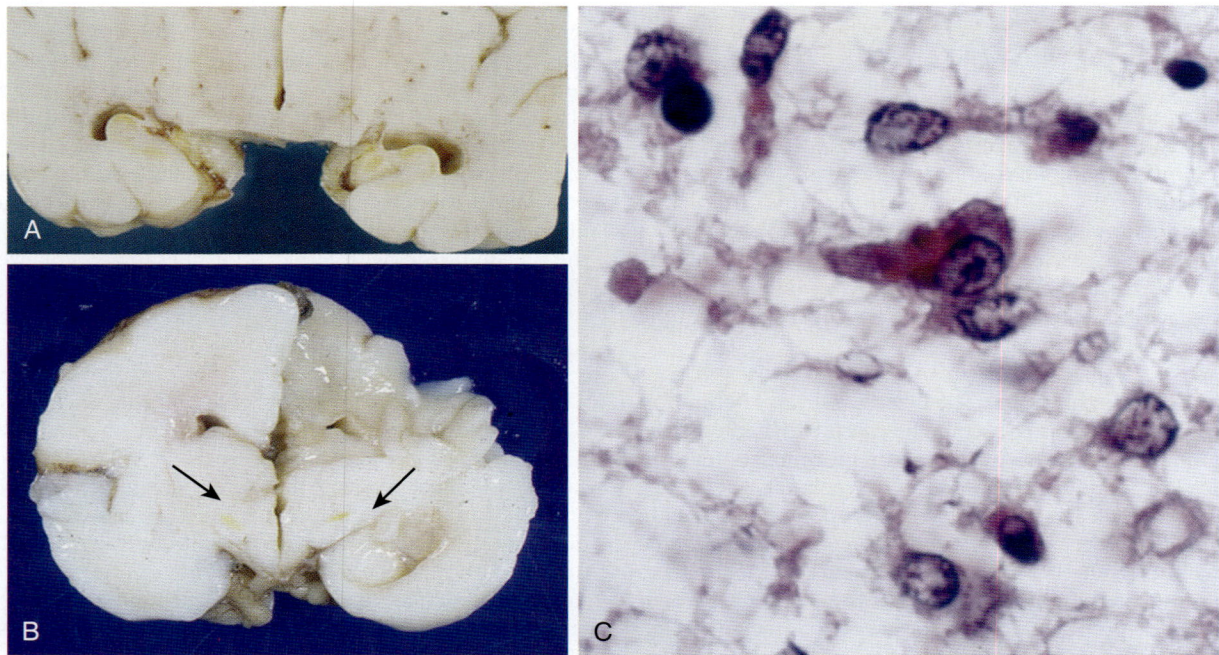

Figure 26.11 Neuronal changes in kernicterus. Bilirubin staining in kernicterus. Note the marked bilirubin staining within the hippocampus (A) and in the subthalamic nuclei (*arrows*) (B). (C) Bilirubin pigment in the cytoplasm of a histologically viable pyramidal neuron (hematoxylin and eosin). ([A and C] From Perlman JM, Rogers BB, Burns D. Kernicteric findings at autopsy in two sick near term infants. *Pediatrics.* 1997;99:612–615. [B] Courtesy Dr. Hannah Kinney.)

TABLE 26.12   Comparative Neuropathology of Acute Bilirubin Encephalopathy or Kernicterus

TOPOGRAPHY OF INJURY	FULL-TERM INFANTS, MARKED HYPERBILIRUBINEMIA	PREMATURE INFANTS, *NO* MARKED HYPERBILIRUBINEMIA	HOMOZYGOUS GUNN RATS
Globus pallidus	+	+	+
Subthalamic nucleus	+	+	+
Hippocampus	+	+	+
Hypothalamus	+	−	+
Substantia nigra	+	+	+
Cranial nerve nuclei[a]	+	+	+
Reticular formation (brain stem)	+	+	
Cerebellum			
Dentate nuclei	+	+	−
Purkinje cells	−	+	+
Spinal cord, anterior horn cells	+	+	+

[a]Includes oculomotor and auditory nuclei; see text for details.

+, Present; −, absent.

Data from Ahdab-Barmada M, Moossy J. The neuropathology of kernicterus in the premature neonate: diagnostic problems. *J Neuropathol Exp Neurol.* 1984;43:45–56.

26.12) and support the concept of the essential neurotoxicity of bilirubin.[103] The period of prominent brain pigmentation lasts for only approximately 7 to 10 days, and this phase is accompanied by the commencement of the neuronal changes that result in chronic (postkernicteric) bilirubin encephalopathy.

Neuronal Injury

Topography. The distribution of neuronal injury corresponds closely with the distribution of the bilirubin staining (see Table 26.12). An intimate relationship between bilirubin deposition and neuronal injury is suggested by this similarity in topography. However, the relationship is not invariable. For example, little or no staining is apparent in Purkinje cells, but impressive neuronal loss is very common in this region, especially in the premature infant. In anticipation of the clinical sequelae of chronic (postkernicteric) bilirubin encephalopathy (see subsequent discussion), it is important to reemphasize that the major regions of neuronal injury include basal ganglia, brain stem nuclei for oculomotor function, and brain stem auditory (cochlear) nuclei and cerebellum in the premature infant.[108]

Cerebellar involvement is not unusual and includes principally the dentate nucleus and Purkinje cells.[110,121] This involvement however, is not as marked as for the structures just described. Nonetheless the possibility has been raised that cerebellar dysfunction contributes to the neuromotor disturbances observed in bilirubin-induced neurotoxicity.[122] It is noteworthy that cerebellar involvement is a prominent feature in the Gunn rat and in the newly described mouse model of neonatal hyperbilirubinemia (vgt1-1-null mutant).[123,124]

Prominent involvement of cerebral cortical neurons is *not* a feature of kernicterus and, when present, appears to be related primarily to concomitant hypoxic-ischemic injury. However, it is possible that a degree of involvement of cerebral cortex would be recognized more commonly if more sophisticated neuropathological techniques than classic light microscopy could be used. Thus, in electron microscopic studies of the Gunn rat, Jew and Sandquist[124] observed qualitatively similar yet clearly less severe ultramicroscopic changes in neurons of cerebral cortex as in those of the cochlear nuclei or hippocampus.

Cytopathology. The cytopathology of kernicterus is distinctive and undergoes a characteristic evolution.[39,117,119] Thus, in the first several days, the early neuronal changes consist of swollen granular cytoplasm, often with microvacuolation and disruption of neuronal and nuclear membranes (see Fig. 26.11). Yellow pigment is often prominent. By the end of the first week, dissolution of affected neurons becomes apparent, and nuclear and plasma membranes become poorly defined. In subsequent days to weeks, neuronal loss, often with mineralization, and astrocytosis are prominent.

Relation to Hypoxic-Ischemic Injury. The neuropathology of kernicterus is clearly different from that of hypoxic-ischemic injury in terms of the topography of the injury (Table 26.13). In addition, the early basophilic, swollen neuron of bilirubin injury differs clearly cytopathologically from the shrunken eosinophilic neuron of hypoxic-ischemic encephalopathy. Although these two encephalopathies may coexist, a hypoxic-ischemic insult sufficient to cause its characteristic encephalopathy is *not* necessary for the resultant neuropathological picture of

TABLE 26.13	Major Differences in Topography of Neuropathology Between Kernicterus and Hypoxic-Ischemic Encephalopathy	
BRAIN REGION	**KERNICTERUS**	**HYPOXIC-ISCHEMIC ENCEPHALOPATHY**
Cerebral cortex and/or periventricular white matter	−	+
Basal ganglia		
Caudate putamen	−	+
Globus pallidus	+	−
Hippocampus	Sectors CA2,3	Sector CA1
Thalamus	Subthalamic nucleus	Anterior and lateral nuclei
Substantia nigra	Reticulata	Compacta
Cochlear nuclei	+	−
Dentate nuclei	+	−

+, Present; −, absent.

kernicterus. This observation supports the aforementioned conclusion that *although asphyxial insults may be important in the pathogenesis of kernicterus in certain infants*, insults sufficient to cause major hypoxic-ischemic brain injury are not obligatory.

Secondary Bilirubin Staining of Brain of Premature Infants

Bilirubin may stain brain regions injured by other insults. Striking examples of such secondary bilirubin staining of discrete hypoxic-ischemic lesions (e.g., periventricular leukomalacia) are well known. The demonstration of more diffuse bilirubin staining of the brain of premature infants (i.e., without the characteristic topography of kernicterus just described) is probably of this variety (see Table 26.11).[125] Thus, although the staining was said to exhibit similarity to that in kernicterus, *no neuronal changes* were seen in the regions observed to have the staining when the fresh brain was examined. Indeed, after fixation, only 2 of 32 brains exhibited any microscopic evidence of bilirubin staining.[125] This lack of retention of bilirubin after brain fixation, and especially the absence of evidence of neuronal injury, indicated that the bilirubin staining of the fresh brain was not that of kernicterus, as described earlier. The principal pathological feature in the premature infants with secondary bilirubin staining was a diffuse, spongy change principally of the cerebral cortex and white matter without associated neuronal injury. Whether this abnormality represented an artifactual change or the effect of concomitant major hypoxic-ischemic or other injury was not clear. At any rate, bilirubin staining did not appear to be related to the structural disturbance and presumably was a secondary phenomenon.

CLINICAL ASPECTS OF ACUTE AND CHRONIC BILIRUBIN ENCEPHALOPATHIES

The clinical features in infants who have sustained bilirubin injury to brain in the neonatal period depend on the

TABLE 26.14   Occurrence of Clinical Features in Acute Bilirubin Encephalopathy

CLINICAL FEATURES	PERCENTAGE OF CASES (%)
No definite neurological signs	15
Equivocal neurological signs	20–30
Definite neurological signs	55–65

Data from Van Praagh R. Diagnosis of kernicterus in the neonatal period. *Pediatrics.* 1961;28:870–876, and Jones MH, Sands R, Hyman CB. Longitudinal study of the incidence of central nervous system damage following erythroblastosis fetalis. *Pediatrics.* 1954;14:346–350.

TABLE 26.15   Major Clinical Features of Acute Bilirubin Encephalopathy

Initial phase
  Slight stupor (*lethargic, sleepy*)
  Slight hypotonia, paucity of movement
  Poor sucking; slightly high-pitched cry
Intermediate phase
  Moderate stupor: irritability
  Tone variable, usually increased; some with retrocollis-opisthotonos
  Minimal feeding; high-pitched cry
Advanced phase
  Deep stupor to coma
  Tone usually increased; pronounced retrocollis-opisthotonos
  No feeding; shrill cry

topography and intensity of the neuropathological findings and their interrelations with brain maturation. Thus, important determining features are the severity of the hyperbilirubinemia (including associated clinical factors), the duration, and the postconceptional age of the infant. These issues are discussed later. In the following, both the clinical features observed in the newborn period (i.e., acute bilirubin encephalopathy associated with kernicterus) and the principal sequelae to this neonatal injury (i.e., chronic postkernicteric bilirubin encephalopathy) are considered. The clinical correlates of both the acute and chronic bilirubin encephalopathies of the *full-term (or premature) infant with marked hyperbilirubinemia* are understood most clearly, and because the disorder in this group of infants serves as the prototype for bilirubin injury to the neonatal nervous system, these correlates are discussed in detail. However, as described earlier (see the section on neuropathology), similar neuropathological findings are observed in the *premature infant without marked hyperbilirubinemia;* the acute and chronic clinical correlates in this important group of infants *remain to be defined fully.* The somewhat limited available data relevant to this group are discussed in the context of the better-defined information available concerning the infants with marked hyperbilirubinemia.

Clinical Features

Acute Bilirubin Encephalopathy-Kernicterus

The occurrence of neonatal clinical features in full-term infants with marked hyperbilirubinemia who either have died with pathologically proven kernicterus or have survived to develop the clinical syndrome of chronic bilirubin encephalopathy of the postkernicteric type was documented in the older literature relative to erythroblastosis fetalis (Table 26.14).[126] Most affected infants exhibited a definite neurological syndrome, although 15% of those with proven kernicterus failed to exhibit any definite neurological signs.

The characteristics of the neonatal neurological syndrome in infants with marked hyperbilirubinemia were defined particularly in older writings and have been supplemented in recent years with experience that included premature infants.[a] The major neurological features involve abnormalities of *(1) level of consciousness, (2) tone and movement,* and *(3) brain stem function, especially relating to feeding and cry* (Table 26.15). It is postulated that the aberrations of level of consciousness relate principally to the involvement of neurons of reticular

[a]References 21, 38, 45, 46, 113, 126, and 127.

formation, aberrations of tone and movement relate to nuclei of the basal ganglia (globus pallidus and subthalamic nucleus), and disorders of brain stem function pertain to the relevant cranial nerve nuclei. The severity of the abnormalities appears to correlate, at least approximately, with both the severity of the hyperbilirubinemia and duration thereof and the gestational age of the infant. In general, overt neurological features are somewhat less common in small premature infants than in full-term or near-term infants, although an increase in apnea and bradycardia has been documented in hyperbilirubinemic premature infants, including late premature infants, versus those without hyperbilirubinemia.[46,47,128] The clinical features of acute bilirubin encephalopathy are best considered in three major phases of increasing severity, which, in marked hyperbilirubinemia, evolve generally over several days (see Table 26.15).

Initial Phase. As the syndrome first evolves, lethargy, stupor, hypotonia, and a paucity of movement are prominent and are usually accompanied by poor sucking and a high-pitched cry (see Table 26.15). These signs clearly are not specific and must raise the question of a variety of primary and secondary disorders of the central nervous system. Recognition of these signs as a signal of acute bilirubin encephalopathy and a need for prompt therapeutic intervention is important because a drastic deterioration in prognosis results if the syndrome progresses markedly.

Intermediate Phase. The cardinal signs of the next phase usually appear within 2 to 3 days and consist of moderate stupor, often with irritability, and a tendency for tone to *increase*, especially with stimulation. The increase in tone involves especially extensor muscle groups, and the infant begins to exhibit backward arching of the neck (retrocollis) or of the back (opisthotonos) (see Table 26.15). In some previous reports, this hypertonia is often referred to as *spasticity*. This term is inaccurate because the increase in tone is probably extrapyramidal rather than corticospinal in origin. (Fever occurred in 80% of the patients studied by Van Praagh,[126] did not relate to any clearly recognized cause, and may have been on a diencephalic basis. Such a high frequency of fever has not been noted in recent descriptions.) If untreated, infants who exhibit the principal features of the intermediate phase, including hypertonia, are highly likely to

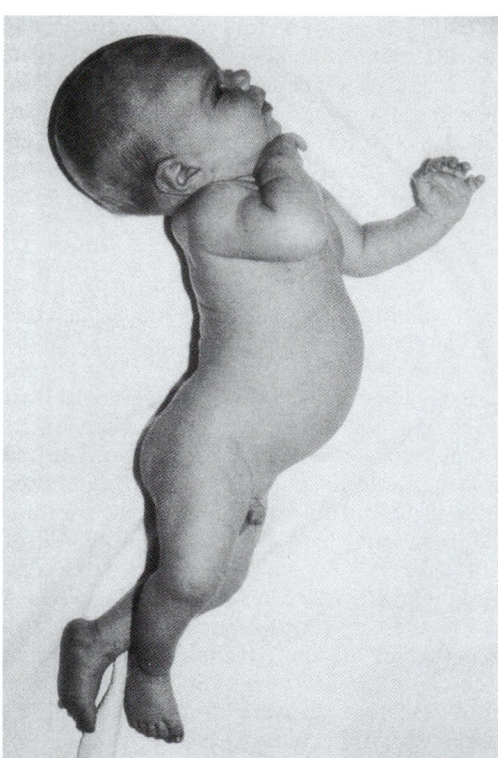

Figure 26.12 Retrocollis and opisthotonos in a 1-month-old infant with kernicterus. The kernicterus was secondary to Crigler-Najjar syndrome. (Courtesy Dr. M. Jeffrey Maisels.)

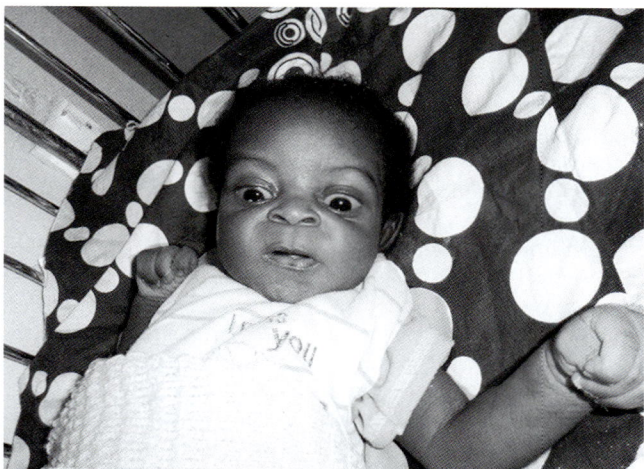

Figure 26.13 Kernicteric facies—photograph of an infant obtained after treatment for and resolution of jaundice on DOL 8 (4 days after presentation). The kernicteric facies can be seen to consist of (1) the setting sun sign, because of paresis of upward gaze, (2) eyelid retraction, and (3) facial dystonia, manifested as a stunned or anxious appearance. (From Slusher TM, Owa JA, Painter MJ, et al. The kernicteric facies: facial features of acute bilirubin encephalopathy. *Pediatr Neurol.* 2011;44:153–154.)

TABLE 26.16	Major Clinical Features of Chronic Postkernicteric Bilirubin Encephalopathy
Extrapyramidal abnormalities, especially athetosis	
Gaze abnormalities, especially of upward gaze	
Auditory disturbance, especially sensorineural hearing loss	
Intellect relatively spared	

progress to the ominous next phase. In the series collected by Johnson and colleagues of 81 infants who appeared to be in the late intermediate phase and who were followed through 18 months of age, 75 (93%) developed "classic kernicteric sequelae."[101,127]

Advanced Phase. In the most severely affected infants, the clinical syndrome evolves, usually after several days, to the advanced phase, characterized by deep stupor or even coma, consistently increased tone, no feeding, and a striking shrill cry (see Table 26.15). Typically, pronounced retrocollis and opisthotonos are easily elicited by stimulation or are observed spontaneously (Fig. 26.12). Some infants will exhibit a distinctive facial appearance, that is, the kernicteric facies (Fig. 26.13),[129] which includes a combination of (1) the setting sun sign, due to paresis of upward gaze; (2) eyelid retraction (which together with the gaze deficit constitutes the "Collier sign"); and (3) facial dystonia, giving the infant a stunned or anxious appearance. Dysconjugate eye movements may also be present. Collier sign relates to involvement of dorsal midbrain, the facial dystonia to globus pallidus and subthalamic nuclei, and the dysconjugate movements to oculomotor brain stem nuclei, all prominent features of kernicteric neuropathology (see earlier) (see Fig. 26.13). Seizures occur in the *minority* of infants with acute bilirubin encephalopathy, although a frequency of 50% was recorded in one older series.[130] When infants reach the advanced phase of the disease, most have irreversible injury and the subsequent development of chronic postkernicteric bilirubin encephalopathy (see later). However, the converse may not be true. In a prospective series of 100

infants with hyperbilirubinemia secondary to erythroblastosis fetalis, approximately 10% of those with no or minimal signs in the newborn period later developed the clinical features of chronic bilirubin encephalopathy.[130] This occurrence may be more common in premature infants.[45]

Chronic Postkernicteric Bilirubin Encephalopathy Following Marked Neonatal Hyperbilirubinemia

Major Features and Temporal Evolution. Chronic bilirubin encephalopathy of the classic postkernicteric type was described particularly well in older studies of infants who experienced marked hyperbilirubinemia secondary to Rh incompatibility (Table 26.16).[118] However, the more recent literature confirms the essential clinical features.[44,45,113,127,131] The temporal evolution of the encephalopathy is particularly interesting. *In the first year of life,* the characteristic features are hypotonia (evolving from the neonatal hypertonia), active deep tendon reflexes, persistent and often obligatory tonic neck reflex (and righting reflex), and delayed acquisition of motor skills. The first three of these features provide an important clue, although not a flagrantly obvious one, of more serious motor disturbances to follow. The constellation of findings particularly characteristic of chronic bilirubin encephalopathy of the postkernicteric type (see Table 26.16) usually does not become apparent until *after the age of 6 months to 1 year.* The extrapyramidal motor disturbances may not be well developed for several years. The major features of the fully developed encephalopathy are extrapyramidal movement abnormalities, gaze disturbances, and auditory deficits. Intellect is relatively spared. Dental dysplasia is a very frequent accompaniment of chronic bilirubin encephalopathy,[21,127] and the term *clinical tetrad of bilirubin injury* is often used to refer to the three neurological features just noted and the dental dysplasia.

Extrapyramidal Movement Abnormalities. The most striking neurological feature of the syndrome is the extrapyramidal disturbance (see Table 26.16). These motor phenomena are present to a variable degree in nearly every case and, in the most severely affected infants, consist principally of athetosis. The slow, writhing movements characteristically involve all limbs, although the upper extremities are usually affected more severely than the lower extremities. Swallowing, phonation, and facial movement are also involved. Dystonic posturing is also a common extrapyramidal feature, and the associated increased tone is often mistakenly termed *spasticity*. In severely affected children, the limb movements may exhibit features of chorea (rapid, jerky movements), ballismus (wide-amplitude flailing movements), or, least commonly, tremor (small-amplitude distal movements). The abnormal movements, especially athetosis, and the increased tone typical of dystonia tend to fluctuate, a dynamic feature more common in the extrapyramidal syndrome of kernicterus than in the syndrome associated with status marmoratus (see Chapter 20).[120] In a minority of cases, the extrapyramidal abnormalities may be apparent only with attempts at skilled movement. The extrapyramidal syndrome reflects the disturbance of basal ganglia, particularly globus pallidus and subthalamic nucleus, the neuropathological hallmark of the encephalopathy.

Gaze Abnormalities. Gaze abnormalities occur in most patients (see Table 26.16) and usually involve vertical gaze, particularly upward gaze, as described earlier for the *kernicteric facies* (see Fig. 26.13). Occasionally both horizontal and vertical movements are affected. In most affected infants, vertical eye movements can be elicited by the doll's-eyes maneuver, thus indicating that the lesion is probably above the level of the oculomotor nuclei. However, a few patients also exhibit apparent paralytic gaze palsies. The neuropathological correlate for the supranuclear palsies is involvement of neurons of upper midbrain,[132] and the nuclear palsies reflect the neuronal injury in appropriate cranial nerve nuclei in the brain stem. Gaze disturbances require careful examination and are frequently overlooked.

Auditory Abnormalities. Disturbances of hearing have been well documented.[46,113,133] In most cases, the auditory disturbance is a high-frequency loss, usually bilateral. The hearing deficit, even when severe, very often escapes clinical detection for months or even longer, and this may be reflected in delayed acquisition of language. In one well-studied series of infants with chronic bilirubin encephalopathy, 63% had moderate or severe hearing loss.[134] Studies of BSAERs[46,47,113,135,136] and morphological data in human infants[116,117] indicate that the pathological substrate for the auditory disturbances resides principally in neurons in the brain stem, particularly the cochlear nuclei and perhaps in the auditory nerve. Thus the hearing disturbance is principally central (brain stem) and to a lesser extent peripheral in origin. The crucial role for bilirubin

in pathogenesis is apparent from experimental studies that established the relationship between the auditory disturbances and bilirubin uptake and deposition.[46,133,137] Studies in human infants have shown a relationship not only with serum bilirubin levels but also with impaired bilirubin albumin binding as well as the combination of bilirubin level and acidosis.[138] The last observation is particularly suggestive of the formation of injurious bilirubin acid in brain (see earlier discussion of determinants of neuronal injury).

Large studies of the associations of hyperbilirubinemia and subsequent hearing loss have provided insight into the relation of bilirubin level to later auditory deficits. Thus a recent systematic review of 19 studies in term infants evaluated the auditory risk of hyperbilirubinemia at levels considered as *low risk* by the current guidelines for treatment of hyperbilirubinemic newborns and reported an incidence of hearing loss at testing that ranged between 13% and 83% initially and 6% to 14% at 3-month follow-up.[135] Five of the studies showed a rising incidence of hearing loss with increasing levels of serum bilirubin. Treatment of hyperbilirubinemia led to a considerable decrease in the incidence of hearing loss.[135] In a recent nested double-cohort design study of infants born at ≥35 weeks' gestation between 1995 and 2011 (n = 525,409) incorporating an exposed cohort of infants with bilirubin levels at or above the level of exchange transfusion therapy (ETT) (>20 mg/dL) and an unexposed cohort of infants with bilirubin levels below the level of ETT,[136] sensorineural hearing loss (SNHL) was found in 11 (0.60%) of the 1834 exposed subjects and 43 (0.23%) of the 19,004 unexposed infants. Only bilirubin levels ≥10 mg/dL above the ETT level were associated with a statistically significant increased risk of SNHL (hazard ratio: 36 [95% confidence interval (CI), 13 to 101]).

In recent years the occurrence of *auditory neuropathy* or *auditory dyssynchrony* has been identified as an important sequela of bilirubin-induced injury.[113,133,139,140] Recognition of auditory dyssynchrony is important because the clinical characteristics and treatment of this disorder differ from those of more typical hearing loss. This auditory disorder is defined as absent or abnormal BSAERs with normal tests of inner ear function. Thus tests of the mechanical integrity of the inner ear (otoacoustic emissions) or of the outer hair cells of the inner ear (cochlear microphonics) are normal with absent BSAERs or abnormal brain stem latencies. *Children with auditory neuropathy may have little or no hearing loss but exhibit abnormal processing of sound.* It appears that conduction in the large, heavily myelinated afferent auditory pathways is not synchronized.[139] Functional effects include difficulties with sound localization and speech discrimination, and although abnormal BSAERs may resolve, this central auditory processing disorder becomes apparent. Importantly, initial data indicate that children with auditory neuropathy and hearing loss appear to respond favorably to cochlear implantation.[139] More data are needed on these issues.

The possibilities that impairment of auditory function is the most consistent abnormality associated with chronic postkernicteric bilirubin encephalopathy—and, as a corollary, that the auditory system is the neural system most sensitive to clinically overt bilirubin injury—have not been clarified decisively. In the acute period, detection of abnormalities of the BSAER is a very sensitive indicator of bilirubin-induced neural dysfunction (see later discussion). Documentation has been made of subsequent hearing impairment secondary to

TABLE 26.17	Intelligence of 19 Patients With Severe Chronic Bilirubin Encephalopathy, Kernicteric Type, Secondary to Hemolytic Disease

INTELLIGENCE QUOTIENT	NO. (PERCENTAGE OF TOTAL [%])
90–100	7 (37)
70–90	4 (21)
50–70	3 (16)
<50	1 (5)
Testing unsatisfactory	4 (21)

Data from Byers RK, Paine RS, Crothers B. Extrapyramidal cerebral palsy with hearing loss following erythroblastosis. *Pediatrics.* 1955;15:248–254.

neonatal bilirubin injury *without* the development of associated athetosis.[46,47,134,139] This observation may be relevant to the possibility of bilirubin auditory neurotoxicity in the premature infant without marked hyperbilirubinemia (see later).

Intellectual Deficits. Marked intellectual deficits occur only in the minority of patients in unselected populations.[141] In patients with athetosis secondary to severe kernicterus (secondary to hemolytic disease) studied decades ago by Byers and coworkers,[141] only approximately 25% of the group had an intelligence quotient (IQ) of less than 70 (Table 26.17). Unfortunately these patients have often been mistakenly considered to be severely cognitively impaired because of their contorted countenance and writhing limbs as well as undetected disturbances in audition. Indeed, more recent studies suggest that intellect is *relatively spared* in chronic bilirubin encephalopathy.[34] In the 81 surviving infants reviewed by Johnson and associates,[127] "intelligence appears to have been spared in almost all infants," although the survivors were not evaluated systematically. The clinician must be alert to the possibility that the movement disorder may mask spared cognitive function or that auditory deficits may disturb language development; thus it is important to recognize that intellectual function is usually relatively spared in this disorder. The *relative* sparing of cerebral cortex on neuropathological examination is compatible with this observation.

Relationship of Neurological Sequelae in Term Infants to Degree of Hyperbilirubinemia. The incidence of cerebral palsy attributable to kernicterus and the relationship of hazardous bilirubin levels (bilirubin >30 mg/dL) to the development of both acute bilirubin encephalopathy (ABE) and subsequent cerebral palsy and sensorineural hearing loss in infants of greater than 35 weeks' gestational age were the subjects of two recent reports from the same large-population database.[142,143] Two important points can be gleaned from these data. First, hazardous bilirubin levels (bilirubin level >30 mg/dL) are uncommon (a higher incidence was noted before universal bilirubin screening vs. that which occurred after; i.e., 11.5 per 100,000 vs. 4.3 per 100,000 live births). Second, the evolution to chronic bilirubin-induced neurotoxicity is likewise *uncommon*; that is, 19% of infants with a peak bilirubin level greater than 35 mg/dL evolved to chronic encephalopathy, whereas no infant developed neurotoxicity

below this value.[143] Factors that increased the susceptibility to neurotoxicity included at least two of the following: late preterm, G6PD deficiency, hypoxia-ischemia, sepsis, hemolytic anemia, acidosis, and hypoalbuminemia, consistent with earlier discussions (see the section on important determinants of neuronal injury by bilirubin). However most of these risk factors were not well defined.[142,143] In a Danish population-based study, acute bilirubin encephalopathy developed in 3 of 11 (27%) of infants with a peak bilirubin value greater than 35 mg/dL and did not occur in any infant with a lower value. The overall risk of acute advanced bilirubin encephalopathy was 0.6 per 100,000 live births.[144]

Further insight into the relationship between bilirubin levels and neurotoxicity is provided by a report from the pilot kernicterus registry (1992–2004), which included 125 infants of greater than 35 weeks' gestational age with acute bilirubin encephalopathy and/or kernicterus, all of whom had serum bilirubin levels greater than 20 mg/dL (range 20.7 to 59.9 mg/dL).[37] Only eight of the infants had no neurological sequelae. Importantly, no clear serum total bilirubin threshold coincided with the onset of acute bilirubin encephalopathy. Conversely, any infant with signs of acute bilirubin encephalopathy and peak total serum bilirubin levels greater than 35 mg/100 mL sustained postkernicteric sequelae. Associated risk factors included late preterm infants, rapid rate of bilirubin increase (>0.2 mg/dL per hour), hemolytic disease, G6PD deficiency, and infection. In another recent report involving 249 newborns admitted with a peak total serum bilirubin level of ≥25 mg/dL, the interaction of peak total serum bilirubin and risk factors as determinants of acute bilirubin encephalopathy was assessed. Peak total serum bilirubin on admission ranged from 25 to 76.4 mg/dL; 44 newborns had moderate or severe acute bilirubin encephalopathy at admission and 35 of the 249 (14%) had evidence of bilirubin encephalopathy at the time of discharge or death.[94] Acute bilirubin encephalopathy risk was increased with Rh incompatibility (OR: 48.6), sepsis (OR: 20.6), and low birth weight, whereas ABO incompatibility with anemia was not related. This observation indicates that the risk for bilirubin encephalopathy in hemolytic disease varies with etiology. The threshold peak total serum bilirubin level that identified 90% of infants with acute bilirubin encephalopathy when risk factors were present was 25.4 mg/dL. By contrast, in the absence of risk factors for neurotoxicity, no cases of acute bilirubin encephalopathy were observed at discharge below a peak total serum bilirubin level of 31.8 mg/dL.[94] This great variation in the response of the brain to total bilirubin levels indicates that biological factors other than serum bilirubin values are extremely important in the pathogenesis of acute bilirubin encephalopathy and highlights the difficulty of defining a target serum bilirubin level above which irreversible brain injury is likely to occur.[145-147]

To summarize, hazardous bilirubin levels (bilirubin level >30 mg/dL) are uncommon and can be reduced by universal bilirubin screening[145] and other measures, as outlined later in the section on management. The risk of developing acute advanced bilirubin encephalopathy (invariably with a bilirubin >30 mg/dL) ranges from 0.6 to 0.9 per 100,000 live births.[142-144,146,147] The risk for acute bilirubin encephalopathy increases with associated risk factors, including late preterm birth, G6PD deficiency, hypoxia-ischemia, sepsis, hemolytic anemia, acidosis, rapid rate of bilirubin increase (>0.2 mg/dL per hour) and

TABLE 26.18   Importance of Associated Risk Factors in Outcome of Infants With Neonatal Bilirubin Encephalopathy With Maximum Total Serum Bilirubin ≥30 mg/dL

CASE	GA	MAX TSB LEVEL	ASSOCIATED RISK FACTOR	NEONATAL CLINICAL SIGNS	LONGER TERM OUTCOME
1	40	38	ABO incompatibility	Opisthotonus, retrocollis, apnea coma	Dystonic CP
2	39	42.9	ABO incompatibility	Opisthotonus, retrocollis, apnea, seizures	Dystonic CP, hearing loss
3	37	57.6	G6PD def	Opisthotonus, retrocollis, apnea, seizures	Athetoid CP
4	41	41	Sepsis	Opisthotonus, retrocollis, seizures	Died
5	37	35.8	Hemolysis (not defined)	Opisthotonus, retrocollis, seizures, ↓ LOC	Hearing loss
6	36	38.7	G6PD def	Opisthotonus, retrocollis, seizures, ↓ LOC	Athetoid CP
7	39	32.9	ABO in compatibility G6PD def	Opisthotonus, ↓ LOC	Normal
8	40	46.9	G6PD def	Seizures, ↓ LOC	Normal
9	36	32.8	Cephalhematoma	Seizures	Hemiparesis
10	39	43.3	G6PD def	Opisthotonus, seizures, ↓ LOC	Athetoid CP
11	37	31.6	Dehydration	Opisthotonus, seizures	Normal
12	40	40.8	Omphalitis	↓ LOC	Died
13	37	31.9	ABO incompatibility	Opisthotonus, seizures, ↓ LOC	CP, severe hearing loss
14	38	30.0	None	Opisthotonus, ↓ LOC	Visual delay
15	36–37	>45	Sepsis, G6PD def	—	CP (quadriplegia)
16	36–37	>45	G6PD def	—	CP (quadriplegia)
17	>37	25–30	Hypoxia-ischemia Albumin <3 mg/dL	—	CP (quadriplegia)

↓ LOC, Decreased level of consciousness; CP, cerebral palsy; GA, gestational age; GSPD def, glucose 6 phosphate dehydrogenase deficiency; TSB, total serum bilirubin.

Cases 1–3: From Ebbesen F, Bjerre JV, Vandborg PK. Relation between serum bilirubin levels ≥450 µmol/L and bilirubin encephalopathy; a Danish population-based study. *Acta Paediatr.* 2012;101:384-385.

Cases 4–14: From Manning D, Todd P, Maxwell M, et al. Prospective surveillance study of severe hyperbilirubinaemia in the newborn in the UK and Ireland. *Arch Dis Child Fetal Neonatal Ed.* 2007;92:F342.

Cases 15–17: From Wu YW, Kuzniewicz MW, Wickremasinghe AC, et al. Risk for cerebral palsy in infants with total serum bilirubin levels at or above the exchange transfusion threshold: a population-based study. *JAMA Pediatr.* 2015;169:239.

hypoalbuminemia (Table 26.18). Such risks lower the threshold for developing acute bilirubin encephalopathy.[94,143]

Chronic Bilirubin Encephalopathies Without Marked Neonatal Hyperbilirubinemia

The striking syndrome of classic chronic postkernicteric bilirubin encephalopathy after marked hyperbilirubinemia led to the postulate that neurological involvement may be less severe, caused by less than marked neonatal hyperbilirubinemia, shorter durations of hyperbilirubinemia, prematurity, or a combination of these factors. In this context, then, we refer to chronic bilirubin encephalopathies that generally do not conform fully to the classic postkernicteric type just described. It is most useful to formulate two questions in this context. *First*, do full-term infants *without marked* hyperbilirubinemia experience subsequent neurological deficits secondary to bilirubin neurotoxicity? *Second*, do premature infants without marked hyperbilirubinemia experience a different spectrum of neurological deficits than do term infants without marked hyperbilirubinemia? As will become apparent, these questions are interrelated but are considered separately in the following discussion.

Neurological Sequelae in Term Infants Without Marked Hyperbilirubinemia. The possibility that brain injury may occur secondary to intermediate levels of bilirubin and without a recognizable neonatal neurological syndrome in term infants has been the subject of numerous reports.[21,34,35,113,134] Results of these studies are variable; several documented an early delay in motor development but most detected no significant ultimate effect on neurological development or cognition at ages 4 to 13 years.[21,35,134] More recent studies also provide variable results. In a study of 43 term babies with a bilirubin ≥220 µmol/L (≥13 mg/dL) compared with those with a bilirubin level less than 220 µmol/L (13 mg/dL) evaluated at 18 months, the rates of minimal brain dysfunction was comparable between groups.[144] However, bilirubin levels of ≥300 µmol/L (≥17 mg/dL) (n = 10) were associated with an increased risk of "complex minimal neurologic dysfunction" (OR: 4.21; 95% CI, 1.02 to 17.37). Specifically, higher hyperactivity scores were observed (effect 0.32; 95% CI, 0.08 to 0.56).[148] A Danish study, which included 167 exposed children at gestational age ≥35 weeks with a total serum bilirubin ≥450 µmol/L (26.3 mg/dL) and examined at a mean age of 7.7 years, found that no child had a diagnosis of cerebral palsy, significant hearing impairment, attention deficit hyperactivity disorder (ADHD), or autism spectrum disorder as recorded in national registries.[149] In a Canadian study of healthy term and late preterm infants, the outcome of infants with peak total serum bilirubin levels of ≥325 mol/L (≥19 mg/dL) was compared with that of infants with less severe or no hyperbilirubinemia. *Softer* neurological adverse effects previously associated with hyperbilirubinemia were not found with the exception of increases in the rates of ADHD (relative risk [RR], 1.9 [1.1 to 3.3]), which remained significant even when adjustment was made for confounders.[150] Finally, in a Finnish study, the long-term consequences of neonatal hyperbilirubinemia were prospectively evaluated in 128 cases (≥2500 g birth weight and ≥37 weeks of gestation) with bilirubin concentrations greater than 340 μmol/L (>19.6 mg/dL) or who required exchange transfusion. Subjects were seen at discharge and at 5, 9 and 16 years of life when parents' and teachers' assessments were recorded. At 30 years the subjects filled out a questionnaire about academic and occupational achievement, life satisfaction, and somatic and psychiatric symptoms including an ADHD self-rating score. Compared with controls, the odds for a child with hyperbilirubinemia having neurobehavioral symptoms at 9 years was increased approximately 4.5-fold. About 45% of the hyperbilirubinemia group were affected by cognitive abnormalities in childhood and continued to experience significant problems in adulthood, including in academic achievement and the ability to complete secondary and tertiary education. In addition, they continued to report persisting cognitive complaints, such as problems with reading, writing, and mathematics. Childhood symptoms of hyperactivity/impulsivity and inattention ($P < .02$) did not persist into adulthood.[151] *Nevertheless, even in these reports, the effects, when present and although statistically significant, are modest.* In view of recent data concerning auditory dyssynchrony (see earlier) in infants with normal or nearly normal hearing,[113] the possibility of previously undetected deficits in central auditory processing after moderate hyperbilirubinemia cannot be excluded.

Neurological Sequelae in Premature Infants Without Marked Hyperbilirubinemia. Several syndromes of chronic bilirubin encephalopathy appear established in premature infants without marked hyperbilirubinemia (Table 26.19). Thus autopsy (see earlier) and imaging studies (see later) have demonstrated *classic kernicterus* in premature infants with bilirubin levels less than 20 mg/dL. Most commonly the hyperbilirubinemia was nonhemolytic but complicated by such factors as sepsis, acidosis, and other features that increase the risk of bilirubin neurotoxicity.

Of great interest has been the possibility that moderate hyperbilirubinemia in very-low-birth-weight infants can lead

to *partial forms* of chronic bilirubin encephalopathy. The most compelling data are available for a *predominantly auditory* partial form.[152,153] Thus a study of hearing loss in surviving premature infants suggests that auditory impairment may be the principal neurological manifestation of bilirubin neurotoxicity in the premature infant without marked hyperbilirubinemia. In one detailed study of 30 premature infants with documented hearing loss on follow-up, multivariate testing demonstrated a peak serum bilirubin concentration (12 mg/dL) to be positively associated and exchange transfusion to be negatively associated with subsequent hearing loss.[152] Only one of the infants exhibited choreoathetosis (and impaired upgaze), and approximately 60% had hearing loss as their only subsequent abnormality. Similarly, moderate hyperbilirubinemia was associated with hearing loss in preterm infants in other reports,[138,151] and in one of these reports the additional association of duration of hyperbilirubinemia and associated acidosis with the occurrence of hearing loss lent further credence to bilirubin (perhaps bilirubin acid) as the neurotoxic agent. In a study of 221 surviving infants of less than 1000 g birth weight, peak serum bilirubin levels greater than 10 mg/dL were predictive of deafness (OR, 4.80; 95% CI, 1.46 to 15.73) but not of the motor deficits of "cerebral palsy" or of developmental delay. Other studies attest to abnormalities of the neonatal BSAERs in premature infants with only moderate hyperbilirubinemia,[46,47,113] although often the abnormalities resolve with treatment of the hyperbilirubinemia. *However, the data indicate the particular sensitivity of the auditory nuclei of the brain stem in the premature infant.* Consistent with this conclusion, one report concerning 2575 surviving infants of less than 1000 g birth weight showed a direct correlation of peak serum bilirubin concentrations with hearing impairment (Fig. 26.14).[113,153] In view of the observations regarding classic

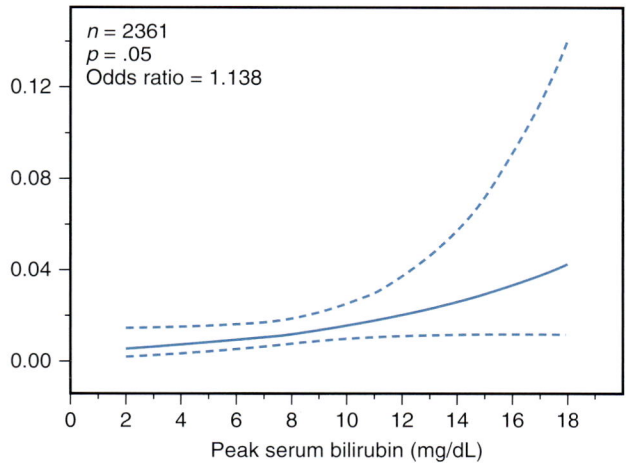

$n = 2361$
$p = .05$
Odds ratio = 1.138

Peak serum bilirubin (mg/dL)

Figure 26.14 Proportion of infants requiring hearing aids as a function of peak serum bilirubin level in the neonatal period. Population consisted of 2575 infants of 401 to 1000 g birth weight and followed until 18 to 22 months of postconceptional age. The peak serum bilirubin level during the neonatal period is shown on the X-axis, and the proportion of infants with hearing aids is shown on the Y-axis. The dotted lines represent 95% confidence intervals. Rights were not granted to include this figure in electronic media. Please refer to the printed book. (From Oh W, Tyson JE, Fanaroff AA, Vohr BR, et al. Association between peak serum bilirubin and neurodevelopmental outcomes in extremely low birth weight infants. *Pediatrics.* 2003;112: 773–779.)

TABLE 26.19	Chronic Bilirubin Encephalopathy Without Marked Hyperbilirubinemia in Premature Infants

Chronic bilirubin encephalopathy: classic postkernicteric
Chronic bilirubin encephalopathy: partial forms
   Predominantly auditory
   Mixed auditory and motor, often mild
   Predominantly motor (?)

postkernicteric encephalopathy that indicate impairment of the auditory system, when carefully evaluated, to be a most sensitive indication of bilirubin injury, these findings suggest similarly that hearing loss may be the principal manifestation of bilirubin neurotoxicity in the premature infant without marked hyperbilirubinemia. Nevertheless, with more aggressive use of phototherapy and exchange transfusion, more recent data suggest that the frequency of such neurotoxicity is relatively low.[113] Finally, in a still-to-be-defined proportion of premature infants with bilirubin-induced hearing loss, motor abnormalities, often not marked, are present.[113] Thus it is likely that a related partial form of chronic bilirubin encephalopathy in this context is a *mixed auditory and motor form* (see Table 26.19).

The possibility that a third partial form is *predominantly motor* has been suggested.[113] An earlier report of 831 premature infants followed in the Netherlands indicated that moderate hyperbilirubinemia was associated with later neurological impairment manifested primarily by cerebral palsy.[42] Thus, at the age of 2 years, a significant increase in such neurological impairment was observed after neonatal hyperbilirubinemia in the moderate range. A subsequent study of this large Dutch population at 5 years of age showed a relationship between hyperbilirubinemia only in infants with intracranial hemorrhage.[42] The OR for impairment increased from 1.0 for maximum serum bilirubin concentrations of 8.7 to 3.3 mg/dL for concentrations of 11.7 to 14.6 mg/dL and to 5.6 for concentrations of 14.7 to 17.5 mg/dL. However, ultrasonographic data did not allow the potentially confounding effect of periventricular lesions (e.g., echodensities, cysts) to be evaluated. Two subsequent reports of 249 and 494 preterm infants with moderate hyperbilirubinemia did evaluate the confounding effects of both intracranial hemorrhage and periventricular lesions and found no consistent relation between the subsequent occurrence of *cerebral palsy* or *developmental problems* and maximum serum bilirubin concentration. Thus, on balance, a relationship between moderate hyperbilirubinemia in the preterm infant and subsequent major motor deficits is unclear but does not appear likely. Indeed, in view of the apparent sensitivity of the auditory system of the premature infant to bilirubin, it is doubtful that a predominantly motor partial form of chronic bilirubin encephalopathy is likely in the premature infant (see Table 26.19).

Finally, the possibility that cognitive impairment is a feature of neurotoxicity caused by moderate hyperbilirubinemia in the premature infant has been raised. Follow-up of 2575 infants of less than 1000 g birth weight showed a correlation between peak serum bilirubin levels and Psychomotor Developmental Index values less than 70; however, the effect was modest (OR, 1.057; $P = .05$), and the cerebral white matter was evaluated only by cranial ultrasonography. Importantly, confounding factors could not be excluded. Thus it currently seems unlikely that moderate hyperbilirubinemia leads to cognitive impairment in the premature infant. Moreover, an analysis of 224 children with a birth weight less than 2000 g who were followed to 6 years of age showed no associations between IQ and maximum bilirubin level, duration of exposure to bilirubin, or measures of bilirubin-albumin binding at bilirubin levels less than 20 mg/dL (Fig. 26.15).[154] A more recent study of 128 infants of less than 800 g birth weight also showed no statistically significant relationship between moderate hyperbilirubinemia and cognitive impairment.

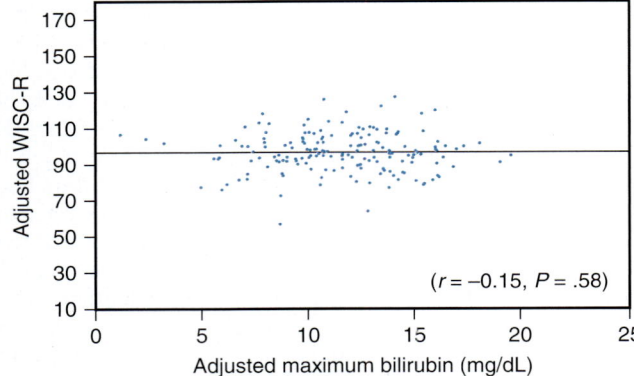

Figure 26.15 Full-scale Wechsler Intelligence Scale for Children-Revised (WISC-R) score at 6 years by maximum bilirubin level for children of less than 2000 g birth weight. Values were obtained using multiple regression analysis. (From Scheidt PC, Graubard BI, Nelson KB, Hirtz DG, et al. Intelligence at six years in relation to neonatal bilirubin level: follow-up of the National Institute of Child Health and Human Development clinical trial of phototherapy. *Pediatrics.* 1991;87:797–806.)

Diagnosis
Serum Bilirubin Measurements

The goal in diagnosis is to identify the infant who is likely to develop brain injury from bilirubin before the occurrence of the neurotoxicity. Toward this goal, certain tests have been devised to determine in an infant's serum the *free* bilirubin, essentially the concentration of unconjugated bilirubin not bound to albumin, the bilirubin binding capacity of albumin, and the bilirubin binding affinity of albumin.[11,21] Although these measures have proved to be of some value in predicting which infants develop kernicterus, the most reproducible tests are not easily applied clinically, and the data are not consistent or conclusive enough to state that one or more of the measures accomplish the goal of identifying the infant susceptible to bilirubin injury before neurotoxicity occurs. However, in a recent randomized study in preterm infants of ≤32 weeks' gestation with hyperbilirubinemia no significant effect of the additional use of bilirubin albumin ratio compared with TSB-based treatment on the neurodevelopmental outcome at 18 to 24 months corrected age was observed.[53] More detailed discussion of these measures is available elsewhere.[11,21,32]

Brain Stem Auditory Evoked Responses and Other Electrophysiological Measures

The more refined laboratory techniques just described indicate the clinical setting for bilirubin neurotoxicity but do not specify whether neuronal injury has occurred or is imminent. Early detection of bilirubin neurotoxicity may be possible by the use of *brain stem evoked response audiometry*. Thus many studies have documented distinct disturbances of the BSAERs with hyperbilirubinemia, and several have documented improvement when bilirubin levels decreased over days or promptly after exchange transfusion (Fig. 26.16).[a] The most consistently observed abnormalities involved the threshold for all waves, latency for wave I, and conduction times between

---

[a]References 21, 46, 47, 113, 133, 135, 136, and 153.

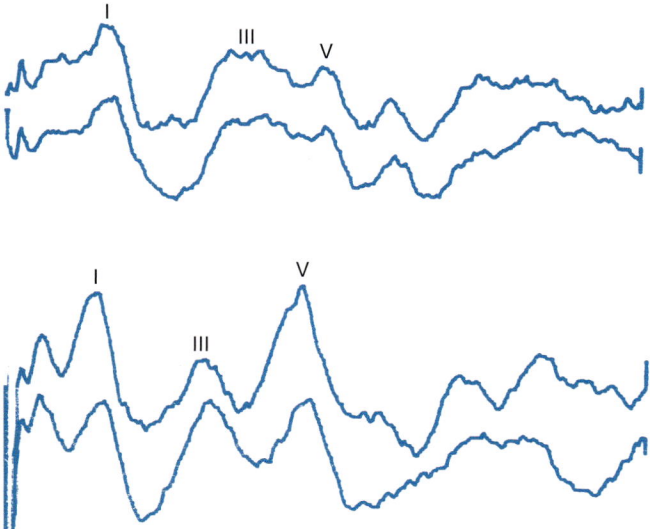

Figure 26.16 Auditory brain stem evoked responses before (*upper tracings*) and after (*lower tracings*) exchange transfusion in an infant with hyperbilirubinemia. The horizontal axis represents time, and the vertical axis represents amplitude. Waves I, III, and V are indicated in both pairs of tracings. Increased wave amplitude and reduced latencies are apparent after exchange transfusion. (From Nwaesei CG, Van Aerde J, Boyden M, Perlman M. Changes in auditory brainstem responses in hyperbilirubinemic infants before and after exchange transfusion. *Pediatrics.* 1984;74:800–803.)

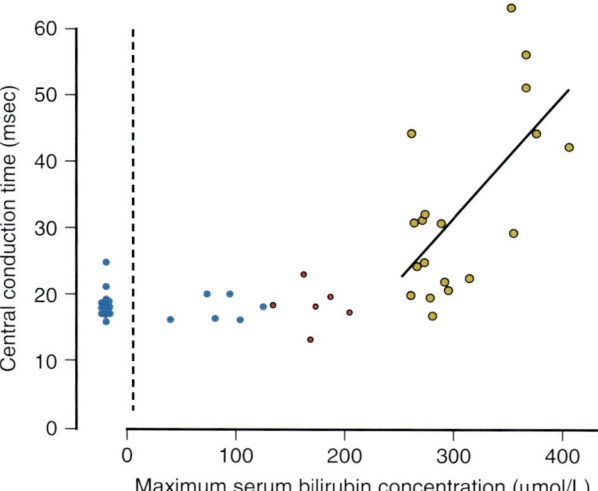

Figure 26.17 Central conduction time of the somatosensory evoked potential as a function of maximum serum bilirubin concentration among term infants. (From Bongers-Schokking JJ, Colon EJ, Hoogland RA, Van Den Brande JL, et al. Somatosensory evoked potentials in neonatal jaundice. *Acta Paediatr Scand.* 1990;79:148–155.)

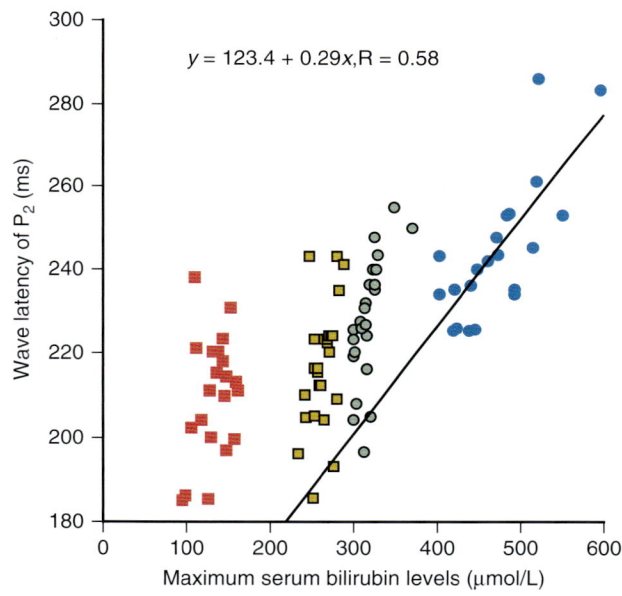

$$y = 123.4 + 0.29x, R = 0.58$$

Figure 26.18 Relationship between the maximal neonatal serum bilirubin level and the latency of wave P_2 of the visual evoked response, obtained on the same day. The four groups were classified according to maximal serum bilirubin level as follows: control (*red squares*) (n = 22), low (*gold squares*) (n = 26), moderate (*green circles*) (n = 25), and severe (*blue circles*) (n = 21). Regression line for the severe group (P < .0001). (From Chen YJ, Kang WM. Effects of bilirubin on visual evoked potentials in term infants. *Eur J Pediatr.* 1995;154:662–666.)

waves I, III, and V. In general, the effects indicated both peripheral and brain stem disturbance, with a predominance of the latter, and correlated with neuropathological findings indicative of injury to the auditory nerve and cochlear nuclei as well as to superior olivary nuclei and inferior colliculi. The adverse electrophysiological effects were observed at serum bilirubin concentrations in the upper teens (i.e., not marked hyperbilirubinemia) in term and near-term infants, with effects at lower concentrations in premature infants. *Reversibility* when the level of serum bilirubin is lowered was consistent. In keeping with the clinical observations reviewed previously concerning the vulnerability of the auditory pathway to bilirubin injury, the data indicate that BSAER audiometry is a sensitive technique for detecting bilirubin neuronal disturbance and, perhaps, imminent neuronal injury. However, the evidence for neuronal *dysfunction* provided by abnormal BSAER audiometry in hyperbilirubinemic infants is not necessarily or even usually followed by evidence of structural *neuronal injury* (i.e., subsequent fixed hearing deficits). Thus the very sensitivity of the technique presents problems in the diagnosis of true bilirubin neurotoxicity. Nevertheless the method holds some promise for the early identification of the infant at risk for neuronal injury.

The possibility that evaluation of *somatosensory evoked responses* may be useful in the assessment of bilirubin neurotoxicity was raised by well-established data.[155] Thus, in a study of 59 term infants, the central conduction time (from cervical cord to cerebral cortex) correlated directly with bilirubin levels above approximately 15 mg/dL (250 μmol/L) (Fig. 26.17). This abnormality disappeared by 5 weeks of age. More data would be of interest.

The possibility that assessment of *visual evoked responses* may be useful in the assessment of bilirubin neurotoxicity was raised by a study of 72 hyperbilirubinemic infants. Earlier reports of 11 hyperbilirubinemic infants and studies of developing Gunn rats suggested that bilirubin may affect the visual system. In the large study of 72 infants, a striking relationship between the major wave latency and maximal serum bilirubin level was observed in the first week of life (Fig. 26.18)[156]; the latencies returned to normal by 8 weeks of age in nearly all infants. Thus this electrophysiological approach, as with the BSAERs, may be too sensitive to distinguish the infant with a fixed deficit from one with a transient deficit.

Transient abnormalities of the *electroencephalogram* were observed in two detailed studies of hyperbilirubinemic term newborns.[157] The disturbances included decreased amplitudes, slowed frequencies, delayed maturation, and multifocal spikes. The changes do not appear consistent enough to be used for diagnostic purposes. Moreover, their clinical significance is unclear.

Magnetic Resonance Imaging

In contrast to common structural imaging modalities, ultrasonography and computed tomography, *MR imaging (MRI)* has been of major value in the identification of both acute and chronic bilirubin encephalopathy (Table 26.20).[38,158] Most infants reported have been term or near-term infants with marked hyperbilirubinemia. However, similar abnormalities were detected in 20 premature infants, most of whom had only moderate hyperbilirubinemia. The principal findings are bilateral and symmetric abnormalities of globus pallidus in approximately 90%, subthalamic nucleus in approximately 40%, and rarely hippocampus. The lesions are seen best in the acute period, during the first several weeks of life, on T1-weighted images (Fig. 26.19) and later, chronic lesions on T2-weighted images (Fig. 26.20). Abnormalities of the globus pallidus and subthalamic nucleus should be distinguished from the typical involvement in hypoxic-ischemic disease of the putamen and thalamus. The acute lesions may be transient and, with clinical recovery, may disappear. Infants who exhibit the chronic abnormality on T2-weighted images consistently exhibit the classic clinical features of chronic postkernicteric

bilirubin encephalopathy (see earlier). However, the converse is not true (i.e., occasional children with the classic clinical syndrome have normal MRI findings).

MR spectroscopy provides additional information in the acute period. A decrease in the *N*-acetylaspartate/choline ratio in "basal ganglia," consistent with neuronal injury, was shown in the first 3 weeks in an infant with a bilirubin concentration greater than 25 mg/dL and later development of athetosis; four other infants with similar bilirubin levels but normal ratios did not develop athetosis, although follow-up was relatively

---

TABLE 26.20   Value of Magnetic Resonance Imaging in the Identification of Acute and Chronic Bilirubin Encephalopathy

Approximately 85 reported cases studied by magnetic resonance imaging; includes 20 premature infants with only moderate hyperbilirubinemia.

Globus pallidus affected bilaterally and symmetrically in approximately 90%, subthalamic nucleus in approximately 40%, and hippocampus in approximately 5%.

In first 3 weeks, lesions seen best on T1-weighted images; chronic lesions seen best on T2-weighted images.

Acute lesions may disappear and not be replaced by chronic lesions; frequency unclear.

Presence of the *chronic* abnormality on magnetic resonance imaging is consistently associated with the classic clinical features of chronic postkernicterus bilirubin encephalopathy; however, a few cases with the classic clinical syndrome do *not* have detectable magnetic resonance imaging abnormality of globus pallidus.

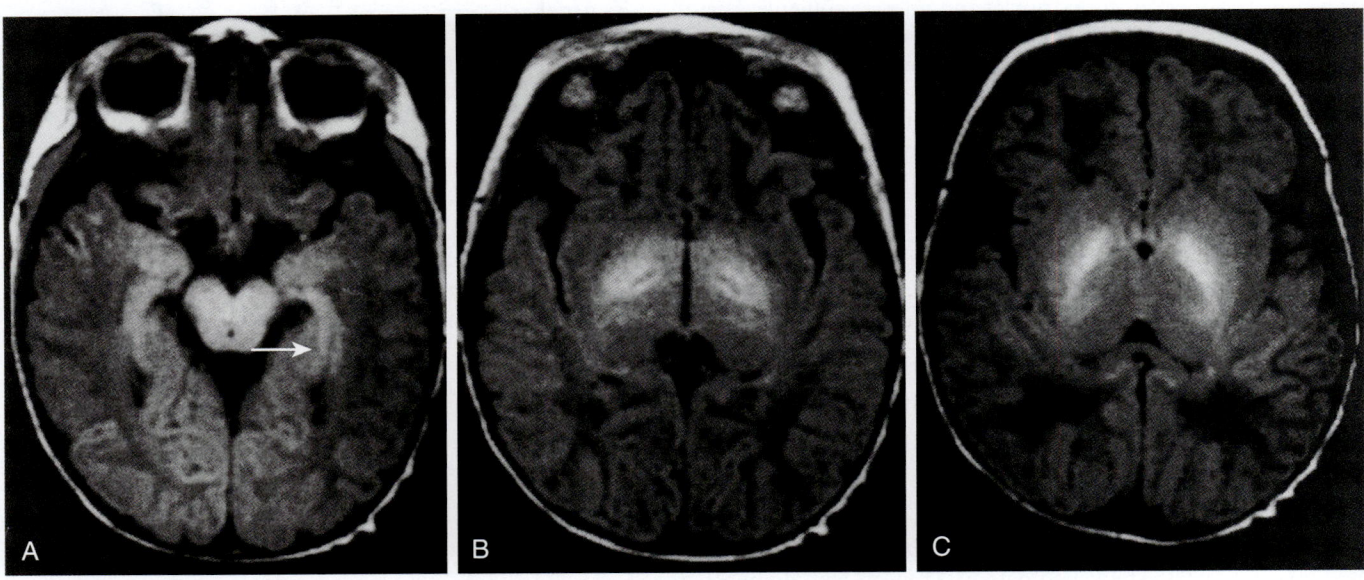

Figure 26.19 Series of three axial T1-weighted magnetic resonance images in a 16-day-old infant with the clinical and biochemical features of acute bilirubin encephalopathy. In A note the abnormal high signal intensity in the hippocampus in the medial temporal lobe (*arrow*). In B and C note the abnormal high signal intensity in the globus pallidus but not putamen. Less prominent high signal intensity is present in the ventroposterolateral nucleus of the thalamus (C). All the findings were less prominent on T2-weighted images (not shown). The topography of the findings is typical of kernicterus. Rights were not granted to include this figure in electronic media. Please refer to the printed book. (From Penn AA, Enzmann DR, Hahn JS, Stevenson DK. Kernicterus in a full-term infant. *Pediatrics.* 1994;93:1003–1006.)

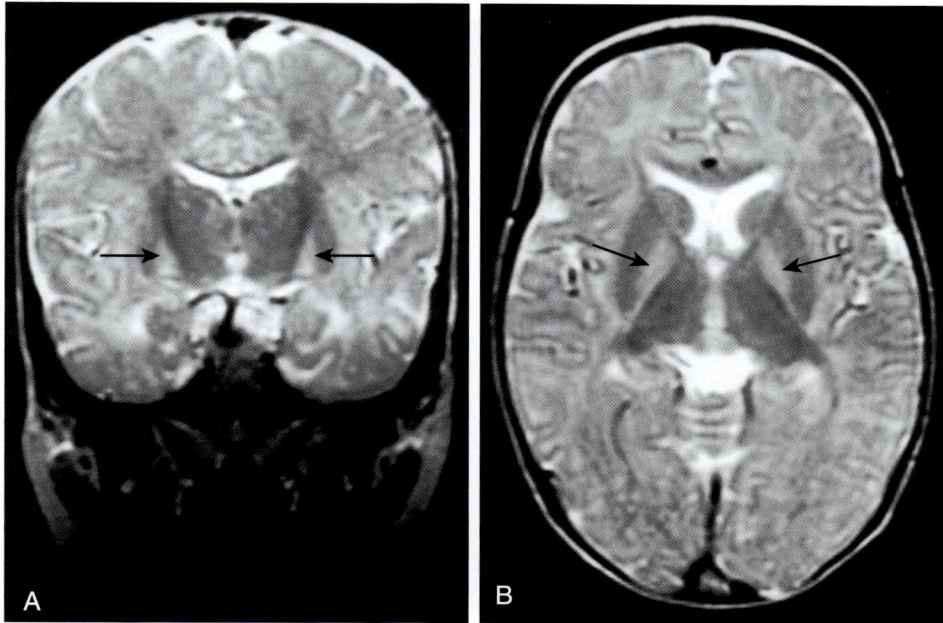

Figure 26.20 MRI scans (T2-weighted). Coronal (A) and axial (B) planes in a 6-month-old infant who had a serum bilirubin concentration of 30 mg/dL at 2 weeks of age. Note the distinct increased signal bilaterally in the globus pallidus (*arrows*), a site of predilection for kernicterus. (Courtesy Drs. Tina Young-Poissants and Charles Barlow.)

brief (12 to 24 months).[159] The single infant with sequelae also exhibited opisthotonus and abnormal signal in the globus pallidus on MRI. Thus it is not clear that the MR spectroscopy results added appreciably to the evaluation of the infant. In another report, six infants with hyperbilirubinemia and MRI findings of kernicterus exhibited, on MR spectroscopy, elevated ratios of glutamate/glutamine to creatine in *basal ganglia*.[160] The authors suggested that the finding reflected an increase in extracellular glutamate, consistent with a role for excitotoxicity in the neuronal injury of kernicterus (see earlier). However, a recent report shows an increased glutamate/glutamine ratio at 3 years in two infants with chronic bilirubin encephalopathy. Persisting excitotoxicity at 3 years seems an unlikely explanation.

Management

The essential aspect of the management of bilirubin encephalopathy is prevention. Although major efforts are directed at prevention and control of neonatal hyperbilirubinemia per se, other factors such as prematurity, acidosis, hypoalbuminemia, hypoxia-ischemia, infection, or other insults to the central nervous system may be as important in the genesis of bilirubin neurotoxicity, at least under certain circumstances (see preceding discussions). These additional deleterious factors must be treated appropriately, when possible, and the search should continue for other such factors that still elude detection.

In this section, the prevention and treatment of neonatal hyperbilirubinemia and, in particular, the choice of therapy as a function of the infant's gestational age, postnatal age, and bilirubin level are briefly addressed. More detailed discussions are available from excellent sources in neonatology.[11,21,45,161] Five major aspects of management of neonatal hyperbilirubinemia should be recognized (Table 26.21): (1) prevention, (2) early

TABLE 26.21	Management of Neonatal Hyperbilirubinemia

Prevention
- Maternal screening for isoimmunization
- Maternal use of anti-Rh immune globulin
- Fetal blood transfusion

Surveillance and early detection of rapid rise of bilirubin

Phototherapy (including high intensity where indicated)

Exchange transfusion

Other therapies
- Intravenous immunoglobulin for hemolytic disease
- Phenobarbital
- Heme oxygenase inhibitors: metalloporphyrins

detection, (3) phototherapy, (4) exchange transfusion, and (5) other therapies.

Prevention

Prevention of hemolytic disease of the newborn begins with maternal screening for isoimmunization. Prevention of the most serious form of hemolytic disease (i.e., that resulting from Rh incompatibility) has been accomplished to a major extent through the widespread use of anti-Rh immune globulin to prevent maternal sensitization.[162] Infants known to be affected in utero have been treated successfully with intrauterine blood transfusion.[163]

Surveillance and Early Detection

Careful surveillance and early detection of the infant at risk for brain injury by bilirubin begin with recognition of infants at risk for severe hyperbilirubinemia. Recognition requires a systematic approach to the infant (Table 26.22) and awareness of major risk factors for the development of severe hyperbilirubinemia (Table 26.23).[11,21,146,161] These issues have been reviewed previously in this chapter. Worthy of emphasis is measurement of total serum bilirubin. In recent years, transcutaneous bilirubin measurements of bilirubin have been developed and have become an important screening tool.[2,21,161] Most importantly, bilirubin levels should be evaluated in the context of hour-specific nomograms (Fig. 26.21).[21,45,161] Those infants in the high-risk zone indicative of a rapid rate of rise

(>0.2 mg/dL per hour) require further evaluation for a cause of their hyperbilirubinemia and phototherapy is invariably indicated (see later). The clinician should be proactive in predicting subsequent bilirubin levels based on the rate of rise and guide management accordingly—that is, either give immediate treatment or institute close follow-up either within the hospital or after discharge.

Identification of the infant *experiencing acute bilirubin encephalopathy* requires *immediate careful clinical assessment* and, if possible, MRI, as discussed earlier. Vigorous therapy should be instituted because the process is potentially reversible.[164]

TABLE 26.22	Selected Key Elements of the American Academy of Pediatrics Guideline on Management of Hyperbilirubinemia in the Newborn of 35 Weeks' Gestation or More

- Measure total serum bilirubin (or transcutaneous bilirubin) on infants jaundiced in the first 24 h.
- Interpret all bilirubin levels according to the infant's age in hours.
- Recognize that infants of less than 38 weeks' gestation, particularly if breast-fed, are at higher risk of developing hyperbilirubinemia and require closer surveillance and monitoring.
- Perform a systematic assessment on all infants before discharge for the *risk* of severe hyperbilirubinemia.
- Provide appropriate follow-up based on risk assessment and time of discharge.
- Treat newborns when indicated with phototherapy or exchange transfusion.

Adapted from Maisels MJ, Baltz RD, Bhutani VK, Newman TB, et al. Management of hyperbilirubinemia in the newborn infant 35 or more weeks of gestation. *Pediatrics.* 2004;114:297–316.

TABLE 26.23	Major Risk Factors for Development of Severe Hyperbilirubinemia in Infants of 35 Weeks' Gestation or More

- Total serum bilirubin (or transcutaneous bilirubin) in the high-risk zone (indicative of a rapid rise of bilirubin >2 mg/dL per hour)
- Jaundice in the first 24 h of life (indicative of a rapid raise rise of bilirubin >0.2 mg/dL)
- Isoimmune or other hemolytic disease (e.g., G6PD deficiency)
- Late preterm gestation (35–36 weeks)
- Exclusive breast-feeding (especially if feeding not going well or weight loss excessive)
- Cephalhematoma or significant bruising
- Sibling with history of phototherapy
- East Asian race

From Maisels MJ, Bhutani VK, Bogen D, Newman TB, Stark AR, Watchko JF. Hyperbilirubinemia in the newborn infant ≥35 weeks' gestation: an update with clarifications. *Pediatrics.* 2009;24:1193–1198.

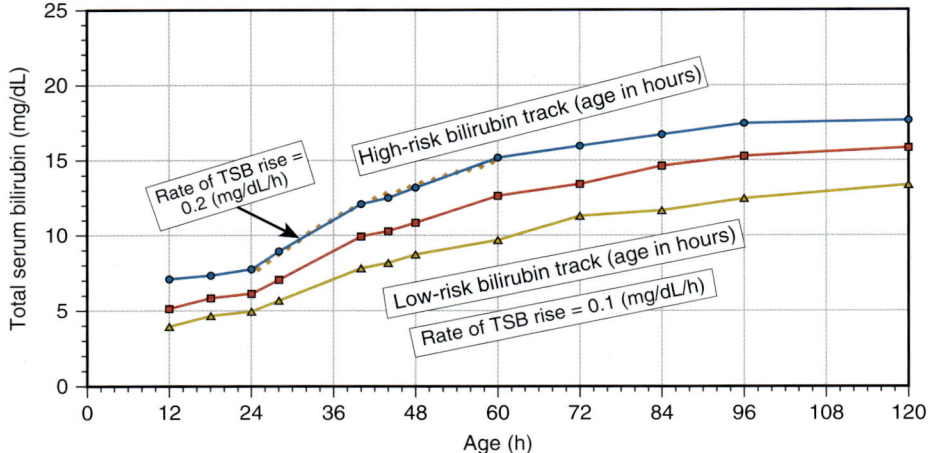

Figure 26.21 Hour-specific bilirubin nomogram for term and near-term healthy infants. The nomogram illustrates the rate of rise in total serum bilirubin (TSB) between 24 and 60 hours of age for the high-risk track (95th percentile) at 0.2 mg/dL per hour, the intermediate-risk track (75th percentile) at 0.15 mg/dL per hour, and the low-risk track (40th percentile) at 0.10 mg/dL per hour. See text for details. (From Bhutani VK, Johnson LH, Keren R: Diagnosis and management of hyperbilirubinemia in the term neonate: for a safer first week. *Pediatr Clin North Am.* 2004;51:843–861.)

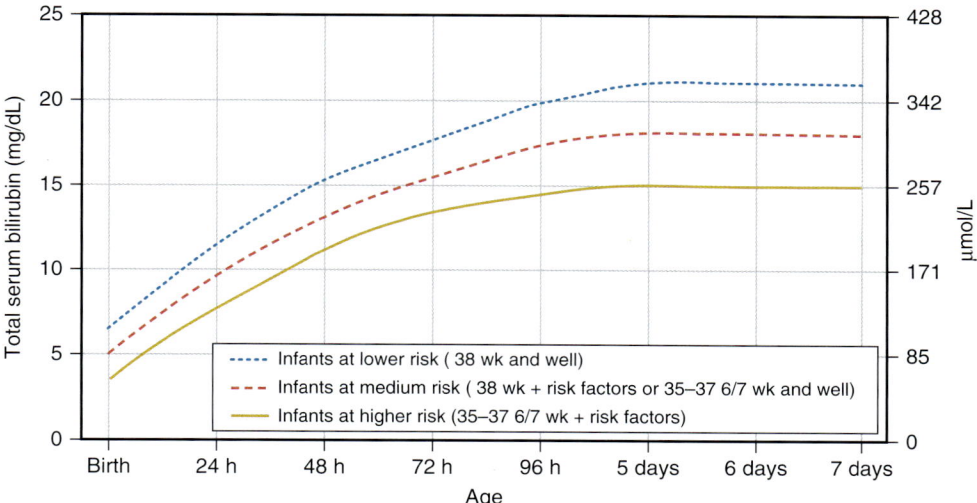

Figure 26.22 Guidelines for phototherapy in hospitalized infants of 35 weeks' gestation or more. The guidelines are based on limited evidence and the levels shown are approximations. The following points are important. Use total serum bilirubin (TSB); do not subtract direct reacting or conjugated bilirubin. Risk factors are isoimmune hemolytic disease, glucose-6-phosphate dehydrogenase deficiency, asphyxia, significant lethargy, temperature instability, sepsis, acidosis, and albumin lower than 3.0 g/dL (if measured). For well infants 35 to 37 6/7 weeks of gestation, TSB levels for intervention can be adjusted around the medium risk line. It is an option to intervene at lower TSB levels for infants closer to 35 weeks and at higher TSB levels for those closer to 37 6/7 weeks. It is an option to provide conventional phototherapy in the hospital or at home at TSB levels of 2 or 3 mg/dL (35 to 50 mmol/L) lower than those shown, but home phototherapy should not be used in any infant with risk factors. Rights were not granted to include this figure in electronic media. (From Maisels MJ, Baltz RD, Bhutani VK, Newman TB, et al. Management of hyperbilirubinemia in the newborn infant 35 or more weeks of gestation. *Pediatrics.* 2004;114:297–316.)

Phototherapy

Phototherapy refers to the exposure of the infant to light with high-energy output near the maximum absorption peak of bilirubin (450 to 460 nm). This procedure exposes the bilirubin circulating in superficial capillaries to the light and stimulates photoisomerization of bilirubin to a form that is water-soluble and can be excreted in bile without conjugation.[11,21,165] This approach is effective as a means of preventing or treating moderate hyperbilirubinemia.[11,21] It has been particularly effective in the premature infant (see later) with nonhemolytic jaundice. With careful attention to temperature, fluid balance, and eye occlusion, this procedure has been considered to be relatively safe and effective even with the use of high-intensity phototherapy (15 to 40 mW/cm² per nanometer).[21,165,166] Currently recommended guidelines for the use of phototherapy for near-term and term infants are shown in Fig. 26.22.

It is important to note that phototherapy has been assumed to be a safe and effective treatment for neonatal jaundice without risk. However, there have been worrying suggestions in the literature that the blue light wavelengths used may cause measurable DNA damage and lead to an increased risk of cancer in later life. This has been evaluated in two large epidemiological studies. The first is the CLIP (California Late Impact of Phototherapy) study, which looked specifically at cancers in infants younger than 1 year using statewide data sets that could link hospital discharge diagnoses.[167] From over 5 million infants born from 1998 to 2007, the investigators identified some 1100 with any form of cancer and 178,000 who had received any form of phototherapy. Those who received phototherapy were 1.6 times more likely to develop cancer (95%

CI, 1.2 to 2.0; P = .002). Owing to many potential confounders, the authors developed a propensity score taking such factors into account, including demographics, chromosomal abnormalities, and gestational age. In propensity-adjusted analyses, associations were seen between phototherapy and overall cancer (adjusted odds ratio [aOR] 1.4; 95% CI, 1.1 to 1.9), myeloid leukemia (aOR 2.6; 95% CI, 1.3 to 5.0), and kidney cancer (aOR 2.5; 95% CI, 1.2 to 5.1). The number of infants needed to be treated with phototherapy to produce an infantile cancer was 10,638. Because of the higher baseline risk of cancer in infants with Down syndrome, the number needed to harm was 1285.

The second study (LIGHT [Late Impact of Getting Hyperbilirubinemia or Phototherapy study]) used a smaller Californian population of 500,000 term infants with a more extensive clinical data set and took account of a cancer diagnosis at any age.[168] In this study there were 60 children with a diagnosis of cancer among 39,403 exposed to phototherapy (25 per 100,000 person-years), compared with 651 of 460,218 unexposed children (18 per 100,000 person-years; incidence rate ratio [IRR] 1.4; P = .01). Phototherapy was associated with increased rates of any leukemia (IRR 2.1; P = .0007), nonlymphocytic leukemia (IRR 4.0; P = .0004), and liver cancer (IRR 5.2; P = .04). With adjustment for a propensity score that incorporated bilirubin levels, chromosomal disorders, congenital anomalies, and other covariates, associations were no longer statistically significant. However, leukemias remained of the highest hazard ratios and children with Down syndrome had upper limits of 95% CIs for adjusted 10-year excess risk as high as 4.4% compared with less than 0.1% for non-Down children.

These studies raise the possibility that phototherapy use may be associated with increased cancer rates (particularly nonlymphocytic leukemia and in infants with Down syndrome); therefore it may be prudent to avoid unnecessary phototherapy.

Phototherapy in the Premature Infant. Chronic bilirubin encephalopathy, including kernicterus at postmortem examination, is currently a very uncommon event in premature neonates but has not disappeared completely. Thus recent case series predominantly from Europe indicate that kernicterus remains a small but important clinical risk.[169-171] The early use of phototherapy is a critical measure in this population. In a recent randomized study evaluating aggressive phototherapy instituted at 23 ± 9 hours after birth and with a target irradiance level between 15 and 40 µW/cm² per nanometer wavelength versus a conservative approach (phototherapy started when the total serum bilirubin level was ≥8 mg/dL (137 µmol/L), showed a slight decrease in neurodevelopmental impairment, including profound impairment and hearing loss (26% vs. 30%; relative risk, 0.86; 95% CI, 0.74 to 0.99) for aggressive versus conservative phototherapy.[166] However, for infants with birth weights of 501 to 750 g in the aggressive phototherapy arm there was a 5% increase in mortality.[166] Although this difference did not achieve statistical significance, post hoc Bayesian analysis estimated an 89% probability that the aggressive phototherapy increased the rate of death in this subgroup. The mechanism potentially accounting for this unanticipated finding remains unclear. Nevertheless, the data suggest some caution when using high intensity phototherapy in this subpopulation.

In premature infants, phototherapy is almost always prophylactic and used to prevent a further increase in total serum bilirubin.[172] Thus intensive phototherapy with high irradiance levels is usually not needed initially. More specifically, in infants ≤1000 g, it is prudent to begin phototherapy at lower irradiance levels. If the total serum bilirubin continues to rise, additional phototherapy should be provided by increasing the surface area exposed and/or by switching to a higher intensity setting. Guidelines for the initiation of phototherapy have been proposed and vary by country.[171,173] However, because the guidelines are largely consensus-derived rather than evidence-based, more conclusive data are needed. It is perhaps most important to determine whether the infant is sick (i.e., clinically unstable, hypotensive, septic) or there is a rapid rise in bilirubin (i.e., >0.2 mg/dL per hour), both of which increase the potential risk for bilirubin neurotoxicity as compared with a stable infant. Despite these caveats, *the overall use of early intensive phototherapy has markedly reduced the need for exchange transfusion in this population.*[166,171]

Intravenous Immunoglobulin. Intravenous immunoglobulin (IVIG) has been used in the treatment of hemolytic disease of the newborn to avoid exchange transfusion for several years. The exact mechanism of action is unknown but the therapy is thought to lead to inhibition of hemolysis by blocking antibody receptors on red blood cells. IVIG occupies the Fc receptor sites and thereby competes with anti-D-sensitized neonatal erythrocytes and prevents further hemolysis. The 2004 American Academy of Pediatrics (AAP) guidelines recommend that in isoimmune hemolytic disease, IVIG (0.5 to 1 g/kg over 2 hours) should be administered if the TSB is rising despite intensive phototherapy or if the TSB level is within 34 to 51 mmol/L (2

to 3 mg/dL) of the exchange level.[161] A recent meta-analysis indicates that IVIG reduces the need for exchange transfusion as well as the duration of phototherapy.[174,175] However, a more recent meta-analysis of 10 trials (*n* = 463) of Rh isoimmunization and 5 trials (*n* = 350) of ABO isoimmunization (3 studies had both populations) has suggested that the impact of IVIG may relate to the bias in measuring factors such as blinded allocation, blinded to therapy, and blinded outcome evaluation.[176] Studies with a high risk of bias showed that IVIG reduced the rate of exchange transfusion in Rh isoimmunization (RR, 0.23, 95% CI, 0.13 to 0.40), whereas studies with a low risk of bias that also used prophylactic phototherapy did not show a statistically significant difference (RR, 0.82, 95% CI, 0.53 to 1.26). For ABO isoimmunization, only studies with a high risk of bias were available, and meta-analysis revealed the efficacy of IVIG in reducing exchange transfusion (RR, 0.31, 95% CI, 0.18 to 0.55). The authors suggested caution regarding the impact of IVIG given that a limited or high-bias study design produced the greatest benefit.

Exchange Transfusion

Exchange transfusion is the treatment of choice for hyperbilirubinemia when the most aggressive intervention is necessary.[11,21] However, in recent years, with the antenatal use of Rhogam, early intensive phototherapy and IVIG, exchange transfusion has been used less frequently. Albumin is a useful adjunct to exchange transfusion and increases the amount of bilirubin removed by the procedure; however, care must be taken to prevent volume overload. In a recent experimental mouse model of severe bilirubin encephalopathy, daily administration of intraperitoneal human serum albumin from birth, without phototherapy, reversed neurological damage and reduced mortality.[177] Albumin infusion increased plasma bilirubin binding capacity and mobilized bilirubin from tissue to plasma. Exchange transfusion lowers the blood bilirubin concentration rapidly, and when performed by experienced personnel, the procedure is relatively free of complications.

A crucial issue is which hyperbilirubinemic infant to treat with exchange transfusion. Current recommendations are shown in Fig. 26.23 for term and near-term infants.[2,161] The guidelines are categorized according to level of "risk," based on such factors as isoimmune hemolytic disease, glucose-6-phosphate dehydrogenase deficiency, asphyxia, sepsis, acidosis, low albumin, or relative immaturity.

Although exchange transfusion in the preterm infant was common historically, with as many as one third of very preterm infants before 1980 receiving an exchange transfusion,[171] more recent data suggest that it is rare, in less than 0.5% of preterm infants.[166] Tradition has suggested that there are no significant differences in the frequency of exchange transfusion–related complications in neonates of less than 1500 g birth weight compared with those weighing greater than 1500 g.[178] Thus, although an uncommon occurrence in modern neonatal practice, exchange transfusion does appear able to be undertaken safely if needed in the very preterm infant.

Other Therapies

Other therapies for neonatal hyperbilirubinemia have been used or are under development.[11,21,115,179,180] These interventions have been directed at several steps in bilirubin metabolism. Thus bilirubin production has been inhibited

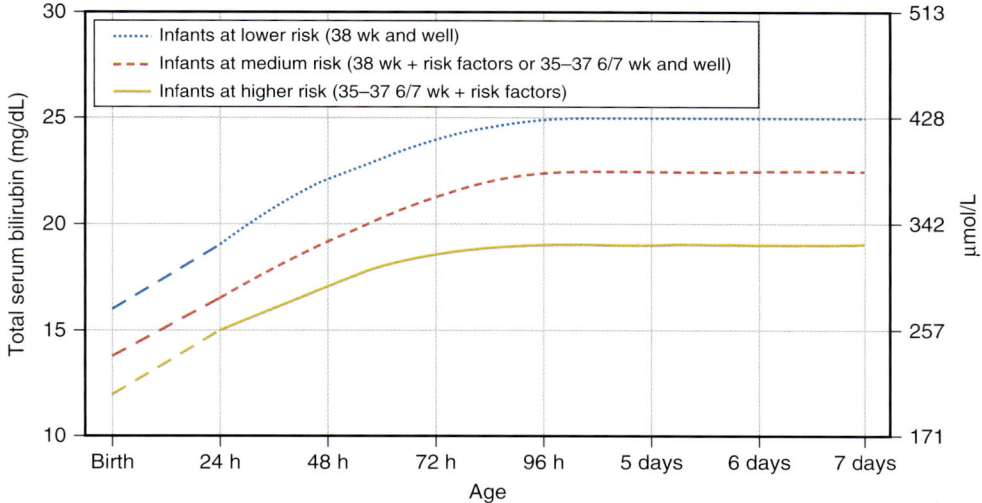

Figure 26.23 **Guidelines for exchange transfusion in infants of 35 weeks' gestation or more.** The guidelines are based on limited evidence, and the levels shown are approximations. The following points are important. The dashed lines for the first 24 hours indicate uncertainty owing to a wide range of clinical circumstances and a range of responses to phototherapy. Immediate exchange transfusion is recommended if infant shows signs of acute bilirubin encephalopathy (hypertonia, arching, retrocollis, opisthotonos, fever, high-pitched cry) or if total serum bilirubin (TSB) is 5 mg/dL (85 μmol/L) or more above these lines. Risk factors are isoimmune hemolytic disease, glucose-6-phosphate dehydrogenase deficiency, asphyxia, significant lethargy, temperature instability, sepsis, and acidosis. Measure serum albumin and calculate the bilirubin/albumin ratio, which can be used as an additional factor in determining for exchange transfusion. Use TSB; do not subtract direct reacting or conjugated bilirubin. If the infant is well and of 35 to 37 6/7 weeks' gestation (median risk), one can individualize TSB levels for exchange based on actual gestational age. Rights were not granted to include this figure in electronic media. Please refer to the printed book. (From Maisels MJ, Baltz RD, Bhutani VK, Newman TB, et al. Management of hyperbilirubinemia in the newborn infant 35 or more weeks of gestation. *Pediatrics.* 2004;114:297–316.)

at the rate-limiting heme oxygenase step by treatment with metalloporphyrins. The hepatic conjugation of bilirubin has been induced by phenobarbital, administered both antenatally and postnatally.[45] Currently none of these therapies is in wide clinical use.

KEY REFERENCES

1. Schmorl G. Zur Kenntnis Des Ikterus Neonatorum, Insbesondere Der Dbei Auftretenden Gehirnerandergungen. *Verh Dtsch Ges Pathol.* 1903;6:109-115.
2. Maisels MJ, Bhutani VK, Bogen D, et al. Hyperbilirubinemia in the newborn infant > or =35 weeks' gestation: an update with clarifications. *Pediatrics.* 2009;124:1193-1198.
3. Kuzniewicz MW, Escobar GJ, Newman TB. Impact of universal bilirubin screening on severe hyperbilirubinemia and phototherapy use. *Pediatrics.* 2009;124:1031-1039.
4. Bhutani VK, Stark AR, Lazzeroni LC, et al. Predischarge screening for severe neonatal hyperbilirubinemia identifies infants who need phototherapy. *J Pediatr.* 2013;162:477-482.e471.
5. Darling EK, Ramsay T, Sprague AE, et al. Universal bilirubin screening and health care utilization. *Pediatrics.* 2014;134:e1017-e1024.
6. Brodersen R. Bilirubin. Solubility and interaction with albumin and phospholipid. *J Biol Chem.* 1979;254:2364-2369.
7. Brodersen R, Stern L. Deposition of bilirubin acid in the central nervous system—a hypothesis for the development of kernicterus. *Acta Paediatr Scand.* 1990;79:12-19.
8. Ostrow JD, Pascolo L, Shapiro SM, et al. New concepts in bilirubin encephalopathy. *Eur J Clin Invest.* 2003;33:988-997.
10. Cashore WJ. Neonatal bilirubin metabolism. In: Polin RA, Fox WW, Abman SH, eds. *Fetal and Neonatal Physiology.* Vol. 2. 4th ed. Philadelphia: Elsevier/Saunders; 2011:1291-1294.
11. Watchko JF, Tiribelli C. Bilirubin-induced neurologic damage—mechanisms and management approaches. *N Engl J Med.* 2013;369:2021-2030.
15. Cashore WJ, Gartner LM, Oh W, et al. Clinical application of neonatal bilirubin-binding determinations: current status. *J Pediatr.* 1978;93:827-833.
16. Watchko JF. Genetics and the risk of neonatal hyperbilirubinemia: commentary on the article by Huang et al. on page 682. *Pediatr Res.* 2004;56:677-678.
17. Bosma PJ, Seppen J, Goldhoorn B, et al. Bilirubin UDP-glucuronosyltransferase 1 is the only relevant bilirubin glucuronidating isoform in man. *J Biol Chem.* 1994;269:17960-17964.
18. Skierka JM, Kotzer KE, Lagerstedt SA, et al. UGT1A1 genetic analysis as a diagnostic aid for individuals with unconjugated hyperbilirubinemia. *J Pediatr.* 2013;162:1146-1152, 1152.e1141-e1142.
19. Travan L, Lega S, Crovella S, et al. Severe neonatal hyperbilirubinemia and UGT1A1 promoter polymorphism. *J Pediatr.* 2014;165:42-45.
20. Huang MJ, Kua KE, Teng HC, et al. Risk factors for severe hyperbilirubinemia in neonates. *Pediatr Res.* 2004;56:682-689.
21. Maisels MJ. Jaundice. In: MacDonald MG, Seshia MMK, Mullett MD, et al., eds. *Avery's Neonatology: Pathophysiology & Management of the Newborn.* Philadelphia: Lippincott Williams & Wilkins; 2005.
22. Gartner LM, Lee KS, Vaisman S, et al. Development of bilirubin transport and metabolism in the newborn rhesus monkey. *J Pediatr.* 1977;90:513-531.
23. Bhutani VK, Johnson L. Kernicterus in late preterm infants cared for as term healthy infants. *Semin Perinatol.* 2006;30:89-97.
24. Raju TN, Higgins RD, Stark AR, et al. Optimizing care and outcome for late-preterm (near-term) infants: a summary of the workshop sponsored by the National Institute of Child Health and Human Development. *Pediatrics.* 2006;118:1207-1214.

25. Engle WA, Tomashek KM, Wallman C, et al. "Late-preterm" infants: a population at risk. *Pediatrics.* 2007;120:1390-1401.

26. Sarici SU, Serdar MA, Korkmaz A, et al. Incidence, course, and prediction of hyperbilirubinemia in near-term and term newborns. *Pediatrics.* 2004;113:775-780.

29. Watchko JF. Vigintiphobia revisited. *Pediatrics.* 2005;115:1747-1753.

30. Ostrow JD, Pascolo L, Brites D, et al. Molecular basis of bilirubin-induced neurotoxicity. *Trends Mol Med.* 2004;10:65-70.

31. Watchko JF. Kernicterus and the molecular mechanisms of bilirubin-induced CNS injury in newborns. *Neuromolecular Med.* 2006;8:513-529.

32. Wennberg RP, Ahlfors CE, Bhutani VK, et al. Toward understanding kernicterus: a challenge to improve the management of jaundiced newborns. *Pediatrics.* 2006;117:474-485.

33. Mollison PL, Cutbush M. Haemolytic disease of the newborn. In: Gairdner D, ed. *Recent Advances in Paediatrics.* New York: The Blakiston Co.; 1954:110-132.

34. Ip S, Chung M, Kulig J, et al. An evidence-based review of important issues concerning neonatal hyperbilirubinemia. *Pediatrics.* 2004;114:e130-e153.

36. Newman TB, Liljestrand P, Jeremy RJ, et al. Outcomes among newborns with total serum bilirubin levels of 25 mg per deciliter or more. *N Engl J Med.* 2006;354:1889-1900.

37. Johnson L, Bhutani VK, Karp K, et al. Clinical report from the pilot USA Kernicterus Registry (1992 to 2004). *J Perinatol.* 2009;29:S25-S45.

38. Penn AA, Enzmann DR, Hahn JS, et al. Kernicterus in a full term infant. *Pediatrics.* 1994;93:1003-1006.

39. Perlman JM, Rogers BB, Burns D. Kernicteric findings at autopsy in two sick near term infants. *Pediatrics.* 1997;99:612-615.

40. Ebbesen F, Andersson C, Verder H, et al. Extreme hyperbilirubinaemia in term and near-term infants in Denmark. *Acta Paediatr.* 2005;94:59-64.

41. Watchko JF. Extreme neonatal hyperbilirubinemia: a view from down under. *J Pediatr.* 2016;168:7-9.

42. van de Bor M, Ens-Dokkum M, Schreuder AM, et al. Hyperbilirubinemia in low birth weight infants and outcome at 5 years of age. *Pediatrics.* 1992;89:359-364.

43. Watchko JF, Claassen D. Kernicterus in premature infants: current prevalence and relationship to NICHD Phototherapy Study exchange criteria. *Pediatrics.* 1994;93:996-999.

44. Okumura A, Hayakawa F, Kato T, et al. Preterm infants with athetoid cerebral palsy: kernicterus? *Arch Dis Child Fetal Neonatal Ed.* 2001;84:F136-F137.

45. Bhutani VK, Johnson LH, Shapiro SM. Kernicterus in sick and preterm infants (1999–2002): a need for an effective preventive approach. *Semin Perinatol.* 2004;28:319-325.

46. Amin SB. Clinical assessment of bilirubin-induced neurotoxicity in premature infants. *Semin Perinatol.* 2004;28:340-347.

47. Amin SB, Charafeddine L, Guillet R. Transient bilirubin encephalopathy and apnea of prematurity in 28 to 32 weeks gestational age infants. *J Perinatol.* 2005;25:386-390.

49. Hansen TW, Bratlid D. Bilirubin and brain toxicity. *Acta Paediatr Scand.* 1986;75:513-522.

51. Oh W, Stevenson DK, Tyson JE, et al. Influence of clinical status on the association between plasma total and unbound bilirubin and death or adverse neurodevelopmental outcomes in extremely low birth weight infants. *Acta Paediatr.* 2010;99:673-678.

52. Sato Y, Morioka I, Miwa A, et al. Is bilirubin/albumin ratio correlated with unbound bilirubin concentration? *Pediatr Int.* 2012;54:81-85.

53. Hulzebos CV, Dijk PH, van Imhoff DE, et al. The bilirubin albumin ratio in the management of hyperbilirubinemia in preterm infants to improve neurodevelopmental outcome: a randomized controlled trial—BARTrial. *PLoS ONE.* 2014;9:e99466.

54. Mreihil K, McDonagh AF, Nakstad B, et al. Early isomerization of bilirubin in phototherapy of neonatal jaundice. *Pediatr Res.* 2010;67:656-659.

55. McDonagh AF, Vreman HJ, Wong RJ, et al. Photoisomers: obfuscating factors in clinical peroxidase measurements of unbound bilirubin? *Pediatrics.* 2009;123:67-76.

57. Calligaris SD, Bellarosa C, Giraudi P, et al. Cytotoxicity is predicted by unbound and not total bilirubin concentration. *Pediatr Res.* 2007;62:576-580.

60. Meisel P, Jahrig D, Beyersdorff E, et al. Bilirubin binding and acid-base equilibrium in newborn infants with low birthweight. *Acta Paediatr Scand.* 1988;77:496-501.

62. Robertson A, Karp W, Brodersen R. Bilirubin displacing effect of drugs used in neonatology. *Acta Paediatr Scand.* 1991;80:1119-1127.

63. Ritter DA, Kenny JD. Bilirubin binding in premature infants from birth to 3 months. *Arch Dis Child.* 1986;61:352-356.

64. Hansen RL, Hughes GG, Ahlfors CE. Neonatal bilirubin exposure and psychoeducational outcome. *J Dev Behav Pediatr.* 1991;12:287-293.

65. Bender GJ, Cashore WJ, Oh W. Ontogeny of bilirubin-binding capacity and the effect of clinical status in premature infants born at less than 1300 grams. *Pediatrics.* 2007;120:1067-1073.

67. Hegyi T, Kathiravan S, Stahl GE, et al. Unbound free fatty acids from preterm infants treated with intralipid decouples unbound from total bilirubin potentially making phototherapy ineffective. *Neonatology.* 2013;104:184-187.

70. Wennberg RP, Gospe SM Jr, Rhine WD, et al. Brainstem bilirubin toxicity in the newborn primate may be promoted and reversed by modulating PCO_2. *Pediatr Res.* 1993;34:6-9.

73. Mayor F Jr, Pages M, Diez-Guerra J, et al. Effect of postnatal anoxia on bilirubin levels in rat brain. *Pediatr Res.* 1985;19:231-236.

74. Vazquez J, Garcia-Calvo M, Valdivieso F, et al. Interaction of bilirubin with the synaptosomal plasma membrane. *J Biol Chem.* 1988;263:1255-1265.

75. Daood M, Tsai C, Ahdab-Barmada M, et al. ABC transporter (P-gp/ABCB1, MRP1/ABCC1, BCRP/ABCG2) expression in the developing human CNS. *Neuropediatrics.* 2008;39:211-218.

76. Gazzin S, Berengeno AL, Strazielle N, et al. Modulation of Mrp1 (ABCc1) and Pgp (ABCb1) by bilirubin at the blood-CSF and blood-brain barriers in the Gunn rat. *PLoS ONE.* 2011;6:e16165.

77. Watchko JF, Daood MJ, Hansen TW. Brain bilirubin content is increased in P-glycoprotein-deficient transgenic null mutant mice. *Pediatr Res.* 1998;44:763-766.

78. Ohsugi M, Sato H, Yamamura H. Transfer of bilirubin covalently bound to ^{125}I-albumin from blood to brain in the Gunn rat newborn. *Biol Neonate.* 1992;62:416-423.

79. Lee C, Oh W, Stonestreet BS, et al. Permeability of the blood brain barrier for ^{125}I-albumin-bound bilirubin in newborn piglets. *Pediatric Res.* 1989;25:452-456.

80. Labrune PH, Myara A, Francoual J, et al. Cerebellar symptoms as the presenting manifestations of bilirubin encephalopathy in children with Crigler-Najjar type I disease. *Pediatrics.* 1992;89:768-770.

82. Burgess GH, Oh W, Bratlid D, et al. The effects of brain blood flow on brain bilirubin deposition in newborn piglets. *Pediatr Res.* 1985;19:691-696.

83. Wennberg RP, Hance AJ. Experimental bilirubin encephalopathy: importance of total bilirubin, protein binding, and blood-brain barrier. *Pediatr Res.* 1986;20:789-792.

84. Hansen TW. Bilirubin entry into and clearance from rat brain during hypercarbia and hyperosmolality. *Pediatr Res.* 1996;39:72-76.

85. Rapoport SI, Hori M, Klatzo I. Reversible osmotic opening of the blood-brain barrier. *Science.* 1971;173:1026-1028.

86. Burgess GH, Stonestreet BS, Cashore WJ, et al. Brain bilirubin deposition and brain blood flow during acute urea-induced hyperosmolality in newborn piglets. *Pediatr Res.* 1985;19:537-542.

87. Ives NK, Bolas NM, Gardiner RM. The effects of bilirubin on brain energy metabolism during hyperosmolar opening of the blood-brain barrier: an in vivo study using ^{31}P nuclear magnetic resonance spectroscopy. *Pediatr Res.* 1989;26:356-361.

89. Lending M, Slobody LB, Mestern J. The relationship of hypercapnia to the production of kernicterus. *Dev Med Child Neurol.* 1967;9:145-151.

90. Bratlid D, Cashore WJ, Oh W. Effect of acidosis on bilirubin deposition in rat brain. *Pediatrics.* 1984;73:431-434.

92. Silver S, Kapitulnik J, Sohmer H. Contribution of asphyxia to the induction of hearing impairment in jaundiced Gunn rats. *Pediatrics.* 1995;95:579-583.

93. Pearlman MA, Gartner LM, Lee K, et al. The association of kernicterus with bacterial infection in the newborn. *Pediatrics.* 1980;65:26-29.

94. Gamaleldin R, Iskander I, Seoud I, et al. Risk factors for neurotoxicity in newborns with severe neonatal hyperbilirubinemia. *Pediatrics.* 2011;128:e925-e931.

96. Silva RF, Rodrigues CM, Brites D. Rat cultured neuronal and glial cells respond differently to toxicity of unconjugated bilirubin. *Pediatr Res.* 2002;51:535-541.

97. Falcao AS, Fernandes A, Brito MA, et al. Bilirubin-induced inflammatory response, glutamate release, and cell death in rat cortical astrocytes are enhanced in younger cells. *Neurobiol Dis.* 2005;20:199-206.

98. Fernandes A, Silva RF, Falcao AS, et al. Cytokine production, glutamate release and cell death in rat cultured astrocytes treated with unconjugated bilirubin and LPS. *J Neuroimmunol.* 2004;153:64-75.

100. Lakovic K, Ai J, D'Abbondanza J, et al. Bilirubin and its oxidation products damage brain white matter. *J Cereb Blood Flow Metab.* 2014;34:1837-1847.

101. Genc S, Genc K, Kumral A, et al. Bilirubin is cytotoxic to rat oligodendrocytes in vitro. *Brain Res.* 2003;985:135-141.

102. Barateiro A, Vaz AR, Silva SL, et al. ER stress, mitochondrial dysfunction and calpain/JNK activation are involved in oligodendrocyte precursor cell death by unconjugated bilirubin. *Neuromolecular Med.* 2012;14:285-302.

103. Bortolussi G, Baj G, Vodret S, et al. Age-dependent pattern of cerebellar susceptibility to bilirubin neurotoxicity in vivo in mice. *Dis Model Mech.* 2014;7:1057-1068.

104. Brito MA, Vaz AR, Silva SL, et al. *N*-Methyl-aspartate receptor and neuronal nitric oxide synthase activation mediate bilirubin-induced neurotoxicity. *Mol Med.* 2010;16:372-380.

105. Brito MA, Lima S, Fernandes A, et al. Bilirubin injury to neurons: contribution of oxidative stress and rescue by glycoursodeoxycholic acid. *Neurotoxicology.* 2008;29:259-269.

107. Roseth S, Hansen TW, Fonnum F, et al. Bilirubin inhibits transport of neurotransmitters in synaptic vesicles. *Pediatr Res.* 1998;44:312-316.

108. Brito MA, Pereira P, Barroso C, et al. New autopsy findings in different brain regions of a preterm neonate with kernicterus: neurovascular alterations and up-regulation of efflux transporters. *Pediatr Neurol.* 2013;49:431-438.

109. Palmela I, Sasaki H, Cardoso FL, et al. Time-dependent dual effects of high levels of unconjugated bilirubin on the human blood-brain barrier lining. *Front Cell Neurosci.* 2012;6:22.

110. Wennberg RP, Johansson BB, Folbergrova J, et al. Bilirubin-induced changes in brain energy metabolism after osmotic opening of the blood-brain barrier. *Pediatr Res.* 1991;30:473-478.

111. Ives NK, Cox DW, Gardiner RM, et al. The effects of bilirubin on brain energy metabolism during normoxia and hypoxia: an in vitro study using ^{31}P nuclear magnetic resonance spectroscopy. *Pediatr Res.* 1988;23:569-573.

112. Vaz AR, Delgado-Esteban M, Brito MA, et al. Bilirubin selectively inhibits cytochrome *c* oxidase activity and induces apoptosis in immature cortical neurons: assessment of the protective effects of glycoursodeoxycholic acid. *J Neurochem.* 2010;112:56-65.

113. Shapiro SM. Definition of the clinical spectrum of kernicterus and bilirubin-induced neurologic dysfunction (BIND). *J Perinatol.* 2005;25:54-59.

114. Hanko E, Hansen TW, Almaas R, et al. Synergistic protection of a general caspase inhibitor and MK-801 in bilirubin-induced cell death in human NT2-N neurons. *Pediatr Res.* 2006;59:72-77.

115. Lin S, Wei X, Bales KR, et al. Minocycline blocks bilirubin neurotoxicity and prevents hyperbilirubinemia-induced cerebellar hypoplasia in the Gunn rat. *Eur J Neurosci.* 2005;22:21-27.

116. Larroche J-C. *Developmental Pathology of the Neonate.* Amsterdam: Excerpta Medica; 1977.

117. Ahdab-Barmada M, Moossy J. The neuropathology of kernicterus in the premature neonate: diagnostic problems. *J Neuropathol Exp Neurol.* 1984;43:45-56.

118. Connolly AM, Volpe JJ. Clinical features of bilirubin encephalopathy. *Clin Perinatol.* 1990;17:371-379.

119. Turkel SB. Autopsy findings associated with neonatal hyperbilirubinemia. *Clin Perinatol.* 1990;17:381-396.

120. Hayashi M, Satoh J, Sakamoto K, et al. Clinical and neuropathological findings in severe athetoid cerebral palsy: a comparative study of globo-Luysian and thalamo-putaminal groups. *Brain Dev.* 1991;13:47-51.

121. Watchko JF, Painter MJ, Panigrahy A. Are the neuromotor disabilities of bilirubin-induced neurologic dysfunction disorders related to the cerebellum and its connections? *Semin Fetal Neonatal Med.* 2015;20:47-51.

124. Fujiwara R, Nguyen N, Chen SJ, et al. Developmental hyperbilirubinemia and CNS toxicity in mice humanized with the UDP glucuronosyltransferase 1 (UGT1) locus. *Proc Natl Acad Sci U S A.* 2010;107:5024-5029.

125. Turkel SB, Miller CA, Guttenberg ME, et al. A clinical pathologic reappraisal of kernicterus. *Pediatrics.* 1982;69:267-272.

126. Van Praagh R. Diagnosis of kernicterus in the neonatal period. *Pediatrics.* 1961;28:870-876.

127. Johnson LH, Bhutani VK, Brown AK. System-based approach to management of neonatal jaundice and prevention of kernicterus. *J Pediatr.* 2002;140:396-403.

128. Amin SB, Bhutani VK, Watchko JF. Apnea in acute bilirubin encephalopathy. *Semin Perinatol.* 2014;38:407-411.

129. Slusher TM, Owa JA, Painter MJ, et al. The kernicteric facies: facial features of acute bilirubin encephalopathy. *Pediatr Neurol.* 2011;44:153-154.

130. Jones MH, Sands R, Hyman CB, et al. Longitudinal study of the incidence of central nervous system damage following erythroblastosis fetalis. *Pediatrics.* 1954;14:346-350.

131. Shapiro SM. Bilirubin toxicity in the developing nervous system. *Pediatr Neurol.* 2003;29:410-421.

132. Hoyt CS, Billson FA, Alpins N. The supranuclear disturbances of gaze in kernicterus. *Ann Ophthalmol.* 1978;10:1487-1492.

133. Shapiro SM, Popelka GR. Auditory impairment in infants at risk for bilirubin-induced neurologic dysfunction. *Semin Perinatol.* 2011;35:162-170.

134. Hyman CB, Keaster J, Hanson V, et al. CNS abnormalities after neonatal hemolytic disease or hyperbilirubinemia. A prospective study of 405 patients. *Am J Dis Child.* 1969;117:395-405.

135. Akinpelu OV, Waissbluth S, Daniel SJ. Auditory risk of hyperbilirubinemia in term newborns: a systematic review. *Int J Pediatr Otorhinolaryngol.* 2013;77:898-905.

136. Wickremasinghe AC, Risley RJ, Kuzniewicz MW, et al. Risk of sensorineural hearing loss and bilirubin exchange transfusion thresholds. *Pediatrics.* 2015;136:505-512.

137. Shapiro SM. Somatosensory and brainstem auditory evoked potentials in the Gunn rat model of acute bilirubin neurotoxicity. *Pediatr Res.* 2002;52:844-849.

138. de Vries LS, Lary S, Dubowitz LM. Relationship of serum bilirubin levels to ototoxicity and deafness in high-risk low-birth-weight infants. *Pediatrics.* 1985;76:351-354.

139. Shaia WT, Shapiro SM, Spencer RF. The jaundiced gunn rat model of auditory neuropathy/dyssynchrony. *Laryngoscope.* 2005;115(12):2167-2173.

140. Unal M, Vayisoglu Y. Auditory neuropathy/dyssynchrony: a retrospective analysis of 15 cases. *Int Arch Otorhinolaryngol.* 2015;19:151-155.

141. Byers RK, Paine RS, Crothers B. Extrapyramidal cerebral palsy with hearing loss following erythroblastosis. *Pediatrics.* 1955;15:248-254.

142. Wu YW, Kuzniewicz MW, Wickremasinghe AC, et al. Risk for cerebral palsy in infants with total serum bilirubin levels at or above the exchange transfusion threshold: a population-based study. *JAMA Pediatr.* 2015;169:239-246.

143. Kuzniewicz MW, Wickremasinghe AC, Wu YW, et al. Incidence, etiology, and outcomes of hazardous hyperbilirubinemia in newborns. *Pediatrics.* 2014;134:504-509.

144. Ebbesen F, Bjerre JV, Vandborg PK. Relation between serum bilirubin levels ≥450 μmol/L and bilirubin encephalopathy; a Danish population-based study. *Acta Paediatr.* 2012;101:384-389.

145. Sgro M, Kandasamy S, Shah V, et al. Severe neonatal hyperbilirubinemia decreased after the 2007 Canadian guidelines. *J Pediatr.* 2016;171:43-47.

146. McGillivray A, Polverino J, Badawi N, et al. Prospective surveillance of extreme neonatal hyperbilirubinemia in Australia. *J Pediatr.* 2016;168:82-87.e83.

147. Manning D, Todd P, Maxwell M, et al. Prospective surveillance study of severe hyperbilirubinaemia in the newborn in the UK and Ireland. *Arch Dis Child Fetal Neonatal Ed.* 2007;92:F342-F346.

148. Lunsing RJ, Pardoen WF, Hadders-Algra M. Neurodevelopment after moderate hyperbilirubinemia at term. *Pediatr Res.* 2013;73: 655-660.

149. Vandborg PK, Hansen BM, Greisen G, et al. Follow-up of extreme neonatal hyperbilirubinaemia in 5- to 10-year-old children: a Danish population-based study. *Dev Med Child Neurol.* 2015;57: 378-384.

150. Jangaard KA, Fell DB, Dodds L, et al. Outcomes in a population of healthy term and near-term infants with serum bilirubin levels of >or=325 micromol/L (>or=19 mg/dL) who were born in Nova Scotia, Canada, between 1994 and 2000. *Pediatrics.* 2008;122:119-124.

151. Hokkanen L, Launes J, Michelsson K. Adult neurobehavioral outcome of hyperbilirubinemia in full term neonates—a 30 year prospective follow-up study. *PeerJ.* 2014;2:e294.

152. Bergman I, Hirsch RP, Fria TJ, et al. Cause of hearing loss in the high-risk premature infant. *J Pediatr.* 1985;106:95-101.

153. Smith CM, Barnes GP, Jacobson CA, et al. Auditory brainstem response detects early bilirubin neurotoxicity at low indirect bilirubin values. *J Perinatol.* 2004;24:730-732.

154. Scheidt PC, Graubard BI, Nelson KB, et al. Intelligence at six years in relation to neonatal bilirubin levels: follow-up of the National Institute of Child Health and Human Development Clinical Trial of Phototherapy. *Pediatrics.* 1991;87:797-805.

155. Bongers-Schokking JJ, Colon EJ, Hoogland RA, et al. Somatosensory evoked potentials in neonatal jaundice. *Acta Paediatr Scand.* 1990;79:148-155.

156. Chen YJ, Kang WM. Effects of bilirubin on visual evoked potentials in term infants. *Eur J Pediatr.* 1995;154:662-666.

157. Gurses D, Kilic I, Sahiner T. Effects of hyperbilirubinemia on cerebrocortical electrical activity in newborns. *Pediatr Res.* 2002;52:125-130.

158. Gkoltsiou K, Tzoufi M, Counsell S, et al. Serial brain MRI and ultrasound findings: relation to gestational age, bilirubin level, neonatal neurologic status and neurodevelopmental outcome in infants at risk of kernicterus. *Early Hum Dev.* 2008;84: 829-838.

159. Groenendaal F, van der Grond J, de Vries LS. Cerebral metabolism in severe neonatal hyperbilirubinemia. *Pediatrics.* 2004;114:291-294.

160. Oakden WK, Moore AM, Blaser S, et al. 1H MR spectroscopic characteristics of kernicterus: a possible metabolic signature. *AJNR Am J Neuroradiol.* 2005;26:1571-1574.

161. American Academy of Pediatrics Subcommittee on Hyperbilirubinemia. Management of hyperbilirubinemia in the newborn infant 35 or more weeks of gestation. *Pediatrics.* 2004;114:297-316.

162. MacKenzie IZ, Bowell P, Gregory H, et al. Routine antenatal Rhesus D immunoglobulin prophylaxis: the results of a prospective 10 year study. *Br J Obstet Gynaecol.* 1999;106:492-497.

163. Liley HG. Rescue in inner space: management of Rh hemolytic disease. *J Pediatr.* 1997;131:340-342.

164. Hansen TW, Nietsch L, Norman E, et al. Reversibility of acute intermediate phase bilirubin encephalopathy. *Acta Paediatr.* 2009;98:1689-1694.

165. Maisels MJ, McDonagh AF. Phototherapy for neonatal jaundice. *N Engl J Med.* 2008;358:920-928.

166. Morris BH, Oh W, Tyson JE, et al. Aggressive vs. conservative phototherapy for infants with extremely low birth weight. *N Engl J Med.* 2008;359:1885-1896.

169. Moll M, Goelz R, Naegele T, et al. Are recommended phototherapy thresholds safe enough for extremely low birth weight (ELBW) infants? A report on 2 ELBW infants with kernicterus despite only moderate hyperbilirubinemia. *Neonatology.* 2011;99: 90-94.

170. Govaert P, Lequin M, Swarte R, et al. Changes in globus pallidus with (pre)term kernicterus. *Pediatrics.* 2003;112:1256-1263.

171. Maisels MJ, Watchko JF, Bhutani VK, et al. An approach to the management of hyperbilirubinemia in the preterm infant less than 35 weeks of gestation. *J Perinatol.* 2012;32:660-664.

172. Okwundu CI, Okoromah CA, Shah PS. Prophylactic phototherapy for preventing jaundice in preterm or low birth weight infants. *Cochrane Database Syst Rev.* 2012;(1):CD007966.

173. Bratlid D, Nakstad B, Hansen TW. National guidelines for treatment of jaundice in the newborn. *Acta Paediatr.* 2011;100: 499-505.

174. Cortey A, Elzaabi M, Waegemans T, et al. [Efficacy and safety of intravenous immunoglobulins in the management of neonatal hyperbilirubinemia due to ABO incompatibility: a meta-analysis]. *Arch Pediatr.* 2014;21:976-983.

175. Walsh S, Molloy EJ. Is intravenous immunoglobulin superior to exchange transfusion in the management of hyperbilirubinaemia in term neonates? *Arch Dis Child.* 2009;94:739-741.

177. Vodret S, Bortolussi G, Schreuder AB, et al. Albumin administration prevents neurological damage and death in a mouse model of severe neonatal hyperbilirubinemia. *Sci Rep.* 2015;5:16203.

179. Schulz S, Wong RJ, Vreman HJ, et al. Metalloporphyrins—an update. *Front Pharmacol.* 2012;3:68.

180. Suresh GK, Martin CL, Soll RF. Metalloporphyrins for treatment of unconjugated hyperbilirubinemia in neonates. *Cochrane Database Syst Rev.* 2003;(2):CD004207.

Full references for this chapter can be found at www.expertconsult .com.

Amino Acids

Jeffrey M. Perlman • Joseph J. Volpe

Since the late 1950s, numerous disorders of amino acid metabolism have been described, with major implications for the developing nervous system. Although each of the disorders is rare, collectively they are important for two major reasons. First, they represent causes of devastating disturbances of neurological development that are potentially treatable, and second, they provide insight into normal and abnormal brain metabolism. *Disorders of amino acid metabolism* are defined, in this context, as those in which the major accumulating metabolite is an amino acid and the enzymatic defect involves the initial step (or, in one case, the second step) in the metabolism of the amino acid. In this chapter, those disorders of amino acid metabolism of especial importance in the neonatal period (e.g., maple syrup urine disease, nonketotic hyperglycinemia, and the urea cycle defects) are discussed in detail. Because urea cycle defects are characterized particularly by hyperammonemia, they are discussed in the larger context of neonatal hyperammonemia.

OVERVIEW OF AMINOACIDOPATHIES WITH NEONATAL NEUROLOGICAL MANIFESTATIONS

Disorders of amino acid metabolism associated with neurological manifestations in the first month of life are shown in Table 27.1. Many other disorders manifest later in infancy and childhood, including variants of most of those conditions listed in the table. The major clinical features include altered level of consciousness, seizures, vomiting (and impaired feeding), and delayed neurological development. In the following sections, maple syrup urine disease, nonketotic hyperglycinemia, and hyperammonemia, including the urea cycle defects, are emphasized because these represent the most common disorders. The other disorders in Table 27.1 are very rare and are noted only briefly (see the section on miscellaneous amino acid disorders later). Pyridoxine dependency is discussed in Chapter 12.

MAPLE SYRUP URINE DISEASE

Maple syrup urine disease, in its classic form, is a fulminating neonatal neurological disorder caused by a disturbance in the metabolism of the branched-chain essential amino acids, leucine, isoleucine, and valine. The disturbance involves the second step in the degradation of these compounds (i.e., oxidative decarboxylation).[1]

Normal Metabolic Aspects
Transamination

The first two steps in the degradation of the branched-chain amino acids (BCAAs) are shown in Fig. 27.1. The initial transamination is thought to occur via a single transaminase.[1] The usual amino acceptor for the transamination is alpha-ketoglutarate, which is converted to glutamate.

Oxidative Decarboxylation

The transaminations result in the formation of the three branched-chain ketoacids (BCKAs), which then undergo oxidative decarboxylation via a dehydrogenase complex to the corresponding short-chain fatty acids (see Fig. 27.1).[1,2] Oxidative decarboxylation of the three alpha-ketoacids is particularly active in liver, kidney, heart, and brain. This reaction is a multistep sequence that requires thiamine pyrophosphate and lipoic acid. The former is of clinical importance because of the occurrence of thiamine-responsive varieties of maple syrup urine disease.[1]

Biochemical Aspects of Disordered Metabolism
Enzymatic Defect and Essential Consequences

The enzymatic defect in maple syrup urine disease involves the oxidative decarboxylation of the BCKAs. The obvious consequence is a marked elevation in body fluid levels of the BCKAs and the BCAAs. The importance of these accumulated materials in the genesis of the short-term and long-term neurological abnormalities associated with maple syrup urine disease is indicated by the favorable response to diets low in the BCAAs.[1,3,4] Available data suggest that both the BCAAs and the BCKAs have deleterious effects on brain and that the precise effect depends in considerable part on the nature of the experimental system examined.

Biochemical Effects of Excess Branched-Chain Amino Acids, Ketoacids, or Both

Neurochemical effects associated with excessive quantities of BCAAs, BCKAs, or both appear to be caused primarily by *alterations of brain amino acids* and *energy failure* (Table 27.2). The alterations of amino acids include a marked increase in BCAAs and a depletion of non-BCAAs. The latter depletion results in part because of impaired amino acid transport across the blood-brain barrier caused by the large quantities of competing BCAAs. However, *cellular* depletion also occurs secondary to the large influx of leucine, which enters brain from blood more readily than any other amino acid.[5,6] Leucine

TABLE 27.1   Disorders of Amino Acid Metabolism Associated With Neurological Manifestations in the First Month of Life

DISORDER	MAJOR CLINICAL FEATURES	ENZYMATIC DEFECT
Urea cycle defects[a]	Vomiting, stupor, seizures	Carbamyl phosphate synthase, ornithine transcarbamylase, argininosuccinic acid synthetase, argininosuccinase
Maple syrup urine disease[a]	Stupor, seizures, dystonia, odor of maple syrup	Branched-chain ketoacid decarboxylase
Nonketotic hyperglycinemia[a]	Stupor, seizures, hiccups	Glycine decarboxylase
Hypervalinemia	Stupor, delayed development	Valine transaminase
Phenylketonuria	Vomiting, musty odor	Phenylalanine hydroxylase
Lysinuric protein intolerance	Vomiting, hypotonia	Transport of cationic amino acids (lysine, arginine, ornithine)
Pyridoxine dependency[b]	Seizures	Glutamic acid decarboxylase (pyridoxal phosphate action), decreased gamma-aminobutyric acid synthesis

[a]Most common disorders and discussed in this chapter.
[b]See Chapter 12.

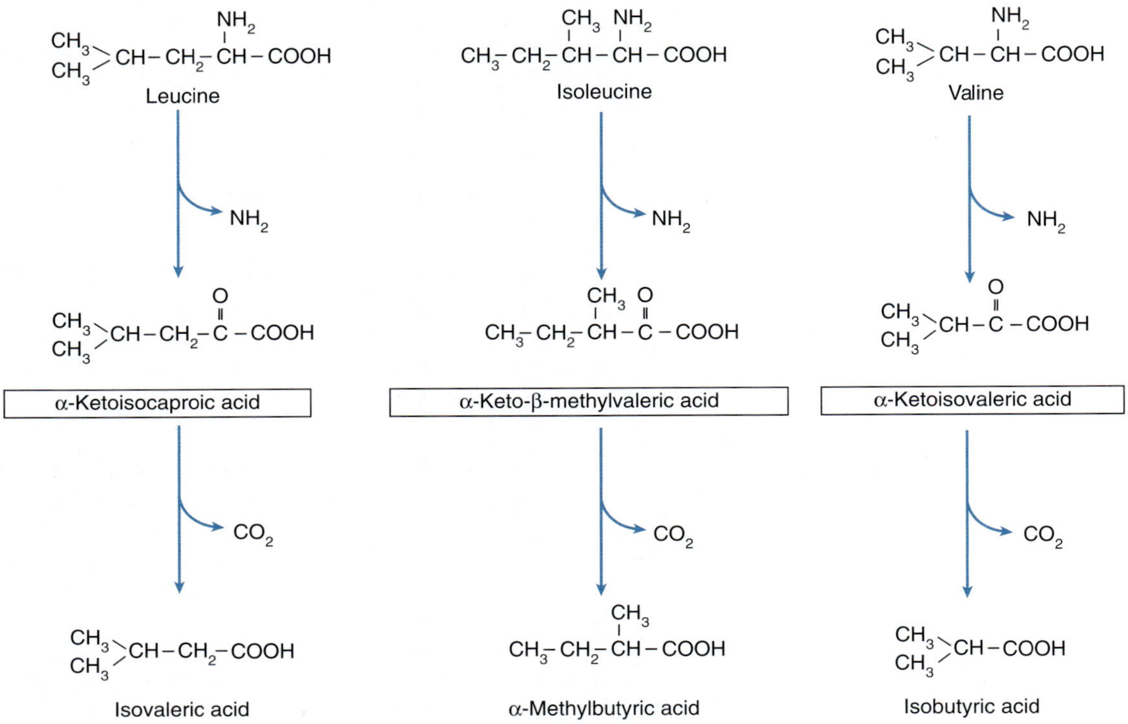

Figure 27.1 Metabolism of branched-chain amino acids. The first step is a transamination, and the second step is an oxidative decarboxylation. The latter is defective in maple syrup urine disease; the ketoacids (enclosed in boxes) accumulate in body fluids.

first enters astrocytes, which surround brain capillaries and is metabolized by the BCAA transaminase to the alpha-ketoacid called alpha-ketoisocaproate (KIC; see Fig. 27.1). KIC enters neurons, and a BCAA transaminase, which uses an amino group of glutamate, reaminates KIC to leucine, forming alpha-ketoglutarate, thereby consuming glutamate. The alpha-ketoglutarate becomes available for the aminotransferase of aspartate and thus consumes aspartate. The result of this process is a diminution in the malate-aspartate shuttle for providing reducing equivalents to the mitochondrion. The consequence is diminished function of the electron transport chain coupled with a direct effect of BCAAs on the chain and

on creatine kinase.[6-9] Indeed, experimental studies of the effects of BCAA on energy metabolism in the cerebral cortex have shown that all the BCAAs reduced energy metabolism and inhibited respiratory chain activity. This effect on respiratory chain activity was prevented by alpha-tocopherol and creatine, suggesting a role for the involvement of free radicals.[7] The disturbance in mitochondrial metabolism results not only in energy failure but also in impaired pyruvate metabolism and increased lactate (see later).

The principal consequences of the altered amino acids and energy failure are multiple (see Table 27.2). Consequences of the amino acid abnormalities include alterations of neurotransmitters

TABLE 27.2 Neurochemical Consequences of Excessive Branched-Chain Amino Acids and Ketoacids

Principal causes
    Alterations of amino acids
    Accumulation of BCAAs, especially leucine
    Impaired transport of non-BCAAs
    Excessive consumption of amino acids, especially glutamate
    Energy failure
    Impaired electron transport
    Impaired creatine kinase
Principal consequences
    Alteration of neurotransmitters
    Reduced gamma-aminobutyric acid
    Reduced glutamate
    Reduced serotonin
    Impaired protein synthesis
    Decreased myelin synthesis
    Increased cytosolic calcium
    Cytoskeletal disturbance
    Free radical generation
    Cell edema
Osmotic effects of BCAAs (especially leucine, and of BCKAs, especially KIC)
    Altered membrane properties
    Cell death

BCAAs, Branched-chain amino acids; *BCKAs*, branched-chain ketoacids; *KIC*, alpha-ketoisocaproate.

TABLE 27.3 Common Features of Maple Syrup Urine Disease

Clinical features
    Vomiting
    Stupor, coma
    Dystonia
    Seizures
    Odor of maple syrup (burnt sugar)
    Full fontanelle
Metabolic features
    Acidosis
    Branched-chain amino acidemia (or aciduria)
    Branched-chain ketoacidemia (or aciduria)
    Hypoglycemia
Neuropathological features
    Myelin disturbance
    Dendritic abnormalities

derived from amino acids (i.e., reduced gamma-aminobutyric acid [GABA], glutamate, and serotonin).[10,11] A second effect of the amino acid abnormalities is disturbed protein synthesis, with multiple effects including myelin synthesis (see later)[12,13] The energy failure likely initiates a cascade to cell death that begins with an increase in cytosolic calcium.[14] The deleterious effects of cytosolic calcium are reviewed in Chapter 13 and include the generation of free radicals, which experimental models of maple syrup urine disease have shown to be involved in cell death.[15-19] A deleterious calcium-mediated effect on the cytoskeleton also has been shown.[20-22] The cell edema that is a prominent feature of classic maple syrup urine disease (see later) appears to relate in part to the osmotic effect of the large accumulation of BCAAs, especially leucine, and BCKAs, especially KIC. In addition, recent data suggest that the energy failure results in a failure of the adenosine triphosphate (ATP)-dependent Na^+K^+ ion pump and, as a consequence, cell edema.[23] Cell death is the final result.

Importance of Branched-Chain Ketoacids

Many of the demonstrated deleterious effects of maple syrup urine disease in animal models in vivo and in other systems in vitro have been associated with the branched-chain *keto*acids. Of these, the ketoacid of leucine (i.e., KIC) is the most critical (see Fig. 27.1). Thus clinical neurological deficits in human infants are correlated best with leucine administration or with blood leucine levels (KIC not measured directly).[1,24-28] Of the branched-chain ketoacids, only KIC inhibits myelination in cultures of cerebellum. Indeed, other adverse effects described in Table 27.2 involving energy failure, free radical generation,

cytosolic calcium accumulation, cytoskeletal disturbance, and cell death have been shown in experimental models particularly or exclusively with KIC. If the ketoacids and especially KIC are critical endogenous toxins, this will have major implications for brain because the transamination of the BCAAs is particularly active in brain (unlike the decarboxylation of the alpha-ketoacids) and would facilitate formation of the ketoacids at the site of greatest sensitivity.

Clinical Features

Of the five types of maple syrup urine disease (lassic, intermediate, intermittent, thiamine-responsive, and lipoamide dehydrogenase deficiency), the classic variety consistently manifests in the newborn period. The onset is in the latter part of the first week and is characterized by poor feeding, vomiting, and stupor (Table 27.3).[1,25-27,29-33] Abnormalities of tone appear; initial fluctuations between hypotonia and hypertonia are followed quickly by dystonic posturing. Opisthotonos, jaw rigidity, and dysphagia become apparent. Seizures occur in approximately half of the symptomatic infants. The characteristic odor of maple syrup may not be present in the early neonatal period. Cerumen is the best source of the odor. Approximately half of infants exhibit a bulging anterior fontanel and signs of increased intracranial pressure. If the disease is not recognized and treated appropriately, death in the first weeks of life is common. The disorder is more fulminating and malignant than phenylketonuria. In phenylketonuria the clinical presentation is usually delayed for several weeks and is insidious in onset, perhaps because the ketoacids of phenylalanine metabolism are derived from a minor pathway, whereas the ketoacids of BCAA metabolism are derived from the major metabolic pathway.

Interesting and helpful clinical signs in acute maple syrup urine disease are *ocular abnormalities*.[25,26,29] These have consisted of fluctuating ophthalmoplegias, including internuclear ophthalmoplegia. Ophthalmoplegia may be total, and oculocephalic and oculovestibular reflexes may be absent. In addition, we have seen two infants with maple syrup urine disease who had opsoclonus. Fluctuating ophthalmoplegias and related eye signs should always raise the possibility of a serious metabolic encephalopathy in the newborn period. These findings are not confined to maple syrup urine disease; similar observations have been made in nonketotic hyperglycinemia (see later). The ocular abnormalities may be associated with signs of lower cranial nerve dysfunction, including facial diplegia, absent gag reflex, and weak cry. *This constellation of ocular and other cranial nerve signs is often initially mistaken for hypoxic-ischemic encephalopathy or a myopathic disorder.*

Neurodiagnostic Studies

The diagnosis of maple syrup urine disease is made on the basis of clinical and metabolic features, but neurodiagnostic studies of value include electroencephalography (EEG) and brain imaging. The EEG during the first 2 weeks demonstrates a characteristic *comb-like* rhythm, consisting of bursts and runs of 5 to 7 Hz, and primarily monophasic negative activity in the central and central-parasagittal regions during both wakefulness and sleep, especially quiet sleep (Fig. 27.2).[34] The abnormality disappears by 40 days after the initiation of dietary therapy. This rhythm may be present on a background of burst suppression, which also disappears after the onset of therapy. This rhythm on the

EEG differs from the alpha and theta bursts of normal infants (see Chapter 10) in their presence during both wakefulness and sleep; in neurologically normal infants, the bursts are present only in quiet and transitional sleep.[34] Because of the prominent involvement of brain stem (see later), brain stem auditory evoked responses show impaired brain stem latencies (between waves 1 and 5) with a normal wave 1.[35]

Brain imaging techniques of value in evaluating the infant with maple syrup urine disease include cranial ultrasonography and especially, magnetic resonance imaging (MRI). Cranial ultrasonography, often of minimal value in acute neonatal metabolic disorders, shows increased echogenicity in periventricular white matter, basal ganglia, and thalami as well as by imaging through the squamosal *temporal window* in brain stem.[36,37] Used previously, computed tomography (CT) shows decreased attenuation, especially in cerebral white matter and deep nuclear structures (Fig. 27.3).[38] MRI, especially diffusion-weighted MRI, is most valuable. The consistent abnormality on T2-weighted images is symmetrical

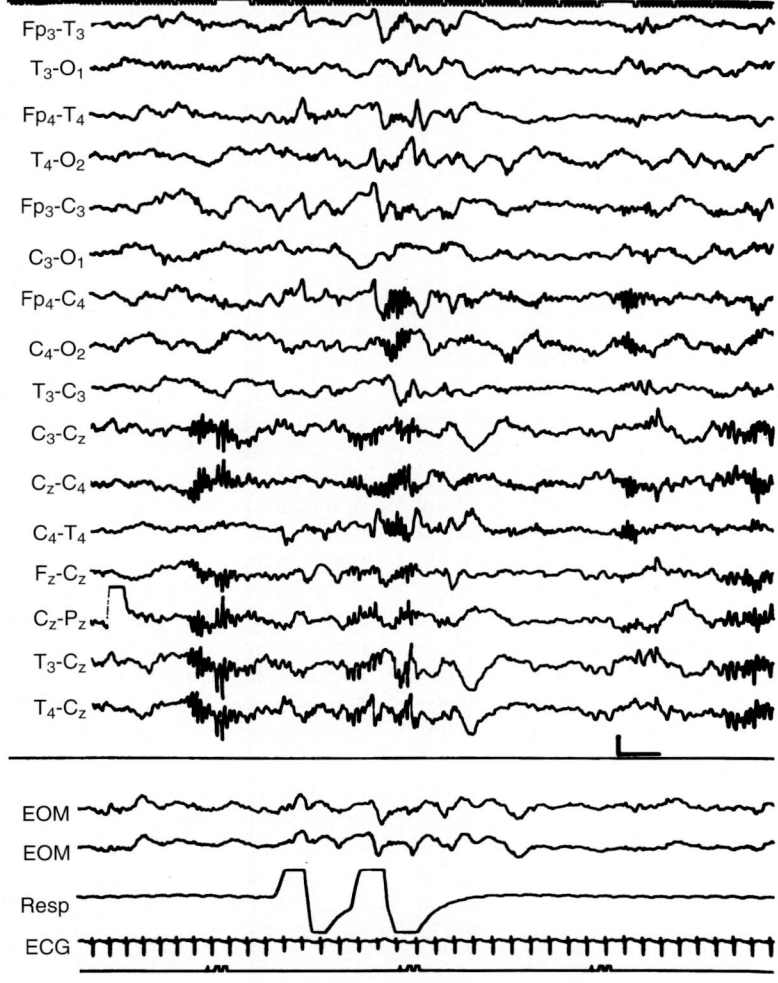

Figure 27.2 Unique electroencephalographic (EEG) pattern in maple syrup urine disease depicting bursts of 4- to 5-Hz *comb-like* activity in active sleep at 13 days of age. Bursts are abundant in the central parasagittal region (C_z), with occasional spread to the right central region (C_4); they also appear independently in C_4. Note also the abnormal respirations (Resp). Calibration: 50 μV, 1 second. *ECG*, Electrocardiogram; *EOM*, extraocular muscles. (From Tharp BR. Unique EEG pattern (comb-like rhythm) in neonatal maple syrup urine disease. *Pediatr Neurol.* 1992;8:65–68.)

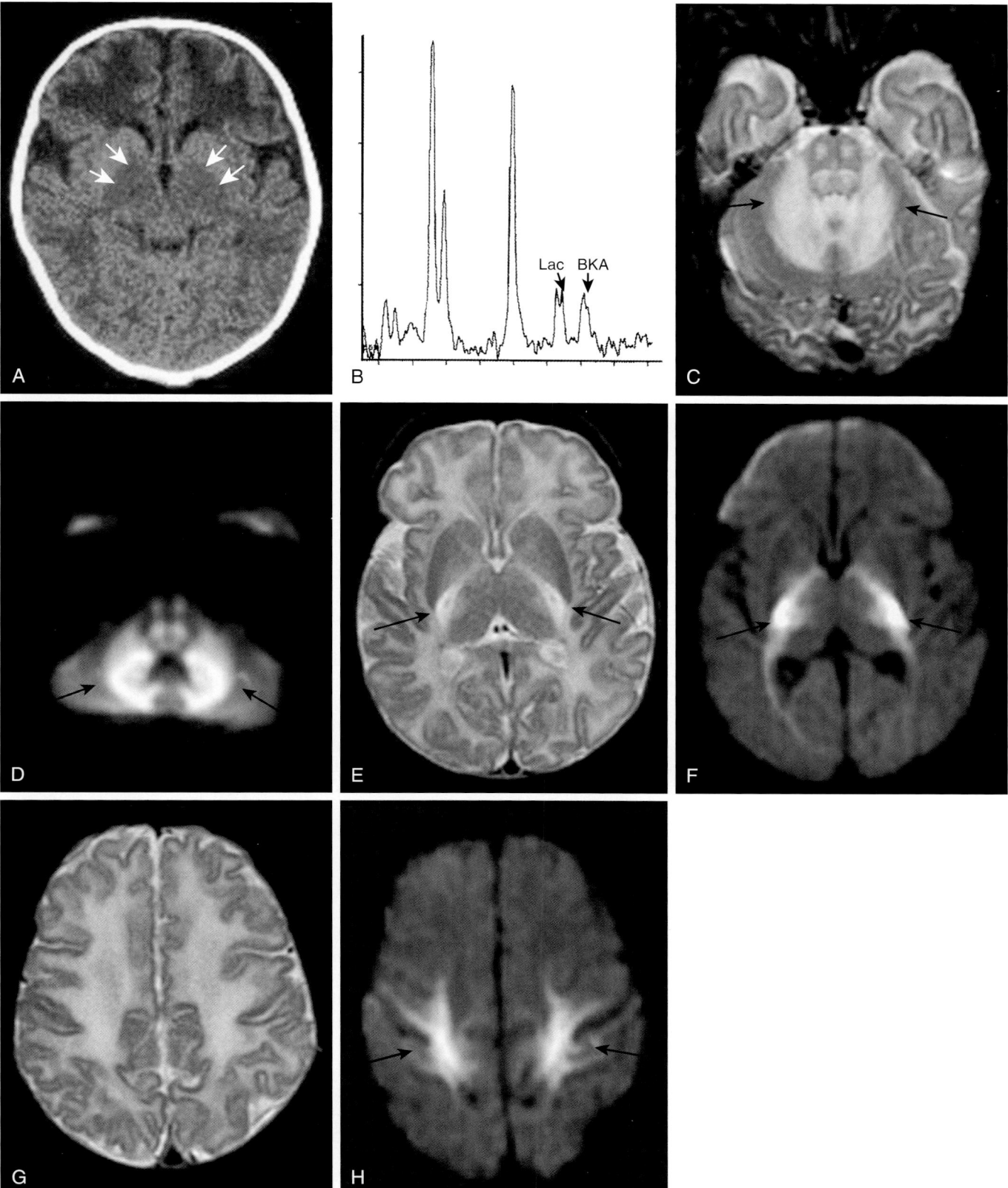

Figure 27.3 Maple syrup urine disease, acute neonatal phase. (A) Axial computed tomography image shows low attenuation (*arrows*) in the globi pallidi and posterior limbs of the internal capsules. (B) Proton magnetic resonance imaging with TE = 288 milliseconds shows abnormal peak at 0.9 ppm (BKA) representing branched-chain amino acids and branched-chain alpha-ketoacids and an abnormal peak at 1.33 ppm (Lac) representing lactate. (C, E, and G) Axial T2-weighted images show abnormal T2 prolongation (*arrows*) in the brain stem, cerebellar white matter, posterior limb of the internal capsule, and centrum semiovale. (D, F, and H) Axial diffusion-weighted images show hyperintensity representing reduced diffusion in the area of T2 prolongation (*arrows*). The diffusion abnormality is more conspicuous than the T2 change in the centrum semiovale. (From Barkovich AJ. *Pediatric Neuroimaging*. 4th ed. Philadelphia: Lippincott Williams & Wilkins; 2005.)

hyperintensity in cerebellar white matter, dorsal brain stem, cerebral peduncles, thalamus, posterior limb of the internal capsule, globus pallidus, and perirolandic cerebral white matter.[38-46] Still more striking than findings on T2-weighted images, diffusion-weighted MRI shows a striking increased signal (decreased diffusion) in the same areas (see Fig. 27.3). The diffusion values are reduced by 70% to 80%. The abnormality is reversible with prompt treatment of the metabolic disorder. However, a subsequent abnormal signal indicative of abnormal myelin is a sequela,[47] and overt volume loss is noted in infants not effectively or promptly treated. The diffusion-weighted MRI findings are consistent with *cytotoxic edema*, particularly affecting myelinated regions. The findings are consistent with the neuropathology (see later). Principal abnormalities on MR spectroscopy include elevated lactate as well as elevated BCAAs and BCKAs, consistent with the adverse effects of the latter on energy metabolism (see earlier) (see Fig. 27.3).

Genetics

Genetic data indicate autosomal recessive inheritance. Thus familial occurrence, affected male and female infants who are products of consanguineous marriages, and biochemical investigations indicating heterozygosity in parents have been documented.[1] The molecular genetic data thus far do not show a straightforward correlation between genotype and phenotype. Most cases of neonatal onset have involvement of the E1 catalytic component (i.e., the thiamine pyrophosphate–dependent decarboxylase).[48] An exception to the variation in molecular defects in general populations, in which the incidence of the disease is 1 in 185,000 newborns, is the single mutation in nearly all Mennonite cases in the United States, in which the incidence is 1 in 176 newborns.[1,33]

Metabolic Features

The major metabolic correlates of maple syrup urine disease are metabolic acidosis, branched-chain aminoacidemia and aminoaciduria, branched-chain ketoacidemia and ketoaciduria, and hypoglycemia (see Table 27.3). Hypoglycemia appears in approximately 50% of the affected infants.

As indicated earlier, the enzymatic defect involves the oxidative decarboxylation of the BCKAs (see Fig. 27.1), which causes the accumulation of the BCAAs and BCKAs. This enzymatic defect can be identified in fresh leukocytes and cultured skin fibroblasts or lymphocytes for diagnosis.[1]

The genesis of the secondary metabolic defects appears to be related principally to the massive accumulation of BCAAs and BCKAs, especially leucine and KIC, its alpha-ketoacid. The ketoacids result in the ketoacidosis, and hypoglycemia is thought to relate principally to the accumulation of leucine.[27] The precise mechanism of the hypoglycemia seen in this disorder is probably multifactorial; a deficiency in gluconeogenic substrates, especially alanine, may be most important.[49] A contributory role of leucine in increasing insulin secretion seems possible but is unproven (see Chapter 25).

Neuropathology

The neuropathological features vary with the onset and severity of disease, the type of therapy, and the age at death. Several general conclusions seem warranted.[1,27,49-56] The *younger infant* may exhibit a slightly enlarged and edematous brain. Neuronal changes are minimal and nonspecific. The most prominent parenchymal disturbance involves myelin and consists of vacuolation (*spongy state*). This last abnormality is most marked in the youngest patients, especially in regions of white matter that myelinate rapidly and near the time of active disease. *Older patients* show a diminution of myelin. A reduction of oligodendrocytes parallels the extent of myelin deficiency. Signs of myelin breakdown are minimal or absent. Because a similar progression from myelin vacuolation to disturbed myelin deposition is seen in several mutant mice with metabolic defects in myelin formation,[57-59] it has been considered that the major brain defect observed in maple syrup urine disease and related states (e.g., nonketotic hyperglycinemia, phenylketonuria, and ketotic hyperglycinemia) involves myelin formation. It is likely that such a myelin defect in metabolic disorders could be caused by disturbances of the synthesis of myelin lipids (e.g., certain fatty acids, as in ketotic hyperglycinemia) or of myelin proteins (as in the amino acid disorders).

The *chemical correlates* of the neuropathological findings are diminutions in the levels of myelin lipids as well as myelin proteolipid protein (Table 27.4). The neuropathological and chemical findings of disturbed myelination and the later evidence of such disturbance on MRI scans are less apparent or absent in patients treated from early infancy (see Table 27.4).[54,60-62]

An additional neuropathological feature involves *neuronal development* and consists primarily of deficiencies in dendritic development and in quantities of dendritic spines, sites of synaptic contacts (Fig. 27.4).[56] Additional abnormalities included aberrant orientation of cerebral cortical neurons. Neuronal loss, although not a prominent feature of this disease, is usually apparent in cerebellar granule cells.

TABLE 27.4 Alterations of White Matter Lipids and Proteolipid Protein in Maple Syrup Urine Disease

AGE OF INFANT	PERCENTAGE OF CONTROL OF		
	TOTAL LIPID	CEREBROSIDES	PROTEOLIPID PROTEIN
16 days	90	50	67
25 days	66	—	64
20 months	82	66	57
36 months[a]	81	93	79

[a]Treated with diet low in branched-chain amino acids from 35 days of age. Data from Prensky AL, Carr S, Moser HW. Development of myelin in inherited disorders of amino acid metabolism. *Arch Neurol.* 1968;19:552–558.

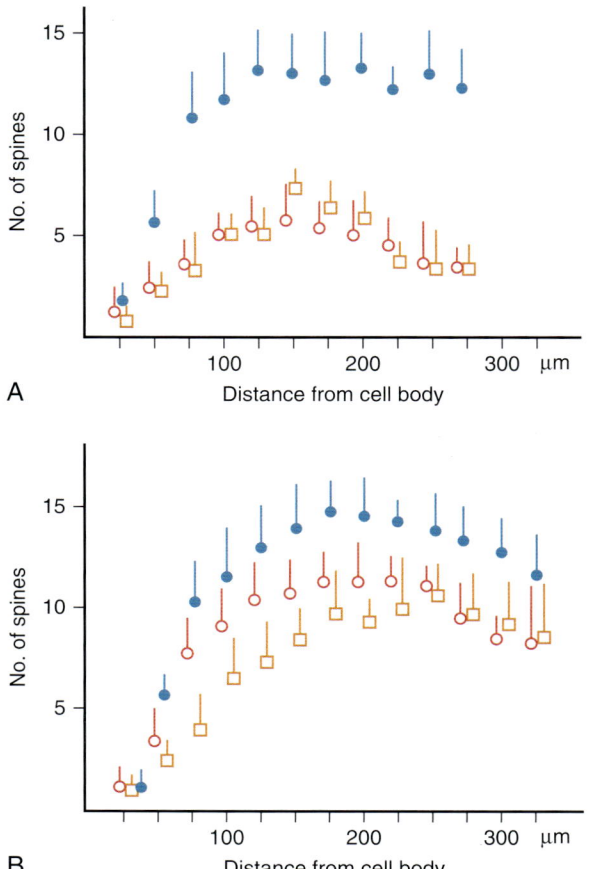

A
Distance from cell body

B
Distance from cell body

Figure 27.4 Diminished number of synaptic spines in maple syrup urine disease (MSUD). Distribution of synaptic spines on basal dendrites of pyramidal neurons in the (A) visual and (B) motor cortex of a patient with MSUD and age-matched control. A marked reduction of spine density in MSUD is noted compared with the control. *Open circles*, layer 5 of MSUD; *open squares*, layer 3 of MSUD; *closed circles*, layer 5 of control. (From Kamei A, Takashima S, Chan F, Becker LE. Abnormal dendritic development in maple syrup urine disease. *Pediatr Neurol.* 1992;8:145–147.)

Management

Prevention

Prenatal diagnosis and prevention of maple syrup urine disease by therapeutic abortion are well-established approaches.[1,27,32] Cultured cells[3,63] derived from chorionic villus biopsy have allowed diagnosis in the first trimester of gestation.[1]

Early Detection

After birth of an affected child, early detection is critical.[1,3-5,28,64] Institution of aggressive therapy at 5 days of age or less with close monitoring of leucine levels has been followed by normal intellectual outcome (see earlier discussion).[28] On the other hand, institution of therapy after 14 days of age is very uncommonly followed by normal intellectual development. Distinction from other causes of metabolic acidosis in the neonatal period is important (see Chapter 28). The early clinical features and odor of maple syrup, especially in cerumen, are most helpful in making the clinical diagnosis. Neonatal blood screening by tandem mass spectrometry to quantify amino acids in whole blood filter paper specimens is highly sensitive, accurate, and rapid and is the currently preferred approach.[65]

Acute Therapy

Acute episodes are managed by correcting dehydration, lowering toxic levels of BCAAs and BCKAs, limiting protein catabolism, and promoting protein anabolism.[1,4,33] A combination of enteral and parenteral therapy is used, including high-dose intravenous thiamine. Intravenous dextrose and intralipid are useful to prevent further protein catabolism, and branched-chain amino acid–free parenteral and enteral preparations help diminish leucine levels promptly. Hemodialysis can be lifesaving.[66,67] Continuous hemofiltration by a pump-assisted, high-flow venovenous system may be as effective and more convenient, albeit somewhat slower than conventional intermittent hemodialysis.[1,68] Signs of brain edema have been managed with mannitol, furosemide, and intravenous sodium supplementation to replace urinary sodium losses and maintain a serum sodium level greater than 140 mg/L.[33]

Long-Term Therapy

Subsequent therapy includes a diet that initially contains no BCAAs.[1,3,4,27] Control of plasma leucine levels is especially crucial, and the adequacy of this control correlates with intellectual outcome in infants with classic maple syrup urine disease.[69] More recent approaches include optimizing specific amino acids (e.g., phenylalanine, tyrosine, tryptophan, histidine, methionine, threonine) that compete with BCAAs for entry into brain via a common transporter (LAT1), providing glutamine, glutamate, and alanine to replenish episodic depletion caused by reverse transamination and correcting deficiencies of omega-3 essential fatty acids, zinc, and selenium in a special formula.[69] Close supervision is mandatory because relapses may occur with minor infections or for no apparent reason. A more favorable outcome is related particularly to early onset of therapy, careful biochemical monitoring, and early introduction of natural foods to provide adequate nutrition, especially protein anabolism.[a]

When dietary therapy is instituted before the onset of symptoms (detected because of an earlier affected sibling), a normal neurological outcome can be achieved.[4,5,28,33] In infants who develop symptoms, the time of detection and institution of therapy are very important. In one earlier study, those detected and treated at 5 days of age or less had a mean intelligence quotient (IQ) of 97 ± 13 versus 65 ± 20 in those detected and treated at 6 or more days of age.[5] In a more recent study, with particularly vigorous metabolic care, most infants with onset of therapy in the second week had favorable neurological outcomes.[33]

NONKETOTIC HYPERGLYCINEMIA (GLYCINE ENCEPHALOPATHY)

Nonketotic hyperglycinemia is an inborn error of metabolism in which large amounts of glycine accumulate in body fluids and a serious neonatal neurological disorder occurs. The disturbance involves the cleavage of glycine to carbon dioxide and a one-carbon fragment. This disorder is approximately twice as common as ketotic hyperglycinemia (see Chapter 28),

---

[a]References 4, 5, 24, 28, 62, and 70.

from which it should be distinguished. Because nonketotic hyperglycinemia involves the central nervous system directly, the term *glycine encephalopathy* may be more appropriate.

Normal Metabolic Aspects

Glycine, the simplest of amino acids, is nonessential because it can be synthesized in numerous ways in humans.[71,72] It is abundant in most proteins and, indeed, approximately 50% of ingested glycine is involved in the *synthesis of protein* (Fig. 27.5).[71,72] In addition, however, a large portion of glycine is *converted to serine,* which, in turn, is involved in the synthesis of phospholipids as well as oxidation to carbon dioxide through the citric acid cycle (see Fig. 27.5). Glycine is also cleaved to a one-carbon fragment that is then used in a wide variety of synthetic reactions. In addition, glycine is the precursor of such other critical compounds as purines, glutathione, and porphyrins.

The major roles of glycine as a *neurotransmitter* are almost certainly crucial for the neurological features of nonketotic hyperglycinemia. It is now clear that glycine has *two* neurotransmitter roles in the central nervous system, one inhibitory and one excitatory, that are influenced by maturation (Table 27.5).[72-79] The *classic* glycine receptor is inhibitory and located primarily in spinal cord and brain stem. This receptor is inhibited by strychnine. However, like the GABA_A receptor, it appears to be excitatory during early brain development in animal models.[72,80] The basis of such early excitatory characteristics may be similar to that for the early excitatory GABA_A receptors (see Chapter 12); thus the immature brain appears to have increased intracellular chloride because of delayed maturation of the chloride exporter.[81,82] The result would be chloride efflux and depolarization (excitation) rather than chloride influx and hyperpolarization (inhibition) when glycine activation of its receptor opens the chloride channel. Whether all or a portion of these classic glycine receptors is also excitatory in the human newborn brain is unknown. The possibility that both inhibitory and excitatory receptors are present in the brain stem is suggested by the frequency of both apnea and hiccups in newborns with nonketotic hyperglycinemia. In addition, glycine acts at a second receptor site associated with the N-methyl-D-aspartate (NMDA) receptor-channel complex and potentiates the action of glutamate at this receptor. This receptor is located throughout the central nervous system, including cerebrum and cerebellum. Thus glycine acting at this second receptor is excitatory and indeed can lead to glutamate-induced excitotoxic neuronal death (see later). The excitation may be reflected clinically in the recalcitrant seizures in newborns with nonketotic hyperglycinemia. Because the neonatal nervous system is particularly sensitive to NMDA receptor–mediated neuronal death (see Chapter 13), it is clear that characteristics of the immature central nervous system cause glycine to be both excitatory and neurotoxic.[76] In addition, the binding of glycine to the NMDA receptor increases postnatally in human cerebral cortical neurons by 100% from term to 6 months.[83] These issues are directly relevant to the clinical, neuropathological, and therapeutic aspects of nonketotic hyperglycinemia (see later discussions).

Biochemical Aspects of Disordered Metabolism
Enzymatic Defect and Essential Consequences

The enzymatic defect in nonketotic hyperglycinemia involves the glycine cleavage enzyme system, which converts the C_1

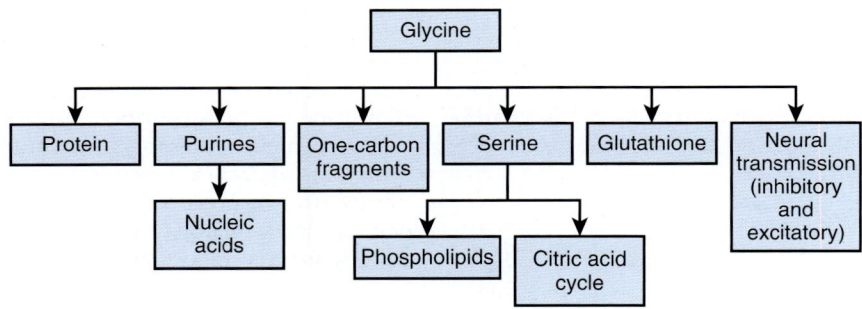

Figure 27.5 Major metabolic fates of glycine.

TABLE 27.5   Glycine Receptors Involved in Neurotransmission and Their Relation to Nonketotic Hyperglycinemia

	GLYCINE RECEPTORS	
	CLASSIC	**NMDA**
Major sites in central nervous system	Spinal cord, brain stem	Diffuse, including cerebral cortex, basal ganglia, cerebellum
Primary action	Inhibitory	Excitatory
Mechanism of action	Opens chloride channel	Potentiates activation of NMDA receptor by glutamate
Developmental feature	Excitatory early in brain development (?)	Most abundant early in development
Antagonist	Strychnine	NMDA antagonist (MK-801), glycine site antagonist (HA-966)
Potential clinical correlates	Respiratory failure, weakness, hypotonia	Seizures, myoclonus, neuronal toxicity

NMDA, N-methyl-D-aspartate.

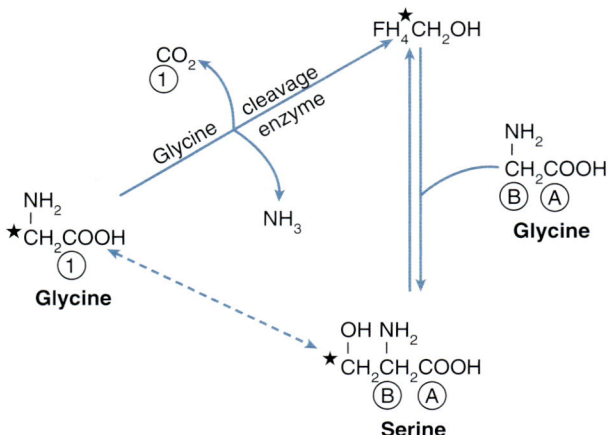

Figure 27.6 Glycine cleavage enzyme system. The glycine that serves as substrate for the cleavage enzyme is shown on the left of the figure; the C_1 is marked with the *circled numeral* and the C_2 with a *star*. A defect in the glycine cleavage enzyme is accompanied by a defect in the formation of (*1*) carbon dioxide from the C_1 of glycine and (2) the C_3 of serine from the C_2 of glycine. (Adapted from Nyhan WL. Nonketotic hyperglycinemia. In: Scriver CR, Beaudet AL, Sly WS, et al., eds. *The Metabolic Basis of Inherited Disease.* 6th ed. New York: McGraw-Hill; 1989.)

of glycine to carbon dioxide and results in the formation of a hydroxymethyl derivative of tetrahydrofolate, the key one-carbon donor (Fig. 27.6).[71,72,84-86] A potential particular importance of the glycine cleavage system in early brain development is suggested by the finding of threefold to fivefold higher activities in brain of the first-trimester fetus than in brain of the adult.[87] The enzyme is expressed early in development in neural stem/progenitor cells in the germinative zones and then later in radial glial cells.[88] Moreover, glycine receptors in developing cerebrum are important in early neuronal development and differentiation.[89] These considerations could partly explain the disturbances in axonal and later myelin development that likely underlie the defects in corpus callosum observed in nonketotic hyperglycinemia (see later).

Abnormalities of two of the four component proteins of the glycine cleavage enzyme complex (i.e., P-protein [the pyridoxal-dependent decarboxylase] encoded by the GLDC gene and T-protein [a tetrahydrofolate-requiring component] encoded by the AMT gene) have been identified as the molecular abnormality in the severe neonatal cases.[71,72,79,90-92] In one study of 30 cases, 87% exhibited a defect of the P-protein, and the remainder had a defect of the T-protein.[79] These data clarified the earlier in vivo observations in affected infants of defects in the formation of carbon dioxide from the C_1 of glycine and in the formation of the C_3 of serine from the C_2 of glycine (see Fig. 27.6).[71,93-95]

This aminoacidopathy is distinctive in that the enzymatic defect has been shown to occur in *brain*,[a] and, indeed, this fact is probably critical in the pathogenesis of the functional and structural features of the disorder. The immediate result is markedly elevated brain concentrations of glycine. Hyperglycinemia from other causes, including *ketotic* hyperglycinemia, is *not* associated with elevated levels of glycine

in brain or with disturbance of glycine cleavage in brain.[85,98] Several lines of evidence suggest that the presence of the defect in *brain* and the resulting accumulation of *glycine in brain* are critical in the neurotoxicity. First, a deficiency of the product of the glycine cleavage reaction (i.e., the one-carbon tetrahydrofolate derivative) is not likely to be highly important because this compound can be generated by other pathways. Second, administration to very young patients with nonketotic hyperglycinemia of sodium benzoate, which is effective in lowering the *plasma* glycine level (through the formation of a water-soluble excretable conjugate) but not the cerebrospinal fluid (CSF) glycine level, does not have consistently beneficial neurological effects (see later). Third, strychnine, a centrally acting antagonist of glycine, is effective in improving certain aspects of the neurological status of at least some affected patients (see later discussion).

Biochemical Effects of Excessive Brain Glycine

The mechanism of the deleterious effect of glycine on neurological *function* may relate to glycine's neurotransmitter roles. Both inhibitory and excitatory actions likely occur. Concerning *inhibition,* the classic inhibitory glycine receptor may account in part for the apparent suppression of ventilation through action on the brain stem neurons crucial for respiratory drive as well as for the hypotonia and weakness through action on spinal cord neurons. Concerning *excitation,* three factors may be relevant. First, as noted earlier, early in brain development some classic inhibitory glycine receptors may be excitatory. Hiccups, which likely represent a brain stem excitatory effect, may relate to paradoxically excitatory glycine receptors (see earlier). Second, any existing inhibitory glycine receptors could exhibit desensitization with persistent exposure to high concentrations of glycine. Indeed, experimental evidence indicates that excess glycine may result in a desensitization of glycine receptors at the postsynaptic membrane, which would result in diminished inhibition of certain pathways.[99] Third, probably the most potent excitatory influence of glycine is exerted at the NMDA receptor, as described earlier. The result of these excitatory influences could include seizures, hyperexcitability, and myoclonus.

The mechanism of the deleterious effect of glycine on neural *structure* may relate to a disturbance in myelin proteins and to excitotoxic neuronal effects. Neuropathological observations demonstrate a striking *myelin disturbance* in nonketotic hyperglycinemia, similar to that observed with maple syrup urine disease and other aminoacidopathies. Because protein synthesis is disturbed when one amino acid is present in markedly abnormal quantities, one possibility is that excessive brain glycine leads to the myelin disturbance by causing a defect in the synthesis of one or more myelin proteins. In addition, *neuronal loss* in cerebrum and cerebellum may be excitotoxic (see later discussion). Disturbances in cerebral development, of prenatal origin (see later), may relate to both the deficient action of the glycine cleavage enzyme and the excessive action of glycine on glycine and NMDA receptors. Thus, as noted earlier, the glycine cleavage system is important in developing neuroepithelium in stem/progenitor cells and radial glial cells. The action of glycine on both the glycine and NMDA receptors is important in brain development; in excess these actions could be deleterious. One such deleterious effect could be excitotoxicity mediated by the NMDA receptor.

[a]References 71-74, 79, 84, 85, 96, and 97.

Clinical Features

The onset of nonketotic hyperglycinemia in the typical case is in the first days of life, most commonly the first 2 days of life, with ineffective suck, impaired ventilatory effort (or apnea), stupor, hypotonia, seizures, multifocal myoclonus, and hiccups (Table 27.6).[24,71-73,79,97,100-114] Approximately two thirds of infants exhibit the onset before 48 hours of life; onset in the first hours of life is not unusual, and abnormal fetal movements suggestive of myoclonus or hiccups have been observed.[72,110,115-120] Seizures occur on the first postnatal day in approximately 15%, by day 3 in nearly 50%, and by day 30 in approximately 70% of patients.[112] Hiccups are a particularly helpful and frequent clinical sign. A mother of one of the affected newborns volunteered before the diagnosis was suspected that she felt that her fetus experienced frequent

TABLE 27.6	Common Features of Nonketotic Hyperglycinemia (Glycine Encephalopathy)

Clinical features
    Seizures
    Stupor, coma
    Myoclonus
    Hiccups
    Ventilatory failure
Metabolic features
    Hyperglycinemia (hyperglycinuria)
Neuropathological features
    Myelin disturbance
    Neuronal excitotoxicity

hiccups. It is important to specifically ask the mother about such fetal movement. As with maple syrup urine disease, interesting and useful neurological signs include a variety of ophthalmoplegias, which may be fluctuating in character. Of particular importance is the need for mechanical ventilation in approximately two thirds of patients. Rapid evolution of intractable seizures, stimulus-sensitive myoclonus, and coma is common.

The *neonatal EEG* is abnormal in at least 90% of infants. The most common finding is the burst-suppression pattern, and nonketotic hyperglycinemia is the most common metabolic cause of the syndrome of early myoclonic encephalopathy (myoclonic seizures, burst-suppression EEG; see Chapter 12). Brain stem auditory evoked responses are characterized by delayed brain stem conduction times (e.g., wave I to V latency).[107,121]

Brain imaging is notable in the neonatal period for the relatively frequent findings of agenesis or hypoplasia of the corpus callosum and abnormalities of cerebral white matter, with subsequent evidence for hypomyelination and to a lesser extent, cerebral cortical atrophy. The CT scan may demonstrate decreased attenuation of the cerebral white matter (Fig. 27.7A) and partial or complete agenesis of the corpus callosum.[122-125] MRI is superior to CT in demonstrating these features (see Figs. 27.7B and 27.8) and is the recommended neuroimaging modality. Thus, decreased attenuation of cerebral white matter may be observed, but, more strikingly, on diffusion-weighted MRI, one sees increased signal (decreased diffusion) in dorsal brain stem, cerebral peduncles, and posterior limbs of the internal capsule (see Fig. 27.8).[43,126-129] These features are consistent with the vacuolating myelinopathy observed at neuropathological examination (see later), as is also seen with maple syrup urine disease (see earlier). The abnormalities of

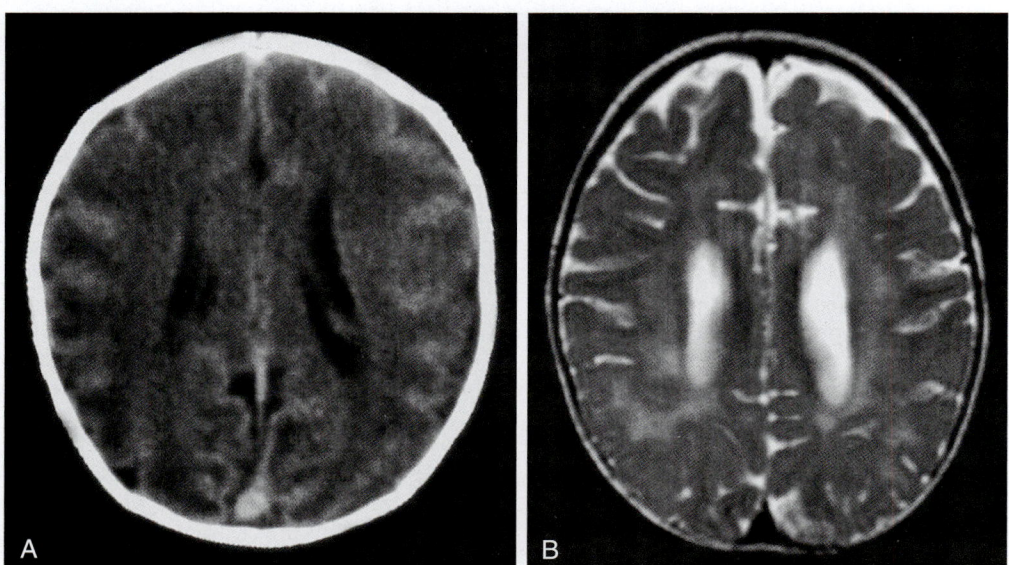

Figure 27.7 Computed tomography (CT) and magnetic resonance imaging (MRI) features of nonketotic hyperglycinemia. (A) CT scan obtained at 4 days of age in an affected infant with refractory seizures. Note the marked and diffuse decrease in attenuation in cerebral white matter. (B) T2-weighted MRI scan obtained at 2 years of age, when the child exhibited severe seizures and mental retardation. Note the increased signal in cerebral white matter, the enlarged ventricles, and the marked paucity of myelin. Atrophy of cerebral cortex is manifested by enlarged subarachnoid spaces.

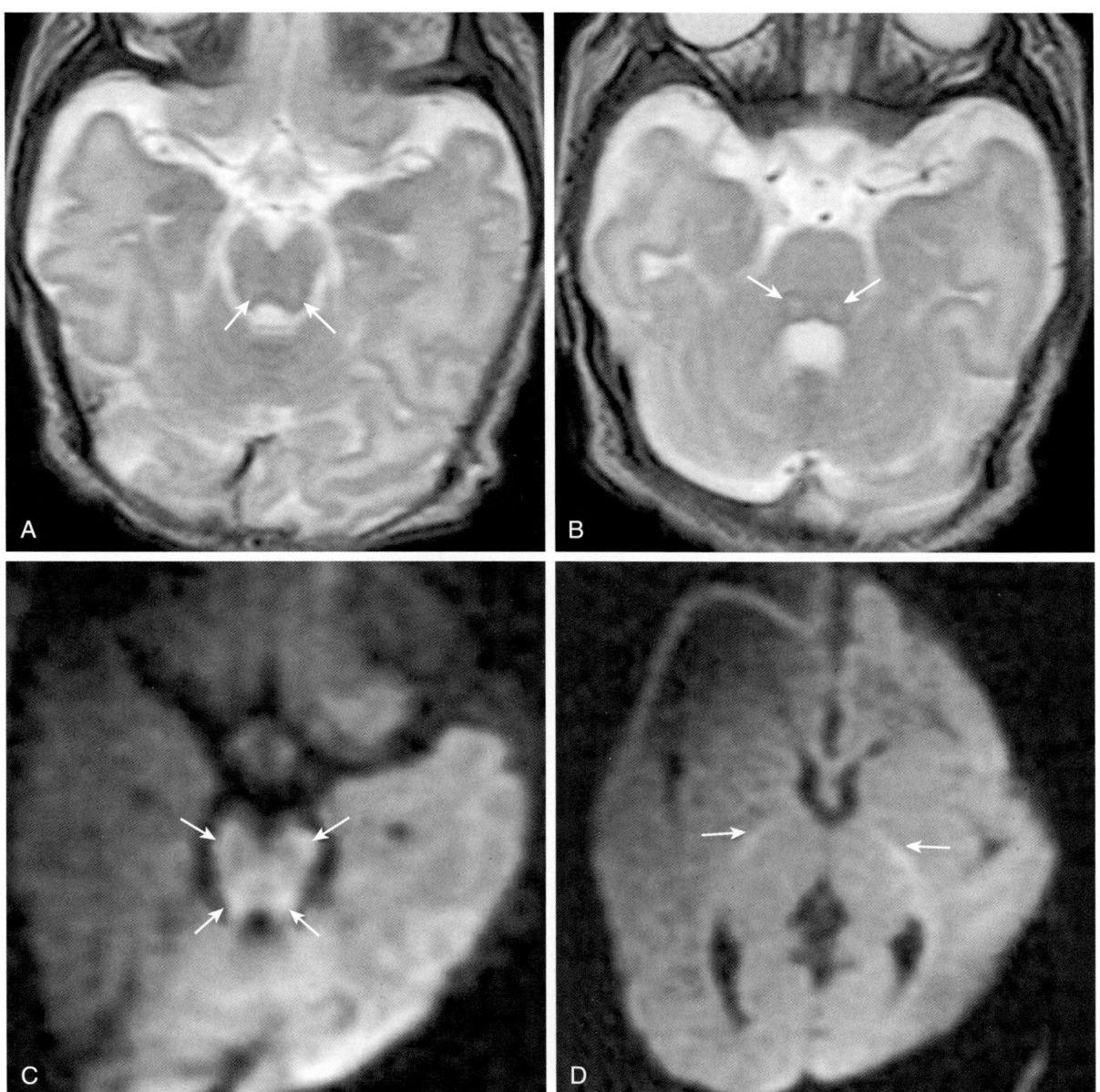

Figure 27.8 Nonketotic hyperglycinemia, conventional and diffusion-weighted (DWI) magnetic resonance imaging (MRI). The infant was 15 days old and had nonketotic hyperglycinemia. Note in A and B T2-weighted MRI scans, hyperintense lesions in the dorsal midbrain and pons (*arrows*). DWI of the middle-to-upper brain stem, C shows more conspicuous and additional hyperintense (restricted diffusion) lesions (*arrows*). DWI at the level of the cerebral hemispheres, D shows prominent hyperintensity in the posterior limbs of the internal capsules (*arrows*). (From Khong PL, Tse C, Wong IY, Lam BC, et al. Diffusion-weighted imaging and proton magnetic resonance spectroscopy in perinatal hypoxic-ischemic encephalopathy: association with neuromotor outcome at 18 months of age. *J Child Neurol.* 2004;19:872–881.)

corpus callosum are best visualized in vivo by MRI and occur in nearly 50% of newborns with severe disease.[a] Progression of findings to abnormal signal and then atrophy of cerebral white matter and, to a lesser extent, cerebral cortex is common.[108,129,130] MR spectroscopy shows a striking increase in brain glycine levels, consistent with the locus of the enzymatic defect (see earlier) (Fig. 27.9).[38,128,130,133,134] In conventional short-echo spectra, glycine cannot be distinguished from the normal

myoinositol peak; with long-echo spectra, the elevation of glycine is seen clearly (see Fig. 27.9).[133]

A syndrome of *transient neonatal nonketotic hyperglycinemia,* which clinically can be indistinguishable from the better-known classic neonatal form first described, has been elucidated.[72,95,135-140] The clinical presentation has been characterized by onset of seizures in the first days of life with hypotonia and depressed level of consciousness; one infant exhibited coma and respiratory failure. All infants survived, and six of eight were normal neurologically on follow-up. The diagnosis was made by the

[a]References 38, 92, 108, 125, 128, and 130.

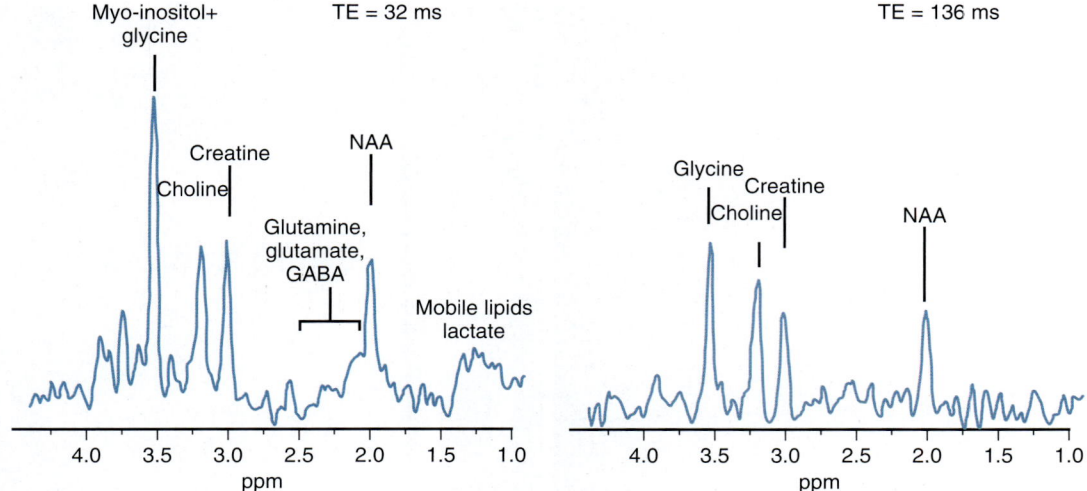

Figure 27.9 Nonketotic hyperglycinemia, magnetic resonance (MR) spectroscopy. On postnatal day 7, proton MR spectroscopy from parieto-occipital white matter of an infant with nonketotic hyperglycinemia shows the high intensity of glycine at 3.55 ppm. With conventional short echo times (TE = 32 ms) glycine and myoinositol cannot be separated, whereas with long echo times (TE = 136 ms), the elevation of glycine is readily distinguished. *GABA*, Gamma-aminobutyric acid; *NAA*, N-acetylaspartate. (From Huisman TA, Thiel T, Steinmann B, Zeilinger G, et al. Proton magnetic resonance spectroscopy of the brain of a neonate with nonketotic hyperglycinemia: in vivo–in vitro (ex vivo) correlation. *Eur Radiol.* 2002;12:858–861.)

finding of increased concentrations of glycine in the CSF, urine, and plasma, with the most consistent elevation in the CSF. The metabolic abnormalities disappeared within 2 to 8 weeks. A transient defect in the glycine cleavage enzyme is presumed but has not been documented. The existence of this syndrome with a markedly better outcome than that associated with the more typical persistent form raises difficult ethical issues in the management of classic nonketotic hyperglycinemia. In the latter disorder, cessation of life support is often considered in the severely ill infant early in the clinical course because of the very poor prognosis despite the typical occurrence of recovery of ventilatory function later in the neonatal period.

Clinical distinction of transient nonketotic hyperglycinemia from *atypical variants of nonketotic hyperglycinemia* is also difficult.[141-144] These infants present clinically like those with classic nonketotic hyperglycinemia, and the outcome has ranged from normal neurological status to death early in infancy. The distinction of this milder variant from transient neonatal nonketotic hyperglycinemia is based on resolution of the metabolic defects in the latter but not fully in the former. Moreover, the milder forms have been shown to be associated with considerable (20% to 30%) residual glycine cleavage enzyme activity. Decisive distinction from true transient disease requires determination of molecular genetic analysis of the glycine cleavage system.

The *outcome* of the severe neonatal form of nonketotic hyperglycinemia has been generally poor.[72,92] Overall approximately 30% to 35% of infants die, often in the neonatal period, and most survivors have serious neurological disturbances, including severe developmental failure, recurrent seizures, and severe abnormalities (e.g., hypsarrhythmia) on the EEG. In one recent series only 25% of infants evaluated at 15 months were able to smile, 4%, to sit alone, and none to babble or speak words.[112,114] Infants who present in the neonatal period or very early infancy, generally without severe signs at

TABLE 27.7	Outcome of Neonatal Nonketotic Hyperglycinemia: Notable Gender Differences[a]

Mortality
  Neonatal mortality: 12% overall, *0% in male patients*, 28% in female patients
  Median age of death: *2–6 years in male patients,* <1 month in female patients
  Overall mortality (neonatal and later): 34% (similar for male and female patients)
Outcome (survivors ≥3 years)
  "Walk and say/sign words": 40% overall, *71% of male patients,* 0% of female patients
  Severe deficits: 60% overall, *29% of male patients, 100% of female patients*

[a]Starting population: n = 65; 36 males and 29 females.
Data from Hoover-Fong JE, Shah S, Van Hove JL, Applegarth D, et al. Natural history of nonketotic hyperglycinemia in 65 patients, *Neurology.* 2004;63: 1847–1853.

onset, have a less dire outcome but do exhibit notable gender differences in outcome (Table 27.7). Thus, in one series of 65 infants, although overall 12% died in the neonatal period, the gender-specific mortality rates were 28% for female patients and 0% for male patients. Indeed overall median age at death was 2.6 years for male patients versus less than 1 month for female patients. The male advantage was noted also for outcome in survivors. Of survivors 3 years or older, although severe deficits occurred overall in 60%, gender-specific rates of poor outcome were 100% for female patients and 29% for male patients. Of the original 65 infants, 10 infants (15%) could walk and say or sign words, and these were all male. None

TABLE 27.8   Nonketotic Versus Ketotic Hyperglycinemia

	NONKETOTIC	KETOTIC
Severe neonatal illness	+	+
Seizures	+	+
Hiccups	+	–
Ketoacidosis	–	+
Neutropenia-thrombocytopenia	–	+
Primary defect in glycine metabolism	+	–
Dietary therapy effective	–	+

+, Present; –, absent.

of these 10 were neurologically normal, however. In a recent mixed series of 124 cases of nonketotic hyperglycinemia with onset in the neonatal period and early infancy, *the best predictors of poor outcome* were CSF glycine level greater than 230 μM, markedly elevated CSF/plasma glycine ratio (median 0.22), and genetic mutations expected to allow no residual activity.[92] Therapeutic intervention may modify the unfavorable outcome in nonketotic hyperglycinemia (see later).

Distinction From Ketotic Hyperglycinemia

It is important to distinguish nonketotic hyperglycinemia from ketotic hyperglycinemia, particularly in view of the observation that not all patients with ketotic hyperglycinemia exhibit consistent ketosis.[71,145] Early therapeutic intervention may be particularly beneficial in ketotic hyperglycinemia. Although this is not yet clearly the case with severe nonketotic hyperglycinemia, some observations raise the hope that specific therapy will become available (see later). Features helpful in the distinction of nonketotic and ketotic hyperglycinemia are included in Table 27.8.

Genetics

Genetic data indicate autosomal recessive inheritance.[72,79] Thus familial occurrence, parental consanguinity, and intermediate molecular defects in heterozygotes have been recorded. More recent data show extensive intragenic molecular heterogeneity in classic NKH, including 78 novel mutations in *GLDC* and 18 novel mutations in *AMT*.[92] In particular, nonsense mutations, frameshift mutations, exonic deletions, and duplications, which result in no residual activity, were more frequent in patients with severe neurodevelopmental outcomes than in those with attenuated outcomes.[92]

Metabolic Features

The major biochemical correlate of nonketotic hyperglycinemia is marked accumulation of glycine in blood, urine, and CSF.[72,106,146] Particularly characteristic is the accumulation of glycine in the CSF. Values generally range between 85 and 280 μmol/L, with control subjects generally having values less than 10 μmol/L.[a] In a recent large series, the median value among severely affected newborns was 213.[92] The ratio of the concentration of glycine in CSF to that in plasma, an important diagnostic measure, generally ranges from 0.09 to 0.25 μmol/L, with control values approximately 0.02 μmol/L.[71,72] The median ratio in a recent large series in severely affected newborns was 0.22.[92] This pronounced elevation of CSF glycine level is not observed in other varieties of hyperglycinemia[84,85] and presumably relates to the presence of the enzymatic defect in brain in the patients with nonketotic hyperglycinemia. As noted earlier, a distinct correlation exists between the degree of elevation of the ratio of CSF glycine to plasma glycine and the severity of the clinical phenotype. The defect in the glycine cleavage reaction (see Fig. 27.6) in brain, liver, and probably other tissues adequately explains the accumulation of glycine in all body fluids. As noted earlier, elevated levels of glycine in the brain of living infants with the disease have been demonstrated by MR spectroscopy.

Neuropathology

Neuropathological findings from studies of more than 20 infants have been described.[a] The dominant abnormality has involved myelin, and the nature of the disturbance is similar to that noted for ketotic hyperglycinemia, maple syrup urine disease, and various other aminoacidopathies.[72,97] The essential features are vacuolation of and diminution in myelin (Fig. 27.10). No striking involvement of neurons or sign of myelin breakdown is noted. Vacuolation is more common in younger patients, and myelin diminution is more common in older patients, findings suggesting that myelin formation is deranged and that the early sign of this derangement is vacuolation. Ultrastructural studies support the notion of origin of the vacuoles from newly formed myelin sheaths (Fig. 27.11).[100,107,150] Involvement is greatest in those systems that myelinate around the time of birth. A prenatal onset of the process is supported by the frequent finding of partial or total agenesis of the corpus callosum (see earlier discussion). MRIs have also shown abnormalities of gyral development in occasional cases.[38,128] Whether such abnormalities could be related to the expression during development of the glycine cleavage system in radial glial cells (see earlier) is an intriguing possibility. More detailed MRI studies will be of interest.

Neuronal injury in cerebrum has not been described consistently at autopsy. The possibility of excitotoxic neuronal injury initiated at the NMDA receptor (see earlier discussion) has not been defined clearly, although this occurrence seems likely. As noted earlier, apparent cerebral cortical atrophy is a common feature on brain imaging studies in infants who survive beyond the neonatal period.

Management
Prevention

Demonstration of very low or no activity of the glycine cleavage system in biopsy samples of chorionic villus has allowed diagnosis in the first trimester.[72,79,87,90] On the basis of such prenatal identification, prevention by therapeutic abortion has been carried out.

Early Detection

Early detection is important because institution of therapy in the neonatal period provides the best opportunity to ameliorate,

---

[a]References 71, 72, 79, 85, 94, and 147.

[a]References 71-73, 94, 97, 100, 102, 107, and 147-153.

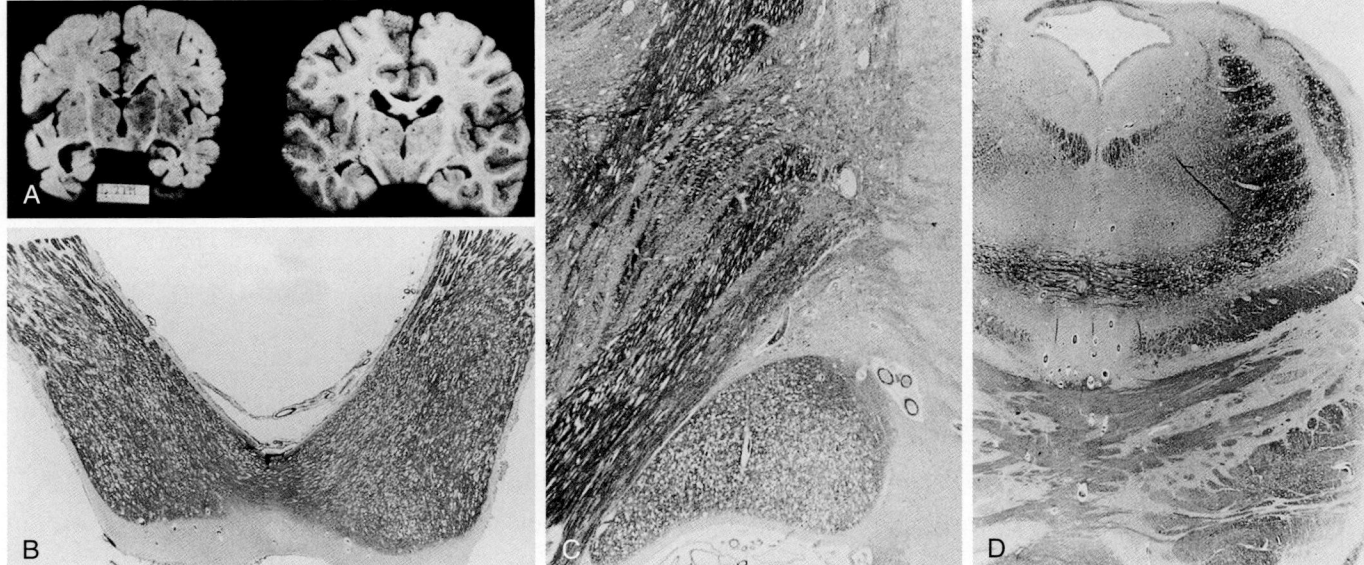

Figure 27.10 Myelin disturbance in nonketotic hyperglycinemia. These sections were obtained from a 24-month-old infant who exhibited lethargy and poor feeding from the first day of life, onset of seizures in the second week, and subsequent failure of neurological development. (A) Coronal section of cerebrum from the patient (*left*) and from an age-matched control (*right*). Note the differences in bulk of cerebral white matter, corpus callosum, and internal capsules. (B) Optic nerves and chiasm; note the vacuolated myelin. (C) Coronal section of the internal capsule. Note vacuolation in the fibers of the capsule (upper portion of the figure) and also of the optic tract (lower portion of the figure). (D) Horizontal section of the midbrain. Note vacuolation of the medial longitudinal fasciculus, the superior cerebellar peduncle, and the lateral lemniscus. (From Shuman RM, Leech RW, Scott CR. The neuropathology of the nonketotic and ketotic hyperglycinemias: three cases. *Neurology.* 1978;28:139–146.)

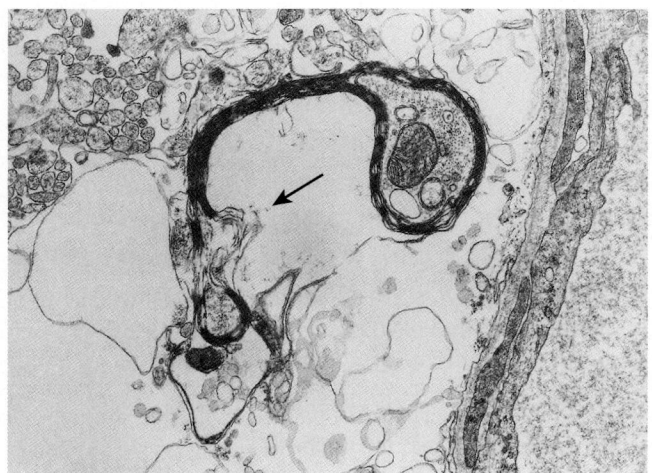

Figure 27.11 Myelin vacuolation in nonketotic hyperglycinemia. This electron micrograph of the pontine tegmentum demonstrates that the microvacuolation is splitting the myelin lamellae (*arrow*). (Epon-embedded lead citrate and uranyl acetate–stained ultrathin section, ×20,650.) (From Scher MS, Bergman I, Ahdab-Barmada M, Fria T. Neurophysiological and anatomical correlations in neonatal nonketotic hyperglycinemia. *Neuropediatrics.* 1986;17:137–143.)

albeit only partially, the very unfavorable neurological outcome (see later discussion). A serious ethical issue arises with the severely affected infant who requires ventilatory support. With the unfavorable prognosis characteristic of this disease, the decision to discontinue life support frequently arises. Because the severe respiratory failure often resolves later in the neonatal

period (see earlier discussion), the continuation of early life support may result in the recovery of ventilatory function but a very poor neurological outcome. With the recognition of *transient* nonketotic hyperglycinemia, however, the decision to discontinue ventilatory support early in the neonatal period in infants with nonketotic hyperglycinemia is especially difficult. Moreover, recent therapeutic attempts provide some reason for hope in this disorder (see next section).

Therapeutic Attempts

The three fundamental aims of therapy in this disorder are to (1) lower tissue glycine levels, (2) treat seizures, and (3) ameliorate excitotoxicity at the NMDA receptor. The available interventions have attained these aims with reasonable success for the first, with moderate success for the second, and with limited success for the third.

Sodium Benzoate. Sodium benzoate has been used to lower glycine in *blood* because an amide bond between glycine and benzoate is formed and the resulting hippuric acid is excreted. The plasma glycine levels are reduced to near normal but, unfortunately, *CSF* glycine levels are often not similarly affected.[a] However, with doses as high as 750 mg/kg per day, a substantial decline in CSF glycine levels has been effected and a decrease in seizures reported.[71,72] Moreover, with doses nearly as high, a decrease in brain (as well as CSF) glycine levels has been shown by MR spectroscopy.[157] High-dose benzoate therapy may result

---

[a]References 71, 72, 94, 119, and 154-156.

in carnitine deficiency, and carnitine supplementation may be necessary. Unfortunately, however, thus far no beneficial effect on cognitive development has been reported with benzoate therapy.

Strychnine. The initial therapeutic approach directed at the effects of glycine in the central nervous system was the use of strychnine.[a] The rationale for administration of this drug is its role as a specific antagonist of the inhibitory glycine receptor at the postsynaptic membrane.[159,160] In general, severely affected neonatal patients have not had apparent benefit, despite onset of therapy from the first hours or days of life.[103,121,153] Nevertheless, some apneic infants have responded to strychnine sufficiently to allow extubation.[114] The principal reason for the lack of major benefit from strychnine presumably relates to the finding that the drug has no effect on glycine's allosteric activation of the NMDA receptor and thereby excitotoxicity.

Benzodiazepines. A class of agents that acts principally by enhancing GABA receptor inhibitory function, the benzodiazepines, has been used in infants with nonketotic hyperglycinemia.[71,118,161] A beneficial response on seizure frequency, often at relatively high doses, has been observed in some patients. However, antiepileptic effects have been inconstant, and no beneficial effect on neurological development has been observed. The latter failure probably relates in part to a lack of effect of benzodiazepines at the NMDA receptor and the concept that GABA_A receptors in the newborn may be largely excitatory (see Chapter 12).

Excitatory Amino Acid Antagonists. A theoretically promising therapy in nonketotic hyperglycinemia involves agents that are excitatory amino acid antagonists.[b] In general, the most commonly used agents have been dextromethorphan or ketamine in combination with sodium benzoate.[165] A beneficial effect on seizures has been documented. However, amelioration of cognitive deficits has generally not been achieved. Further improvements in development of NMDA antagonists, with specific action at the glycine site on the NMDA receptor, may lead to more favorable effects on outcome. A recent report of three infants with neonatal nonketotic hyperglycinemia and early myoclonic encephalopathy with poor seizure control using standard pharmacological therapy (dextromethorphan and sodium benzoate) describes a dramatic reduction of seizures and improved quality of life when treatment with a ketogenic diet was instituted.[166] *Antenatal therapy* with an effective excitatory amino acid antagonist may be necessary for optimal benefit. The findings of hypoplastic corpus callosum, elevated levels of CSF glycine at *birth,* the absence of glycine cleavage activity in *fetal brain,* and the occurrence of severe neurological signs in the first hour of life all support this contention (see earlier).

Conclusions. The data just reviewed are disappointing concerning effective therapy of nonketotic hyperglycinemia. Use of sodium benzoate and an NMDA antagonist theoretically is the best current combination. Additional anticonvulsant

therapy may be required. Nevertheless, it does not appear that this approach, even if improved with newer agents, will correct all the deficits in this disorder. The reasons for this prediction relate to several factors. First, it is likely that brain injury, maldevelopment, or both occur in utero because of the locus of the enzymatic defect in brain (i.e., a locus unavailable to the benefits of placental function). Second, the role of the disturbance of myelination in the genesis of the intellectual failure and some of the other neurological disturbances in nonketotic hyperglycinemia presumably is largely separate from the neurotransmitter effects of glycine.

HYPERAMMONEMIA

Hyperammonemia in the neonatal period may result in serious derangements of neurological function and structure. The Krebs-Henseleit urea cycle is the major pathway of ammonia elimination in mammals; thus defects in the enzymes catalyzing the five steps of this pathway are important causes of hyperammonemia. Neonatal hyperammonemia results from defects of the first four of these five steps. Elevations of blood ammonia levels occur in certain other inborn errors of metabolism and have also been demonstrated in a significant proportion of premature and asphyxiated infants (Table 27.9). In the last two instances, the hyperammonemia is not secondary to an inborn error of ammonia metabolism. (Not listed in Table 27.9 is hyperammonemia with hepatic failure or with total parenteral nutrition, because the severity of the hyperammonemia is rarely marked and clinical phenomena referable to the hyperammonemia are most unusual in these settings.) In the following discussion, the normal aspects of ammonia metabolism, the biochemical aspects of disordered metabolism, and the principal clinical syndromes associated with neonatal hyperammonemia are reviewed. Emphasis is placed not only on the deficits in the urea cycle enzymes but also on the disturbance observed in premature infants. Hyperammonemia associated with perinatal asphyxia is discussed in Chapter 20.

TABLE 27.9   Major Causes of Hyperammonemia in the Neonatal Period

Urea cycle defects
  Carbamyl phosphate synthetase
  Ornithine transcarbamylase
  Argininosuccinic acid synthetase
  Argininosuccinase
Organic acid disorders
  Propionic acidemia
  Methylmalonic acidemia
  Isovaleric acidemia
  Beta-ketothiolase deficiency
  Pyruvate dehydrogenase deficiency
  Mitochondrial (electron transport) disorders
  Glutaric aciduria type II
  Multiple carboxylase deficiency
  Fatty acid oxidation defect
Lysine protein intolerance
Hyperornithinemia, hyperammonemia, and homocitrullinemia
Transient hyperammonemia of prematurity
Perinatal asphyxia

[a]References 101, 103, 104, 121, 153, and 158.
[b]References 72, 79, 91, 95, 114-116, 118-120, 156, and 162-165.

Normal Metabolic Aspects

Major Sources and Fates of Ammonia

The major sources of ammonia in mammals are amino acids and purine nucleotides (amino groups of adenine, guanine, and their derivatives).[145] Although small amounts of ammonia are used for the synthesis of certain amino acids (primarily by transamination) and pyrimidines, the principal fate of ammonia is biosynthesis of urea through the urea cycle for waste nitrogen disposal (Fig. 27.12).

Urea Cycle

The urea cycle consists of five steps, the first two of which are catalyzed by the mitochondrial enzymes carbamyl phosphate synthetase and ornithine transcarbamylase and the latter three of which are catalyzed by the cytosolic enzymes argininosuccinic acid synthetase, argininosuccinase, and arginase (see Fig. 27.12).[145,166,167] An important obligatory positive effector of carbamyl phosphate synthetase is *N*-acetylglutamate, which is synthesized in the mitochondrion from acetyl-coenzyme A and glutamate. The liver is the only organ that is quantitatively important in urea synthesis.[145,168] In human neonatal brain, only argininosuccinic acid synthetase is present in significant

quantities (i.e., 155% of the hepatic activity), whereas activities of carbamyl phosphate synthetase, ornithine transcarbamylase, argininosuccinase, and arginase are present in relatively small quantities (3%, 0.2%, 14%, and 2% of the respective hepatic activities).[166,169]

Ammonia Disposal in Brain

Ammonia is formed constantly in brain and, indeed, ammonia concentrations in brain in adult animals are 60% to 100% higher than in blood.[170-172] Ammonia in brain is eliminated by diffusion and by conversion to glutamate and, particularly, to glutamine (see Fig. 27.10). Glutamine also may diffuse from brain. At least one mode of glutamine transport from brain involves a transporter shared with tryptophan, so glutamine efflux from brain is accompanied by tryptophan influx into brain (see later discussion).[166,173]

Biochemical Aspects of Disordered Metabolism

Enzymatic Defects and Essential Consequences

Of the major causes of hyperammonemia in the perinatal period (see Table 27.9), those studied in most detail involve the enzymes catalyzing the reactions of the urea cycle. These disorders affect the hepatic enzymes and, to a variable extent, the enzymes in

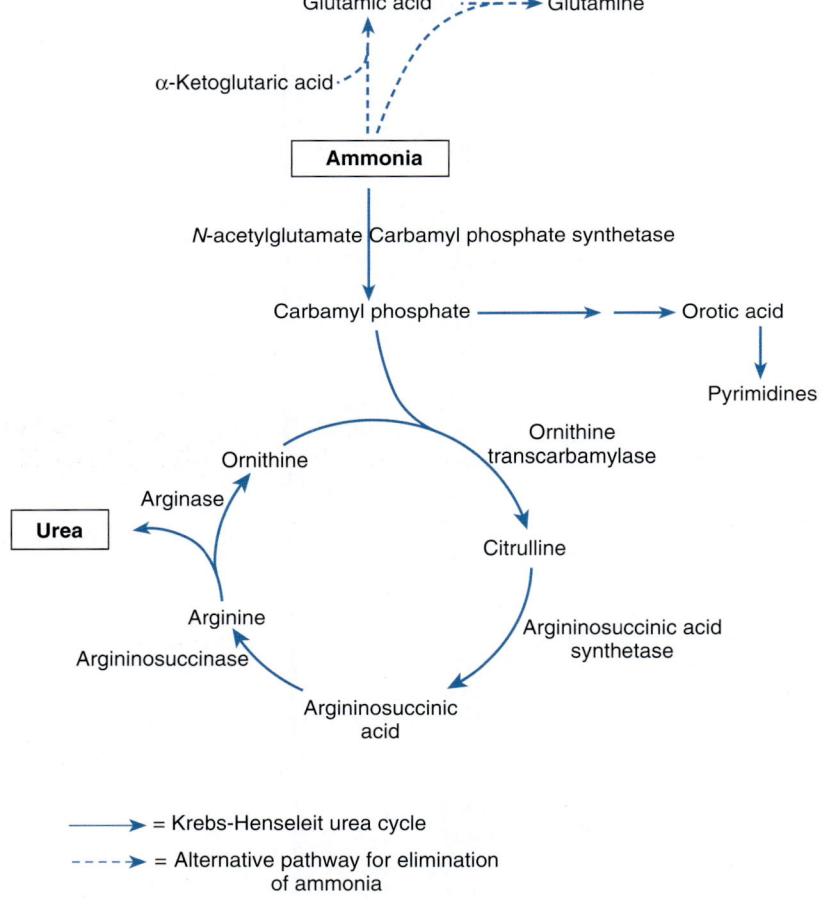

Figure 27.12 Major aspects of ammonia metabolism, particularly in liver. See text for details. The upper portion, depicted by dotted arrows, indicates ammonia metabolism in brain, that is, utilization of two molecules of ammonia for the sequential transamination of alpha-ketoglutarate to form glutamic acid and of the latter, by glutamine synthetase, to form glutamine.

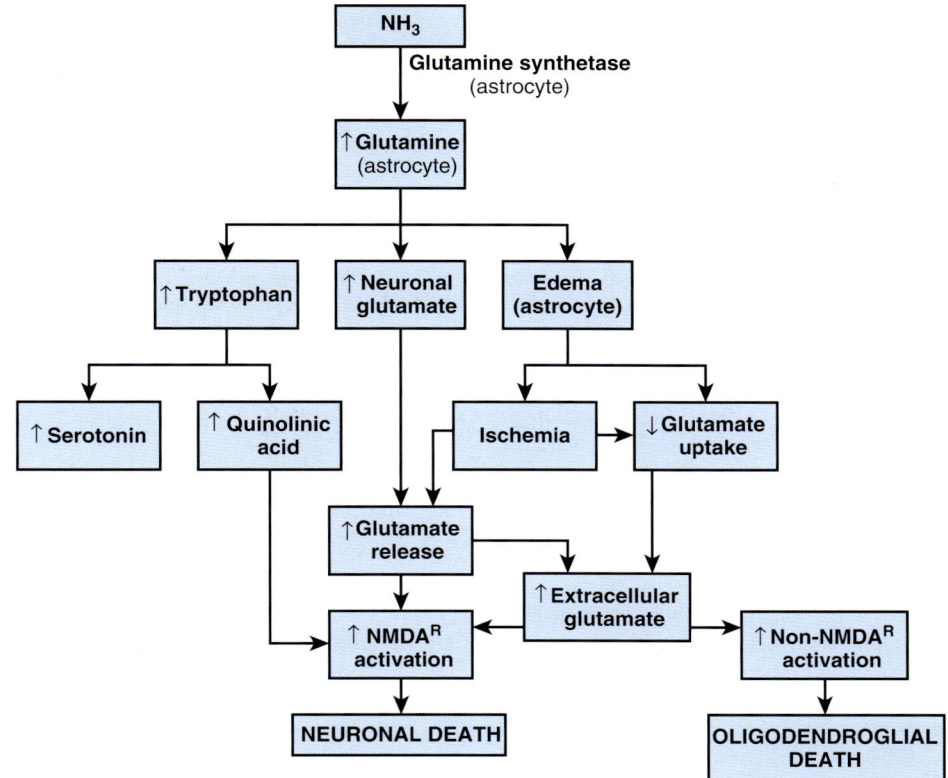

Figure 27.13 Principal mechanisms by which ammonia (NH₃) is toxic to developing brain. *NMDA^R*, Receptor for *N*-methyl-ᴅ-aspartate. See text for details.

other tissues. Hyperammonemia is a prominent consequence and, depending on the site of the enzymatic block, so are aberrations of amino acids in blood or urine. The causes for the striking disturbances in function and structure of the central nervous system observed with these hyperammonemic states are not entirely understood. Mechanisms that are supported by some experimental and clinical evidence are displayed in Fig. 27.13 and discussed in the next sections.

Biochemical Effects of Excessive Ammonia

Ammonia may have a variety of toxic effects on brain (see Fig. 27.13). These effects involve several neurotransmitter molecules and thereby result in major perturbations of neural function.[173-176] Moreover, because such excitatory neurotransmitter molecules as glutamate and quinolinic acid can lead to neuronal and perhaps oligodendroglial death, these effects result in serious structural lesions as well.

The metabolism of ammonia to glutamine appears to be of particular importance in the acute toxicity of hyperammonemia (see Fig. 27.13).[a] Thus, with hyperammonemia, the brain glutamine level increases because of glutamine synthesis from glutamate through the glutamine synthetase reaction with ammonia (see Figs. 27.12 and 27.13). In one animal model, when glutamine synthesis is blocked by inhibition of the synthetase, hyperammonemia is no longer toxic.[179] Marked increases in brain glutamine levels were documented by MR spectroscopy during acute hyperammonemia in several infants

with ornithine transcarbamylase deficiency.[38,182,185] Moreover, a newborn with arginase deficiency and only a slightly elevated blood ammonia level but a markedly elevated CSF glutamine level was severely symptomatic (including coma) and died.[186] The functional effects of increased brain glutamine may be marked. A major functional effect, induction of stupor or coma, is a well-documented result of elevated brain glutamine.

Of still greater importance are the *likely structural consequences* of increased glutamine synthesis (see Fig. 27.13). Perhaps most critically, increased glutamine efflux from brain is accompanied by increased tryptophan influx, because these two amino acids share a common transporter.[167,174,175] This increased tryptophan is metabolized to *serotonin* and to *quinolinic acid.* Serotonin may contribute to the genesis of the stupor and coma. Quinolinic acid is a neurotoxin that activates the NMDA type of glutamate receptor to lead to excitotoxic neuronal death. Batshaw and co-workers[174,187] documented 2-fold to 10-fold elevations of quinolinic acid in newborns with hyperammonemic coma.[174,187] Moreover, the peak toxicity of quinolinic acid in developing rat brain has been shown to occur at 7 postnatal days, a maturational age comparable with that of the human newborn infant.[188] Quinolinic acid administered to late gestation fetal sheep resulted in widespread lipid peroxidation in brain;[189] this result could relate in part to NMDA excitotoxicity, calcium influx, and the generation of reactive oxygen species (see Chapter 13). Related additional deleterious effects of increased brain glutamine include an increase in neuronal levels of glutamate because of the action of the astrocytic-neuronal glutamine-glutamate cycle, in which glutamine diffuses from astrocytes to neurons and is converted

ᵃReferences 146, 167, 168, 174, 175, and 177-184.

to glutamate. The elevated neuronal glutamate then leads to increased glutamate release and the potential for excitotoxic neuronal death (see Fig. 27.13). Another related deleterious effect of the elevated glutamine levels in astrocytes is the induction of astrocytic swelling (see Fig. 27.13) and thereby impaired microcirculatory blood flow with resulting ischemia. This would lead to excitotoxic neuronal death because of excessive glutamate release and decreased glutamate uptake, as described in Chapter 13 regarding ischemia. Reports of a sharp decline in mortality and in ATP depletion resulting from acute ammonia toxicity by administration of MK-801 before the infusion of ammonium acetate in animal models support the possibility of excitotoxicity mediated by NMDA receptors.[174,175,190,191] Thus neuronal injury in hyperammonemia may relate to excitotoxic effects at the NMDA receptor provoked by quinolinic acid and by glutamate. In view of the receptor-mediated toxicity of glutamate to oligodendroglia (see Chapter 13), glutamate-induced injury also may be relevant to the deficit in oligodendroglia (see Fig. 27.13) and myelin observed in hyperammonemic brain injury (see the section on neuropathology, later).

A disturbance in energy metabolism may help initiate some of the excitotoxic effects just described and may be important in contributing to additional later effects of hyperammonemia. Thus, with prolonged hyperammonemia, an *impairment in brain energy* reserves becomes apparent, especially in brain stem and cerebellum.[171,173,191-193] The cause of the disturbance in brain energy production is unknown. A disturbance in pyruvate utilization (see earlier discussion) may be important in this context and may account in part for the small increases in brain lactate documented in animal models and on proton MR spectroscopy in some affected infants.[38,173,194,195] Of additional importance is an apparent *disturbance in transport of reducing equivalents (reduced nicotinamide adenine dinucleotide [NADH] from cytosol to mitochondria).*[173] This disturbance could result in a deficit of NADH for the mitochondrial electron transport chain, inhibit oxidative energy coupling, and lead to a fall in ATP levels.[173] Moreover, in one animal model of hyperammonemia, the NMDA antagonist MK-801 blocked the decline in ATP levels, a finding thereby suggesting that the energy impairment was *caused* by the excitotoxic effects.[191] Nevertheless, only very marked hyperammonemia, prolonged hyperammonemia, or both, will cause appreciable changes in brain energy levels.[195,196] *On balance, therefore, the deleterious effects on neurotransmitter molecules just discussed seem more crucial than do primary alterations in energy metabolism in the genesis of the functional and structural effects of hyperammonemia.*

Urea Cycle Defects

The best-documented causes of severe neonatal hyperammonemia are deficiencies in the urea cycle enzymes. The overall incidence of these disorders is approximately 1 in 30,000 live births.[167,197,198] Although certain differences in clinical and metabolic features occur, the neonatal forms of these defects of the urea cycle exhibit distinct similarities in clinical, metabolic, and neuropathological features (Table 27.10). The *clinical syndrome* consists almost invariably of onset most commonly between 24 and 72 hours of life, poor feeding (sometimes with vomiting), disturbed level of consciousness (i.e., stupor or coma), hyperventilation, and seizures. Highly distinctive is tachypnea (and occasionally respiratory alkalosis),

TABLE 27.10   Common Features of Neonatal Hyperammonemic States
Clinical features
Vomiting, poor feeding
Stupor, coma
Hyperventilation
Seizures
Metabolic features
Marked hyperammonemia
Aminoacidemia (aminoaciduria)
Respiratory alkalosis
Neuropathological features
Acute
Brain swelling
Alzheimer type II astrocytes
Variable neuronal injury
Spongy change in white matter
Chronic
Neuronal loss
Myelin deficiency

presumably a central effect of hyperammonemia and reminiscent of the central hyperventilation noted in hepatic coma.[199,200] This finding may lead to suspicion of respiratory illness. In one large series of newborn male infants with ornithine transcarbamylase deficiency ($n = 74$), at the time of onset of symptoms at approximately 60 hours of age, mean pH was 7.5 and mean carbon dioxide pressure was 24 mm Hg.[201] Hyperammonemia in the neonatal disorders is marked, the course is fulminating, and mortality is high. Approximately 70% die, and at least 60% to 80% of survivors are mentally retarded despite neonatal diagnosis and intervention.[146,177,201-206] Infants treated from birth (detected because of affected siblings) and *before development of hyperammonemic coma* have had IQs within the low normal range.[177] Neuropathological features have included, acutely, brain swelling, swollen astrocytes with the appearance of Alzheimer type II protoplasmic glia (the hallmark of hyperammonemic encephalopathy),[207-209] variable overt neuronal injury, and mild spongy change in white matter. The chronic neuropathology consists of marked cerebral neuronal loss and myelin deficiency. Management of the affected infants is similar in most respects and is considered separately after discussion of the individual entities. The diagnostic flow chart for neonatal hyperammonemia shown in Fig. 27.14 is cited in the discussion of the separate disorders.

Carbamyl Phosphate Synthetase Deficiency (Congenital Hyperammonemia Type I)

Clinical Features. Carbamyl phosphate synthetase deficiency results in hyperammonemia in the first days of life.[a] The onset has been as early as 24 hours of life and consists principally of vomiting, stupor or coma, and seizures. Infants usually exhibit hypotonia, although hypertonia and opisthotonos have been observed as well. The *respiratory distress* frequently reported may represent the tachypnea of hyperammonemia.

The *clinical course* has been fulminating. Approximately 65% to 75% of reported patients have died, usually in the neonatal

---

[a]References 145, 167, 168, 173, 202, 205, 206, and 210-223.

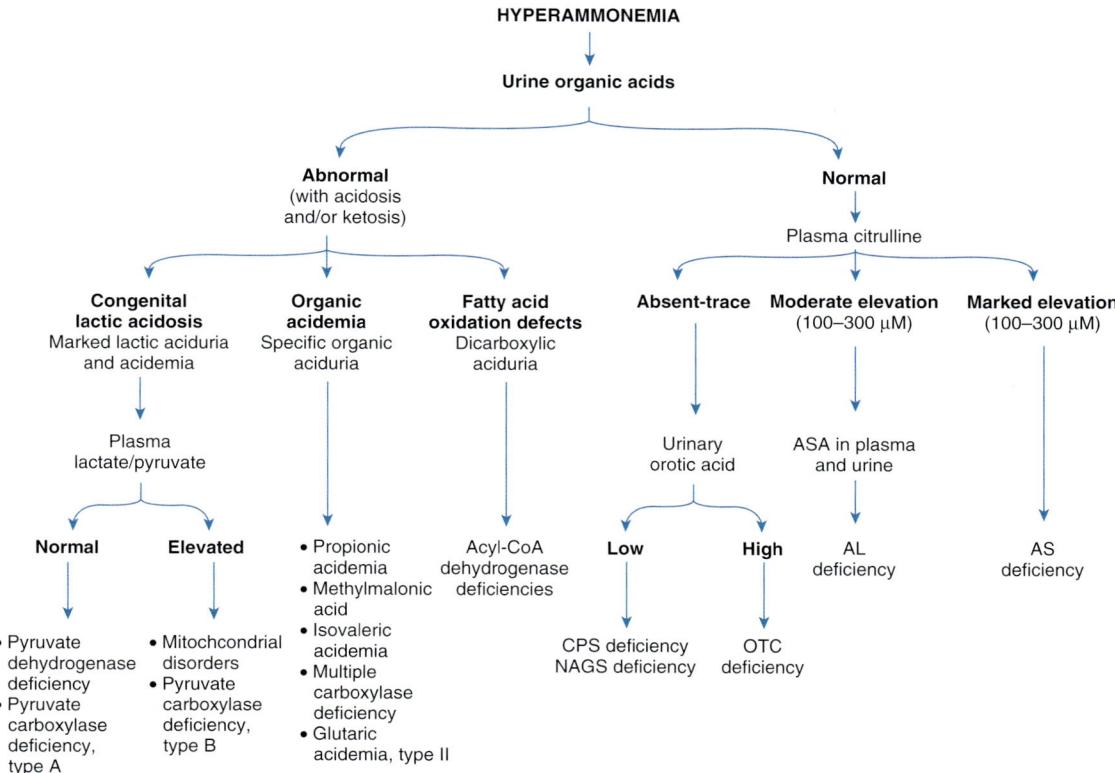

Figure 27.14 Scheme for major diagnostic considerations in hyperammonemia in the newborn. Plasma levels of amino acids and lactate and urinary levels of organic acids and orotic acid are important in the diagnostic scheme. *AL*, Argininosuccinate lyase; *AS*, argininosuccinate synthetase; *ASA*, argininosuccinic acid; *CoA*, coenzyme A; *CPS*, carbamyl phosphate synthetase; *CSF*, cerebrospinal fluid; *NAGS*, N-acetylglutamate synthetase; *OTC*, ornithine transcarbamylase.

period. Of the survivors, only a few have been free of mental retardation on follow-up.[a] Early detection and treatment by dietary and other means are mandatory to preserve significant brain function.

On CT, *brain imaging* has shown findings consistent with severe diffuse cerebral edema. MRI shows particularly bilateral injury to lentiform nuclei (globus pallidus more than putamen), insular and perirolandic cerebral cortex, and subjacent white matter.[38,209,223] The thalamus is relatively spared, a finding helpful in the distinction from hypoxic-ischemic encephalopathy.

The *enzymatic defect* is inherited as an autosomal recessive trait. In several large series of cases of urea cycle disorders with neonatal onset, 10% to 20% had carbamyl phosphate synthetase deficiency.[146,198,203,205,206]

Metabolic Features. Hyperammonemia is moderate to marked in most patients, although levels only two to three times normal have been reported. Other biochemical characteristics include elevated blood glutamine level, absent or trace plasma citrulline level, and normal or diminished urine orotic acid level (see Fig. 27.14). These abnormalities are understandable in view of the pathways of ammonia metabolism (see Fig. 27.12). The occurrence of absent or trace quantities of plasma citrulline is helpful in distinguishing carbamyl phosphate synthetase

deficiency from the more distal deficits of the urea cycle.[146,167] However, citrulline levels may be very low in the first days of life in unaffected infants with very low protein intakes.[167,225] The lack of elevated urinary orotic acid also is useful in distinction from more distal defects (see Fig. 27.14).

Carbamyl phosphate synthetase activity is severely depressed in liver (i.e., none to ≈20% of control values).[146] The enzymatic defect is also detectable in biopsy specimens of duodenal and rectal tissue.[222,226] The deficiency in enzymatic activity is related to a disturbance of enzyme quantity with neither immunoreactive enzyme protein nor mRNA for the enzyme detectable.[227,228] The gene is located on the distal long arm of chromosome 2 (2q35), and mutations have been identified.[146,229,230]

Rare infants with a *defect in synthesis of* N-*acetylglutamate*, the allosteric activator of carbamyl phosphate synthetase, and thereby with deficient activity of the enzyme have been reported.[168,231-236] This disorder at later ages appears to be amenable to treatment with *N*-carbamyl-L-glutamate.[236] The latter substance is a structural analogue of *N*-acetylglutamate that activates carbamyl phosphate synthetase in vitro and is resistant to hepatic degradation.

Neuropathology. Neuropathological data are few.[209,237] The most consistent findings are the presence acutely of swollen astrocytes with the characteristics of Alzheimer type II glia and brain swelling. The findings of brain swelling and swollen astrocytes were reproduced by acute hyperammonemia in the young

---

[a]References 145, 167, 168, 173, 202, 205, 206, and 210-223.

monkey.[238] Neuronal injury can be severe acutely and may reflect excitotoxic injury secondary to hyperammonemia (see earlier discussion). Subsequent brain imaging findings suggest both cortical neuronal and cerebral white matter atrophy.[146,209,213,215,223] Among deep nuclear structures a predilection for putamen and globus pallidus, with relative sparing of thalamus, was noted earlier. The possibility that the oligodendroglial-myelin disturbance also could be related, at least in part, to excitatory amino acids, was discussed earlier.

Ornithine Transcarbamylase Deficiency (Congenital Hyperammonemia Type II)

Clinical Features. Ornithine transcarbamylase deficiency, the most common of the urea cycle defects, results in a severe neonatal syndrome in male infants.[a] The disease in female patients is later in onset and is less severe. However, neonatal onset has been reported in approximately 2% of affected female patients, and approximately 50% of male patients with ornithine transcarbamylase deficiency present after the neonatal period.[203,205,246,250,251] Among neonatal-onset urea cycle disorders, ornithine transcarbamylase deficiency accounts for 55% to 60% of cases.[146,198,204-206] As with carbamyl phosphate synthetase deficiency, the affected infant, a boy in nearly all cases, is normal at birth and appears well for the first day or so after birth. The characteristic syndrome of feeding difficulty, stupor, seizures, hypotonia (more often than hypertonia), and tachypnea then appears and evolves rapidly. If their condition is not detected promptly and treated, such infants progress to coma and death in the first week of life.[146,198,201,203] In one large series, 46% of infants died in the neonatal period.[201] However, with very early detection and therapy (see following sections), most infants survive the neonatal period; of long-term survivors, 30% to 60% are not overtly mentally retarded on follow-up.[201,202] However, normal cognitive outcome is rare.

Brain imaging shows findings consistent with diffuse cerebral edema during the acute period. MRI also shows injury in cerebral cortex, especially depths of sulci, basal ganglia, globus pallidus and putamen, and subcortical white matter (Fig. 27.15).[38]

The *enzymatic defect* is inherited as an X-linked trait.[146,248,252] In general, severe neonatal disease occurs in hemizygous male infants, and heterozygous female infants exhibit later onset and generally milder disease. In affected families, ornithine transcarbamylase deficiency was complete in the male patients and partial in the female patients. Fathers were normal, and mothers exhibited partial enzymatic deficiency. The gene is located on the short arm of the X-chromosome (Xp21.1), and more than 340 different mutations and polymorphisms have been identified.[146,168,247]

Metabolic Features. Hyperammonemia and elevated blood glutamine levels occur, as with carbamyl phosphate synthetase deficiency; however, in addition, orotic acid (and related pyrimidine metabolites) appears in the blood and is excreted in large amounts in the urine.[146,167,201,243] This feature reflects overproduction because of the excessive amounts of carbamyl phosphate available (see Fig. 27.12) and is helpful in distinguishing ornithine transcarbamylase deficiency from

carbamyl phosphate synthetase deficiency (see Fig. 27.14). The prominent respiratory alkalosis was noted earlier.

Most male infants affected with the malignant neonatal form of ornithine transcarbamylase deficiency have less than 2% of normal hepatic enzymatic activity.[146] The enzymatic defect is also demonstrable in leukocytes and duodenal or rectal tissue.[222,226,247,253]

Neuropathology. The relatively scant neuropathological data provide evidence of brain swelling and Alzheimer type II astrocytes with acute encephalopathy. The occurrence of symmetrical infarcts, with cavitation, particularly at the base of sulci and located at the junction of gray and white matter, is of particular interest (Fig. 27.16) because this lesion is considered characteristic of diminished cerebral perfusion in the context of brain swelling and increased intracranial pressure.[254,255] In severe cases, the neuropathological features evolve promptly to neuronal necrosis in cerebral cortex and basal ganglia and to spongiform change of cerebral white matter.[256-258] The chronic neuropathological sequelae are cortical neuronal and cerebral white matter atrophy. The earlier cysts subsequently may evolve to areas of cortical ulegyria.[258]

Two detailed neuropathological studies of infants who died 1 and 6 years after severe neonatal disease demonstrated almost total destruction of cerebral cortex and subjacent cerebral white matter, with numerous Alzheimer type II astrocytes throughout.[258,259] Because the patients died long after the neonatal period and had numerous seizures, it is difficult to determine how much of the brain injury related solely to the metabolic defect. In another case, *mild sponginess* of the cerebral white matter with numerous Alzheimer type II astrocytes was observed.[245] As noted earlier, the astrocytic change is a characteristic abnormality of the hyperammonemic encephalopathy observed in older patients with hepatic disease and in experimental animals.[207,208] Neuronal abnormalities of the type observable after hypoxic-ischemic insult have been reported,[245] and these findings raise the possibility of excitotoxic neuronal death (see earlier discussion).

Argininosuccinic Acid Synthetase Deficiency (Citrullinemia)

Clinical Features. Argininosuccinic acid synthetase deficiency occurs in several clinical forms, including a severe neonatal variety. In several large series, argininosuccinic acid synthetase deficiency accounted for approximately 15% to 20% of cases of urea cycle disorders with neonatal onset, and approximately 80% of cases of argininosuccinic acid synthetase deficiency were of neonatal onset.[146,168,198,203-205] In the neonatal-onset cases, following a brief symptom-free period after birth, the clinical syndrome begins in the first few days of life. Onset on the first postnatal day, before the institution of feeding, has been reported.[146,167] Most commonly, however, onset is between 24 and 72 hours of age. Poor feeding, vomiting, tachypnea, alteration of muscle tone, and seizures are the most common features.[71,146,202,260-272] A careful study of the EEG in three affected infants showed the burst-suppression pattern typical of neonatal hyperammonemia and a close correlation of the severity of the EEG pattern (i.e., the length of the interburst interval) on the EEG with both the degree of hyperammonemia and depression of level of consciousness (Figs. 27.17 and 27.18).[268] Brain imaging shows findings similar to those described for carbamyl phosphate synthetase deficiency and ornithine transcarbamylase

---

[a]References 146, 167, 168, 201-203, 205, 206, 211, and 239-249.

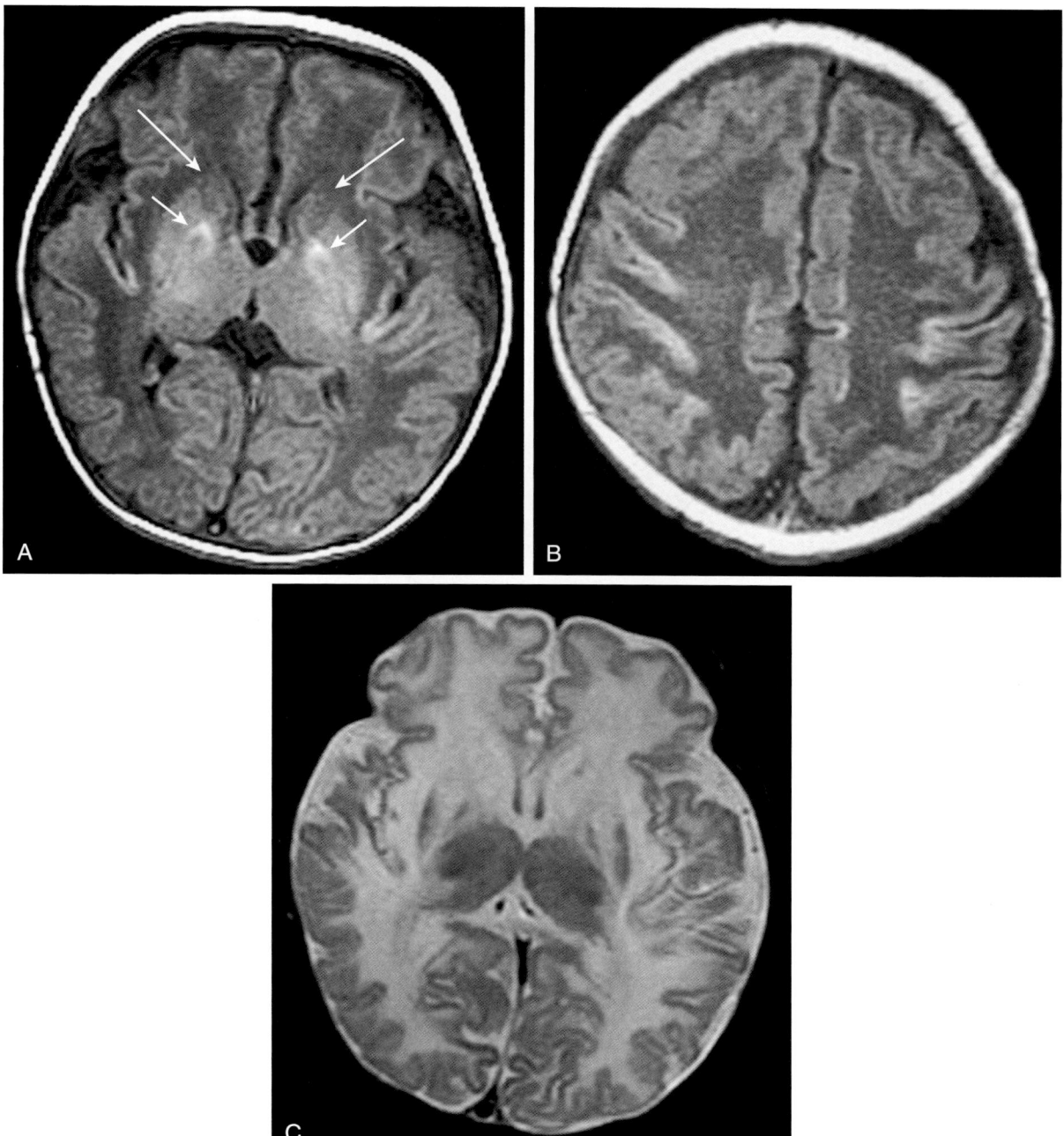

Figure 27.15 Ornithine transcarbamylase deficiency, magnetic resonance imaging scans. (A and B) Short-echo 550/16 images show hyperintensity in the lentiform nuclei, particularly the globi pallidi (*small white arrows*), insular cortex, and perirolandic cortex, in addition to hypointensity of the caudate heads (*large white arrows*). (C) Axial T2-weighted image shows diffusely abnormal hyperintensity of the white matter (which is isointense to cerebrospinal fluid and the basal ganglia, indicating diffuse edema). (From Barkovich AJ. *Pediatric Neuroimaging*. 5th ed. Philadelphia: Lippincott Williams & Wilkins; 2012.)

deficiency (see earlier). In the initial series of reported cases, nearly all infants died in the neonatal period. In two relatively large later series, only 1 of 23 infants died, but 16 of the 18 survivors were mentally retarded on follow-up.[202,203] The mode of inheritance is autosomal recessive.[146]

Metabolic Features. Hyperammonemia with citrullinemia is often not as marked as in carbamyl phosphate synthetase

and ornithine transcarbamylase deficiencies.[146,261-263,270] A massive increase in plasma concentration of citrulline is characteristic (see Fig. 27.14). Orotic aciduria may also occur (see Fig. 27.12).

Affected newborns have exhibited hepatic activities of argininosuccinic acid synthetase that are less than 20% of normal values. The enzymatic defect can be demonstrated readily in cultured skin fibroblasts and in lymphocytes.[266,273,274]

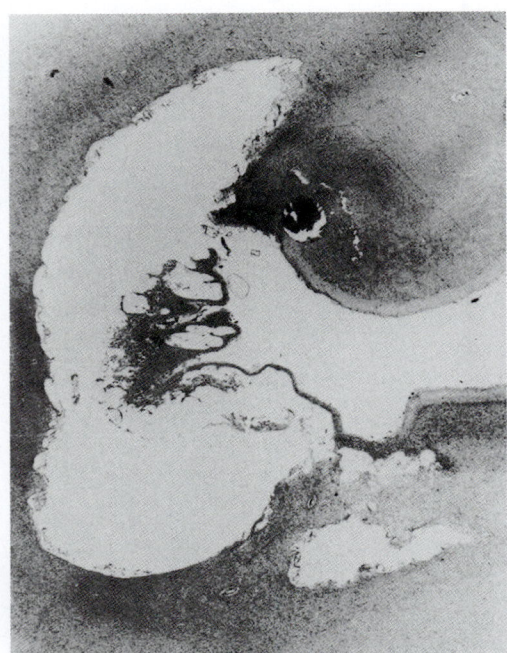

Figure 27.16 Cystic necrosis of cerebral cortex and immediately subjacent subcortical white matter in ornithine transcarbamylase deficiency. The infant died at 17 days of age. (From Filloux F, Townsend JJ, Leonard C. Ornithine transcarbamylase deficiency: neuropathologic changes acquired in utero. *J Pediatr.* 1986;108:942–945.)

Many different mutations of the gene, located on chromosome 9q, have been identified.[146]

Neuropathology. Infants who have died with the fulminating neonatal disorder have exhibited signs of brain edema. Indeed, in one report, marked elevations of intracranial pressure were documented and shown to correlate with the severity of the neurological features.[270] Moreover, the characteristic cortical-subcortical cystic infarcts observed with severe neonatal ornithine transcarbamylase deficiency and considered pathognomonic of diminished cerebral perfusion secondary

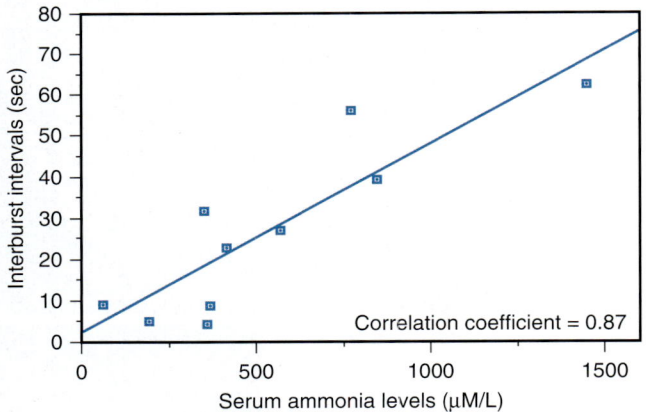

Figure 27.18 Correlation of serum ammonia levels and interburst intervals in three newborns with citrullinemia. Note the significant linear relationship between the serum ammonia levels and the interburst durations in three newborns with citrullinemia. (From Clancy RR, Chung HJ. EEG changes during recovery from acute severe neonatal citrullinemia. *Electroencephalogr Clin Neurophysiol.* 1991;78:222–227.)

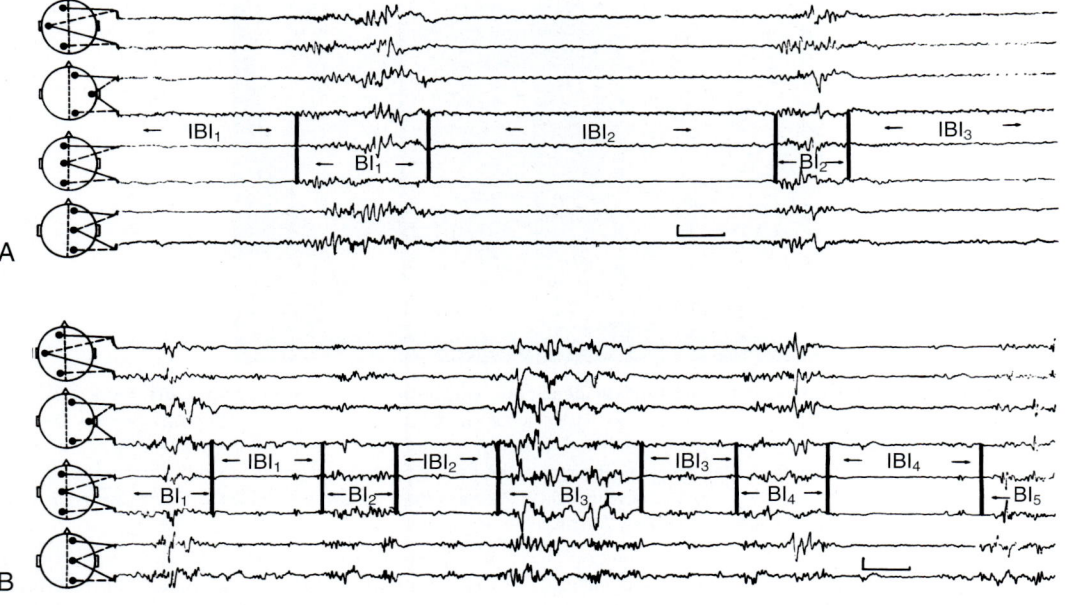

Figure 27.17 Burst-suppression electroencephalogram (EEG) in hyperammonemia caused by severe neonatal citrullinemia. (A) Segment of burst-suppression EEG recorded in an infant when the serum ammonia level was 1445 μmol/L. A 10-minute continuous epoch was chosen for quantitative analysis of the burst (e.g., BI_1, BI_2) and interburst (e.g., IBI_1, IBI_2) intervals. (B) The same patient recorded during recovery after the serum ammonia level fell to 355 μmol/L. Note the markedly decreased duration of the interburst intervals. Calibration: 50 μV, 2 seconds. (From Clancy RR, Chung HJ. EEG changes during recovery from acute severe neonatal citrullinemia. *Electroencephalogr Clin Neurophysiol.* 1991;78:222–227.)

to elevated intracranial pressure have been documented in neonatal citrullinemia.[266] Patients with survival beyond the acute period exhibit features of neuronal loss, impaired myelin formation, and Alzheimer type II glial cells.[260,261,263,266]

Argininosuccinase Deficiency (Argininosuccinic Aciduria)

Clinical Features. One of the several clinical forms of argininosuccinase (argininosuccinic acid lyase) deficiency is a severe neonatal type.[146,167,168,203] In several series, approximately 10% to 15% of patients with urea cycle disorders of neonatal onset exhibited this enzyme deficiency, and approximately 80% of patients with argininosuccinic deficiency had a neonatal onset.[146,198,203,205,206] As in the other neonatal forms of urea cycle defects, apparently normal newborn infants develop symptoms after approximately 24 hours of life. Poor feeding, stupor, and tachypnea, progressing to vomiting, seizures, and coma, constitute the clinical syndrome.[a] Abnormally fragile hair, characterized by dry, brittle strands with microscopically visible nodular swellings of the shafts (trichorrhexis nodosa), has been observed at as early as 2 weeks of age.[282] Although most of the initially reported patients died in the neonatal period, later experience has indicated that only the minority of patients whose condition is detected and treated from the neonatal period die.[202,203,205] However, nearly all survivors are mentally retarded on follow-up examinations. The neonatal form of argininosuccinase deficiency is inherited as an autosomal recessive trait.[227]

Metabolic Features. Hyperammonemia and increased levels of argininosuccinic acid and, to a lesser extent, citrulline in blood and urine are present in the neonatal cases (see Fig. 27.14). Elevated blood glutamine levels and prominent orotic aciduria reflect the alternate pathways of ammonia metabolism (see Fig. 27.12).

Argininosuccinase activity is uniformly severely depressed in liver.[146] The enzymatic defect is detectable in cultured skin fibroblasts as well. Enzyme activity in brain is relatively spared.[283] The gene is located on chromosome 7q.

Neuropathology. The acute neuropathology is likely to be similar to that described earlier for the other defects of the urea cycle but, to my knowledge, has not been reported. Impressive disturbances of myelination have been described in chronic cases.[276,284] In the study of Solitare and co-workers,[284] a patient 8 months of age had an extensive deficit in myelin, the only significant myelin having been observed in the dorsal columns of the spinal cord. The likelihood that this observation reflected a disturbance in myelin *formation* rather than myelin destruction is indicated by the absence of myelin breakdown products or of gliosis in the affected areas. The earlier discussion of potential glutamate-induced oligodendroglial injury may be relevant in this context. In addition to these deficits, the patient had numerous astrocytes of the Alzheimer type II variety.

Arginase Deficiency (Hyperargininemia)

Arginase deficiency, although identified at birth by measurement of the plasma arginine level in siblings of a previously affected patient, generally is not characterized by distinct clinical

---

abnormalities in the newborn period.[146,285,286] In a series of 92 cases of urea cycle disorders of neonatal onset, only a single case of arginase deficiency was found.[203] In a recent neonatal case, blood ammonia levels were only modestly elevated (194 µg/dL [114 µmol/L] with normal <100 µg/dL).[186] However the infant evolved on the second to third day from tachypnea to multiple seizures to apnea and coma. MRI showed diffuse edema, and CSF *glutamine* was markedly elevated (9587 µmol/L, with the upper limit of normal 771 µmol/L). The infant died despite hemodialysis. A postmortem examination revealed acute neuronal injury throughout cerebral cortex, with Alzheimer type II astrocytes and diffuse gliosis of cerebral white matter. The findings strongly support the role of *glutamine* as the toxic factor in this and other urea cycle disorders.[186] In the more common later-onset cases of arginase deficiency, the clinical syndrome becomes apparent later in infancy and is characterized particularly by spastic diplegia, which is slowly progressive.[145,146,284,286,288-291] Cognitive impairment is common, and epilepsy may occur. The typical later-onset syndrome is often mistakenly characterized as *cerebral palsy*.

Other Inherited Metabolic Disorders With Neonatal Hyperammonemia

Various other inherited metabolic disorders may result in hyperammonemia (see Table 27.9). Although metabolic features other than hyperammonemia (particularly acidosis, ketosis, or both) usually predominate, the hyperammonemia may dominate the clinical syndrome and strongly raise the possibility of a primary defect in the urea cycle. These disorders are considered briefly in the following sections.

Organic Acid Disorders

Disorders of organic acid metabolism are discussed in Chapter 28, but it is appropriate here to note that significant hyperammonemia may occur in the neonatal period in several of these disorders, particularly propionic acidemia, methylmalonic acidemias, and beta-ketothiolase deficiency, but also isovaleric acidemia, glutaric aciduria type II, multiple carboxylase deficiency, pyruvate dehydrogenase deficiency, and fatty acid oxidation defects. These disorders are accompanied by acidosis, ketosis, or both (see Fig. 27.14) and are discussed in Chapter 28. The mechanism of the hyperammonemia in the organic acid disorders is unknown, but available data indicate that the coenzyme A derivatives of the accumulated organic acids are potent inhibitors of human liver carbamyl phosphate synthetase (see Chapter 28 for details).[167,292] This observation imparts particular importance to the report of undetectable carbamyl phosphate synthetase activity in liver homogenates from a patient with methylmalonic acidemia.[293]

Lysinuric Protein Intolerance

Lysinuric protein intolerance may have its clinical onset in the neonatal period with poor feeding, vomiting, hypotonia, and hyperammonemia (see Table 27.9).[294] The molecular defect is in the membrane transport of the cationic amino acids lysine, arginine, and ornithine. The mechanism of the hyperammonemia is unknown, although a deficiency of ornithine and perhaps arginine and thereby dysfunction of the urea cycle is possible. Consistent with such a formulation, citrulline, which is transported by a different mechanism in the intestine, abolishes hyperammonemia when it is administered orally. Treatment consists of a low-protein diet and oral citrulline supplementation. Neurological development is generally normal in adequately treated patients.

Hyperornithinemia, Hyperammonemia, and Homocitrullinemia

The clinical features of hyperornithinemia, hyperammonemia, and homocitrullinemia may appear in the first weeks of life with protein intolerance, stupor, and seizures (see Table 27.9).[295-298] Subsequent neurological development may be impaired, but early detection and treatment of hyperammonemia and long-term dietary therapy have been associated with normal neurological development.[296,298] The major biochemical findings include hyperornithinemia and homocitrullinemia in addition to hyperammonemia and orotic aciduria. The basic defect involves transport of ornithine into the mitochondrion through the ornithine transporter protein,[297,299-301] with ammonia metabolism affected secondarily because of functional impairment at the ornithine transcarbamylase step.

ACQUIRED DISORDERS WITH NEONATAL HYPERAMMONEMIA

Most recognized cases of severe neonatal hyperammonemia have exhibited inherited disorders of the urea cycle or organic acid metabolism. However, other inherited metabolic defects (as just discussed), as well as a variety of acquired disorders, may result in severe neonatal hyperammonemia (see Table 27.9). Hepatic failure and total parenteral nutrition are uncommon examples of the noninherited disorders.[146,302] Worthy of particular attention is *a syndrome of significant hyperammonemia in the preterm infant that appears to be transient and reversible but can be fatal if undetected or inadequately treated.*[303-312] This syndrome is reviewed next. Possibly a related syndrome is hyperammonemia observed after perinatal asphyxia, as discussed in Chapter 20.

Transient Hyperammonemia of the Preterm Infant

Clinical Features

Transient *symptomatic* hyperammonemia of the preterm infant has been described in over 100 infants (Table 27.11).[303-309,312-314] Radiographic and clinical evidence of respiratory distress syndrome, albeit often mild, has been consistent. Many patients are near-term premature infants. The onset of central nervous system phenomena is the first or second postnatal day in most patients, often before any protein-containing

---

TABLE 27.11   Transient Hyperammonemia of the Preterm Infant

Clinical features
  Stupor, coma
  Seizures
  Fixed, dilated (>midposition) pupils
Metabolic features
  Marked hyperammonemia
Pathogenesis
  Combination of slow development of urea cycle function
    with disturbance in hepatic blood flow or oxygen
    supply (?)

---

feeding or intravenous solution has been provided. This very early onset differs from that seen in urea cycle disorders. Seizures are a common presenting sign. Stupor progresses rapidly to coma. Pupils frequently are fixed to light, and eyes are not movable by oculocephalic stimulation. Indeed, the combination of coma with absent pupillary responses and eye movements suggested advanced hypoxic-ischemic injury or severe intracranial hemorrhage before the diagnosis of transient symptomatic hyperammonemia was sought and discovered. A dramatic response to exchange transfusion, hemodialysis, or peritoneal dialysis has been observed repeatedly. Spontaneous recovery occurs over days to a week or so.

The *prognosis* for transient hyperammonemia is not clear, in part because the spectrum of the disorder has not been defined precisely. *In more recent years, for unknown reasons, this disorder has been much less common.* In view of the fulminating course and the clinical features of transient hyperammonemia of the preterm infant, it is likely that infants with this disorder in the past have died with the diagnosis of severe perinatal asphyxia, intracranial hemorrhage, sepsis, and so forth. Conversely, it is also likely that less severely affected patients recovered before the correct diagnosis was established. In reported cases, mortality rates of approximately 20% to 30% and rates of neurological sequelae in survivors of approximately 35% to 45% were documented.[309,312-314] With early detection and appropriate therapy, survival without sequelae is an appropriate and attainable goal in this disorder.

Metabolic Features

Hyperammonemia has been marked (see Table 27.11); initial values range from 844 to 3400 mg/dL, and peak values are as high as 7640 mg/dL. Elevations of plasma glutamine level and orotic acid excretion have been observed. Analysis of the urea cycle enzymes in liver of several infants revealed normal values.

Pathogenesis

The pathogenesis of transient hyperammonemia is unknown. Possible mechanisms include deficiency in the development of urea cycle function, either because of insufficient levels of urea cycle intermediates or enzymatic activities, inadequate hepatic blood flow, platelet aggregation with impairment of the hepatic microcirculation, and hypoxia-ischemia.[303,307-311,313,315] The possibility that the normal delay in development of the urea cycle is exacerbated in certain infants because of hypoxic-ischemic insult or other causes of impaired hepatic blood flow is raised by available data.

With regard to the possibility of limiting substrate quantities, investigators have shown that approximately 50% of (asymptomatic) preterm infants have an approximately twofold increase in blood ammonia level, accompanied by a decrease in blood arginine and ornithine levels, and that the hyperammonemia can be lowered by the oral administration of arginine.[307,316] One explanation for this *asymptomatic arginine-responsive hyperammonemia* in the preterm infant is inadequate activation by arginine of the synthesis of *N*-acetylglutamate, which is necessary for carbamyl phosphate synthetase activity (see Fig. 27.12). The cause of the decreased levels of arginine is unclear. Whether this defect in normal preterm infants is exacerbated greatly by illness, such as respiratory disease, and then results in the massive hyperammonemia of the symptomatic syndrome just

TABLE 27.12   Management of Neonatal Hyperammonemia

Antenatal diagnosis and prevention
　Early neonatal detection
Ammonia removal
　Hemodialysis, peritoneal dialysis
Alternate pathways
　Benzoate, phenylacetate, phenylbutyrate,
　　glyceroltriphenylbutyrate citrulline, arginine
Dietary measures
　Protein restriction, essential amino acids, nonprotein caloric
　　sources
Gene therapy
　Liver transplantation

described remains to be determined. A detailed study showed that transient *asymptomatic* hyperammonemia, whether or not treated with arginine in the neonatal period, is followed by normal neurological outcome at 30 months of age.[307]

Management of Neonatal Hyperammonemia

The basic elements in the management of the infant with hyperammonemia are shown in Table 27.12. Not all aspects of management are applicable to every patient, and these differences are discussed subsequently.

Antenatal Diagnosis and Prevention

Antenatal diagnosis is of particular value with defects of the urea cycle. Each of the four defects of the urea cycle discussed earlier can be identified antenatally.[146] Techniques include measurement of an abnormal metabolite in amniotic fluid (the metabolite proximal to the enzymatic defect), analysis of DNA from chorionic villus samples or cultured amniocytes, and enzyme analysis of cultured amniocytes or liver biopsy samples obtained in utero. Details are provided in standard sources.[146] These data can be used to provide either information with regard to therapeutic abortion or early institution of postnatal therapeutic measures.

Early Detection

Detection of the aforementioned disorders as rapidly as possible cannot be overemphasized. The fulminating course of serious neonatal hyperammonemia is observed in all the disorders discussed previously, including transient hyperammonemia of the preterm infant. Early detection and prompt institution of therapy may make the difference between the onset of irreversible central nervous system injury and recovery.

A striking demonstration of the importance of prompt intervention is derived from a study of two large series consisting of 116 infants with neonatal hyperammonemic coma secondary to congenital defects of the urea cycle.[202,203] Survival rates were 34% and 92% in the two studies. In the series with the better survival rate, although 92% of infants survived the neonatal period, approximately 80% of the survivors were mentally retarded (mean IQ, 43) and 17% had seizure disorders despite careful management of diet and the utilization of supplements to increase alternative pathways of waste nitrogen excretion. The most distinct correlate of outcome was *duration of neonatal coma;* four of five infants with coma for less than 3 days had a

normal IQ on follow-up versus none of seven with coma for more than 5 days. Subsequent work confirmed the importance of duration of severe hyperammonemia.[177,198,206,317]

The *initial or peak ammonia level* may contribute prognostic information; in one large series of 88 patients with urea cycle disorders, when plasma ammonia concentrations exceeded 300 µmol/L initially or 480 µmol/L at peak, none of the patients had a normal cognitive outcome.[204] However, these data were obtained by questionnaires and treatment was carried out to a considerable degree at *local hospitals*. Moreover, peak ammonia values were not correlated with neurocognitive outcome in other work.[177] Therefore the threshold values should be interpreted cautiously. I consider *duration* more important than absolute levels of blood ammonia in the determination of outcome.

Careful observations of 15 infants with defects of the urea cycle *treated prospectively from birth* indicated a distinctly more favorable prognosis than that observed in infants treated because of hyperammonemic coma.[318] Thus, of the 12 survivors studied, only 1 was mentally retarded, 4 were within the range of normal intelligence, and the remaining 7 had only mild deficits. The only newborns who died were three of the eight with ornithine transcarbamylase deficiency.

Ammonia Removal

The major therapeutic approaches for the rapid removal of ammonia (and glutamine) are hemodialysis, peritoneal dialysis, and hemofiltration techniques (see Table 27.12).[a] In the late 1980s, the major choice for therapy was between *peritoneal dialysis* and *exchange transfusion*.[227] A large study showed that peritoneal dialysis is the more effective procedure.[324] The superiority of dialysis over exchange transfusion in the removal of water-soluble metabolites (ammonia and glutamine) versus a metabolite confined to the intravascular space (e.g., bilirubin bound to albumin) is perhaps not surprising. Survival rates were 20% in those newborns treated with exchange transfusion, 50% in those treated with peritoneal dialysis after exchange transfusion, and 100% in those treated only with peritoneal dialysis.

Later work demonstrated the superiority of *hemodialysis* relative to peritoneal dialysis, and this approach is now the recommended procedure.[b] Indeed, the ammonia clearance is approximately 10-fold greater by hemodialysis than by peritoneal dialysis. Hemodialysis is a complicated procedure, requiring expensive equipment and considerable skilled personnel, but its superior benefits warrant this intervention.

Alternate Pathways of Waste Nitrogen Excretion

The value of specific supplements in stimulating alternate pathways of waste nitrogen excretion has been established (see Table 27.12 and Fig. 27.19).[c] Thus *(sodium) benzoate* results in acylation of glycine, the latter formed from ammonia and bicarbonate, and the resulting hippuric acid is readily excreted. Similarly, *(sodium) phenylacetate* acetylates glutamine, the latter formed from ammonia by the transamination of glutamate, which itself is formed by transamination of alphaketoglutarate. The resulting phenylacetylglutamine is

[a]References 66, 68, 146, 167, 201, 317, and 319-323.
[b]References 66, 146, 167, 168, 201, 317-319, 322, 325, and 326.
[c]References 65, 146, 167, 168, 177, 198, 202, 206, 271, 319-321, and 327-332.

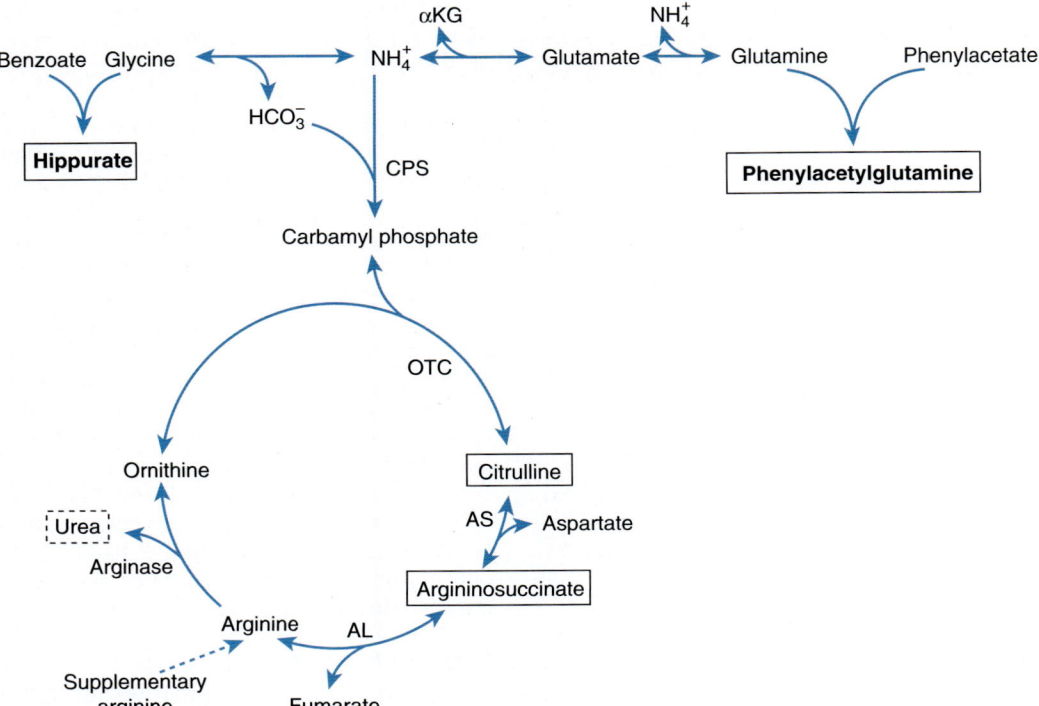

Figure 27.19 Alternate pathways of waste nitrogen excretion in disorders of the urea cycle. Complete deficiencies in carbamyl phosphate synthetase (CPS), ornithine transcarbamylase (OTC), argininosuccinate synthetase (AS), and argininosuccinase (AL) lead to decreased urea synthesis and neonatal hyperammonemic coma. Alternative pathways of nitrogen excretion are as follows: Arginine supplementation stimulates the synthesis and excretion of citrulline in citrullinemia (AS deficiency) and of argininosuccinate in argininosuccinic aciduria (AL deficiency). In all urea cycle disorders, sodium benzoate acylates glycine to form hippurate and sodium phenylacetate acetylates glutamine to form phenylacetylglutamine. (More recently sodium phenylacetate; see text.) Both waste nitrogen products *(boxed compounds)* are readily excreted in urine. HCO₃⁻, bicarbonate; *α*KG, alpha-ketoglutarate; HCO₄⁺, ammonium. (From Msall M, Batshaw ML, Suss R. Neurologic outcome in children with inborn errors of urea synthesis: outcome of urea-cycle enzymopathies. *N Engl J Med.* 1984;310:1500.)

readily excreted. Phenylacetate has been largely superseded by the congener *phenylbutyrate*,[65,330,331] and some data suggest that high-dose monotherapy with phenylbutyrate (without sodium benzoate) may provide the best survival rates.[146] Most recently, *glyceroltriphenylbutyrate*, a further modification of phenylbutyrate, has been shown to be at least as effective as the latter in controlling ammonia levels and is more readily tolerated.[332] In carbamyl phosphate deficiency and ornithine transcarbamylase deficiency, *citrulline* supplementation promotes the formation of argininosuccinate and provides a source of arginine. *Arginine* supplementation stimulates the synthesis and excretion of citrulline in argininosuccinic acid synthetase deficiency and of argininosuccinate in argininosuccinase deficiency (in addition to correcting the hypoargininemia in these two disorders).

Excitatory Amino Acid Antagonists(?)

The observations described earlier (see the section on biochemical effects of excessive ammonia) suggest that deleterious effects of elevated glutamine levels, with increased tryptophan influx and metabolism to the excitotoxin quinolinic acid, and the accumulation of extracellular glutamate, both acting at the NMDA receptor, could be crucial in the induction of neuronal death in congenital hyperammonemia. The potential value of administration of an NMDA antagonist, such as

dextromethorphan (see earlier sections on biochemical effects of excessive ammonia and nonketotic hyperglycinemia), is raised by experimental and clinical data. However, such therapy will require careful study in a relevant animal model; in a study of quinolinate-induced brain injury in developing rat brain, *pretreatment* with MK-801, the NMDA receptor antagonist, led to enhanced neuronal injury, although treatment with the antagonist *minutes after* quinolinate exposure blocked the injury.[188] More information is needed concerning the issue of excitatory amino acid antagonists in hyperammonemia.

Gene Therapy

Gene therapy in urea cycle disorders has consisted of adenovirally mediated gene transfer, hepatocyte infusion, or liver transplantation.[146,333-337] *Management of neonatal-onset urea cycle disorders has consisted of isolated hepatocyte infusion and especially liver transplantation.*[338] Orthoptic liver transplantation has been of limited long-term neurological benefit in neonatal onset cases when transplantation has been instituted after the first year of life. It was speculated that early transplantation would result in a more favorable neurological outcome. However, a review of a national sharing database suggests that children transplanted at the youngest ages appear to have the highest risk of graft loss, often related to technically difficult vessel anastomoses with subsequent thrombosis. While posttransplant mortality was low, the risk of death was higher in the younger children.[339] *Nevertheless, aggressive early metabolic management followed by liver transplantation in early infancy may ultimately prove to be preferred therapy.*

Dietary Therapy

The emergency procedures for ammonia removal described earlier for the newborn with severe hyperammonemia should be followed by appropriate dietary therapy.[a] The cornerstone of the diet is *low protein content.*[b] In addition, abundant *nonprotein calories* and *essential amino acids* are important to prevent protein catabolism. As noted earlier, in carbamyl phosphate deficiency and ornithine transcarbamylase deficiency, supplementation with *citrulline,* the important metabolite of the urea cycle just distal to the two enzymatic blocks, is important. Similarly, in argininosuccinic acid synthetase and argininosuccinase deficiencies, *arginine* is the crucial distal amino acid added.

MISCELLANEOUS AMINO ACID DISORDERS

As indicated earlier in this chapter, other disorders of amino acid metabolism have been reported to occur in the newborn period, albeit very rarely (see Table 27.1). Thus *hypervalinemia,* secondary to a defect in valine transaminase, has been described in an infant with vomiting, stupor, and delayed development.[27,62,342] *Phenylketonuria* now rarely manifests clinically in the first month of life because of neonatal screening and early intervention[343,344]; vomiting and a peculiar musty odor to the infant's urine, skin, and hair were prominent signs.[345] The enzymatic defect involves phenylalanine hydroxylase. *Lysinuric protein intolerance* is discussed earlier in the section on hyperammonemia because this rare disorder may have its onset in the newborn period with prominent hyperammonemia. The molecular defect involves transport of cationic amino acids. *Pyridoxine dependency* results in neonatal seizures, sometimes with intrauterine onset, and is discussed in Chapter 12. The defect involves synthesis of GABA. Rare isolated cases of neonatal seizures, other neurological deficits, or both have been reported with hyperbeta-alaninemia, sarcosinemia, and carnosinemia.[345-354]

KEY REFERENCES

1. Chuang DT, Shih VE. Maple syrup urine disease (branched-chain ketoaciduria). In: Schriver CR, Beaudet AL, Sly WS, et al., eds. *The Metabolic and Molecular Bases of Inherited Disease.* Vol. 2. 8th ed. New York: McGraw-Hill; 2001:1971-2005.
2. Harris RA, Joshi M, Jeoung NH, et al. Overview of the molecular and biochemical basis of branched-chain amino acid catabolism. *J Nutr.* 2005;135:1527S-1530S.
4. Strauss KA, Wardley B, Robinson D, et al. Classical maple syrup urine disease and brain development: principles of management and formula design. *Mol Genet Metab.* 2010;99:333-345.
5. Kaplan P, Mazur A, Field M, et al. Intellectual outcome in children with maple syrup urine disease. *J Pediatr.* 1991;119:46-50.
6. Yudkoff M, Daikhin Y, Nissim A, et al. Brain amino acid requirements and toxicity: the example of leucine. *J Nutr.* 2005;135:1531S-1538S.
7. Ribeiro CA, Sgaravatti AM, Rosa RB, et al. Inhibition of brain energy metabolism by the branched-chain amino acids

accumulating in maple syrup urine disease. *Neurochem Res.* 2008;33:114-124.
8. Sgaravatti AM, Rosa RB, Schuck PF, et al. Inhibition of brain energy metabolism by the alpha-keto acids accumulating in maple syrup urine disease. *Biochim Biophys Acta.* 2003;1639:232-238.
9. Pilla C, Cardozo RF, Dutra-Filho CS, et al. Creatine kinase activity from rat brain is inhibited by branched-chain amino acids in vitro. *Neurochem Res.* 2003;28:675-679.
10. Görtz P, Köller H, Schwahn B, et al. Disturbance of cultured rat neuronal network activity depends on concentration and ratio of leucine and alpha-ketoisocaproate: implication for acute encephalopathy of maple syrup urine disease. *Pediatr Res.* 2003;53:320-324.
11. Fernstrom JD. Branched-chain amino acids and brain function. *J Nutr.* 2005;135:1539S-1546S.
14. Funchal C, Zamoner A, dos Santos AQ, et al. Evidence that intracellular Ca^{2+} mediates the effect of alpha-ketoisocaproic acid on the phosphorylating system of cytoskeletal proteins from cerebral cortex of immature rats. *J Neurol Sci.* 2005;238:75-82.
15. Fontella FU, Gassen E, Pulrolnik V, et al. Stimulation of lipid peroxidation in vitro in rat brain by the metabolites accumulating in maple syrup urine disease. *Metab Brain Dis.* 2002;17:47-54.
16. Bridi R, Araldi J, Sgarbi MB, et al. Induction of oxidative stress in rat brain by the metabolites accumulating in maple syrup urine disease. *Int J Dev Neurosci.* 2003;21:327-332.
17. Bridi R, Latini A, Braum CA, et al. Evaluation of the mechanisms involved in leucine-induced oxidative damage in cerebral cortex of young rats. *Free Radic Res.* 2005;39:71-79.
18. Bridi R, Braun CA, Zorzi GK, et al. alpha-keto acids accumulating in maple syrup urine disease stimulate lipid peroxidation and reduce antioxidant defences in cerebral cortex from young rats. *Metab Brain Dis.* 2005;20:155-167.
19. Mescka CP, Rosa AP, Schirmbeck G, et al. L-carnitine prevents oxidative stress in the brains of rats subjected to a chemically induced chronic model of MSUD. *Mol Neurobiol.* 2016;53:6007-6017.
20. Funchal C, Gottfried C, De Almeida LM, et al. Evidence that the branched-chain alpha-keto acids accumulating in maple syrup urine disease induce morphological alterations and death in cultured astrocytes from rat cerebral cortex. *Glia.* 2004;48:230-240.
21. Funchal C, Dos Santos AQ, Jacques-Silva MC, et al. Branched-chain alpha-keto acids accumulating in maple syrup urine disease induce reorganization of phosphorylated GFAP in C6-glioma cells. *Metab Brain Dis.* 2005;20:205-217.
22. Funchal C, Gottfried C, de Almeida LM, et al. Morphological alterations and cell death provoked by the branched-chain alpha-amino acids accumulating in maple syrup urine disease in astrocytes from rat cerebral cortex. *Cell Mol Neurobiol.* 2005;25:851-867.
23. Rosa L, Galant LS, Dall'Igna DM, et al. Cerebral oedema, blood-brain barrier breakdown and the decrease in Na(+), K(+)-ATPase activity in the cerebral cortex and hippocampus are prevented by dexamethasone in an animal model of maple syrup urine disease. *Mol Neurobiol.* 2016;53:3714-3723.
33. Morton DH, Strauss KA, Robinson DL, et al. Diagnosis and treatment of maple syrup disease: a study of 36 patients. *Pediatrics.* 2002;109:999-1008.
35. Geal-Dor M, Adelman C, Levi H, et al. Changes in the auditory nerve brainstem evoked responses in a case of maple syrup urine disease. *Dev Med Child Neurol.* 2004;46:184-186.
36. Tu YF, Chen CY, Lin YJ, et al. Neonatal neurological disorders involving the brainstem: neurosonographic approaches through the squamous suture and the foramen magnum. *Eur Radiol.* 2005;15:1927-1933.
38. Barkovich AJ. *Pediatric Neuroimaging.* 4th ed. Philadelphia: Lippincott Williams & Wilkins; 2005.
39. Cavalleri F, Berardi A, Burlina AB, et al. Diffusion-weighted MRI of maple syrup urine disease encephalopathy. *Neuroradiology.* 2002;44:499-502.
40. Ha JS, Kim TK, Eun BL, et al. Maple syrup urine disease encephalopathy: a follow-up study in the acute stage using diffusion-weighted MRI. *Pediatr Radiol.* 2004;34:163-166.
41. Jan W, Zimmerman RA, Wang ZJ, et al. MR diffusion imaging and MR spectroscopy of maple syrup urine disease during acute metabolic decompensation. *Neuroradiology.* 2003;45:393-399.

---

[a]References 146, 167, 198, 202, 219, 319, 320, 327, 328, 331, and 340.
[b]References 65, 168, 198, 219, 264, 281, 282, 285, 319, 320, and 341.

42. Righini A, Ramenghi LA, Parini R, et al. Water apparent diffusion coefficient and T2 changes in the acute stage of maple syrup urine disease: evidence of intramyelinic and vasogenic-interstitial edema. *J Neuroimaging*. 2003;13:162-165.

43. Patay Z. Diffusion-weighted MR imaging in leukodystrophies. *Eur Radiol*. 2005;15:2284-2303.

44. Parmar H, Sitoh YY, Ho L. Maple syrup urine disease: diffusion-weighted and diffusion-tensor magnetic resonance imaging findings. *J Comput Assist Tomogr*. 2004;28:93-97.

45. Sakai M, Inoue Y, Oba H, et al. Age dependence of diffusion-weighted magnetic resonance imaging findings in maple syrup urine disease encephalopathy. *J Comput Assist Tomogr*. 2005; 29:524-527.

46. Xia W, Yang W. Diffusion-weighted magnetic resonance imaging in a case of severe classic maple syrup urine disease. *J Pediatr Endocrinol Metabol*. 2015;28:805-808.

47. Schönberger S, Schweiger B, Schwahn B, et al. Dysmyelination in the brain of adolescents and young adults with maple syrup urine disease. *Mol Genet Metab*. 2004;82:69-75.

48. Nellis MM, Kasinski A, Carlson M, et al. Relationship of causative genetic mutations in maple syrup urine disease with their clinical expression. *Mol Genet Metab*. 2003;80:189-195.

52. Silberman JS, Dancis J, Feigin I. Neuropathological observations in maple syrup urine disease. *Arch Neurol*. 1961;5:351.

56. Kamei A, Takashima S, Chan F, et al. Abnormal dendritic development in maple syrup urine disease. *Pediatr Neurol*. 1992;8: 145-147.

60. Prensky AL, Carr S, Moser HW. Development of myelin in inherited disorders of amino acid metabolism. *Arch Neurol*. 1968;19:552.

62. Chuang DT, Shih VE. Disorders of branched chain amino acid and keto acid metabolism. In: Scriver CR, Beaudet AL, Sly WS, eds. *The Metabolic and Molecular Bases of Inherited Disease*. Vol. 1. 7th ed. New York: McGraw-Hill; 1995:1239-1277.

64. Simon E, Fingerhut R, Baumkötter J, et al. Maple syrup urine disease: favourable effect of early diagnosis by newborn screening on the neonatal course of the disease. *J Inherit Metab Dis*. 2006; 29:532-537.

65. Vernon HJ. Inborn errors of metabolism: advances in diagnosis and therapy. *J Am Med Assoc Pediatr*. 2015;169:778-782.

67. Puliyanda DP, Harmon WE, Peterschmitt MJ, et al. Utility of hemodialysis in maple syrup urine disease. *Pediatr Nephrol*. 2002;17:239-242.

69. Hoffmann B, Helbling C, Schadewaldt P, et al. Impact of longitudinal plasma leucine levels on the intellectual outcome in patients with classic MSUD. *Pediatr Res*. 2006;59:17-20.

72. Hamosh A, Johnston MV. Nonketotic hyperglycinemia. In: Schriver CR, Beaudet AL, Sly WS, et al., eds. *The Metabolic and Molecular Bases of Inherited Disease*. Vol. 2. 8th ed. New York: McGraw-Hill; 2001:2065-2078.

81. Dzhala VI, Talos DM, Sdrulla DA, et al. NKCC1 transporter facilitates seizures in the developing brain. *Nat Med*. 2005;11:1205-1213.

82. Kahle KT, Staley KJ. The bumetanide-sensitive Na-K-2Cl cotransporter NKCC1 as a potential target of a novel mechanism-based treatment strategy for neonatal seizures. *Neurosurg Focus*. 2008;25:E22.

88. Ichinohe A, Kure S, Mikawa S, et al. Glycine cleavage system in neurogenic regions. *Eur J Neurosci*. 2004;19:2365-2370.

89. Nguyen MD, Julien J-P, Rivest S. Innate immunity: the missing link in neuroprotection and neurodegeneration? *Nat Rev Neurosci*. 2002;3:216-227.

91. Applegarth DA, Toone JR. Glycine encephalopathy (nonketotic hyperglycinaemia): review and update. *J Inherit Metab Dis*. 2004;27:417-422.

92. Swanson MA, Coughlin CR Jr, Scharer GH, et al. Biochemical and molecular predictors for prognosis in nonketotic hyperglycinemia. *Ann Neurol*. 2015;78:606-618.

97. Shuman RM, Leech RW, Scott CR. The neuropathology of the nonketotic and ketotic hyperglycinemias: three cases. *Neurology*. 1978;28:139-146.

111. Chen PT, Young C, Lee WT, et al. Early epileptic encephalopathy with suppression burst electroencephalographic pattern—an analysis of eight Taiwanese patients. *Brain Dev*. 2001;23:715-720.

112. Hoover-Fong JE, Shah S, Van Hove JL, et al. Natural history of nonketotic hyperglycinemia in 65 patients. *Neurology*. 2004; 63:1847-1853.

113. Applegarth DA, Toone JR. Glycine encephalopathy (nonketotic hyperglycinemia): comments and speculations. *Am J Med Genet A*. 2006;140A:186-188.

114. Hennermann JB, Berger JM, Grieben U, et al. Prediction of long-term outcome in glycine encephalopathy: a clinical survey. *J Inherit Metab Dis*. 2012;35:253-261.

121. Markand ON, Garg BP, Brandt IK. Nonketotic hyperglycinemia: electroencephalographic and evoked potential abnormalities. *Neurology*. 1982;32:151.

125. Nissenkorn A, Michelson M, Ben-Zeev B, et al. Inborn errors of metabolism. A cause of abnormal brain development. *Neurology*. 2001;56:1265-1272.

126. Khong P-L, Lam BC, Chung BHY, et al. Diffusion-weighted MR imaging in neonatal nonketotic hyperglycinemia. *AJNR Am J Neuroradiol*. 2003;24:1181-1183.

127. Paupe A, Bidat L, Sonigo P, et al. Prenatal diagnosis of hypoplasia of the corpus callosum in association with non-ketotic hyperglycinemia. *Ultrasound Obstet Gynecol*. 2002;20:616-619.

128. Shah DK, Tingay DG, Fink AM, et al. Magnetic resonance imaging in neonatal nonketotic hyperglycinemia. *Pediatr Neurol*. 2005;33:50-52.

129. Mourmans J, Majoie CB, Barth PG, et al. Sequential MR imaging changes in nonketotic hyperglycinemia. *AJNR Am J Neuroradiol*. 2006;27:208-211.

130. Sener RN. Nonketotic hyperglycinemia: diffusion magnetic resonance imaging findings. *J Comput Assist Tomogr*. 2003;27: 538-540.

131. Sener RN. Diffusion magnetic resonance imaging patterns in metabolic and toxic brain disorders. *Acta Radiol*. 2004;45:561-570.

133. Huisman TA, Thiel T, Steinmann B, et al. Proton magnetic resonance spectroscopy of the brain of a neonate with nonketotic hyperglycinemia: in vivo-in vitro (ex vivo) correlation. *Eur Radiol*. 2002;12:858-861.

134. Viola A, Chabrol B, Nicoli F, et al. Magnetic resonance spectroscopy study of glycine pathways in nonketotic hyperglycinemia. *Pediatr Res*. 2002;52:292-300.

139. Korman SH, Gutman A. Pitfalls in the diagnosis of glycine encephalopathy (non-ketotic hyperglycinemia). *Dev Med Child Neurol*. 2002;44:712-720.

140. Aliefendioğlu D, Aslan AT, Coşkun T, et al. Transient nonketotic hyperglycinemia: two case reports and literature review. *Pediatr Neurol*. 2003;28:151-155.

141. Kure S, Ichinohe A, Kojima K, et al. Mild variant of nonketotic hyperglycinemia with typical neonatal presentations: mutational and in vitro expression analyses in two patients. *J Pediatr*. 2004;144:827-829.

142. Korman SH, Boneh A, Ichinohe A, et al. Persistent NKH with transient or absent symptoms and a homozygous GLDC mutation. *Ann Neurol*. 2004;56:139-143.

143. Flusser H, Korman SH, Sato K, et al. Mild glycine encephalopathy (NKH) in a large kindred due to a silent exonic *GLDC* splice mutation. *Neurology*. 2005;64:1426-1430.

144. Dinopoulos A, Matsubara Y, Kure S. Atypical variants of nonketotic hyperglycinemia. *Mol Genet Metab*. 2005;86:61-69.

146. Brusilow SW, Horwich AL. Urea cycle enzymes. In: Schriver CR, Beaudet AL, Sly WS, et al., eds. *The Metabolic and Molecular Bases of Inherited Disease*. Vol. 2. 8th ed. New York: McGraw-Hill; 2001:1909-1963.

149. Anderson JM. Spongy degeneration in the white matter of the central nervous system in the newborn: pathological findings in three infants, one with hyperglycinaemia. *J Neurol Neurosurg Psychiatry*. 1969;32:328-337.

164. Chien YH, Hsu CC, Huang A, et al. Poor outcome for neonatal-type nonketotic hyperglycinemia treated with high-dose sodium benzoate and dextromethorphan. *J Child Neurol*. 2004;19:39-42.

165. Suzuki Y, Kure S, Oota M, et al. Nonketotic hyperglycinemia: proposal of a diagnostic and treatment strategy. *Pediatr Neurol*. 2010;43:221-224.

166. Cusmai R, Martinelli D, Moavero R, et al. Ketogenic diet in early myoclonic encephalopathy due to non ketotic hyperglycinemia. *Eur J Paediatr Neurol*. 2012;16:509-513.

168. Lichter-Konecki U, Batshaw ML. Inborn errors of urea synthesis. In: Swaiman KF, Ashwal S, Ferriero DM, Schor NF, eds. *Swaiman's Pediatric Neurology. Principles and Practice*. 5th ed. Philadelphia: Elsevier; 2012:357-367.

177. Gropman AL, Batshaw ML. Cognitive outcome in urea cycle disorders. *Mol Genet Metabol*. 2004;81:S58-S62.

178. de Graaf AA, Deutz NE, Bosman DK, et al. The use of in vivo proton NMR to study the effects of hyperammonemia in the rat cerebral cortex. *NMR Biomed*. 1991;4:31-37.

185. Gropman A. Brain imaging in urea cycle disorders. *Mol Genet Metab*. 2010;100:S20-S30.

186. Picker JD, Puga AC, Levy HL, et al. Arginase deficiency with lethal neonatal expression: evidence for the glutamine hypothesis of cerebral edema. *J Pediatr*. 2003;142:349-352.

189. Yan E, Castillo-Meléndez M, Smythe G, et al. Quinolinic acid promotes albumin deposition in Purkinje cell, astrocytic activation and lipid peroxidation in fetal brain. *Neuroscience*. 2005;134:867-875.

198. Wilcken B. Problems in the management of urea cycle disorders. *Mol Genet Metabol*. 2004;81:S86-S91.

201. Maestri NE, Clissold D, Brusilow SW. Neonatal onset ornithine transcarbamylase deficiency: a retrospective analysis. *J Pediatr*. 1999;134:268-272.

203. Uchino T, Endo F, Matsuda I. Neurodevelopmental outcome of long-term therapy of urea cycle disorders in Japan. *J Inherit Metab Dis*. 1998;21:151-159.

204. Bachmann C. Outcome and survival of 88 patients with urea cycle disorders: a retrospective evaluation. *Eur J Pediatr*. 2003;162:410-416.

205. Nassogne M, Héron B, Touati G, et al. Urea cycle defects: management and outcome. *J Inherit Metabo Dis*. 2005;28:407-414.

206. Enns GM, Berry SA, Berry GT, et al. Survival after treatment with phenylacetate and benzoate for urea-cycle disorders. *N Engl J Med*. 2007;356:2282-2292.

209. Takeoka M, Soman TB, Shih VE, et al. Carbamyl phosphate synthetase 1 deficiency: a destructive encephalopathy. *Pediatr Neurol*. 2001;24:193-199.

211. Leonard JV, Morris AA. Urea cycle disorders. *Semin Neonatol*. 2002;7:27-35.

223. Takanashi J-I, Barkovich AJ, Cheng SF, et al. Brain MR imaging in neonatal hyperammonemic encephalopathy resulting from proximal urea cycle disorders. *AJNR Am J Neuroradiol*. 2003;24:1184-1187.

225. Batshaw ML, Berry GT. Use of citrulline as a diagnostic marker in the prospective treatment of urea cycle disorders. *J Pediatr*. 1991;118:913-918.

230. Díez-Fernández C, Hu L, Cervera J, et al. Understanding carbamoyl phosphate synthetase (CPS1) deficiency by using the recombinantly purified human enzyme: effects of CPS1 mutations that concentrate in a central domain of unknown function. *Mol Genet Metab*. 2014;112:123-132.

232. Schubiger G, Bachmann C, Barben P, et al. *N*-Acetylglutamate synthetase deficiency: diagnosis, management and follow-up of a rare disorder of ammonia detoxication. *Eur J Pediatr*. 1991;150: 353-356.

234. Guffon N, Vianey-Saban C, Bourgeois J, et al. A new neonatal case of *N*-acetylglutamate synthase deficiency treated by carbamylglutamate. *J Inherit Metab Dis*. 1995;18:61-65.

235. Elpeleg O, Shaag A, Ben-Shalom E, et al. *N*-Acetylglutamate synthase deficiency and the treatment of hyperammonemic encephalopathy. *Ann Neurol*. 2002;52:845-849.

236. Caldovic L, Morizono H, Daikhin Y, et al. Restoration of ureagenesis in *N*-acetylglutamate synthase deficiency by *N*-carbamylglutamate. *J Pediatr*. 2004;145:552-554.

245. Kornfeld M, Woodfin BM, Papile L. Neuropathology of ornithine carbamyl transferase deficiency. *Acta Neuropathol*. 1985;65: 261.

246. Pridmore CL, Clarke J, Blaser S. Ornithine transcarbamylase deficiency in females: an often overlooked cause of treatable encephalopathy. *J Child Neurol*. 1995;10:369-374.

248. Gordon N. Ornithine transcarbamylase deficiency: a urea cycle defect. *Eur J Paediatr Neurol*. 2003;7:115-121.

254. Filloux F, Townsend JJ, Leonard C. Ornithine transcarbamylase deficiency: neuropathologic changes acquired in utero. *J Pediatr*. 1986;108:942-945.

256. Harding BN, Leonard JV, Erdohazi M. Ornithine transcarbamy lase deficiency: neuropathological study. *Eur J Pediatr*. 1984;141: 215.

258. Yamanouchi H, Yokoo H, Yuhara Y, et al. An autopsy case of ornithine transcarbamylase deficiency. *Brain Dev*. 2002;24:91-94.

266. Martin JJ, Farriaux JP, De Jonghe P. Neuropathology of citrullinaemia. *Acta Neuropathol*. 1982;56:303.

268. Clancy RR, Chung HJ. EEG changes during recovery from acute severe neonatal citrullinemia. *Electroencephalogr Clin Neurophysiol*. 1991;78:222-227.

272. Majoie CB, Mourmans JM, Akkerman EM, et al. Neonatal citrullinemia: comparison of conventional MR, diffusion-weighted, and diffusion tensor findings. *AJNR Am J Neuroradiol*. 2004;25: 32-35.

286. Prasad AN, Breen JC, Ampola MG, et al. Argininemia: a treatable genetic cause of progressive spastic diplegia simulating cerebral palsy: case reports and literature review. *J Child Neurol*. 1997;12:301-309.

288. Schlune A, Vom Dahl S, Häussinger D, et al. Hyperargininemia due to arginase I deficiency: the original patients and their natural history, and a review of the literature. *Amino Acids*. 2015;47:1751-1762.

289. Oldham MS, vanMeter JW, Shattuck KF, et al. Diffusion tensor imaging in arginase deficiency reveals damage to corticospinal tracts. *Pediatr Neurol*. 2010;42:49-52.

290. Segawa Y, Matsufuji M, Itokazu N, et al. A long-term survival case of arginase deficiency with severe multicystic white matter and compound mutations. *Brain Dev*. 2011;33:45-48.

291. Lee BH, Jin HY, Kim GH, et al. Argininemia presenting with progressive spastic diplegia. *Pediatr Neurol*. 2011;44:218-220.

293. Shapiro LJ, Bocian ME, Raijman L. Methylmalonyl-CoA mutase deficiency associated with severe neonatal hyperammonemia: activity of urea cycle enzymes. *J Pediatr*. 1978;93:986.

294. Simell O. Lysinuric protein intolerance and other cationic aminoacidurias. In: Scriver CR, Beaudet AL, Sly WS, et al., eds. *The Metabolic and Molecular Bases of Inherited Disease*. Vol. 3. 8th ed. New York: McGraw-Hill; 2001:4933-4955.

295. Shih VE, Laframboise R, Mandell R, et al. Neonatal form of the hyperornithinaemia, hyperammonaemia, and homocitrullinura (HHH) syndrome and prenatal diagnosis. *Prenat Diag*. 1992;12: 717-723.

297. Valle D, Simell O. The hyperornithinemias. In: Schriver CR, Beaudet AL, Sly WS, et al., eds. *The Metabolic and Molecular Bases of Inherited Disease*. Vol. 2. 8th ed. New York: McGraw-Hill; 2001:1857-1895.

298. Salvi S, Santorelli FM, Bertini E, et al. Clinical and molecular findings in hyperornithinemia-hyperammonemia-homocitrullinuria syndrome. *Neurology*. 2001;57:911-914.

299. Camacho JA, Obie C, Biery B, et al. Hyperornithinaemia-hy perammonaemia-homocitrullinuria syndrome is caused by mutations in a gene encoding a mitochondrial ornithine transporter. *Nat Genet*. 1999;22:151-158.

300. Tsujino S, Kanazawa N, Ohashi T, et al. Three novel mutations (G27E, insAAC, R179X) in the *ORNT1* gene of Japanese patients with hyperornithinemia, hyperammonemia, and homocitrullinuria syndrome. *Ann Neurol*. 2000;47:625-631.

301. Camacho JA, Mardach R, Rioseco-Camacho N, et al. Clinical and functional characterization of a human ORNT1 mutation (T32R) in the hyperornithinemia-hyperammonemia-homocitrullinuria (HHH) syndrome. *Pediatr Res*. 2006;60:423-429.

303. Ballard RA, Vinocur B, Reynolds JW. Transient hyperammonemia of the preterm infant. *N Engl J Med*. 1978;299:920.

306. Ellison PH, Cowger ML. Transient hyperammonemia in the preterm infant: neurologic aspects. *Neurology*. 1981;31:767.

307. Batshaw ML, Wachtel RC, Cohen L. Neurologic outcome in premature infants with transient asymptomatic hyperammonemia. *J Pediatr*. 1986;108:271-275.

309. Yoshino M, Sakaguchi Y, Kuriya N, et al. A nationwide survey on transient hyperammonemia in newborn infants in Japan: prognosis of life and neurological outcome. *Neuropediatrics*. 1991;22:198-202.

310. Boehm G, Teichmann B, Jung K. Development of urea-synthesizing capacity in preterm infants during the first weeks of life. *Biol Neonate*. 1991;59:1-4.

311. Boehm G, Müller DM, Beyreiss K, et al. Evidence for functional immaturity of the ornithine-urea cycle in very-low-birth-weight infants. *Biol Neonate*. 1988;54:121-125.

312. Giacoia GP, Padilla-Lugo A. Severe transient neonatal hyperammonemia. *Am J Perinatol*. 1986;3:249-254.

313. Hudak ML, Jones MD, Brusilow SW. Differentiation of transient hyperammonemia of the newborn and urea cycle enzyme defects by clinical presentation. *J Pediatr*. 1985;107:712-719.

316. Batshaw ML, Wachtel RC, Thomas GH. Arginine responsive asymptomatic hyperammonemia in premature infants. *J Pediatr*. 1984;105:86.

317. Summar M. Current strategies for the management of neonatal urea cycle disorders. *J Pediatr*. 2001;138:S30-S39.

318. Maestri NE, Hauser ER, Bartholomew D, et al. Prospective treatment of urea cycle disorders. *J Pediatr*. 1991;119.

321. Thoene JG. Treatment of urea cycle disorders. *J Pediatr*. 1999;134:255-256.

322. McBryde KD, Kudelka TL, Kershaw DB, et al. Clearance of amino acids by hemodialysis in argininosuccinate synthetase deficiency. *J Pediatr*. 2004;144:536-540.

323. Hiroma T, Nakamura T, Tamura M, et al. Continuous venovenous hemodiafiltration in neonatal onset hyperammonemia. *Am J Perinatol*. 2002;19:221-224.

326. Wiegand C, Thompson T, Bock GH. The management of life-threatening hyperammonemia: a comparison of several therapeutic modalities. *J Pediatr*. 1980;96:142.

330. Feillet F, Leonard JV. Alternative pathway therapy for urea cycle disorders. *J Inherit Metab Dis*. 1998;21:101-111.

331. Batshaw ML, MacArthur RB, Tuckman M. Alternative pathway therapy for urea cycle disorders: twenty years later. *J Pediatr*. 2001;138:S46-S55.

332. Cederbaum S, Lemons C, Batshaw ML. Alternative pathway or diversion therapy for urea cycle disorders now and in the future. *Mol Genet Metab*. 2010;100:219-220.

333. Whittington PF, Alonso EM, Boyle JT, et al. Liver transplantation for the treatment of urea cycle disorders. *J Inherit Metab Dis*. 1998;21:112-118.

334. Ensenauer R, Tuchman M, ElYoussef M, et al. Management and outcome of neonatal-onset ornithine transcarbamylase deficiency following liver transplantation at 60 days of life. *Mol Genet Metab*. 2005;84:363-366.

335. Horslen SP, McCowan TC, Goertzen TC, et al. Isolated hepatocyte transplantation in an infant with a severe urea cycle disorder. *Pediatrics*. 2003;111:1262-1267.

336. Batshaw ML, Robinson MB, Ye X, et al. Correction of ureagenesis after gene transfer in an animal model and after liver transplantation in humans with ornithine transcarbamylase deficiency. *Pediatr Res*. 1999;46:588-593.

337. McBride KL, Miller G, Carter S, et al. Developmental outcomes with early orthotopic liver transplantation for infants with neonatal-onset urea cycle defects and a female patient with late-onset ornithine transcarbamylase deficiency. *Pediatrics*. 2004;114:e523-e526.

338. Yu L, Rayhill SC, Hsu EK, et al. Liver transplantation for urea cycle disorders: analysis of the United Network for Organ Sharing database. *Transplant Proc*. 2015;47:2413-2418.

339. Perito ER, Rhee S, Roberts JP, et al. Pediatric liver transplantation for urea cycle disorders and organic acidemias: United Network for Organ Sharing data for 2002–2012. *Liver Transpl*. 2014;20:89-99.

340. Tuchman M, Mauer SM, Holzknecht RA, et al. Prospective versus clinical diagnosis and therapy of acute neonatal hyperammonaemia in 2 sisters with carbamyl phosphate synthetase deficiency. *J Inherit Metab Dis*. 1992;15:269-277.

344. Platt LD, Koch R, Azen C, et al. Maternal phenylketonuria collaborative study, obstetric aspects and outcome—the first six years. *Am J Obstet Gynecol*. 1992;166:1150-1162.

345. Scriver CR, Kaufman S. Hyperphenylalaninemia: phenylalanine hydroxylase deficiency. In: Schriver CR, Beaudet AL, Sly WS, et al., eds. *The Metabolic and Molecular Bases of Inherited Disease*. Vol. 2. 8th ed. New York: McGraw-Hill; 2001:1667-1724.

***Full references for this chapter can be found on www.expertconsult
.com.***

Organic Acids

Jeffrey M. Perlman ♦ *Joseph J. Volpe*

A series of metabolic disorders with prominent neurological accompaniments and serious deleterious effects on the developing central nervous system have been described under the designation *organic acid disorders*. The term *organic acid* is particularly imprecise but, unfortunately, appears to be firmly entrenched in the medical literature. Strictly speaking, organic acids should include amino acids, fatty acids, ketoacids, and a variety of other endogenous and exogenous acids. Disorders of amino acids are discussed in Chapter 27. In this chapter, the disorders of organic acids that are associated with prominent neurological phenomena in the neonatal period *and* that have been reported in more than a few infants are discussed.

OVERVIEW OF MAJOR ORGANIC ACID DISORDERS AND NEONATAL METABOLIC ACIDOSIS

The organic acid disorders enumerated in Table 28.1 are important causes of severe neonatal metabolic acidosis. The major acids that accumulate vary according to the site of the metabolic defect, as outlined subsequently. Lactic acidosis is a very frequent accompaniment. A simplified scheme for the differential diagnosis of neonatal lactic acidosis is shown in Fig. 28.1. In the following sections, the disorders of metabolism of propionate and methylmalonate, pyruvate, and branched-chain ketoacids are discussed. The rare other organic acid disorders and a fatty acid oxidation disorder (see Table 28.1) are described briefly at the conclusion of the chapter. The mitochondrial disorders are discussed in Chapter 29. The disorders of carbohydrate metabolism listed in Table 28.1 and renal tubular acidosis either manifest clinically only rarely in the neonatal period or exhibit primarily nonneurological syndromes and are not reviewed further.

DISORDERS OF PROPIONATE AND METHYLMALONATE METABOLISM

Disorders of propionate and methylmalonate metabolism are uncommon but result in serious neonatal neurological disturbances. These disorders are the most common of the so-called organic acid abnormalities. In an earlier large series (105 cases) of patients with organic acidurias with neonatal onset, disorders of propionate and methylmalonate metabolism accounted for 40% of the total.[1] Later reported experiences have been similar.[2-4] These diseases share certain common features (Table 28.2).

Normal Metabolic Aspects

Propionate and methylmalonate are vital intermediates in the catabolism of lipid and protein.[5] The major pathway of the metabolism of propionate and methylmalonate is shown in Fig. 28.2. Although propionyl–coenzyme A (CoA) formation from isoleucine catabolism is depicted, this organic acid is also the product of the catabolism of valine, methionine, threonine, cholesterol (side chain), and odd-chain fatty acids.[5] Involved in the propionate and methylmalonate pathway are two vitamins, biotin and vitamin B_{12}. Biotin is the coenzyme for propionyl-CoA carboxylase, and adenosyl cobalamin (a derivative of vitamin B_{12}) is the coenzyme for methylmalonyl-CoA mutase. Indeed, some of the disorders of this pathway are responsive to large doses of these vitamins (see later section). The product of the pathway, succinyl-CoA, enters the tricarboxylic acid cycle, where pyruvate is formed from reaction with oxaloacetate.

Certain alternate and minor metabolic pathways are important in understanding the disorders of this pathway (see Fig. 28.2). Thus, propionyl-CoA also can be metabolized to lactate and can be used in the synthesis of odd-numbered fatty acids. Methylmalonyl-CoA can be used in the synthesis of methyl-branched fatty acids.

Biochemical Aspects of Disordered Metabolism
Enzymatic Defects and Essential Consequences
The enzymes affected in the disorders of propionate and methylmalonate metabolism are shown in Fig. 28.2. The resulting metabolic consequences (e.g., acidosis, hyperammonemia, and hyperglycinemia) are diverse, and their pathogeneses are now understood to a considerable degree.

Acidosis
The acidosis in disorders of propionate and methylmalonate metabolism results, at least in part, from the accumulation of the acids proximal to the primary enzymatic blocks. However, the degree of acidosis is often greater than can be accounted for by these compounds. Other sources of acidemia include conversion of excessive propionate to lactate by a normally minor metabolic pathway (see Fig. 28.2), inhibition of pyruvate dehydrogenase[5] with resulting increased conversion of pyruvate to lactate, and accumulation of ketone bodies by poorly understood mechanisms.

Hyperammonemia
The *hyperammonemia* that is a nearly consistent feature of the neonatal varieties of propionate and methylmalonate

disturbances appears to result from two closely related mechanisms.[5-7] Both relate to an accumulation of the CoA esters of the acids proximal to the enzymatic blocks (particularly propionyl-CoA, tiglyl-CoA [a metabolite of isoleucine], and methylmalonyl-CoA) and to the effects of these derivatives on the activity of carbamyl phosphate synthetase, the first step in the Krebs–Henseleit urea cycle (see Chapter 27). Thus these CoA esters have been shown to have a direct inhibitory effect on carbamyl phosphate synthetase and an indirect inhibitory effect at this step by inhibiting the synthesis of *N*-acetylglutamate, the important activator of carbamyl phosphate synthetase. Hyperammonemia and acidosis have major deleterious effects on the brain (see Chapter 27) and are thought to be major determinants of the acute neurological dysfunction and brain injury that result in the neonatal period.

Hyperglycinemia

A striking aspect of propionate and methylmalonate metabolism is *hyperglycinemia*. This condition is unlike the nonketotic hyperglycinemia described in Chapter 27 because of the association of ketoacidosis (i.e., ketotic vs. nonketotic hyperglycinemia) and because the glycine abnormality is a secondary and not a primary metabolic phenomenon. Analogous to the cause of the hyperammonemia in these disorders of

---

TABLE 28.1 Major Causes of Metabolic Acidosis in the Neonatal Period

Disorders of propionate-methylmalonate metabolism
- Propionic acidemia
- Methylmalonic acidemia

Disorders of pyruvate and mitochondrial energy metabolism
- Pyruvate dehydrogenase deficiency
- Pyruvate carboxylase deficiency
- Defects of the electron transport chain (complexes I, IV, V)

Disorders of branched-chain amino acid–ketoacid metabolism
- Maple syrup urine disease
- Isovaleric acidemia
- beta-Methylcrotonyl–CoA carboxylase deficiency
- beta-Ketothiolase deficiency
- Hydroxymethylglutaryl-CoA lyase deficiency
- Mevalonic aciduria

Disorders of fatty acid metabolism
- Medium-chain acyl–CoA dehydrogenase deficiency

Other organic acid disorders
- Multiple carboxylase deficiency
- Glutaric acidemia, type II
- Glutathione synthetase deficiency (5-oxoprolinuria)
- Sulfite oxidase deficiency (molybdenum cofactor deficiency)

Disorders of carbohydrate metabolism
- Galactosemia
- Glycogen storage disease, type I (von Gierke glucose-6-phosphatase deficiency)
- Fructose-1,6-diphosphatase deficiency
- Phosphoenolpyruvate carboxykinase deficiency

Renal tubular acidosis

CoA, Coenzyme A.

TABLE 28.2 Common Features of Disorders of Propionate and Methylmalonate Metabolism

Clinical features
- Vomiting
- Tachypnea
- Stupor, coma
- Seizures

Metabolic features
- Acidosis
- Propionic acidemia ± methylmalonic acidemia
- Hyperglycinemia
- Hyperammonemia

Other features
- Neutropenia, anemia, thrombocytopenia

Neuropathological features
- Myelin disturbance
- Basal ganglia injury (caudate, putamen in propionic acidemia; globus pallidus in methylmalonic acidemia)
- Cerebral cortical atrophy (later)

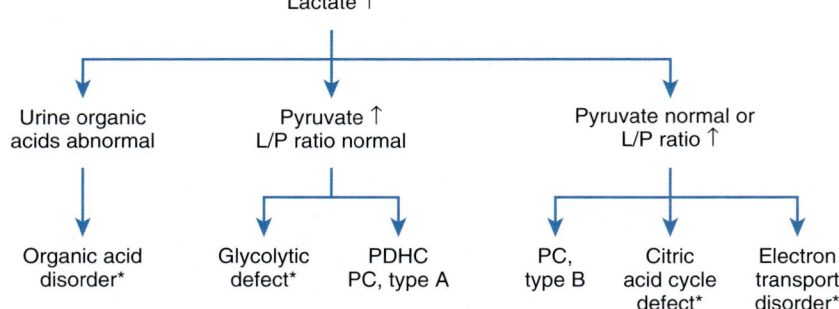

Figure 28.1 Simplified scheme for the differential diagnosis of neonatal lactic acidosis. Note the critical initial role of determinations of urine organic acids and blood lactate and pyruvate levels and ratio. *L/P ratio,* Lactate-to-pyruvate ratio; *PC,* pyruvate carboxylase (deficiency); *PDHC,* pyruvate dehydrogenase complex (deficiency). *Organic acid disorders: propionic acidemia, methylmalonic acidemia, isovaleric acidemia, multiple carboxylase deficiency, fatty acid oxidation defects, among others. *Glycolytic defects: glucose-6-phosphatase, fructose-1,6-diphosphatase, phosphoenolpyruvate carboxykinase deficiencies. *Citric acid cycle defects: fumarase and succinate dehydrogenase deficiencies. *Electron transport disorders: see the section on mitochondrial disorders in Chapter 29.

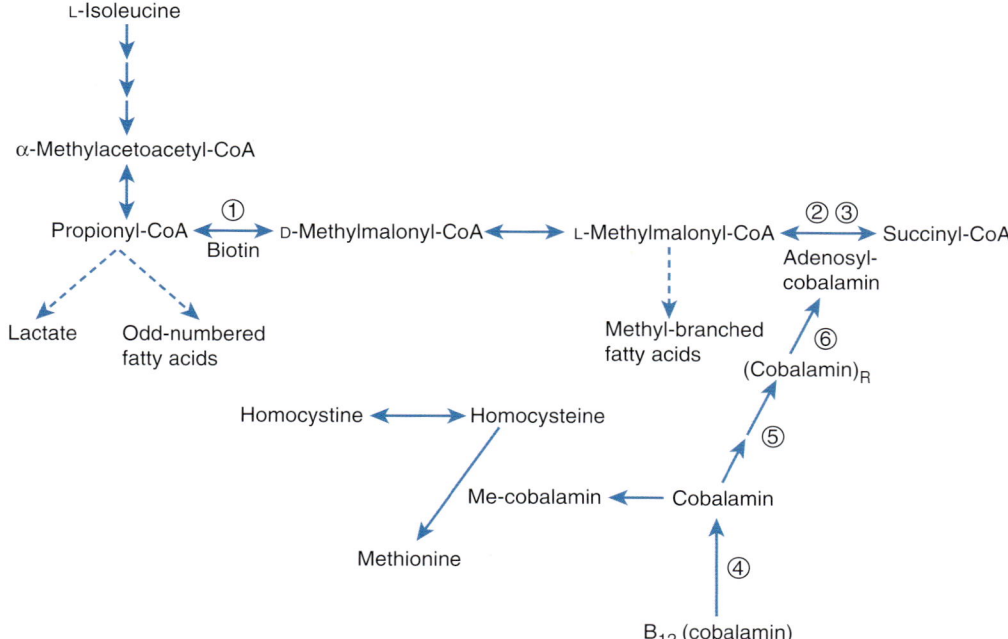

Figure 28.2 Metabolism of propionate and methylmalonate and sites of defects in their metabolism.
Major pathways are shown by solid arrows, and alternate minor pathways by broken arrows. Sites of defects are numbered and include *(1)* propionyl–coenzyme A (CoA) carboxylase, *(2)* and *(3)* methylmalonyl-CoA mutase (two different structural defects), *(4)* cobalamin binding, internalization, lysosomal release and cytosolic reduction, *(5)* mitochondrial cobalamin reductase, and *(6)* mitochondrial adenosyltransferase. See text for details. (Adapted from Fenton WA, Gravel RA, Rosenblatt DS. Disorders of propionate and methylmalonate metabolism. In: Schriver CR, Beaudet AL, Sly WS, et al., eds. *The Metabolic & Molecular Bases of Inherited Disease.* 8th ed. New York: McGraw-Hill; 2001.)

the propionate and methylmalonate pathway, the cause of the hyperglycinemia appears related to an inhibition of glycine cleavage by the accumulation of branched-chain alpha-ketoacids and, more specifically, their CoA derivatives.

A disturbance of glycine cleavage was demonstrated indirectly and directly in studies of patients *with ketotic hyperglycinemia* caused by deficiencies of propionyl-CoA carboxylase and methylmalonyl-CoA mutase, as well as of isovaleryl-CoA dehydrogenase and beta-ketothiolase (the last two disorders of branched-chain amino acid metabolism are discussed later).[8,9] Analyses of the individual protein components of the glycine cleavage system of patients with propionic acidemia and methylmalonic acidemia have shown that the H-protein, one of the four proteins of the system, is the component initially inactivated.[10]

That *the impairment of glycine metabolism* involves the inhibition of the glycine cleavage system *by CoA derivatives* of accumulated metabolites is suggested by data based on studies of rat liver.[11] In vitro studies of the solubilized hepatic glycine cleavage system show marked inhibition by CoA derivatives found in the catabolic pathway for isoleucine. Such derivatives would be expected to accumulate in the disorders of the propionate and methylmalonate pathway (see Fig. 28.2). Coupled with the data referable to the genesis of the hyperammonemia, these observations suggest that the *CoA derivatives of the accumulated organic acids* are responsible for the major critical secondary metabolic effects that accompany the primary enzymatic disorders.

Myelin Disturbance and Fatty Acid Abnormalities

In the disorders associated with the accumulation of propionic and methylmalonic acids, *a disturbance of myelin*, detectable by neuropathological examination (see "Neuropathology"), appears to be important in the genesis of the neurological sequelae.[12,13] Vacuolation of myelin appears in the first months of life and is followed by an apparent disturbance of myelin formation.[12,14] The magnetic resonance imaging (MRI) correlate of the myelin disturbance, present in many reported cases (see later), is, acutely, diffusely swollen T2-hyperintense cerebral white matter, followed later by white matter atrophy. The genesis of the myelin disturbance is not clear but may be related to changes in the fatty acid composition of oligodendroglial membranes. Distinct changes exist in the composition of fatty acids in the brains of patients with disorders resulting in the accumulation of propionate or methylmalonate,[15,16] and these changes can be reproduced in cultured rat glial cells.[17] The major alterations are increases in the amounts of *odd-numbered and methyl-branched fatty acids* (see later). These increases have been demonstrated in phospholipids (i.e., components of all cellular membranes) as well as in myelin lipids (e.g., cerebrosides and sulfatides; Table 28.3).[16] Because the fatty acid composition of membrane lipids is important for not only for structural integrity but also the function of a variety of membrane proteins (e.g., enzymes, transport carriers, surface receptors),[18] these alterations may have major implications for the genesis of neurological dysfunction and the disturbance of myelination.

TABLE 28.3 Fatty Acid Composition of Brain Lipids With Disorder of Propionate-Methylmalonate Metabolism

BRAIN LIPID CLASS	ODD-NUMBERED FATTY ACIDS		METHYL-BRANCHED FATTY ACIDS	
	CONTROL (%)	PATIENT (%)[a]	CONTROL (%)	PATIENT (%)[a]
Choline phospholipid	Trace	9.8	—	2.1
Sphingomyelin	7.5	18.2	—	—
Cerebroside	18.9	29.0	—	—
Sulfatide	21.7	31.1	—	—

[a]Child with methylmalonic aciduria.

Data from Ramsey RB, Scott T, Banik NL. Fatty acid composition of myelin isolated from the brain of patient with cellular deficiency of co-enzyme forms of vitamin B_{12}. *J Neurol Sci.* 1977;34:221–232.

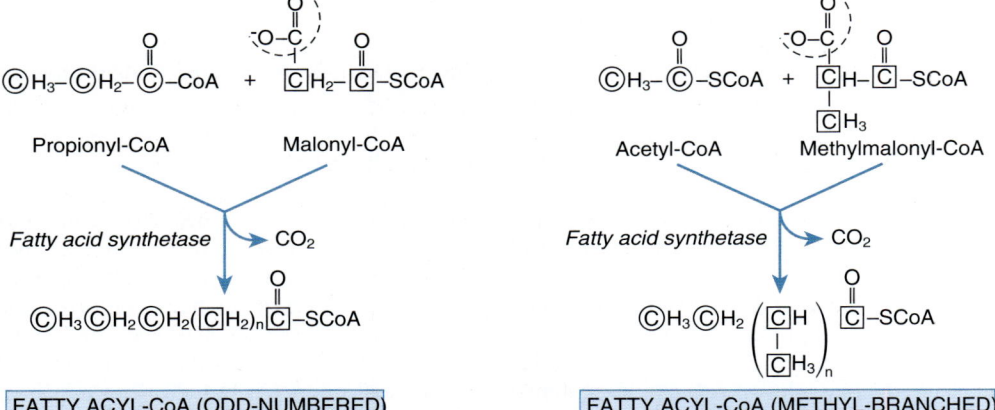

Figure 28.3 Disturbances of fatty acid synthesis in disorders of propionate and methylmalonate metabolism. Under *normal conditions*, the enzyme complex fatty acid synthetase catalyzes the addition of two-carbon fragments from malonyl–coenzyme A (CoA) to the single primer molecule of acetyl-CoA to form even-numbered fatty acids. With *propionyl-CoA accumulation*, this three-carbon compound replaces acetyl-CoA as primer, and therefore with the addition of the two-carbon fragments from malonyl-CoA, odd-numbered fatty acids result. With *methylmalonyl-CoA accumulation*, this branched compound replaces malonyl-CoA, and therefore methyl-branched fatty acids result.

Disturbances of Fatty Acid Synthesis

The fatty acid abnormalities described in the previous section are presumably caused by disturbances of fatty acid synthesis. The nature of the disturbances observed in disorders of propionate and methylmalonate metabolism is depicted in Fig. 28.3. Thus, under normal circumstances, de novo synthesis of fatty acids in brain is catalyzed by the multienzyme complex fatty acid synthetase.[19,20] The first two carbons (i.e., the primer) of the resulting even-numbered fatty acids (primarily the 16-carbon acid, palmitic acid) are derived from acetyl-CoA, whereas the remaining carbons for chain elongation are derived from the two-carbon units obtained from malonyl-CoA (see Fig. 28.3). *When propionyl-CoA is present in excessive amounts,* it can replace acetyl-CoA with a three-carbon fragment as primer; thus an odd-numbered fatty acid results after the addition of the two-carbon units from malonyl-CoA (see Fig. 28.3). *When methylmalonyl-CoA is present in excessive amounts, it can replace malonyl-CoA; thus a methyl-branched unit is derived from malonyl-CoA, resulting in methyl-branched fatty acids* (see Fig. 28.3). These unusual fatty acids are incorporated into cellular membranes, including myelin, as discussed in the previous section.

Propionic Acidemia and Propionyl–Coenzyme A Carboxylase Deficiency

Propionic acidemia is caused by a defect in the first step of the pathway from propionyl-CoA to succinyl-CoA, a step catalyzed by the enzyme propionyl–CoA carboxylase.

Clinical Features

Onset is in the first days of life, with a dramatic clinical syndrome consisting primarily of vomiting, stupor, tachypnea, and seizures (see Table 28.2).[4,5,21-23] The usual time of onset is the second to fourth days of life.[23,24] Infants whose condition is not diagnosed and treated properly rapidly lapse into coma and die. Indeed, in earlier studies, approximately 75% of patients died in early infancy.[2] More recent improvements in management have resulted in improved survival rates.[24] In one series of six infants, all survived the neonatal period. Lethal cerebellar hemorrhage, occurring in association with thrombocytopenia and hyperosmolar bicarbonate therapy, has occasionally been observed in the neonatal period.[25] Survivors of the neonatal period are prone to episodic attacks of vomiting and stupor, with severe ketoacidosis, often precipitated by infection, and to subsequent retardation of neurological development. Of 11 infants reported in one series, no survivor had an intelligence quotient (IQ) higher than 60.[23] In a later series of 38 infants, 95% had "cognitive and neurologic" deficits.[2] In a recent report, the clinical and outcome data of 55 surviving patients with propionic acidemia was evaluated retrospectively (Fig. 28.4). The vast majority of patients (>85%) presented with metabolic decompensation in the neonatal period. Approximately 75% of the study population was mentally retarded, with a median IQ of 55.[3] Chorea or dystonia has been observed in 20% to 40% of surviving children, and such extrapyramidal involvement is common in this disorder (see later discussion of neuropathology).[23,26,27] The genetic data for this disorder indicate *autosomal recessive* inheritance. This conclusion is based in part on the pattern of familial occurrence, partial disturbance of enzymatic activity in parents, and complementation testing of cells in culture.[4,5]

Metabolic Features

Major Findings. The constellation of ketoacidosis, propionic acidemia, hyperglycinemia (and hyperglycinuria), hyperammonemia, neutropenia, anemia, and thrombopenia is characteristic and composes the *ketotic hyperglycinemia syndrome*.[2,5] However, hyperglycinemia with propionic acidemia and propionyl-CoA carboxylase deficiency has occurred in the neonatal period without consistent ketonuria.[28] This finding is important because patients with disorders of propionate and methylmalonate metabolism should be managed differently from those with the more common nonketotic hyperglycinemia described in Chapter 27.

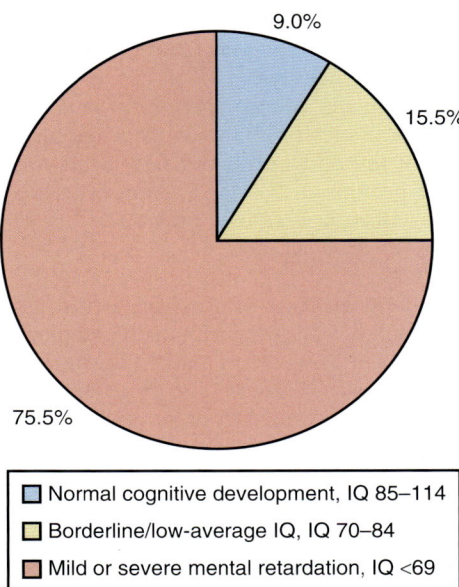

Figure 28.4 Neurocognitive outcome in 45 patients with propionic acidemia. Intelligence quotient (IQ) data were determined for 40 patients, 5 patients could not be tested due to severe cognitive impairment. The last 5 patients were classified with an IQ <69. (From Grunert SC, et al. Propionic acidemia: clinical course and outcome in 55 pediatric and adolescent patients. *Orphanet J Rare Dis.* 2013;8:P6.)

Enzymatic Defect. The enzymatic defect involves propionyl-CoA carboxylase.[5,29] Structural alterations of the two nonidentical subunits (alpha and beta) of the carboxylase molecules account for the enzymatic defect.[5] The enzyme contains four copies each of the alpha and beta subunits, with the gene for the alpha subunit encoded on chromosome 13 and the gene for the beta subunit encoded on chromosome 3.[5] Because this enzyme requires biotin for activity, the possibility of a defect in activation or binding of biotin to the carboxylase apoprotein as the basis of the disturbed activity in certain patients must be considered. The initial observation of a beneficial response of one patient to large amounts of biotin suggested that such an additional defect may occur.[30] The delineation of impaired activity of propionyl-CoA carboxylase (as well as of other carboxylases) in two disorders of biotin metabolism, holocarboxylase synthetase deficiency and biotinidase deficiency, corroborated this suggestion (see later discussion). However, only one of these disorders (holocarboxylase synthetase deficiency) consistently causes prominent clinical phenomena in the newborn, as discussed later.

Pathogenesis of Metabolic Features. The genesis of the various metabolic consequences of this disorder is now understood to a considerable degree. The origins of the *hyperglycinemia* and the *hyperammonemia* relate to the secondary effects of the CoA derivatives of certain of the accumulated metabolites on the pathways of glycine cleavage and ammonia detoxification by the urea cycle (see earlier discussion). The *acidosis* must relate to several factors (i.e., accumulation of the propionic acid proximal to the primary enzymatic block, of lactate produced by the alternate pathway of propionate degradation, and of the various acids that accumulate proximal to propionic acid as a consequence of continuing degradation of branched-chain and other amino acids).

Increased numbers of *odd-numbered fatty acids* have been observed in the tissues of infants with propionic acidemia.[16] The genesis of the odd-numbered fatty acids relates to the utilization of propionyl-CoA as a primer for the fatty acid synthetase reaction, as described previously (see Fig. 28.3).

Neuropathology

A well-studied *neonatal* case of propionic acidemia involved a 1-month-old patient.[12] The dominant neuropathological findings involved myelin and consisted of marked *vacuolation*, with a less striking *diminution* of the amount of myelin. Similar pathological findings have been described in other affected cases.[13,14] The disturbance of myelin is similar to that noted in nonketotic hyperglycinemia and other aminoacidopathies (see Chapter 27). Vacuolation appears to be the early change, occurring principally in systems actively myelinating at the time of the illness (e.g., medial lemniscus, superior cerebellar peduncle, posterior columns, and peripheral nerve in the 1-month-old patient of Shuman and coworkers[12]) (Fig. 28.5). The impaired myelination appears to occur subsequent to the vacuolation.[12] Vacuolation has been observed in oligodendrocytes in areas just

before myelination.[14] The cause of this defect in myelination in ketotic hyperglycinemia may relate to the disturbance of fatty acid synthesis and the resultant altered fatty acid composition of myelin (see earlier discussion). Thus the odd-numbered fatty acids may alter the stability of the oligodendroglial-myelin membrane, thereby impairing oligodendroglial differentiation and rendering the newly formed myelin unstable. Vacuolation and the subsequent deficit of myelin would result. Other possibilities, such as disturbance of synthesis of myelin proteins because of the amino acid imbalance (e.g., the elevated glycine levels) must be considered as well.[12]

An interesting additional feature of the neuropathology of propionic acidemia is the *prominence of involvement of the basal ganglia* in patients who survive for several or more years.[31,32] Thus neuronal loss and gliosis are prominent and, in one case, the addition of aberrant myelin bundles caused a *marbled* appearance, reminiscent of status marmoratus of perinatal asphyxia. In contrast to methylmalonic acidemia (see later), caudate and putamen, rather than globus pallidus, are preferentially involved.[33] The importance of excitotoxicity in the basal ganglia neuronal injury and the potential role of glycine in the genesis of excitotoxic neuronal injury (see discussion of nonketotic hyperglycinemia in Chapter 27) are of interest in this context.[34,35] The involvement of basal ganglia in

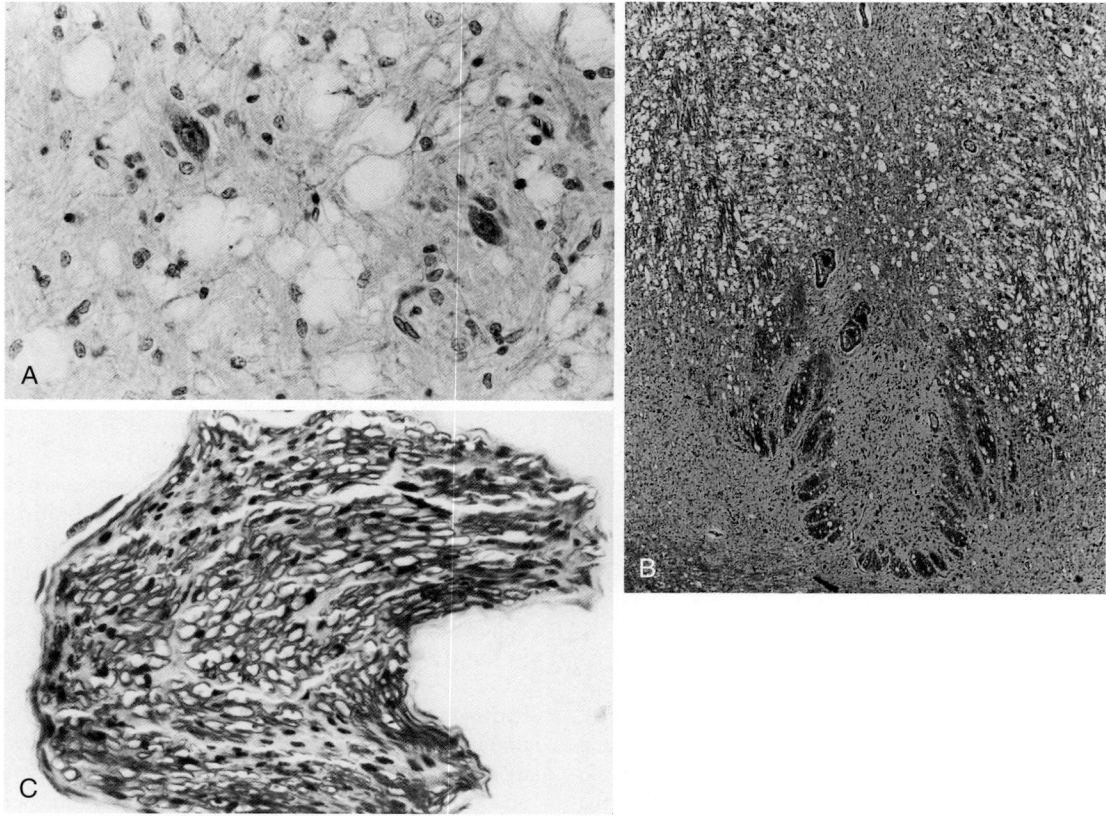

Figure 28.5 Myelin disturbance in propionic acidemia in a 26-day-old infant who exhibited lethargy, poor feeding, tachypnea, profound metabolic acidosis in the first week of life, and generalized seizures in the third week. (A) Vacuolation of myelinated fibers traversing the globus pallidus. (B) Vacuolation of the medial longitudinal fasciculus just rostral to the trochlear nucleus. (C) Demyelination and endoneurial fibrosis of a mixed spinal nerve of the lumbosacral plexus. (From Shuman RM, Leech RW, Scott CR. The neuropathology of the nonketotic and ketotic hyperglycinemias: three cases. *Neurology.* 1978;28:139–146.)

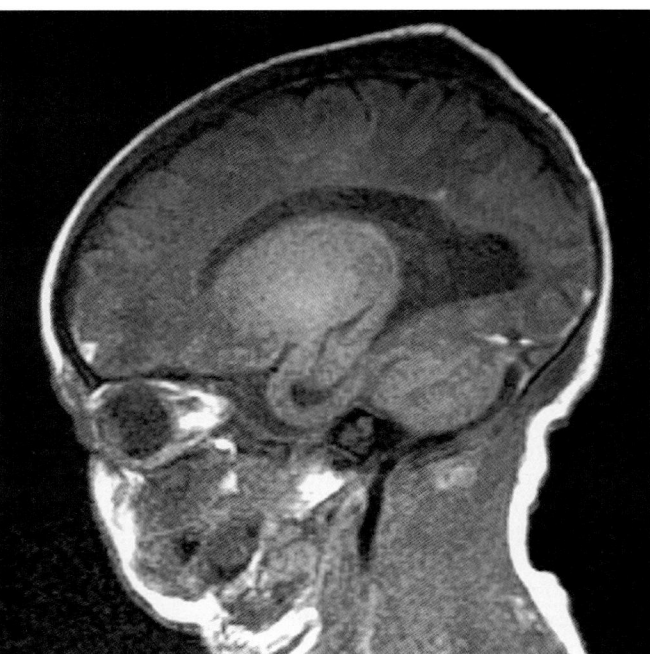

Figure 28.6 Propionic acidemia, magnetic resonance imaging (MRI) scan. An infant with severe lactic acidosis was scanned on the sixth day of life. This T1-weighted MRI scan shows absence of the corpus callosum. (Courtesy Dr. Omar Khwaja.)

older infants and children has been documented repeatedly by brain imaging.[22] Finally, this derangement of basal ganglia may underlie the relative frequency of extrapyramidal movement disorders observed subsequently in infants with propionic acidemia.[23] Cerebral cortical atrophy is noted in survivors of several years or more.[33,36]

As with several other metabolic disorders in which the enzymatic defect is present in brain (see later), agenesis or hypoplasia of the corpus callosum may result (Fig. 28.6). Indeed, the presence of callosal abnormalities without an obvious syndromic or other cause should raise the possibility of a metabolic disorder.

Management

Antenatal Diagnosis. Antenatal diagnosis has been accomplished by measuring propionyl-CoA carboxylase activity chorionic villus samples, by analyzing metabolites in amniotic fluid, and by molecular genetic testing of DNA extracted from fetal cells.[4,5,37] Thus the possibility of preventing the disorder is real.

Early Detection. Early diagnosis, particularly in distinguishing this disorder from other causes of severe metabolic acidosis in the neonatal period (see Table 28.1), is critical. Identification of the accompanying metabolic features is particularly valuable in this regard. Organic acid analysis of urine by tandem mass spectrometry is especially useful.[38] Recent evidence suggests that heptadecanoylcarnitine (C17) is a novel biomarker specific for the identification of patients with propionic acidemia and methyl malonic aciduria. Thus 21 out of 23 neonates (22 with methylmalonic aciduria, and 1 with propionic acidemia) exhibited significantly higher levels of C17 compared with controls.[39] Definitive diagnosis is established by measurement of propionyl-CoA carboxylase activity in leukocytes or cultured fibroblasts.[40]

Acute and Long-Term Therapy. Acute episodes should be treated by withdrawing all protein and administering sodium bicarbonate parenterally. Hyperammonemia may be severe enough to require specific measures for ammonia removal, such as hemolysis, as described in Chapter 27. Subsequently, a low-protein diet (restricted especially in isoleucine, valine, methionine, and threonine) is administered.[5,21] The use of gastrostomy feeding to guarantee nutritional intake has been valuable.[21] Supplementation with L-carnitine may be indicated, because the excretion of carnitine as propionyl carnitine may lead to decreased plasma levels of free carnitine, and supplementation with carnitine has produced beneficial clinical and metabolic responses in isolated patients.[5,21] Oral antibiotic therapy to reduce propionate production by bacteria in the gastrointestinal tract may also be useful later.[5,21]

Biotin. Because some biochemical benefit was observed in an infant treated with biotin, large doses of this vitamin are worthy of a trial in affected patients.[21,30] Biotin responsiveness should be assessed by observation of changes in metabolite levels in blood and urine and in enzyme activity in white blood cells. The effect of biotin in vitro on the enzyme in cultured fibroblasts may be useful in determining the likelihood of a beneficial response in vivo.[13,41] Marked biotin responsiveness is characteristic of multiple carboxylase deficiency (see later discussion).

Gene Therapy. Liver transplantation early in infancy may be of value in the management of neonatal-onset propionic acidemia.[4] Initial mortality rates after transplantation exceeded 50%; thus the number of infants followed sufficiently long after transplant is small. Moreover, in a recent report of 12 treated patients with propionic acidemia, mortality was still high (58%). When cardiomyopathy was present before transplantation, it resolved; but renal failure, present in 50% of the patients before transplantation, worsened in all following transplantation.[42] A beneficial effect on neurological development remains to be defined.

Methylmalonic Acidemias

Methylmalonic acidemias constitute the single most frequent group of organic disorders.[4,5] The accumulation of large quantities of methylmalonic acid in blood and urine is associated with at least five discrete metabolic defects (see Fig. 28.2): (1 and 2) defects of methylmalonyl-CoA mutase (two different defects of the mutase apoenzyme, one resulting in complete deficiency and the other in partial deficiency of the mutase), (3 and 4) defects in the synthesis of adenosylcobalamin, and (5) defective synthesis of both adenosylcobalamin and methylcobalamin (Table 28.4).[4,5,43] The last three defects of vitamin B_{12} metabolism result in diminished activity of methylmalonyl-CoA mutase, for which adenosylcobalamin is a coenzyme. In addition, the last of these defects also results in diminished activity of the methyltransferase required for methylation of homocysteine; the formation of the methyltransferase requires methylcobalamin. In one series of 45 carefully studied patients with methylmalonic acidemia (without homocystinuria), 15 had complete mutase deficiency, 5 had partial mutase deficiency, 14 had deficient

TABLE 28.4   Methylmalonic Acidemias: Biochemical and Metabolic Features[a]

	METABOLIC ACCUMULATION	
DEFECTIVE ENZYME	METHYLMALONIC ACID	HOMOCYSTEINE
Methylmalonic acid mutase	+	−
Mitochondrial cobalamin reductase (cblA)	+	−
Mitochondrial cobalamin adenosyltransferase (cblB)	+	−
Abnormal lysosomal or cytosolic cobalamin metabolism (cblC, cblD, cblF)	+	+

[a]See text for references.

TABLE 28.5   Time of Onset and Outcome in Methylmalonic Acidemias According to Type of Metabolic Defect

	METABOLIC DEFECT			
ONSET OR OUTCOME	mut•	mut⁻	cblA	cblB
Age at onset				
0–7 days	80%	40%	42%	33%
8–30 days	7%	20%	—	22%
>30 days	13%	40%	58%	55%
Outcome				
Dead	60%	40%	8%	30%
Impaired	40%	20%	23%	40%
Well	—	40%	69%	30%

cblA, Deficiency of mitochondrial cobalamin reductase; cblB, deficiency of cobalamin adenosyltransferase; mut•, complete mutase deficiency; mut⁻, partial mutase deficiency.

Data from Rosenberg LE, Fenton WA. Disorders of propionate and methylmalonate metabolism. In: Scriver CR, Beaudet AL, Sly WS, et al., eds. The Metabolic Basis of Inherited Disease. 6th ed. New York: McGraw-Hill; 1989.

mitochondrial cobalamin reductase, and 11 had deficient cobalamin adenosyltransferase (the latter two defects resulting in defective synthesis of adenosylcobalamin).[44] These disorders are discussed collectively.

Clinical Features

The clinical features are similar to those noted for disorders of propionate metabolism (i.e., vomiting, stupor, tachypnea, and seizures; see Table 28.2).[21] Onset of these features in the neonatal period depends on the nature of the enzymatic defect (Table 28.5). Neonatal onset is most likely with complete mutase deficiency, and nearly all neonates with this severe enzymatic lesion present in the first 7 days of life. Fewer than half of all patients with the other three metabolic defects present in the first 7 days. The outcome also is related to the type of metabolic defect (see Table 28.5). The gravity of outcome correlates approximately with the frequency of neonatal onset. Thus infants with complete mutase deficiency nearly invariably die or exhibit subsequent neurological impairment. In earlier series, mortality rates for such patients were approximately 60%, although in more recent series, approximately 30% of

infants have died.[4,5] In a series of 35 infants, of whom 6 were cobalamin-responsive and 29 were cobalamin-nonresponsive (20 were early-onset and 9 late-onset cases), the median range of subsequent full-scale IQ score was 100 for the cobalamin-responsive, 75 for the early-onset cases, and 101 for late-onset non–cobalamin responsive patients, respectively.[45] One infant with severe mutase deficiency detected at 3 weeks of age by neonatal screening was reported to be normal at the age of 5 years after treatment with a low-protein diet.[46] Patients with methylmalonic acidemias who survive are subject to episodic decompensation, especially with minor intercurrent infections. *Brain imaging* reveals the abnormalities of myelin, as noted earlier for propionic acidemia. Involvement of basal ganglia, similarly, is very common, but in the case of methylmalonic acidemia, it involves the *globus pallidus* rather than the caudate/putamen, as in propionic acidemia.[33,47]

The smaller number of infants, approximately 35, reported with a defect in cobalamin metabolism characterized by impaired synthesis of *both* methylcobalamin *and* adenosylcobalamin (see Table 28.4) (see the next section, "Metabolic Features") and onset in the first month of life also had a generally unfavorable neurological outcome (not shown in Table 28.5).[48,49] The clinical and neuroradiological features were similar, albeit milder than those observed in patients with the mutase deficiencies, and the metabolic features included *homocystinuria* as well as methylmalonic acidemia. At least 80% subsequently exhibited major developmental deficits, and completely normal intellectual functioning was very unusual. Available genetic data indicate that these disorders all exhibit *autosomal recessive* inheritance.[5]

Metabolic Features

Major Findings. The constellation of severe ketoacidosis, methylmalonic acidemia, hyperglycinemia, hyperammonemia, neutropenia, and thrombopenia is characteristic. Approximately 40% of neonatal patients have also exhibited significant hypoglycemia with their attacks of ketoacidosis.[21]

As noted earlier, approximately 35 infants were observed with a genetic defect resulting in impaired synthesis of *both* methylcobalamin and adenosylcobalamin and the additional metabolic feature of homocysteinemia/homocystinuria.[5,48,49] However, unlike the classic homocystinuria resulting from cystathionine synthase deficiency (which is associated with elevated levels of methionine and depressed levels of cystathionine), this type is associated with *hypomethioninemia and cystathioninuria* (the product of homocysteine and serine) (see Fig. 28.2).

Enzymatic Defects. The enzymatic defects in methylmalonic acidemias involve the methylmalonyl-CoA mutase apoenzyme (two major defects) and the metabolism of vitamin B_{12} (three major defects), as noted in the introduction to this section (see Table 28.4). The defects have been demonstrated primarily in liver and in cultured fibroblasts.[4,5,50,51]

The two major defects of the mutase apoenzyme result, as noted earlier, in either complete or partial deficiency of enzyme activity. In most reported examples of complete deficiency of mutase activity, little or no immunoreactive enzyme protein was present.[5,52] In the cases with partial deficiency of activity, a presumably altered enzyme with defective catalytic function was present, because the amount of immunologically reactive protein varied from 20% to 100% of control values.[5,52]

The three major sites of the defects in vitamin B_{12} metabolism are shown in Fig. 28.2. Under normal circumstances, vitamin B_{12}, bound to a carrier protein, is internalized by the cell through endocytosis; the endosome is taken up by the lysosome, proteases of which degrade the carrier protein, and the cobalamin is released into the cytosol, where reduction and methylation take place. A portion of the cobalamin released into the cytosol enters the mitochondrion for reduction and adenosylation. The defect that results in impaired synthesis of both methylcobalamin and adenosylcobalamin involves an event after binding and internalization (i.e., after cellular uptake).[5] The defects of vitamin B_{12} metabolism have been defined through studies of cultured fibroblasts from affected patients.[5,53,54]

Pathogenesis of Metabolic Features. The causes of the various metabolic consequences of the methylmalonic acidemias are similar in many ways to those described for other disorders in the propionate and methylmalonate pathway, especially regarding the *hyperglycinemia* and the *hyperammonemia*. The *ketoacidosis* is not as readily accounted for because it is more severe than would be expected from the accumulation of methylmalonic acid. Methylmalonyl-CoA is an inhibitor of pyruvate carboxylase, and its product, succinyl-CoA, is involved in gluconeogenesis by conversion to pyruvate (see earlier discussion). Together, these effects could lead to an impairment of gluconeogenesis to account for the *hypoglycemia* in nearly half of the neonatal cases and, secondarily, to increased catabolism of lipid, with resultant ketosis and acidosis.[55]

The accumulation of *odd-numbered and methyl-branched fatty acids* in neural and other tissues of affected patients[16] relates, respectively, to substitution of propionyl-CoA for acetyl-CoA as primer for the fatty acid synthetase reaction and to the substitution of methylmalonyl-CoA for malonyl-CoA for chain elongation in the same reaction (see Fig. 28.3). The genesis of the defects of sulfur amino acid metabolism in the disorder with impaired synthesis of both methylcobalamin and adenosylcobalamin relates to a disturbance of the methylation of homocysteine to form methionine; the enzyme for this reaction, methionine synthase, requires methylcobalamin (see Fig. 28.2). The consequences of the disturbance of homocysteine methylation, as noted earlier, are *homocystinuria, hypomethioninemia,* and *cystathioninuria*, the last resulting because some of the accumulated homocysteine is converted to cystathionine.

Neuropathology

The neuropathological features of the methylmalonic acidemias suggest a derangement of myelination.[56,57] An abnormality of myelin with features similar to those described for propionic acidemia has been observed.[58] Particular involvement of spinal nerve roots rather than central myelin was noted in one premature infant studied.[56] Whether the myelin defect relates to the abnormal accumulation of odd-numbered and methyl-branched fatty acids in glial membranes, as discussed earlier, remains to be established.

A carefully studied infant of 36 weeks of gestation (death at 4 days of age) exhibited selective death of immature neurons (i.e., residual neuronal cells in germinal matrix), migrating neuroblasts, and neurons of the external granule cell layer of cerebellum (Fig. 28.7).[56] The cytological characteristics, marked karyorrhexis, were compatible with apoptotic cell death and suggested that the toxic effect of the metabolites of methylmalonic acidemia particularly involved provocation of apoptosis of immature neuronal cells. Involvement of the external granule cell layer of cerebellum may be related etiologically to the occasional occurrence of cerebellar hemorrhage with methylmalonic acidemia.[25]

As noted earlier, as with propionic acidemia, evidence for basal ganglia lesions has been obtained by brain imaging later in infancy and childhood. In methylmalonic acidemias, the globus pallidus is preferentially affected. This finding is consistent with the occurrence of dystonia and extrapyramidal features on follow-up in approximately 20% to 25% of cases of methylmalonic acidemia of neonatal onset.[45,47]

Management

Antenatal Diagnosis. Antenatal detection of the methylmalonic acidemias has been accomplished primarily by detecting elevated methylmalonate content in the amniotic fluid and maternal urine and by enzymatic assay of cultured amniotic fluid cells (mutase activity and adenosylcobalamin synthesis).[5,21,43,59,60] The possibility of prenatal therapy with cobalamin supplements was shown initially by demonstrating a decrease in maternal excretion of methylmalonic acid after administration of such supplements to the mother of an affected fetus.[43,60] A subsequent case, treated similarly in utero and postnatally, had normal growth and development in early infancy.[61] However, because at least 60% of *neonatal* cases are not cobalamin-responsive,[5,45] this approach may not be highly useful for the majority of affected fetuses.

In the rare infants with the combined defect resulting in both methylmalonic acidemia and homocystinuria, large doses of hydroxycobalamin also are important.[62] Betaine, another methyl donor, may also be beneficial. Follow-up data are too sparse to assess effects on neurological development. It is likely that both prenatal and postnatal therapy will be critical.[62]

Early Detection and Acute and Long-Term Therapy. Early detection in the neonatal period and the importance of acute and long-term therapy are essentially as described for propionic acidemia. Therapy consists of a low-protein diet or a diet low in the amino acid precursors of methylmalonate, supplemented with cobalamin (see next section) and L-carnitine.[5] The possible role of antibiotic therapy to reduce the production of methylmalonate by bacteria in the gastrointestinal tract may also be relevant in this condition.[5,21]

Vitamin B_{12}. Because some patients with isolated methylmalonic acidemias respond to vitamin B_{12} (see earlier discussion), a trial

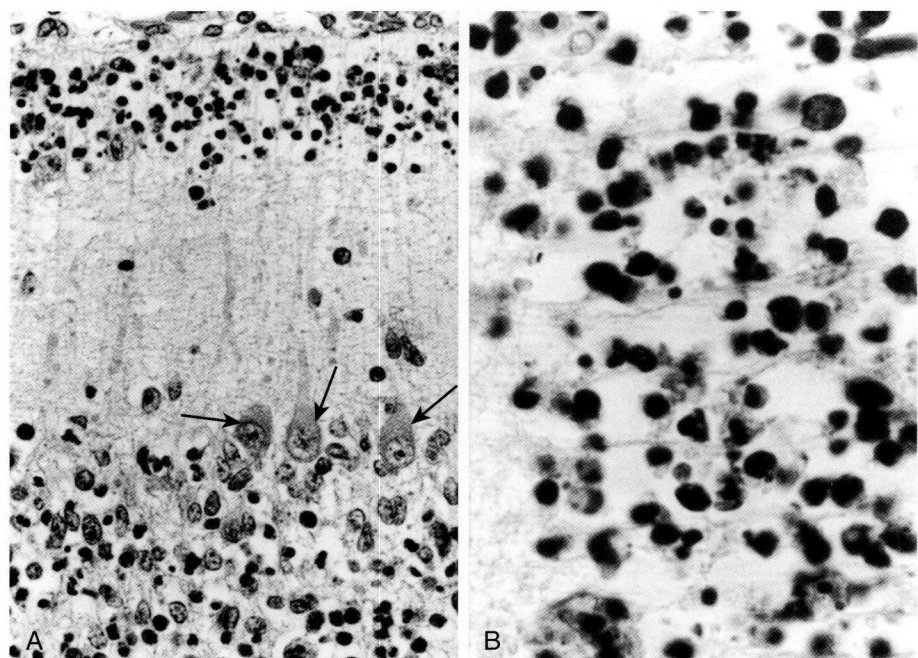

Figure 28.7 **Selective death of immature neurons in a 4-day-old infant with methylmalonic acidemia.** (A) Photomicrograph of the cerebellar cortex shows karyorrhectic immature neuroblasts in the external (*top*) and internal granule cell layers (*bottom*). Purkinje cells (*arrows*) are relatively well preserved. (B) At higher magnification, karyorrhexis in the external granule cell layer is prominent. (From Sum JM, Twiss JL, Horoupian DS. Selective death of immature neurons in methylmalonic acidemia of the neonate: a case report. *Acta Neuropathol [Berl]*. 1993;85:217–221.)

of this vitamin as hydroxycobalamin in high doses is indicated in such patients.[5,21,61] In a series of 21 infants with neonatal-onset methylmalonic acidemia, of the 11 who responded to vitamin B_{12}, 3 were normal on follow-up, whereas of the 10 who did not respond to vitamin B_{12}, none was normal.[63]

Gene Therapy. As with propionic acidemia, liver transplantation has been used in infants with methylmalonic acidemia.[42,60,61] Initial results in transplanted infants were not clearly beneficial. However, recent reports suggest some optimism. First, in a report of 12 infants transplanted at a mean age of 8.2 years, all survived through 3.2 ± 4.2 years and after transplantation had no episodes of hyperammonemia, acidosis, or metabolic decompensation.[64] A second report of two patients, both of whom survived through ages 2 and 12 years, reported similar improvement.[2,3,65] Early transplantation is important, but the youngest infants have the highest risk for graft loss, largely related to technical surgical issues.

Outcome. The long-term outcome of 80 patients with organic aciduria (see earlier) included 38 with methyl malonic acidemia (MMA). Patients with MMA were less likely to have an abnormal neurological examination (24%), a lower abnormal psychometric evaluation at age 3 years (26%), and basal ganglia lesions (i.e., 36%) as compared with patients with propionic acidemia (PA). The prognosis of MMA patients with mutations involving the MMAA (methylmalonic acidemia cblA type) gene has been better than that of patients with mutations involving the MUT (methylmalonyl CoA mutase) gene.[2]

DISORDERS OF PYRUVATE AND MITOCHONDRIAL ENERGY METABOLISM

Disorders of pyruvate and mitochondrial energy metabolism have been the topic of active research in the past several decades and constitute uncommon but serious neonatal neurological disorders. Together with disorders of propionate and methylmalonate metabolism and of branched-chain ketoacid metabolism, these disorders are important examples of organic acid disturbances. In large part because of the difficulties in studying the complex enzyme systems involved, the elucidation of abnormalities of pyruvate and mitochondrial energy metabolism has been relatively recent.

Disorders of pyruvate and mitochondrial energy metabolism may lead to striking metabolic acidosis with lactic acidemia in the neonatal period. Disorders related to *pyruvate metabolism* may involve either the Krebs citric acid cycle or the electron transport system. *Disorders of the citric acid cycle* with neonatal onset include deficiencies of alpha-ketoglutarate decarboxylation (dihydrolipoyl dehydrogenase deficiency), succinate dehydrogenase, or fumarase.[66] However, because only a few well-studied neonatal cases have been documented, these disorders are not discussed in detail. Fumarase deficiency with fumaric acidemia is the most common of these conditions with a neonatal presentation. Reports delineate a rare neonatal or early infantile syndrome of hypotonia, seizures, dysmorphic facial features, frontal bossing, microcephaly, neonatal polycythemia, diffuse polymicrogyria, dysgenetic corpus callosum, hypomyelination, and ventriculomegaly.[67,68] *Disorders*

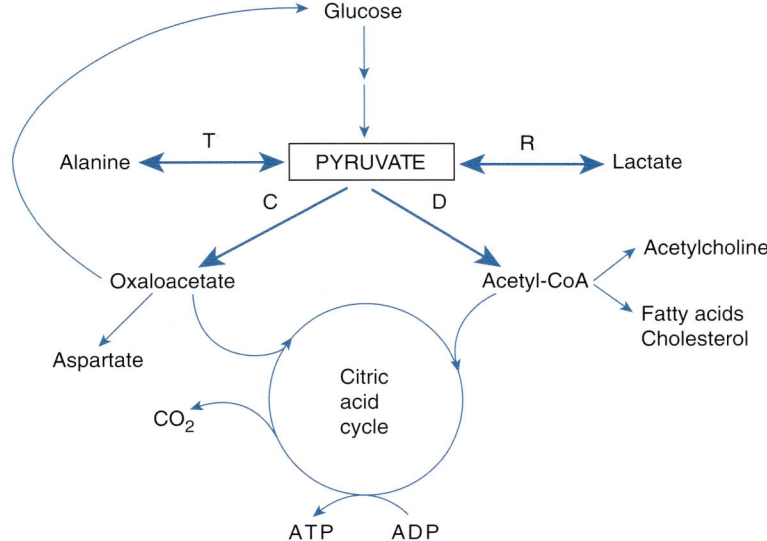

Figure 28.8 **Major metabolic fates of pyruvate.** See text for details. *ADP*, Adenosine diphosphate; *ATP*, adenosine triphosphate; *C*, carboxylation; *CoA*, coenzyme A; *D*, decarboxylation; *R*, reduction; *T*, transamination.

TABLE 28.6   Major Metabolic Fates of Pyruvate
Transamination
• Gluconeogenesis
• Alanine synthesis
Reduction
• Lactate formation
Carboxylation
• Gluconeogenesis
• Aspartate synthesis
• *Prime* citric acid cycle
Decarboxylation
• Energy production
• Lipid synthesis
• Acetylcholine synthesis

of the electron transport chain are more common. In addition to the metabolic abnormalities, the prominent features of these disorders include manifestations of encephalopathy, myopathy, or both; thus they are discussed in Chapters 29 and 33. The focus in this chapter is on disorders of pyruvate metabolism, because the metabolic manifestations, particularly *lactic acidemia*, tend to dominate the neonatal clinical presentation.

Normal Metabolic Aspects

Pyruvate occupies a central position in intermediary metabolism (Fig. 28.8).[66,69,70] It is formed primarily from glucose through the process of glycolysis in brain as in other tissues. The major metabolic fates of pyruvate are shown in Fig. 28.8 and summarized in Table 28.6.

Transamination results in the formation of alanine, used partly for protein synthesis. The reverse reaction is particularly important in liver for gluconeogenesis from alanine.

Reduction to lactate is catalyzed by lactate dehydrogenase. Lactate can be used for gluconeogenesis through the reversal of this reaction.

Pyruvate *carboxylation*, catalyzed by the biotin-dependent enzyme pyruvate carboxylase, results in the formation of oxaloacetate. This step is critical in gluconeogenesis in liver and in several other tissues (but not to any significant extent in brain).[69] Oxaloacetate is also an important intermediate in the citric acid cycle, and this reaction plays a role in priming the cycle. Oxaloacetate transamination results in the formation of aspartate, an excitatory neurotransmitter in brain, a precursor for protein synthesis and an important component of the urea cycle.

Pyruvate *decarboxylation*, catalyzed by the thiamine-dependent pyruvate dehydrogenase complex, is an exceedingly important reaction in all tissues, including brain, in view of the nature of its product, acetyl-CoA. The reaction thereby plays a major role in citric acid cycle function, in adenosine triphosphate synthesis, and in the syntheses of acetylcholine and lipids (i.e., fatty acids and cholesterol).

Biochemical Aspects of Disordered Metabolism
Enzymatic Defects and Essential Consequences

Of the four major fates of pyruvate, impairment of two, decarboxylation and carboxylation, has been described (see later discussion). Defects in the pyruvate dehydrogenase complex and in pyruvate carboxylase have been the enzymatic defects for these disorders. Both defects cause accumulation of pyruvate, lactate, and alanine proximal to the enzymatic block, but obviously the consequences distal to the enzymatic blocks differ to some degree.

Relation to Acute Neurological Dysfunction and to Neuropathology

The mechanisms for brain injury in defects of the pyruvate dehydrogenase complex or of pyruvate carboxylase include acute and more long-lasting effects. The common metabolic feature of these disorders, *lactic acidosis*, may be very important in causing the acute neurological dysfunction. Moreover, an irreversible structural deficit is a likely consequence when the acidosis is severe and prolonged.

A second metabolic feature, important in the genesis of the acute neurological dysfunction associated with disturbances in pyruvate metabolism, is impairment of the synthesis of factors important in *neurotransmission*. Thus, a deficiency of pyruvate dehydrogenase complex activity may be expected to lead to a diminution in the synthesis of acetylcholine (an established and important neurotransmitter).[69,70] A deficiency of pyruvate carboxylase activity, with resulting decreased synthesis of oxaloacetate and function of the citric acid cycle, could lead to a disturbance of the excitatory amino acid transmitters, aspartate (a transamination product of oxaloacetate) and glutamate (a transamination product of the citric acid cycle intermediate alpha-ketoglutarate).

A third metabolic feature, probably important in the genesis of both acute and chronic effects, is impairment of *energy production*.[69] This impairment would be expected with a disturbance of acetyl-CoA synthesis by pyruvate dehydrogenase complex deficiency, but the disturbance of oxaloacetate synthesis by pyruvate carboxylase deficiency may also have a similar consequence.

A fourth metabolic feature, which may be of particular importance in the genesis of the long-term irreversible structural deficits, is a disturbance in the *synthesis of brain lipids and proteins*. Disturbed activity of the pyruvate dehydrogenase complex would be expected to lead to impairment in the synthesis of fatty acids and cholesterol, critical constituents of neural membranes, including myelin, by impairment of acetyl-CoA formation. Experimental support for this notion is available.[71] Deficits of pyruvate dehydrogenase complex and of pyruvate carboxylase also would lead to an alteration in levels of certain amino acids (e.g., alanine and aspartate) and perhaps thereby to a secondary disturbance of protein synthesis. The relative roles of these several factors remain to be defined in the inborn errors of pyruvate decarboxylation and carboxylation.

Pyruvate Dehydrogenase Complex Deficiency
Clinical Features

In general, deficiency in the pyruvate dehydrogenase complex is associated with three major categories of clinical phenotype, divisible according to age of onset: (1) neonatal types, (2) infantile form (onset, 3 to 6 months), and (3) later-onset benign forms with episodic ataxia.[66,69,70,72-76] The infantile form is characterized particularly by hypotonia, cranial nerve signs (especially ophthalmoplegia), ataxia, delayed development, ventilatory disturbance, and other features, and it is most often (≈85% of cases) associated with the neuropathological features of Leigh syndrome (see Chapter 29). The later-onset forms may be punctuated by transient episodes of ataxia or paraparesis, but overall development is normal or only mildly disturbed.

The *clinical features of the neonatal forms of pyruvate dehydrogenase complex deficiency* consist of two basic syndromes: (1) marked lactic acidosis, often with dysmorphic craniofacial features and brain anomalies, and (2) Leigh syndrome. Newborns with Leigh syndrome overlap with those with the infantile forms of pyruvate dehydrogenase complex deficiency with slightly later onset of Leigh syndrome, noted in the previous paragraph and discussed in Chapter 29. In this group, the onset of symptoms is generally in the first week of life and is often within the first 24 hours.[69,73,74,76-78]

The major clinical features of the *more common of the two neonatal forms (i.e., marked lactic acidosis)* include stupor, tachypnea,

---

TABLE 28.7	Common Features of Pyruvate Dehydrogenase Complex Deficiency With Neonatal Onset

Clinical features
- Stupor, coma
- Tachypnea
- Seizures
- Hypotonia
- Dysmorphic facial features

Metabolic features
- Acidosis
- Lactic and pyruvic acidemia
- Hyperalaninemia

Neuropathological features
- Cerebral cortical and white matter atrophy
- Subcortical white matter cysts
- Microcephaly
- Cerebral gyral abnormalities (polymicrogyria, pachygyria)
- Impaired myelination/ventriculomegaly
- Agenesis of the corpus callosum
- Dysgenetic brain stem and cerebellum
- Subacute necrotizing encephalopathy (Leigh syndrome)[a]

[a]See Chapter 29.

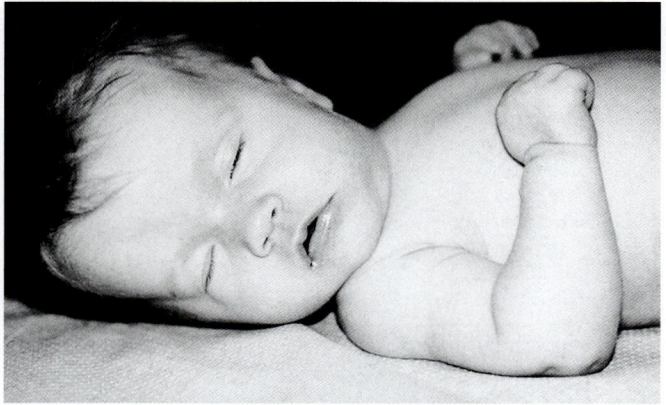

Figure 28.9 Pyruvate dehydrogenase deficiency: craniofacial dysmorphism. This affected girl shows frontal bossing, an upturned nose, a thin upper lip, and low-set ears. (From De Meirleir L, Lissens W, Wayenberg JL, Michotte A, et al. Pyruvate dehydrogenase deficiency: clinical and biochemical diagnosis. *Pediatr Neurol.* 1993;9:216–220.)

hypotonia, and seizures (Table 28.7). The infant's course may be fulminating, with coma evolving in hours to a day or so. Most of the infants with this severe presentation have died in the first year of life. Newborns with pyruvate dehydrogenase complex deficiency may exhibit prominent craniofacial dysmorphic features (Fig. 28.9) and signs of cerebral dysgenesis.[66,68-70,74,76,79] The features of dysgenesis include partial or total agenesis of the corpus callosum, ventricular dilation, gyral abnormalities, subependymal heterotopias, hypoplasia of hindbrain structures (brain stem and cerebellum), and ectopic olivary nuclei. Severe impairment of neurological development, often with microcephaly, is the rule in survivors. Encephaloclastic lesions (see later) often coexist.[72]

Brain imaging, especially MRI, shows the structural features in the cerebrum and posterior fossa.[68,75,76,80,81] Prenatal onset is indicated by the frequent finding of an abnormal corpus callosum (Fig. 28.10). In addition to the callosal anomalies, fetal MRI has detected, in severe cases, such associated encephaloclastic lesions as leukomalacia, basal ganglia calcifications, and pseudocysts in germinal matrix.[72] Moreover, magnetic resonance (MR) spectroscopy has demonstrated an increased pyruvate signal as well as increased lactate.[80]

Genetic data indicate that the disorder is most often inherited in an X-linked dominant fashion. Thus, although nearly equal numbers of male and female patients exhibit defects of the pyruvate dehydrogenase complex, infants with somewhat less severe disease tend to be female. It is likely that severe mutations in hemizygous males are incompatible with life, whereas such severe mutations in females can be tolerated to some extent.[82] Although living male infants tend to exhibit the most severe phenotypes, female infants may also exhibit severe disease. It is now known that most neonatal-onset cases are caused by a defect of the E_{1alpha} subunit of the complex.[66,69,70,73-78,82] The gene for the E_{1alpha} subunit has been localized to the short arms of the X-chromosome (Xp22.1 to 22.2). As noted earlier, hemizygous male infants and heterozygous female infants may exhibit disease. Bias of X-inactivation toward expression of the mutant allele appears to be important in determining the occurrence of the disease and its severity in the heterozygous female infants.[69,78,81]

Metabolic Features

Major Findings. The hallmarks of a disturbance of pyruvate utilization (accumulations in blood of pyruvic and lactic acids and of alanine) are present (see Table 28.7). Distinction from other causes of neonatal metabolic acidosis (see Table 28.1) is aided by the accompanying hyperalaninemia and by the lack of accumulation of propionate or methylmalonic acid. The lactate-to-pyruvate ratio is usually normal (see Fig. 28.1). (Certain patients also exhibit elevated concentrations of alpha-ketoglutarate, branched-chain amino acids, and ketone bodies.[83,84]) The systemic acidosis may be relatively mild in the presence of more marked elevations of cerebrospinal fluid pyruvate and lactate or marked elevations in brain lactate, determined by MR spectroscopy.[76,85] This discrepancy may be more common in female infants and has been attributed to nonrandom X-inactivation with particular affection of brain.[74] The important point concerning the diagnostic evaluation is not to rely exclusively on measurements of lactate in blood.

Enzymatic Defects. The enzymatic defects have included five different components of the pyruvate dehydrogenase complex (Table 28.8). Thus, defects in pyruvate decarboxylase, lipoate acetyltransferase, lipoate dehydrogenase, and the regulatory phosphatase were described in numerous studies.[a] In addition, a protein important in function of both lipoate components, so-called *protein X*, was shown to be defective in approximately 13 neonatal cases.[87] Most neonatal patients have had defects of the E_{1alpha} subunit, the gene located on the X-chromosome.[69,70,76,84] Defective pyruvate dehydrogenase complex activity was demonstrated in brain as well as liver, skeletal muscle, lymphocytes, and cultured fibroblasts.[69,83] However, notably,

---

[a]References 69, 70, 76, 78, 82, 84, and 86.

TABLE 28.8   Pyruvate Dehydrogenase Complex

Pyruvate decarboxylase (thiamine dependent)
Pyruvate → two-carbon unit + carbon dioxide
Lipoate acetyltransferase
Two-carbon unit + reduced lipoate → acetyl-coenzyme A + oxidized lipoate
Lipoate dehydrogenase
Oxidized lipoate → reduced lipoate
Regulatory enzymes
Kinase (adenosine triphosphate dependent): inactivates the first reaction
Phosphatase (magnesium, calcium dependent): activates the first reaction

---

in affected female patients apparently heterozygous for the E_{1alpha} defect, perhaps because of tissue-specific X-inactivation, pyruvate dehydrogenase complex activity may be *normal* in fibroblasts, lymphocytes, and muscle, with the genetic defect clearly present in brain.[74] Thus, because of such tissue-specific expression, a high index of suspicion for the disorder must exist, and multiple tissues (e.g., liver) may require analysis to detect the enzymatic defect.

Pathogenesis of Metabolic Features. The genesis of the metabolic defects relates to the impairment of the conversion of pyruvate to acetyl-CoA. Thus, the *acidosis* is accounted for particularly by the accumulation of pyruvic and lactic acids. The *hyperalaninemia* is related to the accumulation of pyruvate (see Fig. 28.8). Those rare patients with a defect in the lipoate dehydrogenase exhibit elevations of alpha-ketoglutarate and branched-chain ketoacids because the lipoate dehydrogenase in the three complexes (pyruvate dehydrogenase, alpha-ketoglutarate dehydrogenase, and branched-chain ketoacid dehydrogenase) appears to be the same enzyme.[88]

Neuropathology

The neuropathological findings include evidence both of destructive disease and of disturbance in brain development, with onset as early as the first 20 weeks (see Table 28.7). This timing is based on the occurrence of agenesis of the corpus callosum and migrational defects in cerebrum (e.g., gyral abnormalities, heterotopias) and brain stem (e.g., ectopic olivary nuclei, brain stem hypoplasia) (see Figs. 28.10 and 28.11). The gyral and callosal abnormalities have been detected by intrauterine MRI.[72,80,81] Neuropathological findings overall have included cerebral cortical and white matter atrophy and cystic lesions in subcortical white matter in the majority of cases and evidence of disturbance of brain development in at least one third (see Fig. 28.11).[68-70,72,79-81] In approximately one third of predominantly male patients, neuropathological features of Leigh disease, including bilateral putaminal necrosis,[75,81] have been observed, but the full spectrum of Leigh disease is more common in cases with infantile (≈3 to 6 months) onset. The dysgenetic findings tend to be more prominent in female patients[76] and consist of polymicrogyria, pachygyria, cerebral heterotopias, malformed inferior olivary nuclei, and hypoplastic brain stem (including absence of corticospinal tracts), as well as cerebral hypomyelination and absence of

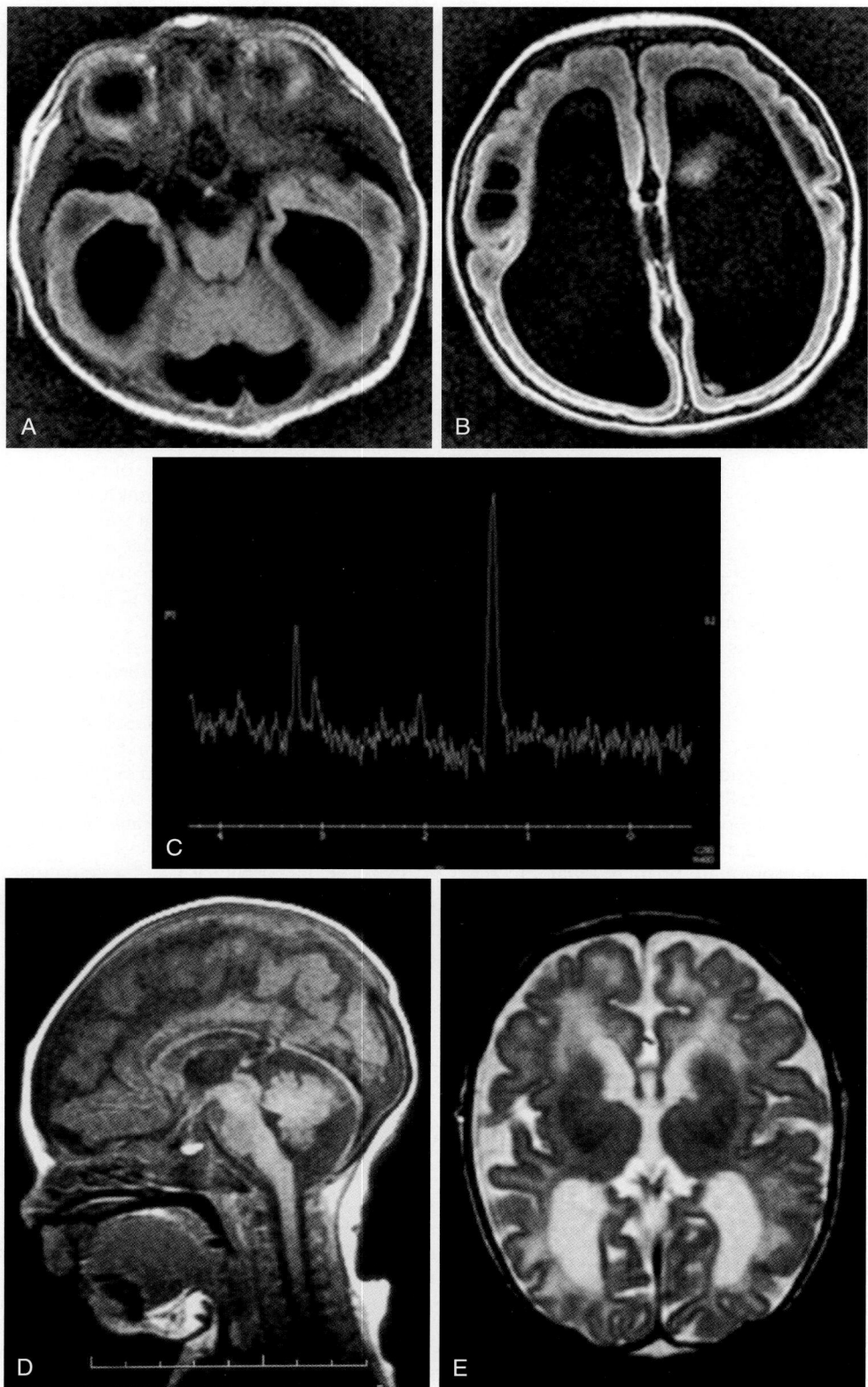

Figure 28.10 Brain abnormalities with pyruvate dehydrogenase complex deficiency. Magnetic resonance imaging (MRI) studies in A–C are from a 4-day-old infant girl and in D and E from a 2-day-old infant girl. (A) T2-weighted MRI shows prominence of the retrocerebellar subarachnoid space with suggestion of cerebellar vermis hypoplasia. (B) Axial flair MRI shows diffuse cortical thinning with lack of normal gyri posteriorly in the parieto-occipital lobes, suggestive of migrational disorder (partial lissencephaly). There are areas of cystic encephalomalacia in the periventricular white matter. (C) MR spectroscopy demonstrates markedly high lactate peak. (D) T1-weighted MRI shows markedly hypoplastic corpus callosum, decreased signal intensity in cerebral white matter, and enlarged subarachnoid spaces. (E) Axial T2-weighted MRI shows markedly increased signal intensity in cerebral white matter, ventriculomegaly, and enlarged subarachnoid spaces. One infant's magnetic resonance spectroscopy (not shown) demonstrated markedly elevated lactate.

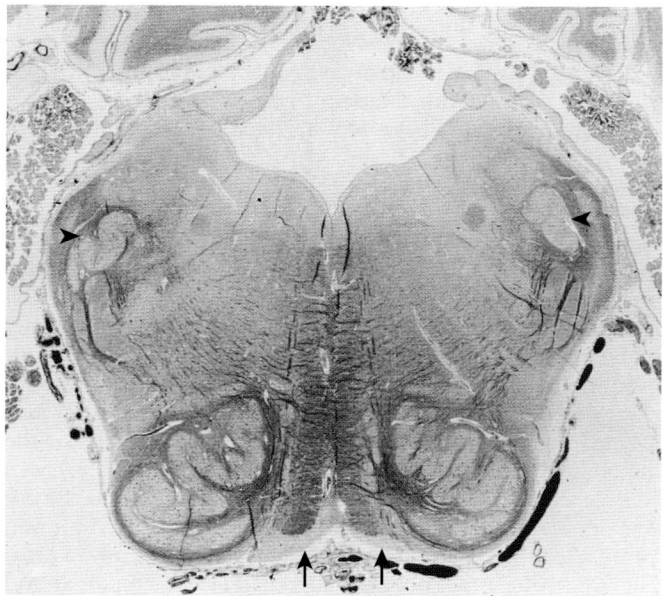

Figure 28.11 Pyruvate dehydrogenase deficiency: neuropathology. Transverse section of the medulla shows dorsal ectopic foci (*arrowheads*) of the inferior olives and absent pyramids (*arrows*). (From De Meirleir L, Lissens W, Wayenberg JL, Michotte A, et al. Pyruvate dehydrogenase deficiency: clinical and biochemical diagnosis. *Pediatr Neurol.* 1993;9:216–220.)

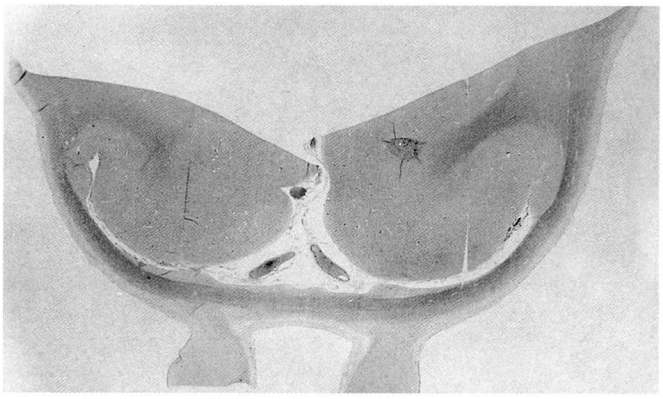

Figure 28.12 Myelin disturbance in pyruvate dehydrogenase complex deficiency. In infancy, this 6-year-old child exhibited hypotonia and impaired neurological development and subsequently manifested spastic quadriplegia, choreoathetosis, seizures, and episodes of severe acidosis. This coronal section was stained for myelin, through the cingulate gyri above and the corpus callosum below. The corpus callosum is very thin, and both the corpus and subcortical white matter are very lightly stained because of the paucity of myelin. (From Cederbaum SD, Blass JP, Minkoff N, Brown WJ, et al. Sensitivity to carbohydrate in a patient with familial intermittent lactic acidosis and pyruvate dehydrogenase deficiency. *Pediatr Res.* 1976;10:713–720.)

hypoplastic corpus callosum. These disturbances suggest abnormalities in neuronal migration, axonal development, and subsequently myelination. Such disturbances have been observed in genetically manipulated mice with pyruvate dehydrogenase deficiency.[89]

Disturbances in myelination have been recognized for many years (Fig. 28.12).[90] Thus, in the initial report, two children

from the same family exhibited considerable diminution in myelin in the cerebrum, brain stem, cerebellum, and spinal cord. No sign of myelin destruction or of neuronal injury was observed. Myelin vacuolation, as observed in infants with various disorders of amino acid and organic acid metabolism, was noted in an infant with onset of disease in the second month and death at 18 months.[91] The nearly uniform occurrence of evidence by brain imaging of diminished cerebral white matter with ventriculomegaly is consistent with an impairment in myelination.[69,70,75,79-81]

Management

Antenatal Diagnosis. Neither antenatal diagnosis nor prevention by therapeutic abortion has been reported. DNA diagnostic techniques hold considerable promise for prenatal diagnosis.[69,74]

Early Detection and Acute Therapy. Early detection and acute therapy are critical. The severe acute acidosis requires treatment with intravenous fluids and sodium bicarbonate and may require peritoneal dialysis. Therapy with dichloroacetate causes a decrease of lactate in both blood and brain.[70,76] This agent inhibits pyruvate dehydrogenase kinase and thereby favors activation of the enzyme. Moreover, the drug also decreases the rate of degradation of the E_{1alpha} subunit and thereby causes an increase in total cellular pyruvate dehydrogenase complex activity.[92] The increased conversion of pyruvate to acetyl-CoA decreases the severity of the lactic acidosis.[93]

Recent evidence suggests that phenylbutyrate may be useful in the treatment of pyruvate dehydrogenase complex deficiency. Thus phosphorylation of specific serine residues of the E_{1alpha} subunit of pyruvate dehydrogenase complex by pyruvate dehydrogenase kinase inactivates the enzyme, whereas dephosphorylation restores pyruvate dehydrogenase complex activity. It was noted that phenylbutyrate enhances the enzymatic activity of the pyruvate dehydrogenase complex in vitro and in vivo by increasing the proportion of unphosphorylated enzyme through inhibition of pyruvate dehydrogenase kinase. Phenylbutyrate given to C57BL/6 wild-type mice results in a significant increase in enzymatic activity of the pyruvate dehydrogenase complex and a reduction of phosphorylated E_{1alpha} in brain, muscle, and liver compared with saline-treated mice. Using recombinant enzymes, it has been shown that phenylbutyrate prevents phosphorylation of E_{1alpha} through binding and inhibition of pyruvate dehydrogenase kinase, providing a molecular explanation for the beneficial effect of phenylbutyrate on the activity of the pyruvate dehydrogenase complex. Phenylbutyrate increases the activity of the pyruvate dehydrogenase complex in fibroblasts from pyruvate dehydrogenase complex–deficient patients harboring various molecular defects and corrects the morphological, locomotor, and biochemical abnormalities in the noa (m631) zebrafish model of pyruvate dehydrogenase complex deficiency.[93]

Long-Term Therapy. Long-term therapy usually includes a diet that is relatively high in fat (e.g., ketogenic diet), because fat, unlike carbohydrate, provides a source of acetyl-CoA (through ketone bodies) that bypasses the pyruvate dehydrogenase step. Particular care must be taken to provide enough calories as fat to make the patient ketonemic but not hypoglycemic or acidotic.[69,71,76,94] Clinical data have shown a beneficial effect of the ketogenic diet on neurological development.[76]

Because thiamine dependence has been reported in some cases of pyruvate dehydrogenase complex deficiency,[69,95] a trial of large doses of *thiamine* is appropriate.[71] Similarly, a therapeutic trial of *lipoic acid* may be considered.[71] In addition, because excretion of carnitine derivatives of metabolic acids may lead to secondary carnitine deficiency, L-carnitine supplementation may be useful.[71] Finally, *dichloroacetate* appears to have value in long-term treatment of pyruvate dehydrogenase complex deficiency, especially if the deficiency is not complete.[69,70,76]

Pyruvate Carboxylase Deficiency
Clinical Features
The clinical presentation of pyruvate carboxylase deficiency consists of two major syndromes: (1) a fulminating syndrome of neonatal onset associated with severe enzyme deficiency caused by absence of the apoenzyme (often termed the French phenotype or type B) and (2) a syndrome usually of slightly later onset, at 2 to 5 months of age, that is somewhat less severe and associated with partial enzyme activity and an alteration in catalytic efficiency of the enzyme (type A).[69,76,78,83,96] (Onset in the neonatal period, however, can occur in the type A cases.) The neonatal syndrome in the type B disorder has been described in approximately 20 infants and is characterized by the clinical features described in Table 28.9.[69,71,96,97] Similarities to the features of pyruvate dehydrogenase complex deficiency are apparent. Macrocephaly may be a distinctive feature of pyruvate carboxylase deficiency, and although the condition is reported commonly, the exact incidence is unclear because of the frequent lack of data on head circumference measurement. A recent report emphasized the high frequency of a movement disorder and unusual ocular behavior.[96] The movement disorder consisted of episodic stimulus-sensitive tremors interspersed with diffuse hypokinesia and lack of facial expression. The ocular findings consisted of fixed gaze interspersed with pendular nystagmus and episodic conjugate eye movements. Both features are reminiscent of the extrapyramidal features observed with inborn defects of monoamine neurotransmitter biosynthesis. Disturbances of neurotransmitter synthesis likely

TABLE 28.9	Common Features of Pyruvate Carboxylase Deficiency With Neonatal Onset

Clinical features
- Stupor, coma
- Tachypnea
- Seizures
- Hypotonia

Metabolic features
- Acidosis
- Lactic and pyruvic acidemia
- Hyperalaninemia
- Low aspartic acid levels
- Hypoglycemia
- Hyperammonemia, citrullinemia, hyperlysinemia
- Ketosis

Neuropathological features
- Cerebral cortical and white matter atrophy
- Periventricular white matter cysts
- Impaired myelination

occur in pyruvate carboxylase deficiency (see later). All the infants died by 4 months of life.

The genetic data available on the neonatal patients indicate *autosomal recessive* inheritance. Intermediate depression of enzymatic activity has been demonstrated in parents of affected patients.[98]

Metabolic Features
Major Findings. The hallmarks of a disorder of pyruvate metabolism, accumulations in blood of pyruvic and lactic acids and alanine, are present. The levels of lactate in the neonatal patients with pyruvate carboxylase deficiency are significantly higher than in the patients with later onsets. The lactate-to-pyruvate ratios in severe (type B) neonatal-onset cases are often normal because of increased cytosolic reduction; in less severely affected type A cases, the ratio is usually normal.[69] Because of the important role of pyruvate carboxylase in hepatic gluconeogenesis (see Fig. 28.8), hypoglycemia is common; median blood glucose was approximately 30 mg/dL in a recent series.[96] Moreover, because of the disturbance in oxaloacetate biosynthesis (see Fig. 28.8), the function of the Krebs cycle is impaired and aspartate is depleted. Aspartate depletion results in impaired function of the urea cycle, which requires this amino acid; thus hyperammonemia, citrullinemia, and hyperlysinemia occur.

Enzymatic Defect. The enzymatic defect involves pyruvate carboxylase and has been demonstrated in brain, liver, kidney, and cultured fibroblasts of affected patients.[a] In the neonatal-onset variety, essentially no enzyme activity can be demonstrated; in most patients, both the pyruvate carboxylase apoenzyme and its mRNA are virtually absent.

Pathogenesis of Metabolic Features. The genesis of the metabolic disturbances relates to the defect in pyruvate carboxylation. As noted earlier, proximal to the enzymatic block, pyruvic and lactic acids accumulate and contribute to the *acidosis*. *Hyperalaninemia* is another proximal consequence of the enzymatic block. *Hyperammonemia*, citrullinemia, and hyperlysinemia occur as a consequence of the disturbance in the urea cycle caused by the depletion of aspartate, in turn caused by the disturbance of oxaloacetate production. An increased conversion of pyruvate to acetyl-CoA occurs as a consequence of the defect in pyruvate carboxylation and, because of the disturbance of the Krebs cycle, acetyl-CoA is converted preferentially to fatty acids and ultimately to ketone bodies, resulting in the ketosis.

In brain, a disturbance in neurotransmitter metabolism is likely; this disturbance involves the astrocyte and particularly glutamate and gamma-aminobutyric acid. Thus pyruvate carboxylase in brain is abundant in astrocytes but not neurons.[69] The resulting deficit in oxaloacetate leads to a defect in the function of the citric acid cycle and thereby alpha-ketoglutarate biosynthesis. The latter is important because, normally, successive transaminations result in formation of glutamate and glutamine. Glutamine then diffuses to neurons, where glutamate is generated and is used as a neurotransmitter and for restoration of the citric acid cycle for energy production and synthetic processes. Failure of this so-called anaplerotic role results in depletion of the neurotransmitters, glutamate, and

[a]References 69, 76, 83, 84, 97, and 98.

its product gamma-aminobutyric acid. The neurotransmitter defects may underlie some of the unusual neonatal neurological features (see earlier),[99] whereas the disturbances of energy production and synthetic processes could lead to neuronal dysgenesis and death.[69]

Neuropathology

Neuropathological features are indicative of both destructive and developmental disturbances (see Table 28.9).[69,76,84,96,97] Thus cerebral cortical neuronal loss, white matter atrophy, and periventricular cysts in cerebral white matter suggest destructive disease. Indeed, the brain imaging picture of apparent periventricular leukomalacia in an infant with lactic acidosis should suggest pyruvate carboxylase deficiency. The white matter lesions have been documented in utero by fetal ultrasonography at 29 weeks of gestation.[100] Vacuolated white matter and subsequent impairment of myelination have been well documented.

Management

Antenatal Diagnosis. Antenatal diagnosis has been accomplished by demonstration of deficient pyruvate carboxylase activity in amniotic fluid cells.[69,98] Prevention by therapeutic abortion is thus possible.

Early Detection and Acute Therapy. Early detection is critical. Treatment of the acute episode with glucose, alkali, and, if necessary, peritoneal dialysis has been lifesaving. However, beneficial effects have been only transient in cases of neonatal onset.

Long-Term Therapy. Dietary therapy is difficult. A relatively high-carbohydrate diet with sufficient amounts of protein for growth is recommended, but no systematic demonstrations of efficacy have been reported.[84] A diet relatively high in fat, as used in pyruvate dehydrogenase complex deficiency, is not indicated in this setting, at least in part because ketosis is a prominent feature of this disorder (see earlier discussion). Aspartic acid supplementation is appropriate, as is a trial of biotin, a critical cofactor for pyruvate carboxylase. Recent reports suggest that triheptanoin, an odd-carbon (seven carbons) triglyceride, and citrate may be useful in improving metabolic status by providing an alternative energy source (ketone bodies).[96,99] Further data will be of interest.

Gene Therapy. Orthoptic liver transplantation in a single case produced partial metabolic improvement but no benefit for neurological development.[101]

DISORDERS OF BRANCHED-CHAIN KETOACID METABOLISM

Branched-chain ketoacids, derived from the branched-chain amino acids leucine, isoleucine, and valine, are involved in several disorders with manifestations in the neonatal period (see Table 28.1). These disorders include classic maple syrup urine disease, isovaleric acidemia, beta-methylcrotonyl-CoA carboxylase deficiency, beta-ketothiolase deficiency, and hydroxymethylglutaryl (HMG)–CoA lyase deficiency.[102] Of these disorders, maple syrup urine disease is the most common and is discussed in Chapter 27 as a disorder of amino acid

metabolism. Isovaleric acidemia is the next most common, accounting for approximately 15% of all organic acidurias in one large series[102]; it is reviewed in detail next. Deficiencies of beta-methylcrotonyl–CoA carboxylase, beta-ketothiolase, and HMG-CoA lyase are very rare in the newborn and are discussed only briefly.

Isovaleric Acidemia

Isovaleric acidemia results from a defect in leucine catabolism at the step immediately distal to that which is the basis for maple syrup urine disease. The defect involves the conversion of isovaleric acid to beta-methylcrotonyl–CoA (Fig. 28.13). This compound is metabolized further by beta-methylcrotonyl–CoA carboxylase (see later discussion).

Clinical Features

Two clinical phenotypes are recognized: an acute, severe neonatal form and a chronic intermittent form with onset later in infancy. The neonatal form accounts for approximately half of all cases, and survivors often develop intermittent episodes later in infancy.[103] Onset of the disease is usually in the first days of life (most often 3 to 6 days of age), and the presenting clinical features are similar to those associated with disorders of propionate and methylmalonate metabolism (see Table 28.2).[2,104] Thus vomiting, tachypnea, and stupor or coma are common (Table 28.10). In addition, the accumulation of isovaleric acid in body fluids (e.g., urine and sweat) imparts a characteristic offensive odor of *sweaty feet*. The course is fulminating. Thrombocytopenia and neutropenia, or pancytopenia, are common. Overall, in earlier studies, more than half of the infants died in the neonatal period, and most of the survivors exhibited mental retardation and other signs of brain injury. However, more recently, earlier detection and more aggressive short-term and long-term therapy (see later discussion) have improved survival rates markedly, and only a minority of survivors have exhibited prominent neurological sequelae.[103] The presence of affected siblings of both sexes and the demonstration of intermediate deficiency of leucine catabolism and levels of dehydrogenase in heterozygotes indicate that inheritance in this disorder is *autosomal recessive*.[103]

Metabolic Features

Major Findings. The characteristic metabolic features are severe acidosis, isovaleric acidemia and aciduria, isovaleryl-glycinuria,

---

TABLE 28.10 Common Features of Isovaleric Acidemia

Clinical features
- Vomiting
- Tachypnea
- Stupor, coma
- Odor of sweaty feet

Metabolic features
- Acidosis
- Isovaleric acidemia (aciduria)
- Isovaleryl-glycinuria, beta-hydroxyisovaleric aciduria
- Hyperammonemia

Other features
- Neutropenia or thrombocytopenia

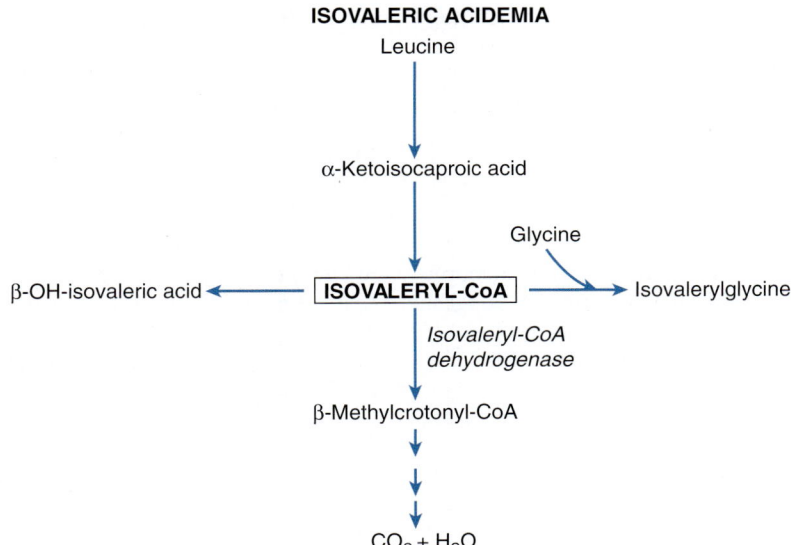

ISOVALERIC ACIDEMIA

Figure 28.13 Metabolic defect in isovaleric acidemia. Isovaleryl–coenzyme A (CoA), a product of leucine catabolism, accumulates because of the impairment of isovaleryl-CoA dehydrogenase.

beta-hydroxyisovaleric acidemia and aciduria, and pancytopenia (see Fig. 28.13). Mild to moderate hyperammonemia is common. Occasionally patients exhibit hypocalcemia, the basis for which is unclear. Mild hyperglycinemia may occur during the acute episodes; thus the ketotic hyperglycinemia syndrome can be caused by this defect.[9]

Enzymatic Defect. The enzymatic defect involves isovaleryl-CoA dehydrogenase. This conclusion was based initially on studies of the accumulated metabolites and the metabolism of leucine in cultured fibroblasts.[105] The enzymatic defect has been demonstrated directly.[103,106] A recently developed enzymatic method allows identification of the defect in only a few hours from the time of initial blood sampling.[107]

Pathogenesis of Metabolic Features. The genesis of the metabolic defects is understood to a considerable degree. The *acidosis* relates partly to the accumulation of isovaleric acid, which, during periods of decompensation, reaches approximately 1000-fold normal concentrations in plasma.[103] In addition, accumulations of ketone bodies and lactate contribute significantly to the acidosis. These accumulations result from a disturbance of mitochondrial function, including pyruvate dehydrogenase, caused by the isovaleric acid (more specifically, the CoA derivative thereof).[108] The mitochondrial disturbance may account for the impairment of brain high-energy phosphates documented in an affected infant by phosphorus MR spectroscopy.[109] *The excessive excretion of isovalerylglycine and of beta-hydroxyisovaleric acid* reflects alternate pathways of isovaleric acid metabolism (see Fig. 28.13).[110] Quantitatively, the more important of these pathways is the conjugation of isovaleric acid with glycine by the enzyme glycine-*N*-acylase to form the water-soluble conjugate, isovalerylglycine. This conjugate is excreted very rapidly; indeed, during periods of remission, very little free isovaleric acid can be detected in the patient's urine. Because this process is so active, *hyperglycinemia* is less likely to develop in this disorder than in other disorders causing the ketotic hyperglycinemia

syndrome, as demonstrated by the only occasional report of hyperglycinemia. By analogy with disorders of the propionate and methylmalonate pathway, the hyperglycinemia is probably caused by inhibition of glycine cleavage by the CoA derivative of the accumulated alpha-ketoisocaproic acid, the ketoacid that is the immediate precursor of isovaleric acid (see Fig. 28.13). Similarly, the moderate *hyperammonemia* that is observed also relates to the effects of the CoA derivative on the carbamyl phosphate step of the Krebs-Henseleit urea cycle.

Neuropathology

No detailed neuropathological study of isovaleric acidemia of neonatal onset has been reported. One infant was reported to have cerebellar hemorrhage at autopsy[104]; the cause may have been analogous to that of the cerebellar hemorrhage of propionic and methylmalonic acidemia (hypertonic sodium bicarbonate, thrombocytopenia, involvement of external granule cell layer; see earlier discussion). *White matter edema and vacuolation have been observed*,[104] but whether these findings are analogous to the myelin disturbance typical of other amino acid and organic acid disturbances is not yet clear.

Management

Antenatal Diagnosis. Prenatal diagnosis has been accomplished by demonstration of either undetectable or minimal isovaleryl dehydrogenase activity in cultured amniocytes or elevated levels of isovalerylglycine in amniotic fluid.[103]

Early Detection. Early detection is critical. Distinction from the other causes of severe metabolic acidosis in the neonatal period is necessary (see Table 28.1). The odor of sweaty feet is the most helpful feature in the clinical detection of isovaleric acidemia.

Acute and Long-Term Therapy. Short-term therapy includes glucose and bicarbonate infusion to reduce endogenous protein catabolism and control acidosis.[103] Later therapy consists of a diet low in protein to decrease the amount of leucine catabolized to isovaleryl-CoA and supplementation with glycine and carnitine.[102,103,111-113] The use of *glycine* has proved to be highly valuable in the treatment of both the acute episode and subsequently. The principle for administering glycine is based on the finding that the isovalerylglycine conjugate, formed from glycine and isovaleryl-CoA, is rapidly excreted by the kidneys. This excretion provides a means for rapid elimination of the accumulated isovaleric acid. Because the Michaelis constant (K_m) of glycine-*N*-acylase is higher than the intracellular concentration of glycine, the provision of exogenous glycine would be expected to increase conjugation of isovaleric acid. Cohn and coworkers[114] initially treated two very sick infants who had isovaleric acidemia in the first month of life with 250 mg/kg of glycine, with dramatic biochemical benefit within 3 days and normalization of the neurological examination within 2 weeks. On a maintenance dosage of glycine (800 mg daily) and a low-protein diet, these infants experienced normal neurological development by 6 and 13 months of age. Subsequent work supports the value of this approach.[103,111]

Supplementation with *carnitine* is based on the finding that, with the accumulation of isovaleric acid and related organic acids, isovalerylcarnitine and carnitine esters of the other acids are markedly excreted, thus resulting in a secondary carnitine deficiency.[103,112] The administration of carnitine corrects the carnitine deficiency and provides a means for the removal of toxic isovaleric acid through easily excreted isovalerylcarnitine.

The importance of *early diagnosis and prompt institution of treatment* is illustrated by a recent evaluation of 12 infants diagnosed within the first week of life.[115] Only 1 infant died in the neonatal period and the other 11 treated survivors had IQs within the normal range

Beta-Methylcrotonyl–Coenzyme A Carboxylase Deficiency

The product of the isovaleryl dehydrogenase reaction, beta-methylcrotonyl–CoA, undergoes carboxylation (see Fig. 28.13) by a specific carboxylase. With widespread use of tandem mass spectroscopy–based neonatal screening programs, deficiency of beta-methylcrotonyl–CoA carboxylase appears to be among the most frequent organic acid abnormalities.[116] However, the phenotype is variable, ranging from neonates with severe onsets to asymptomatic adults. Only about 10 cases have presented in the neonatal period.[103,117,118] The clinical syndrome consisted of stupor, difficulty with feeding, vomiting, tachypnea, and acidosis. Hypoglycemia was a common feature. Several infants died, but the long-term outcome in most survivors is unknown. High-dose biotin therapy has been beneficial.

Hydroxymethylglutaryl–Coenzyme A Lyase Deficiency

HMG–CoA lyase deficiency is a third defect in the catabolism of the branched-chain amino acid leucine.[103,119] The *clinical course* of this autosomal recessive disorder is characterized by onset in the neonatal period in approximately 50% of cases, with stupor, tachypnea, vomiting, and hypotonia.[102,103,119-121] Approximately 10% of infants have had overt seizures. Hepatomegaly is an important finding on physical examination. The course is complicated by severe hypoglycemia and, as a consequence, without prompt intervention, approximately half of the affected infants have died. However, several infants who were promptly

treated have exhibited normal subsequent development, and mortality rates have declined markedly. MRI has shown marked abnormalities of cerebral white matter.[121] Neuropathological data are scant, but one 6½-month-old infant exhibited "diffuse white matter spongiosis" and "gliosis" on a brain biopsy.[122] The *major metabolic features* include metabolic acidosis and severe hypoglycemia. The cause of the hypoglycemia may be related to the enzymatic defect (see next paragraph), which impairs ketone body formation and hence the glucose sparing of these alternative substrates. The combination of severe hypoglycemia and deficient ketone bodies causes the brain to be exquisitely vulnerable to the hypoglycemia because the organ is deprived of a major alternative substrate. The metabolic acidosis is caused by the accumulated organic acids proximal to the enzymatic block. Hyperammonemia, which may be severe, has been observed in approximately half of such infants. A secondary carnitine deficiency, secondary to excessive urinary excretion of acylcarnitines, as in other organic acid disorders, is common. The *enzymatic defect* involves the terminal step in leucine catabolism, the conversion of HMG-CoA to acetoacetate and acetyl-CoA (Fig. 28.14).[103,119,120,123]

Management consists of early detection, prompt and vigorous treatment of both acidosis *and* hypoglycemia, and a subsequent dietary regimen with restriction of leucine and carnitine supplementation. Normal outcome has been reported in several infants identified early and treated effectively.

Mevalonic Aciduria

Mevalonic aciduria, a relatively recently recognized disorder of leucine catabolism, is associated with two clinical phenotypes: a severe neonatal variety and a more commonly recognized later-onset disorder.[103,124,125] The few reported newborns have exhibited dysplastic facial features, cataracts, hepatosplenomegaly, and anemia. Only one of the three carefully studied newborns had metabolic acidosis in the neonatal period, and acidosis does not appear to be a prominent feature of this disease. Subsequent neurological development has been impaired, hypotonia has been prominent, and neuroimaging has shown development of cerebellar atrophy. The level of mevalonic acid in body fluids is elevated. The enzymatic defect involves mevalonate kinase (see Fig. 28.14), which is crucial in the synthesis of cholesterol

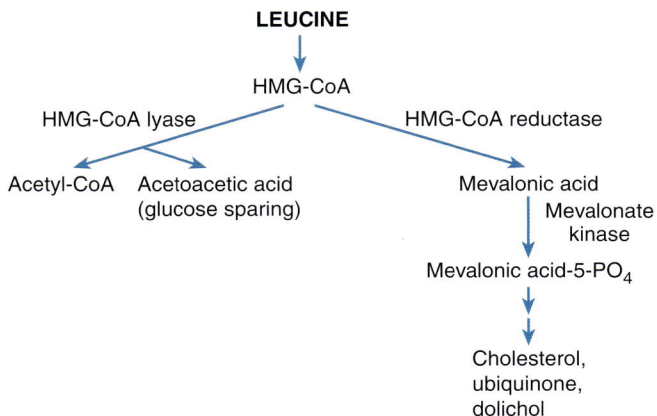

Figure 28.14 Terminal steps in leucine catabolism showing sites of action of hydroxymethylglutaryl (HMG)–coenzyme A (CoA) lyase and mevalonate kinase. *PO₄*, Phosphate.

for cellular membranes, ubiquinone for the electron transport chain, and dolichol for synthesis of the oligosaccharide moieties of glycoproteins. The disorder is autosomal recessive and is classified among disorders of branched-chain organic acid metabolism because the substrate for the reaction, HMG-CoA, is a product of leucine catabolism. Prenatal diagnosis by analysis of mevalonate kinase in a sample of chorionic villus has been accomplished at 12 weeks of gestation.[126] Suitable therapy has not been developed.

Beta-Ketothiolase Deficiency

Beta-ketothiolase deficiency is a defect in the catabolism of the branched-chain amino acid isoleucine.[102,103,119] The autosomal recessive disorder is primarily episodic in *clinical course*, and most patients have had onset months *after* the neonatal period. One infant developed vomiting in the neonatal period that became so severe by 4 weeks of age that a pyloromyotomy was performed[127]—a mistake in diagnosis and treatment not infrequently made with organic acid disorders. Subsequently the infant developed stupor and tachypnea before the correct diagnosis was made and appropriate dietary therapy was instituted.

The *major metabolic features* in the infant reported[127] included ketoacidosis, hyperglycinemia, hyperammonemia, and pancytopenia (i.e., the ketotic hyperglycinemia syndrome). The accumulated CoA derivatives of the ketoacids proximal to the enzymatic block presumably caused the secondary metabolic abnormalities, as described for disorders of propionate and methylmalonate metabolism. Notably, hyperglycinemia has not been a feature of the cases of later onset. The *enzymatic defect* involves the terminal beta-ketothiolase in isoleucine catabolism, the product of which is propionate (see Fig. 28.2).[103,119,127,128]

Management consists of early detection, prompt treatment of acidosis, and subsequent moderate dietary protein restriction. Except for the one neonatal case, normal development has been observed in promptly treated infantile cases.

DISORDERS OF FATTY ACID OXIDATION

Disorders of mitochondrial fatty acid oxidation manifest very uncommonly in the neonatal period. In part this finding may relate to the relatively high carbohydrate feeding of the newborn and the relatively uncommon need for fatty acid oxidation for energy production (e.g., during fasting). Fatty acid oxidation is particularly active in mitochondria of liver and muscle (both cardiac and skeletal) and consists of 20 individual steps. After cellular uptake of the fatty acid and cytosolic generation of the fatty acyl-CoA, the sequence of steps includes transesterification of the acyl-CoA derivative by carnitine palmityltransferase I (CPT I) before mitochondrial translocation by the carnitine acylcarnitine translocase, reesterification of acylcarnitine to acyl-CoA by the mitochondrial CPT II, and then beta-oxidation of the fatty acyl-CoA by the appropriate beta-oxidation series of enzymes.[129]

Because fatty acid oxidation is particularly active in muscle, some fatty acid oxidation disorders manifest in early infancy with prominent hypotonia and weakness, often with signs of cardiomyopathy; these disorders are discussed in Chapter 33. The most common such disorder with neonatal onset, albeit still rare, is carnitine transporter deficiency (primary carnitine deficiency).

TABLE 28.11   Fatty Acid Oxidation Disorders With Neonatal Onset[a]

Carnitine transporter deficiency[a]
  Weakness, hypotonia, cardiomyopathy
Mitochondrial carnitine-acylcarnitine translocase deficiency
  Sudden neonatal death
Carnitine palmityltransferase I deficiency
  Bradycardia, cardiorespiratory arrest
Carnitine palmityltransferase II deficiency
  Apnea, seizures, dysmorphic craniofacial features, cardiomyopathy, cystic dysplasia of brain and kidneys, neonatal death
Mitochondrial trifunctional protein deficiency
  Hypotonia, cardiomyopathy
Medium-chain acyl–coenzyme A dehydrogenase deficiency[a]
  Stupor, hypotonia, poor feeding
Medium-chain 3-ketoacyl–coenzyme A thiolase
  Vomiting, acidosis, rhabdomyolysis, neonatal death
Short-chain acyl–coenzyme A dehydrogenase deficiency
  Seizures, jitteriness
Long-chain hydroxy-acyl–coenzyme A dehydrogenase deficiency
  Hypoglycemia, hypotonia, cardiomyopathy, vomiting
Very-long-chain acyl–coenzyme A dehydrogenase deficiency
  Seizures, stupor, metabolic acidosis, cardiomyopathy

[a]Most common with neonatal onset; carnitine transporter deficiency is discussed in Chapter 33, and medium-chain acyl–coenzyme A dehydrogenase deficiency is discussed in this chapter.

Because fatty acid oxidation is particularly active in liver as well as in muscle, fatty acid oxidation disorders may manifest with striking metabolic disturbances, especially hypoglycemia (without ketones; i.e., hypoketotic hypoglycemia), hyperammonemia, metabolic acidosis (usually mild), and dicarboxylic aciduria (fatty acid intermediates).[129,130] The clinical presentation often includes vomiting, altered level of consciousness, seizures, hypotonia more than hypertonia, and cardiac dysfunction. Sudden death may occur if the diagnosis is not established promptly and therapy instituted. Of all fatty acid oxidation disorders, medium-chain acyl-CoA dehydrogenase deficiency is associated with most cases of neonatal onset (see next paragraph). Rare examples of neonatal onset of the other fatty acid oxidation disorders are included in Table 28.11.[129-135]

Medium-Chain Acyl–Coenzyme A Dehydrogenase Deficiency

Of the inherited defects in the beta-oxidation of fatty acids, impairment of *medium-chain acyl-CoA hydrogenase* has been reported to cause clinical features in the newborn in approximately 10% to 20% of cases.[129,130,134,136-139] The clinical presentation has consisted of stupor, hypotonia, poor feeding, and respiratory difficulties. The onset of the illness has been related to the beginning of breast-feeding, a situation sometimes associated with relative fasting. Metabolic features have included only mild metabolic acidosis, hypoglycemia (without ketones; i.e., hypoketotic hypoglycemia), hyperammonemia, and dicarboxylic aciduria. The ratio of acylcarnitines to free carnitine is markedly elevated. Creatine kinase may be elevated, sometimes markedly. Approximately 45% of infants have died during the acute episode, usually before the correct diagnosis. The diagnosis is established by quantitation of medium-chain fatty acids (C_6 to C_{12}) and demonstration of the enzymatic defect in leukocytes or fibroblasts. The gene for this autosomal recessive disorder is located on the short arm of chromosome 1, and a single mutation accounts for nearly all cases. Therapy includes aggressive treatment of hypoglycemia and avoidance of fasting. Subsequently, a high-carbohydrate, low-fat diet is appropriate. Most infants also receive carnitine supplementation. Normal development has been documented after prompt diagnosis and institution of therapy.

OTHER ORGANIC ACID DISORDERS

Four additional organic acid disorders with manifestations in the newborn do not correspond to the categories described in the preceding sections. These are multiple carboxylase deficiency, multiple acyl-CoA dehydrogenase deficiency (glutaric acid, type II), glutathione synthetase deficiency (5-oxoprolinuria), and sulfite oxidase deficiency. These disorders are associated with metabolic acidosis (see Table 28.1).

Multiple Carboxylase Deficiency

Multiple carboxylase deficiency affects four carboxylases and consists of two essential types (Table 28.12).[102,140-143] The underlying disturbance involves the metabolism of biotin, a vitamin essential for the action of carboxylases. Biotin is attached covalently to the apoenzymes to form the holoenzymes by a holocarboxylase synthetase, and biotin is recovered from the degraded enzyme by biotinidase. A disturbance of the former results in the neonatal form of multiple carboxylase deficiency, and a defect in biotinidase results in a later-onset form of multiple carboxylase deficiency.

Holocarboxylase Synthetase Deficiency

The typical neonatal form of multiple carboxylase deficiency is related to holocarboxylase synthetase deficiency and has been reported in approximately 45 infants.[102,140,143-147] The *clinical course* of this autosomal recessive disorder is characterized by onset in the first days of life of stupor, vomiting, tachypnea, hypotonia, and sometimes seizures. A nonspecific skin rash, often erythematous and desquamating, is a common feature. Several infants have died before diagnosis and institution of appropriate therapy (see later discussion).

The *major metabolic features* include metabolic ketoacidosis, moderate hyperammonemia, hypoglycemia, and an organic acidemia that includes propionate, lactate, and beta-methylcrotonate. The metabolic features are caused principally by

---

TABLE 28.12   Multiple Carboxylase Deficiency

Biotin-dependent carboxylases affected
Propionyl–coenzyme A carboxylase
Pyruvate carboxylase
Beta-methylcrotonyl–coenzyme A carboxylase
Acetyl–coenzyme A carboxylase
Two basic types
Holocarboxylase synthetase deficiency: neonatal onset common
Biotinidase deficiency: neonatal onset uncommon, usually later onset (median, 3 months)

---

deficiencies of the following three carboxylases: propionyl-CoA carboxylase (propionic acidemia and hyperammonemia; see Fig. 28.2), pyruvate carboxylase (lactic acidemia and hypoglycemia; see Fig. 28.8), and beta-methylcrotonyl–CoA carboxylase (beta-methylcrotonic acidemia and beta-methylcrotonylglycinuria; see Fig. 28.13).

The *enzymatic defect* involves holocarboxylase synthetase, the enzyme that catalyzes the covalent linking of biotin to the three apocarboxylases enumerated. As noted earlier, biotin is essential as the carboxyl carrier for the propionyl-CoA, pyruvate, and beta-methylcrotonyl–CoA carboxylases. The mutation usually involves the biotin-binding domain of the apoenzyme, and the resulting enzyme has a markedly increased K_m (i.e., decreased affinity) for biotin. Partial responsiveness to exogenous biotin is thus explained. In rare instances, the mutation involves a different domain, and the resulting enzyme has a less impaired K_m but greatly reduced maximal velocity (maximal carboxylase activity).[140,145] Infants with this enzymatic defect have a poor response to biotin. The defect is demonstrable in cultured fibroblasts and in leukocytes. Prenatal diagnosis is possible by measurement of abnormal organic acids in the amniotic fluid or deficient carboxylase activities in cultured amniocytes.

Therapy of this disorder is principally *biotin* in high doses. This approach has been highly effective, and normal development and growth have been documented in the fetus after therapy commenced in the second or third trimester of pregnancy as well as in newborns treated early postnatally.

Later-Onset Form: Biotinidase Deficiency

Although the second major form of multiple carboxylase deficiency, biotinidase deficiency, typically results in later onset (median age, 3 months), approximately 10% of patients exhibit onset in the first weeks of life.[85,140,141,143,148-151] The clinical features are similar to those observed with holocarboxylase synthetase deficiency, although *seizures* and hypotonia appear to be more common in biotinidase deficiency. Skin rash (dry, squamous appearance) and alopecia are common accompaniments. Subsequent neurological findings include ataxia, hearing loss, optic atrophy, and developmental delay. The diagnosis is suspected by demonstration of the metabolic features described for holocarboxylase synthetase deficiency, but urinary organic acids occasionally are normal and cerebrospinal fluid organic acid analysis may be required to show the metabolic defect.[85] Neuropathological features include vacuolation of white matter, defective myelination, and focal necrotizing lesions with vascular proliferation and gliosis, similar to those observed in Leigh disease but more diffuse in distribution.[140] The vacuolation of myelin is similar to that observed in many other amino acid and organic acid disorders and probably accounts for the abnormalities of white matter observed on reported computed tomography and MRI scans. The diagnosis is made by the detection of low biotinidase in serum, leukocytes, or fibroblasts. Treatment with biotin is effective and should be instituted early in the disease to ensure a favorable outcome. A strikingly favorable response to therapy is illustrated in Fig. 28.15.[142]

Multiple Acyl–Coenzyme A Dehydrogenase Deficiency: Glutaric Acidemia Type II

Only in recent years has it become clear that glutaric acidemia type II is not rare (Table 28.13).[102,152,153] The molecular defect involves a side chain to the main electron transport chain in

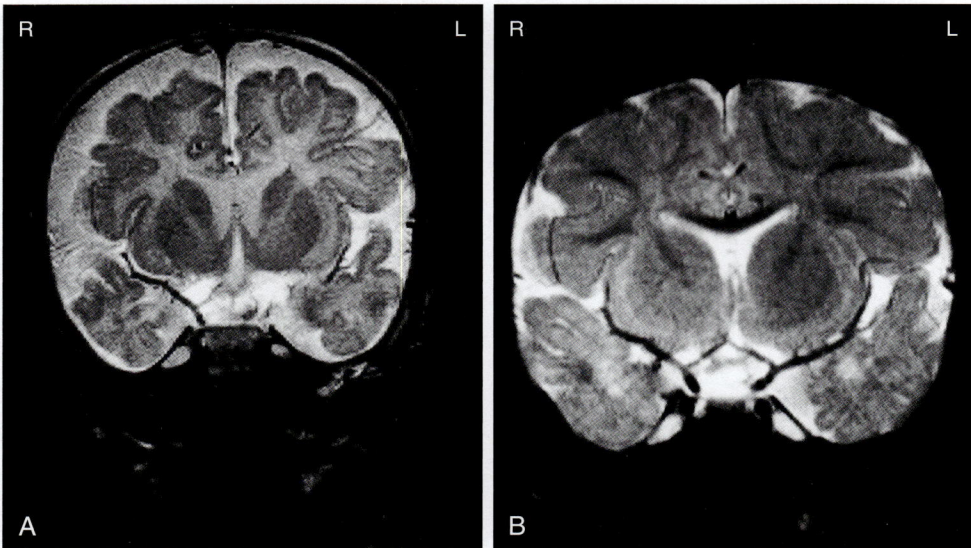

Figure 28.15 **Coronal T2-weighted magnetic resonance imaging scans in an infant with biotinidase deficiency.** (A) Scan performed at 6 weeks of age shows high signal intensity in cerebral white matter and markedly enlarged subarachnoid spaces. The infant had developed a skin rash at 3 weeks and generalized seizures at 6 weeks. (B) Scan performed at 14½ months of age, after 13 months of treatment with oral biotin, is normal. (From Haagerup A, Andersen JB, Blichfeldt S, Christensen MF. Biotinidase deficiency: two cases of very early presentation. *Dev Med Child Neurol.* 1997;39:832–835.)

TABLE 28.13	Multiple Acyl–Coenzyme A Dehydrogenase Deficiency: Glutaric Acidemia Type II

Major acyl–coenzyme A dehydrogenases affected
    Fatty acyl–coenzyme A dehydrogenases (long-chain, medium-chain, short-chain beta-oxidation)
    Isovaleryl–coenzyme A dehydrogenase (branched-chain amino acid catabolism)
    Methylbutyryl–coenzyme A dehydrogenase (branched-chain amino acid catabolism)
    Glutaryl–coenzyme A dehydrogenase (lysine, tryptophan catabolism)
Molecular defects
Electron transport flavoprotein
Electron transport flavoprotein–ubiquinone oxidoreductase (most common defect in neonatal form with congenital anomalies)

the mitochondrion for the coupling of electron transport to the synthesis of adenosine triphosphate. The side chain is composed of electron transfer flavoprotein (ETF) and ETF-ubiquinone oxidoreductase (ETF-QO), which are involved in the transfer of electrons from multiple flavoprotein acyl-CoA and other dehydrogenases to the main respiratory chain. A defect of this side chain thus affects multiple dehydrogenase reactions, including fatty acid oxidation, branched-chain amino acid catabolism, and glutaryl-CoA catabolism, among other processes (see Table 28.13).

Three basic clinical phenotypes are recognized[102,152-154]: (1) a severe neonatal onset form with congenital anomalies, (2) a rarer neonatal onset form without anomalies, and (3) a milder, later-onset variety. The *clinical features* of the classic neonatal syndrome include a high frequency of premature birth and onset in the first 24 to 48 hours of stupor, tachypnea, vomiting, hypotonia, and sometimes seizures. Hepatomegaly, enlarged kidneys, facial dysmorphism, rocker-bottom feet, muscular defects of the anterior abdominal wall, abnormal external genitalia, and the odor of sweaty feet (involvement of isovaleryl dehydrogenase) are characteristic. The hypotonia may be so severe as to suggest a neuromuscular disorder. Infants without anomalies are less commonly seen but are otherwise similar. Rapid progression and death within a week are characteristic of the neonatal disease with anomalies, and survival for a few months is more common in the neonatal disease without anomalies.

The *pathological features* are interesting and characteristic. Thus microvesicular fatty change is prominent in liver, kidney, and myocardium. The kidneys are enlarged and cystic, a diagnosis made in life by ultrasonography or computed tomography. The *brain* shows focal cortical dysplasia with changes indicative of impaired neuronal migration. Warty protrusions over cerebral cortex, especially in the temporoparietal regions, have been demonstrated. In addition, dysgenesis of the corpus callosum has been described.[68] MRI has shown hypoplasia of temporal lobes, abnormal signal in the basal ganglia (especially caudate and putamen) and periventricular white matter, and cerebellar vermian hypoplasia.[33,155]

The *major metabolic features* consist of severe metabolic acidosis, severe hypoglycemia (without ketonemia or ketonuria), moderate hyperammonemia, and organic and fatty acidemia. The fatty acids include glutaric, isobutyric, and isovaleric acids. These fatty acids accumulate because of deficiencies of the dehydrogenases responsible for the degradation of the CoA derivatives of these compounds. Acylcarnitines, as a consequence, are usually elevated. The mitochondrial disturbance in brain is reflected by the finding by MR spectroscopy of elevated lactate.[153]

The *enzymatic defect* involves multiple dehydrogenases and is based on a deficiency of either ETF-QO or ETF. Severe disease with anomalies is associated much more commonly with ETF-QO deficiency than with ETF deficiency.[152] The defect is demonstrable in cultured fibroblasts. Prenatal diagnosis is accomplished most readily by demonstration of abnormal organic acids, usually glutarate, in amniotic fluid. However, diagnosis in the 17th week of gestation has been accomplished by immunoblot analysis and pulse-chase experiments.[156]

Therapy for this disorder requires vigorous supplementation acutely with glucose and alkali. Despite neonatal onset of therapy, outcome has been generally poor.[157] The demonstration of multiple systemic anomalies (e.g., polycystic kidneys and dysmorphic features) and cerebral dysplasia suggestive of migrational defect in many patients indicates that intrauterine disturbance may occur; thus fetal therapy may be required. Treatment with a diet restricted in fat and protein and supplemented with riboflavin and L-carnitine has been generally unsuccessful in infants with the common severe disease and variably effective in those with less severe disease, usually of later onset.[157] A riboflavin-responsive form of glutaric acidemia type II, manifesting later in infancy with severe white matter disease, has been reported.[158]

Glutaric Acidemia Type I

The syndrome of multiple acyl-CoA dehydrogenase deficiency, glutaric acidemia type II, should be distinguished from glutaric acidemia type I, which is caused by an isolated deficiency of glutaryl-CoA dehydrogenase.[159] This disorder typically has its onset in later infancy or early childhood with an extrapyramidal syndrome, especially with dystonia and dyskinesia, and developmental delay.[102,160-163] However, notably, *macrocephaly is present at birth* or in very early infancy in nearly all patients. (Macrocephaly and rapid head growth in early infancy may also herald the occurrence of a rarer but related disorder, L-2-hydroxyglutaric aciduria.[164,165] Perhaps similarly related to glutaric acidemia type I is a separate rare disorder, D-2-hydroxyglutaric aciduria, in which macrocephaly occurs, but only in the minority of infants, whereas neonatal seizures and hypotonia occur in the majority.[166]) Initially, in glutaric acidemia type I, the macrocephaly may be only relative, but head growth that crosses percentile lines is characteristic. Subtle neurological signs (e.g., hypotonia, irritability, and jitteriness) are present frequently before the onset of the overt disease at approximately 1 year. MRI scan in early infancy shows frontotemporal atrophy and delayed myelination (Fig. 28.16). The overt clinical presentation at approximately 1 year of age is characterized in 75% of cases by an acute encephalopathic syndrome in association with infection and accompanied by vomiting, seizures, and coma. Following the acute event, the infant develops a progressive neurological syndrome characterized especially by dystonia and other extrapyramidal manifestations. MRI at this time shows destruction and atrophy of basal ganglia, decreased attenuation of cerebral white matter, and frontotemporal atrophy, severe and progressive. Neuropathological findings include striatal necrosis and spongy myelinopathy. The importance of early detection (i.e., in the first months of life before the occurrence of the acute encephalopathy and subsequent neurological deterioration) and of institution of therapy (oral carnitine, dietary therapy, and vigorous supportive therapy with intercurrent infection) is emphasized by the report of normal development in 20 of

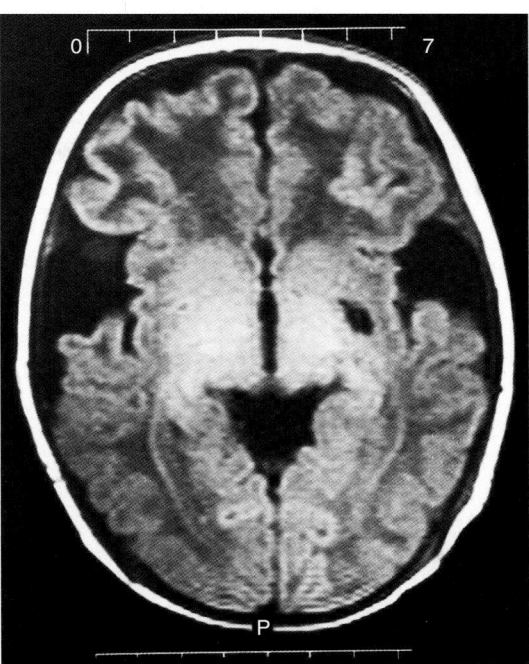

Figure 28.16 Axial T1-weighted magnetic resonance imaging scan performed on a 2-month-old infant with glutaric acidemia type I. The scan, ordered because of macrocephaly and subtle neurological signs (hypotonia, irritability, jitteriness), shows very prominent sylvian fissures with marked frontotemporal atrophy and decreased signal intensity in cerebral white matter. Small subdural effusions are also apparent in the frontotemporal regions. (From Hoffman GF, Athanassopoulos S, Burlina AB, Duran M, et al. Clinical course, early diagnosis, treatment and prevention of disease in glutaryl-CoA dehydrogenase deficiency. *Neuropediatrics*. 1996;27:115–123.)

21 such managed *presymptomatic* infants with the disease.[162] Early detection may require repeated determinations of urinary organic acids because single measurements may be normal or nearly normal.[159,162] Determination of cerebrospinal fluid organic acids may be a more reliable analysis in such situations.[85]

5-Oxoprolinuria

5-Oxoprolinuria has been described in approximately 60 patients, of whom approximately 50% are newborns.[102,167,168] This disorder manifests in the *first days of life* with severe metabolic acidosis and evidence of hemolysis. Approximately half of the reported patients exhibited neurological signs, usually stupor or coma. The *major metabolic features* are 5-oxoprolinemia and 5-oxoprolinuria as well as acidosis. The *enzymatic defect* involves glutathione synthetase, which catalyzes the formation of the tripeptide glutathione from glutamylcysteine and glycine. An increase in glutamylcysteine results, and, as a consequence, excessive amounts of 5-oxoproline, involved in the formation of the former, accumulate in blood and urine. The defect is demonstrable in cultured fibroblasts and erythrocytes. The glutathione deficiency in erythrocytes may account for the hemolysis and jaundice that may occur in the neonatal period. *Therapy* with glucose and sodium bicarbonate is crucial acutely, and subsequently vitamins E and C are administered as free radical scavengers. The latter are used because it is postulated that affected infants have increased sensitivity to oxidative stress. Approximately 25% of affected newborns have died during

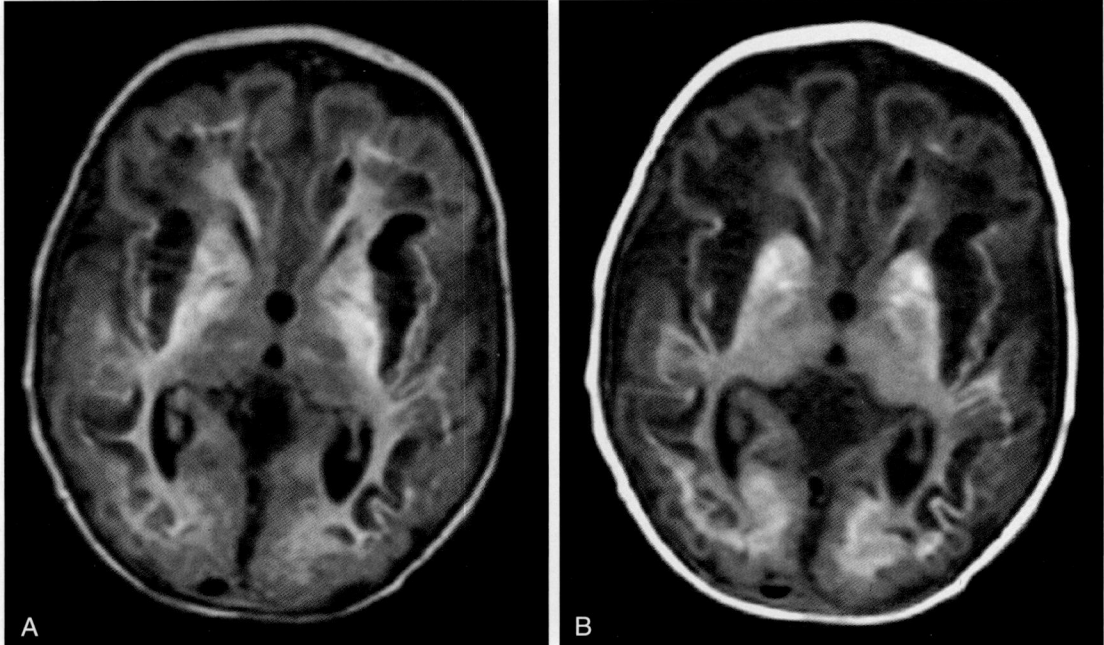

Figure 28.17 Sulfate oxidase deficiency (isolated), magnetic resonance imaging (MRI) scans. (A and B) Axial MRI scans obtained in an affected infant at 31 days show striking cystic lesions diffusely within the white matter, with accompanying abnormal signal and thinning of the cerebral cortex, most marked in the perisylvian regions. Note also the involvement of basal ganglia bilaterally. (From Dublin AB, Hald JK, Wootton-Gorges SL. Isolated sulfite oxidase deficiency: MR imaging features. *AJNR Am J Neuroradiol.* 2002;23:484–485.)

acute episodes. Infants may remain well between intermittent episodes of acidosis, provoked most often by infection.

Sulfite Oxidase Deficiency/Molybdenum Cofactor Deficiency

Sulfite oxidase deficiency may occur as an isolated enzymatic defect or in combination with xanthine dehydrogenase deficiency as part of molybdenum cofactor (MOCO) deficiency. MOCO is essential for the action of both enzymes (as well as aldehyde oxidase, involved in xanthine biosynthesis). Sulfite oxidase catalyzes the oxidation of sulfite to sulfate; the sources of sulfite are the metabolism of sulfur-containing amino acids (e.g., taurine, homocysteine). At least 100 cases of sulfite oxidase deficiency have been reported; approximately 75% have been related to MOCO deficiency.[169-174] Because the neurological features and neuropathology in both forms of sulfite oxidase deficiency are identical, it is assumed that sulfite oxidase deficiency per se is the enzymatic defect responsible for the neural phenomena. Studies with genetically manipulated mice defective in synthesis of MOCO support this conclusion.[175]

The *clinical presentation* is usually in the first days of life, with feeding difficulties, vomiting, and seizures.[169-177] Seizures are often difficult to control. Approximately 75% of infants exhibit facial dysmorphisms (puffy cheeks, small nose, long philtrum). A course involving progression to spasticity, severe mental retardation, and microcephaly occurs in survivors. Dislocated lenses and a seborrheic rash appear later in infancy, but their presence is a clue to the correct diagnosis. Dislocated lenses have been observed as early as 2 months of age.

Brain imaging studies show progressive destruction of neuronal structures (i.e., cerebral cortex, basal ganglia, thalamus,

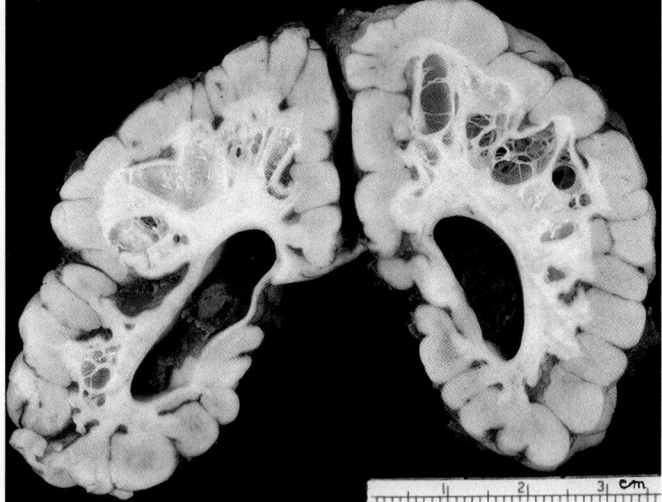

Figure 28.18 Sulfite oxidase deficiency secondary to molybdenum cofactor deficiency: neuropathology. This infant died at 9 months of age. Note the striking and diffuse cystic change in white matter, with atrophic cortical gyri and widening of sulci. Compare with Fig. 28.17. (From Salman MS, Ackerley C, Senger C, Becker L. New insights into the neuropathogenesis of molybdenum cofactor deficiency. *Can J Neurol Sci.* 2002;29:91–96.)

and cerebellum) and of white matter with widespread diminution of and cystic changes within myelin (Fig. 28.17). *Neuropathological evaluation* confirms a widespread destructive process of neurons and white matter with astrocytic gliosis (Fig. 28.18). The disease has resulted in death in approximately 75% of the neonatal-onset cases, usually in infancy. *Metabolic features* are notable for excretion of sulfite, S-sulfocysteine, taurine, and xanthine (the last of these accumulates in MOCO deficiency but not in isolated sulfite oxidase deficiency because aldehyde oxidase for xanthine biosynthesis is spared). Lactic acidosis is not unusual and may raise the possibility of one of the other disorders noted in Table 28.1. The *diagnosis* should be considered in the newborn with seizures of unknown origin; a sulfite strip test on a *fresh* urine sample is a simple screening procedure.[178] However, false-negative and false-positive results can occur. Mass spectrometry is a more sensitive approach for diagnosis. The level of blood uric acid, the product of the xanthine dehydrogenase reaction, is depressed in the MOCO deficiency form of the disease, and detection of hypouricemia thus is a second valuable and simple screening test. A third test is detection of low plasma homocysteine. The *enzymatic defect* involves sulfite oxidase, either in isolation or more commonly, secondary to MOCO deficiency (when xanthine dehydrogenase is also impaired) and is detectable in cultured fibroblasts, cultured amniocytes, and chorionic villus samples. In general no clearly effective *therapy* is available. Administration of diets low in sulfur-containing amino acids (the upstream sources for sulfites) and supplementation with sulfate (the product of sulfite oxidase) have produced positive biochemical responses but no lasting clinical improvement.[178] A recent experimental report suggested benefit with administration of a precursor of MOCO distal to the most common MOCO synthetic block.[175]

KEY REFERENCES

1. Rousson R, Guibaud P. Long term outcome of organic acidurias: survey of 105 French cases (1967–1983). *J Inherit Metab Dis*. 1984;7: 10-12.
2. Nizon M, Ottolenghi C, Valayannopoulos V, et al. Long-term neurological outcome of a cohort of 80 patients with classical organic acidurias. *Orphanet J Rare Dis*. 2013;8:148.
3. Grunert SC, Mullerleile S, De Silva L, et al. Propionic acidemia: clinical course and outcome in 55 pediatric and adolescent patients. *Orphanet J Rare Dis*. 2013;8:6.
4. Deodato F, Boenzi S, Santorelli FM, et al. Methylmalonic and propionic aciduria. *Am J Med Genet C Semin Med Genet*. 2006;142C: 104-112.
5. Fenton WA, Gravel RA, Rosenblatt DS. Disorders of propionate and methylmalonate metabolism. In: Scriver CR, Beaudet AL, Sly WS, et al., eds. *The Metabolic and Molecuar Bases of Inherited Disease*. 8th ed. New York: McGraw-Hill; 2001:2165-2192.
11. Kolvraa S. Inhibition of the glycine cleavage system by branched-chain amino-acid metabolites. *Pediatr Res*. 1979;13: 889-893.
12. Shuman RM, Leech RW, Scott CR. The neuropathology of the nonketotic and ketotic hyperglycinemias: three cases. *Neurology*. 1978;28:139-146.
13. Friede RL. *Developmental neuropathology*. 2nd rev. and expanded ed. Berlin; New York: Springer-Verlag; 1989.
14. Prosenc N, Stoltenburgdidinger G. Spongy encephalopathy in ketotic hyperglycinemia. *Brain Dev*. 1994;16:445-449.
16. Wendel U. Abnormality of odd-numbered long-chain fatty-acids in erythrocyte-membrane lipids from patients with disorders of propionate metabolism. *Pediatr Res*. 1989;25:147-150.
19. Volpe JJ, Kishimoto Y. Fatty acid synthetase of brain: development, influence of nutritional and hormonal factors and comparison with liver enzyme. *J Neurochem*. 1972;19:737-753.
20. Volpe JJ, Vagelos PR. Fatty acid synthetase of mammalian brain, liver and adipose tissue. Regulation by prosthetic group turnover. *Biochim Biophys Acta*. 1973;326:293-304.
21. Baumgartner MR, Horster F, Dionisi-Vici C, et al. Proposed guidelines for the diagnosis and management of methylmalonic and propionic acidemia. *Orphanet J Rare Dis*. 2014;9:130.

22. Bergman AJ, Van der Knaap MS, Smeitink JA, et al. Magnetic resonance imaging and spectroscopy of the brain in propionic acidemia: clinical and biochemical considerations. *Pediatr Res*. 1996; 40:404-409.
23. Surtees RA, Matthews EE, Leonard JV. Neurologic outcome of propionic acidemia. *Pediatr Neurol*. 1992;8:333-337.
24. Sass JO, Hofmann M, Skladal D, et al. Propionic acidemia revisited: a workshop report. *Clinical Pediatr*. 2004;43:837-843.
25. Dave P, Curless RG, Steinman L. Cerebellar hemorrhage complicating methylmalonic and propionic acidemia. *Arch Neurol*. 1984;41:1293-1296.
26. Al-Essa M, Bakheet S, Patay Z, et al. ¹⁸Fluoro-2-deoxyglucose (¹⁸FDG) PET scan of the brain in propionic acidemia: clinical and MRI correlations. *Brain Dev*. 1999;21:312-317.
27. Martinez Alvarez L, Jameson E, Parry NR, et al. Optic neuropathy in methylmalonic acidemia and propionic acidemia. *Br J Ophthalmol*. 2016;100:98-104.
29. Hsia YE, Scully KJ, Rosenberg LE. Inherited propionyl-CoA carboxylase deficiency in "ketotic hyperglycinemia." *J Clin Invest*. 1971;50:127-130.
30. Barnes ND, Hull D, Balgobin L, et al. Biotin-responsive propionicacidaemia. *Lancet*. 1970;2:244-245.
31. Hamilton RL, Haas RH, Nyhan WL, et al. Neuropathology of propionic acidemia: a report of two patients with basal ganglia lesions. *J Child Neurol*. 1995;10:25-30.
32. Haas RH, Marsden DL, Capistrano-Estrada S, et al. Acute basal ganglia infarction in propionic acidemia. *J Child Neurol*. 1995;10: 18-22.
33. Barkovich AJ. *Pediatric Neuroimaging*. 4th ed. Philadelphia: Lippincott Williams & Wilkins; 2005.
34. Kandel A, Amatya SK, Yeh EA. Reversible diffusion weighted imaging changes in propionic acidemia. *J Child Neurol*. 2013;28: 128-131.
35. Broomfield A, Gunny R, Prabhakar P, et al. Spontaneous rapid resolution of acute basal ganglia changes in an untreated infant with propionic acidemia: a clue to pathogenesis? *Neuropediatrics*. 2010;41:256-260.
36. Feliz B, Witt DR, Harris BT. Propionic acidemia: a neuropathology case report and review of prior cases. *Arch Pathol Lab Med*. 2003;127: e325-e328.
37. Perez-Cerda C, Perez B, Merinero B, et al. Prenatal diagnosis of propionic acidemia. *Prenatal Diag*. 2004;24:962-964.
38. Vernon HJ. Inborn errors of metabolism: advances in diagnosis and therapy. *JAMA Pediatr*. 2015;169:778-782.
39. Malvagia S, Haynes CA, Grisotto L, et al. Heptadecanoylcarnitine (C17) a novel candidate biomarker for newborn screening of propionic and methylmalonic acidemias. *Clin Chim Acta*. 2015;450: 342-348.
40. Guenzel AJ, Hofherr SE, Hillestad M, et al. Generation of a hypomorphic model of propionic acidemia amenable to gene therapy testing. *Mol Ther*. 2013;21:1316-1323.
41. Wolf B, Hsia YE, Sweetman L, et al. Propionic acidemia: a clinical update. *J Pediatr*. 1981;99:835-846.
42. Charbit-Henrion F, Lacaille F, McKiernan P, et al. Early and late complications after liver transplantation for propionic acidemia in children: a two centers study. *Am J Transplant*. 2015;15:786-791.
43. Matsui SM, Mahoney MJ, Rosenberg LE. The natural history of the inherited methylmalonic acidemias. *N Engl J Med*. 1983;308: 857-861.
45. Nicolaides P, Leonard J, Surtees R. Neurological outcome of methylmalonic acidaemia. *Arch Dis Child*. 1998;78:508-512.
46. Treacy E, Clow C, Mamer OA, et al. Methylmalonic acidemia with a severe chemical but benign clinical phenotype. *J Pediatr*. 1993;122:428-429.
47. Gropman AL. Patterns of brain injury in inborn errors of metabolism. *Semin Pediatr Neurol*. 2012;19:203-210.
48. Biancheri R, Cerone R, Schiaffino MC, et al. Cobalamin (Cbl) C/D deficiency: clinical, neurophysiological and neuroradiologic findings in 14 cases. *Neuropediatrics*. 2001;32:14-22.
49. Ricci D, Pane M, Deodato F, et al. Assessment of visual function in children with methylmalonic aciduria and homocystinuria. *Neuropediatrics*. 2005;36:181-185.
52. Tanpaiboon P. Methylmalonic acidemia (MMA). *Molec Genet Metabol*. 2005;85:2-6.

56. Sum JM, Twiss JL, Horoupian DS. Selective death of immature neurons in methylmalonic acidemia of the neonate—a case report. *Acta Neuropathol*. 1993;85:217-221.

57. Kanaumi T, Takashima S, Hirose S, et al. Neuropathology of methylmalonic acidemia in a child. *Pediatr Neurol*. 2006;34:156-159.

59. Mahoney MJ, Rosenberg LE, Lindblad B, et al. Prenatal diagnosis of methylmalonic aciduria. *Acta Paediatr Scand*. 1975;64:44-48.

60. Ampola MG, Mahoney MJ, Nakamura E, et al. Prenatal therapy of a patient with vitamin-B12-responsive methylmalonic acidemia. *N Engl J Med*. 1975;293:313-317.

61. van der Meer SB, Spaapen LJ, Fowler B, et al. Prenatal treatment of a patient with vitamin B12-responsive methylmalonic acidemia. *J Pediatr*. 1990;117:923-926.

62. Rosenblatt A. Inherited disorders of folate and cobalamin transport and metabolism. In: Scriver CR, Beaudet AL, Sly WS, et al., eds. *The Metabolic & Molecular Bases of Inherited Disease*. 8th ed. New York: McGraw-Hill; 2001:3897-3933.

63. Hori D, Hasegawa Y, Kimura M, et al. Clinical onset and prognosis of Asian children with organic acidemias, as detected by analysis of urinary organic acids using GC/MS, instead of mass screening. *Brain Dev*. 2005;27:39-45.

64. Niemi AK, Kim IK, Krueger CE, et al. Treatment of methylmalonic acidemia by liver or combined liver-kidney transplantation. *J Pediatr*. 2015;166:1455-1461. e1451.

65. Spada M, Calvo PL, Brunati A, et al. Early liver transplantation for neonatal-onset methylmalonic acidemia. *Pediatrics*. 2015;136:E252-E256.

66. Pithukpakorn M. Disorders of pyruvate metabolism and the tricarboxylic acid cycle. *Molec Genet Metabol*. 2005;85:243-246.

67. Kerrigan JF, Aleck KA, Tarby TJ, et al. Fumaric aciduria: clinical and imaging features. *Ann Neurol*. 2000;47:583-588.

68. Nissenkorn A, Michelson M, Ben-Zeev B, et al. Inborn errors of metabolism—a cause of abnormal brain development. *Neurology*. 2001;56:1265-1272.

69. Robinson BH. Lactic acidemia: disorders of pyruvate carboxylase and pyruvate dehydrogenase. In: Scriver CR, Beaudet AL, Sly WS, et al., eds. *The Metabolic & Molecular Bases of Inherited Disease*. 8th ed. New York: McGraw-Hill; 2001:2275-2295.

70. De Vivo DC. Complexities of the pyruvate dehydrogenase complex. *Neurology*. 1998;51:1247-1249.

71. Volpe JJ, Marasa JC. Role for thiamine in regulation of fatty-acid and cholesterol-biosynthesis in cultured cells of neural origin. *J Neurochem*. 1978;30:975-981.

72. Pirot N, Crahes M, Adle-Biassette H, et al. Phenotypic and neuropathological characterization of fetal pyruvate dehydrogenase deficiency. *J Neuropathol Exper Neurol*. 2016;75:227-238.

73. Patel KP, O'Brien TW, Subramony SH, et al. The spectrum of pyruvate dehydrogenase complex deficiency: clinical, biochemical and genetic features in 371 patients. *Molec Genet Metabol*. 2012;106:385-394.

74. De Meirleir L, Lissens W, Denis R, et al. Pyruvate dehydrogenase deficiency: clinical and biochemical diagnosis. *Pediatr Neurol*. 1993;9:216-220.

75. DeBrosse SD, Okajima K, Zhang S, et al. Spectrum of neurological and survival outcomes in pyruvate dehydrogenase complex (PDC) deficiency: lack of correlation with genotype. *Molec Genet Metabol*. 2012;107:394-402.

76. De Meirleir L. Defects of pyruvate metabolism and the Krebs cycle. *J Child Neurol*. 2002;17:3S26-3S33, discussion 3S33-3S34.

77. Old SE, Devivo DC. Pyruvate-dehydrogenase complex deficiency—biochemical and immunoblot analysis of cultured skin fibroblasts. *Ann Neurol*. 1989;26:746-751.

78. Robinson BH, MacKay N, Chun K, et al. Disorders of pyruvate carboxylase and the pyruvate dehydrogenase complex. *J Inherit Metab Dis*. 1996;19:452-462.

79. Cross JH, Connelly A, Gadian DG, et al. Clinical diversity of pyruvate dehydrogenase deficiency. *Pediatr Neurol*. 1994;10:276-283.

80. Zand DJ, Simon EM, Pulitzer SB, et al. In vivo pyruvate detected by MR spectroscopy in neonatal pyruvate dehydrogenase deficiency. *AJNR Am J Neuroradiol*. 2003;24:1471-1474.

81. Ah Mew N, Loewenstein JB, Kadom N, et al. MRI features of 4 female patients with pyruvate dehydrogenase E_{1alpha} deficiency. *Pediatr Neurol*. 2011;45:57-59.

82. Cameron JM, Levandovskiy V, Mackay N, et al. Deficiency of pyruvate dehydrogenase caused by novel and known mutations in the E_{1alpha} subunit. *Am J Med Genet A*. 2004;131:59-66.

84. De Vivo DC. The expanding clinical spectrum of mitochondrial diseases. *Brain Dev*. 1993;15:1-22.

85. Hoffmann GF, Surtees RA, Wevers RA. Cerebrospinal fluid investigations for neurometabolic disorders. *Neuropediatrics*. 1998;29:59-71.

86. Elpeleg ON, Ruitenbeek W, Jakobs C, et al. Congenital lacticacidemia caused by lipoamide dehydrogenase deficiency with favorable outcome. *J Pediatr*. 1995;126:72-74.

87. Brown RM, Head RA, Morris AA, et al. Pyruvate dehydrogenase E3 binding protein (protein X) deficiency. *Dev Med Child Neurol*. 2006;48:756-760.

88. Taylor J, Robinson BH, Sherwood WG. A defect in branched-chain amino acid metabolism in a patient with congenital lactic acidosis due to dihydrolipoyl dehydrogenase deficiency. *Pediatr Res*. 1978;12:60-62.

89. Pliss L, Pentney RJ, Johnson MT, et al. Biochemical and structural brain alterations in female mice with cerebral pyruvate dehydrogenase deficiency. *J Neurochem*. 2004;91:1082-1091.

92. Morten KJ, Beattie P, Brown GK, et al. Dichloroacetate stabilizes the mutant E_{1alpha} subunit in pyruvate dehydrogenase deficiency. *Neurology*. 1999;53:612-616.

93. Ferriero R, Manco G, Lamantea E, et al. Phenylbutyrate therapy for pyruvate dehydrogenase complex deficiency and lactic acidosis. *Sci Trans Med*. 2013;5:175ra131.

94. Wexler ID, Hemalatha SG, McConnell J, et al. Outcome of pyruvate dehydrogenase deficiency treated with ketogenic diets. Studies in patients with identical mutations. *Neurology*. 1997;49:1655-1661.

96. Garcia-Cazorla A, Rabier D, Touati G, et al. Pyruvate carboxylase deficiency: metabolic characteristics and new neurological aspects. *Ann Neurol*. 2006;59:121-127.

97. Pineda M, Campistol J, Vilaseca MA, et al. An atypical French form of pyruvate carboxylase deficiency. *Brain Dev*. 1995;17:276-279.

100. Brun N, Robitaille Y, Grignon A, et al. Pyruvate carboxylase deficiency: prenatal onset of ischemia-like brain lesions in two sibs with the acute neonatal forum. *Am J Med Genet*. 1999;84:94-101.

101. Nyhan WL, Khanna A, Barshop BA, et al. Pyruvate carboxylase deficiency—insights from liver transplantation. *Molec Genet Metabol*. 2002;77:143-149.

102. Chaves-Carballo E. Detection of inherited neurometabolic disorders. A practical clinical approach. *Pediatr Clin North Am*. 1992;39:801-820.

103. Sweetman L, Williams JC. Branched chain organic acidurias. In: Scriver CR, Beaudet AL, Sly WS, et al., eds. *The Metabolic & Molecular Bases of Inherited Disease*. 8th ed. New York: McGraw-Hill; 2001:2125-2164.

104. Fischer AQ, Challa VR, Burton BK, et al. Cerebellar hemorrhage complicating isovaleric acidemia: a case report. *Neurology*. 1981;31:746-748.

106. Hyman DB, Tanaka K. Isovaleryl-CoA dehydrogenase activity in isovaleric acidemia fibroblasts using an improved tritium release assay. *Pediatr Res*. 1986;20:59-61.

107. Tajima G, Sakura N, Yofune H, et al. Establishment of a practical enzymatic assay method for determination of isovaleryl-CoA dehydrogenase activity using high-performance liquid chromatography. *Clin Chim Acta*. 2005;353:193-199.

108. Gregersen N. The specific inhibition of the pyruvate dehydrogenase complex from pig kidney by propionyl-CoA and isovaleryl-Co-A. *Biochem Med*. 1981;26:20-27.

109. Lorek AK, Penrice JM, Cady EB, et al. Cerebral energy metabolism in isovaleric acidaemia. *Arch Dis Child Fetal Neonat Ed*. 1996;74:F211-F213.

110. Solano AF, Leipnitz G, De Bortoli GM, et al. Induction of oxidative stress by the metabolites accumulating in isovaleric acidemia in brain cortex of young rats. *Free Radical Res*. 2008;42:707-715.

111. Berry GT, Yudkoff M, Segal S. Isovaleric acidemia: medical and neurodevelopmental effects of long-term therapy. *J Pediatr*. 1988;113:58-64.

112. Mayatepek E, Kurczynski TW, Hoppel CL. Long-term L-carnitine treatment in isovaleric acidemia. *Pediatr Neurol*. 1991;7:137-140.

113. Naglak M, Salvo R, Madsen K, et al. The treatment of isovaleric acidemia with glycine supplement. *Pediatr Res*. 1988;24:9-13.

115. Grunert SC, Wendel U, Lindner M, et al. Clinical and neurocognitive outcome in symptomatic isovaleric acidemia. *Orphanet J Rare Dis.* 2012;7:9.

116. Dantas MF, Suormala T, Randolph A, et al. 3-Methylcrotonyl-CoA carboxylase deficiency: mutation analysis in 28 probands, 9 symptomatic and 19 detected by newborn screening. *Hum Mutat.* 2005;26:164.

117. Oude Luttikhuis HG, Touati G, Rabier D, et al. Severe hypoglycaemia in isolated 3-methylcrotonyl-CoA carboxylase deficiency: a rare, severe clinical presentation. *J Inherit Metab Dis.* 2005;28:1136-1138.

118. Baykal T, Gokcay GH, Ince Z, et al. Consanguineous 3-methylcrotonyl-CoA carboxylase deficiency: early-onset necrotizing encephalopathy with lethal outcome. *J Inherit Metab Dis.* 2005;28:229-233.

119. Mitchell GA, Fukao T. Inborn errors of ketone body catabolism. In: Scriver CR, Beaudet AL, Sly WS, et al., eds. *The Metabolic & Molecular Bases of Inherited Disease.* New York: McGraw-Hill; 2001: 2327-2356.

120. Gibson KM, Breuer J, Nyhan WL. 3-Hydroxy-3-methylglutaryl-coenzyme A lyase deficiency: review of 18 reported patients. *Eur J Pediatr.* 1988;148:180-186.

121. Yalcinkaya C, Dincer A, Gunduz E, et al. MRI and MRS in HMG-CoA lyase deficiency. *Pediatr Neurol.* 1999;20:375-380.

122. Zoghbi HY, Spence JE, Beaudet AL, et al. Atypical presentation and neuropathological studies in 3-hydroxy-3-methylglutaryl-CoA lyase deficiency. *Ann Neurol.* 1986;20:367-369.

123. Barash V, Mandel H, Sella S, et al. 3-Hydroxy-3-methylglutaryl-coenzyme A lyase deficiency: biochemical studies and family investigation of four generations. *J Inherit Metab Dis.* 1990;13: 156-164.

124. Hoffmann G, Gibson KM, Brandt IK, et al. Mevalonic aciduria—an inborn error of cholesterol and nonsterol isoprene biosynthesis. *N Engl J Med.* 1986;314:1610-1614.

125. Hoffmann GF, Charpentier C, Mayatepek E, et al. Clinical and biochemical phenotype in 11 patients with mevalonic aciduria. *Pediatrics.* 1993;91:915-921.

126. Rolland MO, Cuisset L, Le Bozec J, et al. First-trimester enzymatic and molecular prenatal diagnosis of mevalonic aciduria. *J Inherit Metab Dis.* 2005;28:1141-1142.

128. Yamaguchi S, Sakai A, Fukao T, et al. Biochemical and immunochemical study of seven families with 3-ketothiolase deficiency: diagnosis of heterozygotes using immunochemical determination of the ratio of mitochondrial acetoacetyl-CoA thiolase and 3-ketoacyl-CoA thiolase proteins. *Pediatr Res.* 1993;33: 429-432.

129. Roe CR, Ding J. Mitochondrial fatty acid oxidation disorders. In: Scriver CR, Beaudet AL, Sly WS, et al., eds. *The Metabolic & Molecular Bases of Inherited Disease.* 8th ed. New York: McGraw-Hill; 2001:2297.

130. Riudor E. Neonatal onset in fatty acid oxidation disorders: how can we minimize morbidity and mortality? *J Inherit Metab Dis.* 1998;21:619-623.

131. Tyni T, Palotie A, Viinikka L, et al. Long-chain 3-hydroxyacyl-coenzyme A dehydrogenase deficiency with the G1528C mutation: clinical presentation of thirteen patients. *J Pediatr.* 1997;130:67-76.

132. Tamaoki Y, Kimura M, Hasegawa Y, et al. A survey of Japanese patients with mitochondrial fatty acid beta-oxidation and related disorders as detected from 1985 to 2000. *Brain Dev.* 2002;24: 675-680.

133. Vladutiu GD, Quackenbush EJ, Hainline BE, et al. Lethal neonatal and severe late infantile forms of carnitine palmitoyltransferase II deficiency associated with compound heterozygosity for different protein truncation mutations. *J Pediatr.* 2002;141:734-736.

134. Derks TG, Reijngoud DJ, Waterham HR, et al. The natural history of medium-chain acyl CoA dehydrogenase deficiency in the Netherlands: clinical presentation and outcome. *J Pediatr.* 2006; 148:665-670.

135. Mikati MA, Chaaban HR, Karam PE, et al. Brain malformation and infantile spasms in a SCAD deficiency patient. *Pediatr Neurol.* 2007;36:48-50.

136. Catzeflis C, Bachmann C, Hale DE, et al. Early diagnosis and treatment of neonatal medium-chain acyl-CoA dehydrogenase deficiency: report of two siblings. *Eur J Pediatr.* 1990;149:577-581.

137. Wilcken B, Carpenter KH, Hammond J. Neonatal symptoms in medium chain acyl coenzyme A dehydrogenase deficiency. *Arch Dis Child.* 1993;69:292-294.

138. Iafolla AK, Thompson RJ Jr, Roe CR. Medium-chain acyl-coenzyme A dehydrogenase deficiency: clinical course in 120 affected children. *J Pediatr.* 1994;124:409-415.

139. Ziadeh R, Hoffman EP, Finegold DN, et al. Medium chain acyl-CoA dehydrogenase deficiency in Pennsylvania: neonatal screening shows high incidence and unexpected mutation frequencies. *Pediatr Res.* 1995;37:675-678.

140. Wolf B. Disorders of biotin metabolism. In: Scriver CR, Beaudet AL, Sly WS, et al., eds. *The Metabolic & Molecular Bases of Inherited Disease.* New York: McGraw-Hill; 2001:3935-3962.

141. Bousounis DP, Camfield PR, Wolf B. Reversal of brain atrophy with biotin treatment in biotinidase deficiency. *Neuropediatrics.* 1993;24:214-217.

142. Haagerup A, Andersen JB, Blichfeldt S, et al. Biotinidase deficiency: two cases of very early presentation. *Dev Med Child Neurol.* 1997;39:832-835.

143. Enns GM, Cowan TM, Klein O, et al. Aminoacidemias and organic acidemias. In: Swaiman KF, Ashwal S, Ferriero DM, eds. *Swaiman's Pediatric Neurology: Principles and Practice.* 5th ed. Philadelphia: Elsevier Saunders; 2012:328-356.

144. Morrone A, Malvagia S, Donati MA, et al. Clinical findings and biochemical and molecular analysis of four patients with holocarboxylase synthetase deficiency. *Am J Med Genet.* 2002;111: 10-18.

145. Wilson CJ, Myer M, Darlow BA, et al. Severe holocarboxylase synthetase deficiency with incomplete biotin responsiveness resulting in antenatal insult in samoan neonates. *J Pediatr.* 2005;147:115-118.

146. Wolf B, Hsia YE, Sweetman L, et al. Multiple carboxylase deficiency: clinical and biochemical improvement following neonatal biotin treatment. *Pediatrics.* 1981;68:113-118.

147. Roth KS, Yang W, Allan L, et al. Prenatal administration of biotin in biotin responsive multiple carboxylase deficiency. *Pediatr Res.* 1982;16:126-129.

148. Suormala TM, Baumgartner ER, Wick H, et al. Comparison of patients with complete and partial biotinidase deficiency: biochemical studies. *J Inherit Metab Dis.* 1990;13:76-92.

149. Moslinger D, Muhl A, Suormala T, et al. Molecular characterisation and neuropsychological outcome of 21 patients with profound biotinidase deficiency detected by newborn screening and family studies. *Eur J Pediatr.* 2003;162:S46-S49.

150. Grunewald S, Champion MP, Leonard JV, et al. Biotinidase deficiency: a treatable leukoencephalopathy. *Neuropediatrics.* 2004;35:211-216.

151. Weber P, Scholl S, Baumgartner ER. Outcome in patients with profound biotinidase deficiency: relevance of newborn screening. *Dev Med Child Neurol.* 2004;46:481-484.

152. Loehr JP, Goodman SI, Frerman FE. Glutaric acidemia type II: heterogeneity of clinical and biochemical phenotypes. *Pediatr Res.* 1990;27:311-315.

153. Shevell MI, Didomenicantonio G, Sylvain M, et al. Glutaric acidemia type II: neuroimaging and spectroscopy evidence for developmental encephalomyopathy. *Pediatr Neurol.* 1995;12:350-353.

155. Takanashi J, Fujii K, Sugita K, et al. Neuroradiologic findings in glutaric aciduria type II. *Pediatr Neurol.* 1999;20:142-145.

156. Yamaguchi S, Shimizu N, Orii T, et al. Prenatal diagnosis and neonatal monitoring of a fetus with glutaric aciduria type II due to electron transfer flavoprotein (beta-subunit) deficiency. *Pediatr Res.* 1991;30:439-443.

157. Frerman FE, Goodman SI. Defects of electron transfer falavoprotein and electron transfer flavoprotein-ubiquinone oxidoreductase: glutaric acidemia type II. In: Scriver CR, Beaudet AL, Sly WS, et al., eds. *The Metabolic & Molecular Bases of Inherited Disease.* 8th ed. New York: McGraw-Hill; 2001:2357-2365.

158. Uziel G, Garavaglia B, Ciceri E, et al. Riboflavin-responsive glutaric aciduria type II presenting as a leukodystrophy. *Pediatr Neurol.* 1995;13:333-335.

159. Goodman SI, Frerman FE. Organic acidemias due to defects in lysine oxidation: 2-ketoadipic acidemia and glutaric acidemia. In: Scriver CR, Beaudet AL, Sly WS, et al., eds. *The Metabolic &*

Molecular Bases of Inherited Disease. 8th ed. New York: McGraw-Hill; 2001:2195-2204.

160. Kolker S, Christensen E, Leonard JV, et al. Diagnosis and management of glutaric aciduria type I—revised recommendations. *J Inherit Metab Dis.* 2011;34:677-694.

161. Haworth JC, Booth FA, Chudley AE, et al. Phenotypic variability in glutaric aciduria type I: report of fourteen cases in five Canadian Indian kindreds. *J Pediatr.* 1991;118:52-58.

162. Hoffmann GF, Athanassopoulos S, Burlina AB, et al. Clinical course, early diagnosis, treatment, and prevention of disease in glutaryl-CoA dehydrogenase deficiency. *Neuropediatrics.* 1996;27:115-123.

163. Kolker S, Garbade SF, Greenberg CR, et al. Natural history, outcome, and treatment efficacy in children and adults with glutaryl-CoA dehydrogenase deficiency. *Pediatr Res.* 2006;59: 840-847.

164. Chen E, Nyhan WL, Jakobs C, et al. L-2-Hydroxyglutaric aciduria: neuropathological correlations and first report of severe neurodegenerative disease and neonatal death. *J Inherit Metab Dis.* 1996;19:335-343.

165. D'Incerti L, Farina L, Moroni I, et al. L-2-Hydroxyglutaric aciduria: MRI in seven cases. *Neuroradiology.* 1998;40:727-733.

166. van der Knaap MS, Jakobs C, Hoffmann GF, et al. D-2-Hydroxyglutaric aciduria: biochemical marker or clinical disease entity? *Ann Neurol.* 1999;45:111-119.

167. Divry P, Roulaud-Parrot F, Dorche C, et al. 5-Oxoprolinuria (glutathione synthetase deficiency): a case with neonatal presentation and rapid fatal outcome. *J Inherit Metab Dis.* 1991;14: 341-344.

168. Ristoff E, Mayatepek E, Larsson A. Long-term clinical outcome in patients with glutathione synthetase deficiency. *J Pediatr.* 2001;139:79-84.

169. Johnson JL, Duran M. Molybdenum cofactor deficiency and isolated sulfite oxidase deficiency. In: Scriver CR, Beaudet AL, Sly WS, et al., eds. *The Metabolic & Molecular Bases of Inherited Disease.* 8th ed. New York: McGraw-Hill; 2001:3163-3177.

170. Dublin AB, Hald JK, Wootton-Gorges SL. Isolated sulfite oxidase deficiency: MR imaging features. *AJNR Am J Neuroradiol.* 2002;23:484-485.

171. Salman MS, Ackerley C, Senger C, et al. New insights into the neuropathogenesis of molybdenum cofactor deficiency. *Can J Neurol Sci.* 2002;29:91-96.

172. Sass JO, Gunduz A, Araujo Rodrigues Funayama C, et al. Functional deficiencies of sulfite oxidase: differential diagnoses in neonates presenting with intractable seizures and cystic encephalomalacia. *Brain Dev.* 2010;32:544-549.

173. Carmi-Nawi N, Malinger G, Mandel H, et al. Prenatal brain disruption in molybdenum cofactor deficiency. *J Child Neurol.* 2011;26:460-464.

174. Vijayakumar K, Gunny R, Grunewald S, et al. Clinical neuroimaging features and outcome in molybdenum cofactor deficiency. *Pediatr Neurol.* 2011;45:246-252.

175. Reiss J, Bonin M, Schwegler H, et al. The pathogenesis of molybdenum cofactor deficiency, its delay by maternal clearance, and its expression pattern in microarray analysis. *Molec Genet Metabol.* 2005;85:12-20.

176. Hansen LK, Wulff K, Dorche C, et al. Molybdenum cofactor deficiency in two siblings: diagnostic difficulties. *Eur J Pediatr.* 1993;152:662-664.

177. Boles RG, Ment LR, Meyn MS, et al. Short-term response to dietary therapy in molybdenum cofactor deficiency. *Ann Neurol.* 1993;34:742-744.

178. Johnson JL, Wadman SK. Molybdenum cofactor deficiency and isolated sulfite oxidase deficiency. In: Scriver CR, Beaudet AL, Sly WS, et al., eds. *The Metabolic & Molecular Bases of Inherited Disease.* 7th ed. New York: McGraw-Hill; 1995:2271-2283.

Full references for this chapter can be found at www.expertconsult .com.

UNIT VII

DEGENERATIVE DISORDERS

Degenerative Disorders of the Newborn

Christopher M. Elitt ◆ Joseph J. Volpe

Certain degenerative disorders of the developing nervous system may be clinically manifested in the neonatal period. Because most of these disorders are related to a disturbance in the metabolism of a lipid or some other compound, they are discussed most appropriately in this series of chapters concerned with metabolic disorders. Indeed, clinical overlap of some of these degenerative disorders with some of the metabolic disorders discussed in previous chapters will be apparent. Nevertheless, the diseases discussed in this chapter are best considered as a more or less distinct group. Early diagnosis is important for the delineation of prognosis, genetic counseling, and, in a few instances, the institution of specific therapy. Because these are relatively rare disorders, discussion of each entity is brief.

MAJOR DISORDERS

From the clinical standpoint, we find it useful to separate the degenerative disorders into those that primarily affect gray matter and those that primarily involve white matter (Table 29.1). (At later ages, disorders that affect specific regions of the brain [e.g., basal ganglia in Huntington or Wilson disease, or cerebellum in ataxia telangiectasia], so-called system degenerations, comprise a third major category.) In general, disorders of gray matter are characterized by the appearance early in the disease of seizures, myoclonus, spikes, or sharp activity on the electroencephalogram, failure of cognitive development (*dementia*), and retinal disease; whereas disorders of white matter are characterized by the appearance early in the disease of marked motor deficits and slow activity on the electroencephalogram. Although overlap in the clinical features and even in the topography of the neuropathology between the two broad categories is considerable, we retain the separation. There are a few disorders involving specific subcellular organelles (e.g., peroxisomes, mitochondria) or other, still-to-be-defined defects that affect *both* gray *and* white matter prominently, and these must be considered separately (see Table 29.1). This chapter focuses only on those diseases for which the recording of more than a few cases with neonatal manifestations is available. The salient features of the disorders are outlined in Tables 29.2 to 29.5. Many of these disorders are abnormalities of degradation of sphingolipids (Fig. 29.1), as noted in the individual discussions later.

DISORDERS PRIMARILY AFFECTING GRAY MATTER

Disorders primarily affecting gray matter are best discussed according to the presence or absence of accompanying

| TABLE 29.1 | Degenerative Diseases of the Nervous System With Manifestations in the Newborn |

Gray matter
No visceral storage
Tay-Sachs disease (GM$_2$ gangliosidosis)
Congenital neuronal ceroid-lipofuscinosis
Alpers disease
Menkes disease

With visceral storage
GM$_1$ gangliosidosis
GM$_2$ gangliosidosis (Sandhoff variant)
Niemann-Pick disease
Gaucher disease
Farber disease
Infantile sialic acid storage disease

White matter
Canavan disease
Alexander disease
Krabbe disease
Pelizaeus-Merzbacher disease
Leukodystrophy with cerebral calcifications and cerebrospinal fluid pleocytosis (Aicardi-Goutieres disease)

Gray and white matter
Peroxisomal disorders: neonatal adrenoleukodystrophy, Zellweger syndrome
Mitochondrial disorder: Leigh syndrome, other mitochondrial encephalopathies
Disorders with cerebellar ± pontine hypoplasia
• Congenital disorders of glycosylation
• Pontocerebellar hypoplasia
Neurotransmitter defects
• Serine synthesis deficiency
Rett syndrome (males)

visceral storage. Visceral storage is clinically identified by hepatosplenomegaly and is often accompanied by abnormalities of the long bones and by coarse facial features.

No Visceral Storage

Tay-Sachs Disease

Tay-Sachs disease is the prototype of a degenerative disease of gray matter in infancy (see Table 29.2). Onset in the first few weeks of life, although uncommon, may occur. (More commonly, onset is at approximately 3 months.) The principal initial *clinical features* are irritability and hypersensitivity to auditory and often other sensory inputs. A cherry-red spot, caused by

TABLE 29.2   Degenerative Diseases Primarily of Gray Matter (No Visceral Storage)

DISEASE	CLINICAL FEATURES	METABOLIC-ENZYMATIC FEATURES	PATHOLOGY
Tay-Sachs disease (GM$_2$ gangliosidosis)	Stimulus-sensitive myoclonus, irritability, hypotonia, weakness, cherry-red macula (virtually all); later seizures, blindness, and macrocephaly	GM$_2$ ganglioside accumulation in brain; hexosaminidase A deficiency	Neurons distended by GM$_2$ ganglioside throughout the CNS
Congenital neuronal ceroid-lipofuscinosis	Neonatal seizures (severe), apnea, microcephaly, developmental arrest, followed by regression and vegetative state	Cathepsin D deficiency	Marked brain atrophy; diffuse neuronal loss with gliosis, autofluorescent granular material in neurons, glia, and macrophages, electron microscopy— osmiophilic granules
Alpers disease	Myoclonus (often stimulus-sensitive), seizures (severe), developmental arrest followed by regression, visual and auditory deficits common, evidence of hepatic dysfunction late	Elevated lactate/pyruvate levels in cerebrospinal fluid (and blood); deficient catalytic subunit of mitochondrial DNA polymerase gamma (mutated gene *POLG*) with mitochondrial DNA depletion and impaired function of electron transport chain at multiple sites; POLG-negative cases (with apparent defect in mitochondrial tRNA metabolism) now recognized especially in the perinatal period	Marked brain atrophy; severe neuronal loss with astrocytosis, spongiosis, and capillary proliferation, especially in the cerebral cortex, and particularly occipital (striate) cortex
Menkes disease (kinky hair disease)	Hypothermia, hypotonia, poor feeding, poor weight gain, seizures, developmental arrest and then regression; cherubic face; colorless, friable, *steely* hair	Low serum copper and ceruloplasmin levels; cultured fibroblasts: reduced efflux of copper; elevated copper content; deficient activity of many copper-containing enzymes; molecular defect of a cation transporting ATPase	Neuronal loss with gliosis in cerebral cortex and cerebellum, marked proliferation of dendritic tree (especially of Purkinje cells), focal axonal swellings (*torpedoes*); myelin loss with gliosis and arterial changes

CNS, Central nervous system; *POLG,* polymerase γ.

ganglioside storage in retinal ganglion cells imparting a yellowish tint around the normally red fovea, is apparent on funduscopic examination. This abnormality has been identified as early as 2 days of age.[1,2] The subsequent course is characterized by myoclonic seizures, motor deterioration, hypotonia, blindness, macrencephaly, and death in the third or fourth year of life, which are the features confirmed in a recent natural history study of more than 200 infantile Tay-Sachs patients.[3] (A clinical variant with organomegaly and bony abnormalities similar to those in generalized GM$_1$ gangliosidosis [see later discussion] is termed a *Sandhoff variant* of Tay-Sachs disease.[1]) The *diagnosis* is established by identification of the enzymatic defect in white blood cells or fibroblasts, which involves hexosaminidase A (see Fig. 29.1). In cases where enzyme testing is indeterminate molecular analysis may be necessary. (In the Sandhoff variant, both hexosaminidase A and B are deficient.) The disorder is inherited in an autosomal recessive manner and is especially common in Ashkenazi Jews, although the majority of cases in North America are now of non-Jewish ancestry.[3] *Neuropathology* is characterized by generalized neuronal storage of the GM$_2$ ganglioside and by markedly dilated neuronal processes (meganeurites).[2,4] *Neuroimaging (magnetic resonance imaging [MRI])* shows an abnormal signal in the thalamus and,

subsequently, marked atrophy of the cerebral cortex and deep nuclear structures; cerebral white matter shows an increased T2 signal.[5] Although no known therapy exists, genetically engineered neural progenitor cells have been shown to correct the enzymatic defect in co-cultured human Tay-Sachs fibroblasts and to secrete active enzyme throughout the fetal and neonatal mouse brain after cellular transplantation.[6]

Recent gene therapy studies are also encouraging. A single intravenous (IV) injection of recombinant adeno-associated virus 9 encoding the hexosaminidase B gene administered to the neonatal Sandhoff disease mouse reduces GM$_2$ ganglioside storage and inflammation, corrects motor function, and prolongs long-term survival.[7] Similar beneficial findings have been shown with intracranial viral injections in a feline model.[8-10] The serendipitous finding of a naturally occurring mutation in the hexosaminidase A gene in Jacob sheep[11,12] offers a unique opportunity to study gene therapy for Tay-Sachs disease in a large animal model. Because clinical trials could follow in humans, the urgency is increased for early diagnosis. *Prenatal diagnosis* can be made readily by enzymatic analysis for hexosaminidase A in cultured amniotic fluid cells or chorionic villus samples.[1] DNA analysis of the hexosaminidase A gene is also possible if disease-causing mutations have been identified in both parents.

TABLE 29.3 Neonatal Seizure Disorders That May Mimic Gray Matter Degenerations at Presentation

Epileptic syndromes (see Chapter 12)
Early infantile epileptic encephalopathy (Ohtahara syndrome)
Early myoclonic epilepsy
Pyridoxine-dependent seizures/folinic acid-responsive seizures
Pyridoxal-5-phosphate-responsive seizures
DEND syndrome
Hyperinsulinism/hyperammonemia syndrome
Malignant migrating partial seizures of infancy
Metabolic disorders
Glucose transporter deficiency[a]
Serine synthesis deficiency[b]
Nonketotic hyperglycinemia (see Chapter 27)
Sulfite oxidase deficiency: molybdenum cofactor deficiency (see Chapter 28)
Multiple carboxylase deficiency: biotinidase deficiency (see Chapter 28)
Multiple acyl-coenzyme A dehydrogenase deficiency (glutaric aciduria type II) (see Chapter 28)

[a]Described in this chapter in the section on neonatal seizure disorders that mimic gray matter degeneration at presentation.
[b]Described in this chapter later among diseases affecting gray and white matter (see Table 29.7).
DEND, Developmental delay, epilepsy, and neonatal diabetes.

TABLE 29.4 Value of Cerebrospinal Fluid Examination in Metabolic and Degenerative Neonatal Neurological Disorders

PARAMETER	DISEASE
Cells (increased)	Aicardi-Goutiere leukodystrophy
Glucose (decreased)	Glucose transporter defect
Protein (increased)	Krabbe disease
Lactate (increased)	Mitochondrial disease, organic acid disorder, fatty acid disorder (Chapters 27 and 28)
Glycine (increased)	Nonketotic hyperglycemia (Chapter 27)
Serine (decreased)	Serine synthesis deficiency
Neurotransmitter metabolites (variably increased)	Neurotransmitter defects
AASA (increased)	Pyridoxine-dependent seizures (Chapter 12)
Folinic acid metabolites (increased)	Folinic-acid responsive seizures (Chapter 12)
Pyridoxal-5-phosphate (increased)	Pyridoxal-5-phosphate dependent seizures (Chapter 12)

AASA, Alpha-amino adipic acid semialdehyde.

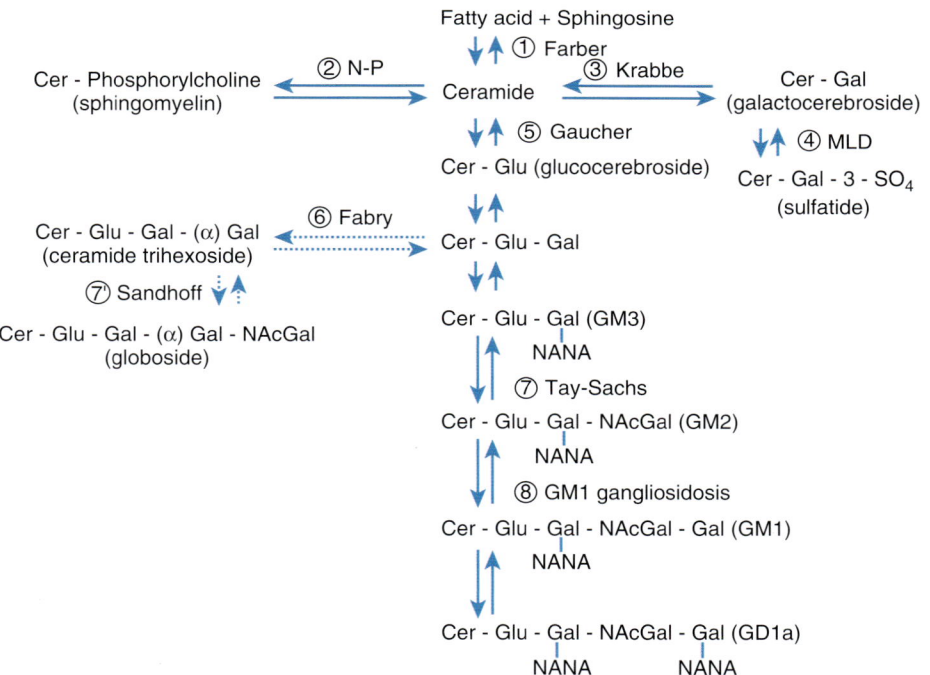

Figure 29.1 Sphingolipid metabolism and disorders. The disorders of sphingolipid metabolism involve degradative enzymes: *(1)* Farber disease, ceramidase deficiency; *(2)* Niemann-Pick disease, sphingomyelinase deficiency; *(3)* Krabbe disease, galactocerebrosidase deficiency; *(4)* metachromatic leukodystrophy (MLD), arylsulfatase A deficiency; *(5)* Gaucher disease, glucocerebrosidase deficiency; *(6)* Fabry disease, ceramide trihexosidase deficiency; *(7)* Tay-Sachs disease, hexosaminidase A deficiency; *(7′)* Sandhoff disease, hexosaminidase A and B deficiencies; *(8)* GM₁ gangliosidosis, beta-galactosidase deficiency. *NANA,* N-acetylneuraminic acid.

TABLE 29.5   Degenerative Diseases Primarily of Gray Matter (With Visceral Storage)

DISEASE	CLINICAL FEATURES	METABOLIC-ENZYMATIC FEATURES	PATHOLOGY
GM₁ gangliosidosis	Sucking and swallowing impairment, hypotonia, decreased movement; edema, coarse facies, hepatosplenomegaly, cherry-red macula (50%)	GM₁ ganglioside accumulation in brain, beta-galactosidase deficiency	Neurons distended by GM₁ ganglioside throughout the CNS
GM₂ gangliosidosis (Sandhoff variant)	See Tay-Sachs disease; also hepatosplenomegaly	See Tay-Sachs disease; also globoside accumulates in viscera, hexosaminidase A and B deficiency	See Tay-Sachs disease
Niemann-Pick disease (type IA, *infantile*)	Feeding impairment, failure to thrive, developmental arrest and then regression, cherry-red macula (50%), hepatosplenomegaly	Sphingomyelin (and cholesterol) accumulate in brain; sphingomyelinase deficiency	Neurons distended with sphingomyelin throughout the CNS; foam cells in leptomeningeal and perivascular spaces
Gaucher disease (type 2, *acute neuronopathic* or *infantile*)	Retrocollis, strabismus, trismus, dysphagia, aspiration, spasticity, hepatosplenomegaly, hydrops fetalis	Glucocerebroside accumulates in brain; glucocerebrosidase (beta-glucosidase) deficiency	Gaucher cells (lipid-laden histiocytes) in perivascular spaces and in parenchyma; neuronal death and neuronophagia throughout the CNS, especially in the brain stem
Farber disease (lipogranulomatosis) type I, classic	Painful swelling of joints, (later periarticular nodules), hoarse cry, feeding disturbance, failure to thrive, hypotonia, muscle atrophy, areflexia or hyporeflexia, and hepatomegaly (50%)	Ceramide accumulates in tissues; ceramidase deficiency	Neurons distended by glycolipid (ceramide?), especially in anterior horn cells, less prominently in brain stem, basal ganglia, and least in cortex
Infantile sialic acid storage disease (also sialidosis type II, and galactosialidosis)	Fetal ascites/hydrops, neonatal hypotonia, impaired feeding, developmental arrest followed by regression; ascites, coarse facies, white hair, and hepatosplenomegaly	Sialic acid accumulates in tissues, including the brain, and in body fluids; defect of sialic acid transport across lysosomal membrane; similar phenotype with sialidosis secondary to deficiency of alpha-neuraminidase (sialidosis type II) or of alpha-neuraminidase and beta-galactosidase (galactosialidosis)	Neurons distended with sialic acid, especially in the diencephalon, brain stem, and spinal cord; prominent axonal spheroids; myelin deficiency

CNS, Central nervous system.

Attempted *therapy* with bone marrow transplantation has not altered the course of the disease.[13]

Congenital Neuronal Ceroid-Lipofuscinosis

Neuronal ceroid-lipofuscinosis consists of a group of neuronal degenerative disorders characterized by an accumulation of the lipopigments ceroid and lipofuscin. At least 13 mutant genes and 6 clinical forms are now recognized.[14-21] The form of most relevance in this context is congenital neuronal ceroid-lipofuscinosis (Norman-Wood disease, CLN-10). This form should be distinguished from the more common and well-known early infantile disorder (Haltia-Santavuori disease, CLN-1). In the latter disorder, the usual age of onset is 6 to 18 months. The rarer congenital form is apparent at birth (see Table 29.2), and at least 11 cases have been reported.[22-27] The clinical phenotype is dramatic. Postnatal respiratory insufficiency, severe neonatal seizures, and microcephaly are nearly consistent *clinical features.* Failure of neurological development and the development of a vegetative state, usually with recalcitrant seizures, are followed by death, usually in the first days or weeks of life. The absence of electroretinographic responses and the development of an isoelectric electroencephalogram are characteristic. Neuroimaging (MRI) shows marked and progressive atrophy of the cerebral cortex, thalamus, and striatum (Fig. 29.2). The diagnosis should be considered in a newborn with severe seizures and microcephaly of unknown origin. *Diagnosis* is initially based on the identification of autofluorescent lipopigments in lymphocytes, skin, or rectal mucosa, which present as granular material on an electron microscopic examination. DNA sequencing is available to confirm the diagnosis. *Neuropathological findings* are characterized by diffuse neuronal loss (Fig. 29.3) with an accumulation of the lipopigment granules of ceroid-lipofuscin in neurons, glia, and macrophages. Marked infiltration with astrocytes and

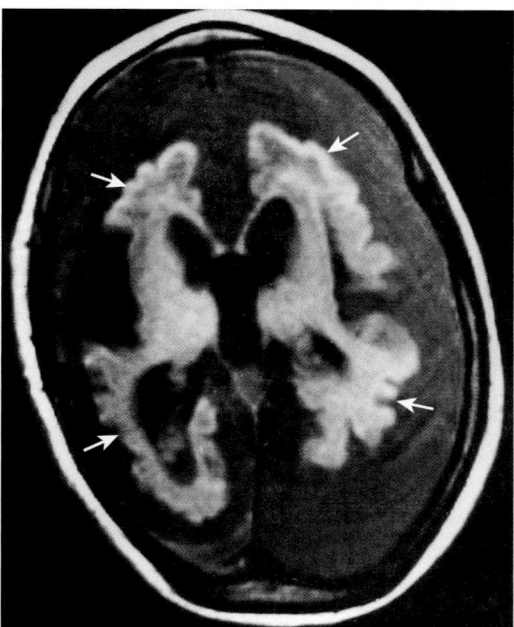

Figure 29.2 Early infantile neuronal ceroid-lipofuscinosis: magnetic resonance imaging (MRI) scan. This T1-weighted MRI scan, performed at 4 years of age, shows striking cortical atrophy and markedly dilated lateral ventricles, secondary to atrophy. The shriveled cortical surface is marked by arrows; the low signal intensity surrounding the brain is extracerebral fluid. In congenital neuronal ceroid-lipofuscinosis, the atrophy is present in the first weeks and months of life (see Fig. 29.3). (From Confort-Gouny S, Chabrol B, Vion-Dury J, Mancini J, et al. MRI and localized proton MRS in early infantile form of neuronal ceroid-lipofuscinosis. *Pediatr Neurol.* 1993;9:57–60.)

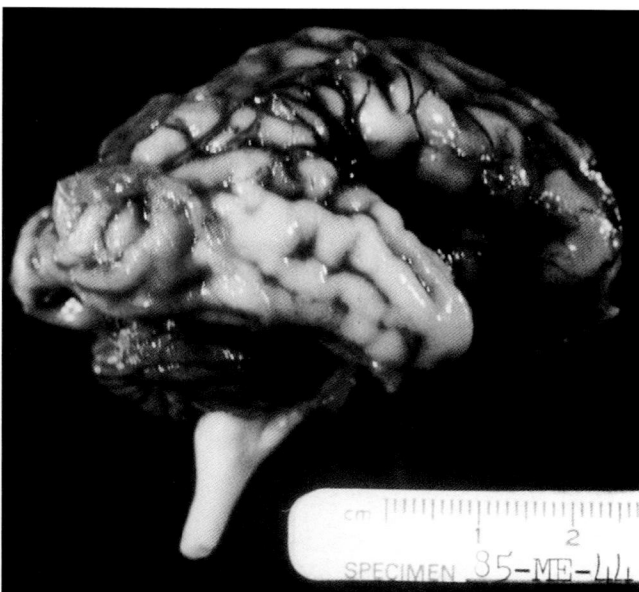

Figure 29.3 Congenital infantile neuronal ceroid-lipofuscinosis: neuropathology. This infant was microcephalic at birth, developed status epilepticus, died at 36 hours of age, and exhibited microscopic findings of neuronal ceroid-lipofuscinosis. Note the marked cerebral cortical atrophy with shriveled gyri and marked widening of the sylvian fissure. (From Barohn RJ, Dowd DC, Kagan-Hallet KS. Congenital ceroid-lipofuscinosis. *Pediatr Neurol.* 1992;8:54–59.)

microglia is apparent. The *molecular defect* involves the cathepsin D gene, which is present in a homozygous form in patients.[17] The encoded protein, cathepsin D, is a lysosomal protease, which is important for proper degradation and clearance in lysosomes. Although the infantile form is caused by mutations in the CLN1 gene-encoding palmitoyl-protein thioesterase-1, there is a secondary deficiency in cathepsin D, thereby biochemically linking the infantile and congenital forms of the disease.[28]

Alpers Disease

The term *Alpers disease*, inappropriately applied in the past to a heterogeneous group of disorders, refers to those relatively uncommon examples, usually familial and consistent with autosomal recessive inheritance, of a progressive degenerative disease of gray matter without neuronal storage or other pathognomonic cytological features, and with subsequent hepatic disease.[29-42] Affected infants exhibit the *clinical hallmarks* of gray matter disease, seizures, and myoclonus (often stimulus sensitive) in the first weeks and months of life (see Table 29.2). Hypotonia and vomiting are also prominent features. In one series, 4 of 26 infants had clear onset within the first 2 months of life. Hepatic disease becomes apparent usually after 9 months of age (mean age, 35 months), but a more frequent assessment of serum transaminase levels before the appearance of hepatomegaly demonstrates hepatic dysfunction earlier.[34] Most infants die by 3 years of age. MRI shows extensive cerebral atrophy (Fig. 29.4).

Neuropathological study shows striking cortical neuronal loss with spongy change and gliosis, which is worse in the deeper cortical layers and is especially prominent in the striate cortex (Fig. 29.5). Frequently, capillary proliferation is apparent, and the constellation of pathological change resembles that of Leigh disease, a mitochondrial disorder (see later discussion). Earlier data suggested that Alpers disease was a *mitochondrial disorder* because of the findings in several study series of patients of elevated blood and cerebrospinal fluid (CSF) lactate and various abnormalities of the electron transport chain.[36-40,43-52] More recently, some cases have been shown to involve mutations in the gene encoding the catalytic subunit of mitochondrial DNA polymerase γ (*POLG*).[37-39] The result is mitochondrial DNA depletion and impaired function of the electron transport chain at multiple sites. However, POLG1-negative cases exist and, notably, these appear to have especially a perinatal onset characterized by seizures, spasticity, progressive microcephaly, and severe intellectual disability.[53] The genetic etiology of the POLG1-negative cases remains largely unknown, although whole exome sequencing has identified mutations in mitochondrial tRNA synthetases, which are critical for efficient mitochondrial protein synthesis.[54,55] Most recently, it has been suggested that the use of the term *Alpers syndrome* be confined to the POLG1-negative infantile form, and that cases with POLG1 mutations, hepatic dysfunction, and typically later onset be better termed *Alpers-Huttenlocher syndrome*.

Menkes Disease

Menkes disease (kinky or steely-hair disease, trichopoliodystrophy) is an X-linked disorder of copper metabolism with onset in the severe form of the disease characteristically in the neonatal period.[56-64] Premature delivery, a cherubic face, hypothermia,

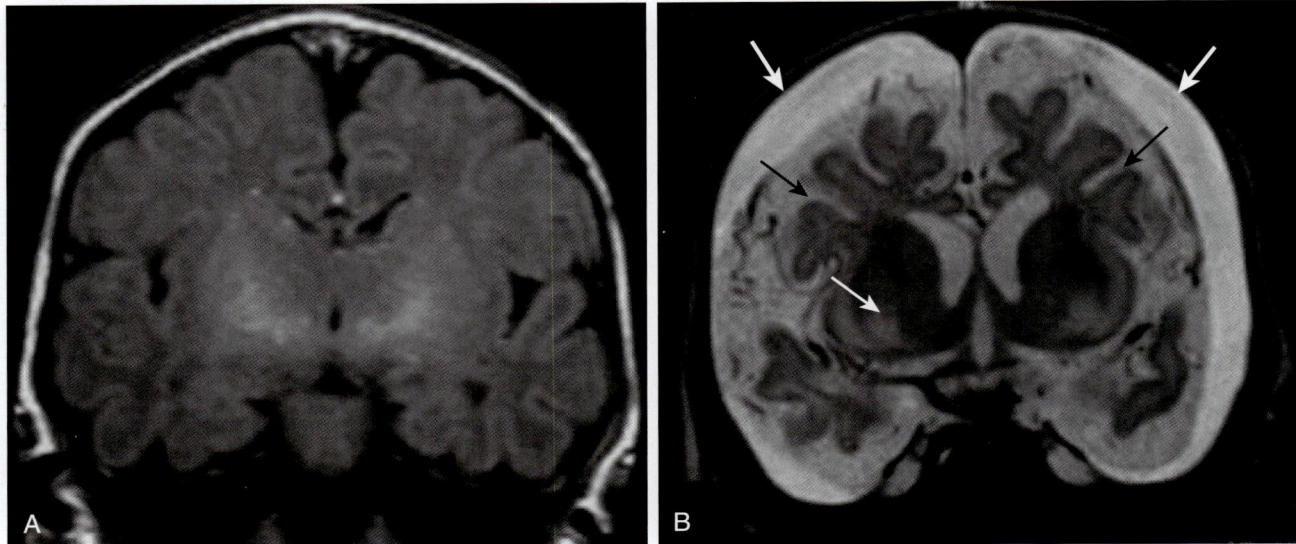

Figure 29.4 Alpers disease: magnetic resonance imaging. T1-weighted image at age of 4 days with no cortical atrophy or abnormal findings (A). Same patient (B) imaged 3 months later. T2-weighted image shows extensive brain atrophy with widened sulci *(black arrows)* and compensatory fluid accumulation around the cerebrum *(white, thick arrows)*. Note increased signal in the putamen *(white, thin arrow)*. (From Elo JM, Yadavalli SS, Euro L, et al. Mitochondrial phenylalanyl-tRNA synthetase mutations underlie fatal infantile Alpers encephalopathy. *Hum Mol Genet.* 2012;21:4521–4529.)

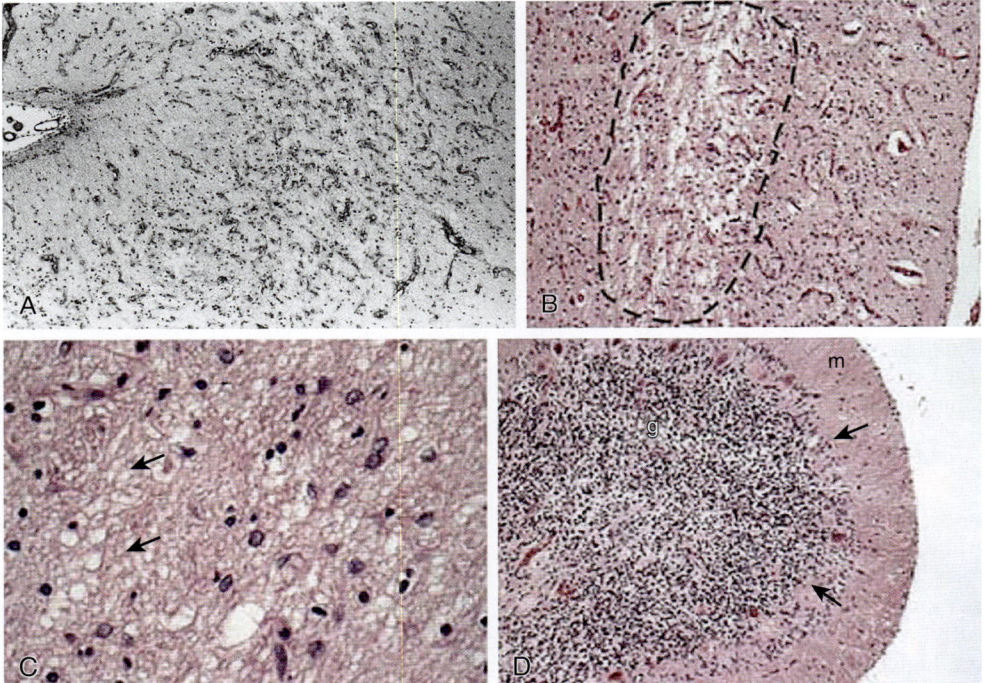

Figure 29.5 Alpers disease: neuropathology. (A) This photomicrograph of the cerebral cortex was obtained at autopsy from a 21-month-old infant with poor feeding and hypotonia in the neonatal period, subsequent development of myoclonic seizures with hypsarrhythmia, minimal neurological development, and, finally, microcephaly, spastic quadriparesis, and an isoelectric electroencephalogram. The cerebral cortex was devoid of neuronal elements and exhibited pronounced spongy changes involving the lower cortical layers and capillary proliferation, which are shown in extreme form in the figure. (Courtesy Dr. Hart Lidov.) (B to D) 8-month-old infant with Alpers disease. (B) Microscopic view of the frontal cortex showing practically no remaining pyramidal neurons, and the mid-laminar region is transformed into a microcystic track with gliosis and capillary proliferation *(dotted line)*. (C) Neuronal loss, spongiosis *(arrows)*, and gliosis can be seen in the medial/reticular thalamus *(higher power)*. (D) The top of an atrophic cerebellar cortical folium shows narrowed molecular layer *(m)*, Purkinje-cell drop out *(arrows)*, Bergmann gliosis, and a sparse granular layer *(g)*. (From Elo JM, Yadavalli SS, Euro L, et al. Mitochondrial phenylalanyl-tRNA synthetase mutations underlie fatal infantile Alpers encephalopathy. *Hum Mol Genet.* 2012;21:4521–4529.)

and hyperbilirubinemia are common neonatal *clinical features* (see Table 29.2). Hypotonia, lethargy, poor feeding, neurological deterioration, and seizures develop promptly. In the neonatal period, the hair is usually fine and colorless, but shortly thereafter, the more characteristic, friable, kinky appearance (feeling like fine sandpaper) develops (Fig. 29.6). We have noted the sandpaper feel in the neonatal period, however. Recalcitrant seizures and neurological deterioration lead to death, usually in the second year. *Diagnosis* is confirmed by the finding of low serum copper and ceruloplasmin levels; in the early neonatal period, serum values may be normal or elevated but decline over the ensuing weeks, whereas in normal infants, serum values increase postnatally. Because of the partial deficiency of dopamine-β-hydroxylase in Menkes disease, the measurement of plasma neurometabolites (dopamine, norepinephrine, dihydroxyphenylacetic acid, and dihydroxyphenylglycol) can be diagnostic in the neonatal period.[65] Definitive molecular diagnosis is now available, supporting the clinical and biochemical results, particularly in neonatal cases where interpretation sometimes can be challenging. Studies of cultured fibroblasts show increased retention and reduced efflux of labeled copper, which are features that can be used for *prenatal diagnosis* by the study of cultured amniotic fluid cells (second trimester) or chorionic villus samples (first trimester).[61,66] However, the preferred method is molecular testing for specific mutations identified in the parents.

Neuropathological examination shows striking cortical neuronal loss, gliosis, and subcortical myelin loss associated with severe axonal degeneration (see Table 29.2). Axonal changes are especially marked in cerebellum. The evolution of the cerebral parenchymal changes is followed best by MRI scans (Figs. 29.7 and 29.8). Intracranial arterial abnormalities are characteristic (see Fig. 29.8). The latter have been identified as striking tortuosities around the circle of Willis by MR angiography as

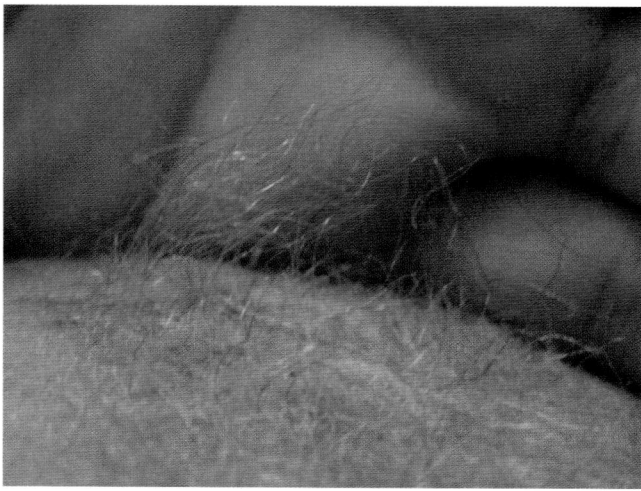

Figure 29.6 Scalp hair in Menkes disease. Hair is sparse, short, thin, fragile, and light-colored with a sandpaper feel. (From Seshadri R, Bindu PS, Gupta AK. Teaching NeuroImages: Menkes kinky hair syndrome. *Neurology.* 2013;81:e12–e13.)

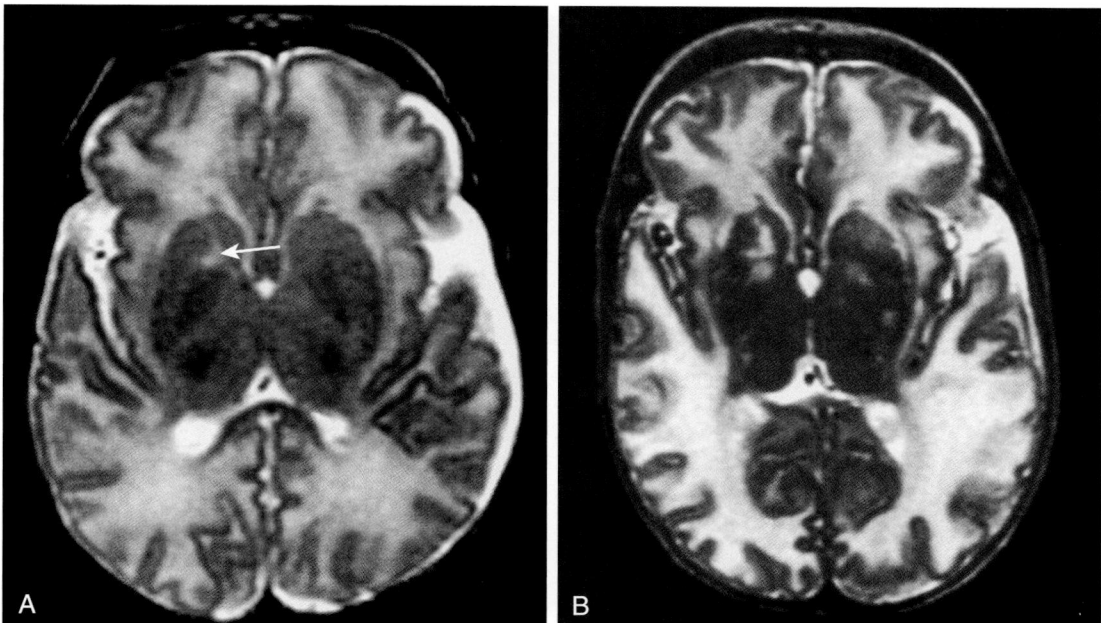

Figure 29.7 Evolution of cerebral parenchymal changes in Menkes disease, as shown by magnetic resonance imaging (MRI). The infant presented with severe refractory seizures at 6 weeks of age, after premature delivery at 30 weeks of gestation. (A) Axial T2-weighted MRI at 8 weeks of age shows a moderate degree of cerebral cortical atrophy, a focal area of high signal intensity in the right putamen *(arrow)*, and moderately high signal intensity in cerebral white matter. (B) Axial T2-weighted MRI at 14 weeks of age shows marked progression with multiple lesions in the basal ganglia and thalami, more cortical atrophy, and markedly higher signal intensity in cerebral white matter. MR spectroscopy at the time of the second MRI showed markedly elevated lactate and markedly depressed N-acetylaspartic acid in the basal ganglia and cerebral white matter.

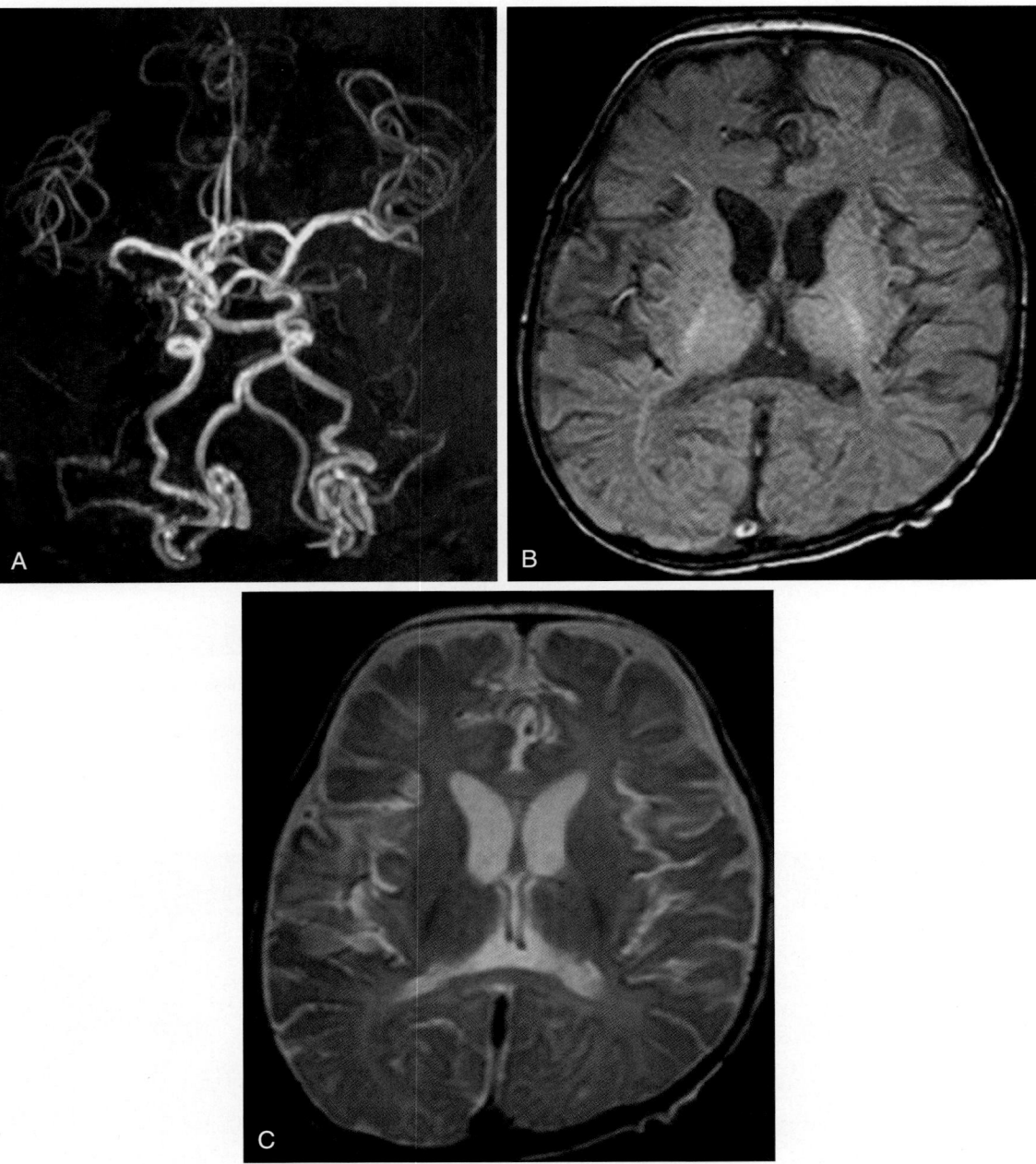

Figure 29.8 **Characteristic magnetic resonance imaging and magnetic resonance angiography in Menkes disease.** There are highly tortuous arteries in the brain (A). T1 sequences (B) and T2 sequences (C) demonstrate diffuse atrophy and delayed myelination in a 6-month-old infant. (From Seshadri R, Bindu PS, Gupta AK. Teaching NeuroImages: Menkes kinky hair syndrome. *Neurology.* 2013;81:e12–e13.)

early as 5 weeks of age.[58,59] The essential *biochemical defect* in the disease involves copper transport across specific cellular compartments (i.e., the placenta, gastrointestinal tract, and blood-brain barrier), with a resulting failure of formation of copper-containing enzymes. The latter include tyrosinase (causing depigmentation of hair), lysyl oxidase (causing defective elastin-collagen cross-linking, and arterial intimal defects), superoxide dismutase (causing vulnerability to free radicals), cytochrome oxidase (causing impaired energy production), and dopamine-beta-hydroxylase (causing impaired

catecholamine synthesis). The latter three defects perhaps are most important for the neurological phenomena. The responsible gene is located on the X-chromosome (Xq13), and the mutant protein is a cation transporting adenosine triphosphatase (ATP7A).[61,67] More than 300 unique mutations have been identified thus far (http://www.LOVD.nl/ATP7A).[68] Attempts to correct the copper deficiency in brain have included parenteral administration of copper histidine. Clinical response, although inconsistent, has been occasionally promising.[59-61,69-71] Response to therapy depends on the ATP7A genotype and the initiation of treatment in the neonatal period enhances survival and neurodevelopmental outcome.[65] However, severe ATP7A mutations still have a poor prognosis even when therapy is initiated in utero.[72]

Disorders Mimicking Gray Matter Degeneration

Several neonatal disorders in which seizures are a prominent manifestation may mimic onset of a gray matter degeneration (with no visceral storage) (see Table 29.3). It is critical to recognize these disorders partly because early management may require specific interventions. The group is best divided into recognized epileptic syndromes and certain metabolic disorders (see Table 29.3). The epileptic syndromes are reviewed in Chapter 12, and the metabolic disorders are primarily discussed in Chapters 27 or 28. One metabolic disorder, the glucose transporter defect, will be discussed here. Another metabolic disorder, serine synthesis deficiency, exhibits prominent white matter abnormalities, in addition to seizures, and thus is discussed later in this chapter (see Disorders Affecting Gray and White Matter).

Glucose Transporter Defect

Defects in the glucose transporter 1 cause inadequate shuttling of glucose from the blood to the brain, resulting in hypoglycorrhachia (low CSF glucose) in the setting of adequate serum glucose, ultimately leading to energy failure in the brain (see Table 29.4).[73-75] The majority of patients present in the first few months of life with seizures, and notably, diagnosis can be considerably delayed without measuring fasting CSF and blood glucose concentrations. Initial clinical features include intractable seizures, eye movement abnormalities, changes in muscle strength or tone, and breathing abnormalities.[76] In the absence of treatment, the disorder progresses to spasticity, dystonia, ataxia, intellectual disability, and acquired microcephaly with a broad phenotypic spectrum.[77,78] In addition to measuring CSF glucose, diagnosis now can be confirmed by DNA sequencing of the SLC2A1 gene encoding Glut1 protein. Brain imaging is not usually informative, although it may be useful in monitoring improvements in myelination after the initiation of treatment.[79] Treatment with the ketogenic diet is effective at controlling seizures and may also have a neuroprotective effect leading to improved developmental outcomes.[78,80] By converting brain energy metabolism to ketosis, the need for glucose is circumvented. Thus, this metabolic disorder can mimic many features of gray matter degeneration, but is largely reversed with the early initiation of the ketogenic diet.

Gray Matter Degenerations With Visceral Storage

Six neuronal degenerations with infantile onset are accompanied by prominent visceral storage (see Tables 29.1 and 29.5). Although these disorders may eventually exhibit the hallmark of a neuronal process (seizures), this feature often appears later in the course of the disease or even not at all. Thus, in this group of disorders, it is often difficult in the neonatal period or in early infancy to recognize the disease as one primarily affecting neurons. However, other clinical features are usually distinctive enough to lead to a high degree of suspicion of the correct diagnosis (see later discussions).

GM₁ Gangliosidosis

Manifestations of the generalized form of *GM₁ gangliosidosis* commonly appear in the first weeks of life (see Table 29.5).[2,81-83]

Clinical features include abnormalities of sucking and swallowing, hypotonia, and a cherry-red spot. Seizures, the hallmark of gray matter disease, are usually not present until after 1 year of age. Generalized edema is a striking early feature.[81,83] Because of the systemic storage of mucopolysaccharide, coarse facies, subperiosteal bony abnormalities, and hepatosplenomegaly are present. Dermal melanocytosis also can be observed because the accumulation of the GM₁ ganglioside in neural crest cells causes the aberrant migration of melanocytes into the dermis (Fig. 29.9).[84,85] Progression to death in the second year is characteristic. *Diagnosis* is based on the identification of the enzymatic defect in white blood cells or fibroblasts, which involves beta-galactosidase (see Fig. 29.1). The gene is located on chromosome 3, and an increasing number of mutations have been identified, but no clear genotype–phenotype relationship has been established.[86] The disorder is inherited in an autosomal recessive manner. *Neuropathology* is characterized by the generalized neuronal storage of the GM₁ ganglioside and by the meganeurites noted for Tay-Sachs disease. *Neuroimaging (MRI)*, as for Tay-Sachs GM₂ gangliosidosis, initially shows an abnormal signal in the thalamus, and subsequently marked cerebral cortical and deep nuclear atrophy; cerebral white matter shows an increased T2 signal.[5] Neuronal storage and elevated brain ganglioside content have been observed as early as 22 weeks of gestation.[87,88] This observation has important implications concerning the need for intervention during fetal life with enzyme or gene replacement therapy, when such therapy is further developed. Intracranial gene therapy in a feline model of GM₁ gangliosidosis increases survival and normalizes neurological symptoms when administered before disease onset,[89] and similar results have been observed

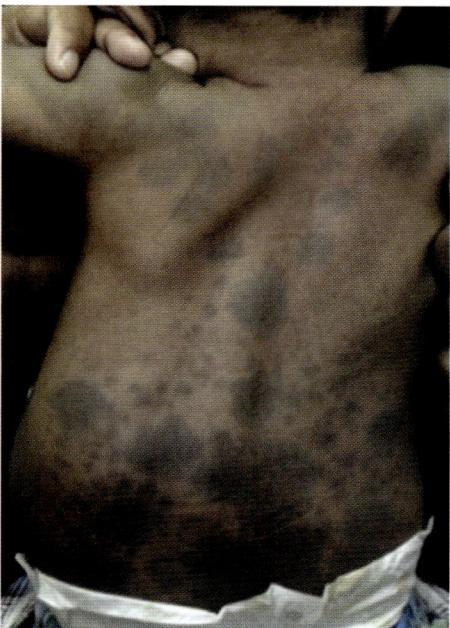

Figure 29.9 Dermal melanocytosis in GM1 gangliosidosis. Infant with extensive dermal melanocytosis (Mongolian spots) is an important supportive diagnostic clue in infants with other clinical features of GM1 gangliosidosis. Accumulation of GM1 gangliosides in neural crest cells leads to aberrant migration of melanocytes into the dermis. (From Sidhu A, Misra VK. Dermal melanocytosis: more than meets the eye. *J Pediatr.* 2014;165:1060.)

in adult mouse models with systemic viral injections.[90] Recently, a small prospective study of six patients suggested that combined therapy with miglustat (a small molecule that reduces GM_1 and GM_2 gangliosides) and the ketogenic diet may have a small benefit on survival but will need to be replicated.[90a] *Prenatal diagnosis* of the enzymatic defect is possible by the analysis of cultured amniotic fluid cells or by the DNA sequencing of previously identified mutations.

GM₂ Gangliosidosis (Sandhoff Variant)

GM₂ gangliosidosis, or the Sandhoff variant of Tay-Sachs disease, is clinically similar to Tay-Sachs disease except for the addition of visceromegaly. The major features were reviewed earlier in relation to Tay-Sachs disease. In this disorder, not only is GM_2 ganglioside stored in the brain because of the defect in hexosaminidase A, but also globoside is stored in the viscera, because the enzymatic defect involves both hexosaminidase A and B. Both isoforms are required for the removal of the terminal *N*-acetylglucosamine from globoside (see Fig. 29.1).

Niemann-Pick Disease

The acute infantile form of *Niemann-Pick disease* may be noted in the first weeks of life (see Table 29.5).[2,91,92] Feeding difficulties are common, and a cherry-red spot is apparent in nearly 50% of cases. Hepatosplenomegaly, caused primarily by the storage of sphingomyelin, is prominent. Neurological features are often not pronounced until several weeks or months of age, when developmental arrest and then regression occur. Seizures are not a common feature early in the disease. Death occurs most frequently in the first several years. This form of disease is classically referred to as type A. *Diagnosis* is established by identification of the enzymatic defect in white blood cells or fibroblasts, which involves a diminution of acid sphingomyelinase (ASM) activity to less than 10% of normal (see Fig. 29.1). The disorder is inherited in an autosomal recessive manner. *Neuropathology* is characterized by neuronal storage of sphingomyelin, which is most prominent in the cerebellum, brain stem, and spinal cord. Foam cells, laden with lipid and representing macrophages, are prominent in the meninges and perivascular spaces. *Prenatal diagnosis* is possible by the identification of the enzymatic defect in cultured amniotic fluid cells or chorionic villus samples or by DNA analysis if pathogenic mutations have been previously identified in the parents. Attempted *therapy* with bone marrow transplantation has not altered the course of the disease.[13] Recent studies suggest that recombinant heat shock protein (HSP) 70 stabilizes the lysosomal membrane and increases the activity of sphingomyelinase, but preliminary work needs validation in an animal model.[93]

Gaucher Disease

The infantile neuronopathic form of *Gaucher disease* (type 2) is noted in the neonatal period in 10% of cases.[94-97] The most common presenting *clinical features* are retrocollis (hyperextension of neck), strabismus (or other oculomotor abnormalities), and spasticity (see Table 29.5). Other brain stem signs, dysphagia and trismus, are common. Hepatosplenomegaly secondary to the storage of glucocerebroside is present. Dermatological findings, particularly thin, reflective skin characterized as collodion, cellophane, or ichthyosis, are common in neonatal cases

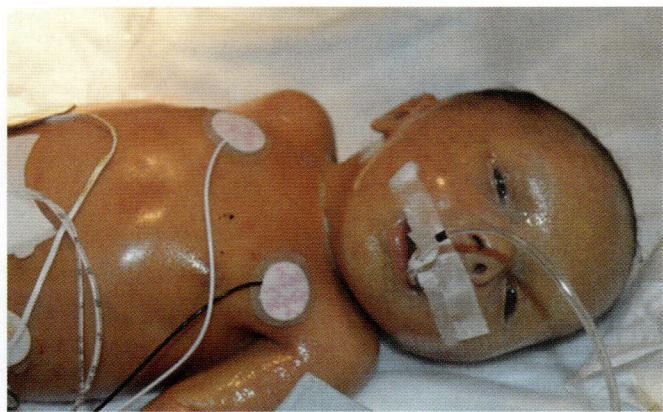

Figure 29.10 **Dermatologic manifestations of Gaucher disease.** Collodion membrane *(thin, reflective skin)* produced from an abnormal ratio of glucosyl-ceramide to ceramide ratio in the epidermis of an infant with Gaucher disease. (From Carr PC, Casamiquela KM, Jacks SK. Gaucher disease type 2 presenting with collodion membrane and blueberry muffin lesions. *Pediatr Dermatol.* 2016;33:e20–e22.)

(Fig. 29.10).[98] A particularly severe form with hydrops fetalis and arthrogryposis has been recognized.[99] The subsequent course of infants with neonatal Gaucher disease generally fulminates with death by 2 or 3 months of age. *Diagnosis* is based on identification of the enzymatic defect in the white blood cells, fibroblasts, or liver, which involves beta-glucosidase (see Fig. 29.1), produced by mutations in the glucocerebrosidase gene (GBA). DNA sequencing is now available, with more than 300 GBA mutations identified.[100] The disorder is inherited in an autosomal recessive manner. *Neuropathology* is characterized by little or no neuronal storage of glucocerebroside, but neuronal loss is present, especially in the brain stem. The basal ganglia and the cerebellum also are particularly involved. Gaucher cells, lipid-laden histiocytes, often with the cytoplasmic appearance of wrinkled tissue paper, are present in perivascular spaces and are free in brain parenchyma. Neuronal death with microglial nodules and gliosis appears to occur in proximity to these cells, a finding suggesting the possibility of a toxic effect from the stored lipid or a product thereof (glucosylsphingosine?). *Prenatal diagnosis* is possible by the identification of the enzymatic defect in cultured amniotic fluid cells or chorionic villus specimens. Molecular genetic testing is also available when both disease-causing mutations in a family are known. The possibility of *therapy* in less severely affected infants is suggested by successes in patients with the nonneuronopathic forms of Gaucher disease who were treated with recombinant human macrophage-targeted glucocerebrosidase.[13,101,102] Other approaches in nonneuronopathic cases have included drugs that decrease glucocerebroside biosynthesis, bone marrow transplantation, or the introduction of somatic cells (e.g., fibroblasts) into the bone marrow or other sites into which the normal gene for glucocerebrosidase was introduced by retrovirally mediated gene transfer.[13,94,101,102] Theoretically, the correction or arrest of the neurological disease can be accomplished because this disorder involves the reticuloendothelial system, particularly the bone marrow, and thus entry of the transplanted cells into the central nervous system (CNS) (i.e., the major limitation of gene therapy of other lysosomal disorders) may not be required.[94] However, a novel mouse model of this disorder suggests that while the microglia of hematopoietic origin might influence disease progression, a deficient enzyme in CNS cells underlies the neuronopathic disorder.[103] Bone marrow approaches are therefore unlikely to be curative. Gene therapy directed at the brain will be necessary and has been successful in mouse models.[104] A recent study has also suggested the involvement of programmed necrosis (necroptosis), which is dependent on receptor-interacting protein kinase-3 (RIPK3) as a primary mechanism of neuronal death in animal models of Gaucher. The autopsy of a single patient with infantile-onset type 2 showed increased RIPK3 in neurons, suggesting that targeted inhibition of RIPK3 may be a novel therapeutic approach.[105] Chemical chaperone drug therapy is another area of active investigation involving the drug binding of misfolded glucocerebrosidase, allowing proper function and trafficking to lysosomes.[106,107]

Farber Disease

In the classic type 1 form of *Farber disease*, as with most other neuronal degenerations with visceral storage, determining that gray matter is primarily involved may be difficult. Thus, the initial *clinical features* are primarily painful swelling of joints, subcutaneous nodules, and hoarse cry (see Table 29.5).[108] Subsequently, feeding disturbance leading to failure to thrive is prominent. Perhaps the most pronounced neurological features are hypotonia, weakness, muscle atrophy, and areflexia or hyporeflexia, which probably reflect the involvement of anterior horn cells and peripheral nerve roots. Consistent with the latter involvement is the finding of elevated CSF protein levels in nearly all cases, and electromyographic findings of denervation. Hepatomegaly is prominent in approximately 75% of cases. Disturbances of swallowing, aspiration, and pulmonary disease lead to death at 1 to 2 years of age. Ceramide accumulates in tissue. *Neuronal storage* occurs, especially in the anterior horn cells and the brain stem. *Diagnosis* is established by detection of the marked defect in ceramidase in cultured fibroblasts (see Fig. 29.1). Genetic characterization of mutations in the ASAH1 gene (which codes for ceramidase) are under way and have primarily identified missense mutations,[109] although deletions have also been found.[110] Interestingly, mutations in this gene have also been found in patients with spinal muscular atrophy with myoclonic epilepsy,[111,112] raising the possibility that there may be more Farber disease patients than previously recognized. *Prenatal diagnosis* is possible by the analysis of cultured amniotic fluid cells or by molecular genetic testing. Attempted *therapy* by bone marrow transplantation has provided some benefit for the regression of nodules (which contain ceramide-laden macrophages) and associated joint pain, but has no apparent neurological benefit.[13,14,44]

Insertion of a human ASAH1 mutation into mice has created a model of Farber disease that recapitulates many characteristics of the human disease.[113] Studies with this model demonstrated that systemic (but not CNS) manifestations of disease could be corrected by neonatal IV injection of a lentiviral vector expressing human acid ceramidase. This novel tool may provide new avenues to study mechanisms and interventions for the neurological symptoms. Finally, recombinant acid ceramidase is currently under development by Plexcera Therapeutics but requires validation in planned clinical trials[114] and is not expected to ameliorate disease in the CNS.

Infantile Sialic Acid Storage Disease (and Sialidoses)

Sialic acid is a critical component of the oligosaccharide portion of many glycoproteins. Two varieties of disturbance of sialic acid metabolism may result in neonatal disease with neuronal storage. One of these is related to a disorder of sialic acid transport and is sometimes referred to as *infantile sialic acid storage disease* or *sialuria*. The other disturbance is related to a defect in the lysosomal enzyme that degrades the oligosaccharides containing sialic acid (i.e., neuraminidase or sialidase) and is often referred to as *sialidosis*.[2,82,115-123] The prototypical *clinical presentation* of both infantile sialic acid storage disease and sialidosis with onset in utero or the neonatal period includes generalized edema (including fetal ascites/hydrops), feeding disturbance, marked hepatosplenomegaly, hypotonia, coarse dysmorphic facies, and radiographic abnormalities of the long bones (Fig. 29.11). In infantile sialic acid storage disease, thin, white hair is a consistent feature (see Fig. 29.11), not noted in the sialidoses. Severe anemia, failure to thrive, developmental arrest, and then regression subsequently develop. *Diagnosis* of the infantile sialic acid storage disorder or sialuria (i.e., the disorder of lysosomal transport of sialic acid) is made by the identification of large increases in free sialic acid in plasma and urine, and normal activity in fibroblasts of alpha-neuraminidase activity. The responsible gene is SLC17A5 and most patients identified thus far harbor a missense mutation.[124] The diagnosis of sialidosis can be suspected by identification of sialic acid–containing oligosaccharides and glycoproteins in urine, but it is made definitively by the demonstration of deficient alpha-neuraminidase activity and/or genetic sequencing. In a subtype of sialidosis, *galactosialidosis,* beta-galactosidase activity is also impaired, and the defect involves another lysosomal protein necessary for the activity of both enzymes (cathepsin A). *Neuropathology* of these disorders is characterized by neuronal storage of either free sialic acid in infantile sialic acid storage disease or sialic acid-containing oligosaccharides and glycoproteins in the sialidoses. Hypomyelination is also a prominent feature, and a SLC17A5 knockout mouse demonstrated an increased oligodendrocyte apoptosis and a decreased number of mature myelinating oligodendrocytes,[125] which suggests that transporter function may be necessary for proper oligodendrocyte maturation. *Prenatal diagnosis* is made by the identification of elevated free sialic acid levels in cultured amniotic fluid cells in the infantile sialic acid storage disorder and of deficient alpha-neuraminidase activity in the sialidoses.[126] DNA analysis is also possible for previously identified familial mutations. (Other disorders of glycoprotein degradation [i.e., mannosidosis and fucosidosis] have their onset beyond the neonatal period.)

DISORDERS PRIMARILY AFFECTING WHITE MATTER

Many neurological disorders affect developing white matter (see Fig. 1 in van den Bosch et al.[127]) but are not degenerative disorders. The principal MRI differences between leukodystrophies and other white matter abnormalities are that the former usually exhibit prominent and confluent T2 hyperintensities on MRI. The discussion here is confined to progressive disorders that principally affect myelin.

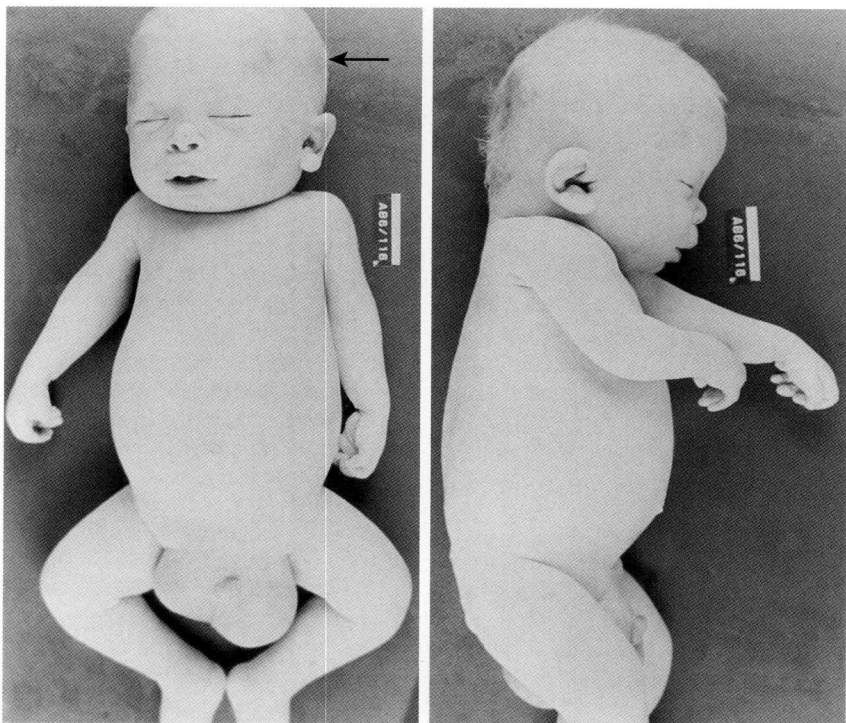

Figure 29.11 **Infantile sialic acid storage disease: postmortem photographs.** Note the coarse dysmorphic facies, generalized edema, abdominal distention, inguinal hernias, bilateral hydroceles, and white hair *(arrow).* (From Pueschel SM, O'Shea PA, Alroy J, Ambler MW, et al. Infantile sialic acid storage disease associated with renal disease. *Pediatr Neurol.* 1988;4:207–212.)

Canavan Disease

Canavan disease, the spongy degeneration of the white matter, is an autosomal recessive disorder that commonly begins in the first days and weeks of life; approximately 20% of patients exhibit first signs at birth, an additional 10% in the first month, and a further 10% to 20% by the end of the second month.[35,128-143] *Clinical features* documented in the first days and weeks of life include poor visual fixation, irritability, and poor suck (see Table 29.6). These features are followed over the ensuing weeks by marked hypotonia, weakness, nystagmus, and failure to attain motor milestones. Macrocephaly becomes apparent in the first 6 to 12 months of life in more than 50% of cases and ultimately in 90% of affected infants. As the disease progresses, hypotonia gives way to spasticity, decorticate posture, intellectual failure, optic atrophy, and then death in early to late childhood. Visual evoked responses are abnormal early in the disease, and these neurophysiological abnormalities precede the onset of blindness. *Diagnosis* is suspected by the clinical features. Although the computed tomography (CT) scan shows decreased attenuation of the white matter, MRI is preferable and shows a strikingly increased signal on the T2-weighted images (Fig. 29.12). The particular involvement of subcortical white matter, especially early in the disease, distinguishes Canavan disease from Krabbe disease (see later discussion). Also characteristic is the involvement of the thalamus and especially the globus pallidus with relative sparing of the putamen (see Fig. 29.12).[5] Elevation of *N*-acetylaspartate (NAA) levels in brain is detected by proton MR spectroscopy.[5,139,144] *Diagnosis* is established by the demonstration of *increased levels of NAA in urine and of decreased activity of N-acetylaspartoacylase (ASPA) activity in cultured fibroblasts.*[137-139,142,143,145-151] Elevated levels of NAA have been documented in Canavan disease early in infancy, in the urine of a mother with an affected 4-month fetus, and in the brain of 5- and 8-month-old fetuses.[150] Deficient aspartoacylase activity has been detected in brain postmortems.[137-139,147] NAA is normally present in high concentration in the neurons, whereas the acylase activity is predominantly localized in the oligodendrocyte. Studies in a mouse model of Canavan disease indicated that NAA is synthesized in the neurons and is transported to the oligodendrocytes, where the action of ASPA generates acetate critical for myelin lipid synthesis (Fig. 29.13).[152] Consistent with this notion is the demonstration that the developmental increase of ASPA in oligodendrocytes parallels cerebral myelination,[153] and deficiency in ASPA impairs proper oligodendrocyte maturation.[154] The hypothesis of *acetate starvation* is supported by observations that dietary acetate supplementation improves motor function and partially reverses myelin vacuolation in a rat model of Canavan disease.[155] A second major hypothesis of oligodendroglial/myelin disease proposes that the accumulated NAA in oligodendrocytes acts as an osmolyte to lead to intramyelinic edema. Thus, studies in a newer Canavan disease mouse model, APSA[nur7/nur7] (harboring a clinically relevant nonsense mutation in the ASPA gene),[156] which also lacks the NAA synthase gene, suggest that NAA-derived acetate is not essential for myelin production. Complete ablation of NAA synthesis by deleting the NAA synthase Nat8L gene (see Fig. 29.13) does not disrupt

TABLE 29.6   Degenerative Diseases Primarily of White Matter

DISEASE	CLINICAL FEATURES	METABOLIC-ENZYMATIC FEATURES	PATHOLOGY
Canavan disease (spongy degeneration of the white matter)	Macrocephaly with rapid head growth, poor visual fixation, hypotonia and later spasticity, developmental arrest, seizures and then regression, spasticity	N-acetylaspartic acid accumulates in brain and in urine and plasma; N-acetylaspartoacylase deficiency detectable in fibroblasts	Myelin deficiency, spongy vacuolation of white matter, especially subcortical, with involvement of globus pallidus and thalamus
Alexander disease (leukodystrophy with diffuse Rosenthal fiber formation)	Macrocephaly with rapid head growth, developmental arrest, seizures, and then regression, spasticity	De novo, dominant gain-of-function mutation of GFAP	Myelin deficiency, Rosenthal fiber formation in fibrillary astrocytes, especially in subpial, perivascular, and subependymal loci
Krabbe disease (globoid cell leukodystrophy)	Irritability, poor feeding, stimulus-sensitive tonic spasms, hypertonia, opisthotonos, developmental arrest and later regression, blindness, decerebration	Galactosylsphingosine accumulates in brain; galactosylceramidase I deficiency (a beta-galactosidase)	Myelin deficiency, multinucleated globoid cells (macrophages), and diminished oligodendroglia; peripheral neuropathy (segmental demyelination)
Pelizaeus-Merzbacher disease	Abnormal eye movements (nystagmus), laryngeal stridor, head titubation, jerky movements, hypotonia (later spasticity), developmental arrest (later deterioration), seizures (2/3); X-linked recessive (PMLD; autosomal recessive)	Defect in gene (duplication, mutation or deletion) encoding myelin proteolipid protein (PMLD; defect in genes encoding connexin 47 and monocarboxylate transporter 8)	Severe myelin deficiency, usually total but occasionally with preserved islands of myelin; decreased number of mature oligodendrocytes; gliosis, occasional sudanophilic material
Leukodystrophy with cerebral calcifications and cerebrospinal fluid pleocytosis (Aicardi-Goutieres syndrome)	Irritability, poor feeding, ocular abnormalities, hypertonia or hypotonia, weakness, jitteriness, dystonia, oral-facial dyskinesias, occasionally seizures, developmental arrest, microcephaly, and spasticity	Defect in TREX1, gene encoding a DNA exonuclease, and at least six other genes involved in nucleic acid metabolism (see text)	Severe myelin deficiency, marked fibrillary gliosis, diffuse/focal calcifications, focal collections of inflammatory cells, microangiopathy

GFAP, Glial fibrillary acidic protein; *PMLD*, Pelizaeus-Merzbacher–like disease.

normal myelination and is protective against leukodystrophy in the APSA[nur7/nur7] model of Canavan disease, further adding to the NAA osmotic toxicity hypothesis.[157] A second group of investigators using identical animals (deletion of Nat8L in APSA knockout mice) similarly demonstrated that the ablation of NAA production prevents myelin and axonal degeneration; however, they unexpectedly found that the survival time of the mice is not prolonged. Interestingly, they showed that the knockdown of Nat8L (using heterozygotes for the mutation) develops less severe pathology, behavioral improvements, and nearly normal survival time.[158] Taken together, these recent mouse results add further support to the NAA toxicity hypothesis and suggest that *partial* inhibition of NAA synthase could be a therapeutic strategy with the development of CNS-permanent Nat8L inhibitors. The major *neuropathological features* are strikingly deficient in myelin and the widespread vacuolization (spongy degeneration) of white matter, especially in the subcortical regions.

More recent attempts at *therapy* have included virally and nonvirally mediated gene transfer methods and lithium (which causes a decrease in elevated brain NAA levels by unknown mechanisms).[143,159-161] The initial findings are encouraging, but more data are needed. Long-term follow-up (up to 10 years) in 13 patients treated with an adeno-associated viral vector

carrying the ASPA gene demonstrated reductions in elevated brain NAA levels, less brain atrophy, improvement in seizure frequency, and stabilization of clinical status.[162] Newer viral constructs, some specifically targeting oligodendrocytes, show promise after single IV injections in animal models.[163,164] A less complex approach may be acetate supplementation, in view of the importance of NAA as an acetate source in the oligodendrocyte/myelin unit,[152] although the recent mouse studies discussed earlier cast some doubt on the utility of this approach. Enzyme replacement therapy has been hampered by blood-brain barrier and immunological limitations, but a modified version of ASPA appears to overcome these barriers in mice.[165] *Prenatal diagnosis* has been made by the detection of elevated NAA levels in amniotic fluid and deficient ASPA activity in cultured amniotic fluid cells or chorionic villus samples. However, the most reliable method of diagnosis is DNA analysis.

Alexander Disease

Alexander disease may have its onset in the first weeks of life (≈30% of infantile cases), and the most frequent initial *clinical features* are macrocephaly, failure to attain early motor milestones and, interestingly, seizures (see Table 29.6).[35,166-179] Progressive spastic quadriparesis, seizures, and failure of neurological

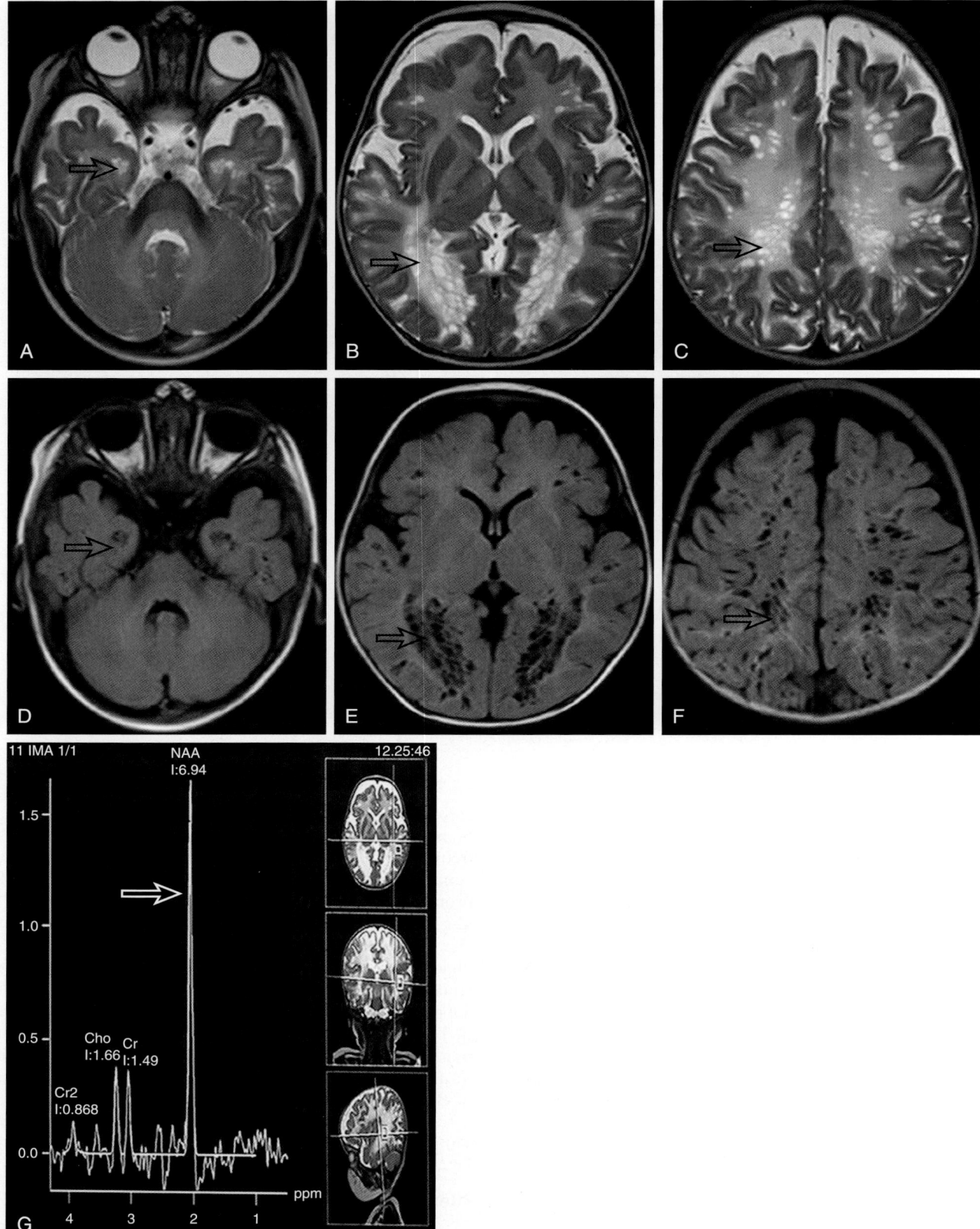

Figure 29.12 Magnetic resonance imaging and magnetic resonance spectroscopy in Canavan disease. Axial T2-weighted (A to C) and axial fluid-attenuated inversion recovery (D to F) magnetic resonance images showing symmetrical hyperintensities in the bilateral white matter, internal capsule, globus pallidi, and thalamus. The small cysts (hollow black arrows) seen in the white matter in the temporal lobes, parieto-occipital and frontal white matter, and centrum semiovale give the spongy appearance. G, Large *N*-aspartylaspartate peak (hollow white arrow) at 2.0 suggesting a diagnosis of Canavan disease. (From Kamate M, Kabate V, Malhotra M. Spongy white matter: a novel neuroimaging finding in Canavan disease. *Pediatr Neurol.* 2016;56:92–93.)

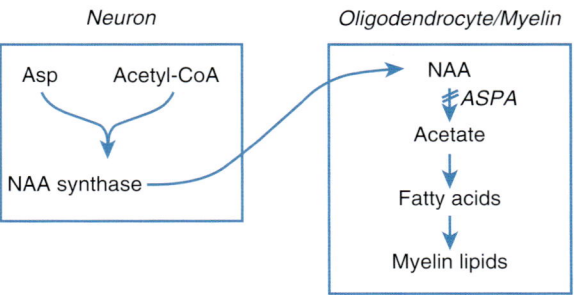

Figure 29.13 Metabolism of *N*-acetylaspartic acid (NAA) in the neuron and oligodendrocyte/myelin. NAA is synthesized in the neuron from aspartate (Asp) and acetyl coenzyme A (Acetyl-CoA) by N-acetyl synthase (NAA), encoded by the Nat8L gene. It is then transported to the oligodendrocyte, where NAA is metabolized by *N*-acetylaspartoacylase (ASPA), the enzyme that is deficient in Canavan disease.

development later become prominent, and death after a median survival of 3.5 years is most common. *Diagnosis* is suggested by the clinical features and brain imaging findings. CT shows decreased attenuation especially in frontal white matter, and after a contrast injection, the areas of increased attenuation (most notably subependymal) are noted early in the disease, particularly around the tips of the frontal horns.[a] Cranial ultrasonography has been reported to show increased echogenicity of cerebral white matter early in the disease.[182] MRI study is preferable and characteristic, showing an increased signal in the frontal white matter, with posterior extension, with abnormalities of the basal ganglia also, especially caudate heads and anterior putamina, and of the brain stem tegmentum and the periaqueductal regions (Fig. 29.14).[183,184] The brain stem changes coupled with the occasional finding of elevated lactate on MR spectroscopy may initially suggest Leigh disease.[171] MRI changes can be evident even before the development of significant clinical symptoms.[184] The major *neuropathological features* are a severe deficiency of myelin and eosinophilic deposits within the fibrillary astrocytes (Rosenthal fibers). These deposits have been shown by electron microscopy to be associated with an accumulation of disordered glial filaments.[175,185,186] The Rosenthal fibers in Alexander disease are enriched in a protein—crystallin—which is characteristic of the eye lens, but is also synthesized in astrocytes.[168,187-189] The crystallin molecules are ubiquitinated, and this modification appears to have altered their biophysical properties to result in insoluble aggregates of abnormally large ubiquitinated crystallin molecules.[168] Interestingly, the TAR DNA binding protein of 43 kDa (TDP-43), a major pathological protein in the neurodegenerative diseases amyotrophic lateral sclerosis and frontotemporal lobar degeneration, becomes mislocalized to the cytoplasm of astrocytes in human and mouse Alexander disease brains. It is then pathologically phosphorylated and becomes increasingly insoluble, which is coincident with an increase in ubiquitinated proteins. The burden of phosphorylated TDP-43 is particular high in the youngest, most severely affected patients, suggesting that the pathophysiology of Rosenthal fibers may be similar to some adult neurodegenerative disorders.[190] The fibers represent the intermediate filaments of astrocytes, which are composed of glial fibrillary acidic protein (GFAP). The

molecular defect has been shown to be a de novo, dominant (i.e., heterozygous), missense mutation of the gene for GFAP.[175-178,186,191,192] The latter results in a so-called toxic gain of function. Mutations continue to be identified (see http://www.waisman.wisc.edu/alexander-disease/) but nearly one-third involve two amino acids (R79 and R239). With the increasing diagnostic accuracy provided by GFAP sequencing, there is now the ability to correlate the age of onset, the genotype, and the clinical outcome.[193] A recent analysis of 215 patients indicates that there are likely two classes of Alexander disease: type 1 with early onset, seizures, macrocephaly, encephalopathy, paroxysmal deterioration, failure to thrive, developmental delay, and classic radiologic features; type 2 with ages across the life span, autonomic dysfunction, bulbar symptoms, ocular movement abnormalities, palatal myoclonus, and atypical radiological features.[193] Notably, cases with the R239 mutation had the most aggressive course. The finding of elevated levels of GFAP in the CSF and blood of affected infantile patients is consistent with the molecular defect and suggests potential value for diagnosis.[174,194]

Exciting experimental studies have suggested two new avenues for potential treatment. A *Drosophila* model of Alexander disease has suggested that increased nitric oxide synthase (iNOS) in astrocytes leads to oxidative stress in glia and neurons, which could be blocked with oral pharmacological inhibitors of nitric oxide production. Importantly, similar upregulation in iNOS was observed in Alexander disease mouse models and patient brains.[195] An in vivo pharmacological screen using the same model identified the upregulation of muscarinic cholinergic receptors that were contributing to GFAP toxicity, which was also observed in mouse models and postmortem patient tissue. Importantly, the muscarinic antagonist glycopyrrolate could block oxidative stress observed in the models and slightly reduce the number of seizures in the flies.[196] Further validation of these drug candidates is necessary, but promising nonetheless.

Krabbe Disease

Krabbe disease, an *autosomal recessive disorder*, has its onset in the first weeks of life, before the median age of onset at 4 months of age, in approximately 25% of cases.[167,197-203] The early *clinical features* are characteristic and consist of irritability, hypersensitivity to stimulation, startle responses, and increased tone (see Table 29.6). Poor feeding and unexplained, recurrent fever are common. Marked spasticity, severe stimulus-sensitive tonic extensor spasms, and decerebration then develop.[197-205] Although macrocephaly has been reported to occur, small head size is more common. The CSF protein level is markedly elevated, which is consistent with the accompanying peripheral neuropathy, and may aid in the initial diagnosis (see Table 29.4). The neuropathy may be detected in the neonatal period by the measurement of nerve conduction velocities.[206,207] As a result, deep tendon reflexes may be absent in advanced disease. A recent World-Wide Krabbe Registry has confirmed these features and the natural history of the disorder with a median survival of 25 months.[208] *Diagnosis* is based on identification in white blood cells or fibroblasts of the enzymatic defect, which involves a beta-galactosidase, galactosylceramidase I (see Fig. 29.1).[198,202,209] *Neuroimaging* findings, by CT, include increased attenuation in the thalamus relatively early in the disease.[5] MRI is preferable and notable for showing particular involvement of cerebellar white matter and periventricular and

---

[a]References 5, 168-170, 177, 178, 180, and 181.

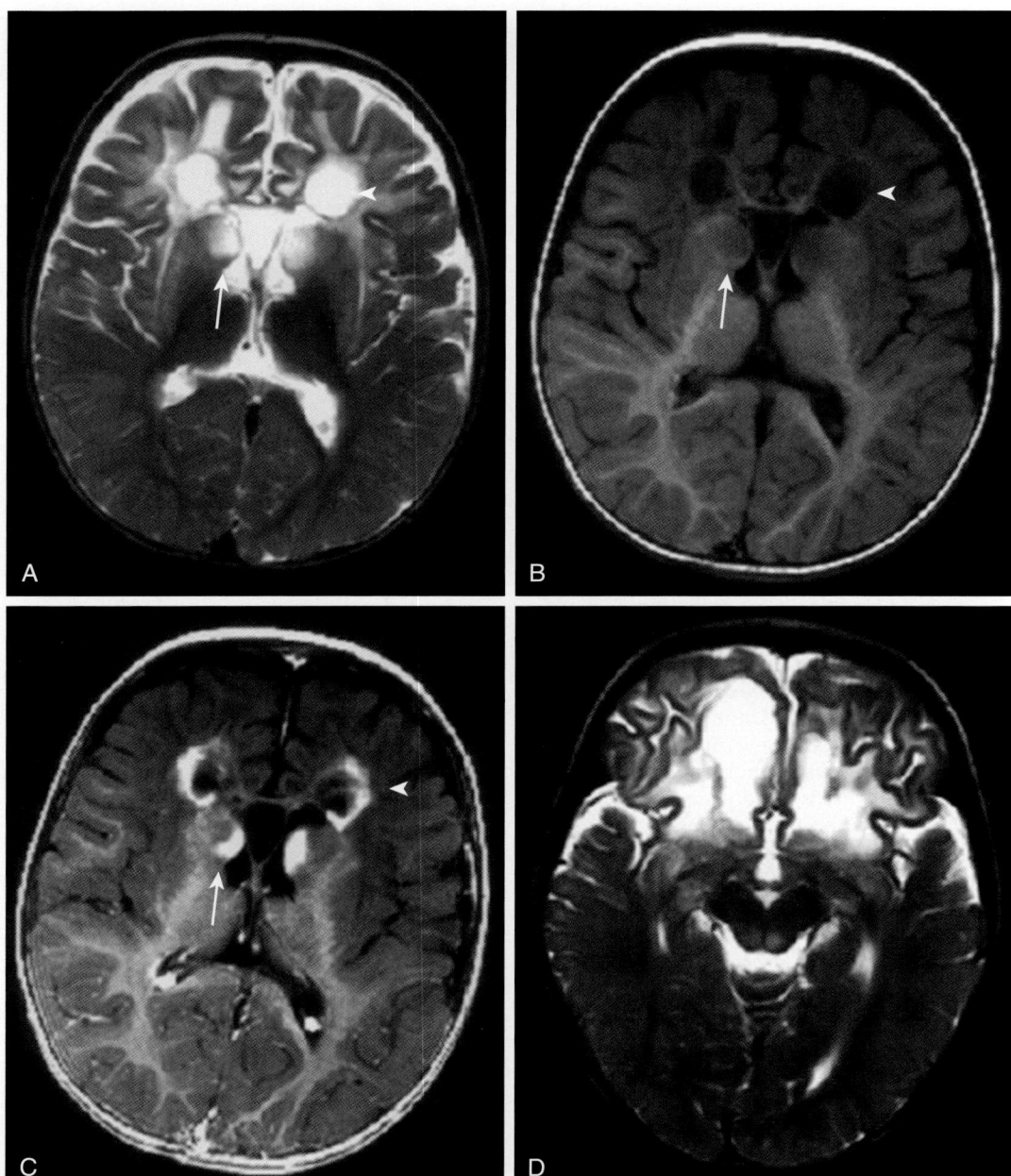

Figure 29.14 Alexander disease: magnetic resonance imaging (MRI) scans. On axial T2-weighted MRI (A and D), signal prolongation is seen in the frontal white matter, caudate nucleus, and putamen bilaterally (A) and in the midbrain (D). A periventricular rim *(arrow)* of slightly high signal intensity on an axial T1-weighted image (B) is low in T2-weighted images (A) and enhanced in T1-weighted images (C). In addition, there are subcortical cysts *(arrowhead)* in the frontal lobes (A to C) and enhanced pericystic regions (C). (From Murakami N, Tsuchiya T, Kanazawa N, Tsujino S, Nagai T. Novel deletion mutation in GFAP gene in an infantile form of Alexander disease. *Pediatr Neurol.* 2008;38:50–52.)

central cerebral white matter, sparing subcortical myelin (in contrast to Canavan disease) (Fig. 29.15).[5,210] Abnormalities on diffusion tensor imaging correlate with the neurodevelopmental outcome and are important biomarkers for assessing the efficacy of the interventions.[211-213]

Suzuki and co-workers[198,209,214] clarified the *basic biochemical nature* of this disease (Fig. 29.16). Because brain

galactosylceramide (galactocerebroside) concentrations were found *not* to be elevated in Krabbe disease, it became apparent that the degradation of galactosylceramide is not the essential defect. However, psychosine (galactosylsphingosine) is elevated in the brain in Krabbe disease. Suzuki and co-workers showed that the enzyme missing in infantile Krabbe disease is galactosylceramidase I, which catalyzes the removal of galactose

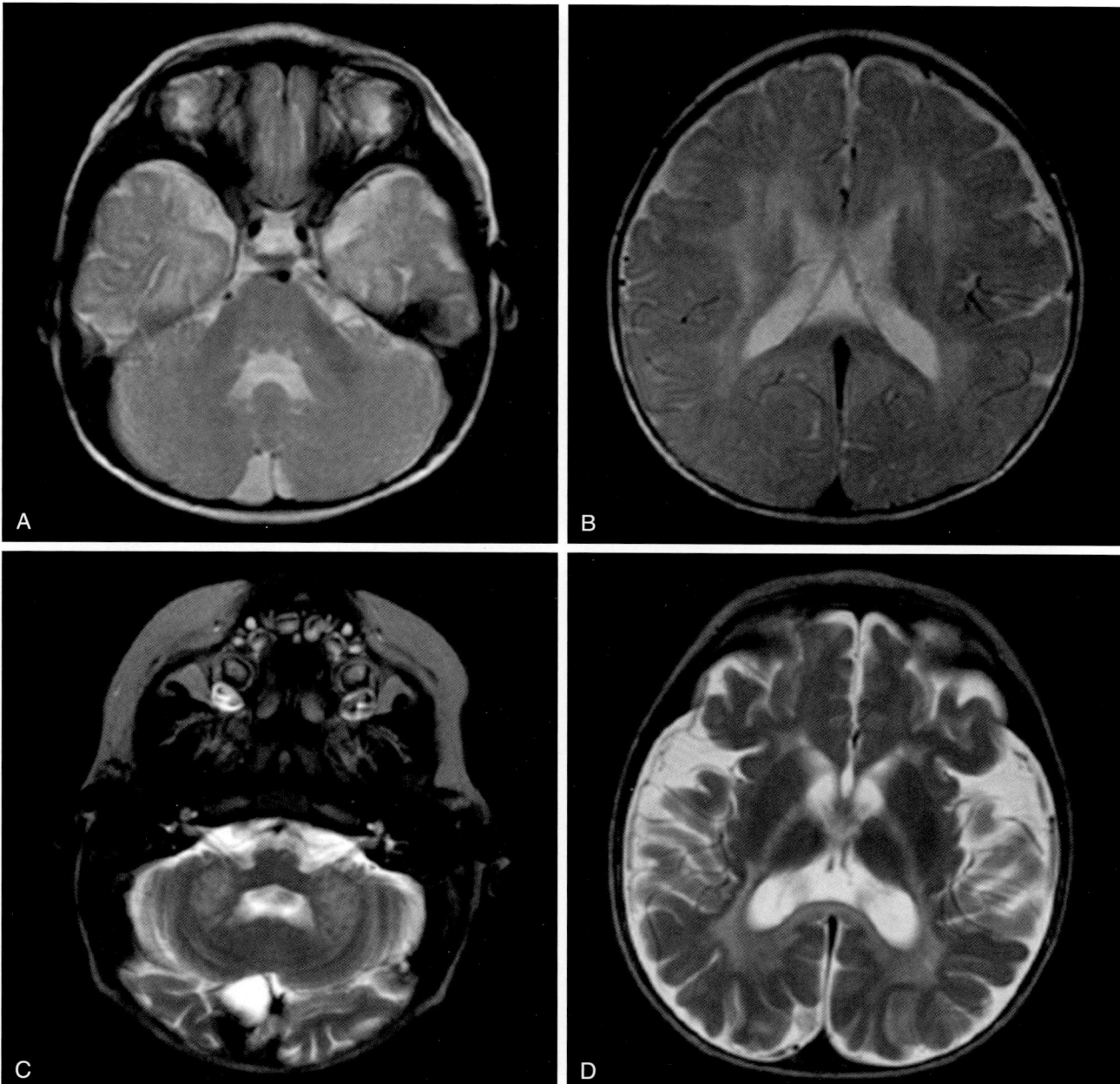

Figure 29.15 Krabbe disease: magnetic resonance imaging (MRI) scans. Infant who presented with crying, irritability, poor feeding, stiffness, fisted hands, poor head control, arching, and loss of developmental milestones. (A) Axial T2-weighted image initially shows no abnormality at the level of the dentate. (B) Axial T2-weighted image shows increased T2 signal in the deep cerebral white matter. MRI at 19 months: (C) axial T2-weighted image shows volume loss and increased T2 signal in the cerebellar white matter bilaterally. (D) Axial T2-weighted image shows extensive volume loss and bilateral T2 hyperintensity in the deep cerebral white matter and the internal and external capsules. (From Abdelhalim AN, Alberico RA, Barczykowski AL, Duffner PK. Patterns of magnetic resonance imaging abnormalities in symptomatic patients with Krabbe disease correspond to phenotype. *Pediatr Neurol.* 2014;50:127–134.)

from galactosylsphingosine (psychosine) as well as from galactosylceramide (see Fig. 29.16). Psychosine is highly toxic to oligodendroglia, and injections of psychosine into the brain lead to the neuropathology of Krabbe disease. Galactosylceramidase II, which is not defective in Krabbe disease, can degrade galactosylceramide but not psychosine, thus explaining the

failure of galactosylceramide concentrations to increase (see Fig. 29.16). The major *neuropathological features* include severe deficiencies of oligodendroglia and myelin, and collections of large, multinucleated globoid cells (Fig. 29.17).[35] These cells are essentially macrophages. The deficiency of galactosylceramidase has been demonstrated in the brain.[198,214,215] *Prenatal diagnosis* is

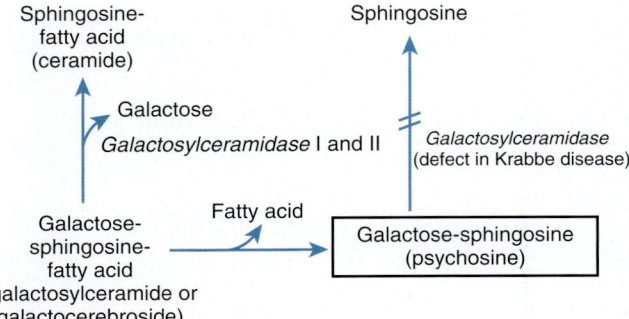

Figure 29.16 Mechanism for the increase in galactose-sphingosine (psychosine) in Krabbe disease. Galactosylceramidase I, the isoform absent in Krabbe disease, is required for the metabolism of psychosine to sphingosine. Galactosylceramidase II, present in Krabbe disease, provides some activity for conversion of galactosylceramide to ceramide.

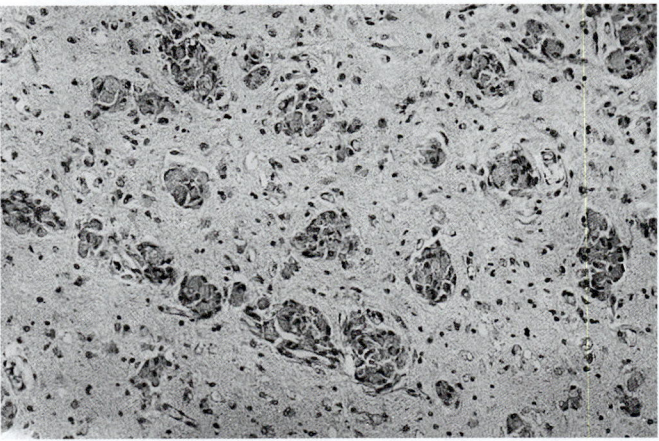

Figure 29.17 Krabbe disease: neuropathology. This photomicrograph of the cerebral white matter in an affected infant shows the large, multinucleated globoid cells. (Courtesy Dr. Kunihiko Suzuki.)

accomplished by assay of the enzyme in cultured amniotic fluid cells or chorionic villus samples. DNA analysis is also available if both pathogenic alleles in an affected family are known. Recent work has suggested a major advance in *therapy* of this disorder. Previous research showed that bone marrow transplantation is beneficial in the late-onset disease but not in the early-onset infantile disease.[13,101] Because of the importance of very early initiation of therapy in the infantile disease, transplantation of umbilical cord blood was carried out after myeloablative chemotherapy in asymptomatic newborns ($n = 11$; 12 to 44 days) and symptomatic infants ($n = 14$; 142 to 352 days) with Krabbe disease.[216] Donor cell engraftment and survival were 100% and 100%, respectively, in the asymptomatic newborns, and 100% but only 43% in the symptomatic newborns, respectively. The surviving infants had restoration of blood galactocerebrosidase levels. In the *asymptomatic* infants, over a median follow-up of 3 years, progressive cerebral myelination and normal cognitive development occurred, and mild to moderate motor disturbances were present. Children who underwent transplantation after the onset of symptoms had minimal neurological improvement. *The findings indicate the importance of transplantation as early as possible*

and the value of umbilical cord blood. New York State now includes Krabbe as part of the newborn screen,[217,218] and measurement of psychosine may make this more reliable and cost effective.[219,219a] However, the benefits and potential harms from false positives remain vigorously debated.[220] Experimental studies that suggest a combination of bone marrow therapy with CNS-directed gene modalities and substrate reduction may have additive benefits[221] that will likely inform future clinical trials.

Pelizaeus-Merzbacher Disease

One form of the three basic varieties of *Pelizaeus-Merzbacher disease* (PMD) typically has its onset in utero or during the first weeks of life. This so-called *connatal form* is distinguished from *classic disease* primarily on the basis of rate of progression (faster in the connatal cases), age at death (first decade in connatal cases vs. second decade or later in classic cases), and in severity of the neuropathology (total demyelination in connatal cases vs. partial demyelination with a tigroid appearance in the classic cases). *Transitional* cases are intermediate in severity. Because the molecular genetics and the clinical features of these three forms considerably overlap, distinction among them can be difficult, especially in infants with onset in the first weeks of life. At least 50 neonatal-onset, apparent connatal cases have been reported.[222-245]

The most consistent initial *clinical features* have been nystagmus, horizontal or rotatory, and inspiratory stridor (see Table 29.6). Head titubation, jerky movements of the head or limbs, and hypotonia are prominent. Seizures occur in approximately 75% of patients with neonatal-onset cases, thereby suggesting a gray matter disorder and a confusing establishment of diagnosis. Visual evoked responses are usually abnormal, which is consistent with the disturbance of the central myelin. *Diagnosis* is suspected on clinical grounds. *MRI shows a striking absence of myelin*, with increased signal on T2-weighted images (Fig. 29.18).[246] CT may show decreased attenuation of cerebral white matter, but findings are not as consistently abnormal as with MRI. MR spectroscopy is distinctive; notable findings include the elevation of choline-containing compounds, NAA and N-acetylaspartyl glutamate, glutamine, and myoinositol.[242-244] The findings are consistent, respectively, with reduced oligodendroglia with dysmyelination, increased axonal packing, and astrogliosis. *Neuropathology* is striking; myelin is virtually absent, with diminished oligodendroglia and gliosis (Fig. 29.19). Small amounts of sudanophilic material, reflecting myelin breakdown products, may be present. *X-linked recessive* inheritance is consistent. The defect involves the gene on the X-chromosome encoding proteolipid protein *(PLP)*,[235,238-241,245,247-254] a crucial structural protein of myelin accounting for 50% of myelin protein. PMD in all its forms is caused by mutations in *PLP*, with approximately 60% to 70% of cases related to duplications of the gene, 15% to 20% with point mutations, and the remainder being deletions. The neonatal-onset cases have been associated with duplications and deletions. The result of the former is multiple copies of PLP, and of the latter, deletion of both PLP and its post-transcriptional alternatively spliced protein product DM20.[245,255] While the clinical phenotype of this disorder correlates with the degree of dysmyelination observed on MRI, specific mutations or size of duplications do not appear to impact the phenotype.[246,256-258]

There are no therapies for PMD, but there are multiple areas of active investigation. A possible role for dietary cholesterol

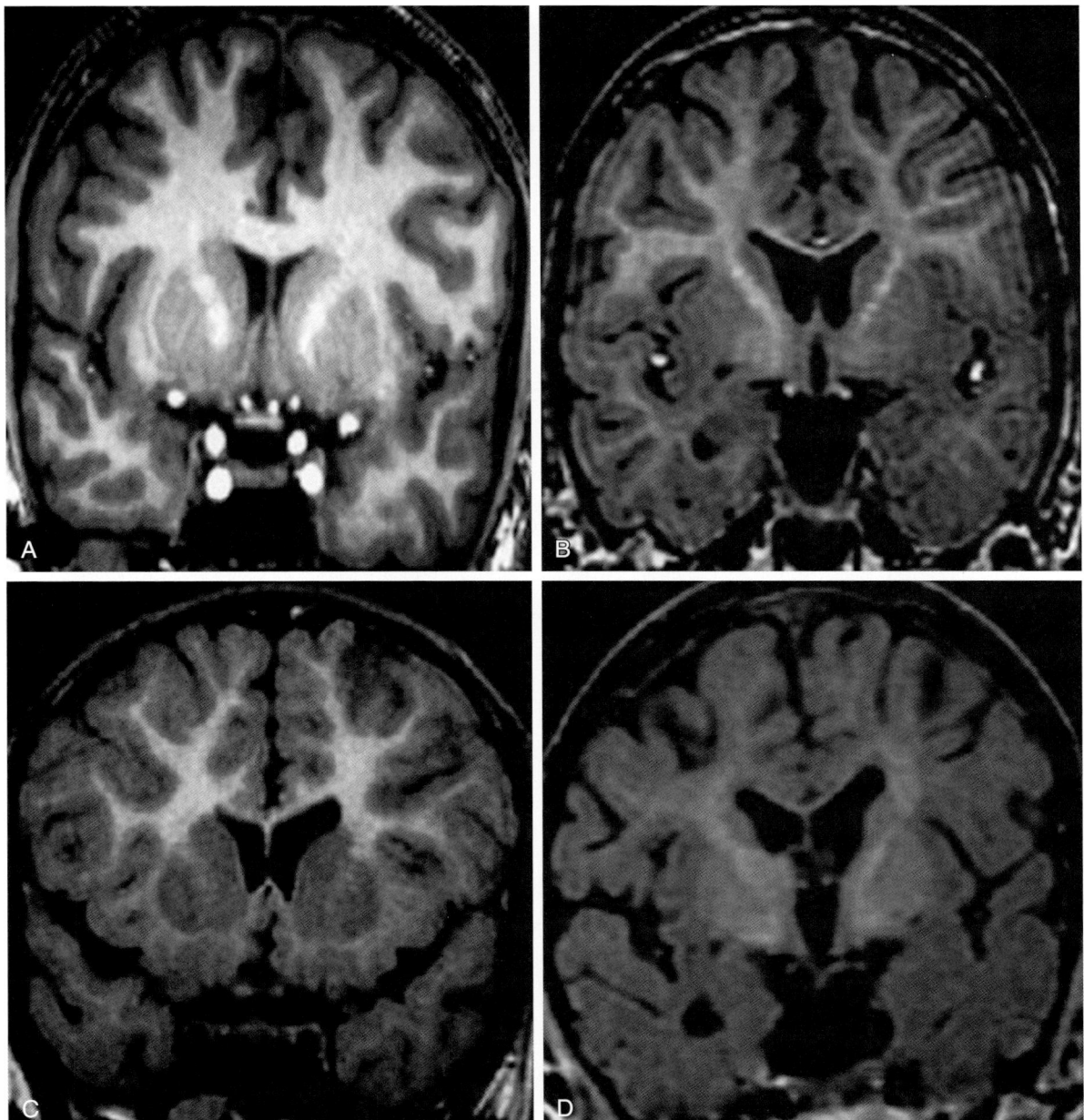

Figure 29.18 Pelizaeus-Merzbacher disease (PMD): magnetic resonance imaging scan. Comparison of gray matter–white matter contrast in patients with PMD. (A) Control showing normal myelination. (B) PMD patient with mild disease. Subcortical white matter is isointense with a gradual decrease in hyperintensity of the internal capsule. (C) PMD patient with moderate disease. The subcortical white matter is thin and the signal is hypointense in the temporal lobe and internal capsule. (D) PMD patient with severe disease. There is a diffusely reduced signal in the subcortical white matter, internal capsule, and temporal lobes with enlargement of the lateral ventricles. (From Laukka JJ, Stanley JA, Garbern JY, et al. Neuroradiologic correlates of clinical disability and progression in the X-linked leukodystrophy Pelizaeus-Merzbacher disease. *J Neurol Sci.* 2013;335:75–81.)

is suggested by recent studies in mouse models of PMD showing that increased dietary cholesterol prevented disease progression. The mechanism involved the promotion of normal PLP trafficking, and thereby oligodendrocyte differentiation and myelination.[259] Preliminary data following implantation of neural stem cells in human patients with early onset disease suggest production of donor-derived myelin.[260] Longer-term

benefits are less clear, and the need for immunosuppression is a limitation. Umbilical cord blood transplantation after myeloablative chemotherapy performed in two young boys with PMD appears to have prevented disease progression.[261] The two patients have been followed for 1 year and 7 years, respectively. Although initial results are encouraging, longer-term follow-up is needed.

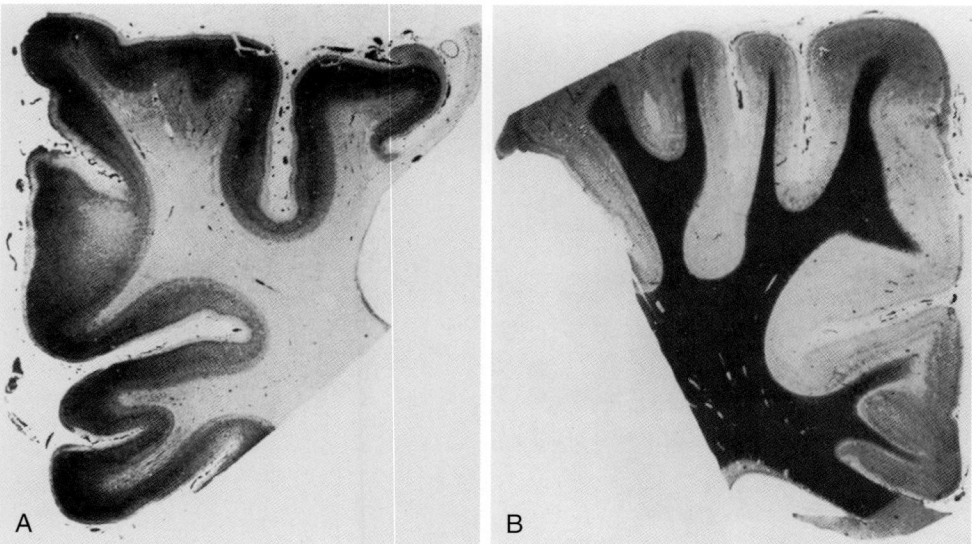

Figure 29.19 Pelizaeus-Merzbacher disease: neuropathology. The infant died at 6 months of age with a history of onset of seizures at 1 month of age, followed by failure of neurological development, hypotonia, hyper-reflexia, and clonus. (A) Frontal white matter is absent. Compare with (B) an age-matched control infant. (From Scheffer IE, Baraitser M, Wilson J, Harding B, et al. Pelizaeus-Merzbacher disease: classical or connatal? *Neuropediatrics.* 1991;22:71–78.)

A disorder phenotypically closely related to PMD, with a hypomyelinative leukoencephalopathy but *autosomal recessive inheritance*, has been termed *Pelizaeus-Merzbacher-like disease* (PMLD).[262] Like connatal PMD, PMLD manifests with nystagmus during the newborn period. However, the subsequent course in PMLD differs from that of connatal, X-linked PMD (i.e., exhibits slower progression with a greater preservation of cognitive functions and the development of at least partial myelination of the corticospinal tracts by MRI). One molecular defect in PMLD involves the *GJA12* gene, which encodes connexin 47, although mutations in this gene account for a minority of patients.[263,264] The connexins are a family of proteins that form intercellular channels of gap junctions, between multiple cell types, including oligodendrocytes. Mutations in the monocarboxylase transporter 8 gene (MCT8) encoding a thyroid hormone transporter have also been identified in PMLD, suggesting that screening T3 and T4 concentrations may be useful in patients with the PMLD phenotype.[265] The exact molecular mechanism of the transporter deficiency remains to be elucidated, but thyroid hormone is essential for proper oligodendrocyte differentiation, and hypothyroidism leads to motor and cognitive disabilities that are attributed to deficits in both gray and white matter.[266-268]

Other rare sudanophilic hypomyelinative/dysmyelinative leukodystrophies may be related to PMD and perhaps may be secondary to defects of other structural proteins of myelin.[232,269-272] The best established of these is *Cockayne syndrome*, an autosomal recessive disorder with the neuropathological finding of patchy tigroid demyelination, as in classic PMD. In the classic form, Cockayne syndrome type I, the development of postnatal growth failure, a *cachectic, elfin, progeroid* facial appearance, pigmentary retinopathy, impaired neurological development, sensorineural hearing loss, and cutaneous photosensitivity become apparent *after* the first months of life.[273-276] In the less common severe form, Cockayne syndrome

type II, *newborns* have already exhibited growth failure in utero, have markedly impaired postnatal somatic and head growth, and have poor to absent neurological development. Congenital cataracts and more rapid development of auditory and cutaneous complications are features of this severe form. The disturbance of myelination in Cockayne syndrome affects the peripheral nervous system as well as the CNS, and is manifested by elevated CSF protein levels, slow nerve conduction velocities, and nerve biopsy specimens showing segmental demyelination. In the CNS, in addition to the myelin disturbance, imaging studies show the calcification of basal ganglia, which is a helpful diagnostic feature. The basic *biochemical disturbance* in the disease involves DNA metabolism and ultrasensitivity to ultraviolet light, with abnormal DNA repair mechanisms detectable in cultured skin fibroblasts. Infants with the severe form of the disease usually die by the age of 6 or 7 years.

Leukodystrophy With Cerebral Calcifications (Aicardi-Goutieres Syndrome)

Leukodystrophy with cerebral calcifications, a rare autosomal recessive disorder initially clearly described by Aicardi and Goutieres, has been identified in approximately 100 cases.[277-298]

Approximately one-third of patients have had the onset of the disease within the first postnatal month (see Table 29.5). *Clinical features* include irritability, poor feeding, ocular abnormalities (especially ocular *jerking*), hypertonia more than hypotonia, weakness, jitteriness, dystonia, oral-facial dyskinesias, and, occasionally, seizures. Developmental arrest, microcephaly, and spastic quadriparesis follow, with death often in the first several years of life. Persistent *CSF pleocytosis* has been consistent (see Table 29.4). CSF protein levels are slightly elevated in fewer than 50% of patients. *Elevated CSF levels of interferon-alpha* also are a consistent finding. *Brain imaging* is distinctive. Ultrasonography shows echogenicity of periventricular white matter, a frequent finding in early infantile white matter degenerations.[282] CT

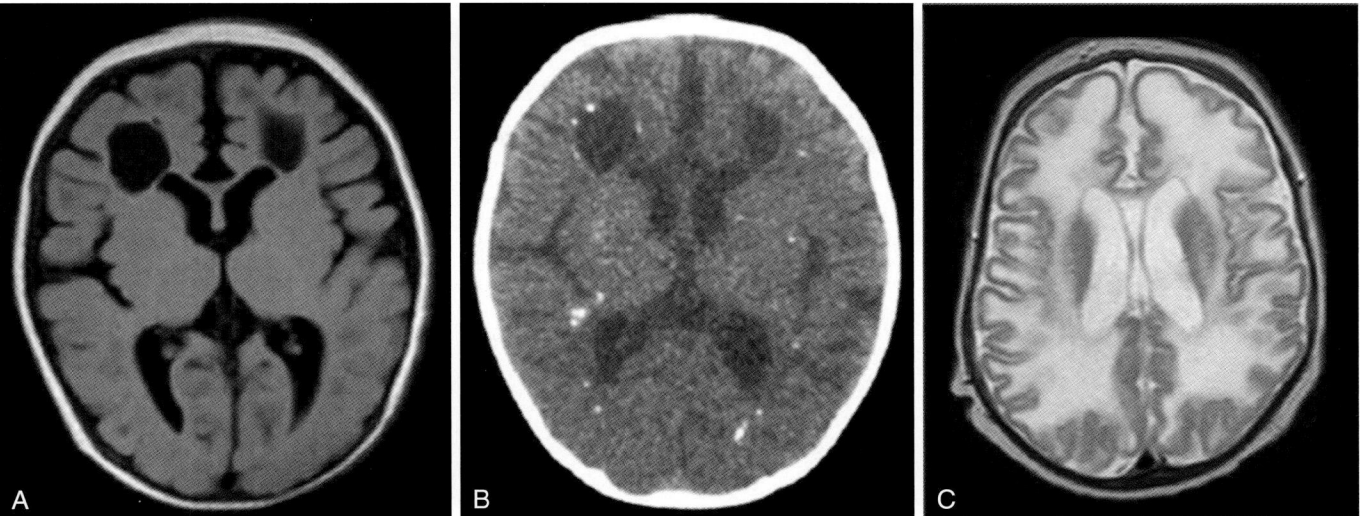

Figure 29.20 Aicardi-Goutieres syndrome: magnetic resonance imaging and computed tomography (CT) scans. (A) Axial T2-weighted fluid-attenuated inversion recovery shows deep frontal white matter cystic lesions in a 4-month-old patient. (B) CT scan shows calcifications along the walls of the cysts. (C) Axial T2-weighted image shows diffuse pattern and swollen frontal poles in another 4-month-old patient. (From La Piana R, Uggetti C, Roncarolo F, et al. Neuroradiologic patterns and novel imaging findings in Aicardi-Goutieres syndrome. *Neurology*. 2016;86:28–35.)

demonstrates decreased attenuation of cerebral white matter and calcifications, which may be diffuse, periventricular, or in basal ganglia (Fig. 29.20). Characteristically, the calcification mostly affects the putamen and cerebellar dentate nuclei. MRI shows diffuse hyperintensity of cerebral white matter on T2-weighted images (see Fig. 29.20).[299] Cerebellar atrophy is a common accompaniment. Severity of frontal and temporal lobe leukoencephalopathy correlates with the early age of onset[300] and is associated with TREX1 mutations.[299] Specific findings of temporal lobe swelling or temporal horn dilation, with progressive frontal lobe atrophy, and evidence of calcifications may also help differentiate infantile Aicardi-Goutieres syndrome from other leukodystrophies.[301] *Neuropathology* consists of a marked decrease of myelin, striking fibrillary gliosis, and the calcifications, which are located primarily in the walls of the blood vessels. Perivascular collections of inflammatory cells have been noted, but no viral particles or other evidence of viral infection has been detected. The microangiopathy may be accompanied by thromboses and microinfarction. Large vessel arteriopathy has also been observed in patients with Aicardi-Goutieres syndrome caused by SAMHD1 mutations and may lead to stenosis, aneurysms, thrombosis, and intracerebral hemorrhage.[302] This genetic subclass of patients (see later) may require unique intracranial arteriopathy screening and treatment. The elevated CSF levels of interferon-alpha raise the possibility that the cytokine is causally related to the cerebral disorder,[303,304] and a recent case control study confirmed that six interferon-stimulated genes could differentiate cases from controls.[305] Transgenic animals with astrocyte-targeted interferon-alpha showed neuropathological features mimicking those found in Aicardi-Goutieres syndrome. Further supporting a direct pathogenetic role of this cytokine, interferon-alpha can directly produce calcifying microangiopathy in smooth muscle cells in vitro.[306] Some infants with the syndrome exhibit cutaneous vascular lesions similar to those observed in patients

treated with interferon-alpha.[297] Interferon-alpha treatment of young infants with vascular malformations has been associated with the development of spastic diplegia, a finding that suggests injury to developing white matter by the cytokine.[307] Recent work shows mutations in Aicardi-Goutieres syndrome involving at least seven different genes, including TREX1, RNASEH2A, RNASHE2B, RNASEH2C, SAMHD1, ADAR, and IFIH1,[308] involved in nucleic acid metabolism and signaling, which lead to an interferon-mediated innate immune response. Other proinflammatory cytokines and chemokines may have distinct patterns of abnormality and be useful biomarkers for diagnostic and therapeutic monitoring.[309] A variety of systemic and brain-reactive autoantibodies also have been identified,[310] further suggesting a likely autoimmune mechanism and supporting current studies of immunosuppressive and immunomodulatory therapies.[311]

DISORDERS AFFECTING BOTH GRAY AND WHITE MATTER

Several disorders with neonatal onset exhibit prominent features of both gray matter and white matter disease (Table 29.7; see also Table 29.1). Two of these affect subcellular structures present in all cells; that is, disorders of peroxisomes and of mitochondria. The peroxisomal disorders are represented in the newborn primarily by *Zellweger (cerebrohepatorenal) syndrome* and *neonatal adrenoleukodystrophy*, and the mitochondrial disorders in this context are represented primarily by *Leigh syndrome* (and related encephalopathies). (The other mitochondrial disorder with possible neonatal presentation, Alpers disease, manifests as a gray matter degeneration, as discussed earlier.) Another disorder in this broad category involves synthesis of an amino acid, serine, which is important in all cells, and includes prominent gray matter (e.g., seizures) and white matter (neuroimaging appearance of *periventricular leukomalacia*) signs (see Table

TABLE 29.7 Degenerative Diseases Affecting Both Gray and White Matter

DISEASE	CLINICAL FEATURES	METABOLIC-ENZYMATIC FEATURES	PATHOLOGY
Zellweger syndrome (cerebrohepatorenal syndrome)	Craniofacial dysmorphism, hypotonia, weakness, impaired feeding, seizures, optic atrophy, renal cysts, calcific stippling, later blindness, deafness, relative macrocephaly, moderately rapid progression to vegetative state	Evidence of deficiency of multiple peroxisomal functions: elevated very-long-chain fatty acids, pipecolic acid, and bile acid intermediate levels, deficient synthesis of plasmalogens; a disorder of peroxisomal biogenesis; molecular defect affecting proteins involved in peroxisomal biogenesis (peroxins), encoded by specific genes (PEX), or rarely single enzyme defects (ACOX1, HSD17B4)	Severe neuronal migrational defects; major features include pachygyria (especially parasagittal region) and microgyria (especially lateral convexity), with heterotopias also involving the cerebellum and inferior olivary nuclei; myelin disturbance as described next for neonatal adrenoleukodystrophy, although less severe
Neonatal adrenoleukodystrophy	Similar to Zellweger syndrome (above), but less severe, course is less rapid, and absence of renal cysts and calcific stippling	Similar to Zellweger syndrome (above), except findings are generally less severe; molecular defect affects proteins involved in peroxisomal biogenesis (peroxins) encoded by specific genes (PEX)	Myelin deficiency and loss, diffuse but especially marked in cerebellum; sudanophilic material, perivascular mononuclear cells, trilamellar inclusions in macrophages; neuronal migrational defects, although less prominent and consistent than in Zellweger syndrome
Leigh syndrome	Hypotonia, weakness, respiratory abnormalities, impaired feeding, oculomotor abnormalities, facial weakness, seizures, developmental arrest with development later of movement disorders and regression	Elevated lactate-pyruvate in cerebrospinal fluid, variably in serum; deficiency in pyruvate dehydrogenase complex, cytochrome c oxidase (complex IV), reduced nicotinamide adenine dinucleotide-coenzyme Q reductase (complex I), or adenosine triphosphatase subunit 6 (complex V)	Focal, symmetrical, spongiform necrosis especially in diencephalon and brain stem, particularly surrounding third ventricle, aqueduct, and fourth ventricle, characterized by necrosis (relative sparing of neurons), demyelination, vascular proliferation, and astrocytosis
Other mitochondrial encephalopathies	Various combinations of the above manifestations	Elevated lactate-pyruvate as for Leigh syndrome; enzymatic defects overlap (see text)	Cellular pathology similar to Leigh syndrome, but regions affected differ; may be principally cerebral white matter and various combinations of the regions involved in Leigh syndrome
Serine synthesis deficiency	Congenital microcephaly, intrauterine growth restriction, refractory seizures, psychomotor delay		Global atrophy and enlarged ventricles
CDG type 1a (CDG1a): carbohydrate-deficient glycoprotein syndrome	Facial dysmorphisms, abnormal subcutaneous fat, abnormal eye movements, hypotonia, joint contractures, cardiac-liver-renal abnormalities; subsequent developmental arrest, seizures, ataxia, strokelike episodes	Abnormally glycosylated transferrin, coagulation factors, hormones, lysosomal enzymes, other glycoproteins; phosphomannomutase deficiency (CDG1a)	Cerebellar hypoplasia; often with pontine hypoplasia (i.e., pontocerebellar hypoplasia); neuronal loss and gliosis, especially in the cerebellum but also in the cerebral cortex, basal ganglia, thalamus, pons, inferior olives, and spinal cord; polyneuropathy
Pontocerebellar hypoplasia type 2	Impaired sucking and swallowing, jitteriness; later progressive microcephaly, extrapyramidal dyskinesias, epilepsy, severe mental retardation	Unknown	Neuronal loss and gliosis, especially in ventral pons and cerebellum, less so in inferior olivary nuclei; moderate cerebral cortical neuronal degeneration and atrophy
Neurotransmitter Disorders	Encephalopathy, epilepsy, pyramidal and extrapyramidal motor features, autonomic changes, and later neuropsychiatric features		

CDG, Congenital disorder of glycosylation.

29.7). Two disorders exhibit a strong regional predilection for cerebellar and brain stem structures; that is, congenital disorders of glycosylation and pontocerebellar hypoplasia (see Table 29.7). A regional predilection involving basal ganglia and related connections is apparent in neurotransmitter defects, which, in the newborn, are accompanied by both gray and white matter signs (see Table 29.7). Finally, Rett syndrome in males—a rare fulminating disorder with seizures and a variety of other neurological signs—involves a transcriptional mechanism present in both neuronal and glial cells (see Table 29.7).

Peroxisomal Disorders

Peroxisomal functions include both *catabolic activities* (e.g., beta-oxidation of very-long-chain fatty acids, degradation of hydrogen peroxide by catalase, pipecolic acid metabolism, oxidation of phytanic acid) and *anabolic* activities (e.g., biosynthesis of plasmalogens and of bile acids).[312-316] Peroxisomal disorders are divided into two broad groups: disorders of peroxisomal assembly, in which there is a decrease in the number or structure of peroxisomes with multiple peroxisomal enzymes affected (group I); and disorders of single peroxisomal enzymes, with normal peroxisomal number and structure (group II) (Table 29.8).

More than 90% of the cases of peroxisomal disorders with consistent and prominent onset in the neonatal period consist of Zellweger syndrome and neonatal adrenoleukodystrophy. Single enzyme deficiencies with consistent and prominent onset in the newborn period include peroxisomal D-bifunctional protein deficiency and acyl-CoA oxidase deficiency, which exhibit many features comparable to those of Zellweger syndrome.[313,314,316-320] The fundamental defect in the disorders of peroxisome biogenesis involves mutations in genes (PEX) involved in peroxisomal biogenesis.[315,316,321-327] A growing list of mutations in 13 PEX genes have been identified (see http://www.dbpex.org and http://www.peroxisomedb.org/home.jsp).[328,329] These genes principally encode for the integral peroxisome membrane, or matrix proteins or receptors involved in targeting cytosolic proteins to the peroxisome.

Zellweger Syndrome

Zellweger syndrome is the prototypical disorder of peroxisome biogenesis that characteristically manifests in the neonatal period.[312,313,315,316,330-346] The *clinical features* include a distinctively dysmorphic craniofacial appearance (Fig. 29.21), cataracts,

pigmentary retinopathy, hepatomegaly, glomerulocystic disease of kidneys, and calcific stippling of patellae, hips, and other epiphyses (Table 29.7; see also Table 29.9). The neurological syndrome is striking and includes severe visual and auditory impairments as well as marked hypotonia and weakness. The latter two features are accompanied by areflexia and may be sufficiently severe to raise the possibility of Werdnig-Hoffmann disease.[347] Neonatal seizures are characteristic. Neurological deterioration is marked, and death by 6 months of age is common.[315,344] The basic *biochemical defect* involves peroxisome biogenesis; peroxisomal membrane *ghosts* are present, but the organelle's enzymes are absent. Because of the failure of importing enzymes into the peroxisome, the proteins are degraded in the cytosol. Catalase is not degraded but it is found in the cytosol, an abnormal site for this enzyme. The total number of peroxisomes is markedly decreased.[315,327]

Diagnosis is based on the clinical features and the finding of deficiency of multiple peroxisomal functions manifested particularly by marked elevations in the plasma of very-long-chain fatty acids, pipecolic acid, and bile acid intermediates, and by a deficiency of plasmalogens in red blood cells (see Table 29.9). If biochemical testing is normal but clinical suspicion remains high, cultured fibroblasts for further biochemical, enzymatic, and immunofluorescence studies should be pursued. Molecular analysis of PEX genes is necessary to pinpoint specific mutations and to differentiate from single enzyme defects (i.e., acyl-CoA oxidase deficiency and D-bifunctional protein deficiency caused by mutations in ACOX1 and HSD17B4, respectively).[345] MRI is effective for the demonstration of the neuropathology (Fig. 29.22).[5,348,349] The *neuropathology* is characterized especially by neuronal migration defects, especially pachygyria and polymicrogyria (see Chapter 6).[315,350,351] In addition to the neuronal migrational defects, the cerebral white matter is abnormal. The accumulation of sudanophilic

TABLE 29.8 Classification of Peroxisomal Disorders
Group I: Disorders of peroxisomal assembly: activities of multiple peroxisomal enzymes deficient
Zellweger cerebrohepatorenal syndrome
Neonatal adrenoleukodystrophy
Infantile Refsum disease
Rhizomelic chondrodysplasia punctate
Group II: Activity of only one peroxisomal enzyme deficient: peroxisomes normal in number and structure
X-linked adrenoleukodystrophy
D-bifunctional protein deficiency
Acyl-coenzyme A oxidase deficiency
beta-Ketothiolase deficiency
Other

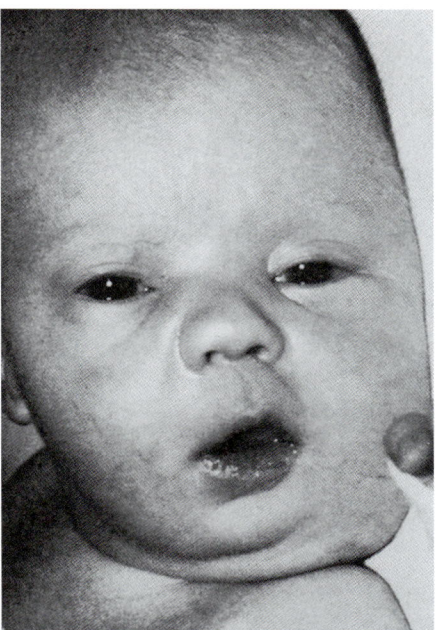

Figure 29.21 Zellweger syndrome: craniofacial appearance. This infant, at 2 weeks of age, exhibits a high and wide head (turribrachycephaly), a high brow, flat supraorbital ridges, *jowly* cheeks, wide-set eyes, and a small mouth.

TABLE 29.9   Clinical, Morphological, and Biochemical Features of Zellweger Syndrome and Neonatal Adrenoleukodystrophy in the Neonatal Period

FEATURE	ZELLWEGER SYNDROME	NEONATAL ADRENOLEUKO-DYSTROPHY
Clinical		
Dysmorphic craniofacial appearance	++	+
Hypotonia and weakness	++	+
Seizures	++	+
Cataracts	++	+
Pigmentary retinopathy	++	+
Visual and auditory impairment	++	+
Hepatomegaly	++	+
Renal cysts	+	−
Calcific stippling	+	−
Mean age at death	6 months	3 years
Morphological		
Neuronal migrational defect	++	+
Myelin disturbance	+	++
Adrenal atrophy	−	++
Biochemical		
↑ Very-long-chain fatty acids	++	+
↑ Bile acid intermediates	++	+
↓ Plasmalogen synthesis	++	+
↑ Pipecolic acid	++	+
↓ Phytanic acid oxidase	+	+
↑ Phytanic acid	−[a]	−[a]

[a]Develops later in first year.

+, Usually present; ++, prominent; −, absent; ↑, increased; ↓, decreased.

of peroxisome biogenesis, because of the defect in oxidation of saturated very-long-chain fatty acids of 26 carbons to 22 carbons. The *molecular defect* in Zellweger syndrome involves the genes encoding proteins necessary for peroxisome biogenesis, termed *peroxins (PEX)*.[315,316] Peroxisome biogenesis begins with the synthesis of the peroxisomal matrix and membrane proteins on cytosolic ribosomes, post-translational targeting, docking at the peroxisomal membrane surface, and importing into the organelle. In Zellweger syndrome, *PEX1* is the most commonly affected gene and is involved in the import of peroxisomal matrix proteins. As noted earlier, single enzyme defects related to ACOX1 or HSD17B4 abnormalities are rarely responsible.

No effective *therapy* has been described for Zellweger syndrome. A report of a beneficial effect of dietary supplementation of docosahexaenoic acid on retinal function, myelination, and perhaps clinical features in five patients with disorders of peroxisomal biogenesis[324,356] was not validated in a double-blind, randomized trial, which showed no significant benefit of DHA.[357] Moreover, somewhat promising is the demonstration that treatment of Zellweger syndrome fibroblasts with the peroxisome proliferator, sodium 4-phenylbutyrate, resulted in an increase in peroxisomal number.[327] Nevertheless, the fact that Zellweger syndrome involves a marked disturbance of brain development that occurs before 20 weeks of gestation suggests that postnatal therapies are not likely to be markedly beneficial.

Neonatal Adrenoleukodystrophy

Neonatal leukodystrophy, unlike the X-linked disease of older children, is an autosomal recessive disorder with a characteristic *clinical presentation* (see Tables 29.7 and 29.9).[a] Infants exhibit a dysmorphic craniofacial appearance, which is similar to, but not as marked as, that seen in Zellweger syndrome (see later discussion). Neurological features include hypotonia, weakness, impaired feeding, and optic atrophy—findings that are probably largely secondary to white matter disease—and seizures, consistent with gray matter disease. Relative macrocephaly, visual and auditory impairment, and neurological deterioration to death at approximately 3 years of age are typical. *Diagnosis* is based on the clinical features and the finding of deficiency of multiple peroxisomal functions, manifested particularly by elevations in plasma of very-long-chain fatty acids, pipecolic acid, and bile acid intermediates and by the deficiency of plasmalogens in red blood cells (see Table 29.9). As with the clinical features, the metabolic abnormalities are not as marked as in Zellweger syndrome.[313,315,364] The basic *biochemical defect* involves peroxisome biogenesis, as in Zellweger syndrome; peroxisomal membrane *ghosts* are present, but the organelle's enzymes are absent or severely deficient.[315,365] The total number of peroxisomes is markedly decreased.[327] As in Zellweger syndrome, the *molecular defect* involves peroxins encoded by specific *PEX* genes. The several defects that lead to the disease have involved the targeting of cytosolic proteins, docking, and importing into the peroxisome.[316]

Neuropathology is characterized by marked and diffusely decreased myelin, perivascular mononuclear *inflammatory* cells, trilamellar inclusions in macrophages, and sudanophilic lipid in reactive astrocytes. The myelin disturbance is somewhat more severe than in Zellweger syndrome.[312] Peripheral nerve

lipids and the deficiency of myelin suggest sudanophilic leukodystrophy.[312] MRI may show signal abnormalities in the hilus of dentate, cerebellar peduncles, and parieto-occipital white matter and thereby suggest underlying peroxisomal disorders in the Zellweger spectrum.[352,353] The molecular basis for the neuronal migrational and the myelin abnormalities may principally relate to the disorder of very-long-chain fatty acid oxidation. Thus, levels of these fatty acids are particularly high in the peroxisomal disorders with migrational abnormalities (i.e., Zellweger syndrome, neonatal adrenoleukodystrophy, and the single enzyme defects, D-bifunctional protein deficiency and acyl-CoA oxidase deficiency).[315-318,354,355] D-bifunctional protein deficiency is also accompanied by the elevation of bile acid intermediates, but these are probably an unlikely perturbant of neuronal migration. Concerning the potential role of very-long-chain fatty acids in the myelin disturbance, an apparent beneficial effect of dietary supplementation of docosahexaenoic acid (22:6n3) on cerebral myelin, as visualized by MRI, is supportive.[356] Thus, levels of this polyunsaturated fatty acid are decreased in the brain of patients with disorders

[a]References 312, 315, 316, 330-335, 343, 344, and 358-363.

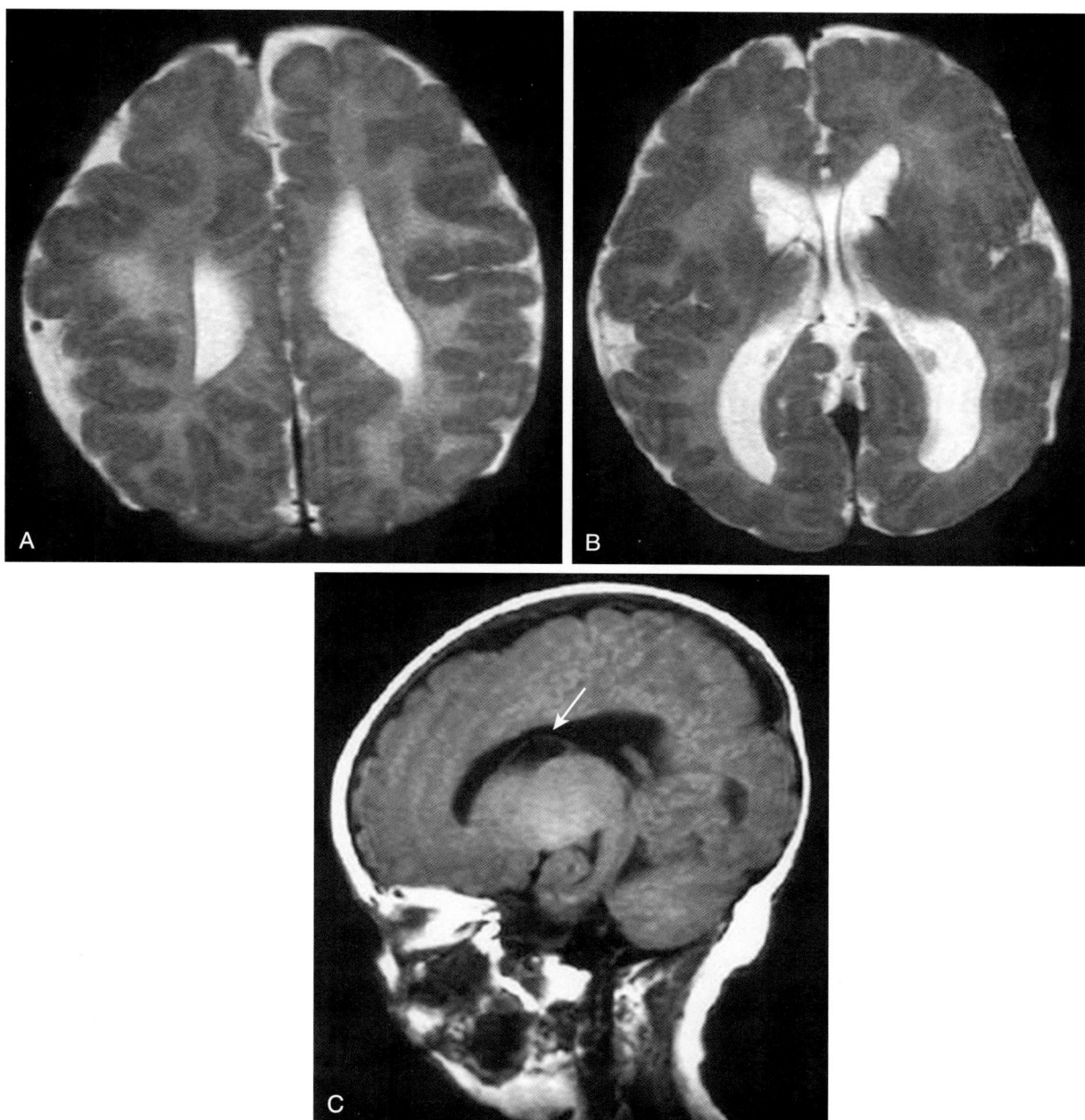

Figure 29.22 Zellweger syndrome: magnetic resonance imaging (MRI). (A and B) T2-weighted images showing severe generalized internal atrophy and mild widening of the Sylvian fissures, severe perisylvian polymicrogyria, and moderate frontoparietal pachygyria in a 6-week-old infant. (C) Sagittal T1-weighted MRI with germinolytic cyst from caudate nucleus protruding into the ventricle *(arrow)*. (From Weller S, Rosewich H, Gartner J. Cerebral MRI as a valuable diagnostic tool in Zellweger spectrum patients. *J Inherit Metab Dis.* 2008;31:270–280.)

myelin is also involved. In addition to the central white matter disease, evidence of the neuronal migration defect is present (see discussion of Zellweger syndrome). The migrational defect in neonatal adrenoleukodystrophy is not as severe as in Zellweger syndrome. MRI identifies both the white matter disease and the neuronal migrational defects.[352] As discussed in relation to Zellweger syndrome, the relation of the biochemical disturbances to the migrational abnormalities is not entirely clear, but evidence suggests that the abnormality of very-long-chain fatty acids is crucial (see also Chapter 6). Consistent with

this notion is the finding that plasma levels of very-long-chain fatty acids in neonatal adrenoleukodystrophy, although markedly elevated, are not as high as in Zellweger syndrome.[316,364]

No effective *therapy* has been described in the neonatal form of adrenoleukodystrophy. However, attempts to correct the elevated very-long-chain fatty acid levels in X-linked adrenoleukodystrophy by dietary restriction and by decreasing endogenous synthesis through administration of the monounsaturated fatty acids, oleate and erucate (Lorenzo's oil),[366-370] led to inconsistent evidence of biochemical and neurophysiological improvement. The initiation of treatment *before the onset of symptoms* has clearly been beneficial.[371] Whether such an approach would be beneficial in neonatal adrenoleukodystrophy is less clear because of the prenatal onset of the neuropathology and the wider spectrum of the biochemical disturbance. When cultured fibroblasts from patients with neonatal adrenoleukodystrophy are treated with sodium 4-phenylbutyrate, an increase in peroxisomal number and an improvement in peroxisomal biochemical functions are observed.[327] Whether similar peroxisomal proliferating agents are effective in vivo will be important to determine.[326,327] *Prenatal diagnosis* is possible by assaying very-long-chain fatty acid levels in cultured amniotic fluid cells or chorionic villus samples.

Mitochondrial Disorders

Five clinical disorders related to mitochondrial disease cause striking encephalopathic syndromes in the pediatric age group: Leigh syndrome; Alpers disease; myoclonic epilepsy with ragged red fibers (MERRF); mitochondrial encephalomyopathy, lactic acidosis, stroke-like episodes (MELAS); and Kearns-Sayre syndrome (progressive external ophthalmoplegia plus).[49,372-381] Of these, *Leigh syndrome* and *Alpers disease* (see earlier discussion of gray matter degenerations) are observed relatively frequently in the neonatal period. Moreover, it is now clear that *other mitochondrial encephalopathies* also occur in the newborn period and in early infancy and do not conform to the classic features of Leigh syndrome or Alpers disease. Because the overlap among these other mitochondrial encephalopathies seems greater with Leigh syndrome than with Alpers disease, we include these conditions here in the discussion of Leigh syndrome. Among other neonatal-onset mitochondrial disorders, an important mitochondrial myopathy secondary to cytochrome c oxidase deficiency is described in Chapter 33, and the defects in pyruvate metabolism with predominant lactic acidosis are described in Chapter 28.

Leigh Syndrome and Other Mitochondrial Encephalopathies

Leigh syndrome is characterized most commonly by clinical onset later in infancy and in early childhood, but neonatal onset is well documented.[374,380,382-413] The principal *clinical features* have been hypotonia, weakness, respiratory abnormalities (including central neurogenic hypoventilation [Ondine's curse]), oculomotor abnormalities, facial weakness, and impaired feeding (see Table 29.7). Seizures, developmental arrest, and then disorders of movement (especially dystonia) and deterioration to death in the first year or so of life have been typical of neonatal-onset cases. Recent natural history studies have largely confirmed this phenotype.[414,415] Onset later in infancy is associated with slower deterioration, and approximately 50% of cases survive for 5 years.[398] *Diagnosis* is suspected on the basis of the clinical features, including (1) clinical evidence of brain stem and/or basal ganglia dysfunction; (2) intellectual and motor developmental delay; and (3) biochemical indicators of abnormal energy metabolism, which are manifested by a severe defect in oxidative phosphorylation or pyruvate dehydrogenase complex activity, a molecular diagnosis involving a gene related to mitochondrial energy generation, or elevated serum or CSF lactate (see Table 29.4).[413] Brain imaging is notable for decreased attenuation of the putamen on CT and, on T2-weighted images of MRI, increased signal in putamen, accompanied also by

TABLE 29.10	Leigh Syndrome: Major Molecular Defects Identified[a]	
MOLECULAR DEFECT	**PERCENTAGE OF TOTAL (%)**	**USUAL INHERITANCE[b]**
Complex I	32	Autosomal recessive, maternal, or X-linked
Complex IV (cytochrome oxidase)	37	Autosomal recessive
Complex V (ATP synthase, subunit 6-mtDNA mutation)	17	Maternal
Pyruvate dehydrogenase complex (E_{1alpha} subunit)	14	X-linked

[a]See text for references. Rare cases have been reported secondary to pyruvate carboxylase deficiency; mitochondrial encephalomyopathy, lactic acidosis, stroke-like episodes (MELAS) mutation; mitochondrial DNA depletion; mitochondrial DNA deletions; complex II deficiency; and complex III deficiency.
[b]Many cases are not familial (i.e., they represent new mutations in the affected infant).

abnormalities in globus pallidus, caudate, periventricular white matter, corpus callosum, midbrain (especially the periaqueductal region), and lower brain stem (Fig. 29.23).[5,398,406,410,416-422] Cranial ultrasonography may show increased echogenicity in the putamen and caudate.[418] Spatially localized proton MR spectroscopy has detected elevated levels of lactate in areas shown to be involved on T2-weighted images.[5,406,419,423,424] A single report has suggested that diffusion imaging may be useful in the preclinical stages of disease in infants.[425] CSF lactate levels are elevated almost uniformly, whereas ratios of blood lactate to pyruvate may or may not be elevated.[43,44,398,426] Fibroblast cultures or tissue samples (muscle, liver, other tissues) have shown *biochemical defects* most commonly involving the pyruvate dehydrogenase complex, particularly the nuclear-encoded gene for the E_{1alpha} subunit, cytochrome c oxidase (complex IV), reduced nicotinamide adenine dinucleotide-coenzyme Q reductase (complex I), or ATP synthase subunit 6 (complex V) (Table 29.10).[a] More than 75 distinct genes have been identified, with a rapid expansion in the last several years related to whole exome sequencing, but these genes only explain about 50% of cases.[413,436] Genetic panels including many of these genes are commercially available and are suggested as a first step before invasive muscle biopsy, a particular challenge in sick neonates with low muscle mass.[412] A common defect is impaired cytochrome oxidase activity (complex IV), involving not the oxidase itself but usually a nuclear-encoded protein, SURF-1, critical in the assembly of cytochrome oxidase activity.[b] A second assembly gene, *SCO2*, has been implicated, especially

---

[a]References 374, 377-381, 386, 390-392, 394, 397-400, 405, 408, and 427-435.
[b]References 379, 380, 404, 420, 428, and 431.

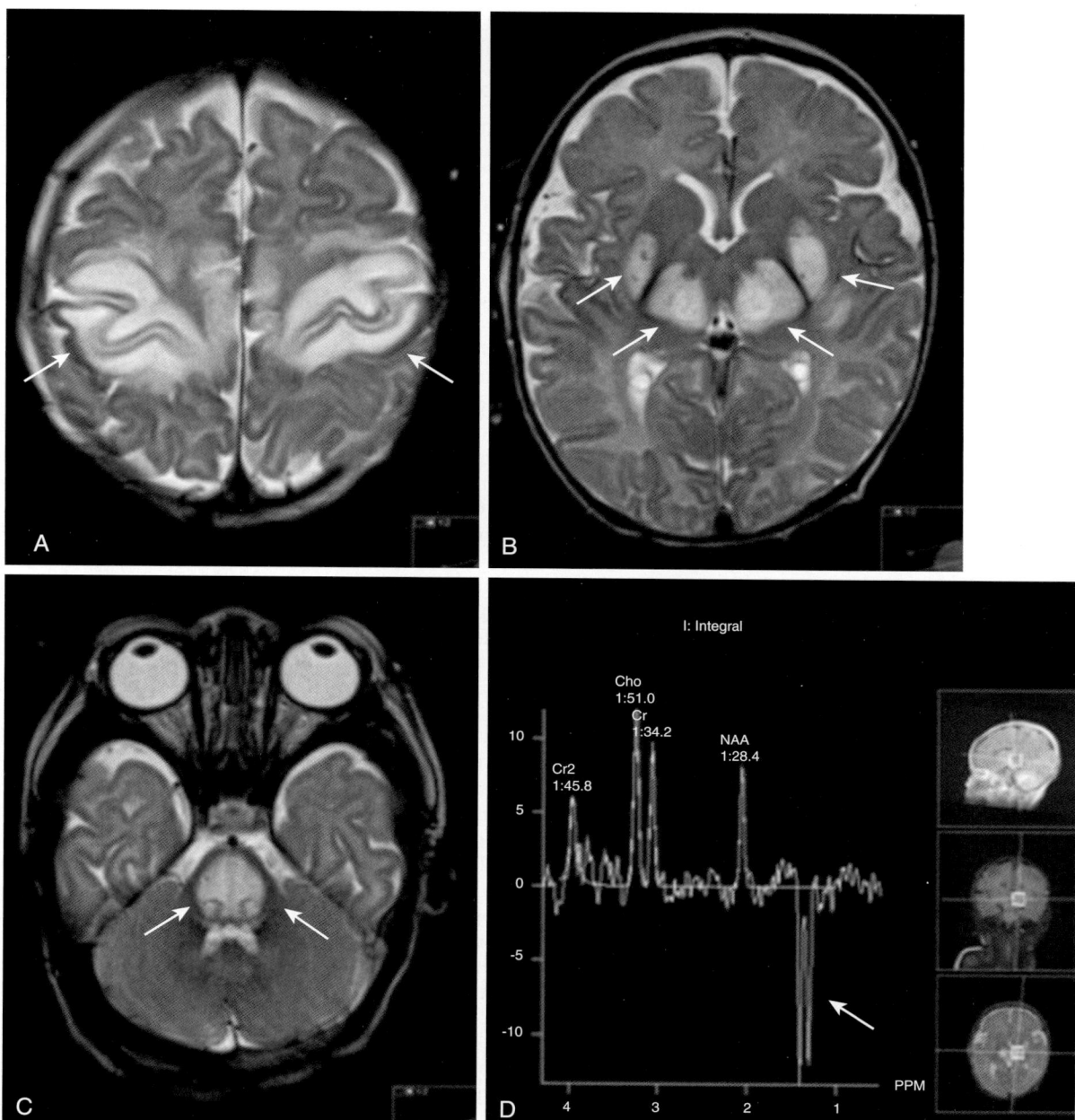

Figure 29.23 **Leigh syndrome: magnetic resonance imaging and magnetic resonance spectroscopy.** (A to C) T2-weighted images demonstrating bilateral hyperintensity in cortical areas (A), basal ganglia (B), and brain stem (C), in a newborn. Abnormalities are indicated with white arrows. (D) Single voxel spectroscopy showing an intense lactate peak at 1.35 ppm *(white arrow)* and reduced *N*-acetylaspartate peak. (From Haack TB, Klee D, Strom TM, et al. Infantile Leigh-like syndrome caused by SLC19A3 mutations is a treatable disease. *Brain.* 2014;137:e295.)

in neonatal-onset cases.[380,431,437] However, in the latter cases, the topography of the abnormalities on brain imaging is not typical for Leigh syndrome, and fulminating hypertrophic cardiomyopathy is distinctive.[380,431,437] The distribution of the major biochemical defects and their usual mode of inheritance in infants with Leigh syndrome in one large series is shown in Table 29.10. In one series based on molecular genetic analyses, the four most common genes involved in neonatal or early infantile onset cases were NDUFS4 (encodes a subunit of Complex I), NDUFV1 (encodes a subunit of Complex II),

PET100 (encodes a subunit of Complex IV), and SUCLA2 (involved in mitochondrial DNA maintenance).[413] Rare cases of Leigh syndrome have been associated with pyruvate carboxylase deficiency, MELAS mutation, mitochondrial DNA depletion, mitochondrial DNA deletions, complex II deficiency, and complex III deficiency.[379,402,403,438,439] Another less common but treatable cause is a mutation in SLC19A3, which encodes the thiamine transporter-2 and leads to impaired cerebral thiamine metabolism and an early-infantile lethal phenotype if not recognized rapidly.[440,441] Cases have been described as young as 1 month and respond well to early administration of thiamine and biotin.[422,442,443] The *neuropathology* of Leigh syndrome is distinctive and is characterized by symmetrical focal necrotic lesions with demyelination, spongy change, vascular proliferation, and gliosis. The areas especially involved are in the periventricular and periaqueductal regions of the brain stem and the diencephalic regions around the third ventricle, especially the thalamus, the basal ganglia (especially putamen), and the subcortical white matter.[444] *Therapy* has included dichloroacetate (to activate the pyruvate dehydrogenase complex), respiratory chain components (e.g., coenzyme Q10), artificial electron acceptors (e.g., ascorbate), free radical scavengers (e.g., vitamin E, idebenone, and the synthetic quinone EPI-743), and metabolites or cofactors (e.g., L-carnitine).[a] Strikingly beneficial responses have not been observed in patients with Leigh syndrome of neonatal onset, *except* in cases of thiamine transporter-2 deficiency.

Other mitochondrial encephalopathies with onset in the newborn period or early infancy do not conform to the classic features of Leigh syndrome, but they sometimes overlap enough to be characterized as *Leigh-like* disorders.[b] However, these other mitochondrial encephalopathies may exhibit quite different topographic features (e.g., cerebral white matter changes suggestive of leukodystrophy,[448-453] or evidence of cerebral or cerebellar atrophy, or both).[454] The clinical features often include fragments of those seen in Leigh syndrome. Mitochondrial disease is established by the findings of elevated lactate in CSF and brain, enzymatic, and molecular genetic features indicative of disturbances of mitochondrial proteins (especially in the electron transport chain), and *cellular* pathology comparable to that described for Leigh syndrome. *The principal difference is the topography of the lesions. The essential clinical point is that newborns and very young infants with evidence for encephalopathy of diverse topographies accompanied by elevated CSF or brain lactate should be investigated carefully for a mitochondrial disorder.* The presence of systemic phenomena (e.g., cardiomyopathy, nephropathy, hepatopathy) should enhance the suspicion of such a disorder.

Serine Synthesis Deficiency

L-serine is an amino acid that is essential for brain development and metabolism. It plays critical roles in the synthesis of proteins, nucleotides, neurotransmitters, and lipids.[455] It is synthesized from the glycolytic intermediate 3-phosphoglycerate in three enzymatic steps. Deficiencies in any of these enzymes can lead to L-serine deficiency, but phosphoglycerate dehydrogenase (PGDH) deficiency is best characterized. Clinical features include congenital microcephaly, intrauterine growth restriction, intractable seizures, and severe psychomotor delay.[456,457,457a] The variable degree refers to glycine alone. Low concentrations of serine and, to a variable degree, glycine in serum and CSF are helpful for diagnosis (see Table 29.4). The measurement of PGDH in cultured fibroblasts or the identification of mutations in the PHGDH gene can provide further confirmation. MRI shows atrophy and enlarged ventricles secondary to severe hypomyelination (Fig. 29.24).[458,459] Oral serine replacement therapy begun postnatally reduces or eliminates seizures but does not appear to improve development.[456,459] A single case of *prenatal* treatment prevented microcephaly, eliminated seizures,

and promoted normal development through to at least 4 years of age.[460]

Disorders With Cerebellar and Pontine Hypoplasia

Other degenerative disorders with neonatal onset and involvement of both gray and white matter are linked by the occurrence of hindbrain hypoplasia, especially in the pontocerebellar regions (see Table 29.7). However, the two disorders, CDG1a (previously termed carbohydrate-deficient glycoprotein syndrome) and pontocerebellar hypoplasia (PCH), differ considerably in clinical features, genetics, and apparent underlying biochemical disturbance.

Congenital Disorders of Glycosylation Type 1a (Carbohydrate-Deficient Glycoprotein Syndromes)

CDGs, previously termed carbohydrate-deficient glycoprotein syndromes, comprise a family of multisystemic disorders, of which one variety, CDG1a, is by far the most common and best characterized.[461-478] The following discussion focuses on CDG1a (see Table 29.7). This *autosomal recessive* disorder exhibits a characteristic *clinical presentation*, which includes mild facial dysmorphism (large, dysplastic ears), abnormal subcutaneous fat distribution (fat pads over buttocks, *orange peel* skin), inverted nipples, and joint contractures (Figs. 29.25 and 29.26).[474,476] Neurological features include *rolling* vertical or horizontal eye movements, alternating internal strabismus, hypotonia, and hyporeflexia. Subsequently, developmental failure, stroke-like episodes, ataxia, moderate to severe cognitive defects, epilepsy, and retinal pigmentary degeneration are prominent. Although the neuropathology appears to progress, in a strict sense the lack of a progressively deteriorating course and frequent survival to adulthood, albeit in a disabled state, argue against a relentlessly progressive degenerative disorder of the nervous system. The multisystem involvement includes cardiac (cardiomyopathy, pericardial effusions, hydrops fetalis), hepatic (hepatomegaly, liver dysfunction), renal (nephrotic syndrome), and, later, reproductive (hypogonadism) effects. Approximately 20% of infants die in the first years of life because of systemic failure or status epilepticus.[467] The *biochemical defect* involves glycosylation of proteins (i.e., synthesis of glycoproteins), and the most common defect (i.e., that for CDG1a) involves the phosphomannomutase (PMM2) involved in the conversion of mannose-6-phosphate to mannose-1-phosphate, an early intermediate key in dolichol-linked glycoprotein synthesis. Dolichol-linked glycoprotein synthesis is *N*-linked; that is, the glycan is attached to the protein by the formation of an amide group with an amino group of asparagine on the protein. *N*-linked glycoprotein synthesis is involved in CDG, whereas the other major pathway of glycoprotein synthesis in mammals, *O*-linked synthesis, which involves linkage of the glycan to the hydroxyl moiety of serine or threonine, is involved in certain congenital muscular dystrophies (see Chapter 33). *Diagnosis* of CDG1a is established on the basis of the clinical features and the biochemical consequences of the basic defect. These abnormalities include reduction in blood levels of various compounds because of the lack of their glycosylated transport proteins (albumin, thyroxine-binding globulin, thyroxine, cholesterol, and coagulation factors, especially factor XI and antithrombin). The diagnosis is usually made by the demonstration of deficiently glycosylated transferrin by isoelectrofocusing. *Neuropathology* includes

---

[a]References 49, 376, 379, 419, 436, and 445-447.
[b]References 379-381, 398, 406, 407, 409, and 431.

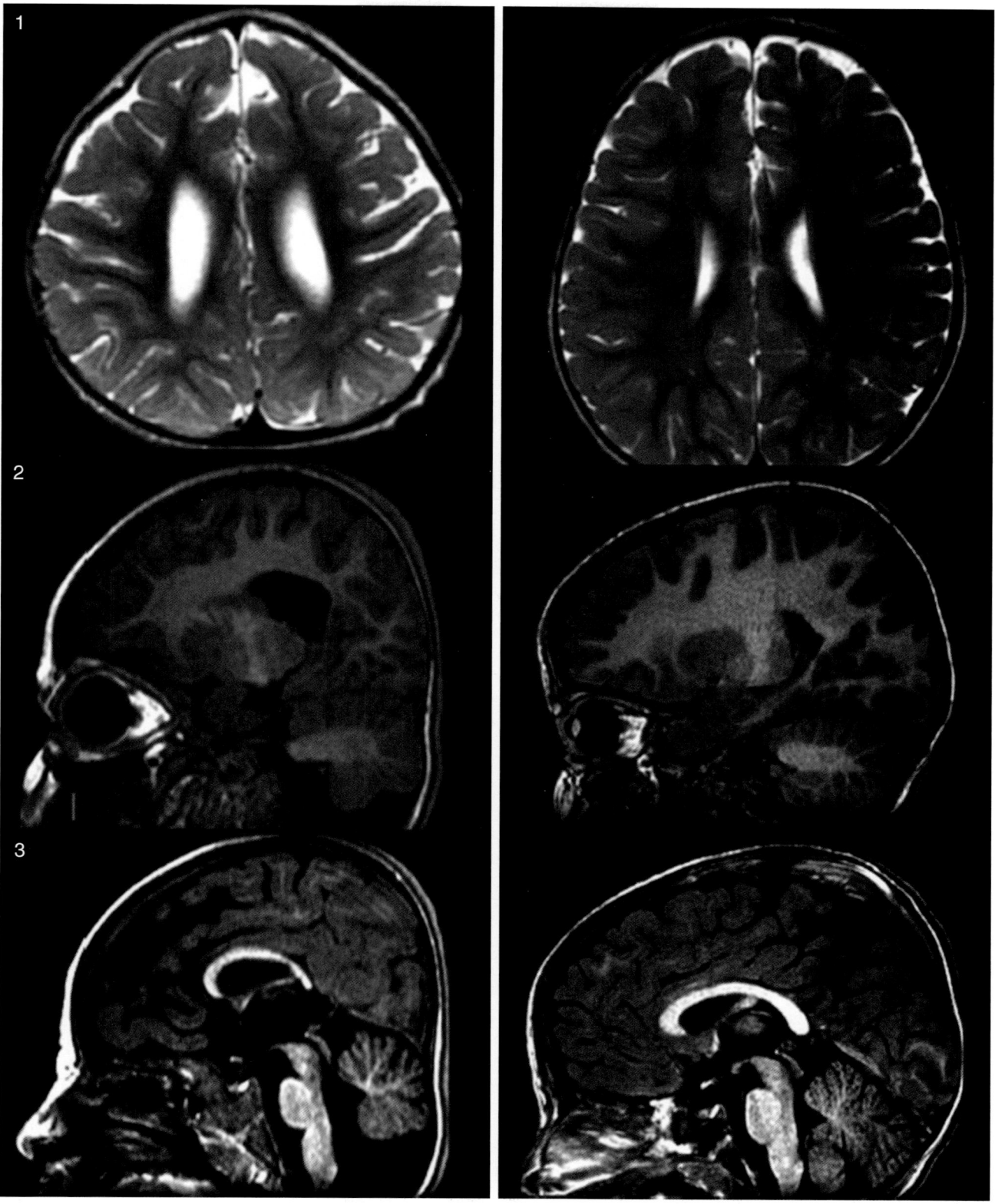

Figure 29.24 Serine deficiency disorder: magnetic resonance imaging. Infant diagnosed at 2 months of age with L-serine deficiency after intrauterine growth restriction, progressive microcephaly, feeding difficulties, dystonic posturing, hyperexcitability, and decreased cerebrospinal fluid serine concentration *(left panels)*. Axial T2-weighted image at 2.7 years *(1)* and parasagittal T1-weighted fast spoiled gradient-echo (FSPGR) images *(2)* show moderate ventricular dilation and global reduction in white matter volume compared to the age-matched control brain on the right. There is reduced volume of the frontal lobes and the frontoparietal sulci are decreased in number, but are normally organized in thickness and depth when present. Median sagittal T1-weighted FSPGR images *(3)* show that the corpus callosum is short and hypoplastic, and there is moderate atrophy of the cerebellar vermis. (From Brassier A, Valayannopoulos V, Bahi-Buisson N, et al. Two new cases of serine deficiency disorders treated with L-serine. *Eur J Paediatr Neurol.* 2016;20:53–60.)

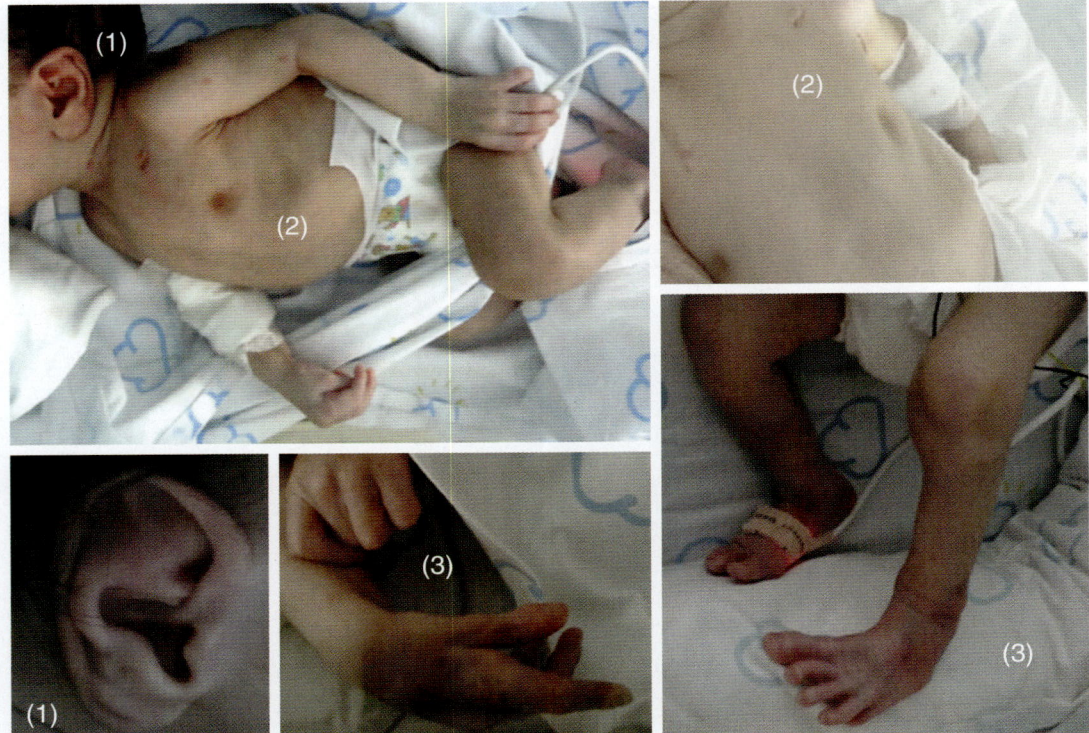

Figure 29.25 Congenital disorders of glycosylation type 1a: clinical features. Newborn with CDG-1a showing dysplastic ear *(1)*, inverted nipples *(2)*, and arachnodactyly and leg joint contractures *(3)*. (From Resende C, Carvalho C, Alegria A, et al. Congenital disorders of glycosylation with neonatal presentation. *BMJ Case Rep.* 2014;2014:bcr2013010037.)

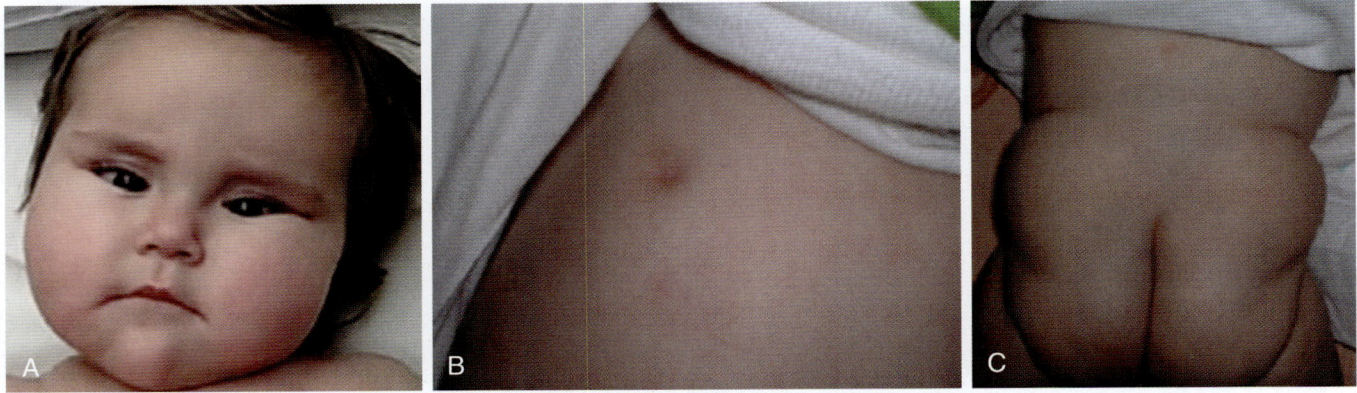

Figure 29.26 Congenital disorders of glycosylation type 1a: clinical features. Infants with CDG-1a frequently present with facial dysmorphism and esotropia (A), nipple inversion (B), and supragluteal fat pads (C). (From Freeze HH, Eklund EA, Ng BG, Patterson MC. Neurology of inherited glycosylation disorders. *Lancet Neurol.* 2012;11:453–466.)

pontocerebellar hypoplasia, with neuronal loss and gliosis, especially in the cerebellum but also in the cerebral cortex, basal ganglia, thalamus, and brain stem. The involvement of neurons in the brain stem and cerebellum particularly affects the pons, inferior olives, and the Purkinje and granule cells of the cerebellum. Pontocerebellar hypoplasia is readily detected by MRI (Fig. 29.27) and often associated with cerebellar cortex and subcortical white matter hyperintensities on T2-weighted imaging.[479] The severity of cerebellar atrophy on imaging correlates with the degree of cerebellar involvement (ataxia) on examination in older children.[480] Polyneuropathy with decreased myelin is also apparent and accounts for decreased motor nerve conduction velocities and hyporeflexia. No known *therapy* exists, although prenatal mannose treatment in a mouse model of CDG1a suggests that early rescue of hypoglycosylation may be beneficial and applicable to at-risk families with appropriate preconception counseling.[481] A zebrafish model, a drosophila model, and patient-derived induced pluripotent stem cells are now available to allow further investigation of the molecular phenotype of this disorder.[482-484]

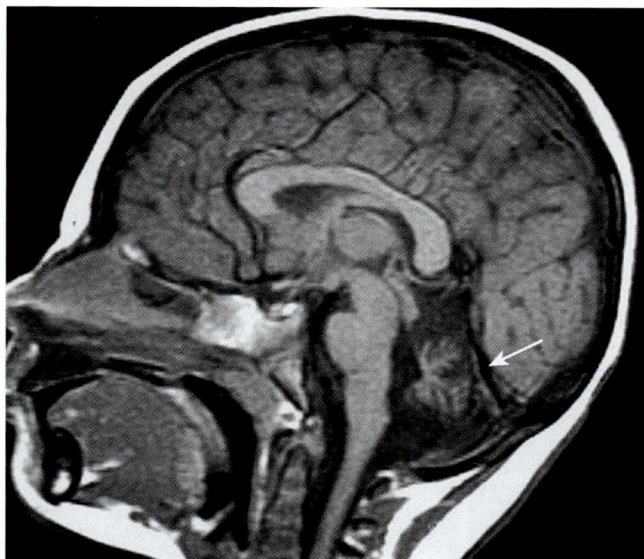

Figure 29.27 Congenital disorder of glycosylation type Ia: magnetic resonance imaging (MRI) scan. Sagittal T1-weighted MRI shows very small cerebellar vermis with shrunken folia and enlarged fissures *(arrow)*. Note that the pons is relatively preserved, unlike in pontocerebellar hypoplasia type 2. (From Barkovich AJ. *Pediatric Neuroimaging*. 4th ed. Philadelphia: Lippincott Williams & Wilkins; 2005.)

TABLE 29.11	Major Forms of Pontocerebellar Hypoplasia Encountered in the Neonatal Period[a]

Pontocerebellar hypoplasia types 1–8
Congenital disorder of glycosylation type Ia
Cerebromuscular dystrophies (see Chapter 33)
Walker-Warburg syndrome
Muscle-eye-brain disease
Mitochondrial disorder

[a]Excludes intrauterine or early postnatal destructive disorders and several other rare syndromic disorders exhibiting pontocerebellar hypoplasia and other distinctive dysmorphic features.

ATP, Adenosine triphosphate.

Pontocerebellar Hypoplasia Type 2

PCH is a heterogeneous group of disorders with the common feature of hypoplasia of the cerebellum and brain stem, especially the pons (Table 29.11), and there are now eight subtypes identified.[485,486] (Because the inferior olivary nuclei are also often involved, the term *olivopontocerebellar hypoplasia* is sometimes used.) Thus far, nearly all the disorders have exhibited autosomal recessive inheritance. PCH type 1 is associated with the severe degeneration of anterior horn cells and is noted in Chapters 31 and 32 in relation to arthrogryposis multiplex congenita and spinal muscular atrophy (Werdnig-Hoffman disease). Cerebromuscular dystrophies with prominent cerebellar and, to a lesser extent, brain stem hypoplasia are discussed in Chapter 33. Some examples of mitochondrial disorders, especially involving the electron transport chain, may be

associated with pontocerebellar hypoplasia (see earlier).[487,488] The loss of function mutations in the X-linked calcium/calmodulin-dependent serine protein kinase (CASK) has been reported, primarily in females, resulting in brain stem and cerebellar hypoplasia, microcephaly, sensorineural hearing loss, and severe intellectual disability.[489,490] Proportionate involvement of both the cerebellar vermis and hemispheres may differentiate this disorder from the other PCH disorders, which disproportionately affect the hemispheres over the vermis. Because PCH type 2 exhibits the clinical characteristics of a degenerative disorder of the CNS most, it is discussed here.

Type 2 PCH exhibits a striking *clinical presentation* apparent from the first days of life.[491-501] The neonatal neurological syndrome consists particularly of abnormalities of sucking and swallowing, and jitteriness. Seizures are less common. Subsequently, head circumference, which is within the normal range at birth, increases at a markedly reduced rate, such that progressive microcephaly develops. A striking extrapyramidal syndrome (chorea, athetosis, dystonia) is characteristic. In addition, epilepsy, severe cognitive deficits, and markedly impaired visual responses ensue. Approximately 40% to 50% of patients have died in childhood. The clinical presentation and mortality rates were confirmed in a recent natural history study of 33 patients.[501] *Diagnosis* of PCH type 2 is suspected from the clinical features. MRI shows the hypoplasia of pons and cerebellum, both vermis and hemispheres, particularly the latter (Fig. 29.28).[502] A moderate degree of cerebral cortical atrophy is also apparent later in the course. Genetic evaluation suggests the involvement of transfer RNA splicing endonuclease subunit genes, specifically TSEN54 (up to 90%) and much less commonly TSEN2, TSEN34, and SEPSECS.[500,501,503-505] *Neuropathology* is striking.[502,506] Pontine hypoplasia with severe reduction of ventral pontine neurons, cerebellar hypoplasia with marked involvement of internal granule cells and dentate nuclei, and a moderate loss of neurons in the inferior olivary nuclei are the prominent features. Gliosis accompanies the neuronal changes. Some degree of cerebral cortical neuronal degeneration also is apparent. No *therapy* is known for this disorder; the biochemical basis (or bases) for which remains to be established.

Several other disorders characterized by autosomal recessively inherited pontocerebellar hypoplasia, with some features resembling PCH type 2, have been reported.[507] Infants with pontocerebellar hypoplasia, but with the addition of optic atrophy, have been designated as having PCH type 3; those with relative preservation of vermis have PCH type 4; and those with relative preservation of cerebellar hemispheres have PCH type 5. PCH type 6 has been reported in several families associated with mitochondrial respiratory chain abnormalities, encephalopathy, optic-atrophy, and hypsarrhythmia with causative mutations in the mitochondrial arginyl transfer RNA synthetase gene (RARS2).[508-510] Type 4 has been associated with a combination of missense and nonsense mutations in TSEN54, producing more severe symptoms than PCH type 2 (which shares the same gene) and earlier death.[502,511] Type 5 is associated with TSEN54 mutations, and type 3 results from a mutation in the PCLO gene.[512] A single case of PCH type 7 has been reported with distinguishing features of testicular regression, micropenis, and death by 5 weeks, but a defining gene mutation has yet to be identified.[513] PCH type 8 has unique features of joint contractures and growth retardation and involves mutations in

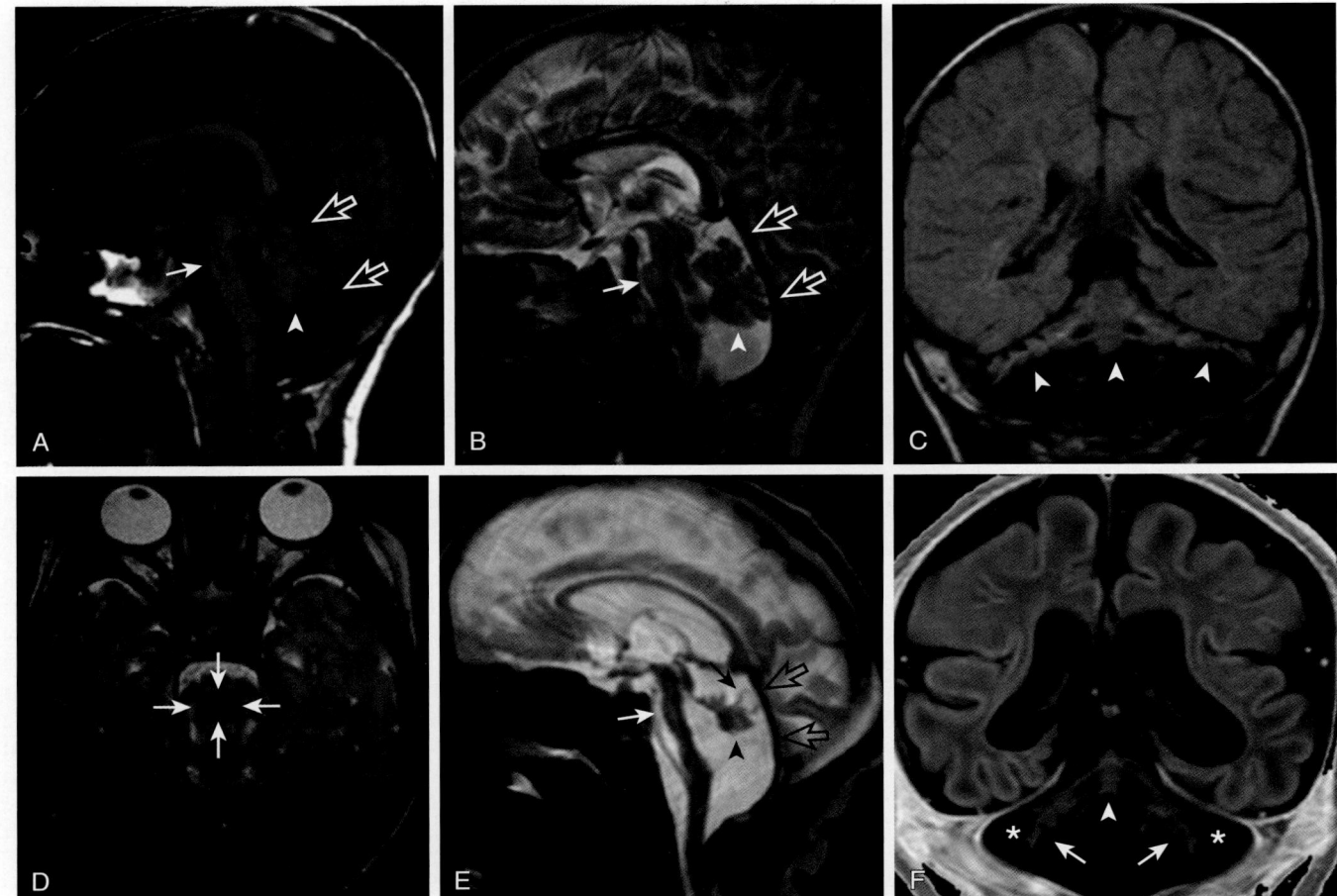

Figure 29.28 Pontocerebellar hypoplasia: magnetic resonance imaging (MRI). Sagittal T1-weighted (A) and T2-weighted images (B) show hypoplastic inferior vermis *(arrowhead)* associated with a small pons *(arrow)*. The posterior fossa is small with verticalization of the tentorium and straight sinus *(open arrows)*. Coronal fluid-attenuated inversion recovery image shows markedly hypoplastic cerebellum *(arrowheads)* occupying the superior portion of the posterior cranial fossa and abutting the tentorium, with dilation of the cisterna magna inferiorly. Mild neocortical atrophy (C) is present. Axial T2-weighted image (D) shows hyperintensity of the median raphe and transverse pontine fibers, generating the sign of the cross *(arrows)*. In a more severely affected patient, sagittal T2-weighted images (E) show markedly hypoplastic vermis *(arrowhead)* with partial cavitation *(black arrow)*. There is concurrent marked hypoplasia of the brain stem, which is particularly severe in the pons *(white arrow)*. The posterior fossa is small with verticalization of the tentorium *(open arrows)*. Coronal inversion recovery image (F) shows markedly hypoplastic cerebellar hemispheres *(arrows)* and vermis *(arrowhead)*. There is central cavitation within the substance of the cerebellar hemispheres *(asterisks)*. Cavitations of the cerebellar white matter are unusual. There is severe neocortical atrophy, and this infant died at age 1 month. (From Cassandrini D, Biancheri R, Tessa A, et al. Pontocerebellar hypoplasia: clinical, pathologic, and genetic studies. *Neurology.* 2010;75:1459–1464.)

the CHMP1A gene, which is important in the proliferation of CNS precusors.[514] Additional subtypes will likely be identified as molecular characterization improves.

Neurotransmitter Disorders

Disorders of monoamine neurotransmitters (dopamine, serotonin, norepinephrine, epinephrine) may present in the neonatal period because of impaired synthesis, degradation, or transport of these neurotransmitters (see Table 29.7).[515-517] Clinical features can include neonatal encephalopathy, epilepsy, pyramidal and extrapyramidal motor features, autonomic changes, and later neuropsychiatric features. A prototypical disorder is deficiency in L-aromatic acid decarboxylase (AADC), a pyridoxal-5α-phosphate-dependent enzyme that

converts L-dopa to dopamine and 5-hydroxytryptophan to serotonin.[518-522] This autosomal recessive disorder is caused by mutations in the dopa-decarboxylase gene (DDC). Fewer than 100 cases have been reported[522] with a large number of unique mutations (see database of pediatric neurotransmitter disorders at http://www.biopku.org/BioPKU_DatabasesJAKE.asp). Infants typically have hypotonia, global developmental delay, oculogyric crises, and dystonia. Most patients have normal brain imaging and electroencephalograms. Around 25% of patients have cerebral atrophy and leukodystrophy-like white matter changes. Diagnosis is made by the interrogation of CSF neurotransmitters that show decreased downstream metabolites (homovanillic acid, 5-hydroxyindoleacetic acid, 3-methoxy-4-hydroxphenylglycol) and increased upstream precursors (L-dopa, 5-hydroxytryptophan, 3-O-methyldopa). Urinary vanillactic acid also may be increased in some patients. Treatment with dopamine agonists, pyridoxal-5-phosphate, and other drugs attempting to circumvent the enzyme deficiency is beneficial in a minority of patients. A phase 1 clinical trial demonstrated that adeno-associated viral transduction of the human AADC gene into the putamen of four patients aged 4 to 6 years increased the deficient CSF neurotransmitters (dopamine and serotonin) and improved motor function at 12 months post-injection.[523] AADC highlights the importance of CSF analysis in encephalopathic infants (see Table 29.4).

Rett Syndrome

Rett syndrome, an X-linked disorder caused by a mutation in the gene encoding methyl-CpG-binding protein 2 *(MECP2)*, is a well-known, clinically defined disorder of female patients, with clinical onset in the first year of life, initially with deceleration of head growth. However, in recent years, more than 30 male patients with the *MECP2* mutation have been recognized, and approximately half of these patients have had a neonatal encephalopathy.[524-536] Although the phenotype is variable, most of the patients with neonatal onset have had seizures, often with apnea, followed by the development of microcephaly, intellectual disability, motor deficits, and autonomic dysfunction, including apneic spells. Most of the infants with neonatal onset have died in the first 2 years of life. The diagnosis is made by DNA analysis of the *MECP2* gene.

KEY REFERENCES

1. Gravel RA, Kalback MM, Proia RL, et al. The G_{M2} gangliosidoses. In: Scriver CR, Beaudet MD, Sly WS, et al., eds. *The Metabolic & Molecular Bases of Inherited Disease*. Vol. 2. 8th ed. New York: McGraw-Hill; 2001:3827-3876.
2. Suzuki K, Suzuki K. Lysosomal diseases. In: Graham DI, Lantos PL, eds. *Greenfield's Neuropathology*. Vol. 1. 7th ed. London: Arnold Publishers; 2002:653-735.
3. Bley AE, Giannikopoulos OA, Hayden D, et al. Natural history of infantile G(M2) gangliosidosis. *Pediatrics*. 2011;128:e1233-e1241.
7. Walia JS, Altaleb N, Bello A, et al. Long-term correction of Sandhoff disease following intravenous delivery of rAAV9 to mouse neonates. *Mol Ther*. 2015;23:414-422.
8. McCurdy VJ, Rockwell HE, Arthur JR, et al. Widespread correction of central nervous system disease after intracranial gene therapy in a feline model of Sandhoff disease. *Gene Ther*. 2015;22:181-189.
9. Rockwell HE, McCurdy VJ, Eaton SC, et al. AAV-mediated gene delivery in a feline model of Sandhoff disease corrects lysosomal storage in the central nervous system. *ASN Neuro*. 2015;7:1759091415569908.
10. Bradbury AM, Gray-Edwards HL, Shirley JL, et al. Biomarkers for disease progression and AAV therapeutic efficacy in feline Sandhoff disease. *Exp Neurol*. 2015;263:102-112.
11. Torres PA, Zeng BJ, Porter BF, et al. Tay-Sachs disease in Jacob sheep. *Mol Genet Metab*. 2010;101:357-363.
12. Wessels ME, Holmes JP, Jeffrey M, et al. GM2 gangliosidosis in British Jacob sheep. *J Comp Pathol*. 2014;150:253-257.
14. Wisniewski KE, Zhong N, Philippart M. Pheno/genotypic correlations of neuronal ceroid lipofuscinoses. *Neurology*. 2001;57:576-581.
15. Mole SE. The genetic spectrum of human neuronal ceroid-lipofuscinoses. *Brain Pathol*. 2004;14:70-76.
20. Kousi M, Lehesjoki AE, Mole SE. Update of the mutation spectrum and clinical correlations of over 360 mutations in eight genes that underlie the neuronal ceroid lipofuscinoses. *Hum Mutat*. 2012;33:42-63.

21. Warrier V, Vieira M, Mole SE. Genetic basis and phenotypic correlations of the neuronal ceroid lipofusinoses. *Biochim Biophys Acta*. 2013;1832:1827-1830.
28. Chandra G, Bagh MB, Peng S, et al. Cln1 gene disruption in mice reveals a common pathogenic link between two of the most lethal childhood neurodegenerative lysosomal storage disorders. *Hum Mol Genet*. 2015;24:5416-5432.
35. Harding BN, Surtees R. Metabolic and neurodegenerative diseases of childhood. In: Graham DI, Lantos PL, eds. *Greenfield's Neuropathology*. Vol. 1. 7th ed. London: Arnold Publishers; 2002:485-517.
36. Tesarova M, Mayr JA, Wenchich L, et al. Mitochondrial DNA depletion in Alpers syndrome. *Neuropediatrics*. 2004;35:217-223.
37. Naviaux RK, Nguyen KV. POLG mutations associated with Alpers' syndrome and mitochondrial DNA depletion. *Ann Neurol*. 2004;55:706-712.
39. Ferrari G, Lamantea E, Donati A, et al. Infantile hepatocerebral syndromes associated with mutations in the mitochondrial DNA polymerase-gamma A. *Brain*. 2005;128:723-731.
40. Davidson G, Mancuso M, Ferraris S, et al. POLG mutations and Alpers syndrome. *Ann Neurol*. 2005;57:921-923.
41. Saneto RP, Cohen BH, Copeland WC, et al. Alpers-Huttenlocher syndrome. *Pediatr Neurol*. 2013;48:167-178.
42. Hunter MF, Peters H, Salemi R, et al. Alpers syndrome with mutations in POLG: clinical and investigative features. *Pediatr Neurol*. 2011;45:311-318.
49. Shoffner JM. Oxidative phosphorylation diseases. In: Scriver CR, Beaudet MD, Sly WS, et al., eds. *The Metabolic & Molecular Bases of Inherited Disease*. Vol. 2. 8th ed. New York: McGraw-Hill; 2001:2367-2423.
50. Flemming K, Ulmer S, Duisberg B, et al. MR spectroscopic findings in a case of Alpers-Huttenlocher syndrome. *AJNR Am J Neuroradiol*. 2002;23:1421-1423.
51. Sarzi E, Bourdon A, Chretien D, et al. Mitochondrial DNA depletion is a prevalent cause of multiple respiratory chain deficiency in childhood. *J Pediatr*. 2007;150:531-534.
52. Sarzi E, Goffart S, Serre V, et al. Twinkle helicase (PEO1) gene mutation causes mitochondrial DNA depletion. *Ann Neurol*. 2007;62:579-587.
53. Sofou K, Moslemi AR, Kollberg G, et al. Phenotypic and genotypic variability in Alpers syndrome. *Eur J Paediatr Neurol*. 2012;16:379-389.
54. Sofou K, Kollberg G, Holmstrom M, et al. Whole exome sequencing reveals mutations in NARS2 and PARS2, encoding the mitochondrial asparaginyl-tRNA synthetase and prolyl-tRNA synthetase, in patients with Alpers syndrome. *Mol Genet Genomic Med*. 2015;3:59-68.
55. Elo JM, Yadavalli SS, Euro L, et al. Mitochondrial phenylalanyl-tRNA synthetase mutations underlie fatal infantile Alpers encephalopathy. *Hum Mol Genet*. 2012;21:4521-4529.
59. Menkes JH. Menkes disease and Wilson disease: two sides of the same copper coin. Part I: Menkes disease. *Eur J Paediatr Neurol*. 1999;3:147-158.
63. Borm B, Moller LB, Hausser I, et al. Variable clinical expression of an identical mutation in the ATP7A gene for Menkes disease/Occipital horn syndrome in three affected males in a single family. *J Pediatr*. 2004;145:119-121.
64. Bindu PS, Taly AB, Kothari S, et al. Electro-clinical features and magnetic resonance imaging correlates in Menkes disease. *Brain Dev*. 2013;35:398-405.
72. Haddad MR, Macri CJ, Holmes CS, et al. In utero copper treatment for Menkes disease associated with a severe ATP7A mutation. *Mol Genet Metab*. 2012;107:222-228.
74. Wang D, Pascual JM, Yang H, et al. Glut-1 deficiency syndrome: clinical, genetic, and therapeutic aspects. *Ann Neurol*. 2005;57:111-118.
76. Akman CI, Yu J, Alter A, et al. Diagnosing glucose transporter 1 deficiency at initial presentation facilitates early treatment. *J Pediatr*. 2016;171:220-226.
77. Pearson TS, Akman C, Hinton VJ, et al. Phenotypic spectrum of glucose transporter type 1 deficiency syndrome (Glut1 DS). *Curr Neurol Neurosci Rep*. 2013;13:342.
78. Alter AS, Engelstad K, Hinton VJ, et al. Long-term clinical course of Glut1 deficiency syndrome. *J Child Neurol*. 2015;30:160-169.

79. Klepper J, Engelbrecht V, Scheffer H, et al. GLUT1 deficiency with delayed myelination responding to ketogenic diet. *Pediatr Neurol.* 2007;37:130-133.

80. Pong AW, Geary BR, Engelstad KM, et al. Glucose transporter type I deficiency syndrome: epilepsy phenotypes and outcomes. *Epilepsia.* 2012;53:1503-1510.

84. Sidhu A, Misra VK. Dermal melanocytosis: more than meets the eye. *J Pediatr.* 2014;165:1060.

86. Sperb F, Vairo F, Burin M, et al. Genotypic and phenotypic characterization of Brazilian patients with GM1 gangliosidosis. *Gene.* 2013;512:113-116.

89. McCurdy VJ, Johnson AK, Gray-Edwards HL, et al. Sustained normalization of neurological disease after intracranial gene therapy in a feline model. *Sci Transl Med.* 2014;6:231ra248.

90. Weismann CM, Ferreira J, Keeler AM, et al. Systemic AAV9 gene transfer in adult GM1 gangliosidosis mice reduces lysosomal storage in CNS and extends lifespan. *Hum Mol Genet.* 2015;24:4353-4364.

98. Carr PC, Casamiquela KM, Jacks SK. Gaucher disease type 2 presenting with collodion membrane and blueberry muffin lesions. *Pediatr Dermatol.* 2016;33:e20-e22.

100. Hruska KS, LaMarca ME, Scott CR, et al. Gaucher disease: mutation and polymorphism spectrum in the glucocerebrosidase gene (GBA). *Hum Mutat.* 2008;29:567-583.

104. Cabrera-Salazar MA, Bercury SD, Ziegler RJ, et al. Intracerebroventricular delivery of glucocerebrosidase reduces substrates and increases lifespan in a mouse model of neuronopathic Gaucher disease. *Exp Neurol.* 2010;225:436-444.

105. Vitner EB, Salomon R, Farfel-Becker T, et al. RIPK3 as a potential therapeutic target for Gaucher's disease. *Nat Med.* 2014;20: 204-208.

106. Aflaki E, Stubblefield BK, Maniwang E, et al. Macrophage models of Gaucher disease for evaluating disease pathogenesis and candidate drugs. *Sci Transl Med.* 2014;6:240ra273.

109. Bashyam MD, Chaudhary AK, Kiran M, et al. Molecular analyses of novel ASAH1 mutations causing Farber lipogranulomatosis: analyses of exonic splicing enhancer inactivating mutation. *Clin Genet.* 2014;86:530-538.

110. Alves MQ, Le Trionnaire E, Ribeiro I, et al. Molecular basis of acid ceramidase deficiency in a neonatal form of Farber disease: identification of the first large deletion in ASAH1 gene. *Mol Genet Metab.* 2013;109:276-281.

112. Gan JJ, Garcia V, Tian J, et al. Acid ceramidase deficiency associated with spinal muscular atrophy with progressive myoclonic epilepsy. *Neuromuscul Disord.* 2015;25:959-963.

113. Alayoubi AM, Wang JC, Au BC, et al. Systemic ceramide accumulation leads to severe and varied pathological consequences. *EMBO Mol Med.* 2013;5:827-842.

114. Frohbergh M, He X, Schuchman EH. The molecular medicine of acid ceramidase. *Biol Chem.* 2015;396:759-765.

121. Lemyre E, Russo P, Melancon SB, et al. Clinical spectrum of infantile free sialic acid storage disease. *Am J Med Genet.* 1999;82: 385-391.

122. Froissart R, Cheillan D, Bouvier R, et al. Clinical, morphological, and molecular aspects of sialic acid storage disease manifesting in utero. *J Med Genet.* 2005;42:829-836.

123. Lines MA, Rupar CA, Rip JW, et al. Infantile sialic acid storage disease: two unrelated inuit cases homozygous for a common novel SLC17A5 mutation. *JIMD Rep.* 2014;12:79-84.

124. Aula N, Salomaki P, Timonen R, et al. The spectrum of SLC17A5-gene mutations resulting in free sialic acid-storage diseases indicates some genotype-phenotype correlation. *Am J Hum Genet.* 2000;67:832-840.

125. Prolo LM, Vogel H, Reimer RJ. The lysosomal sialic acid transporter sialin is required for normal CNS myelination. *J Neurosci.* 2009;29:15355-15365.

127. Schiffmann R, van der Knaap MS. Invited article: an MRI-based approach to the diagnosis of white matter disorders. *Neurology.* 2009;72:750-759.

141. Gordon N. Canavan disease: a review of recent developments. *Eur J Paediatr Neurol.* 2001;5:65-69.

143. Kumar S, Mattan NS, de Vellis J. Canavan disease: a white matter disorder. *Ment Retard Dev Disabil Res Rev.* 2006;12:157-165.

152. Madhavarao CN, Arun P, Moffett JR, et al. Defective N-acetylaspartate catabolism reduces brain acetate levels and myelin lipid synthesis in Canavan's disease. *Proc Natl Acad Sci U S A.* 2005;102:5221-5226.

153. Kirmani BF, Jacobowitz DM, Namboodiri MAA. Developmental increase of aspartoacylase in oligodendrocytes parallels CNS myelination. *Brain Res Dev Brain Res.* 2003;140:105-115.

154. Mattan NS, Ghiani CA, Lloyd M, et al. Aspartoacylase deficiency affects early postnatal development of oligodendrocytes and myelination. *Neurobiol Dis.* 2010;40:432-443.

155. Arun P, Madhavarao CN, Moffett JR, et al. Metabolic acetate therapy improves phenotype in the tremor rat model of Canavan disease. *J Inherit Metab Dis.* 2010;33:195-210.

156. Traka M, Wollmann RL, Cerda SR, et al. Nur7 is a nonsense mutation in the mouse aspartoacylase gene that causes spongy degeneration of the CNS. *J Neurosci.* 2008;28:11537-11549.

157. Guo F, Bannerman P, Mills Ko E, et al. Ablating N-acetylaspartate prevents leukodystrophy in a Canavan disease model. *Ann Neurol.* 2015;77:884-888.

158. Maier H, Wang-Eckhardt L, Hartmann D, et al. N-acetylaspartate synthase deficiency corrects the myelin phenotype in a canavan disease mouse model but does not affect survival time. *J Neurosci.* 2015;35:14501-14516.

160. Janson CG, Assadi M, Francis J, et al. Lithium citrate for Canavan disease. *Pediatr Neurol.* 2005;33:235-243.

161. Assadi M, Janson C, Wang DJ, et al. Lithium citrate reduces excessive intra-cerebral N-acetyl aspartate in Canavan disease. *Eur J Paediatr Neurol.* 2010;14:354-359.

162. Leone P, Shera D, McPhee SW, et al. Long-term follow-up after gene therapy for canavan disease. *Sci Transl Med.* 2012;4:165ra163.

163. von Jonquieres G, Mersmann N, Klugmann CB, et al. Glial promoter selectivity following AAV-delivery to the immature brain. *PLoS ONE.* 2013;8:e65646.

164. Ahmed SS, Li H, Cao C, et al. A single intravenous rAAV injection as late as P20 achieves efficacious and sustained CNS Gene therapy in Canavan mice. *Mol Ther.* 2013;21:2136-2147.

165. Zano S, Malik R, Szucs S, et al. Modification of aspartoacylase for potential use in enzyme replacement therapy for the treatment of Canavan disease. *Mol Genet Metab.* 2011;102:176-180.

170. Springer S, Erlewein R, Naegele E, et al. Alexander disease—classification revisited and isolation of a neonatal form. *Neuropediatrics.* 2000;31:86-92.

174. Kyllerman M, Rosengren L, Wiklund LM, et al. Increased levels of GFAP in the cerebrospinal fluid in three subtypes of genetically confirmed Alexander disease. *Neuropediatrics.* 2005;36: 319-323.

179. Messing A, Brenner M, Feany MB, et al. Alexander disease. *J Neurosci.* 2012;32:5017-5023.

183. Zafeiriou DI, Dragoumi P, Vargiami E. Alexander disease. *J Pediatr.* 2013;162:648.

193. Prust M, Wang J, Morizono H, et al. GFAP mutations, age at onset, and clinical subtypes in Alexander disease. *Neurology.* 2011;77:1287-1294.

194. Jany PL, Agosta GE, Benko WS, et al. CSF and blood levels of GFAP in Alexander disease(1,2,3). *eNeuro.* 2015;2:ENEURO.0080-15.2015.

195. Wang L, Hagemann TL, Kalwa H, et al. Nitric oxide mediates glial-induced neurodegeneration in Alexander disease. *Nat Commun.* 2015;6:8966.

196. Wang L, Hagemann TL, Messing A, et al. An in vivo pharmacological screen identifies cholinergic signaling as a therapeutic target in glial-based nervous system disease. *J Neurosci.* 2016;36:1445-1455.

203. Sahai I, Baris H, Kimonis V, et al. Krabbe disease: severe neonatal presentation with a family history of multiple sclerosis. *J Child Neurol.* 2005;20:826-828.

204. Hagberg B, Kollberg H, Sourander P, et al. Infantile globoid cell leucodystrophy (Krabbe's disease). A clinical and genetic study of 32 Swedish cases 1953–1967. *Neuropadiatrie.* 1969;1: 74-88.

208. Duffner PK, Barczykowski A, Jalal K, et al. Early infantile Krabbe disease: results of the World-Wide Krabbe Registry. *Pediatr Neurol.* 2011;45:141-148.

210. Abdelhalim AN, Alberico RA, Barczykowski AL, et al. Patterns of magnetic resonance imaging abnormalities in symptomatic patients with Krabbe disease correspond to phenotype. *Pediatr Neurol.* 2014;50:127-134.

211. Gupta A, Poe MD, Styner MA, et al. Regional differences in fiber tractography predict neurodevelopmental outcomes in neonates with infantile Krabbe disease. *Neuroimage Clin.* 2015;7: 792-798.

212. Escolar ML, Poe MD, Smith JK, et al. Diffusion tensor imaging detects abnormalities in the corticospinal tracts of neonates with infantile Krabbe disease. *AJNR Am J Neuroradiol.* 2009;30:1017-1021.

216. Escolar ML, Poe MD, Provenzale JM, et al. Transplantation of umbilical-cord blood in babies with infantile Krabbe's disease. *N Engl J Med.* 2005;352:2069-2081.

218. Kemper AR, Knapp AA, Green NS, et al. Weighing the evidence for newborn screening for early-infantile Krabbe disease. *Genet Med.* 2010;12:539-543.

219. Turgeon CT, Orsini JJ, Sanders KA, et al. Measurement of psychosine in dried blood spots—a possible improvement to newborn screening programs for Krabbe disease. *J Inherit Metab Dis.* 2015;38:923-929.

220. Dimmock DP. Should states adopt newborn screening for early infantile Krabbe disease? *Genet Med.* 2016;18:217-220.

221. Hawkins-Salsbury JA, Shea L, Jiang X, et al. Mechanism-based combination treatment dramatically increases therapeutic efficacy in murine globoid cell leukodystrophy. *J Neurosci.* 2015;35:6495-6505.

225. Scheffer IE, Baraitser M, Wilson J, et al. Pelizaeus-Merzbacher disease: classical or connatal? *Neuropediatrics.* 1991;22:71-78.

241. Golomb MR, Walsh LE, Carvalho KS, et al. Clinical findings in Pelizaeus-Merzbacher disease. *J Child Neurol.* 2004;19:328-331.

242. Plecko B, Stockler-Ipsiroglu S, Gruber S, et al. Degree of hypomyelination and magnetic resonance spectroscopy findings in patients with Pelizaeus Merzbacher phenotype. *Neuropediatrics.* 2003;34:127-136.

246. Shimojima K, Inoue T, Hoshino A, et al. Comprehensive genetic analyses of PLP1 in patients with Pelizaeus-Merzbacher disease applied by array-CGH and fiber-FISH analyses identified new mutations and variable sizes of duplications. *Brain Dev.* 2010;32:171-179.

254. Garbern JY. Pelizaeus-Merzbacher disease: pathogenic mechanisms and insights into the roles of proteolipid protein 1 in the nervous system. *J Neurol Sci.* 2005;228:201-203.

255. Percy AK. Pelizaeus-Merzbacher disease. Splice sites are nice sites for disease expression. *Neurology.* 2000;55:1072-1073.

256. Sumida K, Inoue K, Takanashi JI, et al. The magnetic resonance imaging spectrum of Pelizaeus-Merzbacher disease: a multicenter study of 19 patients. *Brain Dev.* 2016;38:571-580.

257. Sarret C, Lemaire JJ, Tonduti D, et al. Time-course of myelination and atrophy on cerebral imaging in 35 patients with PLP1-related disorders. *Dev Med Child Neurol.* 2016;58:706-713.

258. Laukka JJ, Stanley JA, Garbern JY, et al. Neuroradiologic correlates of clinical disability and progression in the X-linked leukodystrophy Pelizaeus-Merzbacher disease. *J Neurol Sci.* 2013;335:75-81.

259. Saher G, Rudolphi F, Corthals K, et al. Therapy of Pelizaeus-Merzbacher disease in mice by feeding a cholesterol-enriched diet. *Nat Med.* 2012;18:1130-1135.

260. Gupta N, Henry RG, Strober J, et al. Neural stem cell engraftment and myelination in the human brain. *Sci Transl Med.* 2012;4:155ra137.

261. Wishnew J, Page K, Wood S, et al. Umbilical cord blood transplantation to treat Pelizaeus-Merzbacher Disease in 2 young boys. *Pediatrics.* 2014;134:e1451-e1457.

271. Wolf NI, Willemsen MAAP, Engelke UF, et al. Severe hypomyelination associated with increased levels of N-acetylaspartylglutamate in CSF. *Neurology.* 2004;62:1503-1508.

272. Uhlenberg B, Schuelke M, Ruschendorf F, et al. Mutations in the gene encoding gap junction protein alpha 12 (Connexin 46.6) cause Pelizaeus-Merzbacher-like disease. *Am J Hum Genet.* 2004;75:251-260.

275. Kubota M, Ohta S, Ando A, et al. Nationwide survey of Cockayne syndrome in Japan: Incidence, clinical course and prognosis. *Pediatr Int.* 2015;57:339-347.

284. Tolmie JL, Shillito P, Hughesbenzie R, et al. The Aicardi-Goutieres syndrome (familial, early onset encephalopathy with calcifications of the basal ganglia and chronic cerebrospinal fluid lymphocytosis). *J Med Genet.* 1995;32:881-884.

289. Barth PG. The neuropathology of Aicardi-Goutieres syndrome. *Eur J Paediatr Neurol.* 2002;6:A27-A31.

290. Rasmussen M, Skullerud K, Bakke SJ, et al. Cerebral thrombotic microangiopathy and antiphospholipid antibodies in Aicardi-Goutieres syndrome—report of two sisters. *Neuropediatrics.* 2005;36: 40-44.

292. Abdel-Salam GMH, Zaki MS, Lebon P, et al. Aicardi-Goutieres syndrome: clinical and neuroradiological findings of 10 new cases. *Acta Paediatr.* 2004;93:929-936.

297. Goutieres F. Aicardi-Goutieres syndrome. *Brain Dev.* 2005;27:201-206.

299. La Piana R, Uggetti C, Roncarolo F, et al. Neuroradiologic patterns and novel imaging findings in Aicardi-Goutieres syndrome. *Neurology.* 2016;86:28-35.

304. Crow YJ, Manel N. Aicardi-Goutieres syndrome and the type I interferonopathies. *Nat Rev Immunol.* 2015;15:429-440.

308. Crow YJ, Chase DS, Lowenstein Schmidt J, et al. Characterization of human disease phenotypes associated with mutations in TREX1, RNASEH2A, RNASEH2B, RNASEH2C, SAMHD1, ADAR, and IFIH1. *Am J Med Genet A.* 2015;167A:296-312.

311. Crow YJ, Vanderver A, Orcesi S, et al. Therapies in Aicardi-Goutieres syndrome. *Clin Exp Immunol.* 2014;175:1-8.

317. Ferdinandusse S, Denis S, Mooyer PA, et al. Clinical and biochemical spectrum of D-bifunctional protein deficiency. *Ann Neurol.* 2006;59:92-104.

319. Nascimento J, Mota C, Lacerda L, et al. D-bifunctional protein deficiency: a cause of neonatal onset seizures and hypotonia. *Pediatr Neurol.* 2015;52:539-543.

320. Masson R, Guerra S, Cerini R, et al. Early white matter involvement in an infant carrying a novel mutation in ACOX1. *Eur J Paediatr Neurol.* 2016;20:431-434.

330. Percy AK. Metabolic disease with central nervous system involvement. *Curr Opin Pediatr.* 1991;3:950-958.

331. Moser HW. New approaches in peroxisomal disorders. *Dev Neurosci.* 1987;9:1-18.

345. Klouwer FC, Berendse K, Ferdinandusse S, et al. Zellweger spectrum disorders: clinical overview and management approach. *Orphanet J Rare Dis.* 2015;10:151.

346. Lee PR, Raymond GV. Child neurology: Zellweger syndrome. *Neurology.* 2013;80:e207-e210.

350. Volpe JJ, Adams RD. Cerebro-hepato-renal syndrome of Zellweger: an inherited disorder of neuronal migration. *Acta Neuropathol.* 1972;20:175-198.

357. Paker AM, Sunness JS, Brereton NH, et al. Docosahexaenoic acid therapy in peroxisomal diseases: results of a double-blind, randomized trial. *Neurology.* 2010;75:826-830.

358. Kelley RI, Datta NS, Dobyns WB, et al. Neonatal adrenoleukodystrophy: new cases, biochemical studies, and differentiation from Zellweger and related peroxisomal polydystrophy syndromes. *Am J Med Genet.* 1986;23:869-901.

370. Moser HW, Smith KD, Watkins PA, et al. X-linked adrenoleukodystrophy. In: Scriver CR, Beaudet MD, Sly WS, et al., eds. *The Metabolic & Molecular Bases of Inherited Disease.* Vol. 2. 8th ed. New York: McGraw-Hill; 2001:3257-3301.

378. Zeviani M, Di Donato S. Mitochondrial disorders. *Brain.* 2004;127:2153-2172.

379. DiMauro S, Hirano M. Mitochondrial encephalomyopathies: an update. *Neuromuscul Disord.* 2005;15:276-286.

400. Kirby DM, Crawford M, Cleary MA, et al. Respiratory chain complex I deficiency. An underdiagnosed energy generation disorder. *Neurology.* 1999;52:1255-1264.

410. Bonfante E, Koenig MK, Adejumo RB, et al. The neuroimaging of Leigh syndrome: case series and review of the literature. *Pediatr Radiol.* 2016;46:443-451.

411. Lee IC, Lee NC, Lu JJ, et al. Mitochondrial depletion causes neonatal-onset Leigh syndrome, myopathy, and renal tubulopathy. *J Child Neurol.* 2013;28:404-408.

413. Lake NJ, Compton AG, Rahman S, et al. Leigh syndrome: one disorder, more than 75 monogenic causes. *Ann Neurol.* 2016;79: 190-203.

436. Gerards M, Sallevelt SC, Smeets HJ. Leigh syndrome: resolving the clinical and genetic heterogeneity paves the way for treatment options. *Mol Genet Metab.* 2016;117:300-312.

441. Gerards M, Kamps R, van Oevelen J, et al. Exome sequencing reveals a novel Moroccan founder mutation in SLC19A3 as a new cause of early-childhood fatal Leigh syndrome. *Brain.* 2013;136:882-890.

443. Ortigoza-Escobar JD, Molero-Luis M, Arias A, et al. Free-thiamine is a potential biomarker of thiamine transporter-2 deficiency: a treatable cause of Leigh syndrome. *Brain.* 2016;139:31-38.

444. Lake NJ, Bird MJ, Isohanni P, et al. Leigh syndrome: neuropathology and pathogenesis. *J Neuropathol Exp Neurol.* 2015;74:482-492.

474. Resende C, Carvalho C, Alegria A, et al. Congenital disorders of glycosylation with neonatal presentation. *BMJ Case Rep.* 2014;2014:bcr2013010037.

476. Freeze HH, Eklund EA, Ng BG, et al. Neurology of inherited glycosylation disorders. *Lancet Neurol.* 2012;11:453-466.

479. Feraco P, Mirabelli-Badenier M, Severino M, et al. The shrunken, bright cerebellum: a characteristic MRI finding in congenital disorders of glycosylation type 1a. *AJNR Am J Neuroradiol.* 2012;33:2062-2067.

480. Serrano M, de Diego V, Muchart J, et al. Phosphomannomutase deficiency (PMM2-CDG): ataxia and cerebellar assessment. *Orphanet J Rare Dis.* 2015;10:138.

483. Thiesler CT, Cajic S, Hoffmann D, et al. Glycomic characterization of induced pluripotent stem cells derived from a patient suffering from phosphomannomutase 2 congenital disorder of glycosylation (PMM2-CDG). *Mol Cell Proteomics.* 2016;15:1435-1452.

486. Namavar Y, Barth PG, Poll-The BT, et al. Classification, diagnosis and potential mechanisms in pontocerebellar hypoplasia. *Orphanet J Rare Dis.* 2011;6:50.

499. Steinlin M, Klein A, Haas-Lude K, et al. Pontocerebellar hypoplasia type 2: variability in clinical and imaging findings. *Eur J Paediatr Neurol.* 2007;11:146-152.

503. Battini R, D'Arrigo S, Cassandrini D, et al. Novel mutations in TSEN54 in pontocerebellar hypoplasia type 2. *J Child Neurol.* 2014;29:520-525.

509. Lax NZ, Alston CL, Schon K, et al. Neuropathologic characterization of pontocerebellar hypoplasia type 6 associated with cardiomyopathy and hydrops fetalis and severe multisystem respiratory chain deficiency due to novel RARS2 mutations. *J Neuropathol Exp Neurol.* 2015;74:688-703.

515. Kurian MA, Gissen P, Smith M, et al. The monoamine neurotransmitter disorders: an expanding range of neurological syndromes. *Lancet Neurol.* 2011;10:721-733.

517. Ng J, Papandreou A, Heales SJ, et al. Monoamine neurotransmitter disorders—clinical advances and future perspectives. *Nat Rev Neurol.* 2015;11:567-584.

518. Helman G, Pappa MB, Pearl PL. Widening phenotypic spectrum of AADC deficiency, a disorder of dopamine and serotonin synthesis. *JIMD Rep.* 2014;17:23-27.

522. Brun L, Ngu LH, Keng WT, et al. Clinical and biochemical features of aromatic L-amino acid decarboxylase deficiency. *Neurology.* 2010;75:64-71.

536. Tarquinio DC, Hou W, Neul JL, et al. The changing face of survival in Rett syndrome and MECP2-related disorders. *Pediatr Neurol.* 2015;53:402-411.

Full references for this chapter can be found on www.expertconsult.com

UNIT VIII

NEUROMUSCULAR DISORDERS

Evaluation, Special Studies

Basil T. Darras ◆ *Joseph J. Volpe*

Neuromuscular disorders may cause dramatic disability in the neonatal period. The dominant features of these disorders are muscle weakness and hypotonia. In this context, neuromuscular disorders are considered those that predominantly involve the motor system, from its origins in the cerebral cortex to its termination in the muscle.

This chapter and the next three chapters are concerned with neuromuscular disorders. In this chapter, the motor system is described in terms of its anatomical and physiological organization; special additional emphasis is placed on the development and biochemical features of muscle. Also, the evaluation of disorders of the motor system in the newborn and the diagnostic studies used in their diagnostic investigation are reviewed in detail.

MOTOR SYSTEM

The control of movement and tone in the human nervous system is highly complex, and there are major lacunae in our understanding of this control in the neonatal period. Nevertheless it is reasonable to expect that the anatomical systems critical for the control of movement and tone in the mature nervous system are operative, although undoubtedly to varying extents, in the immature nervous system. In the following discussion, the major components of the central and peripheral nervous systems that are important for the control of movement and tone are briefly reviewed. The discussion is organized in the framework used in the next three chapters for the categorization of diseases that disturb muscle power and tone in the human infant.

Levels Above the Lower Motor Neuron

Control of muscle power and tone begins in the central nervous system at levels above the lower motor neuron (Box 30.1). This control is mediated in large part by the major motor efferent system—the corticospinal and corticobulbar tracts—often termed the *pyramidal system* because most of these tracts originate in the pyramidal cells of the motor cortex of the cerebrum. Also important in control, primarily through effects on cerebral cortical motor centers, are the basal ganglia and cerebellum. Certain other descending tracts that have an impact on the lower motor neurons involved in muscle power and tone are the rubrospinal, reticulospinal, and vestibulospinal tracts, sometimes collectively referred to as the *bulbospinal tracts*.

Corticospinal and Corticobulbar Tracts

The corticospinal tract is the major efferent system concerned with the movement of the axial and appendicular musculature; the corticobulbar tract is concerned with the movement of muscles innervated by the cranial nerves. The origin of

this system in the mature subhuman primate is principally from pyramidal cells, with the following distributions: motor cortex, 31%; premotor cortex, 29%; and parietal lobe, 40%.[1] The topographic representation of the homunculus on the contralateral cerebral cortex (see Fig. 18.9) provides an estimate of the somatotopic origin of these fibers. This system descends through the posterior limb of the internal capsule, the cerebral peduncles, and the pontine tegmentum; it decussates in the ventral medulla and then descends in the lateral column of the spinal cord. A small portion of the system does not decussate and descends uncrossed in the anterior column of the spinal cord. The corticospinal tract subserves refined volitional movements, although its precise contribution to movement in the human newborn is not entirely known.

Basal Ganglia

The system of basal ganglia, sometimes categorized by the less precise term *extrapyramidal system*, principally consists of five major nuclear masses: caudate, putamen, globus pallidus, subthalamic nucleus, and substantia nigra.[1] These nuclei do not project to the lower motor neuron directly but rather influence muscle power and tone primarily by effects on the corticospinal system. The major afferent centers are the caudate and putamen (the corpus striatum), and the major efferent center is the globus pallidus. Output from the globus pallidus is relayed to the cortical motor neurons principally by way of the thalamus.

Cerebellum

The cerebellum is a complex system of neurons concerned with the coordination of somatic motor activity, regulation of muscle tone, and mechanisms that influence and maintain posture and equilibrium.[1] Afferent connections are derived from muscle and tendon stretch receptors and the visual, auditory, vestibular, and somesthetic sensory systems; these connections are conveyed principally through the inferior and middle cerebellar peduncles in the brain stem. Efferent connections are conveyed principally through the superior cerebellar peduncle to the red nucleus (and then to the rubrospinal tract), the vestibular nuclei (and then to the vestibulospinal tract), and the thalamus (and then to cerebral cortical motor neurons). Thus the control of movement and tone by the cerebellum is ultimately by way of other motor systems. The hypotonia observed in cerebellar disease may be mediated primarily by decreased muscle fusimotor activity.[2,3]

Other Components

The other major components of the motor system include the rubrospinal, reticulospinal, and vestibulospinal tracts, sometimes collectively known as the bulbospinal tracts. *The nerve fibers of*

Levels Above the Lower Motor Neuron
Corticospinal-corticobulbar tracts
Basal ganglia
Cerebellum
Other components ("bulbospinal")
    Rubrospinal tracts
    Reticulospinal tracts
    Vestibulospinal tracts
Lower Motor Neuron
Cranial nerve motor nuclei
Anterior horn cells
Peripheral Nerve
Neuromuscular Junction
Presynaptic
Postsynaptic
Muscle

these tracts, unlike most other fibers of the motor system, are myelinated in the third trimester and may play a particularly important role in the control of movement and tone in both the premature and full-term newborn.[2,3]

Rubrospinal Tract. The rubrospinal tract originates in the red nucleus of the midbrain, decussates, and then descends in the lateral aspect of the spinal cord. Major afferents are from the cerebellar and cerebral cortices, and the rubrospinal tract projects to nuclei in the brain stem and cerebellum before reaching the spinal cord. The most important function of the rubrospinal tract is the control of muscle tone in *flexor* muscle groups.[1] It is tempting to speculate that this system is particularly important in the term newborn because of the impressive flexor tone in the limbs (see Chapter 9).

Reticulospinal Tracts. Reticulospinal tracts emanate from neurons of the reticular formation in the pontine and medullary tegmentum and descend in the anterior aspect of the spinal cord. Afferents are derived from all sensory systems and the cerebral cortex. This system has *major* functional effects on muscle activity and tone, principally through action on the gamma motor neurons in the anterior horn of the spinal cord, which innervate the contractile portions of the muscle spindle.[1] Indeed, the reticulospinal system presumably mediates the impressive changes in tone observed in infants according to their level of alertness.

Vestibulospinal Tract. The vestibulospinal tract arises from the lateral vestibular nucleus and descends in the anterolateral aspect of the spinal cord. Afferents are derived primarily from the labyrinth (and vestibular portion of the eighth nerve) and the cerebellum. An increase in *extensor* muscle tone is observed with stimulation of the lateral vestibular nucleus. This system may play a role in the newborn in the mediation of reflex activity associated with vestibular input and extensor muscle activity (e.g., tonic neck and Moro reflexes).[4]

Lower Motor Neuron

The suprasegmental influences just described play on the final common pathway of the motor system, the motor unit. The term *motor unit* refers to the lower motor neuron (i.e., *anterior horn cell* or *brain stem neuron of the cranial nerve nucleus*), the peripheral nerve (or cranial nerve), the neuromuscular junction, and the innervated muscle.

In the spinal cord, anterior horn cells are arranged so that neurons subserving the function of extensor muscles are located ventrally, those subserving flexor muscles are located dorsally, those subserving proximal muscles are located laterally, and those subserving distal muscles are located medially. The two major types of efferent neurons are the predominant large cells that innervate striated muscle and the less abundant small cells that innervate the fibers of the muscle spindle, the stretch receptors. The latter are important in determining the activity of stretch ("tendon") reflexes and receive input from the aforementioned suprasegmental tracts.

Peripheral Nerve

The large anterior horn cells, concerned with the innervation of skeletal muscle, exit through the anterior roots to the *peripheral nerve.* The nerve fibers conduct the nerve impulse with a velocity directly proportional to their diameter and the size of their myelin sheaths. (In addition to transmission of the nerve impulse, these fibers also transport a variety of compounds, including enzymes, neurotransmitters, organelles, and nutrient materials, to the distal aspect of the fiber.) The terminal aspect of the nerve fiber ramifies into a variable number of smaller fibers that form motor endplates at the neuromuscular junction. The axon of one motor nerve supplies a variable number of skeletal muscle fibers. In the larger muscles involved in postural control, a single anterior horn cell may provide motor endplates to more than 100 muscle fibers.[1] In smaller muscles (e.g., of the thumb) concerned with highly skilled movement, a single anterior horn cell provides endplates for only a few fibers.

Neuromuscular Junction

The neuromuscular junction contains the terminal nerve branch with its specialized *presynaptic ending,* which lies in a specialized trough of the postsynaptic *muscle* plasma membrane (sarcolemma). A synaptic cleft separates the two membranes. When a nerve impulse arrives at the presynaptic site, calcium enters the presynaptic axoplasm and causes the release of vesicles of acetylcholine. The neurotransmitter then diffuses across the synaptic cleft, binds with a specific postsynaptic receptor on the sarcolemma, and alters the permeability of the muscle membrane. Depolarization and a muscle action potential result if enough receptors are activated. This electrical signal is transmitted along the muscle membrane and then internally by a system of invaginations of the sarcolemma to provoke the events leading to muscle contraction. The coupling of excitation and contraction is discussed in more detail subsequently.

Muscle
Development

The chronology and major features of the development of skeletal muscle in the human are summarized in Table 30.1. These features provide information of value in interpreting the pathological significance of specific findings of the muscle biopsy in the newborn and in establishing anatomical correlates for certain developmental changes in muscle function (see subsequent discussion).

TABLE 30.1   Human Muscle Development

DEVELOPMENTAL STAGE	TIME (WEEK OF GESTATION)	MAJOR DEVELOPMENTAL EVENTS
Premyoblastic	0–5	Differentiation of mesenchymal cells to myoblasts
Myoblastic	5–8	Proliferation of myoblasts
Myotubular	8–15	Formation of syncytium with central nuclei, myofibrils, sarcotubular system, and early endplates
Myocyte	15–20	Movement of nuclei to periphery
		Continued synthesis of myofibrils
Early histochemical differentiation	20–24	Differentiation of fiber types I and II; type II fibers predominate
Intermediate histochemical differentiation	24–34	Increase in size of type II fibers
Late histochemical differentiation	34–38	Development of equal numbers of fiber types I and II due to marked increase in small type I fibers
Mature myocyte	>38	Increase in size of all muscle fibers

Data from Sarnat HB. Ontogenesis of striated muscle. In: Polin RA, Fox WW, Abman SH, eds. *Fetal and Neonatal Physiology*. 4th ed. Philadelphia: Elsevier; 2001:1924-1947 and Schloon H, Schlottmann J, Lenard HG, Goebel HH. The development of skeletal muscles in premature infants. *Eur J Pediatr*. 1979;131:49-60.

Premyoblastic Stage. The premyoblastic stage, occurring in the first 5 weeks of gestation, is characterized principally by the differentiation of primitive mesenchymal cells to myoblasts.

Myoblastic Stage. The myoblastic stage, which follows in the next 3 to 8 weeks, is dominated by the active proliferation and migration of myoblasts along programmed pathways in synchrony with neural crest migration. Synthesis of the contractile proteins begins at this stage.

Myotubular Stage. During the myotubular stage, from approximately 8 to 15 weeks of gestation, myoblasts fuse to form the syncytium characteristic of human skeletal muscle. Nuclei are located centrally, unlike the peripheral location of mature muscle. Myofilaments of the contractile proteins, actin and myosin, develop the longitudinal organization necessary for the formation of myofibrils. The sarcotubular system, the invaginations of the sarcolemma so important in excitation-contraction coupling, is formed. Axonal terminals contact muscle at 9 to 11 weeks, and motor endplates begin to appear at 14 weeks of gestation. The genes *myogenin* and *myomaker* are the primary mediators of myoblast fusion; *myomaker* is known as a late membrane activator of that process.[5,6]

Myocytic Stage. The myocytic stage, occurring from 15 to 20 weeks, is characterized by migration of nuclei to the periphery of the myotube. Active synthesis of myofibrils continues at this stage.

Early Histochemical Differentiation. In the stage of early histochemical differentiation, during the period from 20 to 24 weeks, approximately 5% to 10% of fibers develop prominent quantities of oxidative enzymes and correspond to type I fibers; these are distinctly large fibers[7] and are called *Wohlfart b-fibers* (Fig. 30.1). The remaining, smaller fibers, designated *Wohlfart a-fibers* or type II because of their adenosine triphosphatase (ATPase) concentration, predominate (Fig. 30.2).[8] These small fibers are relatively undifferentiated and categorized as type IIc fibers, to be distinguished from the differentiated type IIa and IIb fibers that develop in the ensuing weeks and months.[9]

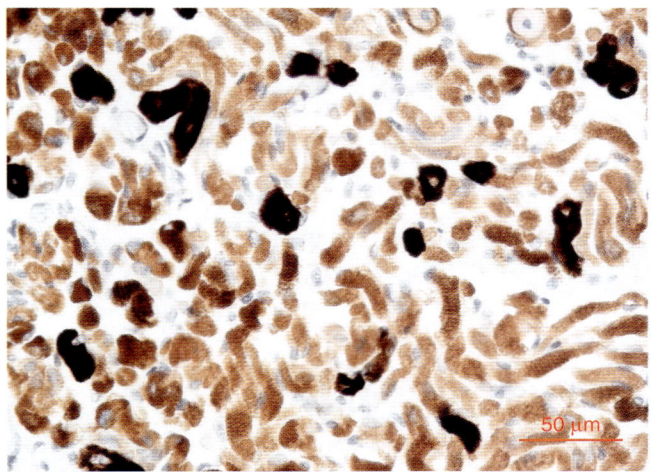

Figure 30.1 Quadriceps femoris muscle from the autopsy of a 22-week fetus. About 10% of total myofibers are larger than the rest, scattered and not grouped, and react as type I fibers (*dark*): these are designated *Wohlfart b-fibers*. Most fibers are smaller, rounded without angularity, and react as type II (*light*); these are *Wohlfart a-fibers*. With further maturation, more a-fibers convert to b-fibers, and the remaining a-fibers grow in size, adding myofibrils until distinction by size is no longer evident; the ratio of fiber types thus becomes relatively equal. At the top of the figure, two fibers with central nuclei and a thin rim of myofibrils represent scattered, persistent myotubular forms still found at this gestational age. The oblique orientation of some fibers is artifactual and unavoidable in autopsied fetal muscle because of the delicate endomysium. Paraffin section with antibody against slow myosin (corresponds to myofibrillar ATPase preincubated at acid pH in frozen sections). (Reprinted with permission from Sarnat HB, Carpenter S. Muscle biopsy for diagnosis of neuromuscular and metabolic diseases. In: Darras BT, Jones HR Jr, Ryan MM, De Vivo DC, eds. *Neuromuscular Disorders of Infancy, Childhood and Adolescence: A Clinician's Approach*. 2nd ed. San Diego: Academic Press; 2015.)

Intermediate Histochemical Differentiation. In the stage of intermediate histochemical differentiation, between 24 and 34 weeks of gestation, the predominant change is a modest increase in size of type II fibers.[8] No significant changes in type I fiber size occur during this period.

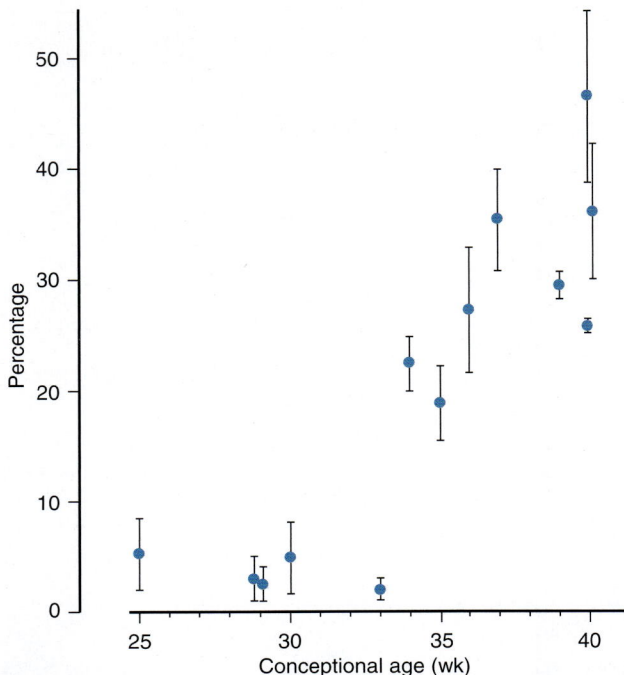

Figure 30.2 Type I fibers as a percentage of total fiber population from the autopsy specimens of several muscles of infants of the gestational ages shown. Percentages were calculated from all the muscles studied for each subject and are given as means ± SD. Note the very low percentage of type I fibers before 34 weeks of gestation and the onset of a dramatic increase in percentage at that time. (From Schloon H, Schlottmann J, Lenard HG, Goebel HH. The development of skeletal muscles in premature infants. *Eur J Pediatr.* 1979;131:49-60.)

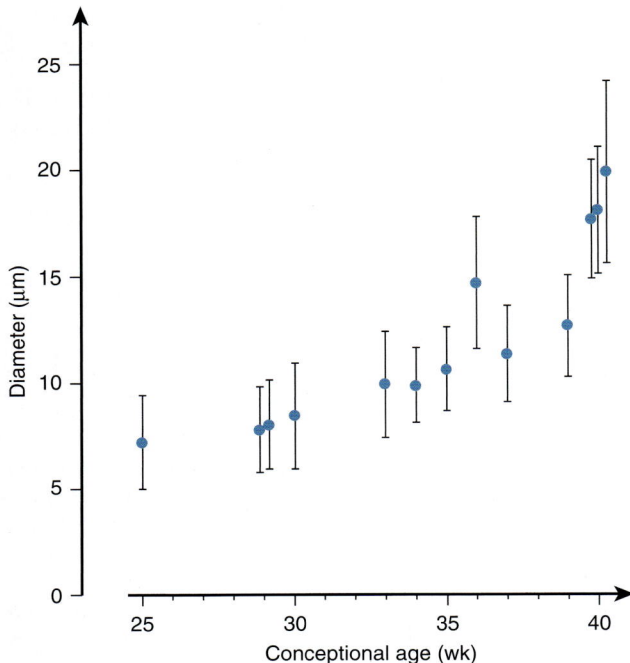

Figure 30.3 Increase in muscle fiber diameter with maturation from autopsy specimens of muscle as described in Fig. 30.2. Means ± SD of fiber diameter were calculated from all the muscles studied for each subject. Note the increase in diameter in the last weeks of gestation, especially after 38 weeks. (From Schloon H, Schlottmann J, Lenard HG, Goebel HH. The development of skeletal muscles in premature infants. *Eur J Pediatr.* 1979;131:49-60.)

Late Histochemical Differentiation. In the stage of late histochemical differentiation, during a relatively brief period from 34 to 38 weeks, a dramatic change occurs.[8] Small type I fibers appear in large numbers (see Fig. 30.2).[8] Near the end of this stage, almost equal numbers of the two muscle fiber types are observed.

Mature Myocytic Stage. Subsequent development (i.e., the mature myocytic stage), after 38 weeks, is characterized particularly by the increasing size of individual muscle fibers (Fig. 30.3). Indeed, with the continued synthesis of myofibrillar components, the mean diameter of muscle fibers increases approximately fourfold from term (15 µm) to 13 years of age (65 µm).[10]

Importance of Motor Innervation. The factors governing the developmental sequence of myogenesis are not entirely understood, although motor innervation likely plays an important role. *Denervation* of the soleus muscle in the newborn rat, when myogenesis is at the myotubular stage, results in a *severe maturational delay*, with persistence of myotubes and the failure of histochemical differentiation.[11] The role of the motor neuron in the *determination of muscle fiber type* has been demonstrated by cross-innervation and reinnervation after denervation experiments.[12,13] Thus muscle fiber type can be changed according to the motor innervation. In addition to its roles in differentiation, motor innervation also plays an

TABLE 30.2	Major Contractile Elements: Myofibrillar Proteins	
PROTEIN	**LOCATION**	**FUNCTION**
Myosin	Thick filament	Contraction
Actin	Thin filament	Contraction
Tropomyosin, troponin	Thin filament	Regulation of actin-myosin interaction; provision of calcium requirement

important trophic role in that disturbances of motor innervation also result in the defective growth of affected fibers.

Contractile Elements

The major contractile elements of skeletal muscle are the longitudinally oriented filaments, two sets of which can be recognized: thick and thin. These filaments are arranged in repeating units, imparting its striated appearance to the muscle cell. The two sets of filaments in each repeating unit become cross-linked only on excitation; contraction of muscle then is effected by a relative sliding motion of the cross-linked filaments.

The major myofibrillar proteins that make up the thin and thick filaments are shown in Table 30.2. The principal protein of the thin filament is actin and that of the thick filament is myosin. The interaction of these filamentous proteins is regulated by proteins in the thin filaments, the tropomyosin-troponin complex. Troponin itself is a complex of three proteins, one of which binds calcium and, in so doing, allows tropomyosin to change its position within the thin filament to permit myosin to combine with actin, which then leads to contraction.

Excitation and Contraction Coupling

Major insight into the coupling of muscle excitation and contraction has been gained.[14] The major events in this fascinating sequence are depicted in Box 30.2. The initial event is the release of the prepackaged vesicles of acetylcholine from the presynaptic nerve ending, provoked by the arrival of the nerve action potential and the subsequent influx of calcium. Acetylcholine traverses the synaptic cleft and binds to a specific postsynaptic receptor on the sarcolemma, thus initiating depolarization of the muscle membrane. Propagation of depolarization occurs along the sarcolemma as well as interiorly. This penetration of depolarization into the interior of the cell occurs by way of the transverse tubules, which are continuous with the outer membrane. In close contact with these tubules is the sarcoplasmic reticulum, membranous sacs rich in calcium. With the inward propagation of depolarization, calcium is released from the sarcoplasmic reticulum and binds with a peptide of the troponin complex. This allows the movement of tropomyosin within the thin filament alluded to previously, the result of which is the interaction of actin and myosin necessary for contraction. Contraction results when actin combines with myosin, thereby stimulating myosin ATPase activity and hydrolysis of adenosine triphosphate (ATP). This occurrence is critical because ATP serves to dissociate actin-myosin cross-links. With a decrease in ATP, the cross-links occur, and the relative sliding motion of the filaments causes contraction. Relaxation is associated with the return of calcium into the sarcoplasmic reticulum, an event mediated by an ATP-dependent calcium pump.

Biochemical Features

Energy is required for the work of muscle contraction; thus the major task of muscle metabolism is to generate ATP. However, the synthesis of structural, contractile, and other components is obviously also of great importance, particularly during myogenesis. The major metabolic mechanisms for energy production in muscle differ primarily according to the functional requirements of a given fiber.

Two essential fiber types can be recognized by histochemical criteria (Table 30.3). *Type I fibers* are generally concerned with slow, sustained activities and are rich in oxidative enzymes. *Type II fibers* are generally concerned with rapid bursts of activity and are rich in glycogenolytic (phosphorylase) and glycolytic enzymes. Although the metabolic and physiological correlates are complex, it appears that fibers involved in rapid bursts of activity derive their ATP principally from carbohydrate metabolism (i.e., glycogenolysis and glycolysis). When more sustained activity is needed, glycogen stores are not adequate and another source of ATP is needed; in largest part, this source is lipid (i.e., fatty acid).[15]

Carbohydrate Metabolism. Glucose and glycogen metabolism and the operation of the citric acid cycle are discussed in Chapters 13 and 25. (The disorders of carbohydrate metabolism associated with muscle disease are noted in Chapters 32 and 33.)

Fatty Acid Utilization. The utilization of lipid for energy is particularly characteristic of muscle. The free fatty acid that serves as a source of energy is derived primarily from blood. To be used for the production of high-energy phosphate, free fatty acids initially must be activated to their respective coenzyme A (CoA) derivatives (Box 30.3). The enzyme involved is fatty

---

TABLE 30.3 Muscle Fiber Types

TYPE	MAJOR ENZYMATIC FEATURES	MAJOR PHYSIOLOGICAL FEATURES
I	Oxidative enzymes (e.g., NADH-tetrazolium reductase)	Slow sustained activity
II	Glycolytic enzymes (e.g., phosphorylase; ATPase [high pH])	Rapid bursts of activity

ATPase, Adenosine triphosphatase; *NADH*, nicotinamide adenine dinucleotide.

BOX 30.2 Major Events in Excitation-Contraction Coupling

The motor nerve action potential causes the release of acetylcholine at the neuromuscular junction.

Acetylcholine initiates depolarization of the muscle cell membrane.

Depolarization penetrates into the interior of the muscle cell through the transverse tubules.

The adjacent sarcoplasmic reticulum releases calcium.

Calcium binds to the troponin component, thus allowing tropomyosin to change position within the thin filament and, in turn, actin to interact with myosin.

The interaction of actin and myosin causes sliding movement of the thin and thick filaments and contraction.

BOX 30.3 Fatty Acid Utilization in Muscle

Activation of fatty acid: *fatty acyl-CoA synthase*
  Fatty acid + CoA + ATP → fatty acyl-CoA + ADP + P_i
Transfer to carnitine: *carnitine-palmitoyltransferase I*
  Fatty acyl-CoA + carnitine → fatty acyl-carnitine + CoA
Transfer to intramitochondrial CoA: *carnitine-palmitoyl transferase II*
  Fatty acyl-carnitine + CoA → fatty acyl-CoA + carnitine
Oxidation to acetyl-CoA: *beta-oxidation system*
  Fatty acyl-CoA + O_2 + ADP + P_i → acetyl-CoA + ATP (by electron equivalents)
Oxidation of acetyl-CoA: *citric acid cycle*
  Acetyl-CoA + O_2 + ADP + P_i → CO_2 + H_2O + ATP
For palmitic acid:
  Palmityl-CoA + 23 O_2 + 131 ADP + 131 P_i → CoA + 16 CO_2 + 146 H_2O + 131 ATP

ADP, Adenosine diphosphate; *ATP*, adenosine triphosphate; *CoA*, coenzyme A; *P_i*, inorganic phosphate.

acyl-CoA synthase, located primarily on the outer surface of the mitochondrial membrane.[16] Fatty acyl-CoA derivatives do not cross the mitochondrial membrane. Carnitine, the obligatory carrier of these derivatives across this membrane, is actively transported into muscle.[17] At the outer surface of the mitochondrial membrane, carnitine-palmitoyl transferase I catalyzes the formation of the carnitine derivative of the long-chain fatty acid (usually palmitic acid). This compound then traverses the mitochondrial barrier, and, on the inner surface, the enzyme carnitine-palmitoyl transferase II regenerates the CoA derivative. The intramitochondrial fatty acyl-CoA then undergoes beta oxidation to acetyl-CoA, a process during which electron equivalents (in the form of reduced flavin adenine dinucleotide and reduced nicotinamide adenine dinucleotide [NADH]) are produced; the latter are used by the electron transport system in the production of ATP (see Chapter 13). Acetyl-CoA is then oxidized by the citric acid cycle and electron transport system with the formation of additional ATP. As shown in Box 30.3, the complete oxidation of palmityl-CoA through this sequence results in 131 molecules of ATP. Because one molecule of ATP is used for the formation of palmityl-CoA, *a net synthesis of* 130 *molecules of ATP* results from the utilization of one molecule of palmitic acid by the system. The importance of lipids for energy production in muscle is emphasized by the occurrence of certain myopathies associated with derangements in this pathway (see Chapter 33).

EVALUATION OF DISORDERS OF THE MOTOR SYSTEM

History

The importance of acquiring a careful history is frequently overlooked in the evaluation of the infant with a motor disorder. The pertinent historical features wi1ll become apparent in the subsequent discussions of the various disorders. However, certain findings that initially may not be considered relevant to a motor abnormality (e.g., polyhydramnios) may prove to be valuable clues to diagnosis (e.g., myotonic dystrophy). Moreover, the family history should be supplemented by examination of the infant's parents. The myotonia and facial weakness of myotonic dystrophy or the pes cavus and leg weakness of familial polyneuropathy are easily overlooked in many affected adults.

Physical Examination

The physical examination must be performed carefully and completely. As will become apparent later, dysmorphic features, cardiac abnormalities, respiratory insufficiency, hepatomegaly, and the like may be features of certain disorders of the motor system. Congenital hip dislocation and other joint contractures are particularly common features in neonatal motor disorders; these and related joint abnormalities are discussed in more detail later.

The neurological evaluation of the motor system is discussed in detail in Chapter 9. As explained later, the anatomical site of a disorder of the motor system is best ascertained by careful determination of muscle bulk, power, tone, tendon reflexes, primary neonatal reflexes, and the presence or absence of myotonia, myasthenia, and fasciculations. Other neurological features, such as abnormalities of cranial nerve function, sensory discrimination, or the occurrence of seizures, provide useful supplementary information in selected instances.

Laboratory Studies

Although the major emphasis of this and the next two chapters is on disorders of the *motor unit* that result in hypotonia and weakness in the neonatal period, disorders of the brain and descending motor tracts in the spinal cord nearly always enter into the differential diagnosis. These disorders and their evaluation are discussed in other chapters, but appropriate diagnostic procedures may include the following: computed tomography (CT), magnetic resonance imaging (MRI), and ultrasound scanning of the brain as well as CT, MRI, or conventional radiography of the spine. Simple radiographs of the ribs and long bones often show marked thinning, hypomineralization, and, occasionally, diaphyseal fractures, caused most probably by intrauterine immobility.[18-20]

The *major laboratory investigations* for evaluation of disorders of the *motor unit* involve (1) examination of the cerebrospinal fluid (CSF), (2) serum enzyme levels, (3) nerve conduction velocities, (4) electromyography (EMG), (5) muscle biopsy, and (6) genetic analysis. Nerve biopsy is necessary in selected cases. Also, examinations of the function of cardiac muscle (electrocardiogram, echocardiogram) and even smooth muscle (barium swallow and upper gastrointestinal series) may be helpful adjuncts. Furthermore, muscle or nerve imaging by ultrasound and/or MRI may be used as well.

Cerebrospinal Fluid

The major value of the examination of CSF in the evaluation of disorders of the motor unit is determination of the protein concentration. Elevations are common accompaniments of polyneuropathy.

Serum Enzyme Levels

The enzymes most consistently elevated in blood in diseases of muscle are creatine kinase (CK), aldolase, aspartate aminotransferase (AST, formerly known as serum glutamic-oxaloacetic transaminase [SGOT]), and alanine aminotransferase (ALT, formerly known as serum glutamic-pyruvic transaminase [SGPT]).

Creatine Kinase. The most useful of the serum enzymes is CK, specific isozymes of which are found in skeletal (and cardiac) muscle and in the brain. Interpretation of serum CK values must be made with the awareness that levels are usually elevated severalfold in the first few days after vaginal delivery. Because such elevations are not observed after elective cesarean section, investigators have suggested that muscle compression during vaginal delivery causes leakage of the enzyme into the bloodstream.[21-23]

CK levels are not elevated in disorders of the peripheral nerve and neuromuscular junction but may be modestly elevated in diseases of the anterior horn cell. Indeed, CK values are not elevated in all disorders of muscle. Values within normal limits are usually observed with neonatal myotonic dystrophy and frequently with congenital myopathies. Moreover, CK levels do not necessarily correlate with muscle weakness. CK levels may be exceedingly high in infants with preclinical Duchenne muscular dystrophy or with certain types of congenital muscular dystrophy (see later). Nevertheless, in general, this highly sensitive test is a useful indicator of muscle disease.

Aldolase. Aldolase levels change in a manner similar to CK. In neonatal neurology, evaluation of the quantity of this enzyme generally adds little information and is not necessary.

Aspartate and Alanine Aminotransferases. Determinations of *AST and ALT levels* may add useful information because these enzymes, unlike CK, are not confined to muscle and brain; rather, they are also concentrated in liver. Thus, in the evaluation of a neuromuscular disorder with hepatic involvement (e.g., Pompe glycogen storage disease), the levels of AST and ALT may be elevated and that of CK may be normal because of minimal muscle disease (although with marked disturbance of the anterior horn cell) but prominent hepatic disease. In general, however, in muscle diseases with significantly elevated CK levels such as congenital muscular dystrophies, AST and ALT levels may be elevated as well in the absence of liver involvement.

Nerve Conduction Studies

Estimation of nerve conduction velocity is a valuable and relatively simple technique in determining the presence of a disorder of the peripheral nerve. The median, ulnar, tibial, and peroneal nerves are usually studied initially; surface electrodes are sufficient for adequate measurements. Determining the distal sensory nerve action potential in the median nerve is important in the assessment of peripheral neuropathy because the finding of a normal sensory nerve action potential is sufficient to exclude an abnormality between the dorsal root ganglion and the distal sensory nerve.[24-27] Because the conduction velocity of motor nerves depends on the diameter of the nerve and thickness of the myelin sheath, it is not surprising that motor nerve conduction velocities are lower in the newborn than in the adult (see Chapter 10). Nerve conduction velocity is particularly depressed in disorders associated with demyelination or failure of myelination and is less severely depressed in disorders of the axon (see Chapter 18). Infants with anterior horn cell disease (e.g., Werdnig-Hoffmann disease) have normal nerve conduction velocities, although a modest decrease in the velocity may occur later in the course of the disease, presumably because of selective loss of the anterior horn cells of large, well-myelinated nerve fibers.[26,28] It should be noted that the amplitude of the compound muscle action potentials is decreased significantly in infants with anterior horn cell disease, whereas the amplitude of the sensory nerve action potentials is normal, a finding to be expected in a pure motor neuron process such as spinal muscular atrophy. Nerve conduction velocities are normal in disorders of the neuromuscular junction as well as in disorders of muscle.

Electromyography

Basic Features. Examination of the electrical activity of muscle provides useful information about every level of the motor unit. Methodological details concerning performance of the EMG in the newborn have been delineated[24-27]; patience, flexibility, and skill are crucial for obtaining useful data. A concentric needle electrode is used, and potentials are displayed on a monitor. Important information is obtained with the muscle *at rest* and with *spontaneous or elicited* (e.g., movement of needle)

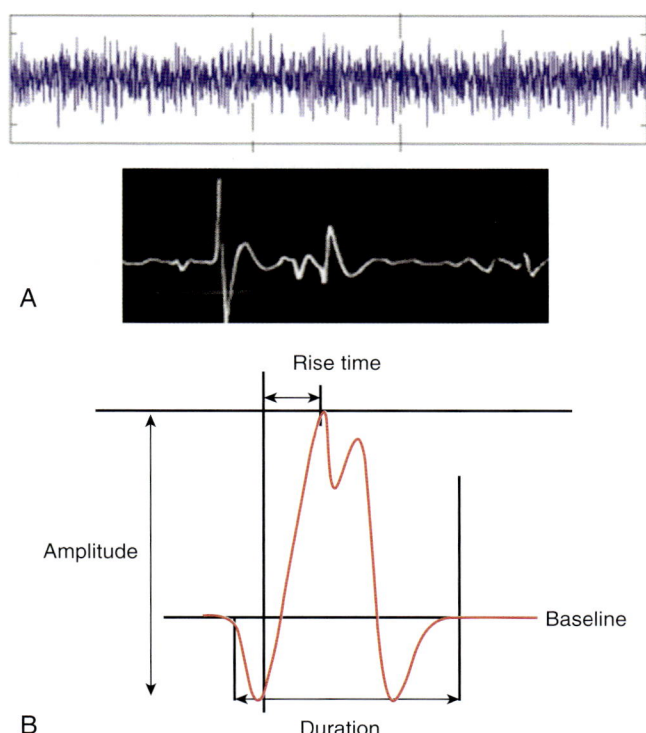

Figure 30.4 (A) Normal electromyogram. The *upper trace* shows a normal "interference pattern" resulting from the summation of motor unit action potentials on contraction; the baseline is obliterated. The *lower trace* shows a normal single triphasic motor unit action potential (note that the time scale is faster). The various components of the motor unit action potential are shown in B. (A [upper trace] adapted from Guo J-Y, Zheng Y-P, Xie H-B, Chen X. Continuous monitoring of electromyography (EMG), mechanomyography (MMG), sonomyography (SMG) and torque output during ramp and step isometric contractions. *Med Eng Phys.* 2010;32:1032-1042. A [lower trace] adapted from Dubowitz V. *Muscle Disorders in Childhood.* 2nd ed. Philadelphia: Saunders; 1978. B from Weiss LD, Weiss JM. Electromyography. In: Weiss JM, Weiss LD, eds. *Easy EMG.* Chapter 5. 2nd ed. Elsevier; 2016:37-68.)

contraction. No electrical activity occurs in normal muscle at rest. With contraction, electrical activity appears. The normal potential is summated and is derived from individual muscle fiber potentials of a motor unit (i.e., the motor unit potential). The *amplitude, duration, number, and conformation* of the motor unit potential are observed. The normal potential in the newborn is usually biphasic or triphasic, with an amplitude of 100 to 700 µV and a duration of 5 to 9 ms (Fig. 30.4).[24-26,28] The number of potentials increases with vigorous contraction and obscures the baseline (i.e., normal interference pattern; see Fig. 30.4). The *amplitude and duration* of the motor unit potential relate to the number of muscle fibers innervated by the anterior horn cell for that motor unit. The *number* of motor unit potentials observed is determined principally by the number of functioning anterior horn cells. *Polyphasic potentials*, normal in small amounts, occur when the muscle fibers of the motor unit are unusually numerous, are separated by increased distance, or both. Abnormalities of the EMG in neuromuscular disorders are summarized in Table 30.4.[24-26,29]

Anterior Horn Cell Disorders. In disorders of the anterior horn cell, spontaneous fibrillations (i.e., short-duration, low-amplitude

TABLE 30.4 Electromyographic Findings in Neuromuscular Disorders

STATE OF MUSCLE EXAMINED	OBSERVED ACTIVITY[a]	SITE OF LESION		
		ANTERIOR HORN CELL	PERIPHERAL NERVE	MUSCLE
Rest	Fibrillation	+	+	$-^{b}$
	Fasciculation	+	$-^{c}$	−
Contraction	Amplitude[d]	↑	N–↑	↓
	Duration[d]	↑	N–↑	↓
	Number[d]	↓	N–↓	N (–↓)
	Polyphasia[d]	More and of larger size	More and of normal or larger size	More and of smaller size

[a]No activity is observed in normal muscle at rest. With voluntary or elicited contraction, the four listed characteristics of the summated motor unit potential are observed.

[b]Fibrillations occasionally may be observed in polymyositis, myotonic dystrophy, myotubular myopathy, nemaline myopathy, congenital fiber type disproportion, and glycogen storage myopathies (types II, V, and VII); the other electromyographic features of myopathy aid in the distinction from anterior horn cell or peripheral nerve disease.

[c]Fasciculations are observed occasionally in peripheral neuropathies with presumed involvement of the anterior horn cell.

[d]Motor unit action potentials (see Fig. 30.7).

+, Present; −, absent; N, normal; ↑, increased; ↓, decreased.

Adapted from sources listed in the text.

potentials) and fasciculations (i.e., high-amplitude, long-duration, often polyphasic potentials) appear at rest (see Table 30.4; Figs. 30.5 and 30.6). Fibrillation potentials are small because they are derived from denervated muscle fibers. Fasciculation potentials, which originate from "irritable" anterior horn cells, are large and are of long duration because the territory of the affected motor neuron is expanded, secondary to reinnervation of adjacent denervated muscle fibers by terminal axonal sprouts.

With contraction, the number of motor unit potentials is decreased because of the reduced number of anterior horn cells (see Table 30.4). The amplitude is large and the duration is long because of the collateral reinnervation noted previously. Polyphasic potentials are abundant and large for the same reason (Fig. 30.7).

Peripheral Nerve Disorders. In disorders of the peripheral nerve, spontaneous fibrillations appear at rest because of the presence of denervated muscle fibers (see Table 30.4). However, fasciculations do not generally occur because the anterior horn cells are not the primary site of disease.

With contraction, motor unit potentials are not strikingly altered in amplitude and duration until later in the course of disease. The number of motor unit potentials is decreased because of the loss of enough terminal fibers to denervate whole motor units.

Muscle Disorders. In disorders of muscle, neither fasciculations nor fibrillations should appear at rest because disease of the anterior horn cell and denervation of muscle fibers are not present. However, in some infantile myopathies, fibrillations may be seen (see Table 30.4).

With contraction, motor unit potentials are decreased in amplitude and duration because the size of the motor unit is decreased (see Table 30.4 and Figs. 30.6 and 30.7). The number of motor unit potentials, however, is relatively less affected because the anterior horn cells are intact. This relative sparing of the number of motor unit potentials is a helpful point in

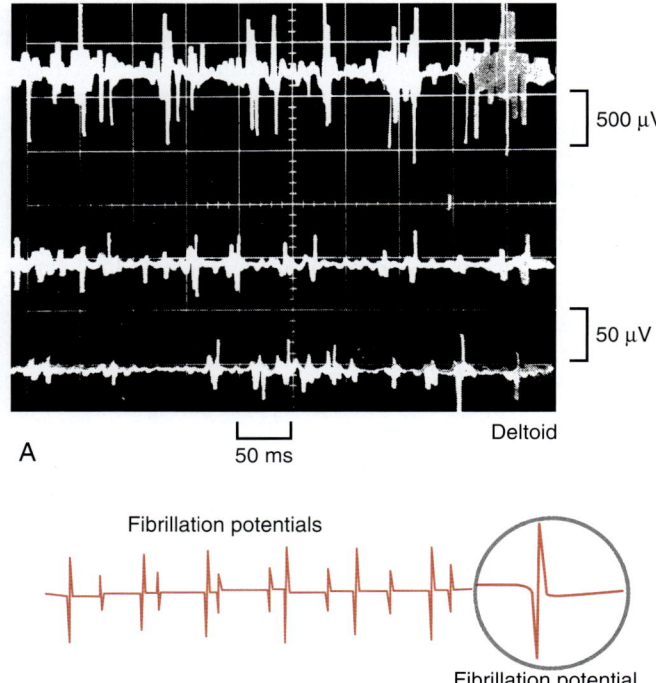

Figure 30.5 Electromyogram showing fibrillation potentials from an infant with anterior horn cell (Werdnig-Hoffmann) disease. In *the upper trace* of A, note the reduced interference pattern and visible baseline between potentials. The *lower traces* show spontaneous biphasic, small (≈50 to 100 µV) potentials at rest (i.e., fibrillation potentials), indicative of denervation, shown better in B. (A from Dubowitz V. *Muscle Disorders in Childhood.* 2nd ed. Philadelphia: Saunders; 1978. B from Weiss LD, Weiss JM. Electromyography. In: Weiss JM, Weiss LD, eds. *Easy EMG.* Chapter 5. 2nd ed. Elsevier; 2016:37-68.)

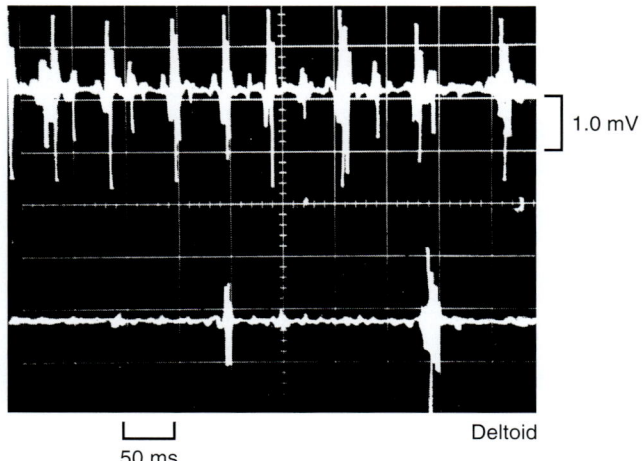

1.0 mV

50 ms   Deltoid

Figure 30.6 Electromyogram showing fasciculation potentials from a child with anterior horn cell disease. The *upper trace* shows a reduced interference pattern and large-amplitude polyphasic potentials (the scale is twice that of the *upper trace* of Fig. 30.5A). The *lower trace* shows the spontaneous, large-amplitude polyphasic potentials at rest (i.e., fasciculation potentials) characteristic of anterior horn cell disease (the scale is 20 times that of the *lower trace* of Fig. 30.5A, which shows fibrillation potentials). (From Dubowitz V. *Muscle Disorders in Childhood*. 2nd ed. Philadelphia: Saunders; 1978.)

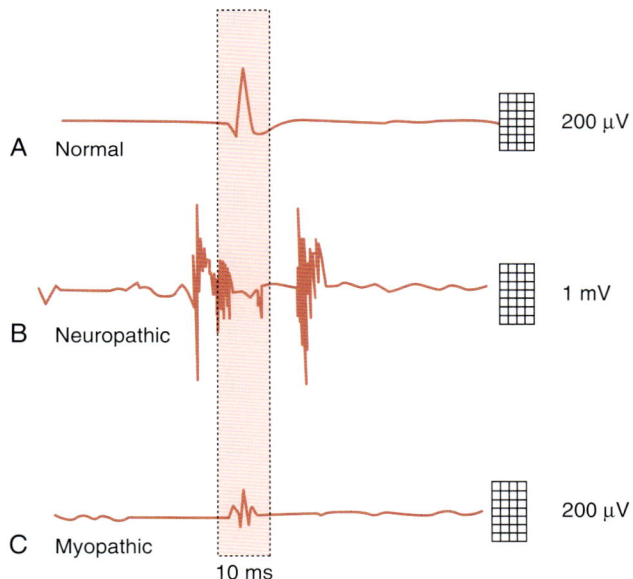

A Normal   200 µV

B Neuropathic   1 mV

C Myopathic   200 µV

10 ms

Figure 30.7 Motor unit action potential (MUAP) patterns; normal, neuropathic, and myopathic. (A) Normal: MUAPs are generally triphasic; the amplitude is measured peak to peak. (B) Neuropathic: in motor neuron diseases and chronic motor axonal neuropathies, because of reinnervation, the number of muscle fibers per motor unit is increased, resulting in high-amplitude, long-duration, polyphasic MUAPs (the scale is 5 times that of the upper and lower traces). (C) Myopathic: in myopathies, the number of functioning muscle fibers per motor unit is decreased, resulting in low-amplitude, short-duration, polyphasic MUAPs. (From Weiss LD, Weiss JM. Electromyography. In: Weiss JM, Weiss LD, eds. *Easy EMG*. Chapter 5. 2nd ed. Elsevier; 2016:37-68.)

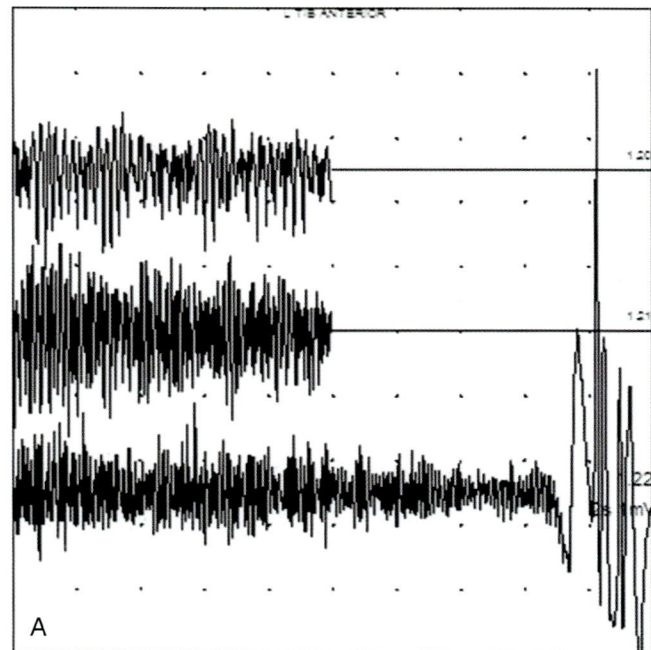

A

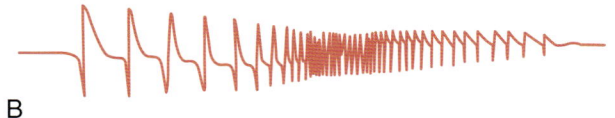

B

Figure 30.8 (A) Electromyograms showing myotonia from a child with congenital myotonic dystrophy. Note the characteristic burst of spontaneous repetitive motor unit potentials with waxing and waning features. (B) Schematic of myotonic discharges with gradual waning. (B from Weiss LD, Weiss JM. Electromyography. In: Weiss JM, Weiss LD, eds. *Easy EMG*. Chapter 5. 2nd ed. Elsevier; 2016:37-68.)

the identification of muscle disease. Polyphasic potentials are abundant because of the increased separation of the individual muscle fibers of the motor unit, a result of random fiber loss.

Myotonia. *Myotonia*, the electrical phenomenon characteristic of myotonic dystrophy, is difficult to demonstrate in the young infant. The classic myotonic pattern consists of a spontaneous burst of potentials in rapid succession with gradual waning (Fig. 30.8). When the electrical pattern is broadcast, the acoustic pattern is characteristic and resembles the sound of a "dive bomber."

Myasthenia. The *myasthenic phenomenon* is striking and characteristic. This electrical correlate of the clinical fatigability of muscle is demonstrable by repetitive nerve stimulation and observation of the waning in size of the motor unit potential (Fig. 30.9). Improvement after the injection of an anticholinesterase drug (e.g., neostigmine or edrophonium) establishes the diagnosis. However, the converse is not true (i.e., in some types of congenital myasthenic syndromes, no improvement occurs after anticholinesterase treatment; see Chapter 32).

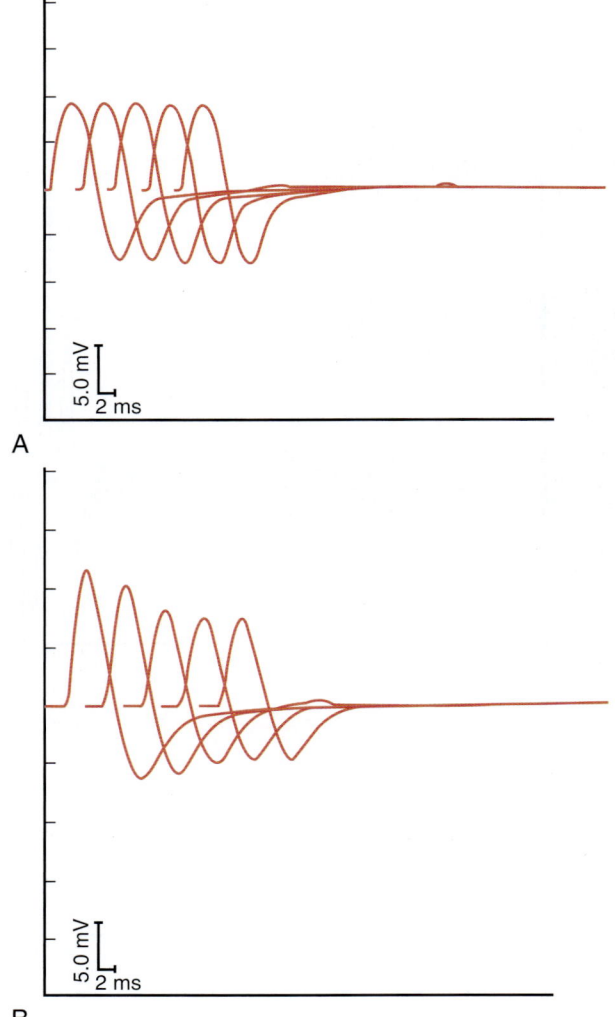

A

B

Figure 30.9 Electromyogram in myasthenia gravis. (A) Normal repetitive motor nerve stimulation; (B) decrement in amplitude noted from the first to the fifth stimulations. (From Weiss LD, Weiss JM. Neuromuscular junction disorders. In: Weiss JM, Weiss LD, eds. *Easy EMG*. Chapter 23. 2nd ed. Elsevier; 2016:193-196.)

Muscle Biopsy

Value and Indications. Examination of a biopsy specimen of muscle is usually the single most definitive diagnostic procedure in the evaluation of the infant with a disorder of the motor unit. The definition of specific diagnosis provides important information for several reasons: (1) determination of prognosis; (2) genetic counseling; and (3) institution of specific therapy, if available, and appropriate supportive therapy (e.g., physical therapy, occupational therapy, and orthopedic intervention).

The indications for muscle biopsy in the neonatal period must be determined for each individual case. Occasionally clinical features, family history, determination of serum enzyme levels, electrophysiological data, or DNA analysis may establish a diagnosis (e.g., myotonic dystrophy, myasthenia gravis, or Werdnig-Hoffman disease). However, often the diagnosis remains uncertain, and the need for examination of muscle is apparent. Although biopsy in the neonatal period is feasible

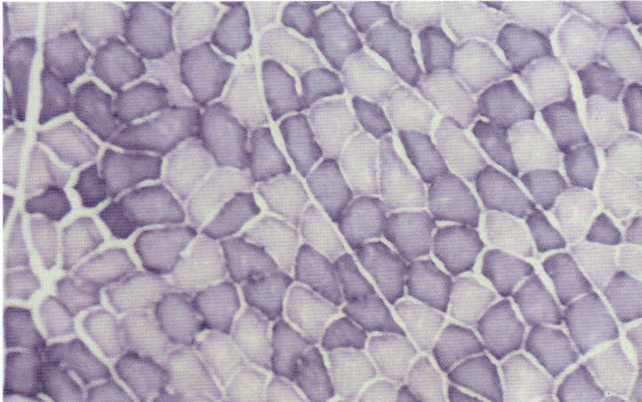

Figure 30.10 Fiber types of normal muscle in transverse section. Note the checkerboard appearance of the different fiber types. Type I fibers are dark in this section, stained for oxidative enzyme activity (reduced nicotinamide adenine dinucleotide [NADH]-tetrazolium reductase stain, ×200).

and probably preferable,[30,31] the difficulties of interpreting the muscle biopsy specimen have led others to suggest deferring the procedure for a few months if possible.[32] We prefer early biopsy despite the occasional problems in interpretation.

Technique. Two basic techniques have been used in newborn infants: open biopsy and needle biopsy.[28,30,33-35] We prefer open biopsy. Both procedures are performed while the patient is under local anesthesia and have been effective.

Muscle specimens should be prepared for histological, histochemical, electron microscopic, and, perhaps, biochemical studies. Histological and histochemical studies are performed on frozen specimens. A separate sample for electron microscopy must be fixed in glutaraldehyde. Biochemical studies are performed on either fresh or frozen material.

For histological study, hematoxylin and eosin and Gomori trichrome stains are used most often. As the clinical situation dictates, periodic acid–Schiff is used for glycogen, and oil red O is used for lipid. For histochemical studies the most common stains are NADH-tetrazolium reductase (oxidative enzyme), phosphorylase (glycogenolytic enzyme), and myosin ATPase (at high and low pH). Type I fibers are rich in oxidative enzyme activity and low in glycogenolytic and glycolytic activity; they exhibit low ATPase activity at high pH. Type II fibers are relatively low in oxidative enzyme activity and rich in glycogenolytic and glycolytic activity; they exhibit high ATPase activity at high pH.

Major Abnormalities. As reviewed previously (see Table 30.1), normal human skeletal muscle is nearly mature from a histological and histochemical standpoint by the latter part of the third trimester. Subsequent development consists principally of an increase in the size of fibers. The full-term newborn has a checkerboard or mosaic distribution of approximately equal numbers of type I and II fibers (Fig. 30.10).[30] Muscle fibers are approximately equal in size and are in close approximation (Fig. 30.11). The major abnormalities observed through histological and histochemical examinations of the muscle biopsy specimen are reviewed in Box 30.4. *No specific abnormalities* of muscle are observed in newborn infants with disorders of the motor system at *levels above the lower motor neuron* (except perhaps for

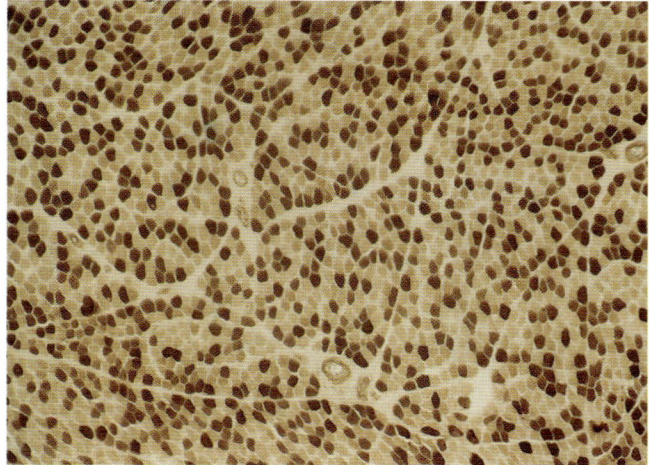

Figure 30.11 Normal muscle in transverse section. Note the polygonal fibers, closely approximated to each other, with peripherally placed subsarcolemmal nuclei and only slight variation in fiber size (ATPase stain, ×100, pH 9.4, dark fibers are type II fibers).

BOX 30.4   Major Histological-Histochemical Abnormalities in the Muscle Biopsy in Disorders of the Motor System

Levels Above the Lower Motor Neuron
None[a]

Anterior Horn Cell
Loss of checkerboard appearance with type grouping[b]
Grouped atrophy[b]
Panfascicular atrophy[b]

Peripheral Nerve
Grouped atrophy, although grouping often not marked

Neuromuscular Junction
None

Muscle
Nongrouped atrophy
Degenerated fibers
Variations in fiber size
Central nuclei
Increased connective tissue and fat
With or without more distinctive changes (e.g., central cores, rods, storage of glycogen or lipid, absence of enzyme [cytochrome *c* oxidase])

---

[a]Fiber type disproportion may be observed.
[b]Classic early features of anterior horn cell involvement (i.e., loss of checkerboard appearance followed by grouped atrophy) are usually not observed with severe Werdnig-Hoffmann disease; marked panfascicular atrophy with involvement of both fiber types is prominent.

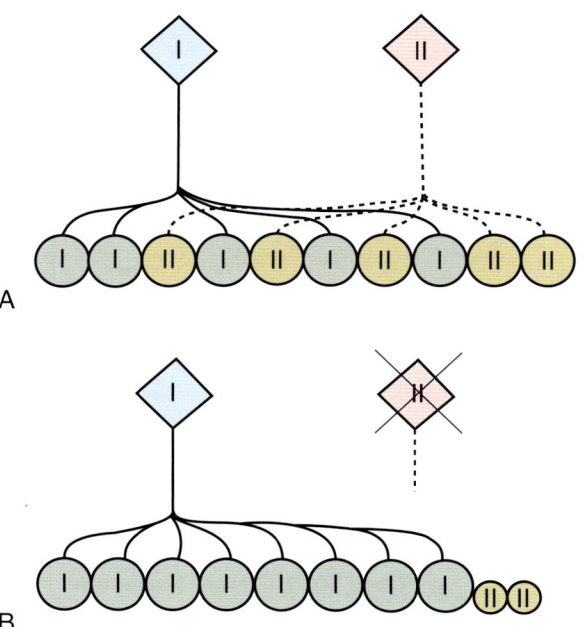

Figure 30.12 Evolution of type grouping with denervation. (A) Normal. The checkerboard distribution of type I and type II fibers is determined by the corresponding pattern of innervation of the fibers by different anterior horn cells. (B) Denervation. The anterior horn cell innervating the type II fibers has degenerated, and many of the corresponding fibers have been reinnervated by terminal axonal sprouts of the surviving anterior horn cell. A group of type I fibers results.

fiber type disproportion, discussed in Chapter 33) or at the *neuromuscular junction*.

The pattern of *denervation* is observed with disease of the anterior horn cell. In older infants, this pattern consists initially of a loss of the normal checkerboard appearance with type grouping by histochemical study; the fibers of the motor unit initially denervated by loss of its anterior horn cell are reinnervated by axon terminals from adjacent anterior horn cells (Fig. 30.12). When the anterior horn cells are then lost,

atrophy of a *group* of fibers, the hallmark of denervation (i.e., *grouped atrophy*), occurs (Fig. 30.13). However, in newborns with severe anterior horn cell disease, type grouping and grouped atrophy are observed very uncommonly, and the characteristic finding is severe *panfascicular atrophy* with involvement of both fiber types (see discussion of Werdnig-Hoffmann disease in Chapter 32). This rarity of type grouping and grouped atrophy may relate to the rapidity and severity of the anterior horn cell disorder in the fetus and newborn, with resulting lack of time or capacity for the axonal sprouting and reinnervation required to produce the classic denervation myohistological features of older infants with less severe disease. Similarly, with severe polyneuropathies of fetal onset, diffuse atrophy is more likely than type grouping and grouped atrophy.

The basic denervation pattern is to be contrasted with the *myopathic* pattern. In the latter instance, the involvement of muscle fibers is more or less random; thus *nongrouped atrophy* is the essential feature (Fig. 30.14). Variations in fiber size, central nuclei, and increased connective tissue and fat are common to most myopathies. In the newborn, degenerative changes in muscle fibers are less obvious than at later ages, and signs of arrested maturation (e.g., persistent myotubes) may occur (see especially the discussion of congenital myotonic dystrophy in Chapter 33). Histochemical stains may demonstrate certain very distinctive changes (e.g., central cores, rod bodies), discussed in more detail in Chapter 33. Similarly, glycogen and lipid stains may suggest a glycogenosis or lipid storage myopathy, and electron microscopy may yield signs of a mitochondrial or related myopathy.

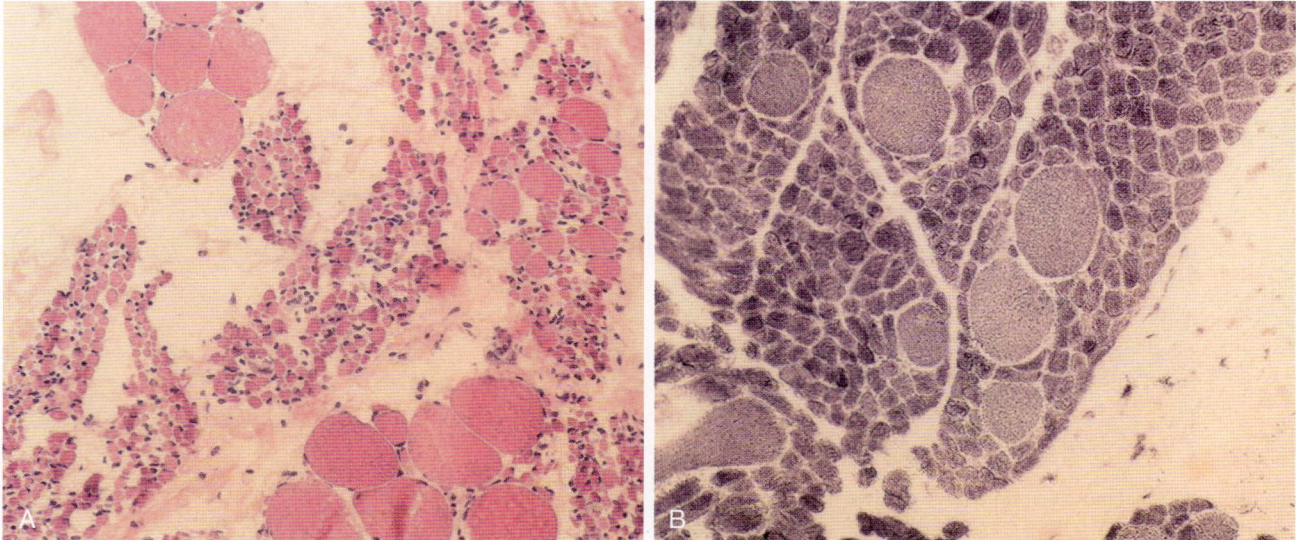

Figure 30.13 Grouped atrophy with denervation from a child with anterior horn cell disease. Note the large groups of uniformly atrophic fibers in both figures (i.e., grouped atrophy), with a few large hypertrophic fibers interspersed. (A) Hematoxylin and eosin stain, ×100. (B) Reduced NADH reductase stain, ×100.

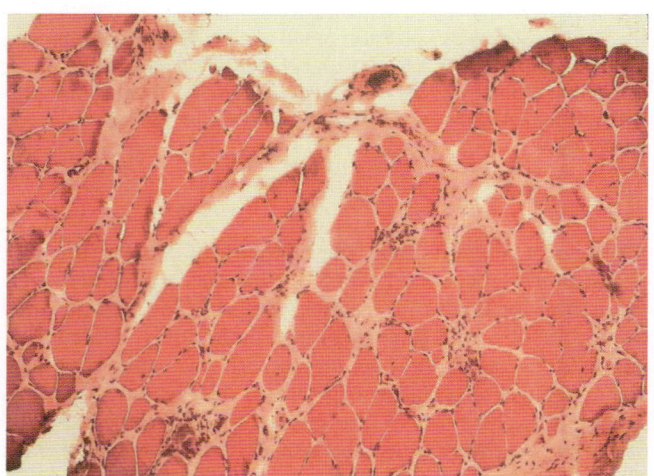

Figure 30.14 Nongrouped atrophy with myopathy from a child with Duchenne dystrophy. Note the nongrouped random abnormalities throughout the section consisting of variation in fiber size, central nuclei, degenerating fibers undergoing phagocytosis *(lower left)*, and separation of fibers by increased connective tissue. Hematoxylin and eosin stain, ×200.

Genetic Testing

Advances in the field of molecular genetics have led to the development of new diagnostic tests, which in certain situations have superseded the use of some of the tests discussed earlier. However, all these advances in DNA diagnostics have added to the complexity of a challenging clinical field and have left physicians uncertain, sometimes, about the indications for traditional tests such as EMG and muscle biopsy. At the same time, the complexity of genetic analysis has also increased over time and requires a level of expertise that most clinicians do not have. In addition to the examination of metabolites in urine, blood, and CSF as a part of a genetic analysis, molecular genetic testing has become widely available and can be performed noninvasively on blood or saliva. Although the cost of genetic testing is rapidly decreasing, cost and the ability to obtain approval from insurance carriers continue to act as potential barriers to testing. Current molecular genetic diagnostic methodology can be divided into "macro" and "micro" techniques.[36]

Chromosomal Microarrays. Whole-genome screening for large mutations can be performed with macro genetic analysis, which mostly includes chromosomal microarrays; the latter technique surveys the genome for copy-number variations (deletions and duplications) and is routinely available through most clinical laboratories. This technology uses oligonucleotide microarrays, which provide a probe density from 4000 to more than 2.5 million oligonucleotides and thus create a higher-resolution molecular karyotype. If a newborn exhibits multiple congenital anomalies or dysmorphic features or the newborn appears to have a syndromic form of arthrogryposis, chromosomal microarray analysis should be considered before other types of genetic testing.

Single-Gene Testing. Micro methods target changes in the DNA sequence down to individual nucleotides. For example, in suspected triple repeat disorders such as congenital myotonic dystrophy, targeted DNA testing should be performed to confirm or exclude the diagnosis. If the phenotype is obvious, as in an infant with spinal muscular atrophy, single-gene genetic testing can be performed to detect either known or private unique mutations.

Gene Panels. Today the clinician has the choice of ordering genetic testing of a defined panel of genes for conditions such as congenital myopathies or peripheral motor and sensory neuropathies. If the clinical sensitivity of a targeted gene panel is high, it is probably preferable to order a specific panel of genes, such as those involved in the pathogenesis of congenital myasthenic syndromes, instead of an exome test, to diminish the cost and also increase the probability of detecting the mutation. The cost of these tests, however, continues to change rapidly, and some but not all exome tests may be less expensive than the respective gene panels.

Whole-Exome or Genome Sequencing. If the sensitivity of the targeted gene panel is less than 50%, it may be preferable to proceed with an exome test, using either next-generation sequencing or whole-exome sequencing, with an initial focus on known disease genes such as the group of congenital muscular dystrophies and/or congenital myopathies. If the results of the exome test, or "exome slice" as it is referred to by certain laboratories, are negative, the clinician has the option of proceeding with a more comprehensive exome test, which, for example, would include all the genes for neuromuscular disorders known to date.

If a mutation is not identified, the next option would be to analyze the remainder of the exome with next-generation sequencing technology, which analyzes the entire human genome or more commonly the whole exome—that is, the collection of all the exons of all known genes in the human genome. The latter is also known as *whole-exome sequencing* and covers approximately 2% of the genome that encodes the exons of all human genes.

If the clinical and laboratory evaluation, including creatine phosphokinase (CPK) testing and electromyography, suggests the possibility of a congenital myopathy, for example, I (*B.T.D.*) am often asked to advise on whether a congenital myopathy panel or exome slice should be ordered instead of a muscle biopsy. As cost now has become an important parameter in the practice of medicine, the ability to understand the intricacies of molecular genetic diagnosis and to use these tests cost-effectively has become of paramount importance for the neonatal neurologist, neonatologist, and neuromuscular specialist practicing in a tertiary care center.

REFERENCES

1. Parent A. *Carpenter's Human Neuroanatomy.* 9th Sub ed. Baltimore: Williams & Wilkins; 1996.
2. Sarnat HB. Cerebral dysgeneses and their influence on fetal muscle development. *Brain Dev.* 1986;8:495-499.
3. Sarnat HB. Do the corticospinal and corticobulbar tracts mediate functions in the human newborn? *Can J Neurol Sci.* 1989;16:157-160.
4. Pasternak JF, Volpe JJ. Neuromuscular problems. In: Paxson CL, ed. *Van Leeuwen's Newborn Medicine.* Chicago: Year Book; 1979.
5. Bentzinger CF, Wang YX, Rudnicki MA. Building muscle: molecular regulation of myogenesis. *Cold Spring Harb Perspect Biol.* 2012;4:a008342.
6. Millay DP, O'Rourke JR, Sutherland LB, et al. Myomaker is a membrane activator of myoblast fusion and muscle formation. *Nature.* 2013;499:301-305.
7. Sarnat HB. Ontogenesis of striated muscle. In: Polin RA, Fox WW, Abman SH, eds. *Fetal and Neonatal Physiology.* Philadelphia: Elsevier; 2011:1924-1947.
8. Schloon H, Schlottmann J, Lenart HG, Goebel HH. The development of skeletal muscles in premature infants. *Eur J Pediatr.* 1979;131:49.
9. Banker BQ. Arthrogryposis multiplex congenita: spectrum of pathologic changes. *Hum Pathol.* 1986;17:656-672.
10. Brooke MH, Engel WK. The histographic analysis of human muscle biopsies with regard to fiber types. 4. Children's biopsies. *Neurology.* 1969;19:591.
11. Engel WK, Karpati G. Impaired skeletal muscle maturation following neonatal neurectomy. *Dev Biol.* 1968;17:713.
12. Karpati G, Engel WK. Type grouping in skeletal muscles after experimental reinnervation. *Neurology.* 1968;18:447.
13. Romanul ICA, Van der Meulen JP. Slow and fast muscles after cross innervation. Enzymatic and physiologic changes. *Arch Neurol.* 1967;17:387.
14. Pascual JM, Darras BT. Disorders of muscle excitation. In: Siegel GJ, Albers RW, Brady ST, Price DL, eds. *Basic Neurochemistry: Molecular, Cellular and Medical Aspects.* San Diego: Elsevier; 2006:713-730.
15. Akman HO, Oldfors A, DiMauro S. Glycogen storage diseases of muscle. In: Darras BT, Jones HRJ, Ryan MM, De Vivo DC, eds. *Neuromuscular Disorders of Infancy, Childhood and Adolescence: A Clinician's Approach.* 2nd ed. San Diego: Academic Press; 2015: 735-760.
16. Tein I. Lipid storage myopathies due to fatty oxidation defects. In: Darras BT, Jones HRJ, Ryan MM, De Vivo DC, eds. *Neuromuscular Disorders of Infancy, Childhood and Adolescence: A Clinician's Approach.* 2nd ed. San Diego: Academic Press; 2015:761-795.
17. De Vivo DC, Paradas C, DiMauro S. Mitochondrial encephalomyopathies. In: Darras BT, Jones HRJ, Ryan MM, De Vivo DC, eds. *Neuromuscular Disorders of Infancy, Childhood and Adolescence: A Clinician's Approach.* 2nd ed. San Diego: Academic Press; 2015:796-833.
18. Osborne JP, Murphy EG, Hill A. Thin ribs on chest X-ray: a useful sign in the differential diagnosis of the floppy newborn. *Dev Med Child Neurol.* 1983;25:343.
19. Rodriguez JI, Palacios J, Garcia-Alix A, Pastor I, Paniagua R. Effects of immobilization on fetal bone development. A morphometric study in newborns with congenital neuromuscular diseases with intrauterine onset. *Calcif Tissue Int.* 1988;43:335-339.
20. Rodriguez JI, Garcia-Alix A, Palacios J, Paniagua R. Changes in the long bones due to fetal immobility caused by neuromuscular disease. A radiographic and histological study. *J Bone Joint Surg Am.* 1988;70:1052-1060.
21. Bodenstein J, Zellweger H. Creatine phosphokinase in normal neonates and young infants. *J Lab Clin Med.* 1971;77:853.
22. Drummond LM. Creatine phosphokinase levels in the newborn and their use in screening for Duchenne muscular dystrophy. *Arch Dis Child.* 1979;54:362.
23. Sutton TM, O'Brien FJ, Kleinberg F. Serum levels of creatine phosphokinase and its isoenzymes in normal and stressed neonates. *Mayo Clin Proc.* 1981;56:150.
24. Jones HR. EMG evaluation of the floppy infant: differential diagnosis and technical aspects. *Muscle Nerve.* 1990;13:338-347.
25. Jones HR. Pediatric electromyography. In: Brown WF, Bolton CF, eds. *Clinical Electromyography.* 2nd ed. Boston: Butterworth-Heinemann; 1993:693-758.
26. Jones HR, Bolton CF, Harper C Jr. *Pediatric Clinical Electromyography.* Philadelphia: Lippincott-Raven; 1996.
27. Pitt M, Kang PB. Electromyography in pediatrics. In: Darras BT, Jones HRJ, Ryan MM, De Vivo DC, eds. *Neuromuscular Disorders of Infancy, Childhood and Adolescence: A Clinician's Approach.* 2nd ed. San Diego: Elsevier; 2015:32-45.
28. Dubowitz V. *Muscle Disorders in Childhood.* 2nd ed. Philadelphia: WB Saunders; 1978.
29. Cohen HL, Brumlik J. *Manual of Electroneuromyography.* Hagerstown: Harper and Row; 1976.
30. Sarnat HB. Diagnostic value of the muscle biopsy in the neonatal period. *Am J Dis Child.* 1978;132:782.
31. Sarnat HB. Pathology of spinal muscular atrophy. In: Gamstorp I, Sarnat HB, eds. *Progressive Spinal Muscular Atrophies.* New York: Raven Press; 1984.
32. Brooke MH, Carroll JE, Ringel SP. Congenital hypotonia revisited. *Muscle Nerve.* 1979;2:84.
33. Curless RG, Nelson MB. Needle biopsies of muscles in infants for diagnosis and research. *Dev Med Child Neurol.* 1975;17: 592.
34. Dubowitz V. *Muscle Disorders in Childhood.* 2nd ed. Philadelphia: WB Saunders; 1995.
35. Anthony DC, De Girolami U, Shapiro F. Muscle biopsy. In: Jones HR Jr, DeVivo DC, Darras BT, eds. *Neuromuscular Disorders of Infancy, Childhood, and Adolescence. A Clinician's Approach.* Philadelphia: Butterworth Heinemann; 2003:75-90.
36. Chung W. Genetics of neuromuscular disorders. In: Darras BT, Jones HR Jr, Ryan MM, De Vivo DC, eds. *Neuromuscular Disorders of Infancy, Childhood, and Adolescence: A Clinician's Approach.* 2nd ed. San Diego: Elsevier; 2015:17-31.

Chapter 31

Arthrogryposis Multiplex Congenita

Partha S. Ghosh ◆ *Joseph J. Volpe*

Arthrogryposis multiplex congenita refers to a syndrome, apparent at birth, characterized by fixed positions of multiple joints and an associated limitation of movement. The term *arthrogryposis* is derived from the Greek and literally means *bent joint*. Arthrogryposis multiplex congenita is a *syndrome,* not a disease entity, and is discussed in this section because, *albeit frequently syndromic, it can also be a manifestation of many nonsyndromic fetal and neonatal disorders of the motor system.* Indeed, disturbances at each of the major levels of the nervous system listed in Box 30.1 have been associated with arthrogryposis. Overall, arthrogryposis multiplex congenita is not rare; the incidence is generally approximately 1 in 3000 live births.[1] The intrauterine frequency may be higher because multiple congenital contractures are common among spontaneous abortions and stillbirths.[2]

CLINICAL FEATURES

The essential clinical features of this syndrome are fixed position and limitation of movement of the affected joints. Distal joints are more frequently and more severely affected than proximal joints. Most common manifestations are talipes equinovarus and flexion deformities of the wrists (Fig. 31.1), but involvement of more proximal joints is also frequent. Both the upper and lower extremities are most commonly affected; lower extremities only, slightly less commonly; and upper extremities only, least commonly. Webbing of affected joints, especially the knee, may be present, and congenital dislocations of the hips are also common.

Muscles are usually atrophic, thus giving a fusiform appearance to the joints. Hypotonia and weakness of the preserved movement occur. Tendon reflexes are depressed and often absent. Elicitation of tendon reflexes is often hindered by the joint contractures.

At least half of patients with arthrogryposis multiplex congenita exhibit *congenital anomalies* of other organs, craniofacial structures, other parts of the musculoskeletal system, or the central nervous system.[1,3-6] Indeed, more than 150 syndromes are known in which arthrogryposis is a predominant sign.[1,5,6] Some of the associated extraneural anomalies are relatively minor (e.g., clinodactyly and undescended testes), whereas others are lethal (e.g., pulmonary hypoplasia and renal agenesis). Certain of the abnormalities of the jaw (micrognathia), tongue, and palate may underlie the approximately 60% incidence of subsequent feeding disturbances.[7] Some of the constellations of anomalies (severe arthrogryposis, camptodactyly, pulmonary hypoplasia) have been designated eponymically (e.g., Pena-Shokeir phenotype).[8-10]

Banker[3] has emphasized particularly the strong relation among the *congenital anomalies* usually observed with arthrogryposis multiplex congenita and their nearly consistent pathogenetic basis as a disturbance of intrauterine movement rather than a primary disturbance of development (Table 31.1).

PATHOGENESIS

Relation to Impaired Intrauterine Motility

In arthrogryposis, the joints themselves are usually normal, but the lack of fetal movements results in the development of extra connective tissue around the joints. Thus the development of fixed joints with limitation of movement in most cases is secondary *to impaired intrauterine motility, almost invariably the result of muscle weakness.*[1,3,11-14] The postural deformities are caused by contractures of muscle with fibrous (not bony) ankylosis of the joints. The time of onset of the paralytic process determines in part the severity of the arthrogryposis; onset in the first trimester may be associated with pterygium formation at the neck and elbows.[15] The positions of the deformities are related in large part to muscle imbalance around the joints involved; neuropathological data support this notion.[12] The intrauterine position of the fetus may also play a role in determining the configuration of the deformities.

The basic concept that impaired motility secondary to muscle weakness is the critical common denominator is supported by experiments with developing chicks and with fetal rats, in which infusion of the neuromuscular blocker curare either into incubating eggs or into the fetal animals resulted in fixed postures of the neck and limbs that corresponded to intrauterine position.[16,17] Pulmonary hypoplasia, micrognathia, polyhydramnios, short umbilical cord, and fetal growth retardation were documented in the fetal rats as in the human[17]—findings further supporting the notion that intrauterine impairments of movement underlie most of the *congenital anomalies* often observed with arthrogryposis (see Table 31.1). An illustrative example is the Pena-Shokeir syndrome (Box 31.1), characterized by (1) arthrogryposis, (2) polyhydramnios, (3) pulmonary hypoplasia, (4) short umbilical cord, (5) intrauterine growth restriction, (6) osteoporosis, and (7) craniofacial abnormalities.[18] Pena-Shokeir syndrome is lethal because, as a result of the fetal akinesia, the lungs are hypoplastic, thus leading to respiratory failure and death after birth. However, because the causes of the Pena-Shokeir phenotype are multiple, the designation of such a syndrome appears to serve little clear purpose.

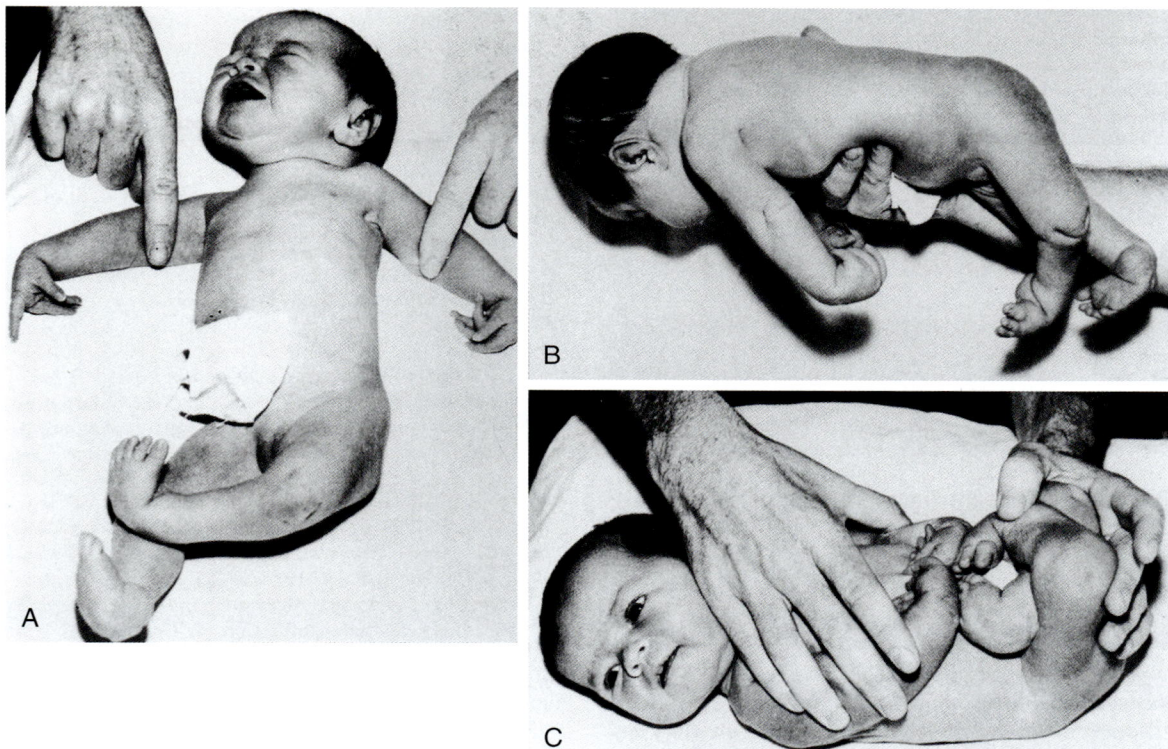

Figure 31.1 Arthrogryposis multiplex congenita in a newborn with congenital fiber-type disproportion.
(A) Deformities of the hands, ankles, and knees. (B) Good posture of the head and trunk in ventral suspension.
(C) Arms and legs folded into a presumptive intrauterine posture. (From Dubowitz V. *Muscle Disorders in Childhood.*
2nd ed. Philadelphia: Saunders; 1978.)

TABLE 31.1 "Congenital Anomalies" Commonly Observed in Severe Arthrogryposis Multiplex Congenita and Likely Pathogeneses

ANOMALY[a]	LIKELY PATHOGENESIS
Micrognathia	Impaired facial and masticatory movements
Retrognathia	Impaired masticatory movements
High-arched or cleft palate	Impaired tongue movement and micrognathia
Wide flat nose	Impaired head and facial movements (?)
Low-set ears	Impaired head movements (?)
Short neck	Impaired neck movements
Pulmonary hypoplasia	Impaired breathing movements
Clinodactyly, camptodactyly	Impaired finger movements
Polyhydramnios	Impaired swallowing

[a]Anomalies present in approximately 10%–40% cases of arthrogryposis multiplex congenita studied at autopsy by Banker BQ. Arthrogryposis multiplex congenita: spectrum of pathologic changes. *Hum Pathol.* 1986;17:656–672.

BOX 31.1   Features of Pena-Shokeir Syndrome

Craniofacial abnormalities (hypertelorism, low-set malformed ears, depressed tip of the nose)
Arthrogryposis (hip and ankle ankyloses, club feet, camptodactyly)
Pulmonary hypoplasia
Polyhydramnios
Short umbilical cord
Intrauterine growth restriction
Osteoporosis

woman that cause diminished motor activity.[19] Disturbance of intrauterine movement is also presumed to be the cause of those unusual cases of arthrogryposis multiplex congenita occurring with intrauterine mechanical restrictions, such as amniotic band, small or malformed maternal pelvis or uterus, or oligohydramnios.[13,20,21]

Two Major Subgroups—Genetic and Nongenetic

Arthrogryposis multiplex congenita can be subdivided into two major subgroups, *genetic and nongenetic.*[22,23] *The vast majority of the disorders have a genetic basis.*[23] Genetic disorders include single gene defects (autosomal recessive, autosomal dominant, and X-linked recessive), chromosomal disorders (e.g., trisomy 18, chromosomal mosaicism), and mitochondrial defects.[22,23] Autosomal recessive disorders are frequently associated with central nervous system dysfunction and severe fetal akinesia sequence (see earlier), whereas autosomal dominant inheritance is frequent in the distal arthrogryposes.[24] Amyoplasia appears to

Other supporting clinical data linking reduced fetal movement to arthrogryposis include the usual association of the disorder with neuromuscular diseases of intrauterine onset (see following discussion) as well as the occurrence of the disorder after the administration of drugs to a pregnant

TABLE 31.2   Distal Arthrogryposes

BAMSHAD CLASSIFICATION	CLINICAL MANIFESTATIONS	KNOWN GENE MUTATIONS
Type 1	Medially overlapping fingers, clenched fists, ulnar deviation of the fingers when extended, camptodactyly, foot contractures	*TPM2, MYBPC1, TNN12, TNNT3*
Type 2A (Freeman-Sheldon syndrome)	*Whistling face* syndrome (see later)	*MYH3*
Type 2B (Sheldon-Hall syndrome)	Clinical features of type 1 and some features of type 2A	*TNNT3, TNN12, MYH3, TPM2*
Type 3 (Gordon syndrome)	Autosomal dominant condition; distal arthrogryposes of hands and feet, short stature, cleft palate	*PIEZO2*
Type 4	Contractures with severe scoliosis	
Type 5	Dominant and recessive inheritance; arthrogryposis, ocular abnormalities (ptosis, ophthalmoplegia, and/or strabismus), occasional pulmonary hypertension due to restrictive lung disease	*PIEZO2* (AD) *ECEL1* (AR)
Type 6	Deafness, camptodactyly	*FGFR3*
Type 7	Trismus, pseudocamptodactyly	*MYH8*
Type 8	Autosomal dominant multiple pterygium syndrome	
Type 9 (Beals syndrome)	Contractural arachnodactyly, phenotypically resembles Marfan syndrome but without cardiovascular and ocular abnormalities	*Fibrillin 2*

be predominantly sporadic (see later).[24] The sites of involvement of the motor system among familial cases of arthrogryposis are diverse, although the lower motor neuron is most commonly affected.[a]

Distal Arthrogryposes

The distal arthrogryposes are a heterogeneous group of genetic disorders in which the joint contractures primarily involve the distal limbs (Table 31.2).[6] Distal arthrogryposis type 1 is an autosomal condition due to mutations in various sarcolemmal proteins (troponin I *[TNNI2]* gene; troponin T3, fast skeletal type *[TNNT3]* gene; myosin binding protein C, slow type *[MYBPC1]* gene; and tropomyosin 2, beta *[TPM2]* gene).[34] Common clinical features include medially overlapping fingers, clenched fists, ulnar deviation of the fingers when extended, contractures of the fingers (camptodactyly), and foot contractures (Fig. 31.2). These deformities appear to be due to misplaced tendons. Mutation in piezo-type mechanosensitive ion channel component 2 *(PIEZO2)* gene causes distal arthrogryposis type 3 (Gordon syndrome), an autosomal dominant condition characterized by distal arthrogryposes of hands and feet, short stature, and cleft palate.[35] Distal arthrogryposis type 5 is heterogeneous and can have both dominant and recessive inheritance. In addition to arthrogryposis, these patients have ocular abnormalities (ptosis, ophthalmoplegia, and/or strabismus). Some may have pulmonary hypertension as a result of restrictive lung disease.[36] Distal arthrogryposis type 6 is similar to types 3 and 4 but very rare and associated with deafness. It is caused by a mutation of the fibroblast growth factor receptor 3 *(FGFR3)* gene.[23,24] Distal arthrogryposis type 7 is characterized by trismus, pseudocamptodactyly, palmar flexion at the wrists, extension at the metacarpophalangeal joints, short stature, and flexion contractures at the knees. It is caused by a mutation of the myosin heavy chain 8 *(MHY8)* gene.[23,24] Distal arthrogryposis type 8 is described as autosomal

dominant multiple pterygium syndrome.[23] Distal arthrogryposis type 9 (Beals syndrome) causes contractural arachnodactyly (see later).[25]

PATHOLOGY

The basis for the weakness that leads to arthrogryposis multiplex congenita can reside at every major level of the motor system. However, many cases of arthrogryposis, such as those related to mutations in connective tissue genes, do not have a neural basis; thus weakness is not always the mechanism for restricted joint movements (Table 31.3).

Cerebrum or Brain Stem

Major intrauterine disorders of the cerebrum, brain stem, or both have resulted in arthrogryposis multiplex congenita (see Table 31.3).[a] The proportion of cases with *exclusive* involvement of cerebrum or brain stem (and not also of the spinal cord) is approximately 10% to 35%. When the spinal cord is evaluated, particularly postmortem but also by electromyography (EMG) in vivo, concomitant involvement of anterior horn cells is often discovered to accompany the more conspicuous central disorders.[b] This combination of findings is apparent particularly with pontocerebellar hypoplasia type I, characterized by atrophy of neurons of the pons, cerebellum, and anterior horn cells (see Chapter 32). Although dysgenetic anomalies account for the majority of this category of cases, encephaloclastic lesions (e.g., ischemic or infectious in origin) and intrauterine hydrocephalus have also been causative. Severity of the disturbance of the motor system has been marked in the infants with central disorders; thus, not unexpectedly (see earlier discussion), the resulting severe arthrogryposis with pulmonary hypoplasia has often led to the designation of Pena-Shokeir syndrome in this group. In a series of 15 infants with arthrogryposis multiplex

---

[a]References 1, 3, 5, 10, 14, 15, 18, 21, and 25-33.

[a]References 1, 3, 11, 14, 25, and 37-61.
[b]References 3, 44, 51-53, 55, 58, 59, 61, and 62.

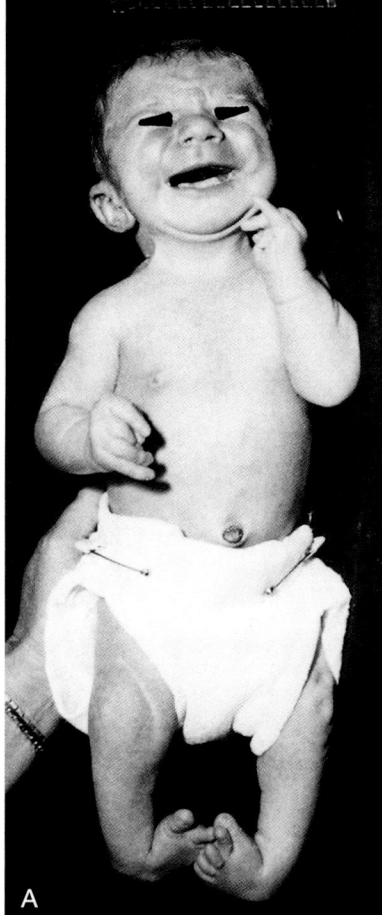
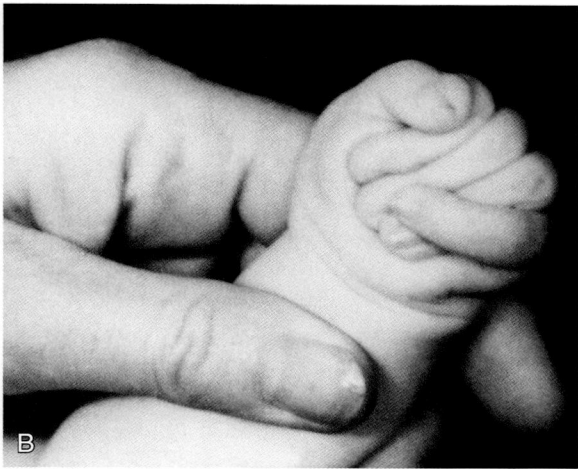

Figure 31.2 Distal arthrogryposis type 1. (A) An infant with distal arthrogryposis type I. Note primarily hand and foot involvement. The hand has a characteristic appearance when clasped. Here the hands are open, with ulnar drift of the fingers. (B) Characteristic positioning of the clasped hand in the newborn period with overlapping fingers—the little finger over third and fourth. Often the second finger and thumb overlap the third finger as well. As the hand opens with use and therapy, the fingers develop an ulnar drift. The fingers often lack well-developed flexion creases. These positional changes seem to be related to misplaced tendons. (From Hall JG, Vincent A. Arthrogryposis. In: Darras BT, Jones HR Jr, Ryan MM, De Vivo DC, eds. *Neuromuscular Disorders of Infancy, Childhood and Adolescence: A Clinician's Approach.* 2nd ed. San Diego: Academic Press; 2015:chap 7, 96–114.)

congenita *and* ventilator dependence in the neonatal period, 9 had severe disease of cerebrum, brain stem, or both.[59] In a carefully studied series of 68 infants identified retrospectively, 23 (34%) had cerebral lesions.[46]

Anterior Horn Cell

Disease of the anterior horn cell has been demonstrated many times (see Table 31.3); this may be the most common single site of disease in arthrogryposis multiplex congenita (Jones HR, personal communication, 1993).[a] This diverse group of disorders appears to account for at least 20% to 25% of cases of arthrogryposis multiplex congenita (Jones HR, personal communication, 1993).[3,46,74,78] The proportion increases considerably when anterior horn cell disturbances occurring in association with abnormalities at higher levels of the central nervous system are included. The basic abnormalities of anterior horn cell are dysgenetic, destructive, or degenerative. *Dysgenetic abnormalities*, which are associated with disturbances of number or migration of neurons of the anterior horns, predominate (Fig. 31.3).[3] A likely example of this category is amyoplasia congenita (see later). *Destructive disorders* consist primarily of apparent intrauterine ischemic events. The association of arthrogryposis with maternal misoprostol exposure (oral or vaginal) may relate to ischemic injury to anterior horn cells.[1,89] *Degenerative disorders* include anterior horn cell degenerations with anatomical features often similar to those of Werdnig-Hoffmann disease (spinal muscular atrophy [SMA] type 1) (see Chapter 32). However, with one exception (SMA type 0 or 1A) (see Chapter 32), when involvement of chromosome 5q in arthrogryposis multiplex congenita has been sought specifically, no relationship with the gene locus of SMA has been found (see later).[a]

---

[a]References 3, 12, 15, 18, 28, 30, 37, 46, 51, 59, 61, and 63-88.

[a]References 66, 70, 71, 76, and 86.

TABLE 31.3   Major Causes of Arthrogryposis Multiplex Congenita

SITE OF MAJOR PATHOLOGICAL FINDINGS	DISORDER
Cerebrum–brain stem	Microcephaly; migrational disorders: lissencephaly-pachygyria (e.g., Zellweger syndrome), schizencephaly, polymicrogyria, agenesis of corpus callosum; fetal alcohol syndrome; cytomegalovirus infection; pontocerebellar hypoplasia (type I); dentato-olivary dysplasia; leptomeningeal angiomatosis; encephaloclastic processes: neuronal destruction, porencephalies, hydranencephaly, multicystic encephalomalacia; hydrocephalus
Anterior horn cell	Developmental agenesis–hypoplasia–dysgenesis (amyoplasia congenita); destructive disorders (apparent intrauterine ischemic events); degenerative disorders (severe Werdnig-Hoffmann disease [SMA type 0 or IA], lethal congenital contracture syndrome, spinal muscular atrophy with pontocerebellar hypoplasia, spinal muscular atrophy with respiratory distress, X-linked infantile spinal muscular atrophy, early-onset non-5q spinal muscular atrophy); Möbius syndrome; cervical spinal atrophy; lumbar spinal atrophy; lumbosacral meningomyelocele; sacral agenesis; other
Peripheral nerve or root	Hypomyelinative polyneuropathy; axonal polyneuropathy; neurofibromatosis
Neuromuscular junction	Infant of myasthenic mother; congenital myasthenic syndromes; multiple pterygium syndrome (Escobar type); infant of mother with multiple sclerosis (?)
Muscle	Congenital muscular dystrophy (merosin-positive and merosin-negative); congenital myotonic dystrophy; myotubular myopathy; central core disease; nemaline myopathy; congenital myopathy due to sodium channel mutation; congenital polymyositis; congenital fiber-type disproportion; glycogen storage myopathy (muscle phosphorylase deficiency, phosphofructokinase deficiency); mitochondrial myopathy; Freeman-Sheldon syndrome
Primary disorder of joint or connective tissue	Marfan syndrome; contractural arachnodactyly; other disorders of connective tissue; intrauterine periarticular inflammation
Intrauterine mechanical obstruction	Uterine abnormality; amniotic bands; oligohydramnios; twin pregnancy; extrauterine pregnancy

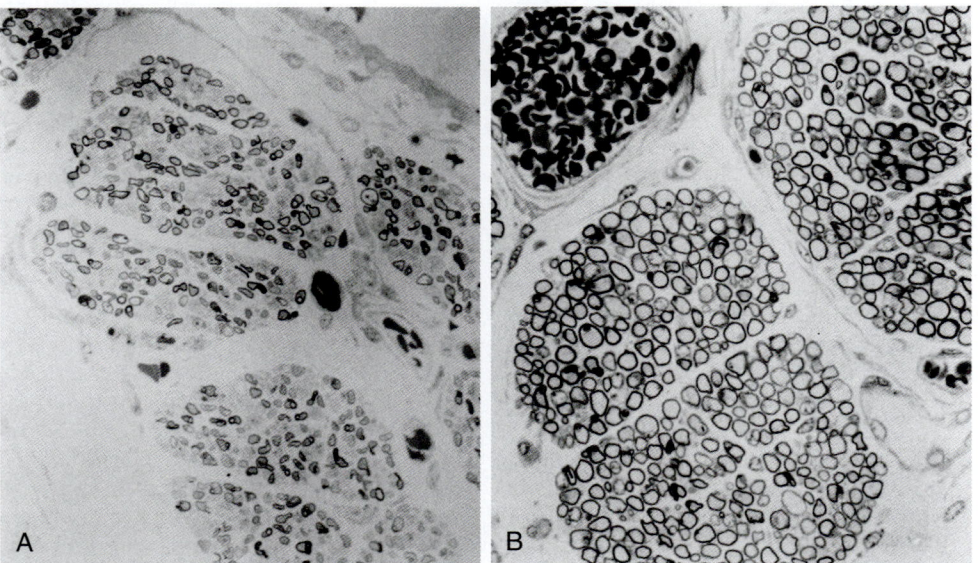

Figure 31.3 Arthrogryposis and dysgenesis of the anterior horns compared with normal findings. Alterations in (A) the anterior root of a newborn infant with arthrogryposis and dysgenesis of the anterior horns, compared with (B) the anterior root of an age-matched control infant. Note in the root from the arthrogryotic infant (A) the large areas devoid of myelinated fibers, without evidence of degeneration. Concordance between the severity of the alteration in the anterior roots and the absence or dysgenesis of the anterior horn cells (not shown) was noted. (From Banker BQ. Arthrogryposis multiplex congenita: spectrum of pathologic changes. *Hum Pathol.* 1986;17:656–672.)

TABLE 31.4	Non-5q Spinal Muscular Atrophy Syndromes With Arthrogryposis	
TYPE	**CLINICAL MANIFESTATIONS**	**KNOWN GENE MUTATIONS**
Lethal congenital contracture syndrome (LCCS)	Autosomal recessive, intrauterine hydrops, growth retardation, fetal death	Type 1: *GLE1* Type 2: *ERBB3* Type 3: *PIP5K1C* Type 4: *MYBPC1* Type 5: *DNM2* Type 6: *ZBTB42*
Spinal muscular atrophy with pontocerebellar hypoplasia (PCH)	Pontocerebellar hypoplasia, infantile spinal muscular atrophy, microcephaly, mental retardation, early death	Type 1A: *VRK1* Type 1B: *EXOSC3*
Spinal muscular atrophy with respiratory distress (SMARD1)	Mild contractures, diaphragmatic paralysis, lethal course	*IGHMBP2*
X-linked infantile spinal muscular atrophy (SMAX2)	Arthrogryposis, facial weakness, cryptorchidism, bone fractures	*UBA1*
Early onset non-5q spinal muscular atrophy	Autosomal dominant, primary involvement of the lower limbs	Scapuloperoneal spinal muscular atrophy: *TRPV4*. Lower extremity–predominant spinal muscular atrophy-1: *DYNC1H*. Lower extremity–predominant spinal muscular atrophy-2: *BICD2*.

Autosomal recessive, X-linked recessive, or autosomal dominant syndromes involving the anterior horn cells (non-5q SMA) have been identified with arthrogryposis (Table 31.4).[a] *Lethal congenital contracture syndrome (LCCS)* is an autosomal recessive form of arthrogryposis associated with intrauterine hydrops, growth retardation, and fetal death; severe neuronal loss in the anterior horns and extreme atrophy of skeletal muscle are present.[61,66,75] LCCS is genetically heterogeneous with mutations in six genes identified to date (see Table 31.4), each of which has a role in the innervation of the contractile apparatus of the skeletal muscles.[90] LCCS1 is caused by mutations in *GLE1*, an RNA export mediator *(GLE1)* gene thought to be involved in the survival of the anterior horn cell neurons.[99] LCCS2 is caused by a mutation of erb-b2 receptor tyrosine kinase 3 *(ERBB3)* gene,[98] and LCCS3, by a mutation of phosphatidylinositol 4-phosphate 5-kinase type-1 gamma *(PIP5K1C)* gene.[93] Both of these genes are involved in the synthesis of inositol hexaphosphate, which binds with GLE1. LCCS4 is caused by a mutation of the myosin binding protein C, slow type *(MYBPC1)* gene,[95] and LCCS5, caused by a mutation of the dynamin 2 *(DNM2)* gene.[94] LCCS6 is due to a mutation of the zinc finger and BTB domain containing the 42 *(ZBTB42)* gene.[90] *Spinal muscular atrophy with pontocerebellar hypoplasia*, also known as pontocerebellar hypoplasia type 1 [PCH1]), is caused by a mutation of either the vaccinia-related kinase 1 *(VRK1)* gene (PCA 1A) or exosome component 3 *(EXOSC3)* gene (PCA 1B) (see Table 31.4). Both genetic forms are characterized by pontocerebellar hypoplasia, infantile spinal muscular atrophy, microcephaly, mental retardation, and early death.[91,97] An autosomal recessive disorder with severe weakness and hypotonia as well as mild contractures, it is also associated with diaphragmatic paralysis, the need for mechanical ventilation, and a generally lethal course *(often designated SMARD1, for spinal muscular atrophy with respiratory*

distress) (see Table 31.4). The disorder is genetically distinct from Werdnig-Hoffman disease and is caused by mutation of the gene encoding the immunoglobulin μ-binding protein 2 *(IGHMBP2)* gene (see Chapter 32).[71]

A severe form of *infantile spinal muscular atrophy inherited as an X-linked recessive disorder (SMAX2)* is caused by a mutation of the ubiquitin-like modifier activating enzyme 1 *(UBA1)* gene (see Table 31.4). Clinical manifestations include severe hypotonia, areflexia, arthrogryposis, facial weakness, cryptorchidism, and frequently bone fractures.[96,100]

A *group of early-onset non-5q spinal muscular atrophy disorders with primary involvement of the lower limbs* have autosomal dominant inheritance (see Table 31.4).[92] These are scapuloperoneal spinal muscular atrophy (due to mutation of the transient receptor potential cation channel, subfamily V, member 4 *TRPV4* gene), lower extremity–predominant spinal muscular atrophy-1 (due to mutation of the dynein cytoplasmic 1 heavy chain 1 *DYNC1H1* gene), and lower extremity–predominant spinal muscular atrophy-2 (due to mutation of the bicaudal D homolog 2 *BICD2* gene).[92]

The *clinical distinction* of the three major categories of anterior horn cell involvement (dysgenetic, destructive, or degenerative) in an infant with arthrogryposis is difficult. The findings of neurological deterioration, fasciculations, and grouped atrophy suggest active degenerative disease rather than a dysgenetic or a completed destructive process. *Among probable dysgenetic types*, the relatively common clinical entity termed *amyoplasia* or *amyoplasia congenita* is perhaps the prototype.[1] This disorder has been said to account for as many as one third of all newborns with arthrogryposis and occurs once in approximately 10,000 live births.[1] In a large series of infants with arthrogryposis, of 16 with anterior horn cell involvement, 14 had amyoplasia.[46] Clinically, these infants are distinctive and exhibit symmetrical involvement of all four limbs, with the upper extremities characteristically in a "waiter's tip" position (Fig. 31.4). The latter relates to internally rotated, adducted shoulders, extended elbows, pronated forearms, and flexed wrists and fingers. Talipes

[a]References 61, 66, 67, 70, 71, 73, 75-77, 80, 86, and 90-100.

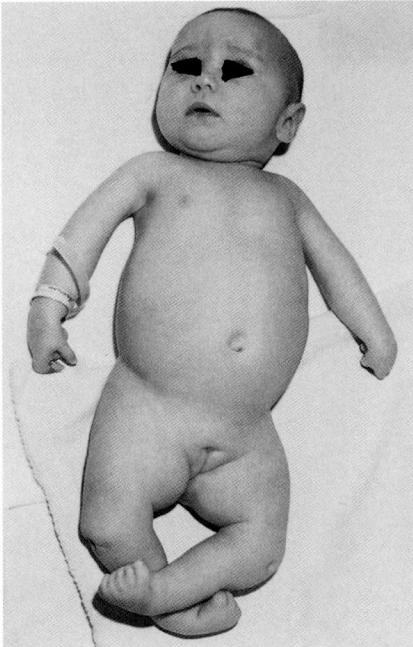

Figure 31.4 Amyoplasia. Infant with amyoplasia; note fixed extension deformity of the elbow and severe equinovarus deformity of the feet. (From Hall JG, Vincent A. Arthrogryposis. In: Darras BT, Jones HR Jr, Ryan MM, De Vivo DC, eds. *Neuromuscular Disorders of Infancy, Childhood and Adolescence: A Clinician's Approach.* 2nd ed. San Diego: Academic Press; 2015:chap 7, 96–114.)

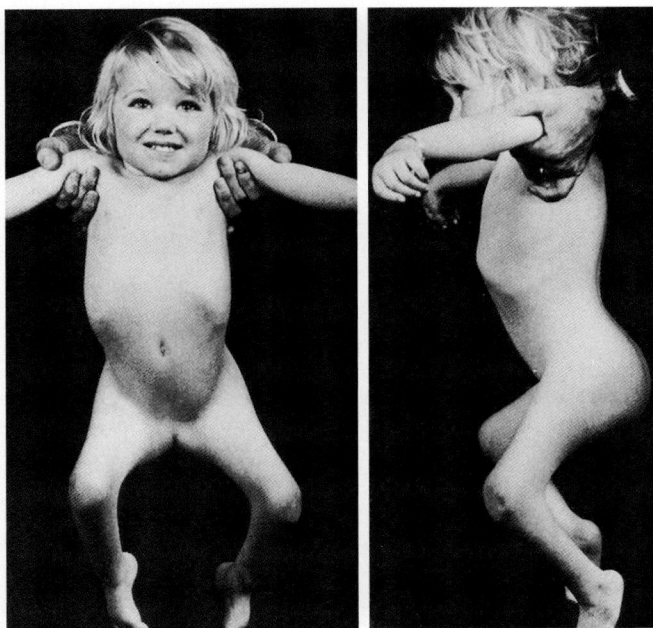

Figure 31.5 Arthrogryposis multiplex congenita in a child with congenital peripheral neuropathy. Note the fixed flexion of the hips and knees, equinus of feet, and ulnar deviation of hands. (From Dubowitz V. *Muscle Disorders in Childhood.* 2nd ed. Philadelphia: Saunders; 1978.)

equinovarus is nearly invariable. Common associations are facial hemangioma as well as abdominal wall and digital defects. The EMG shows a reduced number of motor units but no fasciculations. Muscle biopsy (see later) is nondiagnostic, with affected muscles replaced by fatty and fibrous tissue.[101]

Among the degenerative disorders, the clinical features of various principal genetic disorders involving the anterior horn cell (and genetically distinct from Werdnig-Hoffman disease) were described earlier in relation to the pathological features (see the section on pathology). Particular note should be made of the *relative lack of arthrogryposis in typical Werdnig-Hoffman disease (SMA type 1).* Thus only approximately 10% to 20% of infants with typical chromosome 5q–linked Werdnig-Hoffmann disease exhibit contractures, which are mild and usually restricted to distal limbs.[65] In a series of 68 infants with overt arthrogryposis, only 1 infant had Werdnig-Hoffman disease.[46] The reason for the relatively low incidence of joint deformity in such a severe intrauterine disorder of movement is not known definitely, but it may relate to the uniformity of the disturbance of anterior horn cells, unlike the relative preservation of some anterior horn cells in dysgenetic or destructive disorders, and hence the possibility of contracture formation.[12] The important clinical point is that severe generalized arthrogryposis multiplex congenita, even related to anterior horn cell degeneration, is extremely unlikely to represent typical chromosome 5q–linked (survival motor neuron) spinal muscular atrophy (see Chapter 32). *An exception,* as noted earlier, is the small group of very severe chromosomal 5q–linked cases of prenatal onset (SMA type 0 or 1a) described in Chapter 32.

As many as one third to one half of infants with Möbius syndrome may exhibit arthrogryposis, a finding reflecting involvement of the lower motor neuron in the spinal cord as well

as in the brain stem in this disorder.[a] Fixed contractures of the lower limbs are frequent accompaniments of disorders of neural tube development (e.g., lumbosacral meningomyelocele and sacral agenesis).[103,104] Isolated cervical or lumbar arthrogryposis secondary to nonprogressive anterior horn cell involvement, not defined more clearly, has also been reported.[b]

Peripheral Nerve

Disorder of the peripheral nerve has been shown to result in arthrogryposis multiplex congenita (Fig. 31.5 and see Table 31.3).[c] However, peripheral neuropathy is relatively rare as the basis for arthrogryposis; in the series of Banker,[3] only 2 of 96 patients with arthrogryposis had peripheral nerve disease. In a series of 15 ventilator-dependent newborns with arthrogryposis, 1 infant had congenital (hypomyelinative) neuropathy.[59] In a well-studied retrospective series of 68 infants, only 1 infant had (hypomyelinative) neuropathy.[46] In virtually all reported cases, the neuropathy was hypomyelinative (see Chapter 32).

Neuromuscular Junction

Disorder of the neuromuscular junction is a rare cause of arthrogryposis multiplex congenita (Table 31.5). About 10% of infants born to mothers with myasthenia gravis develop *transient neonatal myasthenia* due to transplacental transfer of maternal acetylcholine receptor antibodies (see Chapter 32). These infants are weak at or shortly after birth but usually recover within a few weeks. More rarely, children are born with arthrogryposis multiplex congenita and other signs of fetal immobility (e.g., pulmonary hypoplasia).[d] In these women, a high proportion of the circulating autoantibodies are directed against

---

[a]References 1, 13, 14, 37, and 102.
[b]References 14, 69, 72, 81, 83, and 88.
[c]References 3, 14, 46, 59, 82, 101, and 105-114.
[d]References 1, 14, 28, 101, 105, and 115-123.

TABLE 31.5 Neuromuscular Junction Disorders With Arthrogryposis

DISORDERS	KNOWN GENE MUTATIONS
Neonatal myasthenia (transplacental transfer of maternal antibodies against fetal acetylcholine receptor subtype)	
Congenital myasthenic syndrome	
Presynaptic	
Choline acetyltransferase deficiency	*CHAT*
Synaptic basal lamina–associated	
Endplate acetylcholinesterase deficiency	*COLQ*
Postsynaptic	
Acetylcholine receptor deficiency	*CHRNA, CHRNB, CHRND, CHRNE*
Kinetic abnormality	*CHRNA, CHRNB, CHRND, CHRNE*
Primary kinetic abnormality:	*CHRNA, CHRND, CHRNE*
Slow-channel syndrome	
Fast-channel syndrome	
Defects of endplate development and maintenance:	
Rapsyn deficiency (most commonly associated with arthrogryposis)	*RAPSN*
DOK-7 myasthenia	*DOK7*
Multiple pterygium syndrome (Escobar type)	*CHRNA, CHRNB, CHRND, CHRNE, CHRNG, RAPSN, DOK7*

the fetal acetylcholine receptor. *A relationship of transplacentally transferred antiacetylcholine receptor antibody with fetal immobility* was suggested by the correlation of maternal antibody titers with the fetal abnormalities in several patients as well as by the improvement in fetal motility and the onset of fetal breathing in a woman after treatment with plasmapheresis and prednisone caused a decrease in antibody titers.[122] The woman, who had had two previous pregnancies complicated by arthrogryposis and pulmonary hypoplasia, delivered an infant with no contractures (although transient neonatal myasthenia gravis did occur).[122] In one sibship of six affected infants, the mother's myasthenia gravis was asymptomatic and previously undetected.[121] For this reason, even if the mother is clinically asymptomatic for myasthenia gravis, maternal acetylcholine receptor antibodies should be assessed if two or more consecutive fetuses have reduced fetal movements or arthrogryposis.[1] *Congenital myasthenic syndromes* have also been associated with the occurrence of arthrogryposis multiplex congenita.[59,124-129] The most common such defect resulting in arthrogryposis is *endplate acetylcholine receptor deficiency caused by a mutation of rapsyn (receptor-associated protein at the synapse),* which is critical for receptor clustering (see Chapter 32). The clinical spectrum of rapsyn-associated congenital myasthenic syndrome is variable. Two distinct phenotypes are known. The first is an early-onset type presenting at birth or in infancy characterized by arthrogryposis, hypotonia, apnea, bulbar symptoms, and neck and proximal limb weakness. Interestingly, respiratory insufficiency diminishes after 6 years of age. The less common late-onset phenotype presents during childhood or adulthood with weakness and sometimes wasting of distal upper limb muscles.[130,131] The response to anticholinesterase medication is good in both phenotypes. 3,4-Diaminopyridine has been found to provide additional benefit in these patients.[131]

Multiple pterygium syndrome (Escobar type) is a clinically and genetically heterogeneous disorder characterized by pterygia of the neck, elbows and/or knees, arthrogryposis, and other features, such as short stature, genital abnormalities, craniofacial abnormalities, clubfoot, kyphoscoliosis, and cardiac abnormalities.[132,133] Specific genes involved in various congenital myasthenic syndromes have been implicated in this syndrome, including *CHRNA1, CHRNB1, CHRND, CHRNG, and CHRNE,* which encode the acetylcholine receptor subunits of a1, b1, d, g, and ε, respectively (see Table 31.5).[132,133] In addition, mutations in *RAPSN* (see earlier) and downstream of the muscle-specific tyrosine kinase *(DOK-7)* gene have also been implicated.[132]

A congenital myasthenic syndrome, though rare, should be considered in the differential diagnosis of hypotonic infants with arthrogryposis, as these are treatable disorders. For example, in a series of 15 ventilator-dependent newborns with arthrogryposis, the only infant with a treatable disorder had a congenital myasthenic syndrome, an observation emphasizing the importance of an edrophonium test in infants with arthrogryposis of unknown origin, especially before elective cessation of ventilator support.[59]

Arthrogryposis of varying severity was reported in seven infants born to mothers with multiple sclerosis.[134,135] The EMG and muscle biopsy were normal. The cause of the fetal immobility is unclear, but a reasonable speculation is that the disturbance was at the level of the neuromuscular junction. This occurrence must be very rare, because a more recent review of 649 births to women with multiple sclerosis did not report any cases of arthrogryposis.[136]

Muscle

Disorders of muscle are well-recognized causes of arthrogryposis multiplex congenita (see Table 31.3). Differences in the incidence of myopathic causes are apparent between series of arthrogryposis studied during life and postmortem. Thus, in the series of 96 autopsy cases studied by Banker,[3] only 6 had myopathic disorders. However, in more than 200 well-studied *living* cases evaluated by EMG, muscle biopsy, or both, approximately 20% to 40% of cases of arthrogryposis were related to myopathy (Jones HR, personal communication, 1993).[46,101,137] Some of the myopathies associated with arthrogryposis are congenital muscular dystrophy, congenital myotonic dystrophy, congenital myopathies, and metabolic myopathy (see Table 31.3). Dominant and recessive central

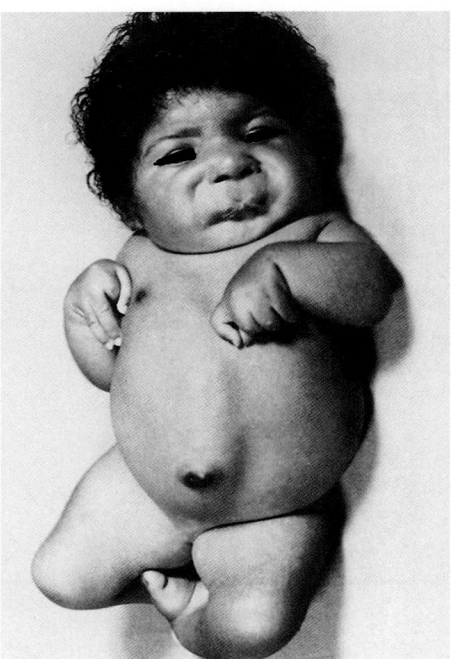

Figure 31.6 Freeman-Sheldon syndrome. Note ulnar drift of fingers, puckered appearance of face, pursed lips, small mouth (which will just barely open), equinovarus deformity of feet, scoliosis, and diastasis rectus. The neck and trunk appear shortened. The face is immobile. (From Hall JG, Vincent A. Arthrogryposis. In: Darras BT, Jones HR Jr, Ryan MM, De Vivo DC, eds. *Neuromuscular Disorders of Infancy, Childhood and Adolescence: A Clinician's Approach.* 2nd ed. San Diego: Academic Press; 2015:chap 7, 96–114.)

core disease associated with *RYR1* mutations and fetal akinesia have been described.[138] Homozygous or compound heterozygous *SCN4A* mutations (α-subunit of the skeletal muscle voltage-gated sodium channel) have recently been implicated in congenital myopathy of variable severity. Those patients at the severe end of the spectrum have manifestations of fetal akinesia/hypokinesia, resulting in intrauterine or early postnatal death.[139]

Freeman-Sheldon syndrome (*whistling face syndrome*) has been associated with both autosomal dominant and autosomal recessive inheritance (severe and at times lethal).[140-142] This disorder is a form of arthrogryposis in which involvement of oral-buccal and chin muscles is severe. Affected individuals tend to have a mask-like face with whistling mouth appearance, high-arched palate, small tongue, H-shaped cutaneous dimpling of the chin, and midface hypoplasia. There is overlapping, flexion, and ulnar deviation of the fingers, equinovarus feet with contracted toes, kyphosis, and scoliosis (Fig. 31.6). Mutations in the myosin heavy chain 3 *(MYH3)* gene have been described for this syndrome.[1] Moreover, several other myopathies have been reported in association with arthrogryposis (see Table 31.3) (Jones HR, personal communication, 1993).[a] These disorders are described in detail in Chapter 33.

Primary Disorder of Joint or Connective Tissue

Approximately 10% of cases of arthrogryposis multiplex congenita appear to relate to a primary disorder of joint or associated connective tissue (see Table 31.3).[1,5,6,13] Such is the

case for Marfan syndrome and related congenital contractural arachnodactyly disorders, usually classified among the nine types of distal arthrogryposis.[a] Contractural arachnodactyly (Beals syndrome) is an autosomal dominant condition due to mutation of the fibrillin gene (different from Marfan syndrome). Affected individuals have congenital contractures, are unusually long and thin, and have crumpling or overfolding of the ear.[154,155] Although the condition of these patients resembles Marfan syndrome, they do not have the typical cardiovascular and ocular abnormalities seen in Marfan syndrome. Experimental and clinical observations suggest a possible role for intrauterine inflammatory disease of muscle or of periarticular tissue as rare causes of arthrogryposis.[156,157]

Intrauterine Mechanical Obstruction

Mechanical constriction of fetal movement may lead to a variety of joint contractures (see Table 31.3). Important causes include uterine structural abnormalities, amniotic bands, oligohydramnios, and multiple fetuses. Although these contractures may be generalized and may simulate arthrogryposis multiplex congenita, they are often focal and restricted, reflecting the specific nature of the mechanical obstruction.

DIAGNOSIS

The occurrence of arthrogryposis multiplex congenita is an indication for a careful evaluation to determine the presence and nature of a disorder of the motor system; as with any such search, genetic studies are likely to be indicated (see Chapter 30). For example, if arthrogryposis is associated with multiple organ system involvement, chromosomal microarray (see Chapter 30) studies should be done to detect chromosomal abnormalities.[1] If the phenotype is characteristic of a particular syndrome, single-gene genetic testing can be performed to detect either known or novel mutations. However, in cases falling into a certain group of genetically heterogeneous arthrogryposes (e.g., distal arthrogryposes), testing a small or large panel of genes may be a more cost-effective approach.

Accurate diagnosis is important for definition of prognosis, genetic counseling, and plan of therapy (Box 31.2). Concerning identification of the level of the motor system affected, careful assessment of the *central nervous system* with clinical examination and brain imaging is critical because of the relatively high frequency of central disorders, especially with severe arthrogryposis multiplex congenita. Evaluation of the *neuromuscular apparatus* requires serum enzyme analysis, EMG, and a study of nerve conduction velocities. Examinations of the cerebrospinal fluid (CSF) or muscle/nerve biopsy may also be appropriate. In a study of 38 patients with arthrogryposis, the investigators concluded that when history, examination, and genetic evaluation for causes of arthrogryposis are unrevealing, EMG and muscle biopsy done together provide valuable diagnostic information.[101] In some cases, when a muscle biopsy is done, the muscle is found to be relatively well preserved; in such cases the prognosis may be good.[105] However, even in some disorders that have a pronounced abnormality of muscle (e.g., amyoplasia), the prognosis for useful function, including walking, is also very good.[1] Similarly, certain

---

[a]References 14, 31, 32, 46, 47, 78, 82, 101, 105, 137, and 143-153.

[a]References 1, 6, 14, 62, 154, and 155.

History and Examination

Antenatal history (maternal illnesses, medication/drug exposure, fetal movements)

Birth history (presentation, abnormal uterine shape, trauma during delivery)

Family history

Types of contractures

Search for other deformities/malformations and organ system involvement

Investigations

Consider chromosomal microarray (associated with multiple organ system involvement)

Single-gene test (characteristic phenotype) or genetic panel (e.g., distal arthrogryposes)

Brain imaging to identify central disorders (common with severe arthrogryposis)

Evaluation of neuromuscular disorders (serum creatine kinase [CK] analysis, electromyography [EMG], muscle and/or nerve biopsy)

BOX 31.3 Management of Arthrogryposis

Early specific diagnosis is crucial for management plan

Outcome better if therapies started early in life

Physical therapy (excellent response usual in first 3–4 months)

Serial casting and splints

Combination of stretching, casting, and splinting

Surgical intervention (newer orthopedic techniques may improve outcome remarkably)

Potential in utero therapy in familial cases can be helpful (encouraging the baby in utero to move, stretch, and extend joints)

Early delivery (after lungs mature) can improve outcome in babies with multiple contractures

varieties of congenital myopathy (e.g., congenital fiber-type disproportion) are often associated with a favorable prognosis, whereas others (e.g., congenital myotonic or severe congenital muscular dystrophy) have a less favorable outlook. Two myopathic patterns commonly observed with arthrogryposis (i.e., *fiber-type predominance* and *disproportion* and aplasia of muscle [*amyoplasia*]) should be discussed further. *Fiber-type predominance*, which is an increase in the percentage of one fiber type, or *fiber-type disproportion*, which is a reduction in diameter of one fiber type (usually type 1 fibers), or both predominance and disproportion may occur. These findings may indicate congenital myopathy (see Chapter 33), but often (20 of 96 cases in the Banker series[3]) they are observed in arthrogrypotic infants with no evidence of myopathy or neurogenic disturbance. Investigators have postulated that such patients have had an intrauterine disturbance in the neural modulation of muscle differentiation—secondary to either undetected central nervous system or anterior horn cell abnormality—as the cause for the fiber-type predominance or disproportion.[3,158,159] The pattern of *amyoplasia* also reflects a disturbance of muscle formation related to neural (i.e., anterior horn cell) disturbance. Most probably, amyoplasia represents the severe end of a continuum of disturbance of neural induction of muscle proliferation and growth and is related to severe anterior horn cell maldevelopment with very early onset (Figs. 31.7 and 31.8). Whenever possible, careful quantitative analysis of the number and organization of anterior horn cells in cases of arthrogryposis of unknown cause is needed. Consistent with these considerations, in a series of five children with amyoplasia, EMG showed evidence of anterior horn cell disease in four.[160]

MANAGEMENT

Determination of a diagnosis that is as specific as possible is an important starting point in patient management (Box 31.3). The basic elements of management and their usual sequence of progression are (1) passive stretching, (2) serial casting, and (3) surgical release procedures.[1,105,161-168] Passive stretching exercises, often augmented by flexible supports, should be instituted first.

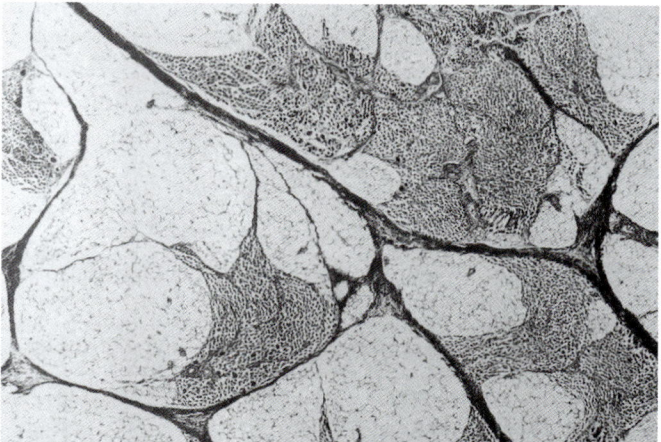

Figure 31.7 Amyoplasia in an infant with arthrogryposis and dysgenesis of the central nervous system that included the anterior horn cells. The muscle fibers are very small in cross section. Portions of fasciculi or whole fasciculi have been replaced by adipose tissue. Hematoxylin and eosin stain, ×70. (From Banker BQ. Arthrogryposis multiplex congenita: spectrum of pathologic changes. *Hum Pathol.* 1986;17:656–672.)

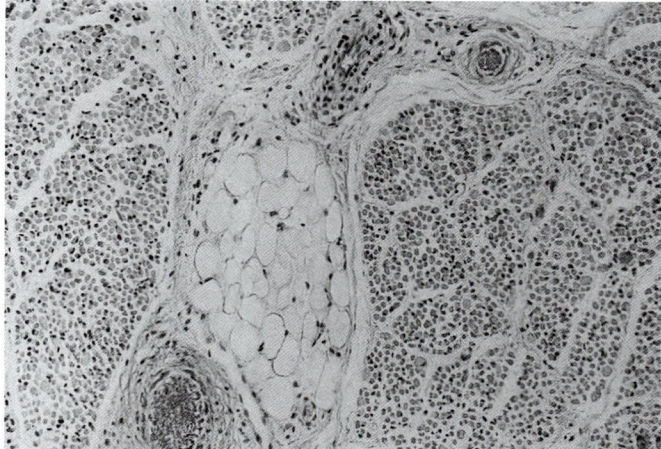

Figure 31.8 Hypoplasia of muscle in an infant with arthrogryposis and dysgenesis of the anterior horns. The muscle fibers are small, as is the entire muscle. Hematoxylin and eosin stain, ×180. (From Banker BQ. Arthrogryposis multiplex congenita: spectrum of pathologic changes. *Hum Pathol.* 1986;17:656–672.)

Because the best responses to physical therapy are usually achieved in the first few months, the onset of such intervention should not be delayed. When needed, these initial procedures are followed by serial casting with lightweight splints. Because the rigidity of joints results from fibrous and not bony ankylosis, these procedures may be particularly beneficial. Marked and persistent deformities can be improved by the surgical release of periarticular tendons and ligaments. Even with major degrees of deformity, a surprising amount of improvement in functional capabilities may be achieved. Infants with progressive disorders, severe central nervous system involvement, or both (see Table 31.3), respond to therapy in only a limited fashion if at all.

Acknowledgement

I am grateful to Dr. Basil T. Darras for his critical review of the manuscript and valuable suggestions. My sincere thanks to Shaye Moore and Irene Miller for their editorial support and help.

KEY REFERENCES

1. Hall JG, Vincent A. Arthrogryposis. In: Darras BT, Jones HR Jr, Ryan MM, et al., eds. *Neuromuscular Disorders of Infancy, Childhood and Adolescence: A Clinician's Approach.* 2nd ed. San Diego: Academic Press; 2015:96-114.
2. Christianson C, Huff D, McPherson E. Limb deformations in oligohydramnios sequence: effects of gestational age and duration of oligohydramnios. *Am J Med Genet.* 1999;86:430-433.
3. Banker BQ. Arthrogryposis multiplex congenita: spectrum of pathologic changes. *Hum Pathol.* 1986;17:656-672.
5. Hall JG. Genetic aspects of arthrogryposis. *Clin Orthop.* 1985;194:44.
6. Hall JC. Overview of arthrogryposis. In: Staheli LT, Hall JG, Jaffe KM, et al., eds. *Arthrogryposis.* Cambridge: Cambridge University Press; 1998:1-25.
7. Robinson RO. Arthrogryposis multiplex congenita; feeding, language and other health problems. *Neuropediatrics.* 1990;21:177-178.
8. Pena CE, Miller F, Budzilovich GN, et al. Arthrogryposis multiplex congenita: report of two cases of radicular type with familial incidence. *Neurology.* 1968;18:92-930.
9. Lavi E, Montone KT, Rorke LB, et al. Fetal akinesia deformation sequence (Pena-Shokeir phenotype) associated with acquired intrauterine brain damage. *Neurology.* 1991;41:1467-1468.
10. Pena SDJ, Shokeir MHK. Syndrome of campodactyly, multiple ankyloses, facial anomalies, and pulmonary hypoplasia: a lethal condition. *J Pediatr.* 1974;85:373-375.
11. Swinyard CA. Concepts of multiple congenital contractures (arthrogryposis) in man and animals. *Teratology.* 1982;25:247.
12. Clarren SK, Hall JG. Neuropathologic findings in the spinal cords of 10 infants with arthrogryposis. *J Neurol Sci.* 1983;58:8-102.
13. Swinyard CA, Bleck EE. The etiology of arthrogryposis (multiple congenital contractures). *Clin Orthop.* 1985;194:15.
14. Gordon N. Arthrogryposis multiplex congenita. *Brain Dev.* 1998;20:507-511.
15. Herva R, Conradi NG, Kalimo H, et al. A syndrome of multiple congenital contractures: neuropathological analysis on five fetal cases. *Am J Med Genet.* 1988;29:67-76.
16. Drachman DB, Coulombre AJ. Experimental clubfoot and arthrogryposis multiplex congenita. *Lancet.* 1962;2:523.
17. Moessinger AC. Fetal akinesia deformation sequence: an animal model. *Pediatrics.* 1983;72:857-863.
18. Sul YC, Mrak RE, Evans OB, et al. Neurogenic arthrogryposis in one identical twin. *Arch Neurol.* 1982;39:717.
19. Jago RH. Arthrogryposis following treatment of maternal tetanus with muscle relaxants. *Arch Dis Child.* 1970;45:277.
22. Haliloglu G, Topaloglu H. Arthrogryposis and fetal hypomobility syndrome. *Handb Clin Neurol.* 2013;113:1311-1319.
23. Kowalczyk B, Felus J. Arthrogryposis: an update on clinical aspects, etiology, and treatment strategies. *Arch Med Sci.* 2016;12:10-24.
24. Hall JG. Arthrogryposis (multiple congenital contractures): diagnostic approach to etiology, classification, genetics, and general principles. *Eur J Med Genet.* 2014;57:464-472.
25. Lindhout D, Hageman G, Beemer FA, et al. The Pena-Shokeir syndrome: report of nine Dutch cases. *Am J Med Genet.* 1985;21:655-668.
30. Herva R, Leisti J, Kirkinen P, et al. A lethal autosomal recessive syndrome of multiple congenital contractures. *Am J Med Genet.* 1985;20:431.
32. Hennekam RCM, Barth PG, Van Lookeren CW, et al. A family with severe X-linked arthrogryposis. *J Pediatr.* 1991;150:656-660.
33. Rosemann A, Arad I. Arthrogryposis multiplex congenita: neurogenic type with autosomal recessive inheritance. *J Med Genet.* 1974;11:91.
34. Bamshad M, Watkins WS, Zenger RK, et al. A gene for distal arthrogryposis type I maps to the pericentromeric region of chromosome 9. *Am J Hum Genet.* 1994;55:1153-1158.
35. McMillin MJ, Beck AE, Chong JX, et al. Mutations in PIEZO2 cause Gordon syndrome, Marden-Walker syndrome, and distal arthrogryposis type 5. *Am J Hum Genet.* 2014;94:734-744.
36. Bamshad M, Van Heest AE, Pleasure D. Arthrogryposis: a review and update. *J Bone Joint Surg Am.* 2009;91(suppl 4):40-46.
37. Banker BQ. Neuropathologic aspects of arthrogryposis multiplex congenita. *Clin Orthop.* 1985;194:30.
38. Hageman G, Willemse J, van Ketel BA, et al. The heterogeneity of the Pena-Shokeir syndrome. *Neuropediatrics.* 1987;18:45-50.
39. Davis JE, Katousek DK. Fetal akinesia deformation sequence in previable fetuses. *Am J Med Genet.* 1988;29:77-87.
41. Bisceglia M, Zelante I, Bosman C, et al. Pathologic features in two siblings with the Pena-Shokeir I syndrome. *Eur J Pediatr.* 1987;146:283-287.
42. Massa G, Casaer B, Ceulemans B, et al. Arthrogryposis multiplex congenita associated with lissencephaly: a case report. *Neuropediatrics.* 1988;19:24-26.
43. Choi BH, Ruess WR, Kim RC. Disturbances in neuronal migration and laminar cortical organization associated with multicystic encephalopathy in the Pena-Shokeir syndrome. *Acta Neuropathol.* 1986;69:177-183.
44. Hageman G, Hoogenraad TU, Prevo RL. The association of cortical dysplasia and anterior horn arthrogryposis: a case report. *Brain Dev.* 1995;16:463-466.
45. Castro-Gago M, Iglesias-Meleiro JM, Blanco-Barca MO, et al. Neurogenic arthrogryposis multiplex congenita and velopharyngeal incompetence associated with chromosome 22q11.2 deletion. *J Child Neurol.* 2005;20:76-78.
46. Darin N, Kimber E, Kroksmark A-K, et al. Multiple congenital contractures: birth prevalence, etiology, and outcome. *J Pediatr.* 2002;140:61-67.
47. Witters I, Moerman P, Fryne J-P. Fetal akinesia deformation sequence: a study of 30 consecutive in utero diagnoses. *Am J Med Genet.* 2002;113:23-28.
48. Charollais A, Lacroix C, Nouyrigat V, et al. Arthogryposis and multicystic encephalopathy after acute fetal distress in the end stage of gestation. *Neuropediatrics.* 2001;32:49-52.
49. Saito Y, Hayashi M, Miyazono Y, et al. Arthrogryposis multiplex congenita with callosal agenesis and dentato-olivary dysplasia. *Brain Dev.* 2006;28:261-264.
50. Takano T, Aotani H, Takeuchi Y. Asymmetric arthrogryposis multiplex congenita with focal pachygyria. *Pediatr Neurol.* 2001;25:247-249.
51. Muntoni F, Goodwin F, Sewry C, et al. Clinical spectrum and diagnostic difficulties of infantile ponto-cerebellar hypoplasia type 1. *Neuropediatrics.* 1999;30:243-248.
52. Gorgen-Pauly U, Sperner J, Reiss I, et al. Familial pontocerebellar hypoplasia type 1 with anterior horn cell disease. *Eur J Paediatr Neurol.* 1999;3:33-38.
53. Hevner RF, Horoupian DS. Pena-Shokeir phenotype associated with bilateral opercular polymicrogyria. *Pediatr Neurol.* 1996;15:348-351.
54. Baker EM, Khorasgani MG, Gardner-Medwin D, et al. Arthrogryposis multiplex congenita and bilateral parietal polymicrogyria in association with the intrauterine death of a twin. *Neuropediatrics.* 1996;27:54-56.

55. Razavi FE, Larroche JC, Roume J, et al. Lethal familial fetal akinesia sequence (FAS) with distinct neuropathological pattern: type III lissencephaly syndrome. *Am J Med Genet*. 1996;62:16-22.
56. Perlman J, Burns DK, Twickler DM, et al. Fetal hypokinesia syndrome in the monochorionic pair of a triplet pregnancy secondary to severe disruptive cerebral injury. *Pediatrics*. 1995;96:521-523.
57. Sztriha L, Al-Gazali LI, Varady E, et al. Autosomal recessive microencephaly with simplified gyral pattern, abnormal myelination and arthrogryposis. *Neuropediatrics*. 1999;30:141-145.
58. Brodtkorb E, Torbergsen T, Nakken KO, et al. Epileptic seizures, arthrogryposis, and migrational brain disorders: a syndrome? *Acta Neurol Scand*. 1994;90:232-240.
59. Bianchi DW, Van Marter LJ. An approach to ventilator dependent neonates with arthrogryposis. *Pediatrics*. 1994;94:682-686.
61. Vuopala K, Leisti J, Herva R. Lethal arthrogryposis in Finland—a clinco-pathological study of 83 cases during thirteen years. *Neuropediatrics*. 1995;25:308-315.
62. Rudnik-Schoneborn S, Sztriha L, Aithala GR, et al. Extended phenotype of pontocerebellar hypoplasia with infantile spinal muscular atrophy. *Am J Med Genet*. 2003;117A:10-17.
63. Moerman P, Fryns JP, Coddeeris P, et al. Multiple ankylosis, facial anomalies, and pulmonary hypoplasia associated with severe antenatal spinal muscular atrophy. *J Pediatr*. 1983;103:238.
64. Amick LD, Johnson WW, Smith HL. Electromyographic and histopathologic correlations in arthrogryposis. *Arch Neurol*. 1967;16:512.
65. Byers RK, Banker BQ. Infantile muscular atrophy. *Arch Neurol*. 1961;5:140.
66. Vuopala K, Makela-Bengs P, Suomalainen A, et al. Lethal congenital contracture syndrome, a fetal anterior horn cell disease is not linked to the SMA 5q locus. *J Med Genet*. 1995;32:36-38.
67. Vuopala K, Ignatius J, Herva R. Lethal arthrogryposis with anterior horn cell disease. *Hum Pathol*. 1995;26:12-19.
68. Frijns C, Vandeutekom J, Frants RR, et al. Dominant congenital benign spinal muscular atrophy. *Muscle Nerve*. 1994;17:192-197.
69. Hageman G. Congenital brachial arthrogryposis. *J Neurol Neurosurg Psychiatry*. 1993;56:365-368.
70. Mercuri E, Messina S, Kinali M, et al. Congenital form of spinal muscular atrophy predominantly affecting the lower limbs: a clinical and muscle MRI study. *Neuromuscul Disord*. 2004;14:125-129.
71. Rudnik-Schoneborn S, Stolz P, Varon R, et al. Long-term observations of patients with infantile spinal muscular atrophy with respiratory distress type 1 (SMARD1). *Neuropediatrics*. 2004;35:174-182.
72. Kaiboriboon K, Hayat GR. Congenital cervical spinal atrophy: an intrauterine hypoxic insult. *Neuropediatrics*. 2001;32:330-334.
73. Mercuri E, Goodwin F, Sewry C, et al. Diaphragmatic spinal muscular atrophy with bulbar weakness. *Eur J Paediatr Neurol*. 2000;4:69-72.
74. Torres AR, Jones HR, Darras BT. Electromyography and biopsy correlation study of infants with arthrogryposis multiplex congenita. *Ann Neurol*. 1999;46:535.
75. Makela-Bengs P, Jarvinen N, Vuopala K, et al. Assignment of the disease locus for lethal congenital contracture syndrome to a restricted region of chromosome 9q34, by genome scan using five affected individuals. *Am J Hum Genet*. 1998;63:506-516.
76. Rudnik-Schoneborn S, Forkert R, Hahnen E, et al. Clinical spectrum and diagnostic criteria of infantile spinal muscular atrophy: further delineation on the basis of SMN gene deletion findings. *Neuropediatrics*. 1996;27:8-15.
77. Greenberg F, Fenolio KR, Hejtmancik F, et al. X-linked infantile spinal muscular atrophy. *Am J Dis Child*. 1988;142:217-219.
78. Strehl E, Vanasse M. EMG and needle muscle biopsy studies in arthrogryposis multiplex congenita. *Neuropediatrics*. 1985;16:225-227.
79. Drachman DB, Banker BQ. Arthrogryposis multiplex congenita. Case due to disease of the anterior horn cells. *Arch Neurol*. 1961;5:77.
80. Hall JG, Reed SD, Scott CI. Three distinct types of X-linked arthrogryposis seen in six families. *Clin Genet*. 1982;21:81-97.
81. Fleury P, Hageman G. A dominantly inherited lower motor neuron disorder presenting at birth with associated arthrogryposis. *J Neurol Neurosurg Psychiatry*. 1985;48:1037-1048.
82. Hageman G, Jennekens FGI, Vette JK, et al. The heterogeneity of distal arthrogryposis. *Brain Dev*. 1984;6:273.
83. Tsukamoto H, Inagaki M, Tomita Y, et al. Congenital caudal spinal atrophy—a case report. *Neuropediatrics*. 1992;23:260-262.
84. Robertson WL, Glinski LP, Kirkpatrick SJ, et al. Further evidence that arthrogryposis multiplex congenita in the human sometimes is caused by an intrauterine vascular accident. *Teratology*. 1992;45:345-351.
86. Kizilates SU, Talim B, Sel K, et al. Severe lethal spinal muscular atrophy variant with arthrogryposis. *Pediatr Neurol*. 2005;32:201-204.
87. Imamura M, Yamanaka N, Nakamura F, et al. Arthrogryposis multiplex congenita: an autopsy case of a fatal form. *Hum Pathol*. 1981;12:699.
88. Darwish H, Sarnat H, Archer G. Congenital cervical spinal atrophy. *Muscle Nerve*. 1981;4:106.
89. Coelho KEFA, Sarmento MV, Veiga CM, et al. Misoprostol embryotoxicity: clinical evaluation of fifteen patients with arthrogryposis. *Am J Med Genet*. 2000;95:297-301.
90. Patel N, Smith LL, Faqeih E, et al. ZBTB42 mutation defines a novel lethal congenital contracture syndrome (LCCS6). *Hum Mol Genet*. 2014;23:6584-6593.
91. Renbaum P, Kellerman E, Jaron R, et al. Spinal muscular atrophy with pontocerebellar hypoplasia is caused by a mutation in the VRK1 gene. *Am J Hum Genet*. 2009;85:281-289.
92. Peeters K, Chamova T, Jordanova A. Clinical and genetic diversity of SMN1-negative proximal spinal muscular atrophies. *Brain*. 2014;137:2879-2896.
93. Narkis G, Ofir R, Landau D, et al. Lethal contractural syndrome type 3 (LCCS3) is caused by a mutation in PIP5K1C, which encodes PIPKI gamma of the phophatidylinsitol pathway. *Am J Hum Genet*. 2007;81:530-539.
94. Koutsopoulos OS, Kretz C, Weller CM, et al. Dynamin 2 homozygous mutation in humans with a lethal congenital syndrome. *Eur J Hum Genet*. 2013;21:637-642.
95. Markus B, Narkis G, Landau D, et al. Autosomal recessive lethal congenital contractural syndrome type 4 (LCCS4) caused by a mutation in MYBPC1. *Hum Mutat*. 2012;33:1435-1438.
96. Jedrzejowska M, Jakubowska-Pietkiewicz E, Kostera-Pruszczyk A. X-linked spinal muscular atrophy (SMAX2) caused by de novo c.1731C>T substitution in the UBA1 gene. *Neuromuscul Disord*. 2015;25:661-666.
97. Rudnik-Schoneborn S, Senderek J, Jen JC, et al. Pontocerebellar hypoplasia type 1: clinical spectrum and relevance of EXOSC3 mutations. *Neurology*. 2013;80:438-446.
98. Narkis G, Ofir R, Manor E, et al. Lethal congenital contractural syndrome type 2 (LCCS2) is caused by a mutation in ERBB3 (Her3), a modulator of the phosphatidylinositol-3-kinase/Akt pathway. *Am J Hum Genet*. 2007;81:589-595.
99. Nousiainen HO, Kestila M, Pakkasjarvi N, et al. Mutations in mRNA export mediator GLE1 result in a fetal motoneuron disease. *Nat Genet*. 2008;40:155-157.
100. Sakonju A, Crawford TO. Acquired presynaptic neuromuscular junction disorders: infant botulism and Lambert-Eaton myasthenic syndrome. In: Darras BT, Jones HR Jr, Ryan MM, et al., eds. *Neuromuscular Disorders of Infancy, Childhood and Adolescence: A Clinician's Approach*. 2nd ed. San Diego: Academic Press; 2015:445-455.
101. Kang PB, Lidov HGW, David WS, et al. Diagnostic value of electyromyography and muscle biopsy in arthrogryposis multiplex congenita. *Ann Neurol*. 2003;54:790-795.
102. Henderson JL. The congenital facial diplegia syndrome: clinical features, pathology and etiology. *Brain*. 1939;62:381.
103. Sarnat HB, Case ME, Graviss R. Sacral agenesis. Neurology and neuropathologic features. *Neurology*. 1976;26:1124.
105. Dubowitz V. *Muscle Disorders in Childhood*. 2nd ed. London: WB Saunders; 1995.
106. Takada E, Koyama N, Ogawa Y, et al. Neuropathology of infant with Pena-Shokeir I syndrome. *Pediatr Neurol*. 1994;10:241-243.
107. Folkerth RD, Guttentag SH, Kupsky WJ, et al. Arthrogryposis multiplex congenita with posterior column degeneration and peripheral neuropathy: a case report. *Clin Neuropathol*. 1993;12:25-33.
108. Seitz RJ, Wechsler W, Mosny DS, et al. Hypomyelination neuropathy in a female newborn presenting as arthrogryposis multiplex congenita. *Neuropediatrics*. 1986;17:132-136.

109. Boylan KB, Ferriero DM, Greco CM, et al. Congenital hypomyelination neuropathy with arthrogryposis multiplex congenita. *Ann Neurol.* 1992;31:337-340.

110. Yuill GM, Lynch PG. Congenital non-progressive peripheral neuropathy with arthrogryposis multiplex. *J Neurol Neurosurg Psychiatry.* 1974;37:316-323.

112. Gibson DA, Urs NDK. Arthrogryposis multiplex congenita. *J Bone Joint Surg Br.* 1970;3:483-493.

113. Hooshmand H, Martinez AJ, Rosenblum WI. Arthrogryposis multiplex congenita. Simultaneous involvement of peripheral nerve and skeletal muscle. *Arch Neurol.* 1971;24:561.

114. Moore BH. Some orthopedic relationships of neurofibromatosis. *J Bone Joint Surg.* 1941;23:109.

115. Shepard MK. Arthrogryposis multiplex congenita in sibs. *Birth Defects Orig Artic Ser.* 1971;7:127.

116. Moutard-Codou ML, Delleur MM, Doulac O, et al. Myasthenic neo-natale servere avec arthrogrypose. *Press Med.* 1987;16:615-618.

117. Dulitzky F, Sirota L, Landman J, et al. An infant with multiple deformations born to a myasthenic mother. *Helv Paediatr Acta.* 1987;42:173-176.

118. Pasternak JF, Hageman J, Adams MA. Exchange transfusion in neonatal myasthenia. *J Pediatr.* 1981;99:644.

119. Dalton P, Clover L, Wallerstein R, et al. Fetal arthrogryposis and maternal serum antibodies. *Neuromuscul Disord.* 2006;16:481-491.

120. Hoff JM, Daltveit AK, Gilhus NE. Myasthenia gravis. Consequences for pregnancy, delivery, and the newborn. *Neurology.* 2003;61:1362-1366.

121. Brueton LA, Huson SM, Cox PM, et al. Asymptomatic maternal myasthenia as a cause of the Pena-Shokeir phenotype. *Am J Med Genet.* 2000;92:1-6.

122. Carr SR, Gilchrist JM, Abuelo DN, et al. Treatment of antenatal myasthenia gravis. *Obstet Gynecol.* 1991;78:485-489.

123. Holmes LB, Driscoll SG, Bradley WG. Contractures in a newborn infant of a mother with myasthenia gravis. *J Pediatr.* 1980;96:1067.

124. Vajsar J, Sloane A, MacGregor DL, et al. Arthrogryposis multiplex congenita due to congenital myasthenic syndrome. *Pediatr Neurol.* 1995;12:237-241.

125. Barisic N, Muller JS, Paucic-Kirincic E, et al. Clinical variability of CMS-EA (congenital myasthenic syndrome with episodic apnea) due to identical CHAT mutations in two infants. *Eur J Paediatr Neurol.* 2005;9:7-12.

126. Harper CM. Congenital myasthenic syndromes. *Semin Neurol.* 2004;24:111-123.

127. Burke G, Cossins J, Maxwell S, et al. Distinct phenotypes of congenital acetylcholine receptor deficiency. *Neuromuscul Disord.* 2004;14:356-364.

129. Smit LME, Barth PG. Arthrogryposis multiplex congenita due to congenital myasthenia. *Dev Med Child Neurol.* 1980;22:371.

130. Milone M, Shen XM, Selcen D, et al. Myasthenic syndrome due to defects in rapsyn: clinical and molecular findings in 39 patients. *Neurology.* 2009;73:228-235.

131. Natera-de Benito D, Bestue M, Vilchez JJ, et al. Long-term follow-up in patients with congenital myasthenic syndrome due to RAPSN mutations. *Neuromuscul Disord.* 2016;26:153-159.

132. Chen CP. Prenatal diagnosis and genetic analysis of fetal akinesia deformation sequence and multiple pterygium syndrome associated with neuromuscular junction disorders: a review. *Taiwan J Obstet Gynecol.* 2012;51:12-17.

133. Robinson KG, Viereck MJ, Margiotta MV, et al. Neuromotor synapses in Escobar syndrome. *Am J Med Genet A.* 2013;161A:3042-3048.

134. Livingstone IR, Sack GH. Arthrogryposis multiplex congenita occurring with maternal multiple sclerosis. *Arch Neurol.* 1984;41:1216-1217.

135. Hall JG, Reed SD. Teratogens associated with congenital contractures in humans and in animals. *Teratology.* 1982;25:173-191.

136. Dahl J, Myhr KM, Daltveit AK, et al. Pregnancy, delivery, and birth outcome in women with multiple sclerosis. *Neurology.* 2005;65:1961-1963.

137. Vasta I, Kinali M, Messina S, et al. Can clinical signs identify newborns with neuromuscular disorders? *J Pediatr.* 2005;146:73-79.

138. Romero NB, Monnier N, Viollet L, et al. Dominant and recessive central core disease associated with RYR1 mutations and fetal akinesia. *Brain.* 2003;126:2341-2349.

139. Zaharieva IT, Thor MG, Oates EC, et al. Loss-of-function mutations in SCN4A cause severe foetal hypokinesia or 'classical' congenital myopathy. *Brain.* 2016;139:674-691.

140. Illum N, Reske-Nielsen E, Skovby F, et al. Lethal autosomal recessive arthrogryposis multiplex congenita with whistling face and calcifications of the nervous system. *Neuropediatrics.* 1988;19:186-192.

141. Alves AFP, Azevedo ES. Recessive form of Freeman-Sheldon's syndrome or "whistling face". *J Med Genet.* 1977;14:139-141.

142. Sauk JJ, Delaney JR, Reaume C, et al. Electromyography of oral-facial musculature in cranio-carpaltarsal dysplasia (Freeman-Sheldon syndrome). *Clin Genet.* 1974;6:132-137.

143. Banker BQ, Victor M, Adams RD. Arthrogryposis multiplex due to congenital muscular dystrophy. *Brain.* 1957;80:319.

144. Sells JM, Jaffe KM, Hall JG. Amyoplasia, the most common type of arthrogryposis: the potential for good outcome. *Pediatrics.* 1996;97:225-231.

146. Sarnat HB, Silbert SW. Maturational arrest of fetal muscle in neonatal myotonic dystrophy. *Arch Neurol.* 1976;33:466.

147. Pearson CM, Fowler WG. Hereditary non-progressive muscular dystrophy inducing arthrogryposis multiplex. *Brain.* 1963;86:75.

148. Kirschner J, Hausser I, Zou YQ, et al. Ullrich congenital muscular dystrophy: connective tissue abnormalities in the skin support overlap with Ehlers-Danlos syndromes. *Am J Med Genet A.* 2005;132A:296-301.

149. Philpot J, Counsell S, Bydder G, et al. Neonatal arthrogryposis and absent limb muscles: a muscle developmental gene defect? *Neuromuscul Disord.* 2001;11:489-493.

150. Vielhaber S, Feistner H, Schneider W, et al. Mitochondrial complex I deficiency in a female with multiplex arthrogryposis congenita. *Pediatr Neurol.* 2000;22:53-56.

151. Laubscher B, Janzer RC, Kruhenbuhl S, et al. Ragged-red fibres and complex I deficiency in a neonate with arthrogryposis congenita. *Pediatr Neurol.* 1997;17:249-251.

152. Tajsharghi H, Kimber E, Holmgren D, et al. Distal arthrogryposis and muscle weakness associated with a beta-tropomyosin mutation. *Neurology.* 2007;68:772-775.

153. Vuopala K, Pedrosadomellof F, Herva R, et al. Familial fetal akinesia deformation sequence with a skeletal muscle maturation defect. *Acta Neuropathol.* 1995;90:176-183.

154. Hecht F, Beals RK. New syndrome of congenital contractual arachnodactyly originally described by Marfan in 1896. *Pediatrics.* 1972;49:574.

158. Adams C, Becker L, Murphy EG. Neurogenic arthrogryposis multiplex congenita: clinical and muscle biopsy findings. *Pediatr Neurosci.* 1988;14:97-102.

159. Uchida T, Nonaka I, Yokochi K, et al. Arthrogryposis multiplex congenita: histochemical study of biopsied muscles. *Pediatr Neurol.* 1985;1:169-173.

160. Gaitanis JN, McMillan HJ, Wu A, et al. Electrophysiologic evidence for anterior horn cell disease in amyoplasia. *Pediatr Neurol.* 2010;43:142-147.

161. Hahn G. Arthrogryposis: pediatric review and habilitative aspects. *Clin Orthop.* 1985;194:104.

162. Palmer PM, MacEwen GD, Bowen JR, et al. Passive motion therapy for infants with arthrogryposis. *Clin Orthop.* 1985;194:54.

163. Carlson WO, Speck GJ, Vicari V, et al. Arthrogryposis multiplex congenita: a long-term followup study. *Clin Orthop.* 1985;194:115.

164. Staheli LT. Orthopedic management principles. In: Staheli LT, Hall JG, Jaffe KM, et al., eds. *Arthrogryposis.* Cambridge: Cambridge University Press; 1998:27-43.

165. Bach A, Almquist L, LaGrone M. Upper limb and spine. In: Staheli LT, Hall JG, Jaffe KM, et al., eds. *Arthrogryposis.* Cambridge: Cambridge University Press; 1998:45-53.

166. Staheli LT. Lower extremity management. In: Staheli LT, Hall JG, Jaffe KM, et al., eds. *Arthrogryposis.* Cambridge: Cambridge University Press; 1998:55-73.

167. Jaffe KM. Rehabilitation: scope and principles. In: Staheli LT, Hall JG, Jaffe KM, et al., eds. *Arthrogryposis.* Cambridge: Cambridge University Press; 1998:75-85.

168. Graubert CS, Chaplin DL, Jaffe KM. Physical and occupational therapy. In: Staheli LT, Hall JG, Jaffe KM, et al., eds. *Arthrogryposis.* Cambridge: Cambridge University Press; 1998:87-113.

Full references for this chapter can be found on www.expertconsult .com.

Levels Above Lower Motor Neuron to Neuromuscular Junction

Basil T. Darras ◆ *Joseph J. Volpe*

An effective means of attaining an understanding of the major disorders of the neonatal motor system is to organize the approach to these disorders on the basis of the major affected anatomical site within the motor system. Thus in this chapter and in Chapter 33, we review disorders of the neonatal motor system according to the following specific anatomical levels: levels above the lower motor neuron and at the lower motor neuron, the peripheral (and cranial) nerve, the neuromuscular junction, and, finally, the muscle.

The major unifying clinical manifestations of the disorders are hypotonia and weakness, not necessarily occurring with similar severity, as discussed later. In this chapter, all disorders, except those related to the involvement of muscle (see Chapter 33), are reviewed, principally in terms of clinical features, results of pertinent laboratory studies, pathological features, pathogenesis and etiology, and management.

LEVELS ABOVE THE LOWER MOTOR NEURON

Disorders leading to hypotonia and weakness that are secondary to the involvement of anatomical levels above the lower motor neuron are summarized in Box 32.1. These disorders are best discussed here as a group, because most are reviewed in detail in other sections of this book. Although the group is rather diverse, three features are generally useful in establishing the locus of the hypotonia at an anatomical level above the lower motor neuron. First, in these so-called central disorders, hypotonia is usually more severe than weakness, and indeed some affected infants, although *floppy*, exhibit strong movements when stimulated. Second, tendon reflexes are usually preserved, although it is unusual to observe the hallmark of central hypotonia, as seen after the first weeks and months of life: hyperactive tendon reflexes. Thus, as with weakness, hypotonia is more marked than is involvement of the tendon reflexes. Third, other signs of central involvement are frequently present; particular note should be made of seizures.

Congenital Encephalopathies

For the purposes of this section, congenital encephalopathies are defined as those with onset before or during the perinatal period and affecting principally cerebrum, brain stem, or cerebellum (see Box 32.1). In contrast to degenerative encephalopathies, these disorders are not progressive, although worsening may occur if infectious, metabolic, or endocrine disturbance is not corrected.

Hypoxia-Ischemia

Hypoxic-ischemic encephalopathy is by far the most common cause of hypotonia in the newborn period. Other features of this disorder are described in Chapters 16 and 20. In patients with minor degrees of this encephalopathy, hypotonia may be the principal neurological abnormality.

Intracranial Hemorrhage and Infection

Intracranial hemorrhage (see Chapters 22–24) and intracranial infection (bacterial and nonbacterial; see Chapters 34 and 35) are relatively uncommon causes of hypotonia in the absence of other features that distinguish these disorders.

Metabolic Disorders

The metabolic disturbances that can result in hypotonia in the newborn period are extremely diverse. Abnormal increases or decreases in electrolyte levels, acidemia, hypoglycemia, increases in divalent cation levels, severe hyperbilirubinemia, aminoacidopathies (including syndromes with hyperammonemia), organic acid disturbances, sepsis, and intoxication of the fetus by administration (usually intrapartum) of analgesics, sedatives, or anesthetics to the mother are the most common of these metabolic disturbances (see Chapters 25–28).

Other rarer metabolic disorders should also be considered. An important category encompasses disturbances in central neurotransmission, the most common of which is aromatic l-amino acid decarboxylase deficiency (see Chapter 29).[1] Neonatal onset occurs in more than 50% of cases, and hypotonia and feeding difficulties are prominent early findings.[2-6] Diagnosis is suggested by the finding of reduced catecholamine metabolites in cerebrospinal fluid (CSF), and it is established by the demonstration of markedly reduced plasma aromatic l-amino acid decarboxylase activity. Subsequent findings include hypokinesia, oculogyric crises, movement disorders, and autonomic disturbances.

Endocrine Disorders

Hypothyroidism is an important endocrine disorder that may produce neonatal hypotonia. A large tongue, temperature instability, feeding problems, constipation, hoarse cry, dry mottled skin, prolonged jaundice, and delayed skeletal maturation should suggest hypothyroidism.[7,8] Neonatal screening of filter paper blood samples has proved superior to clinical recognition and is of considerable value in early detection of hypothyroidism.[7-12] It is critical to identify and to treat hypothyroidism promptly

---

BOX 32.1   Hypotonia and Weakness: Levels Above the Lower Motor Neuron

Congenital (Nonprogressive) Encephalopathies
Hypoxia-ischemia[a]
Intracranial hemorrhage
Intracranial infection
Metabolic
    Multiple (see text)
Endocrine
    Hypothyroid
Trauma
Developmental disturbance
    Cerebral[a] (e.g., Prader-Willi syndrome, neuronal migration
        disorders)
    Cerebellar
Degenerative (Progressive) Encephalopathies
See Chapter 29
Spinal Cord Disorders
Trauma
Developmental

[a]The two most common causes.

BOX 32.2   Major Neonatal Features of Prader-Willi Syndrome[a]

Hypotonia with diminished tendon reflexes
Poor feeding with poor weight gain
Weak cry: often *squeaky*, not sustained
Craniofacial characteristics
    Dolichocephaly, narrow bifrontal diameter
    Almond-shaped eyes
    Small mouth with thin upper lip and downturned corners of mouth
Hypogonadism (male: undescended testes; scrotal hypoplasia; female:
    absence or severe hypoplasia of labia minora and/or clitoris)
History of fetal inactivity
Normal neuromuscular studies
Neuropathological and molecular genetic studies suggesting disturbed
    neuronal and axonal development
Chromosomal disturbance: deletion of the proximal long arm of
    chromosome 15 (15q11–q13 region) in 65%–75%; uniparental
    (maternal) disomy in 20%–30%; imprinting defect in 2%–3%.

[a]See text for references.

---

because of the deleterious effect of the thyroid deficiency on brain development (see Chapters 5–8).

Trauma

Trauma may result in hemorrhagic and nonhemorrhagic lesions of brain, which are uncommon causes of hypotonia, particularly in the absence of other features that dominate the clinical syndrome. Details are provided in Chapters 22, 23, and 36.

Developmental Disturbance

Aberrations of brain development are relatively frequent findings among the neonatal causes of hypotonia referable to anatomical levels above the lower motor neuron. Cerebrum and cerebellum are the principal sites of involvement in these cases. Developmental disturbances of cerebrum, which may result in striking hypotonia, are reviewed in Chapters 6 to 8. Disturbances of neuronal migration are the most prominent cerebral causes. Important examples of cerebral hypotonia are the cerebrohepatorenal syndrome of Zellweger, the oculocerebrorenal syndrome of Lowe, and Prader-Willi syndrome (PWS). The cerebrohepatorenal syndrome of Zellweger is discussed in Chapter 6, along with disorders of neuronal migration.

The oculocerebrorenal syndrome of Lowe is an X-linked recessive disorder, characterized by ocular abnormalities (cataracts and congenital glaucoma), marked hypotonia, cryptorchidism, and renal abnormalities (proteinuria and generalized aminoaciduria). Subsequent development is markedly retarded. The cerebral abnormality has not been defined clearly.

PWS is characterized by striking neonatal hypotonia, accompanied by diminished deep tendon reflexes, poor feeding, weak cry, and often a history of fetal inactivity.[13-27] Careful attention to the clinical and other features described in Box 32.2 allows diagnosis in the neonatal period before development of the complete syndrome of hyperphagia, morbid

obesity, short stature, and cognitive impairment.[13,28-30] The intelligence quotient is less than 70 in 85% of cases, most commonly (75%) in the 40 to 69 range, and is always less than 84.[30] Normal neuromuscular studies such as muscle biopsy and the associated later clinical features (e.g., cognitive impairment) support the conclusion that the hypotonia is on a central basis. The limited neuropathological studies thus far conducted indicate frequent abnormalities of gyral development, hypoplasia of corpus callosum, and minor cerebral, brain stem, and cerebellar migrational anomalies.[26,27] A careful magnetic resonance imaging (MRI) study also showed gyral anomalies reminiscent of polymicrogyria.[31] Two of the proteins deficient in PWS (i.e., NECDIN and MAGEL2) are critically involved in neuronal differentiation and axonal outgrowth.[32] PWS results from three main molecular mechanisms: paternal deletion, maternal uniparental disomy (UPD) 15, and imprinting defect (ID). In addition to NECDIN and MAGEL2, the PWS critical region on chromosome 15 also includes another three paternal-only origin expressed genes that encode MKRN3 and SNURF-SNRPN proteins. The adjacent UBE3A and ATP10A genes are expressed only in the maternally derived chromosome and are involved in the pathogenesis of Angelman syndrome (AS). The diagnosis is established by detection of the chromosome 15 deletion by fluorescent in situ hybridization (FISH) or by chromosomal microarray (CMA) analysis in the 65% to 75% of patients so affected. The approximately 20% to 30% of patients with UPD have normal deletion studies but an abnormal DNA methylation test. The risk of recurrence in large interstitial 5 to 6 Mb 15q11.2–q13 deletion and pure maternal UPD (without predisposing parental translocation) is less than 1%. The 2% to 3% of cases associated with an ID are detected by DNA methylation studies; recurrence risk in this small group could be as high as 50% if the father also has an imprinting center (IC) deletion. ID without IC deletion carries less than 1% recurrence risk. Advanced DNA methylation techniques such as MS-MLPA (methylation-specific multiplex ligation-dependent probe amplification) can detect deletions, UPD, and ID in more than 99% of PWS patients;

this technique can distinguish between deletion and UPD but will not distinguish UPD from ID.[33] Various other probable disturbances of cerebral development (e.g., eponymic syndromes and chromosomal aberrations), some alluded to in Chapters 1 to 8, may cause neonatal hypotonia, but more distinguishing features usually dominate the clinical syndrome.

Developmental disturbance of cerebellum may lead to neonatal hypotonia (see Chapter 4). In one carefully studied series of seven such cases, neonatal hypotonia, occasionally severe, occurred without weakness.[34] Jerky eye movements were prominent, and truncal titubation was apparent within a few weeks. Ataxia and intention tremor appeared later in the first year. Computed tomography scans or pneumoencephalograms demonstrated a strikingly enlarged cisterna magna with symmetrical hypoplasia of the cerebellum. The combination of hypotonia, jerky eye movements, and radiographic findings was diagnostic. Pathological study showed nearly complete absence of internal granule cells, with relatively preserved numbers of Purkinje cells. I (JJV) have seen several similar cases and have been impressed by the hypotonia present in early infancy with Dandy-Walker malformation and Joubert syndrome and related disorders, all disorders of cerebellar development (see Chapter 4).

Degenerative Encephalopathies

Most degenerative disorders of infancy manifest after the first weeks of life. However, many of these disorders may cause hypotonia in the newborn period (see Chapter 29).

Spinal Cord Disorders

Disorders of the spinal cord are frequently overlooked causes of hypotonia and weakness in newborn (see Box 32.1). Traumatic injury is a relatively common cause, and the traumatic event may go undetected in the absence of a careful history (see Chapter 36). Developmental disorders (e.g., dysraphic states) are associated usually with signs restricted to lower or, less commonly, upper extremities and are recognized more readily (see Chapter 1).

LEVEL OF THE LOWER MOTOR NEURON

Disorders affecting the lower motor neuron are the most frequent causes of severe hypotonia and weakness in the neonatal period. The major disorders to be distinguished are listed in Box 32.3. Of these, type 1 spinal muscular atrophy (SMA) or Werdnig-Hoffmann disease is the most common and most important.

BOX 32.3   Hypotonia and Weakness: Level of the Lower Motor Neuron

Spinal muscular atrophy type 1 (Werdnig-Hoffmann disease; also type 0 or type 1A)
Spinal muscular atrophy variants (anterior horn cell disorders not linked to chromosome 5q, non-5q spinal muscular atrophies)
Neurogenic arthrogryposis multiplex congenita
Glycogen storage disease type II (Pompe disease)
Hypoxic-ischemic injury
Neonatal poliomyelitis (other enteroviruses?)

Spinal Muscular Atrophy Type 1 (Werdnig-Hoffmann Disease)

Type 1 SMA or Werdnig-Hoffmann disease refers to the severe, infantile, hereditary form of anterior horn cell disease. This disorder is autosomal recessively inherited. The earliest descriptions of hereditary degeneration of anterior horn cell with onset in infancy were by Werdnig in Austria and Hoffmann in Germany from 1891 to 1900.[35-39] Although the original cases described by Werdnig and Hoffmann did not have their onset in the first weeks of life, the severe, early onset form of SMA type 1 is often referred to as Werdnig-Hoffmann disease. This severe form of SMA (i.e., type 1) is defined by onset before 6 months of age, failure to develop the ability to sit unsupported, and death usually by less than 2 years of age (see later discussion).[24] (This definition contrasts with that for SMA type 2, which is defined as onset less than 18 months of age, ability to sit unsupported, failure to develop the ability to walk, and death after 2 years of age, and with that for SMA type 3, which is defined as onset after 18 months of age, ability to stand and walk, and death in adulthood.)

The recognition of several very severe cases of SMA with clear prenatal onset, multiple joint contractures, ventilatory compromise at birth, early deficits of facial movement, bone fractures, and death by 3 months led to the recognition of an additional type, termed type 0 or type 1A.[40-42] Although these cases occur rarely, it is critical to recognize that the diagnosis of SMA is not excluded by the findings of overt arthrogryposis, respiratory failure at birth, or bone fractures. SMA type 1 has been further divided into type 1B with onset of symptoms before 3 months of age and type 1C with onset between 3 and 6 months of age.

Pathogenesis and Etiology

The acute, early-onset, type 1 form of SMA (Werdnig-Hoffmann disease) as well as the rare, very severe type 0 form and the later-onset, chronic forms (types 2 and 3) are all related to a genetic defect that involves the q13 region of chromosome 5.[24,43-58] The SMA region consists of a large (500 kb) inverted duplication containing two copies of the gene deleted (or mutated) in SMA (i.e., the survival motor neuron [SMN] gene; Fig. 32.1). Thus on each chromosome 5 are two copies of SMN: telomeric (SMN1) and centromeric (SMN2) copies. The deletions involve the telomeric copy. Homozygous deletions involving exon 7 of the SMN1 gene occur in approximately 95% of cases of SMA, with the remaining cases harboring a deletion in one allele and a heterozygous point mutation in the other allele (compound heterozygotes; Table 32.1).[50,57-64] The nearly identical SMN2 gene, which contains a single nucleotide change in exon 7 (a C-to-T transition) that profoundly influences splicing, produces primarily 90% to 95% of a truncated protein lacking exon 7 and having a short half-life and only approximately 5% to 10% of the normal full-length protein. Because of the genomic instability of this duplicated region of chromosome 5, SMN2 copy number may increase or decrease in the presence of the deleted SMN1 gene. The importance of this phenomenon in this context is that abundant evidence in animal models and now in humans shows that the copy number of SMN2 is the most critical determinant of the severity of the SMA phenotype.[a]

---

[a]References 40, 41, 57, 58, 60, and 61.

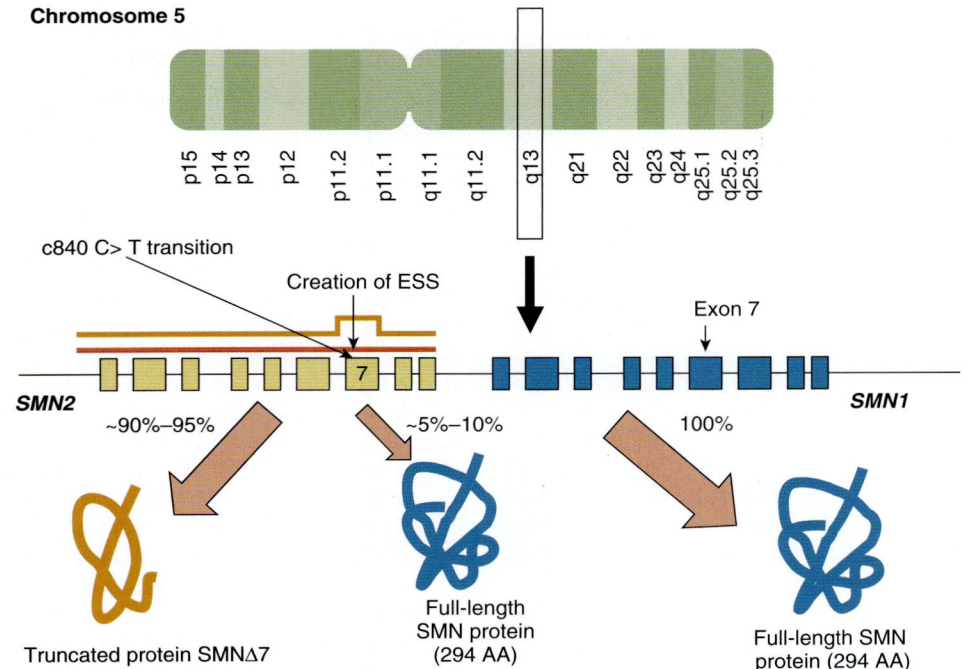

Figure 32.1 Schematic diagram of human *SMN1* and *SMN2* genes on chromosome 5. Patients with spinal muscular atrophy have deletions or mutations in both copies of SMN1. A C-to-T transition at position 6 of SMN2 creates an exonic splicing suppressor (ESS) that leads to skipping of exon 7 during transcription and production of truncated, nonfunctional SMN protein. However, a small amount (~5% to 10%) of full-length messenger RNA is produced from the SMN2 gene, resulting in functional, full-length SMN protein. *AA,* Amino acids; *SMN,* survival motor neuron. (Modified with permission from Darras BT, Markowitz JA, Monani UR, De Vivo DC. Spinal muscular atrophies. In: Darras BT, Jones HR Jr, Ryan MM, De Vivo DC, eds. *Neuromuscular Disorders of Infancy, Childhood and Adolescence: A Clinician's Approach.* 2nd ed. San Diego: Academic Press; 2015:chap 8, 117–145.)

Children with SMA carry various SMN2 copy numbers: of SMA type 1 patients, 80% to 96% carry one or two SMN2 copies (more than 70% carry two SMN2 copies) and 4% to 20% have three copies; of SMA type 2 patients, 82% have three copies of SMN2; and of SMA type 3 patients, 96% to 100% have three or four copies of SMN2 (Fig. 32.2).[65,66] However, the SMN2 copy number is not an accurate predictor of phenotype. Other contributing factors may include modifier genes affecting the motor neurons, and mutations in the SMN2 gene that alter the amount of full length SMN protein it produces. Even among family members who carry the same number of SMN2 copy numbers, variation is observed, suggesting that modulators of SMN2 splicing and other modifier genes may be involved.[67]

The biological functions of SMN1 and its relationship with SMA have been elucidated.[57,58,61,68-73] The SMN protein interacts with other proteins in a multimolecular complex and appears to be involved principally in RNA metabolism. The most critical function of SMN is in the assembly of the ribonucleoproteins of the so-called spliceosome, which is critically involved in the removal of introns from pre-RNA and splicing together of exons in mature RNA, for many proteins. The biological functions potentially affected are many, but most recent work suggests that axonal growth and maintenance are key roles. Spinal cord motor neurons are selectively vulnerable to decreased SMN protein. These neurons (as well as others) have long axons and many targets, particularly in large muscles, and may heavily depend on axonal mRNA transport; SMN protein plays a role in axonal mRNA trafficking. Whether the pathogenesis of SMA is due to a splicing defect caused by SMN protein deficiency, disruption of an additional axonal SMN function, an unknown function, or a combination of the above is still unknown.[74] Absence of SMN protein in cells is embryonic lethal in mice and other organisms.[75] Why partial SMN deficiency specifically affects motor neurons in the spinal cord and brain stem remains unclear.

Clinical Features

Onset. SMA type 1 is clinically apparent at birth or in the first several months of life.[57,60,76,77] In one large series, clinical onset was at birth in 35%, in the first month in 16%, in the second month in 23%, and from the end of the second month to the sixth month in 26%.[78] The finding of onset before 6 months with a median age of onset of 1 to 2 months is consistent.[50,76-84] Onset in utero is supported by the observation that in most patients with SMA type 1 presenting at birth or in the early neonatal period, decreased and weak fetal movements in the last trimester are reported by the patients' mothers.[77] Neuropathological data (see later) have documented prenatal onset.[85] In particularly severely affected infants, neonatal asphyxia or respiratory distress may occur.[86] As just noted, some particularly severely affected infants (type 0) also may exhibit early deficits of facial movement, arthrogryposis, severe diffuse weakness, and early death.[40-42] In those infants whose disease is not apparent at birth, onset in the first weeks is often acute.[87] Indeed, clinical progression to severe disability

TABLE 32.1   Genetic Diagnostic Testing in Spinal Muscular Atrophy

TYPE OF MUTATION	TEST APPLIED	MUTATION DETECTION RATE
Homozygous deletion of exon 7[a]	SMN1 Targeted mutation analysis PCR/restriction enzyme analysis or multiplex ligation probe amplification methodologies	~95%–98%
Compound heterozygosity (Deletion of SMN1 exon 7 [allele 1] and an intragenic mutation of SMN1[b] [allele 2])	Targeted mutation analysis combined with SMN1 gene sequence analysis[c]	2%–5%
SMN2 copy number[d]	Quantitative PCR analysis and other methodologies[e]	N/A

[a]Testing for exon 8 deletion is not necessary.

[b]Small intragenic deletions/insertions and nonsense, missense, and splice site mutations.

[c]Whole-gene deletions/duplications are not detected.

[d]SMN2 copy number ranges from 0 to 5.

[e]MLPA, long-range PCR, chromosomal microarray (CMA) that includes the SMN1, SMN2 chromosomal segment.

PCR, Polymerase chain reaction; SMN, survival motor neuron.

Reprinted with permission from Darras BT, Markowitz JA, Monani UR, De Vivo DC. Spinal muscular atrophies. In: Darras BT, Jones HR Jr, Ryan MM, De Vivo DC, eds. Neuromuscular Disorders of Infancy, Childhood and Adolescence: A Clinician's Approach. 2nd ed. San Diego: Academic Press; 2015:chap 8, 117–145.

BOX 32.4   Type 1 Spinal Muscular Atrophy (Werdnig-Hoffmann Disease): Common Clinical Features

Hypotonia: severe, generalized (floppy infant)
Weakness: severe, generalized, or proximal > distal
Areflexia
Characteristic posture
Bell-shaped thorax, paradoxical or see-saw breathing
Weak cry
Difficulty sucking and swallowing
Relatively preserved facial movements
Normal extraocular movements
Preserved sensory function and sensorium
Normal sphincter function

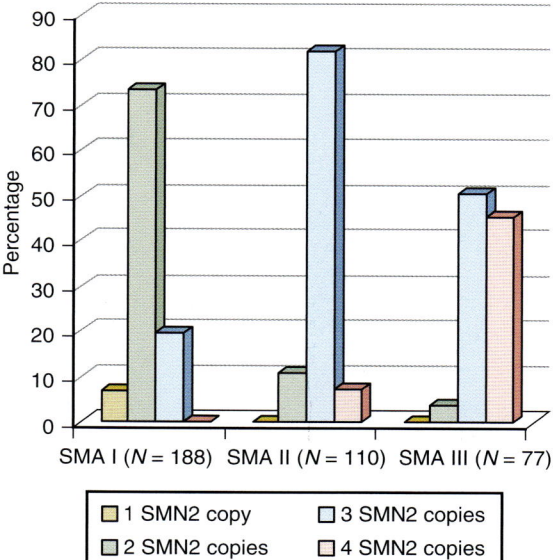

Figure 32.2 **Diagram of frequency of patients with SMA type I, II, and III by SMN2 copy number.** In 80% of children with SMA type I, one or two copies of SMN2 were found but the majority (>70%) had two copies, 82% of patients with SMA type II carried three SMN2 copies, and 96% of patients with SMA type III carried three or four copies of SMN2. SMA, Spinal muscular atrophy; SMN, survival motor neuron. (Modified with permission from Feldkotter M, Schwarzer V, Wirth R, Wienker TF, Wirth B. Quantitative analyses of SMN1 and SMN2 based on real-time lightCycler PCR: fast and highly reliable carrier testing and prediction of severity of spinal muscular atrophy. Am J Hum Genet. 2002;70(2):358–368.)

generalized. Unlike the situation with disorders of the cerebrum and other central causes of hypotonia, weakness is similarly severe. Most infants exhibit generalized weakness, but when it is possible to make a distinction between proximal and distal muscles, a proximal more than distal distribution is discernible. Only minimal movements at hips and shoulders may be elicited in the presence of active movements of hands and feet. The lower extremities are affected more severely than the upper extremities. Involvement of the axial musculature of the trunk and neck is particularly severe, and the resulting deficits are obvious with vertical suspension and pull-to-sit maneuvers (Fig. 32.3A–C). Muscle atrophy is also severe and generalized, although the severity may be difficult to appreciate fully in the newborn. Indeed the replacement of atrophied muscle by connective tissue may further hinder the appreciation of atrophy. Fasciculations of limbs are observed rarely, but an analogous phenomenon may be the characteristic fine rhythmic *tremor* of the extended fingers (polyminimyoclonus) most commonly observed in types 2 and 3 SMA.[77] Total areflexia is the rule, although rarely some reflex response, albeit depressed, can be elicited.

The pattern of weakness of limbs leads to a characteristic posture, characterized particularly by a frog-leg posture with the upper extremities abducted and either externally rotated or internally rotated (*jug handle*) at the shoulders (Fig. 32.4). The chest is almost always anteriorly collapsed and bell shaped, with an associated distention of the abdomen and intercostal recession during inspiration (see Fig. 32.4), known as *paradoxical* breathing. These features relate to weakness of the intercostal

characteristically occurs over a time course measured in days to a week or so. These clinical findings have a correlate from electrophysiological studies that show marked deterioration of motor function over a 1-week to 2-week period postnatally.[60]

Neurological Features. The neurological features are highly consistent and striking (Box 32.4).[a] Hypotonia is severe and

[a]References 40, 41, 50, 58, 76-78, 81-83, and 87-89.

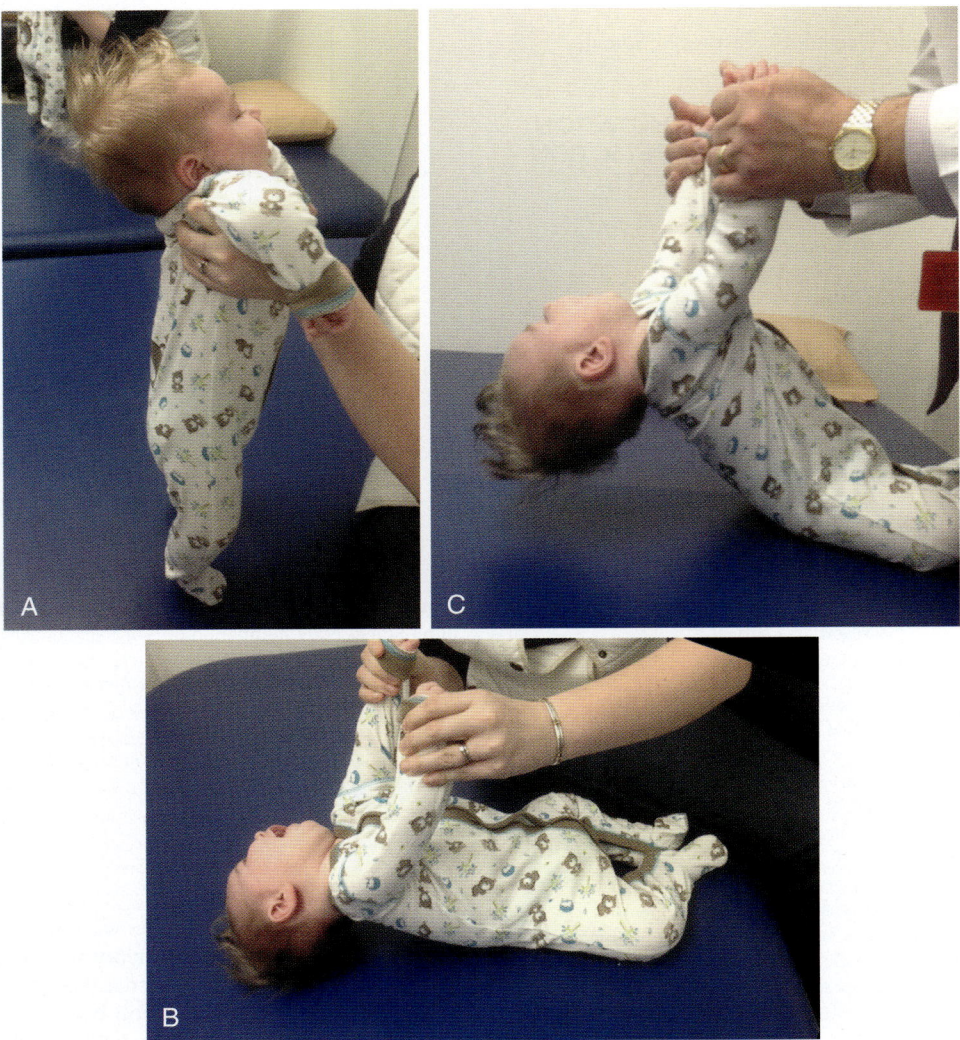

Figure 32.3 Type I spinal muscular atrophy (Werdnig-Hoffmann disease): clinical manifestations of weakness of limb and axial musculature in a 4-month-old infant with severe weakness and hypotonia. With vertical suspension (A), note the dangling lower limbs with lack of hip flexion, tendency of upper limbs to slip through the examiner's hands, and lack of neck flexion with resulting head lag. When subject is supine, note the *frog-leg* positioning of the legs and the lack of traction response (B) and the lag of head (C), with attempts by the examiner to pull the infant to a sitting position. (Reprinted with permission from Oskoui M, Darras BT, De Vivo DC. Spinal muscular atrophy: 125 years later and on the verge of a cure. In: Sumner CJ, Paushkin S, Ko C-P, eds. *Spinal Muscular Atrophy: Disease Mechanisms and Therapy.* San Diego: Academic Press; 2017:chap 1, 3–19.)

muscles and the relatively preserved diaphragmatic function. Contractures of the limbs, usually only at wrists and ankles, are evident in 10% to 20% of infants with onset in utero or in the first month of life.[76,88,90-92]

Involvement of cranial nerve nuclei is less striking than of anterior horn cells, at least early in the clinical course. Thus extraocular movements are normal, and facial motility is relatively well preserved. Indeed, the pathetic picture of a bright-eyed, nearly totally paralyzed infant is characteristic of Werdnig-Hoffmann disease. Sucking and swallowing are affected early in the course in approximately half of cases. Fasciculations and atrophy of the tongue, clinical signs in anterior horn cell disorders of slightly later onset, are apparent in only about one-third to one-half of patients, with the disease occurring at birth or in the first month.[82,88]

Particularly noteworthy differential diagnostic features in the neurological examination include the presence of normal sphincter and sensory functions. Both these functions would be expected to be affected with major spinal cord disease, and sensory function with peripheral nerve disease. The patient's alert state with normal visual and auditory responses rules against a central disorder. Total areflexia and absence of ptosis, ophthalmoplegia, and facial weakness rule against a variety of primary diseases of muscle. Distinction from type II glycogen storage disease (Pompe disease) can be most difficult, but this much less common disease is usually accompanied by prominent involvement of the heart and enlargement of the tongue.

Several rare genetic variants of infantile SMA should be distinguished from the type 1 SMA just described. These SMA

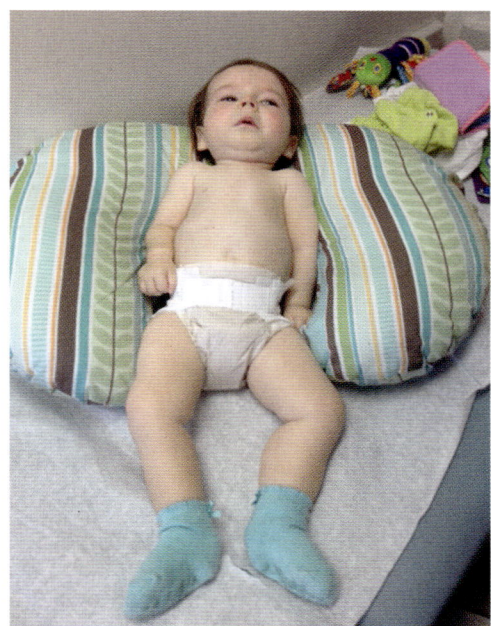

Figure 32.4 Type I spinal muscular atrophy (Werdnig-Hoffmann disease): characteristic posture. Ten-month-old girl with SMA Type I, who became symptomatic at about 1.5 to 2 months of age. Note the floppy appearance with *frog-leg* positioning of the legs. As is the case with the majority of infants with SMA Type I, this infant had no antigravity movement in her legs, only limited distal movement in the arms, and was areflexic throughout. She had two copies of SMN2. She did not receive noninvasive ventilator support (BiPAP) and passed away at 16.5 months of age. *SMA,* Spinal muscular atrophy; *SMN,* survival motor neuron. (Reprinted with permission from Oskoui M, Darras BT, De Vivo DC. Spinal muscular atrophy: 125 years later and on the verge of a cure. In: Sumner CJ, Paushkin S, Ko C-P, eds. *Spinal Muscular Atrophy: Disease Mechanisms and Therapy.* San Diego: Academic Press; 2017:chap 1, 3–19.)

variants and their mode of inheritance include the association of SMA with (1) diaphragmatic SMA or SMA with respiratory distress 1 (SMARD1; autosomal recessive), (2) pontocerebellar atrophy (type 1 pontocerebellar atrophy; see Chapter 29) (autosomal recessive), and (3) congenital arthrogryposis, both with and without bone fractures (autosomal recessive and X-linked, respectively).[24,50,93-96] None of these disorders are linked to the genetic region on chromosome 5 involved in type 1 SMA (see later discussion).

Course. The course of type 1 SMA is a close function of the age of onset.[a] Infants with clear prenatal onset of very severe disease with respiratory failure at birth, marked diffuse weakness, and early deficits of facial movement (i.e., type 0 SMA) usually die by 3 months of age.[40-42] Those infants with clinical onset in the first 2 months of life have a range of median age at death of 4 to 8 months, with maximum survival rarely exceeding 12 to 18 months. Infants with clinical onsets after 2 months of age have clearly longer median and maximum survival times. Authors use various methodologies to report survival in SMA type 1 patients, as seen in Table 32.2.[97,99-107] Survival improves with aggressive pulmonary care and nutritional support.[99,103] The very high survival rates noted in certain groups of type

1 patients (see Table 32.2) may be related to those factors, specifically invasive ventilation via tracheostomy and aggressive *proactive* care; however, these rates may also be related to the small number of patients in the reports.[99,100,103]

Although infants who ultimately prove to have type 2 SMA have a peak age at onset between 8 and 14 months,[83] an occasional infant exhibits onset before 6 months and has a chronic course, including attainment of sitting or even walking, with prolonged survival.[a] This portion of the type 2 SMA cases usually can be distinguished from type 1 SMA in the early stages of the disease because of a more insidious onset and slower initial deterioration. Death in type 1 SMA usually relates to intercurrent respiratory complications. These complications are caused by aspiration because of defective swallowing, hypoventilation because of impaired intercostal muscle function, and impaired clearing of tracheal secretions secondary to weak or absent cough because of weak abdominal muscles.

Laboratory Studies

Serum Enzymes. The creatine kinase (CK) level is usually normal in type 1 SMA[24] or slightly elevated.

Electromyography. The electromyogram (EMG) may be difficult to perform in the young infant, but with patience the major features of anterior horn cell disease are usually observed (see Table 30.4). Thus, at rest, fibrillation potentials are apparent. With muscle contraction, one sees a reduced number of fast-firing motor unit potentials that are usually of normal amplitude and duration because of failure to reinnervate efficiently in SMA type 1. In general, although no simple relationship exists between features on the EMG and outcome,[24,111,112] one study showed a strong correlation between the degree of depression of the compound muscle action potential and functional outcome.[60]

Nerve Conduction Studies. Motor nerve conduction velocities are usually normal, although in particularly severe disease, a slight reduction may be observed.[113] This finding suggests a disproportionate loss of anterior horn cells that give rise to the largest, fastest conducting fibers. The compound muscle action potentials (CMAPs) have very low amplitude because of significant loss of anterior horn neurons and/or axons. In contrast, the sensory nerve action potentials are normal, which underscores the motor neuron nature of the disease. Nevertheless, some patients with particularly severe cases of type 1 SMA have exhibited signs of severe motor and sensory neuropathy.[114-116]

Muscle Biopsy. The muscle biopsy of a patient with Werdnig-Hoffmann disease, with clinically apparent findings at birth or in the first month, usually exhibits advanced changes of denervation (see Chapter 30). Characteristically, pronounced atrophy of all fibers of both types within entire fascicles of muscle (i.e., *panfascicular atrophy*) or large group atrophy occurs (Fig. 32.5). The early signs of denervation (i.e., loss of checkerboard appearance, type grouping, or small group atrophy; see Chapter 30), features of anterior horn cell disease

---

[a]References 40, 41, 45, 50, 60, 76-78, 81, 82, 84, 88, 97, and 98.

[a]References 24, 77, 81, 82, 87-89, 97, 103, and 108-110.

TABLE 32.2   Survival Data of Patients With Spinal Muscular Atrophy Type I

	SURVIVAL PROBABILITY (%)					
	1 YEAR	2 YEARS	4 YEARS	5 YEARS	10 YEARS	20 YEARS
Zerres and Rudnik-Schoneborn[97] (1995)	—	32	18	—	8	0
Mannaa et al.[99] (2009)	—	62	62	—	8	—
Ge et al.[101] (2012)	44.9	38.1	—	29.3	—	—
Farrar et al.[102] (2013)	40	25	6	—	0	—

	AGE AT DEATH: MEDIAN
	(range, unless otherwise noted)
Oskoui et al.[103] (2007)	
1980–1994	7.3 m (1.0–193.5 m)
1995–2006	10.0 m (2.5–112.0 m)
Cobben et al.[106] (2008)	6 m (95% CI: 5–7 m)
Rudnik-Schoneborn et al.[105] (2009)[a]	
All patients	6.1 m (0.0–34.0 m)
2 copies SMN2	6.5 m (0.5–30 m)
3 copies SMN2	Alive at 10–55 m
Ge et al.[101] (2012)	7.0 m
Finkel et al.[107] (2014)[b]	13.5 m (IQR: 81–22 m)
2 SMN2 copies	10.5 m (IQR: 8.1–13.6 m)

[a]Age of all patients at death/permanent ventilation.
[b]Age at death or requiring >16 h of BiPAP per day.
SMN, Survival motor neuron.

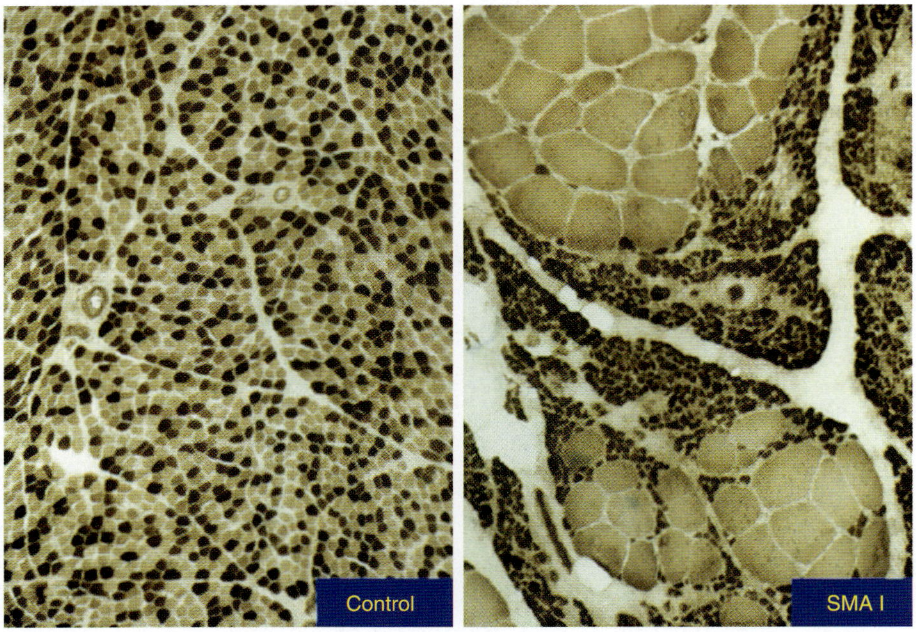

Figure 32.5 **Type I spinal muscular atrophy (Werdnig-Hoffmann disease): muscle biopsy showing diffuse, panfascicular atrophy in an affected infant.** Skeletal muscle biopsy from a patient with SMA type I showing large group atrophy. The small fibers have staining characteristics of both types (I and II), whereas the large hypertrophic fibers all stain as type I (ATPase stain, pH 9.4). A control muscle biopsy is shown on the left for comparison. *SMA,* Spinal muscular atrophy.

later in childhood, are nearly absent (Fig. 32.6). This virtual absence of signs of terminal axonal sprouting and reinnervation (see Chapter 30) is probably indicative of the severe, fulminating process involving anterior horn cells that causes widespread elimination before such compensatory attempts can occur. A consistent increase in connective tissue is associated with the marked atrophy of muscle (see Fig. 32.6). Hypertrophy of predominantly type I fibers, often in clusters, is an additional characteristic feature. The finding that these hypertrophic fibers often occur in clusters suggests the possibility of reinnervation. The distribution of the histopathological findings parallels the generalized pattern of muscle weakness; the diaphragm is

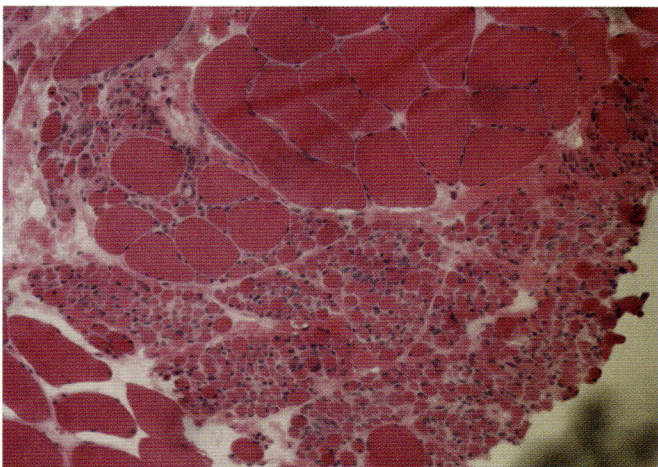

Figure 32.6 Type I spinal muscular atrophy (Werdnig-Hoffmann disease): muscle biopsy showing grouped atrophy. Note the clear neurogenic pattern of grouped atrophy and hypertrophic fibers, with modest increase in endomysial connective tissue. (Reprinted with permission from Oskoui M, Darras BT, De Vivo DC. Spinal muscular atrophy: 125 years later and on the verge of a cure. In: Sumner CJ, Paushkin S, Ko C-P, eds. *Spinal Muscular Atrophy: Disease Mechanisms and Therapy.* San Diego: Academic Press; 2017:chap 1, 3–19.)

conspicuously less affected.[88] Diagnosis by genetic testing has obviated the need for muscle biopsy in most cases (see later).

Other Studies. The identification of the q11.2–13.3 region of chromosome 5 as the site of the genetic defect in Werdnig-Hoffmann disease led to the development of molecular diagnostic techniques (see "Pathogenesis and Etiology" earlier). Radiographs of the chest are useful in demonstrating the chest deformity, the thin ribs characteristic of severe congenital neuromuscular disease,[117-119] and the marked atrophy of muscle. In the rare, very severe type 0 disease, long bone fractures may be observed.[42]

Studies with real-time ultrasonography of limbs have demonstrated several types of changes (i.e., an increase in the intensity of echoes from muscle and the degree of muscle atrophy).[24,120] The echogenicity of muscle correlates well with the severity of histopathological changes observed in biopsy specimens.

Neuropathology

Essential Cellular Changes. The major neuropathological changes are confined to the anterior horn cells of the spinal cord and the motor nuclei of cranial nerves (Box 32.5).[24,46,85,88,121-123] The essential cellular changes in infantile cases are (1) depletion of the number of neurons, (2) degenerative changes of neurons, (3) neuronophagia, and (4) infiltration with microglia and astrocytes (Fig. 32.7A and B). Enhanced apoptosis of anterior horn cell neurons is the most prominent feature during fetal life.[53,85] Some workers also described cytological findings indicative of immaturity of neurons and suggested impaired development, as well as degeneration, of neurons.[80,121] The depletion of neurons may be so marked that few, if any, remain in an anterior horn or cranial nerve nucleus. The degenerative changes consist particularly of central chromatolysis, characterized by rounded and distended neuronal cell bodies with eccentric nuclei and Nissl substance displaced to the periphery. Neuronophagia

is not prominent, although it is readily demonstrated. The glial response consists of both microglia and astrocytes and is particularly prominent in the ventral aspect of the anterior horns.

Topography. In severe Werdnig-Hoffmann disease, anterior horn cells are affected diffusely, with a particularly prominent affection of the ventromedial group. Cranial nerve nuclei involved invariably and markedly are of cranial nerves VII, IX, X, XI, and XII. The motor nucleus of nerve V is affected in approximately 70% of cases, and the abducens nucleus is involved in fewer than 50% of cases.[88]

Other areas of the motor system are not consistently involved. Hypoxic changes are occasionally observed in hippocampal neurons and Purkinje cells of cerebellum.[88] As noted later, associated degenerative changes in pontocerebellar structures are a feature of an SMA variant that is genetically distinct from type 1 SMA.

The motor nerves exhibit the changes expected from a loss of anterior horn cells (i.e., a decrease in number of myelinated fibers particularly and an increase in connective tissue).[88] Striking atrophy with glial proliferation may be apparent in the proximal anterior roots. Indeed, the glial proliferation may be so conspicuous that some workers have attributed to it a pathogenetic role.[124] The view that the glial infiltration is a secondary event is more widely accepted.[46,57,58,121,125] Perhaps of greater interest is the demonstration of changes typical of axonal neuropathy in some severe cases.[46,114-116,126] Such changes have led to the suggestion that the anterior horn cell degeneration is a secondary phenomenon, although the most prevalent view is that the neuropathic abnormalities are secondary. Kariya et al. also demonstrated structural and functional abnormalities at the level of the neuromuscular junction that precede symptoms in mice, as well as structural abnormalities in the neuromuscular junctions of humans with SMA, and hence proposed that SMA may be a *synaptopathy.*[127]

Management. Type 1 SMA that is apparent at birth or in the first month of life is usually accompanied by serious disturbances of sucking and swallowing early in infancy. Frequent aspiration of the oropharynx is needed, and usually cessation of oral feedings and institution of tube feeding are required before long to ensure adequate nutrition. Indeed, when dysphagia becomes severe enough to preclude reasonable nutrition and is complicated by frequent aspirations, many clinicians recommend gastrostomy or gastrojejunostomy feeding. This maneuver is carried out not to prolong life but to improve

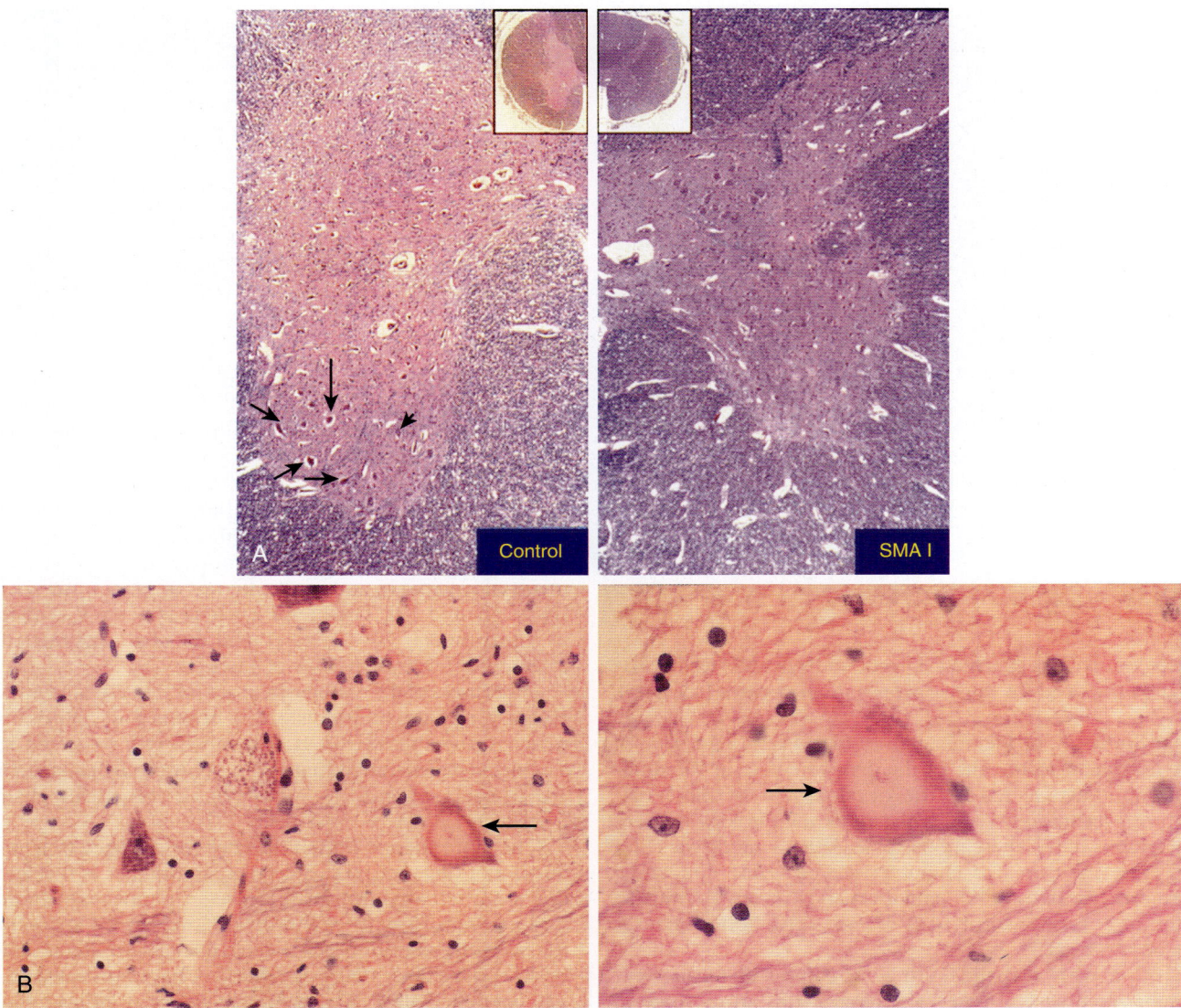

Figure 32.7   The neuropathology of spinal muscular atrophy. (A) Spinal cord. Loss of large motor neurons (*arrows*) in the anterior horns of the spinal cord in tissue obtained from autopsy material from a patient with SMA type I (stained with cresyl echt violet). A control spinal cord section is shown on the left for comparison. Small arrows indicate motor neurons. (B) Motor neuron undergoing chromatolysis appears swollen at lower and higher magnification (*arrows*). (Reprinted with permission from Darras BT, Markowitz JA, Monani UR, De Vivo DC. Spinal muscular atrophies. In: Darras BT, Jones HR Jr, Ryan MM, De Vivo DC eds. *Neuromuscular Disorders of Infancy, Childhood and Adolescence: A Clinician's Approach.* 2nd ed. San Diego: Academic Press; 2015:chap 8, 117–145.)

the patient's quality of life and particularly to reduce parental anxiety associated with attempts at oral feeding. Surveillance for respiratory infection must be diligent, because this complication is the usual mode of demise for these unfortunate babies. The intensity of therapy (e.g., antibiotics, chest physical therapy, postural drainage, noninvasive positive pressure ventilation, and even tracheostomy and long-term mechanical ventilation) sometimes is difficult to determine decisively.[128-135] Tracheostomy and mechanical ventilation have been associated with survival into childhood,[84,97] although longer survival occurs, albeit rarely, without such invasive intervention.[24] The quality of life in such bedridden infants and children is a grave concern. More important, range-of-motion exercises are used to prevent contractures and, I feel (JJV), to help the parents "do something"

for their infant. In severe Werdnig-Hoffmann disease, my approach is foremost to provide emotional support to the parents and to ensure as much comfort as possible for the infant. I indicate to the family our current understanding of the dire outcome and recommend careful attention to oral-pharyngeal secretions, measures to ensure adequate nutrition, and diligent therapy of respiratory infections. I discuss the complex issues related to *long-term* mechanical ventilation.

The clinical trials pipeline for SMA over the past 15 years has been developing several therapeutic agents.[136,137] With the goal of increasing SMN transcript, histone deacetylase inhibitors (such as valproic acid and sodium phenylbutyrate) were tested in randomized trials, but neither was effective[139]; nonhistone deacetylase inhibitors (such as hydroxyurea) were ineffective in a randomized trial; albuterol showed promise in two pilot studies; however, the mechanism of action remains unknown. Ionis Pharmaceuticals has conducted phase 3 clinical trials of an intrathecally delivered antisense oligonucleotide (SMNRx, or Nusinersen) targeting SMN2 exon 7 inclusion. Interim analysis of a phase 3 Nusinersen SMA type 1 study (ENDEAR) showed that infants receiving the medication intrathecally experienced a statistically significant improvement in the acquisition of motor milestones, compared with a control cohort,[138] and led to the approval of nusinersen (Spinraza) by the FDA in December 2016. Early phase clinical trials are testing other orally administered small molecules that modulate SMN2 alternative splicing. Roche-PTC-SMA Foundation partnership put on hold clinical studies of RG7800, an orally administered molecule, after an unexpected safety finding at higher long-term doses in an animal study. They have recently announced phase 1 trials for a new molecule, RG7916. Novartis has entered phase 2 of a clinical trial for the orally administered molecule LM1070. The goal of stabilizing the SMN protein has led to preclinical studies of aminoglycosides, proteasome inhibitors, and indoprofen. Among neuroprotectors, olesoxime, a mitochondrial pore modulator that enhances motor neuron survival in culture, may be effective in stabilizing the disease, but riluzole and gabapentin have shown mixed results.[139] Cell therapy through stem cells is under development; gene replacement therapy with a scAAV9/SMN1 gene construct in type 1 infants is in progress, and preliminary results seem promising.[140] The goal of enhancing muscle function is on the horizon, with new potential therapeutic targets such as myostatin, follistatin, and other molecules.[139]

Spinal Muscular Atrophy Variants

At least four disorders with primary involvement of anterior horn cells, clinical presentation at birth, and subsequent course of progressive deterioration (or severe static disability) mimic SMA in the neonatal period. However, these disorders are not linked to chromosome 5q and do not involve SMN. Thus the term *SMA variants* or *non-5q SMAs* seems most appropriate until the molecular bases are further clarified. At least four disorders should be distinguished (Table 32.3).

SMA with respiratory distress type 1 (SMARD1) is a striking disorder.[96,141-145] From the first days of life, intrauterine growth retardation, mild hypotonia, weak cry, and mild distal contractures are noted. Between 1 and 6 months of age, respiratory distress secondary to diaphragmatic paralysis becomes obvious, and progressive primary distal lower limb weakness ensues. Motor, sensory, and autonomic disturbances develop; these infants become ventilator dependent. A report from the Netherlands of 10 patients with SMARD1 noted significant phenotypic variability and no clear phenotype-genotype correlations.[146] CPK is usually normal; there is no cardiac involvement. Life expectancy in children with SMARD1 is limited; however, patients rarely can have only mild sleep hyperventilation.[147] The responsible gene (IGHMBP2) encodes immunoglobulin mu-binding protein 2, the function of which is unclear.

Pontocerebellar hypoplasia type 1 (PCH1) manifests clinically at birth with arthrogryposis, hypotonia, weakness, and bulbar deficits (swallowing difficulty, stridor).[148-151] Subsequent features include progressive bulbar deficits, nystagmus, microcephaly, and cognitive deficits. Brain imaging shows pontocerebellar hypoplasia and cerebral atrophy. PCH1, linked to mutations

TABLE 32.3	Spinal Muscular Atrophy Variants: Progressive or Severe Neonatal Anterior Horn Cell Disease Not Linked to Survival Motor Neuron Gene[a]
VARIANT	**MAJOR FEATURES**
SMA with respiratory distress type 1 (SMARD1)	Mild hypotonia, weak cry, distal contractures initially; respiratory distress from diaphragmatic paralysis 1–6 months, progressive distal weakness; autosomal recessive, locus 11q13.3, gene: immunoglobulin mu-binding protein 2 (IGHMBP2)
Pontocerebellar hypoplasia type 1 (PCH1)	Arthrogryposis, hypotonia, weakness, bulbar deficits early; later, microcephaly, extraocular defects, cognitive deficits: pontocerebellar hypoplasia; molecular defect unknown; autosomal recessive, genes VRK1 and EXOCS3
X-linked infantile SMA with arthrogryposis ± bone fractures (SMAX2)	Arthrogryposis, hypotonia, weakness, congenital bone fractures, respiratory failure, lethal course as in severe type 1 SMA: most cases X-linked (Xp11.1–3, gene UBA1); a few cases likely autosomal recessive
Congenital SMA with predominant lower limb involvement	Arthrogryposis, hypotonia, weakness, especially distal lower limbs early; nonprogressive but severe disability; autosomal dominant or sporadic; locus 12q24, gene TRPV4

[a]See text for references.
SMA, Spinal muscular atrophy.

in the VRK1 gene,[152] is an unusual phenotype wherein a characteristic brain malformation combines with abnormalities of spinal cord motor neurons. EXOCS3 was recently sequenced in a cohort of 27 families with PCH1; mutations were found in 37%.[153] A common c.395A>C, p.D132A mutation was present in about half of these families. Despite some variation in clinical features, phenotype-genotype correlation underscored the continued usefulness of PCH1 as a clinical category.

X-linked infantile SMA with arthrogryposis ± congenital fractures (SMAX2) manifests clinically in the neonatal period with arthrogryposis, hypotonia, areflexia and weakness.[57,58,61,154-156] Congenital fractures of long bones and ribs are common. Respiratory failure and progressive weakness lead to death in the first days to weeks in most infants. Anterior horn cell loss is marked. Approximately 80% of cases have been in male infants, and linkage to Xp11.3 has been shown. However, some cases with predominance of bone fractures likely are autosomal recessive. The lethal X-linked form of SMA (SMAX2) can be confused with SMA type 1A; mutations in the UBA1 gene have been detected in this group of patients.[157] A clinical and pathological study of a UBA1 gene mutation-positive SMAX2 case showed white matter abnormalities on MRI brain imaging, prominent motor and sensory system disturbance, as well as cerebellar involvement and widespread inflammatory changes on muscle biopsy.[158]

Congenital distal SMA predominantly affecting the lower limbs is the only autosomal dominant disorder of this group.[57,58,61,159] Presentation at birth is with talipes equinovarus and lower limb hypotonia. EMG and muscle biopsy show signs of anterior horn cell disease. The subsequent course is marked by severe weakness of the lower extremities, although it is generally nonprogressive. The disorder is linked to chromosome 12q24.11, and the molecular defect involves mutations in the TRPV4 gene.[160]

Neurogenic Arthrogryposis Multiplex Congenita

Generalized and Localized Types

The term *neurogenic* has been applied to cases of arthrogryposis multiplex congenita secondary to involvement of either anterior horn cell or peripheral nerve (see Chapter 31). Obvious overlap exists with type 0 SMA and with the SMA variants just discussed. I prefer to use the term *neurogenic arthrogryposis multiplex congenita* for the clearly *nonprogressive* forms of arthrogryposis related to anterior horn cell or peripheral nerve disease. By far the most common variety is amyoplasia congenita, probably related in most cases to a dysgenetic disturbance of anterior horn cells, described in Chapter 31. Thus because this and other generalized forms of arthrogryposis multiplex congenita secondary to anterior horn cell have been discussed, I consider in this section only the localized forms.

Cervical Form. A group of infants with a cervical form of anterior horn cell disease and arthrogryposis was described.[161-164] The striking findings in the neonatal period were signs of severe symmetrical lower motor neuron deficit in the upper extremities in the absence of a history suggestive of traumatic injury of spinal cord or brachial plexus. Atrophy and flaccid weakness of upper extremities and the proximal and distal muscle groups were marked, and flexor contractures at the elbow and interphalangeal joints were apparent. Bulbar muscles were not affected. Lower extremities were normal. The course was nonprogressive. Onset in utero was suggested by the presence of flexion contractures, and onset in the first trimester was suggested by the presence of poorly formed palmar creases. The nature of the intrauterine insult to cervical anterior horn cells was not clear. One patient with a clinically similar case had intramedullary telangiectasia.[165]

Caudal Form. A caudal form of anterior horn cell disease with arthrogryposis was described as an apparently sporadic disorder with involvement localized to the lower extremities.[166,167] Weakness, hypotonia, areflexia, and multiple joint contractures were the major features. A few patients later developed signs in the upper extremities and fasciculations of the tongue after several years.[166] Whether these cases represent a different disorder from the SMA variant with predominant lower limb weakness described earlier (see Table 32.3), or are related to intrauterine infections of the anterior horn cells,[168] is unknown.

Laboratory Studies. EMG and muscle biopsy in both the generalized and local forms of neurogenic arthrogryposis multiplex congenita usually demonstrate signs of denervation (see Chapter 30). In the localized forms, the possibility of a correctable structural lesion of the cervical cord or the lumbosacral cord and cauda equina should be ruled out by appropriate studies.

Type II Glycogen Storage Disease (Pompe Disease)

Type II glycogen storage disease, Pompe disease, is an inherited disorder, transmitted in an autosomal recessive manner. The disease is associated with glycogen deposition in anterior horn cells (as well as in skeletal and cardiac muscle, liver, and brain), and with striking weakness and hypotonia in early infancy.

Clinical Features

Onset. Onset of the Pompe disease may be apparent in the first days of life, although the median age at symptom onset in the largest series (*n* = 168) was 2.0 months.[24,169-174]

Neurological Features. Initially, the weakness and hypotonia may be so severe that type 1 SMA is considered the probable diagnosis. The concurrence of fasciculations of the tongue and difficulty sucking, crying, and swallowing further mimics this primary anterior horn cell degeneration. However, several clinical features help distinguish Pompe disease from Werdnig-Hoffmann disease. First, cardiac involvement, resulting from accumulation of glycogen, is prominent in Pompe disease; radiographs demonstrate an enlarged globular heart, and electrocardiograms demonstrate evidence of myocardiopathy with shortened PR interval, giant QRS complexes, and inverted T waves. Second, the tongue, although weak and perhaps even fasciculating, is usually *large* in Pompe disease because of the glycogen accumulation, unlike the small, atrophic tongue of Werdnig-Hoffmann disease. Third, the skeletal muscles, although weak, are usually prominent in Pompe disease, because of glycogen accumulation (i.e., a true hypertrophy), and they have a characteristic rubbery feel. This finding is unlike the atrophy of Werdnig-Hoffmann disease. Fourth, the liver usually is enlarged and readily palpable in Pompe disease. Tendon reflexes are variable in glycogen storage disease. Most patients have preserved tendon reflexes early in the clinical course and later have total areflexia.

A recent report described a delay in myelination, determined by MRI, in five patients with infantile-onset Pompe disease.[175] The clinical correlates of this disturbance remain to be clarified. Deposition of glycogen is a feature of human oligodendroglial development.

Clinical Course. The clinical course is malignant. Infants require ventilatory support at a median age of 6 months, and death in one large series (*n* = 168) occurred at a median age of approximately 9 months.[174] In another series (*n* = 153), the median age at death was 6 months.[173] Survival rates at 12 months of age are approximately 25%, with only 17% ventilator free; at 18 months, the respective values are 12% and 7%.[174] Death is related usually to a combination of cardiac involvement and respiratory complications caused by thoracic muscle weakness and bulbar paralysis.

Laboratory Studies. The serum CK level is elevated because of cardiac and skeletal muscle involvement, and the serum transaminases also are usually elevated because of the combination of muscle and hepatic disease, with the former predominating.[169,173] Muscle biopsy reveals large amounts of periodic acid–Schiff–positive material. Large vacuoles, often confluent, are apparent when standard fixation procedures

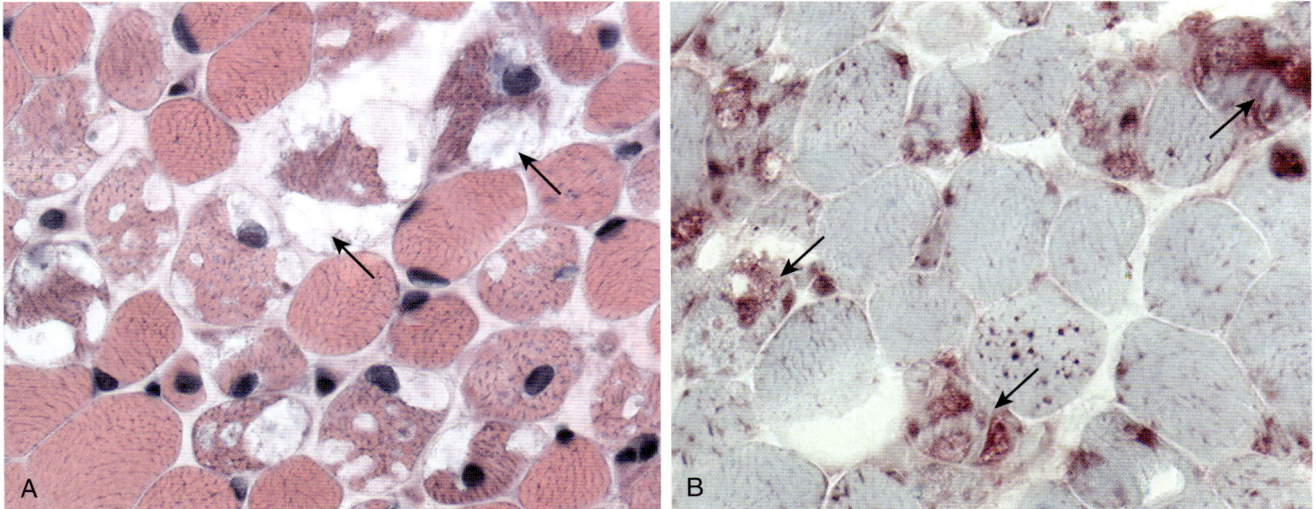

Figure 32.8 Muscle biopsy from an infant with acid maltase (GAA) deficiency (Pompe disease, GSD II). H&E shows large vacuoles in all fibers (A, *arrows*) that stain intensely with the acid phosphatase reaction (B). (Reprinted with permission from Akman HO, Oldfors A, DiMauro S. Glycogen storage diseases of muscle. In: Darras BT, Jones HR Jr, Ryan MM, De Vivo DC eds. *Neuromuscular Disorders of Infancy, Childhood and Adolescence: A Clinician's Approach.* 2nd ed. San Diego: Academic Press; 2015:chap 39, 735–760.)

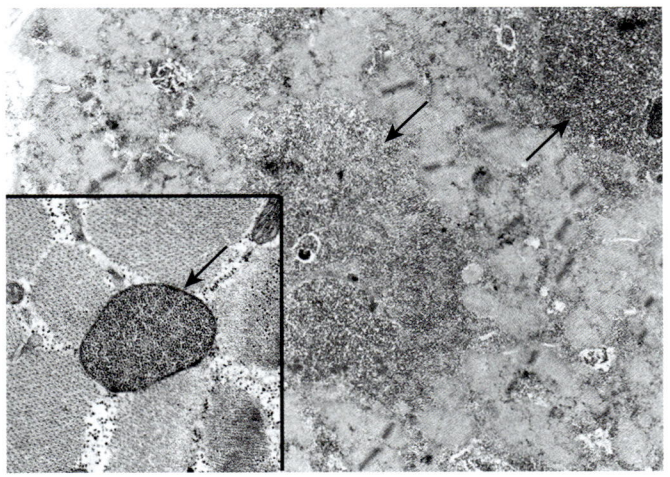

Figure 32.9 Electron microscopy of muscle in infantile Pompe disease, showing large accumulation of free cytoplasmic glycogen *(arrows)* together with intralysosomal glycogen *(inset)*. (Reprinted with permission from Akman HO, Oldfors A, DiMauro S. Glycogen storage diseases of muscle. In: Darras BT, Jones HR Jr, Ryan MM, De Vivo DC eds. *Neuromuscular Disorders of Infancy, Childhood and Adolescence: A Clinician's Approach.* 2nd ed. San Diego: Academic Press; 2015:chap 39, 735–760.)

are used.[176] The confluent vacuoles, often resulting in a *lacework* appearance, are lysosomes filled with PAS-positive diastase-digestible material; they stain positively for acid-phosphatase. Also, free glycogen can be seen in the cytoplasm with electron microscopy (Figs. 32.8A and B and 32.9).[177] The EMG reveals fibrillations but often also signs of myopathic disorder because of prominent muscle involvement (see Chapter 33). An additional characteristic feature is *irritability* of muscle with the occurrence of pseudomyotonic bursts of discharges. The large R waves on electrocardiography are particularly helpful signs in diagnosis.

Neuropathology. The neuropathology of Pompe disease is characterized by a striking increase in glycogen throughout the central and peripheral nervous systems (including the myenteric plexus of rectal mucosa). The accumulation of glycogen in the anterior horn cells is the most striking change.[178]

Pathogenesis and Etiology. The biochemical defect involves acid alpha-glucosidase (GAA; acid maltase) activity (Fig. 32.10).[171,179,180] This enzyme catalyzes the *lysosomal* pathway of glycogen degradation, presumably used during normal turnover of cellular constituents. (The major pathway of glycogen degradation, used for glucose-6-phosphate production, occurs in the *cytosol* and is catalyzed by phosphorylase.) Thus, in Pompe disease, the largest accumulation of glycogen is apparent in lysosomal structures. The enzymatic defect is demonstrable in muscle or cultured fibroblasts.[180,181] Moreover, the enzyme is also present in fibroblasts grown from amniotic fluid cells, and this procedure can be used for prenatal diagnosis.[172,182]

There is good correlation between GAA gene mutations and severity of the phenotype. Infants tend to have deletion or nonsense mutations in the GAA gene, leading to significant enzyme deficiency, whereas older children and adults have milder, *leaky* mutations.[183-185]

Management. Attempts to replenish alpha-glucosidase by bone marrow transplantation have been unsuccessful.[186] Very promising results are available for the use of enzyme replacement therapy (ERT), involving recombinant human alpha-glucosidase, at least for survival and cardiac and skeletal muscle function.[187-189] In addition, a study of five infants treated from a median age of 6 months showed improvement in myelination by MRI in four of the patients.[175] However, the response of infants with Pompe disease has been variable,[190,191] with some infants surviving for more than 11 years but being paralyzed and ventilator-dependent; early treatment seems to improve the outcome.[192] In a series of 20 infants treated in

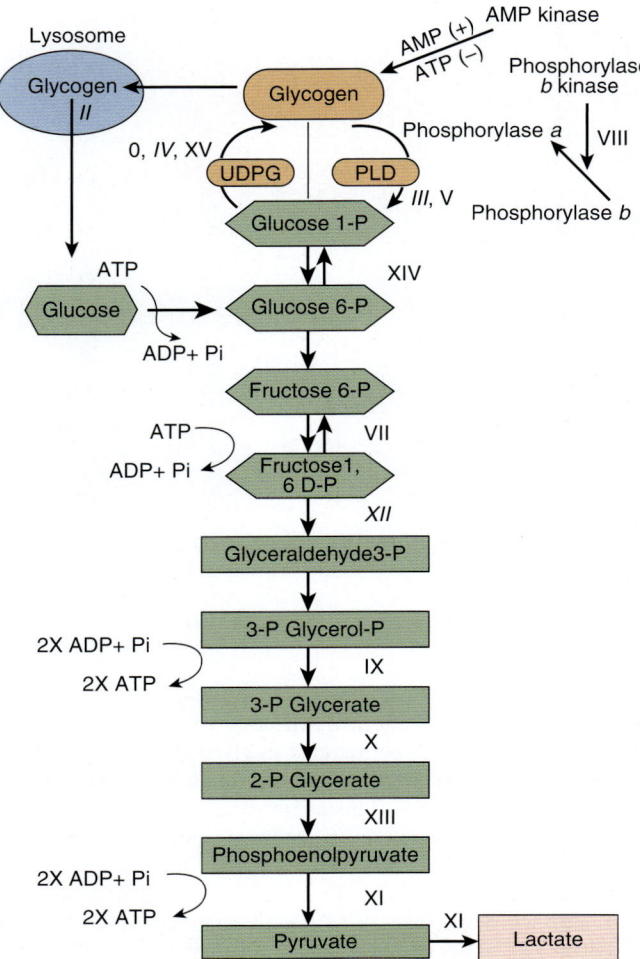

Figure 32.10 Scheme of glycogen metabolism and glycolysis. Roman numerals indicate enzymes whose deficiencies are associated with muscle glycogenosis: II, acid maltase (GAA, Pompe disease); III, debrancher (GDE, Cori-Forbes disease); IV, brancher (GBE, Andersen disease); V, myophosphorylase (PYGM, McArdle disease); VII, phosphofructokinase (PFK, Tarui disease); VIII, phosphorylase kinase (PHK); IX, phosphoglycerate kinase (PGK); X, phosphoglycerate mutase (PGAM); XI, lactate dehydrogenase (LDH); XII, aldolase A; XIII, beta-enolase (ENO3); XIV, phosphoglucomutase (PGM); XV, glycogenin (GYG1); 0, glycogen synthase (GYS1). *AMP,* Adenosine monophosphate; *ATP,* adenosine trisphosphate; *P,* inorganic phosphate; *PLD,* phosphorylase-limit dextrin; *UDPG,* iridine diphosphate glucose. (Reprinted with permission from Oldfors A, DiMauro S. New insights in the field of muscle glycogenoses. *Curr Opin Neurol.* 2013;26: 544–553.)

the UK between 2000 and 2009, the overall ventilator-free survival was 35%; 30% were alive and ventilator-dependent, and 35% died at a median age of 10 months.[193] Further, questions regarding cognitive outcome have been raised in surviving infants because the recombinant GAA does not cross the blood-brain barrier.[194-196]

Neonatal Poliomyelitis

Neonatal poliomyelitis in this section refers to infection with poliovirus acquired either in utero or in the first 4 weeks of life. Only one case has been reported in the United States in the approximately 40 years since the widespread use of

live oral poliovirus vaccine (Sabin vaccine).[197] An additional infantile case with onset at 3 months of age occurred 1 month after administration of live oral polio vaccine.[198] However, poliomyelitis at later ages is still observed, not only in other parts of the world but in the United States among certain religious groups that prohibit vaccination of children. In addition, approximately nine cases per year of poliomyelitis caused by *vaccine-related* poliovirus still occur in the United States. Indeed, the single neonatal case reported in the past 3 decades in this country acquired the infection by contact with a recently vaccinated infant with diarrhea.[197] Moreover, other enteroviruses rarely cause a paralytic syndrome in older patients and, theoretically at least, could cause a neonatal disorder comparable to poliomyelitis. For these reasons, brief attention to neonatal poliomyelitis is warranted here.

Clinical Features

Onset. The disorder may be apparent at birth or may develop in the first weeks of life.[197,199-203] Because the incubation period of the disease is approximately 10 days, infants affected at birth or in the first week presumably were affected in utero.

Neurological Features. Most patients present with diffuse flaccid paralysis that is usually asymmetrical.[88] Apnea may be the initial clinical feature.[197] Not uncommonly, encephalitic involvement results in cerebral signs, including seizures. Respiratory failure may ensue promptly. Moreover, contractures can evolve rapidly, and care must be taken to avoid the postnatal development of arthrogryposis multiplex. Asymmetrical paresis is a common sequel.

Laboratory Studies. The diagnosis is established by viral isolation from the stool. CSF pleocytosis with elevated protein content occurs.

Neuropathology. The neuropathological features in the newborn are often more severe than in the adult. The qualitative features are similar. Neuronal necrosis, neuronophagia, and perivascular cuffing with inflammatory cells involve neurons of the anterior horns, motor nuclei of the brain stem, roof nuclei of the cerebellum, diencephalon, and motor cortex of the cerebrum.

Pathogenesis and Etiology. Neonatal poliomyelitis is caused by infection of neurons by poliovirus, a classic neurotropic virus. The acquisition of virus may occur prenatally or early postnatally. The demonstration of maternal viremia and placental infection and the recovery of virus from meconium of stillborn infants of diseased mothers support the concept of intrauterine infection by transplacental mechanisms. Because of the incubation period for poliomyelitis, infants affected after approximately 10 days of age presumably were infected during delivery by contamination with infected stool or by postnatal exposure.

Management. Management is entirely supportive.

LEVEL OF THE PERIPHERAL NERVE

Disorders affecting the peripheral nerve are the least defined of those leading to hypotonia and weakness in the neonatal

BOX 32.6 Hypotonia and Weakness: Level of the Peripheral Nerve

Chronic Motor-Sensory Polyneuropathy
Myelin
Hypomyelination[a]
   Autosomal recessive
   Sporadic
Hypomyelination and demyelination-remyelination (onion bulbs)
   Autosomal recessive[a]
   Autosomal dominant[a]
   Sporadic
   Other (associated with axonal disease or focal hypermyelination)
Chronic inflammatory demyelinating polyneuropathy

Neuronal-Axonal (Rare)
Autosomal recessive
Autosomal dominant
Sporadic

Subcellular
Mitochondrial: disorders of electron transport chain complex subunits, pyruvate dehydrogenase
Cytoskeletal structures: intermediate filaments (i.e., giant axonal neuropathy), neurofilaments (i.e., infantile neuroaxonal dystrophy)
Lysosomal: Krabbe disease

Hereditary Congenital Sensory and Autonomic Neuropathies
Familial dysautonomia, congenital insensitivity to pain with or without anhidrosis and cognitive impairment

Acute Polyneuropathy
Guillain-Barré syndrome

[a]Each accounts for approximately 25% of all chronic infantile motor-sensory polyneuropathies.

TABLE 32.4 Congenital Polyneuropathy With Hypomyelination and Clinical Onset at Birth[a]

CLINICAL FEATURES	PERCENTAGE OF TOTAL
Neurological deficits	
Severe weakness and hypotonia (at birth)	70
Arthrogryposis multiplex congenita	17
Age of walking	
None (most died; see below)	70
With help (1½–5 years)	19
Unassisted (2–6 years)	11
Outcome	
Dead (1 h–4½ years)	40
Alive (14 months–26 years)	60
Motor nerve conduction velocity	
≤10–12 m/s or unrecordable	96
Onion bulbs	
Absent[b]	33
Present[c]	67
Major genes involved	
Myelin protein (MPZ), peripheral myelin protein 22 (PMP22), early growth response element 2 (EGR2), myotubularin-related protein 2 (MTMR2), ganglioside-induced differentiation-associated protein 1 (GDAP1), periaxin (PRX), neurofilament protein (NEFL).	

[a]See text for references; values shown are percentages of total number of cases for which data are available. All infants had neonatal clinical features and congenital neuropathy with hypomyelination, with or without onion bulbs, on nerve biopsy.
[b]Approximately 85% died (ages, 1 hr–4.5 yr).
[c]Of these, 81% survived (14 mo–21 yr).

period. However, the more frequent consideration of disorders of peripheral nerve as the cause of motor deficits in neonatal patients, the more frequent use of refined techniques for studying nerve histology, such as electron microscopy, and the explosion in application of molecular genetics lead to the conclusion that disease at this level is probably considerably more common than was previously suspected. The major disorders to be considered in the neonatal period are shown in Box 32.6. The categorization is somewhat arbitrary because available reports suggest some overlap, as well as the need for more definitive means of study.

Chronic Motor-Sensory Polyneuropathy: Myelin Disease

In chronic motor-sensory polyneuropathies (see Box 32.6), we include several groups of cases, somewhat heterogeneous in basic type but readily identified as affected with a disorder of peripheral nerve myelin. The disorders are categorized best as those that appear to involve a failure of the Schwann cell's role of synthesis and maintenance of myelin (i.e., characterized by *hypomyelination*). In many cases, an additional feature, related to proliferation of Schwann cells and fibroblasts, is *"onion bulb" formation*, with evidence of demyelination-remyelination. In a rare third group, the disturbance of myelin is *inflammatory*. I discuss the two most commonly recognized of these three categories, the hypomyelinative and the hypomyelinative-demyelinating-remyelinating polyneuropathies, together, because their clinical

features overlap, and in many respects the disorders are interrelated.

Congenital Polyneuropathies With Hypomyelination, With or Without Demyelination and Remyelination

In this group I include those neuropathies associated with hypomyelination alone and those with hypomyelination and evidence of demyelination-remyelination (i.e., onion bulb formation). Those disorders with onion bulb formation were previously termed *Dejerine-Sottas disease* (DSD) or *hereditary motor sensory neuropathy* (HMSN) *type III*, and those with hypomyelination alone were termed *congenital hypomyelinating neuropathy* (CHN). The designation *Charcot-Marie-Tooth disease type 4* (CMT4) has been used inconsistently in the past to denote autosomal recessive demyelinating neuropathies, some of them with early onset. However, this series of terms was coined before the availability of genetic testing and now may cause confusion.[204] The principal overall features of the entire group are summarized in Table 32.4.[205-260]

Pathogenesis and Etiology

The pathogenesis of congenital hypomyelinative neuropathies is diverse but in general involves a disturbance of myelin formation or maintenance. The major genes involved, myelin protein zero *(MPZ)*, peripheral myelin protein 22 *(PMP22)*, early growth

TABLE 32.5   Clinical Clues to the Diagnosis of Infantile Demyelinating Neuropathies

CLINICAL FEATURE	CLINICAL PHENOTYPE	GENE
Pupillary abnormalities	CHN, DSD, CMT1B	MPZ
	CMT4C	SH3TC2
Multiple cranial neuropathies	CHN, DSD, CMT4E	EGR2
Prominent foot and hand deformities	CMT4A, CMT2H/K	GDAP1
	CMT4C	SH3TC2
Severe spinal deformities	CMT4C	SH3TC2
Asymmetric weakness	DSD, CMT4J	FIG4
	GBS/CIDP	—
Posttraumatic rapid progression of weakness	DSD, CMT4J	FIG4
Vocal cord paresis	CMT4A, CMT2H/K	GDAP1
	CMT4B1	MTMR2
Diaphragmatic involvement	CMT4A, CMT2H/K	GDAP1
Glaucoma	CMT4B2	SBF2
Prominent sensory involvement	DSD, CMT4F	PRX
Congenital cataracts	HCC	DRCTNNBIA
	CCFDN	CTDP1
Raised creatine kinase	Merosin-deficient CMD	LAMA2

CCFDN, Congenital cataracts facial dysmorphism neuropathy syndrome; CHN, congenital hypomyelinating neuropathy; CMD, congenital muscular dystrophy; CMT, Charcot-Marie-Tooth disease; DSD, Déjerine-Sottas disease; EGR2, early growth response element 2; GBS/CIDP, Guillain-Barré syndrome/chronic inflammatory demyelinating polyneuropathy; GDAP1, ganglioside-induced differentiation-associated protein 1; HCC, hypomyelination and congenital cataract; MTMR, myotubularin-related protein.

Modified from Yiu EM, Ryan MM. Demyelinating prenatal and infantile developmental neuropathies. J Peripher Nerv Syst. 2012;17(1):32–52, with permission from Wiley.

response element 2 *(EGR2),* myotubularin-related protein 2 *(MTMR2),* ganglioside-induced differentiation-associated protein 1 *(GADP1),* periaxin *(PRX),* and neurofilament protein *(NEFL),* are either structural myelin or Schwann cell proteins or transcription factors.[240,242,246-262] Nevertheless, mutations in many other genes have been linked to the pathogenesis of these disorders (Table 32.5), including SH3TC2, a frequent cause of autosomal recessive CMT4. Mutations in SH3TC2 account for the etiology in 12% of congenital neuropathies, which is the highest frequency of all genes involved.[263]

Congenital hypomyelinative neuropathies overall have occurred sporadically and by autosomal recessive, autosomal dominant, or X-linked recessive inheritance. The last of these is related to a connexin-32 defect and nearly always presents clinically in childhood. The *purely hypomyelinative* cases are caused by either de novo dominant or autosomal recessive mutations. Among the *hypomyelinative group with onion bulb formation* (DSD or HMSN III), autosomal recessive inheritance is most common, but autosomal dominant inheritance has also been defined (often categorized as a subtype of HMSN I or Charcot-Marie-Tooth disease, CMT1).

Autosomal dominant inheritance may be more common than suspected. Thus when nerve conduction velocity determinations

have been performed in apparently unaffected parents of some affected infants, clear evidence of disease has been detected. Indeed, in the series of 20 patients with congenital polyneuropathy described by Hagberg and Lyon,[205,237] five had clear evidence of autosomal dominant inheritance and appeared to represent the HMSN I or CMT1. The most common genetic defect for the latter phenotype is a duplication of the chromosomal 17p region that contains PMP22.[241,257] Although neonatal electrophysiological abnormalities have been identified in 17p duplication cases, clinical neonatal onset is unusual, but it does occur.[252] Autosomal dominant point mutations of both PMP22 and P0 have been shown to lead to CHN and could have accounted for the earlier observations of Hagberg and Lyon.[240,242,243,246-250]

Less commonly, hypomyelinative-demyelinating-remyelinating forms are associated with axonal disease or with focal areas of hypermyelination, in addition to onion bulbs.[257,264] These focal myelin thickenings or *tomacula* presumably reflect a separate defect in the Schwann cell that differs from those seen in the more typical cases described in Table 32.4.

Clinical Features

In most cases, the disorder has its *onset* in utero and manifests at birth. The dominant *neurological features* in the neonatal period are hypotonia and weakness. Involvement usually is generalized, and the distal more than proximal involvement characteristic of peripheral nerve disease has been difficult to demonstrate in the newborn period. This pattern of weakness, however, usually becomes obvious after several months. Muscle atrophy is usually marked. Tendon reflexes are very hypoactive or, more often, absent. Arthrogryposis multiplex congenita has been a feature in a number of cases and may be very prominent (see Table 32.4).

The involvement of musculature innervated by *cranial nerves* has been variable. Impairment of feeding is common, but the nature of the disturbance is not usually characterized. Clear involvement of facial movement is not common, and extraocular abnormalities have not been reported.

Involvement of the *sensory system* is a valuable feature to elicit for identification of neuropathy. Elicitation of sensory deficits in the neonatal patient requires very careful examination (see Chapter 9). Definitive evaluation of the sensory system usually also requires electrophysiological data (see later discussion). Most patients (70%) never walk, and only 11% eventually do so unassisted (see Table 32.4). Approximately 40% of infants die, and a clear relation to severity of disease, as reflected in the presence or absence of evidence for demyelination-remyelination (i.e., onion bulbs on nerve biopsy), is apparent. Thus approximately 85% of infants with absence of onion bulbs have died, whereas 81% of those with onion bulbs survive (see Table 32.4).

Three reports of infants with the clinical electrophysiological and pathological features of congenital hypomyelinating polyneuropathy who improved spontaneously after months and were normal or markedly improved at 18 or 19 months and 9 years, respectively, raised the possibility of a transient, reversible form of this disorder.[244,245,248] These observations suggest the need for some caution in rendering a dismal prognosis with the neonatal diagnosis of this form of neuropathy.

Some clinical clues to the diagnosis of congenital hypomyelinating polyneuropathies, and associated genes and phenotypes, are shown in Table 32.5.

Laboratory Studies
Serum Enzymes. The CK level is normal.

Electromyography. The EMG indicates changes of denervation, as outlined in Table 30.4.

Nerve Conduction Velocity. Determination of nerve conduction velocity is critical and is too frequently overlooked in the evaluation of the hypotonic and weak newborn. In most severely affected infants, a drastic reduction in motor nerve conduction velocity has been demonstrated, and values of less than 10 to 12 m/second are recorded in nearly all cases (see Table 32.4). In many infants (including several of my patients), impulse transmission could not be detected. The absence of sensory nerve action potentials is also common.[265]

Muscle Biopsy. Muscle biopsy usually shows evidence of denervation (see Box 30.4), but the muscle histology occasionally may appear remarkably preserved in the presence of severe disease of nerve. The correct diagnosis may be suggested by examination of intramuscular nerves within the biopsy specimen of muscle. Changes seen in full form on nerve biopsy (see later discussion) may be suggested from such examination.

Other Studies. The CSF protein concentration is a valuable adjunct to the diagnosis of infantile polyneuropathy. The CSF protein concentration is almost always elevated, even in the first weeks of life. The elevation usually becomes more marked with age, and occasionally a CSF protein concentration that is only marginally elevated in the first weeks of life becomes markedly elevated later in infancy.

Neuropathology
The diagnosis of peripheral nerve disease is established by examination of a nerve biopsy specimen. The sural nerve, which has a limited distribution over the skin of the foot, is usually chosen for biopsy. The major abnormalities are *hypomyelination* and *onion bulb formation*. Also, the discovery of mutations in a large number of genes in patients with congenital polyneuropathies has allowed for molecular diagnosis of these disorders (see earlier).

Hypomyelination. In the congenital hypomyelinative neuropathies, the essential feature has been the virtual absence of myelin sheaths (Fig. 32.11). If any myelin is present, large-diameter nerve fibers, which normally are heavily myelinated, are conspicuous by the paucity of myelination. The normal proportion between diameter size and thickness of myelin sheath thus is lost. No signs of myelin destruction can be discerned; the lack of a demyelinating process is supported by biochemical studies, which showed no accumulation of cholesterol ester, the chemical hallmark of demyelination. Accompanying these changes may be a modest proliferation of Schwann cells and endoneurial fibroblasts.

Onion Bulb Formation. In many cases, so-called *onion bulb formation* has been detected. This morphological change is associated with the proliferation of Schwann cells and, to a lesser extent, endoneurial fibroblasts. Individual axons become invested by multiple Schwann cells. The multiple concentric lamellae of Schwann cell processes and, to a lesser

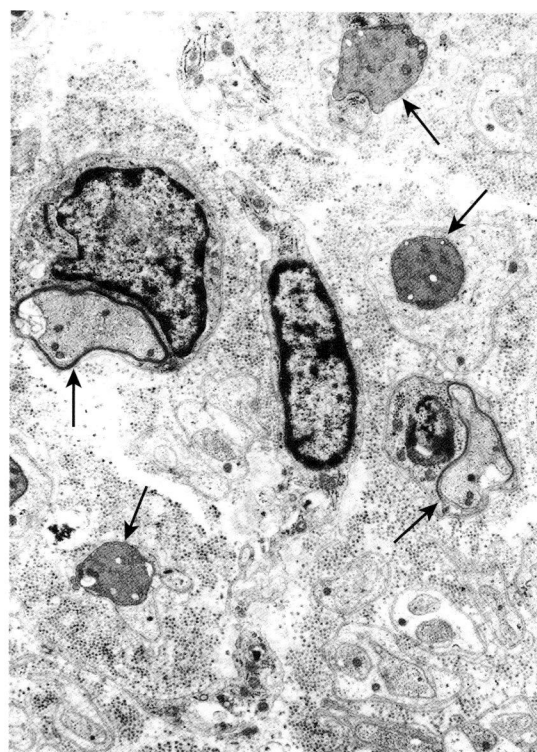

Figure 32.11 Hypomyelination polyneuropathy. This infant had severe, generalized hypotonia and weakness of facial movement, sucking, swallowing, and limb movement from the first days of life. The CSF protein level was slightly elevated on several occasions, and motor nerve conduction velocities were markedly reduced to 2 to 3 m/second. The infant died at 9½ months of age. The electron micrograph shows several axons (*arrows*), each surrounded by a Schwann cell, one of which is sectioned through its nucleus (N). Note the marked paucity of myelin lamellae. No onion bulb formation is present. *CSF,* Cerebrospinal fluid. (Courtesy Dr. Andrew W. Zimmerman.)

extent, collagen fibers render the onion bulb appearance (Fig. 32.12A–D). In the youngest and most severely affected patients, the concentric lamellae consist principally of basement membrane of Schwann cells, there remaining little of Schwann cell plasma membrane.[220] In older and usually less severely affected patients, the proliferative changes cause considerable separation of nerve fibers and an increase in the transverse diameter of the nerve; hence the term *interstitial hypertrophy*. In such patients, nerves may be palpable, particularly the posterior auricular in the neck, the ulnar at the elbow, and the peroneal at the fibular head.

Management
Supportive measures (see the earlier discussion of Werdnig-Hoffmann disease) are important, particularly because many patients live for years. It is critical to prevent contractures, scoliosis, and recurrent pulmonary infection and to optimize the motor function that is retained.

Chronic Inflammatory Demyelinating Polyneuropathy

Chronic inflammatory demyelinating polyneuropathy (CIDP) is a relatively common acquired neuropathy of older children and adults. The disorder is important to recognize because it

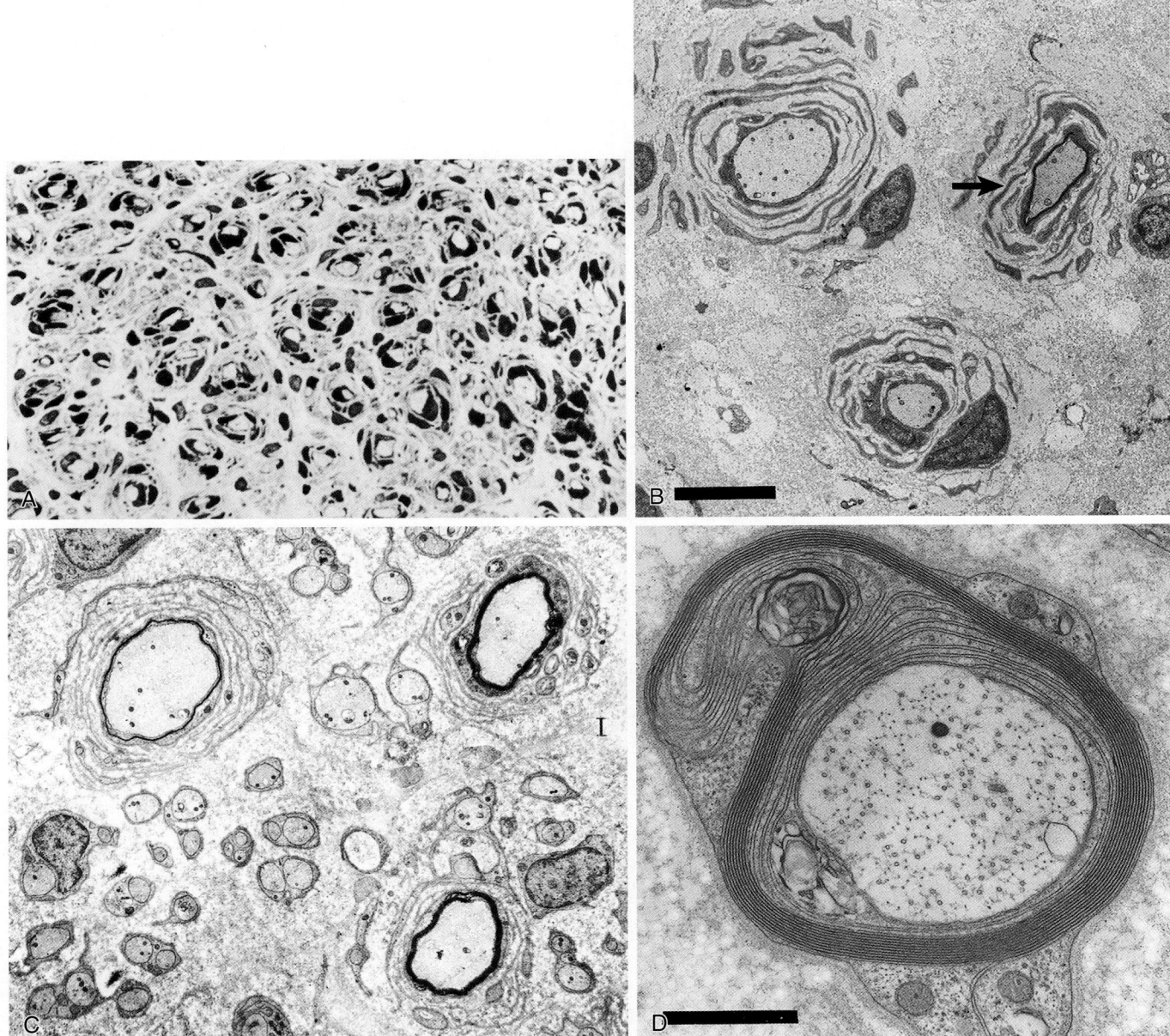

Figure 32.12 Chronic polyneuropathy with onion bulb formation. (A) From an infant with hypotonia and weakness from birth, elevated CSF protein level, and motor nerve conduction velocities markedly reduced to approximately 2 m/second. The sural nerve (which underwent biopsy when the child was 5½ years of age) shows total lack of myelin sheaths and, around individual axons, an increase in the number of Schwann cells arranged concentrically, assuming an onion bulb pattern (toluidine blue–O stain, ×500). (B) Sural nerve biopsy of 4½ year old girl with a DSD phenotype due to a *PMP22* missense mutation. Large onion bulbs are seen around demyelinated and remyelinated *(arrow)* fibers. Marked increase in endoneural collagen. Bar = 5 μm. (C) From an infant with delayed motor development, areflexia, and distal muscular atrophy. This electron micrograph of the sural nerve, which underwent biopsy in the child at 2½ years of age, shows nerve fibers separated by an increased amount of collagen. Note particularly the three poorly myelinated nerve fibers with onion bulb formations. (D) Uncompacted myelin lamellae in sural nerve biopsy of 12-year-old girl with a missense mutation in the extracellular domain of *MPZ*. Bar = 1 μm. (A From Kennedy WR, Sung JH, Berry JF. A case of congenital hypomyelination neuropathy. *Arch Neurol.* 1977;34:337–345. B and D, From Yiu EM, Baets J, Congenital and early infantile neuropathies. In: Darras BT, Jones HR Jr, Ryan MM, De Vivo DC eds. *Neuromuscular Disorders of Infancy, Childhood and Adolescence: A Clinician's Approach.* 2nd ed. San Diego: Academic Press; 2015:chap 16, 289–318. C From Anderson RM, Dennett X, Hopkins IJ, Shield LK. Hypertrophic interstitial polyneuropathy in infancy. *J Pediatr.* 1973;82:619–624.)

is treatable. It may be apparent in the neonatal period.[266-270] Decrease in fetal movement and the occurrence of contractures indicate that prenatal onset may occur. The newborn exhibits a poor suck and is hypotonic and weak. Weakness is either in a distal more than proximal or distal equal to proximal distribution. Areflexia is common. The diagnosis is suggested by the finding of elevated CSF protein level, delayed motor nerve conduction velocities (<70% of normal and usually considerably less), and electrophysiological evidence of an acquired neuropathy (multifocal disease with conduction block and temporal dispersion). Nerve biopsy shows diminution in myelin and evidence of segmental demyelination and remyelination, but especially subperineurial and endoneurial edema with inflammatory cells. Treatment with corticosteroids has been markedly beneficial. Thus in infants with signs of demyelinating neuropathy and no evidence of a familial disorder, this disorder should be considered seriously, because therapy can lead to major clinical improvement. Notably, one reported patient[269] began to improve *without therapy* by 2 months and fully recovered by age 6 months. It should be noted, however, that certain genetic forms of demyelinating neuropathies, such as CMT4J (FIG4 gene mutations), may present during infancy with a clinical and electrophysiologic phenotype of Guillain-Barré syndrome or CIDP (Table 32.5). Lack of response to immunotherapy should alert the clinician to the possibility of an underlying genetic defect.

Chronic Motor-Sensory Neuropathy: Neuronal-Axonal Disease

A rare cause of hypotonia and weakness in the newborn period is peripheral nerve disease on the basis of neuronal-axonal involvement. Two groups of patients with neuronal-axonal neuropathy should be distinguished: those with and those without associated Werdnig-Hoffmann disease. Of note, the term DSD also includes axonal forms of CMT with early onset.

Axonal polyneuropathy unassociated with Werdnig-Hoffmann disease has been reported only rarely.[a] In the series of 20 cases of congenital polyneuropathy studied by Hagberg and Lyon,[205] only a single case was of the neuronal-axonal type. Neonatal features have included marked hypotonia and weakness and respiratory distress. Arthrogryposis multiplex congenita may be present. The clinical course is usually static or subject to improvement. Results of the EMG and muscle biopsy indicate denervation. Nerve conduction velocities are normal or only modestly depressed, in contrast to the markedly depressed velocities in hypomyelinative neuropathy (see later discussion). Sural nerve biopsy shows axonal degeneration (Fig. 32.13). Secondary changes in myelin surrounding the degenerating axons may occur (see Fig. 32.13). Sporadic cases have been most common, although autosomal dominant inheritance has been recorded.[271] A subset of these cases, with a more severe course, consists of infants with *SMARD1*, discussed earlier, because of accompanying anterior horn cell disease (see "Spinal Muscular Atrophy Variants").[141,144,145,277] Most sporadic cases are related to de novo dominant mutations in various genes such as mitofusin 2 (MFN2), TPRV4, DYNC1H1, GDAP1, and NEFL.[204] Mitochondrial genes have also been linked to the pathogenesis of infantile, primarily axonal, neuropathies.

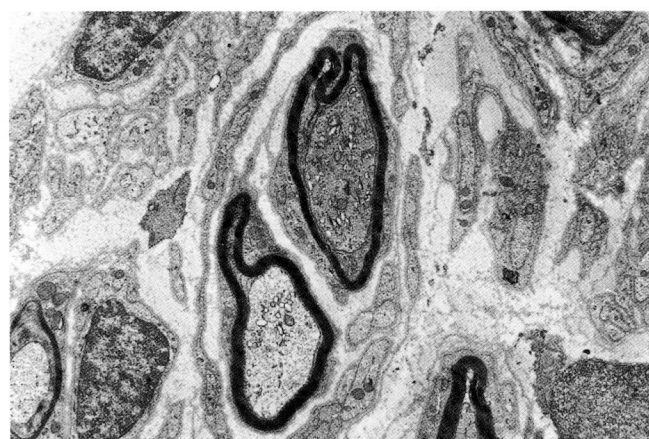

Figure 32.13 Congenital axonal neuropathy with hypomyelination-demyelination. Electron micrograph of onion bulb surrounding two fibers with axonal alterations (×6000). (From Guzzetta F, Ferrière G. Congenital neuropathy with prevailing axonal changes. *Acta Neuropathol [Berl]*. 1985;68: 185–190.)

Neuronal-axonal polyneuropathy associated with Werdnig-Hoffmann disease has been described in numerous reports.[114-116,278-288] The infants studied generally have died in the first year of life with the clinical features of Werdnig-Hoffmann disease and with loss of axons noted at postmortem examination, in addition to the characteristic changes of anterior horn cells. Whether the degree of axonal loss is greater than that expected from the involvement of anterior horn cells of Werdnig-Hoffmann disease is difficult to judge from published data. However, of greater interest, disturbance of *sensory* nerve conduction velocity has been demonstrated, and axonal loss and glial infiltration have been reported in *dorsal* as well as ventral roots and in dorsal root ganglia at postmortem examination. Indeed, in one study, impairment of sensory nerve conduction velocities was said to be present in approximately 40% of cases of infantile SMA, but the diagnosis in these cases was not molecularly confirmed.[285] In two severely affected sibships, associated with homozygous deletions of the SMN1 gene region, sensory as well as motor nerves were inexcitable on electrophysiological testing.[114,288] In one sibship, the deletion was large and probably involved genes neighboring the SMN1 gene. However, in clinical practice SMA type 1 cases with sensory nerve or dorsal root ganglion cell involvement are extremely rare; one of the authors (BTD) has never seen such a case in 20 years of clinical and EMG practice.

Chronic Motor-Sensory Polyneuropathy: Subcellular

Various other neurological disorders, in which a specific *subcellular structure* or biochemical component thereof is affected, occasionally are recognizable in the first month of life and may have associated disease of peripheral nerve (see Box 32.6), including mitochondrial disease, cytoskeletal disorders (giant axonal neuropathy [intermediate filaments], infantile neuroaxonal dystrophy [neurofilaments]), and certain lysosomal disorders (Krabbe disease). Infantile neuroaxonal dystrophy is not a disorder of the neonatal period; the pathology of peripheral nerve has been defined.[289] For practical purposes, Krabbe disease does not deserve serious consideration here because central

---

[a]References 141, 144, 145, 205, 237, and 271-277.

nervous system phenomena usually dominate the clinical presentation and course (see Chapter 29). However, impaired motor nerve conduction velocities have been documented in the second month in Krabbe disease.[290] Thus in this section, we review briefly only the neuropathic aspects of mitochondrial disease, as well as giant axonal neuropathy.

Mitochondrial Disease

Peripheral neuropathy is a common feature of *mitochondrial disease*. As discussed in Chapter 29 in relation to degenerative diseases of the central nervous system, mitochondrial disease, such as Leigh disease, may lead to hypotonia and weakness on the basis of disease above the lower motor neuron. However, in addition, some infants with mitochondrial disease have had electrophysiological and histological evidence of peripheral nerve involvement.[291-295] In a well-studied series of 43 cases of congenital lactic acidosis related primarily to deficiency of pyruvate dehydrogenase activity or various elements of the electron transport chain (complexes I to IV, isolated or in combination), all exhibited neonatal hypotonia.[295] Nerve conduction studies carried out later in infancy provided evidence of neuropathic disease in 42 of the 43. Approximately 70% exhibited signs indicative of both axonal and demyelinative disease. The EMG may reveal fibrillation potentials, findings supporting the concept of an ongoing denervating process.[292,293] Nerve conduction velocities generally are reduced by approximately 15%, more consistent with axonal than myelin disease. No such studies of neonatal patients are available. Histological abnormalities of the nerve system have included evidence for axonal and myelin involvement.[291-293] Several genes, such as *SCO2, DGUOK, TK2,* and others, have been found to be mutated in patients with infantile, primarily axonal neuropathies.[204] The co-occurrence of neuropathy and CNS involvement, cardiomyopathy, hepatopathy, or ophthalmoparesis with or without lactic acidosis should raise the possibility of mitochondrial disease.

Giant Axonal Neuropathy

The unusual disorder of *giant axonal neuropathy* is characterized by onset after the first year of life of chronic, slowly progressive, primarily motor neuropathy.[296-306] However, onset in the neonatal period with marked hypotonia, weakness, and areflexia has been reported.[300,306-308] A nearly constant accompaniment is tightly curled, kinky, poorly pigmented scalp hair that may be apparent in the neonatal period (the hair abnormality is usually more obvious after the first months of life, and its absence is associated with a milder phenotype[309]). Nerve histology is striking: axons are greatly enlarged (giant axons) and are filled with disarrayed neurofilaments. Accumulation of filaments in Schwann cells may account for the associated demyelination.[297] Involvement of neurons and oligodendroglia of the central nervous system may cause progressive cognitive and motor deficits and striking abnormality of cerebral white matter, especially on MRI scans.[298,302,303,306] The demonstrations of disordered filaments in astrocytes and fibroblasts[306,310] involving the principal proteins of intermediate filaments (i.e., glial fibrillary acidic protein [astrocytes] and vimentin [fibroblasts]) led to the suggestion that the disease represents a disturbance of organization of intermediate filaments.[300,311] The genetic defect has been localized to chromosome 16q24, and the giant axonal neuropathy gene *(GAN)* encodes the protein gigaxonin.[304,305,312,313] Gigaxonin appears to play an important role in the integrity of the cytoskeletal structure through interaction with a microtubule-associated protein.

Hereditary Sensory and Autonomic Neuropathies

Currently, *hereditary sensory and autonomic neuropathies* (HSAN) with clinical presentation in the neonatal period include at least four basic disorders: congenital insensitivity to pain (two types), a similar congenital neuropathy with anhidrosis, and familial dysautonomia (Riley-Day syndrome; see Box 32.6). The four disorders are inherited in an autosomal recessive manner and are classified as HSAN types II and V (congenital insensitivity to pain), III (familial dysautonomia), and IV (congenital insensitivity to pain with anhidrosis) in the classic classification system of Dyck and Ohta.[314] Recently, the identification of genes associated with HSANs has led to a genotype-based classification system (Table 32.6).[315] Hereditary sensory radicular neuropathy type I usually exhibits clinical presentation in late childhood to early adulthood, but congenital onset has also been reported.[316]

TABLE 32.6   Hereditary Sensory and Autonomic Neuropathies Pattern of Inheritance and Associated Genes

TYPE	OTHER NAMES	INHERITANCE	GENES	OMIM
I	Hereditary sensory radicular neuropathy	Autosomal dominant	*SPTLC1, SPLTC2*	162400
			ATL1	613640
			RAB7	613708
			DNMT1	600882
				126375
IIA	Congenital insensitivity to pain	Autosomal recessive	*WNK1*	201300
IIB			*FAM134B*	613115
IIC			*KIF1A*	614213
III	FD/Riley-Day	Autosomal recessive	*IKBKAP*	223900
IV	CIPA	Autosomal recessive	*TrK A/NGF R*	256800
V	Congenital insensitivity to pain	Autosomal recessive	*NGF B*	608654

CIPA, Congenital insensitivity to pain with anhidrosis; *FD,* familial dysautonomia; *HSAN,* hereditary sensory and autonomic neuropathy; *OMIM,* Online Mendelian Inheritance in Man.

Reprinted with permission from Axelrod FB, Kaufmann H. Hereditary sensory and autonomic neuropathies. In: Darras BT, Jones HR Jr, Ryan MM, De Vivo DC, eds. *Neuromuscular Disorders of Infancy, Childhood and Adolescence: A Clinician's Approach.* 2nd ed. San Diego: Academic Press; 2015:chap 18, 340–352.

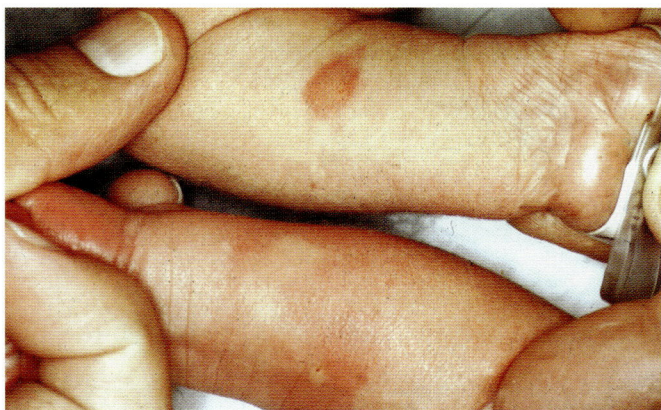

Figure 32.14 Histamine test. The top forearm displays the abnormal reaction to intradermal histamine that is characteristic for HSAN. Only a narrow areola surrounds the wheal. Lower forearm displays normal reaction to histamine test with diffuse axon flare around a central wheal. *HSAN*, Hereditary sensory and autonomic neuropathies. (Reprinted with permission from Axelrod FB, Kaufmann H. Hereditary sensory and autonomic neuropathies. In: Darras BT, Jones HR Jr, Ryan MM, De Vivo DC, eds. *Neuromuscular Disorders of Infancy, Childhood and Adolescence: A Clinician's Approach.* 2nd ed. San Diego: Academic Press; 2015:chap 18, 340–352.)

Because autonomic phenomena are common in all these disorders, the term *hereditary sensory autonomic neuropathies* is preferred.[317,318] These sensory disorders are discussed in this chapter on motor abnormalities, because hypotonia and areflexia are very common features.

HSAN Types II and V

The designation of *congenital insensitivity to pain* has been applied to a variety of cases of sensory neuropathy with onset in infancy and either slow or no progression of disease. Of these cases, patients with onset in the neonatal period consistently have exhibited the *nonprogressive* course.[318-322] Because evaluation of sensory and autonomic nerve function, the prominent sites of involvement, is difficult in the newborn, the clinical presentation often suggests a motor disturbance because of the presence of *hypotonia, areflexia, feeding disturbance*, and occasionally, *limb weakness.* Gag and corneal reflexes are diminished. These deficits are presumably related to the disturbance of afferent input from muscle and the muscle spindle. With careful examination and with maturation of the infant, marked impairment of pain, touch, and temperature develops. Less consistently recorded have been disturbances of hearing, smell, and taste, although more careful testing probably would indicate that such disturbances are common. Although less commonly evaluated, such autonomic disturbances as defective lacrimation, impaired axonal flare after stimulation with intradermal histamine phosphate (Fig. 32.14), and absence of fungiform papillae have been recorded. However, in HSAN type II sweating is normal, and cognitive function varies greatly. Infants with dysmorphic facies[323,324] and with skeletal dysplasia[325] have been described. In HSAN type V, cognitive impairment is not typical, and the degree of hypohidrosis is variable compared with anhidrosis in HSAN type IV. Mutations in four genes have been detected in patients with HSAN types II and V or congenital insensitivity to pain (see Table 32.6).[316,326-329]

Diagnosis is supported by demonstration of a normal EMG and normal motor nerve conduction velocities but grossly

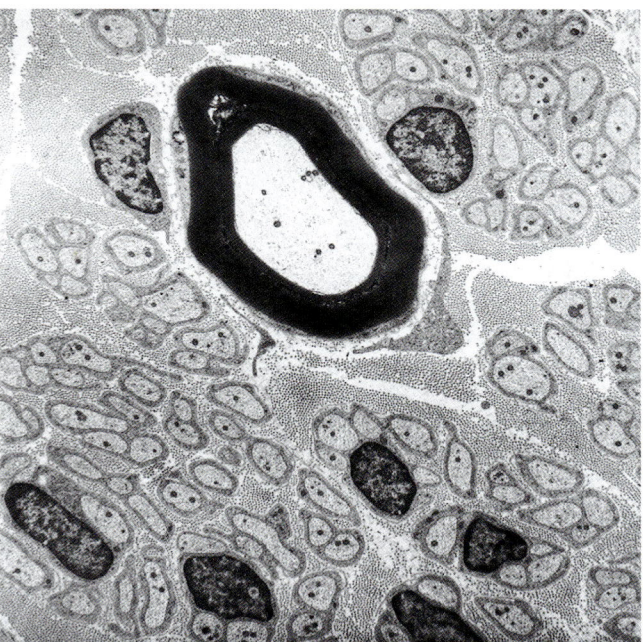

Figure 32.15 Congenital sensory neuropathy from an infant with the clinical features described in the text as characteristic of this disorder. This electron micrograph shows many small unmyelinated fibers but, importantly, only a single myelinated fiber *(upper center)*; the myelin sheath is normal. The unmyelinated small fibers exhibit no signs of axonal disease. Several normal Schwann cell nuclei are visible in the lower portion of the micrograph. (Courtesy Drs. Franco Guzzetta and Gerard Ferrière.)

impaired or absent sensory nerve conduction responses. *Sural nerve biopsy* demonstrates most characteristically a marked reduction in *myelinated fibers* (Fig. 32.15) but without evidence of myelin degeneration or defective myelin formation around the few remaining observable large fibers, which have normal-appearing myelin sheaths (in contrast to congenital hypomyelinative motor neuropathies, in which the many large fibers have little or no myelin sheaths). The essential pathogenesis is unclear, but a defect in the *formation of nerve fibers* destined for myelination seems possible; no cutaneous nerve fibers or receptors are seen.[321,330]

HSAN IV, Congenital Insensitivity to Pain With Anhidrosis

Congenital insensitivity to pain with anhidrosis is a clinical disorder with many similarities to that just recorded but with profound insensitivity to pain, complete lack of sweating, and cognitive impairment.[331-341] (This disorder is sometimes termed *congenital insensitivity to pain with anhidrosis.*) Both autosomal recessive inheritance and sporadic occurrence have been recorded. Nerve biopsy has shown an almost complete absence of *small myelinated and unmyelinated fibers.*[333,335,336,338-343] The particular absence of small fibers accounts for the defect of sweating; the cause of the intellectual impairment is unknown. The molecular genetic defect involves loss of function mutations in the NTRK1 gene, which encodes the tyrosine kinase receptor A gene (TRKA; Table 32.6). The TRKA protein is a receptor tyrosine kinase that is phosphorylated in response to nerve growth factor (NGF)[340,341] and mediates the normal binding of NGF. NGF is critical for the survival of sympathetic ganglion neurons and nociceptive sensory neurons in the dorsal root ganglia.[315]

TABLE 32.7   Common Neonatal Abnormalities in Familial Dysautonomia[a]

ABNORMALITY	PERCENTAGE OF TOTAL (%)
Poor or no suck reflex	62
Gavage feeding in nursery	32
Hypotonia	44
Hypothermia	26
Aspiration	20

[a]Based on 49 cases with (later) proven familial dysautonomia; in only five was the diagnosis made in the neonatal period, and each of these patients had affected siblings.

Adapted from Axelrod FB, Porges RF, Sein ME. Neonatal recognition of familial dysautonomia. *J Pediatr*. 1987;110:946–948.

HSAN III, Familial Dysautonomia (Riley-Day Syndrome)

Familial dysautonomia, a rare, autosomal recessive disorder, usually becomes apparent in the first year of life, although recognition in the neonatal period, albeit very uncommon, is possible.[252,321,343-350] Because of the serious implications for prognosis and genetic counseling, diagnosis early in infancy is important.

The most helpful *clinical features* in the neonatal period include Ashkenazi Jewish parents, feeding difficulty with tracheal aspiration, abnormal *rolling* tongue movements, nasal cry, peculiar jerky limb movements, hypotonia, and episodes of marked irritability with retrocollis and opisthotonos (Table 32.7).[344,348] A report has described unexplained episodic somnolence (duration, 4 to 15 hours) in a newborn with familial dysautonomia.[350] Corneal reflexes are absent, and tendon reflexes are depressed. Absent fungiform papillae, miosis after dilute methacholine, lack of axonal flare after intradermal histamine (see Fig. 32.14), and defective lacrimation complete the syndrome. Clinical progression is common, although variable in severity.

Sural nerve biopsy distinguishes Riley-Day syndrome from those just described. Thus a drastic reduction in *unmyelinated* fibers is observed; much less disturbance of myelinated fibers is present.[345,349]

The genetic defect is localized to chromosome 9q31–33, and the responsible gene *(IKBKAP)* encodes an I kappa-beta kinase–associated protein (see Table 32.6).[343] The protein appears critical for development as well as continued survival of the sensory and autonomic neurons involved. Although three mutations have been reported in the *IKBKAP* gene, 99.5% of the familial dysautonomia patients are homozygous for the IVS2O + 6 T_C splicing mutation in intron 20; this mutation leads to skipping of exon 20 in the *IKBKAP* mRNA, which results in a truncated and thus nonfunctional protein.[351-353]

Acute Polyneuropathy

The evolution of *acute, predominantly motor polyneuropathy* with hypotonia and weakness has been documented in infants in the first weeks of life.[354-361] In four cases, diminished fetal movement was noted. Because of the self-limited course, it seems possible that neonatal cases have been mistaken for other transient causes of hypotonia and weakness. A recognizable

BOX 32.7   Hypotonia and Weakness: Level of the Neuromuscular Junction

Myasthenia
Neonatal transient
Arthrogryposis, fetal akinesia syndrome
Fetal acetylcholine receptor inactivation syndrome
Congenital (hereditary) myasthenic syndromes (see Table 32.9)
Toxic-Metabolic Conditions
Hypermagnesemia
Antibiotics, aminoglycosides
Infantile Botulism

infection may be apparent a week or more previously. In two cases, the mother had Guillain-Barré syndrome during her pregnancy. In affected infants, hypotonia and weakness evolve over days. Two other mothers had inflammatory bowel disease and anti-GM1 neuropathy. Areflexia and involvement of cranial nerves (especially VII) are common. Respiratory failure may ensue.

The diagnosis is suggested by an elevated CSF protein concentration in the absence of pleocytosis (i.e., albuminocytological dissociation). Nerve conduction velocities are severely depressed: in five patients, motor nerve conduction velocities were less than 8 m/second.[354,355,358,359,361]

If respiratory support is accomplished, recovery is the rule, often within 1 to 2 months. Recovery in acute infantile polyneuropathy may be more rapid than in the analogous Guillain-Barré syndrome of older patients, but more data are needed on this point. One infant treated with intravenous immunoglobulin began improvement within 48 hours, but complete recovery did not occur for several months.[361]

LEVEL OF THE NEUROMUSCULAR JUNCTION

Disorders of the neuromuscular junction (Fig. 32.16A) are infrequent causes of neonatal hypotonia and weakness. However, such disorders are critical to recognize because therapeutic intervention is usually beneficial and, indeed, lifesaving. Those disorders that are observed in the neonatal period are listed in Box 32.7. The prototype is myasthenia.

Myasthenia

Myasthenia is characterized principally by muscle weakness provoked by activity and relieved by rest. In an analysis of nearly 500 patients with myasthenia gravis, 11% were observed to have their first symptom in infancy or childhood,[362] 8% were affected after the age of 1 year, and 3% were affected before the age of 1 year. The last group was composed of 2% who were born of myasthenic mothers and experienced *transient* neonatal myasthenia gravis and 1% who were born of nonmyasthenic mothers and possibly had a congenital myasthenic syndrome.

Later work demonstrated that congenital myasthenic syndromes are heterogeneous in clinical presentation and course and, in general, are characterized by inherited defects in neuromuscular transmission (see later discussion). Thus these syndromes are intrinsically different from the typical autoimmune disorder recognized as myasthenia gravis in older infants, children, and adults; indeed, the youngest age

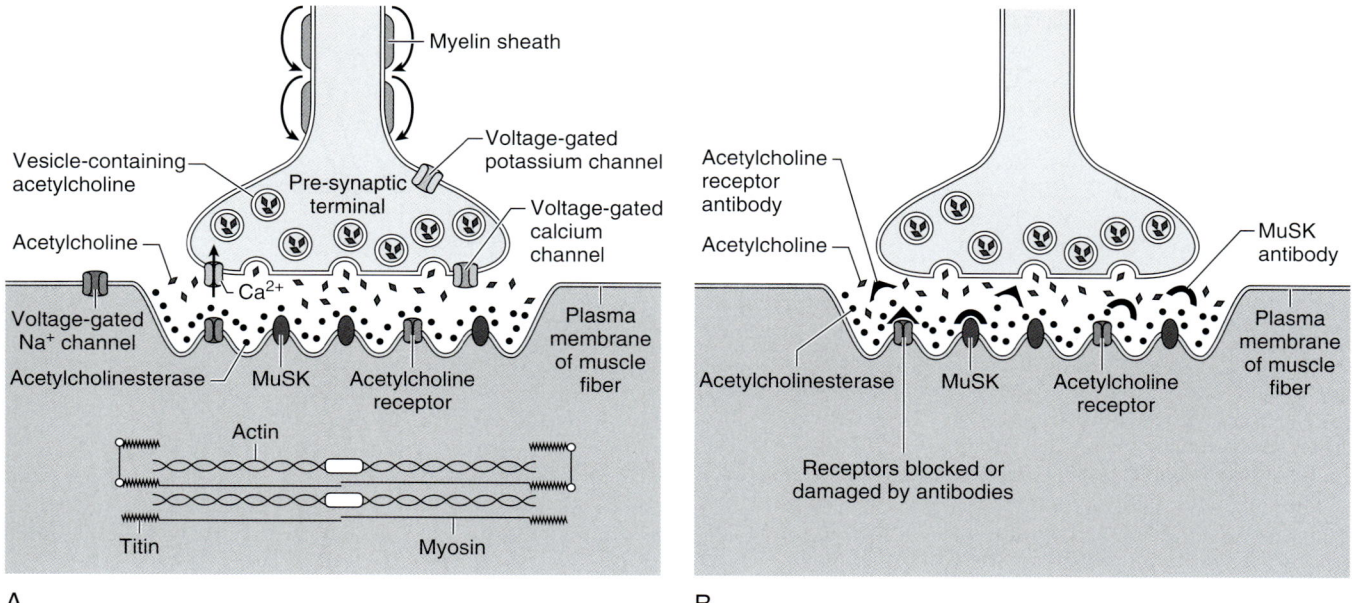

Figure 32.16 Schematic diagrams of (A) a normal neuromuscular junction illustrating locations of the presynaptic vesicles, acetylcholine within the synapse, and the postsynaptic acetylcholine receptors, as well as (B) a neuromuscular junction affected by myasthenia gravis, with antibodies that interfere with the binding and/or structure of the acetylcholine receptors and muscle-specific kinase (MuSK) (note that antibodies to both proteins are not typically present in the same individual, though this phenomenon has been reported on occasion). (Reprinted with permission from Kang PB, Liew WKM, Oskoui M, Vincent A. Juvenile and neonatal myasthenia gravis. In: Darras BT, Jones HR Jr, Ryan MM, De Vivo DC, eds. *Neuromuscular Disorders of Infancy, Childhood and Adolescence: A Clinician's Approach.* 2nd ed. San Diego: Academic Press; 2015:chap 27, 482–496.)

at onset of autoimmune myasthenia gravis reported is 6 to 12 months.[363] Interestingly, 55% of reported infants with onset of autoimmune myasthenia gravis before the age of 3 years were born prematurely.[364,365]

Neonatal Transient Myasthenia Gravis

The dramatic myasthenic syndrome of *neonatal transient myasthenia gravis*, described initially in 1942, occurs in approximately 10% to 20% of infants born to myasthenic mothers.[362,366-372] The disorder has important implications for the pathogenesis of myasthenia gravis (see later discussion).

Clinical Features. The *onset* of neonatal transient myasthenia gravis in approximately two-thirds of the cases is within the first hours after birth, although this often occurs *after* an apparently normal period immediately following delivery.[24,367,368] In nearly 80% of patients, onset is apparent by 24 hours, and the latest onset is 3 days.[367] Thus if an infant of a myasthenic mother has an onset of hypotonia and weakness on the fourth postnatal day or beyond, some other condition should be suspected.

The *neurological features* are usually dramatic and may evolve very rapidly (Table 32.8).[a] Disturbance of cranial nerve musculature is prominent. Nearly all patients exhibit feeding difficulties with weakness of sucking and swallowing. Gavage feedings are required in approximately one-third of patients. Respiratory difficulties occur in two-thirds and result from an inability to handle pharyngeal secretions and from weakness

TABLE 32.8	Clinical Manifestations of Neonatal Transient Myasthenia Gravis
CLINICAL MANIFESTATION	**PERCENTAGE OF TOTAL (%)**
Feeding disturbance	87
Gavage feeding required	31
Respiratory disturbance	65
Weak cry	60
Facial weakness	54
Generalized muscle weakness	69
Hypotonia (marked)[a]	48
Ptosis	15
Oculomotor disturbance	8

[a]Hypotonia of some degree is essentially a constant feature.

Data from Namba T, Brown SB, Grob D. Neonatal myasthenia gravis: report of two cases and review of the literature. *Pediatrics.* 1970;45:488–504.

of respiratory muscles. Ventilation is required in approximately 30% of cases. The cry is weak, and facial diplegia is obvious in approximately 60% of affected infants. Generalized muscle weakness is readily recognized in approximately 70% of cases, and hypotonia is marked in approximately 50%. Hypotonia of some degree is nearly a constant feature. However, tendon reflexes are usually normally active, and no fasciculations can be discerned. In contrast to the most common congenital myasthenic syndrome (see subsequent section), eye signs are *uncommon*; ptosis is apparent in only 15% of patients, and

---

[a]References 24, 87, 362, 367, 368, and 373-379.

oculomotor disturbance is seen in fewer than 10% of these infants.

A few infants exhibit signs of intrauterine onset of weakness manifested especially by arthrogryposis and craniofacial anomalies (hypertelorism, micrognathia, low-set ears; see Chapter 31).[a] Polyhydramnios, short umbilical cord, pulmonary hypoplasia, and neonatal death are common in these more severely affected infants, who have clinical features of *fetal akinesia sequence* (see Chapter 31).

Another severe and less frequent variant is the fetal acetylcholine receptor (AChR) inactivation syndrome.[388] These infants present with facial diplegia, velopharyngeal incompetence, high-arched palate, conductive hearing loss, and cryptorchidism.[388-390] The mothers are not always symptomatic but have very high AChR titers; however, the antibodies are not always specific to the fetal AChR subunit.[390] It is crucial to make the diagnosis because the recurrence risk is near 100%.[388,391]

Most infants (≈80%) with the typical neonatal onset require anticholinesterase therapy for the disorder, and the mean duration of the illness in survivors is 18 days.[367,368] In previous years, approximately 10% of infants died with the disease, most often because of delayed, inadequate, or absent therapy.[367] Neonatal death now is rare.[368]

Diagnosis at the Bedside. Diagnosis is usually readily apparent in the presence of the clinical syndrome in the infant of a myasthenic mother. Occasionally, the mother's disease is not known to her physician or to her, and the diagnosis may be less obvious. There is a recent report of transient neonatal myasthenia gravis in an infant born to a seronegative mother with ocular myasthenia gravis.[392] Observation of the infant's response to anticholinesterase medication is the important diagnostic test. The choice of drug for the test is somewhat controversial. Neostigmine methylsulfate, 0.04 mg/kg, administered intramuscularly or subcutaneously, is commonly used. The maximum effect occurs after approximately 15 to 30 minutes. Muscarinic effects (e.g., diarrhea and excessive tracheal secretions) may require atropine. An advantage of neostigmine is the relatively long duration of beneficial effect (1 to 3 hours). If edrophonium is used, a suitable dose is 0.15 mg/kg, administered intramuscularly or subcutaneously, or 0.15 mg/kg administered intravenously in fractional amounts over several minutes, after a test dose of 0.03 mg/kg. A beneficial effect is apparent within 3 to 5 minutes and persists for approximately 10 to 15 minutes. In evaluation of the clinical response to anticholinesterase medication, it is important to choose a quantifiable clinical feature (e.g., sucking or swallowing ability, ventilatory function, facial or limb movement, or crying volume).

Laboratory Studies. The serum CK level, standard EMG (amplitude, duration, and number of motor unit potentials), nerve conduction velocities, and CSF protein concentration are normal. Muscle biopsy, studied by conventional techniques, is also normal.

The diagnosis is confirmed by demonstration of the *myasthenic* phenomenon on electrophysiological testing (see Chapter 30). Thus, in one careful study, repetitive nerve stimulation at a frequency of 10 impulses/second resulted in

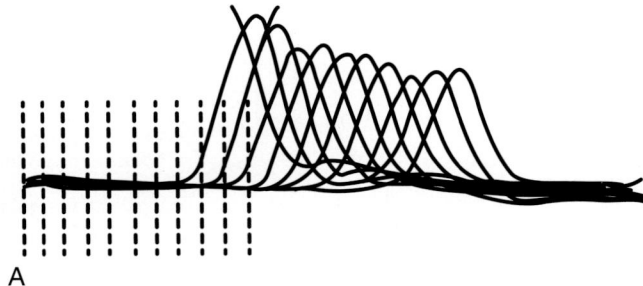

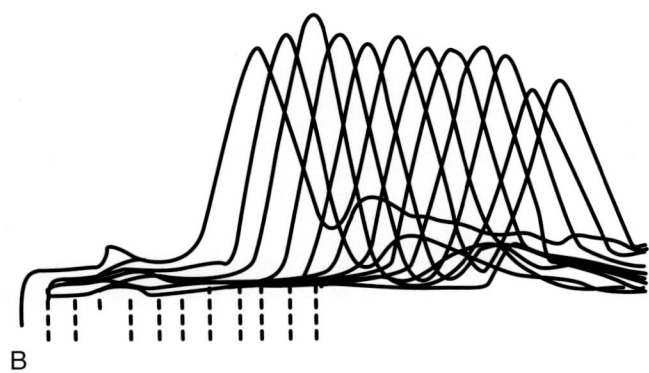

Figure 32.17 Electromyogram in neonatal transient myasthenia gravis: beneficial effect of edrophonium. (A) Repetitive stimulation of the median motor nerve with supramaximal stimulus intensity at a rate of 3 Hz demonstrated a decremental response of 23% between the first and fifth responses. (B) A 10-minute rest period followed to eliminate any possibility of postexercise facilitation. Edrophonium was infused intravenously (0.15 mg/kg). Repetitive stimulation within 120 seconds of infusion revealed complete repair of the decremental response. (From Hays RM, Michaud LJ. Neonatal myasthenia gravis: specific advantages of repetitive stimulation over edrophonium testing. *Pediatr Neurol.* 1988;4:245–247.)

a 40% decrement of the amplitude of the motor unit potential within 1 second.[393] With faster frequencies (e.g., 50 impulses/second), a nearly 50% decrement was observed within 100 milliseconds. Measurable improvement in this decrement can be observed after the injection of anticholinesterase medication (Fig. 32.17). Studies of the muscle response to repetitive nerve stimulation must be interpreted with the awareness that newborn infants exhibit less neuromuscular reserve than do older children, and premature infants have less reserve than do full-term infants. Thus Koenigsberger and co-workers[394] demonstrated an average decrement of 24% in 12 of 17 normal infants at the end of a 15-second train of 20 impulses/second, and an average decrement of 51% in all 17 infants at the end of a similar train of 50 impulses/second.[394] However, with 10 impulses/second, no decrement occurred in these normal infants either during or at the end of the train, in contrast to the observations in neonatal transient myasthenia gravis, as noted earlier. Most commonly used is a 5-second train of 2 to 3 impulses/second with supramaximal stimuli.[368,376]

Pathology. No data in regard to pathology are available for neonatal myasthenia gravis. By conventional techniques, no consistent histological abnormality is observed in myasthenia gravis in older patients.

Pathogenesis and Etiology. The essential defect in autoimmune myasthenia gravis is considered to be a decrease in available acetylcholine receptors at the postsynaptic muscle membrane.[368,395] This decrease is related to a circulating antibody to acetylcholine receptor protein.[396] These antibodies bind to a subunit of the extracellular domain of the acetylcholine receptor and lead to the myasthenic physiological defect in vivo and in vitro.[368,379,396-401] The mechanisms by which the antibodies produce the decrease in available receptors are as follows: (1) acceleration of degradation of receptors; (2) blocking of acetylcholine access to acetylcholine receptors; and (3) induction of local deposition of complement, including the membrane attack complement complex (Fig. 32.16B).[a]

The occurrence of myasthenia in infants of myasthenic mothers for many years stimulated a search for a humoral factor transmitted across the placenta. Antiacetylcholine receptor antibody appears to be the factor. Thus affected infants nearly invariably exhibit elevated antibody levels, and clinical improvement has been associated with lowering of antibody levels by exchange transfusion.[268,378,404-410] Moreover, fetal breathing movements have become apparent when maternal antibody levels are lowered by plasmapheresis,[380] and transient myasthenia gravis has been documented in an infant with neonatal lupus erythematosus and antiacetylcholine receptor antibodies.[411] Moreover, in one careful study, a relationship between the maternal antibody titer and the occurrence of transient neonatal myasthenia gravis was shown.[373,412]

The relationship between maternal antibody level and transmission of the transient neonatal disorder level has been refined by determination of ratio of antibody levels to the fetal (gamma, γ) versus the adult (epsilon, ε) type of acetylcholine receptor. Thus a high ratio in the pregnant woman is associated with a high likelihood for transmission (Fig. 32.18).[377] This observation may have pathogenetic implications because the newborn may have a relatively high proportion of fetal-type acetylcholine receptors.[377] Nevertheless, several observations indicate that host factors also must play an important role in pathogenesis: (1) only 10% to 20% of all infants of myasthenic mothers develop the transient neonatal syndrome; (2) among mothers who have had an affected infant, the incidence of recurrence rises markedly to approximately 75%[367,368,373]; (3) no invariable correlation exists between occurrence of symptoms and the level of neonatal antibodies[369,409,413]; and (4) asymptomatic myasthenic mothers in either spontaneous remission or remission induced by thymectomy have given birth to infants who had similar antibody titers to those of the mother and who developed typical transient neonatal myasthenia gravis.[408,414] Thus factors referable to the infant may govern the impact of the antiacetylcholine receptor antibody. The findings of both marked prolongation of elevated antibody levels and immunochemical differences between the antibody of mother and infant in symptomatic versus asymptomatic infants suggest that symptomatic infants synthesize antiacetylcholine receptor antibodies in addition to receiving passively transferred maternal antibody.[409] Consistent with this notion, antibody levels in affected newborns have been shown to increase after the lowering induced by exchange transfusion.[378] Finally, the possibility of a genetic predisposition to the disorder in

---

[a]References 24, 379, 396, 398, 402, and 403.

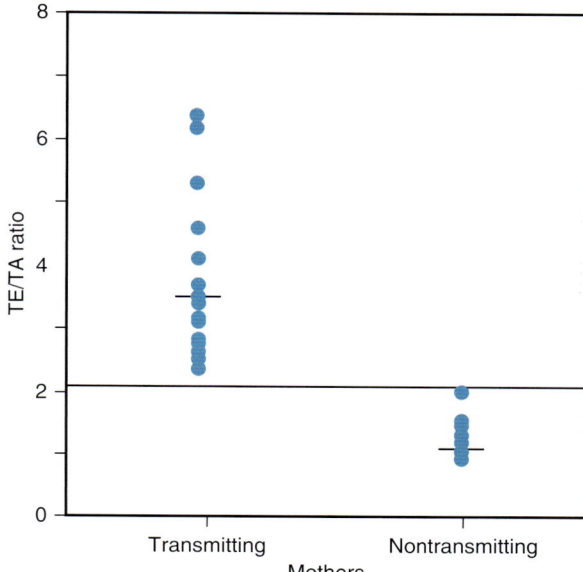

Figure 32.18 Distribution of antifetal (TE) and antiadult (TA) muscle acetylcholine receptor antibody titer ratio (TE/TA) in mothers transmitting or not transmitting neonatal transient myasthenia gravis. (From Gardnerova M, Eymard B, Morel E, Faltin M, et al. The fetal/adult acetylcholine receptor antibody ratio in mothers with myasthenia gravis as a marker for transfer of the disease to the newborn. *Neurology.* 1997;48:50–54.)

certain infants is raised by the observation that infants with the same composition of certain myasthenia-related human leukocyte antigens (HLAs) as exhibited by their mothers develop symptomatic disease, whereas infants with a different HLA composition do not.[368] More data are needed on these issues.

In the fetal AChR inactivation syndrome, the selective muscle involvement and persistence of weakness may be related to the timing and intensity of the antibody response during pregnancy. The distribution and density of the fetal ACh receptors may be the reason for the differential susceptibility of the midline muscles involved in oro-bucco-lingual function.[391]

Management. The management of neonatal transient myasthenia gravis is based on careful surveillance of the infant at risk and prompt diagnosis with the early signs of disease. The strong possibility that the infant likely to be affected can be identified prenatally by determination of the ratio of antibody levels to the fetal versus the adult type of acetylcholine receptor is raised by the work described earlier. Therapy is primarily twofold: supportive care and anticholinesterase medication.

Supportive therapy is critical and is addressed principally to the difficulties with feeding and respiration. Frequent feedings of small volumes are helpful to avoid fatigue and the possibility of aspiration. Tube feeding should be provided in patients with severe disease. Pharyngeal secretions should be suctioned and respiratory support provided as needed. The condition of these infants can deteriorate very rapidly. Aminoglycoside antibiotics should be avoided, if possible, because of their deleterious effect on neuromuscular function (see later section).

Anticholinesterase therapy has been used in approximately 80% of patients. In previous years, approximately 50% of those infants who died did not receive therapy. It is better to treat an infant with marginal deficits than to risk serious deterioration.

TABLE 32.9   Major Congenital Myasthenic Syndromes[a]

BASIC ABNORMALITY	USUAL INHERITANCE	NEONATAL ONSET COMMON	EXTRAOCULAR MUSCLE WEAKNESS COMMON	RESPONSE TO AChE INHIBITOR
Presynaptic abnormalities				
Defects in ACh synthesis (congenital choline acetyltransferase deficiency or familial infantile myasthenia)	Recessive	+	−	+
Paucity of synaptic vesicles	Recessive	+	−	+
Synaptic abnormalities				
AChE deficiency[b]	Recessive	+	+	−
Postsynaptic abnormalities				
ACh receptor deficiency (subunit defect)	Recessive	+	+	+
ACh receptor deficiency (rapsyn mutation)	Recessive	+	−	+
Slow-channel syndrome[b]	Dominant	±	+	−
Fast-channel syndrome	Dominant	±	+	+

[a]Most common congenital myasthenic syndromes.

[b]Avoid pyridostigmine: ineffective or harmful.

ACh, Acetylcholine; *AChE*, acetylcholinesterase; +, present; −, absent; ±, variable.

Neostigmine is the drug of choice and is best administered initially intramuscularly or subcutaneously as the methylsulfate derivative in a dose of 0.04 mg/kg, approximately 20 minutes before feedings. Nasogastric administration of 0.4 mg/kg 30 minutes before feedings is an alternative. Pyridostigmine bromide, in a dose of 4 to 10 mg, also could be used by gavage before feeding. Conversion to oral administration can be accomplished when the infant is stable and is swallowing well.

Exchange transfusion may be an adjunct in management. Thus three reports described clinical improvement in association with decrease in levels of antiacetylcholine receptor antibody caused by exchange transfusion.[268,378,410] Exchange transfusion did not produce clinical benefit in three other reported infants.[409,415] Moreover, when it does produce benefit, the response is transient. Thus the possible role of exchange transfusion is not yet entirely clear. In two reports, high-dose intravenous immunoglobulin was highly effective in one case and not clearly effective in another.[378,415]

To prevent recurrence in future pregnancies of the neonatal myasthenia gravis spectrum diseases, antenatal immunomodulatory treatment has been reported to lead to improved outcomes,[380,388] albeit not invariably.[416] Salbutamol has been shown to be effective in infants with fetal acetylcholine receptor inactivation syndrome[417]; the mechanism is not known, but it has been shown to improve AChR cluster assembly and neuromuscular junction architecture in a mouse model.[418]

Congenital Myasthenic Syndromes: Overview

Congenital (hereditary) myasthenic syndromes are caused by a variety of defects of the neuromuscular junction and are characterized by weakness and fatigability and by the phenomenon on the EMG of myasthenia from the first days or weeks of life. The disorders differ in a central way from later-onset myasthenia gravis and its transient neonatal counterpart; thus the congenital syndromes are *not* related to an immune process but are caused by *genetic defects of the neuromuscular junction*. The latter are described subsequently, but the development of new morphological, electrophysiological, biochemical, and

---

BOX 32.8   Congenital Myasthenic Syndromes: Common Features

Familial occurrence
Autosomal recessive > autosomal dominant
Early ocular involvement: ptosis > ophthalmoparesis
Early facial and bulbar involvement
Response to anticholinesterase drugs[a]
Diagnosis often requires the following: single-fiber electromyogram; single-nerve stimulation; specific staining for acetylcholine receptors, receptor subunits, acetylcholinesterase; electron microscopy of motor endplate; in vitro electrophysiological studies; molecular genetic analyses

[a]Except for acetylcholinesterase deficiency syndrome and slow-channel syndrome.

---

molecular genetic techniques for study of the neuromuscular junction is leading to definitions of new disorders. Although at least 16 congenital myasthenic syndromes are recognized,[419-424] relatively few exhibit *overt* neonatal onset. The major congenital myasthenic syndromes, including those with neonatal onset as a common feature, are reviewed in Table 32.9. Although phenotypic variability and some overlap exist, several clinical features are common to these syndromes (Box 32.8).[24,419,422-441] As a group, these disorders are rare, but the following two categories are the most common among the group.

Congenital Myasthenic Syndromes: Acetylcholine Receptor Deficiency (Congenital Myasthenia)

The designation *congenital myasthenia* previously referred to the most common of the congenital myasthenic syndromes. This disorder (or, better, group of disorders) was described initially by Bowman[442] in 1948. The disorder is related to deficiency of endplate acetylcholine receptors (see later discussion) and now is most commonly referred to as *endplate acetylcholine receptor deficiency*. Two subtypes should be recognized; the more common is related to a defect of a subunit of the acetylcholine receptor, and the somewhat less common is caused by a defect of a protein involved in clustering of the receptors (see later and Table 32.9).

Clinical Features. Although *onset* of this type of myasthenia is in the first weeks of life, the identification of the disorder is often made after that time. From available data, it seems likely that the correct diagnosis would be established in many cases in the newborn period if the physician's index of suspicion were higher.

The *neurological features* of the form associated with a *subunit deficiency* are characterized by prominent ptosis and ophthalmoplegia (see Table 32.9).[a] Ptosis is usually the prominent feature in the first weeks of life, and ophthalmoplegia becomes obvious in the ensuing months. Facial weakness and weak sucking and crying are common, but feeding difficulties are not usually marked. Hypotonia and weakness often are not apparent, except after considerable activity. The *clinical course*, with some exceptions, is benign. Anticholinesterase medication is useful for treating the facial weakness, feeding difficulties, and limb weakness, but is not particularly effective for treating the ophthalmoplegia, which tends to persist.

The *neurological features* of the form of endplate acetylcholine receptor deficiency related to a *mutation of rapsyn* (receptor-associated protein at the synapse), important for clustering of the receptors, is usually more severe than is the case for subunit deficiency (see Table 32.9).[423,441,447-449] In the early-onset cases of rapsyn deficiency, *arthrogryposis multiplex congenita*, severe *bulbar symptoms*, and the frequent need for assisted ventilation are prominent. The *clinical course* is more severe with rapsyn deficiency than with a subunit mutation, and frequent, severe exacerbations result in respiratory failure.

Diagnosis at the Bedside. Diagnosis of both forms of endplate acetylcholine receptor deficiency is made best by observation of the response to parenteral anticholinesterase drugs, as described previously for neonatal transient myasthenia gravis.

Laboratory Studies. The initial laboratory evaluation is similar to that described for neonatal transient myasthenia gravis. The decremental response of muscle action potentials with repetitive stimulation has been documented in endplate acetylcholine receptor deficiency or congenital myasthenia.[363,422-427,441,450,451] However, more detailed analysis is required for definitive diagnosis (see Box 32.8).

Pathology. No morphological abnormality at the site of the defect (i.e., the neuromuscular junction) has been described.

Pathogenesis and Etiology. Two major types of molecular defects underlying endplate acetylcholine receptor deficiency have been described, and both are inherited in an autosomal recessive manner.[b] Thus occurrence in siblings in approximately 50% of families and with consanguineous parents has been documented. Earlier studies indicated that the inherited defects at the neuromuscular junction involved the endplate acetylcholine receptor (see Table 32.9).[426,427,451,452] Thus a deficiency of the number or function of acetylcholine receptors, measured by alpha-bungarotoxin binding studies and electrophysiologically, was defined. The two molecular forms underlying this defect involve a *mutation in a subunit protein* or in *rapsyn*, active in receptor clustering. Of the four subunits of the acetylcholine receptor, the epsilon subunit of the receptor is involved in most cases.[a] The clustering of mutations in the epsilon subunit is related to the low-level expression of the fetal type gamma subunit, which compensates partially for the absence of the epsilon subunit[455-457]; patients with nonsense mutations in other AChR subunits may not survive because of lack of a compensating subunit.[424] The disorder is usually related to a mutation in the coding region of the gene for the epsilon subunit and less commonly in the promoter for this subunit. Rapsyn deficiency is only slightly less common than the subunit deficiency.

Management. The essential aspects of management involve the use of anticholinesterase medications, as discussed for neonatal transient myasthenia gravis. Anticholinesterase medication is not invariably beneficial.[422-424,426,427,441,458] 3,4-Diaminopyridine (DAP), which increases nerve terminal acetylcholine release, may be beneficial alone or in combination with anticholinesterase medication,[459] but only one-third of patients benefit from the addition of 3,4-DAP.[424] Steroid therapy and thymectomy have not been useful, in accordance with the nonimmune basis of the disorder. The nonimmune basis is evidenced by the lack of circulating acetylcholine receptor antibodies.[363,451] Recently, in patients responding poorly to anticholinesterase medication, albuterol treatment was reported to be effective.[460]

Congenital Myasthenic Syndromes: Congenital Choline Acetyltransferase Deficiency (Familial Infantile Myasthenia or Congenital Myasthenic Syndrome With Episodic Apnea)

Congenital choline acetyltransferase deficiency, formerly referred to as *familial infantile myasthenia* or, more recently, *congenital myasthenic syndrome with episodic apnea*, is a presynaptic defect, and the second most common type of congenital myasthenic syndrome with onset in the neonatal period (see Table 32.9). In contrast to endplate acetylcholine receptor deficiency, this disorder is based on a *presynaptic defect*. Like endplate acetylcholine receptor deficiency, the disorder is inherited in an autosomal recessive manner and has its onset in the neonatal period.[b] However, several features, readily delineated at the patient's bedside, help distinguish this form of myasthenia from the transient form and from acetylcholine receptor deficiency (see later discussion).

Clinical Features. *At birth*, infants are hypotonic and cyanotic and require resuscitative efforts. Episodes of apnea occur, and prominent feeding difficulties result from deficits of sucking and swallowing. Facial weakness is prominent, but eye movements are normal and usually remain so. Ptosis may be present but is not striking. Generalized weakness is common. After the serious neonatal course, appropriately treated infants (anticholinesterase medication) improve, and *spontaneous remission* often ensues in the first months of life. However, the disease may *recur* later in infancy and, indeed, develop so abruptly with respiratory

[a]References 24, 362, 363, 419, 422-424, 426, 427, 433, 435, 441, and 443-446.
[b]References 24, 363, 419, 422-424, 426, 427, 435, 438, 441, 444, 449, and 451.

[a]References 24, 419, 420, 422-424, 435, 438, 441, 453, and 454.
[b]References 24, 363, 422-424, 426, 427, 431, 440, 443, 451, and 461-467.

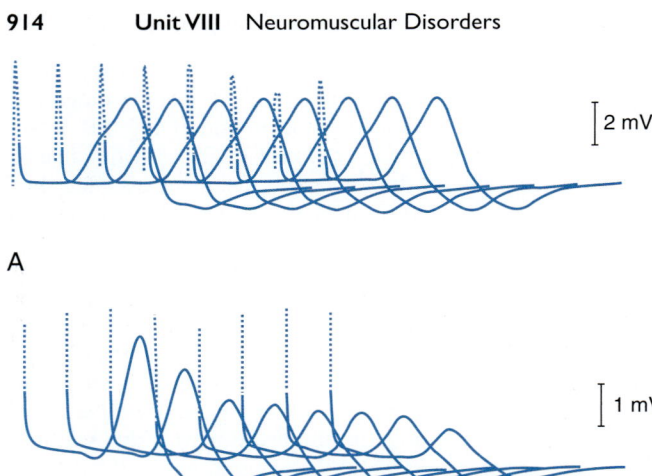

A

B

| | 2 ms |

Figure 32.19 Electromyogram in familial infantile myasthenia. In this repetitive nerve stimulation study, recordings were obtained from the left abductor digiti minimi with surface stimulating and recording electrodes. (A) A 3-Hz stimulation at rest shows no decrement. (B) At 4 minutes after 2 minutes of continuous stimulation of ulnar nerve at 10 Hz, a decrement of 54% (fifth/first response) occurred. (From Matthes JW, Kenna AP, Fawcett PRW. Familial infantile myasthenia: a diagnostic problem. *Dev Med Child Neurol.* 1991;33:912–929.)

infection that apnea and death may result.[468-470] A family history of sudden infant death syndrome in previously born siblings is not uncommon. In general, despite the episodic course, *improvement* with age is the rule.

Diagnosis at the Bedside. Diagnosis is suspected by observation of a beneficial response to parenteral anticholinesterase medication. A decremental response of the muscle to repetitive nerve stimulation requires more prolonged stimulation (several minutes) and more rapid rates (10 Hz) than required for other neonatal myasthenias (Fig. 32.19A and B). This electrophysiological aspect relates to the fundamental *presynaptic* defect, which involves acetylcholine synthesis or release (see later discussion).

Laboratory Studies. Although decremental responses to repetitive stimulation are present in this disorder, as in the other myasthenic disorders, elicitation of the abnormality may require more prolonged stimulation in familial infantile myasthenia.[451,463]

Pathology. No morphological abnormality is demonstrable at the neuromuscular junction.

Pathogenesis and Etiology. The inherited defect at the neuromuscular junction is presynaptic in location and in the gene that codes for choline acetyltransferase *(CHAT)*, the rate-limiting enzyme in resynthesis of acetylcholine from acetyl–coenzyme A and choline within the nerve terminal (see Table 32.9).[422-424]

Management. Anticholinesterase drugs form the cornerstone of therapy. Moreover, therapy should be continued despite improvement or apparent remission, to avoid the occurrence of

apnea and sudden death. DAP may produce transient benefit but then may worsen symptoms, as acetylcholine stores are depleted and are not replenished sufficiently quickly. Midazolam has been reported to resolve severe episodes of apnea in an infant with the disease, but this treatment needs further study.[469] Close surveillance is necessary indefinitely, because serious respiratory exacerbations have been reported, even in adults with this disorder.[465]

Toxic-Metabolic Defects of the Neuromuscular Junction

Various exogenous and endogenous toxins and metabolites may disturb the function of the neuromuscular junction. Of these, the most important for neonatal patients are magnesium and certain antibiotics (see Box 32.7).

Hypermagnesemia

Neonatal hypermagnesemia may result in a striking paralytic syndrome. The disorder most often is secondary to administration to the mother of large quantities of intravenous magnesium sulfate for the treatment of eclampsia before delivery.

Clinical Features. The clinical syndrome is usually apparent at birth with hypoventilation or apnea, severe weakness and hypotonia, and hyporeflexia or areflexia.[471-473] In addition to manifestations relating to *skeletal muscular involvement*, evidence of depression of the *central nervous system* (e.g., stupor or coma) and disturbed function of *smooth muscle* (e.g., abdominal distention and absent bowel sounds) may occur. The smooth muscle dysfunction may be so severe that meconium plug syndrome develops.[473] Infants provided supportive therapy recover within approximately 3 days, although serum magnesium levels may remain elevated longer.

In a retrospective cohort study of 242 neonates of ≥35 weeks' gestation, who were exposed to antenatal magnesium sulfate, 52 (21.1%) were admitted to the neonatal intensive care unit (NICU).[474] There was an association between NICU admission and dose of magnesium sulfate, as well as with duration of exposure; the risk of admission was higher with doses more than 30 grams and with more than 12 hours of exposure.

Laboratory Studies. The diagnosis is confirmed by the observation of elevated serum magnesium levels (usually >4.5 mEq/L). Electrophysiological studies with repetitive stimulation demonstrate impaired neuromuscular function.[473] Prolonged posttetanic facilitation and absent posttetanic exhaustion are characteristic findings.[475]

Pathogenesis and Etiology. The pathogenesis of weakness and hypotonia with hypermagnesemia relates to the effect of magnesium at the presynaptic side of the neuromuscular junction, in contrast to the postsynaptic disturbance in neonatal transient myasthenia or endplate acetylcholine receptor deficiency. Hypermagnesemia results in an impairment of release of acetylcholine from the presynaptic nerve ending. This effect is a result of antagonism of the releasing effect of calcium, and indeed calcium counteracts the toxic effects of magnesium to a variable degree.

Management. Management of hypermagnesemia is based on vigorous support. A clearly beneficial role for calcium supplementation was not supported by the few clinical trials available.[472] *Hypocalcemia, however, should be particularly avoided.* Exchange transfusion has been useful in the management of the very severely affected infant who is not responsive to supportive therapy.[476]

Antibiotics

Certain antibiotics, particularly the aminoglycosides, may disturb neuromuscular function. The drugs reported to have toxic effects include kanamycin, gentamicin, neomycin, colimycin, streptomycin, and polymyxin.[477-479] Drug-induced cases have been recorded in the neonatal period.[477,480] Although this disorder has not been recognized in infants with myasthenia, the particular sensitivity of older patients with myasthenia to these drugs[478,481] makes it imperative in infants with myasthenia to avoid their use or, when necessary, to use such drugs under carefully controlled conditions. A similar conclusion applies to infants with botulism (see subsequent discussion).

Clinical Features. The clinical syndrome in otherwise neurologically normal infants has occurred most commonly with the administration of large quantities of drug, such as at the time of abdominal surgery (intraperitoneal lavage) or pulmonary surgery (intrapleural lavage), retrograde pyelography, and intravenous therapy. Postoperative occurrence has been associated with the combined use of a curare-type drug during anesthesia and an aminoglycoside antibiotic following surgery. Evolution to apnea, bulbar paralysis, and generalized flaccid paralysis occurs within 2 hours.[477] Additional diagnostic signs, when present, include pupillary dilation, atonic bladder, and paralytic ileus.

Laboratory Studies. The diagnosis is based usually on clinical evidence, although electrophysiological studies demonstrate impaired neuromuscular transmission.[478]

Pathogenesis and Etiology. The pathogenesis of the neuromuscular disturbance is impairment of presynaptic mobilization of acetylcholine caused by the antibiotic per se.[479]

Management. Management principally consists of recognition of the syndrome and elimination of the source of the excessive amount of drug. Support of respiration is critical. Neostigmine has been used with benefit.[477] Calcium may play an adjunct role, and in the least, hypocalcemia should be corrected promptly.

Infantile Botulism

Clearly recognized for the first time in 1976,[482] *infantile botulism* is a relatively common disorder. The infantile disease is the result of intestinal infection by *Clostridium botulinum*, rather than ingestion of preformed toxin, as in the more common form of botulism observed in older patients. Previously reported infants with *acute polyneuropathy* probably include those with botulism.[483] More than 1000 cases have been identified in the United States, and currently approximately 70 to 100 cases per year are reported. The disorder has been identified in countries around the world.[57,484-503] Many other infants with transient hypotonia and weakness may represent unidentified cases of infantile botulism.

TABLE 32.10 Infantile Botulism Versus Congenital Myasthenic Syndrome

	INFANTILE BOTULISM	CONGENITAL MYASTHENIC SYNDROME
Generalized hypotonia and weakness	+	±
Facial weakness, ptosis	+	+
Pupillary abnormality	+	−
Constipation	+	−
Response to anticholinesterase	−	+
Electromyogram	Incremental response	Decremental response

+, Present; −, absent; ±, variable.

Clinical Features

Onset. Infantile botulism has a characteristic time of onset, between approximately 2 weeks and 6 months of age, with a median age of 10 weeks.[a] Thus, although most cases have occurred after the neonatal period, approximately 15% manifest in the first month, and infants as young as 54 hours and 6 days of age have been symptomatic with the disease.[490-494,497,498] The patient's presenting problems are usually constipation, poor feeding, hypotonia, and weakness.

Neurological Features. A striking neurological syndrome evolves over days, usually within a week after initial constipation, floppiness, and feeding problems. Almost invariable features include facial diplegia, weak suck, weak cry (*mewlike* or *sheeplike*), impaired swallowing and gag, peripheral weakness, and hypotonia. The resulting paucity of facial expression and minimal limb movement also gives the appearance of *lethargy*. The paralytic process usually progresses in a descending direction (in contrast to the ascending direction in Guillain-Barré syndrome) and is generally symmetrical (in contrast to the asymmetrical flaccid paralysis in poliomyelitis). Ptosis is relatively common, but disturbances of extraocular function occur only in the minority of patients. Particularly helpful in diagnosis are the nearly invariable abnormalities of pupillary function. Pupillary size is most often midposition or dilated, and reaction to light is *absent* or is recognizably *impaired*. The pupillary abnormality is accentuated readily (or made apparent when not clear) by repetitive elicitation of the pupillary light reflex. Thus an initially nearly normal response fatigues rapidly. Pupillary abnormality is the most helpful clinical feature distinguishing this disorder from congenital myasthenic syndromes (Table 32.10).

Clinical Course. The course of the disorder is variable, and with increasing recognition of the illness, less severely affected cases have been recognized.[b] Evolution usually occurs over several or more days, except in rare cases in which evolution to a nadir in hours or a day or so can occur (see botulinum serotype F, later). In most cases, tube feeding is required. Ventilatory

---

[a]References 57, 482-486, 488, 489, 495, 496, 498, 499, 501, 502, and 504-511.
[b]References 57, 484, 485, 487-489, 491, 498, 499, 501, and 502.

support is needed in approximately 70% of cases, from a few days to months.[489,491,504] The duration of the illness has been as long as 4 months, but 1 to 2 months is more common.[a] In earlier reports, among approximately 200 confirmed cases, the fatality rate was approximately 2%.[486,489] A later study of 57 infants found no fatalities.[491] Approximately 5% of infants experience a relapse within 1 to 2 weeks,[512,513] but in general the disorder is self-limiting.

A role for this disorder in the genesis of sudden infant death syndrome was suggested by epidemiological and microbiological data. Thus Arnon and co-workers,[506] in 280 autopsy studies in infants, isolated *C. botulinum* from 10. Of these infants, nine suffered sudden infant death syndrome and represented 4.3% of all cases of the syndrome in the series. Subsequent observations added support for a relationship between infantile botulism and sudden infant death syndrome,[498,514,515] although the possibility that the relationship does not hold for all regions was suggested by other data.[57,58,498,516,517] More importantly, these observations emphasize the suddenness and rapidity with which the disease may evolve.[498,506,514,515] The abrupt onset of apnea or need for mechanical ventilation near the onset of this disease, or both, is common in neonatal cases.[57,493-495,498,501]

Laboratory Studies. With few exceptions, serum enzyme levels, CSF protein concentration, nerve conduction velocities, and muscle biopsy have been normal. The diagnosis is established by observing, *in this clinical setting*, three consistent EMG findings. The first, observed in more than 90% of cases, is an *incremental response* in the compound muscle action potential produced by high rates (20 and 50 Hz) of repetitive nerve stimulation, a finding characteristic of a presynaptic neuromuscular blockade (Figs. 32.20 and 32.21).[57,475,501,510] This so-called *tetanic facilitation* results from enhanced acetylcholine release as a consequence of increased intracellular calcium concentration at the presynaptic terminal. The related posttetanic facilitation is also a feature of the disorder. The second consistent finding consists of the presence of prolonged posttetanic facilitation (>120 seconds) and the absence of posttetanic exhaustion.[475] The third consistent finding is the *brief-duration, small-amplitude, overly abundant motor unit potentials (BSAP) pattern on needle electromyography* (Fig. 32.22A and B).[57,58,475,510] This pattern is caused by presynaptic block of many motor units but not of all the axonal terminals in the units.[518] (Additional findings include abnormal spontaneous activity [e.g., fibrillations], observed in approximately 50% of cases and caused by functional denervation of the muscle fibers.[265,510]) The EMG may be normal initially,[491,492] but usually a repeat study shows the characteristic findings. Indeed, if *all three* of the consistent EMG findings are present, and hypermagnesemia is excluded, the diagnosis of infantile botulism is considered the only possibility.[475] Isolation of *C. botulinum* bacteria and toxin from the stool is an important diagnostic adjunct.[519] Stool usually remains positive for *C. botulinum* organisms and toxin over periods of 1 week to as long as 3 months, although clearance within a month has been reported.[519]

Pathology. Muscle biopsy is normal.[504] This observation is to be expected in view of the nature of the defect (see the following discussion).

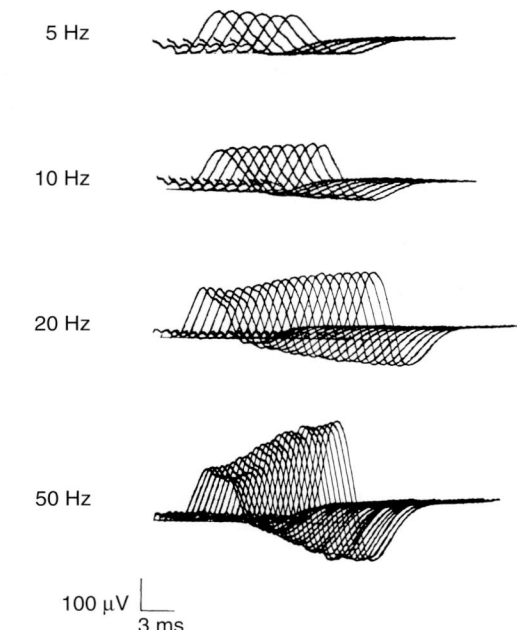

Figure 32.20 Electromyogram in infantile botulism: incremental response obtained with repetitive stimulation of the left median nerve from the innervated abductor pollicis brevis at the rates shown. A striking incremental response is observable at the higher rates of stimulation, especially at 50 Hz. (From Cornblath DR, Sladky JT, Sumner AJ. Clinical electrophysiology of infantile botulism. *Muscle Nerve.* 1983;6:448.)

Pathogenesis and Etiology. The defect at the neuromuscular junction is *presynaptic* in location. The botulinum toxin impairs acetylcholine release from cholinergic nerve terminals.[57,58,498,520-524] The neurotoxin is composed of a heavy chain (100 kDa) and a light chain (50 kDa). The heavy chain binds to specific gangliosides on the nerve terminal, the toxin then enters the nerve ending, and the light chain separates and carries out proteolytic attack on specific proteins involved in synaptic vesicle docking and exocytosis. Botulinum neurotoxin types A and B, produced by *C. botulinum*, account for nearly all cases of infantile botulism, whereas neurotoxin types E and F, produced by *Clostridium butyricum* and *Clostridium baratii*, respectively, account for isolated cases. The cases caused by types E and F evolve more rapidly and recover more promptly than do the cases caused by types A and B.[525] In the United States, cases caused by type A neurotoxin are most prevalent west of the Mississippi River, and those caused by type B neurotoxin are more common east of the Mississippi River.

As just noted, the source of the toxin is *C. botulinum* (or rarely *C. baratii* or *C. butyricum*) infection in the gastrointestinal tract.[a] Thus this disorder is a *toxic infection*, in contrast to the more widely recognized type of botulism observed in older patients (i.e., ingestion of preformed toxin, or toxic ingestion). The source of the organism has been difficult to establish, in part because of its wide distribution in soil and dust.

After the initial recognition of infantile botulism, epidemiological and laboratory investigations, particularly of hospitalized patients with infantile botulism in California, led to

---

[a]References 57, 58, 491, 498, 504, and 511.

[a]References 57, 58, 482, 498, 504-506, and 508.

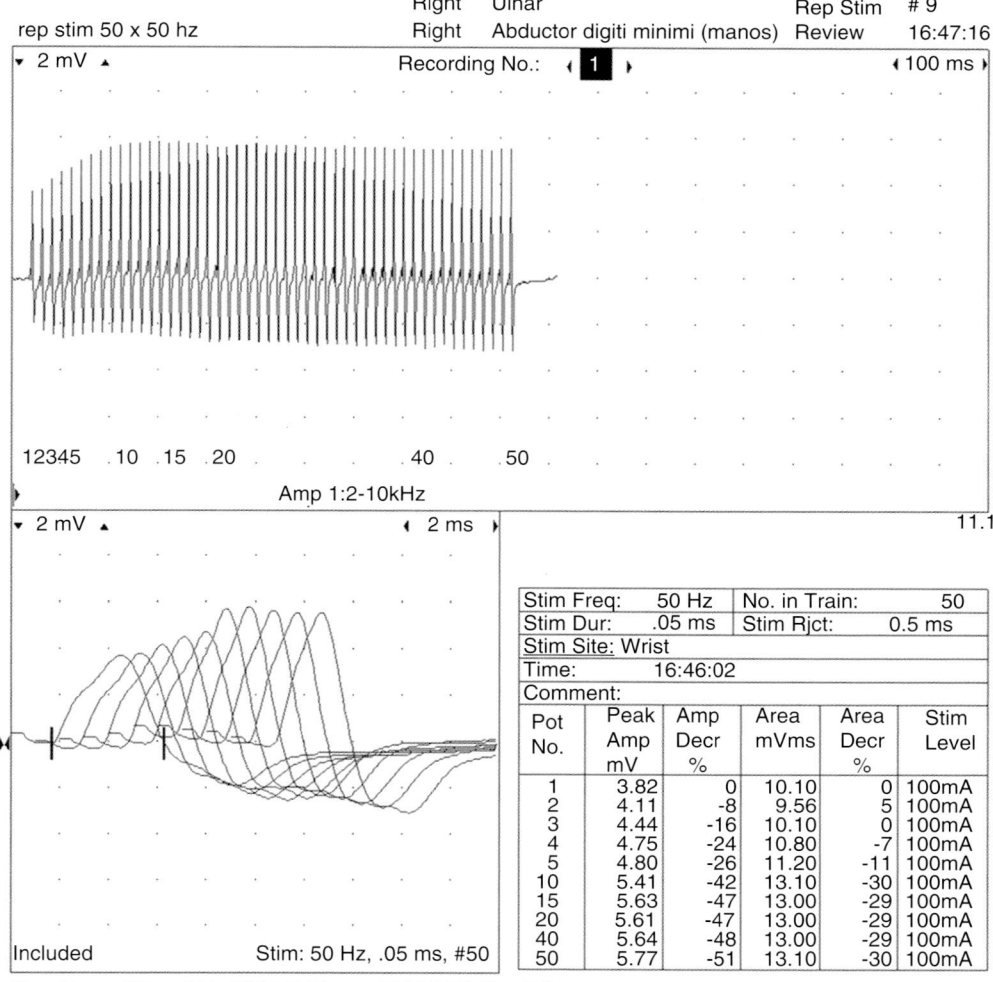

| rep stim 50 x 50 hz | Right   Ulnar | Rep Stim   # 9 |
| | Right   Abductor digiti minimi (manos) | Review   16:47:16 |

Figure 32.21 Tracing derived from patient with confirmed type A infantile botulism. Recording of the right abductor digitus minimus (ADM) muscle with 50 Hz repetitive nerve stimulation shows >50% facilitation of the baseline compound muscle action potential (CMAP). (Reprinted with permission from Sakonju A, Crawford TO. Acquired presynaptic neuromuscular junction disorders: infant botulism and Lambert-Eaton myasthenic syndrome. In: Darras BT, Jones HR Jr, Ryan MM, De Vivo DC, eds. *Neuromuscular Disorders of Infancy, Childhood, and Adolescence: A Clinician's Approach.* 2nd ed. San Diego: Academic Press; 2015:chap 25, 445–455.)

the conclusion that 35% of the cases were caused by ingestion of honey.[508] *The honey was found to harbor* C. botulinum *spores.* Subsequent data confirmed the initial observation.[484] These findings led to the recommendation that infants less than 1 year of age not be given honey. Later work implicated honey as the source of the organism in only approximately 16% of all cases, and more important, in infants less than 2 months of age, honey was not a statistically significant factor.[57,58,490] A more recent study of 122 infants reported honey exposure in only 5% to 7%.[511] Other patients have had similar *Clostridium* strains isolated from both their stool and dust in their immediate environment (vacuum cleaners and soil). Indeed, in careful studies in Pennsylvania, honey was not an important source of the organism, but contact with soil and dust was critical.[489] Residence near an active residential construction site occurred in 87% of cases in a recent series of 34 cases.[499] In two series of infants less than 2 months of age, living in a rural area or on a farm was the only significant predisposing factor, a finding further supporting environmental contact with soil and dust as crucial.[57,58,490,494,498] My most recent patient was a 2-week-old infant whose father was a landscaper. An interesting recent report described an infant presenting at 54 hours of life with *C. baratii* infection and type F botulinum neurotoxin who was born to parents in a rural setting.[497]

Remaining to be determined are the host factors (e.g., intestinal flora and immunological status) that allow the infection to become established in the young infant and not in the similarly exposed older child. Early data attributed particular importance to the first few weeks of exposure to food after a diet of only human breast milk.[57,58,488,489] The combination of loss of immunological factors of a human breast milk diet and the dramatic perturbation of gut flora caused by the change to other food may make the infant particularly vulnerable, for the first several weeks after this change, to colonization

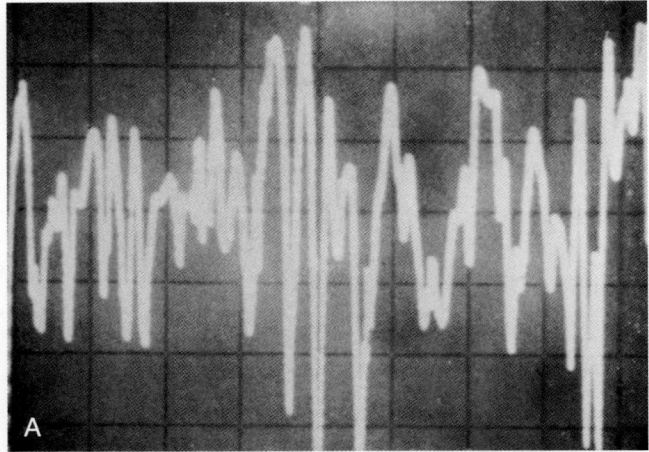

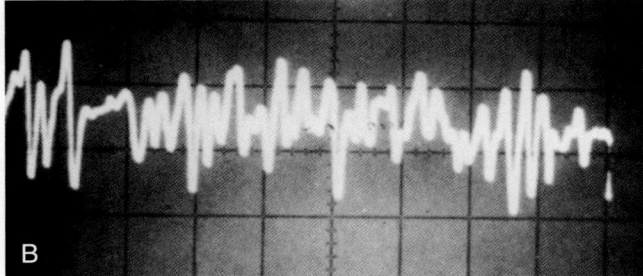

Figure 32.22 Electromyogram in infantile botulism: brief-duration, small-amplitude, overly abundant motor unit potentials (BSAP). (A) Normal pattern of infant muscle. (B) Brief-duration, small-amplitude, overly abundant (for the amount of power exerted) motor unit potentials (i.e., BSAP pattern) from an infant with botulism. (From Johnson RO, Clay SA, Arnon SS. Diagnosis and management of infant botulism. *Am J Dis Child.* 1979;133: 586–593.)

by the botulinum organism. Clinical and experimental data support this formulation.[488,489] However, more important in the youngest infants is poorly developed anaerobic fecal flora, which is important in protection from colonization by *C. botulinum*.[490]

Management. The most critical aspects of management are early recognition of infantile botulism, careful surveillance, particularly of respiratory status, and intervention at the early signs of ventilatory compromise. The disease can evolve exceedingly rapidly. Tube feeding and ventilatory support may be required for many days or weeks. Aminoglycosides should be avoided particularly; these antibiotics have been shown to potentiate muscular weakness and to precipitate respiratory failure in infantile botulism because of their effect on acetylcholine release at the neuromuscular junction.[57,58,498,526]

A major advance in therapy has been the use of human botulism immune globulin (BabyBIG) for use in infant botulism.[498,499,511,527-531] This preparation is derived from the pooled plasma of adults immunized with pentavalent botulinum toxoid and selected for high titers of antibodies versus type A and B toxin. When this preparation is administered early in the course of the disease, marked reductions in hospital stay (2.6 weeks vs. 5.7 weeks), length of mechanical ventilation (1.8 vs. 4.4 weeks), and length of tube feeding (3.6 weeks vs. 10 weeks) have been observed.[498,511] The cost of BabyBIG is high (approximately

$45,000 per treatment per infant); however, the reduction in length of hospital stay and morbidity amounted to an estimated $34.2 million in overall savings.[532] BIG seems to be most effective if administered within the first 3 days after the admission to the hospital.[530,531,533,534]

KEY REFERENCES

1. Volpe JJ. Neonatal hypotonia. In: Darras BT, Jones HR Jr, Ryan MM, De Vivo DC, eds. *Neuromuscular Disorders of Infancy, Childhood, and Adolescence. A Clinician's Approach.* 2nd ed. San Diego: Academic Press; 2015:85-95.
3. Korenke GC, Christen HJ, Hyland K, et al. Aromatic L-amino acid decarboxylase deficiency: an extrapyramidal movement disorder with oculogyric crises. *Eur J Paediatr Neurol.* 1997;1:67-71.
4. Swoboda KJ, Hyland K, Goldstein DS, et al. Clinical and therapeutic observations in aromatic L-amino acid decarboxylase deficiency. *Neurology.* 1999;53:1205-1211.
5. Pons R, Ford B, Chiriboga CA, et al. Aromatic L-amino acid decarboxylase deficiency: clinical features, treatment, and prognosis. *Neurology.* 2004;62:1058-1065.
14. Aughton DJ, Cassidy SB. Physical features of Prader-Willi syndrome in neonates. *Am J Dis Child.* 1990;144:1251-1254.
19. Butler MG. Prader-Willi syndrome: current understanding of cause and diagnosis. *Am J Med Genet.* 1990;35:319-332.
24. Dubowitz V. *Muscle Disorders in Childhood.* 2nd ed. London: WB Saunders; 1995.
26. L'Hermine AC, Aboura A, Brisset S, et al. Fetal phenotype of Prader-Willi syndrome due to maternal disomy for chromosome 15. *Prenat Diagn.* 2003;23:938-943.
32. Lee S, Walker CL, Karten B, et al. Essential role for the Prader-Willi syndrome protein necdin in axonal outgrowth. *Hum Mol Genet.* 2005;14:627-637.
34. Sarnat HB, Alcalá H. Human cerebellar hypoplasia: a syndrome of diverse causes. *Arch Neurol.* 1980;37:300-305.
37. Hoffmann J. Ueber chronische spinale Muskelatrophie im Kindesalter auf familiarer Basis. *Dtsch Z Nervenheilkd.* 1893;3:427.
40. Dubowitz V. Very severe spinal muscular atrophy (SMA type 0): an expanding clinical phenotype. *Eur J Paediatr Neurol.* 1999;3:49-51.
41. Macleod MJ, Taylor JE, Lunt PW, et al. Prenatal onset spinal muscular atrophy. *Eur J Paediatr Neurol.* 1999;3:65-72.
43. Brzustowicz LM, Lehner T, Castilla LH. Genetic mapping of childhood-onset spinal muscular atrophy to chromosome 5q11.2–13.3. *Nature.* 1990;344:540-541.
45. Munsat TL, Skerry L, Korf B, et al. Phenotypic heterogeneity of spinal muscular atrophy mapping to chromosome 5q11.2–13.3 (SMA 5q). *Neurology.* 1990;40:1831-1836.
54. Matthijs G, Devriendt K, Fryns JP. The prenatal diagnosis of spinal muscular atrophy. *Prenat Diagn.* 1998;18:607-610.
58. Darras BT, Markowitz JA, Monani UR, et al. Spinal muscular atrophies. In: Darras BT, Jones HR Jr, Ryan MM, et al., eds. *Neuromuscular Disorders of Infancy, Childhood and Adolescence: A Clinician's Approach.* 2nd ed. San Diego: Academic Press; 2015:117-145.
59. Cusco I, Barcelo J, del Rio E, et al. Detection of novel mutations in the SMN tudor domain in type I SMA patients. *Neurology.* 2004;63:146-149.
60. Swoboda KJ, Prior TW, Scott CB, et al. Natural history of denervation in SMA: relation to age, SMN2 copy number, and function. *Ann Neurol.* 2005;57:704-712.
61. Monani UR. Spinal muscular atrophy: a deficiency in a ubiquitous protein; a motor neuron-specific disease. *Neuron.* 2005;48:885-896.
63. Sumner CJ. Molecular mechanisms of spinal muscular atrophy. *J Child Neurol.* 2007;22:979-989.
64. Prior TW. Spinal muscular atrophy diagnostic. *J Child Neurol.* 2007;22:952-956.
65. Arkblad E, Tulinius M, Kroksmark AK, et al. A population-based study of genotypic and phenotypic variability in children with spinal muscular atrophy. *Acta Paediatr.* 2009;98:865-872.
66. Feldkotter M, Schwarzer V, Wirth R, et al. Quantitative analyses of SMN1 and SMN2 based on real-time lightCycler PCR: fast and highly reliable carrier testing and prediction of severity of spinal muscular atrophy. *Am J Hum Genet.* 2002;70:358-368.

67. Mailman MD, Heinz JW, Papp AC, et al. Molecular analysis of spinal muscular atrophy and modification of the phenotype by SMN2. *Genet Med.* 2002;4:20-26.

73. Kolb SJ, Battle DJ, Dreyfuss G. Molecular functions of the SMN complex. *J Child Neurol.* 2007;22:990-994.

74. Arnold WD, Burghes AH. Spinal muscular atrophy: development and implementation of potential treatments. *Ann Neurol.* 2013;74:348-362.

75. Monani UR, Sendtner M, Coovert DD, et al. The human centromeric survival motor neuron gene (SMN2) rescues embryonic lethality in Smn(-/-) mice and results in a mouse with spinal muscular atrophy. *Hum Mol Genet.* 2000;9:333-339.

78. Thomas NH, Dubowitz V. The natural history of type 1 (severe) spinal muscular atrophy. *Neuromuscul Disord.* 1994;4:497-502.

80. Munsat TL. International SMA collaboration. *Neuromuscul Disord.* 1991;1:81.

81. Russman BS, Iannacone ST, Buncher CR, et al. Spinal muscular atrophy: new thoughts on the pathogenesis and classification schema. *J Child Neurol.* 1992;7:347-353.

82. Iannaccone ST, Browne RH, Samaha FJ, et al. Prospective study of spinal muscular atrophy before age 6 years. *Pediatr Neurol.* 1993;9:187-193.

87. Dubowitz V. *Muscle Disorders in Chilhood.* 2nd ed. Philadelphia: WB Saunders; 1978.

88. Byers RK, Banker BQ. Infantile muscular atrophy. *Arch Neurol.* 1961;5:140.

93. Novelli G, Capon F, Tamisari L, et al. Neonatal spinal muscular atrophy with diaphragmatic paralysis is unlinked to 5q11.2–q13. *J Med Genet.* 1995;32:216-219.

94. Rudnik-Schoneborn S, Forkert R, Hahnen E, et al. Clinical spectrum and diagnostic criteria of infantile spinal muscular atrophy: further delineation on the basis of SMN gene deletion findings. *Neuropediatrics.* 1996;27:8-15.

95. Gorgen-Pauly U, Sperner J, Reiss I, et al. Familial pontocerebellar hypoplasia type 1 with anterior horn cell disease. *Eur J Paediatr Neurol.* 1999;3:33-38.

96. Mercuri E, Goodwin F, Sewry C, et al. Diaphragmatic spinal muscular atrophy with bulbar weakness. *Eur J Paediatr Neurol.* 2000;4:69-72.

97. Zerres K, Rudnik-Schoneborn S. Natural history in proximal spinal muscular atrophy. Clinical analysis of 445 patients and suggestions for a modification of existing classifications. *Arch Neurol.* 1995;52:518-523.

98. Russman BS. Spinal muscular atrophy: clinical classification and disease heterogeneity. *J Child Neurol.* 2007;22:946-951.

102. Farrar MA, Vucic S, Johnston HM, et al. Pathophysiological insights derived by natural history and motor function of spinal muscular atrophy. *J Pediatr.* 2013;162:155-159.

103. Oskoui M, Levy G, Garland CJ, et al. The changing natural history of spinal muscular atrophy type 1. *Neurology.* 2007;69:1931-1936.

105. Rudnik-Schoneborn S, Berg C, Zerres K, et al. Genotype-phenotype studies in infantile spinal muscular atrophy (SMA) type I in Germany: implications for clinical trials and genetic counselling. *Clin Genet.* 2009;76:168-178.

106. Cobben JM, Lemmink HH, Snoeck I, et al. Survival in SMA type I: a prospective analysis of 34 consecutive cases. *Neuromuscul Disord.* 2008;18:541-544.

107. Finkel RS, McDermott MP, Kaufmann P, et al. Observational study of spinal muscular atrophy type I and implications for clinical trials. *Neurology.* 2014;83:810-817.

108. Dubowitz V. Infantile muscular atrophy: a prospective study with particular reference to a slowly progressive variety. *Brain.* 1964;87:707.

112. Jones HR, Bolton CF, Harper C Jr. *Pediatric Clinical Electromyography.* Philadelphia: Lippincott-Raven; 1996.

116. Anagnostou E, Miller SP, Guiot MC, et al. Type I spinal muscular atrophy can mimic sensory-motor axonal neuropathy. *J Child Neurol.* 2005;20:147-150.

117. Osborne JP, Murphy EG, Hill A. Thin ribs on chest X-ray: a useful sign in the differential diagnosis of the floppy newborn. *Dev Med Child Neurol.* 1983;25:343.

120. Wu JS, Darras BT, Rutkove SB. Assessing spinal muscular atrophy with quantitative ultrasound. *Neurology.* 2010;75:526-531.

127. Kariya S, Park GH, Maeno-Hikichi Y, et al. Reduced SMN protein impairs maturation of the neuromuscular junctions in mouse models of spinal muscular atrophy. *Hum Mol Genet.* 2008;17:2552-2569.

129. Iannaccone ST, Guilfoile T. Long-term mechanical ventilation in infants with neuromuscular disease. *J Child Neurol.* 1988;3:30-32.

134. Wang CH, Finkel RS, Bertini ES, et al. Consensus statement for standard of care in spinal muscular atrophy. *J Child Neurol.* 2007;22:1027-1049.

137. O'Hagen JM, Glanzman AM, McDermott MP, et al. An expanded version of the Hammersmith Functional Motor Scale for SMA II and III patients. *Neuromuscul Disord.* 2007;17:693-697.

138. Darras BT, Finkel RS, Kuntz N, et al. Primary efficacy and safety results from the Phase 3 ENDEAR study of nusinersen in infants diagnosed with spinal muscular atrophy (SMA). [Poster.] Muscular Dystrophy Association 2017 Scientific Conference. Arlington, VA: March 19-22, 2017.

139. Darras BT, Monani UR, De Vivo DC. Genetic disorders affecting the motor neuron: spinal muscular atrophy. In: Swaiman KF, Ashwal S, Ferriero DM, et al., eds. *Swaiman's Pediatric Neurology: Principles and Practice.* 6th ed. Philadelphia: Elsevier; 2017.

140. Singh P, Liew WK, Darras BT. Current advances in drug development in spinal muscular atrophy. *Curr Opin Pediatr.* 2013;25:682-688.

141. Grohmann K, Varon R, Stolz P, et al. Infantile spinal muscular atrophy with respiratory distress type 1 (SMARD1). *Ann Neurol.* 2003;54:719-724.

144. Rudnik-Schoneborn S, Stolz P, Varon R, et al. Long-term observations of patients with infantile spinal muscular atrophy with respiratory distress type 1 (SMARD1). *Neuropediatrics.* 2004;35:174-182.

145. Tachi N, Kikuchi S, Kozuka N, et al. A new mutation of IGHMBP2 gene in spinal muscular atrophy with respiratory distress type 1. *Pediatr Neurol.* 2005;32:288-290.

146. Stalpers XL, Verrips A, Poll-The BT, et al. Clinical and mutational characteristics of spinal muscular atrophy with respiratory distress type 1 in The Netherlands. *Neuromuscul Disord.* 2013;23:461-468.

148. Muntoni F, Goodwin F, Sewry C, et al. Clinical spectrum and diagnostic difficulties of infantile ponto-cerebellar hypoplasia type 1. *Neuropediatrics.* 1999;30:243-248.

149. Ryan MM, Cooke-Yarborough CM, Orocopis PG, et al. Anterior horn cell disease and olivopontocerebellar hypoplasia. *Pediatr Neurol.* 2000;23:180-184.

153. Rudnik-Schoneborn S, Senderek J, Jen JC, et al. Pontocerebellar hypoplasia type 1: clinical spectrum and relevance of EXOSC3 mutations. *Neurology.* 2013;80:438-446.

157. Ramser J, Ahearn ME, Lenski C, et al. Rare missense and synonymous variants in UBE1 are associated with X-linked infantile spinal muscular atrophy. *Am J Hum Genet.* 2008;82:188-193.

160. Berciano J, Baets J, Gallardo E, et al. Reduced penetrance in hereditary motor neuropathy caused by TRPV4 Arg269Cys mutation. *J Neurol.* 2011;258:1413-1421.

170. DiMauro S, Eastwood AB. Disorders of glycogen and lipid metabolism. In: Griggs RC, Moxley RT, eds. *Treatment of Neuromuscular Diseases.* New York: Raven Press; 1977.

171. Howell RR, Williams JC. The glycogen storage diseases. In: Stanbury JB, Wyngaarden JB, Frederickson DS, eds. *The Metabolic Basis of Inherited Diseases.* New York: McGraw-Hill; 1983.

172. Hirschhorn R. Glycogen storage disease type II: acid a-glucosidase (acid maltase) deficiency. In: Scriver CR, Beaudet AL, Sly WS, et al., eds. *The Metabolic and Molecular Bases of Inherited Disease.* vol. 2. 7th ed. New York: McGraw-Hill; 1995:2443-2464.

174. Kishnani PS, Hwu W-L, Mandel H, et al. A retrospectivde, multinational, multicenter study on the natural history of infantile-onset Pompe disease. *J Pedaitr.* 2006;148:671-676.

177. Akman HO, Oldfors A, DiMauro S. Glycogen storage diseases of muscle. In: Darras BT, Jones HRJ, Ryan MM, et al., eds. *Neuromuscular Disorders of Infancy, Childhood and Adolescence: A Clinician's Approach.* 2nd ed. San Diego Academic Press; 2015:735-760.

183. Nascimbeni AC, Fanin M, Tasca E, et al. Molecular pathology and enzyme processing in various phenotypes of acid maltase deficiency. *Neurology.* 2008;70:617-626.

188. Kishnani PS, Corzo D, Nicolino M, et al. Recombinant human acid [alpha]-glucosidase: major clinical benefits in infantile-onset Pompe disease. *Neurology.* 2007;68:99-109.

191. Van den Hout JM, Reuser AJ, de Klerk JB, et al. Enzyme therapy for Pompe disease with recombinant human alpha-glucosidase from rabbit milk. *J Inherit Metab Dis.* 2001;24:266-274.

192. van der Ploeg AT. Where do we stand in enzyme replacement therapy in Pompe's disease? *Neuromuscul Disord.* 2010;20:773-774.

194. Ebbink BJ, Aarsen FK, van Gelder CM, et al. Cognitive outcome of patients with classic infantile Pompe disease receiving enzyme therapy. *Neurology.* 2012;78:1512-1518.

195. Kishnani PS, Beckemeyer AA, Mendelsohn NJ. The new era of Pompe disease: advances in the detection, understanding of the phenotypic spectrum, pathophysiology, and management. *Am J Med Genet C Semin Med Genet.* 2012;160C:1-7.

196. van Gelder CM, van Capelle CI, Ebbink BJ, et al. Facial-muscle weakness, speech disorders and dysphagia are common in patients with classic infantile Pompe disease treated with enzyme therapy. *J Inherit Metab Dis.* 2012;35:505-511.

201. Bates T. Poliomyelitis in pregnancy, fetus, and newborn. *Am J Dis Child.* 1955;90:189.

204. Yiu E, Baets J. Congenital and early infantile neuropathies. In: Darras BT, Jones HR Jr, Ryan MM, et al., eds. *Neuromuscular Disorders of Infancy, Childhood and Adolescence: A Clinician's Approach.* 2nd ed. San Diego: Academic Press; 2015.

219. Ulrich J, Hirt HR, Kleihues P, et al. Connatal polyneuropathy—a case with proliferated microfilaments in Schwann cells. *Acta Neuropathol.* 1981;55:39-46.

229. Ouvrier RA, McLeod JG. Conchin TE. The hypertrophic forms of herediatry motor and sensory neuropathy. *Brain.* 1987;110:121-148.

247. Marques W, Thomas PK, Sweeney MG, et al. Dejerine-Sottas neuropathy and PMP22 point mutations: a new base pair substitution and a possible "Hot Spot" on Ser72. *Ann Neurol.* 1998;43:680-683.

252. Wilmshurst JM, Pollard JD, Nicholson G, et al. Peripheral neuropathies of infancy. *Dev Med Child Neurol.* 2003;45:408-414.

256. Nelis E, Erdem S, Van den Bergh PYK, et al. Mutations in *GDAP1.* Autosomal recessive CMT with demyelination and axonopathy. *Neurology.* 2002;59:1865-1872.

257. Gabreels-Festen A, Gabreels F. Congenital and early infantile neuropathies. In: Jones HR Jr, DeVivo DC, Darras BT, eds. *Neuromuscular Disorders of Infancy, Childhood, and Adolescence. A Clinician's Approach.* Philadelphia: Butterworth Heinemann; 2003:361-388.

258. Kochanski A, Drac H, Kabzinska D, et al. A novel MPZ gene mutation in congenital neuropathy with hypomyelination. *Neurology.* 2004;62:2122-2123.

262. Goikhman I, Meer J, Zelnik N. Hereditary neuropathy with liability to pressure palsies in infancy. *Pediatr Neurol.* 2003;28:307-309.

264. Gabreels-Festen AAW, Joosten EMG, Gabreels FJM, et al. Congenital demyelinating motor and sensory neuropathy with focally folded myelin sheaths. *Brain.* 1990;113:1629-1643.

265. Jones HR. Pediatric Electromyography. In: Brown WF, Bolton CF, eds. *Clinical Electromyography.* 2nd ed. Boston: Butterworth-Heinemann; 1993:693-758.

268. Pasternak JF, Hageman J, Adams MA. Exchange transfusion in neonatal myasthenia. *J Pediatr.* 1981;99:644.

270. Pearce J, Pitt M, Martinez A. A neonatal diagnosis of congenital chronic inflammatory demyelinating polyneuropathy. *Dev Med Child Neurol.* 2005;47:489-492.

274. Goebel HH, Zeman W, DeMyer W. Peripheral motor and sensory neuropathy of early childhood, simulating Werdnig-Hoffmann disease. *Neuropaediatrie.* 1976;7:182-195.

285. Swift TR. Commentary: electrophysiology of progressive spinal muscular atrophy. In: Gamstorp I, Sarnat HB, eds. *Progressive Spinal Muscular Atrophies.* New York: Raven Press; 1984.

288. Korinthenberg R, Sauer M, Ketelsen UP, et al. Congenital axonal neuropathy caused by deletions in the spinal muscular atrophy region. *Ann Neurol.* 1997;42:364-368.

295. Stickler DE, Valenstein E, Neiberger RE, et al. Peripheral neuropathy in genetic mitochondrial diseases. *Pediatr Neurol.* 2006;34(2):127-131.

301. Kumar K, Barre P, Nigro M, et al. Giant axonal neuropathy: clinical, electrophysiologic, and neuropathologic features in two siblings. *J Child Neurol.* 1990;5:229-234.

311. Pena SDJ. Giant axonal neuropathy: an inborn error of organization of intermediate filaments. *Muscle Nerve.* 1982;5:166.

315. Axelrod FB, Kaufmann H. Hereditary sensory and autonomic neuropathies. In: Darras BT, Jones HR Jr, Ryan MM, et al., eds. *Neuromuscular Disorders of Infancy, Childhood and Adolescence: A Clinician's Approach.* 2nd ed. San Diego: Academic Press; 2015:340-352.

316. Rotthier A, Baets J, De Vriendt E, et al. Genes for hereditary sensory and autonomic neuropathies: a genotype-phenotype correlation. *Brain.* 2009;132:2699-2711.

317. Dyck PJ, Mellinger JF, Reagan TJ. Not "indifference to pain" but varieties of hereditary sensory and autonomic neuropathy. *Brain.* 1983;106:373-390.

322. Suarez GA. Autonomic neuropathies. In: Jones HR Jr, DeVivo DC, Darras BT, eds. *Neuromuscular Disorders of Infancy, Childhood, and Adolescence. A Clinician's Approach.* Philadelphia: Butterworth Heinemann; 2003:529-543.

327. Kurth I, Pamminger T, Hennings JC, et al. Mutations in FAM134B, encoding a newly identified Golgi protein, cause severe sensory and autonomic neuropathy. *Nat Genet.* 2009;41:1179-1181.

338. Berkovitch M, Copeliovitch L, Tauber T, et al. Hereditary insensitivity to pain with anhidrosis. *Pediatr Neurol.* 1998;19:227-229.

341. Barone R, Lempereur L, Anastasi M, et al. Congenital insensitivity to pain with anhidrosis (NTRK1 mutation) and early onset renal disease: clinical report on three sibs with a 25-year follow-up in one of them. *Neuropediatrics.* 2005;36:270-273.

355. Al-Qudah AA, Shahar E, Logan WJ, et al. Neonatal Guillain-Barre syndrome. *Pediatr Neurol.* 1988;4:255-256.

357. Luijckx GJ, Vies J, de Baets M, et al. Guillain-Barre syndrome in mother and newborn child. *Lancet.* 1997;349:27.

358. Jackson AH, Baquis GD, Shah BL. Congenital Guillain-Barre syndrome. *J Child Neurol.* 1996;11:407-410.

361. Bamford N, Trojaborg W, Sherbany AA, et al. Congenital Guillain-Barre syndrome associated with maternal inflammatory bowel disease is responsive to intravenous immunoglobulin. *Eur J Paediatr Neurol.* 2002;6:115-119.

362. Millichap JG, Dodge PR. Diagnosis and treatment of myasthenia gravis in infancy, childhood, and adolescence. *Neurology.* 1960;10:1007.

363. Seybold ME, Lindstrom JM. Myasthenia gravis in infancy. *Neurology.* 1981;31:476.

364. Roach ES, Buono G, McLean WT. Early-onset myasthenia gravis. *J Pediatr.* 1986;108:193-197.

379. Andrews PI, Sanders DB. Juvenile myasthenia gravis. In: Jones HR Jr, DeVivo DC, Darras BT, eds. *Neuromuscular Disorders of Infancy, Childhood, and Adolescence. A Clinician's Approach.* Philadelphia: Butterworth Heinemann; 2003:575-597.

387. Midelfart Hoff J, Midelfart A. Maternal myasthenia gravis: a cause for arthrogryposis multiplex congenita. *J Child Orthop.* 2015;9:433-435.

388. Oskoui M, Jacobson L, Chung WK, et al. Fetal acetylcholine receptor inactivation syndrome and maternal myasthenia gravis. *Neurology.* 2008;71:2010-2012.

390. Hacohen Y, Jacobson LW, Byrne S, et al. Fetal acetylcholine receptor inactivation syndrome: a myopathy due to maternal antibodies. *Neurol Neuroimmunol Neuroinflamm.* 2015;2:e57.

391. Kang PB, Liew WKM, Oskoui M, et al. Juvenile and neonatal myasthenia gravis. In: Darras BT, Jones HR Jr, Ryan MM, et al., eds. *Neuromuscular Disorders of Infancy, Childhood and Adolescence: A Clinician's Approach.* 2nd ed. San Diego: Academic Press; 2015:482-496.

394. Koenigsberger MR, Patten B, Lovelace RE. Studies of neuromuscular function in the newborn. I. A comparison of myoneural function in full term and premature infants. *Neuropaediatrie.* 1973;4:350.

401. Lennon VA, Lambert EH. Myasthenia gravis induced by monoclonal antibodies to acetylcholine receptors. *Nature.* 1980;285:238.

406. Donaldson JO, Penn AS, Lisak RP. Anti-acetylcholine receptor antibody in neonatal myasthenia gravis. *Am J Dis Child.* 1981;125:222.

409. Lefvert AK, Osterman PO. Newborn infants to myasthenic mothers: a clinical study and an investigation of acetylcholine receptor antibodies in 17 children. *Neurology*. 1983;33:133.

415. Tagber RJ, Baumann R, Desai N. Failure of intravenously administered immunoglobulin in the treatment of neonatal myasthenia gravis. *J Pediatr*. 1999;134:233-235.

417. Allen NM, Hacohen Y, Palace J, et al. Salbutamol-responsive fetal acetylcholine receptor inactivation syndrome. *Neurology*. 2016;86:692-694.

423. Harper CM. Congenital myasthenic syndromes. *Semin Neurol*. 2004;24:111-123.

424. Engel AG. Congenital myasthenic syndromes. In: Darras BT, Jones HR Jr, Ryan MM, et al., eds. *Neuromuscular Disorders of Infancy, Childhood and Adolescence: A Clinician's Approach*. 2nd ed. San Diego: Academic Press; 2015:456-481.

429. Vajsar J, Sloane A, MacGregor DL, et al. Arthrogryposis multiplex congenita due to congenital myasthenic syndrome. *Pediatr Neurol*. 1995;12:237-241.

432. Ohno K, Hutchinson DO, Milone M, et al. Congenital myasthenic syndrome caused by prolonged acetylcholine receptor channel openings due to a mutation in the M2 domain of the e subunit. *Proc Natl Acad Sci*. 1995;92:758-762.

437. Zafeiriou DI, Pitt M, de Sousa C. Clinical and neurophysiological characteristics of congenital myasthenic syndromes presenting in early infancy. *Brain Dev*. 2004;26:47-52.

438. Gurnett CA, Bodnar JA, Neil J, et al. Congenital myasthenic syndrome: presentation, electrodiagnosis, and muscle biopsy. *J Child Neurol*. 2004;19:175-182.

442. Bowman JR. Myasthenia gravis in young children. *Pediatrics*. 1948;1:472.

448. Ioos C, Barois A, Richard P, et al. Congenital myasthenic syndrome due to rapsyn deficiency: three cases with arthrogryposis and bulbar symptoms. *Neuropediatrics*. 2004;35:246-249.

453. Nichols P, Croxen R, Vincent A, et al. Mutation of the acetylcholine receptor e-subunit promotor in congenital myasthenic syndrome. *Ann Neurol*. 1999;45:439-443.

456. Engel AG, Ohno K, Bouzat C, et al. End-plate acetylcholine receptor deficiency due to nonsense mutations in the epsilon subunit. *Ann Neurol*. 1996;40:810-817.

465. Gieron MA, Korthals JK. Familial infantile myasthenia gravis: report of three cases with follow-up until adult life. *Arch Neurol*. 1985;42:143.

474. Greenberg MB, Penn AA, Thomas LJ, et al. Neonatal medical admission in a term and late-preterm cohort exposed to magnesium sulfate. *Am J Obstet Gynecol*. 2011;204:515 e511-515 e517.

478. McQuillen MP, Cantor HE, O'Rourke JF. Myasthenic syndrome associated with antibiotics. *Arch Neurol*. 1968;18:402.

489. Long SS, Gajewski JL, Brown LW, et al. Clinical, laboratory, and environmental features of infant botulism in Southeastern Pennsylvania. *Pediatrics*. 1985;75:935.

490. Spika JS, Shaffer N, Hargrett-Bean N. Risk factors for infant botulism in the United States. *Am J Dis Child*. 1989;143:828-832.

496. Sheth RD, Lotz BP, Hecox KE, et al. Infantile botulism: pitfalls in electrodiagnosis. *J Child Neurol*. 1999;14:156-158.

500. Koepke R, Sobel J, Arnon SS. Global occurrence of infant botulism, 1976–2006. *Pediatrics*. 2008;122:e73-e82.

501. Sakonju A, Crawford TO. Acquired presynaptic neuromuscular junction disorders: infant botulism and Lambert-Eaton myasthenic syndrome. In: Darras BT, Jones HR Jr, Ryan MM, et al., eds. *Neuromuscular Disorders of Infancy, Childhood, and Adolescence: A Clinician's Approach*. 2nd ed. San Diego: Academic Press; 2015:445-455.

502. Rosow LK, Strober JB. Infant botulism: review and clinical update. *Pediatr Neurol*. 2015;52:487-492.

508. Arnon SS, Midura TJ, Damus K. Honey and other environmental risk factors for infant botulism. *J Pediatr*. 1979;94:331.

511. Arnon SS, Schechter R, Maslanka SE, et al. Human botulism immune globulin for the treatment of infant botulism. *N Engl J Med*. 2006;354:462-471.

526. L'Hommedieu C, Stough R, Brown L. Potentiation of neuromuscular weakness in infant botulism by aminoglycosides. *J Pediatr*. 1979;95:1065.

527. Arnon SS. Creation and development of the public service orphan drug Human Botulism Immune Globulin. *Pediatrics*. 2007;119:785-789.

530. Chalk CH, Benstead TJ, Keezer M. Medical treatment for botulism. *Cochrane Database Syst Rev*. 2014;(2):CD008123.

532. California Department of Health Services. *Summary Basis of Approval: Botulism Immune Globulin Intravenous (Human) (BIG-IV)*. California: California Department of Health Services; 2003.

533. Arnon SS. Infant botulism. In: Cherry J, Demmler-Harrison GJ, Kaplan SL, et al., eds. *Feigin and Cherry's Textbook of Pediatric Infectious Diseases*. 7th ed. Philadelphia: Elsevier Saunders; 2014:1801-1809.

534. Pifko E, Price A, Sterner S. Infant botulism and indications for administration of botulism immune globulin. *Pediatr Emerg Care*. 2014;30:120-124, quiz 125-127.

Full references for this chapter can be found at www.expertconsult .com.

Muscle Involvement and Restricted Disorders

Basil T. Darras ◆ *Joseph J. Volpe*

Muscle, the final component of the motor system, is the site of abnormalities with those essential clinical manifestations of hypotonia and weakness that unify the other disorders of the motor system (see Chapter 32). In this chapter, we deal with important myopathic disorders in the neonatal patient. In addition, certain restricted disorders of the motor system are reviewed.

LEVEL OF THE MUSCLE

Disorders of muscle account for a substantial proportion of infants affected with hypotonia and weakness. Although a relatively large number of myopathic disorders may cause manifestations in the neonatal period, only a few disorders account for most of the cases observed. Myotonic dystrophy is the most frequent (see subsequent sections). However, more of the myopathic disorders can be detected in the neonatal period if the physician's index of suspicion is appropriately high. Detection is valuable for purposes of genetic counseling, determination of prognosis, and institution of therapy.

The major myopathic disorders of interest in newborns may be categorized into two broad groups: those in which the histology, although sometimes impressive, is not distinctive enough to be diagnostic, and those in which the histology is distinctive enough to be diagnostic (with some qualifications) (Box 33.1). In the following discussions, major emphasis is placed on the most common disorders.

Myopathic Disorders With Nondiagnostic Histology

Several disorders are characterized by neonatal hypotonia and weakness and by muscle histological findings that are sometimes impressive, although not distinctive enough to be diagnostic. This category includes the most frequently encountered examples of myopathic disease with clinical manifestations evident in the neonatal period. Myotonic dystrophy is the most common of all, although congenital muscular dystrophy (CMD) is not rare (see Box 33.1). Facioscapulohumeral dystrophy (FSHD) rarely manifests in the neonatal period but is important to recognize. Polymyositis is a rare but treatable muscle disorder in the newborn. Congenital myopathy with minimal or no change as determined by current laboratory investigation (i.e., minimal change myopathy) represents a shrinking group as diagnostic techniques improve.

Congenital Myotonic Dystrophy

Congenital myotonic dystrophy is an inherited disorder of muscle that exhibits numerous distinctive differences from myotonic dystrophy type 1 (DM1) of adult patients. The disorder may be associated with muscle weakness so severe that death results in the newborn period. The hallmark of congenital myotonic dystrophy is hypotonia, rather than myotonia, as observed in adult patients. The congenital form of myotonic dystrophy was first described clearly by Vanier in 1960.[1]

Clinical Features. The disorder is usually apparent in the first hours and days of life. Certain characteristics of the pregnancy often precede the neonatal disorder (Table 33.1) and tend to be prominent in the most severely affected cases. Thus, spontaneous abortion or premature birth with the associated increased risk of germinal matrix/intraventricular hemorrhage occurs in the most severely affected infants.[2-7] Polyhydramnios is a common characteristic of the pregnancy (see Table 33.1). Indeed, this sign is almost invariable in the most severely affected infants and is thought to be caused by the disturbance in swallowing.[3,8-12] Polyhydramnios in a mother with myotonic dystrophy is a fairly reliable indicator of serious involvement of the fetus. Abnormalities of labor, which may be either prolonged or abbreviated, have been attributed to maternal uterine muscle involvement.[2,9]

The *clinical features in the neonatal* period are usually marked and characteristic (see Table 33.1).[1,3-5,8,12-28] In the well-established case, the most striking clinical features are facial diplegia, respiratory and feeding difficulties, arthrogryposis (especially of the lower extremities), and hypotonia. The facial diplegia imparts the characteristic tent-shaped appearance to the upper lip (Fig. 33.1). The respiratory difficulties relate to weakness of respiratory muscles, impaired swallowing and handling of secretions, and occasionally diaphragmatic disturbance (Fig. 33.2). At least 80% of patients require mechanical ventilation. The respiratory impairment may be so severe that the newborn infant fails to establish adequate ventilation and suffers an asphyxial episode that so dominates the clinical syndrome that the myopathic origin of the respiratory failure is overlooked. The feeding difficulties involve both sucking and swallowing and are related particularly to weakness of the facial, masticatory, and pharyngeal musculature. (A role for myotonia of pharyngeal muscles is possible.[11]) A disturbance of gastric motility, a manifestation of the smooth muscle involvement

Histology Not Diagnostic
Congenital myotonic dystrophy
Congenital muscular dystrophy
Facioscapulohumeral dystrophy
Polymyositis
Minimal change myopathy
Histology Diagnostic
Central core disease
Nemaline (rod body) myopathy
Myotubular (centronuclear) myopathy
Congenital fiber type disproportion
Multiminicore disease
Mitochondrial myopathies
    Cytochrome c oxidase deficiency
    Mitochondrial DNA depletion
Metabolic myopathies
    Glycogen disorders
    Lipid disorders

TABLE 33.1 Clinical Features of Congenital Myotonic Dystrophy

CLINICAL FEATURE	CASES EXHIBITING FEATURE[a] (%)
Reduced fetal movements	68
Polyhydramnios	80
Premature birth (<36 weeks)	52
Facial diplegia	100
Feeding difficulties	92
Hypotonia	100
Muscle atrophy	100
Hyporeflexia or areflexia	87
Respiratory distress	88
Arthrogryposis	82
Edema	54
Elevated right hemidiaphragm	49
Transmission by mother	100[b]
Neonatal mortality	41
Intellectual disability in survivors	100

[a]See text for references.
[b]Paternal transmission has been documented, albeit very rarely.

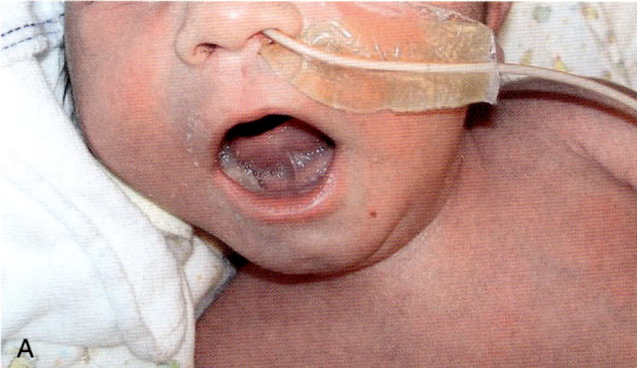
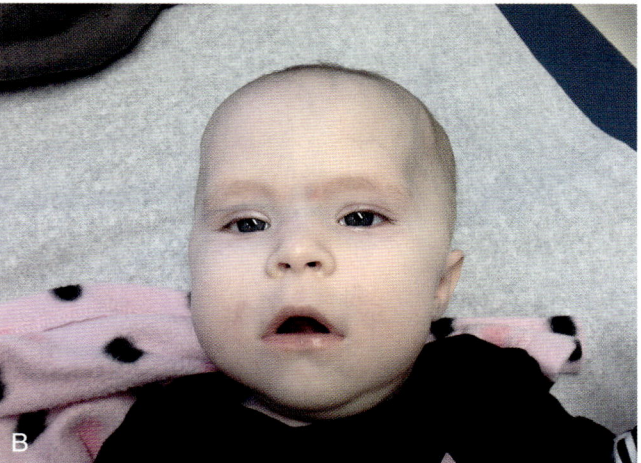

Figure 33.1 Congenital myotonic dystrophy: facial appearance in the neonatal and infantile period. (A) Note the facial diplegia with tent-shaped appearance of upper lip in this newborn. (B) Same affected infant at an older age; note the facial diplegia, tented upper lip, and temporalis muscle atrophy.

Less severely affected infants may go undetected in the newborn period. Facial weakness and hypotonia are the two most common manifestations in such patients.

The *clinical course* relates clearly to the severity of the disease. Neonatal mortality is generally approximately 15% to 20%, but it is as high as approximately 40% in severely affected patients. Feeding difficulties, which initially may require institution of tube feedings, usually improve, at least in reported survivors.[a] However, approximately 20% of infants surviving to adolescence and young adulthood have major gastrointestinal symptoms (e.g., diarrhea and abdominal pain), presumably reflecting smooth muscle involvement.[2,17,32] Moreover, the persistence of some degree of pharyngeal and palatal weakness leads to recurrent otitis media in approximately 25%, occasionally with accompanying hearing loss.[17] Like the neonatal feeding difficulties, the respiratory difficulties subside over the ensuing weeks. However, approximately one third of patients require mechanical ventilation for longer than 30 days.[25] Even after cessation of mechanical ventilation, ventilatory reserve may be compromised in severely affected infants, and death secondary to respiratory complications in association with anesthesia

in this disorder, may contribute in a major way to the feeding difficulties in some infants.[29] Arthrogryposis (Fig. 33.3) is almost invariable and usually involves at least the ankles, leading to clubfoot deformity. Indeed, in one large series of arthrogryposis multiplex congenita, 50% of the patients with cases related to muscle disease had congenital myotonic dystrophy.[30] Hypotonia is also essentially invariable, accompanied by weakness and, in approximately 90% of the cases, by areflexia or marked hyporeflexia. Atrophy is usually obvious, especially after the first days of life, when edema, which is often excessive in these infants, subsides.[3] Clinical myotonia, elicited by percussion of such muscles as the deltoid, has been detected as early as 3 hours of age,[14] but it is usually not readily elicited until much later in infancy.

[a]References 4, 5, 8, 11, 12, 25, 28, and 31.

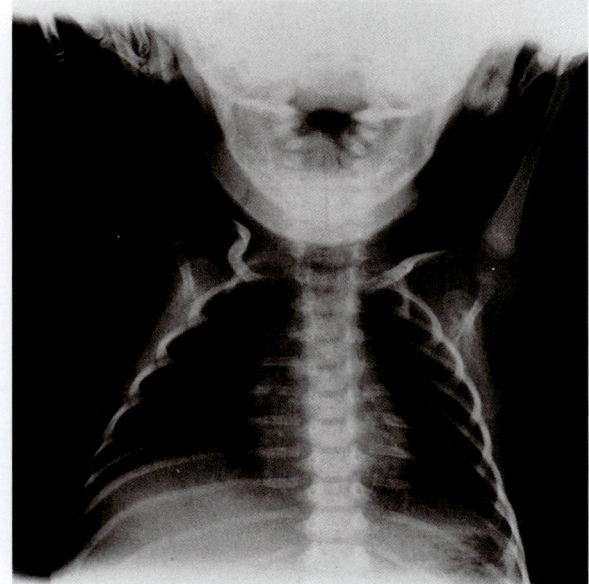

Figure 33.2 Congenital myotonic dystrophy: diaphragmatic involvement. This radiograph of the chest is from a newborn with congenital myotonic dystrophy. The right hemidiaphragm is elevated and paralyzed. Note also the thin ribs, characteristic of severe congenital neuromuscular disease. (From Sarnat HB. Neuromuscular disorders in the neonatal period. In: Korobkin R, Guilleminault C, eds. *Advances in Perinatal Neurology.* Vol 1. New York: Spectrum Publications; 1978.)

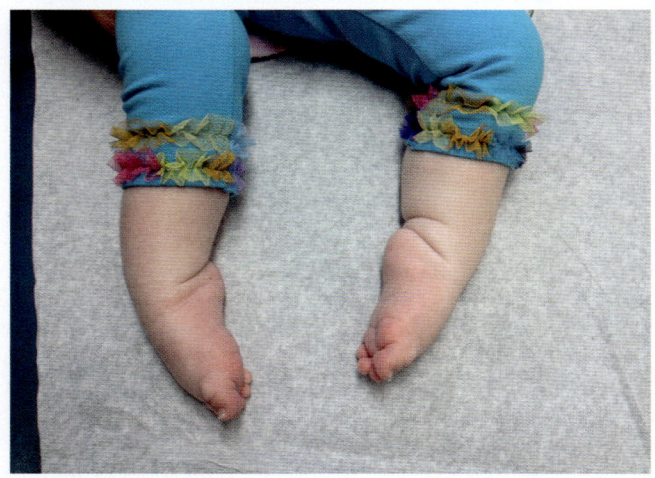

Figure 33.3 Congenital myotonic dystrophy: club feet. This affected infant exhibits contractures at the ankles (club feet).

or aspiration may occur later in infancy.[5,17,25] Unlike the general improvement in neonatal feeding and in respiratory difficulties, facial diplegia usually becomes more obvious as *baby fat* disappears; ptosis often becomes apparent as well. Muscle weakness, which is initially generalized or more marked proximally, begins to assume the *distal* preponderance characteristic of the adult disease. However, in many patients, truncal and appendicular muscle strength improves gradually over time; thus they acquire the ability to sit independently, bear weight on their legs, and eventually walk (Fig. 33.4). Clinical

myotonia becomes elicitable later in infancy (Fig. 33.5) and is present in the majority of patients after the age of 5 years.[15] Cardiac muscle involvement, manifested by electrocardiographic abnormalities, also becomes more prominent later in infancy. However, in very severely affected newborns, cardiomyopathy may be apparent in the newborn period and may contribute to neonatal demise.[33,34] (Cataracts, baldness, gonadal atrophy, and marked facial atrophy develop later in adult life.)

Impairment of motor and intellectual development is apparent in the first weeks of life (see Table 33.1). Intellectual disability is essentially invariable in infants with congenital myotonic dystrophy who survive the neonatal period.[4,5,12,35] Intelligence quotient (IQ) scores in the 50 to 65 range have generally been observed. The disturbance of intellectual development is nonprogressive. The only available data on relatively long-term follow-up (i.e., ≈10–30 years) indicated that only 2 of 42 patients managed *normal education*, and only one was *gainfully employed.*[17] Some improvement in motor function occurs in late infancy and childhood.[25]

Transmission of myotonic dystrophy in patients with the neonatal form of the disease is essentially *always through the mother* (see Table 33.1). Only approximately seven cases of congenital myotonic dystrophy transmitted through an affected father have been reported.[36-41] At any rate, it is critical for the physician to be cognizant of the disorder as it appears in adults. Indeed, it is common for the mother with an affected infant to be unaware that she has the disease.[3-5,28,42] Most helpful in recognition of the disease in the mother is the typical facies of myotonic dystrophy (Fig. 33.6), characterized by atrophy of the masseter and temporalis muscles, ptosis, and a straight, stiff smile. Myotonia is prominent and readily elicited. Thus active myotonia is seen in the affected woman when she closes her eyes tightly and then is unable to open them fully for several seconds or more, or when she clenches her fist tightly and then cannot extend her fingers immediately on command. Passive myotonia is demonstrable by percussion of such muscles as the deltoid, thenar eminence, and tongue and by observation of the prolonged dimpling caused by sustained muscle contraction (Videos 33.1 to 33.4). Other characteristics (e.g., cataracts, disturbance of intellect, and cardiac abnormality) may also be present. The essential point is that the physician should examine the mother when this diagnosis is considered in a newborn.

Laboratory Studies. Serum creatine kinase (CK) level, cerebrospinal fluid (CSF) protein concentration, and nerve conduction studies are normal. Slender ribs are commonly observed on chest radiographs (see Fig. 33.2) and may suggest the diagnosis in an infant thought initially to have primary asphyxia.[43,44] This finding can be observed with other congenital myopathic disorders as well as with Werdnig-Hoffmann disease.[44]

The diagnosis is supported particularly by demonstrating myotonic discharges on the electromyogram (EMG). These discharges are difficult to elicit in the neonatal period, although they have been observed as early as 5 days of age.[14,42] Electrical myotonia is elicited by movement of the recording needle or by direct percussion of the recorded muscle; this procedure results in repetitive electrical potentials of up to 100/second that wax and wane in frequency and amplitude (Fig. 33.7).[4,14,28] These potentials produce the characteristic *dive bomber* sound. Later in infancy, particularly after the age of 2 to 3 years, myotonia is

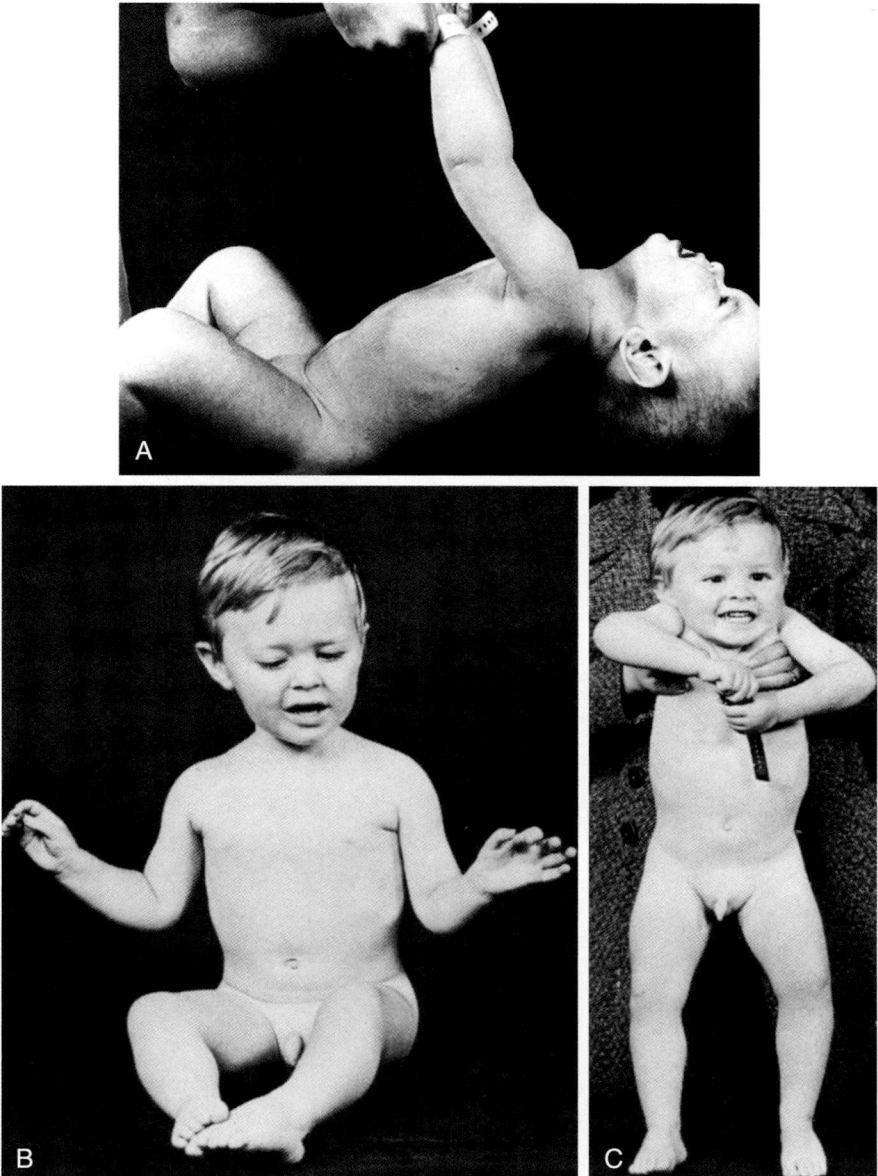

Figure 33.4 Clinical improvement in congenital muscular dystrophy. (A) A 9-month-old boy with weakness and hypotonia from birth. Note the marked head lag with pull to sit. The infant cannot sit without support or support his body weight on his legs. (B and C) The same child at 2 years of age. He can sit without support and can bear considerable weight when standing with support. (From Dubowitz V. *Muscle Disorders in Childhood*. Philadelphia: Saunders; 1978.)

elicited more easily, and small-amplitude, short-duration, and polyphasic potentials, typical of myopathic disease, can also be demonstrated.[16] Fibrillation potentials may also be observed.[28]

Ventricular dilation has been observed in approximately 80% of newborns studied by ultrasonography, computed tomography (CT), or magnetic resonance imaging (MRI).[4,5,45-47] In one study, macrocephaly was present in approximately 70% of the infants in the presence or absence of ventricular dilation.[46] However, head circumference within the upper half of the normal range is more common than is overt macrocephaly.[5] The ventricular dilation is nonprogressive and is not accompanied by rapid head growth or signs of increased intracranial pressure. The

occasional occurrence of periventricular echodensities on ultrasound scans or hyperintensity on subsequent T2-weighted MRI scans may reflect periventricular leukomalacia occurring in association with neonatal respiratory disturbance.[45-49] However, this white matter change could also reflect an abnormality of myelination. A small corpus callosum was documented by MRI in four of seven infants in another study.[47] The possibility of an abnormality in neuronal development was raised by the demonstration by magnetic resonance (MR) spectroscopy of decreased levels of *N*-acetylaspartic acid, a neuronal marker (see Chapter 4), in 5 infants and children with congenital myotonic dystrophy.[50]

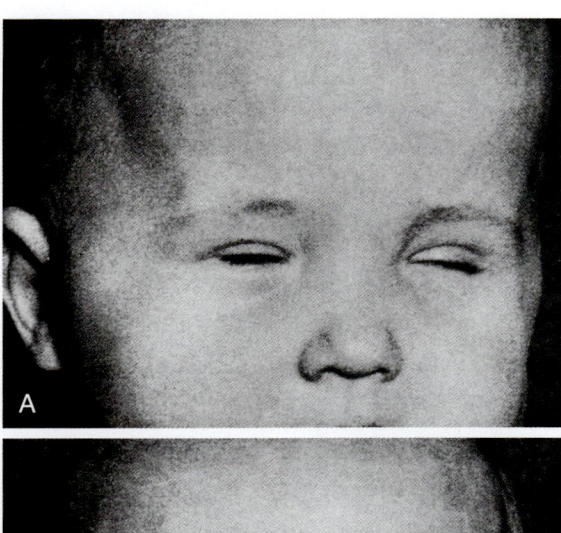

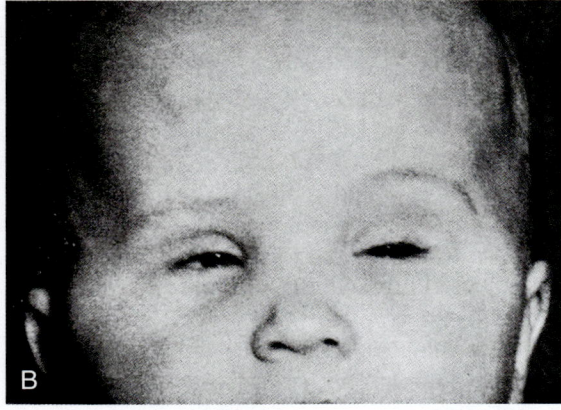

Figure 33.5 Clinical myotonia in an 11-month-old infant. (A) Blinking was precipitated by a bright flash of light. (B) This photograph was taken approximately 15 seconds later. Note the persisting partial closure of the eyelids caused by myotonia of the orbicularis oculi muscles and also the temporal hollowing, suggesting atrophy. (From Dodge PR, Gamstorp I, Byers RK, Russell P. Myotonic dystrophy in infancy and childhood. *Pediatrics.* 1965;35:3–19.)

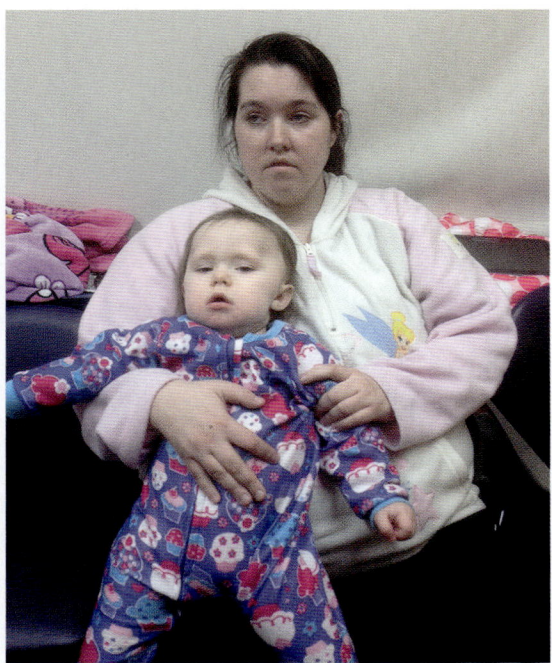

Figure 33.6 Congenital myotonic dystrophy: infant and mother. The mother exhibits some of the typical facial features of myotonic dystrophy, as described in the text. Note also in the affected infant the facial diparesis with a tent-shaped upper lip. Additional features of congenital myotonic dystrophy may be seen in Videos 33.1 to 33.4.

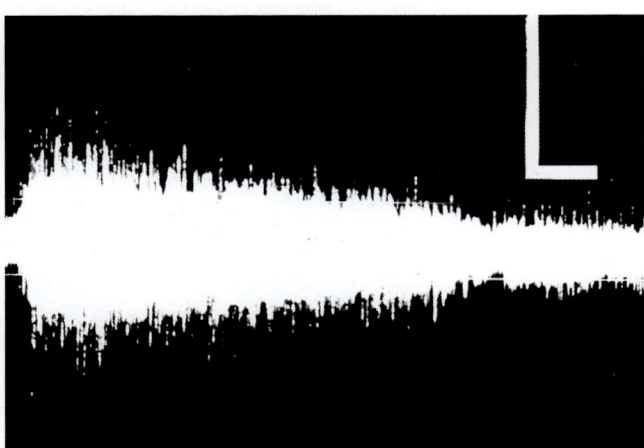

Figure 33.7 Electromyogram from an infant with congenital myotonic dystrophy at 5 days of age. The movement of the needle produces a burst of electrical discharges that then subside over several seconds. Calibration: 200 μV, 1 second. See also Chapter 30 and Figs. 30.8A–B. (From Swift TR, Ignacio OJ, Dyken PR. Neonatal dystrophia myotonica. *Am J Dis Child.* 1975;129:734–737.)

Pathology. *Muscle pathology* in congenital myotonic dystrophy is different from that observed in the adult with the disease and consists particularly of features of immaturity.[4,28,33,51,52] In a detailed postmortem analysis of three infants, Sarnat and Silbert and others[51,53-55] demonstrated particular involvement of limb muscles around arthrogrypotic joints, pharyngeal muscles, and the diaphragm. The features indicative of a disturbance of maturation included small round muscle fibers with large internal nuclei and sparse myofibrils, reminiscent of fetal myotubes (Fig. 33.8). Moreover, differentiation of fibers into distinct histochemical types was incomplete. Similarly, electron microscopy showed dilated transverse tubules that were aligned longitudinally, like fetal myotubes, as well as poorly formed Z-bands, simple mitochondria, peripheral halo of absent mitochondria, and many satellite cells, which are also features of immature muscle. Investigators have suggested that these changes principally represent an arrest in fetal muscle maturation.[51,54] Others have viewed these changes as signs of abnormal development.[33] Pathological findings in pancreas (nesidioblastosis), kidney (persistent renal blastema), and other organs (cryptorchidism and patent ductus arteriosus) support the concept of a disturbance of maturation.[56]

The *neuropathological substrate* for the intellectual failure is unclear. A study of three adult patients with subnormal IQ scores by Rosman and Rebeiz[57] revealed pachygyria in two and disordered cortical architectonics with neuronal heterotopias in all three. These findings were not observed in a later study of four infants from the same institution.[56] However, another report from a different institution also described cerebral cortical neuronal heterotopias in four infants and neuronal heterotopias in two studied postmortem.[46] Thus the neuropathological basis for the consistent impairment of intellect is not currently

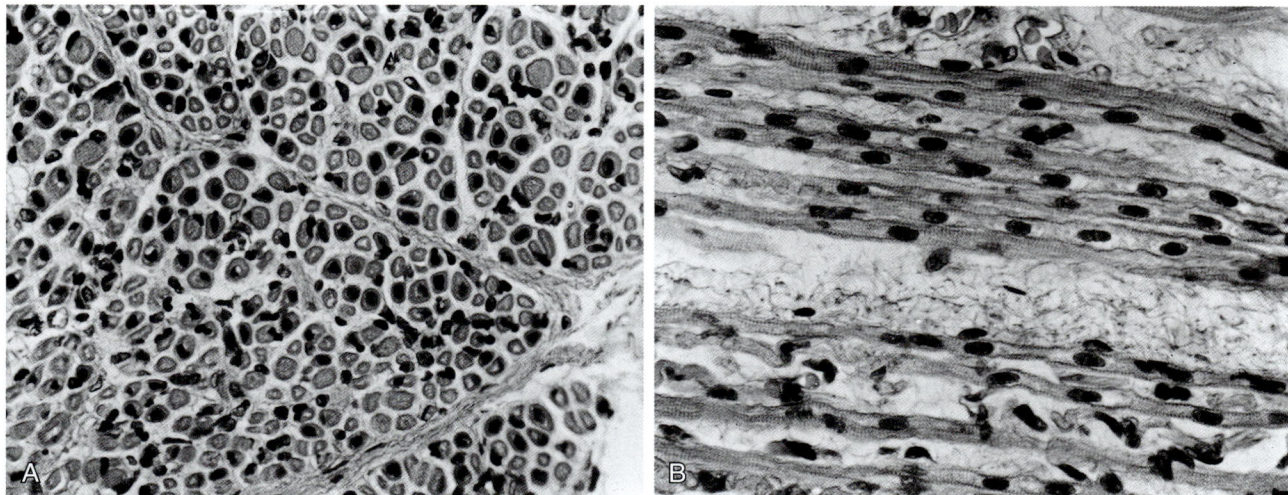

Figure 33.8 Congenital myotonic dystrophy: muscle pathology. These specimens were obtained at autopsy from an affected infant who never established spontaneous respiration and died at 14 days of age. Many of the histological features are those of immature muscle. (A) Cross section of rectus abdominis. The muscle fibers are small, round, and loosely arranged, and most contain a single large internal nucleus or a central pale space (hematoxylin and eosin [H&E] stain, ×400). (B) Longitudinal section of diaphragm. The large vesicular internal nuclei are aligned in rows within the muscle fibers with clear vacuolated spaces between them. The sarcomeric striations are poorly distinguished (H&E stain, ×400). (From Sarnat HB, Silbert SW. Maturational arrest of fetal muscle in neonatal myotonic dystrophy. *Arch Neurol.* 1976;33:466–474.)

established conclusively. It seems reasonable to postulate that an aberration of maturation, as in muscle and other organs, is present. A study of the organizational aspects of brain development (see Chapter 7) would be of interest.

Pathogenesis and Etiology. The disorder is inherited as an *autosomal dominant* trait through *the mother* in virtually every case. In addition, the risk of congenital myotonic dystrophy bears a distinct relationship with the disease in the mother.[58] The earlier the onset and the more severe the maternal disease, the greater is the risk for the severe congenital form of myotonic dystrophy in the child. This phenomenon is consistent with *anticipation* (i.e., the occurrence of progressively earlier onset and more severe disease in successive generations).[58,59]

Molecular genetic studies have provided major insight into the reasons for anticipation and related aspects of congenital myotonic dystrophy (Box 33.2).[4,23,24,28,58-72] Thus myotonic dystrophy has been shown to be associated with an increase in the number of specific (CTG [cytosine-thymine-guanine]) trinucleotide repeats in an unstable DNA region of the 3′ untranslated region of the myotonic dystrophy gene, which is located at chromosome 19q13.3. Moreover, the number of repeats increases with maternal transmission of the gene and a correlation of the number of repeats (i.e., the extent of the so-called expansion of the triplet repeat region on chromosome 19) exists with severity and early onset of the disease in the infant. This molecular genetic phenomenon underlies anticipation. Current data suggest that *paternal* transmission of the unstable trinucleotide repeat is associated with reduced amplification or even contraction of the region of repeats, in contrast to the situation with maternal transmission.[39,73] This feature of paternal transmission may be related to negative selection of sperm with large repeat numbers and may explain the exclusively maternal transmission of congenital myotonic

---

BOX 33.2   Molecular Genetics of Congenital Myotonic Dystrophy[a]

The disease is associated with an abnormally high number of CTG trinucleotide repeats, usually more than a thousand, in the 3′-untranslated region of the myotonic dystrophy protein kinase gene (*MDPK*) on chromosome 19q13.3.

The increased number of repeats correlates approximately with earlier onset and more severe disease.

The mutation is *dynamic* (i.e., does not remain of constant size within a pedigree or across generations).

Maternal transmission is associated with expansion (i.e., increased number) of the repeat region (1000–4000 repeats) and with more severe disease in the infant (i.e., *anticipation*).

The extent of repeat expansion varies among tissues (i.e., *somatic mosaicism*); thus determination of the number of repeats in DNA in blood or chorionic villus cannot predict severity of disease in muscle or other tissues with absolute accuracy.

Sequestration of multiple RNA- and DNA-binding proteins by the region of multiple repeats leads to dysregulation of splicing of pre-mRNAs, such as the insulin receptor and skeletal muscle chloride channel, resulting in insulin resistance and myotonia.

[a]See text for references.

---

dystrophy. At any rate, determination of the number of repeats from a DNA sample of a woman can be used to estimate the likelihood of transmitting severe congenital myotonic dystrophy, and, in an affected infant, such a determination can be used to estimate the likely severity of the disorder. However, correlations are not perfect, in part because of somatic mosaicism (i.e., the extent of repeat expansion varies from tissue to tissue, even in postmitotic tissue).[74] Somatic mosaicism has been documented in congenital myotonic dystrophy,[33,75] although it is less pronounced than in the adult form of the disease.

The gene affected in myotonic dystrophy *(MDPK)* encodes a serine-threonine protein kinase; myogenin, the beta-subunit of the L-type calcium channels, and phospholemman are the substrates for this enzyme, which appears to function normally in patients with DM1. Normal leukocyte DNA contains 5 to 37 copies of the CTG trinucleotide. In *permutation carriers*, the size of the unstable CTG array is 30 to 50 repeats; however, it varies between 50 and 4000 repeats in symptomatic individuals. Infants with congenital myotonic dystrophy are likely to have more than 1000 repeats in their leukocyte DNA, although a number of these patients may have CTG expansions of less than 1000 repeats.[26,76-78] The features of congenital myotonic dystrophy appear to be related to a toxic RNA gain-of-function effect.[72] Thus the trinucleotide repeats appear to bind and sequester multiple RNA- and DNA-binding proteins, such as the muscleblind-like (MBNL) protein family, thereby leading to multiple deleterious effects (see Box 33.2), including dysregulation of alternative splicing of pre-mRNAs. Sequestration of MBNL1 leads to increased synthesis of the less responsive neonatal isoform of the insulin receptor and overproduction of the neonatal isoform of the skeletal muscle chloride channel; this imbalance results in insulin resistance and a significant reduction in chloride conductance, causing myotonia.[24,28,79-82]

The diagnosis is suspected if the mother has clinical or EMG features of DM1 or if she has a confirmed genetic diagnosis; the diagnosis is made in the neonate by identifying the abnormally expanded CTG repeat in the DMPK gene.

Management. Management of the affected infant is, in considerable part, an ethical decision. For optimal development, adequate nutrition and ventilation must be ensured, and respiratory support and tube feedings may be needed for days to weeks.[4,12,25] Survivors are usually able to suck and swallow adequately for oral nutrition by 8 to 12 weeks of age.[4,12] When ventilatory support is required for more than 3 to 4 weeks, the mortality rate exceeds 25%.[12,18,25,83] However, the use of nasal continuous positive airway pressure has facilitated weaning in affected infants after such prolonged mechanical ventilation.[84] In infants with particularly poor gastric motility, metoclopramide, which decreases the smooth muscle threshold for the action of acetylcholine, may be especially useful.[29]

Subsequent problems relate to both the muscle and central nervous system (CNS). Supportive measures for the myopathy are required. Most of the joint deformities can often be managed with a nonsurgical approach, although more aggressive management of the foot and ankle deformities may prevent gait disturbances.[17]

Congenital Muscular Dystrophy

The term *CMD* refers to a group of disorders that share clinical and myopathological features. In older patients, the term *muscular dystrophy* has been used for a group of progressive, inherited disorders of muscle that share a striking myopathology. Although some of the reported cases of CMD do not exhibit definite progression and a familial nature cannot always be established, the disorder indeed does generally conform to an inherited involvement of muscle, progressing prenatally (and ultimately also postnatally) and sharing a myopathology similar to that of later-onset dystrophies.

The classification of CMDs has become particularly difficult because, in the past 20 years or so, largely through molecular genetic studies, increasing numbers of clinical phenotypes and responsible genes have been recognized.[85,86] We have elected to use a fundamentally clinical categorization, and we focus on those disorders that may manifest in the neonatal period (Table 33.2). We find it most useful to distinguish those CMD disorders that involve primarily muscle (i.e., without overt CNS abnormalities, such as those manifested by major neurological deficits) from those CMD disorders that are accompanied by overt CNS abnormalities (with such associated deficits as intellectual disability). Recently, however, CMDs have been classified using a combination of clinical, biochemical, pathological, and genetic features (see Table 33.2). Table 33.2 lists the genes mutated in various CMDs and the respective phenotypes. We focus on those disorders that are most likely to be associated with a clear neonatal presentation: primary, merosin-deficient CMD, and the three major CMDs with overt CNS abnormalities: Walker-Warburg syndrome (WWS), muscle-eye-brain disease (MEB), and Fukuyama CMD (FCMD). We describe only briefly those disorders that are particularly unusual or that do not generally result in marked neonatal features (i.e., Ullrich syndrome, congenital laminopathy, and rigid spine syndrome).

Congenital Muscular Dystrophy Without Overt Structural or Functional Brain Abnormalities. *CMD caused by a primary deficiency of merosin* (i.e., laminin alpha-2 chain; see later), MDC1A, accounts for approximately 20% to 30% of cases of CMD (see Table 33.2).[87,88] In 1979, an initial series of five infants with CMD was reported with no clinical sign of CNS disease (except for one with seizures) but with marked hypodensity of cerebral white matter on CT.[89] Over the next decade, subsequent reports of a similar relationship between CMD and abnormal cerebral white matter, primarily on CT scans, were published.[90-101] With the discovery that this disorder is associated with a deficiency of a critical basal lamina component (i.e., the laminin alpha-2 chain), recognition of the relative frequency of this disorder increased dramatically.[85,86,102-121] The clinical presentation with weakness and hypotonia in merosin-deficient CMD is more severe than that in other merosin-positive CMDs. Indeed, motor function usually does not evolve past sitting or standing with orthotic support; ambulation is hardly ever achieved (Table 33.3). Contractures are common and involve the hips, knees, elbows, and ankles, although severe neonatal arthrogryposis is rare. Nevertheless, in our experience, merosin-deficient CMD and congenital myotonic dystrophy are the two most common muscle disorders leading to multiple congenital contractures. Weakness tends to affect the upper limbs more severely than the lower limbs.[122] Facial weakness is often prominent. A typical clinical sign is limitation of eye movements, particularly of the upgaze, but this is often noted in the second decade of life.[123] Disturbance of chewing and swallowing, with a tendency for aspiration, is very common; a feeding tube may be needed. As many as 20% to 30% die of cardiopulmonary complications in the first year or so of life. A less severe phenotype, associated with *partial deficiency of merosin*, has been reported.[a] However, these patients usually have normal milestones in the first

---

[a]References 109, 112, 113, 120, 121, and 124-128.

TABLE 33.2   Classification of Congenital Muscular Dystrophies: Clinical, Biochemical, and Genetic Characteristics[a]

BIOCHEMICAL DEFECT	LOCUS	GENE	DISEASE PHENOTYPE(S)
Extracellular matrix proteins			
	6q22-23	*LAMA2*	Primary merosin deficiency (MDC1A)
	21q22.3	*COL6A1*	Ullrich CMD
	2q37	*COL6A2*	
		COL6A3	
External sarcolemmal proteins			
	12q13	*ITGA7*	Integrin α7–related CMD
	3p23-21	*ITGA9*	Integrin α9–related CMD
Dystroglycan and glycosyltransferase enzymes			
	9q34.1	*POMT1*	WWS, MEB, CMD with cerebellar involvement, CMD with intellectual disability and microcephaly
	1q32-34	*POMGnT1*	WWS, MEB, CMD with cerebellar involvement
	14q24.3	*POMT2*	WWS, MEB, CMD with cerebellar involvement, CMD with intellectual disability and microcephaly
	19q13.3	*FKRP*	WWS, MEB, CMD with cerebellar involvement, CMD with intellectual disability and microcephaly, CMD with no intellectual disability and normal brain MRI
	9q31	*FCMD*	Fukuyama CMD
	22q12.3-13.1	*LARGE*	WWS, MEB, white matter changes
	1q12-q21	*DPM2/DPM3*	CMD with intellectual disability and severe epilepsy
	7p21.2	*ISPD*	WWS, LGMD
	3p22.1	*GTDC2*	WWS
	11q13.2	*B3GALNT2*	WWS, MEB
	3p21.23	*GMPPB*	CMD with intellectual disability and severe epilepsy, LGMD
	3p21	*DAG1*	Primary dystroglycanopathy, LGMD with early onset and intellectual disability, normal brain MRI
	8p11.21	*SGK196*	MEB
	1q42	—	MDC1B
Endoplasmic reticulum protein			
	1p35-36	*SEPN1*	CMD with spinal rigidity (RSMD1)
Nuclear envelope proteins			
	6q25	*SYNE1 (nesprin 1)*	CMD with adducted thumbs
	1q21.2	*LMNA*	Congenital laminopathy
Sarcolemmal and mitochondrial membrane protein			
	22q13	*CHKB*	Mitochondrial CMD (CMDmt)
	21q22.3	*COL6A1*	Ullrich CMD
		COL6A2	
	2q37.3	*COL6A3*	Ullrich CMD

[a]The classification is based on combined clinical, genetic, and pathological data.

CMD, Congenital muscular dystrophy; *CMDmt,* CMD with mitochondrial structural abnormalities; *LGMD,* limb girdle muscular dystrophy; *MDC,* muscular dystrophy congenital; *MEB,* muscle eye brain; *MRI,* magnetic resonance imaging; *RSMD1,* rigid spine muscular dystrophy 1; *WWS,* Walker-Warburg syndrome.

Reprinted with permission from Mercuri E, Muntoni F. Congenital muscular dystrophy. In: Darras BT, Jones HR Jr, Ryan MM, De Vivo DC, eds. *Neuromuscular Disorders of Infancy, Childhood and Adolescence: A Clinician's Approach.* San Diego: Academic Press; 2015:chap 29, 538–550.

years of life and usually do not require enteral feeding and/or ventilator support.[129]

Despite the uniform occurrence of diffusely abnormal cerebral white matter by brain imaging in merosin-deficient CMD (see later discussion), clinical neurological abnormalities are unusual. Approximately 20% to 30% of patients develop seizure disorders, usually later in childhood, and approximately 5% to 10% of patients exhibit cognitive deficits.

Muscle biopsy shows dystrophic changes, and immunofluorescence with antimerosin antibodies demonstrates decreased or absent staining; in severe infantile cases, there is total absence or only traces of the laminin alpha-2 chain protein. Sometimes an extensive inflammatory infiltrate may be seen.

The diagnosis of merosin-deficient CMD is confirmed by detecting a recessive mutation(s) (homozygous or compound heterozygous state) in the laminin alpha-2 chain (*LAMA2*) gene.

Partial merosin deficiency may occur in the setting of other CMDs, such as dystroglycanopathies. *CMD with secondary deficiency of merosin* is rare in the neonatal period and likely represents a heterogeneous disorder. Formerly, the best characterized of this group was CMD related to *FKRP* mutations (see later). However, the more recent recognition that this disorder may be associated with overt CNS abnormalities makes it more appropriate to discuss later.

Merosin-positive CMD encompasses multiple clinical phenotypes, but the three most likely to be encountered in the neonatal period are Ullrich syndrome, congenital laminopathy, and rigid spine syndrome (see Table 33.2). The term *classic merosin-positive CMD* has become obsolete as molecular genetic studies characterize distinct disorders.

Ullrich CMD is a type of merosin-positive CMD with a characteristic clinical phenotype.[85,86,130-138] Neonatal presentation with hypotonia, weakness, proximal joint contractures, torticollis, hip dislocation, spine kyphosis, and marked distal hyperlaxity is characteristic. In older infants and children, other typical features include prominent calcanei, keratosis pilaris, and hypertrophic scars (keloids).[138] Subsequent motor development is severely delayed, and walking independently occurs only in the minority. The defect involves the gene *(COL6A)* for collagen VI, an extracellular matrix protein. Most cases of neonatal onset are autosomal recessive. Collagen VI is composed of three alpha chains encoded by three genes: *COLA1*, *COLA2*, and *COLA3*.

Congenital laminopathy is another CMD (L-CMD) related to recessive or dominant de novo mutations in the lamin A/C gene *(LMNA)* (Table 33.4). *LMNA* mutations cause the dominant form of Emery-Dreifuss muscular dystrophy.[139] Early onset in infancy has been described with severe axial weakness, wasting of cervicoaxial muscles, limited spontaneous movement, and *dropped head* syndrome as well as cardiac arrhythmias and feeding and respiratory difficulties.[140-143] Muscle biopsy usually shows a dystrophic pattern and sometimes inflammatory infiltrates.[144]

Rigid spine syndrome is a third merosin-positive CMD that usually presents clinically after the neonatal period with hypotonia and axial weakness.[85,86] Neonatal onset has been reported. Subsequently, the characteristic spinal extensor contractures become apparent, with resulting spinal rigidity, scoliosis, and restrictive respiratory disease.[145] The defect involves the gene *(SEPN1)* for an endoplasmic reticulum protein, selenoprotein N, the function of which is unknown.

Congenital Muscular Dystrophy With Overt Structural or Functional Brain Abnormalities. CMD may be accompanied by prominent involvement of the CNS, manifested by severe neurological deficits (e.g., intellectual disability; see Table 33.2). Although primary merosin deficiency is associated with a morphological disturbance of cerebral white matter (see later), no clinical neurological abnormalities occur in most cases. Because these disorders are related to abnormalities of glycosylation of alpha-dystroglycan, they are often grouped as *dystroglycanopathies*. The term *dystroglycanopathies* includes a group of muscle diseases, with hypoglycosylation of alpha-dystroglycan on muscle biopsy, often associated with central nervous system structural abnormalities and less frequently with eye pathology.[122] Some of the entities in this category are associated with disorders of neuronal migration, cerebral white matter abnormalities, hindbrain anomalies, and marked clinical neurological abnormalities; they are termed FCMD, WWS, and MEB. There are also mild dystroglycanopathies with late onset and no structural or functional brain or eye involvement;

TABLE 33.3   Clinical and Laboratory Features: Merosin-Deficient Congenital Muscular Dystrophy[a]

FEATURES	
Clinical severity	Marked
Ambulation	Rare
Creatine kinase elevation	Marked
Myopathology	Severe
Nerve conduction velocity	Slow
White matter abnormality	Marked
Structural brain abnormalities	≈<10%
Epilepsy	≈20%
Chromosomal locus	6q2
Laminin alpha-2 (merosin)	Absent[b]

[a]See text for references.
[b]Partial but not total deficiency of laminin alpha-2 chain is associated with less severe phenotype (see text).

TABLE 33.4   Distinguishing Features Among Major Syndromes of Congenital Muscular Dystrophy With Overt Structural or Functional Brain Abnormalities

	TYPE OF CMD		
CLINICAL FEATURE	FUKUYAMA	WALKER-WARBURG	MUSCLE-EYE-BRAIN
Neurological deficits	+	+	+
Microcephaly	+	−	−
Macrocephaly	−	+	+
Hypotonia	+	+	+
Ocular abnormalities (severe)	−	+	+
White matter abnormality on neuroimaging (persistent or progressive)	+	+	−
Lissencephaly-pachygyria	+	+	+
Cortical mantle thin	±	+	−
Corpus callosum absent	±	+	−
Hydrocephalus	−	+	±
Encephalocele	−	+[a]	−
Cerebellar malformation	−	+	±

[a]Characteristic when present but described in less than 50% of cases.
+, Prominent feature; −, not a prominent feature; ±, variable feature; *CMD*, congenital muscular dystrophy.

these are not discussed here. The Online Mendelian Inheritance in Man (OMIM) database subdivides the group of muscular dystrophies with deficit of dystroglycan glycosylation or muscular dystrophy-dystroglycanopathy (MDDG) into three broad phenotypical groups: A, B, and C. Primarily the type A severe phenotypes are discussed here.[146]

FCMD (see Tables 33.2 and 33.4) has been described in several hundred Japanese children and in a much smaller number of children in North America, Europe, and Australia.[85,86,109,147-165] The disorder exhibits the same basic clinical features referable to muscle involvement as the CMDs without CNS involvement: (1) onset in the neonatal period, (2) marked diffuse weakness and hypotonia, (3) facial weakness, and (4) joint contractures that develop particularly in infancy after the neonatal period. The *clinical course* of the motor function is generally characterized by slow acquisition of skills, usually the ability to crawl or to stand with support, until approximately the age of 8 years, when motor functions begin to deteriorate, ultimately to a lower level. The progression relates both to worsening of contractures and to apparent increasing weakness. Most patients become bedridden by the age of 10 years, and life expectancy is usually approximately 20 years.[109]

The hallmark of FCMD is the evidence of major CNS disease. *Intellectual disability* is essentially constant, and the usual IQ level is between 30 and 50.[a] Moreover, *febrile and afebrile seizures* occur in approximately 60% of the cases. CT and especially MRI scanning and neuropathological studies (see subsequent discussions of diagnosis and pathology) establish the causes of these neural phenomena (i.e., major neuronal migrational and other abnormalities).

WWS is the more severe of the two CMDs, with prominent ocular as well as CNS abnormalities (see Tables 33.2 and 33.4; see Chapter 6).[85,86,166] Indeed, the life expectancy in this disorder is less than 3 years. In the newborn, the muscle disorder is often overshadowed by the severe CNS (cobblestone lissencephaly, pontocerebellar hypoplasia, severe white matter abnormality) and ocular (microphthalmia, hypoplastic optic nerves, colobomata, retinal detachment) abnormalities. Severe disturbances of feeding and tube or gastrostomy feeding are nearly invariable.

MEB is a similar CMD, with ocular and CNS abnormalities, although it is milder than WWS (see Tables 33.2 and 33.4). Thus an initial report from Finland describes 18 affected patients with the clinical features referable to CMD, intellectual disability of variable severity in 15 of the 18 reported patients, *occasional* seizures, and, distinctively, a wide variety of ocular abnormalities.[167] These ocular defects include high myopia, congenital or infantile glaucoma, hypoplasia of the retina and optic nerve, coloboma of the optic nerve, and cataracts.[167,168] Many subsequent reports further delineate this type of CMD.[b]

Although patients with MEB that is overt at birth may exhibit severe abnormalities, in general the features of this disorder are milder than those observed with WWS, and both of these cerebro-ocular types of CMD exhibit differences from FCMD (see Table 33.4).

There is also a fourth group of CMD patients (OMIM classification type B) with posterior fossa/cerebellar abnormalities on imaging or a normal MRI; these patients may be intellectually normal or have an associated intellectual disability. In this group, cerebellar abnormalities may be the only structural brain defects; they include cerebellar cysts and hypoplasia or dysplasia. Albeit supratentorial defects may also occur, cerebellar cysts in the absence of supratentorial white matter or cortical involvement have been described mostly in patients with mutations in the fukutin-related protein (FKRP) gene. Although FKRP-related CMD usually manifests beyond the neonatal period and is not considered in detail, neonatal onset is well documented.[85,86,121,191,192] Weakness and hypotonia are apparent in the first weeks or months of life, although a phenotype as severe as primary deficiency of merosin has been observed. Subsequent motor development is markedly impaired, and respiratory muscle weakness leading to ventilatory failure occurs in the first or second decade of life. In neonatal-onset cases, severe cognitive deficits are common. Muscle biopsy shows a partial deficiency of laminin alpha-2 protein; thus this disorder was previously classified as CMD with secondary deficiency of merosin. However, the principal defect involves FKRP, presumed to be a glycosyl transferase, with alpha-dystroglycan the likely substrate. More than half of 25 reported cases with *FKRP* mutations have had prominent CNS abnormalities and thus should be included with the CMD group with overt CNS abnormalities.[193,194] The neurological abnormalities have included intellectual disability, and the CNS structural deficits have included subependymal heterotopias, focal pachygyria, white matter abnormalities, cerebellar cysts, marked cerebellar dysplasia, and pontine hypoplasia. These CNS deficits are consistent, at least in part, with neuronal migrational disturbance and overlap with those observed in FCMD, WWS, and MEB. This similarity is noteworthy because, as discussed earlier, the last three types of CMD with overt CNS abnormalities all also involve disturbances of glycosylation of alpha-dystroglycan.

Laboratory Studies. When all types of CMD (see Table 33.2) are considered, the serum CK level is elevated in most cases, particularly early in the course of the disease. However, the presence and degree of elevation vary with the type of disorder. In the largest series of cases (*n* = 50) of the now obsolete entity known as *merosin-positive classic (pure) CMD*, 54% of infants had elevated CK levels, and the average elevation was approximately three times the upper limit of normal.[195] In another series of 24 cases, CK elevation was 2.5-fold above the normal upper limit.[196] The important clinical point is that a normal CK level does not exclude the diagnosis. By contrast, in *merosin-negative CMD*, the CK levels are consistently and markedly elevated to approximately 10-fold to 20-fold higher than the upper limit of normal.[102-106,108,109,122,159] In FCMD, CK levels generally range from 10-fold to 50-fold higher than the normal upper limit. Levels are similarly very high in MEB and in WWS. In all cases, CK levels tend to decline with the patient's age. The EMG reveals the changes of myopathy (see Table 30.4), including small-amplitude, brief-duration, and polyphasic motor unit potentials.

CT and, preferably, MRI scans of the head are useful in identifying the cerebral white matter abnormality characteristic of primary *merosin-deficient CMD* (Fig. 33.9). The appearance on CT is decreased attenuation of cerebral white matter and, on MRI, increased signal on T2-weighted images. The cerebral white matter is affected diffusely, whereas the cerebellar white matter

---

[a]References 85, 86, 147, 159, 161, 162, and 165.
[b]References 85, 86, 109, 159, 166, and 169-190.

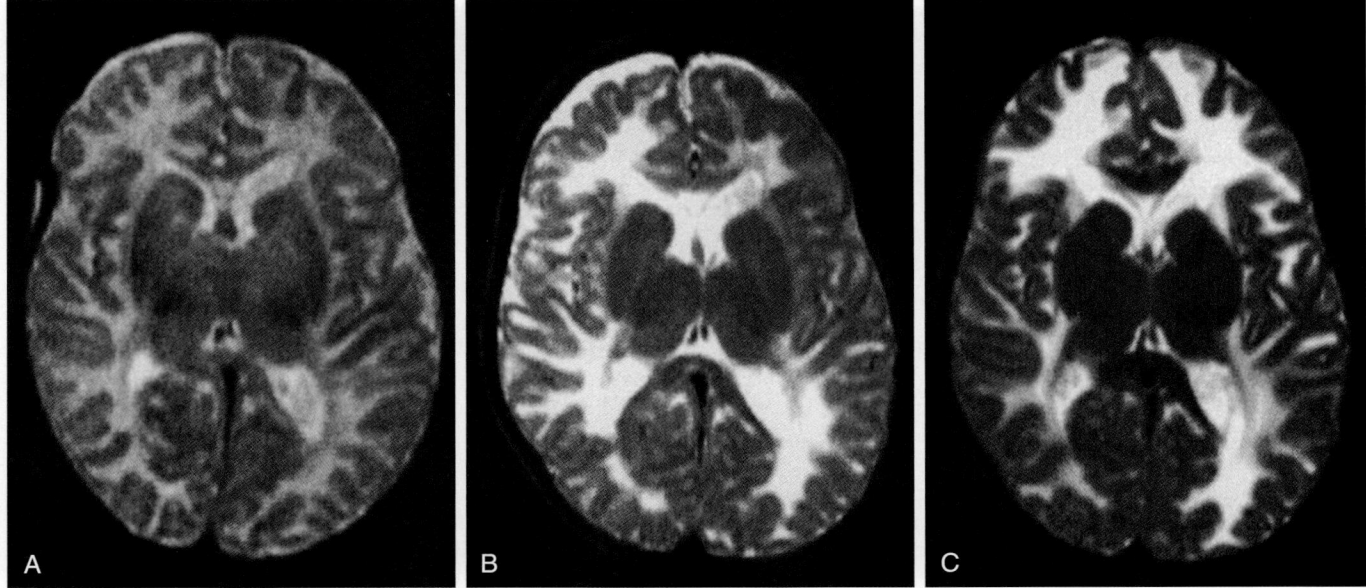

Figure 33.9 Evolution of cerebral white matter abnormality in merosin-deficient congenital muscular dystrophy, as demonstrated by magnetic resonance imaging (T2-weighted images). (A) At 3 weeks of age, the appearance of cerebral white matter was within normal limits. (B) At 6 months of age, abnormal signal intensity in cerebral white matter was clearly apparent. (C) At 12 months of age, the white matter was extremely abnormal. (From Mercuri E, Pennock J, Goodwin F, Sewry C, et al. Sequential study of central and peripheral nervous system involvement in an infant with merosin-deficient congenital muscular dystrophy. *Neuromuscul Disord.* 1996;6:425–429.)

is unaffected. The cerebral white matter abnormality is generally not apparent in the first weeks of life and becomes apparent by approximately 6 months of age (see Fig. 33.9).[85,86,108,197] However, utilization of T2-weighted images with a fast spin-echo sequence has demonstrated the white matter abnormality at 5 days of age.[198] The abnormal white matter signal is most prominent in structures myelinated after birth (e.g., cerebral white matter) rather than in those structures that are myelinated before birth (e.g., brain stem and cerebellar white matter).[199] Thus the abnormality may reflect a delay or arrest in myelination, and the finding in the affected white matter of abnormally increased apparent diffusion coefficients, characteristic of immature white matter, is perhaps consistent with this notion.[200] Although the cerebral white matter abnormality is the unifying feature of the primary merosin-negative cases, several reports document the occurrence of cortical gyral dysplasia, especially in the occipital region, in isolated cases (~ <10%).[118,186,201-205] Hypoplasia of the cerebellum was observed by MRI to varying degrees in 6 of 14 well-studied cases,[116] and associated cerebellar cysts have also been described.[206]

In *FCMD*, the most striking abnormality is the gyral disturbance (Fig. 33.10). The two major findings detectable by MRI are as follows: (1) a thick cortex with shallow sulci in the frontal regions, consistent with polymicrogyria, and (2) a thick cortex with a smooth surface in the temporo-occipital regions, consistent with lissencephaly-pachygyria.[163] These findings correlate well with the neuropathology (see later discussion). Additional consistent features are white matter changes similar to those described earlier for merosin-deficient CMD. However, distinction of these two entities by MRI is straightforward because of the marked gyral abnormalities in

FCMD. Moreover, the white matter abnormality in the latter diminishes with age. The corpus callosum is slightly hypoplastic in most of the Fukuyama cases.[162]

In *WWS and MEB*, the dominant finding is the gyral abnormality. In its full form, as in WWS, the appearance of type II lissencephaly (*cobblestone* lissencephaly) and pachygyria is striking and is associated with diffuse white matter abnormality of the type observed in merosin-deficient CMD. Again, the distinction by MRI from the latter disorder is straightforward because of the presence of the gyral disturbance as well as marked dysgenesis of cerebellum and hypoplasia of the pons, especially in WWS.

Additional laboratory studies of interest include measurements of cerebral visual and somatosensory evoked responses and of peripheral nerve conduction velocities in merosin-deficient CMD (see Table 33.3). Thus, for somatosensory evoked responses, latencies have been delayed in all patients studied, and for visual evoked responses, latencies have been delayed in approximately 90% of patients.[85,86,197,207,208] Nerve conduction velocity studies have shown moderately slow values in more than 80% of merosin-deficient cases studied thus far.[197,209,210] One infant studied in the newborn period had normal values but exhibited slowed conduction when studied again at 6 months of age.[197] No abnormalities in cerebral evoked responses or motor nerve conduction velocities have been observed in merosin-positive CMD.

The demonstration of laminin alpha-2 deficiency in skin biopsy and in cultured fibroblasts in primary merosin-deficient cases indicates the potential value of this approach for the diagnosis of merosin-deficient CMD. In addition, the prenatal demonstration of merosin deficiency in trophoblastic tissue

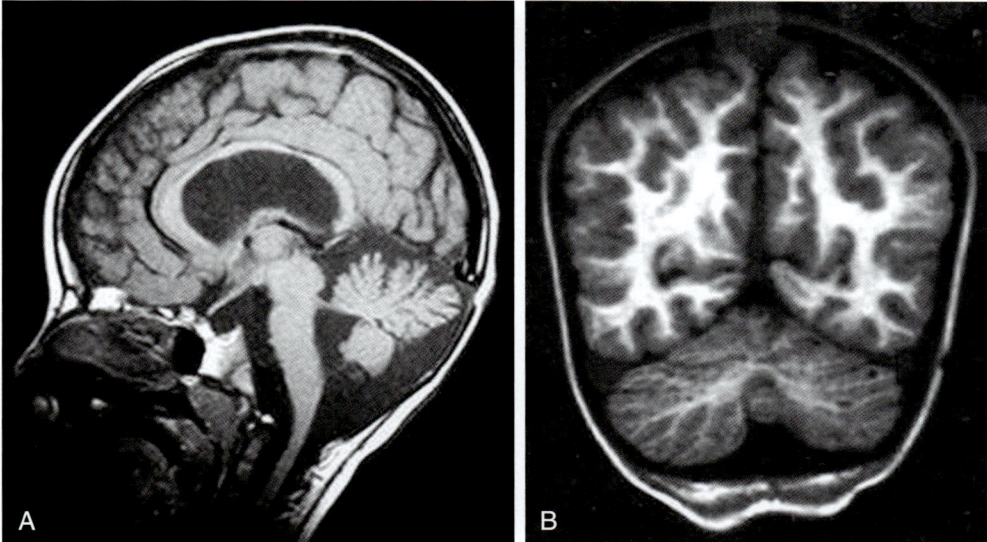

Figure 33.10 Congenital muscular dystrophy and cerebellar abnormalities with POMT2 mutations. (A) Enlarged cisterna magna and mild cerebellar vermis hypoplasia in a 16-month-old child with POMT2 mutations (sagittal T1-weighted brain MR image). (B) Cerebellar cysts in a 7-year-old with POMT2 mutations (coronal T1-weighted MR image). *MR,* Magnetic resonance. (Adapted with permission from Messina S, et al. POMT1 and POMT mutations in CMD patients: a multicentric Italian study. *Neuromusc Disord.* 2008;18:565–571.)

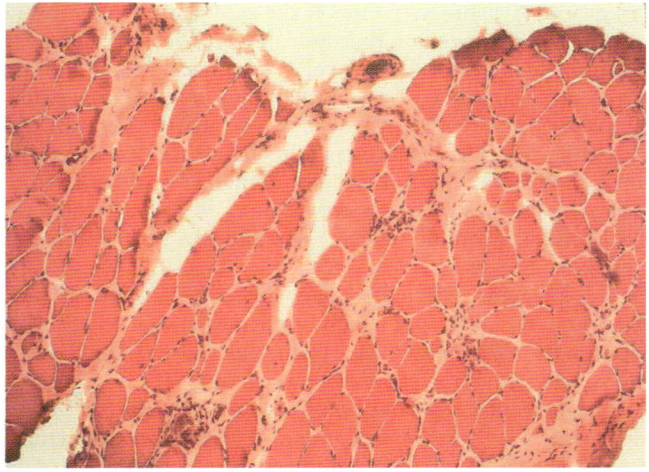

Figure 33.11 Congenital muscular dystrophy: muscle pathology. Note nongrouped changes with marked variation in fiber size and extensive replacement of muscle by connective tissue *(light brown areas)* and fat *(clear areas).* Hematoxylin and eosin stain, ×400.

obtained from chorionic villus samples indicates the value of this approach (with simultaneous linkage analysis) in prenatal diagnosis.[211-213]

Pathology. *Muscle biopsy* in all types of CMDs shows striking changes, consistent with a dystrophic process.[4,16,159] Notable are marked variations in fiber size in a nongrouped distribution, internal nuclei, and marked replacement of muscle by fat and connective tissue (Fig. 33.11).[a] Necrosis of fibers and evidence of regeneration are common. Striking changes not apparent on initial biopsies may appear on subsequent biopsies. The fiber-type pattern is retained; the muscle does not exhibit the prominent signs of maturational disturbance observed in myotonic dystrophy (see earlier discussion). Although comparisons are difficult, the myopathic changes reported in primary merosin-deficient CMD are more striking than those in merosin-positive CMD.[4,106,107,216,217] Several reports have emphasized the presence of inflammatory cellular infiltrates, especially early in the disease and perhaps related to necrosis[218-220]; this finding should not lead to the mistaken diagnosis of infantile polymyositis, a treatable and self-limited disorder (see later discussion). The diagnostic feature critical for merosin-deficient CMD is the lack of staining for this molecule on immunocytochemical study (Fig. 33.12). Partial absence is observed in the infants with the less severe, partial type of merosin-deficient CMD or in secondary merosin deficiencies.[a]

The *neuropathology* in infants with the *merosin-deficient CMD with cerebral white matter abnormalities* is not clearly known. The little neuropathological information available is inconclusive.[91,92] The findings that the white matter abnormality becomes most apparent later in infancy and is associated with disturbances of visual and somatosensory evoked potentials and the MRI findings suggesting a defect in postnatal myelin development (see earlier discussions) suggest that myelination is altered in some way. Laminin alpha-2 chain is expressed in the basement membrane of blood vessels that form the blood-brain barrier and also along developing axonal tracts, where interaction with oligodendrocytes may occur.[86] Disturbances at either or both loci could lead to disturbed myelin development and the abnormal signal with increased water diffusion on MRI or the *edema* by MR spectroscopy.

---

[a]References 4, 85, 86, 107, 122, 147, 159, 160, 196, 214, and 215.

[a]References 85, 86, 110, 112, 113, and 124-126.

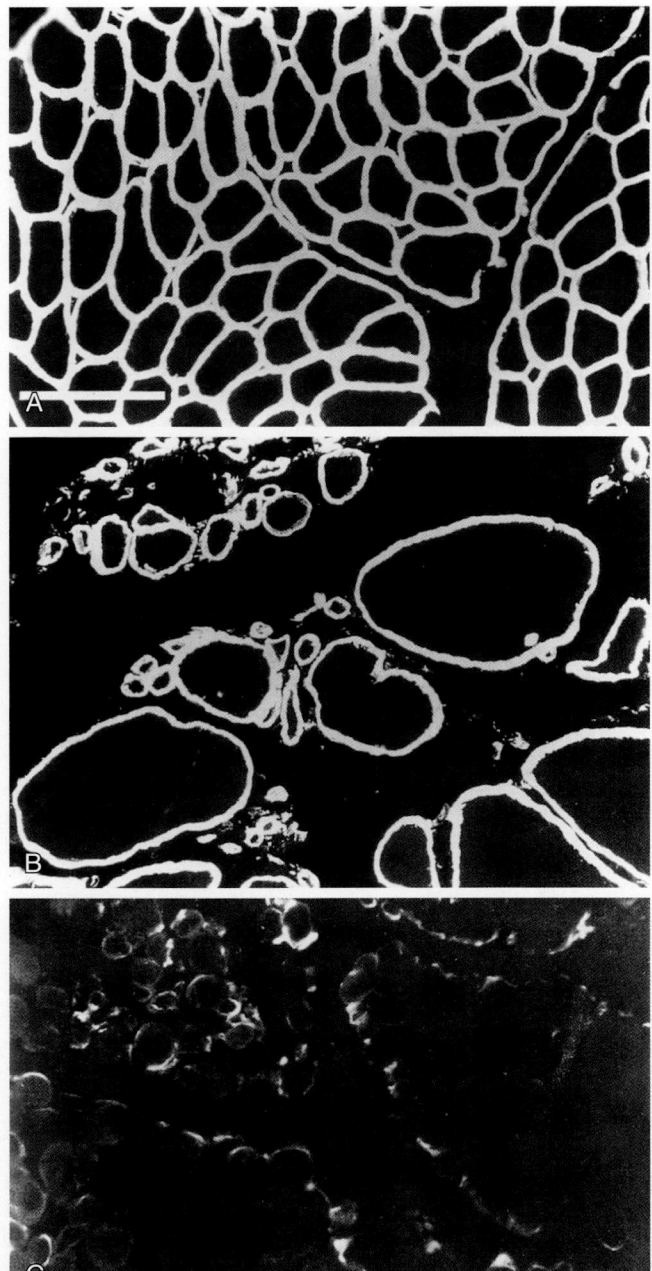

Figure 33.12 Immunofluorescence analysis for merosin. (A) Normal muscle. (B and C) Muscle from two infants with congenital muscular dystrophy. (A) Normal muscle shows strong, continuous staining around the periphery of the myofibers. (B) Similar staining is evident in one of the infants with congenital muscular dystrophy, despite the marked variation in fiber size and increased connective tissue. Thus, this infant has classic merosin-positive congenital muscular dystrophy. In C, however, minimal staining for merosin is apparent. This infant has merosin-deficient congenital muscular dystrophy. (From North KN, Specht LA, Sethi RK, Shapiro F, et al. Congenital muscular dystrophy associated with merosin deficiency. *J Child Neurol.* 1996;11:291–295.)

The *neuropathology* in infants with *FCMD* is striking.[a] The dominant finding is cerebral gyral abnormality, most consistently polymicrogyria (Fig. 33.13A), pachygyria, or agyria (type II lissencephaly). The disorder indicates a disturbance of neuronal migration, as described in Chapter 2. Other neuropathological abnormalities include subpial neuronal–glial heterotopias, cerebellar polymicrogyria (see Fig. 33.13B), aberrant myelinated fascicles over the surface of the cerebellum, hypoplasia and aberrant course of the pyramidal tracts, leptomeningeal thickening, and occasional hydrocephalus. No distinct changes have been described in cerebral white matter except for a delay in myelination; hence the basis for the white matter abnormality detected by CT or MRI is unclear (see earlier discussion).

The *neuropathology* in *the two CMDs with prominent ocular and brain abnormalities* has been described.[b] The findings bear similarities to those described in FCMD, including the following: type II lissencephaly; polymicrogyria, pachygyria, and heterotopias in the basal meninges; hypoplasia of the pyramidal tracts; and aqueductal stenosis. Distinguishing features in the more severe form of cerebro-ocular CMD, WWS, include more severe cortical migrational disturbances, hydrocephalus, cerebellar dysplasia-hypoplasia (including absence of vermis), and encephalocele (see Table 33.4). In general the findings in MEB are milder than in WWS.

Pathogenesis and Etiology. The pathogenesis and etiology of this group of disorders focus on the sarcolemmal membrane and the related proteins that link the extracellular matrix to the actin filaments of the myocytic cytoskeleton.[c] The key sarcolemmal protein involved in linking to the extracellular matrix is alpha-dystroglycan; it interacts with laminin, the key extracellular matrix protein, which, in turn, interacts with collagen type VI. The intracellular connection is mediated by the interaction of alpha-dystroglycan with sarcoglycans, the sarcolemmal proteins, which are linked to dystrophin and thereby to the actin cytoskeleton (Fig. 33.14). In the CMDs, the key proteins affected are *alpha-dystroglycan, laminin,* and *collagen type VI,* defects of which interrupt the vital relationship between the extracellular matrix and the muscle cytoskeleton and result in the muscle degeneration of CMD.

The molecular basis of primary *merosin-deficient CMD* is well established.[85,86,108-110,122,230-232] Laminin-2 or merosin is the critical alpha-dystroglycan–binding basement membrane protein of the muscle extracellular matrix. The critical laminin alpha-2 chain of laminin 2 is encoded by the *LAMA2* gene on chromosome 6q2; this is the gene that is defective in merosin-deficient CMD. Laminin alpha-2 chain is also present in basement membrane of Schwann cells, and thus its lack may underlie the defect of peripheral nerve described earlier. Moreover, as noted earlier, laminin alpha-2 is present in blood vessels and along developing axons in human brain (see earlier). How these observations relate to the cerebral white matter abnormality remains to be clearly elucidated. Demonstration of the deficient protein in muscle and skin facilitates diagnosis in the infant, and demonstration of the defect in chorionic villus samples facilitates prenatal diagnosis.

---

[a]References 147, 149-152, 157, 159, 178-180, and 221-229.
[b]References 85, 86, 169, 170, 174, 175, 178-180, and 185.
[c]References 85, 86, 109, 110, 230, and 231.

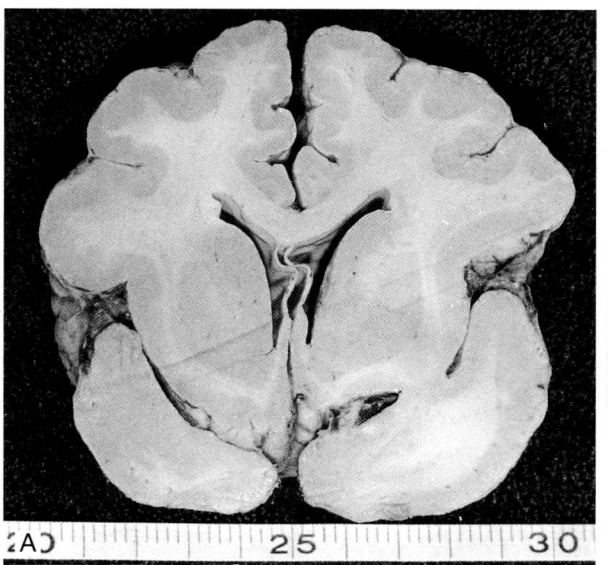
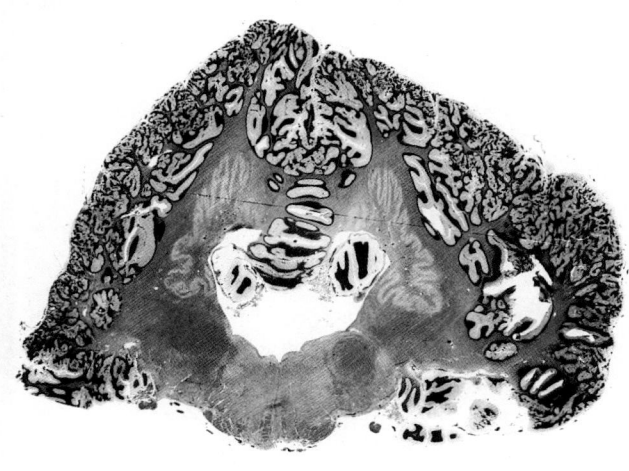

Figure 33.13 Fukuyama congenital muscular dystrophy with associated encephalopathy (migrational disturbance). This cerebrum and cerebellum are from a child with severe hypotonia and weakness from birth and severe intellectual disability. The child died at 6 years, 5 months of age; the muscle pathology was consistent with congenital muscular dystrophy. (A) Coronal section of cerebrum. Note the polymicrogyric cortex involving the superomedial and lateral convexity, the pachygyric cortex involving the lateral convexity, and the agyric cortex involving the temporal lobes. (B) Horizontal section of cerebellum and brain stem. Note the marked and diffuse polymicrogyria involving the cerebellar cortex. (From Kamoshita S, Konishi Y, Segawa M, Fukuyama Y. Congenital muscular dystrophy as a disease of the central nervous system. *Arch Neurol.* 1976;33:513–516.)

The molecular basis of *classic (pure) merosin-positive CMD* is heterogeneous and reflects the nature of the underlying genetic defects.

As discussed earlier, the molecular basis of *Ullrich CMD* involves the three genes *(COL6A1, COL6A2, COL6A3)* for collagen VI (see earlier). This defect results in a prominent loss of the basal lamina of muscle fibers and interrupts the vital link between the extracellular space and the intracellular cytoskeleton, as described earlier.

The molecular basis of *rigid spine syndrome* involves a deficiency of the gene *(SEPN1)* selenoprotein N, an endoplasmic reticulum protein (see earlier). The function of this protein remains elusive; however, it may be involved in protecting cells against oxidative stress.[233]

The molecular bases for the CMDs with overt CNS abnormalities (i.e., *FCMD, WWS, MEB* and others), the dystroglycanopathies, all involve defects in dystroglycan and multiple glycosyl transferase genes catalyzing the *O*-linked glycosylation of alpha-dystroglycan (see Table 33.2).[a] *POMT1* encodes the protein *O*-mannosyl transferase; *POMGnT1* encodes the protein *O*-mannosyl-*N*-acetylglucosaminyl transferase. Multiple *O*-linked glycosylation sites are present in certain serine-threonine–rich domains of alpha-dystroglycan. FCMD is caused by a defect in a gene *(FCMD)* that encodes fukutin (FKTN), a putative glycosyltransferase, the exact function of which is yet unclear.

Mutations in the *FKTN, FKRP,* and *ISPD* genes can result in severe WWS or MEB phenotypes, in intermediate phenotypes such as those associated with cerebellar cysts or normal brain

MRI, or even in milder limb-girdle muscular dystrophies. Although the mutated gene cannot be predicted from the clinical phenotype, there are certain features that may suggest a particular gene or number of genes.

- In WWS, although POMT1 was the first genetic defect to be described, mutations in all known dystroglycanopathy genes have been described.
- In MEB, mutations have been identified in POMGnT1 (the first linked to MEB), POMT1, POMT2, ISPD, and FKRP.
- Cerebellar cysts have been described in association with mutations in FKRP, POMGnT1, and ISPD genes but may rarely also be seen with POMT1 and POMT2 mutations.[122,235]

Disturbances in the glycosylation of alpha-dystroglycan impair its interaction with laminin and sarcolemmal proteins, especially beta-dystroglycan. Muscle degeneration is the result. Because alpha-dystroglycan is also present in the basement membrane of the glia limitans in the developing cerebral cortex, defective glycosylation results in the disturbances in neuronal migration that underlie the occurrence of cobblestone lissencephaly (see Chapter 6). As noted earlier, more than half of the cases of CMD related to *FKRP* mutations and FKRP deficiency, which exhibit CNS abnormalities milder but mechanistically similar to those of the three main disorders discussed here (WWS, MEB, FCMD), are relevant in this context, because the FKRP also appears to be a glycosyltransferase for alpha-dystroglycan.[193]

Management. Because the course in most patients with any of the types of CMD is nonprogressive for months to years, it is important to attempt to correct existing contractures by physical therapy (i.e., passive stretching or serial splints) and to prevent the development of contractures by active and passive exercises. The development of fixed deformities is often more deleterious

[a]References 85, 86, 122, 189, 227, 228, and 234.

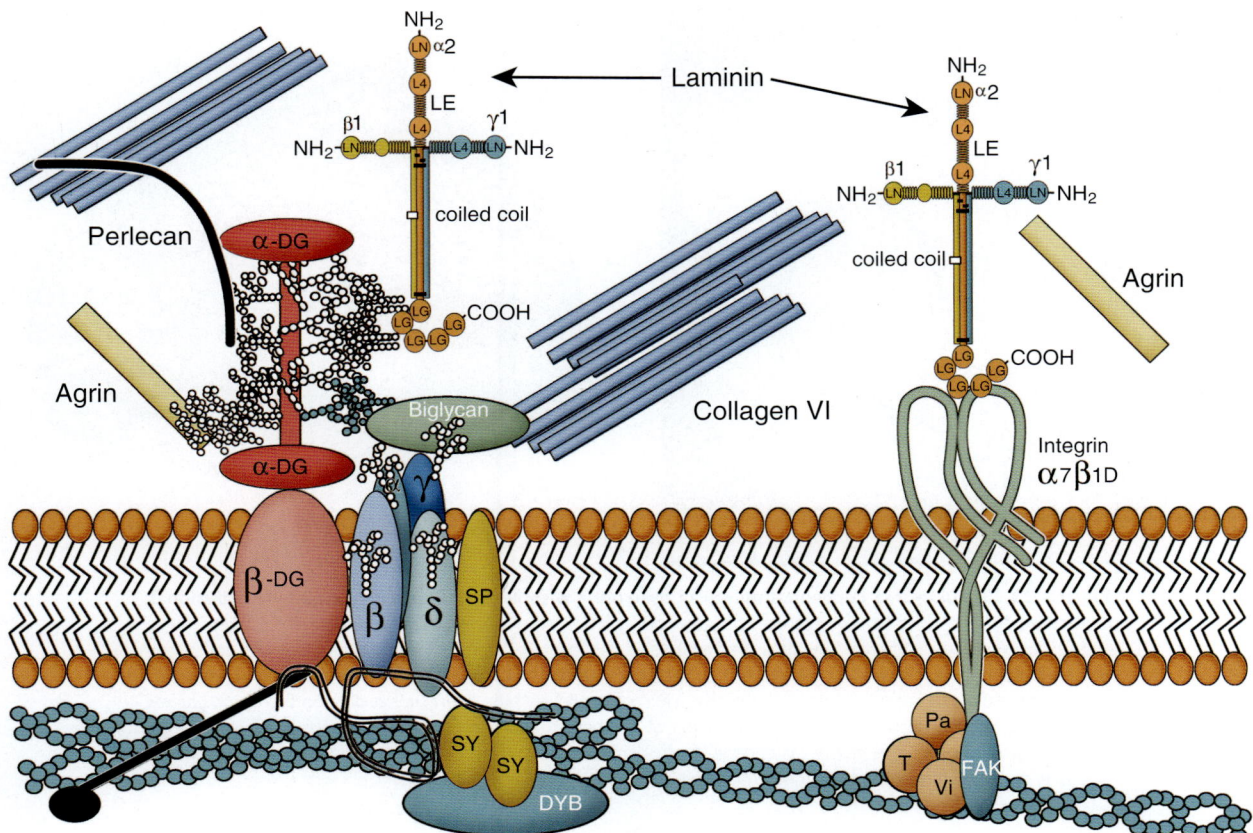

Figure 33.14 The dystrophin-associated protein complex. This schematic shows the location of key proteins involved in the extracellular matrix–dystroglycan–dystrophin axis; a number of these proteins are described in this chapter, in particular α-dystroglycan (α-DG), the laminin α2 chain of the merosin trimer, the integrin complex and collagen VI. (Adapted with permission from Muntoni F, Voit T. The congenital muscular dystrophies in 2004: a century of exciting progress. *Neuromusc Disord.* 2004;14:635–649.)

to future motor abilities than is muscle weakness. Although no specific therapies are available, more details concerning supportive management are available in specialized sources.[122]

Facioscapulohumeral Dystrophy

FSHD is usually recognized as an autosomal dominantly inherited myopathy with prominent involvement of the face and upper extremities, onset in adolescence or early adulthood, and a slowly progressive or apparently static course.[4,236] A rare type of FSHD with onset in early infancy and a more severe course have been delineated.[236-248]

Clinical Features. The infantile *clinical syndrome*, first described by Carroll and Brooke in 1979,[237] is characterized by the onset of facial weakness in early infancy.[236-248] The weakness is distinctive in that most patients are unable to move the upper lip and later have a peculiar horizontal smile. Difficulty in closing the eyes is prominent, and the infant may sleep with the eyes open. The whole face tends to be smooth and expressionless. Difficulty in sucking is common. However, motor milestones are usually not significantly delayed, and 8 of 11 patients in the largest series walked alone by 15 months of age.[237] Later, in infancy and early childhood, progressive weakness and wasting of axial and limb muscles supervene, particularly in

the proximal upper extremities but then also in the lower ones. Of five patients who had reached 15 years of age or more, four were no longer walking, and the remaining patient was walking with difficulty. A similarly progressive disease course has been documented by other investigators.[239,241,244,245] In a report of seven infantile-onset cases, the age at onset was between infancy and 4.5 years and the mean duration between onset of first symptoms and wheelchair dependency was 9.9 years.[248] In a recently reported series of patients enrolled in the Italian FSHD registry, 54.5% showed clinical signs during the first 10 years; however, no patients had perinatal onset.[249] The other clinical accompaniment, observed in the series of Carroll and Brooke,[237] was sensorineural hearing loss in 6 of 11 children; this loss was severe in 2 children. Approximately 50% of subsequently reported cases have exhibited sensorineural hearing loss.[236,241-246] Later in childhood, some patients have developed retinal telangiectasia, exudation, and detachment (Coats syndrome) in addition to sensorineural hearing loss.[240,241,243,245,250] Intellectual disability was observed in 30% of cases in one series[241]; it was also documented with epilepsy in other cases.[246,251,252]

Pathology. Muscle pathology was striking in six of the nine patients studied in detail by Carroll and Brooke,[237] and it

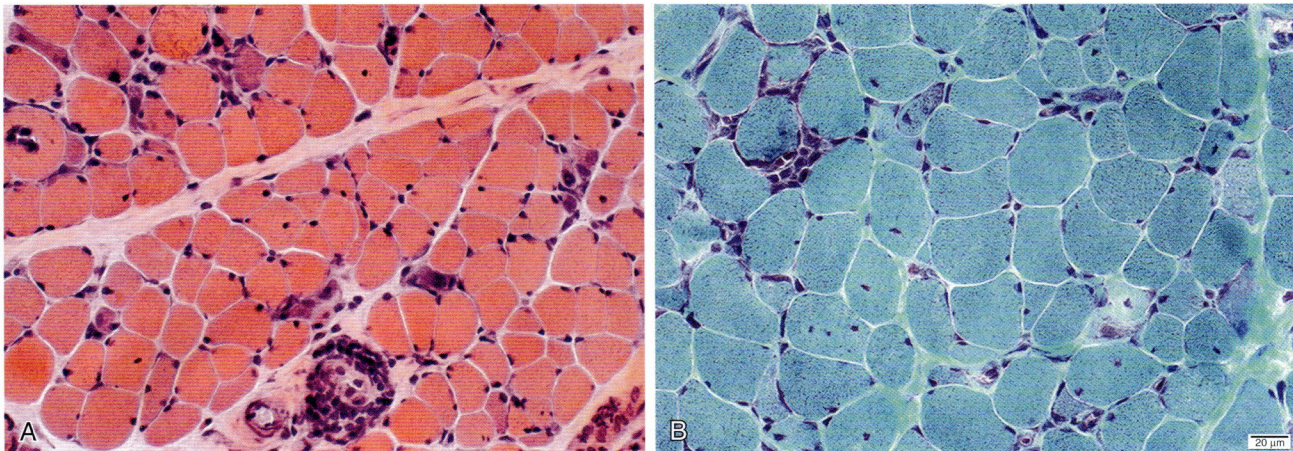

Figure 33.15 **Congenital facioscapulohumeral dystrophy.** (A) Hematoxylin and eosin stain. (B) Gomori trichrome stain. Note striking inflammatory response in muscle and significant variation in fiber size and many small basophilic fibers. In A, note mononuclear inflammatory cells around perimysial blood vessels. (Courtesy Alan Pestronk, MD. http://neuromuscular.wustl.edu/pathol/fsh.htm.)

exhibited an *inflammatory* response suggestive of polymyositis (Fig. 33.15). Inflammatory changes in FSHD have been noted by others.[a] This finding may lead to treatment with steroids, which results in no objective benefit. Indeed, it is clear from the relative frequencies of infantile FSHD and of polymyositis (see later) that inflammatory changes in muscle in an infant should raise the question of FSHD (or other congenital myopathy) rather than polymyositis, especially if the face is particularly involved.

Pathogenesis and Etiology. The genetic abnormality in this dominantly inherited disease is located at chromosome 4q35.[241,242,244,245,248] The frequency of de novo mutations is high. However, on careful examination, as many as half of the apparently sporadic cases were found to have an affected parent. Frequently parents are carriers with somatic mosaicism of the mutation and thus may appear unaffected. The defect is particularly interesting and involves a reduction in the number of repeats of a 3.3-kb repeat sequence, D4Z4, at the 4q35 locus. Normal individuals carry 11 or more D4Z4 repeats; patients with FSHD have 1 to 10 copies.[236] There is an inverse and coarse relationship between the onset and severity of the disease and the size of the D4Z4 repeat array. Most patients with 1 to 3 D4Z4 units are usually severely affected with seizures, cognitive delay, and hearing loss and are typically sporadic cases.[242,255,257,258] However, only about half of the contractions are pathogenic, because the array needs to be on an FSHD-permissive chromosome 4 that contains a polyadenylation signal for *DUX4*. This gene is embedded within each D4Z4 repeat and encodes a germline transcription factor.[259-262] In somatic cells, the D4Z4 repeat is epigenetically repressed, which results in silencing of the DUX4 gene. When the repeat contracts in FSHD1 patients, the epigenetic silencing is released, causing the expression of the DUX4 gene and protein, which is toxic to mature skeletal muscle.[262-264] Normal-sized D4Z4 repeat arrays can also be depressed by heterozygous

mutations in the structural maintenance of chromosomes flexible hinge domain containing protein 1 *(SMCHD1)* gene on chromosome 18, which encodes for a chromatin modifier; this explains the pathogenesis of FSHD2, in which the D4Z4 repeat is of normal size.[265] SMCHD1 mutations in patients with FSHD1-sized D4Z4 repeat arrays of 9 to 10 units cause a more severe phenotype (Fig. 33.16).[266]

Laboratory Studies. The serum CK level is moderately elevated in nearly all patients.[237-241,244-246] The EMG reveals low-amplitude and short-duration motor unit potentials, indicative of myopathy. Nerve conduction studies are normal. However, these tests have become obsolete because, in suspected cases, the diagnosis can be confirmed by examining the leukocyte DNA for the D4Z4 repeat contraction and SMCHD1 mutations.

Management. Management is similar to that for progressive myopathy in late childhood and adolescence.[4] Of importance for the physician evaluating the newborn with facial weakness is the recognition that FSHD may be present; family members must be examined and perhaps have their leukocyte DNA evaluated. The parents should be counseled that, although the disorder in the affected parent is mild, a distinct possibility exists of a more severe form in the child (i.e., the phenomenon of anticipation).[a]

Polymyositis

Previously reported in infants no younger than 3 months of age, *polymyositis* was described in two newborns in 1982.[267] The newborns exhibited marked hypotonia and weakness, weak cry, and poor sucking and feeding ability. Neck flexors were affected markedly, as in older patients with polymyositis. Particularly striking were markedly elevated levels of creatine phosphokinase (CK; 2500 and 3600 mU/mL) and muscle biopsy findings that included lymphocytic infiltration as well as myopathic changes. Improvement in overall strength and a decrease in CK levels

[a]References 237, 240, 243, 246, 253, and 254.

[a]References 236, 237, 240, 242, 245, and 247.

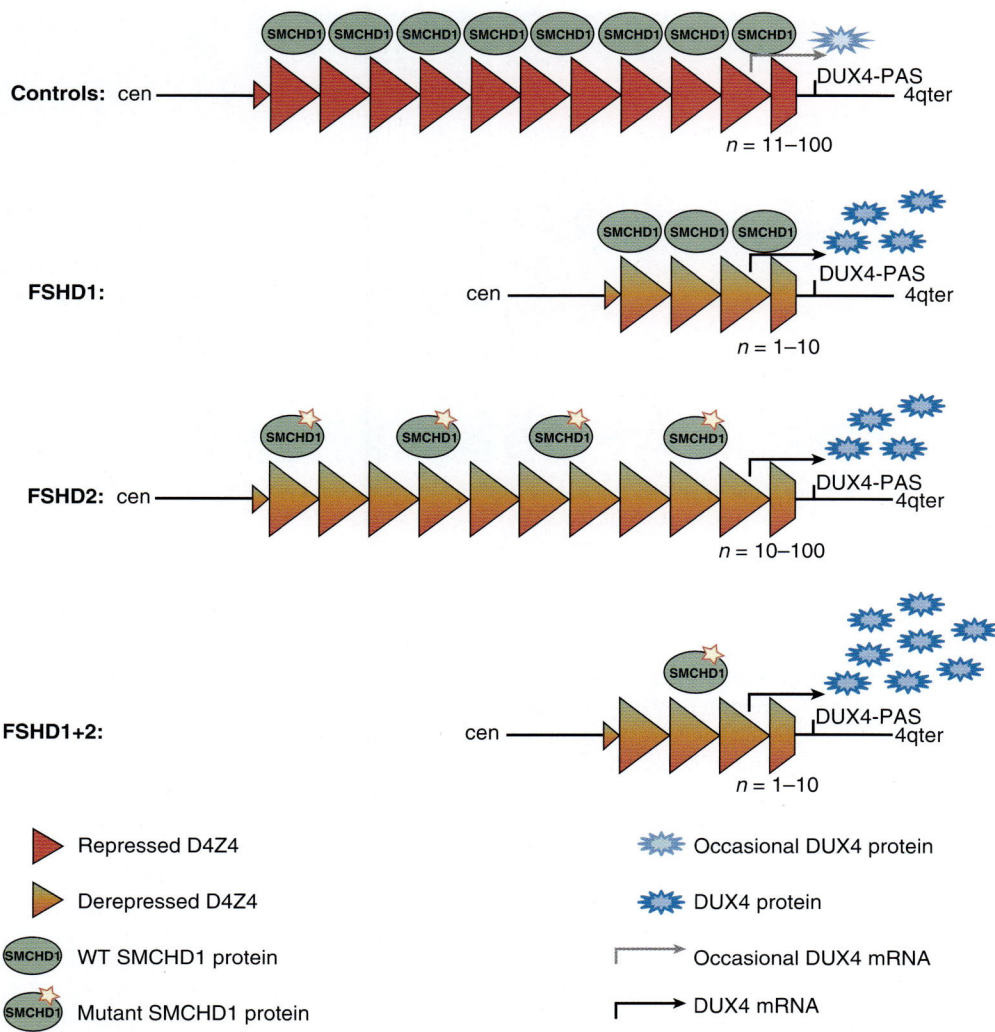

Controls: cen —— DUX4-PAS / 4qter
$n = 11–100$

FSHD1: cen —— DUX4-PAS / 4qter
$n = 1–10$

FSHD2: cen —— DUX4-PAS / 4qter
$n = 10–100$

FSHD1+2: cen —— DUX4-PAS / 4qter
$n = 1–10$

Repressed D4Z4

Derepressed D4Z4

SMCHD1 WT SMCHD1 protein

SMCHD1 Mutant SMCHD1 protein

Occasional DUX4 protein

DUX4 protein

Occasional DUX4 mRNA

DUX4 mRNA

Figure 33.16 Facioscapulohumeral dystrophy (FSHD) is characterized by a greater likelihood of expression of the germline transcription factor *DUX4* in skeletal muscle. Normally, the D4Z4 repeat array contains 11 to 100 units of D4Z4, each encoding a copy of the *DUX4* gene. These long D4Z4 arrays have a repressive chromatin structure; rarely, traces of *DUX4* expression can be observed only on FSHD-permissive chromosomes that contain a *DUX4* polyadenylation signal (*DUX4-PAS*). In the common FSHD1 form, a contraction of the D4Z4 repeat array to a size of 1 to 10 units results in a less repressive chromatin structure and a greater likelihood of *DUX4* expression in skeletal muscle. *SMCHD1* is a chromatin modifier involved in the establishment and maintenance of a repressed D4Z4 chromatin structure in somatic cells. Mutations in *SMCHD1* in FSHD2 also lead to a less repressive D4Z4 chromatin structure and an increase in *DUX4* expression. In some families, FSHD1 and FSHD2 can cosegregate and the combination of both genetic defects leads to greater levels of *DUX4* expression and a more severe phenotype. (Reprinted with permission from Liew WKM, van der Maarel SM, Tawil R. Facioscapulohumeral dystrophy. In: Darras BT, Jones HR Jr, Ryan MM, De Vivo DC, eds. *Neuromuscular Disorders of Infancy, Childhood and Adolescence: A Clinician's Approach.* 2nd ed. San Diego: Academic Press; 2015:chap 32, 620–630.)

followed treatment with steroids at 6 and 15 months of age. The observations suggested that polymyositis may occur in the newborn, that the diagnosis should be suspected with the findings of markedly elevated CK levels and inflammatory cells in the muscle biopsy specimens, and that treatment with steroids may be beneficial. Subsequent reports supported these general conclusions.[268-273] The myopathic changes are consistent with an inflammatory myopathy with an immunological basis (Fig. 33.17). The finding of perifascicular myopathy, generally considered a feature of such autoimmune myopathies as dermatomyositis, is particularly characteristic.[271-273] It is

important to rule out other neonatal myopathic disorders with inflammatory changes (e.g., FSHD, merosin-deficient CMD, or infantile-onset LMNA-associated myopathy),[144] but other features of these latter disorders should make this distinction possible (see earlier discussions).

Minimal Change Myopathy

Minimal change myopathy, or *nonspecific congenital myopathy,* is the designation used for those infants with congenital hypotonia and weakness who exhibit minor (or even no) abnormalities of serum enzyme levels, EMG, or muscle biopsy.[4,274,275] Myopathic

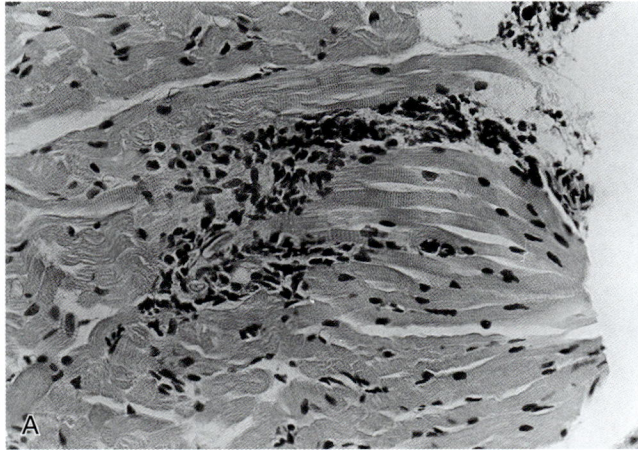

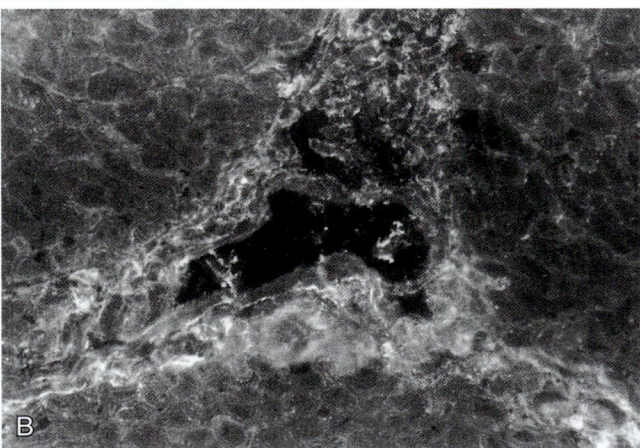

Figure 33.17 Congenital polymyositis: muscle pathology. (A) Muscle biopsy shows focal inflammation. (B) Immunofluorescence microscopy for immunoglobulin G documents immune complex deposition in a ring-like pattern around individual atrophic muscle fibers. (From Roddy SM, Ashwal S, Peckham N. Infantile myositis: a case diagnosed in the neonatal period. *Pediatr Neurol.* 1986;2:241–244.)

illness is inferred from the clinical features (e.g., proximal more than distal weakness, preserved tendon reflexes, normal sensation, and absence of fasciculations) as well as from the occasional myopathic changes observed on the EMG (e.g., small-amplitude, brief duration, and polyphasic motor unit potentials) and abnormal muscle biopsy (e.g., modest variation in fiber size). The clinical features are not as prominent as those observed in more common myopathies (e.g., congenital myotonic dystrophy) and in most cases of CMD. Many of these infants have good prognoses and improve over time. Considering the lack of pathological markers, the molecular basis for most of these myopathies may become easier to delineate with the use of extensive panel-based genetic testing. Therefore this category will become increasingly less common.

Myopathic Disorders With Diagnostic Histology

The *histology-diagnostic* myopathic disorders are characterized by histological changes so striking and distinctive that a specific diagnosis can usually be made. An enormous literature has developed in this area since the 1970s, and several books and reviews deal with the details and complexities of the

problem.[4,250,276-286] Because most of the designations for these disorders are derived from histological and not clinical criteria, the clinical syndromes associated with each histological change vary. Moreover, considerable overlap exists among the disorders on both clinical and histological grounds. Nevertheless, certain specific congenital myopathies are well defined clinically, morphologically, and genetically, and several conclusions relevant to the neonatal patient can be drawn.

In the following discussion, we emphasize the most common features of each disorder, particularly those disorders with prominent clinical manifestations in the neonatal period. Of the seven categories listed in Box 33.1, the first five refer to the disorders with morphologically distinctive changes by standard histological and histochemical techniques (i.e., *specific congenital myopathies*) (Fig. 33.18). Certain features are commonly observed among these disorders (Box 33.3). Central core disease (CCD), nemaline myopathy, myotubular myopathy, and congenital fiber-type disproportion are emphasized because, albeit uncommon, they are the most common in this category. Multiminicore myopathy is rare in the newborn and is described only briefly. The *mitochondrial myopathies* may be suspected by standard histological techniques, but electron microscopic studies are needed to define the distinctive mitochondrial abnormalities if present. Biochemical studies may identify a specific abnormality of a mitochondrial enzyme. The *metabolic myopathies* may show no distinctive morphological change; thus one could argue that these myopathies should be classified as *histology not diagnostic*. However, they are included here because the biopsy specimen may indicate glycogen or lipid deposition in muscle, which is usually the critical initial finding in the definition of the specific biochemical lesion.

Core Myopathies

In core myopathies, the defining pathological feature is the presence of large regions devoid of oxidative staining in the center of myofibers (in CCD) or the presence of multiple smaller *minicores* (in multiminicore disease). Central cores or minicores may be seen in association with other pathological findings, such as nemaline rods, in the so-called core-rod myopathies often associated with mutations in various genes, including *RYR1* (Table 33.5).

Central Core Disease. *Central core disease*, originally described by Shy and Magee in 1956,[287] was the first of the specific congenital myopathies to be defined. Subsequent reports further delineated a fairly discrete clinical syndrome.[4,276,277,280-285,288-297]

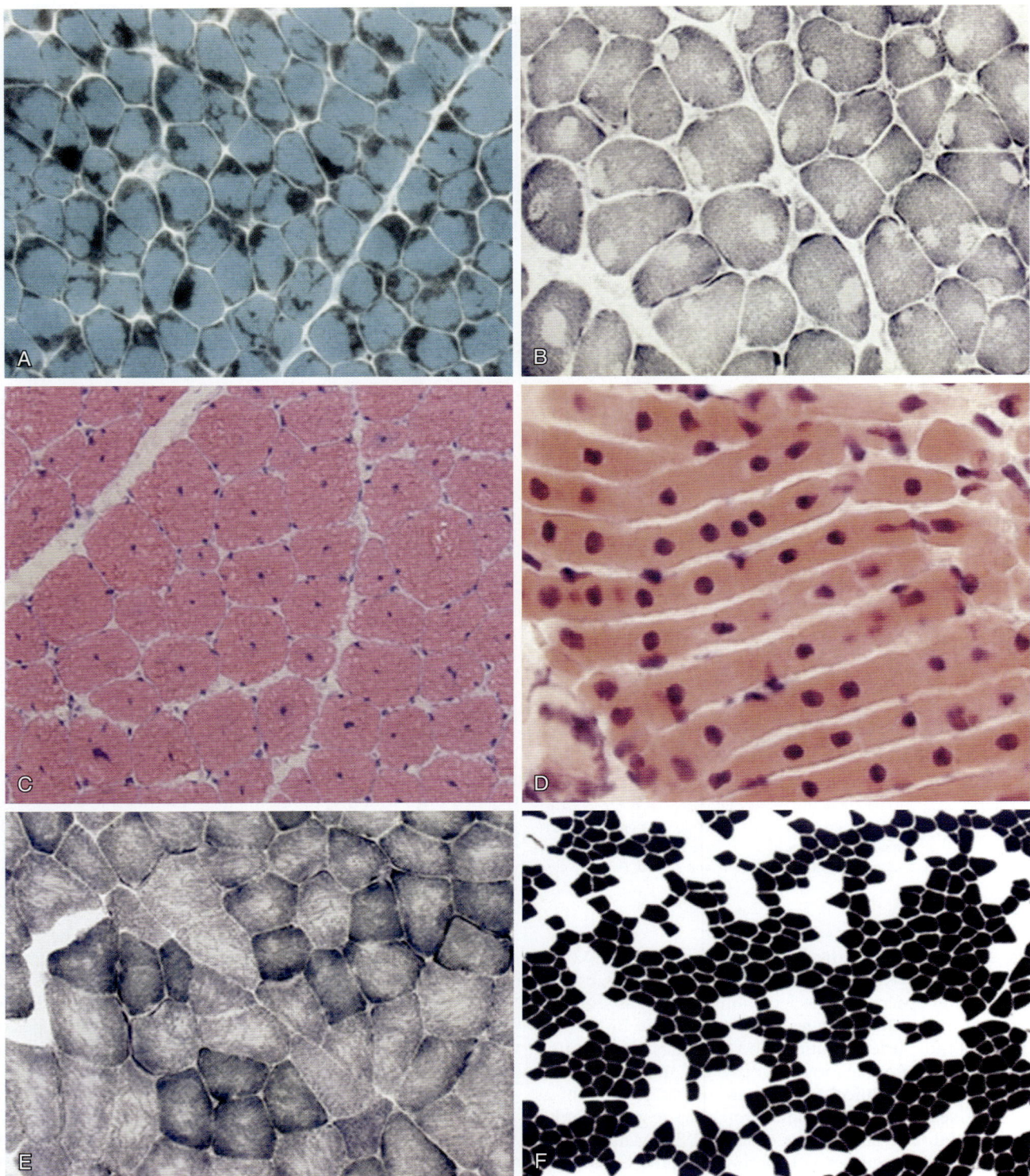

Figure 33.18 Pathological features that define the major subtypes of congenital myopathy. (A) Nemaline rods: Biopsy from patient with nemaline myopathy with a dominant mutation in the *ACTA1* gene, showing clusters of purple-staining rods at the periphery of most fibers and some rods located internally within fibers (Gomori trichrome). (B) Central cores: Biopsy of the quadriceps from a 3-year-old patient with central core disease with a dominant mutation in the ryanodine receptor gene showing mild variation in fiber size (fiber diameter range 15–65 mm), fiber type uniformity, and numerous cores of varying size centrally or peripherally (oxidative enzyme stain succinic dehydrogenase). (C) Central nuclei: Quadriceps biopsy from a 28-year-old patient with autosomal dominant centronuclear myopathy due to a *DNM2* mutation. The biopsy demonstrates small type 1 fibers and centrally placed nuclei in the majority of fibers (hematoxylin and eosin). (D) Central nuclei (longitudinal section): Quadriceps biopsy from an 8-month-old patient with X-linked myotubular myopathy showing large central nuclei. Note the widely spaced nuclei, which affects the number seen in transverse section Most fibers are less than 10 mm in diameter. (E) Multiminicores: Areas in both fiber types of varying size and number devoid of oxidative enzyme stain in a quadriceps biopsy from an 11-year-old patient with multiminicore disease with recessive mutations in the *SEPN1* gene (NADH-TR). (F) Congenital fiber type disproportion with mutation in *ACTA1*: The only apparent pathology in this case was the small size of the dark-staining type 1 fibers and the predominance of type 1 fibers (ATPase preincubated at pH 4.3). Fiber diameter 25 to 70 mm. (Reprinted with permission from North KN, Wang CH, Clarke N, et al.; International Standard of Care Committee for Congenital Myopathies. Approach to the diagnosis of congenital myopathies. *Neuromuscul Disord.* 2014;24:97–116.)

TABLE 33.5   Congenital and Structural Myopathies and Their Identified Gene Loci

SUBTYPE	GENE	OMIM DESIGNATION	CHROMOSOME LOCATION	INHERITANCE PATTERN
Nemaline myopathy	ACTA1	NEM3	1q42.1	AD, AR
	CFL2	NEM7	14q13.1	AR
	KBTBD13	NEM6	15q22.31	AD
	KLHL40	NEM8	3p33.1	AR
	KLHL41	NEM9	2q31.1	AR
	NEB	NEM2	2q23.3	AR
	RYR1		19q13.2	AR
	TNNT1	NEM5	19q13.42	AR
	TPM2	NEM4	9p13.3	AD
	TPM3	NEM1	1q21.3	AD, AR
	LMOD3	NEM10	3p14.1	AR
Cap disease (NM variant)	ACTA1			AD
	TPM2			AD
	TPM3			AD
Zebra body myopathy	ACTA1			AD
Hyaline body myopathy (myosin storage myopathy)	MYH7		14q11.2	AD
Core-rod myopathy	KBTBD13			AD
	NEB RYR1			AR
				AD, AR
	TPM2			AD
Central core disease	RYR1	CCD	19q13.2	AD, AR
Multiminicore disease	RYR1			AR
	SEPN1		1p36.11	AR
	MYH7			AD
Centronuclear myopathy	BIN1	CNM2	2q14.3	AR
	CCDC78	CNM4	16p13.3	AD
	DNM2	CNM1	19p13.2	AD
	MTM1	CNMX	Xq28	XL
	MYF6	CNM3	12q21.31	AD
	RYR1		19q13.2	AR
	TTN		2q31.2	AR
Congenital fiber-type disproportion	ACTA1			AD
	MYH7			AD
	RYR1			AR
	SEPN1			AR
	TPM2			AD
	TPM3			AD
Autophagic vacuolar myopathies	VMA21	MEAX	Xq28	XL
	LAMP2	Danon disease	Xq24	XL
	GAA	Pompe disease	17q25.3	AR
Myofibrillar myopathies	DES	MFM1	2q35	AD, AR
	CRYAB	MFM2	11q23.1	AD
	MYOT	MFM3	5q31.2	AD
	ZASP	MFM4	10q23.2	AD
	FLNC	MFM5	7q32.1	AD
	BAG3	MFM6	10q26.11	AD

AD, Autosomal dominant; *AR,* autosomal recessive; *OMIM,* Online Mendelian Inheritance in Man; *XL,* X-linked.

Adapted with permission from Dowling JJ, North KN, Goebel HH, Beggs AH. Congenital and other structural myopathies. In: Darras BT, Jones HR Jr, Ryan MM, De Vivo DC, eds. *Neuromuscular Disorders of Infancy, Childhood and Adolescence: A Clinician's Approach.* 2nd ed. San Diego: Academic Press; 2015:chap 28, 499–537.

Clinical Features. The *clinical syndrome* consists of hypotonia and weakness, apparent usually in the neonatal period. However, many infants are not recognized as exhibiting muscle disease until months later. Muscle weakness is usually more prominent in the lower limbs and the proximal muscles (Fig. 33.19A), and tendon reflexes are usually preserved, although diminished or absent in proportion to the weakness. Congenital hip dislocation is also common. Mild facial weakness is not unusual. Ptosis,

extraocular muscle weakness, dysphagia, and respiratory difficulties have *not* been features. However, severe neonatal weakness, arthrogryposis, and respiratory failure have been described in a subset of infants with CCD.[298,299]

With the exception of the last subgroup of infants with severe neonatal presentation who do not walk independently and continue to require respiratory support, the *course* of the disease is usually nonprogressive, and infants attain motor

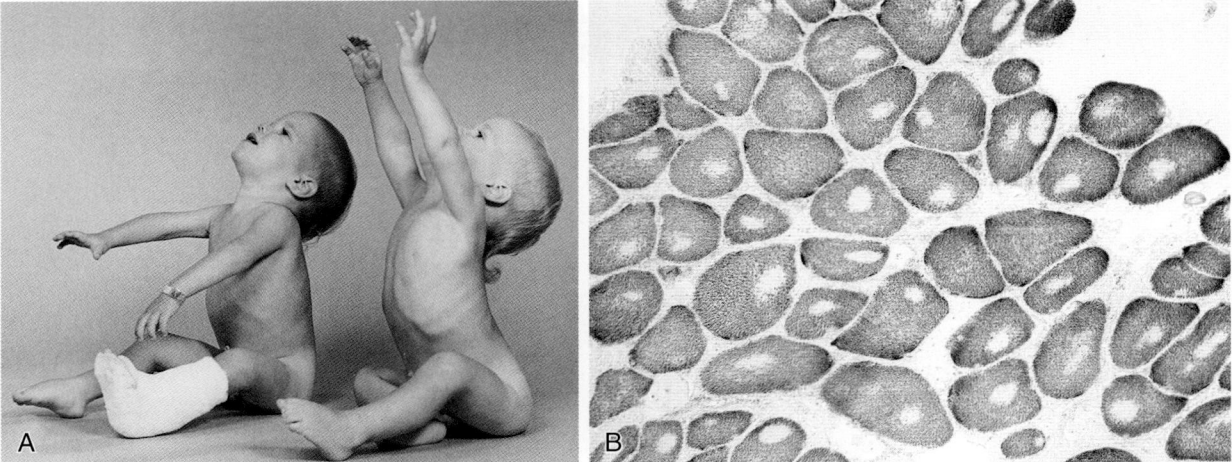

Figure 33.19 Central core disease. (A) Photograph of twins, one of whom has the disease. Note the weakness of the proximal upper extremities. (B) Transverse section stained for NADH (nicotinamide adenine dinucleotide) shows absence of enzyme activity in large central cores. ([A] Reprinted with permission from Cohen ME, Duffner PK, Heffner R. Central core disease in one of identical twins. *J Neurol Neurosurg Psychiatry.* 1978;41:659–663. [B] Reprinted with permission from Dowling JJ, North KN, Goebel HH, Beggs AH. Congenital and other structural myopathies. In: Darras BT, Jones HR Jr, Ryan MM, De Vivo DC, eds. *Neuromuscular Disorders of Infancy, Childhood and Adolescence: A Clinician's Approach.* 2nd ed. San Diego: Academic Press; 2015:chap 28, 502–537.)

milestones albeit at a slow rate. Slow progression of weakness may occur, but even without this progression, contractures, pes cavus or planus, and kyphoscoliosis may result. In a series of 11 patients followed to the age of 4 to 20 years, 2 were unable to walk alone and 2 had difficulty climbing stairs.[294] An increased risk of malignant hyperthermia (e.g., during anesthesia) must be recognized to avoid unexpected death.

Laboratory Studies. Laboratory investigations, aside from muscle biopsy and genetic testing, are not particularly helpful. The serum CK level is usually normal or slightly raised, and the EMG is usually normal or shows myopathic changes, although frequently minor.

Pathology. Muscle pathology is distinctive and diagnostic in the presence of the clinical findings.[4,276,285] Many muscle fibers (20%–100%) exhibit cores that are central or somewhat eccentric in location (see Fig. 33.19B). Single or multiple cores may be observed in a given fiber and are well demonstrated with the histochemical stains for oxidative enzymes (e.g., reduced nicotinamide adenine dinucleotide-tetrazolium reductase [NADH-TR] or succinic dehydrogenase [SDH]), which are absent in the core region. Indeed, electron microscopy shows an absence of mitochondria and sarcoplasmic reticulum in the core region. The cores contain densely packed and disorganized myofibrils. They have a particular predilection for type I fibers and, in some cases, type I fibers predominate or are the only fiber type observable.

Pathogenesis and Etiology. The *pathogenesis relates to a genetic defect* that is usually inherited in an autosomal dominant manner, although rarely autosomal recessive inheritance has been documented.[283-285,296,297,300,301] The gene involved is *RYR1*, which is located on chromosome 19q13.2 and encodes the skeletal muscle ryanodine receptor (see Table 33.5). The latter is a ligand-related release channel for internally stored calcium and thereby plays a crucial role in excitation-contraction coupling.

More than 90% of CCD patients have mutations in *RYR1*, which are most commonly dominant or de novo dominant; de novo dominant and autosomal recessive mutations are more common in the severe cases.[302]

Management. Management is the same as that of nonprogressive or slowly progressive myopathy. The prevention of contractures is important.

Multiminicore Disease. *Multiminicore disease* (MmD) should be discussed briefly in this context of core myopathies. The classic form of MmD typically has its clinical onset in the neonatal period or early infancy.[283-285,303-305] Neonatal hypotonia and weakness, although generalized, tend to predominate in the axial muscles. Mild facial weakness is common. Respiratory difficulties generally appear later, as do spinal abnormalities, especially scoliosis. Some patients with MmD become ventilator-dependent while still ambulant. Motor development is prominently delayed. The clinical course is static in most patients, although approximately 20% of patients exhibit mild progression. The pathology is distinctive and consists of the occurrence of multifocal core-like areas, best seen as areas of reduced activity on oxidative enzyme stains (Fig. 33.20).

Pathogenesis is likely heterogeneous, with primarily sporadic and autosomal recessive cases reported. In separate cohorts, defects in the *SEPN1* gene,[306] the gene mutated in rigid spine syndrome (see discussion of CMD earlier) and in some later-onset forms of congenital fiber-type disproportion,[307] and in the *RYR1* gene,[305,308] the gene mutated in CCD, have been identified. In addition, mutations in the beta-myosin heavy chain gene (*MYH7*)[309] and the giant sarcomeric protein titin (TTN) have been described in patients with MmD (see Table 33.5).[310] The clinical overlap with CMD with rigid spine syndrome and the histological overlap with CCD are consistent with these initial genetic findings.

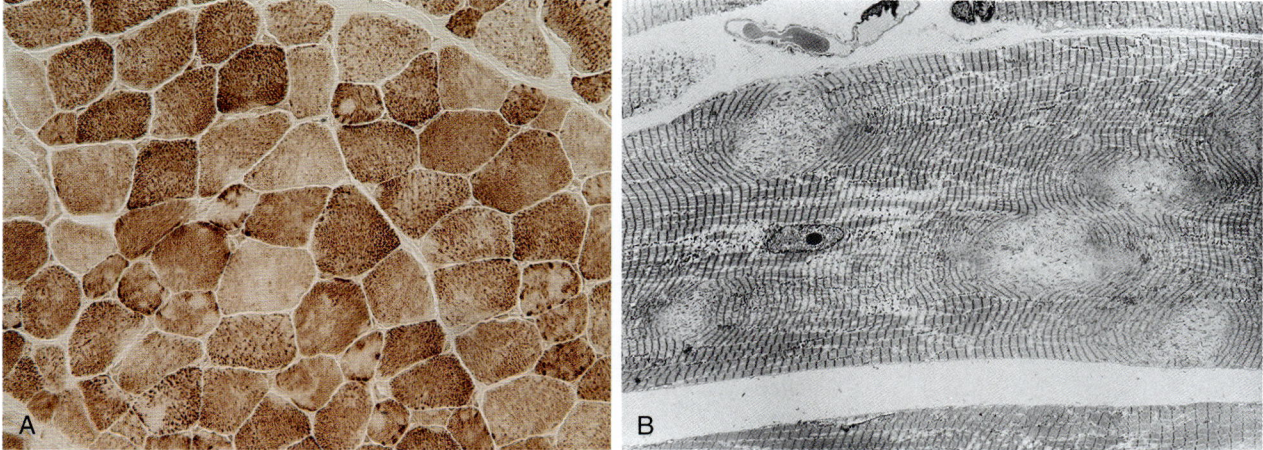

Figure 33.20 Multiminicore myopathy. (A) Transverse section stained with NADH (nicotinamide adenine dinucleotide) demonstrates foci of decreased oxidative enzyme activity throughout the muscle fiber. (B) Low-power electron microscopic view of longitudinal muscle sections demonstrates focal loss of cross striations, corresponding to areas of decreased mitochondrial enzyme activity. (Reprinted with permission from Dowling JJ, North KN, Goebel HH, Beggs AH. Congenital and other structural myopathies. In: Darras BT, Jones HR Jr, Ryan MM, De Vivo DC, eds. *Neuromuscular Disorders of Infancy, Childhood and Adolescence: A Clinician's Approach.* 2nd ed. San Diego: Academic Press; 2015:chap 28, 502–537.)

Nemaline Myopathy

Nemaline (rod body) myopathy, described initially by Shy and colleagues in 1963,[311] was the second of the specific congenital myopathies to be defined. The term *nemaline* is derived from the Greek word *nema*, meaning "thread." Numerous subsequent reports emphasize a considerable variation in clinical expression.[4,276,277,280-285,312-355]

Clinical Features. The *clinical presentation* in infants with manifestations from the neonatal period can be divided into three syndromes. First, as in typical CCD, hypotonia and weakness are relatively mild and are sometimes even overlooked in the newborn period. This variety is termed the *typical congenital or classical form of nemaline myopathy.* Second, marked neonatal hypotonia and weakness occur with no spontaneous movements or respiration at birth. Severe contractures or arthrogryposis and sometimes fractures complete this syndrome of *severe congenital nemaline myopathy.* Cardiac involvement in the form of dilated or hypertrophic cardiomyopathy may occur rarely, but in general cardiac contractility is normal.[356,357] The pregnancy may be complicated by decreased fetal movements and polyhydramnios, and death in utero associated with fetal akinesia may occur.[343] Third, marked neonatal hypotonia and weakness occur, but with some movement and respiratory effort and no severe contractures. This serious disorder, although not so marked as the *severe* cases, is termed *intermediate congenital nemaline myopathy.* In one large series of nemaline myopathy (*n* = 143), approximately 50% of patients presented in the neonatal period; of these, 35% had the severe congenital form, 45% had the intermediate congenital form, and 20% had the typical congenital form.[350] Accompanying the severe and intermediate forms were marked facial diplegia and feeding disturbances. The milder, typical form is associated with varying degrees of facial diparesis and feeding difficulties as well as distal involvement in addition to the proximal muscle weakness.[285] Various skeletal anomalies—including high-arched palate, long dysmorphic face, prognathism malocclusion, pectus excavatum, and *pigeon chest*—may be seen. In surviving infants, pes cavus, kyphoscoliosis, and lumbar lordosis evolve.

The *course* of the typical, milder nemaline myopathy is generally considered to be nonprogressive or slowly progressive.[285] However, in a study with a 5- to 25-year follow-up, 10 of 12 patients exhibited clinical deterioration, and only 8 of 12 were walking unsupported.[324] Ten of 12 patients had developed scoliosis. Similar findings with 3- to 24-year follow-up were reported in a later study.[294]

The *course* in those infants with the two more severe forms of the disease (i.e., the severe and intermediate forms) is generally unfavorable.[284,350-355] Thus, in one series, 74% of patients with severe congenital disease died, generally before 1 year of age, and 28% of patients with intermediate congenital disease died.[350] Among the infants with the severe form, a requirement for ventilation at birth or in the first month was followed by death in more than 90% of cases. Such infants fail to establish adequate ventilation after birth because of their weak respiratory muscles. This weakness results in failure of full expansion of the lungs, and aspiration is often added secondary to difficulty with secretions. Infants usually die in the neonatal period or in the first months of life. However, long-term survival in these patients, who are usually bedridden and receiving mechanical ventilation, has been observed.[320,323,329] Moreover, rare affected infants with the need for mechanical ventilation at birth, severe weakness, and markedly impaired feeding have improved over the ensuing 2 to 3 years to become independent of mechanical ventilation and to achieve the ability to stand or even walk.[327,339]

Laboratory Studies. Laboratory investigations have included either normal or slightly elevated values for the serum CK level.

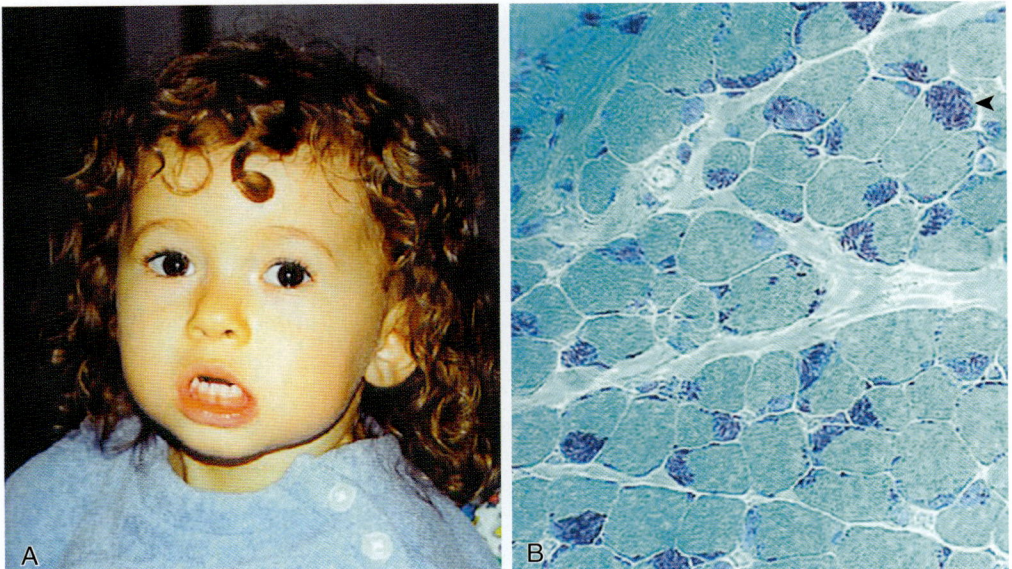

Figure 33.21 Case example of nemaline myopathy. (A) Photograph of patient at age 3. The classical facial appearance, particularly of lower facial weakness, of nemaline myopathy is depicted. (B) Photomicrograph of the muscle biopsy from the patient MLL. Abundant nemaline rods (*arrowhead*), principally subsarcolemmal in location, are present, confirming the histopathologic diagnosis of nemaline myopathy. Stain, modified Gomori trichrome. (Reprinted with permission from Dowling JJ, North KN, Goebel HH, Beggs AH. Congenital and other structural myopathies. In: Darras BT, Jones HR Jr, Ryan MM, De Vivo DC, eds. *Neuromuscular Disorders of Infancy, Childhood and Adolescence: A Clinician's Approach.* 2nd ed. San Diego: Academic Press; 2015:chap 28, 502–537.)

The EMG may be normal but often exhibits short-duration and small-amplitude potentials of myopathy; signs of denervation have also been observed, particularly late in the disease,[a] but nerve conduction studies are normal. Ultrasonography usually shows increased echogenicity in affected muscles.[285] MRI reveals fatty infiltration of muscle tissue and can be valuable in the selection of a muscle to biopsy.[358]

Pathology. Muscle pathology is distinctive and diagnostic in the presence of the clinical features.[4,276,282,285,345] Although the rod bodies are readily overlooked on routine hematoxylin and eosin staining, Gomori trichrome, toluidine blue, and other selected stains demonstrate them well (Fig. 33.21). Predominance of type I fibers, which are also small, is consistent.[b]

The rod body is derived from lateral expansion of the Z-disk, the band found normally at either end of the sarcomere.[c] Thus the rod bodies have been shown by electron microscopy to be in structural continuity with the Z-disk (Fig. 33.22). The rod's major protein component is alpha-actin, the main protein of the Z-disk, and the bodies are penetrated by actin filaments, which normally penetrate the Z-disk. The rods are surrounded by desmin, the structural component of muscle-specific intermediate filaments.[345] A combination of cores and rods has been reported in certain patients (core-rod myopathy).[363] Intranuclear rods have been detected in some severe fatal neonatal cases (Fig. 33.23).[285,338,352,364-366] In general the severity of the myopathological features correlates only imperfectly with the clinical course.[352] However, in nebulin-related nemaline

myopathy a correlation between the severity of the disease and genotype has been reported.[367]

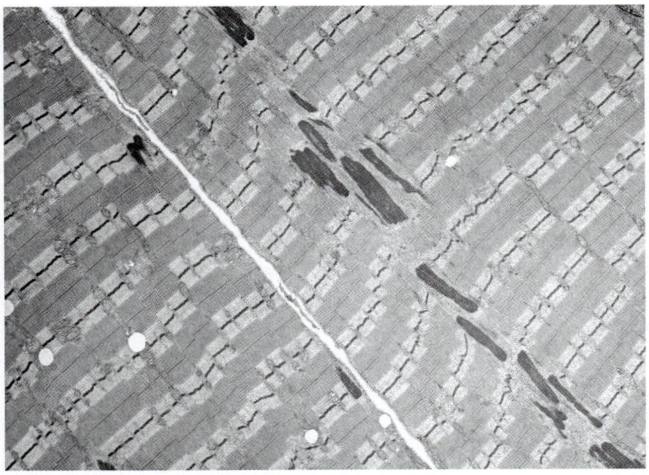

Pathogenesis and Etiology. The pathogenesis of nemaline myopathy relates to defects in one of 11 genes, 7 of which encode proteins of skeletal muscle thin filaments (see Table

Figure 33.22 Nemaline myopathy. Electron microscopy of nemaline bodies. The rods have the same electron density as the Z-lines of adjacent sarcomeres (×28,350). (Reprinted with permission from Dowling JJ, North KN, Goebel HH, Beggs AH. Congenital and other structural myopathies. In: Darras BT, Jones HR Jr, Ryan MM, De Vivo DC, eds. *Neuromuscular Disorders of Infancy, Childhood and Adolescence: A Clinician's Approach.* 2nd ed. San Diego: Academic Press; 2015:chap 28, 502–537.)

---

[a]References 4, 276, 285, 318, 321, 330, 337, and 345.
[b]References 16, 276, 280, 281, 285, 320, 322, 329, and 345.
[c]References 280, 281, 285, 313, 329, 345, 352, and 359-362.

TABLE 33.6   Specific Congenital Myopathies: Distinguishing Clinical Features

	NEONATAL HYPOTONIA AND WEAKNESS	SEVERE FORM WITH NEONATAL DEATH	FACIAL WEAKNESS	PTOSIS	EXTRAOCULAR MUSCULAR WEAKNESS
Central core disease	+	0	±	0	0
Nemaline myopathy	+	+	+	0	0
Myotubular myopathy	+	+	+	+	+
Congenital fiber-type disproportion	+	±	±	0	+

+, Often a prominent feature; ±, variably a prominent feature; 0, not a prominent feature.

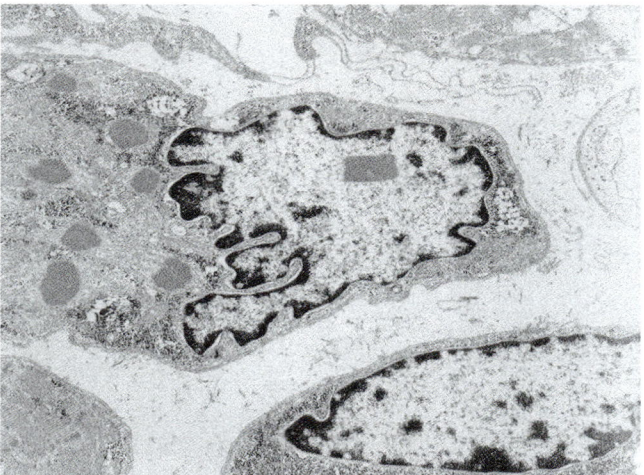

Figure 33.23 Nemaline myopathy. Electron micrograph showing intranuclear rod in a single nucleus. Rods are also present in the adjacent muscle fiber, where there is loss of the regular sarcomeric structure (×36,000). (Reprinted with permission from Dowling JJ, North KN, Goebel HH, Beggs AH. Congenital and other structural myopathies. In: Darras BT, Jones HR Jr, Ryan MM, De Vivo DC, eds. *Neuromuscular Disorders of Infancy, Childhood and Adolescence: A Clinician's Approach.* 2nd ed. San Diego: Academic Press; 2015:chap 28, 502–537.)

33.5).[345,346,348,349,351-355] Approximately 60% to 75% of cases of severe congenital nemaline myopathy are related to defects of *ACTA1*, the gene for alpha-actin.[353,354,368] Most of the remaining cases are related to nebulin, KLHL40, KLHL41, and leiomodin-3 defects and are principally autosomal recessive.[369-371] Mutations in the genes for alpha-tropomyosin, beta-tropomyosin, and troponin are rare causes of severe disease. KLHL40 and KLHL41, which belong to the kelch protein family, are thought to be involved in ubiquitination and protein degradation, while leiomodin-3 is considered essential for the organization of sarcomeric thin filaments (Fig. 33.24).[370,371]

Management. Management of the typical nonprogressive or slowly progressive form of nemaline myopathy depends principally on physical therapy and related techniques. However, respiratory failure may occur during infancy, rapidly and unexpectedly, with a fatal outcome, even in apparently stable or improving patients.[a] Thus, careful follow-up is necessary. Infants

with the severe neonatal form require prompt recognition and vigorous ventilatory and nutritional support if they are to survive. However, on the basis of the data available, appreciable improvement, despite diligent supportive care, is unlikely.

Myotubular Myopathy

Myotubular myopathy, described initially in 1966 by Spiro and co-workers,[372] was the third specific congenital myopathy to be described. The name is derived from the morphological appearance of the affected muscle fibers, which resemble fetal myotubes. Subsequent reports describe considerable variation in clinical expression.[a]

Clinical Features. The clinical features of myotubular myopathy can be divided roughly into two syndromes. Less commonly, hypotonia and weakness are relatively mild and are sometimes overlooked in the newborn period. These autosomal varieties, also known as centronuclear myopathies, generally do not manifest frequently in the neonatal period. The more common disorder affects male infants and is characterized by marked hypotonia and weakness with respiratory failure. Many examples of this severe, malignant, X-linked neonatal form of myotubular myopathy (XLMTM) have been described.[b]

Polyhydramnios and decreased movement are noted in 50% to 60% of these fetuses during pregnancy. Failure to breathe effectively at birth often leads to asphyxia (and the mistaken diagnosis of hypoxic-ischemic encephalopathy for the subsequent motor deficits), and striking impairments of neonatal axial, appendicular, and facial movements well as sucking and breathing are apparent. Family history may reveal miscarriages and neonatal deaths in the maternal line.[285] Ptosis is common, and extraocular muscle weakness is also often present. Indeed, the constellation of marked facial weakness, ptosis, and ophthalmoplegia with generalized hypotonia and weakness is highly suggestive of myotubular myopathy rather than other congenital myopathies (Table 33.6) of either the mild or severe varieties. Cardiomyopathy does not occur, and cognition is normal in survivors.

The *course* in the severely affected male infants with the X-linked syndrome has been considered to be nearly uniform evolution to a fatal outcome. However, a more recent series of 55 affected male infants shows that 64% survived beyond 1 year of age, although 60% of these long-term survivors were entirely ventilator-dependent.[400] Only 13% of the long-term survivors

---

[a]References 285, 319, 322, 323, 332, 333, and 342.

[a]References 4, 276, 277, 281, 282, and 373-395.
[b]References 283-285, 294, 346, 373, 376, 378-390, 392, and 394-402.

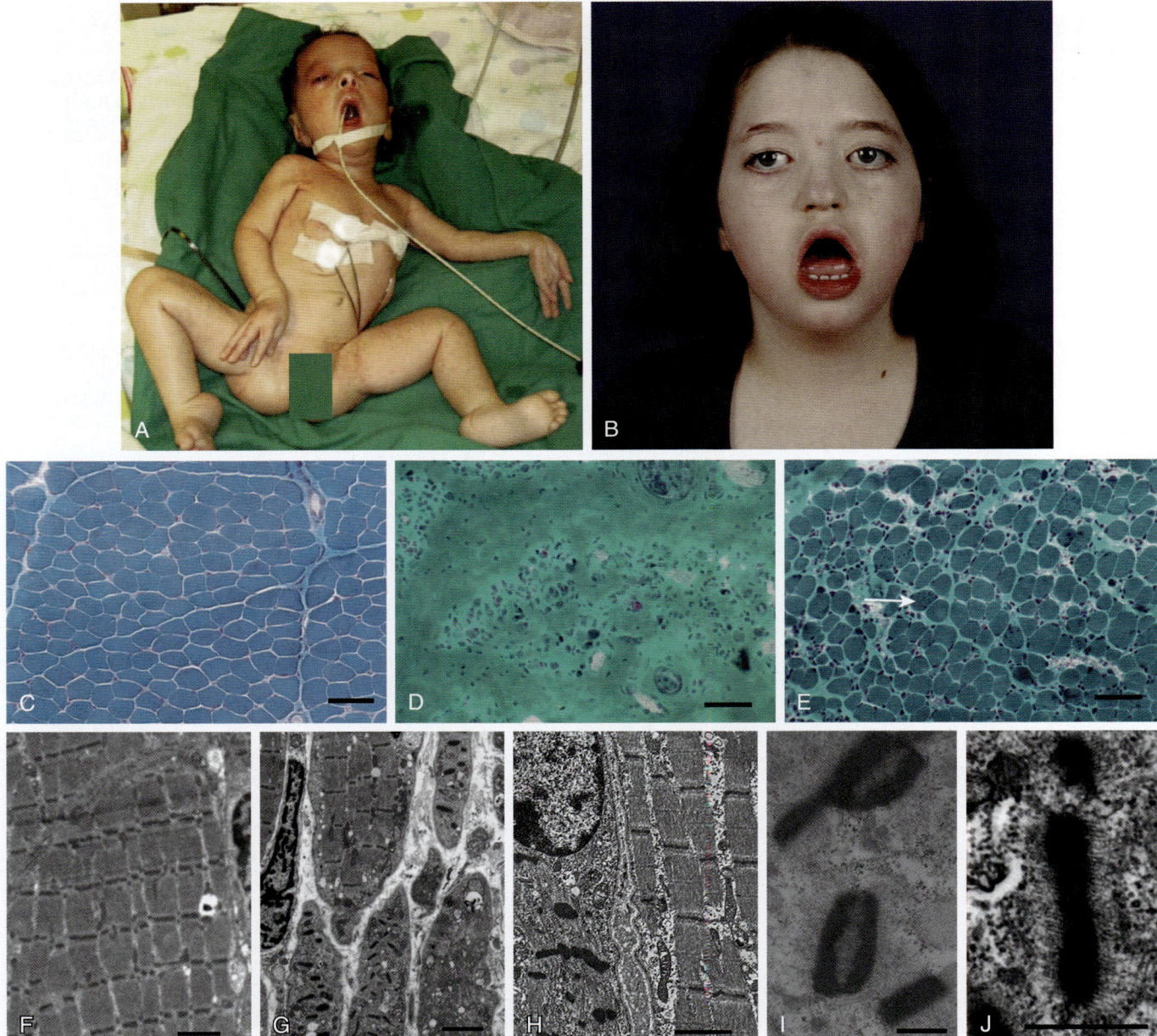

Figure 33.24　Clinical and histological features in nemaline myopathy due to _LMOD3_ mutations. (A and B) Photographs of patients with LMOD3 nemaline myopathy. (A) Most affected individuals had severe generalized muscle weakness and hypotonia at birth and died in infancy (female patient with severe congenital nemaline myopathy, deceased at 4 months). (B) Female patient has less severe weakness and has survived into childhood (alive at 10 years). Note the severe facial and jaw weakness. (C) Control Gomori trichrome image (5-month-old child). (D and E) Skeletal muscle biopsy findings in D female patient alive at 1 year 7 months and (E) male patient alive at 4 months. (D) Some biopsies had only a few scattered atrophic myofibers within abundant connective tissue. Nemaline bodies appear as purple or blue inclusions (_arrow_). (F) Control electron microscopy (EM) image (6-week-old child, rectus abdominis muscle). (G and H) EM images from some patient biopsies show myofibers with ordered sarcomeres adjacent to myofibers with disordered sarcomeres and thickened Z-discs. (I and J) Many nemaline bodies appear as thickened Z-discs, (I) sometimes in pairs interconnected by thin filaments. Some nemaline bodies resemble thickened Z-discs surrounded by a short thin filament _fringe_. Scale bar: 50 μm (C–E); 2 μm (F–H); 500 nm (I and J). (Reprinted with permission from Yuen M, Sandaradura SA, Dowling JJ,, et al. Leiomodin-3 dysfunction results in thin filament disorganization and nemaline myopathy. _J Clin Invest._ 2014;124:4693–4708. Erratum in _J Clin Invest._ 2015;125:456–457.)

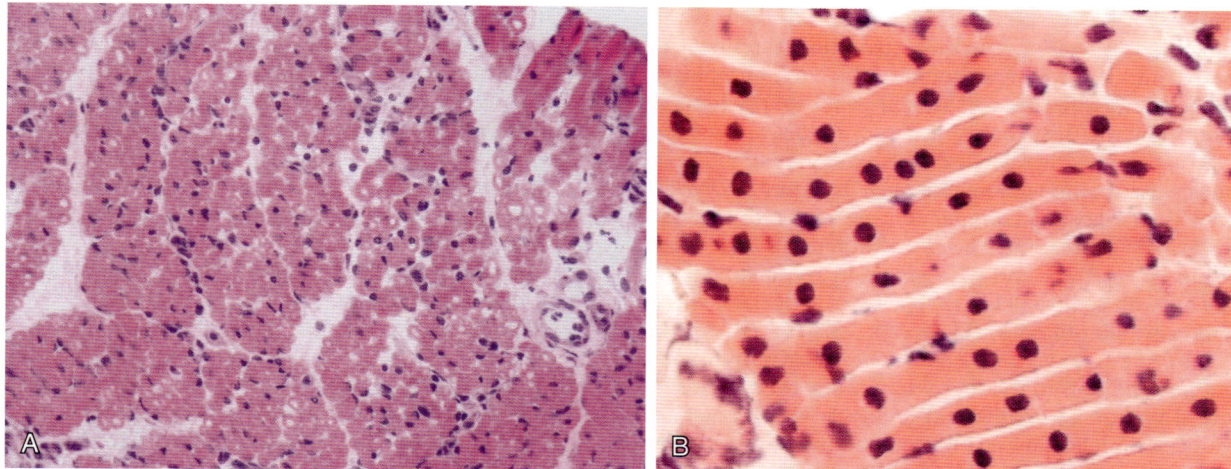

Figure 33.25 Myotubular myopathy. (A) Muscle biopsy from a patient with X-linked myotubular myopathy. Note the histologic resemblance of muscle to fetal myotubes. (B) Central nuclei (longitudinal section): quadriceps biopsy from an 8-month-old patient with X-linked myotubular myopathy showing large central nuclei. Note the widely spaced nuclei, which affects the number seen in transverse section. Most fibers are less than 10 mm in diameter. ([B] Reprinted with permission North KN, Wang CH, Clarke N, et al.; International Standard of Care Committee for Congenital Myopathies. Approach to the diagnosis of congenital myopathies. *Neuromuscul Disord.* 2014;24:97–116.)

did not require at least intermittent mechanical ventilation. Similar data have been reported in other series.[401] In the severely affected infant, because of the failure of lung expansion and the superimposed aspiration secondary to swallowing difficulties, atelectasis and pneumonia are the usual causes of death in the first days or weeks of life. Motor outcome in long-term survivors is very unfavorable in most, who are often bedridden or in wheelchairs. However, in a series of 36 patients, 3 were said to exhibit "no significant disability at 6 months, 5 years, and 7 years, respectively,"[396] and in another group of 55 cases, 7 had only slightly delayed motor milestones.[400] Several patients have developed other medical conditions—such as gallstones, nephrocalcinosis, vitamin K-responsive bleeding diathesis, spherocytosis, and hepatic peliosis—with associated fatal abdominal hemorrhages.[400]

Pathology. The muscle pathology is distinctive and diagnostic in the presence of the clinical findings.[a] Muscle fibers contain one or more centrally placed nuclei, usually surrounded by an area devoid of myofibrils. With adenosine triphosphatase staining, the region around the nucleus appears as a clear zone or halo (Fig. 33.25). Ultrastructurally, the muscle fibers bear some resemblance to fetal myotubes, with each fiber containing a longitudinal chain of central nuclei (Fig. 33.26). Consistent with these findings suggestive of a disturbance of maturation are other features characteristic of fetal but not mature muscle (i.e., abundant vimentin and desmin [filamentous proteins], neural cell adhesion molecules, and intracytoplasmic distribution of dystrophin).[397-399] Type I fibers tend to be small, and this type I fiber hypotrophy is usually a very prominent feature.[b]

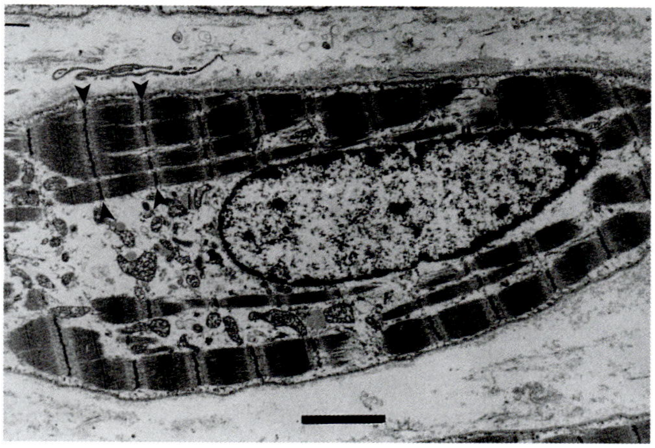

---

[a]References 4, 55, 276, 285, 386, 388, 391, 396-399, 401, and 403.
[b]References 280, 281, 373, 386, 388, 401, and 403.

Figure 33.26 Myotubular myopathy. This electron micrograph is from a muscle biopsy of a term infant with myotubular myopathy. A central nucleus surrounded by mitochondria is shown. Z-bands are in register (*arrowheads*), unlike fetal myotubes. (From Sarnat HB. Myotubular myopathy: arrest of morphogenesis of myofibers associated with persistence of fetal vimentin and desmin. Four cases compared with fetal and neonatal muscle. *Can J Neurol Sci.* 1990;17:109–123.)

Pathogenesis and Etiology. The pathogenesis of myotubular myopathy is not entirely understood; a maturational arrest has been suggested because of the resemblance of the abnormal fibers to fetal myotubes and the persistence of other features of fetal myotubes, as noted in the previous section. Insight into the potential mechanism of this maturational defect has been gained by identification of the gene at Xq28 *(MTM1). MTM1* encodes a protein, myotubularin, that is a phosphatidylinositol phosphatase.[401,404,405] Mutations in *MTM1* are the most common cause of XLMTM. Myotubularin is involved in diverse and numerous cellular processes, including excitation-contraction coupling, neuromuscular junction structure, satellite cell proliferation and survival, endosomal trafficking, autophagy, and cytoskeletal organization.[406] Which of these functions is altered and how the disturbance leads to the disease remain unclear. Mutations in other genes can also cause myotubular or centronuclear myopathy, with mutations in dynamin-2 (DNM2) recognized as an autosomal dominant cause of the disease (see Table 33.5).[407,408] Autosomal recessive mutations have been identified in BIN1, RYR1, and TTN genes. In an Italian cohort of 30 patients with centronuclear myopathy of congenital onset, mutations were identified in 25 (83%): 15 in MTM1, 6 in DNM2, 3 in RYR1, and 1 in TTN.[409] The DNM2 mutations causing a presentation in the first years of life are de novo.[407] The clinical picture of infants and children with autosomal recessive centronuclear myopathy may be indistinguishable from the X-linked form, hence the need for genetic diagnosis, especially in the case of male infants.[285]

Laboratory Studies. Laboratory investigations have included only an occasionally elevated serum CK level. The EMG is usually myopathic, although not impressively so; as with nemaline myopathy, fibrillation potentials are occasionally observed.[285,382,387] Chest radiographs often show very thin ribs.[44,388,389] A histological diagnosis is usually made by muscle biopsy, and genetic testing is then undertaken to detect a mutation in one of the genes associated with centronuclear myopathy. However, if the phenotype is obvious, the clinician may not order a muscle biopsy and instead proceed directly with genetic testing.

Management. Management of the severe X-linked form of myotubular myopathy is as discussed for the severe congenital forms of nemaline myopathy (see previous section). The ethical issues concerning ventilatory support of the severely affected infants are obvious.

Congenital Fiber-Type Disproportion

Congenital fiber-type disproportion (CFTD), initially described by Brooke in 1973,[410] was the fourth identified among the relatively common specific congenital myopathies. Subsequent reports confirmed and amplified the original observations of Brooke.[a] Indeed, variability of the clinical spectrum has been demonstrated conclusively.

Clinical Features. The clinical syndrome of the more than 70 reported cases has included particularly hypotonia and weakness of limb, neck, respiratory, trunk, facial, bulbar, and extraocular muscles. The last feature, ophthalmoparesis, is present in more than half of the patients who are overtly symptomatic in the neonatal period but in fewer than 10% of those who present later.[432] In most cases the deficits in the cases of early neonatal onset are severe. Other musculoskeletal abnormalities are common, such as a long thin face, a high-arched palate, a tented upper lip, limb contractures, short stature, congenital hip dislocations, foot deformities, torticollis, and, later, scoliosis. These abnormalities represent primarily postural deformities, generated either prenatally or postnatally.

The course is variable, but in general it varies according to the time of onset. Thus, among the infants with overt disease of neonatal onset, fully 40% have died because of the combination of bulbar and respiratory muscle weakness. Most surviving infants have had a static course, with generally severe weakness. Infants with slightly later onset are more likely to have the static and then improving course, often considered characteristic of the disorder or, more precisely, group of disorders.

Laboratory Studies. The serum CK level is usually normal. The EMG can be normal, but it usually exhibits myopathic changes, albeit often not severe.

Pathology. Muscle pathology establishes the diagnosis. The essential features are the predominance of type I fibers (i.e., type I fibers account for more than 55% of the total [normally, type I fibers account for 30%–55% of the total]) and the small size of type I fibers (i.e., a disparity of 12% or more in the mean diameters of type I and II fibers [normally, the diameters are approximately equal]; Fig. 33.27). Subsequently, hypertrophy of type II fibers appears to occur, and the discrepancy between the size of the fibers may become marked. (In several cases, type II fibers were hypotrophic.[422,423,426,427])

Fiber-type disproportion of the variety observed with CFTD may be observed with other congenital myopathies, particular nemaline myopathy, myotubular myopathy, and congenital myotonic dystrophy. However, in these disorders, additional changes in muscle coexist and serve to emphasize the nosological status of the disorders as well as to lead to the correct diagnosis. Moreover, fiber-type disproportion has been observed in spondyloepimetaphyseal dysplasia and in CNS disorders, such as Krabbe leukodystrophy, adrenoleukodystrophy, and perinatal asphyxia[436]; in one series, cerebellar hypoplasia was the most common CNS abnormality.[420] Once the known causes of CFTD have been excluded on clinical and pathological grounds, there appears to remain a group of patients in which CFTD is the primary pathological condition.[285]

Pathogenesis and Etiology. The pathogenesis of CFTD is likely heterogeneous. A functional abnormality in maturation of the motor unit has been suggested for several reasons: (1) similar myopathology can be produced by denervation or cross innervation; (2) type IIc fibers, the fetal precursor of types IIa and IIb fibers, are often present in increased numbers; and (3) fiber-type disproportions of various types may occur with developmental disturbances of brain.[418,420] The nature of the postulated disturbance in motor unit development is unclear. Numerous documentations of normal anterior horn cells and peripheral nerves in congenital fiber-type disproportion are available.[415,420]

Approximately 45% of cases have a positive family history; approximately two thirds of these suggest autosomal dominant inheritance, and one third suggest autosomal recessive.[432,435] In a series of neonatal-onset cases (n = 3), mutations in the ACTA1 gene (different from those for nemaline myopathy) were detected (see Table 33.5).[433] The clinical features were similar to those in the severely affected cases noted earlier except for the absence of ophthalmoparesis. A report of eight cases with onset in the first year or later in infancy and childhood noted defects in the SEPN1 gene (see the description of MmD, next).[307] Mutations of the TPM3 gene, which encodes slow

---

[a]References 4, 253, 281, 282, 294, and 411-435.

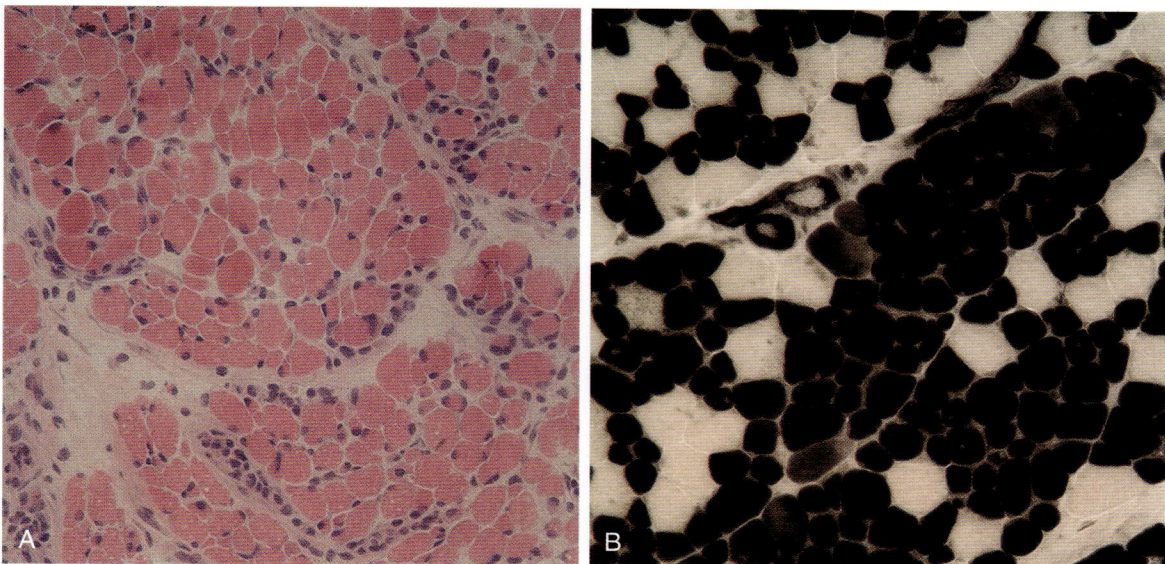

Figure 33.27 Congenital fiber-type disproportion. Two muscle biopsies from an affected child. (A) First biopsy. Note the striking disparity in size of fibers (hematoxylin and eosin stain, ×150). (B) Second biopsy. Histochemical preparation shows many small fibers that stain dark with adenosine triphosphatase reaction at pH 4.3 (i.e., type I fibers) (ATPase stain, pH 4.3, ×250). (Courtesy Peter Kang, MD, University of Florida, Gainesville, Florida.)

alpha-tropomyosin, are the most common cause of CFTD.[437-439] This may explain the selective involvement of type 1 fibers in CFTD, since TPM3 is a type 1 fiber–specific protein.[352,437] Although the mechanism remains unknown, recessive mutations in *RYR1* have also been detected in a relatively large subset of CFTD patients with extreme fiber-size disproportion[440] and may be responsible for the observed ophthalmoparesis in certain cases. In several Japanese patients with CFTD, mutations of the *LMNA* gene were recently identified[441]; such patients may be at risk for developing cardiomyopathy.

Management. The most essential aspect of management is recognition that this disorder may be associated with improvement. Thus even severely affected infants should receive vigorous supportive care, and every effort should be made to prevent contractures.

Mitochondrial Myopathies

Mitochondrial myopathy, in this context, refers to a disorder with prominent involvement of muscle and a *primary* (not secondary) abnormality of mitochondrial structure and function. Abnormalities of mitochondrial structure can sometimes be demonstrated initially on muscle biopsy by the modified Gomori trichrome stain, which reveals accumulations of red-staining material within the fibers (i.e., *ragged-red* fibers) (Fig. 33.28A and B).[4,442,443] Further definition of the structural disturbance in mitochondrial number, configuration, or both is made by electron microscopy.[443-447] Of additional importance is documentation of the abnormalities in mitochondrial biochemical *function* that occur in mitochondrial myopathies.[443,447-452] Finally, as discussed later, study of the ratio of mitochondrial to nuclear DNA is important in identifying the mitochondrial DNA depletion syndrome.

Classification of mitochondrial myopathies according to biochemical defects is valuable, and clear definition of such defects has

progressed rapidly. The major metabolic functions of mitochondria in muscle can be categorized relatively simply as follows: (1) substrate transport, (2) substrate utilization, (3) function of the Krebs cycle, and (4) function of the respiratory (electron transport) chain (Table 33.7 and Fig. 33.29).[443,445,447-455] Of these, only myopathic disease related to defects in the respiratory chain is clearly relevant to the newborn (see subsequent discussion).

Substrate Transport. Of particular importance is transport into mitochondria of the two major substrates for energy production through acetyl-coenzyme A (i.e., pyruvate from glucose metabolism and fatty acids). Disturbance of fatty acid transport occurs with carnitine deficiency; this is discussed later with lipid myopathies because the lipid deposition dominates the myopathology.

Substrate Utilization. Pyruvate dehydrogenase deficiency usually results in a disorder with prominent CNS phenomena, rather than myopathic features (see Chapter 28). However, the enzymatic defect is demonstrable in muscle.[456] A major disorder of fatty acid utilization with occasional clinical presentation in the newborn period is medium-chain acyl-coenzyme A dehydrogenase deficiency. In addition to hypotonia, encephalopathic features are also usually present. This disorder is discussed in Chapter 28.

Krebs Cycle. No such disease primarily of muscle has yet been described in the newborn. However, fumarase deficiency has been reported in infants with encephalopathic features and hepatic involvement.[457,458]

Respiratory Chain. Disturbances of the mitochondrial respiratory chain may lead to a striking neonatal myopathy syndrome with hypotonia and weakness. Defects primarily

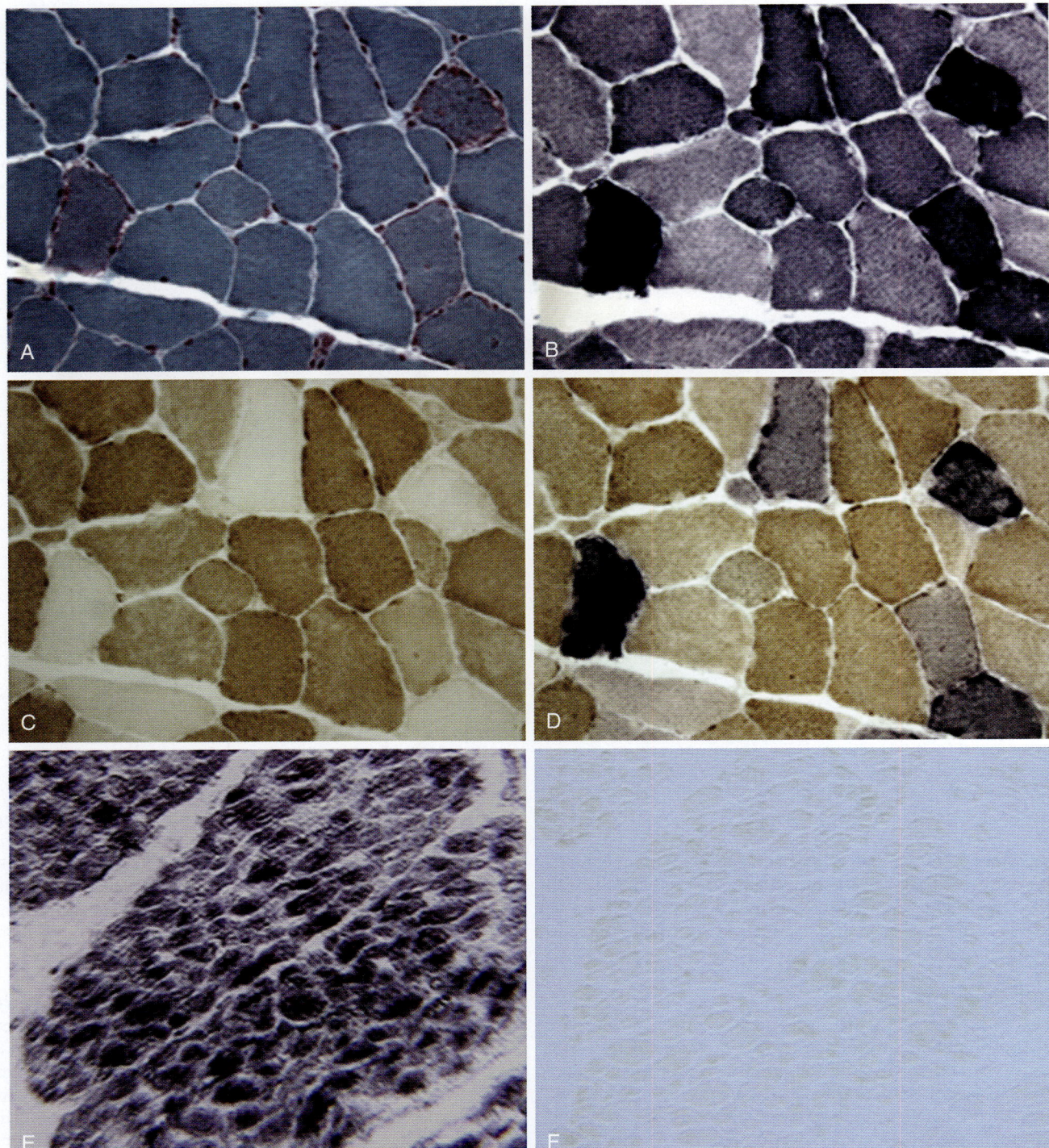

Figure 33.28 Serial sections from the muscle biopsy of a patient with MERRF (myoclonus epilepsy with ragged-red fibers) syndrome. With the modified Gomori trichrome stain (A), two ragged-red fibers are evident. The same fibers appear *ragged-blue* with the succinate dehydrogenase (SDH) stain (B); they are pale with the cytochrome *c* oxidase (COX) stain (C) and appear more or less intensely blue with the combined COX/SDH stain (D). In contrast to the checkerboard appearance of the muscle biopsy in a mtDNA-related disease, the biopsy from a patient with mutations in *SCO2*, a nDNA assembly gene of COX, shows normal fiber type–related variable intensity with the SDH stain (E) but uniformly lacking reaction with the COX stain (F). (Reprinted with permission from: De Vivo DC, Paradas C, DiMauro S. Mitochondrial encephalomyopathies. In: Darras BT, Jones HR Jr, Ryan MM, De Vivo DC, eds. *Neuromuscular Disorders of Infancy, Childhood and Adolescence: A Clinician's Approach.* 2nd ed. San Diego: Academic Press; 2015:chap 41, 796–833.)

TABLE 33.7 Mitochondrial Disorders Characterized by Presentation With Hypotonia or Weakness in the Neonatal Period

	CLINICAL FEATURES	
BIOCHEMICAL DISORDER	PRIMARILY MYOPATHY	PRIMARILY ENCEPHALOPATHY
Substrate transport		
Carnitine deficiency	+	−
Substrate utilization		
Pyruvate carboxylase	−	+
Pyruvate dehydrogenase complex	−	+
Fatty acid oxidation	−	+
Krebs cycle		
Fumarase deficiency	−	+
Respiratory chain		
Complex I	+	+
Complex II	+	+
Complex III	+	+
Complex IV (cytochrome c oxidase)	+	+
Complex V (adenosine triphosphate synthase)	+	+
Multiple defects (mitochondrial DNA depletion)	+	+

BOX 33.4 Major Features of Infantile Cytochrome c Oxidase Deficiency

Onset, first days or weeks
Hypotonia and weakness: axial, appendicular, and facial
Hyporeflexia, areflexia
Respiratory failure, death in early infancy
Hepatomegaly, cardiomyopathy
de Toni-Fanconi-Debré syndrome
Leigh syndrome
Lactic acidosis
Ragged-red fibers, mitochondrial abnormalities, and absent staining for cytochrome c oxidase

of complex IV (cytochrome *c* oxidase [COX]) but also of complexes I, II, III, and V, sometimes in combination, and mitochondrial DNA depletion with impairment of multiple enzymes of the respiratory chain have been associated with this syndrome[4,446,448-452,459-503] Disturbance of *COX* is the most common cause of this serious neonatal syndrome.[504] The clinical features have been striking (Box 33.4): onset in the first days or weeks of life of severe hypotonia and weakness with involvement of limbs, trunk, face, and sucking but only rarely of eye movements. Tendon reflexes are usually absent. Hepatomegaly is common. Additional features have included de Toni-Fanconi-Debré renal syndrome in approximately two thirds, Leigh syndrome, and occasionally myocardiopathy. Macroglossia has also sometimes been noted. The *course* has been progressive, with death in the first year.

A remarkable *benign form* of COX deficiency has been delineated.[448-452,464,473-475,491,505] The newborns present clinically as in the fatal form of the disease but then, over the ensuing weeks and months, exhibit clinical, myopathological, and biochemical improvement.[506] By 2 to 4 years of age, the infants are normal. Distinction of this benign form from the fatal form of COX deficiency in the *newborn period*, crucial for determining prognosis and formulating therapy, requires

muscle immunohistochemistry (see discussion of muscle biopsy, which follows).

Laboratory studies have consistently demonstrated lactic acidosis (see Box 33.4), an important clue to the diagnosis. When evaluated, the serum pyruvate level has also been elevated. The serum CK level is only slightly elevated, and the EMG is usually normal. In those patients with the Fanconi renal abnormality, glycosuria, proteinuria, phosphaturia, and generalized aminoaciduria are present.

Muscle biopsy reveals abnormal accumulations of red-staining material on modified Gomori trichrome stain (*ragged-red* fibers) and abnormalities of mitochondrial structure on electron microscopy. Accumulations of lipid and glycogen are also readily detected by appropriate stains (these *secondary* metabolic changes separate this disorder from the primary abnormalities of lipid and glycogen metabolism, described later). Histochemical staining for COX demonstrates the enzymatic deficiency (see Fig. 33.28). In infants with the benign form of COX deficiency, the deficiency of staining resolves instead of worsening (Fig. 33.30).[452]

The *pathogenesis* of the myopathic disturbance relates to the impairment of energy production caused by the defect in COX. DiMauro and co-workers[470] used immunochemical techniques to demonstrate that the deficiency of enzymatic activity results from a decrease in the quantity of enzyme protein due to incorrect COX assembly rather than a disturbance in catalytic efficiency. The defect in the respiratory chain results in the lactic acidosis because of decreased utilization of pyruvate (which is converted to lactate by lactate dehydrogenase) and in the accumulation of lipid and glycogen because of decreased utilization of fatty acids and glycogen.

The enzymatic defect in the infantile form of COX deficiency appears to be inherited as an *autosomal recessive* disorder. Thus children of both sexes have been affected, parents have been asymptomatic, and siblings with the disorder have been identified in several families. With advances in molecular testing, it has been shown that mutations in mtDNA COX genes

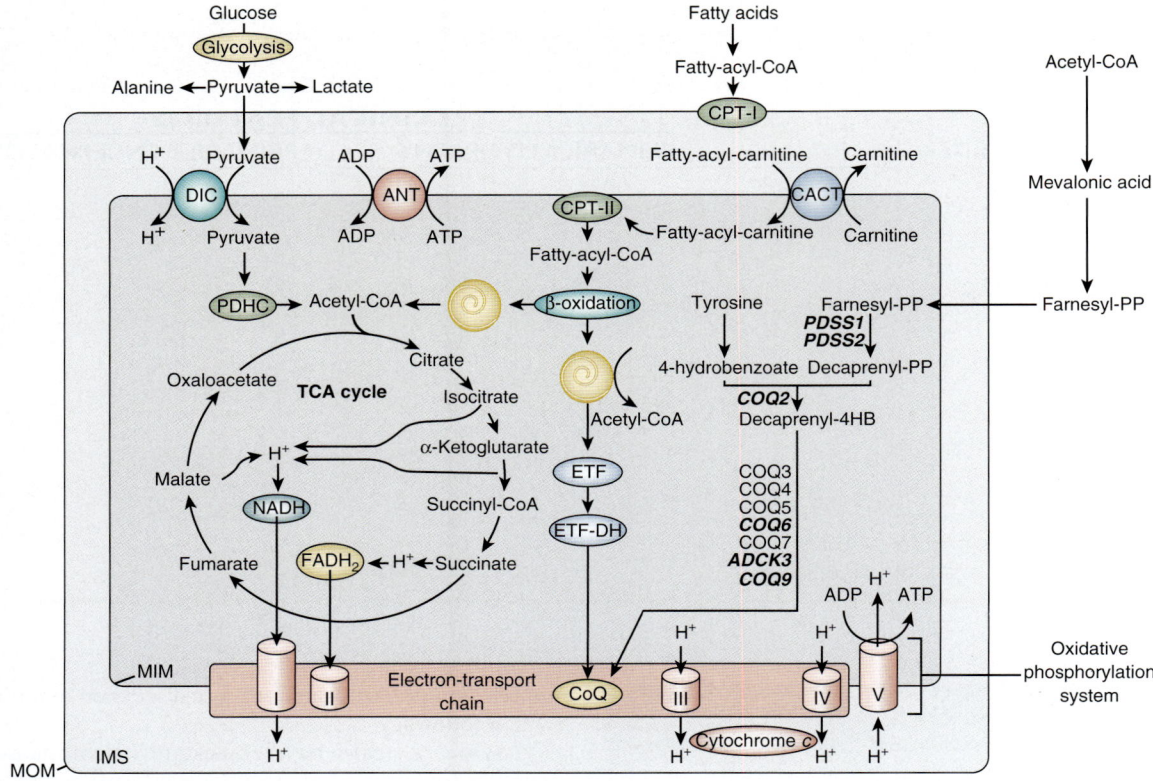

Figure 33.29 Schematic view of mitochondrial metabolism. The respiratory chain is highlighted in red. Electrons from dehydrogenases in the Krebs cycle and in beta-oxidation spirals are passed *horizontally* along four protein complexes and two small carriers (the electron-transport chain) embedded in the MIM. The electrons travel from complex I (an NADH dehydrogenase) and complex II (a succinate dehydrogenase) to CoQ_{10} (a small mobile electron carrier also known as ubiquinone), then to complex III (ubiquinone oxidoreductase), cytochrome c (another small mobile electron carrier), and complex IV (cytochrome c oxidase), ultimately producing water. Concomitant with this horizontal flow of electrons, there is a *vertical* vectorial transport of dehydrogenase-derived protons from the matrix across the MIM into the intermembrane space. This process creates an electrochemical proton gradient across the MIM that is used to drive complex V (F_0F_1 ATPsynthase), a tiny *turbine* that converts adenosine diphosphate (*ADP*) to adenosine trisphosphate (*ATP*). Conventionally, the five complexes compose the oxidative phosphorylation system. The biosynthetic pathway of CoQ_{10}, beginning with acetyl-CoA, is shown. *ANT,* Adenine nucleotide translocator; *CACT,* carnitine-acylcarnitine translocator; *CoA,* coenzyme A; *CoQ_{10},* coenzyme Q_{10}, *CPT,* carnitine palmitoyltransferase; *DIC,* dicarboxylate carrier; *ETF,* electron-transfer flavoprotein; *ETF-DH,* ETF dehydrogenase; *FAD,* flavin adenine dinucleotide; *IMS,* intermembrane space; *MIM,* mitochondrial inner membrane; *MOM,* mitochondrial outer membrane; *PDHC,* pyruvate dehydrogenase complex; *TCA,* tricarboxylic acid. (Reprinted with permission from De Vivo DC, Paradas C, DiMauro S. Mitochondrial encephalomyopathies. In: Darras BT, Jones HR Jr, Ryan MM, De Vivo DC, eds. *Neuromuscular Disorders of Infancy, Childhood and Adolescence: A Clinician's Approach.* 2nd ed. San Diego: Academic Press; 2015:chap 41, 796–833.)

cause mild and later-onset clinical symptoms (heteroplasmy). Infantile onset and severe phenotypes are rarely the result of mutations in nuclear DNA-encoded COX subunits (*direct hits*) but are more frequently due to mutations affecting assembly proteins (*indirect hits*) such as SURF1[507] and SCO2.[504,508,509] Both homozygous and compound heterozygous SCO2 mutations have been linked to a phenotype that simulates spinal muscular atrophy with stridor and respiratory insufficiency.[510-512]

The reversible COX-deficiency myopathy has been reclassified from a primary mtDNA defect to a defect of mtDNA translation.[452] It is genetically heterogeneous because mutations in both mt-tRNA[Glu] (m.1467 T > C or T > G) and the TRMU (5-methyl-aminomethyl-2-thiouridylate methyltransferase) have been described to date.[506,513] mt-tRNA[Glu] is thiouridylated by TRMU.[514-516] Because TRMU is physiologically downregulated

during the symptomatic phase of the disease, the effects of the tRNA[Glu] mutation become exacerbated and result in an mtDNA translation defect.[515] Patients who do not have the mt-tRNA[Glu] mutations may have mutations in the TRMU gene.[506]

Management requires intensive supportive therapy, particularly because of the possibility of the reversible form of COX deficiency. Infants afflicted with the latter disorder in early infancy are severely affected clinically, morphologically, and biochemically. Muscle immunohistochemistry is needed to distinguish the reversible and fatal forms *in the neonatal period.*

Mitochondrial DNA depletion is a disorder with features similar to those just described for COX deficiency.[a] Thus approximately 65% of infants with the reported disease have presented in the

---

[a]References 463, 485, 486, 492, 493, 503, and 517–523.

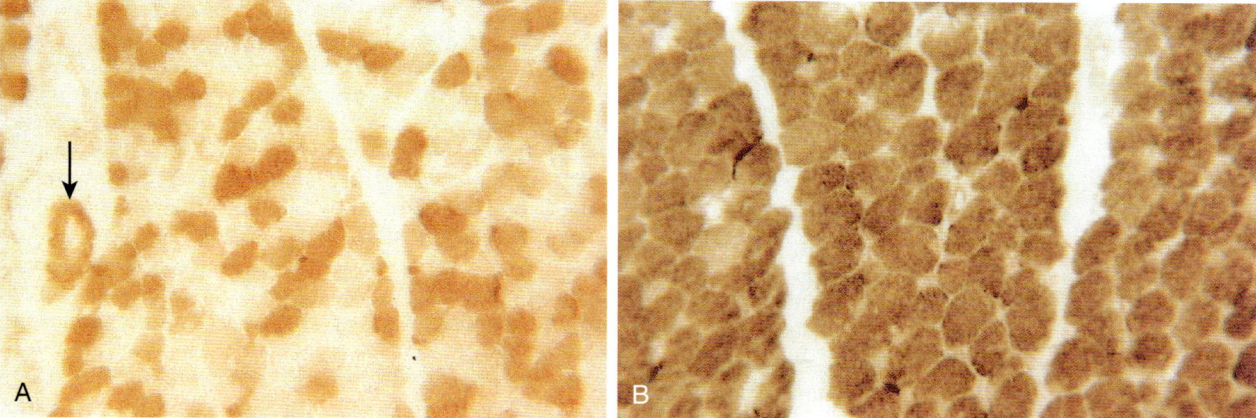

Figure 33.30 Benign cytochrome c oxidase (COX) deficiency. Histochemical reaction for COX activity. (A) At age 2 months, when the patient required assisted ventilation, the histochemical stain shows a mosaic of COX-positive and COX-deficient fibers. In addition, COX activity is seen in the wall of an intramuscular arteriole (*black arrow*). (B) At age 8 months, when the patient had recovered from respiratory distress, COX activity is seen in all muscle fibers (×180). (Reprinted with permission from De Vivo DC, Bonilla E, DiMauro S. Mitochondrial diseases. In: Jones HR Jr, De Vivo DC, Darras BT, eds. *Neuromuscular Disorders of Infancy, Childhood and Adolescence: A Clinician's Approach.* 1st ed. Philadelphia: Butterworth-Heinemann; 2003:chap 46, 867–899.)

neonatal period with weakness (limbs and face), hypotonia, and hyporeflexia. Occasional features have been ophthalmoplegia, liver failure, Fanconi syndrome, and seizures. Lactic acidosis has been noted in approximately 50% of cases. Approximately 60% have had elevated values for CK, ranging from 2 to as high as 30 times the upper limit of normal. Of patients with neonatal onset, most have died in the first year of life. Muscle biopsy shows ragged-red fibers in the minority of cases, but consistent features are a decrease in the content of mitochondrial DNA and a deficiency of multiple mitochondrial enzymes, especially COX (complex IV) and combinations of complexes I, II, or III. In most infantile-onset cases, the disorder appears to be autosomal recessive. The molecular genetic disturbances are likely multiple. Multiple genes are involved in mtDNA maintenance (i.e., thymidine kinase 2 *[TK2]*).[450,503] Infantile myopathy or encephalomyopathy is common in patients with *TK2, SUCLA2, SUCLG1, and RRM2B* mutations.[523-526] Most patients with *TK2* mutations have exceptionally high serum CK values, an unusual finding in other mitochondrial diseases, and certain mutations can closely simulate the clinical and histological phenotype of SMA.[493,527] Other examples will likely be delineated. Recall that Alpers syndrome can be caused by mitochondrial DNA depletion resulting from a mitochondrial DNA–specific polymerase gamma gene (*POLG1;* see Chapter 29).

Metabolic Myopathies

Metabolic myopathy, in this context, refers to a disorder with prominent involvement of muscle and a *primary* abnormality of glycogen or lipid metabolism. Because glycogen and lipid metabolism are also affected *secondarily* by mitochondrial abnormalities (see previous section), a certain overlap of clinical and morphological features is to be expected. Glycogen (through glucose) and lipid (through fatty acids) are important for energy production and for structural maintenance and growth in muscle (see Chapter 30). Disorders of glycogen and lipid metabolism are classified here among myopathies that have

BOX 33.5   Neonatal Neuromuscular Disease and Disordered Glycogen Metabolism
Acid maltase deficiency (type II, Pompe disease)
Debrancher deficiency (type III)
Brancher deficiency (type IV)
Muscle phosphorylase deficiency (type V)
Muscle phosphorylase kinase deficiency (type VIII)
Phosphofructokinase deficiency (type VII)

diagnostic histology because appropriate fixation and staining (e.g., periodic acid–Schiff [PAS] for glycogen and oil red O for lipid) usually demonstrate accumulation of the appropriate material and stimulate the search for the specific metabolic defect. The amount of glycogen can also be quantitated in muscle tissue; however, a specific diagnosis for disorders of glycogen and lipid metabolism is usually made by enzymatic analysis in muscle tissue, skin fibroblasts, or leukocytes and/or genetic testing of the respective genes.[528] Decreased enzymatic activity and/or identification of pathogenic sequence variants confirms the diagnosis.

Disorders of Glycogen Metabolism. Disorders of glycogen metabolism are shown in Fig. 33.31.[528-531] Disorders known to exhibit neuromuscular disease in early infancy are alpha-glucosidase (acid maltase) deficiency or Pompe disease (type II), debrancher deficiency (type III), brancher deficiency (type IV), muscle phosphorylase deficiency (type V), phosphorylase kinase deficiency (type VIII), and phosphofructokinase deficiency (type VII; Box 33.5). Other glycogenoses may be associated with hypotonia secondary to hypoglycemia (e.g., glucose-6-phosphatase deficiency, Von Gierke disease type I, glycogen synthetase deficiency).

Type II Glycogen Storage Disease (Pompe Disease). This disease is the prototype of the glycogenoses with onset in the first weeks of life and is discussed in detail in Chapter 32 regarding disorders

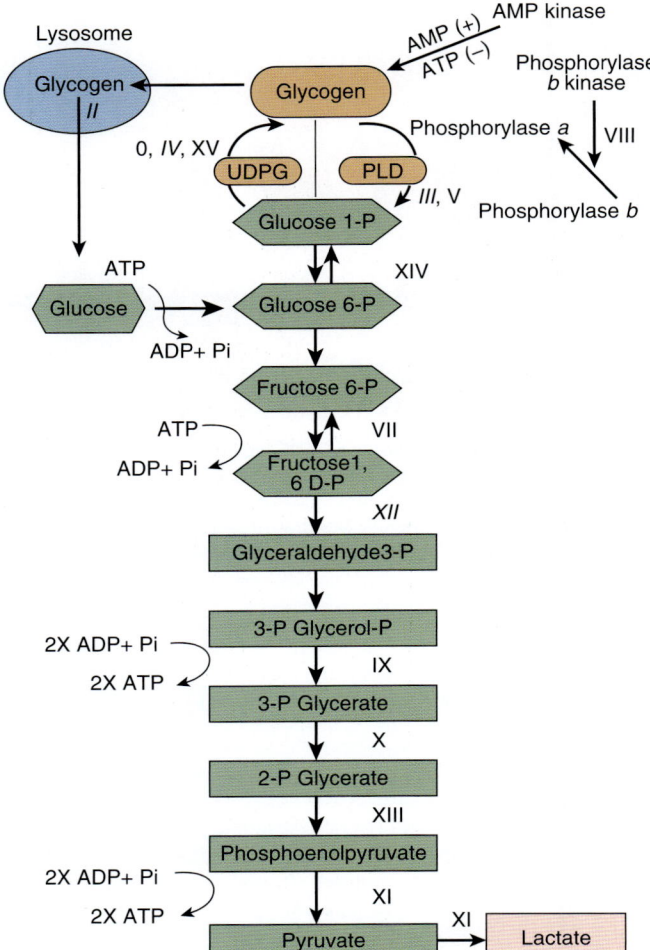

Figure 33.31 Scheme of glycogen metabolism and glycolysis. Roman numerals indicate enzymes whose deficiencies are associated with muscle glycogenosis: II, acid maltase (GAA, Pompe disease); III, debrancher (GDE, Cori-Forbes disease); IV, brancher (GBE, Andersen disease); V, myophosphorylase (PYGM, McArdle disease); VII, phosphofructokinase (PFK, Tarui disease); VIII, phosphorylase kinase (PHK); IX, phosphoglycerate kinase (PGK); X, phosphoglycerate mutase (PGAM); XI, lactate dehydrogenase (LDH); XII, aldolase A; XIII, beta-enolase (ENO3); XIV, phosphoglucomutase (PGM); XV, glycogenin (GYG1); 0, glycogen synthase (GYS1). *AMP,* Adenosine monophosphate; *ATP,* adenosine triphosphate; *P,* inorganic phosphate; *PLD,* phosphorylase-limit dextrin; *UDPG,* uridine diphosphate glucose. (Reprinted with permission from Akman HO, Oldfors A, DiMauro S. Glycogen storage diseases of muscle. In: Darras BT, Jones HR Jr, Ryan MM, De Vivo DC, eds. *Neuromuscular Disorders of Infancy, Childhood and Adolescence: A Clinician's Approach.* 2nd ed. San Diego: Academic Press; 2015:chap 39, 735–760.)

at the level of the lower motor neuron. The disorder involves skeletal muscle, but involvement of anterior horn cells tends to dominate the clinical syndrome.

Type III Glycogen Storage Disease (Debrancher Deficiency). This disorder affects liver as well as muscle. Because debrancher enzyme is involved in the major metabolic pathway for the degradation of glycogen to glucose, ketotic hypoglycemia may occur and may be a prominent aspect of the clinical syndrome. Hepatomegaly is impressive, and hepatic disease may be severe.[532] Hypotonia and weakness from the neonatal period have been reported, albeit rarely.[4,533] Muscle biopsy findings are illustrated

in Fig. 33.32. The gene encoding this enzyme (*AGL*) has been sequenced and mutations have been identified.[534]

Type IV Glycogen Storage Disease (Brancher Deficiency). This disorder classically presents in infancy as progressive cirrhosis of the liver. However, several cases of glycogen storage disease type IV, brancher enzyme deficiency, have been associated with lethal infantile myopathy, sometimes with cardiomyopathy, fetal akinesia deformation sequence, and anterior horn cell glycogen accumulation.[535-538]

Type V Glycogen Storage Disease (Muscle Phosphorylase Deficiency). This disorder, better known as McArdle disease, usually manifests around the time of puberty with exercise intolerance, muscle cramps, fatigue, and myoglobinuria. However, three patients with a fatal infantile form were reported.[539-541] The infants exhibited severe generalized weakness and hypotonia from the neonatal period. Two infants had evidence of prenatal onset because of congenital contractures at the elbows, hips, and knees.[540,541] In all three infants, the disorder progressed rapidly to death by respiratory failure at 16 days, 12 weeks, and 13 weeks.[539,540] The diagnosis of glycogen myopathy was suggested by the finding of subsarcolemmal vacuoles on muscle biopsy (Fig. 33.33), which were PAS-positive. Electron microscopy demonstrated large subsarcolemmal deposits of glycogen that were not membrane-bound (unlike the lysosomal-bound deposits of Pompe disease). No phosphorylase staining was apparent on histochemical reaction of muscle. In two cases studied biochemically, the glycogen content of muscle was found to be increased threefold.[539,541] Other enzymes of glycogen metabolism were normal, and immunochemical techniques demonstrated absence of phosphorylase protein. The occurrence of parental consanguinity in one of the two cases suggests that the disorder is autosomal recessive.[540]

Type VIII Glycogen Storage Disease (Muscle Phosphorylase Kinase Deficiency). A different defect at the phosphorylase step has been described in two infants. One had moderate hypotonia and weakness and delayed motor development from birth (sitting but not walking at 19 months of age[542]). Although total phosphorylase activity was normal in vitro in both cases, the proportion of the active ("a") form was markedly depressed, thus indicating that in vivo most of muscle phosphorylase was present as the inactive ("b") form. A defect in the phosphorylase kinase necessary for activation of phosphorylase caused the disorder. A second infant exhibited more severe weakness and hypotonia and died at 7 months of age.[543] Infants with congenital hypertrophic cardiomyopathy, glycogen storage, and "pseudo-phosphorylase kinase deficiency" in skeletal muscle are now known to harbor de novo mutations in the gamma-2 subunit of the adenosine monophosphate (AMP)-activated protein kinase.[544,545]

Type VII Glycogen Storage Disease (Phosphofructokinase Deficiency). This disorder, like McArdle disease, is associated characteristically with a later onset of exercise intolerance, muscle cramps, fatigue, and myoglobinuria. However, several examples of a severe infantile form of phosphofructokinase deficiency have been reported.[546-550] In the initial report, two siblings, born to related parents, were described with hypotonia and weakness, worse in the upper extremities, from the first days of life. Muscle contractures developed rapidly. One infant died at 6 months of age with respiratory complications and the other, alive at 14 months at the time of report, could not sit without support. In subsequent reports, three infants were described

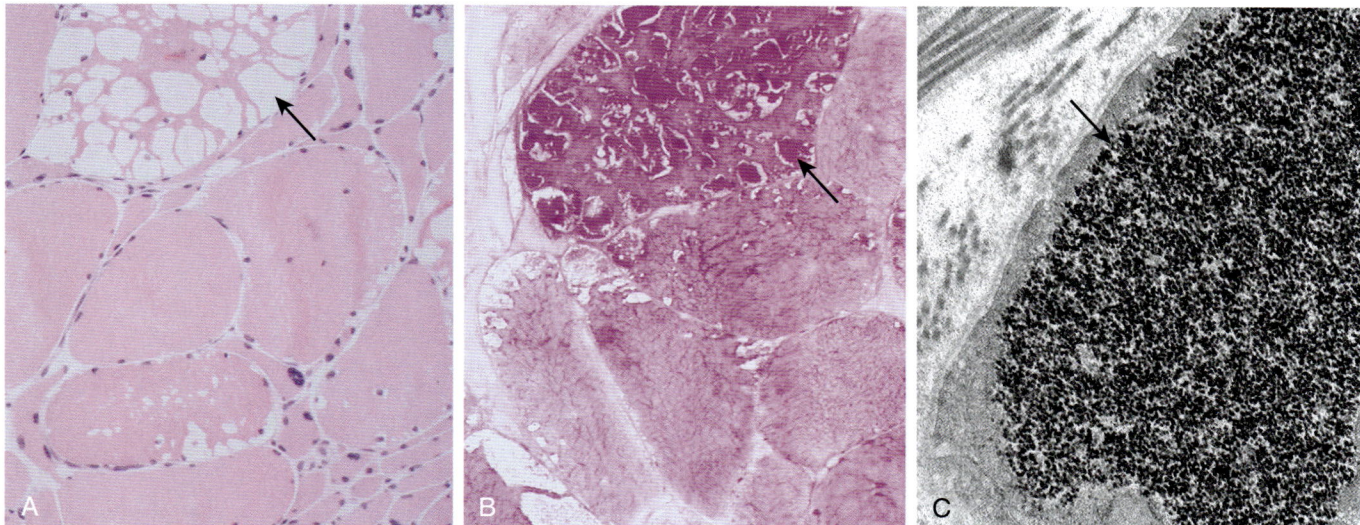

Figure 33.32 Muscle biopsy from a patient with debrancher enzyme (DBE) deficiency (glycogen storage disease [GSD] III). (A) Hematoxylin-eosin reveals large vacuoles in muscle fibers (arrows), and the periodic acid–Schiff stain (B) shows that they are filled with glycogen with apparently normal ultrastructural beta-particle structure (C). (Reprinted with permission from: Akman HO, Oldfors A, DiMauro S. Glycogen storage diseases of muscle. In: Darras BT, Jones HR Jr, Ryan MM, De Vivo DC, eds. *Neuromuscular Disorders of Infancy, Childhood and Adolescence: A Clinician's Approach.* 2nd ed. San Diego: Academic Press; 2015:chap 39, 735–760.)

with progressive weakness and hypotonia, with death at 7, 21, and 21 months, respectively.[548,549] One infant exhibited cortical blindness and seizures, and another had intellectual disability.[547,548] The third infant was treated with a ketogenic diet from 4 months of age and was alive and improving at 2 years of age.[550] Muscle specimens showed subsarcolemmal vacuoles that were PAS-positive. Glycogen accumulation was demonstrated by biochemical techniques, and muscle phosphofructokinase activity was severely depressed. However, despite the lack of enzymatic activity in a series of infants with myopathy and death before the age of 2 years, a molecular defect in the *PFKM* gene was not documented, raising the possibility of an alternative pathogenetic mechanism(s).[551]

Disorders of Lipid Metabolism. Defects in the utilization of fatty acids, the steps for which are outlined in Box 33.6, result in several disorders with hypotonia and weakness in the neonatal period or early infancy.[4,443,531,552-564]

Most of the patients reported with all the defects listed in Box 33.6 exhibit clinical features long after the neonatal period. Even those with neonatal onset manifest, in addition to hypotonia, more prominent features such as stupor or coma, cardiac failure, or congenital malformations (see Chapter 28). Moreover, all but one of the disorders include features more characteristic of a metabolic disorder (hypoketotic hypoglycemia, hyperammonemia) and are discussed as such in Chapter 28. However, the defect of the carnitine transporter (i.e., primary carnitine deficiency) manifests clinically primarily as myopathy involving skeletal and cardiac muscle; thus it is discussed here.

Primary Systemic Carnitine Deficiency (Carnitine Transporter Deficiency). This disorder is usually characterized by the onset of cardiomyopathy in late infancy or early childhood, but onset in the first 2 months of life is well documented.[443,554,555,564-567] The major features of this disorder are weakness, hypotonia,

---

BOX 33.6 Metabolic Defects in Fatty Acid Oxidation[a]

Carnitine transporter[b]
Carnitine palmitoyltransferase I
Carnitine-acylcarnitine translocase
Carnitine palmitoyltransferase II
Very-long-chain acyl-CoA dehydrogenase[b]
Medium-chain acyl-CoA dehydrogenase[b]
Short-chain acyl-CoA dehydrogenase[b]
Multiple acyl-CoA dehydrogenase[b]
Long-chain 3-hydroxy acyl-CoA dehydrogenase
Short-chain 3-hydroxy acyl-CoA dehydrogenase
Acetoacetyl-CoA thiolase (beta-ketothiolase)[b]
3-Oxoacid: CoA transferase
Hydroxymethylglutaryl-CoA lyase[b]

[a]See text for references.
[b]Prominent hypotonia and weakness may occur in the neonatal period.
CoA, Coenzyme A.

---

hepatomegaly, cardiomyopathy, and Reye-syndrome–like encephalopathy. Decreasing fasting ketosis or hypoketotic hypoglycemia may develop. Progression to metabolic decompensation and death may occur if treatment with carnitine is not instituted. Muscle histology demonstrates subsarcolemmal and intermyofibrillar vacuoles that contain lipid (Fig. 33.34). Carnitine levels in muscle, liver, and serum are depressed significantly (<10% of normal).

The nature of the defect in primary systemic carnitine deficiency involves impairment of transport of carnitine into muscle.[553] Studies of cultured fibroblasts showed a defect in the specific high-affinity, carrier-mediated carnitine uptake mechanism (i.e., the OCTN2 carnitine transporter).[443,554,556,564,566-569] This autosomal recessive disease is caused by mutations in the

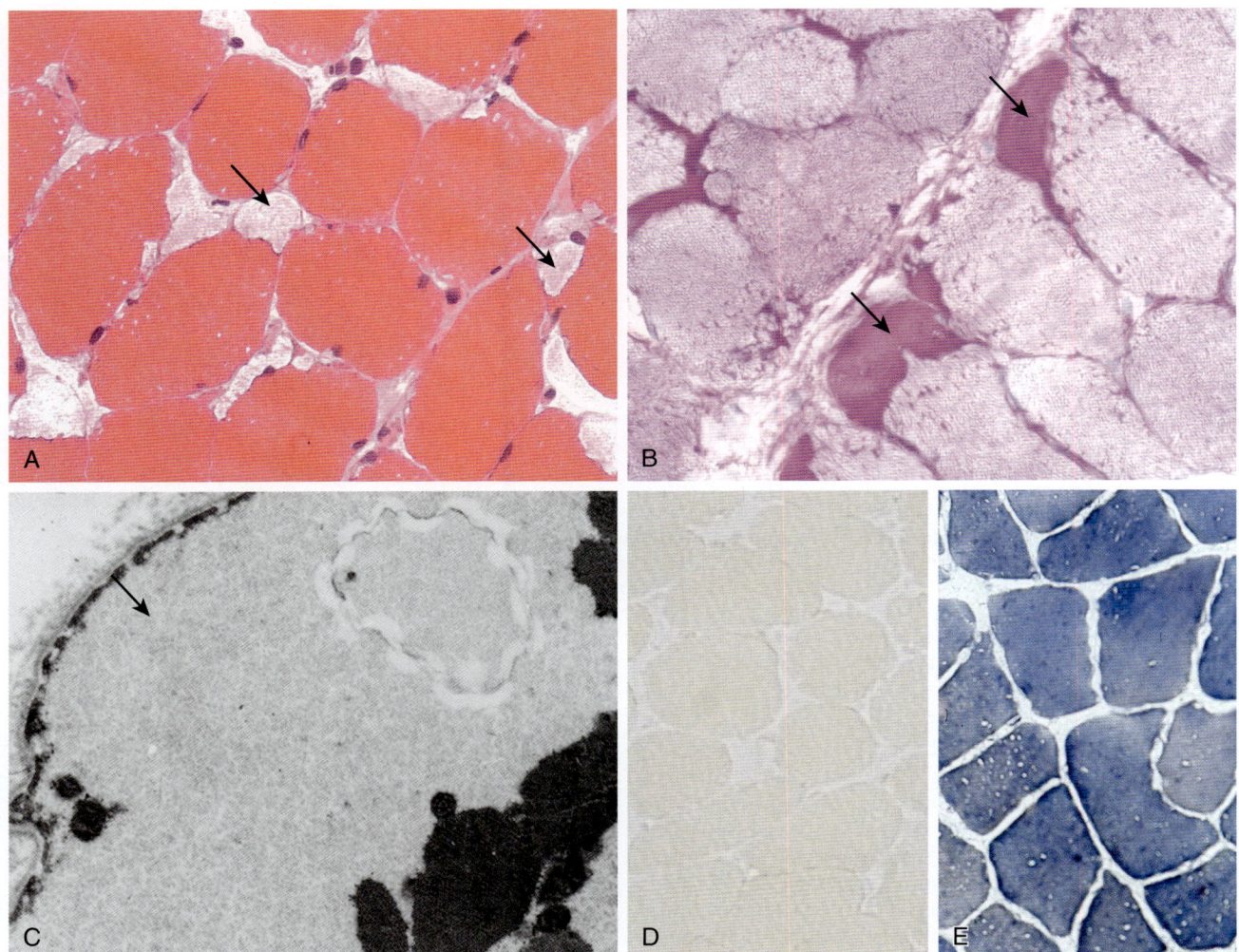

Figure 33.33 Muscle biopsy from a patient with McArdle disease (glycogen storage disease [GSD] V).
(A) Staining with hematoxylin and eosin reveals subsarcolemmal vacuoles (*arrows*). (B) The vacuoles contain glycogen, as shown by the periodic acid–Schiff stain. (C) Electron microscopy documents the presence of glycogen beta particles in the vacuoles. (D) Negative histochemical reaction for phosphorylase in the patient's muscle. (E) Positive histochemical reaction in a control muscle. (Reprinted with permission from Akman HO, Oldfors A, DiMauro S. Glycogen storage diseases of muscle. In: Darras BT, Jones HR Jr, Ryan MM, De Vivo DC, eds. *Neuromuscular Disorders of Infancy, Childhood and Adolescence: A Clinician's Approach.* 2nd ed. San Diego: Academic Press; 2015:chap 39, 735–760.)

SLC22A5 gene encoding for the transporter protein OCTN2. Since carnitine mediates the transport of long-chain fatty acids into mitochondria, the result is defective fatty acid oxidation in muscle, liver, heart, and other tissues. The existence of a distinct primary muscle carnitine deficiency syndrome is disputed and remains unproven. *Management* of primary systemic carnitine deficiency is based particularly on treatment with large doses of oral or intravenous (IV) carnitine.[443,554,557] Prolonged therapy is necessary.

RESTRICTED NEUROMUSCULAR DISORDERS

Several disorders of the neuromuscular apparatus are restricted to a small portion of the motor system. Some restricted disorders are clearly related to traumatic insults and are discussed in Chapter 36. *Restricted disorders that are not established as caused principally by trauma are considered next.*

Congenital Ptosis

Clinical Features

Ptosis is the most common of the congenital nonprogressive neuromuscular syndromes restricted to the ocular region that are likely to manifest in the newborn period (Box 33.7). The disorder is usually familial and is transmitted in an autosomal dominant or X-linked dominant manner. In both cases male and female infants are affected equally. Involvement is unilateral in approximately 75% of cases. Patterns of weakness are consistent within families; thus, in one pedigree, left unilateral predominance was striking.[570] In a large pedigree of 96 people, 49 had congenital ptosis, and 92% of those had bilateral involvement.[571] Superior rectus weakness may also be present;

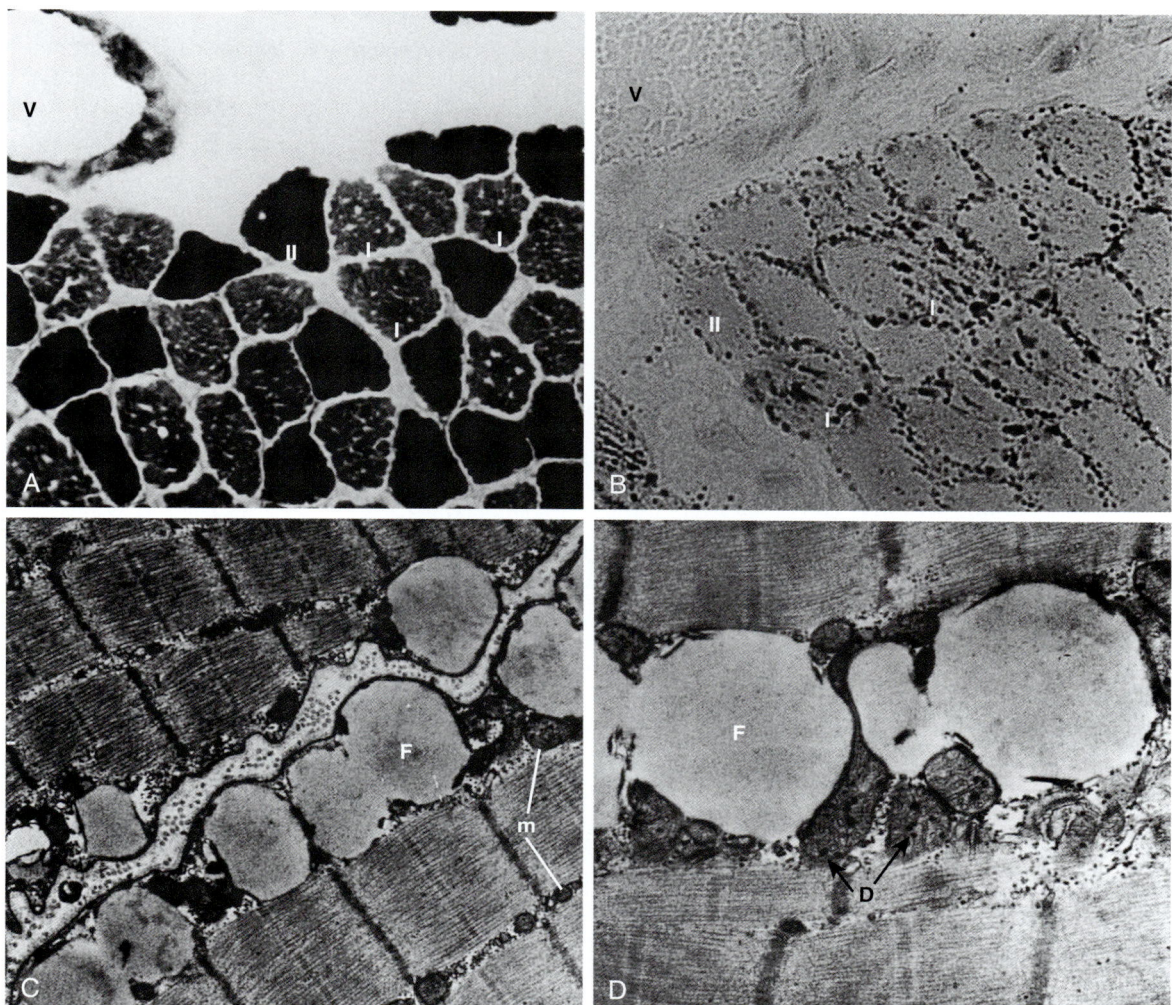

Figure 33.34 Muscle carnitine deficiency with lipid myopathy: muscle biopsy from an affected infant who died at 28 months of age. (A) Histochemical preparation shows that vacuoles are predominantly in type I fibers (II, type II fibers; V, blood vessels) (adenosine triphosphatase stain, pH 9.3, ×200). (B) Vacuoles stain positively for lipid (oil red O stain, ×200). (C) Electron micrograph shows numerous fat vacuoles in the subsarcolemmal area (F, fat; m, mitochondria). (×14,600.) (D) Electron micrograph shows rows of lipid vacuoles (F) in intermyofibrillar spaces. Multiple electron-dense granules (D) are visible in some of the mitochondria (×45,000). (From Hart ZH, Chang CH, DiMauro S, Farooki Q, et al. Muscle carnitine deficiency and fatal cardiomyopathy. *Neurology.* 1978;28:147–151.)

BOX 33.7   Congenital Nonprogressive Ocular Syndromes

Ptosis
Unilateral third nerve palsy
Congenital fibrosis of the extraocular muscles
Duane retraction syndrome
Other ocular disorders (see text)

---

when this weakness accompanies the ptosis, it is on the same side as the levator palpebrae weakness.

Pathology

The anatomical locus of the defect is generally considered to be in the muscle of the levator palpebrae rather than in the third nerve or nucleus thereof. In support of the myogenic theory are the histological abnormalities in the levator muscle and the lack of abnormalities in other structures (e.g., pupil) innervated by the third nerve.[572,573] However, the possibility that the primary abnormality involves an impairment of the caudal central subnucleus of the third nerve with secondary changes in muscle has not been clarified.

Pathogenesis and Etiology

The pathogenesis of the disorder in the typical autosomal dominant case involves a gene on chromosome 1 *(PTOS1).*[574,575] The X-linked locus is at chromosome Xq24-q27.1 *(PTOS2).*[574,575] In addition, in a sporadic case, a balanced chromosomal translocation t(1;8) has been reported, which disrupts the ZFHX4 (zinc finger homeodomain 4) gene at 8q21.12, suggesting a third PTOS locus at that site.[576] However, the causative mutations at these loci remain unknown. Recently, recessive COL25A1 mutations have been reported in two families with probands presenting with either isolated congenital ptosis or exotropic Duane syndrome.[577]

Management

No specific therapy exists. In examples of severe congenital ptosis with the risk of secondary amblyopia, a surgical corrective procedure for the lid is carried out between 6 months and 5 years of age.[575,578]

Congenital Unilateral Third Nerve Palsy

Clinical Features

The designation *congenital unilateral third nerve palsy* refers to those cases of unilateral and isolated third nerve palsies apparent from birth. This lesion is not common, although it is frequently not recognized until after the neonatal period. In contrast to congenital ptosis, congenital third nerve palsy is only rarely familial (2 of 16 cases in one series). A very small proportion of cases can be related to orbital trauma (1 of 16 cases in one series).[579] The lateral deviation of the affected eye may be confused with comitant exotropia. The usual position of the eye, however, is downward as well as outward. The oculomotor deficits involve medial and upward gaze particularly; in addition, ptosis and pupillary dilation are present in the majority of cases. Later in infancy, signs of aberrant reinnervation of third nerve structures are apparent (e.g., constriction of pupil on attempted upward gaze or widening of the palpebral fissure on attempted medial gaze).

Pathology

The anatomical locus of the lesion in the common unilateral case is often considered to be outside the brain stem because of the general absence of other signs of brain-stem involvement (e.g., contralateral hemiparesis) and the presence of aberrant regeneration.[579] However, a disturbance of development of the neurons of the nucleus, as in the congenital fibrosis syndromes (see later), is certainly possible. The usual involvement of the entire third nerve complex excludes a lesion after the bifurcation within the orbit, and the absence of concomitant involvement of the fourth and sixth nerves also suggests that the portion within the cavernous sinus is not the site. Thus the lesion probably involves the third nerve nucleus or nerve between its exit from the brain stem and its entrance into the cavernous sinus. The pathological substrate is unclear. Rarely, a prenatal mesencephalic infarct produces a congenital nuclear syndrome of the oculomotor nerve, with contralateral hemiparesis and aberrant regeneration.[580] In addition, a rare bilateral case of congenital partial third nerve palsy secondary to a mesencephalic malformation has been reported.[581]

Pathogenesis and Etiology

The pathogenesis of the usual case is unknown, but the possibility has been raised that the nerve is injured by cranial deformations during labor and delivery, perhaps at the site of its course over the tentorial edge.[579] As just noted, a prenatal ischemic lesion of the brain stem or mesencephalic anomaly is rarely responsible.[580,581]

Management

Management may include surgical correction of the ptosis, which can be severe, and of the lateral eye deviation. It is critical in the neonatal period to be sure that an intracranial process, such as a supratentorial lesion (e.g., hematoma) leading to herniation of temporal lobe through the tentorial notch and compression of the third nerve, is not present.

Congenital Fibrosis of the Extraocular Muscles

Clinical Features

Syndromes involving congenital fibrosis of the extraocular muscles (CFEOM) are characterized by congenital bilateral ptosis and a *restrictive* external ophthalmoplegia, with eyes partially or completely fixed in a strabismic position.[574,575,582-584] Limitation of extraocular movement in both eyes is pronounced, and forced duction tests reveal marked restriction of globe movement in all directions. The limitations are nonprogressive. When affected infants develop consistent visual fixation and following, the head is held in an extended position to compensate for the marked ptosis. Three clinical phenotypes, designated CFEOM1, CFEOM2, and CFEOM3, are most common. CFEOM1 is characterized by congenital bilateral ptosis and external ophthalmoplegia, (with pupillary sparing; that is, not internal ophthalmoplegia). The primary position of the eyes is downward, and patients have a restricted upward gaze and a variably restricted horizontal gaze. In CFEOM2, in addition to the bilateral ptosis, marked exotropia occurs, with severely limited horizontal and vertical eye movements. The only normally functioning extraocular muscle is the abducens-innervated lateral rectus, which allows outward movement of each eye. In CFEOM3 the phenotypic spectrum is much broader; it includes individuals with severe CFEOM whose eyes are fixed in an infraducted and exotropic position but also those without bilateral ptosis and/or with preserved primary gaze and some ability to elevate one or both eyes above midline.[575]

Pathology

Because of the marked fibrosis of the extraocular muscles, it was assumed until the past 10 years that these disorders were basically myopathic. In CFEOM1, careful neuropathological study showed an absence of the superior divisions of the third cranial nerves and corresponding alpha motor neurons in midbrain, with presumably secondary abnormalities of the superior rectus and levator palpebrae superioris muscles, which are normally innervated by this branch and responsible for elevation of the eye and eyelid.[582,584] In CFEOM2, it appears likely that abnormal development of both the oculomotor and trochlear nuclei is responsible for all eye movements except abduction.[584]

Pathogenesis and Etiology

The pathological defects suggest that these disorders reflect an *abnormality in the development of the lower motor neuron system of the extraocular muscles*[582,584]; they have been categorized as congenital cranial dysinnervation disorders (CCDDs). CFEOM1, an autosomal dominant disorder, is related to heterozygous mutations in *KIF21A*, a developmental kinesin.[584] Kinesins are molecular motors that transport molecules along microtubules. The CFEOM1 defect appears to be in axonal targeting to the extraocular muscles. CFEOM2, an autosomal recessive disorder, is caused by mutations in *PHOX2A*, which encodes a homeodomain transcription factor necessary for development of the oculomotor and trochlear nerves. Autosomal dominant mutations in the neuron-specific beta-tubulin genes *TUBB3* and

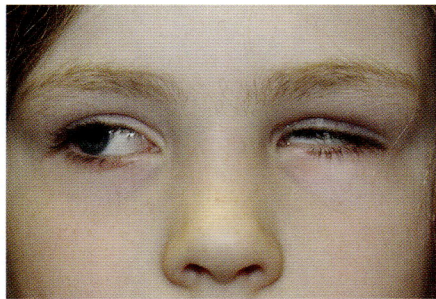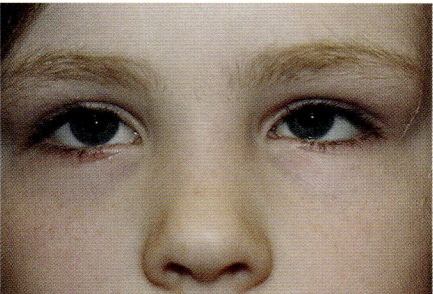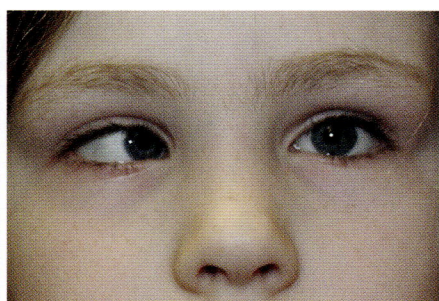

Figure 33.35 Patient with Duane's retraction syndrome attempting to look to her right (*left photo*), straight ahead (*middle photo*), and to her left (*right photo*). Her left eye has restricted lateral movement on attempted abduction and upshoot with narrowing of the palpebral fissure secondary to cocontraction on attempted adduction. (Reprinted with permission from Ryan MM, Engle EC. Disorders of the ocular motor nerves and extraocular muscles. In: Darras BT, Jones HR Jr, Ryan MM, De Vivo DC, eds. *Neuromuscular Disorders of Infancy, Childhood and Adolescence: A Clinician's Approach.* 2nd ed. San Diego: Academic Press; 2015:chap 46, 922–957.)

TUBB2B have been linked to various CFEOM3 phenotypes[585,586]; one *TUBB2B* mutation was found to segregate with CFEOM and polymicrogyria,[587] and two missense *TUBB3* mutations have been shown to cause both CFEOM3 and cortical malformations.[588]

Management

Management is difficult and primarily involves surgical attempts to improve the bilateral ptosis.

Duane Retraction Syndrome

Clinical Features

Duane syndrome is an uncommon congenital disorder of ocular motility with the following characteristics: (1) limitation of abduction of the eye and (2) retraction of the eye into the orbit and consequent narrowing of the palpebral fissure on adduction (Fig. 33.35).[573,575,589] Thus this disorder is another type of congenital *restrictive* ophthalmoparesis, akin to CFEOM. Additional oculomotor findings may include protrusion of the globe and widening of the palpebral fissure on attempted abduction and downward or upward deviation of the eyes with adduction. Approximately 80% of cases are unilateral. The left eye is involved approximately twice as commonly as the right.[573] Approximately 5% to 10% of cases are familial, and inheritance in such cases is autosomal dominant.[590,591]

At least one other congenital malformation accompanies approximately 33% of cases, and 8% of patients have three or more additional anomalies.[591] The anomalies are principally skeletal, auricular, or ocular.[591-593] Major skeletal anomalies include vertebral, palatal and upper extremity defects (e.g., Klippel-Feil anomaly, cervical spina bifida, cleft palate, and anomalies of thumb, radius, and ulna). Auricular anomalies include malformed pinnas, auricular appendages, and malformed inner ear with accompanying deafness. Ocular defects include microphthalmia, coloboma, heterochromia iridis, and congenital cataract. Several syndromes are recognized with varying combinations of these anomalies in association with Duane syndrome.[574,575,584]

Pathology

Analogous to the abnormality in CFEOM (see earlier discussion), Duane syndrome is associated with an absence of the abducens nerve and its corresponding abducens nucleus in the pons, with presumably secondary abnormalities in the lateral rectus muscle, the abductor of the eye.[584,594,595] The fibrosis of the lateral rectus has been thought to cause retraction of the globe on attempted adduction. The Chiari I malformation was reported in two episodic cases of Duane retraction syndrome, perhaps through involvement of the abducens nerve.[584,596,597]

Pathogenesis and Etiology

As in CFEOM, the pathological defect suggests that Duane retraction syndrome and its several variants are related to an abnormality in the development of the lower motor neuron system of the extraocular muscle. The occasional familial occurrence and not infrequent association with anomalies of certain skeletal, auricular, and ocular structures are also consistent with a defect in embryogenesis. Cross and Pfaffenbach[592] emphasize that the sixth nerves and nuclei are developing between the fourth and eighth weeks of gestation, during a period when the eyes, auditory structures, palate, vertebrae, and distal upper extremities are also evolving. Identification of the genes (*HOXA1, CHN1, SALL4,* and *ROBO3*) responsible for several of the syndromic variants of Duane syndrome suggests that the disorders relate to disturbances of nuclear development and axonal targeting.[584,598-603]

Management

Management should include a careful evaluation of skeletal, auditory, and ocular structures to detect accompanying abnormalities.

Other Ocular Disorders

Other ocular disorders may be observed in the neonatal period but are generally rare. Congenital Horner syndrome, unassociated with brachial plexus palsy (see Chapter 36), may occur[604]; association with cervical neuroblastoma has been reported.[605,606] Congenital abducens (lateral rectus palsy) may be observed as an isolated finding, although association with Duane retraction syndrome or Möbius syndrome is common.[607] Congenital fourth nerve palsy usually escapes detection in the neonatal period (the eye is deviated vertically and medially); anomaly of the brain stem may be present.[608]

TABLE 33.8   Clinical Features of Möbius Syndrome[a]

CLINICAL FEATURE	PERCENTAGE OF TOTAL
Congenital facial diplegia	100
Upper = lower[b]	35
Upper > lower	63
Lower > upper	2
Abducens palsy	100
Horizontal ophthalmoplegia[c]	10
Oculomotor palsy	20
Ptosis (bilateral)	10
Tongue weakness	75
Talipes equinovarus	30
Hand or arm malformation	40
Pectoralis hypoplasia	10

[a]See text for references.
[b]Usually complete or near-complete facial paralysis.
[c]Vertical gaze is full.

Möbius Syndrome

Clinical Features

Möbius syndrome, or *congenital facial diplegia syndrome*, described in 1888 by Möbius,[609] consists of unilateral or bilateral nonprogressive facial weakness and abducens palsies, which are usually bilateral, in the presence of full vertical gaze (Table 33.8).[610] Although the essential features of the syndrome are rather restricted, the disorder is accompanied by a variety of neuromuscular and other abnormalities. At first glance, confusion may exist with other disorders of the motor unit with prominent facial weakness (e.g., myasthenias, congenital myotonic dystrophy, CMD, FSHD, nemaline myopathy, myotubular myopathy, congenital fiber-type disproportion, and COX deficiency [mitochondrial myopathy]). However, associated features usually allow clinical distinction in the newborn period.

The *clinical findings* are striking (see Table 33.8).[611-633] The *facial weakness* is essentially always bilateral and severe. In approximately one third of patients, the face is essentially immobile. In at least 60% of patients, the upper part of the face is affected more severely than the lower. The eyes cannot be closed, and the face is smooth and expressionless. The severe involvement of the face prevents formation of a proper seal around the nipple; therefore, feeding difficulty in the newborn period is a major problem.

Abducens palsy, present essentially invariably, is almost always bilateral. In a smaller percentage of cases, external ophthalmoplegia in the form of lateral gaze palsies (i.e., conjugate weakness) appears to be present, but vertical gaze is full.[610] Oculomotor nerve involvement is apparent in 20% and bilateral ptosis in 10% of patients. Involvement of tongue is relatively common, associated with atrophy, and bilateral in approximately half of patients.

Other neuromuscular abnormalities are frequent. Thus, talipes equinovarus occurs in approximately one third; in a few patients, more widespread arthrogryposis may be present. Hypoplasia of the pectoralis muscle, always unilateral, occurs in approximately 10% to 15% of patients; when it is associated with syndactyly of the hand, it constitutes *Poland syndrome*. Hand and arm malformations (e.g., brachydactyly and syndactyly) are present

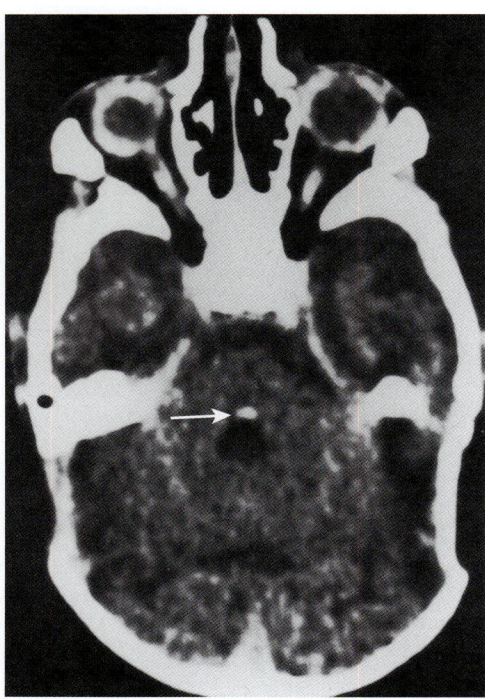

Figure 33.36 Möbius syndrome. This computed tomography scan shows symmetrical dorsal pontine calcifications (*arrow*). (From D'Cruz OF, Swisher CN, Jaradeh S, Tang T, et al. Möbius syndrome: evidence for a vascular etiology. *J Child Neurol.* 1993;8:260–265.)

in approximately 40% of patients. Rarer patients with Möbius syndrome have the marked micrognathia of the Robin sequence, congenital myopathy, developmental delay, and other features of Carey-Fineman-Ziter syndrome.[634-637] Central respiratory dysfunction requiring mechanical ventilation was observed in 13 patients with Möbius syndrome, 7 of whom died because of respiratory failure.[628] Intellectual disability has been reported in 10% to 30% of infants. Autism spectrum disorders have been observed in 25% to 40%.[632] This finding is of particular note because brain-stem disturbance has been postulated as a pathogenic mechanism in autism.[631]

Pathology

The anatomical sites of the pathological features are diverse and may include cranial nerve nuclei, roots, nerves, or muscle. Involvements of cranial nerve nuclei have included apparent developmental hypoplasia or aplasia and destructive lesions.[a] By far the leading abnormalities have been aplasia or hypoplasia of cranial nerve nuclei, sometimes in combination with brain-stem hypoplasia or focal necrosis, usually with calcification involving cranial nerve nuclei. Primary involvement of peripheral nerve or muscle is very uncommon. Abnormalities of brain-stem conduction times with testing of brain-stem auditory evoked responses and other electrophysiological measurements have provided in vivo functional correlates of the neuropathology.[612,626,649] CT may show calcification at the site of ischemic necrosis in the brain stem, usually in the region of the dorsal pons (Fig. 33.36). MRI provides details of brain-stem morphology, including hypoplasia or necrosis. Involvement of

[a]References 612, 613, 615, 618-620, 624-626, 629, 631, 633, and 638-648.

cranial nerves has included apparent developmental hypoplasia or aplasia (with normal cranial nerve nuclei) and possible demyelinative neuropathy.[650,651] Involvement of muscle has included apparent primary hypoplasia or aplasia.[652]

Pathogenesis and Etiology

The pathogenesis of the syndrome is undoubtedly heterogeneous, which is understandable in view of the multiple sites of pathology. Both developmental aberrations and destructive processes appear to be operative. The latter appear to be more common and include intrauterine ischemic brain-stem injury, for which neuropathological and brain imaging data are abundant (see earlier discussion). An ischemic event at approximately 5 to 6 weeks of gestation appears to be very important. Thus one case occurred after a maternal overdose of ergotamine on day 39 of gestation. Exposure to a similar agent in the first 2 months of gestation was associated with Möbius syndrome, limb reduction deficits, or both in seven other cases.[653] Also supportive of an insult during the fourth to eighth weeks, especially at 5 to 6 weeks of gestation, is the presence of muscle, limb defects, and heart anomalies. It is relevant in this context that the brain stem forms and differentiates rapidly during weeks 5 and 6 and that blood flow changes from the primitive trigeminal circulation to the vertebral arteries. Investigators have hypothesized that, during this period, the pontomesencephalic and pontomedullary tegmental areas, the sites of the affected cranial nerve nuclei, become watershed areas and are thereby vulnerable to ischemic insult.[626] It is quite possible that most cases are related to vascular disturbance, with hypoplasias and aplasias the response early in utero and necrosis and calcification later, when fetal inflammatory mechanisms develop. Other agents implicated in the pathogenesis of Möbius syndrome following in utero exposure include thalidomide[653,654] and misoprostol.[655]

A few cases have been familial, including autosomal dominant and, perhaps, autosomal recessive inheritance.[574,656,657] A pedigree described with seven affected members and a reciprocal translocation between chromosomes 1 and 13, demonstrable by banding techniques, suggested that cytogenetic investigation should be considered in the evaluation of affected patients.[658] Several other loci have been identified, but not the responsible genes.[659] A disturbance of rhombencephalic development is suggested by some of the neuropathological features, and such lesions represent good candidates for defects in homeobox genes. This notion received support by the description of a rare, Möbius-like syndrome characterized by bilateral Duane syndrome, facial weakness, sensorineural hearing loss, hypoventilation, intellectual disability, and autism spectrum disorder in association with aberrant hindbrain segmentation. The gene involved was *HOXA1*, which functions in hindbrain patterning.[584,660,661] As postulated in Möbius syndrome, abnormalities of vascular development were demonstrated.[660] Mutations in HXOB1 and TUBB3 genes, particularly the E410K amino acid substitution in TUBB3, have been reported in patients with Möbius syndrome.[661] However, HXOB1 mutations cause congenital facial paresis, esotropia, and deafness; hence they do not meet the strict criteria for Möbius syndrome.[662]

Management

Management requires particular attention to feeding techniques. In addition, poor eye closure may result in conjunctival irritation, and thus appropriate eye drops are needed. Later, surgical correction for the severe facial paralysis may be beneficial.[575,663,664]

Congenital Hypoplasia of Depressor Anguli Oris Muscle

Clinical Features

Congenital hypoplasia of the depressor anguli oris muscle is characterized by an asymmetrical crying facies (Fig. 33.37). The defect is present in approximately 0.5% to 1.0% of newborn infants.[665-667] The essential clinical finding is a failure of one corner of the mouth to move downward and outward, particularly during cry or grimace.[667-671] Other functions of the facial muscles, such as frowning, eye closure, and nasolabial fold depth, are normal. The left side of the face is affected in nearly 80% of cases.[671] The appearance of the face during cry or grimace may lead to the mistaken notion that the patient has facial palsy on the side *opposite* the defect, because the normally functioning muscles, in pulling the corner of the mouth downward and outward, may cause the appearance of lower facial drooping on that normal side. On follow-up, the defect may be less obvious as smiling and other aspects of facial expression become more prominent. A very broad smile or grimace is necessary to elicit the defect in the older child or adult.

The major clinical significance relates to an *association of the lesion with major congenital anomalies*, especially in the cardiovascular system.[652,665,667,671-680] Although the reported incidence of the facial defect and the associated anomalies have varied according to the selection of patients, a prospective study of 6487 newborn infants resulted in 44 cases.[666] Of these, 3 (6.8%) had cardiac defects (vs. 0.45% of controls). The total number with congenital anomalies was 9 (20%), compared with 2.7% of controls. In a hospital-based population, the incidence of anomalies was 70%; the most common of these were generally minor anomalies of ear and face.[671] The proportion with cardiac anomalies in this more selected population was 44%. The cardiac anomalies have been diverse; approximately 50% have consisted of ventricular septal defect (15%–25%), tetralogy of Fallot, patent ductus arteriosus, and coarctation of the aorta.[670,673] Most of the remaining 50% have been atrial septal defects. Other reported anomalies include genitourinary, musculoskeletal (especially vertebral), and, rarely, CNS defects. These last include agenesis of the corpus callosum, mega cisterna magna, and cerebral and cerebellar atrophy.[667,675,678]

The occurrence of the defect in 5% to 10% of infants with congenital heart disease led to the designation *cardiofacial syndrome*.[652] Cayler cardiofacial syndrome is one of a group of conditions linked to a microdeletion in the long arm of chromosome 22.[676,677,681] These syndromes are grouped by the term *CATCH22* (Cardiac defects, Abnormal facies, Thymic hyperplasia, Cleft palate, and Hypocalcemia) and include DiGeorge velocardiofacial and Takas syndromes.[676,682]

Pathology

The anatomical locus of the defect is the depressor anguli oris muscle and probably represents hypoplasia, although no pathological documentation is available. The EMG reveals a paucity of motor units but no fibrillations or other signs of disease of nerve or anterior horn cell. The likelihood of muscle hypoplasia or aplasia is supported further by the occurrence in

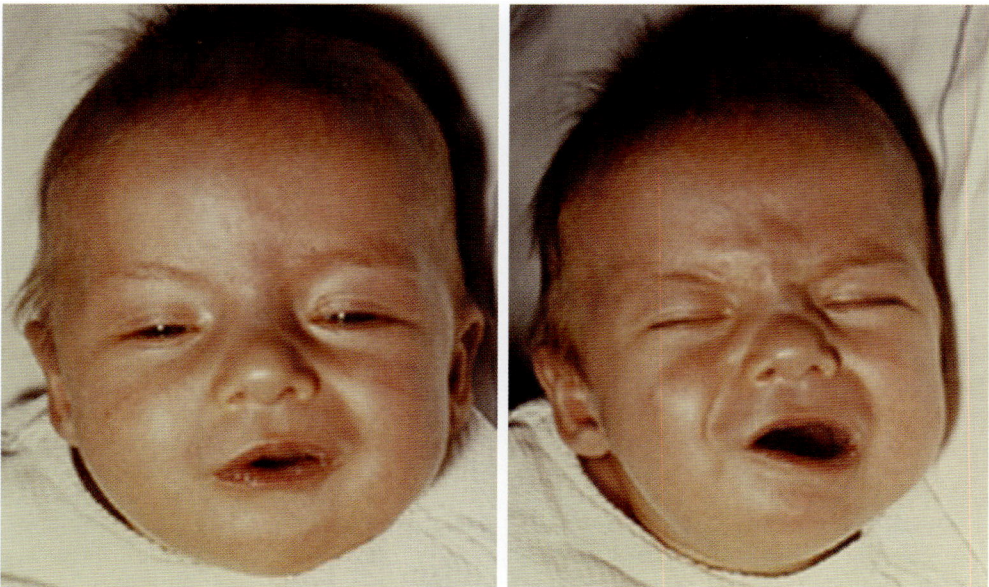

Figure 33.37 Asymmetrical crying facies due to hypoplasia of the depressor anguli oris muscle in a full-term boy at 20 days of age. The face is symmetrical at rest; when the child is crying, the lower lip is asymmetrical but the upper face and nasolabial folds remain symmetrical. (Used with permission from Renault F, Quijano-Roy S. Congenital and acquired facial palsies. In: Darras BT, Jones HR Jr, Ryan MM, De Vivo DC, eds. *Neuromuscular Disorders of Infancy, Childhood and Adolescence: A Clinician's Approach.* 2nd ed. San Diego: Academic Press; 2015:chap 13, 225–242.)

one family of a mother with aplasia of the left tensor fasciae latae muscle, a child with right hemidiaphragmatic hypoplasia, and another child with aplasia of left depressor anguli oris muscle.[670]

Pathogenesis and Etiology

The pathogenesis is unclear. The possibility of an inherited defect was suggested by reports of familial occurrence with autosomal dominant characteristics.[666] This defect is readily overlooked unless family members are specifically examined for the lesion. Moreover, the occurrence in one family of a mother and two children with aplasia or hypoplasia of different muscles (including the depressor anguli oris; see previous section) further supports the possibility of autosomal dominant inheritance with variable expression. In Cayler syndrome, 94% of probands have a de novo deletion of 22q11.2, and 6% have inherited the deletion from a parent.[676,683] Thus fluorescent in situ hybridization analysis should be carried out on patients with asymmetrical crying facies and cardiac anomalies, and the parents' karyotypes should be evaluated if a deletion is found in the infant.

Management

Management is essentially based on ensuring that no other major congenital anomaly is present. An abdominal ultrasound scan to look for a visceral anomaly or neuroblastoma may also be appropriate.

Vocal Cord Paralysis

Vocal cord paralysis, or so-called *laryngeal paralysis*, is a relatively common neonatal disorder.[684-688] Most descriptions of clinical features, etiology, natural history, and therapy are contained in

the literature on otolaryngology; surprisingly few descriptions are contained in the pediatric literature. Data for newborn patients, distinct from older patients, are difficult to obtain, but a reasonable synthesis of current information follows.

Clinical Features

The major presenting signs are stridor, which is inspiratory, and crowing and are present in approximately 70% of cases. Severe airway obstruction with a need for immediate intubation occurs in approximately 45% of affected infants. Dysphonia, notable with crying, dysphagia, and aspiration, is less common. Approximately 40% to 50% of cases are unilateral; when unilateral, the left side is affected in 80% to 90% of cases. The course of the disorder relates largely to cause (see the section on pathogenesis and etiology, which follows). The diagnosis is established by laryngoscopy.

Pathology

The anatomical locus of the pathology is diverse, although few precise data are available. Consideration of probable causes (Table 33.9) suggests that disease at several levels of the neuraxis may be responsible, and levels vary from bilateral upper motor neuron, cranial nuclear (nucleus ambiguus), cranial nerve root (vagal nerve roots), and peripheral nerve (vagus nerve and laryngeal branches).

Pathogenesis and Etiology

The major causes of vocal cord paralysis in the newborn are shown in Table 33.9. Most commonly, no clear cause is apparent. Most such cases resolve spontaneously over a period of weeks or months.[684] Chiari type 2 malformation associated with myelomeningocele accounts for approximately 20% of

TABLE 33.9	Etiology of Vocal Cord Paralysis in the Newborn[a]
CAUSE	**PERCENTAGE OF TOTAL**
Unknown	35
Chiari type 2 malformation with myelomeningocele	20
Associated with miscellaneous neurological disorders	20
Associated with laryngeal anomalies	10
Birth trauma	10
Other	5

[a]Based on 208 cases.
Data from Holinger LD, Holinger PC, Holinger PH. Etiology of bilateral abductor vocal cord paralysis: a review of 389 cases. *Ann Otol Rhinol Laryngol.* 1976;85:428–436; and Cohen SR, Birns JW, Geller KA, Thompson JW. Laryngeal paralysis in children: a long-term retrospective study. *Ann Otol Rhinol Laryngol.* 1982;91:417–424.

cases. In these patients, the syndrome most often evolves several weeks after birth, after correction of the myelomeningocele, in association with the development of hydrocephalus with intracranial hypertension. Vocal cord paralysis often improves after placement of a ventriculoperitoneal shunt and is presumably related to the deformation of the lower brain stem (see Chapter 1). Approximately 20% of infants with vocal cord paralysis have miscellaneous neurological disorders (e.g., cerebral developmental anomalies and Möbius syndrome), which appear to account for the paralysis (see Table 33.9). The 10% of affected infants with associated laryngeal anomalies presumably have a developmental disturbance of the peripheral neuromuscular apparatus in the larynx. The infants with birth trauma usually exhibit signs earliest (i.e., in the first days of life[685]). The likelihood of recovery is good (see Chapter 36). Among other causes worthy of note are the association of unilateral vocal cord paralysis with congenital heart defects complicated by pulmonary hypertension and presumed compression of the recurrent laryngeal nerve by the enlarged, tense pulmonary artery *(cardiovocal syndrome or Ortner syndrome).*[689,690] Injury to the recurrent laryngeal nerve, vagus nerve, or both in association with the neck dissection required for the institution of extracorporeal membrane oxygenation has been reported in approximately 3% of infants undergoing this procedure.[686] In this circumstance, the paralysis is on the right side (i.e., the side of the dissection), unlike the predominantly left-sided paralysis in most cases of unilateral vocal cord paralysis (see earlier discussion). Familial cases are rare, but autosomal dominant, X-linked recessive and autosomal recessive examples have been observed.[688]

Management

Unilateral paralysis generally requires no treatment; even when recovery does not occur, compensation by the normal vocal cord allows adequate phonation. Bilateral paralysis requires very close surveillance. An artificial airway should be placed if ventilatory compromise appears imminent. Infants with bilateral vocal cord paralysis may die unexpectedly, particularly if the lesion is taken lightly. A need for long-term tracheostomy is not unusual.

Congenital Isolated Pharyngeal Dysfunction
Clinical Features

Severe impairment of swallowing in a newborn is life-threatening. Causes of such impairment include structural malformations of the nasal-oral cavity (e.g., choanal atresia, cleft palate), esophageal or tracheoesophageal anomalies (e.g., tracheoesophageal fistula, esophageal stenosis, aberrant vessels related to the aortic arch), and a variety of neurological disorders (e.g., bilateral cerebral disorder, Chiari type II malformation, Möbius syndrome, myasthenia, merosin-deficient CMD, myotonic dystrophy, nemaline myopathy, myotubular myopathy). Nearly all the neurological disorders are characterized by other, generally obvious neurological abnormalities. However, one striking defect (i.e., congenital isolated pharyngeal dysfunction) is confined to the pharyngeal musculature. Approximately 30 cases have been reported,[680,691-694] but the disorder may frequently be overlooked. Approximately half of all reported cases have involved premature infants. Because the disorder is transient, with spontaneous recovery reported in 2 to 40 months, it is crucial to recognize its presence and to institute measures to prevent aspiration and pneumonia, which have resulted in the death of several of the reported infants.

The usual presentation is the development of cyanosis and respiratory distress at the first attempts at feeding. The neurological examination is entirely unremarkable except for the total lack of spontaneous or elicited movements of the pharyngeal muscles and soft palate. Video fluoroscopy of swallowing demonstrates a normal oral propulsive phase but no pharyngeal movement and passive aspiration of contrast medium into the trachea. MRI has revealed no abnormality. The EMG of pharyngeal muscles has been normal.

Pathology

Careful study of the brain-stem nuclei crucial for swallowing (e.g., nucleus ambiguus, dorsal nucleus of the vagus, nuclei of cranial nerves V, X, and XII, nucleus of the tractus solitarius, and adjacent ventromedian reticular formation in the medulla) has revealed no abnormality. Moreover, no abnormality of other central structures, cranial nerves, or muscles has been detected.

Pathogenesis and Etiology

The basic nature of congenital isolated pharyngeal dysfunction is unclear. An abnormality in the functioning of the nucleus ambiguus appears most likely. The abnormality may be at the receptor level, as shown by Kinney and co-workers in the arcuate nucleus of the ventral medulla in sudden infant death syndrome.[694]

Management

Cessation of attempts at oral feeding and institution of nasogastric tube feedings are crucial. We recommend a period of observation of at least 3 to 6 months with a nasogastric tube before placement of a gastrostomy or jejunostomy tube because more than half of all affected infants, especially premature infants, recover within 6 months. Clinical improvement precedes radiological improvement; thus follow-up studies with barium swallow or video fluoroscopy may not provide an early indication of recovery.[694]

Congenital Torticollis

Clinical Features

Congenital torticollis is characterized by contracture of the sternocleidomastoid muscle, with resultant lateral flexion of the neck toward the lesion and slight rotation of the neck with the chin away from the side of the lesion.[4,696-703] The prominent feature of the syndrome is the head tilt. In association with the tilt of the head, asymmetries of the face and skull usually evolve and include flattening of the face and ear on the side of the lesion and flattening of the occiput on the opposite side (the side of contact of the skull with the bed; see Chapter 9). The rhomboidal skull (i.e., plagiocephaly) usually improves spontaneously with rapid brain and skull growth in the first 5 to 6 months of life if active motility and physical therapy supervene. Most infants can hold the head in the midline position after several weeks.[704] Only occasionally do patients have localized swelling of the sternocleidomastoid muscle in the neonatal period, but this fusiform mass, when present, may be quite prominent after 2 to 4 weeks. Although the mass is not usually apparent in the newborn, ultrasonography reveals findings consistent with fibrosis.[702] The mass usually disappears gradually by approximately 6 to 8 months of age. In the neonatal period, the muscle often appears shortened, may feel fibrous, and may resist stretch.

Pathology

The anatomical locus of the disease is usually confined to the sternocleidomastoid muscle, although occasionally the deep cervical muscles and trapezius appear to be involved (manifested by retraction of the head and elevation of the shoulder). The pathological features consist of fibrotic replacement of muscle tissue, but the remaining muscle appears normal.

Pathogenesis and Etiology

The pathogenesis of the disorder in previous years was considered most often to be hemorrhage within the muscle with subsequent fibrosis, but no histological proof of hemorrhage exists. The cause of such hemorrhage is not clear, although birth trauma is often cited. In a study of 311 infants, among those who presented within the first 6 weeks of life with a sternomastoid mass ($n = 195$), 52% had a history of breech presentation, forceps delivery, or vacuum extraction.[703] In another study of 510 infants, the infants with the most severe degree of torticollis had been born after breech presentation in 25% and after "vacuum extraction/forceps delivery" in 41%.[701] However, trauma is often difficult to document, and Eng[696] suggests that any difficulties observed with delivery relate to the already established intrauterine deformity secondarily disturbing engagement of the head during labor. This possibility could underlie the high frequency of breech presentations reported. In a careful study of 34 patients with congenital torticollis, good evidence indicated that the deformity resulted from *aberrant intrauterine positioning* in 29%, and evidence was suggestive in an additional 41%.[704] Further support for intrauterine constraint as the major cause of congenital torticollis is derived from a well-studied infant born to a mother with a large uterine leiomyoma.[705] Hemorrhage into the sternocleidomastoid from vascular anomaly may account for the 18% of infants with congenital torticollis with cavernous hemangioma of face and neck in one series.[704]

Management

Management consists of physical therapy, with emphasis on two basic exercises: (1) stretching of the clavicular portion of the sternocleidomastoid muscle by lateral flexion of the head to the opposite side and (2) stretching of the sternal portion of the muscle by rotation of the chin toward the affected side. Performance of the exercises in the prone position is easier than in the supine position and is preferable.[4] Active stretching exercises may be tolerated more readily than the passive stretching exercises just described; the former exercises involve encouraging the infant to rotate the neck to bottle or breast (when the infant's shoulders are stabilized) through visual cues of the nipple or bottle and the rooting reflex.[704] Faithful physical therapy is successful in preventing facial and skull deformities and in relieving the contracture in most cases. In one large series ($n = 311$), 95% of infants experienced total resolution by 6.5 months.[703] Early onset of physical therapy with manual stretching, applied before 3 to 6 months, is important and appears to result in a generally good outcome.[706,707] Rarely, botulinum toxin (Botox) injections maybe considered. Neglected patients may require tenotomy and develop deformities. Plagiocephaly that persists after 5 to 6 months can be improved markedly by fitting the infant with an individualized plastic helmet to redirect head growth over approximately the next 6 months (see Chapter 9).[704] In a recent study, however, patients with thicker affected sternocleidomastoid muscles, lower birth weight, and breech presentation required longer rehabilitation.[708]

Isolated Diaphragmatic Myopathy

Although most examples of isolated diaphragmatic paralysis in the newborn are related to trauma (see Chapter 36) or aplasia, at least one case has been described in which a disorder of muscle appeared to be restricted to the diaphragm.[709] The infant exhibited respiratory distress with excessive movement of the ribs but no movement of the diaphragm. The EMG and the serum CK level were normal. Plication of the diaphragm was attempted at 2 months of age, but the infant died at 3 months. At postmortem examination, no abnormality of anterior horn cells, spinal nerve roots, or phrenic nerves could be found. Histological examination of a variety of peripheral muscles was normal. However, the diaphragm, which was very atrophic, exhibited marked random variation in fiber size and degenerating and necrotic muscle fibers. The findings were compatible with a myopathic process. Seven similar cases have recently been described. The possibility of myopathy restricted to the diaphragm should thus be considered in infants with respiratory distress secondary to diaphragmatic dysfunction.

Congenital Central Hypoventilation Syndrome

Congenital central hypoventilation syndrome (CCHS), or *Ondine's curse*, is a disorder of ventilation, particularly during sleep, and is categorized here because the syndrome is manifested as a restricted defect of a motor function. However, the essential defect involves a critical *afferent* component of the ventilatory system rather than of the neuromuscular apparatus per se. Many cases have been recorded in the literature.[710-736]

Clinical Features

The essential *clinical features* are as follows: (1) decreased ventilatory drive during sleep, with an impaired response to hypercarbia and hypoxemia, and (2) no recognizable disease of brain stem (e.g., myelomeningocele), spinal cord (e.g., traumatic transection), or cardiopulmonary system to account for the ventilatory defect. Most patients present in the first days of life with the respiratory disturbance (i.e., hypoventilation), apnea with cyanosis, or both, particularly during sleep. Blood gas studies confirm the presence of hypoxemia and hypercarbia. The respiratory disturbance is most apparent during quiet (non–rapid eye movement [REM]) sleep, when the ventilatory drive is most dependent on the response of medullary chemoreceptors to carbon dioxide. This basic defect of unresponsiveness of medullary chemoreceptors to carbon dioxide, however, is also often apparent in these infants during REM sleep. Indeed, some patients also hypoventilate during wakefulness.

Associated abnormalities have included Hirschsprung disease in at least 20% of cases and ganglioneuroblastoma or neuroblastoma in approximately 5%. Indeed CCHS, Hirschsprung disease, and neural crest–derived tumors constitute the major neurocristopathies (see later). Associated disturbances of swallowing—sometimes preceded by polyhydramnios, sensorineural hearing loss, and various ocular abnormalities (e.g., ptosis, pupillary dilation)—occur in a distinct minority of infants. In addition, careful studies of heart rate variability delineated abnormalities in all 12 cases in a series.[730] These findings enhance the notion of a disturbance in derivatives of the neural crest (i.e., autonomic neurons, sensory neurons, adrenal medullary neurons).

The relationship of the ventilatory syndrome with Hirschsprung disease is an excellent example of this common pathogenesis, and the combination probably accounts for more cases than previously suspected.[731] Indeed, CCHS complicates 1.5% of all cases of Hirschsprung disease and fully 10% of *severe* cases with total colonic aganglionosis. Approximately 15% to 20% of patients with CCHS and Hirschsprung disease have an associated neuroblastoma or ganglioneuroblastoma.[731]

Diagnosis

The diagnosis is established by the characteristic clinical features and by documentation of the ventilatory abnormalities and resulting blood gas derangements. In contrast to the lack of responsiveness of medullary chemoreceptors to carbon dioxide, the ventilatory response to oxygen through peripheral chemoreceptors is normal. Detailed evaluation to rule out structural disease of brain stem, spinal cord, phrenic nerves, diaphragm, intercostal muscles, and cardiopulmonary system is important. A search for neuroblastoma or ganglioneuroblastoma is also appropriate. Any suggestion of gastrointestinal dysfunction should lead to rectal biopsy to evaluate the possibility of Hirschsprung disease. Functional MRI studies have shown deficits in pontomedullary regions.[737] Neurodevelopmental testing (Bayley) has indicated cognitive impairment in preschool-aged children with CCHS.[738]

Etiology

Pathological studies in general have demonstrated no consistent abnormalities. In a few cases, an ill-defined decrease in the number of medullary neurons or medullary gliosis has been noted. Recently, in two lethal neonatal cases with confirmed polyalanine repeat expansion (PARM) or non-PARM (PHOX2BΔ8) mutations in PHOX2b, neuronal losses were noted within the locus coeruleus, a finding that suggests dysregulation of central noradrenergic signaling in CCHS.[739]

Molecular genetic studies have clarified the *etiology* of the disorder. Thus the gene involved is *PHOX2B* (a homeobox gene), which is crucial in the development of all autonomic neural crest derivatives. Although most cases are related to sporadic de novo mutations, the heterozygous genetic defect behaves as an autosomal dominant. *PHOX2B* is involved in Hirschsprung disease and in neuroblastoma. A novel heterozygous deletion mutation in the *PHOX2B* gene has been identified in a 1-day-old infant with CCHS, Hirschsprung disease, and neuroblastoma.[740]

Management

Management must begin with prompt detection and careful surveillance. It is important to correct both the hypoxemia and the hypercarbia to prevent the development of pulmonary hypertension and cor pulmonale. Treatment has commonly consisted of *mechanical ventilation*, particularly during sleep. *Diaphragmatic pacing* by stimulation of phrenic nerves has improved treatment while allowing the patient normal mobility and the parents convenient management at home. The apparatus consists of an external radiofrequency transmitter, a subcutaneously implanted receiver to convert the radio frequency signal to an electrical current, and a stimulatory electrode on the phrenic nerve.[720,727,741] The effectiveness of this approach has been improved by using bilateral rather than unilateral pacing, by minimizing electrical injury to the phrenic nerve, and by using pacing only when necessary (e.g., during sleep) rather than continuously.[a] In the largest experience with diaphragmatic pacing, emphasis was placed on the complementary roles of phrenic nerve pacing and intermittent positive pressure ventilation; the latter was used in patients with superimposed respiratory illness or inadequate ventilation while awake as well as asleep.

DISTINGUISHING FEATURES OF DISORDERS OF THE MOTOR SYSTEM

Definition of the anatomical level of the abnormality and of the likely pathology in neonatal disorders of the motor system is possible when one keeps in mind the relatively few distinguishing features (Table 33.10). Thus the levels to be defined include those above the lower motor neuron (i.e., central), the anterior horn cell, the peripheral nerve, the neuromuscular junction, and the muscle. Distinguishing clinical features include the pattern of weakness, the activity of tendon reflexes, the presence of fasciculations or sensory loss, CSF findings, the level of muscle enzymes in serum, the pattern on the EMG, nerve conduction velocities, and the histological appearance of the muscle biopsy (or, less commonly, nerve biopsy).

Disorders related to *central* causes (e.g., hypoxic-ischemic encephalopathy) are characterized by weakness of limbs (degree of weakness usually less striking than degree of hypotonia), relatively preserved tendon reflexes (which become hyperactive after the first months of life), and absence of fasciculations or abnormalities on examination of CSF, serum enzymes, EMG,

---

[a]References 713, 715, 718, 720, 722, and 727.

TABLE 33.10 Distinguishing Features of Disorders of the Motor System

| LOCUS OF LESION | WEAKNESS | | | | DEEP TENDON REFLEXES | EMG | MUSCLE BIOPSY | OTHER |
	FACE	ARMS	LEGS	PROXIMAL–DISTAL				
Central	0	+	+	> or =	Normal or increased	Normal	Normal	Seizures, hemiparesis, and delayed development
Anterior horn cell	Late Tongue fasciculations	+++	++++	> or =	0	Neuropathic pattern and fibrillations	Denervation pattern	Fasciculations (tongue)
Peripheral nerve	0	+++	+++	<	Decreased	Neuropathic pattern and fibrillations	Denervation pattern	Sensory deficit, elevated cerebrospinal fluid protein, abnormal nerve conduction studies, abnormal nerve biopsy
Neuromuscular junction	+++	+++	+++	=	Normal	Decremental response (myasthenia); incremental response and BSAP (botulism)	Normal	Response to neostigmine or edrophonium (myasthenia); constipation and fixed pupils (botulism)
Muscle	Variable (+ to ++++)	++	+	>	Decreased	BSAP and myopathic polyphasic potentials	Myopathic pattern[a]	Elevated muscle enzyme levels (variable)

[a]May also show unique features, such as in central core disease, nemaline myopathy, myotubular myopathy, congenital fiber type disproportion, and multiminicore disease.

+ to ++++, Varying degrees of severity; *BSAP,* brief-duration, small-amplitude motor unit potentials; *EMG,* electromyography.

nerve conduction velocities, and muscle biopsy. Other indicators of central disease (e.g., seizures, hemiparesis, and developmental failure) are important to identify. Disease of the *anterior horn cell (especially spinal muscular atrophy type I or Werdnig-Hoffmann disease)* is characterized by generalized weakness, *absent* reflexes, and *fasciculations* (especially of tongue) but normal sensory function and CSF examination; serum enzyme levels may be mildly elevated. The EMG shows fasciculations, fibrillations, and other signs of denervation, and muscle biopsy demonstrates marked panfascicular atrophy (only rarely type-grouping or grouped atrophy). Disease of *peripheral nerve* is characterized by weakness that often has a distal preponderance, depressed reflexes, *abnormal sensory examination, elevated CSF protein concentration*, and *abnormal nerve conduction studies*. Muscle biopsy demonstrates signs of denervation, and *nerve biopsy* usually shows hypomyelinative changes with or without onion-bulb formation. Disease of *neuromuscular junction* (e.g., myasthenia gravis) is characterized by weakness involving the *face* and, perhaps, *extraocular* muscles; but normal reflexes (usually), sensory function, CSF examination, and serum enzyme levels are present. The *EMG* reveals the characteristic decremental response to repetitive stimulation. In botulism, the absence of *pupillary* reactions and the presence of an incremental response (facilitation), the pattern of brief-duration, small-amplitude, overly abundant motor unit potentials, or both on the *EMG* are characteristic. Disease of *muscle* is characterized by weakness that often is greater in *proximal* limbs. Involvement of the *face* is prominent in several such disorders (e.g., myotonic dystrophy, CMDs, FSHD, CCD, nemaline myopathy, myotubular myopathy, congenital fiber-type disproportion, and COX deficiency [mitochondrial myopathy]). Tendon reflexes are depressed in proportion to the weakness and thus absent in very weak muscles; no fasciculations or sensory or CSF abnormalities are present. *Muscle enzyme* concentrations in serum may be elevated, although this often is not detectable in the slowly progressive disorders. The *EMG* exhibits myopathic changes and, perhaps, more distinctive abnormalities (e.g., myotonia). *Muscle biopsy* demonstrates myopathic changes and, in certain disorders, abnormalities that are diagnostic (e.g., central cores, rod bodies, myotubular fibers, disproportionate distribution and size of muscle fiber types, multiminicores, abnormal mitochondria, or accumulation of glycogen or lipid).

Thus, with the aforementioned distinguishing features in mind, the clinician should be able to define the level of the lesion in the neuromuscular apparatus that accounts for the hypotonia and weakness in the infant. This critical initial accomplishment usually leads rapidly to the correct pathological and etiological diagnosis. Appropriate therapeutic intervention, specific or nonspecific, then becomes a relatively straightforward next step.

KEY REFERENCES

2. Sarnat HB, O'Connor T, Byrne PA. Clinical effects of myotonic dystrophy on pregnancy and the neonate. *Arch Neurol.* 1976;33:459.
4. Dubowitz V. *Muscle Disorders in Childhood.* 2nd ed. London: WB Saunders; 1995.
5. Roig M, Balliu P-R, Navarro C, et al. Presentation, clinical course, and outcome of the congenital form of myotonic dystrophy. *Pediatr Neurol.* 1994;11:208-213.
8. Dodge PR, Gamstorp I, Byers RK, et al. Myotonic dystrophy in infancy and childhood. *Pediatrics.* 1965;35:3.

10. Dunn LJ, Dierker LI. Recurrent hydramnios in association with myotonia dystrophica. *Obstet Gynecol.* 1973;42:104.
22. Wesstrom G, Bensch J, Schollin J. Congenital myotonic dystrophy. *Acta Paediatr Scand.* 1986;75:849-854.
25. Campbell C, Sherlock R, Jacob P, et al. Congenital myotonic dystrophy: assisted ventilation duration and outcome. *Pediatrics.* 2004;113:811-816.
26. Echenne B, Rideau A, Roubertie A, et al. Myotonic dystrophy type I in childhood: long-term evolution in patients surviving the neonatal period. *Eur J Paediatr Neurol.* 2008;12:210-223.
31. Campbell C, Levin S, Siu VM, et al. Congenital myotonic dystrophy: Canadian population-based surveillance study. *J Pediatr.* 2013;163:120-125.e121-123.
44. Osborne JP, Murphy EG, Hill A. Thin ribs on chest X-ray: a useful sign in the differential diagnosis of the floppy newborn. *Dev Med Child Neurol.* 1983;25:343.
49. Kuo HC, Hsiao KM, Chen CJ, et al. Brain magnetic resonance image changes in a family with congenital and classic myotonic dystrophy. *Brain Dev.* 2005;27:291-296.
57. Rosman NP, Rebeiz JJ. The cerebral defect and myopathy in myotonic dystrophy. *Neurology.* 1976;17:1106.
61. Hunter A, Jacob P, Ohoy K, et al. Decrease in the size of the myotonic dystrophy CTG repeat during transmission from parent to child: implications for genetic counselling and genetic anticipation. *Am J Med Genet.* 1993;45:401-407.
68. Aslanidis C, Jansen G, Amemiya C, et al. Cloning of the essential myotonic dystrophy region and mapping of the putative defect. *Nature.* 1992;355:548-551.
74. Udd B, Krahe R. The myotonic dystrophies: molecular, clinical, and therapeutic challenges. *Lancet Neurol.* 2012;11:891-905.
76. Angeard N, Jacquette A, Gargiulo M, et al. A new window on neurocognitive dysfunction in the childhood form of myotonic dystrophy type 1 (DM1). *Neuromuscul Disord.* 2011;21:468-476.
78. Ekstrom AB, Hakenas-Plate L, Samuelsson L, et al. Autism spectrum conditions in myotonic dystrophy type 1: a study on 57 individuals with congenital and childhood forms. *Am J Med Genet B Neuropsychiatr Genet.* 2008;147B:918-926.
81. Lueck JD, Mankodi A, Swanson MS, et al. Muscle chloride channel dysfunction in two mouse models of myotonic dystrophy. *J Gen Physiol.* 2007;129:79-94.
84. Keller C, Reynolds A, Lee B, et al. Congenital myotonic dystrophy requiring prolonged endotracheal and noninvasive assisted ventilation: not a uniformly fatal condition. *Pediatrics.* 1998;101:704-706.
87. Bonnemann CG. Congenital muscular dystrophy. In: Squire LR, ed. *Encyclopedia of Neuroscience.* Oxford: Academic Press; 2009:67-74.
95. Topaloglu H, Yalaz K, Renda Y, et al. Occidental type cerebromuscular dystrophy: a report of eleven cases. *J Neurol Neurosurg Psychiatry.* 1991;54:226-229.
109. Voit T. Congenital muscular dystrophies: 1997 update. *Brain Dev.* 1998;20:65-74.
114. Caro PA, Scavina M, Hoffman E, et al. MR imaging findings in children with merosin-deficient congenital muscular dystrophy. *AJNR Am J Neuroradiol.* 1999;20:324-326.
116. Philpot J, Cowan F, Pennock J, et al. Merosin-deficient congenital muscular dystrophy: the spectrum of brain involvement on magnetic resonance imaging. *Neuromuscul Disord.* 1999;9:81-85.
122. Mercuri E, Muntoni F, et al. Congenital muscular dystrophy. In: Darras BT, Jones HR Jr, Ryan MM, eds. *Neuromuscular Disorders of Infancy, Childhood and Adolescence: A Clinician's Approach.* 2nd ed. San Diego: Academic Press; 2015:538-550.
123. Philpot J, Muntoni F. Limitation of eye movement in merosin-deficient congenital muscular dystrophy. *Lancet.* 1999;353:297-298.
125. Tachi N, Kamimura S, Ohya K, et al. Congenital muscular dystrophy with partial deficiency of merosin. *J Neurol Sci.* 1997;151:25-27.
129. Geranmayeh F, Clement E, Feng LH, et al. Genotype-phenotype correlation in a large population of muscular dystrophy patients with LAMA2 mutations. *Neuromuscul Disord.* 2010;20:241-250.
132. Ishikawa H, Sugie K, Murayama K, et al. Ullrich disease due to deficiency of collagen VI in the sarcolemma. *Neurology.* 2004;62:620-623.

134. Baker NL, Morgelin M, Peat R, et al. Dominant collagen VI mutations are a common cause of Ullrich congenital muscular dystrophy. *Hum Mol Genet.* 2005;14:279-293.

137. Pepe G, Lucarini L, Zhang RZ, et al. COL6A1 genomic deletions in Bethlem myopathy and Ullrich muscular dystrophy. *Ann Neurol.* 2006;59:190-195.

138. Nadeau A, Kinali M, Main M, et al. Natural history of Ullrich congenital muscular dystrophy. *Neurology.* 2009;73:25-31.

142. Quijano-Roy S, Mbieleu B, Bonnemann CG, et al. De novo LMNA mutations cause a new form of congenital muscular dystrophy. *Ann Neurol.* 2008;64:177-186.

143. Bonati U, Bechtel N, Heinimann K, et al. Congenital muscular dystrophy with dropped head phenotype and cognitive impairment due to a novel mutation in the LMNA gene. *Neuromuscul Disord.* 2014;24:529-532.

144. Komaki H, Hayashi YK, Tsuburaya R, et al. Inflammatory changes in infantile-onset LMNA-associated myopathy. *Neuromuscul Disord.* 2011;21:563-568.

146. Godfrey C, Clement E, Mein R, et al. Refining genotype phenotype correlations in muscular dystrophies with defective glycosylation of dystroglycan. *Brain.* 2007;130:2725-2735.

147. Fukuyama Y, Osawa M, Suzuki H. Congenital progressive muscular dystrophy of the Fukuyama type-clinical, genetic and pathological considerations. *Brain Dev.* 1981;3:1.

160. Banker BQ. The congenital muscular dystrophies. In: Engel AG, Franzini-Armstrong C, eds. *Myology.* New York: McGraw-Hill;1994.

163. Aida N, Tamagawa K, Takada K, et al. Brain MR in Fukuyama congenital muscular dystrophy. *AJNR Am J Neuroradiol.* 1996;17:605-613.

174. Santavuori P, Somer H, Sainio K, et al. Muscle-eye-brain diseae (MEB). *Brain Dev.* 1989;1989:147-153.

176. Leyten QH, Renkawek K, Reiner WO, et al. Neuropathological findings in muscle-eye-brain disease (MEB-D). *Acta Neuropathol.* 1991;83:55-60.

181. Wewer UM, Durkin ME, Zhang X, et al. Laminin β2 chain and adhalin deficiency in the skeletal muscle of Walker-Warburg syndrome (cerebro-ocular dysplasia—muscular dystrophy). *Neurology.* 1995;45:2099-2101.

183. Warburg M. Muscle-eye brain disease and Wlaker-Warburg syndrome: phenotype-genotype speculations. Commentary to Pihko's paper (pp. 57-61). *Brain Dev.* 1995;17:62-63.

189. Vervoort VS, Holden KR, Ukadike KC, et al. POMGnT1 gene alterations in a family with neurological abnormalities. *Ann Neurol.* 2004;56:143-148.

191. Topaloglu H, Brockington M, Yuva Y, et al. *FKRP* gene mutations cause congenital muscular dystrophy, mental retardation, and cerebellar cysts. *Neurology.* 2003;60:988-992.

193. Mercuri E, Topaloglu H, Brockington M, et al. Spectrum of brain changes in patients with congenital muscular dystrophy and FKRP gene mutations. *Arch Neurol.* 2006;63:251-257.

198. Mercuri E, Rutherford M, DeVile C, et al. Early white matter changes on brain magnetic resonance imaging in a newborn affected by merosin-deficient congenital muscular dystrophy. *Neuromuscul Disord.* 2001;11:297-299.

204. Tsao C-Y, Mendell JR, Rusin J, et al. Congenital muscular dystrophy with complete laminin-α2-deficiency, cortical dysplasia, and cerebral white-matter changes in children. *J Child Neurol.* 1998;13:253-256.

209. Shorer Z, Philpot J, Muntoni F, et al. Demyelinating peripheral neuropathy in merosin-deficient congenital muscular dystrophy. *J Child Neurol.* 1995;10:472-475.

219. Pegararo E, Mancias P, Swerdlow SH, et al. Congenital muscular dystrophy with primary laminin α2 (merosin) deficiency presenting as inflammatory myopathy. *Ann Neurol.* 1996;40:782-791.

221. Takada K, Nakamura H, Tanaka J. Cortical dysplasia in congenital muscular dystrophy with central nervous system involvement (Fukuyama type). *J Neuropathol Exp Neurol.* 1984;43:395.

224. Itoh M, Houdou S, Kawahara H, et al. Morphological study of the brainstem in Fukuyama type congenital muscular dystrophy. *Pediatr Neurol.* 1996;15:327-331.

227. Saito Y, Mizuguchi M, Oka A, et al. Fukutin protein is expressed in neurons of the normal developing human brain but is reduced in Fukuyama-type congenital muscular dystrophy brain. *Ann Neurol.* 2000;47:756-764.

229. Yamamoto T, Kato Y, Kawaguchi M, et al. Expression and localization of fukutin, POMGnT1, and POMT1 in the central nervous system: consideration for functions of fukutin. *Med Electron Microsc.* 2004;37:200-207.

231. Muntoni F, Sewry CA. Congenital muscular dystrophy. *Neurology.* 1998;51:14-16.

233. Arbogast S, Beuvin M, Fraysse B, et al. Oxidative stress in SEPN1-related myopathy: from pathophysiology to treatment. *Ann Neurol.* 2009;65:677-686.

234. Biancheri R, Bertini E, Falace A, et al. POMGnT1 mutations in congenital muscular dystrophy: genotype-phenotype correlation and expanded clinical spectrum. *Arch Neurol.* 2006;63:1491-1495.

235. Messina S, Mora M, Pegoraro E, et al. POMT1 and POMT2 mutations in CMD patients: a multicentric Italian study. *Neuromuscul Disord.* 2008;18:565-571.

236. Liew WKM, van der Maarel SM, Tawil R, et al. Facioscapulohumeral dystrophy. In: Darras BT, Jones HR Jr, Ryan MM, eds. *Neuromuscular Disorders of Infancy, Childhood and Adolescence: A Clinician's Approach.* 2nd ed. San Diego: Academic Press; 2015:620-630.

237. Carroll JE, Brooke MH. Infantile facioscapulohumeral dystrophy. In: Serratrice G, Roux TH, eds. *Peroneal Atrophies and Related Disorders.* Vol 305. New York: Masson; 1979.

239. Korf BR, Bresnan MJ, Shapiro F. Facioscapulohumeral dystrophy presenting in infancy with facial diplegia and sensorineural deafness. *Ann Neurol.* 1985;17:513.

242. Tawil R, Forrester J, Griggs RC, et al. Evidence for anticipation and association of deletion size with severity in facioscapulohumeral muscular dystrophy. The FSH-DY Group. *Ann Neurol.* 1996;39:744-748.

244. Okinaga A, Matsuoka T, Umeda J, et al. Early-onset facioscapulohumeral muscular dystrophy: two case reports. *Brain Dev.* 1997;19:563-567.

245. Statland JM, Tawil R. Facioscapulohumeral muscular dystrophy. *Continuum (Minneap Minn).* 2016;22(6, Muscle and Neuromuscular Junction Disorders):1916-1931.

248. Klinge L, Eagle M, Haggerty ID, et al. Severe phenotype in infantile facioscapulohumeral muscular dystrophy. *Neuromuscul Disord.* 2006;16:553-558.

249. Nikolic A, Ricci G, Sera F, et al. Clinical expression of facioscapulohumeral muscular dystrophy in carriers of 1-3 D4Z4 reduced alleles: experience of the FSHD Italian National Registry. *BMJ Open.* 2016;6:e007798.

250. Dubowitz V. *The Floppy Infant.* Philadelphia: JB Lippincott; 1980.

251. Bindoff LA, Mjellem N, Sommerfelt K, et al. Severe facioscapulohumeral muscular dystrophy presenting with Coats' disease and mental retardation. *Neuromuscul Disord.* 2006;16:559-563.

252. Funakoshi M, Goto K, Arahata K. Epilepsy and mental retardation in a subset of early onset 4q35-facioscapulohumeral muscular dystrophy. *Neurology.* 1998;50:1791-1794.

258. Scionti I, Greco F, Ricci G, et al. Large-scale population analysis challenges the current criteria for the molecular diagnosis of facioscapulohumeral muscular dystrophy. *Am J Hum Genet.* 2012;90:628-635.

259. Snider L, Asawachaicharn A, Tyler AE, et al. RNA transcripts, miRNA-sized fragments and proteins produced from D4Z4 units: new candidates for the pathophysiology of facioscapulohumeral dystrophy. *Hum Mol Genet.* 2009;18:2414-2430.

262. Lemmers RJ, van der Vliet PJ, Klooster R, et al. A unifying genetic model for facioscapulohumeral muscular dystrophy. *Science.* 2010;329:1650-1653.

263. Snider L, Geng LN, Lemmers RJ, et al. Facioscapulohumeral dystrophy: incomplete suppression of a retrotransposed gene. *PLoS Genet.* 2010;6:e1001181.

265. Lemmers RJ, Tawil R, Petek LM, et al. Digenic inheritance of an SMCHD1 mutation and an FSHD-permissive D4Z4 allele causes facioscapulohumeral muscular dystrophy type 2. *Nat Genet.* 2012;44:1370-1374.

266. Sacconi S, Lemmers RJ, Balog J, et al. The FSHD2 gene SMCHD1 is a modifier of disease severity in families affected by FSHD1. *Am J Hum Genet.* 2013;93:744-751.

268. Shevell M, Rosenblatt B, Silver K, et al. Congenital inflammatory myopathy. *Neurology.* 1990;40:1111-1114.

271. Vajsar J, Jay V, Babyn P. Infantile myositis presenting in the neonatal period. *Brain Dev.* 1996;18:415-419.

272. Nevo Y, Pestronk A. Neonatal perifascicular myopathy. *Pediatr Neurol.* 1996;15:150-152.

275. Jong YJ, Shishikura K, Aoyama M, et al. Nonspecific congenital myopathy (minimal change myopathy): a case report. *Brain Dev.* 1987;9:61-64.

284. Sewry CA, Wallgren-Pettersson C. Myopathology in congenital myopathies. *Neuropathol Appl Neurobiol.* 2017;43:5-23.

285. Dowling JJ, North KN, Goebel HH, et al. Congenital and other structural myopathies. In: Darras BT, Jones HR Jr, Ryan MM, et al., eds. *Neuromuscular Disorders of Infancy, Childhood, and Adolescence: A Clinician's Approach.* 2nd ed. San Diego: Academic Press; 2015:502-537.

286. North KN, Wang CH, Clarke N, et al. Approach to the diagnosis of congenital myopathies. *Neuromuscul Disord.* 2014;24:97-116.

293. Cohen ME, Duffner PK, Heffner R. Central core disease in one of identical twins. *J Neurol Neurosurg Psychiatry.* 1978;41:659.

297. Wu S, Ibarra MC, Malicdan MC, et al. Central core disease is due to RYR1 mutations in more than 90% of patients. *Brain.* 2006;129:1470-1480.

301. Ferreiro A, Monnier N, Romero NB, et al. A recessive form of central core disease, transiently presenting as multi-minicore disease, is associated with a homozygous mutation in the ryanodine receptor type 1 gene. *Ann Neurol.* 2002;51:750-759.

304. Jungbluth H, Sewry C, Brown SC, et al. Minicore myopathy in children: a clinical and histopathological study of 19 cases. *Neuromuscul Disord.* 2000;10:264-273.

306. Moghadaszadeh B, Petit N, Jaillard C, et al. Mutations in SEPN1 cause congenital muscular dystrophy with spinal rigidity and restrictive respiratory syndrome. *Nat Genet.* 2001;29:17-18.

310. Chauveau C, Bonnemann CG, Julien C, et al. Recessive TTN truncating mutations define novel forms of core myopathy with heart disease. *Hum Mol Genet.* 2014;23:980-991.

314. Karpati G, Carpenter S, Andermann F. A new concept of childhood nemaline myopathy. *Arch Neurol.* 1971;24:291.

321. Norton P, Ellison P, Sulaiman AR, et al. Nemaline myopathy in the neonate. *Neurology.* 1983;33:351.

324. Wallgren-Pettersson C. Congenital nemaline myopathy. A clinical follow-up study of twelve patients. *J Neurol Sci.* 1989;89:1-14.

326. Schmalbruch H, Kamieniecka Z, Arroe M. Early fatal nemaline myopathy: case report and review. *Dev Med Child Neurol.* 1987;29:784-804.

334. Van Antwerpen CL, Gospe SM, Dentinger MP. Nemaline myopathy associated with hypertrophic cardiomyopathy. *Pediatr Neurol.* 1988;4:306-308.

336. Laing NG, Majda BT, Akkari PA, et al. Assignment of a gene (NEMI) for autosomal dominant nemaline myopathy to chromosome-I. *Am J Hum Genet.* 1992;50:576-583.

345. North KN, Laing NG, Wallgren-Pettersson C, et al. Nemaline myopathy: current concepts. *J Med Genet.* 1997;34:705-713.

350. Ryan MM, Schnell C, Strickland CD, et al. Nemaline myopathy: a clinical study of 143 cases. *Ann Neurol.* 2001;50:312-320.

352. Ryan MM, Ilkovski B, Strickland CD, et al. Clinical course correlates poorly with muscle pathology in nemaline myopathy. *Neurology.* 2003;60:665-673.

358. Ennis J, Dyment DA, Michaud J, et al. Congenital nemaline myopathy: the value of magnetic resonance imaging of muscle. *Can J Neurol Sci.* 2015;42:338-340.

363. Park YE, Shin JH, Kang B, et al. NEB-related core-rod myopathy with distinct clinical and pathological features. *Muscle Nerve.* 2016;53:479-484.

366. Kawase K, Nishino I, Sugimoto M, et al. Hypoxic ischemic encephalopathy in a case of intranuclear rod myopathy without any prenatal sentinel event. *Brain Dev.* 2015;37:265-269.

368. Waisayarat J, Suriyonplengsaeng C, Khongkhatithum C, et al. Severe congenital nemaline myopathy with primary pulmonary lymphangiectasia: unusual clinical presentation and review of the literature. *Diagn Pathol.* 2015;10:27.

371. Yuen M, Sandaradura SA, Dowling JJ, et al. Leiomodin-3 dysfunction results in thin filament disorganization and nemaline myopathy. *J Clin Invest.* 2015;125:456-457.

372. Spiro AJ, Shy GM, Gonatas NK. Myotubular myopathy. *Arch Neurol.* 1966;14:1.

380. Barth PG, van Wijngaarden GK, Bethlem J. X-linked myotubular myopathy with fatal neonatal asphyxia. *Neurology.* 1975;25:531.

386. Sarnat HB, Roth SI, Jimenez JF. Neonatal myotubular myopathy: neuropathy and failure of postnatal maturation of fetal muscle. *Can J Neurol Sci.* 1981;8:313.

396. Wallgren-Pettersson C, Clarke A, Samson F, et al. The myotubular myopathies: differential diagnosis of the X linked recessive, autosomal dominant, and autosomal recessive forms and present state of DNA studies. *J Med Genet.* 1995;32:673-679.

406. Lawlor MW, Beggs AH, Buj-Bello A, et al. Skeletal muscle pathology in X-linked myotubular myopathy: review with cross-species comparisons. *J Neuropathol Exp Neurol.* 2016.

408. Das S, Dowling J, Pierson CR. X-linked centronuclear myopathy. In: Pagon RA, Adam MP, Ardinger HH, eds. *GeneReviews® [Internet].* Seattle, WA: University of Washington, Seattle, 1993–2016; 2002 Available from: http://www.ncbi.nlm.nih.gov/books/NBK1432/; Updated 06.10.11.

409. Fattori F, Maggi L, Bruno C, et al. Centronuclear myopathies: genotype-phenotype correlation and frequency of defined genetic forms in an Italian cohort. *J Neurol.* 2015;262:1728-1740.

427. Muranaka H, Osari S-I, Fujita H, et al. Congenital familial myopathy with type 2 fiber hypoplasia and type 1 fiber predominance. *Brain Dev.* 1997;19:362-365.

432. Clarke NF, North KN. Congenital fiber type disproportion—30 years on. *J Neuropathol Exp Neurol.* 2003;62:977-989.

437. Lawlor MW, Dechene ET, Roumm E, et al. Mutations of tropomyosin 3 (TPM3) are common and associated with type 1 myofiber hypotrophy in congenital fiber type disproportion. *Hum Mutat.* 2010;31:176-183.

438. Clarke NF, Kolski H, Dye DE, et al. Mutations in TPM3 are a common cause of congenital fiber type disproportion. *Ann Neurol.* 2008;63:329-337.

439. Munot P, Lashley D, Jungbluth H, et al. Congenital fibre type disproportion associated with mutations in the tropomyosin 3 (TPM3) gene mimicking congenital myasthenia. *Neuromuscul Disord.* 2010;20:796-800.

440. Clarke NF, Waddell LB, Cooper ST, et al. Recessive mutations in RYR1 are a common cause of congenital fiber type disproportion. *Hum Mutat.* 2010;31:E1544-E1550.

441. Kajino S, Ishihara K, Goto K, et al. Congenital fiber type disproportion myopathy caused by LMNA mutations. *J Neurol Sci.* 2014;340:94-98.

443. DeVivo DC. The expanding clinical spectrum of mitochondrial diseases. *Brain Dev.* 1993;15:1-22.

446. DiMauro S, Bonilla E, Zeviani M. Mitochondrial myopathies. *Ann Neurol.* 1985;17:521-538.

449. DiMauro S, Schon EA. Mechanisms of disease: mitochondrial respiratory-chain diseases. *N Engl J Med.* 2003;348:2657-2668.

450. Zeviani M, Di Donato S. Mitochondrial disorders. *Brain.* 2004;127:2153-2172.

452. De Vivo DC, Paradas C, DiMauro S, et al. Mitochondrial encephalomyopathies. In: Darras BT, Jones HRJ, Ryan MM, eds. *Neuromuscular Disorders of Infancy, Childhood and Adolescence: A Clinician's Approach.* 2nd ed. San Diego: Academic Press; 2015:796-833.

457. Saini AG, Singhi P. Infantile metabolic encephalopathy due to fumarase deficiency. *J Child Neurol.* 2013;28:535-537.

461. Heiman-Patterson TD, Bonilla E, DiMauro S. Cytochrome *c* oxidase deficiency in a floppy infant. *Neurology.* 1982;32:898.

464. DiMauro S, Nicholson JF, Hays AP. Benign infantile mitochondrial myopathy due to reversible cytochrome *c* oxidase deficiency. *Ann Neurol.* 1983;14:226.

473. Salo MK, Rapola J, Somer H, et al. Reversible mitochondrial myopathy with cytochrome *c* oxidase deficiency. *Arch Dis Child.* 1992;67:1033-1035.

481. Oldfors A, Sommerland H, Holme E, et al. Cytochrome *c* oxidase deficiency in infancy. *Acta Neuropathol.* 1989;77:267-275.

487. Rubio-Gozalbo ME, Smeitink JAM, Ruitenbeek W, et al. Spinal muscular atrophy-like picture, cardiomyopathy, and cytochrome *c* oxidase deficiency. *Neurology.* 1999;52:383-386.

497. Meulemans A, Lissens W, Coster RV, et al. Analysis of the mitochondrial encoded subunits of complex I in 20 patients with a complex I deficiency. *Eur J Paediatr Neurol.* 2004;8:299-306.

503. Galbiati S, Bordoni A, Papadimitriou D, et al. New mutations in TK2 gene associated with mitochondrial DNA depletion. *Pediatr Neurol.* 2006;34:177-185.

504. DiMauro S, Tanji K, Schon EA. The many clinical faces of cytochrome *c* oxidase deficiency. *Adv Exp Med Biol.* 2012; 748:341-357.

506. Uusimaa J, Jungbluth H, Fratter C, et al. Reversible infantile respiratory chain deficiency is a unique, genetically heterogenous mitochondrial disease. *J Med Genet.* 2011;48:660-668.

512. Pronicki M, Kowalski P, Piekutowska-Abramczuk D, et al. A homozygous mutation in the SCO2 gene causes a spinal muscular atrophy like presentation with stridor and respiratory insufficiency. *Eur J Paediatr Neurol.* 2010;14:253-260.

513. Zeharia A, Shaag A, Pappo O, et al. Acute infantile liver failure due to mutations in the TRMU gene. *Am J Hum Genet.* 2009; 85:401-407.

514. Horvath R, Kemp JP, Tuppen HA, et al. Molecular basis of infantile reversible cytochrome *c* oxidase deficiency myopathy. *Brain.* 2009;132:3165-3174.

515. Boczonadi V, Smith PM, Pyle A, et al. Altered 2-thiouridylation impairs mitochondrial translation in reversible infantile respiratory chain deficiency. *Hum Mol Genet.* 2013;22:4602-4615.

516. Mimaki M, Hatakeyama H, Komaki H, et al. Reversible infantile respiratory chain deficiency: a clinical and molecular study. *Ann Neurol.* 2010;68:845-854.

524. Chanprasert S, Wang J, Weng SW, et al. Molecular and clinical characterization of the myopathic form of mitochondrial DNA depletion syndrome caused by mutations in the thymidine kinase (TK2) gene. *Mol Genet Metab.* 2013;110:153-161.

525. Bornstein B, Area E, Flanigan KM, et al. Mitochondrial DNA depletion syndrome due to mutations in the RRM2B gene. *Neuromuscul Disord.* 2008;18:453-459.

528. Akman HO, Oldfors A, DiMauro S. Glycogen storage diseases of muscle. In: Darras BT, Jones HRJ, Ryan MM, et al., eds. *Neuromuscular Disorders of Infancy, Childhood and Adolescence: A Clinician's Approach.* 2nd ed. San Diego: Academic Press; 2015: 735-760.

538. Taratuto AL, Akman HO, Saccoliti M, et al. Branching enzyme deficiency/glycogenosis storage disease type IV presenting as a severe congenital hypotonia: muscle biopsy and autopsy findings, biochemical and molecular genetic studies. *Neuromuscul Disord.* 2010;20:783-790.

564. Tein I. Lipid storage myopathies due to fatty oxidation defects. In: Darras BT, Jones HRJ, Ryan MM, et al., eds. *Neuromuscular Disorders of Infancy, Childhood and Adolescence: A Clinician's Approach.* 2nd ed. San Diego: Academic Press; 2015:761-795.

575. Ryan MM, Engle EC. Disorders of the ocular motor cranial nerves and extraocular muscles. In: Darras BT, Jones HR Jr, Ryan MM, et al., eds. *Neuromuscular Disorders of Infancy, Childhood and Adolescence: A Clinician's Approach.* 2nd ed. San Diego: Academic Press; 2015:922-957.

588. Whitman MC, Andrews C, Chan WM, et al. Two unique TUBB3 mutations cause both CFEOM3 and malformations of cortical development. *Am J Med Genet A.* 2016;170:297-305.

600. Chan WM, Miyake N, Zhu-Tam L, et al. Two novel CHN1 mutations in 2 families with Duane retraction syndrome. *Arch Ophthalmol.* 2011;129:649-652.

610. MacKinnon S, Oystreck DT, Andrews C, et al. Diagnostic distinctions and genetic analysis of patients diagnosed with Moebius syndrome. *Ophthalmology.* 2014;121:1461-1468.

676. Rioja-Mazza D, Lieber E, Kamath V, et al. Asymmetric crying facies: a possible marker for congenital malformations. *J Matern Fetal Neonatal Med.* 2005;18:275-277.

680. Renault F, Quijano-Roy S. Congenital and acquired facial palsies. In: Darras BT, Jones HR Jr, Ryan MM, et al., eds. *Neuromuscular Disorders of Infancy, Childhood and Adolescence: A Clinician's Approach.* 2nd ed. San Diego: Academic Press; 2015.

706. Lee YT, Park JW, Lim M, et al. A clinical comparative study of ultrasound-normal versus ultrasound-abnormal congenital muscular torticollis. *PM R.* 2016;8:214-220.

739. Nobuta H, Cilio MR, Danhaive O, et al. Dysregulation of locus coeruleus development in congenital central hypoventilation syndrome. *Acta Neuropathol.* 2015;130:171-183.

740. Szymonska I, Borgenvik TL, Karlsvik TM, et al. Novel mutation-deletion in the PHOX2B gene of the patient diagnosed with Neuroblastoma, Hirschsprung's Disease, and Congenital Central Hypoventilation Syndrome (NB-HSCR-CCHS) Cluster. *J Genet Syndr Gene Ther.* 2015;6.

Full references for this chapter can be found on www.expertconsult .com.

UNIT IX

INTRACRANIAL INFECTIONS

Viral, Protozoan, and Related Intracranial Infections

Linda S. de Vries ◆ *Joseph J. Volpe*

The central nervous system (CNS) and its covering membranes may become involved in a variety of infectious processes, with devastating effects on structure and function. Infections may occur during intrauterine development, in association with the birth process, or in the first postnatal days or weeks. Microbial organisms implicated include several viruses, a protozoan *(Toxoplasma gondii)*, a spirochete *(Treponema pallidum)*, and numerous bacteria and fungi. In this and the following chapter, the major features of infections caused by these agents will be reviewed. Because some excellent sources review the microbiological aspects of these infections,[1] the emphasis of the following discussion is principally on the neurological, neuroimaging and neuropathological features.

In this chapter, infections of the CNS by viruses, *Toxoplasma*, and *Treponema* are reviewed. The major infections in this group are frequently designated by the term *TORCH syndrome*, in which *T* stands for toxoplasmosis, *O* is for others (i.e., syphilis and human immunodeficiency virus [HIV] infection), *R* is for rubella, *C* is for cytomegalovirus (CMV) infection, and *H* represents herpes simplex. We prefer the term *SCRATCHEZ*, in which *S* stands for syphilis, *C* is for CMV infection, *R* is for rubella, *A* is for acquired immunodeficiency syndrome (AIDS) or HIV infection, *T* is for toxoplasmosis, *C* is for chickenpox or varicella, *H* stands for herpes simplex, *ES* is for enterovirus (EV) infections, and *Z* stands for Zika virus. Some of the essential features of this group are described in Table 34.1. Most are examples of infection by transplacental passage of the microorganism, usually consequent to infection within the maternal bloodstream. Serious illness resulting from herpes simplex virus (HSV) infection is an exception to this rule, because most such cases are contracted around the time of birth, either as an ascending infection just before birth or during passage through an infected birth canal. HIV is transmitted to the fetus by both mechanisms; the relative importance is not entirely clear. With most infections within each group, patients are asymptomatic in the neonatal period, although the neonatal neurological syndromes that do occur are quite dramatic.

In addition to the TORCH group of microbes, infections caused by enterovirus, parechovirus (HPeV), parvovirus B19, rotavirus, varicella, lymphocytic choriomeningitis, mosquito-borne alphaviruses (West Nile, chikungunya), and flaviviruses (dengue virus and Zika virus [ZIKV]) may cause fetal or neonatal illness, with significant neurological consequences. The neonatal disorders caused by these organisms are reviewed after the discussion of the TORCH syndromes.

DESTRUCTIVE VERSUS TERATOGENIC EFFECTS

Although the mechanisms involved in the production of the neuropathological processes associated with these nonbacterial disorders are discussed in more detail in relation to specific infections, two different types of lesions can be distinguished. The first relates to *inflammatory, destructive effects* and the second to *developmental derangements* (i.e., *teratogenic effects*). It may be difficult to separate these two types of effects, because destructive processes affecting the developing brain often cause *coincident* tissue loss *and* subsequent anomalous development. The distinction is made still more difficult by the relatively limited capacity of early fetal brain to respond to injury; thus the neuropathologist, evaluating the brain later, finds it difficult to identify signs of parenchymal inflammation and destruction.

Although destructive and teratogenic effects overlap, and the precise quantitative contributions of each effect are not always clear, a separation of these two basic concepts is retained in this discussion. The recurring theme regarding destructive effects is varying degrees of inflammation, often with tissue injury (i.e., meningoencephalitis). Regarding teratogenic effects, the theme is more varied, although aberrations of neuronal proliferation and migration have been recognized. Defects in organizational events may be significant but require further study for documentation.

TORCH INFECTIONS

Cytomegalovirus Infection

CMV infection of the infant occurs in utero by transplacental mechanisms (congenital infection). CMV infection is the most common and serious congenital infection, with a higher prevalence in developing countries and among persons of lower socioeconomic status in developed nations. In the United States, approximately 35,000 to 45,000 infants with CMV infection are born yearly.[2,3] This number could increase in societies similar to the United States, where mothers with young children work and have their children in day care. Approximately 25% to 75% of such children acquire CMV infection, and 50% of all family members then acquire the infection from them.[3,4] By late adulthood, about 90% of individuals have experienced a CMV infection.[5] A substantial percentage of women of reproductive age are CMV-seronegative and thus at risk of primary CMV infection during pregnancy. Several

TABLE 34.1   Central Nervous System Involvement by the TORCH Group

ORGANISM OR DISEASE	MAJOR ROUTE OF INFECTION	USUAL TIME OF INFECTION[a]	NEONATAL NEUROLOGICAL ILLNESS	
			SYMPTOMATIC	ASYMPTOMATIC
Cytomegalovirus	Transplacental	T1, T2	+	++++
Herpes simplex	Ascending and/or parturitional	Birth	++++	+
Rubella	Transplacental	T1	++	+++
Toxoplasmosis	Transplacental	T1, T2	+	++++
Syphilis	Transplacental	T2, T3	+	++++
Human immunodeficiency virus	Transplacental/parturitional	T2, T3, birth	+	++++

[a]For occurrence of neonatal neurological disease; T1, T2, and T3 refer to the first, second, and third trimesters of gestation, respectively.

+, 0% to 25%; ++, 26% to 50%; +++, 51% to 75%; ++++, 76% to 100%; *TORCH: T,* toxoplasmosis; *O,* others (i.e., syphilis and human immunodeficiency virus); *R,* rubella; *C,* cytomegalovirus; *H,* herpes simplex.

studies support the provision of information concerning hygiene measures to prevent infection during pregnancy. For example, in one series, more than half (217 of 362, or 60%) of the pregnant women had heard of congenital CMV infection, and most of them (72%) knew the hygiene measures to use to prevent it. Knowledge was noted to depend on the hospital's policy concerning CMV infection information, the mother's educational level, parity, and employment in health care. When information was provided, 74% of the recipients exhibited some knowledge about congenital CMV infection, compared with only 34% when no information was given.[6] In a mixed interventional and observational controlled study, the effectiveness of hygiene information among pregnant women at risk for primary CMV infection was again shown.[7] Thus, when hygiene information was provided, seroconversion was observed significantly less often than when mothers did not receive specific hygiene information.

A minority (about 10%) of infants infected in utero exhibit overt neurological or systemic signs in the neonatal period, and most of these will develop important adverse neurological sequelae. About 10% to 15% of asymptomatic infants with a congenital CMV (cCMV) infection also develop sequelae, including especially sensorineural hearing loss (SNHL). Still larger numbers of infants acquire CMV infection at the time of birth, during passage through an infected birth canal, or in the first weeks of life through breast milk or, less commonly, through blood transfusion or other sources.[3,8-10] These infants appear to survive without serious neurological injury. Postnatally acquired CMV (pCMV) infection has also been reported in about 15% of very preterm infants and the majority of these infants do not develop serious neurological sequelae.[11-13]

Pathogenesis

Fetal Infection. Clinically significant infection with CMV occurs during intrauterine life by transplacental passage of the virus.[14,15] The organism is transmitted to the fetus usually during a primary maternal infection (less commonly during recurrent infection) with viremia and subsequent placentitis.[16] Recent data, however, suggest that maternal immunity before pregnancy cannot be viewed as protective in terms of altering long-term outcome and that the outcome of infants infected following primary and nonprimary infections is remarkably similar.[17] The maternal infection is usually asymptomatic but

TABLE 34.2   Cytomegalovirus Transmission Rates Before and During Pregnancy

Preconceptional	7/58 (12.1%)
Periconceptional	25/107 (23.3%)
First trimester	47/155 (30.3%)
Second trimester	43/115 (37.3%)
Third trimester	32/51 (62.7%)
Overall	154/486 (31.6%)

Data from references: Picone O, Vauloup-Fellous C, Cordier AG, et al. A series of 238 cytomegalovirus primary infections during pregnancy: description and outcome. *Prenat Diagn.* 2013;33:751-758; Enders G, Daiminger A, Bader U, et al. Intrauterine transmission and clinical outcome of 248 pregnancies with primary cytomegalovirus infection in relation to gestational age. *J Clin Virol.* 2011;52:244-246.

may be manifested by a mononucleosis-like illness (≈10%) or a more serious systemic illness. Maternal infection is very common; cytomegaloviruria occurs in 3% to 6% of unselected pregnant women.[18] Cervical CMV infection is several times more common than cytomegaloviruria but tends to occur late in pregnancy and is probably less likely to result in significant fetal infection. Clinically significant fetal CMV infection probably occurs principally in the first or second trimesters, particularly if CNS disease is the outcome measure.[14,19-21] The possibility of CNS involvement after CMV infection in the third trimester was suggested by a study of seven children but the exact timing of the fetal infection was established in only one case (at 27 weeks of gestation).[22] Moreover, the nature of the neuropathological features in some infected infants is also consistent with CNS involvement secondary to infection relatively late in pregnancy (see later discussion).[20,21,23]

Two recent studies evaluated intrauterine transmission rates following primary CMV infection in the pre- and periconceptional period, first, second, or third trimester in 248 and 238 pregnancies respectively (Table 34.2).[20,24] The overall transmission rates were very similar in both studies and significantly increased with the trimester of pregnancy, with the highest transmission rate in the third trimester. There was a significantly higher risk of *cranial ultrasound* abnormalities when maternal infection occurred during the preconceptional or periconceptional periods and the first trimester, compared with risk with infection acquired in later trimesters. No symptomatic neonatal infection was noted when maternal infection occurred after 14 weeks of gestation. Hearing loss developed in 5% to 10% of asymptomatic infants.

Approximately 30% to 40% of infants whose mothers experience primary infection during pregnancy develop congenital infection.[15,18,25,26] Cytomegaloviruria has been observed in approximately 0.5% to 2% of infants in the neonatal period.[2,27-30] Because a period of approximately 4 to 8 weeks is required between the time of infection and the viruria,[31] these neonatal examples reflect intrauterine infection and not perinatal acquisition from parturitional or postnatal exposure. In these cases of congenital CMV infection, involvement of the CNS may be overt in the neonatal period or may not become apparent for months or years thereafter (see later discussion). In a prospective series of more than 117,986 infants screened, the overall CMV birth prevalence estimate was 0.7%.[18] The percentage of infected children with CMV-specific symptoms at birth was 12.7%. The percentage of symptomatic children with permanent sequelae was 40% to 58%. The percentage of children without symptoms at birth who developed permanent sequelae was estimated to be 13.5%. The true burden of congenital CMV infection is unclear because data on important outcomes, such as visual impairment, are lacking and follow-up of infected children has been too short to fully identify late-onset sequelae.[18,32] Clinically apparent congenital infection following recurrent (nonprimary) maternal infection (i.e., infection in women with preexisting seroimmunity) is no longer considered a rare event because of the large prevalence of latent maternal CMV infection among women of childbearing age and the failure of maternal antibodies to prevent transmission during pregnancy.[3,19,33-35] This phenomenon of intrauterine transmission in the presence of substantial maternal immunity has been attributed to reactivation of endogenous virus in some cases and to reinfection with different strains of CMV in other instances.[36] A higher prevalence was found in developing countries than for Europe and North America owing to the higher maternal CMV seroprevalence.[32] According to data derived from 11 studies from Africa, Asia, and Latin America and involving numbers of newborns tested ranging from 317 to 12,195, maternal CMV seroprevalence ranged from 84% to 100%. CMV birth prevalence varied from 0.6% to 6.1%.

Parturitional and Postnatal Infections. Parturitional and postnatal exposures cause an additional 10% to 15% of infants to acquire CMV infection in the first 4 to 8 weeks of life.[1,37] Clinical signs and symptoms of pCMV infection in very or extremely preterm infants include pneumonia, enteritis, cholestasis, hepatosplenomegaly, sepsis-like syndrome (SLS), thrombocytopenia, and neutropenia. Postnatal CMV infection has also been associated with an increased risk for bronchopulmonary dysplasia (BPD).[38,39] In one study, 42% of infected infants developed clinical or laboratory abnormalities (neutropenia and thrombocytopenia).[40,41] Another study showed a mean incubation time of 42 days (95% confidence interval [CI] 28 to 69) with symptoms in about 50% of the infected infants and 4 of 33 with sepsis-like symptoms.[41] In a study from the Netherlands, the majority of CMV-infected infants (85%) did not develop any symptoms of pCMV infection. The most important independent risk factors for pCMV infection were

nonnative Dutch maternal origin (OR 9.6 [95% confidence interval (CI) 4.3 to 21.5]) and breast milk (OR 13.2 [95% CI 1.7 to 104.5]). The risk of pCMV infection significantly decreased for each additional week of gestational age (GA) (OR 0.7 [95% CI 0.5 to 0.9]). Lenticulostriate vasculopathy (LSV) was significantly more often present at term-equivalent age in infants with pCMV infection (OR 4.1 [95% CI 1.9 to 8.8]).[11] Breast milk is probably the single most important source of CMV exposure in premature infants.[11,42-46] It has been documented that 96% of CMV-seropositive women have CMV reactivation with shedding of virus or the presence of CMV DNA in breast milk within several days after delivery. In a meta-analysis, among 299 infants fed untreated breast milk, 19% (11% to 32%) acquired pCMV infection and 4% (2% to 7%) developed pCMV-SLS.[47] Among 212 infants fed frozen breast milk, 13% (7% to 24%) developed CMV infection and 5% (2% to 12%) an SLS, yielding slightly lower rates of breast milk–acquired CMV infection (4.4%; 2.4% to 8.2%) but similar rates of CMV-SLS (1.7%; 0.7% to 4.1%). The benefits of breast milk are still considered to outweigh the risks of severe disease from breast milk–acquired CMV infection in the neonatal period, which has so far not been associated with delayed development, SNHL, or clear cognitive impairment.[41]

Although the results of one study raised the possibility of an increased risk of neurological sequelae in premature infants who acquire pCMV infection during the first 8 weeks of life,[8] most data have indicated that CNS involvement does not occur with parturitional or early postnatal infection.[8,9,14,46] However, recent long-term outcome studies raise some concern. Although no effect of pCMV infection was obvious at assessments between 2 and 4.5 years of age, differences in outcome were noted when 42 children were assessed again during adolescence (n = 42, 11.6 to 16.2 years, mean = 13.9; 15 girls; 19 with and 23 without an early pCMV infection).[13,48] Assessed with the German version of the Wechsler Intelligence Scale and the Developmental Test for Visual Perception, adolescents born preterm with early pCMV infection scored significantly lower than those without this infection regarding overall cognitive abilities (92.67 [14.71] vs. 102.75 [13.67], P = .03) but not visuoperceptive abilities (91.22 [10.88] vs. 98.96 [13.45], P > .05). However, the group of children was small, and the data were not adjusted for known independent risk factors such as postnatal corticosteroids, duration of mechanical ventilation, sepsis, other congenital infections, necrotizing enterocolitis, surgery, or socioeconomic status. The last of these is predictive of poor cognitive outcome and could be an important confounder. The reasons for the difference in propensity to affect the CNS between early prenatal versus natal or postnatal acquisition of CMV remain to be determined.

Blood transfusion has been a particularly important source in low-birth-weight infants, but with the introduction of transfusion of CMV-seronegative and leukoreduced blood products, transmission of CMV to very-low-birth-weight infants has been effectively prevented.[10,41]

Neuropathology

Congenital CMV infection may be associated with asymptomatic or symptomatic neurological presentations in the neonatal period (see subsequent discussion). The symptomatic presentation is uncommon but serves as the prototype for the neuropathology produced by primary infection of the developing CNS by this

TABLE 34.3   Neuropathology of Congenital Cytomegalovirus Infection Symptomatic in the Neonatal Period

Meningoencephalitis
Germinal matrix necrosis/cysts
Periventricular cerebral calcification
Cerebral white matter cysts/calcification with atrophy and
   ventriculomegaly
Cerebral cortical atrophy
Microcephaly
Migrational disturbances: polymicrogyria, lissencephaly/
   pachygyria, schizencephaly
Cerebellar hypoplasia

TABLE 34.4   Neuropathological Features of Congenital Cytomegalovirus Infection in 15 Preterm Infants

NEUROPATHOLOGICAL FEATURE	PERCENTAGE OF INFANTS AFFECTED (%)
Microcephaly	87
Meningoencephalitis	75
Calcifications	80
Periventricular	73
Cortical	40
Both	40
Polymicrogyria	33
Lissencephaly	7
Ventriculomegaly	27
Cerebellar hypoplasia	33
Periventricular leukomalacia or porencephaly	20

Nine infants (mean birth weight, 2350 g; mean gestational age, 33 weeks) died in the neonatal period; six infants (mean birth weight, 1145 g; mean gestational age, 33 weeks) were stillborn.

Data from Perlman JM, Argyle C. Lethal cytomegalovirus infection in preterm infants: clinical, radiological, and neuropathological findings. *Ann Neurol.* 1992;31:64-68.

virus. Evidence both for inflammation and destruction and for teratogenicity can be observed (Table 34.3). The spectrum of the neuropathology was well illustrated by a large neuropathological study of 15 premature infants who died with congenital CMV infection (Table 34.4). A more recent study of 16 infected human fetal brains of GA between 23 and 28.5 weeks showed a correlation of density of CMV-immunolabeled cells with the presence of microcephaly and the extent of brain abnormalities.[49] Nine were microcephalic, 10 had extensive cortical lesions, 8 had hippocampal abnormalities, and 5 cases showed infection of the olfactory bulb. CMV infected all cell types but showed higher tropism for stem cells/radial glial cells.

Meningoencephalitis. *Meningoencephalitis* is characterized by the following features: (1) inflammatory cells in the meninges; (2) perivascular infiltrates with inflammatory cells; (3) necrosis of brain parenchyma, with all cellular elements affected, especially in the periventricular region, and often associated with

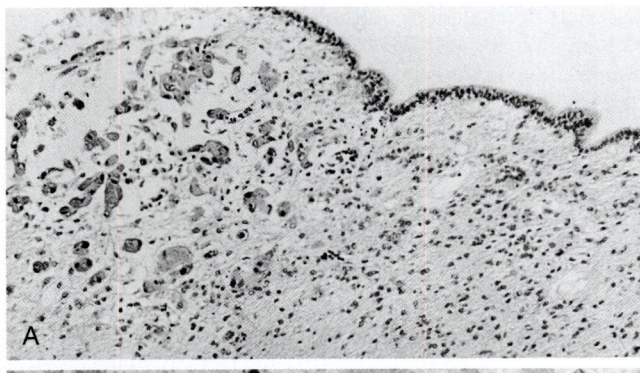
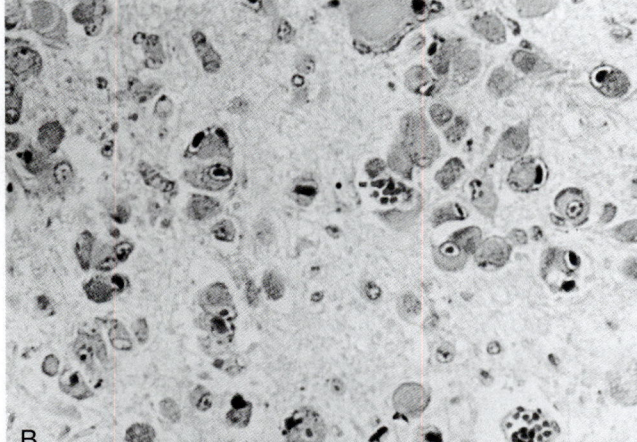
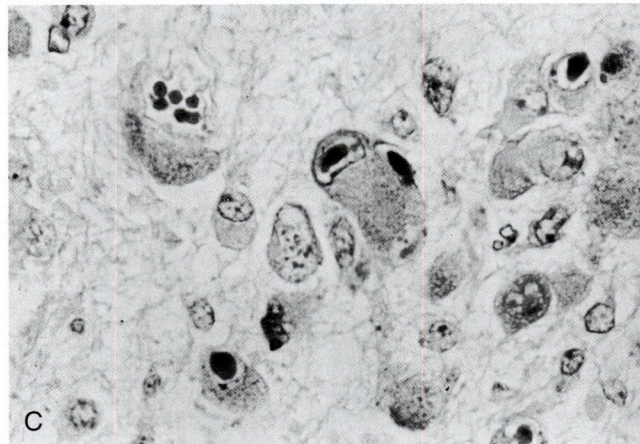

Figure 34.1 Congenital cytomegalovirus infection: encephalitis, from an infant who died at 10 weeks of age. (A) Region of necrosis in the subependymal germinal matrix (ependyma is at the upper right). Note enlargement of cells, many with intranuclear inclusions. (B) Higher-power view of the same region showing the enlarged cells with prominent intranuclear inclusions. (C) A closer view of the inclusions; note the clear halo around the inclusions and the nuclear chromatin displaced to the periphery (Cowdry type A inclusions). (From Bell WE, McCormick WF. *Neurologic Infections in Children.* Philadelphia: Saunders; 1975.)

calcification; (4) reactive microglial and astroglial proliferation; and (5) the occurrence of enlarged cells (neuronal and glial elements) with intranuclear inclusions (Fig. 34.1).[25,31,50] Electron microscopic studies have revealed virions in brain tissue, a finding attesting to primary infection of the CNS by the organism.[51] Recovery of virus from brain confirmed this conclusion. A role for the inflammatory response itself in causing tissue destruction is suggested by the disparity between the detection of cytomegaloviral DNA by in situ hybridization and the extent of the tissue necrosis.[52]

The *cellular and regional targets of the meningoencephalitis* include especially the *germinative ventricular–subventricular zones, radial glial cells, cerebral white matter, subplate neurons, and cerebral cortex.*[25,31,50,53-59] Germinal matrix necrosis and cysts are prominent. Subsequent matrix calcification is important in determining the *periventricular* distribution of *calcifications*. The particular tropism for progenitor cells in the ventricular-subventricular zones, radial glial cells, and subplate neurons has recently been identified.[49] Periventricular cerebral white matter is also a site of injury, sometimes with cyst formation and subsequent calcification. A predilection for the *parietal white matter* may mimic periventricular leukomalacia (PVL). In addition, a predilection for *anterior temporal white matter* is particularly suggestive of CMV infection. Cerebrocortical atrophy is a later feature.

Microcephaly. *Microcephaly* is a common feature in the neonatal period and is still more prominent later in infancy. The small size of the brain appears to relate to the encephaloclastic effects of the virus and probably also to a disturbance of cell proliferation in the developing brain. The latter disturbance relates to the propensity of the virus to affect progenitor cells in the ventricular and subventricular zones (see earlier). A predilection for involvement of proliferative cells is also suggested by the frequency of intrauterine growth retardation in congenital CMV infection and by the observation in a variety of tissues of a decrease in absolute number of cells.[60,61]

Disturbances of Neuronal Migration. Disturbances of neuronal migration have been described repeatedly in congenital CMV infection.[a] Indeed, polymicrogyria has been documented in approximately 65% of well-studied cases. The polymicrogyria may involve cerebellar (Fig. 34.2) as well as cerebral cortex. Although polymicrogyria has been observed most commonly, lissencephaly, pachygyria, schizencephaly, and neuronal heterotopias have also been reported.[50,62,66,70-73] These observations demonstrate the teratogenic potential of CMV and suggest the occurrence of infection in the latter part of the first trimester and in the second trimester, when neuronal migration begins and then becomes active (see Chapter 3). The usual coexistence of inflammatory, destructive lesions indicates persistent infection by the organism. These cases may also be relevant to the notion that cerebrocortical neuronal injury late in the second trimester may underlie other examples of polymicrogyria (see Chapter 2). One careful study of four affected brains from infants with congenital CMV infection provided evidence of neuronal destruction in the lower cortical layers within areas of polymicrogyria and suggested that the cortical neuronal injury led ultimately to the gyral abnormality.[74] At any rate, CMV infection was until recently the only congenital infection associated with overt disturbances of gyral development, and the pathogenesis thereof may include a combination of teratogenic and encephaloclastic mechanisms. ZIKV infection (see later) may exhibit similar disturbances of gyral development.

---

[a]References 49, 50, 53, 55-57, 59, 62-73.

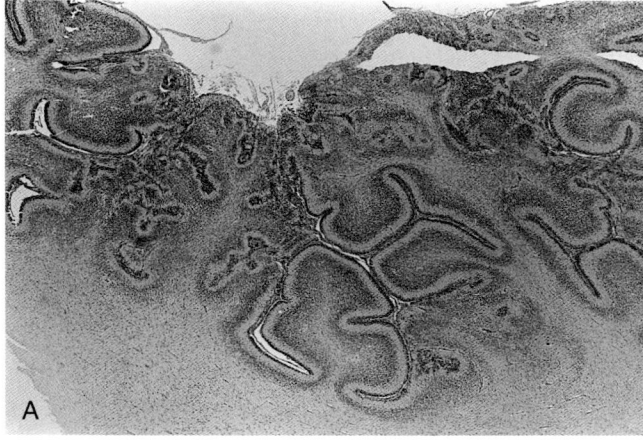

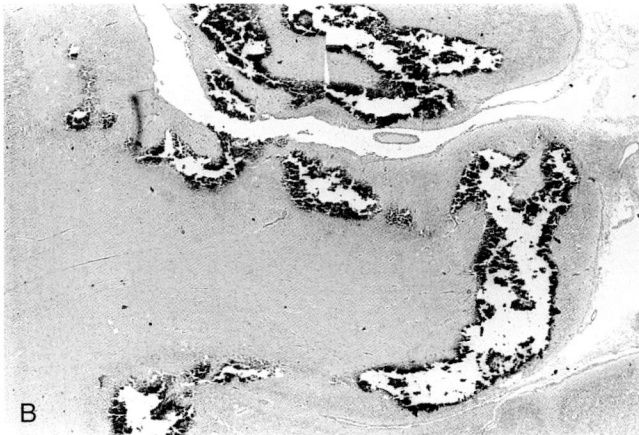

Figure 34.2 Congenital cytomegalovirus infection: neuronal migrational disturbance. (A) Microgyric cerebellar cortex from a preterm infant with congenital cytomegalovirus infection. (B) Section of the same microgyric cerebellar cortex shown in (A), illustrating the distribution of calcification within the malformed cerebellar cortex and suggesting the coexistence of destructive and teratogenic effects. (From Perlman JM, Argyle C. Lethal cytomegalovirus infection in preterm infants: clinical, radiological, and neuropathological findings. *Ann Neurol.* 1992;31:64-68.)

Cerebellar Hypoplasia. *Cerebellar hypoplasia*, best detected by magnetic resonance imaging (MRI), is a feature in at least 50% of symptomatic cases. This finding likely is primarily a proliferative disturbance, although, as noted earlier, migrational disturbances may also be seen in the cerebellum. The finding of cerebellar hypoplasia in the clinical setting of an intrauterine infection is highly suggestive of congenital CMV.

Other Findings. Porencephaly, hydranencephaly, hydrocephalus, focal subcortical cysts, impaired myelination, and more diffuse cerebral calcifications have also been described to variable extents in congenital CMV infection.

Clinical Aspects

Incidence of Clinically Apparent Infection. Although congenital CMV infection occurs frequently, its clinical manifestations do not. Indeed, available data indicate that approximately 90% of affected infants are asymptomatic in the newborn period.[18,28,75-81]

Clinical Features. The most frequent clinical features of symptomatic congenital CMV infection are shown in

TABLE 34.5 Clinical Features of Symptomatic Congenital Cytomegalovirus Infection

CLINICAL FEATURE	APPROXIMATE FREQUENCY (%)
Pregnancy	
Fetal growth restriction	21–50
Premature birth	21–50
Central nervous system	
Meningoencephalitis	51–75
Microcephaly	21–50
Cerebral calcification	51–75
Eye	
Chorioretinitis	0–20
Reticuloendothelial system	
Hepatosplenomegaly	51–75
Hyperbilirubinemia	51–75
Hemolytic and other anemias	21–50
Thrombocytopenia	51–75
Petechiae or ecchymoses	51–75
Other	
Inguinal hernias	21–50
Pneumonitis	0–20

See text for references.

Table 34.5.[14-16,76,77,82,83] The most common findings relate to disturbance of the reticuloendothelial system. Hepatosplenomegaly and a petechial rash, usually related to thrombocytopenia, are encountered very frequently. Infants are often small for GA; moreover, approximately one third of affected infants have a GA of 37 weeks or less. Inguinal hernia is a helpful clinical sign when present ($\approx$25% of cases).

The neurological syndrome is variable in presentation. Seizures may be prominent, although only approximately 10% of symptomatic patients exhibit overt neonatal seizures. Microcephaly is a consistent manifestation in patients with severe disease and appears in approximately 50% of all symptomatic patients.[75] Cerebral calcification, usually periventricular in location, occurs in 50% to 60% of cases. Germinolytic cysts and LSV are also suggestive of CMV infection. Cerebrospinal fluid (CSF) findings of encephalitis (e.g., pleocytosis, elevated protein content) are found in the majority of patients, but precise data are not available. In a recent study, CSF β2-microglobulin levels were increased and of prognostic value for neurodevelopmental outcome.[75]

The *clinical course* is most commonly that of a static process. Rare evidence of progressive encephaloclastic disease, documented by computed tomography (CT) scan, was provided by a report of two such cases.[84] Similarly, postnatal evolution of cerebral calcification and of subependymal necrosis has been documented.[50,85] Progression of hearing loss during infancy and early childhood has been clearly described (see later).[a] The observation that virus is still recoverable in urine in 50% of cases at 5 years of age[89] demonstrates persistence of infection and further raises the possibility of progressive disease.

[a]References 15, 18, 77, 81, 83, 86-88.

Clinical Diagnosis. The diagnosis of congenital CMV infection may be suspected with a high degree of accuracy on the basis of certain clinical features. These features include the periventricular locus of the cerebral calcification, the presence of germinolytic cysts, and LSV—best seen with *ultrasonography*—microcephaly, CSF pleocytosis, and intrauterine growth retardation.[75] Cerebellar hypoplasia and neuronal migrational abnormalities are also distinctive features and are best recognized with MRI.[63] The absence of the "salt and pepper" chorioretinitis of congenital rubella and the relative infrequency of the grossly scarring chorioretinitis of congenital toxoplasmosis are also helpful.

Laboratory Evaluation

Diagnosis During Pregnancy. Most CMV infections encountered during pregnancy are asymptomatic. In about 5% there is a history of a flu-like episode. Only CMV serology (negative for immunoglobulin M [IgM] and immunoglobulin G [IgG]) can exclude a congenital CMV infection. Both primary as well as nonprimary CMV infections (reinfection/reactivation) can lead to congenital CMV infection. The diagnosis of a primary CMV infection can be made by the detection of seroconversion. In most countries women are not routinely screened for CMV antibodies before their pregnancy. The presence of anti-CMV IgM antibodies is considered to be a good indicator of an acute or recent CMV infection, but IgM antibodies are present in only 70% of infected babies and in only fewer than 10% of IgM-positive women is the fetus infected.[90] When the infection takes place before conception or very early in the pregnancy, IgM may have become negative by the time the suspicion of congenital CMV infection is raised. Pregnant women can also produce IgM during reactivation or reinfection, and false-positive results are not uncommon because IgM may be found in mothers who have another viral illness, such as Parvovirus B19 or Epstein-Barr virus. A relationship between low total IgM values and clinical symptoms in newborns with congenital CMV infection has also been reported.[91] This relationship can be explained by the longer period since the occurrence of the CMV infection early in pregnancy, resulting in lower total IgM in symptomatic cases. Severe fetal sequelae were also reported in six fetuses despite maternal immunity for CMV, confirmed by the detection of IgG with no IgM in previous pregnancies or early in the current pregnancy. Cranial ultrasound showed ventriculomegaly, calcification, and LSV, and amniocentesis confirmed the presence of CMV by polymerase chain reaction (PCR) in all six.[92]

The anti-CMV IgG avidity test is the most reliable procedure to identify primary infection in pregnant women.[93,94] The avidity indices may vary with the tests used. Low avidity indices indicate low-avidity IgG antibodies in serum caused by acute or recent primary CMV infection, whereas high avidity indices (high-avidity serum IgG) indicate no current or recent primary infection. The determination of anti-CMV IgG avidity, performed before the 16th to 18th week of pregnancy, identifies all women who will have an infected fetus/newborn (sensitivity 100%). After 20 weeks' gestation, sensitivity is drastically reduced (62.5%). A high avidity index during the first 12 to 16 weeks' gestation can be considered a good indicator of past infection. The presence of true IgM combined with a low/moderate avidity index has the same diagnostic value as seroconversion.[90] Although not quite as powerful as a high-avidity result, an intermediate-avidity result during the first trimester also indicates a low risk of intrauterine transmission. In contrast, an intermediate-avidity or high-avidity result during the second or third trimester does not rule out postconception primary infection and is associated with an increased risk of transmission.[94]

A reliable prenatal diagnosis is obtained by performing a PCR on the amniotic fluid. Amniocentesis is best performed between the 21st and 22nd weeks of gestation. CMV is a slowly replicating virus, and 6 to 9 weeks are required after maternal infection for the virus to be eliminated in the fetal urine in amounts sufficient to be detected in the amniotic fluid. There is a risk of a false-negative test, as can occur when the amniocentesis is carried out earlier, when little amounts of virus have been shed by the fetal kidney. The sensitivity and specificity (90% to 98% and 92% to 98%, respectively) for PCR analysis in the amniotic fluid are high with respect to viral transmission from mother to fetus.[95] The risk of a severe infection with a high risk of severe sequelae occurs when the infection is contracted in the first 12 to 16 weeks of gestation.

Diagnosis of Cytomegalovirus Infection in the Newborn

Serological Studies. Many serological tests have been used, but these tests have become less important with the use of PCR.[1,37] The commonly used complement fixation test depends on IgG, and because this fraction is primarily derived by passive transfer from the infected mother, titers are high in the neonatal period. *Persistence* of an elevated titer in the neonate suggests infection of the infant, because passively transferred maternal antibody is degraded with an approximate half-life of 21 to 23 days.[1] A faster and more useful test depends on the detection of CMV-specific IgM, which is primarily derived from the infected fetus and infant.[1,14]

Isolation of Virus. The gold standard for the diagnosis of congenital CMV infection in the newborn remains viral isolation in the urine and/or saliva within the first 2 to 3 weeks of life. The organism is cultured most readily from the urine but can also be grown from the throat and occasionally from the CSF. The detection of virus in urine remains a highly specific and sensitive test for the diagnosis of congenital CMV infection. The urine is retained after storage at 4°C (not at room temperature and not frozen) for as long as 7 days.[96] A period of 2 to 4 weeks is required to detect the characteristic cytopathic effects in tissue culture. The detection of DNA of CMV in urine by PCR allows for the diagnosis of infection in 1 day.[97] The increase in sensitivity of this test to virtually 100% by the removal of inhibitory materials in urine by glass filter paper absorption helped make this technique the ideal test for detection of infection. PCR has also been shown to detect the virus in CSF, serum, saliva, and specimens of umbilical cord; the use of saliva especially has recently been recommended for screening.[98-102] In a comparison of reverse transcriptase PCR (rtPCR) assays of liquid and dried saliva specimens with the rapid culture of saliva specimens obtained at birth in a prospective, multicenter screening study of newborns,[101] 85 infants (0.5%) had positive results on both culture and PCR assay. The sensitivity and specificity of the liquid saliva PCR assay were 100% (95% CI 95.8 to 100) and 99.9% (95% CI 99.9 to 100), respectively. Seventy-four newborns screened by means of the dried saliva PCR assay were positive for CMV, whereas 76 (0.4%) were found to be CMV-positive on rapid culture. Sensitivity and specificity

of the dried saliva PCR assay were 97.4% (95% CI 90.8 to 99.7) and 99.9% (95% CI 99.9 to 100), respectively. Because rtPCR assays of both liquid and dried saliva specimens showed high sensitivity and specificity for detecting CMV infection, the investigators suggested the use of saliva-rtPCR as a potential screening tool for CMV in newborns. In another study enrolling 73,239 infants screened for CMV, 284 (0.4%) tested positive by rtPCR or rapid culture of saliva, with a 94.7% concordance between rtPCR and rapid culture of saliva. Of 14 infants with discordance, 13 were correctly identified with saliva rtPCR but were missed with rapid culture.[103] This discrepancy might be due to a decrease in the amount of infectious virus during storage, which occurs after 1 week even when stored at 4°C. The discordance could not be explained by a difference in viral load. Use of rtPCR in the saliva in preterm infants with *postnatal* CMV infection was recently reported to be less reliable.[102] The virus was detected in 42 saliva samples (sensitivity 89.4%; CI 76.9 to 96.5) among 47 infants with pCMV infection. Of 214 children without pCMV infection, one saliva sample tested positive for CMV (specificity 99.5%; CI 97.4 to 99.9). Screening saliva for CMV-DNA by rtPCR is inferior to the use of urine to diagnose pCMV infections in preterm infants. This could be because of the lower mean viral shedding in infants with pCMV versus those with cCMV infection.[104]

Diagnostic Studies. *CSF* characteristically exhibits the findings of meningoencephalitis. In a study of 18 infants with neurological manifestations, the mean white blood cell (WBC) count was 42 cells/μL including predominantly lymphocytes, and the mean protein content was 192 mg/dL.[105] In a later series of nine newborns with neurological involvement, all had elevated WBC counts and protein levels.[106] In another study of 56 infants (which included 30% with no CT abnormalities), CSF protein exceeded 120 mg/dL in 50%.[76]

Skull radiographs were formerly used to demonstrate the periventricular calcifications (Fig. 34.3). CT scanning is more sensitive than skull radiography for detection of calcifications (Fig. 34.4). In a series of 41 infants with symptomatic congenital CMV infection, a CT-detected abnormality was present in 78%. Of those with abnormalities, periventricular calcifications occurred in 75%, varying degrees of cortical and white matter abnormalities were seen in 30%, and ventriculomegaly was reported in 40%.[107] CT scanning was recommended in the past as the gold standard to assess cerebral involvement in infants with cCMV infection, but CT scanning is no longer recommended in such infants. Cranial ultrasound and MRI are safer, reliable alternatives.

Cranial ultrasound scans frequently demonstrate abnormalities.[50,53,63,105,108-114] These findings consist of periventricular cysts—especially in the region of the subependymal germinal matrix (Figs. 34.5 and 34.6)—ventriculomegaly, periventricular (and more diffuse) calcifications, and periventricular echolucencies (consistent with cerebral white matter cysts) (see Fig. 34.6). The correlations with neuropathological findings (see previous discussion) are obvious. An additional ultrasonographic finding, overt in approximately one third of cases, is the presence of *branched echodensities in basal ganglia and thalamus* (see Fig. 34.6).[108,112-114] That the echodensities are alongside the lenticulostriate arteries has been shown by Doppler ultrasound examination (see Fig. 34.6).[113-115] In two series, 15% to 40% of infants with such echodensities had CMV infection. (Other diagnoses included

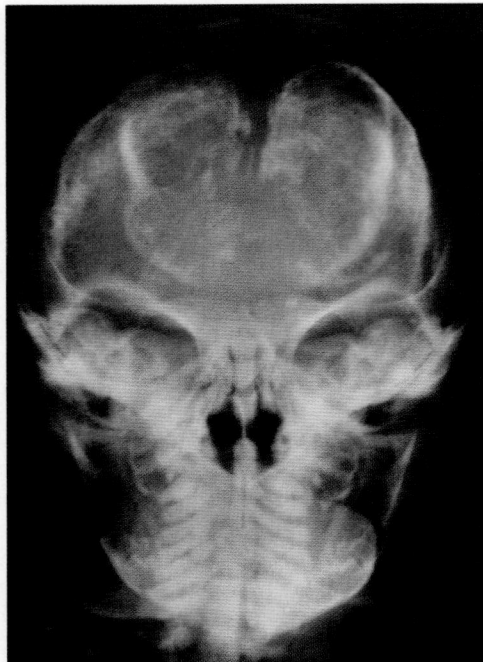

Figure 34.3 Congenital cytomegalovirus infection: periventricular calcification. This skull radiograph is from an affected 5-day-old infant with microcephaly. (From Bell WE, McCormick WF. *Neurologic Infections in Children.* 2nd ed. Philadelphia: Saunders; 1981.)

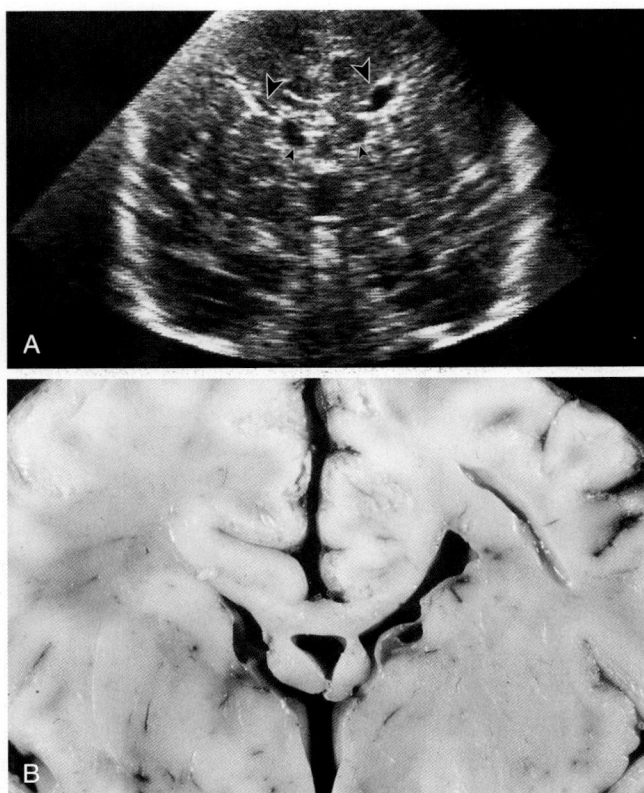

Figure 34.5 Congenital cytomegalovirus infection: periventricular cyst in subependymal germinal matrix: cranial ultrasound. (A) This scan, performed at 1 day of age, demonstrates the bilateral cysts *(small arrowheads).* The ventricles are indicated by the large arrowheads. (B) Coronal section of brain shows both cysts in the subependymal regions. (Courtesy Dr. Gary Shackelford.)

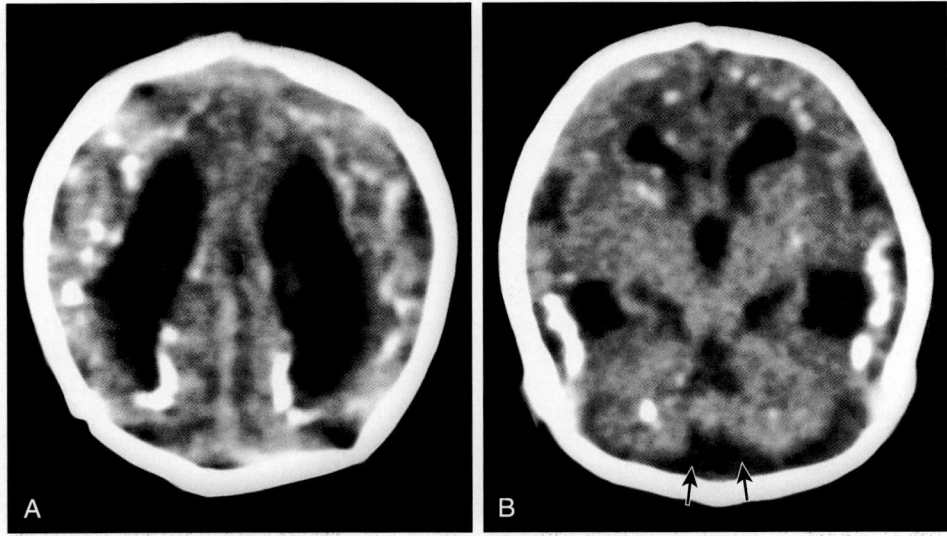

Figure 34.4 Congenital cytomegalovirus infection: computed tomography. These scans are from a 5-day-old infant with congenital cytomegalovirus infection. (A) Periventricular and diffuse cerebral calcifications and ventriculomegaly are apparent. (B) In addition to calcifications and ventriculomegaly, note the cerebellar hypoplasia and large cisterna magna *(arrows).*

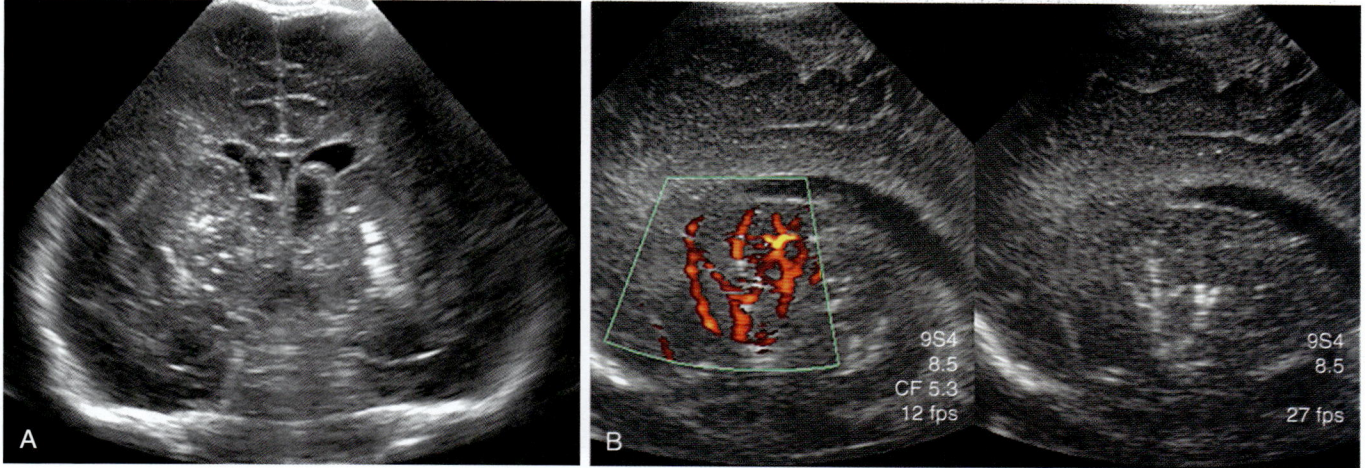

Figure 34.6 Congenital cytomegalovirus infection: cranial ultrasound. Coronal (A) and parasagittal (B) views showing large bilateral germinolytic cysts and lenticulostriate vasculopathy. Using power Doppler (B), it is clear that the echogenic linear abnormalities follow the lenticulostriate arteries.

congenital rubella, congenital syphilis, trisomy 13, trisomy 21, fetal alcohol spectrum disorder, metabolic disorders, and *neonatal asphyxia*.) One pathological study defined hypercellular vessel walls and a mineralizing vasculopathy, probably secondary to perivascular inflammation (Fig. 34.7).[112]

MRI is of particular value for detecting the disorders of neuronal migration, cerebral parenchymal destruction, delays in myelination, and cerebellar hypoplasia observed with congenital CMV (Figs. 34.8–34.10).[a] In a large study of 40 infants with cCMV infection cranial ultrasound and cardiac MRI were performed within the first month of life.[116] Six newborns showed pathological cardiac MRI and cranial ultrasound findings (pseudocysts, ventriculomegaly, calcifications, cerebellar hypoplasia), but MRI provided additional information (white matter abnormalities in three cases, lissencephaly/polymicrogyria in one, and a cyst of the temporal lobe in another); cerebral calcifications were detected in three of six infants by cranial ultrasound but in only two of six by MRI. Four of these six infants showed severe neurodevelopmental impairment and five showed deafness on follow-up. Three newborns had a normal cranial ultrasound, but MRI documented white matter abnormalities and in one case also cerebellar hypoplasia; all showed neurodevelopmental impairment and two were deaf at follow-up. In another study, 36 infants with cCMV infection were studied, with MRI available in 20, allowing comparison of cranial ultrasound and MRI.[63] Migrational disorders were diagnosed only with MRI in 9 of the 20 infants assessed with this technique. Of 10 infants infected during the first trimester, 7 had severe abnormalities on cranial ultrasound (5 confirmed on MRI) and adverse sequelae; 3 had no or mild abnormalities on cranial ultrasound/MRI and a normal outcome. Of seven infants infected during the second or third trimester with no/mild abnormalities on cranial ultrasound/MRI, six had a normal outcome; one with mild cranial ultrasound and MRI abnormalities developed SNHL. As expected, the worst outcome was seen in 16 of 26 symptomatic infants with severe cranial

ultrasound/MRI abnormalities (neuronal migration disorders seen only on MRI: cerebellar hypoplasia, ventriculomegaly, extensive periventricular calcifications, and white matter cysts). In 1 of 16 infants with only mild abnormalities on cranial ultrasound (germinolytic cysts and LSV), occipital cysts as well as extensive polymicrogyria were noted with MRI (see Fig. 34.8), highlighting the need for MRI even in the absence of severe cranial ultrasound abnormalities. The study again showed that infants with cCMV infection acquired during the first trimester of pregnancy are at increased risk of symptomatic presentation with severe cerebral abnormalities and the subsequent development of adverse sequelae such as cerebral palsy, SNHL, and mortality.[62,70]

In a carefully studied series of 11 infants with congenital CMV infection, polymicrogyria was present in 5 and lissencephaly in 4.[62] In a series of MRI-documented cases of lissencephaly-pachygyria, CMV infection was present in 6 of 23 infants.[70] In a related study of 10 infants with MRI-identified migrational disorders, especially polymicrogyria, 4 were found to have CMV.[57] Delays in myelination and increased signal on T2-weighted images (see Figs. 34.8 and 34.9) have been observed in approximately half of the infants with CMV studied by MRI.[a] Indeed, the predilection of abnormal cerebral white matter signal, including cystic change, for posterior parietal regions may mimic PVL. Thus, in an MRI series of 152 infants (mean age 22 months) with "static leukoencephalopathy of unknown etiology," 10% were found to have congenital CMV, based on retrospective PCR testing of neonatal blood spots.[58] Cerebellar hypoplasia, a finding in 40% to 70% of infants with cCMV infection, is detected best by MRI scanning (see Fig.34.10). Notably, MRI is *less* sensitive than CT and cranial ultrasound for the detection of cerebral calcifications.[53,63]

Antenatal neuroimaging combining cranial ultrasound and MRI has shown characteristic findings, also seen on postnatal imaging. Many of the common findings in cCMV are illustrated in a recent review by Averill and colleagues.[119] Dilated occipital

---

[a]References 53, 59, 62, 63, 70-73, 116-118.

[a]References 53, 58, 59, 62, 63, 70, 72, 73.

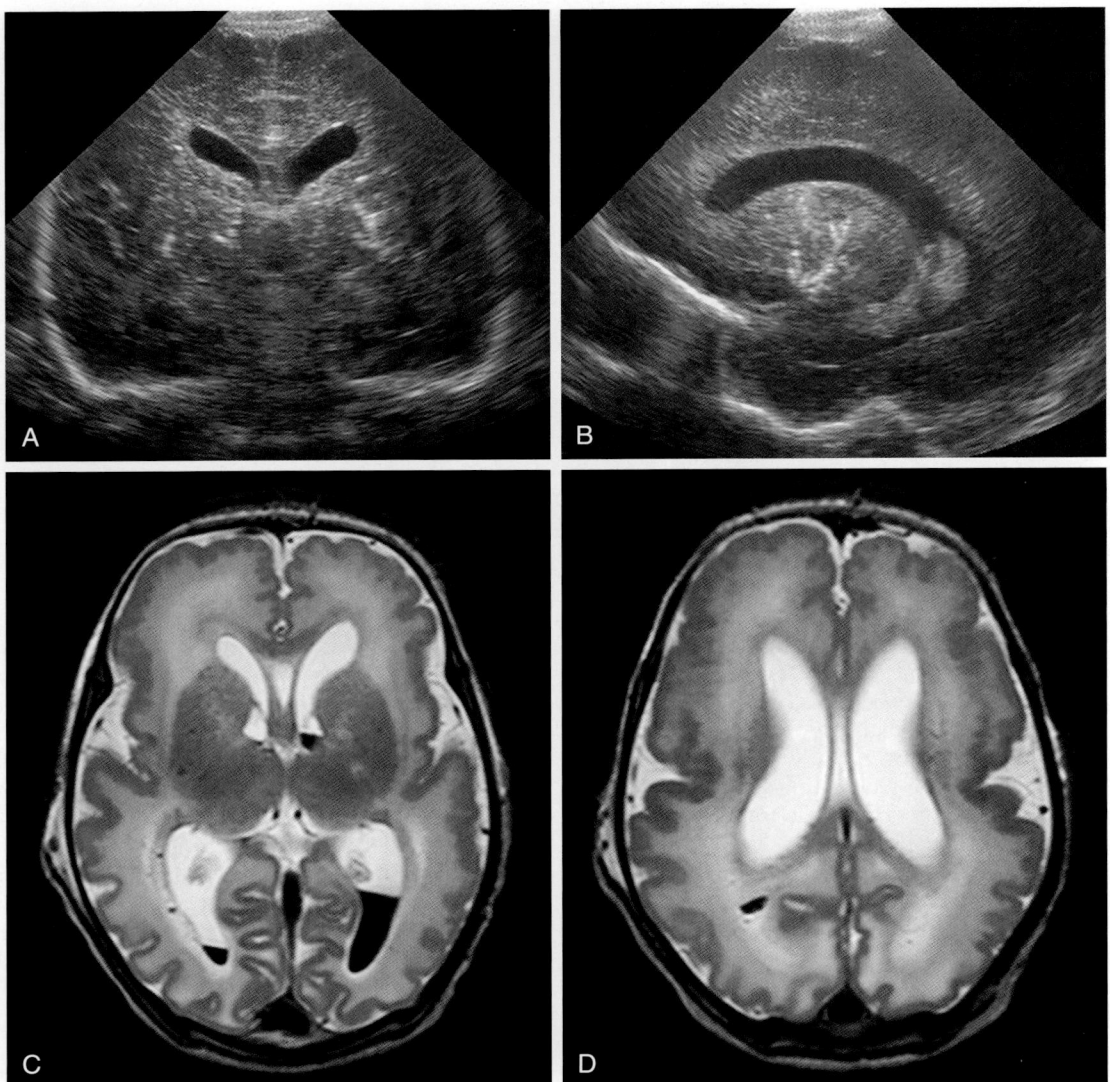

Figure 34.7 Congenital cytomegalovirus infection: cranial ultrasound. Coronal (A) and parasagittal (B) views showing small bilateral germinolytic cysts, lenticulostriate vasculopathy, and mild ventriculomegaly. Magnetic resonance imaging, axial T2-weighted images of the same infant (C and D) additionally show an intraventricular hemorrhage (C), a hemorrhagic lesion in the parietal white matter (D), and extensive polymicrogyria. (From Gunkel J, van der Knoop BJ, Nijman J et al. Congenital cytomegalovirus infection in the absence of maternal cytomegalovirus-IgM antibodies. *Fetal Diagn Therapy.* 2017; DOI: 10.1159/000456615.)

horns of the lateral ventricles with thin septations can be well visualized with cranial ultrasound as well as MRI. These characteristic occipital *cysts* are usually bilateral and will become less conspicuous with time (see Figs. 34.10 and 34.11). Polymicrogyria is likely to be missed with cranial ultrasound and is easier to detect on postnatal MRI, but it is often seen or at least suspected on fetal MRI. In a study by Doneda et al.,[120] prenatal cranial ultrasound and MRI findings were compared in 30 fetuses with a proven cCMV infection. Fetal MRI did show higher sensitivity than cranial ultrasound in predicting symptomatic infection (83% vs. 33%). However, both modalities showed low positive predictive values (36% with MRI vs. 29% with cranial ultrasound). In another study of fetal cranial ultrasound and MRI in 38 cases of cCMV infection, MRI was shown to add important details, especially with regard to the detection of gyrational anomalies, cerebellar

hypoplasia, and white matter abnormalities.[118] In both studies and a more recent study, a negative fetal brain MRI finding was reassuring for a good clinical outcome, although the hearing loss may still develop with time.[121,122]

Hearing loss caused by cCMV infection was first reported in 1964 and is the most common sequela of cCMV infection.[123,124] Hearing loss is thought to be due to cytopathic effects and localized inflammatory responses. This infection is now known to be the most common cause of nonhereditary SNHL, involving 10% to 20% of hearing-impaired children. Testing of *brain stem auditory evoked responses in the neonatal period and subsequently* demonstrates the high likelihood of SNHL, including the delayed onset and postnatal progression of this loss. In four series of 281 infants with symptomatic congenital CMV infections, 50% to 75% exhibited hearing loss on follow-up.[83,87,107,125] Although approximately 60% of those

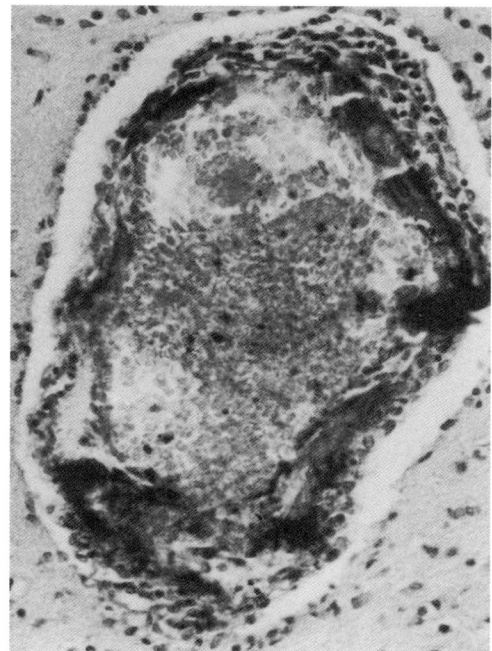

Figure 34.8 Congenital cytomegalovirus infection: photomicrograph of a small vessel. Note the thickened wall, focal globular subendothelial deposits of mineralized material, mononuclear infiltrates in adventitia, and perivascular reactive astrocytosis (hematoxylin and eosin, Luxol fast blue, ×250). (From Teele RL, Hernanz-Schulman M, Sotrel A. Echogenic vasculature in the basal ganglia of neonates: a sonographic sign of vasculopathy. *Radiology.* 1988;169:423-427.)

with hearing loss had hearing loss at birth or in the neonatal period, fully 40% had *delayed-onset* loss (i.e., not apparent until months after the neonatal period). In addition, *progressive* hearing loss was noted in approximately 60% of the infants with hearing loss.[87] Progression of hearing loss has also been observed in infants with *asymptomatic* CMV infection. Thus, in one series, 3% of such patients had hearing loss detected in the neonatal period, but by the age of 6 years, 11% of the previously asymptomatic patients had hearing loss.[83] A recent meta-analysis described findings from 14 longitudinal and 13 retrospective studies.[126] The researchers were able to show that of infants with a proven cCMV infection 12.6% (95% CI, 10.2 to 16.5) will have hearing loss; 1 of 3 symptomatic children and 1 of 10 asymptomatic children. Bilateral hearing loss was present in most children with symptomatic cCMV infection, whereas unilateral hearing was more common in those with asymptomatic cCMV infection. Hearing loss may have a delayed onset and can vary over time. Foulon et al. showed that the risk of cCMV-related SNHL was highest when the infection occurred during the first trimester (4 of 5; 80%), rare following an infection during the second trimester (1 of 12; 8%), and nonexistent in 11 children with cCMV acquired during the third trimester.[21] Fluctuation and improvement of SNHL were seen regardless of the trimester of pregnancy during which the mother's primary infection occurred. The risk of delayed hearing loss was shown to be associated with the presence of symptoms at birth[127]; children who passed initial audiological examinations but had cCMV-related symptoms at birth (e.g., jaundice, petechiae, and microcephaly) were nearly 6 times more likely to develop hearing loss than children who were asymptomatic at birth. A longer duration of viral shedding may also be a predictor of delayed hearing loss. *The value and importance of serial studies throughout infancy are obvious.*

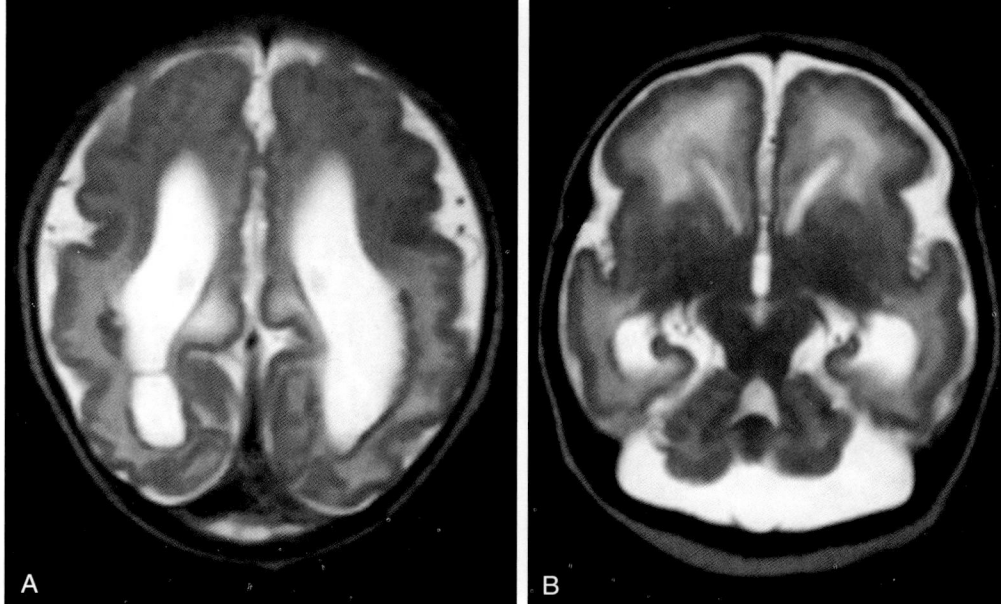

Figure 34.9 Congenital cytomegalovirus infection: magnetic resonance imaging. Axial T2-weighted images showing ventriculomegaly, a loculated area in the right occipital horn, periventricular calcification (low signal intensity), extensive polymicrogyria (A), and cerebellar hypoplasia as well as increased signal intensity in the white matter (B).

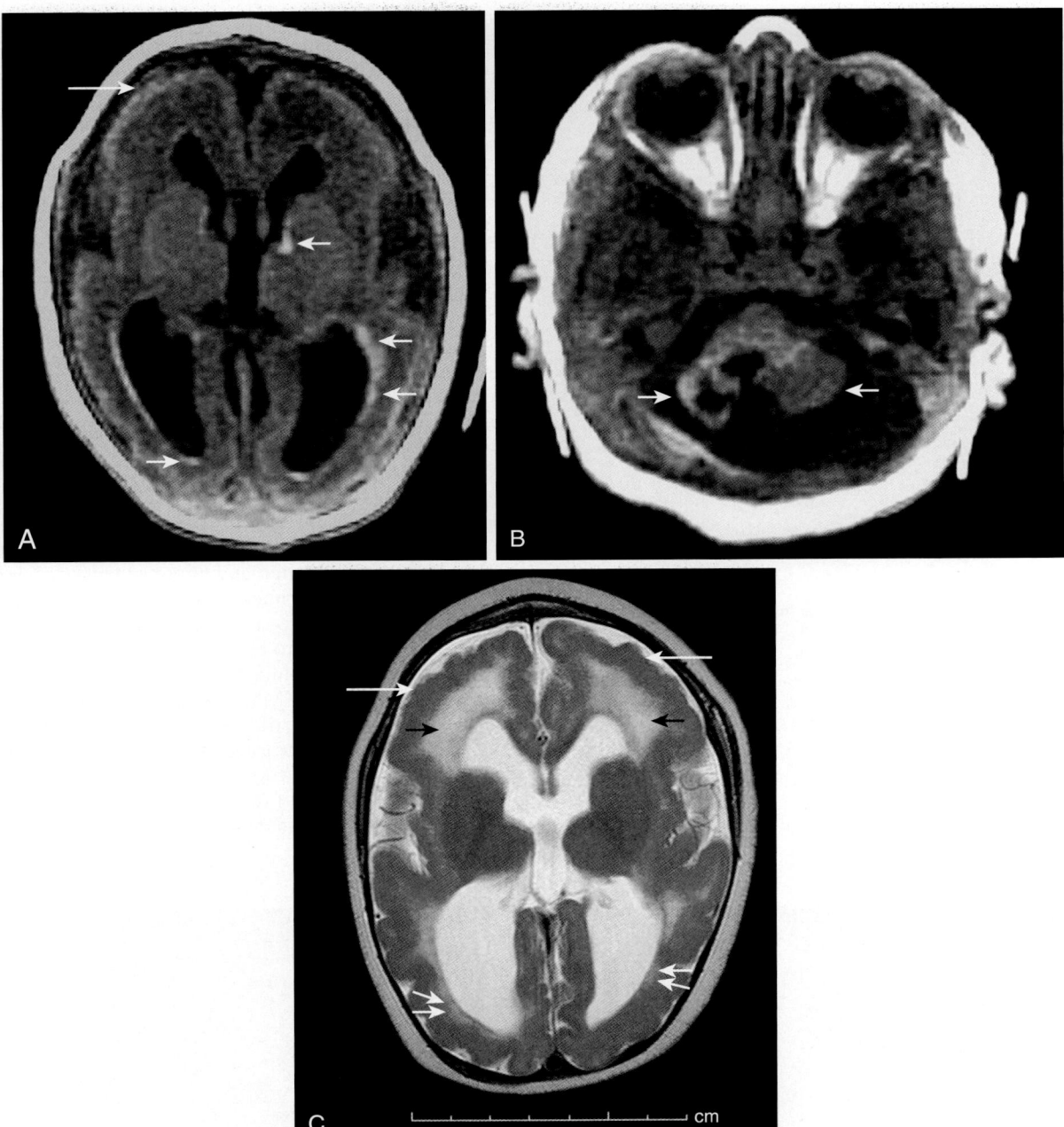

Figure 34.10 Congenital cytomegalovirus infection, magnetic resonance imaging. This 16-day-old infant was born after a 31-week gestation with congenital cytomegalovirus infection identified in utero. The axial T1-weighted magnetic resonance images show (A) increased signal in the periventricular regions *(short arrows)*, consistent with calcification, and diffuse polymicrogyria *(long arrow)*; in B, note the striking cerebellar hypoplasia *(arrows)*. At 6 months of age, the axial T2-weighted image (C) shows diffuse frontal polymicrogyria *(long arrows)*, abnormal high signal intensity in cerebral white matter *(short black arrows)*, and marked paucity of parieto-occipital cerebral white matter *(double white arrows)*. (Courtesy Dr. Omar Khwaja.)

Prognosis

Relation to Time of Onset of Fetal Infection and Antenatal Neuroimaging Findings. In a large prospective study that enrolled 145 fetuses during pregnancy—with a primary CMV infection obtained during the first and second trimesters of pregnancy in 71 and 74 patients, respectively—the risk of an adverse outcome was significantly higher when the infection occurred during the first trimester and when imaging abnormalities were found as well (Table 34.6).[121] Abnormal prenatal findings on ultrasound examination were associated with an increased risk of sequelae. In a recent study of 121 fetuses, MRI was performed at 27 and/or 33 weeks (51 at both time points). A five-grade classification was used: (1) for normal findings, (2) the presence of isolated frontal or parieto-occipital

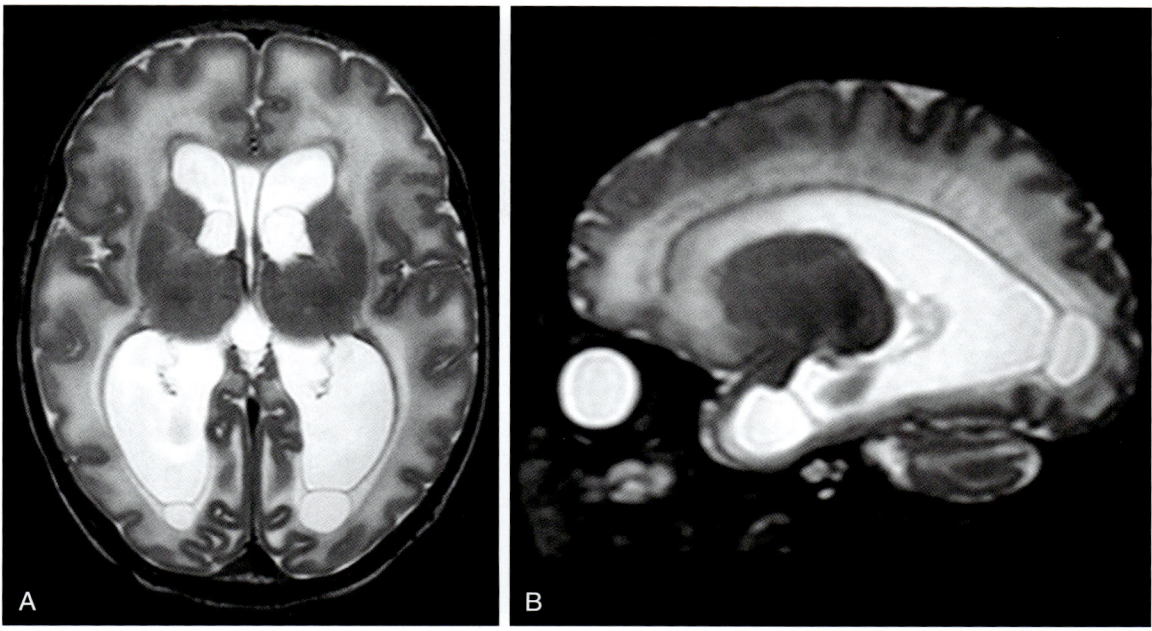

Figure 34.11 Congenital cytomegalovirus infection, magnetic resonance imaging. Axial T2-weighted (A) and parasagittal (B) images showing large germinolytic cysts as well as loculated areas within the occipital and temporal horns of the enlarged lateral ventricles. Signal intensity in the white matter is diffusely increased.

TABLE 34.6 Cytomegalovirus-Associated Sequelae in Relation to Time of Onset of Maternal Infection		
	FIRST TRIMESTER	**SECOND TRIMESTER**
Abnormal fetal ultrasound	15/71 (21.1%)	3/74 (4.1%)
Abnormal fetal MRI	21/56 (37.5%)	11/66 (16.6%)
Termination of pregnancy	4/71 (5.6%)	3/74 (4.1%)
Death in the neonatal period	1/71 (1.4%)	0
Deafness	5/66 (7.6%)	0
Hearing loss	5/66 (7.6%)	1/71 (1.4%)
Neurodevelopmental delay	6/66 (9.1%)	3/71 (4.2%)
Clinical sequelae	13/66 (19.7%)	4/71 (5.6%)

Modified from Lipitz S, Yinon Y, Malinger G, et al. Risk of cytomegalovirus-associated sequelae in relation to time of infection and findings on prenatal imaging. *Ultrasound Obstet Gynecol.* 2013;41:508-514.

periventricular T2-weighted signal hyperintensity, (3) the presence of isolated temporal periventricular T2-weighted signal hyperintensity, (4) the presence of cysts and/or septa in the temporal and/or occipital lobe, and (5) the presence of migration disorders, cerebellar hypoplasia, and/or microcephaly. Isolated periventricular T2-weighted signal hyperintensity is a very common finding in cCMV infection (41%) but was not associated with adverse postnatal outcome except for 3 of the 21 neonates (14.3%) with isolated hyperintensity of the temporal lobes who had SNHL. The negative predictive value (NPV) was especially high: 96% in the absence of any MRI abnormalities.[128]

Relation to Neonatal Clinical Syndrome. The outcome relates to the severity of the neuropathological findings, and these findings correlate with the neonatal clinical syndrome (Table 34.7).[14] Although the data depicted in Table 34.7 are based on a sample that was selected to a certain degree, the observations are useful regarding the relationship between the neonatal clinical signs and the neurological outcome in congenital CMV infection. Thus, of those infants with the overt neurological syndrome (i.e., microcephaly, intracranial calcifications, or chorioretinitis), approximately 95% had major neurological sequelae (e.g., mental retardation, seizures, deafness, and motor deficits) or died. Infants with less obvious (*other*) neurological phenomena had slightly better prognoses. Approximately 70% of these infants with neonatal neurological signs also experienced systemic phenomena. In the large series (*n* = 80) of MacDonald and Tobin,[129] of the group of infants with systemic signs but no neonatal neurological deficits, approximately 50% were normal and only 16% exhibited major neurological sequelae or died (see Table 34.7). Further insight into the spectrum of cCMV infection is provided by the results of a recent study of 178 infants by Dreher et al. Comparison was made between a group of 78 recognized by newborn screening and 100 infants referred with clinical symptoms leading to a diagnosis of cCMV

TABLE 34.7   Relationship Between Neonatal Clinical Signs and Neurological Outcome in Congenital Cytomegalovirus Infection

	NEUROLOGICAL SEQUELAE[a]			
NEONATAL SIGNS	NORMAL (%)	MINOR (%)	MAJOR (%)	DEATH (%)
Neurological				
Microcephaly, intracranial calcifications, or chorioretinitis	7	0	79	14
Other	40	0	50	10
Systemic				
Jaundice, hepatosplenomegaly, or purpura, but no neurological signs	48	36	12	4
No neurological or systemic signs	81	16	3	0

Based on 80 infants.

[a]Expressed as a percentage of those with designated neonatal clinical signs.

Data from MacDonald H, Tobin JO. Congenital cytomegalovirus infection: a collaborative study on epidemiological, clinical and laboratory findings. *Dev Med Child Neurol.* 1978;20:471-478.

infection.[130] Two or more clinical findings were detected at birth in 91% of referred infants and only 58% of screened infants (*P* <.001). Significantly more children in the referred group had hearing loss compared with screened infants (*P* = .009). Of the screened children, 51% were free of sequelae at follow-up compared with only 28% of the referred group (*P* <.003).

For a more reliable prediction of neurological sequelae, MRI is currently recommended, especially in the presence of any cranial ultrasound abnormality. MRI allows assessment of additional migrational abnormalities not recognized with cranial ultrasound (see Fig. 34.8). The major neurological deficits include pronounced cognitive deficits, most commonly with intelligence quotient (IQ) scores lower than 70; spastic motor deficits; seizure disorders; and bilateral hearing loss.[a] In two series of 97 infants with symptomatic congenital CMV infection, mental retardation (IQ < 70) developed in 45% (IQ < 50 in 36%), cerebral palsy in 45%, seizures in 11%, and SNHL in 60%.[76,107] Outcome was accurately predicted based on abnormal cranial ultrasound findings in 12 of 57 (21%) neonates.[133] Cranial ultrasound lesions were more frequent in newborns with clinical and laboratory signs of congenital CMV infection at birth (10 of 18) than in newborns who had no symptoms at birth (2 of 39; *P* <.001). Cranial ultrasound abnormalities consisted of a combination of calcifications, LSV, ventriculomegaly, cysts, and cerebellar abnormalities. Additional neuroimaging, including MRI, performed in 8 infants provided more information in 6, including migrational disorders and white matter abnormalities. At least one sequela developed in all symptomatic neonates who had abnormal cranial ultrasound results, whereas none of the neonates with symptoms without cranial ultrasound abnormalities had long-term sequelae (*P* < .001). In the population without symptoms, SNHL developed in 3 of 37 (8.1%) neonates with normal cranial ultrasound results, whereas severe sequelae developed in 1 of 2 neonates with abnormal cranial ultrasound results. Another study of symptomatic infants showed relative microcephaly, CSF–β2-m concentrations, and grade 2 to 3 neuroimaging abnormalities:

TABLE 34.8   Subsequent Hearing Loss in Infants With Asymptomatic Congenital Cytomegalovirus Infection

HEARING LOSS		AFFECTED
TYPE	SEVERITY[a]	(%)
Bilateral		11
	Mild	5
	Moderate to profound	6
Unilateral		8
	Mild	4
	Moderate to profound	4

[a]Mild hearing loss, 22 to 55 dB; moderate to profound, ≥55 dB.

Data from references 121-124,134,135,137,138.

(grade 1) single punctate calcification and/or LSV; (grade 2) multiple discrete periventricular calcifications and/or moderate to severe ventriculomegaly; and (grade 3) extensive periventricular calcifications and/or brain atrophy. Grade 3 was shown to be significantly associated with an unfavorable outcome.[75] The combination of CSF β2-m greater than 7.9 mg/L and moderate to severe neuroimaging alterations improved predictive ability (area under the curve, 0.92 ± 0.06; sensitivity, 87%; specificity, 100%).

Outcome With Asymptomatic Congenital Infection. The asymptomatic group has been the particular focus of numerous investigators.[a] In these studies, the most consistent sequela was SNHL (Table 34.8). Approximately 11% of the infants developed bilateral hearing loss, with moderate to profound loss in 6%. Often, hearing deficits were not detected until serious impairment of language development occurred. Indeed, as noted with symptomatic disease, with more frequent serial measurements, it became clear that hearing impairment often did not become clearly apparent until infancy and early

---

[a]References 14, 52, 76, 81, 86, 87, 107, 131, 132.

[a]References 35, 77, 83, 86, 88, 134-141.

childhood, during which it progressed (see earlier discussion). In a large longitudinal study of 307 infants, 7.2% exhibited SNHL, and among these infants, 50% exhibited progression (median age at onset of progression, 18 months), and 18% exhibited delayed onset (median age of detection, 27 months).[140] Of 580 children, 77 had hearing loss at birth and 38 developed delayed hearing loss by the end of follow-up.[127] In multivariate analyses, delayed hearing loss was strongly associated with symptomatic infection at birth (OR = 5.9, 95% CI: 1.8 to 18.9) and modestly associated with older age at last culture-positive visit (OR = 1.6, 95% CI: 1.1 to 2.0, comparing 1-year age differences). Between the ages of 6 months and 8 years, delayed hearing loss can be expected to occur in 6.9% of asymptomatic children and in 33.7% of symptomatic children. In a study of 388 infants, as noted earlier, 3% of asymptomatic infants had SNHL in the first month and 11% had hearing loss by 6 years of age.[77] In a more recent series of 300 affected infants born after nonprimary (n = 124) or primary (n = 176) infection, although bilateral hearing loss occurred equally in both groups (10% to 11%), infants born after primary maternal infection were more likely to have severe or profound hearing loss (63% vs. 15%).[88] The diagnosis of hearing loss was made earlier in the infants born after primary maternal infection (mean age, 13 months vs. 39 months). Histopathological and immunofluorescent studies of the inner ear in two affected infants revealed destruction of cells of the organ of Corti and the neurons of the eighth nerve as well as the presence of viral antigen.[138] Thus, in view of the prevalence of the infection, involvement of cochlear structures with congenital CMV infection and the consequent disturbance of hearing may be an enormous public health problem. Assessment of the viral load in blood at birth may aid in predicting the development of late-onset sequelae in asymptomatic congenital CMV infection. This conclusion was supported by a study of 33 newborns with asymptomatic cCMV infection born to women with primary CMV infection during pregnancy.[142] Of these 33 newborns, 10 showed postnatal sequelae, including isolated SNHL in 7; these sequelae were significantly related to DNAemia at birth, with a risk of hearing deficit apparent at a blood viral load of ≥17,000 copies per milliliter.

The possibility of subtle disturbances of intellectual function was initially suggested by studies conducted by Hanshaw et al.,[135] who demonstrated a statistically significant lower mean IQ score in asymptomatic patients versus matched controls (102 vs. 112). Subsequent large-scale studies did not document definite impairment of intellectual function in asymptomatic infants,[122,134,137] particularly when hearing-impaired children were excluded.[136,139] Intellectual outcome in hearing-impaired children has not yet been studied in detail; it is important to define outcome in this setting separately because the virus clearly has entered the CNS in this subgroup of infected infants. Nevertheless, several reports suggest that an asymptomatic neonatal period may be followed by varying combinations of developmental delay, microcephaly, ataxia, SNHL, and seizures, usually recognized in the first year of life.[22,57-59,62] CT or MRI has shown cerebral calcification, abnormal cerebral white matter signal, delayed myelination, polymicrogyria, focal subcortical areas of abnormality, or cerebellar hypoplasia. The possibility of late intrauterine acquisition of infection has been suggested in some of these asymptomatic infants, but most studies indicate that although the risk of intrauterine transmission following

primary maternal infection in the third trimester is high, the risk of neonatal disease is low.[20,121] In the study by Enders and colleagues, no symptoms were observed in infected newborns of mothers with primary infection in the preconceptional period and in the third trimester.

The important clinical point is that CMV infection should be considered later in infancy in the presence of such neurological or neuroradiological features or both, even if the neonatal period was unremarkable. More data are needed on these issues.

Management

Prevention. Congenital CMV infection is related to primary infection of the pregnant woman, presumably early in pregnancy. Two preventive approaches may be used: one to prevent or treat the primary infection and the other to terminate the pregnancy. Prevention of the primary maternal infection by vaccination has received initial investigation, with variable results.[143,144] However, more information is needed about the effectiveness, hazards, and feasibility of this approach.[145-147] Treatment of the primary maternal infection with hyperimmune gamma globulin is a possibility, but the difficulty in detecting most maternal infections has been a major problem with this approach. The results of the first randomized trial with hyperimmune gamma globulin or placebo enrolled 124 women with primary CMV infection.[148] There was no difference in viral load in the amniotic fluid and newborn urine and no difference in cCMV infection. There was a nonsignificant increase in adverse obstetrical events, including preterm birth, preeclampsia, and fetal growth restriction. One other trial (NCT01376778) with hyperimmune gamma globulin is still in progress. Termination of a pregnancy complicated by a primary maternal infection has been difficult because the exact risks of fetal infection are not entirely known. Detection of the infected fetus by amniocentesis and identification of the virus or DNA by culture or PCR, respectively, constitute the principal approach.[54,144,149-152] The sensitivity for detection of fetal infection increases markedly after 21 weeks of gestation. The fetal condition can then be assessed further by ultrasonography, which may show intracranial calcification or other evidence of parenchymal disease, and, if desired, by cordocentesis, with evaluation of fetal blood for abnormal liver function tests, CMV-specific IgM, anemia, or thrombocytopenia. In one series, the risk of identification of *neonatal* neurological abnormality by neurological examination, cranial ultrasonography, or hearing assessment was only 19% when no *prenatal* ultrasonographic abnormalities were present.[54] Ultrasonographic abnormalities were detected prenatally in 21%, and nearly all of these pregnancies were terminated.

Supportive Therapy. From the neonatal neurological standpoint, supportive therapy consists principally of control of seizures.

Antimicrobial Therapy. Prenatal therapy with CMV-specific hyperimmune immunoglobulin is controversial, with a recent phase 2 clinical trial study refuting earlier claims of improved outcomes.[153] Investigation of maternal oral treatment with valganciclovir is currently in clinical trials as well.[154,155] Treatment in the neonatal period is more established and is instituted in infants with evidence of brain involvement including SNHL as well as other serious end-organ disease. Several antiviral agents—including adenine arabinoside (Ara-A),

TABLE 34.9   Effect of 6 Weeks of Ganciclovir and 6 Weeks or 6 Months of Valganciclovir Therapy on Hearing in Symptomatic Cytomegalovirus Disease

HEARING FROM NEONATAL PERIOD TO ≥1 YEAR	NO TREATMENT n = 19 (%)	GANCICLOVIR 6 WEEKS n = 24 (%)	VALGANCICLOVIR 6 WEEKS n = 43 (%)	VALGANCICLOVIR 6 MONTHS n = 43 (%)
No deficit, both periods	22	23	52	66
Deficit improved	0	25	5	8
Deficit unchanged	17	31	30	19
Deficit worsened	61	21	13	8

Values are percentages of all ears tested in each group.
Data from Kimberlin DW, Lin CY, Sanchez PJ, et al. Effect of ganciclovir therapy on hearing in symptomatic congenital cytomegalovirus disease involving the central nervous system: a randomized, controlled trial. J Pediatr. 2003;143:16-25; Kimberlin DW, Jester PM, Sanchez PJ, et al. Valganciclovir for symptomatic congenital cytomegalovirus disease. N Engl J Med. 2015;372:933-943.

5-iodo-2′-deoxyuridine (IDU), cytosine arabinoside (Ara-C), and acyclovir—have been studied because of their effectiveness in vitro.[146,156] Ara-A and acyclovir are the least toxic of these agents, but early trials did not provide reason for optimism. Ganciclovir, an acyclovir derivative, has been shown to be effective in the prophylaxis and treatment of CMV infections in immunocompromised adults and children.[157-160] Initial data with infants are promising.[161,162] An earlier study of 12 infants with congenital CMV infection suggested distinct clinical benefit (e.g., loss of hepatosplenomegaly, improvement in tone) with a 3-month course of therapy.[106] The most impressive data with ganciclovir involved a randomized controlled trial of the effect of the agent on hearing in symptomatic congenital CMV disease involving the CNS (Table 34.9).[125] The treated infants received ganciclovir, 6 mg/kg per dose, administered intravenously every 12 hours for 6 weeks. Hearing deficits either improved or remained static in 56% of the ears of treated infants versus only 17% of those of the control infants (see Table 34.9). Progression of deficits occurred in only 21% in the ganciclovir group versus 61% in the control group. The beneficial effect of ganciclovir was accompanied by significant neutropenia in approximately 65% of treated infants. These findings were supported by an observational study enrolling 23 asymptomatic children with cCMV infection.[163] Twelve children were treated just after diagnosis of cCMV infection in the newborn period, with ganciclovir 10 mg/kg bodyweight for 21 days. The other 11 children were observed without therapy. All 23 children had normal sensorineural hearing at 1-year follow-up. In all, 18 children were seen over the 4- to 11-year follow-up period. SNHL occurred in 2 (11.1%) children who did not receive ganciclovir in the newborn period. None of the nine ganciclovir-treated children developed SNHL. During ganciclovir therapy, moderate neutropenia occurred as a side effect in 2 out of 12 (16.6%) treated children.

The experience with ganciclovir illustrates the need for an agent that has less toxicity and can be administered orally. Valganciclovir, shown to be effective in adults with CMV retinitis, may prove to be such an agent. In a recent randomized, placebo-controlled trial of valganciclovir therapy in 96 neonates with symptomatic cCMV disease, the effect of 6 months of therapy was compared with that resulting from 6 weeks of therapy (Table 34.9).[164] The primary end point was the change in hearing in the better ear (best ear) hearing from baseline to 6 months. Secondary end points included the change in hearing from baseline to follow-up at 12 and 24 months and neurodevelopmental outcomes, with each end point adjusted for CNS involvement at baseline. Of the initial 96 neonates, 86 could be evaluated at 6 months. There was no difference for best-ear hearing at 6 months. Total-ear hearing (hearing in one or both ears that could be evaluated) was more likely to be improved or to remain normal at 12 months in the 6-month treatment group compared with the 6-week treatment group (73% vs. 57%, P = .01). This benefit was still present at 24 months (77% vs. 64%, P = .04). At 24 months, the 6-month group, as compared with the 6-week group, had better neurodevelopmental scores on the language-composite component (P = 0.004) and the receptive-communication scale (P = .003) of the Bayley Scales of Infant and Toddler Development (3rd ed.). Neutropenia was not uncommon and occurred in 27% of those in the 6-week treatment group. In the 6-month treatment group, neutropenia occurred in 19% of the infants during the first 6 weeks and in 21% during the next 4.5 months. Because migrational disorders are associated with the most severe adverse neurological sequelae and evolve in utero, it is unlikely that either 6 weeks or 6 months of treatment with valganciclovir will have a positive effect on such neurological sequelae. Preservation of hearing, however, would be of benefit, and the policy of 6 months of therapy is now recommended. Treatment for 12 months with a combination of ganciclovir and valganciclovir was recently reported.[165] Hearing impairment was diagnosed at birth in 54 (36%) of the 149 infants diagnosed with symptomatic cCMV; it was unilateral in 31 (57%) and bilateral in 23 (43%). After 1 year of antiviral treatment and a long-term follow-up of the 77 affected ears at baseline, 50 (65%) had improved, 22 (29%) remained unchanged, and 5 (6%) had deteriorated. Most improved ears (38 of 50 = 76%) returned to normal hearing. Improvement was most likely to occur in infants born with mild or moderate hearing loss and less in those with severe impairment.

There is at present no agreement about the beneficial role of treatment with valgancyclovir in *preterm* infants with *pCMV* infection. Most clinicians are reluctant to use a potentially toxic drug in preterm infants and restrict therapy to those with a sepsis-like illness.[39] Ultimately, treatment of asymptomatic infants would be ideal if the risk-to-benefit ratio of the agent were favorable.

TABLE 34.10 Relationship Between the Incidence and Severity of Congenital Toxoplasmosis and the Time of Maternal Infection

MATERNAL INFECTION: TRIMESTER OF PREGNANCY	INFANTS INFECTED (%)	CONGENITAL TOXOPLASMOSIS[a]	
		SEVERE (%)	ASYMPTOMATIC OR MILD (%)
First	17	60	40
Second	25	30	70
Third	65	0	100

Based on 145 pregnancies.

[a]Percentage of infected infants with severe disease (central nervous system and ocular involvement) or those with asymptomatic disease or isolated ocular involvement (mild).

Data from Desmonts G, Couvreur J. Toxoplasmosis in pregnancy and its transmission to the fetus. *Bull N Y Acad Med.* 1974;50:146-159.

Toxoplasmosis

Intrauterine infection with *T. gondii*, a protozoan parasite, causes congenital toxoplasmosis. It is estimated that more than a third of the world's population has been infected with the parasite, but seroprevalence is not evenly distributed across countries and different socioeconomic strata. Pregnant women may become infected by ingesting or dealing with raw or undercooked meat containing tissue cysts or water or food containing oocysts excreted in the feces of infected cats.[166] This congenital infection is second only to congenital CMV infection in terms of frequency and clinical importance. As with infection with CMV, congenital toxoplasmosis is acquired in utero by transplacental mechanisms, and most affected newborn infants (85%) are asymptomatic. However, with careful clinical evaluation and a high index of suspicion, this infection is more readily identified in the infected newborn than is CMV infection. Congenital toxoplasmosis can be prevented and treated during gestation. The disease tends to be less severe in countries where prenatal screening and treatment have been systematically implemented.

Pathogenesis

Fetal Infection. Clinically significant infection with toxoplasmosis occurs during intrauterine life by transplacental passage of the parasite.[167] The sequence of events is (1) primary infection of the mother, (2) parasitemia, (3) placentitis, and (4) hematogenous spread to the fetus.[168,169] The organism can be cultured consistently from the placenta when the fetus is infected.[170] As with CMV, the mother infected with toxoplasmosis is usually asymptomatic.[168,171] The most common clinical presentation of the mother is localized or generalized lymphadenopathy, sometimes with fever and other features suggestive of infectious mononucleosis.[168]

The incidence of primary maternal infection during pregnancy varies around the world. In Paris, when consumption of undercooked meat was relatively common, the value was as high as 5 per 100 pregnancies.[168-170] At a comparable time, the rate in the United States was approximately 1.1 per 1000 pregnancies.[171] More recent incidences are 0.5 to 2.0 per 1000 pregnancies in Western Australia, Europe, and the United States.[172-174] These rates should be contrasted with the approximately tenfold-higher rates for CMV infection during pregnancy (see earlier discussion). A study of congenital infection, based on a serological investigation of filter paper blood specimens

TABLE 34.11 Neuropathology of Congenital Toxoplasmosis Overtly Symptomatic in the Neonatal Period

Meningoencephalitis, granulomatous
Diffuse cerebral necrosis, sometimes with porencephaly and hydranencephaly
Diffuse cerebral calcifications
Periventricular inflammation and necrosis, especially periaqueductal
Hydrocephalus

for neonatal metabolic screening in Massachusetts, yielded an incidence of only approximately 1 per 10,000.[175,176] In a study from Switzerland using enzyme-linked immunosorbent assay (ELISA) (IgM and/or IgA antibodies) of the cord blood, seroprevalence of congenital toxoplasmosis declined from 0.08% to 0.012% from 1982 to 1999.[177] Despite increasing maternal age, seroprevalence for toxoplasmosis decreased steadily from 53% to 35% during this period. The unusual susceptibility of the human fetus and newborn to severe infection with *T. gondii* appears to relate in large part to inadequate cellular defenses.[178] Mononuclear phagocytes are the principal defense against such infection, and a decreased generation of macrophage-activating material by fetal lymphocytes has been demonstrated. Moreover, the response to this activating material by macrophages in the neonate is also deficient. Uncontrolled replication of the organism is the expected result.

Importance of Time of Maternal Infection. The likelihood and severity of congenital toxoplasmosis bear a distinct relation to the time of maternal infection (Table 34.10). Only approximately 20% to 25% of infants will be infected if the maternal infection occurs in the first or second trimester, especially the second to sixth months of gestation, versus approximately 65% if maternal infection occurs in the third trimester.[168,179] In a large series of 603 women with confirmed maternal toxoplasmosis, the maternal-fetal transmission rate was only 6% with infection at 13 weeks but increased to 72% with infection at 36 weeks.[179] However, although fetal infection is less likely earlier in pregnancy, the *severity* of the disease is greater. Indeed, most infants infected in the first trimester exhibit severe disease, manifested by CNS and ocular involvement (Table 34.11). As a result of these counterbalancing effects, in one large series the highest risk of bearing an infected infant with early clinical manifestations (10%) occurred in women who seroconverted at 24 to 30 weeks of gestation.[179] A CT study of 31 infants further documented the severity of the CNS lesions as a function of the time of intrauterine infection.[180] Therefore it appears that although a fetal-maternal barrier to infection may be operative early in pregnancy, once fetal infection is established at that time, it is a potentially devastating disease. Treatment of the infected mother alters both the likelihood of fetal transmission and the severity of the disease (see later discussion). Following the introduction of prenatal screening in France in 1992, a significant reduction in the rate of congenital infection and a better outcome at 3 years of age in infected children was reported.[181] Among 2048 mother-infant pairs, 93% of mothers received prenatal treatment and 513 (25%) fetuses were infected. Probabilities of congenital infection were less than 10% for maternal infections before 12 weeks of gestation, 20% at 19 weeks, and to 52% and almost 70% at 28 and 39 weeks' GA, respectively.

Neuropathology

As with CMV infection, congenital toxoplasmosis may be associated with asymptomatic or symptomatic neurological presentations in the newborn period (see later discussion). Although the symptomatic neurological presentation is relatively uncommon, it is described here because it serves as the prototype for the neuropathology produced by infection with this organism. Toxoplasmosis does not appear to possess the teratogenic potential of CMV infection, and essentially all the neuropathological features are related to tissue inflammation and destruction (see Table 34.11).[182-184]

Meningoencephalitis. The meningoencephalitis of toxoplasmosis has a striking multifocal, necrotizing, granulomatous quality and is characterized by the following: (1) inflammatory cells in the meninges, especially over focal lesions; (2) perivascular infiltrates with inflammatory cells, the latter often including eosinophils; (3) multifocal and diffuse necroses of brain parenchyma, with all cellular elements affected, involving cerebrum, brain stem, and spinal cord and often associated with calcification; (4) reactive microglial and astroglial proliferation; and (5) miliary granulomas, containing large epithelioid cells and free, intracellular, or encysted organisms (Fig. 34.12).

Porencephaly and Hydranencephaly. With particularly severe, diffuse, cerebral destructive disease, porencephalic cysts or hydranencephaly may develop.[185] Of the 33 fetuses with congenital toxoplasmosis studied by Hohlfeld et al.,[182] all exhibited areas of brain necrosis, the initial lesions that evolve to porencephaly and hydranencephaly. The development of these large areas of tissue destruction is particularly likely if aqueductal block and increased intraventricular pressure are associated.

Hydrocephalus. Two processes appear to be operative in the periventricular region with toxoplasmosis and may underlie the propensity for aqueductal block and consequent hydrocephalus in this disorder. First, the inflammation with toxoplasmosis has a predilection for the periventricular region, as with CMV infection (although in toxoplasmosis more severe

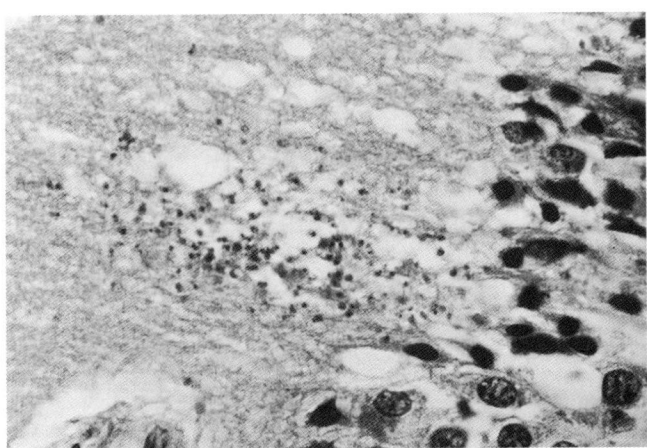

Figure 34.12 Congenital toxoplasmosis: encephalitis. Photomicrograph of a region of necrosis containing many free *Toxoplasma* organisms (note small, darkly stained nuclei to the left of larger, preserved neurons). Although this lesion was from an older child with *Toxoplasma* encephalitis who was receiving immunosuppressive therapy, the organisms are identical in appearance to those of the congenital form. (From Bell WE, McCormick WF. *Neurologic Infections in Children.* Philadelphia: Saunders; 1975.)

diffuse disease is present elsewhere, and calcified areas of necrosis are present throughout the cerebrum). Second, it is believed that *Toxoplasma* organisms enter the ventricular system from the parenchymal lesions and disseminate there. This highly antigenic ventricular fluid then seeps through the damaged ependyma to periventricular blood vessels, where an antigen-antibody reaction may occur at the vessel wall, thereby causing thrombosis and periventricular infarction. This additional necrosis apparently causes the serious aqueductal block that results in hydrocephalus, the common complication. Among 33 infected fetuses identified in utero by Hohlfeld et al.,[182] 19 (58%) had ventricular dilation at autopsy after elective termination of pregnancy.

Microcephaly. Although hydrocephalus is a more common result of congenital infection with *T. gondii* and is more frequent in this variety of congenital infection than in any other, microcephaly does occur in a significant percentage of patients, approximately 15% (see subsequent discussion). The microcephaly relates to the multifocal necrotizing encephalitis, particularly of the cerebral hemispheres. Indeed, even in patients with hydrocephalus, it is clear that a serious loss of brain substance, in addition to the effects of the hydrocephalus, has invariably occurred.

Clinical Aspects

Incidence of Clinically Apparent Infection. As with CMV, clinically asymptomatic cases of congenital toxoplasmosis outnumber symptomatic cases. However, a larger proportion of infants with congenital toxoplasmosis than with congenital CMV infection can be detected clinically in the newborn period.

Of 156 children with congenital toxoplasmosis who were monitored prospectively from the time of maternal infection, approximately 18% had CNS and ocular involvement, 2% had CNS involvement without ocular involvement, 12% had ocular involvement only, and 68% were asymptomatic.[1] Thus 20% of infants with congenital toxoplasmosis had observable CNS

TABLE 34.12	Clinical Features of Symptomatic Congenital Toxoplasmosis	
CLINICAL FEATURE		**APPROXIMATE FREQUENCY (%)**
Pregnancy		
Prematurity, fetal growth restriction, or both		0–20
Central nervous system		
Seizures		21–50
Meningoencephalitis		51–75
Intracranial calcification		51–75
Hydrocephalus		21–50
Microcephaly		0–20
Eye		
Chorioretinitis		76–100
Reticuloendothelial system		
Hepatosplenomegaly		21–50
Hyperbilirubinemia		21–50
Anemia		51–75
Petechiae		0–20
Other		
Pneumonitis		0–20

Data from Remington JS, McLeod R, Thulliez P, Desmonts G. Toxoplasmosis. In: Remington JS, Klein JO, Wilson CB, et al., eds. *Infectious Diseases of the Fetus and Newborn Infant.* 6th ed. Philadelphia: Elsevier Saunders; 2006; Eichenwald H. A study of congenital toxoplasmosis. In: Siim JC, ed. *Human Toxoplasmosis.* Copenhagen: Munksgaard; 1970.

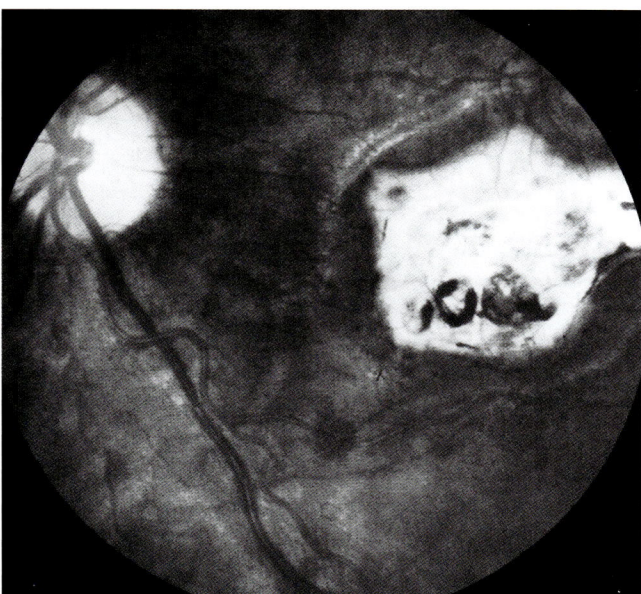

Figure 34.13 Congenital toxoplasmosis: chorioretinitis. Note the striking lesion at the macula *(right)* as well as optic atrophy *(left)*. (From Bell WE, McCormick WF. *Neurologic Infections in Children.* Philadelphia: Saunders; 1975.)

involvement in the newborn period in this study. The incidence of subclinical infection is higher in infants of women treated during pregnancy than in infants of women not treated (see later discussion). The findings are quite similar when compared with a more recent prospective study covering a 20-year period (1985–2005), where all mothers received spiramycin, alone or associated with pyrimethamine-sulfadoxine, and underwent amniocentesis and monthly ultrasound screening.[186] Of 666 liveborn children, 112 (17%) had congenital toxoplasmosis and 107 were followed for 12 to 250 months: 79 were asymptomatic (74%) and 28 had chorioretinitis (26%). There was only one infant with serious neurological involvement.

Clinical Features. Symptomatic patients (not treated in utero) can often be divided into those with predominantly neurological syndromes and those with predominantly systemic syndromes (Table 34.12 shows combined data for both syndromes).[184,187] The *neurological syndrome* accounts for approximately two thirds of the cases and consists principally of abnormal CSF and other signs of meningoencephalitis, seizures, diffuse intracranial calcification, hydrocephalus, or, less commonly, microcephaly (see Table 34.12). At least 90% of these patients exhibit chorioretinitis (also termed retinochoroiditis). In congenital toxoplasmosis, chorioretinitis is typically bilateral and prominent in the macular regions (Fig. 34.13) and is of major diagnostic importance.[1] Initially, the lesion appears in the fundus as yellowish white, cotton-like patches with indistinct margins.[182] These patches evolve over the ensuing months into sharply demarcated, *punched-out*, pigmented lesions, often accompanied by optic atrophy. Although the chorioretinitis is

most commonly apparent in the newborn period, particularly by indirect ophthalmoscopy, it may not develop for months or even years.[181,182] These ocular lesions may relapse after birth despite pre- and postnatal treatment. In a recent study by Wallon and colleagues, 477 cases of confirmed congenital toxoplasmosis were followed for a median of 10.5 years (75th percentile: 15.0 years).[183] Almost one third (29.8%) showed at least one ocular lesion. The lesion was unilateral in about two thirds (69.0%) and lesions were first manifested at a median age of 3.1 (0.0 to 20.7) years. In one third (33.8%) of the children, recurrences or new ocular lesions occurred up to 12 years after the appearance of the first lesion. Early maternal infection, prematurity, and nonocular congenital toxoplasmosis lesions at the time of diagnosis of congenital toxoplasmosis were associated with a higher risk of chorioretinitis.

The *systemic syndrome* of congenital toxoplasmosis is dominated by signs referable to the reticuloendothelial system, especially hepatosplenomegaly, hyperbilirubinemia, and anemia (see Table 34.12). A petechial rash may occur but is less common than with CMV infection. Overt clinical evidence of neurological involvement is often lacking in these patients, but CSF abnormalities, frequently with a disproportionately elevated protein content for the degree of pleocytosis, occur in approximately 85% and reflect concomitant meningoencephalitis.[1,37] Chorioretinitis is observed in at least two thirds of patients with systemic infections, a finding that underscores the importance of careful evaluation of the fundus, especially by indirect ophthalmoscopy, when congenital toxoplasmosis is possible.

An unknown but probably very considerable number of infants with no neurological or systemic signs of congenital toxoplasmosis (i.e., *asymptomatic disease*) will exhibit chorioretinitis, detectable in the newborn period by indirect ophthalmoscopy. Although most of the retinal lesions observed later probably develop in the weeks and months after delivery (see subsequent discussion), further data are needed regarding the proportion detectable in the newborn period. In a series of 48 asymptomatic infants in whom infection was detected by newborn blood screening, 2 had active chorioretinitis and 7 others had retinal scars; thus 19% had retinal disease.[175] Moreover, approximately 20% had cerebral calcifications detectable by CT and 25% had CSF findings consistent with encephalitis. The later development of neurological deficits and visual loss is appreciable and is discussed in the section on prognosis.

The *clinical course* of the disease is not readily predicted; indeed, evidence of progression of retinal and cerebral disease has been presented.[181,182,188,189] Because many patients with symptomatic congenital toxoplasmosis exhibit very severe neurological deficits from the neonatal period, the frequency of progression is difficult to quantitate.

Clinical Diagnosis. Certain clinical features are helpful in suggesting the diagnosis of congenital toxoplasmosis. A particularly noteworthy constellation of features includes evidence of meningoencephalitis, focal and multifocal cerebral necroses, diffuse cerebral calcification, hydrocephalus, and scarring chorioretinopathy in the macular regions. Fetal growth restriction or prematurity is generally not a prominent feature, as in infants with congenital CMV or rubella infections, and microcephaly is less common than in congenital CMV infection. The systemic syndrome may cause confusion in differentiating toxoplasmosis from other congenital infections, but a petechial rash is relatively less common in congenital toxoplasmosis.

Laboratory Evaluation

Isolation of *Toxoplasma*. Determination of *T. gondii* as the responsible microbe in the newborn with congenital toxoplasmosis depends principally on serological tests rather than isolation of the organism per se. Nevertheless, the organism or associated DNA can be isolated from placental tissue, ventricular or lumbar CSF, blood, and amniotic fluid.[1] The tissue extracts or fluids can be injected into either mice or tissue culture preparations.[190,191] Parasitemia is more readily demonstrated in the first week after birth (71%) than in the second to fourth weeks (33%), and it is detected most easily in generalized rather than in neurological disease.[1] The isolation procedures for toxoplasmosis require specialized techniques and an experienced, skilled laboratory staff. Detection of *T. gondii* in amniotic fluid by PCR with a sensitivity of 80% has suggested that this rapid test (result available in ≤6 hours) could become very important in the diagnosis when the technique is applied to biological fluids of the newborn infant.[192] Even better overall sensitivity of 92.2% (95% CI 81% to 98%) was reported in another study, where PCR was performed on 261 amniotic fluid samples.[192] There were four negative results in fetuses that were infected. PCR performed in the CSF was found to be positive in 27 of the 58 (46.5%) congenitally infected infants and negative in each of the 103 infants without congenital toxoplasmosis.[193] The CSF PCR was positive in 70.9%, 53.3%, and 50.9% of those with hydrocephalus, cerebral calcifications, and/or eye disease, respectively. Of six infants who were negative for both IgM and IgA antibodies, three had a positive PCR in their CSF as the confirmatory test for diagnosis of congenital toxoplasmosis. IgM and IgA antibodies and CSF PCR, when combined, yielded a higher sensitivity for

diagnosis of congenital toxoplasmosis when compared with the performance of each test alone. The sensitivity of PCR on placental tissue is only approximately 60%.[194]

Serological Studies. The identification of most cases of congenital toxoplasmosis is established by serological techniques. The two most commonly used tests are the Sabin-Feldman dye test and the IgM-fluorescent antibody test. The *Sabin-Feldman dye test*, perhaps the single most reliable test, is performed by mixing live organisms with the test serum (and a human serum component, the accessory factor) and then exposing the mixture to methylene blue. Parasites exposed to the antibody-containing serum are modified and stained. The antibodies for the dye test are passively transferred, and the maternal component does not decrease significantly for several months after birth. Persistence of high titers is necessary for diagnosis and obviously is time-consuming. Moreover, the dye test requires the use of hazardous live organisms, and the accessory factor is sometimes difficult to obtain. The Sabin-Feldman dye test, immunofluorescent antibody test, ELISA, IgG avidity test, and agglutination and differential agglutination test can be used for the detection of IgG antibodies. These tests are positive within 1 to 2 weeks after the infection and persist indefinitely. IgM antibodies arise within the first week of infection, rapidly increase, and thereafter decline and disappear at highly variable rates. A negative IgM test essentially rules out a recently acquired infection. However, it should be noted that commercial kits used to detect IgM antibodies in nonreference laboratories may be unreliable, with false-positive rates as high as 60%. The avidity test for IgG antibodies helps to discriminate between a recently acquired infection and one obtained in the more distant past. The presence of high-avidity antibodies essentially rules out infection acquired in the preceding 3 to 4 months. Reactivation can be seen in immunocompromised women, and this has been reported in HIV-infected women.[195] The *Toxoplasma-specific IgM-fluorescent antibody technique* is faster and more specific. This test measures fetally produced IgM antibody to the organism. Killed organisms are used to bind specific IgM, which is then detected by exposure to fluorescein-antiserum to human IgM. The reliability of this test is hindered by certain factors that impair both sensitivity and specificity.[173,196] The more recently developed *IgM-capture ELISA*, which isolates and concentrates the infant's IgM, increases the sensitivity markedly (90% of infected infants are detected), and false-positive reactions are unusual.[197] This test has been adapted to filter paper blood specimens. More recent data suggest value for the analysis of IgA or IgE in neonatal blood.[194] However, sensitivities for all these last tests are very low for infants infected in the first 20 weeks of gestation, when severe disease is the most likely result. Finally, the use of a comparative analysis of mother–newborn Ig-G and Ig-M by western blot, first described by Remington et al.,[198] has also been advocated. Tissot Dupont et al.[199] reported a sensitivity of 82.6% for the detection of IgG, IgM, and IgA by western blot within the first 3 months of life, whereas at birth the same combination had a sensitivity of 65.2%.[199] The combination of IgG and IgM yielded the best score, whereas IgA detection was the least sensitive. The combination of western blot and conventional serological analysis increased the sensitivity at birth to 78% and within the first 3 months of life to 85%.[200]

Neurodiagnostic Studies. Neurodiagnostic studies that particularly suggest congenital toxoplasmosis are evaluations of CSF and brain imaging. Pleocytosis and elevated protein content of CSF indicate meningoencephalitis and may be observed in asymptomatic as well as symptomatic patients. Particularly characteristic of congenital toxoplasmosis is the finding of a very high protein content in the ventricular fluid, usually reflecting the aqueductal obstruction and stagnation of infection within the lateral ventricles. Although skull radiographs are effective in demonstrating the diffuse and periventricular cerebral calcification (Fig. 34.14), *CT scan* is more effective and allows identification of calcification more distant from the lateral ventricles, in contrast to CMV, in which calcifications are mostly adjacent to the lateral ventricles (Fig. 34.15).[180] CT data indicate that calcifications of the basal ganglia are more common than previously suspected.[180] The calcifications associated with congenital toxoplasmosis, especially of the periventricular type or of the basal ganglia, can also be detected by *cranial ultrasound* (see Figs. 34.15 and 34.16).[109] In contrast to cCMV, data on MRI in congenital toxoplasmosis are limited. In a small study of eight cases with antenatal imaging, MRI was performed before and after 3 weeks of spiramycin treatment, showing similar findings.[201] *MRI scan* provides the most detailed assessment of parenchymal necroses (Fig. 34.17).

Prognosis

Relation to the Neonatal Clinical Syndrome. As with CMV, the outcome of untreated congenital toxoplasmosis relates to the severity of the neuropathology, which correlates to a modest extent with the neonatal clinical syndrome (Table 34.13). Infants with congenital toxoplasmosis with prominent neonatal *neurological* features do poorly; only 9% are normal on follow-up. Most of the remaining infants exhibit serious disturbances of cerebral function (i.e., mental retardation,

seizures, and spastic motor deficits). Essentially all such patients have chorioretinitis and may also have optic atrophy; as a consequence, approximately 70% have severe visual impairment.

Somewhat unlike congenital CMV infection, congenital toxoplasmosis with a neonatal syndrome characterized by

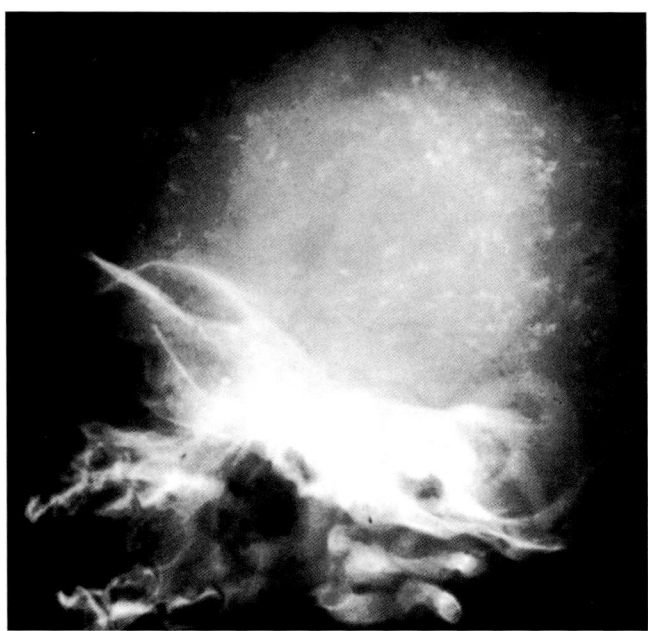

Figure 34.14 **Congenital toxoplasmosis: diffuse calcification shown on skull radiograph.** This is a lateral skull film of an infant with hydrocephalus, chorioretinitis, and multiple, punctate calcifications scattered diffusely in brain. (From Bell WE, McCormick WF. *Neurologic Infections in Children.* Philadelphia: Saunders; 1975.)

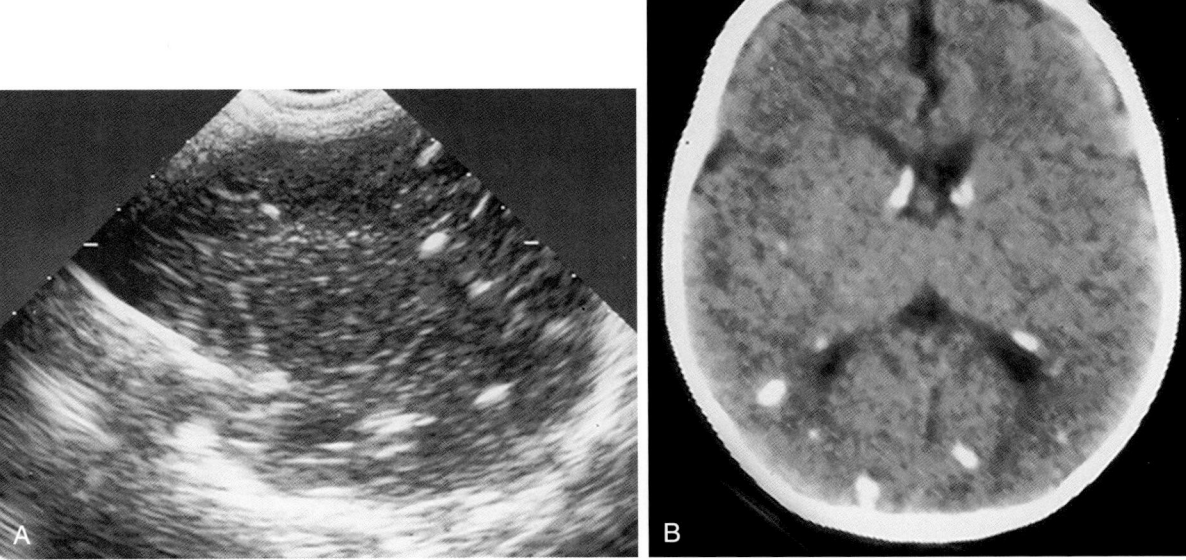

Figure 34.15 **Congenital toxoplasmosis: ultrasonography and computed tomography.** Parasagittal ultrasound (A) showing widespread areas of calcification, confirmed with axial computed tomography (B), showing periventricular as well as subcortical and cortical calcifications.

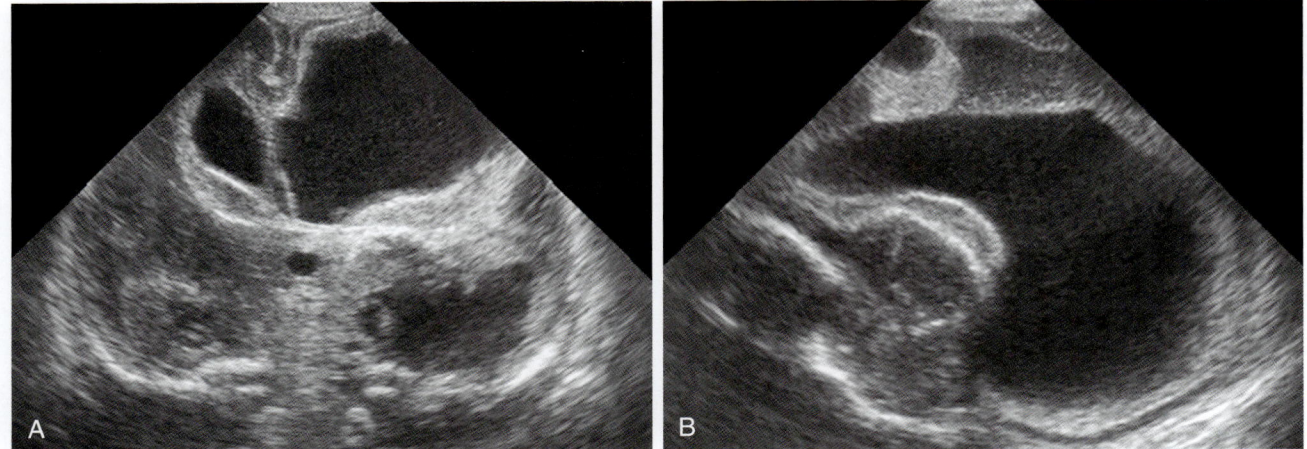

Figure 34.16 Congenital toxoplasmosis: cranial ultrasound. Coronal (A) and parasagittal (B) ultrasound scans showing severely enlarged ventricles and a large left-sided porencephaly. The germinal layer is also very echogenic bilaterally, most likely due to calcification.

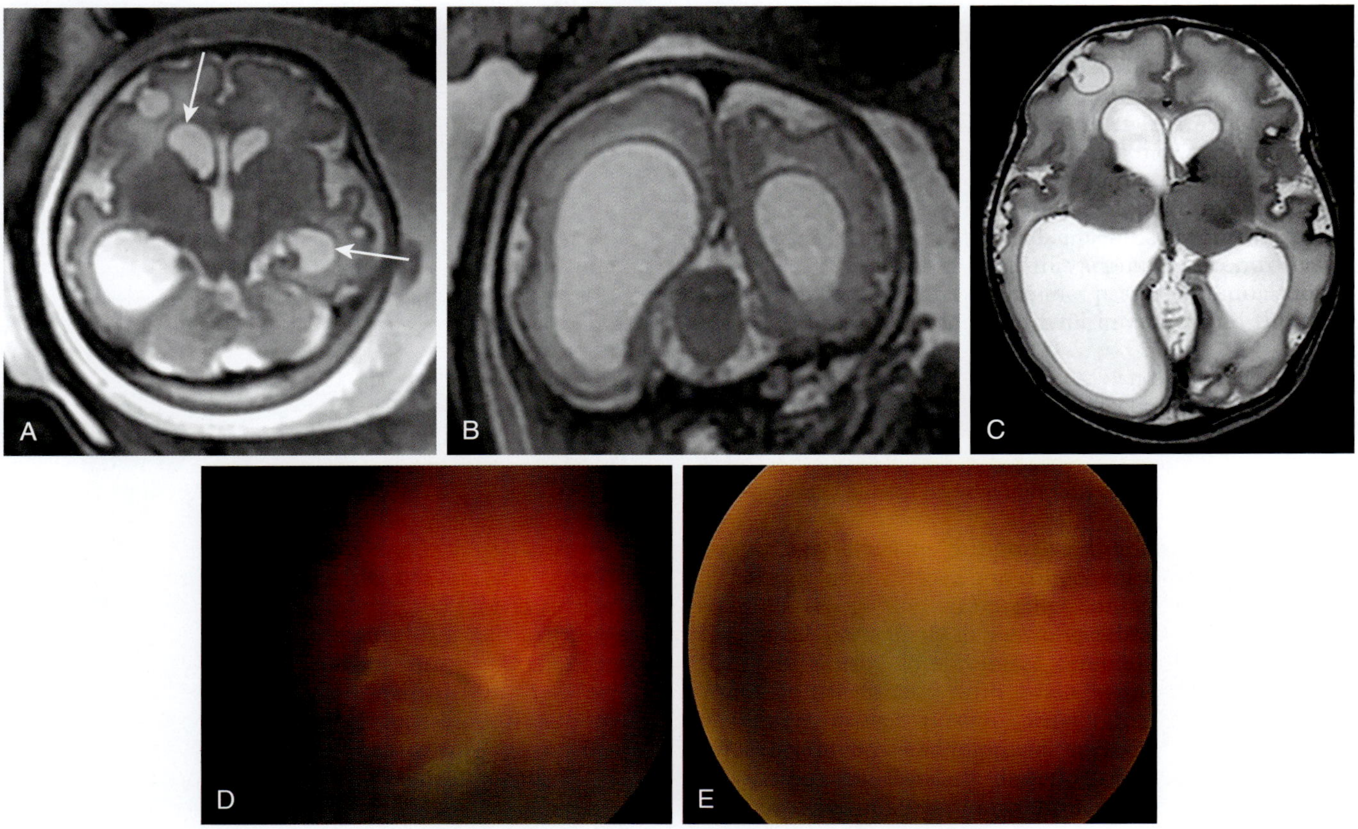

Figure 34.17 Congenital toxoplasmosis: antenatal and postnatal magnetic resonance imaging. Antenatal T2-weighted images obtained at 32 weeks of gestation in axial (A) and coronal (B) planes showing severe ventriculomegaly, subcortical cysts in the right frontal and left temporal lobe, and migrational disturbances *(arrows)*. The postnatal image (C) obtained at 34 weeks of gestation confirmed the antenatal findings and showed more subcortical cysts and areas of calcification. (D) Fundoscopy *(left eye)* shows severe vitritis; the active lesions are seen as whitish foci of retinochoroiditis. (E) Fundoscopy of the right eye shows "headlight in the fog" appearance as a result of intense vitritis. (D and E, courtesy Elsbeth Voskuil-Kerkhof.)

TABLE 34.13   Relationship Between Neonatal Clinical Signs and Neurological Outcome in Symptomatic Congenital Toxoplasmosis

NEUROLOGICAL OUTCOME	NEONATAL SIGNS[a]	
	NEUROLOGICAL (%)	SYSTEMIC (%)
Mental retardation	89	81
Seizures	83	77
Spastic motor deficits	76	58
Severe visual impairment	69	42
Deafness	17	10
Normal	9	16

[a]Values for each neurological outcome are expressed as percentage of infants who exhibited the designated neonatal signs (i.e., neurological [n = 108] or systemic [n = 44]).

Data from Remington JS, McLeod R, Thulliez P, Desmonts G. Toxoplasmosis. In: Remington JS, Klein JO, Wilson CB, et al., eds. *Infectious Diseases of the Fetus and Newborn Infant.* 6th ed. Philadelphia: Elsevier Saunders; 2006; Eichenwald H. A study of congenital toxoplasmosis. In: Siim JC, ed. *Human Toxoplasmosis.* Copenhagen: Munksgaard; 1970.

TABLE 34.14   Subsequent Deficits With Asymptomatic Congenital Toxoplasmosis

SUBSEQUENT DEFICIT	NUMBER AFFECTED (TOTAL n = 13)[a]
None	2
Chorioretinitis	11
Bilateral	8
Unilateral	3
Neurological sequelae	5
Major	1
Minor	4
Mean intelligence quotient	89 ± 23
Sensorineural hearing loss	3

[a]Based on 13 infants identified by serological screening in the newborn period and studied prospectively.

Data from Wilson CB, Remington JS, Stagno S, Reynolds DW. Development of adverse sequelae in children born with subclinical congenital toxoplasma infection. *Pediatrics.* 1980;66:767-774.

prominent *systemic* signs, if untreated, also results in a poor neurological outcome. Approximately 50% of such patients with CMV are normal on follow-up, whereas only approximately 16% of patients with congenital toxoplasmosis are normal (see Table 34.13). Although the nature of the study populations differs, it seems reasonable to conclude that CNS involvement in congenital toxoplasmosis is more prominent than in congenital CMV infection when nonneurological features dominate the neonatal syndrome. Again, chorioretinitis is found in the majority of such patients with toxoplasmosis, and severe visual impairment occurs in approximately 40%. Antiparasitic treatment begun in the first 2½ months of life has a beneficial effect on outcome in symptomatic congenital toxoplasmosis (see later discussion).

Outcome With Asymptomatic Congenital Infection. Infants with subclinical infection (i.e., the majority [about 85%] of cases of congenital toxoplasmosis) comprise an important group. For example, in the United States, approximately 400 to 4000 such infants are affected yearly.[202] Previous studies have emphasized that such infants had a relatively high frequency of chorioretinitis and a modest impairment of intellect.[203] A prospective study of 13 asymptomatic infants identified by serological screening in the newborn period and evaluated by particularly detailed serial, ocular, neurological, and audiological follow-up studies indicated that few such asymptomatic children survive without deficits (Table 34.14).[188] Thus 11 infants in this study developed chorioretinitis (3 with unilateral blindness) and 5 had neurological sequelae (1 with severe mental retardation and microcephaly). The neurological sequelae were always associated with retinochoroiditis. The mean IQ score for the group was only 89. SNHL occurred in 3 of 10 infants tested, although in none was moderate or severe bilateral loss observed. However, diagnosis by neonatal screening and prompt institution of therapy can result in a markedly better outcome (see later discussion).

Management

Prevention. Three major approaches to prevention include (1) avoidance of primary maternal infection, (2) treatment of maternal infection, (3) abortion in the presence of maternal infection, and (4) treatment of the affected fetus. The first of these approaches is the most important. Pregnant women who have seronegative test results *must avoid primary acquisition of Toxoplasma* infection; the two measures necessary are avoiding the ingestion of infective cysts (e.g., in raw meat) and contact with sporulating oocysts (e.g., in animal intestine and feces).[202,204] Ingestion of infective cysts occurs when infected meat is undercooked. It is recommended that consumption of raw or undercooked meat be completely avoided and that handling of raw meat be done with gloves on or followed by careful hand washing. Contact with sporulating oocysts is principally through household cats that carry oocysts in their intestines. It is recommended that pregnant women avoid contact with cat feces and that contact with soil or other materials potentially contaminated with cat feces be avoided or performed while wearing gloves. Cost-to-benefit analyses (relative to other approaches to prevention) demonstrate the particular desirability of a health education campaign to encourage these practices. In a study performed in Finland, the total annual costs of congenital toxoplasmosis without screening amounted, in US dollars, to $128 per pregnancy per year; with systematic serological screening, the cost was $95 per pregnancy per year, thus reducing the cost by 25%. Thus screening for *Toxoplasma* infections during pregnancy is economically worthwhile even in a country with a low incidence. The investigators recommended systematic screening for maternal primary *Toxoplasma* infections combined with health education for prevention.[205]

Primary maternal infection has been treated with the antibiotic spiramycin.[169,189] In one large series, a significant reduction in cases of congenital infection was observed in treated (24%) versus untreated (45%) mothers.[169] The approximately 50% decrease in the incidence of congenital toxoplasmosis was confirmed by subsequent data.[182,189,202] Moreover, a multicenter study showed a marked decrease in the incidence of neonatal

TABLE 34.15 Neonatal Outcome of Liveborn Infants With Congenital Toxoplasma Infection in the Periods Before (1972–1981) and After (1982–1988) Fetal Treatment

| NEONATAL OUTCOME[a] | TIME OF MATERNAL INFECTION (TRIMESTER) | | | | | |
| | FIRST | | SECOND | | THIRD | |
	1972–1981 (%)	1982–1988 (%)	1972–1981 (%)	1982–1988 (%)	1972–1981 (%)	1982–1988 (%)
Subclinical	10	67	37	77	68	100
Benign	50	22	45	23	29	0
Severe	40	11	18	0	3	0

See text for details of prenatal and postnatal treatment. Groups are not entirely comparable, and study was not controlled; data, however, provide an approximation of the effect in the second epoch of prenatal and postnatal treatment with spiramycin (100%) plus pyrimethamine and sulfonamide (85%).

[a]Subclinical, no symptoms. Benign form, infants with chorioretinitis but no visual impairment or with intracerebral calcifications but no neurological impairment. Severe form, infants with hydrocephalus, microcephaly, bilateral chorioretinitis with visual impairment, and abnormal neurological status.

Data from Hohlfeld P, Daffos F, Thulliez P, et al. Fetal toxoplasmosis: outcome of pregnancy and infant follow-up after in utero treatment. *J Pediatr.* 1989;115:765-769.

chorioretinitis and intracranial lesions when prenatal treatment (spiramycin) was instituted *within but not after* 4 weeks of diagnosis of maternal infection.[206] Treatment varies across countries. Spiramycin is continued throughout pregnancy in the United States and France. In Austria and Germany, spiramycin prophylaxis is followed by a 4-week course of pyrimethamine plus sulfadiazine at 17 weeks of gestation.[166]

Abortion has been performed in women who have exhibited serological evidence of primary infection during early pregnancy. This approach is less desirable for several reasons, one of which is the finding that only 17% to 25% of women infected in the first and second trimesters transmit the infection to the fetus (see Table 34.10). However, initial work by Desmonts et al.[170] and subsequently by others[182,183,207-212] demonstrated the feasibility of prenatal diagnosis of congenital toxoplasmosis. Sampling of fetal blood by cordocentesis under ultrasound guidance for serological indicators of infection is less useful, and evaluation of pregnant women for possible fetal infection with toxoplasmosis is based principally on the sampling of amniotic fluid by amniocentesis and detection of the organism's DNA by PCR. It is recommended to carry out amniocentesis after 18 weeks of gestation and at least 4 weeks after the estimated date of maternal infection to minimize the risk of a false-negative result because of the late passage of the parasite across the placenta into the fetus.[182] Ultrasonography of the fetal cranium at approximately 19 to 20 weeks of gestation provides information concerning cerebral abnormality. Fetal cranial ultrasonography may show ventriculomegaly, evidence of tissue necrosis, and cerebral calcifications. The diagnosis of fetal infection has also been made by isolation of the organism from fetal blood or from amniotic fluid and by identification in fetal blood of hematological abnormalities (e.g., eosinophilia, thrombocytopenia), elevated gamma-glutamyltransferase activity, and *Toxoplasma*-specific IgM.

The positive identification of fetal infection provides the possibility of *treatment of the fetus*.[182,183,189] In the classic study of Hohlfeld et al.,[182] fetal treatment consisted of administration to the mother of alternating 3-week courses of spiramycin and of pyrimethamine, sulfadiazine, and folinic acid (see later discussion). (The last three agents are not used before the 18th week of gestation because of the teratogenic potential of pyrimethamine.) The beneficial effect on the *severity* of fetal infection was dramatic (Table 34.15). Although, as in

TABLE 34.16 Postnatal Evolution of Chorioretinitis in 327 Children With Congenital Toxoplasmosis Treated From Birth

TIME OF ASSESSMENT	DIAGNOSIS OF FIRST LESION (%)
1st month	3
2nd–12th month	9
2nd year	2
3rd–6th year	5
7th–9th year	4
9th–13th year	1
Total	24

Infants were treated for approximately the first postnatal year, as described in the text. Eighty-four percent of the mothers had also received therapy in utero.

Data from Wallon M, Kodjikian L, Binquet C, et al. Long-term ocular prognosis in 327 children with congenital toxoplasmosis. *Pediatrics.* 2004;113:1567-1572.

pretreatment years, the incidence of severe fetal infection increased the earlier in pregnancy the infection was acquired, only 11% of first-trimester infections treated in utero resulted in severe manifestations in the neonatal period. Moreover, of the third-trimester fetal infections treated in utero, all resulted in *asymptomatic* newborns. Continuation of antimicrobial therapy postnatally in 53 infants was accompanied, after relatively short-term follow-up, by normal neurological development and examination in 52 (98%) infants and by the development of peripheral chorioretinitis with no visual impairment in 5 (9%) infants. These favorable outcomes represent a dramatic improvement as compared with outcomes in the pretreatment era (see Table 34.13). A larger study (n = 112) also showed a beneficial effect of fetal treatment. The mothers were treated during pregnancy with pyrimethamine-sulfadoxine. Follow-up was available in 107 for 12 to 250 months; 79 were asymptomatic (74%) and 28 had chorioretinitis (26%). Only one child had a serious neurological involvement.[186] A longer-term study confirmed the favorable effects of combined fetal and postnatal therapy, although delayed onset of chorioretinitis was shown (Table 34.16).[181] During follow-up, almost one third of the 142 patients (29.8%) manifested at least 1 ocular lesion. Lesions were unilateral in 98 individuals (69%) and caused no visual loss in 81%. Lesions were first manifested at a median age of 3.1 (0.0 to 20.7) years. In 48 (34%) of the children, recurrences or new ocular lesions were seen up to 12 years after the appearance of the first lesion. However, severe bilateral visual impairment did not occur. Nevertheless, careful long-term follow-up is imperative.

Supportive Therapy. Such therapy is carried out as described for congenital CMV infection.

Antimicrobial Therapy. Although significant injury has already occurred in many cases of untreated congenital toxoplasmosis by the time of birth, good evidence indicates that some of this injury is reversible and that continuing postnatal injury is preventable by therapy directed against the organism.[a] The drugs of choice are pyrimethamine and sulfadiazine, with the addition of folinic acid to counteract the folic acid antagonistic effect of pyrimethamine on the bone marrow. Pyrimethamine is highly effective in experimental infection with *Toxoplasma* and, because of its high lipid solubility, appears to be concentrated in the brain.[1] Sulfadiazine acts synergistically with pyrimethamine such that their combined activity is 8 times what would be expected if additive effects were operative.[215,216] Caution must be exercised with sulfadiazine, particularly in infants with hyperbilirubinemia since sulfonamides compete with bilirubin for binding to serum albumin, causing a rise in free bilirubin levels, which might result in bilirubin-induced neurologic dysfunction (BIND). The combination of pyrimethamine and sulfadoxine (Fansidar) is more convenient because it can be administered every 2 weeks rather than daily. Thrombocytopenia is a particularly early manifestation of pyrimethamine toxicity, and folinic acid is particularly effective in correcting this phenomenon. These antimicrobials kill actively multiplying parasites but not resistant cyst stages. Therefore treatment must begin promptly and must continue until the infant's immune system has matured sufficiently to control the infection. The total recommended duration of therapy in both symptomatic and asymptomatic disease is 1 year.[182,183] In infants with evidence of severe inflammation, as manifested by markedly elevated CSF protein (≥1 g/dL) or severe chorioretinitis, corticosteroids have been recommended. Doses and modes of administration of these various agents are discussed elsewhere. The beneficial effects of postnatal onset of therapy in congenital toxoplasmosis, either clinically symptomatic or detected by newborn blood screening (*asymptomatic*), are illustrated by the data in Table 34.17.

Rubella

Congenital infection of the infant with rubella occurs in utero by transplacental mechanisms. Before the institution of rubella vaccination, congenital rubella, especially in epidemic years, was a common and devastating disease of the newborn. With the widespread use of rubella vaccination, the frequency of the disorder has diminished markedly. For example, the incidence in the United States is less than 1 per 1 million live births.[217] There were 47 cases reported in the United States in 1991, and 22 of these occurred in a cluster in southern California.[218] Nevertheless, rubella remains a common illness in many parts

[a]References 175, 181, 182, 184, 203, 208, 213, 214.

TABLE 34.17	Effect of Postnatal Treatment on Clinically Symptomatic and Asymptomatic Congenital Toxoplasmosis	
Clinically symptomatic[a]		
Motor deficits	20%–25%	
Intelligence quotient <70	25%	
Retinopathy	90% (81% present in neonatal period)	
Asymptomatic[b]		
Motor deficits	2%	
Severe cognitive deficits	2%	
Retinopathy	29% (19% present in neonatal period)	

[a]Data from Roizen N, Swisher CN, Stein MA, et al. Neurologic and developmental outcome in treated congenital toxoplasmosis. *Pediatrics.* 1995;95:11-20 (n = 34); McLeod R, Boyer K, Karrison T, et al. Outcome of treatment for congenital toxoplasmosis, 1981-2004: The National Collaborative Chicago-Based, Congenital Toxoplasmosis Study. *Clin Infect Dis.* 2006;42:1383-1394 (n = 120).
[b]Data from Guerina NG, Hsu HW, Meissner HC, et al. Neonatal serologic screening and early treatment for congenital *Toxoplasma gondii* infection. *N Engl J Med.* 1994;330:1858-1863 (n = 50).

of the world; as a consequence, congenital rubella syndrome (CRS) is not rare (e.g., in Morocco annual rates of CRS are approximately 1 per 10,000 live births).[219] The relationship between intrauterine infection with rubella and congenital defects was first clearly recognized in 1941 by Gregg.[220] Rubella-containing vaccine (RCV) had been introduced in 140 (72%) countries as of December 2014, an increase from 99 (51%) WHO member states in 2000. Reported rubella cases declined by 95%, from 670,894 cases in 102 countries in 2000 to 33,068 cases in 162 countries in 2014, although reporting is inconsistent.[221] The incidence of rubella has remained below 1 case per 10 million population since 2004 in the United States, and the CRS incidence has been below 1 case per 5 million births. About half (54%) of rubella cases were internationally imported or epidemiologically or virologically linked to importation. Owing to the vaccination coverage, the level of population immunity to rubella is high.[222]

Pathogenesis

Fetal Infection. Clinically significant infection with rubella virus occurs during intrauterine life by transplacental passage of the virus.[1,37] As with CMV infection and toxoplasmosis, the sequence of events is primary maternal infection, viremia, placental infection, and, finally, fetal infection. Cases of asymptomatic maternal infection are common, outnumbering those of symptomatic infection by nearly 2 to 1.[1,37] Viremia occurs during the week before the onset of clinical manifestations, which include fever, cervical adenopathy, and a maculopapular rash lasting 3 days.

Importance of Time of Maternal Infection. The likelihood and severity of fetal infection are functions of the time of maternal infection.[223,224] The risk to the fetus begins when the rash in the mother appears at least 12 days after the last menstrual period (i.e., the likely time of conception); in a series of 38

TABLE 34.18   Relationship Between the Clinical Manifestations of Congenital Rubella and the Time of Maternal Infection

CLINICAL MANIFESTATION	MATERNAL INFECTION: MONTH OF PREGNANCY[a]				
	FIRST (%)	SECOND (%)	THIRD (%)	FOURTH (%)	>FOURTH (%)
Ocular defect	50	29	7	0	0
Cardiac defect	57	58	21	5	6
Deafness	83	72	67	49	0
Neurological deficit	57	59	24	26	0

[a]Values for each clinical manifestation are expressed as the percentage of infants affected after maternal infection during the designated month.
Data from Cooper LZ, Ziring PR, Ockerse AB, et al. Rubella. *Am J Dis Child.* 1969;118:18-29.

carefully studied pregnancies in the periconceptional period, no cases of fetal infection occurred when the rash appeared at 11 days or less after the last menstrual period.[225] In general, *both* the frequency of occurrence of infection *and* the severity of clinical disease are greater the earlier in pregnancy the maternal infection occurs (Table 34.18). Thus it differs from the situation with toxoplasmosis, in which the likelihood of infection is less but the severity of disease greater when it is acquired early in pregnancy. With congenital rubella, *ocular* and *cardiac* defects are particularly common when infection occurs in the first and second months, but they become essentially nonexistent when infection occurs after the first trimester. However, *hearing loss*, although most common with early infection, is still found in approximately half of infants infected in the fourth month; later maternal infection appears not to be dangerous in this regard. *Neurological deficits*, especially intellectual retardation and motor deficits, are most common with infection in the first 2 months and are not observed with infection past the fourth month.

The *most critical gestational periods* concerning the major defects have been defined particularly closely.[224] In a series of 55 children from carefully dated, affected pregnancies, cataracts were observed with maternal infection between 26 and 57 days of GA; heart disease occurred in maternal infection between 25 and 93 days of GA; deafness occurred in maternal infection between 16 and 131 days of GA; and severe mental retardation occurred in maternal infection between 26 and 45 days of GA. The placenta may play the greatest role in determining the decreasing incidence of fetal infection with progression of gestation. Maturational factors of host tissue may be most important in determining the concomitant changes in organ susceptibility.

Neuropathology

As with congenital CMV infection and toxoplasmosis, the neuropathology of congenital rubella is characterized by considerable inflammation and tissue necrosis (Table 34.19).[226-228] In addition, rubella also appears to interfere with cellular proliferation in the developing brain and, as a consequence, causes microcephaly and, perhaps, impaired myelination.

Meningoencephalitis. The meningoencephalitis of rubella infection is similar in certain respects to the other neonatal encephalitides and is characterized by the following: (1) inflammatory cells in the meninges; (2) perivascular infiltrates

TABLE 34.19   Neuropathology of Congenital Rubella Symptomatic in the Neonatal Period

Meningoencephalitis
Vasculopathy with focal ischemic necrosis
Microcephaly
Delayed myelination

with inflammatory cells; (3) necrosis of brain parenchyma, with all cellular elements affected; and (4) reactive microglial and astroglial proliferation.

Vasculopathy. An additional, prominent, and distinctive feature of rubella infection is vasculopathy. Involvement of blood vessels is observed in many organs and prominently in the brain.[226] In the well-studied series of Rorke and Spiro,[226] involvement of large leptomeningeal vessels and, particularly, smaller intraparenchymal vessels and capillaries was defined. Destruction of one or more layers of the vessel wall occurs, with replacement by deposits of amorphous granular material (Fig. 34.18). Associated with these vascular lesions are focal areas of ischemic necrosis, especially in the cerebral white matter (centrum semiovale, periventricular regions, and corpus callosum) and in the basal ganglia. The vascular abnormalities may account for the echogenic vessels observable on cranial ultrasonography of the affected newborn (see later discussion) (Fig. 34.19).

Microcephaly and Impaired Myelination. Two additional features of congenital rubella (i.e., microcephaly and impaired myelination) may relate to the effect of the virus on cellular replication. Microcephaly does not appear to be accounted for readily by destructive disease and, indeed, is often not prominent until months after birth. The possibility that the decreased brain mass is related to a decrease in the number of neurons and glia is supported by the observations that rubella disturbs mitotic activity of human fetal cells in culture and also causes a reduced number of cells in a variety of organs in affected infants.[229,230] In addition to the microcephaly, a cellular deficit may account for the moderately impaired myelination observed by Rorke and Spiro[226] and by Kemper et al.[231] Indeed, although quantitative data are lacking, an apparent decrease in oligodendrocytes has been observed in association with the delay in myelination.[226]

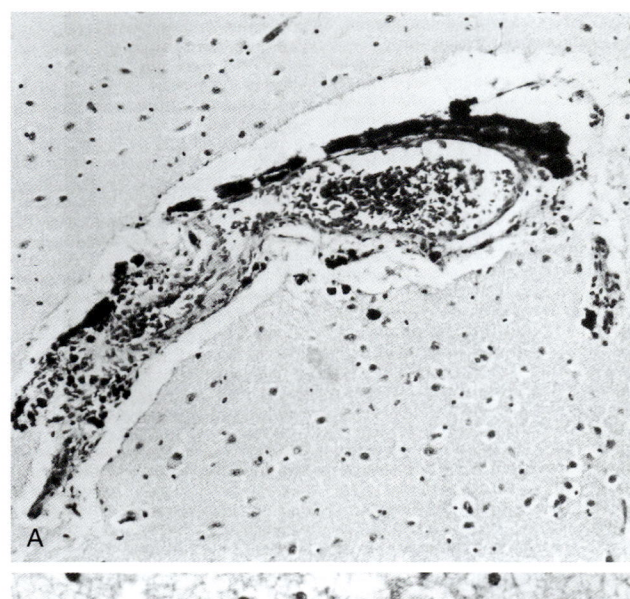

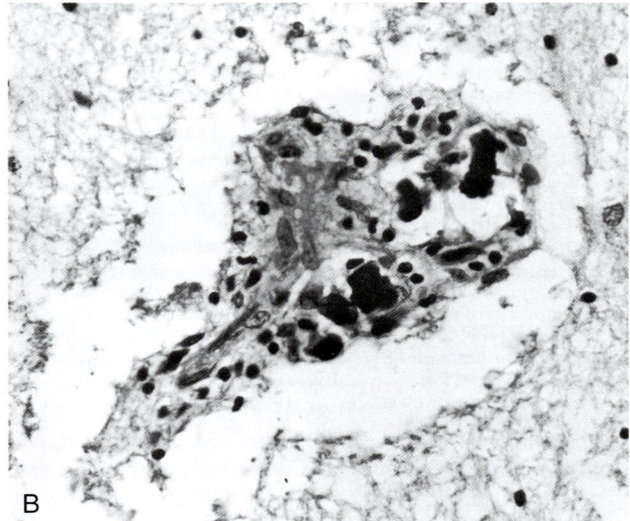

Figure 34.18 Congenital rubella infection: vasculopathy. (A and B) Cerebral vessels from a 10-week-old infant with a birth weight of 2250 g and involvement of multiple organs. Note the destruction of vessel walls with replacement by deposits of amorphous granular material, which is evident especially in A. Surrounding ischemic changes are also present, especially in B. (From Bell WE, McCormick WF. *Neurologic Infections in Children*. Philadelphia: Saunders; 1975.)

Clinical Aspects

Incidence of Clinically Apparent Infection. The devastating rubella pandemic of the mid-1960s made it possible to define the enormous clinical spectrum of congenital rubella.[232-243] Because the largest portion of available data was derived from studies of infants identified at birth, the spectrum of manifestations as a function of *maternal infection* has been more difficult to define than for congenital CMV infection or toxoplasmosis. Nevertheless, it does appear that the likelihood of asymptomatic congenital rubella infection is more nearly comparable to that of congenital toxoplasmosis than to that of congenital CMV infection. Thus approximately two thirds of patients are asymptomatic in the neonatal period. However, most of these infants do develop evidence of disease in the first several years

TABLE 34.20	Clinical Features of Symptomatic Congenital Rubella	

CLINICAL FEATURE	APPROXIMATE FREQUENCY (%)
Pregnancy	
Intrauterine growth retardation	51–75
Central nervous system	
Meningoencephalitis	51–75
Full anterior fontanelle	21–50
Lethargy	21–50
Irritability	21–50
Hypotonia	21–50
Opisthotonos-retrocollis	0–20
Seizures	0–20
Eye	
Cataracts	21–50
Chorioretinitis	21–50
Microphthalmia	0–20
Hearing	
Suspected or definite hearing loss	21–50
Cardiovascular system	
Peripheral pulmonary stenoses	51–75
Patent ductus arteriosus	21–50
Myocardial necrosis	0–20
Reticuloendothelial system	
Hepatosplenomegaly	51–75
Hyperbilirubinemia	0–20
Thrombocytopenia ± purpura	21–50
Anemia	0–20
Dermal erythropoiesis ("blueberry muffin")	0–20
Other	
Bony radiolucencies	21–50
Pneumonitis	21–50

Data from Alford CA Jr. Chronic congenital and perinatal infections. In: Avery GB, ed. *Neonatology: Pathophysiology and Management of the Newborn*. 3rd ed. Philadelphia: JB Lippincott; 1987; Desmond MM, Wilson GS, Melnick JL, et al. Congenital rubella encephalitides. *J Pediatr*. 1967;71:311-331.

of life, a finding imparting clinical significance to observations that prolonged viral replication is an important feature of this disease.[236,243]

Clinical Features. The clinical features in symptomatic patients are shown in Table 34.20.[235] Intrauterine growth retardation (followed by postnatal growth failure) is a particularly common feature. Disturbances of the reticuloendothelial system are also prominent and are characterized particularly by hepatosplenomegaly and thrombocytopenia with or without purpura. The purpura should be distinguished from the peculiar dermal erythropoiesis that results in the small purple lesions of the "blueberry muffin" syndrome. Cardiovascular defects are characteristic and consist principally of peripheral pulmonary stenoses and patent ductus arteriosus.[233,238] Myocardial injury can be demonstrated in a few patients by abnormal electrocardiographic findings as well as pathologically,[239] and it may contribute to the occurrence of congestive heart failure. Other lesions, apparent in 20% to 50% of patients, are linear areas of radiolucency of the metaphyses of long bones (i.e., *celery stalk lesions*), prominent especially around the knee, and

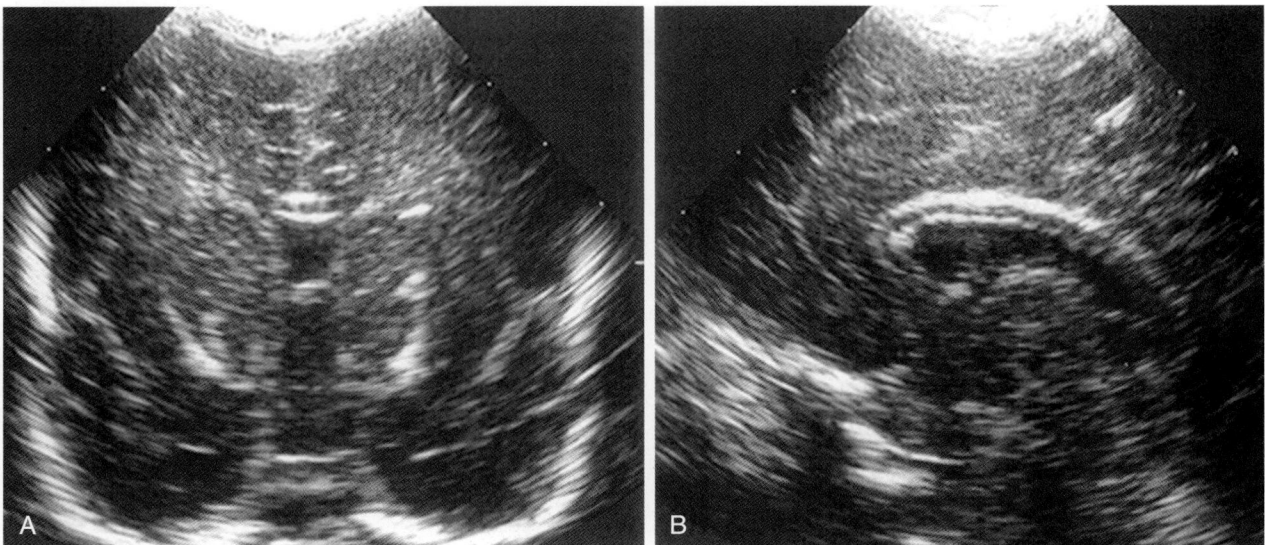

Figure 34.19 Rubella: cranial ultrasound. Coronal (A) and parasagittal (B) scans showing lenticulostriate vasculopathy in both thalami (A) and calcification within the corpus callosum (B).

interstitial pneumonitis.[242] These abnormalities usually subside in the first few months of life.

Neurological phenomena in the newborn period are prominent in approximately 50% to 75% of cases (see Table 34.20).[31,235] The most common manifestations relate to meningoencephalitis, seen most clearly in most patients by elevated levels of CSF protein and mononuclear cells.[235] The anterior fontanelle is full in 25% to 50% of patients. The most common initial neurological features are "lethargy" and hypotonia, accompanied and followed shortly by prominent irritability. The irritability may relate to meningeal irritation, which probably also accounts for the occurrence of retrocollis and opisthotonos. These signs of meningeal irritation may worsen in the first weeks or months of life. Seizures appear in approximately 10% to 15% of infants.[235] Definite microcephaly is unusual at birth. Most of the acute clinical features subside over the first several months and evolve to the sequelae outlined subsequently.

The *ocular lesions* consist principally of cataracts, usually white or pearly, especially centrally, and chorioretinitis, which may be more common than was previously appreciated. Indirect ophthalmoscopy is especially helpful to demonstrate the characteristic spotty pigmentation (i.e., "salt and pepper") appearance, which may be particularly prominent peripherally.[241] Microphthalmia is sometimes difficult to appreciate when it is bilateral and is associated particularly with cataract.

The *auditory lesion* may be difficult to demonstrate in the newborn, although the application of brain stem evoked response audiometry (BERA) has improved detection. In one series, approximately 20% of infants had suspected or definite hearing loss by behavioral testing in the neonatal period.[234] The basis for the hearing loss in congenital rubella is a cochlear inflammatory and destructive lesion.[237] A significant minority of infants will subsequently exhibit disturbances in response to sound that appear to be on a *central* basis,[232] although the locus of this central pathology is unclear. In a detailed study of hearing loss in children with congenital rubella, the hearing deficit was usually uniform over all frequencies, symmetrical, and severe (mean threshold, 93 dB).[244] As many as 60% to 80% of

infants with congenital rubella are found later to have hearing loss as children.[235,244] This increase in incidence from early infancy to childhood relates to a combination of inadequate testing in infancy with delayed diagnosis and progression of disease in the auditory apparatus; the relative importance of each of these factors remains unclear.

Clinical Diagnosis. Clinical features that favor the diagnosis of congenital rubella are intrauterine growth retardation, CSF pleocytosis, salt-and-pepper chorioretinopathy, cataracts, cardiovascular defects, and skeletal lesions. The absences of prominent cerebral calcification, hydrocephalus, overt microcephaly, and vesicular rash are the clinical features that best differentiate congenital rubella from congenital toxoplasmosis, CMV infection, and HSV infection. Following a recent outbreak in Vietnam, a peak incidence of 7.8 per 1000 live births was seen, and 38 infants could be studied in detail.[245] Low birth weight (71%), cardiovascular defects (72%), suspected hearing impairment (93%), hepatosplenomegaly (68%), thrombocytopenia (76%), and developmental delays (73%) were noted. Fully 84% of the patients presented with characteristic hemorrhagic purpuric eruptions, the "blueberry muffin baby" syndrome. Twenty-four of the infants (67%) had a significant persistent ductus arteriosus, and notably this finding was associated with pulmonary hypertension in 16 of the 24 infants. Thirteen infants (34%) died. Pulmonary hypertension, hepatosplenomegaly, and severe thrombocytopenia were more frequently observed among those who died.[245]

Laboratory Evaluation

Isolation of Virus. Determination of rubella virus as the responsible microbe depends particularly on isolation of the virus and serological tests.[228] The virus can be isolated best from the nasopharynx and urine, but it can also be isolated from stool and CSF (and various tissues, including lens and brain). Approximately 55% to 85% of patients exhibit positive cultures.[235] Performance of multiple cultures increases the yield appreciably. The virus has been isolated from approximately

30% to 45% of CSF samples examined.[235,239] This relatively high frequency of isolation of virus from CSF is unlike other congenital viral encephalitides. The chronicity of rubella infection is emphasized by the finding of positive CSF cultures in infants as old as 18 months.[235] A similar conclusion can be derived from isolation of virus from the cataractous lens of a child aged 2 years, 11 months.[240] Moreover, as many as one third of infants with congenital rubella are still excreting virus at 8 months of age.[246,247]

Serological Studies.

All women of childbearing age should have been vaccinated against rubella as children or before conception. Women who have been vaccinated should be considered immune. As seroconversion is not 100%, serological testing is indicated in vaccinated women who have a known exposure or a rash and illness consistent with rubella to rule out acute primary infection or reinfection.[248] Serological diagnosis during pregnancy may be based on maternal blood studies. If negative for IgM (IgM–), the IgG results determine if the woman is seropositive (immune) or seronegative (not immune). If a pregnant woman is IgG-negative at the first visit, she should be retested monthly for seroconversion until the end of the fifth month of pregnancy. If the maternal blood is positive for IgM (IgM+) and IgG (IgG+), the next step would be an IgG avidity assay on the same blood sample to estimate the time of infection, with low avidity indicative of recent primary infection. The same tests should be repeated on a second blood sample obtained 2 to 3 weeks later. If the results remain the same (IgM+ IgG–), the IgM result is considered nonspecific, indicating that the woman has not been infected; however, she is seronegative and should be followed until the end of the fifth month. If the woman has seroconverted (IgM+ IgG+), recent primary infection is confirmed and a prenatal evaluation should be performed, followed by a discussion to see whether the woman wishes to continue her pregnancy.[249] After birth, the fastest and most useful test is determination of IgM-specific antibody; this is the most definitive serological diagnostic test in the first few weeks of life. IgM antibody can be detected in the infant's cord blood or serum and persists for about 6 to 12 months.

Neurodiagnostic Studies.

No specific neurodiagnostic tests are available, although a high rate of viral isolation from the CSF and the frequency of *CSF signs of inflammation* are very helpful in diagnosis. *CT and ultrasound* are useful in the detection of the focal areas of ischemic necrosis secondary to the vasculopathy and the less common calcification in the basal ganglia.[72,250] CT scans obtained between 1 and 3 years of age have demonstrated cerebral white matter hypodensity and multiple calcified nodules in the centrum semiovale,[251] presumably reflecting the impaired myelination and focal ischemic lesions described earlier in the section on neuropathology. *MRI* is most useful for detection of the presumed ischemic lesions in cerebral white matter and impairment of myelination.[250] *Cranial ultrasound* may show focal areas of calcification,[1] subependymal cysts,[110,250,252] and echogenic vessels in the basal ganglia and thalamus (see Fig. 34.19).[110,112,253] In a series of 12 infants with echogenic vessels in basal ganglia, 2 patients had congenital rubella.[112]

Prognosis

Relation to Neonatal Clinical Syndrome.

Although outcome is related to neonatal clinical features, the relationships are not as

TABLE 34.21   Outcome at Age 18 Months of Survivors of Congenital Rubella Syndrome

OUTCOME	PERCENTAGE AFFECTED (%)
Neuromotor deficits	
None	31
Mild	22
Severe	47
Microcephaly	81
Hearing loss	
None	28
Definite	45
Poor speech, inconsistent response to sound	27
Ocular manifestations	
Cataract	47
Chorioretinitis	31
No hearing, speech, or visual problem	9

Data from Desmond MM, Wilson GS, Melnick JL, et al. Congenital rubella encephalitides. *J Pediatr.* 1967;71:311-331.

obvious as with congenital CMV infection and toxoplasmosis. This fact may relate to the particular chronicity of congenital rubella as well as to the relative infrequency of completely asymptomatic neonatal disease. In a population of 100 carefully studied infants, 90% of whom were overtly symptomatic in the neonatal period and very early infancy, only 9% appeared to be free of deficits at 18 months (Table 34.21).[235] Neuromotor deficits (i.e., spastic motor deficits and delayed neurological development) were severe in approximately 50% of the patients. Fully 81% of these infants had microcephaly, and 72% had definite hearing loss or other apparent disturbances related to auditory perception. In a subsequent report on the same population, of patients followed to 16 to 18 years of age, 28% exhibited mental retardation, and an additional 25% exhibited low-average intelligence.[254] Of 14 children with *suspected* hearing loss at 18 months, 13 were definitely hearing impaired. In another prospective series of infants with congenital rubella, approximately similar outcomes were observed; approximately 45% of such infants exhibited *psychomotor retardation*, and 50% of these infants were moderately or severely affected.[217]

Long-Term Hearing Deficits and Other Sequelae.

Even those infants who appear to be less severely affected often show evolution of disabling auditory, motor, behavioral, and learning deficits as they grow older (Table 34.22).[234] A multidisciplinary longitudinal study of 29 *nonretarded* infants with congenital rubella demonstrated definite hearing loss in 1 infant in the first 2 months, in 12 infants by 12 months, in 22 infants by 24 months, in 25 infants by 48 months, and in an additional 2 infants by 11 years, for a total of 27, or 93% of the children. This accretion of patients with definite hearing loss may reflect continuing cochlear injury. The analogy with the delayed onset of hearing loss in congenital CMV infection and of chorioretinopathy in congenital toxoplasmosis is apparent.

In the longitudinal study just mentioned, early disturbances of motor development and of tone were followed by impairments of motor coordination and muscle weakness in approximately

TABLE 34.22	Identification of Hearing Loss in 29 Nonretarded, Longitudinally Studied Children With Congenital Rubella Syndrome	
	HEARING LOSS	
AGE	**SUSPECTED**	**DIAGNOSED**
Birth–2 months	5	1
3–12 months	10	11
13–24 months	2	10
25–48 months	2	3
4–11 years	—	2
		27 (93%)

Data from Desmond MM, Fisher ES, Vorderman AL, et al. The longitudinal course of congenital rubella encephalitis in nonretarded children. *J Pediatr.* 1978;93:584-591.

50% of the children.[234] Behavioral disturbances, which in the early years included impaired attention span and hyperkinesis, evolved to emotional irritability and persisting distractibility in approximately 50%. A propensity for congenital rubella infection to lead to impairment of behavioral and emotional development is also apparent in other studies by a 6% incidence of subsequent autism. Moreover, although IQ scores remained within the normal range in the study of Desmond et al.,[234] learning deficits and visual-perceptual-motor deficits were prominent in approximately 50%. These abnormalities had major impacts on the children's adaptation to educational and home environments and underscore the necessity for careful follow-up and appropriate interventions in infants with congenital rubella.

An interesting relationship between the rate of linear growth and cognitive outcome was apparent in a 20-year follow-up of 105 cases of CRS.[255] Children with normal growth had normal cognitive development, and those whose linear growth was at less than the fifth percentile exhibited moderate to severe mental retardation.

Late Progressive Panencephalitis. A rare complication of congenital rubella, the precise frequency and importance of which are not clear, is the occurrence of progressive panencephalitis with onset, usually in the second decade, of intellectual and motor deterioration, elevated CSF protein levels, and elevated antibody titers to rubella virus in serum and CSF.[256] The virus has been isolated from the brain.[257] Whether this disorder represents reactivated infection, bears a relation to the role of measles virus in subacute sclerosing panencephalitis, or both remains to be determined.

Management

Prevention. Preventive measures present the realistic hope of eradicating CRS. Of the three major approaches to prevention (avoidance of maternal infection, treatment of maternal infection, and abortion in the presence of maternal infection), the first has been accomplished in large part through vaccination.

Active immunization with a live attenuated rubella vaccine has been accomplished by two major approaches.[258] In the United States, mass vaccination of all children aged 1 year to puberty has been used to limit the spread of infection to the pregnant woman by curtailing circulation of virus in the community. In the United Kingdom and in many other European countries, selected immunization, especially of girls from ages 11 to 14 years, was used initially to provide protection for the childbearing years. Mass vaccination of all children in the second year of life was instituted in the United Kingdom in 1988. The policy in the United States has been effective; the incidence of congenital rubella declined by approximately fivefold in the decade following the initiation of this vaccination regimen. Since 2004, the rubella incidence has remained below 1 case per 10 million population, and the incidence of the CRS has been below 1 case per 5 million births.[222,258] However, some questions still remain concerning how long vaccine-induced protection will last or whether inapparent reinfection of the mother with transmission to the fetus may occur. In 1996, it was estimated that 110,000 infants with CRS were born annually in developing countries.[259] In 2000, the World Health Organization (WHO) published the first rubella vaccine position paper to guide introduction of RCV in national childhood immunization schedules. From 1996 to 2009, the number of countries that introduced RCV into their national routine childhood immunization programs increased by 57%, from 83 countries in 1996 to 130 countries in 2009. Also during this time period, the number of rubella cases reported decreased from 670,894 in 2000 to 121,344 in 2009. Rubella control and prevention of CRS can be accelerated by integrating with current global measles mortality reduction and regional elimination activities. *All women identified to be seronegative during pregnancy should be vaccinated postpartum.*[260,261]

Passive immunization with immune globulin may be useful in the special case of a susceptible pregnant woman exposed to rubella. The effectiveness of this approach is controversial, but it is necessary to recognize that passive immunization is useful to prevent viremia and fetal infection and therefore must be given promptly.

Abortion in the woman infected with rubella requires understanding of the risks of fetal infection as they relate to the timing of the infection in pregnancy. The demonstration of prenatal diagnosis by fetal blood sampling in the 20th week of gestation may help to prevent abortion of the unaffected fetus.[262]

Supportive Therapy. Supportive therapy is carried out principally as described for congenital CMV infection. In addition, recognition and prompt control of cardiac failure are critical, particularly in view of cerebral vasculopathy and therefore already compromised cerebral perfusion. Careful auditory assessment, with brain stem evoked response audiometry as well as with behavioral studies, is critical to detect hearing loss and to provide appropriate intervention as early as possible. Similarly, detection of cataract is important because delay of surgery into the second and third years of life prevents useful vision. Opinions differ about the optimal time of therapy. Nevertheless the infant with auditory and visual deficits is at great risk for subsequent disturbances of language and other aspects of neurological development, and the earliest interventions regarding vision and audition are critical.

Antimicrobial Therapy. No known effective chemotherapeutic agents of value exist in the treatment of congenital (or postnatal) rubella infection.

Herpes Simplex

HSV-1 and HSV-2 are members of the alpha herpesvirus subfamily of the family *Herpesviridae*.[263-266] The virus can establish lifelong latency in sensory neural ganglia. Neonates develop three types of infections, which are classified according to the clinical extent of disease: localized involving the skin, eyes, or mouth (SEM disease); CNS infection; and disseminated infection (DIS), which involves several organs (e.g., lungs, liver, and adrenal glands) with or without CNS involvement. Since effective antiviral drugs, such as vidarabine and especially acyclovir, have become available, the prognosis for neonatal HSV infection has improved considerably. However, the mortality for patients with DIS is still relatively high and adverse sequelae are still not uncommon (see later). Neonatal HSV infection, in most cases, is acquired during passage through an infected birth canal. Less commonly, ascending infection near the time of birth is the means of acquisition of the virus. Still less commonly, transplacental passage of virus causes intrauterine infection, or postnatal acquisition of virus from infected adults or infants causes severe postnatal illness. Neonatal HSV infection is very much less common than CMV infection, the other major neonatal infection caused by a herpesvirus. However, unlike CMV infection, essentially all examples of neonatal HSV infection are symptomatic, often with serious neurological concomitants apparent in the newborn period. The premature infant is apparently more susceptible than the full-term infant and accounts for as many as 25% to 35% of cases.[264,267-270]

The incidence of neonatal HSV infection increased pari passu with the increase in incidence of genital HSV infection in adults in the United States over the several decades before the decline in incidence of recent years.[267,270] The incidence of neonatal herpes varies considerably from 5.8 to 60 per 100,000 births.[263,271] The National Health and Nutrition Examination Survey (NHANES) serological data from 1988 to 2004 estimated that 22% of pregnant women were seropositive for HSV-2, 63% for HSV-1, and 13% for both HSV-1 and HSV-2.[271] The epidemiology of HSV disease is changing; in a recent study, HSV-1 was more common than HSV-2 as a cause of oral and genital mucosal infections in young women.[272] Younger participants (18 to 22 years) were more likely to acquire HSV-1 infections and less likely to develop recognized disease than older participants. Overall, 84% of recognized disease cases were genital. No differences were noted in the clinical manifestations of genital HSV-1 versus genital HSV-2 disease.

Pathogenesis

Parturitional and Ascending Infection. Most infants with neonatal HSV infection acquire the infection during passage through an infected birth canal near or at the time of birth (85%). The markedly higher rate of neonatal HSV infection in infants born to mothers shedding virus at delivery when delivery is by the vaginal route than by cesarean section is consistent with this notion (Table 34.23).[267] In the classic case, the virus is acquired by direct contact of the infant's skin, eye, or oral cavity with the virus in the mother's birth canal. Overt maternal herpetic lesions are uncommonly present. Because of the importance of direct contact, it is understandable that the vesicular lesions of the infant's infection are usually over the scalp and face in cephalic presentations and over the buttocks in breech presentations.[268] Vivid demonstrations of the relation

TABLE 34.23   Risk Factors for Development of Neonatal Herpes Simplex Virus Infection

RISK FACTOR	NUMBER OF INFANTS WITH NEONATAL HERPES SIMPLEX VIRUS INFECTION/NUMBER OF DELIVERIES	P VALUE
Type of delivery		
Cesarean	1/85 (1.2%)	.47
Vaginal	9/117 (7.7%)	
Invasive monitors		
Yes	8/79 (10.1%)	.02
No	2/123 (1.6%)	
Type isolated		
HSV-1	5/16 (31.3%)	<.001
HSV-2	5/186 (2.7%)	
First episode		
Yes	8/26 (30.8%)	<.001
No	2/151 (1.3%)	

Based on study of 40,023 deliveries with cultures. Data shown concern the 202 deliveries complicated by neonatal herpes simplex virus infection.

Data from Brown ZA, Wald A, Morrow RA, et al. Effect of serologic status and cesarean delivery on transmission rates of herpes simplex virus from mother to infant. *JAMA.* 2003;289:203-209.

of contact with the sites of herpetic lesions are provided by several reports of vesicular lesions (and serious neonatal disease) at the sites of placement of fetal scalp electrodes for intrapartum monitoring.[264,273-278] In a large study of women with asymptomatic HSV infection at delivery, fetal scalp electrodes were used in 25 infants, of whom 5 developed neonatal herpes, versus zero cases of neonatal herpes in the 25 deliveries in which fetal scalp electrodes were not used.[273] A larger study later confirmed the role of invasive monitoring.[267] The risk of transmission to the newborn is more than 10-fold greater when the mother is shedding HSV-1 versus HSV-2 at delivery (see Table 34.23).[267] The five most important factors known to have an effect on transmission of HSV from mother to neonate are type of maternal infection (primary vs. recurrent), maternal antibody status, duration of rupture of membranes, integrity of mucocutaneous barriers (use of scalp electrodes, for instance), and mode of delivery (cesarean vs. vaginal).[263]

Large-scale studies of neonatal HSV infection in relation to the type of maternal infection have been of great interest.[264,267,273,279-281] It is clear that in most cases neonatal infection occurs in children of *asymptomatic* rather than symptomatic mothers. Moreover, the serological status of the mother is a critical determinant of the risk of neonatal infection (Fig. 34.20).[267,273] It is important to make a distinction between a primary and a recurrent infection. A first-episode primary HSV infection occurs when a person with no prior HSV-1 or HSV-2 antibodies acquires either virus in the genital tract. If a person with preexisting HSV-1 antibodies acquires an HSV-2 genital infection, a first-episode nonprimary infection ensues. A recurrent infection can occur when reactivation of the virus occurs, affecting the skin and mucosal membranes. Of 177 women with positive HSV cultures within 48 hours of delivery, 26 (15%) had evidence of a recently acquired first episode of infection. *Nearly one third of these pregnancies resulted in neonatal HSV infection, and fully 80% of neonatal HSV infection in the entire cohort occurred in this subset of infected women.* No difference in risk of transmission was noted in the first-episode group whether the infection was primary (mother had no antibodies to HSV) or nonprimary (mother had antibodies to HSV-1 with HSV-2 infection or to HSV-2 with HSV-1 infection). In the large group of women (n = 151) with reactivated infection, or 85% of the total group, the risk of transmission of neonatal HSV infection was very low (i.e., only ≈1%). Although most of the reactivated maternal infections involved HSV-2, the risk of transmission of virus to the infant was confined to the small group with reactivated HSV-1 (see Table 34.23). Indeed, none of 140 reactivated maternal HSV-2 infections resulted in neonatal HSV, whereas 2 of 11 reactivated maternal HSV-1 infections were transmitted.

Symptomatic primary infection is characterized by fever, pain, and vesiculoulcerative lesions of the vagina and cervix. The risk of infection for a newborn delivered vaginally in the presence of clinically visible maternal genital infection in an antibody-negative woman may approach 50% to 60% (a much higher risk than in the much more common circumstance of an antibody-positive woman),[267,282] a 25% risk in infants born to women with first-episode nonprimary infection, and a 2% risk increase in those born to women with recurrent genital herpes.

Ascending infection of the fetus can occur after rupture of the membranes. Indeed, available data suggest that the risk of fetal infection in the presence of *clinically visible* maternal genital infection is greater by the ascending route than by parturitional contact (see Table 34.24). This finding may relate to a larger inoculum of virus and exposure at multiple sites with ascending versus parturitional infection.[1,37] The current rarity of this clinical situation is illustrated by a study of 58 cases of neonatal HSV infection in which only 1 mother had intrapartum genital lesions.[264]

Fetal (Transplacental) Infection. Prenatal acquisition of HSV through transplacental mechanisms is a rare cause of fetal infection (5%). Isolated examples have been reported in single case reports.[279,283-288] However, in a study of 155 cases of neonatal HSV infection, 8 (5%) had evidence of acquisition

TABLE 34.24	Risk of Herpes Simplex Virus Infection of the Infant as a Function of the Type of Delivery From a Mother With Clinically Apparent Genital Infection
TYPE OF DELIVERY	**NUMBER OF INFANTS INFECTED/TOTAL NUMBER OF DELIVERIES**
Vaginal	10/20
Cesarean section	
After membrane rupture (>6 hours)	6/7
Before or within 4 hours of membrane rupture	1/16

The antibody status of these women was not known, and the risk of neonatal infection depends markedly on this status (see text for details).
Data from Whitley RJ, Nahmias AJ, Visintine AM, et al. The natural history of herpes simplex virus infection of mother and newborn. *Pediatrics.* 1980;66:489-494.

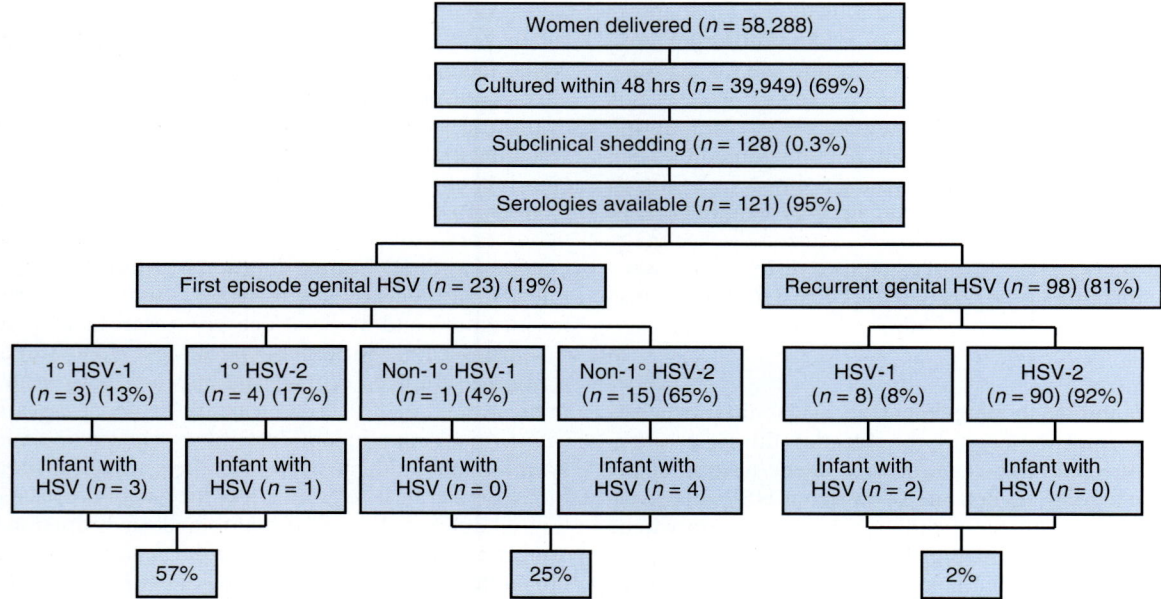

Figure 34.20 Neonatal herpes simplex virus (HSV) infection in relation to asymptomatic maternal infection at the time of labor. Type of maternal infection and risk of HSV transmission to the neonate. A total of 39,949 samples from women without clinical evidence of genital HSV infection were cultured within 48 hours of delivery; 121 were found to be shedding. For the latter, sera were available for analysis. Outcomes for these 121 women are illustrated. (Modified from Brown ZA, Wald A, Morrow RA, et al. Effect of serologic status and cesarean delivery on transmission rates of herpes simplex virus from mother to infant. *JAMA.* 2003;289:203-209. See also Kimberlin 2005; reference 292.)

TABLE 34.25   Clinical Features of Intrauterine Herpes Simplex Virus Infection

	PRESUMED TIMING OF INFECTION	
	FIRST OR SECOND TRIMESTER	LATE SECOND TO THIRD TRIMESTER
Number of infants	6	14
Premature delivery	60%	75%
Organ involvement at birth		
Skin	84%	100%
Brain	84%[a]	29%[a]
Eye	84%	29%
Microcephaly	100%	—
Outcome		
Neonatal death	20%	46%
Developmental delay	80%	16%
Normal	—	38%

[a]Includes hydranencephaly, porencephalies, multicystic leukomalacia, and cerebral calcification.

Data from Christie JD, Rakusan TA, Martinez MA, et al. Hydranencephaly caused by congenital infection with herpes simplex virus. *Pediatr Infect Dis.* 1986;5:473-478.

of infection during early gestation[289] and all were premature. Clinical manifestations have included skin lesions at birth, chorioretinitis, microphthalmia, microcephaly, hydranencephaly, multicystic encephalomalacia, cerebral calcifications, and other CNS abnormalities evident on CT scans. The clinical features of intrauterine HSV infection as a function of estimated time of acquisition of the virus are summarized in Table 34.25. A definable clinical triad includes (1) cutaneous findings (active lesions, scarring, aplasia cutis, hyperpigmentation or hypopigmentation), (2) neurologic findings (microcephaly, intracranial calcifications, hydranencephaly), and (3) ocular findings (chorioretinitis, microphthalmia, optic atrophy).[290]

In a recent review of 64 cases of intrauterine herpes infection,[291] more than two thirds did not have this triad and the cutaneous lesions were the most common presentation. Interestingly the cutaneous lesions seen were not restricted to vesicles or bullae and included aplasia cutis in three. Two thirds (n = 43) had CNS manifestations and 29 of the 43 had more than one neurological finding. Ocular findings were found in 25 (39%), mostly retinal disease (18) as well as microphthalmia (4) and cataracts (4). Subsequent outcome was poor, with death in 29 (45%), including 4 intrauterine deaths. Outcome was not reported in all, but 13 were said to have developmental delay and 8 were doing well at the age of 6 months.

Postnatal Infection. Postnatal acquisition of HSV by the newborn is an uncommon but documented occurrence (10%) and is almost always due to HSV-1.[292,293] Of 24 infants described in a review as having acquired infection shortly after birth, 13 acquired the infection from mothers with oral herpetic lesions, 9 from other adults (including hospital personnel), and 2 from other infected infants.[293] As in other examples of HSV infection of the newborn, the infection was serious, and 67% of the children died. These data have important implications for the prevention of exposure of the newborn to sources of HSV.

Role of Host Factors. Host factors must play some role in explaining the malignancy of HSV infection in the perinatal period. Indeed, in older patients who are immunologically competent, severe disseminated disease is rare. The likelihood of neonatal disturbances in response to HSV infection has been delineated.[294-298] Defects in the infant's response to herpes simplex infection can be divided into those response mechanisms involved in the initial "containment" phase, during which the virus is localized to a limited anatomical area, and those mechanisms active in the later specific *curative* phase, during which localized infection is eliminated.[296,298] Defects in the initial containment phase involve the operation of the alveolar-macrophage barrier, expression of natural killer cytotoxicity, and production of interferon-alpha and tumor necrosis factor. Defects in the later elimination phase involve antibody production, both of the neutralizing type and that responsible for antibody-dependent cellular (leukocyte) cytotoxicity; T-cell proliferation; and the production of interferon-gamma.

Although the two serotypes of HSV are genetically closely related and share many clinical features, their ability to modulate host responses can differ substantially.[299] The systemic inflammatory response was evaluated in a study of 19 infants with HSV infection, 9 of whom had a DIS.[300] Concentrations of inflammatory cytokines and markers of apoptosis were noted to be significantly higher in infants with disseminated HSV infection and were correlated with HSV load. Toll-like receptors (TLRs) constitute a family of innate immune receptors that recognize and respond to a wide spectrum of microorganisms, including viruses (see Chapters 13 and 14). These receptors are located on the plasma membrane or intracellular membranes. TLRs 3, 7, 8, and 9 are localized almost exclusively on intracellular membranes and are activated by nucleic acids of viral and bacterial origin. TLR3 is triggered by viral double-stranded RNA, leading to the activation of specific transcription factors that stimulate the production of antiviral interferons and other cytokines.[301] Human TLR3 deficiency has been associated with childhood herpes simplex encephalitis (HSE), with mutations in TLR3 and TLR3 pathway genes identified in a number of patients, in particular those with HSE recurrence.[302,303] Cord blood natural killer (NK) cells have been reported to have deficient TLR3 expression, which might explain why newborns are especially sensitive to neonatal HSV infections.[304] Ligands for TLR3 (and TLR9) induce potent innate immune antiviral responses against herpes simplex virus type 2 (HSV-2). Among these responses is induction of the expression of type I interferon genes, which are cytokines known to inhibit viral replication. Production of beta interferon but not of alpha interferon, gamma interferon, or tumor necrosis factor alpha was found to be correlated with innate immune protection against HSV-2.[305]

Neuropathology

Neonatal HSV infections may result in a wide range of involvement of the CNS, from no abnormality to devastating brain destruction. Significant involvement is most common and consists of inflammation and destruction (Table 34.26). Whether the few infants with intrauterine infection by transplacental acquisition have, in addition, aberrations of developmental events remains to be established. In this regard, microcephaly is a consistent feature of early intrauterine infection (see Table 34.25).

Meningoencephalitis. Meningoencephalitis is characterized by (1) inflammatory cells in the meninges, (2) perivascular infiltrates with inflammatory cells, (3) severe multifocal necrosis of all cellular elements of brain parenchyma, often with some degree of hemorrhage, (4) reactive microglial and astroglial proliferation, and (5) occurrence of Cowdry type A intranuclear inclusions in neuronal and glial, especially oligodendroglial, cells. The nucleus containing the inclusions is characteristically distorted, with clumping of nuclear chromatin and undulation of the nuclear membrane.[1] These pathological findings are often accompanied by a considerable degree of brain swelling, and hemorrhage in the areas of necrosis may occur, in part because of associated endothelial involvement. A detailed MRI study of 12 infants with neonatal HSV encephalitis showed multilobar cerebral involvement, including temporal and frontal regions and deep gray matter structures.[306]

Neuropathological Sequelae. The result of HSV infection of the perinatal brain most commonly is a devastating effect on neural structure and function. Subsequent failure of brain growth and microcephaly (after the neonatal period) are the rule. Multicystic encephalomalacia has been documented repeatedly (Fig. 34.21).[294,307-312] Indeed, the destruction may be so complete that hydranencephaly is the result. These lesions can be demonstrated readily by cranial ultrasound and especially MRI (see later).

Clinical Aspects

Incidence of Clinically Apparent Infection. Neonatal HSV infection is distinctive among the diseases caused by organisms of the TORCH complex in the essentially uniform occurrence of *symptomatic* disease. The clinical spectrum varies from infections localized to a few vesicles on the skin to those involving dissemination to every major organ (Table 34.27).[a]

A major distinction is made between disseminated and localized HSV disease. Disseminated disease is associated with evidence of involvement of multiple systems, particularly the reticuloendothelial system. Hepatoadrenal necrosis is the hallmark of the disorder.[1,37] Localized disease is associated with involvement confined to a single site; if multiple sites are involved, the term *localized* is still used if the reticuloendothelial system and other visceral organs are not included. A distinction is made between disease localized to the CNS (a serious form) and that localized to the skin, eye, or mouth—that is, SEM disease (a less serious form). Ten or more years ago, disseminated disease accounted for approximately 40% to 70% of all cases. More recently, the approximate distribution of clinical types has been as follows: disseminated disease, about 25%; localized CNS disease, 30%; and localized SEM disease, 45%.[277,280,313,317,319]

---

[a]References 264, 268, 269, 277, 280, 312-318.

TABLE 34.26	Neuropathology of Neonatal Herpes Simplex Virus Infection

Meningoencephalitis
Multifocal parenchymal necrosis, occasionally hemorrhagic
Brain swelling
Multicystic encephalomalacia

TABLE 34.27 Clinical Spectrum and Outcome of *Untreated* and *Treated* Neonatal Herpes Simplex Virus Infection

CLINICAL TYPE		PLACEBO (%)[a]	Acyclovir 30 mg/kg/day (%)[b]	Acyclovir 60 mg/kd/day (%)[c]
DIS		n = 13	n = 18	n = 34
	Death	85	61	29
	No apparent sequelae	50	43	63
	Abnormal	50	29	13
	Unknown	0	29	25
CNS		n = 6	n = 35	n = 23
	Death	50	14	4
	No apparent sequelae	33	27	18
	Abnormal	67	67	41
	Unknown	0	67	41
SEM		n = 8	n = 54	n = 9
	Death	0	0	0
	No apparent sequelae	62	83	22
	Abnormal	38	2	0
	Unknown	0	15	78

[a]Data from Whitley RJ, Nahmias AJ, Visintine AM, et al. The natural history of herpes simplex virus infection of mother and newborn. *Pediatrics.* 1980;66:489-494.
[b]Data from Whitley R, Arvin A, Prober C, et al. Predictors of morbidity and mortality in neonates with herpes simplex virus infections. The National Institute of Allergy and Infectious Diseases Collaborative Antiviral Study Group. *N Engl J Med.* 1991;324:450-454.
[c]Data from Kimberlin DW, Lin CY, Jacobs RF, et al. Natural history of neonatal herpes simplex virus infections in the acyclovir era. *Pediatrics.* 2001;108:223-229.
Data from Kimberlin DW, Gutierrez KM. Herpes simplex virus infections. In: Wilson CB, Nizet V, Maldonado YA, et al. *Remington and Klein's Infectious Diseases of the Fetus and Newborn Infant.* 8th ed. Philadelphia: Saunders; 2016:843-865.
Modified from Kimberlin DW. Advances in the treatment of neonatal herpes simplex infections. *Rev Med Virol.* 2001;11:157-163.

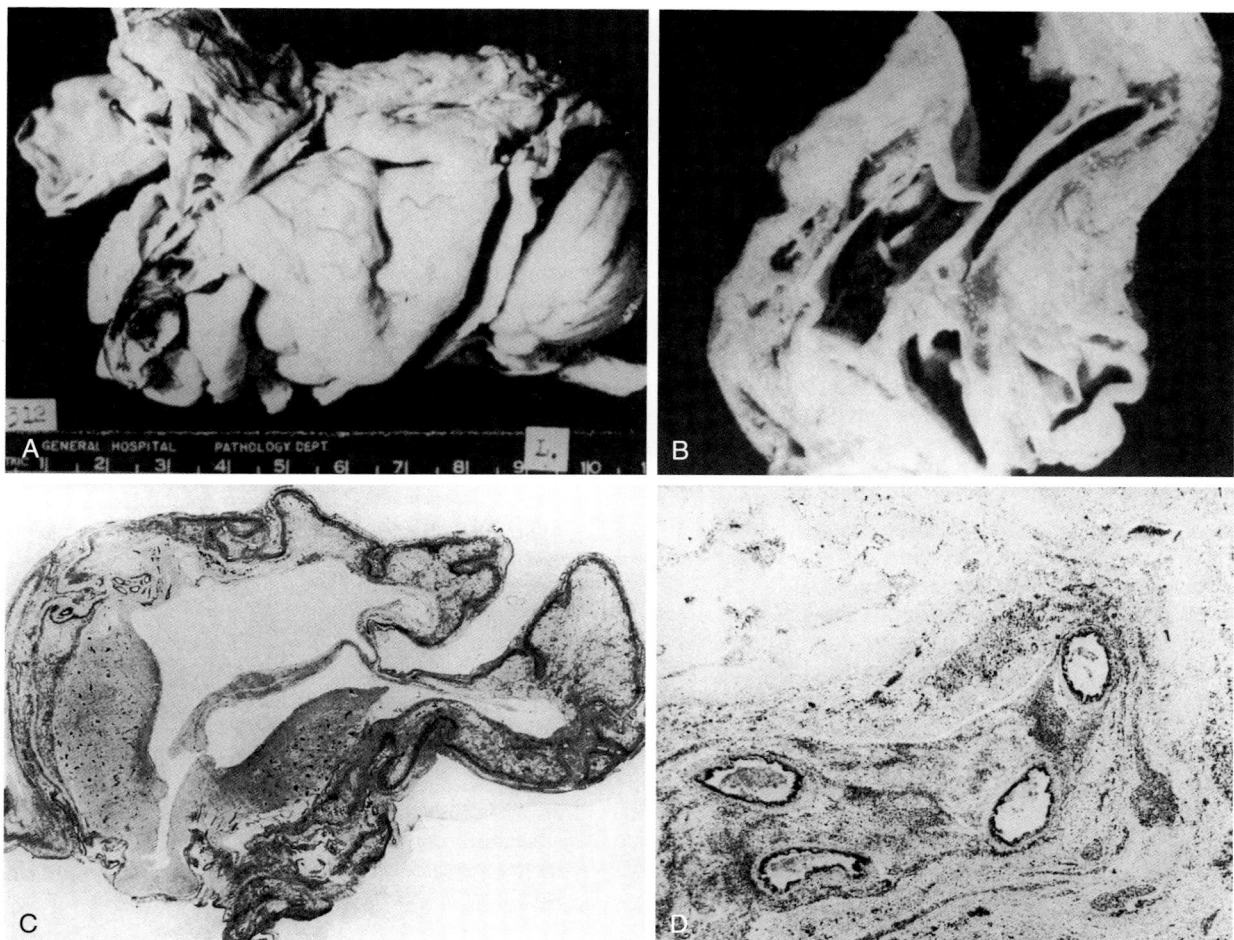

Figure 34.21 Neonatal herpes simplex infection: multicystic encephalomalacia in an infant who died at 24 weeks of age. Onset of recognized disease at approximately 21 days of age with seizures was followed by rapid progression to electrocerebral silence at 34 days of age and subsequent vegetative state. (A) Left lateral view of brain showing thickened covering membranes and severe destruction of cerebral hemispheres. (B) Coronal section of cerebral hemispheres showing parenchymal destruction with cavitation. (C) Photomicrograph of coronal section of cerebral hemispheres stained with hematoxylin and eosin. Note destruction of cerebral cortex and subcortical white matter and replacement by astrocytic glial stroma and dramatic masses of foamy macrophages. The macrophages are particularly striking in the superior aspects of the cerebral convexity. (D) Higher-power view showing the cavitation, necrotic debris, and masses of macrophages, especially around blood vessels. (From Young GF, Knox DL, Dodge PR. Necrotizing encephalitis and chorioretinitis in a young infant: report of a case with rising herpes simplex antibody titers. *Arch Neurol.* 1965;13:15-24.)

Overlap of the latter two localized forms is not uncommon. The relative decrease in disseminated disease and the increase in SEM disease appear to relate to earlier diagnosis and the use of antiviral therapy.

Clinical Features of Disseminated Disease. The early signs of disseminated HSV infection occur in most cases by 10 to 12 days of life.[a] In a series of 186 infected infants, approximately 10% of patients were reported to exhibit signs of illness on the first postnatal day. The usual mode of onset includes lethargy and cessation of feeding. This is followed promptly in approximately half of the cases by a neurological syndrome characterized by stupor, irritability, and seizures (often focal), with progression to coma and opisthotonos (Table 34.28).[1,37,268]

CSF pleocytosis (sometimes with red blood cells) and elevated protein content are present. In approximately one third of patients with disseminated disease, overt CNS signs are not present. However, CSF pleocytosis and elevated protein content may be observed in such cases, and the occurrence of neurological residua in survivors indicates that CNS involvement is frequently present, even though overt neonatal neurological signs are not.

Disseminated HSV infection may involve multiple organ systems including the liver, lungs, adrenals, gastrointestinal tract, and the SEM. Hepatomegaly, hyperbilirubinemia, and bleeding are common (see Table 34.28). The bleeding relates to a combination of hepatic disease and, often, disseminated intravascular coagulation, and it may be very severe. It is important to realize that more than 20% of neonates with disseminated HSV infection do not develop any cutaneous

---

[a]References 268, 269, 273, 277, 313, 314, 316, 317, 320, 321.

TABLE 34.28   Clinical Features of Disseminated Neonatal Herpes Simplex Virus Infection

CLINICAL FEATURE	APPROXIMATE FREQUENCY (%)
Central nervous system	
Meningoencephalitis	51–75
Seizures	21–50
Coma	21–50
Tense anterior fontanelle	0–50
Skin and oral cavity	
Vesicular exanthem	51–75
Vesicular enanthem	0–20
Eye	
Conjunctivitis	0–20
Keratitis	0–20
Chorioretinitis	0–20
Reticuloendothelial system	
Hepatomegaly	21–50
Hyperbilirubinemia	21–50
Bleeding	21–50
Hemolytic and other anemias	0–20
Other	
Fever	21–50
Pneumonitis	0–20
Rapidly fatal course (untreated)	76–100

See text for references.

TABLE 34.29   Major Clinical Features of Localized Neonatal Herpes Simplex Virus Infection of the Central Nervous System

Stupor and irritability
Seizures (often focal)
Vesicular exanthem
Cerebrospinal fluid pleocytosis, elevated protein

vesicles during their illness; the vesicles often appear *after* the clinical onset of the disease and evolve from macules to papules before the vesicles form, which often resemble pustules.[290,292] In a recent study, only 2 of 13 infants (15%) who died had skin lesions at presentation.[322] Disseminated HSV infection is a devastating disorder (see Table 34.27); before the era of therapy, approximately 80% of infected children died, frequently within a few days, and approximately 50% of the survivors exhibited serious neurological sequelae, predictable on the basis of the neuropathology (see the previous section). Mortality has declined to approximately 29% and morbidity to 17% since the introduction of antiviral therapy[263,292] (see Table 34.27).

Clinical Features of Localized Disease. Localized HSV infection is characterized by the absence of clinical or laboratory evidence of visceral involvement.[268,312,315] The sites most commonly affected are the CNS and SEM (see Table 34.29).[264,269,277,313,320] The age of onset of localized involvement of the *CNS* is *later* than for disseminated disease (day 16 to 19).[316,321] Indeed, because relatively more term infants exhibit localized CNS

disease than disseminated disease,[311] the infant with this variety of neonatal HSV infection has usually been discharged from the hospital before the illness begins. The usual signs are stupor and irritability, which evolve to seizures (often focal) and, perhaps, coma. As with disseminated disease, many infants (≈35%) do not exhibit mucocutaneous lesions.[268,312,313,320,321] CSF pleocytosis and elevated protein are characteristic; depressed CSF glucose is also common.[312] The outcome is unfavorable but better than with disseminated disease. Before antiviral therapy, approximately 50% of these infants died, a rate that has declined to 4% following the introduction of antiviral therapy. Similarly, whereas about 70% to 80% of *survivors* exhibited serious neurological sequelae before antiviral therapy, this number has declined to about 40% (see Table 34.27).[263,292] The morbidity among infants with CNS HSV infection is higher among those with HSV-2 infection than among those with HSV-1 infection and may include developmental delay, epilepsy, blindness, and cognitive disabilities.

HSV infection clinically localized to the SEM usually presents in the second week of life (days 10 to 12).[277,292,313] The progression from macules to vesicles occurs over 24 to 48 hours, often at sites of trauma (e.g., site of scalp electrodes or presenting body part). The vesicles may be obscured by overlying hair. The presence of a vesicle in a newborn should be seen as indicating HSV infection until ruled out as soon as possible by appropriate diagnostic studies (see later). Progression to CNS or disseminated disease occurs in 75% of untreated cases. Indeed, clinical localization of lesions to the SEM does not imply that the CNS is not also affected (see Table 34.27). Before antiviral therapy, approximately 30% to 40% of such patients exhibited neurological sequelae on follow-up. Currently, with therapy, sequelae are rare.[1]

Clinical Diagnosis. Of the congenital infections, neonatal HSV infection may be the most distinctive. The presence of a vesicular rash, keratoconjunctivitis, seizures, tense anterior fontanelle, and CSF evidence of meningoencephalitis is characteristic. However, the skin and ocular manifestations are present at the *onset* of the illness in only the *minority* of cases. Even in disseminated HSV, classic signs may not be present on admission. Of 49 infants (16%) with HSV, 18 lacked classic signs at hospitalization, 3 had disseminated disease, 4 had CNS involvement, and 1 uncategorized[323]; most of these 18 infants developed signs suggestive of HSV within 24 hours. The majority (84%) presented with seizure, vesicular rash, or critical illness on admission.

Additional information of value is epidemiological, regarding HSV infection in the mother or her sexual contact. Important negative differential diagnostic information includes the rarity *in the neonatal period* of microcephaly, hydrocephalus, intracranial calcification, and cardiovascular defects.

Laboratory Evaluation

Cytological Techniques. Identification of HSV infection is based principally on cytological techniques, isolation of the virus, or detection of viral DNA.[268,321,324-327] A high index of suspicion of the disease is crucial. Cultures may be taken before any clinical symptoms—for instance, in the presence of genital herpes noted during delivery. However, only 20% to 40% of mothers whose children develop HSV infection have had symptomatic genital herpes or sexual contact with a partner with recognized HSV infection during or before the pregnancy. Certainly any infant with a vesicular lesion should be considered to have an HSV infection and should be evaluated appropriately. However, nonspecific signs (e.g., lethargy, cessation of feeding, or other features suggestive of bacterial sepsis) should raise the possibility of neonatal HSV infection. Cytological techniques are readily available and are a rapid means of establishing a presumptive diagnosis of neonatal HSV infection. Scrapings can be obtained from the base of vesicular lesions of the skin or oral cavity or from conjunctival lesions. Smears are fixed in alcohol and stained immediately, according to the Papanicolaou method. The typical morphological changes are multinucleated giant cells and intranuclear inclusions. Viral particles may also be observed by electron microscopic examination of material from lesions and from urine and CSF.[328] HSV antigens have also been detected in CSF leukocytes through the use of immunofluorescence techniques.[329]

Isolation of Virus and Detection of Viral DNA.
Isolation of the virus is a definitive means for establishing the diagnosis and is best accomplished from observable lesions, but isolation is also possible from throat, stool, urine, and CSF. In one series, a pharyngeal swab was the source with the highest detection rate (79%).[316] In appropriate media, samples can be transported at room temperature.[330,331] Cytopathic changes in inoculated tissue cultures are usually detectable within 1 to 3 days.[1] The virus not uncommonly is difficult to isolate from CSF very early in localized CNS disease.

A major advance in the diagnosis of neonatal HSV infection is application of PCR to amplify the very small quantities of viral DNA, which then can be detected by conventional methods (e.g., DNA hybridization).[324,325,332,333] PCR assay has been shown in the newborn to be clearly superior to culture and is highly sensitive and specific for CNS involvement when CSF is studied. However, HSV DNA in CSF may be undetectable in 30% of cases early in the disease, and serial sampling is required to reach nearly 100% sensitivity in HSV encephalitis. In a recent study, HSV PCR results were obtained from plasma ($n = 47$), CSF ($n = 56$), or both ($n = 40$) at the time of diagnosis in 63 infants with SEM ($n = 26$), CNS ($n = 18$), or disseminated disease ($n = 19$) (Table 34.30).[265] Plasma HSV PCR was 100% positive only in infants with disseminated disease. Even in infants with CNS infection, only 72% had positive CSF PCR. This discrepancy could be explained by the pathogenesis of neonatal HSV CNS disease, which is thought to be neuronal transport to the brain resulting in an initially localized encephalitis before involvement of the meninges.[334] Thus early sampling of the CSF may not detect HSV and repeating a lumbar puncture should be considered when the diagnosis is suspected. Mean plasma viral level was 2.8 log10 copies per milliliter in SEM, 2.2 log10 copies per milliliter in CNS, and 7.2 log10 copies per milliliter in infants with disseminated disease. The HSV levels were higher among infants who died compared with surviving infants, 8.1 log10 copies per milliliter (range 7.7 to 8.6) versus 3.8 log10 copies per milliliter (range 0.0 to 8.6), $P = .001$. However, the level of HSV DNA in the CSF or in plasma did not correlate with neurological outcome.[265]

Importance of Maternal Evaluation.
Isolation of the virus from mothers (or their sexual contacts) with genital infection is a valuable adjunct to diagnosis of the neonatal disorder. Because

TABLE 34.30	Polymerase Chain Reaction Results in Neonatal Herpes Simplex Virus Infection		
POSITIVE POLYMERASE CHAIN REACTION	**SEM** $n = 26$	**CNS** $n = 18$	**DIS** $n = 19$
HSV-plasma	14/18 (78)	7/11 (64)	18/18 (100)
HSV-CSF	2/24 (8)	13/18 (72)	9/14 (64)
HSV-surface	24ª/25 (96)	9ª/18 (50)	12/18 (67)

ªTwo infants (1 SEM and 1 CNS) had pooled nasopharyngeal/conjunctival cultures, which were HSV culture–negative, but they had skin lesions that were not cultured. These two infants were considered culture-negative in the analysis.

CSF, Cerebrospinal fluid; *CNS,* central nervous system; *SEM,* skin, eyes, or mouth.

Modified from Melvin AJ, Mohan KM, Schiffer JT, et al. Plasma and cerebrospinal fluid herpes simplex virus levels at diagnosis and outcome of neonatal infection. *J Pediatr.* 2015;166:827-833.

most cases of genital herpes in pregnant women are subclinical, cultures, PCR assays, or both are usually necessary to establish the diagnosis.[1,324,335] Viral cultures of genital secretions and serological studies of maternal serum by western blot are the most convenient and effective approaches.[273,280,335,336] Detection of viral DNA in genital specimens by PCR is a highly sensitive approach, but its value for routine use in obstetrics is not yet established.

Serological Studies.
Serological studies for the diagnosis of neonatal infection with HSV are less useful than for other congenital infections. This finding relates to the masking of the infant's own IgG response by passively transferred maternal antibody and the 1- to 2-week delay in the rise in specific IgM antibody generated by the infant. There are two type-specific antibody assays that allow a distinction between HSV types 1 and 2.[337] Specific HSV IgM antibody can be detected rapidly by an immunofluorescence test.[338] Because the antibody persists for 6 to 12 months, this test is useful in survivors of the neonatal infection.

Neurodiagnostic Studies.
Neurodiagnostic studies of value include particularly examination of the CSF, electroencephalography (EEG), and brain imaging. Brain biopsy is no longer considered for making a diagnosis.

The *CSF* exhibits the findings of meningoencephalitis (i.e., pleocytosis and elevated protein content). Polymorphonuclear cells are occasionally predominant; in severely affected cases, the pleocytosis includes many red blood cells. The CSF glucose level may be depressed.[308,309,312,318,339] In one series, mean CSF glucose in the first week of the disease was 39 mg/dL; in the second week, it was 32 mg/dL; and in the third to fifth weeks, it was 28 mg/dL. Protein level is elevated consistently and often exceeds 100 to 150 mg/dL as the disease progresses. Any infant with a CSF formula suggestive of encephalitis (i.e., pleocytosis and elevated protein) should be considered to have HSV encephalitis until proven otherwise. The virus can be isolated from the CSF, but as noted in the previous subsection, the cultures are often negative early in the disease. *PCR assay* clearly is the optimal method to identify the virus in CSF rapidly. As noted earlier, the sensitivity early in the disease is approximately 50% to 75% and increases to nearly 100% with later CSF samples.[312,324,326]

CT was formerly used to demonstrate the extent and severity of the brain injury (Fig. 34.22). Progression of abnormalities to multicystic encephalomalacia has readily been documented by serial studies. *Cranial ultrasound* is also useful in the detection of parenchymal changes and evolution into multicystic encephalomalacia, but it is likely to miss cortical and brain stem injury. *MRI* is the most useful approach for the identification of parenchymal lesions.[306,340,341] Diffusion-weighted imaging (DWI) MRI is the most sensitive imaging modality for the early detection of CNS disease (Fig. 34.23). The rapid evolution to multicystic encephalomalacia is clearly delineated by MRI (Figs. 34.24 and 34.25). In a relatively large retrospective study of 29 infants with neonatal HSV infection, bilateral multilobar (*n* = 8), pontine (*n* = 3), thalamic (*n* = 6), or internal capsule and corticospinal tract (*n* = 5) involvement was noted on MRI. Additional information, not yet apparent on conventional T1- and T2-weighted imaging, was seen in 6 infants who had DWI. As might be expected, neurodevelopmental outcome was found to correlate with MRI abnormalities.[342] Notably, somewhat reminiscent of adult HSV encephalitis, the temporal lobe was involved in 67% of cases, and in 25% this cerebral structure was exclusively involved.[306]

The *EEG* usually shows striking and characteristic changes (Fig. 34.26).[312,316-318,343] These are principally focal or multifocal paroxysmal, periodic, or quasiperiodic discharges consisting of repetitive sharp slow-wave complexes.[318] The occurrence of prolonged periods (1 to 2 minutes) of such discharges was associated with death or major neurological sequelae in 9 of 10 affected infants in a reported series.[343] A normal EEG was

associated with normal outcome in all five infants in another series.[317] The EEG is one of the most sensitive noninvasive laboratory studies in the diagnosis of herpes infection (Table 34.31). In the study of Mikati et al.,[318] the EEG was abnormal when CT and ultrasonographic studies were normal in the

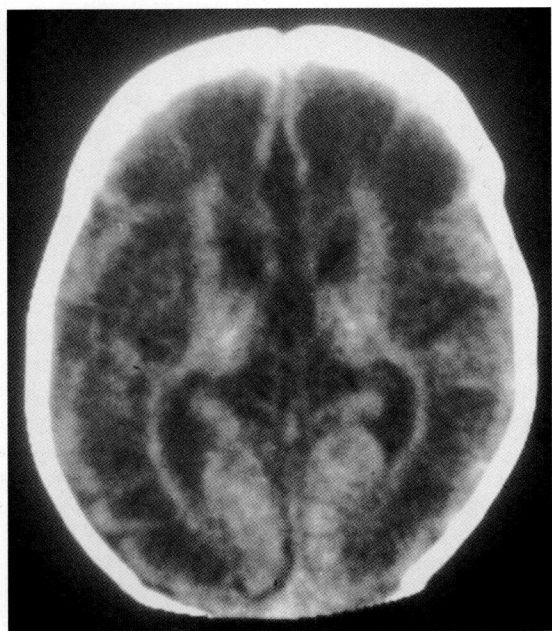

Figure 34.22 Neonatal herpes simplex infection: multicystic encephalomalacia. This computed tomography scan is from an affected 6-week-old infant who had onset of neurological signs at 7 days of age. Note the large lucent areas, representing regions of cystic necrosis, scattered throughout the cerebral hemispheres. (Courtesy Dr. Charles Abramson.)

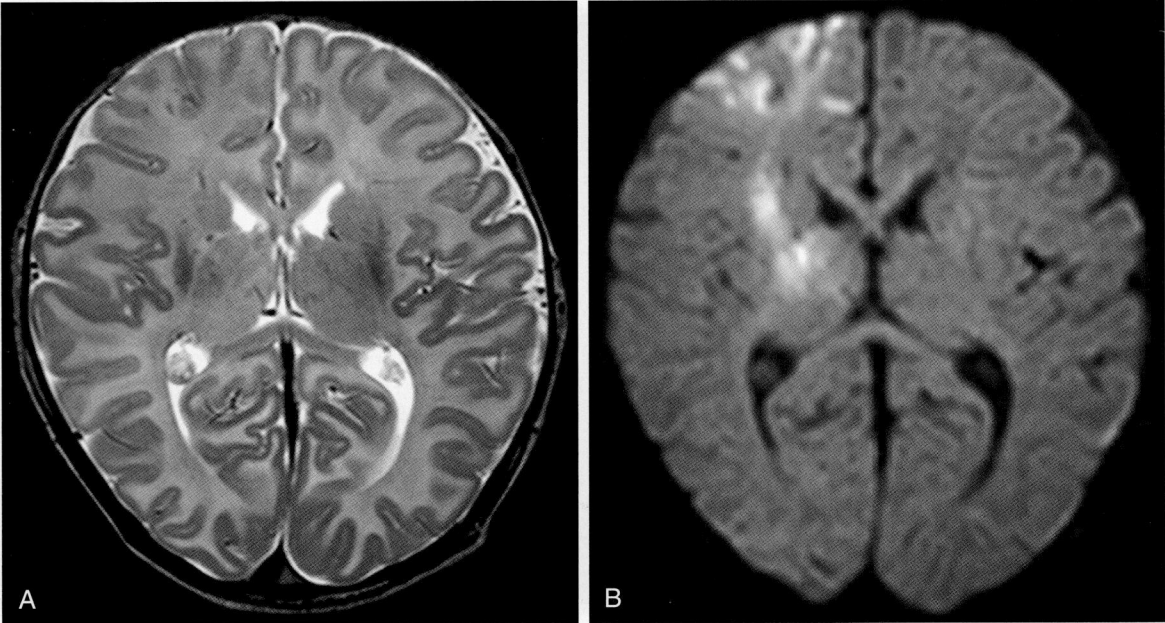

Figure 34.23 Magnetic resonance imaging: axial T2-weighted image (A) and diffusion-weighted image (B) showing restricted diffusion extending from the cortex to the posterior limb of the internal capsule (B), not seen on the T2 sequence (A). The child developed mild unilateral spastic cerebral palsy.

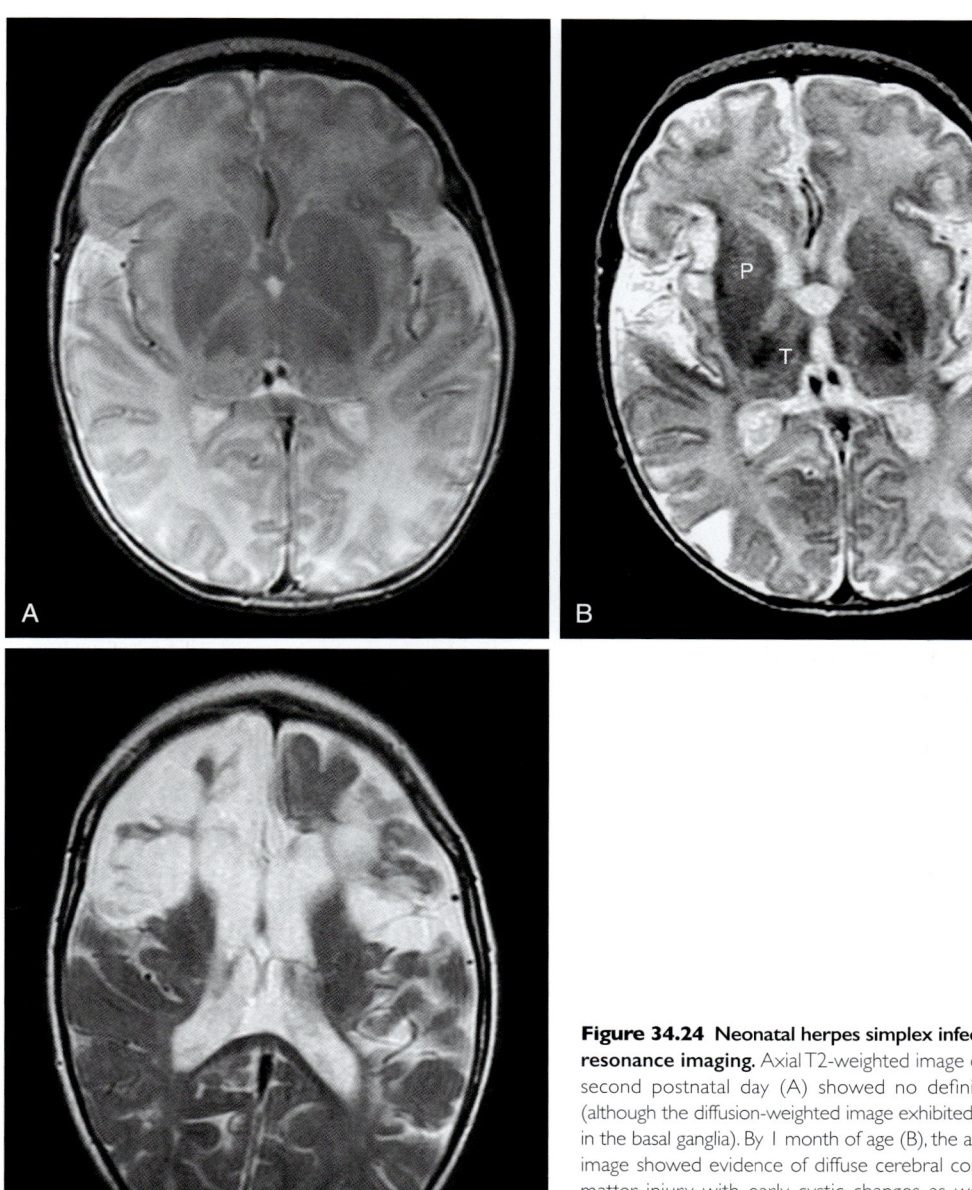

Figure 34.24 Neonatal herpes simplex infection: magnetic resonance imaging. Axial T2-weighted image obtained on the second postnatal day (A) showed no definite abnormality (although the diffusion-weighted image exhibited abnormal signal in the basal ganglia). By 1 month of age (B), the axial T2-weighted image showed evidence of diffuse cerebral cortical and white matter injury with early cystic changes as well as lesions in putamen (P) and thalamus (T). At 6 months of age, an axial T2-weighted image (C) showed multicystic encephalomalacia, most prominent in the right frontal region. (Courtesy Dr. Omar Khwaja.)

TABLE 34.31   Electroencephalographic Findings in Neonatal Herpes Simplex Encephalitis

DAYS OF ILLNESS	NUMBER	FINDINGS	
		ABNORMAL BACKGROUND[a]	PAROXYSMAL[a]
1–4	8	7	7
5–11	13	13	11
≥12	10	9	2

[a]Background abnormalities consisted primarily of low-voltage activity; paroxysmal activity consisted primarily of focal or multifocal periodic abnormalities.
Data from Mikati MA, Feraru E, Krishnamoorthy K, Lombroso CT. Neonatal herpes simplex meningoencephalitis: EEG investigations and clinical correlates. *Neurology.* 1990;40:1433-1437.

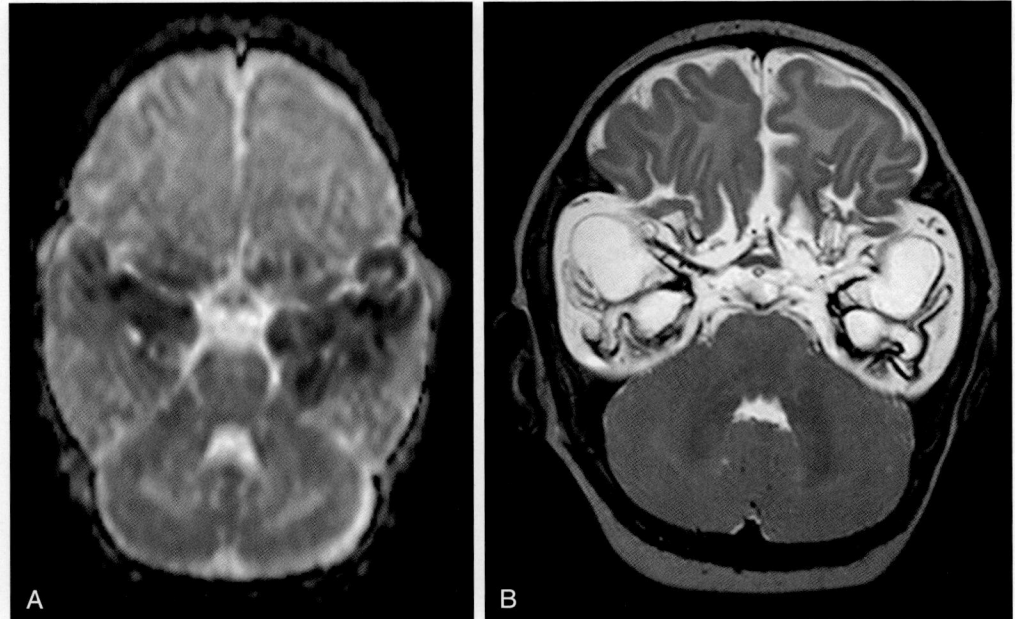

Figure 34.25 Neonatal herpes simplex infection: magnetic resonance imaging. Axial apparent diffusion coefficient (ADC) map (A) 3 days after onset of symptoms and T2-weighted image at 2 months after disease onset (B), showing symmetrical involvement of the temporal lobes, initially seen as restricted diffusion (A) with subsequent cystic evolution.

first 4 days of the illness in seven infants who had both EEG and an imaging study.

Prognosis

Relation to the Neonatal Clinical Syndrome. The outcome in affected infants is clearly related to the nature of the neonatal clinical syndrome (as discussed earlier) and is depicted in Table 34.27 for infants not treated with antiviral therapy. The mortality rate is highest with disseminated disease (≈85%) and lowest with localized skin involvement (no deaths). Survivors exhibit neurological sequelae predictable from the neuropathology (i.e., intellectual retardation, seizures, multifocal spastic motor deficits, and microcephaly). These sequelae are not uncommon in infections clinically localized to sites outside the CNS (e.g., eyes and skin) and indicate subclinical involvement of the CNS. The relatively high rate of neurological sequelae (38%) in patients with SEM disease may relate partly to the direct transmission of virus into the CNS from the eye, as has been demonstrated experimentally.[263] Moreover, the observation that the incidence of chorioretinal scars on follow-up of infants infected with HSV as newborns increased from 4% in the neonatal period to 28% suggests that the virus may continue to cause injury in this region postnatally.[317]

Later data indicate a decrease in the proportion of disseminated HSV infection and an increase in the proportion of disease localized to SEM (see earlier discussion). This change in clinical spectrum relates to both earlier diagnosis and the onset of antiviral therapy.[280] Currently the most favorable outcome is with SEM disease (no mortality, 95% to 100% normal), intermediate with localized CNS disease (4% to 6% mortality, 20% to 30% of survivors normal), and worst with disseminated disease (25% to 30% mortality, although 60% to

80% of survivors were normal; see later).[a] A recent randomized controlled trial suggested that outcome data improve even further with 6 months of antiviral therapy (see further on).[344]

Management

Prevention. Most cases of neonatal HSV infection are acquired close to the time of delivery; thus the major issues are prevention of maternal infection and, if infection is present, detection thereof and management of delivery.[280,282,313,345] *Prevention of maternal infection* currently depends principally on avoidance of unprotected sexual intercourse and unprotected oral–genital contact in late pregnancy, serological testing of pregnant women to identify those at risk for HSV acquisition, and serological testing of pregnant women and their partners to identify those with discordant serological status. Advocates of abstinence in late pregnancy, seeking to prevent neonatal HSV infection, emphasize its universal applicability and low cost. Indeed, current data indicate that prevention of transmission of HSV infection from the male partner to the susceptible pregnant woman can reduce the incidence of neonatal HSV by 60% to 80%.[335]

Because the acquisition of most neonatal HSV infections occurs around the time of delivery, determination of the infected pregnant woman and, in particular, the woman with a *first episode of genital infection* is crucial (see Fig. 34.20).[267,273,282,313,346] Routine screening of pregnant women with viral cultures in the third trimester has failed to identify the women infected at the time of delivery.[313] The optimal approach for screening pregnant women is identification of the mother with primary infection

22 d♀ ; 3rd Day of illness

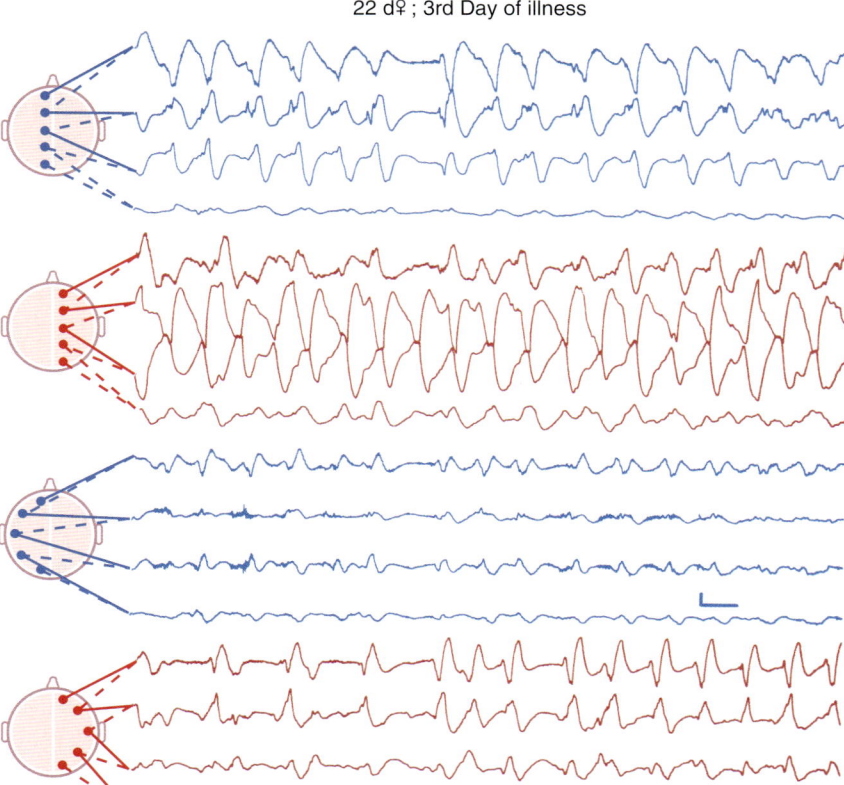

Figure 34.26 Electroencephalographic tracings from an infant with neonatal herpes simplex infection. The tracings were obtained with two different electrode arrays. The upper two tracings were obtained from one array, and the lower two tracings from a second array. Foci of periodic lateralized epileptiform activity are apparent in both hemispheres. (From Mizrahi EM, Tharp BR. A characteristic EEG pattern in neonatal herpes simplex encephalitis. *Neurology.* 1982;32:1215-1220.)

at the time of labor. Serological testing is of importance in this context. Detection of genital shedding of virus can be made by viral cultures or PCR. The latter approach is the most sensitive and rapid.[267,347,348] The risk of HSV transmission in women with a first episode of genital infection is 31% versus 1% in the woman with reactivated infection.[267] Indeed, among women with reactivated infection, those whose infection is with HSV-2 (i.e., the mother has antibodies to HSV-2), although common, *rarely* transmit HSV-2 to their infants. However, reactivated infection with HSV-1 (i.e., mother has antibodies to HSV-1) is followed by transmission to the infant in approximately 20% of cases. These points concerning the risks of a first episode of genital infection and of HSV-1 versus HSV-2 reactivated infection will help to determine whether antiviral suppressive therapy of the mother should be considered. Consideration has been given to the use of antiviral suppressive therapy, commencing at 36 weeks' gestation, with oral acyclovir or valacyclovir in women with active recurrent genital HSV lesions. In a recent multicenter case series, eight infants with HSV infection were reported after antenatal antiviral suppressive therapy. Data were collected between 2005 and 2009 in four states in the United States. Of these mothers, six had a first clinical episode of genital HSV infection during the present pregnancy and two had a recurrent infection. Perinatal transmission of HSV occurred in seven infants, including five who had received antiviral suppressive therapy until the day of delivery. Among these infants, five developed SEM disease, two had CNS disease (one without and one with disseminated disease), and one had intrauterine/disseminated disease. The data suggest that suppressive therapy does not eliminate the risk of perinatal transmission.[266]

The *management of delivery* in the women with genital infection is based, in considerable part, on the markedly lower risk of transmission to the infant with cesarean section versus vaginal delivery (see earlier; also see Table 34.24). Moreover, the risk of ascending infection after membranes have ruptured is significant and time-related (see Table 34.24). Although the risk of neonatal infection increases with duration of ruptured membranes, cesarean section is recommended regardless of duration of amniorrhexis[1] because it cannot be assumed that every infant has already acquired the virus through ascending infection (note the small number for cesarean section more

TABLE 34.32 Outcome of *Untreated* Neonatal Herpes Simplex Virus Infection Manifested Initially by Skin Vesicles Only

NEONATAL CLINICAL COURSE	NUMBER OF PATIENTS	OUTCOME		
		DIED (%)	NEUROLOGICAL SEQUELAE (%)	NO APPARENT SEQUELAE (%)
Vesicles progressed to				
Disseminated disease	21	57	24	19
Local central nervous system disease	10	30	60	10
Local ocular disease	2	0	50	50
Vesicles remained localized to skin	28	0	29	71
Total	61	24	33	43

Infants were managed before availability of antiviral therapy.

Data from Nahmias AJ, Keyserling HL, Kerrick GM. Herpes simplex. In: Remington JS, Klein JO, eds. *Infectious Diseases of the Fetus and Newborn Infant.* 2nd ed. Philadelphia: Saunders; 1983.

than 6 hours after amniorrhexis in Table 34.24). In general, membrane rupture for up to 24 hours has been considered a duration still appropriate for cesarean section.[1] All these comments must be interpreted with the awareness that the serological status of the woman is most crucial in determining the potential value of cesarean section (see Fig. 34.22).

Supportive Therapy. Supportive therapy emphasizes the management of seizures. Although brain swelling is significant with severe involvement of the CNS, there is no evidence to indicate that steroids or hyperosmolar solutions are generally useful. Avoidance of fluid overload, however, is important. Management of disseminated intravascular coagulation, bleeding, ventilation, circulation, and the like is reviewed in standard writings on neonatology.

Antimicrobial Therapy. Specific antiviral therapy is available for neonatal HSV infection. Although the outlook for treated patients remains serious (see subsequent discussion), the value of therapy is established. The decision regarding *whom to treat* is sometimes difficult. Optimal benefit requires prompt institution of therapy.[268,269,314,321] Indeed, in one study, involvement of additional organ systems by HSV was noted in 57% of infants between the time of presentation to medical personnel and diagnosis.[267] In another report, the mean time of onset of therapy was 5 to 6 days after onset of symptoms.[268] The difficulties in establishing the diagnosis rapidly in some infants are described earlier in the section on laboratory evaluation. Antiviral therapy for suspected HSV infection of the newborn should be instituted in the same fashion as antibiotic therapy for suspected bacterial meningitis. Thus treatment should be started after the culture or PCR specimens (including CSF) have been obtained for infants with the suspicious clinical features described previously (e.g., CSF findings suggestive of encephalitis) or vesicles in a clinically sick infant. With proven infection, it is universally recognized that infants with disseminated disease and localized CNS involvement should be treated immediately in view of the potentially poor outcome. It is sometimes not so well recognized that even infants with localized SEM disease also require prompt therapy. Thus infants with localized mucocutaneous or ocular disease on *initial* presentation progress to disseminated disease, overt CNS involvement, or both, in more than 50% of cases

without therapy (Table 34.32).[268,269] Therefore prompt antiviral therapy is indicated even when herpetic disease is apparently localized to mucocutaneous or ocular structures. In addition, because serial assessments of survivors of herpetic disease have demonstrated recurrence of disease in 10% to 30% of cases, including development of chorioretinitis and perhaps of neurological deficits during later infancy, the possibility of *progressive* disease (as with the other infections of the TORCH group) suggests an indication for prolonged initial therapy.[317,324,344,349,350]

Four *antiviral drugs* (iododeoxyuridine [IDU], arabinofuranosylcytosine [Ara-C], arabinofuranosyladenine [Ara-A] or vidarabine, and acyclovir) have been shown to inhibit HSV in vitro by inhibiting DNA synthesis and have been used clinically since the 1980s.[268,321,351-354] IDU and Ara-C proved to be too toxic because of effects on such rapidly dividing cells as the gastrointestinal tract and hemopoietic systems. Moreover, Ara-C has a potent antimitotic effect on dividing brain cells, at least in the rat. A considerable degree of DNA synthesis, especially by glial cells, occurs in human brain in the perinatal period; Ara-C could therefore seriously derange these cells.

Acyclovir represented an advance in therapy because of its limited toxicity, high specificity, and greater activity against the virus than vidarabine.[321,343] The drug is a deoxyguanosine analogue that is activated by a herpes-specific thymidine kinase; it inhibits viral DNA polymerase and thereby viral replication.[321,351] Controlled studies of HSV encephalitis in adults indicated greater benefit in relation to both mortality and morbidity for acyclovir than for vidarabine.[353,355] A controlled multi-institutional study of acyclovir versus vidarabine in the treatment of neonatal HSV infection demonstrated no appreciable difference in efficacy between the two.[321] However, acyclovir is preferred because of its higher solubility and relatively low toxicity. One study compared outcome in infants with neonatal HSV disease treated with acyclovir administered intravenously either in a standard dose (30 mg/kg per day) or high dose (60 mg/kg per day) in three divided doses for 21 days.[319,356] Concerning mortality, a markedly beneficial effect of the high versus the low dose was seen in children with disseminated HSV disease; the mortality rate was 61% for the standard dose (historical controls) versus 29% for the high dose. For CNS disease, a beneficial effect on mortality was suggested

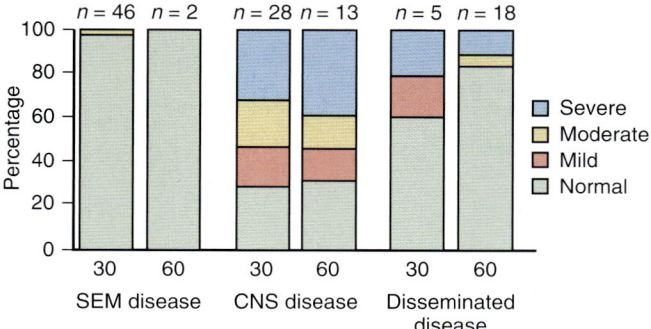

Figure 34.27 Neonatal herpes simplex infection: effect of acyclovir on outcome. Infants were treated with either 30 mg/kg per day (low dose) or 60 mg/kg per day (high dose) of acyclovir. See text for details. *CNS*, Central nervous system; *SEM*, skin-eye-mouth. (From Kimberlin DW, Lin CY, Jacobs RF, et al. Safety and efficacy of high-dose intravenous acyclovir in the management of neonatal herpes simplex virus infections. *Pediatrics.* 2001;108:230-238.)

but did not reach statistical significance; for standard-dose therapy, the mortality rate was approximately 14%, versus 4% for high-dose treatment. Concerning morbidity, both treated groups showed striking beneficial effects compared with untreated historical controls, although outcome was unknown in a subset of infants (Fig. 34.27; see also Table 34.27). Compared with standard-dose therapy, high-dose therapy was associated with a better outcome in disseminated disease; 63% of infants treated with high-dose therapy were normal versus 43% of infants treated with standard-dose therapy. For localized SEM disease, no mortality occurred, and the outcome was essentially uniformly favorable with both therapy groups (see Fig. 34.27). Intravenous high-dose acyclovir is given daily as 60 mg/kg per day (divided into three doses) for 21 days; the dose is lowered in the presence of renal or hepatic dysfunction.

Prolonged antiviral treatment has been shown to be of particular value. Thus, although improved neurodevelopmental outcome in infants surviving CNS disease was not achieved with intravenous acyclovir dosed at 60 mg/kg per day, improved outcomes have been demonstrated with oral suppressive acyclovir therapy given for 6 months following completion of a standard parenteral acyclovir treatment course.[344] In a recent study a total of 74 neonates were enrolled; 45 with CNS involvement and 29 with SEM disease. After completing a regimen of 14 to 21 days of parenteral acyclovir, the infants were randomly assigned to immediate acyclovir suppression (300 mg/m² per dose given orally 3 times daily for 6 months) or placebo. Infants with CNS disease who received suppressive acyclovir therapy for 6 months had better neurodevelopmental outcomes than those who received placebo, and infants with CNS and SEM disease had less frequent recurrences of skin lesions while receiving the suppressive therapy. Of those with CNS disease treated for 6 months, 69% had a normal outcome and 19% severe sequelae. By contrast, only 33% of those in the short-treatment group had a normal outcome and 33% developed severe sequelae.

Congenital Syphilis

Congenital infection with *T. pallidum* occurs by transplacental mechanisms, principally in the second and third trimesters of gestation. In the preantibiotic era, this disorder occurred with exceeding frequency; with the advent of penicillin treatment and improved public health measures, the disease became a rarity. However, in the mid-1980s, associated with some relaxation of surveillance techniques and a variety of social changes, syphilitic infection of women of childbearing age increased in frequency; with this, so did congenital syphilis.[357,358] In the later 1980s and early 1990s, these increases became dramatic and paralleled the increases in the use of illegal drugs, especially cocaine, and in HIV infection.[359-363] The overall rate of reported congenital syphilis in the United States decreased from 10.5 to 8.4 cases per 100,000 live births during 2008–2012; it then increased to 11.6 cases per 100,000 live births in 2014, the highest rate of congenital syphilis reported since 2001.[364] In two European studies the incidence varied from 1.9 to 20 per 100,000 in the United Kingdom and Italy, respectively.[365,366] In the United States, there has been little change in the case fatality ratio over the past several decades. Thus, an overall case fatality of 6.5% was noted during 1999 through 2013 compared with 6.4% from 1992 through 1998. Maternal race/ethnicity was not associated with increased morbidity or mortality, although most cases (83%) of congenital syphilis occurred among black or Hispanic mothers. Although congenital syphilis is rarely associated with *overt* neurological phenomena in the newborn period, involvement of the CNS appears to be relatively common and, in large part, curable. Thus, it is imperative for the perinatal physician to be aware of the features of the disorder.

Pathogenesis

Fetal Infection. Congenital syphilis results from intrauterine infection of the fetus with *T. pallidum* by transplacental mechanisms.[359,367] The fetus is infected during maternal spirochetemia, with resulting placentitis and, then, hematogenous spread of the organisms to multiple fetal organs. Maternal spirochetemia occurs during the primary, secondary, and early latency stages of maternal infection.[359,367,368] The primary infection is represented by a painless chancre at the portal of entry and is followed by the secondary stage of the disease approximately 6 weeks later, when mucocutaneous lesions and generalized lymphadenopathy often occur. This stage is followed by a variable period of 2 to 4 years during which spirochetemia, often asymptomatic, may recur. Most infants acquire the infection in utero from an asymptomatic mother in the early latency stage, when diagnosis by serological testing is a reliable means of detecting the maternal infection.[369] Fetal syphilis can be suspected by the finding in approximately 65% of cases of hepatomegaly on intrauterine ultrasound examination; the diagnosis can be established by the detection of *T. pallidum* DNA by PCR in amniotic fluid or of fetal antitreponemal IgM and abnormal hepatic transaminases in fetal blood.[368]

Importance of Stage and Timing of Maternal Infection. Two factors are of particular importance in determining fetal outcome: the stage of maternal infection and the time of fetal exposure to this infection. The risk to the fetus according to the *stage of untreated maternal infection* is depicted in Table 34.33. The later the stage of the maternal syphilitic process, the better the fetal outcome will be. This finding may relate to a protective effect of maternal immunity acquired with increasing duration of infection. The *time of fetal exposure* to maternal infection is also important; fetal infection rarely occurs before approximately 16 to 20 weeks of gestation. This characteristic has been attributed historically to a protective effect of the Langhans cell layer of

TABLE 34.33   Outcome of Pregnancy as a Function of Stage of Untreated Maternal Syphilis

MATERNAL STATUS	OUTCOME OF PREGNANCY			
	CONGENITAL SYPHILIS (%)	PERINATAL DEATH (%)	PREMATURE INFANT (%)	NORMAL INFANT (%)
Untreated syphilis				
Primary or secondary	50	———— 50 ————		0
Early latency	40	20	20	20
Late	10	11	9	70
No syphilis	0	1	8	91

Modified from Ingall D, Norins L. Syphilis. In: Remington JS, Klein JO, eds. *Infectious Diseases of the Fetus and Newborn Infant.* 2nd ed. Philadelphia: Saunders; 1983.

TABLE 34.34   Neuropathology of Congenital Neurosyphilis

Early
Acute and subacute meningitis
Chronic meningovascular syphilis
    Cranial neuropathies
    Hydrocephalus
    Cerebrovascular lesions, primarily infarction
Late
Optic atrophy and auditory nerve injury
Juvenile general paresis
Juvenile tabes dorsalis

the early placenta and the fact that infection is most likely after approximately 24 weeks, when complete atrophy of this layer is said to occur.[369] More recent electron microscopic studies showed persistence of the Langhans cell layer throughout pregnancy. A role for other factors (e.g., immunological) is likely.

Neuropathology

Congenital syphilis affects the CNS in most cases, although the involvement is generally confined to the meninges. Congenital syphilis is divided, somewhat arbitrarily, into early and late stages: those manifestations apparent in the first 2 years of life are designated *early* and those apparent after 2 years are termed "late." The neuropathological aspects of each stage are shown in Table 34.34.

Acute and Subacute Meningitis. The most common lesion, syphilitic meningitis, which occurs in acute or subacute form, has its onset as early as the newborn period but more often at 4 to 5 months of age.[370,371] It is characterized by inflammatory infiltration of the leptomeninges with mononuclear cells. These cells principally include lymphocytes, plasma cells, and macrophages. The infiltrates are often greatest in the basilar meninges, involving the sheaths of cranial nerves, and around blood vessels. Indeed, the perivascular cellular infiltrates may extend through the Virchow-Robin space into the brain parenchyma. Distinct parenchymal lesions are uncommon, although superficial layers of the cerebral cortex may be involved by the inflammatory infiltrates.

Chronic Meningovascular Syphilis. Presumably an extension of acute-subacute meningitis, chronic meningovascular syphilis, may develop (see Table 34.34). In this disorder, involvement of the basilar meninges becomes marked and may result in two major consequences. The first includes cranial nerve abnormalities (i.e., optic atrophy and involvement of facial, oculomotor, and, probably, auditory nerves). The second consequence of the chronic arachnoiditis is hydrocephalus, usually apparent between approximately the fourth and the ninth months of life.[1,37] The vasculitis may become so severe that obliteration of vessels occurs with resulting cerebral infarction, usually between 1 and 2 years of life. Rarely, involvement of blood vessels results in aneurysm formation and cerebral hemorrhage.

Juvenile General Paresis and Tabes Dorsalis. The late CNS consequences of congenital syphilis, in addition to persistent optic atrophy and auditory nerve injury, are juvenile general paresis and tabes dorsalis. The last two relatively rare parenchymal lesions usually appear at approximately 10 to 15 years of age and are discussed in standard writings on pediatric neurology.[1]

Clinical Aspects

Incidence of Clinically Apparent Infection. Congenital syphilis is particularly likely to be asymptomatic, at least regarding *neurological* illness, *in the neonatal period*.[358,361,363,372] Depending on the mode of ascertainment, between approximately 65% to 90% of cases are totally asymptomatic in the neonatal period.[359,373] Premature infants are more likely to exhibit clinical phenomena (usually hepatosplenomegaly) during their stay in the nursery because of either more severe disease or a longer period in the neonatal unit.[1,37]

Clinical Features: Early Congenital Syphilis. The clinical features of congenital syphilis, symptomatic in the first 2 years of life (i.e., early), include stillbirth (Table 34.35).[358,362,373-375] About 60% of infants are asymptomatic at birth. The major portions of the clinical syndrome are apparent in the first months of life but usually *not until* after the first 2 weeks.[376,377] Two thirds will develop symptoms by 3 to 8 weeks. The most prominent features relate to the skin and reticuloendothelial and skeletal systems. Characteristic rashes include vesiculobullous or papulosquamous lesions, with a predilection for the face and the oral and anogenital regions (Fig. 34.28).[378] A prominent mucocutaneous lesion is associated with a mucopurulent discharge, referred to as *snuffles*. Involvement of the reticuloendothelial system is characterized particularly

TABLE 34.35	Clinical Features of Symptomatic Early Congenital Syphilis

CLINICAL FEATURE	APPROXIMATE FREQUENCY (%)
Pregnancy	
Prematurity	21–50
Central nervous system	
Meningitis	51–75
Seizures	0–20
Cranial nerve palsies	0–20
Hydrocephalus	0–20
Cerebrovascular accident	0–20
Reticuloendothelial system	
Hepatosplenomegaly	51–75
Hyperbilirubinemia	21–50
Lymphadenopathy	51–75
Hemolytic and other anemias	51–75
Skin	
Pleomorphic rashes	51–75
Mucocutaneous lesions	21–50
Bone	
Osteochondritis	76–100
Periostitis	51–75
Other	
Pneumonitis	0–20

See text for references.

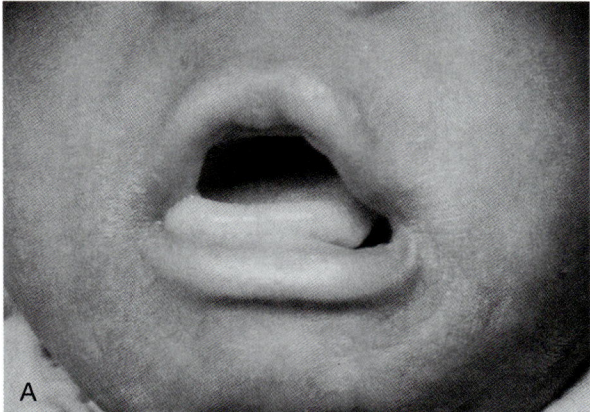
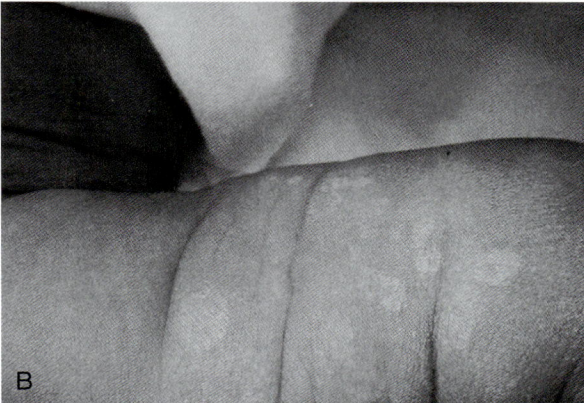

Figure 34.28 A 6-week-old infant with congenital syphilis. (A) Note the papular scaling perioral lesions. Later on, radial scars, termed *rhagades*, developed at this site. (B) Note the ovoid, annular scaly lesions. (From Tunnessen WW. Congenital syphilis. *Am J Dis Child*. 1992;146:115-116.)

by hepatosplenomegaly, lymphadenopathy, and anemia. Hyperbilirubinemia and other signs of hepatic disease are common. Involvement of bone is extremely common and is characterized by diagnostic changes of the distal metaphyses (osteochondritis) with associated periosteal elevations (periostitis).[379-382] In cases with a particularly early onset of clinical disease, bony changes are more common in affected premature infants than in term newborns.[381] Bone changes have also been observed in approximately 20% of clinically asymptomatic newborns.[379]

Involvement of the *CNS* is characterized by CSF pleocytosis and elevated protein content in most symptomatic cases. Among clinically asymptomatic newborns, the incidence of abnormal CSF findings depends on the definition of normal values. Thus nearly all infants identified in large series had CSF leukocyte values of 15/mm³ or higher and protein levels of 150 mg/dL or greater during the first 30 days of life and >5 WBC/mm³ or a CSGF protein >40 mg/dL after the first 30 days of life (Centers for Disease Control and Prevention [CDC] thresholds, 2014).[383,384] However, in a study of 67 infants born to untreated or inadequately treated seropositive women and thereby designated as presumptive congenital syphilis by CDC criteria, mean CSF values of leukocytes (7.7/mm³) and protein content (98 mg/dL) did not differ from values in control infants.[383] Neurological signs are *very* unusual in the first weeks of life and, indeed, such signs are uncommon among all patients with early congenital syphilis. However, the following are occasionally observed: seizures; cranial nerve palsies, especially of cranial nerve VII but also of nerves III, IV, and VI; hydrocephalus; signs of increased intracranial pressure (e.g., bulging anterior fontanelle); and focal neurological deficits (see Table 34.35).

These phenomena are seen in association with acute and subacute syphilitic meningitis and chronic meningovascular syphilis, as described in the section on neuropathology.

Clinical Features: Late Congenital Syphilis. Later clinical manifestations of congenital syphilis usually become apparent near puberty and include the following: abnormalities of the teeth, especially the upper central incisors (Hutchinson teeth) and the first lower molars ("mulberry molars"); interstitial keratitis; optic atrophy and visual loss; sensorineural deafness; and signs of cerebral disease (general paresis) or spinal cord disease (tabes dorsalis).[359] For the most part, these features are unusual and are discussed in standard writings on pediatric neurology.

Clinical Diagnosis. The diagnosis of congenital syphilis in the neonatal period is difficult to establish on clinical grounds because of the paucity of clinical phenomena. Particularly helpful, when present, are vesiculobullous and papulosquamous eruptions, mucocutaneous lesions, hepatosplenomegaly, lymphadenopathy, and osteochondritis. CSF signs of inflammation further support the diagnosis.

Laboratory Evaluation

Identification of *Treponema*. Determination of *T. pallidum* as the responsible microbe in congenital syphilis depends particularly on serological techniques. However, in the evaluation of any infant suspected of having the disease because of clinical phenomena or a history of a mother with a positive serological test for syphilis, a search for the organisms, spirochetal antigen, or DNA should be carried out as well. Dark-field microscopic examination of specimens obtained from skin or mucocutaneous lesions, nasal discharge, placenta, umbilical cord, or amniotic fluid is an effective means for identifying the organism.[385] The most highly sensitive technique for detection is by the inoculation of clinical specimens into rabbits (rabbit infectivity test), but this test is not routinely available.[385] The application of PCR to amniotic fluid, neonatal serum, and CSF to amplify the DNA of the organism has shown a sensitivity of 78% to 86% and a specificity of 100% in the detection of congenital syphilis infection.[370] PCR testing in serum or blood was more sensitive (94%) but not as specific, with a positive predictive value of 73%. Combinations of tests are needed.

Serological Studies. Serological techniques are critical in diagnosis. Two basic types are used: nontreponemal and treponemal.[359,386-388] In the former type, *nonspecific or reagin antigens* are used; the most widely used assay for antibody against these antigens is the Venereal Disease Research Laboratory (VDRL) test. A major disadvantage of assay of these antibodies is, as one would expect, the relative frequency of false-positive reactions.[1,37] *Specific treponemal antibody assays* largely circumvent the problem of false-positive reactions; of the tests available, the fluorescence treponemal antibody-absorbed (FTA-ABS) assay is highly specific and sensitive.[1,37] In this assay, serum antibody is complexed to specific treponemal antigen and is then detected by fluorescein-labeled antihuman gamma globulin. (The term *absorbed* refers to the initial step of removing antibodies directed against treponemes other than *T. pallidum* from the serum.) This test is especially useful for identifying the infected mother at delivery and thereby the infant at risk for congenital syphilis.[387] Because VDRL and FTA-ABS reactivity can be found in the IgG as well as in the IgM classes of antibody, confirmation of fetal infection necessitates the demonstration of persistence of reactivity beyond the time that passively transferred antibody would be expected.[389,390] However, *specific IgM treponemal antibody* is synthesized by the infected fetus and is not passively transferred. A fluorescein-labeled antihuman IgM (FTA-ABSIgM) has been used in a procedure for detecting *specific IgM antibody against T. pallidum*.[391] This test was shown to be sensitive as an indicator of neonatal syphilitic infection.[359,386,388,392-394] Currently, three different methods are used to detect treponemal-specific IgM in neonates suspected of having congenital syphilis: (1) FTA-ABS tests, (2) IgM immunoblots, and (3) IgM ELISAs. More recent improvements in methodology to detect specific IgM antibody have increased the sensitivity to 75% and specificity to 100%. Several rapid or point-of-care (POC) tests have been developed, mainly for resource-limited settings.[395] These tests detect specific antibodies to *T. pallidum* antigen and do not allow the clinician to distinguish between active and past successfully treated infection. When possible, rapid and POC tests should thus be coupled with nontreponemal tests (VDRL). Currently, the CDC defines a *presumptive case* of congenital syphilis as either an infant whose mother had untreated or inadequately treated syphilis at delivery (regardless of findings in the infant) or an infant who has a reactive treponemal test for syphilis and any

of the following: (1) evidence for congenital syphilis on physical examination or on long bone radiographs, (2) reactive CSF VDRL, (3) elevated CSF cell count or protein, (4) nontreponemal serological titers in the infant that are fourfold higher than those in the mother, or (5) a reactive test for fluorescent treponemal antibody absorption IgM antibody.[385]

Neurodiagnostic Studies. The most important neurodiagnostic study is examination of the CSF. The high frequency of CSF pleocytosis and elevated protein content in symptomatic disease has already been mentioned. However, these abnormal CSF findings may not be striking and interpretation in the newborn may be difficult. Another important test is CSF VDRL reactivity; a positive test result is considered diagnostic of CNS involvement whether or not the patient is symptomatic. However, the test is relatively insensitive (22% to 69%). More than one abnormal CSF result (pleocytosis, protein content, VDRL) has an 82% sensitivity.[370] Indeed, because of the poor sensitivity of the available diagnostic tests for neurosyphilis, the CDC has recommended that all infants with systemic evidence of congenital syphilis be treated with crystalline penicillin G 100,000 to 150,000 U/kg per day intravenously every 12 hours during the first 7 days of life and every 8 hours thereafter for a total of 10 days, or procaine penicillin G 50,000 U/kg per dose intramuscularly in a single daily dose for 10 days to ensure sterilization of the CSF. If more than 1 day of therapy is missed, the entire course must be restarted (www.cdc.gov/std/syphilis).

Prognosis

The outlook in congenital syphilis depends principally on the severity of the injury that has been incurred before the onset of therapy. Unfortunately, however, the precise relationships between the *timing* and *adequacy of treatment* of early congenital syphilis and the long-term outcome are not well documented.[1,37] Nevertheless, certain conclusions are justified. Untreated infection in utero may result in abortion or stillbirth in a substantial minority of patients (see the section on clinical aspects). An increase in case fatality has been noted with no or inadequate treatment for maternal syphilis, less than 10 prenatal visits, and elevated maternal nontreponemal titer. Moreover, infants with congenital syphilis born alive at less than 28 weeks' gestation (relative risk, 107.4; P <.001) or born weighing less than 1500 g (relative risk, 43.9; P <.001) were at greatly increased risk of death.[396]

Infection that is symptomatic in the early neonatal period is more likely to result in sequelae than is infection that is not symptomatic until after the first months of life.[1,37] The earlier therapy is initiated, the more likely a satisfactory response.[397] Neurological sequelae are relatively uncommon but can be severe; more important, such sequelae are preventable by early therapy. Indeed, the essential issues regarding outcome in congenital syphilis are early detection and prompt therapy; these aspects are reviewed next.

Management

Prevention. Preventive measures center on three major approaches: avoidance of maternal infection, treatment of maternal infection, and treatment of fetal infection. The first approach is an important public health issue that is not appropriate to discuss in detail here. Particular attention must

TABLE 34.36   Treatment of Infants Born to Mothers With Syphilis

MATERNAL TREATMENT	NEONATAL CLINICAL FINDINGS	PENICILLIN G	DOSE AND DURATION
None or inadequate	Present or absent	Crystalline	100,000–150,000 units/kg per day IV every 8–12 hours for 10–14 days (50,000 units every 12 hours for 7 days; every 8 hours after 7 days)
		Procaine	50,000 units/kg per day IM once daily for 10–14 days
Adequate	Absent	Benzathine (only if follow-up cannot be ensured and cerebrospinal fluid is normal)	500,000 units/kg IM, one dose

IM, Intramuscularly; *IV*, intravenously.

Data from Ingall D, Norins L. Syphilis. In: Remington JS, Klein JO, eds. *Infectious Diseases of the Fetus and Newborn Infant*. 2nd ed. Philadelphia: Saunders; 1983; Ikeda MK, Jenson HB. Evaluation and treatment of congenital syphilis. *J Pediatr*. 1990;117:843-852.

be paid to young, unmarried women of minority groups, who, with no prenatal care, constitute more than 50% of mothers of infants with congenital syphilis in the United States.[370] Prompt detection is begun by assay of maternal serum for reagin antibody (e.g., VDRL) at the first prenatal visit.[387,388] However, such serological tests are poor tools early in the course of maternal disease. More specific antibody studies also miss detection of a significant minority of infected women. Careful examination of women in labor for evidence of primary syphilis is very important. The syphilitic woman should be treated with 2.4 million units of benzathine penicillin; if this therapy is accomplished in the first 16 weeks of pregnancy, fetal infection will be avoided. Of course, this statement is made on the assumption that reinfection does not occur. After the 16th week, eradication of fetal infection is achieved in most cases with the same regimen.[398] In women with late latent syphilis infection or latent syphilis of unknown duration, benzathine penicillin G 7.2 million units total, administered as three doses of 2.4 million units IM each at 1-week intervals, has been recommended (www.cdc.gov/std/syphilis).

Supportive Therapy. From the neurological standpoint, the neonatal syndrome rarely presents therapeutic problems. Supportive measures directed toward involvement of extraneural systems are important.

Antimicrobial Therapy. Penicillin is the drug of choice in the treatment of congenital syphilis. The major questions faced in the neonatal period are *whom to treat and how to treat*. Detection of the infant with congenital syphilis requires a high index of suspicion and a careful evaluation. Particularly important are historical data related to the mother, maternal serology at delivery, and careful clinical radiographic, metabolic, and serological studies of the infant. Because maternal antibody response may occur so late in pregnancy that the infant's VDRL test is negative, positive maternal serology should provoke careful evaluation of the infant and consideration for treatment as outlined in Table 34.36. The mode of penicillin therapy depends largely on the adequacy of treatment of the mother during pregnancy (see Table 34.36). When the mother has had no or inadequate treatment during pregnancy, the infant is treated with a full 10- to 14-day course of either crystalline or procaine penicillin G in the doses shown in Table 34.36,

whether the infant is asymptomatic or symptomatic and whether infection of the infant is confirmed or not. The dose schedule described in Table 34.36 results in adequate spirocheticidal levels in CSF,[399,400] although some data indicate that crystalline penicillin G is superior to procaine penicillin.[401] The importance of treating all confirmed or presumptive cases of congenital syphilis with the higher doses relates to the finding that the CNS may be infected without demonstrable abnormalities of CSF and may serve as an incubating reservoir of infection that culminates in relapse and neurosyphilis.[359]

For infants who are asymptomatic, who have normal physical examinations and laboratory evaluations, and whose mothers have been adequately treated, the risk of congenital syphilis is very low.[359] Treatment is not compulsory if close follow-up can be ensured.[359] However, if follow-up cannot be ensured, administration of a single dose of benzathine penicillin G is recommended (see Table 34.36). Whether follow-up can be ensured or not, the CSF should be examined, and if there is any suspicion of CNS involvement, a 10- to 14-day course of crystalline or procaine penicillin G should be administered.

OTHER VIRUSES

Human Immunodeficiency Virus

HIV infection of the fetus and newborn is a problem of enormous public health importance. Pediatric HIV infection is prevalent around the world. Regions affected most include resource-constrained countries, such as sub-Saharan Africa, many Asian countries, India, and parts of Latin America.[1,37] The median HIV prevalence in antenatal clinics in southern African countries is 24%. In South Africa alone, of a total population of 44 million, 5.3 million have HIV infection. In 2003, some 700,000 children were newly infected with HIV in developing countries.[402] In the United States, approximately 1000 new cases of pediatric AIDS, most acquired perinatally, were recorded in 2002. With the advent of measures to prevent mother-to-child transmission (MTCT) and the development of effective antiretroviral therapeutic programs, the yearly number of children diagnosed with AIDS in the United States has declined to approximately 100. Nevertheless, in the United States currently, more than 1.2 million people have HIV infection, and of individuals older than 13 years with HIV-1,

29% are female. Thus perinatal HIV infection remains an important issue in the United States and other developed countries, but the disorder is of truly extraordinary importance in developing countries.

Transmission of HIV to the fetus accounts for more than 90% of all cases of HIV infection in children in the United States, and mother-to-infant transmission is the principal means of acquisition of pediatric disease worldwide. However, neurological manifestations of HIV infection *in the newborn period* are rare. Indeed, the incidence of symptomatic neurological disease in the HIV-infected newborn is the lowest of all the major infectious disorders described in this chapter. Nevertheless, the importance of the infection for *subsequent* neurological disability and mortality requires its consideration in this chapter.

Pathogenesis

Transmission of HIV from the infected pregnant woman to her fetus is very common. Before major programs to prevent transmission were instituted, published rates varied from 10% to 40%.[403-431] In general, rates were lower in European and North American populations (generally 15% to 20%) than in African, Indian, or Thai populations (generally 25% to 40%). As discussed later, marked decreases in transmission rates, as low as 1% to 2%, have occurred in the last few years, especially in developed countries, with the advent of preventive measures (see later).[1,37] Perinatal HIV-1 transmission is now virtually zero in mothers who start antiretroviral therapy (ART) before conception and maintain suppression of the plasma viral load.[432]

Fetal and Parturitional Infection. Several studies have reported associations between infant gender and in utero transmission, with females having a twofold increased risk of infection at birth as compared with male infants, maybe owing to the higher mortality in males during pregnancy or because the Y antigen, present only in males, activates maternal lymphocytes and either causes cytokine release with anti-HIV effects or limits maternal HIV-infected lymphocyte survival in male infants.[433] The relative importance of direct hematogenous transplacental spread and parturitional mechanisms of infection in the transmission of HIV from mother to infant is not yet established conclusively, but it has been clarified considerably in recent years. Both mechanisms appear to be operative.[a] Concerning *transplacental infection*, although demonstration of virus by PCR is unusual in first trimester specimens, a growing body of data supports the occurrence of infection in the second and third trimesters. The risk of such intrauterine transmission appears greatest with a higher maternal peripheral blood viral RNA load of HIV; thus pregnant women with recently acquired primary HIV infection or those with advanced disease are most at risk for transmission to the fetus. No threshold of viral load has been identified below which transmission does not occur. A higher maternal genital tract viral load is independently associated with higher risk of MTCT of HIV.[438,442,443] Placental inflammation and disruption of the trophoblastic barrier (e.g., by infections such as syphilis) may be additionally important. Overall, approximately 20% of vertically transmitted HIV is thought to occur before 36 weeks of gestation. Detection of HIV in the placenta does not correlate with infant infection.[438,443]

Several copathogens that are also a threat to the developing fetus during gestation, such as CMV, malaria parasites, and *M. tuberculosis* may also facilitate transmission of HIV-1 and increase MTCT in specific patient groups.[444,445] The increase in MTCT may be due to increased proviral load, immune activation, local inflammation, and maternal simulation of fetal CD4 cells to increase cellular susceptibility to HIV-1 infection.[446] A significant reduction of the in utero transmission rate of HIV-1 was seen when nevirapine was added at onset of labor to zidovudine started at 28 weeks of gestation[447] (see later).

Concerning *parturitional infection*, the balance of current data suggests that this mode is the most important mechanism of vertical transmission of this virus and accounts for approximately 80% of cases. For the sake of this discussion, the last several weeks of pregnancy are included in this time period. Infants born to seropositive mothers and subsequently shown to exhibit the clinical and immunological features of HIV infection are negative by PCR in the neonatal period and do not become positive until weeks later. Approximately one third of infant HIV infections in non–breast-fed populations are detected in the first 2 days after birth; around one third are detected beyond the first week and by 6 weeks. Transmission is considered to be during pregnancy in one third and during labor in the other two thirds. The working definition of in utero versus intrapartum HIV infection is based on virus detection during the first 2 days after birth.[448] The period from 36 weeks of gestation to the onset of labor is now considered particularly important, perhaps because the placenta begins to separate from the uterine wall.[436] As much as 50% of MTCT may occur during this period, with less than 4% occurring during the first trimester and less than 20% by 36 weeks of gestation.[449,450] The intrapartum period has long been considered important in transmission. A large study with twins did not find that first-born twins had a greater likelihood of perinatal transmission than second-born twins, supporting the idea that exposure in the birth canal is not the major contributor to the baby's risk.[450] Also consistent with parturitional acquisition is the increased rate of vertical transmission with prolonged rupture of membranes (approximately twofold higher transmission rate if the duration of rupture of membranes was more than 4 hours vs. less than 4 hours, and a rate of nearly 50% when the duration of rupture of membranes was more than 24 hours).[427] Potential mechanisms of parturitional acquisition are ingestion of maternal blood, maternal-fetal placental transfusion, or direct exposure of the fetus to infected cervical and vaginal secretions. Currently at least 30% of vertically transmitted HIV occurs during this brief period.[436] Others consider the intrapartum period to account for more than 50% of all vertically transmitted disease.

Postnatal Infection. MTCT transmission of HIV by breast-feeding is an established means of infection.[a] The additional risk of infection through breast-feeding is between 10% and 25% and in general doubles the overall vertical transmission rate. HIV has been isolated from colostrum and breast milk and has been particularly associated with the macrophages contained in these secretions.[461,462] Because colostrum and early milk are particularly rich in such cells, the danger of transmission to the infant may be greatest in

---

[a]References 402-404, 409, 410, 412, 414, 415, 418, 421, 425-429, 431, 434-441.

[a]References 403, 407, 422, 428, 434, 442, 451-460.

the early phases of breast-feeding. However, infection may also occur months later in the infant breast-fed by a mother who acquires primary infection in the postpartum period or who has established infection and transmits the infection only after many months of breast-feeding. The data clearly have important public health implications. The risk of breast-feeding is associated with a low maternal CD4 count, longer duration of breast-feeding, higher maternal viral load, mastitis, and mixed feeding. The breast-feeding and HIV International Transmission meta-analysis calculated the risk of postnatal HIV transmission after 4 weeks of age to be 8.9 transmissions per 100 child-years of breast-feeding, with a generally constant rate of transmission between 1 and 18 months of infant age.[442] To reduce MTCT, it is recommended by the World Health Organization (WHO) to exclusively breast-feed for 6 months followed by rapid weaning.[463] With this policy the transmission risk could be reduced from 16% to 6%.[464,465]

Neuropathology

The neuropathology of HIV infection differs from that for the TORCH group in that the brain injury primarily occurs without conventional signs of inflammation and appears to relate in considerable part to the immune response of the host to the virus. Moreover, with few exceptions (see later discussion), the brain abnormalities are not apparent for several months or years after the neonatal period. That HIV does infect the brain is apparent from several related findings: recovery of HIV from CSF and brain,[466-468] increased levels of HIV-specific antibody in CSF (indicative of synthesis within the blood-brain barrier),[469] demonstration of HIV nucleotide sequences in brain by in situ hybridization,[467,470] localization of HIV in brain monocytes-macrophages particularly (and to a lesser extent, astrocytes by immunocytochemistry [absence of HIV in neurons, oligodendrocytes, and endothelial cells]),[471-477] identification of viral particles within multinucleated giant cells and macrophages by electron microscopy,[472,478] and demonstration of HIV-DNA by Southern blot analysis[470,472,479] or PCR.[479] It has become clear that HIV-1 invades the CNS early in infection, primarily via infected monocytes/macrophages and CD4+ T lymphocytes.[480] The major neuropathological features of HIV infection in the infant are shown in Table 34.37.

Meningoencephalitis. The pathological manifestations of meningoencephalitis are less prominent in HIV encephalopathy than in infections of brain caused by the TORCH organisms. Thus, although there may be (1) inflammatory cells within the meninges, (2) perivascular infiltration with inflammatory cells,

---

TABLE 34.37   Neuropathology in Infants With Human Immunodeficiency Virus Infection

Meningoencephalitis
Cerebral atrophy: neuronal and myelin loss, dendritic abnormalities
Cerebral calcification: basal ganglia and white matter
Calcific vasculopathy
Spinal cord myelin loss
Rare: central nervous system lymphoma, opportunistic infection, stroke

---

and (3) areas of brain necrosis, these findings are usually not prominent. Indeed, the dominant cellular manifestations of HIV infection are abundant multinucleated giant cells (Fig. 34.29), often in syncytial formations, and macrophages.[466,474,478,481-488] The multinucleated cells appear to be derived from brain macrophages and have been shown to contain the virus. Indeed, macrophages and microglia are the predominant cell types infected by HIV.[467,476] The relative lack of the typical inflammatory characteristics of meningoencephalitis is consistent with the finding of CSF pleocytosis in living infants in only the minority of cases (see later discussion).

Cerebral Atrophy. Cerebral atrophy, secondary to loss of both neurons and myelin, is a prominent feature of the disease (Fig. 34.30). The result is microencephaly, secondary to loss of both gray and white matter.[489,490] Neuronal loss particularly affects basal ganglia and cerebral cortex. The mechanism of the neuronal death is unclear. Experimental studies suggest that products of the immune system (i.e., cytokines) and of the virus may lead to cell death.[472,487,491-502] Similar to all retroviruses, HIV-1 contains the genes for *gag*, which encodes the core nucleocapsid polypeptides (gp24, p17, p9); *env*, which encodes for the surface-coated proteins of the virus (gp120 and gp41), and *pol*, which encodes for the viral reverse transcriptase and other enzymatic activities (i.e., integrase and protease).[503] The coat protein of HIV, gp120, has been shown to be toxic to cultured neurons and to lead to cell death by causing an increase in cytosolic calcium. Moreover, the coat protein appears to sensitize neurons to glutamate-induced cell death mediated at the *N*-methyl-D-aspartate (NMDA) receptor. There are two regulatory (*tat* and *rev*) and four accessory proteins (*vif*, *vpr*, *vpu*, and *nef*) that are essential for viral replication and pathogenicity. The retroviral core also contains two copies of the viral single-stranded RNA associated with enzymes such as the reverse transcriptase, RNase H, integrase, and protease. Tat has a similar neurotoxic effect.[497] The potentiating effect of specific HIV peptides on NMDA-mediated neuronal death has also been shown in vivo in the perinatal rat.[491,497,504] The crucial role of the gp120 coat protein in the genesis of the brain injury in HIV infection is supported particularly by the demonstration, in transgenic mice generated to produce gp120 in brain, of neuronal and glial changes similar to those observed in the disease.[505]

"Neurotoxins" (e.g., arachidonic acid metabolites, reactive oxygen species, glutamate, cytokines) released from infected macrophages and astrocytes have also been shown to lead to activation of the NMDA receptor.[472,487,492-495] Protection of neurons from cell death caused by the HIV coat protein or by the "toxins" released from infected macrophages by NMDA antagonists and by a calcium channel antagonist is consistent with these observations concerning important roles for glutamate and calcium and raises interesting possibilities regarding therapy.[494,497,499,506-508]

The demonstration that inhibitors of nitric oxide synthase prevent the neurotoxicity of gp120 suggests that calcium activation of nitric oxide synthase and the synthesis of nitric oxide may be the final common path to neuronal death.[493,509,510] Thus the sequence in HIV infection would be infection of brain macrophages (and perhaps astrocytes) by HIV; induction by gp120 of release of arachidonic metabolites, reactive oxygen species, and cytokines that act synergistically with endogenous

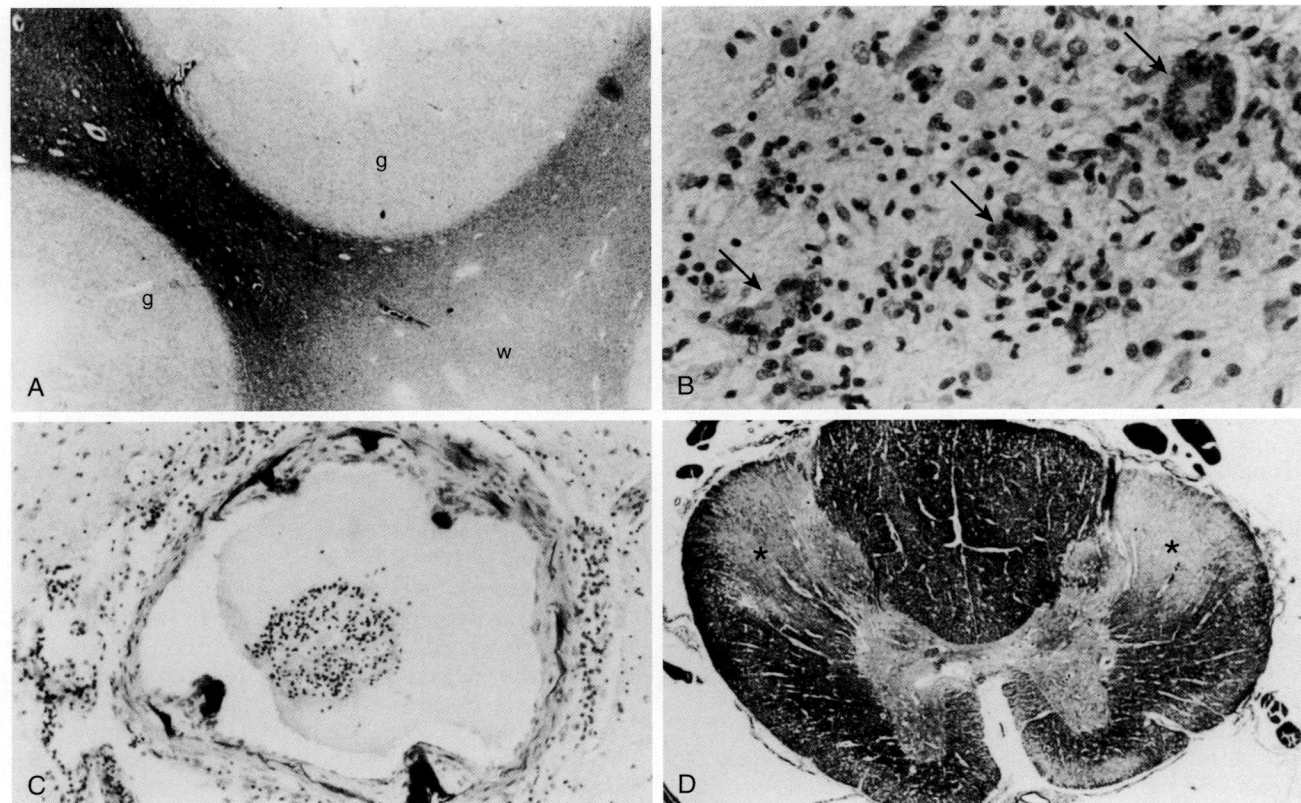

Figure 34.29 Congenital human immunodeficiency virus infection: neuropathology. (A) Section of deep cerebral white matter (w) shows pallor on myelin stain; g indicates gray matter (Luxol fast blue, original magnification ×20). (B) Section of basal ganglia shows three multinucleated giant cells (*arrows*) (hematoxylin and eosin [H & E], original magnification ×320). (C) Large artery in basal ganglia shows multifocal intimal proliferation with dystrophic calcification (H & E, original magnification ×200). (D) Spinal cord cross section with myelin stain shows pallor in both lateral (*asterisks*) and anterior funiculi (Luxol fast blue, original magnification ×8). (From Belman AL, Diamond G, Dickson D, et al. Pediatric acquired immunodeficiency syndrome. *Am J Dis Child.* 1988;142:29-35.)

glutamate to activate glutamate receptors; entry of calcium; nitric oxide synthesis; and cell death by the generation of free radicals from nitric oxide.[509,510]

The cerebrocortical atrophy in HIV infection may also relate to dendritic abnormalities as well as neuronal death.[474,511,512] Such abnormalities have been delineated in adult patients and could be particularly important (and overlooked by conventional neuropathology) in infants in view of the active dendritic development that occurs normally.

White matter loss in HIV encephalopathy can be marked (see Fig. 34.29). The myelin involvement may be diffuse or multifocal.[a] The mechanism of this myelin loss is unclear, although the finding of marked reactive astrocytosis within the areas of myelin loss suggests that the process is destructive rather than a disturbance of myelin formation. The frequent occurrence of calcification in white matter also supports a destructive rather than a developmental abnormality. The demonstration that the HIV coat protein gp120 injures developing oligodendrocytes in culture supports this formulation and links the deleterious role of the coat protein to *both* neuronal *and* oligodendroglial injury. The particular vulnerability of developing oligodendrocytes to

reactive oxygen species further links the final common pathway to cell death in both neurons and oligodendroglia in HIV infection of the brain. As described later (see the section on neurodiagnostic studies), advanced MRI studies of children with HIV show marked disturbances of cerebral white matter volumes and microstructure.

Calcific Vasculopathy. A striking feature of HIV encephalopathy is calcific degeneration of blood vessels (see Fig. 34.29).[a] This finding is most striking in the basal ganglia but is also often prominent in cerebral white matter. Involvement of blood vessels is manifested clinically later in the disease by the occurrence of hemorrhagic or ischemic stroke (see later discussion).

Spinal Cord Myelin Loss. Although relatively uncommonly examined, the spinal cord frequently exhibits myelin loss, particularly of the lateral corticospinal tracts.[482,483,485,513] Indeed, spastic motor deficits are an important component of neurological deficits observed later in some children with HIV infection (see further on).[489] Approximately half of patients appear to exhibit only myelin loss, whereas the other half

---

[a]References 466, 472, 478, 481, 485, 490.   [a]References 466, 472, 478, 481, 483, 485.

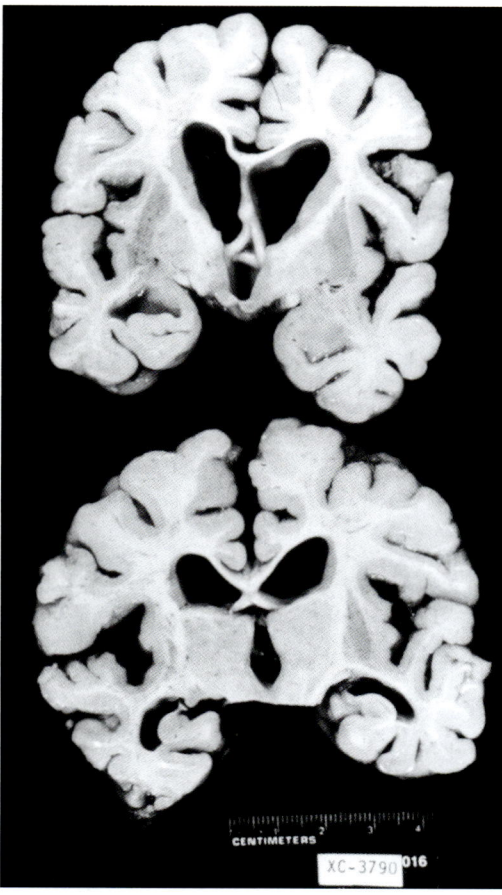

Figure 34.30 Congenital human immunodeficiency virus infection: neuropathology. Coronal sections of cerebrum show atrophy of both cerebral cortex and white matter. Note the marked sulcal widening and dilated ventricles. (From Belman AL, Diamond G, Dickson D, et al. Pediatric acquired immunodeficiency syndrome. *Am J Dis Child.* 1988;142:29-35.)

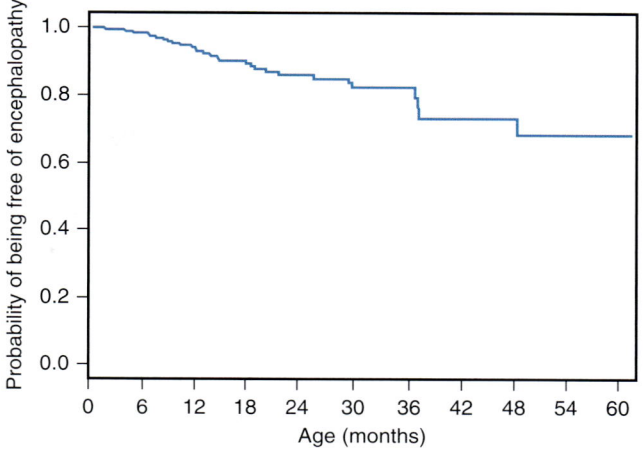

Figure 34.31 Kaplan-Meier plot of development of encephalopathy among human immunodeficiency virus–infected infants (*n* = 128). This study was conducted in the era before antiretroviral therapy. (From Cooper ER, Hanson C, Diaz C, et al. Encephalopathy and progression of human immunodeficiency virus disease in a cohort of children with perinatally acquired human immunodeficiency virus infection. *J Pediatr.* 1998;132:808-812.)

exhibit loss of both myelin and axons. The findings are unlike the vacuolar myelopathy of adults with HIV infection both in microscopic appearance and in topographic distribution (i.e., lateral corticospinal tracts rather than posterior columns, as in vacuolar myelopathy).

Central Nervous System Lymphoma, Opportunistic Infections, Stroke.

Only approximately 10% to 15% of cases of HIV infection of infants examined at autopsy exhibit neoplastic or infectious complications of HIV.[a] Nevertheless, CNS lymphoma or toxoplasmosis, CMV infection, or fungal (especially *Candida*) infection has been described. Evidence of cerebrovascular disease has been reported in up to 25% of autopsy cases[481,485,490,514,515]; lesions have included ischemic and hemorrhagic infarcts associated with arteriopathy and aneurysmal dilation of vessels.

Clinical Aspects

Incidence of Clinically Apparent Infection.

The incidence of clinically recognizable neurological features in the neonatal

period in HIV-infected infants is extremely small. Before the modern era of antiretroviral therapy during pregnancy and infancy, *onset of neurological disease was generally between approximately 2 months and 5 years.*[466,478,482-484,516-529] Approximately 20% of infected infants developed prominent encephalopathy by the age of 5 years, and approximately half of these occurred by the age of 12 months (Fig. 34.31).[519,524] However, single case reports of infants with neonatal meningoencephalitis[530] and neonatal seizures with brain "atrophy" by cranial ultrasonography[488,531] have been recorded. Of 41 infected infants in a reported series, 3 had microcephaly at birth[531]; in large series, mean head circumference is approximately 1 cm lower in HIV-infected newborns than in appropriate control infants.[532] An HIV-infected newborn with cytomegaloviruria in the neonatal period died of fulminating CMV encephalitis at 6 months of age.[533] A 2-month-old infant with HIV exhibited focal seizures and a hemorrhagic infarct in the distribution of the middle cerebral artery.[534]

Clinical Features.

Before the era of antiretroviral therapy during pregnancy and infancy, the major *neurological syndromes* in infants with HIV disease were readily categorized as progressive encephalopathy and static encephalopathy.[a] The progressive encephalopathy is the less common but more serious of the two syndromes.

Progressive HIV-1 encephalopathy (PHE) consists of acquired microcephaly, delay or loss of developmental milestones (motor, mental, and expressive language). Before combination ART became widely available, PHE was reported in the United States in 13% to 35% of children with HIV infection.[466] In approximately 50% of affected infants, the onset was in the first year of life (see Fig. 34.31). The highest incidence rate of HIV-related CNS manifestations occurs in first 2 years

---

[a]References 466, 469, 481, 482, 485, 490.

[a]References 466, 478, 482-484, 489, 516-518, 520, 522, 523, 525, 527, 528, 535-547.

of life, with incidence rates of 9.9% in the first year of life, 4.2% in the second, and less than 1% in the third year of life and thereafter.[519] The syndrome included a dementing process, decreasing rate of head growth, and, ultimately, microcephaly, spastic motor deficits, and, less commonly, extrapyramidal and cerebellar deficits. Seizures were uncommon and often reflected complicating illness, such as opportunistic infection or stroke. Occasionally, CNS lymphoma led to a progressive neurological syndrome.[527,548] Nearly all infants with the progressive encephalopathy exhibited prominent systemic features of HIV, usually apparent at the onset of the encephalopathy. The syndrome, not unexpectedly, was associated with particularly high levels of virus.[489,519,549] Median age of survival after diagnosis was 14 months, and in most infants the neurological syndrome progressed in parallel with the systemic disorder.

With the advent of the use of ART during pregnancy and postnatally (see later), the progressive disorder is now rare. The incidence in most centers with such intervention has declined to less than 2%.[489,537,547,551] Moreover, in the rare instances of occurrence, the disorder presents later, is less severe, and does not progress to severe disability and death.

Before ART during pregnancy and infancy, *static encephalopathy* became apparent in approximately an additional 20% to 25% of infants with HIV infection. The principal clinical characteristic is primarily cognitive impairment and motor dysfunction, usually not severe. The contribution of HIV-related factors (e.g., intrauterine drug exposure, other congenital infection, poor nutrition, systemic illness, poor environment) in the pathogenesis of the static encephalopathy is still unknown. This disorder is less pronounced and has become less common in recent years.[489,527,551-553] However, currently this syndrome is the principal neurological feature of perinatally acquired HIV infection. It is difficult to reliably predict HIV-associated CNS disease. Because many infants with developmental delay and/ or microcephaly are also born preterm or have been exposed to alcohol or drugs, one is not always certain whether the delay is really due to the HIV-1 infection.[489] Infants with intrauterine rather than peripartum or postpartum vertical transmission of infection are more likely to develop early-onset and rapidly progressive PHE; the risk of PHE is also higher among HIV-infected children born to mothers with more advanced disease as measured by CD4+ cell count and viral load at the time of delivery.[538,555]

Laboratory Evaluation

Isolation of Virus. Identification of virus by culture or by testing for viral DNA or RNA (via HIV nucleic acid amplification tests [NAATS]) provides a definitive diagnosis of HIV infection.[a] The HIV DNA PCR array is the preferred test for HIV diagnosis, with 30% to 40% of affected infants testing positive within 48 hours after birth and 93% by 2 weeks of age. However, this test is less sensitive for identifying virus of the non-B subtype.[573] The HIV RNA PCR can also be used and is especially useful for diagnosing the HIV subtype B. However, false-negative HIV RNA results can occur in neonates receiving antiretroviral (ARV) prophylaxis.[574] Viral culture is performed on the infant's peripheral blood mononuclear cells, which are cocultivated with peripheral blood mononuclear cells from an uninfected individual.

The PCR technique, which can be carried out on dried blood spots, detects HIV proviral DNA and is preferable to viral culture because the result is available in 1 day, as opposed to 1 to 4 weeks for viral culture.[a] PCR is slightly more sensitive than culture, but detection at birth is possible in only approximately 25% to 35% of infants later proven to be infected. The detection rate by PCR increases to 80% to 90% at 2 weeks, and to 90% to 95% at 3 weeks, and nearly all cases are detected by 1 month. This delay in the time of first positive result relates less to the difficulties with the PCR technique and more to the finding that approximately 75% of infections are acquired late in pregnancy and in the intrapartum period (see earlier discussion). As a consequence, the early tests are carried out at a previremic phase of the disease or when viral levels are very low. With the use of a PCR that detects viral long terminal repeats rather than gag, it was found that 18% of uninfected infants born to HIV-1 infected mothers had evidence of unintegrated virus in their peripheral blood mononuclear cells. The unintegrated viral intermediate is biologically active, but—in the absence of appropriate activation—decays with time. HIV-1 may therefore enter a virus, but in the absence of activated lymphocytes it might not integrate and establish infection until later if at all.[436,581]

Serological Studies. The serological diagnosis of HIV infection in the newborn is complicated by the passage of maternal IgG across the placenta and by the persistence of this IgG for as long as 15 months.[429,582] Determination of HIV-specific IgM in the newborn has not provided consistent diagnostic information.[428,557,560,569,582] After 18 months of life, detection of antibodies directed at envelope or core proteins is useful diagnostically.

Neurodiagnostic Studies. Detection of involvement of the brain in the neonatal period is very difficult. CSF is usually normal.[1,37] Neuroradiological abnormalities primarily develop after the neonatal period, as may be predicted by the evolution of clinical phenomena (see earlier discussion). *Cranial ultrasound* and *CT* are most useful for detecting basal ganglia and cerebral calcifications (Fig. 34.32), but *MRI* is superior for detecting cerebral atrophy and white matter abnormalities. The neuroradiological hallmarks of PHE include cortical atrophy and basal ganglia calcifications on CT and white matter lesions and central atrophy on MRI.[542,584] An informative recent report of cerebral imaging in perinatally HIV-infected children (median age 13.8 years) studied by advanced 3T-MRI, showed, by volumetric MRI, diminished cortical gray matter and cerebral white matter volumes, and by diffusion tensor MRI, marked disturbances in cerebral white matter fiber tracts.[585] These findings are consistent with the neuropathological disturbances described earlier. It is noteworthy that these children were not begun on combination ART until a mean age of 2.2 years (see management later).

Prognosis

The neurological syndromes just described should be viewed in the context of the overall prognosis of HIV infection of the

---

[a]References 404, 412, 428, 429, 556-572.

[a]References 428, 429, 440, 556, 557, 559, 560, 565, 568, 569, 580.

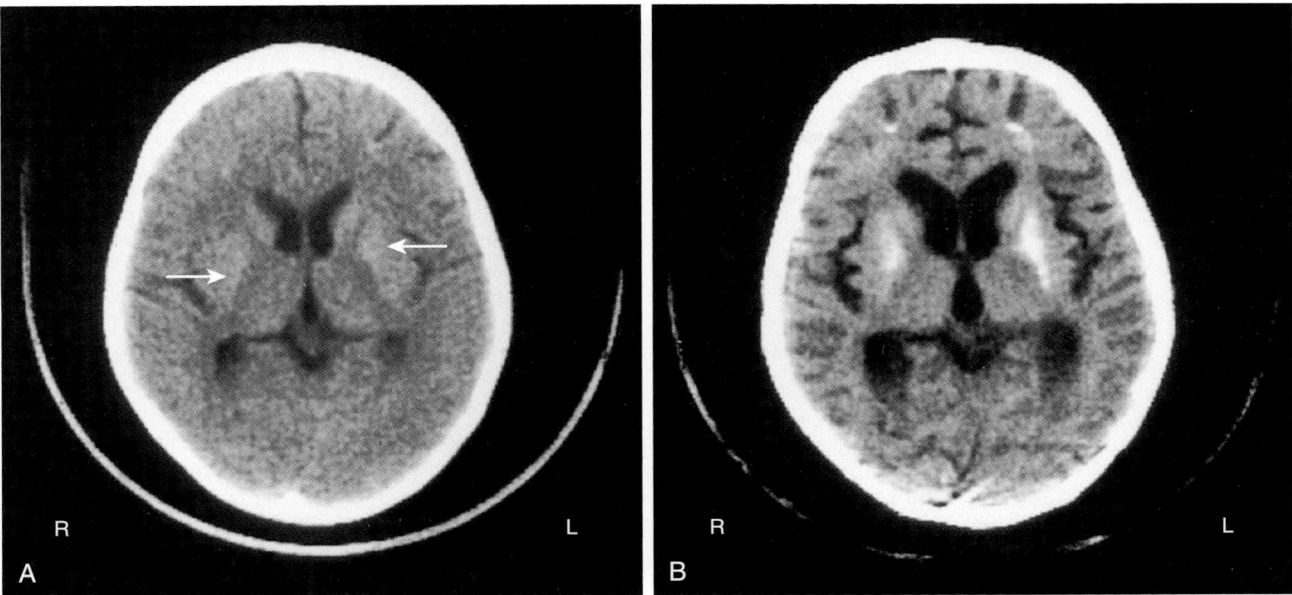

Figure 34.32 Congenital human immunodeficiency virus infection: computed tomography. (A) Computed tomography (CT) shows mild cerebral atrophy and questionable bilateral calcification in basal ganglia *(arrows)* and frontal white matter (at the cortical–white matter junction). (B) Eight months later, CT shows progressive cerebral cortical and white matter atrophy and pronounced basal ganglia calcification. Frontal white matter calcification is now obvious. (From Belman AL, Diamond G, Dickson D, et al. Pediatric acquired immunodeficiency syndrome. *Am J Dis Child.* 1988;142:29-35.)

newborn. Indeed, the overall prognosis now is recognized to be considerably more favorable than that based on earlier studies of selected populations.[a] *In centers where ART during pregnancy and infancy is implemented, approximately 90% of infants with perinatally acquired HIV infection are alive at 6 years. From the neurological perspective, the incidence of the severe progressive encephalopathy has declined to 1% to 2%. Fewer than 25% of infants exhibit overt neurodevelopmental disturbances.* There is an initial regimen of nevirapine plus 2 nucleoside reverse transcriptase inhibitors (NRTIs) for infants aged birth to <14 days. A change from nevirapine to lopinavir/ritonavir should be considered after 14 days of life and 42 weeks' postgestational age.[489]

Management

Prevention. Prevention of transmission of HIV infection from the pregnant woman to her fetus involves prevention of the maternal infection and management of the infected woman. *Prevention of HIV infection* in the woman of childbearing age and detection of that infection are topics beyond the scope of this book.[590]

Management of the infected woman to prevent mother-to-infant transmission focuses most importantly on the use of antiretroviral therapy targeted to cover the major time periods of transmission (i.e., antenatal, intrapartum, and postnatal).[402,428,439,447,591-604] The initial dramatic breakthrough in this area came with the findings of a controlled study of *administration of zidovudine* initiated at 14 to 34 weeks of gestation and continued throughout pregnancy, intravenous zidovudine during labor, and oral zidovudine postpartum for 6 weeks. The result was a reduction

from 26% to 8% in vertical transmission.[605] This beneficial effect was confirmed by several later reports.[606,607] Some reports indicated that benefit from the use of zidovudine is apparent with abbreviated perinatal regimens (Table 34.38).[423,608-610] Moreover, a study in Uganda showed that intrapartum and neonatal single-dose oral administration of the antiretroviral agent nevirapine was nearly 50% more effective than zidovudine in prophylaxis.[608] These exciting data indicated major value for antiretroviral prophylaxis, even when begun in the intrapartum period or the first 2 days of life. Subsequent studies confirmed the benefits of shorter periods of therapy.[601,603] However, the medium- and longer-term side effects are becoming increasingly apparent.[611] Mitochondrial dysfunction has been reported in HIV-negative children perinatally exposed to zidovudine.[612] Evidence for NRTI-associated mitochondrial toxicity is seen in vitro, in animal models, and in NRTI-exposed adults and children. Proposed mechanisms of NRTI mitochondrial toxicity include, among others, impairment of mitochondrial DNA (mtDNA) replication and acquisition of mtDNA point mutations. Alterations in mtDNA synthesis potentially reduce the production of mtDNA-encoded respiratory chain subunits, resulting in impaired oxidative phosphorylation and mitochondrial dysfunction. MRI findings in children with antiretroviral-induced mitochondrial dysfunction are similar to those observed in patients with congenital mitochondrial diseases. The most frequent abnormalities consisted of hyperintensity in the central white matter and in the tegmentum pons.[613] L-Acetylcarnitine was noted to be effective in preventing/ameliorating the neurochemical, neuroendocrine, and behavioral adverse effects induced by azidothymidine (AZT) in the offspring in a mouse model.[614] The enormous benefits of HAART are, however, still considered to outweigh these complications

---

[a]References 489, 516, 518, 519, 523, 525, 529, 532, 537, 544, 545, 547, 552, 587-588.

TABLE 34.38   Prevention of Mother-to-Infant Transmission of Human Immunodeficiency Virus by Zidovudine Prophylaxis

TIME OF INITIATION OF ZIDOVUDINE	RATE OF HIV INFECTION (%)
Prenatal	6.1[a]
Intrapartum	10.0[a]
≤48 hours of birth	9.3[a]
≥3 days of age	18.4
No zidovudine	28.6

n = 939.

[a]*P* <.05 in comparison with no zidovudine.

HIV, Human immunodeficiency virus.

Data from Wade NA, Birkhead GS, Warren BL, et al. Abbreviated regimens of zidovudine prophylaxis and perinatal transmission of the human immunodeficiency virus. *N Engl J Med.* 1998;339:1409-1414.

TABLE 34.39   Prevention of Mother-to-Infant Transmission of Human Immunodeficiency Virus During the Era of Highly Active Antiretroviral Therapy

HAART therapy involves combinations of agents that interrupt both early and late steps in HIV replication.

Usual HAART therapy involves at least a nucleoside analogue (e.g., zidovudine, a reverse transcriptase inhibitor), a nonnucleoside analogue (e.g., nevirapine, a reverse transcriptase inhibitor), and a protease inhibitor (e.g., indinavir).

HAART therapy during pregnancy causes marked reduction in viral load at delivery.

The rate of mother-to-infant transmission is reduced to 1% to 2%.

The addition of elective cesarean section reduces transmission further to 0.5% to 1.0%.

HAART, Highly active antiretroviral therapy; *HIV*, human immunodeficiency virus.

Data primarily from European Collaborative Study. Mother-to-child transmission of HIV infection in the era of highly active antiretroviral therapy. *Clin Infect Dis.* 2005;40:458-465.

(Table 34.39). This approach is designed to use a combination of drugs chosen to affect both early stages of HIV replication (reverse transcriptase inhibitors) and later stages (protease inhibitors). A large collaborative study in Europe indicated that this approach, which causes a remarkable reduction in maternal viral load, leads to a reduction in mother-to-infant transmission to 1% to 2% (see Table 34.39). HAART does not, however, eliminate CNS manifestations, and the risk of CNS disease in children being treated with HAART may be higher among children with moderate abnormalities on CT brain scans and those with CD4+ cell counts below 500. Viral replication in the CNS may be ongoing in spite of virological control in the periphery.[615]

A second approach for the prevention of mother-to-infant HIV transmission is the use of *cesarean section*, before the onset of labor, to avoid many of the critical parturitional factors in viral transmission (see earlier discussion). Several studies showed a beneficial effect, with a reduction in HIV transmission of at least 50%.[a] The beneficial effect of cesarean section generally is not observed in infants who received *emergency* cesarean sections *after complicated labor*.[592,621] In one meta-analysis of 15 prospective studies, among mother-child pairs receiving full antiretroviral prophylaxis, the rates of vertical transmission were only 2.0% among mothers who underwent elective cesarean section versus 7.3% among those with other modes of delivery.[607] With the HAART approach (see Table 34.39), elective cesarean section led to reductions of transmission to 1% or less.

Because postnatal acquisition of HIV by breast-feeding is important in transmission to the infant (see earlier discussion), the US Committee on Pediatric AIDS recommended that "women who are known to be HIV infected must be counseled not to breast-feed or provide their milk for the nutrition of their own or other infants."[451] In many developing countries, no alternatives to breast-feeding exist. Under such circumstances, cessation of breast-feeding by approximately 6 months of age minimizes the *late* postnatal transmission that occurs with prolonged breast-feeding.[454] However, the complicated issue of breast-feeding in relation to HIV infection involves many competing considerations, which are discussed in more specialized sources.[442]

Supportive Therapy. Because neurological phenomena are vanishingly rare in the neonatal period, supportive therapy is confined to nonneural phenomena and is discussed elsewhere.[1,37]

Antimicrobial Therapy. The possibility of specific antimicrobial therapy of the infected newborn (i.e., the infant in whom perinatal transmission was not prevented) was raised initially by the promising findings in studies of treatment of older infants and children with zidovudine.[600,622-630] Improvement of cognition, decreased CT evidence of brain atrophy, decreased CSF protein, improved auditory brain stem responses, and immunological improvement were documented. One infected infant treated from as early as 6 months of age exhibited marked improvement over 6 months in neurological examination, decreased brain stem latencies on testing of auditory brain stem responses, and lessening of brain atrophy by CT.[611] Still more favorable responses have been observed with the combination therapy of the HAART approach (see earlier discussion). A striking reduction of at least 96% in plasma levels of HIV-1 RNA in infected infants 2 to 16 months of age treated with zidovudine, didanosine, and nevirapine was documented.[631] An extended nevirapine regimen for 6 months rather than 6 weeks was studied in a randomized double-blind placebo-controlled trial showing 54% reduction in transmission (*P* = 0.49) but no difference in mortality or combined HIV infection and mortality rates.[632] These data are important from the neurological perspective because zidovudine and nevirapine penetrate the CNS well. This property may explain the marked reduction in HIV encephalopathy in infants treated with HAART (see earlier). The French perinatal cohort study found a significant association of first-trimester zidovudine exposure and congenital heart defects, mostly ventricular septal defects (58%) or atrial septal defects (18%). In the same study a

---

[a]References 402, 428, 439, 592, 596, 616-618, 620.

significant association was also noted for first-trimester efavirenz exposure and neurological defects when using the MACDP classification system of birth defects but not when using the EUROCAT classification.[633] A recent cohort study looked at the association of in utero antiretroviral exposures with congenital anomalies in HIV-exposed uninfected children.[634] No association of first-trimester exposures with congenital anomalies was found for any of the antiretroviral drugs in adjusted models. Among the protease inhibitors, however, higher odds of congenital anomalies for atazanavir sulfate and for ritonavir used as a booster were found. With first-trimester atazanavir exposure, risks were highest for skin and musculoskeletal congenital anomalies. It was concluded that the benefits of recommended antiretroviral therapy use during pregnancy still outweigh the risk of developing a congenital anomaly.

Entero- and Parechoviruses

Enterovirus (EV) is the most common cause of aseptic meningitis in children. Neonatal encephalitis caused by human EV and parechovirus (HPeV), acquired principally by perinatal transmission, have been especially well documented in recent years.[635-639] EV and HPeV belong to the family *Picornaviridae*, a collection of small, nonenveloped viruses with a simple message-sense RNA genome. The family Picornaviridae belongs to the order *Picornavirales* and currently consists of 50 species grouped into 29 genera.[640] *Enteroviruses*, being serologically distinct, were originally distributed into four groups on the basis of their different cytopathic effects in tissue culture and patterns of disease in experimentally infected animals: polioviruses (PV) (causal agents of poliomyelitis), coxsackie A (CBA) viruses (associated with herpangina and human CNS disease), coxsackie B viruses (human CNS and cardiac disease), and echoviruses (initially not linked to human disease).[641] On the basis of their molecular characteristics, these viruses have been reclassified into four EV species, A to D, and the detection of new EV types (numbered) (http://www. picornastudygroup .com). The genus EV consists of 12 species. Species are further classified into serotypes, and there are 118 EV types (within four EV species known to infect humans: A, B, C, and D). *HPeV* was discovered in 1999, originally described as echoviruses 22 and 23 within the EV genus (HPeV1 and -2) because of their similar clinical and morphological properties and cytopathic effect in cell culture; they are considered to belong to the genus *HPeV* in the family Picornaviridae.[642-647] HPeV3 has been associated with neonatal infection presenting with CNS symptoms.[648-650]

As the clinical symptoms and neuroimaging findings are so very similar for EV and HPeV, the two are described together.

Pathogenesis

Fetal Infection. Clinically significant infection with EV and HPeV may occur by transplacental, parturitional, or postnatal mechanisms. Transplacental acquisition of the virus is associated with maternal viremia near the time of delivery and may cause symptoms of infection in the infant at birth.[651-654] No conclusive evidence exists for intrauterine infection during the first or second trimester of pregnancy. Maternal echovirus or coxsackievirus B (CVB) infections were not associated with an increased risk of spontaneous abortions, but stillbirths late in pregnancy have been described. Intrauterine transmission has been documented, but its frequency is unknown.[655] The recent demonstration that CVB targets proliferating neuronal stem cells

in immature mice may be relevant in this context.[656] Moreover, in a study of 28 newborns with congenital hydrocephalus or hydranencephaly, the ventricular fluid of 4 of the infants contained antibody to a CVB serotype.[657] The finding is of interest because hydranencephaly and porencephaly have been identified in neonatal mice after intracranial injection of a CVB. More data are needed.

Parturitional Infections. Perinatal transmission of EV and HPeV from mother to infant is relatively common (30% to 50%) and may occur through contact with maternal secretions or blood during vaginal delivery or through maternal upper respiratory tract secretions.[655] Maternal EV illness around the time of delivery and a lack of maternal antibodies to the infecting serotype increase the risk of perinatal transmission. Onset of disease after perinatal transmission occurs within 1 to 2 weeks after delivery and carries a substantially higher risk for severe illness and death than does postnatally acquired EV infection.

Postnatal Infection. Acquisition of EV and HPeV during the neonatal period is probably common, yet clinical illness is quite uncommon.[1,37] The main factor in the postnatal spread of virus in infants, as in older patients, is human-to-human contact. Taking the time of year into account is helpful, because EV infections are particularly prevalent in the summer and fall in temperate climates. HPeV was noted only in even years in several studies from Europe. Knowledge of exposures and incubation periods is particularly helpful, and careful history of maternal illness, however slight, or illness in nursery personnel is critical to elicit and to document. In a large review of reported cases of fatal neonatal CVB infection, 60% of mothers had signs of a viral-like infection between 10 antepartum and 5 postpartum days.[658]

Several epidemics of CVB infection in neonatal nursery populations have been reported.[655,659-662] The most frequent mode of onset of such nursery infections is transmission from a mother to her infant. This contact is then followed by infant-to-infant transmission through nursery personnel. Although most serious enteroviral nursery epidemics have involved CVB, epidemics associated with neonatal disease have also been described for echovirus infection.[638,661-664]

More recent epidemiological surveillances, using the new classification system, have been reported. Based on a study performed in the Netherlands from 1993 to 1995, a total of 119 (9.5%) of 1273 EV isolates obtained in the study period were from infants less than 30 days of age.[665] The peak season for EV was July to October and approximately 70% of detections occurred during this period. The five most common EV serotypes (CVB1, echovirus 6, echovirus 9, echovirus 18, and CBA9) accounted for 54% of total serotype detections. In another surveillance study performed during 2007 to 2008, there were 1079 reports of EV infection, and CVB1 accounted for 23% of reported cases with known serotype, making it the most commonly reported serotype. Six neonatal deaths due to CVB1 infection were also reported to the CDC.[666,667] In contrast to EV infections, which have a peak season during the summer, HPeV infections are distributed widely across the year. Harvala et al.[668] compared the detection frequencies of EV and HPeV in CSF samples among infants and children presenting with sepsis or CNS disease during a 5-year period. HPeV infections were seen exclusively in children younger than 3 months (31 of 1105, or 2.8%). All but one had serotype HPeV3 and the infections were confined to the spring of even-numbered years.

The investigators witnessed an increase in the incidence of neonatal EV and HPeV infection, which they explained by possible systematic changes in host susceptibility over the past decades.

In several other data sets of newborn infants admitted to a neonatal intensive care unit (NICU) because of suspected sepsis or neurological infection, 8.7% to 11.6% were EV-positive and 3.5% to 9.3% were HPeV3-positive.[642,669-673] The numbers were considerably higher in a multicenter study that prospectively enrolled 84 infants, presenting at less than 1 month with fever of unknown source, sepsis-like illness, and neurological symptoms. As many as 32 were EV-positive (38%) and 9 (11%) HPeV-positive.[674]

Role of Host Factors. Although symptomatic EV infections of the fetus and the newborn are less common than asymptomatic infections, it is apparent that, once established, infections are more severe in younger patients than in older ones.[1,37] The precise reasons for this are unknown. An important role for deficient levels of antiviral antibody in vertically transmitted disease is apparent because illness is more common in the newborn whose mother developed the illness within a week or less of delivery, before transplacental passage of sufficient antibody was possible (Fig. 34.33).[661] Moreover, studies in animals suggest that a critical factor is the inability of cells of the immature animal to elaborate interferon.[675] Other possibilities suggested from experimental work include a relation to transplacentally acquired increased concentrations of adrenocortical hormones or to a progressive, age-related loss of cells with receptors capable of allowing binding and infection by enterovirus.[676-678]

Neuropathology

Neonatal encephalitis caused by EV/HPeV has an apparent predilection for the white matter; at first glance, the involvement of cerebral white matter looks very similar to periventricular leukomalacia (PVL) as typically observed in premature infants. Most of the infants who are affected are, however, near or full term, and it is clear on MRI that the cerebral white matter abnormalities extend into the subcortical white matter and involve entire fiber tracts, such as corpus callosum, optic radiation, as well as gray matter regions (e.g., posterior thalamus). The cause of the injury in the cerebral white matter in EV/HPeV3 encephalitis likely involves activation of microglia, resulting, at least in part, from activation of the intracellular TLRs 7 and 8 by the ssRNA of HPeV or EV. TLRs 7 and especially 8 are involved in the host's immune response to HPeV.[679] Activation of microglia would lead to the release of reactive oxygen and nitrogen species and proinflammatory cytokines, especially tumor necrosis factor α (TNFα) and interleukin-1β (IL1-β), which are toxic to premyelinating oligodendrocytes[680] and probably also to developing axons.[681,682] In view of the very uncommon finding of CSF pleocytosis in PCR-positive HPeV3 CNS infection with white matter injury, it seems unlikely that CNS inflammation is the dominant or at least exclusive feature of the process. TLR 8 has been noted to be localized to neurons and axons.[681,683] Strikingly, this TLR is distributed especially in growth cones and axonal fiber tracts and only in the developing nervous system. Indeed, the axonal expression of TLR 8 correlates closely with that of growth-associated protein (GAP)-43, a marker of axonal growth. Notably, recent study of GAP-43 immunostaining in the developing human brain

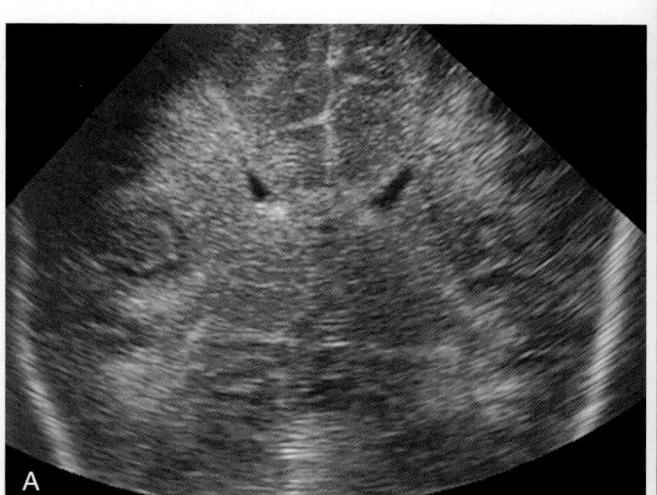 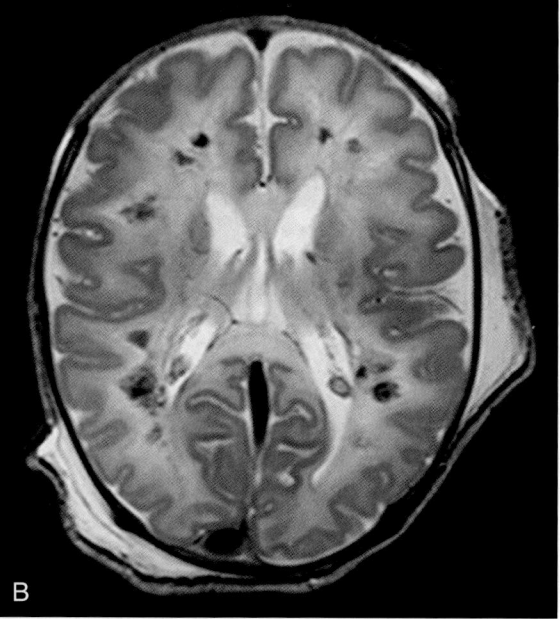

Figure 34.33 Coxsackievirus type B1 infection. Coronal ultrasound (A) and axial T2-weighted magnetic resonance imaging (B) in a late preterm infant (gestational age 36 weeks, birth weight 2600 g). Mother was suspected to have an appendicitis and had a cesarean section. The baby did well initially but became unwell at home on day 3, with lethargy and seizures and eventually died. Periventricular echogenicity was seen on cranial ultrasound (A) and extensive hemorrhagic white matter involvement was confirmed on magnetic resonance imaging (B). Coxsackievirus type B1 was cultured from the feces.

shows that axonal growth and development are very active in the perinatal period.[684] Activation of TLR 8 results in growth cone collapse, inhibition of axonal outgrowth, and neuronal apoptosis. Thus it appears possible not only that activation of TLR 8 in microglia could lead to premyelinating oligodendrocyte and axonal injury but also that activation of TLR 8 in developing neurons/axons could result in disturbed axonal development with axonal retraction and neuronal apoptosis. The axonal disturbance could be exacerbated by loss of trophic interactions with the developing oligodendrocyte and, in turn, could itself lead to impaired oligodendrocyte development. Thus far the only reported neuropathologic examinations involved two late preterm infants (GA 33 and 34 weeks, respectively) who were initially doing well but developed HPeV3 infection and presented with EEG-confirmed seizures.[635] Both developed the features of severe PVL on MRI. HPeV3 was confirmed on PCR in the CSF, sera, and tissues. HPeV3 in situ hybridization detection of infected cells was limited to the meninges and associated blood vessels in addition to the smooth muscle of pulmonary vessels. Neither of the brains showed T-cell infiltration. Macrophage infiltration and moderate astrocytosis were noted, but no mention was made of preoligodendrocytes or axonal involvement. Which cellular structures are affected in HPeV3 encephalitis therefore still needs to be elucidated.

Clinical Aspects

Clinical Diagnosis. The clinical features of EV and HPeV infection are so diverse that it is difficult to define distinctive features. Indeed, this finding should raise the possibility of such infection in *any patient* presenting with suspected meningitis/encephalitis, sometimes in the presence of a rash, fever, and/or diarrhea. The most prominent systemic signs in one series of 27 newborns with EV infection were fever (93%), diarrhea (81%), and meningitis (62%).[685] In a large sample of infants with EV infection, more severe symptoms were seen in those who developed the infection within 2 weeks of life. Twenty-seven percent (*n*=32) of neonates developed symptomatic infection in the first week of life and 65% (*n*=78) within the first 2 weeks of life. The most frequent signs were fever, seizures, irritability, rash, and feeding problems (Table 34.40).[638,639,665] More than half of the infected infants were male (65.5%). In 77 of the 119 cases (65%) the infection was caused by one of the echoviruses with echovirus 11 as the dominant serotype (18% of cases). CVB was responsible for 24% of the cases and was the second largest class of EV found in the study population.[665]

Neonatal systemic EV disease, characterized by multiorgan involvement, is one of the most serious conditions associated with EV infection. CBV and echovirus 11 (both belong to the EV-B species) are most frequently associated with neonatal infection and typically result in two severe clinical presentations, meningoencephalitis and severe myocarditis, respectively, often accompanied by heart failure and hemorrhage-hepatitis syndrome (overwhelming hepatitis with hepatic failure and disseminated intravascular coagulation).

One possible explanation for the more severe course of the HPeV3 infection is the lower observed seroprevalence of HPeV3 among women of childbearing age compared with close to universal adult seropositivity for HPeV1. HPeV3 is known to occur almost exclusively in infants younger than 3 months. Although the illness does not tend to be severe, several fatal cases have been reported (see Table 34.40).[635,686,687] A newborn with HPeV3 encephalitis and clinical (umbilical hernia, large tongue, and abnormal cry) and biochemical findings of transient central hypothyroidism was recently reported.[688]

EV-related *myocarditis* occurs sporadically, and CVB is the predominant causative agent. It is a severe disease in the neonatal period that often leads to death or results in serious chronic cardiac sequelae like chronic heart failure, aneurysm formation within the left ventricle, and mitral regurgitation (Table 34.41).[689] Chronic cardiac drug therapy is necessary in the majority of these patients. In a series of seven infants, two died; combined with previously described cases, the overall mortality was 31% (11 of 35).[660] Among the survivors, 66% (16 of 24) developed severe cardiac damage. Only 23% (8 of 35) of the infants fully recovered. CVB has also been associated with encephalitis.

Infants with prominent encephalitis related to CVB are of interest for two reasons. First, at least in the isolated fatal cases reported, a predominance of infection in the mothers occurs either just before or at the time of labor.[658,690-692] This finding suggests the possibility that infection acquired in utero during maternal viremia results in particularly severe disease, perhaps due to diffuse dissemination of a large inoculum of virus. Second, a paucity of neurological phenomena is referable to the cerebrum (Table 34.42). In the 12 infants studied in a nursery epidemic by Eilard et al.,[659] seizures were noted

---

TABLE 34.40   Clinical Features of Enterovirus Infection in 119 Infants

CLINICAL FEATURES	NUMBER (FREQUENCY)
Fever	1054 (87%)
Diarrhea	25 (21%)
Meningitis	28 (24%)
Sepsis	42 (35%)

Data from Verboon-Maciolek MA, Krediet TG, van Loon AM, et al. Epidemiological survey of neonatal non-polio enterovirus infection in the Netherlands. *J Med Virol.* 2002;66:241-245.

TABLE 34.41   Clinical Features of Neonatal Coxsackievirus B Myocarditis

CLINICAL FEATURES	FREQUENCY (%)
Feeding difficulty	84
Cardiac signs	81
Respiratory distress	75
Cyanosis	72
Fever	70
Pharyngitis	64
Hepatosplenomegaly	53
Central nervous system signs	27
Jaundice	13
Diarrhea	8

Data from Cherry JD. Enterovirus and parechovirus infections. In: Remington JS, Klein JO, Wilson CB, et al., eds. *Infectious Diseases of the Fetus and Newborn Infant.* 6th ed. Philadelphia: Elsevier Saunders; 2006.

TABLE 34.42   Neurological Features of Neonatal Coxsackievirus B Encephalitis

NEUROLOGICAL FEATURE	APPROXIMATE FREQUENCY
Depressed level of consciousness	Common
Hypotonia	Common
Seizures	Uncommon
Focal motor deficits	Rare

in a single patient with heart failure (a finding suggesting a possible relation of seizures to cerebral ischemia), and the remaining infants exhibited principally a depressed level of consciousness, hypotonia, or both. Similar phenomena have been observed in fatal cases.[635,690-693] Whether the depressed level of consciousness relates to involvement of the brain stem reticular formation and the hypotonia relates to anterior horn cell involvement are intriguing possibilities (see the section on neuropathology), but they remain to be established. The relative paucity of cerebral phenomena (e.g., seizures and focal motor deficits) presumably is associated with the scarcity of cerebral neuropathological changes.

Laboratory Evaluation

Isolation of Virus. The most critical laboratory aid in diagnosis is isolation of the virus or detection of EV and HPeV RNA by PCR. Because disease in newborns tends to be generalized, collection of material from multiple sites is indicated, particularly from the throat, stool, blood, urine, and CSF.[1] Tissue culture evidence of EV infection is documented readily by most clinical laboratories and is apparent usually within a few days, in most cases in less than a week. The detection of EV and HPeV RNA by PCR in the CSF from patients with meningitis is an important diagnostic approach.[694] It has been recommended that "the general workup for febrile neonates hospitalized for possible sepsis should include PCR for both EV as well as HPeV in blood and CSF."[1] A similar recommendation can be made for the general workup of neonatal seizures of unknown cause.

Serological Studies. Serological techniques are usually not of major value in the primary diagnosis of neonatal EV and HPeV disease. The disorder is acquired near or shortly after the time of birth, and a rise in antibody titer over 2 to 4 weeks is needed to demonstrate infection.

Neurodiagnostic Studies. *CSF:* Neurodiagnostic studies should center on the analysis of the CSF. Identification of the CSF formula for meningitis with or without encephalitis and attempts to isolate the virus or genetic material from CSF are important. However, cerebral infection with EV and HPeV rarely results in pleocytosis, and the protein and glucose levels tend to be normal. The routine CSF examination is normal in 90% of HPeV3 cases and in the majority of EV cases as well; therefore, on initial clinical evaluation, encephalitis could easily be overlooked. Thus rtPCR analysis that includes analysis for HPeV3 as well as EV in CSF, blood, stool, or nasopharynx is important in the assessment of newborns with unexplained seizures, especially with any of the other clinical features noted earlier or the distinctive imaging features or both. Diagnostic assays are

not routinely available in clinical practice; the involvement of HPeV may therefore be substantially underestimated.

Serum C-reactive protein and CSF protein values were significantly higher in infants with EV infection than in those with HPeV infection. A specific marker of macrophage activation, neopterin, which is released from macrophages that have been stimulated during acute infection was shown to be increased in the CSF in a recent case of HPeV3 encephalitis.[636]

EEG: As in any newborn with suspected seizures, performing (continuous) conventional or amplitude integrated EEG (aEEG) may be useful in suggesting cerebral involvement.[695] Involvement of the CNS is more common in HPeV3 encephalitis (90%) than in EV encephalitis (40%). Seizures are common symptoms, and more than one anticonvulsant drug is required for seizure control in most infants.[639] Intractable seizures leading to death were reported in two newborn infants.[687]

Neuroimaging: Newborn infants with EV and HPeV meningoencephalitis have been reported to have mild to severe white matter abnormalities. *Cranial ultrasound* may show increased echogenicity in the periventricular and deep white matter. *MRI* is preferable for evaluation of parenchymal disease.[638,639,696,697] Involvement of white matter, suspected on *cranial ultrasound,* confirmed with *MRI,* and most clearly seen with DWI was reported in five infants with EV infection and prominent neurological features, including seizures, onset a few days to weeks after birth, presence of a rash in four infants, positive enteroviral cultures from CSF in four, and CSF pleocytosis in three. Cysts subsequently developed in the white matter in three infants, and this was more likely to occur in the preterm infants (Fig. 34.34).[638,639] Although no pathological material was available, the findings suggest a true encephalitis with a predilection for white matter. Of the five infants, two had spastic motor deficits on follow-up. In another study by the same group, very similar clinical and neuroimaging findings due to HPeV-3 infection were reported in 10 infants.[698] Their GA varied from 29 to 41 weeks, and they presented at 36 to 41 weeks postmenstrual age with clinical seizures.[698] Of these infants, seven had a fever and six had a rash. *Cranial ultrasonography* showed increased echogenicity in the periventricular white matter in all infants. Neonatal *MRI* confirmed white matter changes in nine infants, with signal intensity changes suggestive of gliosis of the white matter on a later MRI (Fig. 34.35). Outcome was variable, with cerebral palsy in one, suspect outcome at 18 months in one, learning disabilities at 7 years of age in one, epilepsy in one, and normal neurodevelopmental outcome in five. Diffuse signal intensity changes of the white matter and punctate white matter lesions, seen as restricted diffusion on DWI, involved the corpus callosum as well as the descending corticospinal tracts (Fig. 34.36). Several case reports, subsequently reported, have shown the value of MRI and especially DWI.[636,637,697,699,700] In a few infants with HPeV meningoencephalitis and an adverse outcome, involvement was not restricted to the white matter but also included the thalami. In the two cases with magnetic resonance spectroscopy (MRS), the findings were reduced N-acetylaspartate (NAA) as well as presence of lactate.[636,637,699,700] As noted for EV infection, cysts may develop in the white matter, especially in the preterm infant (see Fig. 34.33). In one recent review of HPeV3 infection in 12 children, no MRI abnormalities were found. However, only two of these infants were less than 1 month when presenting with HPeV infection

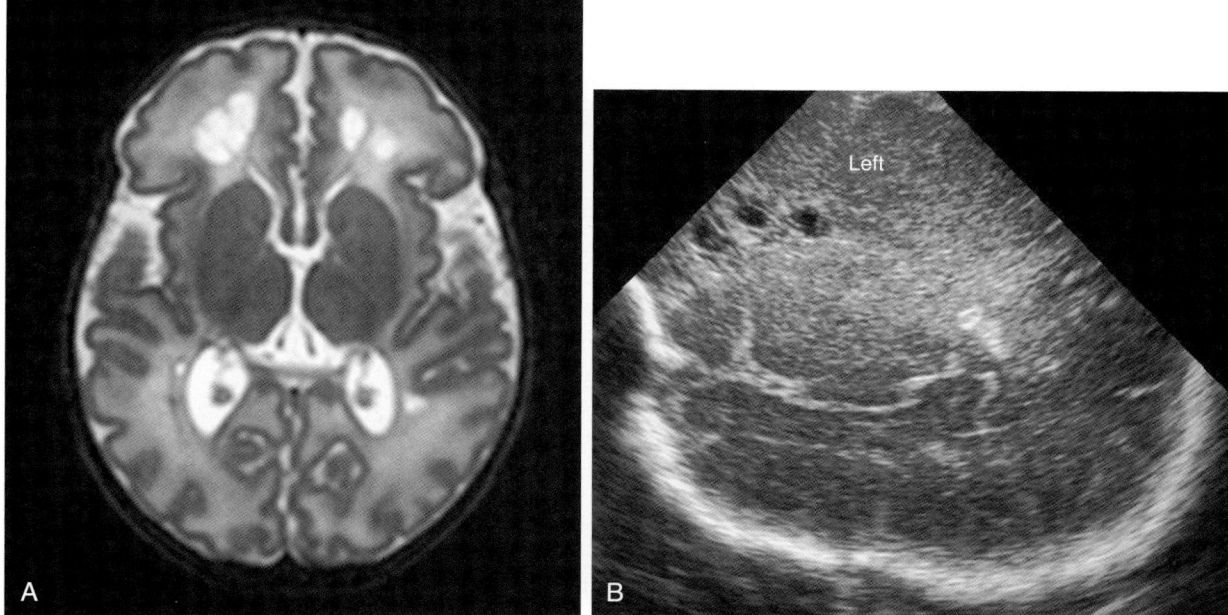

Figure 34.34 Neonatal enteroviral meningoencephalitis: magnetic resonance imaging and ultrasonography.
Axial T2-weighted image (A) obtained 3 weeks after the onset of enteroviral infection shows large cystic lesions in the frontal white matter (detectable by ultrasound [B]) and smaller lesions in the parieto-occipital periventricular region. (From Verboon-Maciolek MA, Groenendaal F, Cowan F, et al. White matter damage in neonatal enterovirus meningoencephalitis. *Neurology.* 2006;66:1267-1269.)

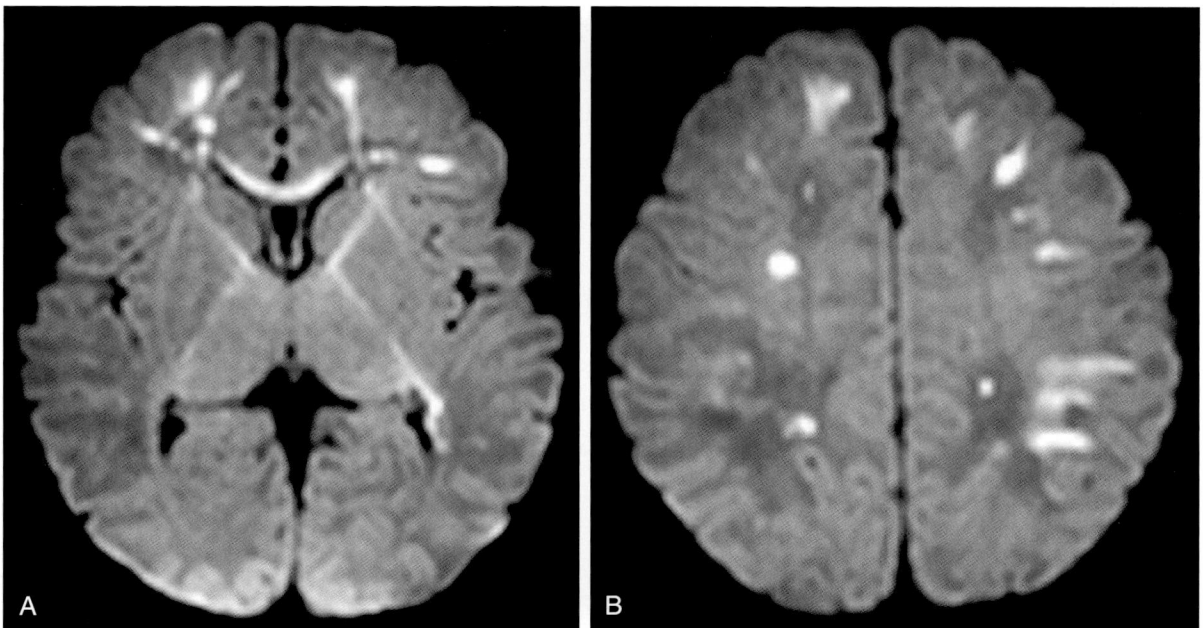

Figure 34.35 Neonatal parechovirus meningoencephalitis: magnetic resonance imaging. Diffusion-weighted images, obtained on day 14, or 4 days after presentation with seizures and a fever. Polymerase chain reaction of the cerebrospinal fluid confirmed parechovirus (HPeV3) infection. The diffusion-weighted images show restricted diffusion throughout the white matter, especially in the corpus callosum and internal capsule as well as optic radiation on the left (A) and in the centrum semiovale (B). Neurodevelopmental outcome at 18 months was normal with a developmental quotient of 99 on the Griffiths mental development test.

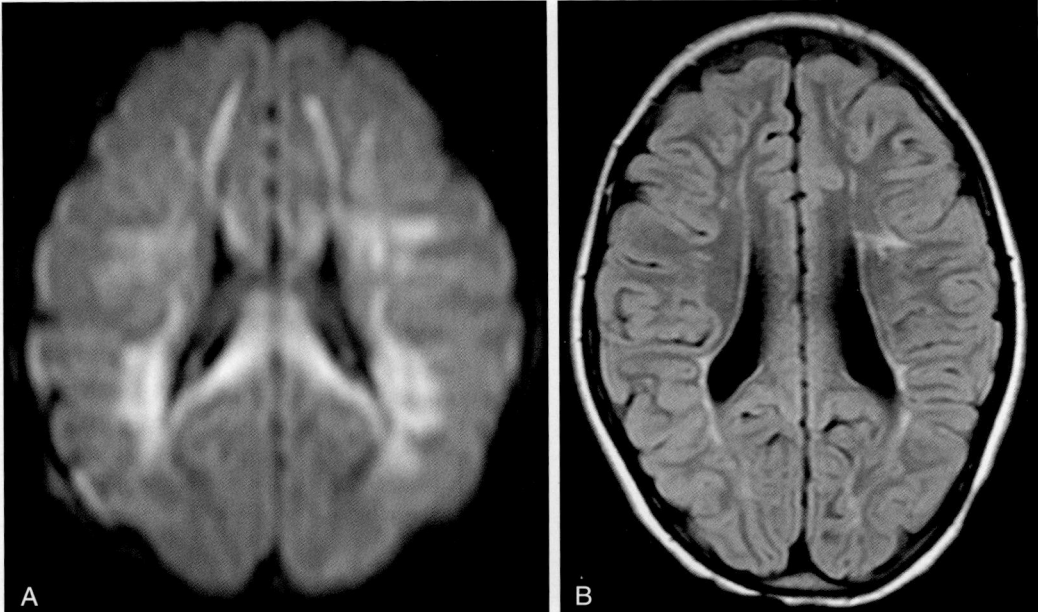

Figure 34.36 Neonatal parechovirus meningoencephalitis: magnetic resonance imaging. A neonatal diffusion-weighted image (A) and FLAIR (B) sequence at 7 years in the same child who, as a full-term infant, presented with a mild rash and seizures on day 7. Polymerase chain reaction of the cerebrospinal fluid confirmed parechovirus (HPeV3) infection. The diffusion-weighted image shows extensive restricted diffusion throughout the periventricular white matter (A). The FLAIR sequence shows mild ventricular dilation with periventricular areas of high signal intensity suggestive of gliosis. Neurodevelopmental outcome at 7 years was within the normal range. The child is left handed with a normal score on the movement ABC test (20th centile) and a total IQ of 98.

and no mention was made of use of DWI, which allows better detection of the white matter abnormalities.[701]

Prognosis

In general, the prognosis with EV and HPeV infections is relatively good. Exceptions are the severe cases of CVB myocarditis and a small number of infants with HPeV encephalitis with a more severe course, which constitute a very small proportion of the total group of affected cases. The possibility of neurological or cognitive deficits after EV and HPeV infection in early infancy has been raised in several relatively *small* studies.[1,37] A study of 45 children in whom EV *meningitis* developed between the ages of 4 days and 12 months found no evidence of impairments of neurological or cognitive function on follow-up.[702] In a group of 15 children who had neonatal meningoencephalitis secondary to CVB infection, only 2 had neurological deficits (spasticity, cognitive deficits) at follow-up at the age of 6 years.[703] In the series of five infants described earlier with apparent neonatal EV white matter necrosis and encephalitis, two subsequently exhibited *cerebral palsy*.[638] The first reported group of 10 infants with neonatal HPeV infection with CNS involvement, confirmed with neuroimaging, had a similar outcome.[639] The largest reported group thus far of 13 infants, including 5 preterm infants, with HPeV meningoencephalitis had outcome measured at only 12 months. Of these, seven patients had characteristic white matter diffusion restriction on neonatal MRI. At 12 months of age, three had severe neurological sequelae, two had developed cerebral palsy, and one developed cerebral visual impairment.[697] Since then, more outcome data have become available, including

several cases with a fatal outcome, and HPeV has also been associated with sudden infant death[a] (Table 34.43).

Management

Prevention. Two major approaches to prevention can be recommended. First, maternal infection should be sought with a high index of suspicion; if infection is present, delivery should not be encouraged. Cesarean section may increase the risk of severe disease by decreasing the time for maternal synthesis and transplacental transfer of protective IgG antibody.[661] Second, nursery procedures should be strict regarding EV infection. For example, infants with suspected disease should be isolated. Nursery personnel who may be infected should be detected and not allowed contact with patients. If illness is demonstrated, the nursery is probably best closed to new admissions.[660]

Supportive Care. The treatment of EV and HPeV infections is primarily supportive. The considerations outlined for other congenital infections are appropriate regarding seizures, which are especially common in HPeV infection and may be resistant to antiepileptic medication.[687]

Antimicrobial Therapy. A recent randomized double-blind placebo-controlled trial of the antiviral agent pleconaril involved 61 subjects who were admitted ≤15 days after birth with suspected EV sepsis (hepatitis, coagulopathy, and/or myocarditis).[706] A 2:1 study drug:placebo randomization with

---

[a]References 636, 637, 686, 699, 700, 704, 705.

TABLE 34.43	Neurodevelopmental Outcome Following Parechovirus Encephalitis
Death	4/21
Cerebral palsy	3/17 (associated with epilepsy in one and with cognitive delay in 2)
Distal hypertonia	1/17 (associated with cognitive delay)
Abnormal outcome <12 months	3/17
Cognitive delay	3/17
Normal outcome	7/17 (2 at 6 months)

Data from Verboon-Maciolek MA, Groenendaal F, Hahn CD, et al. Human parechovirus causes encephalitis with white matter injury in neonates. *Ann Neurol.* 2008;64:266-273; van Zwol AL, Lequin M, Aarts-Tesselaar C, et al. Fatal neonatal parechovirus encephalitis. *BMJ Case Rep.* 2009;2009:bcr0520091883; Gupta S, Fernandez D, Siddiqui A, et al. Extensive white matter abnormalities associated with neonatal Parechovirus (HPeV) infection. *Eur J Paediatr Neurol.* 2010;14:531-534; Belcastro V, Bini P, Barachetti R, et al. Teaching neuroimages: neonatal parechovirus encephalitis: typical MRI findings. *Neurology.* 2014;82:e23; Bissel SJ, Auer RN, Chiang CH, et al. Human parechovirus 3 meningitis and fatal leukoencephalopathy. *J Neuropathol Exp Neurol.* 2015;74:767-777; Renna S, Bergamino L, Pirlo D, et al. A case of neonatal human parechovirus encephalitis with a favourable outcome. *Brain Dev.* 2014;36:70-73; Leow JY, Gupta R, Sohal AP. Human parechovirus central nervous system infection: A rare cause of neonatal encephalitis. *J Paediatr Child Health.* 2015;51:1244; Pariani E, Pellegrinelli L, Pugni L, et al. Two cases of neonatal human parechovirus 3 encephalitis. *Pediatr Infect Dis J.* 2014;33:1191-1193; Brownell AD, Reynolds TQ, Livingston B, et al. Human parechovirus-3 encephalitis in two neonates: acute and follow-up magnetic resonance imaging and evaluation of central nervous system markers of inflammation. *Pediatr Neurol.* 2015;52:245-249.

randomly permuted block sizes was used. Of the 61 infants, 43 received pleconaril and 18 a placebo. EV was confirmed in 43 of 61 infants (31 treatment, 12 placebo). EV-infected subjects in the treatment group became culture-negative from all anatomical sites combined faster than did placebo-group subjects (median 4.0 vs. 7.0 days, $P = .08$). Fewer subjects in the treatment group remained PCR-positive from the oropharynx when last sampled (23% vs. 58%, $P = .02$; median, 14.0 days). By intention to treat, 10 of 43 (23%) subjects in the treatment group and 8 of 18 (44%) in the placebo group died ($P = .02$ for a 2-month survival difference); among EV-confirmed subjects, 7 of 31 (23%) in the treatment group died versus 5 of 12 (42%) in the placebo group ($P = .26$). One subject in the treatment group and three in the placebo group had treatment-related adverse events. An earlier, smaller study randomized 2:1, with pleconaril in 20 infants 12 months of age or less with confirmed EV meningitis (12 pleconaril, 8 placebo),[707] showed no significant differences in duration of positivity by culture or PCR, hospitalization, or symptoms. The larger recent study supports the potential efficacy of pleconaril because of greater survival among pleconaril recipients.[706] Further evaluation of the use of pleconaril is warranted.[706]

Prevention. Development of vaccines against all members of the EV and HPeV genera is not feasible owing to the large quantity of serotypes (more than 250 EVs and 16 HPeVs). A recent review discusses the role of replication of EV and HPeV and the potential value of inhibition by small-molecule inhibitors.[708]

Varicella

Varicella infection of the infant occurs in utero by transplacental mechanisms. Postnatal acquisition of the virus may occur in the newborn period, but this is rare and not of neurological importance. Two syndromes related to intrauterine acquisition of varicella should be distinguished: *congenital varicella syndrome*, caused by maternal-fetal infection primarily in the first 20 weeks of pregnancy, and *perinatal varicella*, caused by maternal-fetal infection within approximately 21 days of delivery (the upper range of the duration of the incubation period for varicella). Both disorders are rare but are important to recognize, in part because appropriate intervention may attenuate or prevent serious disease in the infant (see later discussion).

Following the introduction of routine varicella zoster vaccination, varicella overall has become very uncommon. Vaccination began in Australia in 2005 and resulted in an apparent reduction of congenital varicella and a significant reduction of neonatal varicella.[709] Only two cases of congenital varicella (0.19 per 100,000 live births per annum) and 16 cases of neonatal varicella (2.0 per 100,000 live births per annum) were identified. During 2008 and 2009 no cases of congenital varicella were reported, and neonatal varicella rates declined to 0.7 per 100,000 live births per annum, a significant trend ($P = .005$) and a reduction of more than 85% compared with rates during 1995 to 1997 (the prevaccination era) and the first year of the current surveillance study. Of 16 neonatal cases, 11 followed prenatal maternal infection; 7 of the 11 infections were acquired from children, 4 of whom were living in the same household. A total of 10 (62.5%) infants with neonatal varicella were admitted to hospital, 1 of whom developed varicella pneumonitis requiring ventilatory support, but none died. Only one infecting contact had been vaccinated.

Perinatal Varicella

Perinatal varicella in this context refers to infection of the fetus acquired near the time of delivery and clinically apparent within the first 10 postnatal days. This disorder is rare, principally because varicella infection is rare during pregnancy (most women have natural immunity because of childhood infection). The incidence of varicella during pregnancy has been reported to be 0.7 per 1000 pregnancies.[1,37,710] As noted earlier, this incidence has declined as women who received the vaccine as infants are reaching childbearing age. Approximately 25% of infants born to mothers with varicella during the last 21 days of pregnancy develop the disease.[711-717] The risk of developing perinatal varicella is highest when the rash occurs from 5 days before to 2 days after delivery.[718]

Pathogenesis. The virus is acquired in utero by *transplacental passage* as a consequence of maternal viremia.[1,37] The incubation period, defined as the interval between the onset of the rash in the mother and onset in the newborn (or fetus), is usually 9 to 15 days.[1] The reason for this slightly shorter than usual incubation period is not clearly understood.

Maternal antibody transferred to the fetus has the capacity to modify the disease.[1,37] As discussed subsequently, those infants with early onset of disease (during the first 4 days of life) have milder disease than those with later onset (from 5 to 10 days of life). In later-onset cases, antibody titers at birth are considerable in the mother and are either absent or much

TABLE 34.44   Perinatal Varicella: Relation to Maternal Infection and Outcome

ONSET OF MATERNAL RASH	ONSET OF NEONATAL DISEASE (DAYS)	NO. OF NEONATAL CASES	MORTALITY (%)
≥5 days before delivery	0–4	27	0
≤4 days before delivery	5–10	23	30

See text for references.

TABLE 34.45   Management of the Newborn Exposed to Varicella in Utero

TIME OF MATERNAL INFECTION	NEWBORN MANAGEMENT
6–20 days before delivery	Isolation from mother until no longer clinically infectious
<5 days before delivery	Varicella-zoster immune globulin and isolation from mother[a]
<2 days after delivery	Varicella-zoster immune globulin and isolation from mother[a]

See text for references.
[a]Acyclovir should be considered if varicella develops in the infant (see text).

lower in the infant, whereas in early-onset cases, antibody titers in maternal and cord blood are similar.[719] These data suggest that several days are needed before maternal IgG antibodies against varicella virus cross the placenta and equilibrate with the fetal circulation. This evidence of a protective effect of maternal antibody has implications for the management of the pregnant woman with varicella near the time of delivery (see later discussion).

Neuropathology. The pathological changes in the most severe (i.e., fatal) cases of perinatal varicella include inflammation and necrosis in the lungs, liver, adrenal glands, gastrointestinal tract, kidney, and spleen.[1,37] The predilection for liver and adrenals is reminiscent of neonatal infection with another virus of the herpes group, HSV. Of five brains examined, only one was said to show areas of necrosis; the necrotic areas were associated with dissolution of all tissue elements and with calcification.[720] The lesions were said to be similar to those of toxoplasmosis, but no *Toxoplasma* organisms were seen. No serological studies were available, and the possibility of a dual infection was not excluded. Thus it remains unclear whether a primary viral encephalitis occurs with perinatal varicella; even if so, such an occurrence is exceedingly rare.

Clinical Aspects. Perinatal varicella is characterized by a vesicular rash that may be hemorrhagic in severe cases. The spectrum of severity varies from a few vesicles to a nearly confluent eruption. The severity of disease relates particularly to the time of onset of the maternal illness in relation to delivery (Table 34.44).[a] Early-onset neonatal disease is benign, whereas later-onset disease is associated with a significant mortality (i.e., ≈30%). In a review of 96 cases, nearly 30% of infants with clinically apparent lesions died during the first month of life, and developmental delay occurs in about 12% of survivors.[724] The latter statistic relates to the severe systemic manifestations with necrotizing lung disease resulting in refractory hypoxemia.[725]

The *diagnosis* is usually readily apparent in the presence of a vesicular rash and the maternal history. If the latter is unavailable, confusion with HSV is possible, and the distinction is important. In HSV infection, vesicles tend to occur in clusters rather than in the more even distribution of varicella infection.

Laboratory Evaluation. The laboratory procedures of most value initially are *culture of the virus from the lesion, detection of viral antigen by immunofluorescence, or viral DNA by PCR.* Serological studies also provide diagnostic information; varicella-specific IgM antibodies are usually detectable early in the disease but disappear shortly after birth.

Prognosis. The difference in prognosis as a function of the time of maternal illness has been outlined (see Table 34.44).

Management. Modification of the neonatal disease can be accomplished by *passive immunization* with varicella zoster immune globulin (Table 34.45).[714,722,725,726] Passive immunization, however, does not decrease the clinical attack rate.[714,725] When the onset of maternal varicella is less than 5 days before delivery, a considerable risk exists that (1) varicella was acquired by the fetus too near the time of delivery for significant passive transfer of maternal antibody and (2) serious neonatal disease, with a 30% fatality rate, will result. Thus, for the infant delivered less than 5 days after onset of maternal varicella (some investigators suggest <7 days),[725] varicella zoster immune globulin (1.25 mL) should be administered intramuscularly (see Table 34.45). In case of imminent delivery, acyclovir therapy and tocolysis have been recommended—the latter to allow transplacental passage of maternal IgG, which may help to reduce the risk for the infant yet to be born.[721,727-729] There is consensus regarding the treatment of pregnant women with varicella in late pregnancy, as this is the period of highest risk for maternal complications and neonatal varicella.[730]

Similarly, if the mother contracts varicella within the first few days (2 days is the period recommended by the CDC) after delivery, the infant is at risk for having acquired varicella transplacentally in utero before significant passive transfer of maternal antibody. Such an infant should receive varicella zoster immune globulin and should be isolated from the mother. Finally, if the infant acquires the disease and the manifestations appear to be becoming severe, a course of intravenous acyclovir should be instituted.[1,37]

Congenital Varicella Syndrome

Congenital varicella syndrome is a rare constellation of stigmata caused by intrauterine infection with varicella virus before 20 weeks. Individual case reports have established that a distinctive clinical constellation is associated, albeit rarely, with varicella

---

[a]References 711, 712, 714, 716, 717, 721-723.

TABLE 34.46	Neuropathology of Congenital Varicella Syndrome

Meningoencephalitis
Myelitis, especially affecting anterior horn cells
Dorsal root ganglionitis
Denervation atrophy (and hypoplasia) of muscle in segmental distribution

infection, usually in the first 20 weeks.[713,714,722,731-745] The risk of congenital varicella in most studies is approximately 2% (range, 1% to 2%).[714,718,722,746-748] In a prospective study of 1373 women, the risk of congenital varicella was 0.4% with maternal disease from 0 to 12 weeks of pregnancy and 2% with maternal disease from 13 to 20 weeks.[718] The risk is minimal with maternal infection after 20 weeks.

Pathogenesis. The pathogenesis of the congenital varicella syndrome is presumed to be fetal infection acquired by transplacental passage of virus in association with maternal viremia. Detection of the virus in amniotic fluid and fetal blood has been accomplished by PCR.[746,747] The similarity of some of the neuropathology to later infection by herpes zoster (see later discussion) and the occurrence of disseminated disease with zoster in immunocompromised individuals are of interest because, before 18 to 20 weeks of pregnancy, the fetus exhibits many features of a deficient immune response. Unlike infection with CMV, the fetal infection is not chronic and, indeed, isolation of the virus after birth has not been accomplished. The nature of the lesions indicates that inflammation and destruction of tissue underlie most of the major defects observed.

Neuropathology. The neuropathology was well described in an infant who died at 6½ months of age.[744] The major features included meningoencephalitis, myelitis, dorsal root ganglionitis, and denervation (and hypoplasia) of muscle in a *segmental* distribution (Table 34.46). *Primary viral encephalitis* was suggested by a necrotizing parenchymal process with inflammatory cells in the meninges and throughout the brain. Indeed, the cerebral hemispheres were said to be "replaced by an extensive fluid-filled cyst enclosed by a semilucent yellowish membrane of varying thickness."[744] Evidence of a focal destructive ependymitis in the floor of the fourth ventricle was particularly obvious. Less severe degrees of parenchymal necrosis with perivascular cuffing with inflammatory cells have been described.[736,738] *Dorsal root ganglia* in the lumbar region as well as the lumbar *spinal cord* and, particularly, the anterior horn cells exhibited inflammatory and necrotic changes. In association with the predominant involvement of anterior horn cells of the left lumbar segments was a *marked deficiency of muscle* in the atrophic left lower extremity, the muscular lesion corresponding to the segmental regions particularly affected in the spinal cord. The neuropathological data indicated a severe, inflammatory, destructive process affecting all levels of the CNS, including anterior horn cells and their associated sites of innervation, as well as the dorsal root ganglia of the peripheral nervous system. The involvement of dorsal root ganglia is particularly interesting in view of the tendency for varicella zoster virus to remain latent at that site and to become

TABLE 34.47	Clinical Features of Congenital Varicella Syndrome	
CLINICAL FEATURE		**APPROXIMATE FREQUENCY (%)**
Maternal infection		
8–12 weeks		51–75
13–20 weeks		26–50
>20 weeks		0–25
Small for dates or prematurity or both		51–75
Cutaneous scars (dermatome distribution)		76–100
Ocular abnormality		76–100
Limb abnormality		51–75
Hypoplastic muscle		51–75
Deformity		51–75
Bulbar signs		26–50
Muscle weakness		26–50
Microcephaly		26–50
Seizures (survivors)		26–50
Retarded neurological development (survivors)		51–75
Death in infancy		26–50

See text for references.

reactivated as herpes zoster infection in adult life. Indeed, herpes zoster cutaneous lesions have been observed postnatally at 2 weeks,[749] 3 months,[741] and 17 months[750] of age after intrauterine exposure to varicella.

Although neuropathological information is not available for other cases of congenital varicella, ultrasound or CT in several other infants has revealed such findings as microcephaly, dilated lateral ventricles, and cerebral calcifications indicative of a destructive process.[a] Active inflammation at the time of birth is not common, as evidenced by several patients with normal CSF analysis.[734,742,744] These data further support the notion that congenital varicella syndrome is related to a discrete, acute attack by varicella in utero and is not associated with the type of chronic infection observed with such congenital infections as rubella, CMV, and syphilis.

Clinical Aspects. The clinical presentation is dramatic and distinctive (Table 34.47). In the majority of cases, the mothers of the affected infants had varicella between 8 and 20 weeks of gestation. In a few cases, first- or second-trimester zoster infection was responsible. The mother of the least severely affected infant had varicella in the 28th week of pregnancy.[731] Cutaneous scars, characteristically depressed, are nearly invariably present (Fig. 34.37). The lesions occur in a *segmental* distribution and often exhibit the zigzag appearance observed in herpes zoster infections in adults. The limb abnormalities consist of atrophy or hypoplasia of muscle, usually associated with a limb deformity (e.g., talipes equinovarus, hypoplastic limb). Rarely, patients exhibit hypoplastic muscles of the face, neck, or abdomen and not the limbs.

Neurological features have been prominent in nearly every case. Bulbar signs, especially serious difficulty in swallowing,

[a]References 735-738, 740, 745, 748, 751, 752.

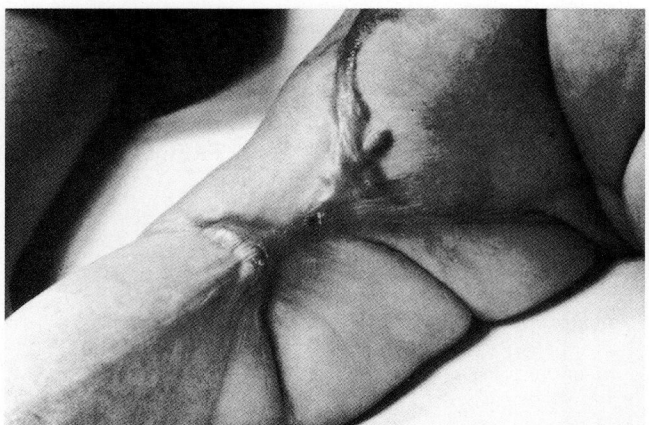

Figure 34.37 Congenital varicella syndrome: cutaneous scar in an infant whose mother had varicella-zoster infection in the 12th week of pregnancy. Note the severe scar over the posterior aspect of the lower extremity in the distribution of the first sacral segment. The limb was also hypoplastic. (From Hanshaw JB, Dudgeon JA. *Viral Disease of the Fetus and Newborn.* Philadelphia: Saunders; 1973.)

have occurred in many patients, thus bringing to mind the neuropathological observation of particular destruction in the floor of the fourth ventricle (see previous discussion). Unilateral laryngeal paralysis with resulting severe respiratory failure has been reported.[753] Muscle weakness is associated with the segmental hypoplasia or atrophy of muscle and presumably is related to anterior horn cell involvement. Sensation was diminished to pinprick in the one case in which this aspect of the neurological examination is mentioned specifically; in view of the involvement of dorsal root ganglia, it is reasonable to suspect that this was present but not elicited in other cases. Cerebral involvement is reflected by the frequent occurrence of microcephaly, seizures, and retarded neurological development (see Table 34.47).

Ocular abnormalities have been present in nearly every case and consist most commonly of chorioretinitis but also microphthalmia, cataracts, optic atrophy, anisocoria, or Horner syndrome.[742,746,751] The presence of Horner syndrome suggests involvement of cervical sympathetic ganglion or cells of the intermediate column of the spinal cord.

The clinical constellation is distinctive enough to suggest the *diagnosis.* The maternal history of varicella confirms the impression.

Laboratory Evaluation. No consistent means of establishing the virological diagnosis in the newborn has been identified. In rare cases, viral particles and multinucleated giant cells obtained from vesicular fluid were compatible with varicella[733,746]; however, the virus was not isolated. Other attempts to isolate virus from CSF, eye, and other tissues have not been successful.[713,733,740,744] However, detection of viral DNA in CSF by PCR has been reported in the newborn.[736] As noted earlier, viral DNA has been detected in amniotic fluid and fetal blood by PCR.[746,747] Detection of varicella-specific IgM in cord blood obtained in utero by cordocentesis also has been reported.[738]

Serological studies, albeit usually not extensive, have been compatible with fetal infection in approximately 75% of cases.[713] In most instances, this conclusion is based on the persistence

of varicella-zoster antibody, measured by complement fixation, beyond the age at which maternal antibody should be expected to have disappeared. A cell-mediated immune response to varicella-zoster virus was detected in two infants. Varicella-specific IgM has also been identified in approximately half of the infants studied.

Prognosis. The unfavorable outlook regarding mortality, retardation of neurological development, occurrence of seizures, and other neurological signs is reviewed in Table 34.47. Nevertheless, approximately 20% of reported patients develop normally in the first year of life.[734] A 27-year-old woman with congenital varicella was normal except for a motor deficit related to limb hypoplasia.[743]

Management. *Prevention* of this disorder is difficult. However, in counseling the parents, the low risk of transmission of infection to the fetus must be considered. Thus the risk for symptomatic intrauterine varicella zoster infection after maternal varicella in the first 20 weeks of gestation is only approximately 2% (see earlier discussion). Intrauterine diagnosis appears to be possible early in pregnancy. Varicella zoster–specific IgM has been detected in fetal blood, and virus has been identified by PCR in amniotic fluid, chorionic villus samples, and fetal blood.[738,746,747] Varicella zoster immune globulin administered to the susceptible mother after exposure to varicella prevents or modifies her disease and decreases the risk of transmission to the fetus.[746] Varicella zoster immune globulin can be administered until 10 days after exposure.[754] There are a few anecdotal reports that acyclovir may reduce MTCT.[755]

Supportive management for the affected infant should include control of seizures. A particular problem is maintenance of adequate nutrition in those infants who have difficulty swallowing. Tube feedings have been required in early infancy. Respiratory support may be needed for the rare case involving laryngeal paralysis.[753] Appropriate training for infants with serious visual impairment secondary to ocular abnormality has been accompanied by normal development.[734]

Rotavirus

Rotaviruses belong to the family *Reoviridae* and are nonenveloped double-stranded RNA viruses. It is the most common cause of gastroenteritis in children worldwide, with near universal exposure to rotavirus by age 5.[756] In 2008, diarrhea attributable to rotavirus infection resulted in 453,000 deaths (95% CI 420,000 to 494,000) worldwide in children younger than 5 years, with 37% of deaths attributable to diarrhea and 5% of all deaths in children younger than 5 years.[757] Rotavirus infection is usually self-limiting and benign, but severe dehydration caused by rotavirus-induced diarrhea and vomiting can be fatal in developing countries, and rotavirus can also be associated with severe complications such as encephalopathy/encephalitis,[758,759] myocarditis,[760] and sudden unexpected death.[761] In developed countries, prematurity, low birth weight, and congenital pathology are important risk factors for rotavirus hospitalization and increased health care needs.[762] Recent studies indicate that rotavirus infection can lead to CNS involvement (see later).[763]

Pathogenesis

Rotavirus is relatively unique in that it contains a transmembrane glycoprotein, NSP4, which functions as a viral enterotoxin capable of inducing diarrhea through complex mechanisms, including interfering with local calcium homeostasis or with tight junctions in the intestine.[764] NSP4 has also been suspected of having a role in rotavirus-associated CNS complications.[764] This viral enterotoxin can induce disruption of calcium homeostasis and release of nitric oxide metabolites in intestinal epithelial cells.[765] In vitro, rotavirus has been shown to infect neurons and to replicate within them, and NSP4 has been detected in dendritic processes.[766] Moreover, recent reports have found that NSP4 triggers the secretion of proinflammatory cytokines from human and murine macrophage-like cell lines via TLR 2. Variability in NSP4 across rotavirus strains in different geographic locations may play a role in the degree of pathogenicity.[764] It has also been suggested that peripheral inflammatory cytokines, such as interleukin-6, released during rotavirus infection, could induce elevated cytokine levels within the CNS, which might result in CNS complications.[767]

Clinical Aspects

While rotavirus replication was initially thought to be limited to the gastrointestinal tract, recent studies have shown that rotavirus infection causes antigenemia and RNAemia,[768,769] which suggests that viral spreading beyond the gastrointestinal tract contributes to systemic infection. Rotavirus antigenemia and viremia are common in children hospitalized for rotavirus gastroenteritis and may be associated with increased severity of fever and vomiting.[768] Although it is far less common for rotavirus to cause an acute encephalopathy or frank encephalitis, neurological complications are not uncommon in older children, occurring in approximately 2% to 3% of all children with rotavirus gastroenteritis, with the most common manifestations being febrile or afebrile seizures.[764] In a large multicenter study of 1359 patients hospitalized with laboratory-confirmed rotavirus in Canada from 2005 to 2007, seizures were reported in 7% of these subjects.[770] The mechanism by which rotavirus causes neurologic complications still needs to be elucidated, although various hypotheses include direct viral invasion causing neuronal injury, viral toxin production, and excitotoxicity.[764] Patients with rotavirus diarrhea and benign or severe convulsions of encephalitis have been found to have evidence of rotavirus in the CSF.[771] However, the significance of this finding is still not clear. The presence of rotavirus in the CSF could be explained as either a cause of convulsions or a result of contamination of the CSF by fecal material introduced during lumbar puncture. Until recently, rotavirus was not considered to be related to encephalopathy in the newborn, but several studies have now shown that rotavirus should be considered in the differential diagnosis of neonatal seizures in late preterm and full-term infants (Table 34.48).[772-774]

Clinical Features. Full-term or near-term infants initially appear well but then present at the end of the first week (days 4 to 6) with apneas and/or seizures.[772,774,775] Diarrhea is present in some but not all. In the study by Oh et al., only 4 of 30 infants had diarrhea and 2 had poor feeding.[775] It is of interest that the onset of seizures in both cohorts, concerning full-term infants, was between days 4 to 6 after birth, which correlates roughly with the amount of time required for rotavirus to become symptomatic. There is a previously demonstrated association between neonatal rotavirus infection and "fifth-day fits."[776] In the latter study, all but 1 of the infants with fifth-day fits (18

TABLE 34.48	Clinical and Diagnostic Features in 56 Newborn Infants With Rotavirus-Associated Encephalitis		
	NUMBER	**FREQUENCY**
Gestation		
Full term	45	80.4%
Late preterm	8	14.2%
Preterm	3	5.4%
Diarrhea	12/56	21.4%
Poor feeding	2/56	3.6%
Apneas	5/56	8.9%
Seizures	51/56	91.1%
CSF Pleocytosis	0/51	0%
Neuroimaging		
MRI-DWI abnormalities	50/50	100%
White matter cysts on repeat imaging	17/32	53.1%

CSF, Cerebrospinal fluid; *DWI,* diffusion-weighted image; *MRI,* magnetic resonance imaging.

Combined data from Lee KY, Oh KW, Weon YC, et al. Neonatal seizures accompanied by diffuse cerebral white matter lesions on diffusion-weighted imaging are associated with rotavirus infection. *Eur J Paediatr Neurol.* 2014;18:624-631; Verboon-Maciolek MA, Truttmann AC, Groenendaal F, et al. Development of cystic periventricular leukomalacia in newborn infants after rotavirus infection. *J Pediatr.* 2012;160:165.e161-168.e161; Yeom JS, Kim YS, Seo JH, et al. Distinctive pattern of white matter injury in neonates with rotavirus infection. *Neurology.* 2015;84:21-27.

of 19, or 95%) had rotavirus in their feces, compared with 12 of 30 (40%) healthy controls. The association between rotavirus and fifth-day fits has not subsequently been replicated, even though significantly more episodes of bradycardia-apnea, often followed by cyanosis, were observed in 114 neonates with diarrhea and rotavirus in their feces, compared with 101 infants with diarrhea but without a confirmed rotavirus infection. These episodes may have been due to seizures, but no EEGs were performed in this study.[777] In a small series of eight predominantly (late) preterm infants with seizures, five presented with gastrointestinal problems, but three had no diarrhea.[773] Further insight into neurological disturbances associated with rotavirus was obtained from a large study from Greece in which stool samples were collected from 415 of 1241 neonatal admissions between April 2009 and April 2013.[778] The stool sample was positive for rotavirus in 126 of 415 samples (30%). The other neonates were not included in the study because they either did not present with symptoms of gastroenteritis, were not simultaneously hospitalized in the same room with a rotavirus case, or had parents who did not consent for a stool sample to be tested. The mean age of neonates at the day of sample collection was 18 days (range 2 to 30 days), and 10 infants were born at a gestation below 37 weeks (7.9%). The most frequent reasons for hospitalization were fever (29%) and diarrhea (15%). Disturbance of consciousness was present in 12%; this was more common in those with community-acquired infection (23%) compared with those with hospital-acquired infection (3%). No mention is made of neuroimaging studies in these infants. *In (late) preterm and full-term infants with neonatal seizures, rotavirus infection should be part of the differential diagnosis even in the absence of diarrhea.*

Laboratory Evaluation

Isolation of Virus. In infants who present with diarrhea, rotavirus is usually cultured from a stool sample. Rotavirus is rarely cultured from the CSF, not even in infants presenting with disturbances in consciousness and/or seizures. Pleocytosis was not present in the CSF in any of the infants studied by Oh et al.,[775] and a weakly positive CSF PCR was found in one of the eight preterm infants studied by Verboon-Maciolek et al.[773]

Neuroimaging Studies. *Cranial ultrasound and MRI* are recommended following any acute neurological deterioration in a preterm infant who is still in the NICU or has been readmitted. In the study by Verboon-Maciolek et al., white matter abnormalities not seen before the rotavirus infection became cystic over the next 10 to 14 days (Fig. 34.38).[773] In the two studies with mainly full-term infants, a distinctive pattern of symmetrical white matter diffusion-restriction was seen on MRI. The MRI was performed because of neonatal seizures and the DWI abnormalities tended to occur in the absence of gastroenteritis or other systemic symptoms.[772,774,775]

These three imaging studies suggest selective vulnerability of the white matter in the late preterm as well as the full-term infant with rotavirus infection, and the pattern of involvement resembles closely the pattern seen in neonatal *EV* and *HPeV* infections (see earlier). For unknown reasons, there is a predilection for the frontal white matter. Even though a weakly

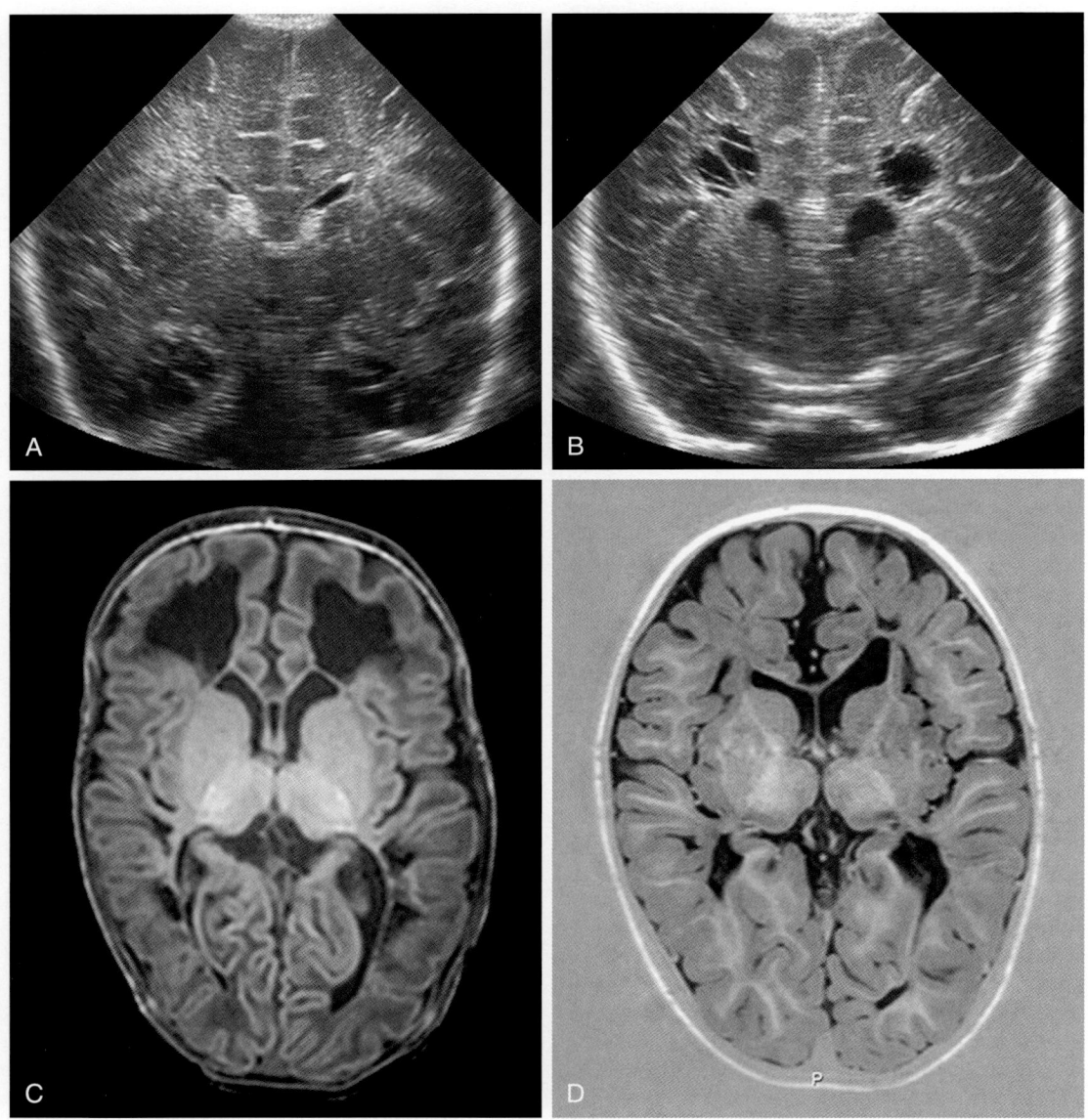

Figure 34.38 Rotavirus infection: cranial ultrasound and MRI. Coronal ultrasound, obtained a few days after an infant presented with seizures (A) and 4 weeks later (B). Echogenic changes in the germinal matrix and extensive echogenicity in the periventricular white matter (A) evolved into extensive cysts, predominantly seen in the anterior white matter (B). T1-weighted axial magnetic resonance images of the same infant obtained at term-equivalent age (C) confirm the extensive cysts seen with ultrasonography and are also seen in the trajectory of the optic radiation. There is some myelination of the posterior limb of the internal capsule bilaterally. The magnetic resonance image at 22 months (D) shows that the cysts are no longer apparent. There is severe white matter loss and delayed myelination.

positive rotavirus PCR in the CSF was present in only one infant thus far, direct CNS infection by rotavirus is still a plausible mechanism of injury, in view of the similarity to other neonatal viral infections (enterovirus, HPeV; see earlier). However, the possibilities of a CNS inflammatory process induced by systemic inflammatory signals or a toxin-mediated process should be considered.

Prognosis

Outcome data are still limited and reported only in the first study, in which three of the eight infants were born preterm, two late preterm, and three at term.[773] A normal outcome was reported for the three full-term infants and one late preterm infant. Outcome was especially poor for the preterm infants, one of whom had cognitive problems; all three developed epilepsy and cerebral palsy. Of the three with epilepsy, two presented with hypsarrythmia.

Management

Prevention. Universal infant vaccination with either the monovalent live-attenuated vaccine (RV1) or the pentavalent human-bovine reassortant vaccine (RV5) has been recommended by professional health care organizations worldwide. Vaccination has been introduced in developing countries and in a limited number of European countries. The vaccination is given as three oral doses at 4- to 10-week intervals with the first dose given to primarily healthy infants aged 6 to 12 weeks.[779]

The value of vaccination was shown by a significant reduction in rotavirus-related seizures in infants and young children following the introduction of rotavirus vaccination. In one study of 250,601 infants, 186,502 who were fully vaccinated (74.4%) were compared with 64,099 (25.6%) who were not vaccinated with rotavirus vaccine.[780] Rates of seizures were associated with rotavirus vaccination status. After adjusting for covariates, a statistically significant protective association was observed between a full course of rotavirus vaccination versus no vaccination for both first-ever seizures (risk ratio [RR] = 0.82; 95% CI, .73 to .91) and all seizures (RR = 0.79; 95% CI, .71 to .88). Overall, compared with no vaccination, there was an 18% to 21% reduction in risk of seizure requiring hospitalization or emergency department care in the year following vaccination.[780]

Because very preterm infants have a lower level of maternal antibody against prevalent rotavirus serotypes, their risk of severe gastroenteritis is increased. In 2006 to 2007, the Advisory Committee on Immunization Practices and the American Academy of Pediatrics supported RV5 vaccination before 84 days of age and recommended the vaccine for "preterm infants who were at least 6 weeks old, discharged or being discharged from the hospital, and clinically well." This recommendation was later revised to no later than 14 weeks and 6 days (104 days).[781] Because viral shedding occurs after vaccination with live-attenuated rotavirus vaccines, some prefer not to administer the vaccine while the infant is still in the NICU, since there is a risk of shedding and potential transmission to other high-risk infants. Shedding appears to be highest after the first dose and among preterm infants.

Parvovirus

Parvovirus B19, which exclusively infects humans, is a small DNA virus of the *Parvoviridae* family. The most common presentation of parvovirus B19 infection is erythema infectiosum, or fifth disease, characterized in children by a prodromal phase of fever and flu-like symptoms followed by a cutaneous eruption several days later, characterized by a "slapped cheek" rash.[782] Parvovirus also has a specific tropism for erythroid precursor cells, causing temporary suppression of erythropoiesis in most patients and triggering aplastic crisis in a subset. Most cases of parvovirus B19 infection are asymptomatic. Parvovirus B19 DNA has been detected in multinucleated reactive microglial cells in fetal white matter, suggesting that immature fetal blood vessels permit CNS infection by parvovirus B19, leading to perivascular changes and white matter damage.[783] Of particular concern in the context of this chapter is intrauterine infection with parvovirus B19, because it can cause several serious complications in the fetus, such as fetal anemia, neurological anomalies, hydrops fetalis, and fetal death.[784-787]

Transmission to the Fetus

Parvovirus B19 infection in pregnancy follows seasonal and annual trend variations and typically occurs in outbreak fashion in the spring in childcare facilities or schools. It may produce a lower frequency of maternal symptoms but a higher rate of fetal loss than previously reported. The estimated risk of transplacental infection among women who are infected with parvovirus B19 during pregnancy is about 30%. The risk of hydrops fetalis is greatest when the infection occurs during the second trimester. Prospective studies performed in the United Kingdom and the United States have reported a 5% to 9% risk of fetal loss.[788,789] The rate of fetal loss depends on the timing of infection acquisition and was 25% (3 of 12) in women who had acute parvovirus B19 infection in early pregnancy (<11 weeks), but there was no fetal loss when infection occurred after a GA of 12 weeks.[790] Parvovirus B19 probably accounts for 10% to 20% of all cases of nonimmune hydrops fetalis.[791] Parvovirus B19 infects the fetal liver, the site of erythrocyte production during early development. Hydrops may occur as the result of severe anemia, and thrombocytopenia may accompany the severe anemia. Congestive heart failure may develop owing to severe anemia, sometimes in combination with myocarditis.

Fetal Infection

Hydrops. In cohort studies, the observed rate of fetal death throughout pregnancy was 6.3%, but it reached as high as 11% for those infected within the first 20 weeks of gestation.[785] Slightly lower percentages were found in another study from the same group (Table 34.49).[784] Fetal death was observed only when maternal parvovirus B19 infection occurred before the completion of 20 weeks of gestation. In this group, 3 of 17 cases with nonsevere hydrops and 13 of 23 cases with severe hydrops received intrauterine transfusions. The proportion of fetuses with severe hydrops that survived following fetal transfusions was 11 of 13 (84.6%). All of the nontransfused fetuses with severe hydrops died.[784,785]

Central Nervous System Involvement. There have been few reports of brain abnormalities detected in fetuses with congenital parvovirus B19 infection. These have included parenchymal calcifications,[783] bilateral hemorrhagic venous infarction in a fetus who was infected shortly before term and was also identified to be heterozygous for factor V Leiden mutation,[792] arterial infarction,[793] and cerebellar hemorrhage,[794] although in some cases additional contributing factors were present. Cortical malformations—including diffuse cortical dysplasia, polymicrogyria, and heterotopia—have been described in several neonates with congenital parvovirus infection, the diagnosis being made after birth in all cases.[795-798]

Prognosis

Data on long-term outcome of fetal parvovirus B19 infection are limited to four studies and focus on those who received antenatal transfusion.[799-801] In the largest sample reported so far concerning 44 cases given intrauterine transfusions,

TABLE 34.49	Risk of Fetal Hydrops and Nonhydropic Late Intrauterine Fetal Death After Gestational Parvovirus B19 Infection		
GESTATIONAL AGE (WEEKS)	**NUMBER OF MOTHERS WITH B19 INFECTION**	**FETAL DEATH**	**HYDROPS FETALIS**
0–8	140	21 (15%)	1 (0.7%)
9–12	168	17 (10.1%)	5 (2.9%)
13–16	199	24 (12%)	16 (8.0%)
17–20	190	10 (5.2%)	15 (7.9%)
>20	557	0	13 (2.3%)
All ≤20 weeks	697	72 (5.7%)	50 (3.9%)

Combined data from Enders M, Weidner A, Zoellner I, et al. Fetal morbidity and mortality after acute human parvovirus B19 infection in pregnancy: prospective evaluation of 1018 cases. *Prenat Diagn.* 2004;24:513-518; Enders M, Klingel K, Weidner A, et al. Risk of fetal hydrops and non-hydropic late intrauterine fetal death after gestational parvovirus B19 infection. *J Clin Virol.* 2010;49:163-168.

there were 6 intrauterine fetal deaths, 1 intrapartum death, 1 termination of pregnancy, and 4 neonatal deaths. The overall survival rate was 73% (*n* = 32).[801] Follow-up data were available in 28 cases. Neurodevelopmental impairment was present in 3 of 28 (11%) children: one child had severe neurodevelopmental delay combined with cerebral palsy (case 1) and two had severe neurodevelopmental delay (cases 2 and 3), one in combination with minor neurological dysfunction. Isolated minor neurological dysfunction was diagnosed in 3 of 28 (11%). Neuroimaging during the neonatal period or during infancy was performed in 8 of the 28 (29%) children. One child with mild delay who presented with headaches at 4 years of age had an MRI showing signal intensity abnormalities in the occipital and frontal lobes. In another infant, MRI performed at the age of 4 weeks showed migrational abnormalities with left frontal polymicrogyria and cortical heterotopias (Fig. 34.39).[797] In one child an MRI performed at 3 years of age because of an unstable gait showed atrophy of the cerebellar vermis. Cerebellar hemorrhages were reported in a case with parvovirus B19; it is therefore likely that the atrophy was related to the parvovirus B19–related problems during pregnancy.[794] Whether disabilities noted at follow-up can be attributed to the parvovirus B19 infection itself or to the sometimes severe fetal anemia and fetal hydrops still needs to be elucidated. Neuroimaging, preferably MRI, is recommended following fetal parvovirus B19 infection, especially when the fetus required fetal transfusion.

Management

Prevention. There is no specific antiviral drug against parvovirus B19 infection and no vaccine can be offered as yet.[802,803] Frequent handwashing is recommended as a practical and probably effective method to reduce the spread of parvovirus B19. There is no consensus recommendation that pregnant

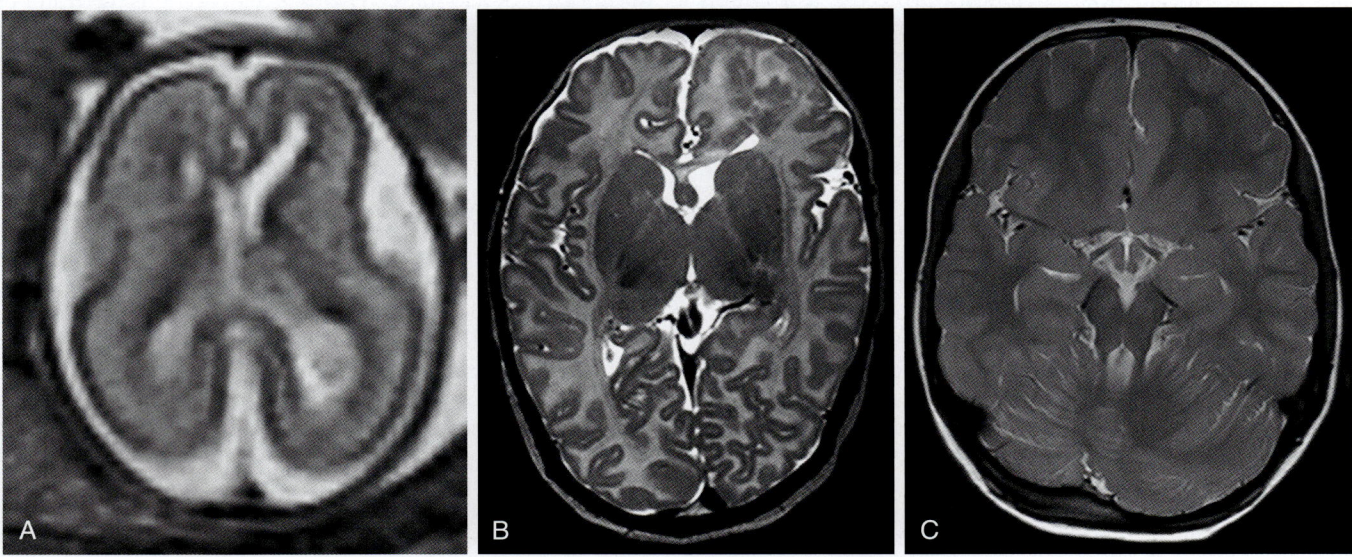

Figure 34.39 Parvovirus infection. Fetal (A), neonatal (B), and childhood (C) magnetic resonance images. Axial T2-weighted images obtained at 23 weeks of gestation show an elongated left frontal horn and mildly dilated left occipital horn. A repeat examination performed during the first postnatal week (B) shows volume loss in the left hemisphere and polymicrogyria and heterotopia in the left frontal lobe. (C) The heterotopia is still apparent at 7 years of age. The child was attending a mainstream school at 8 years of age. (From Pistorius LR, Smal J, de Haan TR et al. Disturbnces of cerebral neuronal migation following congenital parvovirus B19 infection. *Fetal Diagn Ther.* 2008;24:491–494.)

women should routinely be excluded from a workplace where a parvovirus B19 infection outbreak is occurring, although a few European countries have applied such recommendations. The most common exposure is probably from the woman's own children.

Lymphocytic Choriomeningitis

Lymphocytic choriomeningitis virus (LCMV) is an enveloped single-stranded RNA virus that is rodent-borne and within the *Arenaviridae* family.[804] The virus has been associated in approximately 100 cases with intrauterine infection and the development of microcephaly, neuronal migration anomalies, pachygyria, porencephaly, periventricular cysts, hydrocephalus, cerebral calcifications, and chorioretinitis have been reported.[805-813] Studies in a mouse model support several proposed mechanisms for congenital LCMV infection of the CNS involving both destructive effects and impairment of neuronal proliferation and migration. Immune mechanisms may be important.[808,813]

The infection may occur from either vertical transmission across the placenta or from exposure to maternal vaginal secretions or blood during maternal viremia.[813] The maternal infection generally occurs in the first and second trimesters of pregnancy. Acquisition of virus by the mother has been shown or assumed to be related to exposure to domestic or other rodents that commonly harbor the virus.[808]

Clinical Aspects

The *clinical presentation* may become apparent antenatally or postnatally. Antenatal presentation with nonimmune hydrops fetalis has been reported.[814] The clinical features in most of the neonatal cases have included microcephaly (70%) and chorioretinitis (lacunar chorioretinopathy) (100%).[808,814] Gyral abnormalities occur in 45% and periventricular calcifications in 80% of cases. Subsequently visual impairment, motor deficits, seizures, and mental retardation occur in most infants.[808,814] The disorder likely is much more common than previously expected. LCMV seroprevalence in humans is estimated to be between 4.7% and 10%.[804] Thus, in a review of 14 infants identified with chorioretinitis over a 3-year period at a major children's hospital, 3 infants had elevated antibody titers to lymphocytic choriomeningitis but not to CMV, *Toxoplasma*, rubella, or HSV.[811] Moreover, two of four children with chorioretinitis or chorioretinal scars at a home for the severely mentally retarded had similar findings.

The *diagnosis* has been made serologically by determination of LCMV antibody levels by immunofluorescent or ELISA determinations. The use of PCR offers possibilities for both prenatal and postnatal detection of LCMV. However, LCMV is not known to induce persistent infection in humans, and the time course of viral clearance from an infected human fetus is unknown.[815] Substantial brain damage from LCMV may be present, but the virus may have been cleared successfully and LCMV RNA may no longer be detected by PCR in the postnatal period.

Management consists of attempts at prevention by counseling pregnant women to avoid contact with pets, laboratory and household mice, and hamsters as well as avoidance of aerosolized excreta. The possibility of LCMV infection should be considered in all babies with evidence of congenital infection, especially those with prominent neurological signs, such as microencephaly, periventricular calcifications, hydrocephalus, and chorioretinitis.[813]

West Nile Virus

West Nile virus (WNV) is a mosquito-borne arbovirus belonging to the genus *Flavivirus* in the family Flaviviridae. It is found in temperate and tropical regions of the world.[816] WNV, first isolated from a febrile woman in the West Nile province of Uganda in 1937, was recognized in a cluster of cases of encephalitis in New York in 1999. The virus has spread throughout North America.[817]

Maternal-Fetal Transmission

It is now apparent that this virus can be transmitted from mother to fetus and can cause fetal disease. Five cases of maternal-fetal transmission have been documented with maternal infections from 16 to 28 weeks of gestation. One infant exhibited chorioretinitis and cerebral parenchymal destruction.[817] The demonstration that the virus can also be transmitted by breast-feeding further supports an enhanced suspicion of WNV infection in early infancy.[817]

Diagnosis

In the mother, the diagnosis can be made by PCR or serology. In 2002, a previously healthy woman at 27 weeks of gestation developed a febrile illness, followed by lower extremity paresis and meningoencephalitis. At 38 weeks of gestation, she delivered an infant with bilateral chorioretinitis and severe bilateral white matter loss in the temporal and occipital lobes. Maternal, cord, and infant blood samples at birth were positive for WNV-specific IgM and neutralizing antibodies; CSF from the infant was WNV IgM–positive; and the placenta was WNV PCR–positive.[818] Testing of serum to detect WNV-specific IgM antibody is the most commonly available assay.[819] Positive WNV IgM results from serum or CSF provide supportive evidence of WNV infection, but false-positives may occur from cross-reacting IgM due to other flaviviruses or even other nonspecific IgM. Accordingly, positive results should be confirmed with neutralizing antibody testing of acute and convalescent serum, typically available through public health laboratories. WNV IgG is detectable shortly after IgM. Demonstrating a seroconversion from a WNV IgG–negative status to detectable IgG supports recent infection. WNV is capable of evading the innate immune system by blocking TLRs, disrupting type I interferon signaling, and interfering with complement activation pathways. It is unclear how WNV evades the immune system to enter the brain, but once inside the CNS, WNV directly invades neurons. Resultant neuronal damage likely occurs from a combination of direct virus-mediated destruction and indirect host-mediated immune responses. Within the brain, a combination of interferon responses, alongside CD4+ and CD8+ involvement, helps clear WNV.

Prognosis

The consequences of WNV infection during pregnancy have not been well studied.[819] A review of the outcomes of 77 women with WNV infection during pregnancy showed no major difference in the rate or severity of WNV infection in pregnant women as compared with the general population.[820] The outcome was studied in 11 children at 3 years of age, and a mild delay was seen in only 1.[821] Overall, the risk of serious adverse events with WNV infection in pregnancy does not appear large. Transmission of WNV infection from mother to child through breast milk appears to be rare.[822]

Chikungunya Virus

Chikungunya virus (CHIKV) is a mosquito-borne RNA alphavirus genus in the Togaviridae family. The virus is spread by bites of various strains of *Aedes* mosquitoes (*Aedes aegypti* and *Aedes albopictus*) and was first identified in 1952 in Tanzania.[823] Since then several epidemics have been described. In late 2013 CHIKV was first found in the Caribbean islands. *Chikungunya* means "bent man" in East African dialect, which relates to bent posture, one of the clinical signs in infected adults, due to the associated arthralgia. The *Aedes albopictus* mosquito can survive in colder regions and has spread to southern Europe and the United States.

Perinatal Transmission

Following occurrence of CHIKV infection around the time of delivery, perinatal transmission has been described, causing mild to severe disease in the newborn. Ramful and colleagues, studying the Reunion Island epidemic, identified 38 newborn infants with this viral infection diagnosed by RT-PCR detection of the virus in CSF or serum or by virus-specific IgM during the first week of life.[824] Gerardin and colleagues prospectively screened 7504 women who delivered at one hospital for evidence of infection during or immediately after delivery.[825] In both studies, maternal symptoms began during the week before delivery or within 2 days thereafter.

Clinical Aspects

Chikungunya fever in older patients is typically a rapid-onset febrile disease characterized by intense asthenia, arthralgia, myalgia, headache, and rash. The abrupt onset of fever (usually higher than 39°C) follows a mean incubation period of 3 days; less than 15% of patients have asymptomatic seroconversion. A maculopapular rash occurs in 20% to 80% of cases. Severe chikungunya fever can manifest as encephalopathy and encephalitis, myocarditis, hepatitis, and multiorgan failure. Although rare, severe CHIKV fever can be fatal and is typically seen in patients with underlying medical conditions.

The *pregnant mother* may become symptomatic 3 to 12 days following a bite by a contaminated mosquito. About 1 in 4 will acquire an infection, which then tends to follow a more severe course during pregnancy. The incubation period is 2 to 6 days, and the viremia usually lasts for 2 to 7 days.

Neonates are also at risk for developing a severe infection, and the rate of infection of neonates born to viremic mothers and exposed to the virus during birth can be as high as 50%. Onset of symptoms in newborns ranged from days 3 to 7 of life and included fever, poor feeding, gastrointestinal symptoms including diarrhea, melena, and a rash, initially with generalized erythroderma, followed by brownish discoloration of the skin, particularly of the limbs and face.[824] Hemorrhagic conjunctivitis has also been reported. Severe disease and encephalopathy occur in half of the affected newborns, followed by long-term neurological sequelae.[825,826] CNS symptoms have included hypotonia, seizures, and coma, with intracerebral hemorrhage and ischemic white matter injury noted on neuroimaging. Fetal infection, however, appears to be rare.

Laboratory abnormalities included thrombocytopenia (severe in some), lymphopenia, elevated liver enzymes, and hypoprothrombinemia. IgM becomes detectable 3 to 8 days after symptom onset and usually persists for 1 to 3 months. IgG is detectable 4 to 10 days after symptom onset and persists for years. Diagnosis of chikungunya virus infection can best be made using enzyme immunoassay to detect IgM or with PCR detection of viral RNA.

MRI and Neurodevelopmental Outcome. MRI performed in infants with CNS symptoms showed scattered white matter lesions well seen with DWI and very similar to findings in infants with EV and HPeV encephalitis (see earlier). In the initial study by Gerardin and colleagues, 10 of 19 (52.6%) infected infants developed a severe illness that consisted of encephalopathy in 9 (90%).[825] These nine infants had abnormal MRI findings, with DWI white matter abnormalities in all nine and subsequent cystic evolution in two. Additional scattered white matter and intracerebellar hemorrhages were observed in two of these nine infants. Gerardin and colleagues subsequently performed follow-up in 33 children who had a CHIKV infection during the neonatal period and compared their outcome around the age of 2 years with that of 135 uninfected controls. Of the infected children, 51% had global neurodevelopmental delay, compared with 15% of uninfected peers.[826] The mean developmental quotient (DQ) score was 86.3 (95%CI: 81.0 to 91.5) in infected children compared with 100.2 (95%CI: 98.0 to 102.5) in uninfected peers (P <.001). Of the 12 children with CHIKV neonatal encephalopathy, five had microcephaly (head circumference ≤2 standard deviations) and four developed cerebral palsy.

Management

There are no antiviral agents available for treatment and no vaccine has been developed. Treatment of infected infants involves supportive care and management of hemorrhagic, neurological, and cardiac complications.

Zika Virus

ZIKV is another mosquito-borne flavivirus, transmitted by the same vectors (the *Aedes aegypti* and *Aedes albopictus* mosquitoes) as dengue virus; it belongs to the Flaviviridae family.[827-830] ZIKV was first first isolated from a Rhesus monkey in 1947 in the Zika Valley of Uganda. Of major concern is the explosive Brazilian epidemic of microcephaly, manifested by an apparent 20-fold increase in the incidence of microcephaly from 2014 to 2015, which public health officials currently believe was caused by ZIKV infections in pregnant women.[831] Based on a recent review of the available evidence, it has been suggested that there is sufficient evidence to infer a causal relationship between prenatal ZIKV infection and microcephaly and other severe brain anomalies.[832]

Pathogenesis

Transmission to Fetus and Newborn. *Perinatal transmission* has been described, following occurrence of the infection around the time of delivery and causing mild disease in the newborns.[833] Recent reports provide evidence that ZIKV is the only arbovirus linked to sexual transmission to date and that persistent shedding of ZIKV-RNA in semen can occur for as long as 6 months.[834]

Fetal Infection. Clinically significant infection with ZIKV occurs during intrauterine life by transplacental passage of the virus. The ZIKV genome was detected in the amniotic fluid of two pregnant women who had clinical symptoms at 10 and 18 weeks, respectively, and amniocentesis performed at 28 weeks of gestation. The virus was not detected in their urine or serum.[835] In a retrospective analysis of all infants with microcephaly born during a large ZIKV outbreak in French Polynesia in the period from 2013 to 2014, a strong statistical support on the basis of mathematical models was found for the association between ZIKV infection and microcephaly. The fetus is especially at risk to develop microcephaly following ZIKV infection during the first trimester of pregnancy and possibly also the second and third trimesters. An estimated number of microcephaly cases associated with ZIKV was 95 per 10,000 women infected in the first trimester.[836] Five cases with ZIKV infection during the first trimester, who showed severe brain lesions on antenatal ultrasound, have been reported in more detail.[837-840] Fetal ultrasound in all and fetal MRI in two showed brain atrophy with severe ventriculomegaly in all, bandlike calcifications in the subcortical white matter, corpus callosal dysgenesis, vermian dysgenesis, and enlarged cisterna magna. Cataracts and intraocular calcifications were seen in one, with one eye being smaller than the other. Fundoscopic alterations in the macular region have also been reported.[841] Ten infants with ZIKV-associated microcephaly resulted after a symptomatic first trimester infection (malaise, rash and arthralgia) in the mother. Ocular findings included macular alterations (gross pigment mottling and/or chorioretinal atrophy) in 15 eyes (75%) and optic nerve abnormalities (hypoplasia with double-ring sign, pallor, and/or increased cup-to-disk ratio) in 9 eyes (45%).[842,843]

Clinical Aspects

In Brazil in 2015, there were 1248 new suspected cases of microcephaly, a prevalence of 99.7 per 100,000 live births.[502] In a recent study, 88 pregnant women with a rash were enrolled from September 2015 through February 2016[845]; of these, 72 (82%) tested positive for ZIKV in blood, urine, or both. Only 28% had fever (short-term and low-grade). The timing of acute ZIKV infection ranged from 5 to 38 weeks of gestation. Doppler ultrasonography was performed in 42 of the ZIKV-positive women; fetal abnormalities were detected in 12 of these 42 (29%) and in none of the 16 ZIKV-negative women. Adverse findings included fetal deaths at 36 and 38 weeks of gestation (two fetuses), fetal growth restriction with or without microcephaly (five fetuses), ventricular calcifications or other CNS lesions (seven fetuses), and abnormal amniotic fluid volume or cerebral or umbilical artery flow (seven fetuses). Some infants with presumed congenital ZIKV infection have had features that were consistent with fetal brain disruption sequence, a phenotype involving the brain that is characterized by severe microcephaly, overlapping cranial sutures, prominent occipital bone, redundant scalp skin (rugae), and considerable neurological impairment.[846] Because of the typical pattern of abnormalities—including severe microcephaly, intracranial calcifications, migrational disorders sometimes accompanied by eye findings, redundant scalp skin, arthrogryposis, and clubfoot—the term *congenital Zika syndrome* is now being used as well (Fig. 34.40).[843,847,848]

Neuropathology. ZIKV infection in early pregnancy has been associated with severe brain injury, but detailed information is still limited. Tang and colleagues were able to show that MR766, a strain of the ZIKV, serially passaged in monkey and mosquito cells efficiently infects human neural progenitor cells derived from induced pluripotent stem cells. Infected human neural progenitor cells further release infectious ZIKV

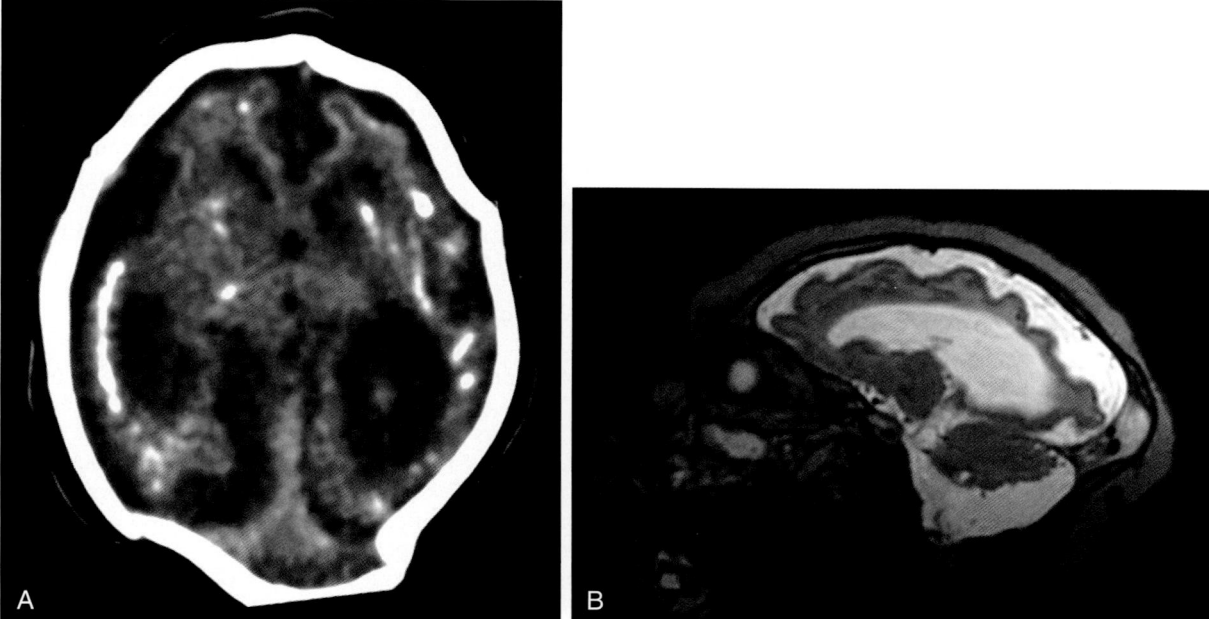

Figure 34.40 Zika virus infection. (A) Axial computed tomography performed on day 2 of life, and (B) sagittal T2-weighted magnetic resonance images obtained at 4 months of age, following infection of the mother during the third month of pregnancy. Cerebrospinal fluid immunoglobulin M was positive for Zika virus. The computed tomography scan (A) shows ventriculomegaly and extensive subcortical band-like calcification as well as calcification in the central gray nuclei. The magnetic resonance image (B) shows enlarged extracerebral space, a simplified gyral pattern, and cerebellar hypoplasia. Note that magnetic resonance imaging does not show the extensive calcification as clearly as computed tomography. (Images courtesy Dr. Vanessa van der Linden.)

particles. Importantly, ZIKV infection increases cell death and dysregulates cell cycle progression, attenuating the growth of human neural progenitor cells. These results identify human neural progenitor cells as a direct ZIKV target.[849] Garcez and colleagues used human-induced pluripotent stem cells cultured as neural stem cells, neurospheres, and brain organoids to study the effect of ZIKV infection during neurogenesis and growth.[850] Human-induced pluripotent-derived neural stem cells were exposed to ZIKV. After 24 hours, ZIKV was detected in neural stem cells and viral RNA was also detected in the supernatant of infected neural stem cells. To investigate the effects of ZIKV during neural differentiation, mock- and ZIKV-infected neural stem cells were cultured as neurospheres. While mock-infected neural stem cells generated round neurospheres after 3 days in vitro, ZIKV-infected neural stem cells generated neurospheres with morphological abnormalities and cell detachment. Apoptotic nuclei, a hallmark of cell death, were observed in all ZIKV-infected neurospheres analyzed. Furthermore, brain organoids derived from human-induced pluripotent stem cells that were exposed to ZIKV and observed for 11 days in vitro showed that the average growth area of ZIKV-exposed organoids was reduced by 40% compared with brain organoids under mock conditions.

Following termination of pregnancy, two fetuses have been described in detail.[838,840] The first pregnancy was terminated at 21 weeks following a ZIKV infection around the 11th week of pregnancy. Microscopy showed abundant apoptosis primarily affecting the intermediately differentiated postmigratory neurons in the neocortex. In contrast, the well-differentiated neurons of the basal ganglia and limbic regions as well as primitive cells in the germinal matrix appeared to be unaffected. There was diffuse infiltration of macrophages in the cerebral cortex, subventricular zone, white matter, and leptomeninges but not in the germinal matrix of the ganglionic eminence. There were no viral inclusions, perivascular inflammatory infiltrates, or signs of ventriculitis or viral encephalitis.[840] The autopsy of the other fetus was performed following termination of pregnancy at 32 weeks of gestation. The maternal infection occurred at 13 weeks of gestation, and antenatal ultrasound at 29 weeks showed severe intracranial pathology. The postmortem examination showed almost complete agyria, hydrocephalus, and multifocal dystrophic calcifications in the cortex and subcortical white matter with mild focal inflammation. Calcifications were also found in the placenta, but no ZIKV was noted in any of the other organs, suggesting a strong neurotropism of the virus.[838] Importantly, ZIKV was found in the fetal brain tissue on rtPCR. The most prominent histopathological features were multifocal collections of filamentous, granular, and neuron-shaped calcifications in the cortex and subcortical white matter with focal involvement of the whole cortical ribbon, occasionally associated with cortical displacement. Diffuse astrogliosis was present with focal astrocytic outburst into the subarachnoid space, mostly on the convexity of the cerebral hemispheres. The cerebellum, brain stem, and spinal cord showed neither inflammation nor dystrophic calcifications.[838] In another series of five cases—including two newborn infants with microcephaly and severe arthrogryposis who died shortly after birth, one 2-month-old infant, and two placentas (from spontaneous abortions)—formalin-fixed paraffin-embedded tissue samples were examined. Histopathological assessment of the brains showed microcalcifications, scattered microglial nodules, cell degeneration, and necrosis. The antigens of ZIKV were localized

in the cytoplasm of degenerating and necrotic neurons and glial cells and were associated with microcalcifications in all three fatal cases with microcephaly. Immunohistochemical testing of first-trimester placental tissue was positive for ZIKV, with immunolocalization in Hofbauer cells in the chorionic villi. Tissues from all five cases were positive for ZIKV.[851,852]

Clinical Diagnosis. Symptoms in women are usually mild; they include fever, a maculopapular rash, conjunctivitis, and arthralgia. Most infections (80%) are said to be asymptomatic. Guillain-Barré syndrome has also now been well documented in affected adults.[853,854] In the largest series reported so far, 602 infants were assessed and classified as definite (76), highly probable (54), moderately probable (181), and somewhat probable (291). Among 183 definite or probable cases whose mothers provided information about the timing of the rash, 141 (77%) of 183 reported occurrence in the first trimester, 33 (18%) in the second trimester, and 9 (5%) in the third trimester. Notably a rash occurring in the third trimester was also associated with brain abnormalities in 9 of the 183 definite or probable cases, whose mothers were able to provide information about the timing of the rash. Brain abnormalities were present in these 9 infants but restricted to calcifications and mild ventriculomegaly (personal communication). Furthermore, in one third of the definite and probable cases, the mother did not have a rash during pregnancy.[855]

Laboratory Diagnosis. During the first 7 days of the illness in the pregnant woman, viral RNA can often be identified in serum, and rtPCR is the preferred diagnostic test. Fragments of ZIKV genome have been identified in saliva, breast milk, urine, and serum of two mothers and their newborn babies within 4 days of delivery, supportive of perinatal transmission.[833] The whole genome of ZIKV has also been isolated directly from the amniotic fluid during pregnancy.[835] Virus-specific IgM antibodies may be detectable more than 3 days after the onset of illness. However, serum collected within 7 days of illness onset may not have detectable virus-specific IgM antibodies; therefore IgM testing should be repeated on a convalescent-phase sample to rule out infection in patients with a compatible clinical syndrome. IgM antibodies against ZIKV, dengue viruses, and other flaviviruses (e.g., yellow fever and WNV) have strong cross-reactivity, possibly generating false-positive results in serological tests.[856]

Neurodiagnostic Studies

A large series was recently reported by the Brazilian Society of Medical Genetics–Zika Embryopathy Task Force (SBGM–ZETF); it included clinical and neuroimaging information on 35 infants with microcephaly (≥2 SD below the mean for GA and sex of the infant at birth) following ZIKV infection.[846] Overall, 26 (74%) mothers of infants with microcephaly reported a rash, 21 during the first trimester and 5 during the second trimester. Twenty-five (74%) infants had severe microcephaly (>3 SD below the mean for GA). *CT* scans and transfontanellar *ultrasonography* showed a consistent pattern of widespread brain calcifications, mainly in periventricular, parenchymal, thalamic, and basal ganglia regions, associated in approximately one third of cases with evidence of neuronal migration abnormalities (e.g., lissencephaly, pachygyria) (Table 34.50). Excessive and redundant scalp skin, reported in 11 (31%) cases, also suggests acute intrauterine arrest in cerebral growth but not in the growth of scalp skin. Of these 11 infants, 4 (11%) had arthrogryposis. Another large CT study comprised 23 infants with congenital microcephaly; here the clinical and epidemiological data were compatible with congenital ZIKV infection.[857] CSF samples were available for serological testing in 7 of the 23 infants, and ZIKV IgM antibodies were positive in all seven samples. Intracranial calcifications were seen in all the infants, mainly involving the frontal and the parietal lobes. The calcifications were mostly punctate with a band-like distribution and located at the corticomedullary junction. In more than half of the infants, calcifications were present in the basal ganglia but were less often seen in the thalami. Ventriculomegaly was seen in all and was severe in more than half of the infants. Cortical hypogyration was present in all infants and cerebellar hypoplasia in 74%. The most detailed case series[858] reported CT and MRI findings in another 23 infants with microcephaly and presumed ZIKV-related infection. Of the 23 infants, 15 underwent CT only, 7 both CT and MRI, and 1 MRI only.

Of the 23 mothers, 22 were able to recall whether they had had a rash during pregnancy; all reported a rash—17 (77%) in the first trimester, 5 (23%) in the second trimester, and none in the third trimester. As for the infants, 20 of the 23 (87%) were born at term and 9 (39%) were small for GA. The anterior fontanelle was closed in 20 (87%) infants at the first clinical examination. Of the 22 children who underwent CT, all had calcifications in the junction between cortical and subcortical white matter, 21 (95%) had malformations of cortical development, 20 (91%) had a decrease in brain volume, 19 (86%) had ventriculomegaly, and 11 (50%) had hypoplasia of the cerebellum or brain stem. Of the eight children who underwent MRI, all had calcifications in the junction between cortical and subcortical white matter, malformations of cortical development occurring predominantly in the frontal lobes, and ventriculomegaly. Of the eight (88%) children who underwent MRI, seven had an enlarged cisterna magna, seven (88%) had delayed myelination, and six (75%) had a moderate to severe decrease in brain volume, simplified gyral pattern, and abnormalities of the corpus callosum (38% hypogenesis and 38% hypoplasia). Malformations were symmetrical in 75% of the cases. The largest series reported so far included 45 infants, 17 with confirmed and 28 with presumed congenital ZIKV infections.[859] Of these, 12 had a fetal MRI, 42 postnatal CT, and 11 a postnatal MRI. Imaging findings were similar for the two groups, with ventriculomegaly in 16 of 17 (94%) and 27 of 28 (96%) infections, respectively; abnormalities of the corpus callosum in 16 of 17 (94%) and 22 of 28 (78%) infections, respectively; and cortical migrational abnormalities in 16 of 17 (94%) and 28 of 28 (100%) infections, respectively. Three infants did not have microcephaly in the presence of severe ventriculomegaly. As previously reported, calcifications were predominantly seen at the gray-white matter junction but were also commonly seen in the central gray nuclei. Notably, septation of the occipital horns of the lateral ventricles was observed in eight infants, an imaging finding that, until now, was considered typical of congenital CMV infection. Imaging data from six studies are summarized in Table 34.51.

TABLE 34.50 Neurological Symptoms in Infants With Microcephaly Following Zika Virus Infection (n = 35)

Neurological examination

Any abnormality	17 (49%)
Hypertonia/spasticity	12 (37%)
Hyperreflexia	7 (20%)
Irritability	7 (20%)
Tremors	4 (11%)
Seizures	3 (9%)

Neuroimaging (n = 27)

Any abnormality	27 (100%)
Calcifications	20 (74%)
Ventricular enlargement	12 (44%)
Neuronal migrational disorders (lissencephaly, pachygyria)	9 (33%)

Adjusted from Schuler-Faccini L, Ribeiro EM, Feitosa IM, et al. Possible association between Zika virus infection and microcephaly—Brazil, 2015. *MMWR Morb Mortal Wkly Rep.* 2016;65:59-62.

TABLE 34.51 Imaging Findings in Infants With Zika Virus Infection (n = 134)

ABNORMALITIES	STUDY 1 n = 27	STUDY 2 n = 23	STUDY 3 n = 23	STUDY 4 n = 45	STUDY 5 n = 13	STUDY 6 n = 3	ALL STUDIES APPROXIMATE FREQUENCIES n = 134
Calcifications	20 (74%)	23 (100%)	23 (100%)	45 (100%)	12 (92%)	3 (100%)	94%
Ventricular enlargement	12 (44%)	23 (100%)	20 (87%)	43 (96%)	13 (100%)	3 (100%)	85%
Migrational abnormalities	9 (33%)	18 (78%)	22 (96%)	44 (98%)	13 (100%)	3 (100%)	81%
Cerebellar hypoplasia	—	17 (74%)	6 (26%)	35 (78%)	0	2 (67%)	56% (107)
Decreased brain volume	—	—	21 (91%)	45 (100%)	13 (100%)	3 (100%)	98% (84)
Septation	—	—	—	8 (18%)	5 (38%)	2 (67%)	24% (61)
Corpus callosum hypoplasia	—	—	6/8 (75%) with MRI	38 (84%)	13 (100%)	1 (33%)	—

Data from Schuler-Faccini L, Ribeiro EM, Feitosa IM, et al. Possible association between Zika virus infection and microcephaly—Brazil, 2015. *MMWR Morb Mort Wkly Rep.* 2016;65:59-62;Hazin AN, Poretti A, Cruz DD, et al. Computed tomographic findings in microcephaly associated with Zika virus. *N Engl J Med.* 2016;374:2193-2195; de Fatima Vasco Aragao M, van der Linden V, Brainer-Lima AM, et al. Clinical features and neuroimaging (CT and MRI) findings in presumed Zika virus related congenital infection and microcephaly: retrospective case series study. *BMJ.* 2016;353:i1901; Soares de Oliveira-Szejnfeld P, Levine D, Melo AS, et al. Congenital brain abnormalities and Zika virus: what the radiologist can expect to see prenatally and postnatally. *Radiology.* 2016;281:203-218; Cavalheiro S, Lopez A, Serra S, et al. Microcephaly and Zika virus: neonatal neuroradiological aspects. *Child Nerv System.* 2016;32:1057-1060; Guillemette-Artur P, Besnard M, Eyrolle-Guignot D, Jouannic JM, Garel C. Prenatal brain MRI of fetuses with Zika virus infection. *Pediatr Radiol.* 2016;46:1032-1039.

Postnatal Infection. There is also evidence that ZIKV may be transmitted through blood transfusion and by sexual transmission.[860,861]

Prognosis

Relation to Time of Infection. Data on outcome are still limited but do indicate a strong relation to the degree of involvement of the CNS, which is most severe when the infection takes place during the first trimester. Termination of pregnancy is considered when antenatal neuroimaging shows severe microcephaly associated with calcifications and migrational disorders. The outcome is likely to be as severe or even more so as seen in infants with a severe CMV infection.

Management. No antiviral agents are available for treatment, and no vaccine has been developed. Pregnant women are advised to avoid mosquito exposure by covering their skin and using mosquito repellent. Moreover, the WHO and the USCDC have cautioned pregnant women to avoid travel to endemic areas. Several countries have suggested that women of childbearing age defer pregnancy.

KEY REFERENCES

7. Revello MG, Tibaldi C, Masuelli G, et al. Prevention of primary cytomegalovirus infection in pregnancy. *EBio Medicine.* 2015;2:1205-1210.

10. Josephson CD, Caliendo AM, Easley KA, et al. Blood transfusion and breast milk transmission of cytomegalovirus in very low-birth-weight infants: a prospective cohort study. *JAMA Pediatr.* 2014;168:1054-1062.

13. Brecht KF, Goelz R, Bevot A, Krageloh-Mann I, Wilke M, Lidzba K. Postnatal human cytomegalovirus infection in preterm infants has long-term neuropsychological sequelae. *J Pediatr.* 2015;166:834. e1-839.e1.

17. Britt W. Controversies in the natural history of congenital human cytomegalovirus infection: the paradox of infection and disease in offspring of women with immunity prior to pregnancy. *Med Microbiol Immunol.* 2015;204:263-271.

18. Dollard SC, Grosse SD, Ross DS. New estimates of the prevalence of neurological and sensory sequelae and mortality associated with congenital cytomegalovirus infection. *Rev Med Virol.* 2007;17:355-363.

20. Enders G, Daiminger A, Bader U, Exler S, Enders M. Intrauterine transmission and clinical outcome of 248 pregnancies with primary cytomegalovirus infection in relation to gestational age. *J Clin Virol.* 2011;52:244-246.

21. Foulon I, Naessens A, Foulon W, Casteels A, Gordts F. Hearing loss in children with congenital cytomegalovirus infection in relation to the maternal trimester in which the maternal primary infection occurred. *Pediatrics.* 2008;122:e1123-e1127.

24. Picone O, Vauloup-Fellous C, Cordier AG, et al. A series of 238 cytomegalovirus primary infections during pregnancy: description and outcome. *Prenat Diagn.* 2013;33:751-758.

32. Lanzieri TM, Dollard SC, Bialek SR, Grosse SD. Systematic review of the birth prevalence of congenital cytomegalovirus infection in developing countries. *Int J Infect Dis.* 2014;22:44-48.

33. Gaytant MA, Rours GI, Steegers EA, Galama JM, Semmekrot BA. Congenital cytomegalovirus infection after recurrent infection: case reports and review of the literature. *Eur J Pediatr.* 2003;162:248-253.

36. Boppana SB, Rivera LB, Fowler KB, Mach M, Britt WJ. Intrauterine transmission of cytomegalovirus to infants of women with preconceptional immunity. *N Engl J Med.* 2001;344:1366-1371.

41. Hamprecht K, Maschmann J, Vochem M, Dietz K, Speer CP, Jahn G. Epidemiology of transmission of cytomegalovirus from mother to preterm infant by breastfeeding. *Lancet.* 2001;357:513-518.

42. Yasuda A, Kimura H, Hayakawa M, et al. Evaluation of cytomegalovirus infections transmitted via breast milk in preterm infants with a real-time polymerase chain reaction assay. *Pediatrics.* 2003;111:1333-1336.

47. Lanzieri TM, Dollard SC, Josephson CD, Schmid DS, Bialek SR. Breast milk-acquired cytomegalovirus infection and disease in VLBW and premature infants. *Pediatrics.* 2013;131:e1937-e1945.

55. Malinger G, Lev D, Zahalka N, et al. Fetal cytomegalovirus infection of the brain: the spectrum of sonographic findings. *AJNR Am J Neuroradiol.* 2003;24:28-32.

58. van der Knaap MS, Vermeulen G, Barkhof F, Hart AA, Loeber JG, Weel JF. Pattern of white matter abnormalities at MR imaging: use of polymerase chain reaction testing of Guthrie cards to link pattern with congenital cytomegalovirus infection. *Radiology.* 2004;230:529-536.

63. Oosterom N, Nijman J, Gunkel J, et al. Neuro-imaging findings in infants with congenital cytomegalovirus infection: relation to trimester of infection. *Neonatology.* 2015;107:289-296.

83. Boppana SB, Fowler KB, Pass RF, et al. Congenital cytomegalovirus infection: association between virus burden in infancy and hearing loss. *J Pediatr.* 2005;146:817-823.

87. Rivera LB, Boppana SB, Fowler KB, Britt WJ, Stagno S, Pass RF. Predictors of hearing loss in children with symptomatic congenital cytomegalovirus infection. *Pediatrics.* 2002;110:762-767.

88. Ross SA, Fowler KB, Ashrith G, et al. Hearing loss in children with congenital cytomegalovirus infection born to mothers with preexisting immunity. *J Pediatr.* 2006;148:332-336.

101. Boppana SB, Ross SA, Shimamura M, et al. Saliva polymerase-chain-reaction assay for cytomegalovirus screening in newborns. *N Engl J Med.* 2011;364:2111-2118.

103. Pinninti SG, Ross SA, Shimamura M, et al. Comparison of saliva PCR assay versus rapid culture for detection of congenital cytomegalovirus infection. *Pediatr Infect Dis J.* 2015;34:536-537.

107. Noyola DE, Demmler GJ, Nelson CT, et al. Early predictors of neurodevelopmental outcome in symptomatic congenital cytomegalovirus infection. *J Pediatr.* 2001;138:325-331.

116. Capretti MG, Lanari M, Tani G, et al. Role of cerebral ultrasound and magnetic resonance imaging in newborns with congenital cytomegalovirus infection. *Brain Dev.* 2014;36:203-211.

118. Picone O, Simon I, Benachi A, Brunelle F, Sonigo P. Comparison between ultrasound and magnetic resonance imaging in assessment of fetal cytomegalovirus infection. *Prenat Diagn.* 2008;28:753-758.

119. Averill LW, Kandula VV, Akyol Y, Epelman M. Fetal brain magnetic resonance imaging findings in congenital cytomegalovirus infection with postnatal imaging correlation. *Semin Ultrasound CT MR.* 2015;36:476-486.

121. Lipitz S, Yinon Y, Malinger G, et al. Risk of cytomegalovirus-associated sequelae in relation to time of infection and findings on prenatal imaging. *Ultrasound Obstet Gynecol.* 2013;41:508-514.

125. Kimberlin DW, Lin CY, Sanchez PJ, et al. Effect of ganciclovir therapy on hearing in symptomatic congenital cytomegalovirus disease involving the central nervous system: a randomized, controlled trial. *J Pediatr.* 2003;143:16-25.

126. Goderis J, De Leenheer E, Smets K, Van Hoecke H, Keymeulen A, Dhooge I. Hearing loss and congenital CMV infection: a systematic review. *Pediatrics.* 2014;134:972-982.

128. Cannie MM, Devlieger R, Leyder M, et al. Congenital cytomegalovirus infection: contribution and best timing of prenatal MR imaging. *Eur Radiol.* 2016;26:3760-3769.

130. Dreher AM, Arora N, Fowler KB, et al. Spectrum of disease and outcome in children with symptomatic congenital cytomegalovirus infection. *J Pediatr.* 2014;164:855-859.

133. Ancora G, Lanari M, Lazzarotto T, et al. Cranial ultrasound scanning and prediction of outcome in newborns with congenital cytomegalovirus infection. *J Pediatr.* 2007;150:157-161.

142. Forner G, Abate D, Mengoli C, Palu G, Gussetti N. High cytomegalovirus (CMV) DNAemia predicts CMV sequelae in asymptomatic congenitally infected newborns born to women with primary infection during pregnancy. *J Infect Dis.* 2015;212:67-71.

153. Revello MG, Lazzarotto T, Guerra B, et al. A randomized trial of hyperimmune globulin to prevent congenital cytomegalovirus. *N Engl J Med.* 2014;370:1316-1326.

164. Kimberlin DW, Jester PM, Sanchez PJ, et al. Valganciclovir for symptomatic congenital cytomegalovirus disease. *N Engl J Med.* 2015;372:933-943.

165. Bilavsky E, Shahar-Nissan K, Pardo J, Attias J, Amir J. Hearing outcome of infants with congenital cytomegalovirus and hearing impairment. *Arch Dis Child.* 2016;101:433-438.

183. Wallon M, Garweg JG, Abrahamowicz M, et al. Ophthalmic outcomes of congenital toxoplasmosis followed until adolescence. *Pediatrics.* 2014;133:e601-e608.

186. Berrebi A, Assouline C, Bessieres MH, et al. Long-term outcome of children with congenital toxoplasmosis. *Am J Obstet Gynecol.* 2010;203:552.e1-552.e6.

189. Thiebaut R, Leproust S, Chene G, Gilbert R. Effectiveness of prenatal treatment for congenital toxoplasmosis: a meta-analysis of individual patients' data. *Lancet.* 2007;369:115-122.

193. Olariu TR, Remington JS, Montoya JG. Polymerase chain reaction in cerebrospinal fluid for the diagnosis of congenital toxoplasmosis. *Pediatr Infect Dis J.* 2014;33:566-570.

201. Malinger G, Werner H, Rodriguez Leonel JC, et al. Prenatal brain imaging in congenital toxoplasmosis. *Prenat Diagn.* 2011;31:881-886.

206. Gras L, Wallon M, Pollak A, et al. Association between prenatal treatment and clinical manifestations of congenital toxoplasmosis in infancy: a cohort study in 13 European centres. *Acta Paediatr.* 2005;94:1721-1731.

214. McLeod R, Boyer K, Karrison T, et al. Outcome of treatment for congenital toxoplasmosis, 1981–2004: the National Collaborative Chicago-Based, Congenital Toxoplasmosis Study. *Clin Infect Dis.* 2006;42:1383-1394.

219. Bloom S, Rguig A, Berraho A, et al. Congenital rubella syndrome burden in Morocco: a rapid retrospective assessment. *Lancet.* 2005;365:135-141.

222. Papania MJ, Wallace GS, Rota PA, et al. Elimination of endemic measles, rubella, and congenital rubella syndrome from the Western hemisphere: the US experience. *JAMA Pediatr.* 2014;168:148-155.

245. Toizumi M, Motomura H, Vo HM, et al. Mortality associated with pulmonary hypertension in congenital rubella syndrome. *Pediatrics.* 2014;134:e519-e526.

259. Reef SE, Strebel P, Dabbagh A, Gacic-Dobo M, Cochi S. Progress toward control of rubella and prevention of congenital rubella syndrome—worldwide, 2009. *J Infect Dis.* 2011;204:S24-S27.

260. Bouthry E, Picone O, Hamdi G, Grangeot-Keros L, Ayoubi JM, Vauloup-Fellous C. Rubella and pregnancy: diagnosis, management and outcomes. *Prenat Diagn.* 2014;34:1246-1253.

263. Corey L, Wald A. Maternal and neonatal herpes simplex virus infections. *N Engl J Med.* 2009;361:1376-1385.

265. Melvin AJ, Mohan KM, Schiffer JT, et al. Plasma and cerebrospinal fluid herpes simplex virus levels at diagnosis and outcome of neonatal infection. *J Pediatr.* 2015;166:827-833.

266. Pinninti SG, Angara R, Feja KN, et al. Neonatal herpes disease following maternal antenatal antiviral suppressive therapy: a multicenter case series. *J Pediatr.* 2012;161:134.e1-3-138.e1-3.

267. Brown ZA, Wald A, Morrow RA, Selke S, Zeh J, Corey L. Effect of serologic status and cesarean delivery on transmission rates of herpes simplex virus from mother to infant. *JAMA.* 2003;289:203-209.

268. Kimberlin DW, Lin CY, Jacobs RF, et al. Natural history of neonatal herpes simplex virus infections in the acyclovir era. *Pediatrics.* 2001;108:223-229.

272. Bernstein DI, Bellamy AR, Hook EW 3rd, et al. Epidemiology, clinical presentation, and antibody response to primary infection with herpes simplex virus type 1 and type 2 in young women. *Clin Infect Dis.* 2013;56:344-351.

284. Duin LK, Willekes C, Baldewijns MM, Robben SG, Offermans J, Vles J. Major brain lesions by intrauterine herpes simplex virus infection: MRI contribution. *Prenat Diagn.* 2007;27:81-84.

290. James SH, Kimberlin DW. Neonatal herpes simplex virus infection: epidemiology and treatment. *Clin Perinatol.* 2015;42:47-59, viii.

291. Marquez L, Levy ML, Munoz FM, Palazzi DL. A report of three cases and review of intrauterine herpes simplex virus infection. *Pediatr Infect Dis J.* 2011;30:153-157.

292. Kimberlin DW. Herpes simplex virus infections in neonates and early childhood. *Semin Pediatr Infect Dis.* 2005;16:271-281.

301. Steiner I, Tyler KL. The toll (like receptor 3) to the pathogenesis of herpes simplex encephalitis. *Neurology.* 2014;83:1882-1883.

302. Lim HK, Seppanen M, Hautala T, et al. TLR3 deficiency in herpes simplex encephalitis: high allelic heterogeneity and recurrence risk. *Neurology.* 2014;83:1888-1897.

306. Vossough A, Zimmerman RA, Bilaniuk LT, Schwartz EM. Imaging findings of neonatal herpes simplex virus type 2 encephalitis. *Neuroradiology.* 2008;50:355-366.

315. Kimura H, Futamura M, Ito Y, et al. Relapse of neonatal herpes simplex virus infection. *Arch Dis Child Fetal Neonatal Ed.* 2003;88:F483-F486.

319. Kimberlin DW, Lin CY, Jacobs RF, et al. Safety and efficacy of high-dose intravenous acyclovir in the management of neonatal herpes simplex virus infections. *Pediatrics.* 2001;108:230-238.

322. Lopez-Medina E, Cantey JB, Sanchez PJ. The mortality of neonatal herpes simplex virus infection. *J Pediatr.* 2015;166:1529.e1-1532.e1.

334. Frenkel LM. Challenges in the diagnosis and management of neonatal herpes simplex virus encephalitis. *Pediatrics.* 2005;115:795-797.

340. Okanishi T, Yamamoto H, Hosokawa T, et al. Diffusion-weighted MRI for early diagnosis of neonatal herpes simplex encephalitis. *Brain Dev.* 2015;37:423-431.

342. Bajaj M, Mody S, Natarajan G. Clinical and neuroimaging findings in neonatal herpes simplex virus infection. *J Pediatr.* 2014;165:404.e1-407.e1.

344. Kimberlin DW, Whitley RJ, Wan W, et al. Oral acyclovir suppression and neurodevelopment after neonatal herpes. *N Engl J Med.* 2011;365:1284-1292.

368. Wendel GD Jr, Sheffield JS, Hollier LM, Hill JB, Ramsey PS, Sanchez PJ. Treatment of syphilis in pregnancy and prevention of congenital syphilis. *Clin Infecti Dis.* 2002;35:S200-S209.

370. Michelow IC, Wendel GD Jr, Norgard MV, et al. Central nervous system infection in congenital syphilis. *N Engl J Med.* 2002;346:1792-1798.

396. Su JR, Brooks LC, Davis DW, Torrone EA, Weinstock HS, Weinstock ML. Congenital syphilis: trends in mortality and morbidity in the United States, 1999 through 2013. *Am J Obstet Gynecol.* 2016;214:381.e1-381.e9.

402. Luzuriaga K, Sullivan JL. Prevention of mother-to-child transmission of HIV infection. *Clin Infect Dis.* 2005;40:466-467.

432. Mandelbrot L, Tubiana R, Le Chenadec J, et al. No perinatal HIV-1 transmission from women with effective antiretroviral therapy starting before conception. *Clin Infect Dis.* 2015;61:1715-1725.

433. Biggar RJ, Taha TE, Hoover DR, Yellin F, Kumwenda N, Broadhead R. Higher in utero and perinatal HIV infection risk in girls than boys. *J Acquir Immune Defic Syndr.* 2006;41:509-513.

436. Kourtis AP, Bulterys M, Nesheim SR, Lee FK. Understanding the timing of HIV transmission from mother to infant. *JAMA.* 2001;285:709-712.

442. Coutsoudis A, Dabis F, Fawzi W, et al. Late postnatal transmission of HIV-1 in breast-fed children: an individual patient data meta-analysis. *J Infect Dis.* 2004;189:2154-2166.

447. Lallemant M, Jourdain G, Le Coeur S, et al. Single-dose perinatal nevirapine plus standard zidovudine to prevent mother-to-child transmission of HIV-1 in Thailand. *N Engl J Med.* 2004;351:217-228.

449. Lehman DA, Farquhar C. Biological mechanisms of vertical human immunodeficiency virus (HIV-1) transmission. *Rev Med Virol.* 2007;17:381-403.

450. Biggar RJ, Cassol S, Kumwenda N, et al. The risk of human immunodeficiency virus-1 infection in twin pairs born to infected mothers in Africa. *J Infect Dis.* 2003;188:850-855.

452. Bulterys M, Fowler MG, Van Rompay KK, Kourtis AP. Prevention of mother-to-child transmission of HIV-1 through breast-feeding: past, present, and future. *J Infect Dis.* 2004;189:2149-2153.

487. Speth C, Dierich MP, Sopper S. HIV-infection of the central nervous system: the tightrope walk of innate immunity. *Mol Immunol.* 2005;42:213-228.

489. Chiriboga CA, Fleishman S, Champion S, Gaye-Robinson L, Abrams EJ. Incidence and prevalence of HIV encephalopathy in children with HIV infection receiving highly active anti-retroviral therapy (HAART). *J Pediatr.* 2005;146:402-407.

525. Tardieu M, Mayaux MJ, Seibel N, et al. Cognitive assessment of school-age children infected with maternally transmitted human immunodeficiency virus type 1. *J Pediatr.* 1995;126:375-379.

527. Van Rie A, Harrington PR, Dow A, Robertson K. Neurologic and neurodevelopmental manifestations of pediatric HIV/AIDS: a global perspective. *Eur J Paediatr Neurol.* 2007;11:1-9.

544. Foster CJ, Biggs RL, Melvin D, Walters MD, Tudor-Williams G, Lyall EG. Neurodevelopmental outcomes in children with HIV infection under 3 years of age. *Dev Med Child Neurol.* 2006;48:677-682.

547. Sanchez-Ramon S, Resino S, Bellon Cano JM, Ramos JT, Gurbindo D, Munoz-Fernandez A. Neuroprotective effects of early antiretrovirals in vertical HIV infection. *Pediatr Neurol.* 2003;29:218-221.

551. Mitchell CD. HIV-1 encephalopathy among perinatally infected children: neuropathogenesis and response to highly active antiretroviral therapy. *Ment Retard Dev Disabil Res Rev.* 2006; 12:216-222.

552. Lindsey JC, Malee KM, Brouwers P, Hughes MD. Neurodevelopmental functioning in HIV-infected infants and young children before and after the introduction of protease inhibitor-based highly active antiretroviral therapy. *Pediatrics.* 2007;119:e681-e693.

553. Willen EJ. Neurocognitive outcomes in pediatric HIV. *Ment Retard Dev Disabil Res Rev.* 2006;12:223-228.

555. Smith R, Malee K, Charurat M, et al. Timing of perinatal human immunodeficiency virus type 1 infection and rate of neurodevelopment. The Women and Infant Transmission Study Group. *Pediatr Infect Dis J.* 2000;19:862-871.

572. Read JS. Diagnosis of HIV-1 infection in children younger than 18 months in the United States. *Pediatrics.* 2007;120:e1547-e1562.

585. Cohen S, Caan MW, Mutsaerts HJ, et al. Cerebral injury in perinatally HIV-infected children compared to matched healthy controls. *Neurology.* 2016;86:19-27.

587. Liu KL, Peters V, Weedon J, Thomas P, Dominguez K. Sex differences in morbidity and mortality among children with perinatally acquired human immunodeficiency virus infection in New York City. *Arch Pediatr Adolesc Med.* 2004;158:1187-1188.

593. Coovadia H. Antiretroviral agents—how best to protect infants from HIV and save their mothers from AIDS. *N Engl J Med.* 2004;351:289-292.

597. Jourdain G, Ngo-Giang-Huong N, Le Coeur S, et al. Intrapartum exposure to nevirapine and subsequent maternal responses to nevirapine-based antiretroviral therapy. *N Engl J Med.* 2004;351:229-240.

603. Taha TE, Kumwenda NI, Gibbons A, et al. Short postexposure prophylaxis in newborn babies to reduce mother-to-child transmission of HIV-1: NVAZ randomised clinical trial. *Lancet.* 2003;362:1171-1177.

604. Tuomala RE, Shapiro DE, Mofenson LM, et al. Antiretroviral therapy during pregnancy and the risk of an adverse outcome. *N Engl J Med.* 2002;346:1863-1870.

611. McComsey GA, Leonard E. Metabolic complications of HIV therapy in children. *AIDS.* 2004;18:1753-1768.

612. Barret B, Tardieu M, Rustin P, et al. Persistent mitochondrial dysfunction in HIV-1-exposed but uninfected infants: clinical screening in a large prospective cohort. *AIDS.* 2003;17:1769-1785.

613. Tardieu M, Brunelle F, Raybaud C, et al. Cerebral MR imaging in uninfected children born to HIV-seropositive mothers and perinatally exposed to zidovudine. *AJNR Am J Neuroradiol.* 2005;26:695-701.

615. Martin SC, Wolters PL, Toledo-Tamula MA, Zeichner SL, Hazra R, Civitello L. Cognitive functioning in school-aged children with vertically acquired HIV infection being treated with highly active antiretroviral therapy (HAART). *Dev Neuropsychol.* 2006;30:633-657.

632. Coovadia HM, Brown ER, Fowler MG, et al. Efficacy and safety of an extended nevirapine regimen in infant children of breastfeeding mothers with HIV-1 infection for prevention of postnatal HIV-1 transmission (HPTN 046): a randomised, double-blind, placebo-controlled trial. *Lancet.* 2012;379:221-228.

633. Sibiude J, Mandelbrot L, Blanche S, et al. Association between prenatal exposure to antiretroviral therapy and birth defects: an analysis of the French perinatal cohort study (ANRS CO1/CO11). *PLoS Med.* 2014;11:e1001635.

634. Williams PL, Crain MJ, Yildirim C, et al. Congenital anomalies and in utero antiretroviral exposure in human immunodeficiency virus-exposed uninfected infants. *JAMA Pediatr.* 2015;169:48-55.

635. Bissel SJ, Auer RN, Chiang CH, et al. Human parechovirus 3 meningitis and fatal leukoencephalopathy. *J Neuropathol Exp Neurol.* 2015;74:767-777.

638. Verboon-Maciolek MA, Groenendaal F, Cowan F, Govaert P, van Loon AM, de Vries LS. White matter damage in neonatal enterovirus meningoencephalitis. *Neurology.* 2006;66:1267-1269.

639. Verboon-Maciolek MA, Krediet TG, Gerards LJ, de Vries LS, Groenendaal F, van Loon AM. Severe neonatal parechovirus infection and similarity with enterovirus infection. *Pediatr Infect Dis J.* 2008;27:241-245.

642. Harvala H, Simmonds P. Human parechoviruses: biology, epidemiology and clinical significance. *JClinVirol.* 2009;45:1-9.

644. Joki-Korpela P, Hyypia T. Parechoviruses, a novel group of human picornaviruses. *Ann Med.* 2001;33:466-471.

649. Boivin G, Abed Y, Boucher FD. Human parechovirus 3 and neonatal infections. *Emerg Infect Dis.* 2005;11:103-105.

650. Benschop KS, Schinkel J, Minnaar RP, et al. Human parechovirus infections in Dutch children and the association between serotype and disease severity. *Clin Infect Dis.* 2006;42:204-210.

656. Feuer R, Pagarigan RR, Harkins S, Liu F, Hunziker IP, Whitton JL. Coxsackievirus targets proliferating neuronal progenitor cells in the neonatal CNS. *J Neurosci.* 2005;25:2434-2444.

660. Freund MW, Kleinveld G, Krediet TG, van Loon AM, Verboon-Maciolek MA. Prognosis for neonates with enterovirus myocarditis. *Arch Dis Child Fetal Neonatal Ed.* 2010;95:F206-F212.

666. Wikswo ME, Khetsuriani N, Fowlkes AL, et al. Increased activity of Coxsackievirus B1 strains associated with severe disease among young infants in the United States, 2007-2008. *Clin Infect Dis.* 2009;49:e44-e51.

667. Centers for Disease Control and Prevention (CDC). Nonpolio enterovirus and human parechovirus surveillance—United States, 2006-2008. *MMWR Morb Mortal Wkly Rep.* 2010;59:1577-1580.

668. Harvala H, McLeish N, Kondracka J, McIntyre CL, et al. Comparison of human parechovirus and enterovirus detection frequencies in cerebrospinal fluid samples collected over a 5-year period in Edinburgh: HPeV type 3 identified as the most common picornavirus type. *J Med Virol.* 2011;83:889-896.

671. Piralla A, Mariani B, Stronati M, Marone P, Baldanti F. Human enterovirus and parechovirus infections in newborns with sepsis-like illness and neurological disorders. *Early Hum Dev.* 2014;90:S75-S77.

673. Wolthers KC, Benschop KS, Schinkel J, et al. Human parechoviruses as an important viral cause of sepsislike illness and meningitis in young children. *Clin Infect Dis.* 2008;47:358-363.

679. Triantafilou K, Vakakis E, Orthopoulos G, et al. TLR8 and TLR7 are involved in the host's immune response to human parechovirus 1. *Eur J Immunol.* 2005;35:2416-2423.

680. Kadhim H, Tabarki B, De Prez C, Rona AM, Sebire G. Interleukin-2 in the pathogenesis of perinatal white matter damage. *Neurology.* 2002;58:1125-1128.

681. Ma Y, Haynes RL, Sidman RL, Vartanian T. TLR8: an innate immune receptor in brain, neurons and axons. *Cell Cycle.* 2007;6:2859-2868.

682. Volpe JJ. Neonatal encephalitis and white matter injury: more than just inflammation? *Ann Neurol.* 2008;64:232-236.

683. Ma Y, Li J, Chiu I, et al. Toll-like receptor 8 functions as a negative regulator of neurite outgrowth and inducer of neuronal apoptosis. *J Cell Biol.* 2006;175:209-215.

684. Haynes RL, Borenstein NS, Desilva TM, et al. Axonal development in the cerebral white matter of the human fetus and infant. *J Comp Neurol.* 2005;484:156-167.

686. Sedmak G, Nix WA, Jentzen J, et al. Infant deaths associated with human parechovirus infection in Wisconsin. *Clin Infect Dis.* 2010;50:357-361.

696. Wu T, Fan XP, Wang WY, Yuan TM. Enterovirus infections are associated with white matter damage in neonates. *J Paediatr Child Health.* 2014;50:817-822.

697. Britton PN, Dale RC, Nissen MD, et al. Parechovirus encephalitis and neurodevelopmental outcomes. *Pediatrics.* 2016;137:1-11.

706. Abzug MJ, Michaels MG, Wald E, et al. A randomized, double-blind, placebo-controlled trial of pleconaril for the treatment of neonates with enterovirus sepsis. *J Pediatr Infect Dis Soc.* 2015;5:53-62.

707. Abzug MJ, Cloud G, Bradley J, et al. Double blind placebo-controlled trial of pleconaril in infants with enterovirus meningitis. *Pediatr Infect Dis J.* 2003;22:335-341.

709. Khandaker G, Marshall H, Peadon E, et al. Congenital and neonatal varicella: impact of the national varicella vaccination programme in Australia. *Arch Dis Child.* 2011;96:453-456.

714. Brunell PA. Varicella in pregnancy, the fetus, and the newborn: problems in management. *J Infect Dis.* 1992;166:S42-S47.
721. Mandelbrot L. Fetal varicella—diagnosis, management, and outcome. *Prenat Diagn.* 2012;32:511-518.
724. Sauerbrei A, Wutzler P. The congenital varicella syndrome. *J Perinatol.* 2000;20:548-554.
728. Huang YC, Lin TY, Lin YJ, Lien RI, Chou YH. Prophylaxis of intravenous immunoglobulin and acyclovir in perinatal varicella. *Eur J Pediatr.* 2001;160:91-94.
738. Petignat P, Vial Y, Laurini R, Hohlfeld P. Fetal varicella-herpes zoster syndrome in early pregnancy: ultrasonographic and morphological correlation. *Prenat Diagn.* 2001;21:121-124.
741. Sauerbrei A, Pawlak J, Luger C, Wutzler P. Intracerebral varicella-zoster virus reactivation in congenital varicella syndrome. *Dev Med Child Neurol.* 2003;45:837-840.
743. Schulze A, Dietzsch HJ. The natural history of varicella embryopathy: a 25-year follow-up. *J Pediatr.* 2000;137:871-874.
757. Tate JE, Burton AH, Boschi-Pinto C, Steele AD, Duque J, Parashar UD. 2008 estimate of worldwide rotavirus-associated mortality in children younger than 5 years before the introduction of universal rotavirus vaccination programmes: a systematic review and meta-analysis. *Lancet Infect Dis.* 2012;12:136-141.
758. Dickey M, Jamison L, Michaud L, Care M, Bernstein DI, Staat MA. Rotavirus meningoencephalitis in a previously healthy child and a review of the literature. *Pediatr Infect Dis J.* 2009;28:318-321.
767. Ge Y, Mansell A, Ussher JE, et al. Rotavirus NSP4 triggers secretion of proinflammatory cytokines from macrophages via toll-like receptor 2. *J Virol.* 2013;87:11160-11167.
769. Sugata K, Taniguchi K, Yui A, et al. Analysis of rotavirus antigenemia and extraintestinal manifestations in children with rotavirus gastroenteritis. *Pediatrics.* 2008;122:392-397.
772. Lee KY, Oh KW, Weon YC, Choi SH. Neonatal seizures accompanied by diffuse cerebral white matter lesions on diffusion-weighted imaging are associated with rotavirus infection. *Eur J Paediatr Neurol.* 2014;18:624-631.
773. Verboon-Maciolek MA, Truttmann AC, Groenendaal F, et al. Development of cystic periventricular leukomalacia in newborn infants after rotavirus infection. *J Pediatr.* 2012;160:165.e1-168.e1.
774. Yeom JS, Kim YS, Seo JH, et al. Distinctive pattern of white matter injury in neonates with rotavirus infection. *Neurology.* 2015;84:21-27.
775. Oh KW, Moon CH, Lee KY. Association of rotavirus with seizures accompanied by cerebral white matter injury in neonates. *J Child Neurol.* 2015;30:1433-1439.
780. Payne DC, Baggs J, Zerr DM, et al. Protective association between rotavirus vaccination and childhood seizures in the year following vaccination in US children. *Clin Infect Dis.* 2014;58(2):173-177.
782. Young NS, Brown KE. Parvovirus B19. *N Engl J Med.* 2004;350:586-597.
784. Enders M, Klingel K, Weidner A, et al. Risk of fetal hydrops and non-hydropic late intrauterine fetal death after gestational parvovirus B19 infection. *J Clin Virol.* 2010;49:163-168.
785. Enders M, Weidner A, Zoellner I, Searle K, Enders G. Fetal morbidity and mortality after acute human parvovirus B19 infection in pregnancy: prospective evaluation of 1018 cases. *Prenat Diagn.* 2004;24:513-518.
794. Glenn OA, Bianco K, Barkovich AJ, Callen PW, Parer JT. Fetal cerebellar hemorrhage in parvovirus-associated non-immune hydrops fetalis. *J Matern Fetal Neonatal Med.* 2007;20:769-772.
797. Pistorius LR, Smal J, de Haan TR, et al. Disturbance of cerebral neuronal migration following congenital parvovirus B19 infection. *Fetal Diagn Ther.* 2008;24:491-494.
798. Schulert GS, Walsh WF, Weitkamp JH. Polymicrogyria and congenital parvovirus b19 infection. *AJP Rep.* 2011;1:105-110.
799. Nagel HT, de Haan TR, Vandenbussche FP, Oepkes D, Walther FJ. Long-term outcome after fetal transfusion for hydrops associated with parvovirus B19 infection. *Obstet Gynecol.* 2007;109:42-47.
800. Dembinski J, Haverkamp F, Maara H, Hansmann M, Eis-Hubinger AM, Bartmann P. Neurodevelopmental outcome after intrauterine red cell transfusion for parvovirus B19-induced fetal hydrops. *BJOG.* 2002;109:1232-1234.
801. De Jong EP, Lindenburg IT, van Klink JM, et al. Intrauterine transfusion for parvovirus B19 infection: long-term neurodevelopmental outcome. *Am J Obstet Gynecol.* 2012;206:204.e1-205.e1.
804. Bonthius DJ, Nichols B, Harb H, Mahoney J, Karacay B. Lymphocytic choriomeningitis virus infection of the developing brain: critical role of host age. *Ann Neurol.* 2007;62:356-374.
808. Bonthius DJ, Wright R, Tseng B, et al. Congenital lymphocytic choriomeningitis virus infection: spectrum of disease. *Ann Neurol.* 2007;62:347-355.
813. Bonthius DJ. Lymphocytic choriomeningitis virus: an underrecognized cause of neurologic disease in the fetus, child, and adult. *Semin Pediatr Neurol.* 2012;19:89-95.
816. Cao-Lormeau VM, Musso D. Emerging arboviruses in the Pacific. *Lancet.* 2014;384:1571-1572.
818. Centers for Disease Control and Prevention (CDC). Intrauterine West Nile virus infection—New York, 2002. *MMWR Morb Mortal Wkly Rep.* 2002;51:1135-1136.
819. Smith JC, Mailman T, MacDonald NE. West Nile virus: should pediatricians care? *J Infect.* 2014;69:S70-S76.
820. O'Leary DR, Kuhn S, Kniss KL, et al. Birth outcomes following West Nile Virus infection of pregnant women in the United States: 2003-2004. *Pediatrics.* 2006;117:e537-e545.
823. Weaver SC, Lecuit M. Chikungunya virus and the global spread of a mosquito-borne disease. *N Engl J Med.* 2015;372:1231-1239.
825. Gerardin P, Barau G, Michault A, et al. Multidisciplinary prospective study of mother-to-child chikungunya virus infections on the island of La Reunion. *PLoS Med.* 2008;5:e60.
826. Gerardin P, Samperiz S, Ramful D, et al. Neurocognitive outcome of children exposed to perinatal mother-to-child Chikungunya virus infection: the CHIMERE cohort study on Reunion Island. *PLoS Negl Trop Dis.* 2014;8:e2996.
828. Fauci AS, Morens DM. Zika virus in the Americas—yet another arbovirus threat. *N Engl J Med.* 2016;374:601-604.
836. Cauchemez S, Besnard M, Bompard P, et al. Association between Zika virus and microcephaly in French Polynesia, 2013-15: a retrospective study. *Lancet.* 2016;387:2125-2132.
837. Oliveira Melo AS, Malinger G, Ximenes R, Szejnfeld PO, Alves Sampaio S, Bispo de Filippis AM. Zika virus intrauterine infection causes fetal brain abnormality and microcephaly: tip of the iceberg? *Ultrasound Obstet Gynecol.* 2016;47:6-7.
838. Mlakar J, Korva M, Tul N, et al. Zika virus associated with microcephaly. *N Engl J Med.* 2016;374:951-958.
839. Werner H, Fazecas T, Guedes B, et al. Intrauterine Zika virus infection and microcephaly: perinatal imaging correlations with 3D virtual physical models. *Ultrasound Obstet Gynecol.* 2016;47:657-660.
840. Driggers RW, Ho CY, Korhonen EM, et al. Zika virus infection with prolonged maternal viremia and fetal brain abnormalities. *N Engl J Med.* 2016;374:2142-2151.
841. Ventura CV, Maia M, Bravo-Filho V, Gois AL, Belfort R Jr. Zika virus in Brazil and macular atrophy in a child with microcephaly. *Lancet.* 2016;387:228.
842. Ventura CV, Maia M, Ventura BV, et al. Ophthalmological findings in infants with microcephaly and presumable intra-uterus Zika virus infection. *Arq Bras Oftalmol.* 2016;79:1-3.
845. Brasil P, Pereira JP Jr, Raja Gabaglia C, et al. Zika virus infection in pregnant women in Rio de Janeiro—preliminary report. *N Engl J Med.* 2016;375:2321-2334.
849. Tang H, Hammack C, Ogden SC, et al. Zika virus infects human cortical neural progenitors and attenuates their growth. *Cell Stem Cell.* 2016;18:587-590.
857. Hazin AN, Poretti A, Cruz DD, et al. Computed tomographic findings in microcephaly associated with Zika virus. *N Engl J Med.* 2016;374:2193-2195.

Full references for this chapter can be found on www.expertconsult.com.

Bacterial and Fungal Intracranial Infections

Linda S. de Vries ◆ *Joseph J. Volpe*

Bacterial infections of the central nervous system (CNS) in the newborn are common and are of major clinical importance. By far the most frequent of these infections is neonatal bacterial meningitis, and this chapter deals with this disorder in detail. Other bacterial processes include primary intracranial infections (e.g., epidural and subdural empyema and brain abscess) and disorders in which involvement of the CNS is secondary to extraneural infection (e.g., subacute bacterial endocarditis with focal embolic encephalitis, neonatal botulism, and neonatal tetanus). Because most of these bacterial diseases are exceedingly rare, and one (botulism) is discussed in Chapter 32, only brain abscess and neonatal tetanus are discussed in this chapter. Systemic candidiasis, a disseminated fungal infection, is also discussed briefly (rather than in Chapter 34) because the manifestations thereof, which include meningitis and brain abscess, are related more closely to the subject matter of this chapter.

BACTERIAL MENINGITIS

Bacterial meningitis is the most common and serious variety of neonatal intracranial bacterial infection. In most cases, bacterial meningitis is associated with recognizable bacteremia (i.e., sepsis). The disorder is usually fulminating in evolution but is amenable to therapeutic intervention. Indeed, prompt recognition and appropriate therapy of bacterial meningitis are major challenges in the care of the neonatal patient.

Early-Onset and Late-Onset Bacterial Sepsis and Meningitis

Certain basic and common themes recur in any discussion of neonatal bacterial sepsis and meningitis. Perhaps most prominent of these themes is the dual pattern of illness observed with the major etiological agents for neonatal bacterial meningitis (see following discussion). Thus, early-onset and late-onset disease can often be readily distinguished (Table 35.1).[1-20] In *early-onset disease* (i.e., onset usually in the first days of life), infection appears to be derived near the time of delivery from an infected birth canal. Understandably, obstetrical complications are common, and infants are often of low-birth-weight. Multisystemic manifestations are prominent. In *late-onset disease* (i.e., onset usually after the first few days of life), the infection may still have been acquired from the mother but frequently is acquired from contacts with infected medical personnel, other infants, contaminated equipment, and vascular access devices or other materials. Meningitis is often the dominant manifestation of late-onset disease.

The major bacterial causes of early- versus late-onset sepsis are shown in Table 35.2. Group B *Streptococcus* (GBS) is the most prominent early-onset pathogen, whereas *E.coli* has been shown to be the most common pathogen for early-onset sepsis in very-low-birth-weight (VLBW) infants. Coagulase-negative *Staphylococcus* (CONS) becomes very prominent in late-onset sepsis, especially sepsis after very long hospital stays (>30 days). These organisms are part of the normal skin and mucosal flora and induce infection in the presence of prolonged indwelling vascular catheters and related features of neonatal intensive care, especially of very premature infants. *Pseudomonas* and related gram-negative organisms that contaminate moist ventilatory equipment also become prominent in late-onset sepsis. *Escherichia coli* and *Klebsiella* species account for 20% to 25% of both early-onset and late-onset cases. Although the causes of neonatal meningitis reflect the causes of neonatal sepsis, the relative proportions for each organism differ somewhat because of the varying propensity to invade the CNS (see later).

In the ensuing discussion, the etiology, pathogenesis, neuropathology, clinical features, diagnostic aspects, prognosis, and management of neonatal bacterial *meningitis* are reviewed. Particular emphasis is placed on aspects most relevant to neonatal neurology. Where relevant, the discussion centers on specific aspects related to a particular organism, but in general the features of neonatal bacterial meningitis caused by most organisms exhibit more similarities than differences.

Etiology

The major organisms associated with neonatal meningitis and their relative frequency as current etiological agents are shown in Table 35.3.[5,10,12,21-30] Although relative frequencies vary somewhat from one medical center to another and over time, the data are at least representative of cases largely in medical centers in North America. GBS is the single most commonly encountered organism, with *E. coli* second.[19] *Listeria monocytogenes* is the third most common organism and accounts for approximately 5% of cases in most series in North America.[31] The remaining cases are accounted for principally by other streptococcal and staphylococcal species, by other gram-negative enteric bacilli, and by a variety of unusual organisms. Particular note should be made of the role of *Staphylococcus aureus* and *S. epidermidis* (CONS) in the presence of indwelling catheters, particularly in association with neurosurgical procedures, and the role of *Proteus* species, *Pseudomonas aeruginosa*, *Serratia marcescens*, *Bacillus cereus*, and *Flavobacterium meningosepticum* in the presence of respiratory devices using moist inhalation. An occasional newborn infant develops meningitis secondary to

TABLE 35.1 Major Features of Early-Onset and Late-Onset Bacterial Sepsis-Meningitis[a]

MAJOR FEATURE	EARLY-ONSET DISEASE	LATE-ONSET DISEASE
Usual age of onset	First 72 hours	>7 days
Obstetrical complications	Common	Uncommon
Dominant clinical signs referable to sepsis and respiratory disease	Common	Uncommon
Dominant clinical signs referable to meningitis	Uncommon	Common
Mode of transmission	Mother to infant	Mother to infant
		Human contacts, equipment, vascular access devices, and so forth
Specific serotype	Uncommon	Common

[a]See text for references.

TABLE 35.2 Bacterial Etiology of Early-Onset and Late-Onset Neonatal Sepsis[a]

	PERCENTAGE OF TOTAL	
ORGANISM	EARLY-ONSET SEPSIS	LATE-ONSET SEPSIS
Group B beta-hemolytic streptococci	50%	5%
Group D streptococci	5%	10%
Coagulase-negative staphylococci	5%	40%[b]
Staphylococcus aureus	5%	10%
Escherichia coli, Klebsiella species	25%	20%
Pseudomonas, Serratia	0%	10%
Miscellaneous	10%	5%

[a]See text for references.
[b]More common in cases with onset after 30 days, especially in low-birth-weight infants.
Most data from references 14, 16, and 17.

TABLE 35.3 Bacterial Etiology of Neonatal Meningitis[a]

BACTERIAL ETIOLOGY	PERCENTAGE OF TOTAL
Group B Streptococcus	50%
Other streptococci and staphylococci (including especially group D streptococci, Streptococcus pneumoniae, Staphylococcus epidermidis,[b] and Staphylococcus aureus)	5%
Escherichia coli	25%
Other gram-negative enteric bacteria (including Pseudomonas aeruginosa, Klebsiella and Enterobacter species, Proteus species, Citrobacter species, and Serratia marcescens)	10%
Listeria monocytogenes	5%
Other (including Haemophilus influenzae, Salmonella species, and Flavobacterium meningosepticum)	5%

[a]See text for references.
[b]Coagulase-negative staphylococci are particularly common etiologies in very-low-birth-weight infants with late-onset meningitis.

Haemophilus influenzae, Salmonella, Pasteurella multocida, Vibrio cholerae, Mycoplasma hominis, or several other less commonly known organisms.[5,21-27,32-56]

Pathogenesis

Meningitis is more common in premature infants than in full-term infants and in the first months of life than in succeeding months.[34] Because the final common pathway in the pathogenetic sequence is almost always bacteremia leading to meningitis, a close association exists between the causes and rates of neonatal sepsis and neonatal meningitis. The association is not perfect, however, because certain organisms are particularly efficient at invading the CNS (see later). Sepsis occurs at a rate of approximately 1.5 per 1000 live births, and meningitis occurs at a rate of approximately 0.3 per 1000 live births.[52,53] Thus neonatal meningitis is an important problem, and a clear understanding of its pathogenesis will be critical for attempts to reduce the enormity of the problem in the future.

TABLE 35.4 Neonatal Sepsis-Meningitis: Predisposing Factors Related to Pregnancy and Delivery

Complications of labor and delivery
Maternal peripartum infection, especially of the genital or urinary tract
Prolonged rupture of membranes
Chorioamnionitis

Factors Related to Pregnancy and Delivery

Most cases of neonatal sepsis and meningitis, especially those of early onset, are related to acquisition of bacteria during labor or delivery, after rupture of membranes. Acquisition is principally by parturitional exposure or, less commonly, ascending infection (e.g., after prolonged rupture of membranes). Thus, it is not surprising that important factors predisposing to sepsis and meningitis include a variety of complications of labor and delivery (especially fetal distress, obstetrical trauma, and placental abnormalities), maternal peripartum infection (especially of the genital or urinary tracts), prolonged rupture of membranes, and chorioamnionitis (Table 35.4).[a]

Maternal urinary tract infection associated with neonatal sepsis and meningitis is usually gram-negative, and maternal genital infection associated with these neonatal disorders is usually with GBS. Indeed, genital infection secondary to GBS (usually asymptomatic) is identifiable at delivery in approximately 15% to 35% of women.[58,61,65-73] Approximately 40% to 70% of infants delivered to such women become colonized at one or more mucocutaneous sites (e.g., ear, throat, rectum, and umbilicus). Approximately 2% to 4% of such colonized infants exhibit invasive, early-onset GBS disease. The incidence is particularly high (8%) in heavily colonized infants (i.e., those found to have three to four positive mucocutaneous sites). Following the introduction of preventive guidelines in New Zealand, a decrease in the incidence of invasive early onset GBS disease from 0.5 in the late 1990s to 0.23 per 1000 live births in 2009 to 2011 was shown.[74] A decrease by more than 80% from 1.8 cases per 1000 live births in the early 1990s to 0.26 cases per 1000 live births in 2010 was shown in the United States. However, the guidelines had no effect on the incidence of late-onset disease.[75]

Factors related to pregnancy and delivery are also particularly important in the pathogenesis of early-onset neonatal listeriosis.[31,76-84] Thus various obstetrical complications are present in the history of approximately half of such patients, and in most cases maternal isolates of serotypes identical to those infecting the infants have been found. In the majority of cases of early-onset neonatal listeriosis, a maternal history of flu-like syndrome, unexplained fever, or urinary tract symptoms in the several days to weeks before delivery can be elicited. In keeping with probable fecal–oral transmission of this organism, epidemics of maternal infection during pregnancy and subsequent neonatal listeriosis have been associated with the consumption of contaminated foods.[82,84] Indeed, unlike the other varieties of neonatal meningitis, listeriosis probably occurs commonly by transplacental passage, as evidenced by the finding of well-developed placentitis with recognizable organisms in carefully studied cases.[78,81]

Factors Related to the Infant

Significant host factors operative in the newborn period relate particularly to defense mechanisms versus bacterial infection. In early life, immunity is characterized by age-dependent adaptations of both innate and adaptive immune responses. The first-line host defense is formed by innate immune cells recognizing pathogens by unique molecular patterns with pathogen recognition receptors. Innate immune responses include opsonization, complement activation, secretion of inflammatory mediators, and induction of apoptosis.[85-87] The adaptive immune system depends on antigen recognition and comprises particularly the function of T and B cells.[86,87]

Innate Immunity. Age-dependent adaptations of innate immunity include the following: impaired leukocyte chemotaxis, phagocytosis, and bactericidal activity; defective neutrophilic metabolic responses after phagocytosis (e.g., activation of the hexose monophosphate shunt and, especially, oxidative metabolism, with diminished generation of the critical bactericidal hydroxyl radical); impaired costimulatory capacity of antigen-presenting cells (dendritic cell populations and monocytes) and decreased production of proinflammatory cytokines on stimulation of Toll-like receptors (TLRs); lower cytotoxic capacity of neonatal natural killer (NK) cells and γδ–T cells than in adults; and diminished concentrations of several complement components.[57,67,71,88-97] Moreover, lower fibronectin concentrations in the newborn appear to contribute to diminished opsonization and phagocytosis.[98,99] These adaptations are accentuated and especially affect immune function in premature infants and in infants subjected to illnesses of diverse types.

Adaptive Immunity. Studies of T cells in cord blood demonstrate qualitative and quantitative differences in immune responses compared with adult T cells, and these differences are diminished only gradually during infancy.[100-103] T cells generally express a naive phenotype but differentiate easily into regulatory T cells.[104,105] In addition, T-cell lineage differentiation begins in utero and is highly controlled by epigenetic regulation, which is interestingly influenced by environmental factors.[104,106,107]

Neonatal B cells have a naïve phenotype and have only a partially developed surface immunoglobulin repertoire. Deficiencies of specific humoral immunity have involved the immunoglobulin M (IgM) and immunoglobulin G (IgG) classes of antibodies.[108-112] The latter are transferred passively across the placenta, particularly in the third trimester.[108] Thus some premature infants may have decreased levels of IgG antibodies.[112] IgM and immunoglobulin A (IgA) are not transferred passively across the placenta and are in very low concentrations in the normal newborn. IgM antibodies include several antibody types that are important in the defense against gram-negative bacteria; deficiency of these antibodies in the newborn infant may play a role in the susceptibility to gram-negative bacteria.[109] IgA antibodies are abundant at later ages at mucosal surfaces (e.g., the respiratory and gastrointestinal tracts); their deficiency in the newborn may explain in part the relative ease with which mucosal barriers are colonized and penetrated.[110] Newborn infants have diminished production of these antibodies because

---

[a]References 11, 14, 24, 27, 28, and 57-64.

of both immaturity of the antibody-producing B cells and plasma cells and diminished T-cell help for antibody production. The deficiency in immune globulins has led to clinical trials of the use of intravenous immune globulin in the prophylaxis and treatment of bacterial infection in newborns, especially premature newborns.[113-115] This approach has not proven useful for general practice.

Neonates are heavily dependent on innate immune responses for protection against infections. The brain microglial cell, which is derived from monocytes (see Chapter 13), is an important part of this defense. Activation of innate immune cells occurs by way of specific cell-surface receptors (i.e., TLRs), which respond to specific molecular motifs shared by the products of large classes of microorganisms.[116-120] For example, TLR4 is the receptor that recognizes gram-negative bacterial lipopolysaccharide, and TLR2 is the receptor for gram-positive peptidoglycan and lipopeptides. Activation of these receptors triggers an inflammatory response by a mechanism that operates through nuclear factor (NF) kappaB and mitogen-activated protein kinase. A study of newborns has shown that the basal expression of TLR2 (but not TLR4) is slightly lower in neonatal than in adult phagocytes.[120] In infants with sepsis, TLR2 is sharply upregulated, unlike TLR4. A similar disturbance of TLR4 responsiveness was shown in neonatal monocytes as a function of gestational age.[121] Thus the deficits in TLR2 and TLR4 may be relevant to the importance of such gram-positive organisms as GBS and CONS and of such gram-negative organisms as *E. coli* in neonatal sepsis and meningitis. Furthermore, downstream signaling through the MyD88 and p38 pathways is impaired in neonates following TLR2 and TLR4 stimulation.[122,123] High levels of adenosine in neonatal blood may increase cyclic AMP levels and protein kinase A–dependent or independent inhibition of TLR-stimulated TNF-alpha secretion.[85,87,95]

Immunological Aspects of Group B Streptococcal Infection. Immunological studies of perinatal GBS infection illustrated the potential roles of both maternal and host defense factors in pathogenesis.[124-127] Thus, using a sensitive, radioactive antigen-binding assay, Baker and Kasper[128,129] showed that the prevalence of antibody to GBS (capsular polysaccharide of the type III strain) in *mothers* with vaginal colonization was 76% for those whose infants did not develop GBS disease and only 5% for those whose infants did develop GBS sepsis or meningitis. These data suggest that this IgG antibody is important in protecting the infant and that passive transfer across the placenta did not occur because of maternal failure to synthesize the antibody. Moreover, the infants with sepsis or meningitis had low levels of antibody *after* recovery, a finding suggesting that, in addition, these infants also failed to synthesize this IgG component. Similarly, infants who develop GBS sepsis have been shown to exhibit defective humoral (opsonic activity) and neutrophilic responses to their infecting strain.[130]

Factors Related to the Neonatal Environment
Certain factors related to the neonatal environment increase the risk of sepsis and meningitis, including the following: use of inhalation therapy equipment; use of aerosols; use of vascular, umbilical, and intraventricular indwelling catheters; and exposure to nursery personnel, parents, or other infants harboring pathogenic organisms.[3,14,30,127,131-133] Operation of some of these factors may be suggested by the organism causing the sepsis or meningitis, as discussed earlier. Horizontal (or nosocomial) transmission of an organism from human contacts has been studied, particularly for GBS. Thus nosocomial infection rates of up to 40% have been reported, particularly in medical centers where high rates of newborns are already colonized at birth (by vertical transmission from the mother) and where high daily census rates are reported, thereby favoring cross-contamination of infants by nursery personnel.[134,135] The particular importance of factors related to neonatal intensive care is illustrated by the marked increase in CONS infections with increasing time in neonatal intensive care (see Table 35.2). This issue is particularly important in very premature infants, in whom later-onset sepsis is related primarily to CONS and of whom nearly 80% have a central vascular catheter in place at the time of infection.[14] In the subset of very-low-birth-weight infants, CONS are important etiological agents. Indeed, in a series of 134 very-low-birth-weight (<1500 g) infants with meningitis, 76% of whom weighed less than 1000 g at birth, 29% had positive cerebrospinal fluid (CSF) and blood cultures for CONS.[136]

Factors Related to the Microorganism
Specific Serotypes Related to Meningitis. The propensity for specific strains of GBS, *E. coli*, and *L. monocytogenes* to be most commonly responsible for neonatal meningitis suggests important pathogenetic roles for the microorganism itself. (Recall the earlier discussion concerning innate immunity and the risk of infection by gram-negative and gram-positive organisms.) Thus serotype III of GBS, K1 strains of *E. coli*, and serotype IVb of *L. monocytogenes* are the predominant specific types of these three bacteria that cause neonatal meningitis (Table 35.5).[1,63,79,83,137] Approximately 70% to 80% of all cases of neonatal meningitis are caused by these three bacterial types.

TABLE 35.5 Relationship Between Severity of Neonatal Infection and Specific Strain of Group B *Streptococcus*, *Escherichia coli*, and *Listeria monocytogenes*

ORGANISM	CLINICAL DISEASE[a]		
	ASYMPTOMATIC	SEPSIS	MENINGITIS
Group B *Streptococcus* serotype III	36%	32%	85%
Escherichia coli K1 strain	12%	39%	84%
Listeria monocytogenes serotype IVb	?	42% (early-onset disease)	78% (late-onset disease)

[a]Data for each clinical disorder expressed as a percentage of total cases (caused by the indicated bacterium) resulting from the specific serotype.
Data from references 1 and 137 and Remington and Klein's Infectious Diseases of the Fetus and Newborn 2016.

TABLE 35.6   Outcome of Neonatal Meningitis Caused by K1 and Non-K1 Strains of *Escherichia coli*

TYPE OF *ESCHERICHIA COLI*	OUTCOME		
	NORMAL	NEUROLOGICAL SEQUELAE	DEATH
Non-K1 strains	8 (89%)	1 (11%)	0
K1 strains	19 (40%)	14 (29%)	15 (31%)

n = 57.

Data from McCracken GH Jr, Sarff LD, Glode MP, Mize SG, et al. Relation between *Escherichia coli* K1 capsular polysaccharide antigen and clinical outcome in neonatal meningitis. *Lancet.* 1974;2:246–250.

Importance of Capsular Polysaccharides. The likelihood that capsular polysaccharides reflect, to a considerable degree, an intrinsic virulence of these organisms is suggested by in vivo and in vitro observations.[30,126,127,137-141] Studies with immature rats have demonstrated, for K1 strains of *E. coli* relative to other *E. coli* strains, a high virulence, particularly regarding bacteremia and meningitis, that was age-related.[138] The younger the animal, the greater was the likelihood of serious disease. Moreover, investigators showed that GBS type III and K1 strains of *E. coli* have distinctive capsules that contain polysaccharide with sialic acid in high concentration (≥25% of total carbohydrate).[129,137,139,140] (This distinctive polysaccharide for *E. coli* is termed *K1*, hence the name *K1 strain*.) A relation of the capsular polysaccharide antigen to virulence is suggested by the different outcomes of *E. coli* meningitis secondary to K1 and non-K1 strains (Table 35.6).[142] In addition to a marked preponderance of cases secondary to K1 strains, whereas 60% of reported infants with meningitis secondary to K1 strains died or exhibited neurological sequelae, only 11% of infants with meningitis secondary to non-K1 strains exhibited the poor outcome (see Table 35.6). A protein component of the outer membrane of the K1 strain of *E. coli*, OmpA, was also shown to be critical for the capacity of this strain to penetrate brain endothelial cells and thus to cause intracranial infection.[143] The relation of the capsular polysaccharide antigen to virulence is supported further by the studies reviewed previously, relating the occurrence of GBS type III neonatal disease to the deficiency in the mother and in the newborn of antibody against the specific capsular polysaccharide of that organism.

Neuropathology

Major Features

The neuropathology of bacterial meningitis may be considered in terms of acute and chronic changes (Table 35.7). Moreover, certain additional histological features are particularly characteristic of infection with specific organisms; these features are discussed separately.

Acute Changes

The acute changes of bacterial meningitis are dramatic and include arachnoiditis, ventriculitis, vasculitis, cerebral edema, infarction, and associated encephalopathy (see Table 35.7).[89,144-146] Because the hallmark of the disease is arachnoiditis, this aspect is discussed first; however, the neuropathological progression of neonatal bacterial meningitis probably begins with choroid plexitis and ventriculitis (Fig. 35.1). Arachnoiditis is discussed first because it is the dominant feature of bacterial meningitis.

TABLE 35.7   Major Neuropathological Features of Neonatal Bacterial Meningitis

Acute
Arachnoiditis
Ventriculitis: choroid plexitis
Vasculitis
Cerebral edema
Infarction
Associated encephalopathy (cortical neuronal necrosis, periventricular leukomalacia)

Chronic
Hydrocephalus
Multicystic encephalomalacia porencephaly
Cerebral cortical and white matter atrophy
Cerebral cortical developmental (organizational) defects (?)

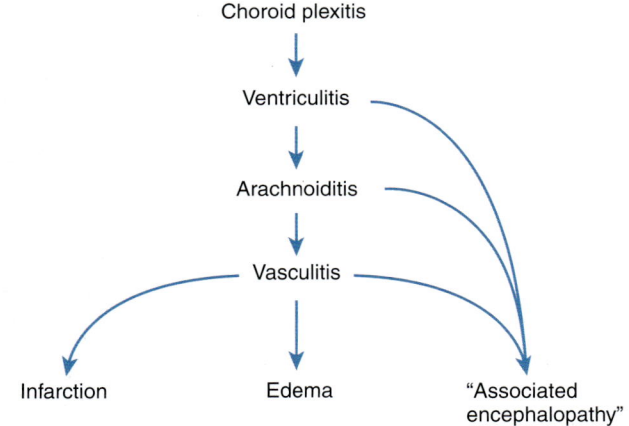

Figure 35.1 Neuropathological progression of neonatal bacterial meningitis. The process probably begins with choroid plexitis and ventriculitis. The pathogenesis of associated encephalopathy, especially cerebral cortical neuronal injury and periventricular leukomalacia, is detailed in Fig. 35.10.

Arachnoiditis. The hallmark of bacterial meningitis is infiltration of the arachnoid with inflammatory cells. The exudate is predominant over the base of the brain in approximately half of the cases and is distributed more evenly in most of the remainder (Fig. 35.2). The evolution of this inflammatory response is well described by Berman and Banker.[89]

In the acute state (i.e., *approximately the first week*), the predominant cells in the arachnoidal (and ventricular) exudate

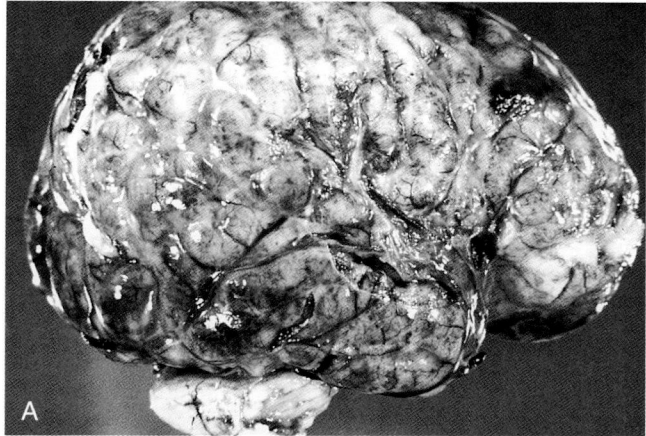

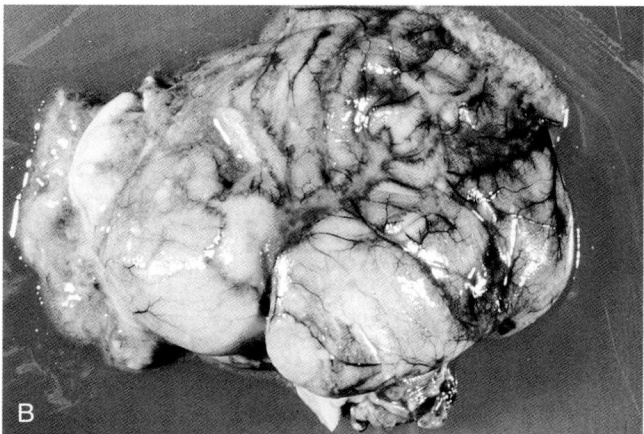

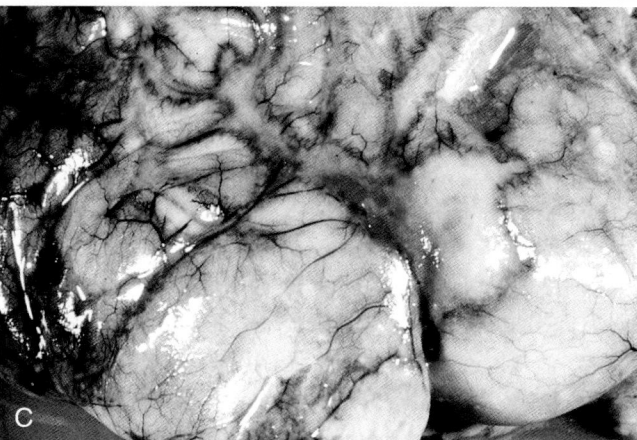

Figure 35.2 Neonatal bacterial meningitis: arachnoidal exudate. (A) From an infant with group B streptococcal meningitis who died at 12 days of age. This right lateral view of the cerebrum shows thick arachnoidal exudate. (B) From an infant who died at 13 days of age with *Escherichia coli* meningitis. This left lateral view of the cerebrum shows thick arachnoidal exudate, especially prominent in the region of the sylvian fissure. (C) Closer view of the exudate in the region of the sylvian fissure. (A, From Bell WE, McCormick WF. *Neurologic Infections in Children*. Philadelphia: Saunders; 1975.)

are polymorphonuclear leukocytes. Bacteria are visible, free, and within polymorphonuclear leukocytes and macrophages. The inflammatory exudate is particularly prominent around blood vessels and extends into the brain parenchyma along the Virchow-Robin space. In *the second and third weeks* of the

disease, the proportion of polymorphonuclear leukocytes decreases gradually and constitutes approximately 25% of the cell population. The predominant cells are now mononuclear, mainly histiocytes and macrophages. Lymphocytes and plasma cells are present in relatively small numbers, and this paucity is a characteristic feature of neonatal meningitis. Whether this apparent deficiency of cells involved in the immunological response plays a role in the relative tenacity of neonatal bacterial meningitis remains to be determined but seems plausible. A prominent feature of this stage of the disease is infiltration of cranial nerve roots by the exudate; particular involvement occurs in the subarachnoid space of the posterior fossa and especially affects cranial nerves III through VIII. This involvement is clinically relevant (see subsequent discussion). *After approximately 3 weeks*, the exudate decreases in amount and consists of mononuclear cells. Thick strands of collagen become apparent as arachnoidal fibrosis begins to develop. This process is probably important in the genesis of the obstructions to CSF flow that result in hydrocephalus.

The characteristics of the arachnoiditis caused by different bacteria vary little. However, *early-onset* GBS meningitis is accompanied by *much less arachnoidal inflammation* than is late-onset meningitis.[126] Indeed, approximately 75% of cases of early-onset meningitis (i.e., positive culture results) are said to exhibit little or no evidence of *leptomeningeal inflammation* at autopsy.[126] It is not clear whether the relative lack of arachnoidal inflammatory response relates to rapidity of death after onset of symptoms or to immaturity of host responses to infection within the CNS of premature infants (who represent the largest proportion of fatal cases of early-onset GBS meningitis).

Ventriculitis. *Ventriculitis* (i.e., inflammatory exudate and bacteria in the ventricular fluid and lining) is a particularly common feature of neonatal meningitis. In the 50 brains studied by Berman and Banker[89] and by Gilles et al.,[146] overt ventriculitis was present in 44 (88%). In a collaborative study of 70 infants with meningitis caused by gram-negative bacteria in whom ventricular tap was performed at the time of diagnosis, 51 (73%) had ventriculitis, as manifested by positive cultures with pleocytosis in the ventricular fluid (comparable data are not available for GBS meningitis). Although precise, controlled data are not available, ventriculitis appears to be more common in neonatal meningitis than in meningitis at later ages.[147]

The ventriculitis is initially characterized by exudate most prominent in the *choroid plexus stroma and just external to the plexus* (Fig. 35.3).[67,89,146] Exudative excrescences from the ventricular surface can be visualized in vivo by cranial ultrasonography (see later discussion). In the second and third weeks of the disease course, the ventricular exudate is associated with active ependymitis, characterized by disruption of the ependymal lining and projections of glial tufts into the ventricular lumen. Later, glial bridges may develop and cause obstruction, particularly at the aqueduct of Sylvius (Fig. 35.4). Less commonly, septations in the lateral ventricle may produce a multiloculated state that is similar to abscess formation. The multiple ventricular obstructions, in fact, may *isolate* portions of the lateral ventricles or the fourth ventricle, cause disproportionate and severe dilation of the affected ventricle, and present a difficult therapeutic problem.[148,149] Ventriculitis with obstructive hydrocephalus may

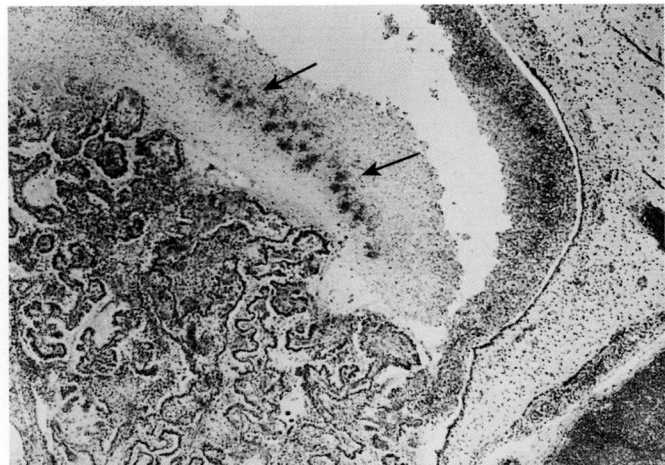

Figure 35.3 Ventriculitis and choroid plexitis from an infant who died of bacterial meningitis in the first month of life. The choroid plexus is in the left lower corner. Plexus stroma is filled with cellular exudate. The lateral ventricle contains a mass of protein-rich cellular exudate and necrotic debris organized into layers. The middle layer *(arrows)* is composed of colonies of bacteria (hematoxylin and eosin, ×60). (From Gilles FH, Jammes JL, Berenberg W. Neonatal meningitis: the ventricle as a bacterial reservoir. *Arch Neurol.* 1977;34:560–562.)

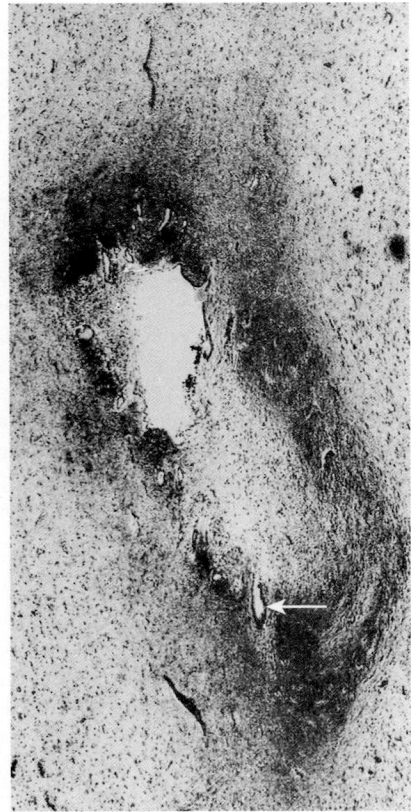

Figure 35.4 Aqueductal obstruction subsequent to ventriculitis from an infant who died of neonatal bacterial meningitis. Stain for glial fibers shows the formation of glial bridges that have narrowed and partially occluded the aqueduct. The lower portion of the aqueduct is reduced to a small slit *(arrow)* (phosphotungstic acid hematoxylin ×100). (From Berman PH, Banker BQ. *Neonatal meningitis: a clinical and pathological study of 29 cases. Pediatrics.* 1966;38:6–24.)

manifest subacutely in newborns (with no history of acute meningitis) after several weeks, especially ventriculitis caused by GBS and *E. coli* meningitis.[150,151]

The nearly uniform occurrence of ventriculitis in acute bacterial meningitis in the newborn has *pathogenetic and therapeutic implications.* Regarding *pathogenesis,* it appears reasonable to suggest that the initial sequence of events in bacterial invasion of the CNS is for hematogenously borne bacteria to localize first in the choroid plexus and to cause choroid plexitis, with subsequent entrance of bacteria into the ventricular system and later movement to the arachnoid through normal CSF flow (see Fig. 35.1). Gilles and co-workers[146] have presented considerable data to support this view, including the high glycogen content of the neonatal choroid plexus, which provides an excellent medium for bacteria. Moreover, an age-related effect is suggested by the postnatal decrease in glycogen content of plexus epithelial cells.[152]

Experimental studies of bacterial meningitis produced in infant rhesus monkeys indicate that infection of the lateral ventricle is a *uniform* feature.[153] Moreover, when discordance between the amount of bacteria in ventricular and subarachnoid CSF samples was observed in these studies of rhesus monkeys, ventricular bacterial densities were greater. These observations further support the notion that the initial events in the genesis of bacterial meningitis are bacteremia and infection of the choroid plexus and lateral ventricles.

The *therapeutic implications* of these data concerning ventriculitis are important and are discussed later, in the section on management. Suffice it to say here that the ventricle may be a major reservoir of bacterial infection, inaccessible either to systemic antibiotics, which are unable to penetrate the purulent covering over the ventricular lining, or to intraventricular antibiotics, which are unable to reach the choroid plexus epithelium (and particularly inaccessible to intrathecal antibiotics, which are unable to reach the ventricles because of normal CSF flow). Moreover, if obstruction of the ventricular system is added (e.g., at the aqueduct), a closed infection, approximating an extraparenchymal abscess, will result.

Vasculitis. Vasculitis is an almost invariable feature of neonatal bacterial meningitis.[89] The involvement of both arteries and veins can be considered an extension of the inflammatory reaction in the arachnoid and within the ventricles. The arteritis is manifested particularly by inflammatory cells in the adventitia; however, involvement of the intima is not uncommon.[26,154] Although the arterial lumen may be narrowed, only rarely is complete occlusion observed. Involvement of veins is severe and includes arachnoidal, cortical, and subependymal veins.[145] In contrast to arterial involvement, phlebitis is frequently complicated by thrombosis and complete occlusion. Multiple fibrin thrombi of adjacent veins are often observed in association with areas of hemorrhagic infarction (see the section on infarction later). The vasculitic changes are apparent in the *first days* of meningitis and become particularly prominent by the second and third weeks.

More similarities than differences exist among various bacteria with regard to the nature and severity of the vascular changes with meningitis. However, vasculitis with thrombosis or even hemorrhage is relatively frequent in early-onset GBS disease, despite the relatively modest arachnoidal inflammation.[126]

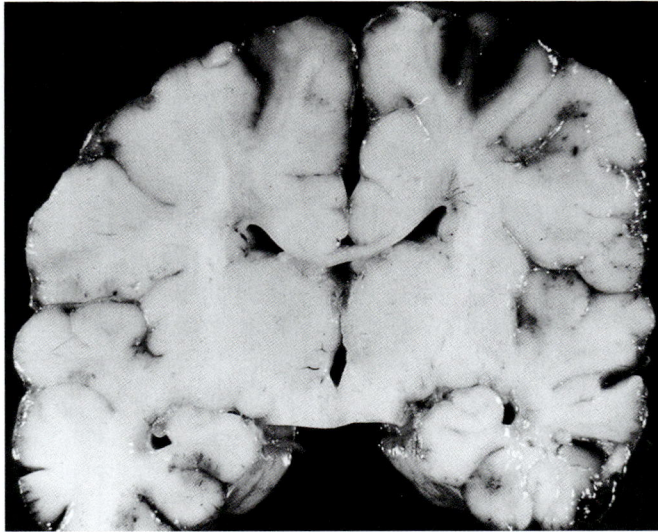

Figure 35.5 Cerebral edema with neonatal bacterial meningitis. Coronal section of the brain from the same infant shown in Fig. 35.2A. Note the diffusely swollen appearance of the cerebral parenchyma, resulting in flattened gyri and small, slit-like ventricles. Purulent material is evident in the ventricles (medial aspect), and a hemorrhagic infarct is apparent in the parasagittal region. (From Bell WE, McCormick WF. *Neurologic Infections in Children*. Philadelphia: Saunders; 1975.)

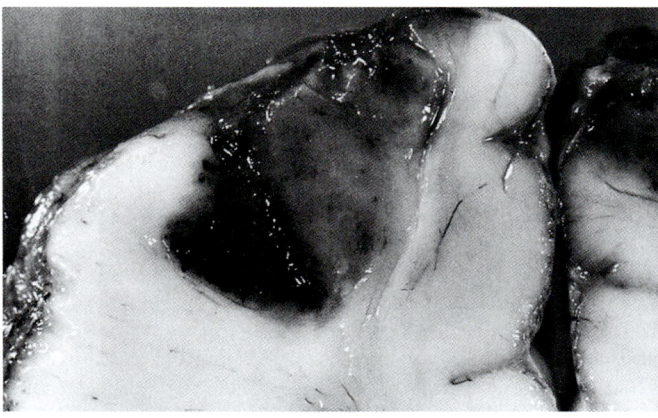

Figure 35.6 Infarction with neonatal bacterial meningitis. Same specimen as shown in Fig. 35.5 but with a higher-power view of the hemorrhagic infarct in the parasagittal region. The lesion was secondary to cortical vein thrombosis. (From Bell WE, McCormick WF. *Neurologic Infections in Children*. Philadelphia: Saunders; 1975.)

TABLE 35.8   Cerebral Infarction in Neonatal Bacterial Meningitis

≈30%–50% of autopsy cases
Associated with thrombi in inflamed meningeal, cortical, and/or subependymal veins; venous sinuses; arteries (*arterial distribution* often suggested by brain imaging findings)
Related to a combination of vasculitis, endothelial injury, thrombotic effects of arachidonic acid metabolites, impaired autoregulation, decreased cerebral perfusion pressure

---

Cerebral Edema. Cerebral edema is a characteristic of the acute stage of neonatal bacterial meningitis (Fig. 35.5). Indeed, the swelling of brain parenchyma is often so severe that the ventricles are reduced to small slits. The difficulty and hazard of performing ventricular puncture in the acute stage are significant because of this phenomenon. The cause of the edema is related primarily to the vasculitis and increased permeability of blood vessels (i.e., vasogenic edema; see Fig. 35.1). This vasogenic component may be complicated by a cytotoxic component, when parenchymal injury occurs (e.g., through infarction), or when impairment of CSF flow results in development of interstitial edema (see later discussion).

Despite the edema, another feature of neonatal bacterial meningitis that is distinctive relative to disease at later ages is the rarity of evidence, clinical or pathological, for herniation of supratentorial structures through the tentorial notch or of cerebellar tonsils into the foramen magnum. This feature may relate to the distensibility of the neonatal cranium, especially because of the separable sutures. This factor may also prevent marked increases in intracranial pressure and therefore impaired cerebral perfusion; studies of intracranial pressure and cerebral blood flow velocity in neonatal bacterial meningitis have supported this suggestion (see later discussion).[155] Nevertheless, lethal uncal and cerebellar tonsillar herniation has been documented in neonatal bacterial meningitis.[156] Moreover, the rare phenomenon of anterior fontanelle herniation has been reported to complicate neonatal meningitis.[157]

Infarction. Infarction may be a prominent and serious feature of neonatal bacterial meningitis (see Fig. 35.1). Studies of autopsy cases indicate an incidence of 30% to 50% (see Table 35.7).[89,144,145] More than half of the infants in Friede's[145] neuropathological series sustained their lesions in the *first week* after the diagnosis of meningitis. Thus, although the vascular lesions become particularly prominent in the second and third weeks, infarction may often be an early event. The lesions are most frequently related to *venous* occlusions and are often hemorrhagic (characteristic of venous infarcts). Occlusion of *multiple adjacent* veins appears to be necessary to result in infarction, as evidenced by the usual demonstration of several thrombosed vessels contiguous to the infarct. The loci of the infarcts are most often cerebral cortex and underlying white matter (Fig. 35.6), although subependymal and deep white matter lesions are not uncommon. Involvement of major cerebral arteries may be more common than previously expected, because brain imaging in living infants not uncommonly demonstrates lesions in an arterial distribution (see later discussion and Table 35.8).[158] In addition, stroke patterns within the distribution of perforating arteries were recently shown to be especially common in neonatal GBS meningitis.[159] The origin of the infarction is related particularly to the vasculitis, in combination with concomitant thrombotic effects of arachidonic acid metabolites (e.g., thromboxanes, platelet-activating factor), impaired cerebrovascular autoregulation, and decreased cerebral perfusion pressure (caused by systemic hypotension, increased intracranial pressure, or both; see later in the section on mechanisms of brain injury). Such a combination of factors presumably could lead to infarction in the presence of vascular narrowing and not necessarily complete thrombotic occlusion.

Although venous or arterial infarction of cerebral structures predominates, involvement of the spinal cord may occur. Indeed, spinal cord necrosis and the clinical picture of a segmental myelopathy may rarely develop. The onset may be delayed, as shown in two infants who developed severe progressive late-onset myelopathy precipitated by a fall following presumed chronic arachnoditis.[160,161]

Associated Encephalopathy. Associated with neonatal bacterial meningitis are parenchymal changes (i.e., *associated encephalopathy*), the causes of which have been elucidated increasingly in recent years (see later in the section on mechanisms of brain injury). The major changes are (1) diffuse gliosis of regions subjacent to inflammatory exudate, (2) neuronal loss in cerebral cortex and several other brain regions, and (3) periventricular leukomalacia. The first change, parenchymal gliosis, is observed in cerebral cortex (molecular layer and superficial cortical layers), cerebellar cortex (molecular layer), brain stem and spinal cord (marginal white matter), and subependymal regions. These various regions are immediately subjacent to the inflammatory exudate and presumably are injured by the toxic and metabolic factors associated with the bacterial process (see later discussion). The clinical significance of the gliosis is not entirely clear. The second and third changes, involving cortical neurons and periventricular white matter, are similar in topography in many ways to hypoxic-ischemic encephalopathy. The cause of these neuronal and white matter lesions probably relates at least in part to *ischemia* (see later discussion and Table 35.9). Moreover, it is likely that concentrations of endotoxin and related cytokines in brain and ventricular fluid are high in gram-negative bacterial meningitis and that the endotoxin could injure cerebral white matter through the *activation of innate immunity* in brain (see later and Chapter 13). A similar conclusion applies to the capsular polysaccharides and proteins of GBS, which have also been shown to be neurotoxic (see Chapter 13). Further data are needed on these issues, because the clinical significance of the neuronal loss and of the white matter injury is almost certainly considerable.

Subdural Effusion and Empyema. One neuropathological feature of neonatal bacterial meningitis, conspicuous by its relative lack of prominence, is subdural effusion.[89,162] The reason for the notable difference in the incidence of significant subdural effusion between meningitis in the newborn and in the infant of 2 to 3 months of age and older is not clear.

Subdural empyema is a very rare acute feature of bacterial meningitis.

TABLE 35.9   Impaired Cerebral Blood Flow in Bacterial Meningitis

Vascular narrowing or obstruction
Vasculitis
Vasospasm
Thrombosis
Increased intracranial pressure
Vasogenic > cytotoxic > interstitial edema
Hydrocephalus
Systemic hypotension
Septic shock
Impaired cerebrovascular autoregulation

Long-Term Changes

The major neuropathological sequelae of neonatal bacterial meningitis are hydrocephalus, multicystic encephalomalacia, and cerebrocortical and white matter atrophy (see Table 35.7).[89,162,163] Experimental observations suggest the possibility of a subsequent impairment in brain development involving organizational events (see later discussion).

Hydrocephalus. In studies of postmortem material, hydrocephalus is apparent in approximately 50% of cases.[89] Of the 14 autopsy cases of hydrocephalus studied carefully by Berman and Banker,[89] the major obstruction to CSF flow appeared to be at the level of the aqueduct in 4, at the outflow of the fourth ventricle in 2, and in the subarachnoid space (i.e., communicating) in 8. Multiple sites of impairment in CSF flow are probable. Ventricular dilation secondary to obstruction to CSF flow should be distinguished from that secondary to loss of cerebral substance. Because both hydrocephalus and cerebral atrophy are usually present concurrently, this distinction may be difficult.

Multicystic Encephalomalacia and Porencephaly. Multicystic encephalomalacia and porencephaly are at the end of the continuum of multifocal parenchymal injury secondary to neonatal bacterial meningitis. The single or multiple cystic areas of destruction in the cerebral hemispheres appear to reflect primarily residua of infarction (Fig. 35.7). In postmortem material, some of the cavities rarely appear to represent abscesses.[145] The implications of multicystic encephalomalacia for neurological outcome are obviously grave.

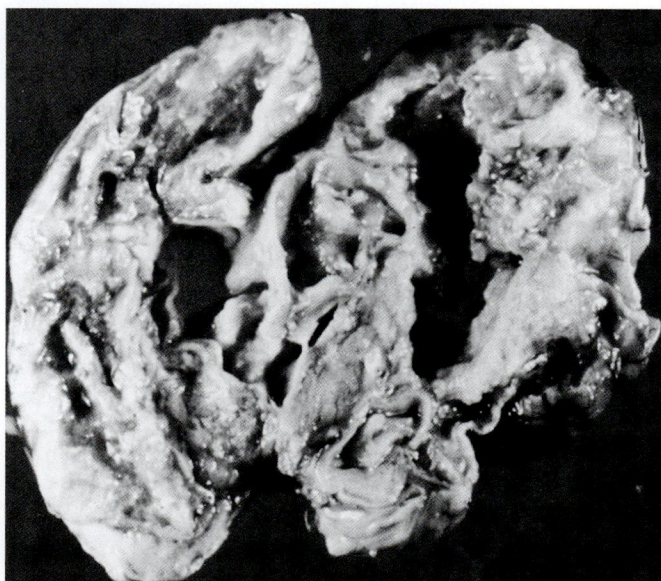

Figure 35.7 Multicystic encephalomalacia following neonatal bacterial meningitis: neuropathology. From an infant with neonatal gram-negative bacterial meningitis who died at 5 weeks of age. This coronal section of the cerebrum shows that the cerebral hemispheres have been converted into a necrotic mass, with many cystic cavities of various sizes. The corpus callosum is necrotic, and the ventricles cannot be delineated from cystic spaces in the brain. (From Bell WE, McCormick WF. *Neurologic Infections in Children.* Philadelphia: Saunders; 1975.)

Cerebral Cortical and White Matter Atrophy. Most commonly, the major neuropathological sequela of neonatal bacterial meningitis is cerebral atrophy, manifested particularly by loss of cerebral cortical neurons and periventricular white matter. This state appears to be a sequela principally of the associated encephalopathy described previously. Neuronal loss in deep cortical layers and myelin loss in the periventricular region, both areas also infiltrated with glial fibers, are the major histological findings.

Possible Cerebral Cortical Developmental (Organizational) Defects. Experimental data suggest that more refined techniques may reveal subsequent aberrations of brain *development* following neonatal bacterial meningitis. In an infant rat model of bacterial meningitis, disturbances of subsequent dendritic arborization and synaptogenesis were observed.[164] Because of the timing of neonatal bacterial meningitis with regard to brain developmental events (see Chapters 5 to 8), it is reasonable to postulate that application of Golgi, immunocytochemical, and electron microscopic techniques to the study of cerebral cortex and myelin of infants who survive the acute state of neonatal meningitis would reveal impairment of cerebral organizational events and perhaps myelination. Further data in this regard would be of particular importance concerning the effects of neonatal bacterial meningitis on subsequent neurological outcome.

Neuropathological Changes Characteristic of Specific Microorganisms

Certain neuropathological changes are particularly characteristic of specific microorganisms (Table 35.10).

***Citrobacter* species, *Serratia marcescens*, *Proteus*, *Pseudomonas*, *Enterobacter*, and *Bacillus cereus* species.** These bacteria have a particular propensity to cause severe cerebral necrosis, usually hemorrhagic (see Table 35.10).[42,163,165-177] In the presence of bacteremia, one consequence of this tissue necrosis is the occurrence of brain abscess. Indeed, the brain abscess may dominate the clinical syndrome, which occasionally may evolve in a less acute fashion than uncomplicated meningitis.[174,176] (The most common organism leading to meningitis complicated by brain abscess is *Citrobacter*, which is discussed later in the section on brain abscess.)

An even more dramatic and malignant form of neonatal bacterial meningitis is caused by *S. marcescens*.[163,178] Widespread hemorrhagic necrosis of cerebral cortex and white matter occurs (Fig. 35.8). Striking invasion of brain parenchyma by bacteria, which can be seen streaming from blood vessels (see Fig. 35.8), is a prominent feature.

A rapid destruction of brain tissue may also occur with *B. cereus* meningoencephalitis, a gram-positive spore-forming rod. The organism has often been considered to be a contaminant but is now recognized as a pathogen in immune-compromised patients.[179] Invasive infections are related to the use of central or peripheral catheters, contaminated dressings, hospital linens, ventilator equipment, balloons used for manual ventilation, and breast milk.[180,181] Following an uneventful initial neonatal period, the infant may become unwell, with signs of sepsis. The disease can be rapidly progressive owing to the production of several toxins (necrotizing enterotoxin, emetic toxin, hemolysin, and phospholipase C), resulting in hemolysis, tissue invasion, and tissue necrosis.[182-184] In a review of 15 newborn infants with neonatal meningitis caused by this organism, the gestational age ranged from 26 to 37 weeks, with birth weights from 830 to 2780 g.[185] Twelve (75%) of the infants died, the majority within 3 days of onset. Of the four who survived infection, one developed cerebral palsy, and the other three had no sequelae. Hemorrhagic necrosis and liquefaction of brain tissue have been reported in postmortem studies. Special stains reveal Gram-variable rods in brain tissue. An important aspect of treatment is recognition that this organism produces beta-lactamase, which renders it resistant to most penicillins and cephalosporins. Treatment involves a combination of vancomycin and an aminoglycoside. Imaging characteristics may show destructive changes of the white matter, cortex, and basal ganglia, which can develop within 12 to 24 hours. Cranial ultrasound shows a typical irregular cauliflower-like pattern with extensive areas of increased echogenicity, followed by rapid cystic evolution (Fig. 35.9). Most infants are unstable and die before they can be transferred to the MR unit. In one study, three infants assessed with MRI showed extensive hemorrhagic lesions in the cerebral white matter on conventional T1- and T2-weighted sequences, as well as areas of restricted diffusion on diffusion-weighted imaging (DWI).[165]

Listeria monocytogenes. Although *L. monocytogenes* may cause typical bacterial meningitis in the newborn, especially in infants with late-onset disease, transplacental infection of the fetus may occur and may produce a particularly fulminating infection.[a] The latter may be manifest in utero and may result in fetal death or in an early-onset, septicemic-type of syndrome. The pathological features of this multifocal variety of listeriosis are miliary granulomatous lesions in many organs, including the CNS (see Table 35.10).[162,163] The characteristic lesion is a necrotizing granuloma, which occurs particularly in the meninges, ventricular walls, and choroid plexus. Granulomata may form microabscesses, and organisms can be demonstrated in the necrotic portions of the lesions. As may be expected, this variety of infection is not readily accessible to antibiotics, and death occurs in 25% to 50% of cases, often in utero. Notably, however, treatment of the *mother* early in her infection can prevent infection and sequelae in the fetus and newborn.[141]

Mechanisms of Brain Injury

The neuropathological features of neonatal bacterial meningitis are caused by the action of a complex series of mechanisms summarized very broadly in Fig. 35.1 and in detail in

---

TABLE 35.10   Additional Neuropathological Changes Caused by Specific Microorganisms

***Citrobacter, Serratia marcescens, Proteus, Pseudomonas, Bacillus cereus, Enterobacter* species**
Tissue necrosis, often hemorrhagic, and/or brain abscess
***Listeria monocytogenes* (transplacental)**
Multifocal granulomata with or without microabscesses

---

aReferences 1, 31, 76-79, 81-84, 141, 162, 163, and 186.

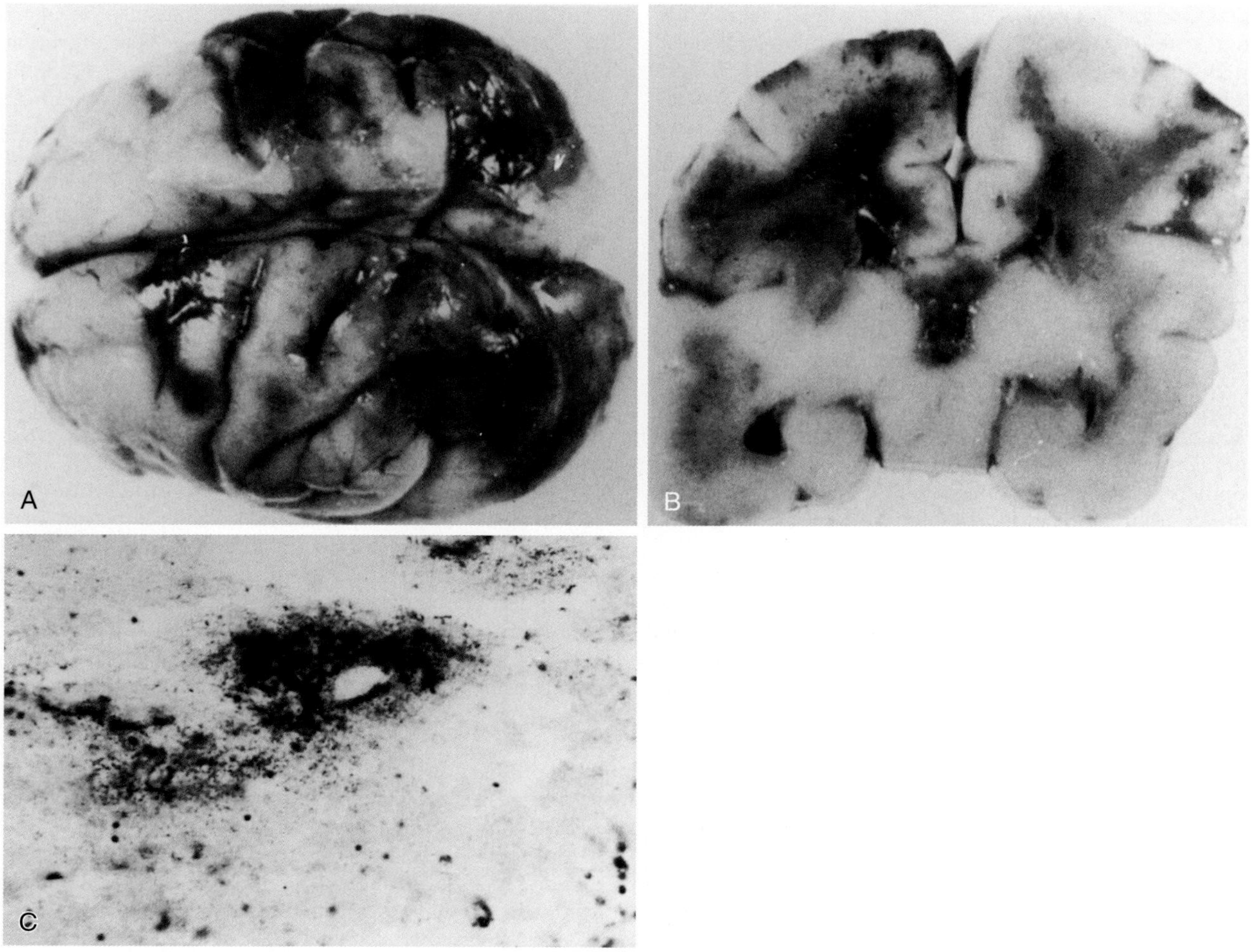

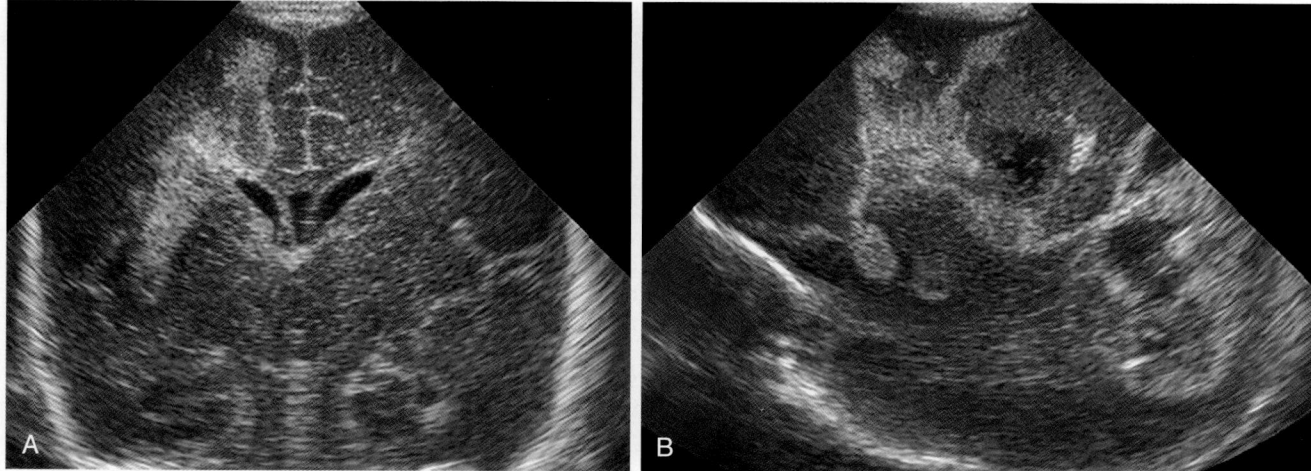

Figure 35.8 Neonatal bacterial meningitis secondary to *Serratia marcescens.* (A and B) Note the regions of hemorrhagic necrosis involving both hemispheres. (C) Gram-negative bacteria can be seen around a small vein and invading the surrounding parenchyma (cresyl violet). (From Larroche JC. *Developmental Pathology of the Neonate.* New York: Excerpta Medica; 1977.)

Figure 35.9 *Bacillus cereus* meningitis. Ultrasound scans coronal (A) and parasagittal views (B) showing an irregular pattern with extensive areas of increased echogenicity in cerebral white matter, with the development of echolucencies seen within 24 hours after the first symptoms of the meningitis.

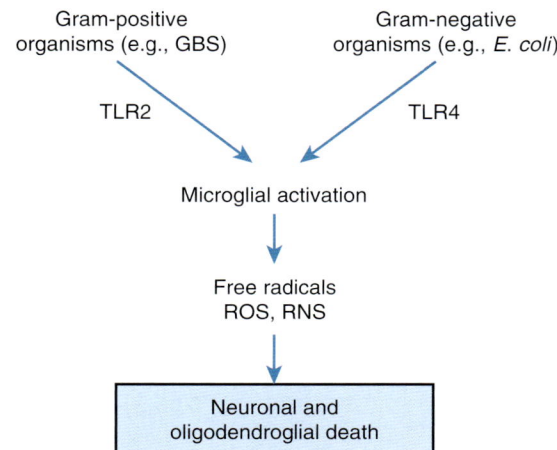

Figure 35.10 Role of the innate immune response in the pathogenesis of neuronal and oligodendroglial death in bacterial meningitis. Microglia contain the two Toll-like receptors that are activated by specific molecular components of gram-positive *(TLR2)* and gram-negative organisms *(TLR4)* (see text). Microglial activation and release of toxic reactive oxygen species *(ROS)* and reactive nitrogen species *(RNS)* lead to cell death in both gray (neuronal) and white (oligodendroglial) matter. *GBS*, Group B streptococci.

Figs. 35.10 and 35.11. The mechanisms shown in Figs. 35.10 and 35.11 represent a summary of more detailed physiological and biochemical processes, described briefly next and based on a variety of studies primarily in animal models and cellular systems but also in human infants.[187-213] The process begins with sepsis, followed by invasion of the CNS; penetration of the bacteria across the blood-brain barrier is one of the most critical steps in the pathogenesis of bacterial meningitis. The role of specific capsular polysaccharides in this invasion is crucial, as discussed earlier. Once the bacteria invade the local tissue barrier and the blood-brain barrier, most pathogens can activate the transcription factor NF-κb, another important feature of bacterial meningitis, resulting in high levels of inflammatory cytokines in the blood and CSF, a result of the stimulation of phagocytic cells. This secretion of proinflammatory cytokines is followed by recruitment of leukocytes into the CNS across the blood-brain barrier.[213] The meningitic process begins with the action of specific bacterial components, especially in gram-positive bacteria, the peptidoglycan layers, the teichoic acid of the cell wall, gram-negative bacteria, and the lipopolysaccharide molecules of the outer cell membrane. Among the early events induced by these products, of particular importance is activation of the immediate immune response (i.e., the *innate immune response*; see Fig. 35.10). As noted earlier, these molecular products of gram-positive organisms (e.g., group B *Streptococcus*) and gram-negative organisms (e.g., *E. coli*) activate specific receptors on brain microglia (the immune cell of the CNS). For gram-positive organisms, the receptor is TLR2, and for gram-negative organisms, it is TLR4. The resulting microglial activation results in several effects, the most important of which is the generation of free radicals, both reactive oxygen and nitrogen species. These reactive compounds ultimately lead to neuronal and oligodendroglial death (see also Chapter 14), the key feature of the associated encephalopathy of neonatal bacterial meningitis. Evidence of

neonatal bacterial meningitis leading to the generation of free radicals and periventricular leukomalacia has been obtained by direct serial measurements of markers of free radical attack in CSF and correlation of elevations of these markers with the occurrence of magnetic resonance imaging (MRI)–documented cerebral white matter lesions.[206]

The myriad deleterious biochemical and physiological events initiated by the bacterial products discussed earlier are shown in Fig. 35.11. Thus these components induce an increase in blood-brain barrier permeability and the early phases of the inflammatory response (i.e., the synthesis and secretion of cytokines, especially tumor necrosis factor from CNS macrophages [microglia] and astrocytes and interleukin-1 beta from astrocytes and endothelial cells). The cytokines lead to the adhesion and interaction of leukocytes with endothelial cells by inducing specific cell-surface molecules on both leukocytes and endothelial cells. The result is the ventriculitis, arachnoiditis, and vasculitis described earlier, the generation of free radicals by leukocytes, and the activated microglia just discussed (see Fig. 35.11). A second crucial effect of the cytokines is the activation of phospholipase A₂ and thereby arachidonic acid release and subsequent metabolism, the products of which include free radicals, platelet-activating factor, prostaglandins, thromboxanes, and leukotrienes. The interaction of these effects—leading to diffuse neuronal injury, periventricular leukomalacia, and thrombotic cerebral infarction—is shown in Fig. 35.11. The importance of impaired cerebral blood flow is substantial, as discussed earlier. Impairment of cerebrovascular autoregulation is suggested by experimental data (Fig. 35.12), and the importance of systemic hypotension is implied by clinical observations. Ischemia as an important final common denominator is suggested further by the demonstration of elevations of extracellular glutamate and reactive oxygen and nitrogen species in experimental models of bacterial meningitis.

Finally, activation of innate immunity and of many of the mechanisms shown in Figs. 35.10 and 35.11 may occur *without* bacterial invasion of the CNS, as discussed in Chapters 13 to 15 concerning the roles of systemic infection in white matter and neuronal injury, especially in the premature infant. *Indeed, in a large study of more than 6000 premature infants (weighing 401 to 1000 g at birth), infants with sepsis alone (without meningitis) had 50% to 100% higher rates of cognitive deficits, cerebral palsy, visual impairment, hearing impairment, and neurodevelopmental disability as compared with the rates of these outcomes in uninfected infants.*[214]

Clinical Features

Two Basic Syndromes

The clinical features of neonatal bacterial meningitis occur in the setting of two basic clinical syndromes, separable principally by age of onset: early-onset disease and late-onset disease (see Table 35.1). Both syndromes have been described with the three major organisms associated with neonatal bacterial meningitis: group B *Streptococcus*, *E. coli*, and *L. monocytogenes*.[10,215-230]

Early-Onset Disease

Early-onset disease is associated with clinical phenomena usually in the first 72 hours of life. As noted earlier, a history of obstetrical complications and premature birth is common and, understandably, the mode of transmission is primarily from mother to infant near the time of delivery. Specific serotypes are

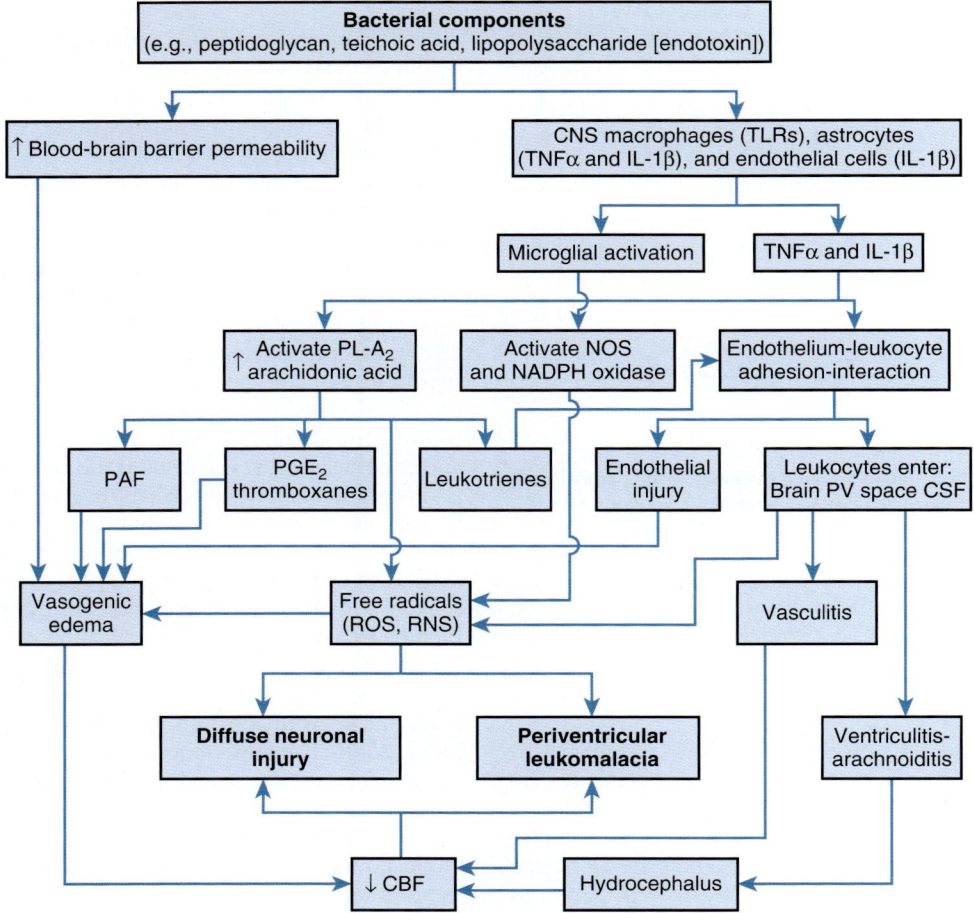

Figure 35.11 Major mechanisms leading to brain injury, especially diffuse cerebral cortical neuronal injury and periventricular white matter injury, in neonatal bacterial meningitis. See text for details. *CBF,* Cerebral blood flow; *CSF,* cerebrospinal fluid; *IL-1 beta,* interleukin-1 beta; *NADPH,* reduced nicotinamide adenine dinucleotide phosphate; *NOS,* nitric oxide synthase; *PL-A2,* phospholipase A2; *PAF,* platelet-activating factor; *PGE2,* prostaglandin E2; *PV space,* perivascular space (Virchow-Robin space); *ROS/RNS,* reactive oxygen species/reactive nitrogen species; *TLR,* Toll-like receptor; *TNF,* tumor necrosis factor.

less likely to be involved, and the course may be fulminating. However, mortality rates in recent years are much lower than previously (see the section on prognosis later).

Dominance of Nonneurological Signs. The clinical presentation is dominated by *nonneurological signs* (i.e., signs related to sepsis and respiratory disease). The most common signs are hyperthermia, apnea, hypotension, disturbances of feeding, jaundice, hepatomegaly, and respiratory distress; less common signs are hypothermia, skin lesions (e.g., petechiae and sclerema), and overt focal infection (e.g., otitis media, omphalitis, arthritis, and osteomyelitis). Neurological signs are generally limited to stupor (usually termed *lethargy*) and irritability. Signs suggestive of meningitis (see later discussion) are unusual, in part because overt meningitis occurs in only approximately 30% of the patients with early-onset disease. Indeed, even those infants with culture-proven meningitis often do not exhibit striking CSF pleocytosis.

The respiratory manifestations of early-onset sepsis-meningitis may be particularly prominent with GBS infection and, indeed, may simultaneously present serious diagnostic problems and important diagnostic clues. Approximately 40% to 60% of infants with early-onset GBS disease have manifestations of prominent respiratory disease in the first 6 hours of life.[28,72,126,231] Only approximately 35% of these infants exhibit radiographic infiltrates suggestive of congenital pneumonia, whereas approximately 50% exhibit radiographic features of respiratory distress syndrome.[126] Distinction from nonbacterial respiratory disease is suggested by the history of premature rupture of membranes, low Apgar scores (<4 at 1 minute in 85%), rapid progression of pulmonary disease, and low or declining absolute neutrophil counts in the first 24 hours of life.[126,232]

Late-Onset Disease

Late-onset bacterial sepsis-meningitis is much more likely to manifest as a neurological syndrome with overt signs of meningitis. Indeed, approximately 80% to 90% of affected infants have CSF findings clearly indicative of meningitis.[1,2,30,126,233] As noted earlier, unlike the case in early-onset disease, obstetrical complications and prematurity are uncommon, and onset is usually after the first week of life. The mode of transmission may be from mother to infant, but often horizontal transmission

TABLE 35.11 Neurological Signs of Neonatal Bacterial Meningitis

NEUROLOGICAL SIGN	APPROXIMATE FREQUENCY
Stupor with or without irritability	76%–100%
Seizures	26%–50%
Bulging or full anterior fontanelle	26%–50%
Extensor rigidity, opisthotonos	26%–50%
Focal cerebral signs	26%–50%
Cranial nerve signs	26%–50%
Nuchal rigidity	0%–25%

TABLE 35.12 Neurological Complications of Neonatal Bacterial Meningitis

Increased intracranial pressure
Ventriculitis with localized, inaccessible infection
Acute hydrocephalus
Intracerebral mass or extracerebral collection

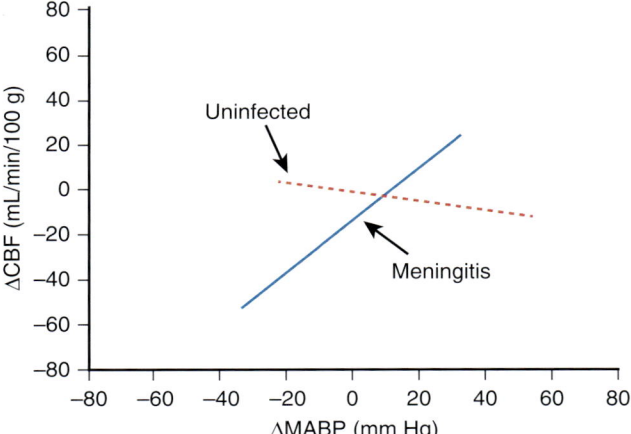

Figure 35.12 Loss of cerebrovascular autoregulation in experimental bacterial meningitis in rabbits. Change in cerebral blood flow (ΔCBF) as a function of change in mean arterial blood pressure (ΔMABP) in control and meningitic rabbits. Changes in MABP result in corresponding changes in CBF in infected rabbits (indicative of impaired autoregulation) but do not cause similar alterations in control (indicative of intact autoregulation). Rights were not granted to include this figure in electronic media. Please refer to the printed book. (From Tureen JH, Dworkin RJ, Kennedy SL, et al. Loss of cerebrovascular autoregulation in experimental meningitis in rabbits. *J Clin Invest.* 1990;85: 577–581.)

from human contacts, indwelling catheters, or contaminated equipment can be documented. Specific serotypes are usually involved (serotype III for GBS, IVb for *L. monocytogenes*, and K1 strains for *E. coli*); the course is not so fulminating as in early-onset disease, and the mortality rate is slightly lower.

Dominance of Neurological Signs. Although *neurological signs* associated with meningitis are *prominent in late-onset disease*, some of the signs prominent in early-onset disease are also common, especially fever and feeding disturbances. Most impressive, however, are the neurological signs (Table 35.11).[30,57,89,226,227] Most patients exhibit *impairment of consciousness*, manifested usually as varying degrees of stupor, with or without irritability. The disturbances of level of consciousness presumably relate to the cerebral edema and, perhaps, the associated encephalopathy (see the section on neuropathology earlier). *Seizures* develop at some time in the illness in nearly 50% of cases, although these seizures may be predominantly subtle. The convulsive

phenomena presumably relate to the cortical effects of the arachnoidal inflammatory infiltration. *Focal seizures* occur in approximately 50% of infants with seizures and may be prominent. These focal episodes may be related to ischemic vascular lesions. Similar bases are probable for the *focal cerebral signs* (e.g., hemiparesis and horizontal deviation of eyes), which are movable with the "doll's eyes maneuver." These signs are reported only uncommonly in the literature, but they can be elicited with careful examination in nearly half of the cases. *Extensor rigidity* occurs in approximately one third of cases and may be so severe that opisthotonos occurs. These phenomena probably relate to the arachnoidal inflammation, especially in the posterior fossa. A similar basis is likely for the nuchal rigidity, which occurs in fewer than 25% of cases. Apparent in most patients, however, is a distinct increase in irritability, elicitable by flexion of the neck; this, presumably, is the neonatal counterpart of more overt nuchal rigidity. *Cranial nerve signs* usually involve the seventh, third, and sixth nerves, in that order of frequency, and are more common than often suggested in the literature. These signs relate to the involvement of cranial nerve roots by the arachnoidal inflammation (see the section on neuropathology earlier). A *bulging or full anterior fontanelle* is present, often later in the course of the disease, in approximately 35% to 50% of patients. This feature relates to an increase in intracranial pressure (see following section). Rarely, anterior fontanelle herniation of cerebral tissue occurs and imparts a *doughy* consistency to the bulging fontanelle.[157] Moreover, very uncommonly, signs of segmental cord involvement (sensory level, flaccidity below the level of the lesion), secondary to myelopathy, may be present.[160,161]

Major Neurological Complications

The clinical course of neonatal bacterial meningitis may be *complicated* by the following four major and often interrelated events: (1) severe increase in intracranial pressure, (2) ventriculitis with localization of infection, (3) acute hydrocephalus, and (4) an intracerebral mass or extraparenchymal collection (e.g., abscess, hemorrhagic infarct, and subdural effusion) (Table 35.12).

Increased Intracranial Pressure. Intracranial pressure, although only uncommonly monitored, may be markedly increased in neonatal bacterial meningitis. Major causes include cerebral edema, hydrocephalus, and, uncommonly, formation of an intracranial mass or extracerebral collection (Table 35.13). Cerebral edema (vasogenic and cytotoxic) is a frequent feature in the first several days of the disease and may be aggravated by water retention secondary to inappropriate antidiuretic hormone secretion.[234–236] Increased intracranial pressure may persist or worsen in the ensuing days, with the development of acute hydrocephalus or an intracranial space-occupying lesion (see subsequent discussion).

TABLE 35.13	Causes of Increased Intracranial Pressure in Neonatal Bacterial Meningitis

Cerebral edema
Vasogenic: endothelial effects of bacterial components, cytokines, arachidonate metabolites, free radicals, vasculitis
Cytotoxic: cellular injury
Water intoxication: inappropriate antidiuretic hormone secretion
Hydrocephalus, secondary to obstruction of cerebrospinal fluid flow
Arachnoiditis and extraventricular block
Ventriculitis and intraventricular block
Intracerebral mass or extracerebral collection
Abscess
Subdural effusion or empyema
Other

The increased intracranial pressure rarely causes signs of transtentorial (e.g., unilateral dilated pupil) or cerebellar (e.g., apnea and bradycardia) herniation, but both these forms of herniation have been reported.[156] Although uncommon, the increased intracranial pressure may interfere with cerebral perfusion and may contribute to the associated encephalopathy described in the section on neuropathology. Clinical signs suggestive of increased intracranial pressure include a full or bulging anterior fontanelle, separated cranial sutures, and deterioration of the level of consciousness.

Ventriculitis With Localization of Infection. Ventriculitis complicated by localization of infection is caused by a particularly exuberant inflammation of the ependymal lining usually in association with obstruction to CSF flow, especially at the aqueduct. Occasionally the formation of glial septa may localize intraventricular infection in a particularly severe manner. There are no reliable clinical signs for these events; the diagnosis must be suspected on the basis of the failure of clinical and bacterial responses to therapy (see the section on management later). Ultrasound scanning may show signs suggestive of ventriculitis (see the section on diagnosis later) and may at least indicate the potential for sequestered infection.

Acute Hydrocephalus. Hydrocephalus occurs in an appreciable proportion of infants with neonatal bacterial meningitis who survive into the second and third weeks of life. The causes of hydrocephalus include obstruction to CSF flow—either inside the ventricular system, secondary to ventriculitis, or outside the ventricular system—secondary to arachnoiditis. The suggestive clinical signs are those of increased intracranial pressure, as just discussed, and acceleration of head growth. Diagnosis is made best with ultrasound or other brain modality (see the section on diagnosis, later), particularly because ventricular dilation develops *before* overt clinical signs.

Intracerebral Mass or Extracerebral Collection. Formation of an intracerebral mass or extracerebral collection of clinical significance is very uncommon in neonatal bacterial meningitis. *Brain abscess* can occur, particularly in necrotic brain tissue (e.g.,

infarction), and it should be suspected if existing clinical signs worsen, despite apparently adequate therapy, and if signs of increased intracranial pressure or focal cerebral disturbance develop (see the later section on brain abscess). Sudden onset of a focal deficit with evidence of a unilateral mass may also occur with a large *hemorrhagic infarct.* Abscess and massive infarction, although clinically very important, are very unusual in neonatal bacterial meningitis. *Subdural effusion* should be suspected in the presence of accelerated head growth and signs of increased intracranial pressure. Increased cranial transillumination can be helpful at the bedside. However, clinically significant subdural effusion is very uncommon in neonatal bacterial meningitis. Similarly, *subdural empyema* is a rare extracerebral collection that may cause signs of increased intracranial pressure in addition to fever and leukocytosis.

Diagnosis

Clinical Evaluation

The clinical suspicion of *sepsis* is based on a wide variety of *very common*, previously discussed clinical signs. It is necessary to consider and distinguish not only virtually all nonbacterial infections (see Chapter 34) but also disorders of other organ systems as common as respiratory distress syndrome. Obstetrical and epidemiological factors are very important to evaluate. Indeed, the most significant point is that *a high index of clinical suspicion is critical* and should provoke the initiation of laboratory studies (reviewed in the next section).

Clinical suspicion of *meningitis*, of course, must always be raised when sepsis is suspected. In addition, certain neurological signs should suggest meningitis (see previous discussion). Unfortunately, too often these signs appear *after* significant disease is well established. Disturbances of the *level of consciousness* are the most nearly constant *initial* neurological signs; indeed, perhaps the most useful early clinical constellation that should lead to the suspicion of neonatal bacterial meningitis is the combination of stupor, even if slight, and irritability.

Laboratory Evaluation

The essential questions to be answered through laboratory studies in the evaluation of the infant suspected of having bacterial meningitis are principally the following:
1. Is meningitis present?
2. What is the cause?
3. What is the status of the CNS?

The answer to the first question is based principally on evaluation of the CSF, the answer to the second is based on the identification of the microorganism, and the answer to the third is based on several important neurodiagnostic studies.

Cerebrospinal Fluid Findings. Examination of the CSF is indicated in any infant with suspected sepsis, even in the absence of overt neurological signs. Indeed, in one series, 37% of cases of primarily early-onset neonatal meningitis would have been missed or the diagnosis delayed if the decision to perform a lumbar puncture had been reserved for infants with *neurological signs* or proven bacteremia.[237] Similarly, in a series of 9461 very-low-birth-weight infants, *one third of those with meningitis had meningitis in the absence of sepsis.*[136] Because CSF cultures were performed only half as often as blood cultures, the discordance in blood and CSF culture results suggested that "meningitis may be underdiagnosed among very-low-birth-weight infants."[136]

Interpretation of the CSF findings in the newborn is difficult, especially when that interpretation is critical in making a diagnosis (i.e., bacterial meningitis) that requires urgent intervention. Among the many reasons for the difficulties in interpretation of the CSF findings, the most important relates to the uncertainty of normal values in the *specific population of infants at risk* for bacterial meningitis (see Chapter 10). Previously published studies dealt with normal or poorly defined populations.

Sarff and co-workers[238] described the *CSF findings in 117 high-risk infants* (87 term and 30 preterm, with 95% examined in the first week of life) without meningitis or other clinical evidence of viral or bacterial disease (Table 35.14). Mean values for term and preterm infants, respectively, were as follows: white blood cell (WBC) count, 8 and 9 cells/mm^3 (60% polymorphonuclear leukocytes); protein concentration, 90 and 115 mg/dL; glucose concentration, 52 and 50 mg/dL;

and ratio of CSF to blood glucose concentration, 81% and 74%. Although the ranges are wide, the values provided a useful framework.[238a] A later study by Rodriguez and co-workers[239] amplified these findings by focusing on very-low-birth-weight infants, 80% of whom were examined *after* the first week of life. CSF findings as a function of postconceptional age were defined (Table 35.15). CSF values for protein and glucose contents are highest in the most immature infants and may reflect an increased permeability of the blood-brain barrier in these infants (see Table 35.15 and Chapter 10).[240] These additional features are important in assessing the CSF in the large numbers of very premature infants evaluated in modern neonatal intensive care units.

The CSF formula for neonatal bacterial meningitis is an elevated WBC count predominantly consisting of polymorphonuclear leukocytes, an elevated protein concentration, and a depressed glucose concentration, particularly in relation to blood glucose concentration. The abnormalities tend to be more severe for late-onset than early-onset disease and for gram-negative enteric than GBS meningitis. Of 119 newborn infants with proven bacterial meningitis, more than 1000 WBCs/mm^3 were observed in the initial sample of CSF in approximately 75% of patients with gram-negative infection but in only approximately 30% of those with GBS infection.[238] Values in excess of 10,000 WBCs/mm^3 were observed in approximately 20% of gram-negative infections but were rare in GBS infections. Evaluation of the other end of the continuum is still more informative (Table 35.16). Thus, using the *ranges* determined in their high-risk newborns (see Table 35.14), Sarff and co-workers[238] showed that CSF values for WBC count were within the *normal* range for approximately 30% of infants with culture-proven GBS meningitis versus only 4% of infants with gram-negative meningitis. Values for CSF protein concentration and the ratio of CSF to blood glucose were within the *normal* range in nearly 50% of the infants with GBS meningitis versus only 15% to 25% of those with gram-negative bacterial meningitis (see Table 35.16). The importance of evaluating *all* the CSF findings, and not just one isolated value, is emphasized by the finding that *only 1 of 119 infants had normal values for all three parameters in the initial lumbar puncture sample.*[238] Thus the CSF findings should be evaluated in toto and in the context of other clinical, epidemiological, and laboratory data in assessing the

---

TABLE 35.14   Cerebrospinal Fluid Findings in High-Risk Newborns Without Bacterial Meningitis^a

CSF FINDINGS	TERM	PRETERM
White blood cell count (cells/mm^3)		
Mean	7	9
Range	1–130	0–29
Protein concentration (mg/dL)		
Mean	90	115
Range	20–170	65–150
Glucose concentration (mg/dL)		
Mean	52	50
Range	34–119	24–63
CSF/blood glucose (%)		
Mean	81	74
Range	44–248	55–105

^{a}Ninety-five percent of infants were examined in the first week of life.

CSF, Cerebrospinal fluid.

Data from Ahmed A, Hickey SM, Ehrett S, et al. Cerebrospinal fluid values in the term neonate. *Pediatr Infect Dis J.* 1996;15:298–303.

TABLE 35.15   Cerebrospinal Fluid Findings in Infants Weighing Less Than 1500 g as a Function of Postconceptional Age^a

POSTCONCEPTIONAL AGE (WEEK)	CSF FINDINGS		
	WBCs/mm^3 (MEAN ± SD)	GLUCOSE (mg/dL) (MEAN ± SD)	PROTEIN (mg/dL) (MEAN ± SD)
26–28 (n = 17)	6 ± 10	85 ± 39	177 ± 60
29–31 (n = 23)	5 ± 4	54 ± 18	144 ± 40
32–34 (n = 18)	4 ± 3	55 ± 21	142 ± 49
35–37 (n = 8)	6 ± 7	56 ± 21	109 ± 53
38–40 (n = 5)	9 ± 9	44 ± 10	117 ± 33

^{a}Eighty percent of infants were examined after the first week of life.

CSF, Cerebrospinal fluid; *WBCs,* white blood cells.

Data from Rodriguez AF, Kaplan SL, Mason EO Jr. Cerebrospinal fluid values in the very-low-birth-weight infant. *J Pediatr.* 1990;116:971–974.

TABLE 35.16 Cerebrospinal Fluid Findings in Neonatal Bacterial Meningitis

CSF FINDING	BACTERIAL ETIOLOGY OF MENINGITIS[a]	
	GROUP B *STREPTOCOCCUS*	GRAM-NEGATIVE ORGANISM
WBC count	29%	4%
Protein concentration <170 mg/dL	47%	23%
CSF/blood glucose >44%	45%	15%

[a]Data expressed as percentage of total patients with indicated type of meningitis.

CSF, Cerebrospinal fluid; *WBC*, white blood cell.

From Sarff LD, Platt LH, McCracken GH Jr. Cerebrospinal fluid evaluation in neonates: comparison of high-risk infants with and without meningitis. *J Pediatr.* 1976;88:473–477.

possibility of meningitis. In the rare patient with a totally normal CSF examination but a continuing suspicion of meningitis, a second lumbar puncture is indicated.

Identification of the Microorganism in Cerebrospinal Fluid. Determination of the bacterial cause of meningitis obviously is made most readily and decisively by *culture of the CSF.* The yield in the previously untreated patient whose CSF is cultured promptly on the various media necessary to isolate the different microorganisms responsible for neonatal bacterial meningitis (including *Listeria*) approaches 100%. The result is usually available within 48 hours.

Faster techniques available for identifying microorganisms include Gram-stained smears, countercurrent immunoelectrophoresis, limulus lysate assay, and latex particle agglutination. *Stained smears* demonstrated bacteria on the initial CSF evaluation of 119 newborn infants with meningitis in 83% of patients with GBS meningitis and in 78% of those with gram-negative bacterial meningitis.[238] This universally available, simple procedure should be performed on every CSF sample. *Countercurrent immunoelectrophoresis* is a sensitive and rapid technique that demonstrates the presence of bacterial antigen within approximately 2 hours. The test was formerly widely used, particularly in the previously treated patient with possible nonviable bacteria in the CSF. Countercurrent immunoelectrophoresis requires specific antiserum, which is available for type III GBS and K1 *E. coli* (among the common pathogens for neonatal meningitis).[30,233,241-245] Rapid detection of meningitis caused by gram-negative enteric organisms was formerly based particularly on the *limulus lysate assay.*[30,246] These last two tests have been largely replaced by *latex particle agglutination tests,*[247] which is based on the agglutination of specific antibody-coated latex particles by bacterial antigen. The test is particularly useful for GBS and *E. coli* K1. The assay can provide a result in minutes.

Identification of the Microorganism From Other Sites. Valuable supporting data and occasionally the only information concerning the precise bacterial cause of meningitis are derived from isolation of the organism or its antigens in body fluids other than CSF. *Blood cultures* are positive in approximately 50% to 80% of cases of neonatal bacterial meningitis.[a] Detection of bacterial antigen by *latex particle agglutination tests* can be

made with serum or urine as well as with CSF. *Concentrated urine* specimens are the most productive for detection of GBS antigen.[126,250] In a cumulative series, 88% of concentrated urine specimens were antigen positive by countercurrent immunoelectrophoresis, and 96% were antigen positive by latex particle agglutination. Moreover, when urine, CSF, and serum are all studied, the likelihood of missing the infection is minimal. In the unusual case in which a suppurative focus (e.g., otitis media, arthritis, or skin abscess) is the source of the meningitic infection, *cultures and stains of aspirated material* are of obvious value. Isolation of an organism from surface cultures (e.g., skin, nose, throat, rectum, and umbilicus) indicates *colonization* but does not establish active systemic infection. Recent data suggest that rapid fluorescent real-time polymerase chain reaction testing for GBS DNA is highly sensitive for rapid detection of colonization by this organism.[251]

Adjunct Tests. Adjunct tests that support the diagnosis of bacterial infection include an increase in the absolute neutrophilic band count and particularly the ratio of immature to total neutrophils.[30,127,245,252-254] Neutrophilic leukocytosis or leukopenia is demonstrable in 50% to 75% of cases. Other tests (e.g., determination of C-reactive protein, erythrocyte sedimentation rate, and IgM level) are somewhat less sensitive.[203,255] Several studies raise the possibility that detection of certain proinflammatory cytokines, chemokines, adhesion molecules, and cell surface markers may have value in early identification of neonatal bacterial sepsis (determinations in serum) or meningitis (determinations in CSF), even before the onset of clinical disease.[203,210,255-258] More data will be important.

Neurodiagnostic Studies

The status of the CNS in neonatal bacterial meningitis is evaluated best by careful clinical examination and by selected neurodiagnostic studies. Choice of studies depends particularly on the stage of the disease and, as a corollary, the neuropathological features to be assessed. The three neurodiagnostic tests, in addition to examination of CSF, that are considered most valuable are (1) measurement of CSF pressure, (2) ventricular puncture (in highly selected cases), and (3) brain imaging studies (primarily by ultrasound and MRI scans). The electroencephalogram is of definite adjunct value (see the section on prognosis later).

Cerebrospinal Fluid Pressure. CSF pressure may be a critical factor in determining outcome, and measurements of pressure,

---

[a]References 28, 57, 131, 136, 248, and 249.

TABLE 35.17   Ventriculitis

Definition: Ventricular inflammation with infection (often apparently inaccessible to systemically administered antibiotics)
Suspect if (1) persistence of infection in lumbar CSF at 4 days or (2) clinical deterioration or failure of clinical improvement, even with improvement of CSF pleocytosis and CSF sterilization

CSF, Cerebrospinal fluid.

especially in the acute stage, can be valuable. The initial lumbar puncture should include CSF pressure measurement, and CSF pressure in excess of normal (i.e., ≈50 mm H_2O) should be cause for concern. Continual or frequent intermittent monitoring of CSF pressure with an anterior fontanelle sensor, when available (see Chapter 10), can be useful in the evaluation of the degree of cerebral edema, the development of obstructive hydrocephalus, and the occurrence of a major intracerebral mass or extracerebral collection. Clear elevations of intracranial pressure should provoke further, more definitive diagnostic studies and appropriate intervention (see the section on management later). Our initial studies of this issue demonstrated that intracranial hypertension with impaired cerebral blood flow velocity, measured at the anterior fontanelle by the Doppler technique (see Chapter 10), was more commonly a complication of bacterial meningitis *of older infants than of newborns.*[155] This observation concerning intracranial hypertension was confirmed in a later study.[259]

Ventricular Puncture. Ventricular puncture provides valuable information concerning intraventricular pressure and the presence of ventriculitis, particularly when associated with serious localized infection (Table 35.17). *Although only uncommonly necessary,* ventricular puncture should be performed in any newborn with bacterial meningitis who is not responding favorably to apparently appropriate antibiotic therapy in terms *either* of clinical signs *or* of sterilization of lumbar CSF (see the section on management later). Severe ventriculitis may be present in an infant with improved or even a normal *lumbar* CSF WBC count. Indeed, the constellation of a deteriorating clinical state (e.g., apnea, bradycardia, or both and persistent fever) in the presence of decreasing CSF pleocytosis or even CSF sterilization should raise the suspicion of clinically important ventriculitis. Moreover, ventriculitis may evolve in a subacute fashion, with signs of increased intracranial pressure, either de novo or after apparent recovery from bacterial meningitis.[260] The presence in ventricular fluid of bacteria (Gram stain or culture) or bacterial antigen (latex particle agglutination) and a WBC count in excess of approximately 100/mm³ indicates ventriculitis. Cranial ultrasonography often shows excrescences associated with the ependymal surface. Whether ventricular infection is localized and inaccessible to antibiotics depends on evaluation of a variety of factors. Favoring such a possibility is the presence of marked pleocytosis in ventricular CSF or evidence of intraventricular block of CSF flow (e.g., elevated intraventricular pressure and dilated ventricles) or both pleocytosis and CSF block. Management of such a situation is reviewed in subsequent discussions.

Ventricular puncture should be performed by a physician with expertise in the procedure and awareness of its hazards. In acute bacterial meningitis, the lateral ventricles are often small and may be tapped only with considerable difficulty. An ultrasound scan before the procedure is important. Indeed, ventricular puncture with ultrasound guidance is recommended if the ventricles are small. Ventricular puncture may be followed by the development of a cystic cavity.[147,261] This development is particularly likely to occur if obstruction to CSF flow and increased intraventricular pressure, common complications of bacterial ventriculitis, are present. The subsequent cavitation along the needle track relates most probably to the combination of disruption of edematous, poorly myelinated, readily separable brain parenchyma and transmission of elevated intraventricular pressure. In the large, older series studied by Lorber and Emery,[261] the approximately 50% of infants subjected to *multiple* ventricular punctures for the treatment of bacterial ventriculitis subsequently developed cystic cavities, demonstrable by ventriculography, at the sites of the taps. The incidence of significant cavity formation in infants with ventriculitis after a *single tap* is unknown but is probably relatively low. Although small diverticula from the lateral ventricles into the needle track are common after single taps, major cavity formation is very unusual.

Ultrasound Scan. Cranial ultrasound scan has proved very useful in the evaluation of infants with bacterial meningitis.[262-270] The spectrum of abnormalities has included both acute changes (e.g., evidence of ventriculitis [intraventricular strands attached to the ventricular surface and echogenic ependyma] [Fig. 35.13], echogenic sulci, abnormal parenchymal echogenicities [periventricular or focal cerebral] [Figs. 35.14 and 35.15], and extracellular fluid collection) and chronic changes (e.g., ventricular dilation [see Fig. 35.13] and multicystic parenchymal change). The neuropathological correlates of the sonographic changes include essentially the entire spectrum of the neuropathology (see previous discussion). The particular value of cranial ultrasonography is the capacity to perform serial studies safely and at the patient's bedside and thus to define progression of complications. Such definition is of major benefit in formulating rational management. Cranial ultrasonography of the thoracolumbar spine might reveal debris within the spinal subarachnoid space. This finding has been associated with an increased risk of subsequent hydrocephalus.[271]

Magnetic Resonance Imaging. As for nearly all other forms of neonatal neuropathology, MRI provides important structural information.[159,210,272,273] In the largest study so far, 75 infants were studied and only 19% had a normal MRI.[273] The most common abnormalities noted were leptomeningeal enhancement (57%) (Fig. 35.16), infarction (43%) (Figs. 35.17 and 35.18), subdural empyema (52%), cerebritis (25%) (Fig. 35.19), hydrocephalus (20%), and abscess (11%) (Table 35.18). All the acute and chronic lesions of neonatal bacterial meningitis are delineated very well by MRI (Figs. 35.20 and 35.21; see also Fig. 35.17). Different patterns of injury were recognized in a study of 63 patients with bacterial meningitis (25 neonates and 38 infants), including GBS (n = 32, mean age 4.7 months), and *E. coli* (n = 9, mean age 1.2 months). Ventriculomegaly was especially common in *E. coli* meningitis compared with GBS meningitis (64% vs. 22%), while infarcts were commonly seen in GBS meningitis (13/32, 41%) and rarely seen with other organisms

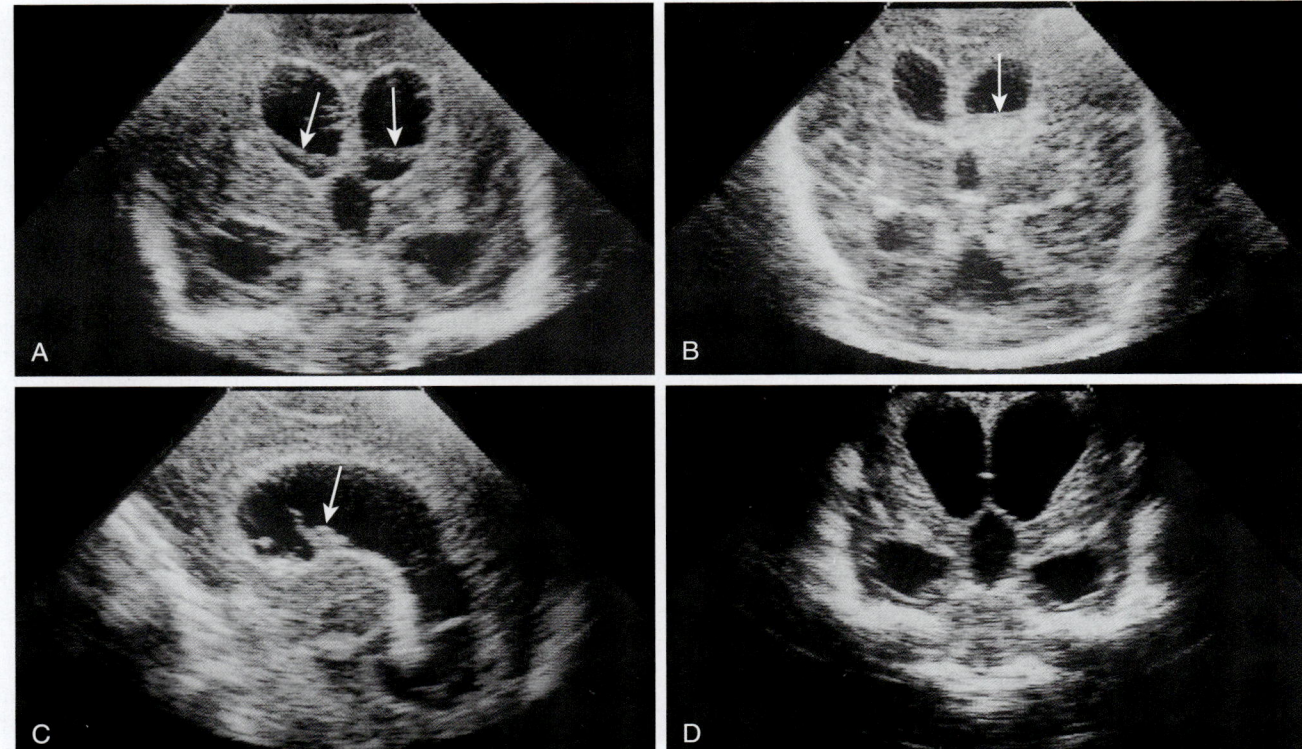

Figure 35.13 Cranial ultrasound scans in neonatal bacterial meningitis. (A) Coronal scan obtained from a 27-day-old infant with group B streptococcal meningitis on the third hospital day. Note dense linear strands of echogenic material in the lateral ventricles *(arrows)*, apparently attached to the ependymal surface, and diffuse low-level echoes in both lateral ventricles. (B) Coronal scan on the fourth hospital day. Note the collection of intraventricular material apparently attached to the ventricular wall *(arrow)*. (C) Parasagittal view of the same scan as in (B). Note abnormal intraventricular echoes *(arrow)* apparently contiguous with ventricular surface and choroid plexus. (D) Note later development of hydrocephalus and disappearance of abnormal echoes.

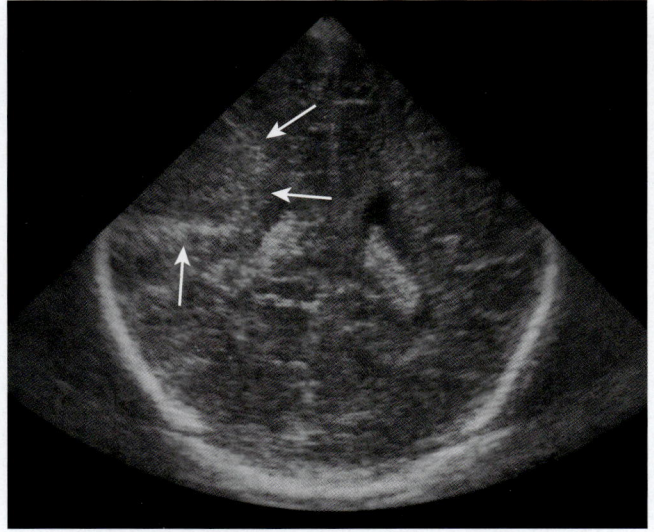

Figure 35.14 Neonatal bacterial meningitis: ultrasound. This coronal scan obtained from an infant with *Escherichia coli* meningitis shows an area of increased echogenicity *(arrows)* in the distribution of the middle cerebral artery, consistent with an infarction.

TABLE 35.18	MRI Findings in 75 Infants With Culture-Proven Meningitis
Normal MRI	19%
Leptomeningeal enhancement	57%
Infarction	43%
Subdural empyema	52%
Cerebritis	25%
Hydrocephalus	20%
Abscess	11%

MRI, Magnetic resonance imaging.
Data from Oliveira CR, et al. Brain magnetic resonance imaging of infants with bacterial meningitis. *J Pediatr.* 2014;165:134–139.

(2 of 31, 6%, *P* = .001). There were also three cases with a *Serratia* meningitis, and these infants had large parenchymal abscesses.[272] The association of GBS meningitis and a pattern of perforator infarction (see Fig. 35.20) was also shown in another study.[159] Involvement of the cerebellar tissue can also be present in GBS meningitis and is also better recognized with MRI than with mastoid window ultrasonography (see Fig. 35.21).[274]

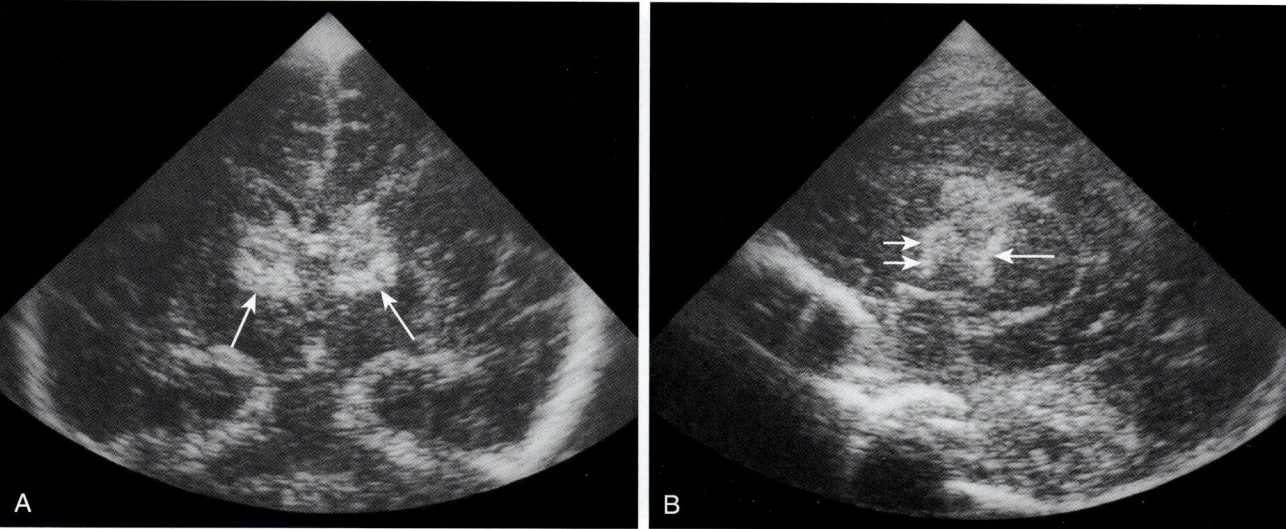

Figure 35.15 Neonatal bacterial meningitis: ultrasound. (A and B) Coronal and parasagittal ultrasound scans from a 2-week-old infant with bacterial meningitis showing areas of echogenicity, most consistent with deep venous infarction. Note on the coronal scan (A) bilateral symmetrical areas of involvement in the region of the basal ganglia (putamen and globus pallidus) *(arrows)*. On the parasagittal scan (B), the involvement is seen not only in basal ganglia *(small arrows)* but also in thalamus *(large arrow)*.

TABLE 35.19	Outcome of Meningitis Caused by Group B Streptococcal Infection[a]	
STATUS	**PERCENTAGE OF SURVIVORS**	**PERCENTAGE OF TOTAL**
Dead		10%–15%
Normal	50%	
Mild or moderate sequelae (borderline or mild mental retardation, unilateral sensorineural hearing loss, arrested hydrocephalus, and spastic monoparesis)	40%	
Severe sequelae (uncontrolled seizures, cortical blindness, spastic quadriparesis, mental retardation [excluding mild cases], severe microcephaly, and hydrocephalus)	10%	

[a]See text for references.

In addition, diffusion-weighted MRI shows ischemic lesions and brain edema effectively early (see Figs. 35.20 and 35.21). Pus within the lateral ventricles can be seen as restricted diffusion as well. Diffusion restriction of the extra-axial fluid is consistent with meningeal edema or pus (see Fig. 35.17).[270]

Prognosis

Reservations Concerning Available Data

The prognosis for neonatal bacterial meningitis depends on the rapidity of diagnosis and the institution of appropriate therapy. Therapy is not perfect; indeed, in certain types of meningitis it is often inadequate. In any assessment of outcome, it is necessary to recognize the inherent difficulty in extrapolating to a given infant with meningitis data that are generalized from large-scale studies, which are often based on populations with a broad spectrum of bacterial causes and followed for relatively brief durations.

Duration of follow-up is particularly important for two reasons. The first is obvious: disturbances of higher cortical function may not become apparent until the child is of school age. Similarly, deficits in certain sensory discriminations, particularly hearing, may be difficult to detect in infancy. The second reason for the importance of duration of follow-up relates to the not infrequent *transient* nature of neurological deficits after neonatal meningitis. Infants may improve for many months, and deficits that were striking shortly after the neonatal period may decrease markedly in severity or may disappear totally. The relation of these observations to the plasticity of developing brain is an interesting topic for future research. Nevertheless, with these reservations, useful estimates of prognosis can be derived from available data (see next sections).

Group B Streptococcal Infection

By far the most common gram-positive organism causing meningitis is GBS, the outcome for which is shown in Table 35.19.[a] These data, derived from several large populations,

---

[a]References 10, 12, 29, 126, 214, 226, and 227.

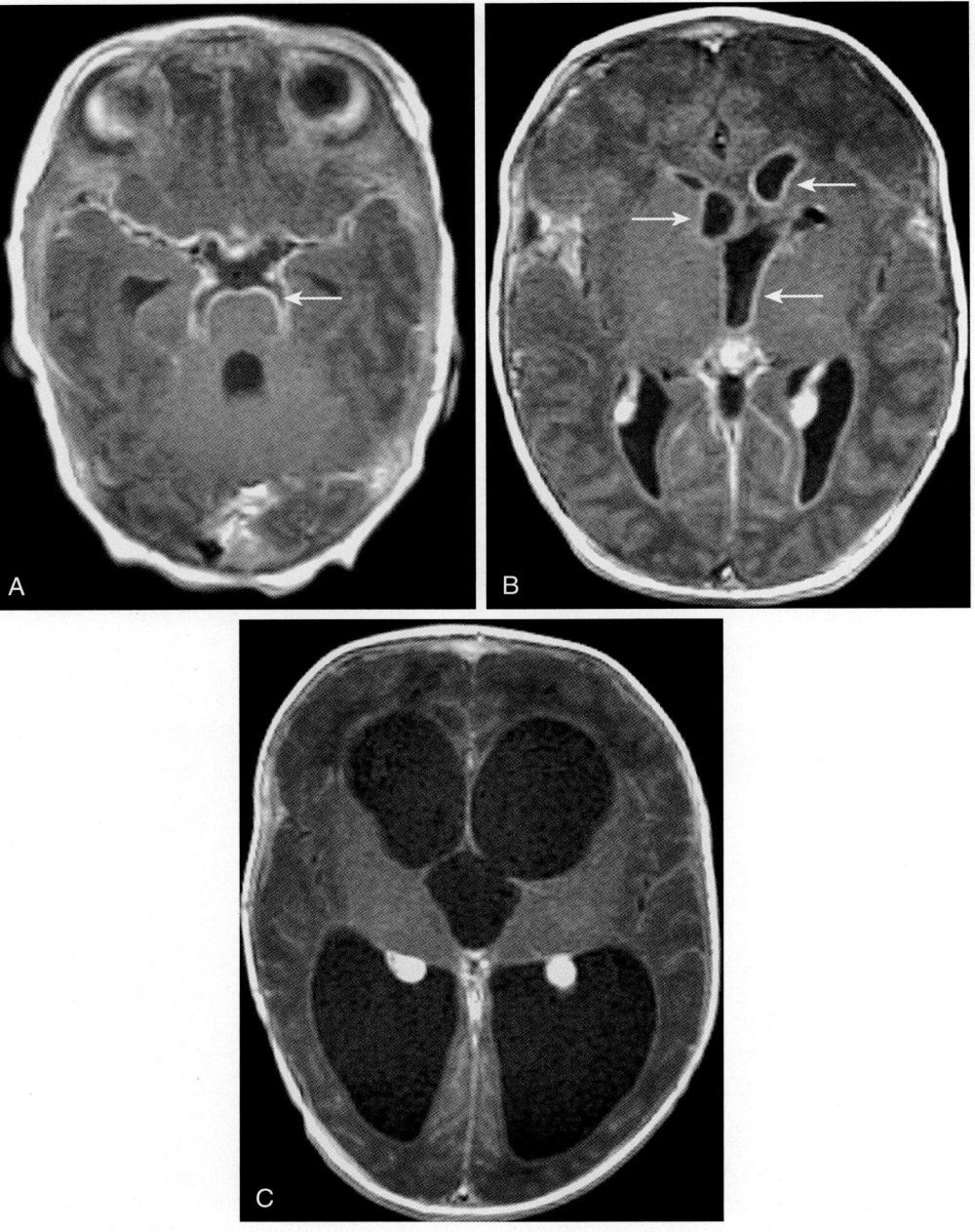

Figure 35.16 Neonatal bacterial meningitis: magnetic resonance imaging (MRI). (A and B) The initial MRI scan, obtained during the acute period, shows, after administration of gadolinium, leptomeningeal enhancement (*arrow* in A), consistent with leptomeningitis, ependymal enhancement (*arrows* in B), consistent with ventriculitis (with loculation), and evidence of diffuse cerebral white matter injury and more focal bifrontal lesions, possibly infarcts. Three weeks later (C), note marked dilation of the lateral and third ventricles, indicative of hydrocephalus (with a likely block at the aqueduct) and diffuse cerebral cortical and white matter injury, especially bifrontally. (Courtesy Dr. Omar Khwaja.)

included more later-onset cases and term infants than early-onset cases and premature infants. The overall fatality rate has declined in recent years to approximately 10% to 15%, with slightly higher rates for early-onset disease or premature infants and slightly lower rates for later-onset cases or term infants. Fifty percent of survivors are normal; approximately 40% have mild

or moderate sequelae, and 10% to 20% exhibit severe deficits. In a recent study of 90 infants, 56% were normal, 25% had mild to moderate impairment, and 19% had severe impairment. A failed hearing screen ($P = .004$), abnormal neurological examination ($P < .001$), and abnormal brain imaging ($P = .038$) at discharge were associated with late death or severe impairment.[275] These

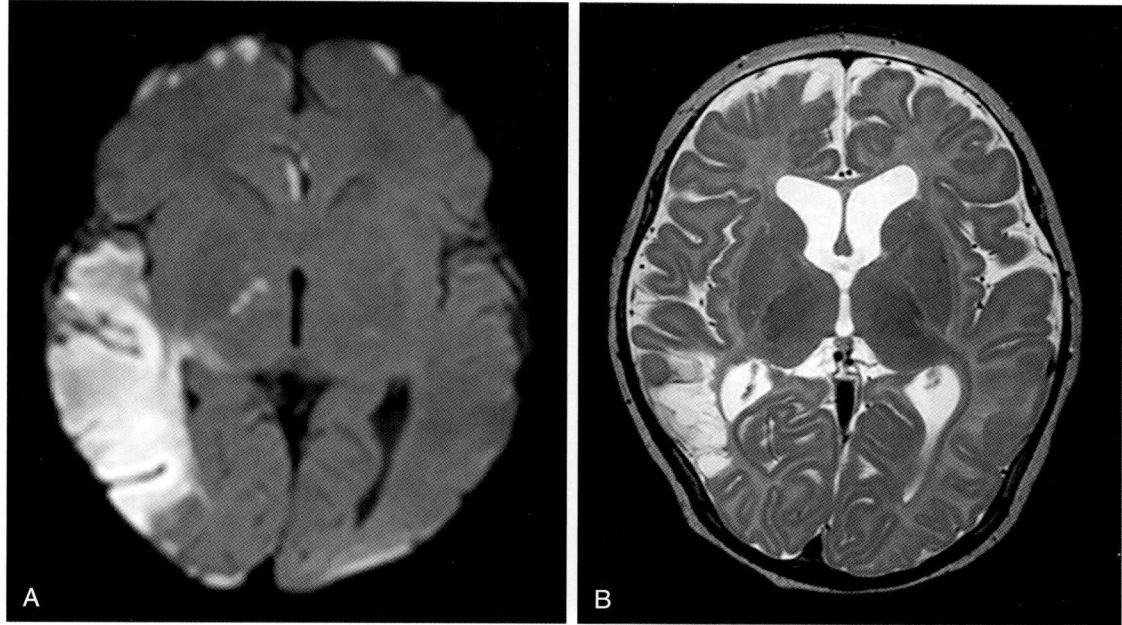

Figure 35.17 Neonatal bacterial meningitis (group B *Streptococcus*): magnetic resonance imaging. Axial neonatal diffusion-weighted (A) and T2-weighted 3-month (B) images showing increased signal intensity in the frontal cortex and the posterior branch of the middle cerebral artery territory and right posterior limb of the internal capsule in the neonatal period. At 3 months, an area of cavitation is seen in the middle cerebral artery distribution as well as a small cyst in the right frontal region. Ex vacuo dilatation is also seen.

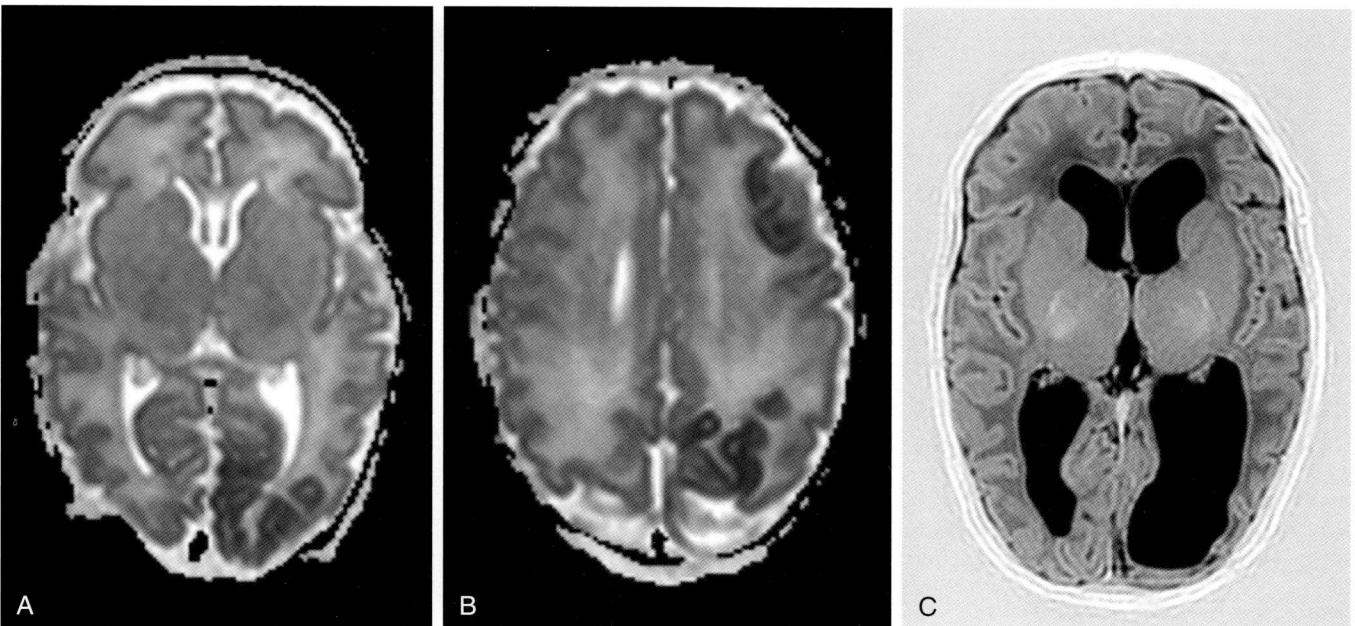

Figure 35.18 Neonatal bacterial meningitis (group B *Streptococcus*), magnetic resonance imaging (MRI). Axial apparent diffusion coefficient maps (ADC) (A and B) at 35 weeks postmenstrual age, following GBS infection at 34 weeks in a preterm infant with a gestational age of 32 weeks. Low ADC values were present in the posterior cerebral artery distribution and in the left anterior middle cerebral artery distribution. A repeat MRI is performed at term-equivalent age (C). This T1-weighted sequence shows ex vacuo dilation in the left occipital lobe.

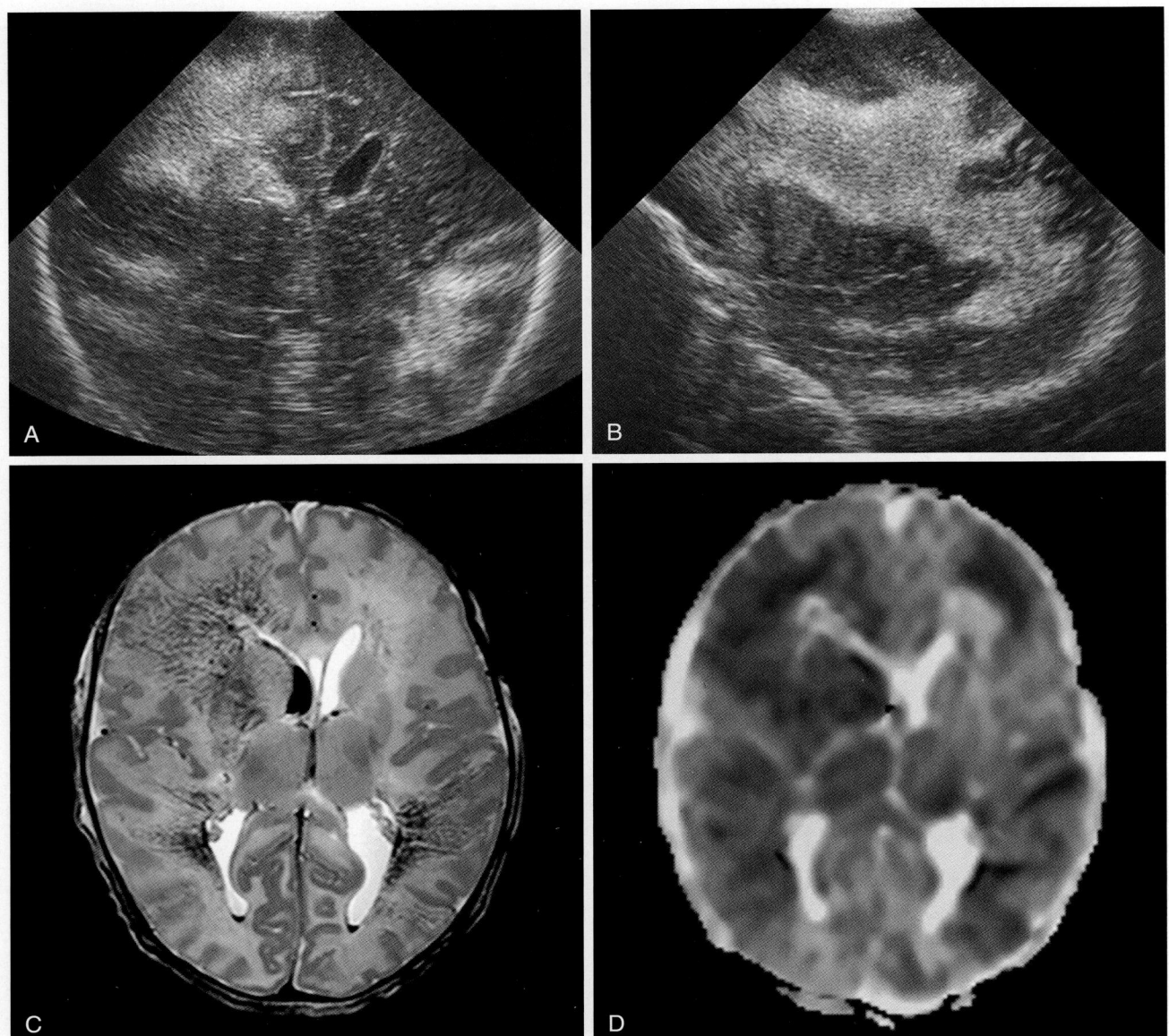

Figure 35.19 Neonatal cerebritis (*Citrobacter koseri*) ultrasound. Cranial ultrasound, coronal (A) and parasagittal views (B), showing irregular areas of increased echogenicity in the periventricular white matter and blood in the right ventricle. Magnetic resonance imaging of the same infant, T2-weighted sequence (C), and apparent diffusion coefficient map (D), confirming the intraventricular hemorrhage and showing a mild midline shift and large areas of low ADC values suggestive of cytotoxic edema with petechial hemorrhages.

outcomes represent a decline in mortality rates and in morbidity among survivors as compared with results of earlier reports.[a]

Gram-Negative Enteric Infections

Neonatal meningitis secondary to gram-negative enteric organisms has been considered more ominous than neonatal meningitis secondary to gram-positive organisms, particularly GBS. More recent data suggest that this distinction may no longer be obvious (Table 35.20).[10,12,136,226,227] Thus findings suggest that the outcome is nearly similar to that for GBS

meningitis, especially among later-onset cases. Mortality rates and the incidence of sequelae in survivors are slightly higher in early-onset cases, premature infants, or both. The most striking change in neonatal outcome with gram-negative bacterial meningitis in recent years has been continuation of a sharp decrease in mortality rate.[a]

Selected Prognostic Factors

Certain factors, readily identified in the newborn period, may have prognostic importance, at least regarding the likelihood of

---

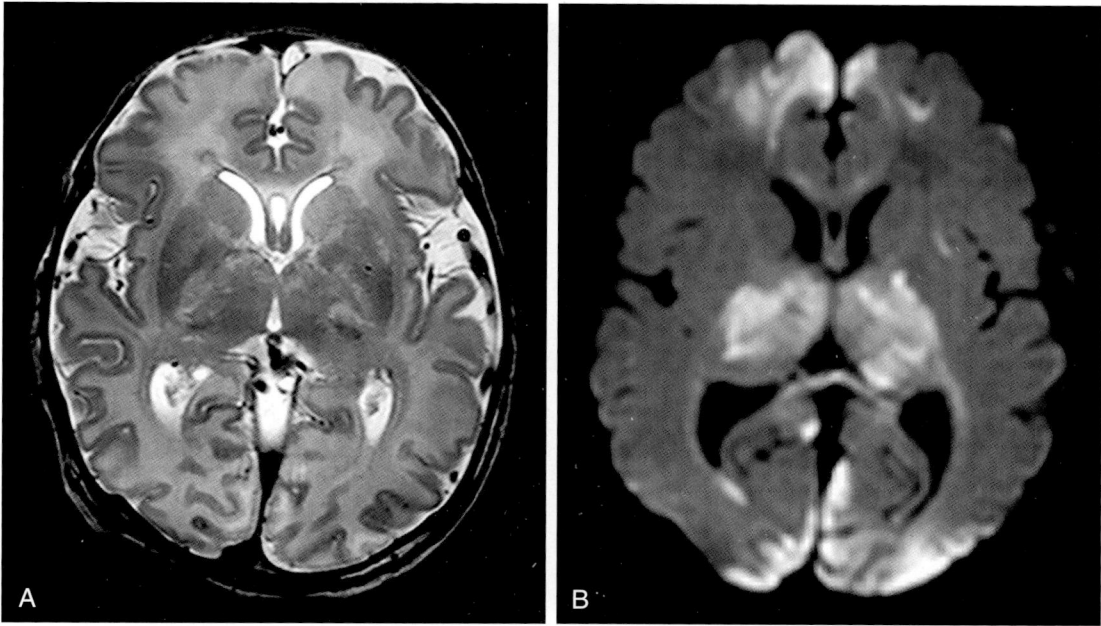

Figure 35.20 Neonatal bacterial meningitis (group B *Streptococcus*): magnetic resonance imaging scans. Axial T2-weighted (A) and diffusion-weighted (B) images showing increased signal intensity in the frontal and occipital cortex and the thalami.

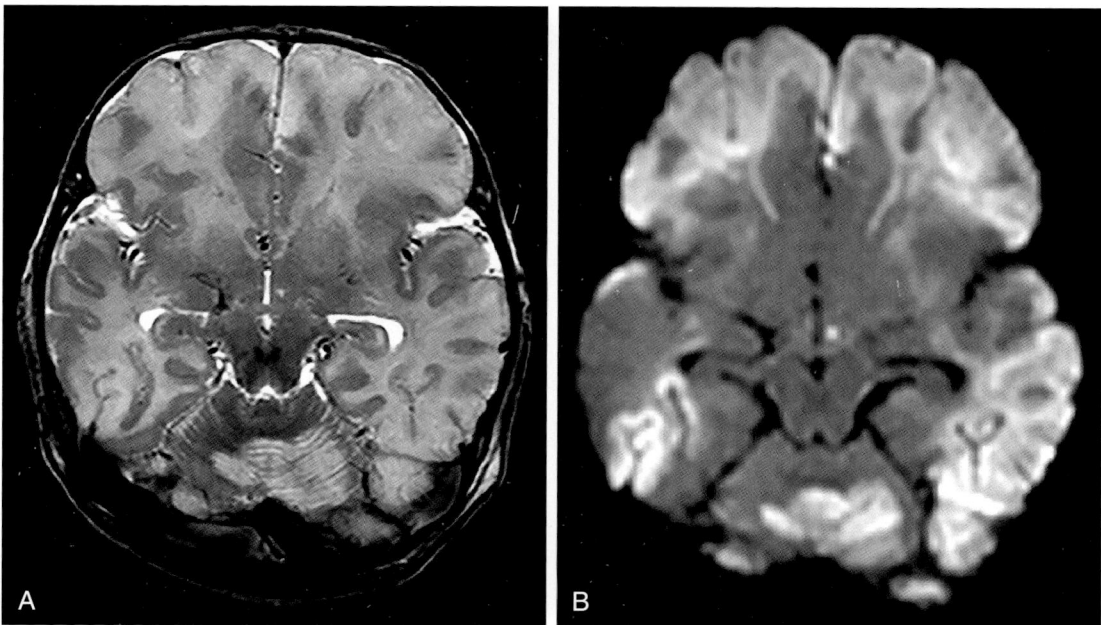

Figure 35.21 Neonatal bacterial meningitis: magnetic resonance imaging. Axial T2-weighted (A) and diffusion-weighted (B) images showing increased signal intensity in the frontal cortex and temporal lobes as well as the cerebellum.

a fatal outcome or survival with severe neurological sequelae.[a] Thus decreased survival rates and higher incidences of severe sequelae are associated with low-birth-weight, marked leukopenia or neutropenia or both, coma or opisthotonos, persistent seizures (>12 hours), and markedly elevated CSF

protein content. Also of value with specific infections are the quantitative levels in CSF of the type III GBS or the K1 *E. coli* antigenic markers; these levels correlate directly with prognosis.[233] A careful study of the electroencephalogram during bacterial meningitis in 29 infants indicated value for the degree of background abnormality in prediction of outcome (Table 35.21).[293] A more recent study confirmed these initial

[a]References 10, 12, 29, 136, 226, 229, 233, 248, 280, 284, 287, and 292.

TABLE 35.20   Outcome of Meningitis Caused by Gram-Negative Enteric Organisms[a]

STATUS	PERCENTAGE OF SURVIVORS	PERCENTAGE OF TOTAL
Dead		15%
Normal	50%	
Mild or moderate sequelae (see Table 35.19)	40%	
Severe sequelae (see Table 35.19)	10%	

[a]See text for references.

TABLE 35.21   Relationship Between Electroencephalographic Background Activity and Outcome[a]

MOST ABNORMAL BACKGROUND	OUTCOME		
	NORMAL OR MILDLY ABNORMAL	SEVERELY ABNORMAL	DEATH
Normal or mildly abnormal	9	0	0
Moderately abnormal	5	3	1
Markedly abnormal[b]	0	5	6

[a]From a study of 29 infants, 15 of whom were less than 38 weeks of gestational age.

[b]Markedly abnormal: markedly excessive discontinuity for postconceptional age, burst suppression, markedly excessive interhemispheric asynchrony or asymmetry, diffusely slow background, extremely low voltage (<5 μV for all states), or isoelectric.

Data from Chequer RS, Tharp BR, Dreimane D, Hahn JS, et al. Prognostic value of EEG in neonatal meningitis: retrospective study of 29 infants. *Pediatr Neurol.* 1992;8:417–422.

findings.[29] Amplitude integrated electroencephalography (EEG) was also shown to be useful, with the presence of background abnormalities and persistent seizures associated with an adverse outcome.[294] Although not systematically analyzed, the degree of injury on MRI scan performed in the infant's course appears to be useful prognostically. However, although these various associations are valuable, outcome in neonatal bacterial meningitis depends on the interplay of so many factors that prognostic judgments in every case must be carefully individualized. Indeed, in perhaps no other variety of neonatal neurological disease is dramatic recovery from a devastated clinical state more likely to be observed than in an infant with neonatal bacterial meningitis.

Management

The major issues in the management of neonatal bacterial meningitis relate to prevention, supportive care, neurological complications, antibiotics, and ventriculitis. Although many aspects of management are surrounded by unresolved problems, the basic fact remains that neonatal bacterial meningitis is a treatable disease.

Prevention (Group B Streptococcal Infection)

The most critical and challenging problem in the prevention of neonatal bacterial meningitis relates to GBS disease. GBS is the single most common organism implicated in many medical centers (see earlier). The enormity of the public health problem associated with neonatal sepsis and meningitis caused by GBS has been alluded to earlier (see the section on pathogenesis). Two basic approaches to prevention of neonatal disease have been proposed: chemoprophylaxis and immunoprophylaxis.

Chemoprophylaxis. Historically, chemoprophylaxis has been an attractive approach because of the susceptibility of GBS to penicillin in vitro and the relative ease of administering such a relatively safe and well-known antibiotic. The three major chemoprophylactic approaches used since the late 1980s have included treatment of a colonized woman in the third trimester or at delivery and treatment of the newborn at birth.[65,66,126,295-305]

Among these approaches, *treatment of the colonized woman at delivery* has become the approach of choice.[a] The findings in several controlled studies showed conclusively that intravenous ampicillin or penicillin during labor leads to a marked reduction in colonization of infants born to infected mothers and to a virtual elimination of early-onset GBS sepsis-meningitis. The most difficult issue has been whom to treat. The data depicted in Table 35.22 emanated from a classic study and showed the value of intrapartum chemoprophylaxis, especially in certain high-risk groups.[297] Indeed, in the years since the advent of widespread intrapartum chemoprophylaxis, the incidence of GBS disease has declined markedly: for early-onset sepsis-meningitis, it has declined from 1.7 in 1000 births to approximately 0.3 in 1000; and for late-onset disease, it has declined from 0.5 per 1000 births to 0.3 per 1000 births.[74,126,297,309] These and similar observations have led to the current recommendations of the Centers for Disease Control and Prevention: (1) a screening strategy with culture of pregnant women for GBS at 35 to 37 weeks of gestation and administration of intrapartum penicillin G (or ampicillin) to all culture-positive women, whether or not they have a risk factor (see next); or (2) a nonscreening approach with administration of intrapartum penicillin G (or ampicillin) to all women with a risk factor (previous delivery of an infant with GBS disease, history of GBS during pregnancy, preterm labor at less than 37 weeks of gestation, rupture of membranes 18 hours or more before delivery, or intrapartum fever).

[a]References 65, 66, 126, 295-300, 302, 304, and 306-308.

TABLE 35.22 Effect of Intrapartum Chemoprophylaxis on Early-Onset Neonatal Group B Streptococcal Disease

PERINATAL RISK FACTOR	NEONATAL EARLY-ONSET DISEASE	
	AMPICILLIN	CONTROL
None	0/85 (0%)	5/1170 (0.4%)
Gestation <37 wk or membrane rupture >12 h	0/167 (0%)	12/305 (4.0%)
Intrapartum fever	0/80 (0%)	3/23 (13.0%)
Total	0/320 (0%)	20/1493 (1.3%)

Data from Boyer KM, Gotoff SP. Prevention of early-onset neonatal group B streptococcal disease with selective intrapartum chemoprophylaxis. *N Engl J Med.* 1986;314:1665–1669, with permission.

Immunoprophylaxis. Immunoprophylaxis is potentially of greater value than chemoprophylaxis because the approach would be less complex and would be most likely to prevent late-onset as well as early-onset disease.[126,304,310,311] Because of the protective value of antibody directed against the capsular polysaccharide of GBS, *passive immunization* of antibody-deficient women or newborns with intravenous gamma globulin is a reasonable consideration.[126] Given that transplacental transfer of antibody does not occur until after the 34th week of gestation, this approach requires timing late in pregnancy. The value of intravenous human globulin administration was demonstrated in a newborn animal model of GBS sepsis. Of greatest promise is *active immunization* with purified GBS polysaccharide. Currently, the most prevalent types causing global GBS perinatal disease are III and Ia. The type III polysaccharide was shown to be immunogenic in adult volunteers, including pregnant women, and to be protective of neonatal infection in a mouse model of maternal immunization.[126,295,310-313] More refined vaccines are under development.[126] The identification of pilus-like structures on the surface of GBS, their potential importance in GBS colonization and pathogenicity, and the ubiquitous presence of their coding loci in the GBS genome make these structures important candidates in the development of a vaccine.[314] More data are needed about the optimal vaccine preparation, the degree of immunogenicity, and the prophylactic benefit of available vaccine preparations before widespread use can be recommended, but the approach appears to be very promising.

Supportive Care

Because most infants with neonatal bacterial meningitis exhibit bacteremia and, to varying degrees, multisystem disease, vigorous supportive care is often a major factor in determining outcome. Diligent attention must be paid to ventilation, perfusion, temperature, metabolic state, and complications such as disseminated intravascular coagulation and the development of focal areas of suppurative infection.

Particular importance for vigorous treatment of systemic hypotension relates to the danger of decreases in cerebral blood flow and the consequent occurrence of ischemic neuronal and white matter injury. Thus the combination of increased intracranial pressure (see Table 35.13) and impaired cerebrovascular autoregulation (see Fig. 35.11) may lead to impaired cerebral blood flow particularly easily with systemic hypotension. A careful clinical study of the occurrence of periventricular leukomalacia in infants with GBS infection supported this conclusion.[279]

Neurological Disturbances

The major neurological disturbances that must be dealt with in these infants are seizures, inappropriate antidiuretic hormone secretion, cerebral edema, acute hydrocephalus, subdural effusion, and brain abscess.

Seizures. Seizures associated with neonatal bacterial meningitis are notoriously difficult to manage, particularly in the early phases of the disease. Seizures that occur later in the disease, often related to vasculitis and ischemic events, are controlled more readily. In the newborn, phenobarbital is the drug of choice; the dosage regimen, mode of administration, and other aspects of anticonvulsant management are described in Chapter 12.

Inappropriate Antidiuretic Hormone Secretion. Inappropriate antidiuretic hormone secretion should be suspected in the infant who exhibits hyponatremia and hypo-osmolality with inappropriately concentrated urine. The diagnosis can be suggested by measurements of serum and urine osmolality, urine volume, fluid intake, and body weight. A radioimmunoassay for antidiuretic hormone can corroborate the diagnosis.[234,235]

The syndrome may lead to a degree of hyponatremia and hypo-osmolality that results in deterioration of the level of consciousness and seizures as well as aggravation of increased intracranial pressure. Therapy consists principally of fluid restriction.

Cerebral Edema. Cerebral edema is common early in the disease but is rarely severe enough to cause life-threatening herniation of the temporal lobe through the tentorial notch or cerebellar tonsils through the foramen magnum. However, this occurrence has been documented in the newborn.[156] Elevation of intracranial pressure is a common accompaniment, but when arterial blood pressure is maintained, the degree of intracranial hypertension alone is not usually severe enough to raise the likelihood of impaired cerebral perfusion. Measurements of cerebral blood flow velocity in patients with neonatal bacterial meningitis support this conclusion.[155] Nevertheless, intracranial pressure should be determined and, as noted earlier, control of arterial blood pressure is crucial.

Specific treatment of suspected cerebral edema must not be instituted without good reason. Indeed, considerable concern exists that use of hyperosmolar solutions (e.g., mannitol) could cause more difficulties than benefits because of increased movement of the material across the inflamed and permeable blood-brain barrier. Nevertheless, study of a rabbit model of bacterial meningitis showed, after bolus infusion of mannitol, not only a decline in elevated intracranial pressure but also a decrease in elevated CSF lactate and hypoxanthine concentrations, consistent with an improvement in cerebral perfusion.[315] More data are needed on this issue.

Corticosteroids (dexamethasone) are worthy of consideration because of their value in management of some forms of vasogenic edema (e.g., in association with brain tumors) and bacterial meningitis in older infants and children (particularly that caused by H. influenzae).[315-319] In the latter situation, corticosteroids (dexamethasone) administered at the onset of antibiotic therapy have been associated with a decreased incidence of neurological or audiological sequelae, perhaps through inhibition of cytokine production and action. However, a randomized clinical trial of 54 infants with neonatal meningitis showed no apparent benefit of dexamethasone (0.15 mg/kg every 6 hours for 4 days from onset of antibiotic treatment).[320] In a Cochrane review, only two randomized controlled trials of very low quality were available; these suggested some reduction in death and hearing loss from use of adjunctive steroids with standard antibiotic therapy for the treatment of patients with neonatal meningitis. There was no reduction in neurological sequelae.[321] Administration of fluids at minimal maintenance levels is usually adequate in the management of cerebral edema with neonatal bacterial meningitis.

Acute Hydrocephalus. *Acute* hydrocephalus is a serious, although uncommon, complication. This complication should be suspected when signs of increased intracranial pressure appear in the latter part of the first week and in the second and third weeks of the disease (see also the sections on clinical signs and diagnosis later). When prompt decompression is needed, ventriculostomy is the most effective and safest treatment. Because acute hydrocephalus is often related to marked ventriculitis with localized infection that may be inaccessible to systemic antibiotics, ventriculostomy may also be used for instillation of antibiotic (see the section on ventriculostomy later). Occasionally intraventricular infection and inflammation subside, and the hydrocephalus does not progress after removal of the ventriculostomy. More commonly, a ventriculoperitoneal shunt is subsequently required for long-term treatment of the hydrocephalic state.

Subdural Effusion. Subdural effusion is rarely of clinical significance in neonatal meningitis (i.e., it is not associated with increased intracranial pressure, localized infection, or development of craniocerebral disproportion).[233,322,323] This complication can be detected from the clinical evaluation, coupled with transillumination, or, in the more suggestive case, by computed tomography (CT) or preferably MRI. In the absence of signs of increased intracranial pressure, localized infection, or imminent development of craniocerebral disproportion, a patient with subdural effusion detected by imaging should not be subjected to repeated taps because the natural history of the lesion is to resolve spontaneously.[322,323]

Brain Abscess. Brain abscess may occur with neonatal bacterial meningitis (see earlier discussion); its management is discussed in a separate section later. The diagnosis is best made by MRI,

and the use of contrast enhancement (gadolinium) can be used to better delineate the lesion.

Pneumocephalus. Gas-containing encephalitis is rarely associated with neonatal meningitis.[169,324-327] Intracranial anaerobic and aerobic infections may produce gas by putrefaction of the intracellular protein derived from autolysis and by decomposition of glucose. Gas production has been reported in a few cases with such gram-negative bacteria as *Citrobacter koseri*, *Proteus*, and *Enterobacter*. In one infant this occurrence was associated with pneumatosis oculi.[169] All reported cases have been fatal.

Antibiotics

The central goal in the treatment of neonatal bacterial meningitis is eradication of microorganisms from the CSF. To accomplish this, the appropriate antibiotic must be chosen and administered in adequate doses and by an effective route. In general the CSF in meningitis secondary to gram-positive organisms (e.g., GBS and *L. monocytogenes*) is more readily sterilized than in meningitis secondary to gram-negative organisms. Thus, with GBS or *L. monocytogenes*, negative cultures are usually attained after 24 to 48 hours of treatment, whereas with coliform bacilli, negative cultures generally are not obtained until after 2 to 5 days of treatment.[245,328,329] To a considerable degree, this time difference relates to the relative ease of attaining adequate CSF concentrations of ampicillin versus an aminoglycoside.

Initial Treatment. Initial empirical therapy for suspected bacterial meningitis within the first 3 to 6 days of age is ampicillin and an aminoglycoside, usually gentamicin.[a] An alternative regimen of ampicillin and an expanded spectrum third-generation cephalosporin (such as cefotaxime) can be used if *Listeria monocytogenes* or enterococci are unlikely. Adding cefotaxime to the regimen broadens empirical coverage for gram-negative organisms. High rates of ampicillin resistance among *E. coli* isolates and a link between maternal intrapartum ampicillin and *E. coli* resistance have been reported in very-low-birth-weight (VLBW) infants (birth weight [BW] <1500 g) but not in near-term or term infants. For infants who are still admitted or have been recently discharged, the antibiotic therapy should take into account the resistance patterns of pathogens present within the unit and previously cultured from the baby. In the neonatal intensive care unit (NICU) setting, cephalosporin use should be restricted to neonates with suspected bacterial meningitis based on CSF parameters and/or clinical findings. When cefotaxime is routinely used (e.g., when it is used more broadly for all neonates treated for "rule out sepsis"), rapid emergence of cephalosporin-resistant strains (especially *Enterobacter cloacae*, *Klebsiella pneumoniae*, and *Serratia* species) may occur. Carbapenem would be selected when the baby is known to be colonized with extended-spectrum beta lactamase (ESBL) producing strains or cefotaxim-resistant bacteria. The drugs can be administered intramuscularly, but intravenous administration is preferred. Standard sources should be consulted for recent changes in preferred antibiotics and dosing. Time to sterilization of the CSF has an impact on neurodevelopmental outcome.

Specific Treatment. When a definitive bacteriological diagnosis is established and appropriate susceptibilities are determined,

---

[a]References 30, 126, 127, 133, 233, 245, and 330-334.

TABLE 35.23 Antibiotics Preferred in Neonatal Meningitis According to Organism

ORGANISM	ANTIBIOTICS
Group B *Streptococcus*	Ampicillin (or penicillin G) and aminoglycoside (gentamicin)
Escherichia coli and other coliforms	Aminoglycoside and ampicillin or third-generation cephalosporin (cefotaxime) with or without aminoglycoside
Aminoglycoside-resistant coliforms	Third-generation cephalosporin (cefotaxime)
Listeria monocytogenes	Ampicillin with or without aminoglycoside
Group D *Streptococcus* (nonenterococcal)	Ampicillin
Group D *Streptococcus* (enterococcal)	Ampicillin and aminoglycoside
Staphylococcus epidermidis	Vancomycin
Staphylococcus aureus	Methicillin or vancomycin
Pseudomonas aeruginosa	Ceftazidime and aminoglycoside
Citrobacter diversus	Third-generation cephalosporin (cefotaxime), gentamicin, trimethoprim-sulfamethoxazole (or meropenem or imipenem-cilastatin)

more specific antibiotic treatment can be instituted. The usual organisms and the respective, preferred antibiotics are shown in Table 35.23.[a] Thus a penicillin (ampicillin or penicillin G) and an aminoglycoside (see later section) are preferred for group B *Streptococcus*, ampicillin and an aminoglycoside or cefotaxime with or without an aminoglycoside are preferred for *E. coli* and most other coliforms, a third-generation cephalosporin (e.g., cefotaxime) is preferred for aminoglycoside-resistant coliform bacteria, ampicillin alone or with an aminoglycoside is preferred for *L. monocytogenes* and nonenterococcal group D *Streptococcus* (ampicillin and an aminoglycoside are used for enterococcal group D *Streptococcus*), vancomycin is used for *S. epidermidis* (a common organism in infants with indwelling vascular catheters) infections, methicillin or vancomycin is given for *S. aureus* (almost always beta-lactamase positive) infections, and a third-generation cephalosporin (ceftazidime) and an aminoglycoside are preferred for *P. aeruginosa*. Treatment of *Citrobacter diversus* is very difficult and consists of a third-generation cephalosporin (cefotaxime), gentamicin, and trimethoprim-sulfamethoxazole; imipenem-cilastatin may be a useful alternative to the last of these agents. Standard sources should be consulted for recent changes in preferred antibiotics and dosing.

Duration of Treatment. The duration of treatment in neonatal bacterial meningitis is based on the clinical condition of the patient, as well as on the bacteriological response to therapy. The latter is monitored by the sampling of CSF approximately every 2 to 3 days in the first week after initiation of therapy or until the CSF is sterile. In general meningitis caused by gram-negative organisms is treated for at least 2 weeks after sterilization of the CSF or for a total of 3 weeks, whichever is greater. Meningitis resulting from gram-positive organisms is most prudently treated also for 3 weeks, although the infant with a rapid bacteriological response and good clinical status could be treated for 2 weeks after bacteria can no longer be cultured from the CSF. A repeat examination of the CSF is indicated 48 hours after discontinuation of antibiotic therapy.

Treatment Failure. Treatment failure, for the purposes of this discussion, refers to abnormal persistence of a positive CSF culture, clinical deterioration, or both. Failure to sterilize the CSF in meningitis is much more common with gram-negative

than with gram-positive organisms and is related principally to (1) inadequate delivery of antibiotic to the site of the infection within the subarachnoid and ventricular spaces, (2) the presence of an organism that is not sensitive to the usually attainable concentration of antibiotic in the CSF, (3) the presence of a site of infection that is inaccessible to antibiotic, and (4) host factors. Evaluation of these factors requires the assessment of antibiotic levels in at least lumbar (and perhaps ventricular) CSF, of inhibitory and bactericidal susceptibilities of the organism to the antibiotics used and of a possible site of sequestered infection (e.g., ventriculitis; see the next section).

Ventriculitis

Ventriculitis is considered an important cause of the difficulty in sterilizing the CSF and, as a corollary, of the relatively poor prognosis in neonatal bacterial meningitis, particularly that resulting from infection with gram-negative organisms, for two major reasons. First, as described earlier, involvement of the ventricular lining is a nearly uniform occurrence.[89,146] Second, as noted by experienced clinicians and as reported in earlier uncontrolled series of infants with ventriculitis and persistence of infection in the CSF after treatment with systemic antibiotics, intraventricular instillation of antibiotics appears to be beneficial in *selected* cases.[147,245,343-345]

Inadequacy of Intrathecal Therapy. Intrathecal antibiotic therapy is not an adequate means of sterilizing ventricular CSF or improving outcome in gram-negative neonatal bacterial meningitis. In a controlled study of 117 infants with meningitis caused by gram-negative organisms, the effect of the addition of intrathecal gentamicin to a regimen of systemic ampicillin and gentamicin was evaluated.[328] No benefit of intrathecal antibiotic was observed. The failure to demonstrate any benefit from the intrathecal therapy was considered to suggest that adequate concentrations of antibiotic were not delivered throughout the CNS and, particularly, the ventricular system. Failure of intrathecal administration of antibiotics to enter and sterilize the ventricular CSF has been demonstrated in older patients.[346,347] These observations are entirely compatible with the unidirectional flow of CSF out of the ventricular system.

Inadequacy of Routine Intraventricular Therapy. A cooperative study of 70 infants with meningitis caused by gram-negative organisms was carried out to evaluate the role of *intraventricular*

[a]References 127, 133, 215, 228, 229, 233, 245, 287, 332, 335, and 337-342.

TABLE 35.24   Effect of Intraventricular Therapy on Neonatal Meningitis and Ventriculitis Caused by Gram-Negative Enteric Organisms[a]

MODE OF THERAPY	DAYS CSF CULTURE POSITIVE	MORTALITY RATE	NORMAL (PERCENTAGE OF SURVIVORS)
Parenteral[b]	3.6	13%	54%
Parenteral[b] and intraventricular[c]	3.4	44%	60%

CSF, Cerebrospinal fluid.
[a]Based on 51 cases.
[b]Ampicillin and gentamicin.
[c]Gentamicin.
Data from McCracken GH Jr, Mize SG, Neonatal Cooperative Study Group. Intraventricular therapy of neonatal meningitis caused by gram-negative enteric bacilli. *Pediatr Res.* 1979;13:464.

instillation of gentamicin (in addition to systemic ampicillin and gentamicin).[328] Fifty-one infants had evidence of ventriculitis (i.e., ventricular CSF containing more than 200 WBCs/mm³ or organisms on stained smear or culture); the results of treatment of that group are displayed in Table 35.24. No difference between the two groups in the time required to sterilize the CSF was observed. Still more impressive, the mortality rate in the infants treated with parenteral therapy alone was lower than in those treated with parenteral therapy and intraventricular therapy. Thus, *routine* intraventricular therapy of meningitis produced by gram-negative organisms had no beneficial effect and may have had a deleterious effect. If the latter is true, the cause of such a deleterious effect is unclear, although injury to myelin and axons in the brain stem of an adult human patient and in brain stem and spinal cord of rabbits administered gentamicin by the intrathecal route has been described.[348] Deleterious neurological and neuropathological effects of gentamicin have also been demonstrated in rabbits administered gentamicin intraventricularly.[349] However, in view of the generally favorable outcome in the control group, it is apparent that ventriculitis only very uncommonly results in a site of infection inaccessible to systemic antibiotics. Nevertheless, recent Cochrane review showed a threefold higher mortality in the group who were randomized to intraventricular gentamicin compared with those who received intravenous antibiotics, and it was not recommended to perform any further randomized trials to study this issue.[300,305,350-352]

Indications for Diagnostic Ventricular Puncture. The failure to improve the prognosis of meningitis caused by gram-negative bacteria with routine intraventricular therapy raises two important questions in the management of neonatal bacterial meningitis:
1. When should the lateral ventricle be tapped?
2. How should the information obtained be used?

As discussed earlier in the section on diagnosis, the indications for evaluating the lateral ventricles in the infant are as follows: (1) bacteriological (i.e., persistence of infection in the lumbar CSF at 4 days) or (2) clinical (i.e., failure of clinical improvement or, still more importantly, the appearance of clinical deterioration even if lumbar CSF cell count is improving and CSF sterilization occurs). If these indications are present and *antibiotic therapy has been appropriate in terms of susceptibilities of the organism, doses of the drugs, and, if available, concentrations of the critical drugs in the CSF,* an ultrasound or MRI scan should be obtained. If the ventricles are not too small,

TABLE 35.25   Intraventricular Antibiotics for Ventriculitis

ANTIBIOTIC	DOSE (mg)	DESIRED PEAK CEREBROSPINAL FLUID CONCENTRATION (µg/mL)
Gentamicin	1–5	80–120[a]
Vancomycin	4–5	80–100
Polymyxin	1–2	Unknown

[a]Histological change in white matter observed with concentrations >150 µg/mL.
Data from Smith AL, Haas J. Neonatal bacterial meningitis. In: Scheld WM, Whitley RJ, Durack DT, eds. *Infections of the Central Nervous System.* New York: Raven Press; 1991.

a ventricular tap should be performed. If the ventricular fluid exhibits marked pleocytosis and organisms demonstrable on smear or culture, it is likely that the systemically administered antibiotics, usually aminoglycosides in meningitis caused by gram-negative bacteria, are not eradicating a reservoir of infection within the ventricular system.

Ventriculostomy. Ventriculostomy with external drainage may be required in neonatal bacterial meningitis when ventriculitis has caused obstruction to CSF flow and acute hydrocephalus manifested by increased intracranial pressure and dilated lateral ventricles. This condition may develop despite eradication of the ventricular infection by the systemic antibiotics (Table 35.25) and therefore with a sterile ventricular CSF. In such a circumstance, intraventricular instillation of antibiotic is not needed and the task is management of the intracranial hypertension by CSF drainage, as described in Chapter 24 in relation to rapidly progressive posthemorrhagic hydrocephalus.

BRAIN ABSCESS

Brain abscess is an uncommon and devastating, although potentially treatable, disorder in the neonatal period (Table 35.26). Most examples of neonatal brain abscess occur as a complication of bacterial meningitis, especially that resulting from particularly virulent gram-negative organisms.[42,170,177,351-374] However, *S. aureus* was cultured from the abscess in several cases: two preterm infants and two infants who were 1 month

TABLE 35.26 Brain Abscess in the Newborn[a]

Occurrence without bacterial meningitis
≈33% of cases of neonatal brain abscess *not* accompanied by
bacterial meningitis
Relation to bacterial meningitis
≈15% of *gram-negative* bacterial meningitis complicated by
abscess
Most common organisms
Citrobacter diversus, Proteus species, *Serratia* species
Neuropathology
Abscesses usually large, multiple (≈60%), frontal (≈70%), and
not well encapsulated
Onset of clinical features
Average age, 9 days
Clinical presentation
Seizures > nonspecific signs of sepsis > increasing head
circumference
Complications
Hydrocephalus requiring shunt placement (35%): only in
patients with meningitis
Treatment
Aspiration (ultrasound-guided) and antibiotics generally
effective; antibiotics alone may lead to cure
Prognosis
Mortality rate, ≈15%; cognitive deficits, ≈75%; epilepsy, ≈60%

[a]See text for references.

and 3 months of age, respectively.[375-378] Approximately 30 cases of neonatal brain abscesses have been reported that were apparently not the consequence of meningitis.[a] However, lumbar punctures were not always performed, or were performed following administration of antibiotics, and the organism was cultured only following puncturing the abscess.[361,376,377]

Etiology

The most commonly reported organisms associated with brain abscess have been those with the particular capacity to invade nervous tissue and cause necrosis. Gram-negative organisms have been implicated most often, especially *Citrobacter* but also *Proteus, Pseudomonas, Serratia, Klebsiella,* and other coliform bacilli (see previous discussion of bacterial meningitis).[b] *Citrobacter* and, to a lesser extent, *Proteus* and *Serratia* are the most commonly identified pathogens. Gram-positive organisms are involved much less often, although GBS and *S. aureus* have been identified in isolated cases.[375-377,383,388-391] Spinal epidural abscess and a cerebellar abscess secondary to *S. aureus* also have been reported.[377,392] Still rarer, three cases of neonatal brain abscess secondary to *M. hominis* have been recorded.[384,385,389] Finally, as noted in the following section, certain fungi, especially *Candida*, may cause brain abscess, usually multiple and small, especially in very-low-birth-weight infants.

Pathogenesis

The common conditions for the development of brain abscess are *cerebral necrosis and bacteremia*. In bacterial meningitis, the parenchymal necrosis that may become infected to form an abscess is usually caused initially by vasculitis with infarction. It is not surprising, then, that the organisms associated with brain abscess are those that produce severe vasculopathy with the meningitis. This point was demonstrated vividly by the study of Foreman and co-workers.[393] Severe vasculitis with infarction and with numerous organisms present around inflamed blood vessels and in cerebral parenchyma was shown in two infants who died within 2 days of clinical onset of meningitis caused by *Citrobacter*.[393] Presumably the next phase of the illness would have been infection of necrotic tissue and abscess formation, a feature of approximately 50% to 80% of reported cases of *Citrobacter* meningitis.[a] In the rarer cases of brain abscess not associated with primary meningitis, the initial injury to brain is not always clear but has often appeared to be hypoxic-ischemic cerebral injury, periventricular hemorrhagic infarction, or septic embolus.

Neuropathology

The distinguishing features of brain abscess in the newborn have been threefold: (1) relatively large size of lesions, (2) relatively poor capsule formation, and (3) multiple number. The lesions have been located almost uniformly in the cerebral hemispheres, most often the frontal lobes, and have often encompassed several lobes. Occasionally the abscess has been tapped inadvertently at the time of ventricular or subdural puncture. Detailed microscopic data are not available, but hemorrhage and necrosis have usually been noted with the purulence.

Clinical Features

Two major clinical syndromes have been described with neonatal brain abscess: (1) an acute to subacute evolution of signs of cerebral parenchymal involvement, especially seizures (less commonly, hemiparesis), often accompanied by signs of increased intracranial pressure (vomiting, bulging anterior fontanelle, separated sutures, and an enlarging head); and (2) an acute onset of fulminating bacterial meningitis. The *first syndrome* is more common, has its onset from the first few days to weeks of life, and often occurs in association with acute or ongoing bacterial meningitis. The initial diagnosis has occasionally been congenital hydrocephalus. The *second syndrome* differs little from later-onset neonatal bacterial meningitis (see previous section).

Diagnosis

Clinical Evaluation

The diagnosis of brain abscess should be considered in any infant with the acute or subacute evolution of signs of increased intracranial pressure or possible hydrocephalus. In the absence of meningitis, fever is not a feature; in the six well-studied cases of Hoffman and co-workers,[380] four infants were afebrile. In an infant with bacterial meningitis, brain abscess should be suspected when seizures or prominent focal cerebral signs develop, a poor clinical response to antibiotic therapy occurs, or the CSF formula does not appear to be compatible with the clinical syndrome (e.g., several hundred WBCs in the CSF of a gravely ill infant, or, in a child with "meningitis" and a few hundred WBCs in the initial CSF, the sudden appearance of

[a]References 170, 176, 366, 370, 373, 377, and 379-385.
[b]References 42, 170, 173, 177, 353-355, 358, 359, 361-364, 366-370, 386, and 387.

[a]References 170, 353, 354, 357-359, 362, 367, and 386.

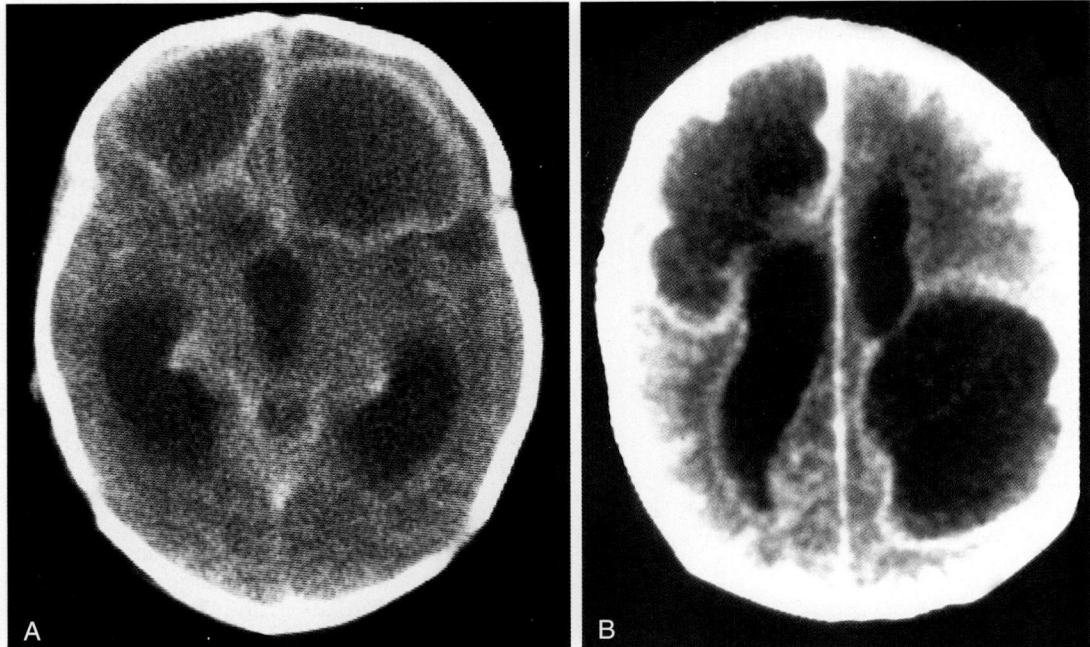

Figure 35.22 Brain abscess: computed tomography. After injection of contrast material, scans were obtained from infants with *Citrobacter diversus* meningitis. Note the areas of decreased attenuation surrounded by a rim of increased attenuation in (A) bilateral frontal areas and (B) right frontal and left parietal areas. (Courtesy Dr. Mark W. Kline.)

several thousand polymorphonuclear WBCs in a subsequent CSF examination and marked clinical deterioration). (The latter occurrence develops with rupture of the brain abscess into the lateral ventricle or subarachnoid space.)

Laboratory Evaluation

Peripheral White Blood Cell Count. The combination of clinical features just described, without fever but with a high peripheral WBC count, is common in brain abscess without meningitis. In the series of Hoffman and co-workers,[380] the peripheral WBC count ranged from 18,000 to 34,000.

Cerebrospinal Fluid. In the infant without bacterial meningitis, the CSF usually contains pleocytosis consisting predominantly of mononuclear cells, usually numbering less than a few hundred. CSF protein content is elevated, usually to approximately 75 to 150 mg/100 mL. Unless bacterial meningitis is also present, the organism will not be apparent on Gram stain or culture. The sudden appearance of clinical deterioration and thousands of polymorphonuclear leukocytes in the CSF is characteristic of rupture of the abscess into the ventricular system.

Brain Imaging. The diagnosis of brain abscess is usually raised by ultrasound or, especially, MRI. CT is no longer the first diagnostic method of choice; when used, however, it shows a variably circumscribed region of decreased attenuation, often much greater in extent than the abscess itself, because of the presence of cerebritis with surrounding edema. The rim of the abscess usually enhances after the injection of contrast material (Fig. 35.22). MRI provides better resolution than does CT and is preferred (Figs. 35.23 and 35.24).

Cranial ultrasound is often useful in diagnosing cerebral abscess in the newborn, especially since the frontal lobes are well within the field of view (Fig. 35.25; see also Fig. 35.23). Thus, in experimental brain abscess, ultrasound scanning was as effective as CT in identifying the early stages. An echogenic rim with a hypoechogenic center was characteristic.[394] Such an appearance has been observed in neonatal brain abscess.[a]

Identification of the Organism. The organism can occasionally be isolated from blood, but aspiration of the abscess cavity is usually necessary to obtain a definite bacteriological diagnosis. (In the presence of meningitis, the organism can be isolated from the CSF.) Aspiration can be carried out with ultrasonographic guidance (see the section on management). Because some of the responsible organisms require special techniques for isolation and identification, the material should be handled in an especially careful manner.

Prognosis

The prognosis has been poor for those infants in whom correct diagnosis and appropriate treatment were delayed. Overall, approximately 15% of newborns with brain abscess have died of the acute illness; of the survivors, 75% have experienced mental deficiency (intelligence quotient or development quotient <80), and 60% have developed epilepsy.[b] Perhaps the most unfavorable outcome has been in infants with abscess and *C. diversus* meningitis; the mortality rate has been 30%, and only 20% of survivors have been normal on follow-up.

Management

The most essential issue concerning management is prompt diagnosis. In the infant with meningitis, particularly that caused

[a]References 361, 363, 365, 388, 395, and 396.
[b]References 170, 173, 353-356, 358, 359, 361-363, 365, 380, and 383.

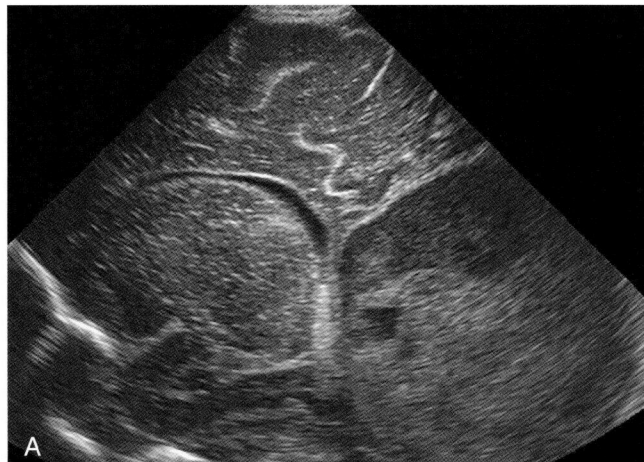

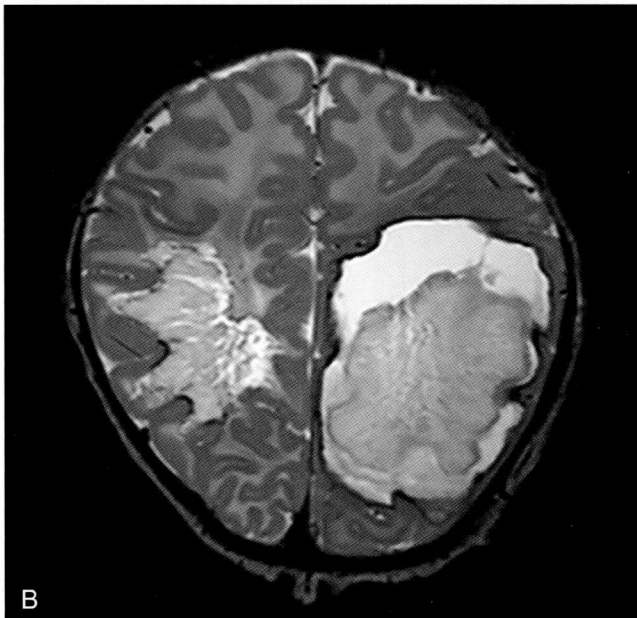

Figure 35.23 Neonatal brain abscess, ultrasound and magnetic resonance imaging (MRI). Left parasagittal cranial ultrasound (A) and axial MRI, T2-weighted sequence (B), showing a large left sided abscess and a smaller one on the right. The cerebrospinal fluid culture was negative but *Proteus mirabilis* was cultured from the abscess.

Figure 35.24 Brain abscess: magnetic resonance imaging (MRI) after gadolinium contrast. This 5-week-old infant had focal seizures, *Proteus* sepsis, and a complicated congenital cardiac lesion, including an atrioventricular canal defect. This axial MRI scan shows a striking ring-enhancing cerebral lesion, consistent with brain abscess. Craniotomy with drainage of the abscess was performed. (Courtesy Dr. Omar Khwaja.)

and good penetration into the CNS (e.g., third-generation cephalosporins) will prove most useful in this regard remains to be determined. In the case of *C. diversus*, the addition to the antibiotic regimen of a drug that is concentrated in phagocytes (i.e., trimethoprim-sulfamethoxazole) or to which the organism is especially sensitive (i.e., meropenem or imipenem) may be particularly important.[354,358,359]

Despite the multiple reports of *medical cure* of brain abscess, drainage is necessary in selected cases. Of the two approaches to drainage (i.e., serial aspirations and open surgical drainage), the advent of ultrasound-guided aspiration suggests that this method is of particular value, even for multiple lesions.[395,396] CT-guided aspiration can also be used, but this approach is less convenient. Needle aspiration is useful not only for initial diagnosis and drainage but also for determining antibiotic levels in the abscess cavity.

Open surgical drainage is the most definitive therapeutic approach for brain abscess. However, if the infant's condition is not deteriorating and the responsible organism has been identified, a trial of intensive antibiotic therapy, followed, if necessary, by serial ultrasound-guided needle aspiration, is reasonable. Careful serial brain imaging should be performed to ensure that the lesion (or lesions) is (are) not worsening. In such a circumstance, prompt open surgical drainage is necessary.

DISSEMINATED FUNGAL INFECTION

Invasive candidiasis (*Candida* infections of the blood and other body fluids) is the second most common cause of infectious disease–related death in the extremely premature infant. Despite antifungal treatment, 20% of infants who develop invasive

by *Citrobacter, Proteus, Klebsiella,* or *Serratia,* serial brain imaging is indicated to detect abscess as early as possible. In the infant without meningitis, a high index of clinical suspicion is critical and appropriate imaging procedures are essential.

No consensus exists for therapy for brain abscess in the neonatal period. The three principal approaches are (1) medical therapy alone, (2) aspirations through a burr hole or by the percutaneous route, and (3) open surgical drainage and extirpation. The demonstration of cure with systemic antibiotics early in the disease has been observed in newborns as well as in older children.[a] Whether antibiotics with potent bactericidal activity, broad antibacterial spectrum,

[a]References 177, 355, 356, 361, 377, 384, 388, and 397-401.

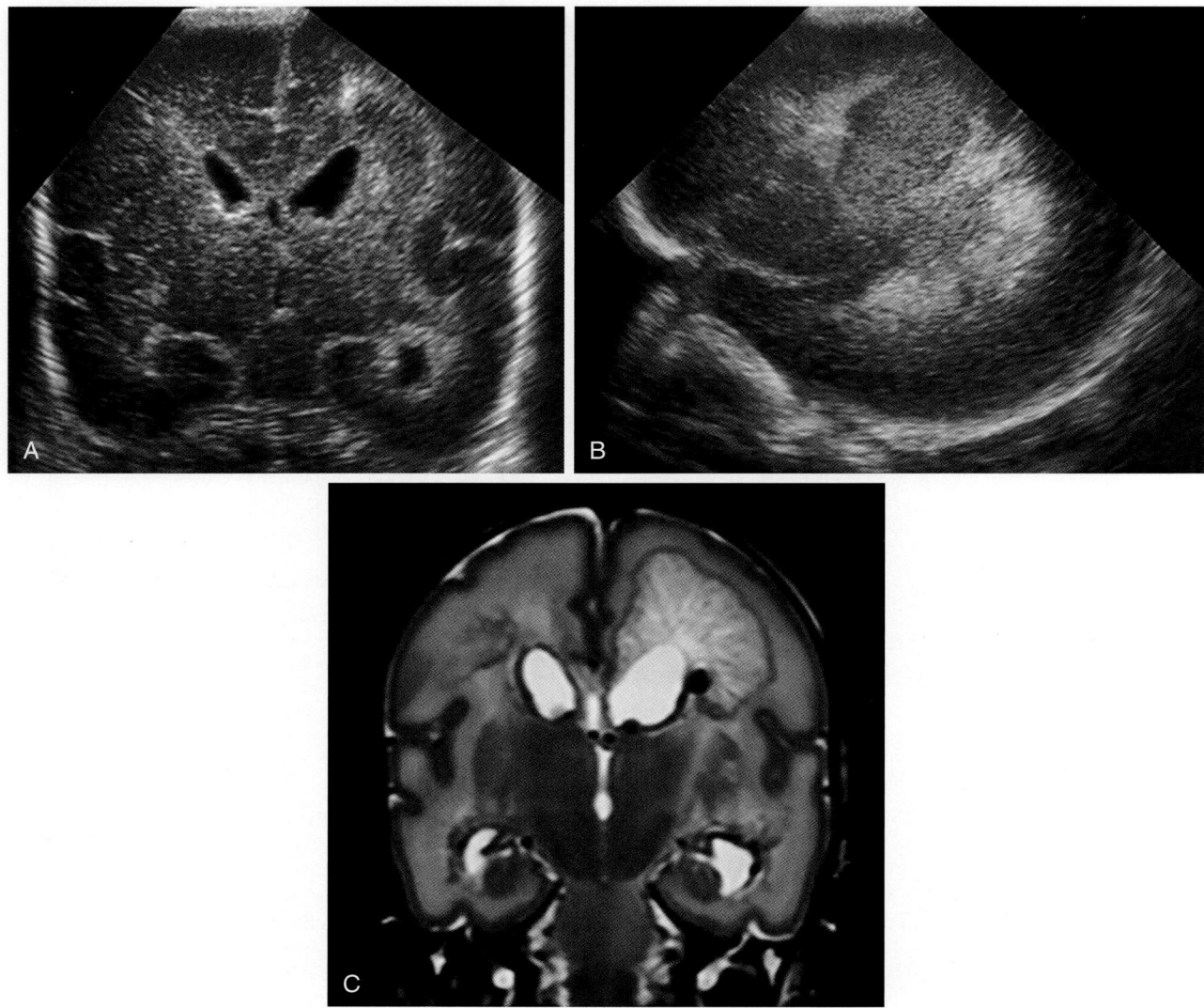

Figure 35.25 Coronal (A) and parasagittal (B) cranial ultrasound in a preterm infant (28 weeks' gestational age) with *Serratia marcescens* infection. On the parasagittal view (B) extensive areas of increased echogenicity are seen adjacent to the round area of relative echolucency. The coronal magnetic resonance images, T2-weighted sequence (C), confirm the large left-sided abscess.

candidiasis die, and neurodevelopmental impairment occurs in nearly 60% of survivors.[214,402] Disseminated fungal infection in the newborn may cause meningitis, often with microabscesses. This category of nonbacterial disease is discussed here rather than in Chapter 34 because the clinical features often mimic those of bacterial sepsis and the neuropathological features are similar to those of bacterial meningitis and brain abscess. Although several fungi (e.g., *Cryptococcus*, *Coccidioides*, and *Aspergillus*) have been reported to cause meningitis, abscess, or both, in the newborn systemic infection by *Candida*, especially *Candida albicans* and, more recently, *Candida parapsilosis*, particularly in the very-low-birth-weight newborn, is by far the most common neonatal disseminated fungal infection.[402-424] Earlier studies of somewhat selected cases indicate that at least one third of cases of systemic candidiasis in premature infants exhibited involvement of the CNS.[403,410,411] More recent data show that approximately 10% to 25% of cases exhibit CNS

involvement.[402,405,414,417] However, the magnitude of the problem is substantial because approximately 10% to 20% of all infants weighing less than 1000 g at birth develop candidiasis, as do approximately 25% of infants of 23 to 24 weeks of gestational age.[402,419,425,426] The major features of systemic candidiasis in the newborn are summarized in Table 35.27.

Pathogenesis

The reasons that the newborn, particularly the premature newborn, is vulnerable to disseminated fungal infection are not entirely known but involve a combination of multiple immune deficiencies and insufficient anatomical barriers to infection in a setting of intensive medical interventions for systemic illness.[404,411,426,427] The common historical findings of intrapartum antibiotics, prolonged use of indwelling vascular catheters often with receipt of intravenous lipid emulsion, endotracheal intubation, administration of broad-spectrum antibiotics, and the use of steroids and gastric acid–suppressing agents in the week prior to culture, necrotizing enterocolitis, and surgery indicate possible portals of entry for the organism.[a] The retrograde medication syringes of total parenteral nutrition systems were important sites for infection in one large study.[427] The prior use of multiple courses of broad-spectrum antibiotics in most patients is a likely cause of disrupted microbial flora and enhances the potential for fungal infection.[411,426,427,430]

Neuropathology

Neuropathological studies of neonatal systemic candidiasis are not abundant.[417,426] However, the principal features have included meningitis, ventriculitis, and cerebral or cerebellar microabscesses. The abscesses are characterized by a necrotic center with a rim of inflammatory cells and edema (Figs. 35.26 and 35.27). Fungal filaments are common in the lesion. With subacute lesions, a more granulomatous appearance

---

[a]References 404, 408, 411, 418, 423, and 426-429.

---

develops, and endothelial proliferation is often prominent. The microabscesses may become confluent and may create prominent mass lesions. A subdural empyema was reported in a preterm infant who had a malpositioned central venous catheter such that the tip of the catheter migrated into the epidural space.[431]

Clinical Features

Like bacterial sepsis, systemic candidiasis does not produce a distinct clinical syndrome. However, certain features are common (see Table 35.27), such as insidious more often than abrupt onset, mean age of approximately 2 to 4 weeks (albeit with an overall wider range), respiratory deterioration (often requiring reinstitution of ventilatory therapy), apnea and bradycardia, abdominal signs suggestive of necrotizing enterocolitis (e.g., abdominal distention and guaiac-positive stools), and carbohydrate intolerance with hyperglycemia and glycosuria.[a] Many infants exhibit a generalized macular erythematous rash shortly after onset of the systemic illness; skin abscesses are apparent somewhat less commonly.[403,411,427]

Diagnosis

A high index of suspicion and a persistent approach to diagnosis are critical. *Identification of the organism in blood, CSF, or urine* is the most common means of establishing the diagnosis.[b] Gram stain of urine or CSF, especially urine, is a useful means of diagnosis. The presence of gram-positive, small, oval, budding yeast cells and sometimes hyphae with budding yeast cells attached along their length is typical.[423] Culture then results in growth of the organism in 2 to 3 days; however, cultures may be positive only intermittently, and frequent cultures are necessary. The use of *Candida*-specific PCR was initially limited by unacceptably high rates of contamination, resulting in false-positive tests; but newer assays are more specific and sensitive and allow rapid detection, within hours, of *Candida* DNA in the blood samples of infants at risk for candidemia.[433]

---

[a]References 402, 410-412, 414, 417, 418, 423, 426-428, and 432.
[b]References 403, 411, 418, 423, 426, 427, and 432.

TABLE 35.27 Major Features of Systemic Candidiasis
Very-low-birth-weight infant (<1500 g), especially extremely low-birth-weight infant (<1000 g)
History of *broad-spectrum antibiotic therapy* and *indwelling vascular catheters*; also, total parenteral nutrition, steroid therapy, necrotizing enterocolitis, and abdominal or cardiac surgery
Acute or subacute evolution of respiratory deterioration, temperature instability, apnea and bradycardia, abdominal distention, guaiac-positive stools, and hyperglycemia
Diagnosis by identification of organism (usually *Candida albicans*) by Gram stain and culture
Neuropathology of meningitis and brain abscesses
Treatment by combination of amphotericin B and flucytosine
Outcome in promptly identified and treated patients improving: 70%–85% survive but ≈50% of survivors have neurodevelopmental impairments

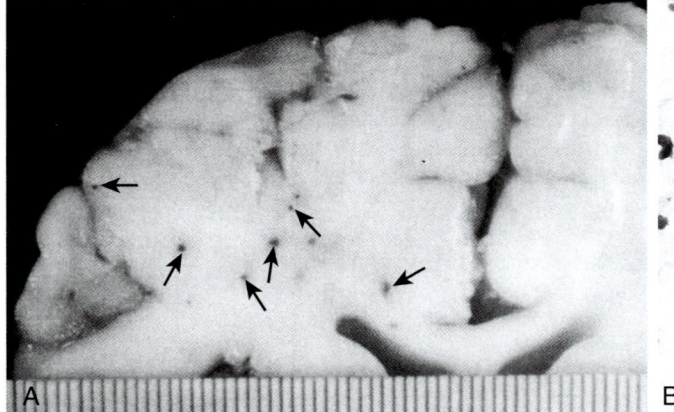
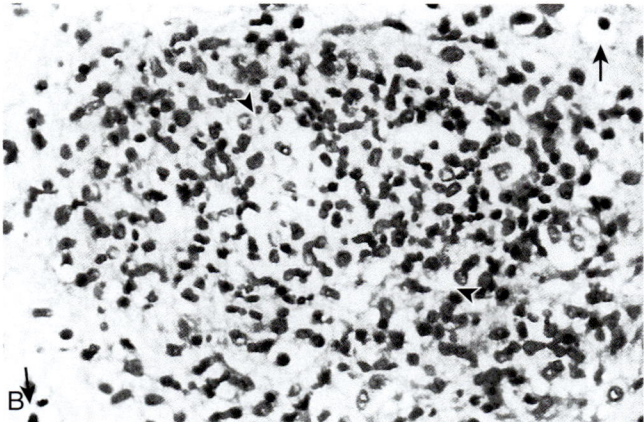

Figure 35.26 Neuropathology of disseminated candidiasis in a premature infant (29 weeks' gestation) who died at 3 months of age. Note the microabscesses *(arrows)* in (A), a coronal section of cerebrum. (B) Photomicrograph of a microabscess shows a slightly necrotic center with infiltrating leukocytes *(arrowheads)* and surrounding swollen astrocytes *(arrows)*. (From Huang CC, Chen CY, Yang HB, Wang SM, et al. Central nervous system candidiasis in very low-birth-weight premature neonates and infants: US characteristics and histopathologic and MR imaging correlates in five patients. *Radiology.* 1998;209:49–56.)

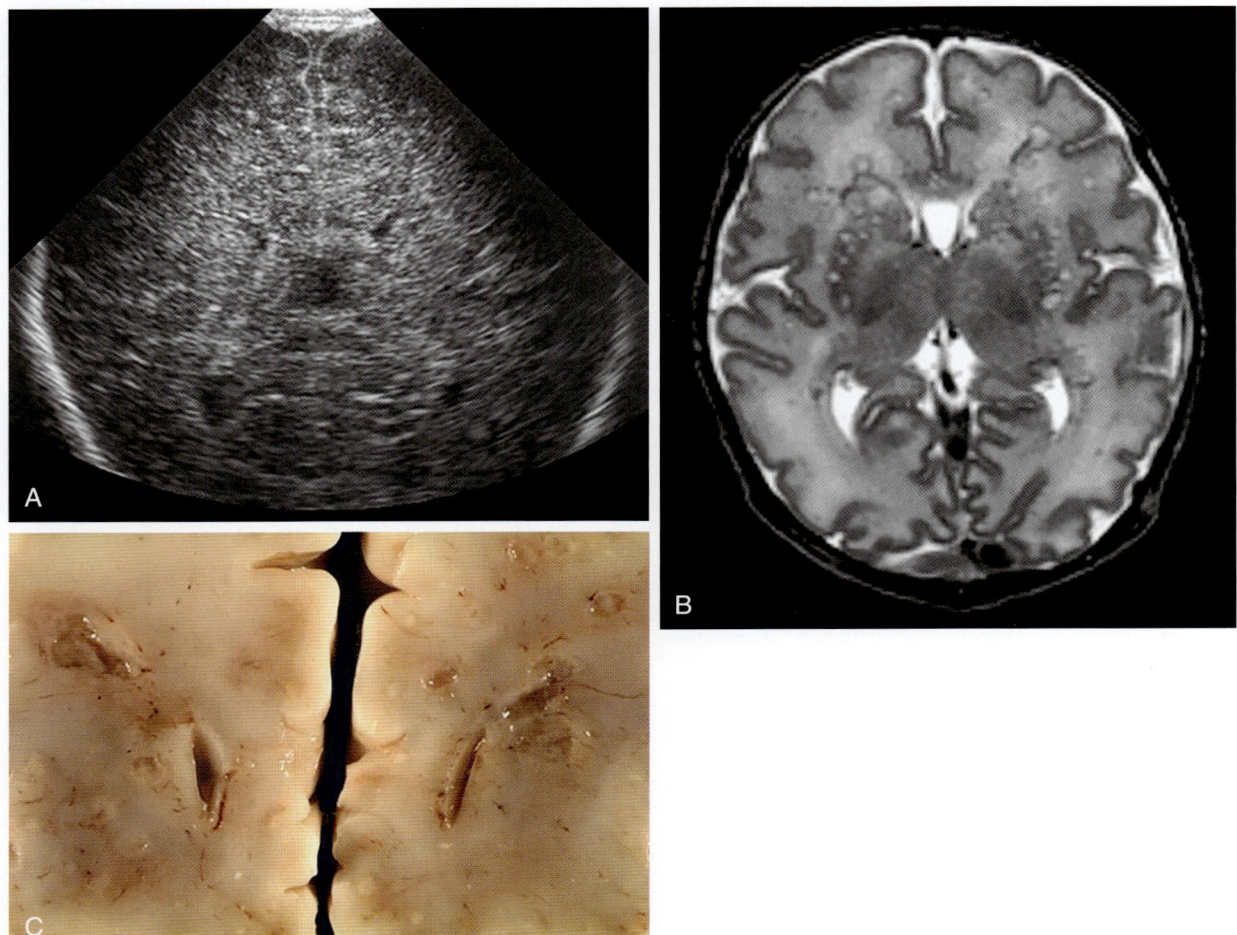

Figure 35.27 Disseminated candidiasis: ultrasound, magnetic resonance imaging (MRI), and neuropathology. Coronal cranial ultrasound (A) and axial MRI, T2-weighted sequence (B) in a preterm infant with disseminated candidiasis. Cranial ultrasound (A) shows severe, diffuse echogenicity throughout the white matter. On MRI (B), small round microabscesses can be recognized in the basal ganglia. (C) Neuropathology of the same infant showing a coronal brain section with multiple microabscesses as well as some larger abscesses. (Courtesy Dr. P.G. Nikkels.)

Careful *study of the CSF* shows abnormalities, albeit often not marked, in most patients with CNS involvement.[434] In a study of 13 patients, the WBC count was greater than 10/mm³ in 10 patients (range, 2 to 260/mm³), the protein concentration was greater than 100 mg/dL in 11 (range, 84 to 825 mg/dL), and the CSF-to-serum glucose ratio was less than 0.60 in 4 patients (range, 0.35 to 0.70).[410] At least one of these abnormalities was present in all 13 patients. In a later study of 5 infants, the CSF WBC count ranged from 31 to 399/mm³, the protein concentration ranged from 127 to 259 mg/dL, and the glucose concentration ranged from 10 to 58 mg/dL.[417] In a study of 16 infants, the median WBC count was 52/mm³ and the protein level 226 mg/dL.[412] However, it is not unusual to observe overt *Candida* meningitis by cranial imaging with unremarkable CSF findings. Moreover, cerebral abscesses have been reported in multiple infants with negative CSF cultures, negative CSF examinations, and often both.[414,416,428]

The structural pathology is shown particularly well by ultrasound and MRI.[417,435] Ultrasonography is especially effective in demonstrating the intraventricular septae and periventricular echogenicity of the ventriculitis (Fig. 35.28). Moreover, the

multiple echogenic foci of microabscesses may be seen in cerebral parenchyma, basal ganglia, and cerebellum. They are usually not seen in the first days of candidemia but rather within a week after onset of the infection.[435] MRI is particularly sensitive for the demonstration of the microabscesses and meningitis, especially in the posterior fossa, and even better when gadolinium is used (Figs. 35.29 and 35.30). The additional value of diffusion-weighted imaging (DWI) was noted in eight preterm infants by showing hyperintense signal on DWI consistent with diffuse or multiple miliary nodules at a time when T1- and T2-weighted imaging failed to show clear abnormalities in signal intensity. DWI abnormalities were present for a period of about 3 weeks. Signal changes on T1- and T2-weighted imaging became more obvious within 2 to 4 weeks following the CNS infection, with ring-shaped lesions consisting of a hyperintense border and lower signal in the center on T1-weighted imaging.[436]

Prognosis

Once the blood culture is positive for *Candida*, further investigations should be performed including the assessment

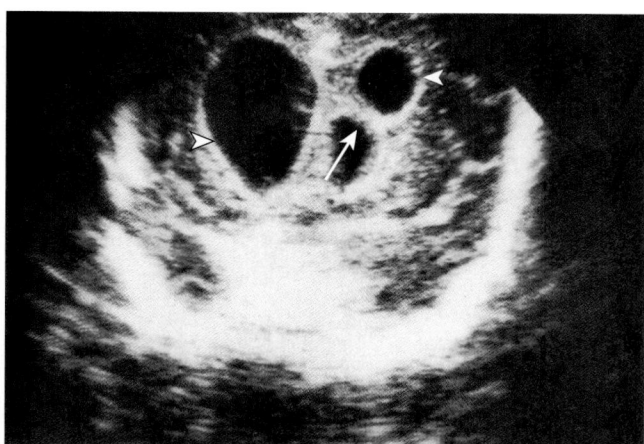

Figure 35.28 Disseminated candidiasis: coronal ultrasound in a premature infant. Note the echogenic ependyma *(arrowheads)* and the intraventricular septa *(arrow)*, both consistent with ventriculitis. (From Huang CC, Chen CY, Yang HB, Wang SM, et al. Central nervous system candidiasis in very-low-birth-weight premature neonates and infants: US characteristics and histopathologic and MR imaging correlates in five patients. *Radiology.* 1998;209:49–56.)

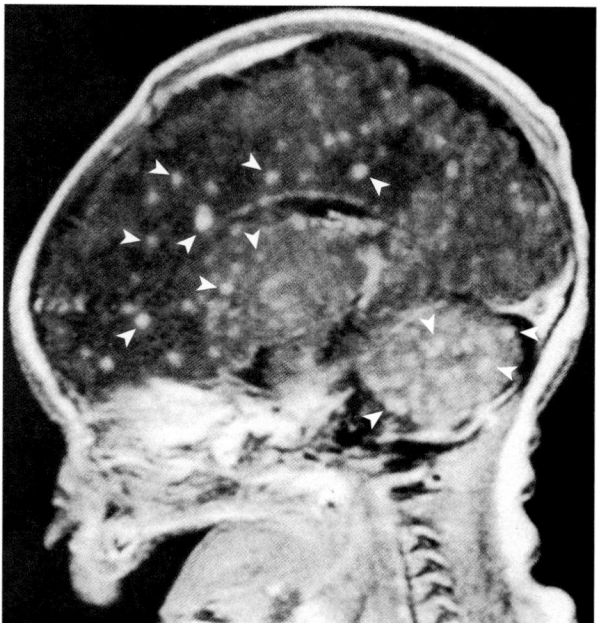

Figure 35.29 Disseminated candidiasis: magnetic resonance imaging **(MRI).** This parasagittal T1-weighted MRI scan after gadolinium injection shows disseminated enhancing nodules *(arrowheads)*, consistent with microabscesses. (From Huang CC, Chen CY, Yang HB, Wang SM, et al. Central nervous system candidiasis in very-low-birth-weight premature neonates and infants: US characteristics and histopathologic and MR imaging correlates in five patients. *Radiology.* 1998;209:49–56.)

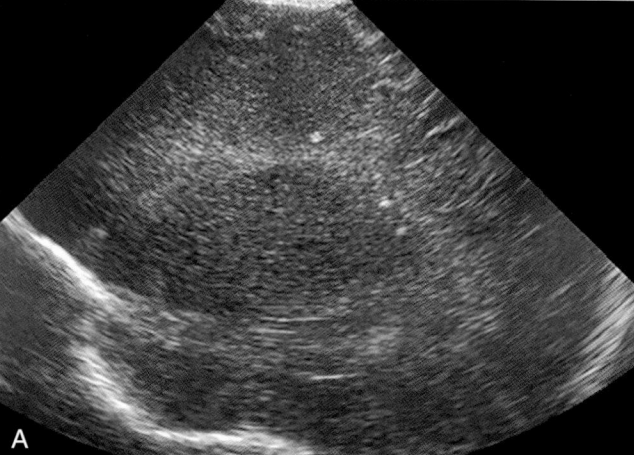

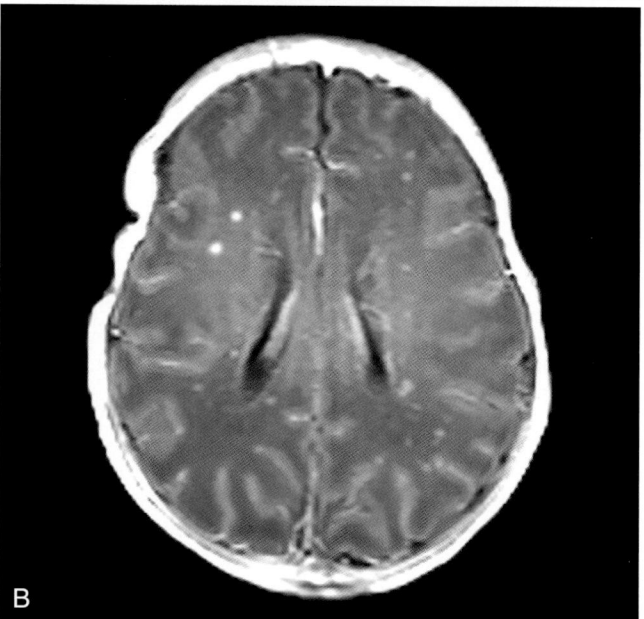

Figure 35.30 Disseminated candidiasis: ultrasound and magnetic resonance imaging **(MRI).** Parasagittal cranial ultrasound (A) and axial MRI, gadolinium-enhanced T1-weighted sequence (B) in a preterm infant with systemic *Candida albicans* infection. Microabscesses are apparent as small foci of echogenicity with both imaging techniques.

of the involvement of other organs. This should include ophthalmological examination, echocardiography, abdominal ultrasound, and urine analysis. The outcome is not entirely clear because of the relatively recent advent of prompt diagnosis and therapy. In previous years, most affected infants with CNS involvement were either first detected at postmortem examination or died before therapy could be instituted. However, with prompt diagnosis and therapy (see

following section), approximately 70% to 85% of premature infants have survived, although approximately 40% to 50% of survivors exhibit cognitive deficits, motor deficits, or both.[a] Friedman and colleagues[414] found a higher incidence in infected infants versus matched noninfected controls of periventricular leukomalacia (26% vs. 12%), severe retinopathy of prematurity (ROP) (22% vs. 9%), and adverse neurological outcomes at 2 years of corrected age (60% vs. 35%). Characteristic unilateral or bilateral, yellow-white, fluffy retinal or vitreal balls with frequent hemorrhage or inflammatory vitreous haze may be seen on indirect fundoscopy. Systemic antifungal therapy for such endophthalmitis usually results in a good visual outcome but there may be some subsequent decrease in visual acuity.[439] Mortality was found to be highest (57%) in infants from whom

---

[a]References 410, 411, 413, 414, 417, 418, 427, 428, 437, and 438.

Candida was isolated from multiple sources (e.g., urine and blood or urine and CSF), compared with 28% when the organism was isolated only from blood and 26% when isolated only from urine.[429] The outcome is distinctly better in term than in premature infants.[a] Substantial numbers of deaths in the premature infants have been related to complicating illnesses (e.g., chronic pulmonary disease).

Management

Prevention is a major goal, and surely injudicious use of indwelling vascular catheters and broad-spectrum antibiotics should be avoided. In recent years, promising data have been presented concerning the use of fluconazole prophylaxis in premature infants in neonatal intensive care units (NICUs).[425,437,440-442] Prophylaxis in extremely preterm infants has been shown to be safe without adverse effects on long-term outcome.[441] In NICUs with moderate (5% to 10%) or high (>10%) rates of invasive candidiasis, fluconazole prophylaxis has been recommended.[443] A reduction in colonization and systemic *Candida* infection and decreased rates of progression from initial colonization to systemic disease have been shown. In one study, prophylactic fluconazole was targeted to infants administered broad-spectrum antibiotics for more than 3 days; the incidence of invasive fungal infection was 6.3% in the control group versus 1.1% in the treated group.[437] The use of fluconazole prophylaxis has not led to an increase in fungal resistance.[444]

Treatment of documented infection should be prompt. It is critical to remove central catheters immediately.[402] Amphotericin B remains the drug of choice for systemic candidiasis.[426,432] The initial dose is 1 mg/kg intravenously every 24 hours.[445] CSF concentrations are variable, ranging from 40% to 90% of plasma levels in one study of preterm infants.[403] Penetration of CSF and brain tissue is generally better in neonates than in adults.[445] For CNS disease, a cumulative dose of 25 to 30 mg/kg is usually necessary. The major adverse effect in newborns is renal toxicity; hepatic toxicity is much less common in infants than in older patients. Serial monitoring of serum potassium and magnesium levels and of renal, liver, and bone marrow function is required. Reduction in dosage at the first signs of toxicity is important and effective.[419,423] The addition of 5-fluorocytosine (flucytosine 50 to 100 mg/kg per day) has been advocated for patients with CNS disease.[403,407,419,423,426] This agent exhibits hepatotoxicity but acts synergistically with amphotericin B in treatment of the disease. Moreover, the excellent penetration into the CSF of flucytosine as opposed to amphotericin B suggests that this is the particularly critical drug for intracranial disease. More recent reports, however, suggest no added therapeutic benefit when 5-fluorocytosine is combined with amphotericin B.[446] In apparently resistant infection, caspofungin and micafungin, newer antifungal agents, have been used.[447,448]

TETANUS NEONATORUM

Neonatal tetanus is a rare disorder in the United States, primarily because of widespread immunization programs and effective obstetrical care. Four cases have been reported in the United States in the past 25 years.[449,450] However, the disease is very common in many developing countries and is a major cause

of neonatal death. In a careful study conducted in a town in Sudan, 1 in every 110 infants died of neonatal tetanus.[451,452] In Bangladesh, Pakistan, and India, the rate of deaths caused by neonatal tetanus has been reported to be more than 20 per 1000 live births.[452,453] Such worldwide mortality rates from neonatal tetanus suggest that at least 260,000 lives are lost each year from neonatal tetanus in developing countries.[453-457] In 2010 an estimated 1% of global neonatal deaths were attributed to tetanus.[458]

Pathogenesis

Neonatal tetanus is caused by the exotoxin of the anaerobe *Clostridium tetani*, which usually gains entry through the umbilical stump. The umbilical cord has usually been cut at the time of birth with an unsterile instrument and occasionally has even been smeared with a variety of unsterile foreign materials. Any degree of passive transfer of immunity to the infant during gestation is rare. In an older series of 54 affected infants reported from the United States, only 3 of the mothers had any form of tetanus toxoid immunization.[459] A similar experience, albeit of much greater magnitude, has been reported from developing countries.[452,454-457,460-462] In one large study in Bangladesh, the apparent risk of neonatal tetanus initially appeared to be no less in infants of mothers who had received tetanus toxoid previously; subsequent to the survey, it was discovered by a reference laboratory that the tetanus vaccine had "no potency."[456]

Tetanus toxin, a protein of 150,000 molecular weight, selectively inhibits *inhibitory* synaptic activity within the CNS.[463-465] The tetanus neurotoxin has been shown to be a zinc-dependent protease, the substrate for which is a membrane protein localized to the presynaptic nerve ending.[465] This protein serves as a docking site of synaptic vesicles before vesicular release. The proteolytic action of the tetanus neurotoxin on this vesicle-associated membrane protein releases the latter into the cytosol and prevents docking and thereby release of the neurotransmitter-containing vesicles. The *synaptic release* of inhibitory transmitters, particularly glycine and gamma-aminobutyric acid, is affected. The synapses are those of interneurons of polysynaptic pathways, especially in spinal cord and brain stem. Once fixed at the presynaptic membrane site, the toxin cannot be neutralized by antitoxin, and clinical recovery depends on the slow process of membrane turnover and synthesis of vesicle-associated membrane protein. The enhanced excitatory activity that characterizes the neurological features of neonatal tetanus presumably relates to an impairment of the normal balance between inhibitory and excitatory influences on the lower motor neurons in the brain stem and spinal cord.

Clinical Features

The major clinical features, depicted in Table 35.28, have been derived from the study of hundreds of affected infants reported from developing countries.[454,460,466-476] The usual incubation period is 5 to 10 days; thus it is not surprising that most cases of neonatal tetanus begin in the latter part of the first week or early in the second week of life. The earlier the onset, the more severe the clinical features and the greater the risk of death. In the moderate to severe case, the course is characteristic. Diminished sucking or refusal to suck, impaired feeding, excessive crying, irritability, and rigid abdomen are the initial features. Fever is common and is a risk factor for a poor outcome. These signs are followed within 24 to 48

---

[a]References 402, 405, 412, 414, 426, and 427.

TABLE 35.28 Major Clinical Features of Neonatal Tetanus

Home delivery of infant
Deficient or absent maternal immunization
Fever
Diminished suck or refusal to suck
Impaired feeding
Abnormal crying
Rigid abdomen
Trismus
Cyanosis
Facial rigidity (risus sardonicus)
Opisthotonos
Generalized rigidity
Flexed toes; muscular spasms

hours by the hallmarks of the disease, which are related to enhanced muscular activity (i.e., trismus, facial rigidity [risus sardonicus], generalized rigidity [retrocollis and opisthotonos in severe cases], and spasms). The trismus impairs feeding, and the infant exhibits certain features particularly characteristic of neonatal tetanus (i.e., the jaw is often held open, only to close tightly when stimulated by attempts to feed the infant orally). The generalized rigidity is usually accompanied by a characteristic, persistent flexion of the toes. The spasms are exacerbated by stimulation, may occur many times an hour, and may be mistaken for seizures. Commonly, the spasms are accompanied by apnea and cyanosis. Indeed, respiratory failure resulting from repeated spasms is the most common cause of mortality and morbidity in this disease. The usual duration of disease in the patient with a moderate to severe case and who is effectively supported therapeutically is 3 to 5 weeks.

Diagnosis
Clinical Evaluation

The diagnosis of neonatal tetanus is based primarily on clinical findings. The setting of birth at home, inadequate management of the umbilical stump, nonimmunized mother, and characteristic neurological features should raise the suspicion of the diagnosis of tetanus. Initially, nuchal rigidity may suggest meningeal irritation and hence meningitis or intracranial hemorrhage. Moreover, the spasms are readily mistaken for convulsions and therefore a variety of cerebral conditions. These disorders should be ruled out because more specific therapy may be needed urgently (e.g., therapy for bacterial meningitis).

Laboratory Evaluation

No convenient laboratory test identifies neonatal tetanus. Cultures of the umbilical stump, even when handled carefully for anaerobic organisms, are usually negative. Electromyographic findings of increased insertional activity in the form of trains of motor unit discharges can be helpful in diagnosing the difficult case.[468]

Prognosis

Until recently, the mortality of neonatal tetanus in large series varied from 60% to 85%.[459,466,470,474,475] In an earlier study of 196 cases in India in the 1950s, the mortality rate was approximately 85%.[474] More recent studies suggest that, with improved management, mortality can be decreased to approximately 10%.[472,473,477,478] However, in many underdeveloped areas, the mortality rate remains high (i.e., 30% to 80%).[a] Comparing data from the 1990s and the last decade in Turkey, the number of infected infants decreased from 55 cases admitted between 1991 and 1996 to only 12 patients admitted in the last decade.[479] Twenty-eight (41.8%) of the 67 infants died during their follow-up.[479] Lower birth weight, younger age at onset of symptoms and at the time admission, the presence of opisthotonos, and risus sardonicus were associated with a higher mortality rate. In a systemic review and meta-analysis, low-birth-weight showed a significantly increased risk of mortality.[480] Approximately 10% to 30% of survivors exhibit neurological sequelae (e.g., mental retardation and spastic motor deficits), which are apparently secondary to hypoxic-ischemic injury sustained in association with severe muscular spasms. In a cumulative series of 138 infants, 19 (14%) exhibited mental retardation or an intelligence quotient lower than 80 on long-term follow-up.[471,476,478,481] However, in addition to this cerebral involvement, the demonstration of flaccid quadriparesis and a muscle biopsy indicative of denervation in one child raised the possibility of anterior horn cell injury by the toxin, at least in isolated cases.[482]

Management
Prevention

The most essential feature of management of tetanus neonatorum is prevention. This goal has been accomplished to a major degree in many countries by the widespread active immunization of the population, such that transplacental transfer of antitoxin is adequate. Immunization of women during pregnancy has proved highly effective in preventing the occurrence of disease in the infant.[461,462] Also of particular importance are delivery of infants and management of the newborn and the umbilical cord under aseptic conditions.[483] In a recent case control study enrolling 26 cases and 52 controls, maternal education and immunization status, birth site, and lack of a skilled birth attendant were identified as independent risk factors of tetanus in the newborn.[484] In another study from Vietnam, similar risk factors for a poor outcome were identified in 107 newborn infants with neonatal tetanus. In settings with critical care facilities, younger age, lower weight, delay in admission, and leukocytosis were independent risk factors of a poor outcome.[485]

Treatment

The improved outcome for the newborn with tetanus in recent years appears to be related primarily to improved supportive care.[467,471-473,477,486] The major aspects of management are depicted in Table 35.29. In a recent study, a 66% reduction in mortality was achieved by the introduction of a new management regimen including antibiotic therapy, muscle relaxation, and invasive monitoring.[486] Improved spasm control was achieved by combining continuous midazolam and neuromuscular blockade. Invasive blood pressure monitoring enabled early detection of autonomic nervous system dysfunction and timely intervention.[486]

Supportive Care. Supportive care is paramount in the management of neonatal tetanus, and maintenance of adequate

---

[a]References 451, 454, 460, 467, 469, and 471.

TABLE 35.29   Management of Neonatal Tetanus

Intravenous fluids
Enteric feeding
Temperature control
Respiratory support, including mechanical ventilation and neuromuscular blockade
Sedation and muscle relaxation, especially with high-dose diazepam
Tetanus immune globulin
Penicillin G

---

ventilation is most important of all. Nasotracheal intubation (rather than tracheostomy), mechanical ventilation, and a degree of muscular paralysis sufficient to allow smooth ventilatory control have been shown to be highly effective.[477,486] Important therapeutic adjuncts include administration of intravenous fluids, enteric feeding by indwelling nasogastric tube, and control of temperature. These various measures are designed to prevent the respiratory failure, pulmonary disease, hyperpyrexia, pneumonia, and dehydration, which may result in death.

The *sedative* drugs chosen to alleviate the muscular spasms most commonly have included primarily phenobarbital, chlorpromazine, and diazepam.[487] The use of doses of diazepam as high as 20 to 40 mg/kg per day (in association with intragastric phenobarbital) has been associated with a 90% survival.[473,478] The need for such doses has been shown in pharmacokinetic and clinical studies.[471,488] Although management of infants not requiring mechanical ventilation should include reduction of environmental stimulation and some form of sedation, it appears that the most effective approach is to use mechanical ventilation early in the course of the disease and in association with the administration of a paralytic agent. This approach requires a skilled neonatal intensive care team, and, indeed, when rapid transfer of such infants to an appropriate facility can be accomplished, the use of dangerously high levels of sedative drugs can be avoided. Nevertheless, a skilled neonatal intensive care team with sophisticated equipment is usually unavailable in developing countries, where high-dose diazepam without routine use of mechanical ventilation is the mainstay of therapy.[471,473]

Antitoxin and Antimicrobial Therapy. The umbilical infection does not usually require local surgical therapy, but penicillin G is administered intravenously in a dose of 10,000 units/kg per day for 10 days.[477] Tetanus immune globulin, 500 units, is administered intramuscularly in divided doses to neutralize any unbound toxin. A controlled study demonstrated equivalent benefit for human tetanus immune globulin, 500 units, and equine tetanus antitoxin, 10,000 units.[489] Because tetanus immune globulin has a more sustained effect (i.e., half-life of ≈4 to 5 weeks vs. 1 to 2 weeks for equine tetanus antitoxin) and is less frequently associated with adverse side effects, this preparation is preferred, when available.

ACKNOWLEDGMENT

Dr. de Vries acknowledges the assistance of Saane B. Hoeks, MD, Department of Neonatology, UMCU, Utrecht, the Netherlands, in the preparation of this chapter.

KEY REFERENCES

19. Okike IO, Ribeiro S, Ramsay ME, et al. Trends in bacterial, mycobacterial, and fungal meningitis in England and Wales 2004-11: an observational study. *Lancet Infect Dis.* 2014;14:301-307.
159. Hernandez MI, Sandoval CC, Tapia JL, et al. Stroke patterns in neonatal group B streptococcal meningitis. *Pediatr Neurol.* 2011;44: 282-288.
165. Lequin MH, Vermeulen JR, van Elburg RM, et al. *Bacillus cereus* meningoencephalitis in preterm infants: neuroimaging characteristics. *AJNR Am J Neuroradiol.* 2005;26:2137-2143.
213. Wang S, Peng L, Gai Z, et al. Pathogenic triad in bacterial meningitis: pathogen invasion, NF-kappaB activation, and leukocyte transmigration that occur at the blood-brain barrier. *Front Microbiol.* 2016;7:148.
214. Stoll BJ, Hansen NI, Adams-Chapman I, et al. Neurodevelopmental and growth impairment among extremely low-birth-weight infants with neonatal infection. *JAMA.* 2004;292:2357-2365.
251. Natarajan G, Johnson YR, Zhang F, et al. Real-time polymerase chain reaction for the rapid detection of group B streptococcal colonization in neonates. *Pediatrics.* 2006;118:14-22.
254. Harris MC, D'Angio CT, Gallagher PR, et al. Cytokine elaboration in critically ill infants with bacterial sepsis, necrotizing enterocolitis, or sepsis syndrome: correlation with clinical parameters of inflammation and mortality. *J Pediatr.* 2005;147:462-468.
270. Yikilmaz A, Taylor GA. Sonographic findings in bacterial meningitis in neonates and young infants. *Pediatr Radiol.* 2008;38:129-137.
272. Jaremko JL, Moon AS, Kumbla S. Patterns of complications of neonatal and infant meningitis on MRI by organism: a 10 year review. *Eur J Radiol.* 2011;80:821-827.
273. Oliveira CR, Morriss MC, Mistrot JG, et al. Brain magnetic resonance imaging of infants with bacterial meningitis. *J Pediatr.* 2014;165:134-139.
275. Libster R, Edwards KM, Levent F, et al. Long-term outcomes of group B streptococcal meningitis. *Pediatrics.* 2012;130:e8-e15.
294. ter Horst HJ, van Olffen M, Remmelts HJ, et al. The prognostic value of amplitude integrated EEG in neonatal sepsis and/or meningitis. *Acta Paediatr.* 2010;99:194-200.
314. Martins ER, Andreu A, Melo-Cristino J, et al. Distribution of pilus islands in *Streptococcus agalactiae* that cause human infections: insights into evolution and implication for vaccine development. *Clin Vaccine Immunol.* 2013;20:313-316.
321. Ogunlesi TA, Odigwe CC, Oladapo OT. Adjuvant corticosteroids for reducing death in neonatal bacterial meningitis. *Cochrane Database Syst Rev.* 2015;(11):CD010435.
334. Polin RA. Management of neonates with suspected or proven early-onset bacterial sepsis. *Pediatrics.* 2012;129:1006-1015.
350. Shah SS, Ohlsson A, Shah VS. Intraventricular antibiotics for bacterial meningitis in neonates. *Cochrane Database Syst Rev.* 2012;(7):CD004496.
402. Benjamin DK Jr, Stoll BJ, Fanaroff AA, et al. Neonatal candidiasis among extremely low birth weight infants: risk factors, mortality rates, and neurodevelopmental outcomes at 18 to 22 months. *Pediatrics.* 2006;117:84-92.
405. Benjamin DK Jr, Poole C, Steinbach WJ, et al. Neonatal candidemia and end-organ damage: a critical appraisal of the literature using meta-analytic techniques. *Pediatrics.* 2003;112:634-640.
412. Fernandez M, Moylett EH, Noyola DE, et al. Candidal meningitis in neonates: a 10-year review. *Clin Infect Dis.* 2000;31:458-463.
417. Huang CC, Chen CY, Yang HB, et al. Central nervous system candidiasis in very-low-birth-weight premature neonates and infants: US characteristics and histopathologic and MR imaging correlates in five patients. *Radiology.* 1998;209:49-56.
424. Pammi M, Holland L, Butler G, et al. Candida parapsilosis is a significant neonatal pathogen: a systematic review and meta-analysis. *Pediatr Infect Dis J.* 2013;32:e206-e216.
425. Manzoni P, Arisio R, Mostert M, et al. Prophylactic fluconazole is effective in preventing fungal colonization and fungal systemic infections in preterm neonates: a single-center, 6-year, retrospective cohort study. *Pediatrics.* 2006;117:e22-e32.
429. Benjamin DK Jr, Stoll BJ, Gantz MG, et al. Neonatal candidiasis: epidemiology, risk factors, and clinical judgment. *Pediatrics.* 2010;126:e865-e873.

433. Wellinghausen N, Siegel D, Winter J, et al. Rapid diagnosis of candidaemia by real-time PCR detection of *Candida* DNA in blood samples. *J Med Microbiol.* 2009;58:1106-1111.

434. Cohen-Wolkowiez M, Smith PB, Mangum B, et al. Neonatal *Candida* meningitis: significance of cerebrospinal fluid parameters and blood cultures. *J Perinatol.* 2007;27:97-100.

438. Adams-Chapman I, Bann CM, Das A, et al. Neurodevelopmental outcome of extremely low birth weight infants with *Candida* infection. *J Pediatr.* 2013;163:961-967.e963.

441. Kaufman DA, Cuff AL, Wamstad JB, et al. Fluconazole prophylaxis in extremely low birth weight infants and neurodevelopmental outcomes and quality of life at 8 to 10 years of age. *J Pediatr.* 2011;158: 759-765.e751.

458. Liu L, Johnson HL, Cousens S, et al. Global, regional, and national causes of child mortality: an updated systematic analysis for 2010 with time trends since 2000. *Lancet.* 2012;379:2151-2161.

479. Dikici B, Uzun H, Yilmaz-Keskin E, et al. Neonatal tetanus in Turkey: what has changed in the last decade? *BMC Infect Dis.* 2008;8:112.

480. Lambo JA, Anokye EA. Prognostic factors for mortality in neonatal tetanus: a systematic review and meta-analysis. *Int J Infect Dis.* 2013;17:e1100-e1110.

485. Lam PK, Trieu HT, Lubis IN, et al. Prognosis of neonatal tetanus in the modern management era: an observational study in 107 Vietnamese infants. *Int J Infect Dis.* 2015;33:7-11.

Full references for this chapter can be found on www.expertconsult .com.

UNIT X

PERINATAL TRAUMA

Injuries of Extracranial, Cranial, Intracranial, Spinal Cord, and Peripheral Nervous System Structures

Joseph J. Volpe

This chapter focuses on injuries of extracranial, cranial, intracranial, spinal cord, and peripheral nervous system structures. In particular, the emphasis is on those disorders that appear to be related primarily to mechanical trauma. The adverse mechanical events occur principally during labor and delivery. Unfortunately such events often lead to criticism of obstetrical management. Such criticism generally is unwarranted, because the mechanical factors are most often beyond the control of the obstetrician. Indeed, in many well-documented instances, apparent *traumatic* lesions are related to unknown antepartum events or to developmental or acquired lesions evolving in utero. Nevertheless perinatal mechanical traumatic events do occur, result in well-defined clinical syndromes, and require recognition and appropriate management. The chapter is organized into extracranial, cranial, intracranial, spinal cord, and peripheral nervous system lesions.

A brief caveat concerning terminology is important to note in the introduction to this chapter. The terms *perinatal trauma* and *birth injury* have been given definitions so broad as to be confusing and nearly meaningless. Indeed, a commonly used definition of birth injury is considered to be any condition that affects the fetus adversely during labor or delivery. In this discussion, however, *perinatal trauma* refers to those adverse effects on the fetus during labor or delivery and in the neonatal period that, as noted earlier, appear to be caused *primarily* by *mechanical* factors. Thus specifically excluded are the disturbances of labor and delivery that lead principally to *hypoxic-ischemic* brain injury (see Chapters 17 to 20). (Nevertheless, potential overlap between mechanical trauma and the occurrence of hypoxic-ischemic cerebral injury is important to recognize because perinatal mechanical insults may result also in hypoxic-ischemic cerebral injury, perhaps secondary to disturbances of placental or cerebral blood flow. The precise mechanistic relationships remain largely unknown.)

The incidence of traumatic brain injury is difficult to establish conclusively. Nevertheless, it is clear that there have been drastic reductions in the occurrence of traumatic injuries to central and peripheral nervous structures, primarily because of improved obstetrical management. Specific examples are apparent in the subsequent discussions, but recurring themes are the rational use of cesarean section and improved techniques of manual and instrumental vaginal deliveries.

MAJOR VARIETIES OF PERINATAL TRAUMA

The major varieties of perinatal trauma are outlined in Table 36.1. These include extracranial hemorrhage, skull fracture, intracranial hemorrhage, cerebral contusion, cerebellar contusion, spinal cord injury, and several types of injuries to the peripheral nervous system—for example, nerve roots and cranial or peripheral nerves. The injuries to extracranial, cranial, and central nervous system structures are discussed first.

INJURY TO EXTRACRANIAL, CRANIAL, AND CENTRAL NERVOUS SYSTEM STRUCTURES

Extracranial Hemorrhage

The three major varieties of extracranial hemorrhage are caput succedaneum, subgaleal hemorrhage, and cephalhematoma. These lesions occur in different tissue planes between the skin and the cranial bone (Fig. 36.1 and Table 36.2).

Caput Succedaneum

This term refers to the hemorrhagic edema that is very commonly observed after vaginal delivery. Compression on the presenting part, exerted by the uterus or cervix, is the most common pathogenesis. Caput and related scalp injuries have been reported in 10% to 20% of deliveries by vacuum extraction.[1] The usual site of caput formation is the vertex, and marked molding of the head is a common accompaniment. The edema is soft, superficial, and pitting in nature and crosses sites of suture lines (see Table 36.2). The lesion steadily resolves over the first days of life, and no intervention is necessary.

Subgaleal Hemorrhage

Subgaleal hemorrhage refers to hemorrhage beneath the aponeurosis covering the scalp and connecting the frontal and occipital components of the occipitofrontalis muscle (see Fig. 36.1).[2] (Understandably this lesion also is termed *subaponeurotic* hemorrhage.) Blood may spread beneath the entire scalp and even dissect into the subcutaneous tissue of the neck. The pathogenesis of subgaleal hematoma is related to a combination of external compressive and dragging

TABLE 36.1   Perinatal Traumatic Lesions

Extracranial hemorrhage	**Cerebral contusion**
Caput succedaneum	**Cerebellar contusion**
Subgaleal hemorrhage	**Spinal cord injury**
Cephalhematoma	**Peripheral nervous**
Skull fracture	**system injury**
Linear	Brachial plexus
Depressed	Phrenic nerve
Occipital osteodiastasis	(diaphragmatic paralysis)
Intracranial hemorrhage	Facial nerve
Epidural	Laryngeal nerve
Subdural	Median nerve
Primary subarachnoid	Radial nerve
Intraventricular	Lumbosacral plexus
Intracerebral	Sciatic nerve
Intracerebellar	Peroneal nerve

forces, occasionally aided by a coagulation disturbance (e.g., vitamin K deficiency).[3-5] A strong association with delivery by vacuum extraction is suggested by available data.[4-7] In one series approximately 90% of the lesions were associated with vacuum extraction.[8] In a prospective series of 71 infants with subgaleal hemorrhage and delivery by vacuum extraction, a strong relationship was observed with maternal nulliparity and placement of the vacuum cup over the sagittal suture or less than 3 cm from the anterior fontanel.[5] The last two factors would cause the vacuum extractor to exert traction forces with a slanting or shearing effect on the scalp, considered to be central to the rupture of the emissary veins in the subgaleal space. The infants presented at 1 hour of age and had an appreciable incidence of hypovolemic shock (10%), requirement for volume expansion or inotropic support (35%), need for transfusion for anemia (35%), secondary coagulopathy (50%), and hyperbilirubinemia (35%). In a unique study of 27

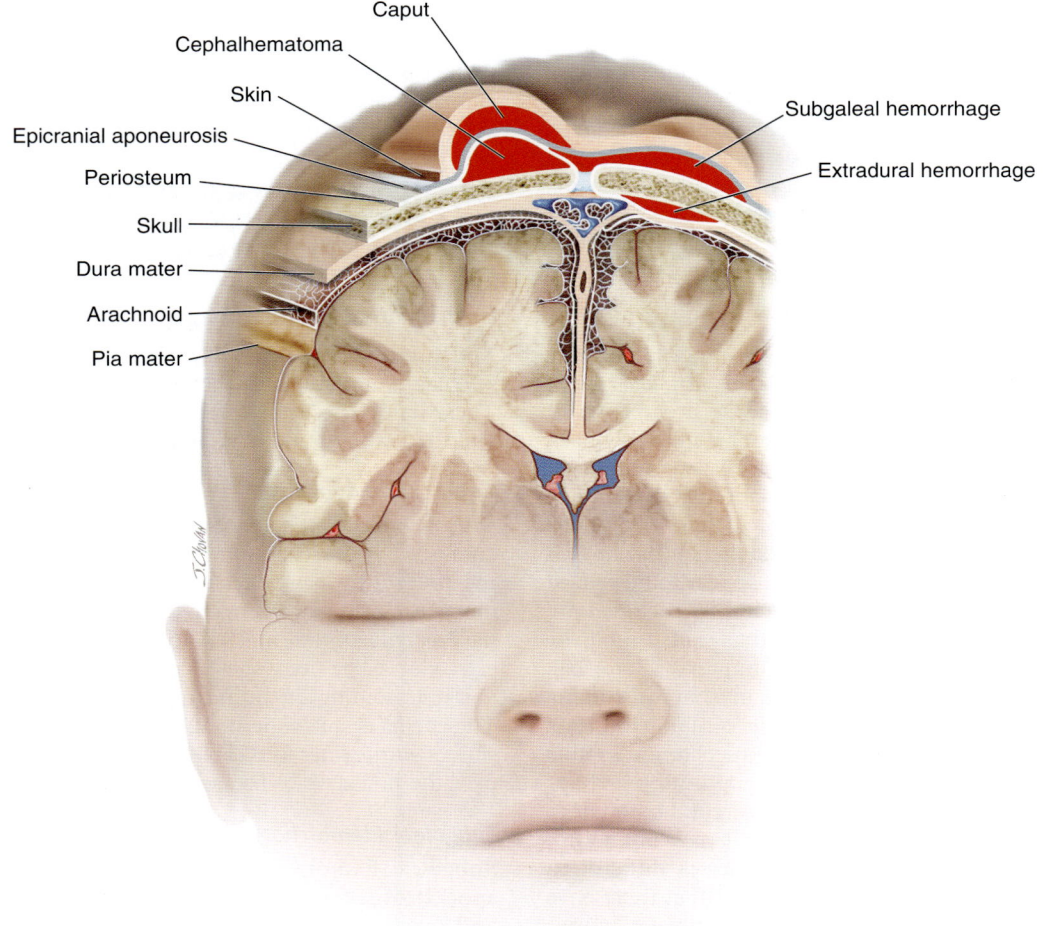

Figure 36.1   Sites of extracranial (and extradural) hemorrhages in the newborn. Schematic diagram of important tissue planes from skin to dura. (Adapted from Pape KE, Wigglesworth JS. *Haemorrhage, Ischaemia and the Perinatal Brain*. Philadelphia: JB Lippincott; 1979.)

TABLE 36.2   Major Varieties of Traumatic Extracranial Hemorrhage

LESION	FEATURES OF EXTERNAL SWELLING	INCREASES AFTER BIRTH	CROSSES SUTURE LINES	MARKED ACUTE BLOOD LOSS
Caput succedaneum	Soft, pitting	No	Yes	No
Subgaleal hematoma	Firm, fluctuant	Yes	Yes	Yes
Cephalhematoma	Firm, tense	Yes	No	No

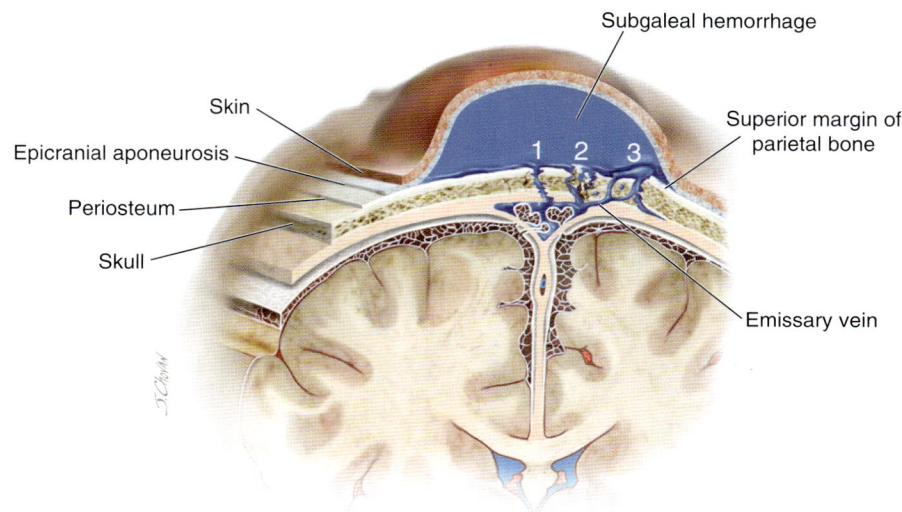

Figure 36.2 Schematic drawing of the potential events that lead to subgaleal hemorrhage. *1*, Suture diastasis, *2*, skull fracture, and, *3*, fragmentation of the superior margin of the parietal bone with ruptured emissary vein. (From Govaert P, Vanhaesebrouch P, De Praeter C, Moens K, Leroy J. Vacuum extraction, bone injury and neonatal subgaleal bleeding. *Eur J Pediatr.*1992;151:532.)

affected infants by computed tomography (CT) scan, 14 infants demonstrated various angulation abnormalities of the parietal bones; such abnormalities suggest that the lesion can result from bleeding caused by one or more of three mechanisms (linear skull fracture, suture diastasis, and fragmentation of the superior margin of the parietal bone) illustrated in Fig. 36.2.[6] This lesion is much less common than caput succedaneum, although the precise incidence is unknown. In contrast to uncomplicated caput, subgaleal hematoma presents as a firm, fluctuant mass, increases in size after birth, and may be present in the subcutaneous tissue of the posterior neck (see Table 36.2). Because of the findings noted earlier, infants must be watched carefully for signs of blood loss, coagulopathy, and the development of hyperbilirubinemia. Urgent blood transfusion may be necessary. After the acute phase, the lesion resolves over 2 to 3 weeks.

Cephalhematoma

Cephalhematoma refers to a circumscribed region of hemorrhage overlying the skull and confined by cranial sutures.

Incidence. Cephalhematoma occurs in approximately 1% to 2% of live births.[6,7,9] The lesion is nearly twice as common in males as in females and is more frequent in children of primiparous than multiparous mothers. The use of forceps or vacuum extraction in delivery sharply increases incidence.[1,7,10-13] In one large earlier series the incidence of cephalhematoma after the use of outlet forceps was 4.3%; after low forceps, 7.4%; and after midforceps, 9.5%.[11] More recent data indicate that these incidences have declined considerably.[13] Vacuum extraction increases the likelihood of cephalhematoma over threefold relative to the incidence with forceps deliveries.[13] In one careful series of term infants, cephalhematoma occurred in approximately 10% of vacuum-assisted deliveries.[1] Among premature infants the incidence was 20%.[1]

Pathology. The hemorrhage is subperiosteal in cephalhematoma, as opposed to the edema and blood in caput succedaneum and subgaleal hemorrhage, which are located over the periosteum in either the subcutaneous or subaponeurotic spaces (see Fig. 36.1). The subperiosteal locus explains the confinement of the hematoma by cranial sutures (see Table 36.2). By far the most common locus of cephalhematoma is over the parietal bone and unilateral. The rare occipital cephalhematoma, midline in location because of confinement by the lambdoid sutures, may mimic occipital encephalocele (cranial ultrasound scan is a convenient means to make this distinction). An underlying linear skull fracture is detected in 10% to 30% of cases of

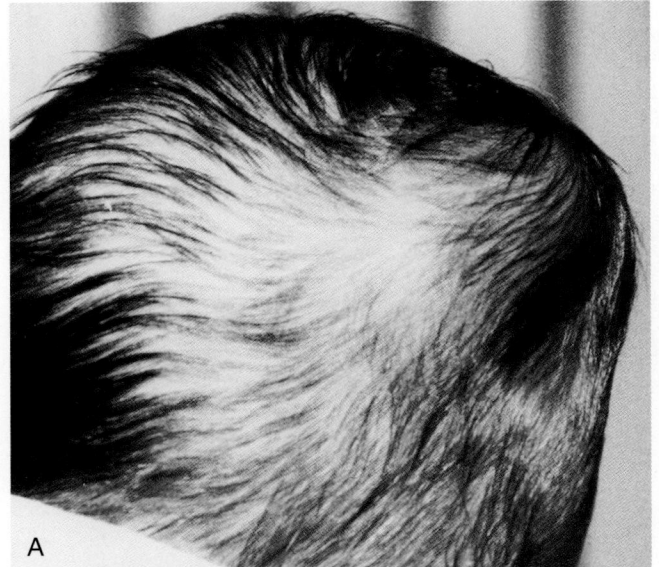

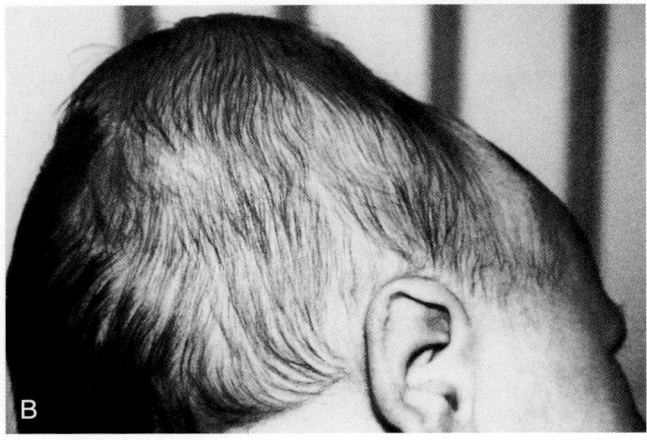

Figure 36.3 Parietal cephalhematoma. Clinical appearance from a 10-day-old infant delivered with the aid of midforceps. (A) Posterior view. (B) Right lateral view. Note prominent swelling that extends medially to the sagittal suture, posteriorly to the lambdoid suture, and laterally to the squamosal suture.

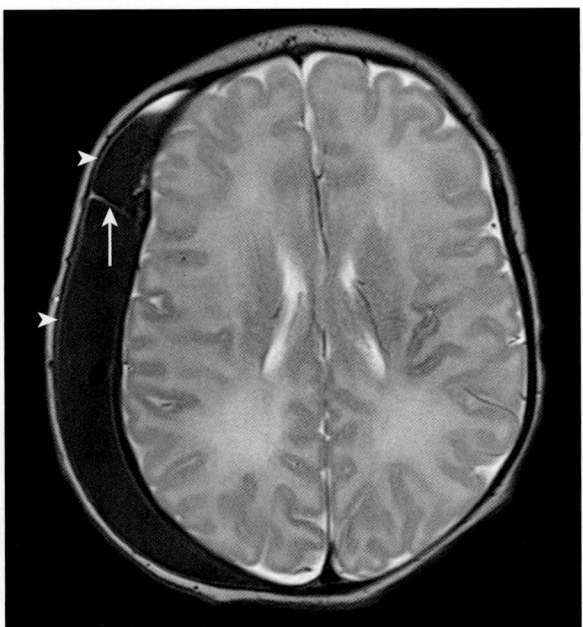

Figure 36.4 Frontal and parietal cephalhematomas. Magnetic resonance imaging (MRI) scan in a 1-day-old infant delivered by vacuum extraction. Clinical diagnosis was subgaleal hemorrhage, because the scalp mass crossed the coronal suture line. However, the MRI shows separate frontal and parietal cephalhematomas. The arrowheads indicate the periosteum external to the (subperiosteal) hematoma. The arrow indicates stripped periosteum at the coronal suture, leading to the external clinical appearance suggestive of a subgaleal hematoma. The intracerebral structures are normal. (MRI courtesy Dr. Jeffrey Neil.)

cephalhematoma.[9,14] The presence of a skull fracture increases the possibility of accompanying intracranial hemorrhage. In one series, 9 of 10 infants with cephalhematoma associated with skull fracture also had intracranial hemorrhage, including subdural and epidural hemorrhage.[9]

Pathogenesis. Cephalhematoma is caused by mechanical forces—that is, is clearly a traumatic lesion in nearly all cases. The most reasonable formulation for pathogenesis implicates generally unavoidable obstetrical factors relating to the size of the skull and birth canal and to the use of forceps or vacuum, causing tight apposition of subcutaneous structures to the periosteum but separation of periosteum from bone by external dragging forces.[15]

Clinical Features. The lesion usually increases in size after birth and presents as a firm, tense mass that does not transilluminate (see Table 36.2 and Fig. 36.3). The elevated periosteum palpable at the margin of the hematoma causes

the palpating finger to appreciate a ridge at the margin of the lesion and a recessed center. This finding is readily mistaken for a depressed skull fracture. Rarely, contiguous cephalhematomas will appear to cross suture lines and thus will be mistaken for subgaleal hematoma (Fig. 36.4). Cephalhematoma is rarely of clinical significance from the neurological standpoint unless a complicating intracranial lesion is present. As noted earlier, linear skull fracture is an occasional accompaniment of cephalhematoma, and in this setting there is a clear association of linear skull fracture and intracranial hemorrhage. I have seen one infant with an infected cephalhematoma and meningitis. Rare additional complications are hyperbilirubinemia, late-onset anemia, and osteomyelitis.[16-19]

Essentially all cephalhematomas resolve in a few weeks to months. The few that calcify and result initially in hard skull protuberances gradually disappear over many months of skull growth and remodeling.

Management. No specific therapy is indicated. The degree of acute blood loss rarely requires urgent intervention. Evacuation of the lesion is contraindicated. Treatment of unusual complications, especially large intracranial hemorrhage, may be necessary.

Skull Fracture

Three principal bony lesions of the newborn are categorized appropriately under the designation *skull fracture*. These lesions are linear and depressed skull fractures and occipital osteodiastasis (see Table 36.1). In fact, only with linear skull

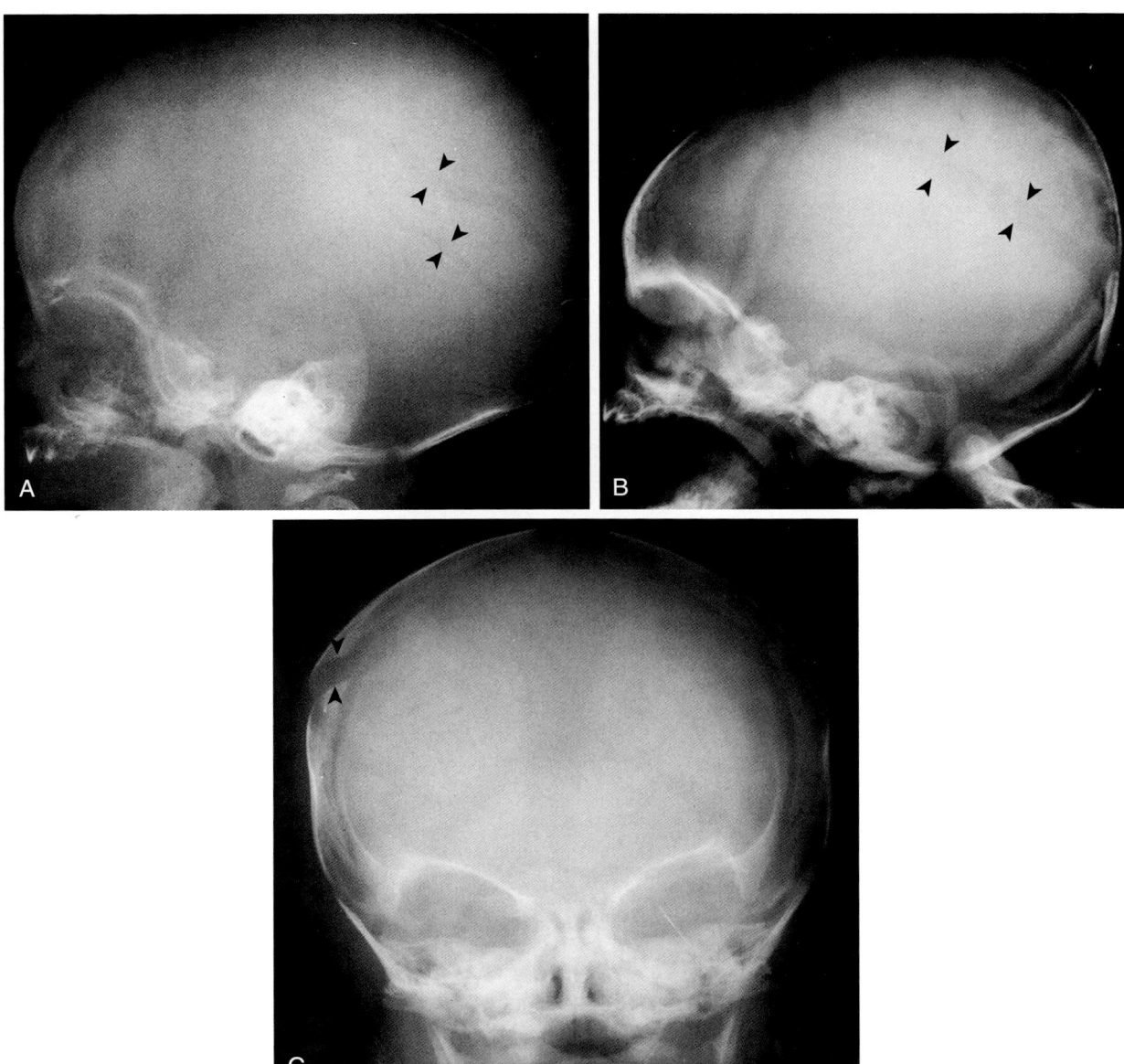

Figure 36.5 X-rays from a newborn show linear skull fractures. (A–C) Lesions are identified by arrowheads. (Courtesy Dr. Gary Shackelford.)

fracture is there loss of bony continuity and therefore true fracture.

Linear Fracture

Linear skull fracture refers to a nondepressed fracture and is most commonly parietal in location (Fig. 36.5).

Incidence. Linear skull fractures are relatively common in newborns; however, incidence is difficult to determine precisely because identification of the lesion depends particularly on the frequency of radiographic studies and the diligence of examination. In one older series (1975), the incidence was 10%,[14] but more recent data indicate an incidence less than 3%.[7,13] The incidence after vacuum-assisted delivery is approximately 5%.[1]

Pathology. Linear skull fracture may be associated with extracranial (e.g., cephalhematoma) and intracranial (e.g., epidural and subdural hemorrhage and cerebral contusion) complications. It should be emphasized, however, that the more serious, intracranial complications are *uncommon* concomitants of linear skull fracture in the newborn. Also rarely, the fracture is associated with a tear of the dura and subsequent development of a leptomeningeal cyst. Leptomeningeal cyst may also occur after an unusual type of linear fracture—that is, coronal suture diastasis, particularly secondary to vacuum extraction.[20]

Pathogenesis. Linear skull fracture is principally a traumatic lesion. Direct compressive effects are probably most important in genesis of the fracture.

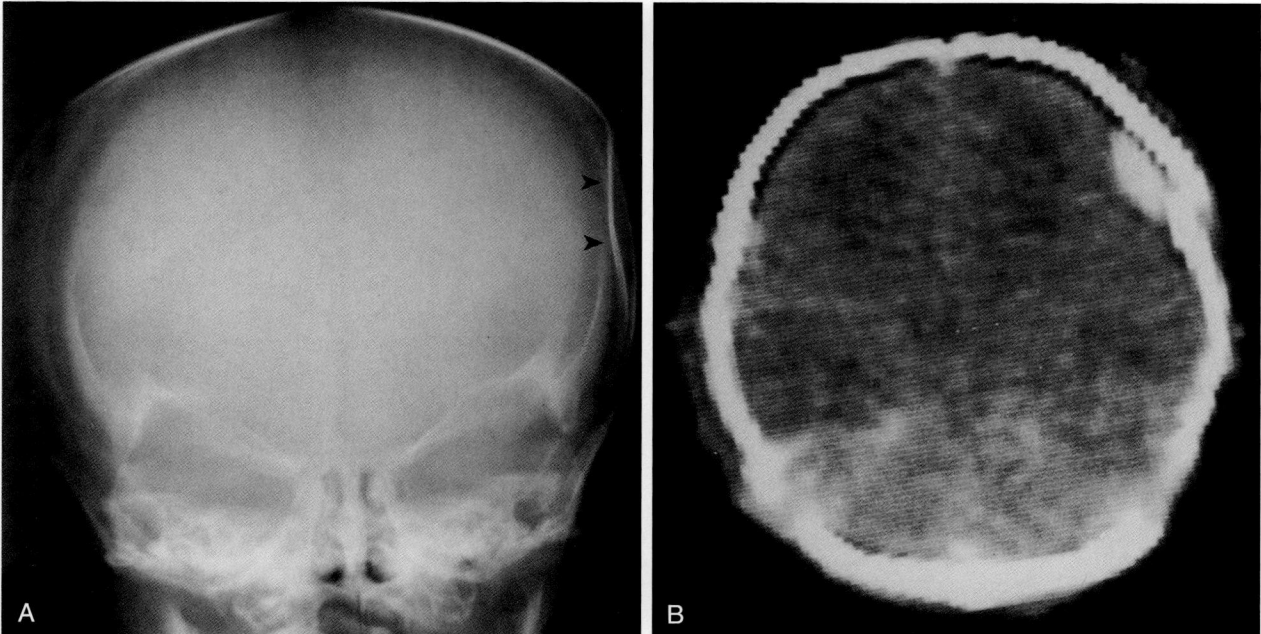

Figure 36.6 Depressed skull fracture: x-ray and computed tomography. (A) Conventional skull x-ray showing the typical depressed, "ping-pong" fracture of the newborn (*arrowheads*). (B) Computed tomography scan from another infant showing a less common depressed *fracture* in which the right coronal suture has been disrupted, causing the parietal bone to be sharply depressed. There is an underlying small epidural hematoma that exhibits the characteristic convex configuration. (A, Courtesy Dr. Gary Shackelford.)

Clinical Features. No clinical feature is associated with the fracture per se. The important clinical point is that the fracture should alert the physician to the possibility, however remote, of a more serious intracranial traumatic lesion. The development of a leptomeningeal cyst over the weeks or months subsequent to fracture can be suspected at the bedside by the finding of increased transillumination of the affected region and defined in more detail by CT or MRI.

Management. No therapy is indicated. Follow-up skull radiographs at several months of age are useful to document that healing has occurred and that a widened defect indicative of an enlarging leptomeningeal cyst has not developed.

Depressed Fracture

Depressed skull fracture in the newborn usually refers to the "ping-pong" lesion associated with inward buckling of the unusually resilient neonatal bone, usually without loss of bony continuity (Fig. 36.6).

Incidence. In one large series of 270 infants "injured at birth," 32 exhibited depressed skull fracture.[21] The use of forceps was common; thus, in 28 of these 32, forceps were known to have been used. In a more recent series, 50 of 68 cases of depressed skull fracture occurred after instrument-related delivery.[22]

Pathology. The most common site of depressed fracture is the parietal bone. Although in the vast majority of cases there is no visible fracture, occasionally bone fragments may be seen. Rarely, epidural or subdural hemorrhage or cerebral contusion is associated.

Pathogenesis. Depressed fracture is almost certainly a result of localized compression of the skull. The compressing force is generated by either forceps or pressure against maternal pelvic structures during labor. A prolonged second stage of labor followed by forceps delivery was the most common sequence in one large series.[22] Rarely, depressed skull fracture may occur in utero.[23]

Clinical Features. The obvious and palpable bony defect calls immediate attention to the lesion (Fig. 36.7). Neurological accompaniments are unusual and relate to associated intracranial traumatic complications. Neurological complications are rare in spontaneous depressed skull fracture but are relatively common in fractures related to forceps deliveries. Indeed, in the latter group, epidural or subdural hemorrhage complicates 30% of cases and subsequent neurological sequelae occur in 4%.[22]

Management. Traditionally depressed fractures were considered an indication for neurosurgical elevation.[24] This view has been challenged by the observation in several cases of spontaneous elevation of the deformity.[25-27] Indeed, the natural history of neonatal depressed skull fracture is unclear and the incidence of spontaneous elevation unknown. This fact and the reports of elevation by digital pressure[28] or the use of a breast pump[29] or obstetrical vacuum extractor[30-33] suggest that neurosurgical intervention may be indicated less commonly than is currently done. The combination of a transparent breast pump shield attached to a vacuum extractor appears to be particularly useful (Fig. 36.8). Nevertheless 85% of 68 cases in one series were said to "require neurosurgery."[22]

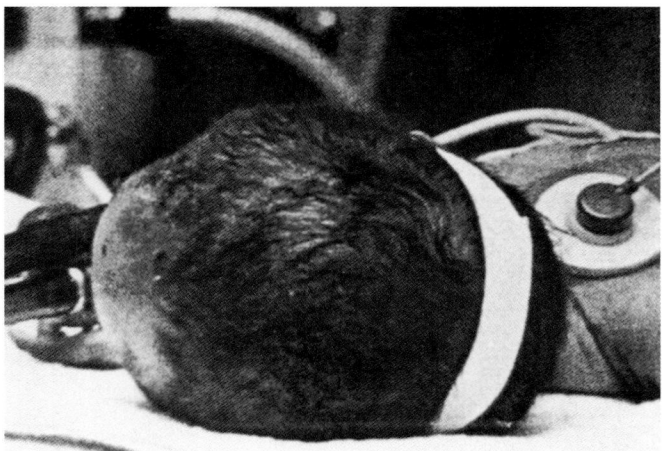

Figure 36.7 Depressed skull fracture: clinical appearance. From an infant with the typical "ping-pong" fracture shown in Fig. 36.6A. Note the depression in the right parietal region. (From Saunders BS, Lazoritz S, McArtor RD, Marshall P, Bason WM. Depressed skull fracture in the neonate. Report of three cases. *J Neurosurg.* 1979;50:512.)

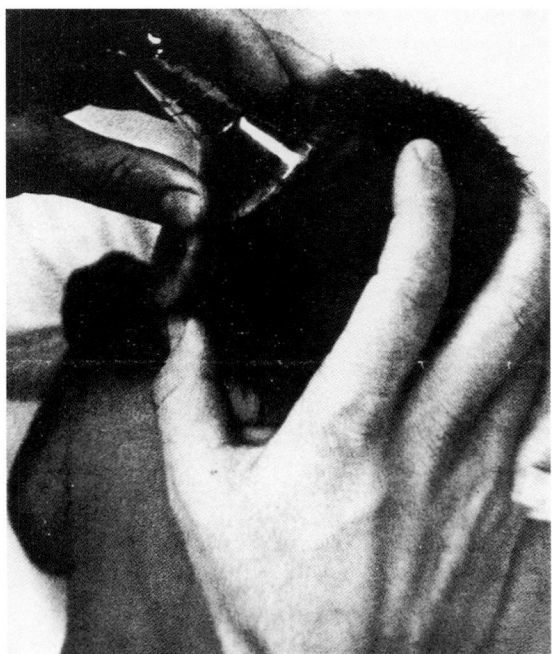

Figure 36.8 Depressed skull fracture: nonsurgical treatment. Infant with a "ping-pong" fracture is shown with a transparent plastic breast pump shield applied over the left frontal lesion. The transparent shield, which allows visualization of the elevation of the depression, is attached to an obstetrical vacuum extractor. (From Saunders BS, Lazoritz S, McArtor RD, Marshall P, Bason WM. Depressed skull fracture in the neonate. Report of three cases. *J Neurosurg.* 1979;50:512.)

The most reasonable approach to depressed fracture is careful radiological assessment of the lesion—including CT, MRI, or both—to rule out the presence of extradural or subdural clot or bone fragments, as well as careful neurological surveillance to ensure that acute complications do not develop. This approach could then be followed by a trial of the nonsurgical modalities

noted previously. If that is unsuccessful, consideration of neurosurgical intervention is then appropriate. However, small uncomplicated "ping-pong" fractures, on the basis of current information, do not seem to warrant prompt neurosurgical intervention.

Occipital Osteodiastasis

Occipital osteodiastasis, or separation of the squamous and lateral parts of the occipital bone, may result in posterior fossa subdural hemorrhage, cerebellar contusion, and cerebellar-medullary compression without hemorrhage or gross contusion.[2] The evolution of the lesion by skull radiography is shown in Fig. 36.9.[34] Its consequences are discussed primarily in Chapter 23.

Intracranial Hemorrhage

Major Varieties

The major varieties of intracranial hemorrhage associated with cranial trauma in the perinatal period include epidural hemorrhage, subdural hemorrhage (acute, subacute, and chronic), primary subarachnoid hemorrhage, intraventricular hemorrhage, intracerebral hemorrhage, and intracerebellar hemorrhage (see Table 36.1). Pathogeneses other than trauma play more important roles in several of these varieties of intracranial hemorrhage. Trauma appears to play the dominant pathogenetic role in epidural and subdural hemorrhage and may contribute to pathogenesis of the other varieties of intracranial hemorrhage. Except for epidural hemorrhage, the neuropathology, clinical features, management, and other features of neonatal intracranial hemorrhage are discussed in detail in Chapters 22 to 24.

Epidural Hemorrhage

An epidural hemorrhage refers to hemorrhage in the plane between the bone and the periosteum on the inner surface of the skull (see Fig. 36.1). It represents the intracranial analogue of a cephalhematoma (which is often associated).

Incidence. Epidural hemorrhage is a rare lesion in the newborn and constitutes only about 2% of all cases of neonatal intracranial hemorrhage observed at autopsy.[35] This relative rarity may relate to the fact that in the newborn the dura is unusually thick and largely contiguous with the inner periosteum.[35]

Pathology. Bleeding into the epidural space stems either from branches of the middle meningeal artery or from major veins or venous sinuses. Fractures across suture lines are likely to be associated with the venous sinuses. Linear skull fracture is present in the majority of cases but not all.[35] Cephalhematoma is also a frequent accompaniment.[9,36,37]

Pathogenesis. When epidural hemorrhage is accompanied by linear skull fracture, overriding of fracture segments and tearing of branches of the middle meningeal artery or a large venous sinus are the probable reasons for the hemorrhage. In the infant without fracture, the reason for the hemorrhage is unclear. The dura can be separated from the bone when "the skull is bent inward or outward" at autopsy, and it is possible that this separation in vivo could cause tears of arteries running in the richly vascularized dural-periosteal layer of the neonatal

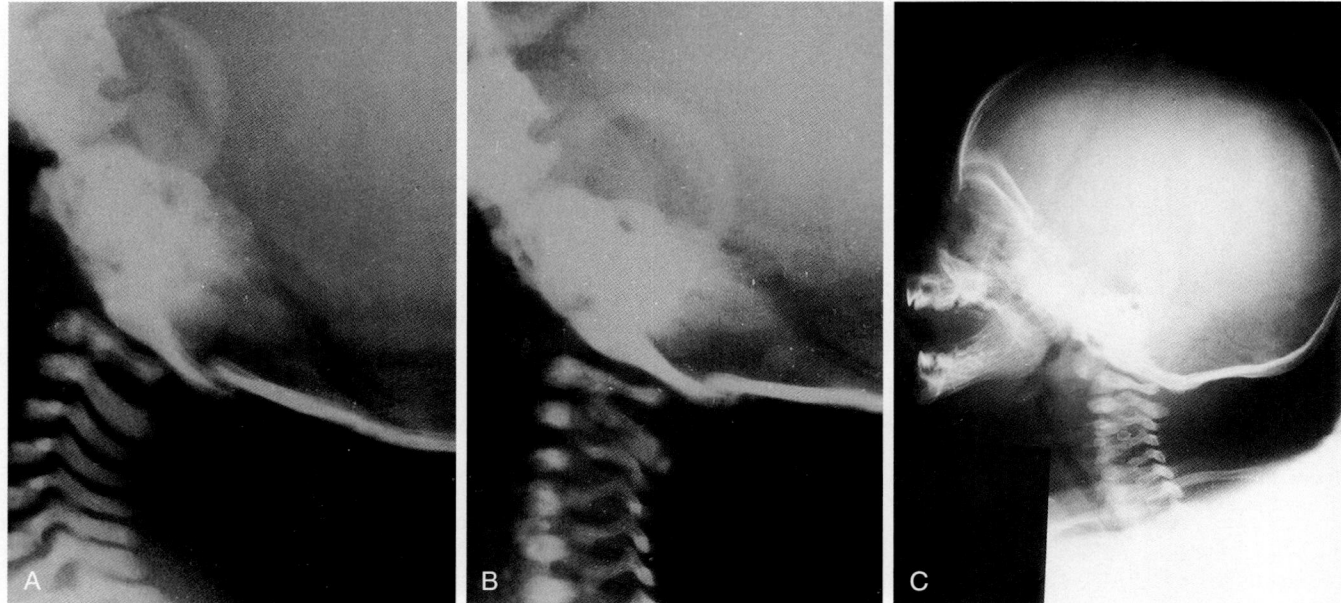

Figure 36.9 Lateral skull radiographs showing occipital osteodiastasis. (A) In the seventh day of life; (B) at 2 1/2 months; and, C, at 1 year. Note gradual improvement in the neonatal period and normal appearance at 1 year. (From Roche MC, Velez A, García Sanchez PG, Pascual Castroviejo I. Occipital osteodiastasis. A rare complication in cephalic delivery. *Acta Paediatr Scand.* 1990;79:380.)

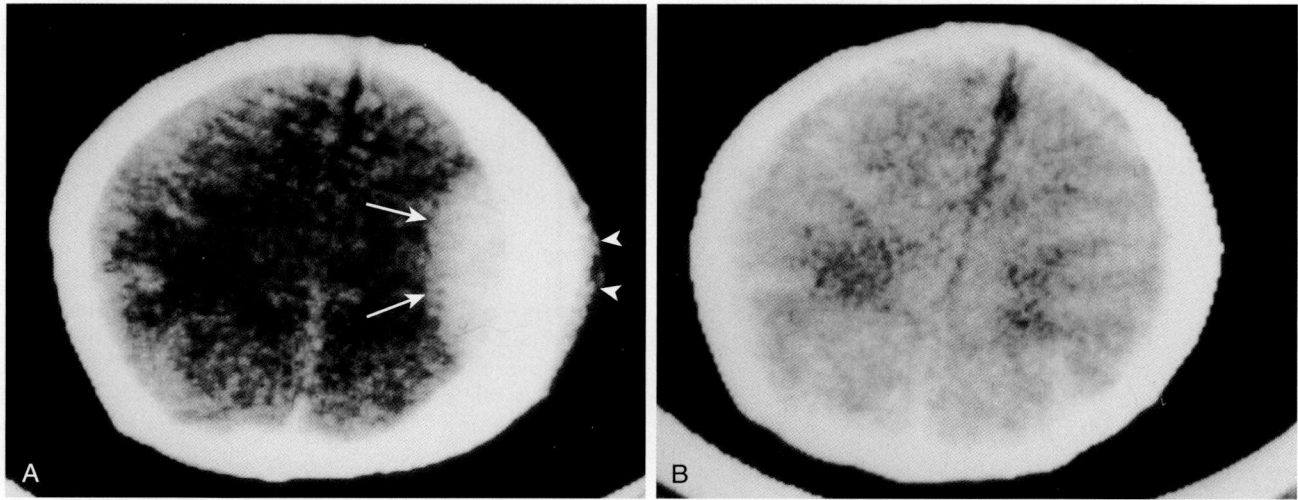

Figure 36.10 Computed tomography scans of a newborn with epidural hematoma. (A) Before and (B) after aspiration of an overlying cephalhematoma. The epidural hematoma, apparent as a lentiform high-density area (*arrows*), disappeared after aspiration of the cephalhematoma (*arrowheads*). A similar resolution occurred without aspiration in another infant with no cephalhematoma. (From Negishi H, Lee Y, Itoh K, et al. Nonsurgical management of epidural hematoma in neonates. *Pediatr Neurol.* 1989;5:253.)

cranium.[35] Several cases have been associated with neonatal in-hospital falls.[38,39]

Clinical Features. Most affected infants have experienced a traumatic labor or delivery and exhibit signs of increased intracranial pressure (bulging anterior fontanel) from the first hours of life. A delay in onset of signs also may occur,[37] perhaps when a venous origin is present. In approximately half of the reported cases, seizures were also present.[9,35] Signs of uncal herniation—for example, a fixed, dilated ipsilateral pupil—may occur. Suspicion of the lesion is an indication for emergency CT or MRI, which will demonstrate the hemorrhage effectively. The convex, lentiform appearance of the lesion is characteristic (see Figs. 36.6B and 36.10A). Untreated infants often die within 24 to 48 hours. Surgical evacuation and survival, often with normal outcome, have been reported frequently.[9,35,36] Moreover, survival after nonsurgical therapy has also been documented (see Fig. 36.10).[9,37]

Management. Although epidural hemorrhage is a rare lesion, it should be considered in any infant who has experienced a traumatic labor or delivery or exhibits signs of increased intracranial pressure in the first day of life. Rapid diagnosis by CT or MRI and prompt intervention should improve the outcome. Although surgical evacuation has been the most common therapy, in one series three infants treated by aspiration of an accompanying cephalhematoma recovered without sequelae.[37] In each case the epidural hematoma disappeared after aspiration of the cephalhematoma, apparently because of communication of the two lesions through a fracture site (see Fig. 36.10). In a fourth case without cephalhematoma, the hematoma resolved with no direct therapy.[37] In a recent series of four infants, all were normal on follow-up, two after surgical evacuation, one after needle aspiration, and one after *conservative* therapy.[9]

Cerebral Contusion

Cerebral contusion refers to a focal region of necrosis and hemorrhage usually involving the cerebral cortex and subcortical white matter.[2]

Incidence

Cerebral contusion is an apparently uncommon lesion in the newborn, although the precise incidence is unknown because of past difficulty in establishing the diagnosis in vivo. The reason for the relatively low incidence perhaps relates to the uncommon occurrence in the perinatal period of focal blunt trauma and to the relative resiliency of the neonatal cranium and cerebral mantle. These properties render less likely acceleration-deceleration movements of brain, which result in cerebral contusion at later ages.

Pathology

The term *cerebral contusion* describes the pathology of focal necrosis and hemorrhage, typically observed in older children, involving particularly cerebral cortex and subcortical white matter. Such lesions are usually found in coup and contrecoup, as well as inferior orbital, frontal, and temporal locations. This characteristic topography is observed only rarely in the newborn. Another variety of cerebral contusion described in newborns and young infants, albeit rarely, consists of slit-like tears in hemispheric white matter that may extend into the cerebral cortex or even the walls of the lateral ventricle.[40]

Pathogenesis

Focal areas of cortical necrosis and hemorrhage result from direct compressive effects in the newborn. Studies in neonatal rat pups implicate excitotoxic effects, mediated at the *N*-methyl-D-aspartate (NMDA) receptor, in the final pathway to tissue injury and show protective effects of NMDA antagonists administered 30 minutes or 1 hour after the insult.[41] The tears of white matter are attributed to shearing forces within subcortical cerebral parenchyma produced by rapid and extreme deformation of brain.[40] The latter is made possible by the pliability of the newborn skull. An additional predisposing factor may relate to the relative lack of myelin in the developing cerebral white matter.

Clinical Features

Cerebral contusion probably constitutes the substrate for some of the focal cerebral signs associated with serious perinatal traumatic injury. Thus seizures, often focal, motor deficits, especially hemiparesis or monoparesis, and deviation of eyes to the side of the lesion (but movable with the "doll's eyes" maneuver) represent particularly characteristic cerebral signs. Diagnosis is made best by MRI.

Management

No specific therapy is indicated.

Cerebellar Contusion

Cerebellar contusion may occur with occipital osteodiastasis. More often the contusion that results is associated with infratentorial subdural hematoma or intracerebellar hemorrhage. These lesions are discussed in Chapters 22 and 23.

Spinal Cord Injury

Spinal cord injury incurred during delivery results from excessive traction or rotation and is unlike the compression injury that is characteristic of most cord injuries encountered in older patients. Spinal cord injury secondary to obstetrical disturbances and apparent mechanical trauma is readily distinguished from the rare spinal cord injuries that occur postnatally in association with vascular occlusion, observed with umbilical artery catheterization or accidental injection of air into a peripheral vein.[42-45] More difficult to distinguish are the intrauterine cord injuries related to a variety of vascular, malformative, and other factors (see the section on diagnosis, later). These last disorders occur in infants born after *atraumatic* vaginal or cesarean deliveries.

Incidence

The true incidence of spinal cord injury is difficult to determine, in part because the spinal cord is examined at autopsy only uncommonly. It is likely that injury to the spinal cord is more common than expected. Indeed, in one early series Pierson[46] identified intraspinal hemorrhages in 46% of infants of breech deliveries examined at autopsy. The clinical significance of such lesions is not clear. The most widely cited neuropathological observations are those of Towbin,[47,48] who concluded in the 1960s that spinal cord injury was a causal factor in approximately 10% of neonatal deaths. Friede[49] cautions against overinterpretation of these data and suggests distinguishing clearly clinically significant lesions from "the often observed minor perivascular petechiae in the cord and from the extreme congestion or hemorrhagic imbibition of the epidural adipose tissue of newborns," which are presumably of little clinical importance.

Pathology

Two major sites of injury can be identified (Table 36.3). One site occurs principally with breech delivery and involves the lower cervical and upper thoracic regions[49-54]; the other site occurs principally with cephalic delivery and involves the upper to midcervical regions.[49,51,52,54-60] In one large series, the latter site was involved more than twice as often as the former.[52]

The dominant *acute lesions* are hemorrhages, especially epidural and intraspinal, and edema. The intraspinal hemorrhages particularly involve dorsal and central gray matter. These hemorrhagic lesions are usually associated with varying degrees of stretching, laceration, disruption, or total transection. The dura not infrequently is torn, but complete cord transection

TABLE 36.3	Pathology of Neonatal Spinal Cord Injury

Major sites of injury
Lower cervical and upper thoracic regions (especially breech delivery)
Upper and midcervical regions (especially cephalic delivery)
Major neuropathological changes
Acute: hemorrhage (epidural and intraspinal), edema, laceration, disruption, and/or transection of cord
Chronic: fibrosis of dura, arachnoid, and cord; focal areas of necrosis, often cystic; syringomyelia; disrupted architecture; and vascular occlusions with infarction

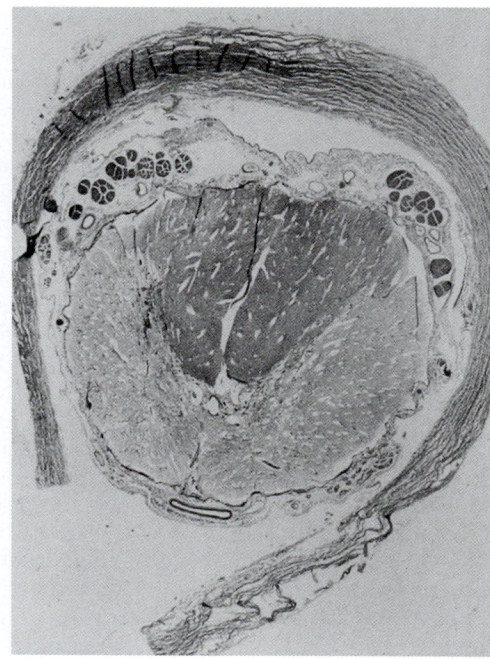

Figure 36.11 Neonatal spinal cord injury. Neuropathology of ischemic infarction below the level of the traumatic lesion. Horizontal section of spinal cord at the upper thoracic level from an infant who died at 6 months of age after a neonatal cervical cord transection at the level of C-2. Note the striking pallor, consistent with infarction, in the distribution of the anterior spinal artery.

may occur with an intact dura.[50] Only uncommonly do lesions of the vertebral column appear.[49,53] Such lesions consist of vertebral fractures or dislocations and separation of the vertebral epiphysis.[53,54,61]

The acute lesions of the spinal cord are followed by striking subacute and *chronic changes*—for example, formation of fibrotic adhesions between dura, leptomeninges, and cord; focal areas of necrosis with cystic cavities within the cord; syringomyelia; drastically disrupted architecture of the cord; and, often, total separation of transected cord segments. Vascular occlusions, perhaps developing as a posttraumatic event, may cause ischemic infarction of cord segments caudal to the level of the primary lesion (Fig. 36.11).[62,63] This *posttraumatic vasopathy* may be related causally to the persistence of the clinical state of *spinal shock* in certain patients (see subsequent section).

Pathogenesis

Central to the pathogenesis of neonatal spinal cord injury is the fact that the large majority of cases are associated with *excessive longitudinal or lateral traction of the spine or excessive torsion*. (The term *excessive* must be interpreted cautiously because spinal cord injury has been described in multiple reports after apparently atraumatic deliveries [see earlier].) Traction is more important in breech deliveries, which account now for the minority of cases, and torsion in cephalic deliveries, which account now for the majority of cases.

The critical factors in pathogenesis relate to the *relative elasticities* of the vertebral column with its associated ligamentous and muscular structures, the dura, and the spinal cord. In the newborn the bony vertebral column is nearly entirely cartilaginous and very elastic, as are the associated ligaments.[64-66] Similarly, the muscles are relatively hypotonic, and the tone may be depressed further by maternal drugs or anesthesia. The dura is somewhat less elastic. However, least elastic is the neonatal spinal cord, which is anchored above by the medulla and the roots of the brachial plexus and below by the cauda equina. Thus it is easy to understand why excessive longitudinal traction results in marked stretching of the vertebral column and rupture of the dura (the *snap* often heard at delivery of the aftercoming head in such cases) and the spinal cord. The cord ruptures at the sites of particular mobility and anchoring—that is, in the lower cervical to upper thoracic region. With extreme rotational maneuvers, as with forceps rotation in difficult cephalic deliveries, the site of particular cord mobility and most frequent rupture is in the upper to midcervical region. In a series of 15 cases of high cervical cord injury, the nearly invariable feature was a forceps rotation of 90 degrees or more from the occipitoposterior to occipitotransverse position.[59] The infant's spine is particularly susceptible to rotational forces because the bony processes ("uncinate processes") of one vertebral body that articulate with corresponding processes of the adjacent vertebral body and thereby limit rotation are not well developed in the newborn.[51]

Recent insight into pathogenesis at the vascular, cellular, and molecular levels has been gained from studies of adult animals and humans.[67-77] Thus an early posttraumatic disturbance in cord perfusion may result from local disturbances in cord microcirculation and from systemic hypotension. Release of excitatory amino acids from injured neurons may lead to local excitotoxic mechanisms of cell death, as described in Chapter 13. The final common pathway of ischemic and neurotransmitter injury includes increases in cytosolic calcium, release of arachidonic acid, production of vasoactive prostanoids and free radicals, lipid peroxidation, membrane injury, and cell death. Potential interventions (e.g., glutamate blockers, corticosteroids, lipid peroxidation inhibitors) are suggested from these findings, and one such intervention, early steroid therapy, has been shown to be of modest benefit in human adults (see the section on management, further on).

Clinical Features

Clinical Settings. Of paramount importance in the clinical setting are obstetrical factors, particularly breech or midforceps deliveries, which are present in the majority of recognized neonatal spine injuries.[51-54,60,78-82] In addition, a frequent contributing feature is fetal depression secondary to maternal drugs or anesthesia or to intrauterine asphyxia.[60,83]

TABLE 36.4	Neonatal Clinical Features of Spinal Cord Injury

Three basic clinical syndromes
Stillbirth or rapid neonatal death
Neonatal respiratory failure
Neonatal weakness and hypotonia → spasticity ("cerebral palsy")
Neurological features
Motor: weakness, hypotonia, areflexia of lower extremities (perhaps also upper extremities), and diaphragmatic breathing (or paralysis)
Sensory: sensory level
Sphincters: distended bladder and patulous anus
Other: Horner syndrome

Basic Clinical Syndromes. The clinical syndromes of spinal cord injury in the newborn are principally threefold (Table 36.4).[53,54,60,84] First, stillbirth or rapid neonatal death with failure to establish adequate respiratory function occurs, particularly in cases with lesions involving the upper cervical cord, lower brain stem, or both. Second, severe respiratory failure may develop in the first days of life and lead to death. (This development may be delayed by mechanical ventilation, which presents major ethical difficulties in the ensuing weeks.) Third, the infant may exhibit neurological phenomena in the neonatal period but survive, with weakness and hypotonia of limbs as the prominent features. The nature of the *neonatal* neurological syndrome may not be recognized, and the possibility of a neuromuscular disorder or transient hypoxic-ischemic encephalopathy is often considered. Most of these infants later develop spasticity and may be mistakenly considered to have cerebral lesions ("cerebral palsy").

Neurological Features. The typical infant is born after a difficult delivery. In the lower cervical–upper thoracic injury, the following neurological features are apparent to varying degrees in the first hours or days of life: flaccid weakness with areflexia of lower extremities and variable involvement of upper extremities (see subsequent discussion); sensory level in the region of the lower neck or upper trunk; respiratory disturbance with diaphragmatic breathing and *paradoxical* respiratory movements or even diaphragmatic paralysis; paralyzed abdominal muscles with a soft, sometimes bulging abdomen; atonic anal sphincter; and distended bladder that usually empties with gentle suprapubic pressure (see Table 36.4).[a] Involvement of the upper extremities may reflect concomitant brachial plexus injuries or, if only distal portions of the upper extremities are affected, injury to anterior horn cells at the segmental levels of the spinal cord injury. Horner syndrome is occasionally present and relates to involvement of either cord neurons in the intermediate column of gray matter or exiting roots (especially T-1) destined for the sympathetic ganglia. The major additional neurological feature with mid- or upper-cervical injury is respiratory failure and the need for mechanical ventilation because innervation of the diaphragm emanates from cervical segments 3, 4, and 5, especially 4.

[a]References 51, 52, 55, 60, 66, 85.

Detection of a sensory level is critical and is accomplished readily if the examiner observes both the quantity and quality of movement and the presence of grimace or affective facial response elicited by pinprick. Stimulation should be performed slowly, and low-level reflex movements without facial response, probably mediated at a spinal level, should be recognized.

Coexistence of the clinical features of hypoxic-ischemic encephalopathy (see Chapter 20) in the acute neonatal period is not unusual in those infants with upper cervical lesions and the need for mechanical ventilation. In the largest series of such cases reported to date ($n = 14$), 9 infants exhibited such signs.[52] Similarly, cognitive deficits, presumably of cerebral origin, were observed later in approximately 40% of infants with upper cervical spinal injury who survived more than 3 months.[52] With improvements in mechanical ventilation, these sequelae appear to be less frequent.[54]

Subsequent Course. The neonatal neurological syndrome is followed primarily by one of two courses. First, and less commonly, the state just described, sometimes characterized as spinal shock, persists. This state may relate to secondary ischemia (see the section on posttraumatic vasopathy, described earlier) or to degenerative changes in the caudal segment of cord. Second and more commonly, as edema and hemorrhage subside over the ensuing several weeks to months, the state of spinal shock subsides and evolves to a state of enhanced reflex activity. Tendon reflexes become hyperactive and Babinski signs appear. Hypotonia gives way to spasticity, and lower limbs may assume a position of *triple flexion*—that is, flexion of the hips, knees, and ankles. However, newborns usually do not develop spasticity as severe as that observed later in older children and adults with spinal cord injury.[86] Changes in the upper extremities depend on the level of the lesion. If anterior horn cells or the brachial plexus is involved, these limbs remain flaccid and areflexic. If the lesion is at the midcervical level or higher, spasticity and hyperreflexia supervene in upper extremities as in lower extremities. Persistent respiratory failure and a need for mechanical ventilation also are present in such mid- or upper cervical cases. Reflex emptying of the bladder occurs, often as part of mass reflex activity elicited by cutaneous or other stimulation. Higher-level motor or affective responses to sensory stimulation below the level of the lesion, however, do not develop. Disturbances of autonomic function—for example, sweating and vasomotor phenomena—may lead to wide fluctuations in body temperature, especially in young infants. Trophic disturbances of muscle and bone may become prominent. The orthopedic and urinary tract complications that dominate the clinical course of these patients in the years after infancy are appropriately discussed in other texts.

Diagnosis

Diagnosis is often not difficult in the typical case. In less severely affected newborns or infants born after an apparently atraumatic delivery, differentiation is necessary from an occult dysraphic state (see Chapter 1); cervical arachnoid cyst[87]; an intravertebral, extramedullary mass, such as abscess, neuroblastoma, or hemorrhage[88]; an intramedullary lesion, such as syringomyelia, hemangioblastoma, or hemorrhage[89,90-92]; bony abnormalities[93]; apparent intrauterine traumatic lesions related to maternal abdominal trauma[94,95]; infarction occurring prenatally or caused postnatally by a vascular catastrophe associated with an indwelling catheter[42-45,96]; or a neuromuscular disorder (see Chapters 32 and 33).[52,66,82,97] Radiographs of the spine and a search for cutaneous dimples, sinus tracts, hemangioma, and abnormal hair should aid in the differential diagnosis of occult dysraphic state, cervical arachnoid cyst, or bony abnormality. Demonstration of a sensory level rules out a neuromuscular disorder, such as Werdnig-Hoffmann disease. Differentiation from other extramedullary or intramedullary lesions requires an imaging study.

The principal choices for imaging of the cord are ultrasonography, CT, or MRI. Ultrasonography is useful because the infant need not be moved, and the modality demonstrates cord size and configuration and echogenic blood or edema within the cord or blood in the extramedullary space.[52,80,82,98,99] Although blood is more echogenic than is edema, this critical distinction can be difficult with ultrasonography. Serial studies are carried out readily. I consider ultrasonography the *initial* imaging modality of choice in the acute situation. However, MRI provides superior resolution and should be used promptly subsequently.[52,60,81,99-101] In the acute period, hemorrhage and edema can be distinguished by utilization of gradient-echoacquisition sequences.[60] In the subacute and chronic periods, MRI provides superb resolution of parenchymal changes (Figs. 36.12 and 36.13A). CT is useful when bony detail is required. CT or air myelography is generally not used now because of the superiority of MRI. Diffusion tensor MRI techniques show promise for the delineation of fiber tracts in the neonatal spinal cord.[102] Current MRI data indicate that the worst *prognosis* for subsequent cord function in the infant with traumatic spinal cord injury is associated with the finding

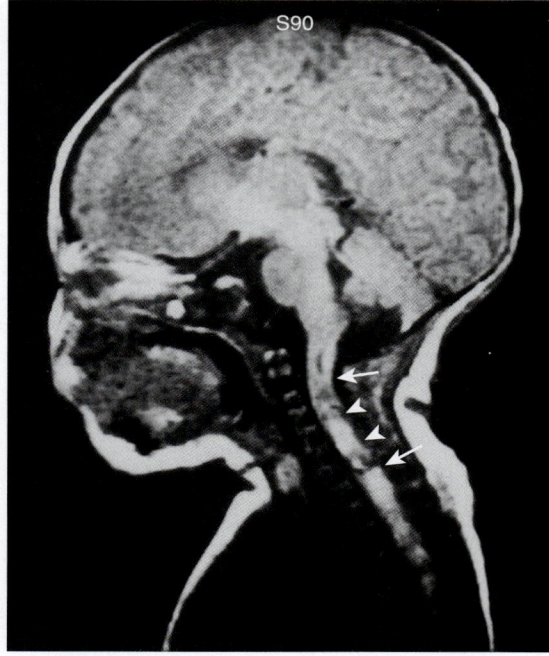

Figure 36.12 Neonatal spinal cord injury. Magnetic resonance imaging scan obtained at 5 days of age. Sagittal plane of cervical cord on T1-weighted scan. Oval high-intensity areas *(arrows)* and surrounding low-intensity areas *(arrowheads)* are observed in the lower cervical cord. (From Minami T, Ise K, Kukita J, Koyanagi T, Ueda K. A case of neonatal spinal cord injury: magnetic resonance imaging and somatosensory evoked potentials. *Brain Dev.* 1994;16:57.)

of intramedullary hemorrhage.[99] The prognosis is better with edema over several segments and best with edema involving one segment or less.[60,99]

Management

Prevention. The most important element of management is prevention (Table 36.5). Of paramount importance is *appropriate management of breech presentations* and any other obstetrical situation that might lead to *dysfunctional labor.* Particularly, pharmacological augmentation of dysfunctional labor, ill-advised use of instrumentation, and the production of *fetal depression* by inappropriate use of maternal drugs or anesthesia should be avoided. Because a substantial proportion of neonatal spinal cord injuries are associated with breech delivery, careful radiographic assessment of fetal position and size and of the maternal pelvis is necessary.

Hyperextension of the fetal head represents a fetal position that carries a very high risk for the development of spinal cord injury if the infant is delivered by the vaginal route.[103-108] It is critical to recognize that approximately 5% of all breech presentations are associated with a hyperextended fetal head.[108-110] (This dangerous fetal position may also be present with a transverse lie.) Vaginal delivery of a fetus with a hyperextended head and breech presentation is associated with death or survival with severe spinal cord injury in approximately 20% to 25% of cases. Thus, in a composite series of 73 such infants delivered vaginally, 15 experienced significant spinal cord injury, whereas none of 35 infants delivered by cesarean section experienced such injury.[108] That is, the beneficial role of cesarean section in preventing spinal cord injury is exemplified exceptionally well in this clinical setting. Nevertheless, a small minority of fetuses with hyperextended heads in utero may sustain serious cord injury *before* delivery and exhibit quadriplegia and respiratory failure despite cesarean section.[51,111-115] A decrease in fetal movement in the last weeks of gestation may herald the occurrence of cord injury in the fetus with a hyperextended head.[51] The cord lesions have been upper cervical in location, and one careful neuropathological study suggests intrauterine vascular injury.[114] The likely intrauterine mechanism (see the section on pathogenesis, earlier) is subluxation and dislocation of upper cervical vertebrae, shown at autopsy to occur with hyperextension of the head with compromise of the vertebral arteries, the vascular supply for upper cervical cord via the anterior spinal artery.[116] Thus, although cesarean section for the fetus in breech position with hyperextended head is critically important, spinal cord injury may, uncommonly, already have occurred. Indeed, as noted earlier, other examples of spinal

TABLE 36.5	Management of Spinal Cord Injury in the Neonatal Period

Prevention
Appropriate management of breech presentations and dysfunctional labor
Avoidance of fetal depression
Cesarean section for hyperextension of fetal head
Therapy
Rule out surgically correctable lesion
Supportive care

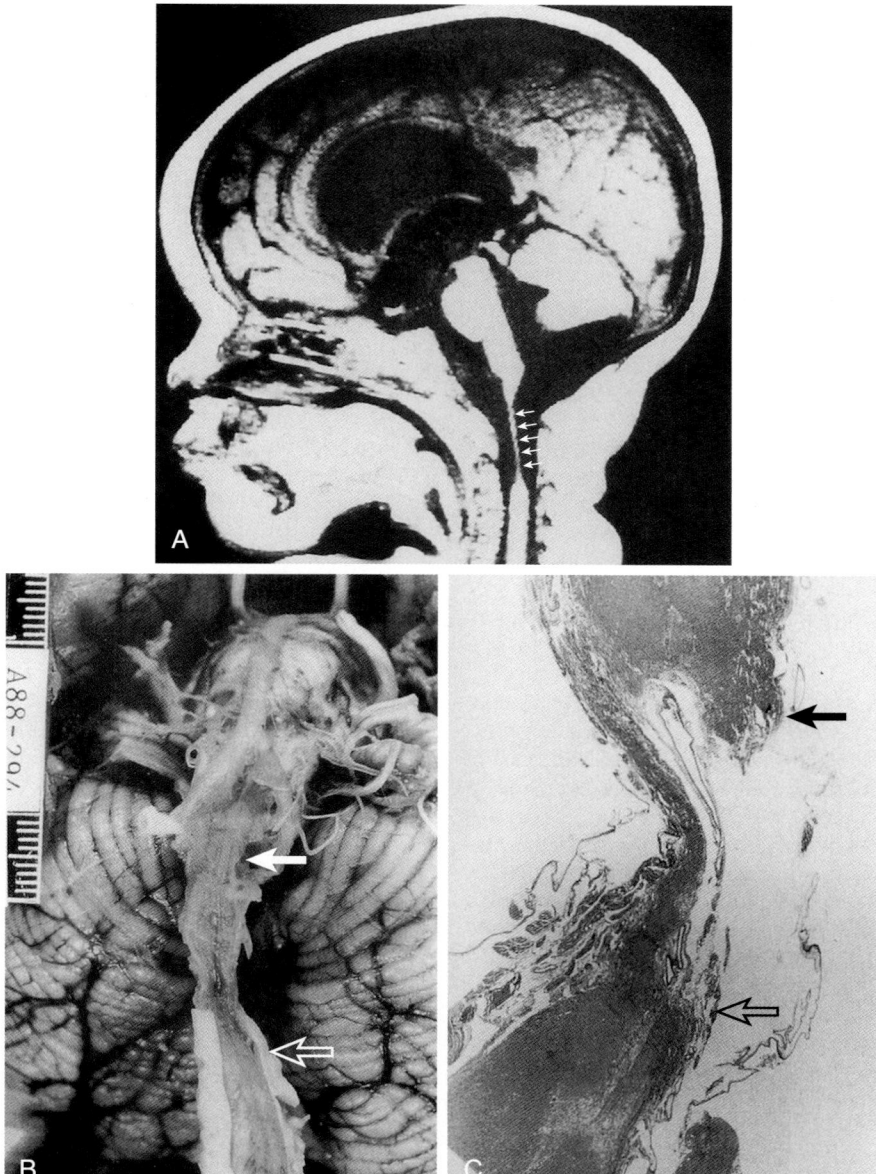

Figure 36.13 (A) Neonatal spinal cord injury: magnetic resonance imaging (MRI) scan at 4 months of age. Midline sagittal T1-weighted (TR, 500 ms; TE, 15 ms) MRI showing marked attenuation of cord caliber from the level of the caudal medulla to the level of C3 to C4 *(arrows)*. (B and C) Pathological specimen of infant whose MRI is shown in A. Infant died at 15 months of age. In B, note gross specimen demonstrating complete disruption between the lower medulla *(arrow)* and the upper cervical cord *(open arrow)*. In C, note microscopic section of upper cervical cord showing discontinuity between the lower medulla *(arrow)* and the upper cervical cord *(open arrow)*. The segment between the two arrows contains no neural elements, only leptomeninges and minimal scar tissue. (H & E, original magnification ×1.5.) (From Lanska MJ, Roessmann U, Wiznitzer M. Magnetic resonance imaging in cervical cord birth injury. *Pediatrics.* 1990;85:760.)

cord injury occurring in utero and *observed after cesarean section* have been recorded.[88,91,93-95,115]

Therapy. When a newborn infant has already sustained a serious cord injury, no specific therapy can be offered (see Table 36.5). It is critical to rule out a surgically approachable lesion—such as an occult dysraphic state, vertebral fracture, dislocation, or other extramedullary lesion—as previously discussed. A careful

history, physical examination, radiographs of the spine, and ultrasonography may be sufficient to rule out such lesions. However, when there is any doubt about the nature of the lesion or the possible presence of an extramedullary block, MRI should be carried out promptly. Intramedullary block, secondary usually to marked cord edema, is demonstrable in a small minority of cases, but surgical intervention is generally not indicated. In the rare case of extramedullary block, exploration may be reasonable to rule out a surgically remediable lesion or a major epidural hemorrhage that might be contributing seriously to a traumatic lesion of the cord. Nevertheless, it must be emphasized that there is little evidence that laminectomy and decompression have anything to offer these unfortunate infants in view of the basic nature of the cord lesion. Further data, however, are needed on this issue.

A potential role for methylprednisolone in the acute management of spinal cord injury was suggested by the results of randomized, controlled trials in adult patients.[70,71,76,117] However, on balance, the increased likelihood of complications and the modest beneficial effects have led to a lack of enthusiasm for this approach.[117,118] Many other interventions, suggested by study of experimental models—for example, GM-1 ganglioside, neurotrophic factors, antiexcitotoxic agents, antiinflammatory drugs, neural stem cells, and others—have either not yet been studied in humans or have not shown clear benefit.[77,117,119,120] Proof of benefit (without major risk)[121] is difficult to obtain in infants because of the relatively small number of cases available for study. Moreover, the correct diagnosis is usually delayed for many hours or days in infants (see earlier discussion).

Supportive therapy is important and is directed at ventilation, maintenance of body temperature, maintenance of perfusion, and prevention of urinary tract infection and contractures.

Major ethical issues are raised when infants are unable to sustain adequate ventilation without mechanical support. *Prediction of outcome in the neonatal period* is very difficult and clearly essential for decisions to withdraw life support. Certain tentative conclusions can be reached at 24 hours of age and 30 days of age. Thus, in one series of nine infants with spinal cord injury above the level of C-4 and requiring mechanical ventilation *and who had survived at least 3 months,* the only two patients who survived with a favorable outcome (independent daytime breathing, good motor function) had *breathing movements on day 1.*[52] Of the seven survivors who took their first breath after the first day of life, all still required mechanical ventilation (although one infant required only nocturnal mechanical ventilation) 8 months to 9 years later.[52] All four survivors who were *totally apneic beyond 30 days of age* required long-term mechanical ventilation and had severe motor disability.[52] It should also be noted that in this study five additional patients with upper cervical lesions had no respiratory movements in the first days of life and had life support withdrawn at 4 to 10 days of age. Nevertheless, although these data are useful in predicting outcome, the numbers of infants studied is relatively small and conclusions remain tentative. Moreover, some rehabilitative centers report that improvements in home mechanical ventilatory systems have been associated with relatively low long-term mortality rates and intercurrent morbidities and with successful reintegration into schools and the community.[54,122] Additionally, newer rehabilitative approaches—such as peripheral sensory level electrical stimulation and surface electromyography (EMG) triggered stimulation—have been reported to lead to surprising improvements in motor function.[86]

INJURY TO PERIPHERAL NERVOUS SYSTEM STRUCTURES

Traumatic injury to peripheral structures—for example, nerve roots, plexuses, and peripheral and cranial nerves—may result in serious and sometimes fatal disorders. In this section I review,

first, the four most common or serious of these injuries—that is, brachial plexus palsies, diaphragmatic paralysis, facial paralysis, and median nerve injury. Next, a variety of less common peripheral traumatic injuries of nerve roots, plexuses, and trunks are discussed.

Brachial Plexus Injury

Brachial plexus injury is weakness or total paralysis of muscles innervated by the nerve roots that supply the brachial plexus—that is, cervical roots 5 to 8 (C-5 to C-8) and thoracic root 1 (T-1) (Fig. 13.14).

Incidence

Brachial plexus injury is distinctly more common than spinal cord injury. In the largest reported series of traumatic birth injuries, brachial plexus injuries occurred 10 to 20 times more commonly than did spinal cord injuries.[123,124] The incidence has varied generally between 0.5 and 2.5 per 1000 live births.[125-146] Attesting further to the relatively common occurrence of brachial plexus injury, albeit not necessarily severe, I have been impressed with the relative frequency with which subtle but definite evidence for plexus injury can be ascertained by meticulous examination of infants at risk for such traumatic injury (see the section on pathogenesis, later). My observations have not been made in a systematic or quantitative fashion; indeed, the clinical significance is probably minimal because the subtle deficits invariably resolve in a matter of days.

Pathology

Although the term *brachial "plexus" injury* is consistently used, it should be recognized that the major pathology often involves the nerve *roots* that supply the plexus, particularly at the site where the roots form the trunks of the plexus (a similar site is observed in *stretch* injuries to the brachial *plexus* in adults) (see Fig. 36.14).[147] In the most severe neonatal lesions, actual avulsion of the root from the cord and, often, associated cord injury are present. A collection of cerebrospinal fluid (CSF) not confined by dura—that is, pseudomeningocele—usually accompanies avulsion. In the much more common, less severe lesions, hemorrhage and edema consequent to injury to the nerve sheath or axon are prominent.[66,132,148,149] In the most common form of brachial plexus palsy, the involvement of the proximal upper extremity, or Erb palsy, is caused particularly by a lesion at the point (Erb's point), where the fifth and sixth cervical nerve roots unite to form the upper trunk of the brachial plexus. Involvement of the distal upper extremity, that is, Klumpke palsy, is caused particularly by a lesion at the point where the eighth cervical and first thoracic nerve roots unite to form the lower trunk of the plexus.

The general relationships between the nature of the gross pathology and outcome are summarized in Table 36.6. Injury to the nerve sheath with associated hemorrhage and edema but with intact axons (*neurapraxia*) secondarily impairs axonal function, primarily by compression, but recovery is complete. *Severance of axons or roots is more serious.* Rupture of roots is associated with essentially no chance of spontaneous recovery. Similarly, axonal rupture when associated with severance of the nerve sheath and thus loss of a *guide* for regenerating axons ("neurotmesis") is associated with a poor spontaneous outcome. However, axonal rupture with an intact nerve sheath is intermediate in severity; axonal regeneration occurs at a rate

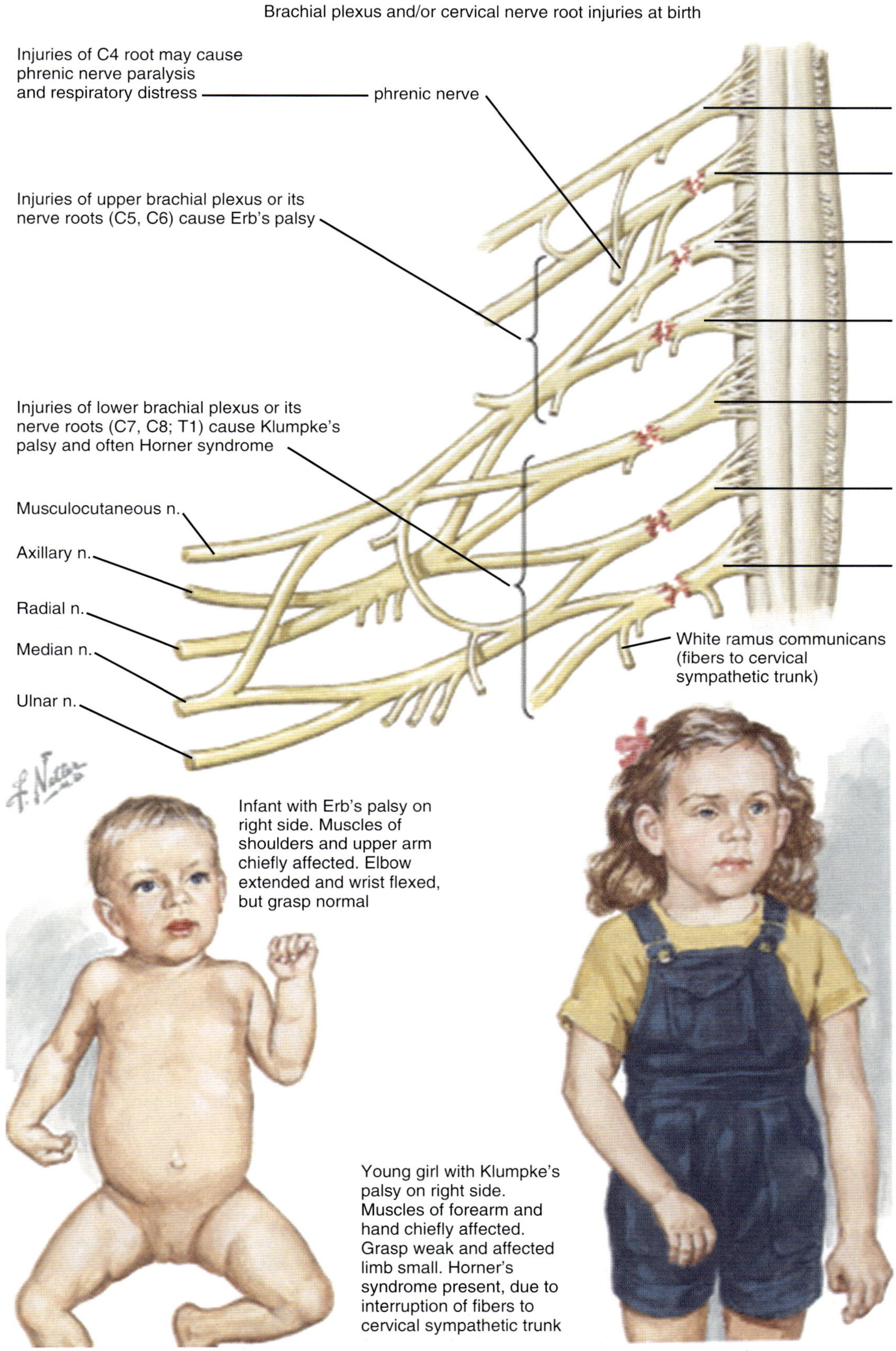

Brachial plexus and/or cervical nerve root injuries at birth

Injuries of C4 root may cause phrenic nerve paralysis and respiratory distress —— phrenic nerve

Injuries of upper brachial plexus or its nerve roots (C5, C6) cause Erb's palsy

Injuries of lower brachial plexus or its nerve roots (C7, C8; T1) cause Klumpke's palsy and often Horner syndrome

Musculocutaneous n.

Axillary n.

Radial n.

Median n.

Ulnar n.

C3

C4

C5

C6

C7

C8

T1

White ramus communicans (fibers to cervical sympathetic trunk)

Infant with Erb's palsy on right side. Muscles of shoulders and upper arm chiefly affected. Elbow extended and wrist flexed, but grasp normal

Young girl with Klumpke's palsy on right side. Muscles of forearm and hand chiefly affected. Grasp weak and affected limb small. Horner's syndrome present, due to interruption of fibers to cervical sympathetic trunk

Figure 36.14 Schematic representation of the brachial plexus with its terminal branches. The major sites of brachial plexus injury are shown; see text for details. (From Jones HR, Ryan MM, Levin KH. Radiculopathies and plexopathies. In: Darras BT, Jones HR, Ryan MM, De Vivo DC, eds. *Neuromuscular Disorders of Infancy, Childhood, and Adolescence.* 2nd ed. Elsevier; 2015 with permission.)

TABLE 36.6   Relation of Pathology to Likelihood of Spontaneous Recovery in Brachial Plexus Injury

SEVERITY OF LESION	NERVE SHEATH	AXONS	ROOTS	LIKELIHOOD OF SPONTANEOUS RECOVERY
Mild	Intact[a]	Intact	Intact	Good
Moderate	Intact	Severed	Intact	Fair
Severe	Severed	Severed	Intact	Poor
Severe	Intact	Intact	Severed	Poor

[a]Nerve sheath intact but injured; injury usually consists of edema and hemorrhage with secondary impairment of axonal function.

of approximately 1.8 mm per day,[150] somewhat faster than the rate of approximately 1 mm/day in older individuals.

Pathogenesis

Brachial plexus injury is thought to result from stretching of the brachial plexus, with its roots anchored to the cervical cord, by downward lateral traction. The forces underlying injurious lateral traction may be endogenous, or related to strong maternal and uterine expulsion forces and an impacted shoulder, or they may be exogenous, or related to the process of delivering the head, or likely commonly, by both endogenous and exogenous forces. Endogenous forces are considered generally to be stronger than exogenous forces.[151] With delivery, the traction is exerted via the shoulder in the process of delivering the head with breech deliveries and via the head in the process of delivering the shoulder in cephalic deliveries. The upper roots of the plexus are most vulnerable, but with marked traction all roots are affected and total paralysis results. The relatively uncommon occurrences of *intrauterine* injury to the brachial plexus have been secondary to abnormalities of fetal position or of uterine structure, congenital cervical bone abnormalities, congenital tumors, or, most commonly, unknown intrauterine factors.[134,141,145,152-157]

The most common pathogenetic events just mentioned occur secondary to especially, *obstetrical factors* and *large fetal size*.[a] (It should be noted that *obstetrical* factors relate principally to such issues as fetal position, forces of labor, and characteristics of delivery; they should not be construed as those factors that are always under the control of the obstetrician.) In Gordon's[126] large, essentially unselected series, abnormal presentations occurred in 56% of cases; this group consisted of 14% breech and 42% abnormal vertex presentations (occiput posterior and occiput transverse). Shoulder dystocia was present in 51% of all vertex deliveries and in 30% of all breech deliveries. Labor was augmented in 50% of these cases. In a large series (n = 276) studied in the United Kingdom and Ireland, 65% had shoulder dystocia.[136] In several earlier series of shoulder dystocia, approximately 20% of infants sustained some degree of brachial plexus injury.[131,140,161] More recent studies suggest that this value is less than 10%.[143,163] Birth weight of affected infants exceeds 3500 g in 50% to 85% of cases.[b] In a large Swedish series, the incidence of brachial plexus palsy was 45-fold greater at a birth weight of greater than 4500 g than at a birth weight of less than 3500 g.[133] In a careful earlier study, intrauterine asphyxia with fetal depression was suggested by the signs of fetal distress in 44% and Apgar score at 1 minute of less than 4 in 39%.[126] Thus a large depressed infant with an abnormal labor and delivery appears to be at particular risk.

Clinical Features

Clinical Setting. The typical clinical setting comprises obstetrical and fetal factors that predispose the infant to traumatic injury, particularly by downward lateral traction. Thus, as noted previously, abnormal presentations, dysfunctional labor, augmented labor, large fetal size, and perhaps fetal depression occur to varying degrees in most cases of brachial plexus injury.

Neonatal Varieties. In standard writings on brachial plexus injury, two basic types are recognized: the upper type, or Erb palsy, and the lower type, or Klumpke palsy (Figs. 36.15 and 36.16). In neonatal patients, approximately 90% of cases of brachial plexus injury involve the proximal upper limb and correspond to Erb palsy.[a] A true Klumpke palsy—that is, weakness of distal upper extremity *only*—in my experience does not occur in the newborn period; infants with distal involvement *also* exhibit proximal involvement. These neonatal patients with essentially *total* brachial plexus palsy often are described, appropriately or not, as Klumpke palsy.

The nerve roots involved in the common, upper Erb palsy emanate from cervical segments 5 and 6 in at least 50% of such cases, with the addition of cervical segment 7 in the remainder.[146,159] The additional roots involved in the patients with total brachial plexus injury emanate from cervical segment 8 to thoracic segment 1. In Erb palsy, affection of the diaphragm may be associated if involvement extends to cervical roots 4 and, perhaps, 3. (The innervation to the diaphragm, as noted previously, is from cervical segments 3, 4, and 5, with most input from C-4.) Affection of the ipsilateral diaphragm is present in approximately 5% of cases of Erb palsy. In total plexus injury, affection of sympathetic outflow from thoracic root 1 may result in Horner syndrome, manifested in the newborn by ptosis and miosis. An additional complication of this deficit of sympathetic innervation of the iris is a disturbance in pigment formation. Thus the affected eye remains unpigmented (i.e., blue) for many months or years.[66]

Major Neurological Features. The major neurological features of Erb and total plexus palsies are best considered in terms of effects on muscle function, tendon reflexes (especially

---

[a]References 12, 126, 128-131, 133-141, 143, 144, 148, 156-162.
[b]References 126, 130, 131, 136, 138-140, 159, 161, 164, 165.

[a]References 126, 128, 136, 159, 166, 167.

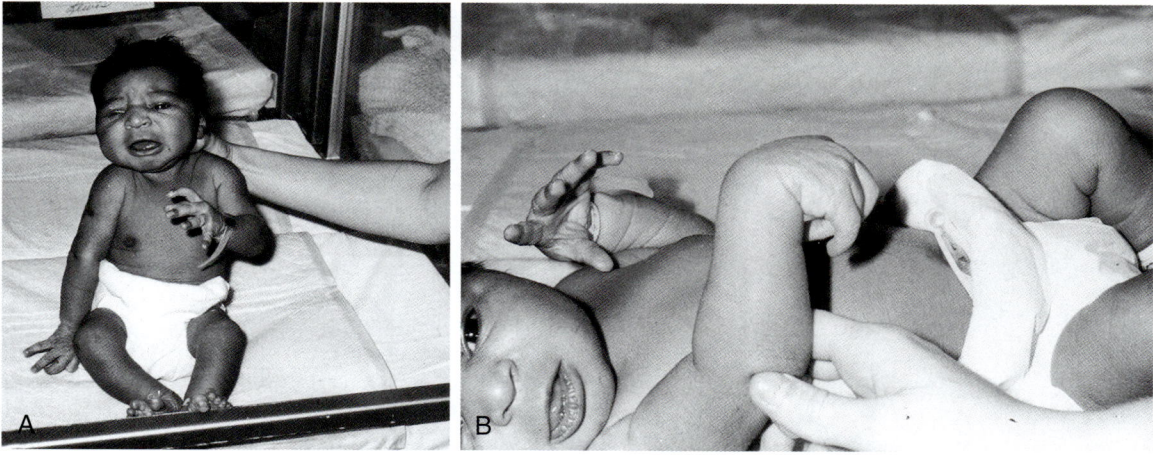

Figure 36.15 Brachial plexus injury, upper or Erb type: clinical appearance. (A) Infant holds upper extremity adducted, internally rotated, and pronated. (B) *Waiter's tip* position of affected wrist and fingers. (From Painter MJ, Bergman I. Obstetrical trauma to the neonatal central and peripheral nervous system. *Semin Perinatol.*1982;6:89.)

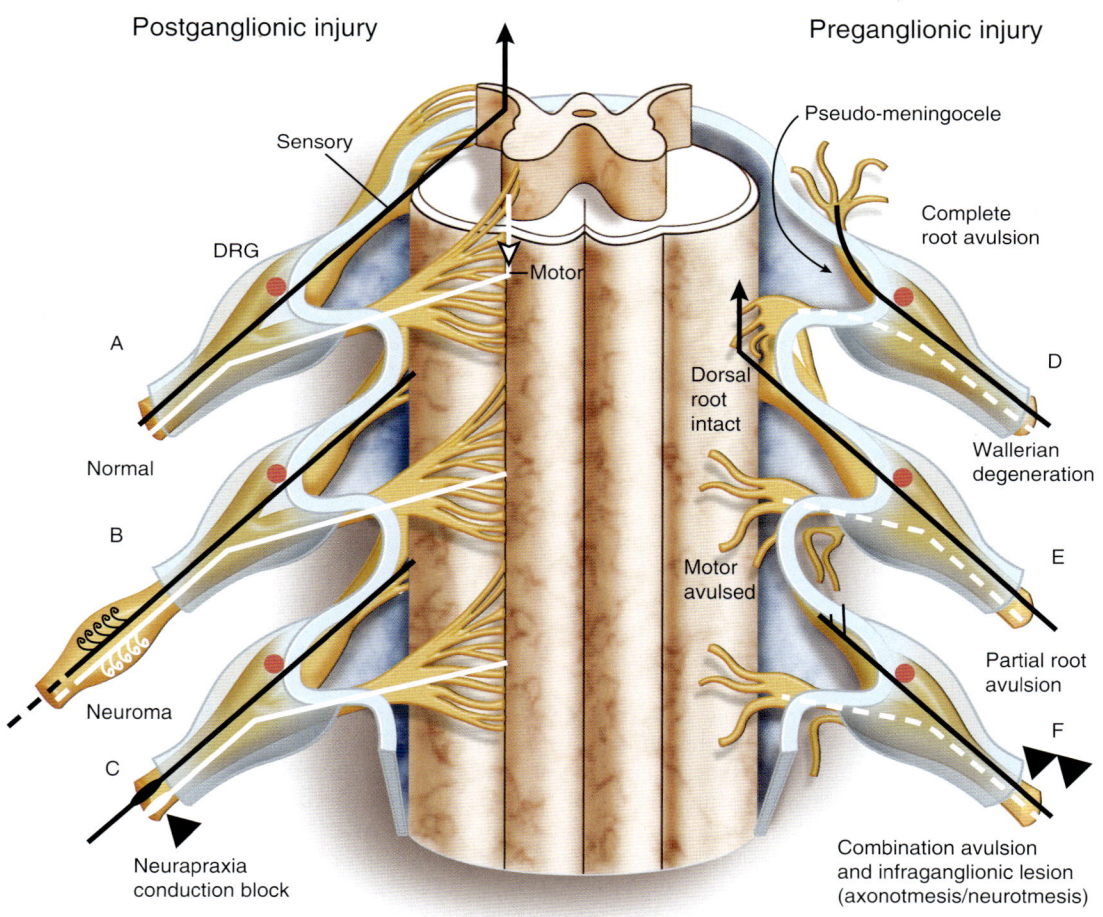

Figure 36.16 Brachial plexus injury in the newborn: pathology and clinical appearance. *DRG,* Dorsal root ganglion. (From Jones HR, Ryan MM, Levin KH. Radiculopathies and plexopathies. In: Darras BT, Jones HR, Ryan MM, De Vivo DC, eds. *Neuromuscular Disorders of Infancy, Childhood, and Adolescence.* 2nd ed. Elsevier; 2015, with permission.)

TABLE 36.7   Major Pattern of Weakness With Erb (Upper) Brachial Plexus Palsy

WEAK MOVEMENT	SPINAL CORD SEGMENT	RESULTING POSITION
Shoulder abduction	C-5	Adducted
Shoulder external rotation	C-5	Internally rotated
Elbow flexion	C-5,6	Extended
Supination	C-5,6	Pronated
Wrist extension	C-6,7	Flexed
Finger extension	C-6,7	Flexed
Diaphragmatic descent	C-4,5	Elevated

TABLE 36.8   Major Additional Pattern of Weakness With Total Brachial Plexus Palsy

WEAK MOVEMENT	SPINAL CORD SEGMENT	RESULTING POSITION
Wrist flexion	C-7,8, T-1	Extended
Finger flexion	C-7,8, T-1	Extended
Finger abduction	C-8, T-1	Neutral position
Finger adduction	C-8, T-1	Neutral position
Dilator of iris	T-1	Miosis
Full lid elevation	T-1	Ptosis

TABLE 36.9   Reflex Abnormalities in Erb (Upper) and Total Brachial Plexus Palsies

REFLEX	SPINAL CORD SEGMENT	RESPONSE UPPER PALSY	RESPONSE TOTAL PALSY
Biceps	C-5,6	Absent	Absent
Moro	—	—	—
Shoulder abduction	C-5	Absent	Absent
Hand movement	C-8, T-1	Present	Absent
Palmar grasp	C-8, T-1	Present	Absent

the biceps), Moro and grasp reflexes, and sensory function (Tables 36.7–36.9). In general the motor deficits are much more striking than the sensory deficits because of the overlapping innervation of sensory dermatomes, the greater affection of anterior than posterior roots, and the difficulty of precise assessment of sensation in the newborn. Based on clinical features, the lesion is bilateral in approximately 5% of cases.[a] Interestingly, a careful electrophysiological study of 18 cases showed *neurophysiological* abnormalities in the clinically unaffected arm in 5 cases.[168]

Erb Palsy. In Erb (upper) palsy, there is weakness at the shoulder of abduction (deltoid, C-5) and external rotation (spinati, C-5), at the elbow of flexion (biceps, brachioradialis, C-5, C-6) and

supination (biceps, supinator, C-5, C-6), and to a variable extent at the wrist and fingers of extension (extensors of the wrist and long extensors of the fingers, C-6, C-7) (see Table 36.7). Thus the limb assumes the characteristic "waiter's tip" posture because of preservation of shoulder abduction and internal rotation, elbow extension and pronation, and wrist and finger flexion (see Fig. 36.13). The biceps (C-5, C-6) reflex is absent (see Table 36.9). The brachioradialis and triceps reflexes (C-6, C-7, C-8), which are sometimes difficult to elicit in the newborn, might be expected to be inconsistently disturbed. The Moro reflex is disturbed because of the deficit in shoulder abduction (although hand movement is present). The grasp reflex is present because of the preserved finger flexion. I have found *sensory deficits* to pinprick (assessed primarily by observation of facial response) to be relatively common, contrary to the experience recorded by many others. The most consistent hypesthesia is over the lateral aspect of the proximal upper extremity (C-5). *Diaphragmatic paralysis,* which should be looked for specifically, was associated with Erb palsy in 3 of the 55 cases studied by Gordon and co-workers.[126]

Total Plexus Palsy. In total plexus palsy, with involvement of lower as well as upper roots, the paralysis extends to the intrinsic muscles of the hand (C-8, T-1) (see Table 36.8). (I have never seen a case of involvement of hand *alone,* although a report recorded one case among 57 cases of neonatal brachial plexus palsy.[129]) The grasp reflex is *absent* (see Table 36.8). The sensory loss is more extensive in these patients with total plexus involvement because of the loss of the overlapping sensory innervation. *Horner syndrome* has been reported in about 30% of these severely affected infants.[126,128,136,159,166]

Other Traumatic Lesions. Other traumatic lesions may be associated with brachial plexus injury. Thus the approximate proportions of associated lesions are as follows: fractured clavicle (10%), fractured humerus (10%), subluxation of the shoulder (5% to 10%), subluxation of cervical spine (5%), cervical cord injury (< 5%), and facial palsy (10%).[129,136,140,159,169]

Diagnosis

Delineation of the *clinical features* can be accomplished effectively by meticulous neurological examination. *Electromyographic studies* have been recommended as adjuncts to the evaluation at approximately 1 and 3 months of age.[a] Signs of denervation— that is, fibrillations—appear about 2 to 3 weeks after the injury. If fibrillations are absent, the likely lesion is *neurapraxia* and the outlook is favorable. Nerve root avulsion and a poor outcome are indicated on the first study by diffuse fibrillations, unrecordable or scanty motor unit potentials, no muscle response with stimulation of motor nerves and no improvement on the second EMG examination. Definition of diaphragmatic paralysis can be made conclusively by *real-time ultrasound,* which demonstrates high placement of the diaphragm on the affected side and *seesaw* movements of the whole diaphragm with respiration. The latter results because on inspiration the paralyzed side ascends while the intact side descends; the opposite occurs with expiration. *MRI* may demonstrate pseudomeningoceles and other findings suggesting partial or complete avulsion of roots and thus a poor prognosis for spontaneous recovery

[a]References 107, 136, 141, 159, 160, 166.

[a]References 128, 146, 159, 166, 167, 170, 171.

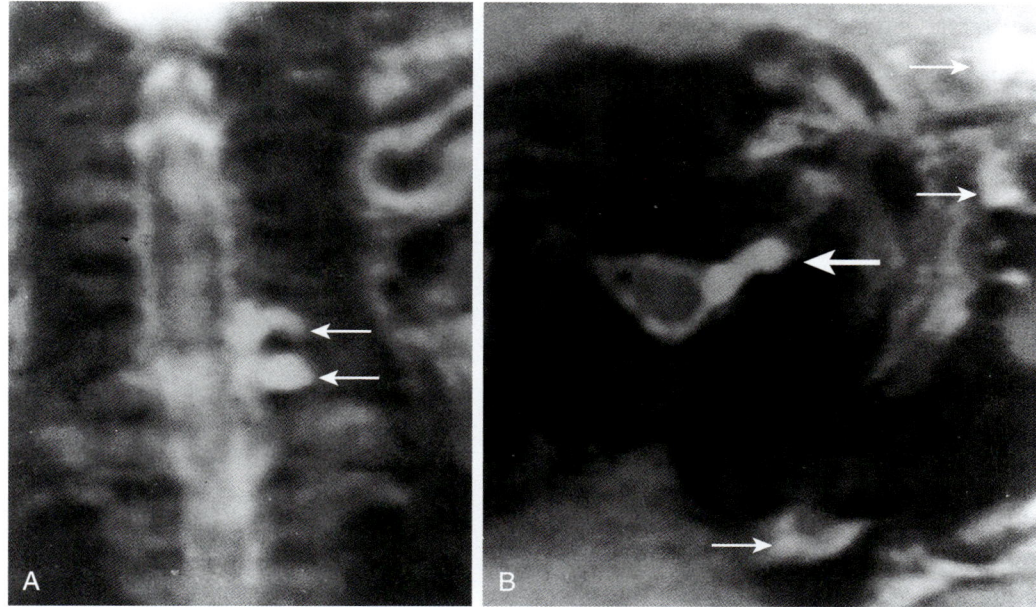

Figure 36.17 **MRI in a 6-day-old infant with left brachial plexus injury.** (A) Reconstructed coronal T2-weighted image shows pseudomeningoceles of left C-7 and C-8 roots (*arrows*). (B) Axial T2-weighted image shows pseudo-meningoceles of left C-8 root (*large arrow*). Note also soft-tissue swelling and fluid in fascial planes of left lower neck and shoulder (*small arrows*). (From Francel PC, Koby M, Park TS, et al. Fast spin-echo magnetic resonance imaging for radiological assessment of neonatal brachial plexus injury. *J Neurosurg.* 1995;83:461–466.)

(Figs. 36.17 and 36.18).[172-175] However, pseudomeningoceles may be absent in infants who ultimately have a poor outcome, and their presence is not invariably followed by a poor outcome.[167] The total constellation of MRI findings may allow distinction of root avulsion from axonal rupture and thereby aid in surgical planning (generally nerve reconstruction for the former and nerve grafting for the latter).[175] Occasionally, differentiation of brachial plexus injury from *pseudoparalysis* secondary to bony lesions presents a diagnostic problem. *Radiographs of the cervical spine, clavicles, and humerus* are of value in this regard.

Prognosis

Prognosis relates to the severity and extent of the lesion. Reported rates of full recovery generally range from 65% to 90%.[a] The variation in rates depends particularly on whether the population has been followed from the neonatal period and whether full recovery is based on careful clinical examination and excludes good functional recovery, albeit with residual weakness. In populations followed from the neonatal period, recovery rates are generally higher than in populations referred later to a tertiary center. For example, in two series followed from the neonatal period, approximately 90% of infants were said to be normal at 6 months of age.[126,131] More recent studies with rigorous assessments of function found approximately 70% of infants normal at 6 months of age.[142,185] Recovery continues to approximately 12 to 18 months of age, when 80% to 90% of infants are normal.[142,185] This prolonged duration of recovery is illustrated in a more severely affected referral population. Thus, in a carefully studied population followed at a

---

[a]References 126, 131, 133, 136, 137, 140, 142, 146, 159, 162, 176-185.

TABLE 36.10   Outcome of Neonatal Brachial Plexus Palsy Relative to Examination at 6 Months

MUSCLE STRENGTH AT 6 MONTHS	PATIENTS n (%)	FINAL OUTCOME
≥3/5 in BTD (*also at 4.5 months*)	53 (66)	Complete recovery
≥3/5 in BTD	9 (11)	Mild weakness
≥3/5 in B, T, or both, *but not D*	7 (9)	Moderate weakness
0-1/5 WE and/or ≤2/5 in BTD	11 (14)	Severe weakness

B, Biceps; *D*, deltoid; *T*, triceps; *WE*, wrist extensors.
Muscle strength scale: *0*, No contraction; *1*, trace contraction; *2*, active movement with gravity eliminated; *3*, active movement against gravity, *4*, active movement against gravity and resistance; *5*, normal.
Data derived from Noetzel MJ, Park TS, Robinson S, Kaufman B. Prospective study of recovery following neonatal brachial plexus injury. *J Child Neurol.* 2001;16:488–492.

children's hospital (*n* = 116), only 33% were normal at 6 months of age, 45% at 9 months, and 66% at 15 months.[178] Early onset of recovery—that is, within 2 to 4 weeks—is an excellent prognostic sign; in one series, all patients who recovered fully showed some improvement in arm function by 2 weeks.[186] The importance of serial assessments and in particular the findings at 6 months in prediction of final outcome after 12 months is illustrated by the data in Table 36.10. Thus, infants with

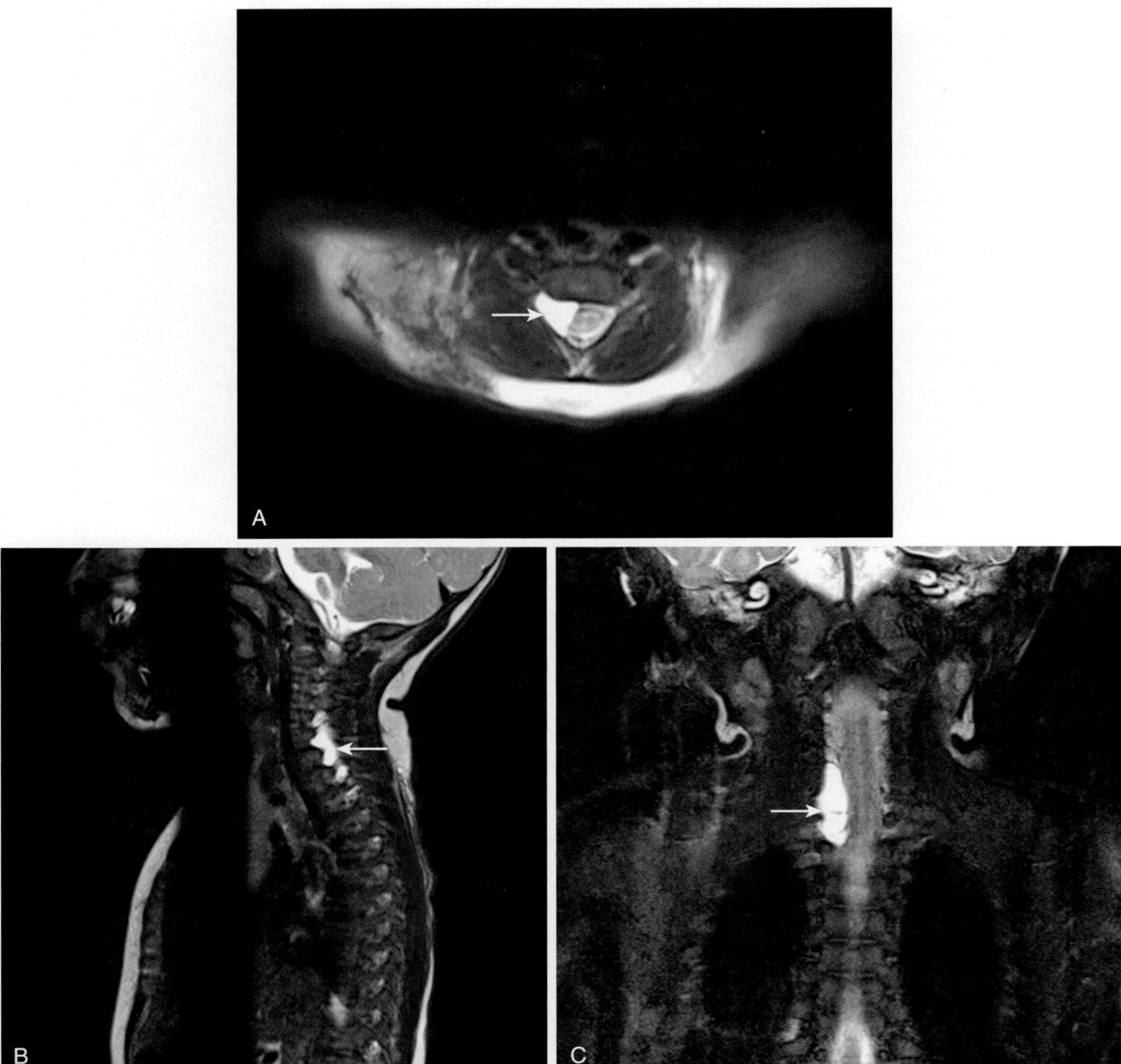

Figure 36.18 Magnetic resonance imaging in neonatal brachial plexus injury. (A) Axial T2-weighted MRI shows a pseudomeningocele from nerve root avulsion (*arrow*). (B), Sagittal T2-weighted image shows multiple pseudomeningoceles in the cervical spine from C-5 to T-1 (*arrow*). (C) Coronal T2 fat suppression MRI scan indicative of multiple pseudomeningoceles secondary to nerve root avulsions on the right (*arrow*). (From Jones HR, Ryan MM, Levin KH. Radiculopathies and plexopathies. In: Darras BT, JonesHR, Ryan MM, De Vivo DC, eds. *Neuromuscular Disorders of Infancy, Childhood, and Adolescence.* 2nd ed. Elsevier; 2015, with permission.)

a final outcome of complete recovery recovered antigravity movement of biceps, triceps, and deltoid by 4.5 months (80% by 3 months); those with a final outcome of mild residual weakness did not recover antigravity movement until 6 months; those with ultimate moderate residual weakness had failure of antigravity recovery at least in the deltoid at 6 months; and those with later severe residua had no or trace recovery of wrist extensors at 6 months. Clearly the last group comprised those with extensive plexus lesions. In an obstetrical series of 19 infants with C-5 to T-1 lesions, none made a full recovery, 68% made a partial recovery, and fully 32% failed to recover.[136]

Management

There are two major aspects to the management of brachial plexus injury in the neonatal period. The first is prevention and the second is care of the affected infant.

Prevention. Prevention of brachial plexus injury must be based on eliminating the opportunity for traction injury (see the section on pathogenesis, earlier). Reasoned obstetrical management of abnormal presentations and deliveries and judicious use of maternal drugs and anesthesia to avoid fetal depression, especially with a large fetus, are critical. A recent study showed a pronounced (75%) decrease of brachial plexus palsy at birth in the setting of shoulder dystocia after institution of a consistent, detailed approach to obstetrical management.[163]

Therapy. Management of the infant, once affected, is directed particularly toward prevention of the development of contractures, which worsen the degree of functional disability. After the diagnosis is made, the limb should be immobilized gently across the upper abdomen. Therapy should begin in the early part of the first week with gentle, passive range-of-motion exercises at the shoulder, elbow, wrists, and small joints of the hands.[128,159,166,171] Supportive wrist splints to prevent flexion contractures and stabilize the fingers are important. Not recommended is the former "Statue of Liberty" splint, which placed the limb in a position at shoulder, elbow, and wrist that was opposite from that assumed by the unsupported limb. This type of splint carries considerable risk of causing contractures in the new position. Trophic disturbances of skin, muscle, and bone are particularly likely to develop in infants with *total* plexus involvement (which usually includes marked sensory involvement); these disturbances are difficult to treat effectively. In addition, a few infants, even some with good sensorimotor recovery, "ignore and refuse to use" the affected limb.[159,171] This state has been attributed to a failure of development of appropriate cerebral motor patterns and organization of body image secondary to the transient interruption of peripheral pathways, which has some experimental support.[187] Eng's considerable clinical experience led to the following conclusion: "Attempts at sensory stimulation, massage, calling the infant's attention to the arm have been questionably successful in minimizing this problem."[159] Orthopedic problems at the shoulder and elbow may require surgical intervention, discussed elsewhere.[188]

The possibility of *surgical treatment* should be considered in selected patients after careful serial assessments over the first 6 months. The advent of the operating microscope and recent success in microsurgical repair of brachial plexus lesions in adults have led to the surgical management of severely affected infants.[a] Surgical options depend on the specific findings but include removal of disruptive fibrous tissue at the site of the lesion, excision of neuroma, sural nerve graft at the site of axonal rupture, and local root grafts from intact roots at the sites of root avulsions.[132,139,148,188] Improvement in function has been reported in the majority of operated infants.[132,139,146,148] The critical issue concerning *timing of the decision* to proceed to surgery is unresolved.[b] I consider particularly rational the approach based in considerable part on the data shown in Table 36.10.[178] Thus infants with upper plexus palsies who attain antigravity movements of biceps, triceps and deltoid by 6 months of age have a very high likelihood of excellent spontaneous recovery. However, the families of those infants destined for a poor outcome (see "severe weakness"

in Table 36.10), including more severe upper plexus palsies and total plexus palsies, should be apprised of neurosurgical interventions at 4 to 6 months of age. EMG and MRI can provide additional useful information (see earlier). Neurosurgical intervention is often best considered for ages 6 to 9 months.[178] However, a recent neurosurgical review of cases of upper brachial plexus (C-5 to C-7) palsies suggests that delaying surgical repair to 12 months of age markedly increases the proportion of infants who will experience spontaneous recovery without need for surgery.[185] A controlled trial will likely be necessary to resolve the issue of optimal timing for surgery. For the small group of total plexus palsies, some advocate neurosurgical intervention before 6 months.[182]

Diaphragmatic Paralysis

Diaphragmatic paralysis secondary to traumatic injury to cervical nerve roots supplying the phrenic nerve occurs primarily in association with brachial plexus injury (Table 36.11). Other varieties of neonatal diaphragmatic paralysis may occur, albeit rarely (see later).

Incidence

The incidence of neonatal diaphragmatic paralysis is related to the incidence of brachial plexus injury because approximately 80% to 90% of cases are associated with such plexus injury and approximately 5% of cases of brachial plexus injury are associated with diaphragmatic paralysis.[a]

Pathology

The pathogenesis of diaphragmatic paralysis appears to be similar in most cases to that described for brachial plexus injury. This conclusion is supported by the high frequency of similar obstetrical and fetal factors and of extreme lateral traction in the delivery of affected infants. Phrenic nerve injury is more common after breech than after cephalic deliveries. The major sites of injury defined in anatomical studies are shown in Fig. 36.19.[208]

Clinical Features

Clinical Syndrome. Although the clinical syndrome is somewhat variable, the most typical features can be summarized as follows.[97,192-203,205,208-211] The birth occurs in a clinical setting

| TABLE 36.11 | Diaphragmatic Paralysis in the Newborn: Clinical and Related Features |

Relation to brachial plexus injury
Approximately 80%–90% of cases have associated plexus injury; approximately 5% of plexus injuries have diaphragmatic paralysis
Cervical roots involved
C-3 to C-5, especially C-4
Onset
First hours after birth
Diagnosis
Ultrasonography, chest fluoroscopy
Prognosis
Mortality in composite series approximately 10%–15%

[a]References 132, 139, 146, 148, 171, 177, 182, 188-191.
[b]References 146, 171, 182, 185, 190, 191.
[a]References 97, 136, 160, 166, 192-207.

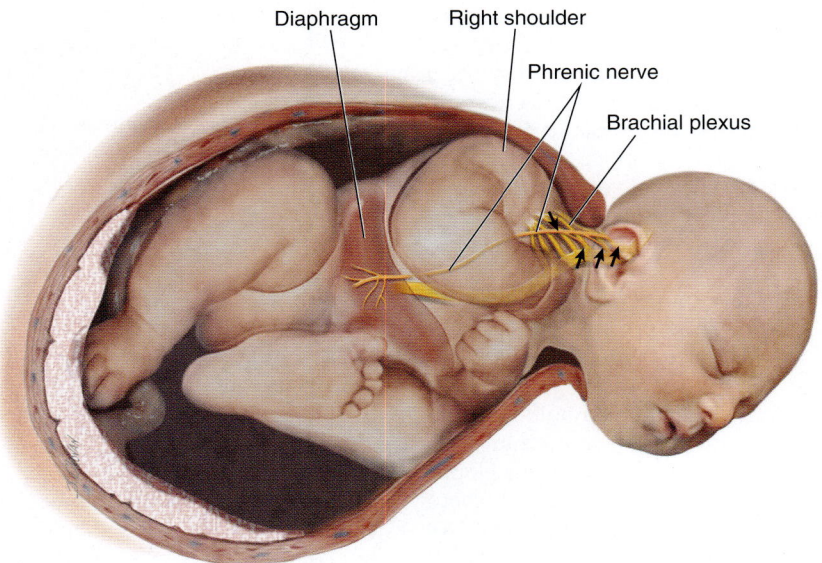

Diaphragm   Right shoulder   Phrenic nerve   Brachial plexus

Figure 36.19 Schematic appearance of infant during vaginal delivery before downward lateral traction of the head and neck to deliver the right shoulder (uppermost in the figure). Sites where the phrenic nerve can be stretched and injured are indicated by the four arrows. (From Alvord EC, Austin EJ, Larson CP. Neuropathologic observations in congenital phrenic nerve palsy. *J Child Neurol.* 1990;5:205.)

that includes the obstetrical and fetal factors conducive to traumatic injury, particularly difficult breech delivery, as described previously for brachial plexus injury, and where Erb palsy is evident. The hemidiaphragm on the same side as an Erb palsy is affected. Often there appears to be a biphasic course with diaphragmatic paralysis. *In the first hours after birth* the infant experiences respiratory difficulty, often with tachypnea, but with blood gas values suggestive of hypoventilation—for example, hypoxemia, hypercapnia, and acidosis. (In some cases signs of gross ventilation-perfusion unevenness are suggested by hypoxemia without significant hypercapnia.[197]) The occurrence of cyanosis with the respiratory difficulty often raises the possibility of congenital heart disease or primary pulmonary disease. *Over the next several days,* with oxygen therapy and varying degrees of ventilatory support, the infant may improve or at least stabilize. The diagnosis of diaphragmatic paralysis may be missed during this period, despite radiographs of the chest, because the elevated hemidiaphragm commonly is not present or prominent early in the course, especially with positive-pressure ventilation. In more severely affected infants, deterioration, sometimes insidious, of respiratory status occurs over the next days to weeks, often provoked by atelectasis or pulmonary infection. Indeed, in some infants,[212] the diagnosis may not be made for several weeks. Of course in the most severely affected infants, those with bilateral involvement, respiratory failure is obvious from birth.

In the uncommon infants without accompanying Erb palsy, the diaphragmatic paralysis may be an isolated finding and related to diaphragmatic muscle hypoplasia.[213] Additionally, several neuromuscular disorders may present at birth with unilateral or bilateral diaphragmatic paralysis—for example, congenital myasthenic syndromes, congenital myotonic dystrophy, congenital muscular dystrophies, congenital myopathies (nemaline or myotubular myopathy), and the

syndrome of spinal muscular atrophy with respiratory distress (SMARD) (see Chapters 32 and 33).[213,214] Accompanying these disorders are other signs of neuromuscular disease, especially generalized hypotonia and weakness (see Chapters 32 and 33). In medical centers that carry out substantial numbers of major cardiac surgeries in newborns, diaphragmatic paralysis secondary to phrenic nerve injury may be encountered in the absence of brachial plexus injury.[215] Finally, chest drains abutting the mediastinum may rarely lead to phrenic nerve injury in the newborn.[216]

Diagnosis

The diagnosis is established by ultrasonographic or fluoroscopic examination of the chest, which reveals the elevated hemidiaphragm and the paradoxical movement of the affected side with breathing (see previous section titled brachial plexus injury). It should be remembered that these radiographic abnormalities will not be present if the infant is receiving positive-pressure ventilation. Real-time ultrasonography is particularly useful in assessing diaphragmatic function because of the lack of radiation and the capacity for serial study.[215,217] Approximately 80% of the lesions involve the right side and less than 10% are bilateral.

Diagnosis of the forms of diaphragmatic paralysis without Erb palsy, as noted, may include diaphragmatic muscle biopsy for diaphragmatic hypoplasia or the variety of tests for neuromuscular disorders described in Chapter 30.

Prognosis

The subsequent course of the infant's condition in typical diaphragmatic paralysis related to phrenic nerve injury depends in part on the severity of the injury but particularly on the quality of supportive care. The mortality rate for the common unilateral lesions in composite series has been approximately

10% to 15%. The large majority of the infants, however, recover, usually in the first 6 to 12 months of life.[196,202,205,211,212] Clinical recovery may occur despite persistence of considerable weakness demonstrable by radiography.[212] Outcome is predictably poorer for the small number of infants with bilateral diaphragmatic paralysis[202-205,209,210,218]; mortality has approached 50% with the prolonged ventilatory support required. However, advancements in management are improving outcome (see the following section on management).

Management

Prevention. The comments on prevention of brachial plexus injury are appropriate here because the mechanism of production of the root lesions is similar.

Therapy. Once diaphragmatic paralysis is documented in the newborn infant, careful surveillance of respiratory status and intervention, when appropriate, are critical. Clinical experience suggests that the newborn infant tolerates diaphragmatic paralysis less well than does the older child or adult. Reasons suggested for this difference in vulnerability in the newborn include the usual recumbent posture, which leads to a greater reduction in vital capacity than does the upright posture; the relatively weaker intercostal muscles; the relatively greater risk of airway obstruction secondary to proportionately smaller airways; and the relatively longer time spent in rapid-eye-movement sleep, when tone in such postural muscles as the intercostals is inhibited.[209,215,219] Management of the newborn with diaphragmatic paralysis may be divided into *nonsurgical, so-called expectant modalities* and *surgical plication of the diaphragm.*

The *nonsurgical modalities* have been characterized as *expectant* because their major purpose is to stabilize the infant and provide adequate ventilation for a temporary period, until natural improvement of the neural injury occurs. These modalities have included oxygen supplementation, continuous positive airway pressure, intermittent negative-pressure ventilation, and intermittent positive-pressure ventilation (Table 36.12). Oxygen supplementation via a nasal cannula or hood may be beneficial. If more substantial support is needed, *continuous positive airway pressure* via a nasal cannula (with the infant in a semiupright position) has been associated with some benefit and merits a trial because it obviates the need for endotracheal intubation.[218] *Intermittent negative-pressure ventilation* has also been useful[209]; this approach has the advantages of avoiding intubation and avoiding trauma to airways. In recalcitrant cases, *intubation and intermittent positive-pressure breathing* have been advocated.[202] In general it has been suggested that the trial of positive-pressure ventilation be continued for approximately 1 to 2 months until

it is clear that no recovery is occurring.[207,209,211,220] If the latter is the case, then *plication of the affected diaphragm* is appropriate. A satisfactory respiratory outcome was achieved in 86% of surgically treated infants in one series.[211] In cases of bilateral lesions, it is recommended that, if possible, only the more severely involved hemidiaphragm be plicated.[209] Autologous nerve transplantation has been associated with improved diaphragmatic function in one reported bilateral case.[205]

Phrenic nerve stimulation (percutaneous) with surface recordings of diaphragmatic action potentials may provide important information for appropriate management.[97,205,221,222] Thus very prolonged conduction latencies or a marked reduction in amplitude or absence of diaphragmatic action potentials suggests that spontaneous recovery will not occur and that surgical plication is necessary.

Facial Paralysis

Facial paralysis involves the weakness of facial muscles and, in this context of perinatal trauma, indicates facial nerve injury; it therefore means involvement of the muscles of the upper as well as lower parts of the face.

Incidence

Facial weakness secondary to injury to the facial nerve is a common neurological manifestation of perinatal trauma. In an older study reported in 1951 of 875 term infants examined specifically for facial paresis on the second day of life, the incidence was 6.4%.[223] In a later series, the incidence was 0.75% of term infants,[158] and in still more recent series, the incidence was approximately 0.18% (Table 36.13).[224]

Pathology

The pathological basis for the typical traumatic injury to the facial nerve is unknown. It is likely that, in view of the generally favorable prognosis, the pathology in most infants consists of hemorrhage or edema into the nerve sheath rather than the disruption of nerve fibers (see the section on prognosis, later). The site of the lesion is almost certainly at or near the exit of the nerve from the stylomastoid foramen (Fig. 36.20). Shortly after the exit from the foramen, the nerve divides into its two major branches: the temporofacial, to the zygomatic region,

TABLE 36.12	Management of Diaphragmatic Paralysis in the Newborn
Nonsurgical modalities	
Supplemental oxygen by hood or nasal cannula	
Continuous positive airway pressure	
Intermittent negative pressure ventilation	
Intermittent positive pressure ventilation	
Surgical plication	
Timing—if no spontaneous recovery within 1–2 months	

TABLE 36.13	Incidence and Major Features of Facial Paresis

Total births: 44,292
Newborns with facial palsy: 92
    Acquired (presumed trauma): 81
        Incidence: 1.8 per 1000 births
    Developmental: 11
        Möbius syndrome, malformation, etc.
Acquired facial palsy
    Forceps delivery: 91%
    Signs of external trauma to scalp, head or face: 79%
    Follow-up
        Complete recovery: 89%
        Partial recovery: 11%

Data from Falco NA, Ericksson E. Facial nerve palsy in the newborn: incidence and outcome. *Plast Reconstr Surg.* 1990;85:1–4.

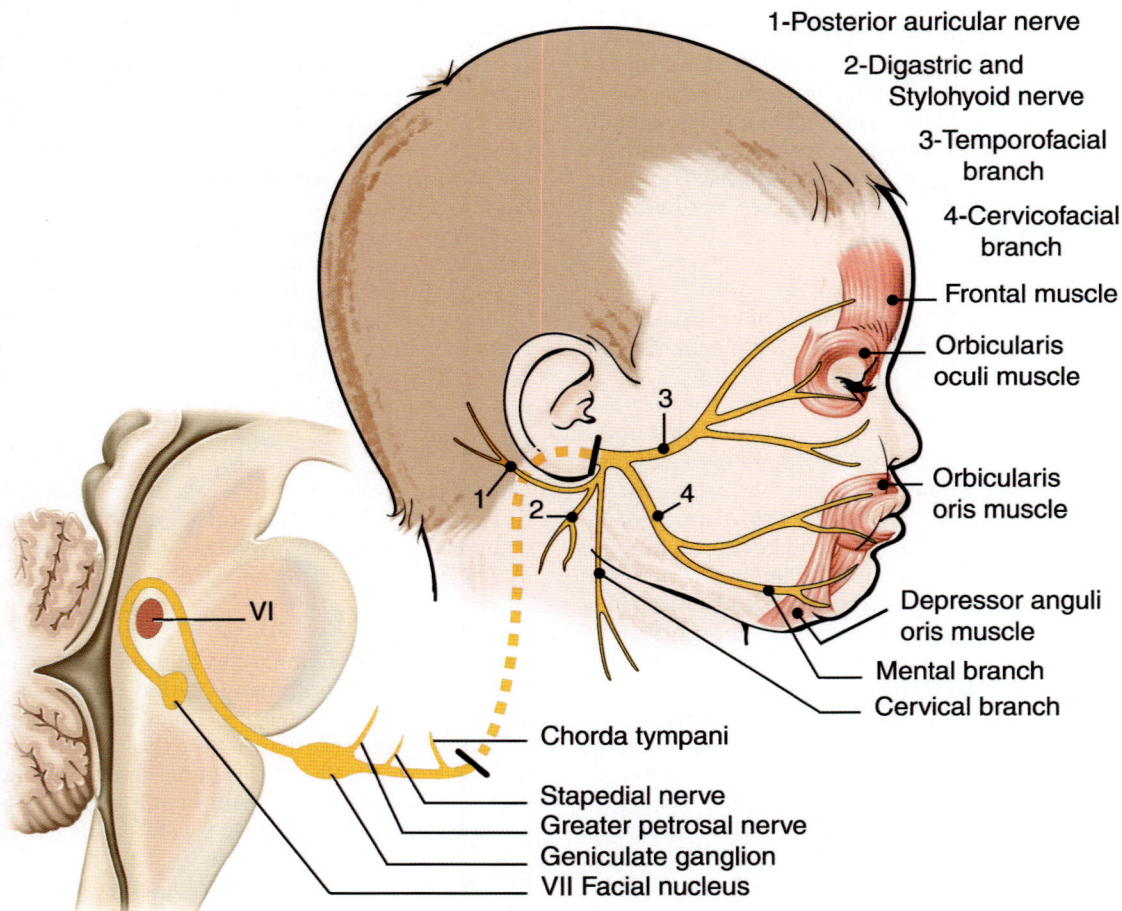

1-Posterior auricular nerve
2-Digastric and Stylohyoid nerve
3-Temporofacial branch
4-Cervicofacial branch

Frontal muscle
Orbicularis oculi muscle
Orbicularis oris muscle
Depressor anguli oris muscle
Mental branch
Cervical branch

Chorda tympani
Stapedial nerve
Greater petrosal nerve
Geniculate ganglion
VII Facial nucleus

VI

Figure 36.20 **Anatomy of the facial nerve.** (From Renault F, Quijano-Roy S. Congenital and acquired facial palsies. In: Darras BT, Jones HR, Ryan MM, De Vivo DC, eds. *Neuromuscular Disorders of Infancy, Childhood, and Adolescence.* 2nd ed. Elsevier; 2015, with permission.)

eye, and upper face, and the cervicofacial, to the mandibular region and platysma. Involvement of the nerve at more proximal sites—for example, in the facial canal or posterior fossa—is rare in the newborn infant. However, compression against a fracture of the petrous temporal bone, identified at surgery, has been reported in two infants.[225,226]

Pathogenesis

Two prinicipal pathogenetic mechanisms are operative to produce injurious compression of the facial nerve (i.e., intrauterine compression against the sacral promontory or intrapartum compression by forceps blade) (see Table 36.13).[13,223,224,227] Hepner's[223] interesting study in 1951 of 875 term infants examined on the second postnatal day presents strong evidence for the pathogenetic importance of intrauterine pressure on the facial nerve by the sacral promontory (Table 36.14).[223] There was a direct correlation between the side of the face affected and the position of the head in utero (see Table 36.14). Thus the 40 infants with left facial paresis were born from the obstetrical positions, occiput left transverse or left anterior, and the 16 infants with right facial paresis

TABLE 36.14	Relation of Side of Facial Paresis to Intrauterine Position		
INFANTS (n)	**TYPE OF DELIVERY**	**SIDE OF FACIAL PARESIS**	**INTRAUTERINE POSITION**
6	Natural	Left	Occiput left transverse
4	Natural	Right	Occiput right transverse
34	Forceps	Left	Occiput left transverse or anterior
12	Forceps	Right	Occiput right anterior, transverse, or posterior

Data from Hepner WR. Some observations on facial paresis in the newborn infant: etiology and incidence. *Pediatrics.* 1951;8:494.

TABLE 36.15	Incidence of Facial Paresis as a Function of Level of Forceps Delivery		
	LEVEL OF FORCEPS DELIVERY[a]		
	OUTLET	**LOW**	**MID**
No. of infants	116	178	63
Percent with facial palsy	0.8	1.7	9.5

[a]The level of forceps delivery is based on the revised definition of level in which midforceps is the highest level, that is, the term *high forceps* is not used. Data from Hagadorn-Freathy AS, Yeomans ER, Hankins GD. Validation of the 1988 ACOG forceps classification system. *Obstet Gynecol.* 1991;77:356–360.

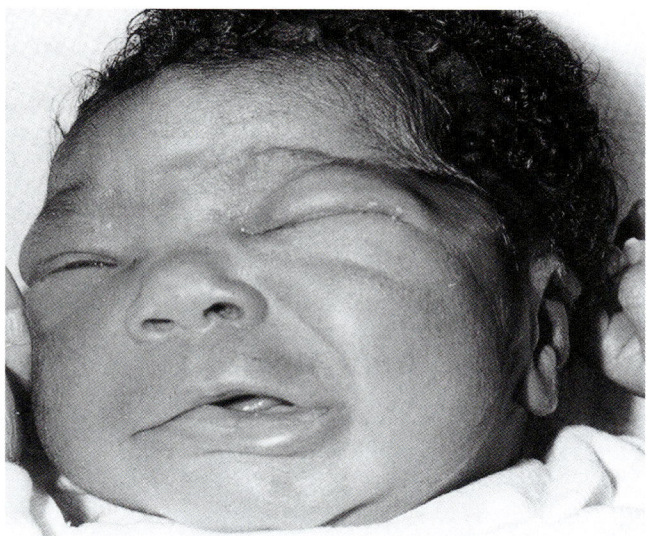

Figure 36.21   Right facial paralysis: clinical appearance. Note that lack of movement on the right leads to the appearance of the face being *pulled* to the left with cry. The right nasolabial fold is flattened. (From Painter MJ, Bergman I. Obstetrical trauma to the neonatal central and peripheral nervous system. *Semin Perinatol.* 1982;6:89.)

were born from similar obstetrical positions on the right. The common denominator was the position of the face on the sacral promontory. Thus compression of the nerve as the face is pressed against this bony protuberance appeared to cause the injury.

A forceps blade is frequently the source of compression of the facial nerve (see Table 36.13).[11,158,224] In an older study of nearly 14,000 singleton live term infants at a major teaching hospital, those with facial nerve injury were delivered with forceps in 72% of cases (midforceps in 28%) versus 33% (midforceps in 4%) in the control group.[158] A later study of 357 vertex deliveries by forceps extraction shows clearly the relation of the incidence of facial palsy to the level of forceps delivery (Table 36.15).[11] In the largest series of cases of traumatic facial palsy, 74 of the 81 cases (91%) were associated with forceps deliveries (see Table 36.13).[224] (It should be noted that 8500 infants were delivered with forceps assist in the overall cohort[224]; thus the vast majority of forceps deliveries were unaccompanied by facial palsy.) Birth weight greater than 3500 g and primiparity were additional risk factors for facial nerve palsy.[224] The role of mechanical factors is emphasized further by the accompanying findings of shoulder dystocia in 10% and brachial plexus palsy in 9%.[224] Consistent with these findings, one study of over 4000 infants delivered by forceps or vacuum extraction showed a fourfold higher risk of facial nerve palsy in the forceps-delivered infants.[228] In a more recent review of 33,000 infants, an 11-fold higher risk in forceps- versus vacuum-delivered infants was found.[13]

Clinical Features

Clinical Setting. The clinical setting is not necessarily that of an overtly traumatic birth, although forceps deliveries, above average birth weight, and primiparity are overrepresented (see the section on pathogenesis, earlier). The traumatic nature of the lesion is emphasized by the almost invariable relationship between the side of the facial weakness and the side of the face that was apposed in utero to the sacral promontory or that was encountered by a forceps blade. The forceps blade may leave a distinct mark on the face near the underlying stylomastoid foramen. Approximately 80% of affected infants in one large series had signs of external trauma to the head or face (ecchymosis, lacerations, molding, cephalhematoma) (see Table 36.13).[224,227] Less commonly the infant appeared to exhibit evidence for an abnormal fetal posture—that is, firm apposition of the angle of the jaw to the shoulder.

Clinical Syndrome. By far the most common syndrome of neonatal facial nerve palsy is related to affection of the nerve after exit from the stylomastoid foramen; therefore the typical features include weakness of both upper and lower facial muscles (Fig. 36.21). At rest the palpebral fissure is wider on the affected side, the nasolabial fold is flattened, and the subtle nuances of facial expression are absent. With elicited movement it is apparent that the infant is unable to wrinkle the brow, close the eye firmly, or move the corner of the mouth or lower face into an effective grimace. Moreover, there is often dribbling of liquid from the corner of the mouth with feeding. Approximately 75% of cases involve the left side of the face, perhaps in part reflecting the relative frequencies of intrauterine positions (see previous discussion).

Diagnosis

Differential diagnosis of the newborn with facial palsy is discussed in Chapter 9. It should only be emphasized here that the vast majority of infants with overt paralysis of the *upper and lower* face—that is, a *peripheral* lesion—have sustained the apparently traumatic injury discussed in this section. Peripheral facial nerve lesions at other sites—for example, posterior fossa subdural or intracerebral hemorrhage, lesions within the brain stem (e.g., hemorrhage, ischemia), and central lesions (e.g., hypoxic-ischemic injury and cerebral contusions)—are distinctly uncommon or exhibit other identifying neurological features. Disorders of muscle (e.g., myotonic dystrophy), the myoneural junction (myasthenia gravis), and nucleus of the facial nerve (Möbius syndrome), although potentially involving both the upper and lower face, are usually bilateral and exhibit the ancillary features described in Chapters 32 and 33. A miscellaneous and rare group of newborns with congenital facial nerve palsy, occasionally familial, of unknown etiology has also been reported.[229-231] The syndrome of unilateral weakness of the depressor of the corner of the mouth (see Chapter 33) is a more restricted deficit and readily distinguished from typical peripheral facial paralysis.

I generally do not use electrodiagnostic tests to evaluate these infants. However, in infants with marked involvement, such testing may be useful.[225,226,229] Thus, in typical traumatic facial nerve paresis, transdermal stimulation of the facial nerve at the stylomastoid foramen usually reveals normal facial nerve function in the first 48 hours of life because the distal nerve is still capable of conduction. The percentage decrease of this facial nerve function over time provides useful prognostic information.[229] The presence of fibrillations after 2 to 3 weeks indicates denervation of muscle fibers. However, these abnormalities do not necessarily preclude excellent functional recovery; thus electrodiagnostic abnormalities must be interpreted with caution and in the context of personal experience.

Prognosis

The prognosis of affected infants is very good. The large majority of infants recover completely within 1 to 3 weeks, and only rarely do infants have any detectable deficit after several months.[11,97,224,227,232] In one large series ($n = 67$) recovery was complete for 89% (in most, within 2 weeks of life) and partial in the remaining 11% (mean age at follow-up, 34 months).[224] Regeneration of the nerve in the unusual case with severe degeneration takes place at the rate of approximately 1 inch a month. Unusual sequelae of facial paralysis include contracture and synkinesis (mass facial motion).[233]

Management

Therapy is generally restricted to the use of artificial tears and, if necessary, taping of the involved eye to prevent corneal injury. No controlled data exist to indicate a value for massage, electrical stimulation, or early surgical intervention. Some have advocated surgical exploration in cases with severe persistent findings of denervation; rarely, a petrous temporal fracture may compress the nerve.[234] I have not encountered this occurrence. Indeed, the lesion usually resolves before any therapy can be attempted.

Laryngeal Nerve Palsy

Disturbance of branches of the laryngeal nerve may affect swallowing and breathing; this occurrence has led to the descriptive term *duosyndrome of the laryngeal nerve*.[235] The disorder appears, in many cases, to result from an intrauterine posture in which the head is rotated slightly and flexed laterally. It is also likely that similar head and neck movements during delivery, when marked, may injure the laryngeal nerve and account for the approximately 10% of examples of vocal cord paralysis attributed to *birth trauma* (see the discussion of all varieties of newborn vocal cord paralysis in Chapter 33).[236-238] Similarly, such head and neck movements may occur during deliveries that result in brachial plexus injuries because approximately 2% of the latter are accompanied by evidence of laryngeal nerve involvement (e.g., stridor).[166] The lateral neck flexion causes the rigid thyroid cartilage of the larynx to compress the superior branch of the laryngeal nerve against the hyoid bone above or the recurrent branch against the cricoid cartilage below. The result is disturbance of swallowing (because of involvement of the superior branch) or of vocal

cord closure with resulting dyspnea (because of involvement of the recurrent branch). A similar syndrome may be observed because of direct trauma during the cannulation of neck vessels for extracorporeal membrane oxygenation, ligation of a patent ductus arteriosus, repair of a tracheoesophageal atresia, or cardiac surgery, especially procedures involving the vicinity of the aortic arch.[239-244] In the last instance as many as 20% of infants are affected.[241] In the context of perinatal traumatic injury, the vocal cord paralysis is the dominant and most dangerous feature of the syndrome. Because rotation of the head causes the face to be compressed against the pelvic wall, a contralateral facial paresis may be associated. Moreover, if the lateral flexion of the neck is severe, the phrenic nerve may be affected and diaphragmatic paresis may occur.[212,235] Similarly, the nearby hypoglossal nerve may be injured, resulting in paralysis of the tongue.[245,246] The diagnosis of the laryngeal involvement is best made by direct laryngoscopic examination.

Treatment is *symptomatic*. In severe lesions, gavage feeding or tracheotomy may be required. Noisy breathing and the threat of aspiration may last a year or longer, although affected patients usually recover by 6 to 12 months of life.[235]

Median Nerve Injury

Injury to the median nerve has been described at two sites, the antecubital fossa and the wrist, both related to percutaneous punctures of the brachial and the radial arteries, respectively (Table 36.16).[247] The median nerve is derived from the brachial plexus and courses through the antecubital fossa into the forearm, where it supplies muscles that principally pronate the forearm and flex the wrist and fingers; it then proceeds over the radial aspect of the wrist and through the carpal tunnel to the hand, where it supplies muscles that oppose, flex, and adduct the thumb.

Antecubital Fossa and Brachial Artery

Injury to the median nerve in the antecubital fossa was described in one study in 13% of low-birth-weight infants ($\leq$1500 g) examined at 18 months postterm.[248] Median nerve dysfunction was identified clinically on the basis of impaired pincer grasp, which depends on flexion of the index finger and adduction, opposition, and flexion of the thumb. A characteristic posture of the hand was observed in affected patients (Fig. 36.22). Evidence of injury was most frequent in the smallest infants; 30% of infants weighing less than 1000 g were affected versus 8% of infants weighing 1000 to 1500 g.

Two observations suggested that injury to the median nerve in the antecubital fossa was responsible for the clinical deficits. First, all affected infants had obviously visible scarring in the antecubital fossa related to frequent percutaneous brachial artery punctures. Because the right brachial artery is preferred for arterial puncture (to avoid contamination from ductal shunting),

TABLE 36.16	Arterial Puncture and Median Nerve Injury in the Neonatal Period
SITE OF INJURY	**ARTERY PUNCTURED**
Antecubital fossa	Brachial (usually right)
Wrist	Radial

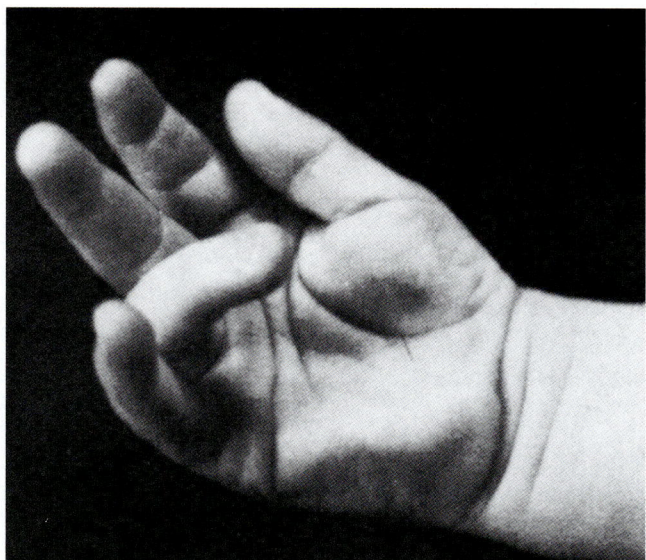

Figure 36.22 Median nerve injury: clinical appearance. The right hand of an infant, approximately 24 months of age, who weighed less than 1500 g at birth and sustained median nerve injury secondary to brachial artery puncture in the neonatal period. Note the position of the hand, assumed because there is weakness of flexion of the proximal phalanx of the first three fingers and the distal phalanx of the thumb, and of adduction and opposition of the thumb; all of these functions are mediated by the median nerve. Note also the slight atrophy of the thenar eminence. (From Pape KE, Armstrong DL, Fitzhardinge PM. Peripheral median nerve damage secondary to brachial arterial blood gas sampling. *J Pediatr.* 1978;93:852.)

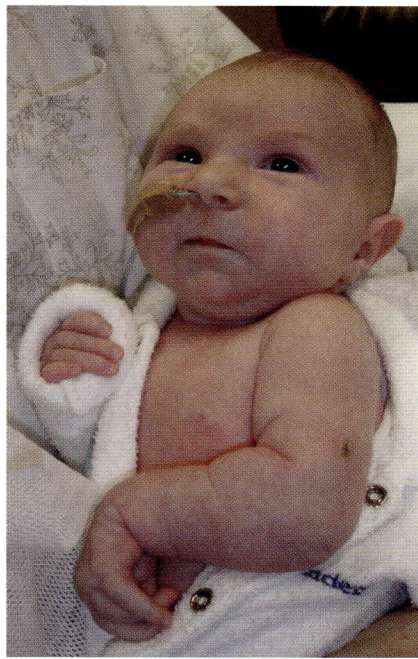

Figure 36.23 Radial nerve injury in a newborn: clinical features. Note evidence of weakness of finger and hand extension, with the appearance of *wrist drop*. Because the lesion in this case was proximal to the triceps branch of the nerve, the limb also is held in flexion at the elbow. An area of subcutaneous fat necrosis due to compressive injury sustained during a prolonged labor (see dark spot above elbow) overlies the radial nerve. The child recovered completely within 3 months. (From Jones HR, Ryan MM, Levin KH. Radiculopathies and plexopathies. In: Darras BT, Jones HR, Ryan MM, De Vivo DC, eds. *Neuromuscular Disorders of Infancy, Childhood, and Adolescence.* 2nd ed. Elsevier; 2015, with permission.)

the right hand and antecubital fossa were affected in all 18 infants. In 5 of these infants bilateral deficits were present, as were bilateral scarring and histories of left as well as right punctures. The second observation was derived from block sections of the cubital fossa at autopsy on 12 randomly selected low-birth-weight infants who had one or more percutaneous brachial artery punctures during life; perineural hemorrhage and axonal injury with wallerian degeneration were observed in 8.

In the current era of care for the very low birth-weight infant, further data are needed to define the frequency of the aforementioned deficits of the *dominant* hand, and, more importantly, the long-term functional consequences. The data suggest that percutaneous brachial artery puncture should be avoided, if possible, in the very small infant.

Wrist and Radial Artery

Radial artery puncture has been shown to cause injury to the median nerve in the newborn infant. Two infants exhibited prolonged median nerve conduction velocity and distal motor latency after radial artery punctures for determination of arterial blood gas values.[249] Postmortem examination in one infant demonstrated compression of the median nerve by hematoma. The other infant had a diminished grasp on the affected side, but electrical and clinical functions became normal after 4 weeks. This compressive neuropathy could go undetected in the neonatal period without careful clinical and electrical testing. These data again raise the question of whether long-term effects on hand function occur in graduates of neonatal intensive care facilities as a result of median nerve injury.

Radial Nerve Injury

Injury to the radial nerve has been associated most often with apparent compression of the nerve, the latter caused by restricted fetal position in utero (e.g., secondary to passively acquired sedative drugs or constricting uterine bands); during difficult labor, delivery by forceps, or both; and postnatally by such factors as blood pressure cuffs.[66,97,247,250-257] An indurated area with underlying fat necrosis, usually over the distal course of the nerve around the humerus above the radial epicondyle, often marks the site of compression. Less common etiological factors are humeral fracture or subcutaneous abscess. The clinical features are distinctive and consist of weakness of the extensors of wrist, fingers, and thumb, the normal distal innervations of the radial nerve (Fig. 36.23). Thus a *wrist drop* calls attention to the injury. On cursory examination, the patient's deficits could be mistaken for a lower brachial plexus lesion, but the preservation of grasp and function of other intrinsic muscles of the hand rules out this diagnosis. EMG indicates fibrillations in the affected muscles after an interval yet to be defined although probably at least 1 week.[254] Of the approximately 21 reported patients with adequate follow-up data, all except 1 recovered in the first weeks or months of life. The single exception had an apparently long-standing intrauterine compression.

Lumbosacral Plexus Injury

Injury to lumbosacral roots is exceedingly uncommon.[247] In Eng's[258] series of "128 neonatal peripheral palsies," only 3 such cases were observed. The injury involves roots of both the lumbar (L-2 to L-4) and sacral (L-4 to S-3) plexuses and is related to traction, primarily with frank breech deliveries. The clinical features include essentially a total paralysis of the involved lower extremity. An infant with involvement principally of the lumbar component exhibited particular weakness of knee extension (quadriceps function) and an absent knee jerk.[259] Differentiation of lumbosacral plexus injury from sciatic nerve injury and occult dysraphic state with asymmetry is necessary (see the following section on sciatic nerve injury). Sciatic nerve injury spares motor functions of the femoral and obturator nerves (L-2 to L-4); thus hip flexion, adduction, and external rotation are present. Occult dysraphic states in the vast majority of cases exhibit cutaneous, subcutaneous, and skeletal stigmata and are rarely, if ever, entirely confined to one limb. The outcome in an infant with lumbosacral plexus injury is difficult to generalize from the small numbers reported, but in Eng's[258] series, "none of the recoveries … was complete." In the single patient that I have studied, although only minimal function was present at 2 months of age, rapid recovery commenced thereafter, and at 3 years of age only minor disability remained.

Sciatic Nerve Injury

Sciatic nerve injury in the newborn has been observed principally after misplaced injection of drugs into the buttocks but also after prolonged paralysis (induced by pancuronium) with pressure necrosis of the skin overlying the buttock[247,255,256] and after injection of hypertonic glucose or certain other agents into the umbilical artery.[97,260-263] The mechanism of the effect in the last instance is presumed to be spasm or thrombosis in the inferior gluteal artery that supplies the sciatic nerve. Traction injury with difficult breech deliveries may also lead to sciatic nerve injury.[247] The clinical features include deficits of abduction at the hip and of all movements at more distal joints. (Necrosis of buttock tissue may be an obvious accompaniment.) Distinction from lumbosacral plexus injury is based primarily on the sparing of hip flexion, adduction, and external rotation in sciatic nerve injury. Distinction from peroneal nerve injury (see next section) may be difficult because preferential affection of the superficially and laterally placed fibers destined for the peroneal nerve often occurs, and a *foot drop* may be the prominent neurological abnormality.

Prognosis is variable. Many infants have failed to recover after misplaced intramuscular injections, whereas the prognosis appears to be better for the small number of cases reported secondary to umbilical artery injections.

Peroneal Nerve Injury

Several reports of injury to the peroneal nerve of the newborn have been recorded.[247,264-270] The common pathogenetic factor has been compression, whether in utero by uterine bands or postnatally by footboard or infiltrated intravenous solution. The site of injury is the superficial course of the nerve around the fibular head. The clinical feature that calls attention to the lesion is *foot drop*, which is caused by weakness of ankle dorsiflexion and eversion, functions of the peroneal nerve.

Determinations of nerve conduction velocities can establish the site of the injury.[265,267] The demonstration of fibrillations on the first day of life established the intrauterine timing of the injury in two cases.[268,269] The reported patients recovered within 3 to 6 months.

KEY REFERENCES

1. Simonson C, Barlow P, Dehennin N, et al. Neonatal complications of vacuum-assisted delivery. *Obstet Gynecol.* 2007;109:626-633.
2. Pape KE, Wigglesworth JS. *Haemorrhage, Ischaemia and the Perinatal Brain.* Philadelphia: JB Lippincott; 1979.
4. Fortune PM, Thomas RM. Sub-aponeurotic haemorrhage: a rare but life-threatening neonatal complication associated with ventouse delivery. *Br J Obstet Gynaecol.* 1999;106(8):868-870.
5. Boo NY, Foong KW, Mahdy ZA, et al. Risk factors associated with subaponeurotic haemorrhage in full-term infants exposed to vacuum extraction. *Br J Obstet Gynaecol.* 2005;112:1516-1521.
6. Govaert P, Vanhaesebrouck P, Depraeter C, et al. Vacuum extraction, bone injury and neonatal subgaleal bleeding. *Eur J Pediatr.* 1992;151:532-535.
7. Reichard R. Birth injury of the cranium and central nervous system. *Brain Pathol.* 2008;18:565-570.
9. Kim HM, Kwon SH, Park SH, et al. Intracranial hemorrhage in infants with cephalohematoma. *Pediatr Int.* 2014;56:378-381.
11. Hagadorn-Freathy AS, Yeomans ER, Hankins GD. Validation of the 1988 ACOG forceps classification system. *Obstet Gynecol.* 1991;77:356-360.
12. Hankins GDV, Leicht T, Van Hook J, et al. The role of forceps rotation in maternal and neonatal injury. *Am J Obstet Gynecol.* 1999;180:231-234.
13. Werner EF, Janevic TM, Illuzzi J, et al. Mode of delivery in nulliparous women and neonatal intracranial injury. *Obstet Gynecol.* 2011;118:1239-1246.
20. Djientcheu VD, Rilliet B, Delavelle J, et al. Leptomeningeal cyst in newborns due to vacuum extraction: report of two cases. *Childs Nerv Syst.* 1996;12:399-403.
21. Harwood-Nash DC, Hendrick EB, Hudson AR. The significance of skull fracture in children. A study of 1,187 patients. *Radiology.* 1971;101:151.
22. Dupuis O, Silveira R, Dupont C, et al. Comparison of "instrument-associated" and "spontaneous" obstetric depressed skull fractures in a cohort of 68 neonates. *Am J Obstet Gynecol.* 2005;192:165-170.
23. Nakahara T, Sakoda K, Uozumi T, et al. Intrauterine depressed skull fracture. *Pediatr Neurosci.* 1989;15:121-124.
24. Matson D. *Neurosurgery of Infancy and Childhood.* Springfield: Charles C. Thomas; 1969.
26. Loeser JD, Kilburn HL, Jolley T. Management of depressed skull fracture in the newborn. *J Neurosurg.* 1976;44:62.
29. Schrager GO. Elevation of depressed skull fracture with a breast pump. *J Pediatr.* 1970;77:300.
32. Amin AA, Al-Zeky AM, El-Azm M. Vacuum extraction as a treatment modality of neonatal skull depression in a twin infant. *Saudi Med J.* 2007;28:1122-1124.
33. de Paul Djientcheu V, Njamnshi AK, Ongolo-Zogo P, et al. Depressed skull fractures in children: treatment using an obstetrical vacuum extractor. *Pediatr Neurosurg.* 2006;42:273-276.
34. Roche MC, Velez A, Garcia Sanchez P. Occipital osteodiastasis. A rare complication in cephalic delivery. *Acta Paediatr Scand.* 1990;79:380-382.
35. Takagi T, Nagai R, Wakabayashi S. Extradural hemorrhage in the newborn as a result of birth trauma. *Childs Brain.* 1978;4:306.
37. Negishi H, Lee Y, Itoh K, et al. Nonsurgical management of epidural hematoma in neonates. *Pediatr Neurol.* 1989;5:253-256.
38. King J, Haddock G. Neonatal head injuries revisited. *Scott Med J.* 2009;54:34-36.
39. Josephsen JB, Kemp J, Elbabaa SK, et al. Life-threatening neonatal epidural hematoma caused by precipitous vaginal delivery. *Am J Case Rep.* 2015;16:50-52.
40. Lindenberg R, Freytag E. Morphology of brain lesions from blunt trauma in early infancy. *Arch Pathol.* 1969;87:298.

41. Ikonomidou C, Qin Q, Labruyere J, et al. Prevention of trauma-induced neurodegeneration in infant rat brain. *Pediatr Res.* 1996;39:1020-1027.

45. Munoz ME, Roche C, Escriba R, et al. Flaccid paraplegia as complication of umbilical artery catheterization. *Pediatr Neurol.* 1993;9:401-403.

46. Pierson RN. Spinal and cranial injuries of the baby in breech deliveries. A clinical and pathological study of thirty-eight cases. *Surg Gynecol Obstet.* 1923;37:802.

51. Rossitch E, Oakes WJ. Perinatal spinal cord injury: clinical, radiographic and pathologic features. *Pediatr Neurosurg.* 1992;18:149-152.

52. MacKinnon JA, Perlman M, Kirpalani H, et al. Spinal cord injury at birth: diagnostic and prognostic data in twenty- two patients. *J Pediatr.* 1993;122:431-437.

53. Caird MS, Reddy S, Ganley TJ, et al. Cervical spine fracture-dislocation birth injury: prevention, recognition, and implications for the orthopaedic surgeon. *J Pediatr Orthop.* 2005;25:484-486.

54. Vialle R, Pietin-Vialle C, Vinchon M, et al. Birth-related spinal cord injuries: a multicentric review of nine cases. *Childs Nerv Syst.* 2008;24:79-85.

59. Menticoglou SM, Perlman M, Manning FA. High cervical spinal cord injury in neonates delivered with forceps: report of 15 cases. *Obstet Gynecol.* 1995;86:589-594.

60. Mills JF, Dargaville PA, Coleman LT, et al. Upper cervical spinal cord injury in neonates: the use of magnetic resonance imaging. *J Pediatr.* 2001;138:105-108.

63. Yamano T, Fujiwara S, Matsukawa S, et al. Cervical cord birth injury and subsequent development of syringomyelia: a case report. *Neuropediatrics.* 1992;23:327-328.

64. Crothers B. The effect of breech extraction on the central nervous system of the fetus. *Med Clin North Am.* 1922;5:1287.

67. Tator CH, Fehlings MG. Review of the secondary injury theory of acute spinal cord trauma with emphasis on vascular mechanisms. *J Neurosurg.* 1991;75:15-26.

70. Bracken MD, Shepard MJ, Collins WF, et al. A randomized, controlled trial of methylprednisolone or naloxone in the treatment of acute spinal-cord injury. *N Engl J Med.* 1990;322:1405-1411.

76. Bracken MB, Shepard MJ, Holford TR, et al. Administration of methylprednisolone for 24 or 48 hours or Tirilazad Mesylate for 48 hours in the treatment of acute spinal cord injury. *JAm Med Assoc.* 1997;277:1597-1604.

77. Boulland JL, Lambert FM, Zuchner M, et al. A neonatal mouse spinal cord injury model for assessing post-injury adaptive plasticity and human stem cell integration. *PLoS ONE.* 2013;8:e71701.

86. Pape KE. Developmental and maladaptive plasticity in neonatal SCI. *Clin Neurol Neurosurg.* 2012;114:475-482.

87. Jain L. School outcome in late preterm infants: a cause for concern. *J Pediatr.* 2008;153:5-6.

88. Blount J, Doughty K, Tubbs RS, et al. In utero spontaneous cervical thoracic epidural hematoma imitating spinal cord birth injury. *Pediatr Neurosurg.* 2004;40:23-27.

89. Berck DJ, Mussalli GM, Manning FA. Atraumatic fetal cervical spinal cord injury and cruciate paralysis. *Obstet Gynecol.* 1998;91(5 Pt 2):833-834.

91. Coulter DM, Zhou H, Rorke-Adams LB. Catastrophic intrauterine spinal cord injury caused by an arteriovenous malformation. *J Perinatol.* 2007;27:186-189.

92. Goetz E. Neonatal spinal cord injury after an uncomplicated vaginal delivery. *Pediatr Neurol.* 2010;42:69-71.

93. Fenger-Gron J, Kock K, Nielsen RG, et al. Spinal cord injury at birth: a hidden causative factor. *Acta Paediatr.* 2008;97:824-826.

94. Morgan C, Newell SJ. Cervical spinal cord injury following cephalic presentation and delivery by Caesarean section. *Dev MedChild Neurol.* 2001;43:274-276.

95. Hedderly T, Chalmers S, Fox G, et al. Extensive cervical spinal cord lesion with late foetal presentation. *Acta Paediatr.* 2005;94:245-247.

96. Ebinger F, Boor R, Bruhl K, et al. Cervical spinal cord atrophy in the atraumatically born neonate: one form of prenatal or perinatal ischaemic insult? *Neuropediatrics.* 2003;34:45-51.

98. Simanovsky N, Stepensky P, Hiller N. The use of ultrasound for the diagnosis of spinal hemorrhage in a newborn. *Pediatr Neurol.* 2004;31:295-297.

99. Barkovich AJ, Raybaud C. *Pediatric Neuroimaging.* 5th ed. Philadelphia: Lippincott Williams & Wilkins; 2012.

102. Murphy BP, Zientara GP, Huppi PS, et al. Line scan diffusion tensor MRI of the cervical spinal cord in preterm infants. *J Magn Reson Imaging.* 2001;13:949-953.

104. Hellstrom B, Sallmander U. Prevention of spinal cord injury in hyperextension of the fetal head. *JAm Med Assoc.* 1968;204:1041-1044.

115. Kobayashi S, Kanda K, Yokochi K, et al. A case of spinal cord injury that occurred in utero. *Pediatr Neurol.* 2006;35:367-369.

116. Gilles FH, Bina M, Sotrel A. Infantile atlanto-occipital instability: the potential danger of extreme extension. *Am J Dis Child.* 1979;133:30.

117. Yilmaz T, Kaptanoglu E. Current and future medical therapeutic strategies for the functional repair of spinal cord injury. *World J Orthop.* 2015;6:42-55.

118. Grant RA, Quon JL, Abbed KM. Management of acute traumatic spinal cord injury. *Curr Treat Options Neurol.* 2015;17:334.

119. All AH, Gharibani P, Gupta S, et al. Early intervention for spinal cord injury with human induced pluripotent stem cells oligodendrocyte progenitors. *PLoS ONE.* 2015;10:e0116933.

120. Stenudd M, Sabelstrom H, Frisen J. Role of endogenous neural stem cells in spinal cord injury and repair. *J Am Med Assoc Neurol.* 2015;72:235-237.

121. Ramer LM, Ramer MS, Bradbury EJ. Restoring function after spinal cord injury: towards clinical translation of experimental strategies. *Lancet Neurol.* 2014;13:1241-1256.

122. Gilgoff RL, Gilgoff IS. Long-term follow-up of home mechanical ventilation in young children with spinal cord injury and neuromuscular conditions. *J Pediatr.* 2003;142:476-480.

123. Crothers B, Putnam MC. Obstetrical injuries of the spinal cord. *Medicine (Baltimore).* 1927;6:41.

132. Laurent JP, Lee RT. Birth-related upper brachial plexus injuries in infants: operative and nonoperative approaches. *J Child Neurol.* 1994;9:111-117.

133. Bager B. Perinatally acquired brachial plexus palsy—a persisting challenge. *Acta Paediatr.* 1997;86:1214-1219.

134. Gherman RB, Ouzounian JG, Goodwin TM. Brachial plexus palsy: an in utero injury? *Am J Obstet Gynecol.* 1999;180:1303-1307.

135. Donnelly V, Foran A, Murphy J, et al. Neonatal brachial plexus palsy: an unpredictable injury. *Am J Obstet Gynecol.* 2002;187:1209-1212.

136. Evans-Jones G, Kay SPJ, Weindling AM, et al. Congenital brachial palsy: incidence, causes, and outcome in the United Kingdom and Republic of Ireland. *Arch Dis Child.* 2003;88:185-189.

137. Pondaag W, Malessy MJA, van Dijk JG, et al. Natural history of obstetric brachial plexus palsy: a systematic review. *Dev Med Child Neurol.* 2004;46:138-144.

138. Mollberg M, Hagberg H, Bager B, et al. Risk factors for obstetric brachial plexus palsy among neonates delivered by vacuum extraction. *Obstet Gynecol.* 2005;106:913-918.

139. Piatt JH. Birth injuries of the brachial plexus. *Pediatr Clin North Am.* 2004;51:421-440.

140. Chauhan SP, Rose CH, Gherman RB, et al. Brachial plexus injury: a 23-year experience from a tertiary center. *Am J Obstet Gynceol.* 2005;192:1795-1802.

141. Zafeiriou DI, Psychogiou K. Obstetrical brachial plexus palsy. *Pediatr Neurol.* 2008;38:235-242.

142. Lagerkvist AL, Johansson U, Johansson A, et al. Obstetric brachial plexus palsy: a prospective, population-based study of incidence, recovery, and residual impairment at 18 months of age. *Dev Med Child Neurol.* 2010;52:529-534.

143. Walsh JM, Kandamany N, Ni Shuibhne N, et al. Neonatal brachial plexus injury: comparison of incidence and antecedents between 2 decades. *Am J Obstet Gynecol.* 2011;204:324, e321–e326.

144. Chauhan SP, Blackwell SB, Ananth CV. Neonatal brachial plexus palsy: incidence, prevalence, and temporal trends. *Semin Perinatol.* 2014;38:210-218.

145. Executive summary: neonatal brachial plexus palsy. Report of the American College of Obstetricians and Gynecologists' task force on neonatal brachial plexus palsy. *Obstet Gynecol.* 2014;123:902-904.

146. Jones HR Jr, Ryan MM. Radiculopathies and plexopathies. In: Darras BT, Jones HR Jr, Ryan MM, De Vivo DC, eds. *Neuromuscular*

Disorders of Infancy, Childhood, and Adolescence. A Clinician's Approach. 2nd ed. San Diego: Academic Press; 2014:199-224.

148. Laurent JP, Shenaq S, Lee R, et al. Upper brachial plexus birth injuries: a neurosurgical approach. *Concepts Pediatr Neurosurg.* 1990;10:156-178.

149. Vredeveld JW, Blaauw G, Slooff BAC, et al. The findings in paediatric obstetric brachial palsy differ from those in older patients: a suggested explanation. *Dev Med Child Neurol.* 2000;42:158-161.

151. Gonik B, Walker AM, Grimm M. Mathematic modeling of forces associated with shoulder dystonia: a comparison of endogenous and exogenous sources. *Am J Obstet Gynecol.* 2000;182:689-691.

152. Gherman RB, Goodwin TM, Ouzounian JG, et al. Brachial plexus palsy associated with cesarean section: an in utero injury? *Am J Obstet Gynecol.* 1997;177:1162-1164.

153. Alfonso I, Papazian O, Shuhaiber H, et al. Intrauterine shoulder weakness and obstetric brachial plexus palsy. *Pediatr Neurol.* 2004;31:225-227.

154. Alfonso I, Diaz-Arca G, Alfonso DT, et al. Fetal deformations: a risk factor for obstetrical brachial plexus palsy? *Pediatr Neurol.* 2006;35:246-249.

155. Tierney TS, Tierney BJ, Rosenberg AE, et al. Infantile myofibromatosis: a nontraumatic cause of neonatal brachial plexus palsy. *Pediatr Neurol.* 2008;39:276-278.

156. Torki M, Barton L, Miller DA, et al. Severe brachial plexus palsy in women without shoulder dystocia. *Obstet Gynecol.* 2012;120:539-541.

157. Ouzounian JG. Risk factors for neonatal brachial plexus palsy. *Semin Perinatol.* 2014;38:219-221.

160. Ubachs JMH, Slooff ACJ, Peters LLH. Obstetric antecedents of surgically treated obstetric brachial plexus injuries. *Br J Obstet Gynaecol.* 1995;102:813-817.

161. Gherman RB, Ouzounian JG, Satin AJ, et al. A comparison of shoulder dystocia-associated transient and permanent brachial plexus palsies. *Obstet Gynecol.* 2003;102:544-548.

162. Mollberg M, Lagerkvist AL, Johansson U, et al. Comparison in obstetric management on infants with transient and persistent obstetric brachial plexus palsy. *J Child Neurol.* 2008;23:1424-1432.

163. Grobman WA, Miller D, Burke C, et al. Outcomes associated with introduction of a shoulder dystocia protocol. *Am J Obstet Gynecol.* 2011;205:513-517.

164. Jennett RJ, Tarby TJ, Kreinick CJ. Brachial plexus palsy: an old problem revisited. *Am J Obstet Gynecol.* 1992;166:1673-1677.

165. Poggi SH, Stallings SP, Ghidini A, et al. Intrapartum risk factors for permanent brachial plexus injury. *Am J Obstet Gynecol.* 2003;189:725-729.

166. Eng GD, Binder H, Getson P, et al. Obstetrical brachial plexus palsy (OBPP) outcome with conservative management. *Muscle Nerve.* 1996;19:884-891.

167. Yilmaz K, Caliskan M, Oge E, et al. Clinical assessment, MRI, and EMG in congenital brachial plexus palsy. *Pediatr Neurol.* 1999;21:705-710.

168. Scarfone H, McComas AJ, Pape K, et al. Denervation and reinnervation in congenital brachial palsy. *Muscle Nerve.* 1999;22:600-607.

169. Wall LB, Mills JK, Leveno K, et al. Incidence and prognosis of neonatal brachial plexus palsy with and without clavicle fractures. *Obstet Gynecol.* 2014;123:1288-1293.

171. Yang LJ. Neonatal brachial plexus palsy—management and prognostic factors. *Semin Perinatol.* 2014;38:222-234.

174. Tse R, Nixon JN, Iyer RS, et al. The diagnostic value of CT myelography, MR myelography, and both in neonatal brachial plexus palsy. *AJNR Am J Neuroradiol.* 2014;35:1425-1432.

175. Somashekar D, Yang LJ, Ibrahim M, et al. High-resolution MRI evaluation of neonatal brachial plexus palsy: a promising alternative to traditional CT myelography. *AJNR Am J Neuroradiol.* 2014;35:1209-1213.

176. Sundholm LK, Eliasson A-C, Forssberg H. Obstetric brachial plexus injuries: assessment protocol and functional outcome at age 5 years. *Dev Med Child Neurol.* 1998;40:4-11.

177. Strombeck C, Krumlinde-Sundholm L, Forssberg H. Functional outcome at 5 years in children with obstetrical brachial plexus palsy with and without microsurgical reconstruction. *Dev Med Child Neurol.* 2000;42:148-157.

178. Noetzel MJ, Park TS, Robinson S, et al. Prospective study of recovery following neonatal brachial plexus injury. *J Child Neurol.* 2001;16:488-492.

179. DiTaranto P, Campagna L, Price AE, et al. Outcome following nonoperative treatment of brachial plexus birth injuries. *J Child Neurol.* 2004;19:87-90.

180. Hoeksma AF, ter Steeg AM, Nelissen RG, et al. Neurological recovery in obstetric brachial plexus injuries: an historical cohort study. *Dev Med Child Neurol.* 2004;46:76-83.

181. Smith NC, Rowan P, Benson LJ, et al. Neonatal brachial plexus palsy. Outcome of absent biceps function at three months of age. *J Bone Joint Surg Am.* 2004;86-A:2163-2170.

182. Grossman JA. Early operative intervention for selected cases of brachial plexus birth injury. *Arch Neurol.* 2006;63:1031-1032.

183. Strombeck C, Krumlinde-Sundholm L, Remahl S, et al. Long-term follow-up of children with obstetric brachial plexus palsy. I: functional aspects. *Dev Med Child Neurol.* 2007;49:198-203.

184. Strombeck C, Remahl S, Krumlinde-Sundholm L, et al. Long-term follow-up of children with obstetric brachial plexus palsy. II: neurophysiological aspects. *Dev Med Child Neurol.* 2007;49:204-209.

185. Ali ZS, Bakar D, Li YR, et al. Utility of delayed surgical repair of neonatal brachial plexus palsy. *J Neurosurg Pediatr.* 2014;13:462-470.

190. Roach ES. Surgery for brachial plexus palsy: does timing matter? *Arch Neurol.* 2006;63:1034-1035.

191. Sparagana SP, Ezaki M. Microneurosurgery for neonatal brachial plexus palsy: the need for more information. *Arch Neurol.* 2006;63:1033-1034.

205. Zifko U, Hartmann M, Girsch W, et al. Diaphragmatic paresis in newborns due to phrenic nerve injury. *Neuropediatrics.* 1995;26:281-284.

206. Al-Qattan MM, Clarke HM, Curtis CG. The prognostic value of concurrent phrenic nerve palsy in newborn children with Erb's palsy. *J Hand Surg [Br].* 1998;23:225.

207. Murty VS, Ram KD. Phrenic nerve palsy: a rare cause of respiratory distress in newborn. *J Pediatr Neurosci.* 2012;7:225-227.

208. Alvord EC, Austin EJ, Larson CP. Neuropathologic observations in congenital phrenic nerve palsy. *J Child Neurol.* 1990;5:205-209.

211. Stramrood CA, Blok CA, van der Zee DC, et al. Neonatal phrenic nerve injury due to traumatic delivery. *J Perinat Med.* 2009;37:293-296.

213. Renault F, Nicot F, Liptai Z, et al. Congenital diaphragm weakness without neuromuscular disease. *Muscle Nerve.* 2008;38:1201-1205.

214. Gitiaux C, Bergounioux J, Magen M, et al. Diaphragmatic weakness with progressive sensory and motor polyneuropathy: case report of a neonatal IGHMBP2-related neuropathy. *J Child Neurol.* 2013;28:787-790.

215. Epelman M, Navarro OM, Daneman A, et al. M-mode sonography of diaphragmatic motion: description of technique and experience in 278 pediatric patients. *Pediatr Radiol.* 2005;35:661-667.

216. Williams O, Greenough A, Mustfa N, et al. Extubation failure due to phrenic nerve injury. *Arch Dis Child.* 2003;88:F72-F73.

220. de Vries TS, Koens BL, Vos A. Surgical treatment of diaphragmatic eventration caused by phrenic nerve injury in the newborn. *J Pediatr Surg.* 1998;33:602-605.

223. Hepner WR. Some observations on facial paresis in the newborn infant: etiology and incidence. *Pediatrics.* 1951;8:494.

224. Falco NA, Eriksson E. Facial nerve palsy in the newborn: incidence and outcome. *Plast Reconstr Surg.* 1990;85:1-4.

225. Renault F, Quijano-Roy S. Congenital and acquired facial palsies. In: Darras BT, Jones HR Jr, Ryan MM, De Vivo DC, eds. *Neuromuscular Disorders of Infancy, Childhood, and Adolescence. A Clinician's Approach.* San Diego: Academic Press; 2014:225-242.

226. Renault F. Facial electromyography in newborn and young infants with congenital facial weakness. *Dev Med Child Neurol.* 2001;43:421-427.

227. Malik S, Bhandekar HS, Korday CS. Traumatic peripheral neuropraxias in neonates: a case series. *J Clin Diagn Res.* 2014;8:PD10-PD12.

228. Caughey AB, Sandberg PL, Zlatnik MG, et al. Forceps compared with vacuum—rates of neonatal and maternal morbidity. *Obstetr Gynecol.* 2005;106:908-912.

229. Shapiro NL, Cunningham MJ, Parikh SR, et al. Congenital unilateral facial paralysis. *Pediatrics.* 1996;97:261-264.

230. Kondev L, Bhadelia RA, Douglass LM. Familial congenital facial palsy. *Pediatr Neurol*. 2004;30:367-370.
231. Toelle SP, Boltshauser E. Long-term outcome in children with congenital unilateral facial nerve palsy. *Neuropediatrics*. 2001;32:130-135.
232. Hamish J, Laing E, Harrison DH, et al. Is permanent congenital facial palsy caused by birth trauma? *Arch Dis Child*. 1996;74:56-58.
238. Nisa L, Holtz F, Sandu K. Paralyzed neonatal larynx in adduction. Case series, systematic review and analysis. *Int J Pediatr Otorhinolaryngol*. 2013;77:13-18.
239. Skinner ML, Halstead LA, Rubinstein CS, et al. Laryngopharyngeal dysfunction after the Norwood procedure. *J Thorac Cardiovasc Surg*. 2005;130:1293-1301.
240. Morini F, Iacobelli BD, Crocoli A, et al. Symptomatic vocal cord paresis/paralysis in infants operated on for esophageal atresia and/or tracheo-esophageal fistula. *J Pediatr*. 2011;158:973-976.
241. Dewan K, Cephus C, Owczarzak V, et al. Incidence and implication of vocal fold paresis following neonatal cardiac surgery. *Laryngoscope*. 2012;122:2781-2785.
242. Kang SL, Samsudin S, Kuruvilla M, et al. Outcome of patent ductus arteriosus ligation in premature infants in the East of England: a prospective cohort study. *Cardiol Young*. 2013;23:711-716.
243. Clement WA, El-Hakim H, Phillipos EZ, et al. Unilateral vocal cord paralysis following patent ductus arteriosus ligation in extremely low-birth-weight infants. *Arch Otolaryngol Head Neck Surg*. 2008;134:28-33.
244. Benjamin JR, Smith PB, Cotten CM, et al. Long-term morbidities associated with vocal cord paralysis after surgical closure of a patent ductus arteriosus in extremely low birth weight infants. *J Perinatol*. 2010;30:408-413.
245. Haenggeli CA, Lacourt G. Brachial plexus injury and hypoglossal paralysis. *Pediatr Neurol*. 1989;5:197-198.
246. Greenberg SJ, Kandt RS, D'Souza BJ. Birth injury-induced glossolaryngeal paresis. *Neurology*. 1987;37:533-535.
247. Ryan MM, Jones R Jr. Mononeuropathies. In: Darras BT, Jones HR Jr, Ryan MM, De Vivo DC, eds. *Neuromuscular Disorders of Infancy, Childhood, and Adolescence. A Clinician's Approach*. 2nd ed. San Diego: Academic Press; 2014:243-273.
255. Jones HR. Compressive neuropathy in childhood: a report of 14 cases. *Muscle Nerve*. 1986;9:720-723.
257. Hayman M, Roland EH, Hill A. Newborn radial nerve palsy: report of four cases and review of published reports. *Pediatr Neurol*. 1999;21:648-651.
261. Gilles FH, Matson DD. Sciatic nerve injury following misplaced gluteal injection. *J Pediatr*. 1970;76:247.
267. Kreusser KL, Volpe JJ. Peroneal palsy produced by intravenous fluid infiltration in a newborn. *Dev Med Child Neurol*. 1984;26:522-524.
268. Jones HR, Herbison GJ, Jacobs SR, et al. Intrauterine onset of a mononeuropathy: peroneal neuropathy in a newborn with electromyographic findings at age one day compatible with prenatal onset. *Muscle Nerve*. 1996;19:88-91.
269. Yilmaz Y, Oge AE, Yilmaz-Degpirmenci S, et al. Peroneal nerve palsy: the role of early electromyography. *Eur J Paediatr Neurol*. 2000;4:239-242.

Full references for this chapter can be found on www.expertconsult.com.

UNIT XI

INTRACRANIAL MASS LESIONS

Brain Tumors and Vein of Galen Malformations

Shenandoah Robinson ◆ *Joseph J. Volpe*

In this chapter, space-occupying lesions—including brain tumors, vein of Galen malformations, and arachnoid cysts—are discussed. These disorders are considered in the same chapter because they represent important intracranial mass lesions and share certain clinical features. We do not review management in detail; this is considered in depth in standard neurosurgical writings. Improvements in management in recent years have made the prognosis of these serious disorders considerably more favorable than in the past. But although the prognosis has improved, very few children with neonatal mass lesions will survive without unfavorable consequences, which can include hydrocephalus, intractable seizures, or significant developmental delay. Because the risks of interventions, such as anesthesia and blood loss, are tolerated better by infants older than 3 months, definitive treatment may be deferred until later in infancy. Arachnoid cysts are an exception, since they are now often treated with minimally invasive techniques.

BRAIN TUMORS

Brain tumors manifesting either at birth or in utero or within the first 2 months of life account for approximately 1% to 2% of all brain tumors encountered in the pediatric age group, or 1 to 3 cases per million live births.[1-10] Although in most major reviews neonatal brain tumors are grouped with tumors manifesting in the first 1 to 2 years of life, brain tumors appearing at birth or in utero or in the first 2 postnatal months are sufficiently distinctive in histological and clinical characteristics to be considered separately. In this chapter, we discuss only tumors manifesting at birth or in utero and in the first 2 postnatal months.

The diagnosis, treatment, and prognosis of neonatal brain tumors have progressed markedly since Raskind and Beigel attributed congenital brain tumors to *cell rests* in 1964.[11] Genetic and molecular subtyping of pediatric brain tumors then began to transform the field. Derangements in the control of cell proliferation and differentiation are central to etiology, and abnormalities of genes encoding proteins that function as growth factors (e.g., platelet-derived growth factor), as stimulators of cell proliferation (e.g., oncogenes) or as suppressors of cell proliferation (e.g., tumor suppressor genes) have been identified in various tumors.[4] Additionally, abnormal genetic material inserted into the human genome by certain viruses may induce tumor formation; polymerase chain reaction technology has been used to show the presence of DNA sequences of simian virus 40, one member of a family of viruses (polyomaviruses) that induces tumors in laboratory animals.[12]

These sequences were observed in 10 of 20 choroid plexus tumors and in 10 of 11 ependymomas in children; both of these tumors are relatively common in the neonatal period (see later discussion). Molecular classification of ependymal tumors[13] and atypical teratoid rhabdoid tumors (ATRTs)[14] were recently proposed. For example, a tumor suppressor protein that regulates chromatin remodeling is missing in some ATRTs.[15] Additional mutations in the chromatin remodeling complex gene *SMARCB1/HSNF5/INI1* (*SWI/SNF*-related matrix-associated actin-dependent regulator of chromatin subfamily B member 1 gene, also known as *INI1*) are present in 23% to 35% of infants with ATRT.[16] Similarly, tumor suppressor p53 mutations have been found in 50% of choroid plexus tumors.[17] Although in many instances progress is still limited to case reports, drugs targeting specific mutations can be effective in situations in which traditional chemotherapy has failed.[18] The pace of genetic discoveries is accelerating with technical advances, and it is anticipated that the field will change markedly over the next decade.

Neuropathology
Histological Types

The histological types of neonatal brain tumors differ considerably according to the time of clinical presentation (Table 37.1).[2-8,11,19-36] Thus teratomas are the predominant tumors in infants who present clinically in fetal life or at birth, whereas tumors of neuroepithelial origin predominate in the first 2 postnatal months. The high proportion of teratomas shown in Table 37.1 is based on two large series (cumulative total, 425).[4,8] These lesions are usually very large (Fig. 37.1). Indeed, approximately 35% to 60% are so large that the site of origin in the supratentorial compartment cannot be determined.[2,4,8] Nearly 20% of neonatal teratomas originate from the region of the lateral ventricle, and another approximately 10% to 20% originate from the region of the third ventricle. Only uncommonly do neonatal teratomas originate from the pineal region, the site of most intracranial teratomas that manifest clinically after the neonatal period.

The major types of *nonteratomatous tumors* (i.e., neuroepithelial and mesenchymal tumors) are shown in Table 37.2.[4,8] Astrocytoma is the most common single category.[34,37-48] Medulloblastoma,[49] ATRT,[14,16,49] choroid plexus papilloma (and carcinoma),[31-33,50-53] and ependymoma[13,37] are also relatively common.[43] The remaining tumors encountered include other primitive neuroectodermal tumors (not medulloblastoma)[49,54] and desmoplastic infantile ganglioglioma.[55-58] Desmoplastic infantile gangliogliomas (DIGs) account for approximately 16% of infantile tumors[57] and must be distinguished from

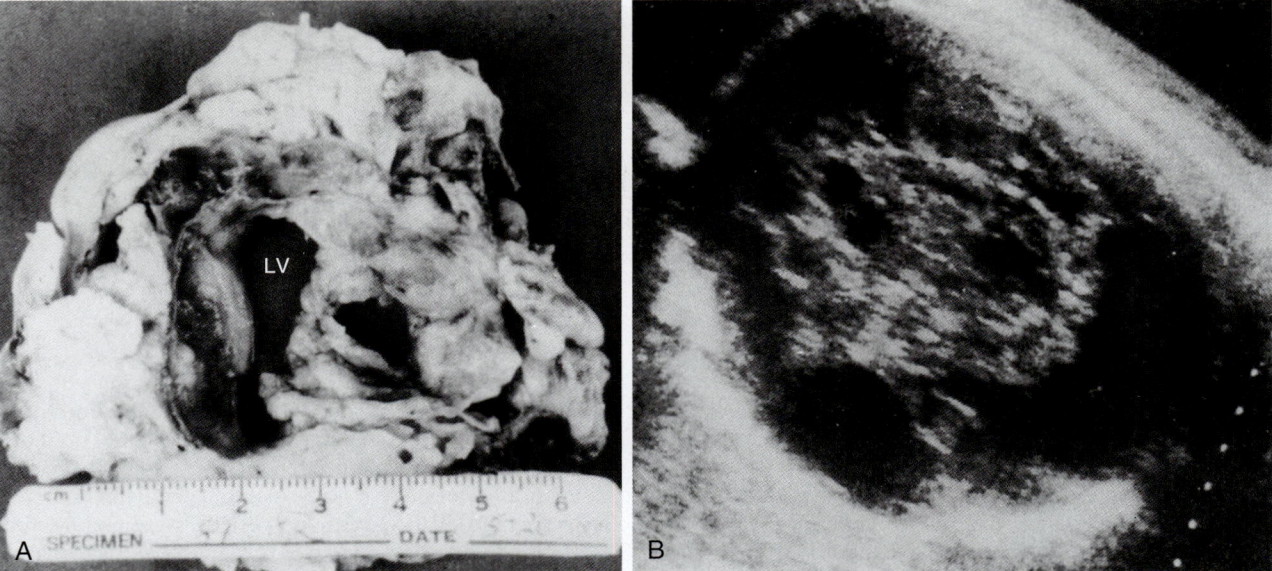

Figure 37.1 Intracranial teratoma: gross neuropathology. (A) Multicystic mass replaces most of normal brain; the dilated lateral ventricle (LV) is visible. (B) Intrauterine ultrasound scan shows a multicystic mass replacing normal brain; no normal intracranial structures could be identified. (From Lipman SP, Pretorius DH, Rumack CM, Manco-Johnson ML. Fetal intracranial teratoma: US diagnosis of three cases and a review of the literature. *Radiology.* 1985;157:491–494.)

TABLE 37.1   Neonatal Brain Tumors: Histological Types[a]

	PERCENTAGE OF TUMORS WITH PRESENTATION AT BIRTH OR IN UTERO	PERCENTAGE OF TUMORS WITH PRESENTATION IN FIRST 2 MONTHS
Teratoma	47	26
Neuroepithelial tumor	40	65
Other	13	9

[a]n = 200 in study of Wakai and colleagues.
Data from Wakai S, Arai T, Nagai M. Congenital brain tumors. *Surg Neurol.* 1984;21:597–609 and Isaacs HI. Perinatal brain tumors: a review of 250 cases. *Pediatr Neurol.* 2002;27:249–261.

glioblastomas (GBMs) owing to the marked difference in prognosis (Fig. 37.2). Both occur supratentorially, have cystic and solid components, and have similar features on magnetic resonance imaging (MRI).[59-61] The prognosis for DIG is generally favorable, although a few more aggressive cases have been reported.[55] Of the neuroepithelial tumors, choroid plexus papilloma has the most consistent site of origin (i.e., the lateral ventricle in most cases). Among other tumors, craniopharyngioma is the most common single type, although sarcoma, fibroma, hemangioblastoma, hemangioma, and meningioma have all been documented.[a]

Particularly unusual, additional examples of neonatal brain tumors include intracranial chordoma, derived from midline remnants of notochord, gliomatosis cerebri, mixed neural tissue masses extending into the oropharynx, hypothalamic hamartoma, lipoma of corpus callosum, multiple lipomata, and subependymal giant cell astrocytoma associated with tuberous sclerosis.[a] The astrocytomas associated with tuberous sclerosis are usually accompanied in the newborn by cardiac rhabdomyoma, and, indeed, this may be the principal clue to the diagnosis of tuberous sclerosis in the neonatal period in such patients. The cardiac tumor may lead to cardiac complications (e.g., arrhythmia) that can be life-threatening at the time of surgery for the subependymal astrocytoma. The mTOR inhibitor everolimus has shown benefit in a few infants with TSC tumors.[73]

Location

The *location of neonatal brain tumors* is distinctly different from that observed in pediatric patients in late infancy and childhood (Table 37.3).[2-6,8,20] Thus, *supratentorial* predominance is apparent, with 60% to 70% being supratentorial.[74] This predominance is marked for teratomas, which are nearly always supratentorial in location. In contrast, medulloblastoma is the one type of neonatal brain tumor with consistent predominance in the infratentorial compartment. If only neuroepithelial tumors are considered, the ratio of supratentorial to infratentorial lesions is 1.7:1 for tumors manifesting at birth and 2.4:1 for those appearing in the first 2 postnatal months. If all neonatal brain tumors are considered (i.e., teratomas and mesenchymal tumors as well as neuroepithelial tumors), the supratentorial predominance is even more marked (see Table 37.3).

---

[a]References 3, 4, 8, 47, 58, and 62-65.

[a]References 3, 4, 8, 38, 39, 41, 44, and 66-72.

| **TABLE 37.2** | Types of Nonteratomatous Neonatal Brain Tumors |

A. Classification of nonteratomatous brain tumors[a]

Neuroepithelial tumor
Astrocytoma
Choroid plexus papilloma and carcinoma
Desmoplastic infantile tumors (DIT)
 Desmoplastic infantile ganglioglioma (DIG)
 Desmoplastic infantile astrocytoma (DIA)
Embryonal
 Medulloblastoma (currently often classified by additional
  molecular subtyping)
  Desmoplastic tumor
  Medulloblastoma with extensive nodularity
 Anaplastic tumor
 Large cell tumor
 CNS primitive neuroectodermal tumor (PNET)
  CNS neuroblastoma
  CNS ganglioneuroblastoma
  Medulloepithelioma
  Ependymoblastoma
 Atypical teratoid/rhabdoid tumor (ATRT)
 Other
  Embryonal tumor with multilayered rosettes (ETMR)
  Embryonal tumor with abundant neuropil and true
   rosettes (ETANTR)
Ependymoma
 Ependymoma (WHO grade I)
 Anaplastic ependymoma (WHO grade III)
Miscellaneous
Other
 Craniopharyngioma
Mesenchymal (carcinoma)
Miscellaneous

B. Relative location of nonteratomatous neonatal brain tumors in modern series[b]

Supratentorial	66%
Infratentorial	34%

C. Relative frequency of nonteratomatous neonatal brain tumors in modern case series[c]

Astrocytoma (WHO grades I–IV)	27%
Atypical teratoid/rhabdoid tumor	18%
Choroid plexus papilloma/carcinoma	16%
Ependymoma (WHO grades I–III)	13%
Desmoplastic infantile ganglioglioma	9%
Medulloblastoma/PNET	8%
Glioneuronal tumor	4%
Poorly differentiated carcinoma	4%
Craniopharyngioma	1%

[a]Adapted from references 49, 60, 82, 85, and 90.
[b]From references 82 and 90.
[c]From references 60, 82, and 90.

Clinical Features

The clinical features of neonatal brain tumors can be divided essentially into four major syndromes (Table 37.4).[a] The *first syndrome* is characterized by a mass lesion that is so large in fetal life that severe macrocrania results in cranial-pelvic disproportion, dystocia, stillbirth, or premature labor. This *obstetrical* syndrome is characteristic of teratomas (Fig. 37.3), but it may also be observed with large neuroepithelial tumors (see Table 37.4). Commonly, other features related to displacement of intracranial tissue by tumor (e.g., local skull swelling, proptosis, or epignathus) may be present in this syndrome. The *second syndrome* is characterized predominantly by macrocrania and bulging fontanelle, often secondary to hydrocephalus, and is observed in approximately 50% of newborns with CNS tumors.[82] Seizures and progressive macrocephaly are observed with DIG tumors.[56] This syndrome also may accompany the features just described for teratomas and may occur for tumors that manifest at birth or in the first 2 postnatal months (see Table 37.4). The *third syndrome* consists of specific neurological features related to the particular type and location of the tumor and is particularly characteristic of tumors manifesting after birth, in the first 2 postnatal months. These neurological features include seizures, present in 15% to 25% of patients with neonatal brain tumors; hemiparesis or quadriparesis; cranial nerve abnormalities; and signs of increased intracranial pressure, often secondary to hydrocephalus. The last of these characteristics is a consistent feature of choroid plexus papilloma. Specific neurological features of spinal cord tumors include torticollis with high cervical spinal cord lesions, usually astrocytoma, and weakness of lower extremities with disturbance of sphincter function in lumbosacral-coccygeal lesions, usually teratoma.[2,80,81,83] The spinal cord lesions are particularly important to identify promptly, because abrupt neurological deterioration may occur spontaneously or after mild trauma (e.g., neck manipulation). The *fourth clinical syndrome* associated with neonatal brain tumors is abrupt onset of intracranial hemorrhage (Figs. 37.4 and 37.5).[a] Hemorrhage with brain tumor is more common in neonatal lesions than in tumors at later ages and develops in approximately 8% to 18% of cases, more commonly in patients with neuroepithelial lesions or vascular tumors (e.g., cavernous hemangioma) than in patients with teratomas (Table 37.5). More often, the hemorrhage is an incidental finding at the time of diagnostic brain imaging, surgery, or autopsy, but occasionally it is large enough to be the presenting clinical feature. Indeed, any infant with an intraparenchymal hemorrhage with no readily identifiable cause (see Chapter 22) should be evaluated for the presence of brain tumor.

Diagnosis

The diagnosis is based on a high index of clinical suspicion. Notably, only 18% of neonatal brain tumors reported are identified by prenatal ultrasound.[9] The majority of congenital tumors undergo rapid growth during the third trimester.[85] The need for evaluation for brain tumor is straightforward in the infant with macrocrania, bulging anterior fontanelle, hydrocephalus of unknown cause, or focal neurological deficit. Sometimes overlooked is the need to consider tumor in the infant with unexplained intracranial hemorrhage (see earlier discussion), seizures, irritability, or persistent vomiting. The diagnostic approach should begin with a brain imaging procedure, and cranial ultrasonography is the best initial choice. This noninvasive modality demonstrates tumors in and near the lateral and third ventricles especially well

---

[a]References 2-5, 7, 8, 10, 20, 24, 26, 27, 30, 35, 45, 46, 52, 53, 67, and 75-81.

[a]References 2-4, 8, 20, 28, 31, 46, 75, 79, and 84.

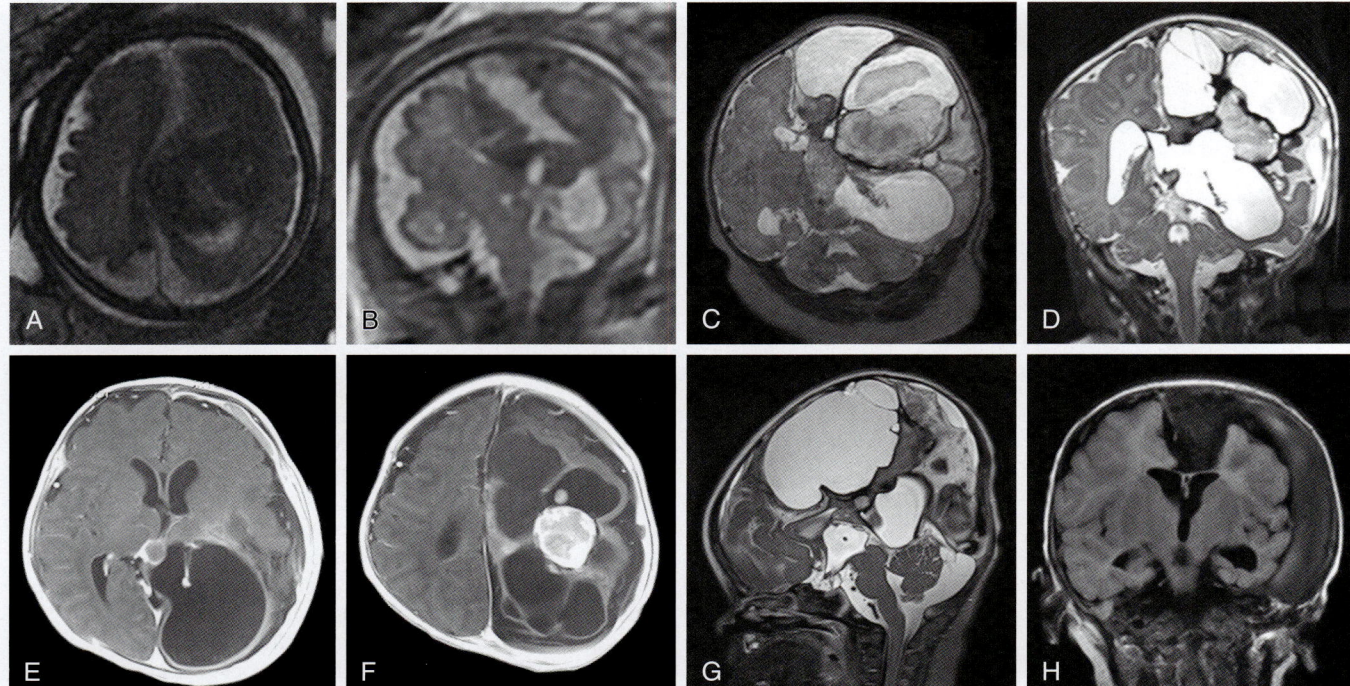

Figure 37.2 Low-grade (WHO grade I) glioneuronal tumor that was initially considered a high-grade glioma based on fetal and newborn magnetic resonance imaging (MRI) scans. (A) Fetal axial and (B) coronal images show a large frontoparietal tumor in the left hemisphere. (C) Coronal MRI obtained on first day of life reveals an extensive cystic and solid tumor with significant mass effect. (D) Coronal MRI at 2 months, prior to resection, demonstrates persistent mass effect, which is also seen on axial images E and F. (G) Preoperative sagittal MRI at 2 months emphasizes the extent of tumor involvement. (H) Coronal MRI at 4 months, approximately 6 weeks after resection, shows some reconstitution of the left hemisphere. (Courtesy Alan R. Cohen, MD.)

TABLE 37.3   Supratentorial and Infratentorial Locations of Neonatal Brain Tumors

	PRESENTATION AT BIRTH		PRESENTATION IN FIRST 2 MONTHS	
	SUPRATENTORIAL	INFRATENTORIAL	SUPRATENTORIAL	INFRATENTORIAL
Teratoma	44	0	18	1
Neuroepithelial tumor				
Medulloblastoma	2	7	1	8
Astrocytoma	5	3	9	2
Choroid plexus papilloma	6	0	9	0
Ependymoma, ependymoblastoma	4	0	7	2
Other neuroepithelial tumors	10	6	8	2
Total of all neuroepithelial tumors	27	16	34	14
Supratentorial-to-infratentorial ratio for neuroepithelial tumors	1.7:1		2.4:1	
Supratentorial-to-infratentorial ratio for all tumors (teratoma, neuroepithelial, mesenchymal)	5.2:1		3.4:1	

Data from Wakai S, Arai T, Nagai M. Congenital brain tumors. *Surg Neurol.* 1984;21:597–609.

TABLE 37.4 Neonatal Brain Tumors: Initial Signs and Symptoms[a]

SIGNS AND SYMPTOMS	PRESENTATION AT BIRTH (%)		PRESENTATION IN FIRST 2 MONTHS (%)
	TERATOMA	OTHERS	
Dystocia	45	20	–
Stillborn	40	15	–
Prematurity	30	20	–
Large head and/or bulging fontanelle	70	55	70
Epignathus	10	–	–
Local skull swelling	10	5	2
Proptosis	8	1	–
Seizure	–	2	15
Vomiting	–	1	30

[a]n = 200 in reference 1, n = 250 in reference 7, and n = 534 in reference 9. Numbers are rounded off. Data from references 1, 7, and 9.

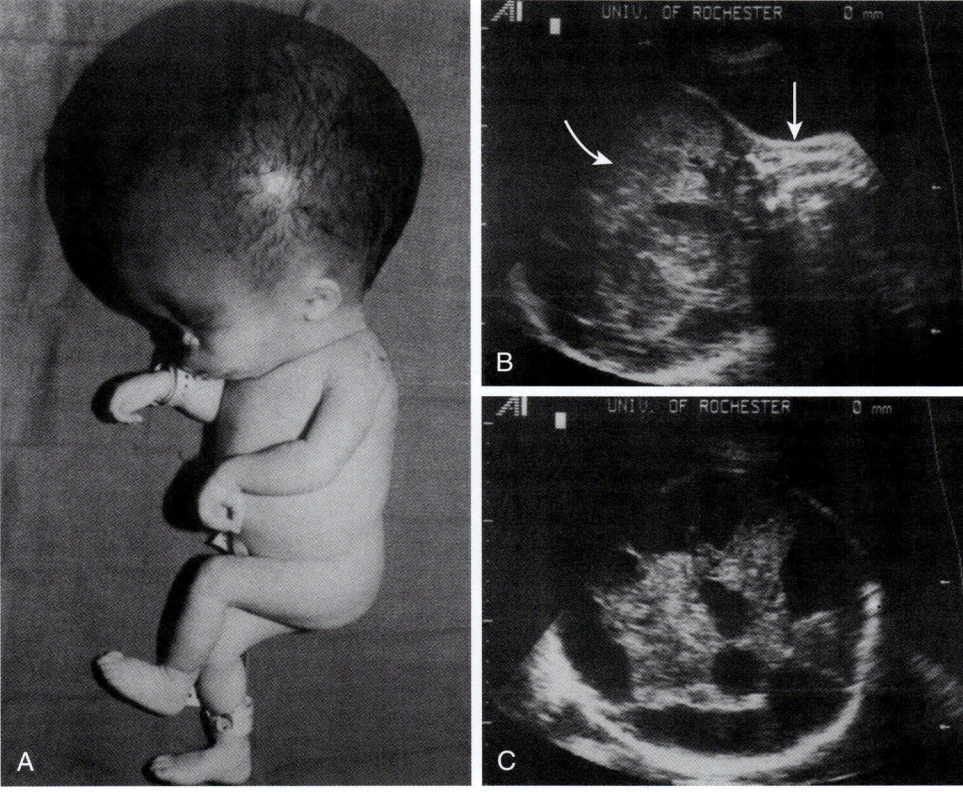

Figure 37.3 Teratoma with intrauterine presentation. (A) Newborn exhibits massive craniomegaly secondary to intracranial teratoma. The infant died at 90 minutes of age. (B and C) Intrauterine ultrasonography of the same infant. Note in B a midsagittal view of the fetus, the solid echogenic mass *(curved arrow)* in the cranium above the level of the cervical spine *(straight arrow)*. In C a transverse view of fetal vertex shows the absence of normal symmetrical intracranial anatomy and the presence of a solid echogenic core surrounded by cystic structures. (From Sherer DM, Abramowicz JS, Eggers PC, Metlay LA, et al. Prenatal ultrasonographic diagnosis of intracranial teratoma and massive craniomegaly with associated high-output cardiac failure. *Am J Obstet Gynecol.* 1993;168:97–99.)

(Figs. 37.6 and 37.7).[3,4,41,63] The addition of Doppler evaluation of blood flow within the tumor is useful in the identification of choroid plexus papilloma, a strikingly hypervascular tumor (Fig. 37.8).[86] In general, however, MRI is the mainstay of the diagnostic evaluation (see Fig. 37.4; Figs. 37.9 to 37.13).[10,31,87] MRI is preferred for all lesions, especially for those in the posterior fossa and spinal cord (see Fig. 37.13). Computed tomography (CT) is currently reserved for use in neonates when emergent neurosurgical intervention is indicated and a timely MRI is not available.

Prognosis

The outcome of patients with neonatal brain tumors depends on the size and location of the lesion, the time of diagnosis,

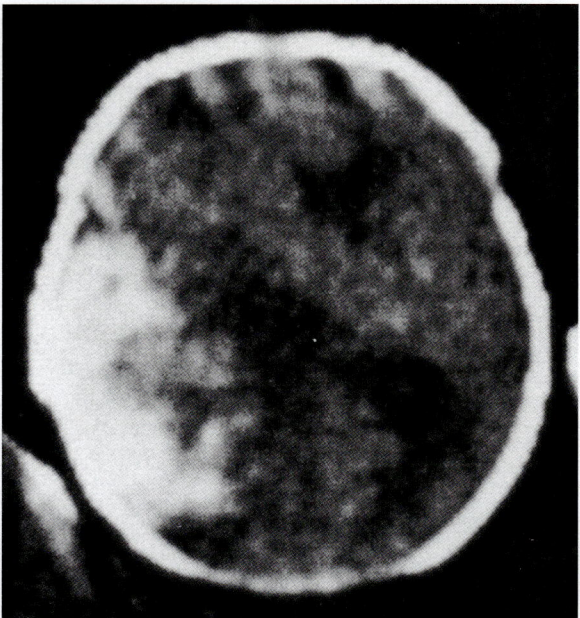

Figure 37.4 Intracerebral hemorrhage associated with an astrocytoma: computed tomography scan from a 2-week-old infant with a 9-day history of vomiting, left focal seizures, and left hemiparesis. Note the large hemorrhagic mass in the right cerebral hemisphere with surrounding edema and shift of ventricles to the left. A fibrillary astrocytoma was identified at surgery. (From Rothman SM, Nelson JS, DeVivo DC, Coxe WS. Congenital astrocytoma presenting with intracerebral hematoma. *J Neurosurg.* 1979;51: 237–239.)

and particularly the histological type of the tumor. General conclusions concerning prognosis of the most common neonatal brain tumors are summarized in Table 37.6.[a]

Teratomas are associated with a poor outcome. Mortality rates in these patients generally exceed 90%, principally because the lesions are usually very extensive at the time of identification. In the largest reported experience (n = 73), the 1-year survival rate for patients with teratomas was 7.2%.[8] Long-term survivors of large embryonal tumors have significant deficits, with 54% exhibiting an IQ less than 70. In addition, 85% show motor deficits; 50% have vision, hearing, and/or speech delay; and 25% demonstrate feeding and endocrine abnormalities.[90]

Medulloblastoma manifesting at birth or in the first 2 postnatal months is also associated with a poor outcome,

[a]References 2-5, 8, 19, 20, 24, 26, 27, 30-32, 35, 51, 53, 75, 78, 79, 83, 88, and 89.

TABLE 37.5 Association of Hemorrhage With Neonatal Brain Tumors[a]

HISTOLOGICAL TYPE	INCIDENCE OF HEMORRHAGE (%)
Teratoma	8
Neuroepithelial and other	18
All tumors	14

[a]See text for references.

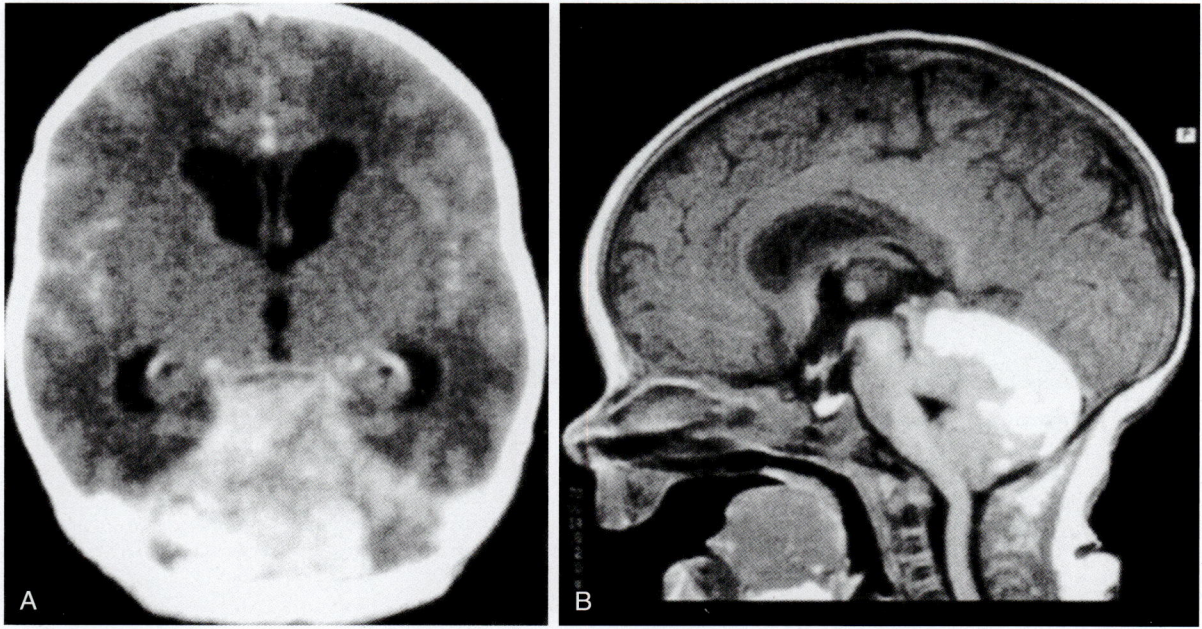

Figure 37.5 Posterior fossa hemorrhage in a newborn with a medulloblastoma. (A) Axial computed tomography scan shows an apparent posterior fossa hemorrhage in a term infant who presented at 6 hours of age with signs of brain-stem compression. (B) Sagittal magnetic resonance imaging scan shows posterior fossa subdural hemorrhage, apparently originating in the cerebellar vermis. Six months later, a large midline medulloblastoma was detected. Rights were not granted to include this figure in electronic media. Please refer to the printed book. (From Perrin RG, Rutka JT, Drake JM, Meltzer H, et al. Management and outcomes of posterior fossa subdural hematomas in neonates. *Neurosurgery.* 1997;40:1190–1200.)

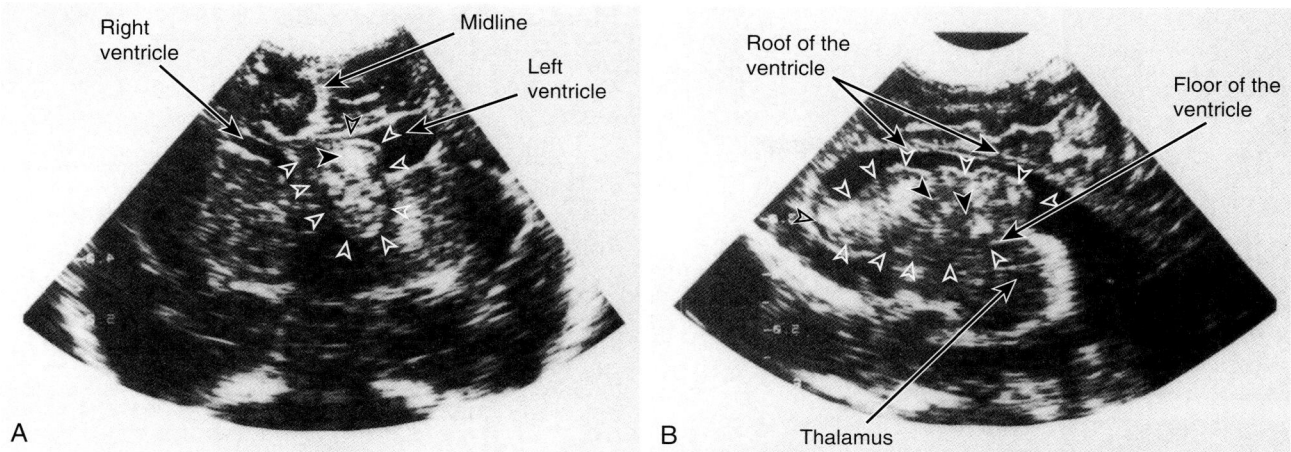

Figure 37.6 Cranial ultrasonography: neonatal subependymal astrocytoma. (A) Coronal and (B) sagittal ultrasound scans obtained from the anterior fontanelle show a large intraventricular mass in the left lateral ventricle *(outlined with open arrowheads)* with midline shift and dilation of the left lateral ventricle. Closed arrowheads indicate some areas of calcification. This infant had tuberous sclerosis. (From Hahn JS, Bejar R, Gladson CL. Neonatal subependymal giant cell astrocytoma associated with tuberous sclerosis: MRI, CT, and ultrasound correlation. *Neurology.* 1991;41:124–128.)

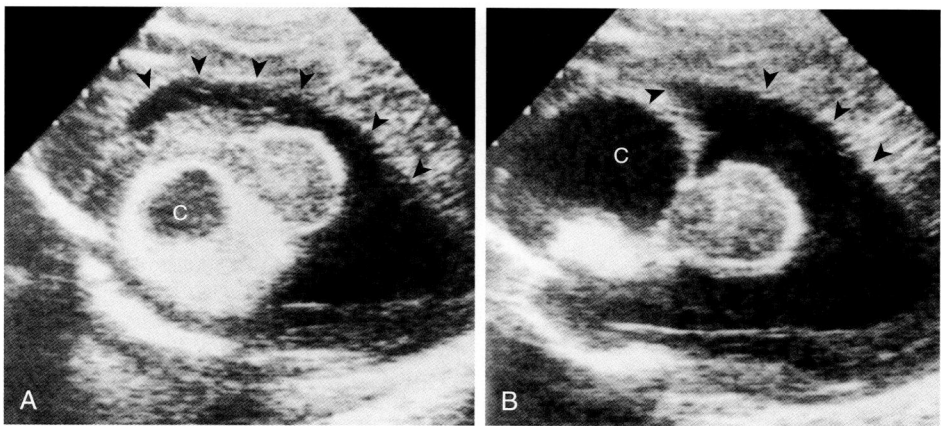

Figure 37.7 Cranial ultrasonography: neonatal craniopharyngioma. (A and B) Sagittal ultrasound scans show cyst-like regions of tumor (C) with internal echoes. Adjacent to the cyst-like regions are focal echogenic areas with shadowing, consistent with calcification. The lateral ventricle *(arrowheads)* is dilated. (From Hurst RW, McIlhenny J, Park TS, Thomas WO. Neonatal craniopharyngioma: CT and ultrasonographic features. *J Comput Assist Tomogr.* 1988;12:858–861.)

with mortality rates exceeding 80%. In a series of 19 cases of perinatal medulloblastoma, only 1 survivor was reported.[4]

Choroid plexus papilloma has the most favorable outcome. With rare exceptions, all infants are cured and have a normal outcome. Choroid plexus carcinoma, which accounts for approximately 5% to 10% of neonatal choroid plexus tumors, had been associated with a poor chance for survival until recently, when improvements in chemotherapy appreciably increased the chance of prolonged survival.[50] Desmoplastic infantile ganglioma is often curable with resection.

Astrocytomas and ependymomas are associated with variable outcomes, depending primarily on the degree of differentiation of the tumor and its location. Markedly anaplastic lesions and deep diencephalic and brain-stem locations are rarely curable.[40]

Management

Major Modalities of Treatment

Major modalities of treatment of brain tumors in children are surgery, chemotherapy, and radiation therapy. Surgery is by far the most important of these modalities in the management of neonatal brain tumors. Indeed, improvements in the localization of lesions by modern brain imaging, advances in pediatric neuroanesthesia and intensive care, and the advent of microneurosurgical techniques have markedly reduced the operative mortality of patients with even large tumors. Indeed, aggressive resection, including subtotal hemispherectomy, has been advocated for large tumors.[3,4,24,79,91] Long-term survival with satisfactory outcomes has been reported, especially when gross total resection of a favorable pathology is present.[92]

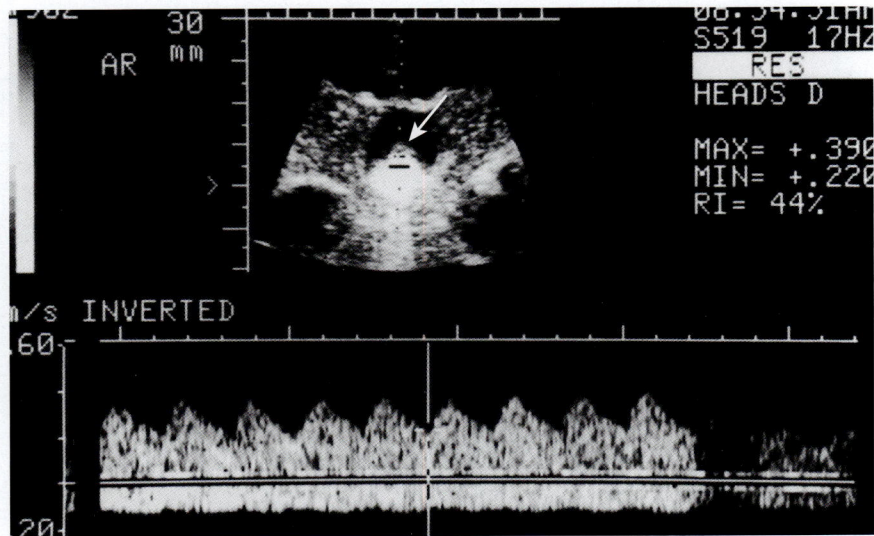

Figure 37.8 Cranial Doppler and ultrasonographic study of choroid plexus papilloma. This coronal study shows a dilated third ventricle within which is an echogenic mass (arrow). Dilated lateral ventricles and temporal horns also are visible. The Doppler tracing (lower portion of figure) from the mass indicates hypervascularity with high blood flow. (From Harmon BH, Yap MA. One-month-old infant with increasing head size. Invest Radiol. 1990;25:862-864.)

TABLE 37.6	General Conclusions Concerning Prognosis of Most Common Neonatal Brain Tumors

Teratomas
  >90% mortality rate
Astrocytoma
  Variable mortality rate: potentially curable for WHO grade I to very poor for WHO grades III–IV
Medulloblastoma
  Varies with molecular subtype
Choroid plexus papilloma
  Minimal mortality rate and high likelihood of normal outcome
Ependymoma
  Variable prognosis, as stated for astrocytoma, but less commonly curable
Atypical teratoid/rhabdoid tumor
  >90% mortality rate
Desmoplastic infantile ganglioglioma
  Often curable with resection

Chemotherapy in the neonatal period is hindered by the immaturity of the infant's hepatic and renal mechanisms for the metabolism and excretion of these agents.[88] However, in recent years improved *multiagent chemotherapy after surgery* has been advocated to delay or obviate the need for radiation therapy, a modality of high risk in the young infant.[93,94] In selected patients, neoadjuvant chemotherapy is used to reduce tumor bulk and neovascularity prior to surgical resection.[95,96]

Radiation therapy is the most problematic and controversial approach in the treatment of neonatal brain tumors.[a] Indeed, few data are available for newborns and very young infants,

but in a series of 13 infants treated for brain tumors at less than 2 years of age, 10 later had below-normal intelligence quotients and impaired growth.[98] Such adverse neurological and endocrinological effects have been replicated in infants and young children treated with craniospinal irradiation for prophylaxis for acute lymphoblastic leukemia.[99-101] Indeed, many clinicians consider radiation to be "absolutely contraindicated in the neonate"[79] and to be used only for recurrent disease after aggressive surgery and, when indicated, chemotherapy.[24] The advent of stereotactically applied, highly focused radiation (radiation surgery), which provides radiation to the tumor with a minimum of involvement of normal brain in the management of pediatric brain tumors, raises the possibility of ultimate application of this technique to young infants.[102,103] Unfortunately the frequent presence of infiltrating tumor borders in neonatal brain tumors may limit the applicability of even this promising approach.

Hematopoietic stem cell transplantation (HSCT) has been added to the armamentarium for treating neonates and infants. With HSCT, more aggressive chemotherapy can be administered. In a recent Toronto series comprising three infants, an infant with ATRT and another with choroid plexus carcinoma had long-term survival while the third died.[104]

Treatment of Specific Tumors

Concerning the *treatment of specific tumors*, teratomas are managed essentially entirely by surgery. Unfortunately only partial resections are usually possible because of the very large size of these lesions. Medulloblastoma is treated with partial or total resection and, in recent years, by chemotherapy. Radiation therapy, if used at all, is instituted most often later in infancy for recurrent disease. Choroid plexus papilloma is treated with total surgical resection, and choroid plexus carcinoma is treated with surgery and chemotherapy. Astrocytomas and ependymomas are treated with aggressive surgery, the former with more success than the latter, particularly because of more

[a]References 24, 79, 93, 94, 97, and 98.

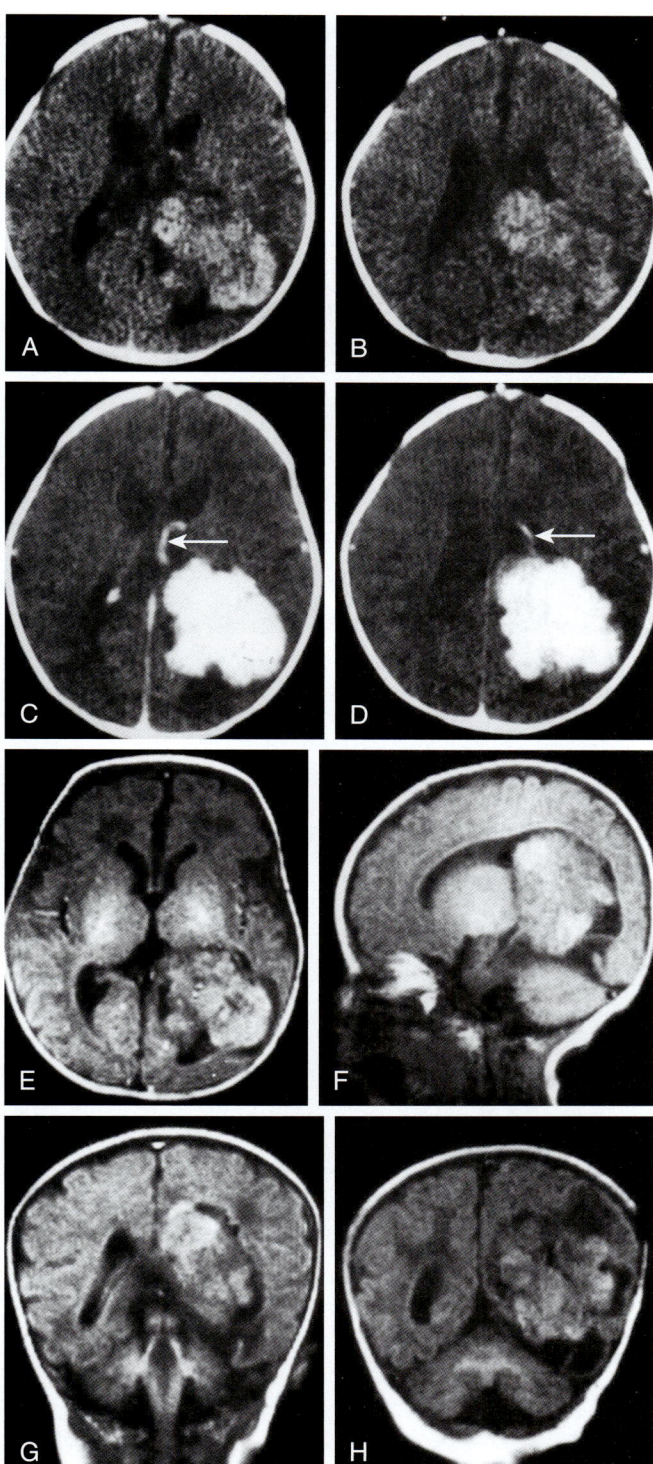

Figure 37.9 Choroid plexus papilloma: computed tomography (CT) and magnetic resonance imaging (MRI) scans from an 11-day-old infant with macrocrania. (A–D) Axial CT sections before (A and B) and after (C and D) contrast enhancement reveal a large, lobulated, partially calcified, hyperdense mass that is near a dilated choroidal vessel (*arrows* in C and D). The mass expands the ventricle and extends into the surrounding parenchyma. (E–H) Spin-echo T1-weighted MRI scans in axial (E), sagittal (F), and coronal (G and H) planes demonstrate mixed high and low signal intensity of the mass within the ventricle and periventricular tissue. (From Radkowski MA, Naidich TP, Tomita T, Byrd SE, et al. Neonatal brain tumors: CT and MR findings. *J Comput Assist Tomogr.* 1988;12:10–20.)

TABLE 37.7   Vein of Galen Malformation With Presentation in the Neonatal Period

Neonatal presentation
≈60% of all pediatric cases of vein of Galen malformation
Most common arterial feeding vessels
Choroidal arteries (posterior and anterior), anterior and middle cerebral arteries, and proximal posterior cerebral arteries
Clinical presentation
High-output congestive heart failure in virtually all neonatal cases; hydrocephalus present in ≈15%
Diagnosis
Made most readily by ultrasonography, Doppler studies of cerebral vessels and peripheral arteries, computed tomographic angiography, and magnetic resonance imaging
Outcome
In previous years, nearly 100% mortality; more recently, ≈40%–65% have favorable outcomes
Therapy
Most commonly embolization, either by selective arterial infusion with liquid adhesive agents or microcoils or by transvenous-transtorcular embolization with metallic coils

favorable locations with astrocytoma. Multiagent chemotherapy has had some postoperative benefit for anaplastic astrocytomas but not particularly for ependymomas.[93,94] Limited-volume radiation therapy is under investigation for these lesions.[93,94]

VEIN OF GALEN MALFORMATION

Vein of Galen malformation is discussed best in this context because, like brain tumor, the disorder constitutes an intracranial mass lesion and manifests in the newborn in approximately 60% of all pediatric examples of this malformation (Table 37.7).[105-109] Moreover, certain features of the clinical presentation (e.g., macrocephaly and hydrocephalus) can be similar to the clinical presentation of brain tumors. Notably, however, the clinical presentation more commonly does not mimic brain tumor and is quite distinctive (see later discussion). Because of fetal screening and increased use of fetal MRI, vein of Galen malformations are increasingly diagnosed prenatally, allowing the opportunity for prenatal counseling.[110] Vein of Galen malformation continues to be a great therapeutic challenge. Despite advances in radiological diagnosis, neonatal intensive care, and microneurosurgical and endovascular techniques, this disorder, when severe enough to appear in the newborn, remains a major therapeutic problem.

Neuropathology

The essential feature of the vein of Galen malformation is aneurysmal dilation of the venous structure generally characterized as the vein of Galen. The most common arterial vessels feeding into this dilated venous structure are, in order of frequency, the posterior choroidal artery, the anterior cerebral (pericallosal) artery, the middle cerebral artery (especially thalamoperforating branches), the anterior choroidal artery, and the posterior cerebral artery (see Table 37.7).[106,108,111,112] Although the vein of Galen is considered in most writings to be the vein that is dilated, careful anatomical study suggests that the so-called *median prosencephalic vein of Markowski*, a transitory

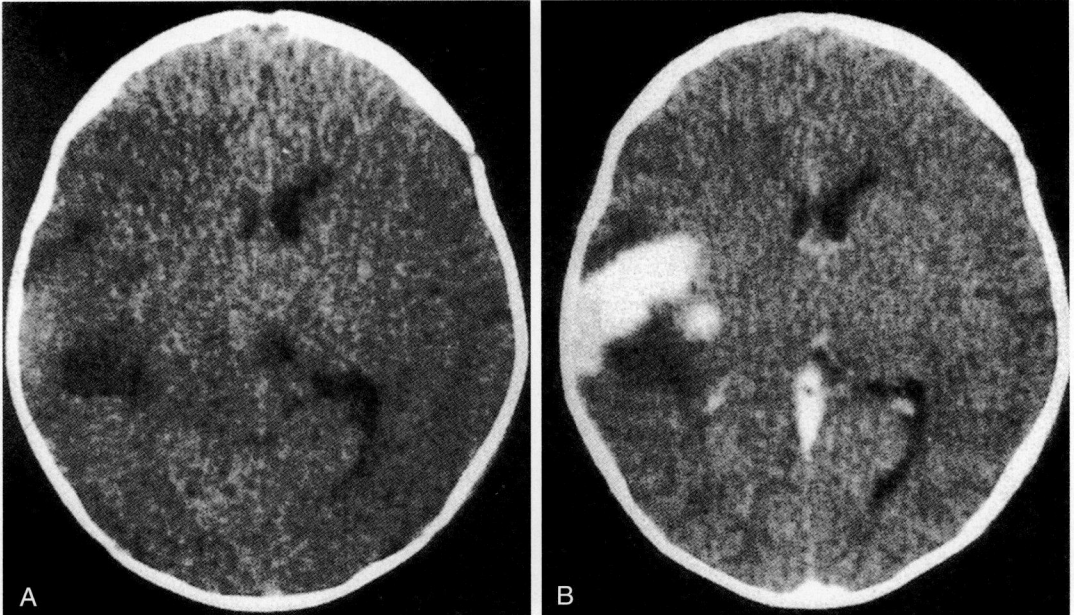

Figure 37.10 Gliosarcoma in a 26-day-old infant: computed tomography (CT) scan. Axial CT sections before (A) and after (B) contrast enhancement reveal an isodense, densely enhancing temporoparietal mass, associated edema, and compression of the right lateral ventricle. The tumor itself reaches the pial surface of the brain (confirmed by surgery). (From Radkowski MA, Naidich TP, Tomita T, Byrd SE, et al. Neonatal brain tumors: CT and MR findings. *J Comput Assist Tomogr.* 1988;12:10–20.)

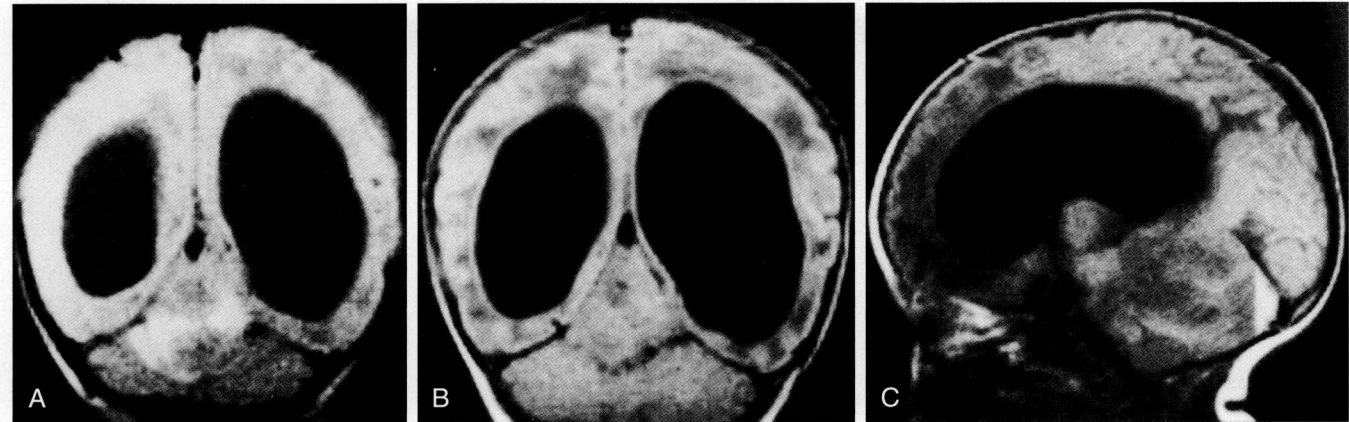

Figure 37.11 Medulloblastoma in a 49-day-old infant: magnetic resonance imaging (MRI) scans. (A–C) Spin-echo MRI scans in the coronal plane at TR 1000, TE 30 ms (A and B) and in the sagittal plane at TR 550, TE 30 ms (C) reveal a large superior vermian mass that compresses the fourth ventricle and brain stem, invades the tectum to obliterate the aqueduct (causing hydrocephalus), and grows exophytically to overlie the cerebellar hemispheres. (From Radkowski MA, Naidich TP, Tomita T, Byrd SE, et al. Neonatal brain tumors: CT and MR findings. *J Comput Assist Tomogr.* 1988;12:10–20.)

venous structure that normally disappears by the 11th week of gestation, is the vein involved (Figs. 37.14 and 37.15).[111] During early development, this vein drains directly into the vein of Galen; after 11 weeks, it is replaced by the internal cerebral veins. The median prosencephalic vein is involved particularly in venous drainage from the choroid plexus.[111,113] The frequent position of the aneurysmally dilated vein anterior to the position of the vein of Galen further supports the notion that the involved vein is the primitive median prosencephalic vein. The frequent association of abnormal venous channels, including

the so-called *falcine sinus*, a normally transient fetal vessel, is additionally consistent with this hypothesis.[111] Nevertheless, the term *vein of Galen malformation* is entrenched in the medical literature, and we continue to use it to characterize this entity.

The *associated neuropathological findings* observed with vein of Galen malformation consist of a variety of ischemic, hemorrhagic, and mass effects of the malformation.[106-108,111-125] Thus, in a carefully analyzed series of 13 infants who died in the first 6 weeks of life, *ischemic lesions* included cerebral infarction (focal vascular and border zone lesions) in 4 infants, basal

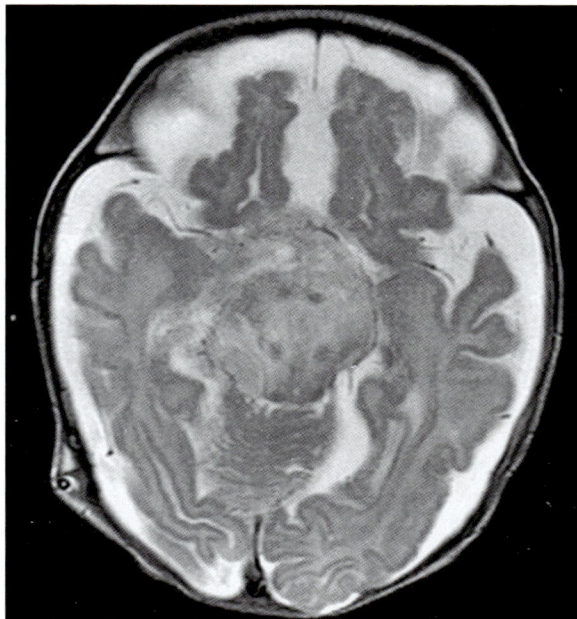

Figure 37.12 Glioma: magnetic resonance imaging scan. This 2-month-old infant had a large, heterogeneous mass (undifferentiated glioma) in the diencephalic–upper midbrain region. Disseminated tumor was present in extracerebral spaces, which are markedly widened. (Courtesy Dr. Omar Khwaja.)

ganglia or other infarction in 3, periventricular leukomalacia in 7, pontosubicular necrosis in 3, and selective neuronal necrosis of cerebral cortex, brain stem, or both in 4 infants. *Hemorrhagic lesions* included subarachnoid hemorrhage in three infants, germinal matrix–intraventricular hemorrhage in two, and intracerebral hemorrhage in two. Venous thrombosis was present in three infants. *Mass effects* included hydrocephalus secondary to obstruction, usually at the level of quadrigeminal plate and the aqueduct, in two infants, and compression of other structures (e.g., cerebral peduncles) in one infant. The mechanisms of these lesions are multifactorial and are summarized in Table 37.8.

TABLE 37.8	Major Mechanisms of Brain Injury With the Vein of Galen

Intracranial *steal* phenomena because of diastolic *runoff*, resulting in cerebral ischemia

Congestive heart failure (secondary to high cardiac output and myocardial ischemia, because of low diastolic pressure and, as a consequence, impaired coronary flow), resulting in cerebral ischemia

Thrombosis of the dilated vein of Galen with hemorrhagic infarction, intraventricular hemorrhage, or both

Vascular rupture with massive hemorrhage

Atrophy secondary to compression of adjacent structures by the dilated vein of Galen

Hydrocephalus secondary to aqueductal obstruction (by compression)

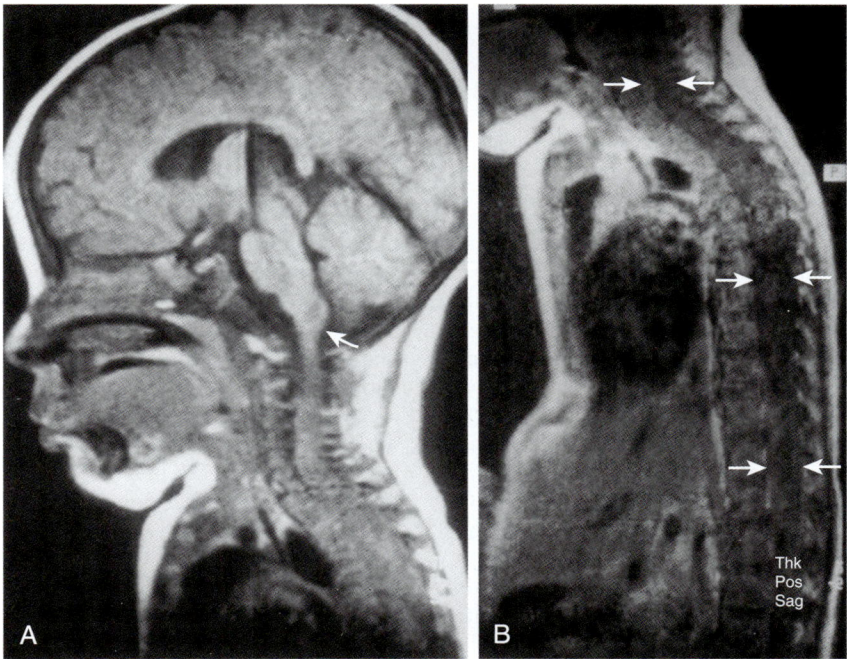

Figure 37.13 Spinal cord and medullary astrocytoma: magnetic resonance imaging (MRI) scan. (A) Midsagittal MRI, T1-weighted (TR 600/TE 15), unenhanced. The tumor can be appreciated in the medulla *(arrow)*. Additional signal sequences (not shown) had no indication of a fluid cavity or enhancement. (B) Midsagittal MRI, T1-weighted (TR 770, TE 15), gadolinium-enhanced. The entire spinal cord is diffusely expanded by a nonenhancing, noncystic mass *(arrows)*. Rights were not granted to include this figure in electronic media. Please refer to the printed book. (From Kaufman BA, Park TS. Congenital spinal cord astrocytomas. *Childs Nerv Syst.* 1992;8: 389–393.)

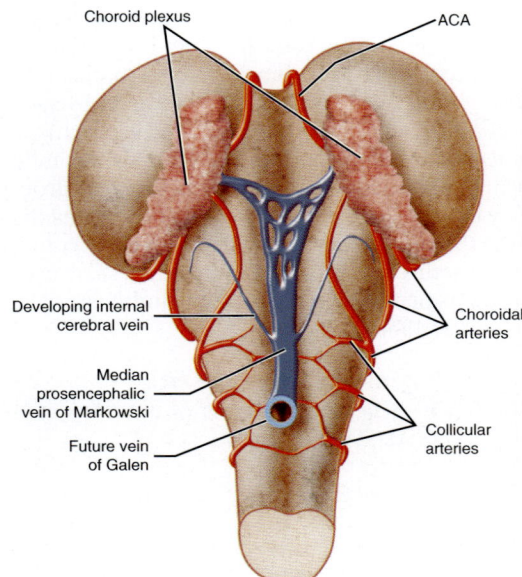

Figure 37.14 Artist's rendering of the early vascularization of the choroid plexuses. Just before the growth of the neural tube induces the development of the intrinsic vascularization, the meninx primitiva invaginates into the ventricular lumen to produce the choroid plexuses. The arterial afferents are the choroidal arteries, including the terminal branch of the anterior cerebral artery (ACA). The venous blood drains through the median prosencephalic vein of Markowski. This single midline vein forms by collecting blood from the plexuses at the level of the paraphysis and courses backward toward the dorsal (interhemispheric) dural plexus. Simultaneously, the development of the collicular plate is accompanied by development of quadrigeminal (collicular) arteries. Later, when the intrinsic vascularization develops in the basal ganglia and thalamus, the internal cerebral veins develop to drain them. These join with the posterior end of the median prosencephalic vein to form what will become the vein of Galen. Progressively, the internal cerebral veins replace the median prosencephalic vein for choroidal venous drainage; the median prosencephalic vein attenuates and disappears, and the vein of Galen develops. Rights were not granted to include this figure in electronic media. Please refer to the printed book. (From Raybaud CA, Strother CM, Hald JK. Aneurysms of the vein of Galen: embryonic considerations and anatomical features relating to the pathogenesis of the malformation. *Neuroradiology.* 1989;31:109–128.)

The ischemic phenomena are related primarily to a combination of intracranial *steal* phenomena, caused by the absence or even the reversal of diastolic cerebral blood flow, and congestive heart failure. The heart failure is caused principally by the remarkably high cardiac output, secondary to both the marked decrease in cerebrovascular resistance and the increased venous return to the heart and to marked cardiac ischemia. The latter results from decreased coronary blood flow, which normally occurs predominantly during diastole, because of the low diastolic pressure associated with the vein of Galen malformation.

As genetic understanding of developmental lesions progresses, some vein of Galen and other high-flow congenital vascular lesions have been associated with genetic mutations. For example, three infants with RASA1 mutations have been reported with high-flow shunts, including one with a vein of Galen malformation.[126]

Clinical Features

The clinical manifestations of the vein of Galen malformation in the neonatal period reflect the large size of the lesions and consist

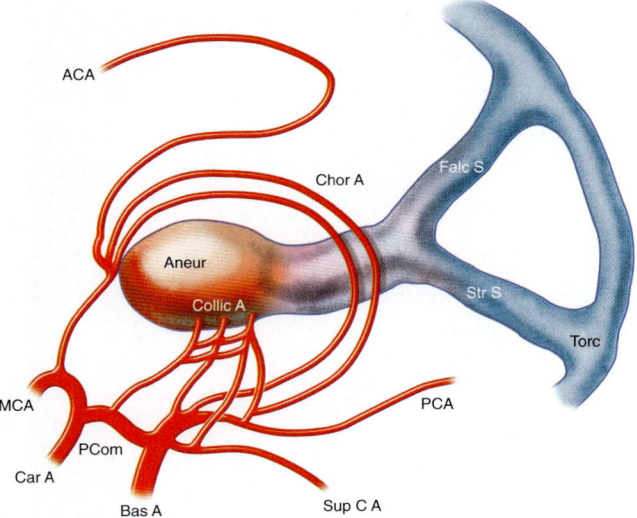

Figure 37.15 Artist's rendering of a vein of Galen malformation. This drawing is based on two anatomical dissections. Two fistula sites are present in the aneurysmal sac (Aneur). The anterior fistula receives blood from the choroidal vessels (anterior cerebral artery [ACA], choroidal branches [Chor A] of the posterior cerebral artery [PCA]) and from posterior perforators of the middle cerebral artery (MCA). The inferior fistula receives blood from an arterioarterial subarachnoid maze formed by anastomoses between the collicular arteries (branches of the superior cerebellar arteries [Sup C A], the PCA, and the posteromedial choroidal arteries). Posterior thalamoperforating arteries also may be involved. The aneurysmal sac is usually drained by dural sinuses, either the normal straight sinus (Str S) or a persistent fetal falcine sinus (Falc S), or both, as shown here. *Bas A,* Basilar artery; *Car A,* carotid artery; *PCom,* posterior communicating artery; *Torc,* torcular. Rights were not granted to include this figure in electronic media. Please refer to the printed book. (From Raybaud CA, Strother CM, Hald JK. Aneurysms of the vein of Galen: embryonic considerations and anatomical features relating to the pathogenesis of the malformation. *Neuroradiology.* 1989;31:109–128.)

predominantly of congestive heart failure (see Table 37.7).[a] Thus, of the approximately 130 cases with adequate clinical data, 80% to 95% of infants presented with congestive heart failure. The remaining infants presented with hydrocephalus, subarachnoid hemorrhage, or intraventricular hemorrhage. The features accompanying the congestive failure aid in diagnosis and include a cranial bruit and bounding carotid pulses. The cranial bruit differs from the benign systolic bruit of infancy and early childhood by its continuous nature and by the frequent localization over the posterior rather than the anterior cranium. The marked carotid pulses may be accompanied by prominent peripheral pulses, but in the presence of overt congestive heart failure the peripheral pulses may be depressed whereas the carotid pulses remain prominent. A consequence of congestive heart failure, prerenal azotemia, was observed in 11 of 15 infants in a reported series.[105] Seizures and other neurological signs are very unusual.

The clinical presentation of neonatal cases differs from that in older infants and children with vein of Galen malformation. Thus, older infants present most commonly with hydrocephalus, and children present most commonly with neurological signs (perhaps secondary to intracranial *steal* phenomena), headache, and occasionally subarachnoid hemorrhage.

---

[a]References 105-109, 112, 120, 122-125, and 127-136.

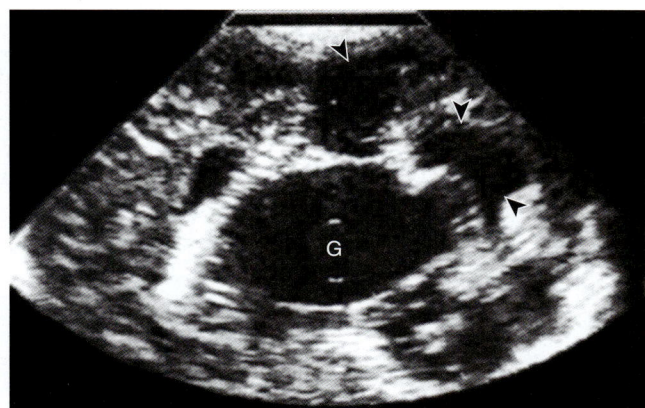

Figure 37.16 Ultrasound scan of an arteriovenous malformation in an infant with cardiac failure. This coronal ultrasound scan shows large, circular, midline, aneurysmal vein of Galen (G); the areas of echolucency in the left hemisphere represent regions of necrosis (*arrowheads*). (Courtesy Dr. Gary D. Shackelford.)

TABLE 37.9	Outcome of Neonatal Vein of Galen Malformation After Endovascular Treatment[a]

OUTCOME	PERCENTAGE OF TOTAL
Death	19
Developmental evaluation	
No permanent disability	43[b]
Permanent disability	57
Neurological examination	
No/mild abnormality	43
Severe abnormality	57
Epilepsy	33

[a]$n = 21$. The median length of follow-up was 4.5 years.
[b]Value was 38% for the 16 infants who had congestive heart failure and 60% for the 5 infants without congestive heart failure.
Data from Fullerton HJ, Aminoff AR, Ferriero DM, Gupta N, et al. Neurodevelopmental outcome after endovascular treatment of vein of Galen malformations. *Neurology.* 2003;61:1386–1390.

The subsequent course in newborns with an untreated vein of Galen malformation who survive the neonatal period and whose congestive heart failure is stabilized medically is dominated by the development of neurological disturbances and progressive hydrocephalus. The neurological disturbances include delayed development and evolution of major neurological deficits, presumably secondary to the intracranial ischemic and hemorrhagic phenomena (see later discussion).

Diagnosis

The vein of Galen malformation should be suspected in any newborn with unexplained congestive heart failure, especially high-output heart failure, or with unexplained intracranial hemorrhage or hydrocephalus. The initial diagnostic evaluation should be performed using cranial ultrasonography.[a] The aneurysmally dilated vein appears as a large, echolucent region in the region of the vein of Galen (Fig. 37.16). The addition of Doppler study of flow velocity in the arterial feeders and in the vein further defines the hemodynamics and the anatomy of the lesion.[142,144] The resistance index (RI) may be useful to follow changes in blood flow shunting.[145]

MRI has largely replaced CT in diagnosis; it is especially effective not only in the evaluation of the brain parenchyma and the aneurysmally dilated vein but also in the demonstration of major arterial feeding vessels (Fig. 37.17). MR angiography is also an effective noninvasive means of delineating both the arterial supply and venous drainage of the malformation (Fig. 37.18).

CT can be useful for the assessment of parenchymal ischemic injury or intracranial hemorrhage (Figs. 37.19 and 37.20) but has largely been supplanted by MRI. A discussion with the neuroradiology team should be held prior to obtaining CT scans in neonates. In infants with intraventricular hemorrhage, a clue that a vein of Galen malformation may be the source of the hemorrhage is a dilated third ventricle filled with blood in the absence of a large amount of blood in the lateral ventricles.[131] The major current value of CT is to identify vascular details with spiral CT angiography.[112]

Angiography is used to define the anatomical details of the vein of Galen malformation. Delineation of the crucial arterial feeders and of the size and location of the aneurysmally dilated vein is important for the determination of intervention (see later discussion). In many cases the diagnostic study may be combined with the initial interventional procedure. Thus invasive studies may be deferred until the newborn has been transferred to a center with neonatal neurointerventional expertise. Radiation exposure during diagnostic and interventional procedures should be kept in mind.

Prognosis

The natural history of the vein of Galen malformation with clinical presentation in the newborn period is apparent from the review of Hoffman and co-workers[106] in 1982, prior to the modern era of endovascular neurointervention, of 16 cases and 45 reported by others. No difference in outcome between those treated and not treated was reported. Overall, of the 61 cases, 51 (84%) died, usually in early infancy, 8 (13%) survived with neurological impairment, and only 2 (3%) were normal on follow-up. Survival with neurological impairment principally reflected the ischemic and hemorrhagic phenomena that complicate the lesion. Some of these pathological features were shown to occur in utero, and infants were left with severe neurological impairments.

The development and application of endovascular therapies for this lesion in the late 1980s and 1990s brought an increasing improvement in outcome.[107,108,133,135] The outcome in the largest neonatal series ($n = 21$) with the longest duration of follow-up (4.5 years) after neonatal endovascular therapy is shown in Table 37.9. Thus 80% of the infants survived, and nearly half had a normal or nearly normal outcome.[124] This series was recently updated.[146] Similarly promising results have been reported by other investigators.[79,90,92] Outcomes have continued to improve as neurointerventional techniques and critical care for these patients have been refined (reviewed by Khullar and co-workers).[147] Thus, in a series of 33 neonates and infants treated at Great Ormond Street, 5 who were not treated died, whereas only 2 of the 28 who had endovascular treatment failed

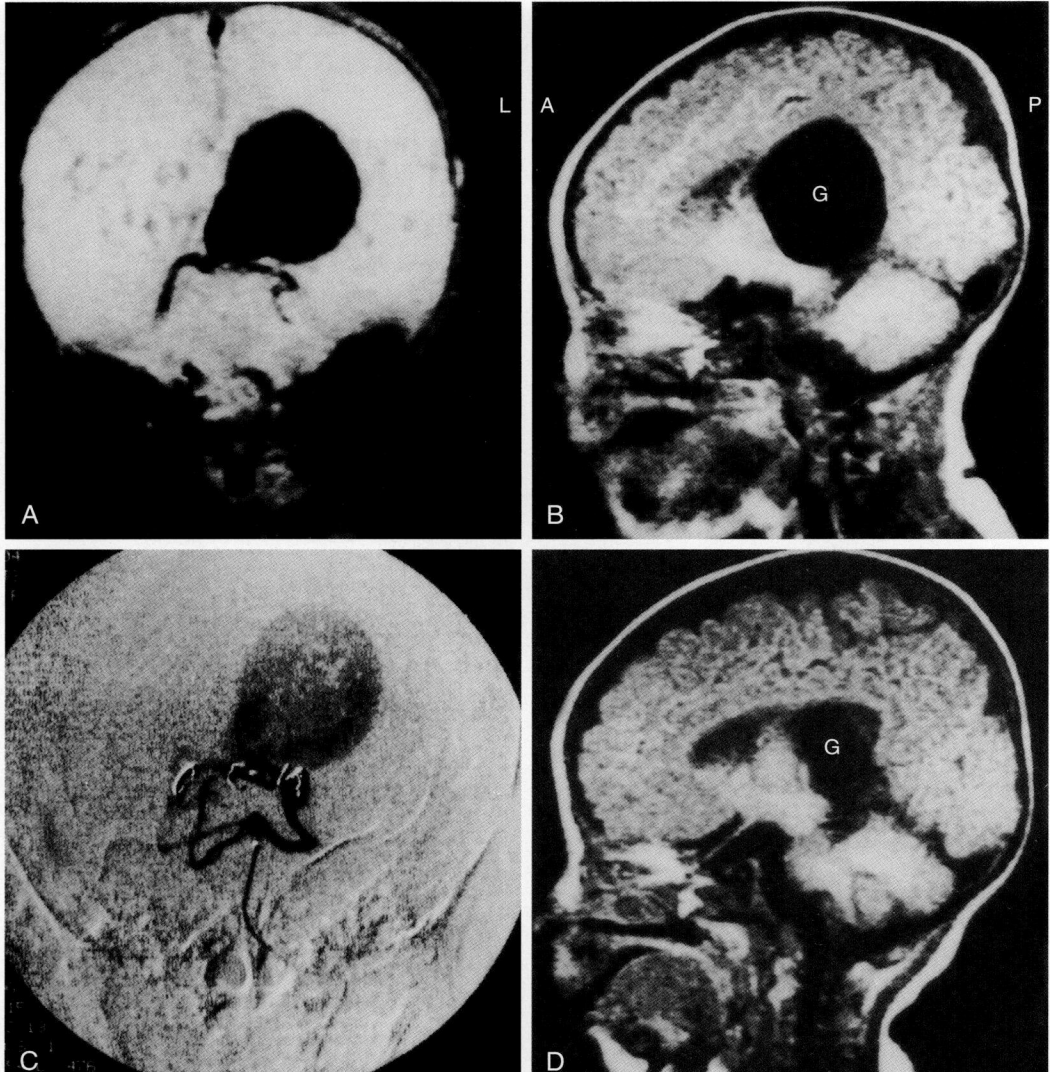

Figure 37.17 Vein of Galen malformation: magnetic resonance imaging (MRI) scans. (A) Coronal and (B) sagittal MRI scans of a newborn before and (D) 2 months after embolization show a marked decrease in the size of the aneurysmal dilation (G). In A feeding arteries are demonstrated in the coronal plane. (C) Anteroposterior view of a left vertebral angiogram showing microcoils within feeding arteries from the posterior cerebral arteries (8 days of age). Rights were not granted to include this figure in electronic media. Please refer to the printed book. (From Yamashita Y, Abe T, Ohara N, Maruoka T, et al. Successful treatment of neonatal aneurysmal dilation of the vein of Galen: the role of prenatal diagnosis and trans-arterial embolization. *Neuroradiology.* 1992;34:457–459.)

to survive. At a median follow-up at the age of 2 years, 39% of the survivors were considered neurologically intact, 21% had mild impairments, and 18% had severe impairments.[148] Similar results were reported from a Toronto series, with 71% survival for neonates with congestive heart failure who underwent endovascular treatment.[149] In Berenstein's recent series of nine treated neonates, one preterm infant died; at long-term follow-up, two of the eight survivors had mild deficits and only one child had severe impairment and seizures.[150]

Management

Management of a vein of Galen malformation large enough to manifest clinically in the neonatal period is a major

therapeutic challenge. Medical management requires vigorous therapy of cardiac failure. Aggressive use of beta-adrenergic agents (dobutamine, dopamine) may worsen cardiac output. Best results appear to occur with the use of low-dose dopamine in combination with a systemic vasodilator (e.g., a phosphodiesterase inhibitor).[125]

Concerning the approach to the vein of Galen malformation, in many centers no intervention is chosen if the infant already exhibits evidence of severe cerebral injury.[108] Direct operative intervention is made extraordinarily difficult by the large size and complicated nature of the lesions and by the vulnerability of the infant in congestive heart failure with a compromised myocardium (see earlier discussion) as well as the small

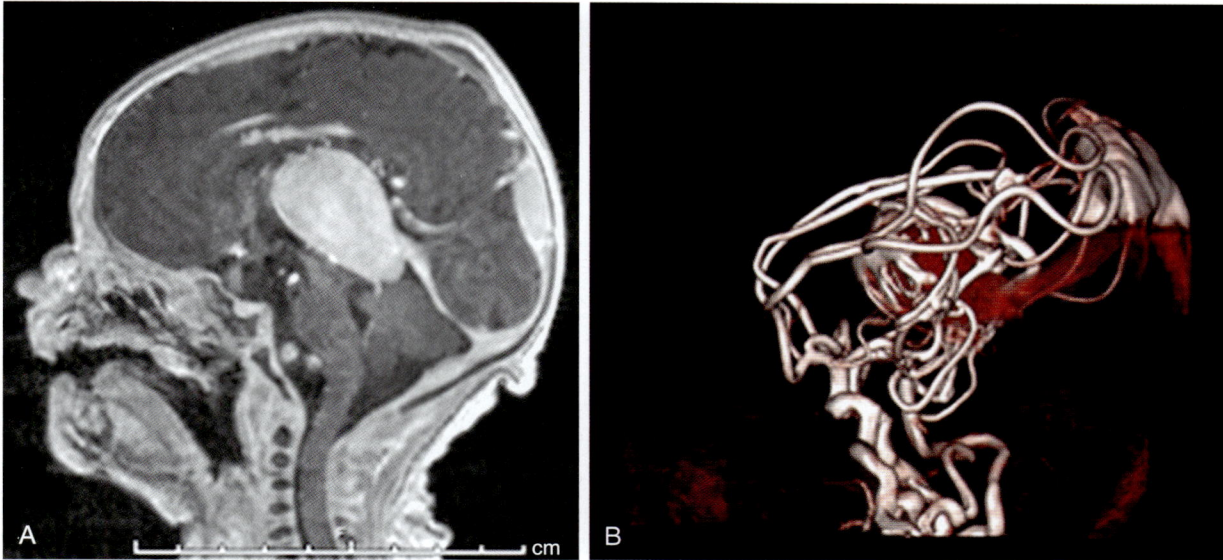

Figure 37.18 Vein of Galen malformation: magnetic resonance imaging (MRI) scans prior to treatment. (A) Sagittal MRI of a newborn with significant cardiac instability noted soon after birth. (B) MR angiogram shows shunting of arterial flow from the internal carotid and vertebral arteries to the venous drainage.

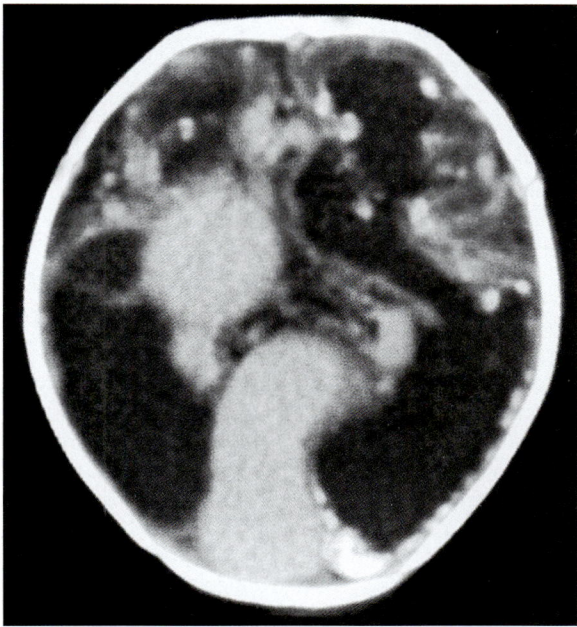

Figure 37.19 Computed tomography scan of an arteriovenous malformation from an infant with cardiac failure. The scan shows the midline aneurysmal vein of Galen and large areas of necrosis and calcification in both hemispheres, probably secondary to a *steal* phenomenon.

circulatory volume. Indeed, the possibility of hypotension in association with surgery greatly increases the risk of fatal myocardial ischemia because of the already low diastolic flow and thereby impaired coronary circulation resulting from the malformation. Currently the treatment of choice is an endovascular approach (see next).

The *principal approaches to treatment* in the newborn involve attempts to eliminate the high flow through the vascular lesion, either by arterial embolization, usually with a liquid adhesive (glue-forming) agent (e.g., bucrylate or related polymerizing compound) or microcoils, or by venous embolization, usually by retrograde catheterization through femoral or jugular access or by a transtorcular approach with placement of microcoils.[a] Technological advances may further improve treatment and outcome. Currently the most common initial therapeutic intervention is the transarterial femoral approach with delivery of a liquid adhesive agent.[112] Multiple staged procedures are usually necessary. In the large series shown in Table 37.9, three procedures per patient, on average, were required.[124]

ARACHNOID CYSTS

Arachnoid cysts, although fundamentally developmental anomalies, are best discussed briefly in the present context because their clinical presentation in the newborn most closely mimics a space-occupying lesion. These *congenital* or *primary* arachnoid cysts should be distinguished from arachnoid cystic collections secondary to hemorrhage or infection. The clinical distinction is usually straightforward. Recognition of arachnoid cysts in the neonatal period has increased markedly in recent years because of the widespread use of fetal cranial ultrasonography and MRI as well as of neonatal imaging, especially with MRI.

Pathology

Arachnoid cysts are derived from the developing arachnoid and appear to arise by splitting or duplication of the arachnoid.[155] The fine structure of the lining is similar to that of normal arachnoid cells, which secrete cerebrospinal fluid and cause the expansion often observed in vivo. In some cases, a one-way

---

[a]References 105, 107-109, 112, 117, 118, 120, 122-125, 133, 135, and 151-154.

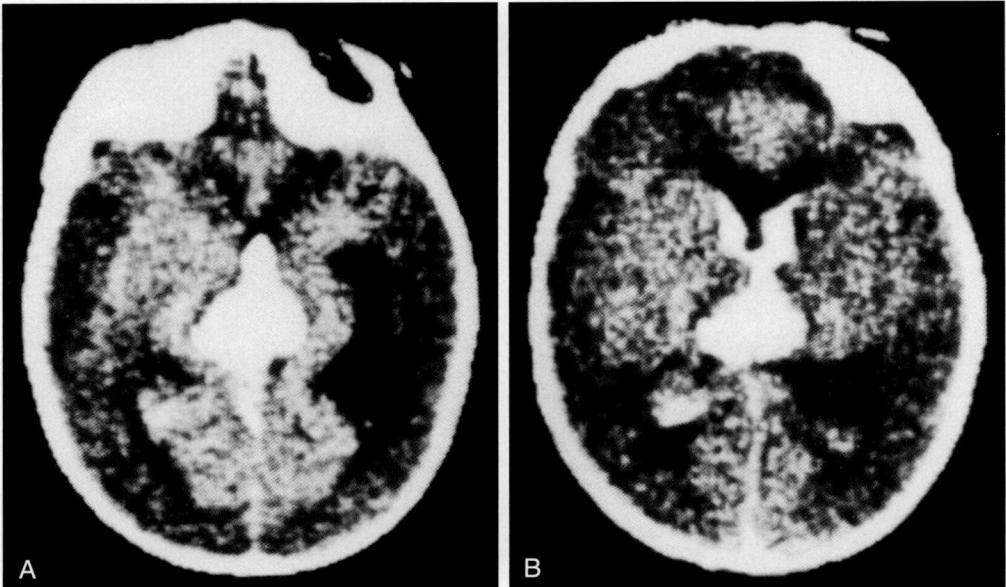

Figure 37.20 Computed tomography scans of intracranial hemorrhage secondary to an arteriovenous malformation involving the vein of Galen. These scans are from a full-term infant with abrupt onset of seizures and opisthotonic posturing on the fourth day of life. (A) Note the large amount of blood distending the posterior third ventricle. (B) A relatively small amount of blood has extended into the lateral ventricles and is visible over the head of the caudate nuclei and in the occipital horns. (From Schum TR, Meyer GA, Grausz JP, Glaspey JC. Neonatal intracranial ventricular hemorrhage due to an intracranial arteriovenous malformation: a case report. *Pediatrics.* 1979;64:242–244.)

ball-valve mechanism between the cyst and the subarachnoid space may contribute to the expansion.[156]

The *principal loci* of arachnoid cysts include regions particularly rich in arachnoid, often cisterns. The reported distribution of loci differs according to the age of the infant or child, the means of identification, and the clinical features if any. Approximately 50% of these cysts are located in the *region of the sylvian fissure* and are often associated with underdevelopment of the anterior superior surface of the temporal lobe.[87,155-158] Whether the temporal abnormality is an associated developmental anomaly or occurs secondary to compression is unknown. Other common sites include the following: the *suprasellar region*, often associated with displacement of the pituitary stalk, hypothalamus, and optic chiasm; the *interhemispheric fissure*, often with agenesis of the corpus callosum; the *supracollicular area*, with tectal compression; the *cerebellopontine angle*, with congenital cranial nerve paralysis and other signs; and *supracerebellar and infracerebellar areas*, sometimes confused with the Dandy-Walker complex (see Chapter 1).[1,87,155-159]

Clinical Features

Arachnoid cysts identified in the fetal and neonatal period most often cause no clinical abnormalities. When present, clinical features usually consist of various combinations of macrocrania, hydrocephalus, signs of increased intracranial pressure, or, least commonly, neurological abnormalities related to the locus of the cyst (see earlier). Slight to moderate hemiparesis related to the presence of a cyst in the region of the sylvian fissure or elsewhere in the middle cranial fossa is the most common of these abnormalities.[156,157]

The *diagnosis* is often suspected by screening intrauterine or neonatal ultrasonography. The finding of a large, fluid-filled space may mimic an epidermoid lesion or a cystic tumor (e.g., cystic astrocytoma) (Fig. 37.21). Because neonates and infants may remain relatively asymptomatic with cyst enlargement, serial imaging is often warranted (Fig. 37.22).

The *prognosis* of arachnoid cysts is largely unknown because the natural history is obscure. Lesions may regress antenatally.[156] Many other cysts remain stationary and do not cause neurological symptoms. Nevertheless, some arachnoid cysts clearly increase in size and lead to macrocephaly, hydrocephalus, or both or to parenchymal signs, progressive hemiparesis, intractable epilepsy, hypothalamic syndromes, or posterior fossa disorders according to the site of the lesion. Some arachnoid cysts may enlarge during the first year and then stabilize or regress.[160] Thus management should be tailored to each infant.

Management

Management of arachnoid cysts is controversial because of uncertainties about their natural history. However, in the neonatal period, the clearest indications for intervention are signs of increased intracranial pressure (vomiting, bulging fontanelle, rapid head growth) and prominent or progressive parenchymal signs. Currently the two leading neurosurgical interventions are fenestration of the cyst to produce communication with the subarachnoid space via either craniotomy or endoscopy and placement of a cyst-peritoneal shunt.[156,157] These approaches have eliminated signs of increased intracranial pressure, have restored normal head growth, and have often reversed or at least halted the progression of parenchymal signs.

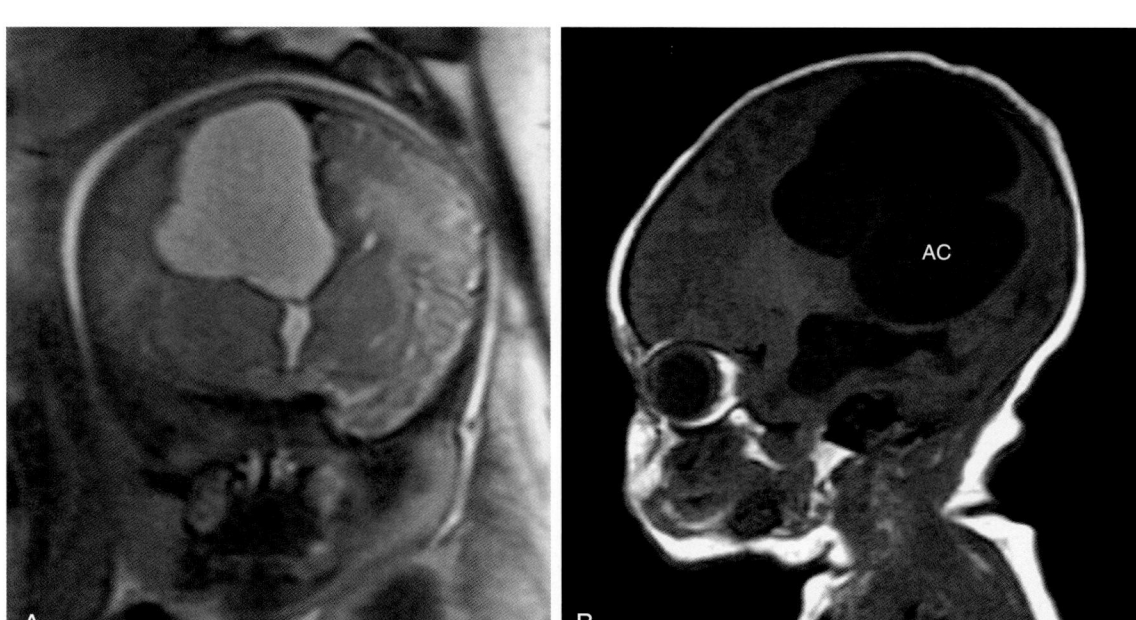

Figure 37.21 Supratentorial arachnoidal cyst, magnetic resonance imaging (MRI) scans. (A) Coronal MRI scan performed in utero at 33 weeks of gestation shows a large arachnoidal cyst in the interhemispheric fissure. (B) On this postnatal sagittal MRI, the lesion was shown to be continuous with a multilobulated cyst (AC) in the suprasellar region.

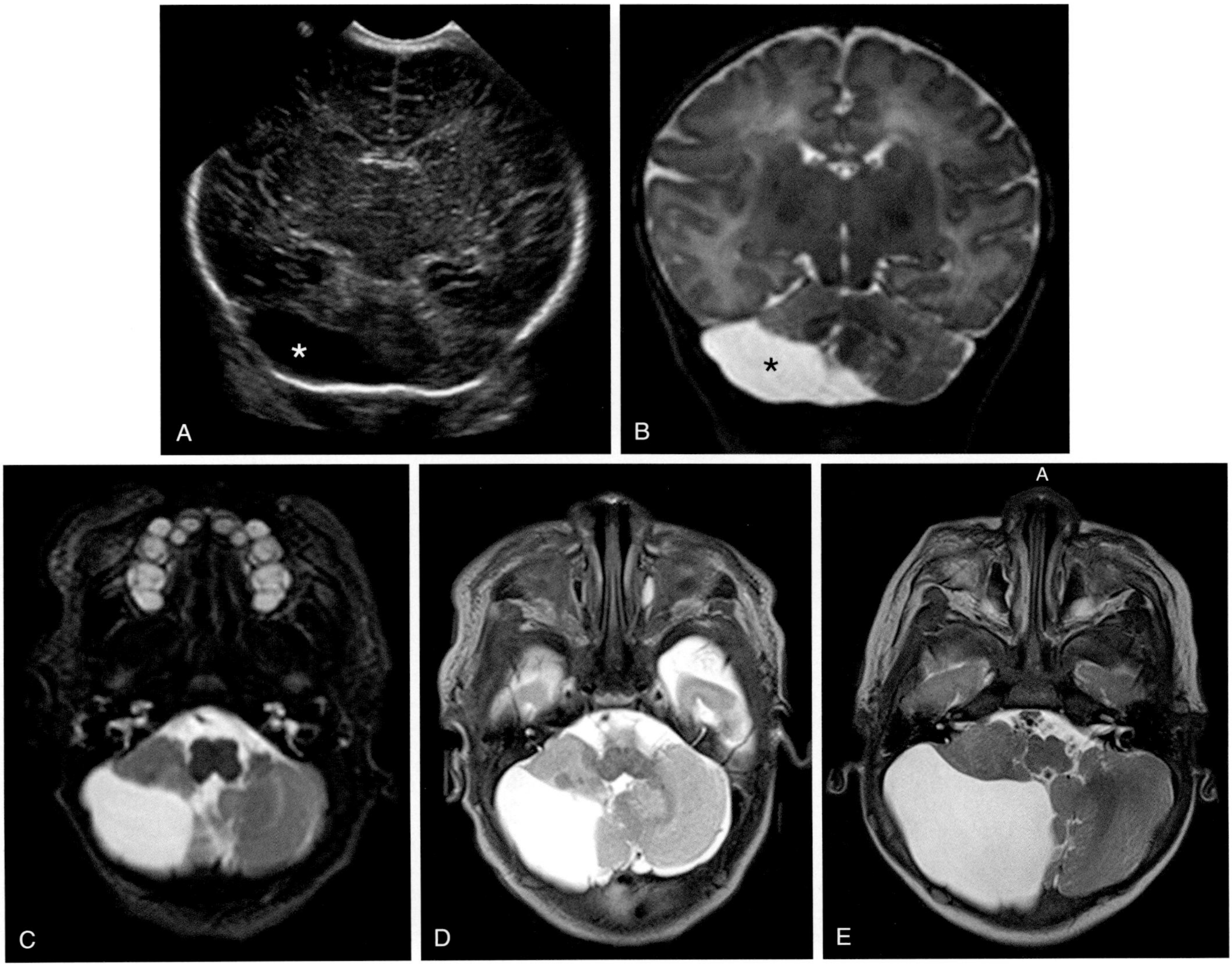

Figure 37.22 Posterior fossa arachnoid cyst, magnetic resonance imaging (MRI) scans. (A) Coronal image of cranial ultrasound from the first day of life shows a right-sided arachnoid cyst (*). (B) Coronal MRI scan on day of life 3 provides more detail. (C) Axial MRI on day of life 3 shows minimal mass effect. (D) Axial MRI on day of life 10 shows mild mass effect. (E) Routine surveillance imaging at 10 months shows cyst enlargement, remodeling of the skull, and moderate mass effect with right-to-left shift of the brain stem. The patient was asymptomatic, illustrating the importance of surveillance imaging for infants.

KEY REFERENCES

1. Erman T, Demirhindi H, Gocer AI, et al. Congenital peripheral facial palsy associated with cerebellopontine angle arachnoid cyst. *Pediatr Neurosurg*. 2004;40:297-300.
2. Isaacs H Jr. Perinatal (fetal and neonatal) germ cell tumors. *J Pediatr Surg*. 2004;39:1003-1013.
3. Isaacs H II. Perinatal brain tumors: a review of 250 cases. *Pediatr Neurol*. 2002;27:333-342.
4. Isaacs H I. Perinatal brain tumors: a review of 250 cases. *Pediatr Neurol*. 2002;27:249-261.
5. Rickert CH. Neuropathology and prognosis of foetal brain tumours. *Acta Neuropathol*. 1999;98:567-576.
6. Rickert CH, Probst-Cousin S, Gullotta F. Primary intracranial neoplasms of infancy and early childhood. *Childs Nerv Syst*. 1997;13:507-513.
7. Fort DW, Rushing EJ. Congenital central nervous system tumors. *J Child Neurol*. 1997;12:157-164.
8. Wakai S, Arai T, Nagai M. Congenital brain tumors. *Surg Neurol*. 1984;21:597-609.
9. Manoranjan B, Provias JP. Congenital brain tumors: diagnostic pitfalls and therapeutic interventions. *J Child Neurol*. 2011;26:599-614.
12. Bergsagel DJ, Finegold MJ, Butel JS, et al. DNA sequences similar to those of simian virus 40 in ependymomas and choroid plexus tumors of childhood. *N Engl J Med*. 1992;326(15):988-993.
13. Pajtler KW, Witt H, Sill M, et al. Molecular classification of ependymal tumors across all CNS compartments, histopathological grades, and age groups. *Cancer Cell*. 2015;27:728-743.
14. Torchia J, Picard D, Lafay-Cousin L, et al. Molecular subgroups of atypical teratoid rhabdoid tumours in children: an integrated genomic and clinicopathological analysis. *Lancet Oncol*. 2015;16:569-582.
15. Haberler C, Laggner U, Slavc I, et al. Immunohistochemical analysis of INI1 protein in malignant pediatric CNS tumors: lack of INI1 in atypical teratoid/rhabdoid tumors and in a fraction of primitive neuroectodermal tumors without rhabdoid phenotype. *Am J Surg Pathol*. 2006;30:1462-1468.
16. Bourdeaut F, Lequin D, Brugieres L, et al. Frequent hSNF5/INI1 germline mutations in patients with rhabdoid tumor. *Clin Cancer Res*. 2011;17:31-38.
17. Tabori U, Shlien A, Baskin B, et al. TP53 alterations determine clinical subgroups and survival of patients with choroid plexus tumors. *J Clin Oncol*. 2010;28:1995-2001.
18. Watanabe Y, Shido K, Niihori T, et al. Somatic BRAF c.1799T>A p.V600E Mosaicism syndrome characterized by a linear syringocystadenoma papilliferum, anaplastic astrocytoma, and ocular abnormalities. *Am J Med Genet*. 2016;170A:189-194.
19. Rickert CH, Probst-Cousin S, Louwen F, et al. Congenital immature teratoma of the fetal brain. *Childs Nerv Syst*. 1997;13:556-559.
20. Erman T, Gocer IA, Erdogan S, et al. Congenital intracranial immature teratoma of the lateral ventricle: a case report and review of the literature. *Neurol Res*. 2005;27:53-56.
24. Haddad SF, Menezes AH, Bell WE, et al. Brain tumors occurring before 1 year of age: a retrospective review of 22 cases in an 11-year period (1977–1987). *Neurosurgery*. 1991;29:8-13.
25. Kumar R, Tekkok IH, Jones RA. Intracranial tumours in the first 18 months of life. *Childs Nerv Syst*. 1990;6:371-374.
26. DiRocco C, Iannelli A, Ceddia A. Intracranial tumors of the first year of life. *Childs Nerv Syst*. 1991;7:150-153.
27. Galassi E, Godano U, Cavallo M, et al. Intracranial tumors during the 1st year of life. *Childs Nerv Syst*. 1989;5:288-298.
30. Sherer DM, Abramowicz JS, Eggers PC, et al. Prenatal ultrasonographic diagnosis of intracranial teratoma and massive craniomegaly with associated high-output cardiac failure. *Am J Obstet Gynecol*. 1993;168:97-99.
31. Anderson DR, Falcone S, Bruce JH, et al. Radiologic-pathologic correlation congenital choroid plexus papillomas. *AJNR Am J Neuroradiol*. 1995;16:2072-2076.
32. DiRocco C, Iannelli A. Poor outcome of bilateral congenital choroid plexus papillomas with extreme hydrocephalus. *Eur Neurol*. 1997;37:33-37.
33. Costa JM, Ley L, Claramunt E, et al. Choroid plexus papillomas of the III ventricle in infants—report of three cases. *Childs Nerv Syst*. 1997;13:244-249.
34. Narita T, Kurotaki H, Hashimoto T, et al. Congenital oligodendroglioma: a case report of a 34th-gestational week fetus with immunohistochemical study and review of the literature. *Hum Pathol*. 1997;28:1213-1217.
35. Chien Y-H, Tsao P-N, Lee W-T, et al. Congenital intracranial teratoma. *Pediatr Neurol*. 2000;22:72-74.
36. Mazouni C, Porcu-Buisson G, Girard N, et al. Intrauterine brain teratoma: a case report of imaging (US, MRI) with neuropathologic correlations. *Prenat Diagn*. 2003;23:104-107.
37. Purdy E, Johnston DL, Bartels U, et al. Ependymoma in children under the age of 3 years: a report from the Canadian Pediatric Brain Tumour Consortium. *J Neuro-oncol*. 2014;117:359-364.
38. Barth PG, Stam FC, Hack W, et al. Gliomatosis cerebri in a newborn. *Neuropediatrics*. 1988;19:197-200.
39. Brat DJ, Shehata BM, Castellano-Sanchez AA, et al. Congenital glioblastoma: a clinicopathologic and genetic analysis. *Brain Pathol*. 2007;17:276-281.
40. Gabel BC, Yoon J, Levy ML, et al. A diffuse intrinsic pontine glioma in a neonate diagnosed by MRI. *BMJ Case Rep*. 2014;2014.
41. Hahn JS, Bejar R, Gladson CL. Neonatal subependymal giant cell astrocytoma associated with tuberous sclerosis: MRI, CT, and ultrasound correlation. *Neurology*. 1991;41:124-128.
42. Kotulska K, Borkowska J, Mandera M, et al. Congenital subependymal giant cell astrocytomas in patients with tuberous sclerosis complex. *Child's Nerv Syst*. 2014;30:2037-2042.
43. Macy ME, Birks DK, Barton VN, et al. Clinical and molecular characteristics of congenital glioblastoma. *Neuro Oncol*. 2012;14:931-941.
44. Oikawa S, Sakamoto K, Kobayashi N. A neonatal huge subependymal giant cell astrocytoma: case report. *Neurosurgery*. 1994;35:748-750.
45. Roosen N, Deckert M, Nicola N, et al. Congenital anaplastic astrocytoma with favorable prognosis. *J Neurosurg*. 1988;69:604-609.
47. Winters JL, Wilson D, Davis DG. Congenital glioblastoma multiforme: a report of three cases and a review of the literature. *J Neurol Sci*. 2001;188:13-19.
48. Zaky W, Dhall G, Khatua S, et al. Choroid plexus carcinoma in children: the head start experience. *Pediatr Blood Cancer*. 2015;62:784-789.
49. McGovern SL, Grosshans D, Mahajan A. Embryonal brain tumors. *Cancer J*. 2014;20:397-402.
50. Dudley RW, Torok MR, Gallegos D, et al. Pediatric choroid plexus tumors: epidemiology, treatments, and outcome analysis on 202 children from the SEER database. *J Neuro-oncol*. 2015;121:201-207.
51. Johnson DL. Management of choroid plexus tumors in children. *Pediatr Neurosci*. 1989;15:195-206.
53. Tomita T, McLone DG, Flannery AM. Choroid plexus papillomas of neonates, infants and children. *Pediatr Neurosci*. 1988;14:23-30.
54. Manjila S, Ray A, Hu Y, et al. Embryonal tumors with abundant neuropil and true rosettes: 2 illustrative cases and a review of the literature. *Neurosurg Focus*. 2011;30:E2.
55. Alghamdi S, Castellano-Sanchez A, Brathwaite C, et al. Strong desmin expression in a congenital desmoplastic infantile ganglioglioma mimicking pleomorphic rhabdomyosarcoma: a case report including ultrastructural and cytogenetic evaluation and review of the literature. *Child's Nerv Syst*. 2012;28:2157-2162.
56. Gelabert-Gonzalez M, Serramito-Garcia R, Arcos-Algaba A. Desmoplastic infantile and non-infantile ganglioglioma. Review of the literature. *Neurosurg Rev*. 2010;34:151-158.
57. Rout P, Santosh V, Mahadevan A, et al. Desmoplastic infantile ganglioglioma—clinicopathological and immunohistochemical study of four cases. *Child's Nerv Syst*. 2002;18:463-467.
58. Trehan G, Bruge H, Vinchon M, et al. MR imaging in the diagnosis of desmoplastic infantile tumor: retrospective study of six cases. *AJNR Am J Neuroradiol*. 2004;25:1028-1033.
59. Jurkiewicz E, Grajkowska W, Nowak K, et al. MR imaging, apparent diffusion coefficient and histopathological features of desmoplastic infantile tumors-own experience and review of the literature. *Child's Nerv Syst*. 2015;31:251-259.
60. Kralik SF, Taha A, Kamer AP, et al. Diffusion imaging for tumor grading of supratentorial brain tumors in the first year of life. *AJNR Am J Neuroradiol*. 2014;35:815-823.
61. Bader A, Heran M, Dunham C, et al. Radiological features of infantile glioblastoma and desmoplastic infantile tumors: British

Columbia's Children's Hospital experience. *J Neurosurg Pediatr.* 2015;16:119-125.

62. Chadduck WM, Boop FA, Blankenship JB, et al. Meningioma and sagittal craniosynostosis in an infant: case report. *Neurosurgery.* 1992;30:441-442.

63. Hurst RW, McIlhenny J, Park TS, et al. Neonatal craniopharyngioma: CT and ultrasonographic features. *J Comput Assist Tomogr.* 1988;12:858-861.

64. Richmond BK, Schmidt JH. Congenital cystic supratentorial hemangioblastoma—case report. *J Neurosurg.* 1995;82:113-115.

65. Hundt C, Auberger K, Munch G, et al. Brain hemangiomas of infancy. *J Neuroimag.* 1997;7:81-85.

66. Oexle K, Dammann O, Bechmann B, et al. Intracranial chordoma in a neonate. *Eur J Pediatr.* 1992;151:336-338.

67. Alfonso I, Lopez PF, Cullen RF, et al. Spinal cord involvement in encephalocranio-cutaneous lipomatosis. *Pediatr Neurol.* 1986;2:380-384.

68. Painter MJ, Pang D, Ahdab-Barmada M, et al. Connatal brain tumors in patients with tuberous sclerosis. *Neurosurgery.* 1984;14:570-573.

69. Boechat MI, Kangarloo H, Diament MJ, et al. Lipoma of the corpus callosum: sonographic appearance. *J Clin Ultrasound.* 1983;11:447-448.

70. Wakai S, Nakamura K, Arai T, et al. Extracerebral neural tissue mass in the middle cranial fossa extending into the oropharynx in a neonate. *J Neurosurg.* 1983;59:692-696.

71. Saxonhouse MA, Yachnis AT, Burchfield DJ, et al. Neonatal hypothalamic hamartoma: a differentiating nonlethal hamartoblastoma. *J Neurosurg.* 2005;103:277-281.

72. Thompson WD Jr, Kosnik EJ. Spontaneous regression of a diffuse brainstem lesion in the neonate. Report of two cases and review of the literature. *J Neurosurg.* 2005;102:65-71.

73. Goyer I, Dahdah N, Major P. Use of mTOR inhibitor everolimus in three neonates for treatment of tumors associated with tuberous sclerosis complex. *Pediatr Neurol.* 2015;52:450-453.

74. Hwang SW, Su JM, Jea A. Diagnosis and management of brain and spinal cord tumors in the neonate. *Semin Fetal Neonat Med.* 2012;17:202-206.

75. Jooma R, Kendall BE, Hayward RD. Intracranial tumors in neonates: a report of seventeen cases. *Surg Neurol.* 1984;21:165-170.

76. Rutledge SL, Snead OC, Morawetz R, et al. Brain tumors presenting as a seizure disorder in infants. *J Child Neurol.* 1987;2:214-219.

77. Ellams ID, Neuhauser G, Agnoli AL. Congenital intracranial neoplasms. *Childs Nerv Syst.* 1986;2:165-168.

78. Asai A, Hoffman HJ, Hendrick EB, et al. Primary intracranial neoplasms in the first year of life. *Childs Nerv Syst.* 1989;5:230-233.

79. Venes JL. A proposal for management of congenital brain tumors. In: Marlin AE, ed. *Concepts in Pediatric Neurosurgery.* Vol. 6. Basal, Switzerland: S Karger; 1985:25-36.

80. Shafrir Y, Kaufman BA. Quadriplegia after chiropractic manipulation in an infant with congenital torticollis caused by a spinal cord astrocytoma. *J Pediatr.* 1992;120:266-269.

81. Pascual-Castroviejo I. Congenital tumors or malformations. In: Pascual-Castroviejo I, ed. *Spinal Tumors in Children and Adolescents.* New York: Raven Press; 1990.

82. Pillai S, Metrie M, Dunham C, et al. Intracranial tumors in infants: long-term functional outcome, survival, and its predictors. *Child's Nerv Syst.* 2012;28:547-555.

83. Kaufman BA, Park TS. Congenital spinal cord astrocytomas. *Child's Nerv Syst.* 1992;8:389-393.

84. Sandbank U. Congenital astrocytoma. *J Pathol Bact.* 1962;84:226.

85. Severino M, Schwartz ES, Thurnher MM, et al. Congenital tumors of the central nervous system. *Neuroradiology.* 2010;52:531-548.

86. Harmon BH, Yap MA. One-month-old infant with increasing head size. In: Brogdon BG, ed. *Cases from A^3CR^2.* Philadelphia: JB Lippincott; 1990.

87. Barkovich AJ. *Pediatric Neuroimaging.* 4th ed. Philadelphia: Lippincott Williams & Wilkins; 2005.

88. Cohen ME, Duffner PK. Brain tumors in children less than 2 years of age. In: Familusi J, Fukuyama Y, eds. *Brain Tumors in Children.* New York: Raven Press; 1984:245.

89. Ventureyra ECG, Herder S. Neonatal intracranial teratoma. *J Neurosurg.* 1983;59:879.

90. Qaddoumi I, Carey SS, Conklin H, et al. Characterization, treatment, and outcome of intracranial neoplasms in the first 120 days of life. *J Child Neurol.* 2011;26:988-994.

91. Rivera-Luna R, Medina-Sanson A, Leal-Leal C, et al. Brain tumors in children under 1 year of age: emphasis on the relationship of prognostic factors. *Child's Nerv Syst.* 2003;19:311-314.

92. Lundar T, Due-Tonnessen BJ, Egge A, et al. Neurosurgical treatment of brain tumors in the first 6 months of life: long-term follow-up of a single consecutive institutional series of 30 patients. *Child's Nerv Syst.* 2015;31:2283-2290.

93. Geyer JR, Sposto R, Jennings M, et al. Multiagent chemotherapy and deferred radiotherapy in infants with malignant brain tumors: a report from the Children's Cancer Group. *J Clin Oncol.* 2005;23:7621-7631.

94. Kalifa C, Grill J. The therapy of infantile malignant brain tumors: current status? *J Neuro-oncol.* 2005;75:279-285.

95. Van Poppel M, Klimo P Jr, Dewire M, et al. Resection of infantile brain tumors after neoadjuvant chemotherapy: the St. Jude experience. *J Neurosurg Pediatr.* 2011;8:251-256.

96. Fukuoka K, Yanagisawa T, Suzuki T, et al. Successful treatment of hemorrhagic congenital intracranial immature teratoma with neoadjuvant chemotherapy and surgery. *J Neurosurg Pediatr.* 2014;13:38-41.

97. Ellenberg L, McComb JG, Siegel SE, et al. Factors affecting intellectual outcome in pediatric brain tumor patients. *Neurosurgery.* 1987;21:638-644.

98. Spunberg JJ, Chang CH, Goldman M, et al. Quality of long-term survival following irradiation for intracranial tumors in children under the age of two. *Int J Radiat Oncol Biol Phys.* 1981;7:727-736.

99. Meadows AT, Massari DJ, Fergusson J, et al. Declines in I.Q. scores and cognitive dysfunctions in children with acute lymphocytic leukaemia treated with cranial irradiation. *Lancet.* 1981;2:1015-1018.

100. Waber DP, Urion DK, Tarbell NJ, et al. Late effects of central nervous system treatment of childhood acute lymphoblastic leukemia are sex-dependent. *Dev Med Child Neurol.* 1990;32:238-248.

101. Waber DP, Gioia G, Paccia J, et al. Sex differences in cognitive processing in children treated with CNS prophylaxis for acute lymphoblastic leukemia (ALL). *J Pediatr Psychol.* 1990;15:105-122.

102. Loeffler JS, Rossitch E, Siddon R, et al. Role of stereotactic radiosurgery with a linear accelerator in treatment of intracranial arteriovenous malformations and tumors in children. *Pediatrics.* 1990;85:774-782.

103. Pollack IF. Brain tumors in children. *N Engl J Med.* 1994;331:1500-1507.

104. Gassas A, Ashraf K, Zaidman I, et al. Hematopoietic stem cell transplantation in infants. *Pediatr Blood Cancer.* 2015;62:517-521.

105. Wisoff JH, Berenstein A, Choi IS, et al. Management of vein of Galen malformations. In: Marlin AE, ed. *Concepts in Pediatric Neurosurgery.* Basal, Switzerland: S Karger; 1990.

106. Hoffman HJ, Chuang S, Hendrick B, et al. Aneurysms of the vein of Galen. *J Neurosurg.* 1982;57:316.

107. Lylyk P, Vinuela F, Dion JE, et al. Therapeutic alternatives for vein of Galen vascular malformations. *J Neurosurg.* 1993;78:438-445.

108. Lasjaunias P. *Vascular Diseases in Neonates, Infants and Children.* Berlin: Springer-Verlag; 1997.

109. Johnston IH, Whittle IR, Besser M, et al. Vein of Galen malformation: diagnosis and management. *Neurosurgery.* 1987;20:747-758.

110. Wagner MW, Vaught AJ, Poretti A, et al. Vein of Galen aneurysmal malformation: prognostic markers depicted on fetal MRI. *Neuroradiol J.* 2015;28:72-75.

111. Raybaud CA, Strother CM, Hald JK. Aneurysms of the vein of Galen: embryonic considerations and anatomical features relating to the pathogenesis of the malformation. *Neuroradiology.* 1989;31:109-128.

112. Gailloud P, O'Riordan DP, Burger I, et al. Diagnosis and management of vein of Galen aneurysmal malformations. *J Perinatol.* 2005;25:542-551.

113. Lasjaunias P, Garcia-Monaco R, Rodesch G, et al. Deep venous drainage in great cerebral vein (vein of Galen) absence and malformations. *Neuroradiology.* 1991;33:234-238.

114. Takashima S, Becker LE. Neuropathology of cerebral arteriovenous malformations in children. *J Neurol Neurosurg Psychiatr*. 1980;43: 380-385.

115. Norman MG, Becker LE. Cerebral damage in neonates resulting from arteriovenous malformations in the vein of Galen. *J Neurol Neurosurg Psychiatr*. 1974;37:252-258.

116. Yamashita Y, Nakamura Y, Okudera T, et al. Neuroradiological and pathological studies on neonatal aneurysmal dilation of the vein of Galen. *J Child Neurol*. 1990;5:45-48.

117. Yamashita Y, Abe T, Ohara N, et al. Successful treatment of neonatal aneurysmal dilation of the vein of Galen: the role of prenatal diagnosis and trans-arterial emboilization. *Neuroradiology*. 1992;34:457-459.

118. Lasjaunias P, Garcia MR, Rodesch G, et al. Vein of Galen malformation. Endovascular management of 43 cases. *Childs Nerv Syst*. 1991;7:360-367.

119. Baenziger O, Martin E, Willi U, et al. Prenatal brain atrophy due to a giant vein of Galen malformation. *Neuroradiology*. 1993; 35:105-106.

120. Horowitz BM, Jungreis CA, Quisling RG, et al. Vein of Galen aneurysms: a review and current perspectivew. *AJNR Am J Neuroradiol*. 1994;15:1486-1496.

121. de Koning TJ, Meijboom EJ, de Vries LS, et al. Arteriovenous malformation of the vein of Galen in three neonates: emphasis on associated early ischaemic brain damage. *Eur J Pediatr*. 1997;156:228-229.

122. Nakano S, Agid R, Klurfan P, et al. Limitations and technical considerations of endovascular treatment in neonates with high-flow arteriovenous shunts presenting with congestive heart failure: report of two cases. *Child's Nerv Syst*. 2006;22:13-17.

123. Wong FY, Mitchell PJ, Tress BM, et al. Hemodynamic disturbances associated with endovascular embolization in newborn infants with vein of Galen malformation. *J Perinatol*. 2006;1-7.

124. Fullerton HJ, Aminoff AR, Ferrierio DM, et al. Neurodevelopmental outcome after endovascular treatment of vein of Galen malformations. *Neurology*. 2003;61:1386-1390.

125. Frawley GP, Dargaville PA, Mitchell PJ, et al. Clinical course and medical management of neonates with severe cardiac failure related to vein of Galen malformation. *Arch Dis Child*. 2002;87:F144-F149.

126. Grillner P, Soderman M, Holmin S, et al. A spectrum of intracranial vascular high-flow arteriovenous shunts in RASA1 mutations. *Child's Nerv Syst*. 2016;32:709-715.

127. Hirano A, Solomon S. Arteriovenous aneurysm of the vein of Galen. *Arch Neurol*. 1960;3:589.

128. Gomez MR, Shitten CF, Nolke A. Aneurysmal malformation of the great vein of Galen causing heart failure in early infancy. Report of five cases. *Pediatrics*. 1963;31:400-411.

129. Watson DG, Smith RR, Brann AW. Arteriovenous malformation of the vein of Galen. *Am J Dis Child*. 1976;130:520.

130. Iannucci AM, Buonanno F, Rizzuto N. Arteriovenous aneurysm of the vein of Galen. *J Neurol Sci*. 1979;40:29.

131. Schum TR, Meyer GA, Grausz JP, et al. Neonatal intracranial ventricular hemorrhage due to an intracranial arteriovenous malformation: a case report. *Pediatrics*. 1979;64:242.

132. O'Donnabhain D, Duff DF. Aneurysms of the vein of Galen. *Arch Dis Child*. 1989;64:1612-1617.

133. Rodesch G, Hui F, Alvarez H, et al. Prognosis of antenatally diagnosed vein of Galen aneurysmal malformations. *Childs Nerv Syst*. 1994;10:79-83.

134. Lasjaunias PL, Alvarez H, Rodesch G, et al. Aneurysmal malformations of the vein of Galen. *Interven Neuroradiol*. 1996;2: 15-26.

135. Friedman DM, Verma R, Madrid M, et al. Recent improvement in outcome using transcatheter embolization techniques for neonatal aneurysmal malformations of the vein of Galen. *Pediatrics*. 1993;91:583-586.

136. Meyers PM, Halbach VV, Phatouros CP, et al. Hemorrhagic complications in vein of Galen malformations. *Ann Neurol*. 2000;47:748-755.

137. Mullaart RA, Daniels O, Hopman JCW. Ultrasound detection of congenital arteriovenous aneurysm of the great cerebral vein of Galen. *Eur J Pediatr*. 1982;139:195.

138. Schwechheimer K, Kuhl G. Arteriovenous angioma of the vein of Galen causing cardiac failure in the neonate. *Neuropediatrics*. 1983;14:184.

139. Cubberley DA, Jaffe RB, Nixon GW. Sonographic demonstration of galenic arteriovenous malformations in the neonate. *AJNR Am J Neuroradiol*. 1982;3:435-439.

140. Langer R, Kaufmann HJ. Arteriovenous malformation of the great cerebral vein of Galen in a newborn. *Eur J Pediatr*. 1987;146:87-89.

141. Abbitt PL, Hurst RW, Ferguson RDG, et al. The role of ultrasound in the management of vein of Galen aneurysms in infancy. *Neuroradiology*. 1990;32:86-89.

142. Deeg KH, Scharf J. Colour Doppler imaging of arteriovenous malformation of the vein of Galen in a newborn. *Neuroradiology*. 1990;32:60-63.

143. Vaksmann G, Decoulx E, Mauran P, et al. Evaluation of vein of Galen arteriovenous malformations in newborns by two dimensional ultrasound, pulsed and colour Doppler method. *Eur J Pediatr*. 1989;148:510-512.

144. Tessler FN, Dion J, Vinuela F, et al. Cranial arteriovenous malformations in neonates: color Doppler imaging with angiographic correlation. *AJR Am J Radiol*. 1989;153:1027-1030.

145. Meila D, Lisseck K, Jacobs C, et al. Cranial Doppler ultrasound in vein of Galen malformation. *Neuroradiology*. 2015;57:211-219.

146. Chow ML, Cooke DL, Fullerton HJ, et al. Radiological and clinical features of vein of Galen malformations. *J Neurointervention Surg*. 2015;7:443-448.

147. Khullar D, Andeejani AM, Bulsara KR. Evolution of treatment options for vein of Galen malformations. *J Neurosurg Pediatr*. 2010;6:444-451.

148. McSweeney N, Brew S, Bhate S, et al. Management and outcome of vein of Galen malformation. *Arch Dis Childhood*. 2010;95(11):903-909.

149. Li AH, Armstrong D, terBrugge KG. Endovascular treatment of vein of Galen aneurysmal malformation: management strategy and 21-year experience in Toronto. *J Neurosurg Pediatr*. 2011;7:3-10.

150. Berenstein A, Fifi JT, Niimi Y, et al. Vein of Galen malformations in neonates: new management paradigms for improving outcomes. *Neurosurgery*. 2012;70:1207-1213. discussion 1213-1214.

151. McCord FB, Shields MD, McNeil A, et al. Cerebral arteriovenous malformation in a neonate: treatment by embolisation. *Arch Dis Child*. 1987;62:1273-1275.

152. King WA, Wackym PA, Vinuela F, et al. Management of vein of Galen aneurysms. Combined surgical and endovascular approach. *Childs Nerv Syst*. 1989;5:208-211.

153. Miller VS, Roach ES. Embolization and radiosurgical treatment of cerebral arteriovenous malformations. *Int Pediatr*. 1992;7:173-180.

154. Swanstrom S, Flodmark O, Lasjaunias P. Conditions for treatment of cerebral arteriovenous malformation associated with ectasia of the vein of Galen in the newborn. *Acta Paediatr*. 1994;83:255-257.

155. Harding BN, Surtees R. Metabolic and neurodegenerative diseases of childhood. In: Graham DI, Lantos PL, eds. *Greenfield's Neuropathology*. Vol. 1. 7th ed. London: Arnold Publishers; 2002: 485-517.

156. Gosalakkal JA. Intracranial arachnoid cysts in children: a review of pathogenesis, clinical features, and management. *Pediatr Neurol*. 2002;26:93-98.

157. Germano A, Caruso G, Caffo M, et al. The treatment of large supratentorial arachnoid cysts in infants with cyst-peritoneal shunting and Hakim programmable valve. *Child's Nerv Syst*. 2003;19:166-173.

158. Arriola G, Castro P, Verdu A. Familial arachnoid cysts. *Pediatr Neurol*. 2005;33:146-148.

159. Balsubramaniam C, Laurent J, Rouah E, et al. Congenital arachnoid cysts in children. *Pediatr Neurosci*. 1989;15:223-228.

160. Lee JY, Kim JW, Phi JH, et al. Enlarging arachnoid cyst: a false alarm for infants. *Child's Nerv Syst*. 2012;28:1203-1211.

Full references for for this chapter can be found at www.expertconsult .com.

DRUGS AND THE DEVELOPING NERVOUS SYSTEM

Passive Addiction and Teratogenic Effects

Lianne J. Woodward ◆ Christopher C. McPherson ◆ Joseph J. Volpe

Drugs can exert major effects on the developing central nervous system (CNS). In the broadest sense, drugs may disturb specific developmental events in the brain and, in turn, produce teratogenic effects. In addition, maternal ingestion of certain drugs can result in passive addiction of the fetus, and postnatally lead to a neonatal withdrawal or abstinence syndrome. The capacity for teratogenicity was first recognized in the late 1950s and early 1960s with the recognition of the adverse effects of thalidomide. Believed to be safe, thalidomide was prescribed to large numbers of pregnant women as a treatment for morning sickness but was later found to result in a number of birth defects. The most notable of these was phocomelia, in which the bones of the arms and, in some cases, other limbs were extremely shortened or absent.[1] With this medical tragedy came an increased awareness of the potential teratogenic risks of fetal exposure to prescribed and recreational drugs.

Evidence suggests that prenatal exposure to both licit and illicit drugs can have short-term and long-lasting effects on the structure and function of the developing CNS. These effects vary in severity, from profound effects on morphological structure to more subtle, but nonetheless clinically significant, neurological effects. Some of the latter may include a striking neonatal abstinence syndrome (NAS) or include a range of neonatal neurobehavioral difficulties (Table 38.1). Further, few of these effects are transient, with most persisting in some form into childhood and adolescence. Multiple systems are often affected spanning cognition, motor function, language, and behavior. Fig. 38.1 provides a conceptual overview of the factors and processes involved in the effects of drug exposure in utero on child neurological development.

MAJOR FACTORS INVOLVED IN NEUROLOGIC DISTURBANCES ASSOCIATED WITH INTRAUTERINE DRUG EXPOSURE

Almost all drugs unbound to protein move freely across the placenta, enter the fetal bloodstream, and can affect fetal brain development, either directly or indirectly (Fig. 38.2). The direct effects of a drug on the developing brain will vary depending on the type of drug, the gestational timing of exposure, dose, the extent of drug distribution, and the number of drugs. The developmental stage of the fetus at the time of exposure as well as the sensitivity of different brain regions to different chemical agents also likely play a role. For prescribed drugs, information about timing and extent of exposure is typically known, whereas for alcohol and other illicit drugs, such information is harder

to obtain accurately, thereby posing additional challenges for clinical assessment and diagnosis.

In addition to these direct effects, drugs can have indirect effects on fetal brain development via their impact on other organ and physiological systems. Numerous drugs impact fetal blood flow and nutritional exposure. For example, cocaine impairs fetal oxygen and nutrient transfer via profound vasoconstriction of the umbilical vein. Acutely, these alterations may contribute to cerebral infarction and intracranial hemorrhage. Chronically, these perturbations may contribute to the documented impact of cocaine on cortical neuronal migration and differentiation.

It is also increasingly recognized that maternal and fetal genotypes may interact with a drug exposure to determine phenotypic effects (Fig. 38.1). Functional polymorphisms in alcohol metabolism may best exemplify this phenomenon. The offspring of individuals with normal metabolism experience long-term impacts from in utero alcohol exposure, whereas the offspring of rapid metabolizers avoid these effects.[2] Fetal genetic susceptibility has also been observed, with concordance in the manifestations of fetal alcohol spectrum disorder (FASD) between monozygotic twins but not dizygotic twins. Finally, there is also growing evidence to suggest epigenetic influences on outcome.[3] These epigenetic modifications may even be transgenerational, placing subsequent generations at increased risk of drug dependence, even in the absence of direct exposure during gestation.

In addition to these drug- and infant-related factors, several other maternal and environmental factors may play a role in determining the clinical presentation of an infant and are therefore important to consider. Comorbid physical and mental health conditions in the mother, combined with the underlying disease state, may complicate the interpretation of prenatal drug effects and exacerbate risks for the infant. In addition, maternal life style factors, such as pregnancy, nutrition, and social disadvantage, which are correlated with substance use, may also contribute to later risks, including poor growth and neurodevelopmental impairment.

DEVELOPMENTAL CONSEQUENCES FOR THE INFANT

As a result of the various factors noted previously, considerable heterogeneity in the nature and severity of outcomes may be observed, including death, malformations, neurodevelopmental disability, and impaired neurobehavioral functioning (see Table 38.1). A distinction can also be made between drugs that are associated with congenital malformations in the newborn infant

TABLE 38.1   Nature of Outcomes Related to Intrauterine Drug Exposure

OUTCOME	ALCOHOL	AEDs	STIMULANTS	OPIOIDS	SSRIs	MARIJUANA
Congenital malformations	X	X				
Neonatal abstinence	X	X	X	X	X	
Newborn neurobehavioral difficulties	X		X	X	X	X
Global cognitive deficits/delay	X	X				
Executive function						X
Language problems	X	X				X
Attention problems	X		X			X
Externalizing problems	X					
Internalizing problems						X

AEDs, Antiepileptic drugs; *SSRIs,* selective serotonin reuptake inhibitors.

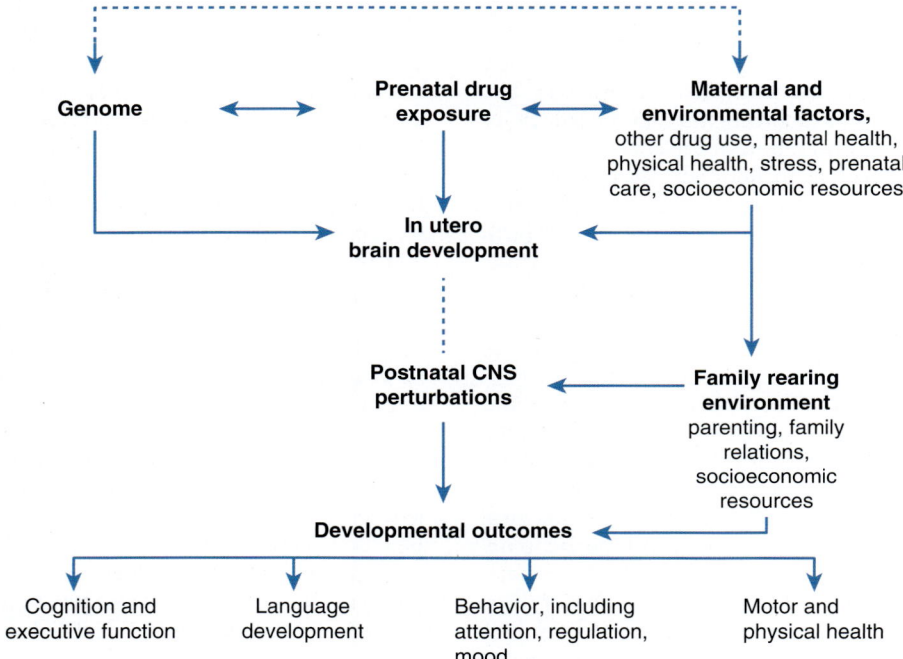

Figure 38.1 Schematic model of factors involved in the effects of drug exposure in utero on child neurological developmental outcome. *CNS,* Central nervous system.

versus those that have more subtle but nonetheless clinically significant neurobehavioral effects, with or without withdrawal symptoms that may require medical management (Table 38.2). In the following, we discuss fetal exposure to alcohol, antiepileptic drugs (AEDs), stimulants, opioids, selective serotonin reuptake inhibitors (SSRIs), sedatives, anesthetics, and marijuana.

ALCOHOL

FASD includes a range of possible diagnoses that may result from a woman drinking alcohol during pregnancy. These diagnoses, which vary in the severity of later abnormalities or impairment, include fetal alcohol syndrome (FAS), partial FAS, alcohol-related birth defects (ARBDs), alcohol-related neurodevelopmental disorder (ARND), and neurobehavioral disorder associated with prenatal alcohol exposure (ND-PAE). At the severe end of the spectrum is the clinical diagnosis

of FAS, which was first described in 1968 by Lemoine and colleagues and then reported in further detail by Jones and colleagues.[4-6] This disorder refers to a specific constellation of neural and extraneural anomalies that include abnormal facial features (Fig. 38.3), poor body growth, and CNS abnormalities that are in turn associated with later cognitive, learning, and behavioral impairments.[7,8] However, even in the absence of the full features of FAS, it is now also recognized that prenatal alcohol exposure can result in a range of less pronounced dysmorphic, cognitive, and behavioral effects of varying severity, termed *fetal alcohol effects* (with terminology noted previously).[9]

Prevalence

The prevalence of maternal alcohol use during pregnancy and FASD varies with the drinking patterns of a population. The accurate estimation of these rates is hindered by a number of methodological problems. These include (1) reliance on

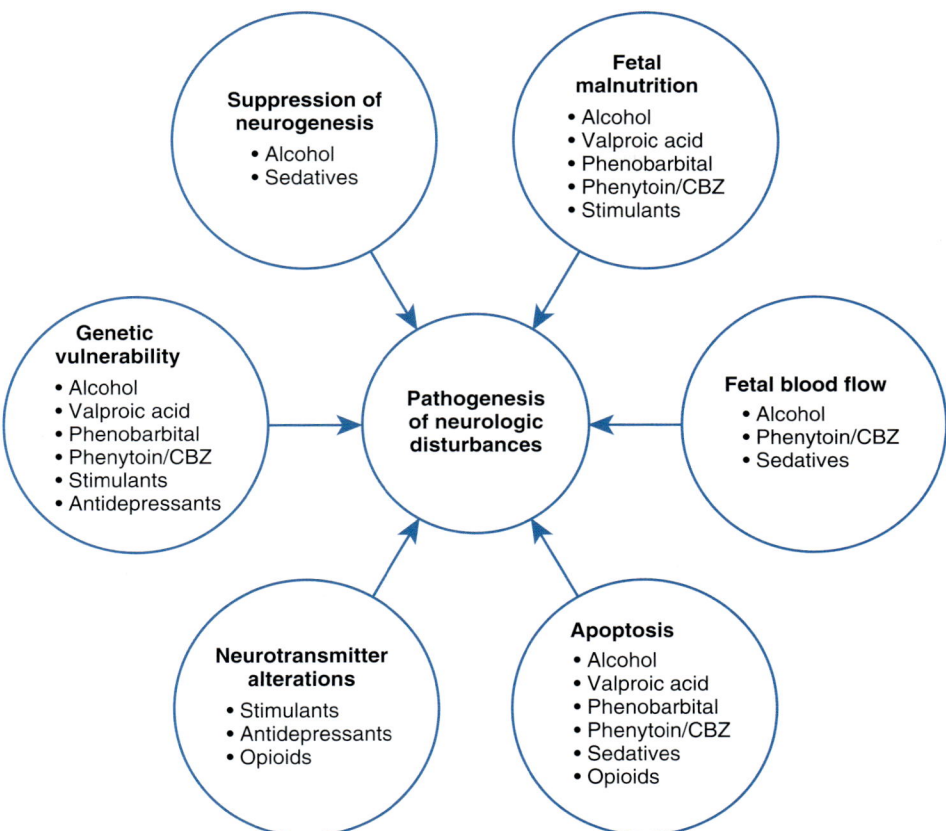

Figure 38.2 Pathogenesis of neurologic disturbances from intrauterine drug exposure. *CBZ,* Carbamazepine.

TABLE 38.2	Major Drugs Associated With Teratogenic Effects, Congenital Malformations, and Neonatal Neurobehavioral Effects

Teratogenic effects
Alcohol
Antiepileptic drugs such as valproate, hydantoins, barbiturates, and carbamazepine
Stimulants (cocaine, amphetamines)
Neonatal neurobehavioral effects (including neonatal abstinence syndrome)
Stimulants (cocaine, amphetamines)
Opioids
Selective serotonin reuptake inhibitors
Benzodiazepines

---

maternal recall and underreporting due to stigma and a fear of potential punitive consequences; (2) limitations of toxicological measures, such as urine and meconium; and (3) differences in the diagnostic criteria used to define FAS and FASD.[10-12] Nonetheless, findings generally suggest that in the United States, approximately one-half of all women of childbearing age report having consumed alcohol in the past month, with 15% likely to have had a binge-drinking episode, defined as more than five standard alcoholic drinks on at least one occasion. Although most women reduce their alcohol intake during pregnancy, 8% to 11% continue to drink and 1% to 2% binge drink.[13] Even higher rates of drinking during pregnancy are reported in the United Kingdom, Ireland, Australia, and New Zealand, with prevalence estimates ranging from 20% to 80%.[14] Importantly, these rates were pervasive across all social groups. Finally, one of the most affected regions of the world is Africa, where binge drinking is reported by around one in four women, and in some cases half of all pregnant women.[15-17]

The prevalence of FAS in the United States ranges from 6 to 9 cases per 1000 live births in the general population, with the risk increasing to 1% to 2% for infants from socioeconomically disadvantaged families and infants in foster care.[18,19] Rates of FASD, which are more common but harder to detect because of their more subtle presentation, are even higher in the United States, ranging from 24 to 48 cases per 1000 live births or up to 5% of all live-born infants.[20,21] A lower rate of FASD was found in Alberta, Canada (8.2 to 15.1 cases per 1000 live births),[22] whereas a similar rate was reported for Lazio, Italy (20.3 to 40.5 cases per 1000 live births).[23] Current rates in the United Kingdom are not available. It is important to note that these rates are widely regarded to *underestimate the extent of this problem* for the methodological reasons listed previously, as well as difficulties with both misdiagnosis and underdiagnosis.

Clinical Features

The diagnostic features of FAS are distinctive and include growth disturbance, characteristic facial anomalies, and neurological

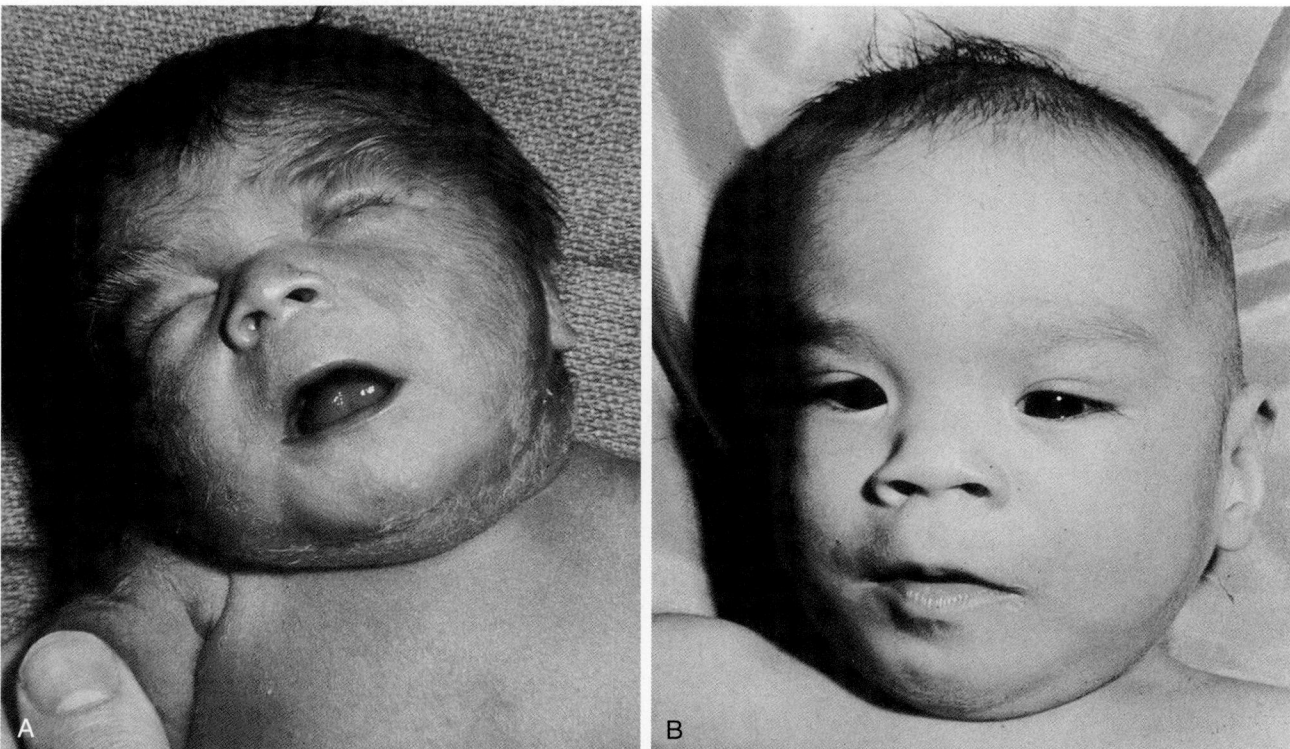

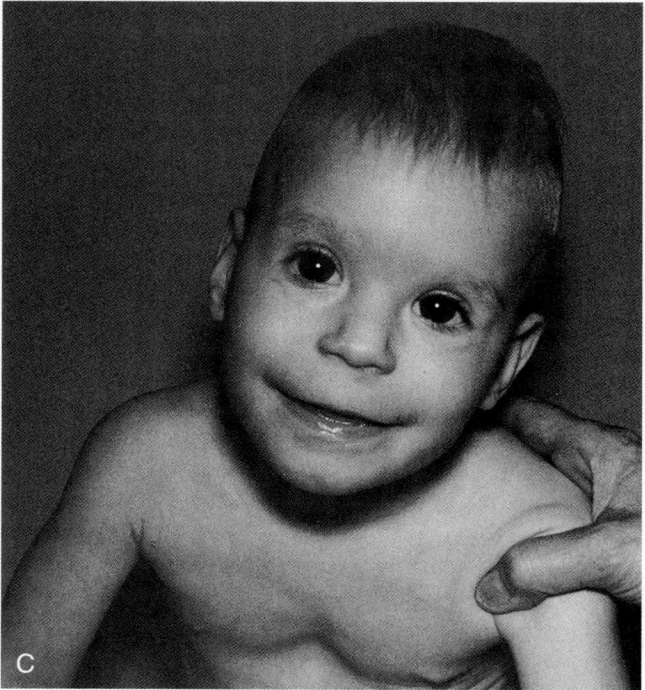

Figure 38.3 Fetal alcohol syndrome: clinical appearance. Two children: one (A) in the newborn period and (B) at the age of 6 months, and (C) the other at the age of 16 months. Note the short palpebral fissures, especially prominent in the newborn (A), and the low nasal bridge with short, upturned nose, epicanthal folds, long, hypoplastic philtrum, and convex upper lip with narrow vermilion border. (A and B, From Jones KL, Smith DW. Recognition of the fetal alcohol syndrome in early infancy. *Lancet.* 1973;2:999–1001; C, from Hanson JW, Jones KL, Smith DW. Fetal alcohol syndrome: experience with 41 patients. *JAMA.* 1976;235:1458–1460.)

abnormalities.[9,21,24,25] Growth disturbance is the hallmark of the disorder, with microcephaly present in nearly all cases. At birth, infants have a distinct pattern of growth restriction, with length often affected more than weight, which is a pattern different from that expected with intrauterine undernutrition. This poor growth persists postnatally, but weight gain is more disturbed than linear growth.

For a diagnosis of FAS, three criteria must be met: (1) *prenatal and/or postnatal growth deficiency*; (2) *the presence of three key facial features—short palpebral fissures, hypoplastic philtrum, and a narrow vermilion lip border* (see Fig. 38.3); and (3) *evidence of structural or functional CNS impairment* (discussed later).[8,9,24,25] Confirmation of prenatal alcohol exposure through maternal report or infant toxicology strengthens, but is not required, for a FAS diagnosis. As with all recreational drugs, it is also important to clarify the extent of prenatal exposure to other drugs, such as tobacco, illicit substances, and any prescribed medications. The possibility of other genetic and environmental conditions that share similar dysmorphic features with FAS (e.g., Williams syndrome, fetal hydantoin syndrome, and trisomy 21) or present at older ages with a similar behavioral phenotype (e.g., attention-deficit/hyperactivity disorder [ADHD]) should also be considered.

In addition to the three previously noted defining criteria, a number of other clinical features may also aid FAS diagnosis (Table 38.3). For example, a variety of limb anomalies can be observed in around one-half of these infants. These include abnormal palmar creases and minor joint abnormalities, such as

an inability to completely extend the elbows, camptodactyly, and clinodactyly. Cardiac lesions occur in approximately one-half, but these lesions are usually not severe and mostly consist of septal defects, with atrial defects more common than ventricular defects. Minor ear anomalies occur in approximately one-fourth of the children, and hearing loss, primarily conductive and of a mild nature, occurs in 75% of infants. Optic nerve hypoplasia affects 75% of infants, but disturbances of visual acuity are not marked. Other less common anomalies include strabismus, ptosis, micrognathia, cleft palate, railroad track ears (prominent horizontal crus of the helix with prominent and parallel inferior crus of the antihelix), decreased elbow pronation/supination, joint contractures (most commonly incomplete extension of one or more digits), and palmar crease abnormalities.[26]

The less severe FASD conditions are more difficult to diagnose because only some of the features are present. For example, ARND requires confirmation of prenatal alcohol exposure and evidence of structural or functional CNS impairment, such as learning and/or behavior problems, but not facial anomalies. When prenatal alcohol exposure is confirmed but all other criteria for FASD are not met, an infant can be described as exhibiting partial FAS or fetal alcohol effects. These diagnoses may be needed to ensure that a child receives ongoing developmental surveillance in view of high rates of neurodevelopmental impairment in children exposed to alcohol in utero.

Neurodevelopmental Consequences

The nature of a child's later neurobehavioral problems and their manifestation varies depending on a number of factors. These include (1) the extent of prenatal alcohol exposure (dose, timing) and the severity of the condition (i.e., FAS or fetal alcohol effects); (2) the presence of other developmental risk factors in the child, mother, or family situation; and (3) the age of the child at the time of evaluation. Genetic factors also likely play a role. Nonetheless, reasonable consensus exists regarding the neurobehavioral profile of children with FASD. These problems span a number of developmental domains, including (1) *cognition and executive impairment*; (2) *language*; (3) *behavioral and regulatory problems, especially ADHD*; and (4) *motor and visuospatial deficits*. The most disabling of these subsequent problems are the intellectual and behavioral impairments. A brief description of the neurobehavioral profile of children with FASD across each impairment domain is provided next.

Cognition and Executive Functioning

Children exposed prenatally to alcohol typically have intelligence quotient (IQ) scores in the low average to borderline range. Children with more dysmorphic features tend to have lower IQ scores, but cognitive problems are not limited to this group.[27] Of those with FAS, around 25% to 50% will experience severe cognitive delay (IQ score <70), with the pooled prevalence of cognitive disability being 97 times higher in infants with FAS than the general population.[28,29] In addition to global cognitive impairment, deficits in executive function and memory are also evident on neuropsychological testing. Executive deficits include problems with planning and organization, cognitive flexibility/set shifting, working memory, and behavioral inhibition, with parents reporting the greatest difficulty with inhibitory control and problem solving.[30-33] In terms of memory deficits, problems encoding or memorizing information appear more

TABLE 38.3	Clinical Features of the Fetal Alcohol Syndrome[a]
CLINICAL FEATURES	**APPROXIMATE FREQUENCY (%)**
Growth	
Prenatal growth deficiency	95
Postnatal deficiency	95%
Central nervous system	
Microcephaly	95
Developmental delay	90
Facial	
Short palpebral fissures	90
Epicanthal folds	50
Midfacial hypoplasia	65
Short, upturned nose	75
Hypoplastic long or smooth philtrum	90
Thin vermilion of upper lip	90
Limb	
Abnormal palmar creases	55
Joint abnormalities	50
Cardiac	
Cardiac defects	50
Other	
Ear anomalies	25
Conductive hearing loss	75
Sensorineural hearing loss	10
Optic nerve hypoplasia	75
External genital anomalies	30
Cutaneous hemangioma	25

[a]See text for references.

Numbers are rounded off to nearest 5%.

prominent than problems with recall.[34] Not surprisingly, given this constellation of cognitive impairments, learning problems are very common at school, even after controlling for IQ.[35,36]

Language Development

Children with FASD are characterized by delays in the acquisition of language and understanding of spoken language. Common difficulties include word comprehension, naming ability, phonological processing, speech production, and articulation errors, resulting in poorer performance on tests of both receptive and expressive language development.[28,29,37]

Behavior and Regulatory Problems

Virtually all infants with FASD exhibit serious attentional and behavioral problems, with 70% subsequently meeting clinical criteria for a diagnosis of ADHD.[35,38,39] The next most common condition is oppositional defiant/conduct disorder, with children with FASD showing less guilt after misbehaving, less behavioral maturity for their age, and higher levels of antisocial behavior, including cruelty and stealing. Longer-term substance abuse and mood disorders, such as anxiety and depression, are also common. For example, relative to the general population, adults with FASD have more hospital admissions for alcohol abuse (9% vs. 2%) and psychiatric disorders (33% vs. 5%), and are also more likely to be prescribed psychotropic medications (57% vs. 27%).[40]

Motor and Visual Function

Finally, deficits in both fine and gross motor development have been reported in children with FASD and include tremors, weak grasp, poor hand-eye coordination, and impaired postural balance.[5,41,42] Visuospatial performance indicates poorer saccadic control, which results in the processing of visual stimuli in a disorganized way.[43]

Neuropathology

The essential nature of the neural disturbance in FASD is an impairment of brain development (Table 38.4). Several aspects of the developmental program appear to be involved, on the basis of neuropathological analysis of brain tissue from children with FAS who died in infancy.[44-51] In keeping with the microcephaly, micrencephaly is common. The most striking additional abnormalities reported appear to involve neuronal and glial migration. Thus, in the series of infants studied by Clarren and colleagues,[44] the most frequent abnormality was a leptomeningeal neuroglial heterotopia that

took the form of a sheet of aberrant neuronal and glial cells covering portions of the cerebral, cerebellar, and brain stem surfaces (Fig. 38.4). Aberrations of brain stem and cerebellar development, in large part related to faulty migration, also have been particularly frequent.[44,45] Schizencephaly and polymicrogyria are other migrational disturbances observed.[45] In addition, disordered midline prosencephalic formation (e.g., agenesis of the corpus callosum, septo-optic dysplasia, and incomplete holoprosencephaly) has been documented.[47,49,51] Other developmental defects have included anencephaly, lumbar meningomyelocele, lumbosacral and sacral meningomyelocele, absent olfactory bulbs or *arrhinencephaly*, and disturbances of dendritic development.[45,48,52,53]

Thus it appears that multiple aspects of CNS development can be affected in severe cases. In chronological order, these include

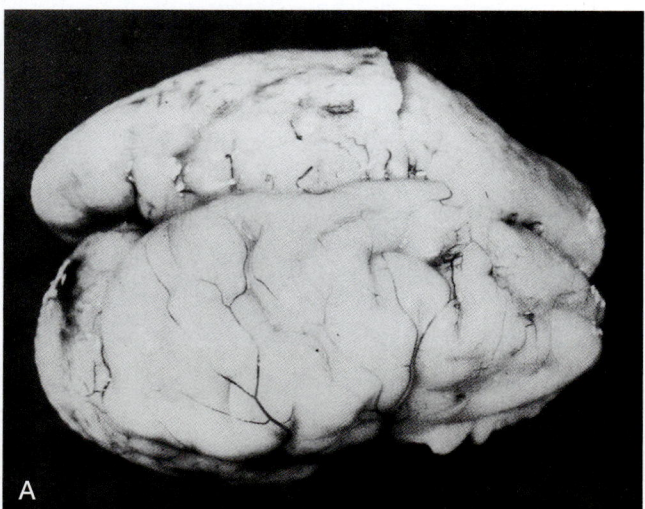

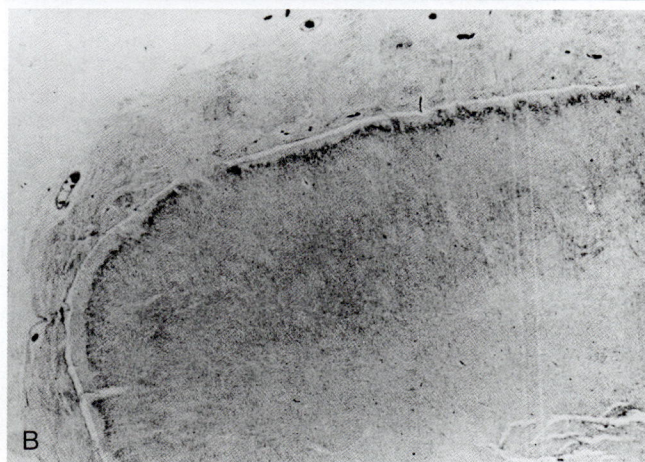

Figure 38.4 Fetal alcohol syndrome: neuropathology. Brain from a 6-week-old infant who was born after a 32-week gestation. (A) Right superolateral view of the cerebrum. Note that nearly all of the left hemisphere is covered by a massive sheet of tissue that crosses the midline and extends onto the superior and medial aspects of the right frontal lobe. (B) Section through the cerebral cortex covered by the aberrant tissue. Extending through a break in the pial surface (upper left of cortex) is the heterotopic sheet of tissue composed of neuronal, glial, and pial elements that have covered the true cortex. (A much smaller break in the pial surface is evident in the *lower left* of the figure.) (From Jones KL, Smith DW. The fetal alcohol syndrome. *Teratology.* 1975;12:1–10.)

TABLE 38.4   Major Neuropathological Features of Fetal Alcohol Syndrome[a]
In order of decreasing frequency:
Micrencephaly
Migrational abnormalities: neuronal > glial
Midline prosencephalic abnormalities: agenesis of the corpus callosum, septo-optic dysplasia, incomplete holoprosencephaly
Dendritic abnormalities
Disorders of neural tube formation

[a]See text for references.

TABLE 38.5 Major Central Nervous System Alterations Defined by Magnetic Resonance Imaging in Fetal Alcohol Spectrum Disorders

- Decreased brain size including lower white and gray matter volumes with enlarged ventricles
- Disproportionately lower cortical volume of parietal, temporal and frontal lobes
- Abnormal corpus callosum: partial or complete agenesis or hypoplasia, splenium most affected
- Decreased volume of basal ganglia, especially caudate nucleus, and hippocampus
- Decreased volume of cerebellum
- Lower fractional anisotropy values in regions showing reduced volume suggesting altered microstructure

neurulation, canalization and retrogressive differentiation, prosencephalic development, neuronal proliferation, neuronal migration, and organizational events (see Chapters 1 to 7). The time periods of the most frequently reported occurrences (i.e., disorders of neuronal proliferation and migration and of midline prosencephalic development) range from the second to the fifth months of gestation, suggesting that teratogens could be acting either during these time periods or, of course, earlier.

Advanced magnetic resonance imaging (MRI) techniques have helped further define the neuropathology of FASD in the human infant (Table 38.5).[54-58] Key findings from studies using different imaging modalities are summarized next. However, it is important to note that almost all studies have been conducted in older children, thus limiting information about structural and functional brain abnormalities during infancy, or the way in which prenatal alcohol exposure affects the developing brain over time and age.[54]

Volumetric MRI studies indicate both global and regional disturbances in cortical and subcortical development, alterations in cortical thickening, and specific regional vulnerability of the corpus callosum, cerebellum, and basal ganglia, especially the caudate nucleus.[54-62] Findings confirm smaller brain size, with both white and gray matter volumes affected.[63-65] In terms of regional abnormalities, a highly consistent finding across studies is the altered shape and area of the corpus callosum, further supporting the vulnerability of midline brain structures to the effects of alcohol. Abnormalities include partial or complete agenesis, underdevelopment, and corpus callosal thinning, particularly in the splenium which is involved in communication between the parietal and temporal lobes.[5,51,66,67] Fig. 38.5 illustrates several examples of corpus callosum abnormalities.[57] These imaging abnormalities have been related to motor function, attention, verbal learning, and executive function.[68-72] Other subcortical structures affected by prenatal alcohol exposure include the cerebellum and caudate nucleus, which may help explain deficits seen in balance, bimanual coordination, memory, and attention among children with FASD.

At the microstructural level, diffusion tensor imaging (DTI) studies indicate that white matter abnormalities also extend to other brain regions beyond the corpus callosum, including the anterior-posterior fiber bundles and the cerebellum.[54,57,73-77] White matter abnormalities have also been seen in the frontal and temporal lobes, as well as several subcortical structures (i.e., globus pallidus, thalamus, and putamen), suggesting more widespread impacts on white matter integrity.[78-81] While these abnormalities may contribute to the attention, executive function, and other neurobehavioral impairments of children with FASD, studies addressing these links are, as of yet, rare and insufficient to draw clear conclusions.

Taken together, these findings suggest prenatal alcohol exposure has global and regional effects on the development of the CNS. These abnormalities appear to reflect both the adverse effects of alcohol on different organizational events during fetal development, but also the cascading effects of early brain abnormalities on brain growth, myelination, and pruning, suggesting an altered trajectory of brain development in children with prenatal alcohol exposure.[81]

Pathogenesis

The pathogenesis of these disturbances of CNS development has been studied in both clinical and experimental models—primarily the latter. Findings indicate that the adverse effects of alcohol and acetaldehyde, its major metabolite, likely result from some combination of (1) effects on fetal blood flow, (2) fetal malnutrition, (3) direct deleterious molecular effects, and (4) genetic/epigenetic alterations within the rapidly developing CNS. A brief review of each of these processes is given in the following sections.

Fetal Blood Flow

Maternal alcohol exposure has a variable impact on uterine blood flow, depending on the gestation of the fetus as well as the pattern of exposure.[82] However, there is converging evidence to suggest that alcohol alters the development of new blood vessels and vascular remodeling, which are both essential to normal uteroplacental circulation during gestation. There is also evidence that alcohol may alter cerebral oxygen and glucose consumption in the fetus near term gestation, but these effects do not appear earlier in gestation.[83,84] Further studies are needed to better understand how alcohol consumption affects uteroplacental hemodynamics during different maturational periods of pregnancy.

Fetal Malnutrition

The quality of maternal nutrition as well as the direct physiologic effects of alcohol on the fetus are also likely involved in the pathogenesis of FASD. Specifically, poor maternal nutritional status and vitamin deficiencies are common comorbidities of chronic alcoholism.[85] Alcohol also interferes directly with the absorption, digestion, and utilization of nutrients. Retinol (vitamin A), folate, and zinc, three nutrients that are important for fetal brain development, have been shown to be directly affected by maternal alcohol use. First, retinoic acid, the oxidized form of retinol, plays a pivotal role in the development of the nervous system as well as limb morphogenesis.[86] Alcohol competitively inhibits the oxidation of retinol in the liver.[87] In mouse models, deficiencies in retinoic acid early in gestation alter the expression of the sonic hedgehog gene, resulting in the classic craniofacial and corpus callosum abnormalities characterizing severe FAS.[88] Second, folic acid has numerous roles in the developing nervous system, especially neural tube closure (see Chapter 1). Alcohol interferes with folic acid absorption, inhibits its metabolism, and increases excretion.[89]

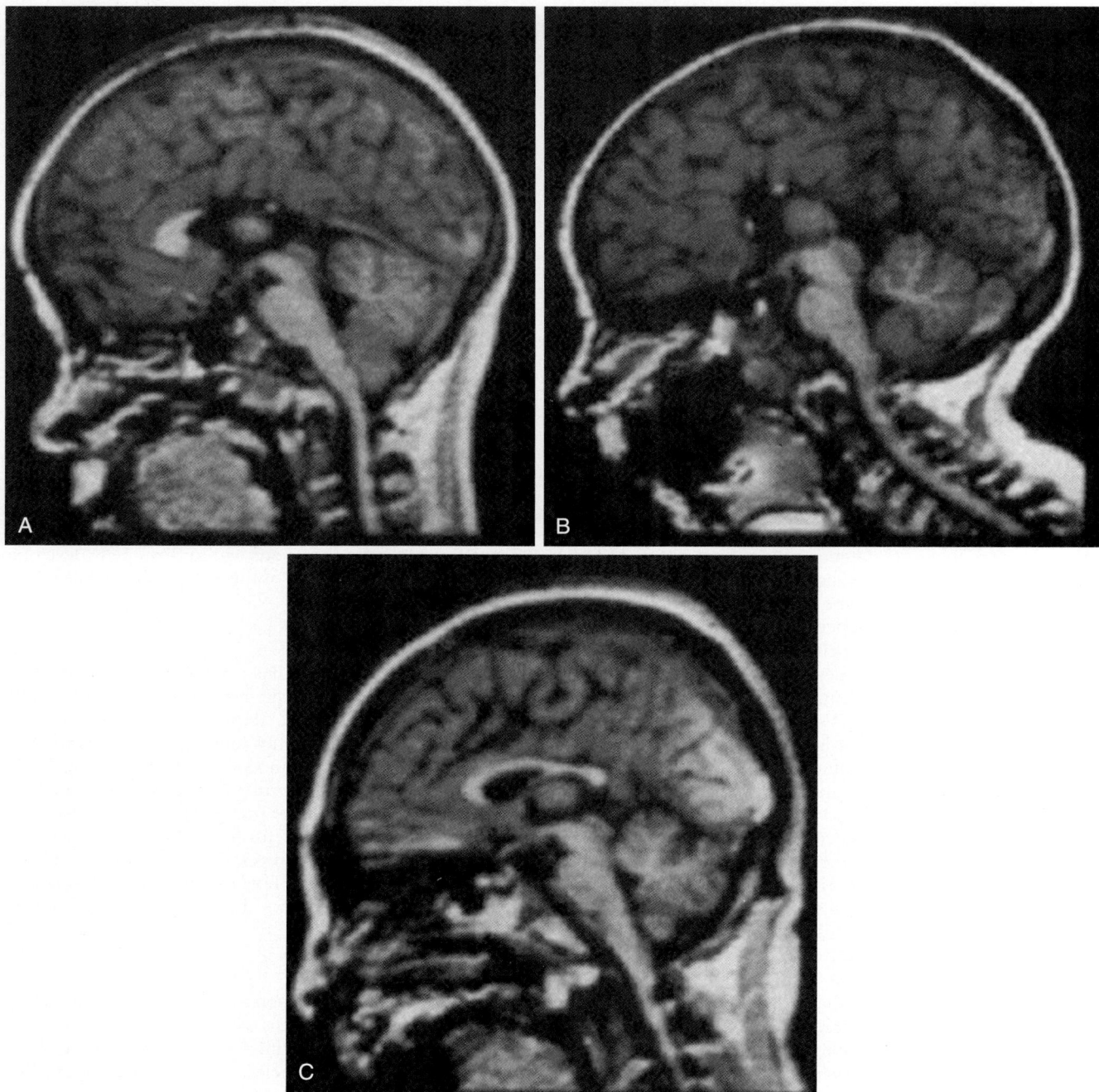

Figure 38.5 Corpus callosum abnormalities in newborns with prenatal alcohol exposure. Severe malformations, including partial agenesis (A and B) and hypoplasia (C) of the corpus callosum, observed in cases of very heavy prenatal alcohol exposure. More subtle callosal abnormalities are observed in most cases of fetal alcohol spectrum disorders. (From Johnson VP, Swayze VW II, Sato Y, Andreasen NC. Fetal alcohol syndrome: craniofacial and central nervous system manifestations. *Am J Med Genet.* 1996;61:329–339.)

Clinical research has shown a significant reduction in fetal-to-maternal folate ratios associated with chronic maternal alcohol use.[90] Third, zinc is necessary for neurogenesis, neuronal migration, and synaptogenesis. Alcohol induces the zinc binding protein metallothionein in the maternal liver, which sequesters zinc and results in fetal deficiency.[91] Although other primary and secondary nutritional deficiencies may exist in the fetuses of mothers who consume alcohol during pregnancy, the relative importance of these perturbations in the overall pathogenesis of FASD requires additional investigation.

Molecular Effects

Major contributors to the cascade of developmental damage associated with fetal alcohol exposure include (1) excessive cell death (apoptosis), (2) deficient cell proliferation, (3) impaired cell migration, and (4) altered differentiation. In experimental models, neuronal and oligodendrocyte degeneration is a prominent feature of prenatal alcohol toxicity.[92,93] In particular, alcohol induces two types of cell death in the developing fetal brain. These include apoptosis and necrosis. Necrosis appears to represent a minority of cell death associated with alcohol exposure, typically occurring following binge drinking or alcohol withdrawal.[94] Even low levels of alcohol exposure early in gestation appear to promote apoptosis, via elevation of phospholipase C activity, promotion of intracellular calcium transit, and repression of the transcriptional effector, β-catenin.[95,96] This is an abnormal process during this stage of development. Later in gestation, apoptosis naturally occurs in approximately one-third of postmitotic neurons.[97] However, in experimental models, alcohol exposure may increase the extent of apoptosis, most likely through N-methyl-D-aspartate (NMDA) receptor blockade and hyperactivation of γ-aminobutyric acid type A (GABA$_A$) receptors.[92]

Experimental models of fetal alcohol exposure during the equivalent of the human second trimester demonstrate a profound impact on neuronal proliferation, migration, and differentiation. Organization of neural circuitry relies on ongoing electrochemical activity, allowing firing neurons to locate and synapse with other cells as part of activity-dependent network formation.[98] Neurosuppression via NMDA antagonism/GABA$_A$ agonism depresses electrochemical activity, suppressing neurogenesis and triggering apoptotic neuronal death in the developing brain.[99] In addition, alcohol impairs the function of insulin-like growth factor receptors, potentially via inhibition of cyclins and cyclin-dependent kinases.[100] This inhibition may help explain delays in progression through the neuronal cell cycle that have been observed in experimental models.[101] Alcohol induces errors in neuronal migration, perhaps through disruption of L1 cell adhesion molecule and interference with glial fibers.[102] Alcohol phosphorylates the cytoplasmic domain of L1 cell adhesion molecule, thus altering the conformation and function of the extracellular domain.[103] These changes not only affect neuronal migration, but also promote aberrant dendritic morphology.[104]

Genetic and Epigenetic Alterations

Maternal and fetal genetics play a prominent role in susceptibility to FASD. Alcohol is metabolized in the liver to acetaldehyde by alcohol dehydrogenase (ADH). Functional polymorphisms in the locus encoding the beta subunit of the Class I ADH (ADH1B) alter the rate of alcohol metabolism. Alcohol is more rapidly metabolized in individuals with the ADH1B*3 allele (15% to 20% of African Americans) compared with individuals with the more common ADH1B*1 allele. This finding appears to have functional significance because prenatal alcohol exposure has been associated with increased attention problems and externalizing behavior in adolescents born to mothers with two ADH1B*1 alleles. In contrast, these differences were not observed in adolescents whose mothers had at least one ADH1B*3 allele.[2]

Fetal genetic differences may also play an important role in outcome. After prenatal alcohol exposure, monozygotic twins are more concordant in outcome than dizygotic twins.[105] Neuronal nitric oxide synthase (nNOS) and oxyguanine glycosylase 1 (OGG1) protect the developing brain from injury induced by alcohol. Mice homozygous for null nNOS or OGG1 have more severe neuronal damage and functional deficiencies following alcohol

exposure compared with wild-type mice.[106,107] In contrast, homozygous mutation of the tissue plasminogen activator and Bax genes are protective against the effects of alcohol on fetal brain development.[108,109] Further research is required to determine the array of genes that influence the spectrum of fetal alcohol disorders.

Changes in gene expression after prenatal alcohol exposure represent a relatively new field of study. However, there is evidence to suggest that alcohol alters the sequence of genes involved in methylation, chromatin remodeling, protein synthesis, and mRNA splicing.[110] Alcohol also promotes epigenetic changes, including alterations in methylation and acetylation, that give rise to phenotypic changes in animal models.[111,112] As noted earlier, there is also evidence that epigenetic modifications associated with prenatal alcohol exposure may be transgenerational, placing subsequent generations at increased risk of alcohol dependence.[113] Further study of the mechanisms underlying these important transgenerational effects is needed.

Prevention

Consensus guidelines recommend that the safest choice for a woman is to not drink alcohol during pregnancy.[8] Given that malformation risks are greatest when the fetus is exposed to alcohol during the first weeks and months of gestation, it is critical that women be advised about the risks to their infant as early as possible in the pregnancy. Indeed, advice should ideally be given before pregnancy because most women do not begin prenatal care until after the first important weeks of pregnancy have passed. As discussed previously, most women of childbearing age in the United States consume alcohol, and a small percentage continue during pregnancy.[13] Reduction or cessation of alcohol consumption during any stage of pregnancy benefits the developing fetus. When this cessation is initiated very early in pregnancy, malformations as well as cognitive and motor impairment may be avoided or at least minimized.[114,115] When it is carried out in midpregnancy, although malformations are not prevented, growth retardation is clearly diminished.[116] Thus there is benefit to be gained, even if cessation of drinking is delayed.

Supplementation to correct the nutritional deficiencies of the fetus (discussed previously) has been investigated. Supplementation with retinoids reduces alcohol-induced ocular phenotypes in experimental models.[117] Similarly, folic acid supplementation may prevent alcohol-induced cardiac defects.[118,119] Supplementation with other vitamins having a vital role in normal human development also may hold promise, despite the unknown direct impact of alcohol on these molecules. Choline, a B-complex vitamin, has been considered, given that it is the methyl donor for DNA methylation and the precursor for acetylcholine and essential cell membrane constituents. Alcohol induces hypermethylation in the hippocampus and prefrontal cortex, resulting in long-term functional abnormalities; choline may be helpful in competitively reducing these effects.[120] Vitamin E (α-tocopherol) encourages antioxidant activity, with deficiencies in vitamin E having an established role in developmental and behavioral deficits.[121] Oxidative stress has a well-established role in the teratogenic effects of alcohol, promoting caspase-3 activity and subsequent cell death.[122] In multiple experimental models, supplementation with vitamin E reduces cell loss within the brain following prenatal alcohol exposure.[123,124] Importantly, however, none of the interventions described previously independently eliminate the full spectrum of fetal alcohol effects.[125,126] In addition, the identification of at-risk women and the challenges of compliance in this population limit the feasibility of these interventions.

Treatment

Newborns with FASD represent a complex, high-risk population. Nutritional supplementation after fetal alcohol exposure has been proposed. As noted earlier, postnatal choline supplementation reduces cognitive deficits and behavioral outcomes in experimental models.[127] Optimizing an infant's postnatal experiences, educating parents, engaging social support, and mobilizing developmental and educational interventions may improve outcomes.[128] These interventions demonstrate promise in mitigating some of the negative effects of fetal alcohol exposure.

ANTIEPILEPTIC DRUGS

AEDs are among the most common teratogenic drugs prescribed to women of childbearing age.[129] Their primary use is in the treatment of epilepsy, but over half of AED prescriptions are for neuropathic pain, migraine headaches, and psychiatric disorders. A large number of drugs fall into this class, and prescription patterns have changed considerably in the last 2 decades as knowledge about the teratogenic effects of AEDs on the developing fetus and child have increased.[130,131] Older drugs, such as valproate, phenytoin, phenobarbital, and carbamazepine, have declined in use among women of childbearing age and increasingly have been replaced with newer therapies, such as gabapentin, lamotrigine, levetiracetam, and topiramate.[131] Because all of these drugs are still in use, and with more neonatal and outcome data available for such older drugs as valproate, we review these as exemplars. However, drugs such as trimethadione and paramethadione, which are no longer in clinical use because of their severe teratogenic effects, are not considered.

Prevalence

Approximately a third of individuals treated with AEDs are women of reproductive age.[132] In the United States alone, recent estimates suggest that more than 4 million prescriptions for AEDs are written each year for women of childbearing age.[133] Of these, approximately 17% were for valproate, and two-thirds were for conditions other than epilepsy—most notably psychiatric disorders. Consistent with these national trends, the prevalence of AED treatment for epilepsy and other indications during pregnancy is about 2%.[134] Moreover, there is evidence to suggest that AED prescriptions during pregnancy are increasing. Analysis of data from the US Medication Exposure in Pregnancy Risk Evaluation Program found that in a cohort of almost 580,000 pregnant women, AED prescriptions more than tripled from 1996 to 2007. This change was driven primarily by a fivefold increase in the number of prescriptions for newer AEDs. In contrast, the use of older AEDs such as valproate and benzodiazepines was relatively stable, which was somewhat unexpected given contraindications for the use of these drugs in pregnancy.[134] The most common indications were psychiatric disorders (48%), followed by epilepsy (21%) and pain disorders (22%), regardless of AED type (older vs. newer), year of conception, or gestational timing of exposure.

Finally, 13% of deliveries involved AED *combination therapy* during pregnancy.

Clinical Features
Maternal-Fetal Effects

In addition to the risks of major congenital malformations (see later), a recent meta-analysis of 38 studies across both low and high income countries found that infants born to pregnant women who were treated with AEDs for epilepsy had increased odds of preterm (<37 weeks gestation) birth (OR = 1.16, 95% CI 1.01 to 1.34) and fetal growth restriction (OR = 1.26, 95% CI 1.20 to 1.33).[135] Fetal and neonatal mortality were not increased. However, this finding is contrasted by recent observational data suggesting a higher incidence of intrauterine death associated with maternal AED polytherapy.[136] Microcephaly has also been noted in about 12% of cases.[137-140] For example, a prospective longitudinal study of 329 pregnant women with epilepsy reported an increased risk of microcephaly at birth and at 12 months of age (12%), but which normalized by 24 months.[137] More research is needed to examine other potential neonatal neurobehavioral outcomes, as well as the extent to which these risks vary by AED, dose, epilepsy type, and therapy regimen (monodrug vs. polydrug exposure).

Major Congenital Malformations

AED exposure in pregnancy results in a constellation of fetal and developmental effects that range in severity from major congenital malformations to subtle variations in normal development.[129,141-143] Early, large-scale retrospective studies in the 1970s and 1980s were the first to document the teratogenic effects of AEDs on the developing fetus. Findings suggested a more than twofold increased risk of major malformations in offspring of epileptic women on AEDs versus those not on medication or nonepileptic women.[144-158] Subsequent studies in the 1990s supported this initial work.[159-167] These studies focused largely on *fetal valproate syndrome* and *fetal hydantoin syndrome*; the latter is a syndrome associated with phenytoin exposure or structurally similar agents, such as phenobarbital, carbamazepine, and oxcarbazepine. The clinical features of these syndromes are reviewed in Table 38.6 and Figs. 38.6 and 38.7.

More recently, given the increased use of AEDs and a growing awareness of adverse effects on the cognition and behavior of children born to treated women, a number of new important data sources have been established. These include (1) large registries of pregnant epileptic women in North America, Scandinavia, the United Kingdom, India, and Australia[168-170]; (2) pharmaceutical company registries for specific drugs; (3) the European Surveillance of Congenital Anomalies (EUROCAT) database across 14 countries[171]; (4) the US National Birth Defects Prevention Study (NBDPS)[172]; and (5) prospective cohort studies of pregnant women treated with AEDs and their infants. Although not without methodological challenges, including limited information on newer AEDs, insufficient follow-up data, and variable methods used, these efforts have helped advance understanding of the neonatal and longer-term effects of AED exposure during pregnancy.

It is clear from this work that *several factors* have an influence on the teratogenic effects of AEDs (Table 38.7). First, *fetal effects differ for each AED.* Valproate appears to be the most teratogenic, followed by phenobarbital and topiramate that carry moderate risks.[173] Newer drugs, at least based on current

TABLE 38.6   Clinical Features of 63 Cases of the Fetal Hydantoin Syndrome

CLINICAL FEATURES	PERCENTAGE AFFECTED[a]
Growth	
Prenatal growth deficiency	19
Postnatal growth deficiency	26
Central nervous system	
Microcephaly	29
Developmental delay or mental deficiency	38[b]
Craniofacial	
Large anterior and posterior fontanel	42
Metopic ridging	27
Medial epicanthal folds	46
Ocular hypertelorism	23
Broad and/or depressed nasal bridge	54
Cleft lip and/or palate	5
Limb	
Nail and/or distal phalangeal hypoplasia	32
Fingerlike thumb	14
Other	
Short neck with or without low hairline	18
Inguinal hernia	14
Bifid or shawl scrotum	33
Cardiac defect	8

[a]Data are expressed as percentage of those patients for whom information is available.
[b]Includes only those patients 4 years of age or older.
Data from Hill RM, Verniaud WM, Horning MG, McCulley LB, Morgan NF. Infants exposed in utero to antiepileptic drugs. *Am J Dis Child.* 1974;127:645–653; and Hanson JW, Smith DW. The fetal hydantoin syndrome. *J Pediatr.* 1975;87:285–290.

TABLE 38.7   Factors Influencing Teratogenic Effects of Antiepileptic Drugs

- Mechanism of the specific drug
- Dose
- Timing of exposure during pregnancy
- Type of epilepsy and level of seizure control
- Monotherapy versus polytherapy
- Presence of comorbid conditions and polytherapy
- Maternal genetic factors

TABLE 38.8   Relative Risk of Major Malformations Associated With Different Antiepileptic Drugs Used During Pregnancy

AGENT	RELATIVE RISK OF MAJOR MALFORMATIONS COMPARED WITH UNEXPOSED
Valproate (N = 323)	9.0 (3.4–23.3)
Hydantoins and agents with similar structure	
Phenytoin (N = 416)	2.6 (0.9–7.4)
Phenobarbital (N = 199)	5.1 (1.8–14.9)
Carbamazepine (N = 1033)	2.7 (1.0–7.0)
Oxcarbazepine (N = 182)	2.0 (0.5–7.4)
Newer agents	
Topiramate (N = 359)	3.8 (1.4–10.6)
Lamotrigine (N = 1562)	1.8 (0.7–4.6)
Levetiracetam (N = 450)	2.2 (0.8–6.4)
Gabapentin (N = 145)	0.6 (0.07–5.2)

Adapted from Hernandez-Diaz S, Smith CR, Shen A, et al. Comparative safety of antiepileptic drugs during pregnancy. *Neurology.* 2012;78:1692–1699.

endocrine disorders, and the potential for polypharmacy (e.g., antidepressants) may further increase the risk for the infant born to a woman with epilepsy. Sixth and relatedly, fetal effects can vary depending on *whether one or multiple AEDs are prescribed.* Delineation of the teratogenic potential of each drug or drug combination is very difficult based on current evidence, especially for newer drugs. However, clear evidence exists to show that polydrug therapy is associated with a higher risk of congenital malformations than monotherapy, especially if polydrug therapy includes valproate.[180,187-189] Additional evidence is needed to characterize the impacts of different polytherapy combinations, to assist the clinical management of women (and their infants) when monotherapy is ineffective for seizure control. Finally, there is increasing evidence to suggest that *maternal genetic factors* relating to the cerebral disorder underlying the epilepsy or other heritable conditions in the family increase the risk of congenital malformations. For example, a parental history of major congenital malformations increases the fetal risk more than fourfold, and the birth of a previous child with malformations when on the same AED increases the risk 17-fold.[180,190,191]

With respect to individual AEDs, while the data are not perfectly consistent, several conclusions appear justified regarding the malformation and neurobehavioral risks associated with AED exposure during pregnancy. The most common *major malformations* reported in recent large series are neural tube defects, cardiac anomalies, oral clefts, hypospadias and other genitourinary anomalies, gastrointestinal anomalies, and skeletal deficits (Table 38.9).[130,168,173,189,192-195] The incidence of these malformations ranges from 2% to 10%, depending on the AED used, in contrast to a malformation rate of 1% to 3% in the general population.

Neonatal Effects

In relation to the neonatal effects of AEDs, neonatal withdrawal has been described. This has been reported most extensively with phenobarbital.[196] Onset generally occurs around 7 days

evidence, appear to be generally less harmful, although not all are completely risk-free (Table 38.8).[141,142,168,171,174-179] Second, *the dose of drug* has been found to influence outcome.[180,181] Higher maternal doses tend to carry more risk.[181-183] Third, *the timing of AED exposure during pregnancy* is also important. This fact poses challenges, given that neural tube closure occurs between weeks 3 and 4 of gestation and systemic organogenesis between weeks 4 and 10. This early period of vulnerability is a time when women are often unaware of their pregnancy. Fourth, the *type of epilepsy* can further complicate outcomes for the fetus. Specifically, breakthrough seizures during pregnancy may result directly in fetal hypoxia, and consequent falls may increase the risk of premature labor and fetal death.[184-186] Fifth, the *presence of other comorbid conditions*, such as psychiatric and

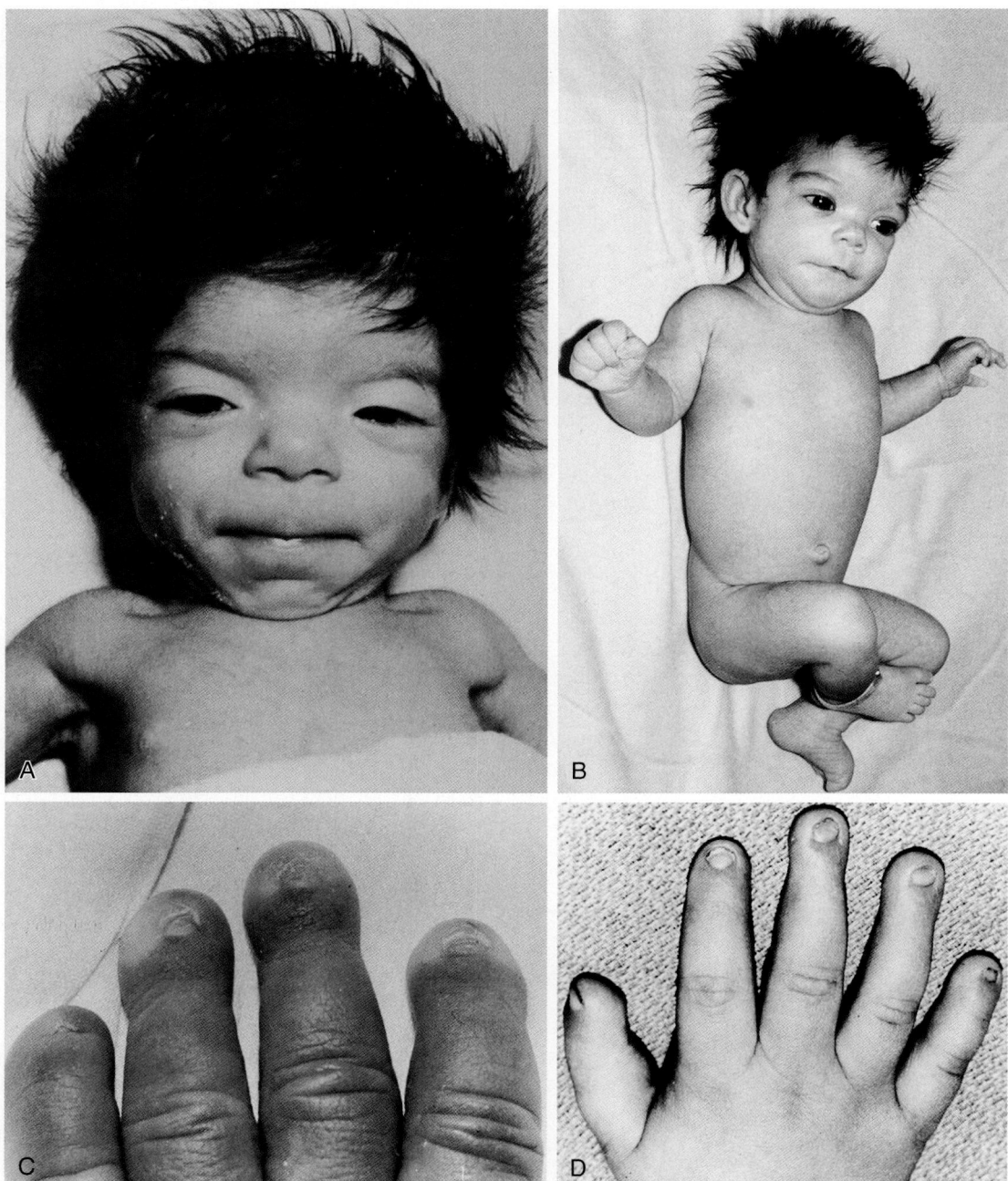

Figure 38.6 Fetal hydantoin syndrome: clinical appearance. (A and B) Two different infants with the syndrome; note the similar facial appearance, especially the broad, depressed nasal bridge, the widely spaced eyes, the epicanthal folds, the low hairline at the forehead, and the short neck. (C) Hand of an affected newborn. Note hypoplasia of nails and distal phalanges. (D) Hand of an affected child at 1 year of age; some nail growth is evident. (From Hill RM, Verniaud WM, Horning MG, McCulley LB, Morgan NF. Infants exposed in utero to antiepileptic drugs. *Am J Dis Child.* 1974;127:645–653.)

of age, which is understandable in view of the slow elimination of phenobarbital in the immediate neonatal period due to its half-life of several days. The major features consist primarily of CNS phenomena, including jitteriness, overactivity, disturbed sleeping, excessive crying, hyperreflexia, and disturbed sucking. Overt gastrointestinal phenomena, such as diarrhea, may occur but usually are not prominent. The symptoms may appear after the infant is discharged from the hospital, and the infant's irritability may be mistaken for colic or some other extraneural cause. Symptoms often worsen over several weeks and persist for several *months*.

Neonatal withdrawal from other AEDs has been less extensively described. Recent reports describe withdrawal symptoms after prolonged in utero exposure to gabapentin.[197,198] Symptoms developed within 24 hours of life, including sneezing, irritability, jitteriness, and loose stools. Given the increasing

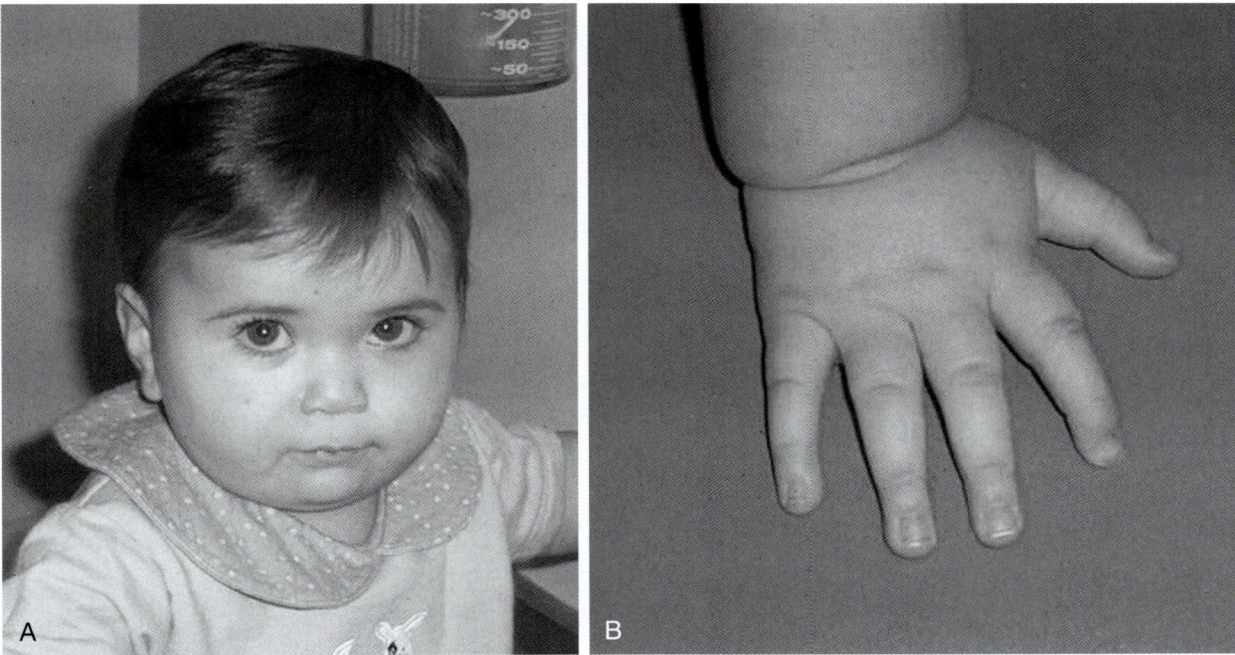

Figure 38.7 Fetal valproate syndrome, clinical appearance. Infant (10 months old) whose gestation was complicated by administration of 2000 mg of valproate daily to the mother: note the microbrachycephaly, apparent hypertelorism, broad flat nasal bridge, small mouth with thin lips (A), and thin, tapering fingers (B). (From Schorry EK, Oppenheimer SG, Saal HM. Valproate embryopathy: clinical and cognitive profile in 5 siblings. *Am J Med Genet A*. 2005;133:202–206.)

TABLE 38.9 Types of Major Congenital Malformation by Antiepileptic Drugs

DRUG	HYPOSPADIAS[a]	NEURAL TUBE DEFECTS	CARDIOVASCULAR ANOMALIES	ORAL CLEFTS
No antiepileptic drugs (N = 206,224)	0.04	0.12	0.33	0.11
Valproate (N = 323)	3.1	1.2	2.5	1.2
Hydantoins and agents with similar structure				
Phenytoin (N = 416)	0.0	0.0	0.96	0.48
Phenobarbital (N = 199)	0.97	0.0	2.5	2
Carbamazepine (N = 1033)	0.19	0.29	0.29	0.48
Newer agents				
Lamotrigine (N = 1562)	0.0	0.13	0.19	0.45
Levetiracetam (N = 450)	0.0	0.22	0.22	0.0
Topiramate (N = 359)	1.1	0.0	0.28	1.4

[a]Excludes mild glandular hypospadias. Restricted to male infants.

Restricted for malformations identified before 5 days of age, including elective terminations. Confirmed by review of medical records. Some infants had more than one defect.

Adapted from Hernandez-Diaz S, Smith CR, Shen A, et al. Comparative safety of antiepileptic drugs during pregnancy. *Neurology*. 2012;78:1692–1699.

utilization of other novel AEDs, withdrawal should remain in the differential diagnosis for exposed infants presenting with similar symptomatology.

An additional potential complication for the newborn infant associated with maternal AED treatment using a select group of AEDs is *neonatal hemorrhage*. The drugs incriminated are hepatic enzyme inducers and have included *hydantoins*, *barbiturates*, *primidone* (which is metabolized to phenobarbital in vivo), and *carbamazepine*. In one series of 111 infants born to epileptic women treated with phenytoin or phenobarbital, 8 exhibited *severe* bleeding.[199] In this syndrome, the infant developed hemorrhage shortly after birth. This *early onset* is unlike hemorrhagic disease of the newborn secondary to vitamin K deficiency. Sites of hemorrhage are, in order of decreasing frequency, skin, liver, gastrointestinal tract, intracranial sites, and thorax. *Intracranial hemorrhage* has been reported in 20% to 25% of the cases with any bleeding. The course may be fulminating, and approximately 40% of reported

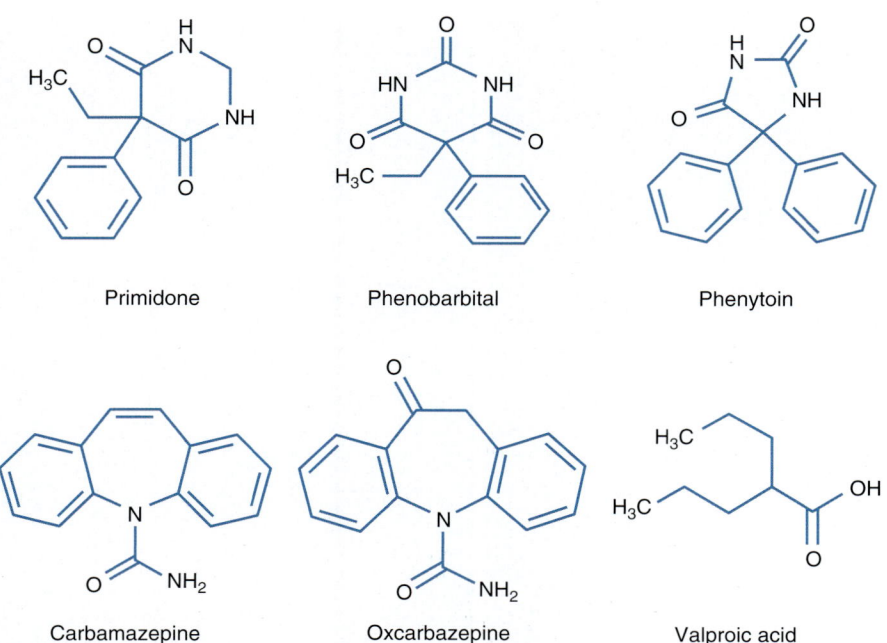

Figure 38.8 Chemical structure of important anticonvulsant drugs. Note the structural similarities of phenobarbital, phenytoin, and carbamazepine; each is composed of a basic five- or six-membered ring and a side chain substitution containing phenol groups. Valproic acid differs markedly from the other anticonvulsant drugs and is essentially a short-chain fatty acid.

infants have died. Clotting studies demonstrate diminution of the vitamin K–dependent clotting factors (factors 2, 7, 9, and 10), with prolongation of either the prothrombin time or partial thromboplastin time, or both. Vitamin K levels in cord blood are depressed, as evidenced by the presence of PIVKA-II (a protein, induced by vitamin K absence, of factor II), an incompletely carboxylated, functionally defective form of factor II (prothrombin).[200,201] Indeed, in one study of 24 infants born to mothers on antiepileptic therapy during pregnancy, 13 (54%) had detectable levels of PIVKA-II, and of the four infants exposed to valproate (none of whom had detectable levels of PIVKA-II), the incidence was 65%. Moreover, vitamin K levels also were depressed in the infants.[200,201] These findings suggested increased degradation of vitamin K with impaired action of vitamin K on hepatic production of prothrombin. The latter occurs because of insufficient carboxylation of the glutamic acid residues of prothrombin, a posttranslational event that requires vitamin K. The pathogenetic mechanism by which some AEDs lead to vitamin K deficiency may relate primarily to increased degradation of vitamin K by fetal hepatic microsomal mixed-function oxidase enzymes, known to be inducible by phenytoin, phenobarbital, primidone, and carbamazepine. The similarity in structure of these so-called enzyme-inducible AEDs is shown in Fig. 38.8. Nevertheless, *in recent years this disorder appears to have become rare.*[202-204] Three reports (*n* totals = 105, 204, and 662) have shown no increased incidence of hemorrhagic complications among women treated with various combinations of phenobarbital, phenytoin, primidone, and carbamazepine during pregnancy. The women were not treated with vitamin K during pregnancy, although the infants did receive vitamin K at birth. Whether the decline in incidence in this disorder relates to the diminishing use of polytherapy or increasing use of carbamazepine or related factors is unclear.

Neurodevelopmental Consequences

Longitudinal follow-up data describing the longer-term outcomes of children exposed prenatally to AEDs is limited to a few studies.[167,183,205-208] As illustrated in Table 38.10, sample sizes tend to be small for individual AEDs and especially some newer AEDs. Outcomes are also incomplete, with an emphasis on early global cognitive development assessed using the Griffth and Bayley Scales, and/or general intelligence at later ages. While helpful in evaluating general function and risk, these measures provide no or limited information about other important aspects of neurodevelopmental functioning, such as executive function, memory, attention, and language, at least until recently.[177] With this in mind, existing research relating to each outcome domain is summarized as follows.

Cognition and Executive Functioning

Prospective studies have consistently documented the negative effects of valproate on cognitive development, with an 8- to 9-point IQ decrement.[183,208,209] Of note, significant effects appear to relate largely to high-dose valproate exposure (>800 mg daily). The NEAD study also found that higher doses of valproate exposure during pregnancy were associated with poorer memory and executive function in offspring at age 6.[208] In addition, evidence consistently suggests that monotherapy may be less harmful than polytherapy, although historically polytherapy has generally included valproate (see Table 38.10).[176] Findings for other AEDs or combinations are mixed and insufficient.

Language Development

There is some suggestion that, based on IQ, verbal abilities may be more impaired than nonverbal abilities in children born to mothers treated with valproate.[183,208] Of note, lower doses

TABLE 38.10 Impact of Antiepileptic Drugs on Early Childhood Development and Intelligence Quotient

DRUG	EARLY CHILDHOOD DEVELOPMENT			SCHOOL AGE INTELLIGENCE QUOTIENT		
	N DRUG EXPOSED	N NOT DRUG EXPOSED	MEAN DIFF (95% CF)	N DRUG EXPOSED	N NOT DRUG EXPOSED	MEAN DIFF (95% CF)
Valproate	42[a]	230	−8.00 (−12.79 to −3.21)	76	552	−8.94 (−11.96 to −5.92)
Hydantoins and agents with similar structure						
Phenytoin	20	44	−0.12 (−7.54–7.30)	5	201	4.80 (−4.10–13.70)
Phenobarbital	—	—	—	14	201	−6.80 (−12.90 to −0.70)
Carbamazepine	50[a]	79	−5.5 (0.34–10.83)	150	552	−0.03 (−3.08–3.01)
Newer agents						
Levetiracetam	51[a]	97	1.09 (−2.81–4.99)	—	—	—
Lamotrigine	34[a]	230	−1.0 (−5.75–3.75)	29	210	−4.0 (−8.32–0.32)
Monotherapy	138[a]	230	−4.00 (−6.86 to −1.14)	182	391	−1.30 (−4.12–1.51)
Polytherapy	30[a]	230	−6.00 (−13.27–1.27)	105		−8.57 (−11.77–5.38)

General development assessed with either Griffiths or Bayley depending on measure used most commonly across studies, with the largest N. Measure is Bayley unless otherwise marked ([a]). Intelligence quotient was assessed with age appropriate standardized measures of intelligence.

Data from Bromley R, Weston J, Adab N, et al. Treatment for epilepsy in pregnancy: neurodevelopmental outcome in the child. *Cochrane Database Syst Rev.* 2014;CD010236.

of valproate appear to be associated with less severe effects, although performance is still negatively affected compared with controls. Carbamazepine appears to exert similar negative effects as lower doses of valproate.[183] In contrast, studies suggest that language abilities are comparable to control children for other AEDs, including phenytoin, lamotrigine, topiramate, gabapentin, and levetiracetam.[183,210] However, these conclusions are based on studies with small sample sizes and unstandardized language measures.

Behavior and Regulatory Problems

A small series of studies suggest that children exposed prenatally to valproate are at increased risk of behavior problems based on screening measures, such as the Vineland Adaptive Behavior Scales and Strengths and Difficulties Questionnaire.[207,211-213] Virtually nothing is known about specific risks for mental health problems, such as ADHD and anxiety disorders. One exception is a population-based Danish study that has linked valproate to an increased risk of autism spectrum disorder (ASD).[214]

Motor and Visual Function

There is little evidence to suggest that prenatal AED exposure is associated with later motor problems, at least on global measures of psychomotor development.[211] The one exception is a small study of 56 AED-exposed and 77 nonexposed newborns which found that exposed infants had lower limb and axial tone, and were less irritable than nonexposed infants.[215] However, little evidence exists to suggest that prenatal AED exposure is associated with later motor problems, at least on global measures of psychomotor development.[211]

Neuropathology

The nature of the neural disturbance associated with intrauterine AED exposure in the human infant has yet to be well characterized. Experimental models have shown decreased brain weight after phenobarbital, phenytoin, valproic acid, or benzodiazepine exposure.[216] In contrast, these morphologic effects have not been observed after exposure to clinically relevant doses of carbamazepine, lamotrigine, or levetiracetam. Neuroimaging studies with human infants or older children exposed prenatally to AED have not been reported. A recent study examining early cortical activity with electroencephalography (EEG) in a small series of AED exposed newborns (N = 56; predominantly oxcarbazepine/carbamazepine monotherapy or polytherapies containing these agents) found both individual alpha oscillatory bouts and wider band spectra in these infants, as well as differences in interhemispheric synchrony, suggesting that functional brain networks may be altered as a result of prenatal AED exposure.[215]

Pathogenesis

As with alcohol exposure, direct effects on fetal perfusion, fetal malnutrition, direct molecular effects of individual agents or their metabolite(s), and genetic variables are all likely contributors to the developmental anomalies associated with intrauterine exposure to AEDs (Table 38.11). These impacts may be further modulated by genetic factors. While the mechanisms of adverse effects of older agents, such as phenobarbital and phenytoin, have been evaluated extensively, less insight exists regarding newer agents, such as levetiracetam and lamotrigine, which are now more widely used in the management of epilepsy during pregnancy.

Fetal Blood Flow

AEDs have been found to have *direct cardiotoxic effects* in fetal experimental models. Phenytoin and phenobarbital, specifically, inhibit the potassium channel IKr at clinically relevant concentrations.[217] Via this mechanism, phenytoin induces bradycardia and transient ventricular arrhythmias in experimental models.[218] These fetal cardiac effects may result in episodic hypoxia, leading to hemorrhage and necrosis of developing tissues.[219] Preliminary data suggest lamotrigine has similar potential.[220] The relevance of this adverse effect for other AEDs requires further investigation.

TABLE 38.11 Pathogenesis of Anomalies Associated With Intrauterine Exposure to Antiepileptic Drugs

Valproate
Inhibition of folate utilization
Neuronal apoptosis
Generation of reactive oxygen species
Generation of epoxides
Hydantoins and agents with similar structure (phenytoin, phenobarbital, carbamazepine, oxcarbazepine)
Direct cardiotoxic effects
Increased degradation of vitamin K
Inhibition of folate uptake
Neuronal apoptosis
Generation of reactive oxygen species
Generation of epoxides
Newer antiepileptic drugs (lamotrigine, levetiracetam, topiramate, gabapentin)
Inhibition of folate utilization
Generation of epoxides

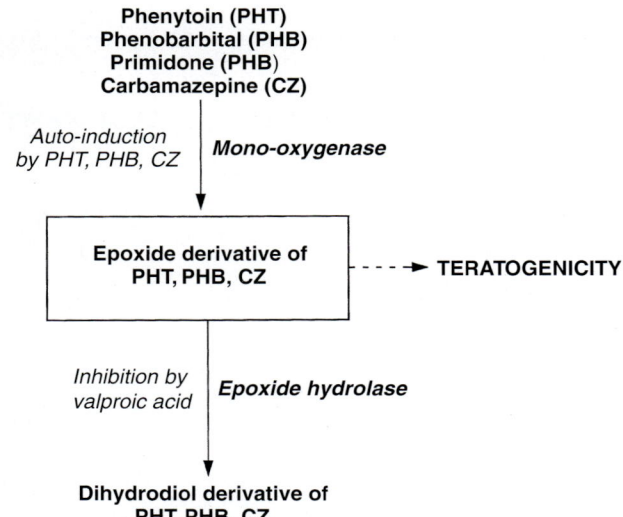

Figure 38.9 **Potential mechanism of teratogenic effect of major anticonvulsant drugs.** Generation of epoxide derivative is catalyzed by a mono-oxygenase that is induced by the drugs themselves (i.e., autoinduction). The potentially teratogenic epoxide derivative must be degraded by a hydrolase to the apparently harmless dihydrodiol derivative. Impaired activity of the hydrolase, because of either genetic variability or exogenous factors (e.g., valproic acid), could cause the epoxide derivative to accumulate and exert teratogenic effects.

Fetal Malnutrition

There is also a suggestion that *nutritional deficiencies* may potentially modulate the teratogenic effects of AEDs. As discussed previously, hepatic enzyme inducers, including phenytoin, phenobarbital, and carbamazepine, have been implicated as a risk factor for neonatal hemorrhage. This effect may relate to increased degradation of vitamin K by fetal hepatic microsomal mixed-function oxidases inducible by these agents.[200,201]

Women with epilepsy and abnormal pregnancy outcomes also have significantly lower blood folate concentrations.[221] Valproic acid functions as a noncompetitive inhibitor of cellular folate receptors and increases methylenetetrahydrofolate reductase activity, which is a crucial determinant of folate utilization in the methyl cycle.[222,223] Phenobarbital and carbamazepine decrease the expression of reduced folate carrier (RFC), potentially reducing folate uptake and transfer to the fetus.[224] Newer AEDs also alter folate uptake and transfer. Specifically levetiracetam and lamotrigine decrease placental expression of RCF and folate receptor α, respectively.[225] In rodent models of fetal valproic acid or hydantoin exposure, treatment with folate reduces the risk of congenital malformation.[226,227] Unfortunately, studies in women with epilepsy do not suggest any protective benefits of folic acid supplementation before conception.[228] In this context, preconceptional folic acid supplementation is recommended in a similar fashion as it is for all women of childbearing age for the prevention of neural tube defects (see Chapter 1). The role of higher doses in women with epilepsy has yet to be determined.

Molecular Effects

Several AEDs induce widespread *neuronal apoptosis* in a manner similar to fetal alcohol exposure.[229] As described in detail earlier, the mechanism of alcohol-induced apoptotic neurodegeneration is likely mediated through *NMDA receptor blockade and hyperactivation of GABA$_A$ receptors*. Similar neuronal apoptosis has been described in newborn rodents after exposure to phenytoin, phenobarbital, diazepam, and valproic acid, all of which directly activate GABA$_A$ receptors or increase levels of GABA through sodium channel blockade or inhibition of catabolism.[229] Of concern, recent in vitro data suggest similar potential with oxcarbazepine.[230] Interestingly, although carbamazepine appears to exert antiepileptic activity through a similar mechanism, apoptosis is only augmented in rat pups exposed at postnatal day 7 at concentrations that far exceed those used in clinical practice.[231] Notably, AEDs with a less clear impact on GABA, including levetiracetam and lamotrigine, appear to induce little to no apoptosis in experimental models.[232-234] However, with the exception of levetiracetam, these *safer* agents do potentiate cell death when used in combination with proapoptotic AEDs.[216]

An additional mechanism of teratogenesis may be the *generation of reactive oxygen species* (ROS). Experimental models demonstrate the ability of fetal peroxidases to rapidly bioactivate hydantoin derivatives (phenytoin and carbamazepine) to free radical intermediates that initiate the formation of ROS.[235,236] Valproic acid also increases the formation of ROS in embryos, although the mechanism has not been clearly described.[237] In vitro models demonstrate ROS generation in astrocytes after exposure to gabapentin, oxcarbazepine, and topiramate, but minimal effects from levetiracetam and lamotrigine.[238,239] ROS generation interferes with development by direct oxidative damage to cellular macromolecules, including DNA and RNA. In addition, ROS generation leads to dysregulation of signal transduction, thereby triggering apoptotic or necrotic cell death.[240]

Later in gestation, the fetus develops an additional ability to generate *toxic metabolites via the cytochrome P-450 enzyme system* (Fig. 38.9). Several AEDs, including phenytoin, phenobarbital, carbamazepine, lamotrigine, and valproic acid, undergo metabolism in multiple phases. The first phase is generally a two-step hydroxylation catalyzed by cytochrome P-450. The first step produces a highly reactive epoxide that can bind nucleic acids and impair developmental processes.[241] Multiple systems exist to detoxify harmful epoxides, including epoxide hydrolase, resulting in a hydroxylated molecule. Glucuronidation of these molecules in a later phase produces a highly water-soluble metabolite suitable for urinary excretion.[242] Increased exposure to epoxides in experimental models increases the risk of teratogenesis. For example, exogenous inhibition of microsomal epoxide hydrolase produces a higher incidence of fetal demise and anatomical abnormalities after phenytoin exposure in mice.[243] Importantly, several AEDs (carbamazepine, oxcarbazepine, phenobarbital, phenytoin, valproic acid) induce the cytochrome P-450 system, increasing the generation of reactive epoxides, and valproic acid specifically inhibits microsomal epoxide hydrolase (see Fig. 38.9).[244] Many investigators have proposed these interactions as a potential explanation for the increased incidence of teratogenesis observed with polytherapy compared with monotherapy.[130] Of note, inhibitors of the cytochrome P-450 system decrease the incidence of teratogenesis in experimental models.[245] Importantly, this modulatory effect of polytherapy does not occur when using agents with no impact on the cytochrome P-450 system.[246]

However, recent evidence suggests apoptosis may not be the fundamental mechanism of neurodevelopmental alterations from AEDs. These experimental models in mice highlight the importance of neocortical dysgenesis through alteration of proliferation and differentiation of neural progenitor cells.[247] Specifically, valproic acid inhibits histone deacetylase, alters the expression of G1-phase regulatory proteins, inhibits neural progenitor cells from exiting the cell cycle during neocortical histogenesis, and increases the production of projection neurons in superficial neocortical layers. These findings highlight our incomplete understanding of the fundamental mechanisms underpinning well-described syndromes associated with valproic acid and other AEDs.

Genetic Factors

Genetic factors appear to mediate the incidence and severity of anomalies after prenatal AED exposure. Syndromic features are dramatically more likely to recur in children born to mothers with a previously affected offspring compared with mothers whose previous offspring showed no observable effects.[191] Maternal metabolic variability may explain this observation to some extent. Cytochrome P-450 polymorphisms are common and result in more rapid production of toxic epoxides in some individuals.[248] In addition, epoxide hydrolase exhibits polymorphisms that result in large variability in the capacity to detoxify metabolic intermediates.[249] Observational studies of pregnant females taking phenytoin have found that lower epoxide hydrolase activity correlates with fetal hydantoin syndrome in offspring (Fig. 38.10).[250,251] However, the fact that these reactive hydrophilic metabolites most likely do not cross the placenta raises questions regarding these associations.[240] In this case, maternal genetics may represent a proxy for fetal genetics, which clearly play a role in the risk of adverse outcomes associated with prenatal AED exposure.[252,253] Children with major congenital anomalies after phenytoin exposure are also characterized by abnormal metabolite detoxification in experimental tests conducted in vitro after birth.[254] Additional fetal genetic factors may include a sensitivity to the cardiac effects of AED exposure.[255]

Prevention

As described, AED exposure during pregnancy increases the risk of congenital anomalies. However, maternal seizures put

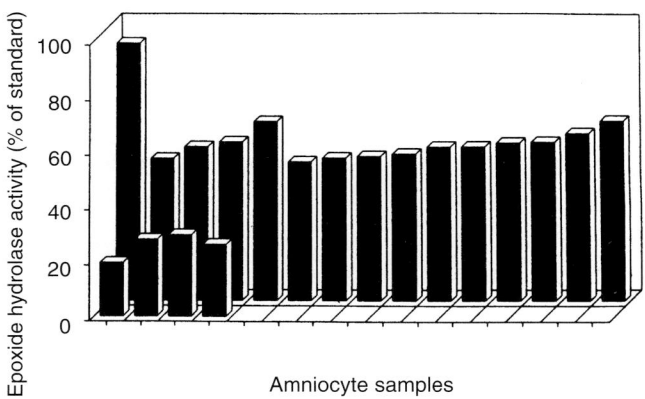

Figure 38.10 Epoxide hydrolase activity in amniocyte samples from 19 prospectively monitored fetuses whose mothers were administered phenytoin during the pregnancy. The samples from the four fetuses subsequently noted postnatally to exhibit the clinical features of fetal hydantoin syndrome are shown in the front row of bars, and the 15 samples from fetuses subsequently confirmed not to have the characteristic features of the syndrome are shown in the rear row of bars. Note the markedly lower epoxide hydrolase activities in the fetal samples from infants who exhibited the clinical features of fetal hydantoin syndrome. (From Buehler BA, Delimont D, Van Waes M, Finnell RH. Prenatal prediction of risk of the fetal hydantoin syndrome. *N Engl J Med.* 1990;322:1567–1572.)

both the mother and fetus at risk for physical injury. Therefore preconception planning is ideal to allow careful consideration of the risks and benefits of transitioning the mother to a less teratogenic treatment plan. Expert recommendations suggest the avoidance of valproic acid, phenytoin, and phenobarbital. In addition, the avoidance of AED polytherapy is recommended if possible.[256] However, experts emphasize that polytherapy may be preferable to monotherapy with valproic acid and may be necessary with newer AEDs to achieve seizure control. Based on available evidence, it appears levetiracetam and lamotrigine are the preferred AEDs in pregnancy, followed by carbamazepine and oxcarbazepine.[141]

Treatment

Newborns with withdrawal from phenobarbital respond well to postnatal phenobarbital therapy, starting on a dose of 3 to 5 mg/kg per day and then tapering very slowly, over months, as symptoms are controlled.[196] A single case report describing gabapentin withdrawal noted a positive response to postnatal gabapentin therapy, at a maximum dose of 5 mg/kg every 12 hours, followed by gradual weaning over 48 days.[197] As discussed previously, the incidence as well as treatment of withdrawal from other AEDs is less clear. Similar to newborns with FASD, newborns exposed to any AED in utero may benefit from developmental care.

The *management* of newborn infants whose mothers have been on AEDs during pregnancy to prevent neonatal hemorrhage has previously been recommended as follows: (1) consideration of delivery by cesarean section *if* a difficult or traumatic delivery is anticipated, (2) administration of oral vitamin K (10 mg/day) to the mother before delivery during the last month of pregnancy (parenteral vitamin K should be administered as soon as possible after the onset of labor if oral vitamin K was not given), (3) administration of vitamin K to the infant intravenously immediately after birth, (4) administration of fresh frozen plasma to the infant if clotting studies are distinctly abnormal, and (5) consideration of exchange transfusion if hemorrhage ensues. Oral supplementation of vitamin K_1 to the mother for 2 to 4 weeks before delivery prevented neonatal coagulation defects in one study. However, in view of the recent studies showing no increase in the risk of hemorrhage in infants whose mothers did not receive vitamin K during pregnancy, its use has been questioned.[199,257] A more selective approach may be preferable, such as in pregnancies where there is a higher likelihood of hemorrhage due to trauma, prematurity, or other related risk factors. At least based on current evidence, prenatal vitamin K appears to pose no risks to the fetus, but may have potential benefits.

STIMULANTS

Two classes of stimulants that are used recreationally and have been shown to affect fetal development are discussed here. These include *cocaine* and *methamphetamines*. The effect of cocaine on the fetus became an important issue during the crack cocaine epidemic of the 1980s. Cocaine is benzoylmethylecgonine, an alkaloid derived from the leaves of the *Erythroxylon* plant species.[258,259] It is available in two forms: cocaine hydrochloride and highly purified cocaine alkaloid (free base).[258-267] The latter is derived from the former principally by alkali extraction. Cocaine hydrochloride is heat labile but water soluble, and therefore is generally administered by nasal insufflation, orally, or intravenously. Cocaine alkaloid is heat stable but highly water insoluble and therefore is generally administered by inhalation (smoking). The cocaine alkaloid preparation is also called *crack* because of the popping sound made by the heated crystals.

In response to early concerns about the possibility of a "crack baby" syndrome, several large prospective longitudinal studies were initiated.[268-273] These clinical studies, as well as experimental observations, have helped inform understanding of the neurological and developmental effects of prenatal cocaine exposure on the developing fetus and infant. Findings from these studies demonstrate that cocaine has the potential to cause, directly and indirectly, alterations in brain structure and associated behavioral functions in the child. However, in general, these effects were more subtle than first suggested. These longitudinal studies were also very important for the field in general because they helped advance methods and models of studying prenatal drug effects. Specifically, these studies helped (1) develop improved strategies for addressing the effects of confounding polydrug use and lifestyle factors; (2) establish more reliable and valid measures of drug exposure(s) and child outcomes assessments; (3) highlight the importance of postnatal environmental influences; and (4) emphasize the need for a life course perspective.[274]

Because prenatal methamphetamine abuse is relatively recent, less is known about the outcomes of newborns after methamphetamine (Desoxyn in medical use; "meth" in the illicit setting) or amphetamine (Adderall, Dexedrine, Dextrostat, and Vyvanse in medical use; "speed" in the illicit setting) exposure. In contrast to cocaine, fewer studies have examined the effects of prenatal methamphetamine exposure on pregnancy, infant, and child outcomes. With the exception of a Swedish cohort ($n = 66$ exposed infants) and the US–New Zealand Infant Development, Environment, and Lifestyle (IDEAL) study ($n = 204$ exposed and 208 unexposed infants), most research in this area is cross-sectional and/or based on retrospective chart review.[275-290]

Thus, especially for longer-term outcomes, conclusions are heavily dependent on one, if not two, longitudinal studies (see later). The mechanism of action of methamphetamine is similar to cocaine, *promoting dopamine release* through inhibition of reuptake transporters.[291] However, there are also several important differences between the two drugs. First, the half-life of methamphetamine is nearly four times longer than cocaine, resulting in a greater window of drug exposure for the fetus during pregnancy. Second, although both amphetamines and cocaine exert their effect by blocking the reuptake of dopamine, amphetamines also *increase the release of dopamine*. Despite these differences and based on available information, there appears to be significant overlap between the pathologic and developmental effects observed after exposure to these agents.

Prevalence

The exact prevalence of crack/cocaine use in pregnancy is not known, although estimates generally suggest that rates are declining relative to the rates for other drugs of abuse.[292,293] Estimates vary widely depending on the method used to assess drug exposure, with hair and meconium analysis yielding higher rates than either self-report (which is susceptible to underreporting) or urine analysis (which captures only a short window of time during the pregnancy). For example, 11% of women self-reported illicit drug use in a large local cohort of 3000 urban women in Detroit; however, a 31% prevalence of cocaine was detected on the basis of infant meconium analysis shortly after delivery.[294] These rates and discrepancies are not confined to urban areas (Table 38.12).[295] More recent studies suggest a declining rate nationally (~10% prevalence by meconium; ~7.5% by self-report), but demonstrate that cocaine remains a common drug of abuse, especially in some urban areas of the United States.[274,296,297]

Although amphetamine-based stimulants have a long history of use for fatigue and weight loss, it was not until the 1990s and early 2000s that methamphetamine abuse became a public health problem.[298] This largely occurred as a consequence of the advent of illicit *home* manufacturing of the drug. Commonly known as *ice* or *crystal*, this crystallized form is heated and inhaled as a vapor, intensifying the euphoric (and addictive) effects of the drug. These home-based manufacturing laboratories initially emerged on the West Coast and in deprived rural areas of the United States, but then quickly spread across the North American continent and to regions of Southeast and East Asia, Australasia, South Africa, and parts of Europe, such as the Czech and Slovak Republics.[299]

TABLE 38.12	Incidence of Cocaine Use in a Suburban US Hospital	
	PRIVATE ($n = 366$)	CLINIC ($n = 134$)
Cocaine use (meconium)	6.3%	26.9%
Cocaine use (maternal report)	0%	4.0%

Data from Schutzman DL, Frankenfield CM, Clatterbaugh HE, Singer J. Incidence of intrauterine cocaine exposure in a suburban setting. *Pediatrics.* 1991;88:825–827.

Limited information exists regarding the prevalence of methamphetamine use during pregnancy. Estimates in the United States vary from 0.7% to 5.2%.[300] Importantly, many of these women are also subject to high levels of social and psychological disadvantage. For example, a large study of United States (*n* = 127) and New Zealand (*n* = 97) women, who either reported using methamphetamine during pregnancy or whose infant's meconium tested positive for the drug, found that social disadvantage, single motherhood, and delayed prenatal care were relatively common. A large proportion also had comorbid psychiatric (48% United States, 43% New Zealand) and other substance abuse disorders (71% in both United States and New Zealand women), highlighting the complex presentation of these women and infants.[301]

Clinical Features

Maternal-Fetal Effects

Cocaine use during pregnancy has deleterious effects on both the mother and the fetus (Table 38.13).[273,302-314] The specific features and the magnitude of these effects are relatively consistent across studies. A recent meta-analysis of 31 studies found that cocaine use during pregnancy was associated with significantly higher odds of *preterm birth* (OR = 3.4), *low birth weight* (OR = 3.7), and *being born small for gestational age* (OR = 3.2).[315] On average, cocaine-exposed infants were born 1.5 weeks earlier and were almost 500 g lighter than nonexposed infants. Findings are mixed as to whether these infants catch up in growth, with one study finding no differences in the height and weight of exposed children between the ages of 1 and 6 years, and another reporting that they were in fact heavier at age 13 months, potentially indicating some postnatal compensation for intrauterine growth deficiencies.[316,317]

Similarly, a recent meta-analysis of 10 studies found that methamphetamine exposure during pregnancy was associated with increased risks of preterm birth (OR = 4.1), low birth weight (OR = 4.0), and being born small for gestational age (OR = 5.8; see Table 38.13).[318] Only three studies, two of which were from the same cohort, examined the extent to which these risks persisted after other confounding factors were taken into account.[319-321] Findings from these studies showed that while risks were lower (OR range = 1.3 to 2.5), they remained statistically significant and consistent with unadjusted findings.

Neonatal Effects

The neonatal features of infants exposed to cocaine in utero are not characterized by a distinct constellation of craniofacial or other anomalies, but neurobehavioral features are common.[272,297,322-346] The most consistent findings from both experimental and human infant studies indicate neurobehavioral and motor abnormalities.[347-354] These consist principally of poorer state regulation, impaired arousal and altered sleep-wake states, poorer visual and auditory attentiveness, and increased periods of excitable and agitated behavior.[355-359] Additional motor features include extensor and flexor hypertonicity, hyperreflexia, coarse tremor, and increased motor activity. Neither set of problems generally requires therapy, but rather appears to improve with time, especially the motor features.[351,360,361] These adverse effects are even more evident when the fetus is exposed to other drugs of abuse, such as opioids, in addition to cocaine.[357] The likelihood that these neurobehavioral characteristics are related to a direct effect of cocaine is supported by the demonstration of a dose-response relationship between the extent of maternal cocaine use during

---

TABLE 38.13   Odds of Selected Neonatal Outcomes Associated With Intrauterine Cocaine and Methamphetamine Exposure

	COCAINE		AMPHETAMINE	
	N INFANTS (EXPOSED AND NOT EXPOSED)	OR (95% CI)	N INFANTS (EXPOSED AND NOT EXPOSED)	OR (95% CI)
Birth characteristics[a]				
Preterm birth (<37 weeks' gestation)	39,860	3.4 (2.7–4.2)	62,070	4.1 (3.1–5.6)
Low birth weight (<2500 grams)	38,796	3.7 (2.9–4.6)	26,132	4.0 (2.5–6.4)
Small for gestational age (<10th percentile for weight)	28,098	3.2 (2.4–4.3)	4,383	5.8 (1.4–24.1)
Neurobehavioral features[b]	123,101	*Birth—3 days* No differences *3 weeks old* ↑ Excitability ↓ State regulation	291,268	*Birth—5 days* ↑ Stress abstinence ↓ Quality of movement

[a]Data from Gouuin K, Murphy K, Shah PS. Effects of cocaine use during pregnancy on low birthweight and preterm birth: systematic review and metaanalyses. *Am J Obstet Gynecol.* 2011;204:340.e1–e12 and Ladhani NN, Shah PS, Murphy KE. Prenatal amphetamine exposure and birth outcomes: a systematic review and metaanalysis. *Am J Obstet Gynecol.* 2011;205:219.e211–e217.

[b]Based on NBAS (Tronick et al.) and NNNS (LaGasse et al.) exam. Findings reported are after adjustment for covariates.

OR, Unadjusted Odds Ratio (95% Confidence Interval).

Data from Tronick EZ, Frank DA, Cabral H, Mirochnick M, Zuckerman B. Late dose-response effects of prenatal cocaine exposure on newborn neurobehavioral performance. *Pediatrics.* 1996;98:76–83 and LaGasse LL, Wouldes T, Newman E, et al. Prenatal methamphetamine exposure and neonatal neurobehavioral outcome in the USA and New Zealand. *Neurotoxicol Teratol.* 2011;33:166–175.

pregnancy and the severity of neonatal neurobehavioral and motor outcomes shortly after birth.[310,361]

Methamphetamine exposed newborns are also characterized by a number of neurobehavioral features similar to those seen in cocaine-exposed infants.[279,283,362] Neonatal intensive care unit (NICU) admission is often required. However, similar to cocaine, maternal methamphetamine use during pregnancy is generally not associated with a withdrawal syndrome that requires pharmacological treatment. Common features of methamphetamine withdrawal include a weaker and less coordinated suck, disorganized-state behavior, poorer quality of movement, and increased physiological/CNS stress.[362] A dose-response relationship has been demonstrated for arousal and excitability. Severe symptoms requiring hospitalization resolve rapidly, with full resolution generally occurring by age 1 month.[279]

An additional complication of prenatal cocaine exposure is *sudden infant death syndrome (SIDS)*, with this risk being approximately three- to sevenfold higher than for healthy unexposed infants. Both clinical and laboratory data suggest that the regulation of respiration and arousal are impaired in cocaine-exposed infants, and that such impairments could presage the occurrence of SIDS.[363-367] Newborns exposed in utero to cocaine also have abnormalities of EEG and brain stem auditory evoked responses, which generally disappear after 1 to 6 months.[340,344,368-372] However, more sophisticated EEG studies, based on quantified EEG, have shown persistence of abnormalities after 12 months.[373] Limited experimental data suggest that the risk of SIDS may not be affected by methamphetamine exposure, although this conclusion requires further investigation.[374]

Destructive Effects on the Central Nervous System

Cocaine appears to have both *destructive effects* (i.e., associated with the histopathological hallmarks of a destructive process, such as dissolution of tissue with a reactive cellular response) and *development effects* (i.e., teratogenic effects). It may be difficult to distinguish developmental from destructive effects in the fetus, because a destructive process that occurs in a rapidly developing tissue may not only have direct effects on already developed structure, but may also perturb the course of future developmental events. In addition, the reactive cellular response to tissue destruction may be less vigorous early in development, and thus evidence for a primarily destructive event may be absent or barely detectable morphologically. Indeed, distinction of the destructive effects from the teratogenic effects is difficult, in part because they may coexist in the same infant.

Cerebral Infarction and Intracranial Hemorrhage. Cocaine and likely amphetamines are distinctive among the drugs that produce teratogenic effects on the CNS in their capacity to lead also to *destructive neural effects*. The first clearly documented example of a destructive lesion in the brain was the demonstration of *infarction* in the distribution of the middle cerebral artery in a newborn infant whose mother used cocaine by nasal insufflation in large doses during the 3 days before delivery.[375] The presence of hemiparesis *at birth* and the computed tomography (CT) appearance of the lesion indicated that the infarct occurred shortly before birth, presumably during the period of cocaine exposure. Subsequently, numerous infants exposed to cocaine or methamphetamine in utero, with cerebral

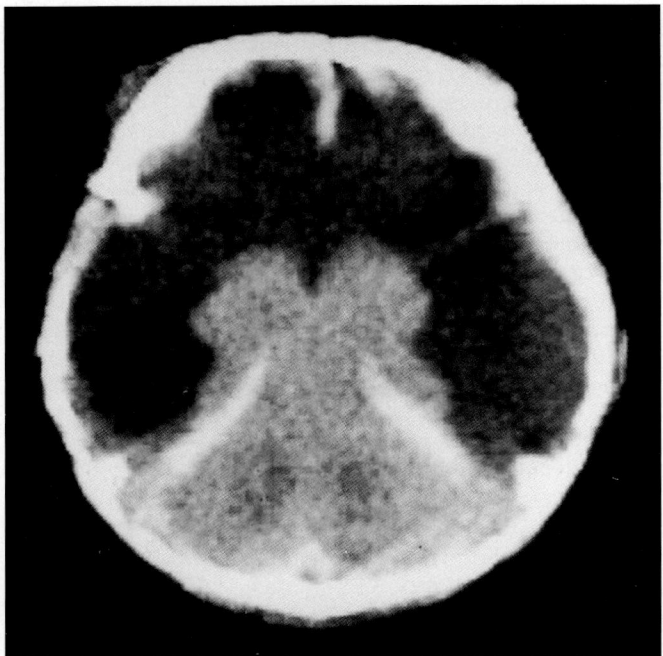

Figure 38.11 Hydranencephaly in an infant exposed to cocaine in utero. This computed tomography scan shows evidence of severe destruction of cerebral hemispheres in the distribution of the middle and anterior cerebral arteries. The appearance is consistent with severe ischemic insult in utero. (Courtesy Dr. Elke Roland.)

infarction in the distribution of major cerebral vessels, usually the middle cerebral artery, have been identified.[a] In one series, 6% of cocaine-exposed infants exhibited cerebral infarction. Although all such lesions appear to have been prenatal in origin, the timing of the infarctions based on radiographical and clinical criteria has varied from hours to months before delivery. Thus, in the four affected newborns in the series of Dominguez and colleagues, three had well-established porencephaly, compatible with an event occurring weeks or months previously, and one had findings (edema) compatible with an acute event.[329] A similar prenatal origin was apparent in an infant with hydranencephaly, related to destruction of the cerebral hemispheres in the distribution of the middle and anterior cerebral arteries, noted at birth after a pregnancy marked by cocaine exposure (Fig. 38.11). However, it must be recognized that the reported cases were selected and were not identified in a prospective manner. In a prospective study of 717 cocaine-exposed infants, cranial ultrasonography, although not the optimal imaging modality, did not identify cerebral infarction.[311] Smaller areas of apparent infarction have been described in basal ganglia, periventricular white matter, and brain stem by some investigators.[332,380-382] However, it is unclear that such lesions are more common in cocaine-exposed infants versus appropriately chosen control infants.[311,383-385]

Intracranial hemorrhage has been described in approximately 10% to 20% of primarily full-term cocaine or methamphetamine-exposed infants in one series, and in approximately 30% to 70% of very low-birth-weight, cocaine-exposed infants in three other series.[332,384,386,387] Lesions

---

[a]References 324, 325, 329, 332, 333, and 376-379.

TABLE 38.14 Major Developmental Disturbances Reported After Intrauterine Cocaine Exposure and Developmental Event Presumably Affected

NEUROANATOMICAL FINDING	DEVELOPMENTAL EVENT PRESUMABLY AFFECTED
Micrencephaly; less gray matter, predominantly in dorsal prefrontal and frontal brain regions with accompanying increases in CSF	Neuronal proliferation
Agenesis of corpus callosum; agenesis of septum pellucidum; septo-optic dysplasia	Prosencephalic development
Schizencephaly, lissencephaly, pachygyria, neuronal heterotopias	Neuronal migration
Abnormal cortical neuronal differentiation	Neuronal differentiation
Myelomeningocele, encephalocele	Neural tube formation

Abnormalities are listed in order of decreasing frequency.
CSF, Cerebrospinal fluid.

appearing in more mature infants are not of major clinical importance. As previously noted, intracranial hemorrhage was not identified disproportionately in a prospective, controlled observational study of very-low-birth-weight infants.[311] In summary, the available data derived from studies of cocaine or methamphetamine-exposed newborns by brain imaging lead to the tentative conclusion that both ischemic and hemorrhagic lesions may occur. However, available data indicate that the infarctions related directly to cocaine are likely exceedingly rare, and the hemorrhagic lesions are likely related largely to the degree of prematurity.

Teratogenic Effects on the Central Nervous System

The major abnormalities of CNS development reported after intrauterine cocaine exposure and the developmental event apparently affected (see Chapters 2, 5, and 6) are summarized in Table 38.14).[302,325-332,381,388-396]

Microcephaly. An impairment of intrauterine brain growth, manifested as diminished head circumference at birth, is the most common brain abnormality in infants of cocaine-abusing mothers.[a] Indeed, in one large study, 16% of newborns exposed to cocaine in utero (compared with 6% of control newborns) had microcephaly.[302] The relationship between cocaine exposure and microcephaly remain after associated factors are taken into account, including maternal undernutrition, intrauterine infection, smoking, and the use of other illicit drugs during pregnancy. Moreover, in one study based on analysis of maternal hair, a clear dose-dependent relationship was shown between the level of cocaine exposure and risk for head size less than 10%.[310] Consistent findings exist for methamphetamine-exposed infants.[318]

---

[a]References 273, 302, 306, 310-312, 326, 328-332, 381, 385, 387, 389-391, and 397-401.

Disturbances of Midline Prosencephalic Development and Neuronal Migration. An earlier study of a selected group of seven infants with abnormal neurological or ocular findings suggested that disorders of midline prosencephalic development or neuronal migration may be associated with intrauterine cocaine exposure.[329] Three of the seven infants had varying combinations of agenesis of the corpus callosum, absence of septum pellucidum, septo-optic dysplasia, schizencephaly, and neuronal heterotopias, and two of the three also had optic nerve hypoplasia and blindness.[329] The remaining four infants had evidence of destructive cerebral lesions. Subsequent reports have confirmed these findings and have documented the occurrence of schizencephaly, lissencephaly, pachygyria, and neuronal heterotopias as manifestations of disorders of neuronal migration.[381,393,395,396] Funduscopic examination of cocaine-exposed infants has revealed optic nerve dysgenesis, coloboma, hypoplasia, and atrophy.[381,394,402] The possibility that both the disorders of midline prosencephalic development and neuronal migration and the disorders of optic nerve development are more common than is currently known is real because cranial ultrasonography and CT may underestimate these abnormalities, and careful funduscopic examinations are not often done in newborn infants. Nevertheless, it is noteworthy that in a recent careful study of 717 cocaine-exposed infants, cranial ultrasonography failed to detect *any abnormalities* of prosencephalic development or overt migrational disturbance.[311] To date, no reports have identified these findings in amphetamine-exposed newborns. In contrast, preliminary studies of methamphetamine exposure found higher rates of facial dysmorphism, skeletal abnormalities, cardiac defects, and respiratory problems in infants.[275] However, these abnormalities were not more common in the IDEAL study of 204 methamphetamine-exposed newborns, which included a matched comparison group.[283] Thus further data are required to fully understand the impact of these agents on midline brain development, and how this may relate to the dose and timing of exposure, alongside other factors.

Neurodevelopmental Consequences

Neurodevelopmental outcomes of infants exposed to cocaine in utero have been addressed in numerous reports, with a number of useful reviews on this topic.[292,403-407] Overall, findings are somewhat mixed, with some studies reporting negative impacts and others reporting small or no effects. However, the weight of evidence generally suggests the presence of a range of adverse impacts on child cognition, language, and behavior. While relatively subtle compared with the teratogenic effects seen with alcohol and AEDs, these impacts are nonetheless developmentally significant and persistent, at least into adolescence.[403]

As discussed with AEDs and alcohol, the nature and severity of child developmental outcomes associated with prenatal cocaine exposure are influenced by a number of factors, including the amount and timing of maternal drug use, maternal and infant genetic factors, and other risk exposures during pregnancy (e.g., other drug use, maternal undernutrition) or at birth that are correlated with maternal cocaine use (e.g., preterm birth). For example, heavier use, although not always easy to interpret given the increased likelihood of polydrug use among these women, tends to be associated with poorer outcomes. The following is a brief overview of key findings across each key neurobehavioral domain (Table 38.15).

TABLE 38.15   Neurodevelopmental Effects of Prenatal Cocaine Exposure in Infants, Children, and Adolescents

DEVELOPMENTAL DOMAIN	INFANCY	CHILDHOOD	ADOLESCENCE
Cognition	Habituation Recognition memory Inhibitory control Auditory working memory Cognitive flexibility	Narrative memory Inhibitory control Visuospatial working memory	Problem solving Learning Educational achievement
Language		Receptive and expressive language (incl. auditory comprehension) Verbal reasoning Syntax Phonology	Educational achievement
Behavior	Arousal, attention Irritability, excitability	Attention and ADHD Conduct disorder Aggressive behavior Internalizing problems, incl. anxiety and depression Early-onset sexual behavior and risk-taking	Attention ADHD Delinquent and risk-taking behavior Emotionally volatile Unempathetic Substance use/abuse
Motor	Seizures, tremors Respiratory distress/SIDS Fine motor Visuospatial abilities		

ADHD, Attention-deficit/hyperactivity disorder; *SIDS*, sudden infant death syndrome.

Cognition and Executive Functioning

Most studies using measures of global cognitive functioning and IQ (e.g., Bayley Scales, Stanford Binet Test of Intelligence) have found that cocaine-exposed children generally perform in the *low average score range*.[403] However, these cognitive effects appear to reflect other adverse exposures during pregnancy and/or in the postnatal environment, rather than the direct effects of cocaine. Similarly, children prenatally exposed to methamphetamine do not appear to be subject to cognitive delay or IQ deficits after covariate adjustment.[284]

In contrast, when *specific neuropsychological abilities* have been examined in more recent studies, these suggest *adverse effects* on a range of abilities, including executive functioning, inhibitory control, working memory, and cognitive flexibility.[a] Subtle effects on measures of executive functioning and attention, including poorer inhibitory control and sustained attention, are also apparent after methamphetamine exposure.[280,424] Longer term, these challenges and related behavior problems (discussed later), combined with an often less than ideal family home situation, predispose these children to impaired problem solving, learning difficulties, educational underachievement, and in turn, reduced life course opportunities.[189,425,426]

Language Development

Global language delays are more common among children and adolescents exposed in utero to cocaine, with problems spanning *both comprehension and receptive abilities*. Importantly, these effects persist after covariate adjustment.[427-430] Specific problems with syntax and phonology have also been reported.[314] In contrast, no significant between-group differences were

found between exposed and nonexposed 3-year-old children on measures of receptive or expressive language development after methamphetamine exposure.[431] However, these children are at increased risk of educational difficulties in mathematics and language at a later age, although the extent to which these learning difficulties reflect direct drug effects or associated family risk exposures remains unclear.[432]

Behavior and Regulatory Problems

Consistent with findings showing impacts on limbic and hypothalamic systems, cocaine exposure is associated with *persistent emotional and behavioral regulatory problems* spanning from infancy through adolescence.[433,434] These difficulties manifest in a number of ways, including attention problems, aggression, and an increased risk of externalizing and internalizing behavior problems, including ADHD, conduct problems, anxiety problems, and depression.[292,314,433-439] During adolescence, risk-taking and delinquent behaviors are common, such as fighting, running away from home, purposefully breaking or damaging things, early sexual behavior, and substance abuse.[426,440-443] These latter problems are independent of other perinatal exposures and have been shown to be exacerbated and, in some cases, mediated by adverse family circumstances, including parental ongoing drug use, family violence, poor parental supervision, and caregiver mental health problems.[436,437,443-445]

Although limited, studies of amphetamine exposure suggest similar long-term challenges. Prenatal methamphetamine exposure places children at increased risk of anxious/depressive problems and emotional reactivity during the preschool period.[282] By school age, externalizing behaviors (aggressive behavior, rule-breaking) and ADHD symptoms are also more common, suggesting the likelihood of higher rates of ADHD later in life.[277,280] Follow-up studies of methamphetamine-exposed adolescents are needed.

---

[a]References 349, 354, 381, 386, 401, and 408-423.

Motor and Visual Function

Findings are mixed with respect to motor outcomes of children exposed to cocaine during pregnancy, with studies largely confined to infants and young children.[351,446,447] Some studies find no enduring effects of cocaine, whereas others report subtle impairments in fine motor and visual perceptual domains, especially for boys.[351,446,447] As with other outcomes, these developmental difficulties frequently occur in the context of family psychosocial disadvantage, which predicts later risk more strongly than prenatal cocaine exposure.[446]

Beyond the neonatal period, little is known about the potential adverse motor effects of prenatal amphetamine exposure. Poor fine motor and, in particular, grasping skills were noted at age 3 in a cohort exposed to methamphetamine.[448] To date, studies in early childhood and beyond have not emerged.

Neuropathology

As suggested by the hallmark microcephaly associated with in utero cocaine or amphetamine exposure, *micrencephaly* is prevalent in neuroimaging studies. Examination of regional brain volumetric differences between infants exposed in utero to cocaine, and those not exposed, suggest that cocaine exposure is associated with *structural alterations in cortical gray and white matter development*.[270,449,450] These alterations were largely confined to prefrontal and frontal brain regions implicated in cognitive and behavioral control. Further analysis using functional connectivity MRI methods revealed both polydrug effects on amygdala-frontal, insular-frontal, and insular-sensorimotor circuits, but left amygdala-frontal functional connectivity alterations associated specifically with cocaine exposure.[451] These results suggest that prenatal drug exposure perturbs functional connections between the amygdala and frontal cortex in a way that may disrupt top-down regulation of amygdala functions by the prefrontal cortex, potentially accounting for some of the difficulties these children experience regulating emotional arousal. These between-group differences remained after controlling for other confounding factors. However, unfortunately, the sample was too small to allow dose-response relations to be examined.

Volumetric studies of methamphetamine-exposed children similarly reveal both thinning of the cortex and reduced tissue volumes in dopamine-rich striatal areas, including the caudate nucleus and associated frontal and parietal areas.[452-455] These findings are consistent with clinical and experimental research showing the neurotoxicity of methamphetamine to striatal neurons.[456] Alterations in white matter microstructure within these areas, as well as the corpus callosum, have also been found in prenatal methamphetamine-exposed children at 3 to 4 years.[457]

The possibility that cocaine or amphetamine exposure *disturbs neuronal differentiation* in cerebral, diencephalic, and brain stem structures is suggested by a series of neuroanatomical, neurobehavioral, neuropharmacological, neurochemical, and physiological studies, primarily in rats, but also in primates and most recently in human infants.[392,458-484] Thus prenatal cocaine exposure in rats and monkeys results in persistent defects in learning and memory. Moreover, Dow-Edwards and colleagues, using radioactive 2-deoxyglucose autoradiography, found that *adult* rats exposed to cocaine *prenatally* had impaired glucose metabolism in the hippocampus, a structure crucial for memory and learning; the nigrostriatal pathway, important in the regulation of movement; the mesolimbic dopaminergic system, important for the reinforcing effects of drugs like cocaine; and the hypothalamus, important for reproductive function, growth regulation, and osmotic balance.[458,459] Thus exposure to cocaine during the earliest phases of neuronal differentiation in the experimental animal can lead to profound and permanent effects on the function of many crucial neuronal systems. These effects should be considered teratogenic, because it appears that a permanent derangement of neuronal development has resulted. The correlate, if any, in humans remains to be defined, but there is one report of disturbances of neuronal differentiation demonstrated by immunocytochemical and histologic techniques in cerebral cortex of three infants exposed to cocaine in utero.[393] Very similar findings have been observed in the cerebral cortex of the newborn rat exposed to cocaine in utero; importantly, these alterations in development persist into adulthood in animal models (Fig. 38.12).[471,472,479]

Pathogenesis

Cocaine and amphetamines produce both acute and chronic disturbances in fetal development. Acute deleterious effects most likely arise from increased levels of multiple monoamines exerting effects on cardiac, vascular, and uterine tissue. Chronic disturbances of CNS development result from a constellation of hemodynamic effects as well as nutritional, molecular, and genetic disturbances (Fig. 38.13).

Fetal Blood Flow

Cocaine and amphetamines act as stimulants by blocking the reuptake of dopamine, serotonin, and norepinephrine, leading to both euphoric and profound cardiovascular effects.[268,485] Tachycardia and vasoconstriction in the mother, including direct vasoconstriction of the umbilical vein, *impair placental blood flow*, disrupting oxygen and nutrient transfer to the fetus.[486,487] These acute alterations in fetal blood flow may contribute to the destructive effects of cocaine in the neonatal CNS. Increases in fetal cerebrovascular resistance have also been documented following cocaine administration.[488] Although global cerebral blood flow is not disturbed, the *state of development of cerebral vessels in the human fetus* may explain the *distribution* of ischemic lesions observed in human studies. The extraparenchymal, leptomeningeal arteries begin to develop a distinct muscularis in the second trimester and have a well-developed muscularis in the third trimester of gestation, the time of occurrence of the cerebral infarcts reported in the cocaine-exposed infants.[489] Thus the middle cerebral artery, the vessel affected in most cocaine-induced strokes, presumably does not develop the capacity to undergo spasm until the third trimester. Intracranial hemorrhage could also occur in the immediate neonatal period secondary to elevation in blood pressure and cerebral blood flow velocity that have been documented on the first and second postnatal day in infants exposed to cocaine in utero.[490,491] Elevated levels of catecholamines in the presence of cocaine also increase uterine contractility, likely resulting in the increased rate of spontaneous abortion, preterm birth, and placental abruption associated with antepartum cocaine use.[492]

Fetal Nutrition

Cocaine and amphetamines have *important impacts on fetal nutrition*, arising from both maternal malnutrition as well as

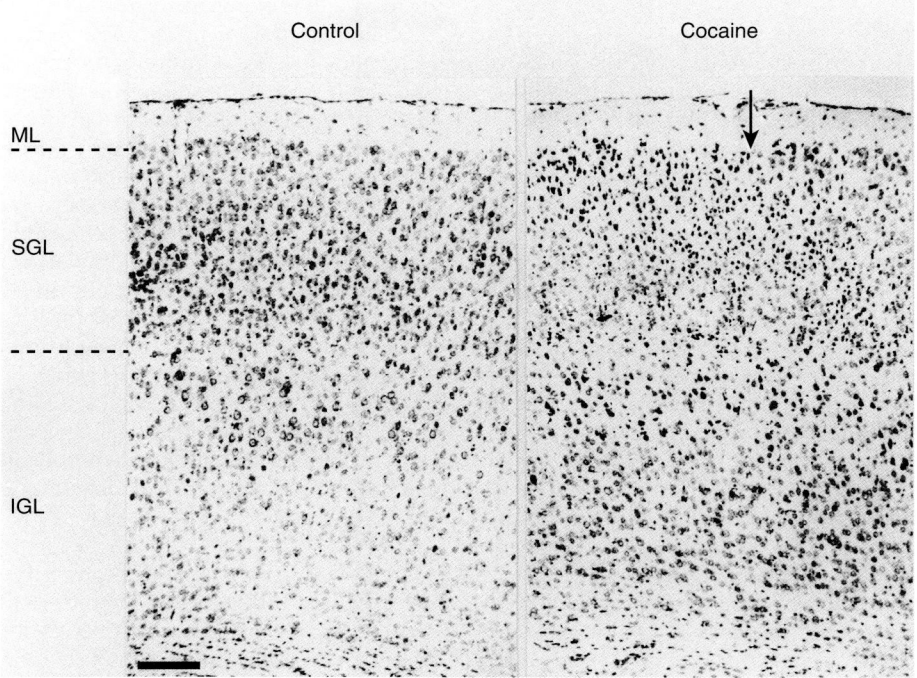

Figure 38.12 Impaired cerebral cortical neuronal organization (in the adult rat) after intrauterine cocaine exposure. Animals were exposed to saline (control) or cocaine from intrauterine day E8 through E18 and sacrificed at 40 days after birth. Cresyl violet staining of the molecular layer (ML), supragranular layers (SGL), and infragranular layers (IGL) of cerebral cortex is shown. The severe disorganization of the cortical layering in the cocaine-exposed animals contrasts with the regular lamination in the control animals. In particular, note the inversion of nuclear staining intensity between the SGL and IGL and the focal heterogeneity of nuclear size within the SGL (*arrow*). (From Nassogne MC, Gressens P, Evrard P, Courtoy PJ. In contrast to cocaine, prenatal exposure to methadone does not produce detectable alterations in the developing mouse brain. *Dev Brain Res.* 1998;110:61–67.)

direct effects. Cocaine and amphetamines are both associated with low body mass index in adults, potentially due in part to their anorexic effects.[493] Cocaine also inhibits the placental transport of specific amino acids, including arginine, phenylalanine, and valine.[494] Of interest, these effects appear to be exacerbated by concurrent exposures, including nicotine. In addition, catecholamines increase metabolism of nutrients, further contributing to fetal depletion.[495]

Molecular Effects

Cocaine administration to neonatal rats results in the inhibition of DNA synthesis and alterations of membrane lipids in all brain regions, consistent with the direct effects shown in nonneural tissues.[496-499] Deleterious effects on neuronal differentiation in rodent models have also been observed.[480,482,484] The disturbances in neuronal number and differentiation have also been observed in primate models.[480,481,483]

The mechanism of the effects of cocaine on neuronal differentiation and on development of crucial neuronal pathways in the cerebrum, diencephalon, and brain stem (subsequent to neuronal proliferation) could relate to the fundamental mechanisms of the effects of cocaine on neurotransmitters. The neuronal pathways involved either use as neurotransmitters several monoamines (e.g., norepinephrine, dopamine, serotonin) or are the targets of neurons that use monoamines as neurotransmitters. The derangements of homeostasis of these neurotransmitters by cocaine are, of course, the principal mechanisms of action of the drug in the adult brain. The specific nature of the derangements in the fetus requires further definition but appears similar. Although increased levels of these neurotransmitters might be expected, at least initially, chronic exposure to cocaine could lead to their depletion, as has been shown in experimental models and in adult humans.[258,500-504] The findings of reduction in striatal dopamine in neonatal rabbits exposed to cocaine in utero and diminished cerebrospinal fluid levels of homovanillic acid, the principal metabolite of dopamine, in cocaine-exposed newborns supports this possibility.[504,505] These neurotransmitters appear very early in brain development and *play important regulatory roles in development of neuronal circuitry.*[475,480,506-516] Indeed, because these monoaminergic systems, which originate especially in the brain stem, have widely distributed contacts in the basal ganglia, cerebral cortex, hypothalamus, and elsewhere, disturbances in their function during development could have very far-reaching effects. For example, neurons containing norepinephrine in the locus ceruleus (a pigmented nucleus in the pons) give rise to ascending monosynaptic pathways that are distributed widely in the cerebral cortex and diencephalon. These pathways are considered to have primarily activating influences. A prominent dopaminergic system originates in the substantia nigra of the midbrain and terminates in the striatum. These connections are important in the regulation of movement and tone. Other dopaminergic systems terminate in limbic and cortical structures and are crucial not only for the reinforcing actions of drugs

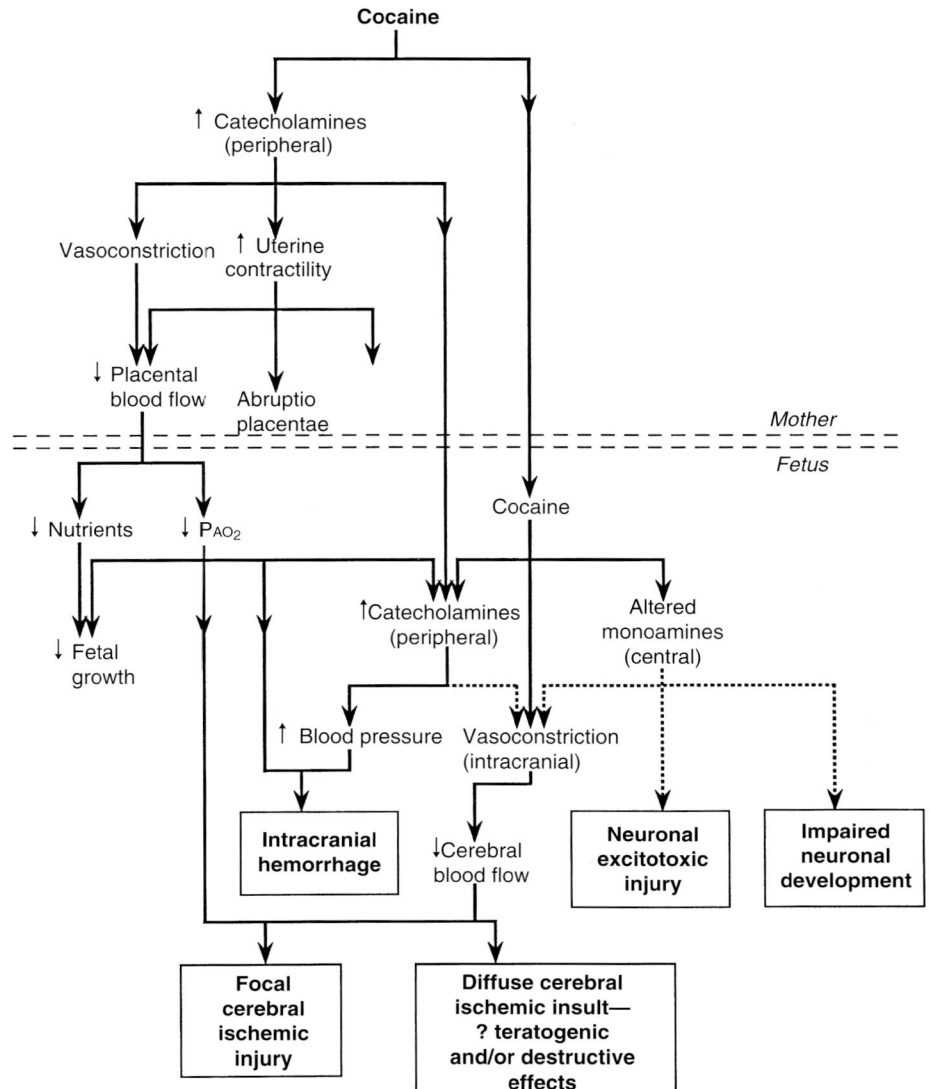

Figure 38.13 Scheme for the potentially deleterious effects of cocaine taken by pregnant women on their fetuses. Effects on the maternal side of the placenta are shown in the upper portion of the figure and on the fetus in the lower portion. Effects that appear plausible on the basis of current information but that require more supporting information are indicated by interrupted lines.

like cocaine but importantly also for motivational-attentional functions. Prominent serotoninergic systems originate in the raphe nuclei of the brain stem, project widely, and are crucial for regulation of sleep and level of alertness. However, because disturbances of the development of neuronal circuitry do not leave a readily identifiable, morphological stamp, and require highly sensitive immunochemical and neuropharmacological techniques for detection, identification of such neural abnormalities in humans is very difficult. However, impairment of subsequent cerebral cortical development by prenatal cocaine exposure during the period in which monoamines influence neural development has been shown in the primate as well as rodent cerebral cortex.[471,475,479,481,483] Careful study of cerebral cortical development in the rat has shown in the *adult* cortex abnormalities of neuronal lamination and dendritic morphology after *prenatal* exposure to cocaine (see Fig. 38.12).[479,482]

Genetic and Epigenetic Alterations

Whether the effects on neuronal proliferation and differentiation relate to *perturbation of the action of critical genes*, including immediate early genes, is an intriguing possibility.[473,474] Cocaine exposure downregulates the placental norepinephrine transporter (NET), responsible for sodium-chloride-dependent reuptake of extracellular norepinephrine.[517] Reduced placental NET expression may lead to increased circulating norepinephrine, downregulation of the steroid metabolic enzyme 11β-HSD-2, and fetal hypercortisolism, resulting in altered activity of the hypothalamic-pituitary-adrenal (HPA) axis.[387] Altered function of the HPA axis has been implicated as a potential contributor to long-term behavioral and emotional disorders observed in children exposed prenatally to cocaine.[518] These changes are associated with hypermethylation of genomic DNA, most profoundly in promoter regions.[519] In adults, chronic cocaine exposure permanently alters brain-derived neurotrophic factor (BDNF) and Cdk5 promoters.[520] Alteration of these and other promoters has the potential to produce profound alterations in development *throughout* life. Of interest, genetic modifications may not be confined to the maternal-fetal dyad, as evidenced by behavioral alterations in offspring after *paternal* cocaine exposure.[521,522]

Prevention

Prevention of prenatal cocaine and illicit methamphetamine exposure is essential. Although human data regarding prescription amphetamine exposure are lacking, caution is warranted, and these agents should be avoided in pregnancy, if possible. Prenatal care among women exposed to cocaine improves birth weight in offspring and may be the first step in a comprehensive rehabilitation program that would ideally extend into longer-term parental drug treatment and family/parenting support.[309,523]

Treatment

Abstinence from both cocaine and amphetamines occurs rapidly in the newborn and resolves relatively quickly. As discussed previously, nearly all exposed infants exhibit symptoms—most consistently hypertonia.[328] However, severe symptoms resolve rapidly without pharmacological intervention.[319] An enriched *postnatal environment* over the first several years appears crucial in modulating any effects of cocaine on the infant's cognitive and behavioral development.[268,413,425,524-526] Early intervention should be used in all high-risk infants, particularly those exposed to illicit stimulants prenatally.

OPIOIDS

Opioids have been used for centuries to manage pain and have a long history of popularity as a recreational drug in view of their additional euphoric effects. Derived from opium, a powdered exudate from the fruit capsule of the poppy plant *Papaver somniferum*, opioids act by binding to opioid receptors throughout the body. The analgesic and euphoric effects of these drugs result through the activation of receptors in the central and peripheral nervous systems, whereas side effects such as respiratory depression, sedation, and reduced intestinal motility arise from peripheral receptors.

Until early this century, the most commonly used opioids were opium and heroin. For pregnant women with an addiction to heroin or other illicit opioids, the most effective mode of therapy has been maintenance with oral methadone since the early 1970s. Evidence shows that methadone maintenance is effective in stabilizing maternal blood opioid concentrations, facilitating engagement in treatment and prenatal care, and reducing lifestyle risks associated with risk-taking and illegal behaviors such as prostitution and criminal offending.[527-530] These methadone programs have been the source of valuable information regarding the effects of opioids on the fetus and newborn.[309,531-557] More recently, the efficacy of maintenance of pregnant women with another synthetic opioid, buprenorphine, has become a further focus of research and clinical interest, because of its longer half-life (>24 hours) and reduced risk of respiratory depression when overdosed.[558] Early findings suggest some short-term neonatal

benefits for the infant, but longer-term outcome research is still needed.

Of great public health significance has been the dramatic surge since the early 2000s in the use and abuse of prescription opioids, including hydrocodone (Vicodin) and oxycodone (Percocet).[559] This increase has been especially noticeable in the United States, with the recognition of pain by the American Pain Society as a *fifth vital sign* and the active marketing of new opioid medications.[560] This increased medical use has dramatically affected the numbers of pregnant women and infants affected by prenatal opioid use. It has also led to increases in the availability and appeal of prescription opioids (and in turn heroin) as a recreational drug of abuse across socioeconomically and demographically diverse groups.[559,561,562]

Prevalence

As noted earlier, while there is evidence worldwide of increasing opioid use during pregnancy,[563] this has been most prominent in the United States.[559,561,564,565] Estimates suggest that on average between 2008 and 2012, 39% of Medicaid insured and 28% of privately insured women of reproductive age (15 to 44 years) filled an outpatient prescription for an opioid each year.[566] These rates were highest in the Southern states, especially rural areas, and among non-Hispanic white women.[566] The rates are somewhat lower during pregnancy, but still are high. A recent analysis of the prevalence and patterns of opioid use among pregnant women enrolled in commercial insurance plans (>500,000) in the United States between 2005 and 2011 found that 14.4% were dispensed an opioid at some time during pregnancy. No variation was found in rates across the three pregnancy trimesters, and the most commonly prescribed drugs were hydrocodone (6.8%), codeine (6.1%), and oxycodone (2%).[561] A small proportion (2.2%) of women were dispensed opioids three or more times during their pregnancy. In general, similar rates and distributions have been reported among pregnant women on Medicaid in New York (9.5%)[564] and in Tennessee (28%).[562] The latter study also showed that women taking prescription opioids were more likely to be white (72.4% vs. 65.8%), have depression (5.3% vs. 2.7%) and anxiety disorders (4.3% vs. 1.6%), use tobacco (41.8% vs. 25.8%), and also be taking an SSRI (4.3% vs. 1.9%). These comorbid difficulties are lower, but similar in profile to those reported among pregnant women enrolled in methadone maintenance treatment programs.[567]

Although the US accounts for more than 80% of the world's consumption of opioid pain relievers, this issue is also of concern for other developed countries.[568] For example, data from a population-based survey in Norway indicate that 6% of pregnant women filled at least one opioid prescription between 2004 and 2006.[569]

The rising prevalence of opioid use in pregnancy has led to an increase in associated neonatal outcomes such as NAS (Fig. 38.14). From 2000 to 2012, the number of newborns in the United States diagnosed with the syndrome increased nearly fivefold, reaching a rate of 5.8%.[562,570-572] This equates on average to one newborn every 30 minutes in the United States.[562] In contrast, estimates of rates of NAS in England and Australia have remained relatively stable, at around 2.7%.[573] Findings from large-scale prevalence studies suggest that the risks of NAS are greatest for infants born to mothers characterized by long-term opioid use (relative risk = 2.1) and use later in pregnancy (relative risk =1.2).[570] The presence of additional risk factors, such as maternal SSRI use (OR = 2.1) and cigarette smoking, was also associated with increased risk.[574]

Clinical Features

There has been an intermittent history of interest in the effects of opioid use during pregnancy on both the mother and infant, with studies primarily of heroin in the 1970s and 1980s, followed by methadone and, more recently, prescribed opioids, in line with population trends.[575] The methodological quality of studies is variable and often limited by retrospective review of clinical databases rather than direct assessment of the infant, lack of an appropriate reference or control group, and examination of a limited range of outcomes. Nonetheless, converging evidence suggests that infants who are born to opioid-dependent mothers are characterized by two major features: poorer intrauterine growth and an increased risk of the *withdrawal syndrome* NAS.[309,538-540,551,576-589]

Maternal-Fetal Effects

Among infants born to heroin-dependent women, the incidence of *low birth weigh*t (i.e., <2500 g) was approximately 40% to 50% among early studies.[578-581] Relatedly, approximately one-third of exposed newborns will be *small for gestational age* (SGA), and approximately 40% will have a head circumference below the

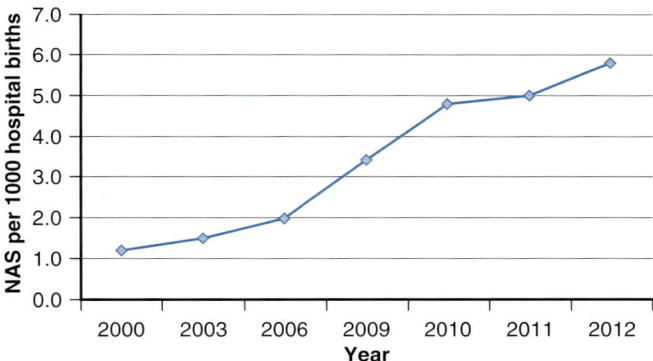

Figure 38.14 US incidence of neonatal abstinence syndrome *(NAS)*, 2000–2012. This trend mirrors the rising prevalence of opioid use in the general population in the United States during this time period. (From Pryor JR, Maalouf F, Krans EE, Schumacher RE, Cooper WO, Patrick SW. The opioid epidemic and neonatal abstinence syndrome in the USA: a review of the continuum of care. *Arch Dis Child Fetal Neonatal Ed.* 2017;102:F183–F187.)

10th percentile for gestational age (Table 38.16).[578-581] This occurrence of intrauterine growth restriction in heroin-exposed infants is reminiscent of experimental studies showing growth retardation in the progeny of female rats given morphine *before* but not after conception.[590] However, it is likely that other factors, related to nutrition and infection, were present in the mothers before and during pregnancy. Unfortunately (and as highlighted earlier), many of the early heroin studies did not examine the relative contribution of these correlated lifestyle factors.

Infants born to methadone-maintained mothers have been shown to be at increased risk of being born early, and even when born close to term, to weigh less, be shorter, and have smaller head circumferences than infants born to non-drug-using mothers.[591-594] Between 10% and 35% are low birth weight (i.e., <2500 g). Of these, two in five infants will be born SGA. Risks of SIDS, strabismus, hyaline membrane disease, vision abnormalities (particularly nystagmus), and congenital birth defects are also higher among infants born to mothers receiving methadone maintenance treatment compared with infants born to non-drug-dependent mothers.[557,595-599] However, findings demonstrate that outcomes associated with maternal methadone use are generally better than for untreated heroin use during pregnancy. The reasons for the disturbances in intrauterine growth are not entirely clear, and the relative roles of intrauterine undernutrition, infection, and toxic effects of other drugs and exogenous materials remain to be elucidated. Although a direct effect of narcotic analgesics on cell number has been suggested by experimental studies (discussed in a later section), findings are mixed with respect to the analysis of human infants. Some studies are more supportive of an indirect effect related to impaired maternal nutrition and other factors, whereas other studies support the persistence of growth differences, even after covariate factors are taken into account.[537,594,600]

Only a few studies have examined the neonatal effects of maternal buprenorphine treatment during pregnancy.[601] Of these, some have found no differences in the risks of fetal death, preterm birth, low birth weight, and SGA/growth restriction, whereas others have reported a lower risk of preterm birth and higher birth weights for buprenorphine-exposed infants compared with methadone-exposed infants.[601-612] A recent meta-analysis of 18 studies (three randomized controlled trials [RCTs] and 15 cohort) found that buprenorphine was associated with lower risk of preterm birth (RR = 0.40 to 0.67), greater birth weight (weighted mean difference = 265 to 277 g), and

TABLE 38.16 Mean Birth Weight and Gestational Age of Infants With Different Drug Exposure During Gestation			
MATERNAL DRUG USE	**NO. OF INFANTS**	**BIRTH WEIGHT: MEAN (g)**	**GESTATIONAL AGE: MEAN (WEEKS)**
Heroin	61	2490	38.0
Ex-addict	33	2616	38.6
Heroin and methadone	59	2535	38.3
Methadone	106	2961	39.4
Control	66	3176	40.0

Adapted from Kandall SR, Albin S, Lowinson J, Berle B, Eidelman AI, Gartner LM. Differential effects of maternal heroin and methadone use on birth weight, *Pediatrics* 58:681–685, 1976.

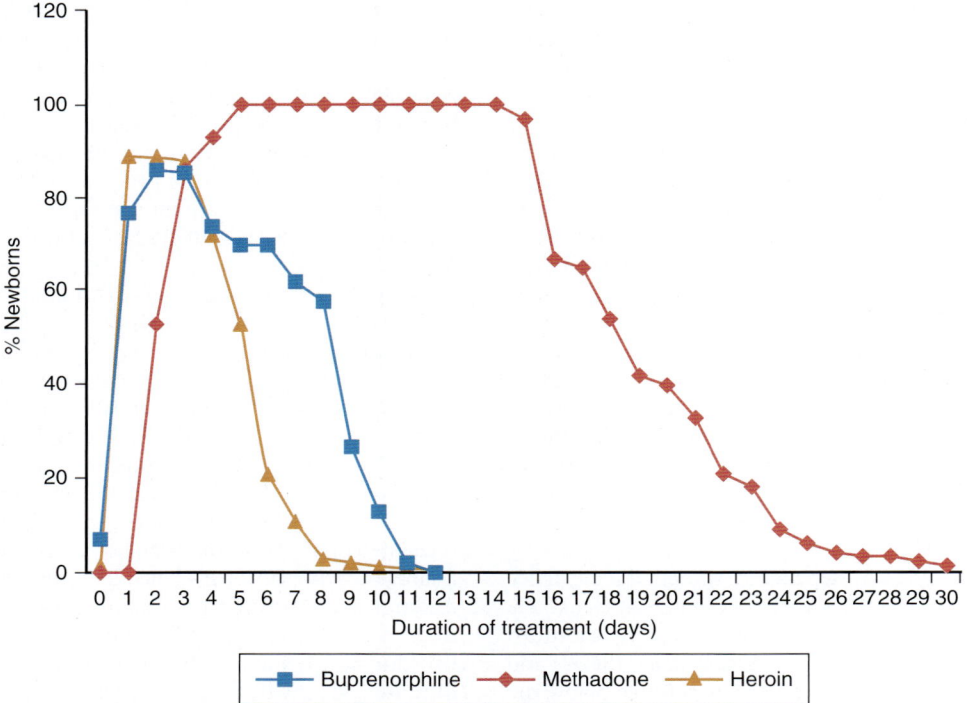

Figure 38.15 Onset and duration of neonatal abstinence syndrome symptoms from heroin, methadone, and buprenorphine. Note the delayed onset and prolonged duration of methadone withdrawal compared to heroin withdrawal. Interestingly, despite a long half-life, buprenorphine withdrawal symptoms appear early and resolve rapidly compared to methadone. (Adapted from Binder T, Vavrinkova B. Prospective randomised comparative study of the effect of buprenorphine, methadone and heroin on the course of pregnancy, birthweight of newborns, early postpartum adaptation and course of the neonatal abstinence syndrome (NAS) in women followed up in the outpatient department. *Neuro Endocrinol Lett.* 2008;29:80–86.)

a larger head circumference (weighted mean difference = 0.68 to 0.90), with bigger differences observed in RCT studies.[613] No differences were found for spontaneous fetal death, fetal congenital anomalies, and other growth measures.

Neonatal Abstinence Syndrome

Early studies suggested that the incidence of NAS in heroin-exposed infants was about 70%, varying from about 50% to 90%.[a] In general, similar rates are reported among infants born to mothers enrolled in methadone maintenance treatment programs, with rates varying widely from 13% to 90%. This variability likely reflects both differences in clinical approaches with respect to maternal and infant management (in-hospital weaning of the infant vs. early discharge with home visiting care vs. in-hospital maternal detoxification during pregnancy and follow-up care) and other factors related to maternal drug use (i.e., maternal nicotine use, other drug exposure, methadone dose).[b] There is some support that maternal maintenance with buprenorphine during pregnancy may be associated with a lower risk of NAS and in turn a shorter length of stay than with methadone.[604]

Concerning the perinatal outcomes associated with maternal prescription opioid use, findings are now emerging but are

exclusively confined to medical record review. For example, an analysis of more than 100,000 pregnant women who filled more than one prescription (28%) in Tennessee found that opioid-exposed infants with and without NAS (the latter implying high levels of exposure) were more likely to be born with low birth weight (no NAS 21.2%, NAS 11.8%) than nonexposed infants (9.9%).[574]

The *clinical presentation* of NAS following opioid exposure consists of an array of signs and symptoms, including increased irritability, hypertonia, tremors, seizures, feeding intolerance, watery stools, emesis, and respiratory distress, with both male and female infants affected equally.[575,619-621] The predominance of signs and symptoms relevant to the CNS and gastrointestinal tract relate to the particular concentration of opioid receptors in these regions (see later). These symptoms tend to emerge between 6 and 48 hours after birth as a result of the sudden discontinuation of exposure to the opioids being used or abused by the mother during pregnancy (Fig. 38.15). The *time of onset* of the withdrawal syndrome in the newborn delivered to a heroin-addicted woman is usually quite early (Table 38.17). Approximately 65% of infants present within the first 24 hours of life; an additional approximately 20% on the second day of life; and the remainder, or about 15%, on the third and fourth days.[581] This contrasts with the *time of onset* of the withdrawal symptoms with methadone. Most infants exposed to methadone have the onset of overt symptoms on the second day of life (Table 38.18), not the first day as with heroin. Median onset

---

[a]References 309, 538-540, 551, 557, 576, 578-584, 587, 588, and 614-616.
[b]References 529, 585, 591, 594, 617, and 618.

TABLE 38.17   Time of Onset of Withdrawal Syndrome in Infants Passively Addicted to Heroin

TIME AFTER BIRTH (H)	NO. OF INFANTS	PERCENTAGE OF TOTAL[a]
0–12	76	29%
12–24	88	34%
24–48	56	21%
48–96	39	15%

[a]Total is all infants with withdrawal syndrome (i.e., 259 of 384, or 67.4% of complete series of infants born to heroin addicts).

Adapted from Zelson C, Rubio E, Wasserman E. Neonatal narcotic addiction: 10-year observation. *Pediatrics.* 1971;48:178–189.

TABLE 38.18   Time of Onset of Withdrawal Syndrome in Infants Passively Addicted to Methadone

TIME AFTER BIRTH (H)	NO. OF INFANTS	PERCENTAGE OF TOTAL[a]
0–12	0	—
12–24	8	27%
24–48	16	53%
48–72	3	10%
>72	3	10%

[a]Total is all infants with withdrawal syndrome.

Adapted from Stimmel B, Adamsons K. Narcotic dependency in pregnancy. *JAMA.* 1976;235:1121–1124.

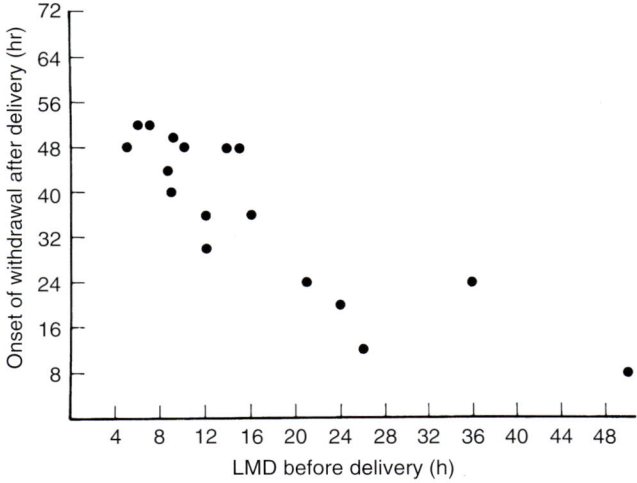

Figure 38.16 Passive addiction to methadone: relation of the time of the last maternal methadone dose *(LMD)* to the time of onset of neonatal withdrawal. The interval between onset of withdrawal and time of last maternal dose did not vary markedly and approximated 48 hours. (From Rosen TS, Pippenger CE. Pharmacologic observations on the neonatal withdrawal syndrome. *J Pediatr.* 1976;88:1044–1048.)

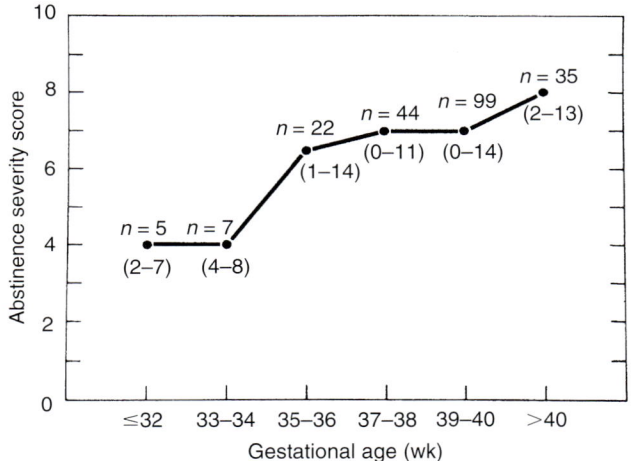

Figure 38.17 Relationship between the severity of the neonatal withdrawal syndrome after passive addiction to methadone and the gestational age of the infant. Scores are expressed as median values, with ranges in parentheses. Note the increase in severity with advancing gestational age. (From Doberczak TM, Kandall SR, Wilets I. Neonatal opiate abstinence syndrome in term and preterm infants. *J Pediatr.* 1991;118:933–937.)

of therapy in a recent study was 35 hours.[555] Ten percent to 15% of infants born to methadone-treated mothers have had onset of their neurological syndrome *after* day 3.[541,622,623] This late onset is rare with infants passively addicted to heroin. The delay in onset correlates with the administration of the last dose of methadone before the time of delivery (Fig. 38.16). Indeed, withdrawal symptoms in infants passively addicted to methadone may occur initially or may recur as late as 2 to 4 weeks or more after birth.[551,623] In fact, an occasional infant has died before the nature of this later syndrome has been recognized.

The reasons for the delayed onset and prolonged duration may relate to the pharmacokinetics of methadone elimination in the newborn.[557,624] It is well known in adults that the withdrawal syndrome in methadone addiction develops more slowly (peak 6 days) and lasts longer than with heroin.[625] Good evidence is available for avid tissue binding of methadone, with gradual and slow release on withdrawal.[626] The critical point is that the clinician must be alert to this possibility of delayed onset in the infant of age 1 week or more who develops jitteriness, diarrhea, and other signs of withdrawal.

The *likelihood of withdrawal symptoms* in an infant exposed to heroin during pregnancy seems to relate primarily to five factors: (1) the amount of the maternal dose; (2) the length of the time from the last dose to birth; (3) the duration of maternal

drug use/abuse; (4) the use of other drugs, particularly nicotine and SSRIs; and (5) the gestational age of the infant at birth.[a] Withdrawal symptoms in the passively addicted newborn are more likely if the maternal dose has been high; if the last dose has been within 24 hours of the time of birth; if the mother has been a long-term user, smokes, or takes SSRIs; and if the infant is born at term.

Similarly, the gestational age of the infant at birth influences the likelihood and severity of neonatal withdrawal after methadone (Fig. 38.17). In contrast to heroin, maternal

---

[a]References 309, 539, 540, 557, 574, 576, 581, and 584.

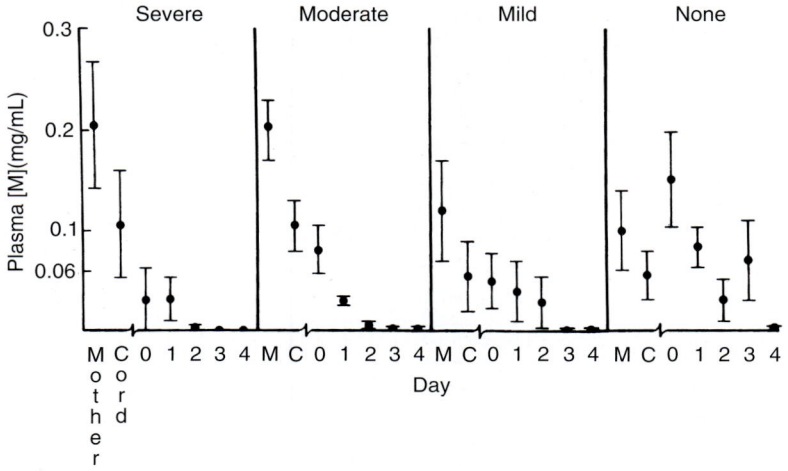

Figure 38.18 **Passive addiction to methadone: relation of occurrence and severity of signs of withdrawal to rate of elimination of methadone.** Data derived from study of 31 infants born to mothers receiving methadone during pregnancy. The fastest declines in plasma methadone (M) concentrations correlated with occurrence of the most severe signs. (From Rosen TS, Pippenger CE. Pharmacologic observations on the neonatal withdrawal syndrome. J Pediatr. 1976;88:1044–1048.)

TABLE 38.19 Signs of Withdrawal From Heroin			
RELATIVE FREQUENCY (PERCENTAGE OF TOTAL)			
75%–100%	**25%–75%**	**<25%**	**RARE**
Jitteriness	Poor feeding	Fever	Seizures
Irritability	Vomiting		
Hyperactivity-hypertonicity	Diarrhea		
Decreased sleeping	Sneezing		
Shrill cry	Tachypnea		
Excessive sucking	Sweating		

methadone dose does *not* appear to be a critical determinant of the likelihood of withdrawal,[554-556] although cord blood levels are inversely related to the occurrence of a neonatal withdrawal syndrome requiring therapy.[555] In fact, the likelihood of neonatal withdrawal features directly correlates with more rapid rates of decline of neonatal methadone levels. Moreover, the *severity* of symptoms also relates particularly to the rate of elimination (Fig. 38.18). This finding is entirely consistent with an observation in adult patients (i.e., a rapid decrease in the drug level in blood causes more frequent and more severe symptoms).

The *initial and dominant symptoms and signs* of the withdrawal syndrome relate primarily to disturbance of the *CNS* (Table 38.19). A virtually invariable feature is jitteriness. As discussed in Chapter 12, the movements of jitteriness are characterized primarily by tremulousness; are exquisitely stimulus-sensitive, rhythmic, and usually of equal rate and amplitude; and can be induced to cease by gentle passive flexion of the limb. Unlike seizure, jitteriness is accompanied neither by abnormalities of gaze or extraocular movement, nor by the clonic jerking of limbs. The tremulous movements in infants passively addicted to heroin are usually quite dramatic and have a coarse, flapping quality. The babies are very irritable and frequently are extremely active and hypertonic. Sleep periods are markedly diminished, and the cry is often high pitched and shrill. Sucking is excessive, and often *frantic sucking* of the fists or fingers has been noted. These frequent clinical features (75% to 100% of symptomatic cases) are very helpful in making the clinical distinction of the jitteriness of drug withdrawal from that resulting from other important causes (e.g., hypoglycemia and hypoxia). Hypoglycemia can cause jitteriness in the first 24 to 48 hours of life, but with hypoglycemia the infant is almost always stuporous as well, quite unlike the hyperalert, hyperactive infant with withdrawal symptoms. Similarly, hypoxic-ischemic encephalopathy characteristically causes jitteriness in the first 24 to 48 hours of life, but such infants almost always have had the characteristic history of a perinatal hypoxic-ischemic insult, are significantly stuporous, and very frequently exhibit seizures. The clinical picture may be complicated by concomitant passive addiction and hypoxic encephalopathy; in several series, 20% to 40% of addicted infants exhibited signs of fetal distress, Apgar scores of six or less at 1 or 5 minutes, or both.[551,622,627]

Next in frequency of occurrence are a series of symptoms relating especially to *gastrointestinal* disturbance (see Table 38.19). Poor feeding is the most prominent of these features (one that in fact may reflect more of a neurological than a gastrointestinal disturbance). Despite the initially excessive sucking described previously, the infant decreases its sucking rapidly with feeding. Poor coordination of sucking, swallowing, and respiration is very common.[589] Regurgitation of feedings is also a relatively common feature. Diarrhea occurs in as many as 30% to 50% of the infants and can contribute to dehydration and electrolyte disturbances. These latter gastrointestinal phenomena tend to appear later (i.e., at days 4 to 6) than those related to the CNS.[539,551,576,580]

Sneezing and tachypnea are less common disturbances (see Table 38.19). Still less common, but disturbing when they do occur, are *fever* and *sweating*. Fever must always raise the possibility of infection, and this possibility should be ruled out by appropriate diagnostic studies. Sweating, while uncommon, can be a helpful diagnostic sign because it is very unusual to see sweating in newborns, especially small newborns.

Seizures are a distinctly uncommon manifestation of neonatal withdrawal to opioids (see Table 38.19). The incidence has been approximately 1% to 2% of cases.[577,581] It is in fact difficult to be convinced from the published data that any of the examples of seizure associated with withdrawal to heroin were not related to complicating factors, such as hypoxia-ischemia or metabolic disease, or were not examples of particularly marked jitteriness. This conclusion is compatible with the fact that seizures are not a feature of withdrawal to heroin in adult patients. Thus it should be emphasized that passive addiction to opioids should be low on the list of considerations when one is faced with a newborn with seizures, and even in the infant definitely passively addicted to heroin, seizure phenomena should raise the possibility of a serious complicating illness and provoke appropriate diagnostic studies.

Neurodevelopmental Consequences

Research examining the longer-term outcomes of children exposed to opioids during pregnancy is even more sparse than the short-term infant outcome studies reviewed earlier. In addition, much of what is known is confined to heroin/methadone exposure, and with a few exceptions, based on older cohorts of children where maternal methadone doses were typically lower than in current practice.[405,575,628] Follow-up rates are also often poor and rarely extend into middle childhood when many cognitive functions are beginning to become apparent. As of yet no studies have examined the effects of maternal prescription opioid use on child development beyond the infancy period. Finally, it is important to note that, as with other drug exposure studies, most pregnant women who use opioids or are in methadone/buprenorphine treatment programs continue to use other drugs.[567] They are also more likely to come from high-risk socioeconomic backgrounds and to raise their children in family circumstances characterized by ongoing drug use and high rates of interpartner violence, child maltreatment and parental dysfunction, poverty, and social risk, making it difficult without large samples to delineate the relative contributions of these factors from the direct effects of the target opioid drug.[567,629,630]

Cognition and Executive Function

Studies examining the cognitive outcomes of children exposed to opioids during pregnancy report conflicting results.[628] While some studies report no difference, others have found that opioid-exposed children perform less well on standardized cognitive measures.[a] In general, cognitive function tends to be within the normal range, although sometimes somewhat lower in opioid-exposed infants than in control infants.[628] Language is also often delayed.[636] At least based on existing methodologically limited evidence, these variations appear to largely reflect the effects of family socioeconomic status and other factors correlated with prenatal opioid exposure.[633] Beyond general cognition, little is known about the extent to which these children are also at risk of executive function and learning problems. The one exception is a study of 35 methadone/buprenorphine-exposed and 31 nonexposed comparison children followed to age 48 to 57 months, which found that exposed children performed less well on behavioral measures of inhibitory control and short-term memory.[638]

---

[a]References 309, 531-537, 539, 540, 549, 551, 576, 614, and 631-637.

Behavior and Regulatory Problems

There is fairly consistent evidence, at least based on parent and teacher report, to show that children exposed to opioids during pregnancy have higher levels of attention, hyperactivity, and impulsivity problems than non-opioid-exposed children.[639-643] There is also some suggestion that these problems may become more problematic with age. However, the proportion of opioid-exposed children who meet either DSM or ICD criteria for a range of potential psychiatric disorders, including anxiety and conduct disorder, is not known.

Motor and Visual Function

There is increasing evidence that infants born to opioid-using mothers may be at increased risk for a range of visual abnormalities, including nystagmus, strabismus, reduced visual acuity, delayed visual maturation (DVM), impaired voluntary eye movements, and absent binocular vision.[598,643-649] A recent study of 81 methadone-exposed and 26 nonexposed comparison infants at age 6 months (retention 79% and 52%, respectively) found that opioid-exposed infants had a fivefold increased risk of failing standardized ophthalmologic assessment, with 40% (32/81) failing and a further 11% (9/81) deemed borderline.[598] Visual abnormalities included horizontal nystagmus (*n* = 9/32), strabismus (*n* = 20/32), and reduced visual acuity (>0.90 logMAR) (*n* = 18/32). The latter was associated with other visual abnormalities in 11 of these infants. Further electrophysiological assessment of visual function using visual evoked potentials (VEP) found that 70% of opioid-exposed infants exhibited abnormal VEP parameters (slower peak times, smaller amplitudes), suggesting that prenatal drug exposure may have altered the functioning of visual pathways and/or cerebral sources of VEPs (see Chapter 10). These adverse clinical and electrophysiological outcomes were independent of other prenatal drug exposures.

Neuropathology

No detailed human neuropathological studies in the setting of fetal opioid exposure are available. However, experimental studies have identified a number of structural alterations that could potentially underlie the effects of maternal opioid use on infant and child outcomes. Although morphologic studies are not entirely uniform, the majority demonstrate decreases in cerebral and cerebellar weight.[479,650-656] Zagon and McLaughlin also found reduced cerebellar area and decreased number and density of internal granular neurons in the cerebellum with perinatal methadone exposure.[654]

Human imaging studies are confined to a small series of studies based on small samples of opioid-exposed infants (*n* = 7 to 16), thus limiting interpretation and generalizability of results. Unfortunately, polydrug use was also common and, given sample size constraints, not able to be taken into account statistically. With these caveats in mind, several volumetric MRI studies suggest that prenatal opioid exposure may be associated with lower overall brain volume shortly after birth, with regions such as the basal ganglia more affected than others.[657,658] Cortical thinning of cingulate and orbitofrontal cortices was also observed.[657] Interestingly, these differences were not found in a cohort of infants born to opioid-dependent mothers who underwent detoxification during pregnancy.[659] Finally, two studies suggest that maturation of white matter tracts may also be affected, with higher mean diffusivity (MD) values found for the superior longitudinal fasciculus.[660,661] Extending this research with more controlled studies of larger samples will be important.

Pathogenesis

Antenatal opioid exposure has both acute and long-term consequences for the newborn. Acute effects occur because of a series of physiological disturbances after withdrawal of chronic opioid receptor stimulation. A cascade of molecular effects appears to be the most important source of long-term alterations in cognition and behavior.

Pathogenesis of Neonatal Abstinence

Opioids act through G protein–coupled receptors μ, κ, and δ; μ-opioid receptors appear to predominate in the developing brain.[662] Neurons in the locus coeruleus of the pons have a high density of noradrenergic μ-opioid receptors, and this nucleus appears to be the principal site that triggers opioid withdrawal.[663] μ-Opioid receptor stimulation suppresses production of cyclic adenosine monophosphate (cAMP), decreasing the release of norepinephrine from neurons in the locus coeruleus. The persistent presence of an opioid stimulus eventually leads to the compensatory release of norepinephrine, possibly through upregulation and/or supersensitization of adenylyl cyclase isoforms (described as *development of alternative pathways* and *disuse hypersensitivity* in the previous edition of this text).[664] Upregulation/supersensitization appears to rely on phosphorylation of the opioid receptor after persistent stimulation, followed by uncoupling from the G protein and receptor colocalization with β-arrestins, protein kinases (including activated Src), and adenylyl cyclases.[665,666] In the absence of depressive opioids, hyperactive neurons in the locus coeruleus release excessive amounts of norepinephrine, resulting in hyperthermia, hypertension, tremors, and tachycardia.[667]

Other sites of altered enzymatic activity include the ventral tegmental area of the midbrain, the medial habenula of the thalamus, the hypothalamus, and the dorsal raphe nucleus of the brain stem. The ventral tegmental area releases less dopamine during opioid withdrawal, resulting in hyperirritability and anxiety.[668] The midbrain and medial habenula release increased amounts of acetylcholine, contributing to diarrhea, vomiting, and diaphoresis.[669] The hypothalamus releases increased amounts of corticotrophin, leading to increased stress and hyperphagia.[670] The dorsal raphe nucleus releases decreased amounts of serotonin during opioid withdrawal, leading to sleep disturbances.[671] Decreased levels of brain-derived neurotrophic factor and corticotrophin releasing-factor appear to underlie the latter; however, the mechanisms of all of these alterations remain incompletely elucidated.

Pathogenesis of Potential Long-Term Consequences

The molecular effects of opioid exposure include apoptosis as well as altered patterns of myelination. In vitro studies demonstrate the apoptotic effect of even a single dose of opioid on neural progenitor cells, increasing levels of caspase-3 in these proliferating cells.[672] Opioids disrupt myelination through multiple mechanisms. Opioids *accelerate* maturation of preoligodendrocytes in the developing brain, a phenomenon that appears to disrupt the synchronized sequence of events contributing to normal connectivity.[673] In addition, opioids suppress neuronal migration to the cortical plate, and alter dendritic growth and branching patterns.[674] The underlying mechanisms of these effects are not completely understood, although they likely reflect, at least to some degree, suppression of activity-dependent network formation as well as phosphorylation and uncoupling of the opioid receptor after persistent stimulation. Receptor colocalization and binding with β-arrestin activates signal transduction, recruiting kinases. Formation of a receptor/β-arrestin/extracellular signal-regulated kinase (Erk) aggregate inhibits the growth-promoting effects of Erk. Alternatively, receptor/β-arrestin may bind to c-Jun N-terminal kinase and apoptosis signal-regulating kinase, increasing the activity of these mediators of cell death.[675] In addition, chronic opioid exposure results in lower levels of BDNF in the hippocampus. Decreased levels of BDNF precipitate decreased activation of tropomyosin receptor kinase (Trk) receptors, expressed widely in this brain region. Trk receptors are responsible for the release of Akt serine/threonine kinase, an essential inhibitor of the apoptotic caspase cascade.[676] Cumulatively these, and likely other perturbations, result in the phenotypic neurodevelopmental manifestations of fetal opioid exposure.

Prevention

As discussed earlier, complete abstinence represents the safest choice for optimal fetal development. In mothers with an opioid addiction, maintenance treatment offers an opportunity to minimize and stabilize the effects of opioid exposure on the fetus. *Methadone* is the historic mainstay of maintenance therapy. Benefits of methadone over continued use of illicit drugs include improved adherence to obstetric care, decreased risk of HIV infection, and increased fetal growth.[677] *Buprenorphine*, a partial μ-opioid agonist, has emerged as a potential alternative maintenance therapy. Buprenorphine possesses greater affinity for the μ-opioid receptor, but causes less activation. Buprenorphine also has very low transplacental transfer.[678] Randomized controlled trials (RCTs) have demonstrated shorter hospitalization and decreased dose and duration of morphine therapy for NAS with buprenorphine in comparison to methadone.[604] Disadvantages of buprenorphine include the difficulty of initiating this therapy in pregnancy, with a higher early dropout rate observed in a recent randomized controlled trial.[604] In addition, there is a lack of long-term data describing childhood outcomes after fetal buprenorphine exposure. Although such long-term data are lacking, preliminary data are hopeful. Experimental data suggest a lower impact on myelination in the developing brain.[679] In clinical studies, neonatal head circumference is larger, and neonatal neurobehavior is improved with buprenorphine exposure compared with methadone.[680,681] Four-month-old infants have a significantly shorter latency of peak response to pattern-reversal VEPs.[682] These promising early findings suggest potential, but must be confirmed by long-term follow-up studies.

Pharmacological treatment of mothers aimed at modifying withdrawal in newborns has been explored recently. *Ondansetron* represents such a promising therapy. The Htr3a gene, which encodes the 5-HT3 receptor, has been identified as a modulator of the response to precipitated withdrawal in mice. In susceptible mice, administration of ondansetron, a 5-HT3 antagonist, reduces the physical symptoms of withdrawal.[683] Ondansetron rapidly crosses the placenta in humans, raising the possibility

TABLE 38.20   Management of Withdrawal Syndrome in Infants Passively Addicted to Opioids

Recognition
Supportive therapy
Drug therapy
Opioid[a]: morphine or methadone
Clonidine[b]
Phenobarbital[c]

[a]Treatment of first choice.

[b]Combination of opioid and clonidine may be superior to opioid alone (see text).

[c]Adjunctive therapy reserved for infants exposed to barbiturates or benzodiazepines in addition to opioids.

of antenatal therapy to blunt NAS.[684] This therapy requires further evaluation, including examination of the impact of antenatal intervention on developmental outcome. It is also unclear how long the modification of withdrawal symptoms will last after birth.

Treatment

The three important components in the clinical management of NAS secondary to opioids are recognition, supportive therapy, and drug therapy (Table 38.20).

Recognition

First, the diagnosis must be considered. Perhaps it is trite to include this discussion, but so often the diagnosis is overlooked for a day or more because of incomplete maternal history. All pregnant women should be screened by their obstetrician using a standardized screening tool.[685] A maternal history of hepatitis, thrombophlebitis, or other complications of illicit drug usage should also be sought. The newborn's physician must confirm that screening has occurred and, if necessary, ask the specific question of drug use, preferably directly to the mother. Suitable screening of urine and especially meconium is useful if not recommended. Infants at risk for NAS should be carefully monitored for signs of withdrawal for an appropriate duration depending on the exposure (i.e., 3 days for short half-life opiates and 5 to 7 days for opiates with a prolonged half-life).[686] Each nursery should adopt a standardized abstinence assessment tool (commonly the Lipsitz tool or modified Finnegan's tool) and ensure staff are trained in correct use.[687,688]

Supportive Therapy

Supportive therapy is clearly the most critical aspect of the management of these infants. Optimal supportive therapy includes minimization of environmental stimuli (dark, quiet environment), avoiding autostimulation (careful swaddling), optimized positioning and comfort technique, and frequent small-volume feeding.[686] Additional nonpharmacologic therapies, including laser acupuncture, have been used with some success.[689] Notably, rooming in with family may provide a superior environment for care compared with the NICU.[690] In the absence of specific contraindications, mothers who adhere to a supervised drug treatment program should be encouraged to breastfeed.[691]

Drug Therapy

The third major aspect of the therapeutic program is the choice of the drug to be used for the treatment of severe CNS and gastrointestinal disturbances. Of particular concern are marked jitteriness and hyperactivity, minimal sleeping, impaired feeding, persistent vomiting, and diarrhea. Currently evidence is lacking to define unequivocally optimal pharmacological therapy for NAS. Research regarding the optimal treatment threshold as well as the long-term neurodevelopmental outcomes of newborns treated with various strategies is urgently needed. The following represents our best assessment of the current literature.

Opioids, specifically morphine or methadone, form the backbone of therapy for NAS secondary to opioid exposure.[692,693] These agents have replaced paregoric and tincture of opium because of variable concentrations and toxic ingredients, including a high concentration of alcohol in both products. Opioids appear to provide superior symptom resolution with a shorter overall duration of therapy compared with monotherapy with sedatives, including phenobarbital and diazepam.[692] Morphine is generally initiated at 0.05 to 0.1 mg/kg every 3 to 4 hours. The short half-life of morphine allows for rapid titration to clinical effect. Methadone was traditionally given at a similar dose, with an interval of 12 hours. However, recent reports have leveraged the long half-life of methadone with short initial intervals (every 4 to 6 hours) to gain rapid control, followed by aggressive weaning, resulting in a shorter length of stay compared with morphine.[694-696]

Adjunctive therapy has traditionally been used after the failure of monotherapy. More recently, adjunctive agents have been explored to reduce the magnitude and duration of opioid exposure. *Phenobarbital* has traditionally been the adjunct of choice and remains the preferred second agent for newborns with polydrug exposure.[616] Loading doses of 20 mg/kg are generally followed by 5 mg/kg per day, with the maintenance dose adjusted by symptoms. However, concerns regarding the long-term impact of phenobarbital exposure have led to the consideration of alternative adjunctive agents.[698] *Clonidine*, an α_2-adrenergic receptor agonist, has been proposed because of promising clinical data, as well as evidence for neuroprotection in experimental studies.[699,700] Recent work suggests value for clonidine, initiated at 0.5 to 3 mcg/kg every 3 to 6 hours, as adjunctive therapy to opioid.[698] Moreover, clonidine has recently been evaluated as *monotherapy*, in an effort to eliminate opioid exposure during the initial period of rapid postnatal brain development.[701] A small pilot trial demonstrated a decreased duration of clonidine monotherapy compared with morphine monotherapy, with better neurobehavioral scores at 1 week and 2 to 4 weeks after initiation of treatment. No difference was noted in motor, cognitive, or language scores at 1 year of age.[702] A larger randomized controlled trial appears warranted and will inform the rapidly evolving effort to optimize pharmacotherapy in newborns exposed to opioids in utero. Regardless of the agents chosen, *staff education and standardized treatment protocols* have been clearly shown to decrease length of stay.[703-706]

ANTIDEPRESSANTS

SSRIs are the most commonly prescribed pharmacological treatment for major depressive disorder. The most common SSRIs include sertraline and fluoxetine. These drugs exert their effect by binding to the serotonin transporter (SERT) to prevent the uptake of serotonin by the presynaptic neuron. As a neurotransmitter, serotonin plays a central role in both the developing and mature brain. Developmentally, it is involved in neuronal proliferation, neuronal migration, and synaptogenesis.[707] There is also some suggestion that it may contribute to neuroplasticity in the developing brain, with higher levels of serotonin increasing the brain's sensitivity to the influence of both harmful and beneficial environmental exposures.[708] Although the efficacy of SSRIs in treating depression is well established, less is known about their effects on fetal brain development.

Prevalence

For women, the risk of developing a depressive episode is highest during the childbearing years.[709] Pregnancy and motherhood are also associated with increased risk.[710] As a result, an estimated 14% to 23% of pregnant women will experience clinically significant depressive symptoms, with up to a half of this group receiving treatment with an SSRI.[711,712] In line with general population trends suggesting increases in the use of prescription medications by pregnant women, antidepressant use is also trending upward, rising in the United States from 2% in 1996 to more than 7% by 2008.[713,714]

Clinical Features

Similar to other prescription drugs reviewed, a methodological challenge in understanding the short- and long-term effects of prenatal SSRI exposure is determining the relative contributions of an underlying maternal medical condition, in this case depressive symptomatology, and the drug used to treat the condition. Despite these challenges, large epidemiologic studies have increased our understanding of the potential impacts of exposure.

Maternal-Fetal Effects

Based on a recent systematic review of eight studies involving more than a million women, SSRI treatment during pregnancy has been linked with a small increase in the risk of preterm birth, even after controlling for other risk factors (OR = 1.24).[715] Relatedly, there is also an increased risk of low birth weight and a lower APGAR score at birth.[716-719] However, of particular significance, SSRIs do not appear to increase the risk of congenital malformations in the infant.[720,721] One exception may be a slight elevation in the risk of cardiovascular malformations (OR = 1.36), although this finding may reflect the higher rate of diagnostic tests in exposed women.[722-724]

Neonatal Effects

Although congenital malformations do not appear to be a major concern, there is consistent evidence of short-term adverse neurobehavioral effects of antidepressant exposure, with motor and autonomic systems most affected (Table 38.21). Specifically, infants are characterized by greater agitation, irritability, tremors, spasms, hypertonia, hypotonia, respiratory problems, and sleep disturbance.[719,725-729] For about 30% of infants, these difficulties may be sufficiently severe to present in a manner that is somewhat similar to NAS. This occurrence is often referred to as *poor neonatal adaptation syndrome*.[730]

In addition, SSRIs have been linked to the pathophysiology of persistent pulmonary hypertension of the newborn (PPHN).[731]

TABLE 38.21	Clinical Phenomena in Newborns Exposed to SSRIs in Utero[a]	
CLINICAL FEATURE	**SSRI-EXPOSED INFANTS** ($n = 60$)	**CONTROL INFANTS** ($n = 60$)
Neonatal abstinence syndrome[a]	18	0
High-pitched cry	18	0
Sleep disturbance	21	2
Tremor	37	11
Hypertonicity or myoclonus	14	1
Convulsions	2	0
Tachypnea	12	0
Gastrointestinal disturbance	34	2
Hypoglycemia	3	0

[a]Finnegan score of 4 or higher.
SSRIs, Selective serotonin reuptake inhibitors.
Data from Levinson-Castiel R, Merlob P, Linder N, Sirota L, Klinger G. Neonatal abstinence syndrome after in utero exposure to selective serotonin reuptake inhibitors in term infants. *Arch Pediatr Adolesc Med.* 2006;160:173–176.

Initially, smaller epidemiologic studies suggested a dramatic impact.[732] More recently, larger studies have confirmed the significance of this association, but emphasize a smaller relative risk than previously suggested (OR = 1.51). They also emphasize that PPHN, even in SSRI-exposed newborns, was relatively rare, affecting 32 infants per 10,000 live births.[733]

Neurodevelopmental Consequences

Compared with other drug exposures during pregnancy, follow-up studies of children born to mothers treated with antidepressants during pregnancy are limited. These studies also are subject to challenges associated with differentiating direct drug effects from maternal mental health effects, both during pregnancy and after birth. In addition, few studies have extended beyond infancy and early childhood, thereby precluding study of developmental functions yet to emerge. In general, findings suggest few adverse effects, with the exception of perhaps some suggestion of elevated risks of anxiety and depression.

Cognition and Executive Functioning

No association has been found between prenatal SSRI exposure and children's general cognitive development on either standardized measures, such as the Bayley scales, or parent reports.[716,734-738] Executive abilities have not been examined.

Language Development

One study of 178 mother-infant dyads found a small five-point decrement in children's expressive language scores during early childhood but a large representative control group was not included.[734] Thus further replication is needed.

Behavior

This functional domain appears to be most affected by prenatal SSRI exposure. Findings suggest some persistence of regulatory difficulties, with slightly elevated levels of anxiety during early childhood, even after adjusting for maternal and familial factors.[738-741] These difficulties are also observed into early adolescence, with a recent large national registry study in Finland showing that prenatal SSRI exposure was associated with increased cumulative rates of the diagnosis of depression (8.2% vs. 1.9% among infants born to nonpharmacologically treated women with a psychiatric disorder). No association with ASD or ADHD was observed.[742] However, other registry studies have noted a significant link between prenatal SSRI exposure and ASD, even after controlling for maternal depression.[743] Replication is needed with potential adverse consequences balanced against the significant risks associated with untreated maternal depression.[744,745] Longer-term follow-up will also be important, as the risk of depression increases over the course of adolescence.

Motor Function

There is some evidence for slower psychomotor and fine motor development among infants prenatally exposed to SSRIs based on parent report screening measures.[738,746] However, the difficulties are subtle and appear to resolve by age 2 years. These findings also require replication with standardized tools administered by blinded testers before firm conclusions can be established.

Neuropathology

No human neuropathological data are available. A recent structural MRI study compared 27 infants prenatally exposed to an SSRI, 41 who were born to mothers with a history of depression but no prenatal SSRI use, and 54 unexposed comparison infants.[747] At age 1 month, no differences were found between infants born to depressed mothers treated with an SSRI and either those whose mother had a history of depression but no prenatal SSRI use or control infants. However, SSRI-exposed infants exhibited lower fractional anisotropy (FA) and increased MD values across multiple white matter tracts. These results suggest widespread alterations in white matter microstructural development. There was also some evidence of lower volumes of right thalamic gray matter tissue, despite no differences in total brain tissue volumes. These findings are interesting but clearly demand further replication. Although inclusion of a group of infants born to mothers with a history of depression but who were not being treated with an SSRI is a clear strength, it is also likely that these mothers would have had a less severe disorder, which may account at least in part for study findings. There is also a need for future studies to control for other pregnancy factors, such as maternal nutrition, that may also affect fetal brain development.

Pathogenesis

SSRIs inhibit serotonin uptake at the presynaptic nerve ending by the SERT, resulting in an increased serotonin concentration in the synaptic cleft and thereby potentiated serotonergic neurotransmission.[748]

Pathogenesis of Poor Neonatal Adaptation Syndrome

The etiology of the neonatal neurobehavioral disturbances after SSRI exposure remains unknown. *Intoxication* in the early postpartum period may be important. The symptoms observed in newborns are similar to those associated with serotonin toxicity in adults.[749] Some newborns whose symptoms occur immediately after birth have had serum SSRI concentrations and cord blood markers of increased SSRI activity.[750,751] However, in most infants, symptoms begin approximately 8 hours after birth and persist for 2 to 4 days.[752] Notably, irritability, tremors, and sleep disturbances are also observed in adult *SSRI withdrawal.*[753] It seems likely that the neurobehavioral symptoms of neonatal SSRI exposure may occur because of withdrawal and/or toxicity. Genetic factors, including polymorphisms in CYP450 2D6 and 3A4, alter SSRI metabolism in mothers and may influence the incidence and severity of neurobehavioral symptoms in the newborn.[754] In addition, polymorphisms in the promoter region of the SERT gene (SLC6A4) are known to influence susceptibility to SSRIs in adults and have been shown to influence neurobehavioral symptoms after exposure in the newborn.[755]

Pathogenesis of Potential Long-Term Effects

During development, *serotonin plays a vital role in neurogenesis, neuronal migration and differentiation, and synaptogenesis.*[707] In experimental models, prenatal exposure to SSRIs disrupts thalamocortical afferents and dendritic organization and results in aberrant axonal morphology, abnormal raphe circuitry, and altered cortical function.[756-759] However, some alterations in brain morphology resolve in adulthood after withdrawal of the drug.[760] The mechanisms underlying these perturbations in early life are unclear. Throughout life, serotonin is a fundamental modulator of many cognitive and behavioral functions. Experimental models suggest that exposure to SSRIs during development reduces the expression of the 5-HT$_{1A}$ receptor gene in the midbrain and increases the expression of SERT in the hypothalamus and hippocampus in adulthood.[761] These longstanding disruptions in gene expression may explain alterations in the risk of psychiatric disorders observed in epidemiological studies of SSRI exposure.

Prevention

The decision to use pharmacological antidepressants in pregnancy is complex and multifactorial. The negative effects of untreated depression to mother and child must be weighed against the possible negative effects of medications on the developing fetus. Untreated maternal depression is associated with low birth weight and prematurity, as well as alterations in neonatal neurobehavior.[762] In addition, maternal-child attachment exerts influence on learning and behavior later in life.[763] Behavioral cognitive therapy should be considered as the first line of therapy for depression.[764,765] For women on medication with mild or no symptoms for longer than 6 months, it may be appropriate to taper or discontinue medication. Withholding or discontinuing medication is most likely not appropriate in women with a history of severe, recurrent depression or other psychiatric illnesses requiring medication. As paroxetine has been most consistently associated with adverse effects in newborns, alternative agents should be used with women requiring pharmacological therapy.[766,767]

Treatment

Recovery from the neurobehavioral effects of prenatal SSRI exposure generally occurs over days. Hospitalization is often prolonged, although specific interventions to reduce the length of stay or the severity of symptoms have not been defined.[768] Supportive therapy, as described for opioid exposure, should be used. Chlorpromazine has been described as a successful treatment for severe symptoms in newborns exposed to SSRIs, although many experts recommend phenobarbital.[768,769] In view of the uncertainty regarding the long-term impact of these agents, referral to early intervention therapy is not common. However, careful follow-up of the infant is recommended.[712,770,771] Further research regarding the value of both short-term and long-term interventions is needed because of the increasing prevalence of this exposure in the population.

SEDATIVES

Hypnotic or sedating medications can be used to treat insomnia, anxiety, and panic disorders, as well as restless leg syndrome during pregnancy. This section predominantly focuses on *benzodiazepines*, most commonly lorazepam, diazepam, or alprazolam, which are $GABA_A$ receptor agonists. Newer sedatives, including such *commonly prescribed sleep aids* as eszopiclone (Lunesta), zaleplon (Sonata), and zolpidem (Ambien), act as selective agonists of the α_1 subunit of the $GABA_A$ receptor.[772] The use of these agents during pregnancy raises concerns about their impact on the developing fetus.[773]

Prevalence

There has been a decline in the prescribing of benzodiazepines in the general population in recent years.[774] This downward trend has also been seen with respect to their use during pregnancy. An epidemiological study from 1988 to 1990 across 22 countries found that 3% of pregnant women were prescribed benzodiazepines and 3.5% some form of psychotropic drug.[775] The primary reasons given for benzodiazepine use were anxiety and insomnia, with chronic use being rare. More recent estimates suggest rates ranging from 0.1% to 2%, depending on the sample studied.[776-779]

In contrast to benzodiazepines, the use of prescription sleep aids has become more common, with recent data suggesting that about 5% of women are using these medications.[773] This population trend has resulted in increased exposure during pregnancy, with a recent report showing that 2.4% of pregnant women are likely to be treated with a prescription sleep aid.[780]

Clinical Features
Maternal-Fetal Effects
Data on the potential teratogenic effects of benzodiazepines and other sedative drug use during pregnancy are scarce and limited to retrospective registry studies. Based on this research, evidence suggests that maternal sedative use during pregnancy *does not increase the risk of major congenital anomalies* in the infant.[776,778,781-783] However, these drugs have been linked with an increased risk of *preterm birth, low birth weight*, and other adverse neonatal outcomes.[778,779,781,784] For example, a Swedish national birth registry study found that the maternal use of benzodiazepines and benzodiazepine receptor agonists was associated with modest increases in the odds of preterm birth (OR = 1.5) and low birth weight (OR = 1.3).[778] Although less common, these odds were even greater for infants born to mothers who were taking these drugs later in their pregnancy (preterm OR = 2.6, LBW OR = 1.9), suggesting that use was for a chronic as opposed to short-term problem. No increased risks were observed on infant Apgar scores or for respiratory problems.

In contrast to this Swedish study, similar but higher odds of preterm birth and having a low-birth-weight infant were found in a cohort of more than 2500 pregnant women in the United States, where benzodiazepine use was somewhat more common (3% vs. Sweden's 2.3%).[779] After taking into account a range of maternal (age, race, pregnancy smoking, preeclampsia) and infant (parity, multiple birth) factors, infants born to women who used benzodiazepines had clearly increased odds of preterm birth (OR = 6.8) and a low birth weight infant (OR = 7.4). However, in contrast to the Swedish study noted previously, the risk of a low (<7) Apgar score (OR = 3.9), intensive care admission (OR = 4.3), and respiratory distress syndrome (OR = 3.7) was also elevated. One potential explanation for these study differences could be the greater use of lorazepam in the US cohort, highlighting the need for larger data sets that allow the effects of different drugs to be compared in the same population.

Neonatal Effects

In terms of *neurobehavioral characteristics*, some but not all infants exhibit either a floppy infant syndrome or neonatal withdrawal symptoms to varying degrees. Features of the floppy infant syndrome include mild sedation, hypothermia, hypotonia, poor suck, hyperbilirubinemia, and CNS depression.[785-790] There are also several published reports of a withdrawal syndrome, with symptoms being largely neurologic, including jitteriness, irritability, hyperactivity, hypertonicity, and an impaired metabolic response to cold stress.[551,789-792] Diarrhea and vomiting are also not typical. These difficulties persist for approximately 2 to 6 weeks and respond well to phenobarbital therapy.[792] The occurrence of neonatal withdrawal to diazepam is understandable in view of the fact that the drug is a small, highly lipid-soluble molecule that readily crosses the placenta and accumulates in fetal tissues, especially adipose tissue.[551,793] The drug, with a half-life of 54 hours, is eliminated slowly by the newborn.[794] The reason for the early onset of symptoms, despite the relatively long half-life, probably relates to the interval from the last maternal dose of the drug to the time of birth, which has varied from 2 to 14 days.[792] The limited ability of the newborn to mobilize, metabolize, and excrete diazepam results in the appearance of drug metabolites in the urine for many weeks[794] and probably accounts for the prolonged duration of symptoms.

Neurodevelopmental Consequences

Virtually nothing is known about the longer-term outcomes of infants exposed prenatally to sedative drugs. Of the small number of studies that do exist, results suggest that infants may catch up in weight by age 8 months.[796] Early differences in muscle tone and general body movements, as well as lower general development scores, have also been reported.[797-799] However, the interpretation of these findings is challenging because of small sample sizes, the use of global measures that were not administered by *blinded* examiners, and the lack of control for other confounding maternal and infant factors.

Neuropathology

No neuroimaging studies of infants or children prenatally exposed to sedatives are available. A study of 138 very preterm infants found that higher mean doses of midazolam administered in the NICU were associated with poorer hippocampal development at term equivalent age, based on MRI measures of hippocampal volume and diffusivity.[800] Hippocampal measures were in turn predictive of lower cognitive scores on the Bayley at corrected age 18 months.

Pathogenesis

Despite limited clinical research, the impact of sedatives on the developing brain has been a focus of experimental research for more than 3 decades. Findings from this body of work indicate that GABA agonists induce significant apoptotic degeneration of oligodendrocytes and suppress neurogenesis in the immature brain.[801,802] These findings may be a function of the paradoxical excitatory nature of $GABA_A$ receptors within the immature CNS (see Chapter 12), although this functionality is most prominent in the perinatal period.[803] Alternatively, $GABA_A$ receptor-mediated neurosuppression may also suppress activity-dependent network formation (as discussed previously).

In contrast, virtually nothing is known about the impact of the newer sleep aid drugs, α_1-selective $GABA_A$ receptor agonists, on the fetal and infant brain. Studies in adult experimental models suggest that these agents may protect against hypoxia-induced apoptosis,[804] but similar effects cannot be presumed in the immature brain, given the paradoxical action of GABA receptors in this setting. Given their growing use in pregnancy, and related findings for benzodiazepines and anesthetic agents (see later), there is a need for both experimental and clinical research examining both their mechanisms of action and short- and longer-term effects on fetal development.

Prevention

Disturbed sleep may be an independent risk factor for adverse pregnancy outcomes, highlighting the difficulty of understanding the impacts of treatment per se.[805] Nonpharmacological approaches should form the foundation of treatment—most notably cognitive behavioral therapies.[806] Diphenhydramine is a widely used, over-the-counter medication treating both hyperemesis gravidarum and sleep disturbances during pregnancy.[807,808] Limited data suggest no association with major malformations, although caution and further investigation is warranted.[809]

Treatment

Diazepam is the benzodiazepine described in the vast majority of cases informing the presentation and treatment of perinatal intoxication/withdrawal. Exposure in labor may produce hypothermia, with CNS depression being common.[785,786] The onset of symptoms is highly dependent on the last maternal dose, given the long half-life of diazepam in the newborn.[810] Symptoms are largely neurological, including jitteriness, irritability, hyperactivity, and hypertonicity. Symptoms persist for approximately 2 to 6 weeks and respond well to phenobarbital therapy.[792] Risks are likely to be greater for the infant born to mothers characterized by chronic sedative use during pregnancy.[797]

Sleep aids have not, as of yet, been linked with a neurobehavioral syndrome in exposed newborns. However, withdrawal symptoms have been reported after chronic use in adults.[811] Thus infants exposed chronically to these agents in pregnancy warrant careful monitoring.

ANESTHETICS

As an extension to the discussion of maternal sedative use during pregnancy, the effects of fetal exposure to anesthetic agents also merit discussion in view of growing concerns about their potential teratogenic effects during pregnancy and in early life.[812-818] Surgery and anesthesia may be needed during pregnancy for reasons that may or may not be related to the pregnancy. Pregnancy-related indications for surgery include cervical incompetence, ovarian cysts, fetal anomaly, and cesarean section, and unrelated reasons including acute abdominal infections, maternal trauma, and tumor removal.[812,813] Anesthetic agents used in these procedures include inhalational anesthetics, such as nitrous oxide, desflurane, isoflurane, and sevoflurane; barbiturates; benzodiazepines; ketamine; and propofol. The chemical properties and mechanisms of action of these drugs overlap with those for alcohol and sedative drugs reviewed earlier. Specifically, inhalational anesthetics are combined NMDA antagonists/GABA agonists, among other actions, whereas barbiturates, benzodiazepines, and propofol are potent GABA agonists. Finally, ketamine is an NMDA antagonist. However, for surgical purposes, they are administered at much higher doses over a shorter period of time, ranging from 1 to 12 hours.

Prevalence

Estimates suggest that between 0.5% and 4% of women require nonobstetric surgery at some point during their pregnancy.[812] In terms of timing, these procedures most commonly occur early in pregnancy, with 42% in the first trimester, 35% in the second trimester, and 23% in the third trimester.[819] The usage of general anesthesia during cesarean delivery (as many as 33% of overall deliveries in developed countries) varies widely, from 5% to 30%, depending heavily on the urgency and setting of delivery.[820]

Clinical Features

Based on extensive experimental and limited human data, several factors have been shown to influence the extent to which prenatal anesthetic exposure has adverse effects on the developing fetal brain. These include (1) the duration of exposure, (2) the concentration of the drug used, (3) the number of times anesthetics were used during pregnancy, (4) the number of anesthetics used, and (5) the developmental timing of fetal exposure to the anesthetic agent.[817,821] Increasing duration, drug dose, number of drugs, and frequency of use are therefore likely to be associated with increasing neurodevelopmental risk for the infant. However, a major challenge of clinical studies examining the potential teratogenic effects of anesthetic agents is distinguishing direct drug effects from the effects of the underlying maternal condition making surgery necessary, as well as the indirect effects associated with respiratory depression, hypotension, and hypothermia, secondary to general anesthesia, that may also result in teratogenic consequences for the fetus.

Maternal and Neonatal Effects

As noted previously, with the exception of a few studies of pregnant women at risk of anesthetic exposure because of their occupations (e.g., veterinary staff), almost all studies examining maternal and neonatal effects of prenatal anesthetic exposure are retrospective registry studies.[822] One systematic review of pregnancy and neonatal outcomes for women undergoing elective or emergency surgery during pregnancy found an *increased risk of preterm birth* and, for first trimester surgeries only, a small increased risk of pregnancy loss and congenital malformations.[823] The anesthetic agent used was not specified. More recently, a 10-year retrospective chart review of 235 pregnant women undergoing adnexal mass surgery found a significantly higher rate of preterm birth (7.7% vs. 4.8% in the general population).[824] Risk was higher for women undergoing regional anesthesia for laparotomy (29.6%) than for women given inhalational anesthesia for either laparotomy (5.8%) or laparoscopy (0%). There is a clear need for more detailed measurement of the effects of different anesthetic agents, doses, and exposure durations, with consideration of the impacts of maternal and surgical factors.

Neurodevelopmental Consequences

Only two studies have examined the longer-term outcomes associated with prenatal anesthetic exposure, with both focusing on cesarean section, a late and relatively mild exposure.[825,826] In a review of the medical and educational records of children living in five towns across Minnesota, the investigators found no increased risk of learning disability among children born by cesarean section with anesthetic assistance, compared with those born vaginally. A second study also found no link with ASD.[826] Longer-term outcome studies of pregnant women and their anesthetic-exposed infants are critically needed to understand the possible effects of more prolonged anesthetic exposure and/or multiple exposures on measures of neurodevelopmental function such as attention, behavior, and executive function.

Neuropathology and Pathophysiology

Animal data indicate that the *window of vulnerability* to the neurotoxic effects of anesthetics particularly involves the period of *synaptogenesis*. As described in Chapter 7, this period extends from approximately the third trimester to around 3 to 4 years of age. Anesthetic exposure during synaptogenesis in rodents and nonhuman primates consistently produces *neurodegeneration, particularly apoptosis, and impairment of proper synapse formation*.[827-830] These morphologic changes result in long-term alterations in synaptic transmission.[831] Although the pathologic (as well as therapeutic) mechanisms of inhalational anesthetics have not been completely described, the combination of NMDA antagonism/GABA agonism appears to contribute significantly.[832] In fact, initial interest in the apoptotic potential of anesthetics was driven largely by existing knowledge of the impact of alcohol on the fetus. Although the differences in duration and magnitude of exposure limit extrapolation to anesthetics, some of the pathogenic mechanisms for alcohol and anesthetics appear to overlap substantially (see the discussion of molecular effects in the section on alcohol pathogenesis).[833] However, in view of the pleiotropic nature of inhalational anesthetics, numerous points of developmental disruption have been identified both during neurogenesis and synaptogenesis, with their relevance for the human infant yet to be established (Table 38.22).[821]

Prevention

In obstetric patients requiring surgery, selection of the optimal agent, dose, and duration of anesthesia remains important. Balancing the potential neurotoxic effects of anesthetic agents

TABLE 38.22	Pathogenic Mechanisms of Anesthetic Neurotoxicity During Brain Development

- Apoptotic neurodegeneration
- Suppression of neurogenesis
- Impairment of proper synapse formation
- Alteration of dendritic spine formation
- Deformation of actin, a cytoskeletal protein in neurons and astroglia
- Neuronal mitochondrial dysfunction
- Dysregulation of neuronal calcium

Adapted from Palanisamy A. Maternal anesthesia and fetal neurodevelopment. *Int J Obstet Anesth.* 2012;21;152–162.

with the clear benefits of providing adequate anesthesia during major surgery remains an ongoing challenge in clinical practice. Little to no data exist comparing agents or adding neuroprotective strategies in the setting of antenatal surgery.

MARIJUANA

The prevalence of marijuana use during pregnancy has nearly doubled in the past decade.[834] Given recent trends to decriminalize and, in some states of the United States, legalize its use, marijuana use is expected to increase further. Therefore it is an important drug to consider in the obstetric and neonatal setting.

Prevalence

Marijuana is the most commonly used illicit drug during pregnancy, with prevalence rates ranging from 1% to 11%, depending on the population studied and the method of detection used.[834-841] Although it is the *most widely used illicit drug*, its prevalence is lower than rates reported for such legally obtainable drugs as alcohol and tobacco/nicotine.[839] As with other illicit drugs of abuse, these estimates almost certainly underestimate the prevalence, given their reliance on maternal self-report. Furthermore, in view of the vast body of epidemiological research linking availability and drug use, rates are expected to rise as marijuana becomes more socially acceptable and available, especially in regions where it is currently or soon to be legalized.[835] The use of marijuana during pregnancy is highest in the first trimester (11%) and then declines through the second (3%) and third (2%) trimesters.[839] After birth, women tend to quickly resume use.[842] The demographic and psychosocial profile of women who use marijuana during pregnancy has been characterized in a large sample of more than 12,000 women as part of the UK-based Avon Longitudinal Study of Pregnancy and Childhood.[836] Relative to nonusing pregnant women, those who used marijuana during pregnancy tended to be younger, of lower parity, better educated, and were more likely to also use alcohol, nicotine, and hard drugs. Similar results were reported in a record linkage study which found that close to 50% were concurrent tobacco smokers (>10 cigarettes/day), 12% opioid users, 10% stimulant users, and 4% had an alcohol-related disorder.[843] An even higher rate of marijuana and tobacco co-use was reported in the more recent Generation R study

TABLE 38.23   Relative Risks of Adverse Clinical Outcomes for Infants Exposed to Marijuana During Pregnancy: Results From Two Meta-Analyses

BIRTH CHARACTERISTICS	GUNN ET AL. 2016 RELATIVE RISK		CONNER ET AL. 2016 RELATIVE RISK	
	UNADJUSTED	ADJUSTED	UNADJUSTED	ADJUSTED
Low birth weight (<2500 g)	1.7	—	1.4	ns
Preterm birth (<37 weeks' gestation)	ns	—	1.3	ns
Length	ns	—	—	—
Head circumference	ns	—	—	—
Level II/III NICU admission	2.0	—	ns	—
Neurobehavioral features				
↑ Arousal				
↑ Excitablity				
↓ State regulation				
↑ Tremors, startles				

Adjusted for tobacco use in pregnancy, social background factors, and in some cases, other drug use.

ns, Not significant.

Data sources: Gunn JK, Rosales CB, Center KE, et al. Prenatal exposure to cannabis and maternal and child health outcomes: a systematic review and meta-analysis. *BMJ Open.* 2016;6:e009986 and Conner SN, Bedell V, Lipsey K, Macones GA, Cahill AG, Tuuli MG. Maternal marijuana use and adverse neonatal outcomes: a systematic review and meta-analysis. *Obstet Gynecol.* 2016;128:713–723.

of women in Rotterdam, with four out of five marijuana users also smoking tobacco (85%).[844] These findings emphasize the need for further inquiry about other adverse lifestyle behaviors, should pregnancy marijuana use be disclosed or detected.

Notably, marijuana may also be used during pregnancy for perceived therapeutic indications. Two cannabinoid medications (dronabinol and nabilone) are approved by the U.S. Food and Drug Administration for the treatment of chemotherapy-induced nausea. In addition, nausea is an approved indication for medical marijuana in all states where it is legalized. Low quality evidence supports the efficacy of cannabinoids for this indication.[845] However, this evidence has been extrapolated to the treatment of nausea in pregnancy, including hyperemesis gravidarum. In fact, epidemiological data suggest pregnant women with nausea are significantly more likely to use marijuana compared with other pregnant women.[846] Given current uncertainty about the impact of marijuana on the developing fetus, medical professionals should caution against this practice.[847]

Clinical Features

Maternal-Fetal Effects

There is an increased risk of preeclampsia in women who co-use marijuana and tobacco during pregnancy, even after controlling for confounding factors (adjusted OR = 2.5, 95% CI 1.4 to 5.0).[848] Continued maternal marijuana use has also been linked with an increased fetal pulsatility index and resistance index of the uterine artery, suggesting higher placental resistance during pregnancy.[849] Because the placental circulation is important for fetal growth, these findings may contribute in part to the elevated risks of poor fetal growth reported among chronic marijuana users.

Neonatal Effects

Current data do not indicate that marijuana has major teratogenic effects on the fetus. With respect to growth and other neonatal effects, findings are less consistent. In general studies suggest infants born to mothers who use marijuana during pregnancy may have a small increased risk of poorer fetal growth, low birth weight, and the need for intensive care support.[836,848,850-852] As shown in Table 38.23, results from two recent meta-analyses show that infants born to mothers who used marijuana during pregnancy were 1.4 to 1.7 times more likely to be born low birth weight, 1.3 times more likely to be born preterm, and had double the risk of being admitted to a level II/III NICU than infants born to mothers who did not use marijuana during pregnancy.[852,853] After tobacco use and other factors were taken into account, these differences were attenuated to nonsignificance (relative risks: LBW = 1.2, preterm = 1.1), suggesting, at least based on current data, that maternal marijuana use during pregnancy may not be an independent risk factor for poor neonatal outcomes.[852] However, this research is based almost exclusively on medical record data or assessments at birth. One exception is the Dutch Generation R study that assessed fetal growth in early, mid-, and late pregnancy with a range of fetal ultrasound measures.[854] This cohort was also exposed to higher levels of tetrahydrocannabinol (THC) than previous cohorts. The data show that maternal marijuana use during pregnancy was associated with poorer fetal growth during mid- and late pregnancy, as well as a lower eventual birth weight. This growth restriction consisted of a loss of about 14.4 grams/week and a reduction in head circumference of about 0.21 mm/week. Infants born to mothers who continued to use marijuana throughout their pregnancy showed the poorest growth, suggesting both a dose-response effect and an association with increased neonatal and, potentially, longer-term risk.

An overt NAS has not been reported in any of the prospective longitudinal studies. However, a *reasonably consistent pattern of neurobehavioral effects* is observed.[855] These include increased arousal, excitability, dysregulation, disorganized cry, as well as signs of irritability, such as tremors, startles, and an altered sleep pattern characterized by less quiet sleep.[856-859]

Neurodevelopmental Consequences

Outcome studies of infants born to mothers who use marijuana during pregnancy are subject to many of the methodological difficulties previously reviewed for other illicit drugs of abuse. These include underreporting, lack of toxicology measures, and failure to adequately include consideration of the dual hazard effects of both prenatal drug exposures *and* family environmental factors correlated with maternal marijuana use and/or dependence that may also increase child developmental risk (see Huizink for a fuller discussion).[855] In general, findings suggest that more prolonged exposure is associated with increased developmental risk for the infant.[860,861]

Cognition, Executive Functioning, and Language Development

There is little evidence of developmental differences on global measures of cognitive function before age 2 years.[855,862] Interestingly, however, as children get older, differences are increasingly observed, especially on measures of executive function. Specifically, in preschoolers, prenatal cannabis exposure has been linked with poorer performance on measures of language, memory, and abstract/visual reasoning ability.[859,863] From around ages 8 to 9, problems are increasingly evident in executive functioning and continue into adulthood, with difficulties in visual working memory and response inhibition.[864-866] Related to this finding, Smith also observed increased activation in the left posterior cingulate gyrus during a spatial working memory fMRI task and in the left postcentral gyrus, left precentral gyrus, and left superior frontal gyrus during a go-no-go behavioral inhibition task in prenatally exposed adults, whose task performance was similar to nonexposed same-age peers.[865] These differences suggest a compensatory response whereby more effort and potentially additional brain regions are engaged by marijuana-exposed individuals to achieve the same task success as nonexposed individuals.[865] A structural MRI study also observed increased thickness of the frontal cortex, specifically the left superior frontal cortex and the right frontal pole, in 6- to 8-year-old children whose mothers used marijuana during pregnancy compared with children whose mothers did not.[844] No differences were seen in global brain volumes between the two groups. These findings suggest the possibility of altered maturation of cortical areas involved in higher order cognitive functions, such as executive and attentional control, consistent with reported behavioral findings. However, further replication and earlier MRI assessment are needed to confirm these results. Finally, and not unexpectedly, given the previous findings and the family backgrounds of many of these children, they also perform less well in school, obtaining lower scores on standardized measures of reading and spelling.[867]

Behavior and Regulatory Problems

In addition to executive functioning and potentially also related to these executive difficulties, attention and behavioral adjustment also appear to be affected by prenatal marijuana exposure, with findings indicating elevated risks of attention problems and depressive symptoms.[859,860,866,868] These associations persist even after adjustment for other prenatal drug exposures, family social

risk, and children's concurrent living situation. These findings are consistent with human and experimental studies, suggesting that prenatal cannabis exposure may alter the organization of the dopamine system that has been shown to be involved in the etiology of a number of neuropsychiatric conditions, including depression later in life.[869,870] Further research examining specific psychiatric disorders will be important in clarifying the mental health consequences of prenatal marijuana exposure. Finally, prenatal marijuana exposure has also been associated with an increased risk of early onset drug use and possibly also aggression.[871,872] The latter is consistent with difficulties with behavioral control, but may also reflect the effects of environmental factors correlated with maternal marijuana use in pregnancy, so replication is needed.[873]

Motor and Visual Function

There is little evidence of significant motor or visual problems during infancy and early childhood. However, deficits in visual motor coordination have been reported at age 16.[874]

Pathophysiology

The primary psychoactive compound in marijuana is Δ9-tetrahydrocannabinol (THC), whose metabolites readily cross the placenta and are also found in breast milk. Following maternal marijuana use during pregnancy, its metabolites provide a relatively wide window of exposure for the fetus, with traces evident in a mother's body for up to 30 days.[437] Also relevant to the care of the marijuana-exposed infant and to comparison of findings from older and newer studies is that the potency of marijuana has increased considerably in recent decades.[875-877] For example, between the 1970s and 2000s in the United States, there was a six- to sevenfold increase in the potency of marijuana in the market.[876] These shifts raise the possibility of increased risk of exposure for the developing fetus and emphasize the need for research based on contemporary cohorts of mothers and infants.

Although the precise mechanisms by which marijuana affects fetal brain development are not well understood, experimental and human clinical studies suggest *several likely pathways*.[869] The first is via the endogenous cannabinoid system that is involved in early embryonic development and synaptic brain plasticity. This system is also involved in synaptic pruning later in life.[878] Cannabinoids are naturally expressed within this system from around gestational week 14 and then increase in density through the third trimester.[879,880] Prenatal exposure to exogenous cannabinoids, therefore, has the potential to upregulate this system and in turn disrupt normal signaling, synaptogenesis, and the formation of neuronal connections. A second potential mechanism relates to cannabinoid interference of developing neurotransmitter systems, through the disruption of chemical processes involved in the synthesis of dopamine and other neurotransmitters.[862,869,870] Although human data are scarce, neuroanatomical studies reveal major cannabinoid receptor sites in the prefrontal cortex, amygdala, basal ganglia, striatum, hippocampus, and cerebellum.[851] The involvement of these brain areas in executive functioning, memory, and emotional processing is consistent with findings from longer term outcome studies suggesting the possibility of subtle disturbances in executive and emotional functioning (discussed earlier).

In addition to these direct effects on the cannabinoid system, important *indirect* effects of exogenous cannabinoids could also affect fetal development. Specifically, maternal marijuana use has been shown to affect placental function and maternal respiratory function, which could in turn adversely affect fetal cardiovascular function and cerebral perfusion. For example, serum carbon monoxide levels following marijuana use are about five times higher than those following tobacco use, increasing the likelihood of downstream effects on maternal respiratory and gas exchange physiology that could indirectly affect the fetus.[881]

Prevention

Women of childbearing age should be counseled regarding the potential adverse effects of marijuana exposure during pregnancy and encouraged to discontinue use.[882] THC also appears in breast milk.[883] In the absence of data regarding the safety of marijuana use during breastfeeding, use is discouraged in this setting as well.[884]

DRUG USE AND THE PRETERM INFANT

This chapter has focused primarily on the effects of exposure to a range of licit and illicit drugs during pregnancy on the fetal brain and subsequent neurodevelopment. However, it is important to note that opioids and sedatives are also used in the care of the preterm infant during a stage of brain development equivalent to the late second and third trimester of pregnancy.[885,886] Recent epidemiological data suggest that the use of both opioids and sedatives in the NICU setting are steadily increasing (Fig. 38.19).[885-887] These agents are recommended for painful procedures, including endotracheal intubation and chest drain insertion and removal.[888] However, prolonged utilization of analgesia and/or sedation during mechanical ventilation remains controversial, despite well-designed randomized controlled trials examining this indication.[889-891] As a result, there is considerable variability in clinical practice, with some units hardly using these agents and others reporting relatively high rates of use.[885,886] This degree of clinical variability is understandable. Numerous studies have documented the adverse effects of pain and agitation on brain development and long-term outcomes.[892] However, emerging evidence highlights the potential negative impact of chronic exposure to analgesics and sedatives on the developing preterm brain.[800,893-896] These data highlight the delicate balance clinicians must achieve between adequate pain relief and avoidance of drug toxicities in this high-risk population.[897,898]

In addition, preterm infants often require invasive surgery because of the complications of prematurity. As discussed previously, anesthetic exposure during this vulnerable period of rapid brain development may affect outcome. Several studies have identified an association between surgery during neonatal intensive care and neurodevelopmental impairment in childhood.[899-901] For example, a recent follow-up study of 137 very preterm-born infants found that two or more surgeries before term equivalent age placed infants at increased risk of a lower IQ score at age 4.6 years (mean difference = 20.3 IQ points), even after controlling for the effects of gestational age, prenatal steroid exposure, hypotension, patent ductus arteriosus (PDA), necrotizing enterocolitis (NEC), number of infections, length of mechanical ventilation, white matter injury, and number of sedated MRIs.[902] Although a full discussion of this issue is beyond the scope of this chapter, some caution and further investigation of the impacts of changing pharmacological practices on the developing preterm brain are clearly needed.[818]

CONCLUSIONS

Prenatal exposure to both licit and illicit drugs can have short-term and long-lasting effects on the structure and function of the developing CNS. These effects vary in severity from profound effects on morphological structure to more subtle, but nonetheless clinically significant, neurological effects. Importantly, studies suggest that for all of the drugs reviewed, these effects are not transient but tend to persist into childhood and adolescence. Multiple systems are often affected, spanning cognition, motor function, language, and behavior. These effects appear to arise both directly through the passage of a drug through the placenta to the fetus, as well as indirectly through its effects on maternal systems and health behaviors. Given the significant public health costs associated with the neonatal and longer-term care of these high-risk infants, more precise and mechanistic work is needed to characterize the extent of neurobehavioral alterations and how developmental timing, drug dosage, and genetics affect these processes. Also important is the need to recognize the likely ongoing needs of these infants and their families, given their often complex clinical presentation and, in many cases, disadvantaged family circumstances that are likely to also adversely affect these children's neurodevelopmental outcomes and life-course opportunities.

Full references for this chapter can be found on www.expertconsult.com.

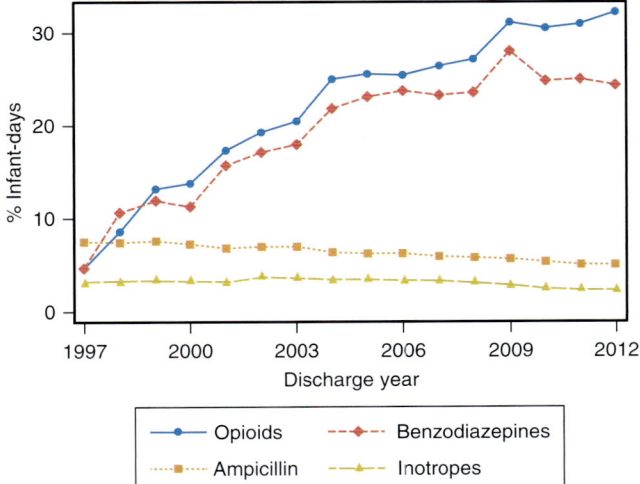

Figure 38.19 Increasing use of opioids and sedatives in the NICU from 1997 to 2012. (From Zimmerman KO, Smith PB, Benjamin DK, et al. Sedation, analgesia, and paralysis during mechanical ventilation of premature infants. *J Pediatr.* 2017;180:99–104.e101

Index

Page numbers followed by *f* indicate figures; *t*, tables, *b*, boxes.